HEMATOLOGY-ONCOLOGY THERAPY

THIRD EDITION

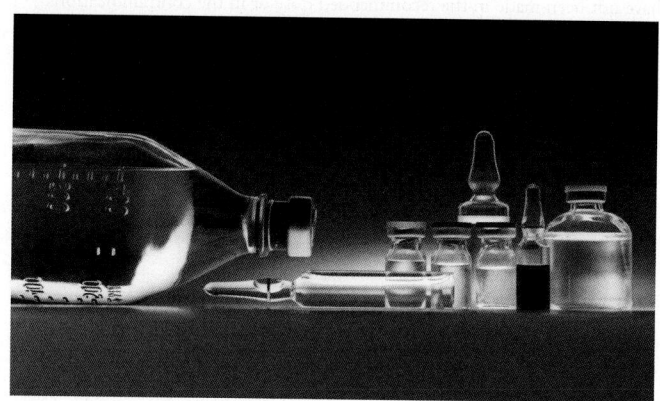

MICHAEL M. BOYIADZIS, MD, MHSc
Professor of Medicine and Clinical and Translational Science
Department of Medicine, Division of Hematology-Oncology
University of Pittsburgh School of Medicine
UPMC Hillman Cancer Center
Pittsburgh, Pennsylvania

TITO FOJO, MD, PhD
Professor of Medicine
Department of Medicine, Division of Hematology-Oncology
Columbia University
Herbert Irving Comprehensive Cancer Center
New York, New York

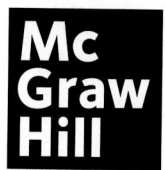

New York   Chicago   San Francisco   Athens   London   Madrid
Mexico City   Milan   New Delhi   Singapore   Sydney   Toronto

1 2 3 4 5 6 7 8 9 DSS 26 25 24 23 22 21

ISBN 978-1-260-11740-0
MHID 1-260-11740-5

Notice

Medicine is an ever-changing science. As new research and clinical experience broaden our knowledge, changes in treatment and drug therapy are required. The authors and the publisher of this work have checked with sources believed to be reliable in their efforts to provide information that is complete and generally in accord with the standards accepted at the time of publication. However, in view of the possibility of human error or changes in medical sciences, neither the authors nor the publisher nor any other party who has been involved in the preparation or publication of this work warrants that the information contained herein is in every respect accurate or complete, and they disclaim all responsibility for any errors or omissions or for the results obtained from use of the information contained in this work. Readers are encourage to confirm the information contained herein with other sources. For example and in particular, readers are advised to check product information sheet included in the package of each drug they plan to administer to be certain that the information contained in this work is accurate and that changes have not been made in the recommended dose or in the contraindications for administration. This recommendation is of particular importance in connection with new or infrequently used drugs.

This book was set in Centaur MT Std by Thomson Digital.
The editors were Jason Malley, Karen Edmonson and Harriet Lebowitz.
The production supervisor was Richard Ruzycka.
The book designer was Eve Siegel.
Project management was provided by Sudhi Singh, Thomson Digital.
Cover art: Chryso Boyiatzi
The cover designer was W2 Design.

Library of Congress Control Number: 2020951231

To the patients our profession has the privilege to serve, and to our colleagues whose compassionate care and research efforts continue to extend the spectrum of hope.

Contents

Online Only Chapters

AccessHemOnc.com

Contents: Regimens Listed by Type of Cancer

Chapter 3. ADRENOCORTICAL CANCER

Chapter 4. ANAL CANCER

Chapter 5. BILIARY: GALLBLADDER CANCER AND CHOLANGIOCARCINOMA

Chapter 6. BLADDER CANCER

Chapter 7. BREAST CANCER

Chapter 8. CARCINOMA OF UNKNOWN PRIMARY

First-Line

Subsequent Therapy

Chapter 9. CENTRAL NERVOUS SYSTEM CANCERS

Glioma, Newly Diagnosed

Anaplastic Oligodendroglioma and Anaplastic Oligoastrocytoma, Newly Diagnosed

Anaplastic Astrocytoma, Newly Diagnosed

Glioblastoma, Newly Diagnosed

Glioblastoma, Recurrent

Primary CNS Lymphoma, Newly Diagnosed

Chapter 14. ENDOMETRIAL CANCER

Chapter 15. ESOPHAGEAL CANCER

Chapter 16. GASTRIC CANCER

Chapter 24. MELANOMA

Authors

David H. Aggen, MD, PhD
Attending
Genitourinary Oncology Service
Memorial Sloan Kettering Cancer Center
New York, New York
Renal Cell Cancer

Ivan Aksentijevich, MD
Virginia Cancer Specialists
Specialist in Medical Oncology and Hematology
Alexandria, Virginia
Acute Lymphoblastic Leukemia; Acute Myeloid Leukemia

Srivandana Akshintala, MBBS, MPH
Assistant Research Physician
Pediatric Oncology Branch
Center for Cancer Research
National Cancer Institute
Bethesda, Maryland
Sarcomas

Tamarah A. Al-Dawoodi, MD
University of Nevada, Las Vegas School of Medicine
University Medical Center
Las Vegas, Nevada
Mesothelioma

Philippe Armand, MD, PhD
Chief, Division of Lymphoma
Harold and Virginia Lash Endowed Chair in Lymphoma Research
Associate Professor of Medicine, Harvard Medical School
Non-Hodgkin Lymphoma

Mohamed M. Azab, MD
University of Nevada, Las Vegas School of Medicine
University Medical Center
Las Vegas, Nevada
Mesothelioma

Carmen Joseph Allegra, MD
Professor and Chief Hematology and Oncology
Department of Medicine
University of Florida Health
Gainesville, Florida
Colorectal Cancer

Jennifer E. Amengual, MD
Herbert Irving Assistant Professor of Medicine
Division of Hematology and Oncology
Herbert Irving Comprehensive Cancer Center
Columbia University Irving Medical Center
New York, New York
Non-Hodgkin Lymphoma

Kenneth C. Anderson, MD
Professor of Medicine, Department of Medicine,
Harvard Medical School
Physician, Oncology, Brigham and Women's Hospital
Medical Director, Kraft Family Blood Center,
Dana-Farber Cancer Institute
Boston, Massachusetts
Multiple Myeloma

Andrea B. Apolo, MD
Investigator and Lasker Scholar
Chief, Bladder Cancer Section
Genitourinary Malignancies Branch
Center for Cancer Research, National Cancer Institute
National Institutes of Health
Bethesda, Maryland
Bladder Cancer

Dean Bajorin, MD
Member and Professor of Medicine
Genitourinary Oncology Service
Memorial Sloan-Kettering Cancer Center
New York, New York
Bladder Cancer

James C. Barton, MD
Medical Director, Southern Iron Disorders Center
Clinical Professor of Medicine
University of Alabama at Birmingham
Birmingham, Alabama
Hemochromatosis

Susan E. Bates, MD
Professor of Medicine
Division of Hematology and Oncology
Department of Medicine
Columbia University
New York, New York
Pancreatic Cancer, Tissue-Agnostic Therapies

Kenneth A. Bauer, MD
Professor of Medicine, Harvard Medical School
Director, Thrombosis Clinical Research,
Beth Israel Deaconess Medical Center
Boston, Massachusetts
The Hypercoagulable State

Sigbjørn Berentsen, MD, PhD
Consultant Hematologist and Senior Researcher
Department of Research and Innovation
Helse Fonna HF, Haugesund Hospital
Haugesund, Norway
Autoimmune Hemolytic Anemia

Ann Berger, MSN, MD
Chief, Pain and Palliative Care Service
National Institutes of Health Clinical Center
Bethesda, Maryland
Cancer Pain: Assessment and Management

Giada Bianchi, MD
Department of Medical Oncology, Instructor in Medicine
Dana Farber Cancer Institute
Harvard Medical School
Boston, Massachusetts
Multiple Myeloma

Michael R. Bishop, MD
Professor of Medicine
Director, Hematopoietic Stem Cell Transplantation Program
The University of Chicago Medicine
Chicago, Illinois
Complications and Follow-Up After Hematopoietic Cell Transplantation

Jean-Yves Blay, MD
Professor of Medicine in Medical Oncology
Head of the Medical Oncology Department
Centre Leon Berard of the Université Claude Bernard
Scientific Director, Canceropole Lyon Rhône Alpes
Lyon, France
Sarcomas

Leslie Boyd, MD
Assistant Professor of Gynecology
Perlmutter Cancer Center
NYU Langone Medical Center
New York, New York
Vaginal Cancer

Michael M. Boyiadzis, MD, MHSc
Professor of Medicine and Clinical and Translational Science
Department of Medicine, Division of Hematology-Oncology
University of Pittsburgh School of Medicine
UPMC Hillman Cancer Center
Pittsburgh, Pennsylvania
Acute Lymphoblastic Leukemia; Acute Myeloid Leukemia; Myelodysplastic Syndromes

Diana Brewer, PA
Physician Assistant
Center for Hematologic Malignancies
Instructor of Medicine, School of Medicine
Oregon Health & Science University
Portland, Oregon
Chronic Myeloid Leukemia

Kathleen A. Calzone, PhD, RN, APNG, FAAN
Senior Nurse Specialist, Research
National Cancer Institute
Center for Cancer Research, Genetics Branch
Bethesda, Maryland
Cancer Screening; Genetics of Common Inherited Cancer Syndromes

Lisa Cordes, PharmD, BCACP, BCOP
Oncology Clinical Pharmacy Specialist & Educator
National Institutes of Health
Bethesda, Maryland
Indications for Bone-Modifying Agents in Hematology-Oncology

Mary Czech, MD
National Institutes of Health
Bethesda, Maryland
Fever and Neutropenia

William L. Dahut, MD
Scientific Director for Clinical Research
Genitourinary Malignancies Branch
Center for Cancer Research
National Cancer Institute
National Institutes of Health
Bethesda, Maryland
Prostate Cancer

Nancy E. Davidson, MD
Senior Vice President, Director and Professor
Clinical Research Division, Fred Hutch
Raisbeck Endowed Chair for Collaborative Research
Fred Hutch
President and Executive Director
Seattle Cancer Care Alliance
Seattle, Washington
Breast Cancer

Michael W.N. Deininger, MD, PhD
M.M. Wintrobe Professor of Medicine
Chief, Division of Hematology and Hematologic Malignancies
Senior Director for Transdisciplinary Research
University of Utah
Huntsman Cancer Institute
Salt Lake City, Utah
Chronic Myeloid Leukemia

Volker Diehl, MD
Emeritus Professor of Medicine, Hematology, Oncology
University of Cologne
Cologne, Germany
Hodgkin Lymphoma

David L. Diuguid, MD
Professor of Medicine
Department of Medicine, Division of Hematology and Oncology
Columbia University
New York, New York
Heparin-Induced Thrombocytopenia

Don S. Dizon, MD, FACP, FASCO
Professor of Medicine, Brown University
Director, Women's Cancers and Hematology-Oncology Outpatient Clinics, Lifespan Cancer Institute
Director, Medical Oncology and the Oncology Sexual Health Program
Rhode Island Hospital
Providence, Rhode Island
Endometrial Cancer

Brian J. Druker, MD
Professor of Medicine, Division of Hematology and Medical Oncology
Director, Oregon Health & Science University Knight Cancer Institute
JELD-WEN Chair of Leukemia Research
Oregon Health & Science University
Portland, Oregon
Chronic Myeloid Leukemia

Brian J. Druker, MD
Professor of Medicine, Division of Hematology and Medical Oncology
Director, Oregon Health & Science University Knight Cancer Institute
JELD-WEN Chair of Leukemia Research
Oregon Health & Science University
Portland, Oregon
Chronic Myeloid Leukemia

Jennifer M. Duff, MD
Assistant Chief of Medical Service
Associate Professor of Hematology and Oncology
University of Florida Health
Gainesville, Florida
Colorectal Cancer

Sara Ekeblad, MD, PhD
Uppsala University Hospital
Stockholm, Sweden
Neuroendocrine Tumors

Darren R. Feldman, MD
Member, Department of Medicine
Memorial Sloan Kettering Cancer Center, and
Associate Professor in Medicine, Weill Cornell Medical College
New York, New York
Testicular Cancer

Jonas W. Feilchenfeldt, MD
Attending Physician
FMH Internal Medicine and Medical Oncology
Department of Medical Oncology
Hôpital du Valais
Sion, Switzerland
Gastric Cancer

Enriqueta Felip, MD, PhD
Vall d'Hebron Institute of Oncology
Vall d'Hebron University Hospital
Barcelona, Spain
Lung Cancer

Howard A. Fine, MD
Director of the Brain Tumor Center
New York-Presbyterian Weill Cornell Medical Center
New York, New York
Central Nervous System Cancers

Tito Fojo, MD, PhD
Professor of Medicine
Department of Medicine, Division of Hematology-Oncology
Columbia University
Herbert Irving Comprehensive Cancer Center
New York, New York
Adrenocortical Cancer; Guidelines for Chemotherapy Dosage Adjustment; Indications for Growth Factors in Hematology-Oncology; Oncologic Emergencies; Pheochromocytoma; Tissue-Agnostic Therapies; Indications for Bone-Modifying Agents in Hematology-Oncology

Michael Fuchs, MD
Head of the Trial Coordination Center German Hodgkin Study Group
Department of Internal Medicine
University Hospital of Cologne
Cologne, Germany
Hodgkin Lymphoma

Naseema Gangat, MD
Associate Professor of Medicine
Division of Hematology
Mayo Clinic
Rochester, Minnesota
Myeloproliferative Neoplasms

Juan C. Gea-Banacloche, MD
National Institute of Allergy and Infectious Diseases (NIAID)
Bethesda, Maryland
Fever and Neutropenia; Complications and Follow-Up After Hematopoietic Cell Transplantation

Timothy J. George, PharmD, BCOP
UPMC Shadyside Hospital
Pittsburgh, Pennsylvania
Guidelines for Chemotherapy Dosage Adjustment

Irene M. Ghobrial, MD
Professor of Medicine
Dana-Farber Cancer Institute
Harvard Medical School
Boston, Massachusetts
Multiple Myeloma

Giuseppe Giaccone, MD, PhD
Associate Director for Clinical Research
Sandra and Edward Meyer Cancer Center
Weill-Cornell Medicine
New York, New York
Thymic Malignancies

Mark T. Gladwin, MD
Jack D. Myers Distinguished Professor and Chair
Chairman of the Department of Medicine
UPMC and the University of Pittsburgh School of Medicine
Pittsburgh, Pennsylvania
Sickle Cell Disease: Acute Complications

F. Anthony Greco, MD
Co-Founder, Sarah Cannon Research Institute
Investigator
Tennessee Oncology
Nashville, Tennessee
Carcinoma of Unknown Primary

Tim Greten, MD, PhD
Deputy Branch Chief & Senior Investigator
Thoracic and GI Malignancies Branch
Co-Director, NCI CCR Liver Cancer Program
National Cancer Institute
National Institutes of Health
Bethesda, Maryland
Biliary: Gallbladder Cancer and Cholangiocarcinoma; Hepatocellular Carcinoma

Christine D. Hudak, MD
Hospice & Palliative Medicine for OhioHealth
Columbus, Ohio
Hospice Care and End-of-Life Issues

Thomas E. Hughes, PharmD, BCOP
Oncology Clinical Pharmacy Specialist
Pharmacy Department
National Institutes of Health
Bethesda, Maryland
Prophylaxis and Treatment of Chemotherapy-Induced Nausea and Vomiting

Irfan Jawed, MD
Medical Oncologist
Memorial Hermann Southeast Hospital
Pasadena, Texas
Anal Cancer

Ramasubramanian Kalpatthi, MD
Associate Professor of Pediatrics
UPMC Children's Hospital of Pittsburgh
Pittsburgh, Pennsylvania
Sickle Cell Disease: Acute Complications

Fatima Karzai, MD
Associate Research Physician
Genitourinary Malignancies Branch
National Cancer Institute
National Institutes of Health
Bethesda, Maryland
Prostate Cancer

Lyndon Kim, MD
Division of Neuro-Oncology
Department of Neurological Surgery
Department of Medical Oncology
Thomas Jefferson University Hospital
Philadelphia, Pennsylvania
Central Nervous System Cancers

Sunnie Kim, MD
Assistant Professor
University of Colorado Cancer Center
Aurora, Colorado
Esophageal Cancer

Chul Kim, MD, MPH
Assistant Professor
Medstar Georgetown University Hospital
Washington DC
Thymic Malignancies

John M. Kirkwood, MD
Distinguished Service Professor of Medicine
Usher Professor of Medicine, Dermatology and Translational Science
Co-Director, Melanoma and Skin Cancer Program
University of Pittsburgh School of Medicine
UPMC Hillman Cancer Center
Pittsburgh, Pennsylvania
Melanoma

Joseph E. Kiss, MD
Professor of Medicine
Department of Medicine
Division of Hematology-Oncology
Medical Director, Hemapheresis and Blood Services
University of Pittsburgh School of Medicine
Pittsburgh, Pennsylvania
Transfusion Therapy

Satyajit Kosuri, MD
Clinical Director - Hematopoietic Cellular Therapy Program
Section of Hematology and Oncology
University of Chicago Medical Center
Chicago, Illinois
Complications and Follow-Up After Hematopoietic Cell Transplantation

Livia Lamartina, MD, PhD
Department of Nuclear Medicine and Endocrine Oncology
Gustave Roussy, Université Paris-Saclay
Villejuif, France
Thyroid Cancer

John R. Lurain, MD
Marcia Stenn Professor of Gynecologic Oncology
John I. Brewer Trophoblastic Disease Center
Northwestern University, Feinberg School of Medicine
Chicago, Illinois
Gestational Trophoblastic Neoplasia

Kathryn Lurain, MD, MPH
Center for Cancer Research
National Cancer Institute
Bethesda, Maryland
HIV-Related Malignancies

Mark R. Litzow, MD
Professor of Medicine
Mayo Clinic
Rochester, Minnesota
Acute Lymphoblastic Leukemia

Pier M. Mannucci, MD
Professor
Scientific Direction
IRCCS Ca' Granda Maggiore Policlinico Hospital Foundation
Milano, Italy
von Willebrand Disease

Gerard P. Mascara, PharmD, BCOP
Adjunct Assistant Professor of Pharmacy and Therapeutics
University of Pittsburgh School of Pharmacy
VA Pittsburgh Healthcare System
Pittsburgh, Pennsylvania
Content represents Dr. Mascara's own views, not the views of the US Government or VA
Indications for Growth Factors in Hematology-Oncology;
Guidelines for Chemotherapy Dosage Adjustment;
Drug Preparation and Administration

John Marshall, MD
Director, The Ruesch Center for the Cure of GI Cancers
Chief, Hematology and Oncology
Lombardi Comprehensive Cancer Center
Georgetown University Medical Center
Washington, DC
Anal Cancer; Esophageal Cancer

Dhaval Mehta, MD
Clinical Assistant Professor of Medicine
University of Pittsburgh School of Medicine
UPMC Hillman Cancer Center
Pittsburgh, Pennsylvania
Chronic Lymphocytic Leukemia

Cecilia Monge, MD
Gastrointestinal Malignancy Section
National Cancer Institute
National Institutes of Health
Bethesda, Maryland
Hepatocellular Carcinoma

Franco Muggia, MD
Professor of Medicine (Oncology)
Perlmutter Cancer Center
NYU Langone Medical Center
New York, New York
Vaginal Cancer

Ashok Nambiar, MD
Professor, Laboratory Medicine
Director, Transfusion Medicine
Director, Moffitt-Long & Mt. Zion Hospital Tissue Banks
UCSF Medical Center
University of California, San Francisco
San Francisco, California
Transfusion Therapy

Mariam Nawas, MD
Assistant Professor
Hematopoietic Cellular Therapy Program
Section of Hematology and Oncology
The University of Chicago Medical Center
Chicago, Illinois
Complications and Follow-Up After Hematopoietic Cell Transplantation

Cindy Neunert, MD, MSCS
Assistant Professor of Pediatrics
Section Head, Pediatric Hematology
Columbia University Medical Center
New York, New York
Idiopathic Thrombocytopenic Purpura

Enrico M. Novelli, MD, MS
Associate Professor of Medicine
UPMC and the University of Pittsburgh School of Medicine
Pittsburgh, Pennsylvania
Sickle Cell Disease: Acute Complications

Melanie S. Norris, PharmD
University of Pittsburgh School of Pharmacy
Pittsburgh, Pennsylvania

Kunle Odunsi, MD, PhD
Director of the University of Chicago Medicine Comprehensive Cancer Center
AbbVie Foundation Distinguished Service Professor of Obstetrics and Gynecology
Dean for Oncology, Biological Sciences Division
Chicago, Illinois
Ovarian Cancer

Naomi P. O'Grady, MD
Medical Director, Procedures, Vascular Access, and Conscious Sedation Services
Department of Critical Care Medicine
National Institutes of Health
Bethesda, Maryland
Catheter-Related Bloodstream Infections: Management and Prevention

Karel Pacak, MD, PhD, DSc
Senior Investigator
Chief, Section on Medical Neuroendocrinology
Eunice Kennedy Shriver NICHD, National Institutes of Health
Bethesda, Maryland
Pheochromocytoma

Bhavisha Patel, MD
Staff Clinician
National Heart, Lung, and Blood Institute,
National Institutes of Health
Bethesda, Maryland
Aplastic Anemia

Khilna Patel, PharmD, BCOP, MBA
New York-Presbyterian Hospital | Columbia University Medical Center
New York, New York
Antineoplastic Drugs: Preventing and Managing Extravasation

Justin R. Price, MD
Assistant Professor in Hospice and Palliative care
University of Maryland Medical Center
Baltimore, Maryland
Cancer Pain: Assessment and Management

Sheila Prindiville, MD, MPH
Director, Coordinating Center for Clinical Trials
National Cancer Institute
Bethesda, Maryland
Cancer Screening; Genetics of Common Inherited Cancer Syndromes

Kanti Rai, MD
Professor, The Karches Center for Oncology Research, Feinstein Institutes for Medical Research
Joel Finkelstein Cancer Foundation Professor of Medicine and Molecular Medicine, Donald and Barbara Zucker School of Medicine at Hofstra/Northwell
New Hyde Park, New York
Chronic Lymphocytic Leukemia

Margaret V. Ragni, MD, MPH
Professor of Medicine and Clinical Translational Science
Department of Medicine
Division of Hematology-Oncology
University of Pittsburgh School of Medicine
Director, Hemophilia Center of Western Pennsylvania
Pittsburgh, Pennsylvania
Hemophilia

Ramesh Rengan, MD, PhD, FASTRO
Professor and Chair
Department of Radiation Oncology
Fred Hutchinson Cancer Research Center
University of Washington
Seattle, Washington
Radiation Complications

Aldo Roccaro, MD, PhD
Dana Farber Cancer Institute
Harvard Medical School
Boston, Massachusetts
Multiple Myeloma

Griffin P. Rodgers, MD, MACP
Chief, Molecular and Clinical Hematology Branch
National Heart, Lung and Blood Institute
Director, National Institute of Diabetes, Digestive and Kidney Diseases
National Institutes of Health
Bethesda, Maryland
Sickle Cell Disease: Acute Complication

Peter G. Rose, MD
Section Head Gynecologic Oncology
Cleveland Clinic Foundation
Tenured Professor of Surgery, Oncology and Reproductive Biology
Case Western Reserve University
Cleveland, Ohio
Cervical Cancer

Rafael Rosell, MD
IOR, Quirón-Dexeus
Rosell Molecular and Cellular Oncology Laboratory
Germans Trias i Pujol Research Institute and Hospital (IGTP)
Barcelona, Spain
Lung Cancer

Craig D. Seaman, MD, MS
Assistant Professor of Medicine
Division of Hematology-Oncology
Department of Medicine
University of Pittsburgh School of Medicine
Associate Director, Hemophilia Center of Western Pennsylvania
Pittsburgh, Pennsylvania
Hemophilia

Manish A. Shah, MD
Professor of Medicine
Director, Gastrointestinal Oncology
Weill Cornell Medical College of Cornell University
New York-Presbyterian
New York, New York
Gastric Cancer

Marie Scully, MD
Professor of Hematology
Department of Hematology
University College London Hospitals
London, United Kingdom
Thrombotic Thrombocytopenic Purpura/Hemolytic Uremic Syndrome

Britt Skogseid, MD, PhD
Professor of Endocrine Tumorbiology
Department of Endocrine Oncology
Uppsala University Hospital
Uppsala, Sweden
Neuroendocrine Tumors

Roy E. Smith, MD, MS
Professor of Medicine
Division of Hematology-Oncology
University of Pittsburgh School of Medicine
Pittsburgh, Pennsylvania
Venous Catheter-Related Thrombosis Iron Deficiency Anemia

Pol Specenier, MD, PhD
Department of Oncology
Antwerp University Hospital
Edegem, Belgium
Head and Neck Cancers

Jennifer M. Specht, MD
Associate Professor
Clinical Research Division
Fred Hutchinson Cancer Research Center
Associate Professor of Medicine
University of Washington School of Medicine
Seattle, Washington
Breast Cancer

David R. Spigel, MD
Chief Scientific Officer
Sarah Cannon Research Institute
Director, Lung Cancer Research Program
Principal Investigator
Tennessee Oncology
Nashville, Tennessee
Carcinoma of Unknown Primary

Jason Starr, DO
Department of Medicine
Mayo Clinic Hospital
Jacksonville, Florida
Colorectal Cancer

Maximilian Stahl, MD
Chief Hematology-Oncology Fellow
Memorial Sloan Kettering Cancer Center
Visiting Fellow, Rockefeller University
New York, New York
Hairy Cell Leukemia

J. Brian Szender MD, MPH
START Center for Cancer Care
San Antonio, Texas
Ovarian Cancer

Martin S. Tallman, MD
Chief of the Leukemia Service
Department of Medicine
Memorial Sloan Kettering Cancer Center
Professor of Medicine
Weill Cornell Medical College
New York, New York
Hairy Cell Leukemia; Acute Myeloid Leukemia

Ahmad A. Tarhini, MD, PhD
Director, Cutaneous Clinical and Translational Research
Leader, Cutaneous Neoadjuvant and Adjuvant Translational Science Program
Senior Member, Departments of Cutaneous Oncology and Immunology
H Lee Moffitt Cancer Center and Research Institute
Professor of Oncologic Sciences
University of South Florida Morsani College of Medicine
Tampa, Florida
Melanoma

Ayalew Tefferi, MD
Professor of Medicine
Division of Hematology
Mayo Clinic
Rochester, Minnesota
Myeloproliferative Neoplasms

Susanna Ulahannan, MD, MMed
Associate Director, Oklahoma TSET Phase 1 Program
NCI Early Stage Clinical Investigator
Assistant Professor of Medicine, Medical Oncology/Hematology
Stephenson Cancer Center at Oklahoma University Medicine
Oklahoma City, Oklahoma
Biliary: Gallbladder Cancer and Cholangiocarcinoma

Thomas S. Uldrick, MD, MS
Deputy Head, Global Oncology Program
Associate Professor
Vaccine and Infectious Disease Division
Clinical Research Division
Fred Hutchinson Cancer Research Center
Seattle, Washington
HIV-Related Malignancies

JB Vermorken, MD, PhD
Emeritus Professor of Oncology
Department of Medical Oncology
Antwerp University Hospital
Antwerp, Belgium
Head and Neck Cancers

Nicholas J. Vogelzang, MD
Clinical Professor of Medicine
Hematology-Oncology
University of Nevada, Las Vegas School of Medicine
Las Vegas, Nevada
Mesothelioma

Charles F. von Gunten, MD, PhD
Vice President, Medical Affairs
Hospice and Palliative Medicine for OhioHealth
Columbus, Ohio
Hospice Care and End-of-Life Issues

Daniel D. Von Hoff, MD, FACP
Physician in Chief, Distinguished Professor
Translational Genomics Research Institute
Professor of Medicine, Mayo Clinic
Chief Scientific Officer, Scottsdale Healthcare
Medical Director of Research and Scientific Medical Officer,
US Oncology Research
Senior Investigator
Clinical Professor of Medicine
Translational Genomics Research Institute
University of Arizona Cancer Center
Phoenix, Arizona
Pancreatic Cancer

Martin H. Voss, MD
Clinical Director
Genitourinary Oncology Service
Memorial Sloan Kettering Cancer Center
New York, New York
Renal Cell Cancer

Benjamin A. Weinberg, MD
Assistant Professor of Medicine, Division of Hematology and
Oncology
Attending Physician, MedStar Georgetown University Hospital
Gastrointestinal Medical Oncologist
Lombardi Comprehensive Cancer Center
Georgetown University Medical Center
Georgetown, Wahington DC
Anal Cancer

Emily S. Weg, MD
Assistant Professor, Department of Radiation Oncology
University of Washington School of Medicine
Seattle, Washington
Radiation Complications

Brigitte Widemann, MD
Senior Investigator
Pediatric Oncology Branch
Center for Cancer research
National Cancer Institute, National Institutes of Health
Bethesda, Maryland
Sarcomas

Jacob E. Winschel, MS, PharmD
UPMC Presbyterian Hospital
Pittsburgh, Pennsylvania

Neal S. Young, MD
Chief, Hematology Branch
National Heart, Lung, and Blood Institute
National Institutes of Health
Bethesda, Maryland
Aplastic Anemia; Myelodysplastic Syndromes

Robert Yarchoan, MD
Chief. HIV and AIDS Malignancy Branch
Senior Investigator
Head, Viral Oncology Section
Director, Office of HIV and AIDS Malignancy
Center for Cancer research
National Cancer Institute, National Institutes of Health
Bethesda, Maryland
HIV-Related Malignancies

Rachel Yung, MD
Assistant Professor
Clinical Research Division, Fred Hutchinson Cancer Research
Center
Asistant Professor of Medicine
University of Washington School of Medicine
Seattle, Washington
Breast Cancer

Wenhui Zhu, MD, PhD
Seidman Cancer Center
Southwest General Hospital
Middleburg Heights, Ohio
Prostate Cancer

Jeffrey I. Zwicker, MD
Associate Professor of Medicine
Division of Hematology-Oncology
Beth Israel Deaconess Medical Center, Harvard Medical School
Boston, Massachusetts
The Hypercoagulable State

Preface

The development of *Hematology-Oncology Therapy* was originally inspired by the need for a readily accessible, up-to-date, comprehensive therapy resource, supported by referenced literature. The first and second editions received considerable acclaim and filled a void in the medical literature. Over 800 treatment regimens are presented in a concise and uniform format that includes oncologic disorders, non-neoplastic hematologic disorders, and supportive care.

Due to rapid and extensive advances in the field of hematology-oncology, the third edition has significantly expanded and the entire content is now online at AccessHemOnc.com. The online platform created for the third edition will be continually updated, including newly approved regimens.

The four sections of *Hematology-Oncology Therapy* are:

I. Cancer regimens (Print & Online)
II. Antiemetics, Growth Factors, Dose Modification and Drug Preparation (Print & Online)
III. Supportive Care, Complications, and Screening (Online)
IV. Selected Hematologic Diseases (Online)

Section I provides detailed information about the administration, supportive care, toxicity, dose modification, monitoring, and efficacy of commonly used and recently approved therapeutic regimens. Each chapter is focused on a specific cancer and contains information about epidemiology, pathology, work-up, and staging, as well as survival data. In addition, each chapter has an Expert Opinion section in which experts in the field provide treatment recommendations and guidance on the use of the included regimens. Section II contains chapters on antiemetics, growth factors, and the administration and formulation of anti-cancer drugs. Section III consists of topics commonly encountered in clinical hematology-oncology practice. Section IV provides an authoritative guide to therapy for principal diseases in consultative hematology.

Hematology-Oncology Therapy integrates extensive information that is critical to both office- and hospital-based hematology and oncology clinical practices. This comprehensive approach makes the book invaluable to all practitioners involved in the care of patients with cancer or hematologic diseases and complements other excellent reference books on hematology-oncology.

We wish to express our appreciation to the many contributors to this book, whose expert knowledge in their fields makes *Hematology-Oncology Therapy* a unique addition to the medical literature. They helped us compile the extensive and detailed therapy information contained in this book, which is a testament to the efforts of so many to improve the treatment of patients with oncologic and hematologic diseases. We are profoundly grateful to our outstanding colleague Gerard Mascara, Oncology Clinical Pharmacy Specialist, for his dedication and untiring efforts in reviewing each treatment regimen and confirming the accuracy of dosage administration and to Melanie S. Norris, PharmD and Jacob E. Winschel, MS, PharmD for their assistance for the treatment regimens.

We also wish to thank our editors, Harriet Lebowitz, Karen Edmonson and Jason Malley, at McGraw Hill for their continued support, patience, and faith in our vision and concept for this book. Their professional support has earned our admiration and gratitude. Finally, we would like to thank those with whom we work and those we love for their support during the writing and editing of the third edition.

Michael M. Boyiadzis, MD, MHSc
Tito Fojo, MD, PhD

SECTION I. Treatment Regimens

1. Acute Lymphoblastic Leukemia

Michael M. Boyiadzis, MD, MHSc, Ivan Aksentijevich, MD, and Mark R. Litzow, MD

Epidemiology

Incidence:	6150 (male: 3470; female: 2680. Estimated new cases for 2020 in the United States) The incidence of ALL follows a bimodal distribution, with a peak between the ages of 2 and 4 years and again during the sixth decade
Deaths:	Estimated 1520 in 2020 (male: 860; female: 660)
Median age:	B-cell lymphoblastic leukemia/lymphoma: 12 years T-cell lymphoblastic leukemia/lymphoma: 18 years Lymphoblastic leukemia/lymphoma unknown lineage: 12 years
Male to female ratio:	1.2:1

Dores GM. Blood 2012;119:34–43
Malard F et al. Lancet 2020;395:1146–1162
Siegel R et al. CA Cancer J Clin 2020;70:7–30
Surveillance, Epidemiology and End Results (SEER) Program, available from http://seer.cancer.gov [accessed in 2020]

Pathology

WHO classification of acute leukemia

B-lymphoblastic leukemia/lymphoma
  B-lymphoblastic leukemia/lymphoma, NOS
  B-lymphoblastic leukemia/lymphoma with recurrent genetic abnormalities
  B-lymphoblastic leukemia/lymphoma with t(9;22)(q34.1;q11.2);*BCR-ABL1*
  B-lymphoblastic leukemia/lymphoma with t(v;11q23.3);*KMT2A* rearranged
  B-lymphoblastic leukemia/lymphoma with t(12;21)(p13.2;q22.1); *ETV6-RUNX1*
  B-lymphoblastic leukemia/lymphoma with hyperdiploidy
  B-lymphoblastic leukemia/lymphoma with hypodiploidy
  B-lymphoblastic leukemia/lymphoma with t(5;14)(q31.1;q32.3) *IL3-IGH*
  B-lymphoblastic leukemia/lymphoma with t(1;19)(q23;p13.3);*TCF3-PBX1*
  Provisional entity: B-lymphoblastic leukemia/lymphoma, BCR-ABL1–like
  Provisional entity: B-lymphoblastic leukemia/lymphoma with iAMP21

T-lymphoblastic leukemia/lymphoma
Provisional entity: Early T-cell precursor lymphoblastic leukemia
Provisional entity: Natural killer (NK) cell lymphoblastic leukemia/lymphoma

Arber A et al. Blood 2016;127:2391–2405

Molecular Abnormalities in B-cell ALL

Risk Class	Involved Gene	Frequency Adults
Favorable risk		
Cytogenetic (numerical change)		
Hyperdiploid	*CREBBP*	2–15%
Tetraploid		

Work-up

1. H&P
2. CBC, leukocyte differential, platelets, electrolytes, liver function tests, PT, PTT, fibrinogen, d-dimer, LDH, uric acid, urinalysis, hepatitis serology
3. HLA typing for patients who are candidates for allogeneic hematopoietic cell transplantation
4. Bone marrow biopsy with cytogenetics (karyotype and FISH), immunophenotyping, and molecular studies
5. Testicular exam and scrotal ultrasound if clinical indicated
6. Echocardiogram if therapy with anthracycline is planned, especially if prior cardiac history or prior anthracycline use
7. CT/MRI of head if neurologic symptoms
8. Chest x-ray and CT/MRI scans if clinically indicated

(*continued*)

Pathology (*continued*)

Risk Class	Involved Gene	Frequency Adults
Cytogenetic (translocation)		
t(12;21)(p12;q22)	*ETV6-RUNX1*	<1%
High risk		
Cytogenetic (numerical change)		
Hypodiploid	*RAS, IKZF2, TP53*	5–10%
Near-triploid	Unknown/unidentified	3–5%
Trisomy 8	Unknown/unidentified	10–12%
Monosomy 7	Unknown/unidentified	6–11%
Cytogenetic (translocation)		
t(9;22)(q34;q11)	*BCR-ABL, IKZF, CRLF2*	15–25%
t(4;11); t(9;11); t(19;11); t(3;11)	*MLL* with various partners	5%–10%
t(8;14); t(8;22); t(2;8)	*C-MYC* with various partners	5%
t(17;19)	*E2A-HLF*	<5%
Cytogenetic (other)		
Complex cytogenetic		5–10%
iAMP21	*RUNX1*	—
7 p deletion	Unknown/unidentified	5–10%
17 p deletion	*TP53*	8%
9 p deletion	*CDKN2A, CDKN2B*	7–11%
Molecular genetics		
CRLF2 overexpression	*CRLF2*	5–10%
IGH rearrangement	*IGH*	<3%
JAK mutations	*JAK1, JAK2*	7–18%
Gene expression		
BCR-ABL1-like	*CRLF2, IKZF1, JAK2, ABL1, ABL2, PDGFRB, EPOR, RAS, NTRK3*	25–30%
Intermediate risk		
Cytogenetics		
t(1;14); t(10;14); t(5;14)	TCR with various oncogenes	35%

Hefazi M et al. Blood Lymphat Cancer 2018;8:47–61

(*continued*)

Pathology (continued)

Molecular Abnormalities in T-cell ALL

Gene	Type of Genetic Aberration	Frequency
NOTCH1 signaling pathway		
FBXW7	Inactivating mutations	14
NOTCH1	Chromosomal rearrangements/activating mutations	57
Cell cycle		
CDKN2A	9p21 deletion	55
CKDN2B	9p21 deletion	46
Transcription factors		
BCL11B	Inactivating mutations/deletions	9
ETV6	Inactivating mutations/deletions	14
GATA3	Inactivating mutations/deletions	3
HOXA (CALM-AF10, MLL-ENL and SET-NUP214)	Chromosomal rearrangements/inversions/expression	8
LEF1	Inactivating mutations/deletions	2
LMO2	Chromosomal rearrangements/deletions/expression	21
MYB	Chromosomal rearrangements/duplications	17
RUNX1	Inactivating mutations/deletions	10
TAL1	Chromosomal rearrangements/5' super-enhancer mutations/deletions/expression	34
TLX1	Chromosomal rearrangements/deletions/expression	20
TLX3	Chromosomal rearrangements/expression	9
WT1	Inactivating mutation/deletion	11
Signaling		
AKT	Activating mutations	2
DNM2	Inactivating mutations	13
FLT3	Activating mutations	4
JAK1	Activating mutations	7
JAK3	Activating mutations	12
IL7R	Activating mutations	12
NF1	Deletions	4
KRAS	Activating mutations	0
NRAS	Activating mutations	9
P13KCA	Activating mutations	5
PTEN	Inactivating mutations/deletion	11

(continued)

Pathology *(continued)*

Gene	Type of Genetic Aberration	Frequency
PTPN2	Inactivating mutations/deletion	7
STAT5B	Activating mutations	6
Epigenetic factors		
DNMT3A	Inactivating mutations	14
EED	Inactivating mutations/deletion	5
EZH2	Inactivating mutations/deletion	12
KDM6A/UTX	Inactivating mutations/deletion	7
PHF6	Inactivating mutations/deletion	30
SUZ12	Inactivating mutations/deletion	5
Translation and RNA stability		
CNOT3	Missense mutations	8
RPL5	Inactivating mutations	2
RPL10	Missense mutations	1
RPL22	Inactivating mutations/deletion	0

Girard T et al. Blood 2017;129:1113–1123

Prognostic Factors for Risk Stratification of Adult ALL

Characteristics	Poor Risk Factors
Age	>35 years
Leukocytosis	>30,000 mm^3 (B lineage) >100,000 mm^3 (T lineage)
Karyotype*	Hypodiploidy (<44 chromosomes) *KMT2A* rearranged (t (4;11) or others) t (v;14q32)/IgH t (9;22) (q34;q11.2): *BCR-ABL1* Complex karyotype (5 or more chromosomal abnormalities) Ph-like ALL; intrachromosomal amplification of chromosome 21 (iAMP21)
Therapy response	Time to morphologic CR >4weeks Persistent measurable residual disease (MRD)

*Good-risk cytogenetics: Hyperdiploidy (51–65 chromosomes)
    t (12;21) (p13;q22): ETV6-RUNXI

Expert Opinion

Initial therapy for acute lymphoblastic leukemia (ALL) should be based on several factors, including the patient's performance status, age, comorbidities, cytogenetics, and molecular abnormalities. Treatment regimens for ALL have evolved empirically into complex schemes that use numerous agents in various doses, combinations, and schedules, and few of the individual components have been tested rigorously in randomized trials. However, the backbone of chemotherapy for ALL remains the sequence of induction, consolidation, and maintenance

Remission induction: Most regimens include steroids, vincristine, an anthracycline, and, usually, asparaginase. Cyclophosphamide and cytarabine are often added. The combination of these agents results in CR rates of 80–90%; thus, treating physicians should use a regimen with which they are familiar and have experience for successful supportive care

Rituximab may be incorporated in CD20+ B-cell ALL as part of the induction therapy based on the results of the GRAALL-2005/R study. The study included adults age 18–59 years with Ph-negative, CD20-positive B-ALL. CD20 positivity was defined as expression of CD20 by >20% of leukemia cells by multiparameter flow cytometry with gating for CD45. Patients were randomly assigned to chemotherapy either with or without rituximab. Event-free survival at 4 years was estimated at 55% (95% CI, 46–66) in the rituximab-containing group vs 43% (95% CI, 34–55) in the group without rituximab (HR 0.66; 95% CI, 0.45–0.98; P = 0.04). Overall survival at 4 years was estimated at 71% (95% CI, 62–80) and 64% (95% CI, 55–74), respectively (P = 0.1)

Adolescent and young adult patients with ALL should be treated with a pediatric-based ALL regimen.

A study performed in 423 younger adults, median age 31.2 years (range, 15.2-59.9) with Philadelphia chromosome–negative ALL in first remission (265 B-cell precursor and 158 T-cell ALL) that were treated in the multicenter GRAALL-2003 and GRAALL-2005 trials, demonstrated that a higher specific hazard of relapse was independently associated with postinduction MRD level $\geq 10^{-4}$ and unfavorable genetic characteristics (ie, MLL gene rearrangement or focal IKZF1gene deletion in BCP-ALL and NOTCH1/FBXW7mutation and/or N/K-RAS mutation and/or PTEN gene alteration in T-cell ALL).

MRD positivity at the end of induction predicts high relapse rates and patients should be evaluated for allogeneic hematopoietic cell transplantation (allo-HCT). Therapy aimed at eliminating MRD prior to allo-HCT is preferred, when possible. Blinatumomab, a bispecific CD19-directed CD3 T-cell engager, is approved for B-cell ALL in first remission with measurable/minimal residual disease (MRD)

Consolidation: Eradication of MRD during hematologic remission is the primary aim of the consolidation phase. It is difficult to assess the value of individual components of treatment because the number, schedule, and combination of antineoplastic drugs vary considerably among studies. Consolidation therapy typically consists of several cycles of treatment similar to, but often less intensive than, the drugs, dosages, and administration schedules given during induction, and consolidation is usually better tolerated than induction. Rituximab may be incorporated in CD20 + B-cell ALL as part of the consolidation therapy

Allo-HCT should be considered in high-risk patients. Patients may be considered as high risk if they have positive MRD, presence of poor-risk cytogenetics, or elevated WBC count ($\geq 30 \times 10^9$/L for B-cell lineage, $\geq 100 \times 10^9$/L for B-cell lineage) at diagnosis. Allo-HCT also provides a significant improvement in overall and leukemia-free survival in younger patients (age <35 years), standard risk, and patients with Philadelphia chromosome (Ph)-negative ALL compared with less-intensive chemotherapy regimens

Maintenance: Maintenance therapies are important for patients not undergoing allogeneic hematopoietic cell transplantation (allo-HCT). Maintenance regimens consist of combinations of mercaptopurine, methotrexate, vincristine, and steroids given continually for 2–3 years. Rituximab may be incorporated in CD20+ B-cell ALL as part of the maintenance therapy

Patients with inherited deficiency in the activity of the enzyme thiopurine methyltransferase (TPMT) are more sensitive to the myelosuppressive effects of mercaptopurine and should be considered for testing for *TPMT* gene polymorphisms. Periodic assessment for MRD should be performed (no more than every 3 months) for patients with complete molecular remission. The frequency should be increased if MRD levels are detectable

Philadelphia chromosome–positive acute lymphoblastic leukemia: Patients with Philadelphia chromosome–positive acute lymphoblastic leukemia (Ph+ ALL) are a distinct disease subgroup comprising 20–30% of adults

Tyrosine kinase inhibitors (TKIs) should be combined with induction chemotherapy for Ph+ ALL. The use of TKIs, either alone or in combination with steroids or less intensive chemotherapy, is an alternative treatment option for elderly ALL patients or patients unfit for intensive therapy. The potential benefits of allo-HCT in patients with Ph+ ALL have been described in several studies. For patients who receive allo-HCT, DFS and OS are better than would be expected with chemotherapy alone. Consolidation therapy with a TKI plus chemotherapy can achieve and sustain deep molecular remissions, but studies are needed to determine if this approach can routinely cure adults with Ph+ ALL. For patients without a donor, consolidation/maintenance therapy should include chemotherapy with TKI

Ph-like ALL is a subtype that carries a gene expression signature similar to that of Ph+ ALL without harboring the *BCR-ABL1* translocation. This entity represents 10% of ALL cases in children, 15–20% in AYA, and 25–30% in adults. These patients demonstrate an unfavorable outcome, with a 5-year DFS of only 25% in AYA patients. Approximately 50% of Ph-like patients harbor *CRLF2* rearrangements, with concomitant *JAK* mutations detected in approximately half of *CRLF2* cases

Relapsed ALL: patients with relapsed ALL have a poor prognosis with standard salvage chemotherapy. Response rates to salvage chemotherapy range from 30% to 70% but are generally short-lived with a median survival of 6 months. For Ph+ ALL patients treated with a TKI who relapse, mutation testing for *ABL1* kinase domain should be performed. Second-line therapy with a new TKI alone, or TKI with chemotherapy and/or steroids, should be considered. Patients in second CR should be considered for allo-HCT. Inotuzumab ozogamicin and blinatumomab

(continued)

Expert Opinion (*continued*)

are approved for relapsed ALL. For patients with a high disease burden, inotuzumab ozogamicin should be considered first, followed by blinatumomab for persistent disease or MRD positivity

Tisagenlecleucel is an anti-CD19 CAR T cell therapy, generated via the ex-vivo genetic engineering and expansion of T lymphocytes obtained from the patient's blood to incorporate a novel receptor into the T cell repertoire. Engineered T cells recognize and associate with antigen-positive malignant cells for elimination. In the phase 1/2a ELIANA trial, 75 children and young adults (median age, 11 years; range, 3–23 years) with RR B-ALL were treated with tisagenlecleucel. Of the enrolled patients, 46 (61%) had undergone prior allo-HCT. Before tisagenlecleucel infusion, 72 of 75 patients (96%) received lymphodepleting chemotherapy. The median duration of follow-up among patients who received a tisagenlecleucel infusion was 13.1 months. The overall remission rate within 3 months was 81%, with all patients who had a response to treatment found to be negative for minimal residual disease. The rates of EFS and OS were 73% (95% CI, 60–82) and 90% (95% CI, 81–95), respectively, at 6 months and 50% (95% CI, 35–64) and 76% (95% CI, 63–86) at 12 months. On August 30th, 2017, tisagenlecleucel became the first ever FDA-approved CAR T therapy, gaining approval for the treatment of patients ≤25 years of age with B-ALL who have relapsed or have not responded after two previous lines of therapy

Cytokine release syndrome (CRS) is the most common adverse event reported across all CAR T clinical trials, with an incidence as high as 74–100% for CD19-directed CAR T cells. CRS can present with a variety of symptoms. Mild symptoms of CRS include fever, headache, rash, arthralgia, and myalgia. More severe cases are characterized by hypotension that can progress to an uncontrolled systemic inflammatory response with vasopressor-requiring circulatory shock, vascular leakage, disseminated intravascular coagulation, and multi-organ system failure. Several descriptions of management strategies for CAR T-associated CRS have been published, which generally encompass supportive care and anti–IL-6 therapies to break the cycle of inflammation. The treatment algorithm for CRS secondary to tisagenlecleucel consists of tocilizumab for early symptoms and corticosteroids only as second-line treatment for refractory CRS. Neurotoxicity has been reported in nearly every study involving CD19-directed T cells, including CAR T cells. Unlike CRS, neurotoxicity secondary to CAR T treatment does not respond to tocilizumab

Central nervous system involvement: Up to 10% of adults with ALL present with CNS involvement at the time of diagnosis. The cumulative risk of CNS leukemia in patients who do not receive prophylaxis can be as high as 50%. Factors associated with an increased risk for CNS leukemia in adults include mature B-cell immunophenotype, T-cell immunophenotype, high WBC count at presentation, and elevated serum LDH levels. CNS involvement should be evaluated by lumbar puncture (LP) at the appropriate timing in accordance with the specific treatment protocol used, and when LP is performed intrathecal therapy should be administered. Adult patients with ALL and CNS involvement at diagnosis require CNS-directed therapy starting at the same time as induction therapy. Treatment and prophylaxis of CNS involvement may consist of intrathecally administered methotrexate either alone, or combined with intrathecally administered cytarabine or corticosteroids and/or intravenously administered high-dose cytarabine, high-dose methotrexate. With the incorporation of adequate systemic chemotherapy and intrathecal chemotherapy regimens, it is possible to avoid the use of upfront cranial irradiation except for cases of overt CNS leukemia at presentation and reserve the use of irradiation for salvage therapy settings. CNS prophylaxis should be given to all patients throughout the entire course of treatment, from induction, to consolidation, to the maintenance phase

DeFilipp Z et al. Biol Blood Marrow Transplant 2019;25:2113–2123
Gökbuget N et al. Blood 2018;131:1522–1531
Kantarjian H et al. Cancer 2004;101:2788–2801
Kantarjian H et al. N Engl J Med 2017;376:836–847
Kantarjian HM et al. J Clin Oncol 2000;18:547–561
Kantarjian HM et al. N Engl J Med 2016;375:740–753
Larson RA et al. Blood 1998;92:1556–1564
Linker C et al. J Clin Oncol 2002;20:2464–2471
Malard F et al. Lancet 2020;395:1146–1162
Maude SL et al. N Engl J Med 2018;378:439–448
Maury S et al. N Engl J Med 2016;375:1044–1053
Neelapu SS et al. Nat Rev 2018;15:47–62
Rowe JM et al. Blood 2005;106:3760–3767
Stock W et al. Blood 2019;133:1548–1559
Wetzler M et al. Blood 2007;109:4164–4167
Beldjord K et al, Blood 2014;123:3739–3749

PROPHYLAXIS AGAINST TUMOR LYSIS SYNDROME
HYDRATION, URINARY ALKALINIZATION, AND ALLOPURINOL ADMINISTRATION

Hydration with 2500–3000 mL/m² per day as tolerated; administer intravenously to maintain urine output ≥100 mL/m² per hour (or ≥2 mL/kg per hour in persons whose body weight is <50 kg)

Urinary alkalinization with **sodium bicarbonate** injection added to intravenously administered fluids

• The amount of sodium bicarbonate added to intravenously administered fluids should produce a solution with sodium content not greater than the concentration of sodium in 0.9% sodium chloride injection (≤154 mEq/L):

Sodium Bicarbonate Is Added to a Solution to Increase Urine pH Within a Range of 6.5 to ≤7

Base Solution Sodium Content	Sodium Bicarbonate Additive	Total Sodium Content
0.45% Sodium chloride injection (0.45% NS)		
77 mEq/L	50–75 mEq	127–152 mEq/L
0.2% Sodium chloride injection (0.2% NS)		
34 mEq/L	100–125 mEq	134–159 mEq/L
5% Dextrose injection (D5W)		
0	125–150 mEq	125–150 mEq/L
D5W/0.45% NS		
77 mEq/L	50–75 mEq	127–152 mEq/L
D5W/0.2% NS		
34 mEq/L	100–125 mEq	134–159 mEq/L

Notes:

• Hydration rate may be decreased at the completion of chemotherapy administration

• Urinary alkalization increases the solubility and excretion of uric acid and its oxypurine precursors (hypoxanthine and xanthine) and helps avoid uric acid crystallization in renal tubules; however, alkalinization is not uniformly recommended because:

  1. It favors precipitation of calcium phosphate in renal tubules, a concern in patients with concomitant hyperphosphatemia
  2. A metabolic alkalemia may result from the administration of bicarbonate and can worsen the neurologic manifestations of hypocalcemia

• Discontinue sodium bicarbonate administration (while continuing hydration) if serum bicarbonate concentration is >30 mEq/L (>30 mmol/L) or urine pH >7.5

Allopurinol

• Administer orally or intravenously starting 12 hours to 3 days (preferably, 2–3 days) before starting cytoreductive chemotherapy

• Hyperuricemia develops within 24–48 hours after initiating chemotherapy when the excretory capacity of the renal tubules for uric acid is exceeded

• In the presence of an acidic pH, uric acid crystals form in the renal tubules, leading to intraluminal renal tubular obstruction, an acute renal obstructive uropathy, and renal dysfunction

• *Initial dosage*

  ▪ Allopurinol 100 mg/m² per dose; administer orally every 8 hours (maximum daily dose = 800 mg), *or*
  ▪ Allopurinol 3.3 mg/kg per dose; administer orally every 8 hours (maximum daily dose = 800 mg), *or*
  ▪ Allopurinol 200–400 mg/m² per day; administer intravenously (maximum daily dose = 600 mg) in a volume of 5% dextrose injection or 0.9% sodium chloride injection sufficient to yield a concentration not greater than 6 mg/mL. The duration for administering individual doses should be informed by the volume to be given
    ○ Allopurinol may be administered as a single daily dose, or the total daily dose may be divided equally for administration at 6-, 8-, or 12-hour intervals

• **Maintenance doses** should be based on serum uric acid determinations performed approximately 48 hours after initiation of allopurinol therapy, and periodically thereafter

• Continue administering allopurinol until leukemic blasts have been cleared from the peripheral blood

(continued)

(continued)

Notes:
• Allopurinol dose adjustments for impaired renal function:

Creatinine Clearance	Oral Allopurinol Dose
10–20 mL/min (0.17–0.33 mL/s)	200 mg/day
3–10 mL/min (0.05–0.17 mL/s)	100 mg/day
<3 mL/min (<0.05 mL/s)	100 mg every 36–48 hours

• Allopurinol does not remove uric acid already present
• The incidence of allergic reactions is increased in patients receiving amoxicillin, ampicillin, or thiazide diuretics

Rasburicase

• Rasburicase is recombinant urate oxidase (uricase) produced by genetically modified *Saccharomyces cerevisiae* that express urate oxidase cDNA cloned from a strain of *Aspergillus flavus*
• Uricase enzymes catalyze uric acid oxidation to allantoin, which is at least 5 times more soluble than uric acid
• Rational utilization
  ▪ Rasburicase should be considered among initial interventions against hyperuricemia in patients with high peripheral WBC counts, rapidly increasing blast counts, high uric acid, or evidence of impaired renal function; that is:

Burkitt Leukemia	
WBC count ≥100,000/mm^3	
WBC count <100,000/mm^3 + LDH ≥2 × ULN	
WBC count <100,000/mm^3 + LDH <2 × ULN +	Acute kidney injury *or* Normal renal function + uric acid > ULN, *or* potassium > ULN, *or* phosphorus > ULN

ULN, upper limit of normal

Rasburicase 0.2 mg/kg per dose intravenously in a total volume of 50 mL 0.9% sodium chloride injection over 30 minutes once daily for up to 5 consecutive days is often used, but much lower doses (eg, single fixed doses ranging from 3 to 6 mg) are usually sufficient (dosage and administration recommendations published in U.S. Food and Drug Administration product labeling, December 2019)
• Rasburicase has demonstrated effectiveness in prophylaxis and treatment for hyperuricemia and acute increases in uric acid associated with cytoreductive therapies at dosages <0.2 mg/kg based on body weight, with fixed doses, and after administration of from 1–3 doses

Cairo MS, Bishop M. Br J Haematol 2004;127:3–11
Cairo MS et al. Br J Haematol 2010;149:578–586
Coiffier B et al. J Clin Oncol 2008;26:2767–2778
Klinenberg JR et al. Ann Intern Med 1965;62:639–647

ADOLESCENT/YOUNG ADULT

ACUTE LYMPHOBLASTIC LEUKEMIA: CALGB 10403 INDUCTION (COURSE I)

Stock W et al. Blood 2019;133:1548–1559

The CALGB 10403 regimen is a complex treatment protocol that may be used for adolescents and young adults (age ≥16 years and <40 years) with newly diagnosed Ph-negative B- or T-cell acute lymphoblastic leukemia. The protocol includes several phases of treatment outlined in the table below. For organizational purposes, each phase of the treatment protocol has been separated into an individual regimen within this textbook

CALGB 10403 Regimen General Overview
(See individual regimen descriptions for details)

Course	Treatment	Dose	Schedule
Induction (Course I, 4 weeks)	Cytarabine, IT Vincristine, IV Pegaspargase, IM/IV Prednisone, PO Daunorubicin, IV Methotrexate, IT	70 mg 1.5 mg/m² (2 mg max) 2500 units/m² 30 mg/m²/dose twice per day 25 mg/m² 15 mg	Day 1 Days 1, 8, 15, 22 Day 4 (*or 5 or 6*) Days 1–28 Days 1, 8, 15, 22 Days 8, 29 (CNS3*: +15, 22)
Extended induction† (Course IA, 2 weeks)	Vincristine, IV Pegaspargase, IM/IV Prednisone, PO Daunorubicin, IV	1.5 mg/m² (2 mg max) 2500 units/m² 30 mg/m²/dose twice per day 25 mg/m²	Days 1, 8 Day 4 (*or 5 or 6*) Days 1–14 Day 1
Consolidation (Course II, 8 weeks)	Cyclophosphamide, IV Cytarabine, SQ/IV Mercaptopurine, PO Vincristine, IV Pegaspargase, IM/IV Methotrexate, IT	1000 mg/m² 75 mg/m² 60 mg/m² 1.5 mg/m² (2 mg max) 2500 units/m² 15 mg	Days 1, 29 Days 1–4, 8–11, 29–32, 36–39 Days 1–14, 29–42 Days 15, 22, 43, 50 Days 15, 43 Days 1, 8 (Not CNS3*: +15, 22)
Interim maintenance (Course III, 8 weeks)	Vincristine, IV Methotrexate, IV Pegaspargase, IM/IV Methotrexate, IT	1.5 mg/m² (2 mg max) 100 mg/m²‡ 2500 units/m² 15 mg	Every 10 days × 5 doses Every 10 days × 5 doses Days 2, 22 Days 1, 31
Delayed Intensification (Course IV, 8 weeks)	Vincristine, IV Pegaspargase, IM/IV Dexamethasone, PO Doxorubicin, IV Cytarabine, SQ/IV Cyclophosphamide, IV Thioguanine, PO Methotrexate, IT	1.5 mg/m² (2 mg max) 2500 units/m² 10 mg/m²/day 25 mg/m²/day 75 mg/m²/day 1000 mg/m² 60 mg/m²/day 15 mg	Days 1, 8, 15, 43, 50 Day 4 (*or 5 or 6*), and day 43 Days 1–7, 15–21 Days 1, 8, 15 Days 29–32, 36–39 Day 29 Days 29–42 Days 1, 29, 36
Maintenance (Course V, 12-week cycles§)	Vincristine, IV Dexamethasone, PO Mercaptopurine, PO Methotrexate, PO Methotrexate, IT Radiation therapy∥	1.5 mg/m² (2 mg max) 3 mg/m²/dose twice per day 75 mg/m²/day 20 mg/m²/dose 15 mg Indication-dependent dosing∥	Days 1, 29, 57 Days 1–5, 29–33, 57–61 Daily on days 1–84 Days 8, 15, 22, ±29, 36, 43, 50, 57, 64, 71, 78 Day 1 (+D29 first four cycles) During first cycle only∥

*CNS3 is defined as cerebrospinal fluid with ≥5 WBC/μL with cytospin positive for blasts; or ≥10 RBC/μμL, ≥5 WBC/μL, and positive by Steinherz/Bleyer algorithm; or clinical signs of CNS leukemia such as facial nerve palsy, brain/eye involvement, or hypothalamic syndrome

†Administered only to patients with either an M2 marrow response (ie, >5–25% lymphoblasts) or an M1 marrow response (ie, <5% lymphoblasts) *with* ≥1% lymphoblasts detected by flow cytometry or immunohistochemistry on day 29 of induction (course I)

‡Capizzi methotrexate IV: 100 mg/m² (dose escalated by 50 mg/m² every 10 days for a total of five doses, adjusted for toxicity)

§Total duration of maintenance treatment from start of interim maintenance: females, 2 years; males, 3 years.

∥ *T-cell acute lymphoblastic leukemia:* 2400 cGy (200 cGy × 12 daily fractions) cranial radiation during the first maintenance cycle (course V). *CNS3* leukemia at diagnosis who achieve a complete remission: 1800 cGy (180 cGy × 10 daily fractions) cranial radiation during the first cycle of maintenance (course V). *Testicular involvement at diagnosis persisting at completion of induction (course I):* 2400 cGy (200 cGy × 12 daily fractions) testicular radiation during the first cycle of maintenance (course V) only

IT, intrathecal; IV, intravenous; IM, intramuscular; PO, by mouth; max, maximum; SQ, subcutaneously

(continued)

(continued)

Induction (Course I, 4 weeks):
Cytarabine 70 mg; administer intrathecally via lumbar puncture for 1 dose on day 1 of induction (total dosage/28-day induction course = 70 mg)

• Patients should remain in a horizontal position for ≥30 minutes following intrathecal chemotherapy

Vincristine 1.5 mg/m^2 (maximum dose = 2 mg) per dose; administer by intravenous infusion over 15 minutes in 50 mL 0.9% sodium chloride injection (0.9% NS) for 4 doses on days 1, 8, 15, and 22 of induction (total dosage/28-day induction course = 6 mg/m^2; maximum dosage/28-day induction course = 8 mg)

Daunorubicin 25 mg/m^2 per dose; administer by intravenous injection over 3–5 minutes for 4 doses on days 1, 8, 15, and 22 of induction (total dosage/28-day induction course = 100 mg/m^2)

Prednisone 30 mg/m^2 per dose; administer orally twice per day, with food, for 28 consecutive days on days 1–28 of induction (total dosage/28-day induction course = 1680 mg/m^2)

• *Note:* prednisone should be stopped abruptly without a taper upon the completion of the induction course

Premedications for pegaspargase:
• **Acetaminophen** 650–100 mg; administer orally 30 minutes prior to pegaspargase administration on day 4 (OR day 5 OR day 6)

• **Diphenhydramine** 25–50 mg; administer orally or intravenously 30 minutes prior to pegaspargase administration on day 4 (*or* day 5 *or* day 6)

  ▪ *Note:* pegaspargase may cause anaphylaxis and serious hypersensitivity reactions. An expert panel recommends premedication prior to pegaspargase in adolescent and young adult patients (Stock W et al. Leuk Lymphoma 2011;52:2237–2253). Steroid premedication (eg, hydrocortisone) may be omitted during induction (course I) due to inclusion of prednisone in the regimen. Observe patients for 1 hour after the administration of pegaspargase in a setting with the capability to provide emergency resuscitation and with immediate availability of emergency supplies including epinephrine, oxygen, a histamine receptor [H$_1$]-subtype antagonist (eg, diphenhydramine), and intravenous corticosteroids

Choose one of the following options for pegaspargase:
• **Pegaspargase** 2500 units/m^2; administer by intravenous infusion over 1–2 hours in 100 mL 0.9% NS or 5% dextrose injection (D5W) into a running infusion of either 0.9% NS or D5W (choose the same fluid that was used for dilution of pegaspargase) for one dose on day 4 (*or* day 5 *or* day 6) of induction (total dosage/28-day induction course = 2500 units/m^2), or:

• **Pegaspargase** 2500 units/m^2; administer by intramuscular injection for one dose on day 4 (*or* day 5 *or* day 6) of induction (total dosage/28-day induction course = 2500 units/m^2)

  ▪ Limit the volume at a single injection site to ≤2 mL. If the volume to be administered is >2 mL, multiple injection sites should be used

  ▪ Patients with platelets <50,000/mm^3 may require a platelet transfusion prior to an intramuscular injection

Methotrexate 15 mg; administer intrathecally via lumbar puncture, to all patients, for 2 doses on day 8 and day 29 of induction (total dosage/28-day induction course for patients without CNS 3 disease = 30 mg)

• Patients should remain in a horizontal position for ≥30 minutes following intrathecal chemotherapy

• Additional intrathecal methotrexate is given during induction for patients with CNS 3 disease only. CNS 3 disease is defined as cerebrospinal fluid with ≥5 WBC/μL with cytospin positive for blasts; or ≥10 RBC/μL, ≥5 WBC/μL, and positive by Steinherz/Bleyer algorithm; or clinical signs of CNS leukemia such as facial nerve palsy, brain/eye involvement, or hypothalamic syndrome

  ▪ The Steinherz/Bleyer method should be applied to classify cerebrospinal fluid (CSF) results if the patient has leukemia cells circulating in the peripheral blood and undergoes a traumatic lumbar puncture and CSF is found to have ≥5 WBC/μL with blasts. A patient with this scenario should be considered to have CNS 3 disease if:

$$\frac{CSF\ WBC}{CSF\ RBC} > 2X\ \frac{Blood\ WBC}{Blood\ RBC}$$

  ▪ **Methotrexate** 15 mg; administer intrathecally via lumbar puncture, to patients with CNS3 disease only, for an additional 2 doses on days 15 and 22 of induction (total dosage/28-day induction course for patients with CNS 3 disease = 60 mg)

  ▪ Patients should remain in a horizontal position for ≥30 minutes following intrathecal chemotherapy

  ▪ *Note:* CNS 3 disease is defined as the presence in cerebrospinal fluid of ≥5 WBCs and cytospin positive for blasts, or clinical signs of central nervous system leukemia (eg, facial nerve palsy, brain/eye involvement or hypothalamic syndrome)

Note: consider incorporation of rituximab throughout all phases of treatment for a total of 16 infusions based on the results of the GRAALL-2005/R study

Maury S et al. N Engl J Med 2016;375:1044–1053

Supportive Care
Antiemetic prophylaxis
Emetogenic potential on days 1, 8, 15, and 22 is **MODERATE**

(continued)

(continued)

Emetogenic potential on day of pegaspargase administration (Day 4 or day 5 or day 6) is **MINIMAL**
See Chapter 42 for antiemetic recommendations

Hematopoietic growth factor (CSF) prophylaxis
Primary prophylaxis is **NOT** indicated
See Chapter 43 for more information

Antimicrobial prophylaxis
Risk of fever and neutropenia is **HIGH**
  Antimicrobial primary prophylaxis to be considered:
  • Antibacterial—consider prophylaxis with a fluoroquinolone during periods of prolonged neutropenia only (eg, <500/mm^3 for ≥7 days) until ANC recovery
  • Antifungal—consider prophylaxis with fluconazole or another antifungal medication during periods of prolonged neutropenia only (eg, <500/mm^3 for ≥7 days) until ANC recovery. Note that use of voriconazole, posaconazole, and itraconazole should be avoided with concomitant vincristine use. *Pneumocystis jirovecii* prophylaxis is recommended (eg, cotrimoxazole)
  • Antiviral—anti-herpes antivirals (eg, acyclovir, famciclovir, valacyclovir)

Patient Population Studied

CALGB 10403 was a prospective, cooperative group, single-arm trial conducted in the United States that included 318 adolescent or young adult patients (age 17–39 years) with newly diagnosed precursor B- or T-cell acute lymphoblastic leukemia. The purpose of the trial was to determine the feasibility and efficacy of a pediatric regimen (mirrored after the AALL0232 protocol) in adolescent and young adult patients. Patients were required to have an Eastern Cooperative Oncology Group performance status of ≤2. Patients who were found subsequently to have Philadelphia chromosome–positive leukemia were recommended to receive alternative tyrosine kinase inhibitor–based therapy and were excluded from analysis. Patients with a Burkitt immunophenotype were excluded

Efficacy (N = 295)

Efficacy Variable	(N = 295)
Survival—months (95% CI)	
Median EFS	78.1 (41.8–NR)
Median OS	NR
Median DFS*	81.7 (58.4–NR)
Survival rate—% (95% CI)	
3-year OS	73 (68–78)
3-year EFS	59 (54–65)
3-year DFS*	66 (60–72)
Survival rate by MRD status after induction (N = 80 patients evaluable)—% (95% CI)	
3-year DFS in patients with negative MRD (N = 35)	85 (74–98) ‡
3-year DFS in patients with positive MRD (N = 45)	54 (41–71)
Response	
CR—n/N (%) [95% CI]	263/295 (89) [85–92]
Multivariable analysis of pretreatment characteristics†	
Obesity (BMI >30 kg/m^2)	HR 1.82; P = 0.04 for disease-free survival
Aberrant *CRLF2* expression	HR 2.84; P<0.001 for disease-free survival

*Among 263 patients who achieved a bone marrow response
†Other pre-treatment characteristics that were significant in the univariable model for DFS, but did not maintain independent significance in the multivariable analysis for DFS, included WBC >30 (vs ≤30) in patients with B-cell ALL, Ph-like signature (vs not), and intermediate cytogenetics (vs unfavorable cytogenetics)
‡HR 0.25 (95% CI, 0.10–0.60); P = 0.001 for DFS in patients with negative MRD vs those with detectable MRD
Note: median follow-up was 64 months
CI, confidence interval; EFS, event-free survival; NR, not reached; DFS, disease-free survival; CR, complete remission; MRD, minimal residual disease; BMI, body mass index; HR, hazard ratio

Therapy Monitoring

1. Laboratory monitoring:
   - CBC with differential and platelet count daily during and after induction chemotherapy until recovery of ANC >500/mm^3
   - BUN, serum creatinine, electrolytes, mineral panel, uric acid, and LDH at least daily during active treatment until the risk of tumor lysis is past, and then at least weekly thereafter
   - Liver function tests (ALT, AST, total bilirubin, direct bilirubin, alkaline phosphate) at least once per week prior to daunorubicin and vincristine dosing on days 1, 8, 15, and 22
   - Fasting blood glucose, fasting lipid panel, aPTT, PT/INR, and fibrinogen prior to pegaspargase administration and then at least once per week thereafter during induction therapy. In patients with risk factors for hyperglycemia, increase the frequency of blood glucose monitoring
   - Serum amylase and lipase prior to pegaspargase and then as clinically indicated for abdominal pain
2. *Daunorubicin toxicity:* determination of LVEF by echocardiogram prior to treatment and then as clinically indicated
3. *Vincristine toxicity:* Perform a neurologic exam prior to each dose on days 1, 8, 15, and 22
4. *Pegaspargase toxicity:*
   - *Hypersensitivity:* Monitor for signs of an allergic reaction including bronchospasms, hypotension, laryngeal edema, local erythema or swelling, systemic rash, and urticaria. Monitor vital signs at baseline and every 30 minutes during and for 1 hour following administration of pegaspargase
   - *Pancreatitis and hepatotoxicity:* Advise patients to avoid alcohol during therapy
   - *Hemorrhage/thrombosis:* Avoid the use of oral contraceptives
5. *Response assessment:* Bone marrow aspirate and biopsy on day 15 to assess initial response and on day 29 to assess induction response and minimal residual disease. Repeat testicular exam in male patients with evidence of testicular involvement at diagnosis. With each dose of intrathecal chemotherapy, evaluate cerebrospinal fluid for cell count and cytospin exam

Treatment Modifications

PEGASPARGASE DOSE MODIFICATIONS

Adapted from: Stock W et al. Leuk Lymphoma 2011;52:2237–2253

Toxicity	Grade 2	Grade 3	Grade 4
Hypersensitivity, urticaria, wheezing, laryngospasm, hypotension, etc	For urticaria without bronchospasm, hypotension, edema, or need for parenteral intervention, continue pegaspargase	For wheezing or other symptomatic bronchospasm with or without urticaria, indicated parenteral intervention, angioedema, or hypotension, discontinue pegaspargase. Substitute Erwinia asparaginase 25,000 units/m^2 (if available) by IM injection every other day for 6 doses (including weekends if possible) to replace each dose of pegaspargase	For life-threatening consequences or indicated urgent intervention, discontinue pegaspargase. Substitute Erwinia asparaginase 25,000 units/m^2 (if available) by IM injection every other day for 6 doses (including weekends if possible) to replace each dose of pegaspargase
Hypertriglyceridemia	If serum triglyceride level <1000 mg/dL (<11.3 mmol/L), continue pegaspargase but follow patient closely for evolving pancreatitis	Hold pegaspargase for triglyceride >1000 mg/dL (>11.3 mmol/L); follow closely for pancreatitis; resume pegaspargase at prior dose level after patient's triglyceride level returns to normal range	Hold pegaspargase for triglyceride >1000 mg/dL (>11.3 mmol/L); follow closely for pancreatitis; resume pegaspargase at prior dose level after patient's triglyceride level returns to normal range
Hyperglycemia, ketoacidosis	Continue pegaspargase for uncomplicated hyperglycemia	For hyperglycemia requiring insulin therapy, hold pegaspargase (and glucocorticoid therapy) until blood glucose regulated with insulin; resume pegaspargase at prior dose level	For hyperglycemia with life-threatening consequences or indicated urgent intervention, hold pegaspargase (and glucocorticoid therapy) until blood glucose is regulated with insulin; resume pegaspargase and do not make up for missed doses
Hyperammonemia-related fatigue	Continue pegaspargase	Reduce pegaspargase dose by 25%; resume full dose when toxicity is Grade ≤2; make up for missed doses	Reduce pegaspargase dose 50%; resume full dose when toxicity is Grade ≤2; make up for missed doses

(continued)

Treatment Modifications (*continued*)

Toxicity	Grade 2	Grade 3	Grade 4
Pancreatitis	Continue pegaspargase for asymptomatic amylase or lipase elevation >3 × ULN (chemical pancreatitis) or only radiologic abnormalities; observe closely for rising amylase or lipase levels	Continue pegaspargase for non-symptomatic chemical pancreatitis but observe patient closely for development of symptomatic pancreatitis for early treatment. Temporarily withhold pegaspargase for amylase or lipase elevation >3 × ULN until enzyme levels stabilize or are declining. Permanently discontinue pegaspargase for symptomatic pancreatitis	Permanently discontinue all pegaspargase for clinical pancreatitis (vomiting, severe abdominal pain) with amylase or lipase elevation >3 × ULN for >3 days and/or development of pancreatic pseudocyst
Hyperbilirubinemia	Continue pegaspargase if direct bilirubin ≤3.0 mg/dL (≤51 μmol/L)	If direct bilirubin is 3.1–5.0 mg/dL (53–86 μmol/L), administer pegaspargase with the dose reduced by 50%	If direct bilirubin is >5.0 mg/dL (>86 μmol/L) and ≤6.0 mg/dL (≤103 μmol/L), withhold pegaspargase and administer the next scheduled dose if toxicity has resolved. Do not make up missed doses
Non-CNS thrombosis	For abnormal laboratory findings without clinical correlates, continue pegaspargase	Withhold pegaspargase until acute toxicity and clinical signs resolve and anticoagulant therapy is stable or completed. Do not withhold pegaspargase for abnormal laboratory findings without a clinical correlate	Withhold pegaspargase until acute toxicity and clinical signs resolve and anticoagulant therapy is stable or completed
Non-CNS hemorrhage	For bleeding in conjunction with hypofibrinogenemia, withhold pegaspargase until bleeding is Grade ≤1. Do not withhold pegaspargase for abnormal laboratory findings without a clinical correlate	Withhold pegaspargase until bleeding is Grade ≤1, until acute toxicity and clinical signs resolve, and coagulant replacement therapy is stable or completed	Withhold pegaspargase until bleeding is Grade ≤1, until acute toxicity and clinical signs resolve, and coagulant replacement therapy is stable or completed
CNS thrombosis	For abnormal laboratory findings without a clinical correlate, continue pegaspargase	Discontinue all pegaspargase; if CNS symptoms and signs are fully resolved and significant pegaspargase remains to be administered, may resume pegaspargase therapy at a lower dose and/or longer intervals between doses	Permanently discontinue pegaspargase
CNS hemorrhage	Discontinue pegaspargase; do not withhold pegaspargase for abnormal laboratory findings without a clinical correlate	Discontinue pegaspargase; if CNS symptoms and signs are fully resolved and significant pegaspargase remains to be administered, may resume pegaspargase therapy at a lower dose and/or longer intervals between doses	Permanently discontinue pegaspargase

Grade according to the National Cancer Institute Common Terminology Criteria for Advance Events version 4, with the exception of pancreatitis
IM, intramuscular; ULN, upper limit of normal; CNS, central nervous system

VINCRISTINE DOSE MODIFICATIONS

Hepatic Impairment	
Direct bilirubin <3.1 mg/dL	Administer full dose vincristine
Direct bilirubin 3.1–5.0 mg/dL	Administer vincristine with the dosage reduced by 50%
Direct bilirubin 5.1–6.0 mg/dL	Administer vincristine with the dosage reduced by 75%
Direct bilirubin >6.0 mg/dL	Withhold vincristine and administer the next scheduled dose if toxicity has resolved. Do not make up missed doses

(*continued*)

Treatment Modifications (*continued*)

Neuropathy

G ≥3 peripheral sensory neuropathy (severe symptoms; limiting self-care ADL; or worse)	Withhold vincristine until symptoms resolve to G ≤1, then resume vincristine with the dosage reduced by 50%. If the toxicity remains G ≤1, then consider re-escalating the vincristine dose back to the full dose
G ≥3 jaw pain (severe pain; limiting self-care ADL)	
G ≥3 vocal cord paralysis (severe symptoms; medical intervention indicated, eg, thyroplasty, vocal cord injection; or worse)	
G ≥3 motor neuropathy (severe symptoms; limiting self-care ADL; assistive device indicated; or worse)	

Gastrointestinal Toxicity

G ≥3 constipation (obstipation with manual evacuation indicated; limiting self-care ADL)	Withhold vincristine and optimize laxative regimen. When toxicity improves to G ≤1, resume vincristine with the dosage reduced by 50%. If the toxicity does not recur, then re-escalate the vincristine dose back to full dose
G ≥3 ileus (severely altered GI function; TPN indicated)	

DAUNORUBICIN DOSE MODIFICATIONS

Hepatic Impairment

Direct bilirubin ≥3 mg/dL but <5 mg/dL	Administer daunorubicin with the dosage reduced by 50%
Direct bilirubin ≥5 mg/dL but ≤7 mg/dL	Administer daunorubicin with the dosage reduced by 75%
Direct bilirubin >7 mg/dL	Omit the daunorubicin dose. Do not make up missed doses

Cardiac Toxicity

Congestive heart failure or decline in LVEF to <50%	Discontinue daunorubicin

ADL, activities of daily living; LVEF, left ventricular ejection fraction

Adverse Events (N = 295)

Event*	Induction (Course I) (N = 295)		
Grade (%)	Grade 3	Grade 4	Grade 5
Hypersensitivity	1	0	0
ALT	26	3	0
AST	11	1	0
Hyperbilirubinemia	12	6	0
Death NOS	0	0	<1
Fatigue	5	1	0
Febrile neutropenia	19	3	0
Hyperglycemia	23	8	0
Hemorrhage CNS	<1	1	0
Infection	13	5	1
Liver dysfunction/failure	1	<1	1
Mucositis†	1	<1	0

Event*	Induction (Course I) (N = 295)		
Grade (%)	Grade 3	Grade 4	Grade 5
Motor neuropathy	1	1	0
Sensory neuropathy	2	1	0
Avascular necrosis	<1	0	0
Pancreatitis	1	1	0
Thrombosis	3	3	0
Hypertriglyceridemia	1	1	0
Tumor lysis syndrome	5	0	0
Ventricular arrhythmia	0	<1	<1

*According to the National Cancer Institute Common Terminology Criteria for Adverse Events, version 3.0
†Term also includes stomatitis or esophagitis
Note: the table includes select Grade 3 or worse adverse events that are at least possibly related to protocol therapy that occurred during induction (course I)
ALT, alanine aminotransferase; AST, aspartate aminotransferase; NOS, not otherwise specified; CNS, central nervous system

ADOLESCENT/YOUNG ADULT

ACUTE LYMPHOBLASTIC LEUKEMIA: CALGB 10403 EXTENDED INDUCTION (COURSE IA)

Stock W et al. Blood 2019;133:1548–1559

Note: refer to regimen entitled "CALGB 10403 INDUCTION (COURSE I)" for a table containing an overview of the entire CALGB 10403 treatment regimen. For organizational purposes, each phase of the treatment protocol has been separated into an individual regimen within this textbook

Extended Induction (Course Ia, 2 weeks):

Important *Note:* administer extended induction (course Ia) only to patients with either an M2 marrow response (ie, >5–25% lymphoblasts) or an M1 marrow response (ie, <5% lymphoblasts) *with* ≥1% lymphoblasts detected by flow cytometry or immunohistochemistry on day 29 of induction (course I). If either of these criteria are met, then begin extended induction (course Ia) as soon as possible

Vincristine 1.5 mg/m^2 (maximum dose = 2 mg) per dose; administer by intravenous infusion over 15 minutes in 50 mL 0.9% sodium chloride injection (0.9% NS) for 2 doses on days 1 and 8 of extended induction (total dosage/14-day extended induction course = 3 mg/m^2; maximum dosage/28-day induction course = 4 mg)

Daunorubicin 25 mg/m^2; administer by intravenous injection over 3–5 minutes for 1 dose on day 1 only of extended induction course (total dosage/14-day extended induction course = 25 mg/m^2)

Prednisone 30 mg/m^2 per dose; administer orally twice per day, with food, for 14 consecutive days on days 1–14 of extended induction (total dosage/14-day induction course = 840 mg/m^2)

- *Note:* prednisone should be stopped abruptly without a taper upon the completion of the extended induction course

Premedications for pegaspargase:

- **Acetaminophen** 650–100 mg; administer orally 30 minutes prior to pegaspargase administration on day 4 (*or day 5 or day 6*)
- **Diphenhydramine** 25–50 mg; administer orally or intravenously 30 minutes prior to pegaspargase administration on day 4 (*or day 5 or day 6*)
  - *Note:* pegaspargase may cause anaphylaxis and serious hypersensitivity reactions. An expert panel recommends premedication prior to pegaspargase in adolescent and young adult patients (Stock W et al. Leuk Lymphoma 2011;52:2237–2253). Steroid premedication (eg, hydrocortisone) may be omitted during extended induction (course Ia) due to inclusion of prednisone in the regimen. Observe patients for 1 hour after the administration of pegaspargase in a setting with the capability to provide emergency resuscitation and with immediate availability of emergency supplies including epinephrine, oxygen, a histamine receptor [H$_1$]-subtype antagonist (eg, diphenhydramine), and intravenous corticosteroids

Choose one of the following options for pegaspargase:

- **Pegaspargase** 2500 units/m^2; administer by intravenous infusion over 1–2 hours in 100 mL 0.9% NS or 5% dextrose injection (D5W) into a running infusion of either 0.9% NS or D5W (choose the same fluid that was used for dilution of pegaspargase) for one dose on day 4 (*or day 5 or day 6*) of extended induction (total dosage/14-day induction course = 2500 units/m^2), or:
- **Pegaspargase** 2500 units/m^2; administer by intramuscular injection for one dose on day 4 (*or day 5 or day 6*) of extended induction (total dosage/14-day induction course = 2500 units/m^2)
  - Limit the volume at a single injection site to ≤2 mL. If the volume to be administered is >2 mL, multiple injection sites should be used
  - Patients with platelets <50,000/mm^3 may require a platelet transfusion prior to an intramuscular injection

Note: consider incorporation of rituximab throughout all phases of treatment for a total of 16 infusions based on the results of the GRAALL-2005/R study

Maury S et al. N Engl J Med 2016;375:1044–1053

Supportive Care
Antiemetic prophylaxis
Emetogenic potential on day 1 is **MODERATE**
Emetogenic potential on day 8 is **MINIMAL**
Emetogenic potential on day of pegaspargase administration (Day 4 or day 5 or day 6) is **MINIMAL**
See Chapter 42 for antiemetic recommendations

Hematopoietic growth factor (CSF) prophylaxis
Primary prophylaxis is **NOT** *indicated*
See Chapter 43 for more information

Antimicrobial prophylaxis
Risk of fever and neutropenia is **HIGH**
  Antimicrobial primary prophylaxis to be considered:
- Antibacterial—consider prophylaxis with a fluoroquinolone during periods of prolonged neutropenia only (eg, <500/mm^3 for ≥7 days) until ANC recovery
- Antifungal—consider prophylaxis with fluconazole or another antifungal medication during periods of prolonged neutropenia only (eg, <500/mm^3 for ≥7 days) until ANC recovery. Note that use of voriconazole, posaconazole, and itraconazole should be avoided with concomitant vincristine use. *Pneumocystis jirovecii* prophylaxis is recommended (eg, cotrimoxazole)
- Antiviral—anti-herpes antivirals (eg, acyclovir, famciclovir, valacyclovir)

Patient Population Studied

Refer to regimen entitled "CALGB 10403 INDUCTION (COURSE I)" for a description of the patient population

Efficacy

Refer to regimen entitled "CALGB 10403 INDUCTION (COURSE I)" for efficacy results

Therapy Monitoring

1. *Laboratory monitoring:*
   a. CBC with differential and platelet count daily during and after extended induction chemotherapy until recovery of ANC >500/mm^3
   b. BUN, serum creatinine, electrolytes, mineral panel, uric acid, and LDH at least daily during active treatment until the risk of tumor lysis is past, and then at least weekly thereafter
   c. Liver function tests (ALT, AST, total bilirubin, direct bilirubin, alkaline phosphate) at least once per week during extended induction therapy and prior to daunorubicin and/or vincristine dosing on days 1 and 8
   d. Fasting blood glucose, fasting lipid panel, aPTT, PT/INR, and fibrinogen prior to pegaspargase administration and then at least once per week thereafter during extended induction therapy. In patients with risk factors for hyperglycemia, increase the frequency of blood glucose monitoring
   e. Serum amylase and lipase prior to pegaspargase and then as clinically indicated for abdominal pain
2. *Daunorubicin toxicity:* repeat determination of LVEF as clinically indicated
3. *Vincristine toxicity:* perform a neurologic exam prior to each dose on days 1 and 8
4. *Pegaspargase toxicity:*
   a. *Hypersensitivity:* monitor for signs of an allergic reaction including bronchospasms, hypotension, laryngeal edema, local erythema or swelling, systemic rash, and urticaria. Monitor vital signs at baseline and every 30 minutes during and for 1 hour following administration of pegaspargase
   b. *Pancreatitis and hepatotoxicity:* advise patients to avoid alcohol during therapy
   c. *Hemorrhage/thrombosis:* avoid the use of oral contraceptives
5. *Response assessment:* bone marrow aspirate and biopsy on day 15 of extended induction (course Ia) to assess initial response and minimal residual disease. Repeat testicular exam in male patients with evidence of testicular involvement at diagnosis

Treatment Modifications

PEGASPARGASE DOSE MODIFICATIONS

Refer to regimen entitled "CALGB 10403 INDUCTION (COURSE I)" for pegaspargase dose modification recommendations.

VINCRISTINE DOSE MODIFICATIONS

Hepatic Impairment

Direct bilirubin <3.1 mg/dL	Administer full dose vincristine
Direct bilirubin 3.1–5.0 mg/dL	Administer vincristine with the dosage reduced by 50%
Direct bilirubin 5.1–6.0 mg/dL	Administer vincristine with the dosage reduced by 75%
Direct bilirubin >6.0 mg/dL	Withhold vincristine and administer the next scheduled dose if toxicity has resolved. Do not make up missed doses

Neuropathy

G ≥3 peripheral sensory neuropathy (severe symptoms; limiting self-care ADL; or worse)	Withhold vincristine until symptoms resolve to G ≤1, then resume vincristine with the dosage reduced by 50%. If the toxicity remains G ≤1, then consider re-escalating the vincristine dose back to the full dose
G ≥3 jaw pain (severe pain; limiting self-care ADL)	
G ≥3 vocal cord paralysis (severe symptoms; medical intervention indicated, eg, thyroplasty, vocal cord injection; or worse)	
G ≥3 motor neuropathy (severe symptoms; limiting self-care ADL; assistive device indicated; or worse)	

(continued)

Treatment Modifications (*continued*)

Gastrointestinal Toxicity

G ≥3 constipation (obstipation with manual evacuation indicated; limiting self-care ADL)	Withhold vincristine and optimize laxative regimen. When toxicity improves to G ≤1, resume vincristine with the dosage reduced by 50%. If the toxicity does not recur, then re-escalate the vincristine dose back to full dose
G ≥3 ileus (severely altered GI function; TPN indicated)	

DAUNORUBICIN DOSE MODIFICATIONS

Hepatic Impairment

Direct bilirubin ≥3 mg/dL but <5 mg/dL	Administer daunorubicin with the dosage reduced by 50%
Direct bilirubin ≥5 mg/dL but ≤7 mg/dL	Administer daunorubicin with the dosage reduced by 75%
Direct bilirubin >7 mg/dL	Omit the daunorubicin dose. Do not make up missed doses
Cardiac toxicity	
Congestive heart failure or decline in LVEF to <50%	Discontinue daunorubicin

ADL, activities of daily living; LVEF, left ventricular ejection fraction

Adverse Events

Refer to regimen entitled "CALGB 10403 INDUCTION (COURSE I)" for a table containing a summary of adverse events observed during induction therapy

ADOLESCENT/YOUNG ADULT

ACUTE LYMPHOBLASTIC LEUKEMIA: CALGB 10403 CONSOLIDATION (COURSE II)

Stock W et al. Blood 2019;133:1548–1559

Note: refer to regimen entitled "CALGB 10403 INDUCTION (COURSE I)" for a table containing an overview of the entire CALGB 10403 treatment regimen. For organizational purposes, each phase of the treatment protocol has been separated into an individual regimen within this textbook

Consolidation (course II, 8 weeks); begin within 7 days from remission marrow or when ANC recovers to ≥750/mm³ and platelets recover to ≥75,000/mm³, whichever occurs later:

Hydration prior to cyclophosphamide:
0.9% sodium chloride injection 1000 mL; administer intravenously over 2 hours, starting 2 hours prior to cyclophosphamide on days 1 and 29 of consolidation

Cyclophosphamide 1000 mg/m² per dose; administer intravenously in 25–250 mL 0.9% sodium chloride injection (0.9% NS) or 5% dextrose injection (D5W) over 30 minutes for 2 doses on days 1 and 29 of consolidation (total dosage/56-day consolidation course = 2000 mg/m²)
- Delay day 29 cyclophosphamide until ANC is ≥750/mm³ and platelets are ≥75,000/mm³

Cytarabine 75 mg/m² per dose; administer by subcutaneous or intravenous injection once daily for a total of 16 doses to be administered on days 1–4, 8–11, 29–32, and 36–39 of consolidation (total dosage/56-day consolidation course = 1200 mg/m²)
- Delay the initiation of cytarabine on day 29 until ANC is ≥750/mm³ and platelets are ≥75,000/mm³

Mercaptopurine 60 mg/m² per dose; administer orally, on an empty stomach at least 1 hour after the evening meal, without milk or citrus products, once per day on days 1–14 and on days 29–42 during consolidation (total dosage/56-day consolidation course = 1680 mg/m²)
- Delay the initiation of mercaptopurine on day 29 until ANC is ≥750/mm³ and platelets are ≥75,000/mm³
- Adjust the dose using 50 mg tablets and different doses on alternating days in order to attain a weekly cumulative dose as near to 420 mg/m²/week as possible

Vincristine 1.5 mg/m² (maximum dose = 2 mg) per dose; administer by intravenous infusion over 15 minutes in 50 mL 0.9% NS for 4 doses on days 15, 22, 43, and 50 of consolidation (total dosage/56-day consolidation course = 6 mg/m²; maximum dosage/56-day consolidation course = 8 mg)

Premedications for pegaspargase:
- **Acetaminophen** 650–100 mg; administer orally 30 minutes prior to pegaspargase administration on days 15 and 43 of consolidation
- **Diphenhydramine** 25–50 mg; administer orally or intravenously 30 minutes prior to pegaspargase administration on days 15 and 43 of consolidation
- **Hydrocortisone sodium succinate** 100 mg; administer by intravenous injection 30 minutes prior to pegaspargase administration on days 15 and 43 of consolidation
  - *Note:* pegaspargase may cause anaphylaxis and serious hypersensitivity reactions. An expert panel recommends premedication prior to pegaspargase in adolescent and young adult patients (Stock W et al. Leuk Lymphoma 2011;52:2237–2253). Observe patients for 1 hour after the administration of pegaspargase in a setting with the capability to provide emergency resuscitation and with immediate availability of emergency supplies including epinephrine, oxygen, a histamine receptor [H₁]-subtype antagonist (eg, diphenhydramine), and intravenous corticosteroids

Choose one of the following options for pegaspargase:
- **Pegaspargase** 2500 units/m²; administer by intravenous infusion over 1–2 hours in 100 mL 0.9% NS or D5W into a running infusion of either 0.9% NS or D5W (choose the same fluid that was used for dilution of pegaspargase) for two doses on days 15 and 43 of consolidation (total dosage/56-day consolidation course = 5000 units/m²), *or:*
- **Pegaspargase** 2500 units/m²; administer by intramuscular injection for two doses on days 15 and 43 of consolidation (total dosage/56-day consolidation course = 5000 units/m²)
  - Limit the volume at a single injection site to ≤2 mL. If the volume to be administered is >2 mL, multiple injection sites should be used
  - Patients with platelets <50,000/mm³ may require a platelet transfusion prior to an intramuscular injection

Choose a methotrexate schedule based on CNS status:
For patients *without* CNS 3 disease:
- **Methotrexate** 15 mg; administer intrathecally via lumbar puncture or instillation via Ommaya reservoir for 4 doses on days 1, 8, 15, and 22 of consolidation (total dosage/56-day consolidation course for patients without CNS 3 disease = 60 mg)
  - Patients should remain in a horizontal position for ≥30 minutes following intrathecal chemotherapy

(continued)

(continued)

For patients *with* CNS 3 disease:

- **Methotrexate** 15 mg; administer intrathecally via lumbar puncture or instillation via Ommaya reservoir for 2 doses on days 1 and 8 of consolidation (total dosage/56-day consolidation course for patients with CNS 3 disease = 30 mg)
  - Patients should remain in a horizontal position for ≥30 minutes following intrathecal chemotherapy

Note: CNS 3 disease is defined as cerebrospinal fluid with ≥5 WBC/μL with cytospin positive for blasts; or ≥10 RBC/μL, ≥5 WBC/μL, and positive by Steinherz/Bleyer algorithm; or clinical signs of CNS leukemia such as facial nerve palsy, brain/eye involvement, or hypothalamic syndrome

  - The Steinherz/Bleyer method should be applied to classify cerebrospinal fluid (CSF) results if the patient has leukemia cells circulating in the peripheral blood and undergoes a traumatic lumbar puncture and CSF is found to have ≥5 WBC/μL with blasts. A patient with this scenario should be considered to have CNS 3 disease if:

$$\frac{\text{CSF WBC}}{\text{CSF RBC}} > 2X \frac{\text{Blood WBC}}{\text{Blood RBC}}$$

Note: consider incorporation of rituximab throughout all phases of treatment for a total of 16 infusions based on the results of the GRAALL-2005/R study

Maury S et al. N Engl J Med 2016;375:1044–1053

Supportive Care

Antiemetic prophylaxis
Emetogenic potential on days with cyclophosphamide (days 1 and 29) is **MODERATE**
Emetogenic potential on all other days of treatment besides days 1 and 29 is **MINIMAL**
See Chapter 42 for antiemetic recommendations

Hematopoietic growth factor (CSF) prophylaxis
Primary prophylaxis is **NOT** *indicated*
See Chapter 43 for more information

Antimicrobial prophylaxis
Risk of fever and neutropenia is **HIGH**
  Antimicrobial primary prophylaxis to be considered:
- Antibacterial—consider prophylaxis with a fluoroquinolone during periods of prolonged neutropenia only (eg, <500/mm³ for ≥7 days) until ANC recovery
- Antifungal—consider prophylaxis with fluconazole or another antifungal medication during periods of prolonged neutropenia only (eg, <500/mm³ for ≥7 days) until ANC recovery. Note that use of voriconazole, posaconazole, and itraconazole should be avoided with concomitant vincristine use. *Pneumocystis jirovecii* prophylaxis is recommended (eg, cotrimoxazole)
- Antiviral—anti-herpes antivirals (eg, acyclovir, famciclovir, valacyclovir)

Patient Population Studied

Refer to regimen entitled "CALGB 10403 INDUCTION (COURSE I)" for a description of the patient population

Efficacy

Refer to regimen entitled "CALGB 10403 INDUCTION (COURSE I)" for efficacy results

Therapy Monitoring

1. *Laboratory monitoring:*
   a. CBC with differential and platelet count, BUN, serum creatinine, electrolytes, liver function tests (ALT, AST, total bilirubin, direct bilirubin, alkaline phosphate), fasting blood glucose, fasting lipid panel, aPTT, PT/INR, and fibrinogen at least once per week on days 1, 8, 15, 22, 29, 36, 43, and 50; and as clinically indicated. In patients with risk factors for hyperglycemia, increase the frequency of blood glucose monitoring
   b. Serum amylase and lipase prior to each dose of pegaspargase on days 15 and 43, and then as clinically indicated for abdominal pain
2. *Vincristine toxicity:* perform a neurologic exam prior to each dose on **days 15, 22, 43, and 50**
3. *Pegaspargase toxicity:*
   a. *Hypersensitivity:* monitor for signs of an allergic reaction including bronchospasms, hypotension, laryngeal edema, local erythema or swelling, systemic rash, and urticaria. Monitor vital signs at baseline and every 30 minutes during and for 1 hour following administration of pegaspargase
   b. *Pancreatitis and hepatotoxicity:* advise patients to avoid alcohol during therapy
   c. *Hemorrhage/thrombosis:* avoid the use of oral contraceptives
4. *Response assessment:* with each dose of intrathecal chemotherapy, evaluate cerebrospinal fluid for cell count and cytospin exam

Treatment Modifications

PEGASPARGASE DOSE MODIFICATIONS

Refer to regimen entitled "CALGB 10403 INDUCTION (COURSE I)" for pegaspargase dose modification recommendations.

GENERAL DOSE MODIFICATIONS

Myelosuppression

Day 1 ANC <750/mm^3 or platelets <75,000/mm^3	Delay initiation of consolidation chemotherapy until ANC ≥750/mm^3 and platelets ≥75,000/mm^3, and at least 7 days from the remission marrow, whichever occurs later
Day 29 ANC <750/mm^3 or platelets <75,000/mm^3	Delay initiation of day 29 chemotherapy until ANC ≥750/mm^3 and platelets ≥75,000/mm^3
ANC <750/mm^3 on days 2–28 or on days 30–56 in a patient without a documented infection (*Note:* neutropenic fever without a source of infection is not considered a documented infection)	Continue chemotherapy without interruption
Platelets <75,000/mm^3 on days 2–28 or on days 30–56	
ANC <750/mm^3 (any day) and patient is febrile and proven to be infected	Withhold chemotherapy and then resume at the same point when signs and symptoms of infection have resolved

VINCRISTINE DOSE MODIFICATIONS

Hepatic Impairment

Direct bilirubin <3.1 mg/dL	Administer full dose vincristine
Direct bilirubin 3.1–5.0 mg/dL	Administer vincristine with the dosage reduced by 50%
Direct bilirubin 5.1–6.0 mg/dL	Administer vincristine with the dosage reduced by 75%
Direct bilirubin >6.0 mg/dL	Withhold vincristine and administer the next scheduled dose if toxicity has resolved. Do not make up missed doses

Neuropathy

G ≥3 peripheral sensory neuropathy (severe symptoms; limiting self-care ADL; or worse)	Withhold vincristine until symptoms resolve to G ≤1, then resume vincristine with the dosage reduced by 50%. If the toxicity remains G ≤1, then consider re-escalating the vincristine dose back to the full dose
G ≥3 jaw pain (severe pain; limiting self-care ADL)	
G ≥3 vocal cord paralysis (severe symptoms; medical intervention indicated, eg, thyroplasty, vocal cord injection; or worse)	
G ≥3 motor neuropathy (severe symptoms; limiting self-care ADL; assistive device indicated; or worse)	

Gastrointestinal Toxicity

G ≥3 constipation (obstipation with manual evacuation indicated; limiting self-care ADL)	Withhold vincristine and optimize laxative regimen. When toxicity improves to G ≤1, resume vincristine with the dosage reduced by 50%. If the toxicity does not recur, then re-escalate the vincristine dose back to full dose
G ≥3 ileus (severely altered GI function; TPN indicated)	

CYCLOPHOSPHAMIDE DOSE MODIFICATIONS

Bladder Toxicity

Gross hematuria	Withhold cyclophosphamide until resolution of hematuria. Optimize hydration (eg, administer IV fluids for 24 hours after cyclophosphamide) and add MESNA 200 mg/m^2 per dose given 15 minutes prior to and 3, 6, and 9 hours following the next dose of cyclophosphamide (or alternative MESNA dosing per local practice)
Significant microscopic hematuria (>50 RBCs/HPF)	

(continued)

Treatment Modifications (continued)

MERCAPTOPURINE DOSE MODIFICATIONS

Other Toxicities

G ≥2 creatinine increased (serum creatinine >1.5× ULN)	Withhold mercaptopurine until improvement to G ≤1, then resume mercaptopurine at the same dose
Patient requires treatment with a xanthine oxidase inhibitor (allopurinol or febuxostat)	If concomitant therapy is unavoidable, reduce the starting mercaptopurine dose to 25–33% of the usual starting dose and monitor closely for toxicity
Myelosuppression leading to significant delays (>2 weeks) in therapy or myelosuppression is extremely severe	Perform TPMT genotyping
Patient is known to be a TPMT intermediate metabolizer and has experienced significant myelosuppression	Reduce the mercaptopurine dosage by 30–50%
Patient is known to be a TPMT poor metabolizer	Initiate mercaptopurine with the dosage reduced to 10–20 mg/m² per day given 3 days per week

CYTARABINE DOSE MODIFICATIONS

Cytarabine Syndrome

Cytarabine syndrome (non-infectious fevers considered related to cytarabine, arthralgias, non-severe macular rash)	Continue cytarabine without interruption
G ≥3 rash related to cytarabine (severe, generalized erythroderma or macular, papular, or vesicular eruption; desquamation covering ≥50% BSA)	Withhold cytarabine until improvement to G ≤2, then resume cytarabine

ANC, absolute neutrophil count; ADL, activities of daily living; GI, gastrointestinal; TPN, total parenteral nutrition; RBCs, red blood cells; HPF, high power field; ULN, upper limit of normal; TPMT, thiopurine methyltransferase; BSA, body surface area

Adverse Events (N = 237)

Event[†]	Postremission Consolidation Therapy (Courses II–IV) (N = 237)		
Grade (%)	**Grade 3**	**Grade 4**	**Grade 5**
Hypersensitivity	7	4	0
ALT	39	3	0
AST	23	2	0
Hyperbilirubinemia	8	2	0
Death NOS	0	0	0
Fatigue	12	0	0
Febrile neutropenia	39	5	0
Hyperglycemia	8	3	0
Hemorrhage CNS	0	0	0
Infection	22	3	1
Liver dysfunction/failure	0	0	0
Mucositis[‡]	8	1	0
Motor neuropathy	4	<1	0

Event[†]	Postremission Consolidation Therapy (Courses II–IV) (N = 237)		
Grade (%)	**Grade 3**	**Grade 4**	**Grade 5**
Sensory neuropathy	15	<1	0
Avascular necrosis	<1	0	0
Pancreatitis	4	0	0
Thrombosis	6	3	0
Hypertriglyceridemia	3	9	0
Tumor lysis syndrome	0	0	0
Ventricular arrhythmia	0	0	0

*Includes consolidation, interim maintenance, and delayed intensification
[†]According to the National Cancer Institute Common Terminology Criteria for Adverse Events, version 3.0
[‡]Term also includes stomatitis or esophagitis
Note: the table includes select Grade 3 or worse adverse events that are at least possibly related to protocol therapy that occurred during consolidation, interim maintenance, and/or delayed intensification
ALT, alanine aminotransferase; AST, aspartate aminotransferase; NOS, not otherwise specified; CNS, central nervous system

ADOLESCENT/YOUNG ADULT

ACUTE LYMPHOBLASTIC LEUKEMIA: CALGB 10403 INTERIM MAINTENANCE (COURSE III)

Stock W et al. Blood 2019;133:1548–1559

Note: refer to regimen entitled "CALGB 10403 INDUCTION (COURSE I)" for a table containing an overview of the entire CALGB 10403 treatment regimen. For organizational purposes, each phase of the treatment protocol has been separated into an individual regimen within this textbook

Interim Maintenance (Course III, "Capizzi Methotrexate," 8 weeks); begin when ANC recovers to ≥750/mm³ and platelets recover to ≥75,000/mm³:

Vincristine 1.5 mg/m² (maximum dose = 2 mg) per dose; administer by intravenous infusion over 15 minutes in 50 mL 0.9% NS for 5 doses on days 1, 11, 21, 31, and 41 of interim maintenance (total dosage/56-day interim maintenance course = 7.5 mg/m²; maximum dosage/56-day interim maintenance = 10 mg)

Hydration prior to each methotrexate dose:
- Encourage oral hydration with ≥3000 mL/day of fluids. In patients who cannot hydrate adequately with oral fluids, supplement with intravenous hydration

Urine alkalinization during interim maintenance (goal urine pH≥7):
- **Sodium bicarbonate** 1950 mg per dose; administer orally every 4 hours for 72 hours starting on the evening prior to each dose of intravenous methotrexate
  - If the urine pH is <7 on the day of methotrexate administration, consider supplementing with acetazolamide as follows:
    - **Acetazolamide** 250 mg; administer orally on the day of intravenous methotrexate administration if needed for pH <7

Methotrexate 100 mg/m² *starting* dose; administer by intravenous injection, every 10 days, for 5 doses on days 1, 11, 21, 31, and 41 of interim maintenance (total dosage/56-day interim maintenance course = variable depending on dose adjustments; see "Therapy Monitoring" section)
- **Important:** modify the day 11, 21, 31, and 41 methotrexate doses according to level of myelosuppression and on the basis of renal, hepatic, and gastrointestinal toxicity. See "Treatment Modifications" section for details
- Withhold cotrimoxazole doses on days of intravenous methotrexate administration
- Carefully monitor patients with pleural effusions; patients may experience more severe toxicity due to slow methotrexate clearance
- If it is necessary (due to clinic schedule) to avoid weekend treatments, then it is acceptable to alternate Monday/Tuesday with Thursday/Friday treatments, maintaining 9–11 days between doses

Premedications for pegaspargase:
- **Acetaminophen** 650–100 mg; administer orally 30 minutes prior to pegaspargase administration on days 2 and 22 of interim maintenance
- **Diphenhydramine** 25–50 mg; administer orally or intravenously 30 minutes prior to pegaspargase administration on days 2 and 22 of interim maintenance
- **Hydrocortisone sodium succinate** 100 mg; administer by intravenous injection 30 minutes prior to pegaspargase administration on days 2 and 22 of interim maintenance
  - *Note:* pegaspargase may cause anaphylaxis and serious hypersensitivity reactions. An expert panel recommends premedication prior to pegaspargase in adolescent and young adult patients (Stock W et al. Leuk Lymphoma 2011;52:2237–2253). Observe patients for 1 hour after the administration of pegaspargase in a setting with the capability to provide emergency resuscitation and with immediate availability of emergency supplies including epinephrine, oxygen, a histamine receptor [H₁]-subtype antagonist (eg, diphenhydramine), and intravenous corticosteroids

Choose one of the following options for pegaspargase:
- **Pegaspargase** 2500 units/m²; administer by intravenous infusion over 1–2 hours in 100 mL 0.9% NS or D5W into a running infusion of either 0.9% NS or D5W (choose the same fluid that was used for dilution of pegaspargase) for two doses on days 2 and 22 of interim maintenance (total dosage/56-day interim maintenance course = 5000 units/m²), *or:*
- **Pegaspargase** 2500 units/m²; administer by intramuscular injection for two doses on days 2 and 22 of interim maintenance (total dosage/56-day interim maintenance course = 5000 units/m²)
  - Limit the volume at a single injection site to ≤2 mL. If the volume to be administered is >2 mL, multiple injection sites should be used
  - Patients with platelets <50,000/mm³ may require a platelet transfusion prior to an intramuscular injection

Methotrexate 15 mg; administer intrathecally via lumbar puncture or instillation via Ommaya reservoir for 2 doses on days 1 and 31 of interim maintenance (total dosage/56-day interim maintenance course = 30 mg)
- Patients should remain in a horizontal position for ≥30 minutes following intrathecal chemotherapy

Note: consider incorporation of rituximab throughout all phases of treatment for a total of 16 infusions based on the results of the GRAALL-2005/R study

Maury S et al. N Engl J Med 2016;375:1044–1053

(continued)

(continued)

Supportive Care
Antiemetic prophylaxis
Emetogenic potential on days *1, 11, 21, 31, and 41* is **LOW**
Emetogenic potential on days *2 and 22* is **MINIMAL**
See Chapter 42 for antiemetic recommendations

Hematopoietic growth factor (CSF) prophylaxis
Primary prophylaxis is **NOT** indicated
See Chapter 43 for more information

Antimicrobial prophylaxis
Risk of fever and neutropenia is **HIGH**
  Antimicrobial primary prophylaxis to be considered:
• Antibacterial—consider prophylaxis with a fluoroquinolone during periods of prolonged neutropenia only (eg, <500/mm^3 for ≥7 days) until ANC recovery
• Antifungal—consider prophylaxis with fluconazole or another antifungal medication during periods of prolonged neutropenia only (eg, <500/mm^3 for ≥7 days) until ANC recovery. Note that use of voriconazole, posaconazole, and itraconazole should be avoided with concomitant vincristine use. *Pneumocystis jirovecii* prophylaxis is recommended (eg, cotrimoxazole)
• Antiviral—anti-herpes antivirals (eg, acyclovir, famciclovir, valacyclovir)

Patient Population Studied

Refer to regimen entitled "CALGB 10403 INDUCTION (COURSE I)" for a description of the patient population.

Efficacy

Refer to regimen entitled "CALGB 10403 INDUCTION (COURSE I)" for efficacy results.

Therapy Monitoring

1. *Laboratory monitoring:*
   a. CBC with differential and platelet count, BUN, serum creatinine, liver function tests (ALT, AST, total bilirubin, direct bilirubin, alkaline phosphate), fasting lipid panel, aPTT, PT/INR, fibrinogen, fasting blood glucose, and urine pH prior to each dose of methotrexate on days 1, 11, 21, 31, and 41, and as clinically indicated. In patients with risk factors for hyperglycemia, increase the frequency of blood glucose monitoring
   b. Serum amylase and lipase on days 1 and 21, then as clinically indicated for abdominal pain
   c. For patients with acute kidney injury, evaluate a serum methotrexate level
2. *Methotrexate toxicity:* evaluate for mucositis prior to each dose
3. *Vincristine toxicity:* perform a neurologic exam prior to each dose on **days 1, 11, 21, 31, and 51**
4. *Pegaspargase toxicity:*
   a. *Hypersensitivity:* monitor for signs of an allergic reaction including bronchospasms, hypotension, laryngeal edema, local erythema or swelling, systemic rash, and urticaria. Monitor vital signs at baseline and every 30 minutes during and for 1 hour following administration of pegaspargase
   b. *Pancreatitis and hepatotoxicity:* advise patients to avoid alcohol during therapy
   c. *Hemorrhage/thrombosis:* avoid the use of oral contraceptives
5. *Response assessment:* with each dose of intrathecal chemotherapy, evaluate cerebrospinal fluid for cell count and cytospin exam. In the CALGB 10403 study, a bone marrow aspirate and biopsy was obtained 1 week after completion of course III. If a bone marrow specimen is obtained, evaluate for minimal residual disease

Treatment Modifications

CAPIZZI METHOTREXATE DOSE MODIFICATION GUIDELINES

Note: starting dose of IV methotrexate is 100 mg/m^2

ANC ≥750/mm^3 and platelets ≥75,000/mm^3 on day of IV methotrexate administration (not applicable to day 1)	Increase the IV methotrexate dose by 50 mg/m^2 from the previous dose
ANC ≥500/mm^3 but <750/mm^3 or platelets ≥50,000/mm^3 but <75,000/mm^3 on day of IV methotrexate administration	Administer the same dose of IV methotrexate as previously

(continued)

Treatment Modifications (*continued*)

ANC <500/mm^3 or platelets <50,000/mm^3 on day of IV methotrexate administration	Delay *all* chemotherapy and repeat CBC with differential and platelet count in 4 days: • If after 4 days the ANC recovers to ≥500/mm^3 and platelets ≥50,000/mm^3, then administer vincristine and administer the same dose of IV methotrexate as previously. If the day 22 pegaspargase was held, then reschedule it for administration on the next day • If after 4 days the ANC is still <500/mm^3 or platelets are still <50,000/mm^3, then omit this dose of IV methotrexate (do not make up). Administer vincristine, pegaspargase (if it was delayed) and intrathecal methotrexate (if due) • Repeat a CBC with differential and platelet count in 7 days to begin the next dose of methotrexate
First occurrence of ANC <750/mm^3 or platelets <75,000/mm^3 for ≥7 days after IV methotrexate administration	Discontinue cotrimoxazole temporarily. Upon resolution of hematologic toxicity (ANC ≥750/mm^3 and platelets ≥75,000/mm^3), administer IV methotrexate at the same dose
Recurrence of ANC <750/mm^3 or platelets <75,000/mm^3 for ≥7 days after IV methotrexate administration despite temporary discontinuation of cotrimoxazole (or first occurrence in patients who are not taking cotrimoxazole)	Upon resolution of hematologic toxicity (ANC ≥750/mm^3 and platelets ≥75,000/mm^3), reduce the IV methotrexate dose by 25%. If neutropenia or thrombocytopenia does not recur after 2 doses of intravenous methotrexate at a reduced dose, attempt to resume therapy at the previous higher dose
G ≥3 mucositis	Temporarily withhold IV methotrexate. For severe symptoms, consider administration of IV hydration and a low dose (5 mg) of leucovorin. Upon improvement to G ≤1, resume IV methotrexate with the dosage reduced by 25% from the previous dose. Do not make up missed doses. If G ≥3 mucositis does not recur with the subsequent dose, then attempt to re-escalate to full dose IV methotrexate
ALT <10× ULN on the day of IV methotrexate administration	Continue with therapy as scheduled
ALT ≥10× ULN but <20× ULN on the day of IV methotrexate administration	Discontinue cotrimoxazole and other potentially hepatotoxic drugs (eg, azole antifungals). Administer IV methotrexate as scheduled for one dose
ALT ≥10× ULN but <20× ULN that occurs on two consecutive treatment days prior to IV methotrexate	Discontinue cotrimoxazole and other potentially hepatotoxic drugs (eg, -azole antifungals). Hold IV methotrexate until ALT <10× ULN, and then resume at the previous dose. Make up missed doses
ALT >20× ULN on the day of IV methotrexate administration	Discontinue cotrimoxazole and other potentially hepatotoxic drugs (eg, -azole antifungals). Hold IV methotrexate until ALT <10× ULN, and then resume at the previous dose. Make up missed doses
ALT >20× ULN for > 2 weeks	Exclude viral causes of hepatitis (eg, hepatitis A, hepatitis B, hepatitis C, CMV, EBV). Evaluate lipase, amylase, albumin, and PT/INR. Increase the frequency of ALT, AST, total bilirubin, direct bilirubin, and alkaline phosphatase monitoring. Consider liver biopsy before additional therapy is administered
SCr >1.5× baseline or CrCL <65 mL/1.73m^2/minute	Postpone IV methotrexate dose until improvement in renal function. Provide aggressive IV hydration with alkaline fluids. Obtain a methotrexate level. If the methotrexate concentration is ≥0.1 micromolar initiate leucovorin and continue until methotrexate concentration is <0.1 micromolar. Adjust the leucovorin dose and frequency based upon a standard nomogram (eg, Widemann BC et al. Oncologist. 2006;11:694–703). Consider resuming IV methotrexate if full recovery of renal function occurs

IV, intravenous; CBC, complete blood count; ALT, alanine aminotransferase; AST, aspartate aminotransferase; BUN, blood urea nitrogen; ANC, absolute neutrophil count; ULN, upper limit of normal; CMV, cytomegalovirus; EBV, Epstein-Barr virus

PEGASPARGASE DOSE MODIFICATIONS

Refer to regimen entitled "CALGB 10403 INDUCTION (COURSE I)" for pegaspargase dose modification recommendations

GENERAL DOSE MODIFICATIONS

Myelosuppression

Severe, active infection	Interrupt chemotherapy until infection is controlled

(*continued*)

Treatment Modifications (continued)

VINCRISTINE DOSE MODIFICATIONS

Hepatic Impairment

Direct bilirubin <3.1 mg/dL	Administer full dose vincristine
Direct bilirubin 3.1–5.0 mg/dL	Administer vincristine with the dosage reduced by 50%
Direct bilirubin 5.1–6.0 mg/dL	Administer vincristine with the dosage reduced by 75%
Direct bilirubin >6.0 mg/dL	Withhold vincristine and administer the next scheduled dose if toxicity has resolved. Do not make up missed doses

Neuropathy

G ≥3 peripheral sensory neuropathy (severe symptoms; limiting self-care ADL; or worse)	Withhold vincristine until symptoms resolve to G ≤1, then resume vincristine with the dosage reduced by 50%. If the toxicity remains G ≤1, then consider re-escalating the vincristine dose back to the full dose
G ≥3 jaw pain (severe pain; limiting self-care ADL)	
G ≥3 vocal cord paralysis (severe symptoms; medical intervention indicated, eg, thyroplasty, vocal cord injection; or worse)	
G ≥3 motor neuropathy (severe symptoms; limiting self-care ADL; assistive device indicated; or worse)	

Gastrointestinal Toxicity

G ≥3 constipation (obstipation with manual evacuation indicated; limiting self-care ADL)	Withhold vincristine and optimize laxative regimen. When toxicity improves to G ≤1, resume vincristine with the dosage reduced by 50%. If the toxicity does not recur, then re-escalate the vincristine dose back to full dose
G ≥3 ileus (severely altered GI function; TPN indicated)	

ADL, activities of daily living; GI, gastrointestinal; TPN, total parenteral nutrition

Adverse Events (N = 237)

Note: refer to regimen entitled "CALGB 10403 INDUCTION (COURSE I)" for a table containing a summary of adverse events observed during post-remission consolidation therapy (courses II–IV)

ADOLESCENT/YOUNG ADULT

ACUTE LYMPHOBLASTIC LEUKEMIA: CALGB 10403 DELAYED INTENSIFICATION (COURSE IV)

Stock W et al. Blood 2019;133:1548–1559

Note: refer to regimen entitled "CALGB 10403 INDUCTION (COURSE I)" for a table containing an overview of the entire CALGB 10403 treatment regimen. For organizational purposes, each phase of the treatment protocol has been separated into an individual regimen within this textbook

Delayed intensification (course IV, 8 weeks); begin when ANC recovers to $\geq750/mm^3$ and platelets recover to $\geq75,000/mm^3$:

Vincristine 1.5 mg/m^2 (maximum dose = 2 mg) per dose; administer by intravenous infusion over 15 minutes in 50 mL 0.9% NS for 5 doses on days 1, 8, 15, 43, and 50 of delayed intensification (total dosage/56-day delayed intensification course = 7.5 mg/m^2; maximum dosage/56-day delayed intensification course = 10 mg)

Premedications for pegaspargase:
- **Acetaminophen** 650–100 mg; administer orally 30 minutes prior to pegaspargase administration on day 4 (*or* day 5 *or* day 6) and day 43 of delayed intensification
- **Diphenhydramine** 25–50 mg; administer orally or intravenously 30 minutes prior to pegaspargase administration on day 4 (*or* day 5 *or* day 6) and day 43 of delayed intensification
- **Hydrocortisone sodium succinate** 100 mg; administer by intravenous injection 30 minutes prior to pegaspargase administration on day 43 only of delayed intensification
  - *Note:* pegaspargase may cause anaphylaxis and serious hypersensitivity reactions. An expert panel recommends premedication prior to pegaspargase in adolescent and young adult patients (Stock W et al. Leuk Lymphoma 2011;52:2237–2253). Steroid premedication (eg, hydrocortisone) may be omitted prior to the day 4 (*or* day 5 *or* day 6) dose during delayed intensification (course IV) due to inclusion of dexamethasone in the regimen. Observe patients for 1 hour after the administration of pegaspargase in a setting with the capability to provide emergency resuscitation and with immediate availability of emergency supplies including epinephrine, oxygen, a histamine receptor [H$_1$]-subtype antagonist (eg, diphenhydramine), and intravenous corticosteroids

Choose one of the following options for pegaspargase:
- **Pegaspargase** 2500 units/m^2; administer by intravenous infusion over 1–2 hours in 100 mL 0.9% NS or D5W into a running infusion of either 0.9% NS or D5W (choose the same fluid that was used for dilution of pegaspargase) for two doses on day 4 (*or* day 5 *or* day 6) and day 43 of delayed intensification (total dosage/56-day delayed intensification course = 5000 units/m^2), or:
- **Pegaspargase** 2500 units/m^2; administer by intramuscular injection for two doses on day 4 (*or* day 5 *or* day 6) and day 43 of delayed intensification (total dosage/56-day delayed intensification course = 5000 units/m^2)
  - Limit the volume at a single injection site to ≤2 mL. If the volume to be administered is >2 mL, multiple injection sites should be used
  - Patients with platelets <50,000/mm^3 may require a platelet transfusion prior to an intramuscular injection

Methotrexate 15 mg; administer intrathecally via lumbar puncture or instillation via Ommaya reservoir for 3 doses on days 1, 29, and 36 of delayed intensification (total dosage/56-day delayed intensification course = 45 mg)
- Patients should remain in a horizontal position for ≥30 minutes following intrathecal chemotherapy

Dexamethasone 5 mg/m^2 per dose; administer orally twice per day with food for a total of 14 days (28 doses) to be administered on days 1–7 and on days 15–21 of delayed intensification (total dosage/56-day delayed intensification course = 140 mg/m^2)

Doxorubicin 25 mg/m^2 per dose; administer by intravenous injection over 3–5 minutes for 3 doses on days 1, 8, and 15 of delayed intensification (total dosage/56-day delayed intensification course = 75 mg/m^2)

Hydration prior to cyclophosphamide:
0.9% sodium chloride injection 1000 mL; administer intravenously over 2 hours, starting 2 hours prior to cyclophosphamide on day 29 of delayed intensification

Cyclophosphamide 1000 mg/m^2 per dose; administer intravenously in 25–250 mL 0.9% sodium chloride injection (0.9% NS) or 5% dextrose injection (D5W) over 30 minutes for 1 dose on day 29 of delayed intensification (total dosage/56-day delayed intensification course = 1000 mg/m^2)
- Delay the initiation of day 29 cyclophosphamide until ANC is $\geq750/mm^3$ and platelets are $\geq75,000/mm^3$

Cytarabine 75 mg/m^2 per dose; administer by subcutaneous or intravenous injection once daily for a total of 8 doses to be administered on days 29–32 and days 36–39 of delayed intensification (total dosage/56-day delayed intensification course = 600 mg/m^2)
- Delay the initiation of cytarabine on day 29 until ANC is $\geq750/mm^3$ and platelets are $\geq75,000/mm^3$

Thioguanine 60 mg/m^2 per dose; administer orally, on an empty stomach at least 1 hour after the evening meal, without milk or citrus products, once per day on days 29–42 during delayed intensification (total dosage/56-day delayed intensification course = 840 mg/m^2)
- Delay the initiation of thioguanine on day 29 until ANC is $\geq750/mm^3$ and platelets are $\geq75,000/mm^3$

(continued)

(continued)

- Adjust the thioguanine dose using 40-mg tablets and different doses on alternating days in order to attain a weekly cumulative dose as near to 420 mg/m²/week as possible

Note: consider incorporation of rituximab throughout all phases of treatment for a total of 16 infusions based on the results of the GRAALL-2005/R study

Maury S et al. N Engl J Med 2016;375:1044–1053

Supportive Care

Antiemetic prophylaxis
Emetogenic potential on days 1, 8, 15, and 29 is **MODERATE**
Emetogenic potential on all other days of chemotherapy is **MINIMAL**
See Chapter 42 for antiemetic recommendations

Hematopoietic growth factor (CSF) prophylaxis
Primary prophylaxis is **NOT** *indicated*
See Chapter 43 for more information

Antimicrobial prophylaxis
Risk of fever and neutropenia is **HIGH**
  Antimicrobial primary prophylaxis to be considered:

- Antibacterial—consider prophylaxis with a fluoroquinolone during periods of prolonged neutropenia only (eg, <500/mm³ for ≥7 days) until ANC recovery

- Antifungal—consider prophylaxis with fluconazole or another antifungal medication during periods of prolonged neutropenia only (eg, <500/mm³ for ≥7 days) until ANC recovery. Note that use of voriconazole, posaconazole, and itraconazole should be avoided with concomitant vincristine use. *Pneumocystis jirovecii* prophylaxis is recommended (eg, cotrimoxazole)

- Antiviral—anti-herpes antivirals (eg, acyclovir, famciclovir, valacyclovir)

Patient Population Studied

Refer to regimen entitled "CALGB 10403 INDUCTION (COURSE I)" for a description of the patient population

Efficacy

Refer to regimen entitled "CALGB 10403 INDUCTION (COURSE I)" for efficacy results

Therapy Monitoring

1. *Laboratory monitoring:*
   a. CBC with differential and platelet count, BUN, serum creatinine, liver function tests (ALT, AST, total bilirubin, direct bilirubin, alkaline phosphate), fasting lipid panel, aPTT, PT/INR, fibrinogen, and fasting blood glucose at baseline and then at least once per week throughout delayed intensification. In patients with risk factors for hyperglycemia, increase the frequency of blood glucose monitoring
   b. Serum amylase and lipase prior to each dose of pegaspargase, then as clinically indicated for abdominal pain
2. *Doxorubicin toxicity:* repeat determination of LVEF as clinically indicated
3. *Vincristine toxicity:* perform a neurologic exam prior to each dose on **days 1, 8, 15, 43, and 50**
4. *Pegaspargase toxicity:*
   a. *Hypersensitivity:* monitor for signs of an allergic reaction including bronchospasms, hypotension, laryngeal edema, local erythema or swelling, systemic rash, and urticaria. Monitor vital signs at baseline and every 30 minutes during and for 1 hour following administration of pegaspargase
   b. *Pancreatitis and hepatotoxicity:* advise patients to avoid alcohol during therapy
   c. *Hemorrhage/thrombosis:* avoid the use of oral contraceptives
5. *Response assessment:* with each dose of intrathecal chemotherapy, evaluate cerebrospinal fluid for cell count and cytospin exam. In the CALGB 10403 study, a bone marrow aspirate and biopsy was obtained 1 week after completion of course III. If a bone marrow specimen is obtained, evaluate for minimal residual disease

Treatment Modifications

PEGASPARGASE DOSE MODIFICATIONS

Refer to regimen entitled "CALGB 10403 INDUCTION (COURSE I)" for pegaspargase dose modification recommendations

GENERAL DOSE MODIFICATIONS

Myelosuppression

Day 1 ANC <750/mm³ or platelets <75,000/mm³	Delay initiation of delayed intensification chemotherapy until ANC ≥750/mm³ and platelets ≥75,000/mm³
Day 29 ANC <750/mm³ or platelets <75,000/mm³	Delay initiation of day 29 chemotherapy until ANC ≥750/mm³ and platelets ≥75,000/mm³
ANC <750/mm³ on days 2–28 or on days 30–56 in a patient without a documented infection (*Note:* neutropenic fever without a source of infection is not considered a documented infection)	Continue chemotherapy without interruption
Platelets <75,000/mm³ on days 2–28 or on days 30–56	
ANC <750/mm³ (any day) and patient is febrile and proven to be infected	Withhold chemotherapy and then resume at the same point when signs and symptoms of infection have resolved

DOXORUBICIN DOSE MODIFICATIONS

Direct bilirubin ≥3 mg/dL but <5 mg/dL	Administer doxorubicin with the dosage reduced by 50%
Direct bilirubin ≥5 mg/dL but <7 mg/dL	Administer doxorubicin with the dosage reduced by 75%
Direct bilirubin ≥7 mg/dL	Omit the doxorubicin dose. Do not make up missed doses

Cardiac Toxicity

Congestive heart failure or decline in LVEF to <50%	Discontinue doxorubicin

VINCRISTINE DOSE MODIFICATIONS

Hepatic Impairment

Direct bilirubin <3.1 mg/dL	Administer full dose vincristine
Direct bilirubin 3.1–5.0 mg/dL	Administer vincristine with the dosage reduced by 50%
Direct bilirubin 5.1–6.0 mg/dL	Administer vincristine with the dosage reduced by 75%
Direct bilirubin >6.0 mg/dL	Withhold vincristine and administer the next scheduled dose if toxicity has resolved. Do not make up missed doses

Neuropathy

G ≥3 peripheral sensory neuropathy (severe symptoms; limiting self-care ADL; or worse)	Withhold vincristine until symptoms resolve to G ≤1, then resume vincristine with the dosage reduced by 50%. If the toxicity remains G ≤1, then consider re-escalating the vincristine dose back to the full dose
G ≥3 jaw pain (severe pain; limiting self-care ADL)	
G ≥3 vocal cord paralysis (severe symptoms; medical intervention indicated, eg, thyroplasty, vocal cord injection; or worse)	
G ≥3 motor neuropathy (severe symptoms; limiting self-care ADL; assistive device indicated; or worse)	

(continued)

Treatment Modifications (*continued*)

Gastrointestinal Toxicity

G ≥3 constipation (obstipation with manual evacuation indicated; limiting self-care ADL)	Withhold vincristine and optimize laxative regimen. When toxicity improves to G ≤1, resume vincristine with the dosage reduced by 50%. If the toxicity does not recur, then re-escalate the vincristine dose back to full dose
G ≥3 ileus (severely altered GI function; TPN indicated)	

CYTARABINE DOSE MODIFICATIONS

Cytarabine Syndrome

Cytarabine syndrome (non-infectious fevers considered related to cytarabine, arthralgias, non-severe macular rash)	Continue cytarabine without interruption
G ≥3 rash related to cytarabine (severe, generalized erythroderma or macular, papular, or vesicular eruption; desquamation covering ≥50% BSA)	Withhold cytarabine until improvement to G ≤2, then resume cytarabine

CYCLOPHOSPHAMIDE DOSE MODIFICATIONS

Bladder Toxicity

Patient experienced gross hematuria with a prior dose of cyclophosphamide	Optimize hydration (eg, administer IV fluids for 24 hours after cyclophosphamide) and add mesna 200 mg/m² per dose given 15 minutes prior to and 3, 6, and 9 hours following the dose of cyclophosphamide (or alternative mesna dosing per local practice)
Patient experienced significant microscopic hematuria (>50 RBCs/HPF) with a prior dose of cyclophosphamide	

THIOGUANINE DOSE MODIFICATIONS

Other Toxicities

Myelosuppression leading to significant delays (>2 weeks) in therapy or myelosuppression is extremely severe	Perform TPMT genotyping
Patient is known to be a TPMT intermediate metabolizer and has experienced significant myelosuppression	Reduce the thioguanine dosage by 30–50%
Patient is known to be a TPMT poor metabolizer	Initiate thioguanine with the dosage reduced to 10 mg/m² per day given 3 days per week

ANC, absolute neutrophil count; LVEF, left ventricular ejection fraction; ADL, activities of daily living; GI, gastrointestinal; TPN, total parenteral nutrition; BSA, body surface area; RBCs, red blood cells; HPF, high power field; TPMT, thiopurine methyltransferase

Adverse Events

Note: refer to regimen entitled "CALGB 10403 CONSOLIDATION (COURSE II)" for a table containing a summary of adverse events observed during post-remission consolidation therapy (courses II–IV)

ADOLESCENT/YOUNG ADULT

ACUTE LYMPHOBLASTIC LEUKEMIA: CALGB 10403 MAINTENANCE (COURSE V)

Stock W et al. Blood 2019;133:1548–1559

Note: refer to regimen entitled "CALGB 10403 INDUCTION (COURSE I)" for a table containing an overview of the entire CALGB 10403 treatment regimen. For organizational purposes, each phase of the treatment protocol has been separated into an individual regimen within this textbook

Maintenance (course V, 12 week cycles); begin when ANC recovers to ≥750/mm^3 and platelets recover to ≥75,000/mm^3:

Important *Note:* the total duration of maintenance treatment from the start of interim maintenance is 2 years for females and 3 years for males

Radiation therapy is administered during the initial maintenance cycle to patients with the following indications:
- *T-cell acute lymphoblastic leukemia:* 2400 cGy (200 cGy × 12 daily fractions) cranial radiation during the first maintenance cycle
- *CNS3 leukemia at diagnosis:* 1800 cGy (180 cGy × 10 daily fractions) cranial radiation during the first maintenance cycle
- *Testicular involvement at diagnosis persisting at completion of induction (Course I):* 2400 cGy (200 cGy × 12 daily fractions) testicular radiation during the first maintenance cycle

Mercaptopurine 75 mg/m^2 per dose; administer orally, on an empty stomach at least 1 hour after the evening meal, without milk or citrus products, once daily, continuously on days 1–84, every 84 days until completion of maintenance chemotherapy (total dosage/84-day consolidation course = 6,300 mg/m^2)
- Adjust the dose using 50 mg tablets and different doses on alternating days in order to attain a weekly cumulative dose as near to 525 mg/m^2/week as possible
- See "Treatment Modifications" section for instructions on dose escalation based on CBC results

Vincristine 1.5 mg/m^2 (maximum dose = 2 mg) per dose; administer by intravenous infusion over 15 minutes in 50 mL 0.9% NS for 3 doses on days 1, 29, and 57, every 84 days, until completion of maintenance chemotherapy (total dosage/84-day maintenance cycle = 4.5 mg/m^2; maximum dosage/84-day maintenance cycle = 6 mg)

Dexamethasone 3 mg/m^2 per dose; administer orally twice per day, with food, for 5 consecutive days on days 1–5, 29–33, and 57–61, every 84 days, until completion of maintenance chemotherapy (total dosage/84-day maintenance cycle = 90 mg/m^2)

Note: the doses and schedules of intrathecal and oral methotrexate in the initial 4 cycles of maintenance chemotherapy are different from those in the remaining cycles of maintenance chemotherapy. *Therefore:*
- **During maintenance cycles 1–4:**
  - **Methotrexate** 20 mg/m^2 per dose; administer orally once per week only on days 8, 15, 22, 36, 43, 50, 57, 64, 71, and 78, every 84 days, for 4 initial maintenance cycles (total dosage/84-day cycle during maintenance cycles 1–4 = 200 mg/m^2)
    - *Note:* oral methotrexate is omitted on days of intrathecal methotrexate administration
    - See "Treatment Modifications" section for instructions on dose escalation based on CBC results
  - **Methotrexate** 15 mg per dose; administer intrathecally via lumbar puncture or instillation via Ommaya reservoir for 2 doses on days 1 and 29, every 84 days, for 4 initial maintenance cycles (total dosage/84-day cycle during maintenance cycles 1–4 = 30 mg)
    - Patients should remain in a horizontal position for ≥30 minutes following intrathecal chemotherapy
    - *Note:* omit the weekly oral methotrexate dose on days of intrathecal methotrexate administration
- **During maintenance cycles ≥5:**
  - **Methotrexate** 20 mg/m^2 per dose; administer orally once per week only on days 8, 15, 22, 29, 36, 43, 50, 57, 64, 71, and 78, every 84 days, until completion of maintenance chemotherapy (total dosage/84-day cycle during maintenance cycles ≥5 = 220 mg/m^2)
    - *Note:* oral methotrexate is omitted on days of intrathecal methotrexate administration
    - See "Treatment Modifications" section for instructions on dose escalation based on CBC results
  - **Methotrexate** 15 mg per dose; administer intrathecally via lumbar puncture or instillation via Ommaya reservoir for 1 dose on day 1 only, every 84 days, until completion of maintenance chemotherapy (total dosage/84-day cycle during maintenance cycles ≥5 = 15 mg)
    - Patients should remain in a horizontal position for ≥30 minutes following intrathecal chemotherapy
    - Omit the weekly oral methotrexate dose on the day(s) of intrathecal methotrexate administration

Note: consider incorporation of rituximab throughout all phases of treatment for a total of 16 infusions based on the results of the GRAALL-2005/R study

Maury S et al. N Engl J Med 2016;375:1044–1053

Supportive Care
Antiemetic prophylaxis
Emetogenic potential on all days is **MINIMAL**
See Chapter 42 for antiemetic recommendations

(continued)

(continued)

Hematopoietic growth factor (CSF) prophylaxis
Primary prophylaxis is **NOT** indicated
See Chapter 43 for more information

Antimicrobial prophylaxis
Risk of fever and neutropenia is **INTERMEDIATE**
  Antimicrobial primary prophylaxis to be considered:
  • Antibacterial—not indicated
  • Antifungal—not indicated. Note that use of voriconazole, posaconazole, and itraconazole should be avoided with concomitant vincristine use. *Pneumocystis jirovecii* prophylaxis is recommended (eg, cotrimoxazole)
  • Antiviral—not indicated unless patient previously had an episode of HSV

Patient Population Studied

Refer to regimen entitled "CALGB 10403 INDUCTION (COURSE I)" for a description of the patient population

Efficacy

Refer to regimen entitled "CALGB 10403 INDUCTION (COURSE I)" for efficacy results

Therapy Monitoring

1. *Laboratory monitoring:*
   a. CBC with differential and platelet count, BUN, serum creatinine, electrolytes, liver function tests (ALT, AST, total bilirubin, direct bilirubin, alkaline phosphate), every 4 weeks prior to vincristine administration on **days 1, 29, and 57 of each maintenance cycle,** and as clinically indicated
2. *Vincristine toxicity:* perform a neurologic exam prior to each dose on **days 1, 29, and 57** of each maintenance cycle
3. *Response assessment:* with each dose of intrathecal chemotherapy, evaluate cerebrospinal fluid for cell count and cytospin exam. In the CALGB 10403 clinical trial, a bone marrow biopsy and aspirate was obtained prior to the start of maintenance therapy and then every 6 months during maintenance until 3 months following completion of all chemotherapy. Evaluate each bone marrow specimen for minimal residual disease

Treatment Modifications

GENERAL DOSE MODIFICATIONS

Myelosuppression	
ANC is ≥1500/mm³ on three complete blood counts done over a 6-week period or the ANC is ≥1500/mm³ on two successive monthly complete blood counts	Increase the dose of either methotrexate *or* mercaptopurine by 25% in alternating sequence. If the same parameters are met again following the initial increase in dose of one medication, then subsequently increase the dose of the other drug by 25%. If ANC remains ≥1500/mm³ despite increasing both medications, then continue to alternate 25% increases in the dose of each medication after ruling out non-compliance or oral absorption–related issues
First occurrence of ANC <500/mm³	Increase the frequency of CBC with differential and platelet count monitoring to weekly. Withhold mercaptopurine and oral methotrexate until improvement of ANC to ≥750/mm³, then resume mercaptopurine and oral methotrexate at full doses. Do not make up for missed doses. When resuming methotrexate, resume therapy at the correct point chronologically
Second occurrence of ANC <500/mm³	Increase the frequency of CBC with differential and platelet count monitoring to weekly. Withhold mercaptopurine and oral methotrexate until improvement of ANC to ≥750/mm³, then resume both mercaptopurine and oral methotrexate but with the dosages of either or both drugs reduced by 50% from the previous dose. Gradually increase to 75% of the original dose and then eventually to 100% of the original dose at 2–4 weeks intervals provided that the ANC remains ≥750/mm³. Consider discontinuing cotrimoxazole and using an alternative medication (eg, dapsone or pentamidine) for prophylaxis. Perform TPMT testing if not done previously. Do not make up for missed doses. When resuming methotrexate, resume therapy at the correct point chronologically
First occurrence of platelet count <75,000/mm³	Increase the frequency of CBC with differential and platelet count monitoring to weekly. Withhold mercaptopurine and oral methotrexate until improvement of the platelet count to ≥75,000/mm³, then resume mercaptopurine and oral methotrexate at full doses. Do not make up for missed doses. When resuming methotrexate, resume therapy at the correct point chronologically

(continued)

Treatment Modifications (continued)

Myelosuppression

Second occurrence of platelet count <75,000/mm³	Withhold mercaptopurine and oral methotrexate until improvement of the platelet count to ≥75,000/mm³, then resume both mercaptopurine and oral methotrexate but with the dosages of either or both drugs reduced by 50% from the previous dose. Gradually increase to 75% of the original dose and then eventually to 100% of the original dose at 2–4 weeks intervals provided that the platelet count remains ≥75,000/mm³. Consider discontinuing cotrimoxazole and using an alternative medication (eg, dapsone or pentamidine) for prophylaxis. Perform TPMT testing if not done previously. Do not make up for missed doses. When resuming methotrexate, resume therapy at the correct point chronologically

METHOTREXATE DOSE MODIFICATIONS

General Toxicities

Direct bilirubin >2.0 mg/dL	Increase the frequency of liver function test monitoring to weekly. Withhold oral methotrexate until direct bilirubin improves to ≤2 mg/dL, then resume methotrexate at the previous dose. Do not make up for missed doses. When resuming methotrexate, resume therapy at the correct point chronologically
ALT or AST >20× ULN on 2 determinations at least one week apart	Increase the frequency of liver function test monitoring to weekly. Withhold oral methotrexate until ALT/AST improve to <5× ULN and direct bilirubin is within normal limits, then resume methotrexate at the previous dose. Do not make up for missed doses. When resuming methotrexate, resume therapy at the correct point chronologically
G3 mucositis (severe pain; interfering with oral intake)	Reduce the oral methotrexate dosage by 50%
G4 mucositis (life-threatening consequences; urgent intervention indicated)	Withhold oral methotrexate until resolution of mucositis, then resume oral methotrexate with the dosage reduced by 50% of the previous dose. If tolerated, consider gradually re-escalating the dosage back to full dose
G ≥3 diarrhea or vomiting	Withhold oral methotrexate until improvement in symptoms to G <2 for ≥1 week, then resume oral methotrexate with the dosage reduced by 50% of the previous dose. If tolerated, consider gradually re-escalating the dosage back to full dose
G ≥2 creatinine increased (serum creatinine >1.5× ULN)	Withhold oral methotrexate until improvement to G <1, then resume methotrexate at the previous dose

VINCRISTINE DOSE MODIFICATIONS

Hepatic Impairment

Direct bilirubin <3.1 mg/dL	Administer full dose vincristine
Direct bilirubin 3.1–5.0 mg/dL	Administer vincristine with the dosage reduced by 50%
Direct bilirubin 5.1–6.0 mg/dL	Administer vincristine with the dosage reduced by 75%
Direct bilirubin >6.0 mg/dL	Withhold vincristine and administer the next scheduled dose if toxicity has resolved. Do not make up missed doses

Neuropathy

G ≥3 peripheral sensory neuropathy (severe symptoms; limiting self-care ADL; or worse)	Withhold vincristine until symptoms resolve to G ≤1, then resume vincristine with the dosage reduced by 50%. If the toxicity remains G ≤1, then consider re-escalating the vincristine dose back to the full dose
G ≥3 jaw pain (severe pain; limiting self-care ADL)	
G ≥3 vocal cord paralysis (severe symptoms; medical intervention indicated, eg, thyroplasty, vocal cord injection; or worse)	
G ≥3 motor neuropathy (severe symptoms; limiting self-care ADL; assistive device indicated; or worse)	

(continued)

Treatment Modifications (continued)

Gastrointestinal Toxicity

G ≥3 constipation (obstipation with manual evacuation indicated; limiting self-care ADL)	Withhold vincristine and optimize laxative regimen. When toxicity improves to G ≤1, resume vincristine with the dosage reduced by 50%. If the toxicity does not recur, then re-escalate the vincristine dose back to full dose
G ≥3 ileus (severely altered GI function; TPN indicated)	

MERCAPTOPURINE DOSE MODIFICATIONS

Other Toxicities

G ≥2 creatinine increased (serum creatinine >1.5× ULN)	Withhold mercaptopurine until improvement to G ≤1, then resume mercaptopurine at the same dose
Patient requires treatment with a xanthine oxidase inhibitor (allopurinol or febuxostat)	If concomitant therapy is unavoidable, reduce the starting mercaptopurine dose to 25–33% of the usual starting dose and monitor closely for toxicity
Myelosuppression leading to significant delays (>2 weeks) in therapy or myelosuppression is extremely severe	Perform TPMT genotyping
Patient is known to be a TPMT intermediate metabolizer and has experienced significant myelosuppression	Reduce the mercaptopurine dosage by 30–50%
Patient is known to be a TPMT poor metabolizer	Initiate mercaptopurine with the dosage reduced to 10–20 mg/m^2 per day given 3 days per week

ANC, absolute neutrophil count; CBC, complete blood count; TPMT, thiopurine methyltransferase; ALT, alanine aminotransferase; AST, aspartate aminotransferase; ULN, upper limit of normal; ADL, activities of daily living; GI, gastrointestinal; TPN, total parenteral nutrition

Adverse Events (N = 173)

Event* Grade (%)	Maintenance Therapy (Course V) (N = 173)		
	Grade 3	Grade 4	Grade 5
Hypersensitivity	0	0	0
ALT	40	1	0
AST	15	1	0
Hyperbilirubinemia	9	1	0
Death NOS	0	0	0
Fatigue	3	0	0
Febrile neutropenia	15	2	0
Hyperglycemia	11	1	0
Hemorrhage CNS	1	0	0
Infection	14	2	0
Liver dysfunction/failure	0	0	0
Mucositis†	2	1	0

Event* Grade (%)	Maintenance Therapy (Course V) (N = 173)		
	Grade 3	Grade 4	Grade 5
Motor neuropathy	2	0	0
Sensory neuropathy	9	0	0
Avascular necrosis	6	1	0
Pancreatitis	1	0	0
Thrombosis	0	1	0
Hypertriglyceridemia	1	1	0
Tumor lysis syndrome	0	0	0
Ventricular arrhythmia	<1	0	0

ALT, alanine aminotransferase; AST, aspartate aminotransferase; NOS, not otherwise specified; CNS, central nervous system
*According to the National Cancer Institute Common Terminology Criteria for Adverse Events, version 3.0
†Term also includes stomatitis or esophagitis
Note: the table includes select Grade 3 or worse adverse events that are at least possibly related to protocol therapy that occurred during consolidation, interim maintenance, and/or delayed intensification

ADULT
ACUTE LYMPHOBLASTIC LEUKEMIA: LARSON

Larson RA et al. Blood 1998;92:1556–1564
Wetzler M et al. Blood 2007;109:4164–4167
Supplemental data to: Wetzler M et al. Blood 2007;109:4164–4167

Course I, Induction (1 course, 4 weeks in duration)

Treatment Stratified by Patient Age	
<60 Years	**≥60 Years**
Cyclophosphamide 1200 mg/m^2; administer intravenously in 100–250 mL 0.9% sodium chloride injection (0.9% NS) or 5% dextrose injection (D5W) over 15–30 minutes on day 1 (total dosage/course = 1200 mg/m^2)	**Cyclophosphamide** 800 mg/m^2; administer intravenously in 100–250 mL 0.9% sodium chloride injection (0.9% NS) or 5% dextrose injection (D5W) over 15–30 minutes on day 1 (total dosage/course = 800 mg/m^2)
Daunorubicin 45 mg/m^2 per day; administer by intravenous injection over 3–5 minutes for 3 consecutive days, on days 1–3 (total dosage/course = 135 mg/m^2)	**Daunorubicin** 30 mg/m^2 per day; administer by intravenous injection over 3–5 minutes for 3 consecutive days, on days 1–3 (total dosage/course = 90 mg/m^2)
Prednisone 60 mg/m^2 per day; administer orally, continually, for 21 consecutive days, on days 1–21 (total dosage/course = 1260 mg/m^2)	**Prednisone** 60 mg/m^2 per day; administer orally, continually, for 7 consecutive days, on days 1–7 (total dosage/course = 420 mg/m^2)

All Patients

Vincristine 2 mg per dose; administer by intravenous infusion over 15 minutes in 50 mL 0.9% NS for 4 doses, on days 1, 8, 15, and 22 (total dose/course = 8 mg)

Asparaginase 6000 IU/m^2 per dose; administer intramuscularly, or intravenously in 10–50 mL 0.9% NS or D5W over at least 30 minutes for 6 doses, on days 5, 8, 11, 15, 18, and 22 (total dosage/course = 36,000 IU/m^2)

Note: in the United States, asparaginase was withdrawn from the market in December 2012. Consider substituting with pegaspargase as follows:

Premedications for pegaspargase (if being used *instead of* asparaginase):
- Acetaminophen 650–100 mg; administer orally 30 minutes prior to pegaspargase administration on days 5 and 22
- Diphenhydramine 25–50 mg; administer orally or intravenously 30 minutes prior to pegaspargase administration on days 5 and 22

  - *Note:* pegaspargase may cause anaphylaxis and serious hypersensitivity reactions. An expert panel recommends premedication prior to pegaspargase in adult patients (Stock W et al. Leuk Lymphoma 2011;52:2237–2253). Steroid premedication (eg, hydrocortisone) may be omitted during induction (course I) due to inclusion of prednisone in the regimen. Observe patients for 1 hour after the administration of pegaspargase in a setting with the capability to provide emergency resuscitation and with immediate availability of emergency supplies including epinephrine, oxygen, a histamine receptor [H$_1$]-subtype antagonist (eg, diphenhydramine), and intravenous corticosteroids

Choose one of the following options for pegaspargase (if being used *instead of* asparaginase):
- **Pegaspargase** 2000 units/m^2 (maximum dose = 3750 units); administer by intravenous infusion over 1–2 hours in 100 mL 0.9% NS or 5% dextrose injection (D5W) into a running infusion of either 0.9% NS or D5W (choose the same fluid that was used for dilution of pegaspargase) for 2 doses on days 5 and 22 (total dosage/course = 4000 units/m^2; maximum dosage/course = 7500 units), *or:*
- **Pegaspargase** 2000 units/m^2 (maximum dose = 3750 units); administer by intramuscular injection for 2 doses on days 5 and 22 (total dosage/course = 4000 units/m^2; maximum dosage/course = 7500 units)

  - Limit the volume at a single injection site to ≤2 mL. If the volume to be administered is >2 mL, multiple injection sites should be used.
  - Patients with platelets <50,000/mm^3 may require a platelet transfusion prior to an intramuscular injection.

Filgrastim 5 μg/kg per day; administer by subcutaneous injection for at least 7 consecutive days. Start on day 4, at least 12 hours after the last dose of daunorubicin, and continue after the ANC nadir until the ANC is ≥1000/mm^3 on 2 consecutive days (measurements ≥24 hours apart)

Note: consider incorporation of rituximab throughout all phases of treatment for a total of 16 infusions based on the results of the GRAALL02005/R study

Maury S et al. N Engl J Med 2016;375:1044–1053

Supportive Care
Antiemetic prophylaxis
*Emetogenic potential on day 1 is **HIGH**. Potential for delayed symptoms*
*Emetogenic potential on days 2 and 3 is **MODERATE***
*Emetogenic potential on days with (peg-)asparaginase ± vincristine is **MINIMAL***
See Chapter 42 for antiemetic recommendations

(continued)

(*continued*)

Hematopoietic growth factor (CSF) prophylaxis
Primary prophylaxis is indicated with:

Filgrastim (G-CSF) 5 µg/kg per day, by subcutaneous injection
- Begin use on day 4
- Continue daily filgrastim use for at least 7 days, and until ANC ≥1000/mm³ on 2 measurements separated temporally by ≥24 hours
- Discontinue daily filgrastim use at least 24 hours before administering myelosuppressive treatment

See Chapter 43 for more information

Antimicrobial prophylaxis
Risk of fever and neutropenia is **HIGH**
  Antimicrobial primary prophylaxis is recommended:
- Antibacterial—consider fluoroquinolone prophylaxis; *Pneumocystis jirovecii* prophylaxis is recommended (eg, cotrimoxazole)
- Antifungal—recommended
- Antiviral—antiherpes antivirals (eg, acyclovir, famciclovir, valacyclovir)

Courses IIA and IIB, early intensification (2 courses, each is 4 weeks in duration)
Methotrexate 15 mg; administer intrathecally via lumbar puncture in 3–15 mL *preservative-free* 0.9% sodium chloride injection (PF 0.9% NS) on day 1, every 4 weeks for 2 courses (total dose/course = 15 mg)
Cyclophosphamide 1000 mg/m²; administer intravenously in 100–250 mL 0.9% NS or D5W over 15–30 minutes on day 1, every 4 weeks for 2 courses (total dosage/course = 1000 mg/m²)
Mercaptopurine 60 mg/m² per day, administer orally, continually, for 14 consecutive days, days 1–14, every 4 weeks for 2 courses (total dosage/course = 840 mg/m²)
Cytarabine 75 mg/m² per dose; administer by subcutaneous injection for 8 doses on days 1–4 and days 8–11, every 4 weeks for 2 courses (total dosage/course = 600 mg/m²)
Vincristine 2 mg per dose; administer by intravenous infusion over 15 minutes in 50 mL 0.9% NS for 2 doses, on days 15 and 22, every 4 weeks for 2 courses (total dose/course = 4 mg)
Asparaginase 6000 IU/m² per dose; administer intramuscularly, or intravenously in 10–50 mL 0.9% NS or D5W over at least 30 minutes for 4 doses, on days 15, 18, 22, and 25, every 4 weeks for 2 courses (total dosage/course = 24,000 IU/m²)

Note: in the United States, asparaginase was withdrawn from the market in December 2012. Consider substituting with pegaspargase as follows:

Premedications for pegaspargase (if being used *instead of* asparaginase):
- **Acetaminophen** 650–100 mg; administer orally 30 minutes prior to pegaspargase administration on day 15, every 4 weeks for 2 courses
- **Diphenhydramine** 25–50 mg; administer orally or intravenously 30 minutes prior to pegaspargase administration on day 15, every 4 weeks for 2 courses
- **Hydrocortisone** sodium succinate 100 mg; administer by intravenous injection 30 minutes prior to pegaspargase administration on day 15, every 4 weeks for 2 courses

Choose one of the following options for pegaspargase (if being used *instead of* asparaginase):
- **Pegaspargase** 2000 units/m² (maximum dose = 3750 units); administer by intravenous infusion over 1–2 hours in 100 mL 0.9% NS or D5W into a running infusion of either 0.9% NS or D5W (choose the same fluid that was used for dilution of pegaspargase) for 1 dose on day 15, every 4 weeks for 2 courses (total dosage/course = 2000 units/m²; maximum dosage/course = 3750 units), *or:*
- **Pegaspargase** 2000 units/m² (maximum dose = 3750 units); administer by intramuscular injection for 1 dose on day 15, every 4 weeks for 2 courses (total dosage/course = 2000 units/m²; maximum dosage/course = 3750 units)
  - Limit the volume at a single injection site to ≤2 mL. If the volume to be administered is >2 mL, multiple injection sites should be used
  - Patients with platelets <50,000/mm³ may require a platelet transfusion prior to an intramuscular injection

Note: in the CALGB 9511 study, it is stated that pegaspargase was administered subcutaneously in the text, which is an unapproved route of administration for pegaspargase. In the supplemental data, the route of administration is noted to be by intramuscular injection

Filgrastim 5 µg/kg per day; administer by subcutaneous injection for at least 14 consecutive days. Start on day 2, and continue after the ANC nadir until the ANC is ≥5000/mm³ on 2 consecutive days (measurements ≥24 hours apart)

Note: in all cases, filgrastim should be discontinued at least 2 days before cyclophosphamide administration resumed on the first day of the second early intensification course

Supportive Care
Antiemetic prophylaxis
Emetogenic potential on Day 1 is **MODERATE**
Emetogenic potential on days with cytarabine is **LOW**
Emetogenic potential on days with mercaptopurine alone is **MINIMAL–LOW**
Emetogenic potential on days with (peg-)asparaginase ± vincristine is **MINIMAL**
See Chapter 42 for antiemetic recommendations

(*continued*)

(continued)

Hematopoietic growth factor (CSF) prophylaxis
Primary prophylaxis is indicated with:

Filgrastim (G-CSF) 5 μg/kg per day, by subcutaneous injection

- Begin use on day 2
- Continue daily filgrastim use for at least 14 days, and until ANC ≥5000/mm^3 on 2 measurements separated temporally by ≥24 hours
- Priority was given to starting the second course (course IIB) 28 days after the first began
  - For patients whose ANC recovers to ≥1000/mm^3 and platelet count ≥50,000/mm^3 28 days after starting the first course (course IIA), the second course of therapy began on the 29th day of course IIA even if they had not yet recovered an ANC ≥5000/mm^3 by day 27
- Discontinue daily filgrastim use at least 2 days before restarting myelosuppressive treatment

See Chapter 43 for more information

Antimicrobial prophylaxis
Risk of fever and neutropenia is **HIGH**
Antimicrobial primary prophylaxis is recommended:

- Antibacterial—consider fluoroquinolone prophylaxis; *P. jirovecii* prophylaxis is recommended (eg, cotrimoxazole)
- Antifungal—recommended
- Antiviral—antiherpes antivirals (eg, acyclovir, famciclovir, valacyclovir)

Course III, CNS prophylaxis and interim maintenance (1 course, 12 weeks in duration)
Cranial irradiation 2400 cGy (total dose), delivered during 12 consecutive days, days 1–12

Methotrexate 15 mg per dose; administer intrathecally via lumbar puncture in 3–15 mL preservative-free 0.9% sodium chloride injection for 5 doses, on days 1, 8, 15, 22, and 29 (total dose/course = 75 mg)
Mercaptopurine 60 mg/m^2 per day; administer orally, continually, for 70 consecutive days, days 1–70 (total dosage/course = 4200 mg/m^2)
Methotrexate 20 mg/m^2 per dose; administer orally, for 5 doses, on days 36, 43, 50, 57, and 64 (total dosage/course = 100 mg/m^2)

Supportive Care
Antiemetic prophylaxis
Emetogenic potential is **MINIMAL–LOW**
See Chapter 42 for antiemetic recommendations

Hematopoietic growth factor (CSF) prophylaxis
Primary prophylaxis is **NOT** *indicated*
See Chapter 43 for more information

Antimicrobial prophylaxis
Risk of fever and neutropenia is **HIGH**
Antimicrobial primary prophylaxis is recommended:

- Antibacterial—*P. jirovecii* prophylaxis is recommended (eg, cotrimoxazole)
- Antifungal—recommended
- Antiviral—antiherpes antivirals (eg, acyclovir, famciclovir, valacyclovir)

Course IV, late intensification (1 course, 8 weeks in duration)
Doxorubicin 30 mg/m^2 per dose; administer by intravenous injection over 3–5 minutes for 3 doses, on days 1, 8, and 15 (total dosage/course = 90 mg/m^2)
Vincristine 2 mg per dose; administer by intravenous infusion over 15 minutes in 50 mL 0.9% NS for 3 doses, on days 1, 8, and 15 (total dose/course = 6 mg)
Dexamethasone 10 mg/m^2 per day; administer orally, continually, for 14 consecutive days, days 1–14 (total dosage/course = 140 mg/m^2)
Cyclophosphamide 1000 mg/m^2; administer intravenously in 100–250 mL 0.9% NS or D5W over 15–30 minutes on day 29 (total dosage/course = 1000 mg/m^2)
Thioguanine 60 mg/m^2 per day; administer orally, continually, for 14 consecutive days, days 29–42 (total dosage/course = 840 mg/m^2)
Cytarabine 75 mg/m^2 per dose; administer by subcutaneous injection for 8 doses on days 29–32 and days 36–39 (total dosage/course = 600 mg/m^2)

Supportive Care
Antiemetic prophylaxis
Emetogenic potential on Days 1, 8, 15, and 29 is **MODERATE**
Emetogenic potential on Days 30–32 and 36–39 is **LOW**
Emetogenic potential on days with thioguanine alone is **MINIMAL–LOW**
See Chapter 42 for antiemetic recommendations

(continued)

(continued)

Hematopoietic growth factor (CSF) prophylaxis
Primary prophylaxis may be indicated
• During the intervals between doses of doxorubicin, and the interval from days 16 through 28
• Discontinue daily filgrastim use at least 24 hours before administering myelosuppressive treatment
See Chapter 43 for more information

Antimicrobial prophylaxis
Risk of fever and neutropenia is **HIGH**
  Antimicrobial primary prophylaxis is recommended:
  • Antibacterial—consider fluoroquinolone prophylaxis; *P. jirovecii* prophylaxis is recommended (eg, cotrimoxazole)
  • Antifungal—recommended
  • Antiviral—antiherpes antivirals (eg, acyclovir, famciclovir, valacyclovir)

Course V, prolonged maintenance (courses are 4 weeks in duration and are repeated until 24 months after diagnosis)
Vincristine 2 mg per dose; administer by intravenous infusion over 15 minutes in 50 mL 0.9% NS, on day 1, every 4 weeks (total dose/course = 2 mg)
Prednisone 60 mg/m^2 per day; administer orally, continually, for 5 consecutive days, on days 1–5, every 4 weeks (total dosage/course = 300 mg/m^2)
Mercaptopurine 60 mg/m^2 per day; administer orally, continually, for 28 consecutive days, days 1–28, every 4 weeks (total dosage/course = 1680 mg/m^2)
Methotrexate 20 mg/m^2 per dose; administer orally, for 4 doses, on days 1, 8, 15, and 22, every 4 weeks (total dosage/course = 80 mg/m^2)

Supportive Care
Antiemetic prophylaxis
Emetogenic potential is **MINIMAL–LOW**
See Chapter 42 for antiemetic recommendations

Hematopoietic growth factor (CSF) prophylaxis
Primary prophylaxis is **NOT** indicated
See Chapter 43 for more information

Antimicrobial prophylaxis
Risk of fever and neutropenia is **HIGH**
  Antimicrobial primary prophylaxis is recommended:
  • Antibacterial—*P. jirovecii* prophylaxis is recommended (eg, cotrimoxazole)
  • Antifungal—recommended
  • Antiviral—antiherpes antivirals (eg, acyclovir, famciclovir, valacyclovir)

Efficacy (N = 102)

Induction Course

Complete CR (n = 97*)	90%
≥60 years (n = 21)	81%
<60 years (n = 76)	89%
Refractory disease (n = 102)	8%
Died during induction (n = 102)	5%
DFS, median	2.3 years
DFS Ph+ patients, median	0.8 years
Overall survival, median	2.4 years

*Among 102 patients randomly assigned to receive filgrastim during induction and early intensification courses, 97 patients were eligible for comparison with patients who did not receive filgrastim

(continued)

Patient Population Studied

102 patients (median age 35 years) with newly diagnosed ALL

Efficacy (N = 102) *(continued)*

Adverse Effects of Remission Induction

	Grades 3 and 4 or Grade 5 Toxicity
WBC (<1000/mm³)	98
Platelets (<25,000/mm³)	97
Hemoglobin (<6.5 g/dL)	93
Infection	78
Nausea	23
Bilirubin (>1.5 × NL)	44
Transaminase (>5 × NL)	35
Malaise/fatigue (PS >2)	16
Motor neuropathy	18
Pain	21
Hyperglycemia (>250 mg/dL)	33
Hypofibrinogenemia (<0.5 × NL)	26

Adverse Effects of Intensification and Maintenance

Grades 3 and 4 Toxicities	Intensification	Maintenance
Leukopenia	97	75
Thrombocytopenia	84	32
Anemia	84	26
Hemorrhage	4	0
Infection	49	25
Nausea/vomiting	17	8
Stomatitis	9	7
Diarrhea	3	1
Hepatic	28	30
Pulmonary	5	4
Cardiac	1	6
Genitourinary	2	1
CNS	13	6
Peripheral nervous system	12	7
Skin	1	2
Allergy	1	1

Data from 197 newly diagnosed ALL patients who were treated with the same chemotherapy regimen but did not receive filgrastim. Larson RA et al. Blood 1995;85:2025–2037

Therapy Monitoring

1. CBC with differential daily during and after chemotherapy until recovery of ANC >500/mm³. Platelets every day while in hospital until patients no longer require platelet transfusions

2. Serum electrolytes, mineral panel, and uric acid, at least daily during active treatment until the risk of tumor lysis is past

3. *Anthracycline toxicity:* determination of LVEF by echocardiogram prior to treatment and then as clinically indicated

4. *(Peg-)asparaginase clinical toxicity monitoring:*
   a. *Hypersensitivity:* monitor for signs of an allergic reaction including bronchospasms, hypotension, laryngeal edema, local erythema or swelling, systemic rash, and urticaria. Monitor vital signs frequently during and for 1 hour following administration
   b. *Pancreatitis and hepatotoxicity:* advise patients to avoid alcohol during therapy
   c. *Hemorrhage/thrombosis:* avoid the use of oral contraceptives

5. *Asparaginase toxicity laboratory monitoring:*
   a. Amylase, lipase, fibrinogen, fasting blood glucose, aPTT, PT/INR, and liver function tests prior to each dose of asparaginase. If fibrinogen level is <100 mg/dL (<1 g/L) consider prophylactic administration of cryoprecipitate. Fasting lipid panel prior to each course of asparaginase

6. *Pegaspargase toxicity laboratory monitoring:*
   a. Fasting blood glucose, fasting lipid panel, aPTT, PT/INR, liver function tests, and fibrinogen prior to pegaspargase administration and then at least once per week for at least 4 weeks after each dose. In patients with risk factors for hyperglycemia, increase the frequency of blood glucose monitoring. Serum amylase and lipase prior to pegaspargase and then as clinically indicated for abdominal pain

Treatment Modifications

Adverse Events	Treatment Modifications
Creatinine 1.5–2 mg/dL (133–177 μmol/L)	Reduce methotrexate dosage by 25%
Creatinine >2 mg/dL (>177 μmol/L)	Reduce methotrexate dosage by 50%
Creatinine >3 mg/dL (>265 μmol/L)	Reduce daunorubicin dosage by 50%
Total bilirubin 3–5 mg/dL (51–86 μmol/L)	Reduce daunorubicin dosage by 50%
	Reduce methotrexate dosage by 25%
Total bilirubin >3 mg/dL (>51 μmol/L)	Reduce vincristine dosage by 50%
Total bilirubin >5 mg/dL (>86 μmol/L)	Hold daunorubicin Hold methotrexate

(PEG-)ASPARAGINASE DOSE MODIFICATIONS

Adapted from: Stock W et al. Leuk Lymphoma 2011;52:2237–2253

Toxicity	Grade 2	Grade 3	Grade 4
Hypersensitivity, urticaria, wheezing, laryngospasm, hypotension, etc.	For urticaria without bronchospasm, hypotension, edema, or need for parenteral intervention, continue (peg-)asparaginase	For wheezing or other symptomatic bronchospasm with or without urticaria, indicated parenteral intervention, angioedema, or hypotension, discontinue (peg-)asparaginase. Substitute Erwinia asparaginase 25,000 units/m² (if available) by IV or IM for each scheduled dose of native *E. coli* asparaginase	For life-threatening consequences or indicated urgent intervention, discontinue (peg-)asparaginase. Substitute Erwinia asparaginase 25,000 units/m² (if available) by IV or IM for each scheduled dose of native *E. coli* asparaginase
Hypertriglyceridemia	If serum triglyceride level <1000 mg/dL (<11.3 mmol/L), continue (peg-)asparaginase but follow patient closely for evolving pancreatitis	Hold (peg-)asparaginase for triglyceride >1000 mg/dL (>11.3 mmol/L); follow closely for pancreatitis; resume (peg-)asparaginase at prior dose level after patient's triglyceride level returns to normal range	Hold (peg-)asparaginase for triglyceride >1000 mg/dL (>11.3 mmol/L); follow closely for pancreatitis; resume (peg-)asparaginase at prior dose level after patient's triglyceride level returns to normal range
Hyperglycemia, ketoacidosis	Continue (peg-)asparaginase for uncomplicated hyperglycemia	For hyperglycemia requiring insulin therapy, hold (peg-)asparaginase (and glucocorticoid therapy) until blood glucose regulated with insulin; resume (peg-)asparaginase at prior dose level	For hyperglycemia with life-threatening consequences or indicated urgent intervention, hold (peg-)asparaginase (and glucocorticoid therapy) until blood glucose is regulated with insulin; resume (peg-)asparaginase and do not make up for missed doses
Hyperammonemia-related fatigue	Continue (peg-)asparaginase	Reduce (peg-)asparaginase dose by 25%; resume full dose when toxicity is Grade ≤2; make up for missed doses	Reduce (peg-)asparaginase dose 50%; resume full dose when toxicity Grade 2; make up for missed doses
Pancreatitis	Continue (peg-)asparaginase for asymptomatic amylase or lipase elevation >3 × ULN (chemical pancreatitis) or only radiologic abnormalities; observe closely for rising amylase or lipase levels	Continue pegaspargase for non-symptomatic chemical pancreatitis but observe patient closely for development of symptomatic pancreatitis for early treatment. Hold native asparaginase for amylase or lipase elevation >3 ×ULN until enzyme levels stabilize or are declining. Permanently discontinue asparaginase for symptomatic pancreatitis	Permanently discontinue all (peg-)asparaginase for clinical pancreatitis (vomiting, severe abdominal pain) with amylase or lipase elevation >3 × ULN for >3 days and/or development of pancreatic pseudocyst
Hyperbilirubinemia	Continue (peg-)asparaginase if direct bilirubin ≤3.0 mg/dL (≤51 μmol/L)	If direct bilirubin is 3.1–5.0 mg/dL (53–86 μmol/L), administer (peg-)asparaginase with the dose reduced by 50%	If direct bilirubin is >5.0 mg/dL (>86 μmol/L) and ≤6.0 mg/dL (≤103 μmol/L), withhold (peg-)asparaginase and administer the next scheduled dose if toxicity has resolved. Do not make up missed doses

(continued)

Treatment Modifications (*continued*)

Toxicity	Grade 2	Grade 3	Grade 4
Non-CNS thrombosis	For abnormal laboratory findings without clinical correlates, continue (peg-)asparaginase	Withhold (peg-)asparaginase until acute toxicity and clinical signs resolve and anticoagulant therapy is stable or completed. Do not withhold (peg-)asparaginase for abnormal laboratory findings without a clinical correlate	Withhold (peg-)asparaginase until acute toxicity and clinical signs resolve and anticoagulant therapy is stable or completed
Non-CNS hemorrhage	For bleeding in conjunction, with hypofibrinogenemia, withhold (peg-)asparaginase until bleeding is Grade ≤1. Do not withhold (peg-)asparaginase for abnormal laboratory findings without a clinical correlate	Withhold (peg-)asparaginase until bleeding is Grade ≤1, until acute toxicity and clinical signs resolve, and coagulant replacement therapy is stable or completed	Withhold (peg-)asparaginase until bleeding is Grade ≤1, until acute toxicity and clinical signs resolve, and coagulant replacement therapy is stable or completed
CNS thrombosis	For abnormal laboratory findings without a clinical correlate, continue (peg-)asparaginase	Discontinue all (peg-)asparaginase; if CNS symptoms and signs are fully resolved and significant (peg-)asparaginase remains to be administered, may resume (peg-)asparaginase therapy at a lower dose and/or longer intervals between doses	Permanently discontinue (peg-)asparaginase
CNS hemorrhage	Discontinue (peg-)asparaginase; do not withhold (peg-)asparaginase for abnormal laboratory findings without a clinical correlate	Discontinue (peg-)asparaginase; if CNS symptoms and signs are fully resolved and significant (peg-)asparaginase remains to be administered, may resume (peg-)asparaginase therapy at a lower dose and/or longer intervals between doses	Permanently discontinue (peg-)asparaginase

Grade according to the National Cancer Institute Common Terminology Criteria for Advance Events version 4, with the exception of pancreatitis

IV, intravenous; IM, intramuscular; ULN, upper limit of normal; CNS, central nervous system

Notes

1. An additional group of 96 patients in a study reported by Larson et al (Blood 1998;92:1556–1564) did not receive filgrastim after assignment to treatment. The median time to recover neutrophils ≥1000/mm³ during the remission induction course was 16 days for patients assigned to receive filgrastim and 22 days for patients assigned to placebo. Patients who received filgrastim had significantly shorter durations of neutropenia and thrombocytopenia and fewer days in hospital compared with patients who received placebo

2. Among patients assigned to receive filgrastim, more achieved CR and fewer experienced death during remission induction than those who received placebo. Overall toxicity was not lessened by the use of filgrastim. After a median follow-up of 4.7 years, there was no significant difference in the overall survival between the two groups

3. Larson et al (Blood 1995:85:2025–2037) performed lumbar puncture at diagnosis of ALL only in symptomatic patients. Patients with CNS leukemia should receive intrathecal therapy via lumbar puncture or an intraventricular reservoir (eg, Ommaya) weekly until CNS clearance with methotrexate 15 mg + hydrocortisone sodium succinate 50 mg per dose; administer intrathecally once weekly, alternating with cytarabine 100 mg + hydrocortisone sodium succinate 50 mg per dose; administer intrathecally once weekly

   • Doses may be given in a volume of 0.9% sodium chloride injection *without* antimicrobial preservatives (preservative-free) equal to the volume of CSF removed for chemical or cytologic evaluations

   • Intrathecal chemotherapy is given twice weekly; alternating doses of either methotrexate + hydrocortisone or cytarabine + hydrocortisone

   • Alternating intrathecal chemotherapy doses are separated by at least 3 days

4. Patients should continue systemic treatment as specified in the regimen

ADULT

ACUTE LYMPHOBLASTIC LEUKEMIA: HYPER-CVAD

Kantarjian H et al. Cancer 2004;101:2788–2801
Kantarjian HM et al. J Clin Oncol 2000;18:547–561

Dose-intensive chemotherapy

The dose-intensive phase consists of 8 cycles of hyper-CVAD alternating with high-dose methotrexate and cytarabine every 3–4 weeks (when the WBC count is >3000/mm^3 and platelet count is >60,000/mm^3)

Hyper-CVAD (cycles 1, 3, 5, and 7)

Cyclophosphamide 300 mg/m^2 per dose; administer intravenously over 3 hours in 500 mL 0.9% sodium chloride injection (0.9% NS) or 5% dextrose injection (D5W) every 12 hours for 6 doses on days 1–3, for 4 cycles, cycles 1, 3, 5, and 7 (total dosage/cycle = 1800 mg/m^2)

Mesna 600 mg/m^2 per 24 hours; administer by continuous intravenous infusion in 1000 mL 0.9% NS for approximately 69 hours for 4 cycles, cycles 1, 3, 5, and 7 (total dosage/cycle ~1725 mg/m^2)
• Mesna administration starts concurrently with cyclophosphamide on day 1 and continues until 6 hours after the last dose of cyclophosphamide is completed (69 hours)

Vincristine 2 mg/dose; administer by intravenous infusion over 15 minutes in 50 mL 0.9% NS for 2 doses, on days 4 and 11, for 4 cycles, cycles 1, 3, 5, and 7 (total dose/cycle = 4 mg)

Doxorubicin 50 mg/m^2; administer intravenously via central venous access in 25–250 mL 0.9% NS or D5W over 2 hours on day 4, for 4 cycles, cycles 1, 3, 5, and 7 (total dosage/cycle = 50 mg/m^2)

Dexamethasone 40 mg per day; administer orally, or intravenously in 25–150 mL 0.9% NS or D5W over 15–30 minutes for 8 doses, on days 1–4 and days 11–14, for 4 cycles, cycles 1, 3, 5, and 7 (total dose/cycle = 320 mg)

Supportive Care

Antiemetic prophylaxis
Emetogenic potential on Days 1–4 is **MODERATE**
Emetogenic potential on Days 11 is **MINIMAL**
See Chapter 42 for antiemetic recommendations

Hematopoietic growth factor (CSF) prophylaxis
Primary prophylaxis is indicated with:
  Filgrastim (G-CSF) 5 µg/kg per dose; administer by subcutaneous injection every 12 hours, starting on day 5 (24 hours after doxorubicin)
  • Continue filgrastim administration until postnadir WBC count >3000/mm^3 and platelet count is >60,000/mm^3. If platelet recovery is delayed, filgrastim is continued until the WBC count >30,000/mm^3
  • Discontinue daily filgrastim use at least 24 hours before administering myelosuppressive treatment
See Chapter 43 for more information

Antimicrobial prophylaxis
Risk of fever and neutropenia is **HIGH**
  Antimicrobial primary prophylaxis is recommended:
  • Antibacterial—consider fluoroquinolone prophylaxis; *P. jirovecii* prophylaxis is recommended (eg, cotrimoxazole)
  • Antifungal—recommended
  • Antiviral—antiherpes antivirals (eg, acyclovir, famciclovir, valacyclovir)

High-dose methotrexate + cytarabine (cycles 2, 4, 6, and 8)

Hydration: with a solution containing a total amount of sodium not >0.9% NS (ie, ≤154 mEq sodium/1000 mL) by intravenous infusion during methotrexate administration and for at least 24 hours afterward
• Commence fluid administration 2–12 hours before starting methotrexate, depending on patient's fluid status
• Urine output should be at least 100 mL/hour before starting methotrexate infusion
• Maintain hydration at a rate that maintains urine output ≥100 mL/hour until the serum methotrexate concentration is <0.1 µmol/L
• Urine pH should be increased within the range ≥7.0 to ≤8.0 to enhance methotrexate solubility and ensure elimination
• Adverse effects attributable to methotrexate are related to systemic methotrexate concentrations *and* the duration for which concentrations are maintained

(continued)

(continued)

Sodium bicarbonate 50–150 mEq/1000 mL is added to parenteral hydration solutions to maintain urine pH ≥7.0 to ≤8.0

Base Solution Sodium Content	Sodium Bicarbonate Additive	Total Sodium Content
0.45% Sodium chloride injection (0.45% NS)		
77 mEq/L	50–75 mEq	127–152 mEq/L
0.2% Sodium chloride injection (0.2% NS)		
34 mEq/L	100–125 mEq	134–159 mEq/L
5% Dextrose injection (D5W)		
0	125–150 mEq	125–150 mEq/L
D5W/0.45% NS		
77 mEq/L	50–75 mEq	127–152 mEq/L
D5W/0.2% NS		
34 mEq/L	100–125 mEq	134–159 mEq/L

Methotrexate 200 mg/m²; administer intravenously over 2 hours, on day 1, *followed by:*
Methotrexate 800 mg/m²; administer intravenously over 24 hours, on day 1, for 4 cycles, cycles 2, 4, 6, and 8 (total dosage/cycle, bolus + infusion = 1000 mg/m²)

Note: for logistical practicality and efficiency, parenteral admixtures containing methotrexate may include a portion or all of the fluid and sodium bicarbonate needed to meet hydration and urinary alkalinization requirements during methotrexate administration

Leucovorin calcium 15 mg per dose; administer intravenously in 25–250 mL 0.9% NS or D5W over 15–30 minutes, starting 48 hours after methotrexate administration began (22 hours after methotrexate administration ends), every 6 hours for 8 doses (total dosage/cycle = 120 mg)

Note: if serum methotrexate concentrations are:

Hours After *Starting* Methotrexate	Methotrexate Concentration	Leucovorin Regimen
Hour 24	>20 μmol/L (>2 × 10⁻⁵ mol/L)	Increase leucovorin dosages to 50 mg/dose; administer intravenously in 25–250 mL 0.9% NS or D5W over 15–30 minutes every 6 hours until serum methotrexate concentrations are <0.1 μmol/L (<1 × 10²⁷ mol/L)
Hour 48	>1 μmol/L (>1 × 10⁻⁶ mol/L)	
Hour 72	>0.1 μmol/L (>1 × 10⁻⁷ mol/L, *or* >100 nmol/L)	

Cytarabine
 Patient age <60 years: **Cytarabine** 3000 mg/m² per dose; administer intravenously in 50–500 mL 0.9% NS or D5W over 2 hours every 12 hours for 4 doses on days 2 and 3, for 4 cycles, cycles 2, 4, 6, and 8 (total dosage/cycle [not including intrathecal cytarabine] = 12,000 mg/m²)
 Patient age ≥60 years: **Cytarabine** 1000 mg/m² per dose; administer intravenously in 50–500 mL 0.9% NS or D5W over 2 hours every 12 hours for 4 doses on days 2 and 3, for 4 cycles, cycles 2, 4, 6, and 8 (total dosage/cycle [not including intrathecal cytarabine] = 4000 mg/m²)

Methylprednisolone 50 mg; administer intravenously twice daily for 6 doses, on days 1–3 (total dose/cycle = 300 mg)

Filgrastim 5 μg/kg per dose; administer subcutaneously, every 12 hours, starting on day 4 (24 hours after the last dose of chemotherapy) and continue until postnadir WBC count >3000/mm³ and platelet count is >60,000/mm³. If platelet recovery is delayed, filgrastim is continued until the WBC count >30,000/mm³

Supportive Care
Antiemetic prophylaxis
Emetogenic potential on Days 1–3 is **MODERATE**
See Chapter 42 for antiemetic recommendations

Hematopoietic growth factor (CSF) prophylaxis
Primary prophylaxis is indicated with:
 Filgrastim (G-CSF) 5 μg/kg per dose; administer by subcutaneous injection every 12 hours, starting on day 4 (24 hours after the last dose of cytarabine)
 • Continue filgrastim administration until postnadir WBC count >3000/mm³ and platelet count is >60,000/mm³. If platelet recovery is delayed, filgrastim is continued until the WBC count >30,000/mm³
 • Discontinue daily filgrastim use at least 24 hours before administering myelosuppressive treatment
See Chapter 43 for more information

(continued)

(continued)

Antimicrobial prophylaxis
Risk of fever and neutropenia is **HIGH**
Antimicrobial primary prophylaxis is recommended:
- Antibacterial—consider fluoroquinolone prophylaxis; *P. jirovecii* prophylaxis is recommended (eg, cotrimoxazole)
- Antifungal—recommended
- Antiviral—antiherpes antivirals (eg, acyclovir, famciclovir, valacyclovir)

Keratitis prophylaxis
Steroid ophthalmic drops (prednisolone 1% or dexamethasone 0.1%); administer by intraocular instillation daily until 24 hours after high-dose cytarabine is completed

Maintenance phase
Mercaptopurine 50 mg/dose; administer orally on an empty stomach, continually, 3 times daily for 2 years (total dose/4 weeks = 4200 mg)
Methotrexate 20 mg/m^2 per dose; administer orally, once weekly for 2 years (total dosage/4 weeks = 80 mg/m^2)
Vincristine 2 mg; administer by intravenous infusion over 15 minutes in 50 mL 0.9% NS, once monthly for 2 years (total dose/month = 2 mg)
Prednisone 200 mg per day; administer orally, continually, for 5 consecutive days every month, starting on the day vincristine is given (total dose/month = 1000 mg)

Supportive Care
Antiemetic prophylaxis
Emetogenic potential is **MINIMAL–LOW**
See Chapter 42 for antiemetic recommendations

Hematopoietic growth factor (CSF) prophylaxis
Primary prophylaxis is **NOT** *indicated*
See Chapter 43 for more information

Antimicrobial prophylaxis
Risk of fever and neutropenia is **HIGH**
Antimicrobial primary prophylaxis is recommended:
- Antibacterial—consider fluoroquinolone prophylaxis; *P. jirovecii* prophylaxis is recommended (eg, cotrimoxazole)
- Antifungal—recommended
- Antiviral—antiherpes antivirals (eg, acyclovir, famciclovir, valacyclovir)

Patient Population Studied

288 newly diagnosed ALL patients (median age: 40 years)

Efficacy (N = 288)

CR	92%
CR <30 years	99%
CR >60 years	80%
Resistant disease	3%
Died during induction	5%
5-year estimated survival rate	38%
5-year CR rate	38%
CR for Ph+ ALL	91%
5-year survival for Ph+ ALL	12%

Dose Modifications During the Induction Phase

Adverse Effect	Dose Modification
Total bilirubin >2 mg/dL (>34 μmol/L)	Reduce vincristine doses to 1 mg
Total bilirubin 2–3 mg/dL (34–51 μmol/L)	Reduce doxorubicin dosage by 25%
Total bilirubin 3–4 mg/dL (51–68 μmol/L)	Reduce doxorubicin dosage by 50%
Total bilirubin 3–5 mg/dL (51–86 μmol/L)	Reduce methotrexate dosage by 25%
Total bilirubin >4 mg/dL (>68 μmol/L)	Reduce doxorubicin dosage by 75%
Total bilirubin >5 mg/dL (>86 μmol/L)	Hold methotrexate
Creatinine 1.5–2 mg/dL (133–177 μmol/L)	Reduce methotrexate dosage by 25%
Bilirubin level 3–5 mg/dL (51–86 μmol/L)	Reduce methotrexate dose by 25%
Bilirubin >5 mg/dL (>86 μmol/L)	Hold methotrexate
Creatinine >2 mg/dL (>177 μmol/L)	Reduce methotrexate dosage by 50% Reduce cytarabine dosage to 1000 mg/m^2

Toxicity (N = 288)

Induction Chemotherapy (First Course of Hyper-CVAD Therapy)

Myelosuppression	
Median time to ANC >1000/mm^3	19 days
Median time to platelets >100,000/mm^3	22 days
Hospitalization	54%
Sepsis	11%
Pneumonia	16%
Fungal infection	4%
Fever of unknown origin	37%
Neurotoxicity	64%
Moderate–severe mucositis	4%
Moderate–severe diarrhea	3%
Disseminated intravascular coagulopathy	3%
Induction deaths	5%

Consolidation Courses (Second Course of Hyper-CVAD Therapy)

Pneumonia	4%
Hospitalization	16%
Neurotoxicity	7%
Mucositis	1%
Diarrhea	1%
Sepsis	10%
Fever of unknown origin	8%

High-Dose Methotrexate + Cytarabine Therapy

Sepsis	8%
Pneumonia	5%
Fever of unknown origin	22%
Neurotoxicity	5%
Minor infections	4%
Hospitalization	36
Mucositis	4%
Rash and desquamation of palms and feet	2%
Diarrhea	1%

Therapy Monitoring

1. CBC with differential daily during and after chemotherapy during induction therapy until recovery of ANC >500/mm^3. Platelets every day while in hospital until patient no longer requires platelet transfusions
2. *Pretreatment evaluation:* determination of LVEF by echocardiogram
3. Serum electrolytes, mineral panel, and uric acid, at least daily during active treatment until the risk of tumor lysis is past
4. Bone marrow aspirate and biopsy after the initial induction course upon recovery of peripheral blood counts. After patient achieves a CR, bone marrow biopsy and aspirate should be performed at least following completion of consolidation therapy

Notes

1. In the studies reported by Kantarjian et al (J Clin Oncol 2000;18:547–561), patients underwent a diagnostic LP on day 2 of the first course of treatment
   a. Patients with CNS disease at the time of diagnosis receive intrathecal therapy with:
      - **Methotrexate;** administer intrathecally 12 mg/dose via lumbar puncture *or* 6 mg/dose intraventricularly via indwelling ventricular reservoir catheter (eg, Ommaya) twice weekly until cerebrospinal fluid cell counts normalize and cytology becomes negative for malignant disease, *then:*
      - **Methotrexate;** administer intrathecally 12 mg/dose via lumbar puncture *or* 6 mg/dose intraventricularly via indwelling ventricular reservoir catheter on day 2 of each remaining treatment cycle, plus
      - **Cytarabine** 100 mg/dose; administer intrathecally via lumbar puncture *or* intraventricularly via indwelling ventricular reservoir catheter on day 8 of each remaining treatment cycle
   b. Patients with cranial nerve root involvement received radiation 24–30 Gy in 10–12 fractions to the base of the skull or whole brain
   c. Patients with no evidence of CNS disease should receive intrathecal prophylaxis based on prognostic factors for CNS leukemia

CNS Prophylaxis

Risk Factors	Risk Categories		
	High	**Low**	**Unknown**
LDH	>600 units/L	Within normal limits	unknown
Proliferative index (% S+G$_2$M)	≥14%		
Histology	Mature B-cell ALL	Not applicable	

Regimen for Intrathecal Prophylaxis	Administration Schedule by Risk Category		
	High Risk	**Unknown Risk**	**Low Risk**
Methotrexate; administer intrathecally 12 mg/dose via lumbar puncture *or* 6 mg/dose intraventricularly (via Ommaya reservoir) on day 2 of each cycle indicated, *plus* **Cytarabine** 100 mg administer; intrathecally via lumbar puncture or intraventricularly on day 8 of each cycle indicated	For 8 cycles, cycles 1–8	For 4 cycles, cycles 1–4	For 2 cycles, cycles 1 & 2

(*continued*)

Notes (*continued*)

2. Patients with mature B-cell ALL received no maintenance therapy

3. Patients who receive high-dose cytarabine need to be closely monitored for changes in renal function. Renal dysfunction is highly correlated with increased risk of cerebellar toxicity associated with cytarabine. Patients need to be monitored for nystagmus, dysmetria, and ataxia before each cytarabine dose

4. Hyper-CVAD + rituximab (Thomas DA et al. J Clin Oncol 2010;28:3880–3889): two hundred eighty-two adolescents and adults with de novo Philadelphia chromosome (Ph)–negative precursor B-lineage ALL were treated with standard or modified hyper-CVAD regimens. The latter incorporated standard-dose rituximab if CD20 expression ≥20%. The complete remission (CR) rate was 95% with 3-year rates of CR duration (CRD) and survival (OS) of 60% and 50%, respectively. In the younger (age <60 years) CD20-positive subset, rates of CRD and OS were superior with the modified hyper-CVAD and rituximab regimens compared with standard hyper-CVAD (70% vs 38%; P <.001% and 75% vs 47%, P = 0.003). In contrast, rates of CRD and OS for CD20-negative counterparts treated with modified versus standard hyper-CVAD regimens were similar (72% vs 68%, P = not significant [NS] and 64% vs 65%, P = NS, respectively). Older patients with CD20-positive ALL did not benefit from rituximab-based chemoimmunotherapy (rates of CRD 45% vs 50%, P = NS and OS 28% vs 32%, P = NS, respectively), related in part to deaths in CR. The incorporation of rituximab into the hyper-CVAD regimen improves outcome for younger patients with CD20-positive Ph-negative precursor B-lineage ALL

ADULT

ACUTE LYMPHOBLASTIC LEUKEMIA: LINKER

Linker C et al. J Clin Oncol 2002;20:2464–2471
Wieduwilt MJ et al. Blood 2018;132(suppl_1):4018

Treatment consisted of a total of 7 courses given in the order 1A → 1B → 1C → 2A → 2B → 2C → 3C, followed by maintenance chemotherapy

Induction (course 1A): DVP/Asp
Daunorubicin 60 mg/m^2 per day; administer by intravenous injection over 3–5 minutes for 3 consecutive days, on days 1–3 (total dosage/course after 3 doses = 180 mg/m^2)

Note: if day 14 bone marrow evaluation reveals residual leukemia, give a fourth dose of daunorubicin on day 15 (total dosage/course after 4 doses = 240 mg/m^2)

Vincristine

   Patient age ≤40 years: **Vincristine** 1.4 mg/m^2 per dose; administer by intravenous infusion over 15 minutes in 50 mL 0.9% NS for 4 doses on days 1, 8, 15, and 22 (total dosage/course = 5.6 mg/m^2)

   Patient age >40 years: **Vincristine** 1.4 mg/m^2 per dose (maximum single dose = 2 mg), administer by intravenous infusion over 15 minutes in 50 mL 0.9% NS for 4 doses on days 1, 8, 15, and 22 (total dosage/course = 5.6 mg/m^2; maximum dose/course = 8 mg)

Prednisone 60 mg/m^2 per day; administer orally, continually, for 28 consecutive days, on days 1–28 (total dosage/course = 1680 mg/m^2)

Asparaginase 6000 IU/m^2 per day; administer intramuscularly, or intravenously in 10–50 mL 0.9% sodium chloride injection or 5% dextrose injection over at least 30 minutes for 12 consecutive days on days 17–28 (total dosage/course = 72,000 IU/m^2)

Note: in the United States, asparaginase was withdrawn from the market in December 2012. Consider substituting with pegaspargase as follows:

Premedications for pegaspargase (if being used *instead of* asparaginase):
• **Acetaminophen** 650–100 mg; administer orally 30 minutes prior to pegaspargase administration on day 15
• **Diphenhydramine** 25–50 mg; administer orally or intravenously 30 minutes prior to pegaspargase administration on day 15

   ▪ *Note:* pegaspargase may cause anaphylaxis and serious hypersensitivity reactions. An expert panel recommends premedication prior to pegaspargase in adult patients (Stock W et al. Leuk Lymphoma 2011;52:2237–2253). Steroid premedication (eg, hydrocortisone) may be omitted during induction (course 1A) due to inclusion of prednisone in the regimen. Observe patients for 1 hour after the administration of pegaspargase in a setting with the capability to provide emergency resuscitation and with immediate availability of emergency supplies including epinephrine, oxygen, a histamine receptor [H$_1$]-subtype antagonist (eg, diphenhydramine), and intravenous corticosteroids

Choose one of the following options for pegaspargase (if being used *instead of* asparaginase):
• **Pegaspargase** age ≤50 years, 2000 units/m^2 (maximum dose = 3750 units); age >50 years, 1000 units/m^2 (maximum dose = 1875 units); administer by intravenous infusion over 1–2 hours in 100 mL 0.9% NS or 5% dextrose injection (D5W) into a running infusion of either 0.9% NS or D5W (choose the same fluid that was used for dilution of pegaspargase) for 1 dose on day 15 (total dosage/course = 2000 units/m^2; maximum dosage/course = 3750 units [age ≤50 years] or 1000 units/m^2; maximum dosage/course =1875 units [age >50 years]), *or:*
• **Pegaspargase** 2000 units/m^2 (maximum dose = 3750 units); administer by intramuscular injection for 1 dose on day 15 (total dosage/course = 2000 units/m^2; maximum dosage/course = 3750 units [age ≤50 years] or 1000 units/m^2; maximum dosage/course =1875 units [age >50 years])

   ▪ Limit the volume at a single injection site to ≤2 mL. If the volume to be administered is >2 mL, multiple injection sites should be used
   ▪ Patients with platelets <50,000/mm^3 may require a platelet transfusion prior to an intramuscular injection

CNS Prophylaxis and Treatment
1. Patients received CNS prophylaxis with methotrexate administered intrathecally during the initial diagnostic lumbar puncture. Five additional doses began with the first course of postremission chemotherapy with repeated doses delivered at weekly intervals as tolerated
2. Patients with CNS disease at diagnosis received intensified CNS therapy: 10 intrathecal treatments, and cranial irradiation 18 Gy was given after bone marrow remission was achieved

Methotrexate 12 mg per dose; administer intrathecally via lumbar puncture in 3–12 mL preservative-free 0.9% sodium chloride injection

	Prophylaxis	Treatment
Methotrexate (12 mg/dose)		
Total number of doses	6*	10*
Total dose/all courses	72 mg	120 mg
Cranial irradiation	None	1800 cGy after bone marrow CR

*First dose is given at the start of induction course 1A
Second and subsequent doses start concurrently with post-CR chemotherapy and continue on a weekly schedule

(*continued*)

(continued)

Note: consider incorporation of rituximab throughout all phases of treatment for a total of 16 infusions based on the results of the GRAALL-2005/R study

Maury S et al. N Engl J Med 2016;375:1044–1053

Supportive Care
Antiemetic prophylaxis
Emetogenic potential on days when daunorubicin is given is **MODERATE–HIGH**

Emetogenic potential on days when vincristine or (peg-)asparaginase ± vincristine are given is **MINIMAL**

See Chapter 42 for antiemetic recommendations

Hematopoietic growth factor (CSF) prophylaxis
Primary prophylaxis is indicated with:

Filgrastim (G-CSF) 5 µg/kg per day, by subcutaneous injection
- If only 3 doses of daunorubicin are given, begin filgrastim use on day 14. If a fourth dose of daunorubicin is given (on day 15), postpone instituting filgrastim use until 24 hours after daunorubicin was administered
- Continue daily filgrastim use until ANC >1500/mm^3 on two measurements separated temporally by ≥24 hours
- Discontinue daily filgrastim use at least 24 hours before commencing the next course of myelosuppressive treatment

See Chapter 43 for more information

Antimicrobial prophylaxis
Risk of fever and neutropenia is **HIGH**

Antimicrobial primary prophylaxis is recommended:
- Antibacterial—consider fluoroquinolone prophylaxis; *P. jirovecii* prophylaxis is recommended (eg, cotrimoxazole)
- Antifungal—recommended
- Antiviral—antiherpes antivirals (eg, acyclovir, famciclovir, valacyclovir)

Consolidation (courses 1B and 2B): high-dose cytarabine + etoposide (HDAC/etoposide)

Cytarabine 2000 mg/m^2 per day; administer intravenously in 100–1000 mL 0.9% sodium chloride injection (0.9% NS) or 5% dextrose injection (D5W) over 2 hours for 4 consecutive days on days 1–4 (total dosage/course = 8000 mg/m^2)

Etoposide 500 mg/m^2 per day; administer intravenously diluted in 0.9% NS or D5W to a concentration within the range of 0.2–0.4 mg/mL over 3 hours for 4 consecutive days on days 1–4 (total dosage/course = 2000 mg/m^2)

Note: consider incorporation of rituximab throughout all phases of treatment for a total of 16 infusions based on the results of the GRAALL-2005/R study

Maury S et al. N Engl J Med 2016;375:1044–1053

Supportive Care
Antiemetic prophylaxis
Emetogenic potential is at least **MODERATE**

See Chapter 42 for antiemetic recommendations

Hematopoietic growth factor (CSF) prophylaxis
Primary prophylaxis is indicated with one of the following:

Filgrastim (G-CSF) 5 µg/kg per day, by subcutaneous injection, *or*

Pegfilgrastim (pegylated filgrastim) 6 mg/0.6 mL, by subcutaneous injection for 1 dose
- Begin use from 24–72 hours after myelosuppressive chemotherapy is completed
- Continue daily filgrastim use until ANC >1500/mm^3 on 2 measurements separated temporally by ≥24 hours
- Discontinue daily filgrastim use at least 24 hours before commencing the next course of myelosuppressive treatment. Do not administer pegfilgrastim within 14 days before administering myelosuppressive treatment

See Chapter 43 for more information

Antimicrobial prophylaxis
Risk of fever and neutropenia is **HIGH**

Antimicrobial primary prophylaxis is recommended:
- Antibacterial—consider fluoroquinolone prophylaxis; *P. jirovecii* prophylaxis is recommended (eg, cotrimoxazole)
- Antifungal—recommended
- Antiviral—antiherpes antivirals (eg, acyclovir, famciclovir, valacyclovir)

Keratitis prophylaxis
Steroid ophthalmic drops (prednisolone 1% or dexamethasone 0.1%); administer by intraocular instillation daily until 24 hours after high-dose cytarabine is completed

(continued)

(continued)

Consolidation (course 2A): DVP/Asp

Daunorubicin 60 mg/m^2 per day; administer by intravenous injection over 3–5 minutes for 3 consecutive days on days 1–3 (total dosage/course = 180 mg/m^2)

Vincristine
> *Patients age ≤40 years:* **Vincristine** 1.4 mg/m^2 per dose; administer by intravenous infusion over 15 minutes in 50 mL 0.9% NS for 3 doses on days 1, 8, and 15 (total dosage/course = 4.2 mg/m^2)
> *Patients age >40 years:* **Vincristine** 1.4 mg/m^2 per dose (maximum single dose = 2 mg); administer by intravenous infusion over 15 minutes in 50 mL 0.9% NS for 3 doses on days 1, 8, and 15 (total dosage/course = 4.2 mg/m^2; maximum dose/course = 6 mg)

Prednisone 60 mg/m^2 per day; administer orally, continually, for 21 consecutive days on days 1–21 (total dosage/course = 1260 mg/m^2)

Asparaginase 12,000 IU/m^2 per dose; administer intramuscularly, or intravenously in 10–50 mL 0.9% sodium chloride injection or 5% dextrose injection over at least 30 minutes, for 3 doses/week (eg, Monday, Wednesday, and Friday), for a total of 6 doses during 2 consecutive weeks (total dosage/course = 72,000 IU/m^2)

Note: in the United States, asparaginase was withdrawn from the market in December 2012. Consider substituting with pegaspargase as follows:

Premedications for pegaspargase (if being used *instead of* asparaginase):
- **Acetaminophen** 650–100 mg; administer orally 30 minutes prior to pegaspargase administration on day 4
- **Diphenhydramine** 25–50 mg; administer orally or intravenously 30 minutes prior to pegaspargase administration on day 4

Choose one of the following options for pegaspargase:
- **Pegaspargase** age ≤50 years, 2000 units/m^2 (maximum dose = 3750 units); age >50 years, 1000 units/m^2 (maximum dose = 1875 units); administer by intravenous infusion over 1–2 hours in 100 mL 0.9% NS or 5% dextrose injection (D5W) into a running infusion of either 0.9% NS or D5W (choose the same fluid that was used for dilution of pegaspargase) for 1 dose on day 4 (total dosage/course = 2000 units/m^2; maximum dosage/course = 3750 units [age ≤50 years] or 1000 units/m^2; maximum dosage/course =1875 units [age >50 years]), *or:*
- **Pegaspargase** 2000 units/m^2 (maximum dose = 3750 units); administer by intramuscular injection for 1 dose on day 4 (total dosage/course = 2000 units/m^2; maximum dosage/course = 3750 units [age ≤50 years] or 1000 units/m^2; maximum dosage/course =1875 units [age >50 years])
  - Limit the volume at a single injection site to ≤2 mL. If the volume to be administered is >2 mL, multiple injection sites should be used
  - Patients with platelets <50,000/mm^3 may require a platelet transfusion prior to an intramuscular injection

Note: consider incorporation of rituximab throughout all phases of treatment for a total of 16 infusions based on the results of the GRAALL-2005/R study

Maury S et al. N Engl J Med 2016;375:1044–1053

Supportive Care
Antiemetic prophylaxis
Emetogenic potential on days when daunorubicin is given is **MODERATE–HIGH**
Emetogenic potential on days when vincristine or (peg-)asparaginase ± vincristine are given is **MINIMAL**
See Chapter 42 for antiemetic recommendations

Hematopoietic growth factor (CSF) prophylaxis
Primary prophylaxis is indicated with one of the following:
> **Filgrastim** (G-CSF) 5 µg/kg per day, by subcutaneous injection, *or*
> **Pegfilgrastim** (pegylated filgrastim) 6 mg/0.6 mL by subcutaneous injection for 1 dose
- Begin use from 24–72 hours after myelosuppressive chemotherapy is completed
- Continue daily filgrastim use until ANC >1500/mm^3 on 2 measurements separated temporally by ≥24 hours
- Discontinue daily filgrastim use at least 24 hours before commencing the next course of myelosuppressive treatment. Do not administer pegfilgrastim within 14 days before administering myelosuppressive treatment

See Chapter 43 for more information

Antimicrobial prophylaxis
Risk of fever and neutropenia is **HIGH**
> *Antimicrobial primary prophylaxis is recommended:*
- Antibacterial—consider fluoroquinolone prophylaxis; *P. jirovecii* prophylaxis is recommended (eg, cotrimoxazole)
- Antifungal—recommended
- Antiviral—antiherpes antivirals (eg, acyclovir, famciclovir, valacyclovir)

Consolidation (courses 1C, 2C, and 3C): high-dose methotrexate + mercaptopurine
Hydration with methotrexate:
Administer 1500–3000 mL/m^2 per day. Use a solution containing a total amount of sodium not greater than 0.9% sodium chloride injection (ie, 154 mEq/1000 mL); administer by intravenous infusion during methotrexate administration *and* for at least 24 hours afterward

(continued)

(continued)

- Commence fluid administration 2–12 hours before starting methotrexate, depending upon a patient's fluid status
- Urine output should be at least 100 mL/hour before starting methotrexate infusion
- Maintain hydration at a rate that maintains urine output of at least 100 mL/hour until the serum methotrexate concentration is <0.05 μmol/L
- Adverse effects attributable to methotrexate are related to systemic methotrexate concentrations and the duration for which concentrations are maintained

Sodium bicarbonate 50–150 mEq/1000 mL is added to parenteral hydration solutions to maintain urine pH ≥7.0 to ≤8.0

Base Solution Sodium Content	Sodium Bicarbonate Additive	Total Sodium Content
0.45% Sodium chloride injection (0.45% NS)		
77 mEq/L	50–75 mEq	125–152 mEq/L
0.2% Sodium chloride injection (0.2% NS)		
34 mEq/L	100–125 mEq	134–159 mEq/L
5% Dextrose injection (D5W)		
0	125–150 mEq	125–150 mEq/L
D5W/0.45% NS		
77 mEq/L	50–75 mEq	125–152 mEq/L
D5W/0.2% NS		
34 mEq/L	100–125 mEq	134–159 mEq/L

Methotrexate 220 mg/m^2; administer intravenously over 1 hour (loading dose, or *bolus*), every 2 weeks on days 1 and 15, *followed by*
Methotrexate 60 mg/m^2 per hour; administer by continuous intravenous infusion for 36 hours, every 2 weeks on days 1 and 15 (total dosage/administration event, bolus + infusion = 2380 mg/m^2; total dosage/course = 4760 mg/m^2)
Note: for logistical practicality and efficiency, parenteral admixtures containing methotrexate may include a portion or all of the fluid and sodium bicarbonate needed to meet hydration and urinary alkalinization requirements during methotrexate administration

Leucovorin calcium 50 mg/m^2 per dose; administer intravenously in 25–250 mL 0.9% NS or D5W over 15–30 minutes starting immediately after methotrexate is completed (37 hours after methotrexate administration began), every 6 hours for 3 doses, every 2 weeks on days 2 and 16, *and then:*

Leucovorin calcium 50 mg/dose; administer orally starting 6 hours after the last intravenously administered dose of leucovorin. Continue administration every 6 hours until serum methotrexate concentrations are <0.05 μmol/L (<5 ×10^{-8} mol/L, or <50 nmol/L), every 2 weeks

Mercaptopurine 75 mg/m^2 per day; administer orally, continually, for 28 consecutive days on days 1–28 (total dosage/course = 2100 mg/m^2)

Note: consider incorporation of rituximab throughout all phases of treatment for a total of 16 infusions based on the results of the GRAALL-2005/R study

Maury S et al. N Engl J Med 2016;375:1044–1053

Supportive Care
Antiemetic prophylaxis
Emetogenic potential on days when methotrexate is given is MODERATE
Emetogenic potential on days when mercaptopurine alone is given is MINIMAL–LOW
See Chapter 42 for antiemetic recommendations

Hematopoietic growth factor (CSF) prophylaxis
Primary prophylaxis is NOT indicated
See Chapter 43 for more information

Antimicrobial prophylaxis
Risk of fever and neutropenia is HIGH
  Antimicrobial primary prophylaxis is recommended:
- Antibacterial—consider fluoroquinolone prophylaxis; *P. jirovecii* prophylaxis is recommended (eg, cotrimoxazole)
- Antifungal—recommended
- Antiviral—antiherpes antivirals (eg, acyclovir, famciclovir, valacyclovir)

(continued)

Maintenance Therapy

Mercaptopurine 75 mg/m² per day; administer orally, continually, until complete remission is sustained for 30 months (total dosage/week = 525 mg/m²)

Methotrexate 20 mg/m² per dose; administer orally once weekly until complete remission is sustained for 30 months (total dosage/week = 20 mg/m²)

Note: consider incorporation of rituximab throughout all phases of treatment for a total of 16 infusions based on the results of the GRAALL-2005/R study

Maury S et al. N Engl J Med 2016;375:1044–1053

Supportive Care
Antiemetic prophylaxis
Emetogenic potential is MINIMAL–LOW
See Chapter 42 for antiemetic recommendations

Hematopoietic growth factor (CSF) prophylaxis
Primary prophylaxis is NOT indicated
See Chapter 43 for more information

Antimicrobial prophylaxis
Risk of fever and neutropenia is HIGH
  Antimicrobial primary prophylaxis is recommended:
  • Antibacterial—*P. jirovecii* prophylaxis is recommended (eg, cotrimoxazole)
  • Antifungal—not indicated
  • Antiviral—antiherpes antivirals (eg, acyclovir, famciclovir, valacyclovir)

Patient Population Studied

Eighty-four newly diagnosed ALL adult patients (median age 27 years)

Efficacy (N = 84)

Induction	
Complete remission (CR) 1 Treatment-related death 5 Patients had resistant disease	93%
5-Year event-free survival	48% ± 13%
Overall survival	47%
5-Year event-free survival for patients achieving remission	52%
5-Year DFS for patients achieving remission	54%

Therapy Monitoring

1. CBC with differential daily during and after chemotherapy until recovery of ANC >500/mm³. Platelets every day while in hospital until patients no longer require platelet transfusions

2. Electrolytes, mineral panel, and uric acid at least daily during active treatment until the risk of tumor lysis is past

3. *Anthracycline toxicity:* determination of LVEF by echocardiogram prior to treatment and then as clinically indicated

4. *(peg-)asparaginase clinical toxicity monitoring:*
   a. *Hypersensitivity:* Monitor for signs of an allergic reaction including bronchospasms, hypotension, laryngeal edema, local erythema or swelling, systemic rash, and urticaria. Monitor vital signs frequently during and for 1 hour following administration
   b. *Pancreatitis and hepatotoxicity:* Advise patients to avoid alcohol during therapy
   c. *Hemorrhage/thrombosis:* Avoid the use of oral contraceptives

5. *Asparaginase toxicity laboratory monitoring:*
   a. Amylase, lipase, fibrinogen, fasting blood glucose, aPTT, PT/INR, and liver function tests prior to each dose of asparaginase. If fibrinogen level is <100 mg/dL (<1 g/L), consider prophylactic administration of cryoprecipitate. Fasting lipid panel prior to each course of asparaginase

6. *Pegaspargase toxicity laboratory monitoring:*
   a. Fasting blood glucose, fasting lipid panel, aPTT, PT/INR, liver function tests, and fibrinogen prior to pegaspargase administration and then at least once per week for at least 4 weeks after each dose. In patients with risk factors for hyperglycemia, increase the frequency of blood glucose monitoring. Serum amylase and lipase prior to pegaspargase and then as clinically indicated for abdominal pain

7. Bone marrow aspirate and biopsy after the initial induction course upon recovery of peripheral blood counts. After patient achieves a CR, bone marrow biopsy and aspirate should be performed at least following completion of consolidation therapy

Treatment Modifications

Adverse Events	Treatment Modifications
Creatinine 1.5–2 mg/dL (133–177 µmol/L)	Reduce methotrexate dosage by 25%
Creatinine >2 mg/dL (>177 µmol/L)	Reduce methotrexate dosage by 50%
Creatinine >3 mg/dL (>265 µmol/L)	Reduce daunorubicin dosage by 50%
Total bilirubin 3–5 mg/dL (51–86 µmol/L)	Reduce daunorubicin dosage by 50% Reduce methotrexate dosage by 25%
Total bilirubin >3 mg/dL (>51 µmol/L)	Reduce vincristine dosage by 50%
Total bilirubin >5 mg/dL (>86 µmol/L)	Hold daunorubicin Hold methotrexate

Adverse Effects

Median Number of Days to Hematologic Recovery

	Courses			
	Induction 1A DVP/Asp n = 84	1B HDAC/Etoposide n = 79	2A DVP/Asp n = 59	2B HDAC/Etoposide n = 53
ANC >500/mm³	18	19	16	20
ANC >1000/mm³	23	20	17	20
No. of days with ANC <500/mm³	14	12	5	12
Platelets				
>20,000/mm³	15	19	1	22
>50,000/mm³	18	21	20	27
>100,000/mm³	22	24	29	29
No. of platelet transfusions	4	3	0	4
No. of RBC transfusions	6	7	2	6

Eleven patients experienced a peak serum total bilirubin >3 mg/dL, and 1 had a peak total bilirubin >10 mg/dL

(Peg-)asparaginase Toxicity Management

Stock W et al. Leuk Lymphoma 2011;52:2237–2253

(PEG-)ASPARAGINASE DOSE MODIFICATIONS

Adapted from: Stock W et al. Leuk Lymphoma 2011;52:2237–2253

Toxicity	Grade 2	Grade 3	Grade 4
Hypersensitivity, urticaria, wheezing, laryngospasm, hypotension, etc.	For urticaria without bronchospasm, hypotension, edema, or need for parenteral intervention, continue (peg-)asparaginase	For wheezing or other symptomatic bronchospasm with or without urticaria, indicated parenteral intervention, angioedema, or hypotension, discontinue (peg-)asparaginase. Substitute Erwinia asparaginase 25,000 units/m² (if available) IV or IM for each scheduled dose of native *E. coli* asparaginase	For life-threatening consequences or indicated urgent intervention, discontinue (peg-)asparaginase. Substitute Erwinia asparaginase 25,000 units/m² (if available) IV or IM for each scheduled dose of native *E. coli* asparaginase
Hypertriglyceridemia	If serum triglyceride level <1000 mg/dL (<11.3 mmol/L), continue (peg-)asparaginase but follow patient closely for evolving pancreatitis	Hold (peg-)asparaginase for triglyceride >1000 mg/dL (>11.3 mmol/L); follow closely for pancreatitis; resume (peg-)asparaginase at prior dose level after patient's triglyceride level returns to normal range	Hold (peg-)asparaginase for triglyceride >1000 mg/dL (>11.3 mmol/L); follow closely for pancreatitis; resume (peg-)asparaginase at prior dose level after patient's triglyceride level returns to normal range
Hyperglycemia, ketoacidosis	Continue (peg-)asparaginase for uncomplicated hyperglycemia	For hyperglycemia requiring insulin therapy, hold (peg-)asparaginase (and glucocorticoid therapy) until blood glucose regulated with insulin; resume (peg-)asparaginase at prior dose level	For hyperglycemia with life-threatening consequences or indicated urgent intervention, hold (peg-)asparaginase (and glucocorticoid therapy) until blood glucose is regulated with insulin; resume (peg-)asparaginase and do not make up for missed doses

(continued)

(Peg-)asparaginase Toxicity Management (continued)

Toxicity	Grade 2	Grade 3	Grade 4
Hyperammonemia-related fatigue	Continue (peg-)asparaginase	Reduce (peg-)asparaginase dose by 25%; resume full dose when toxicity is Grade ≤2; make up for missed doses	Reduce (peg-)asparaginase dose 50%; resume full dose when toxicity Grade 2; make up for missed doses
Pancreatitis	Continue (peg-)asparaginase for asymptomatic amylase or lipase elevation >3 × ULN (chemical pancreatitis) or only radiologic abnormalities; observe closely for rising amylase or lipase levels	Continue pegaspargase for non-symptomatic chemical pancreatitis but observe patient closely for development of symptomatic pancreatitis for early treatment. Hold native asparaginase for amylase or lipase elevation >3 ×ULN until enzyme levels stabilize or are declining. Permanently discontinue asparaginase for symptomatic pancreatitis	Permanently discontinue all (peg-)asparaginase for clinical pancreatitis (vomiting, severe abdominal pain) with amylase or lipase elevation >3 × ULN for >3 days and/or development of pancreatic pseudocyst
Hyperbilirubinemia	Continue (peg-)asparaginase if direct bilirubin ≤3.0 mg/dL (≤51 μmol/L)	If direct bilirubin is 3.1–5.0 mg/dL (53–86 μmol/L), administer (peg-)asparaginase with the dose reduced by 50%	If direct bilirubin is >5.0 mg/dL (>86 μmol/L) and ≤6.0 mg/dL (≤103 μmol/L), withhold (peg-)asparaginase and administer the next scheduled dose if toxicity has resolved. Do not make up missed doses
Non-CNS thrombosis	For abnormal laboratory findings without clinical correlates, continue (peg-)asparaginase	Withhold (peg-)asparaginase until acute toxicity and clinical signs resolve and anticoagulant therapy is stable or completed. Do not withhold (peg-)asparaginase for abnormal laboratory findings without a clinical correlate	Withhold (peg-)asparaginase until acute toxicity and clinical signs resolve and anticoagulant therapy is stable or completed
Non-CNS hemorrhage	For bleeding in conjunction, with hypofibrinogenemia, withhold (peg-)asparaginase until bleeding is Grade ≤1. Do not withhold (peg-)asparaginase for abnormal laboratory findings without a clinical correlate	Withhold (peg-)asparaginase until bleeding is Grade ≤1, until acute toxicity and clinical signs resolve, and coagulant replacement therapy is stable or completed	Withhold (peg-)asparaginase until bleeding is Grade ≤1, until acute toxicity and clinical signs resolve, and coagulant replacement therapy is stable or completed
CNS thrombosis	For abnormal laboratory findings without a clinical correlate, continue (peg-)asparaginase	Discontinue all (peg-)asparaginase; if CNS symptoms and signs are fully resolved and significant (peg-)asparaginase remains to be administered, may resume (peg-)asparaginase therapy at a lower dose and/or longer intervals between doses	Permanently discontinue (peg-)asparaginase
CNS hemorrhage	Discontinue (peg-)asparaginase; do not withhold (peg-)asparaginase for abnormal laboratory findings without a clinical correlate	Discontinue (peg-)asparaginase; if CNS symptoms and signs are fully resolved and significant (peg-)asparaginase remains to be administered, may resume (peg-)asparaginase therapy at a lower dose and/or longer intervals between doses	Permanently discontinue (peg-)asparaginase

Grade according to the National Cancer Institute Common Terminology Criteria for Advance Events version 4, with the exception of pancreatitis

IV, intravenous; IM, intramuscular; ULN, upper limit of normal; CNS, central nervous system

ADULT
ACUTE LYMPHOBLASTIC LEUKEMIA: MRC UKALL XII/ECOG E2993

Rowe JM et al. Blood 2005;106:3760–3767

Induction therapy
Induction—phase 1 (weeks 1–4)
Daunorubicin 60 mg/m² per dose; administer by intravenous injection over 3–5 minutes for 4 doses on days 1, 8, 15, and 22 (total dosage/4-week course = 240 mg/m²)

Vincristine 1.4 mg/m² per dose; administer by intravenous infusion over 15 minutes in 50 mL 0.9% NS for 4 doses on days 1, 8, 15, and 22 (total dosage/4-week course = 5.6 mg/m²)

Prednisone 60 mg/m² per day; administer orally, continually, for 28 consecutive days on days 1 to 28 (total dosage/4-week course = 1680 mg/m²)
• Daily prednisone doses may be given in a single dose or ≥2 divided doses

Methotrexate 12.5 mg; administer intrathecally in 3–12 mL preservative-free 0.9% sodium chloride injection on day 15 (total dose/4-week course = 12.5 mg)

Asparaginase 10,000 IU/dose; administer intramuscularly, or intravenously in 10–50 mL 0.9% sodium chloride injection (0.9% NS) or 5% dextrose injection (D5W) for 12 consecutive days, on days 17 to 28 (total dose/4-week course = 120,000 IU)

Induction—phase 2 (weeks 5–8)
(Regardless of whether residual leukemia is present at the end of phase 1)
Cyclophosphamide 650 mg/m²; administer intravenously in 100–1000 mL 0.9% NS or D5W over 15–60 min for 3 doses on days 1, 15, and 29 (total dosage/4-week course = 1950 mg/m²)

Cytarabine 75 mg/m² per dose; administer intravenously in 25–250 mL 0.9% NS or D5W over 15–60 min for 16 doses on days 1–4, 8–11, 15–18, and 22–25 (total dosage/4-week course = 1200 mg/m²)

Mercaptopurine 60 mg/m² per day; administer orally, continually, for 28 consecutive days on days 1 to 28 (total dosage/4-week course = 1680 mg/m²)

Methotrexate 12.5 mg per dose; administer intrathecally in 3–12 mL preservative-free 0.9% sodium chloride injection for 4 doses on days 1, 8, 15, and 22 (total dose/4-week course = 50 mg)

Notes: A diagnostic spinal tap was performed on all patients. If CNS leukemia was present at diagnosis, methotrexate was administered intrathecally via lumbar puncture or through a ventricular reservoir (eg, Ommaya) every week until blast cells were no longer present in the spinal fluid. In addition, 2400 cGy of cranial irradiation and 1200 cGy to the spinal cord were administered concurrently during induction, phase 2. For patients with CNS leukemia at presentation, intrathecal methotrexate was not administered during phase 2

Intensification therapy
Hydration for methotrexate: 6–18 hours before the anticipated start of methotrexate, start intravenous hydration containing sodium bicarbonate (NaHCO₃) to alkalinize a patient's urine to pH ≥7.0, but ≤8.0, at a rate that achieves a urine output ≥100 mL/hour
Options recommended to initially produce an alkaline urine, include:

Fluid	Administration Rate	Sodium Bicarbonate Content (per 1000 mL)
0.45% NS	150–250 mL/hour	50–75 mEq
0.2% NS		100–125 mEq
D5W/0.45% NS		50–75 mEq
D5W/0.2% NS		100–125 mEq
D5W		150 mEq

D5W, 5% dextrose injection; NS, sodium chloride injection

Notes: Urine alkalinization to pH ≥7.0 to ≤8.0 and urine output ≥100 mL/hour often initially require more NaHCO₃ and more rapid hydration rates than will be required to maintain either or both parameters after they are achieved
The amount of sodium bicarbonate added to intravenously administered fluids should produce a solution with sodium content not greater than the concentration of sodium in 0.9% sodium chloride injection (≤154 mEq/L)

Methotrexate 3000 mg/m²; administer intravenously in one of the solutions identified above in admixture with 25–75 mEq NaHCO₃ over 4 hours after urine pH ≥7.0 to ≤8.0 and urine output >100 mL/hour are confirmed for 3 doses on days 1, 8, and 22 (total dosage/course = 9000 mg/m²)
• Temporarily interrupt hydration while methotrexate is administered
  ▪ The methotrexate product should contain volume and sodium bicarbonate content equivalent to what was being given in intravenous hydration to maintain urine pH ≥7.0 to ≤8.0 and output >100 mL/hour

(continued)

(continued)

- Order daily serum methotrexate levels timed to start 24 hours after methotrexate administration begins and continue daily measurements until the serum methotrexate level is ≤0.05 μmol/L
- Continue hydration with urine alkalinization (pH ≥7.0 to ≤8.0) until serum methotrexate level is ≤0.05 μmol/L

Leucovorin calcium 100 mg/m^2 per dose (preferred), or **levoleucovorin calcium** 50 mg/m^2 per dose; administer intravenously in 25–250 mL 0.9% NS or D5W over 10–30 minutes every 6 hours starting 24 hours after methotrexate administration began, and continue for at least 6 doses or until serum methotrexate concentrations are ≤0.5 μmol/L, whichever occurs later

When the methotrexate level is <0.5 μmol/L, parenterally administered leucovorin or levoleucovorin may be replaced with leucovorin administered orally (10 mg/m^2, or a fixed 25-mg dose for patients whose body surface area is <2.5 m^2), until the serum methotrexate level is ≤0.05 μmol/L

Asparaginase 10,000 IU/dose; administer intramuscularly, or intravenously in 10–50 mL 0.9% NS or D5W intravenously or intramuscularly for 3 doses on days 2, 9, and 23 (total dose/course = 30,000 IU)

Consolidation therapy
Cytarabine 50 mg/dose; administer intrathecally in 3–12 mL preservative-free 0.9% sodium chloride injection weekly for 4 weeks, *with:*
Cranial irradiation 2400 cGy
Consolidation—cycle 1
Cytarabine 75 mg/m^2 per day; administer intravenously in 25–250 mL 0.9% NS or D5W over 15–60 minutes for 5 consecutive days on days 1–5 (total dosage/cycle = 375 mg/m^2)
Etoposide 100 mg/m^2 per day; administer intravenously in a volume of 0.9% NS or D5W sufficient to produce a concentration within the range, 0.2–0.4 mg/mL over at least 60 minutes for 5 consecutive days on days 1–5 (total dosage/cycle = 500 mg/m^2)
Vincristine 1.4 mg/m^2 per dose; administer by intravenous infusion over 15 minutes in 50 mL 0.9% NS for 4 doses on days 1, 8, 15, and 22 (total dosage/cycle = 5.6 mg/m^2)
Dexamethasone 10 mg/m^2 per day; administer orally, continually, for 28 consecutive days on days 1 to 28 (total dosage/cycle = 280 mg/m^2)
Consolidation—cycle 2 (starts 4 weeks after cycle 1)
Cytarabine 75 mg/m^2 per day; administer intravenously in 25–250 mL 0.9% NS or D5W over 15–60 minutes for 5 consecutive days on days 1–5 (total dosage/cycle = 375 mg/m^2)
Etoposide 100 mg/m^2 per day; administer intravenously in a volume of 0.9% NS or D5W sufficient to produce a concentration within the range, 0.2–0.4 mg/mL over at least 60 minutes for 5 consecutive days on days 1–5 (total dosage/cycle = 500 mg/m^2)
Consolidation—cycle 3 (starts 4 weeks after cycle 2)
Daunorubicin 25 mg/m^2 per dose; administer by intravenous injection over 3–5 minutes for 4 doses on days 1, 8, 15, and 22 (total dosage/4-week course = 100 mg/m^2)
Cyclophosphamide 650 mg/m^2; administer intravenously in 100–1000 mL 0.9% NS or D5W over 15–60 min on day 29 (total dosage/4-week course = 650 mg/m^2)
Cytarabine 75 mg/m^2 per dose; administer intravenously in 25–250 mL 0.9% NS or D5W over 15–60 minutes for 8 doses on days 31–34 and 38–41 (total dosage/4-week course = 600 mg/m^2)
Thioguanine 60 mg/m^2 per day; administer orally, continually, for 14 consecutive days on days 29–42 (total dosage/4-week course = 840 mg/m^2)
Consolidation—cycle 4 (8 weeks after the conclusion of cycle 3)
Cytarabine 75 mg/m^2 per day; administer intravenously in 25–250 mL 0.9% NS or D5W over 15–60 minutes for 5 consecutive days on days 1–5 (total dosage/cycle = 375 mg/m^2)
Etoposide 100 mg/m^2 per day; administer intravenously in a volume of 0.9% NS or D5W sufficient to produce a concentration within the range, 0.2–0.4 mg/mL over at least 60 minutes for 5 consecutive days on days 1–5 (total dosage/cycle = 500 mg/m^2)

Maintenance therapy (continues for a total of 2.5 years after the start of intensification therapy)
Cytarabine 50 mg/dose; administer intrathecally in 3–12 mL preservative-free 0.9% sodium chloride injection on 4 occasions 3 months apart during maintenance therapy (total of 4 doses = 200 mg)
Vincristine 1.4 mg/m^2; administer by intravenous infusion over 15 minutes in 50 mL 0.9% NS every 3 months (total dosage/3-month period = 1.4 mg/m^2)
Prednisone 60 mg/m^2; administer orally for 5 consecutive days every 3 months (total dosage/3-month period = 300 mg/m^2)
Mercaptopurine 75 mg/m^2; administer orally, continually each day (total dosage/week = 525 mg/m^2)
Methotrexate 20 mg/m^2; administer orally or intravenously once a week (total dosage/week = 20 mg/m^2)

Supportive Care
Antiemetic Prophylaxis During Induction—phase 1
Emetogenic potential on days 1, 8, and 15 is **MODERATE**
Emetogenic potential on days with asparaginase (days 17–28) is **MINIMAL**

Antiemetic Prophylaxis During Induction—phase 2
Emetogenic potential on days with cyclophosphamide (days 1, 15, and 29) is **MODERATE**
Emetogenic potential on days with cytarabine without cyclophosphamide is **LOW**
Emetogenic potential on days with mercaptopurine alone is **MINIMAL–LOW**

(continued)

(continued)

Antiemetic Prophylaxis During Intensification
Emetogenic potential on days with methotrexate (days 1, 8, and 22) is **MODERATE**
Emetogenic potential on days with asparaginase (days 2, 9, and 23) is **MINIMAL**

Antiemetic Prophylaxis During Consolidation, Cycle 1
Emetogenic potential on days 1–5 is **LOW**
Emetogenic potential on days 8 and 15 is **MINIMAL**

Antiemetic Prophylaxis During Consolidation, Cycle 2
Emetogenic potential on days 1–5 is **LOW**

Antiemetic Prophylaxis During Consolidation, Cycle 3
Emetogenic potential on days 1, 8, 15, and 29 is **MODERATE**
Emetogenic potential on days with cytarabine is **LOW**
Emetogenic potential on days with thioguanine alone is **LOW**

Antiemetic Prophylaxis During Consolidation, Cycle 4
Emetogenic potential on days 1–5 is **LOW**

Antiemetic Prophylaxis During Maintenance
Emetogenic potential on days methotrexate is given is **MINIMAL–LOW**
Emetogenic potential all other days is **MINIMAL**
See Chapter 42 for antiemetic recommendations

Hematopoietic growth factor (CSF) prophylaxis
Primary prophylaxis is **NOT** *indicated*
See Chapter 43 for more information

Antimicrobial prophylaxis
Risk of fever and neutropenia is **HIGH**
  Antimicrobial primary prophylaxis is recommended:
  • Antibacterial—consider fluoroquinolone prophylaxis; *Pneumocystis jirovecii* prophylaxis is recommended (eg, cotrimoxazole)
  • Antifungal—recommended
  • Antiviral—antiherpes antivirals (eg, acyclovir, famciclovir, valacyclovir)

Population Studied

Of patients from 15 to 59 years of age newly diagnosed with ALL, 1521 received identical induction therapy, irrespective of risk assessment, including central nervous system (CNS) prophylaxis and treatment of CNS disease, if present at diagnosis. Philadelphia chromosome (Ph)-positive patients were considered the highest-risk group. Patients who were Ph-negative were considered at high risk if any of the following were present: age ≥35 years; time to CR >4 weeks or WBC count >30 × 10^9/L for B-lineage ALL and >100 × 10^9/L for T-lineage ALL. Ph-negative patients who had none of these risk factors were considered at standard risk. After induction therapy, all patients younger than 50 years of age who had a human leukocyte antigen (HLA)–compatible sibling were assigned to undergo allogeneic transplantation. All other patients were randomly assigned between autologous transplantation and standard consolidation/maintenance therapy. Patients who were Ph-positive were offered a search for a matched unrelated donor if they did not have a histocompatible family donor

Efficacy

	No.	CR, %	5-Year Survival, %	5-Year Survival for Patients in CR, %
All patients	1521	91	38	41
Ph+	293	83	25	28
Ph–	1153	93	41	44
Standard risk*	533	97	54	57
High risk*	590	90	29	35

	No.	CR, %	5-Year Survival, %	5-Year Survival for Patients in CR, %
Unknown risk	30	84	23	

*Risk stratification at diagnosis based on age and WBC count only
Overall survival (OS) rates at 5 years in this study were 38% for all patients, 41% for Ph-negative patients, and 25% for Ph-positive patients
In subsequent reports (Goldstone AH et al. Blood 2008;111:1827–1833), the 5-year OS in 1913 ALL patients was 39% and 43% for patients with Ph-negative ALL. In Ph-positive patients (Fielding AK et al. Blood 2009;113:4489–4496), the OS was 44% after sib allo-HSCT, 36% after MUD, and 19% after chemotherapy

Treatment Modifications

Adverse Events	Treatment Modifications
Creatinine 1.5–2 mg/dL (133–177 µmol/L)	Reduce methotrexate dosage by 25%
Creatinine >2 mg/dL (>177 µmol/L)	Reduce methotrexate dosage by 50%
Creatinine >3 mg/dL (>265 µmol/L)	Reduce daunorubicin dosage by 50%
Total bilirubin 3–5 mg/dL (51–86 µmol/L)	Reduce daunorubicin dosage by 50% Reduce methotrexate dosage by 25%
Total bilirubin >3 mg/dL (>51 µmol/L)	Reduce vincristine dosage by 50%
Total bilirubin >5 mg/dL (>86 µmol/L)	Hold daunorubicin Hold methotrexate

Toxicity

Overall mortality rates for induction therapy were 4.7% (54 of 1153 patients) for Ph-negative patients and 5.5% (16 of 293 patients) for Ph-positive patients. Twenty-nine patients died of infection, most significantly caused by *Aspergillus* (7 patients). Five patients died of hemorrhage (3 pulmonary, 2 cerebral), 2 patients died of thromboses (possibly related to asparaginase), and 1 patient died from tumor lysis. The remaining 10 patients died of causes described as multiorgan failure, which might also have been related to an infectious etiology

Asparaginase Toxicity Management

Stock W et al. Leuk Lymphoma 2011;52:2237–2253

Toxicity	Grade 2	Grade 3	Grade 4
Hypersensitivity, urticaria, wheezing, laryngospasm, hypotension, etc.	For urticaria without bronchospasm, hypotension, edema, or need for parenteral intervention, continue asparaginase	For wheezing or other symptomatic bronchospasm with or without urticaria, indicated parenteral intervention, angioedema, or hypotension, discontinue asparaginase. If Erwinia asparaginase is available, replace asparaginase with Erwinia asparaginase	For life-threatening consequences or indicated urgent intervention, discontinue asparaginase. If Erwinia asparaginase is available, replace asparaginase with Erwinia asparaginase
Hypertriglyceridemia	If serum triglyceride level <1000 mg/dL (<11.3 mmol/L), continue asparaginase but follow patient closely for evolving pancreatitis	Hold asparaginase for triglyceride >1000 mg/dL (>11.3 mmol/L); follow closely for pancreatitis; resume asparaginase at prior dose level after patient's triglyceride level returns to normal range	Hold asparaginase for triglyceride >1000 mg/dL (>11.3 mmol/L); follow closely for pancreatitis; resume asparaginase at prior dose level after patient's triglyceride level returns to normal range
Hyperglycemia, ketoacidosis	Continue asparaginase for uncomplicated hyperglycemia	For hyperglycemia requiring insulin therapy, hold asparaginase (and glucocorticoid therapy) until blood glucose regulated with insulin; resume asparaginase at prior dose level	For hyperglycemia with life-threatening consequences or indicated urgent intervention, hold asparaginase (and glucocorticoid therapy) until blood glucose is regulated with insulin; resume asparaginase and do not make up for missed doses
Hyperammonemia-related fatigue	Continue asparaginase	Reduce asparaginase dose by 25%; resume full dose when toxicity is Grade ≤2; make up for missed doses	Reduce asparaginase dose 50%; resume full dose when toxicity Grade 2; make up for missed doses
Pancreatitis	Continue asparaginase for asymptomatic amylase or lipase elevation >3 ×ULN (chemical pancreatitis) or only radiologic abnormalities; observe closely for rising amylase or lipase levels	Continue pegaspargase for non-symptomatic chemical pancreatitis but observe patient closely for development of symptomatic pancreatitis for early treatment. Hold native asparaginase for amylase or lipase elevation >3 ×ULN until enzyme levels stabilize or are declining. Permanently discontinue asparaginase for symptomatic pancreatitis	Permanently discontinue all asparaginase for clinical pancreatitis (vomiting, severe abdominal pain) with amylase or lipase elevation >3 ×ULN for >3 days and/or development of pancreatic pseudocyst
Increased hepatic transaminases	For alanine or glutamine aminotransferase elevation >3–5 ×ULN, continue asparaginase	For alanine or glutamine aminotransferase elevation >5–20 ×ULN, delay next dose of asparaginase until transaminasemia is Grade <2	For alanine or glutamine aminotransferase elevation >20 ×ULN, discontinue asparaginase if toxicity reduction to Grade <2 takes >1 week

(continued)

Asparaginase Toxicity Management (continued)

Toxicity	Grade 2	Grade 3	Grade 4
Hyperbilirubinemia	Continue asparaginase if direct bilirubin <3.0 mg/dL (<51 μmol/L)	If direct bilirubin is 3.1–5.0 mg/dL (53–86 μmol/L), hold asparaginase and resume when direct bilirubin is <2.0 mg/dL Consider switching to native asparaginase	If direct bilirubin is >5.0 mg/dL (>86 μmol/L), discontinue all asparaginase and do not make up for missed doses
Non-CNS thrombosis	For abnormal laboratory findings without clinical correlates, continue asparaginase	Withhold asparaginase until acute toxicity and clinical signs resolve and anticoagulant therapy is stable or completed. Do not withhold asparaginase for abnormal laboratory findings without a clinical correlate	Withhold asparaginase until acute toxicity and clinical signs resolve and anticoagulant therapy is stable or completed
Non-CNS hemorrhage	For bleeding in conjunction with hypofibrinogenemia, withhold asparaginase until bleeding is Grade ≤1. Do not withhold asparaginase for abnormal laboratory findings without a clinical correlate	Withhold asparaginase until bleeding is Grade ≤1, until acute toxicity and clinical signs resolve, and coagulant replacement therapy is stable or completed	Withhold asparaginase until bleeding is Grade ≤1, until acute toxicity and clinical signs resolve, and coagulant replacement therapy is stable or completed
CNS thrombosis	For abnormal laboratory findings without a clinical correlate, continue asparaginase	Discontinue all asparaginase; if CNS symptoms and signs are fully resolved and significant asparaginase remains to be administered, may resume asparaginase therapy at a lower dose and/or longer intervals between doses	Permanently discontinue all asparaginase
CNS hemorrhage	Discontinue asparaginase; do not withhold asparaginase for abnormal laboratory findings without a clinical correlate	Discontinue all asparaginase; if CNS symptoms and signs are fully resolved and significant asparaginase remains to be administered, may resume asparaginase therapy at a lower dose and/or longer intervals between doses	Permanently discontinue all asparaginase

Grade according to the National Cancer Institute Common Terminology Criteria for Advance Events version 4, with the exception of pancreatitis

Monitoring Therapy

1. CBC with differential daily during and after chemotherapy until recovery of ANC >500/mm^3. Platelets every day while in hospital until patient no longer requires platelet transfusions

2. Metabolic panel and uric acid, at least daily during active treatment until the risk of tumor lysis is past

3. *Asparaginase monitoring:*

   a) Amylase, lipase, fibrinogen, fasting blood glucose, aPTT, PT/INR, and liver function tests prior to each dose of asparaginase. If fibrinogen level is <100 mg/dL (<1 g/L), consider prophylactic administration of cryoprecipitate. Fasting lipid panel prior to each course of asparaginase

   b) *Hypersensitivity:* monitor for signs of an allergic reaction including bronchospasms, hypotension, laryngeal edema, local erythema or swelling, systemic rash, and urticaria. Monitor vital signs frequently during and for 1 hour following administration

   c) *Pancreatitis and hepatotoxicity:* advise patients to avoid alcohol during therapy

   d) *Hemorrhage/thrombosis:* avoid the use of oral contraceptives

4. *Anthracycline toxicity:* determination of LVEF by echocardiogram prior to treatment with anthracycline

5. Bone marrow aspirate and biopsy after phase 1 and phase 2 of induction therapy. After a patient achieves a CR, bone marrow biopsy and aspirate should be performed at the end of each consolidation cycle (or at the very least, every other cycle), and every 3 months during maintenance therapy

Notes: A diagnostic spinal tap was performed on all patients

(continued)

Monitoring Therapy (*continued*)

If CNS leukemia was present at diagnosis, methotrexate administered intrathecally via lumbar puncture or through a ventricular reservoir (eg, Ommaya) was given weekly until blast cells were no longer present in the spinal fluid. In addition, 2400 cGy of cranial irradiation and 1200 cGy to the spinal cord were administered concurrently during phase 2. For patients with CNS leukemia at presentation, intrathecal methotrexate was not administered during phase 2

In a subsequent analysis (Fielding AK et al. Blood 2007;109:944–950) of the MRC UKALL XII/ECOG E2993 study, among 1372 patients with ALL who entered remission, 609 (44%) relapsed at a median of 11 months after the start of treatment. Most (556 [91%]) patients relapsed within the bone marrow, the sole site of relapse in most (90%) of those patients. A group of 45 (8%) patients relapsed solely at extramedullary sites

Most patients (81%) relapsed within 2 years after diagnosis, although a significant minority (19%) relapsed >2 years after diagnosis. Of the 440 chemotherapy-treated patients, 349 relapsed within 2 years after diagnosis, and 87 relapsed later. Those on chemotherapy who relapsed within 2 years can be considered "relapses on therapy" because the duration of therapy was set to be 18 months from the point of initiation of the consolidation therapy (ie, 23 months)

The median survival after relapse was 24 weeks. Survival at 1 year was 22% (95% CI = 18–25%), and 7% (95% CI = 4–9%) at 5 years. Only 42 of 609 patients who relapsed remain alive without further relapse

Factors predicting a good outcome after salvage therapy were young age (OS of 12% in patients <20 years vs OS of 3% in patients >50 years; 2P <0.001) and short duration of first remission (CR1) (OS of 11% in those with a CR1 >2 years vs OS of 5% in those with a CR1 <2 years; 2P <0.001). Patients treated with HSCT had a superior OS (15% [95% CI, 0–35%] for autograft [n = 13], 16% [95% CI, 7–26%] for matched unrelated donor transplantation [n = 65], and 23% [95% CI, 10–36%] for sibling allograft [n = 42]) to those receiving chemotherapy alone (n = 182) whose OS was only 4% (95% CI, 1–7%) at 5 years

ADULT

ACUTE LYMPHOBLASTIC LEUKEMIA: HYPER-CVAD + DASATINIB

Kantarjian H et al. Cancer 2004;101:2788–2801
Ravandi F et al. Blood Adv 2016;1:250–259
Ravandi F et al. Blood 2010;116:2070–2077

Dose-intensive chemotherapy
The dose-intensive phase consists of 8 cycles of hyper-CVAD alternating with high-dose methotrexate and cytarabine every 3–4 weeks (when the WBC count is >3000/mm^3 and platelet count is >60,000/mm^3)

Dasatinib (cycle 1)
Dasatinib 100 mg per dose; administer orally, once daily, with or without a meal for 14 consecutive days on days 1–14 during cycle 1 of dose-intensive chemotherapy (total dosage/cycle = 1400 mg)

Dasatinib (cycles 2, 3, 4, 5, 6, 7, and 8)
Dasatinib 70 mg per dose; administer orally, once daily, continually, with or without a meal, beginning with the start of hyper-CVAD cycle 2 and continuing through the remainder of the dose-intensive chemotherapy phase (total dosage/week = 490 mg)

Hyper-CVAD (cycles 1, 3, 5, and 7)
Cyclophosphamide 300 mg/m^2 per dose; administer intravenously over 3 hours in 500 mL 0.9% sodium chloride injection (0.9% NS) or 5% dextrose injection (D5W) every 12 hours for 6 doses on days 1–3, for 4 cycles, cycles 1, 3, 5, and 7 (total dosage/cycle = 1800 mg/m^2)

Mesna 600 mg/m^2 per 24 hours; administer by continuous intravenous infusion in 1000 mL 0.9% NS for approximately 69 hours for 4 cycles, cycles 1, 3, 5, and 7 (total dosage/cycle ~1725 mg/m^2)
• Mesna administration starts concurrently with cyclophosphamide on day 1 and continues until 6 hours after the last dose of cyclophosphamide is completed (69 hours)

Vincristine 2 mg/dose; administer by intravenous infusion over 15 minutes in 50 mL 0.9% NS for 2 doses, on days 4 and 11, for 4 cycles, cycles 1, 3, 5, and 7 (total dose/cycle = 4 mg)

Doxorubicin 50 mg/m^2; administer intravenously via central venous access in 25–250 mL 0.9% NS or D5W over 2 hours on day 4, for 4 cycles, cycles 1, 3, 5, and 7 (total dosage/cycle = 50 mg/m^2)

Dexamethasone 40 mg per day; administer orally, or intravenously in 25–150 mL 0.9% NS or D5W over 15–30 minutes for 8 doses, on days 1–4 and days 11–14, for 4 cycles, cycles 1, 3, 5, and 7 (total dose/cycle = 320 mg)

Supportive Care
Antiemetic prophylaxis
Emetogenic potential on Days 1–4 is **MODERATE**
Emetogenic potential on Days 11 is **MINIMAL**
See Chapter 42 for antiemetic recommendations

Hematopoietic growth factor (CSF) prophylaxis
Primary prophylaxis is indicated with:
Filgrastim (G-CSF) 5 μg/kg per dose; administer by subcutaneous injection every 12 hours, starting on day 5 (24 hours after doxorubicin)
• Continue filgrastim administration until postnadir WBC count >3000/mm^3 and platelet count is >60,000/mm^3. If platelet recovery is delayed, filgrastim is continued until the WBC count >30,000/mm^3
• Discontinue daily filgrastim use at least 24 hours before administering myelosuppressive treatment
See Chapter 43 for more information

Antimicrobial prophylaxis
Risk of fever and neutropenia is **HIGH**
Antimicrobial primary prophylaxis is recommended:
• Antibacterial—consider fluoroquinolone prophylaxis; *P. jirovecii* prophylaxis is recommended (eg, cotrimoxazole)
• Antifungal—recommended
• Antiviral—antiherpes antivirals (eg, acyclovir, famciclovir, valacyclovir)

High-dose methotrexate + cytarabine (cycles 2, 4, 6, and 8)
Hydration: with a solution containing a total amount of sodium not >0.9% NS (ie, ≤154 mEq sodium/1000 mL) by intravenous infusion during methotrexate administration and for at least 24 hours afterward
• Commence fluid administration 2–12 hours before starting methotrexate, depending on patient's fluid status
• Urine output should be at least 100 mL/hour before starting methotrexate infusion
• Maintain hydration at a rate that maintains urine output ≥100 mL/hour until the serum methotrexate concentration is <0.1 μmol/L
• Urine pH should be increased within the range ≥7.0 to ≤8.0 to enhance methotrexate solubility and ensure elimination

(continued)

(continued)

- Adverse effects attributable to methotrexate are related to systemic methotrexate concentrations *and* the duration for which concentrations are maintained

Sodium bicarbonate 50–150 mEq/1000 mL is added to parenteral hydration solutions to maintain urine pH ≥7.0 to ≤8.0

Base Solution Sodium Content	Sodium Bicarbonate Additive	Total Sodium Content
0.45% Sodium chloride injection (0.45% NS)		
77 mEq/L	50–75 mEq	127–152 mEq/L
0.2% Sodium chloride injection (0.2% NS)		
34 mEq/L	100–125 mEq	134–159 mEq/L
5% Dextrose injection (D5W)		
0	125–150 mEq	125–150 mEq/L
D5W/0.45% NS		
77 mEq/L	50–75 mEq	127–152 mEq/L
D5W/0.2% NS		
34 mEq/L	100–125 mEq	134–159 mEq/L

Methotrexate 200 mg/m^2; administer intravenously over 2 hours, on day 1, *followed by:*
Methotrexate 800 mg/m^2; administer intravenously over 24 hours, on day 1, for 4 cycles, cycles 2, 4, 6, and 8 (total dosage/cycle, bolus + infusion = 1000 mg/m^2)

Note: for logistical practicality and efficiency, parenteral admixtures containing methotrexate may include a portion or all of the fluid and sodium bicarbonate needed to meet hydration and urinary alkalinization requirements during methotrexate administration

Leucovorin calcium 15 mg per dose; administer intravenously in 25–250 mL 0.9% NS or D5W over 15–30 minutes, starting 48 hours after methotrexate administration began (22 hours after methotrexate administration ends), every 6 hours for 8 doses (total dosage/cycle = 120 mg)

Note: if serum methotrexate concentrations are:

Hours After *Starting* Methotrexate	Methotrexate Concentration	Leucovorin Regimen
Hour 24	>20 µmol/L (>2 × 10^{-5} mol/L)	Increase **leucovorin** dosages to 50 mg/dose; administer intravenously in 25–250 mL 0.9% NS or D5W over 15–30 minutes every 6 hours until serum methotrexate concentrations are <0.1 µmol/L (<1 × 10^{27} mol/L)
Hour 48	>1 µmol/L (>1 × 10^{-6} mol/L)	
Hour 72	>0.1 µmol/L (>1 × 10^{-7} mol/L, *or* >100 nmol/L)	

Cytarabine
  Patient ages <60 years: **Cytarabine** 3000 mg/m^2 per dose; administer intravenously in 50–500 mL 0.9% NS or D5W over 2 hours every 12 hours for 4 doses on days 2 and 3, for 4 cycles, cycles 2, 4, 6, and 8 (total dosage/cycle [not including intrathecal cytarabine] = 12,000 mg/m^2)
  Patient ages ≥60 years: **Cytarabine** 1000 mg/m^2 per dose; administer intravenously in 50–500 mL 0.9% NS or D5W over 2 hours every 12 hours for 4 doses on days 2 and 3, for 4 cycles, cycles 2, 4, 6, and 8 (total dosage/cycle [not including intrathecal cytarabine] = 4000 mg/m^2)

Methylprednisolone 50 mg; administer intravenously twice daily for 6 doses, on days 1–3 (total dose/cycle = 300 mg)

Supportive Care
Antiemetic prophylaxis
Emetogenic potential on Days 1–3 is **MODERATE**
See Chapter 42 for antiemetic recommendations

Hematopoietic growth factor (CSF) prophylaxis
Primary prophylaxis is indicated with:
  Filgrastim (G-CSF) 5 µg/kg per dose; administer by subcutaneous injection every 12 hours, starting on day 4 (24 hours after the last dose of cytarabine)
  - Continue filgrastim administration until postnadir WBC count >3000/mm^3 and platelet count is >60,000/mm^3. If platelet recovery is delayed, filgrastim is continued until the WBC count >30,000/mm^3
  - Discontinue daily filgrastim use at least 24 hours before administering myelosuppressive treatment
See Chapter 43 for more information

(continued)

(*continued*)

Antimicrobial prophylaxis
Risk of fever and neutropenia is **HIGH**
Antimicrobial primary prophylaxis is recommended:
- Antibacterial—consider fluoroquinolone prophylaxis; *P. jirovecii* prophylaxis is recommended (eg, cotrimoxazole)
- Antifungal—recommended
- Antiviral—antiherpes antivirals (eg, acyclovir, famciclovir, valacyclovir)

Keratitis prophylaxis
Steroid ophthalmic drops (prednisolone 1% or dexamethasone 0.1%); administer 2 drops by intraocular instillation into each eye every 6 hours starting prior to the first cytarabine dose and continuing until 48 hours after high-dose cytarabine is completed

Maintenance phase
Dasatinib 100 mg per dose; administer orally, once daily, with or without a meal, continually until disease progression (total dosage/week = 700 mg)
Vincristine 2 mg; administer by intravenous infusion over 15 minutes in 50 mL 0.9% NS, once monthly for 2 years (total dose/month = 2 mg)
Prednisone 200 mg per day; administer orally, continually, for 5 consecutive days every month, starting on the day vincristine is given, for 2 years (total dose/month = 1000 mg)
Note: the protocol allowed two cycles of intensification with hyper-CVAD during months 6 and 13 of maintenance to be administered at the discretion of the treating physician based on the results of minimal residual disease testing and tolerability. After completion of 2 years of maintenance therapy, dasatinib was continued as monotherapy

Supportive Care
Antiemetic prophylaxis
Emetogenic potential is **MINIMAL**
See Chapter 42 for antiemetic recommendations

Hematopoietic growth factor (CSF) prophylaxis
Primary prophylaxis is NOT indicated
See Chapter 43 for more information

Antimicrobial prophylaxis
Risk of fever and neutropenia is **LOW**
Antimicrobial primary prophylaxis is recommended:
- Antibacterial—*P. jirovecii* prophylaxis is recommended (eg, cotrimoxazole)
- Antifungal—not indicated
- Antiviral—antiherpes antivirals (eg, acyclovir, famciclovir, valacyclovir)

Patient Population Studied

NCT00792948 was an intergroup phase 2 study conducted in the United States that involved 94 evaluable adult (age 18–60 years) patients with Philadelphia chromosome–positive (Ph+) acute lymphoblastic leukemia (ALL) who were either untreated (n = 60) or who had undergone 1 prior cycle of ALL-type induction therapy prior to determination of Ph+ status (n = 34). Patients were required to have a performance status of ≤3 and adequate organ function. Patients who had an available matched donor were encouraged to undergo protocol-specified hematopoietic stem cell transplantation in first complete remission (N = 41). The median age of patients was 44 years (range, 20–60). Three percent of patients had central nervous system involvement at diagnosis. Thirty-six percent of patients had received prior treatment before enrollment (n = 16 previously treated, achieved complete remission [CR] or CR with incomplete peripheral blood recovery [CRi]; n = 7 previously treated, unknown remission status; and n = 11 previously treated, refractory disease)

Efficacy (N = 94)

Efficacy Variable	Hyper-CVAD + Dasatinib (N = 94, Total Cohort)	
Survival Outcomes		
Outcome	*Event incidence—n/N (%)*	*Outcome at 3 years—% (95% CI)*
EFS, whole cohort	41/94 (44)	55 (46–66)
RFS, whole cohort	30/83 (36)	62 (52–74)
OS, whole cohort	28/94 (30)	69 (52–79)

(*continued*)

Efficacy (N = 94) *(continued)*

Outcome	Event incidence—n/N (%)	Outcome at 3 years—% (95% CI)
RFS, no protocol-specified transplant in CR1	21/44 (48)	51
OS, no protocol-specified transplant in CR1	22/53 (42)	56

Survival Outcomes with Protocol-Specified HCT

Outcome	Event incidence—n/N (%)	Outcome at 12 months—% (95% CI)	Outcome at 3 years—% (95% CI)
RFS after protocol transplant	9/40 (23)	83 (72–95)*	76 (63–91)
OS after protocol transplant	6/40 (15)	NR	NR

Landmark Analysis Performed at 175 days after Achieving CR or CRi

Outcome	Event incidence—n/N (%)	Comparison
RFS, protocol transplant	8/38 (22)	HR 0.42 (95% CI, 0.18–0.97); P = 0.038
RFS, no protocol transplant	17/40 (43)	
OS, protocol transplant	5/38 (13)	HR 0.35 (95% CI, 0.12–0.97); P = 0.037
OS, no protocol transplant	13/40 (33)	

Response Rate

CR—n/N (%)	81/94 (86)
CRi—n/N (%)	2/94 (2)
Unresponsive to treatment—n/N (%)	8/94 (9)
Response unknown—n/N (%)	1/94 (1)

*The primary end point of the study was 12-month RFS after transplant measured from date of transplant to the first relapse or death from any cause. The 12-month RFS rate of 83% (95% CI, 72–95) was higher than the historical rate of 40% (P <0.001)
CI, confidence interval; EFS, event-free survival; RFS, relapse-free survival; HCT, hematopoietic stem cell transplantation; OS, overall survival; CR1, first complete remission; CR, complete remission; CRi, complete remission with incomplete peripheral blood recovery; HR, hazard ratio

Treatment Modifications

DOSE-INTENSIVE CHEMOTHERAPY TREATMENT MODIFICATIONS

Adverse Effect	Dose Modification
Total bilirubin >2 mg/dL (>34 μmol/L)	Reduce vincristine doses to 1 mg
Total bilirubin 2–3 mg/dL (34–51 μmol/L)	Reduce doxorubicin dosage by 25%
Total bilirubin 3–4 mg/dL (51–68 μmol/L)	Reduce doxorubicin dosage by 50%
Total bilirubin 3–5 mg/dL (51–86 μmol/L)	Reduce methotrexate dosage by 25%
Total bilirubin >4mg/dL (>68 μmol/L)	Reduce doxorubicin dosage by 75%
Total bilirubin >5 mg/dL (>86 μmol/L)	Hold methotrexate
Creatinine 1.5–2 mg/dL (133–177 μmol/L)	Reduce methotrexate dosage by 25%
Bilirubin level 3–5 mg/dL (51–86 μmol/L)	Reduce methotrexate dose by 25%
Bilirubin >5 mg/dL (>86μmol/L)	Hold methotrexate
Creatinine >2 mg/dL (>177 μmol/L)	Reduce methotrexate dosage by 50%. Reduce cytarabine dosage to 1000 mg/m²

(continued)

Treatment Modifications (continued)

DASATINIB TREATMENT MODIFICATIONS

Dasatinib Dose Levels

Starting dose	100 mg daily (hyper-CVAD cycle 1 and maintenance therapy) 70 mg daily (hyper-CVAD cycles 2–8)
Dose level –1	80 mg daily
Dose level –2	50 mg once daily

Nonhematologic Toxicity

G1	No dose modifications
G2/3	Hold dasatinib until toxicity resolves to Grade 1, then restart with the dosage reduced by 1 dose level
G4	Hold dasatinib until toxicity resolves to Grade 1, then restart with the dosage reduced by 1–2 dose levels
Recurrent G4	Discontinue dasatinib

Toxicity (N = 92)

Toxicity During Dose-Intensive Phase

Event*	Hyper-CVAD + Dasatinib (N = 92)			
Grade (%)	Grade 1–2	Grade 3	Grade 4	Grade 5
Diarrhea	33	4	0	0
Gastrointestinal	24	2	2	0
Hemorrhage	19	3	0	0
Infection	5	48	9	2
Liver function tests	29	25	4	0
Mucositis	24	4	0	0
Nausea/vomiting	72	9	0	0
Neurologic	45	8	2	0
Pericardial effusion	0	1	0	0
Pleural effusion	10	1	0	0
Renal	14	4	0	0
Sudden death	—	—	—	1

Note: percentages are approximated based on the graphical representation in the original publication in Ravandi F et al. Blood Adv 2016;1:250–259

Toxicity During Maintenance Phase

Event*	Maintenance Treatment (N = 22)	
Grade (%)	Grade 1–2	Grade 3
Diarrhea	14	0
Gastrointestinal	23	5
Infection	14	14
LFTs	50	9
Mucositis	9	0
Nausea/vomiting	46	5
Neurologic	50	14
Pleural effusion	5	5
Renal	5	0

Note: percentages are approximated based on the graphical representation in the original publication in Ravandi F et al. Blood Adv 2016;1:250–259

Therapy Monitoring

1. CBC with differential daily during and after chemotherapy during induction therapy until recovery of ANC >500/mm^3. Platelets every day while in hospital until patient no longer requires platelet transfusions

2. *Pretreatment evaluation:* determination of LVEF by echocardiogram

3. Serum electrolytes, mineral panel, and uric acid, at least daily during induction therapy until the risk of tumor lysis is past

4. CMP and CBC with differential and platelet count prior to each cycle of consolidation therapy

5. Monitor serum methotrexate levels 24, 48, and 72 hours after the start of each methotrexate infusion. In patients with delayed clearance, monitor daily methotrexate levels thereafter until the methotrexate concentration declines to <0.1 micromolar

6. Patients who receive high-dose cytarabine need to be closely monitored for changes in renal function. Renal dysfunction is highly correlated with increased risk of cerebellar toxicity associated with cytarabine. Patients need to be monitored for nystagmus, dysmetria, and ataxia before each cytarabine dose

7. Monitor for signs and symptoms of pleural effusion and fluid overload periodically during therapy with dasatinib and prior to each even cycle of intensive therapy. If there is concern for pleural effusion, perform additional work-up (ie, chest x-ray) prior to administration of methotrexate

8. In patients at risk for dasatinib-induced QT prolongation, monitor electrocardiogram for QTc interval. Monitor electrolytes periodically

9. Bone marrow aspirate and biopsy after the initial induction course upon recovery of peripheral blood counts. After patient achieves a CR, bone marrow biopsy and aspirate should be performed at least following completion of consolidation therapy

Notes

In the study reported by Ravandi F et al. (Blood Adv. 2016;1:250–259), patients underwent a diagnostic LP on day 2 of the first course of treatment

- Patients with no evidence of CNS disease at the time of diagnosis should receive prophylactic intrathecal therapy with:
  - **Methotrexate;** administer intrathecally 12 mg/dose via lumbar puncture *or* 6 mg/dose intraventricularly via indwelling ventricular reservoir catheter (eg, Ommaya) on day 2 of courses 1–4 of intensive induction therapy, *and:*
  - **Cytarabine** 100 mg/dose; administer intrathecally via lumbar puncture *or* intraventricularly via indwelling ventricular reservoir on day 8 of courses 1–4 of intensive induction therapy

- Patients with CNS disease at the time of diagnosis receive intrathecal therapy with:
  - **Methotrexate;** administer intrathecally 12 mg/dose via lumbar puncture *or* 6 mg/dose intraventricularly via indwelling ventricular reservoir catheter (eg, Ommaya) once per week, *and:*
  - **Cytarabine** 100 mg/dose; administer intrathecally via lumbar puncture *or* intraventricularly via indwelling ventricular reservoir once per week
    - Twice-weekly intrathecal chemotherapy doses should be separated by at least 72 hours
    - Continue twice per week intrathecal chemotherapy until cerebrospinal fluid cell counts normalize and cytology becomes negative for malignant disease, then revert back to the usual prophylactic schedule outlined above

- Patients with cranial nerve root involvement may be considered for radiation 24–30 Gy in 10–12 fractions to the base of the skull or whole brain

ADULT
ACUTE LYMPHOBLASTIC LEUKEMIA: HYPER-CVAD + IMATINIB

Daver N et al. Haematologica 2015;100:653–661
Supplementary appendix to: Daver N et al. Haematologica 2015;100:653–661
Thomas DA et al. Blood 2004;103:4396–4407
Lee S et al. Blood 2005;105:3449–3457

Dose-intensive chemotherapy
The dose-intensive phase consists of 8 cycles of hyper-CVAD alternating with high-dose methotrexate and cytarabine every 3–4 weeks (when the WBC count is >3000/mm^3 and platelet count is >60,000/mm^3)

Imatinib (cycle 1)
Imatinib 600 mg/day; administer orally, with the largest meal of the day, once daily for 14 consecutive days on days 1–14 during cycle 1 of dose-intensive chemotherapy (total dosage in cycle 1 = 8400 mg)

Imatinib (cycles 2, 3, 4, 5, 6, 7, and 8)
Imatinib 600 mg/day; administer orally, once daily, continually, with the largest meal of the day, beginning with the start of hyper-CVAD cycle 2 and continuing through the remainder of the dose-intensive chemotherapy phase (total dosage/week during cycles 2–8 = 4,200 mg)

Hyper-CVAD (cycles 1, 3, 5, and 7)
Cyclophosphamide 300 mg/m^2 per dose; administer intravenously over 2 hours in 500 mL 0.9% sodium chloride injection (0.9% NS) or 5% dextrose injection (D5W) every 12 hours for 6 doses on days 1–3, for 4 cycles, cycles 1, 3, 5, and 7 (total dosage/cycle = 1800 mg/m^2)

Mesna 600 mg/m^2 per 24 hours; administer by continuous intravenous infusion in 1000 mL 0.9% NS for approximately 68 hours for 4 cycles, cycles 1, 3, 5, and 7 (total dosage/cycle ~1725 mg/m^2)
• Mesna administration starts concurrently with cyclophosphamide on day 1 and continues until 6 hours after the last dose of cyclophosphamide is completed (68 hours)

Vincristine 2 mg/dose; administer by intravenous infusion over 15 minutes in 50 mL 0.9% NS for 2 doses, on days 4 and 11, for 4 cycles, cycles 1, 3, 5, and 7 (total dose/cycle = 4 mg)

Doxorubicin 50 mg/m^2; administer intravenously via central venous access in 25–1000 mL 0.9% NS or D5W by continuous infusion over 24 hours on day 4, for 4 cycles, cycles 1, 3, 5, and 7 (total dosage/cycle = 50 mg/m^2)
• *Note:* in patients with left ventricular ejection fraction <50%, each doxorubicin dose was infused over 48 hours rather than over 24 hours

Dexamethasone 40 mg per day; administer orally, or intravenously in 25–150 mL 0.9% NS or D5W over 15–30 minutes for 8 doses, on days 1–4 and days 11–14, for 4 cycles, cycles 1, 3, 5, and 7 (total dose/cycle = 320 mg)

Supportive Care
Antiemetic prophylaxis
Emetogenic potential on Days 1–4 is **MODERATE**
Emetogenic potential on Days 11 is **MINIMAL**
See Chapter 42 for antiemetic recommendations

Hematopoietic growth factor (CSF) prophylaxis
Primary prophylaxis is indicated with:
Filgrastim (G-CSF) 5 µg/kg per dose; administer by subcutaneous injection every 12 hours, starting on day 6 (24 hours after completion of doxorubicin)
• Continue filgrastim administration until postnadir WBC count >3000/mm^3 and platelet count is >60,000/mm^3. If platelet recovery is delayed, filgrastim is continued until the WBC count >30,000/mm^3
• Discontinue daily filgrastim use at least 24 hours before administering myelosuppressive treatment
See Chapter 43 for more information

Antimicrobial prophylaxis
Risk of fever and neutropenia is **HIGH**
Antimicrobial primary prophylaxis is recommended:
• Antibacterial—consider fluoroquinolone prophylaxis; *P. jirovecii* prophylaxis is recommended (eg, cotrimoxazole)
• Antifungal—recommended
• Antiviral—antiherpes antivirals (eg, acyclovir, famciclovir, valacyclovir)

High-dose methotrexate + cytarabine (cycles 2, 4, 6, and 8)
Hydration: with a solution containing a total amount of sodium not >0.9% NS (ie, ≤154 mEq sodium/1000 mL) by intravenous infusion during methotrexate administration and for at least 24 hours afterward
• Commence fluid administration 2–12 hours before starting methotrexate, depending on patient's fluid status

(continued)

(continued)

- Urine output should be at least 100 mL/hour before starting methotrexate infusion
- Maintain hydration at a rate that maintains urine output ≥100 mL/hour until the serum methotrexate concentration is <0.1 μmol/L
- Urine pH should be increased within the range ≥7.0 to ≤8.0 to enhance methotrexate solubility and ensure elimination
- Adverse effects attributable to methotrexate are related to systemic methotrexate concentrations *and* the duration for which concentrations are maintained

Sodium bicarbonate 50–150 mEq/1000 mL is added to parenteral hydration solutions to maintain urine pH ≥7.0 to ≤8.0

Base Solution Sodium Content	Sodium Bicarbonate Additive	Total Sodium Content
0.45% Sodium chloride injection (0.45% NS)		
77 mEq/L	50–75 mEq	127–152 mEq/L
0.2% Sodium chloride injection (0.2% NS)		
34 mEq/L	100–125 mEq	134–159 mEq/L
5% Dextrose injection (D5W)		
0	125–150 mEq	125–150 mEq/L
D5W/0.45% NS		
77 mEq/L	50–75 mEq	127–152 mEq/L
D5W/0.2% NS		
34 mEq/L	100–125 mEq	134–159 mEq/L

Methotrexate 200 mg/m^2; administer intravenously over 2 hours, on day 1, *followed by:*
Methotrexate 800 mg/m^2; administer intravenously over 24 hours, on day 1, for 4 cycles, cycles 2, 4, 6, and 8 (total dosage/cycle, bolus + infusion = 1000 mg/m^2)

Note: for logistical practicality and efficiency, parenteral admixtures containing methotrexate may include a portion or all of the fluid and sodium bicarbonate needed to meet hydration and urinary alkalinization requirements during methotrexate administration

Leucovorin calcium 50 mg; administer intravenously in 25–250 mL 0.9% NS or D5W over 15–30 minutes for 1 dose given 36 hours after methotrexate administration began (12 hours after methotrexate administration ends), *followed 6 hours later by:*
Leucovorin calcium 15 mg per dose; administer intravenously in 25–250 mL 0.9% NS or D5W over 15–30 minutes, every 6 hours for 8 doses (total dosage [including loading dose]/cycle = 170 mg)

Note: if serum methotrexate concentrations are:

Hours After *Starting* Methotrexate	Methotrexate Concentration	Leucovorin Regimen
Hour 24	>20 μmol/L (>2 × 10^{-5} mol/L)	Increase **leucovorin** dosages to 50 mg/dose; administer intravenously in 25–250 mL 0.9% NS or D5W over 15–30 minutes every 6 hours until serum methotrexate concentrations are <0.1 μmol/L (<1 × 10^{27} mol/L)
Hour 48	>1 μmol/L (>1 × 10^{-6} mol/L)	
Hour 72	>0.1 μmol/L (>1 × 10^{-7} mol/L, *or* >100 nmol/L)	

Cytarabine
  Patient ages <60 years: **Cytarabine** 3000 mg/m^2 per dose; administer intravenously in 50–500 mL 0.9% NS or D5W over 2 hours every 12 hours for 4 doses on days 2 and 3, for 4 cycles, cycles 2, 4, 6, and 8 (total dosage/cycle [not including intrathecal cytarabine] = 12,000 mg/m^2)
  Patient ages ≥60 years: **Cytarabine** 1000 mg/m^2 per dose; administer intravenously in 50–500 mL 0.9% NS or D5W over 2 hours every 12 hours for 4 doses on days 2 and 3, for 4 cycles, cycles 2, 4, 6, and 8 (total dosage/cycle [not including intrathecal cytarabine] = 4000 mg/m^2)

Methylprednisolone 50 mg; administer intravenously twice daily for 6 doses, on days 1–3 (total dose/cycle = 300 mg)

Supportive Care
Antiemetic prophylaxis
Emetogenic potential on Days 1–3 is **MODERATE**
See Chapter 42 for antiemetic recommendations

(continued)

(continued)

Hematopoietic growth factor (CSF) prophylaxis
Primary prophylaxis is indicated with:

Filgrastim (G-CSF) 5 μg/kg per dose; administer by subcutaneous injection every 12 hours, starting on day 4 (24 hours after the last dose of cytarabine)

- Continue filgrastim administration until postnadir WBC count >3000/mm³ and platelet count is >60,000/mm³. If platelet recovery is delayed, filgrastim is continued until the WBC count >30,000/mm³
- Discontinue daily filgrastim use at least 24 hours before administering myelosuppressive treatment

See Chapter 43 for more information

Antimicrobial prophylaxis
Risk of fever and neutropenia is **HIGH**

Antimicrobial primary prophylaxis is recommended:

- Antibacterial—consider fluoroquinolone prophylaxis; *P. jirovecii* prophylaxis is recommended (eg, cotrimoxazole)
- Antifungal—recommended
- Antiviral—antiherpes antivirals (eg, acyclovir, famciclovir, valacyclovir)

Keratitis prophylaxis
Steroid ophthalmic drops (prednisolone 1% or dexamethasone 0.1%); administer 2 drops by intraocular instillation into each eye every 6 hours starting prior to the first cytarabine dose and continuing until 48 hours after high-dose cytarabine is completed

Maintenance phase
Imatinib 400 mg per dose; administer orally, twice per day with meals, continually until disease progression (total dosage/week during maintenance = 5600 mg)
Vincristine 2 mg; administer by intravenous infusion over 15 minutes in 50 mL 0.9% NS, once monthly for 2 years (total dose/month = 2 mg)
Prednisone 200 mg per day; administer orally, continually, for 5 consecutive days every month, starting on the day vincristine is given, for 2 years (total dose/month = 1000 mg)
Note: the protocol allowed two cycles of intensification with hyper-CVAD + imatinib during months 6 and 13 of maintenance to be administered at the discretion of the treating physician. After completion of 2 years of maintenance therapy, imatinib was continued as monotherapy

Supportive Care
Antiemetic prophylaxis
Emetogenic potential is **MINIMAL**
See Chapter 42 for antiemetic recommendations

Hematopoietic growth factor (CSF) prophylaxis
Primary prophylaxis is **NOT** *indicated*
See Chapter 43 for more information

Antimicrobial prophylaxis
Risk of fever and neutropenia is **LOW**

Antimicrobial primary prophylaxis is recommended:

- Antibacterial—*P. jirovecii* prophylaxis is recommended (eg, cotrimoxazole)
- Antifungal—not indicated
- Antiviral—antiherpes antivirals (eg, acyclovir, famciclovir, valacyclovir)

Patient Population Studied

NCT00038610 was a single-arm, single-center study conducted at the University of Texas M.D. Anderson Cancer Center that involved 54 adult (age ≥15 years) patients with Philadelphia chromosome–positive (Ph+) acute lymphoblastic leukemia (ALL) who were untreated (n = 39), or who were in complete remission after having undergone 1–2 prior cycles of ALL-type therapy without a tyrosine kinase inhibitor (TKI) (n = 9), or who were refractory to a single course of induction therapy without a TKI (n = 6). Patients were required to have an Eastern Cooperative Oncology Group performance status of ≤2 and adequate organ function. Patients could optionally undergo an allogeneic stem cell transplant in first complete remission if they had a matched donor available. The median (range) age of patients was 51 years (17–84). Thirteen percent of patients had central nervous system involvement at diagnosis

Efficacy (N = 54)

Efficacy Variable	Hyper-CVAD + Imatinib (N = 54, Total Cohort)		
Survival outcomes			
Outcome	*Event incidence—n/N*	*Outcome at 5 years—%*	*Median—months*
OS	35/54	43	31
DFS	33/51	43	22
OS censored for AHCT	27/54	35	27
DFS according to AHCT			
Outcome	*Event incidence—n/N*	*Outcome at 5 years—%*	*Comparison*
DFS with transplant, age <60 years	6/16	63	P = 0.52
DFS with no transplant, age <60 years	14/23	43	
DFS with transplant, age ≤40 years	4/11	82	P = 0.16
DFS with no transplant, age ≤40 years	4/6	33	
DFS with transplant, age 41–60 years	4/5	20	P = 0.19
DFS with no transplant, age 41–60 years	10/17	47	
Survival outcomes according to molecular remission status at 3 months			
DFS, CMR/MMR status at 3 months	10/20	60	P = 0.05
DFS, BCR/ABL >0.1 at 3 months	7/8	25	
Response rate (N = 45 patients who were not in CR at enrollment)			
CR—n/N (%)	42/45 (93)		
CRp—n/N (%)	1/45 (2)		
PR—n/N (%)	1/45 (2)		
Induction death—n/N (%)	1/45 (2)		

OS, overall survival; DFS, disease-free survival; AHCT, allogeneic hematopoietic stem cell transplantation; CMR, complete molecular response; MMR, major molecular response; CR, complete remission; CRp, complete remission except platelet count <100,000/mm³; PR, partial remission

Treatment Modifications

DOSE-INTENSIVE CHEMOTHERAPY TREATMENT MODIFICATIONS

Adverse Effect	Dose Modification
Total bilirubin >2 mg/dL (>34 µmol/L)	Reduce vincristine doses to 1 mg
Total bilirubin 2–3 mg/dL (34–51 µmol/L)	Reduce doxorubicin dosage by 25%
Total bilirubin 3–4 mg/dL (51–68 µmol/L)	Reduce doxorubicin dosage by 50%
Total bilirubin 3–5 mg/dL (51–86 µmol/L)	Reduce methotrexate dosage by 25%
Total bilirubin >4mg/dL (>68 µmol/L)	Reduce doxorubicin dosage by 75%
Total bilirubin >5 mg/dL (>86 µmol/L)	Hold methotrexate
Creatinine 1.5–2 mg/dL (133–177 µmol/L)	Reduce methotrexate dosage by 25%

Treatment Modifications (*continued*)

Adverse Effect	Dose Modification
Bilirubin level 3–5 mg/dL (51–86 μmol/L)	Reduce methotrexate dose by 25%
Bilirubin >5 mg/dL (>86μmol/L)	Hold methotrexate
Creatinine >2 mg/dL (>177 μmol/L)	Reduce methotrexate dosage by 50%. Reduce cytarabine dosage to 1000 mg/m²

IMATINIB TREATMENT MODIFICATIONS

Imatinib Dose Levels

	Dose Intensive Phase	Maintenance Phase
Starting dose	600 mg once daily	400 mg twice per day
Dose level −1	400 mg once daily	600 mg once daily
Dose level −1	300 mg once daily	400 mg once daily

Hematologic Toxicity

ANC <500/mm³ and/ or platelets <10,000/ mm³	Consider whether cytopenia is related to leukemia; perform a marrow aspirate or biopsy as clinically indicated. If cytopenia is unrelated to leukemia, reduce the dosage by 1 dose level. If the cytopenia persists for ≥2 weeks, then reduce the dosage further by another dose level. If the cytopenia persists ≥4 weeks and is still unrelated to leukemia, withhold imatinib until ANC ≥1000/mm³ and platelets ≥20,000/ mm³ and then resume treatment at 300 mg once daily

Nonhematologic Toxicity

Bilirubin >3× ULN or ALT/AST >5× ULN	Withhold imatinib until bilirubin improves to <1.5× ULN and ALT/AST improve to <2.5× ULN, then resume imatinib with the dosage reduced by 1 dose level
Other severe nonhematologic adverse reaction	Withhold imatinib until improvement of the adverse reaction to G ≤1, then resume imatinib (if clinically appropriate) at a reduced dosage

Therapy Monitoring

1. CBC with differential daily during and after chemotherapy during induction therapy until recovery of ANC >500/mm³. Platelets every day while in hospital until patient no longer requires platelet transfusions
2. *Pretreatment evaluation:* determination of LVEF by echocardiogram
3. Serum electrolytes, mineral panel, and uric acid, at least daily during induction therapy until the risk of tumor lysis is past
4. CMP and CBC with differential and platelet count prior to each cycle of consolidation therapy
5. Monitor serum methotrexate levels 24, 48, and 72 hours after the start of each methotrexate infusion. In patients with delayed clearance, monitor daily methotrexate levels thereafter until the methotrexate concentration declines to <0.1 micromolar
6. Patients who receive high-dose cytarabine need to be closely monitored for changes in renal function. Renal dysfunction is highly correlated with increased risk of cerebellar toxicity associated with cytarabine. Patients need to be monitored for nystagmus, dysmetria, and ataxia before each cytarabine dose
7. Bone marrow aspirate and biopsy after the initial induction course upon recovery of peripheral blood counts. After patient achieves a CR, bone marrow biopsy and aspirate should be performed at least following completion of consolidation therapy

Toxicity (N = 54)

Median time to hematologic recovery and pattern and incidence of severe toxicities was similar to that observed in prior studies of conventional chemotherapy for the treatment of Ph+ B-ALL. Treatment-emergent Grade 3/4 adverse events included infections (52% in induction, 70% in consolidation), hyperglycemia (43%), hypophosphatemia (59%), hyperbilirubinemia (17%), fluid retention (2%), left ventricular dysfunction (2%), arrythmia (4%), myocardial infarction (4%), peripheral neuropathy (4%), confusion (2%), syncope (4%), constipation (2%), diarrhea (9%), nausea (6%), deep-vein thrombosis (7%), pulmonary embolism (2%). There was 1 death reported during induction

Notes

In the study reported by Daver N et al. (Haematologica. 2015;100:653–661), patients underwent a diagnostic LP on day 2 of the first course of treatment

- Patients with CNS disease at the time of diagnosis receive intrathecal therapy with:
  - **Methotrexate;** administer intrathecally 12 mg/dose via lumbar puncture *or* 6 mg/dose intraventricularly via indwelling ventricular reservoir catheter (eg, Ommaya) once per week, *and:*
  - **Cytarabine** 100 mg/dose; administer intrathecally via lumbar puncture *or* intraventricularly via indwelling ventricular reservoir once per week
  - Twice-weekly intrathecal chemotherapy doses should be separated by at least 72 hours
  - Continue twice per week intrathecal chemotherapy until cerebrospinal fluid cell counts normalize and cytology becomes negative for malignant disease, then revert back to the usual prophylactic schedule outlined below
- Patients with cranial nerve root involvement may be considered for radiation 24–30 Gy in 10–12 fractions to the base of the skull or whole brain

CNS Prophylaxis

Risk Factors	Risk Categories		
	High	Low	Unknown
LDH	>600 units/L	Within normal limits	unknown
Proliferative index (% S+G$_2$M)	≥14%		
Histology	Mature B-cell ALL	Not applicable	

Regimen for Intrathecal Prophylaxis	Administration Schedule by Risk Category		
	High Risk	Unknown Risk	Low Risk
Methotrexate; administer intrathecally 12 mg/dose via lumbar puncture *or* 6 mg/dose intraventricularly (via Ommaya reservoir) on day 2 of each cycle indicated, *plus* **Cytarabine** 100 mg administer; intrathecally via lumbar puncture or intraventricularly on day 7 of each cycle indicated	For 4 cycles, cycles 1–4	For 4 cycles, cycles 1–4	For 3 cycles, cycles 1–3

MINIMAL RESIDUAL DISEASE-POSITIVE
ACUTE LYMPHOBLASTIC LEUKEMIA: BLINATUMOMAB

Gökbuget N et al. Blood 2018;131:1522–1531
Supplemental appendix to: Gökbuget N et al. Blood 2018;131:1522–1531
BLINCYTO (blinatumomab) prescribing information. Amgen Inc.: Thousand Oaks, CA; April 2019

The regimen consists of 1 cycle of blinatumomab induction therapy followed by up to 3 identical cycles of consolidation therapy. Triple intrathecal chemotherapy (dexamethasone *plus* methotrexate *plus* cytarabine) is recommended for central nervous system prophylaxis prior to cycle 1, on day 29 of cycle 2 and cycle 4, and every 3 months following treatment for up to 18 months; the provision of intrathecal chemotherapy may be done per institutional guidelines and is not described below. Patients may proceed to hematopoietic stem cell transplantation at any time after the first treatment cycle at the discretion of the medically responsible health care provider. In the study, patients who completed the initial 4-cycle treatment achieving an MRD response lasting ≥4 weeks who subsequently experienced a minimal residual disease relapse within 18 months of the start of treatment were eligible for blinatumomab retreatment

Premedication for each cycle of blinatumomab:
- **Dexamethasone** 16 mg; administer intravenously once, 1 hour prior to initiation of blinatumomab on day 1

For patients who weigh ≥45 kg:
Blinatumomab 28 μg per day; administer by continuous intravenous infusion for 28 consecutive days using any suitable combination of prepared 24-hour, 48-hour, and/or 168-hour intravenous infusion bags, on days 1–28, followed by no treatment for 14 days during days 29–42, every 42 days for up to 4 cycles (total dosage/42-day cycle in patients who weigh ≥45 kg = 784 μg)

For patients who weigh <45 kg:
Blinatumomab 15 μg/m^2 per day (maximum dose = 28 μg per day); administer by continuous intravenous infusion for 28 consecutive days using any suitable combination of prepared 24-hour, 48-hour, and/or 168-hour intravenous infusion bags, on days 1–28, followed by no treatment for 14 days during days 29–42, every 42 days for up to 4 cycles (total dosage/42-day cycle in patients who weigh <45 kg = 420 μg/m^2; maximum dosage/42-day = 784 μg)

Blinatumomab Notes:
- Administer blinatumomab through a dedicated intravenous catheter or dedicated lumen of a multi-lumen catheter at a constant flow rate using a programmable, lockable, non-elastomeric, alarm-capable infusion pump. A sterile, non-pyrogenic, low-protein-binding, 0.2-μm in-line filter must be used for 24-hour and 48-hour infusion preparations, but is not required with 168-hour infusion preparations
- Hospitalization is recommended to monitor for neurotoxicity and cytokine release syndrome during cycle 1 on days 1–3 and then during days 1–2 of the next cycle. Subsequent cycles may be initiated either in the hospital or in an outpatient setting with appropriate supervision by a health care professional
- If an infusion interruption lasting ≥4 hours occurs, then resumption of the blinatumomab infusion must occur either in a hospital setting or in an outpatient setting with appropriate supervision by a health care professional
- Blinatumomab must be prepared using aseptic technique by trained personnel in an ISO class 5 or better laminar flow hood in a USP 797–compliant facility
- Blinatumomab solutions may be incompatible with intravenous infusion tubing sets, infusion bags, or infusion cassettes containing Di(2-ethylhexyl)phthalate (DEHP) due to the possibility of particle formation leading to formation of a cloudy solution. Therefore, use only materials (ie, infusion bags, infusion cassettes, and intravenous tubing sets) made of polyolefin, DEHP-free polyvinyl chloride (PVC), or ethyl vinyl acetate (EVA)
- The pre-infusion dexamethasone dose listed applies to adult patients
- Blinatumomab preparation errors have occurred; carefully follow the preparation instructions described in the most current U.S. Food and Drug Administration (FDA)-approved prescribing information
- Neurotoxicity may occur with blinatumomab. Advise patients to refrain from driving, operating dangerous machinery, or performing activities where an unexpected episode of neurologic toxicity might lead to injury
- Cytokine release syndrome may occur with blinatumomab. There is a theoretical risk that inadvertent bolus administration of blinatumomab may precipitate blinatumomab toxicity. Therefore, avoid rapid flushing of the blinatumomab infusion catheter, especially when changing infusion bags, as this may result in an excessive rate of blinatumomab administration. When the catheter must be flushed, administer a volume of intravenous solution sufficient to replace the catheter priming volume at a rate less than or equal to the rate at which the blinatumomab infusion was being administered
- Do not administer live viral vaccines within 2 weeks prior to initiation of blinatumomab therapy, during blinatumomab therapy, or following blinatumomab therapy until demonstration of adequate immune recovery

(continued)

(*continued*)

Blinatumomab Infusion Options (for Patients Who Weigh ≥45 kg)

Intended Infusion Duration	Blinatumomab Dose	Volume 0.9% Sodium chloride Injection, USP	Volume Bacteriostatic 0.9% Sodium chloride Injection, USP (containing 0.9% Benzyl Alcohol)	IV Solution Stabilizer* Volume	Reconstituted Blinatumomab Solution Volume (Blinatumomab Content)	Final Bag Volume†	Infusion Rate, Duration, and Delivered Dose of Blinatumomab
24-hour bag	9 μg per day	270 mL	Not applicable	5.5 mL	0.83 mL (10.375 μg)	276.33 mL	10 mL/hour intravenously, for 24 hours only, to deliver a dose of 9 μg over 24 hours‡
48-hour bag	9 μg per day	270 mL	Not applicable	5.5 mL	1.7 mL (21.25 μg)	277.2 mL	5 mL/hour intravenously, for 48 hours only, to deliver an approximate dose of 18 μg over 48 hours§
24-hour bag	28 μg per day	270 mL	Not applicable	5.5 mL	2.6 mL (32.5 μg)	278.1 mL	10 mL/hour intravenously, for 24 hours only, to deliver a dose of 28 μg over 24 hours‡
48-hour bag	28 μg per day	270 mL	Not applicable	5.5 mL	5.2 mL (65 μg)	280.7 mL	5 mL/hour intravenously, for 48 hours only, to deliver an approximate dose of 56 μg over 48 hours§
168-hour bag	28 μg per day	1 mL	90 mL	2.2 mL	16.8 mL (210 μg)	110 mL	0.6 mL/hour intravenously, for 168 hours only, to deliver an approximate dose of 196 μg over 168 hours‖

* The sterile, preservative-free IV solution stabilizer is provided with the product package; each 10-mL vial contains 52.5 mg citric acid monohydrate, 2283.8 mg lysine HCl, 10 mg polysorbate 80, sodium hydroxide to adjust pH to 7.0, and water for injection. The specified volume of IV solution stabilizer is transferred to the IV bag containing either 0.9% sodium chloride injection, USP (for 24-hour and 48-hour bags) or bacteriostatic 0.9% sodium chloride injection, USP (containing 0.9% benzyl alcohol) (for 168-hour bags) before the transfer of the specified volume of reconstituted blinatumomab. The IV solution stabilizer is *not* to be used for reconstitution of blinatumomab

† Remove air from final infusion preparation, especially when intended to be used with an ambulatory infusion pump. The infusion line must be primed with the final blinatumomab solution

‡ Bag contains overfill; discard remaining solution after 24 hours of infusion have elapsed

§ Bag contains overfill; discard remaining solution after 48 hours of infusion have elapsed

‖ Bag contains overfill; discard remaining solution after 168 hours of infusion have elapsed

(*continued*)

(continued)

Blinatumomab Infusion Options (for Patients Who Weigh <45 kg)

Intended Infusion Duration	Blinatumomab Dose	IV Solution Stabilizer* Volume	Volume Bacteriostatic 0.9% Sodium chloride Injection, USP (Containing 0.9% Benzyl Alcohol)	BSA (m²) Range	Volume 0.9% Sodium chloride Injection, USP	Reconstituted Blinatumomab Solution Volume (Blinatumomab Content)	Final Bag Volume†	Infusion Rate, Duration, and Delivered Dose of Blinatumomab
24-hour bag	5 μg/m² per day	5.5 mL	Not applicable	1.5–1.59	270 mL	0.7 mL (8.75 μg)	276.2 mL	10 mL/hour intravenously, for 24 hours only, to deliver an approximate dose of 5 μg/m² over 24 hours‡
				1.4–1.49	270 mL	0.66 mL (8.25 μg)	276.16 mL	
				1.3–1.39	270 mL	0.61 mL (7.625 μg)	276.11 mL	
				1.2–1.29	270 mL	0.56 mL (7 μg)	276.06 mL	
				1.1–1.19	270 mL	0.52 mL (6.5 μg)	276.02 mL	
				1–1.09	270 mL	0.47 mL (5.875 μg)	275.97 mL	
				0.9–0.99	270 mL	0.43 mL (5.375 μg)	275.93 mL	
				0.8–0.89	270 mL	0.38 mL (4.75 μg)	275.88 mL	
				0.7–0.79	270 mL	0.33 mL (4.125 μg)	275.83 mL	
				0.6–0.69	270 mL	0.29 mL (3.625 μg)	275.79 mL	
				0.5–0.59	270 mL	0.24 mL (3 μg)	275.74 mL	
				0.4–0.49	270 mL	0.2 mL (2.5 μg)	275.7 mL	
48-hour bag	5 μg/m² per day	5.5 mL	Not applicable	1.5–1.59	270 mL	1.4 mL (17.5 μg)	276.9 mL	5 mL/hour intravenously, for 48 hours only, to deliver an approximate dose of 10 μg/m² over 48 hours§
				1.4–1.49	270 mL	1.3 mL (16.25 μg)	276.8 mL	
				1.3–1.39	270 mL	1.2 mL (15 μg)	276.7 mL	
				1.2–1.29	270 mL	1.1 mL (13.75 μg)	276.6 mL	
				1.1–1.19	270 mL	1 mL (12.5 μg)	276.5 mL	
				1–1.09	270 mL	0.94 mL (11.75 μg)	276.44 mL	
				0.9–0.99	270 mL	0.85 mL (10.625 μg)	276.35 mL	
				0.8–0.89	270 mL	0.76 mL (9.5 μg)	276.26 mL	
				0.7–0.79	270 mL	0.67 mL (8.375 μg)	276.17 mL	
				0.6–0.69	270 mL	0.57 mL (7.125 μg)	276.07 mL	
				0.5–0.59	270 mL	0.48 mL (6 μg)	275.98 mL	
				0.4–0.49	270 mL	0.39 mL (4.875 μg)	275.89 mL	

(continued)

(continued)

Intended Infusion Duration	Blinatumomab Dose	IV Solution Stabilizer* Volume	Volume Bacteriostatic 0.9% Sodium chloride Injection, USP (Containing 0.9% Benzyl Alcohol)	BSA (m²) Range	Volume 0.9% Sodium chloride Injection, USP	Reconstituted Blinatumomab Solution Volume (Blinatumomab Content)	Final Bag Volume†	Infusion Rate, Duration, and Delivered Dose of Blinatumomab
24-hour bag	15 µg/m² per day	5.5 mL	Not applicable	1.5–1.59	270 mL	2.1 mL (26.25 µg µg)	277.6 mL	10 mL/hour intravenously, for 24 hours only, to deliver an approximate dose of 15 µg/m² over 24 hours‡
				1.4–1.49	270 mL	2 mL (25 µg)	277.5 mL	
				1.3–1.39	270 mL	1.8 mL (22.5 µg)	277.3 mL	
				1.2–1.29	270 mL	1.7 mL (21.25 µg)	277.2 mL	
				1.1–1.19	270 mL	1.6 mL (20 µg)	277.1 mL	
				1–1.09	270 mL	1.4 mL (17.5 µg)	276.9 mL	
				0.9–0.99	270 mL	1.3 mL (16.25 µg)	276.8 mL	
				0.8–0.89	270 mL	1.1 mL (13.75 µg)	276.6 mL	
				0.7–0.79	270 mL	1 mL (12.5 µg)	276.5 mL	
				0.6–0.69	270 mL	0.86 mL (10.75 µg)	276.36 mL	
				0.5–0.59	270 mL	0.72 mL (9 µg)	276.22 mL	
				0.4–0.49	270 mL	0.59 mL (7.375 µg)	276.09 mL	
48-hour bag	15 µg/m² per day	5.5 mL	Not applicable	1.5–1.59	270 mL	4.2 mL (52.5 µg)	279.7 mL	5 mL/hour intravenously, for 48 hours only, to deliver an approximate dose of 30 µg/m² over 48 hours§
				1.4–1.49	270 mL	3.9 mL (48.75 µg)	279.4 mL	
				1.3–1.39	270 mL	3.7 mL (46.25 µg)	279.2 mL	
				1.2–1.29	270 mL	3.4 mL (42.5 µg)	278.9 mL	
				1.1–1.19	270 mL	3.1 mL (38.75 µg)	278.6 mL	
				1–1.09	270 mL	2.8 mL (35 µg)	278.3 mL	
				0.9–0.99	270 mL	2.6 mL (32.5 µg)	278.1 mL	
				0.8–0.89	270 mL	2.3 mL (28.75 µg)	277.8 mL	
				0.7–0.79	270 mL	2 mL (25 µg)	277.5 mL	
				0.6–0.69	270 mL	1.7 mL (21.25 µg)	277.2 mL	
				0.5–0.59	270 mL	1.4 mL (17.5 µg)	276.9 mL	
				0.4–0.49	270 mL	1.2 mL (15 µg)	276.7 mL	

(continued)

(*continued*)

Intended Infusion Duration	Blinatumomab Dose	IV Solution Stabilizer* Volume	Volume Bacteriostatic 0.9% Sodium chloride Injection, USP (Containing 0.9% Benzyl Alcohol)	BSA (m²) Range	Volume 0.9% Sodium chloride Injection, USP	Reconstituted Blinatumomab Solution Volume (Blinatumomab Content)	Final Bag Volume†	Infusion Rate, Duration, and Delivered Dose of Blinatumomab
168-hour bag‖	15 µg/m² per day	2.2 mL	90 mL	1.5–1.59	3.8 mL	14 mL (175 µg)	110 mL	0.6 mL/hour intravenously, for 168 hours only, to deliver an approximate dose of 105 µg/m² over 168 hours˻
				1.4–1.49	4.7 mL	13.1 mL (163.75 µg)	110 mL	
				1.3–1.39	5.6 mL	12.2 mL (152.5 µg)	110 mL	
				1.2–1.29	6.5 mL	11.3 mL (141.25 µg)	110 mL	
				1.1–1.19	7.4 mL	10.4 mL (130 µg)	110 mL	
				1–1.09	8.3 mL	9.5 mL (118.75 µg)	110 mL	
				0.9–0.99	9.2 mL	8.6 mL (107.5 µg)	110 mL	

* The sterile, preservative-free IV solution stabilizer is provided with the product package; each 10-mL vial contains 52.5 mg citric acid monohydrate, 2283.8 mg lysine HCl, 10 mg polysorbate 80, sodium hydroxide to adjust pH to 7.0, and water for injection. The specified volume of IV solution stabilizer is transferred to the IV bag containing either 0.9% sodium chloride injection, USP (for 24-hour and 48-hour bags) or bacteriostatic 0.9% sodium chloride injection, USP (containing 0.9% benzyl alcohol) (for 168-hour bags) before the transfer of the specified volume of reconstituted blinatumomab. The IV solution stabilizer is *not* to be used for reconstitution of blinatumomab
† Remove air from final infusion preparation, especially when intended to be used with an ambulatory infusion pump. The infusion line must be primed with the final blinatumomab solution
‡ Bag contains overfill; discard remaining solution after 24 hours of infusion have elapsed
§ Bag contains overfill; discard remaining solution after 48 hours of infusion have elapsed
‖ 168-hour bag is not recommended for patients who weigh <22 kg
˻ Bag contains overfill; discard remaining solution after 168 hours of infusion have elapsed

Supportive Care
Antiemetic prophylaxis
Emetogenic potential is **LOW**
See Chapter 42 for antiemetic recommendations

Hematopoietic growth factor (CSF) prophylaxis
Primary prophylaxis is **NOT** indicated
See Chapter 43 for more information

Antimicrobial prophylaxis
Risk of fever and neutropenia is **MODERATE**
Antimicrobial primary prophylaxis to be considered:
- Antibacterial—consider prophylaxis with a fluoroquinolone during periods of prolonged neutropenia only (eg, <500/mm³ for ≥7 days), or no prophylaxis, until ANC recovery
- Antifungal—consider prophylaxis with fluconazole or another azole antifungal medication during periods of prolonged neutropenia only (eg, <500/mm³ for ≥7 days) until ANC recovery
- Antiviral—antiherpes antivirals (eg, acyclovir, famciclovir, valacyclovir)

Patient Population Studied

This international, multicenter, open-label, single-arm, phase 2 trial involved 116 patients with B-cell precursor acute lymphoblastic leukemia in hematologic complete remission with persistent or recurrent minimal residual disease. Patients received up to four 6-week cycles of 4-weeks continuous infusion of blinatumomab 15 µg/day and 2 weeks with no treatment

Efficacy (N = 113)

Complete minimal residual disease response after cycle 1	78%
Any minimal residual disease response	88%
18-months hematologic relapse-free survival	54%

Therapy Monitoring

1. *Prior to initiation of blinatumomab:* CBC with differential, serum chemistries, total bilirubin, alkaline phosphatase, alanine aminotransferase, aspartate aminotransferase, gamma-glutamyl transferase, fibrinogen, D-dimer, PT, aPTT, and bone marrow biopsy and aspirate

2. *During infusion with blinatumomab:*
   a. Hospitalization is recommended during days 1–3 of the first cycle and during days 1–2 of the second cycle. Subsequent cycles may be initiated either in the hospital or in the outpatient setting with appropriate supervision by a health care professional
      i. *Daily while hospitalized:* CBC with differential, serum chemistries, total bilirubin, alkaline phosphatase, alanine aminotransferase, aspartate aminotransferase, gamma-glutamyl transferase, fibrinogen, D-dimer, PT, and aPTT
      ii. *1–2 times per week, as clinically indicated, during outpatient therapy:* CBC with differential, serum chemistries, total bilirubin, alkaline phosphatase, alanine aminotransferase, aspartate aminotransferase, gamma-glutamyl transferase
         1. *As clinically indicated, if concerned for disseminated intravascular coagulation:* fibrinogen, D-dimer, PT, and aPTT
   b. Monitor for signs and symptoms of cytokine release syndrome (CRS), infusion-related reaction, and/or anaphylaxis, which may include fever or hypothermia, hypotension, tachycardia, hypoxia, headache, asthenia, nausea, increased aspartate aminotransferase, increased alanine aminotransferase, increased bilirubin, macrophage activation syndrome, and disseminated intravascular coagulation. Advise outpatients to notify a health care professional immediately for signs and symptoms of CRS. In the minimal residual disease study, CRS occurred in 4/116 (3%) of patients (G1, n = 2; G3, n = 2), all during cycle 1
   c. Monitor for signs and symptoms of neurologic toxicity, which may include tremor, dizziness, confusion, encephalopathy, ataxia, somnolence, aphasia, or convulsions. Advise outpatients and caregivers to notify a health care professional immediately for signs and symptoms of neurologic toxicity. Advise patients to refrain from driving, operating dangerous machinery, or performing activities where an unexpected episode of neurologic toxicity might lead to injury. In the minimal residual disease study, all-grade neurologic toxicity occurred in approximately 53% of patients. The incidence of neurologic toxicity decreased with subsequent treatment cycles (cycle 1, 47%; cycle 2, 24%; cycle 3, 15%; cycle 4, 15%). Grade 3 or higher neurologic toxicity occurred in 13% of patients. Neurologic toxicity is almost always reversible

3. Advise patients to report symptoms of pancreatitis or infection during blinatumomab therapy. Consider administration of antimicrobial prophylaxis and surveillance for infection as clinically indicated

4. *Response assessment:* CBC with differential, bone marrow aspirate, and biopsy (with minimal residual disease assessment) on day 29 of each cycle and then as clinically indicated

Treatment Modifications

BLINATUMOMAB

Cytokine Release Syndrome	
G3 CRS (hypotension managed with 1 pressor; hypoxia requiring ≥40% O_2)	Withhold blinatumomab In addition to providing other supportive care as clinically indicated, administer dexamethasone 8 mg (patients ≥45 kg) or 5 mg/m² (maximum dose = 8 mg; patients <45 kg) orally or intravenously every 8 hours until resolution of CRS and for up to 3 days, followed by a step-wise taper over an additional 4 days Evaluate for a possible infectious etiology and consider administration of broad-spectrum antibiotic therapy, as clinically indicated Upon resolution of CRS, restart blinatumomab at 9 μg/day (patients ≥45 kg) or at 5 μg/m²/day (patients <45 kg).* Escalate to 28 μg/day (patients ≥45 kg) or to 15 μg/m²/day (patients <45 kg) after 7 days if the toxicity does not recur

(continued)

Treatment Modifications (continued)

Cytokine Release Syndrome

G4 CRS (life-threatening consequences; urgent intervention indicated)	Permanently discontinue blinatumomab In addition to providing other supportive care as clinically indicated, administer dexamethasone 8 mg (patients ≥45 kg) or 5 mg/m² (maximum dose = 8 mg; patients <45 kg) orally or intravenously every 8 hours until resolution of CRS and for up to 3 days, followed by a step-wise taper over an additional 4 days Due to the short half-life of blinatumomab (2.1 hours), most patients will improve rapidly following discontinuation of blinatumomab and administration of dexamethasone. However, in case of refractory and life-threatening symptoms, consider administration of tocilizumab 8 mg/kg (maximum dose = 800 mg) intravenously over 1 hour. Tocilizumab doses may be repeated, if necessary, every 8 hours for up to a maximum of 4 total doses Evaluate for possible infectious etiology and consider administration of broad-spectrum antibiotic therapy, as clinically indicated

Neurologic Toxicities

G3 neurologic toxicity occurring during the blinatumomab infusion at a dose of 9 μg/day (patients ≥45 kg) or 5 μg/m² day (patients <45 kg)	Permanently discontinue blinatumomab In addition to providing other supportive care as clinically indicated, consider administering dexamethasone 8 mg (patients ≥45 kg) or 5 mg/m² (maximum dose = 8 mg; patients <45 kg) orally or intravenously every 8 hours until resolution of toxicity, followed by a step-wise taper over 4 days
G3 neurologic toxicity occurring during the blinatumomab infusion at a dose of 28 μg/day (patients ≥45 kg) or 15 μg/m² day (patients <45 kg)	Withhold blinatumomab until toxicity improves to G ≤1 and for at least 3 days In addition to providing other supportive care as clinically indicated, consider administering dexamethasone 8 mg (patients ≥45 kg) or 5 mg/m² (maximum dose = 8 mg; patients <45 kg) orally or intravenously every 8 hours until resolution of toxicity, followed by a step-wise taper over 4 days If the neurologic toxicity was a seizure, then administer therapeutic doses of a prophylactic anticonvulsant (eg, phenytoin or levetiracetam) during subsequent infusions of blinatumomab, if applicable Consider additional diagnostic investigations, as clinically indicated, to exclude other causes of neurologic symptoms If the toxicity improves to G ≤1 within 7 days, then restart blinatumomab at 9 μg/day (patients ≥45 kg) or at 5 μg/m²/day (patients <45 kg).* Escalate to 28 μg/day (patients ≥45 kg) or to 15 μg/m²/day (patients <45 kg) after 7 days if the toxicity does not recur
G3 neurologic toxicity does not improve to G ≤1 within 7 days	Permanently discontinue blinatumomab
Second occurrence of seizure	Permanently discontinue blinatumomab

Hematologic Toxicity

Prolonged G4 neutropenia (ANC <500/mm³) occurs during blinatumomab infusion in a patient in morphologic remission (<5% bone marrow blasts)	Interrupt blinatumomab until improvement of ANC to >1500/mm³ or post-remission baseline value. If the ANC improves to >1500/mm³ or to post-remission baseline value within 14 days, then restart blinatumomab at 9 μg/day (patients ≥45 kg) or at 5 μg/m²/day (patients <45 kg).* Escalate to 28 μg/day (patients ≥45 kg) or to 15 μg/m²/day (patients <45 kg) after 7 days if the toxicity does not recur

Hepatic Toxicity

ALT >5× ULN, AST >5× ULN, GGT >5× ULN, or total bilirubin >3× ULN	Interrupt blinatumomab until improvement of ALT and AST to ≤3× ULN and improvement of GGT and total bilirubin to ≤2.5× ULN If improvement to the above values occurs within 14 days, then restart blinatumomab at 9 μg/day (patients ≥45 kg) or at 5 μg/m²/day (patients <45 kg).* Escalate to 28 μg/day (patients ≥45 kg) or to 15 μg/m²/day (patients <45 kg) after 7 days if the toxicity does not recur If improvement to the above values does not occur within 14 days, then permanently discontinue blinatumomab

Vaccinations

Vaccination with a live virus vaccine is contemplated	Do not administer live viral vaccines within 2 weeks prior to initiation of blinatumomab therapy, during blinatumomab therapy, or following blinatumomab therapy until demonstration of adequate immune recovery

(continued)

Treatment Modifications (*continued*)

Other Clinically Relevant Adverse Reactions

Other clinically relevant G3 adverse reaction	Withhold blinatumomab until toxicity improves to G ≤1. If the toxicity improves to G ≤1 within 14 days, then restart blinatumomab at 9 μg/day (patients ≥45 kg) or at 5 μg/m²/day (patients <45 kg).* Escalate to 28 μg/day (patients ≥45 kg) or to 15 μg/m²/day (patients <45 kg) after 7 days if the toxicity does not recur
Other clinically relevant G3 adverse reaction which does not resolve to G ≤1 within 14 days	Permanently discontinue blinatumomab
Other clinically relevant G4 adverse reaction	Consider permanently discontinuing blinatumomab If the decision is made to continue blinatumomab, then withhold blinatumomab until toxicity improves to G ≤1. If the toxicity improves to G ≤1 within 14 days, then restart blinatumomab at 9 μg/day (patients ≥45 kg) or at 5 μg/m²/day (patients <45 kg).* Escalate to 28 μg/day (patients ≥45 kg) or to 15 μg/m²/day (patients <45 kg) after 7 days if the toxicity does not recur

*If the interruption after an adverse event is ≤7 days, then continue the same cycle to a total of 28 days of infusion inclusive of days before and after the interruption in that cycle. If an interruption due to an adverse event is longer than 7 days, start a new cycle

CRS, cytokine release syndrome; O₂, oxygen; ANC, absolute neutrophil count; ALT, alanine aminotransferase; ULN, upper limit of normal; AST, aspartate aminotransferase; GGT, gamma-glutamyl transferase

Adverse Events (N = 116)

Grade (%)*	Grade 3	Grade 4
Neutropenia	2	14
Pyrexia	8	0
Leukopenia	4	2
Elevated alanine aminotransferase level	2	3
Thrombocytopenia	2	3
Encephalopathy	3	2
Tremor	5	0
Elevated aspartate aminotransferase level	1	3
Anemia	3	1
Headache	3	0

*According to the National Cancer Institute Common Terminology Criteria for Adverse Events, version 4.0
Note: Grade ≥3 adverse events that occurred in ≥3% patients during the treatment period and subsequent 30 days are included, regardless of causality. All patients experienced at least one adverse event. One treatment-related death was reported (atypical pneumonitis with H1N1 influenza)

RELAPSED/REFRACTORY DISEASE
ACUTE LYMPHOBLASTIC LEUKEMIA: BLINATUMOMAB

Kantarjian H et al. N Engl J Med 2017;376:836–847
Protocol for: Kantarjian H et al. N Engl J Med 2017;376:836–847
Supplementary appendix to: Kantarjian H et al. N Engl J Med 2017;376:836–847
BLINCYTO (blinatumomab) prescribing information. Amgen Inc.: Thousand Oaks, CA; April 2019

The regimen consists of 1–2 cycles of blinatumomab induction therapy (blinatumomab continuous IV infusion on days 1–28 of each 42-day induction cycle). Patients who achieve morphologic remission following induction therapy may receive up to 3 cycles of consolidation blinatumomab therapy (blinatumomab continuous IV infusion on days 1–28 of each 42-day consolidation cycle) followed by up to 4 cycles of maintenance blinatumomab therapy (blinatumomab continuous IV infusion on days 1–28 of each 84-day maintenance cycle). Triple intrathecal chemotherapy (dexamethasone *plus* methotrexate *plus* cytarabine) is recommended for central nervous system prophylaxis prior to cycle 1, and between days 29–42 of each subsequent induction and consolidation cycle; the provision of intrathecal chemotherapy may be done per institutional guidelines and is not described below. Patients may proceed to hematopoietic stem cell transplantation at any time after the first treatment cycle at the discretion of the medically responsible health care provider

Induction cycle 1:
Pre-phase treatment to prevent cytokine release syndrome (recommended in patients with blasts representing >50% of bone marrow cellularity, or with an absolute peripheral blast count ≥15,000/mm3, or with lactate dehydrogenase levels indicative of rapidly progressive disease, or with high extramedullary disease burden):
• **Dexamethasone** 10 mg/m²/day (maximum dose, 24 mg per day); administer orally or intravenously once daily for up to 5 days prior to the initiation of blinatumomab

Premedication for blinatumomab during induction cycle 1:
• **Dexamethasone** 20 mg; administer intravenously once, 1 hour prior to initiation of blinatumomab on day 1
• **Dexamethasone** 20 mg; administer intravenously once, 1 hour prior to escalation of the blinatumomab dose on day 8

For patients who weigh ≥45 kg:
    Blinatumomab 9 μg per day; administer by continuous intravenous infusion for 7 consecutive days using any suitable combination of prepared 24-hour and/or 48-hour intravenous infusion bags, on days 1–7, *followed by:*
    Blinatumomab 28 μg per day; administer by continuous intravenous infusion for 21 consecutive days using any suitable combination of prepared 24-hour, 48-hour, and/or 168-hour intravenous infusion bags, on days 8–28, followed by no treatment for 14 days during days 29–42 (total dosage/induction cycle 1 in patients who weigh ≥45 kg = 651 μg)

For patients who weigh <45 kg:
    Blinatumomab 5 μg/m² per day (maximum dose = 9 μg per day); administer by continuous intravenous infusion for 7 consecutive days using any suitable combination of prepared 24-hour and/or 48-hour intravenous infusion bags, on days 1–7 of induction cycle 1, *followed by:*
    Blinatumomab 15 μg/m² per day (maximum dose = 28 μg per day); administer by continuous intravenous infusion for 21 consecutive days using any suitable combination of prepared 24-hour, 48-hour, and/or 168-hour intravenous infusion bags, on days 8–28, followed by no treatment for 14 days during days 29–42 (total dosage/induction cycle 1 in patients who weigh <45 kg = 350 μg/m²; maximum dosage/induction cycle 1 = 651 μg)

Induction cycle 2 (administer only if >5% bone marrow blasts after induction cycle 1):
Premedication for blinatumomab during induction cycle 2:
• **Dexamethasone** 20 mg; administer intravenously once, 1 hour prior to initiation of blinatumomab on day 1

For patients who weigh ≥45 kg:
    Blinatumomab 28 μg per day; administer by continuous intravenous infusion for 28 consecutive days using any suitable combination of prepared 24-hour, 48-hour, and/or 168-hour intravenous infusion bags, on days 1–28, followed by no treatment for 14 days during days 29–42 (total dosage/induction cycle 2 in patients who weigh ≥45 kg = 784 μg)

For patients who weigh <45 kg:
    Blinatumomab 15 μg/m² per day (maximum dose = 28 μg per day); administer by continuous intravenous infusion for 28 consecutive days using any suitable combination of prepared 24-hour, 48-hour, and/or 168-hour intravenous infusion bags, on days 1–28, followed by no treatment for 14 days during days 29–42 (total dosage/induction cycle 2 in patients who weigh <45 kg = 420 μg/m²; maximum dosage/induction cycle 2 = 784 μg)

Consolidation cycles (administer only if ≤5% bone marrow blasts after completion of induction therapy):
Premedication for blinatumomab during each consolidation cycle:
• **Dexamethasone** 20 mg; administer intravenously once 30 minutes prior to initiation of blinatumomab on day 1

For patients who weigh ≥45 kg:
    Blinatumomab 28 μg per day; administer by continuous intravenous infusion for 28 consecutive days using any suitable combination of prepared 24-hour, 48-hour, and/or 168-hour intravenous infusion bags, on days 1–28, followed by no treatment for 14 days during days 29–42, every 42 days for 3 consolidation cycles (total dosage/42-day consolidation cycle in patients who weigh ≥45 kg = 784 μg)

(continued)

(continued)

For patients who weigh <45 kg:
   Blinatumomab 15 μg/m² per day; administer by continuous intravenous infusion for 28 consecutive days using any suitable combination of prepared 24-hour, 48-hour, and/or 168-hour intravenous infusion bags, on days 1–28, followed by no treatment for 14 days during days 29–42, every 42 days for 3 consolidation cycles (total dosage/42-day consolidation cycle in patients who weigh <45 kg = 420 μg/m²; maximum dosage/42-day consolidation cycle = 784 μg)

Maintenance cycles (administer only if patient is in continued morphologic complete remission):
   Premedication for blinatumomab during each maintenance cycle:
   • **Dexamethasone** 20 mg; administer intravenously once, 1 hour prior to initiation of blinatumomab on day 1

For patients who weigh ≥45 kg:
   Blinatumomab 28 μg per day; administer by continuous intravenous infusion for 28 consecutive days using any suitable combination of prepared 24-hour, 48-hour, and/or 168-hour intravenous infusion bags, on days 1–28, followed by no treatment for 56 days during days 29–84, every 84 days for 4 maintenance cycles (total dosage/84-day maintenance cycle in patients who weigh ≥45 kg = 784 μg)

For patients who weigh <45 kg:
   Blinatumomab 15 μg/m² per day; administer by continuous intravenous infusion for 28 consecutive days using any suitable combination of prepared 24-hour, 48-hour, and/or 168-hour intravenous infusion bags, on days 1–28, followed by no treatment for 56 days during days 29–84, every 84 days for 4 maintenance cycles (total dosage/84-day maintenance cycle in patients who weigh <45 kg = 420 μg/m²; maximum dosage/84-day maintenance cycle = 784 μg)

Blinatumomab Notes:
• Administer blinatumomab through a dedicated intravenous catheter or dedicated lumen of a multi-lumen catheter at a constant flow rate using a programmable, lockable, non-elastomeric, alarm-capable infusion pump. A sterile, non-pyrogenic, low-protein-binding, 0.2-μm in-line filter must be used for 24-hour and 48-hour infusion preparations, but is not required with 168-hour infusion preparations
• Hospitalization is recommended to monitor for neurotoxicity and cytokine release syndrome during induction cycle 1 on days 1–9 and then during days 1–2 of the next cycle. Subsequent cycles may be initiated either in the hospital or in an outpatient setting with appropriate supervision by a health care professional
• If an infusion interruption lasting ≥4 hours occurs, then resumption of the blinatumomab infusion must occur either in a hospital setting or in an outpatient setting with appropriate supervision by a health care professional, and following readministration of premedication as follows:
   ▪ **Dexamethasone** 20 mg; administer intravenous once 1 hour prior to resumption of the blinatumomab infusion following an interruption lasting ≥4 hours
• Blinatumomab must be prepared using aseptic technique by trained personnel in an ISO class 5 or better laminar flow hood in a USP 797–compliant facility
• Blinatumomab solutions may be incompatible with intravenous infusion tubing sets, infusion bags, or infusion cassettes containing Di(2-ethylhexyl)phthalate (DEHP) due to the possibility of particle formation leading to formation of a cloudy solution. Therefore, use only materials (ie, infusion bags, infusion cassettes, and intravenous tubing sets) made of polyolefin, DEHP-free polyvinyl chloride (PVC), or ethyl vinyl acetate (EVA)
• The pre-infusion dexamethasone doses listed apply to adult patients
• Blinatumomab preparation errors have occurred; carefully follow the preparation instructions described in the most current U.S. Food and Drug Administration (FDA)-approved prescribing information
• Neurotoxicity may occur with blinatumomab. Advise patients to refrain from driving, operating dangerous machinery, or performing activities where an unexpected episode of neurologic toxicity might lead to injury
• Cytokine release syndrome may occur with blinatumomab. There is a theoretical risk that inadvertent bolus administration of blinatumomab may precipitate blinatumomab toxicity. Therefore, avoid rapid flushing of the blinatumomab infusion catheter, especially when changing infusion bags, as this may result in an excessive rate of blinatumomab administration. When the catheter must be flushed, administer a volume of intravenous solution sufficient to replace the catheter priming volume at a rate less than or equal to the rate at which the blinatumomab infusion was being administered
• Do not administer live viral vaccines within 2 weeks prior to initiation of blinatumomab therapy, during blinatumomab therapy, or following blinatumomab therapy until demonstration of adequate immune recovery

(continued)

(*continued*)

Blinatumomab Infusion Options (for Patients Who Weigh ≥45 kg)

Intended Infusion Duration	Blinatumomab Dose	Volume 0.9% Sodium chloride Injection, USP	Volume Bacteriostatic 0.9% Sodium chloride Injection, USP (Containing 0.9% Benzyl Alcohol)	IV Solution Stabilizer* Volume	Reconstituted Blinatumomab Solution Volume (Blinatumomab Content)	Final Bag Volume[†]	Infusion Rate, Duration, and Delivered Dose of Blinatumomab
24-hour bag	9 μg per day	270 mL	Not applicable	5.5 mL	0.83 mL (10.375 μg)	276.33 mL	10 mL/hour intravenously, for 24 hours only, to deliver a dose of 9 μg over 24 hours[‡]
48-hour bag	9 μg per day	270 mL	Not applicable	5.5 mL	1.7 mL (21.25 μg)	277.2 mL	5 mL/hour intravenously, for 48 hours only, to deliver an approximate dose of 18 μg over 48 hours[§]
24-hour bag	28 μg per day	270 mL	Not applicable	5.5 mL	2.6 mL (32.5 μg)	278.1 mL	10 mL/hour intravenously, for 24 hours only, to deliver a dose of 28 μg over 24 hours[‡]
48-hour bag	28 μg per day	270 mL	Not applicable	5.5 mL	5.2 mL (65 μg)	280.7 mL	5 mL/hour intravenously, for 48 hours only, to deliver an approximate dose of 56 μg over 48 hours[§]
168-hour bag	28 μg per day	1 mL	90 mL	2.2 mL	16.8 mL (210 μg)	110 mL	0.6 mL/hour intravenously, for 168 hours only, to deliver an approximate dose of 196 μg over 168 hours[∥]

*The sterile, preservative-free IV solution stabilizer is provided with the product package; each 10-mL vial contains 52.5 mg citric acid monohydrate, 2283.8 mg lysine HCl, 10 mg polysorbate 80, sodium hydroxide to adjust pH to 7.0, and water for injection. The specified volume of IV solution stabilizer is transferred to the IV bag containing either 0.9% sodium chloride injection, USP (for 24-hour and 48-hour bags) or bacteriostatic 0.9% sodium chloride injection, USP (containing 0.9% benzyl alcohol) (for 168-hour bags) before the transfer of the specified volume of reconstituted blinatumomab. The IV solution stabilizer is *not* to be used for reconstitution of blinatumomab
[†]Remove air from final infusion preparation, especially when intended to be used with an ambulatory infusion pump. The infusion line must be primed with the final blinatumomab solution
[‡]Bag contains overfill; discard remaining solution after 24 hours of infusion have elapsed
[§]Bag contains overfill; discard remaining solution after 48 hours of infusion have elapsed
[∥]Bag contains overfill; discard remaining solution after 168 hours of infusion have elapsed

Blinatumomab Infusion Options (for Patients Who Weigh <45 kg)

Intended Infusion Duration	Blinatumomab Dose	IV Solution Stabilizer* Volume	Volume Bacteriostatic 0.9% Sodium chloride Injection, USP (Containing 0.9% Benzyl Alcohol)	BSA (m²) Range	Volume 0.9% Sodium chloride Injection, USP	Reconstituted Blinatumomab Solution Volume (Blinatumomab Content)	Final Bag Volume[†]	Infusion Rate, Duration, and Delivered Dose of Blinatumomab
24-hour bag	5 μg/m² per day	5.5 mL	Not applicable	1.5–1.59	270 mL	0.7 mL (8.75 μg)	276.2 mL	10 mL/hour intravenously, for 24 hours only, to deliver an approximate dose of 5 μg/m² over 24 hours[‡]
				1.4–1.49	270 mL	0.66 mL (8.25 μg)	276.16 mL	
				1.3–1.39	270 mL	0.61 mL (7.625 μg)	276.11 mL	
				1.2–1.29	270 mL	0.56 mL (7 μg)	276.06 mL	
				1.1–1.19	270 mL	0.52 mL (6.5 μg)	276.02 mL	
				1–1.09	270 mL	0.47 mL (5.875 μg)	275.97 mL	
				0.9–0.99	270 mL	0.43 mL (5.375 μg)	275.93 mL	
				0.8–0.89	270 mL	0.38 mL (4.75 μg)	275.88 mL	
				0.7–0.79	270 mL	0.33 mL (4.125 μg)	275.83 mL	

(*continued*)

(*continued*)

Intended Infusion Duration	Blinatumomab Dose	IV Solution Stabilizer* Volume	Volume Bacteriostatic 0.9% Sodium chloride Injection, USP (Containing 0.9% Benzyl Alcohol)	BSA (m²) Range	Volume 0.9% Sodium chloride Injection, USP	Reconstituted Blinatumomab Solution Volume (Blinatumomab Content)	Final Bag Volume†	Infusion Rate, Duration, and Delivered Dose of Blinatumomab
				0.6–0.69	270 mL	0.29 mL (3.625 μg)	275.79 mL	
				0.5–0.59	270 mL	0.24 mL (3 μg)	275.74 mL	
				0.4–0.49	270 mL	0.2 mL (2.5 μg)	275.7 mL	
48-hour bag	5 μg/m² per day	5.5 mL	Not applicable	1.5–1.59	270 mL	1.4 mL (17.5 μg)	276.9 mL	5 mL/hour intravenously, for 48 hours only, to deliver an approximate dose of 10 μg/m² over 48 hours§
				1.4–1.49	270 mL	1.3 mL (16.25 μg)	276.8 mL	
				1.3–1.39	270 mL	1.2 mL (15 μg)	276.7 mL	
				1.2–1.29	270 mL	1.1 mL (13.75 μg)	276.6 mL	
				1.1–1.19	270 mL	1 mL (12.5 μg)	276.5 mL	
				1–1.09	270 mL	0.94 mL (11.75 μg)	276.44 mL	
				0.9–0.99	270 mL	0.85 mL (10.625 μg)	276.35 mL	
				0.8–0.89	270 mL	0.76 mL (9.5 μg)	276.26 mL	
				0.7–0.79	270 mL	0.67 mL (8.375 μg)	276.17 mL	
				0.6–0.69	270 mL	0.57 mL (7.125 μg)	276.07 mL	
				0.5–0.59	270 mL	0.48 mL (6 μg)	275.98 mL	
				0.4–0.49	270 mL	0.39 mL (4.875 μg)	275.89 mL	
24-hour bag	15 μg/m² per day	5.5 mL	Not applicable	1.5–1.59	270 mL	2.1 mL (26.25 μg μg)	277.6 mL	10 mL/hour intravenously, for 24 hours only, to deliver an approximate dose of 15 μg/m² over 24 hours‡
				1.4–1.49	270 mL	2 mL (25 μg)	277.5 mL	
				1.3–1.39	270 mL	1.8 mL (22.5 μg)	277.3 mL	
				1.2–1.29	270 mL	1.7 mL (21.25 μg)	277.2 mL	
				1.1–1.19	270 mL	1.6 mL (20 μg)	277.1 mL	
				1–1.09	270 mL	1.4 mL (17.5 μg)	276.9 mL	
				0.9–0.99	270 mL	1.3 mL (16.25 μg)	276.8 mL	
				0.8–0.89	270 mL	1.1 mL (13.75 μg)	276.6 mL	
				0.7–0.79	270 mL	1 mL (12.5 μg)	276.5 mL	
				0.6–0.69	270 mL	0.86 mL (10.75 μg)	276.36 mL	
				0.5–0.59	270 mL	0.72 mL (9 μg)	276.22 mL	
				0.4–0.49	270 mL	0.59 mL (7.375 μg)	276.09 mL	

(*continued*)

(continued)

Intended Infusion Duration	Blinatumomab Dose	IV Solution Stabilizer* Volume	Volume Bacteriostatic 0.9% Sodium chloride Injection, USP (Containing 0.9% Benzyl Alcohol)	BSA (m²) Range	Volume 0.9% Sodium chloride Injection, USP	Reconstituted Blinatumomab Solution Volume (Blinatumomab Content)	Final Bag Volume†	Infusion Rate, Duration, and Delivered Dose of Blinatumomab
48-hour bag	15 μg/m² per day	5.5 mL	Not applicable	1.5–1.59	270 mL	4.2 mL (52.5 μg)	279.7 mL	5 mL/hour intravenously, for 48 hours only, to deliver an approximate dose of 30 μg/m² over 48 hours§
				1.4–1.49	270 mL	3.9 mL (48.75 μg)	279.4 mL	
				1.3–1.39	270 mL	3.7 mL (46.25 μg)	279.2 mL	
				1.2–1.29	270 mL	3.4 mL (42.5 μg)	278.9 mL	
				1.1–1.19	270 mL	3.1 mL (38.75 μg)	278.6 mL	
				1–1.09	270 mL	2.8 mL (35 μg)	278.3 mL	
				0.9–0.99	270 mL	2.6 mL (32.5 μg)	278.1 mL	
				0.8–0.89	270 mL	2.3 mL (28.75 μg)	277.8 mL	
				0.7–0.79	270 mL	2 mL (25 μg)	277.5 mL	
				0.6–0.69	270 mL	1.7 mL (21.25 μg)	277.2 mL	
				0.5–0.59	270 mL	1.4 mL (17.5 μg)	276.9 mL	
				0.4–0.49	270 mL	1.2 mL (15 μg)	276.7 mL	
168-hour bag‖	15 μg/m² per day	2.2 mL	90 mL	1.5–1.59	3.8 mL	14 mL (175 μg)	110 mL	0.6 mL/hour intravenously, for 168 hours only, to deliver an approximate dose of 105 μg/m² over 168 hours⁋
				1.4–1.49	4.7 mL	13.1 mL (163.75 μg)	110 mL	
				1.3–1.39	5.6 mL	12.2 mL (152.5 μg)	110 mL	
				1.2–1.29	6.5 mL	11.3 mL (141.25 μg)	110 mL	
				1.1–1.19	7.4 mL	10.4 mL (130 μg)	110 mL	
				1–1.09	8.3 mL	9.5 mL (118.75 μg)	110 mL	
				0.9–0.99	9.2 mL	8.6 mL (107.5 μg)	110 mL	

*The sterile, preservative-free IV solution stabilizer is provided with the product package; each 10-mL vial contains 52.5 mg citric acid monohydrate, 2283.8 mg lysine HCl, 10 mg polysorbate 80, sodium hydroxide to adjust pH to 7.0, and water for injection. The specified volume of IV solution stabilizer is transferred to the IV bag containing either 0.9% sodium chloride injection, USP (for 24-hour and 48-hour bags) or bacteriostatic 0.9% sodium chloride injection, USP (containing 0.9% benzyl alcohol) (for 168-hour bags) before the transfer of the specified volume of reconstituted blinatumomab. The IV solution stabilizer is *not* to be used for reconstitution of blinatumomab
†Remove air from final infusion preparation, especially when intended to be used with an ambulatory infusion pump. The infusion line must be primed with the final blinatumomab solution
‡Bag contains overfill; discard remaining solution after 24 hours of infusion have elapsed
§Bag contains overfill; discard remaining solution after 48 hours of infusion have elapsed
‖168-hour bag is not recommended for patients who weigh <22 kg
⁋Bag contains overfill; discard remaining solution after 168 hours of infusion have elapsed

Supportive Care
Antiemetic prophylaxis
Emetogenic potential is **LOW**
See Chapter 42 for antiemetic recommendations

Hematopoietic growth factor (CSF) prophylaxis
Primary prophylaxis is **NOT** *indicated*
See Chapter 43 for more information

(continued)

(*continued*)

Antimicrobial prophylaxis
Risk of fever and neutropenia is **HIGH**
  Antimicrobial primary prophylaxis to be considered:
  • Antibacterial—consider prophylaxis with a fluoroquinolone during periods of prolonged neutropenia only (eg, <500/mm³ for ≥7 days), or no prophylaxis, until ANC recovery
  • Antifungal—consider prophylaxis with fluconazole or another azole antifungal medication during periods of prolonged neutropenia only (eg, <500/mm³ for ≥7 days) until ANC recovery
  • Antiviral—antiherpes antivirals (eg, acyclovir, famciclovir, valacyclovir)

Patient Population Studied

This prospective, international, multicenter, randomized, open-label, phase 3 trial involved 405 patients with advanced acute lymphoblastic leukemia. Eligible patients were aged ≥18 years and had Eastern Cooperative Oncology Group (ECOG) performance status score ≤2, >5% blasts in the bone marrow, and Ph-negative, B-cell precursor, acute lymphoblastic leukemia that was refractory either to primary induction therapy or to salvage with intensive combination chemotherapy, first relapse with the first relapse lasting <12 months, second or greater relapse, or relapse at any time after allogeneic stem-cell transplantation. Patients with active disease involving the central nervous system or testes were excluded. Patients were randomly assigned 2:1 to receive blinatumomab or standard chemotherapy. Patients received up to two cycles of induction therapy; those in morphologic remission then received up to three cycles of consolidation therapy and, if still in morphologic remission, up to 12 months of maintenance therapy. In the blinatumomab group, induction and consolidation therapy consisted of 6-week cycles of 4 weeks continuous infusion of blinatumomab (9 μg/day in week 1 of induction cycle 1 and 28 μg/day thereafter) and 2 weeks with no treatment; maintenance therapy consisted of 12-week cycles of 4-weeks continuous infusion of blinatumomab (28 μg/day) and 8 weeks with no treatment

Efficacy (N = 405)

	Blinatumomab (N = 271)	Standard Chemotherapy (N = 134)	
Median overall survival	7.7 months	4.0 months	HR 0.71, 95% CI 0.55–0.93; P = 0.01
Complete remission with full hematologic recovery within 12 weeks after initiation of treatment	34%	16%	P <0.001
Complete remission with full, partial, or incomplete hematologic recovery within 12 weeks after initiation of treatment	44%	25%	P <0.001
6-month event-free survival	31%	12%	HR 0.55, 95% CI 0.43–0.71; P <0.001

Note: median follow-up was 11.7 months in the blinatumomab group and 11.8 months in the controls

Therapy Monitoring

1. *Prior to initiation of blinatumomab:* CBC with differential, serum chemistries, electrolytes, uric acid, LDH, total bilirubin, alkaline phosphatase, alanine aminotransferase, aspartate aminotransferase, gamma-glutamyl transferase, fibrinogen, D-dimer, PT, aPTT, and bone marrow biopsy and aspirate
   a. Consider pre-phase treatment with dexamethasone for up to 5 days prior to initiation of blinatumomab to reduce the incidence of cytokine release syndrome in patients with blasts representing >50% of bone marrow cellularity, or with an absolute peripheral blast count ≥15,000/mm³, or with lactate dehydrogenase levels indicative of rapidly progressive disease, or with high extramedullary disease burden
2. *During infusion with blinatumomab:*
   a. Hospitalization is recommended during days 1–9 of the first cycle and during days 1–2 of the second cycle. Subsequent cycles may be initiated either in the hospital or in the outpatient setting with appropriate supervision by a health care professional
      i. *Daily while hospitalized:* CBC with differential, serum chemistries, electrolytes, uric acid, LDH, total bilirubin, alkaline phosphatase, alanine aminotransferase, aspartate aminotransferase, gamma-glutamyl transferase, fibrinogen, D-dimer, PT, and aPTT

(*continued*)

(continued)

    1. *In patients at high risk for tumor lysis syndrome (eg, high tumor burden, renal dysfunction, rapidly progressing disease, markedly elevated LDH, baseline abnormalities in laboratory indices of tumor lysis syndrome [potassium, phosphate, uric acid, calcium, serum creatinine]):* consider frequent monitoring of laboratory indices of tumor lysis syndrome, intravenous hydration, and prophylaxis with a xanthine oxidase inhibitor (eg, allopurinol) during the induction course

   ii. *1–3 times per week, as clinically indicated, during outpatient therapy:* CBC with differential, serum chemistries, total bilirubin, alkaline phosphatase, alanine aminotransferase, aspartate aminotransferase, gamma-glutamyl transferase

    1. *As clinically indicated, if concerned for disseminated intravascular coagulation:* fibrinogen, D-dimer, PT, and aPTT

    2. *As clinically indicated, if patient is at continued risk for tumor lysis syndrome:* blood urea nitrogen, serum creatinine, calcium, phosphorus, uric acid, LDH, potassium

  b. Monitor for signs and symptoms of cytokine release syndrome (CRS), infusion-related reaction, and/or anaphylaxis which may include fever or hypothermia, hypotension, tachycardia, hypoxia, headache, asthenia, nausea, increased aspartate aminotransferase, increased alanine aminotransferase, increased bilirubin, macrophage activation syndrome, and disseminated intravascular coagulation. Advise outpatients to notify a heath care professional immediately for signs and symptoms of CRS. All-grade CRS occurred in 14.2% of patients with a median onset of 2 days. Grade 3 or higher CRS or macrophage activation syndrome occurred in 4.9% of patients. CRS or infusion reactions resulted in treatment interruption in 8% of patients and in treatment discontinuation in 1% of patients

  c. Monitor for signs and symptoms of neurologic toxicity, which may include tremor, dizziness, confusion, encephalopathy, ataxia, somnolence, aphasia, or convulsions. Advise outpatients and caregivers to notify a heath care professional immediately for signs and symptoms of neurologic toxicity. Advise patients to refrain from driving, operating dangerous machinery, or performing activities where an unexpected episode of neurologic toxicity might lead to injury. All-grade neurologic toxicity occurred in approximately 65% of patients with a median onset of <2 weeks. Grade 3 or higher neurologic toxicity occurred in 9.4% of patients. Neurologic toxicity is almost always reversible. Neurologic toxicity resulted in treatment interruption in 6% of patients and in treatment discontinuation in 4% of patients

3. Advise patients to report symptoms of pancreatitis or infection during blinatumomab therapy. Consider administration of antimicrobial prophylaxis and surveillance for infection as clinically indicated

4. *Response assessment:* CBC with differential, bone marrow aspirate, and biopsy after each cycle (between days 29–37) of induction therapy and then as clinically indicated

Treatment Modifications

BLINATUMOMAB

Cytokine Release Syndrome	
G3 CRS (hypotension managed with 1 pressor; hypoxia requiring ≥40% O$_2$)	Withhold blinatumomab In addition to providing other supportive care as clinically indicated, administer dexamethasone 8 mg (patients ≥45 kg) or 5 mg/m² (maximum dose = 8 mg; patients <45 kg) orally or intravenously every 8 hours until resolution of CRS and for up to 3 days, followed by a step-wise taper over an additional 4 days Evaluate for a possible infectious etiology and consider administration of broad-spectrum antibiotic therapy, as clinically indicated Upon resolution of CRS, restart blinatumomab at 9 μg/day (patients ≥45 kg) or at 5 μg/m²/day (patients <45 kg).* Escalate to 28 μg/day (patients ≥45 kg) or to 15 μg/m²/day (patients <45 kg) after 7 days if the toxicity does not recur
G4 CRS (life-threatening consequences; urgent intervention indicated)	Permanently discontinue blinatumomab In addition to providing other supportive care as clinically indicated, administer dexamethasone 8 mg (patients ≥45 kg) or 5 mg/m² (maximum dose = 8 mg; patients <45 kg) orally or intravenously every 8 hours until resolution of CRS and for up to 3 days, followed by a step-wise taper over an additional 4 days Due to the short half-life of blinatumomab (2.1 hours), most patients will improve rapidly following discontinuation of blinatumomab and administration of dexamethasone. However, in case of refractory and life-threatening symptoms, consider administration of tocilizumab 8 mg/kg (maximum dose = 800 mg) intravenously over 1 hour. Tocilizumab doses may be repeated, if necessary, every 8 hours for up to a maximum of 4 total doses Evaluate for possible infectious etiology and consider administration of broad-spectrum antibiotic therapy, as clinically indicated

(continued)

Treatment Modifications (*continued*)

Neurologic Toxicities

G3 neurologic toxicity occurring during the blinatumomab infusion at a dose of 9 μg/day (patients ≥45 kg) or 5 μg/m² day (patients <45 kg)	Permanently discontinue blinatumomab In addition to providing other supportive care as clinically indicated, consider administering dexamethasone 8 mg (patients ≥45 kg) or 5 mg/m² (maximum dose = 8 mg; patients <45 kg) orally or intravenously every 8 hours until resolution of toxicity, followed by a step-wise taper over 4 days
G3 neurologic toxicity occurring during the blinatumomab infusion at a dose of 28 μg/day (patients ≥45 kg) or 15 μg/m² day (patients <45 kg)	Withhold blinatumomab until toxicity improves to G ≤1 and for at least 3 days In addition to providing other supportive care as clinically indicated, consider administering dexamethasone 8 mg (patients ≥45 kg) or 5 mg/m² (maximum dose = 8 mg; patients <45 kg) orally or intravenously every 8 hours until resolution of toxicity, followed by a step-wise taper over 4 days If the neurologic toxicity was a seizure, then administer therapeutic doses of a prophylactic anticonvulsant (eg, phenytoin or levetiracetam) during subsequent infusions of blinatumomab, if applicable Consider additional diagnostic investigations, as clinically indicated, to exclude other causes of neurologic symptoms If the toxicity improves to G ≤1 within 7 days, then restart blinatumomab at 9 μg/day (patients ≥45 kg) or at 5 μg/m²/day (patients <45 kg).* Escalate to 28 μg/day (patients ≥45 kg) or to 15 μg/m²/day (patients <45 kg) after 7 days if the toxicity does not recur
G3 neurologic toxicity does not improve to G ≤1 within 7 days	Permanently discontinue blinatumomab
Second occurrence of seizure	Permanently discontinue blinatumomab

Hematologic Toxicity

Prolonged G4 neutropenia (ANC <500/mm³) occurs during blinatumomab infusion in a patient in morphologic remission (<5% bone marrow blasts)	Interrupt blinatumomab until improvement of ANC to >1500/mm³ or post-remission baseline value. If the ANC improves to >1500/mm³ or to post-remission baseline value within 14 days, then restart blinatumomab at 9 μg/day (patients ≥45 kg) or at 5 μg/m²/day (patients <45 kg).* Escalate to 28 μg/day (patients ≥45 kg) or to 15 μg/m²/day (patients <45 kg) after 7 days if the toxicity does not recur

Hepatic Toxicity

ALT >5× ULN, AST >5× ULN, GGT >5× ULN, or total bilirubin >3× ULN	Interrupt blinatumomab until improvement of ALT and AST to ≤3× ULN and improvement of GGT and total bilirubin to ≤2.5× ULN If improvement to the above values occurs within 14 days, then restart blinatumomab at 9 μg/day (patients ≥45 kg) or at 5 μg/m²/day (patients <45 kg).* Escalate to 28 μg/day (patients ≥45 kg) or to 15 μg/m²/day (patients <45 kg) after 7 days if the toxicity does not recur If improvement to the above values does not occur within 14 days, then permanently discontinue blinatumomab

Vaccinations

Vaccination with a live virus vaccine is contemplated	Do not administer live viral vaccines within 2 weeks prior to initiation of blinatumomab therapy, during blinatumomab therapy, or following blinatumomab therapy until demonstration of adequate immune recovery

Other Clinically Relevant Adverse Reactions

Other clinically relevant G3 adverse reaction	Withhold blinatumomab until toxicity improves to G ≤1. If the toxicity improves to G ≤1 within 14 days, then restart blinatumomab at 9 μg/day (patients ≥45 kg) or at 5 μg/m²/day (patients <45 kg).* Escalate to 28 μg/day (patients ≥45 kg) or to 15 μg/m²/day (patients <45 kg) after 7 days if the toxicity does not recur
Other clinically relevant G3 adverse reaction which does not resolve to G ≤1 within 14 days	Permanently discontinue blinatumomab
Other clinically relevant G4 adverse reaction	Consider permanently discontinuing blinatumomab If the decision is made to continue blinatumomab, then withhold blinatumomab until toxicity improves to G ≤1. If the toxicity improves to G ≤1 within 14 days, then restart blinatumomab at 9 μg/day (patients ≥45 kg) or at 5 μg/m²/day (patients <45 kg).* Escalate to 28 μg/day (patients ≥45 kg) or to 15 μg/m²/day (patients <45 kg) after 7 days if the toxicity does not recur

*If the interruption after an adverse event is ≤7 days, then continue the same cycle to a total of 28 days of infusion inclusive of days before and after the interruption in that cycle. If an interruption due to an adverse event is longer than 7 days, start a new cycle. Administer dexamethasone premedication as clinically indicated or for infusion interruptions lasting ≥4 hours

CRS, cytokine release syndrome; O₂, oxygen; ANC, absolute neutrophil count; ALT, alanine aminotransferase; ULN, upper limit of normal; AST, aspartate aminotransferase; GGT, gamma-glutamyl transferase

Adverse Events (N = 376)

All-grade* adverse events:

(%)	Blinatumomab (N = 267)	Standard Chemotherapy (N = 109)
Pyrexia	60	45
Headache	29	29
Anemia	26	42
Febrile neutropenia	24	39
Diarrhea	22	35
Neutropenia	20	30
Nausea	19	42
Thrombocytopenia	18	29
Hypokalemia	17	28
Cough	15	6
Peripheral edema	15	15
Cytokine release syndrome	14	0
Back pain	13	9
Constipation	13	26
Fatigue	13	13
Vomiting	12	24
Hypotension	12	12
Bone pain	11	7
Hypomagnesemia	11	17
Insomnia	10	9

Note: all-grade adverse events that occurred in >10% of the blinatumomab group are included

Grade ≥3* adverse events:

(%)	Blinatumomab (N = 267)	Standard Chemotherapy (N = 109)
Neutropenia	38	58
Infection	34	52
Elevated liver enzyme	13	15
Neurologic event	9	8
Cytokine release syndrome	5	0
Infusion reaction	3	<1

*According to the National Cancer Institute Common Terminology Criteria for Adverse Events, version 4.0
Note: grade adverse events that occurred in ≥3% of the blinatumomab group are included. Treatment discontinuation owing to any adverse event was reported for 12% of the blinatumomab group and 8% of the controls. Treatment-related fatal adverse events were reported for 3% of the blinatumomab group and 7% of the controls

RELAPSED/REFRACTORY DISEASE

ACUTE LYMPHOBLASTIC LEUKEMIA: INOTUZUMAB OZOGAMICIN

Kantarjian HM et al. N Engl J Med 2016;375:740–753
Protocol for: Kantarjian HM et al. N Engl J Med 2016;375:740–753
Supplementary appendix to: Kantarjian HM et al. N Engl J Med 2016;375:740–753
Kebriaei P et al. Bone Marrow Transplant 2018;53:449–456
BESPONSA (inotuzumab ozogamicin) prescribing information. Wyeth, Pharmaceuticals Inc: Philadelphia, PA; August 2017

Induction inotuzumab ozogamicin:
Premedications for each dose of inotuzumab ozogamicin:
- **Methylprednisolone** 1 mg/kg per dose; administer intravenously 30 minutes prior to each inotuzumab ozogamicin dose on days 1, 8, and 15, *plus:*
- **Acetaminophen** 650 mg per dose; administer orally 1 hour prior to each inotuzumab ozogamicin dose on days 1, 8, and 15, *plus:*
- **Diphenhydramine** 50 mg per dose; administer orally or intravenously 1 hour prior to each inotuzumab ozogamicin dose on days 1, 8, and 15

Inotuzumab ozogamicin (see table for dose); administer intravenously over 1 hour in 50 mL of 0.9% sodium chloride according to the schedule in the table below

Inotuzumab Ozogamicin Dosing and Schedule Based on Cycle and Response to Treatment				
	Day 1	**Day 8***	**Day 15***	**Total Dosage per Cycle**
Dosing regimen for cycle 1				
Dose	0.8 mg/m^2	0.5 mg/m^2	0.5 mg/m^2	Total dosage during cycle 1 for *all* patients = 1.8 mg/m^2
Cycle length	21 days†			
Dosing regimen for subsequent cycles depending on response to treatment				
Patients who *have* achieved a CR or CRi:				
Dose	0.5 mg/m^2	0.5 mg/m^2	0.5 mg/m^2	Total dosage during subsequent cycles for patients *with* CR or CRi = 1.5 mg/m^2
Cycle length‡	28 days			
Patients who *have not* achieved a CR or CRi:				
Dose	0.8 mg/m^2	0.5 mg/m^2	0.5 mg/m^2	Total dosage during subsequent cycles for patients *without* CR or CRi = 1.8 mg/m^2
Cycle length‡	28 days			

*± 2 days (maintain a minimum of 6 days between doses)
†Cycle length may be extended up to 28 days to allow for recovery from toxicity and for patients who achieve a complete remission (CR) or CR with incomplete count recovery (CRi)
- CR is defined as <5% blasts in the bone marrow, absence of peripheral blood leukemic blasts, resolution of extramedullary disease (if applicable), and recovery of ANC to ≥1000/mm^3 and platelet count to ≥100,000/mm^3
- CRi is defined as <5% blasts in the bone marrow, absence of peripheral blood leukemic blasts, resolution of extramedullary disease (if applicable), but with incomplete recovery of peripheral blood counts (ie, ANC <1000/mm^3 and/or platelet count <100,000/mm^3)
‡If the patient is planned to undergo a future hematopoietic stem cell transplant (HSCT), then administer up to 2 cycles. If CR or CRi with measurable residual disease (MRD) negativity has not been achieved after 2 cycles, then consider administering a third cycle. If no HSCT is planned, then administer up to a maximum of 6 cycles

Notes:
- The maximum number of cycles depends on whether the patient will proceed to HSCT. See note ‡ in the above table for details
- The methylprednisolone dosage used for infusion-related reaction prophylaxis is not specified in the U.S. Food and Drug Administration-approved prescribing information, in the article by Kantarjian and colleagues, or in the accompanying protocol or supplementary appendix. Thus, the medically responsible heath care provider may use discretion when choosing the methylprednisolone dose
- Patients with circulating lymphoblasts should undergo cytoreduction (eg, with a combination of hydroxyurea, steroids, and/or vincristine) to achieve a peripheral blast count ≤10,000/mm^3 prior to the initial dose of inotuzumab ozogamicin to reduce the risk of an infusion-related reaction
- Infusion-related reactions, all of which were Grade 2 severity, occurred in 2% of patients in the study by Kantarjian and colleagues. Signs and symptoms of infusion-related reactions may include chills, fever, rash, hypoxia, and/or bronchospasm. Reactions typically occurred during cycle 1 shortly after completion of the inotuzumab ozogamicin infusion and were either self-limiting or responded to supportive care. See therapy monitoring and therapy modification sections for further details

(continued)

(continued)

Supportive Care
Antiemetic prophylaxis
Emetogenic potential is LOW
See Chapter 42 for antiemetic recommendations

Hematopoietic growth factor (CSF) prophylaxis
Primary prophylaxis is indicated with one of the following:
Filgrastim (G-CSF) 5 μg/kg per dose; administer by subcutaneous injection once daily starting on day 16 (24 hours after inotuzumab ozogamicin), *or:*
- Continue daily filgrastim administration until postnadir WBC count >3000/mm³
- Discontinue daily filgrastim use at least 24 hours before administering myelosuppressive treatment

Pegfilgrastim 6 mg per dose; administer by subcutaneous injection once on day 16 (24 hours after inotuzumab ozogamicin)
- Do not administer myelosuppressive treatment within 14 days following a dose of pegfilgrastim

See Chapter 43 for more information

Veno-occlusive disease (VOD) prophylaxis
Consider administration of ursodiol for VOD prophylaxis as follows:
Ursodiol 12 mg/kg per day; administer orally daily, in two to three divided doses, starting prior to initiation of inotuzumab ozogamicin
- *For patients planned to undergo HSCT:* continue through at least day +90 following HSCT
- *For patients in whom HSCT is not planned:* continue at least through completion of the final cycle of inotuzumab ozogamicin

Antimicrobial prophylaxis
Risk of fever and neutropenia is HIGH
Antimicrobial primary prophylaxis to be considered:
- Antibacterial—consider prophylaxis with a fluoroquinolone during periods of prolonged neutropenia only (eg, <500/mm³ for ≥7 days), or no prophylaxis, until ANC recovery
- Antifungal—consider prophylaxis with fluconazole or another azole antifungal medication during periods of prolonged neutropenia only (eg, <500/mm³ for ≥7 days) until ANC recovery
- Antiviral—antiherpes antivirals (eg, acyclovir, famciclovir, valacyclovir)

Patient Population Studied

This international, multicenter, randomized, open-label, phase 3 trial (INO-VATE ALL) involved 326 patients with relapsed/refractory, CD22-positive, acute lymphoblastic leukemia. Patients were randomly assigned 1:1 to receive inotuzumab ozogamicin or standard chemotherapy. In the inotuzumab ozogamicin group, therapy consisted of one 21-day cycle followed by up to five 28-day cycles of intravenous inotuzumab ozogamicin (0.8 mg/m² on day 1, and 0.5 mg/m² on days 8 and 15; day 1 dose reduced to 0.5 mg/m² when patient had achieved complete remission)

Efficacy (N = 326)

	Inotuzumab Ozogamicin	Standard Chemotherapy	
Complete remission rate	80.7%	29.4%	P <0.001
Median overall survival	7.7 months	6.7 months	P = 0.04
Median progression-free survival	5.0 months	1.8 months	P <0.001

Therapy Monitoring

1. *Prior to initiation of inotuzumab ozogamicin therapy:* CBC with differential, baseline chemistries, electrolytes, uric acid, LDH, total bilirubin, alkaline phosphatase, alanine aminotransferase, aspartate aminotransferase, pregnancy test (women of reproductive potential only), electrocardiogram for QTc interval measurement, signs and symptoms of bleeding, signs and symptoms of infection
   a. In addition to baseline monitoring, consider interval monitoring of the electrocardiogram for QTc interval measurement as clinically indicated, especially in patients with a predisposition for QTc prolongation, with congenital long QTc syndrome, with congestive heart failure, with hypokalemia or hypomagnesemia, or who are taking concurrent medications that have a potential to prolong the QTc interval
2. *Prior to each dose of inotuzumab ozogamicin:* CBC with differential, baseline chemistries, electrolytes, uric acid, LDH, total bilirubin, alkaline phosphatase, alanine aminotransferase, and aspartate aminotransferase, signs and symptoms of bleeding, signs and symptoms of infection
3. *In patients at high risk for tumor lysis syndrome (eg, high tumor burden, renal dysfunction, rapidly progressing disease, markedly elevated LDH, baseline abnormalities in laboratory indices of tumor lysis syndrome [potassium, phosphate, uric acid, calcium, serum creatinine]):* consider frequent monitoring of laboratory indices of tumor lysis syndrome, intravenous hydration, and prophylaxis with a xanthine oxidase inhibitor (eg, allopurinol) during the induction course
4. *At least 1–2 times per week following each dose of inotuzumab ozogamicin, until recovery:*
   a. CBC with differential, chemistries, electrolytes, uric acid, LDH, total bilirubin, alkaline phosphatase, alanine aminotransferase, and aspartate aminotransferase
   b. Monitor for signs and symptoms of hepatic sinusoidal obstruction syndrome (SOS)/veno-occlusive disease (VOD) (elevations in ALT, AST, total bilirubin, painful hepatomegaly, weight gain, ascites). The incidence of any-grade SOS/VOD was 13% and the incidence of G ≥4 SOS/VOD was 11% in the inotuzumab ozogamicin arm of the study. The median (range) time to onset of SOS/VOD following the initial inotuzumab ozogamicin dose was 30 (14–238) days. Among patients who proceeded to hematopoietic stem cell transplant (HSCT), the median onset of VOD was 15 days after HSCT. The incidence of SOS/VOD after transplant increased with more cycles of inotuzumab ozogamicin (8% after 1 cycle, 19% after 2 cycles, and 29% after 3 or more cycles)
5. *At least every 30 minutes during each inotuzumab ozogamicin infusion and for 1 hour post-infusion completion:* Monitor vital signs and monitor for signs and symptoms of an infusion-related reaction (chills, fever, rash, hypoxia, respiratory failure, and/or bronchospasm)
6. *Response assessment:* CBC with differential, bone marrow aspirate, and biopsy after induction therapy (clinical trial protocol performed between days 16–28), then as clinically indicated

Treatment Modifications

INOTUZUMAB OZOGAMICIN

Hematologic Toxicities*

Peripheral blast count is >10,000/mm³ prior to the first dose of inotuzumab ozogamicin	Delay initiation of inotuzumab ozogamicin until the peripheral blast count is ≤10,000/mm³. Consider cytoreduction with a combination of hydroxyurea, corticosteroids, and/or vincristine
Day 1 ANC <1,000/mm³ in a patient with a baseline ANC ≥1000/mm³ prior to inotuzumab ozogamicin treatment	Delay the start of the next cycle of treatment until recovery of ANC to ≥1000/mm³. Do not modify the dose. If ANC does not recover within 28 days and neutropenia is thought to be related to inotuzumab ozogamicin, then discontinue inotuzumab ozogamicin
Day 1 platelet count <50,000/mm³ in a patient with a baseline platelet count ≥50,000/mm³ prior to inotuzumab ozogamicin treatment	Delay the start of the next cycle of treatment until recovery of platelet count to ≥50,000/mm³ (independent of platelet transfusions). Do not modify the dose. If the platelet count does not recover within 28 days and thrombocytopenia is thought to be related to inotuzumab ozogamicin, then discontinue inotuzumab ozogamicin
Day 1 ANC <1000/mm³ and/or platelet count <50,000/mm³ in a patient with baseline ANC <1000/mm³ and/or platelet count <50,000/mm³ prior to inotuzumab ozogamicin treatment	Delay the start of the next cycle until at least one of the following criteria are met: • ANC and platelet counts recover to at least baseline values (independent of platelet transfusions) for the prior cycle, *or:* • ANC recovers to ≥1000/mm³ and platelet count recovers to greater than 50,000/mm³ (independent of platelet transfusions), *or:* • Stable or improved disease (based on most recent bone marrow assessment) and the ANC and platelet count decrease is considered to be due to the underlying disease and not due to toxicity from inotuzumab ozogamicin
G ≥3 infection	Delay inotuzumab ozogamicin dose (applies to day 1, 8, or 15) until infection is controlled; then, depending on the severity of the infection, consider either treating at the same dose, treating with each subsequent dose reduced by 25%, or permanently discontinuing inotuzumab ozogamicin

(continued)

Treatment Modifications (continued)

Hematologic Toxicities*

G ≥3 bleeding	Delay inotuzumab ozogamicin dose (applies to day 1, 8, or 15) until resolution of bleeding; then, depending on the severity of the bleeding, consider either treating at the same dose, treating with each subsequent dose reduced by 25%, or permanently discontinuing inotuzumab ozogamicin

*Note: inotuzumab ozogamicin doses within a cycle (ie, days 8 and/or 15) do not need to be interrupted due to uncomplicated neutropenia or thrombocytopenia

Hepatic Toxicity or Hepatic Impairment

Hepatic SOS/VOD	Discontinue inotuzumab ozogamicin
Patient treated with inotuzumab ozogamicin is planned to undergo subsequent HSCT	Plan to administer no more than 2 cycles of inotuzumab ozogamicin prior to HSCT. If the patient has not achieved a CR or CRi with negative measurable residual disease after 2 cycles, then consider administering a third cycle of inotuzumab ozogamicin. Continue ursodiol prophylaxis (12 mg/kg/day in 2–3 divided doses daily) through the transplant period until at least day +90. Avoid conditioning regimens consisting of dual alkylating agents (eg, busulfan plus another alkylating agents) or thiotepa. Monitor for signs and symptoms of hepatic SOS/VOD and LFTs frequently, especially during the first month following transplant
Total bilirubin >1.5× ULN and AST/ALT >2.5× ULN	Interrupt inotuzumab ozogamicin treatment until total bilirubin ≤1.5× ULN, AST ≤2.5× ULN, and ALT ≤2.5× ULN prior to each dose of inotuzumab ozogamicin unless due to Gilbert syndrome or hemolysis
	Consider increasing the frequency of monitoring of liver function tests and for sign/symptoms of hepatotoxicity
	If total bilirubin, AST, and ALT do not recover to the above values, then permanently discontinue inotuzumab ozogamicin

Infusion Reactions

G1 infusion-related reaction (mild transient reaction; infusion interruption not indicated; intervention not indicated)	Interrupt the inotuzumab ozogamicin infusion immediately for any grade reaction and institute appropriate supportive medical management
	Depending on the severity of the reaction, consider repeating administration of acetaminophen and diphenhydramine (if >4 hours has transpired since administration of the premedication doses) and consider repeating administration of corticosteroids (eg, methylprednisolone 1 mg/kg intravenously × 1 dose)
G2 infusion-related reaction (therapy or infusion interruption indicated but responds promptly to symptomatic treatment [eg, antihistamines, NSAIDs, narcotics, IV fluids]; prophylactic medications indicated for ≤24 hours)	Once symptoms resolve, depending on the severity of the reaction, consider resuming the infusion at a reduced rate (eg, reduced by 50%), or discontinuing inotuzumab ozogamicin
G3 infusion-related reaction (prolonged [eg, not rapidly responsive to symptomatic medication and/or brief interruption of infusion]; recurrence of symptoms following initial improvement; hospitalization indicated for clinical sequelae)	Permanently discontinue inotuzumab ozogamicin. Institute appropriate supportive medical management
G4 infusion related reaction (life-threatening consequences; urgent intervention indicated)	

Other Toxicities

Other nonhematologic toxicity G ≥2	Delay inotuzumab ozogamicin administration until recovery to G ≤1 or pre-treatment grade levels prior to each dose. Then, at the discretion of the medically responsible heath care provider and depending on the severity of the toxicity, consider resuming treatment at the same dose

ANC, absolute neutrophil count; SOS, sinusoidal obstruction syndrome; VOD, veno-occlusive disease; CR, complete remission; CRi, complete remission with incomplete count recovery; LFTs, liver function tests; AST, aspartate aminotransferase; ALT, alanine aminotransferase; ULN, upper limit of normal; NSAIDs, non-steroidal anti-inflammatory drugs

Adverse Events (N = 259)

Serious Adverse Event	Inotuzumab Ozogamicin (N = 139)		Standard Chemotherapy (N = 120)	
	Grade 1–2 (%)	Grade ≥3 (%)	Grade 1–2 (%)	Grade ≥3 (%)
Febrile neutropenia	<1	11	<1	18
Veno-occlusive disease	1	9	0	<1
Disease progression	0	4	0	2
Pneumonia	0	4	<1	0
Pyrexia	1	1	2	<1
Sepsis	0	2	0	5
Neutropenic sepsis	0	2	0	2
Abdominal pain	<1	1	0	<1
Asthenia	0	1	0	0
Bacteremia	0	1	0	<1
Clostridium difficile colitis	0	1	0	<1
Influenza	0	1	0	0
Nausea	0	1	0	0
Septic shock	0	1	0	<1
Stomatitis	0	1	0	<1
Acute renal failure	<1	<1	0	0
Tumor lysis syndrome	<1	<1	0	0
Respiratory failure	0	<1	0	3
Escherichia sepsis	0	<1	0	2
Multiorgan failure	0	<1	0	2
Hyperbilirubinemia	0	0	<1	2
Hypotension	0	0	<1	2
Fungal pneumonia	0	0	0	2
Klebsiella infection	0	0	0	2
Pancytopenia	0	0	0	2

Note: serious adverse events that occurred during treatment are included. During treatment, four deaths in the inotuzumab ozogamicin group and two deaths in the control group were deemed to be treatment-related. Two treatment-related deaths resulting from veno-occlusive disease occurred after post-trial transplantation in the inotuzumab ozogamicin group

RELAPSED/REFRACTORY DISEASE

ACUTE LYMPHOBLASTIC LEUKEMIA: MINI-HYPER-CVD + INOTUZUMAB OZOGAMICIN

Jabbour E et al. JAMA Oncol 2018:230–234
Revised protocol for: Jabbour E et al. JAMA Oncol 2018:230–234
Supplementary online content for: Jabbour E et al. JAMA Oncol 2018:230–234

Regimen overview: The dose-intensive phase consists of 8 total cycles of mini-hyper-CVD alternating with methotrexate and cytarabine for a total of 8 cycles. Inotuzumab ozogamicin is given for a total of 4 doses during cycles 1–4. Rituximab is administered to patients with CD20 expression in ≥20% of leukemia cells for a total of 8 doses during cycles 1–4. Cycles are administered every 4 weeks. Patients receive POMP maintenance after completion of the dose-intensive phase

Inotuzumab Ozogamicin (Cycles 1–4 of Dose-intensive Phase Only; Cycle Length = 28 days)

Premedications (cycles 1–4)	• **Methylprednisolone** 1 mg/kg per dose; administer intravenously 30 minutes prior to each inotuzumab ozogamicin dose • **Acetaminophen** 650 mg per dose; administer orally 1 hour prior to each inotuzumab ozogamicin dose • **Diphenhydramine** 50 mg per dose; administer orally or intravenously 1 hour prior to each inotuzumab ozogamicin dose
Cycle 1	**Inotuzumab ozogamicin** 1.3 mg/m^2; administer intravenously over 1 hour in 50 mL of 0.9% sodium chloride (0.9% NS) on day 3 of cycle 1 only (total dosage/cycle in cycle 1 = 1.3 mg/m^2)
Cycles 2, 3, and 4	**Inotuzumab ozogamicin** 1 mg/m^2; administer intravenously over 1 hour in 50 mL of 0.9% NS for 1 dose per cycle on day 2 OR day 3, every 28 days, during cycles 2, 3, and 4 (total dosage/cycle in cycles 2–4 = 1 mg/m^2)

Notes:

• The methylprednisolone dosage used for infusion-related reaction prophylaxis is not specified in the product label. Thus, the medically responsible heath care provider may use discretion when choosing the methylprednisolone dose. May substitute dexamethasone 20 mg orally or intravenously (part of mini-hyper-CVD) instead of methylprednisolone for premedication during odd cycles (ie, cycles 1 and 3)
• Patients with circulating lymphoblasts should undergo cytoreduction if necessary to achieve a peripheral blast count ≤10,000/mm^3 prior to the initial dose of inotuzumab ozogamicin
• Infusion-related reactions may occur. Signs and symptoms may include chills, fever, rash, hypoxia, and/or bronchospasm. Reactions typically occurred during cycle 1 shortly after completion of the infusion and either were self-limiting or responded to supportive care. See therapy monitoring and therapy modification sections for further details

Rituximab (Cycles 1–4 of Dose-intensive Phase Only; Restricted to Patients with CD20 Expression in ≥20% of Leukemia Cells; Cycle Length = 28 days)

Premedications (cycles 1–4)	• **Acetaminophen** 650–1000 mg per dose; administer orally 30–60 minutes prior to each rituximab dose • **Diphenhydramine** 25–50 mg per dose; administer orally or intravenously 30–60 minutes prior to each rituximab dose
Cycles 1–4	**Rituximab** 375 mg/m^2 per dose; administer intravenously in 0.9% NS or 5% dextrose injection (D5W), diluted to a concentration within the range 1–4 mg/mL, on days 2 and 8, every 28 days, for 4 cycles (total dosage/28-day cycle = 750 mg/m^2) *Rituximab administration:* • Infuse initially at 50 mg/hour. If hypersensitivity or infusion reactions do not occur during the first 30 minutes, increase the rate by 50 mg/hour every 30 minutes as tolerated to a maximum rate of 400 mg/hour. During subsequent treatments if previous rituximab administration was well tolerated, start at 100 mg/hour and increase by 100 mg/hour every 30 minutes as tolerated to a maximum rate of 400 mg/hour • Interrupt rituximab administration for fever, chills, edema, congestion of the head and neck mucosa, hypertension, and other serious adverse events. Resume rituximab administration after adverse events abate

Mini-hyper-CVD (Cycles 1, 3, 5, and 7 of Dose-intensive Phase Only; Cycle Length = 28 days)

Cyclophosphamide 150 mg/m^2 per dose; administer intravenously over 3 hours in 500 mL 0.9% or D5W every 12 hours for 6 doses on days 1–3, for 4 cycles, cycles 1, 3, 5, and 7 (total dosage/cycle = 900 mg/m^2)

Mesna 300 mg/m^2 per 24 hours; administer by continuous intravenous infusion in 1000 mL 0.9% NS for 3 days on days 1–3, for 4 cycles, cycles 1, 3, 5, and 7 (total dosage/cycle 900 mg/m^2)

• Mesna administration starts concurrently with cyclophosphamide on day 1 and continues until approximately 9 hours after the last dose of cyclophosphamide is completed

(continued)

(continued)

Vincristine 2 mg/dose; administer by intravenous infusion over 15 minutes in 50 mL 0.9% NS for 2 doses, on days 1 and 8, for 4 cycles, cycles 1, 3, 5, and 7 (total dosage/cycle = 4 mg)

Dexamethasone 20 mg per day; administer orally, or intravenously in 25–150 mL 0.9% NS or D5W over 15–30 minutes for 8 doses, on days 1–4 and days 11–14, for 4 cycles, cycles 1, 3, 5, and 7 (total dose/cycle = 160 mg)

Methotrexate/Cytarabine (Cycles 2, 4, 6, and 8 of Dose-intensive Phase Only; Cycle Length = 28 days)

Hydration: with a solution containing a total amount of sodium not >0.9% NS (ie, ≤154 mEq sodium/1000 mL) by intravenous infusion during methotrexate administration and for at least 24 hours afterward
- Commence fluid administration 2–12 hours before starting methotrexate, depending on patient's fluid status
- Urine output should be at least 100 mL/hour before starting methotrexate infusion
- Maintain hydration at a rate that maintains urine output ≥100 mL/hour until the serum methotrexate concentration is <0.1 μmol/L
- Urine pH should be increased within the range ≥7.0 to ≤8.0 to enhance methotrexate solubility and ensure elimination

Adverse effects attributable to methotrexate are related to systemic methotrexate concentrations *and* the duration for which concentrations are maintained

Sodium Bicarbonate 50–150 mEq/1000 mL Is Added to Parenteral Hydration Solutions to Maintain Urine pH ≥7.0 to ≤8.0

Base Solution Sodium Content	Sodium Bicarbonate Additive	Total Sodium Content
0.45% Sodium chloride injection (0.45% NS)		
77 mEq/L	50–75 mEq	127–152 mEq/L
0.2% Sodium chloride injection (0.2% NS)		
34 mEq/L	100–125 mEq	134–159 mEq/L
5% Dextrose injection (D5W)		
0	125–150 mEq	125–150 mEq/L
D5W/0.45% NS		
77 mEq/L	50–75 mEq	127–152 mEq/L
D5W/0.2% NS		
34 mEq/L	100–125 mEq	134–159 mEq/L

Methotrexate 50 mg/m²; administer intravenously over 2 hours, on day 1, *followed by:*
Methotrexate 200 mg/m²; administer intravenously over 22 hours, on day 1, for 4 cycles, cycles 2, 4, 6, and 8 (total dosage/cycle, bolus + infusion = 250 mg/m²)

Note: for logistical practicality and efficiency, parenteral admixtures containing methotrexate may include a portion or all of the fluid and sodium bicarbonate needed to meet hydration and urinary alkalinization requirements during methotrexate administration

Leucovorin calcium 50 mg; administer intravenously in 25–250 mL 0.9% NS or D5W over 15–30 minutes for 1 dose administered 36 hours after methotrexate administration began (12 hours after methotrexate administration ends), *followed 6 hours later by:*
Leucovorin calcium 15 mg per dose; administer orally or intravenously in 25–250 mL 0.9% NS or D5W over 15–30 minutes, every 6 hours for 8 doses (total dosage/cycle = 170 mg)

Note: adjust regimen if needed according to the results of methotrexate concentration measurements as outlined in the table below. Note that leucovorin may be escalated to even higher doses for elevated methotrexate levels or delayed clearance as clinically appropriate

Hours After *Starting* Methotrexate	Methotrexate Concentration	Regimen Adjustments
Hour 24	>20 μmol/L (>2 × 10⁻⁵ mol/L)	Withhold cytarabine and repeat methotrexate level. If confirmed >20 μmol/L, then reduce each cytarabine dose to 250 mg/m² IV over 2 hours every 12 hours for 4 doses on days 2 and 3. Continue with leucovorin as outlined above

(continued)

(continued)

| Hour 48 | >1 µmol/L (>1 × 10⁻⁶ mol/L) | Increase **leucovorin** dosages to 50 mg/dose; administer intravenously in 25–250 mL 0.9% NS or D5W over 15–30 minutes every 6 hours until serum methotrexate concentrations are <0.1 µmol/L (<1 × 10²⁷ mol/L) |
| Hour 72 | >0.1 µmol/L (>1 × 10⁻⁷ mol/L, *or* >100 nmol/L) | |

Cytarabine 500 mg/m² per dose; administer intravenously in 50–500 mL 0.9% NS or D5W over 3 hours every 12 hours for 4 doses on days 2 and 3, for 4 cycles, cycles 2, 4, 6, and 8 (total dosage/cycle [not including intrathecal cytarabine] = 2000 mg/m²)

Keratitis prophylaxis for cytarabine
Steroid ophthalmic drops (**prednisolone 1% or dexamethasone 0.1%**); administer 2 drops by intraocular instillation into each eye every 6 hours starting prior to the first cytarabine dose and continuing until 48 hours after cytarabine is completed

Maintenance Therapy (Initiate After Completion of Dose-intensive Phase; Cycle Length = 28 days)

Vincristine 2 mg/dose; administer by intravenous infusion over 15 minutes in 50 mL 0.9% NS for 1 doses, on day 1, every 28 days, for 1 year (total dosage/28-day cycle = 2 mg)

Prednisone 50 mg per day; administer orally, for 5 consecutive days every month, on days 1–5, every 28 days, for 1 year (total dosage/28-day cycle = 250 mg)

Mercaptopurine 50 mg per dose; administer orally twice per day, continuously on days 1–28, every 28 days, for 3 years (total dosage/28-day cycle = 2800 mg)

Methotrexate 10 mg/m² per dose; administer orally, once per week for 4 doses on days 1, 8, 15, and 22, every 28 days, for 3 years (total dosage/28-day cycle = 40 mg/m²)

Supportive Care for Dose-Intensive Phase
Antiemetic prophylaxis for cycles 1, 3, 5, and 7
Emetogenic potential on Days 1–3 is **MODERATE**
Emetogenic potential on Day 8 is **MINIMAL**
See Chapter 42 for antiemetic recommendations

Antiemetic prophylaxis for cycles 2, 4, 6, and 8
Emetogenic potential on Days 1–3 is **MODERATE**
See Chapter 42 for antiemetic recommendations

Hematopoietic growth factor (CSF) prophylaxis for cycles 1–8
Primary prophylaxis is indicated with:
   Filgrastim (G-CSF) 5 µg/kg per dose; administer by subcutaneous injection once per day, *or:*
   Pegfilgrastim (pegylated filgrastim) 6 mg/0.6 mL, by subcutaneous injection for one dose
   • Begin use from 24–72 h after myelosuppressive chemotherapy is completed
   • Continue daily filgrastim use until ANC ≥5000/mm³ after the leukocyte nadir
   • Discontinue daily filgrastim use at least 24 hours before administering myelosuppressive treatment. Do not administer pegfilgrastim within 14 days before administering myelosuppressive treatment
See Chapter 43 for more information

Antimicrobial prophylaxis for Cycles 1–8
Risk of fever and neutropenia is **HIGH**
   Antimicrobial primary prophylaxis is recommended:
   • Antibacterial—consider fluoroquinolone prophylaxis; *P. jirovecii* prophylaxis is recommended (eg, cotrimoxazole)
   • Antifungal—recommended
   • Antiviral—antiherpes antivirals (eg, acyclovir, famciclovir, valacyclovir)
Veno-occlusive Disease (VOD) prophylaxis for cycles 1–4
   VOD prophylaxis is recommended with:
   Ursodiol 300 mg per dose; administer orally three times per day starting prior to administration of the first dose of inotuzumab ozogamicin and continuing for at least 28 days after the last dose, or longer in patients who are candidates for an allogeneic hematopoietic stem cell transplant

(continued)

(*continued*)

Supportive Care for Maintenance Phase
Antiemetic prophylaxis for Maintenance Therapy
Emetogenic potential is **MINIMAL**
See Chapter 42 for antiemetic recommendations

Hematopoietic growth factor (CSF) prophylaxis for Maintenance Therapy
Primary prophylaxis is **NOT** *indicated*
See Chapter 43 for more information

Antimicrobial prophylaxis for Maintenance Therapy
Risk of fever and neutropenia is **LOW**
 Antimicrobial primary prophylaxis is recommended:
 • Antibacterial—*P. jirovecii* prophylaxis is recommended (eg, cotrimoxazole)
 • Antifungal—not indicated
 • Antiviral—antiherpes antivirals (eg, acyclovir, famciclovir, valacyclovir)

Patient Population Studied

NCT01371630 was a single-center, single-arm, phase 2 study involving 59 adult patients with relapsed or refractory CD22-positive B-cell acute lymphoblastic leukemia that evaluated the combination of mini-hyper-CVD plus inotuzumab ozogamicin. Patients were required to have normal organ function and a performance status of ≤3

Patient Characteristics (N = 59)		
Characteristic	Category	N (%)/Median [Range]
Age (years)		35 [18–87]
Gender	Male	29 (49)
ECOG PS	≥2	7 (12)
WBC (x 10⁹ /L)	Median	3.7 [0.1–194.7]
	≥50	1 (2)
PB blasts percentage		4 [0–93]
BM blasts ≥50%		42 (71)
Karyotype	Diploid	12 (20)
	MLL	10 (17)
	Miscellaneous	28 (47)
	ND/IM	9 (15)

Patient Characteristics (N = 59)		
Characteristic	Category	N (%)/Median [Range]
CD22 expression	Median	95 [20–100]
CD20 expression	≥20%	12 (20)
Prior ASCT		15 (25)
Salvage status	Salvage 1	33 (56)
	Salvage 1, primary refractory	5 (8)
	Salvage 1, CRD1	15 (25)
	Salvage 1, CRD1 ≥12 months	13 (22)
	Salvage 2	13 (22)
	≥Salvage 3	13 (22)

ECOG PS, Eastern Cooperative Oncology Group performance status; BM, bone marrow; WBC, white blood cell; PB, peripheral blast; ND, not determined; IM, insufficient metaphases; CRD, complete remission duration

Efficacy (N = 59)

Best Overall Response to Therapy		
Response	n/N (%)	
Morphologic response		
CR	35/59 (59)	
CRp	10/59 (17)	
CRi	1/59 (2)	
ORR	46/59 (78)	
MRD negativity		
At response	23/44 (52)	
Overall	36/44 (82)	
No response	6/59 (10)	
Early death	7/59 (12)	
Response by salvage status		
Salvage 1	30/33 (91)	
Salvage 1, primary refractory	5/5 (100)	
Salvage 1, CRD1 <12 months	12/15 (80)	
Salvage 1, CRD1 ≥12 months	13/13 (100)	
Salvage 2	8/13 (62)	
Salvage ≥3	8/13 (62)	
MRD negativity		
Salvage 1	28/30 (93)	
Salvage ≥2	8/14 (57)	
Survival		
Median OS, months (N = 59)	11	
OS rate at 1 year (95% CI)	46 (33–58)	
OS rate at 2 years (95% CI)	34 (22–47)	
Median RFS, months (N = 46)	8	
RFS rate at 1 year (95% CI)	40 (26–54)	
RFS rate at 2 years (95% CI)	32 (19–46)	
Median OS, months (N = 33 in salvage 1)	17	
Median OS, months (N = 13 in salvage 2)	6	
Median OS, months (N = 13 in salvage ≥3)	5	
Median OS, months (N = 36 MRD-negative)	25	P = 0.05
Median OS, months (N = 8 MRD-positive)	9	

CR, complete response; CRp, CR without platelets recovery; CRi, CR with incomplete hematologic recovery; ORR, overall response rate; MRD, minimal residual disease; CRD, complete remission duration; OS, overall survival; RFS, relapse-free survival

Note: median follow-up was 24 months. Twenty-six patients (44%) proceeded to allogeneic stem cell transplantation; these patients had a median OS of 25 months

Treatment Modifications

DOSE-INTENSIVE CHEMOTHERAPY TREATMENT MODIFICATIONS

Adverse Effect	Dose Modification
Day 1 WBC count is <3000/mm³ or platelet count is <60,000/mm³	WBC count is >3000/mm³ and platelet count is >60,000/mm³
Total bilirubin >2.6 and ≤3.9 mg/dL	Reduce vincristine doses to 1 mg
Clinically significant G2 peripheral neuropathy for >2 weeks	
G ≥3 peripheral neuropathy	Discontinue vincristine
G ≥3 ileus related to vincristine	
Total bilirubin >3.9 mg/dL	
G ≥3 mucositis with prior methotrexate course	Consider a 25–50% reduction in the methotrexate dose
Calculated creatinine clearance 10–50 mL/min	Reduce methotrexate dose by 50%
Calculated creatinine clearance <10 mL/min	Discontinue methotrexate
Delayed excretion and/or nephrotoxicity with prior methotrexate course	Reduce methotrexate dose by 25–75%
Pleural effusion or ascites	Reduce methotrexate dose by 50% and drain effusion, if possible

INOTUZUMAB OZOGAMICIN TREATMENT MODIFICATIONS

Hematologic Toxicities*

Peripheral blast count is >10,000/mm³ prior to the first dose of inotuzumab ozogamicin	Delay initiation of inotuzumab ozogamicin until the peripheral blast count is ≤10,000/mm³

Hepatic Toxicity or Hepatic Impairment

Hepatic veno-occlusive disease	Discontinue inotuzumab ozogamicin
Patient is planned to undergo subsequent HSCT	Continue ursodiol prophylaxis through the transplant period until at least day +90. Avoid conditioning regimens consisting of dual alkylating agents (eg, busulfan plus another alkylating agents) or thiotepa. Monitor for signs and symptoms of hepatic veno-occlusive disease and LFTs frequently, especially during the first month following transplant
Total bilirubin >1.5× ULN and AST/ALT >2.5× ULN	Interrupt inotuzumab ozogamicin treatment until total bilirubin ≤1.5× ULN, AST ≤2.5× ULN, and ALT ≤2.5× ULN prior to each dose of inotuzumab ozogamicin unless due to Gilbert syndrome or hemolysis Consider increasing the frequency of monitoring of liver function tests and for sign/symptoms of hepatotoxicity If total bilirubin, AST, and ALT do not recover to the above values, then permanently discontinue inotuzumab ozogamicin

Infusion Reactions

G1 infusion-related reaction (mild transient reaction; infusion interruption not indicated; intervention not indicated)	Interrupt the inotuzumab ozogamicin infusion immediately for any grade reaction and institute appropriate supportive medical management Depending on the severity of the reaction, consider repeating administration of acetaminophen and diphenhydramine (if >4 hours has transpired since administration of the premedication doses) and consider repeating administration of corticosteroids (eg, methylprednisolone 1 mg/kg intravenously × 1 dose)
G2 infusion-related reaction (therapy or infusion interruption indicated but responds promptly to symptomatic treatment [eg, antihistamines, NSAIDs, narcotics, IV fluids]; prophylactic medications indicated for ≤24 hours)	Once symptoms resolve, depending on the severity of the reaction, consider resuming the infusion at a reduced rate (eg, reduced by 50%), or discontinuing inotuzumab ozogamicin

(continued)

Treatment Modifications (*continued*)

Infusion Reactions

G3 infusion-related reaction (prolonged [eg, not rapidly responsive to symptomatic medication and/or brief interruption of infusion]; recurrence of symptoms following initial improvement; hospitalization indicated for clinical sequelae)	Permanently discontinue inotuzumab ozogamicin. Institute appropriate supportive medical management
G4 infusion related reaction (life-threatening consequences; urgent intervention indicated)	

Other Toxicities

Other nonhematologic toxicity G ≥2 related to inotuzumab ozogamicin	Delay inotuzumab ozogamicin administration until recovery to G ≤1 or pre-treatment grade levels prior to each dose. Then, at the discretion of the medically responsible health care provider and depending on the severity of the toxicity, consider resuming treatment at the same dose

LFTs, liver function tests; AST, aspartate aminotransferase; ALT, alanine aminotransferase; ULN, upper limit of normal; NSAIDs, non-steroidal anti-inflammatory drugs

RITUXIMAB TREATMENT MODIFICATIONS

Rituximab Infusion-Related Toxicities

Onset of infusion-related events (fevers, chills, rigors, edema, congestion of the head and neck mucosa, hypotension)

1. Interrupt rituximab infusion

2. *For fever, chills:* Give additional dose of acetaminophen 650 mg orally and diphenhydramine 25–50 mg by intravenous push

3. *For rigors:* Give meperidine 12.5–25 mg by intravenous push ± promethazine 12.5–25 mg by intravenous infusion in at least 10 mL 0.9% NS or D5W over 5–15 minutes. If after 15–20 minutes the response to a single dose is considered inadequate, the dose may be repeated

4. After symptoms resolve, resume rituximab infusion at a minimum of 50% reduction in the rate at which the event occurred. If no further infusion-related events, increase the rate by 50 mg/hour every 30 minutes, as tolerated, up to a maximum rate of 400 mg/hour

Dyspnea or wheezing, without allergic findings (urticaria, or tongue or laryngeal edema)

1. Interrupt rituximab infusion immediately

2. Give hydrocortisone 100 mg by intravenous push (or glucocorticoid equivalent)

3. Give an additional dose of diphenhydramine 25–50 mg by intravenous push and a histamine H_2-antagonist (ranitidine 50 mg or famotidine 20 mg) by intravenous push

4. After symptoms resolve, resume rituximab infusion at a minimum of 50% reduction in the rate at which the event occurred. If no further infusion-related events, increase the rate by 50 mg/hour every 30 minutes, as tolerated, up to a maximum rate of 400 mg/hour

Note: medications and equipment for the treatment of hypersensitivity reactions should be available for immediate use in the event of a reaction during rituximab administration (eg, intravenous fluids, epinephrine, antihistamines, glucocorticoids, and oxygen)

POMP MAINTENANCE TREATMENT MODIFICATIONS

POMP Dose Levels

Level	Vincristine	Prednisone	Mercaptopurine	Methotrexate
Starting dose	2 mg	50 mg	50 mg twice per day	10 mg/m² per week
−1	1 mg	40 mg	50 mg once per day	7.5 mg/m² per week
−2	Discontinue	30 mg	50 mg once per day	5 mg/m² per week
−3	Discontinue	Discontinue	Discontinue	Discontinue

Adverse Effect	Dose Modification
Steroid myopathy or other significant toxicity related to prednisone (excluding hyperglycemia)	Reduce prednisone dose by ≥1 dose level

(*continued*)

Treatment Modifications (*continued*)

Adverse Effect	Dose Modification
G2 peripheral neuropathy for >2 weeks	Reduce vincristine dosage by 1 dose level
G ≥3 peripheral neuropathy for >2 weeks	Discontinue vincristine
G ≥3 myelosuppression	Reduce mercaptopurine and methotrexate dosages by 1 dose level
G ≥3 nonhematologic toxicity related to mercaptopurine and/or methotrexate	Reduce the dosage of the applicable medication(s) by ≥1 dose level

Toxicity (N = 59)

Event	Mini-Hyper-CVD + Inotuzumab Ozogamicin (N = 59)
Grade (%)	Grade 3/4 Toxicities
Infections	73
Hyperglycemia	17
VOD	15
Increased bilirubin	14
Increased LFTs	12
Hypokalemia	12
Hemorrhage	12

Note: treatment-related toxicities encountered in ≥10% of patients regardless of causality are included in the table. Most adverse effects were Grades 1–2. Overall, 48 patients (81%) had prolonged thrombocytopenia lasting >6 weeks. VOD occurred in 9 patients (15%) after a median (range) of 3 cycles (1–5). All 9 patients had received an allogeneic hematopoietic stem cell transplant (N = 3 prior to inotuzumab ozogamicin, N = 5 after, and N = 1 both before and after)

VOD, veno-occlusive disease; LFTs, liver function tests

Therapy Monitoring

1. CBC with differential daily during and after chemotherapy during induction therapy until recovery of ANC >500/mm^3. Platelets every day while in hospital until patient no longer requires platelet transfusions
2. *Pretreatment evaluation:* determination of LVEF by echocardiogram; hepatitis B core antibody (IgG or total) and hepatitis B surface antigen for patients who will receive rituximab
3. Serum electrolytes, mineral panel, and uric acid, at least daily during induction therapy until the risk of tumor lysis is past
4. *During each inotuzumab ozogamicin and rituximab infusion and for at least 1 hour after infusion completion:* signs and symptoms of infusion-related reaction, vital signs every 30 minutes
5. CMP and CBC with differential and platelet count prior to each cycle of consolidation therapy
6. Monitor serum methotrexate levels 24, 48, and 72 hours after the start of each methotrexate infusion. In patients with delayed clearance, monitor daily methotrexate levels thereafter until the methotrexate concentration declines to <0.1 micromolar
7. Patients who receive high-dose cytarabine need to be closely monitored for changes in renal function. Renal dysfunction is highly correlated with increased risk of cerebellar toxicity associated with cytarabine. Patients need to be monitored for nystagmus, dysmetria, and ataxia before each cytarabine dose
8. Monitor for signs and symptoms of pleural effusion and fluid overload prior to each even cycle of intensive therapy. If there is concern for pleural effusion, perform additional work-up (ie, chest x-ray) prior to administration of methotrexate
9. Bone marrow aspirate and biopsy after the initial induction course upon recovery of peripheral blood counts. After patient achieves a CR, bone marrow biopsy and aspirate should be performed at least following completion of consolidation therapy

Notes

In the study reported by Jabbour E et al. (JAMA Oncol 2018;4:230–234), patients underwent a diagnostic LP on day 2 of the first course of treatment

a. *Patients with no evidence of CNS disease at the time of diagnosis should receive prophylactic intrathecal therapy with:*

Methotrexate; administer intrathecally 12 mg/dose via lumbar puncture *or* 6 mg/dose intraventricularly via indwelling ventricular reservoir catheter (eg, Ommaya) on day 2 of courses 1–4 of intensive induction therapy, *and:*

Cytarabine 100 mg/dose; administer intrathecally via lumbar puncture *or* intraventricularly via indwelling ventricular reservoir on day 8 of courses 1–4 of intensive induction therapy

b. *Patients with CNS disease at the time of diagnosis receive intrathecal therapy with:*

Methotrexate; administer intrathecally 12 mg/dose via lumbar puncture *or* 6 mg/dose intraventricularly via indwelling ventricular reservoir catheter (eg, Ommaya) once per week, *and:*

Cytarabine 100 mg/dose; administer intrathecally via lumbar puncture *or* intraventricularly via indwelling ventricular reservoir once per week

i. Twice-weekly intrathecal chemotherapy doses should be separated by at least 72 hours

ii. Continue twice-weekly intrathecal chemotherapy until cerebrospinal fluid cell counts normalize and cytology becomes negative for malignant disease and for at least 4 weeks, then reduce the frequency to once per week for 2 months, then every other week for 2 months, then once per month to complete a total of 1 year of therapy

RELAPSED/ REFRACTORY DISEASE

ACUTE LYMPHOBLASTIC LEUKEMIA: LIPOSOMAL VINCRISTINE SULFATE

O'Brien S et al. J Clin Oncol 2013;31:676–683

Vincristine sulfate liposome injection
2.25 mg/m^2 per dose; administer intravenously in (total volume [QS]) 100 mL 0.9% sodium chloride or 5% dextrose injection over 60 minutes for 4 doses on days 1, 8, 15, and 22, every 28 days (total dosage/cycle = 9 mg/m^2)
• Liposomal vincristine sulfate doses are calculated from actual body surface area, and are not capitated

Supportive Care
Antiemetic prophylaxis
Emetogenic potential is **MINIMAL**
See Chapter 42 for antiemetic recommendations

Hematopoietic growth factor (CSF) prophylaxis
Primary prophylaxis is **NOT** *indicated*
See Chapter 43 for more information

Antimicrobial prophylaxis
Risk of fever and neutropenia is **LOW**
   Antimicrobial primary prophylaxis to be considered:
   • Antibacterial—not indicated
   • Antifungal—not indicated
   • Antiviral—not indicated unless patient previously had an episode of HSV

Patient Population Studied

Sixty-five adults (median age, 31 years; range, 19–83 years) with Ph-negative ALL in second or greater relapse, or whose disease had progressed following 2 or more leukemia therapies

Efficacy

CR/CRi rate was 20% and overall response rate was 35%
Median OS, overall, 4.6 months (range, <1 month to >25 months), and 7.7 months (range, 2.4 to >23.3 months) among patients who achieved a CR/CRi

Treatment Modifications

G ≥3 adverse effects (severe symptoms; limiting self-care activities of daily living [ADL]*) or persistent G2 (moderate symptoms; limiting instrumental ADL)† peripheral neuropathy	Interrupt liposomal vincristine sulfate If the peripheral neuropathy remains at G ≥3, discontinue liposomal vincristine sulfate If the peripheral neuropathy recovers to G ≤2, continue treatment with liposomal vincristine sulfate dosage decreased to 2 mg/m^2 per dose
Persistent G2 peripheral neuropathy after the first dose reduction to 2 mg/m^2	Interrupt liposomal vincristine sulfate for up to 7 days If the peripheral neuropathy increases to G ≥3, discontinue liposomal vincristine sulfate If peripheral neuropathy recovers to G ≤1, continue treatment with liposomal vincristine sulfate dosage decreased to 1.825 mg/m^2 per dose
Persistent G ≥2 peripheral neuropathy after a second dose reduction to 1.825 mg/m^2	Interrupt liposomal vincristine sulfate for up to 7 days If the peripheral increases to G ≥3, discontinue liposomal vincristine sulfate If the toxicity recovers to G ≤1, continue treatment with liposomal vincristine sulfate dosage decreased to 1.5 mg/m^2 per dose

If neutropenia, thrombocytopenia, or anemia G ≥3 develop, consider dose modification or reduction as well as supportive care measures

Reduce liposomal vincristine sulfate dosages or interrupt treatment for hepatic toxicity

Severity grading for adverse events is based on the National Cancer Institute (NCI) Common Terminology Criteria for Adverse Events (CTCAE) v3.0. Available at: http://ctep.cancer.gov/protocolDevelopment/electronic_ applications/ ctc.htm [accessed December 7, 2013]
*Self-care ADL refers to bathing, dressing and undressing, feeding self, using the toilet, taking medications, and not bedridden
†Instrumental ADL refers to preparing meals, shopping for groceries and clothes, using telephone, managing money, etc

Therapy Monitoring

CBC with differential leukocyte count, as well as renal and hepatic function tests, prior to each dose of liposomal vincristine sulfate
Bone marrow biopsy on day 28 of treatment courses 1 and 2 and every second treatment course thereafter

Toxicity

	All Grades %	G3 %	G4 %
Any treatment-related adverse event	82	39	19
Nervous system disorders	63	19	2
Neuropathy peripheral	29	15	0
Hypoesthesia	25	2	0
Paresthesia	20	2	0
Areflexia	9	2	0
Hyporeflexia	8	0	0

Toxicity (continued)

	All Grades %	G3 %	G4 %
GI disorders	51	12	0
Constipation	34	3	0
Nausea	22	0	0
Vomiting	11	0	0
Abdominal pain	9	3	0
Diarrhea	6	2	0
Blood and lymphatic system disorders	29	9	12
Neutropenia	17	8	8
Anemia	12	5	0
Thrombocytopenia	9	2	5
Febrile neutropenia	8	3	0
General disorders and administration site conditions	25	8	0
Fatigue	11	3	0
Asthenia	9	3	0
Pyrexia	9	2	0
Metabolism and nutrition disorders	22	6	3
Decreased appetite	12	2	0
Tumor lysis syndrome	8	2	3
Investigations	19	8	2
Weight decreased	11		

Notes:
- Liposomal vincristine sulfate is a vinca alkaloid indicated for the treatment of adult patients with Philadelphia chromosome-negative (Ph−) acute lymphoblastic leukemia (ALL) in second or subsequent relapse, or whose disease has progressed following two or more antileukemia therapies
- Liposomal vincristine sulfate is contraindicated in patients with demyelinating conditions including Charcot-Marie-Tooth syndrome
- Neurologic toxicity: Monitor patients for peripheral, motor, sensory, central, and autonomic neuropathy, and reduce, interrupt, or discontinue treatment if signs or symptoms present
  - Patients with preexisting severe neuropathy should be treated with liposomal vincristine sulfate only after careful risk-benefit assessment

RELAPSED/REFRACTORY DISEASE

ACUTE LYMPHOBLASTIC LEUKEMIA: NELARABINE

Gökbuget N et al. Blood 2011;118:3504–3511

Nelarabine 1500 mg/m^2 per dose; administer intravenously (without dilution) over 2 hours for 3 doses on days 1, 3, and 5, every 21 days (total dosage/cycle = 4500 mg/m^2)

Supportive Care
Antiemetic prophylaxis
Emetogenic potential is **MINIMAL**
See Chapter 42 for antiemetic recommendations

Hematopoietic growth factor (CSF) prophylaxis
Primary prophylaxis is **NOT** *indicated*
See Chapter 43 for more information

Antimicrobial prophylaxis
Risk of fever and neutropenia is **LOW**
  Antimicrobial primary prophylaxis to be considered:
  • Antibacterial—not indicated
  • Antifungal—not indicated
  • Antiviral—not indicated unless patient previously had an episode of HSV

Patient Population Studied

Study of 126 relapsed/refractory patients (85% T-cell acute lymphoblastic leukemia [T-ALL], 15% T-cell lymphoblastic lymphoma), median age 33 years (range, 18–81 years) treated with nelarabine

Treatment Modifications

Nelarabine administration should be discontinued for Grade ≥2 neurologic adverse reactions of NCI Common Terminology Criteria for Adverse Events. Treatment may be delayed for other toxicities

Therapy Monitoring

1. *Weekly and before a treatment cycle:* CBC with differential, as well as renal and hepatic function
2. *Response evaluation:* bone marrow biopsy every 2 cycles

Efficacy (N = 126)

	Result After Cycle 1 (%)	Overall Result After 1–3 Cycles (%)
CR	32	36
PR	19	10
Failure	47	52
Death on therapy	1	1
Withdrawal	2	2

Toxicity

Hematologic	G 3–4 (%)
Leukopenia	41
Granulocytopenia	37
Thrombocytopenia	17

• Patients with CR after 1 cycle (N = 36) tended to have a better 3-year survival (32% ± 8%) compared with those who later achieved a CR (N = 9; 11% ± 10%; P = 0.06)
• The probability of survival after 1 year was 24% (SE ± 3%) and after 3 years 12% (SE ± 3%) with a median survival of 6 months
• The 3-year survival of patients with failure or PR after nelarabine (N = 81) compared with patients who achieved a CR (N = 45) was 4% (SE ± 2%) versus 28% (SE ± 7%), respectively (P <0.0001)
• A total of 36 of 45 patients (80%) who achieved a CR after nelarabine subsequently received stem cell transplantation (SCT) in continuous CR. Four patients died in CR (11%) related to transplantation (GVHD N = 1, infection N = 3) and 20 patients relapsed (56%). The probability of survival 3 years after transplantation in 36 patients transplanted in CR after nelarabine was 31% (SE ± 8%), and the relapse-free survival at 3 years was 37% (SE ± 9%). The median time to relapse after SCT was 4 months (range, 1–24) months. In patients alive after SCT, the median survival was 41 months (range, 13–85 months)
• Survival probability at 3 years was 36% (SE ± 8%) in the 36 patients transplanted in CR after nelarabine. In comparison, CR patients without transplantation in CR after nelarabine (N = 9) survival probability was zero and failure or PR was 4% (SE ± 2%; N = 81) after 3 years (P <0.0001)

Neurotoxicity

Incidence, N (%) of Cycles		G 1	G 2	G 3	G 4
		Number of Cycles			
Cognitive disturbance	9 (4)	3	0	1	5
Confusion	9 (4)	3	0	3	3
Consciousness impaired	1 (0.5)	0	0	1	0
Dizziness	13 (6)	7	2	2	2
Fatigue	1 (0.5)	1	0		0
Guillain-Barré–like syndrome	1 (0.5)	0	0	1	0
Hallucination	4 (2)	0	0	2	2
Insomnia	2 (1)	1	0	1	0
Memory impaired	7 (3)	2	1	1	3
Mood alteration	12 (6)	7	1	4	0
Neuropathy increased	5 (2)	2	2	1	0
Restlessness	4 (2)	1	2	0	1
Somnolence	1 (0.5)	0	0	1	0
Tremor	4 (2)	1	1	2	0

- Neurologic toxicities of any degree were observed after 26 cycles (13%) in 20 patients (16%). The majority of events were G1 or G2. In 4% of the cycles (N = 4) and 7% of the patients (N = 9), G3/4 neurotoxicities were observed
- In 1 patient, treatment had to be stopped because of a Guillain-Barré–like syndrome with tetraparesis, hallucinations, and reduced vigilance, which developed at day 3 of the first cycle. The symptoms improved slowly after nelarabine was withdrawn

Notes

- Nelarabine is indicated for the treatment of patients with T-cell acute lymphoblastic leukemia and T-cell lymphoblastic lymphoma whose disease has not responded to or has relapsed following treatment with at least 2 chemotherapy regimens
- Severe neurologic adverse reactions have been reported with the use of nelarabine, including altered mental states such as severe somnolence, central nervous system effects such as convulsions, and peripheral neuropathy ranging from numbness and paresthesias to motor weakness and paralysis. There have also been reports of adverse reactions associated with demyelination, and ascending peripheral neuropathies similar to Guillain-Barré syndrome. Full recovery from adverse reactions has not always occurred with cessation of therapy with nelarabine. Close monitoring for neurologic adverse reactions is strongly recommended
- DeAngelo DJ et al (Blood 2007;109: 5136–5142) also reported their experience with 26 refractory/relapsed patients with T-cell acute lymphoblastic leukemia (T-ALL) and 13 patients with T-cell lymphoblastic lymphoma whose median age was 34 years (range, 16–66 years). Treatment consisted of **nelarabine** 1500 mg/m² per dose intravenously over 2 hours for 3 doses on days 1, 3, and 5, every 21 days (total dosage/cycle = 4500 mg/m²). The investigators reported a complete remission rate of 31% (95% CI, 17–48), and an overall response of 41% (95% CI, 26–58). The principal toxicities were G3 or G4 neutropenia and thrombocytopenia, which occurred in 37% and 26% of patients, respectively. Only one G4 neurologic adverse event occurred, a reversible depressed level of consciousness. The median disease-free survival (DFS) was 20 weeks (95% CI, 11–56), and the median overall survival was 20 weeks (95% CI, 13–36%). The 1-year overall survival was 28% (95% CI, 15–43)

2. Acute Myeloid Leukemia

Michael M. Boyiadzis, MD, MHSc, Ivan Aksentijevich, MD, and Martin S. Tallman, MD

Epidemiology

Incidence: 19,940 (male: 11,090; female: 8850. Estimated new cases for 2020 in the United States)
4.3 per 100,000 male and female per year

Deaths: Estimated 11,180 in 2020 (male: 6470; female: 4710)

Median age: 68 years (median age for acute promyelocytic leukemia: 40 years)

Male to female ratio: 1.48

Dores GM. Blood 2012;119:34–43
Siegel R et al. CA Cancer J Clin 2020;70:7–30
Surveillance, Epidemiology and End Results (SEER) Program, available from http://seer.cancer.gov (accessed in 2020)

Work-up

- H&P
- CBC and leukocyte differential counts, platelets, electrolytes, liver function tests, PT, PTT, INR, fibrinogen, LDH, uric acid
- Bone marrow biopsy with cytogenetics (karyotype and FISH), immunophenotyping, and molecular studies (including c-KIT, FLT3 [ITD and TDK], NPM1, CEBPA [biallelic], IDH1, IDH2, TP53)
- HLA typing for patients who are candidates for allogeneic hematopoietic stem cell transplantation
- Chest x-ray and CT/MRI scans if clinically indicated to rule out infection or myeloid sarcoma
- Echocardiogram if therapy with anthracycline is planned, especially if prior cardiac history or prior anthracycline use
- Lumbar puncture if neurologic symptoms (LP should be performed if a mass/lesion is not detected on imaging studies)

Pathology

WHO Classification of Acute Myeloid Leukemia

1. **AML with recurrent genetic abnormalities**
   - AML with t(8;21)(q22;q22) (RUNX1-RUNX1T1)
   - AML with inv(16)(p13.1q22) or t(16;16)(p13.1;q22) (CBFB-MYH11)
   - Acute promyelocytic leukemia with *PML-RARA*
   - AML with t(9;11)(p21.3;q23.3); MLLT3-KMT2A
   - AML with t(6;9)(p23;q34.1); DEK-NUP214
   - AML with inv(3)(q21q26.2) or t(3;3) (q21.3;q26.2); GATA2, MECOM (EVI1)
   - AML (megakaryoblastic) with t(1;22) (p13.3;q13.3); RBM15-MKL1
   - *Provisional entity: AML with BCR-ABL1*
   - AML with mutated NPM1
   - AML with biallelic mutations of CEBPA
   - *Provision entity: AML with mutated RUNX1*
2. **AML with MDS-related changes**
3. **Therapy-related myeloid neoplasms**
4. **AML not otherwise specified**
   - AML minimal with differentiation
   - AML without maturation
   - AML with maturation
   - Acute myelomonocytic leukemia
   - Acute monoblastic/monocytic leukemia
   - Pure erythroid leukemia
   - Acute megakaryoblastic leukemia
   - Acute basophilic leukemia
   - Acute panmyelosis with myelofibrosis
5. **Myeloid sarcoma**
6. **Myeloid proliferation related to Down syndrome**
   - Transient abnormal myelopoiesis (TAM)
   - Myeloid leukemia associated with Down syndrome

(continued)

Response Criteria for Acute Myeloid Leukemia

Morphologic leukemia-free state
Bone marrow <5% blasts in an aspirate with spicules
No blasts or Auer rods or persistence of extramedullary disease; no hematologic recovery required

Complete remission (CR)
Patient achieves a morphologic leukemia-free state, *and*
Absolute neutrophil count >1000/mm^3
Platelets ≥100,000/mm^3
No residual evidence of extramedullary disease

CR with incomplete hematologic recovery (CR$_i$)—All CR criteria except for residual neutropenia (ANC <1000/mm^3) or thrombocytopenia (platelet count <100,000/mm^3)

CR without minimal residual disease (C$_{MRD-}$)—All CR criteria met and also negative for a genetic marker by RT-qPCR (if studied pretreatment) or negative by multiparameter flow cytometry

Partial remission (PR): All hematologic criteria of CR; decrease of bone marrow blast percentage to 5% to 25%; and decrease of pretreatment bone marrow blast percentage by at least 50%

Hematologic relapse—reappearance of leukemic blasts in the peripheral blood or the finding of >5% blasts in the bone marrow; or the development of extramedullary disease following CR, CR$_i$, or CR$_{MRD-}$

Molecular relapse—if studied pretreatment, reoccurrence of minimal residual disease as assessed by RT-qPCR or by multiparameter flow cytometry

Döhner H et al. Blood 2017;129:424–447

Risk Stratification

Risk Category	Genetic Abnormality
Favorable	t(8;21)(q22;q22.1); *RUNX1-RUNX1T1*
	inv(16)(p13.1q22) or t(16;16)(p13.1;q22); *CBFB-MYH11*
	Mutated NPM1 without *FLT3*-ITD or with *FLT3*-ITD^{low*}
	Biallelic mutated *CEBPA*
Intermediate	Mutated *NPM1* and *FLT3*-ITD^{high*}
	Wild-type *NPM1* without *FLT3*-ITD or with *FLT3*-ITD^{low*} (without adverse-risk genetic lesions)
	t(9;11)(p21.3;q23.3); *MLLT3-KMT2A*†
	Cytogenetic abnormalities not classified as favorable or adverse
Adverse	t(6;9)(p23;q34.1); *DEK-NUP214*
	t(v;11q23.3); *KMT2A* rearranged
	t(9;22)(q34.1;q11.2); *BCR-ABL1*
	inv(3)(q21.3q26.2) or t(3;3)(q21.3;q26.2); *GATA2, MECOM(EVI1)*
	−5 or del(5q); −7; −17/abn(17p)
	Complex karyotype‡, monosomal karyotype§
	Wild-type *NPM1* and *FLT3*-ITD^{high*}
	Mutated *RUNX1*$^|$
	Mutated *ASXL1*$^|$
	Mutated *TP53*$^\epsilon$

*Low, low allelic ratio (<0.5); high, high allelic ratio (≥0.5)
†Presence of t(9;11) (p21.3;q23.3) takes precedence over rare, concurrent adverse-risk gene mutations
‡Three or more unrelated chromosome abnormalities in the absence of 1 of the WHO-designated recurring translocations or inversions, that is t(8;21), inv(16) or t(16;16), t(9;11), t(v;11)(v;q23.3), t(6;9), inv(3) or t(3;3); AML with *BCR-ABL1*
§Defined as the presence of 1 single monosomy (excluding loss of X or Y) in associated with at least 1 additional monosomy or structure chromosome abnormalities (excluding core-binding factor AML)
$^|$These markers should not be used as an adverse prognostic marker if they co-occur with favorable-risk AML subtypes
$^\epsilon$TP53 mutations are significantly associated with AML with complex and monosomal karyotype
Döhner H et al. Blood 2017;129:424–447

Pathology (*continued*)

Blastic plasmacytoid dendritic cell neoplasms

Acute leukemias of ambiguous lineage
- Acute undifferentiated leukemia
- Mixed phenotype acute leukemia with t(9;22)(q34.1;q11.2); BCR-ABL1
- Mixed phenotype acute leukemia with t(v;11q23.3); KMT2A rearranged
- Mixed phenotype acute leukemia, B/myeloid, not otherwise specified
- Mixed phenotype acute leukemia, T/myeloid, not otherwise specified

Myeloid neoplasms with germ-line predisposition without a pre-existing disorder or organ dysfunction
- AML with germ line *CEBPA* mutation
- Myeloid neoplasms with germ line *DDX41* mutation

Myeloid neoplasms with germ line predisposition and pre-existing platelet disorders
- Myeloid neoplasms with germ line *RUNX1* mutation
- Myeloid neoplasms with germ line *ANKRD26* mutation
- Myeloid neoplasms with germ line *ETV6* mutation

Myeloid neoplasms with germ line predisposition and other organ dysfunction
- Myeloid neoplasms with germ line *GATA2* mutation
- Myeloid neoplasms associated with bone marrow failure syndromes
- Juvenile myelomonocytic leukemia associated with neurofibromatosis, Noonan syndrome, or Noonan syndrome–like disorders
- Myeloid neoplasms associated with Noonan syndrome
- Myeloid neoplasms associated with Down syndrome

Arber DA et al. Acute myeloid leukaemia with recurrent genetic abnormalities. In: Swerdlow S et al. editors. World Health Organization Classification of Tumours of Haematopoietic and Lymphoid Tissues. Update to 4th Edition. Lyon, France: World Health Organization; in press

Peterson L et al. Myeloid neoplasms with germline predisposition. In: Swerdlow S et al. editors. World Health Organization Classification of Tumours of Haematopoietic and Lymphoid Tissues. Update to 4th Edition. Lyon, France: World Health Organization; in press

Arber DA et al. Blood 2016;127:2391–2405

Expert Opinion

Initial work-up for AML requires pre-treatment evaluation for appropriate risk stratification. Guidance from the recently updated WHO and ELN classifications incorporating cytogenetic and molecular data can allow for stratification into favorable, intermediate, and unfavorable risk of disease

New drug approvals for AML have led to a change in the landscape for the treatment of AML. Initial therapy for AML should be based on several factors including patient's performance status, age, comorbidities, cytogenetics, and molecular abnormalities

Induction chemotherapy should be considered in young patients with good performance status and patients eligible for allogeneic cell transplantation (allo-HCT). An anthracycline combined with cytarabine is a common initial induction chemotherapy regimen. A higher dose of daunorubicin has been shown to improve survival compared with a lower dose of daunorubicin (45 mg/m^2). Gemtuzumab ozogamicin should be combined with an anthracycline + cytarabine induction regimen in patients with core-binding factor leukemia (t 8;21, inv 16). The addition of gemtuzumab ozogamicin to the induction regimen leads to improvement in overall survival. Patients with FLT–3 ITD/TDK mutations should receive an FLT–3 inhibitor with initial induction chemotherapy. Midostaurin combined with daunorubicin and cytarabine has been approved for FLT+3 leukemia. Patients with therapy-related acute myeloid leukemia (t-AML) or AML with myelodysplasia-related changes can also be treated with CPX–351, a liposomal combination of daunorubicin and cytarabine

Bone marrow biopsy/aspirate should be performed 7–10 days after completion of induction therapy with anthracycline + cytarabine. If midostaurin is added to the initial induction regimen, a bone marrow biopsy is performed on day 21 after therapy was started. If the bone marrow is hypoplastic (defined as cellularity <10–20% and residual blasts <5–10%), a repeated bone marrow biopsy should be performed until count recovery when the remission status can be assessed. If the bone marrow has residual blasts, then a second course of therapy can be administered; this can be identical to the first induction course, escalation to high-dose cytarabine, or non–cross-resistant antileukemic regimens (eg, mitoxantrone and etoposide)

Clinical trial enrollment should be considered for patients with primary refractory AML. Young patients with primary refractory AML with no significant co-morbidities and adequate organ function should be evaluated for allogeneic hematopoietic transplantation (allo-HCT). The 3-year overall survival for primary refractory AML following allo-HCT is 19% and the mortality rate at 100 days after transplantation is 39%

For older patients or patients not eligible for induction chemotherapy, a combination of venetoclax with a hypomethylating agent, ozogamicin gemtuzumab, a combination of venetoclax with low-dose cytarabine, IDH inhibitor (ivosidenib), or hedgehog pathway inhibitor (glasdegib) combined with low-dose cytarabine are treatment options. Combining these targeted agents may prove to improve CR rates and overall survival.

Patients in first relapse after a CR duration >6–12 months can be retreated with either the induction regimen they last received or a high-dose cytarabine-containing regimen; after a second CR, patients should be considered for an allo-HCT. For patients in first relapse after a short CR duration (<6 months), a non-cross-resistant antileukemic regimen should be used, and after a second CR, patients should be considered for an allo-HCT

Relapsed AML patients not eligible for re-induction therapy can be treated with enasidenib (IDH2 mutated), ivosidenib (IDH1 mutated), gilteritinib (FLT-3 mutated), hypomethylating agents, or low-dose cytarabine.

The choice of post-remission therapy must be determined by the prognostic group and, most importantly, the cytogenetics/molecular studies at presentation. In patients with favorable cytogenetics/molecular studies, intensive post-remission therapy with cytarabine should be administered. Midostaurin has been approved with cytarabine in FLT-3 AML during consolidation. Allo-HCT should be performed in high-risk AML patients and should be considered in patients with intermediate risk. There is no added benefit to receiving additional high-dose post-remission therapy prior to allo-HCT if there is no delay in the HCT

The role of maintenance therapy after consolidation therapy with hypomethylating agents or FLT–3 inhibitors is under investigation

Acute promyelocytic leukemia (APL)

- APL is a medical emergency primarily because of bleeding, which continues to represent a major cause of early death. Once a diagnosis is suspected on the basis of clinical findings and the peripheral blood smear (even without waiting for a bone marrow examination), and before the diagnosis is confirmed by molecular studies, tretinoin (all *trans*-retinoic acid; ATRA) should be given emergently, both to resolve the coagulopathy and to initiate induction therapy. Patients with WBC >10,000/mm³ at presentation are considered at high risk

- Induction therapy for APL: a combination of ATRA + arsenic trioxide (ATO) has provided the opportunity to minimize and even eliminate standard cytotoxic chemotherapy from initial treatment regimens without compromising the excellent outcomes achieved by anthracycline-containing protocols. For low-risk APL (WBC <10,000/mm³ at presentation), patients should be treated with induction therapy with ATRA + ATO. For high-risk APL, patients can be treated with different induction regimens including ATRA + ATO + GO, ATRA plus daunorubicin and cytarabine, and ATRA + idarubicin. A bone marrow biopsy should be performed after peripheral blood counts recover from induction therapy to determine whether a CR by morphology has been achieved. Cytogenetic analysis is usually normal, but molecular remission is achieved after at least two cycles of consolidation therapy

- Consolidation therapy: The goal of consolidation therapy for APL is the conversion of a morphologic and cytogenetic remission into a durable molecular remission. The choice of regimen should be influenced by risk group, age, and cardiovascular risk. Patients should be treated according to regimens established from large clinical trials, and one should use a regimen consistently through all components, not mixing induction from one trial with consolidation from a different trial

- Maintenance therapy: ATRA combined with mercaptopurine + methotrexate has been used as maintenance therapy, which continues for 1–2 years. The addition of ATRA to maintenance therapy improved disease-free survival and relapse rates

(continued)

Expert Opinion (continued)

- Relapsed APL: Therapy depends on the timing of relapse and prior therapies. For patients who relapse early (<6 months of initial CR) from first-line therapy with ATRA + ATO, an anthracycline-based regimen should be considered. For patients who relapse early from ATRA + anthracycline-based regimen, patients can be treated with ATO ± ATRA ± GO. For patients with late relapse ATO ± ATRA ± anthracycline or GO should be considered

CNS Leukemia

- Leptomeningeal involvement is much less frequent (<5%) in AML than in ALL; thus, routine lumbar puncture is not recommended during routine diagnostic work-up. However, if neurologic symptoms are present at diagnosis, an initial MRI/CT should first be performed to rule out bleeding or mass effect. If the lumbar puncture is positive, intrathecal chemotherapy with cytarabine (cytarabine 100 mg [fixed dose] in 3–12 mL preservative-free 0.9% sodium chloride injection) alternating with methotrexate (methotrexate 12 mg [fixed dose] in 3–12 mL preservative-free 0.9% sodium chloride injection) is recommended, concurrent with induction chemotherapy. Intrathecal chemotherapy is given twice per week until cerebrospinal fluid cytology shows no blasts, and then weekly for 4–6 weeks. Screening for occult CNS should be considered for AML patients in remission with M4 or M5 morphology, biphenotypic leukemia, presence of myeloid sarcoma, or WBC >100,000/mm^3 at diagnosis

- For high-risk APL patients, intrathecal chemotherapy with cytarabine alternating with methotrexate 4–6 doses should be given during consolidation

Supportive Care

- **Hyperleukocytosis in AML**

- The frequency of hyperleukocytosis (conventionally and arbitrarily defined as a WBC count >100,000/mm^3) ranges from 5% to 13% in adult patients with AML. Symptoms may arise from the involvement of any organ, but intracranial hemorrhages and respiratory failure account for the majority of deaths. In many patients, leukostasis becomes evident a few days after diagnosis, and sometimes after the first leukocytoreduction. Clinical deterioration and death may occur after the blast count has been significantly reduced, which suggests that although leukocytoreduction is an important step in the management of leukostasis, additional measures are needed to prevent leukostasis-related deaths. Leukocytoreduction can be achieved with the use of hydroxyurea. Hydroxyurea can be given at dosages up to 50–60 mg/kg per day orally

- Leukapheresis is also an option for the initial management of hyperleukocytosis. The disadvantage of leukapheresis is that it requires the placement of a large-caliber central venous catheter in patients who may be thrombocytopenic and coagulopathic, and it may also worsen their thrombocytopenia. There are no guidelines that identify the absolute WBC count to be achieved by leukapheresis that correlates with reversal of the signs and symptoms of leukostasis.

Coagulopathy in APL

- For patients with clinical coagulopathy, provide platelet transfusion to maintain a platelet count of 50,000/μL, fibrinogen replacement with cryoprecipitate/fresh-frozen plasma to maintain a level >150 mg/dL, and maintenance of normal prothrombin and partial thromboplastin times

Differentiation syndrome in APL

- Patients who develop differentiation syndrome should be treated with dexamethasone 10 mg twice a day for 3–5 days. ATRA may need to be withheld and restarted once symptoms of differentiation syndrome improve

Abaza Y et al. Blood 2017;129:1275–1283
Amadori S et al. J Clin Oncol 2016;34:972–979
Castaigne S et al. Lancet 2012;379:1508–1516
Coco F et al. N Engl J Med 2016;374:1197–1198
Cortes JE et al. Leukemia 2019;33:379–389
DiNardo CD et al. Blood 2019;133:7–17
DiNardo CD et al. N Engl J Med 2018;378:2386–2398
Döhner H et al. N Engl J Med 2015;373:1136–1152
Duval et al. J Clin Oncol 2010;28:3730–3738
Fernandez HF et al. N Engl J Med 2009;361:1249–1259
Hills RK et al. Lancet Oncol 2014;115:986–996
Lancet JE et al. J Clin Oncol 2018;36:2684–2692
Mayer RJ et al. N Engl J Med 1994;331:896–903
Perl AE et al. N Engl J Med 2019;381:1728–1740
Roboz GJ et al. Blood 2020;135:463–471
Sanz MA et al. Blood 2019;133:1630–1643
Stein EM et al. Blood 2019;133:676–687
Soignet SL et al. J Clin Oncol 2001;19:3852–3860
Stone RM et al. N Engl J Med 2017;377:454–464
Taksin AL et al. Leukemia 2007;21:66–71
Vogler WR et al. J Clin Oncol 1992;10:1103–1111
Wei A et al. J Clin Oncol. 2019;37:1277–1284

PROPHYLAXIS AGAINST TUMOR LYSIS SYNDROME
HYDRATION + URINARY ALKALINIZATION + ADMINISTRATION OF ALLOPURINOL

Hydration with 2500–3000 mL/m^2 per day as tolerated; administer intravenously to maintain urine output ≥100 mL/hour (or ≥2 mL/kg per hour in persons whose body weight is <50 kg)

Urinary alkalinization with sodium bicarbonate injection added to intravenously administered fluids

- The amount of sodium bicarbonate added to intravenously administered fluids should produce a solution with sodium content not greater than the concentration of sodium in 0.9% sodium chloride injection (≤154 mEq/L):

Sodium Bicarbonate Is Added to a Solution to Increase Urine pH Within a Range of 6.0 to ≤7

Base Solution Sodium Content	Sodium Bicarbonate Additive	Total Sodium Content
0.45% Sodium Chloride Injection (0.45% NS)		
77 mEq/L	50–75 mEq	127–152 mEq/L
0.2% Sodium Chloride Injection (0.2% NS)		
34 mEq/L	100–125 mEq	134–159 mEq/L
5% Dextrose Injection (D5W)		
0	125–150 mEq	125–150 mEq/L
D5W/0.45% NS		
77 mEq/L	50–75 mEq	127–152 mEq/L
D5W/0.2% NS		
34 mEq/L	100–125 mEq	134–159 mEq/L

Notes:
- Hydration rate may be decreased at the completion of chemotherapy administration
- Urinary alkalization increases the solubility and excretion of uric acid and its oxypurine precursors (hypoxanthine and xanthine) and helps avoid uric acid crystallization in renal tubules; however, alkalinization is not uniformly recommended because:
  1. It favors precipitation of calcium/phosphate in renal tubules, a concern in patients with concomitant hyperphosphatemia
  2. A metabolic alkalemia may result from the administration of bicarbonate that can worsen the neurologic manifestations of hypocalcemia

Allopurinol
- Administer orally or intravenously starting 12 hours to 3 days (preferably 2–3 days) before starting cytoreductive chemotherapy
- Hyperuricemia develops within 24–48 hours after initiating chemotherapy when the excretory capacity of the renal tubules is exceeded
- In the presence of an acid pH, uric acid crystals form in the renal tubules, leading to intraluminal renal tubular obstruction, an acute renal obstructive uropathy, and renal dysfunction

Initial dosage
- Allopurinol 100 mg/m^2 per dose; administer orally every 8 hours (maximum daily dose = 800 mg), *or*
- Allopurinol 3.3 mg/kg per dose; administer orally every 8 hours (maximum daily dose = 800 mg), *or*
- Allopurinol 200–400 mg/m^2 per day; administer intravenously (maximum daily dose = 600 mg) in a volume of 5% dextrose injection or 0.9% sodium chloride injection sufficient to yield a concentration not greater than 6 mg/mL. The duration for administering individual doses should be informed by the volume to be given
  - Allopurinol may be administered as a single daily dose, or the total daily dose may be divided equally for administration at 6-, 8-, or 12-hour intervals
- **Maintenance doses** should be based on serum uric acid determinations performed approximately 48 hours after initiation of allopurinol therapy, and periodically thereafter
- Continue administering allopurinol until leukemic blasts have been cleared from the peripheral blood

(*continued*)

(*continued*)

Notes:

• Allopurinol dose adjustments for impaired renal function:

Creatinine Clearance	Oral Allopurinol Dose
10–20 mL/min (0.17–0.33 mL/s)	200 mg/day
3–10 mL/min (0.05–0.17 mL/s)	100 mg/day
<3 mL/min (<0.05 mL/s)	100 mg every 36–48 hours

• The incidence of allergic reactions is increased in patients receiving amoxicillin, ampicillin, or thiazide diuretics

Rasburicase is recombinant urate oxidase (uricase) produced by genetically modified *Saccharomyces cerevisiae* that express urate oxidase cDNA cloned from a strain of *Aspergillus flavus*

• Uricase enzymes catalyze uric acid oxidation to allantoin, which is at least 5 times more soluble than uric acid

Rasburicase should be considered among initial interventions against hyperuricemia in patients with high peripheral WBC counts, rapidly increasing blasts counts, high uric acid, or evidence of impaired renal function—that is:

WBC ≥100,000/mm³	
WBC ≥25,000 to <100,000/mm³ *or* WBC <25,000/mm³ + LDH ≥2× ULN	+ Acute kidney injury *or* + Normal renal function uric acid >ULN potassium or phosphorus >ULN

ULN, upper limit of normal

Rasburicase 0.2 mg/kg per dose intravenously in a total volume of 50 mL 0.9% sodium chloride injection over 30 minutes once daily for up to 5 consecutive days is often used, but much less is usually sufficient

• Rasburicase has demonstrated effectiveness in prophylaxis and treatment for hyperuricemia and acute increases in uric acid associated with cytoreductive therapies at dosages <0.2 mg/kg based on body weight, with fixed doses, and after administration of from 1–3 doses

Cairo MS et al. Br J Haematol 2010;149:578–586
Coiffier B et al. J Clin Oncol 2008;26:2767–2778
Döhner H et al. Blood 2010;115:453–474
Döhner H, Gaidzik VI. Hematology Am Soc Hematol Educ Program 2011;2011:36–42
O'Donnell MR et al. J Natl Compr Canc Netw 2011;9:280–317
Rowe JM, Tallman MS. Blood 2010;116:3147–3156
Sanz MA et al. Blood 2009;113:1875–1891
Tallman MS, Altman JK. Blood 2009;114:5126–5135

INTENSIVE INDUCTION THERAPY • FIRST-LINE

ACUTE MYELOID LEUKEMIA REGIMEN: CYTARABINE + DAUNORUBICIN

Fernandez HF et al. N Engl J Med 2009;361:1249–1259

Cytarabine 100 mg/m^2 per day; administer by continuous intravenous infusion in 100–1000 mL 0.9% sodium chloride injection or 5% dextrose injection over 24 hours for 7 consecutive days on days 1–7 (total dosage/cycle = 700 mg/m^2)

Daunorubicin 60–90 mg/m^2 per day; administer by intravenous injection over 3–5 minutes for 3 consecutive days on days 1–3 (total dosage/cycle = 180–270 mg/m^2)

Supportive Care
Antiemetic prophylaxis
Emetogenic potential on days 1–3 is **MODERATE**
Emetogenic potential on days 4–7 is **LOW**
See Chapter 42 for antiemetic recommendations

Hematopoietic growth factor (CSF) should be considered in patients with severe infection or in elderly patients or in patients with slow bone marrow recovery. Begin use after bone marrow aplasia is confirmed and continue use until ANC recovers

Primary prophylaxis is indicated with one of the following:
   Filgrastim (G-CSF) 5 mcg/kg per day; administer by subcutaneous injection, *or*
   Sargramostim (GM-CSF) 250 mcg/m^2 per day; administer by subcutaneous injection
See Chapter 43 for more information

Antimicrobial prophylaxis
Risk of fever and neutropenia is **HIGH**
   Antimicrobial primary prophylaxis is recommended:
   • Antibacterial—consider prophylaxis with a fluoroquinolone during periods of prolonged neutropenia only (eg, ANC <500/mm^3 for ≥7 days) until ANC recovery
   • Antifungal—consider prophylaxis with posaconazole or another antifungal medication during periods of prolonged neutropenia only (eg, <500/mm^3 for ≥7 days) until ANC recovery
   • Antiviral—antiherpes antivirals (eg, acyclovir, famciclovir, valacyclovir)

Patient Population Studied

Study of 657 patients who had untreated AML (age 17–60 years) who were randomized to receive 3 once-daily doses of daunorubicin at either the standard dose (45 mg/m^2 of body-surface area per day) or a high dose (90 mg/m^2 per day), combined with 7 daily doses of cytarabine 100 mg/m^2 per day by continuous intravenous infusion

Efficacy

Induction therapy: 57% in the standard-dose group vs 71% in the high-dose group
In the standard-dose group, patients younger than the age of 50 years had a CR of 59.4% in comparison with CR of 74.3% in the high-dose group
High-dose daunorubicin (90 mg/m^2 per day) did not provide benefit in patients older than 50 years or those with unfavorable cytogenetic profile
The median overall survival was 15.7 months in the standard-dose group and 23.7 months in the high-dose group

Toxicity

Adverse Events	Standard Dose (45 mg/m^2 per Day) n = 318		High Dose (90 mg/m^2 per Day) n = 315	
	G3	**G4**	**G3**	**G4**
Low hemoglobin	67	11	63	13
Low Blood Count				
Leukocytes	2	95	<1	98
Neutrophils	3	93	18	80
Platelets	16	81	18	80
Transfusions Required				
Platelets	55	5	57	6
PRBC	59	1	59	<1
Fatigue	5	<1	3	3
Fever	5	1	5	3
Rash or desquamation	5	<1	5	0
Anorexia	4	4	5	5
Nausea	6	<1	5	0
Hemorrhage with G3/4 low platelet count	8	1	10	1
Febrile neutropenia	32	3	31	4
Infection with G3/4 neutropenia	40	7	39	<1
Dyspnea	4	2	<1	3
Cardiac event*	5	2	4	3

*A reduced left ventricular ejection fraction was reported in none of 318 patients in the standard group and in 4 of 315 patients in the high-dose group

Note: The death rates during induction therapy were 4.5% in the standard-dose group and 5.5% in the high-dose group (P = 0.60). Causes of death were infection (14 patients), pulmonary failure (6 patients), cardiac failure (4 patients), hemorrhage (3 patients), hypotension (2 patients), and ileus (1 patient)

Treatment Modifications

Adverse Events	Treatment Modifications
Creatinine >3 mg/dL (>265 μmol/L)	Reduce daunorubicin dosage by 50%
Total bilirubin 2.5–5 mg/dL (42.8–85.5 μmol/L)	
Total bilirubin >5 mg/dL (>85.5 μmol/L)	Hold daunorubicin

Therapy Monitoring

1. CBC with differential daily during induction chemotherapy and following therapy until neutrophil recovery (>500/mm^3) and patients achieve independence from platelet transfusions
2. *Pretreatment evaluation:* determination of LVEF by echocardiogram
3. Electrolytes, mineral panel, liver function tests daily, and uric acid at least daily during active treatment until risk of tumor lysis is past
4. Bone marrow aspirate/biopsy 7–10 days after chemotherapy is completed

INTENSIVE INDUCTION THERAPY • FIRST-LINE

ACUTE MYELOID LEUKEMIA REGIMEN: CYTARABINE + IDARUBICIN

Vogler WR et al. J Clin Oncol 1992;10:1103–1111

Cytarabine 100 mg/m^2 per day; administer by continuous intravenous infusion in 100–1000 mL 0.9% sodium chloride injection (0.9% NS) or 5% dextrose injection (D5W) over 24 hours for 7 consecutive days, on days 1–7 (total dosage/cycle = 700 mg/m^2)

Idarubicin 12 mg/m^2 per day; administer intravenously diluted to a concentration >0.01 mg/mL with 0.9% NS or D5W over 15–30 minutes for 3 consecutive days, on days 1–3 (total dosage/cycle = 36 mg/m^2)

Supportive Care
Antiemetic prophylaxis
Emetogenic potential on Days 1–3 is **MODERATE**
Emetogenic potential on Days 4–7 is **LOW**
See Chapter 42 for antiemetic recommendations

Hematopoietic growth factor (CSF) should be considered in patients with severe infection or in elderly patients or in patients with slow bone marrow recovery. Begin use after bone marrow aplasia is confirmed and continue use until ANC recovers

Primary prophylaxis is indicated with one of the following:
   Filgrastim (G-CSF) 5 mcg/kg per day by subcutaneous injection, *or*
   Sargramostim (GM-CSF) 250 mcg/m^2 per day by subcutaneous injection
See Chapter 43 for more information

Antimicrobial prophylaxis
Risk of fever and neutropenia is **HIGH**
   Antimicrobial primary prophylaxis is recommended:
- Antibacterial—consider prophylaxis with a fluoroquinolone during periods of prolonged neutropenia only (eg, ANC <500/mm^3 for ≥7 days) until ANC recovery
- Antifungal—consider prophylaxis with posaconazole or another antifungal medication during periods of prolonged neutropenia only (eg, <500/mm^3 for ≥7 days) until ANC recovery
- Antiviral—antiherpes antivirals (eg, acyclovir, famciclovir, valacyclovir)

Patient Population Studied

Study of 111 patients (median age: 60 years) with newly diagnosed AML

Efficacy (N = 105)

Response by Age Group

Ages		
	15–50 years (N = 29):	86%
	51–60 years (N = 24):	71%
	>60 years (N = 52):	63%

Induction CR: 69%
Number in CR with 1 course: 77 %
Median time to CR: 42 days

Toxicity (N = 105)

Adverse Events	G1/2 %	G3/4 %
Nausea and vomiting	76	6
Diarrhea	57	16
Mucositis	43	7
Total bilirubin	36	9
SGOT (AST)	47	5
Alkaline phosphatase	52	5
Creatinine	29	2
Skin rash	41	5
Cardiac	5	11
Hair loss	37	40

	Mean Duration of Aplasia (Days)
WBC <1000/mm^3	31.2
Platelets <50,000/mm^3	35.1

Therapy Monitoring

1. CBC with differential daily during induction chemotherapy and following therapy until neutrophil recovery (>500/mm^3), and until patients achieve independence from platelet transfusions
2. *Pretreatment evaluation:* determination of LVEF by echocardiogram
3. Electrolytes, mineral panel, liver function tests daily, and uric acid at least daily during active treatment until risk of tumor lysis is past
4. Bone marrow aspirate/biopsy 7–10 days after chemotherapy is completed

Treatment Modifications

Adverse Events	Treatment Modifications
Creatinine >3 mg/dL (>265 µmol/L)	Reduce idarubicin dosage by 50%
Total bilirubin 2.6–5 mg/dL (44.5–85.5 µmol/L)	Reduce idarubicin dosage by 50%
Total bilirubin >5 mg/dL (>85.5 µmol/L)	Hold idarubicin

INTENSIVE POST-REMISSION THERAPY

ACUTE MYELOID LEUKEMIA REGIMEN: HIGH-DOSE CYTARABINE

Mayer RJ et al. N Engl J Med 1994;331:896–903

Cytarabine 3000 mg/m² per dose; administer intravenously in 100–1000 mL 0.9% sodium chloride injection or 5% dextrose injection over 3 hours, every 12 hours for 6 doses (2 doses/day) on days 1, 3, and 5, every 28 days for 4 cycles (total dosage/cycle = 18,000 mg/m²)

Notes: Repeated cycles were initiated no sooner than 28 days after a previously administered cycle, or 1 week after patients achieved postnadir ANC >1500/mm³ and platelet counts >100,000/mm³, with the expectation the maximal interval between consecutive cycles would be ≤35 days

Supportive Care
Antiemetic prophylaxis
Emetogenic potential on days of treatment is **MODERATE–HIGH**
See Chapter 42 for antiemetic recommendations

Hematopoietic growth factor (CSF) prophylaxis
Primary prophylaxis with one of the following may be indicated in patients who have a documented complete remission with infection, in elderly patients, or in patients with a history of slow bone marrow recovery:
Filgrastim (G-CSF) 5 mcg/kg per day by subcutaneous injection, *or*
Pegfilgrastim (pegylated filgrastim) 6 mg/0.6 mL, by subcutaneous injection for one dose
- Begin use from 24–72 h after myelosuppressive chemotherapy is completed
- Continue daily filgrastim use until ANC ≥5000/mm³ after the leukocyte nadir
- Discontinue daily filgrastim use at least 24 hours before administering myelosuppressive treatment. Do not administer pegfilgrastim within 14 days before administering myelosuppressive treatment

See Chapter 43 for more information

Antimicrobial prophylaxis
Risk of fever and neutropenia is **HIGH**
  Antimicrobial primary prophylaxis is recommended:
- Antibacterial—consider prophylaxis with a fluoroquinolone during periods of prolonged neutropenia only (eg, ANC <500/mm³ for ≥7 days) until ANC recovery
- Antifungal—consider prophylaxis with fluconazole or another azole antifungal during periods of prolonged neutropenia only (eg, <500/mm³ for ≥7 days) until ANC recovery
- Antiviral—antiherpes antivirals (eg, acyclovir, famciclovir, valacyclovir)

Keratitis prophylaxis
Steroid ophthalmic drops (prednisolone 1% or dexamethasone 0.1%); administer 2 drops by intraocular instillation into each eye every 6 hours starting prior to the first cytarabine dose and continuing until 48 hours after each course of high-dose cytarabine is completed

Treatment Modifications

Adverse Events	Treatment Modifications	
Neurologic toxicity	Hold cytarabine. Patients who develop CNS symptoms should not receive subsequent high-dose cytarabine	
The risk of neurotoxicity with high-dose cytarabine therapy is directly related to renal function throughout therapy	**Serum Creatinine**	**Cytarabine Dosage**
	<1.5 mg/dL (<133 µmol/L)	2000 mg/m²
	1.5–1.9 mg/dL (133–168 µmol/L), or an increase from baseline by 0.5–1.2 mg/dL (44–106 µmol/L)	1000 mg/m²
	≥2 mg/dL (≥177 µmol/L), or an increase of >1.2 mg/dL (>106 µmol/L)	100 mg/m² per day by continuous intravenous infusion over 24 hours for up to 6 days
In patients exhibiting rapidly rising creatinine as a result of tumor lysis	Hold cytarabine	

Patient Population Studied

Study of 596 patients in CR after induction chemotherapy (daunorubicin + cytarabine) who were randomly assigned to receive 4 cycles of cytarabine on one of three 5-day dosage schedules: low-dose or moderate-dose cytarabine administered by continuous intravenous infusion, or high-dose cytarabine administered intravenously intermittently

Efficacy

The likelihood of remaining alive and disease-free (DFS) after 4 years was 21% among subjects who received low-dose continuous infusion cytarabine, 25% in the moderate-dose group, and 39% among those who received high-dose cytarabine
The probability of remaining alive (survival) for 4 years after randomization was 31% for the group assigned to receive low-dose continuous infusion cytarabine, 35% for the group assigned to receive moderate-dose intermittent infusions, and 46% among patient who received high-dose cytarabine
The probability of remaining in continuous complete remission after 4 years among patients ≤60 years of age was 24% in the low-dose group, 29% in the moderate-dose group, and 44% in the high-dose group
In contrast, for patients older than 60 years of age, the probability of remaining disease-free after 4 years was ≤16% in each group
Subsequent analysis showed a disease-free survival rate of 60% for patients with good-risk cytogenetics, 30% with intermediate-risk cytogenetics, and 12% with poor-risk cytogenetics in patients who received high-dose cytarabine

Bloomfield CD et al. Cancer Res 1998;58:4173–4179

Toxicity

% of Patients Who Received 4 Planned Cycles	Cytarabine Regimens		
	LD CIVI	MD CIVI	High-Dose
All patients	76%	74%	56%
Patients aged ≤60 years	78%	76%	62%

Cytarabine Regimens	Cycles During Which Patients Were Hospitalized	Serious CNS Toxicity	Deaths During Remission
LD CIVI	16%	0	1%
MD CIVI	59%	0	6%
High-Dose	71%	12%	5%

LD CIVI, cytarabine 100 mg/m² per day by continuous intravenous infusion over 24 hours for 5 consecutive days on days 1–5; MD CIVI, cytarabine 400 mg/m² per day by continuous intravenous infusion over 24 hours for 5 consecutive days on days 1–5; High-Dose, 3000 mg/m² per dose by intravenous infusion over 3 hours, twice daily on days 1, 3, and 5, for 6 doses

Therapy Monitoring

1. CBC with differential and platelet counts daily during chemotherapy; electrolytes, LFTs, and mineral panel, daily during chemotherapy
2. *Outpatient monitoring postchemotherapy:* CBC with differential, platelets, and electrolytes, 2–3 times weekly until counts recovery
3. *Between cycles:* Bone marrow biopsy/ aspirate if peripheral blood counts are abnormal, or patients' failure to recover counts after therapy. Bone marrow biopsy after recovery of counts following the last course of therapy

Notes:
1. This trial of postremission therapy for AML demonstrated a significant dose–response effect for cytarabine. Patients 60 years of age or younger who received high-dose cytarabine were more likely to remain in remission and to survive longer than patients in the same age group who received lower doses. Serious CNS abnormalities were reported only in the group given high-dose cytarabine, and they were especially common in patients older than 60 years of age
2. Patients who receive high-dose cytarabine need to be closely monitored for changes in renal function. Renal dysfunction is highly correlated with an increased risk of cerebellar toxicity. Patients need to be monitored for nystagmus, dysmetria, and ataxia before each dose of cytarabine

INTENSIVE INDUCTION THERAPY AND POST-REMISSION THERAPY • FIRST-LINE

ACUTE MYELOID LEUKEMIA REGIMEN: DAUNORUBICIN + CYTARABINE + GEMTUZUMAB OZOGAMICIN

Castaigne S et al. Lancet 2012;379:1508–1516
Supplementary appendix to: Castaigne S et al. Lancet 2012;379:1508–1516
Hills RK et al. Lancet Oncol 2014;115:986–996
Supplementary appendix to: Hills RK et al. Lancet Oncol 2014;115:986–996
MYLOTARG (gemtuzumab ozogamicin) prescribing information. Philadelphia, PA: Wyeth Pharmaceuticals Inc; 2018 April

Induction, course 1: daunorubicin, cytarabine, and gemtuzumab ozogamicin
Premedications for each dose of gemtuzumab ozogamicin:

- **Methylprednisolone** 1 mg/kg per dose; administer intravenously 30 minutes prior to each gemtuzumab ozogamicin dose on days 1, 4, and 7, *plus:*

- **Acetaminophen** 650 mg per dose; administer orally 1 hour prior to each gemtuzumab ozogamicin dose on days 1, 4, and 7, *plus:*

- **Diphenhydramine** 50 mg per dose; administer orally or intravenously 1 hour prior to each gemtuzumab ozogamicin dose on days 1, 4, and 7

Gemtuzumab ozogamicin 3 mg/m^2 (maximum dose 4.5 mg) per dose; administer intravenously over 2 hours in a volume of 0.9% sodium chloride (0.9% NS) sufficient to produce a gemtuzumab ozogamicin concentration within the range 0.075–0.234 mg/mL, for 3 doses on days 1, 4, and 7 (total dosage/first induction course = 9 mg/m^2; maximum total dosage/first induction course = 13.5 mg)
Notes:

- Administer gemtuzumab ozogamicin with an administration set that contains an in-line polyethersulfone filter with pore size of 0.2 μm. Protect the infusion bag or syringe from light using a light-blocking cover during infusion

- Consider cytoreduction (eg, with hydroxyurea) in patients with WBC ≥30,000/mm^3 prior to gemtuzumab ozogamicin administration

- Although the report by Castaigne et al. states that each dose of gemtuzumab ozogamicin was not to exceed 5 mg, the U.S. Food and Drug Administration–approved prescribing information states that the maximum dose of gemtuzumab ozogamicin when used in combination with daunorubicin and cytarabine is 4.5 mg, which corresponds to the available vial size

- Doses <3.9 mg must be prepared and administered in a syringe. Doses ≥3.9 mg may be prepared and administered in either a syringe or an infusion bag

- Life-threatening and/or fatal infusion-related reactions consisting of chills, fever, tachycardia, hypotension, hypoxia, respiratory failure, and/or bronchospasm may occur infrequently, up to 24 hours following infusion of gemtuzumab ozogamicin. See therapy monitoring and therapy modification sections for further details

Cytarabine 200 mg/m^2 per day; administer by continuous intravenous infusion in 100–1000 mL 0.9% NS or 5% dextrose injection (D5W) over 24 hours for 7 consecutive days on days 1–7 (total dosage/induction = 1400 mg/m^2)

Daunorubicin 60 mg/m^2 per dose; administer by intravenous injection over 3–5 minutes once daily for 3 consecutive days on days 1–3 (total dosage/induction = 180 mg/m^2)

Induction, course 2, if applicable: daunorubicin and cytarabine (administer only if persistent leukemic blasts >10% observed on day 15 bone marrow biopsy following initial induction)

Daunorubicin 60 mg/m^2 per dose; administer by intravenous injection over 3–5 minutes once daily for 2 consecutive days on days 1–2 (total dosage/induction course 2 = 120 mg/m^2)

Cytarabine 1000 mg/m^2 per dose; administer intravenously in 100–1000 mL 0.9% NS or D5W over 2 hours, every 12 hours, for 6 doses (2 doses/day) on days 1, 2, and 3 (total dosage/induction course 2 = 6000 mg/m^2)

Filgrastim 5 mcg/kg/dose; administer subcutaneously once daily, starting on day 4 twenty-four hours after completion of chemotherapy, until post-nadir absolute neutrophil count improves to ≥2000/mm^3
- *Note:* the report by Castaigne et al. indicates that lenograstim 263 mcg/dose may be used, if available

Keratitis prophylaxis
- Steroid ophthalmic drops (prednisolone 1% or dexamethasone 0.1%); administer 2 drops by intraocular instillation into each eye every 6 hours starting prior to the first cytarabine dose and continuing until 48 hours after high-dose cytarabine is completed

Consolidation daunorubicin, cytarabine, and gemtuzumab ozogamicin (administer to patients who achieve a complete remission [CR] or complete remission with residual thrombocytopenia [platelet count <100,000/mm^3]). Omit gemtuzumab ozogamicin from consolidation cycles if there was persistent thrombocytopenia (platelet count <100,000/mm^3) by day 45 of induction therapy

Consolidation, course 1 (begin upon hematologic recovery following induction therapy):

Daunorubicin 60 mg/m^2; administer by intravenous injection over 3–5 minutes once on day 1 (total dosage/first consolidation course = 60 mg/m^2)

Cytarabine 1000 mg/m^2 per dose; administer intravenously in 100–1000 mL 0.9% NS or D5W over 2 hours, every 12 hours, for 8 doses (2 doses/day) on days 1, 2, 3, and 4 (total dosage/first consolidation course = 8000 mg/m^2)

Keratitis prophylaxis
- Steroid ophthalmic drops (prednisolone 1% or dexamethasone 0.1%); administer 2 drops by intraocular instillation into each eye every 6 hours starting prior to the first cytarabine dose and continuing until 48 hours after high-dose cytarabine is completed

(continued)

(*continued*)

Premedications for gemtuzumab ozogamicin:
- **Methylprednisolone** 1 mg/kg; administer intravenously 30 minutes prior to gemtuzumab ozogamicin on day 1 *plus:*
- **Acetaminophen** 650 mg; administer orally 1 hour prior to gemtuzumab ozogamicin on day 1, *plus:*
- **Diphenhydramine** 50 mg; administer orally or intravenously 1 hour prior to gemtuzumab ozogamicin on day 1

Gemtuzumab ozogamicin 3 mg/m^2 (maximum dose 4.5 mg); administer intravenously over 2 hours in a volume of 0.9% NS sufficient to produce a gemtuzumab ozogamicin concentration within the range 0.075–0.234 mg/mL, once on day 1 (total dosage/first consolidation course = 3 mg/m^2; maximum total dosage/first consolidation course = 4.5 mg)

Notes:
- Omit gemtuzumab ozogamicin from consolidation cycles in patients with persistent thrombocytopenia (platelet count <100,000/mm^3) by day 45 from induction therapy
- Administer gemtuzumab ozogamicin with an administration set that contains an in-line polyethersulfone filter with pore size of 0.2 μm. Protect the infusion bag or syringe from light using a light-blocking cover during infusion
- Consider cytoreduction (eg, with hydroxyurea) in patients with WBC ≥30,000/mm^3 prior to gemtuzumab ozogamicin administration
- Although the report by Castaigne et al. states that each dose of gemtuzumab ozogamicin was not to exceed 5 mg, the U.S. Food and Drug Administration–approved prescribing information states that the maximum dose of gemtuzumab ozogamicin when used in combination with daunorubicin and cytarabine is 4.5 mg, which corresponds to the available vial size
- Doses <3.9 mg must be prepared and administered in a syringe. Doses ≥3.9 mg may be prepared and administered in either a syringe or an infusion bag

Consolidation, course 2 (begin upon hematologic recovery following consolidation course 1):

Daunorubicin 60 mg/m^2 per dose; administer by intravenous injection over 3–5 minutes once daily for 2 consecutive days on days 1–2 (total dosage/second consolidation course = 120 mg/m^2)

Cytarabine 1000 mg/m^2 per dose; administer intravenously in 100–1000 mL 0.9% NS or D5W over 2 hours, every 12 hours, for 8 doses (2 doses/day) on days 1, 2, 3, and 4 (total dosage/second consolidation course = 8000 mg/m^2)

Keratitis prophylaxis
- Steroid ophthalmic drops (prednisolone 1% or dexamethasone 0.1%); administer 2 drops by intraocular instillation into each eye every 6 hours starting prior to the first cytarabine dose and continuing until 48 hours after high-dose cytarabine is completed

Premedications for gemtuzumab ozogamicin:
- **Methylprednisolone** 1 mg/kg; administer intravenously 30 minutes prior to gemtuzumab ozogamicin on day 1 *plus:*
- **Acetaminophen** 650 mg; administer orally 1 hour prior to gemtuzumab ozogamicin on day 1, *plus:*
- **Diphenhydramine** 50 mg; administer orally or intravenously 1 hour prior to gemtuzumab ozogamicin on day 1

Gemtuzumab ozogamicin 3 mg/m^2 (maximum dose 4.5 mg); administer intravenously over 2 hours in a volume of 0.9% NS sufficient to produce a gemtuzumab ozogamicin concentration within the range 0.075–0.234 mg/mL, once on day 1 (total dosage/second consolidation course = 3 mg/m^2; maximum total dosage/second consolidation course = 4.5 mg)

Notes:
- Omit gemtuzumab ozogamicin from consolidation cycles in patients with persistent thrombocytopenia (platelet count <100,000/mm^3) by day 45 from induction therapy
- Administer gemtuzumab ozogamicin with an administration set that contains an in-line polyethersulfone filter with pore size of 0.2 μm. Protect the infusion bag or syringe from light using a light-blocking cover during infusion
- Consider cytoreduction (eg, with hydroxyurea) in patients with WBC ≥30,000/mm^3 prior to gemtuzumab ozogamicin administration
- Although the report by Castaigne et al. states that each dose of gemtuzumab ozogamicin was not to exceed 5 mg, the U.S. Food and Drug Administration–approved prescribing information states that the maximum dose of gemtuzumab ozogamicin when used in combination with daunorubicin and cytarabine is 4.5 mg, which corresponds to the available vial size
- Doses <3.9 mg must be prepared and administered in a syringe. Doses ≥3.9 mg may be prepared and administered in either a syringe or an infusion bag
- Life-threatening and/or fatal infusion-related reactions consisting of chills, fever, tachycardia, hypotension, hypoxia, respiratory failure, and/or bronchospasm may occur infrequently, up to 24 hours following infusion of gemtuzumab ozogamicin. See therapy monitoring and therapy modification sections for further details

Supportive Care

Antiemetic prophylaxis

Emetogenic potential with induction course 1 on days 1–3 is **MODERATE** *and on days 4–7 is* **LOW**

Emetogenic potential with induction course 2 on days 1–3 is **MODERATE**

Emetogenic potential with consolidation courses 1 and 2 (with or without gemtuzumab ozogamicin) on days 1–4 is **MODERATE**

See Chapter 42 for antiemetic recommendations

Hematopoietic growth factor (CSF) prophylaxis

Primary prophylaxis with one of the following may be indicated following consolidation therapy cycles in patients who have a documented complete remission with infection, in elderly patients, or in patients with a history of slow bone marrow recovery:

(*continued*)

(*continued*)

Filgrastim (G-CSF) 5 mcg/kg per day by subcutaneous injection, *or*
Pegfilgrastim (pegylated filgrastim) 6 mg/0.6 mL, by subcutaneous injection for one dose
- Begin use from 24–72 h after myelosuppressive chemotherapy is completed
- Continue daily filgrastim use until ANC ≥5000/mm³ after the leukocyte nadir
- Discontinue daily filgrastim use at least 24 hours before administering myelosuppressive treatment. Do not administer pegfilgrastim within 14 days before administering myelosuppressive treatment

See Chapter 43 for more information

Antimicrobial prophylaxis
Risk of fever and neutropenia is **HIGH**
  Antimicrobial primary prophylaxis to be considered:
- Antibacterial—consider prophylaxis with a fluoroquinolone during periods of prolonged neutropenia only (eg, <500/mm³ for ≥7 days), or no prophylaxis, until ANC recovery
- Antifungal—fluconazole or another azole antifungal medication is recommended during periods of prolonged neutropenia only (eg, <500/mm³ for ≥7 days) until ANC recovery
- Antiviral—antiherpes antivirals (eg, acyclovir, famciclovir, valacyclovir)

Patient Population Studied

Castaigne S et al. Lancet 2012;379:1508–1516
ALFA-0701 was a multicenter, randomized, open-label, phase 3 trial involving 278 patients with previously untreated acute myeloid leukemia. Eligible patients were aged 50–70 years and had normal cardiac function. Patients with central nervous system involvement, or previous myeloproliferative or myelodysplastic syndrome, or exposure to chemotherapy or radiotherapy, were ineligible. Patients were randomly assigned 1:1 to receive chemotherapy with or without gemtuzumab ozogamicin. Patients received induction therapy of intravenous daunorubicin and intravenous cytarabine with or without intravenous gemtuzumab ozogamicin in cases of >10% persistent leukemic blasts on day 15, patients received a second cycle of induction therapy consisting of intravenous daunorubicin and intravenous cytarabine without gemtuzumab ozogamicin, followed by daily granulocyte colony-stimulating factor until neutrophil recovery. Patients with complete remission after induction therapy received two courses of consolidation therapy with intravenous daunorubicin and intravenous cytarabine with or without intravenous gemtuzumab ozogamicin according to their initial random assignment

Hills RK et al. Lancet Oncol 2014;115:986–996
This was a meta-analysis that included individual patient data collected from 5 randomized controlled trials (ALFA-0701, GOELAMS AML 2006 IR, NCRI AML16, SWOG S0106, and MRC AML15) evaluating the addition of gemtuzumab ozogamicin to induction chemotherapy in adult patients with acute myeloid leukemia. Patients with favorable cytogenetics benefit most from the addition of gemtuzumab ozogamicin

Efficacy

	Control Group	Gemtuzumab Ozogamicin Group	Point Estimate (95% CI)
All patients	139	139	
CR + CRp	104 (75%)	113 (81%)	1.46 (0.82–2.59) P = 0.25
Induction courses			
1	104 (75%)	113 (81%)	
2	35 (25%)	25 (18%)	
Death during induction	5 (4%)	9 (6%)	
Resistant disease (no CR or CRp)	29 (21%)	17 (12%)	
CR	100 (72%)	102 (73%)	
CRp	4 (3%)	11 (8%)	

CR, complete remission; CRp, complete remission with incomplete platelet recovery

Castaigne S et al. Lancet 2012;379:1508–1516

	Standard Chemotherapy + Gemtuzumab Ozogamicin (n = 139)	Standard Chemotherapy Only (n = 139)	
Median event-free survival	15.6 months	9.7 months	HR 0.58, 95% CI 0.43–0.78; P = 0.0003
Median overall survival	34.0 months	19.2 months	HR 0.69, 95% CI 0.49–0.98; P = 0.0368
Median relapse-free survival	28.1 months	11.4 months	HR 0.52, 95% CI 0.36–0.75; P = 0.0003

Note: Median follow-up was 14.8 months overall and 20.0 months on survivors

Efficacy (continued)

Hills RK et al. Lancet Oncol 2014;115:986–996

Outcome	Induction Chemotherapy + Gemtuzumab Ozogamicin	Chemotherapy Without Gemtuzumab Ozogamicin	Between-group Comparison
	Events/Patients		
Overall survival	1024/1660	1084/1663	OR 0.90 (95% CI, 0.82–0.98); P = 0.01
Overall survival in patients with favorable cytogenetics	30/122	54/124	OR 0.47 (95% CI, 0.31–0.73); Difference 20.7% (SD 6.5); Log-rank P = 0.0006
Overall survival in patients with intermediate cytogenetics	506/911	559/916	OR 0.84 (95% CI, 0.75–0.95); Difference 5.7% (SD 2.8); Log-rank P = 0.005
Overall survival in patients with adverse cytogenetics	260/299	258/284	OR 0.99 (95% CI, 0.83–1.18); Difference 2.2% (SD 9.8); Log-rank P = 0.9
Relapse-free survival	819/1306	874/1282	OR 0.84 (95% CI, 0.76–0.92); P = 0.0003
Survival after achieving remission	690/1306	736/1282	OR 0.85 (95% CI, 0.77–0.94); P = 0.002
Relapse	659/1306	721/1282	OR 0.81 (95% CI, 0.73–0.90); P = 0.0001
Death in complete remission	160/1306	153/1282	OR 0.97 (95% CI, 0.77–1.21); P = 0.8

Therapy Monitoring

1. *Prior to induction therapy:* CBC with differential, baseline chemistries, electrolytes, uric acid, LDH, liver function tests, pregnancy test (women of reproductive potential only), left ventricular ejection fraction (LVEF), electrocardiogram for QTc interval measurement (only in patients with a predisposition for QTc prolongation, with congenital long QTc syndrome, with congestive heart failure, with hypokalemia or hypomagnesemia, or who are taking concurrent medications that have a potential to prolong the QTc interval)

   • In addition to baseline monitoring, evaluate LVEF during daunorubicin treatment if clinical symptoms of heart failure are present

   • *In patients at high risk for tumor lysis syndrome (eg, high tumor burden, renal dysfunction, rapidly progressing disease, markedly elevated LDH, baseline abnormalities in laboratory indices of tumor lysis syndrome [potassium, phosphate, uric acid, calcium, serum creatinine]):* consider frequent monitoring of laboratory indices of tumor lysis syndrome, intravenous hydration, and prophylaxis with a xanthine oxidase inhibitor (eg, allopurinol) during induction therapy

2. *Prior to induction course 2 (if applicable), consolidation course 1, and consolidation course 2:* CBC with differential, baseline chemistries, electrolytes, uric acid, LDH, liver function tests, left ventricular ejection fraction (LVEF)

3. *Prior to each dose of cytarabine in induction course 2 and consolidation courses 1–2:* monitor for signs of cerebellar toxicity (nystagmus, dysmetria, and ataxia)

4. *At least 3 times per week following each course of therapy, until recovery:*

   • Chemistries, electrolytes, uric acid, LDH, and liver function tests

   • Monitor for signs and symptoms of hepatic sinusoidal obstruction syndrome/veno-occlusive disease (elevations in ALT, AST, total bilirubin, painful hepatomegaly, weight gain, ascites)

   • CBC with differential daily during induction chemotherapy and following therapy until neutrophil recovery (>500/mm^3) and patients achieve independence from platelet transfusions

(continued)

Treatment Modifications

INDUCTION COURSE 1*

Cytarabine 200 mg/m^2 days 1–7; daunorubicin 60 mg/m^2 days 1–3; gemtuzumab ozogamicin 3 mg/m^2 (maximum 4.5 mg) days 1, 4, 7
*See dedicated section of table for gemtuzumab ozogamicin dose modifications

Adverse Events	Treatment Modifications
Creatinine >3 mg/dL	Reduce daunorubicin dosage by 50%
Total bilirubin 2.5–5 mg/dL	Reduce daunorubicin dosage by 50%
Total bilirubin >5 mg/dL	Hold daunorubicin; consider alternative regimen

INDUCTION COURSE 2 (WHEN APPLICABLE)

Cytarabine 1000 mg/m^2 intravenously over 2 hours, every 12 hours, days 1–3; daunorubicin 60 mg/m^2 days 1–2

CONSOLIDATION COURSE 1*

Cytarabine 1000 mg/m^2 intravenously over 2 hours, every 12 hours, days 1–4; daunorubicin 60 mg/m^2 day 1; gemtuzumab ozogamicin 3 mg/m^2 (maximum 4.5 mg) day 1

CONSOLIDATION COURSE 2*

Cytarabine 1000 mg/m^2 intravenously over 2 hours, every 12 hours, days 1–4; daunorubicin 60 mg/m^2 days 1–2; gemtuzumab ozogamicin 3 mg/m^2 (maximum 4.5 mg) day 1
*See dedicated section of table for gemtuzumab ozogamicin dose modifications

Adverse Events	Treatment Modifications
Creatinine >3 mg/dL	Reduce daunorubicin dosage by 50%
CrCl 46–60 mL/minute	Reduce each cytarabine dose to 600 mg/m^2/dose
CrCl 31–45 mL/minute	Reduce each cytarabine dose to 500 mg/m^2/dose
CrCl <30 mL/minute	Hold cytarabine; consider alternative regimen
Total bilirubin 2.5–5 mg/dL	Reduce daunorubicin dosage by 50%
Total bilirubin >5 mg/dL	Hold daunorubicin; consider alternative regimen
LVEF is ≤40%, or is 40% to 45% with a ≥10% absolute decrease below the pre-treatment value	Hold daunorubicin; consider alternative regimen
Fever, myalgia, bone pain, occasionally chest pain, maculopapular rash, conjunctivitis, and malaise 6–12 hours following drug administration (cytarabine syndrome)	Corticosteroids beneficial in treating or preventing this syndrome. If the symptoms are deemed treatable, continue therapy with cytarabine and pre-treat with corticosteroids
Neurologic (cerebellar) toxicity	Hold cytarabine. Patients who develop CNS symptoms should not receive subsequent high-dose cytarabine

GEMTUZUMAB OZOGAMICIN

Myelosuppression

Adverse Events	Treatment Modifications
Persistent thrombocytopenia (platelet count <100,000/mm^3) within 14 days after hematologic recovery from the prior cycle of chemotherapy	Withhold gemtuzumab ozogamicin from consolidation courses
Persistent neutropenia (ANC <500/mm^3) within 14 days after hematologic recovery from the prior cycle of chemotherapy	Withhold gemtuzumab ozogamicin from consolidation courses

Therapy Monitoring
(continued)

5. *At least every 30 minutes during each gemtuzumab ozogamicin infusion and for 1 hour post-infusion completion:* monitor vital signs and monitor for signs and symptoms of an infusion-related reaction (chills, fever, tachycardia, hypotension, hypoxia, respiratory failure, and/or bronchospasm)

6. *Periodically:*
   - Advise patient to report signs or symptoms of bleeding
   - Electrocardiogram for QTc interval measurement as clinically indicated, especially in patients with a predisposition for QTc prolongation, with congenital long QTc syndrome, with congestive heart failure, with hypokalemia or hypomagnesemia, or who are taking concurrent medications that have a potential to prolong the QTc interval

7. *Response assessment:* bone marrow aspirate, and biopsy at day 15 of each induction course and then repeated upon recovery of peripheral blood counts, CBC with differential

(continued)

Treatment Modifications (*continued*)

Hepatic Toxicity or Hepatic Impairment

Hepatic sinusoidal obstruction syndrome/veno-occlusive disease	Discontinue gemtuzumab ozogamicin
Patient treated with gemtuzumab ozogamicin undergoes subsequent hematopoietic stem cell transplant	Monitor for signs and symptoms of hepatic sinusoidal obstruction syndrome/veno-occlusive disease and liver function tests frequently
Total bilirubin >2× ULN, or AST >2.5× ULN, or ALT >2.5× ULN	Delay gemtuzumab ozogamicin treatment until total bilirubin ≤2× ULN, AST ≤2.5× ULN, and ALT ≤2.5× ULN Consider increasing the frequency of monitoring of liver function tests and for signs/symptoms of hepatotoxicity Omit the scheduled dose if delay is required more than 2 days between sequential infusions

Infusion Reactions

Infusion-related reaction	Interrupt the infusion immediately and institute appropriate supportive medical management Administer acetaminophen and diphenhydramine (if >4 hours has transpired since administration of the premedication doses) Administer methylprednisolone 1 mg/kg intravenously × 1 dose For mild, moderate, or severe infusion-related reactions, once symptoms resolve, consider resuming the infusion at no more than half the rate at which the reaction occurred. Repeat the procedure in the event of recurrent symptoms Permanently discontinue gemtuzumab ozogamicin in patients who experience a life-threatening infusion reaction
Anaphylactic reaction suspected (eg, severe respiratory symptoms or clinically significant hypotension) or life-threatening infusion reaction	Permanently discontinue gemtuzumab ozogamicin

Other Toxicities

Other severe or life-threatening nonhematologic toxicities	Delay gemtuzumab ozogamicin administration until recover to G ≤1. Omit the scheduled dose if delayed more than 2 days between sequential infusions

CrCl, creatinine clearance; LVEF, left ventricular ejection fraction; CNS, central nervous system; ANC, absolute neutrophil count; ULN, upper limit of normal; AST, aspartate aminotransferase; ALT, alanine aminotransferase

Adverse Events

	Control Group (n = 139)	Gemtuzumab Ozogamicin Group (n = 139)	Point Difference (95% CI)	P Value
Duration of treatment-induced cytopenias (days)	Neutropenia (<0.5 × 10⁹ cells per L)			
After induction	22 (18–27)	22 (20–26)	–0.4 (–2.6 to –1.8)	0.68
After first consolidation	10 (8–15)	13 (10–18)	–2.9 (–5.4 to –0.6)	0.0017
After second consolidation	13 (10–16)	15 (12–20)	–3.7 (–6.2 to –1.4)	0.0021
Thrombocytopenia (<50 × 10⁹ cells per L)				
After induction	21 (18–25)	25 (20–30)	–3.3 (–5.8 to –0.8)	0.0006
After first consolidation	9 (6–13)	17 (11–27)	–9.5 (–16.4 to –2.8)	<0.0001
After second consolidation	13 (9–20)	24 (15–35)	–9.5 (–13.5 to –5.4)	<0.0001
Persistent thrombocytopenia (<50 × 10⁹ cells per L)				
By day 45 after induction	0/139	4/139 (3%)	0 (0 to 0.9)	0.12
By day 45 after first consolidation	2/98 (2%)	9/99 (9%	0.2 (0.1 to 0.9)	0.0582
By day 45 after second consolidation	2/90 (2%)	9/85 (11%)	0.2 (0.1 to 0.8)	0.0289
Grade 3 and 4 adverse events				
Hemorrhage	4/139 (3%)	12/139 (9%)	0.33 (0.12–0.95)	0.068
Cardiac	9/139 (6%)	11/139 (8%)	0.82 (0.36–1.87)	0.82
Liver	9/139 (6%)	18/139 (13%)	0.50 (0.24–1.05)	0.10
Skin or mucosa	25/139 (18%)	32/139 (23%)	0.11 (0.03–0.42)	0.37
Gastrointestinal	14/139 (10%)	22/139 (16%)	0.64 (0.34–1.18)	0.21
Pulmonary	16/139 (12%)	16/139 (12%)	1.00 (0.53–1.90)	1.00
Grade 3 and 4 infections				
During induction	50/131 (38%)	59/129 (46%)	0.83 (0.62–1.11)	0.26
During first consolidation	38/95 (40%)	48/97 (49%)	0.80 (0.59–1.11)	0.19
During second consolidation	38/82 (46%)	38/81 (47%)	0.99 (0.71–1.37)	0.99

INTENSIVE INDUCTION THERAPY AND POST-REMISSION THERAPY • FIRST-LINE

ACUTE MYELOID LEUKEMIA REGIMEN: DAUNORUBICIN + CYTARABINE + MIDOSTAURIN

Stone RM et al. N Engl J Med 2017;377:454–464
Supplementary appendix to: Stone RM et al. N Engl J Med 2017;377:454–464
Protocol for: Stone RM et al. N Engl J Med 2017;377:454–464
RYDAPT (midostaurin capsules) prescribing information. East Hanover, NJ: Novartis Pharmaceuticals Corporation; 2018 June

Induction daunorubicin, cytarabine, and midostaurin (may repeat once for persistent disease evident on bone marrow biopsy performed on day 21):
   Cytarabine 200 mg/m^2 per day; administer by continuous intravenous infusion in 100–1000 mL 0.9% sodium chloride (0.9% NS) or 5% dextrose injection (D5W) over 24 hours for 7 consecutive days on days 1–7 (total dosage/induction = 1400 mg/m^2)
   Daunorubicin 60 mg/m^2 per dose; administer by intravenous injection over 3–5 minutes once daily for 3 consecutive days on days 1–3 (total dosage/induction = 180 mg/m^2)
   Midostaurin 50 mg per dose; administer orally, every 12 hours, with food for 14 consecutive days on days 8–21 (total dosage/induction = 1400 mg)

Consolidation cytarabine and midostaurin (four 28-day cycles, begin upon documentation of complete remission following induction therapy):
   Cytarabine 3000 mg/m^2 per dose; administer intravenously in 100–1000 mL 0.9% NS or D5W over 3 hours, every 12 hours, for a total of 6 doses (2 doses/day) on days 1, 3, and 5 only, every 28 days, for 4 cycles (total dosage/28-day consolidation cycle = 18,000 mg/m^2)
   Keratitis prophylaxis
   • Steroid ophthalmic drops (prednisolone 1% or dexamethasone 0.1%); administer 2 drops by intraocular instillation into each eye every 6 hours starting prior to the first cytarabine dose and continuing until 48 hours after high-dose cytarabine is completed
   Midostaurin 50 mg per dose; administer orally, every 12 hours, with food for 14 consecutive days on days 8–21, every 28 days, for 4 cycles (total dosage/28-day consolidation cycle = 1400 mg)

Maintenance midostaurin (twelve 28-day continuous cycles; begin upon hematologic recovery from the final cycle of consolidation and not sooner than 14 days following the last dose of midostaurin administered during consolidation):
   Midostaurin 50 mg per dose; administer orally, every 12 hours, with food, continuously on days 1–28, every 28 days, for 12 cycles (total dosage/28-day maintenance cycle = 2800 mg)

Midostaurin treatment notes:
• The FDA-approved prescribing information recommends that patients receive prophylactic antiemetics prior to midostaurin treatment
• Midostaurin area under the curve AUC extrapolated to infinity (AUC$_{inf}$) increased by 1.2-fold and by 1.6-fold when administered with a standard meal or high-fat meal, respectively, compared with administration in a fasting state. The clinical trial protocol (Stone et al.) and FDA-approved prescribing information specify that doses should be administered with food
• Advise patients to not consume grapefruit products, as they may inhibit CYP3A in the gut wall and increase the bioavailability of midostaurin
• Midostaurin capsules should be swallowed whole. Do not open or crush midostaurin capsules
• Patients who delay taking midostaurin at a regularly scheduled time or who vomit a dose of midostaurin should not make up the missed or vomited dose; the next dose should be administered at the next usual scheduled time
• Advise patients to keep midostaurin in its original package to protect from moisture
• A pungent odor may be noticed when the blister packaging is opened. The odor is caused by ethyl thioglycolate, a substance formed due to an interaction between ethanol within the capsules and the blister pack foil thermostabilizer. Advise patients that allowing the odor to dissipate prior to attempted administration may reduce nausea
• If concomitant use of another QTc prolonging medication in addition to midostaurin is unavoidable, then consider performing interval electrocardiograms to assess the QTc interval
• Midostaurin is primarily metabolized by the cytochrome P450 (CYP) 3A4 isoform to two active metabolites, CGP62221 (representing a mean 28% of circulating radioactivity in a mass-balance study) and CGP52421 (representing a mean 38% of circulating radioactivity). In vitro studies suggest that midostaurin and its metabolites are also inducers of CYP1A2, CYP2B6, CYP2C8, CYP2C9, CYP2C19, and CYP3A4. Therefore, midostaurin is capable of inducing its own metabolism and exhibits time-dependent pharmacokinetics
• Coadministration of midostaurin with strong CYP3A inhibitors may increase midostaurin concentrations and therefore potentially increase the risk of toxicity, with the effect being most prominent when the CYP3A inhibitor is administered during the first week of midostaurin administration. If the strong CYP3A4 inhibitor cannot be avoided, then monitor patients closely for increased risk of toxicity, especially during the first week of midostaurin administration
• Thus, coadministration of CYP3A inducers with midostaurin may decrease midostaurin exposure and potentially reduce efficacy and should be avoided

Supportive Care
Antiemetic prophylaxis
Emetogenic potential with induction on days 1–3 is **MODERATE** *and on days 4–7 is* **LOW**
Emetogenic potential with consolidation on days 1, 3, and 5 is **MODERATE**
Emetogenic potential on days with midostaurin is **MODERATE–HIGH**
See Chapter 42 for antiemetic recommendations

(continued)

(continued)

Hematopoietic growth factor (CSF) prophylaxis

Primary prophylaxis with one of the following may be indicated following consolidation therapy cycles in patients who have a documented complete remission with infection, in elderly patients, or in patients with a history of slow bone marrow recovery:

Filgrastim (G-CSF) 5 mcg/kg per day by subcutaneous injection, *or*

Pegfilgrastim (pegylated filgrastim) 6 mg/0.6 mL, by subcutaneous injection for one dose

- Begin use from 24–72 h after myelosuppressive chemotherapy is completed
- Continue daily filgrastim use until ANC ≥5000/mm^3 after the leukocyte nadir
- Discontinue daily filgrastim use at least 24 hours before administering myelosuppressive treatment. Do not administer pegfilgrastim within 14 days before administering myelosuppressive treatment

See Chapter 43 for more information

Antimicrobial prophylaxis

Risk of fever and neutropenia is **HIGH**

Antimicrobial primary prophylaxis to be considered:

- Antibacterial—consider prophylaxis with a fluoroquinolone during periods of prolonged neutropenia only (eg, <500/mm^3 for ≥7 days), or no prophylaxis, until ANC recovery
- Antifungal—fluconazole or another antifungal medication such as an echinocandin (eg, caspofungin) is recommended during periods of prolonged neutropenia only (eg, <500/mm^3 for ≥7 days) until ANC recovery. Note that certain azole antifungals (eg, posaconazole, voriconazole, itraconazole, and ketoconazole) are strong CYP3A4 inhibitors and, in the case of itraconazole and ketoconazole, are also major CYP3A4 substrates, and may have the potential to interact with midostaurin
- Antiviral—antiherpes antivirals (eg, acyclovir, famciclovir, valacyclovir)

Patient Population Studied

This international, multicenter, randomized, phase 3 trial involved 717 patients with newly diagnosed acute myeloid leukemia with a *FLT3* (internal tandem duplication or point mutation). Eligible patients had a diagnosis of acute myeloid leukemia that was not related to therapy, bilirubin less than 2.5 times the upper limit of the normal range, age ≥18 to <60 years, and absence of other major coexisting illnesses. Patients with acute promyelocytic leukemia were ineligible. Patients were randomly assigned 1:1 to receive standard chemotherapy plus either placebo or midostaurin. Patients received induction therapy of daunorubicin cytarabine and either oral placebo or oral midostaurin in cases of definitive evidence of clinically significant residual leukemia, patients received a second, identical cycle of induction therapy. Patients with complete remission after induction therapy received four 28-day cycles of consolidation therapy with high-dose cytarabine and either oral placebo or oral midostaurin. Patients remaining in remission after consolidation therapy received twelve 28-day cycles of maintenance therapy with continuous oral placebo or oral midostaurin

Efficacy

	Midostaurin Group n = 360	Placebo Group n = 357	P Value
Complete remission	212 (59%)	191 (54%)	0.15

	Chemotherapy + Midostaurin (n = 360)	Chemotherapy + Placebo (n = 357)	
Median overall survival	74.7 months	25.6 months	HR 0.78, 95% CI 0.63–0.96; P = 0.009
Median event-free survival	8.2 months	3.0 months	HR 0.78, 95% CI 0.66–0.93; P = 0.002
Median disease-free survival	26.7 months	15.5 months	P = 0.01

Note: Median follow-up was 59 months.

Therapy Monitoring

1. *Prior to induction therapy:* CBC with differential, baseline chemistries, electrolytes, uric acid, LDH, liver function tests, pregnancy test (women of reproductive potential only), left ventricular ejection fraction (LVEF), electrocardiogram for QTc interval measurement (only in patients with a predisposition for QTc prolongation or who are taking concurrent medications that have a potential to prolong the QTc interval)
    a. In addition to baseline monitoring, evaluate LVEF during daunorubicin treatment if clinical symptoms of heart failure are present
    b. *In patients at high risk for tumor lysis syndrome (eg, high tumor burden, renal dysfunction, rapidly progressing disease, markedly elevated LDH, baseline abnormalities in laboratory indices of tumor lysis syndrome [potassium, phosphate, uric acid, calcium, serum creatinine]):* consider frequent monitoring of laboratory indices of tumor lysis syndrome, intravenous hydration, and prophylaxis with a xanthine oxidase inhibitor (eg, allopurinol) during induction therapy
2. *Prior to each cycle of consolidation:* CBC with differential, baseline chemistries, electrolytes, liver function tests
3. *Prior to each administration of high-dose cytarabine during consolidation:* monitor for signs of cerebellar toxicity (nystagmus, dysmetria, and ataxia)
4. Serum chemistry daily and CBC with differential daily during induction chemotherapy and following therapy until neutrophil recovery (>500/mm^3) and patients achieve independence from platelet transfusions
5. *Periodically:*
    a. Monitor for signs and symptoms of interstitial lung disease or pneumonitis (new cough, chest discomfort, or shortness of breath)
    b. Advise patients to report signs or symptoms of hypersensitivity reactions. Hypersensitivity reactions were not reported in patients treated with midostaurin for AML, but were reported in 4% of patients receiving midostaurin for advanced systemic mastocytosis (including 1 case of anaphylaxis)
    c. Advise patient to report signs or symptoms of bleeding
    d. Electrocardiogram for QTc interval measurement as clinically indicated, especially in patients with a predisposition for QTc prolongation or who are taking concurrent medications that have a potential to prolong the QTc interval
6. *Response assessment:* bone marrow aspirate, and biopsy at day 21 of induction therapy, upon recovery of peripheral blood counts following induction, and as clinically indicated; CBC with differential

Treatment Modifications

INDUCTION THERAPY*

Cytarabine 200 mg/m^2 days 1–7; daunorubicin 60 mg/m^2 days 1–3; midostaurin 50 mg twice daily days 8–21
*See separate dedicated section for midostaurin dose modifications

Adverse Events	Treatment Modifications
Interstitial lung disease or pneumonitis is suspected	Interrupt midostaurin until pulmonary status is clarified. Do not make up missed doses
Interstitial lung disease or pneumonitis is confirmed	Permanently discontinue midostaurin
Hypersensitivity reaction to midostaurin	Permanently discontinue midostaurin
QTc interval >450 ms and ≤470 ms	Check magnesium and potassium levels and correct any abnormalities. Minimize concurrent use of other medications with the potential to prolong the QTc interval if possible. Continue midostaurin at the same dose
QTc interval >470 ms and ≤500 ms	Check magnesium and potassium levels and correct any abnormalities. Minimize concurrent use of other medications with the potential to prolong the QTc interval if possible. Reduce the dose of midostaurin to 50 mg by mouth once daily for the remainder of the cycle. If the QTc interval improves to ≤470 ms prior to the next cycle, then resume midostaurin at the initial dose in that cycle. If the QTc interval remains >470 and ≤500 ms prior to the next cycle, then continue midostaurin at a dose of 50 mg once daily for that cycle and reassess prior to the next cycle
QTc interval >500 ms	Check magnesium and potassium levels and correct any abnormalities. Minimize concurrent use of other medications with the potential to prolong the QTc interval if possible. Interrupt midostaurin administration for the remainder of the current cycle. If the QTc interval improves to ≤470 ms prior to the next cycle, then resume midostaurin at the initial dose. If the QTc interval remains >470 ms, then withhold midostaurin during that cycle and reassess prior to the next cycle. Do not make up missed doses of midostaurin
G ≥3 nonhematologic toxicity possibly related to midostaurin	Interrupt midostaurin. At the discretion of the medically responsible health care provider, resume midostaurin at the same dose upon resolution of the toxicity to G ≤2. Do not make up missed doses of midostaurin
Creatinine >3 mg/dL	Reduce daunorubicin dosage by 50%
Total bilirubin >2 to ≤3 mg/dL	Reduce daunorubicin dosage by 25%
Total bilirubin >3 mg/dL	Reduce daunorubicin dosage by 50%

(continued)

Treatment Modifications (continued)

Adverse Events	Treatment Modifications
LVEF is ≤40%, or is 40% to 45% with a ≥10% absolute decrease below the pre-treatment value and the patient requires a second course of induction therapy	Hold daunorubicin. Consider an alternative regimen for the second induction course

CONSOLIDATION CYCLES*

Cytarabine 3000 mg/m² intravenously over 3 hours, every 12 hours, days 1, 3, and 5; midostaurin 50 mg twice daily days 8–21
*See separate dedicated section for midostaurin dose modifications

Adverse Events	Treatment Modifications
Day 1 ANC <1000/mm³ or platelet count <75,000/mm³	Delay the start of the consolidation cycle until ANC ≥1000/mm³ and platelet count ≥75,000/mm³. For delays of ≥3 weeks due to slow peripheral blood count recovery, consider obtaining a bone marrow biopsy to rule out relapsed leukemia and consider reducing the dose of cytarabine by 25–50% during subsequent cycles
Prior cycle of consolidation therapy complicated by G ≥3 infection or neutropenic fever	Consider either continuing cytarabine at the same dose or reducing the cytarabine dose by 25–50% during subsequent consolidation cycles
CrCl 46–60 mL/minute	Reduce each cytarabine dose to 1800 mg/m²/dose
CrCl 31–45 mL/minute	Reduce each cytarabine dose to 1500 mg/m²/dose
CrCl <30 mL/minute	Withhold cytarabine. Consider an alternative regimen for consolidation
Fever, myalgia, bone pain, occasionally chest pain, maculopapular rash, conjunctivitis, and malaise 6–12 hours following drug administration (cytarabine syndrome)	Corticosteroids beneficial in treating or preventing this syndrome. If the symptoms are deemed treatable, continue therapy with cytarabine and pre-treat with corticosteroids
Neurologic (cerebellar) toxicity	Withhold cytarabine. Patients who develop CNS symptoms should not receive subsequent high-dose cytarabine

MIDOSTAURIN

Hematologic Toxicity

G4 neutropenia (ANC <500/mm³) occurring during single-agent midostaurin maintenance therapy	Evaluate peripheral blood smear. Consider obtaining a bone marrow biopsy to rule out the possibility of relapsed leukemia as clinically appropriate. Withhold midostaurin. If neutropenia is thought to be related to midostaurin, then resume midostaurin upon improvement of the ANC to ≥1000/mm³ at the previous dose. If neutropenia persists for >2 weeks, then consider discontinuing midostaurin
G4 neutropenia (ANC <500/mm³) occurring during induction or consolidation therapy	Continue midostaurin at the same dose without interruption. G4 neutropenia is an expected toxicity following induction and consolidation chemotherapy
Interstitial lung disease or pneumonitis is suspected	Interrupt midostaurin until pulmonary status is clarified. Do not make up missed doses
Interstitial lung disease or pneumonitis is confirmed	Permanently discontinue midostaurin
Hypersensitivity reaction to midostaurin	Permanently discontinue midostaurin
QTc interval >450 ms and ≤470 ms	Check magnesium and potassium levels and correct any abnormalities. Minimize concurrent use of other medications with the potential to prolong the QTc interval if possible. Continue midostaurin at the same dose
QTc interval >470 ms and ≤500 ms	Check magnesium and potassium levels and correct any abnormalities. Minimize concurrent use of other medications with the potential to prolong the QTc interval if possible. Reduce the dose of midostaurin to 50 mg by mouth once daily for the remainder of the cycle. If the QTc interval improves to ≤470 ms prior to the next cycle, then resume midostaurin at the initial dose in that cycle. If the QTc interval remains >470 and ≤500 ms prior to the next cycle, then continue midostaurin at a dose of 50 mg once daily for that cycle and reassess prior to the next cycle
QTc interval >500 ms	Check magnesium and potassium levels and correct any abnormalities. Minimize concurrent use of other medications with the potential to prolong the QTc interval if possible. Interrupt midostaurin administration for the remainder of the current cycle. If the QTc interval improves to ≤470 ms prior to the next cycle, then resume midostaurin at the initial dose. If the QTc interval remains >470 ms, then withhold midostaurin during that cycle and reassess prior to the next cycle. Do not make up missed doses of midostaurin

(continued)

Treatment Modifications (continued)

MIDOSTAURIN

Hematologic Toxicity

G ≥3 nonhematologic toxicity possibly related to midostaurin	Interrupt midostaurin. At the discretion of the medically responsible health care provider, resume midostaurin at the same dose upon resolution of the toxicity to G ≤2. Do not make up missed doses of midostaurin
Concomitant therapy with a strong CYP3A4 inducer is required	Avoid concomitant use of midostaurin with a strong CYP3A4 inducer
Concomitant therapy with a strong CYP3A4 inhibitor is required	Monitor closely for midostaurin toxicity, especially if a strong CYP3A4 inhibitor is used during the first week of midostaurin therapy
Concomitant therapy with a medication that has a potential to increase the QTc interval is required	Consider interval ECG and electrolyte monitoring during periods of combined therapy

LVEF, left ventricular ejection fraction; ANC, absolute neutrophil count; CrCl, creatinine clearance; CNS, central nervous system; ECG, electrocardiogram

Adverse Events (N = 709)

Grade ≥3 Event (%)	Chemotherapy + Midostaurin (n = 355)	Chemotherapy + Placebo (n = 354)
Thrombocytopenia	97	97
Neutropenia	95	96
Anemia	93	88
Febrile neutropenia	82	82
Infection	52	50
Leukopenia	26	30
Lymphopenia	19	22
Diarrhea	16	15
Hypokalemia	14	17
Rash or desquamation	14	8
Pain	13	12
Elevated alanine aminotransferase level	13	9
Fatigue	9	10
Hyponatremia	9	6
Pneumonitis or pulmonary infiltrates	8	8
Hyperbilirubinemia	7	8
Hypocalcemia	7	6
Mucositis or stomatitis	6	8
Nausea	6	10
Hypophosphatemia	5	8
Other blood or bone marrow event	<1	1
Bone marrow hypocellularity	0	<1

Note: Grade ≥3 adverse events are included. The midostaurin group had higher rates of Grade ≥3 anemia (P = 0.03) and rash (P = 0.008). The placebo group had a higher rate of Grade ≥3 nausea (P = 0.05)

INTENSIVE INDUCTION THERAPY AND POST-REMISSION THERAPY • FIRST-LINE

ACUTE MYELOID LEUKEMIA REGIMEN: CPX–351 (CYTARABINE + DAUNORUBICIN) LIPOSOME

Lancet JE et al. J Clin Oncol 2018;36:2684–2692
Data supplement to: Lancet JE et al. J Clin Oncol 2018;36:2684–2692
Protocol for: Lancet JE et al. J Clin Oncol 2018;36:2684–2692
VYXEOS (daunorubicin and cytarabine, liposome for injection) prescribing information. Palo Alto, CA: Jazz Pharmaceuticals, Inc; 2017 August

Initial induction course:

Daunorubicin and cytarabine liposome injection 44 mg/m² per dose and 100 mg/m² per dose, respectively; administer by intravenous infusion through a central venous catheter (CVC) or peripherally inserted central catheter (PICC) in 500 mL 0.9% sodium chloride (0.9% NS) or 5% dextrose injection (D5W) over 90 minutes for 3 doses on days 1, 3, and 5 (total dosage of daunorubicin and cytarabine liposome injection/initial induction course = 132 mg/m² [daunorubicin] and 300 mg/m² [cytarabine])
• *Note:* flush line with 0.9% NS or D5W after each administration of daunorubicin and cytarabine liposome injection

Second induction course (administer 2–5 weeks after the initial course of induction therapy to patients who have unequivocal evidence of persistent leukemia in a bone marrow specimen obtained 14 days after the start of the initial course and in the absence of unacceptable toxicity):

Daunorubicin and cytarabine liposome injection 44 mg/m² per dose and 100 mg/m² per dose, respectively; administer by intravenous infusion through a CVC or PICC in 500 mL 0.9% NS or D5W over 90 minutes for 2 doses on days 1 and 3 (total dosage of daunorubicin and cytarabine liposome injection/second induction course = 88 mg/m² [daunorubicin] and 200 mg/m² [cytarabine])
• *Note:* flush line with 0.9% NS or D5W after each administration of daunorubicin and cytarabine liposome injection

Post-remission consolidation (initiate 5–8 weeks after the start of the last course of induction therapy to patients who have achieved either CR or CRi):

Daunorubicin and cytarabine liposome injection 29 mg/m² per dose and 65 mg/m² per dose, respectively; administer by intravenous infusion through a CVC or PICC in 500 mL 0.9% NS or D5W over 90 minutes for 2 doses on days 1 and 3, every 5–8 weeks, for 2 cycles (total dosage of daunorubicin and cytarabine liposome injection/consolidation course = 58 mg/m² [daunorubicin] and 130 mg/m² [cytarabine])
• *Note:* flush line with 0.9% NS or D5W after each administration of daunorubicin and cytarabine liposome injection

Supportive Care

Antiemetic prophylaxis
Emetogenic potential is **MODERATE**
See Chapter 42 for antiemetic recommendations

Hematopoietic growth factor (CSF) prophylaxis
Primary prophylaxis is **NOT** *indicated*
See Chapter 43 for more information

Antimicrobial prophylaxis
Risk of fever and neutropenia is **HIGH**
  Antimicrobial primary prophylaxis to be considered:
• Antibacterial—consider prophylaxis with a fluoroquinolone during periods of prolonged neutropenia only (eg, <500/mm³ for ≥7 days) until ANC recovery
• Antifungal—consider prophylaxis with posaconazole or another azole antifungal medication during periods of prolonged neutropenia only (eg, <500/mm³ for ≥7 days) until ANC recovery
• Antiviral—antiherpes antivirals (eg, acyclovir, famciclovir, valacyclovir)

Therapy Monitoring

1. *Prior to induction therapy:* CBC with differential, baseline chemistries, electrolytes, uric acid, LDH, liver function tests, pregnancy test (women of reproductive potential only), left ventricular ejection fraction (LVEF), calculate prior cumulative lifetime daunorubicin (or equivalent) exposure
   • In addition to baseline monitoring, evaluate LVEF during daunorubicin and cytarabine liposome treatment if clinical symptoms of heart failure are present
   • *In patients at high risk for tumor lysis syndrome (eg, high tumor burden, renal dysfunction, rapidly progressing disease, markedly elevated LDH, baseline abnormalities in laboratory indices of tumor lysis syndrome [potassium, phosphate, uric acid, calcium, serum creatinine]):* consider frequent monitoring of laboratory indices of tumor lysis syndrome, intravenous hydration, and prophylaxis with a xanthine oxidase inhibitor (eg, allopurinol) during induction therapy

2. *Prior to each cycle of consolidation:* CBC with differential, baseline chemistries, electrolytes, liver function tests, LVEF, calculate prior cumulative lifetime daunorubicin (or equivalent) exposure

3. *During each administration of daunorubicin and cytarabine liposome injection:* monitor for signs and symptoms of hypersensitivity reaction and monitor the site of administration for signs and symptoms of extravasation

4. *Serum chemistry daily and CBC with differential daily during induction chemotherapy and following therapy until neutrophil recovery (>500/mm³) and patients achieve independence from platelet transfusions*

5. *Periodically:* advise patient to report signs or symptoms of bleeding and/or infection throughout regimen

6. *Response assessment:* bone marrow aspirate, and biopsy at day 14 of initial induction course and then repeated upon recovery of peripheral blood counts following induction, and as clinically indicated; CBC with differential

Patient Population Studied

This multicenter, randomized, open-label, phase 3 trial involved 309 patients with newly diagnosed, therapy-related acute myeloid leukemia, acute myeloid leukemia with antecedent myelodysplastic syndrome or chronic myelomonocytic leukemia, or de novo acute myeloid leukemia with myelodysplastic syndrome–related cytogenetic abnormalities. Eligible patients were aged 60–75 years. Patients were randomly assigned 1:1 to receive CPX-351 or conventional cytarabine plus daunorubicin. The CPX-351 cohort received a first induction cycle on days 1, 3, and 5; patients who did not achieve hypoplastic marrow on a day 14 bone marrow assessment underwent a second induction cycle on days 1 and 3; patients who achieved complete response or complete response with incomplete neutrophil or platelet recovery after induction then received up to two consolidation cycles on days 1 and 3. The conventional cytarabine plus daunorubicin cohort received a first induction cycle of cytarabine and daunorubicin a second induction cycle of cytarabine and daunorubicin and consolidation cycles of cytarabine and daunorubicin on days 1 and 2

Efficacy (N = 309)

	CPX-351 (n = 153)	Conventional Cytarabine + Daunorubicin (n = 156)	
Median overall survival	9.56 months	5.95 months	HR 0.69, 95% CI 0.52–0.90; P = 0.003
Remission rate*	47.7%	33.3%	P = 0.016
Median duration of remission	6.93 months	6.11 months	P = 0.291
Median event-free survival	2.53 months	1.31 months	HR 0.74, 95% CI 0.58–0.96; P = 0.021

*Remission rate includes patients with either a complete response or a complete response with incomplete neutrophil or platelet recovery
Note: Median follow-up was 20.7 months

Adverse Events (N = 304)

The median rate of adverse events per patient-year was 75.68 in the CPX-351 group and 87.22 in the conventional cytarabine + daunorubicin group. The most common Grade 3–5 adverse events were febrile neutropenia (68.0% with CPX-351 vs 70.9% with conventional cytarabine + daunorubicin), pneumonia (19.6% vs 14.6%), and hypoxia (13.1% vs 15.2%). Treatment discontinuation owing to adverse events was reported for three patients in the CPX-351 group (due to cardiac failure, cardiomyopathy, and acute renal failure) and two patients in the conventional cytarabine + daunorubicin group (both due to decreased ejection fraction). Early mortality through to day 30 was 5.9% in the CPX-351 group and 10.6% in the conventional cytarabine + daunorubicin group (P = 0.149), and early mortality through to day 60 was 13.7% in the CPX-351 group and 21.2% in the conventional cytarabine + daunorubicin group (P = 0.097)

Treatment Modifications

DAUNORUBICIN AND CYTARABINE LIPOSOME INJECTION

Induction course 1: (daunorubicin and cytarabine liposome injection, 44 mg/m^2 per dose and 100 mg/m^2 per dose, respectively; administered intravenously on days 1, 3, and 5)
Induction course 2 (if needed): (daunorubicin and cytarabine liposome injection, 44 mg/m^2 per dose and 100 mg/m^2 per dose, respectively; administered intravenously on days 1 and 3)
Consolidation (2 cycles): (daunorubicin and cytarabine liposome injection, 29 mg/m^2 per dose and 65 mg/m^2 per dose, respectively; administered intravenously on days 1 and 3)

Adverse Events	Treatment Modifications
Response Assessment	
Bone marrow specimen obtained on day 14 following the initial course of induction therapy demonstrates evidence of aplasia or hypoplasia with <5% blast count	Omit the second course of daunorubicin and cytarabine liposome injection Proceed to consolidation between 5–8 weeks after the start of the last induction course, upon confirmation of complete remission (CR) or complete remission with incomplete count recovery (CRi), and upon recovery of ANC to >500/mm^3 and platelet count to >50,000/mm^3
Bone marrow specimen obtained on day 14 following the initial course of induction therapy demonstrates unequivocal evidence of persistent leukemia	Administer the second induction course of daunorubicin and cytarabine liposome injection (daunorubicin and cytarabine liposome injection, 44 mg/m^2 per dose and 100 mg/m^2 per dose, respectively; administered intravenously on days 1 and 3) between 2–5 weeks after the start of the first course of induction therapy, in the absence of unacceptable toxicity
Bone marrow specimen obtained on day 14 following the initial course of induction therapy demonstrates equivocal evidence of persistent leukemia	Determine the need for a second induction course of daunorubicin and cytarabine liposome injection based upon the results of a repeat bone marrow evaluation performed in 5–10 days

(continued)

Treatment Modifications (continued)

Hematologic Toxicity

Day 1 ANC <500/mm³ prior to a consolidation cycle	Delay the initiation of the consolidation cycle until ANC >500/mm³. If the ANC does not recover to >500/mm³ by 8 weeks from the start of the last course of therapy, then omit consolidation and/or consider other therapies
Day 1 platelet count <50,000/mm³ prior to a consolidation cycle	Delay the initiation of the consolidation cycle until platelet count >50,000/mm³. If the platelet count does not recover to >50,000/mm³ by 8 weeks from the start of the last course of therapy, then omit consolidation and/or consider other therapies

Hepatic Impairment or Renal Impairment

Total bilirubin is ≤3 mg/dL	No dose modification is required for daunorubicin and cytarabine liposome injection
Total bilirubin is >3 mg/dL	Daunorubicin and cytarabine liposome injection has not been evaluated in patients with a bilirubin >3 mg/dL. No dose recommendation is available; consider alternative therapy
Patient with severe renal impairment (CrCl 15 mL/min to 29 mL/min) or with ESRD	Daunorubicin and cytarabine liposome injection has not been evaluated in patients with severe renal impairment or with ESRD. No dose recommendation is available; consider alternative therapy

Cardiac Toxicity

LVEF <50% at any time	Consider alternative therapies; only administer daunorubicin and cytarabine liposome injection therapy after careful consideration of the potential risk of irreversible cardiac toxicity
Prior cumulative daunorubicin exposure >368 mg/m² (or equivalent) prior to initiation of daunorubicin and cytarabine liposome injection therapy*	Patients with >368 mg/m² cumulative daunorubicin exposure (or equivalent) were excluded from the study because these patients would have reached excessive lifetime cumulative doses after receiving the initial course of induction therapy. Consider alternative therapies; only administer daunorubicin and cytarabine liposome injection therapy after careful consideration of the potential risk of irreversible cardiac toxicity
Patient will exceed the lifetime cumulative limit of daunorubicin exposure (550 mg/m²) with the next planned cycle (ie, induction course 2, consolidation cycle 1, or consolidation cycle 2) of daunorubicin and cytarabine liposome injection	Consider alternative therapy. Avoid lifetime daunorubicin exposures exceeding 550 mg/m²; only administer further daunorubicin and cytarabine liposome injection after careful consideration of the potential risk of irreversible cardiac toxicity Note that the second induction course provides a total of 132 mg/m² of daunorubicin and each cycle of consolidation provides a total of 58 mg/m² of daunorubicin

Hypersensitivity Reactions

Mild hypersensitivity reaction	Interrupt the daunorubicin and cytarabine liposome injection infusion. Consider premedication with antihistamine (eg, diphenhydramine 25 mg IV or orally) and corticosteroid (eg, dexamethasone 10 mg IV or orally) prior to resumption of the current infusion, and prior to subsequent infusions Upon resolution of symptoms, resume infusion at 50% of the prior rate for the remainder of the current infusion Subsequent infusions may be initiated at the usual rate (ie, over 90 minutes) as tolerated
Moderate hypersensitivity reaction	Discontinue the current daunorubicin and cytarabine liposome injection infusion and do not attempt to reinitiate the infusion on the same day. Provide supportive care and monitoring until resolution of symptoms Administer premedications prior to subsequent infusions of daunorubicin and cytarabine liposome injection (eg, with antihistamine, such as diphenhydramine 25 mg IV or orally) and corticosteroid (eg, dexamethasone 10 mg IV or orally) and initiate subsequent infusions at the usual rate (ie, over 90 minutes) as tolerated
Severe or life-threatening hypersensitivity reaction	Permanently discontinue daunorubicin and cytarabine liposome injection. Provide supportive care and monitoring until resolution of symptoms
Patient did not receive a planned dose of daunorubicin and cytarabine liposomal injection	Administer the dose as soon as possible and adjust the dosing schedule accordingly to maintain the treatment interval

(continued)

Treatment Modifications (*continued*)

Drug Interactions

Patient is receiving concomitant therapy with a medication that has the potential to cause cardiotoxicity	Consider more frequent cardiac monitoring
Patient is receiving concomitant therapy with a medication that has the potential to cause hepatotoxicity	Consider more frequent monitoring of liver function tests

Copper Toxicity

Patient has Wilson disease or other metabolic disorder related to copper	Therapy with daunorubicin and cytarabine liposome injection may lead to a maximum administration of 106 mg/m² of elemental copper over the entire course of therapy and should be used only if the benefits are thought to outweigh risks. Consider consultation with an expert in the management of acute copper toxicity in patients with Wilson disease who are treated with daunorubicin and cytarabine liposome injection. Monitor total serum copper, serum non-ceruloplasmin bound copper, 24-hour urine copper levels, and serial neuropsychological examinations in these patients
Patient with Wilson disease or other metabolic disorder related to copper exhibiting signs or symptoms of acute copper toxicity after treatment with daunorubicin and cytarabine liposome injection	Permanently discontinue daunorubicin and cytarabine liposome injection

ANC, absolute neutrophil count; CrCl, creatinine clearance; ESRD, end-stage renal disease; LVEF, left ventricular ejection fraction
*The clinical trial protocol used conversion factors to convert prior anthracycline exposure to an equivalent daunorubicin dose. Multiply the total prior cumulative dose (expressed in mg/m²) of the anthracycline by the conversion factor to obtain the total equivalent daunorubicin dose (mg/m²). *Conversion factors:* daunorubicin, 1; doxorubicin, 2; epirubicin, 1; idarubicin, 4; mitoxantrone, 4.4

LOW-INTENSITY THERAPY • FIRST-LINE

ACUTE MYELOID LEUKEMIA REGIMEN: VENETOCLAX + DECITABINE

DiNardo CD et al. Blood 2019;133:7–17
Supplementary materials to: DiNardo CD et al. Blood 2019;133:7–17
Protocol for: DiNardo CD et al. Blood 2019;133:7–17
Venclexta (venetoclax tablets) prescribing information. North Chicago, IL: AbbVie Inc; 2018 November
Dacogen (decitabine injection) prescribing information. Rockville, MD: Otsuka America Pharmaceutical, Inc; 2018 December

Prophylaxis for tumor lysis syndrome (TLS) during ramp-up phase:

0.9% sodium chloride (0.9% NS); administer intravenously at 75–150 mL/hour, as tolerated, starting prior to the first dose of venetoclax on day 1 during cycle 1 only, and continue until at least 24 hours following attainment of the target venetoclax dose. Patients with persistent risk of TLS may require prolonged intravenous hydration

Allopurinol 300 mg; administer orally once daily starting ≥2 days prior to initiation of venetoclax and continue until at least 24 hours following attainment of the target venetoclax dose. Patients with persistent risk of TLS may require extended duration of allopurinol (eg, through day 28 of cycle 1)

Decitabine 20 mg/m^2 per dose; administer intravenously in a volume of cold (2°–8°C) 0.9% NS or cold (2°–8°C) 5% dextrose injection (D5W) sufficient to produce a final concentration between 0.1 mg/mL and 1 mg/mL over 1 hour daily for 5 consecutive days on days 1–5, every 28 days for a minimum of 4 cycles and until disease progression (total dosage/28-day cycle = 100 mg/m^2)
  - *Note:* If decitabine is prepared using cold (2°–8°C) diluent, then the final prepared product may be stored at 2°–8°C for up to 4 hours following preparation before initiation of administration. If decitabine is prepared using room temperature (20°–25°C) diluent, then initiation of administration must occur within 15 minutes of preparation

Venetoclax administration during cycle 1:

Venetoclax 100 mg; administer orally with 240 mL water within 30 minutes of completion of a meal (preferably breakfast) once on day 1 of cycle 1 only, *then:*

Venetoclax 200 mg; administer orally with 240 mL water within 30 minutes of completion of a meal (preferably breakfast) once on day 2 of cycle 1 only, *then:*

Venetoclax 400 mg; administer orally with 240 mL water within 30 minutes of a meal (preferably breakfast) once daily for 26 consecutive days on days 3–28 of cycle 1 only (total dosage in cycle 1= 10,700 mg)

Venetoclax administration during cycle 2 and beyond:
Venetoclax 400 mg; administer orally with 240 mL water within 30 minutes of a meal (preferably breakfast) once daily, continuously, on days 1–28, beginning with cycle 2, every 28 days, until disease progression (total dosage/28-day cycle during cycle ≥2 = 11,200 mg)
  Notes:
  - Venetoclax tablets should be swallowed whole. Do not chew, crush, or break venetoclax tablets
  - Patients who delay taking venetoclax at a regularly scheduled time may administer the missed dose within 30 minutes of completion of a meal if within 8 hours of the usual dosing time. If >8 hours, skip the missed dose and resume treatment at the next regularly scheduled time. Patients who vomit after a dose of venetoclax should not repeat the dose but rather take the next dose at the next regularly scheduled time
  - Venetoclax is a substrate of cytochrome P450 (CYP) CYP3A subfamily enzymes, P-glycoprotein (P-gp), and BCRP. Venetoclax is a weak inhibitor of CYP2C8, CYP2C9, and UGT1A1 in vitro but due to high protein binding is predicted to cause clinically insignificant inhibition of these enzymes in vivo. Venetoclax is a P-gp and BCRP inhibitor and weak OATP1B1 inhibitor in vitro
    - Avoid concurrent use with strong or moderate CYP3A inducers at all times
    - See therapy modification section for venetoclax dose modifications in patients who require concomitant therapy with posaconazole, other strong CYP3A inhibitors, moderate CYP3A inhibitors, or P-glycoprotein (P-gp) inhibitors

(continued)

Patient Population Studied

This multicenter, phase 1b dose-escalation and expansion study involved 145 patients with previously untreated acute myeloid leukemia who were deemed unsuitable for intensive chemotherapy. Eligible patients were aged ≥65 years and had Eastern Cooperative Oncology Group (ECOG) performance status ≤2. Venetoclax was administered with a short ramp-up during cycle 1 from 20 mg daily (in early dose escalation stage) or 100 mg daily (in expansion stage) to a target dose of 400, 800, or 1200 mg daily. In the expansion stage of the study, patients (N = 100) received venetoclax (400 mg or 800 mg) in combination with either decitabine or azacitidine

(*continued*)

- Advise patients to not consume grapefruit products, Seville oranges, or starfruit as they may inhibit CYP3A in the gut wall and increase the bioavailability of venetoclax
- Coadministration of venetoclax with warfarin caused increased exposure to *R*-warfarin and *S*-warfarin. Monitor the international normalized ratio closely in patients coadministered warfarin
- Venetoclax inhibits P-glycoprotein (P-gp). Concomitant use of narrow therapeutic index P-gp substrates (eg, digoxin, everolimus, sirolimus) should be avoided when possible. If use of a P-gp substrate is unavoidable, then administer the P-gp substrate ≥6 hours before venetoclax

- Venetoclax can cause rapid death of leukemic cells leading to rapid onset of tumor lysis syndrome (TLS) during the dose escalation period in some patients. In clinical trials of venetoclax for the treatment of chronic lymphocytic leukemia, fatal cases of tumor lysis syndrome have occurred, leading to the development of a step-wise dose escalation approach to initiation of venetoclax. Notably, no cases of TLS were observed in the phase 1 dose escalation and expansion study of venetoclax plus decitabine or azacitidine in AML patients (DiNardo et al. 2018)

  - Do not initiate venetoclax in patients with acute myeloid leukemia until the white blood cell count is <25,000/mm³. Cytoreduction (eg, with hydroxyurea) may be necessary to meet this criterion
  - Provide appropriate prophylaxis for TLS (ie, hydration, anti-hyperuricemic agents) prior to the first dose and until at least 24 hours following attainment of the target venetoclax dose of 400 mg
  - For patients with risk factors for TLS (eg, circulating blasts, extensive involvement of AML in bone marrow, markedly elevated baseline lactate dehydrogenase levels, or renal insufficiency), consider increased frequency of laboratory monitoring and initiation of venetoclax at a lower dose
  - In the phase 1b dose escalation and expansion study (DiNardo et al. 2018), patients were required to be hospitalized starting on day 1 of cycle 1 and for a minimum of 24 hours following attainment of the target venetoclax dose

Supportive Care

Antiemetic prophylaxis
Emetogenic potential on days with decitabine is **MINIMAL**
Emetogenic potential on days with venetoclax only is **MINIMAL–LOW**
See Chapter 42 for antiemetic recommendations

Hematopoietic growth factor (CSF) prophylaxis
Primary prophylaxis is NOT indicated
See Chapter 43 for more information

Antimicrobial prophylaxis
Risk of fever and neutropenia is **MODERATE**
  Antimicrobial primary prophylaxis to be considered:
- Antibacterial—consider prophylaxis with a fluoroquinolone during periods of prolonged neutropenia only (eg, <500/mm³ for ≥7 days), or no prophylaxis, until ANC recovery
- Antifungal—consider prophylaxis with fluconazole or another azole antifungal medication during periods of prolonged neutropenia only (eg, <500/mm³ for ≥7 days), or no prophylaxis, until ANC recovery. Note that use of azole antifungals necessitates venetoclax dose reduction (see therapy modification section)
- Antiviral—antiherpes antivirals (eg, acyclovir, famciclovir, valacyclovir)

Therapy Monitoring

1. *Prior to initiation of venetoclax:*
   a. Assess tumor burden (CBC with differential, bone marrow aspirate, and biopsy) and baseline chemistries (potassium, uric acid, phosphorus, calcium, serum creatinine, LDH) to determine the risk for tumor lysis syndrome (TLS)
      i. If the white blood cell (WBC) count is ≥25,000/mm³, delay the initiation of venetoclax plus decitabine and administer cytoreductive therapy (eg, hydroxyurea). When the WBC count is reduced to <25,000/mm³, discontinue cytoreductive therapy and proceed with initiation of venetoclax plus decitabine
   b. Verify adherence to the prescribed xanthine oxidase inhibitor regimen (eg, allopurinol) to begin ≥2 days prior to venetoclax initiation
   c. Assess blood chemistry (potassium, uric acid, phosphorus, calcium, bicarbonate, and creatinine) and correct pre-existing abnormalities prior to initiation of treatment with venetoclax
   d. Monitor liver function tests
   e. Screen for the presence of drug-drug interactions involving venetoclax
2. *On days 1, 2, and 3 of cycle 1 only:* monitor potassium, uric acid, phosphorus, calcium, and serum creatinine prior to the venetoclax dose and 6–8 hours following the venetoclax dose
3. *Prior to each cycle:* serum chemistries, liver function tests, CBC with differential
4. *Twice per week until achievement of remission:* CBC with differential and platelet count
5. *Every 1–2 weeks after achievement of remission:* CBC with differential and platelet count
6. *Response assessment following cycle 1, and then every 3–4 cycles:* CBC with differential, bone marrow aspirate, and biopsy (as clinically indicated)

Efficacy

	Composite Response Rate (CR + CRi) [n], n (%)	Overall Response Rate (CR + CRi + PR) [n], n (%)	Leukemia Response Rate (CR + CRi + PR + MLFS) [n], n (%)	Median Duration of CR + CRi (95% CI)	Median OS (95% CI)
Ven 400 mg + Dec n = 31	22 (71)	22 (71)	25 (81)	12.5 (5.1–NR)	14.2 (7.7–NR)

Treatment Modifications

VENETOCLAX + DECITABINE

Starting venetoclax dose	400 mg by mouth once daily on days 1–28 of each 28-day cycle
Venetoclax dose level –1	400 mg by mouth once daily on days 1–21 of each 28-day cycle

*Decitabine doses generally should not be reduced. Follow guidelines below for delaying treatment

Hematologic Toxicities

G4 neutropenia (ANC <500/mm^3) with or without fever or infection; or G4 thrombocytopenia (platelet count <25,000/mm^3) Any occurrence prior to achieving remission	Transfuse blood products, administer prophylactic and treatment antimicrobial agents as clinically indicated In most cases, venetoclax plus decitabine should not be interrupted due to cytopenias prior to achieving remission
G4 neutropenia (ANC <500/mm^3) persisting ≥7 days with or without fever or infection; *or* G4 thrombocytopenia (platelet count <25,000/mm^3) persisting ≥7 days First occurrence after achieving remission	Delay subsequent treatment cycle of venetoclax plus decitabine and monitor blood counts. Consider administering G-CSF for neutropenia Once the toxicity has resolved to G ≤2 (ANC ≥1000/mm^3 and platelet count ≥50,000/mm^3), resume venetoclax plus decitabine at the same doses
G4 neutropenia (ANC <500/mm^3) persisting ≥7 days with or without fever or infection; or G4 thrombocytopenia (platelet count <25,000/mm^3) persisting ≥7 days Subsequent occurrence during cycles after achieving remission	Delay subsequent treatment cycle of venetoclax plus decitabine and monitor blood counts. Consider administering G-CSF for neutropenia Once the toxicity has resolved to G ≤2 (ANC ≥1000/mm^3 and platelet count ≥50,000/mm^3), resume venetoclax at the same dose but with the duration reduced by 7 days per cycle (ie, administer on days 1–21 of each 28-day cycle only). Do not reduce decitabine dose

Drug-Drug Interactions

Concomitant therapy with posaconazole is required	**Ramp Up Venetoclax Dose** Day 1: 10 mg Day 2: 20 mg Day 3: 50 mg Day 4: 70 mg	**Steady Venetoclax Maintenance Dose** Reduce the venetoclax dose to 70 mg
Other strong CYP3A inhibitor (aside from posaconazole) is required	**Ramp Up Venetoclax Dose** Day 1: 10 mg Day 2: 20 mg Day 3: 50 mg Day 4: 100 mg	**Steady Venetoclax Maintenance Dose** Reduce the venetoclax dose to 100 mg
Moderate CYP3A inhibitor or moderate P-glycoprotein inhibitor is required	**Ramp Up Venetoclax Dose** Day 1: ≤50 mg Day 2: ≤100 mg Day 3: ≤200 mg	**Steady Venetoclax Maintenance Dose** Reduce the venetoclax dose by at least 50% (ie, to ≤200 mg per dose)
Concomitant therapy with a strong or moderate CYP3A inducer is required	Do not administer a strong or moderate CYP3A inducer with venetoclax	
Concomitant strong or moderate CYP3A inhibitor, posaconazole, or P-gp inhibitor is subsequently discontinued	Resume the venetoclax dosage that was used prior to concomitant use of a strong or moderate CYP3A4 inhibitor, posaconazole, or P-gp inhibitor 2–3 days after discontinuation of the inhibitor	
Concomitant therapy with warfarin is required	Monitor international normalized ratio frequently	
Concomitant therapy with a P-gp substrate is required	Consider alternative medications. If concomitant use is unavoidable, administer the P-gp substrate at least 6 hours before the administration of venetoclax	
Immunization with a live attenuated vaccine is indicated prior to, during, or after therapy with venetoclax	Do not administer live attenuated vaccines prior to, during, or after treatment with venetoclax until B-cell recovery occurs	

Venetoclax may cause fetal harm. Advise females of reproductive potential of the potential risk to a fetus and to use effective contraception during treatment

ANC, absolute neutrophil count; G-CSF, granulocyte-colony stimulating factor; BUN, blood urea nitrogen; P-gp, P-glycoprotein

Adverse Events

	All-Grade Event (%)*		
	Venetoclax 400 mg	Venetoclax 800 mg	Venetoclax 1200 mg
	Decitabine (n = 31)	Decitabine (n = 37)	Decitabine (n = 5)
Nausea	55	62	80
Diarrhea	42	60	80
Constipation	45	41	40
Febrile neutropenia	61	41	40
Fatigue	39	35	80
Hypokalemia	32	46	60
Decreased appetite	26	35	60
Decreased white blood cell count	42	27	40
Vomiting	32	27	60
Anemia	23	30	40
Cough	32	30	40
Peripheral edema	23	32	20

*According to the National Cancer Institute Common Terminology Criteria for Adverse Events, version 4.0
Note: All-grade treatment-emergent adverse effects that occurred in >25% of patients are included.

LOW-INTENSITY THERAPY • FIRST-LINE
ACUTE MYELOID LEUKEMIA REGIMEN: VENETOCLAX + AZACITIDINE

DiNardo CD et al. Blood 2019;133:7–17
Supplementary materials to: DiNardo CD et al. Blood 2019;133:7–17
Protocol for: DiNardo CD et al. Blood 2019;133:7–17
Venclexta (venetoclax tablets) prescribing information. North Chicago, IL: AbbVie Inc; 2018 November
Vidaza (azacitidine injection) prescribing information. Summit, NJ: Celgene Corporation; 2018 September

Prophylaxis for tumor lysis syndrome (TLS) during ramp-up phase:

0.9% sodium chloride (0.9% NS); administer intravenously at 75–150 mL/hour, as tolerated, starting prior to the first dose of venetoclax on day 1 during cycle 1 only, and continue until at least 24 hours following attainment of the target venetoclax dose. Patients with persistent risk of TLS may require prolonged intravenous hydration

Allopurinol 300 mg; administer orally once daily starting ≥2 days prior to initiation of venetoclax and continue until at least 24 hours following attainment of the target venetoclax dose. Patients with persistent risk of TLS may require extended duration of allopurinol (eg, through day 28 of cycle 1)

Azacitidine 75 mg/m² per dose; administer intravenously in 50–100 mL of 0.9% NS or Lactated Ringer's injection over 10–40 minutes once daily for 7 consecutive days on days 1–7, every 28 days, for a minimum of 4 cycles and until disease progression (total dosage/28-day cycle = 525 mg/m²)
- *Note:* Azacitidine administration must be completed within 1 hour of reconstitution of the azacitidine vial
- Alternatively, may administer azacitidine subcutaneously as follows:
  - **Azacitidine** 75 mg/m² per dose; administer subcutaneously into the thigh, abdomen, or upper arm, in a volume of sterile water for injection (SWFI) sufficient to produce a final concentration of 25 mg/mL, once daily for 7 consecutive days on days 1–7, every 28 days, for a minimum of 4 cycles and until disease progression (total dosage/28-day cycle = 525 mg/m²)
  - Notes:
    - Immediately prior to subcutaneous injection, roll the syringe between the palms until a uniform, cloudy suspension is achieved. Rotate injection sites and administer a new injection at least 2.5 cm from an old site. Avoid administration in areas that are tender, erythematous, sclerotic, or ecchymotic. For total subcutaneous doses >100 mg, divide the dose equally between two syringes and inject into two separate sites
    - If azacitidine for subcutaneous injection is prepared using room-temperature (20°–25°C) SWFI and the prepared product is subsequently stored at room temperature, then administration must occur within 1 hour of reconstitution
    - If azacitidine for subcutaneous injection is prepared using room-temperature (20°–25°C) SWFI and the prepared product is immediately stored in refrigerated conditions (2°–8°C), then administration must occur within 8 hours of reconstitution. Prior to administration, allow the suspension to equilibrate to room temperature for up to 30 minutes following removal from the refrigerator
    - If azacitidine for subcutaneous injection is prepared using cold (2°–8°C) SWFI and is immediately stored in refrigerated conditions (2°–8°C), then administration must occur within 22 hours of reconstitution. Prior to administration, allow the suspension to equilibrate to room temperature for up to 30 minutes following removal from the refrigerator

Venetoclax administration during cycle 1:

Venetoclax 100 mg; administer orally with 240 mL water within 30 minutes of completion of a meal (preferably breakfast) once on day 1 of cycle 1 only, *then:*

Venetoclax 200 mg; administer orally with 240 mL water within 30 minutes of completion of a meal (preferably breakfast) once on day 2 of cycle 1 only, *then:*

Venetoclax 400 mg; administer orally with 240 mL water within 30 minutes of a meal (preferably breakfast) once daily for 26 consecutive days on days 3–28 of cycle 1 only (total dosage in cycle 1= 10,700 mg)

Venetoclax administration during cycle 2 and beyond:

Venetoclax 400 mg; administer orally with 240 mL water within 30 minutes of a meal (preferably breakfast) once daily, continuously, on days 1–28, beginning with cycle 2, every 28 days, until disease progression (total dosage/28-day cycle during cycle ≥2 = 11,200 mg)
  Notes:
- Venetoclax tablets should be swallowed whole. Do not chew, crush, or break venetoclax tablets
- Patients who delay taking venetoclax at a regularly scheduled time may administer the missed dose within 30 minutes of completion of a meal if within 8 hours of the usual dosing time. If >8 hours, skip the missed dose and resume treatment at the next regularly scheduled time. Patients who vomit after a dose of venetoclax should not repeat the dose but rather take the next dose at the next regularly scheduled time
- Venetoclax is a substrate of cytochrome P450 (CYP) CYP3A subfamily enzymes, P-glycoprotein (P-gp), and BCRP. Venetoclax is a weak inhibitor of CYP2C8, CYP2C9, and UGT1A1 in vitro but due to high protein binding is predicted to cause clinically insignificant inhibition of these enzymes in vivo. Venetoclax is a P-gp and BCRP inhibitor and weak OATP1B1 inhibitor in vitro
  - Avoid concurrent use with strong or moderate CYP3A inducers at all times
  - See therapy modification section for venetoclax dose modifications in patients who require concomitant therapy with posaconazole, other strong CYP3A inhibitors, moderate CYP3A inhibitors, or P-glycoprotein (P-gp) inhibitors

(continued)

(continued)

- Advise patients to not consume grapefruit products, Seville oranges, or starfruit as they may inhibit CYP3A in the gut wall and increase the bioavailability of venetoclax
- Coadministration of venetoclax with warfarin caused increased exposure to *R*-warfarin and *S*-warfarin. Monitor the international normalized ratio closely in patients coadministered warfarin
- Venetoclax inhibits P-glycoprotein (P-gp). Concomitant use of narrow therapeutic index P-gp substrates (eg, digoxin, everolimus, sirolimus) should be avoided when possible. If use of a P-gp substrate is unavoidable, then administer the P-gp substrate ≥6 hours before venetoclax

• Venetoclax can cause rapid death of leukemic cells leading to rapid onset of tumor lysis syndrome (TLS) during the dose escalation period in some patients. In clinical trials of venetoclax for the treatment of chronic lymphocytic leukemia, fatal cases of tumor lysis syndrome have occurred, leading to the development of a step-wise dose escalation approach to initiation of venetoclax. Notably, no cases of TLS were observed in the phase 1 dose escalation and expansion study of venetoclax plus decitabine or azacitidine in AML patients (DiNardo et al. 2018)

- Do not initiate venetoclax in patients with acute myeloid leukemia until the white blood cell count is <25,000/mm³. Cytoreduction (eg, with hydroxyurea) may be necessary to meet this criterion
- Provide appropriate prophylaxis for TLS (ie, hydration, anti-hyperuricemic agents) prior to the first dose and until at least 24 hours following attainment of the target venetoclax dose of 400 mg
- For patients with risk factors for TLS (eg, circulating blasts, extensive involvement of AML in bone marrow, markedly elevated baseline lactate dehydrogenase levels, or renal insufficiency), consider increased frequency of laboratory monitoring and initiation of venetoclax at a lower dose
- In the phase 1b dose escalation and expansion study (DiNardo et al. 2018), patients were required to be hospitalized starting on day 1 of cycle 1 and for a minimum of 24 hours following attainment of the target venetoclax dose

Supportive Care
Antiemetic prophylaxis
Emetogenic potential on days with azacitidine is **MODERATE**
Emetogenic potential on days with venetoclax only is **MINIMAL–LOW**
See Chapter 42 for antiemetic recommendations

Hematopoietic growth factor (CSF) prophylaxis
Primary prophylaxis is **NOT** *indicated*
See Chapter 43 for more information

Antimicrobial prophylaxis
Risk of fever and neutropenia is **MODERATE**
Antimicrobial primary prophylaxis to be considered:
- Antibacterial—consider prophylaxis with a fluoroquinolone during periods of prolonged neutropenia only (eg, <500/mm³ for ≥7 days), or no prophylaxis, until ANC recovery
- Antifungal—consider prophylaxis with fluconazole or another azole antifungal medication during periods of prolonged neutropenia only (eg, <500/mm³ for ≥7 days), or no prophylaxis, until ANC recovery. Note that use of azole antifungals necessitates venetoclax dose reduction (see therapy modification section)
- Antiviral—antiherpes antivirals (eg, acyclovir, famciclovir, valacyclovir)

Patient Population Studied

This multicenter, phase 1b dose-escalation and expansion study involved 145 patients with previously untreated acute myeloid leukemia who were deemed unsuitable for intensive chemotherapy. Eligible patients were aged ≥65 years and had Eastern Cooperative Oncology Group (ECOG) performance status ≤2. Venetoclax was administered with a short ramp-up during cycle 1 from 20 mg daily (in early dose escalation stage) or 100 mg daily (in expansion stage) to a target dose of 400, 800, or 1200 mg daily. In the expansion stage of the study, patients (N = 100) received venetoclax (400 mg or 800 mg) in combination with either decitabine or azacitidine

Efficacy

	Composite Response Rate (CR + CRi) [n], n (%)	Overall Response Rate (CR + CRi + PR) [n], n (%)	Leukemia Response Rate (CR + CRi + PR + MLFS) [n], n (%)	Median Duration of CR + CRi (95% CI)	Median OS (95% CI)
Ven 400 mg + Aza n = 29	22 (76)	22 (76)	24 (83)	NR (5.6–NR)	NR (9.0–NR)

Therapy Monitoring

1. *Prior to initiation of venetoclax:*
   - Assess tumor burden (CBC with differential, bone marrow aspirate, and biopsy) and baseline chemistries (potassium, uric acid, phosphorus, calcium, serum creatinine, LDH) to determine the risk for tumor lysis syndrome (TLS)
     i. If the white blood cell (WBC) count is ≥25,000/mm^3, delay the initiation of venetoclax plus azacitidine and administer cytoreductive therapy (eg, hydroxyurea). When the WBC count is reduced to <25,000/mm^3, discontinue cytoreductive therapy and proceed with initiation of venetoclax plus azacitidine
   - Verify adherence to the prescribed xanthine oxidase inhibitor regimen (eg, allopurinol) to begin ≥2 days prior to venetoclax initiation
   - Assess blood chemistry (potassium, uric acid, phosphorus, calcium, bicarbonate, and creatinine) and correct pre-existing abnormalities prior to initiation of treatment with venetoclax
   - Monitor liver function tests
   - Screen for the presence of drug-drug interactions involving venetoclax
2. *On days 1, 2, and 3 of cycle 1 only:* monitor potassium, uric acid, phosphorus, calcium, and serum creatinine prior to the venetoclax dose and 6–8 hours following the venetoclax dose
3. *Prior to each cycle:* serum chemistries, liver function tests, CBC with differential
4. *Twice per week until achievement of remission:* CBC with differential and platelet count
5. *Every 1–2 weeks after achievement of remission:* CBC with differential and platelet count
6. *Periodically:* monitor for injection site reactions (applies to subcutaneous route of azacitidine only)
7. *Response assessment following cycle 1, and then every 3–4 cycles:* CBC with differential, bone marrow aspirate, and biopsy (as clinically indicated)

Treatment Modifications

VENETOCLAX + AZACITIDINE

Starting venetoclax dose	400 mg by mouth once daily on days 1–28 of each 28-day cycle
Venetoclax dose level −1	400 mg by mouth once daily on days 1–21 of each 28-day cycle

*Azacitidine doses generally should not be reduced. Follow guidelines below for delaying treatment

Hematologic Toxicities

G4 neutropenia (ANC <500/mm^3) with or without fever or infection; or G4 thrombocytopenia (platelet count <25,000/mm^3) Any occurrence prior to achieving remission	Transfuse blood products, administer prophylactic and treatment antimicrobial agents as clinically indicated In most cases, venetoclax plus azacitidine should not be interrupted due to cytopenias prior to achieving remission
G4 neutropenia (ANC <500/mm^3) persisting ≥7 days with or without fever or infection; *or* G4 thrombocytopenia (platelet count <25,000/mm^3) persisting ≥7 days First occurrence after achieving remission	Delay subsequent treatment cycle of venetoclax plus azacitidine and monitor blood counts. Consider administering G-CSF for neutropenia Once the toxicity has resolved to G ≤2 (ANC ≥1000/mm^3 and platelet count ≥50,000/mm^3), resume venetoclax plus azacitidine at the same doses
G4 neutropenia (ANC <500/mm^3) persisting ≥7 days with or without fever or infection; or G4 thrombocytopenia (platelet count <25,000/mm^3) persisting ≥7 days Subsequent occurrence during cycles after achieving remission	Delay subsequent treatment cycle of venetoclax plus azacitidine and monitor blood counts. Consider administering G-CSF for neutropenia Once the toxicity has resolved to G ≤2 (ANC ≥1000/mm^3 and platelet count ≥50,000/mm^3), resume venetoclax at the same dose but with the duration reduced by 7 days per cycle (ie, administer on days 1–21 of each 28-day cycle only). Do not reduce the azacitidine dose

Renal Toxicity

Unexplained reduction in serum bicarbonate levels to <20 mEq/L in a patient receiving azacitidine	Reduce the azacitidine dosage by 50% in the subsequent course. If the toxicity does not recur, consider administering full dose azacitidine thereafter
Unexplained elevations of BUN or serum creatinine in a patient receiving azacitidine	Withhold the next cycle of azacitidine until serum creatinine and BUN values return to normal or baseline, then reduce the azacitidine dosage by 50% for the next cycle. If the toxicity does not recur, consider administering full dose azacitidine thereafter

Dermatologic Toxicity

Intolerable injection site adverse reaction (erythema, pain, bruising, reaction) in a patient receiving subcutaneous azacytidine	Consider switching the route of azacitidine administration from subcutaneous to intravenous

Drug-Drug Interactions

Concomitant therapy with posaconazole is required	**Ramp Up Venetoclax Dose** Day 1: 10 mg Day 2: 20 mg Day 3: 50 mg Day 4: 70 mg	**Steady Venetoclax Maintenance Dose** Reduce the venetoclax dose to 70 mg
Other strong CYP3A inhibitor (aside from posaconazole) is required	**Ramp Up Venetoclax Dose** Day 1: 10 mg Day 2: 20 mg Day 3: 50 mg Day 4: 100 mg	**Steady Venetoclax Maintenance Dose** Reduce the venetoclax dose to 100 mg
Moderate CYP3A inhibitor or moderate P-glycoprotein inhibitor is required	**Ramp Up Venetoclax Dose** Day 1: ≤50 mg Day 2: ≤100 mg Day 3: ≤200 mg	**Steady Venetoclax Maintenance Dose** Reduce the venetoclax dose by at least 50% (ie, to ≤200 mg per dose)

(continued)

Treatment Modifications (*continued*)

Drug-Drug Interactions	
Concomitant therapy with a strong or moderate CYP3A inducer is required	Do not administer a strong or moderate CYP3A inducer with venetoclax
Concomitant strong or moderate CYP3A inhibitor, posaconazole, or P-gp inhibitor is subsequently discontinued	Resume the venetoclax dosage that was used prior to concomitant use of a strong or moderate CYP3A4 inhibitor, posaconazole, or P-gp inhibitor 2–3 days after discontinuation of the inhibitor
Concomitant therapy with warfarin is required	Monitor international normalized ratio frequently
Concomitant therapy with a P-gp substrate is required	Consider alternative medications. If concomitant use is unavoidable, administer the P-gp substrate at least 6 hours before the administration of venetoclax
Immunization with a live attenuated vaccine is indicated prior to, during, or after therapy with venetoclax	Do not administer live attenuated vaccines prior to, during, or after treatment with venetoclax until B-cell recovery occurs

Venetoclax may cause fetal harm. Advise females of reproductive potential of the potential risk to a fetus and to use effective contraception during treatment

ANC, absolute neutrophil count; G-CSF, granulocyte-colony stimulating factor; BUN, blood urea nitrogen; P-gp, P-glycoprotein

Adverse Events (N = 145)

	All-Grade Event (%)*		
	Venetoclax 400 mg	Venetoclax 800 mg	Venetoclax 1200 mg
	Azacitidine (n = 29)	Azacitidine (n = 37)	Azacitidine (n = 6)
Nausea	62	62	50
Diarrhea	52	49	67
Constipation	59	49	67
Febrile neutropenia	38	35	50
Fatigue	34	35	33
Hypokalemia	17	30	50
Decreased appetite	28	38	33
Decreased white blood cell count	24	32	17
Vomiting	31	27	33
Anemia	31	30	0
Cough	21	27	33
Peripheral edema	34	27	17

*According to the National Cancer Institute Common Terminology Criteria for Adverse Events, version 4.0
Note: All-grade treatment-emergent adverse effects that occurred in >25% of patients are included.

LOW-INTENSITY THERAPY • FIRST-LINE

ACUTE MYELOID LEUKEMIA REGIMEN: VENETOCLAX + LOW-DOSE CYTARABINE

Wei A et al. J Clin Oncol. 2019;37:1277–1284
Venclexta (venetoclax tablets) prescribing information. North Chicago, IL: AbbVie Inc; 2018 November

Prophylaxis for tumor lysis syndrome (TLS) during ramp-up phase:

0.9% sodium chloride (0.9% NS); administer intravenously at 75–150 mL/hour, as tolerated, starting prior to the first dose of venetoclax on day 1 during cycle 1 only, and continue until at least 24 hours following attainment of the target venetoclax dose. Patients with persistent risk of TLS may require prolonged intravenous hydration

Allopurinol 300 mg; administer orally once daily starting ≥2 days prior to initiation of venetoclax and continue until at least 24 hours following attainment of the target venetoclax dose. Patients with persistent risk of TLS may require extended duration of allopurinol (eg, through day 28 of cycle 1)

Cytarabine 20 mg/m^2 per dose; administer subcutaneously once daily for 10 consecutive days, days 1–10, every 28 days, until disease progression (total dosage/28-day cycle = 200 mg/m^2)

Venetoclax administration during cycle 1:

Venetoclax 100 mg; administer orally with 240 mL water within 30 minutes of completion of a meal (preferably breakfast) once on day 1 of cycle 1 only, *then:*

Venetoclax 200 mg; administer orally with 240 mL water within 30 minutes of completion of a meal (preferably breakfast) once on day 2 of cycle 1 only, *then:*

Venetoclax 400 mg; administer orally with 240 mL water within 30 minutes of a meal (preferably breakfast) once on day 3 of cycle 1 only, *then:*

Venetoclax 600 mg; administer orally with 240 mL water within 30 minutes of a meal (preferably breakfast) once daily for 25 consecutive days on days 4–28 of cycle 1 only (total dosage in cycle 1= 15,700 mg)

Venetoclax administration during cycle 2 and beyond:

Venetoclax 600 mg; administer orally with 240 mL water within 30 minutes of a meal (preferably breakfast) once daily, continuously, on days 1–28, beginning with cycle 2, every 28 days, until disease progression (total dosage/28-day cycle during ≥cycle 2 = 16,800 mg)

Notes:

- Venetoclax tablets should be swallowed whole. Do not chew, crush, or break venetoclax tablets

- Patients who delay taking venetoclax at a regularly scheduled time may administer the missed dose within 30 minutes of completion of a meal if within 8 hours of the usual dosing time. If >8 hours, skip the missed dose and resume treatment at the next regularly scheduled time. Patients who vomit after a dose of venetoclax should not repeat the dose but rather take the next dose at the next regularly scheduled time

- Venetoclax is a substrate of cytochrome P450 (CYP) CYP3A subfamily enzymes, P-glycoprotein (P-gp), and BCRP. Venetoclax is a weak inhibitor of CYP2C8, CYP2C9, and UGT1A1 in vitro but due to high protein binding is predicted to cause clinically insignificant inhibition of these enzymes in vivo. Venetoclax is a P-gp and BCRP inhibitor and weak OATP1B1 inhibitor in vitro

- Avoid concurrent use with strong or moderate CYP3A inducers at all times

- See therapy modification section for venetoclax dose modifications in patients who require concomitant therapy with posaconazole, other strong CYP3A inhibitors, moderate CYP3A inhibitors, or P-glycoprotein (P-gp) inhibitors

- Advise patients to not consume grapefruit products, Seville oranges, or starfruit as they may inhibit CYP3A in the gut wall and increase the bioavailability of venetoclax

- Coadministration of venetoclax with warfarin caused increased exposure to *R*-warfarin and *S*-warfarin. Monitor the international normalized ratio closely in patients coadministered warfarin

- Venetoclax inhibits P-glycoprotein (P-gp). Concomitant use of narrow therapeutic index P-gp substrates (eg, digoxin, everolimus, sirolimus) should be avoided when possible. If use of a P-gp substrate is unavoidable, then administer the P-gp substrate ≥6 hours before venetoclax

(continued)

Patient Population Studied

This open-label, international phase Ib/II study involved 82 patients with previously untreated acute myeloid leukemia who were age 60 years or older and deemed unsuitable for intensive chemotherapy. Eligible patients had Eastern Cooperative Oncology Group (ECOG) performance status ≤2. Venetoclax was administered with a short (4–5-day) ramp-up during cycle 1 from 50 mg or 100 mg daily to a target dose of 600 mg daily. Subcutaneous low-dose cytarabine (20 mg/m^2 daily) was administered on days 1–10 of each 28-day cycle

Efficacy (N = 82)

Complete response or complete response with incomplete blood count recovery	54%
Complete response	26%
Median time to first response	1.4 months
Median duration of response	8.1 months (95% CI, 5.3–14.9)
Median overall survival	10.1 months (95% CI, 5.7–14.2)

(continued)

- Venetoclax can cause rapid death of leukemic cells leading to rapid onset of tumor lysis syndrome (TLS) during the dose escalation period in some patients. In clinical trials of venetoclax for the treatment of chronic lymphocytic leukemia, fatal cases of tumor lysis syndrome have occurred which led to the development of a step-wise dose escalation approach to initiation of venetoclax. Notably, only 2 cases of laboratory TLS (both Grade 3) and no cases of clinical TLS were observed in the phase 1/2 study of venetoclax plus cytarabine in AML patients (Wei et al. 2018). Both patients with TLS were able to reach the target dose of venetoclax

  - Do not initiate venetoclax in patients with acute myeloid leukemia until the white blood cell count is <25,000/mm³. Cytoreduction (eg, with hydroxyurea) may be necessary to meet this criterion

  - Provide appropriate prophylaxis for TLS (ie, hydration, anti-hyperuricemic agents) prior to the first dose and until at least 24 hours following attainment of the target venetoclax dose of 400 mg

  - For patients with risk factors for TLS (eg, circulating blasts, extensive involvement of AML in bone marrow, markedly elevated baseline lactate dehydrogenase levels, or renal insufficiency), consider increased frequency of laboratory monitoring and initiation of venetoclax at a lower dose

  - In the phase 1/2 study (Wei et al. 2018), patients were required to be hospitalized starting on day 1 of cycle 1 and for a minimum of 24 hours following attainment of the target venetoclax dose

Supportive Care
Antiemetic prophylaxis
Emetogenic potential is **MINIMAL–LOW**
See Chapter 42 for antiemetic recommendations

Hematopoietic growth factor (CSF) prophylaxis
Primary prophylaxis is **NOT** indicated
See Chapter 43 for more information

Antimicrobial prophylaxis
Risk of fever and neutropenia is **MODERATE**
Antimicrobial primary prophylaxis to be considered:

- Antibacterial—consider prophylaxis with a fluoroquinolone during periods of prolonged neutropenia only (eg, <500/mm³ for ≥7 days), or no prophylaxis, until ANC recovery

- Antifungal—consider prophylaxis with fluconazole or another azole antifungal medication during periods of prolonged neutropenia only (eg, <500/mm³ for ≥7 days), or no prophylaxis, until ANC recovery. Note that use of azole antifungals necessitates venetoclax dose reduction (see therapy modification section)

- Antiviral—antiherpes antivirals (eg, acyclovir, famciclovir, valacyclovir)

Treatment Modifications

VENETOCLAX + CYTARABINE	
Starting venetoclax dose	600 mg by mouth once daily on days 1–28 of each 28-day cycle
Venetoclax dose level −1	600 mg by mouth once daily on days 1–21 of each 28-day cycle

*The cytarabine dose should generally not be reduced. Follow below guidelines for delaying treatment

Hematologic Toxicities	
G4 neutropenia (ANC <500/mm³) with or without fever or infection; or G4 thrombocytopenia (platelet count <25,000/mm³) Any occurrence prior to achieving remission	Transfuse blood products, administer prophylactic and treatment antimicrobial agents as clinically indicated In most cases, venetoclax plus cytarabine should not be interrupted due to cytopenias prior to achieving remission

(continued)

Therapy Monitoring

1. *Prior to initiation of venetoclax:*
   a. Assess tumor burden (CBC with differential, bone marrow aspirate, and biopsy) and baseline chemistries (potassium, uric acid, phosphorus, calcium, serum creatinine, LDH) to determine the risk for tumor lysis syndrome (TLS)
      i. If the white blood cell (WBC) count is ≥25,000/mm³, delay the initiation of venetoclax plus cytarabine and administer cytoreductive therapy (eg, hydroxyurea). When the WBC count is reduced to <25,000/mm³, discontinue cytoreductive therapy and proceed with initiation of venetoclax plus cytarabine
   b. Verify adherence to the prescribed xanthine oxidase inhibitor regimen (eg, allopurinol) to begin ≥2 days prior to venetoclax initiation
   c. Assess blood chemistry (potassium, uric acid, phosphorus, calcium, bicarbonate, and creatinine) and correct pre-existing abnormalities prior to initiation of treatment with venetoclax
   d. Monitor liver function tests
   e. Screen for the presence of drug-drug interactions involving venetoclax

2. *On days 1, 2, 3, and 4 of cycle 1 only:* monitor potassium, uric acid, phosphorus, calcium, and serum creatinine prior to the venetoclax dose and 6–8 hours following the venetoclax dose

3. *Prior to each cycle:* serum chemistries, liver function tests, CBC with differential

4. *Twice per week until achievement of remission:* CBC with differential and platelet count

5. *Every 1–2 weeks after achievement of remission:* CBC with differential and platelet count

6. *Response assessment following cycle 1, and then every 3–4 cycles:* CBC with differential, bone marrow aspirate, and biopsy (as clinically indicated)

Treatment Modifications (continued)

Hematologic Toxicities

G4 neutropenia (ANC <500/mm³) persisting ≥7 days with or without fever or infection; *or* G4 thrombocytopenia (platelet count <25,000/mm³) persisting ≥7 days First occurrence after achieving remission	Delay subsequent treatment cycle of venetoclax plus cytarabine and monitor blood counts. Consider administering G-CSF for neutropenia Once the toxicity has resolved to G ≤2 (ANC ≥1000/mm³ and platelet count ≥50,000/mm³), resume venetoclax plus cytarabine at the same doses
G4 neutropenia (ANC <500/mm³) persisting ≥7 days with or without fever or infection; or G4 thrombocytopenia (platelet count <25,000/mm³) persisting ≥7 days Subsequent occurrence during cycles after achieving remission	Delay subsequent treatment cycle of venetoclax plus cytarabine and monitor blood counts. Consider administering G-CSF for neutropenia Once the toxicity has resolved to G ≤2 (ANC ≥1000/mm³ and platelet count ≥50,000/mm³), resume venetoclax at the same dose but with the duration reduced by 7 days per cycle (ie, administer on days 1–21 of each 28-day cycle only). Do not reduce the cytarabine dose

Drug-Drug Interactions

Concomitant therapy with posaconazole is required	**Ramp Up Venetoclax Dose** Day 1: 10 mg Day 2: 20 mg Day 3: 50 mg Day 4: 70 mg	**Steady Venetoclax Maintenance Dose** Reduce the venetoclax dose to 70 mg
Other strong CYP3A inhibitor (aside from posaconazole) is required	**Ramp Up Venetoclax Dose** Day 1: 10 mg Day 2: 20 mg Day 3: 50 mg Day 4: 100 mg	**Steady Venetoclax Maintenance Dose** Reduce the venetoclax dose to 100 mg
Moderate CYP3A inhibitor or moderate P-glycoprotein inhibitor is required	**Ramp Up Venetoclax Dose** Day 1: ≤50 mg Day 2: ≤100 mg Day 3: ≤200 mg Day 4: ≤300 mg	**Steady Venetoclax Maintenance Dose** Reduce the venetoclax dose by at least 50% (ie, to ≤300 mg per dose)

Concomitant therapy with a strong or moderate CYP3A inducer is required	Do not administer a strong or moderate CYP3A inducer with venetoclax
Concomitant strong or moderate CYP3A inhibitor, posaconazole, or P-gp inhibitor is subsequently discontinued	Resume the venetoclax dosage that was used prior to concomitant use of a strong or moderate CYP3A4 inhibitor, posaconazole, or P-gp inhibitor 2–3 days after discontinuation of the inhibitor
Concomitant therapy with warfarin is required	Monitor international normalized ratio frequently
Concomitant therapy with a P-gp substrate is required	Consider alternative medications. If concomitant use is unavoidable, administer the P-gp substrate at least 6 hours before the administration of venetoclax
Immunization with a live attenuated vaccine is indicated prior to, during, or after therapy with venetoclax	Do not administer live attenuated vaccines prior to, during, or after treatment with venetoclax until B-cell recovery occurs

Venetoclax may cause fetal harm. Advise females of reproductive potential of the potential risk to a fetus and to use effective contraception during treatment

ANC, absolute neutrophil count; G-CSF, granulocyte-colony stimulating factor; BUN, blood urea nitrogen; P-gp, P-glycoprotein

Adverse Events (N = 82)

AE	Venetoclax 600 mg + LDAC (n = 82)
Any AE	82 (100)
AE with grade ≥3	
Febrile neutropenia	34 (42)
Thrombocytopenia	31 (38)
WBC count decreased	28 (34)
Anemia	22 (27)
Neutropenia	22 (27)
Platelet count decreased	20 (24)
Lymphocyte count decreased	15 (18)
Neutrophil count decreased	14 (17)
Hypophosphatemia	13 (16)
Hypokalemia	12 (15)
Hypertension	9 (11)
Pneumonia	9 (11)
Sepsis	9 (11)
Serious AE	
Anemia	25 (31)
Febrile neutropenia	22 (27)
Pneumonia	8 (10)
AML progression	7 (9)
Sepsis	6 (7)

Data are presented as No. (%). Adverse events (AEs) were listed if they were reported for at least 10% of patients with Grade 3 or higher or at least 5% of patients with serious AEs

LOW-INTENSITY THERAPY • FIRST-LINE
ACUTE MYELOID LEUKEMIA REGIMEN: GLASDEGIB + LOW-DOSE CYTARABINE

Cortes JE et al. Leukemia 2019;33:379–389
Supplementary material to: Cortes JE et al. Leukemia 2019;33:379–389
DAURISMO (glasdegib tablet) prescribing information. New York, NY: Pfizer Labs; 2018 November

Cytarabine 20 mg per dose; administer subcutaneously twice per day for 10 consecutive days, days 1–10, every 28 days, until disease progression (total dosage/28-day cycle = 400 mg)

Glasdegib 100 mg per dose; administer orally once daily at approximately the same time each day, without regard to food, continuously on days 1–28, every 28 days, until disease progression (total dosage/28-day cycle = 2800 mg)

Notes:
- In the absence of disease progression or unacceptable toxicity, continue treatment for at least 6 months to allow sufficient time for a response to take place
- Glasdegib tablets should be swallowed whole. Do not split or crush glasdegib tablets
- Patients who delay taking glasdegib at a regularly scheduled time should be advised to administer the dose as soon as possible and at least 12 hours prior to the next regularly scheduled dose, and return to the normal schedule the following day. Patients who vomit a dose of glasdegib should be advised to not replace the vomited dose and to take the next dose at the next regularly scheduled time
- Glasdegib is associated with concentration-dependent QTc prolongation. At therapeutic glasdegib plasma concentrations in healthy volunteers (n = 36), the largest placebo- and baseline-adjusted QTc interval change was 8 ms (90% CI, 6–10) and at supratherapeutic (two-fold higher) plasma concentrations the largest adjusted QTc interval change was 13 ms (90% CI, 11–16). Of 98 evaluable patients in the clinical trial who received the combination of glasdegib and low-dose cytarabine, 5% of patients had a QTc interval >500 ms and 4% of patients had an increase from baseline QTc of >60 ms.
- Drug interactions:
  - Coadministration of ketoconazole (a strong CYP3A4 inhibitor) with glasdegib increased the glasdegib AUC_{inf} by 2.4-fold and increased the C_{max} by 1.4-fold. Therefore, if concomitant administration of a strong CYP3A4 inhibitor with glasdegib is unavoidable, monitor patients more closely for glasdegib adverse reactions, including QTc interval prolongation
  - Coadministration of rifampin (a strong CYP3A4 inducer) with glasdegib decreased the glasdegib AUC_{inf} by 70% and decreased the C_{max} by 35%. Therefore, avoid coadministration of glasdegib with strong CYP3A4 inducers
  - Coadministration of rabeprazole (a proton pump inhibitor) with glasdegib did not alter the glasdegib AUC_{inf} but decreased the C_{max} by 20%. Therefore, it is not necessary to avoid concomitant administration of glasdegib with medications that increase the gastric pH
  - Patients receiving other medications with a potential to prolong the QTc interval may be at higher risk for QTc interval prolongation. If concomitant administration of another medication with potential to prolong the QTc interval is unavoidable, then more frequent ECG monitoring is recommended
  - In vitro studies suggest that glasdegib is a substrate of P-glycoprotein (P-gp) and that glasdegib is an inhibitor of P-gp, BCRP, multidrug and toxin extrusion (MATE) protein 1, and MATE-2K
- Hepatic and renal dysfunction:
  - Glasdegib has not been studied in patients with severe renal impairment (CrCl 15–29 mL/min) or in patients with moderate (total bilirubin 1.5–3× ULN and any AST) or severe (total bilirubin >3× ULN and any AST) hepatic impairment

Supportive Care
Antiemetic prophylaxis
Emetogenic potential of glasdegib and low-dose cytarabine is **MINIMAL–LOW**
See Chapter 42 for antiemetic recommendations

Hematopoietic growth factor (CSF) prophylaxis
Primary prophylaxis is **NOT** *indicated*
See Chapter 43 for more information

Antimicrobial prophylaxis
Risk of fever and neutropenia is **HIGH**
Antimicrobial primary prophylaxis to be considered:
- Antibacterial—consider prophylaxis with a fluoroquinolone during periods of prolonged neutropenia only (eg, <500/mm³ for ≥7 days), or no prophylaxis, until ANC recovery
- Antifungal—consider prophylaxis with fluconazole or another azole antifungal medication during periods of prolonged neutropenia only (eg, <500/mm³ for ≥7 days), or no prophylaxis, until ANC recovery
- Antiviral—antiherpes antivirals (eg, acyclovir, famciclovir, valacyclovir)

Patient Population Studied

The BRIGHT AML 1003 study is an phase 2, randomized, open-label, international study involving 132 adult (age ≥55 years) patients with newly diagnosed, previously untreated acute myeloid leukemia (AML) or high-risk myelodysplastic syndrome (MDS) who were ineligible for intensive chemotherapy. Patients were randomized 2:1 to receive either the combination of glasdegib plus low-dose cytarabine (LDAC) or LDAC monotherapy. High-risk MDS RAEB-2 (refractory anemia with excess blasts 2) was diagnosed according to the WHO 2008 classification and required bone marrow blasts of 10–19% for eligibility. Ineligibility for intensive chemotherapy was defined as having ≥1 of the following characteristics: age ≥75 years, serum creatinine >1.3 mg/dL, severe cardiac disease (eg, left ventricular ejection fraction <45%), or Eastern Cooperative Oncology Group performance status of 2. Patients were excluded from the study if they had acute promyelocytic leukemia, t(9;22), another active malignancy, known active uncontrolled central nervous system leukemia involvement, a baseline QTc interval >470 ms, or a history of long QT syndrome or uncontrolled cardiovascular disease

Efficacy (N = 132)

Efficacy Variable	Glasdegib + LDAC (n = 88)	LDAC (n = 44)	Between-group Comparison
OS in all patients (n = 88 glasdegib/LDAC arm, n = 44 LDAC arm)			
Median OS—months (80% CI)	8.8 (6.9–9.9)	4.9 (3.5–6.0)	HR 0.513 (80% CI, 0.394–0.666); P = 0.0004
OS rate % (80% CI)			
6 months	59.8 (52.6–66.3)	38.2 (28.6–47.7)	—
12 months	39.5 (32.6–46.3)	9.5 (4.8–16.3)	—
OS in AML patients (n = 78 glasdegib/LDAC arm, n = 38 in LDAC arm)			
Median OS—months (80% CI)	8.3 (6.6–9.5)	4.3 (2.9–4.9)	HR 0.46 (80% CI, 0.35–0.62); P = 0.0002
OS in good/intermediate cytogenetic risk patients (n = 52 glasdegib/LDAC arm, n = 25 LDAC arm)			
Median OS—months (80% CI)	12.2 (8.3–14.4)	4.8 (4.1–6.0)	HR 0.427 (80% CI, 0.300–0.609); P = 0.0008
OS in patients with poor cytogenetic risk (n = 36 in glasdegib/LDAC arm, n = 19 in LDAC arm)			
Median OS—months (80% CI)	4.7 (4.0–7.4)	4.9 (2.3–6.4)	HR 0.633 (80% CI, 0.430–0.934); P = 0.0640
Response*			
CR, all patients—n/N (%) (80% CI)	15/88 (17) (11.9–22.2)	1/44 (2.3) (0.0–5.2)	P = 0.0142[†] OR 5.03 (80% CI, 1.59–15.88); P = 0.0152[‡]
Median DOR—months (range)[§]	9.9 (0.03–28.8)	NR	—
CR, good/intermediate cytogenetic risk—n/N (%) (80% CI)	10/52 (19.2) (12.3–28.1)	0/25 (0) (0.0–8.8)	—
CR, poor cytogenetic risk—n/N (%) (80% CI)	5/36 (13.9) (6.9–24.2)	1/19 (5.3%) (80% CI, 0.6–19.0)	
ORR, AML patients—n/N (%)	21/78 (26.9)	2/38 (5.3)	—
Median DOR—months (range)[|]	6.5 (0.03–28.8)	NR	—

*Investigator-reported
[†]Pearson Chi-square test for all enrolled patients (unstratified)
[‡]Cochran-Mantel-Haenszel test for all enrolled patients stratified by cytogenetics
[§]Among patients in the glasdegib/low-dose cytarabine arm who achieved a complete remission (n = 15)
[|]Among AML patients in the glasdegib/low-dose cytarabine arm who achieved complete remission, complete remission with incomplete count recovery, or a morphologic leukemia-free state (n = 21)
LDAC, low-dose cytarabine; OS, overall survival; CI, confidence interval; HR, hazard ratio; AML, acute myeloid leukemia; CR, complete remission; OR, odds ratio; DOR, duration of response; ORR, overall response rate which includes complete remission + complete remission with incomplete count recovery (CRi) + morphologic leukemia-free state (MLFS)

Note: The efficacy end points were assessed in the intention to treat population (n = 132 randomized patients). At the data cutoff date of 3 January 2017, the median follow-up for overall survival was 21.7 months in the glasdegib/LDAC arm and 20.1 months in the LDAC arm

Therapy Monitoring

1. *Prior to initiation of therapy:* CBC with differential, electrolytes, BUN, serum creatinine, ALT, AST, total bilirubin, alkaline phosphatase, creatine kinase, ECG for QTc interval, urine or serum pregnancy test in females of reproductive potential

2. *At least once weekly for the first month:* CBC with differential, electrolytes, BUN, serum creatinine, ALT, AST, total bilirubin, and alkaline phosphatase

3. *Cardiac monitoring:*
   a. ECG for QTcF interval at baseline (as above), 1 week after initiation of treatment, and then once monthly for the next 2 months. If QTcF is abnormal (>480 ms), repeat the ECG and then follow the instructions outlined in the "Treatment Modifications" section. Note that patients with a baseline QTcF interval >470 ms or with a history of long QT syndrome or uncontrolled cardiovascular disease were excluded from the BRIGHT AML 1003 study

4. *At least monthly for the duration of therapy:* electrolytes, BUN, serum creatinine

5. *As clinically indicated for muscle symptoms:* creatinine kinase

6. *Note on embryo-fetal toxicity:*
   a. Glasdegib can cause embryo-fetal death or severe birth defects when administered to a pregnant woman
   b. Advise females of reproductive potential to use effective contraception during treatment with glasdegib and for ≥30 days after the last dose
   c. Advise males of the potential risk of glasdegib exposure through semen and to use condoms with a pregnant partner or a female partner of reproductive potential during treatment with glasdegib and for ≥30 days after the last dose. Males taking glasdegib should refrain from donating semen during treatment with glasdegib and for ≥30 days after the last dose
   d. Advise patients to refrain from donating blood or blood products while taking glasdegib and for ≥30 days after the last dose

7. *Response assessment:* CBC with differential, bone marrow aspirate, and biopsy (as clinically indicated)

Treatment Modifications

GLASDEGIB + LOW DOSE CYTARABINE (LDAC) DOSE MODIFICATIONS

Dose Level	Glasdegib	LDAC
Starting dose	100 mg by mouth once daily	20 mg subcutaneously twice per day on days 1–10
Dose level −1	50 mg by mouth once daily	15 mg subcutaneously twice per day on days 1–10
Dose level −2	Discontinue*	10 mg subcutaneously twice per day on days 1–10
Dose level −3	—	Discontinue

QTc Interval Prolongation

QTcF interval >480 ms to ≤500 ms†	Continue glasdegib at the current dose. Assess electrolyte levels (eg, magnesium, potassium) and supplement as necessary to achieve a goal magnesium level of ≥2 mg/dL and goal potassium level of ≥4 mmol/L. Review and adjust concomitant medications with known QTc interval-prolonging effects and/or CYP3A4 inhibitory effects as clinically appropriate. Monitor ECGs at least weekly for 2 weeks following resolution of QTc prolongation to ≤480 ms
QTcF interval >500 ms†	Withhold glasdegib. Assess electrolyte levels (eg, magnesium, potassium) and supplement as necessary to achieve a goal magnesium level of ≥2 mg/dL and goal potassium level of ≥4 mmol/L. Review and adjust concomitant medications with known QTc interval-prolonging effects and/or CYP3A4 inhibitory effects as clinically appropriate. Resume glasdegib with the dosage reduced by 1 dose level once the QTc interval has improved to within 30 ms of baseline or to <480 ms. Monitor ECGs at least once per week for 2 weeks following resolution of QTc prolongation. Consider escalating glasdegib back to full dose if an alternative etiology (eg, electrolyte deficiency, concomitant medication therapy) for the QTc prolongation is identified and corrected
QTcF interval prolongation with life-threatening arrhythmia	Permanently discontinue glasdegib*

Hematologic Toxicity

Platelets <10,000/mm³ for >42 days in the absence of disease	Permanently discontinue glasdegib and LDAC
ANC <500/mm³ for >42 days in the absence of disease	Permanently discontinue glasdegib and LDAC

(continued)

Treatment Modifications (*continued*)

Other Nonhematologic Toxicities	
Other G3 nonhematologic toxicity	Withhold glasdegib* and/or LDAC until symptoms improve to G ≤1 or baseline. Resume glasdegib at the same dose level, or with the dosage reduced by 1 dose level, at the discretion of the medically responsible health care provider. Resume LDAC at the same dose level, or with the dosage reduced to 15 mg or 10 mg at the discretion of the medically responsible health care provider. If toxicity recurs, permanently discontinue glasdegib* and LDAC
Other G4 nonhematologic toxicity	Permanently discontinue glasdegib* and LDAC

*If toxicity is attributable to glasdegib only, low-dose cytarabine may be continued
†Confirmed on at least 2 separate ECGs
LDAC, low-dose cytarabine; QTcF, Fridericia corrected QT interval; ECG, electrocardiogram; ANC, absolute neutrophil count

Adverse Events (N = 125)

	Grade (%)					
	Glasdegib + Low-Dose Cytarabine (n = 84)			Low-Dose Cytarabine (n = 41)		
Event*	Grade 1–2	Grade 3–4	Grade 5	Grade 1–2	Grade 3–4	Grade 5
Any adverse event	7.1	64.3	28.6	2.4	56.1	41.5
Anemia	3.6	41.7	0	4.9	36.6	0
Febrile neutropenia	0	35.7	0	0	24.4	0
Nausea	33.6	2.4	0	9.8	2.4	0
Decreased appetite	29.8	3.6	0	7.3	4.9	0
Fatigue	16.7	14.3	0	14.6	4.9	0
Thrombocytopenia	0	31.0	0	2.4	24.4	0
Pneumonia	4.8	16.7	7.1	2.4	14.6	7.3
Diarrhea	22.6	4.8	0	19.5	2.4	0
Pyrexia	25.0	2.4	0	17.1	4.9	0
Edema peripheral	26.2	0	0	14.6	2.4	0
Constipation	23.8	1.2	0	14.6	0	0
Dysgeusia	25.0	0	0	2.4	0	0
Dyspnea	17.9	7.1	0	22.0	4.9	0
Muscle spasms	17.9	4.8	0	4.9	0	0
Cough	21.4	0	0	14.6	2.4	0
Dizziness	20.2	1.2	0	9.8	0	0
Vomiting	19.0	2.4	0	7.3	2.4	0

*Medication Dictionary for Regulatory Activities (MedDRA) version 19.1 coding dictionary applied
Note: Treatment-emergent all-causality adverse events occurring in ≥20% of patients in any treatment arm are included in the table

LOW-INTENSITY THERAPY • FIRST-LINE
ACUTE MYELOID LEUKEMIA REGIMEN: IVOSIDENIB

Roboz GJ et al. Blood 2020;135:463–471
Supplemental data to: Roboz GJ et al. Blood 2020;135:463–471
TIBSOVO (ivosidenib tablets) prescribing information. Cambridge, MA: Agios Pharmaceuticals, Inc; 2019 May

Ivosidenib 500 mg; administer orally once daily, with a low-fat meal or without food, continuously until disease progression (total dosage/week = 3500 mg)

Notes:

- In the absence of disease progression or unacceptable toxicity, continue treatment for at least 6 months to allow sufficient time for a response to take place. In patients with newly diagnosed acute myeloid leukemia, the median (range) time to overall response was 1.9 months (0.9–3.6)

- Ivosidenib tablets should be swallowed whole. Do not split or crush ivosidenib tablets

- Administration of ivosidenib with a high-fat meal (defined as 900–1000 total calories, 500–600 calories from fat, 250 calories from carbohydrates, and 150 calories from protein) increased ivosidenib C_{max} by 95% and area under the curve (AUC) extrapolated to infinity by 25%. Therefore, do not administer ivosidenib with a high-fat meal

- Patients who delay taking ivosidenib at a regularly scheduled time may administer the missed dose if within 12 hours of the usual dosing time. If >12 hours, skip the missed dose and resume treatment at the next regularly scheduled time. Patients who vomit after a dose of ivosidenib should not repeat the dose but rather take the next dose at the next regularly scheduled time

- Ivosidenib is a substrate of cytochrome P450 (CYP) CYP3A subfamily enzymes and P-glycoprotein (P-gp). Ivosidenib induces CYP3A4 (and therefore induces its own metabolism with repeated dosing), CYP2B6, CYP2C8, and CYP2C9. Ivosidenib inhibits OAT3 and P-gp

  - Itraconazole, a strong CYP3A4 inhibitor, increased the single-dose AUC of ivosidenib to 269% of control. Therefore, if concomitant use of a strong CYP3A4 inhibitor with ivosidenib is unavoidable, then reduce the ivosidenib dose to 250 mg orally once daily. If the strong CYP3A4 inhibitor is subsequently discontinued, then increase the ivosidenib dose to 500 mg orally once daily after at least 5 half-lives of the strong CYP3A4 inhibitor have transpired

  - Based on pharmacokinetic modeling, fluconazole, a moderate CYP3A4 inhibitor, is predicted to increase steady state ivosidenib C_{max} to 152% of control and AUC to 190% of control. Therefore, if concomitant use of ivosidenib with a moderate CYP3A4 inhibitor is unavoidable, monitor closely for increased risk of toxicities, especially QTc prolongation

  - Advise patients to not consume grapefruit products as they may inhibit CYP3A in the gut wall and increase the bioavailability of ivosidenib

  - Based on pharmacokinetic modeling, rifampin, a strong CYP3A4 inducer, is predicted to decrease ivosidenib steady-state AUC by 33%. Therefore, avoid concomitant use of strong CYP3A4 inducers with ivosidenib

  - Ivosidenib may decrease the concentrations of sensitive substrates of CYP3A4 and CYP2C9. If concomitant use of a sensitive CYP3A4 substrate with ivosidenib is unavoidable, then monitor closely for loss of efficacy of the sensitive CYP3A4 substrate. Ivosidenib may decrease concentrations of hormonal contraceptives; consider alternative forms of contraception. Ivosidenib may reduce the concentration of itraconazole and ketoconazole; consider alternative antifungal therapies when indicated

- After repeated dosing of ivosidenib 500 mg daily, a concentration-dependent prolongation of the QTc interval by 16.1 ms (90% CI 13.3–18.9) was noted. In clinical trials, among patients treated with ivosidenib, 9% were found to have a QTc interval >500 ms and 14% had an increase in QTc of >60 ms from baseline. Therefore, if concomitant use of another QTc prolonging medication in addition to ivosidenib is unavoidable, then consider increasing the frequency of QTc interval monitoring

Supportive Care
Antiemetic prophylaxis
Emetogenic potential is **MINIMAL–LOW**
See Chapter 42 for antiemetic recommendations

Hematopoietic growth factor (CSF) prophylaxis
Primary prophylaxis is **NOT** indicated
See Chapter 43 for more information

Antimicrobial prophylaxis
Risk of fever and neutropenia is **MODERATE**
Antimicrobial primary prophylaxis to be considered:

- Antibacterial—consider prophylaxis with a fluoroquinolone during periods of prolonged neutropenia only (eg, <500/mm³ for ≥7 days), or no prophylaxis, until ANC recovery. Note that use of fluoroquinolones may increase the risk of QTc prolongation with ivosidenib

- Antifungal—consider prophylaxis with fluconazole or another azole antifungal medication during periods of prolonged neutropenia only (eg, <500/mm3 for ≥7 days), or no prophylaxis, until ANC recovery. Note that use of azole antifungals may increase the risk of QTc prolongation with ivosidenib. Avoid use of ketoconazole and itraconazole due to likelihood of loss of antifungal efficacy when used concomitantly with ivosidenib

- Antiviral—anti-herpes antivirals (eg, acyclovir, famciclovir, valacyclovir)

Patient Population Studied

Study AG120-C-001 (NCT02074839) was a multicenter, open-label, phase 1 dose-escalation and dose-expansion trial that involved 34 patients with newly diagnosed, *IDH1*-mutated acute myeloid leukemia who were ineligible for standard therapy. Eligible patients were aged ≥18 years and had Eastern Cooperative Oncology Group (ECOG) performance status score ≤2. All patients included in the population reported by Roboz et al. received 28-day cycles of oral ivosidenib at a dose of 500 mg daily

Efficacy (N = 33)

Efficacy Variable	Ivosidenib (N = 33*)
CR + CRh rate, n (%) [95% CI]	14 (42.4) [25.5–60.8]
Time to CR/CRh, median (range), mo	2.8 (1.9–12.9)
Duration of CR/CRh, median (95% CI), mo	NE (4.6 to NE)
CR rate, n (%) [95% CI]	10 (30.3) [15.6–48.7]
Time to CR, median (range), mo	2.8 (1.9–4.6)
Duration of CR, median (95% CI), mo	NE (4.2 to NE)
CRh rate, n (%) [95% CI]	4 (12.1) [3.4–28.2]
Time to CRh, median (range), mo	3.7 (1.9–12.9)
Duration of CRh, median (95% CI), mo	6.5 (2.8 to NE)
ORR by IWG, n (%) [95% CI][†]	18 (54.5) [36.4–71.9]
Time to first response, median (range), mo	1.9 (0.9–3.6)
Duration of response, median (95% CI), mo	NE (4.6 to NE)
Best response by IWG, n (%)	
CR	10 (30.3)
CRi or CRp	6 (18.2)
PR	1 (3.0)
MLFS	1 (3.0)
SD	10 (30.3)
PD	3 (9.1)
Not assessed	2 (6.1)
Overall survival	
Median OS—months (95% CI)	12.6 (4.5–25.7)
OS rate at 12 months—%	51.1

CR, complete remission; CRh, complete remission with partial hematologic recovery; CI, confidence interval; mo, months; NE, not estimable; ORR, overall response rate; IWG, 2003 modified International Working Group; CRi, complete remission with incomplete hematologic recovery; CRp, complete remission with incomplete platelet recovery; PR, partial response; MLFS, morphologic leukemia-free state; SD, stable disease; PD, progressive disease; OS, overall survival
*One patient was enrolled based on presence of an *IDH1*-D54N mutation detected locally and was subsequently excluded from the efficacy analyses since the companion diagnostic test was negative for the presence of the *IDH1*-R132 mutation
[†]ORR (overall response rate) = CR + CRi + CRp + PR + MLFS. IWG responses, including CR, were reported by investigators
Note: At the data cutoff date of 2 November 2018, the median follow-up was 23.5 months (range, 0.6–40.9)

Therapy Monitoring

1. *Prior to initiation of ivosidenib:* CBC with differential, baseline chemistries, electrolytes, uric acid, LDH, liver function tests, electrocardiogram for QTc interval measurement

2. Monitor CBC with differential, chemistries, and electrolytes at least weekly during month 1, then at least every 2 weeks during month 2, and then at least monthly thereafter

3. Monitor creatine phosphokinase weekly during the first month of therapy

4. Electrocardiogram for QTc interval measurement once per week for the first 3 weeks of treatment, then at least monthly. Consider more frequent measurement in patients who are receiving concomitant medications that prolong the QTc interval, are receiving concomitant moderate or strong CYP3A4 inhibitors, have congenital long QTc syndrome, have congestive heart failure, or have electrolyte abnormalities (especially hypomagnesemia and/or hypokalemia)

5. Guillain-Barré syndrome occurred in 2 of 258 patients (<1%) treated with ivosidenib. Monitor for and advise patients to promptly report new signs or symptoms of motor and/or sensory neuropathy (ie, weakness, sensory alterations, paresthesias, breathing difficulty)

6. Differentiation syndrome occurred in 6 of 34 newly diagnosed AML patients (18%) treated at a starting ivosidenib dose of 500 mg daily. Among these 6 patients, 3 interrupted ivosidenib. Median onset of differentiation syndrome was 14.5 days (range, 8–82)

   a. Especially during the first 1–2 months of therapy, monitor closely for, and advise patients to promptly report, signs and symptoms of differentiation syndrome (fever, dyspnea, hypoxia, pulmonary infiltrates, weight gain, effusions, peripheral edema, hypotension, renal dysfunction, hepatic dysfunction, or multiorgan dysfunction). In case of suspected differentiation syndrome, institute hemodynamic monitoring, promptly administer corticosteroids, and treat concomitant hyperleukocytosis if present

7. *Response assessment:* CBC with differential, bone marrow aspirate, and biopsy (as clinically indicated)

Treatment Modifications

IVOSIDENIB

Starting dose	500 mg by mouth once daily
Dose level −1	250 mg by mouth once daily

Differentiation Syndrome

Differentiation syndrome is suspected	Promptly administer systemic corticosteroids (ie, dexamethasone 10 mg IV every 12 hours, or equivalent) for a minimum of 3 days or until resolution of symptoms, whichever is longer, and then taper the corticosteroid Initiate hemodynamic monitoring and monitor CBC with differential Continue ivosidenib at the same dose
Severe signs and symptoms of differentiation syndrome persist for >48 hours despite corticosteroid treatment	Interrupt ivosidenib until improvement of severe signs and symptoms of differentiation syndrome to G ≤2, then continue ivosidenib at the same dose
Noninfectious leukocytosis (WBC >25,000/mm³ or absolute increase in total WBC >15,000/mm³ above baseline)	Initiate treatment with hydroxyurea. Consider leukapheresis if clinically indicated. Taper hydroxyurea only after leukocytosis improves or resolves Interrupt ivosidenib if leukocytosis is not improved with hydroxyurea, and then resume ivosidenib at the same dose when leukocytosis has resolved

QTc Interval Prolongation

QTc interval >480 ms to 500 ms	Monitor and replete electrolyte levels. Minimize the use of concomitant medications which may have the potential to prolong the QTc interval. Interrupt ivosidenib until the QTc interval improves to ≤480 ms, then resume ivosidenib at the same dose. Monitor electrocardiograms at least weekly for 2 weeks following resolution of QTc prolongation, and then at least monthly thereafter
QTc interval >500 ms	Monitor and replete electrolyte levels. Minimize the use of concomitant medications which may have the potential to prolong the QTc interval. Interrupt ivosidenib until the QTc interval improves to ≤480 ms or to within 30 ms of baseline, then resume ivosidenib at a reduced dose of 250 mg once daily. Monitor electrocardiograms at least weekly for 2 weeks following resolution of QTc prolongation, and then at least monthly thereafter. Consider re-escalating the dose of ivosidenib to 500 mg once daily if an alternative etiology for QTc prolongation can be identified
QTc interval prolongation with signs/symptoms of life-threatening arrhythmia	Permanently discontinue ivosidenib

Drug-Drug Interactions

Strong CYP3A inhibitor is required	Reduce the ivosidenib dose to 250 mg once daily. Monitor closely for a potential increased risk for toxicity, especially QTc interval prolongation
Strong CYP3A4 inhibitor is discontinued	After 5 half-lives of the strong CYP3A4 inhibitor have transpired, then increase the ivosidenib dose to 500 mg once daily

(continued)

Adverse Events (N = 34)

Event*	Ivosidenib (N = 34)	
	Grade 1–2	Grade ≥3
Diarrhea	47	6
Fatigue	35	12
Nausea	32	6
Decreased appetite	32	3
Thrombocytopenia	12	15
Anemia	15	12
Leukocytosis	24	3
Peripheral edema	26	0
Dyspnea	21	3
Dizziness	24	0
Hypomagnesemia	24	0
Abdominal pain	18	3
Arthralgia	18	3
Constipation	18	3
Epistaxis	21	0
Hypokalemia	18	3
Insomnia	21	0

*According to the National Cancer Institute Common Terminology Criteria for Adverse Events, version 4.0.3
Note: The table includes treatment-emergent adverse events of any grade, irrespective of causality, that were reported in ≥20% of patients. Adverse events of special interest included differentiation syndrome (DS), leukocytosis, and prolonged QT interval. DS occurred in 6 (18%) patients, was G ≥3 in 3 (9%), and led to dose interruptions in 3 (9%). The median (range) time to onset of DS was 14.5 days (8–82). No patient required dose reduction or permanent discontinuation of ivosidenib due to DS. Notably, 5 of the 6 patients who experienced DS achieved CR (n = 3) or CRh (n = 2); the remaining patient was not assessed for response. Leukocytosis occurred in 9 (27%) patients, was deemed treatment-related in 2 (6%), and was G ≥3 in 1 (3%). A prolonged QT interval occurred in 6 (18%) patients, was G ≥3 in 2 (6%), required dose interruption in 4 (12%) patients, required dose reduction in 2 (6%) patients, and required permanent discontinuation in 0 patients

Treatment Modifications (*continued*)

Drug-Drug Interactions	
Moderate CYP3A is required	Do not reduce the ivosidenib dose. Monitor closely for a potential increased risk for toxicity, especially QTc interval prolongation
Strong CYP3A inducer is considered	Do not administer a strong CYP3A inducer with ivosidenib
Concomitant therapy with a sensitive CYP3A4 substrate is required	Monitor closely for loss of efficacy of the sensitive CYP3A4 substrate
Patient is taking hormonal form of contraception	Ivosidenib may decrease concentrations of hormonal contraceptives; consider an alternative form of contraception
Concomitant therapy with a medication that has the potential to prolong the QTc interval is required	Consider more frequent monitoring of electrolytes and of the QTc interval

Other	
Guillain-Barré syndrome	Permanently discontinue ivosidenib
Other G ≥3 treatment-related toxicity	Interrupt ivosidenib until toxicity resolves to G ≤2, then resume ivosidenib at a reduced dose of 250 mg once daily. Consider increasing the dose to 500 mg once daily if the toxicity resolves to G ≤1
Recurrence of the same G ≥3 treatment-related toxicity	Permanently discontinue ivosidenib

CBC, complete blood count; WBC, white blood cell count

LOW-INTENSITY THERAPY • FIRST-LINE
ACUTE MYELOID LEUKEMIA REGIMEN: GEMTUZUMAB OZOGAMICIN

Amadori S et al. J Clin Onc 2016;34:972–979
Protocol for: Amadori S et al. J Clin Onc 2016;34:972–979
Supplementary appendix to: Amadori S et al. J Clin Onc 2016;34:972–979
MYLOTARG (gemtuzumab ozogamicin) prescribing information. Philadelphia, PA: Wyeth Pharmaceuticals Inc; 2018 April

The regimen consists of one course of induction therapy. In the absence of progressive disease, patients could subsequently receive up to eight continuation cycles.

Induction gemtuzumab ozogamicin:
Premedications for each dose of gemtuzumab ozogamicin:
- **Methylprednisolone** 1 mg/kg per dose; administer intravenously 30 minutes prior to each gemtuzumab ozogamicin dose on days 1 and 8, *plus:*
- **Acetaminophen** 650 mg per dose; administer orally 1 hour prior to each gemtuzumab ozogamicin dose on days 1 and 8, *plus:*
- **Diphenhydramine** 50 mg per dose; administer orally or intravenously 1 hour prior to each gemtuzumab ozogamicin dose on days 1 and 8

Gemtuzumab ozogamicin 6 mg/m^2; administer intravenously over 2 hours in a volume of 0.9% sodium chloride (0.9% NS) sufficient to produce a gemtuzumab ozogamicin concentration within the range 0.075–0.234 mg/mL, for 1 dose on day 1, *followed by:*
Gemtuzumab ozogamicin 3 mg/m^2; administer intravenously over 2 hours in a volume of 0.9% NS sufficient to produce a gemtuzumab ozogamicin concentration within the range 0.075–0.234 mg/mL, for 1 dose on day 8 (total dosage during induction = 9 mg/m^2)

> *Notes:*
> - Administer gemtuzumab ozogamicin with an administration set that contains an in-line polyethersulfone filter with pore size of 0.2 μm. Protect the infusion bag or syringe from light using a light-blocking cover during infusion
> - Consider cytoreduction (eg, with hydroxyurea) in patients with WBC ≥30,000/mm^3 prior to gemtuzumab ozogamicin administration
> - Doses <3.9 mg must be prepared and administered in a syringe. Doses ≥3.9 mg may be prepared and administered in either a syringe or an infusion bag
> - There is no maximum gemtuzumab ozogamicin dose when used as a single agent for newly diagnosed acute myeloid leukemia

Continuation gemtuzumab ozogamicin (for patients without evidence of disease progression or significant toxicities following induction):
Premedications for each dose of gemtuzumab ozogamicin:
- **Methylprednisolone** 1 mg/kg per dose; administer intravenously 30 minutes prior to gemtuzumab ozogamicin on day 1, every 28 days, for up to 8 continuation cycles, *plus:*
- **Acetaminophen** 650 mg per dose; administer orally 1 hour prior to gemtuzumab ozogamicin on day 1, every 28 days, for up to 8 continuation cycles, *plus:*
- **Diphenhydramine** 50 mg per dose; administer orally or intravenously 1 hour prior to gemtuzumab ozogamicin on day 1, every 28 days, for up to 8 continuation cycles

Gemtuzumab ozogamicin 2 mg/m^2; administer intravenously over 2 hours in a volume of 0.9% NS sufficient to produce a gemtuzumab ozogamicin concentration within the range 0.075–0.234 mg/mL, for 1 dose on day 1, every 28 days, for up to 8 continuation cycles (total dosage/4-week continuation cycle = 2 mg/m^2)

> *Notes:*
> - Administer gemtuzumab ozogamicin with an administration set that contains an in-line polyethersulfone filter with pore size of 0.2 μm. Protect the infusion bag or syringe from light using a light-blocking cover during infusion
> - Doses <3.9 mg must be prepared and administered in a syringe. Doses ≥3.9 mg may be prepared and administered in either a syringe or an infusion bag
> - There is no maximum gemtuzumab ozogamicin dose when used as a single agent for newly diagnosed acute myeloid leukemia

Supportive Care
Antiemetic prophylaxis
Emetogenic potential is **LOW**
See Chapter 42 for antiemetic recommendations

Hematopoietic growth factor (CSF) prophylaxis
Primary prophylaxis is **NOT** indicated
See Chapter 43 for more information

Antimicrobial prophylaxis
Risk of fever and neutropenia is **MODERATE**
> Antimicrobial primary prophylaxis to be considered:
> - Antibacterial—consider prophylaxis with a fluoroquinolone during periods of prolonged neutropenia only (eg, <500/mm^3 for ≥7 days), or no prophylaxis, until ANC recovery
> - Antifungal—consider prophylaxis with fluconazole or another azole antifungal medication during periods of prolonged neutropenia only (eg, <500/mm^3 for ≥7 days) until ANC recovery
> - Antiviral—antiherpes antivirals (eg, acyclovir, famciclovir, valacyclovir)

Patient Population Studied

This randomized, open-label, phase 3 trial involved 237 patients with previously untreated acute myeloid leukemia who were deemed unsuitable for intensive chemotherapy. Eligible patients were aged ≥61 years. Patients were randomly assigned 1:1 to receive best supportive care with or without a single induction course of intravenous gemtuzumab ozogamicin (6 mg/m² on day 1 plus 3 mg/m² on day 8 and, if benefitting, up to eight monthly 2-mg/m² infusions)

Efficacy

Outcome	GO Arm (n = 111)	
	Induction Response	Best Response
CR + CRi	27 (24.3)	30 (27)
CR	9 (8.1)	17 (15.3)
CRi	18 (16.2)	13 (11.7)
PR	7 (6.3)	6 (5.4)
SD	44 (39.6)	43 (38.7)
Progressive disease	16 (14.4)	16 (14.4)
Induction death	8 (7.2)	8 (7.2)

CR, complete remission; CRi, complete remission with incomplete blood count recovery; GO, gemtuzumab ozogamicin; PR, partial remission; SD, stable disease

	Gemtuzumab Ozogamicin + Best Supportive Care (n = 118)	Best Supportive Care Only (n = 119)	
Median overall survival	4.9 months	3.6 months	HR 0.69, 95% CI 0.53–0.90; P = 0.005

Therapy Monitoring

1. *Prior to initiation of gemtuzumab ozogamicin therapy:* CBC with differential, baseline chemistries, electrolytes, uric acid, LDH, liver function tests, pregnancy test (women of reproductive potential only), electrocardiogram for QTc interval measurement (only in patients with a predisposition for QTc prolongation, with congenital long QTc syndrome, with congestive heart failure, with hypokalemia or hypomagnesemia, or who are taking concurrent medications that have a potential to prolong the QTc interval)

2. *Prior to each dose of gemtuzumab ozogamicin:* CBC with differential, baseline chemistries, electrolytes, uric acid, LDH, liver function tests

3. *In patients at high risk for tumor lysis syndrome (eg, high tumor burden, renal dysfunction, rapidly progressing disease, markedly elevated LDH, baseline abnormalities in laboratory indices of tumor lysis syndrome [potassium, phosphate, uric acid, calcium, serum creatinine]):* consider frequent monitoring of laboratory indices of tumor lysis syndrome, intravenous hydration, and prophylaxis with a xanthine oxidase inhibitor (eg, allopurinol) during the induction course

4. *At least 3 times per week following each dose of gemtuzumab ozogamicin, until recovery:*
   a. CBC with differential, chemistries, electrolytes, uric acid, LDH, and liver function tests
   b. Monitor for signs and symptoms of hepatic sinusoidal obstruction syndrome/veno-occlusive disease (elevations in ALT, AST, total bilirubin, painful hepatomegaly, weight gain, ascites)

5. *At least every 30 minutes during each gemtuzumab ozogamicin infusion and for 1 hour post-infusion completion:* monitor vital signs and monitor for signs and symptoms of an infusion-related reaction (chills, fever, tachycardia, hypotension, hypoxia, respiratory failure, and/or bronchospasm)

6. *Periodically:*
   a. Advise patient to report signs or symptoms of bleeding
   b. Electrocardiogram for QTc interval measurement as clinically indicated, especially in patients with a predisposition for QTc prolongation, with congenital long QTc syndrome, with congestive heart failure, with hypokalemia or hypomagnesemia, or who are taking concurrent medications that have a potential to prolong the QTc interval

7. *Response assessment:* CBC with differential, bone marrow aspirate, and biopsy after recovery from induction therapy (clinical trial protocol performed on day 36), then as clinically indicated

Treatment Modifications

GEMTUZUMAB OZOGAMICIN

Hepatic Toxicity or Hepatic Impairment

Hepatic sinusoidal obstruction syndrome/veno-occlusive disease	Discontinue gemtuzumab ozogamicin
Patient treated with gemtuzumab ozogamicin undergoes subsequent hematopoietic stem cell transplant	Monitor for signs and symptoms of hepatic sinusoidal obstruction syndrome/veno-occlusive disease and liver function tests frequently
Total bilirubin >2× ULN, or AST >2.5× ULN, or ALT >2.5× ULN	Delay gemtuzumab ozogamicin treatment until total bilirubin ≤2× ULN, AST ≤2.5× ULN, and ALT ≤2.5× ULN Consider increasing the frequency of monitoring of liver function tests and for signs/symptoms of hepatotoxicity Omit the scheduled dose if delay is required more than 2 days between sequential infusions

Infusion Reactions

Infusion-related reaction	Interrupt the infusion immediately and institute appropriate supportive medical management Administer acetaminophen and diphenhydramine (if >4 hours has transpired since administration of the premedication doses) Administer methylprednisolone 1 mg/kg intravenously × 1 dose For mild, moderate, or severe infusion-related reactions, once symptoms resolve, consider resuming the infusion at no more than half the rate at which the reaction occurred. Repeat the procedure in the event of recurrent symptoms Permanently discontinue gemtuzumab ozogamicin in patients who experience a life-threatening infusion reaction
Anaphylactic reaction suspected (eg, severe respiratory symptoms or clinically significant hypotension) or life-threatening infusion reaction	Permanently discontinue gemtuzumab ozogamicin

Other Toxicities

Other severe or life-threatening nonhematologic toxicities	Delay gemtuzumab ozogamicin administration until recover to G ≤1. Omit the scheduled dose if delayed more than 2 days between sequential infusions

ULN, upper limit of normal; AST, aspartate aminotransferase; ALT, alanine aminotransferase

Adverse Events (N = 225)

AE	GO (n = 111)		BSC (n = 114)	
	Any Grade	Grade ≥3	Any Grade	Grade ≥3
Infection	49 (44.1)	39 (35.1)	48 (42.1)	39 (34.2)
Febrile neutropenia	20 (18)	20 (18)	27 (23.7)	27 (23.7)
Bleeding	28 (25.2)	14 (12.6)	34 (29.8)	14 (12.3)
Fatigue	51 (45.9)	13 (11.7)	69 (60.5)	24 (21)
Liver	57 (51.3)	8 (7.2)	52 (45.6)	7 (6.1)
Cardiac	31 (27.9)	7 (6.3)	37 (32.5)	16 (14)
Metabolic	18 (16.2)	4 (3.6)	17 (14.9)	7 (6.1)
Renal	7 (6.3)	4 (3.6)	9 (7.9)	5 (4.4)
Death due to any AE	19 (17.1)		23 (20.2)	

AE, adverse event; BSC, best supportive care; GO, gemtuzumab ozogamicin

SUBSEQUENT THERAPY

ACUTE MYELOID LEUKEMIA REGIMEN: GILTERITINIB

Perl AE et al. N Engl J Med 2019;381:1728–1740
Protocol for: Perl AE et al. N Engl J Med 2019;381:1728–1740
Supplementary appendix to: Perl AE et al. N Engl J Med 2019;381:1728–1740
XOSPATA (gilteritinib) prescribing information. Northbrook, IL: Astella Pharma US, Inc; 2019 May

Gilteritinib 120 mg per dose; administer orally once daily, without regard to food, continuously on days 1–28, every 28 days, until disease progression (total dosage/4-week cycle = 3360 mg)

Notes:

- Clinical responses to gilteritinib may be delayed. Mean time to composite complete remission in the ADMIRAL trial was 2.3 ± 1.9 months. In the absence of disease progression or unacceptable toxicity, it is recommended that treatment continue for ≥6 months to allow enough time for a clinical response

- Gilteritinib tablets should be swallowed whole; do not crush or break tablets

- Patients who delay taking gilteritinib at a regularly scheduled time may administer the missed dose as soon as possible on the same day if it is at least 12 hours prior to the next regularly scheduled dose. Patients should then return to the normal schedule the following day. Patients should not administer 2 doses within 12 hours

- Gilteritinib has not been studied in patients with severe hepatic impairment (Child-Pugh class C) or in patients with severe renal impairment (creatinine clearance ≤29 mL/minute)

- Gilteritinib is metabolized predominantly by CYP3A4 and is also a substrate of P-glycoprotein (P-gp)

  - Coadministration of gilteritinib with rifampin, a combined P-gp and strong CYP3A inducer, reduced gilteritinib C_{max} by approximately 30% and AUC by approximately 70%. Therefore, avoid concomitant use of combined P-gp and strong CYP3A inducers with gilteritinib

  - Coadministration of gilteritinib with itraconazole, a strong CYP3A inhibitor, increased gilteritinib C_{max} by approximately 20% and AUC increased by approximately 120%. Therefore, consider alternative therapies that are not strong CYP3A inhibitors. If concomitant use of a strong CYP3A inhibitor with gilteritinib is unavoidable, then increase the frequency of monitoring for gilteritinib adverse reactions

  - Coadministration of gilteritinib with fluconazole, a moderate CYP3A inhibitor, increased gilteritinib C_{max} by 16% and AUC by 40%

- Avoid coadministration of gilteritinib with other drugs that have the potential to prolong the QTc interval. Correct hypokalemia or hypomagnesemia prior to and during gilteritinib therapy

- Gilteritinib inhibits human 5-hydroxytryptamine receptor 2B ($5HT_{2B}$) or sigma nonspecific receptors. Concomitant use of gilteritinib with medications that target the 5HT2B receptor or the sigma nonspecific receptor (eg, escitalopram, fluoxetine, and sertraline) may lead to reduced efficacy of the medications targeting these receptors. Therefore, avoid concomitant use of these medications with gilteritinib when possible

Supportive Care

Antiemetic prophylaxis
Emetogenic potential is **MINIMAL–LOW**
See Chapter 42 for antiemetic recommendations

Hematopoietic growth factor (CSF) prophylaxis
Primary prophylaxis is **NOT** indicated
See Chapter 43 for more information

Antimicrobial prophylaxis
Risk of fever and neutropenia is **MODERATE**

Antimicrobial primary prophylaxis to be considered:

- Antibacterial—consider prophylaxis with a fluoroquinolone during periods of prolonged neutropenia only (eg, <500/mm³ for ≥7 days), or no prophylaxis, until ANC recovery. Note that use of fluoroquinolones may increase the risk of QTc prolongation with gilteritinib

- Antifungal—consider prophylaxis with fluconazole or another azole antifungal medication during periods of prolonged neutropenia only (eg, <500/mm³ for ≥7 days), or no prophylaxis, until ANC recovery. Note that use of azole antifungals may increase the risk of QTc prolongation with gilteritinib

- Antiviral—anti-herpes antivirals (eg, acyclovir, famciclovir, valacyclovir)

Patient Population Studied

The ADMIRAL study (NCT02421939) was a multicenter, international, open-label, phase 3, randomized trial that involved 371 adult patients with relapsed or refractory *FLT3*-mutated (*FLT3* ITD or TKD D835 or I836 with allelic ratio ≥0.05) acute myeloid leukemia. Patients with refractory disease were eligible if their disease was refractory to 1–2 cycles of conventional anthracycline-containing induction chemotherapy. Prior treatment with sorafenib or midostaurin with first-line therapy was allowed (only 5.7% of patients had received prior midostaurin). Patients were randomly assigned 2:1 to receive either gilteritinib or salvage chemotherapy. Salvage chemotherapy was chosen for each patient prior to randomization; choices included mitoxantrone + etoposide + cytarabine (MEC), fludarabine + cytarabine + granulocyte colony-stimulating factor + idarubicin (FLAG-IDA), low-dose cytarabine, and azacitidine. MEC and FLAG-IDA were considered high-intensity options whereas low-dose cytarabine and azacitidine were considered low-intensity

Efficacy (N = 371)

Efficacy Variable	Gilteritinib (n = 247)	Salvage Chemotherapy (n = 124)	Between-group Comparison
Overall survival			
Median OS—months (95% CI)	9.3 (7.7–10.7)	5.6 (4.7–7.3)	HR 0.64 (95% CI, 0.49–0.83); P<0.001
Median EFS—months (95% CI)	2.8 (1.4–3.7)	0.7 (0.2-NE)	HR 0.79 (95% CI, 0.58–1.09); P = NS
Overall survival at 12 months—%	37.1	16.7	—
Response (%)			
CR	21.1	10.5	Risk difference 10.6 (95% CI, 2.8–18.4)
CR or CR with partial hematologic recovery	34.0	15.3	Risk difference 18.6 (95% CI, 9.8–27.4)
CR with partial hematologic recovery	13.0	4.8	ND
CR with incomplete hematologic recovery	25.5	11.3	ND
CR with incomplete platelet recovery	7.7	0	ND
Partial remission	13.4	4.0	ND
No response	26.7	34.7	ND
Composite CR*	54.3	21.8	ND
Overall response	67.6	25.8	Risk difference 32.5 (95% CI, 22.3–42.6)
Duration of remission, median—months (95% CI)	11.0 (4.6-NE)	NE (NE-NE)	NE
Time to composite CR, mean—months ± SD	2.3±1.9	1.3±0.5	NA
Leukemia-free survival, median—months (95% CI)	4.4 (3.6–5.2)	6.7 (2.1–8.5)	NE

OS, overall survival; CI, confidence interval; HR, hazard ratio; EFS, event-free survival; NE, not estimable; NS, not significant; CR, complete remission; ND, not determined; SD, standard deviation; NA, not applicable
*Composite CR = CR + CR with incomplete hematologic recovery + CR with incomplete platelet recovery
Note: At the data cutoff date of 19 October 2018, the median follow-up was 17.8 months. Multiple subgroups were analyzed for overall survival; a particularly noteworthy finding was that gilteritinib benefited patients regardless if they were preselected for a high-intensity regimen (HR 0.66 [95% CI, 0.47–0.93]) or a low-intensity regimen (HR 0.56 [95% CI, 0.38–0.84])

Therapy Monitoring

1. *Within 7 days of initiation of gilteritinib (in females of reproductive potential):* urine or serum pregnancy test
2. *Prior to initiation of gilteritinib and then at least weekly for the first month, at least every other week for the second month, and then at least once monthly for the duration of therapy (or as clinically indicated):* CBC with differential and platelet count, blood chemistries and electrolytes, liver function tests, creatine phosphokinase
   a. Correct hypomagnesemia and hypokalemia prior to initiation of gilteritinib and throughout therapy
3. *Electrocardiogram monitoring for QTcF determination:* prior to initiation; on cycle 1, day 8; on cycle 1, day 15; prior to cycle 2; and prior to cycle 3
4. *In patients considered to be at risk for spontaneous or treatment-related tumor lysis syndrome:* monitor serum creatinine, potassium, calcium, phosphorus, uric acid, and LDH frequently during the period of risk. Consider administration of a xanthine oxidase inhibitor (eg, allopurinol 300 mg by mouth daily) and intravenous or oral hydration
5. *Monitor for the following adverse reactions:*
   a. Signs and symptoms of differentiation syndrome (fever, dyspnea, hypoxia, pulmonary infiltrates, weight gain, effusions, peripheral edema, hypotension, renal dysfunction, hepatic dysfunction, or multiorgan dysfunction). In case of suspected differentiation syndrome, institute hemodynamic monitoring and promptly administer corticosteroids
   b. Signs and symptoms of reversible posterior leukoencephalopathy syndrome (RPLS) such as headache, seizure, lethargy, confusion, blindness, and/or other visual and neurologic disturbances along with hypertension. If RPLS is suspected, evaluate the patient immediately with a brain MRI
   c. Signs and symptoms of hypersensitivity reactions, including anaphylaxis
   d. Signs and symptoms of pancreatitis
6. *Response assessment:* CBC with differential and platelet count and bone marrow biopsy (as clinically indicated)

Treatment Modifications

GILTERITINIB

Starting dose	120 mg by mouth once daily
Dose level −1	80 mg by mouth once daily

Differentiation Syndrome

Differentiation syndrome is suspected	Promptly administer systemic corticosteroids (ie, dexamethasone 10 mg IV every 12 hours, or equivalent) for a minimum of 3 days or until resolution of symptoms, whichever is longer, and then taper the corticosteroid Initiate hemodynamic monitoring and monitor CBC with differential for a minimum of 3 days Continue gilteritinib at the same dose
Severe signs and/or symptoms of differentiation syndrome persist for >48 hours despite corticosteroid treatment	Interrupt gilteritinib until signs and symptoms of differentiation syndrome resolve to G ≤2, then continue gilteritinib at the same dose

Central Nervous System Toxicity

Patient presents with syndrome of headache, and/or altered consciousness, and/or visual disturbances, and/or seizures, and/or hypertension-posterior reversible encephalopathy syndrome is suspected	Interrupt gilteritinib while central nervous system status is clarified. Consider performing magnetic resonance imaging of the brain
Posterior reversible encephalopathy syndrome is confirmed	Permanently discontinue gilteritinib

Cardiac Toxicity

QTcF interval greater than 500 ms	Interrupt gilteritinib. Monitor potassium and magnesium and replete as necessary to maintain levels within the upper end of the normal ranges Review medication list for other medications which have the potential to prolong the QTcF interval and modify as appropriate Monitor serial electrocardiograms until QTcF interval returns to within 30 ms of baseline or ≤480 ms, then resume gilteritinib at a reduced dose of 80 mg by mouth once daily Resume regular electrocardiogram monitoring as described in the therapy monitoring section. If the toxicity developed after initiation of cycle 3, then consider continued electrocardiogram monitoring (eg, prior to each of the next 2 cycles)
QTcF interval increased by >30 ms on electrocardiogram performed on day 8 of cycle 1	Monitor potassium and magnesium and replete as necessary to maintain levels within the upper end of the normal ranges Review medication list for other medications which have the potential to prolong the QTcF interval and modify as appropriate Confirm with electrocardiogram performed on day 9. If QTcF remains >30 ms, then consider dose reduction to 80 mg by mouth once daily Resume regular electrocardiogram monitoring as described in the therapy monitoring section

Gastrointestinal Toxicity

Pancreatitis	Interrupt gilteritinib until pancreatitis is resolved, then resume gilteritinib at a reduced dose of 80 mg by mouth once daily

Other toxicity

Anaphylactic reaction to gilteritinib	Permanently discontinue gilteritinib
Other G ≥3 toxicity considered related to treatment	Interrupt gilteritinib until toxicity resolves or improves to G1, then resume gilteritinib, if appropriate, at a reduced dose of 80 mg by mouth once daily

Adverse Events (N = 355)

Event	Grade (%)*					
	Gilteritinib (n = 246)			Salvage Chemotherapy (n = 109)		
	Grade 1–2	Grade 3–5	Serious AE	Grade 1–2	Grade 3–4	Serious AE
Febrile neutropenia	1	46	30.9	0	37	8.3
Anemia	7	41	3.3	5	30	0
Pyrexia	39	3	13.0	26	4	0.9
ALT increased	28	14	5.3	5	5	0
Diarrhea	29	4	4.1	27	3	0
AST increased	26	15	4.1	10	2	0
Hypokalemia	16	13	0	20	11	0.9
Constipation	30	1	0	15	0	0
Fatigue	26	2	1.6	11	2	0.9
Platelets decreased	1	22	2.0	1	25	0
Cough	29	0	0.8	10	0	0
Thrombocytopenia	3	23	1.6	0	17	0.9
Headache	25	1	2.0	15	0	0
Peripheral edema	24	0	0	12	0	0
Vomiting	21	0	0.4	14	0	0
Dyspnea	20	4	4.1	4	3	1.8
Alkaline phosphatase increased	20	3	0.4	2	0	0

AE, adverse event; ALT, alanine aminotransferase; AST, aspartate aminotransferase
Note: Events shown are those that occurred during treatment in ≥20% of the patients in either treatment group and that had a difference in incidence of ≥2 percentage points between the treatment groups

SUBSEQUENT THERAPY
ACUTE MYELOID LEUKEMIA REGIMEN: IVOSIDENIB

DiNardo CD et al. N Engl J Med 2018;378:2386–2398
Supplementary appendix to: DiNardo CD et al. N Engl J Med 2018;378:2386–2398
Protocol for: DiNardo CD et al. N Engl J Med 2018;378:2386–2398
Tibsovo (ivosidenib tablets) prescribing information. Cambridge, MA: Agios Pharmaceuticals, Inc; 2018 July

Ivosidenib 500 mg; administer orally once daily, with a low-fat meal or without food, continuously until disease progression (total dosage/week = 3500 mg)

Notes:

- In the absence of disease progression or unacceptable toxicity, continue treatment for at least 6 months to allow sufficient time for a response to take place. In patients with relapsed or refractory acute myeloid leukemia, the median time to complete remission was 2.0 (range, 0.9–5.6) months

- Ivosidenib tablets should be swallowed whole. Do not split or crush ivosidenib tablets

- Administration of ivosidenib with a high-fat meal (defined as 900–1000 total calories, 500–600 calories from fat, 250 calories from carbohydrates, and 150 calories from protein) increased ivosidenib Cmax by 95% and area under the curve (AUC) extrapolated to infinity by 25%. Therefore, do not administer ivosidenib with a high-fat meal

- Patients who delay taking ivosidenib at a regularly scheduled time may administer the missed dose if within 12 hours of the usual dosing time. If >12 hours, skip the missed dose and resume treatment at the next regularly scheduled time. Patients who vomit after a dose of ivosidenib should not repeat the dose but rather take the next dose at the next regularly scheduled time

- Ivosidenib is a substrate of cytochrome P450 (CYP) CYP3A subfamily enzymes and P-glycoprotein (P-gp). Ivosidenib induces CYP3A4 (and therefore induces its own metabolism with repeated dosing), CYP2B6, CYP2C8, and CYP2C9. Ivosidenib inhibits OAT3 and P-gp

  - Itraconazole, a strong CYP3A4 inhibitor, increased the single-dose AUC of ivosidenib to 269% of control. Therefore, if concomitant use of a strong CYP3A4 inhibitor with ivosidenib is unavoidable, then reduce the ivosidenib dose to 250 mg orally once daily. If the strong CYP3A4 inhibitor is subsequently discontinued, then increase the ivosidenib dose to 500 mg orally once daily after at least 5 half-lives of the strong CYP3A4 inhibitor have transpired

  - Based on pharmacokinetic modeling, fluconazole, a moderate CYP3A4 inhibitor, is predicted to increase steady state ivosidenib C_{max} to 152% of control and AUC to 190% of control. Therefore, if concomitant use of ivosidenib with a moderate CYP3A4 inhibitor is unavoidable, monitor closely for increased risk of toxicities, especially QTc prolongation

  - Advise patients to not consume grapefruit products as they may inhibit CYP3A in the gut wall and increase the bioavailability of ivosidenib

  - Based on pharmacokinetic modeling, rifampin, a strong CYP3A4 inducer, is predicted to decrease ivosidenib steady-state AUC by 33%. Therefore, avoid concomitant use of strong CYP3A4 inducers with ivosidenib

  - Ivosidenib may decrease the concentrations of sensitive substrates of CYP3A4 and CYP2C9. If concomitant use of a sensitive CYP3A4 substrate with ivosidenib is unavoidable, then monitor closely for loss of efficacy of the sensitive CYP3A4 substrate. Ivosidenib may decrease concentrations of hormonal contraceptives; consider alternative forms of contraception. Ivosidenib may reduce the concentration of itraconazole and ketoconazole; consider alternative antifungal therapies when indicated

- After repeated dosing of ivosidenib 500 mg daily, a concentration-dependent prolongation of the QTc interval by 16.1 ms (90% CI 13.3–18.9) was noted. In the clinical trial, among patients treated with ivosidenib dosed at 500 mg daily, 44 of 179 patients (24.6%) experienced QTc interval prolongation, with 18 of 179 (10.1%) experiencing G ≥3 QTc interval prolongation. Therefore, if concomitant use of another QTc prolonging medication in addition to ivosidenib is unavoidable, then consider increasing the frequency of QTc interval monitoring

Supportive Care
Antiemetic prophylaxis
Emetogenic potential is **MINIMAL–LOW**
See Chapter 42 for antiemetic recommendations

Hematopoietic growth factor (CSF) prophylaxis
Primary prophylaxis is **NOT** indicated
See Chapter 43 for more information

Antimicrobial prophylaxis
Risk of fever and neutropenia is **MODERATE**
Antimicrobial primary prophylaxis to be considered:

- Antibacterial—consider prophylaxis with a fluoroquinolone during periods of prolonged neutropenia only (eg, <500/mm³ for ≥7 days), or no prophylaxis, until ANC recovery. Note that use of fluoroquinolones may increase the risk of QTc prolongation with ivosidenib

- Antifungal—consider prophylaxis with fluconazole or another azole antifungal medication during periods of prolonged neutropenia only (eg, <500/mm³ for ≥7 days), or no prophylaxis, until ANC recovery. Note that use of azole antifungals may increase the risk of QTc prolongation with ivosidenib. Avoid use of ketoconazole and itraconazole due to likelihood of loss of antifungal efficacy when used concomitantly with ivosidenib

- Antiviral—antiherpes antivirals (eg, acyclovir, famciclovir, valacyclovir)

Patient Population Studied

This multicenter, open-label, phase 1 dose-escalation and dose-expansion trial involved 258 patients with relapsed or refractory, *IDH1*-mutated acute myeloid leukemia. Eligible patients were aged ≥18 years and had Eastern Cooperative Oncology Group (ECOG) performance status score ≤2. All patients received 28-day cycles of oral ivosidenib (179 patients had starting dose of 500 mg daily)

Efficacy (N = 125)

Rate of complete remission or complete remission with partial hematologic recovery	30.4%
Rate of complete remission	21.6%
Overall response rate*	41.6%
Median duration of complete remission or complete remission with partial hematologic recovery	8.2 months
Median duration of complete remission	9.3 months
Median duration of response	6.5 months
Median overall survival	8.8 months

Overall response rate includes patients with either a complete or partial response to treatment
Note: The efficacy end points were assessed in 125 patients who received oral ivosidenib at a dose of 500 mg daily and were followed up for ≥6 months. Median follow-up was 14.8 months

Therapy Monitoring

1. *Prior to initiation of ivosidenib:* CBC with differential, baseline chemistries, electrolytes, uric acid, LDH, liver function tests, electrocardiogram for QTc interval measurement
2. Monitor CBC with differential, chemistries, and electrolytes at least weekly during month 1, then at least every 2 weeks during month 2, and then at least monthly thereafter
3. Monitor creatine phosphokinase weekly during the first month of therapy
4. Electrocardiogram for QTc interval measurement once per week for the first 3 weeks of treatment, then at least monthly. Consider more frequent measurement in patients who are receiving concomitant medications that prolong the QTc interval, are receiving concomitant moderate or strong CYP3A4 inhibitors, have congenital long QTc syndrome, have congestive heart failure, or have electrolyte abnormalities (especially hypomagnesemia and/or hypokalemia)
5. Guillain-Barré syndrome occurred in <1% of patients (2/258) treated with ivosidenib. Monitor for and advise patients to promptly report new signs or symptoms of motor and/or sensory neuropathy (ie, weakness, sensory alterations, paresthesias, breathing difficulty)
6. Differentiation syndrome occurred in 10.6% of relapsed/refractory AML patients (19/179) treated at a starting ivosidenib dose of 500 mg daily. Among these 19 patients, 6 patients interrupted ivosidenib, 14 patients recovered without sequelae, 3 patients recovered with sequelae, and 2 patients had ongoing differentiation syndrome. There were no G ≥4 differentiation syndrome events. Median onset of differentiation syndrome was 29 (range, 5–59) days. Of 19 events, 11 (57.9%) occurred between days 1–30, 4 (21.1%) occurred between days 31–45, and 4 (21.1%) occurred between days 46–60
   a. Especially during the first 1–2 months of therapy, monitor closely for, and advise patients to promptly report, signs and symptoms of differentiation syndrome (fever, dyspnea, hypoxia, pulmonary infiltrates, weight gain, effusions, peripheral edema, hypotension, renal dysfunction, hepatic dysfunction, or multiorgan dysfunction). In case of suspected differentiation syndrome, institute hemodynamic monitoring, promptly administer corticosteroids, and treat concomitant hyperleukocytosis if present
7. *Response assessment:* CBC with differential, bone marrow aspirate, and biopsy (as clinically indicated)

Treatment Modifications

IVOSIDENIB	
Starting dose	500 mg by mouth once daily
Dose level −1	250 mg by mouth once daily

Differentiation Syndrome	
Differentiation syndrome is suspected	Promptly administer systemic corticosteroids (ie, dexamethasone 10 mg IV every 12 hours, or equivalent) for a minimum of 3 days or until resolution of symptoms, whichever is longer, and then taper the corticosteroid Initiate hemodynamic monitoring and monitor CBC with differential Continue ivosidenib at the same dose
Severe signs and symptoms of differentiation syndrome persist for >48 hours despite corticosteroid treatment	Interrupt ivosidenib until improvement of severe signs and symptoms of differentiation syndrome to G ≤2, then continue ivosidenib at the same dose
Noninfectious leukocytosis (WBC >25,000/mm³ or absolute increase in total WBC >15,000/mm³ above baseline)	Initiate treatment with hydroxyurea. Consider leukapheresis if clinically indicated. Taper hydroxyurea only after leukocytosis improves or resolves Interrupt ivosidenib if leukocytosis is not improved with hydroxyurea, and then resume ivosidenib at the same dose when leukocytosis has resolved

(continued)

Adverse Events (N = 179)

Grade ≥3* Treatment-related Adverse Event	%
Prolongation of the QT interval on electrocardiography	8
Differentiation syndrome	4
Anemia	2
Decreased platelet count	2
Leukocytosis	2
Thrombocytopenia	2
Hypoxia	1

*According to the National Cancer Institute Common Terminology Criteria for Adverse Events, version 4.0.3
Note: Grade ≥3 treatment-related adverse events that occurred in >1% of patients whose starting dose was 500 mg daily are included. No patients permanently discontinued ivosidenib owing to prolongation of the QT interval, isocitrate dehydrogenase syndrome, or leukocytosis. No deaths owing to treatment-related adverse events were reported for patients whose starting dose was 500 mg daily; one adverse event leading to death (cardiac tamponade) was reported as being possibly related to treatment

Treatment Modifications (continued)

QTc Interval Prolongation

QTc interval >480 ms to 500 ms	Monitor and replete electrolyte levels. Minimize the use of concomitant medications which may have the potential to prolong the QTc interval. Interrupt ivosidenib until the QTc interval improves to ≤480 ms, then resume ivosidenib at the same dose. Monitor electrocardiograms at least weekly for 2 weeks following resolution of QTc prolongation, and then at least monthly thereafter
QTc interval >500 ms	Monitor and replete electrolyte levels. Minimize the use of concomitant medications which may have the potential to prolong the QTc interval. Interrupt ivosidenib until the QTc interval improves to ≤480 ms or to within 30 ms of baseline, then resume ivosidenib at a reduced dose of 250 mg once daily. Monitor electrocardiograms at least weekly for 2 weeks following resolution of QTc prolongation, and then at least monthly thereafter. Consider re-escalating the dose of ivosidenib to 500 mg once daily if an alternative etiology for QTc prolongation can be identified
QTc interval prolongation with signs/symptoms of life-threatening arrhythmia	Permanently discontinue ivosidenib

Drug-Drug Interactions

Strong CYP3A inhibitor is required	Reduce the ivosidenib dose to 250 mg once daily. Monitor closely for a potential increased risk for toxicity, especially QTc interval prolongation
Strong CYP3A4 inhibitor is discontinued	After 5 half-lives of the strong CYP3A4 inhibitor have transpired, then increase the ivosidenib dose to 500 mg once daily
Moderate CYP3A is required	Do not reduce the ivosidenib dose. Monitor closely for a potential increased risk for toxicity, especially QTc interval prolongation
Strong CYP3A inducer is considered	Do not administer a strong CYP3A inducer with ivosidenib
Concomitant therapy with a sensitive CYP3A4 substrate is required	Monitor closely for loss of efficacy of the sensitive CYP3A4 substrate
Patient is taking hormonal form of contraception	Ivosidenib may decrease concentrations of hormonal contraceptives; consider an alternative form of contraception
Concomitant therapy with a medication that has the potential to prolong the QTc interval is required	Consider more frequent monitoring of electrolytes and of the QTc interval

Other

Guillain-Barré syndrome	Permanently discontinue ivosidenib
Other G ≥3 treatment-related toxicity	Interrupt ivosidenib until toxicity resolves to G ≤2, then resume ivosidenib at a reduced dose of 250 mg once daily. Consider increasing the dose to 500 mg once daily if the toxicity resolves to G ≤1
Recurrence of the same G ≥3 treatment-related toxicity	Permanently discontinue ivosidenib

CBC, complete blood count; WBC, white blood cell count

SUBSEQUENT THERAPY

ACUTE MYELOID LEUKEMIA REGIMEN: ENASIDENIB

Fathi AT et al. JAMA Oncol 2018;4:1106–1110
Stein EM et al. Blood 2019;133:676–687
Supplementary material to: Stein EM et al. Blood 2019;133:676–687
IDHIFA (enasidenib tablets) prescribing information. Summit, NJ: Celgene Corporation; 2018 August

Enasidenib 100 mg per dose; administer orally once daily, without regard to food, continuously until disease progression (total dosage/week = 700 mg)

Notes:

- In the absence of disease progression or unacceptable toxicity, continue treatment for at least 6 months to allow sufficient time for a response to take place. In patients with relapsed or refractory acute myeloid leukemia treated with enasidenib at 100 mg per day, the median time to first response was 1.9 (range, 0.5–9.4) months, and median time to best response was 3.7 (range, 0.6–14.7) months
- Enasidenib tablets should be swallowed whole. Do not split or crush enasidenib tablets
- Patients who delay taking enasidenib at a regularly scheduled time should administer the dose as soon as possible on the same day, and return to the normal schedule the following day. Patients who vomit a dose of enasidenib should readminister the dose as soon as possible on the same day, and then return to the normal schedule the following day
- No human drug-drug interaction studies have been performed with enasidenib
  - In vitro studies suggest that enasidenib is a substrate of several cytochrome P450 (CYP) subfamily enzymes including CYP1A2, CYP2B6, CYP2C8, CYP2C9, CYP2C19, CYP2D6, and CYP3A4. Enasidenib is a substrate of several UDP-glucuronosyltransferase enzymes including UGT1A1, UGT1A3, UGT1A4, UGT1A9, UGT2B7, and UGT2B15. A major N-dealkylated metabolite, AGI–16903, is a substrate of CYP1A2, CYP2C19, CYP3A4, UGT1A1, UGT1A3, and UGT1A9
  - In vitro studies suggest that enasidenib inhibits CYP1A2, CYP2B6, CYP2C8, CYP2C9, CYP2C19, CYP2D6, CYP3A4, UGT1A1, P-glycoprotein (P-gp), BCRP, OAT1, OATP1B1, OATP1B3, and OCT2. A major N-dealkylated metabolite, AGI–16903, inhibits CYP1A2, CYP2B6, CYP2C8, CYP2C9, CYP2C19, CYP2D6, BCRP, OAT1, OAT3, OATP1B1, and OCT2
    - Inhibition of UGT1A1 by enasidenib may impede the normal metabolism of bilirubin. Thirty-seven percent of patients were documented to have ≥1 episode of elevation of total bilirubin to at least 2 times the upper limit of normal. In most (89%) cases, there was no concurrent elevation of aminotransferases or other hepatic-related adverse events
  - In vitro studies suggest that enasidenib induces the activity of CYP2B6 and CYP3A4

Supportive Care

Antiemetic prophylaxis
Emetogenic potential is **MODERATE–HIGH**
See Chapter 42 for antiemetic recommendations

Hematopoietic growth factor (CSF) prophylaxis
Primary prophylaxis is **NOT** *indicated*
See Chapter 43 for more information

Antimicrobial prophylaxis
Risk of fever and neutropenia is **MODERATE**
  Antimicrobial primary prophylaxis to be considered:
- Antibacterial—consider prophylaxis with a fluoroquinolone during periods of prolonged neutropenia only (eg, <500/mm³ for ≥7 days), or no prophylaxis, until ANC recovery
- Antifungal—consider prophylaxis with fluconazole or another azole antifungal medication during periods of prolonged neutropenia only (eg, <500/mm³ for ≥7 days), or no prophylaxis, until ANC recovery
- Antiviral—antiherpes antivirals (eg, acyclovir, famciclovir, valacyclovir)

Patient Population Studied

This multicenter, phase 1/2 trial involved 345 patients with relapsed or refractory, *IDH1*-mutated acute myeloid leukemia. All 214 patients in the phase 1 expansion and phase 2 groups received 28-day cycles of oral enasidenib, 100 mg daily

Efficacy (N = 214)

Overall response rate*	38.8%
Median duration of response	5.6 months
Median overall survival	8.8 months
Median event-free survival	4.7 months

*Overall response rate includes patients with either a complete or partial response to treatment or morphologic leukemia-free state
Note: The efficacy end points were assessed in the 214 patients who received oral enasidenib at a dose of 100 mg daily. Median follow-up was 7.8 months

Therapy Monitoring

1. *Prior to initiation of enasidenib:* CBC with differential, baseline chemistries, electrolytes, uric acid, LDH, liver function tests, pregnancy test (women of child-bearing potential only)

2. Monitor CBC with differential, chemistries, electrolytes, liver function tests, uric acid, and LDH at least every 2 weeks during the first 3 months of treatment, and then as clinically indicated

3. Differentiation syndrome occurred in 33 of 281 relapsed/refractory AML patients (11.7%) treated with varying doses of enasidenib in a phase 1/2 study. The median onset of differentiation syndrome was 30 (range, 7–129) days. Patients who developed differentiation syndrome more frequently had ≥20% bone marrow blasts (94% vs 78%, P = 0.04) and had previously undergone fewer prior regimens (median 1 [range, 1–4] vs median 2 [range, 1–14]) compared with patients who did not develop differentiation syndrome. Among these 33 patients, 28 (84.8%) were treated with corticosteroids for a median duration of 12 (range, 4–43) days. Of 13 patients who presented with concomitant leukocytosis, 11 were treated with hydroxyurea for a median duration of 15 (range, 4–71) days. There were no fatal differentiation syndrome events

(continued)

Treatment Modifications

ENASIDENIB

Starting dose	100 mg by mouth once daily
Dose level −1	50 mg by mouth once daily

Differentiation Syndrome

Differentiation syndrome is suspected	Promptly administer systemic corticosteroids (ie, dexamethasone 10 mg IV every 12 hours, or equivalent) for a minimum of 3 days or until resolution of symptoms, whichever is longer, and then taper the corticosteroid Initiate hemodynamic monitoring and monitor CBC with differential Continue enasidenib at the same dose
Severe pulmonary symptoms (ie, requiring intubation or ventilator support) and/or renal dysfunction persist for >48 hours despite corticosteroid treatment	Interrupt enasidenib until signs and symptoms of differentiation syndrome resolve to G ≤2, then continue enasidenib at the same dose
Noninfectious leukocytosis (WBC >30,000/mm³)	Initiate treatment with hydroxyurea. Consider leukapheresis if clinically indicated. Taper hydroxyurea only after leukocytosis improves or resolves Interrupt enasidenib if leukocytosis is not improved with hydroxyurea, and then resume enasidenib at the same dose when leukocytosis has resolved (WBC <30,000/mm³)

Hyperbilirubinemia

Elevation of bilirubin to >3× ULN sustained for ≥2 weeks without elevated transaminases or other hepatic disorders	Reduce the enasidenib dose to 50 mg daily. If the bilirubin elevation improves to <2× ULN, then increase the enasidenib dose to 100 mg daily

Drug-Drug Interaction

Patient is taking hormonal form of contraception	Enasidenib may affect the concentrations of hormonal contraceptives in unpredictable ways; consider an alternative form of contraception

Other

Other G ≥3 treatment-related toxicity	Interrupt enasidenib until toxicity resolves to G ≤2, then resume enasidenib at a reduced dose of 50 mg once daily. Consider increasing the dose to 100 mg once daily if the toxicity resolves to G ≤1
Recurrence of the same G ≥3 treatment-related toxicity	Permanently discontinue enasidenib

CBC, complete blood count; WBC, white blood cell count; ULN, upper limit of normal

Therapy Monitoring
(*continued*)

a. Especially during the first 1–2 months of therapy, monitor closely for, and advise patients to promptly report, signs and symptoms of differentiation syndrome (fever, dyspnea, hypoxia, pulmonary infiltrates, weight gain, effusions, peripheral edema, hypotension, renal dysfunction, hepatic dysfunction, or multiorgan dysfunction). In case of suspected differentiation syndrome, institute hemodynamic monitoring, promptly administer corticosteroids, and treat concomitant hyperleukocytosis if present

4. *Response assessment:* CBC with differential, bone marrow aspirate, and biopsy (as clinically indicated)

Adverse Events (N = 214)

Any Grade* Treatment-related Adverse Event	%
Hyperbilirubinemia	33
Nausea	28
Decreased appetite	19
Vomiting	17
Diarrhea	15
Fatigue	14
Isocitrate dehydrogenase differentiation syndrome	13
Dysgeusia	10
Dyspnea	9
Elevated aspartate aminotransferase level	9
Leukocytosis	8
Elevated alanine aminotransferase level	7
Anemia	7
Rash	6
Hyperuricemia	6

Note: Any-grade treatment-related adverse events that occurred in ≥5% patients who received oral enasidenib at a dose of 100 mg daily are included. The most frequent treatment-related Grade 3–4 adverse events were hyperbilirubinemia (10%), thrombocytopenia (7%), isocitrate dehydrogenase differentiation syndrome (6%), and anemia (6%)

SUBSEQUENT THERAPY

ACUTE MYELOID LEUKEMIA REGIMEN: GEMTUZUMAB OZOGAMICIN

Taksin AL et al. Leukemia 2007;21:66–71
MYLOTARG (gemtuzumab ozogamicin) prescribing information. Philadelphia, PA: Wyeth Pharmaceuticals Inc; 2018 April

Induction gemtuzumab ozogamicin:
Premedications for each dose of gemtuzumab ozogamicin:

- **Methylprednisolone** 1 mg/kg per dose; administer intravenously 30 minutes prior to each gemtuzumab ozogamicin dose on days 1, 4, and 7, *plus:*

- **Acetaminophen** 650 mg per dose; administer orally 1 hour prior to each gemtuzumab ozogamicin dose on days 1, 4, and 7, *plus:*

- **Diphenhydramine** 50 mg per dose; administer orally or intravenously 1 hour prior to each gemtuzumab ozogamicin dose on days 1, 4, and 7

Gemtuzumab ozogamicin 3 mg/m^2 (maximum dose 4.5 mg) per dose; administer intravenously over 2 hours in a volume of 0.9% sodium chloride (0.9% NS) sufficient to produce a gemtuzumab ozogamicin concentration within the range 0.075–0.234 mg/mL, for 3 doses on days 1, 4, and 7 (total dosage/induction course = 9 mg/m^2; maximum total dosage/induction course = 13.5 mg)

> *Notes:*
> - Administer gemtuzumab ozogamicin with an administration set that contains an in-line polyethersulfone filter with pore size of 0.2 μm. Protect the infusion bag or syringe from light using a light-blocking cover during infusion
> - Consider cytoreduction (eg, with hydroxyurea) in patients with WBC ≥30,000/mm^3 prior to gemtuzumab ozogamicin administration
> - Although the report by Taksin et al. does not indicate a maximum dose of gemtuzumab ozogamicin, the U.S. Food and Drug Administration–approved prescribing information states that the maximum dose of gemtuzumab ozogamicin when used as a single agent for the treatment of relapsed or refractory AML is 4.5 mg, which corresponds to the available vial size
> - Doses <3.9 mg must be prepared and administered in a syringe. Doses ≥3.9 mg may be prepared and administered in either a syringe or an infusion bag

Consolidation high-dose cytarabine: refer to separate regimen description within this chapter

Supportive Care
Antiemetic prophylaxis
Emetogenic potential of gemtuzumab ozogamicin is **LOW**
See Chapter 42 for antiemetic recommendations

Hematopoietic growth factor (CSF) prophylaxis
Primary prophylaxis is **NOT** indicated
See Chapter 43 for more information

Antimicrobial prophylaxis
Risk of fever and neutropenia is **MODERATE**
> Antimicrobial primary prophylaxis to be considered:
> - Antibacterial—consider prophylaxis with a fluoroquinolone during periods of prolonged neutropenia only (eg, <500/mm^3 for ≥7 days), or no prophylaxis, until ANC recovery
> - Antifungal—consider prophylaxis with fluconazole or another azole antifungal medication during periods of prolonged neutropenia only (eg, <500/mm^3 for ≥7 days) until ANC recovery
> - Antiviral—antiherpes antivirals (eg, acyclovir, famciclovir, valacyclovir)

Patient Population Studied

The MyloFrance-1 study was a prospective, multicenter, phase 2, uncontrolled trial involving 57 adult patients with a confirmed diagnosis of CD33-positive acute myeloid leukemia (AML). Patients were required to be in first untreated relapse with a duration of first remission lasting ≥3 months but ≤18 months. Patients were required to have an Eastern Cooperative Oncology Group performance status of ≤2, a serum creatinine <180 micromolar (<2 mg/dL), and alanine/aspartate aminotransferase levels less than twice the upper limit of normal. Patients were excluded if they had secondary leukemia, acute promyelocytic leukemia, AML following myelodysplastic syndrome or myeloproliferative disease, or if they had received a prior hematopoietic stem cell transplant as part of their initial treatment

Therapy Monitoring

1. *Prior to initiation of gemtuzumab ozogamicin therapy:* CBC with differential, baseline chemistries, electrolytes, uric acid, LDH, liver function tests, pregnancy test (women of reproductive potential only), electrocardiogram for QTc interval measurement (only in patients with a predisposition for QTc prolongation, with congenital long QTc syndrome, with congestive heart failure, with hypokalemia or hypomagnesemia, or who are taking concurrent medications that have a potential to prolong the QTc interval)

2. *Prior to each dose of gemtuzumab ozogamicin:* CBC with differential, baseline chemistries, electrolytes, uric acid, LDH, liver function tests

3. *In patients at high risk for tumor lysis syndrome (eg, high tumor burden, renal dysfunction, rapidly progressing disease, markedly elevated LDH, baseline abnormalities in laboratory indices of tumor lysis syndrome [potassium, phosphate, uric acid, calcium, serum creatinine]):* consider frequent monitoring of laboratory indices of tumor lysis syndrome, intravenous hydration, and prophylaxis with a xanthine oxidase inhibitor (eg, allopurinol) during the induction course

4. *At least 3 times per week following gemtuzumab ozogamicin, until recovery:*
   a. CBC with differential, chemistries, electrolytes, uric acid, LDH, and liver function tests

(continued)

Efficacy (N = 57)

	Gemtuzumab Ozogamicin (N = 57)	
Response after gemtuzumab ozogamicin treatment		
Early death	4/57 (7%)	—
Blast clearance at day 15	25/46 (54%)	—
Therapeutic failures	36/57 (63.1%)	—
Overall response rate (ORR)	19/57 (33.3%)	—
Complete remission (CR) rate	15/57 (26%)	—
CR with incomplete platelet recovery (CRp)	4/57 (7%)	—
ORR in patients with intermediate risk cytogenetics	15/43 (35%)	P = 0.25
ORR in patients with poor risk cytogenetics	5/22 (22.7%)	
ORR in patients >60 years	14/35 (40%)	P = 0.73
ORR in patients <60 years	5/22 (22.7%)	
ORR in patients with first remission duration <12 months	8/32 (25%)	P = 0.16
ORR in patients with first remission duration >12 months	11/25 (44%)	
Survival		
Median overall survival	8.4 months	—
Median relapse-free survival among 19 patients achieving CR or CRp	11.0 months	—

Therapy Monitoring
(*continued*)

b. Monitor for signs and symptoms of hepatic sinusoidal obstruction syndrome/veno-occlusive disease (elevations in ALT, AST, total bilirubin, painful hepatomegaly, weight gain, ascites)

5. *At least every 30 minutes during each gemtuzumab ozogamicin infusion and for 1 hour post-infusion completion:* monitor vital signs and monitor for signs and symptoms of an infusion-related reaction (chills, fever, tachycardia, hypotension, hypoxia, respiratory failure, and/or bronchospasm)

6. *Periodically:*

   a. Advise patient to report signs or symptoms of bleeding

   b. Electrocardiogram for QTc interval measurement as clinically indicated, especially in patients with a predisposition for QTc prolongation, with congenital long QTc syndrome, with congestive heart failure, with hypokalemia or hypomagnesemia, or who are taking concurrent medications that have a potential to prolong the QTc interval

7. *Response assessment:* CBC with differential, bone marrow aspirate, and biopsy

   a. In the MyloFrance-1 study, a bone marrow aspirate was recommended on day-15 to assess for clearance of blasts and a final determination of remission status was assessed upon normalization of blood counts and/or at a maximum of 43 days from the first dose of gemtuzumab ozogamicin

      i. Of 46 patients who underwent a day-15 bone marrow aspirate, 25 (54%) had less than 5% blast cells. Of these, 13 achieved a complete remission (CR) or CR with incomplete platelet recovery (CRp). Of the 21 patients who had >5% blasts at day 15, three achieved CRp

Treatment Modifications

GEMTUZUMAB OZOGAMICIN

Hepatic Toxicity or Hepatic Impairment

Hepatic sinusoidal obstruction syndrome/veno-occlusive disease	Discontinue gemtuzumab ozogamicin
Patient treated with gemtuzumab ozogamicin undergoes subsequent hematopoietic stem cell transplant	Monitor for signs and symptoms of hepatic sinusoidal obstruction syndrome/veno-occlusive disease and liver function tests frequently
Total bilirubin >2× ULN, or AST >2.5× ULN, or ALT >2.5× ULN	Delay gemtuzumab ozogamicin treatment until total bilirubin ≤2× ULN, AST ≤2.5× ULN, and ALT ≤2.5× ULN Consider increasing the frequency of monitoring of liver function tests and for signs/symptoms of hepatotoxicity Omit the scheduled dose if delay is required more than 2 days between sequential infusions

Infusion Reactions

Infusion-related reaction	Interrupt the infusion immediately and institute appropriate supportive medical management Administer acetaminophen and diphenhydramine (if >4 hours has transpired since administration of the premedication doses) Administer methylprednisolone 1 mg/kg intravenously × 1 dose For mild, moderate, or severe infusio-related reactions, once symptoms resolve, consider resuming the infusion at no more than half the rate at which the reaction occurred. Repeat the procedure in the event of recurrent symptoms Permanently discontinue gemtuzumab ozogamicin in patients who experience a life-threatening infusion reaction
Anaphylactic reaction suspected (eg, severe respiratory symptoms or clinically significant hypotension) or life-threatening infusion reaction	Permanently discontinue gemtuzumab ozogamicin

Other Toxicities

Other severe or life-threatening nonhematologic toxicities	Delay gemtuzumab ozogamicin administration until recover to G ≤1. Omit the scheduled dose if delayed more than 2 days between sequential infusions

ULN, upper limit of normal; AST, aspartate aminotransferase; ALT, alanine aminotransferase

Adverse Events (N = 57)

Event	Gemtuzumab Ozogamicin (N = 57)
Grade (%)*	Grade 3
Grade 3 treatment-emergent adverse events occurring in >1% of patients	
Sepsis	31.5
Fever	15.8
Rash	10.5
Pneumonia	7
Bleeding	7
Mucositis	3.5
Diarrhea	1.75
Headaches	1.75
Tachycardia	1.75
Edema	1.75

*Treatment-emergent adverse events (TEAEs) were graded according to the National Cancer Institute Common Toxicity Criteria (v2)

Adverse events were included in the table if they were Grade 3, deemed treatment-emergent, and occurred in >1% of patients

Among the 19 patients achieving complete remission (CR) or CR with incomplete platelet recovery (CRp), the median time to ANC recovery (ANC >500/mm^3) was 23 days and median time to platelet recovery (platelets >50,000/mm^3) was 20 days. Grade 1–2 hyperbilirubinemia (bilirubin 1.5–3× upper limit of normal [ULN]) occurred in 4 (7%) patients. Grade 1 elevations in aspartate or alanine aminotransferase levels occurred in 23 (40%) of patients, and Grade 2 elevations occurred in 9 (16%) patients. There were no reported episodes of hepatic veno-occlusive disease

LOW/INTERMEDIATE RISK • FIRST-LINE

LEUKEMIA, ACUTE PROMYELOCYTIC REGIMEN: TRETINOIN (ALL TRANS-RETINOIC ACID; ATRA) + ARSENIC TRIOXIDE

Lo-Coco F et al. N Engl J Med 2016;374:1197–1198
Lo-Coco F et al. N Engl J Med 2013;369:111–121
Supplementary appendix to: Lo-Coco F et al. N Engl J Med 2013;369:111–121
Protocol for: Lo-Coco F et al. N Engl J Med 2013;369:111–121
Comment in: N Engl J Med 2013;369:186–187
Sanz MA et al. Blood 2019;133:1630–1643

Induction:

Prednisone 0.5 mg/kg per dose; administer orally once daily, continually, as differentiation syndrome prophylaxis until hematologic complete remission (HCR) *or* a maximum of 60 days (total dosage/week during induction therapy = 3.5 mg/kg)
Arsenic trioxide 0.15 mg/kg per day; administer intravenously in 100–250 mL 0.9% sodium chloride injection (0.9% NS) or 5% dextrose injection (D5W) over 2 hours, daily, continually, until HCR *or* a maximum of 60 days (total dosage/week during induction therapy = 1.05 mg/kg); *plus*
Tretinoin 22.5 mg/m^2 per dose; administer orally twice daily, continually, until HCR *or* for a maximum of 60 days (total dosage/week during induction therapy = 315 mg/m^2)

Note: see "Treatment Modifications" section for instructions on management of leukocytosis occurring during induction therapy

Consolidation:

Arsenic trioxide 0.15 mg/kg per dose; administer intravenously in 100–250 mL 0.9% NS or D5W over 2 hours for 5 days/week, weekly for 4 consecutive weeks (weeks 1–4, 9–12, 17–20, and 25–28), followed by 4 consecutive weeks without arsenic trioxide treatment, for a total of 4 courses (total dosage/week = 0.75 mg/kg; total dosage/4-week consolidation course = 3 mg/kg); *plus*
Tretinoin 22.5 mg/m^2 per dose; administer orally twice daily for 2 consecutive weeks (28 doses during weeks 1–2, 5–6, 9–10, 13–14, 17–18, 21–22, and 25–26) followed by 2 consecutive weeks without tretinoin treatment for a total of 7 courses (total dosage/week = 315 mg/m^2; total dosage/2-week course = 630 mg/m^2)

Supportive Care
Antiemetic prophylaxis
Emetogenic potential when arsenic trioxide is administered is **MODERATE**. *Avoid antiemetics with potential to prolong the QT interval (eg, ondansetron) during arsenic trioxide therapy*
Emetogenic potential when tretinoin alone is administered is **MINIMAL–LOW**
See Chapter 42 for antiemetic recommendations

Hematopoietic growth factor (CSF) prophylaxis
Primary prophylaxis is **NOT** *indicated*
See Chapter 43 for more information

Risk of fever and neutropenia during induction *therapy is* **INTERMEDIATE**
Antimicrobial primary prophylaxis to be considered during induction therapy:

- Antibacterial—consider prophylaxis (eg, cotrimoxazole) during periods of prolonged neutropenia only (eg, <500/mm^3 for ≥7 days), or no prophylaxis, until ANC recovery. Note that routine use of fluoroquinolones for prophylaxis should be avoided due to the risk of QTc prolongation with arsenic trioxide

- Antifungal—consider prophylaxis with an echinocandin (eg, caspofungin) during periods of prolonged neutropenia only (eg, <500/mm^3 for ≥7 days), or no prophylaxis, until ANC recovery. Note that routine use of azole antifungals (eg, fluconazole) for prophylaxis should be avoided due to the risk of QTc prolongation with arsenic trioxide. *Pneumocystis jirovecii* prophylaxis is recommended during prolonged prednisone therapy (eg, cotrimoxazole)

- Antiviral—antiherpes antivirals (eg, acyclovir, famciclovir, valacyclovir)

Risk of fever and neutropenia during consolidation *therapy is* **LOW**
Antimicrobial primary prophylaxis to be considered during consolidation therapy:

- Antibacterial—not indicated

- Antifungal—not indicated

- Antiviral—not indicated unless patient previously had an episode of HSV

Patient Population Studied

A phase 3, multicenter trial comparing ATRA plus chemotherapy with ATRA plus arsenic trioxide in patients with APL classified as low to intermediate risk (white cell count, ≤10,000/mm^3). Patients (18–71 years of age) were randomly assigned to receive either ATRA plus arsenic trioxide for induction and consolidation therapy or standard ATRA-idarubicin induction therapy followed by 3 cycles of consolidation therapy with ATRA, plus chemotherapy and maintenance therapy with low-dose chemotherapy and ATRA

Efficacy (n = 156)

	ATRA–Arsenic Trioxide (n = 77)	ATRA-Chemotherapy (n = 79)	
Hematologic complete remission*	100%	95%	
Two-year event-free survival rate	97%	86%	Difference, 11 percentage points (95% CI, 2–22) P<0.001 for noninferiority P = 0.02 for superiority
Two-year overall survival rate	99% (95% CI, 96–100)	91% (95% CI, 85–97)	P = 0.02
Two-year disease-free survival rate	97% (95% CI, 94–100)	90% (95% CI, 84–97)	P = 0.11
Two-year cumulative incidence of relapse	1% (95% CI, 0–4)	6% (95% CI, 0–11)	P = 0.24
50-month event-free survival rate[†]	96% (95% CI, 92–100)	81% (95% CI, 73–91)	P = 0.003
50-month overall survival rate[†]	99% (95% CI, 96–100)	88% (95% CI, 81–96)	P = 0.006

*The median time to hematologic complete remission was 32 days (range, 22 to 68 days) in the ATRA–arsenic trioxide group and 35 days (range, 26 to 63 days) in the ATRA–chemotherapy group
[†]50-month follow-up data are reported in an updated analysis (Lo-Coco F et al. N Engl J Med 2016;374:1197–1198). Post-remission events in the ATRA-arsenic group included 2 relapses and 1 death in remission. Post-remission events in the ATRA-chemotherapy group included 6 relapses and 5 deaths in remission (1 death related to secondary leukemia)

Therapy Monitoring

During induction therapy:
1. CBC with differential and platelet count, 2–3 times daily until resolution of coagulopathy, then daily
2. Fibrinogen, PT/INR, and aPTT, thrombin time, fibrinogen-fibrin degradation products twice daily until resolution of coagulopathy, then daily
   a. During induction therapy when clinical and laboratory signs of coagulopathy are present:[1]
      i. Platelet transfusion support to maintain platelets ≥30,000 to 50,000/mm³
      ii. Cryoprecipitate and/or fresh frozen plasma transfusions to maintain fibrinogen >100–150 mg/dL and international normalized ratio (INR) <1.5
3. *In patients at high risk for tumor lysis syndrome (eg, high tumor burden, renal dysfunction, rapidly progressing disease, markedly elevated LDH, baseline abnormalities in laboratory indices of tumor lysis syndrome [potassium, phosphate, uric acid, calcium, serum creatinine]):* consider frequent monitoring of laboratory indices of tumor lysis syndrome, intravenous hydration, and prophylaxis with a xanthine oxidase inhibitor (eg, allopurinol) during the induction course
4. *Liver function tests:* obtain ALT, AST, total bilirubin, and alkaline phosphatase prior to induction therapy and then 2–3 times per week
5. *Lipid panel:* obtain a fasting lipid panel prior to therapy and then every 2–4 weeks
6. *Cardiac monitoring (goal QTc <500 ms during arsenic trioxide therapy):*
   a. *During therapy:* maintain serum potassium concentration >4 mEq/L (>4 mmol/L) and maintain serum magnesium concentration >0.74 mmol/L (>1.8 mg/dL, >1.48 mEq/L)[1]
   b. ECG at baseline and at least twice per week during therapy with arsenic trioxide[1]
   c. The QT interval should be corrected for heart rate using the Fridericia, Hodges, or Sagie/Framingham formulae. Avoid using the standard Bazett formula since it may lead to an overestimate of the QTc interval and cause unnecessary interruptions in arsenic trioxide therapy[1,2]
7. *Response assessment:* bone marrow biopsy should be performed on day 28 of induction therapy. Discontinue induction therapy in patients without evidence of morphologic disease (<5% blasts and no abnormal promyelocytes). In patients with evidence of morphologic disease at day 28, repeat a bone marrow examination weekly until clearance of blasts and abnormal promyelocytes. Note that at the end of induction therapy it is expected that patients will have detectable PML-RARA transcripts by polymerase chain reaction and detectable t(15;17) by conventional cytogenetics and/or fluorescence in situ hybridization. Importantly, this does not represent resistant disease but rather slow clearance of terminally differentiating blasts, and therefore detection of PML-RARA and/or t(15;17) should have no impact on treatment decisions during induction therapy[1]

During consolidation therapy:
1. CBC with differential and platelet count and liver function tests (ALT, AST, total bilirubin, and alkaline phosphatase) 1–2 times per week during therapy with arsenic trioxide
2. *Lipid panel:* obtain a fasting lipid panel every 2–4 weeks

(continued)

Therapy Monitoring (continued)

3. *Cardiac monitoring (goal QTc <500 ms during arsenic trioxide therapy):*

   a. *During arsenic trioxide therapy:* maintain serum potassium concentration >4 mEq/L (>4 mmol/L) and maintain serum magnesium concentration >0.74 mmol/L (>1.8 mg/dL, >1.48 mEq/L)[1]

   b. *During arsenic trioxide therapy:* ECG before each course and at least twice per week[1]

   c. The QT interval should be corrected for heart rate using the Fridericia, Hodges, or Sagie/Framingham formulae. Avoid using the standard Bazett formula since it may lead to an overestimate of the QTc interval and cause unnecessary interruptions in arsenic trioxide therapy[1,2]

4. *Response assessment:* bone marrow examination at the completion of consolidation to document molecular remission using a RT-PCR or RQ-PCR assay with a sensitivity of at least 1 in 10[4]. If molecular CR is confirmed, prolonged measurable residual disease (MRD) monitoring can be avoided in low-risk acute promyelocytic leukemia patients treated with tretinoin + arsenic trioxide. Consider obtaining a CBC with differential and platelet count monthly during the first year following attainment of molecular complete remission, and then every 3–4 months for an additional 2 years[1]

1. Sanz MA et al. Blood. 2019 Apr 11;133:1630–1643
2. Roboz GJ et al. J Clin Oncol 2014;32:3723–3728

Treatment Modifications

DOSE MODIFICATIONS FOR ARSENIC TRIOXIDE AND TRETINOIN

	Arsenic Trioxide	Tretinoin
Starting dose	0.15 mg/kg per dose	22.5 mg/m² per dose
Dose level −1	0.11 mg/kg per dose	18.75 mg/m² per dose
Dose level −2	0.1 mg/kg per dose	12.5 mg/m² per dose
Dose level −3	0.075 mg/kg per dose	10 mg/m² per dose

Adverse Event	Treatment Modification
QT prolongation QTc interval >500 ms	For patients with heart rate >60 bpm, ensure that QT interval is corrected using the Fridericia, Hodges, or Sagie/Framingham formulae and not using the Bazett formula. Withhold arsenic trioxide and replete electrolytes. Discontinue any medication known to prolong the QTc interval (eg, ondansetron, haloperidol, fluconazole). Increase frequency of ECG monitoring to daily and strongly consider telemetered ECG monitoring 1. When the QTc improves to approximately ≤460 ms, then resume arsenic trioxide with dosage decreased by 50%: arsenic trioxide 0.075 mg/kg per day 2. If no further QTc prolongation occurs after 7 days of treatment at the reduced dosage, escalate arsenic trioxide dosage to 0.11 mg/kg per day 3. If QTc prolongation does not occur after escalation to 0.11 mg/kg per day for 7 days, arsenic trioxide dosage may again be escalated to 0.15 mg/kg per day (full dose)
Differentiation syndrome (ie, during induction therapy)	Withhold therapy with arsenic trioxide and/or tretinoin only in cases of severe differentiation syndrome. Promptly initiate dexamethasone 10 mg IV every 12 hours at the earliest clinical suspicion of incipient differentiation syndrome until disappearance of signs/symptoms, and for a minimum of 3 days. Consider treatment with loop diuretics (eg, furosemide) when clinically required. If treatment with arsenic trioxide and/or tretinoin were held for severe symptoms, then upon improvement in clinical condition and symptoms, resume treatment with tretinoin and/or arsenic trioxide at 50% of the previous dose during the first 7 days after disappearance of the differentiation syndrome. Thereafter, in absence of worsening of the previous toxicity, tretinoin and/or arsenic trioxide should be resumed at full dosage. In case of reappearance of symptoms, tretinoin and arsenic trioxide will be reduced at the previous dosage
Leukocytosis occurring during induction therapy (WBC >10,000/mm³ to ≤50,000/mm³)	Initiate treatment with **hydroxyurea** 500 mg per dose; administer orally four times per day until WBC <10,000/mm³. Monitor closely for signs and symptoms of differentiation syndrome. Note that an increase in WBC to a level >10,000/mm³ after treatment with tretinoin and/or arsenic trioxide does not reclassify a patient as having high-risk disease

(continued)

Treatment Modifications (continued)

Adverse Event	Treatment Modification
Leukocytosis occurring during induction therapy (WBC >50,000/mm³)	Increase the hydroxyurea dosage as follows: **hydroxyurea** 1000 mg per dose; administer orally four times per day until WBC <50,000/mm³, then reduce the dose to 500 mg four times per day until WBC <10,000/mm³, then discontinue hydroxyurea. Monitor closely for signs and symptoms of differentiation syndrome. Note that an increase in WBC to a level >10,000/mm³ after treatment with tretinoin and/or arsenic trioxide does not reclassify a patient as having high-risk disease For extreme cases of hyperleukocytosis resistant to hydroxyurea, consider a one-time dose of either idarubicin (12 mg/m²) or gemtuzumab ozogamicin (6–9 mg/m²)
Hepatotoxicity (increase in serum bilirubin >5× ULN and/or AST >5× ULN and/or alkaline phosphatase >5× ULN)	Temporarily discontinue tretinoin and/or arsenic trioxide and increase the frequency of liver function test monitoring to once daily After serum bilirubin, AST, and alkaline phosphatase decrease to <4× the upper limit of their normal ranges (ULN), treatment with tretinoin and/or arsenic trioxide may resume at 50% of the dosages previously given for 7 days If toxicity does not recur during the 7 days after resuming ATRA and arsenic trioxide, drug administration may resume at full dosages If hepatotoxicity recurs, the drugs are permanently discontinued
Acute vasomotor reaction during arsenic trioxide infusion	Prolong the arsenic trioxide infusion duration to 4 hours
Significant myelosuppression (ANC <1000 or platelets <50k for >5 weeks after start of a course)	Reduce arsenic trioxide and/or tretinoin dosages by 1 dose level. If myelosuppression lasts >49 days or occurs on 2 consecutive courses, repeat bone marrow aspirate with specimens for RT-PCR or RQ-PCR. In case of molecular remission resume treatment at one dose level lower than previously used dosage
Other intolerable Grade 2 nonhematologic toxicities	Reduce arsenic trioxide and/or tretinoin dosages by 1 dose level
Grades 3–4 nonhematologic toxicity	Withhold tretinoin and arsenic trioxide until toxicities remit to G <2, then resume treatment with both agents with the dosages reduced by 2 dose levels. If the toxicity is definitely related to only 1 agent, then treatment with the other non-offending agent may be continued without interruption and at full dose

Lo-Coco F et al. N Engl J Med 2013;369:111–121
Supplementary appendix to: Lo-Coco F et al. N Engl J Med 2013;369:111–121
Protocol for: Lo-Coco F et al. N Engl J Med 2013;369:111–121
Sanz MA et al. Blood 2019;133:1630–1643

Toxicity

The differentiation syndrome, including moderate and severe forms, developed in 15 patients in the group who received tretinoin (ATRA)–arsenic trioxide (19%) and in 13 patients in the ATRA-chemotherapy group (16%) (P = 0.62)
Four patients in the ATRA-chemotherapy group died during induction therapy: 2 from differentiation syndrome, 1 from ischemic stroke, and 1 from bronchopneumonia. No patients in the tretinoin + arsenic trioxide arm died during induction

Grades 3 or 4 neutropenia lasting >15 days and G3 or G4 thrombocytopenia lasting >15 days occurred with significantly greater frequency during induction therapy and after each consolidation course in the ATRA–chemotherapy group than in the ATRA–arsenic trioxide group

A total of 43 of 68 patients in the ATRA–arsenic trioxide group (63%) and 4 of 69 patients in the ATRA-chemotherapy group (6%) had G3 or G4 hepatic toxic effects during induction or consolidation therapy or during maintenance therapy (only patients in the ATRA-chemotherapy group) (P<0.001)

Prolongation of the QTc interval occurred in 12 patients in the ATRA–arsenic trioxide group (16%) and in no patients in the ATRA-chemotherapy group (P<0.001)

HIGH RISK • FIRST-LINE

LEUKEMIA, ACUTE PROMYELOCYTIC REGIMEN: TRETINOIN (ALL TRANS-RETINOIC ACID; ATRA) + ARSENIC TRIOXIDE + GEMTUZUMAB OZOGAMICIN

Abaza Y et al. Blood 2017;129:1275–1283
Sanz MA et al. Blood 2019;133:1630–1643
MYLOTARG (gemtuzumab ozogamicin) prescribing information. Philadelphia, PA: Wyeth Pharmaceuticals Inc; 2018 April

Induction:

Prednisone 0.5 mg/kg per dose; administer orally once daily, continually as differentiation syndrome prophylaxis until hematologic complete remission (HCR) *or* a maximum of 60 days (total dosage/week during induction therapy = 3.5 mg/kg)

Premedications for gemtuzumab ozogamicin:

• **Methylprednisolone** 1 mg/kg per dose; administer intravenously 30 minutes prior to gemtuzumab ozogamicin on day 1, *plus:*

• **Acetaminophen** 650 mg per dose; administer orally 1 hour prior to gemtuzumab ozogamicin on day 1, *plus:*

• **Diphenhydramine** 50 mg per dose; administer orally or intravenously 1 hour prior to gemtuzumab ozogamicin on day 1

Gemtuzumab ozogamicin 9 mg/m²; administer intravenously over 2 hours in a volume of 0.9% sodium chloride (0.9% NS) sufficient to produce a gemtuzumab ozogamicin concentration within the range 0.075–0.234 mg/mL, for 1 dose on day 1 of induction therapy (total dosage/induction course = 9 mg/m²); *plus:*

Notes:

• Administer gemtuzumab ozogamicin with an administration set that contains an in-line polyethersulfone filter with pore size of 0.2 μm. Protect the infusion bag or syringe from light using a light-blocking cover during infusion

• Doses <3.9 mg must be prepared and administered in a syringe. Doses ≥3.9 mg may be prepared and administered in either a syringe or an infusion bag

• There is no maximum gemtuzumab ozogamicin dose when used in combination with tretinoin and arsenic trioxide for the off-label indication of acute promyelocytic leukemia

• Life-threatening and/or fatal infusion-related reactions consisting of chills, fever, tachycardia, hypotension, hypoxia, respiratory failure, and/or bronchospasm may occur infrequently, up to 24 hours following infusion of gemtuzumab ozogamicin. See therapy monitoring and therapy modification sections for further details

Arsenic trioxide 0.15 mg/kg per day; administer intravenously in 100–250 mL 0.9% NS or 5% dextrose injection (D5W) over 2 hours, daily, continually, until HCR *or* a maximum of 60 days (total dosage/week during induction therapy = 1.05 mg/kg); *plus*

Tretinoin 22.5 mg/m² per dose; administer orally twice daily, continually, until HCR *or* for a maximum of 60 days (total dosage/week during induction therapy = 315 mg/m²)

Consolidation:

Arsenic trioxide 0.15 mg/kg per dose; administer intravenously in 100–250 mL 0.9% NS or D5W over 2 hours for 5 days/week, weekly for 4 consecutive weeks (weeks 1–4, 9–12, 17–20, and 25–28), followed by 4 consecutive weeks without arsenic trioxide treatment, for a total of 4 courses (total dosage/week = 0.75 mg/kg; total dosage/4-week consolidation course = 3 mg/kg); *plus*

Tretinoin 22.5 mg/m² per dose; administer orally twice daily for 2 consecutive weeks (28 doses during weeks 1–2, 5–6, 9–10, 13–14, 17–18, 21–22, and 25–26) followed by 2 consecutive weeks without tretinoin treatment for a total of 7 courses (total dosage/week = 315 mg/m²; total dosage/2-week course = 630 mg/m²)

Supportive Care
Antiemetic prophylaxis
Emetogenic potential of arsenic trioxide is **MODERATE**. *Avoid antiemetics with potential to prolong the QT interval (eg, ondansetron) during arsenic trioxide therapy.*
Emetogenic potential of gemtuzumab ozogamicin is **LOW**
Emetogenic potential when tretinoin alone is administered is **MINIMAL–LOW**
See Chapter 42 for antiemetic recommendations

(continued)

Therapy Monitoring

During induction therapy:
1. CBC with differential and platelet count, 2–3 times daily until resolution of coagulopathy, then daily
2. Fibrinogen, PT/INR, and aPTT, thrombin time, fibrinogen-fibrin degradation products twice daily until resolution of coagulopathy, then daily
   a. During induction therapy when clinical and laboratory signs of coagulopathy are present:[1]
      i. Platelet transfusion support to maintain platelets ≥30,000 to 50,000/mm³
      ii. Cryoprecipitate and/or fresh frozen plasma transfusions to maintain fibrinogen >100–150 mg/dL and international normalized ratio (INR) <1.5
3. *In patients at high risk for tumor lysis syndrome (eg, high tumor burden, renal dysfunction, rapidly progressing disease, markedly elevated LDH, baseline abnormalities in laboratory indices of tumor lysis syndrome [potassium, phosphate, uric acid, calcium, serum creatinine]):* consider frequent monitoring of laboratory indices of tumor lysis syndrome, intravenous hydration, and prophylaxis with a xanthine oxidase inhibitor (eg, allopurinol) during the induction course
4. *Liver function tests:* obtain ALT, AST, total bilirubin, and alkaline phosphatase prior to induction therapy and then 2–3 times per week
5. *Lipid panel:* obtain a fasting lipid panel prior to therapy and then every 2–4 weeks
6. *Cardiac monitoring (goal QTc < 500 ms during arsenic trioxide therapy):*
   a. *During therapy:* maintain serum potassium concentration >4 mEq/L (>4 mmol/L) and maintain serum magnesium concentration >0.74 mmol/L (>1.8 mg/dL, >1.48 mEq/L)[1]
   b. ECG at baseline and at least twice per week during therapy with arsenic trioxide[1]
   c. The QT interval should be corrected for heart rate using the Fridericia, Hodges, or Sagie/Framingham formulae. Avoid using the standard Bazett formula since it may lead to an overestimate of the QTc interval and cause unnecessary interruptions in arsenic trioxide therapy[1,2]

(continued)

(continued)

Hematopoietic growth factor (CSF) prophylaxis
*Primary prophylaxis is **NOT** indicated*
See Chapter 43 for more information

Risk of fever and neutropenia during induction *therapy is **INTERMEDIATE***
Antimicrobial primary prophylaxis to be considered during induction therapy:
- Antibacterial—consider prophylaxis (eg, cotrimoxazole) during periods of prolonged neutropenia only (eg, <500/mm³ for ≥7 days), or no prophylaxis, until ANC recovery. Note that routine use of fluoroquinolones for prophylaxis should be avoided due to the risk of QTc prolongation with arsenic trioxide
- Antifungal—consider prophylaxis with an echinocandin medication (eg, caspofungin) during periods of prolonged neutropenia only (eg, <500/mm³ for ≥7 days), or no prophylaxis, until ANC recovery. Note that routine use of azole antifungals (eg, fluconazole) for prophylaxis should be avoided due to the risk of QTc prolongation with arsenic trioxide. *Pneumocystis jirovecii* prophylaxis is recommended during prolonged prednisone therapy (eg, cotrimoxazole)
- Antiviral—antiherpes antivirals (eg, acyclovir, famciclovir, valacyclovir)

Risk of fever and neutropenia during consolidation *therapy is **LOW***
Antimicrobial primary prophylaxis to be considered during consolidation therapy:
- Antibacterial—not indicated
- Antifungal—not indicated
- Antiviral—not indicated unless patient previously had an episode of HSV

Patient Population Studied

This was a single-center retrospective review of patients with acute promyelocytic leukemia treated at MD Anderson Cancer Center on 3 consecutive clinical trials using a combination of tretinoin and arsenic trioxide with or without gemtuzumab ozogamicin (ID01–014, NCT01409161, and NCT00413166). Eligible patients were aged ≥10 years and had newly diagnosed acute promyelocytic leukemia based on detection of t(15;17) by conventional cytogenetics or detection of *PML-RARA* fusion gene by RT-PCR. Patients were excluded if they had a pretreatment QTc interval (corrected for heart rate using Fridericia's formula) >480 ms unrelated to electrolyte imbalance, or organ dysfunction (bilirubin ≥2× ULN, serum creatinine >2.5× ULN, or AST/ALT >3× ULN) unless related to leukemia, hemolysis, or Gilbert disease. A total of 54 high-risk patients (WBC >10,000/mm³ at presentation) were treated with tretinoin, arsenic trioxide, and a single dose of gemtuzumab ozogamicin 9 mg/m² (n = 45) or idarubicin 12 mg/m² (n = 7) on day 1, the latter used only during a brief period when gemtuzumab ozogamicin was unavailable

Efficacy (n = 54)

	Tretinoin + Arsenic Trioxide + Gemtuzumab Ozogamicin/ Idarubicin (n = 54)*
Five-year overall survival	86%
Five-year event-free survival	81%
Five-year disease-free survival	89%
Hematologic complete remission	96%

*Note that 1 patient with high-risk disease (WBC of 11,100/mm³ at presentation) did not receive cytoreductive therapy with either gemtuzumab ozogamicin or idarubicin
Median duration of follow-up was 47.6 months

Therapy Monitoring
(continued)

7. *At least every 30 minutes during each gemtuzumab ozogamicin infusion and for 1 hour post-infusion completion:* monitor vital signs and monitor for signs and symptoms of an infusion-related reaction (chills, fever, tachycardia, hypotension, hypoxia, respiratory failure, and/or bronchospasm)

8. *Hepatic veno-occlusive disease:* monitor for signs and symptoms of hepatic sinusoidal obstruction syndrome/veno-occlusive disease (elevations in ALT, AST, total bilirubin, painful hepatomegaly, weight gain, and ascites)

9. *Response assessment:* bone marrow biopsy should be performed on day 28 of induction therapy. Discontinue induction therapy in patients without evidence of morphologic disease (<5% blasts and no abnormal promyelocytes). In patients with evidence of morphologic disease at day 28, repeat a bone marrow examination weekly until clearance of blasts and abnormal promyelocytes. Note that at the end of induction therapy it is expected that patients will have detectable PML-RARA transcripts by polymerase chain reaction and detectable t(15;17) by conventional cytogenetics and/or fluorescence in situ hybridization. Importantly, this does not represent resistant disease but rather slow clearance of terminally differentiating blasts and therefore detection of PML-RARA and/ or t(15;17) should have no impact on treatment decisions during induction therapy[1]

During consolidation therapy:
1. CBC with differential and platelet count and liver function tests (ALT, AST, total bilirubin, and alkaline phosphatase) 1–2 times per week during therapy with arsenic trioxide

2. *Lipid panel:* obtain a fasting lipid panel every 2–4 weeks

3. *Cardiac monitoring (goal QTc <500 ms during arsenic trioxide therapy):*
   a. *During arsenic trioxide therapy:* maintain serum potassium concentration >4 mEq/L (>4 mmol/L) and maintain serum magnesium concentration >0.74 mmol/L (>1.8 mg/dL, >1.48 mEq/L)[1]
   b. *During arsenic trioxide therapy:* ECG before each course and at least twice per week[1]

(continued)

Treatment Modifications

DOSE MODIFICATIONS FOR ARSENIC TRIOXIDE AND TRETINOIN

	Arsenic Trioxide	Tretinoin
Starting dose	0.15 mg/kg per dose	22.5 mg/m² per dose
Dose level −1	0.11 mg/kg per dose	18.75 mg/m² per dose
Dose level −2	0.1 mg/kg per dose	12.5 mg/m² per dose
Dose level −3	0.075 mg/kg per dose	10 mg/m² per dose

Adverse Event	Treatment Modification
Infusion-related reaction related to gemtuzumab ozogamicin	Interrupt the gemtuzumab ozogamicin infusion immediately and institute appropriate supportive medical management
Anaphylactic reaction to gemtuzumab ozogamicin is suspected (eg, severe respiratory symptoms or clinically significant hypotension) or life-threatening infusion reaction	Permanently discontinue gemtuzumab ozogamicin
QT prolongation QTc interval >500 ms	For patients with heart rate >60 bpm, ensure that QT interval is corrected using the Fridericia, Hodges, or Sagie/Framingham formulae and not using the Bazett formula. Withhold arsenic trioxide and replete electrolytes. Discontinue any medication known to prolong the QTc interval (eg, ondansetron, haloperidol, fluconazole). Increase frequency of ECG monitoring to daily and strongly consider telemetered ECG monitoring 1. When the QTc improves to approximately ≤460 ms, then resume arsenic trioxide with dosage decreased by 50%: arsenic trioxide 0.075 mg/kg per day 2. If no further QTc prolongation occurs after 7 days of treatment at the reduced dosage, escalate arsenic trioxide dosage to 0.11 mg/kg per day 3. If QTc prolongation does not occur after escalation to 0.11 mg/kg per day for 7 days, arsenic trioxide dosage may again be escalated to 0.15 mg/kg per day (full dose)
Differentiation syndrome (ie, during induction therapy)	Withhold therapy with arsenic trioxide and/or tretinoin only in cases of severe differentiation syndrome. Promptly initiate dexamethasone 10 mg IV every 12 hours at the earliest clinical suspicion of incipient differentiation syndrome until disappearance of signs/symptoms, and for a minimum of 3 days. Consider treatment with loop diuretics (eg, furosemide) when clinically required. If treatment with arsenic trioxide and/or tretinoin were held for severe symptoms, then upon improvement in clinical condition and symptoms, resume treatment with tretinoin and/or arsenic trioxide at 50% of the previous dose during the first 7 days after disappearance of the differentiation syndrome. Thereafter, in absence of worsening of the previous toxicity, tretinoin and/or arsenic trioxide should be resumed at full dosage. In case of reappearance of symptoms, tretinoin and arsenic trioxide will be reduced at the previous dosage
Worsening leukocytosis occurring during induction therapy despite administration of gemtuzumab ozogamicin on day 1 (WBC >10,000/mm³ to ≤50,000/mm³ and increasing)	Initiate treatment with **hydroxyurea** 500 mg per dose; administer orally four times per day until WBC <10,000/mm³. Monitor closely for signs and symptoms of differentiation syndrome

Therapy Monitoring
(continued)

c. The QT interval should be corrected for heart rate using the Fridericia, Hodges, or Sagie/Framingham formulae. Avoid using the standard Bazett formula since it may lead to an overestimate of the QTc interval and cause unnecessary interruptions in arsenic trioxide therapy[1,2]

4. *Response assessment:* bone marrow examination at the completion of consolidation to document molecular remission using a RT-PCR or RQ-PCR assay with a sensitivity of at least 1 in 10⁴. If molecular CR is confirmed, then monitor for measurable residual disease (MRD) by RT-PCR or RQ-PCR on a bone marrow specimen every 3 months for up to 3 years following completion of chemotherapy. Consider also obtaining a CBC with differential and platelet count monthly during the first year following attainment of molecular complete remission, and then every 3–4 months for an additional 2 years[1]

References:
1. Sanz MA et al. Blood. 2019;133:1630–1643
2. Roboz GJ et al. J Clin Oncol 2014;32:3723–3728

(continued)

Treatment Modifications (*continued*)

Adverse Event	Treatment Modification
Worsening leukocytosis occurring during induction therapy despite administration of gemtuzumab ozogamicin on day 1 (WBC >50,000/mm^3 and increasing)	Increase the hydroxyurea dosage as follows: **hydroxyurea** 1000 mg per dose; administer orally four times per day until WBC <50,000/mm^3, then reduce the dose to 500 mg four times per day until WBC <10,000/mm^3, then discontinue hydroxyurea. Monitor closely for signs and symptoms of differentiation syndrome. For very rare, extreme cases of hyperleukocytosis resistant to hydroxyurea and gemtuzumab ozogamicin, consider a one-time dose of idarubicin (12 mg/m^2). Avoid leukapheresis due to the risk of precipitating fatal hemorrhage
Hepatotoxicity (increase in serum bilirubin >5× ULN and/or AST >5× ULN and/or alkaline phosphatase >5× ULN)	Temporarily discontinue tretinoin and/or arsenic trioxide and increase the frequency of liver function test monitoring to once daily After serum bilirubin, AST, and alkaline phosphatase decrease to <4× the upper limit of their normal ranges (ULN), treatment with tretinoin and/or arsenic trioxide may resume at 50% of the dosages previously given for 7 days If toxicity does not recur during the 7 days after resuming ATRA and arsenic trioxide, drug administration may resume at full dosages If hepatotoxicity recurs, the drugs are permanently discontinued
Acute vasomotor reaction during arsenic trioxide infusion	Prolong the arsenic trioxide infusion duration to 4 hours
Significant myelosuppression (ANC <1000 or platelets <50,000 for >5 weeks after start of a course)	Reduce arsenic trioxide and/or tretinoin dosages by 1 dose level. If myelosuppression lasts >49 days or occurs on 2 consecutive courses, repeat bone marrow aspirate with specimens for RT-PCR or RQ-PCR. In case of molecular remission, resume treatment at one dose level lower than previously used dosage
Other intolerable Grade 2 nonhematologic toxicities	Reduce arsenic trioxide and/or tretinoin dosages by 1 dose level
Grade 3–4 nonhematologic toxicity	Withhold tretinoin and arsenic trioxide until toxicities remit to G <2, then resume treatment with both agents with the dosages reduced by 2 dose levels. If the toxicity is definitely related to only 1 agent, then treatment with the other non-offending agent may be continued without interruption and at full dose

Lo-Coco F et al. N Engl J Med 2013;369:111–121
Supplementary appendix to: Lo-Coco F et al. N Engl J Med 2013;369:111–121
Protocol for: Lo-Coco F et al. N Engl J Med 2013;369:111–121
Sanz MA et al. Blood 2019;133:1630–1643

Toxicity (n = 187)

Most severe adverse events occurred during the induction phase of treatment; the most common treatment-related Grade 3–4 adverse events among all patients (including low-risk patients treated with only arsenic trioxide + tretinoin) were infections (23.5%), QT prolongation (7.5%), and hemorrhage (5%). Differentiation syndrome occurred in 11% of patients and was managed successfully by administration of corticosteroids and withholding of tretinoin; arsenic trioxide was continued in cases of differentiation syndrome. Grade 3–4 hepatotoxicity occurred in 14% of patients. Seven patients (4%) died in the midst of induction therapy; the median (range) time to induction death was 12 days (7–24). Causes of death during induction therapy were considered disease-related complications including infection, hemorrhage, and multiorgan failure

HIGH RISK • FIRST-LINE

LEUKEMIA, ACUTE PROMYELOCYTIC REGIMEN: TRETINOIN (ALL TRANS-RETINOIC ACID) + IDARUBICIN

Sanz MA et al. Blood 2010;115:5137–5146

Induction:

Tretinoin 22.5 mg/m^2 per dose; administer orally every 12 hours until hematologic CR (total dosage/week = 315 mg/m^2)

Idarubicin 12 mg/m^2 per dose; administer intravenously diluted to a concentration >0.01 mg/mL in 0.9% sodium chloride injection (0.9% NS) or 5% dextrose injection (D5W) over 15–30 minutes for 4 doses on days 2, 4, 6, and 8 (total dosage/induction course = 48 mg/m^2)
Note: This regimen describes the remission induction phase of treatment only. Post-remission therapy (per Sanz et al. 2010) is risk-adapted; the remainder of this regimen will describe the post-remission strategy for high-risk acute promyelocytic leukemia (APL) patients, defined as WBC >10,000/mm^3 at presentation, who are younger than 60 years of age. For older patients with high-risk APL, or for any-age patients who have low-intermediate-risk APL, refer to the Sanz et al. publication for post-remission regimen details

Supportive Care (induction)
Antiemetic prophylaxis (induction)
Emetogenic potential on days with tretinoin alone is **MINIMAL–LOW**
Emetogenic potential on days with idarubicin is **MODERATE**
See Chapter 42 for antiemetic recommendations

Hematopoietic growth factor (CSF) prophylaxis (induction)
Primary prophylaxis is **NOT** *indicated*
See Chapter 43 for more information

Antimicrobial prophylaxis (induction)
Risk of fever and neutropenia is **HIGH**
  Antimicrobial primary prophylaxis is recommended:
  • Antibacterial—consider prophylaxis with a fluoroquinolone during periods of prolonged neutropenia only (eg, ANC <500/mm^3 for ≥7 days) until ANC recovery
  • Antifungal—consider prophylaxis with fluconazole or another azole antifungal medication during periods of prolonged neutropenia only (eg, <500/mm^3 for ≥7 days) until ANC recovery
  • Antiviral—antiherpes antivirals (eg, acyclovir, famciclovir, valacyclovir)

Consolidation course 1 (high-risk patients age ≤60 years; begin upon hematologic recovery (ANC >1500/mm^3 and platelet count >100,000/mm^3) in patients who achieve a morphologic CR following remission induction therapy):

Idarubicin 5 mg/m^2 per dose; administer intravenously diluted to a concentration >0.01 mg/mL in 0.9% NS or D5W over 15–30 minutes once daily for 4 consecutive days on days 1–4 of a 28-day cycle (total dosage/consolidation course 1 = 20 mg/m^2)
Cytarabine 1000 mg/m^2 per dose; administer intravenously in 100–1000 mL 0.9% NS or D5W over 6 hours, once daily for 4 consecutive days on days 1–4 of a 28-day cycle (total dosage/consolidation course 1 = 4,000 mg/m^2)
Tretinoin 22.5 mg/m^2 per dose; administer orally every 12 hours for 15 consecutive days, on days 1–15 of a 28-day cycle (total dosage/consolidation course 1 = 675 mg/m^2)

Supportive Care (consolidation course 1)
Antiemetic prophylaxis (consolidation course 1)
Emetogenic potential on days with tretinoin alone is **MINIMAL–LOW**
Emetogenic potential on days 1–4 with high-dose cytarabine ± idarubicin is **MODERATE**
See Chapter 42 for antiemetic recommendations

Hematopoietic growth factor (CSF) prophylaxis (consolidation course 1)
Primary prophylaxis is **NOT** *indicated*
See Chapter 43 for more information

(continued)

Patient Population Studied

Study of 437 consecutive patients with genetic diagnosis of APL

Efficacy

Of 402 evaluable patients, 372 achieved morphologic CR (92.5%)*
The median time interval to CR was 39 days (range, 18–81 days)
Patients with WBC counts >10,000/mm^3 and >50,000/mm^3 had poorer response rates (83% and 73%, respectively) compared with those with low- and intermediate-risk patients (99% and 96%, respectively; P<0.001)

*The median time to reach neutrophil counts >1000/mm^3 and platelet counts >50,000/mm^3 was 24 days (range, 6–72 days) and 19 days (range, 4–80 days), respectively

Toxicity

Causes of induction deaths*
Hemorrhage: 3.7%
Infection: 1.5%
Differentiation syndrome: 1%

*Hemorrhage and infection accounted for most of the deaths during induction therapy (15 and 6 patients, respectively). Deaths caused by hemorrhage were caused by intracranial (12 patients, 80%), pulmonary (2 patients, 13%), and gastrointestinal hemorrhages (1 patient, 7%). Differentiation syndrome and acute myocardial infarction were contributing causes of death in 4 and 2 patients, respectively. The remaining 3 deaths were attributable to massive suprahepatic thrombosis, myocarditis, and cardiac failure, each of which occurred in 1 patient

Therapy Monitoring

During induction therapy:
1. *Pretreatment evaluation:* determination of LVEF by echocardiogram
2. CBC with differential and platelet count, 2–3 times daily until resolution of coagulopathy, then daily
3. Fibrinogen, PT/INR, and aPTT, thrombin time, fibrinogen-fibrin degradation products twice daily until resolution of coagulopathy, then daily
   a. During induction therapy when clinical and laboratory signs of coagulopathy are present:[1]
      i. Platelet transfusion support to maintain platelets ≥30,000 to 50,000/mm^3

(continued)

(continued)

Antimicrobial prophylaxis (consolidation course 1)
*Risk of fever and neutropenia is **HIGH***
   Antimicrobial primary prophylaxis is recommended:
   - Antibacterial—consider prophylaxis with a fluoroquinolone during periods of prolonged neutropenia only (eg, ANC <500/mm^3 for ≥7 days) until ANC recovery
   - Antifungal—consider prophylaxis with fluconazole or another azole antifungal medication during periods of prolonged neutropenia only (eg, <500/mm^3 for ≥7 days) until ANC recovery
   - Antiviral—antiherpes antivirals (eg, acyclovir, famciclovir, valacyclovir)

Keratitis prophylaxis
Steroid ophthalmic drops (prednisolone 1% or dexamethasone 0.1%); administer 2 drops by intraocular instillation into each eye every 6 hours starting prior to the first cytarabine dose and continuing until 48 hours after high-dose cytarabine is completed

Consolidation course 2 (high-risk patients age ≤60 years):

Mitoxantrone 10 mg/m^2 per dose; administer intravenously in 50 mL 0.9% NS or D5W over 5–30 minutes once daily for 5 consecutive days on days 1–5 of a 28-day cycle (total dosage/consolidation course 2 = 50 mg/m^2)
Tretinoin 22.5 mg/m^2 per dose; administer orally every 12 hours for 15 consecutive days, on days 1–15 of a 28-day cycle (total dosage/consolidation course 2 = 675 mg/m^2)

Supportive Care (consolidation course 2)
Antiemetic prophylaxis (consolidation course 2)
*Emetogenic potential on days with tretinoin alone is **MINIMAL–LOW***
*Emetogenic potential on days 1–5 with mitoxantrone is **LOW***
See Chapter 42 for antiemetic recommendations

Hematopoietic growth factor (CSF) prophylaxis (consolidation course 2)
*Primary prophylaxis is **NOT** indicated*
See Chapter 43 for more information

Antimicrobial prophylaxis (consolidation course 2)
*Risk of fever and neutropenia is **HIGH***
   Antimicrobial primary prophylaxis is recommended:
   - Antibacterial—consider prophylaxis with a fluoroquinolone during periods of prolonged neutropenia only (eg, ANC <500/mm^3 for ≥7 days) until ANC recovery
   - Antifungal—consider prophylaxis with fluconazole or another azole antifungal medication during periods of prolonged neutropenia only (eg, <500/mm^3 for ≥7 days) until ANC recovery
   - Antiviral—antiherpes antivirals (eg, acyclovir, famciclovir, valacyclovir)

Consolidation course 3 (high-risk patients age ≤60 years):

Tretinoin 22.5 mg/m^2 per dose; administer orally every 12 hours for 15 consecutive days, on days 1–15 of a 28-day cycle (total dosage/consolidation course 3 = 675 mg/m^2)
Idarubicin 12 mg/m^2; administer intravenously diluted to a concentration >0.01 mg/mL in 0.9% NS or D5W over 15–30 minutes once on day 1 only of a 28-day cycle (total dosage/consolidation course 3 = 12 mg/m^2)
Cytarabine 150 mg/m^2 per dose; administer by subcutaneous injection every 8 hours for a total of 12 doses (ie, 3 doses per day) on days 1–4 of a 28-day cycle (total dosage/consolidation course 3 = 1800 mg/m^2)

Supportive Care (consolidation course 3)
Antiemetic prophylaxis (consolidation course 3)
*Emetogenic potential on days with tretinoin alone is **MINIMAL–LOW***
*Emetogenic potential on day 1 with idarubicin is **MODERATE***
*Emetogenic potential on days 1–4 with cytarabine is **LOW***
See Chapter 42 for antiemetic recommendations

Hematopoietic growth factor (CSF) prophylaxis (consolidation course 3)
*Primary prophylaxis is **NOT** indicated*
See Chapter 43 for more information

(continued)

Therapy Monitoring
(continued)

ii. Cryoprecipitate and/or fresh frozen plasma transfusions to maintain fibrinogen >100–150 mg/dL and international normalized ratio (INR) <1.5

4. *In patients at high risk for tumor lysis syndrome (eg, high tumor burden, renal dysfunction, rapidly progressing disease, markedly elevated LDH, baseline abnormalities in laboratory indices of tumor lysis syndrome [potassium, phosphate, uric acid, calcium, serum creatinine]):* consider frequent monitoring of laboratory indices of tumor lysis syndrome, intravenous hydration, and prophylaxis with a xanthine oxidase inhibitor (eg, allopurinol) during the induction course

5. *Liver function tests:* obtain ALT, AST, total bilirubin, and alkaline phosphatase prior to induction therapy and then 2–3 times per week

6. *Response assessment:* bone marrow biopsy should be performed upon recovery of peripheral blood counts to determine whether a CR by morphology has been achieved. Note that at the end of induction therapy it is expected that patients will have detectable PML-RARA transcripts by polymerase chain reaction and detectable t(15;17) by conventional cytogenetics and/or fluorescence in situ hybridization. Importantly, this does not represent resistant disease but rather slow clearance of terminally differentiating blasts and therefore detection of PML-RARA and/or t(15;17) should have no impact on treatment decisions during induction therapy[1]

During consolidation therapy:

1. *Pretreatment evaluation:* consider repeat determination of LVEF by echocardiogram prior to the first cycle of consolidation

2. CBC with differential and platelet count 1–2 times per week during consolidation therapy

3. Liver function tests (ALT, AST, total bilirubin, and alkaline phosphatase), BUN/SCr, and fasting lipid panel prior to each course of consolidation

4. Monitoring for high-dose cytarabine (applicable to consolidation cycle 1 only):
   a. Patients who receive high-dose cytarabine need to be closely monitored for changes in renal function. Renal dysfunction is highly correlated with an increased risk of cerebellar toxicity. Patients need to be monitored for nystagmus, dysmetria, and ataxia before each dose of cytarabine

(continued)

(continued)

Antimicrobial prophylaxis (consolidation course 3)
Risk of fever and neutropenia is **HIGH**
Antimicrobial primary prophylaxis is recommended:
- Antibacterial—consider prophylaxis with a fluoroquinolone during periods of prolonged neutropenia only (eg, ANC <500/mm^3 for ≥7 days) until ANC recovery
- Antifungal—consider prophylaxis with fluconazole or another azole antifungal medication during periods of prolonged neutropenia only (eg, <500/mm^3 for ≥7 days) until ANC recovery
- Antiviral—antiherpes antivirals (eg, acyclovir, famciclovir, valacyclovir)

Maintenance therapy:
Mercaptopurine 50 mg/m^2 per dose; administer orally, on an empty stomach, without milk products, once daily, to complete a total of 2 years of maintenance therapy (total dosage/week = 350 mg/m^2)
- Begin mercaptopurine 1 month following hematologic recovery of the final consolidation course
- Withhold mercaptopurine on days when the patient is administered tretinoin

Methotrexate 15 mg/m^2 per dose; administer orally, once every 7 days, to complete a total of 2 years of maintenance therapy (total dosage/week = 15 mg/m^2)
- Begin weekly methotrexate 1 month following hematologic recovery of the final consolidation course
- Withhold methotrexate on days when the patient is administered tretinoin

Tretinoin 22.5 mg/m^2 per dose; administer orally every 12 hours for 15 consecutive days, on days 1–15, repeated every 3 months (ie, every 13 weeks) to complete a total of 2 years of maintenance therapy (total dosage/3-month course = 675 mg/m^2)
- Begin tretinoin 3 months following completing of the final consolidation course

Supportive Care (consolidation course 3)
Antiemetic prophylaxis (consolidation course 3)
Emetogenic potential on all days of maintenance therapy is **MINIMAL–LOW**
See Chapter 42 for antiemetic recommendations

Hematopoietic growth factor (CSF) prophylaxis (consolidation course 3)
Primary prophylaxis is **NOT** indicated
See Chapter 43 for more information

Antimicrobial prophylaxis (consolidation course 3)
Risk of fever and neutropenia is **LOW**
Antimicrobial primary prophylaxis is recommended:
- Antibacterial—not indicated
- Antifungal—not indicated
- Antiviral—not indicated unless patient previously had an episode of HSV

Therapy Monitoring
(continued)

5. *Response assessment:* bone marrow examination at the completion of consolidation to document molecular remission using a highly sensitive RT-PCR or RQ-PCR assay[1]

During and following maintenance therapy:
1. *Monthly during maintenance therapy:* CBC with differential and platelet count, BUN/serum creatinine, AST, ALT, total bilirubin, alkaline phosphatase, electrolytes, fasting lipid panel
2. *Response assessment:* bone marrow examination every 3 months for a total of 3 years following completion of consolidation therapy in high-risk patients (WBC >10,000/mm^3 at presentation); apply a highly sensitive RT-PCR or RQ-PCR assay for *PML-RARA*[1]

1. Sanz MA et al. Blood 2019;133:1630–1643

Treatment Modifications

Treatment Modifications Induction Therapy: Idarubicin + Tretinoin	
Adverse Events	**Treatment Modifications**
Total bilirubin >3 mg/dL	Reduce idarubicin dose by 25%
ATRA syndrome	Hold ATRA and treat with dexamethasone 10 mg intravenously every 12 hours for 3–5 days, then decrease the dexamethasone dose and administration schedule (taper) over a week to discontinue. Restart ATRA when symptoms and signs improve
Pseudotumor cerebri (severe headaches with nausea, vomiting, and visual disorders; more common in pediatric patients)	Manage pain associated with headache and temporarily withhold ATRA until resolution of symptoms

(continued)

Treatment Modifications (*continued*)

Treatment Modifications

Consolidation Course 1 *(age <60 years; cycle length = 28 days)*
(Idarubicin 5 mg/m²/day on days 1–4, cytarabine 1000 mg/m²/day on days 1–4, tretinoin 45 mg/m²/day on days 1–15)
Consolidation Course 2 *(age <60 years; cycle length = 28 days)*
(Mitoxantrone 10 mg/m²/day on days 1–5, tretinoin 45 mg/m²/day on days 1–15)
Consolidation Course 3 *(age <60 years; cycle length = 28 days)*
(Idarubicin 12 mg/m² on day 1, cytarabine 150 mg/m²/dose every 8 hours on days 1–4, tretinoin 45 mg/m²/day on days 1–15)

LVEF is 40%, or is 40–45% with a ≥10% absolute decrease below the pretreatment	Withhold idarubicin and/or mitoxantrone and continue with remainder of regimen. Repeat LVEF assessment prior to the next cycle of consolidation and carefully weigh the potential risks versus benefits of further future treatment with idarubicin and/or mitoxantrone
Total bilirubin >3 mg/dL	Reduce idarubicin dose by 25%
Fever, myalgia, bone pain, occasionally chest pain, maculopapular rash, conjunctivitis, and malaise 6–12 hours following high-dose cytarabine administration (cytarabine syndrome; applicable to cycle 1 only)	Corticosteroids beneficial in treating or preventing this syndrome. If the symptoms are deemed treatable, continue therapy with cytarabine and pre-treat with corticosteroids
Neurologic (cerebellar) toxicity related to high-dose cytarabine administration (applicable to cycle 1 only)	Hold high-dose cytarabine. Patients who develop CNS symptoms should not receive subsequent high-dose cytarabine
Pseudotumor cerebri related to ATRA (severe headaches with nausea, vomiting, and visual disorders; more common in pediatric patients)	Manage pain associated with headache and temporarily withhold ATRA until resolution of symptoms

Maintenance Therapy (total duration = 2 years)
(Methotrexate 15 mg/m² once per week, mercaptopurine 50 mg/m2/day continuously, tretinoin 45 mg/m²/day on days 1–15 repeated every 3 months)

ANC ≥1000/mm³ and ≤1500/mm³ during maintenance therapy	Reduce the doses of methotrexate and mercaptopurine by 50%
ANC <1000/mm³ during maintenance therapy	Temporarily withhold methotrexate and mercaptopurine. Upon improvement of ANC to >1500/mm³, resume methotrexate and mercaptopurine with the doses of each medication reduced by 50%
Creatinine clearance 10–50 mL/minute	Reduce weekly methotrexate dose to 50% of the usual starting dose and carefully monitor for toxicity
Evidence of acute kidney injury	Withhold methotrexate dose(s) until renal function returns to baseline
Patient requires treatment with a xanthine oxidase inhibitor (allopurinol or febuxostat)	If concomitant therapy is unavoidable, reduce the starting mercaptopurine dose to 25–33% of the usual starting dose and monitor closely for toxicity
Patient is known to be a TPMT intermediate metabolizer	Initiate mercaptopurine with the dosage reduced to between 30–80% of the usual dose and adjust as clinically appropriate for adverse effects
Patient is known to be a TPMT poor metabolizer	Initiate mercaptopurine with the dosage reduced to 10% of the usual dose and with the frequency reduced from once per day to 3 times per week and adjust as clinically appropriate for adverse effects

Relling MV et al. Clin Pharmacol Ther 2011;89:387–391

Notes:
1. ATRA (all *trans*-retinoic acid) syndrome may occur in patients with APL after treatment initiation during induction therapy. It is characterized by fever, peripheral edema, pulmonary infiltrates, hypoxemia, respiratory distress, hypotension, renal and hepatic dysfunction, and serositis, resulting in pleural and pericardial effusions. Considering that this complex of symptoms is not specific to the use of retinoic acid but may occur during therapy with agents such as arsenic trioxide it is now referred as the "APL differentiation syndrome." Early recognition and aggressive management with dexamethasone (10 mg; administer intravenously every 12 hours for ≥3 days) have been effective in most patients. If the symptoms or signs are severe, ATRA is discontinued and resumed at resolution of symptoms and signs, but under the cover of steroids, because the syndrome may recur. Tretinoin can be restarted in most cases
2. Disseminated intravascular coagulation (DIC) is frequently present at diagnosis in patients with APL, or occurs soon after the initiation of cytotoxic chemotherapy. This complication constitutes a medical emergency because, if left untreated, it can cause pulmonary or cerebrovascular hemorrhage in up to 40% of patients with a 10–20% incidence of early hemorrhagic death. Tretinoin therapy appears to shorten the duration of the coagulopathy

RELAPSED

LEUKEMIA, ACUTE PROMYELOCYTIC REGIMEN: ARSENIC TRIOXIDE

Soignet SL et al. J Clin Oncol 2001;19:3852–3860

Induction:
Arsenic trioxide 0.15 mg/kg per day; administer intravenously in 100–250 mL 5% dextrose injection (D5W) or 0.9% sodium chloride injection (0.9% NS) over 2 hours once daily until bone marrow remission or to a cumulative maximum of 60 doses (total dosage/week = 1.05 mg/kg; maximum dosage during induction = 9 mg/kg [60 doses])
or
Arsenic trioxide 0.15 mg/kg per dose administer intravenously in 100–250 mL D5W or 0.9% NS over 2 hours once daily for 5 days/week (eg, Monday through Friday) until bone marrow remission or to a cumulative maximum of 60 doses (total dosage/week = 0.75 mg/kg; maximum dosage during induction = 9 mg/kg [60 doses])

Consolidation/maintenance (up to 5 courses, beginning 3–4 weeks after completion of induction therapy):
Arsenic trioxide 0.15 mg/kg per day; administer intravenously in 100–250 mL 5% dextrose injection (D5W) or 0.9% sodium chloride injection (0.9% NS) over 2 hours once daily for 25 doses (total dosage during consolidation = 3.75 mg/kg [25 doses])
or
Arsenic trioxide 0.15 mg/kg per dose administer intravenously in 100–250 mL D5W or 0.9% NS over 2 hours once daily for 5 days/week (eg, Monday through Friday) for 25 doses (total dosage during consolidation course = 3.75 mg/kg [25 doses])

Treatment notes:
- Patients enrolled on the study were offered to enroll on a maintenance protocol which prescribed up to 4 additional cycles of maintenance arsenic trioxide at a dose and schedule similar to the consolidation cycle described above (Soignet SL et al. J Clin Oncol 2001;19:3852–3860)
- The goal of induction therapy in patients with relapsed acute promyelocytic leukemia is to induce a second complete remission as a bridge to autologous stem cell transplant. Patients who achieve a molecular remission should be considered for consolidation with an autologous stem cell transplant. Patients who fail to achieve a molecular remission should be considered for an allogeneic stem cell transplant. Patients who are not transplant candidates may be considered for repeated cycles of arsenic trioxide ± tretinoin ± chemotherapy (Sanz MA et al. Blood 2019;133:1630–1643)

Supportive Care
Antiemetic prophylaxis
Emetogenic potential is **MODERATE**. *Avoid antiemetics with potential to prolong the QT interval (eg, ondansetron) during arsenic trioxide therapy*
See Chapter 42 for antiemetic recommendations

Hematopoietic growth factor (CSF) prophylaxis
Primary prophylaxis is **NOT** indicated
See Chapter 43 for more information

Risk of fever and neutropenia during induction *therapy is* **INTERMEDIATE**
Antimicrobial primary prophylaxis to be considered during induction therapy:
- Antibacterial—consider prophylaxis (eg, cotrimoxazole) during periods of prolonged neutropenia only (eg, <500/mm³ for ≥7 days) until ANC recovery. Note that routine use of fluoroquinolones for prophylaxis should be avoided due to the risk of QTc prolongation with arsenic trioxide
- Antifungal—consider prophylaxis with an echinocandin (eg, caspofungin) during periods of prolonged neutropenia only (eg, <500/mm³ for ≥7 days), or no prophylaxis, until ANC recovery. Note that routine use of azole antifungals (eg, fluconazole) for prophylaxis should be avoided due to the risk of QTc prolongation with arsenic trioxide
- Antiviral—antiherpes antivirals (eg, acyclovir, famciclovir, valacyclovir)

Risk of fever and neutropenia during consolidation *therapy is* **LOW**
Antimicrobial primary prophylaxis to be considered during consolidation therapy:
- Antibacterial—not indicated
- Antifungal—not indicated
- Antiviral—not indicated unless patient previously had an episode of HSV

Patient Population Studied

Study of 40 patients with either relapsed and/or refractory acute promyelocytic leukemia

Efficacy

CR: 85%
Median time to clinical CR: 59 days

Therapy Monitoring

During induction therapy:
1. CBC with differential and platelet count, 2–3 times daily until resolution of coagulopathy, then daily
2. Fibrinogen, PT/INR, and aPTT, thrombin time, fibrinogen-fibrin degradation products twice daily until resolution of coagulopathy, then daily
   a. During induction therapy when clinical and laboratory signs of coagulopathy are present:[1]
      i. Platelet transfusion support to maintain platelets ≥30,000 to 50,000/mm³
      ii. Cryoprecipitate and/or fresh frozen plasma transfusions to maintain fibrinogen >100–150 mg/dL and international normalized ratio (INR) <1.5
3. *In patients at high risk for tumor lysis syndrome (eg, high tumor burden, renal dysfunction, rapidly progressing disease, markedly elevated LDH, baseline abnormalities in laboratory indices of tumor lysis syndrome [potassium, phosphate, uric acid, calcium, serum creatinine]): consider frequent monitoring of laboratory indices of tumor lysis syndrome, intravenous hydration, and prophylaxis with a xanthine oxidase inhibitor (eg, allopurinol) during the induction course*
4. *Liver function tests:* obtain ALT, AST, total bilirubin, and alkaline phosphatase prior to induction therapy and then 2–3 times per week
5. *Cardiac monitoring (goal QTc < 500 ms during arsenic trioxide therapy):*
   a. *During therapy:* maintain serum potassium concentration >4 mEq/L (>4 mmol/L) and maintain serum magnesium concentration >0.74 mmol/L (>1.8 mg/dL, >1.48 mEq/L)[1]
   b. ECG at baseline and at least twice per week during therapy with arsenic trioxide[1]

Treatment Modifications

DOSE MODIFICATIONS FOR ARSENIC TRIOXIDE AND TRETINOIN

	Arsenic Trioxide
Starting dose	0.15 mg/kg per dose
Dose level −1	0.075 mg/kg per dose

Adverse Event	Treatment Modification
QT prolongation QTc interval >500 ms	For patients with heart rate >60 bpm, ensure that QT interval is corrected using the Fridericia, Hodges, or Sagie/Framingham formulae and not using the Bazett formula. Withhold arsenic trioxide and replete electrolytes. Discontinue any medication known to prolong the QTc interval (eg, ondansetron, haloperidol, fluconazole, etc). Increase frequency of ECG monitoring to daily and strongly consider telemetered ECG monitoring 1. When the QTc improves to approximately ≤460 ms, then resume arsenic trioxide with dosage decreased by 50%: arsenic trioxide 0.075 mg/kg per day 2. If no further QTc prolongation occurs after 3 days of treatment at the reduced dosage, escalate arsenic trioxide dosage to 0.15 mg/kg per day (full dose)
Differentiation syndrome (ie, during induction therapy)	Withhold therapy with arsenic trioxide only in cases of severe differentiation syndrome. Promptly initiate dexamethasone 10 mg IV every 12 hours at the earliest clinical suspicion of incipient differentiation syndrome until disappearance of signs/symptoms, and for a minimum of 3 days. Consider treatment with loop diuretics (eg, furosemide) when clinically required. If treatment with arsenic trioxide was held for severe symptoms, then upon improvement in clinical condition and symptoms, resume treatment with arsenic trioxide at 50% of the previous dose during the first 3 days after disappearance of the differentiation syndrome. Thereafter, in absence of worsening of the previous toxicity, arsenic trioxide should be resumed at full dosage. In case of reappearance of symptoms, arsenic trioxide will be reduced at the previous dosage
Leukocytosis occurring during induction therapy (WBC >10,000/mm³ to ≤50,000/mm³)	Initiate treatment with **hydroxyurea** 500 mg per dose; administer orally four times per day until WBC <10,000/mm³. Monitor closely for signs and symptoms of differentiation syndrome
Leukocytosis occurring during induction therapy (WBC >50,000/mm³)	Increase the hydroxyurea dosage as follows: **hydroxyurea** 1000 mg per dose; administer orally four times per day until WBC <50,000/mm³, then reduce the dose to 500 mg four times per day until WBC <10,000/mm³, then discontinue hydroxyurea. Monitor closely for signs and symptoms of differentiation syndrome. For extreme cases of hyperleukocytosis resistant to hydroxyurea, consider a one-time dose of either idarubicin (12 mg/m²) or gemtuzumab ozogamicin (6–9 mg/m²)
Hepatotoxicity (increase in serum bilirubin >5× ULN and/or AST >5× ULN and/or alkaline phosphatase >5× ULN)	Temporarily discontinue arsenic trioxide and increase the frequency of liver function test monitoring to once daily After serum bilirubin, AST, and alkaline phosphatase decrease to <4× the upper limit of their normal ranges (ULN), treatment with arsenic trioxide may resume at 50% of the dosage previously given for 3 days If toxicity does not recur during the 3 days after resuming arsenic trioxide, drug administration may resume at full dosage
Acute vasomotor reaction during arsenic trioxide infusion	Prolong the arsenic trioxide infusion duration to 4 hours

(continued)

Therapy Monitoring
(*continued*)

c. The QT interval should be corrected for heart rate using the Fridericia, Hodges, or Sagie/Framingham formulae. Avoid using the standard Bazett formula since it may lead to an overestimate of the QTc interval and cause unnecessary interruptions in arsenic trioxide therapy[1,2]

6. *Response assessment:* bone marrow biopsy should be performed on day 28 of induction therapy. Discontinue induction therapy in patients without evidence of morphologic disease (<5% blasts and no abnormal promyelocytes). In patients with evidence of morphologic disease at day 28, repeat a bone marrow examination weekly until clearance of blasts and abnormal promyelocytes. Note that at the end of induction therapy it is expected that patients will have detectable PML-RARA transcripts by polymerase chain reaction and detectable t(15;17) by conventional cytogenetics and/or fluorescence in situ hybridization. Importantly, this does not represent resistant disease but rather slow clearance of terminally differentiating blasts and therefore detection of PML-RARA and/or t(15;17) should have no impact on treatment decisions during induction therapy[1]

During consolidation therapy:
1. CBC with differential and platelet count and liver function tests (ALT, AST, total bilirubin, and alkaline phosphatase) 1–2 times per week during consolidation therapy with arsenic trioxide
2. Cardiac monitoring (goal QTc <500 ms during arsenic trioxide therapy):
   a. During arsenic trioxide therapy: maintain serum potassium concentration >4 mEq/L (>4 mmol/L) and maintain serum magnesium concentration >0.74 mmol/L (>1.8 mg/dL, >1.48 mEq/L)[1]
   b. During arsenic trioxide therapy: ECG before the start of consolidation and at least twice per week[1]
   c. The QT interval should be corrected for heart rate using the Fridericia, Hodges, or Sagie/Framingham formulae. Avoid using the standard Bazett formula since it may lead to an overestimate of the QTc interval and cause unnecessary interruptions in arsenic trioxide therapy[1,2]

(continued)

Treatment Modifications (*continued*)

Adverse Event	Treatment Modification
Other intolerable Grade 2 nonhematologic toxicities	Reduce arsenic trioxide dosage by 1 dose level. If toxicity does not recur during the 3 days after resuming arsenic trioxide, drug administration may resume at full dosage if clinically appropriate
Grades 3–4 nonhematologic toxicity	Withhold arsenic trioxide until toxicity remits to G <2, then resume treatment (if clinically appropriate) with the dosage reduced by 1 dose level

Soignet SL et al. J Clin Oncol 2001;19:3852–3860
Lo-Coco F et al. N Engl J Med 2013;369:111–121
Supplementary appendix to: Lo-Coco F et al. N Engl J Med 2013;369:111–121
Protocol for: Lo-Coco F et al. N Engl J Med 2013;369:111–121
Sanz MA et al. Blood 2019;133:1630–1643

Toxicity (N = 40)

Adverse Events	All Grades	G4
Nausea	75%	—
Vomiting	58%	—
Diarrhea	53%	—
Sore throat	40%	—
Abdominal pain	38%	8%
Cough	65%	—
Dyspnea	38%	10%
Headache	60%	3%
Insomnia	43%	3%
Dermatitis	43%	—
Hypokalemia	50%	13%
Hyperglycemia	45%	13%
Tachycardia	55%	—
Fatigue	63%	—
Fever	63%	—
QTc prolongation	40%	—
APL syndrome*	25%	—
Peripheral neuropathy	43%	—

There were no treatment-related deaths
*Treatment with arsenic trioxide for remission induction is associated with the development of symptoms identical to retinoic acid syndrome. Considering the complex of symptoms is not specific to the use of retinoic acid, it is now referred as the APL syndrome

Therapy Monitoring (*continued*)

3. *Response assessment:* bone marrow examination at the completion of consolidation to document molecular remission using a highly sensitive RT-PCR or RQ-PCR assay

1. Sanz MA et al. Blood 2019;133:1630–1643
2. Roboz GJ et al. J Clin Oncol 2014;32:3723–3728

3. Adrenocortical Cancer

Tito Fojo, MD, PhD

Epidemiology

Incidence: 0.5 to 2.0 cases per 1 million population
Deaths: 0.2% of cancer deaths
Median age: Bimodal median, at age 4 years and ages 40–50 years
Male to female ratio: 1:1.3

Cohn K et al. Surgery 1986;100:1170–1177
Wooten MD, King DK. Cancer 1993;72:3145–3155

Stage at Presentation

Stage I:	3%
Stage II:	29%
Stage III:	19%
Stage IV:	49%

Pathology

1. Unlike renal cell carcinoma, adrenocortical cancer stains positive for vimentin
2. >20 mitoses per HPF—median survival 14 months
   ≤20 mitoses per HPF—median survival 58 months
3. Tumor necrosis—poor prognosis
4. Vascular invasion—poor prognosis
5. Capsular invasion—poor prognosis

Weiss LM et al. Am J Surg Pathol 1989;13:202–206

Survival After Complete Resection

5-Year Actuarial Survival	
Stages I–II	54%
Stage III	24%
1-Year survival	
Stage IV	9%

Icard P et al. Surgery 1992;112:972–980;
discussion 979–980
Icard P et al. World J Surg 1992;16:753–758

Work-up

1. CT scan of chest, abdomen, and pelvis to determine extent of disease
2. MRI of abdomen may help to identify and follow liver metastases
3. If IVC is compressed, consider IVC contrast study, ultrasound, or MRI to assess disease involvement before surgical exploration, although apparent extent of involvement should not deter exploration
4. Serum and 24-hour urinary cortisol; 24-hour urinary 17-ketosteroid
5. Additional studies can be performed to determine the functional status of the tumor, including serum estradiol, estrone, testosterone, dehydroepiandrosterone sulfate (S-DHAS), 17-OH-progesterone, and androstenedione

Staging

Stage I	<5-cm tumor confined to adrenal
Stage II	>5-cm tumor confined to adrenal
Stage III	Positive lymph nodes or local invasion with tumor outside adrenal in fat or adjacent organs
Stage IV	Distant metastasis

Macfarlane DA. Ann R Coll Surg Engl 1958;23:155–186
Sullivan M et al. J Urol 1978;120:660–665

Expert Opinion

1. *Primary therapy:* Primary therapy is complete surgical resection

2. *Surgery, embolization/chemoembolization, and thermal ablation as options for recurrences:* When possible, local recurrences should be addressed surgically. Some advocate surgical resection of metastatic disease, and although it may improve survival, firm evidence is lacking. Embolization/chemoembolization and thermal ablation may be used as alternatives if the recurrence is deemed amenable and has an expendable margin. Just as incomplete resections should not be embarked on, neither should incomplete embolizations/ablations be performed

3. *Management of excess hormone production:* Excess hormone production should not be ignored. Manage severe hypercortisolism aggressively. Because chemotherapy is usually ineffective, treatment of hormonal excess should not be delayed in expectation that chemotherapy will reduce the tumor burden and improve symptoms. Instead, use steroidogenesis inhibitors either singly or in combination. **Mitotane** is the cornerstone of any strategy and should be started as soon as a diagnosis has been made. Use mitotane at the highest tolerable dose. However, because a therapeutic mitotane level and steady state will not be reached for several months, other agents must be initiated concurrently. In patients with LFT results not more than 3 times normal range, begin therapy with **ketoconazole**, mindful of the potential for a pharmacokinetic interaction with other drugs. If LFTs are elevated, if an aggressive ketoconazole dose escalation is unsuccessful in controlling symptoms, or if toxicity develops, use **metyrapone***, either alone or in combination with ketoconazole. Cortisol levels must be monitored frequently to adjust steroidogenesis inhibitor drug doses and to avoid adrenal insufficiency, which occurs infrequently in patients with cortisol-producing tumors. Should adrenal insufficiency occur, hydrocortisone and mineralocorticoid replacement should be instituted as indicated below

   - *Mitotane:* Refer to section describing mitotane as a regimen for ACC
   - *Ketoconazole:* In patients with ACC and frank Cushing syndrome, treatment can start with 200 mg/dose given 3 or 4 times per day. The dose can then be increased by 400 mg/day every few days to a maximum single dose of 1200–1600 mg administered 3 or 4 times per day (ie, total daily doses = 3600–6400 mg) while monitoring liver function. Because ketoconazole requires stomach acidity for absorption, proton pump inhibitors should be avoided, and achlorhydria should be suspected in elderly individuals who do not respond to therapy
   - *Metyrapone*:* Metyrapone is begun at a low dose of 500–1000 mg (250–500 mg 2–4 times daily) and is escalated every few days to the maximum daily dose. The dose needed to inhibit cortisol production ranges from 500 to 6000 mg/day, although little is gained with total daily doses greater than 2000 mg

4. *Chemotherapy for unresectable, advanced, and recurrent disease:* Chemotherapy is recommended for patients with metastatic disease, although evidence of survival benefit is not and will never be available. EDP (etoposide + doxorubicin + cisplatin) plus mitotane or streptozocin plus mitotane should be used as first-line therapy. "Novel targeted therapies" that may seem attractive have not been proved and should not be substituted for these chemotherapies that have known activity in ACC

5. *Adjuvant mitotane:* A recent analysis of 177 patients with ACC compared the outcome in 47 patients treated with adjuvant mitotane therapy with 130 patients who received no additional therapy (Terzolo et al., 2007). Surprisingly, when used at "more tolerable" daily doses of 2000–3000 mg, the authors reported that mitotane demonstrated significant benefit in the adjuvant setting. However, the results of this retrospective nonrandomized study must be viewed cautiously. Because the advantage was confined to time to recurrence and not to overall survival, the value of adjuvant mitotane is diminished. Furthermore, the short follow-up period of patients treated with mitotane leaves the conclusions in doubt. The lack of convincing evidence and the difficulty of administering mitotane has often guided a recommendation that "adjuvant" mitotane therapy should be used only in cases where a tumor cannot be fully removed surgically or in patients with a high likelihood of recurrence; that is, large tumors with extensive necrosis, capsular, lymphatic, or venous invasion, a high mitotic or Ki67 labeling index, and small or questionable surgical margins. Until further data are available, this continues to be the most reasonable approach

6. *Long-term mitotane monotherapy:* Administer mitotane long-term only to patients who tolerate it well and experience a therapeutic response or those who are at high risk for recurrence. The optimal duration of therapy is not known: a recommendation of "indefinite" is most conservative. *Prolonged therapy is often made possible by the fact that after months of therapy body stores are finally saturated, and the dose needed to maintain serum levels is then markedly reduced.* In this case the tolerability improves markedly. However, suboptimal therapy (judged by serum mitotane levels) that is limited by side effects should not be continued; in this setting there is little chance of benefit in the face of continued toxicity. Although suboptimal therapy cannot be accurately defined, blood levels of 10–14 mg/L are often cited as optimal based on two small studies, but lower levels are likely of some value; a clinical observation also noted in the recent retrospective analysis of adjuvant mitotane (Terzolo et al., 2007).

7. *Immunotherapy/checkpoint inhibitors, ie, anti-PD-1 and anti-PD-L1 antibodies:* Despite the novelty of checkpoint inhibitors and the excitement surrounding their use as well as some "encouraging" preliminary data to date only published in abstract form, the value of checkpoint inhibitors in ACC has not been proven. At least two large studies conducted have not been reported and unfortunately may never be published, and the single published study (Le Tourneau et al., 2018) reported 3 partial responses in 50 patients, a disappointing 6% overall response rate, without accompanying molecular analysis that could have helped inform the underpinnings to responses. To be sure, the rare patient with Lynch Syndrome in whom ACC has developed or a patient whose tumors are mismatch repair deficient should receive a checkpoint inhibitor. No one else should receive this initially and should only be treated with a checkpoint inhibitor after standard-of-care options including EDP and streptozocin have been tried in what may be regarded as a "desperation oncology" strategy.

8. *Adjuvant treatment:* There is no evidence that adjuvant therapy is effective; unless there is obvious disease and despite concerns for recurrence, a strategy of careful follow-up is preferred.

(continued)

Expert Opinion (*continued*)

9. ***Radiation therapy:*** While not formally studied, ACC appears to be very responsive to radiation and its use in diverse settings as part of a salvage strategy can be beneficial. There is no evidence for its use as an adjuvant therapy following surgical resection, and as it may complicate the only curative option for a local recurrence—surgical resection—its use in this setting is discouraged unless there is pathologic evidence of positive margins/residual disease.

*At present, metyrapone is not available in pharmacies. To obtain metyrapone (Metopirone), a pharmacist or physician must call Novartis Pharmaceuticals Corporation at 1-800-988-7768

Ho et al. Cancer J. 2013;19:288–294
Le Tourneau C et al. J Immunother Cancer 2018:6:111
Ng L, Libertino JM. J Urol 2003;169:5–11
Terzolo M et al. N Engl J Med 2007;356:2372–2380
Vassilopoulou-Sellin R, Shultz PN. Cancer 2001;92:1113–1121
Veytsman I et al. J Clin Oncol 2009;27:4619–4629
Wajchenberg BL et al. Cancer 2000;88:711–736

ADJUVANT OR METASTATIC

ADRENOCORTICAL CANCER REGIMEN: MITOTANE (*O,P'*-DDD)

Luton J-P et al. N Engl J Med 1990;322:1195–1201

Mitotane 2000–20,000 mg/day; administer orally as a single dose or in 2–4 divided doses

Glucocorticoid replacement is necessary in all patients:
Hydrocortisone 15–20 mg; administer orally every morning, *plus:*
Hydrocortisone 7.5–10 mg; administer orally every afternoon around 4 PM
Mineralocorticoid replacement also is recommended:
Fludrocortisone acetate 100–200 mcg/day; administer orally every morning, *or:*
Fludrocortisone acetate 100 mcg/day; administer orally every morning and every evening

Supportive Care
Antiemetic prophylaxis
Emetogenic potential: **MINIMAL**
See Chapter 42 for antiemetic recommendations

Hematopoietic growth factor (CSF) prophylaxis
Primary prophylaxis is **NOT** *indicated*
See Chapter 43 for more information

Antimicrobial prophylaxis
Risk of fever and neutropenia is **LOW**
  Antimicrobial primary prophylaxis to be considered:
  • Antibacterial—not indicated
  • Antifungal—not indicated
  • Antiviral—not indicated unless patient previously had an episode of HSV

Mitotane is available in the United States for oral administration in tablets that contain 500 mg mitotane. Lysodren (mitotane tablets). Bristol-Myers Squibb Company, Princeton, NJ

Patient Population Studied

A study of 59 patients with adrenocortical carcinoma treated with mitotane at different times in relation to surgery

Efficacy (N = 37)

Overall response rate	22%
Stable disease >12 months	5%
Clinical benefit rate	27%

Complete responses have been reported in other studies but are rare

Toxicity

Adverse Event	% Patients	No. of Patients
Anorexia/nausea	93	
Vomiting	82	
Diarrhea	68	28
Skin rash	32	
Confusion/ sleepiness	100	
Ataxia	39	
Depression	33	
Dysarthria	28	18
Tremor	22	
Visual disturbance	17	
Leukopenia	17	

Van Slooten H et al. Eur J Cancer Clin Oncol 1984;20:47–53

Treatment Modifications

Adverse Event	Dose Modification
General Guidelines:	First step with most side effects, especially if they occur as mitotane dose is advanced: (1) stop mitotane; (2) wait up to 7 days for symptoms to resolve; (3) restart mitotane at lower dose (500–1000 mg/day less than previous dose) or at previously tolerated dose; (4) increase dose in 500-mg/day increments at 1-week intervals
Anorexia Nausea/vomiting	Administer mitotane in divided doses, and/ or most of dose before bedtime. Crush tablets and dissolve in vehicle. Use antiemetics as needed. Reassess adrenal replacement
Diarrhea	Administer as divided doses. Use loperamide or diphenoxylate/ atropine
Altered mental status	Stop therapy. Follow general guidelines. Obtain imaging study only if symptoms persist after 1 week off therapy
Skin rash	If not severe, continue mitotane and treat rash with local measures and antipruritics

Therapy Monitoring

1. Check mitotane level at least every 4 weeks initially. Patients receiving long-term mitotane therapy can have monitoring reduced to every 2–3 months
2. Adrenal function can be monitored by measuring ACTH, but this alone is not reliable and should be interpreted together with clinical assessment
3. *Response assessment:* Initially every 6–8 weeks. Patients receiving long-term mitotane therapy can have monitoring reduced to every 3–6 months

Notes

1. Begin mitotane administration at a low dosage, usually no more than 2000 mg/day

2. Increase dose in increments of 500 mg to a maximum of 1000 mg/day, usually at intervals of not less than 1 week

3. Do not increase mitotane if a patient is experiencing side effects; follow General Guidelines in the Treatment Modifications section. Although mitotane is considered to have low to no emetogenic potential, it often produces low-grade nausea that is difficult to tolerate because it occurs every day. In some patients, chronic administration of antiemetics is required. See Chapter 42

4. The optimal dosage is not known; however, mitotane levels should be monitored with a goal of attaining a level of 14–20 mcg/mL. Levels greater than 20 mcg/mL are usually associated with intolerable side effects

5. A dosage of 4000–6000 mg/day usually results in a therapeutic level of mitotane in most patients after 6–10 weeks; however, some patients tolerate or require doses as high as 10,000–12,000 mg/day

6. Therapeutic levels can be achieved more quickly by administering higher doses and by increasing doses more aggressively, but this strategy usually fails because of side effects that result

7. With long-term administration of mitotane, the dosage required to maintain a therapeutic level may be substantially less, even as low as 500–1000 mg/day

8. Chronic administration results in adrenal insufficiency requiring steroid replacement therapy, as recommended in Regimen. Some physicians prefer to begin replacement therapy at the time mitotane therapy is started; others wait until there is evidence of incipient adrenal insufficiency, usually 6–8 weeks after the start of therapy. Replacement therapy is recommended with twice-daily hydrocortisone and with once- or twice-daily fludrocortisone replacement. Measuring ACTH levels to monitor the adequacy of replacement therapy is of limited value, because normal ACTH levels are difficult if not impossible to achieve. Patients should be instructed to obtain and wear identification that warns health care providers about possible adrenal insufficiency

9. Even without effecting a reduction in tumor size, mitotane may reduce circulating hormone levels, so that mitotane therapy can be continued solely to control the signs and symptoms of hormonal excess. Furthermore, if, after a period of mitotane administration, there is evidence of disease progression, discontinuing mitotane will result in a recurrence of the signs and symptoms of hormonal excess. The latter may appear gradually as mitotane is slowly cleared, but may eventually be worse than before mitotane therapy because of interval growth of the tumor. In these patients, consider continuing mitotane or begin an alternate drug to control hormonal excess

Haak HR et al. Br J Cancer 1994;69:947–951

Hoffman DL, Mattox VR. Med Clin North Am 1972;56:999–1012

Van Slooten H et al. Eur J Cancer Clin Oncol 1984;20:47–53

METASTATIC

ADRENOCORTICAL CANCER REGIMEN: CISPLATIN + MITOTANE

Bukowski RM et al. J Clin Oncol 1993;11:161–165

Hydration: ≥2000 mL 0.9% sodium chloride injection (0.9% NS), at ≥100 mL/hour before and after cisplatin administration. Also encourage increased oral fluid intake. Monitor and replace magnesium/electrolytes as needed

Cisplatin 75–100 mg/m²; administer intravenously in 50–250 mL of 0.9% NS over 30 minutes on day 1 every 3 weeks (total dosage per cycle = 75–100 mg/m²)
Mitotane[*] 4000 mg/day; administer orally, continually

Glucocorticoid replacement is necessary in all patients:
Hydrocortisone 15–20 mg; administer orally every morning, *plus*
Hydrocortisone 7.5–10 mg; administer orally every evening, continually
Mineralocorticoid replacement also is recommended
Fludrocortisone acetate 100–200 mcg/day; administer orally every morning, *or*
Fludrocortisone acetate 100 mcg/day; administer orally every morning and every evening, continually

Supportive Care
Antiemetic prophylaxis
Emetogenic potential on day 1: **HIGH**. *Potential for delayed symptoms*
Emetogenic potential on days with mitotane alone: **MINIMAL**
See Chapter 42 for antiemetic recommendations

Hematopoietic growth factor (CSF) prophylaxis
Primary prophylaxis is **NOT** *indicated*
See Chapter 43 for more information

Antimicrobial prophylaxis
Risk of fever and neutropenia is **LOW**
Antimicrobial primary prophylaxis to be considered:
- Antibacterial—not indicated
- Antifungal—not indicated
- Antiviral—not indicated unless patient previously had an episode of HSV

[*]Mitotane therapy may be better tolerated if started at a dose of 2000 mg/day, increasing by 500–1000 mg/day at 1-week intervals. The total daily mitotane dosage can be taken in 2–4 divided doses or as a single daily dose, which often is best tolerated at bedtime

Mitotane is available in the United States for oral administration in tablets that contain 500 mg mitotane Lysodren (mitotane tablets). Bristol-Myers Squibb Company, Princeton, NJ

Treatment Modifications

Adverse Event	Dose Modification
CrCl 30–50 mL/min (0.5–0.83 mL/s)	Hold cisplatin until CrCl ≥50 mL/min (≥0.83 mL/s), then reduce dose to 75 mg/m² if previous dose was 100 mg/m² or 60 mg/m² if previous dose was 75 mg/m²
CrCl <30 mL/min (<0.5 mL/s)	Discontinue cisplatin
Unacceptable GI or neuromuscular side effects from mitotane	Reduce mitotane to 2000 mg/day
Unacceptable side effects from mitotane at 2000 mg/day	Reduce mitotane to 1000 mg/day
Unacceptable side effects from mitotane at 1000 mg/day	Discontinue mitotane

CrCl, creatinine clearance

Patient Population Studied

A trial of 42 patients with metastatic or residual adrenocortical carcinoma because complete resection was not possible. Prior therapy with mitotane was allowed

Efficacy (N = 37)

Complete response	2.7%
Partial response	27%
Median response duration	7.9 months
Median time to response	76 days

Toxicity (N = 36)

Adverse Event	% G1/2	% G3/4
Hematologic		
Anemia	8	8
Leukopenia	36	6
Thrombocytopenia	—	3
Nonhematologic		
Nausea/vomiting	75	22
Diarrhea	11	—
Mucositis	6	—
Increased bilirubin	6	—
Renal	17	8
Peripheral neuropathy	3	6
Myalgias	17	6

N = 36, but reported as percent of 37 eligible patients

Therapy Monitoring

1. CBC with leukocyte differential count, serum creatinine and electrolytes, serum magnesium, and LFTs on day 1
2. *Response assessment:* Repeat imaging studies every 2 cycles; 24-hour urine cortisol and 17-ketosteroids with each cycle, if abnormal at baseline
3. Mitotane level at least every 4 weeks initially. A level of 14–20 mcg/mL is desirable
4. Adrenal function can be monitored by measuring ACTH, but this alone is not reliable and should be interpreted together with clinical assessment

METASTATIC

ADRENOCORTICAL CANCER REGIMEN: ETOPOSIDE + DOXORUBICIN + CISPLATIN + MITOTANE (EDP-M)

Fassnacht M et al. N Engl J Med 2012;366:2189–2197

Mitotane 500–5000 mg/day; administer orally, continually
- If possible, mitotane is started a minimum of 1 week before cytotoxic treatment is initiated. The ultimate goal is to attain mitotane concentrations in blood of 14–20 mcg/mL over time, as tolerated, trying not to exceed these values as side effects worsen with higher values. Note that side effects may preclude this range from being attained
- Initiate treatment with doses of 1000–1500 mg per day at bedtime to minimize sedative effects during waking hours, and escalate doses as tolerated
- Large daily doses may be divided in ≥2 doses

Doxorubicin 40 mg/m^2; administer by intravenous injection over 3–5 minutes on day 1, every 4 weeks (total dosage/cycle = 40 mg/m^2)

Prehydration for cisplatin: ≥500 mL 0.9% sodium chloride injection (0.9% NS) per day; administer intravenously at ≥100 mL/hour for 2 consecutive days, starting before cisplatin on days 3 and 4

Cisplatin 40 mg/m^2 per day; administer intravenously in 50–500 mL of 0.9% NS over 30–60 minutes for 2 doses on 2 consecutive days, days 3 and 4, every 4 weeks (total dosage/cycle = 80 mg/m^2)

Posthydration for cisplatin: ≥500 mL 0.9% NS per day; administer intravenously at ≥100 mL/hour for 2 consecutive days, after cisplatin on days 3 and 4. Encourage increased oral fluid intake. Monitor and replace magnesium and electrolytes as needed

± *Mannitol diuresis:* May be given to patients who have received adequate hydration

Mannitol 12.5–25 g may be administered by intravenous injection before or during cisplatin administration, *or*

Mannitol 10–40 g; administer intravenously over 1–4 hours before or during cisplatin administration, or may be prepared as an admixture with cisplatin

Note: Diuresis with mannitol requires maintaining hydration with intravenously administered fluid during and for hours after mannitol administration

Etoposide 100 mg/m^2 per dose; administer intravenously diluted to a concentration within the range 0.2–0.4 mg/mL in 5% dextrose injection or 0.9% NS over at least 60 minutes for 3 consecutive days, on days 2, 3, and 4, every 4 weeks (total dosage/cycle = 300 mg/m^2)

Glucocorticoid replacement is necessary in all patients taking mitotane
Hydrocortisone 15–20 mg orally every morning, *plus:*
Hydrocortisone 7.5–10 mg orally every evening
Mineralocorticoid replacement also is recommended:
Fludrocortisone acetate 100–200 mcg/day orally every morning, *or:*
Fludrocortisone acetate 100 mcg/day orally every morning and every evening

Supportive Care
Antiemetic prophylaxis
Emetogenic potential on day 1: **MODERATE**
Emetogenic potential on day 2: **LOW**
Emetogenic potential on days 3 and 4: **HIGH**. *Potential for delayed symptoms*
See Chapter 42 for antiemetic recommendations

Hematopoietic growth factor (CSF) prophylaxis
Primary prophylaxis is **NOT** *indicated*
See Chapter 43 for more information

Antimicrobial prophylaxis
Risk of fever and neutropenia is **LOW**
   Antimicrobial primary prophylaxis to be considered:
- Antibacterial—not indicated
- Antifungal—not indicated
- Antiviral—not indicated unless patient previously had an episode of HSV

Patient Population Studied

Patients with histologically confirmed adrenocortical carcinoma not amenable to radical surgical resection who had not received any previous treatment with cytotoxic drugs, except mitotane, and had an Eastern Cooperative Oncology Group (ECOG) performance status of 0, 1, or 2. A total of 151 patients received etoposide + doxorubicin + cisplatin + mitotane

Age (y)	
Median	51.9
Range	19.0–76.2

Sex—Number (%)	
Male	60 (39.7)
Female	91 (60.3)

Tumor stage—Number (%)	
III	0
IV	151 (100.0)

Endocrine symptoms—Number (%)	
Cushing syndrome ± other symptoms	60 (39.7)
Conn syndrome only	2 (1.3)
Virilization only	6 (4.0)
Feminization only	3 (2.0)
No symptoms	70 (46.4)
Missing data	10 (6.6)

ECOG performance status score—Number (%)	
0	73 (48.3)
1	64 (42.4)
2	13 (8.6)
4	1 (0.7)

Time since primary diagnosis—Months	
Median	7.3
Range	0–183.7

Number of affected sites*	
Median	3
Range	1–7

*The following sites were calculated as separate sites of adrenocortical carcinoma: adrenal gland (including local recurrence), liver, lung, bone, peritoneum, retroperitoneum, pleura, mediastinum, central nervous system, soft tissue, spleen, and ovary

Treatment Modifications

Adverse Event	Dose Modification
Day 1 WBC <1000/mm^3 *or* platelet count <100,000/mm^3 *or* G >2 nonhematologic toxicity	Delay chemotherapy until WBC ≥1000/mm^3 and platelet count ≥100,000/mm^3, or nonhematologic toxicity G ≤1 for a maximum delay of 2 weeks
>2-week delay in reaching WBC >1000/mm^3 or platelet count >100,000/mm^3 *or* for resolution of non-hematologic toxicity to G ≤1	Discontinue therapy
G4 ANC or G ≥3 platelet counts	Reduce dosages of all drugs by 25% except mitotane
Creatinine clearance <50 to 60 mL/min	Hold cisplatin until creatinine clearance >50–60 mL/min

Toxicity

Event	Number of Patients (%)
Any serious adverse event	86 (58.1)
Adrenal insufficiency	5 (3.4)
Bone marrow toxicity	17 (11.5)
Cardiovascular or thromboembolic event	10 (6.8)
Fatigue or general health deterioration	8 (5.4)
Gastrointestinal disorder	6 (4.1)
Impaired liver function	0
Impaired renal function	1 (0.7)
Infection	10 (6.8)
Neurologic toxicity	5 (3.4)
Respiratory disorder	9 (6.1)
Other	15 (10.1)

Efficacy

Efficacy in the Intention-to-Treat Population
Randomized Comparison versus Streptozocin + Mitotane[*]

Variable	EDP-M (N = 151)[†]	Sz-M (N = 153)[†]	P-Value
Type of response—no. (%)			
Complete response	2 (1.3)	1 (0.7)	
Disease-free by time of surgery[‡]	4 (2.6)	2 (1.3)	
Partial response	29 (19.2)	11 (7.2)	
Stable disease[§]	53 (35.1)	34 (22.2)	
Progressive disease	43 (28.5)	88 (57.5)	
Did not receive treatment	3 (2.0)	4 (2.6)	
Not evaluable for response	17 (11.3)	13 (8.5)	
Objective response[ϵ]			
Number of patients	35	14	
% (95% CI)	23.2 (16.7–30.7)	9.2 (5.1–14.9)	<0.001
Disease control[**]			
Number of patients	88	48	
% (95% CI)	58.3 (50.0–66.2)	31.4 (24.1–39.4)	<0.001

	EDP-M (N = 151)[†]	Sz-M (N = 153)[†]	HR [95%CI]; P-Value
Progression-free survival	5.0 months	2.1 months	0.55 [0.42–0.68]; <0.001
Overall survival[††]	14.8 months	12.0 months	0.79 [0.61–1.02]; 0.07

[*]Responses according to Response Evaluation Criteria in Solid Tumors (RECIST)
[†]EDP + M = etoposide + doxorubicin + cisplatin + mitotane; Sz + M = streptozocin + mitotane
[‡]Surgery performed >PR to study treatment; not included in PR category
[§]Stable disease was defined as no disease progression for at least ≥8 weeks and no objective response to treatment. Confirmatory scans were not required for this determination, according to the study protocol
[ϵ]Objective response = CR + PR
[**]Disease control + CR + PR + SD
[††]Patients classified according to first-line therapy, but they were allowed to receive the alternate therapy in second line

Therapy Monitoring

1. CBC with leukocyte differential count, serum creatinine and electrolytes, serum magnesium, and LFTs on day 1 of each cycle
2. *Response assessment:* Repeat imaging studies every 2 cycles; 24-hour urine 17-ketosteroids and cortisol with each cycle if abnormal at baseline
3. Mitotane level at least every 4 weeks initially. A level of 14–20 mcg/mL is desirable but may not be attained
4. Adrenal function can be monitored by measuring ACTH, but this alone is not reliable and should be interpreted together with clinical assessment

METASTATIC

ADRENOCORTICAL CANCER REGIMEN: STREPTOZOCIN + MITOTANE (SZ-M)

Fassnacht M et al. N Engl J Med 2012;366:2189–2197

Mitotane 500–5000 mg/day; administer orally, continually
- If possible, mitotane is started a minimum of 1 week before cytotoxic treatment is initiated. The ultimate goal is to attain mitotane concentrations in blood of 14–20 mcg/mL over time, as tolerated, trying not to exceed these values as side effects worsen with higher values. Note that side effects may preclude this range from being attained
- Initiate treatment with doses of 1000–1500 mg/day at bedtime to minimize sedative effects during waking hours, and escalate doses as tolerated
- Large daily doses may be divided in ≥2 doses

Hydration for streptozocin (all cycles): 1000 mL 0.9% sodium chloride injection (0.9% NS) per day; administer intravenously with 500 mL given before streptozocin and 500 mL given after streptozocin

First cycle: **Streptozocin** 1000 mg/day; administer intravenously in 50–500 mL of 0.9% NS or 5% dextrose injection (D5W) over 30–60 minutes for 5 doses on 5 consecutive days, days 1–5, every 3 weeks (total dose/cycle = 5000 mg)

Second and subsequent cycles: **Streptozocin** 2000 mg; administer intravenously in 50–500 mL of 0.9% NS or D5W over 30–60 minutes on day 1, every 3 weeks (total dose/cycle = 2000 mg)

Glucocorticoid replacement is necessary in all patients taking mitotane
Hydrocortisone 15–20 mg orally every morning, *plus*:
Hydrocortisone 7.5–10 mg orally every evening
Mineralocorticoid replacement also is recommended:
Fludrocortisone acetate 100–200 mcg/day orally every morning, *or*:
Fludrocortisone acetate 100 mcg/day orally every morning and every evening

Supportive Care
Antiemetic prophylaxis
*Emetogenic potential is **HIGH** each day streptozocin is administered. Potential for delayed symptoms*
See Chapter 42 for antiemetic recommendations

Hematopoietic growth factor (CSF) prophylaxis
*Primary prophylaxis is **NOT** indicated*
See Chapter 43 for more information

Antimicrobial prophylaxis
*Risk of fever and neutropenia is **LOW***
   Antimicrobial primary prophylaxis to be considered:
- Antibacterial—not indicated
- Antifungal—not indicated
- Antiviral—not indicated unless patient previously had an episode of HSV

Treatment Modifications

Adverse Event	Dose Modification
Day 1 WBC <1000/mm³ *or* platelet count <100,000/mm³ *or* G >2 nonhematologic toxicity	Delay chemotherapy until WBC ≥1000/mm³ and platelet count ≥100,000/mm³, or nonhematologic toxicity G ≤1 for a maximum delay of 2 weeks
>2-week delay in reaching WBC, >1000/mm³ or platelet count >100,000/mm³, *or* for resolution of nonhematologic toxicity to G ≤1	Discontinue therapy
G4 ANC *or* G ≥3 platelet counts	Reduce streptozocin dose by 25%
Creatinine clearance <50–60 mL/min	Hold streptozocin until creatinine clearance >50–60 mL/min

Patient Population Studied

Patients with histologically confirmed adrenocortical carcinoma not amenable to radical surgical resection who had not received any previous treatment with cytotoxic drugs, except mitotane, and had an Eastern Cooperative Oncology Group (ECOG) performance status of 0, 1, or 2. A total of 153 patients received streptozocin + mitotane

Age (y)	
Median	50.0
Range	18.8–72.8
Sex—Number (%)	
Male	61 (39.9)
Female	92 (60.1)
Tumor stage—Number (%)	
III	1 (0.7)
IV	152 (99.3)
Endocrine symptoms— Number (%)	
Cushing syndrome ± other symptoms	64 (41.8)
Conn syndrome only	3 (2.0)
Virilization only	7 (4.6)
Feminization only	2 (1.3)
No symptoms	68 (44.4)
Missing data	9 (5.9)
ECOG performance status score—Number (%)	
0	72 (47.1)
1	60 (39.2)
2	21 (13.7)
4	0
Time since primary diagnosis—Months	
Median	4.5
Range	0–111.6
Number of affected sites*	
Median	3
Range	1–8

*The following sites were calculated as separate sites of adrenocortical carcinoma: adrenal gland (including local recurrence), liver, lung, bone, peritoneum, retroperitoneum, pleura, mediastinum, central nervous system, soft tissue, spleen, and ovary

Efficacy

Efficacy in the Intention-to-Treat Population
Randomized Comparison vs. Etoposide + Doxorubicin + Cisplatin + Mitotane[*]

Variable	EDP-M (N = 151)[†]	Sz-M (N = 153)[†]	P-Value
Type of response—no. (%)			
Complete response	2 (1.3)	1 (0.7)	
Disease-free by time of surgery[‡]	4 (2.6)	2 (1.3)	
Partial response	29 (19.2)	11 (7.2)	
Stable disease[§]	53 (35.1)	34 (22.2)	
Progressive disease	43 (28.5)	88 (57.5)	
Did not receive treatment	3 (2.0)	4 (2.6)	
Not evaluable for response	17 (11.3)	13 (8.5)	
Objective response[ϵ]			
Number of patients	35	14	
% (95% CI)	23.2 (16.7–30.7)	9.2 (5.1–14.9)	<0.001
Disease control[**]			
Number of patients	88	48	
% (95% CI)	58.3 (50.0–66.2)	31.4 (24.1–39.4)	<0.001
	EDP-M (N = 151)[†]	Sz-M (N = 153)[†]	HR [95% CI]; P-Value
Progression-free survival	5.0 months	2.1 months	0.55 [0.42–0.68]; <0.001
Overall survival[††]	14.8 months	12.0 months	0.79 [0.61–1.02]; 0.07

[*]Responses according to Response Evaluation Criteria in Solid Tumors (RECIST)
[†]EDP + M = etoposide + doxorubicin + cisplatin + mitotane; Sz + M = streptozocin + mitotane
[‡]Surgery performed >PR to study treatment; not included in PR category
[§]Stable disease was defined as no disease progression for at least 8 weeks and no objective response to treatment.
Confirmatory scans were not required for this determination, according to the study protocol
[ϵ]Objective response = CR + PR
[**]Disease control + CR + PR + SD
[††]Patients classified according to first-line therapy, but they were allowed to receive the alternate therapy in second line

Toxicity

Event	Number of Patients (%)
Any serious adverse event	62 (41.6)
Adrenal insufficiency	1 (0.7)
Bone marrow toxicity	3 (2.0)
Cardiovascular or thromboembolic event	0
Fatigue or general health deterioration	7 (4.7)
Gastrointestinal disorder	12 (8.1)
Impaired liver function	7 (4.7)
Impaired renal function	6 (4.0)
Infection	4 (2.7)
Neurologic toxicity	4 (2.7)
Respiratory disorder	5 (3.4)
Other	13 (8.7)

Therapy Monitoring

1. CBC with leukocyte differential count, serum creatinine, electrolytes, and LFTs on day 1; obtain creatinine clearance on day 1 if an elevation in serum creatinine is observed
2. Twenty-four–hour urine for protein on day 1
3. *Response assessment:* Repeat imaging studies every 2 cycles; 24-hour urine 17-ketosteroids and cortisol with each cycle if abnormal at baseline
4. Mitotane level at least every 4 weeks initially. A level of 14–20 mcg/mL is desirable, but may not be attained
5. Adrenal function can be monitored by measuring ACTH, but this alone is not reliable and should be interpreted together with clinical assessment

4. Anal Cancer

Benjamin A. Weinberg, MD, Irfan Jawed, MD, and John Marshall, MD

Epidemiology

Incidence: 8590 (male: 2690; female: 5900. Estimated new cases for 2020 in the United States) 1.6 per 100,000 men per year, 2.2 per 100,000 women per year

Deaths: Estimated 1350 in 2020 (male: 540; female: 810)

Median age at diagnosis: 62 years

Male to female ratio: Female predominance (1:1.5–2)

Stage at Presentation

Stages I/II:	48%
Stage III:	32%
Stage IV:	13%

Shiels MS et al. Cancer Epidemiol Biomarkers Prev 2015;24:1548–1556
Siegel R et al. CA Cancer J Clin 2020;70:7–30
Surveillance, Epidemiology and End Results (SEER) Program, available from http://seer.cancer.gov

Work-up

All stages

1. Digital rectal examination, sigmoidoscopy with biopsy
2. CT scan of chest and abdomen with IV and oral contrast, pelvic CT or MRI with contrast
3. Consider HIV testing and CD4 level if indicated
4. Consider PET-CT scan
5. Gynecologic exam for women, including screening for cervical cancer

NCCN Guidelines Version 2.2017 Anal Carcinoma

Positive inguinal lymph node on imaging

1. Fine-needle aspiration or biopsy of node

Pathology

By convention, anal cancer should now refer only to *squamous cell cancers* arising in the anus. Earlier surgical series often did not make this distinction. *Adenocarcinomas* occurring in the anal canal should be treated according to the same principles applied to rectal adenocarcinoma. Similarly, melanomas and sarcomas should be treated according to the same principles applied to those tumor types at other sites

The distal anal canal is lined by squamous epithelium, and tumors arising in this portion are often keratinizing. Around the dentate line, the mucosa transitions from squamous mucosa to the nonsquamous rectal mucosa. Tumors arising in this transitional zone are often nonkeratinizing and previously were referred to as basaloid or cloacogenic

Clark MA et al. Lancet Oncol 2004;5:149–157
Ryan DP et al. N Engl J Med 2000;342:792–800

Five-Year Relative Survival

Localized	81.7%
Regional	64.9%
Distant	32.2%

Surveillance, Epidemiology and End Results (SEER) Program, available from http://seer.cancer.gov

Poor Prognostic Factors

1. Nodal involvement
2. Skin ulceration
3. Male gender
4. Tumor >5 cm
5. HPV negative and/or p16 negative

Ajani JA et al. JAMA 2008;299:1914–1921
Bartelink H et al. J Clin Oncol 1997;15:2040–2049
Glynne-Jones R et al. Cancer 2013;119:748–755
Rodel F et al. Int J Cancer 2015;136:278–288

Staging

Primary Tumor (T)

TX	Primary tumor not assessed
T0	No evidence of primary tumor
Tis	High-grade squamous intraepithelial lesion (previously termed carcinoma in situ, Bowen disease, anal intraepithelial neoplasia II–III, high-grade anal intraepithelial neoplasia)
T1	Tumor 2 cm or less in greatest dimension
T2	Tumor more than 2 cm but not more than 5 cm in greatest dimension
T3	Tumor more than 5 cm in greatest dimension
T4	Tumor of any size invades adjacent organ(s), eg, vagina, urethra, bladder*

*Direct invasion of the rectal wall, perirectal skin, subcutaneous tissue, or the sphincter muscle(s) is not classified as T4

Regional Lymph Nodes (N)

NX	Regional lymph nodes cannot be assessed
N0	No regional lymph node metastasis
N1	Metastasis in inguinal, mesorectal, internal iliac, or external iliac nodes
N1a	Metastasis in inguinal, mesorectal, or internal iliac lymph nodes
N1b	Metastasis in external iliac lymph nodes
N1c	Metastasis in external iliac with any N1a nodes

Distant Metastasis (M)

M0	No distant metastasis (no pathologic M0; use clinical M to complete stage group)
M1	Distant metastasis

Group	T	N	M
0	Tis	N0	M0
I	T1	N0	M0
IIA	T2	N0	M0
IIB	T3	N0	M0
IIIA	T1	N1	M0
IIIA	T2	N1	M0
IIIB	T4	N0	M0
IIIC	T3	N1	M0
IIIC	T4	N1	M0
IV	Any T	Any N	M1

Amin MB et al, editors. AJCC Cancer Staging Manual. 8th ed. New York: Springer; 2017

Expert Opinion

Locoregional disease *(squamous cell cancers)*
Anal canal cancer

- Concurrent chemoradiation is the recommended primary treatment for patients with anal canal cancer that has not metastasized, with fluorouracil (1000 mg/m^2 per day by continuous intravenous infusion over 24 hours for 4 consecutive days on days 1–4) or capecitabine (825 mg/m^2 by mouth twice daily Monday–Friday on each day radiation is given), *plus* mitomycin 10 mg/m^2 by slow intravenous injection on days 1 and 29 (see Regimens below)
- Long-term update of U.S. GI intergroup RTOG 98-11 phase III trial for anal carcinoma: superior disease-free and overall survival with RT + fluorouracil + mitomycin over RT + fluorouracil + cisplatin

Long-term Update of U.S. GI Intergroup RTOG 98-11

Gunderson LL et al. J Clin Oncol 2012;30:4344–4351

	# Patients	DFS TF	DFS %, 5 Years	OS TF	OS %, 5 Years	CFS TF	CFS %, 5 Years	LRF TF	LRF %, 5 Years	DM TF	DM %, 5 Years	CF TF	CF %, 5 Years
RT + fluorouracil + mitomycin	325	122	67.8	87	78.3	106	71.9	67	20.0	46	13.1	38	11.9
RT + fluorouracil + cisplatin	324	159	57.8	115	70.7	132	65.0	86	26.4	61	18.1	55	17.3
P			0.006		0.026		0.05		0.087		0.12		0.074

CF, colostomy failure; CFS, colostomy-free survival; DFS, disease-free survival; DM, distant metastases; LRF, locoregional failure; OS, overall survival; RT, radiation therapy; TF, total failures

- Locoregional failure rate is 10–30%. If locally persistent or progressive disease is present, consider abdominoperineal resection (APR). If positive lymph nodes are found, perform groin dissection with RT (if RT was not previously administered) or without RT

(continued)

Expert Opinion (continued)

Anal margin cancer
- A well-differentiated anal margin lesion characterized as T1, N0 can be treated with margin negative excision alone with close follow-up
- For T2–T4 or any N, the recommended treatment is chemoradiation: fluorouracil (1000 mg/m^2 per day by continuous intravenous infusion over 24 hours for 4 consecutive days on days 1–4) or capecitabine (825 mg/m^2 by mouth twice daily Monday–Friday on each day radiation is given), *plus* mitomycin 10 mg/m^2 by slow intravenous injection on days 1 and 29 (see Regimens below)

Metastatic anal cancer (*squamous cell cancers*)
Metastatic disease should be treated with cisplatin-based chemotherapy or enrollment in a clinical trial. Although immunotherapy with anti–programmed death 1 (anti-PD-1) checkpoint inhibitors is not FDA-approved for treatment of metastatic anal cancer, nivolumab and pembrolizumab have demonstrated clinical efficacy in phase 2 trials and may be used in an off-label manner. Patients with chemorefractory metastatic anal cancer should be enrolled in clinical trials

Faivre C et al. Bull Cancer 1999;86:861–865
Morris VK et al. Lancet Oncol 2017;18:446–453
Ott PA et al. Ann Oncol 2017;28:1036–1041

Supportive Care/Alternate Treatments
- Radiotherapy might be delivered with less toxicity by means of 3D conformal radiotherapy or IMRT followed by conventional radiotherapy as shown in RTOG 0529 trial (2-year outcomes of RTOG 0529: a phase II evaluation of dose-painted IMRT in combination with fluorouracil and mitomycin for the reduction of acute morbidity in carcinoma of the anal canal). However, IMRT is not recommended in obese patients with nonreproducible external skin contours or patients with a major component of tumor outside the anal canal

Two-Year Outcomes of RTOG 0529

Kachnic LA et al. J Clin Oncol 2011;29(Suppl 4) [abstract 368]

End Point	0529 (N = 52)		9811 (N = 325)	
	Events	2-Year % (95% CI)	Events	2-Year % (95% CI)
LRF	10	20 (9–31)	67	19 (14–23)
CF	4	8 (0.4–15)	38	11 (8–14)
OS	7	88 (75–94)	80	91 (87–94)
DFS	12	77 (62–86)	117	76 (70–80)
CFS	7	86 (73–93)	101	83 (79–87)

CF, colostomy failures; CFS, colostomy-free survival; DFS, disease-free survival; LRF, Locoregional failure; OS, overall survival

- Tolerance to treatment can be maximized with antibiotics, antifungals, antiemetics, analgesia, skincare, advice regarding nutrition, and psychological support

Prevention of Anal Cancer
The U.S. Food and Drug Administration has approved recombinant human papillomavirus nonavalent vaccine (Gardasil® 9) for use in females and males ages 9 through 45 years for indications including (1) the prevention of anal cancer caused by human papillomavirus (HPV) types 16, 18, 31, 33, 45, 52, and 58; and (2) the prevention of anal intraepithelial neoplasia and associated precancerous lesions caused by HPV types 6, 11, 16, 18, 31, 33, 45, 52, and 58

Management of HIV-Positive Patients
HIV-positive patients are generally treated similarly to those without HIV infection; however, dosage may need to be adjusted (or treat without mitomycin) specifically if CD4 count is <200 cells/mm^3 or patients with a history of HIV-related complications as outcomes appear to be comparable but treatment-related toxicity may be worse

Post-treatment Surveillance
There are no prospective trials to guide the post-treatment surveillance strategy for patients treated for anal cancer
- For patients who have a complete remission at 8–12 weeks from initial chemoradiotherapy, guidelines from the NCCN suggest the following every 3–6 months for 5 years:
  - Digital rectal examination
  - Anoscopy
  - Inguinal node palpation
  - If initially T3–4 disease or inguinal node–positive, or for those with persistent disease at the initial post-treatment biopsy who regress on serial examinations, consider imaging of the chest/abdomen and pelvis annually for 3 years

(continued)

Expert Opinion (continued)

- For patients who have persistent disease at 8–12 weeks on DRE, it is recommended to re-evaluate in 4 weeks, and, if regression is observed on serial exams, continue to observe and re-evaluate in 3 months. If progressive disease is documented, perform a biopsy and restage
- For patients who undergo APR for biopsy-proven progressive or recurrent disease, perform inguinal node palpation every 3–6 months for 5 years, and annual radiographic imaging of the chest/abdomen/pelvis for 3 years

Allal AS et al. Cancer 1999;86:405–409
Faivre C et al. Bull Cancer 1999;86:861–865
Glynne-Jones R et al. Int J Radiat Oncol Biol Phys 2008;72:119–126
Gunderson LL et al. J Clin Oncol 2011;29:257s
Kachnic LA et al. J Clin Oncol 2011;29(Suppl 4) [abstract 368]
Kreuter A et al. Br J Dermatol 2010;162:1269–1277
Schiller DE et al. Ann Surg Oncol 2007;14:2780–2789

LOCOREGIONAL DISEASE • CHEMORADIATION

ANAL CANCER REGIMEN: MITOMYCIN + FLUOROURACIL + RADIATION THERAPY (RTOG 8704/ECOG 1289 AND RTOG-0529)

Flam M et al. J Clin Oncol 1996;14:2527–2539
Kachnic LA et al. J Clin Oncol 2011;29(Suppl 4) [abstract 368]

Mitomycin 10 mg/m^2 single dose (maximum dose = 20 mg); administer by intravenous injection over 3–5 minutes on day 1 every 4 weeks for 2 cycles (days 1 and 29 of radiation) (total dosage/cycle = 10 mg/m^2, but *not* greater than 20 mg)

Fluorouracil 1000 mg/m^2 per day (maximum daily dose = 2000 mg); administer by continuous intravenous infusion over 24 hours for 4 consecutive days, on days 1–4 every 4 weeks for 2 cycles (days 1–4 and 29–32 of radiation therapy) (total dosage/cycle = 4000 mg/m^2, but *not* greater than 8000 mg)

External beam radiation therapy 1.8 Gy/fraction; administer daily 5 days/week for 5 weeks (total dose to pelvis/complete course = 45 Gy in 5 weeks)

For patients with T3, T4, or N+ lesions or T2 lesions with residual disease after 45 Gy, current RTOG protocol recommends an additional 10–14 Gy to a reduced field

Alternate RT regimen: dose-painted (DP) IMRT

DP-IMRT prescribed as follows:
- T2N0: 42-Gy elective nodal and 50.4-Gy anal tumor planning target volumes (PTVs), 28 fractions
- T3–4N0–3: 45-Gy elective nodal, 50.4-Gy ≤3 cm, and 54-Gy >3 cm metastatic nodal and 54-Gy anal tumor PTVs, 30 fractions

Note: IMRT is not recommended in obese patients with nonreproducible external skin contours, or patients with a major component of tumor outside the anal canal

Alternative chemotherapy with concurrent RT: capecitabine + mitomycin

Goodman KA et al. Int J Radiat Oncol Biol Phys 2017;98:1087–1095
Thind G et al. Radiat Oncol 2014;9:124

Mitomycin 10 mg/m^2 single dose (maximum dose = 20 mg); administer by intravenous injection over 3–5 minutes on day 1 every 4 weeks for 2 cycles (days 1 and 29 of radiation) (total dosage/cycle = 10 mg/m^2, but *not* greater than 20 mg)

Capecitabine 825 mg/m^2 by mouth twice daily Monday–Friday (on each day RT is given)

External beam radiation therapy 1.8 Gy/fraction; administer daily 5 days/week for 5 weeks (total dose to pelvis/complete course = 45 Gy in 5 weeks)

For patients with T3, T4, or N+ lesions or T2 lesions with residual disease after 45 Gy, current RTOG protocol recommends an additional 10–14 Gy to a reduced field

Note: There is retrospective evidence that chemoradiation with capecitabine and mitomycin has less hematologic toxicity and is associated with fewer treatment interruptions compared to traditional chemoradiation with infusional fluorouracil and mitomycin

Supportive Care

Antiemetic prophylaxis
Emetogenic potential is **LOW**
See Chapter 42 for antiemetic recommendations

Hematopoietic growth factor (CSF) prophylaxis
Primary prophylaxis is **NOT** indicated
See Chapter 43 for more information

Antimicrobial prophylaxis
Risk of fever and neutropenia is **LOW**
  Antimicrobial primary prophylaxis to be considered:
  - Antibacterial—not indicated
  - Antifungal—not indicated
  - Antiviral—not indicated, unless patient previously had an episode of herpes simplex virus (HSV)

(continued)

Treatment Modifications

Adverse Event	Dose Modification
G3/4 Diarrhea or stomatitis	Reduce fluorouracil dosage 50% during second cycle
G3 Radiation dermatitis	
G4 Radiation dermatitis	Do not give second cycle of chemotherapy
ANC <500/mm^3 or platelets <50,000/mm^3	Reduce fluorouracil and mitomycin dosages 50%
G3/4 Hematologic or nonhematologic events	Suspend chemoradiation until recovers to G ≤2

Based on RTOG protocol 98-11

Toxicity (N = 146)

	% G4/5
Acute (≤90 days after starting treatment)	25
Hematologic	18
Nonhematologic (diarrhea, skin, mucositis)	7
Late (>90 days after starting treatment)	5
Any grade 4 adverse event	23
Toxic death rate[*]	2.8

[*]All treatment-related deaths occurred in a setting of neutropenia and sepsis
NCI Common Toxicity Criteria, version 2.0

Efficacy (N = 129–146)

Positive biopsy after induction	8%
5-Year locoregional failure	36%
5-Year colostomy rate	22%
5-Year colostomy-free survival	64%
5-Year disease-free survival	67%
5-Year overall survival	67%

Flam M et al. Cancer Res 1999;3:539–552

(*continued*)

Diarrhea management

Latent or delayed-onset diarrhea*:

 Loperamide 4 mg orally initially after the first loose or liquid stool, *then* 2-4 mg orally every 2-4 hours or **diphenoxylate hydrochloride** 2.5 mg **with atropine sulfate** 0.025 mg (e.g., Lomotil®)

Persistent diarrhea:

 Octreotide 100–150 mcg subcutaneously 3 times daily. Maximum total daily dose is 1500 mcg

Antibiotic therapy during latent or delayed-onset diarrhea:

 A fluoroquinolone (eg, **ciprofloxacin** 500 mg orally every 12 hours) if absolute neutrophil count <500/mm^3 with or without accompanying fever in association with diarrhea

 • Antibiotics should also be administered if patient is hospitalized with prolonged diarrhea and should be continued until diarrhea resolves

Abigerges D et al. J Natl Cancer Inst 1994;86:446–449
*Rothenberg ML et al. J Clin Oncol 2001;19:3801–3807
Wadler S et al. J Clin Oncol 1998;16:3169–3178

Oral care

Standard prophylaxis and treatment for mucositis/stomatitis

Patient Population Studied

A study of 146 patients with localized (nonmetastatic) squamous cell cancer of the anal canal

Therapy Monitoring

1. *Every week:* CBC with differential
2. *Response assessment:* PE 6 weeks after completion of chemoradiotherapy. If there is regression of tumor on exam, then 12 weeks after completion of therapy repeat PE, perform sigmoidoscopy, and obtain CT scan. If there is a residual mass or thickening, a biopsy should be performed. If there is residual disease at 12 weeks or if there is progression of disease on exam, consider salvage abdominoperineal resection

Notes

Severely immunocompromised patients or HIV-positive patients with low CD4 counts should be treated with caution. Consider omitting and/or reducing the dose of chemotherapy

LOCOREGIONAL DISEASE • CHEMORADIATION

ANAL CANCER REGIMEN: FLUOROURACIL + CISPLATIN + RADIATION THERAPY

Doci R et al. J Clin Oncol 1996;14:3121–3125

Fluorouracil 750 mg/m^2 per day; administer by continuous intravenous infusion in 500–1000 mL 0.9% sodium chloride injection (0.9% NS) or 5% dextrose injection (D5W) over 24 hours for 4 consecutive days, on days 1–4, every 21 days for 2 cycles (total dosage/cycle = 3000 mg/m^2)
(Days 1–4 and 21–24 of radiation therapy)
Hydration before cisplatin ≥1000 mL 0.9% NS; administer intravenously over a minimum of 2–4 hours
Cisplatin 100 mg/m^2; administer intravenously in 50–250 mL 0.9% NS over 60 minutes, on day 1 every 21 days for 2 cycles (total dosage/cycle = 100 mg/m^2)
(Days 1 and 21 of radiation therapy)
Hydration after cisplatin ≥1000 mL 0.9% NS; administer intravenously over a minimum of 2–4 hours. Encourage patients to supplement their usual oral hydration with extra non-alcohol-containing fluids for at least 24 hours after receiving cisplatin
External beam radiation therapy 1.8 Gy/fraction; administer daily 5 days/week up to 54–58 Gy

Supportive Care
Antiemetic prophylaxis
Emetogenic potential on days with cisplatin, fluorouracil, and RT is **HIGH**. *Potential for delayed symptoms*
Emetogenic potential on days with fluorouracil and RT is **LOW**
See Chapter 42 for antiemetic recommendations

Hematopoietic growth factor (CSF) prophylaxis
Primary prophylaxis is **NOT** *indicated*
See Chapter 43 for more information

Antimicrobial prophylaxis
Risk of fever and neutropenia is **LOW**
  Antimicrobial primary prophylaxis to be considered:
  • Antibacterial—not indicated
  • Antifungal—not indicated
  • Antiviral—not indicated unless patient previously had an episode of HSV

Diarrhea management
Latent or delayed-onset diarrhea*:
Loperamide 4 mg orally initially after the first loose or liquid stool, *then* 2-4 mg orally every 2-4 hours or **diphenoxylate hydrochloride** 2.5 mg with **atropine sulfate** 0.025 mg (e.g., Lomotil®)

Persistent diarrhea:
Octreotide 100–150 mcg subcutaneously 3 times daily. Maximum total daily dose is 1500 mcg

Antibiotic therapy during latent or delayed-onset diarrhea:
  A fluoroquinolone (eg, **ciprofloxacin** 500 mg orally every 12 hours) if absolute neutrophil count <500/mm^3 with or without accompanying fever in association with diarrhea
  • Antibiotics should also be administered if patient is hospitalized with prolonged diarrhea and should be continued until diarrhea resolves

Abigerges D et al. J Natl Cancer Inst 1994;86:446–449
*Rothenberg ML et al. J Clin Oncol 2001;19:3801–3807
Wadler S et al. J Clin Oncol 1998;16:3169–3178

(continued)

Patient Population Studied

A study of 35 patients with previously untreated basaloid (n = 5) or squamous cell carcinoma (n = 30) of the anus. In all patients, the cancer was located in the anal canal; in 28, the tumor extended to adjacent sites. Nine patients had nodal metastases; no patient had distant metastases

Efficacy (N = 35)

Complete response	94%
Partial response*	6%
Local recurrence	6%
At a median follow-up of 37 months	
No evidence of disease	94%
Colostomy free	86%

Normal anal function preserved in 30 of 35 patients
*Two partial responses in 2 of 5 (40%) patients with T3 tumors

Toxicity (N = 35)

	% G1	% G2	% G3
Hematologic (leukopenia)	40	31	—
Vomiting	40	33	10
Dermatitis, proctitis, diarrhea	8.5	88.5	3
Cardiac	—	3†	—

*Acute toxicities. Chronic toxicities not reported. No grade 4 toxicities reported
†Transient at end of first cycle; resolved WHO criteria

(*continued*)

Oral care
Standard prophylaxis and treatment for mucositis/stomatitis

Note: The RTOG has amended the above regimen as follows:
Two cycles of chemotherapy are given before external beam radiation therapy commences; that is, radiation therapy begins coincident with the start of chemotherapy cycle 3
The chemotherapy regimen used has been modified as follows:
Fluorouracil 1000 mg/m^2 per day; administer by continuous intravenous infusion in 500–1000 mL 0.9% NS or D5W over 24 hours for 4 consecutive days on days 1–4, every 28 days for 4 cycles (total dosage/cycle = 4000 mg/m^2)
Cisplatin 75 mg/m^2; administer intravenously in 250 mL 0.9% NS over 60 minutes on day 1 every 28 days for 4 cycles on days 1, 29, 57, and 85 (total dosage/cycle = 75 mg/m^2)

Ajani JA et al. JAMA 2008;299:1914-1921.

Treatment Modifications

Adverse Event	Dose Modification
ANC <500/mm^3 or platelets <50,000/mm^3	Decrease fluorouracil and cisplatin dosages by 50%
G3/4 diarrhea or stomatitis	Decrease fluorouracil dosage by 50%
G3 radiation dermatitis	
G4 radiation dermatitis	Hold radiation until dermatitis resolves to G ≤2, and do not administer additional fluorouracil
Creatinine 1.5–2.0 mg/dL (133–177 μmol/L)	Decrease cisplatin dosage by 50%
Creatinine >2.0 mg/dL (>177 μmol/L)	Hold cisplatin

Recommended by RTOG 98-11

Therapy Monitoring

1. *Before each cycle:* CBC with differential, BUN, creatinine, magnesium, and electrolytes
2. *Response assessment:* PE 4–6 weeks after completion of chemoradiotherapy. Perform a biopsy only in the absence of a response to therapy. If there has been a response to therapy, reevaluate at 12 weeks with PE, sigmoidoscopy, and CT scan. If residual tumor is suspected, biopsy the affected area. If residual disease is documented at 12 weeks or if there is progression of disease on exam, consider salvage abdominoperineal resection

METASTATIC • FIRST-LINE
ANAL CANCER REGIMEN: CARBOPLATIN + PACLITAXEL

Kim R et al. Oncology 2014;87:125–132
Rao S et al. *J Clin Oncol.* 2020; doi:10.1200/JCO.19.03266 [Epub ahead of print]
Sclafani F et al. J Clin Oncol 2015;33(3_suppl);TPS792

Carboplatin plus paclitaxel is the preferred first-line chemotherapy regimen over cisplatin plus fluorouracil, based on results from the phase 2 InterAACT trial. Paclitaxel may be administered on a weekly schedule (Rao et al., 2018) or on an every-3-week schedule (Kim et al., 2014)

Kim R et al. Oncology 2014;87:125–132
Premedication for paclitaxel:
Dexamethasone 10 mg/dose; administer orally for 2 doses 12 hours and 6 hours before paclitaxel, *or*
Dexamethasone 20 mg/dose; administer intravenously over 10–15 minutes, 30–60 minutes before paclitaxel (total dose/cycle = 20 mg)
Diphenhydramine 50 mg; administer by intravenous injection 30 minutes before paclitaxel
Cimetidine 300 mg (or **ranitidine** 50 mg, **famotidine** 20 mg, or an equivalent histamine receptor [H_2]-subtype antagonist); administer intravenously over 15–30 minutes, 30–60 minutes before paclitaxel

Paclitaxel 175 mg/m²; administer intravenously in a volume of 0.9% sodium chloride injection (0.9% NS) or 5% dextrose injection (D5W) sufficient to produce a concentration within the range 0.3–1.2 mg/mL, over 3 hours, on day 1, every 21 days (total dosage/cycle = 175 mg/m²)

Carboplatin target AUC = 5 mg/mL × min*; administer intravenously in 0.9% NS or D5W 100–500 mL over 60 minutes, on day 1 after completing paclitaxel, every 21 days (total dosage/cycle calculated to achieve a target AUC = 5 mg/mL × min)

Rao S et al. Ann Oncol 2018;29:Abstract LBA21
Premedication for paclitaxel:
Dexamethasone 10 mg/dose; administer orally for 2 doses 12 hours and 6 hours before paclitaxel, *or*
Dexamethasone 20 mg/dose; administer intravenously over 10–15 minutes, 30–60 minutes before paclitaxel (total dose/cycle = 20 mg)
Diphenhydramine 50 mg; administer by intravenous injection 30 minutes before paclitaxel
Cimetidine 300 mg (or **ranitidine** 50 mg, **famotidine** 20 mg, or an equivalent histamine receptor [H_2]-subtype antagonist); administer intravenously over 15–30 minutes, 30–60 minutes before paclitaxel

Paclitaxel 80 mg/m²/dose; administer intravenously in a volume of 0.9% sodium chloride injection (0.9% NS) or 5% dextrose injection (D5W) sufficient to produce a concentration within the range 0.3–1.2 mg/mL, over 1 hour, for 3 doses on days 1, 8, and 15, every 28 days (total dosage/cycle = 240 mg/m²)

Carboplatin target AUC = 5 mg/mL × min*; administer intravenously in 0.9% NS or D5W 100–500 mL over 60 minutes, on day 1 after completing paclitaxel, every 28 days (total dosage/cycle calculated to achieve a target AUC = 5 mg/mL × min)

Carboplatin dose
Carboplatin dose is based on a formula described by Calvert et al. to achieve a target area under the plasma concentration versus time curve (AUC):

$$\text{Total carboplatin dose (mg)} = (\text{target AUC}) (\text{GFR} + 25)$$

In practice, creatinine clearance (CrCl) is used in place of glomerular filtration rate (GFR). CrCl can be estimated from the equation of Cockcroft and Gault, thus:

$$\text{For males, CrCl} = \frac{(140 - \text{age[years]}) \times (\text{body weight [kg]})}{72 \times (\text{serum creatinine [mg/dL]})}$$

$$\text{For females, CrCl} = \frac{(140 - \text{age[years]}) \times (\text{body weight [kg]})}{72 \times (\text{serum creatinine [mg/dL]})}$$

(continued)

Patient Population Studied

In the InterAACT study, 91 patients with advanced anal cancer were randomized to receive treatment with cisplatin 60 mg/m² IV day 1 plus 5-fluorouracil 1000 mg/m²/24 hours days 1-4 every 21 days or carboplatin AUC 5 IV day 1 plus paclitaxel 80 mg/m² IV days 1, 8, and 15 every 28 days. The median age was 61 years; 67% were female; 12% had locally advanced and 88% had metastatic squamous cell carcinoma of the anal canal

Treatment Monitoring

1. *Baseline and before each cycle*: LFTs, serum chemistry, and CBC with differential and platelet count. Complete history and physical examination
2. *Follow-up*: CBC with differential and platelet count at least weekly through leukocyte and platelet count nadirs
3. *Responses assessment*: every 8 weeks

(*continued*)

Calvert AH et al. J Clin Oncol 1989;7:1748–1756
Cockcroft DW , Gault MH. Nephron 1976;16:31–41
Jodrell DI et al. J Clin Oncol 1992;10:520–528
Sorensen BT et al. Cancer Chemother Pharmacol 1991;28:397–401

Note: On October 8, 2010, the U.S. Food and Drug Administration (FDA) identified a potential safety issue with carboplatin dosing based on recent changes in the measurement of serum creatinine. All clinical laboratories in the United States should be using the standardized isotope dilution mass spectrometry (IDMS) method to measure serum creatinine, which could result in an overestimation of the GFR in some patients with normal renal function. A carboplatin dose calculated with an IDMS-measured serum creatinine result using the Calvert formula could exceed an expected exposure (AUC) and result in increased drug-related toxicity. Provided actual GFR measurements are made to assess renal function, carboplatin can be safely dosed according to the Calvert formula described in product labeling. If GFR (or creatinine clearance) is estimated based on serum creatinine measurements by the IDMS method, the FDA recommended for patients with normal renal function capping an estimated GFR at 125 mL/min for any targeted AUC value. No greater estimated GFR values should be used.

Supportive Care
Antiemetic prophylaxis
Emetogenic potential on days with carboplatin is **HIGH**. *Potential for delayed symptoms*
Emetogenic potential on days when only paclitaxel is administered (without carboplatin) is **LOW**
See Chapter 42 for antiemetic recommendations

Hematopoietic growth factor (CSF) prophylaxis
Primary prophylaxis is **NOT** *indicated*
See Chapter 43 for more information

Antimicrobial prophylaxis
Risk of fever and neutropenia is **LOW**
  Antimicrobial primary prophylaxis to be considered:
  • Antibacterial—not indicated

  • Antifungal—not indicated

  • Antiviral—not indicated unless patient previously had an episode of HSV

Treatment Modifications

	Carboplatin	Paclitaxel (every-3-week regimen)	Paclitaxel (weekly regimen)
Starting dose	AUC target = 5 mg/mL × min	175 mg/m²	80 mg/m² per dose
Dose level −1	AUC target = 4 mg/mL × min	135 mg/m²	70 mg/m² per dose
Dose level −2	AUC target = 3 mg/mL × min	110 mg/m²	60 mg/m² per dose

Adverse Event	Dose Modification
At start of a cycle, ANC ≤1000/mm³ or platelets ≤100,000/mm³	Delay start of cycle up to 2 weeks until ANC >1000/mm³ and platelets >100,000/mm³
Febrile neutropenia OR neutrophil count <500/mm³ for ≥5 days OR Thrombocytopenic bleeding OR Platelet count <25,000/mm³ during the previous cycle	Hold treatment until neutrophil count is ≥1,000/mm³ and platelet count is ≥100,000/mm³, then decrease the carboplatin dosage by 1 dose level and decrease the paclitaxel dosage by one dose level
G3 neurotoxicity or non-hematologic toxicity	Hold treatment until toxicities recover to G ≤2, then decrease the carboplatin dosage by 1 dose level and decrease the paclitaxel dosage by 1 dose level

(*continued*)

Treatment Modifications (continued)

Adverse Event	Dose Modification
G4 neurotoxicity or non-hematologic toxicity	Permanently discontinue regimen
Severe hypersensitivity reaction	Discontinue paclitaxel or carboplatin infusion immediately and administer appropriate support. For hypersensitivity reaction ≤G3, initial management includes temporary discontinuation of infusion for 30 minutes, and administration of additional intravenous antihistamines and glucocorticoids. Upon resolution of symptoms, the paclitaxel infusion may be restarted at a slower rate if deemed safe. Re-challenge with carboplatin will require institution of a desensitization regimen If G4 hypersensitivity is experienced, stabilize the cardiorespiratory system and use epinephrine as needed, then permanently discontinue paclitaxel or carboplatin. Re-challenge with carboplatin will require institution of a desensitization regimen

Efficacy (N = 91)

	Cisplatin + 5-Fluorouracil (N = 46)	Carboplatin + Paclitaxel (N = 45)
Overall response rate	57.1%	59.0%
Median progression-free survival	5.7 months	8.1 months
Median overall survival*	12.3 months	20 months

*P = 0.014

Toxicity (N = 91)

	Cisplatin + 5-Fluorouracil (N = 46)	Carboplatin + Paclitaxel (N = 45)
Grade ≥3 adverse events	76%	71%
Serious adverse events*	62%	36%

*P = 0.016

METASTATIC • FIRST-LINE

ANAL CANCER REGIMEN: CISPLATIN + FLUOROURACIL BY CONTINUOUS INTRAVENOUS INFUSION

Faivre C et al. Bull Cancer 1999;86:861–865

Hydration before, during, and after cisplatin administration ± mannitol:

- *Pre-cisplatin hydration* with ≥1000 mL 0.9% sodium chloride injection (0.9% NS); administer intravenously with potassium and magnesium supplementation as needed based on pretreatment values

- *Mannitol diuresis:* May be given to patients who have received adequate hydration. A dose of **mannitol** 12.5–25 g may be administered by intravenous injection or a short infusion before or during cisplatin administration, or prepared as an admixture with cisplatin. Continued intravenous hydration is essential

- *Continued mannitol diuresis:* In an inpatient or day-hospital setting, one may administer additional mannitol in the form of an intravenous infusion: **mannitol** 10–40 g administered intravenously over 1–4 hours. This can be done either during or immediately after cisplatin but requires maintenance of adequate intravenously administered fluids during and for hours after mannitol administration

- Post-cisplatin hydration with ≥1000 mL 0.9% NS; administer intravenously with potassium and magnesium supplementation as needed based on measured values. Encourage patients to supplement their usual oral hydration with extra non-alcohol-containing fluids for at least 24 hours after receiving cisplatin

Cisplatin 100 mg/m^2; administer intravenously in 100–500 mL 0.9% NS over 30–60 minutes on day 2, every 4 weeks (total dosage/cycle = 100 mg/m^2)
Fluorouracil 1000 mg/m^2 per day; administer by continuous intravenous infusion in 50–1000 mL 0.9% NS or 5% dextrose injection over 24 hours for 5 consecutive days, on days 1–5, every 4 weeks (total dosage/cycle = 5000 mg/m^2)

Notes:

- Ten patients received further local treatment
- Carboplatin used instead of cisplatin in the event of renal toxicity

Supportive Care
Antiemetic prophylaxis
Emetogenic potential on days with cisplatin is **HIGH**. *Potential for delayed symptoms*
Emetogenic potential on days with fluorouracil alone is **LOW**
See Chapter 42 for antiemetic recommendations

Hematopoietic growth factor (CSF) prophylaxis
Primary prophylaxis is **NOT** *indicated*
See Chapter 43 for more information

Antimicrobial prophylaxis
Risk of fever and neutropenia is **LOW**
   Antimicrobial primary prophylaxis to be considered:
   - Antibacterial—not indicated
   - Antifungal—not indicated
   - Antiviral—not indicated unless patient previously had an episode of HSV

Diarrhea management
Latent or delayed-onset diarrhea*:
   Loperamide 4 mg orally initially after the first loose or liquid stool, *then* 2-4 mg orally every 2-4 hours or **diphenoxylate hydrochloride** 2.5 mg **with atropine sulfate** 0.025 mg (e.g., Lomotil®)

Abigerges D et al. J Natl Cancer Inst 1994; 86:446–449
Rothenberg ML et al. J Clin Oncol 2001; 19:3801–3807
Wadler S et al. J Clin Oncol 1998; 16:3169–3178

(continued)

Patient Population Studied

Study of 19 patients (3 males, 16 females), median age 58 years, WHO performance status: G0–1 in 68% and G2 in 32%. Metastases were synchronous in 6 patients and metachronous in 13 patients. Metastatic sites included liver (10/19 patients), lymph nodes (11/19 patients: paraaortic 5, iliac 4, and inguinal 2) and pulmonary (3/11 patients). In 9 of 19 patients, lymph node metastases were isolated; in 7 of 19 patients liver metastases were isolated

Toxicity, N = 19

Hematologic	
G3/4 thrombocytopenia	24%
G3/4 neutropenia	13%
Febrile neutropenia	0
Nonhematologic	
G3/4 nausea/vomiting	30%
G3/4 diarrhea	0
G3/4 mucositis	0
Neurotoxicity	0
Ototoxicity	0
G1–2 nephrotoxicity	11.1%

Mean fluorouracil dose intensity during cycles 1 and 2	92.5%
Mean cisplatin dose intensity during cycles 1 and 2	95%

*WHO criteria

(*continued*)

Persistent diarrhea:
Octreotide 100–150 mcg subcutaneously 3 times daily. Maximum total daily dose is 1500 mcg

Antibiotic therapy during latent or delayed-onset diarrhea:
A fluoroquinolone (eg, **ciprofloxacin** 500 mg orally every 12 hours) if absolute neutrophil count <500/mm^3 with or without accompanying fever in association with diarrhea
• Antibiotics should also be administered if patient is hospitalized with prolonged diarrhea and should be continued until diarrhea resolves

Abigerges D et al. J Natl Cancer Inst 1994;86:446–449
*Rothenberg ML et al. J Clin Oncol 2001;19:3801–3807
Wadler S et al. J Clin Oncol 1998;16:3169–3178

Oral care
Standard prophylaxis and treatment for mucositis/stomatitis

Treatment Modifications

Adverse Event	Dose Modification
G3/4 hematologic	Reduce fluorouracil and cisplatin dosages by 20%
Hand-foot syndrome (palmar-plantar erythrodysesthesia)	Interrupt fluorouracil therapy until symptoms resolve. Then, reduce fluorouracil dosage by 20%, or discontinue fluorouracil
Mucositis	Interrupt fluorouracil therapy until symptoms resolve. Then, reduce fluorouracil dosage by 20%
Diarrhea	
Reduction in creatinine clearance* to ≤60% of on study value	Delay therapy for 1 week. If creatinine clearance does not recover to pretreatment values, consider reducing cisplatin dose or replace cisplatin with carboplatin
Creatinine clearance* 40–60 mL/min (0.66–1 mL/s)	Consider reducing cisplatin dose, so that dose in milligrams equals the creatinine clearance* value expressed in mL/min†. Alternatively, replace cisplatin with carboplatin
Creatinine clearance* <40 mL/min (<0.66 mL/s)	Hold cisplatin
Clinically significant ototoxicity	Discontinue cisplatin
Clinically significant sensory loss	Discontinue cisplatin

*Creatinine clearance is used as a measure of glomerular filtration rate
†This also applies to patients with creatinine clearance of 40–60 mL/min before commencing treatment

Efficacy (N = 18)

Overall response rate	66%
Complete response	5.5%
Partial response	61.1%
Stable disease	22.2%
Progressive disease	11.1%
Median number of cycles (range)	4 (2–7)

1-Year survival	62.2%
5-Year survival	32.2%
Overall survival	34.5 months

*WHO criteria
Note: Three patients who were alive at 4, 5, and 7 years, respectively, had received additional local treatment (1 patient received chemotherapy after hepatic resection and 2 patients were treated after response to the FUP regimen with surgery or radiotherapy)

Treatment Monitoring

CBC with diff, electrolytes (including sodium, potassium, magnesium), and serum creatinine and LFTs before each cycle

Assessment evaluation: every 8 weeks

METASTATIC • SUBSEQUENT THERAPY

ANAL CANCER REGIMEN: NIVOLUMAB

Morris VK et al. Lancet Oncol 2017;18:446–453
Supplementary appendix to: Morris VK et al. Lancet Oncol 2017;18:446–453
OPDIVO (nivolumab) prescribing information. Princeton, NJ: Bristol-Myers Squibb Company; revised 2019 September

Nivolumab 3 mg/kg; administer intravenously over 30 minutes in a volume of 0.9% sodium chloride injection (0.9% NS) or 5% dextrose injection (D5W), not to exceed 160 mL and sufficient to produce a nivolumab concentration within the range 1–10 mg/mL, every 2 weeks until disease progression (total dosage/2-week course = 3 mg/kg)

- Administer nivolumab through an administration set that contains a sterile, non-pyrogenic, low protein-binding in-line filter with pore size within the range of 0.2–1.2 μm
- Nivolumab can cause severe infusion-related reactions

Supportive Care

Antiemetic prophylaxis
Emetogenic potential with nivolumab is **MINIMAL**
See Chapter 42 for antiemetic recommendations

Hematopoietic growth factor (CSF) prophylaxis
Primary prophylaxis is **NOT** indicated
See Chapter 43 for more information

Antimicrobial prophylaxis
Risk of fever and neutropenia is **LOW**
Antimicrobial primary prophylaxis to be considered:
- Antibacterial—not indicated
- Antifungal—not indicated
- Antiviral—not indicated unless patient previously had an episode of HSV

Therapy Monitoring

1. Initially at the time of each dose, and eventually every 6–12 weeks, perform a total body skin examination with attention to ALL mucous membranes as well as a complete review of systems

2. Monitor patients for signs and symptoms of pneumonitis. Evaluate patients with suspected pneumonitis with chest x-ray, CT, and pulse oximetry. For ≥2 toxicity may include nasal swab, sputum culture and sensitivity, blood culture and sensitivity, and urine culture and sensitivity

3. Monitor patients for signs and symptoms of colitis. Encourage patients to report diarrhea immediately to any member of the health care team

4. Draw AST, ALT, and bilirubin prior to each infusion and/or weekly if there are grade 1 liver function test elevations. Note, no treatment is recommended for G1 LFT abnormalities. For ≥2 toxicity, work up for other causes of elevated LFTs including viral hepatitis

5. Use basic metabolic panel (Na, K, CO2, glucose) and patient history as screening tools for hypophysitis including hypopituitarism and adrenal insufficiency. If in doubt evaluate AM adrenocorticotropic hormone (ACTH) and cortisol levels. Consider ACTH stimulation test for indeterminate results

6. Measure thyroid function (at the start of treatment, periodically during treatment, and as indicated based on clinical evaluation) and for clinical signs and symptoms of thyroid disorders. Test for TSH and free thyroxine (FT4) every 4–6 weeks as part of routine clinical monitoring on therapy or for case detection in symptomatic patients

7. Measure glucose at baseline and with each treatment during the first 12 weeks and every 6 weeks thereafter

8. Obtain a serum creatinine test prior to every dose. If creatinine is found to be newly elevated consider holding therapy while other potential causes are evaluated. Note, routine urinalysis is not necessary other than to rule out urinary tract infections, etc.

9. Obtain a complete rheumatologic history and perform an examination of all peripheral joints for tenderness, swelling, and range of motion. Examine the spine. Consider plain x-ray/imaging to exclude metastases and evaluate joint damage (erosions), if appropriate

Patient Population Studied

NCI9673 was a multicenter, single-arm, phase 2 study coordinated by the National Cancer Institute's Experimental Therapeutics Clinical Trials Network in the United States. The study involved 37 adult patients who had histologically confirmed squamous cell carcinoma of the anal canal, a life expectancy of ≥6 months, an Eastern Cooperative Oncology Group performance status of ≤1, measurable disease according to RECIST v1.1, adequate organ function, and prior receipt of ≥1 systemic therapy for surgically unresectable or metastatic disease. Patients who developed metastatic disease within 6 months of completion of chemoradiation for locoregional anal carcinoma were also allowed to be enrolled. Key exclusion criteria included adenocarcinoma of the anal canal, prior receipt of immunotherapy drugs, active autoimmune disease, and a condition requiring systemic corticosteroid treatment

Efficacy (N = 37)

	Nivolumab N = 37
CR	5%
PR	19%
ORR	24% (95% CI, 15–33)
Stable disease	47% (95% CI, 30–63)
DCR	72% (95% CI, 53–84)
Median DOR	5.8 months (IQR, 3.9–8.1)
Median PFS	4.1 months (95% CI, 3.0–7.9)
6-month PFS rate	38% (95% CI, 24–60)
Median OS	11.5 months (95% CI, 7.1–NE)
1-year OS rate	48% (95% CI, 32–74)

Data reported are from an analysis conducted with a data cutoff date of 16 May 2016 after a median follow-up of 10.1 months (95% CI, 9.4–12.2)
CR, complete response; PR, partial response; ORR, overall response rate; DCR, disease control rate; DOR, duration of response; PFS, progression-free survival; OS, overall survival; NE, not estimable

Treatment Modifications

RECOMMENDED DOSE MODIFICATIONS FOR NIVOLUMAB

Adverse Event	Grade / Severity	Treatment Modification
Infusion reaction	Clinically significant but not severe infusion reaction	Interrupt the infusion in patients with clinically significant infusion reactions and consider resuming at a slower rate following resolution. If the decision is made to restart, begin at <50% of the rate prior to the reaction and increase in 50% increments every 30 minutes if well tolerated. Infusions may be restarted at the full rate during the next cycle
	G3/4 (severe infusion reaction—pyrexia, chills, flushing, hypotension, dyspnea, wheezing, back pain, abdominal pain, and urticaria). Not rapidly responsive to brief interruption of infusion	Stop infusion and administer appropriate medical therapy (eg, epinephrine, corticosteroids, intravenous antihistamines, bronchodilators, and/or oxygen). Discontinue nivolumab
Colitis	G1	Loperamide 4 mg as starting dose then 2 mg before each meal and after each loose stool until without diarrhea for 12 hours, with a maximum of 16 mg loperamide per day. If G1 diarrhea or colitis persists >14 days, then add prednisolone 0.5–1 mg/kg (non-enteric coated) or consider oral budesonide 9 mg daily if no bloody diarrhea
	G2/3 diarrhea or colitis	Withhold nivolumab. Loperamide 4 mg as starting dose then 2 mg before each meal and after each loose stool until without diarrhea for 12 hours, with a maximum of 16 mg loperamide per day. Administer oral prednisone/prednisolone at a dose of 0.5 to 2 mg/kg/day or its equivalent. When improves to G1 begin a slow corticosteroid taper over at least 4 weeks. Resume nivolumab upon symptom control, or when prednisone/prednisolone daily dose <10 mg
	G4 diarrhea or colitis	Permanently discontinue nivolumab. Loperamide 4 mg as starting dose then 2 mg before each meal and after each loose stool until without diarrhea for 12 hours, with a maximum of 16 mg loperamide per day. Administer 1–2 mg/kg IV (methyl)prednisolone and convert to 0.5–2 mg/kg prednisone/prednisolone orally each day or its equivalent only after a response. Taper over at least 4 weeks when symptoms improve. If does not improve over 72 hours or worsens, perform flexible sigmoidoscopy/colonoscopy to document colitis then begin infliximab 5 mg/kg (if no perforation/sepsis/TB/hepatitis/NYHA III/IV CHF). If no response, add MMF 500–1000 mg twice daily. If worse on MMF, consider addition of tacrolimus or ATG
Pneumonitis	G2	Withhold nivolumab. Consider *Pneumocystis* prophylaxis depending on the clinical context and coverage with empiric antibiotics. Administer oral prednisone/prednisolone at a dose of 1–2 mg/kg/day or its equivalent. When improves to G1 begin a slow corticosteroid taper over at least 4 weeks. If does not respond adequately after 48 hours then administer 2–4 mg/kg IV (methyl)prednisolone and convert to 0.5–2 mg/kg prednisone/prednisolone orally each day or its equivalent only after a response, followed by a taper over at least 6 weeks when symptoms improve to G1, titrating to symptoms. Resume nivolumab upon symptom control, or when prednisone/prednisolone daily dose <10 mg
	G3/4	Permanently discontinue nivolumab. Consider *Pneumocystis* prophylaxis depending on the clinical context; cover with empiric antibiotics. Administer 2-4 mg/kg IV (methyl)prednisolone and convert to 1–2 mg/kg prednisone/prednisolone orally each day or its equivalent only after a response, followed by a taper over at least 8 weeks when symptoms improve to G1, titrating to symptoms. If when initially treated improvement does not occur within 48–72 hours begin infliximab 5 mg/kg (if no perforation/sepsis/TB/hepatitis/NYHA III/IV CHF). If no response to infliximab, add MMF 500–1000 mg twice daily. Consider MMF especially if has concurrent hepatic toxicity

(continued)

Treatment Modifications (continued)

RECOMMENDED DOSE MODIFICATIONS FOR NIVOLUMAB

Adverse Event	Grade / Severity	Treatment Modification
Hepatitis	G2 (AST or ALT >3–5× ULN or total bilirubin >1.5–3× ULN)	Withhold nivolumab. Administer oral prednisone/prednisolone at a dose of 1–2 mg/kg/day or its equivalent. When improves to G1 begin a slow corticosteroid taper over at least 4 weeks. Resume nivolumab upon symptom control, or when prednisone/prednisolone daily dose <10 mg
	G3/4 (AST or ALT >5× ULN or total bilirubin >3× ULN)	Permanently discontinue nivolumab. Administer 1–2 mg/kg IV (methyl)prednisolone and convert to 0.5–2 mg/kg prednisone/prednisolone orally each day or its equivalent only after a response. Taper over at least 6 weeks when symptoms improve. If no response, add MMF 500–1000 mg twice daily. If worse on MMF, consider adding tacrolimus or ATG
Hypophysitis	G2/3 (Moderate symptoms, ie, headache but no visual disturbance or fatigue/mood alteration but hemodynamically stable, no electrolyte disturbance)	Administer analgesia as needed for headache. Withhold nivolumab. Administer oral prednisone/prednisolone at a dose of 0.5–2 mg/kg/day or its equivalent. When improves to G1 begin a slow corticosteroid taper over at least 4 weeks. If no improvement in 48 hours administer 1–2 mg/kg IV (methyl)prednisolone and convert to 0.5–2 mg/kg prednisone/prednisolone orally each day or its equivalent only after a response. Taper over at least 4 weeks when symptoms improve to 5 mg prednisone/prednisolone or equivalent; do not stop steroids. Resume nivolumab upon symptom control, or when prednisone/prednisolone daily dose <10 mg
	G4 (Severe mass effect symptoms, ie, severe headache, any visual disturbance or severe hypoadrenalism, ie, hypotension, severe electrolyte disturbance)	Permanently discontinue nivolumab. Administer analgesia as needed for headache. Administer 1–2 mg/kg IV (methyl)prednisolone and convert to 0.5–2 mg/kg prednisone/prednisolone orally each day or its equivalent only after a response. Taper over at least 4 weeks when symptoms improve to 5 mg prednisone/prednisolone or equivalent; do not stop steroids
Adrenal Insufficiency	G2	Withhold nivolumab. Administer oral prednisone/prednisolone at a dose of 0.5–2 mg/kg/day or its equivalent. When improves to G1 begin a slow corticosteroid taper over at least 4 weeks. Serially assess adrenal function and continue steroids at replacement doses (20–40 mg hydrocortisone daily ~2/3 dose in AM upon awakening and ~1/3 at 4 PM) until recovery of adrenal function is documented. Resume nivolumab upon symptom control, or when prednisone/prednisolone daily dose <10 mg
	G3/4	Permanently discontinue nivolumab. Administer oral prednisone/prednisolone at a dose of 0.5–2 mg/kg/day or its equivalent. When improves to G1 begin a slow corticosteroid taper over at least 4 weeks. Serially assess adrenal function and continue steroids at replacement doses (20–40 mg hydrocortisone daily ~2/3 dose in AM upon awakening and ~1/3 at 4 PM) until recovery of adrenal function is documented
Type 1 diabetes mellitus	G3 hyperglycemia	Withhold nivolumab. Admit to hospital to manage hyperglycemia. Role of corticosteroids in preventing complete loss of insulin-producing cells is unknown and not recommended. Resume nivolumab upon symptom control, or when prednisone/prednisolone daily dose <10 mg
	G4 hyperglycemia	Permanently discontinue nivolumab. Admit to hospital to manage hyperglycemia. The role of corticosteroids in preventing complete loss of insulin-producing cells is unknown and not recommended
Nephritis and renal dysfunction	G2/3 (serum creatinine 1.5–6× ULN)	Withhold nivolumab. Administer oral prednisone/prednisolone at a dose of 0.5–2 mg/kg/day or its equivalent. When improves to G1 begin a slow corticosteroid taper over at least 4 weeks. If does not respond adequately then administer 0.5–1 mg/kg IV (methyl)prednisolone and convert to 0.5–2 mg/kg prednisone/prednisolone orally each day or its equivalent only after a response, followed by a taper over at least 4 weeks when improves to G1. Resume nivolumab upon symptom control, or when prednisone/prednisolone daily dose <10 mg
	G4 (serum creatinine >6× ULN)	Permanently discontinue nivolumab. Administer 0.5–1 mg/kg IV (methyl)prednisolone and convert to 0.5–2 mg/kg prednisone/prednisolone orally each day or its equivalent only after a response, followed by a taper over at least 4 weeks when improves to G1

(continued)

Treatment Modifications (*continued*)

RECOMMENDED DOSE MODIFICATIONS FOR NIVOLUMAB

Adverse Event	Grade / Severity	Treatment Modification
Skin	G1/2	Continue nivolumab. Avoid skin irritants, avoid sun exposure, topical emollients recommended. Topical steroid (mild strength for G1, moderate/potent strength for G2) cream once or twice daily ± oral or topical antihistamines for itching
	G3 rash or suspected SJS or TEN	Withhold nivolumab. Avoid skin irritants, avoid sun exposure, topical emollients recommended. Administer oral or topical antihistamines for itching. Administer oral prednisone/prednisolone at a dose of 0.5–2 mg/kg or its equivalent daily for 3 days followed by a slow corticosteroid taper over at least 4 weeks when the rash improves to G1. If does not respond adequately then administer 0.5–1 mg/kg IV (methyl) prednisolone and convert to 0.5–2 mg/kg prednisone/prednisolone orally each day or its equivalent only after a response, followed by a taper over at least 4 weeks when the rash improves to G1. Resume nivolumab upon symptom control, or when prednisone/ prednisolone daily dose <10 mg
	G4 rash or confirmed SJS or TEN	Avoid skin irritants, avoid sun exposure, topical emollients recommended. Administer oral or topical antihistamines for itching. Administer 1–2 mg/kg IV (methyl)prednisolone and convert to oral steroids 0.5–2 mg/kg prednisone/prednisolone each day or its equivalent only after a response. Taper over at least 4 weeks when the rash improves to G1. Permanently discontinue nivolumab
Encephalitis	Confusion or altered behavior, headaches, alteration in Glasgow Coma Scale, motor or sensory deficits, speech abnormality, may or may not be febrile	Initially withhold nivolumab, but permanently discontinue nivolumab if there is no doubt as to diagnosis. Exclude bacterial and ideally viral infections prior to high-dose steroids. Administer oral prednisone/prednisolone at a dose of 0.5–2 mg/kg/day or its equivalent. When symptoms improve begin a slow corticosteroid taper over at least 4–8 weeks. If symptoms are severe administer 1–2 mg/kg IV (methyl)prednisolone and convert to 0.5–2 mg/kg prednisone/prednisolone orally each day or its equivalent only after a response. Consider concurrent empiric antiviral (IV acyclovir) and antibacterial therapy
Aseptic meningitis	Headache, photophobia, neck stiffness with fever or may be afebrile, vomiting; normal cognition/cerebral function (distinguishes from encephalitis)	
Other syndromes include neurosarcoidosis, posterior reversible leukoencephalopathy syndrome (PRES), Vogt-Koyanagi-Harada syndrome, demyelination, vasculitic encephalopathy, and generalized seizures		
Transverse myelitis	Acute or subacute neurologic signs/ symptoms of motor/sensory/ autonomic origin; most have sensory level; often bilateral symptoms	Initially withhold nivolumab, but permanently discontinue nivolumab if there is no doubt as to diagnosis. Administer 2 mg/kg IV (methyl)prednisolone or consider 1 g/day and convert to 0.5–2 mg/kg prednisone/prednisolone orally each day or its equivalent only after a response. When symptoms improve begin a slow corticosteroid taper over at least 4–8 weeks. Plasmapheresis may be required if steroids do not bring about improvement
Myocarditis	G3	Permanently discontinue nivolumab. Administer 2 mg/kg IV (methyl)prednisolone or consider 1 g/day and convert to 0.5–2 mg/kg prednisone/prednisolone orally each day or its equivalent only after a response. When symptoms improve begin a slow corticosteroid taper over at least 4–8 weeks. If no response, add MMF 500–1000 mg twice daily. If worse on MMF, consider adding tacrolimus
Peripheral neurologic toxicity	Moderate: some interference with ADL, symptoms concerning to patient	Withhold nivolumab. Initial observation reasonable or initiate prednisone/ prednisolone 0.5–1 mg/kg (if progressing, eg, from mild) and/or pregabalin or duloxetine for pain. When symptoms improve begin a slow corticosteroid taper over at least 4 weeks. Resume nivolumab upon symptom control, or when prednisone/ prednisolone daily dose <10 mg
	Severe: limits self-care and aids warranted, life-threatening, eg, respiratory problems	Permanently discontinue nivolumab. Administer 1–2 mg/kg IV (methyl)prednisolone and convert to 0.5–2 mg/kg prednisone/prednisolone orally each day or its equivalent only after a response. Taper over at least 4–8 weeks when symptoms improve to G1

(*continued*)

Treatment Modifications (*continued*)

RECOMMENDED DOSE MODIFICATIONS FOR NIVOLUMAB

Adverse Event	Grade / Severity	Treatment Modification
Guillain-Barré syndrome	Progressive symmetrical muscle weakness with absent or reduced tendon reflexes—involves extremities, facial, respiratory, and bulbar and oculomotor muscles; dysregulation of autonomic nerves	Permanently discontinue nivolumab. Use of steroids not recommended in idiopathic Guillain-Barré syndrome; however, a trial of (methyl)prednisolone 1–2 mg/kg is reasonable, converting to 0.5–2 mg/kg prednisone/prednisolone orally each day or its equivalent only after a response. If no improvement or worsening, plasmapheresis or IVIG indicated
Myasthenia gravis	Fluctuating muscle weakness (proximal limb, trunk, ocular, eg, ptosis/diplopia or bulbar) with fatigability, respiratory muscles may also be involved	Permanently discontinue nivolumab. Administer pyridostigmine at an initial dose of 30 mg three times daily. Administer oral prednisone/prednisolone at a dose of 0.5–2 mg/kg/day or its equivalent or 1–2 mg/kg IV (methyl)prednisolone depending on the severity of symptoms. If began with IV, convert to 0.5–2 mg/kg prednisone/prednisolone orally each day or its equivalent only after a response. If no improvement or worsening, plasmapheresis or IVIG may be considered. Additional immunosuppressants used in myasthenia gravis include azathioprine, cyclosporine, and mycophenolate. Avoid certain medications, eg, ciprofloxacin, beta-blockers, that may precipitate cholinergic crisis
Other syndromes including motor and sensory peripheral neuropathy, multifocal radicular neuropathy/plexopathy, autonomic neuropathy, phrenic nerve palsy, cranial nerve palsies (eg, facial nerve, optic nerve, hypoglossal nerve)		Permanently discontinue nivolumab. Administer oral prednisone/prednisolone at a dose of 0.5–2 mg/kg/day or its equivalent or 1–2 mg/kg IV (methyl)prednisolone depending on the severity of symptoms. If began with IV, convert to 0.5–2 mg/kg prednisone/prednisolone orally each day or its equivalent only after a response
Arthralgia	G1 (Mild pain with inflammation, erythema, or joint swelling)	Continue nivolumab. Administer acetaminophen (paracetamol) and ibuprofen
	G2 (Moderate pain with inflammation, erythema, or joint swelling that limits ADLs)	Withhold nivolumab. Administer higher doses of acetaminophen (paracetamol) and ibuprofen and use diclofenac or naproxen or etoricoxib. If inadequately controlled, consider intra-articular steroid injections for large joints or administer oral prednisone/prednisolone at a dose of 0.5–2 mg/kg/day or its equivalent. When improves to G1 begin a slow corticosteroid taper over at least 4 weeks. If does not respond adequately then administer 0.5–1 mg/kg IV (methyl)prednisolone and convert to 0.5–2 mg/kg prednisone/prednisolone orally each day or its equivalent only after a response, followed by a taper over at least 4 weeks when improves to G1. Resume nivolumab upon symptom control, or when prednisone/prednisolone daily dose <10 mg
	G3 (Severe pain; irreversible joint damage; disabling; limits self-care ADL)	Withhold nivolumab. Administer 0.5–1 mg/kg IV (methyl)prednisolone and convert to 0.5–2 mg/kg prednisone/prednisolone orally each day or its equivalent only after a response, followed by a taper over at least 4 weeks when improves to G1. In severe cases, infliximab or another anti–TNF alpha drug may be required for improvement of arthritis. Resume nivolumab upon symptom control, or when prednisone/prednisolone daily dose <10 mg
Other	First occurrence of other G3	Withhold nivolumab. Administer oral prednisone/prednisolone at a dose of 0.5–2 mg/kg/day or its equivalent. When improves to G1 begin a slow corticosteroid taper over at least 4 weeks. Resume nivolumab upon symptom control, or when prednisone/prednisolone daily dose <10 mg
	Recurrence of same G3	Permanently discontinue nivolumab. Administer 1–2 mg/kg IV (methyl)prednisolone and convert to 0.5–2 mg/kg prednisone/prednisolone orally each day or its equivalent only after a response. Taper over at least 4–8 weeks when symptoms improve to G1
	Life-threatening or G4	
	Requirement for ≥10 mg/day prednisone or equivalent for >12 weeks	Permanently discontinue nivolumab
	Persistent G2/3 adverse reactions lasting ≥12 weeks	

Abbreviations: ADL, activities of daily living; ALT, alanine aminotransferase; AST, aspartate aminotransferase; ATG, anti-thymocyte globulin; SJS, Stevens-Johnson Syndrome; TEN, toxic epidermal necrolysis; ULN, upper limit of normal

Notes on general supportive care:
- Steroid taper in most cases will proceed over a minimum of 1 month, but if symptoms improve rapidly a 2-week taper can be considered. If steroids are administered for more than 4 weeks, consider PCP prophylaxis (cotrimoxazole 480 mg twice daily M/W/F or inhaled pentamidine if has cotrimoxazole allergy), regular random blood glucose, vitamin D level and starting calcium/vitamin D supplementation per guidelines

Adverse Events (N = 37)

Grade (%)	Nivolumab (N = 37)		
	Grade 1	Grade 2	Grade 3
Anemia	35	30	5
Fatigue	46	19	3
Rash	22	5	3
Constipation	22	5	0
Anorexia	14	11	0
Diarrhea	22	0	0
Weight loss	14	3	0
Arthralgia	8	8	0
Hyperglycemia	8	3	0
Hypothyroidism	3	3	3
Lymphedema	3	3	0
Nausea	5	0	0
Pneumonitis	0	3	0

The table includes all adverse events
There were no grade 4 or 5 adverse events reported
Adverse events were graded according to the National Cancer Institute Common Terminology Criteria for Adverse Events, version 4.0

METASTATIC • SUBSEQUENT THERAPY
ANAL CANCER REGIMEN: PEMBROLIZUMAB

Ott PA et al. Ann Oncol. 2017;28:1036–1041

KEYTRUDA (pembrolizumab) injection prescribing information. Whitehouse Station, NJ: Merck & Co., Inc; updated 2020 January

Pembrolizumab 10 mg/kg; administer intravenously over 30 minutes in a volume of 0.9% sodium chloride injection (0.9% NS) or 5% dextrose injection (D5W) sufficient to produce a pembrolizumab concentration within the range 1–10 mg/mL every 2 weeks for up to 24 months (total dose/2-week cycle = 10 mg/kg)

- Administer pembrolizumab with an administration set that contains a sterile, non-pyrogenic, low protein-binding in-line or add-on filter with pore size within the range of 0.2–5 μm
- Pembrolizumab can cause severe or life-threatening infusion-related reactions, including hypersensitivity and anaphylaxis

Supportive Care

Antiemetic prophylaxis

Emetogenic potential is **MINIMAL**

See Chapter 42 for antiemetic recommendations

Hematopoietic growth factor (CSF) prophylaxis

Primary prophylaxis is **NOT** *indicated*

See Chapter 43 for more information

Antimicrobial prophylaxis

Risk of fever and neutropenia is **LOW**

  Antimicrobial primary prophylaxis to be considered:

- Antibacterial—not indicated
- Antifungal—not indicated
- Antiviral—not indicated unless patient previously had an episode of HSV

Patient Population Studied

KEYNOTE-028 was an international, multicenter, open-label, multicohort, phase 1b study evaluating pembrolizumab in adult patients with PD-L1-positive advanced solid tumors. The anal carcinoma cohort (n = 25, n = 24 with squamous cell carcinoma histology) included patients with histologically or cytologically confirmed locally advanced or metastatic anal carcinoma who had failed prior therapy and whose tumors expressed PD-L1. PD-L1 positivity was defined as membrane staining of ≥1% of scorable cells, including neoplastic cells and contiguous mononuclear inflammatory cells, or the presence of a distinctive interface pattern. Patients were also required to have measurable disease based on RECIST v1.1, an Eastern Cooperative Oncology Group performance status of ≤1, and adequate organ function. Patients were excluded if they had a diagnosis of immunodeficiency, if they had received systemic steroids within the past 7 days, if they had an active autoimmune disease, if they had interstitial lung disease, if they had active brain metastases, and if they had received prior treatment with an immune checkpoint inhibitor. Of 43 patients who were screened for PD-L1 expression, 32 (74%) had PD-L1-positive tumors

Efficacy (N = 24)

	Pembrolizumab N = 24
Confirmed CR	0% (95% CI, 0–14)
Confirmed PR	17% (95% CI, 5–37)
Stable disease	42% (95% CI, 22–63)
Progressive disease	38% (95% CI, 19–59)
Not assessed for response	4% (95% CI, 0–21)
Median DOR*†	NR (range, <0.1+ to 9.2+)
Median PFS	3.0 months (95% CI, 1.7–7.3)
6-month PFS rate	31.6%
12-month PFS rate	19.7%
Median OS	9.3 months (95% CI, 5.9–NA)
6-month OS rate	64.5%
12-month OS rate	47.6%

*Includes 1 partial responder with non-squamous histology

CR, complete response; PR, partial response; DOR, duration of response; NR, not reached; PFS, progression-free survival; OS, overall survival; NA, not available

Data reported are from an analysis conducted with a data cutoff date of 1 July 2015 after a median follow-up of 10.6 months (range, 0.3–15.0 months) and median duration of therapy of 92 days (range, 1–449 days)

Therapy Monitoring

1. Initially at the time of each dose, and eventually every 6–12 weeks, perform a total body skin examination with attention to ALL mucous membranes as well as a complete review of systems
2. Monitor patients for signs and symptoms of pneumonitis. Evaluate patients with suspected pneumonitis with chest x-ray, CT, and pulse oximetry. For ≥ 2 toxicity may include nasal swab, sputum culture and sensitivity, blood culture and sensitivity, and urine culture and sensitivity
3. Monitor patients for signs and symptoms of colitis. Encourage patients to report diarrhea immediately to any member of the health care team
4. Draw AST, ALT, and bilirubin prior to each infusion and/or weekly if there are grade 1 liver function test elevations. Note, no treatment is recommended for G1 LFT abnormalities. For ≥ 2 toxicity, work up for other causes of elevated LFTs including viral hepatitis
5. Use basic metabolic panel (Na, K, CO2, glucose) and patient history as screening tools for hypophysitis including hypopituitarism and adrenal insufficiency. If in doubt evaluate AM adrenocorticotropic hormone (ACTH) and cortisol levels. Consider ACTH stimulation test for indeterminate results
6. Measure thyroid function (at the start of treatment, periodically during treatment, and as indicated based on clinical evaluation) and for clinical signs and symptoms of thyroid disorders. Test for TSH and free thyroxine (FT4) every 4–6 weeks as part of routine clinical monitoring on therapy or for case detection in symptomatic patients
7. Measure glucose at baseline and with each treatment during the first 12 weeks and every 6 weeks thereafter
8. Obtain a serum creatinine prior to every dose. If creatinine is found to be newly elevated consider holding therapy while other potential causes are evaluated. Note, routine urinalysis is not necessary other than to rule out urinary tract infections, etc
9. Obtain a complete rheumatologic history and perform an examination of all peripheral joints for tenderness, swelling, and range of motion. Examine the spine. Consider plain x-ray/imaging to exclude metastases and evaluate joint damage (erosions), if appropriate

Treatment Modifications

RECOMMENDED DOSE MODIFICATIONS FOR PEMBROLIZUMAB

Adverse Event	Grade / Severity	Treatment Modification
Infusion reaction	Clinically significant but not severe infusion reaction	Interrupt the infusion in patients with clinically significant infusion reactions and consider resuming at a slower rate following resolution. If the decision is made to restart, begin at <50% of the rate prior to the reaction and increase in 50% increments every 30 minutes if well tolerated. Infusions may be restarted at the full rate during the next cycle
	G3/4 (severe infusion reaction— pyrexia, chills, flushing, hypotension, dyspnea, wheezing, back pain, abdominal pain, and urticaria). Not rapidly responsive to brief interruption of infusion	Stop infusion and administer appropriate medical therapy (eg, epinephrine, corticosteroids, intravenous antihistamines, bronchodilators, and/or oxygen). Discontinue pembrolizumab
Colitis	G1	Loperamide 4 mg as starting dose then 2 mg before each meal and after each loose stool until without diarrhea for 12 hours, with a maximum of 16 mg loperamide per day. If G1 diarrhea or colitis persists >14 days, then add prednisolone 0.5–1 mg/kg (non-enteric coated) or consider oral budesonide 9 mg daily if no bloody diarrhea
	G2/3 diarrhea or colitis	Withhold pembrolizumab. Loperamide 4 mg as starting dose then 2 mg before each meal and after each loose stool until without diarrhea for 12 hours, with a maximum of 16 mg loperamide per day. Administer oral prednisone/prednisolone at a dose of 0.5–2 mg/kg/ day or its equivalent. When improves to G1 begin a slow corticosteroid taper over at least 4 weeks. Resume pembrolizumab upon symptom control, or when prednisone/prednisolone daily dose <10 mg
	G4 diarrhea or colitis	Permanently discontinue pembrolizumab. Loperamide 4 mg as starting dose then 2 mg before each meal and after each loose stool until without diarrhea for 12 hours, with a maximum of 16 mg loperamide per day. Administer 1–2 mg/kg IV (methyl)prednisolone and convert to 0.5–2 mg/kg prednisone/prednisolone orally each day or its equivalent only after a response. Taper over at least 4 weeks when symptoms improve. If does not improve over 72 hours or worsens, perform flexible sigmoidoscopy/colonoscopy to document colitis then begin infliximab 5 mg/kg (if no perforation/sepsis/TB/hepatitis/NYHA III/IV CHF). If no response, add MMF 500–1000 mg twice daily. If worse on MMF, consider addition of tacrolimus or ATG

(continued)

Treatment Modifications (continued)

RECOMMENDED DOSE MODIFICATIONS FOR PEMBROLIZUMAB

Adverse Event	Grade / Severity	Treatment Modification
Pneumonitis	G2	Withhold pembrolizumab. Consider *Pneumocystis* prophylaxis depending on the clinical context and coverage with empiric antibiotics. Administer oral prednisone/prednisolone at a dose of 1–2 mg/kg/day or its equivalent. When improves to G1 begin a slow corticosteroid taper over at least 4 weeks. If does not respond adequately after 48 hours then administer 2–4 mg/kg IV (methyl)prednisolone and convert to 0.5–2 mg/kg prednisone/prednisolone orally each day or its equivalent only after a response, followed by a taper over at least 6 weeks when symptoms improve to G1, titrating to symptoms. Resume pembrolizumab upon symptom control, or when prednisone/prednisolone daily dose <10 mg
	G3/4	Permanently discontinue pembrolizumab. Consider *Pneumocystis* prophylaxis depending on the clinical context; cover with empiric antibiotics. Administer 2–4 mg/kg IV (methyl)prednisolone and convert to 1–2 mg/kg prednisone/prednisolone orally each day or its equivalent only after a response, followed by a taper over at least 8 weeks when symptoms improve to G1, titrating to symptoms. If when initially treated improvement does not occur within 48–72 hours begin infliximab 5 mg/kg (if no perforation/sepsis/TB/hepatitis/NYHA III/IV CHF). If no response to infliximab, add MMF 500–1000 mg twice daily. Consider MMF especially if has concurrent hepatic toxicity
Hepatitis	G2 (AST or ALT >3–5× ULN or total bilirubin >1.5–3× ULN)	Withhold pembrolizumab. Administer oral prednisone/prednisolone at a dose of 1–2 mg/kg/day or its equivalent. When improves to G1 begin a slow corticosteroid taper over at least 4 weeks. Resume pembrolizumab upon symptom control, or when prednisone/prednisolone daily dose <10 mg
	G3/4 (AST or ALT >5× ULN or total bilirubin >3× ULN)	Permanently discontinue pembrolizumab. Administer 1–2 mg/kg IV (methyl)prednisolone and convert to 0.5–2 mg/kg prednisone/prednisolone orally each day or its equivalent only after a response. Taper over at least 6 weeks when symptoms improve. If no response, add MMF 500–1000 mg twice daily. If worse on MMF, consider adding tacrolimus or ATG
Hypophysitis	G2/3 (Moderate symptoms, ie, headache but no visual disturbance or fatigue/mood alteration but hemodynamically stable, no electrolyte disturbance)	Administer analgesia as needed for headache. Withhold pembrolizumab. Administer oral prednisone/prednisolone at a dose of 0.5–2 mg/kg/day or its equivalent. When improves to G1 begin a slow corticosteroid taper over at least 4 weeks. If no improvement in 48 hours administer 1–2 mg/kg IV (methyl)prednisolone and convert to 0.5–2 mg/kg prednisone/prednisolone orally each day or its equivalent only after a response. Taper over at least 4 weeks when symptoms improve to 5 mg prednisone/prednisolone or equivalent; do not stop steroids. Resume pembrolizumab upon symptom control, or when prednisone/prednisolone daily dose <10 mg
	G4 (Severe mass effect symptoms, ie, severe headache, any visual disturbance or severe hypoadrenalism, ie, hypotension, severe electrolyte disturbance)	Permanently discontinue pembrolizumab. Administer analgesia as needed for headache. Administer 1–2 mg/kg IV (methyl)prednisolone and convert to 0.5–2 mg/kg prednisone/prednisolone orally each day or its equivalent only after a response. Taper over at least 4 weeks when symptoms improve to 5 mg prednisone/prednisolone or equivalent; do not stop steroids
Adrenal Insufficiency	G2	Withhold pembrolizumab. Administer oral prednisone/prednisolone at a dose of 0.5–2 mg/kg/day or its equivalent. When improves to G1 begin a slow corticosteroid taper over at least 4 weeks. Serially assess adrenal function and continue steroids at replacement doses (20–40 mg hydrocortisone daily ~2/3 dose in AM upon awakening and ~1/3 at 4 PM) until recovery of adrenal function is documented. Resume pembrolizumab upon symptom control, or when prednisone/prednisolone daily dose <10 mg
	G3/4	Permanently discontinue pembrolizumab. Administer oral prednisone/prednisolone at a dose of 0.5–2 mg/kg/day or its equivalent. When improves to G1 begin a slow corticosteroid taper over at least 4 weeks. Serially assess adrenal function and continue steroids at replacement doses (20–40 mg hydrocortisone daily ~2/3 dose in AM upon awakening and ~1/3 at 4 PM) until recovery of adrenal function is documented

(continued)

Treatment Modifications (continued)

RECOMMENDED DOSE MODIFICATIONS FOR PEMBROLIZUMAB

Adverse Event	Grade / Severity	Treatment Modification
Type 1 diabetes mellitus	G3 hyperglycemia	Withhold pembrolizumab. Admit to hospital to manage hyperglycemia. The role of corticosteroids in preventing complete loss of insulin-producing cells is unknown and not recommended. Resume pembrolizumab upon symptom control, or when prednisone/prednisolone daily dose <10 mg
	G4 hyperglycemia	Permanently discontinue pembrolizumab. Admit to hospital to manage hyperglycemia. The role of corticosteroids in preventing complete loss of insulin-producing cells is unknown and not recommended.
Nephritis and renal dysfunction	G2/3 (serum creatinine 1.5–6× ULN)	Withhold pembrolizumab. Administer oral prednisone/prednisolone at a dose of 0.5–2 mg/kg/day or its equivalent. When improves to G1 begin a slow corticosteroid taper over at least 4 weeks. If does not respond adequately then administer 0.5–1 mg/kg IV (methyl) prednisolone and convert to 0.5–2 mg/kg prednisone/prednisolone orally each day or its equivalent only after a response, followed by a taper over at least 4 weeks when improves to G1. Resume pembrolizumab upon symptom control, or when prednisone/prednisolone daily dose <10 mg
	G4 (serum creatinine >6× ULN)	Permanently discontinue pembrolizumab. Administer 0.5–1 mg/kg IV (methyl) prednisolone and convert to 0.5–2 mg/kg prednisone/prednisolone orally each day or its equivalent only after a response, followed by a taper over at least 4 weeks when improves to G1.
Skin	G1/2	Continue pembrolizumab. Avoid skin irritants, avoid sun exposure, topical emollients recommended. Topical steroid (mild strength for G1, moderate/potent strength for G2) cream once or twice daily ± oral or topical antihistamines for itching.
	G3 rash or suspected SJS or TEN	Withhold pembrolizumab. Avoid skin irritants, avoid sun exposure, topical emollients recommended. Administer oral or topical antihistamines for itching. Administer oral prednisone/prednisolone at a dose of 0.5–2 mg/kg or its equivalent daily for 3 days followed by a slow corticosteroid taper over at least 4 weeks when the rash improves to G1. If does not respond adequately then administer 0.5–1 mg/kg IV (methyl)prednisolone and convert to 0.5–2 mg/kg prednisone/prednisolone orally each day or its equivalent only after a response, followed by a taper over at least 4 weeks when the rash improves to G1. Resume pembrolizumab upon symptom control, or when prednisone/prednisolone daily dose <10 mg
	G4 rash or confirmed SJS or TEN	Avoid skin irritants, avoid sun exposure, topical emollients recommended. Administer oral or topical antihistamines for itching. Administer 1–2 mg/kg IV (methyl)prednisolone and convert to oral steroids 0.5–2 mg/kg prednisone/prednisolone each day or its equivalent only after a response. Taper over at least 4 weeks when the rash improves to G1. Permanently discontinue pembrolizumab
Encephalitis	Confusion or altered behavior, headaches, alteration in Glasgow Coma Scale, motor or sensory deficits, speech abnormality, may or may not be febrile	Initially withhold pembrolizumab, but permanently discontinue pembrolizumab if there is no doubt as to diagnosis. Exclude bacterial and ideally viral infections prior to high-dose steroids. Administer oral prednisone/prednisolone at a dose of 0.5–2 mg/kg/day or its equivalent. When symptoms improve begin a slow corticosteroid taper over at least 4–8 weeks. If symptoms are severe administer 1–2 mg/kg IV (methyl)prednisolone and convert to 0.5–2 mg/kg prednisone/prednisolone orally each day or its equivalent only after a response. Consider concurrent empiric antiviral (IV acyclovir) and antibacterial therapy
Aseptic meningitis	Headache, photophobia, neck stiffness with fever or may be afebrile, vomiting; normal cognition/cerebral function (distinguishes from encephalitis)	
Other syndromes include neurosarcoidosis, posterior reversible leukoencephalopathy syndrome (PRES), Vogt-Koyanagi-Harada syndrome, demyelination, vasculitic encephalopathy, and generalized seizures		

(continued)

Treatment Modifications (*continued*)

RECOMMENDED DOSE MODIFICATIONS FOR PEMBROLIZUMAB

Adverse Event	Grade / Severity	Treatment Modification
Transverse myelitis	Acute or subacute neurologic signs/ symptoms of motor/sensory/ autonomic origin; most have sensory level; often bilateral symptoms	Initially withhold pembrolizumab, but permanently discontinue pembrolizumab if there is no doubt as to diagnosis. Administer 2 mg/kg IV (methyl)prednisolone or consider 1 g/day and convert to 0.5–2 mg/kg prednisone/prednisolone orally each day or its equivalent only after a response. When symptoms improve begin a slow corticosteroid taper over at least 4–8 weeks. Plasmapheresis may be required if steroids do not bring about improvement
Myocarditis	G3	Permanently discontinue pembrolizumab. Administer 2 mg/kg IV (methyl)prednisolone or consider 1 g/day and convert to 0.5–2 mg/kg prednisone/prednisolone orally each day or its equivalent only after a response. When symptoms improve begin a slow corticosteroid taper over at least 4–8 weeks. If no response, add MMF 500–1000 mg twice daily. If worse on MMF, consider adding tacrolimus
Peripheral neurologic toxicity	Moderate: some interference with ADL, symptoms concerning to patient	Withhold pembrolizumab. Initial observation reasonable or initiate prednisone/prednisolone 0.5–1 mg/kg (if progressing, eg, from mild) and/or pregabalin or duloxetine for pain. When symptoms improve begin a slow corticosteroid taper over at least 4 weeks. Resume pembrolizumab upon symptom control, or when prednisone/prednisolone daily dose <10 mg
	Severe: limits self-care and aids warranted, life-threatening, eg, respiratory problems	Permanently discontinue pembrolizumab. Administer 1–2 mg/kg IV (methyl)prednisolone and convert to 0.5–2 mg/kg prednisone/prednisolone orally each day or its equivalent only after a response. Taper over at least 4–8 weeks when symptoms improve to G1
Guillain-Barré syndrome	Progressive symmetrical muscle weakness with absent or reduced tendon reflexes—involves extremities, facial, respiratory, and bulbar and oculomotor muscles; dysregulation of autonomic nerves	Permanently discontinue pembrolizumab. Use of steroids not recommended in idiopathic Guillain-Barré syndrome; however, a trial of (methyl)prednisolone 1–2 mg/kg is reasonable, converting to 0.5–2 mg/kg prednisone/prednisolone orally each day or its equivalent only after a response. If no improvement or worsening, plasmapheresis or IVIG indicated
Myasthenia gravis	Fluctuating muscle weakness (proximal limb, trunk, ocular, eg, ptosis/diplopia or bulbar) with fatigability, respiratory muscles may also be involved	Permanently discontinue pembrolizumab. Administer pyridostigmine at an initial dose of 30 mg three times daily. Administer oral prednisone/prednisolone at a dose of 0.5–2 mg/kg/ day or its equivalent or 1–2 mg/kg IV (methyl)prednisolone depending on the severity of symptoms. If began with IV, convert to 0.5–2 mg/kg prednisone/prednisolone orally each day or its equivalent only after a response. If no improvement or worsening, plasmapheresis or IVIG may be considered. Additional immunosuppressants used in myasthenia gravis include azathioprine, cyclosporine, and mycophenolate. Avoid certain medications, eg, ciprofloxacin, beta-blockers, that may precipitate cholinergic crisis
Other syndromes including motor and sensory peripheral neuropathy, multifocal radicular neuropathy/plexopathy, autonomic neuropathy, phrenic nerve palsy, cranial nerve palsies (eg, facial nerve, optic nerve, hypoglossal nerve)		Permanently discontinue pembrolizumab. Administer oral prednisone/prednisolone at a dose of 0.5–2 mg/kg/day or its equivalent or 1–2 mg/kg IV (methyl)prednisolone depending on the severity of symptoms. If began with IV, convert to 0.5–2 mg/kg prednisone/prednisolone orally each day or its equivalent only after a response
Arthralgia	G1 (Mild pain with inflammation, erythema, or joint swelling)	Continue pembrolizumab. Administer acetaminophen (paracetamol) and ibuprofen
	G2 (Moderate pain with inflammation, erythema, or joint swelling that limits ADLs)	Withhold pembrolizumab. Administer higher doses of acetaminophen (paracetamol) and ibuprofen and use diclofenac or naproxen or etoricoxib. If inadequately controlled, consider intra-articular steroid injections for large joints or administer oral prednisone/prednisolone at a dose of 0.5–2 mg/kg/day or its equivalent. When improves to G1 begin a slow corticosteroid taper over at least 4 weeks. If does not respond adequately then administer 0.5–1 mg/kg IV (methyl)prednisolone and convert to 0.5–2 mg/kg prednisone/ prednisolone orally each day or its equivalent only after a response, followed by a taper over at least 4 weeks when improves to G1. Resume pembrolizumab upon symptom control, or when prednisone/prednisolone daily dose <10 mg
	G3 (Severe pain; irreversible joint damage; disabling; limits self-care ADL)	Withhold pembrolizumab. Administer 0.5–1 mg/kg IV (methyl)prednisolone and convert to 0.5–2 mg/kg prednisone/prednisolone orally each day or its equivalent only after a response, followed by a taper over at least 4 weeks when improves to G1. In severe cases, infliximab or another anti–TNF alpha drug may be required for improvement of arthritis. Resume pembrolizumab upon symptom control, or when prednisone/prednisolone daily dose <10 mg

(*continued*)

Treatment Modifications (*continued*)

RECOMMENDED DOSE MODIFICATIONS FOR PEMBROLIZUMAB

Adverse Event	Grade / Severity	Treatment Modification
Other	First occurrence of other G3	Withhold pembrolizumab. Administer oral prednisone/prednisolone at a dose of 0.5–2 mg/kg/day or its equivalent. When improves to G1 begin a slow corticosteroid taper over at least 4 weeks. Resume pembrolizumab upon symptom control, or when prednisone/prednisolone daily dose <10 mg
	Recurrence of same G3	Permanently discontinue pembrolizumab. Administer 1–2 mg/kg IV (methyl)prednisolone and convert to 0.5–2 mg/kg prednisone/prednisolone orally each day or its equivalent only after a response. Taper over at least 4–8 weeks when symptoms improve to G1
	Life-threatening or G4	
	Requirement for ≥10 mg/day prednisone or equivalent for >12 weeks	Permanently discontinue pembrolizumab
	Persistent G2/3 adverse reactions lasting ≥12 weeks	

Abbreviations: ADL, activities of daily living; ALT, alanine aminotransferase; AST, aspartate aminotransferase; ATG, anti-thymocyte globulin; SJS, Stevens-Johnson Syndrome; TEN, toxic epidermal necrolysis; ULN, upper limit of normal

Notes on general supportive care:
• Steroid taper in most cases will proceed over a minimum of one month but if symptoms improve rapidly a two-week taper can be considered. If steroids are administered for more than 4 weeks, consider PCP prophylaxis (cotrimoxazole 480 mg twice daily M/W/F or inhaled pentamidine if has cotrimoxazole allergy), regular random blood glucose, vitamin D level and starting calcium/vitamin D supplementation per guidelines

Adverse Events (N = 25)

Any-grade adverse events occurring in ≥2 patients	
	Pembrolizumab (N = 25)
Grade (%)	Any Grade
Diarrhea	16
Fatigue	16
Nausea	12
Dry mouth	8
Hypersensitivity	8
Hypothyroidism	8
Night sweats	8
Stomatitis	8
Thrombocytopenia	8
Vomiting	8

Adverse events were graded according to the National Cancer Institute Common Terminology Criteria for Adverse Events, version 4.0

Grade 3–4 adverse events occurring in ≥1 patient	
	Pembrolizumab (N = 25)
Grade (%)	Grade 3–4
Colitis*†	4%
Diarrhea*†	4%
General physical health deterioration*	4%
Increased blood thyroid-stimulating hormone*	4%

*All events were grade 3
†Occurred in the same patient
Adverse events were graded according to the National Cancer Institute Common Terminology Criteria for Adverse Events, version 4.0. As of the data cutoff date of 1 July 2015, there were no treatment-related study discontinuations or treatment-related deaths

5. Biliary: Gallbladder Cancer and Cholangiocarcinoma

Tim Greten, MD, PhD and Susanna Ulahannan, MD, MMed

Epidemiology

Gallbladder Cancer & Other
Biliary Incidence: 11,980 (male: 5600; female: 6380. Estimated new cases for 2020 in the United States)
Deaths: Estimated 4090 in 2020 (male: 1700; female: 2390)
Median age: 71 years
Gallbladder cancer: Women are two to six times more likely to develop gallbladder cancer than men
Cholangiocarcinoma: Slightly more common in men

Siegel R et al. CA Cancer J Clin 2020;70:7–30
Surveillance, Epidemiology and End Results (SEER) Program. Available at: http://seer.cancer.gov [accessed April 6, 2020]

Work-up

1. Early diagnosis of gallbladder or cholangiocellular carcinoma is nearly impossible or can be realized only in exceptional cases

2. In a patient with specific clinical symptoms or ultrasound suspicion of biliary tract cancer, a spiral CT and chest x-ray should be performed

3. Medically fit, nonjaundiced patients whose disease appears *potentially resectable* may proceed directly to surgical exploration without needle biopsy to avoid tumor spread. Consider a laparoscopic evaluation before open surgery owing to the common occurrence of otherwise nonvisible metastatic spread to the peritoneum

4. If the potential to perform a resection remains *uncertain* and for those with jaundice, a more precise assessment of tumor extent and lymph node involvement should be obtained with MRCP ± MRA, which may help to rule out vascular invasion and anomalous anatomic findings for surgical planning

5. If it is obvious that a resection will *not* be possible or if distant metastases are present, fine-needle biopsy for tissue confirmation should be obtained

6. In *nonresectable jaundiced* patients, depending on the location of the biliary obstruction, a percutaneous transhepatic cholangiography (PTC) or an endoscopic retrograde cholangiography (ERC) should be considered to guide placement of a stent

Fong Y et al. Cancer of the liver and biliary tree. In: Principles and Practice of Oncology, 6th ed. Baltimore, MD: Lippincott Williams & Wilkins 2001:1162–1203

Pathology

1. Gallbladder cancer	(60%)
2. Cholangiocarcinoma	(40%)
Intrahepatic	10%
Perihilar (Klatskin tumor)	40–60%
Distal	20–30%
Multifocal	<10%

Histopathology

1. Adenocarcinoma papillary, nodular, tubular, medullary	80–90%
2. Pleomorphic giant cell carcinoma	>10%
3. Squamous cell carcinoma	5%
4. Mucoid carcinoma	<1%
5. Anaplastic carcinoma	<1%
6. Cystadenocarcinoma	<1%
7. Clear cell carcinoma	<1%
8. Other rare forms	<1%

Lazcano-Ponce EC et al. CA Cancer J Clin 2001;51:349–364
Nakeeb A et al. Ann Surg 1996;224:463–475

Five-Year Survival (Intrahepatic Cholangiocarcinoma)

AJCC 8th Edition Stage	5-Year Survival, % (95% CI)
Stage IA	90.0 (47.3–98.5)
Stage IB	50.6 (19.9–75.0)
Stage II	55.1 (34.5–71.7)
Stage IIIA	49.7 (16.6–76.2)
Stage IIIB	16.2 (9.5–24.5)

Spolverato G et al. J Surg Oncol 2017;115:696–703

Staging

Gallbladder Cancer

Primary Tumor (T)

TX	Primary tumor cannot be assessed
T0	No evidence of primary tumor
Tis	Carcinoma in situ
T1	Tumor invades lamina propria or muscular layer
T1a	Tumor invades lamina propria
T1b	Tumor invades muscular layer
T2	Tumor invades the perimuscular connective tissue on the peritoneal side, without involvement of the serosa (visceral peritoneum) or tumor invades the perimuscular connective tissue on the hepatic side, with no extension into the liver
T2a	Tumor invades the perimuscular connective tissue on the peritoneal side, without involvement of the serosa (visceral peritoneum)
T2b	Tumor invades the perimuscular connective tissue on the hepatic side, with no extension into the liver
T3	Tumor perforates the serosa (visceral peritoneum) and/or directly invades the liver and/or one other adjacent organ or structure, such as the stomach, duodenum, colon, pancreas, omentum, or extrahepatic bile ducts
T4	Tumor invades main portal vein or hepatic artery or invades 2 or more extrahepatic organs or structures

Regional Lymph Nodes (N)*

NX	Regional lymph nodes cannot be assessed
N0	No regional lymph node metastasis
N1	Metastases to one to three regional lymph nodes
N2	Metastases to four or more regional lymph nodes

*At least 6 lymph nodes should be harvested and evaluated

Distant Metastasis (M)

M0	No distant metastasis
M1	Distant metastasis

Group	T	N	M
0	Tis	N0	M0
I	T1	N0	M0
IIA	T2a	N0	M0
IIB	T2b	N0	M0
IIIA	T3	N0	M0
IIIB	T1–3	N1	M0
IVA	T4	N0-1	M0
IVB	Any T	N2	M0
	Any T	Any N	M1

(continued)

Staging (continued)

Intrahepatic Bile Duct Staging

Primary Tumor (T)	
TX	Primary tumor cannot be assessed
T0	No evidence of primary tumor
Tis	Carcinoma in situ (intraductal tumor)
T1	Solitary tumor without vascular invasion, ≤5 cm or >5 cm
T1a	Solitary tumor ≤5 cm without vascular invasion
T1b	Solitary tumor >5 cm without vascular invasion
T2	Solitary tumor with intrahepatic vascular invasion or multiple tumors, with or without vascular invasion
T3	Tumor perforating the visceral peritoneum
T4	Tumor involving local extrahepatic structures by direct invasion

Regional Lymph Nodes (N)*	
NX	Regional lymph nodes cannot be assessed
N0	No regional lymph node metastasis
N1	Regional lymph node metastasis present

*At least 6 lymph nodes should be harvested and evaluated

Distant Metastasis (M)

M0	No distant metastasis		
M1	Distant metastasis		
Group	T	N	M
0	Tis	N0	M0
IA	T1a	N0	M0
IB	T1b	N0	M0
II	T2	N0	M0
IIIA	T3	N0	M0
IIIB	T4	N0	M0
	Any T	N1	M0
IV	Any T	Any N	M1

Perihilar Bile Ducts Staging

Primary Tumor (T)	
TX	Primary tumor cannot be assessed
T0	No evidence of primary tumor
Tis	Carcinoma in situ/high-grade dysplasia
T1	Tumor confined to the bile duct, with extension up to the muscle layer or fibrous tissue
T2a	Tumor invades beyond the wall of the bile duct to surrounding adipose tissue
T2b	Tumor invades adjacent hepatic parenchyma
T3	Tumor invades unilateral branches of the portal vein or hepatic artery
T4	Tumor invades the main portal vein or its branches bilaterally, or the common hepatic artery; or unilateral second-order biliary radicals with contralateral portal vein or hepatic artery involvement

Regional Lymph Nodes (N)	
NX	Regional lymph nodes cannot be assessed
N0	No regional lymph node metastasis
N1	One to three positive lymph nodes typically involving the hilar, cystic duct, common bile duct, hepatic artery, posterior pancreatoduodenal, and portal vein lymph nodes
N2	Four or more positive lymph nodes from the sites described for N1

Distant Metastasis (M)

M0	No distant metastasis		
M1	Distant metastasis		
Group	T	N	M
0	Tis	N0	M0
I	T1	N0	M0
II	T2a–b	N0	M0
IIIA	T3	N0	M0
IIIB	T4	N0	M0
IIIC	Any T	N1	M0
IVA	Any T	N2	M0
IVB	Any T	Any N	M1

(continued)

Staging (continued)

Distal Bile Duct Staging

Primary Tumor (T)	
TX	Primary tumor cannot be assessed
T0	No evidence of primary tumor
Tis	Carcinoma in situ/high-grade dysplasia
T1	Tumor invades the bile duct wall with a depth <5 mm
T2	Tumor invades the bile duct wall with a depth of 5–12 mm
T3	Tumor invades the bile duct wall with a depth >12 mm
T4	Tumor involves the celiac axis, superior mesenteric artery, and/or common hepatic artery

Regional Lymph Nodes (N)	
NX	Regional lymph nodes cannot be assessed
N0	No regional lymph node metastasis
N1	Metastasis in one to three regional lymph nodes
N2	Metastasis in four or more regional lymph nodes

Distant Metastasis (M)

M0	No distant metastasis		
M1	Distant metastasis		
Group	**T**	**N**	**M**
0	Tis	N0	M0
I	T1	N0	M0
IIA	T1	N1	M0
	T2	N0	M0
IIB	T2	N1	M0
	T3	N0	M0
	T3	N1	M0
IIIA	T1	N2	M0
	T2	N2	M0
	T3	N2	M0
IIIB	T4	N0	M0
	T4	N1	M0
	T4	N2	M0
IV	Any T	Any N	M1

Amin MB et al, editors. AJCC Cancer Staging Manual. 8th ed. New York: Springer; 2017.

Expert Opinion

Biliary tract malignancies include carcinoma of the gallbladder as well as of the intrahepatic, perihilar, and distal bile ducts. *Complete surgical resection remains the only curative modality for gallbladder cancer* (cholecystectomy, en bloc hepatic resection, and lymphadenectomy with or without bile duct excision). Postoperative (adjuvant) therapy for patients who undergo an operative resection might be considered with adjuvant chemotherapy and/or fluoropyrimidine-based radiochemotherapy, in selected cases. Patients with unresectable tumor without obvious metastatic disease and without jaundice may benefit from a regimen of fluorouracil- or capecitabine-based chemotherapy ± radiation. Metastatic disease is typically treated with systemic chemotherapy. Interventional procedures including brachytherapy and photodynamic therapy represent a therapeutic option for selected patients. However, overall survival of such patients remains poor (Razumilava and Gores, 2013)

Less than 20% of all patients have disease that is deemed resectable, and even after having undergone potential curative resection, recurrence rates are high. Thus for the majority of patients, systemic chemotherapy is the mainstay of treatment. The problem concerning chemotherapy is the fact that most studies conducted in the past have been single-center, nonrandomized, phase 2 studies with relatively small patient numbers (Hezel and Zhu, 2008). Heterogeneous inclusion criteria, inherent difficulties in measuring tumor response, and the lack of studies having applied RECIST (Response Evaluation Criteria in Solid Tumors) methodology for confirmation of treatment effects further contribute to our limited knowledge how to best treat patients with advanced tumors (Eckel and Schmid, 2007)

In the absence of validated data from prospective randomized studies, patients with biliary cancer were usually treated with gemcitabine or fluoropyrimidines ± platinum compounds. This, however, changed with the publication of the results from the ABC-01 trial that evaluated patients with locally advanced or metastatic cholangiocarcinoma, gallbladder cancer, or ampullary cancer (Valle et al, 2010). After a median follow-up of 8.2 months, the median overall survival was 11.7 months in the cisplatin plus gemcitabine group and 8.1 months in the gemcitabine group (hazard ratio, 0.64; 95% CI, 0.52–0.80; P <0.001). The median progression-free survival was 8 months in the cisplatin plus gemcitabine group and 5 months in the gemcitabine-only group (P <0.001). Adverse events were similar in both groups, with the exception of

(continued)

Expert Opinion (continued)

neutropenia—higher in the cisplatin plus gemcitabine group—although the number of neutropenia-associated infections was similar in the two groups. Consequently, a cisplatin + gemcitabine regimen has become the standard of care for this indication. An ongoing phase 3 SWOG trial is looking to assess the value of adding abraxane to gemcitabine plus cisplatin, a combination that in a single-arm phase 2 study reported a mPFS of 11.8 months and a median OS of 19.2 months (Shroff et al, 2019)

Two targets against which novel agents are under development and may receive or have received regulatory approvals are novel agents targeting IDH1 and FGF/FGFR:

- About 15% of patients with intrahepatic cholangiocarcinoma have IDH1 mutations (Weinberg et al, 2019) and about 15% have FGF/FGFR fusions (Jain et al, 2018), and these are mutually exclusive. Thus about 30% of all intrahepatic cholangiocarcinomas have targetable mutations. Because patients with IDH1 or FGF/FGFR fusions also have better prognosis, molecular profiling/genomic testing should become standard of care (Jusakul et al, 2017; Lamarca et al, 2020). The phase 3 ClarIDHy trial examined ivosidenib, an oral drug targeting mutant isocitrate dehydrogenase 1 (IDH1). The results showed a significant improvement in PFS of 1.3 months with a PFS of 2.7 months with ivosidenib compared to 1.4 months with placebo (Abou-Alfa et al, 2019)

- FGFR2 alterations are expected to be found in 9–16% of patients with cholangiocarcinoma. Results from the phase II FIGHT 202 trial looking at pemigatinib, an inhibitor of fibroblast growth factor FGFR 1, 2, and 3, reported a mPFS of 6.9 months and a median duration of response of 7.5 months in the 35% of patients with FGF/FGFR fusions or alterations who achieved a response (Abou-Alfa et al, 2020). These results led to an FDA approval in adults with previously treated, unresectable locally advanced or metastatic cholangiocarcinoma with a fibroblast growth factor receptor 2 (FGFR2) fusion or other rearrangement as detected by an FDA-approved (Foundation Medicine) test. Although the study enrolled patients previously treated with chemotherapy and this formed the basis of the FDA approval, one can expect that agents targeting FGFR2 will now undergo evaluation as front-line therapy alone or in combination

Finally, agents such as epidermal growth factor receptor blockers, HER2, BRAF inhibitors + MEK inhibitors, angiogenesis inhibitors, PARP inhibitors, and immune therapy may hold promise for improving the therapeutic results obtained with conventional chemotherapy alone, but clinical study results are pending (Sasaki et al, 2013). The changing landscape for cholangiocarcinoma will in the near future hopefully impact both prognosis and treatment choices

Intrahepatic cholangiocarcinoma

Patients who have undergone a tumor resection with or without ablation with negative margins may be followed up with observation, because there is no definitive adjuvant regimen to improve their overall survival. For individuals whose disease is resectable but who are left with positive margins after resection, consider (a) additional resection, (b) ablative therapy, or (c) combined radiation with or without chemotherapy using either fluorouracil- or capecitabine-based regimens or gemcitabine (Horgan et al, 2012). For patients with unresectable disease, therapeutic options include, depending on tumor location, extent of disease, and performance status: (a) chemotherapy with cisplatin plus gemcitabine or a fluorouracil- or capecitabine-based regimen, (b) combined radiochemotherapy, or (c) best supportive care

Extrahepatic cholangiocarcinoma

Patients with positive margins after resection should be considered candidates for either cisplatin plus gemcitabine or fluorouracil- or capecitabine-based chemotherapy with radiation (external beam therapy or brachytherapy) (Valero et al, 2012). The addition of adjuvant therapy in patients after potential curative surgical resection remains a subject of clinical investigation. Patients whose disease is deemed unresectable at the time of surgery should undergo biliary drainage if required, ideally nonsurgically; that is, by using a stent. Photodynamic therapy has demonstrated to be even more effective than stenting alone (Ortner et al, 2003). Given their overall poor prognosis, further options for patients with unresectable disease include (a) chemotherapy with cisplatin plus gemcitabine, (b) a clinical trial, (c) chemoradiation (fluorouracil- or capecitabine-based chemotherapy/RT), and (d) best supportive care

Abou-Alfa GK et al. ESMO Congress 2019. Abstract LBA10
Abou-Alfa et al, Lancet Oncol 2020;21:671–684
Eckel F et al. Br J Cancer 2007;96:896–902
Hezel AF et al. Oncologist 2008;13:415–423
Horgan AM et al. J Clin Oncol 2012;30:1934–1940
Jain et al. JCO Precision Oncol, 2018; doi: 10.1200/PO.17.00080 JCO [Epub ahead of print]
Jusakul A et al. Cancer Discov 2017;7:1116–1135
Lamarca A et al. J Natl Cancer Inst 2020;112:200–210
Ortner ME et al. Gastroenterology 2003;125:1355–1363
Razumilava N, Gores GJ. Clin Gastroenterol Hepatol 2013;11:13–21
Sasaki T et al. Korean J Intern Med 2013;28:515–524
Shroff et al. JAMA Oncol 2019;5: 824–830
Valero V et al. Expert Rev Gastroenterol Hepatol 2012;6:481–495
Valle J et al. N Engl J Med 2010;362:1273–1281
Weinberg et al. J Gastrointest Oncol 2019;10:652–662

(continued)

Expert Opinion (continued)

First-Line Chemotherapy in Advanced Biliary Cancer
Phase 3 and Randomized Phase 2 Trials

Regimen	#	%RR	PFS/ TTP*		OS*		References
Phase 3							
GEM + CDDP	204	26.1[†]	8.0	P<0.001	11.7	HR = 0.64 (95% CI, 0.52–0.80); P<0.001	Valle
GEM	206	15.5[†]	5.0		8.1		
GEM + oxaliplatin	26	30.8[‡]	8.5	P<0.001	9.5	P = 0.039	Sharma
5-FU + folinic acid	28	14.3[‡]	3.5		4.6		
BSC	27	0	2.8		4.5		
Randomized Phase 2							
GEM + CDDP	41	19.5	5.8	HR = 0.66 (95% CI, 0.41–1.05); P = 0.077	11.2	HR = 0.69 (95% CI, 0.42–1.13); P = 0.139	Okusaka
GEM	42	11.9	3.7		7.7		
GEM + S-1	30	20.0	5.6	95% CI 2.0–10.5	8.9	95% CI 5.8–11.9	Sasaki
GEM	32	9.4	4.3	95% CI 1.9–5.7	9.2	95% CI 5.2–14.6	
GEM + S-1	51	36.4	7.1	HR = 0.437 (95% CI, 0.286–0.669); P<0.0001	12.5	HR = 0.859 (95% CI, 0.543–1.360); P = 0.52	Morizane
S-1	50	17.4	4.2		9.0		
GEM + CDDP	49	19.6	5.7	HR = 0.85 (95% CI 0.52–1.36); P = 0.488	10.1	HR = 0.72 (95% CI 0.45–1.17); P = 0.187	Kang
S-1 + CDDP	47	23.8	5.4		9.9		

#, number of patients enrolled; %RR, percent response rate; BSC, best supportive care; CDDP, cisplatin; 5FU, fluorouracil; GEM, gemcitabine; S-1, an oral anticancer drug consisting of the fluorouracil prodrug tegafur and 2 biochemical modulators, 5-chloro-2,4-dihydroxypyridine (CDHP) and potassium oxonate (Oxo)
*Median values in months
[†]Not significant
[‡]P<0.001

Kang JH et al. Acta Oncol 2012;51:860–866
Morizane C et al. Cancer Sci 2013;104:1211–1216
Okusaka T et al. Br J Cancer 2010;103(4):469–474
Sasaki T et al. Cancer Chemother Pharmacol 2013;71:973–979
Sharma A et al. J Clin Oncol 2010;28:4581–4586
Valle J et al. N Engl J Med 2010;362:1273–128

ADJUVANT

BILIARY: GALLBLADDER CANCER AND CHOLANGIOCARCINOMA
REGIMEN: ORAL CAPECITABINE [BILCAP]

Primrose JN et al. Lancet Oncol 2019;20:663–673
Supplementary appendix to: Primrose JN et al. Lancet Oncol 2019;20:663–673

Capecitabine 1250 mg/m^2 per dose; administer orally twice daily (approximately every 12 hours, within 30 minutes after a meal) for 14 consecutive days (28 doses) on days 1–14, followed by 7 days without treatment, repeated every 21 days, for 8 cycles (total dosage/3-week cycle = 35,000 mg/m^2)

Notes:

- The median capecitabine dose in the study was 1250 mg/m^2 twice daily (IQR 1060.9–1250.0), and 55% of patients completed eight cycles of capecitabine
- Doses are rounded to use combinations of 500-mg and 150-mg tablets that most closely approximate calculated values
- Patients who miss a dose of capecitabine should be instructed to continue with the usual dosing schedule without making up the missed dose and to contact their physician for further instructions
- Patients who take too much (ie, overdose) capecitabine should contact their doctor immediately and present to the emergency department for further care and consideration for timely treatment with the antidote uridine triacetate
- Initial capecitabine dosage should be decreased by 25% in patients with moderate renal impairment (baseline creatinine clearance = 30–50 mL/min [0.5–0.83 mL/s]). Capecitabine use is contraindicated in persons with severe renal impairment (creatinine clearance <30 mL/min [<0.5 mL/s])
- Although food decreases the rate and extent of drug absorption and the time to peak plasma concentration and systemic exposure (AUC) for both capecitabine and fluorouracil, product labeling recommends giving capecitabine within 30 minutes after the end of a meal because established safety and efficacy data are based on administration with food

Supportive Care
Antiemetic prophylaxis
Emetogenic potential is **MINIMAL–LOW**
See Chapter 42 for antiemetic recommendations

Hematopoietic growth factor (CSF) prophylaxis
Primary prophylaxis is **NOT** indicated
See Chapter 43 for more information

Antimicrobial prophylaxis
Risk of fever and neutropenia is **LOW**
   Antimicrobial primary prophylaxis to be considered:
- Antibacterial—not indicated
- Antifungal—not indicated
- Antiviral—not indicated unless patient previously had an episode of HSV

Diarrhea management
Latent or delayed-onset diarrhea
Loperamide 4 mg orally initially after the first loose or liquid stool, *then*
Loperamide 2 mg orally every 2 hours during waking hours, *plus*
Loperamide 4 mg orally every 4 hours during hours of sleep
- Continue for at least 12 hours after diarrhea resolves
- Recurrent diarrhea after a 12-hour diarrhea-free interval is treated as a new episode
- Rehydrate orally with fluids and electrolytes during a diarrheal episode
- If a patient develops blood or mucus in stool, dehydration, or hemodynamic instability, or if diarrhea persists >48 hours despite loperamide, stop loperamide and hospitalize the patient for IV hydration

Alternatively, a trial of **diphenoxylate hydrochloride 2.5 mg with atropine sulfate** 0.025 mg (eg, Lomotil)
- Initial adult dose is 2 tablets 4 times daily until control has been achieved, after which the dose may be reduced to meet individual requirements. Control may often be maintained with as little as 2 tablets daily
- Clinical improvement of acute diarrhea is usually observed within 48 hours. If improvement of chronic diarrhea after treatment with a maximum daily dose of 8 tablets is not observed within 10 days, control is unlikely with further administration

(continued)

(continued)

Persistent diarrhea:
  Octreotide 100–150 mcg subcutaneously 3 times daily. Maximum total daily dose is 1500 mcg
Antibiotic therapy during latent or delayed-onset diarrhea:
  A fluoroquinolone (eg, **ciprofloxacin** 500 mg orally every 12 hours) if absolute neutrophil count <500/mm^3 with or without accompanying fever in association with diarrhea
  • Antibiotics should also be administered if patient is hospitalized with prolonged diarrhea and should be continued until diarrhea resolves

Abigerges D et al. J Natl Cancer Inst 1994;86:446–449
Rothenberg ML et al. J Clin Oncol 2001;19:3801–3807
Wadler S et al. J Clin Oncol 1998;16:3169–3178

Hand-foot syndrome
For patients who develop a hand-foot syndrome, use topical emollients (eg, Aquaphor), topical or orally administered steroids, antihistamine agents (H$_1$-receptor antagonists), or pyridoxine 50–150 mg/day administered orally

Treatment Modifications

CAPECITABINE DOSE MODIFICATIONS

	Capecitabine dose
Starting dose	1250 mg/m^2/dose twice per day
Dose level −1	1000 mg/m^2/dose twice per day
Dose level −2	750 mg/m^2/dose twice per day

Adverse Event	Treatment Modification
Hematologic Toxicities	
ANC <1500/mm^3 on day 1 of a cycle OR platelet count <75,000/mm^3 on day 1 of a cycle	Delay start of cycle until ANC ≥1500/mm^3 and platelet count ≥75,000/mm^3. Upon recovery, resume capecitabine with any applicable dose reductions as described elsewhere in this table
ANC ≥500/mm^3 and <1000/mm^3 during a cycle OR Platelet count ≥25,000/mm^3 and <50,000/mm^3 during a cycle	Withhold capecitabine until recovery to ANC ≥1500/mm^3 or baseline and platelets to ≥75,000/mm^3 or baseline, then administer one lower dose level in subsequent cycles
ANC <500/mm^3 during a cycle OR Platelet count <25,000/mm^3 during a cycle	Discontinue permanently OR If physician deems it to be in the patient's best interest to continue, interrupt until recovery to ANC ≥1500/mm^3 or baseline and platelets to ≥75,000/mm^3 or baseline, then resume therapy with doses one lower dose level in subsequent cycle(s)
Prior episode of neutropenic fever (single temperature ≥38.3°C or a temperature ≥38.0°C sustained for ≥1 hour with an ANC <500/mm^3 or predicted to be <500/mm^3 within 48 hours)	Withhold capecitabine until recovery, then *permanently* reduce the dosage by one level. Consider use of filgrastim to treat neutropenic fever and/or for secondary prophylaxis with subsequent cycles according to local practice
Other Toxicities	
G2/3/4 diarrhea	Withhold capecitabine; provide supportive care. Do not resume capecitabine until toxicity resolves to G≤1. If toxicity is G4 then *permanently* discontinue capecitabine. Otherwise, in subsequent cycle(s) *permanently* reduce the capecitabine dosage by 1 dose level
G2/3/4 mucositis	
G2/3/4 dehydration	
G2/3 hand-and-foot syndrome or palmar-plantar erythrodysesthesia or chemotherapy-induced acral erythema*	
Stevens-Johnson syndrome and toxic epidermal necrolysis (severe mucocutaneous reactions, some with fatal outcome)	Permanently discontinue capecitabine

(continued)

Treatment Modifications (continued)

CAPECITABINE DOSE MODIFICATIONS

Other Toxicities

Capecitabine-induced coronary vasospasm/cardiac ischemia	Permanently discontinue capecitabine
Creatinine clearance 30–50 mL/minute	Reduce the capecitabine dosage by 1 dose level
Creatinine clearance <30 mL/minute	Withhold capecitabine

ANC, absolute neutrophil count; CBC, complete blood count

Grading of hand-foot syndrome
G1: Numbness, dysesthesia/paresthesia, tingling, painless swelling or erythema of the hands and/or feet and/or discomfort which does not disrupt normal activities
G2: Painful erythema and swelling of the hands and/or feet and/or discomfort affecting the patient's activities of daily living
G3: Moist desquamation, ulceration, blistering or severe pain of the hands and/or feet and/or severe discomfort that causes the patient to be unable to work or perform activities of daily living

Patient Population Studied

Histologically confirmed cholangiocarcinoma or muscle-invasive gallbladder cancer who had undergone a macroscopically complete resection (which includes liver resection, pancreatic resection, or, less commonly, both) with curative intent, and an Eastern Cooperative Oncology Group performance status of <2

Baseline characteristics

Capecitabine group (n = 223)

Sex	
Female	112 (50%)
Male	111 (50%)
Age, years	62 (55–68)

Primary tumor site	
Intrahepatic cholangiocarcinoma	43 (19%)
Hilar cholangiocarcinoma	65 (29%)
Muscle-invasive gallbladder carcinoma	39 (17%)
Mucosal gallbladder carcinoma	0
Lower common bile duct cholangiocarcinoma	76 (34%)

Resection status	
R0	139 (62%)
R1	84 (38%)

ECOG performance status	
0	100 (45%)
1	116 (52%)
2	7 (3%)

Tumor stage	
I	57 (26%)
II	137 (61%)
III	28 (13%)
IV	1 (<1%)

Lymph node status	
N0	115 (52%)
N1	108 (48%)

Disease grade	
Well differentiated	34 (15%)
Moderately differentiated	110 (49%)
Poorly differentiated	64 (29%)
Not determined	12 (5%)
Not known	3 (1%)
Hemoglobin (g/dL)	12 (12–13)

White blood cell count, × 10^9 cells per L	7 (6–8)
Absolute neutrophil count, × 10^9 cells per L	4 (3–5)
Platelet count, × 10^9 per L	279 (231–346)
Glomerular filtration rate, mL/min	92 (77–113)
Aspartate aminotransferase, U/L	27 (22–35)
Alanine aminotransferase, U/L	27 (20–41)
Bilirubin, μmol/L	8 (6–10)
Creatinine, μmol/L	67 (58–76)
Tumor size, mm	25 (19–45)

Resection type	
Liver	129 (58%)
Pancreas	92 (41%)
Other	2 (1%)

Data are n (%) or median (IQR)
ECOG, Eastern Cooperative Oncology Group; N0, negative; N1, positive; R0, negative resection margin; R1, positive resection margin

Efficacy

	Capecitabine	Observation	Statistics
Disease recurrence	134/223 (60%)	146/224 (65%)	—
Intention-to-treat analysis			
Median OS	51.1 months (95% CI 34.6–59.1)	36.4 months (95% CI 29.7–44.5)	HR 0.81 95% CI 0.63–1.04; P = 0.097
Median OS, adjusted for nodal status, grade of disease, and sex	—	—	HR 0.71 95% CI 0.55–0.92; P = 0.010
Median RFS	24.4 months (95% CI 18.6–35.9)	17.5 months (95% CI, 12.0–23.8)	—
Adjusted RFS first 24 months	—	—	HR 0.75 95% CI 0.58–0.98; P = 0.033
Adjusted RFS beyond months	—	—	HR 1.48 95% CI 0.80–2.77; P = 0.21
Per protocol analysis			
Median OS	53 months (95% CI 40–NR)	36 months (95% CI 30–44)	Adjusted HR 0.75 95% CI 0.58–0.97; P = 0.028
Median RFS	25.9 months (95% CI 19.8–46.3)	17.4 months (95% CI, 12.0–23.7)	
Adjusted RFS first 24 months	—	—	HR 0.70 95% CI 0.54–0.92; P = 0.0093
Adjusted RFS beyond 24 months	—	—	HR 1.55 95% CI 0.82–2.93; P = 0.18

NR, not reached; OS, overall survival; RFS, recurrence-free survival

Toxicity

Adverse events in the capecitabine group (n = 213)

	Grades 1 and 2	Grade 3
Hand-foot syndrome	127 (60%)	43 (20%)
Fatigue	159 (75%)	16 (8%)
Diarrhea	121 (57%)	16 (8%)
Gastrointestinal or abdominal pain not otherwise specified	61 (29%)	10 (5%)
Neutrophils or granulocytes	45 (21%)	4 (2%)
Bilirubin	42 (20%)	3 (1%)
Nausea	106 (50%)	2 (1%)
Oral mucositis or stomatitis	94 (44%)	2 (1%)
Skin rash or desquamation (dermatology)	31 (15%)	2 (1%)
Insomnia (constitutional symptoms)	—	2 (1%)
Gastrointestinal ascites	—	2 (1%)

(continued)

Toxicity (continued)

Adverse events in the capecitabine group (n = 213)

	Grades 1 and 2	Grade 3
Biliary sepsis	—	2 (1%)
Vomiting	49 (23%)	1 (<1%)
Fever	30 (14%)	1 (<1%)
Low platelet count	25 (12%)	1 (<1%)
Dry skin (dermatology/skin)	—	1 (<1%)
Lip swelling (dermatology/skin)	—	1 (<1%)
Gastrointestinal dehydration	—	1 (<1%)
Gastrointestinal obstruction	—	1 (<1%)
Infection	—	1 (<1%)
Limb edema (lymphatics)	—	1 (<1%)
Alanine aminotransferase (metabolic/laboratory)	—	1 (<1%)
Aspartate aminotransferase (metabolic/laboratory)	—	1 (<1%)
Alkaline phosphatase (metabolic/laboratory)	—	1 (<1%)
Low serum potassium (metabolic/laboratory)	—	1 (<1%)
γ-glutamyltransferase (metabolic/laboratory)	—	1 (<1%)
Ischemic cardiac pain	—	1 (<1%)
General pain	—	1 (<1%)
Musculoskeletal back pain	—	1 (<1%)
Musculoskeletal joint pain	—	1 (<1%)
Vascular thrombosis or embolism	—	1 (<1%)

Data are n (%). All grade 3 events are reported. Only those grades 1 and 2 events experienced by 10% or more of patients are reported. One (<1%) patient had grade 4 cardiac ischemia or infarction. No grade 5 adverse events were reported

Notes:
- 99 (46%) had at least one dose reduction
- 69 (32%) discontinued treatment because of toxicity, the most common complaints were hand-foot syndrome in ten patients (14%), diarrhea in nine patients (13%), and other (patients could cite more than one toxicity type) in 21 (31%) patients

Therapy Monitoring

1. *Prior to each cycle:* History and physical exam, CBC with differential, BUN, serum creatinine, serum electrolytes, ALT, AST, total bilirubin, and alkaline phosphate
2. *On day 8 and 15:* CBC with differential, BUN, serum creatinine, serum electrolytes, ALT, AST, total bilirubin, and alkaline phosphate
3. Patients receiving concomitant capecitabine and oral coumarin-derivative anticoagulant therapy should have their anticoagulant response (INR or prothrombin time) monitored frequently in order to adjust the anticoagulant dose accordingly
4. Monitor for signs/symptoms of hand-foot syndrome, Stevens-Johnson syndrome and toxic epidermal necrolysis, hydration status, diarrhea, mucositis, coronary vasospasm, and signs of infection

Note: Toxicity in the setting of DPD deficiency occurs early and is characterized by severe mucositis, diarrhea, neutropenia, and neurotoxicity. It occurs in individuals with homozygous or certain compound heterozygous mutations in the DPD gene that result in complete or near complete absence of DPD activity. Discontinue capecitabine permanently. There are insufficient data to recommend a specific dose in patients with partial DPD activity as measured by any specific test

ADVANCED DISEASE

BILIARY: GALLBLADDER CANCER AND CHOLANGIOCARCINOMA
REGIMEN: GEMCITABINE + CISPLATIN

Valle J et al. N Engl J Med 2010;362:1273–1281

Note: Biliary obstruction per se is not considered to be disease progression in the absence of radiologically confirmed disease progression, and treatment can be recommenced after initial or further biliary stenting and normalization of liver function

Hydration before cisplatin: ≥1000 mL 0.9% sodium chloride injection (0.9% NS); administer by intravenous infusion over ≥1 hour

Cisplatin 25 mg/m^2 per dose; administer intravenously in 50–1000 mL 0.9% NS over 1 hour for 2 doses on days 1 and 8, every 3 weeks for 4 cycles (total dosage/cycle = 50 mg/m^2), *followed by:*

Hydration after cisplatin: ≥1000 mL 0.9% NS; administer by intravenous infusion over ≥1 hour

Gemcitabine 1000 mg/m^2 per dose; administer intravenously in 50–250 mL 0.9% NS over 30 minutes for 2 doses on days 1 and 8, every 3 weeks, for 4 cycles (total dosage/cycle = 2000 mg/m^2)

- Gemcitabine may be administered concurrently with hydration after cisplatin administration is completed

Note: In the absence of disease progression at 12 weeks, treatment with the same regimen may continue for an additional 12 weeks

Supportive Care
Antiemetic prophylaxis
Emetogenic potential is **HIGH**
See Chapter 42 for antiemetic recommendations

Hematopoietic growth factor (CSF) prophylaxis
Primary prophylaxis is **NOT** indicated
See Chapter 43 for more information

Antimicrobial prophylaxis
Risk of fever and neutropenia is **LOW**
  Antimicrobial primary prophylaxis to be considered:
- Antibacterial—not indicated
- Antifungal—not indicated
- Antiviral—not indicated, unless patient previously had an episode of HSV

Treatment Modifications

Adverse Event	Dose Modification
Cisplatin	
Any G ≥3 adverse event Hematologic toxicity, abnormal renal function, nausea, vomiting, edema, or tinnitus	Decrease cisplatin dosage by 25%
Reduction in creatinine clearance* to ≤60% of on study value	Delay therapy 1 week. If creatinine clearance does not recover to pretreatment values, then consider reducing cisplatin dose
Creatinine clearance* 40–60 mL/min (0.66–1 mL/s)	Consider reducing cisplatin so that dose in milligrams equals the creatinine clearance value in mL/min (mL/s × 1/0.0166)†
Creatinine clearance <40 mL/min (<0.66 mL/s)	Hold cisplatin
Clinically significant ototoxicity	Discontinue cisplatin
Persistent (>14 days) peripheral neuropathy without functional impairment	Decrease cisplatin dosage by 50%
Clinically significant sensory loss—persistent (>14 days) peripheral neuropathy with functional impairment	Discontinue cisplatin
Day 1 WBC count <2000/mm^3 or platelet count <100,000/mm^3	Delay cisplatin and gemcitabine for 1 week or until myelosuppression resolves
Recurrent treatment delay because of myelosuppression	Delay cisplatin for 1 week, or until myelosuppression resolves, then decrease cisplatin and gemcitabine dosages by 25% during subsequent treatments
Sepsis during an episode of neutropenia	

*Creatinine clearance is used as a measure of glomerular filtration rate
†This also applies to patients with creatinine clearance (GFR) of 40–60 mL/min at the outset of treatment

Patient Population Studied

Patients with a diagnosis of nonresectable, recurrent, or metastatic biliary tract carcinoma (intrahepatic or extrahepatic cholangiocarcinoma, gallbladder cancer, or ampullary carcinoma); an Eastern Cooperative Oncology Group performance status of 0, 1, or 2; and an estimated life expectancy of more than 3 months. Other eligibility criteria included a total bilirubin level ≤1.5 times the upper limit of the normal range; liver-enzyme levels that were ≤5 times the upper limit of the normal range; renal function with levels of serum urea and serum creatinine that were <1.5 times the upper limit of the normal range; and an estimated glomerular filtration rate ≥45 mL/minute (≥0.75 mL/s)

Efficacy (N = 161)*

	All Patients (N = 161)	Gallbladder Tumors[†] (N = 61)	Bile Duct and Ampullary Tumors[†] (N = 100)
Complete response	0.6%	0	1%
Partial response	25.5%	37.7%	18%
Stable disease[‡]	55.3%	47.5%	60%
Progressive disease	18.6%	14.8%	21%
Median progression-free survival	8.0 months	—	—
Median overall survival	11.7 months	—	—

*RECIST (Response Evaluation Criteria in Solid Tumors) (Therasse P et al. J Natl Cancer Inst 2000;92:205–216)
[†]No differences in RR between gallbladder and cholangiocarcinoma subgroups
[‡]Not defined

Toxicity (N = 198)

	% G3/4
Hematologic	
Decreased WBC	15.7
Decreased platelet counts	8.6
Decreased hemoglobin concentration	7.6
Decreased ANC	25.3
Any hematologic toxic effect	32.3
Liver Function	
Increased alanine amino transferase level	9.6
Other abnormal liver function	13.1
Any abnormal liver function	16.7
Nonhematologic	
Alopecia	1
Anorexia	3
Fatigue	18.7
Nausea	4
Vomiting	5.1
Impaired renal function	1.5
Infection	
Without neutropenia	6.1
With neutropenia	10.1
Biliary sepsis	4.0
Any type	18.2
Deep vein thrombosis	2.0
Thromboembolic event	3.5
Other	54.5
Any G3/4 toxic effect	70.7

NCI Common Terminology Criteria for Adverse Events v3.0

Therapy Monitoring

1. *Between days 8 and 10:* CBC with differential
2. *Before each cycle:* Electrolytes, renal function, LFTs
3. *Response assessment:* Every 2–3 cycles

ADVANCED DISEASE

BILIARY: GALLBLADDER CANCER AND CHOLANGIOCARCINOMA
REGIMEN: GEMCITABINE + OXALIPLATIN (GEMOX)

André T et al. Ann Oncol 2004;15:1339–1343

Gemcitabine 1000 mg/m^2; administer by intravenous infusion in 250 mL 0.9% sodium chloride injection at an infusion rate of 10 mg/m^2 per minute (over 100 minutes) on day 1, every 2 weeks (total dosage every 2 weeks = 1000 mg/m^2)

Oxaliplatin 100 mg/m^2; administer by intravenous infusion in 250–500 mL of 5% dextrose injection over 2 hours on day 2, every 2 weeks (total dosage every 2 weeks = 100 mg/m^2)

Supportive Care
Antiemetic prophylaxis
Emetogenic potential with gemcitabine (day 1) is **LOW**
Emetogenic potential with oxaliplatin (day 2) is **MODERATE**
See Chapter 42 for antiemetic recommendations

Hematopoietic growth factor (CSF) prophylaxis
Primary prophylaxis is **NOT** *indicated*
See Chapter 43 for more information

Antimicrobial prophylaxis
Risk of fever and neutropenia is **LOW**
   Antimicrobial primary prophylaxis to be considered:
   • Antibacterial—not indicated
   • Antifungal—not indicated
   • Antiviral—not indicated unless patient previously had an episode of HSV

Toxicity (N = 56)

G3 Neutropenia	12.5%
G3 Thrombocytopenia	9%
Peripheral sensory neuropathy	7.1%
G2 Alopecia	5.3%
G3 Nausea/vomiting	3.5%
G3 Diarrhea	—

NCI, CTC, National Cancer Institute (USA) Common Toxicity Criteria, version 2.0. Available at: http://ctep.cancer.gov/protocolDevelopment/electronic_applications/ctc.htm [accessed December 7, 2013]

Therapy Monitoring

1. *Every week:* CBCs with differential
2. *Before each cycle:* Complete biochemical profile
3. *Response assessment:* Every 2 months

Treatment Modifications

Adverse Event	Dose Modification
Nadir WBC <1000/mm^3, ANC <500/mm^3, or platelets <50,000/mm^3	Decrease gemcitabine and oxaliplatin dosages by 25% in subsequent cycles
G ≥3 nonhematologic adverse event during the previous treatment cycle	
WBC <3000/mm^3 or platelets <75,000/mm^3 on day of treatment	Delay chemotherapy for up to 2 weeks
Treatment delay >2 weeks for recovery from hematologic adverse events	Discontinue treatment

Efficacy (N = 31)*

Overall response rate	35.5%
Stable disease	26%
Progressive disease	38.5%
Median progression-free survival	5.7 months
Overall survival	14.3 months

*André T et al. Ann Oncol 2004;15:1339–1343

Complete response	7.7%
Partial response	23%
Stable disease	38%
Progressive disease	31%
Median overall survival	9.5 months
Median progression-free survival	8.5 months

Sharma A et al. J Clin Oncol 2010;28:4581–4586

Patient Population Studied

A study of 33 patients with advanced biliary tract carcinoma

ADVANCED DISEASE

BILIARY: GALLBLADDER CANCER AND CHOLANGIOCARCINOMA
REGIMEN: GEMCITABINE + CAPECITABINE

Koeberle D et al. J Clin Oncol 2008;26:3702–3708

Gemcitabine 1000 mg/m^2 per dose; administer intravenously in 50–250 mL 0.9% sodium chloride injection over 30 minutes for 2 doses on days 1 and 8, every 3 weeks (total dosage/cycle = 2000 mg/m^2)

Capecitabine 650 mg/m^2 per dose; administer orally twice daily (approximately every 12 hours) for 14 consecutive days (28 doses), days 1–14, every 3 weeks (total dosage/cycle = 18,200 mg/m^2)

Supportive Care
Antiemetic prophylaxis
Emetogenic potential is **LOW**
See Chapter 42 for antiemetic recommendations

Hematopoietic growth factor (CSF) prophylaxis
Primary prophylaxis is **NOT** *indicated*
See Chapter 43 for more information

Antimicrobial prophylaxis
Risk of fever and neutropenia is **LOW**
   Antimicrobial primary prophylaxis to be considered:
   • Antibacterial—not indicated
   • Antifungal—not indicated
   • Antiviral—not indicated, unless patient previously had an episode of HSV

Treatment Modifications

Adverse Event	Dose Modification
Nadir WBC <1000/mm^3, ANC <500/mm^3, or Platelets <50,000/mm^3	Delay chemotherapy for up to 3 weeks until adverse events are G ≤1, then reduce gemcitabine dosage by 25%
Any G3 nonhematologic toxicity during a previous cycle	Delay chemotherapy for up to 3 weeks until adverse events are G ≤1, then decrease gemcitabine and capecitabine dosages by 25%
Any G4 nonhematologic toxicity during a previous cycle	Delay chemotherapy for up to 3 weeks until adverse events are G ≤1, then decrease gemcitabine and capecitabine dosages by 50%

Patient Population Studied

A total of 44 chemotherapy-naïve patients with unresectable, locally advanced or metastatic biliary tract cancer. Patients were required to be symptomatic and have at least 1 of the following characteristics at baseline: Karnofsky performance score 60–80, average analgesic consumption of ≥10 mg of morphine equivalents per day, and average pain intensity score of ≥20 mm out of a maximum of 100 mm based on a linear analog self-assessment (LASA ≥2/10) scale. No prior chemotherapy for advanced disease was allowed

Efficacy (N = 44)

Complete response	1 (2%)
Partial responses	10 (23%)
Stable disease*	24 (55%)
Progression/nonassessable	9 (20%)
Median time to progression	7.2 months
Median overall survival	13.2 months

*Stable disease lasting for ≥8 weeks
RECIST Criteria (Response Evaluation Criteria in Solid Tumors) (Therasse P et al. J Natl Cancer Inst 2000;92:205–216)

Toxicity (N = 44)

	% G1/2	% G3/4
Hematologic		
Anemia	91	2
Leukocytopenia	71	11
Thrombocytopenia	63	7
Nonhematologic		
Nausea	50	5
Vomiting	32	2
Diarrhea	21	2
Stomatitis	9	0
Anorexia	52	7
Fatigue	62	11
Hand-foot syndrome	11	0

NCI, CTC, National Cancer Institute (USA) Common Toxicity Criteria, version 2.0. Available at: http://ctep.cancer.gov/protocolDevelopment/electronic_applications/ctc.htm [accessed December 7, 2013]

Therapy Monitoring

1. *Between days 8 and 10:* CBC with differential
2. *Before each cycle:* Electrolytes, renal function, LFTs
3. *Response assessment:* Every 3 cycles

ADVANCED DISEASE

BILIARY: GALLBLADDER CANCER AND CHOLANGIOCARCINOMA
REGIMEN: CAPECITABINE + OXALIPLATIN

Nehls O et al. Br J Cancer 2008;98:309–315

Capecitabine 1000 mg/m² per dose; administer orally twice daily (approximately every 12 hours) for 14 consecutive days (28 doses) on days 1–14, every 3 weeks (total dosage/cycle = 28,000 mg/m²)

Oxaliplatin 130 mg/m²; administer intravenously in 250–500 mL 5% dextrose injection over 2 hours on day 1, every 3 weeks (total dosage/cycle = 130 mg/m²)

Supportive Care
Antiemetic prophylaxis
Emetogenic potential for oxaliplatin is **MODERATE**
Emetogenic potential on days with capecitabine alone is **LOW**
See Chapter 42 for antiemetic recommendations

Hematopoietic growth factor (CSF) prophylaxis
Primary prophylaxis is **NOT** *indicated*
See Chapter 43 for more information

Antimicrobial prophylaxis
Risk of fever and neutropenia is **LOW**
 Antimicrobial primary prophylaxis to be considered:
 • Antibacterial—not indicated
 • Antifungal—not indicated
 • Antiviral—not indicated, unless patient previously had an episode of HSV

Treatment Modifications

Adverse Event	Dose Modification
Capecitabine	
Any G ≥2 adverse event except alopecia	Interrupt/delay capecitabine until adverse event improves to G ≤1, and decrease capecitabine dosage by 25% during subsequent cycles
Second occurrence of G ≥2 adverse event	Interrupt/delay capecitabine until adverse event improves to G ≤1 and decrease capecitabine dosage by 50% during subsequent cycles
Third occurrence of G ≥2 adverse event	Discontinue capecitabine use permanently
Oxaliplatin	
Any G ≥3 adverse event	Decrease oxaliplatin dosage by 25%
Persistent (>14 days) peripheral neuropathy without functional impairment	Decrease oxaliplatin dosage by 50%
Persistent (>14 days) peripheral neuropathy with functional impairment	Discontinue oxaliplatin use permanently

Patient Population Studied

A study of 65 chemotherapy-naïve patients with advanced biliary tract cancer (adenocarcinomas of the gallbladder [GBC] or the intrahepatic [ICC] or extrahepatic [ECC] biliary tract) not amenable to curative surgical treatment strategies, ECOG performance status ≤2. Patients were stratified prospectively between 2 groups based on location of the primary, that is, gallbladder cancer or extrahepatic cholangiocarcinoma versus intrahepatic cholangiocarcinoma

Efficacy*

	GBC/ECC (N = 47)	ICC (N = 18)
Complete response	2 (4%)	0
Partial response	11 (23%)	0
Stable disease†	23 (49%)	6 (33%)
Progression	11 (23%)	12 (67%)
Median time to progression	6.5 months	2.2 months
Median overall survival	12.8 months	5.2 months

*WHO criteria
†Stable disease was defined as a reduction <50% for an unspecified duration or an increase <25% of measurable lesions according to the previous method, with the absence of any new lesions

Toxicity (N = 65)

	% G2	% G3	% G4
Hematologic			
Anemia	18	0	0
Neutropenia	14	0	2
Thrombocytopenia	20	9	2
Nonhematologic			
Nausea/vomiting	29	6	0
Diarrhea	18	5	2
Stomatitis	2	0	0
Hand-foot syndrome	9	5	NA
Infection	15	0	3
Thromboembolic event	0	0	2
Peripheral neuropathy	35	15	2

NCI, CTC, National Cancer Institute (USA) Common Toxicity Criteria, version 2.0. Available at: http://ctep.cancer.gov/protocolDevelopment/electronic_applications/ctc.htm [accessed December 7, 2013]

Therapy Monitoring

1. *Between days 8 and 10:* CBC with differential
2. *Before each cycle:* Electrolytes, renal function, LFTs
3. *Response assessment:* Every 2–3 cycles

ADVANCED DISEASE

BILIARY: GALLBLADDER CANCER AND CHOLANGIOCARCINOMA
REGIMEN:
GEMCITABINE + NAB-PACLITAXEL + CISPLATIN

Shroff RT et al. JAMA Oncol 2019;5:824–830
Supplement to: Shroff RT et al. JAMA Oncol 2019;5:824–830

Hydration before each dose of cisplatin: ≥1000 mL 0.9% sodium chloride injection (0.9% NS); administer by intravenous infusion over ≥1 hour prior to cisplatin on days 1 and 8

Paclitaxel protein-bound particles for injectable suspension (*nab-paclitaxel*) 100 mg/m^2 per dose intravenously over 30 minutes once weekly for 2 doses on days 1 and 8, every 21 days, until disease progression (total dosage/3-week cycle = 200 mg/m^2), *followed by:*

Cisplatin 25 mg/m^2 per dose; administer intravenously in 50–1000 mL 0.9% NS over 1 hour once weekly for 2 doses on days 1 and 8, every 21 days, until disease progression (total dosage/3-week cycle = 50 mg/m^2), *followed by:*

Gemcitabine HCl 800 mg/m^2 per dose intravenously in 50–250 mL 0.9% NS over 30 minutes once weekly for 2 doses on days 1 and 8, every 21 days, until disease progression (total dosage/3-week cycle = 1600 mg/m^2)

Hydration after cisplatin: ≥1000 mL 0.9% NS; administer by intravenous infusion over ≥1 hour following cisplatin on days 1 and 8

Supportive Care
Antiemetic prophylaxis
Emetogenic potential is **HIGH**. *Potential for delayed symptoms.*
See Chapter 42 for antiemetic recommendations

Hematopoietic growth factor (CSF) prophylaxis
Primary prophylaxis is **NOT** *indicated*
See Chapter 43 for more information

Antimicrobial prophylaxis
Risk of fever and neutropenia is **LOW**
   Antimicrobial primary prophylaxis to be considered:
   • Antibacterial—not indicated
   • Antifungal—not indicated
   • Antiviral—not indicated unless patient previously had an episode of HSV

Diarrhea management
Latent or delayed-onset diarrhea*:
   Loperamide 4 mg orally initially after the first loose or liquid stool, *then* 2-4 mg orally every 2-4 hours or **diphenoxylate hydrochloride** 2.5 mg **with atropine sulfate** 0.025 mg (e.g., Lomotil®)

Persistent diarrhea:
   Octreotide 100–150 mcg subcutaneously 3 times daily. Maximum total daily dose is 1500 mcg
Antibiotic therapy during latent or delayed-onset diarrhea:
   A fluoroquinolone (eg, **ciprofloxacin** 500 mg orally every 12 hours) if absolute neutrophil count <500/mm^3 with or without accompanying fever in association with diarrhea
   • Antibiotics should also be administered if patient is hospitalized with prolonged diarrhea and should be continued until diarrhea resolves

*Abigerges D et al. J Natl Cancer Inst 1994;86:446–449
Rothenberg ML et al. J Clin Oncol 2001;19:3801–3807
Wadler S et al. J Clin Oncol 1998;16:3169–3178

Treatment Modifications

Dose Levels

	nab-Paclitaxel (mg/m²)	Gemcitabine HCl (mg/m²)	Cisplatin (mg/m²)
Starting dose	100	800	25
Dose level −1	75	600	25
Dose level −2	50	600	25
Dose level −3	50	600	20

Dose Adjustments on Day 1 of Each Treatment Cycle for Hematologic Toxicity

ANC		Platelets	Timing
≥1500/mm³	AND	≥100,000/mm³	Treat on time
<1500/mm³	OR	<100,000/mm³	Delay by 1 week intervals until recovery

Dose Adjustments on Day 8 of a Treatment Cycle for Hematologic Toxicity

Blood Counts	*nab*-Paclitaxel, gemcitabine, and cisplatin
ANC >1000/mm³ *and* platelets ≥75,000/mm³	100%
ANC 500–1000/mm³ *or* platelets 50,000–74,999/mm³	Decrease dose by 1 level (treat on time)
ANC <500/mm³ *or* platelets <50,000/mm³	Hold and administer filgrastim*

Note: Febrile patients (regardless of ANC) should have chemotherapy treatment interrupted

Dose Adjustments on Day 1 of Each Treatment Cycle for Nonhematologic Toxicity and/or Dose Hold Based on Previous Cycle Toxicity

Toxicity/Dose Held	*nab*-Paclitaxel + Gemcitabine Dose This Cycle
G1 peripheral neuropathy	Dose adjustment not needed but follow carefully
G2 peripheral neuropathy	Reduce *nab*-paclitaxel one dose level and cisplatin by 5 mg/m² but continue gemcitabine administration
G ≥3 peripheral neuropathy	Hold *nab*-paclitaxel and cisplatin treatment but continue gemcitabine administration if indicated. Resume *nab*-paclitaxel and cisplatin treatment at next lower dose level after the peripheral neuropathy improves to G ≤1
Serum creatinine >1.7 mg/dL	Do not administer cisplatin
Other G1/2 toxicity†	Same as day 1 previous cycle (except for G2 cutaneous toxicity where doses of gemcitabine and *nab*-paclitaxel should be reduced to next lower dose level)
Other G3 toxicity†	Decrease *nab*-paclitaxel and gemcitabine to next lower dose level*
Other G4 toxicity†	Hold therapy†

†The decision as to which drug should be modified depends upon the type of nonhematologic toxicity seen and which course is medically most sound in the judgment of the physician

Dose Adjustments within a Treatment Cycle for Nonhematologic Toxicity

CTC Grade	Percent of Day 1 *nab*-Paclitaxel + Gemcitabine Dose
G1/2, G3 nausea/vomiting and alopecia	100%
G3 (except G3 nausea/vomiting and alopecia)	Hold either 1 or both drugs until resolution to G ≤1. Then resume treatment at the next lower dose level
G ≥3 peripheral neuropathy	Hold *nab*-paclitaxel treatment but continue gemcitabine administration if indicated. Resume *nab*-paclitaxel treatment at next lower dose level after the peripheral neuropathy improves to G ≤1
G4	Hold therapy†

Patient Population Studied

Sixty-two patients with advanced biliary tract cancers

Demographic and Baseline Disease Characteristics of the Intention-to-Treat Population

Characteristic	Patients, No. (%)		
	All (N = 60)	High-Dose Group (n = 32)	Reduced-Dose Group (n = 28)
Age, mean (SD), years	58.4 (11.0)	58.1 (11.1)	58.8 (11.1)
Male/female	33 (55)/27 (45)	16 (50)/16 (50)	17 (61)/11 (39)
ECOG PS			
0	22 (37)	12 (37)	10 (36)
1	38 (63)	20 (63)	18 (64)
Tumor type			
IHCC	38 (63)	24 (75)	14 (50)
EHCC	9 (15)	4 (13)	5 (18)
GBC	13 (22)	4 (13)	9 (32)
Disease stage*			
Metastatic	47 (78)	29 (91)	18 (64)
Locally advanced	13 (22)	3 (9)	10 (36)
Median CA19-9, U/mL (IQR)	99 (15–722)	99 (18–608)	99 (13–1053)

*$P = 0.03$ for the comparison of disease stage distribution between the high-dose and reduced-dose groups
CA19-9, carbohydrate antigen 19-9; ECOG PS, Eastern Cooperative Oncology Group performance status; EHCC, extrahepatic cholangiocarcinoma; GBC, gallbladder cancer; IHCC, intrahepatic cholangiocarcinoma; IQR, interquartile range

Efficacy

Post hoc analyses showed that response rates were not significantly associated with dose group, tumor type, or disease stage.

Best Treatment Responses: Intention-to-Treat Analysis

Response, n (%)	Dose group			Tumor type			Disease stage	
	All Patients (N = 60)	High Dose (n = 32)	Reduced Dose (n = 28)	IHCC (n = 38)	EHCC (n = 9)	GBC (n = 13)	Metastatic Disease (n = 47)	Locally Advanced Disease (n = 13)
DCR	43 (84)	25 (89)	18 (78)	29 (85)	6 (86)	8 (80)	32 (80)	11 (100)
CR	0	0	0	0	0	0	0	0
PR	23 (45)	14 (50)	9 (39)	15 (44)	4 (57)	4 (40)	18 (45)	5 (45)
SD	20 (39)	11 (39)	9 (39)	14 (41)	2 (29)	4 (40)	14 (35)	6 (55)
PD	8 (16)	3 (11)	5 (22)	5 (15)	1 (14)	2 (20)	8 (20)	0
Unknown	9	4	5	4	2	3	7	2

CR, complete response; DCR, disease control rate; EHCC, extrahepatic cholangiocarcinoma; GBC, gallbladder cancer; IHCC, intrahepatic cholangiocarcinoma; ITT, intention-to-treat; PD, progressive disease; PR, partial response; SD, stable disease

(continued)

Efficacy (continued)

PFS		
Median PFS	11.8 (95% CI, 6.0–15.6) months	
12-month PFS rate	45% (95% CI, 30–60)	
PFS, post hoc subgroup analyses		
Median PFS, high-dose treatment	11.4 months (95% CI, 6.0–15.6 months)	P = 0.62
Median PFS, reduced-dose group	14.9 months (95% CI, 3.8 months to not estimable [NE])	
Number of deaths/progressions		
High-dose group	24	
Reduced-dose group	10	
PFS according to tumor type		
Median PFS, IHCC	12.9 months (95% CI, 8.5–16.1)	P = 0.22
Median PFS, EHCC	6.0 months (95% CI, 0.7–NE)	
Median PFS, GBC	4.1 months (95% CI, 2.1–14.9)	
PFS according to disease stage		
Metastatic disease	11.4 months (95% CI, 5.7–14.9)	P = 0.50
Locally advanced disease	16.1 months (95% CI, 3.8–NE)	
OS		
Median OS	19.2 months (95% CI, 13.2–NE)	
12-month OS rate	66% (95% CI, 51–78)	
OS, post hoc subgroup analyses		
Median OS, high-dose treatment	19.5 months (95% CI, 10.0–NE)—15 dead	P = 0.39
Median OS, reduced-dose group	15.7 months (95% CI, 8.7–NE)—10 dead	
OS according to tumor type		
Median OS, IHCC	NE (95% CI, 13.6–NE)	P = 0.13
Median OS, EHCC	13.2 months (95% CI, 1.8–NE)	
Median OS, GBC	15.7 months (95% CI, 3.8–NE)	
OS according to tumor type		
Metastatic disease	18.8 months (95% CI, 10.0–NE)	P = 0.60
Locally advanced disease	NE (95% CI, 4.6–NE)	
Converted from unresectable to resectable and underwent surgery		
High-dose group	5/32 (16%)	
Reduced dose group	7/28 (25%)	

EFFICACY – CA19-9 Values

Median change from baseline to best response	–25 U/mL (95% CI, –95 to –1; P < 0.001)	
Median value decreased	93–27 U/mL	
Post hoc analyses		
Median change, high-dose recipients	–34 U/mL (95% CI, –129 to 0; P = 0.002)	
Median change, reduced-dose recipients	–16 U/mL (95% CI, –280 to 0; P = 0.01)	
Decrease in median values, high-dose recipients	93–27 U/mL	P = 0.86
Decrease in median values, reduced-dose recipients	79–41 U/mL	

Toxicity

Treatment Exposure and Safety Profile of Gemcitabine, Cisplatin, and nab-Paclitaxel in the Safety Population*

	All Patients (n = 57)	High Dose (n = 31)	Reduced Dose (n = 26)
Median treatment cycles, n (IQR)	6 (3–11)	8 (3–15)	5 (3–9)
Patients on starting dose for trial duration, n (%)	26 (46)	11 (35)	15 (58)
Premature withdrawal owing to AEs, n (%)	9 (16)	5 (16)	4 (15)
Discontinued cisplatin, n (%)	4 (7)	4 (13)	0
Discontinued nab-paclitaxel, n (%)	1 (2)	1 (3)	0
Any grade ≥3 AE, na (%)	33 (58)	19 (61)	14 (54)
Grade ≥3 hematologic AEs, na (%)			
Grade 3			
Neutropenia	17 (30)	8 (26)	9 (35)
Anemia	9 (16)	6 (19)	3 (12)
Thrombocytopenia	5 (9)	4 (13)	1 (4)
Febrile neutropenia	3 (5)	1 (3)	2 (8)
Grade 4			
Neutropenia	6 (11)	5 (16)	1 (4)
Thrombocytopenia	2 (4)	1 (3)	1 (4)
Grade 5	0	0	0
Grade ≥3 non-hematologic AEs, na (%)			
Grade 3			
Diarrhea	2 (4)	1 (3)	1 (4)
Elevated ALP	2 (4)	1 (3)	1 (4)
Vomiting	2 (4)	2 (6)	0
Abdominal infection	1 (2)	0	1 (4)
Constipation	1 (2)	1 (3)	0
Cystitis	1 (2)	1 (3)	0
Elevated AST	1 (2)	1 (3)	0
Hypokalemia	1 (2)	0	1 (4)
Hyponatremia	1 (2)	1 (3)	0
Maculopapular rash	1 (2)	1 (3)	0
Nausea	1 (2)	1 (3)	0
Neuropathy	1 (2)	0	1 (4)
Sepsis	1 (2)	0	1 (4)
Thromboembolic event	1 (2)	1 (3)	0
Grade 4	0	0	0
Grade 5			
Sepsis	1 (2)	1 (3)	0

AE, adverse event; ALP, alkaline phosphatase; AST, aspartate aminotransferase; IQR, interquartile range
*n = number of patients with ≥1 event, regardless of relationship to treatment

Treatment Monitoring

1. *Before each cycle:* History and physical examination
2. Where available, consider genotyping for UGT1A1 prior to therapy; patients who are homozygous for the UGT1A1*28 allele may be at higher risk for toxicity related to irinotecan and should initiate therapy at a lower dosage
3. CBC with differential on days 1 and 8, but initially also at day 14
4. Serum bilirubin, AST, ALT, alkaline phosphatase, BUN, serum creatinine, and electrolytes prior to each cycle
5. CA 19-9 and/or CEA prior to each cycle if detectable and being used to monitor disease
6. Every 1–3 months: CT scans to assess response

ADVANCED DISEASE • SUBSEQUENT THERAPY
BILIARY: CHOLANGIOCARCINOMA REGIMEN: PEMIGATINIB

Abou-Alfa GK et al. Lancet Oncol, 2020;21:671-684

PEMAZYRE (pemigatinib) prescribing information. Wilmington, DE: Incyte Corporation; revised 2020 April

Pemigatinib 13.5 mg per dose; administer orally once daily, without regard to food at approximately the same time each day, for 14 consecutive days on days 1–14, followed by 7 days without therapy, every 21 days, until disease progression (total dosage/21-day cycle = 189 mg)

Notes:
- Confirm the presence of an FGFR2 fusion or rearrangement prior to the initiation of pemigatinib
- Patients who delay taking pemigatinib by ≥4 hours and those who vomit after taking a dose should be instructed to take the next regular dose at the regularly scheduled time the next day
- Pemigatinib tablets should be swallowed whole. Do not crush, chew, split, or dissolve tablets
- Pemigatinib is metabolized by cytochrome P450 (CYP) CYP3A4
  - Advise patients to avoid intake of grapefruit juice during therapy with pemigatinib
  - Avoid concurrent use with moderate or strong CYP3A4 inducers
- Pemigatinib is a substrate of P-glycoprotein (P-gp) and BCRP; however, P-gp or BCRP inhibitors are not expected to affect pemigatinib exposure at clinically relevant concentrations
- Pemigatinib is an inhibitor of P-gp, OCT2, and MATE1. Inhibition of OCT2 and MATE1 may result in a reduction of renal tubular secretion of creatinine and therefore an increased serum creatinine level that may not represent a decrease in the glomerular filtration rate
  - Within the first cycle of pemigatinib, serum creatinine increased (mean increase of 0.2 mg/dL) and reached steady state by day 8, and then decreased during the 7 days off treatment

Drug Interactions	
Moderate or strong CYP3A4 inhibitor is unavoidable in a patient taking pemigatinib 13.5 mg per day on days 1–14 of a 21-day cycle	Decrease the pemigatinib dose to 9 mg per day on days 1–14 of a 21-day cycle.
Moderate or strong CYP3A4 inhibitor is unavoidable in a patient taking pemigatinib 9 mg per day on days 1–14 of a 21-day cycle	Decrease the pemigatinib dose to 4.5 mg per day on days 1–14 of a 21-day cycle
Moderate or strong CYP3A4 inhibitor is discontinued	Increase the pemigatinib dose (after 3 plasma half-lives of the inhibitor have transpired) to the dose that was used before starting the inhibitor
Moderate or strong CYP3A4 inducer	Avoid concomitant use of pemigatinib with a moderate or strong CYP3A4 inducer
Medication known to increase serum phosphate levels	In patients with elevated phosphate levels, avoid co-administration of other medications known to increase serum phosphate levels

Supportive Care
Antiemetic prophylaxis
Emetogenic potential is **MINIMAL–LOW**
See Chapter 42 for antiemetic recommendations

Hematopoietic growth factor (CSF) prophylaxis
Primary prophylaxis is **NOT** indicated
See Chapter 43 for more information

Antimicrobial prophylaxis
Risk of fever and neutropenia is **LOW**
  Antimicrobial primary prophylaxis to be **CONSIDERED**:
  - Antibacterial—not indicated
  - Antifungal—not indicated
  - Antiviral—not indicated unless patient previously had an episode of HSV

Ocular care
Prophylaxis and treatment for dry eye
Advise patients to use artificial tears or substitutes, hydrating or lubricating eye gels to prevent or treat dry eyes and to immediately report new-onset visual symptoms.

(continued)

(*continued*)

Oral care
Standard prophylaxis and treatment for mucositis/stomatitis

Diarrhea management
Loperamide 4 mg orally initially after the first loose or liquid stool, *then*
Loperamide 2 mg orally every 2 hours during waking hours, *plus*
Loperamide 4 mg orally every 4 hours during hours of sleep
- Continue for at least 12 hours after diarrhea resolves
- Recurrent diarrhea after a 12-hour diarrhea-free interval is treated as a new episode
- Rehydrate orally with fluids and electrolytes during a diarrheal episode
- If a patient develops blood or mucus in stool, dehydration, or hemodynamic instability, or if diarrhea persists >48 hours despite loperamide, stop loperamide and evaluate urgently in clinic or hospitalize the patient for IV hydration

Alternatively, a trial of **diphenoxylate hydrochloride 2.5 mg with atropine sulfate** 0.025 mg (eg, Lomotil)
- Initial adult dose is 2 tablets 4 times daily until control has been achieved, after which the dose may be reduced to meet individual requirements. Control may often be maintained with as little as 2 tablets daily
- Clinical improvement of acute diarrhea is usually observed within 48 hours. If improvement of chronic diarrhea after treatment with a maximum daily dose of 8 tablets is not observed within 10 days, control is unlikely with further administration

Hand-foot reaction (palmar-plantar erythrodysesthesia, PPE)
- For patients who develop a hand-foot reaction, use topical emollients (eg, Aquaphor), topical or orally administered steroids, antihistamine agents (H_1-receptor antagonists), or pyridoxine
- Pyridoxine may provide relief for discomfort/pain associated with PPE although the mechanism through which this occurs remains unclear
- The suggested pyridoxine starting dose is 50 mg/day, which may be increased to a maximum of 200 mg/day

Treatment Modifications

PEMIGATINIB TREATMENT MODIFICATIONS

Pemigatinib dose levels

Starting dose	13.5 mg orally once daily for first 14 days of each 21-day cycle
Dose level −1	9 mg orally once daily for first 14 days of each 21-day cycle
Dose level −2	4.5 mg orally once daily for first 14 days of each 21-day cycle
Dose level −3	Permanently discontinue pemigatinib

Hyperphosphatemia

Serum phosphate level is between 5.6–6.9 mg/dL	Continue pemigatinib at the same dose and restrict phosphate intake to 600–800 mg daily.*
Serum phosphate level is between 7.0–9.9 mg/d	• Restrict phosphate intake to 600–800 mg daily,* monitor serum phosphate levels weekly, and initiate a phosphate binder (eg, calcium carbonate, calcium acetate, sevelamer, or lanthanum) administered with meals. Continue pemigatinib at the same dose • If phosphate levels do not improve to <7.0 mg/dL within 2 weeks of the initiation of a phosphate binder, then withhold pemigatinib until phosphate levels are <7.0 mg/dL and then resume pemigatinib at the same dose (first occurrence) or with the dosage reduced by 1 dose level (subsequent occurrences).
Serum phosphate level is >10 mg/dL	• Restrict phosphate intake to 600–800 mg daily,* monitor serum phosphate levels weekly, and initiate a phosphate binder (eg, calcium carbonate, calcium acetate, sevelamer, or lanthanum) administered with meals. Continue pemigatinib at the same dose • If phosphate levels do not improve to ≤10 mg/dL within 1 week of the initiation of a phosphate binder, then withhold pemigatinib until phosphate levels are <7.0 mg/dL and then resume pemigatinib with the dosage reduced by 1 dose level
Serum phosphate level is >10 mg/dL while on a pemigatinib dose of 4.5 mg	Permanently discontinue pemigatinib

(*continued*)

Treatment Modifications (continued)

Retinal Pigment Epithelial Detachment (RPED)

RPED, asymptomatic and stable on serial examination	Continue pemigatinib at the same dose and continue serial comprehensive ophthalmologic examinations (including optical coherence tomography); advise the patient to promptly report any new-onset visual symptoms
RPED, symptomatic or worsening on serial examination	Withhold pemigatinib. Increase the frequency of ophthalmologic follow-up (including optical coherence tomography) to every 3 weeks. If asymptomatic and improved on subsequent examination, then resume pemigatinib with the dosage reduced by 1 dose level. If symptoms persist or examination does not improve, then consider permanent discontinuation of pemigatinib based on clinical status

Other toxicities

Any other grade 3[†] toxicity	• Withhold pemigatinib until the toxicity resolves to G ≤1 or baseline. If the toxicity resolves within 2 weeks, then resume pemigatinib with the dosage reduced by 1 dose level • If the toxicity has not resolved within 2 weeks, then permanently discontinue pemigatinib
Recurrent grade 3 toxicity after two dose reductions of any other grade 4[†] toxicity	Permanently discontinue pemigatinib

*Provide information on the phosphorus content of common foods and provide instruction on reading "Nutrition Facts" labels. Foods that have low amounts of phosphorus include fresh fruits and vegetables, unenriched rice milk, breads, pasta, rice, corn and rice cereals, light-colored sodas, and home-brewed iced tea. Foods that contain higher amounts of phosphorus include meat, poultry, fish, dairy foods, beans, lentils, nuts, bran cereal, oatmeal, colas, and some bottled iced teas. National Kidney Disease Education Program (NKDEP). Phosphorus. NIH Publication No. 10-7407 April 2010 [accessed September 9, 2019]
[†]Adverse events graded according to the National Cancer Institute Common Terminology Criteria for Adverse Events, (NCI CTCAE) v4.03

Patient Population Studied

FIGHT-202 was an open-label, phase 2, single-arm study that involved 146 patients with locally advanced or metastatic cholangiocarcinoma who experienced disease progression after ≥1 prior treatment and who had a documented fibroblast growth factor (FGF) and fibroblast growth factor receptor (FGFR) gene status. Patients were assigned to cohort A (FGFR2 gene rearrangements/fusions, n = 107), cohort B (other FGF/FGFR gene alterations, n = 20), or cohort C (no FGF/FGFR gene alterations, n = 19 including 1 patient with undetermined gene status)

Efficacy (N = 146)

Efficacy Variable	Pemigatinib Cohort A* (n = 107)
Centrally confirmed objective response rate, % (95% CI)	35.5 (26.5–45.4)
CR rate, %	2.8
Median DOR, months (95% CI)	7.5 (5.7–14.5)
DCR, % (95% CI)	82 (74–89)
Median PFS, months (95% CI)	6.9 (6.2–9.6)
Median OS, months (95% CI)[†]	21.1 (14.8–NR)

*Patients with FGFR2 gene rearrangements/fusions
[†]Overall survival data were immature at the data cutoff date of March 22, 2019
Note: no patients in cohort B (n = 20) or C (n = 19) achieved an objective response

Adverse Events (N = 146)

Adverse reactions occurring in ≥15% of patients

Grade (%)*	Pemigatinib (N = 146)	
	All grades	Grades ≥3[†]
Metabolism and nutrition disorders		
Hyperphosphatemia[‡]	60	0
Decreased appetite	33	1.4
Hypophosphatemia[§]	23	12
Dehydration	15	3.4
Skin and subcutaneous tissue disorders		
Alopecia	49	0
Nail toxicity[ǀ]	43	2.1
Dry skin	20	0.7
Palmar-plantar erythrodysesthesia syndrome	15	4.1
Gastrointestinal disorders		
Diarrhea	47	2.7
Nausea	40	2.1
Constipation	35	0.7
Stomatitis	35	5
Dry mouth	34	0
Vomiting	27	1.4
Abdominal pain	23	4.8
General disorders		
Fatigue	42	4.8
Edema peripheral	18	0.7
Nervous system disorders		
Dysgeusia	40	0
Headache	16	0
Eye disorders		
Dry eye[¢]	35	0.7
Retinal pigment epithelial detachment (RPED)	6%[¥]	0.6%
Musculoskeletal and connective tissue disorders		
Arthralgia	25	6
Back pain	20	2.7
Pain in extremity	19	2.1
Infections and infestations		
Urinary tract infections	16	2.7
Investigations		
Weight loss	16	2.1

*Graded per the National Cancer Institute Common Terminology Criteria for Adverse Events (NCI CTCAE) v4.03
[†]Only grades 3–4 were identified
[‡]Includes hyperphosphatemia and blood phosphorus increased; graded based on clinical severity and medical interventions taken according to the "investigations-other, specify" category in NCI CTCAE v4.03
[§]Includes hypophosphatemia and blood phosphorus decreased
[ǀ]Includes nail toxicity, nail disorder, nail discoloration, nail dystrophy, nail hypertrophy, nail ridging, nail infection, onychalgia, onychoclasis, onycholysis, onychomadesis, onychomycosis, and paronychia
[¢]Includes dry eye, keratitis, lacrimation increased, pinguecula, and punctate keratitis
[¥]Any grade of RPED occurred in 6% of 466 patients across clinical trials of pemigatinib with a median onset of 62 days
PEMAZYRE (pemigatinib) prescribing information. Wilmington, DE: Incyte Corporation; revised 2020 April

(continued)

Therapy Monitoring

1. *At baseline, periodically, and as clinically indicated*: Monitor serum phosphate levels. If serum phosphate is >7 mg/dL, increase the frequency of monitoring to weekly

2. *At baseline, every 2 months for the first 6 months, every 3 months thereafter, and urgently for new-onset visual symptoms*: Perform a comprehensive ophthalmologic examination, including optical coherence tomography. In patients with visual symptoms, ensure follow-up at least every 3 weeks until symptoms resolution or discontinuation of pemigatinib

3. *Periodically*: Monitor for visual symptoms; symptoms of dry eyes, stomatitis, palmar-plantar erythrodysesthesia syndrome, and diarrhea. Monitor adherence. Advise patients to use artificial tears or substitutes, hydrating or lubricating eye gels to prevent or treat dry eyes

Adverse Events (N = 146) *(continued)*

Select laboratory abnormalities worsening from baseline, occurring in ≥10% of patients

Grade (%)[†]	Pemigatinib (N = 146)*	
	All grades	Grades ≥3
Hematology		
Decreased hemoglobin	43	6
Decreased lymphocytes	36	8
Decreased platelets	28	3.4
Increased leukocytes	27	0.7
Decreased leukocytes	18	1.4
Chemistry		
Increased phosphate[‡]	94	0
Decreased phosphate	68	38
Increased ALT	43	4.1
Increased AST	43	6
Increased calcium	43	4.1
Increased alkaline phosphatase	41	11
Increased creatinine[§]	41	1.4
Decreased sodium	39	12
Increased glucose	36	0.7
Decreased albumin	34	0
Increased urate	30	10
Increased bilirubin	26	6
Decreased potassium	26	5
Decreased calcium	17	2.7
Increased potassium	12	2.1
Decreased glucose	11	1.4

*The denominator varied from 142 to 146 based on the number of patients with a baseline and at least 1 post-treatment value
[†]Graded per the NCI CTCAE v4.03
[‡]Based on NCI CTCAE v5.0 grading
[§]Graded based on comparison to upper limit of normal
ALT, alanine aminotransferase; AST, aspartate aminotransferase; NCI CTCAE, National Cancer Institute Common Terminology Criteria for Adverse Events
Note: Within the first 21-day cycle of pemigatinib, serum creatinine increased (mean increase of 0.2 mg/dL) and reached steady state by day 8, and then decreased during the 7 days off treatment
PEMAZYRE (pemigatinib) prescribing information. Wilmington, DE: Incyte Corporation; revised 2020 April

6. Bladder Cancer

Andrea B. Apolo, MD and Dean Bajorin, MD

Epidemiology

Incidence: Estimated new cases in 2020 in the United States: 81,400 (62,100 in men and 19,300 in women)

Deaths: Estimated in 2020: 17,980 (13,050 in men and 4,930 in women)

Median age: 73 (seventh decade)

Male:female ratio: 3:1

Stage at presentation	
Stage I:	70%
Stages II/III:	25%
Stage IV:	5%

www.cancer.org [accessed 2018]

Pathology

Urothelial carcinoma	90%–95%
Squamous cell carcinoma	5%
Adenocarcinoma	1%–2%
Small cell carcinoma	1%

Histopathologic evaluation should include a description of cell type[s], whether there are areas of differing differentiation and the extent of differentiation, whether the tumor is a micropapillary or nested variant, grade (low [G1] versus high [G2, G3]), presence or absence of lymphatic invasion, depth of invasion, and whether there is muscle in the specimen. Pathologic grade is important in the management of noninvasive tumors

McDougal WS et al. Cancer of the bladder, ureter, and renal pelvis. In: Devita VT, Lawrence TS, Rosenberg SA, eds. Cancer: Principles and Practice of Oncology. Philadelphia: Lippincott Williams and Wilkins, 2008.

Work-up

Stage	
Stage I	H&P, cystoscopy, transurethral resection of the bladder tumor (TURBT), examination under anesthesia (EUA), and cytology. In patients with high-grade and/or invasive tumors, radiologic assessment should be performed with high-resolution CT or magnetic resonance (MR) of the abdomen and pelvis prior to TURBT. The TURBT specimen should include muscle to accurately assess the depth of tumor invasion. A repeat TURBT is recommended in the case of T1 high-grade disease, even if muscle is present in the specimen, as T1 tumors can be understaged by TURBT, and a repeat TURBT has prognostic value in predicting response to intravesical therapy. TURBT is performed with an EUA. Consider upper tract imaging with either CT urogram, retrograde pyelogram, or MR urogram. This full investigation of the upper tracts is especially important in patients with positive cytology and normal cystoscopy.
Stages II/III	H&P, cystoscopy, TURBT, EUA, and cytology. In patients with high-grade and/or invasive tumors, radiologic assessment should be performed with high-resolution CT or MR of the abdomen and pelvis prior to TURBT. The TURBT specimen should include muscle to accurately assess the depth of tumor invasion. A repeat TURBT is recommended in the case of T1 high-grade disease, even if muscle is present in the specimen, as T1 tumors can be understaged by TURBT, and a repeat TURBT has prognostic value in predicting response to intravesical therapy. EUA is important in clinical staging as it can detect locally advanced bladder cancer by assessing for invasion into adjacent organs, extravesical extension, and abdominal or pelvic sidewall extension. A bladder fixed on EUA suggests that it may be surgically unresectable. Also consider a CT chest. A 99mTc bone scan is recommended for patients with elevated blood alkaline phosphatase or bone pain. NaF-PET/CT to assess bone disease is also under investigation in bladder cancer. Consider upper tract imaging with CT urogram, retrograde pyelogram, or MR urogram. This full investigation of the upper tracts is especially important in patients with positive cytology and normal cystoscopy.
Stage IV	H&P, cystoscopy, TURBT, EUA, and cytology. High-resolution CT chest, abdomen, and pelvis with IV contrast or CT chest without contrast and MR of the abdomen and pelvis. Upper tract imaging with either CT urogram, retrograde pyelogram, or MR urogram. A 99mTc bone scan is recommended for patients with elevated blood alkaline phosphatase or bone pain. NaF-PET/CT to assess bone disease is also under investigation in bladder cancer. The value of FDG-PET/CT for initial staging is still under investigation, but it appears to be a good adjunct (not a substitute) to anatomic imaging with high-resolution CT or MR.

Expert Opinion

1. The current standard of care systemic therapy for first-line cisplatin-eligible metastatic bladder cancer is gemcitabine and cisplatin or dose-dense (DD) methotrexate, vinblastine, doxorubicin (Adriamycin), and cisplatin (MVAC). A phase 3 trial demonstrated that the two-drug doublet of gemcitabine and cisplatin (GC) and standard MVAC have similar response and survival rates, but that GC has a better toxicity profile. A phase 3 trial compared DD MVAC plus granulocyte colony-stimulating factor (G-CSF) on 2-week cycles to standard MVAC on a 4-week cycle. Although there was no significant difference in median survival, DD MVAC was superior in response rate, 5-year survival rates, and progression-free survival, making DD MVAC another first-line chemotherapy option for metastatic bladder cancer

   After completion of therapy, imaging with a high-resolution CT chest, abdomen, and pelvis with IV contrast or an MR of the abdomen and pelvis with gadolinium and non-contrast CT chest, along with testing of creatinine and electrolytes is recommended at 3- to 6-month intervals for 3 years and then as clinically indicated

2. MVAC includes doxorubicin, which can cause myocardial damage for cumulative doses of 300–500 mg/m². Assess left ventricular ejection fraction before and regularly during and after treatment with doxorubicin. MVAC should be avoided in patients with pre-existing heart failure; consider a cardiology consult prior to initiating doxorubicin in high-risk cardiac patients

3. Patients with marginal renal function (60–70 mL/min) may benefit from having cisplatin administered in a divided dose over 2 days (either day 1 and 2 for MVAC or day 1 and 8 for GC)

4. Patients with inadequate renal function (creatinine clearance [CrCl] <60 mL/min [<1 mL/s]) and stage IV disease should be treated with carboplatin-based therapy rather than cisplatin. A regimen of gemcitabine and carboplatin has been well-studied in randomized trials and is considered a standard of care based on a higher response rate and less toxicity than carboplatin, vinblastine, and methotrexate

5. In patients with muscle-invasive bladder cancer (T2–T4N0), good performance status, and adequate renal function, use neoadjuvant cisplatin-based chemotherapy (either DD MVAC or GC × 4 cycles) prior to definitive surgery. Adjuvant chemotherapy is a consideration for patients at high risk of relapse after cystectomy if neoadjuvant chemotherapy was not administered. Carboplatin-regimens should not be given in the neoadjuvant or adjuvant setting unless in the context of a clinical trial

   After cystectomy, imaging with CT or MR of the abdomen and pelvis, urine cytology, creatinine, and electrolytes are recommended at 3- to 6-month intervals for 2 years and then as clinically indicated

6. Immunotherapy with checkpoint inhibition of the PD-1/PD-L1 pathway has demonstrated rapid, durable responses in metastatic urothelial carcinoma. Two checkpoint inhibitors, atezolizumab and pembrolizumab, are FDA-approved for first-line treatment of PDL-1 high metastatic urothelial carcinoma in cisplatin-ineligible patients

7. In patients with metastatic urothelial carcinoma that has not progressed with first-line platinum-containing chemotherapy, avelumab can be started after completion of chemotherapy as a maintenance therapy.

8. Five checkpoint inhibitors—atezolizumab, nivolumab, durvalumab, avelumab, and pembrolizumab—have demonstrated clinical efficacy in the second-line setting in patients with metastatic urothelial carcinoma, with comparable overall response rates of 15–20%. Atezolizumab, nivolumab, durvalumab, and avelumab received accelerated FDA approval, while pembrolizumab gained regular approval for the treatment of metastatic urothelial carcinoma refractory to platinum-based chemotherapy

9. In metastatic urothelial carcinoma patients who have progressed on platinum-based chemotherapy and harbor a fibroblast growth factor receptor (FGFR)3 or FGFR2 mutation may receive erdafitinib as a treatment option

10. In metastatic urothelial cancer who have previously received a programmed death receptor-1 (PD-1) or programmed death-ligand 1 (PD-L1) inhibitor, and a platinum-containing chemotherapy in the neoadjuvant/adjuvant, locally advanced or metastatic setting may receive enfortumab vedotin, a nectin-4-directed antibody-drug conjugate

11. Patients with metastatic bladder cancer, as well as those with organ-confined, muscle-invasive bladder cancer, should be considered for clinical trials

Staging

Primary Tumors of the Bladder (T)

TX	Primary tumor cannot be assessed	T3	Tumor invades perivesical tissue
T0	No evidence of primary tumor	pT3a	Microscopically
Ta	Noninvasive papillary carcinoma	pT3b	Macroscopically (extravesical mass)
Tis	Carcinoma in situ (ie, flat tumor)	T4	Tumor invades any of the following: prostatic stroma, seminal vesicles, uterus, vagina, pelvic wall, abdominal wall
T1	Tumor invades subepithelial connective tissue		
T2	Tumor invades muscularis propria	T4a	Tumor invades prostatic stroma, seminal vesicles, uterus, vagina
pT2a	Tumor invades superficial muscularis propria (inner half)		
pT2b	Tumor invades deep muscularis propria (outer half)	T4b	Tumor invades pelvic wall, abdominal wall

Regional Lymph Nodes for Urothelial Tumors (N)

NX	Regional lymph nodes cannot be assessed
N0	No lymph node metastasis
N1	Single regional lymph node metastasis in the true pelvis (hypogastric, obturator, external iliac, or presacral node)
N2	Multiple regional lymph node metastases in the true pelvis (hypogastric, obturator, external iliac, or presacral nodes)
N3	Lymph node metastasis to the common iliac lymph nodes

Distant Metastasis for Urothelial Tumors (M)

M0	No distant metastasis
M1	Distant metastasis
M1a	Distant metastasis limited to lymph nodes beyond the common iliacs
M1b	Non-lymph-node distant metastases

Anatomic Stage

Stage 0a	Ta	N0	M0
Stage 0is	Tis	N0	M0
Stage I	T1	N0	M0
Stage II	T2a	N0	M0
	T2b	N0	M0
Stage IIIA	T3a	N0	M0
	T3b	N0	M0
	T4a	N0	M0
	T1-T4a	N1	M0
Stage IIIB	T1–T4a	N2-3	M0
Stage IVA	T4b	Any N	M0
	Any T	Any N	M1a
Stage IVB	Any T	Any N	M1b

Amin MB et al, editors. AJCC Cancer Staging Manual. 8th ed. New York: Springer; 2017.

Five-year Survival*

Stage 0	98.4%
Stage I	87.7%
Stage II	62.6%
Stage III	45.5%
Stage IV	14.8%

*Lynch CF et al. Chapter 23. Cancer of the urinary bladder. In: Ries LAG et al, editors. SEER Survival Monograph: Cancer Survival Among Adults: U.S. SEER Program, 1988–2001, Patient and Tumor Characteristics. Bethesda, MD, National Cancer Institute, SEER Program, NIH Pub. No. 07-6215, 2007.

NEOADJUVANT

BLADDER CANCER REGIMEN: GEMCITABINE + CISPLATIN (GC)

Dash A et al. Cancer 2008;113:2471–2477

Gemcitabine 1000 mg/m² per dose; administer intravenously in 50–250 mL 0.9% sodium chloride injection (0.9% NS) over 30–60 minutes for 2 doses on days 1 and 8 every 21 days for 4 cycles (total dosage/cycle = 2000 mg/m²)

Hydration before and after cisplatin administration: Administer ≥500 mL 0.9% NS intravenously over a minimum of 1 hour before and after cisplatin. Encourage patients to increase oral intake of non-alcoholic fluids. Monitor serum electrolytes (potassium, magnesium, sodium) and replace as needed

Cisplatin 70 mg/m² single dose; administer intravenously in 100–250 mL 0.9% NS over 60 minutes on day 1 every 21 days for 4 cycles (total dosage/cycle = 70 mg/m²)*

or

Cisplatin 35 mg/m² per dose; administer intravenously in 100–250 mL 0.9% NS over 60 minutes for 2 doses after gemcitabine on days 1 and 8 every 21 days for 4 cycles (total dosage/cycle = 70 mg/m²)†

*Soto Parra H et al. Ann Oncol 2002;13:1080–1086
†Hussain SA et al. Br J Cancer 2004;91:844–849

Supportive Care
Antiemetic prophylaxis
Emetogenic potential on days with cisplatin and gemcitabine: **HIGH**; *potential for delayed symptoms*
Emetogenic potential on days with gemcitabine alone: **LOW**
See Chapter 42 for antiemetic recommendations

Hematopoietic growth factor (CSF) prophylaxis
Primary prophylaxis is **NOT** indicated
See Chapter 43 for more information

Antimicrobial prophylaxis
Risk of fever and neutropenia: **LOW**
  Antimicrobial primary prophylaxis to be considered:
  • Antibacterial—not indicated
  • Antifungal—not indicated
  • Antiviral—not indicated unless patient previously had an episode of HSV

Efficacy (Response at Cystectomy, N = 52)

Cisplatin dose intensity achieved	90%
Gemcitabine dose intensity achieved	90%
Pathologic complete response	26%
< pT2 disease	36%
Median overall survival	Not reached
Median duration of response	9.6 months

Patient Population Studied

Study enrolled 52 patients with locally advanced transitional cell urothelial cancer defined as muscle-invasive (T2–T4a) without evidence of adenopathy (N0) and without prior systemic chemotherapy. Prior local intravesical therapy and/or immunotherapy were allowed. Karnofsky performance status ≥70; CrCl ≥60 mL/min (≥1 mL/s)

Notes

1. Administer 4 cycles followed by CT scan and cystectomy
2. This study randomized patients with multiple malignancies, not just urothelial cancer, to GC for 3 weeks (days 1 and 8) or 4 weeks (days 1, 8, 15)

Treatment Modifications

Adverse Events	Treatment Modifications
Day 1 WBC count <3000/mm³ or platelet count <100,000/mm³	Hold chemotherapy until WBC count >3000/mm³ and platelet count >100,000/mm³
Day 8 WBC count ≤1000/mm³ or platelet count ≤100,000/mm³	Hold chemotherapy and reduce subsequent gemcitabine doses by 10%
Febrile neutropenia or G4 thrombocytopenia	Reduce subsequent gemcitabine doses by 10%

Missed chemotherapy doses are not given later

Toxicity with 21-Day GC (N = 53)

Toxicity	% G3	% G4
Hematologic Toxicities		
Anemia	9.4	0
Thrombocytopenia	3.7	1.8
Neutropenia	16.9	5.6
Nonhematologic Toxicities		
Mucositis	1.8	1.8
Nausea	5.6	0
Alopecia	0	0
Infection	1.8	0
Fatigue	3.0	0
Cardiac	1.8	0
Fever	0	0

Soto Parra H et al. Ann Oncol 2002;13:1080–1086

Therapy Monitoring

1. *Prior to each dose of cisplatin:* CBC with differential count, serum electrolytes, BUN, and creatinine
2. *On all treatment days:* CBC with differential count
3. *Response evaluation after 4 cycles:* CT scan
4. *Follow-up after cystectomy:* CT or MR of abdomen and pelvis, chest x-ray, urine cytology, creatinine, and electrolytes recommended at 3- to 6-month intervals for 2 years, then as clinically indicated

NEOADJUVANT

BLADDER CANCER REGIMEN: METHOTREXATE + VINBLASTINE + DOXORUBICIN + CISPLATIN (MVAC) BEFORE RADICAL CYSTECTOMY*

Grossman HB et al. N Engl J Med 2003;349:859–866. Erratum in: N Engl J Med 2003;349:1880
*Consider DDMVAC or GC instead

Methotrexate 30 mg/m² per dose; administer by intravenous injection over 15–60 seconds on days 1, 15, and 22 every 28 days for 3 cycles (total dosage/cycle = 90 mg/m²)

Vinblastine 3 mg/m² per dose; administer by intravenous injection over 1–2 minutes on days 2, 15, and 22 every 28 days for 3 cycles (total dosage/cycle = 9 mg/m²)

Doxorubicin 30 mg/m²; administer by intravenous injection over 3–5 minutes on day 2 every 28 days for 3 cycles (total dosage/cycle = 30 mg/m²)

Hydration before and after cisplatin administration: Administer intravenously ≥1000 mL 0.9% sodium chloride injection (0.9% NS), at ≥100 mL/hour before and after cisplatin administration. Encourage patients to increase oral intake of non-alcoholic fluids. Monitor serum electrolytes (potassium, magnesium, sodium) and replace as needed

Cisplatin 70 mg/m²; administer intravenously in 100–250 mL 0.9% NS over 70 minutes on day 2 every 28 days for 3 cycles (total dosage/cycle = 70 mg/m²)

Supportive Care
Antiemetic prophylaxis
Emetogenic potential on days 1, 15, and 22: **LOW**
Emetogenic potential on day 2: **HIGH**; *potential for delayed symptoms*
See Chapter 42 for antiemetic recommendations

Hematopoietic growth factor (CSF) prophylaxis
Primary prophylaxis may be indicated between doses of myelosuppressive chemotherapy
See Chapter 43 for more information

Antimicrobial prophylaxis
Risk of fever and neutropenia: **LOW**
  Antimicrobial primary prophylaxis to be considered:
  • Antibacterial—not indicated
  • Antifungal—not indicated
  • Antiviral—not indicated unless patient previously had an episode of HSV

Oral care
Encourage patients to maintain intake of non-alcoholic fluids
  If mucositis or stomatitis is present:
  • Rinse mouth several times a day with ¼ teaspoon (1.25 g) each of baking soda and table salt in 1 quart of warm water. Follow with a plain water rinse
  • Do not use mouthwashes that contain alcohol

Treatment Modifications

Adverse Events	Treatment Modifications
On day 1 if WBC count <3000/mm³ or platelet count <100,000/mm³	Delay chemotherapy for 1 week
On day 15 or 22: WBC count ≤2900/mm³ or platelet count ≤74,000/mm³	Hold dose of methotrexate and vinblastine
Severe mucositis (G3 or G4)*	Reduce methotrexate dose by 33% for all doses and into next cycle
Severe neurotoxicity	Reduce vinblastine dose by 33%
Clinical evidence of congestive heart failure	Discontinue doxorubicin

*Leucovorin may be started 24 hours after methotrexate infusion

Toxicity (N = 150*)

Adverse Event	% G3†	% G4‡
Hematologic Toxicities		
Granulocytopenia	23	33
Thrombocytopenia	5	0
Anemia	6	1
Nonhematologic Toxicities		
Nausea/vomiting	6	0
Stomatitis	10	0
Diarrhea/constipation	4	0
Renal effects	1	0
Neuropathy	2	0
Fatigue, lethargy, malaise	3	0
All Toxicities		
Maximal grade of any adverse event	35	37

*Patients who received any methotrexate, vinblastine, doxorubicin, and cisplatin
†Grade 3 described as adverse event of moderate severity
‡Grade 4 described as severe adverse event

Therapy Monitoring

1. *Prior to each cycle:* CBC with differential count, serum electrolytes, BUN, creatinine, and LFTs
2. *Weekly:* CBC with differential
3. *Response evaluation:* None needed during neoadjuvant therapy
4. *Follow-up after cystectomy:* CT chest, abdomen and pelvis with IV contrast or CT chest without contrast and MR abdomen and pelvis, urine cytology, creatinine, and electrolytes recommended at 3- to 6-month intervals for 2 years, then as clinically indicated

Efficacy (N = 153)

Intention-to-Treat Analysis	
Median survival	77 months
5-year survival	57%

Patient Population Studied

Study enrolled 153 patients with muscle-invasive bladder tumors without nodal or metastatic disease, eligible for radical cystectomy. No previous pelvic radiation; adequate renal, hepatic, hematologic function; ECOG performance status ≤1

METASTATIC • FIRST-LINE

BLADDER CANCER REGIMEN: GEMCITABINE + CISPLATIN (GC)

von der Maase H et al. J Clin Oncol 2000;17:3068–3077

Gemcitabine 1000 mg/m^2 per dose; administer intravenously in 50–250 mL 0.9% sodium chloride injection (0.9% NS) over 30–60 minutes for 3 doses on days 1, 8, and 15 every 28 days for a maximum of 6 cycles, (total dosage/cycle = 3000 mg/m^2).
Hydration before and after cisplatin administration: ≥ 500 mL 0.9% NS intravenously over a minimum of 1 hour before and after cisplatin. Encourage increased oral fluid intake.
Cisplatin 70 mg/m^2; administer intravenously in 100–250 mL 0.9% NS over 1 hour on day 2 every 28 days for a maximum of 6 cycles (total dosage/cycle = 70 mg/m^2).

Supportive Care
Antiemetic prophylaxis
Emetogenic potential on days 1, 8, and 15: **LOW**
Emetogenic potential on day 2: **HIGH**; potential for delayed symptoms
See Chapter 42 for antiemetic recommendations

Hematopoietic growth factor (CSF) prophylaxis
Primary prophylaxis may be indicated between doses of myelosuppressive chemotherapy
See Chapter 43 for more information

Antimicrobial prophylaxis
Risk of fever and neutropenia: **LOW**
  Antimicrobial primary prophylaxis to be considered:
  • Antibacterial—not indicated
  • Antifungal—not indicated
  • Antiviral—not indicated unless patient previously had an episode of HSV

Patient Population Studied

Study enrolled 203 patients with locally advanced or metastatic transitional cell urothelial cancer without prior systemic chemotherapy or immunotherapy. Prior local intravesical therapy, immunotherapy, or RT were allowed. Karnofsky performance status ≥70; CrCl ≥60 mL/minute (≥1 mL/s)

Efficacy (N = 200)

Complete response	12.2%
Partial response	37.2%
Median overall survival	13.8 months
Median time to disease progression	5.4 months
Median time to treatment failure	7.8 months
Median duration of response	9.6 months

Toxicity (N = 203)

(WHO Criteria)

Toxicity	% G3	% G4
Hematologic Toxicities		
Anemia	23.5	3.5
Thrombocytopenia	28.5	28.5
Neutropenia	41.2	29.9
Nonhematologic Toxicities		
Mucositis	1.0	0
Nausea	22	0
Alopecia	10.5	0
Infection	2.0	0.5
Diarrhea	3.0	0
Pulmonary	2.5	0.5
Hematuria	4.5	0
Constipation	1.5	0
Hemorrhage	2.0	0
Altered consciousness	0.5	0
Fever	0	0

Treatment Modifications

Adverse Events	Treatment Modifications
Day 1 WBC count <3000/mm^3 or platelet count <100,000/mm^3	Hold chemotherapy until WBC count is >3000/mm^3 and platelet count is >100,000/mm^3
Days 8 or 15 WBC count ≤1990/mm^3 or platelet count ≤49,000/mm^3	Omit gemcitabine on that day*
Treatment delay >4 weeks	Discontinue treatment

*Missed chemotherapy doses are not given later. If gemcitabine is omitted on day 15, the cycle duration may be shortened to 21 days

Therapy Monitoring

1. *Prior to each of 6 cycles:* CBC with differential count, serum electrolytes, BUN, and creatinine
2. *On all treatment days:* CBC with differential count
3. *Response evaluation every 2–3 cycles:* CT or MR of chest, abdomen or pelvis, or chest x-ray for lung lesions every 2–3 cycles (von der Maase et al, 2000)
4. *Follow-up after completion of therapy:* Imaging with CT or MR of the abdomen and pelvis, chest x-ray or CT of chest, urine cytology (if applicable), creatinine and electrolytes recommended at 3- to 6-month intervals for 2 years, then as clinically indicated

Notes

1. Give 6 cycles unless disease progression can be documented

METASTATIC • FIRST-LINE

BLADDER CANCER REGIMEN: HIGH-DOSE (HD) OR DOSE-DENSE (DD) METHOTREXATE, VINBLASTINE, DOXORUBICIN, AND CISPLATIN

Plimack ER et al. J Clin Oncol 2012;30(suppl):abstract 4526
Sternberg CN et al. J Clin Oncol 2001;19:2638–2646
Sternberg CN et al. Eur J Cancer 2006;42:50–54

Methotrexate 30 mg/m²; administer by intravenous injection over ≤1 minute *or* intravenously in 10–100 mL 0.9% sodium chloride injection (0.9% NS) or 5% dextrose injection (D5W) over 10–30 minutes on day 1 every 14 days (total dosage/14-day cycle = 30 mg/m²)

Hydration before cisplatin: 1000 mL 0.9% NS; administer intravenously over ≥1 hour before cisplatin administration

Vinblastine 3 mg/m²; administer by intravenous injection over 1–2 minutes on day 2 every 14 days (total dosage/14-day cycle = 3 mg/m²)

Doxorubicin 30 mg/m²; administer by intravenous injection over 3–5 minutes on day 2 every 14 days (total dosage/14-day cycle = 30 mg/m²)

Cisplatin 70 mg/m²; administer intravenously in 50–500 mL 0.9% NS over 30–60 minutes on day 2 every 14 days (total dosage/14-day cycle = 70 mg/m²)

Hydration after cisplatin: 1000 mL 0.9% NS; administer intravenously over ≥2 hours. Monitor and replace magnesium and other electrolytes as needed. Encourage patients to increase intake of non-alcoholic fluids

or

2000 mL 0.45% NS; administer intravenously over ≥2 hours

± *Mannitol diuresis:* May be given to patients who have received adequate hydration

Mannitol 37.5 grams; administer intravenously over 1–4 hours before or during cisplatin administration, or may be prepared as an admixture with cisplatin

Note: Diuresis with mannitol requires maintaining hydration with intravenously administered fluid during and for hours after mannitol administration

Filgrastim 240 mcg/m² per dose; administer subcutaneously daily for 7 consecutive days (days 4–10) every 14 days

- Calculated doses may be rounded by ± 10% to use the most economical combination of commercially available products
- Discontinue filgrastim when patient achieves a post-nadir ANC = 30,000/mm³
- Use of filgrastim may be extended to 14 consecutive days if neutrophil recovery is inadequate after a 7-day course

Supportive Care

Antiemetic prophylaxis

Emetogenic potential on day 1: **MINIMAL**

Emetogenic potential on day 2: **HIGH**; *potential for delayed symptoms*

See Chapter 42 for antiemetic recommendations

Hematopoietic growth factor (CSF) prophylaxis

Primary prophylaxis with granulocyte colony-stimulating factor is an integral part of the treatment regimen

Antimicrobial prophylaxis

Risk of fever and neutropenia: **LOW**

Antimicrobial primary prophylaxis to be considered:

- Antibacterial—not indicated
- Antifungal—not indicated
- Antiviral—not indicated unless patient previously had an episode of HSV

Oral care

Encourage patients to maintain intake of non-alcoholic fluids

If mucositis or stomatitis is present:

- Rinse mouth several times a day with ¼ teaspoon (1.25 g) each of baking soda and table salt in 1 quart of warm water. Follow with a plain water rinse
- Do not use mouthwashes that contain alcohol

Dose Modifications

Adverse Event	Treatment Modification
G3/4 hematologic toxicity	Extend filgrastim treatment as needed, up to 14 consecutive days
ANC >30,000/mm³	Discontinue filgrastim
G3/4 mucositis	Reduce methotrexate dose by 33%
G3/4 neurotoxicity	Reduce vinblastine dose by 33%
Clinical evidence of congestive heart failure	Discontinue doxorubicin

Patient Population Studied

A total of 263 patients with metastatic or advanced transitional-cell carcinoma (TCC) were randomly assigned to HD-MVAC (2-week cycles) or MVAC (4-week cycles). Eligibility criteria included TCC of the urinary tract (bladder, ureter, urethra, or renal pelvis) and bi-dimensionally measurable metastatic or locally advanced disease, no prior systemic cytotoxic or biologic treatment, and WHO performance status of 0, 1, or 2 (median: 1). In all, 60–65% of patients were considered low-risk, 30–35% intermediate-risk, and 5% high-risk; 15–20% had prior radiotherapy, and 73–75% had prior surgery. Sites of origin included bladder (82–88%), renal pelvis (8–12%), and other sites (ureter, urethra, or prostatic ducts). Visceral metastases were present in 28–36%. The majority of patients had abdominal masses (pelvic, extranodal, or retroperitoneal) and more than one disease site

Toxicity (WHO Grade)

Toxicity	MVAC (n = 129)		HD-MVAC (n = 134)		P (Trend)
	# Patients	%	# Patients	%	
WBC	2	2	4	3	
0	8	6	46	34	
1	11	8	29	21	
2	28	22	28	21	<0.001
3	59	46	16	12	
4	21	16	11	8	
Platelets	2	2	4	3	
0	80	62	48	43	
1	10	8	22	16	
2	15	12	22	16	0.033
3	14	11	14	11	
4	8	6	14	11	
Mucositis	7	5	10	8	
0	31	24	43	32	
1	43	33	44	33	
2	26	20	24	18	0.034
3	18	14	12	9	
4	4	3	1	1	
Creatinine	2	2	5	4	
0	113	88	118	88	
1	7	5	4	3	0.815
2	3	2	2	2	
3	4	3	5	4	
Nausea and/or vomiting	4	3	7	5	
0	9	7	3	2	
1	27	21	20	15	0.025
2	52	40	55	41	
3	32	25	42	31	
4	5	4	7	5	
Neurotoxicity	7	5	10	8	
0	70	54	63	47	
1	38	30	44	33	
2	12	9	10	8	0.170
3	2	2	5	4	
4	0	0	2	2	
Alopecia	7	5	9	7	
0	11	9	16	12	
1	13	10	19	14	
2	36	28	33	25	0.180
3	62	48	57	43	
4	0	0	0	0	

Efficacy

Response Rates			
	MVAC (n = 129)	HD-MVAC (n = 134)	P Value
Number evaluable	113 (88%)	114 (85%)	
CR + PR	65 (58%)	83 (72%)	0.016 (2-sided)
CR	12 (11%)	28 (25%)	0.006 (2-sided)
PR	53 (47%)	55 (48%)	

Endpoint	Time/Percent (95% CI)	Time/Percent (95% CI)	P Value HR (95% CI)
Progression-free survival	8.1 months (7.0–9.9)	9.5 months (7.6–12.2)	P = 0.017 HR = 0.73 (0.56–0.95)
Overall survival	14.9 months	15.1 months	P = 0.042 HR 0.76 (0.58–0.99)
2-year survival	26.2% (18.4%–34%)	36.7% (28.3%–45%)	
5-year survival	13.5% (7.4%–19.6%)	21.8% (14.5%–29.2%)	P = 0.042
7.3-year survival*	13.2%	24.6%	
Cancer death	76%	64.9%	

*Median follow-up

METASTATIC • FIRST-LINE
BLADDER CANCER REGIMEN: GEMCITABINE + CARBOPLATIN

De Santis M et al. J Clin Oncol 2009;27:5634–5639
De Santis M et al. J Clin Oncol 2012;30(2):191–199

Gemcitabine 1000 mg/m² per dose; administer intravenously 50–250 mL 0.9% sodium chloride injection over 30 minutes for 2 doses on days 1 and 8, every 21 days × 6 cycles (total dosage/cycle = 2000 mg/m²)
Carboplatin* (calculated dose) AUC = 4.5 mg/mL × min; administer intravenously in 50–150 mL 5% dextrose injection over 60 minutes after gemcitabine on day 1, every 21 days × 6 cycles (total dose/cycle calculated to produce an AUC = 4.5 mg/mL × min)

*Carboplatin dose is based on Calvert et al.'s formula to achieve a target area under the plasma concentration versus time curve (AUC) (AUC units = mg/mL × min)

$$\text{Total carboplatin dose (mg)} = (\text{target AUC}) \times (\text{GFR} + 25)$$

In practice, CrCl is used in place of glomerular filtration rate (GFR). CrCl can be calculated from the Cockcroft-Gault Equation:

$$\text{For males, CrCl} = \frac{(140 - \text{age[years]}) \times (\text{body weight [kg]})}{72 \times (\text{serum creatinine [mg/dL]})}$$

$$\text{For females, CrCL} = \frac{(140 - \text{age[years]}) \times (\text{body weight [kg]})}{72 \times (\text{serum creatinine [mg/dL]})} \times 0.85$$

Note: A carboplatin dose calculated with an IDMS-measured serum creatinine result using the Calvert formula could exceed an expected exposure (AUC) and result in increased drug-related toxicity. The FDA recommends capping an estimated GFR at 125 mL/min for any targeted AUC value.
U.S. Food and Drug Administration. Carboplatin dosing. May 23, 2013. Available from: https://www.nccn.org/professionals/OrderTemplates/PDF/appendix_B.pdf [accessed February 26, 2014]

Calvert AH et al. J Clin Oncol 1989;7:1748–1756
Cockcroft DW Gault MH. Nephron 1976;16:31–41
Jodrell DI et al. J Clin Oncol 1992;10:520–528
Sorensen BT et al. Cancer Chemother Pharmacol 1991;28:397–401

Supportive Care
Antiemetic prophylaxis—first regimen
Emetogenic potential on day 1: **HIGH**; *potential for delayed symptoms*
Emetogenic potential on day 8: **LOW**
See Chapter 42 for antiemetic recommendations

Hematopoietic growth factor (CSF) prophylaxis
Primary prophylaxis is NOT indicated
See Chapter 43 for more information

Antimicrobial prophylaxis
Risk of fever and neutropenia: **LOW**
  Antimicrobial primary prophylaxis to be considered:
  • Antibacterial—not indicated
  • Antifungal—not indicated
  • Antiviral—not indicated, unless patient previously had an episode of HSV

Patient Population Studied

Study enrolled 88 patients with either unresectable and measurable transitional cell tumors of the urothelial tract, or patients with metastatic (N+ or M+) tumors. Patients who met any of the following criteria were deemed cisplatin-ineligible: (a) ECOG performance status of 2; (b) GFR <60 mL/min but >30 mL/min and normal cardiovascular and hepatic function

Efficacy (N = 88)

Complete response	3.4%
Partial response	34%
Median overall survival	Too early

Serious Adverse Toxicity (N = 119)

Death	2.3%
G3 mucositis	1.1%
G4 thrombocytopenia plus bleeding	3.4%
Neutropenia and fever	5.7%
Grades 3/4 renal toxicity	3.4%

Data are from the phase 2 portion of a randomized phase 2/3 study. More definitive data will be available upon completion of accrual and maturation of the phase 3 part of the trial

Treatment Modifications

Adverse Events	Treatment Modifications
Day 1 ANC <1500/mm^3, platelets <100,000/mm^3, or mucositis	Hold treatment until ANC >1500/mm^3, platelets >100,000/mm^3, and mucositis resolves
Day 8 ANC 500–1000/mm^3 or platelets 50,000–99,000/mm^3	Reduce gemcitabine dose by 50% on day of treatment
G4 neutropenia and fever, G4 thrombocytopenia >3 days, or thrombocytopenia and active bleeding	Reduce doses of both drugs by 25%

Therapy Monitoring

1. *Day 1:* CBC with differential count, serum electrolytes, BUN, and creatinine
2. *Day 8:* CBC with differential count
3. *Treatment evaluation after C3 and C6:* CT or MR of the initial evaluable/measurable sites
4. *Duration of treatment:* Treat for 6 cycles unless progression documented
5. *Follow-up after completion of therapy:* CT or MR of abdomen and pelvis, chest x-ray or CT of chest, urine cytology (if applicable), creatinine, and electrolytes recommended at 3- to 6-month intervals for 2 years, then as clinically indicated

Notes

1. Give platelet transfusions if platelets <20,000/mm^3
2. Treat for 6 cycles unless progression documented

METASTATIC • FIRST-LINE

BLADDER CANCER REGIMEN: METHOTREXATE + VINBLASTINE + DOXORUBICIN + CISPLATIN (MVAC)

von der Maase H et al. J Clin Oncol 2000;17:3068–3077
von der Maase H et al. J Clin Oncol 2005;21:4602–4608

Methotrexate 30 mg/m² per dose; administer by intravenous injection over 15–60 seconds for 3 doses on days 1, 15, and 22 every 28 days for a maximum of 6 cycles (total dosage/cycle = 90 mg/m²)

Vinblastine 3 mg/m² per dose; administer by intravenous injection over 1–2 minutes for 3 doses on days 2, 15, and 22 every 28 days for a maximum of 6 cycles (total dosage/cycle = 9 mg/m²)

Doxorubicin 30 mg/m²; administer by intravenous injection over 3–5 minutes on day 2 every 28 days for a maximum of 6 cycles (total dosage/cycle = 30 mg/m²)

Hydration before and after cisplatin administration: Administer intravenously ≥1000 mL 0.9% sodium chloride injection (0.9% NS) over at least 2 hours before and after cisplatin administration. Encourage patients to increase oral intake of non-alcoholic fluids. Monitor serum electrolytes (potassium, magnesium, sodium) and replace as needed

Cisplatin 70 mg/m²; administer intravenously in 100–1000 mL 0.9% NS over 1–8 hours on day 2 every 28 days for a maximum of 6 cycles (total dosage/cycle = 70 mg/m²)

Supportive Care: Antiemetic prophylaxis
Emetogenic potential on days 1, 15, and 22: **LOW**
Emetogenic potential on day 2: **HIGH**. *Potential for delayed symptoms*
See Chapter 42 for antiemetic recommendations

Hematopoietic growth factor (CSF) prophylaxis
Primary prophylaxis may be indicated between doses of myelosuppressive chemotherapy
See Chapter 43 for more information

Antimicrobial prophylaxis
Risk of fever and neutropenia: **LOW**
  Antimicrobial primary prophylaxis to be considered:
  • Antibacterial—not indicated
  • Antifungal—not indicated
  • Antiviral—not indicated unless patient previously had an episode of HSV

Oral care: Encourage patients to maintain intake of non-alcoholic fluids
  If mucositis or stomatitis is present:
  Rinse mouth several times a day with ¼ teaspoon (1.25 g) each of baking soda and table salt in 1 quart of warm water. Follow with a plain water rinse
  Do not use mouthwashes that contain alcohol

Patient Population Studied

Study enrolled 202 patients with locally advanced or metastatic transitional cell urothelial cancer without prior systemic chemotherapy or immunotherapy. Prior local intravesical therapy, immunotherapy, or RT were allowed. Karnofsky Performance Status ≥70, CrCl ≥60 mL/min (≥1 mL/s)

Efficacy (N = 196)

Complete response	11.9%
Partial response	33.8%
Median overall survival	14.8 months
Median time to treatment failure	4.6 months
Median time to disease progression	7.4 months
Median duration of response	9.6 months

Therapy Monitoring

1. *Prior to each cycle:* CBC with differential count, serum electrolytes, BUN, creatinine, and LFTs
2. *Days 15 and 22:* CBC with differential count
3. *Response evaluation every 2–3 cycles:* CT or MR of chest, abdomen, or pelvis, or chest x-ray for lung lesions every 2–3 cycles (von der Maase et al, 2000)
4. *Follow-up after completion of therapy:* Imaging with CT or MR of abdomen and pelvis, chest x-ray or CT of chest, urine cytology (if applicable), creatinine and electrolytes recommended at 3- to 6-month intervals for 2 years, then as clinically indicated

Toxicity (N = 202)

(WHO Criteria)

Toxicity	% G3	% G4
Hematologic Toxicities		
Anemia	15.5	2.1
Thrombocytopenia	7.7	12.9
Neutropenia	17.1	65.2
Nonhematologic Toxicities		
Mucositis	17.7	4.2
Nausea	19.2	1.6
Alopecia	54.2	1.0
Infection	9.9	5.2
Diarrhea	7.8	0.5
Pulmonary	2.6	3.1
Hematuria	2.3	0
Constipation	2.6	0.5
Hemorrhage	2.1	0
Altered consciousness	3.1	0.5
Fever	3.1	0

Treatment Modifications

Adverse Events	Treatment Modifications
Day 1 if WBC <3000/mm³ or platelet count <100,000/mm³	Delay chemotherapy for 1 week
Day 15 or 22 if WBC ≤2900/mm³ or platelet count ≤74,000/mm³	Hold dose of methotrexate and vinblastine
G3/4 mucositis*	Reduce methotrexate dose by 33% (all remaining doses and into next cycle)
Severe neurotoxicity	Reduce vinblastine dose by 33%
Clinical evidence of CHF	Discontinue doxorubicin

*Leucovorin may be given 24 hours after methotrexate for patients who experienced G3/4 mucositis after previously administered doses

Notes

1. Give 6 cycles unless there is documented disease progression
2. Avoid this regimen in patients with pre-existing cardiac disease without guidance from a cardiologist familiar with effects of doxorubicin

METASTATIC • FIRST-LINE • SUBSEQUENT THERAPY

BLADDER CANCER REGIMEN: ATEZOLIZUMAB

Balar AV et al. Lancet 2017;389:67–76. Comment in: Lancet 2017;389:6–7
Powles T et al. Nature 2014;515:558–562. Comment in: Eur Urol 2015;67:975. Nat Rev Urol 2015;12:61. Nat Rev Clin Oncol 2015;12:63. J Urol 2015;194:956
Rosenberg JE et al. Lancet 2016;387:1909–1920. Comment in: Nat Rev Clin Oncol 2016;13:266. Lancet 2016; 387:1881–1882

Atezolizumab 1200 mg; administer intravenously in 250 mL 0.9% sodium chloride injection over 60 minutes every 3 weeks (total dosage/cycle = 1200 mg)

Alternative atezolizumab dosage regimens as per the U.S. FDA regimens approved on May 6, 2019:

Atezolizumab 840 mg; administer intravenously in a volume of 0.9% NS sufficient to produce a final concentration within the range 3.2 mg/mL to 16.8 mg/mL over 60 minutes every 2 weeks (total dosage/2-week cycle = 840 mg)

Atezolizumab 1680 mg; administer intravenously in a volume of 0.9% NS sufficient to produce a final concentration within the range 3.2 mg/mL to 16.8 mg/mL over 60 minutes every 4 weeks (total dosage/4-week cycle = 1680 mg)

- Atezolizumab may be administered through an administration set either with or without a low-protein binding in-line filter with pore sizes of 0.2–0.22 μm
- If the initial infusion is well tolerated, subsequent administration may be completed over 30 minutes
- Severe infusion reactions have occurred in patients in clinical trials of atezolizumab
  - Interrupt or slow the administration rate in patients with mild or moderate infusion reactions
  - Permanently discontinue atezolizumab in patients who experience infusion reactions G ≥3

Supportive Care

Antiemetic prophylaxis
Emetogenic potential is **LOW**
See Chapter 42 for antiemetic recommendations

Hematopoietic growth factor (CSF) prophylaxis
Primary prophylaxis is **NOT** indicated
See Chapter 43 for more information

Antimicrobial prophylaxis
Risk of fever and neutropenia is **LOW**
Antimicrobial primary prophylaxis to be considered:
- Antibacterial—not indicated
- Antifungal—not indicated
- Antiviral—not indicated, unless patient previously had an episode of HSV

Patient Population Studied

Two cohorts of patients were enrolled into a multicenter, phase 2 trial (IMvigor210). Cohort 1 contained 119 patients with inoperable, locally advanced, or metastatic urothelial cancer who were not eligible for cisplatin treatment. Eligible patients had measurable disease and Eastern Cooperative Oncology Group (ECOG) performance status ≤2. Patients who had previously received neoadjuvant or adjuvant chemotherapy or radiation were eligible if >12 months had elapsed between treatment and recurrence. Cohort 2 contained 310 patients with inoperable, locally advanced, or metastatic urothelial cancer who had experienced disease progression after platinum-based chemotherapy. Eligible patients had measurable disease, ECOG performance status ≤1, adequate hematologic and end-organ function, and no autoimmune disease or active infections. Patients received intravenous atezolizumab (1200 mg) every 21 days

Efficacy

	Cohort 1 (N = 119) (First-Line Treatment in Cisplatin-Ineligible Patients)	Cohort 2 (N = 310) (Second-Line Treatment)
Objective response rate*	23% (95% CI 16–31%)	15% (95% CI 11–19%)
Median progression-free survival	2.7 months (95% CI 2.1–4.2 months)	2.1 months (95% CI 2.1–2.1 months)
Median overall survival	15.9 months (95% CI 10.4–NE)	7.9 months (95% CI 6.6–9.3 months)
Overall survival at 12 months	57% (95% CI 48–66%)	36% (95% CI 30–41%)

*Per Response Evaluation Criteria in Solid Tumors (RECIST) version 1.1 (central review). Median follow-up of 17.2 months for cohort 1 and 11.7 months for cohort 2. NE, not estimable

Therapy Monitoring

1. Monitor patients for signs and symptoms of infusion-related reactions, including pyrexia, chills, flushing, hypotension, dyspnea, wheezing, back pain, abdominal pain, and urticaria
2. Initially at the time of each dose, and eventually every 6–12 weeks, perform a total body skin examination with attention to *all* mucous membranes, as well as a complete review of systems
3. Monitor patients for signs and symptoms of pneumonitis. Evaluate patients with suspected pneumonitis with chest x-ray, CT scan, and pulse oximetry. For toxicity ≥2, may include nasal swab, sputum culture and sensitivity, blood culture and sensitivity, and urine culture and sensitivity
4. Monitor patients for signs and symptoms of colitis. Encourage patients to report diarrhea immediately to any member of the health care team
5. Draw AST, ALT, and bilirubin prior to each infusion and/or weekly if there are G1 LFT elevations. *Note:* No treatment is recommended for G1 LFT abnormalities. For toxicity ≥2, implement work-up for other causes of elevated LFTs, including viral hepatitis
6. Use basic metabolic panel (Na, K, CO_2, glucose) and patient history as screening tools for hypophysitis, including hypopituitarism and adrenal insufficiency. If in doubt, evaluate morning adrenocorticotropic hormone (ACTH) and cortisol levels. Consider ACTH stimulation test for indeterminate results
7. Assess thyroid function at the start of treatment, periodically during treatment, and as indicated based on clinical evaluation, and for clinical signs and symptoms of thyroid disorders. Test for TSH and free thyroxine (FT4) every 4–6 weeks as part of routine clinical monitoring on therapy or for case detection in symptomatic patients
8. Measure glucose at baseline and with each treatment during the first 12 weeks and every 6 weeks thereafter
9. Obtain a serum creatinine level prior to every dose. If creatinine is found to be newly elevated, consider holding therapy while other potential causes are evaluated. *Note:* Routine urinalysis is not necessary other than to rule out urinary tract infections, etc
10. Obtain a complete rheumatologic history and perform an examination of all peripheral joints for tenderness, swelling, and range of motion. Examine the spine. Consider plain x-ray/imaging to exclude metastases and evaluate joint damage (erosions), if appropriate
11. In patients at high risk for infections and in appropriately selected patients based on an infectious disease evaluation, draw screening laboratories (HIV, hepatitis A and B, and blood QuantiFERON for TB) to prepare patients to start infliximab
12. Response evaluation: Every 2–4 months

Treatment Modifications

RECOMMENDED DOSE MODIFICATIONS FOR ATEZOLIZUMAB

Adverse Event	Grade/Severity	Treatment Modification
Infusion reaction	Clinically significant but not severe infusion reaction	Interrupt the infusion in patients with clinically significant infusion reactions and consider resuming at a slower rate following resolution. If decision is made to restart, begin at ≤50% of the rate prior to the reaction and increase in 50% increments every 30 minutes if well tolerated. Infusions may be restarted at the full rate during the next cycle
	G3/4 (severe infusion reaction—pyrexia, chills, flushing, hypotension, dyspnea, wheezing, back pain, abdominal pain, and urticaria). Not rapidly responsive to brief interruption of infusion	Stop infusion and administer appropriate medical therapy (eg, epinephrine, corticosteroids, intravenous antihistamines, bronchodilators, and/or oxygen). Discontinue atezolizumab
Infection	Severe or life threatening	Withhold atezolizumab
Colitis	G1	Loperamide 4 mg as starting dose, then 2 mg before each meal and after each loose stool until without diarrhea for 12 hours, with maximum of 16 mg loperamide per day. If G1 diarrhea or colitis persists >14 days, add prednisolone 0.5–1 mg/kg (non-enteric-coated) or consider oral budesonide 9 mg daily if no bloody diarrhea
	G2/3 diarrhea or colitis	Withhold atezolizumab. Loperamide 4 mg as starting dose, then 2 mg before each meal and after each loose stool until without diarrhea for 12 hours, with maximum of 16 mg loperamide per day. Administer oral prednisone/prednisolone at a dosage of 0.5–2 mg/kg/day or its equivalent. When symptoms improve to G1, begin a slow corticosteroid taper over at least 4 weeks. Resume atezolizumab upon symptom control, or when prednisone/prednisolone daily dose <10 mg

(continued)

Treatment Modifications (*continued*)

RECOMMENDED DOSE MODIFICATIONS FOR ATEZOLIZUMAB

Adverse Event	Grade/Severity	Treatment Modification
	G4 diarrhea or colitis	Permanently discontinue atezolizumab. Loperamide 4 mg as starting dose, then 2 mg before each meal and after each loose stool until without diarrhea for 12 hours, with maximum of 16 mg loperamide per day. Administer 1–2 mg/kg intravenous (methyl) prednisolone and convert to 0.5–2 mg/kg prednisone/prednisolone orally each day or its equivalent only after a response. Taper over at least 4 weeks when symptoms improve. If symptoms do not improve over 72 hours or worsen, perform flexible sigmoidoscopy/ colonoscopy to document colitis, then begin infliximab 5 mg/kg (if no perforation, sepsis, TB, hepatitis, NYHA III/IV CHF). If no response, add MMF 500–1000 mg twice daily. If worse on MMF, consider addition of tacrolimus or ATG
Pneumonitis	G2	Withhold atezolizumab. Start *Pneumocystis* prophylaxis (while patient is receiving a glucocorticoid dose equivalent to ≥20 mg of prednisone daily for 4 weeks or longer) and coverage with empiric antibiotics. Administer oral prednisone/prednisolone at a dosage of 1–2 mg/kg/day or its equivalent. When symptoms improve to G1, begin a slow corticosteroid taper over at least 4 weeks. If response is not adequate after 48 hours, administer 2–4 mg/kg intravenous (methyl)prednisolone and convert to 0.5–2 mg/kg prednisone/prednisolone orally each day or its equivalent only after a response, followed by a taper over at least 6 weeks when symptoms improve to G1, titrating to symptoms. Resume atezolizumab upon symptom control, or when prednisone/prednisolone daily dose <10 mg
	G3/4	Permanently discontinue atezolizumab. Start *Pneumocystis* prophylaxis (while patient is receiving a glucocorticoid dose equivalent to ≥20 mg of prednisone daily for 4 weeks or longer); cover with empiric antibiotics. Administer 2–4 mg/kg intravenous (methyl) prednisolone and convert to 1–2 mg/kg prednisone/prednisolone orally each day or its equivalent only after a response, followed by a taper over at least 8 weeks when symptoms improve to G1, titrating to symptoms. If, when initially treated, improvement does not occur within 48–72 hours, begin infliximab 5 mg/kg (if no perforation, sepsis, TB, hepatitis, NYHA III/IV CHF). If no response to infliximab, add MMF 500–1000 mg twice daily. Consider MMF, especially if concurrent hepatic toxicity
Hepatitis	G2 (AST or ALT >3–5× ULN or total bilirubin >1.5–3× ULN)	Withhold atezolizumab. Administer oral prednisone/prednisolone at a dosage of 1 mg/ kg/day or its equivalent. When symptoms improve to G1, begin a slow corticosteroid taper over at least 4 weeks. Resume atezolizumab upon symptom control, or when prednisone/ prednisolone daily dose <10 mg
	G3/4 (AST or ALT >5× ULN or total bilirubin >3× ULN)	Permanently discontinue atezolizumab. Administer 1–2 mg/kg intravenous (methyl) prednisolone and convert to 0.5–2 mg/kg prednisone/prednisolone orally each day or its equivalent only after a response. Taper over at least 6 weeks when symptoms improve. If no response, add MMF 500–1000 mg twice daily. If worse on MMF, consider adding tacrolimus or ATG
Hypophysitis	G2/3 (moderate symptoms, ie, headache but no visual disturbance or fatigue/mood alteration but hemodynamically stable, no electrolyte disturbance)	Administer analgesia as needed for headache. Withhold atezolizumab. Administer oral prednisone/prednisolone at a dosage of 0.5–2 mg/kg/day or its equivalent. When symptoms improve to G1, begin a slow corticosteroid taper over at least 4 weeks. If no improvement in 48 hours, administer 1–2 mg/kg intravenous (methyl)prednisolone and convert to 0.5–2 mg/kg prednisone/prednisolone orally each day or its equivalent only after a response. Taper over at least 4 weeks when symptoms improve to 5 mg prednisone/ prednisolone or equivalent; do not stop steroids. Resume atezolizumab upon symptom control, or when prednisone/prednisolone daily dose <10 mg
	G4 (severe mass effect symptoms, ie, severe headache, any visual disturbance; or severe hypoadrenalism, ie, hypotension, severe electrolyte disturbance)	Permanently discontinue atezolizumab. Administer analgesia as needed for headache. Administer 1–2 mg/kg intravenous (methyl)prednisolone and convert to 0.5–2 mg/kg prednisone/prednisolone orally each day or its equivalent only after a response. Taper over at least 4 weeks when symptoms improve to 5 mg prednisone/prednisolone or equivalent; do not stop steroids

(*continued*)

Treatment Modifications (continued)

RECOMMENDED DOSE MODIFICATIONS FOR ATEZOLIZUMAB

Adverse Event	Grade/Severity	Treatment Modification
Adrenal insufficiency	G2	Withhold atezolizumab. Administer oral prednisone/prednisolone at a dosage of 0.5–2 mg/kg/day or its equivalent. When symptoms improve to G1, begin a slow corticosteroid taper over at least 4 weeks. Serially assess adrenal function and continue steroids at replacement doses (20–40 mg hydrocortisone daily, ~2/3 dose in morning upon awakening and ~1/3 at 4 PM) until recovery of adrenal function is documented. Resume atezolizumab upon symptom control, or when prednisone/prednisolone daily dose <10 mg
	G3/4	Permanently discontinue atezolizumab. Administer oral prednisone/prednisolone at a dosage of 0.5–2 mg/kg/day or its equivalent. When symptoms improve to G1, begin a slow corticosteroid taper over at least 4 weeks. Serially assess adrenal function and continue steroids at replacement doses (20–40 mg hydrocortisone daily ~2/3 dose in morning upon awakening and ~1/3 at 4 PM) until recovery of adrenal function is documented
Type 1 diabetes mellitus	G3 hyperglycemia	Withhold atezolizumab. Admit to hospital to manage hyperglycemia. Role of corticosteroids in preventing complete loss of insulin-producing cells is unknown and use is not recommended. Resume atezolizumab upon symptom control, or when prednisone/prednisolone daily dose <10 mg
	G4 hyperglycemia	Permanently discontinue atezolizumab. Admit to hospital to manage hyperglycemia. Role of corticosteroids in preventing complete loss of insulin-producing cells is unknown and use is not recommended
Nephritis and renal dysfunction	G2/3 (serum creatinine 1.5–6× ULN)	Withhold atezolizumab. Administer oral prednisone/prednisolone at a dosage of 0.5–2 mg/kg/day or its equivalent. When symptoms improve to G1, begin a slow corticosteroid taper over at least 4 weeks. If response is not adequate, administer 0.5–1 mg/kg intravenous (methyl)prednisolone and convert to 0.5–2 mg/kg prednisone/prednisolone orally each day or its equivalent only after a response, followed by a taper over at least 4 weeks when symptoms improve to G1. Resume atezolizumab upon symptom control, or when prednisone/prednisolone daily dose <10 mg
	G4 (serum creatinine >6× ULN)	Permanently discontinue atezolizumab. Administer 0.5–1 mg/kg intravenous (methyl)prednisolone and convert to 0.5–2 mg/kg prednisone/prednisolone orally each day or its equivalent only after a response, followed by a taper over at least 4 weeks when symptoms improve to G1
Skin	G1/2	Continue atezolizumab. Avoid skin irritants, avoid sun exposure; topical emollients recommended. Topical steroid (mild strength for G1, moderate/potent strength for G2) cream once or twice daily ± oral or topical antihistamines for itching
	G3 rash or suspected SJS or TEN	Withhold atezolizumab. Avoid skin irritants, avoid sun exposure; topical emollients recommended. Administer oral or topical antihistamines for itching. Administer oral prednisone/prednisolone at a dosage of 0.5–2 mg/kg or its equivalent daily for 3 days followed by a slow corticosteroid taper over at least 4 weeks when the rash improves to G1. If rash does not respond adequately, administer 0.5–1 mg/kg intravenous (methyl)prednisolone and convert to 0.5–2 mg/kg prednisone/prednisolone orally each day or its equivalent only after a response, followed by a taper over at least 4 weeks when the rash improves to G1. Resume atezolizumab upon symptom control, or when prednisone/prednisolone daily dose <10 mg
	G4 rash or confirmed SJS or TEN	Avoid skin irritants, avoid sun exposure; topical emollients recommended. Administer oral or topical antihistamines for itching. Administer 1–2 mg/kg intravenous (methyl)prednisolone and convert to oral steroids 0.5–2 mg/kg prednisone/prednisolone each day or its equivalent only after a response. Taper over at least 4 weeks when the rash improves to G1. Permanently discontinue atezolizumab

(continued)

Treatment Modifications (*continued*)

RECOMMENDED DOSE MODIFICATIONS FOR ATEZOLIZUMAB

Adverse Event	Grade/Severity	Treatment Modification
Encephalitis	Confusion or altered behavior, headaches, alteration in Glasgow Coma Scale, motor or sensory deficits, speech abnormality; may or may not be febrile	Initially withhold atezolizumab, but permanently discontinue atezolizumab if there is no doubt as to diagnosis. Exclude bacterial and ideally viral infections prior to high-dose steroids. Administer 1–2 mg/kg intravenous (methyl)prednisolone for 5 days or oral prednisone/prednisolone at a dosage of 0.5–2 mg/kg/day or its equivalent. When symptoms improve, begin a slow corticosteroid taper over at least 4–8 weeks. If symptoms are severe, administer 1–2 mg/kg intravenous (methyl)prednisolone and convert to 0.5–2 mg/kg prednisone/prednisolone orally each day or its equivalent only after a response. Consider concurrent empiric antiviral (intravenous acyclovir) and antibacterial therapy
Aseptic meningitis	Headache, photophobia, neck stiffness with fever, or may be afebrile, vomiting; normal cognition/cerebral function (distinguishes from encephalitis)	
Other syndromes include neurosarcoidosis, posterior reversible leukoencephalopathy syndrome (PRES), Vogt-Koyanagi-Harada syndrome, demyelination, vasculitic encephalopathy, and generalized seizures		
Transverse myelitis	Acute or subacute neurologic signs/symptoms of motor, sensory, autonomic origin; most have sensory level; often bilateral symptoms	Initially withhold atezolizumab, but permanently discontinue atezolizumab if there is no doubt as to diagnosis. Administer 2 mg/kg intravenous (methyl)prednisolone or consider 1 g/day and convert to 0.5–2 mg/kg prednisone/prednisolone orally each day or its equivalent only after a response. When symptoms improve, begin a slow corticosteroid taper over at least 4–8 weeks. Plasmapheresis may be required if steroids do not bring about improvement
Myocarditis	G3	Permanently discontinue atezolizumab. Administer 2 mg/kg intravenous (methyl)prednisolone or consider 1 g/day and convert to 0.5–2 mg/kg prednisone/prednisolone orally each day or its equivalent only after a response. When symptoms improve, begin a slow corticosteroid taper over at least 4–8 weeks. If no response, add MMF 500–1000 mg twice daily. If worse on MMF, consider adding tacrolimus
Peripheral neurologic toxicity	Moderate: some interference with ADL, symptoms concerning to patient	Withhold atezolizumab. Initial observation reasonable or initiate prednisone/prednisolone 0.5–1 mg/kg (if progressing, eg, from mild) and/or pregabalin or duloxetine for pain. When symptoms improve, begin a slow corticosteroid taper over at least 4 weeks. Resume atezolizumab upon symptom control, or when prednisone/prednisolone daily dose <10 mg
	Severe: limits self-care and aids warranted, life-threatening, eg, respiratory problems	Permanently discontinue atezolizumab. Administer 1–2 mg/kg intravenous (methyl)prednisolone and convert to 0.5–2 mg/kg prednisone/prednisolone orally each day or its equivalent only after a response. Taper over at least 4–8 weeks when symptoms improve to G1
Guillain-Barré syndrome	Progressive symmetrical muscle weakness with absent or reduced tendon reflexes—involves extremities, facial, respiratory, and bulbar and oculomotor muscles; dysregulation of autonomic nerves	Permanently discontinue atezolizumab. Use of steroids not recommended in idiopathic Guillain-Barré syndrome; however, a trial of (methyl)prednisolone 1–2 mg/kg is reasonable, converting to 0.5–2 mg/kg prednisone/prednisolone orally each day or its equivalent only after a response. If no improvement or worsening, plasmapheresis or IVIG indicated
Myasthenia gravis	Fluctuating muscle weakness (proximal limb, trunk, ocular, eg, ptosis/diplopia or bulbar) with fatigability; respiratory muscles may also be involved	Permanently discontinue atezolizumab. Administer pyridostigmine at an initial dose of 30 mg 3 times daily. Administer oral prednisone/prednisolone at a dosage of 0.5–2 mg/kg/day or its equivalent or 1–2 mg/kg intravenous (methyl)prednisolone, depending on the severity of symptoms. If treatment begins with intravenous drug, convert to 0.5–2 mg/kg prednisone/prednisolone orally each day or its equivalent only after a response. If no improvement or worsening, plasmapheresis or IVIG may be considered. Additional immunosuppressants used in myasthenia gravis include azathioprine, cyclosporine, and mycophenolate. Avoid certain medications, eg, ciprofloxacin, beta-blockers, that may precipitate cholinergic crisis

(*continued*)

Treatment Modifications (continued)

RECOMMENDED DOSE MODIFICATIONS FOR ATEZOLIZUMAB

Adverse Event	Grade/Severity	Treatment Modification
Other syndromes, including motor and sensory peripheral neuropathy, multifocal radicular neuropathy/plexopathy, autonomic neuropathy, phrenic nerve palsy, cranial nerve palsies (eg, facial nerve, optic nerve, hypoglossal nerve)		Permanently discontinue atezolizumab. Administer oral prednisone/prednisolone at a dosage of 0.5–2 mg/kg/day or its equivalent or 1–2 mg/kg intravenous (methyl) prednisolone, depending on the severity of symptoms. If treatment begins with intravenous drug, convert to 0.5–2 mg/kg prednisone/prednisolone orally each day or its equivalent only after a response
Arthralgia	G1 (mild pain with inflammation, erythema, or joint swelling)	Continue atezolizumab. Administer acetaminophen (paracetamol) and ibuprofen
	G2 (moderate pain with inflammation, erythema, or joint swelling that limits ADLs)	Withhold atezolizumab. Administer higher doses of acetaminophen (paracetamol) and ibuprofen and use diclofenac or naproxen or etoricoxib. If inadequately controlled, consider intra-articular steroid injections for large joints or administer oral prednisone/prednisolone at a dosage of 0.5–2 mg/kg/day or its equivalent. When symptoms improve to G1, begin a slow corticosteroid taper over at least 4 weeks. If response is not adequate, administer 0.5–1 mg/kg intravenous (methyl)prednisolone and convert to 0.5–2 mg/kg prednisone/prednisolone orally each day or its equivalent only after a response, followed by a taper over at least 4 weeks when symptoms improve to G1. Resume atezolizumab upon symptom control, or when prednisone/prednisolone daily dose <10 mg
	G3 (severe pain; irreversible joint damage; disabling; limits self-care ADL)	Withhold atezolizumab. Administer 0.5–1 mg/kg intravenous (methyl)prednisolone and convert to 0.5–2 mg/kg prednisone/prednisolone orally each day or its equivalent only after a response, followed by a taper over at least 4 weeks when symptoms improve to G1. In severe cases, infliximab or another anti-TNF-alpha drug may be required for improvement of arthritis. Resume atezolizumab upon symptom control, or when prednisone/prednisolone daily dose <10 mg
Other	First occurrence of other G3	Withhold atezolizumab. Administer oral prednisone/prednisolone at a dosage of 0.5–2 mg/kg/day or its equivalent. When symptoms improve to G1, begin a slow corticosteroid taper over at least 4 weeks. Resume atezolizumab upon symptom control, or when prednisone/prednisolone daily dose <10 mg
	Recurrence of same G3	Permanently discontinue atezolizumab. Administer 1–2 mg/kg intravenous (methyl) prednisolone and convert to 0.5–2 mg/kg prednisone/prednisolone orally each day or its equivalent only after a response. Taper over at least 4–8 weeks when symptoms improve to G1
	Life-threatening or G4	
	Requirement for ≥10 mg/day prednisone or equivalent for >12 weeks	Permanently discontinue atezolizumab
	Persistent G2/3 adverse reactions lasting ≥12 weeks	

ADL, activities of daily living; ALT, alanine aminotransferase; AST, aspartate aminotransferase; ATG, antithymocyte globulin; IVIG, intravenous immunoglobulin; MMF, mycophenolate mofetil; NYHA, New York Heart Association; SJS, Stevens-Johnson syndrome; TEN, toxic epidermal necrolysis; ULN, upper limit of normal

Notes on general supportive care:
- Steroid taper in most cases will proceed over a minimum of 1 month, but if symptoms improve rapidly, a 2-week taper can be considered. If steroids are administered for more than 4 weeks, administer PCP prophylaxis (cotrimoxazole 480 mg twice daily M/W/F or inhaled pentamidine if cotrimoxazole allergy), regular random blood glucose, vitamin D level and starting calcium/vitamin D supplementation per guidelines

Notes on pregnancy and breastfeeding:
- Atezolizumab can cause fetal harm. If used during pregnancy, or if the patient becomes pregnant during treatment, apprise the patient of the potential hazard to a fetus. Females of reproductive potential should use highly effective contraception during treatment and for 5 months after the last dose of atezolizumab
- It is not known whether atezolizumab is excreted in human milk. Therefore, it is recommended that women discontinue nursing during treatment with and for 5 months after the final dose of atezolizumab

Adverse Events

Grade (%)*	Cohort 1 (N = 119) (First-Line Treatment in Cisplatin-Ineligible Patients)		Cohort 2 (N = 310) (Second-Line Treatment)	
	Grade 1/2	Grade 3–4	Grade 1/2	Grade 3–4
Fatigue	27	3	28	2
Diarrhea	10	2	7	<1
Pruritus	10	<1	10	<1
Decreased appetite	8	<1	11	<1
Hypothyroidism	7	0	—	—
Anemia	4	<1	2	<1
Rash	4	<1	7	<1
Chills	5	0	—	—
Nausea	5	0	14	0
Pyrexia	5	0	9	<1
Vomiting	5	0	5	<1
Elevated ALT level	<1	3	—	—
Arthralgia	4	0	6	<1
Rash, macropapular	4	0	—	—
Elevated AST level	<1	3	3	<1
Elevated blood bilirubin levels	2	2	—	—
Elevated blood alkaline phosphatase level	3	<1	—	—
Decreased lymphocyte count	3	0	—	—
Dyspnea	3	0	3	<1
Infusion-related reaction	3	0	—	—
Hypophosphatemia	<1	2	—	—
Hypotension	2	<1	<1	<1
Pneumonitis	—	—	2	<1
Asthenia	3	0	—	—
Back pain	3	0	—	—
Dermatitis acneiform	3	0	—	—
Dry mouth	3	0	—	—
Headache	3	0	—	—
Influenza-like illness	3	0	—	—
Muscle spasms	3	0	—	—
Thrombocytopenia	3	0	—	—

(continued)

Adverse Events (*continued*)

Grade (%)*	Cohort 1 (N = 119) (First-Line Treatment in Cisplatin-Ineligible Patients)		Cohort 2 (N = 310) (Second-Line Treatment)	
	Grade 1/2	Grade 3–4	Grade 1/2	Grade 3–4
Renal failure	0	2	—	—
Autoimmune colitis	0	<1	<1	<1
Hypersensitivity	0	<1	—	—
Hypertension	—	—	0	<1
Liver disorder	0	<1	—	—
Multiple organ dysfunction syndrome	0	<1	—	—
Portal vein thrombosis	0	<1	—	—

*According to the National Cancer Institute Common Terminology Criteria for Adverse Events, version 4.0
Note: Treatment-related toxicities are included in the table if all-grade events occurred in ≥3 patients or G3/4 events occurred in ≥1 patient. One patient in cohort 1 had a treatment-related G5 adverse event (sepsis with unidentified source of infection). No patients in cohort 2 had a treatment-related death

METASTATIC • FIRST-LINE • SUBSEQUENT THERAPY
BLADDER CANCER REGIMEN: PEMBROLIZUMAB

Balar AV et al. Lancet Oncol 2017;18:1483–1492
Bellmunt J et al. N Engl J Med 2017;376:1015–1026. Comment in: N Engl J Med 2017;376:2302–2304
Brahmer JR et al. J Clin Oncol 2018;36:1714–1768
Freshwater T et al. J Immunother Cancer 2017;5:43
Haanen JB et al. Ann Oncol 2017;28(suppl 4):iv119–iv142
FDA and EMA prescribing information

The U.S. Food and Drug Administration (FDA)–approved regimen for urothelial carcinoma includes a fixed dose of pembrolizumab, consistent with the regimen approved on May 18, 2017, and consistent with the regimens described by Bellmunt et al and Balar et al, thus:

Pembrolizumab 200 mg; administer intravenously over 30 minutes in a volume of 0.9% sodium chloride injection (0.9% NS) or 5% dextrose injection (D5W) sufficient to produce a pembrolizumab concentration within the range 1–10 mg/mL every 3 weeks for up to 24 months (total dosage/ cycle = 200 mg)

Alternative pembrolizumab dose and schedule as per the U.S. FDA regimens approved on April 28, 2020:

Pembrolizumab 400 mg; administer intravenously over 30 minutes in a volume of 0.9% NS or D5W sufficient to produce a pembrolizumab concentration within the range 1–10 mg/mL every 6 weeks for up to 24 months (total dose/6-week cycle = 400 mg)

- Administer pembrolizumab with an administration set that contains a sterile, nonpyrogenic, low protein-binding in-line or add-on filter with pore size within the range of 0.2–5 μm
- Patients who achieved a confirmed complete response after receiving at least 6 months of pembrolizumab could discontinue treatment after receiving 2 doses beyond the determination of complete response
- Pembrolizumab can cause severe or life-threatening infusion-related reactions, including hypersensitivity and anaphylaxis

Supportive Care
Antiemetic prophylaxis
Emetogenic potential is **MINIMAL**
See Chapter 42 for antiemetic recommendations

Hematopoietic growth factor (CSF) prophylaxis
Primary prophylaxis is **NOT** indicated
See Chapter 43 for more information

Antimicrobial prophylaxis
Risk of fever and neutropenia is **LOW**
  Antimicrobial primary prophylaxis to be considered:
- Antibacterial—not indicated
- Antifungal—not indicated
- Antiviral—not indicated, unless patient previously had an episode of HSV

Patient Population Studied

The multicenter, single-arm phase 2 trial (KEYNOTE-052) involved 370 patients with histologically or cytologically confirmed, locally advanced and inoperable or metastatic urothelial cancer who were not eligible for cisplatin treatment. Eligible patients were aged ≥18 years and had measurable disease and Eastern Cooperative Oncology Group (ECOG) performance status ≤2; life expectancy >3 months; adequate hematologic, renal, and liver function; and had not previously received systemic therapy for advanced disease. Patients who had previously received perioperative, platinum-based chemotherapy were eligible if >12 months had elapsed between treatment and recurrence. Patients received intravenous pembrolizumab (200 mg) every 21 days
The multicenter, open-label, randomized, phase 3 trial (KEYNOTE-045) involved 542 patients with histologically or cytologically confirmed urothelial cancer that showed predominantly transitional-cell features on histology who had experienced disease progression or recurrence after platinum-based chemotherapy. Eligible patients were aged ≥18 years, had measurable disease and ECOG performance status ≤2, and had previously received ≤2 lines of systemic chemotherapy for advanced disease. Patients were randomly assigned (1:1) to receive intravenous pembrolizumab (200 mg) or investigator's choice of paclitaxel (175 mg/m²), docetaxel (75 mg/m²), or vinflunine (320 mg/m²) every 21 days

Efficacy

	Used as First-Line Treatment in Cisplatin-Ineligible Patients (N = 370) (phase 2 trial)	Used as Second-Line Treatment (N = 542) (phase 3 trial)
Objective response rate*	24% (95% CI 20–29)	21.1% (95% CI 16.4–26.5) in pembrolizumab group 11.4% (95% CI 7.9–15.8) in chemotherapy group P = 0.001
Median progression-free survival[†]	2 months (95% CI 2–3)	2.1 months (95% CI 2.0–2.2) in pembrolizumab group 3.3 months (95% CI 2.3–3.5) in chemotherapy group HR for disease progression or death 0.98 (95% CI 0.81–1.19); P = 0.42
Median overall survival[†]	—	10.3 months (95% CI 8.0–11.8) in pembrolizumab group 7.4 months (95% CI 6.1–8.3) in chemotherapy group HR for death 0.73 (95% CI 0.59–0.91); P = 0.002
Overall survival at 12 months	—	43.9% (95% CI 37.8–49.9) in pembrolizumab group 30.7% (95% CI 25.0–36.7) in chemotherapy group
Overall survival at 6 months	67% (95% CI 62–73)	—

*Per Response Evaluation Criteria in Solid Tumors (RECIST) version 1.1 (central review). Primary endpoint in the phase 2 trial, secondary endpoint in the phase 3 trial. Median follow-up of 5 months for the phase 2 trial and 14.1 months for the phase 3 trial
[†]Co-primary endpoint in the phase 3 trial

Therapy Monitoring

1. Monitor patients for signs and symptoms of infusion-related reactions including pyrexia, chills, flushing, hypotension, dyspnea, wheezing, back pain, abdominal pain, and urticaria

2. Initially at the time of each dose, and eventually every 6–12 weeks, perform a total body skin examination with attention to *all* mucous membranes as well as a complete review of systems

3. Monitor patients for signs and symptoms of pneumonitis. Evaluate patients with suspected pneumonitis with chest x-ray, CT scan, and pulse oximetry. For toxicity ≥2, may include nasal swab, sputum culture and sensitivity, blood culture and sensitivity, and urine culture and sensitivity

4. Monitor patients for signs and symptoms of colitis. Encourage patients to report diarrhea immediately to any member of the healthcare team

5. Draw AST, ALT, and bilirubin prior to each infusion and/or weekly if there are G1 LFT elevations. Note, no treatment is recommended for G1 LFT abnormalities. For toxicity ≥2, work up for other causes of elevated LFTs, including viral hepatitis

6. Use basic metabolic panel (Na, K, CO_2, glucose) and patient history as screening tools for hypophysitis, including hypopituitarism and adrenal insufficiency. If in doubt evaluate morning adrenocorticotropic hormone (ACTH) and cortisol levels. Consider ACTH stimulation test for indeterminate results

7. Assess thyroid function at the start of treatment, periodically during treatment, and as indicated based on clinical evaluation, and for clinical signs and symptoms of thyroid disorders. Test for TSH and free thyroxine (FT4) every 4–6 weeks as part of routine clinical monitoring on therapy or for case detection in symptomatic patients

8. Measure glucose at baseline and with each treatment during the first 12 weeks and every 6 weeks thereafter

9. Obtain a serum creatinine level prior to every dose. If creatinine is found to be newly elevated, consider holding therapy while other potential causes are evaluated. *Note:* Routine urinalysis is not necessary other than to rule out urinary tract infections, etc

10. Obtain a complete rheumatologic history and perform an examination of all peripheral joints for tenderness, swelling, and range of motion. Examine the spine. Consider plain x-ray/imaging to exclude metastases and evaluate joint damage (erosions), if appropriate

11. In patients at high risk for infections and in appropriately selected patients based on an infectious disease evaluation, draw screening laboratories (HIV, hepatitis A and B, and blood QuantiFERON for TB) to prepare patients to start infliximab

12. Response evaluation: Every 2–4 months

Treatment Modifications

RECOMMENDED DOSE MODIFICATIONS FOR PEMBROLIZUMAB

Adverse Event	Grade/Severity	Treatment Modification
Infusion reaction	Clinically significant but not severe infusion reaction	Interrupt the infusion in patients with clinically significant infusion reactions and consider resuming at a slower rate following resolution. If decision is made to restart, begin at ≤50% of the rate prior to the reaction and increase in 50% increments every 30 minutes if well tolerated. Infusions may be restarted at the full rate during the next cycle
	G3/4 (severe infusion reaction—pyrexia, chills, flushing, hypotension, dyspnea, wheezing, back pain, abdominal pain, and urticaria). Not rapidly responsive to brief interruption of infusion	Stop infusion and administer appropriate medical therapy (eg, epinephrine, corticosteroids, intravenous antihistamines, bronchodilators, and/or oxygen). Discontinue pembrolizumab
Colitis	G1	Loperamide 4 mg as starting dose, then 2 mg before each meal and after each loose stool until without diarrhea for 12 hours, with maximum of 16 mg loperamide per day. If G1 diarrhea or colitis persists >14 days, add prednisolone 0.5–1 mg/kg (non-enteric-coated) or consider oral budesonide 9 mg daily if no bloody diarrhea
	G2/3 diarrhea or colitis	Withhold pembrolizumab. Loperamide 4 mg as starting dose, then 2 mg before each meal and after each loose stool until without diarrhea for 12 hours, with maximum of 16 mg loperamide per day. Administer oral prednisone/prednisolone at a dosage of 0.5–2 mg/kg/day or its equivalent. When symptoms improve to G1, begin a slow corticosteroid taper over at least 4 weeks. Resume pembrolizumab upon symptom control, or when prednisone/prednisolone daily dose <10 mg
	G4 diarrhea or colitis	Permanently discontinue pembrolizumab. Loperamide 4 mg as starting dose, then 2 mg before each meal and after each loose stool until without diarrhea for 12 hours, with maximum of 16 mg loperamide per day. Administer 1–2 mg/kg intravenous (methyl)prednisolone and convert to 0.5–2 mg/kg prednisone/prednisolone orally each day or its equivalent only after a response. Taper over at least 4 weeks when symptoms improve. If symptoms do not improve over 72 hours or worsen, perform flexible sigmoidoscopy/colonoscopy to document colitis then begin infliximab 5 mg/kg (if no perforation, sepsis, TB, hepatitis, NYHA III/IV CHF). If no response, add MMF 500–1000 mg twice daily. If worse on MMF, consider addition of tacrolimus or ATG
Pneumonitis	G2	Withhold pembrolizumab. Start *Pneumocystis* prophylaxis (while patient is receiving a glucocorticoid dose equivalent to ≥20 mg of prednisone daily for 4 weeks or longer) and coverage with empiric antibiotics. Administer oral prednisone/prednisolone at a dose of 1–2 mg/kg/day or its equivalent. When symptoms improve to G1, begin a slow corticosteroid taper over at least 4 weeks. If response is not adequate after 48 hours, administer 2–4 mg/kg intravenous (methyl)prednisolone and convert to 0.5–2 mg/kg prednisone/prednisolone orally each day or its equivalent only after a response, followed by a taper over at least 6 weeks when symptoms improve to G1, titrating to symptoms. Resume pembrolizumab upon symptom control, or when prednisone/prednisolone daily dose <10 mg
	G3/4	Permanently discontinue pembrolizumab. Start *Pneumocystis* prophylaxis (while patient is receiving a glucocorticoid dose equivalent to ≥20 mg of prednisone daily for 4 weeks or longer); cover with empiric antibiotics. Administer 2–4 mg/kg intravenous (methyl)prednisolone and convert to 1–2 mg/kg prednisone/prednisolone orally each day or its equivalent only after a response, followed by a taper over at least 8 weeks when symptoms improve to G1, titrating to symptoms. If, when initially treated, improvement does not occur within 48–72 hours, begin infliximab 5 mg/kg (if no perforation, sepsis, TB, hepatitis, NYHA III/IV CHF). If no response to infliximab, add MMF 500–1000 mg twice daily. Consider MMF, especially if concurrent hepatic toxicity

(continued)

Treatment Modifications (*continued*)

RECOMMENDED DOSE MODIFICATIONS FOR PEMBROLIZUMAB

Adverse Event	Grade/Severity	Treatment Modification
Hepatitis	G2 (AST or ALT >3–5× ULN or total bilirubin >1.5–3× ULN)	Withhold pembrolizumab. Administer oral prednisone/prednisolone at a dose of 1–2 mg/kg/day or its equivalent. When symptoms improve to G1, begin a slow corticosteroid taper over at least 4 weeks. Resume pembrolizumab upon symptom control, or when prednisone/prednisolone daily dose <10 mg
	G3/4 (AST or ALT >5× ULN or total bilirubin >3× ULN)	Permanently discontinue pembrolizumab. Administer 1–2 mg/kg intravenous (methyl)prednisolone and convert to 0.5–2 mg/kg prednisone/prednisolone orally each day or its equivalent only after a response. Taper over at least 6 weeks when symptoms improve. If no response, add MMF 500–1000 mg twice daily. If worse on MMF, consider adding tacrolimus or ATG
Hypophysitis	G2/3 (moderate symptoms, ie, headache but no visual disturbance or fatigue/mood alteration but hemodynamically stable, no electrolyte disturbance)	Administer analgesia as needed for headache. Withhold pembrolizumab. Administer oral prednisone/prednisolone at a dose of 0.5–2 mg/kg/day or its equivalent. When symptoms improve to G1, begin a slow corticosteroid taper over at least 4 weeks. If no improvement in 48 hours, administer 1–2 mg/kg intravenous (methyl)prednisolone and convert to 0.5–2 mg/kg prednisone/prednisolone orally each day or its equivalent only after a response. Taper over at least 4 weeks when symptoms improve to 5 mg prednisone/prednisolone or equivalent; do not stop steroids. Resume pembrolizumab upon symptom control, or when prednisone/prednisolone daily dose <10 mg
	G4 (severe mass effect symptoms, ie, severe headache, any visual disturbance or severe hypoadrenalism, ie, hypotension, severe electrolyte disturbance)	Permanently discontinue pembrolizumab. Administer analgesia as needed for headache. Administer 1–2 mg/kg intravenous (methyl)prednisolone and convert to 0.5–2 mg/kg prednisone/prednisolone orally each day or its equivalent only after a response. Taper over at least 4 weeks when symptoms improve to 5 mg prednisone/prednisolone or equivalent; do not stop steroids
Adrenal insufficiency	G2	Withhold pembrolizumab. Administer oral prednisone/prednisolone at a dose of 0.5–2 mg/kg/day or its equivalent. When symptoms improve to G1, begin a slow corticosteroid taper over at least 4 weeks. Serially assess adrenal function and continue steroids at replacement doses (20–40 mg hydrocortisone daily ~2/3 dose in morning upon awakening and ~1/3 at 4 PM) until recovery of adrenal function is documented. Resume pembrolizumab upon symptom control, or when prednisone/prednisolone daily dose <10 mg
	G3/4	Permanently discontinue pembrolizumab. Administer oral prednisone/prednisolone at a dose of 0.5–2 mg/kg/day or its equivalent. When symptoms improve to G1, begin a slow corticosteroid taper over at least 4 weeks. Serially assess adrenal function and continue steroids at replacement doses (20–40 mg hydrocortisone daily ~2/3 dose in morning upon awakening and ~1/3 at 4 PM) until recovery of adrenal function is documented
Type 1 diabetes mellitus	G3 hyperglycemia	Withhold pembrolizumab. Admit to hospital to manage hyperglycemia. Role of corticosteroids in preventing complete loss of insulin-producing cells is unknown and use is not recommended. Resume pembrolizumab upon symptom control, or when prednisone/prednisolone daily dose <10 mg
	G4 hyperglycemia	Permanently discontinue pembrolizumab. Admit to hospital to manage hyperglycemia. Role of corticosteroids in preventing complete loss of insulin-producing cells is unknown and use is not recommended
Nephritis and renal dysfunction	G2/3 (serum creatinine 1.5–6× ULN)	Withhold pembrolizumab. Administer oral prednisone/prednisolone at a dose of 0.5–2 mg/kg/day or its equivalent. When symptoms improve to G1, begin a slow corticosteroid taper over at least 4 weeks. If response is not adequate, administer 0.5–1 mg/kg intravenous (methyl)prednisolone and convert to 0.5–2 mg/kg prednisone/prednisolone orally each day or its equivalent only after a response, followed by a taper over at least 4 weeks when symptoms improve to G1. Resume pembrolizumab upon symptom control, or when prednisone/prednisolone daily dose <10 mg

(*continued*)

Treatment Modifications (*continued*)

RECOMMENDED DOSE MODIFICATIONS FOR PEMBROLIZUMAB

Adverse Event	Grade/Severity	Treatment Modification
	G4 (serum creatinine >6× ULN)	Permanently discontinue pembrolizumab. Administer 0.5–1 mg/kg intravenous (methyl)prednisolone and convert to 0.5–2 mg/kg prednisone/prednisolone orally each day or its equivalent only after a response, followed by a taper over at least 4 weeks when symptoms improve to G1
Skin	G1/2	Continue pembrolizumab. Avoid skin irritants, avoid sun exposure; topical emollients recommended. Topical steroid (mild strength for G1, moderate/potent strength for G2) cream once or twice daily ± oral or topical antihistamines for itching
	G3 rash or suspected SJS or TEN	Withhold pembrolizumab. Avoid skin irritants, avoid sun exposure, topical emollients recommended. Administer oral or topical antihistamines for itching. Administer oral prednisone/prednisolone at a dose of 0.5–2 mg/kg or its equivalent daily for 3 days followed by a slow corticosteroid taper over at least 4 weeks when the rash improves to G1. If rash does not respond adequately, administer 0.5–1 mg/kg intravenous (methyl)prednisolone and convert to 0.5–2 mg/kg prednisone/prednisolone orally each day or its equivalent only after a response, followed by a taper over at least 4 weeks when the rash improves to G1. Resume pembrolizumab upon symptom control, or when prednisone/prednisolone daily dose <10 mg
	G4 rash or confirmed SJS or TEN	Avoid skin irritants, avoid sun exposure; topical emollients recommended. Administer oral or topical antihistamines for itching. Administer 1–2 mg/kg intravenous (methyl)prednisolone and convert to oral steroids 0.5–2 mg/kg prednisone/prednisolone each day or its equivalent only after a response. Taper over at least 4 weeks when the rash improves to G1. Permanently discontinue pembrolizumab
Encephalitis	Confusion or altered behavior, headaches, alteration in Glasgow Coma Scale, motor or sensory deficits, speech abnormality; may or may not be febrile	Initially withhold pembrolizumab, but permanently discontinue pembrolizumab if there is no doubt as to diagnosis. Exclude bacterial and ideally viral infections prior to high-dose steroids. Administer 1–2 mg/kg intravenous (methyl)prednisolone for 5 days or oral prednisone/prednisolone at a dosage of 0.5–2 mg/kg/day or its equivalent. When symptoms improve, begin a slow corticosteroid taper over at least 4–8 weeks. If symptoms are severe, administer 1–2 mg/kg intravenous (methyl)prednisolone and convert to 0.5–2 mg/kg prednisone/prednisolone orally each day or its equivalent only after a response. Consider concurrent empiric antiviral (intravenous acyclovir) and antibacterial therapy
Aseptic meningitis	Headache, photophobia, neck stiffness with fever, or may be afebrile, vomiting; normal cognition/cerebral function (distinguishes from encephalitis)	
Other syndromes include neurosarcoidosis, posterior reversible leukoencephalopathy syndrome (PRES), Vogt-Koyanagi-Harada syndrome, demyelination, vasculitic encephalopathy, and generalized seizures		
Transverse myelitis	Acute or subacute neurologic signs/symptoms of motor, sensory, autonomic origin; most have sensory level; often bilateral symptoms	Initially withhold pembrolizumab, but permanently discontinue pembrolizumab if there is no doubt as to diagnosis. Administer 2 mg/kg intravenous (methyl)prednisolone or consider 1 g/day and convert to 0.5–2 mg/kg prednisone/prednisolone orally each day or its equivalent only after a response. When symptoms improve, begin a slow corticosteroid taper over at least 4–8 weeks. Plasmapheresis may be required if steroids do not bring about improvement
Myocarditis	G3	Permanently discontinue pembrolizumab. Administer 2 mg/kg intravenous (methyl)prednisolone or consider 1 g/day and convert to 0.5–2 mg/kg prednisone/prednisolone orally each day or its equivalent only after a response. When symptoms improve, begin a slow corticosteroid taper over at least 4–8 weeks. If no response, add MMF 500–1000 mg twice daily. If worse on MMF, consider adding tacrolimus
Peripheral neurologic toxicity	Moderate: some interference with ADL, symptoms concerning to patient	Withhold pembrolizumab. Initial observation reasonable or initiate prednisone/prednisolone 0.5–1 mg/kg (if progressing, eg, from mild) and/or pregabalin or duloxetine for pain. When symptoms improve, begin a slow corticosteroid taper over at least 4 weeks. Resume pembrolizumab upon symptom control, or when prednisone/prednisolone daily dose <10 mg

(continued)

Treatment Modifications (continued)

RECOMMENDED DOSE MODIFICATIONS FOR PEMBROLIZUMAB

Adverse Event	Grade/Severity	Treatment Modification
	Severe: limits self-care and aids warranted, life-threatening, eg, respiratory problems	Permanently discontinue pembrolizumab. Administer 1–2 mg/kg intravenous (methyl)prednisolone and convert to 0.5–2 mg/kg prednisone/prednisolone orally each day or its equivalent only after a response. Taper over at least 4–8 weeks when symptoms improve to G1
Guillain-Barré syndrome	Progressive symmetrical muscle weakness with absent or reduced tendon reflexes—involves extremities; facial, respiratory, and bulbar and oculomotor muscles; dysregulation of autonomic nerves	Permanently discontinue pembrolizumab. Use of steroids not recommended in idiopathic Guillain-Barré syndrome; however, a trial of (methyl)prednisolone 1–2 mg/kg is reasonable, converting to 0.5–2 mg/kg prednisone/prednisolone orally each day or its equivalent only after a response. If no improvement or worsening, plasmapheresis or IVIG indicated
Myasthenia gravis	Fluctuating muscle weakness (proximal limb, trunk, ocular, eg, ptosis/diplopia or bulbar) with fatigability; respiratory muscles may also be involved	Permanently discontinue pembrolizumab. Administer pyridostigmine at an initial dose of 30 mg 3 times daily. Administer oral prednisone/prednisolone at a dose of 0.5–2 mg/kg/day or its equivalent or 1–2 mg/kg intravenous (methyl)prednisolone, depending on the severity of symptoms. If treatment begins with intravenous drug, convert to 0.5–2 mg/kg prednisone/prednisolone orally each day or its equivalent only after a response. If no improvement or worsening, plasmapheresis or IVIG may be considered. Additional immunosuppressants used in myasthenia gravis include azathioprine, cyclosporine, and mycophenolate. Avoid certain medications, eg, ciprofloxacin, beta-blockers, that may precipitate cholinergic crisis
Other syndromes, including motor and sensory peripheral neuropathy, multifocal radicular neuropathy/plexopathy, autonomic neuropathy, phrenic nerve palsy, cranial nerve palsies (eg, facial nerve, optic nerve, hypoglossal nerve)		Permanently discontinue pembrolizumab. Administer oral prednisone/prednisolone at a dose of 0.5–2 mg/kg/day or its equivalent or 1–2 mg/kg intravenous (methyl)prednisolone, depending on the severity of symptoms. If treatment begins with intravenous drug, convert to 0.5–2 mg/kg prednisone/prednisolone orally each day or its equivalent only after a response
Arthralgia	G1 (mild pain with inflammation, erythema, or joint swelling)	Continue pembrolizumab. Administer acetaminophen (paracetamol) and ibuprofen
	G2 (moderate pain with inflammation, erythema, or joint swelling that limits ADLs)	Withhold pembrolizumab. Administer higher doses of acetaminophen (paracetamol) and ibuprofen and use diclofenac or naproxen or etoricoxib. If inadequately controlled, consider intra-articular steroid injections for large joints or administer oral prednisone/prednisolone at a dosage of 0.5–2 mg/kg/day or its equivalent. When symptoms improve to G1, begin a slow corticosteroid taper over at least 4 weeks. If response is not adequate, administer 0.5–1 mg/kg intravenous (methyl)prednisolone and convert to 0.5–2 mg/kg prednisone/prednisolone orally each day or its equivalent only after a response, followed by a taper over at least 4 weeks when symptoms improve to G1. Resume pembrolizumab upon symptom control, or when prednisone/prednisolone daily dose <10 mg
	G3 (severe pain; irreversible joint damage; disabling; limits self-care ADLs)	Withhold pembrolizumab. Administer 0.5–1 mg/kg intravenous (methyl)prednisolone and convert to 0.5–2 mg/kg prednisone/prednisolone orally each day or its equivalent only after a response, followed by a taper over at least 4 weeks when symptoms improve to G1. In severe cases, infliximab or another anti-TNF-alpha drug may be required for improvement of arthritis. Resume pembrolizumab upon symptom control, or when prednisone/prednisolone daily dose <10 mg
Other	First occurrence of other G3	Withhold pembrolizumab. Administer oral prednisone/prednisolone at a dosage of 0.5–2 mg/kg/day or its equivalent. When symptoms improve to G1, begin a slow corticosteroid taper over at least 4 weeks. Resume pembrolizumab upon symptom control, or when prednisone/prednisolone daily dose <10 mg
	Recurrence of same G3	Permanently discontinue pembrolizumab. Administer 1–2 mg/kg intravenous (methyl)prednisolone and convert to 0.5–2 mg/kg prednisone/prednisolone orally each day or its equivalent only after a response. Taper over at least 4–8 weeks when symptoms improve to G1
	Life-threatening or G4	

(continued)

Treatment Modifications (continued)

RECOMMENDED DOSE MODIFICATIONS FOR PEMBROLIZUMAB

Adverse Event	Grade/Severity	Treatment Modification
	Requirement for ≥10 mg/day prednisone or equivalent for >12 weeks	Permanently discontinue pembrolizumab
	Persistent G2/3 adverse reactions lasting ≥12 weeks	

ADL, activities of daily living; ALT, alanine aminotransferase; AST, aspartate aminotransferase; ATG, anti-thymocyte globulin; IVIG, intravenous immunoglobulin; MMF, mycophenolate mofetil; NYHA, New York Heart Association; SJS, Stevens-Johnson syndrome; TEN, toxic epidermal necrolysis; ULN, upper limit of normal

Notes on general supportive care:
• Steroid taper in most cases will proceed over a minimum of 1 month, but if symptoms improve rapidly, a 2-week taper can be considered. If steroids are administered for more than 4 weeks, administer PCP prophylaxis (cotrimoxazole 480 mg twice daily M/W/F or inhaled pentamidine if cotrimoxazole allergy), regular random blood glucose, vitamin D level and starting calcium/vitamin D supplementation per guidelines

Notes on pregnancy and breastfeeding:
• Pembrolizumab can cause fetal harm. If used during pregnancy, or if the patient becomes pregnant during treatment, apprise the patient of the potential hazard to a fetus. Females of reproductive potential should use highly effective contraception during treatment and for 4 months after the last dose of pembrolizumab
• It is not known whether pembrolizumab is excreted in human milk. Therefore, it is recommended that women discontinue nursing during treatment with and for 4 months after the final dose of pembrolizumab

Adverse Events

	Used as First-Line Treatment in Cisplatin-Ineligible Patients (N = 370) (Phase 2 Trial)		Used as Second-Line Treatment (N = 542) (Phase 3 Trial)			
	Pembrolizumab		Pembrolizumab		Chemotherapy	
Grade (%)*	Grade 1/2	Grade 3–5	Grade 1/2	Grade 3–5	Grade 1/2	Grade 3–5
Pruritus	14	<1	20	0	2	<1
Fatigue	15	2	13	1	24	4
Rash	9	<1	—	—	—	—
Nausea	7	<1	11	<1	23	2
Diarrhea	7	<1	8	1	12	<1
Decreased appetite	8	<1	9	0	15	1
Asthenia	4	<1	5	<1	11	3
Pyrexia	4	<1	—	—	—	—
Anemia	2	<1	3	<1	17	8
Elevated AST level	3	<1	—	—	—	—
Elevated ALT level	2	<1	—	—	—	—
Rash, macropapular	2	<1	—	—	—	—
Arthralgia	2	<1	—	—	—	—

(continued)

Adverse Events (continued)

| Grade (%)* | Used as First-Line Treatment in Cisplatin-Ineligible Patients (N = 370) (Phase 2 Trial) | | Used as Second-Line Treatment (N = 542) (Phase 3 Trial) | | | |
| | Pembrolizumab | | Pembrolizumab | | Chemotherapy | |
	Grade 1/2	Grade 3–5	Grade 1/2	Grade 3–5	Grade 1/2	Grade 3–5
Increased creatinine level	2	<1	—	—	—	—
Constipation	—	—	2	0	17	3
Colitis	<1	1	—	—	—	—
Elevated alkaline phosphatase level	<1	1	—	—	—	—
Muscle weakness	<1	1	—	—	—	—
Dizziness	1	<1	—	—	—	—
Elevated bilirubin level	1	<1	—	—	—	—
Acute kidney injury	<1	<1	—	—	—	—
Arthritis	<1	<1	—	—	—	—
Back pain	<1	<1	—	—	—	—
Dehydration	<1	<1	—	—	—	—
Elevated hepatic enzymes	<1	<1	—	—	—	—
Elevated LFT	<1	<1	—	—	—	—
Hyperglycemia	<1	<1	—	—	—	—
Hyperuricemia	<1	<1	—	—	—	—
Hyponatremia	<1	<1	—	—	—	—
Hypotension	<1	<1	—	—	—	—
Muscle spasms	<1	<1	—	—	—	—
Pneumonitis	<1	<1	—	—	—	—
Thyroiditis	<1	<1	—	—	—	—
Type 1 diabetes	<1	<1	—	—	—	—
Urinary tract infection	<1	<1	—	—	—	—
Aortic thrombosis	0	<1	—	—	—	—
Addison disease	0	<1	—	—	—	—
Adrenal insufficiency	0	<1	—	—	—	—
Autoimmune arthritis	0	<1	—	—	—	—
Autoimmune hepatitis	0	<1	—	—	—	—
Cellulitis	0	<1	—	—	—	—
Chest pain	0	<1	—	—	—	—
Decreased cortisol level	0	<1	—	—	—	—

(continued)

Adverse Events (continued)

Grade (%)*	Used as First-Line Treatment in Cisplatin-Ineligible Patients (N = 370) (Phase 2 Trial)		Used as Second-Line Treatment (N = 542) (Phase 3 Trial)			
	Pembrolizumab		Pembrolizumab		Chemotherapy	
	Grade 1/2	Grade 3–5	Grade 1/2	Grade 3–5	Grade 1/2	Grade 3–5
Decreased neutrophil count	—	—	0	<1	2	12
Diabetic ketoacidosis	0	<1	—	—	—	—
Diverticulitis	0	<1	—	—	—	—
Elevated lipase level	0	<1	—	—	—	—
Eyelid ptosis	0	<1	—	—	—	—
Facial paralysis	0	<1	—	—	—	—
Hepatitis	0	<1	—	—	—	—
Hyperbilirubinemia	0	<1	—	—	—	—
Hypercalcemia	0	<1	—	—	—	—
Hyperhidrosis	0	<1	—	—	—	—
Hyperkalemia	0	<1	—	—	—	—
Hypophosphatasemia	0	<1	—	—	—	—
Hypopituitarism	0	<1	—	—	—	—
Hypophysitis	0	<1	—	—	—	—
Infected skin ulcer	0	<1	—	—	—	—
Lichen planus	0	<1	—	—	—	—
Liver injury	0	<1	—	—	—	—
Lower respiratory tract infection	0	<1	—	—	—	—
Myositis	0	<1	—	—	—	—
Myocarditis	0	<1	—	—	—	—
Pneumonia	0	<1	—	—	—	—
Proctitis	0	<1	—	—	—	—
Renal failure	0	<1	—	—	—	—
Toxic hepatitis	0	<1	—	—	—	—
Peripheral sensory neuropathy	—	—	<1	0	9	2
Peripheral neuropathy	—	—	<1	0	10	<1
Neutropenia	—	—	0	0	2	13
Alopecia	—	—	0	0	37	<1

*According to the National Cancer Institute Common Terminology Criteria for Adverse Events, version 4.0
Note: Treatment-related toxicities are included in the table if all-grade events occurred in ≥10% patients or G3–5 events occurred in any patient. One patient in the phase 2 trial had a treatment-related death (myositis). Four patients in the pembrolizumab group of the phase 3 trial had treatment-related deaths (pneumonitis, urinary tract infection, malignant neoplasm progression, and one unspecified cause). Four patients in the chemotherapy group in the phase 3 trial had treatment-related deaths (2 sepsis, 1 septic shock, and 1 unspecified cause)

METASTATIC • SUBSEQUENT THERAPY
BLADDER CANCER REGIMEN: NIVOLUMAB

Sharma P et al. Lancet Oncol 2016;17:1590–1598

The U.S. Food and Drug Administration (FDA)–approved regimens for urothelial carcinoma include fixed doses of nivolumab and allow for a shortened infusion duration of 30 minutes, consistent with the regimens approved on March 5, 2018, thus:

Nivolumab 240 mg; administer intravenously over 30 minutes in a volume of 0.9% sodium chloride injection (0.9% NS) or 5% dextrose injection (D5W), not to exceed 160 mL and sufficient to produce a nivolumab concentration within the range 1–10 mg/mL, every 2 weeks until disease progression (total dosage/cycle = 240 mg)
- Administer nivolumab through an administration set that contains a sterile, nonpyrogenic, low protein-binding in-line filter with pore size within the range of 0.2–1.2 μm
- Nivolumab can cause severe infusion-related reactions

OR

Nivolumab 480 mg; administer intravenously over 30 minutes in a volume of 0.9% NS or D5W not to exceed 160 mL and sufficient to produce a nivolumab concentration within the range 1–10 mg/mL, every 4 weeks until disease progression (total dosage/cycle = 480 mg)
- Administer nivolumab through an administration set that contains a sterile, nonpyrogenic, low protein-binding in-line filter with pore size within the range of 0.2–1.2 μm
- Nivolumab can cause severe infusion-related reactions

Supportive Care
Antiemetic prophylaxis
Emetogenic potential is **MINIMAL**
See Chapter 42 for antiemetic recommendations

Hematopoietic growth factor (CSF) prophylaxis
Primary prophylaxis is **NOT** indicated
See Chapter 43 for more information

Antimicrobial prophylaxis
Risk of fever and neutropenia is **LOW**
  Antimicrobial primary prophylaxis to be considered:
  - Antibacterial—not indicated
  - Antifungal—not indicated
  - Antiviral—not indicated, unless patient previously had an episode of HSV

Efficacy (N = 78)

Objective response rate*	24.4% (95% CI 15.3–35.4)
Median duration of response	9.4 months
Median overall survival	9.7 months (95% CI 7.3–16.2)
Overall survival at 12 months	46% (95% CI 34–56)
Median progression-free survival	2.8 months (95% CI 1.5–5.9)
Progression-free survival at 12 months	21% (95% CI 12–31)

*Per Response Evaluation Criteria in Solid Tumors (RECIST) version 1.1; the primary endpoint

Patient Population Studied

The nivolumab monotherapy arm of the multicenter, open-label phase 1/2 trial (CheckMate 032) involved 78 patients with histologically or cytologically confirmed metastatic or locally advanced urothelial cancer who had experienced disease progression after platinum-based chemotherapy, or had refused standard treatment with chemotherapy. Eligible patients were aged ≥18 years and had measurable disease and Eastern Cooperative Oncology Group (ECOG) performance status ≤1. Patients with active brain or leptomeningeal metastases, with history of autoimmune disease, or who needed ≥2 weeks of immunosuppressive doses of systemic corticosteroids before the study were not eligible. Patients received intravenous nivolumab (3 mg/kg) every 2 weeks. If they experienced disease progression and met prespecified criteria, patients were allowed to switch to intravenous nivolumab + ipilimumab therapy (1 mg/kg and 3 mg/kg, respectively, or 3 mg/kg and 1 mg/kg) every 3 weeks for four cycles.

Therapy Monitoring

1. Monitor patients for signs and symptoms of infusion-related reactions including pyrexia, chills, flushing, hypotension, dyspnea, wheezing, back pain, abdominal pain, and urticaria
2. Initially at the time of each dose, and eventually every 6–12 weeks, perform a total body skin examination with attention to *all* mucous membranes, as well as a complete review of systems
3. Monitor patients for signs and symptoms of pneumonitis. Evaluate patients with suspected pneumonitis with chest x-ray, CT scan, and pulse oximetry. For toxicity ≥2, may include nasal swab, sputum culture and sensitivity, blood culture and sensitivity, and urine culture and sensitivity
4. Monitor patients for signs and symptoms of colitis. Encourage patients to report diarrhea immediately to any member of the health care team
5. Draw AST, ALT, and bilirubin prior to each infusion and/or weekly if there are G1 LFT elevations. *Note:* No treatment is recommended for G1 LFT abnormalities. For toxicity ≥2, work up for other causes of elevated LFTs, including viral hepatitis
6. Use basic metabolic panel (Na, K, CO_2, glucose) and patient history as screening tools for hypophysitis, including hypopituitarism and adrenal insufficiency. If in doubt, evaluate morning adrenocorticotropic hormone (ACTH) and cortisol levels. Consider ACTH stimulation test for indeterminate results
7. Assess thyroid function at the start of treatment, periodically during treatment, and as indicated based on clinical evaluation, and for clinical signs and symptoms of thyroid disorders. Test for TSH and free thyroxine (FT4) every 4–6 weeks as part of routine clinical monitoring on therapy or for case detection in symptomatic patients
8. Measure glucose at baseline and with each treatment during the first 12 weeks and every 6 weeks thereafter
9. Obtain a serum creatinine level prior to every dose. If creatinine is found to be newly elevated, consider holding therapy while other potential causes are evaluated. *Note:* Routine urinalysis is not necessary other than to rule out urinary tract infections, etc
10. Obtain a complete rheumatologic history and perform an examination of all peripheral joints for tenderness, swelling, and range of motion. Examine the spine. Consider plain x-ray/imaging to exclude metastases and evaluate joint damage (erosions), if appropriate
11. In patients at high risk for infections and in appropriately selected patients based on an infectious disease evaluation, draw screening laboratories (HIV, hepatitis A and B, and blood QuantiFERON for TB) to prepare patients to start infliximab
12. Response evaluation: Every 2–4 months

Treatment Modifications

RECOMMENDED DOSE MODIFICATIONS FOR NIVOLUMAB

Adverse Event	Grade/Severity	Treatment Modification
Infusion reaction	Clinically significant but not severe infusion reaction	Interrupt the infusion in patients with clinically significant infusion reactions and consider resuming at a slower rate following resolution. If decision is made to restart, begin at ≤50% of the rate prior to the reaction and increase in 50% increments every 30 minutes if well tolerated. Infusions may be restarted at the full rate during the next cycle
	G3/4 (severe infusion reaction—pyrexia, chills, flushing, hypotension, dyspnea, wheezing, back pain, abdominal pain, and urticaria). Not rapidly responsive to brief interruption of infusion	Stop infusion and administer appropriate medical therapy (eg, epinephrine, corticosteroids, intravenous antihistamines, bronchodilators, and/or oxygen). Discontinue nivolumab
Colitis	G1	Loperamide 4 mg as starting dose, then 2 mg before each meal and after each loose stool until without diarrhea for 12 hours, with maximum of 16 mg loperamide per day. If G1 diarrhea or colitis persists >14 days, add prednisolone 0.5–1 mg/kg (non-enteric-coated) or consider oral budesonide 9 mg daily if no bloody diarrhea
	G2/3 diarrhea or colitis	Withhold nivolumab. Loperamide 4 mg as starting dose, then 2 mg before each meal and after each loose stool until without diarrhea for 12 hours, with maximum of 16 mg loperamide per day. Administer oral prednisone/prednisolone at a dosage of 0.5–2 mg/kg/day or its equivalent. When symptoms improve to G1, begin a slow corticosteroid taper over at least 4 weeks. Resume nivolumab upon symptom control, or when prednisone/prednisolone daily dose <10 mg

(continued)

Treatment Modifications (continued)

RECOMMENDED DOSE MODIFICATIONS FOR NIVOLUMAB

Adverse Event	Grade/Severity	Treatment Modification
	G4 diarrhea or colitis	Permanently discontinue nivolumab. Loperamide 4 mg as starting dose, then 2 mg before each meal and after each loose stool until without diarrhea for 12 hours, with maximum of 16 mg loperamide per day. Administer 1–2 mg/kg intravenous (methyl) prednisolone and convert to 0.5–2 mg/kg prednisone/prednisolone orally each day or its equivalent only after a response. Taper over at least 4 weeks when symptoms improve. If symptoms do not improve over 72 hours or worsen, perform flexible sigmoidoscopy/colonoscopy to document colitis then begin infliximab 5 mg/kg (if no perforation, sepsis, TB, hepatitis, NYHA III/IV CHF). If no response, add MMF 500–1000 mg twice daily. If worse on MMF, consider addition of tacrolimus or ATG
Pneumonitis	G2	Withhold nivolumab. Start *Pneumocystis* prophylaxis (while patient is receiving a glucocorticoid dose equivalent to ≥20 mg of prednisone daily for 4 weeks or longer) and coverage with empiric antibiotics. Administer oral prednisone/prednisolone at a dosage of 1–2 mg/kg/day or its equivalent. When symptoms improve to G1, begin a slow corticosteroid taper over at least 4 weeks. If response adequate after 48 hours, administer 2–4 mg/kg intravenous (methyl)prednisolone and convert to 0.5–2 mg/kg prednisone/prednisolone orally each day or its equivalent only after a response, followed by a taper over at least 6 weeks when symptoms improve to G1, titrating to symptoms. Resume nivolumab upon symptom control, or when prednisone/prednisolone daily dose <10 mg
	G3/4	Permanently discontinue nivolumab. Start *Pneumocystis* prophylaxis (while patient is receiving a glucocorticoid dose equivalent to ≥20 mg of prednisone daily for 4 weeks or longer); cover with empiric antibiotics. Administer 2–4 mg/kg intravenous (methyl)prednisolone and convert to 1–2 mg/kg prednisone/prednisolone orally each day or its equivalent only after a response, followed by a taper over at least 8 weeks when symptoms improve to G1, titrating to symptoms. If, when initially treated, improvement does not occur within 48–72 hours, begin infliximab 5 mg/kg (if no perforation, sepsis, TB, hepatitis, NYHA III/IV CHF). If no response to infliximab, add MMF 500–1000 mg twice daily. Consider MMF, especially if concurrent hepatic toxicity
Hepatitis	G2 (AST or ALT >3–5× ULN or total bilirubin >1.5–3× ULN)	Withhold nivolumab. Administer oral prednisone/prednisolone at a dosage of 1–2 mg/kg/day or its equivalent. When symptoms improve to G1, begin a slow corticosteroid taper over at least 4 weeks. Resume nivolumab upon symptom control, or when prednisone/prednisolone daily dose <10 mg
	G3/4 (AST or ALT >5× ULN or total bilirubin >3× ULN)	Permanently discontinue nivolumab. Administer 1–2 mg/kg intravenous (methyl) prednisolone and convert to 0.5–2 mg/kg prednisone/prednisolone orally each day or its equivalent only after a response. Taper over at least 6 weeks when symptoms improve. If no response, add MMF 500–1000 mg twice daily. If worse on MMF, consider adding tacrolimus or ATG
Hypophysitis	G2/3 (moderate symptoms, ie, headache but no visual disturbance or fatigue/mood alteration but hemodynamically stable, no electrolyte disturbance)	Administer analgesia as needed for headache. Withhold nivolumab. Administer oral prednisone/prednisolone at a dose of 0.5–2 mg/kg/day or its equivalent. When symptoms improve to G1, begin a slow corticosteroid taper over at least 4 weeks. If no improvement in 48 hours, administer 1–2 mg/kg intravenous (methyl)prednisolone and convert to 0.5–2 mg/kg prednisone/prednisolone orally each day or its equivalent only after a response. Taper over at least 4 weeks when symptoms improve to 5 mg prednisone/prednisolone or equivalent; do not stop steroids. Resume nivolumab upon symptom control, or when prednisone/prednisolone daily dose <10 mg
	G4 (severe mass effect symptoms, ie, severe headache, any visual disturbance or severe hypoadrenalism, ie, hypotension, severe electrolyte disturbance)	Permanently discontinue nivolumab. Administer analgesia as needed for headache. Administer 1–2 mg/kg intravenous (methyl)prednisolone and convert to 0.5–2 mg/ kg prednisone/prednisolone orally each day or its equivalent only after a response. Taper over at least 4 weeks when symptoms improve to 5 mg prednisone/prednisolone or equivalent; do not stop steroids

(continued)

Treatment Modifications (continued)

RECOMMENDED DOSE MODIFICATIONS FOR NIVOLUMAB

Adverse Event	Grade/Severity	Treatment Modification
Adrenal insufficiency	G2	Withhold nivolumab. Administer oral prednisone/prednisolone at a dose of 0.5–2 mg/kg/day or its equivalent. When symptoms improve to G1, begin a slow corticosteroid taper over at least 4 weeks. Serially assess adrenal function and continue steroids at replacement doses (20–40 mg hydrocortisone daily ~2/3 dose in morning upon awakening and ~1/3 at 4 PM) until recovery of adrenal function is documented. Resume nivolumab upon symptom control, or when prednisone/prednisolone daily dose <10 mg
	G3/4	Permanently discontinue nivolumab. Administer oral prednisone/prednisolone at a dose of 0.5–2 mg/kg/day or its equivalent. When symptoms improve to G1, begin a slow corticosteroid taper over at least 4 weeks. Serially assess adrenal function and continue steroids at replacement doses (20–40 mg hydrocortisone daily ~2/3 dose in morning upon awakening and ~1/3 at 4 PM) until recovery of adrenal function is documented
Type 1 diabetes mellitus	G3 hyperglycemia	Withhold nivolumab. Admit to hospital to manage hyperglycemia. Role of corticosteroids in preventing complete loss of insulin-producing cells is unknown and use is not recommended. Resume nivolumab upon symptom control, or when prednisone/prednisolone daily dose <10 mg
	G4 hyperglycemia	Permanently discontinue nivolumab. Admit to hospital to manage hyperglycemia. Role of corticosteroids in preventing complete loss of insulin-producing cells is unknown and use is not recommended
Nephritis and renal dysfunction	G2/3 (serum creatinine 1.5–6× ULN)	Withhold nivolumab. Administer oral prednisone/prednisolone at a dose of 0.5–2 mg/kg/day or its equivalent. When symptoms improve to G1, begin a slow corticosteroid taper over at least 4 weeks. If response is not adequate, administer 0.5–1 mg/kg intravenous (methyl)prednisolone and convert to 0.5–2 mg/kg prednisone/prednisolone orally each day or its equivalent only after a response, followed by a taper over at least 4 weeks when symptoms improve to G1. Resume nivolumab upon symptom control, or when prednisone/prednisolone daily dose <10 mg
	G4 (serum creatinine >6× ULN)	Permanently discontinue nivolumab. Administer 0.5–1 mg/kg intravenous (methyl)prednisolone and convert to 0.5–2 mg/kg prednisone/prednisolone orally each day or its equivalent only after a response, followed by a taper over at least 4 weeks when symptoms improve to G1
Skin	G1/2	Continue nivolumab. Avoid skin irritants, avoid sun exposure; topical emollients recommended. Topical steroid (mild strength for G1, moderate/potent strength for G2) cream once or twice daily ± oral or topical antihistamines for itching
	G3 rash or suspected SJS or TEN	Withhold nivolumab. Avoid skin irritants, avoid sun exposure, topical emollients recommended. Administer oral or topical antihistamines for itching. Administer oral prednisone/prednisolone at a dose of 0.5–2 mg/kg or its equivalent daily for 3 days followed by a slow corticosteroid taper over at least 4 weeks when the rash improves to G1. If rash does not respond adequately, administer 0.5–1 mg/kg intravenous (methyl)prednisolone and convert to 0.5–2 mg/kg prednisone/prednisolone orally each day or its equivalent only after a response, followed by a taper over at least 4 weeks when the rash improves to G1. Resume nivolumab upon symptom control, or when prednisone/prednisolone daily dose <10 mg
	G4 rash or confirmed SJS or TEN	Avoid skin irritants, avoid sun exposure; topical emollients recommended. Administer oral or topical antihistamines for itching. Administer 1–2 mg/kg intravenous (methyl)prednisolone and convert to oral steroids 0.5–2 mg/kg prednisone/prednisolone each day or its equivalent only after a response. Taper over at least 4 weeks when the rash improves to G1. Permanently discontinue nivolumab

(continued)

Treatment Modifications (continued)

RECOMMENDED DOSE MODIFICATIONS FOR NIVOLUMAB

Adverse Event	Grade/Severity	Treatment Modification
Encephalitis	Confusion or altered behavior, headaches, alteration in Glasgow Coma Scale, motor or sensory deficits, speech abnormality; may or may not be febrile	Initially withhold nivolumab, but permanently discontinue nivolumab if there is no doubt as to diagnosis. Exclude bacterial and ideally viral infections prior to high-dose steroids. Administer 1–2 mg/kg intravenous (methyl)prednisolone for 5 days or oral prednisone/prednisolone at a dosage of 0.5–2 mg/kg/day or its equivalent. When symptoms improve, begin a slow corticosteroid taper over at least 4–8 weeks. If symptoms are severe, administer 1–2 mg/kg intravenous (methyl)prednisolone and convert to 0.5–2 mg/kg prednisone/prednisolone orally each day or its equivalent only after a response. Consider concurrent empiric antiviral (intravenous acyclovir) and antibacterial therapy
Aseptic meningitis	Headache, photophobia, neck stiffness with fever, or may be afebrile, vomiting; normal cognition/cerebral function (distinguishes from encephalitis)	
Other syndromes include neurosarcoidosis, posterior reversible leukoencephalopathy syndrome (PRES), Vogt-Koyanagi-Harada syndrome, demyelination, vasculitic encephalopathy, and generalized seizures		
Transverse myelitis	Acute or subacute neurologic signs/symptoms of motor, sensory, autonomic origin; most have sensory level; often bilateral symptoms	Initially withhold nivolumab, but permanently discontinue nivolumab if there is no doubt as to diagnosis. Administer 2 mg/kg intravenous (methyl)prednisolone or consider 1 g/day and convert to 0.5–2 mg/kg prednisone/prednisolone orally each day or its equivalent only after a response. When symptoms improve, begin a slow corticosteroid taper over at least 4–8 weeks. Plasmapheresis may be required if steroids do not bring about improvement
Myocarditis	G3	Permanently discontinue nivolumab. Administer 2 mg/kg intravenous (methyl)prednisolone or consider 1 g/day and convert to 0.5–2 mg/kg prednisone/prednisolone orally each day or its equivalent only after a response. When symptoms improve, begin a slow corticosteroid taper over at least 4–8 weeks. If no response, add MMF 500–1000 mg twice daily. If worse on MMF, consider adding tacrolimus
Peripheral neurologic toxicity	Moderate: some interference with ADL, symptoms concerning to patient	Withhold nivolumab. Initial observation reasonable or initiate prednisone/prednisolone 0.5–1 mg/kg (if progressing, eg, from mild) and/or pregabalin or duloxetine for pain. When symptoms improve, begin a slow corticosteroid taper over at least 4 weeks. Resume nivolumab upon symptom control, or when prednisone/prednisolone daily dose <10 mg
	Severe: limits self-care and aids warranted, life-threatening, eg, respiratory problems	Permanently discontinue nivolumab. Administer 1–2 mg/kg intravenous (methyl)prednisolone and convert to 0.5–2 mg/kg prednisone/prednisolone orally each day or its equivalent only after a response. Taper over at least 4–8 weeks when symptoms improve to G1.
Guillain-Barré syndrome	Progressive symmetrical muscle weakness with absent or reduced tendon reflexes—involves extremities; facial, respiratory, and bulbar and oculomotor muscles; dysregulation of autonomic nerves	Permanently discontinue nivolumab. Use of steroids not recommended in idiopathic Guillain-Barré syndrome; however, a trial of (methyl)prednisolone 1–2 mg/kg is reasonable, converting to 0.5–2 mg/kg prednisone/prednisolone orally each day or its equivalent only after a response. If no improvement or worsening, plasmapheresis or IVIG indicated
Myasthenia gravis	Fluctuating muscle weakness (proximal limb, trunk, ocular, eg, ptosis/diplopia or bulbar) with fatigability; respiratory muscles may also be involved	Permanently discontinue nivolumab. Administer pyridostigmine at an initial dose of 30 mg 3 times daily. Administer oral prednisone/prednisolone at a dose of 0.5–2 mg/kg/day or its equivalent or 1–2 mg/kg intravenous (methyl)prednisolone, depending on the severity of symptoms. If treatment begins with intravenous drug, convert to 0.5–2 mg/kg prednisone/prednisolone orally each day or its equivalent only after a response. If no improvement or worsening, plasmapheresis or IVIG may be considered. Additional immunosuppressants used in myasthenia gravis include azathioprine, cyclosporine, and mycophenolate. Avoid certain medications, eg, ciprofloxacin, beta-blockers, that may precipitate cholinergic crisis
Other syndromes, including motor and sensory peripheral neuropathy, multifocal radicular neuropathy/plexopathy, autonomic neuropathy, phrenic nerve palsy, cranial nerve palsies (eg, facial nerve, optic nerve, hypoglossal nerve)		Permanently discontinue nivolumab. Administer oral prednisone/prednisolone at a dose of 0.5–2 mg/kg/day or its equivalent or 1–2 mg/kg intravenous (methyl)prednisolone, depending on the severity of symptoms. If treatment begins with intravenous drug, convert to 0.5–2 mg/kg prednisone/prednisolone orally each day or its equivalent only after a response

(continued)

Treatment Modifications (*continued*)

RECOMMENDED DOSE MODIFICATIONS FOR NIVOLUMAB

Adverse Event	Grade/Severity	Treatment Modification
Arthralgia	G1 (mild pain with inflammation, erythema, or joint swelling)	Continue nivolumab. Administer acetaminophen (paracetamol) and ibuprofen
	G2 (moderate pain with inflammation, erythema, or joint swelling that limits ADLs)	Withhold nivolumab. Administer higher doses of acetaminophen (paracetamol) and ibuprofen and use diclofenac or naproxen or etoricoxib. If inadequately controlled, consider intra-articular steroid injections for large joints or administer oral prednisone/prednisolone at a dose of 0.5–2 mg/kg/day or its equivalent. When symptoms improve to G1, begin a slow corticosteroid taper over at least 4 weeks. If response is not adequate, administer 0.5–1 mg/kg intravenous (methyl)prednisolone and convert to 0.5–2 mg/kg prednisone/prednisolone orally each day or its equivalent only after a response, followed by a taper over at least 4 weeks when symptoms improve to G1. Resume nivolumab upon symptom control, or when prednisone/prednisolone daily dose <10 mg
	G3 (severe pain; irreversible joint damage; disabling; limits self-care ADLs)	Withhold nivolumab. Administer 0.5–1 mg/kg intravenous (methyl)prednisolone and convert to 0.5–2 mg/kg prednisone/prednisolone orally each day or its equivalent only after a response, followed by a taper over at least 4 weeks when symptoms improve to G1. In severe cases, infliximab or another anti-TNF-alpha drug may be required for improvement of arthritis. Resume nivolumab upon symptom control, or when prednisone/prednisolone daily dose <10 mg
Other	First occurrence of other G3	Withhold nivolumab. Administer oral prednisone/prednisolone at a dose of 0.5–2 mg/kg/day or its equivalent. When symptoms improve to G1, begin a slow corticosteroid taper over at least 4 weeks. Resume nivolumab upon symptom control, or when prednisone/prednisolone daily dose <10 mg
	Recurrence of same G3	Permanently discontinue nivolumab. Administer 1–2 mg/kg intravenous (methyl)prednisolone and convert to 0.5–2 mg/kg prednisone/prednisolone orally each day or its equivalent only after a response. Taper over at least 4–8 weeks when symptoms improve to G1
	Life-threatening or G4	
	Requirement for ≥10 mg/day prednisone or equivalent for >12 weeks	Permanently discontinue nivolumab
	Persistent G2/3 adverse reactions lasting ≥12 weeks	

ADL, activities of daily living; ALT, alanine aminotransferase; AST, aspartate aminotransferase; ATG, anti-thymocyte globulin; IVIG, intravenous immunoglobulin; MMF, mycophenolate mofetil; NYHA, New York Heart Association; SJS, Stevens-Johnson syndrome; TEN, toxic epidermal necrolysis; ULN, upper limit of normal

Notes on general supportive care:
• Steroid taper in most cases will proceed over a minimum of 1 month, but if symptoms improve rapidly, a 2-week taper can be considered. If steroids are administered for more than 4 weeks, administer PCP prophylaxis (cotrimoxazole 480 mg twice daily M/W/F or inhaled pentamidine if cotrimoxazole allergy), regular random blood glucose, vitamin D level and starting calcium/vitamin D supplementation per guidelines

Notes on pregnancy and breastfeeding:
• Nivolumab can cause fetal harm. If used during pregnancy, or if the patient becomes pregnant during treatment, apprise the patient of the potential hazard to a fetus. Females of reproductive potential should use highly effective contraception during treatment and for 5 months after the last dose of nivolumab
• It is not known whether nivolumab is excreted in human milk. Therefore, it is recommended that women discontinue nursing during treatment with nivolumab

Adverse Events (N = 78)

Grade (%)*	Grade 1/2	Grade 3-5
Fatigue	33	3
Pruritus	29	0
Rash, macropapular	15	3
Elevated lipase level	9	5
Nausea	12	1
Arthralgia	12	0
Anemia	10	0
Elevated amylase level	5	4
Dyspnea	5	3
Decreased lymphocyte count	4	3
Hyperglycemia	5	1
Decreased neutrophil count	1	3
Decreased white blood cell count	3	1
Dermatitis acneiform	1	1
Hyponatremia	1	1
Wheezing	1	1
Acute kidney injury	0	1
Back pain	0	1
Colitis	0	1
Elevated AST level	0	1

*According to the National Cancer Institute Common Terminology Criteria for Adverse Events, version 4.0
Note: Treatment-related toxicities are included in the table if all-grade events occurred in ≥10% patients or G3–5 events occurred in any patient, and occurred while on nivolumab monotherapy (not on combination therapy). Two patients discontinued treatment owing to treatment-related adverse events (thrombocytopenia and pneumonitis) and subsequently died as a result of these treatment-related events

METASTATIC • SUBSEQUENT THERAPY

BLADDER CANCER REGIMEN: AVELUMAB

Apolo AB et al. J Clin Oncol 2017;35:2117–2124

Premedications

Acetaminophen 500–650 mg; administer orally 30–60 minutes prior to starting avelumab administration

Diphenhydramine 25–50 mg (or an equivalent H$_1$ antihistamine); administer orally 30–60 minutes *or* intravenously 30 minutes prior to starting avelumab administration

• Primary prophylaxis against infusion-related reactions is given during the first 4 avelumab doses

• Premedication after the fourth avelumab dose may be administered based upon clinical judgment and the presence and severity of infusion-related reactions encountered during previously administered avelumab doses

The U.S. FDA–approved regimen is a fixed dose of avelumab (approved October 19, 2018)

Avelumab 800 m; administer intravenously over 60 minutes in 250 mL 0.9% sodium chloride injection or 0.45% sodium chloride injection, every 2 weeks (total dosage/cycle = 800 mg)

• Administer avelumab with an administration set that contains a sterile, nonpyrogenic, low protein-binding in-line filter with pore size of 0.2 μm

Notes:

• Avelumab can cause severe or life-threatening infusion-related reactions
  ■ Monitor patients for signs and symptoms of infusion-related reactions, including pyrexia, chills, flushing, hypotension, dyspnea, wheezing, back pain, abdominal pain, and urticaria
    ○ Infusion-related reactions have included severe (G3) and life-threatening (G4) reactions after premedication with an antihistamine and acetaminophen
    ○ Infusion-related reactions may occur after avelumab administration is completed
  ■ Interrupt or slow the administration rate for mild or moderate infusion-related reactions
  ■ STOP administration and permanently discontinue avelumab for G ≥3 severity infusion-related reactions
• Hypertension G ≥3, including hypertensive crisis, has been associated with avelumab use

Supportive Care

Antiemetic prophylaxis
Emetogenic potential is **LOW**
See Chapter 42 for antiemetic recommendations

Hematopoietic growth factor (CSF) prophylaxis
Primary prophylaxis is **NOT** *indicated*
See Chapter 43 for more information

Antimicrobial prophylaxis
Risk of fever and neutropenia is **LOW**
  Antimicrobial primary prophylaxis to be considered:
  • Antibacterial—not indicated
  • Antifungal—not indicated
  • Antiviral—not indicated, unless patient previously had an episode of HSV

Patient Population Studied

The multicenter, dose-expansion cohort, phase 1b study involved 44 patients with histologically or cytologically confirmed metastatic urothelial cancer who had experienced disease progression or recurrence after platinum-based chemotherapy. Patients who were not eligible for cisplatin therapy were also included. Eligible patients were aged ≥18 years, had measurable disease and Eastern Cooperative Oncology Group (ECOG) performance status ≤1, life expectancy ≥3 months, and had adequate hepatic, renal, and hematologic function. Patients who were receiving any concurrent chemotherapy, immunosuppressive therapy, or hormonal therapy were not eligible. Patients received intravenous avelumab (10 mg/kg in a 1-hour infusion) every 2 weeks

Efficacy (N = 44)

Objective response rate*	18.2% (95% CI 8.2–32.7)
Median overall survival	13.7 months (95% CI 8.5–not estimable)
Overall survival at 12 months	54.3% (95% CI 37.9–68.1)
Median progression-free survival	11.6 weeks (95% CI 6.1–17.4)

*Per Response Evaluation Criteria in Solid Tumors (RECIST) version 1.1 (central review). Median follow-up was 16.5 months

Therapy Monitoring

1. Premedicate with antihistamine and acetaminophen prior to the first 4 infusions. Monitor patients for signs and symptoms of infusion-related reactions, including pyrexia, chills, flushing, hypotension, dyspnea, wheezing, back pain, abdominal pain, and urticaria

2. Initially at the time of each dose, and eventually every 6–12 weeks, perform a total body skin examination with attention to *all* mucous membranes, as well as a complete review of systems

3. Monitor patients for signs and symptoms of pneumonitis. Evaluate patients with suspected pneumonitis with chest x-ray, CT scan, and pulse oximetry. For toxicity ≥2, may include nasal swab, sputum culture and sensitivity, blood culture and sensitivity, and urine culture and sensitivity

(continued)

Therapy Monitoring (*continued*)

4. Monitor patients for signs and symptoms of colitis. Encourage patients to report diarrhea immediately to any member of the health care team

5. Draw AST, ALT, and bilirubin prior to each infusion and/or weekly if there are G1 LFT elevations. *Note:* No treatment is recommended for G1 LFT abnormalities. For toxicity ≥2, work up for other causes of elevated LFTs, including viral hepatitis

6. Use basic metabolic panel (Na, K, CO_2, glucose) and patient history as screening tools for hypophysitis, including hypopituitarism and adrenal insufficiency. If in doubt, evaluate morning adrenocorticotropic hormone (ACTH) and cortisol levels. Consider ACTH stimulation test for indeterminate results

7. Assess thyroid function at the start of treatment, periodically during treatment, and as indicated based on clinical evaluation, and for clinical signs and symptoms of thyroid disorders. Test for TSH and free thyroxine (FT4) every 4–6 weeks as part of routine clinical monitoring on therapy or for case detection in symptomatic patients

8. Measure glucose at baseline and with each treatment during the first 12 weeks and every 6 weeks thereafter

9. Obtain a serum creatinine level prior to every dose. If creatinine is found to be newly elevated, consider holding therapy while other potential causes are evaluated. *Note:* Routine urinalysis is not necessary other than to rule out urinary tract infections, etc

10. Obtain a complete rheumatologic history and perform an examination of all peripheral joints for tenderness, swelling, and range of motion. Examine the spine. Consider plain x-ray/imaging to exclude metastases and evaluate joint damage (erosions), if appropriate

11. In patients at high risk for infections and in appropriately selected patients based on an infectious disease evaluation, draw screening laboratories (HIV, hepatitis A and B, and blood QuantiFERON for TB) to prepare patients to start infliximab

12. Response evaluation: Every 2–4 months

Treatment Modifications

RECOMMENDED DOSE MODIFICATIONS FOR AVELUMAB

Adverse Event	Grade/Severity	Treatment Modification
Infusion reaction	Clinically significant but not severe infusion reaction	Interrupt the infusion in patients with clinically significant infusion reactions and consider resuming at a slower rate following resolution. If decision is made to restart, begin at ≤50% of the rate prior to the reaction and increase in 50% increments every 30 minutes if well tolerated. Infusions may be restarted at the full rate during the next cycle
	G3/4 (severe infusion reaction—pyrexia, chills, flushing, hypotension, dyspnea, wheezing, back pain, abdominal pain, and urticaria). Not rapidly responsive to brief interruption of infusion	Stop infusion and administer appropriate medical therapy (eg, epinephrine, corticosteroids, intravenous antihistamines, bronchodilators, and/or oxygen). Discontinue avelumab
Colitis	G1	Loperamide 4 mg as starting dose, then 2 mg before each meal and after each loose stool until without diarrhea for 12 hours, with maximum of 16 mg loperamide per day. If G1 diarrhea or colitis persists >14 days, add prednisolone 0.5–1 mg/kg (non-enteric-coated) or consider oral budesonide 9 mg daily if no bloody diarrhea
	G2/3 diarrhea or colitis	Withhold avelumab. Loperamide 4 mg as starting dose, then 2 mg before each meal and after each loose stool until without diarrhea for 12 hours, with maximum of 16 mg loperamide per day. Administer oral prednisone/prednisolone at a dosage of 0.5–2 mg/kg/day or its equivalent. When symptoms improve to G1, begin a slow corticosteroid taper over at least 4 weeks. Resume avelumab upon symptom control, or when prednisone/prednisolone daily dose <10 mg
	G4 diarrhea or colitis	Permanently discontinue avelumab. Loperamide 4 mg as starting dose, then 2 mg before each meal and after each loose stool until without diarrhea for 12 hours, with maximum of 16 mg loperamide per day. Administer 1–2 mg/kg intravenous (methyl)prednisolone and convert to 0.5–2 mg/kg prednisone/prednisolone orally each day or its equivalent only after a response. Taper over at least 4 weeks when symptoms improve. If symptoms do not improve over 72 hours or worsen, perform flexible sigmoidoscopy/colonoscopy to document colitis, then begin infliximab 5 mg/kg (if no perforation, sepsis, TB, hepatitis, NYHA III/IV CHF). If no response, add MMF 500–1000 mg twice daily. If worse on MMF, consider addition of tacrolimus or ATG

(*continued*)

Treatment Modifications (*continued*)

RECOMMENDED DOSE MODIFICATIONS FOR AVELUMAB

Adverse Event	Grade/Severity	Treatment Modification
Pneumonitis	G2	Withhold avelumab. Start *Pneumocystis* prophylaxis (while patient is receiving a glucocorticoid dose equivalent to ≥20 mg of prednisone daily for 4 weeks or longer) and coverage with empiric antibiotics. Administer oral prednisone/prednisolone at a dosage of 1–2 mg/kg/day or its equivalent. When symptoms improve to G1, begin a slow corticosteroid taper over at least 4 weeks. If response is not adequate after 48 hours, administer 2–4 mg/kg intravenous (methyl)prednisolone and convert to 0.5–2 mg/kg prednisone/prednisolone orally each day or its equivalent only after a response, followed by a taper over at least 6 weeks when symptoms improve to G1, titrating to symptoms. Resume avelumab upon symptom control, or when prednisone/prednisolone daily dose <10 mg
	G3/4	Permanently discontinue avelumab. Start *Pneumocystis* prophylaxis (while patient is receiving a glucocorticoid dose equivalent to ≥20 mg of prednisone daily for 4 weeks or longer); cover with empiric antibiotics. Administer 2–4 mg/kg intravenous (methyl)prednisolone and convert to 1–2 mg/kg prednisone/prednisolone orally each day or its equivalent only after a response, followed by a taper over at least 8 weeks when symptoms improve to G1, titrating to symptoms. If, when initially treated, improvement does not occur within 48–72 hours, begin infliximab 5 mg/kg (if no perforation, sepsis, TB, hepatitis, NYHA III/IV CHF). If no response to infliximab, add MMF 500–1000 mg twice daily. Consider MMF, especially if concurrent hepatic toxicity
Hepatitis	G2 (AST or ALT >3–5× ULN or total bilirubin >1.5–3× ULN)	Withhold avelumab. Administer oral prednisone/prednisolone at a dosage of 1–2 mg/kg/day or its equivalent. When symptoms improve to G1, begin a slow corticosteroid taper over at least 4 weeks. Resume avelumab upon symptom control, or when prednisone/prednisolone daily dose <10 mg
	G3/4 (AST or ALT >5× ULN or total bilirubin >3× ULN)	Permanently discontinue avelumab. Administer 1–2 mg/kg intravenous (methyl)prednisolone and convert to 0.5–2 mg/kg prednisone/prednisolone orally each day or its equivalent only after a response. Taper over at least 6 weeks when symptoms improve. If no response, add MMF 500–1000 mg twice daily. If worse on MMF, consider adding tacrolimus or ATG
Hypophysitis	G2/3 (moderate symptoms, ie, headache but no visual disturbance or fatigue/mood alteration but hemodynamically stable, no electrolyte disturbance)	Administer analgesia as needed for headache. Withhold avelumab. Administer oral prednisone/prednisolone at a dosage of 0.5–2 mg/kg/day or its equivalent. When symptoms improve to G1, begin a slow corticosteroid taper over at least 4 weeks. If no improvement in 48 hours, administer 1–2 mg/kg intravenous (methyl)prednisolone and convert to 0.5–2 mg/kg prednisone/prednisolone orally each day or its equivalent only after a response. Taper over at least 4 weeks when symptoms improve to 5 mg prednisone/prednisolone or equivalent; do not stop steroids. Resume avelumab upon symptom control, or when prednisone/prednisolone daily dose <10 mg
	G4 (severe mass effect symptoms, ie, severe headache, any visual disturbance, or severe hypoadrenalism, ie, hypotension, severe electrolyte disturbance)	Permanently discontinue avelumab. Administer analgesia as needed for headache. Administer 1–2 mg/kg intravenous (methyl)prednisolone and convert to 0.5–2 mg/kg prednisone/prednisolone orally each day or its equivalent only after a response. Taper over at least 4 weeks when symptoms improve to 5 mg prednisone/prednisolone or equivalent; do not stop steroids
Adrenal insufficiency	G2	Withhold avelumab. Administer oral prednisone/prednisolone at a dosage of 0.5–2 mg/kg/day or its equivalent. When symptoms improve to G1, begin a slow corticosteroid taper over at least 4 weeks. Serially assess adrenal function and continue steroids at replacement doses (20–40 mg hydrocortisone daily ~2/3 dose in morning upon awakening and ~1/3 at 4 PM) until recovery of adrenal function is documented. Resume avelumab upon symptom control, or when prednisone/prednisolone daily dose <10 mg
	G3/4	Permanently discontinue avelumab. Administer oral prednisone/prednisolone at a dosage of 0.5–2 mg/kg/day or its equivalent. When symptoms improve to G1, begin a slow corticosteroid taper over at least 4 weeks. Serially assess adrenal function and continue steroids at replacement doses (20–40 mg hydrocortisone daily ~2/3 dose in morning upon awakening and ~1/3 at 4 PM) until recovery of adrenal function is documented

(*continued*)

Treatment Modifications (*continued*)

RECOMMENDED DOSE MODIFICATIONS FOR AVELUMAB

Adverse Event	Grade/Severity	Treatment Modification
Type 1 diabetes mellitus	G3 hyperglycemia	Withhold avelumab. Admit to hospital to manage hyperglycemia. Role of corticosteroids in preventing complete loss of insulin-producing cells is unknown and not recommended. Resume avelumab upon symptom control, or when prednisone/prednisolone daily dose <10 mg
	G4 hyperglycemia	Permanently discontinue avelumab. Admit to hospital to manage hyperglycemia. Role of corticosteroids in preventing complete loss of insulin-producing cells is unknown and use is not recommended
Nephritis and renal dysfunction	G2/3 (serum creatinine 1.5–6× ULN)	Withhold avelumab. Administer oral prednisone/prednisolone at a dosage of 0.5–2 mg/kg/day or its equivalent. When symptoms improve to G1 begin a slow corticosteroid taper over at least 4 weeks. If response is not adequate, administer 0.5–1 mg/kg intravenous (methyl) prednisolone and convert to 0.5–2 mg/kg prednisone/prednisolone orally each day or its equivalent only after a response, followed by a taper over at least 4 weeks when symptoms improve to G1. Resume avelumab upon symptom control, or when prednisone/prednisolone daily dose <10 mg
	G4 (serum creatinine >6× ULN)	Permanently discontinue avelumab. Administer 0.5–1 mg/kg intravenous (methyl) prednisolone and convert to 0.5–2 mg/kg prednisone/prednisolone orally each day or its equivalent only after a response, followed by a taper over at least 4 weeks when symptoms improve to G1
Skin	G1/2	Continue avelumab. Avoid skin irritants, avoid sun exposure; topical emollients recommended. Topical steroid (mild strength for G1, moderate/potent strength for G2) cream once or twice daily ± oral or topical antihistamines for itching
	G3 rash or suspected SJS or TEN	Withhold avelumab. Avoid skin irritants, avoid sun exposure; topical emollients recommended. Administer oral or topical antihistamines for itching. Administer oral prednisone/prednisolone at a dosage of 0.5–2 mg/kg or its equivalent daily for 3 days followed by a slow corticosteroid taper over at least 4 weeks when the rash improves to G1. If rash does not respond adequately, administer 0.5 –1 mg/kg intravenous (methyl) prednisolone and convert to 0.5–2 mg/kg prednisone/prednisolone orally each day or its equivalent only after a response, followed by a taper over at least 4 weeks when the rash improves to G1. Resume avelumab upon symptom control, or when prednisone/prednisolone daily dose <10 mg
	G4 rash or confirmed SJS or TEN	Avoid skin irritants, avoid sun exposure; topical emollients recommended. Administer oral or topical antihistamines for itching. Administer 1–2 mg/kg intravenous (methyl)prednisolone and convert to oral steroids 0.5–2 mg/kg prednisone/prednisolone each day or its equivalent only after a response. Taper over at least 4 weeks when the rash improves to G1. Permanently discontinue avelumab
Encephalitis	Confusion or altered behavior, headaches, alteration in Glasgow Coma Scale, motor or sensory deficits, speech abnormality; may or may not be febrile	Initially withhold avelumab, but permanently discontinue avelumab if there is no doubt as to diagnosis. Exclude bacterial and ideally viral infections prior to high-dose steroids. Administer 1–2 mg/kg intravenous (methyl)prednisolone for 5 days or oral prednisone/prednisolone at a dosage of 0.5–2 mg/kg/day or its equivalent. When symptoms improve, begin a slow corticosteroid taper over at least 4–8 weeks. If symptoms are severe, administer 1–2 mg/kg intravenous (methyl)prednisolone and convert to 0.5–2 mg/kg prednisone/prednisolone orally each day or its equivalent only after a response. Consider concurrent empiric antiviral (intravenous acyclovir) and antibacterial therapy
Aseptic meningitis	Headache, photophobia, neck stiffness with fever, or may be afebrile, vomiting; normal cognition/cerebral function (distinguishes from encephalitis)	
Other syndromes include neurosarcoidosis, posterior reversible leukoencephalopathy syndrome (PRES), Vogt-Koyanagi-Harada syndrome, demyelination, vasculitic encephalopathy, and generalized seizures		

(*continued*)

Treatment Modifications (continued)

RECOMMENDED DOSE MODIFICATIONS FOR AVELUMAB

Adverse Event	Grade/Severity	Treatment Modification
Transverse myelitis	Acute or subacute neurologic signs/symptoms of motor, sensory, autonomic origin; most have sensory level; often bilateral symptoms	Initially withhold avelumab, but permanently discontinue avelumab if there is no doubt as to diagnosis. Administer 2 mg/kg intravenous (methyl)prednisolone or consider 1 g/day and convert to 0.5–2 mg/kg prednisone/prednisolone orally each day or its equivalent only after a response. When symptoms improve, begin a slow corticosteroid taper over at least 4–8 weeks. Plasmapheresis may be required if steroids do not bring about improvement
Myocarditis	G3	Permanently discontinue avelumab. Administer 2 mg/kg intravenous (methyl)prednisolone or consider 1 g/day and convert to 0.5–2 mg/kg prednisone/prednisolone orally each day or its equivalent only after a response. When symptoms improve, begin a slow corticosteroid taper over at least 4–8 weeks. If no response, add MMF 500–1000 mg twice daily. If worse on MMF, consider adding tacrolimus
Peripheral neurologic toxicity	Moderate: some interference with ADL, symptoms concerning to patient	Withhold avelumab. Initial observation reasonable or initiate prednisone/prednisolone 0.5–1 mg/kg (if progressing, eg, from mild) and/or pregabalin or duloxetine for pain. When symptoms improve, begin a slow corticosteroid taper over at least 4 weeks. Resume avelumab upon symptom control, or when prednisone/prednisolone daily dose <10 mg
	Severe: limits self-care and aids warranted, life-threatening, eg, respiratory problems	Permanently discontinue avelumab. Administer 1–2 mg/kg intravenous (methyl)prednisolone and convert to 0.5–2 mg/kg prednisone/prednisolone orally each day or its equivalent only after a response. Taper over at least 4–8 weeks when symptoms improve to G1
Guillain-Barré syndrome	Progressive symmetrical muscle weakness with absent or reduced tendon reflexes—involves extremities; facial, respiratory, and bulbar and oculomotor muscles; dysregulation of autonomic nerves	Permanently discontinue avelumab. Use of steroids not recommended in idiopathic Guillain-Barré syndrome; however, a trial of (methyl)prednisolone 1–2 mg/kg is reasonable, converting to 0.5–2 mg/kg prednisone/prednisolone orally each day or its equivalent only after a response. If no improvement or worsening, plasmapheresis or IVIG indicated
Myasthenia gravis	Fluctuating muscle weakness (proximal limb, trunk, ocular, eg, ptosis/diplopia or bulbar) with fatigability; respiratory muscles may also be involved	Permanently discontinue avelumab. Administer pyridostigmine at an initial dose of 30 mg 3 times daily. Administer oral prednisone/prednisolone at a dosage of 0.5–2 mg/kg/day or its equivalent or 1–2 mg/kg intravenous (methyl)prednisolone, depending on the severity of symptoms. If treatment begins with intravenous drug, convert to 0.5–2 mg/kg prednisone/prednisolone orally each day or its equivalent only after a response. If no improvement or worsening, plasmapheresis or IVIG may be considered. Additional immunosuppressants used in myasthenia gravis include azathioprine, cyclosporine, and mycophenolate. Avoid certain medications, eg, ciprofloxacin, beta-blockers, that may precipitate cholinergic crisis
Other syndromes, including motor and sensory peripheral neuropathy, multifocal radicular neuropathy/plexopathy, autonomic neuropathy, phrenic nerve palsy, cranial nerve palsies (eg, facial nerve, optic nerve, hypoglossal nerve)		Permanently discontinue avelumab. Administer oral prednisone/prednisolone at a dosage of 0.5–2 mg/kg/day or its equivalent or 1–2 mg/kg intravenous (methyl)prednisolone, depending on the severity of symptoms. If treatment begins with intravenous drug, convert to 0.5–2 mg/kg prednisone/prednisolone orally each day or its equivalent only after a response
Arthralgia	G1 (mild pain with inflammation, erythema, or joint swelling)	Continue avelumab. Administer acetaminophen (paracetamol) and ibuprofen
	G2 (moderate pain with inflammation, erythema, or joint swelling that limits ADLs)	Withhold avelumab. Administer higher doses of acetaminophen (paracetamol) and ibuprofen and use diclofenac or naproxen or etoricoxib. If inadequately controlled, consider intra-articular steroid injections for large joints or administer oral prednisone/prednisolone at a dosage of 0.5–2 mg/kg/day or its equivalent. When symptoms improve to G1, begin a slow corticosteroid taper over at least 4 weeks. If response is not adequate, administer 0.5–1 mg/kg intravenous (methyl)prednisolone and convert to 0.5–2 mg/kg prednisone/prednisolone orally each day or its equivalent only after a response, followed by a taper over at least 4 weeks when symptoms improve to G1. Resume avelumab upon symptom control, or when prednisone/prednisolone daily dose <10 mg
	G3 (severe pain; irreversible joint damage; disabling; limits self-care ADLs)	Withhold avelumab. Administer 0.5–1 mg/kg intravenous (methyl)prednisolone and convert to 0.5–2 mg/kg prednisone/prednisolone orally each day or its equivalent only after a response, followed by a taper over at least 4 weeks when symptoms improve to G1. In severe cases, infliximab or another anti-TNF-alpha drug may be required for improvement of arthritis. Resume avelumab upon symptom control, or when prednisone/prednisolone daily dose <10 mg

(continued)

Treatment Modifications (continued)

RECOMMENDED DOSE MODIFICATIONS FOR AVELUMAB

Adverse Event	Grade/Severity	Treatment Modification
Other	First occurrence of other G3	Withhold avelumab. Administer oral prednisone/prednisolone at a dosage of 0.5–2 mg/kg/day or its equivalent. When symptoms improve to G1, begin a slow corticosteroid taper over at least 4 weeks. Resume avelumab upon symptom control, or when prednisone/prednisolone daily dose <10 mg
	Recurrence of same G3	Permanently discontinue avelumab. Administer 1–2 mg/kg intravenous (methyl)prednisolone and convert to 0.5–2 mg/kg prednisone/prednisolone orally each day or its equivalent only after a response. Taper over at least 4–8 weeks when symptoms improve to G1
	Life-threatening or G4	
	Requirement for ≥10 mg/day prednisone or equivalent for >12 weeks	Permanently discontinue avelumab
	Persistent G2/3 adverse reactions lasting ≥12 weeks	

ADL, activities of daily living; ALT, alanine aminotransferase; AST, aspartate aminotransferase; ATG, anti-thymocyte globulin; IVIG, intravenous immunoglobulin; MMF, mycophenolate mofetil; NYHA, New York Heart Association; SJS, Stevens-Johnson syndrome; TEN, toxic epidermal necrolysis; ULN, upper limit of normal

Notes on general supportive care:
- Steroid taper in most cases will proceed over a minimum of 1 month, but if symptoms improve rapidly, a 2-week taper can be considered. If steroids are administered for more than 4 weeks, administer PCP prophylaxis (cotrimoxazole 480 mg twice daily M/W/F or inhaled pentamidine if cotrimoxazole allergy), regular random blood glucose, vitamin D level and starting calcium/vitamin D supplementation per guidelines

Notes on pregnancy and breastfeeding:
- Avelumab can cause fetal harm. If used during pregnancy, or if the patient becomes pregnant during treatment, apprise the patient of the potential hazard to a fetus. Females of reproductive potential should use highly effective contraception during treatment and for at least 1 month after the last dose of avelumab
- It is not known whether avelumab is excreted in human milk. Therefore, it is recommended that women discontinue nursing during treatment with and for at least 1 month after the final dose of avelumab

Adverse Events (N = 44)

Grade (%)*	Grade 1/2	Grade 3–4
Fatigue	20	0
Infusion-related reaction	20	0
Asthenia	9	2
Nausea	11	0
Diarrhea	9	0
Rash	9	0
Hypothyroidism	7	0
Pruritus	7	0
Decreased appetite	2	2
Elevated AST level	2	2
Elevated creatine phosphokinase level	0	2
Elevated ALT level	2	0
Pneumonitis	2	0
Rheumatoid arthritis	2	0
Uveitis	2	0

*According to the National Cancer Institute Common Terminology Criteria for Adverse Events, version 4.0
Note: Treatment-related toxicities are included in the table if all-grade events occurred in ≥5% patients or G3–5 events occurred in any patient, or if the event was classified as immune-related in any patient. No treatment-related deaths occurred

METASTATIC • SUBSEQUENT THERAPY
BLADDER CANCER REGIMEN: DURVALUMAB

Massard C et al. J Clin Oncol 2016;34:3119–3125
Powles T et al. JAMA Oncol 2017;3:e172411

Durvalumab 10 mg/kg; administer intravenously over 60 minutes in a volume of 0.9% sodium chloride injection (0.9% NS) or 5% dextrose injection (D5W), sufficient to produce a durvalumab concentration within the range 1–15 mg/mL every 2 weeks for up to 12 months (total dosage/2-week course = 10 mg/kg)

Alternative durvalumab dosage regimen as per the U.S. FDA regimens approved on November 18, 2020:

Durvalumab 1500 mg [note: fixed dose option applies to patients weighing >30 kg only]; administer intravenously over 60 minutes in a volume of 0.9% NS or D5W sufficient to produce a durvalumab concentration within the range 1-15 mg/mL every 4 weeks (total dosage/4-week cycle = 1500 mg)
- Administer durvalumab with an administration set that contains a sterile, nonpyrogenic, low protein-binding in-line filter with pore size of 0.2–0.22 μm

Notes:
- Durvalumab can cause severe or life-threatening infusion-related reactions
  - Monitor patients for signs and symptoms of infusion-related reactions
    - During clinical development, urticaria was reported to have developed within 48 hours after durvalumab administration
  - Interrupt or slow the administration rate for mild (G1) or moderate (G2) infusion-related reactions
  - STOP administration and permanently discontinue durvalumab for severe (G3) and life-threatening (G4) infusion-related reactions

Supportive Care
Antiemetic prophylaxis
Emetogenic potential is **MINIMAL**
See Chapter 42 for antiemetic recommendations

Hematopoietic growth factor (CSF) prophylaxis
Primary prophylaxis is **NOT** indicated
See Chapter 43 for more information

Antimicrobial prophylaxis
Risk of fever and neutropenia is **LOW**
  Antimicrobial primary prophylaxis to be considered:
- Antibacterial—not indicated
- Antifungal—not indicated
- Antiviral—not indicated, unless patient previously had an episode of HSV

Patient Population Studied

The urothelial cancer cohort in the multicenter, open-label, phase 1/2 trial involved 191 patients with histologically or cytologically confirmed metastatic or locally advanced urothelial cancer who had experienced disease progression after platinum-based chemotherapy, or were ineligible for or had refused prior chemotherapy. Eligible patients were aged ≥18 years, had Eastern Cooperative Oncology Group (ECOG) performance status ≤1, and had adequate organ and bone marrow function. Patients who had received any immunotherapy or investigational anticancer agent in the month before study enrollment, or who were receiving any concurrent chemotherapy, immunotherapy, or biologic or hormonal therapy for cancer, were not eligible. Patients received intravenous durvalumab (10 mg/kg) every 2 weeks for up to 12 months.

Efficacy (N = 191)

Objective response rate*	17.8% (95% CI 12.7–24.0)
Median overall survival	18.2 months (95% CI 8.1—NE
Overall survival at 12 months	55% (95% CI 44–65)
Median progression-free survival	1.5 months (95% CI 1.4–1.9)
Progression-free survival at 12 months	16% (95% CI 10–23)

*Per Response Evaluation Criteria in Solid Tumors (RECIST) version 1.1; the primary endpoint. Median follow-up was 5.8 months. NE, not estimable

Therapy Monitoring

1. Monitor patients for signs and symptoms of infusion-related reactions, including pyrexia, chills, flushing, hypotension, dyspnea, wheezing, back pain, abdominal pain, and urticaria

2. Initially at the time of each dose, and eventually every 6–12 weeks, perform a total body skin examination with attention to *all* mucous membranes as well as a complete review of systems

3. Monitor patients for signs and symptoms of pneumonitis. Evaluate patients with suspected pneumonitis with chest x-ray, CT scan, and pulse oximetry. For toxicity ≥2, may include nasal swab, sputum culture and sensitivity, blood culture and sensitivity, and urine culture and sensitivity

4. Monitor patients for signs and symptoms of colitis. Encourage patients to report diarrhea immediately to any member of the health care team

5. Draw AST, ALT, and bilirubin prior to each infusion and/or weekly if there are G1 LFT elevations. Note: No treatment is recommended for G1 LFT abnormalities. For toxicity ≥2, work up for other causes of elevated LFTs, including viral hepatitis

6. Use basic metabolic panel (Na, K, CO_2, glucose) and patient history as screening tools for hypophysitis, including hypopituitarism and adrenal insufficiency. If in doubt, evaluate morning adrenocorticotropic hormone (ACTH) and cortisol levels. Consider ACTH stimulation test for indeterminate results

7. Assess thyroid function at the start of treatment, periodically during treatment, and as indicated based on clinical evaluation, and for clinical signs and symptoms of thyroid disorders. Test for TSH and free thyroxine (FT4) every 4–6 weeks as part of routine clinical monitoring on therapy or for case detection in symptomatic patients

8. Measure glucose at baseline and with each treatment during the first 12 weeks and every 6 weeks thereafter

9. Obtain a serum creatinine level prior to every dose. If creatinine is found to be newly elevated, consider holding therapy while other potential causes are evaluated. Note: Routine urinalysis is not necessary other than to rule out urinary tract infections, etc

10. Obtain a complete rheumatologic history and perform an examination of all peripheral joints for tenderness, swelling, and range of motion. Examine the spine. Consider plain x-ray/imaging to exclude metastases and evaluate joint damage (erosions), if appropriate

11. In patients at high risk for infections and in appropriately selected patients based on an infectious disease evaluation, draw screening laboratories (HIV, hepatitis A and B, and blood QuantiFERON for TB) to prepare patients to start infliximab

12. Response evaluation: Every 2–4 months

Treatment Modifications

RECOMMENDED DOSE MODIFICATIONS FOR DURVALUMAB

Adverse Event	Grade/Severity	Treatment Modification
Infusion reaction	Clinically significant but not severe infusion reaction	Interrupt the infusion in patients with clinically significant infusion reactions and consider resuming at a slower rate following resolution. If decision is made to restart, begin at ≤50% of the rate prior to the reaction and increase in 50% increments every 30 minutes if well tolerated. Infusions may be restarted at the full rate during the next cycle
	G3/4 (severe infusion reaction—pyrexia, chills, flushing, hypotension, dyspnea, wheezing, back pain, abdominal pain, and urticaria). Not rapidly responsive to brief interruption of infusion	Stop infusion and administer appropriate medical therapy (eg, epinephrine, corticosteroids, intravenous antihistamines, bronchodilators, and/or oxygen). Discontinue durvalumab
Infection	Severe or life-threatening	Withhold durvalumab
Colitis	G1	Loperamide 4 mg as starting dose, then 2 mg before each meal and after each loose stool until without diarrhea for 12 hours, with maximum of 16 mg loperamide per day. If G1 diarrhea or colitis persists >14 days, add prednisolone 0.5–1 mg/kg (non-enteric-coated) or consider oral budesonide 9 mg daily if no bloody diarrhea
	G2/3 diarrhea or colitis	Withhold durvalumab. Loperamide 4 mg as starting dose, then 2 mg before each meal and after each loose stool until without diarrhea for 12 hours, with maximum of 16 mg loperamide per day. Administer oral prednisone/prednisolone at a dose of 0.5–2 mg/kg/day or its equivalent. When symptoms improve to G1, begin a slow corticosteroid taper over at least 4 weeks. Resume durvalumab upon symptom control, or when prednisone/prednisolone daily dose <10 mg

(continued)

Treatment Modifications (*continued*)

RECOMMENDED DOSE MODIFICATIONS FOR DURVALUMAB

Adverse Event	Grade/Severity	Treatment Modification
	G4 diarrhea or colitis	Permanently discontinue durvalumab. Loperamide 4 mg as starting dose, then 2 mg before each meal and after each loose stool until without diarrhea for 12 hours, with maximum of 16 mg loperamide per day. Administer 1–2 mg/kg intravenous (methyl)prednisolone and convert to 0.5–2 mg/kg prednisone/prednisolone orally each day or its equivalent only after a response. Taper over at least 4 weeks when symptoms improve. If symptoms do not improve over 72 hours or worsen, perform flexible sigmoidoscopy/colonoscopy to document colitis, then begin infliximab 5 mg/kg (if no perforation, sepsis, TB, hepatitis, NYHA III/IV CHF). If no response, add MMF 500–1000 mg twice daily. If worse on MMF, consider addition of tacrolimus or ATG
Pneumonitis	G2	Withhold durvalumab. Start *Pneumocystis* prophylaxis (while patient is receiving a glucocorticoid dose equivalent to ≥20 mg of prednisone daily for 4 weeks or longer) and coverage with empiric antibiotics. Administer oral prednisone/prednisolone at a dose of 1–2 mg/kg/day or its equivalent. When symptoms improve to G1, begin a slow corticosteroid taper over at least 4 weeks. If response is not adequate after 48 hours, administer 2–4 mg/kg intravenous (methyl)prednisolone and convert to 0.5–2 mg/kg prednisone/prednisolone orally each day or its equivalent only after a response, followed by a taper over at least 6 weeks when symptoms improve to G1, titrating to symptoms. Resume durvalumab upon symptom control, or when prednisone/prednisolone daily dose <10 mg
	G3/4	Permanently discontinue durvalumab. Start *Pneumocystis* prophylaxis (while patient is receiving a glucocorticoid dose equivalent to ≥20 mg of prednisone daily for 4 weeks or longer); cover with empiric antibiotics. Administer 2–4 mg/kg intravenous (methyl)prednisolone and convert to 1–2 mg/kg prednisone/prednisolone orally each day or its equivalent only after a response, followed by a taper over at least 8 weeks when symptoms improve to G1, titrating to symptoms. If, when initially treated, improvement does not occur within 48–72 hours, begin infliximab 5 mg/kg (if no perforation, sepsis, TB, hepatitis, NYHA III/IV CHF). If no response to infliximab, add MMF 500–1000 mg twice daily. Consider MMF, especially if concurrent hepatic toxicity
Hepatitis	G2 (AST or ALT >3–5× ULN or total bilirubin >1.5–3× ULN)	Withhold durvalumab. Administer oral prednisone/prednisolone at a dosage of 1–2 mg/kg/day or its equivalent. When symptoms improve to G1, begin a slow corticosteroid taper over at least 4 weeks. Resume durvalumab upon symptom control, or when prednisone/prednisolone daily dose <10 mg
	G3/4 (AST or ALT >5× ULN or total bilirubin >3× ULN)	Permanently discontinue durvalumab. Administer 1–2 mg/kg intravenous (methyl)prednisolone and convert to 0.5–2 mg/kg prednisone/prednisolone orally each day or its equivalent only after a response. Taper over at least 6 weeks when symptoms improve. If no response, add MMF 500–1000 mg twice daily. If worse on MMF, consider adding tacrolimus or ATG
Hypophysitis	G2/3 (moderate symptoms, ie, headache but no visual disturbance or fatigue/mood alteration but hemodynamically stable, no electrolyte disturbance)	Administer analgesia as needed for headache. Withhold durvalumab. Administer oral prednisone/prednisolone at a dosage of 0.5–2 mg/kg/day or its equivalent. When symptoms improve to G1, begin a slow corticosteroid taper over at least 4 weeks. If no improvement in 48 hours, administer 1–2 mg/kg intravenous (methyl)prednisolone and convert to 0.5–2 mg/kg prednisone/prednisolone orally each day or its equivalent only after a response. Taper over at least 4 weeks when symptoms improve to 5 mg prednisone/prednisolone or equivalent; do not stop steroids. Resume durvalumab upon symptom control, or when prednisone/prednisolone daily dose <10 mg
	G4 (severe mass effect symptoms, ie, severe headache, any visual disturbance or severe hypoadrenalism, ie, hypotension, severe electrolyte disturbance)	Permanently discontinue durvalumab. Administer analgesia as needed for headache. Administer 1–2 mg/kg intravenous (methyl)prednisolone and convert to 0.5–2 mg/kg prednisone/prednisolone orally each day or its equivalent only after a response. Taper over at least 4 weeks when symptoms improve to 5 mg prednisone/prednisolone or equivalent; do not stop steroids

(*continued*)

Treatment Modifications (continued)

RECOMMENDED DOSE MODIFICATIONS FOR DURVALUMAB

Adverse Event	Grade/Severity	Treatment Modification
Adrenal insufficiency	G2	Withhold durvalumab. Administer oral prednisone/prednisolone at a dose of 0.5–2 mg/kg/day or its equivalent. When symptoms improve to G1, begin a slow corticosteroid taper over at least 4 weeks. Serially assess adrenal function and continue steroids at replacement doses (20–40 mg hydrocortisone daily ~2/3 dose in morning upon awakening and ~1/3 at 4 PM) until recovery of adrenal function is documented. Resume durvalumab upon symptom control, or when prednisone/prednisolone daily dose <10 mg
	G3/4	Permanently discontinue durvalumab. Administer oral prednisone/prednisolone at a dose of 0.5–2 mg/kg/day or its equivalent. When symptoms improve to G1, begin a slow corticosteroid taper over at least 4 weeks. Serially assess adrenal function and continue steroids at replacement doses (20–40 mg hydrocortisone daily ~2/3 dose in morning upon awakening and ~1/3 at 4 PM) until recovery of adrenal function is documented
Type 1 diabetes mellitus	G3 hyperglycemia	Withhold durvalumab. Admit to hospital to manage hyperglycemia. Role of corticosteroids in preventing complete loss of insulin-producing cells is unknown, and use is not recommended. Resume durvalumab upon symptom control, or when prednisone/prednisolone daily dose <10 mg
	G4 hyperglycemia	Permanently discontinue durvalumab. Admit to hospital to manage hyperglycemia. Role of corticosteroids in preventing complete loss of insulin-producing cells is unknown, and use is not recommended
Nephritis and renal dysfunction	G2/3 (serum creatinine 1.5–6× ULN)	Withhold durvalumab. Administer oral prednisone/prednisolone at a dose of 0.5–2 mg/kg/day or its equivalent. When symptoms improve to G1, begin a slow corticosteroid taper over at least 4 weeks. If response is not adequate, administer 0.5–1 mg/kg intravenous (methyl)prednisolone and convert to 0.5–2 mg/kg prednisone/prednisolone orally each day or its equivalent only after a response, followed by a taper over at least 4 weeks when symptoms improve to G1. Resume durvalumab upon symptom control, or when prednisone/prednisolone daily dose <10 mg
	G4 (serum creatinine >6× ULN)	Permanently discontinue durvalumab. Administer 0.5–1 mg/kg intravenous (methyl)prednisolone and convert to 0.5–2 mg/kg prednisone/prednisolone orally each day or its equivalent only after a response, followed by a taper over at least 4 weeks when symptoms improve to G1
Skin	G1/2	Continue durvalumab. Avoid skin irritants and sun exposure; topical emollients recommended. Topical steroid (mild strength for G1, moderate/potent strength for G2) cream once or twice daily ± oral or topical antihistamines for itching
	G3 rash or suspected SJS or TEN	Withhold durvalumab. Avoid skin irritants and sun exposure; topical emollients recommended. Administer oral or topical antihistamines for itching. Administer oral prednisone/prednisolone at a dosage of 0.5–2 mg/kg or its equivalent daily for 3 days followed by a slow corticosteroid taper over at least 4 weeks when the rash improves to G1. If rash does not respond adequately, then administer 0.5–1 mg/kg intravenous (methyl)prednisolone and convert to 0.5–2 mg/kg prednisone/prednisolone orally each day or its equivalent only after a response, followed by a taper over at least 4 weeks when the rash improves to G1. Resume durvalumab upon symptom control, or when prednisone/prednisolone daily dose <10 mg
	G4 rash or confirmed SJS or TEN	Avoid skin irritants and sun exposure; topical emollients recommended. Administer oral or topical antihistamines for itching. Administer 1–2 mg/kg intravenous (methyl)prednisolone and convert to oral steroids 0.5–2 mg/kg prednisone/prednisolone each day or its equivalent only after a response. Taper over at least 4 weeks when the rash improves to G1. Permanently discontinue durvalumab

(*continued*)

Treatment Modifications (*continued*)

RECOMMENDED DOSE MODIFICATIONS FOR DURVALUMAB

Adverse Event	Grade/Severity	Treatment Modification
Encephalitis	Confusion or altered behavior, headaches, alteration in Glasgow Coma Scale, motor or sensory deficits, speech abnormality; may or may not be febrile	Initially withhold durvalumab, but permanently discontinue durvalumab if there is no doubt as to diagnosis. Exclude bacterial and ideally viral infections prior to high-dose steroids. Administer 1–2 mg/kg intravenous (methyl)prednisolone for 5 days or oral prednisone/prednisolone at a dosage of 0.5–2 mg/kg/day or its equivalent. When symptoms improve, begin a slow corticosteroid taper over at least 4–8 weeks. If symptoms are severe, administer 1–2 mg/kg intravenous (methyl)prednisolone and convert to 0.5–2 mg/kg prednisone/prednisolone orally each day or its equivalent only after a response. Consider concurrent empiric antiviral (intravenous acyclovir) and antibacterial therapy
Aseptic meningitis	Headache, photophobia, neck stiffness with fever, or may be afebrile, vomiting; normal cognition/cerebral function (distinguishes from encephalitis)	
Other syndromes include neurosarcoidosis, posterior reversible leukoencephalopathy syndrome (PRES), Vogt-Koyanagi-Harada syndrome, demyelination, vasculitic encephalopathy, and generalized seizures		
Transverse myelitis	Acute or subacute neurologic signs/symptoms of motor, sensory, autonomic origin; most have sensory level; often bilateral symptoms	Initially withhold durvalumab, but permanently discontinue durvalumab if there is no doubt as to diagnosis. Administer 2 mg/kg intravenous (methyl)prednisolone or consider 1 g/day and convert to 0.5–2 mg/kg prednisone/prednisolone orally each day or its equivalent only after a response. When symptoms improve, begin a slow corticosteroid taper over at least 4–8 weeks. Plasmapheresis may be required if steroids do not bring about improvement
Myocarditis	G3	Permanently discontinue durvalumab. Administer 2 mg/kg intravenous (methyl)prednisolone or consider 1 g/day and convert to 0.5–2 mg/kg prednisone/prednisolone orally each day or its equivalent only after a response. When symptoms improve, begin a slow corticosteroid taper over at least 4–8 weeks. If no response, add MMF 500–1000 mg twice daily. If worse on MMF, consider adding tacrolimus
Peripheral neurologic toxicity	Moderate: some interference with ADL, symptoms concerning to patient	Withhold durvalumab. Initial observation reasonable or initiate prednisone/prednisolone 0.5–1 mg/kg (if progressing, eg, from mild) and/or pregabalin or duloxetine for pain. When symptoms improve, begin a slow corticosteroid taper over at least 4 weeks. Resume durvalumab upon symptom control, or when prednisone/prednisolone daily dose <10 mg
	Severe: limits self-care and aids warranted, life-threatening, eg, respiratory problems	Permanently discontinue durvalumab. Administer 1–2 mg/kg intravenous (methyl)prednisolone and convert to 0.5–2 mg/kg prednisone/prednisolone orally each day or its equivalent only after a response. Taper over at least 4–8 weeks when symptoms improve to G1
Guillain-Barré syndrome	Progressive symmetrical muscle weakness with absent or reduced tendon reflexes—involves extremities; facial, respiratory, and bulbar and oculomotor muscles; dysregulation of autonomic nerves	Permanently discontinue durvalumab. Use of steroids not recommended in idiopathic Guillain-Barré syndrome; however, a trial of (methyl)prednisolone 1–2 mg/kg is reasonable, converting to 0.5–2 mg/kg prednisone/prednisolone orally each day or its equivalent only after a response. If no improvement or worsening, plasmapheresis or IVIG indicated
Myasthenia gravis	Fluctuating muscle weakness (proximal limb, trunk, ocular, eg, ptosis/diplopia or bulbar) with fatigability; respiratory muscles may also be involved	Permanently discontinue durvalumab. Administer pyridostigmine at an initial dose of 30 mg 3 times daily. Administer oral prednisone/prednisolone at a dose of 0.5–2 mg/kg/day or its equivalent or 1–2 mg/kg intravenous (methyl)prednisolone, depending on the severity of symptoms. If treatment begins with intravenous drug, convert to 0.5–2 mg/kg prednisone/prednisolone orally each day or its equivalent only after a response. If no improvement or worsening, plasmapheresis or IVIG may be considered. Additional immunosuppressants used in myasthenia gravis include azathioprine, cyclosporine, and mycophenolate. Avoid certain medications, eg, ciprofloxacin, beta-blockers, that may precipitate cholinergic crisis
Other syndromes, including motor and sensory peripheral neuropathy, multifocal radicular neuropathy/plexopathy, autonomic neuropathy, phrenic nerve palsy, cranial nerve palsies (eg, facial nerve, optic nerve, hypoglossal nerve)		Permanently discontinue durvalumab. Administer oral prednisone/prednisolone at a dose of 0.5–2 mg/kg/day or its equivalent or 1–2 mg/kg intravenous (methyl)prednisolone, depending on the severity of symptoms. If treatment begins with intravenous drug, convert to 0.5–2 mg/kg prednisone/prednisolone orally each day or its equivalent only after a response

(*continued*)

Treatment Modifications (continued)

RECOMMENDED DOSE MODIFICATIONS FOR DURVALUMAB

Adverse Event	Grade/Severity	Treatment Modification
Arthralgia	G1 (mild pain with inflammation, erythema, or joint swelling)	Continue durvalumab. Administer acetaminophen (paracetamol) and ibuprofen
	G2 (moderate pain with inflammation, erythema, or joint swelling that limits ADLs)	Withhold durvalumab. Administer higher doses of acetaminophen (paracetamol) and ibuprofen and use diclofenac or naproxen or etoricoxib. If inadequately controlled, consider intra-articular steroid injections for large joints or administer oral prednisone/prednisolone at a dosage of 0.5–2 mg/kg/day or its equivalent. When symptoms improve to G1, begin a slow corticosteroid taper over at least 4 weeks. If response is not adequate, administer 0.5–1 mg/kg intravenous (methyl) prednisolone and convert to 0.5–2 mg/kg prednisone/prednisolone orally each day or its equivalent only after a response, followed by a taper over at least 4 weeks when symptoms improve to G1. Resume durvalumab upon symptom control, or when prednisone/prednisolone daily dose <10 mg
	G3 (severe pain; irreversible joint damage; disabling; limits self-care ADLs)	Withhold durvalumab. Administer 0.5–1 mg/kg intravenous (methyl)prednisolone and convert to 0.5–2 mg/kg prednisone/prednisolone orally each day or its equivalent only after a response, followed by a taper over at least 4 weeks when symptoms improve to G1. In severe cases, infliximab or another anti-TNF-alpha drug may be required for improvement of arthritis. Resume durvalumab upon symptom control, or when prednisone/prednisolone daily dose <10 mg
Other	First occurrence of other G3	Withhold durvalumab. Administer oral prednisone/prednisolone at a dosage of 0.5–2 mg/kg/day or its equivalent. When symptoms improve to G1, begin a slow corticosteroid taper over at least 4 weeks. Resume durvalumab upon symptom control, or when prednisone/prednisolone daily dose <10 mg
	Recurrence of same G3	Permanently discontinue durvalumab. Administer 1–2 mg/kg intravenous (methyl) prednisolone and convert to 0.5–2 mg/kg prednisone/prednisolone orally each day or its equivalent only after a response. Taper over at least 4–8 weeks when symptoms improve to G1
	Life-threatening or G4	
	Requirement for ≥10 mg/day prednisone or equivalent for >12 weeks	Permanently discontinue durvalumab
	Persistent G2/3 adverse reactions lasting ≥12 weeks	

ADL, activities of daily living; ALT, alanine aminotransferase; AST, aspartate aminotransferase; ATG, anti-thymocyte globulin; IVIG, intravenous immunoglobulin; MMF, mycophenolate mofetil; NYHA, New York Heart Association; SJS, Stevens-Johnson syndrome; TEN, toxic epidermal necrolysis; ULN, upper limit of normal

Notes on general supportive care:
• Steroid taper in most cases will proceed over a minimum of 1 month, but if symptoms improve rapidly, a 2-week taper can be considered. If steroids are administered for more than 4 weeks, administer PCP prophylaxis (cotrimoxazole 480 mg twice daily M/W/F or inhaled pentamidine if cotrimoxazole allergy), regular random blood glucose, vitamin D level, and starting calcium/vitamin D supplementation per guidelines

Notes on pregnancy and breastfeeding:
• Durvalumab can cause fetal harm. If used during pregnancy, or if the patient becomes pregnant during treatment, apprise the patient of the potential hazard to a fetus. Females of reproductive potential should use highly effective contraception during treatment and for 4 months after the last dose of durvalumab
• It is not known whether durvalumab is excreted in human milk. Therefore, it is recommended that women discontinue nursing during treatment and for 4 months after the final dose of durvalumab

Adverse Events (N = 191)

Grade (%)*	Grade 1/2	Grade 3–5
Fatigue	19	0
Decreased appetite	9	0
Diarrhea	8	<1
Rash	7	0
Nausea	7	0
Arthralgia	6	0
Pyrexia	6	0
Pruritus	5	0
Elevated ALT level	3	1
Elevated AST level	2	2
Elevated gamma glutamyltransferase level	2	1
Elevated blood alkaline phosphatase level	2	<1
Hypertension	<1	1
Anemia	<1	<1
Autoimmune hepatitis	<1	<1
Elevated transaminases	<1	<1
Infusion-related reaction	<1	<1
Rash, macropapular	<1	<1
Tumor flare	<1	<1
Acute kidney injury	0	<1
Atrial fibrillation	0	<1

*According to the National Cancer Institute Common Terminology Criteria for Adverse Events, version 4.03
Note: Treatment-related toxicities are included in the table if all-grade events occurred in ≥5% patients or G3–5 events occurred in any patient. Two patients experienced treatment-related death (associated with autoimmune hepatitis and pneumonitis, respectively)

METASTATIC • SUBSEQUENT THERAPY
BLADDER CANCER REGIMEN: ERDAFITINIB

BALVERSA (erdafitinib) prescribing information. Horsham, PA: Janssen Products, LP; 2019
Loriot Y et al. N Engl J Med 2019;381:338–348
Supplementary appendix to: Loriot Y et al. N Engl J Med 2019;381:338–348
Protocol for: Loriot Y et al. N Engl J Med 2019;381:338–348
Taberno J et al. J Clin Oncol 2015;33:3401–3408

Erdafitinib 8 mg/dose; administer orally once daily, without regard to food, continually on days 1–28, every 28 days, until disease progression (total dosage/28-day cycle = 224 mg)

Notes:
- Erdafitinib can cause hyperphosphatemia via inhibition of *FGFR2* in the renal tubules. The phase 1 study demonstrated an association between hyperphosphatemia (phosphate level >5.5 mg/dL) and improved outcomes (Taberno et al, 2015)
  - After 14–21 days, increase the dose to: erdafitinib 9 mg/dose; administer orally once daily, without regard to food, continually on days 1–28, every 28 days, until disease progression (total dosage/28-day cycle = 252 mg) *if the following 3 criteria are met*:
    - The serum phosphate level is <5.5 mg/dL assessed within 14–21 days after initiation of erdafitinib therapy at 8 mg/day
    - There are no treatment-related ocular disorders
    - There are no other G ≥2 adverse reactions
  - Avoid drugs that can increase serum phosphate levels (eg, potassium phosphate supplements, vitamin D supplements, antacids, and phosphate-containing enemas or laxatives), especially during the initial 2–3 weeks of therapy (ie, especially prior to erdafitinib dose titration)
  - Avoid the use of phosphate binders during the initial 2–3 weeks of therapy (ie, prior to erdafitinib dose titration). After this period, phosphate binders may be prescribed to manage hyperphosphatemia (see treatment modifications section)
  - Advise patients to consume a low-phosphorus diet (goal 600–800 mg of dietary phosphate intake per day) during treatment with erdafitinib. Provide information on the phosphorus content of common foods and provide instruction on reading "Nutrition Facts" labels.*
    - Foods which have low amounts of phosphorus include fresh fruits and vegetables, unenriched rice milk, breads, pasta, rice, corn and rice cereals, light-colored sodas, and home-brewed iced tea
    - Foods which contain higher amounts of phosphorus include meat, poultry, fish, dairy foods, beans, lentils, nuts, bran cereal, oatmeal, colas, and some bottled iced teas
- Patients who delay taking erdafitinib at a regularly scheduled time should take the missed dose as soon as possible on the same day, and then take the next regular dose at the regularly scheduled time the next day. Patients should not take more than the prescribed dose to make up for a missed dose
- Patients who vomit after taking erdafitinib should take the next erdafitinib dose at the next regularly scheduled time on the following day
- Erdafitinib tablets should be swallowed whole
- Erdafitinib is metabolized by cytochrome P450 (CYP) CYP2C9 and CYP3A4
  - Avoid concurrent use with strong CYP2C9 or CYP3A4 inhibitors or monitor more closely for adverse reactions
  - Avoid concurrent use with strong CYP2C9 or CYP3A4 inducers
  - If a moderate CYP2C9 or CYP3A4 inducer must be administered concurrently, then increase the erdafitinib dose up to 9 mg per day
  - Patients known or suspected to be CYP2C9 poor metabolizers (ie, *CYP2C9*3/*3 genotype*) may experience higher erdafitinib exposure and have a higher risk of toxicities. Monitor closely for adverse reactions
- Erdafitinib is a time dependent inhibitor and inducer of CYP3A4 based on *in vitro* studies
  - Avoid concurrent use with sensitive CYP3A4 substrates with narrow therapeutic indices
- Erdafitinib is a substrate and inhibitor of P-glycoprotein (P-gp) based on in vitro studies
  - Separate administration of erdafitinib by at least 6 hours before or after administration of P-gp substrates with narrow therapeutic indices (eg, digoxin and dabigatran)

*National Kidney Disease Education Program (NKDEP). Phosphorus. NIH Publication No. 10-7407 April 2010 [accessed September 9, 2019]

Supportive Care
Antiemetic prophylaxis
Emetogenic potential is **MINIMAL-LOW**
See Chapter 42 for antiemetic recommendations

Hematopoietic growth factor (CSF) prophylaxis
Primary prophylaxis is **NOT** *indicated*
See Chapter 43 for more information

(continued)

(*continued*)

Antimicrobial prophylaxis
Risk of fever and neutropenia is **LOW**
   Antimicrobial primary prophylaxis to be **CONSIDERED**:
   • Antibacterial—not indicated
   • Antifungal—not indicated
   • Antiviral—not indicated unless patient previously had an episode of HSV

Oral care
Standard prophylaxis and treatment for mucositis/stomatitis

Hand-foot reaction (palmar-plantar erythrodysesthesia, PPE)
For patients who develop a hand-foot reaction, use topical emollients (eg, Aquaphor), topical or orally administered steroids, antihistamine agents (H_1-receptor antagonists), or pyridoxine
   Pyridoxine may provide relief for discomfort/pain associated with PPE although the mechanism through which this occurs remains unclear
   • The suggested pyridoxine starting dose is 50 mg/day, which may be increased to a maximum of 200 mg/day

Patient Population Studied

This was an open-label, phase 2 study that involved 99 patients with locally advanced unresectable or metastatic urothelial carcinoma who experienced disease progression during or following ≥1 prior systemic chemotherapy regimen or within 12 months of receiving (neo)adjuvant chemotherapy. Chemotherapy-naïve patients who had a contraindication to cisplatin therapy also were eligible. In all patients, the tumor was required to have at least 1 *FGFR1* mutation or *FGFR2/3* fusion. Eligible patients had Eastern Cooperative Oncology Group (ECOG) performance status ≤2 **and** had normal organ function. Patients were excluded if they had persistent baseline hyperphosphatemia, uncontrolled cardiovascular disease, brain metastases, known hepatitis B or C infection, or known human immunodeficiency virus.

Efficacy (N = 99)

	Erdafitinib (N = 99)
Investigator-assessed confirmed response rate*	40% (95% CI, 31–50)
Complete response	3%
Partial response	37%
Investigator-assessed stable disease rate	39%
Investigator-assessed progressive disease rate	18%
Median time to confirmed response	1.4 months
Median response duration	5.6 months (95% CI, 4.2–7.2)
Objective response rate in patients receiving 8 mg/day	34% (95% CI, 22–47)
Objective response rate in patients receiving 8 mg/day initially with dose escalation to 9 mg/day	49% (95% CI, 34–64)
Independent radiologic assessment confirmed objective response rate*	34% (95% CI, 25–44)
Independent radiologic assessment: Complete response	3%
Independent radiologic assessment: Partial response	31%
Median progression-free survival†	5.5 months (95% CI, 4.2–6.0)
12-month progression-free survival	19% (95% CI, 11–29)
Median overall survival‡	13.8 months (95% CI, 9.8–not reached)
12-month overall survival	55% (95% CI, 43–66)

*Includes complete responses and partial responses; responses were confirmed on repeat imaging within 6 weeks after the initial documentation of response
†After a median follow-up of 11.2 months
‡After a median follow-up of 11.0 months

Therapy Monitoring

1. Erdafitinib can cause hyperphosphatemia via inhibition of *FGFR2* in the renal tubules. Hyperphosphatemia occurred in 76% of patients treated with erdafitinib, with a median onset of 20 days (range, 8–116). In the clinical trial, phosphate binders were initiated in 32% of patients to manage hyperphosphatemia. Advise patients to consume a low-phosphorus diet (goal 600–800 mg of dietary phosphate intake per day) during treatment with erdafitinib
   a. *Prior to treatment, between 14–21 days after start of treatment, and then at least monthly:* monitor serum phosphate levels. Patients with serum phosphate levels ≥7 mg/dL should undergo weekly monitoring until the level improves to <5.5 mg/dL (or baseline)
2. Erdafitinib treatment has been associated with ocular disorders, including central serous retinopathy/retinal pigment epithelial detachment (CSR/RPED) resulting in visual field defect. CSR/RPED occurred in 25% of patients in the clinical trial with a median onset of 50 days
   a. *Monthly during the first 4 months of therapy, then every 3 months, and any time if needed for new-onset visual symptoms:* perform an ophthalmologic exam
3. *Periodically:* Monitor for visual symptoms; symptoms of stomatitis, palmar-plantar erythrodysesthesia, and diarrhea. Monitor adherence
4. Obtain a pregnancy test in females of reproductive potential prior to initiation of treatment. Advise female patients of reproductive potential and male patients with female partners of reproductive potential to use effective contraception during treatment with erdafitinib and for 1 month after the last dose

Treatment Modifications

Erdafitinib

Dose level + 1	9 mg orally once daily
Starting dose	8 mg orally once daily
Dose level −1	6 mg orally once daily
Dose level −2	5 mg orally once daily
Dose level −3	4 mg orally once daily
Dose level −4	Discontinue erdafitinib

Hyperphosphatemia

Restrict phosphate intake to 600–800 mg daily for all patients. If serum phosphate is >7.0 mg/dL, consider adding an oral phosphate binder (eg, calcium carbonate, calcium acetate, sevelamer, or lanthanum) administered with meals

Serum phosphate level is between 5.6–6.9 mg/dL	Continue erdafitinib at the same dose
Serum phosphate level is between 7.0–9.0 mg/dL	Withhold erdafitinib until the serum phosphate level is <5.5 mg/dL (or baseline). Monitor serum phosphate levels weekly. Consider adding a phosphate binder as described above Resume erdafitinib at the same dose if resolution to <5.5 mg/dL (or baseline) occurred in ≤1 week. If resolution required >1 week, then reduce the erdafitinib dosage by 1 dose level
Serum phosphate level is between 9.1–10.0 mg/dL	Withhold erdafitinib until the serum phosphate level is <5.5 mg/dL (or baseline). Monitor serum phosphate levels weekly. Consider adding a phosphate binder as described above Resume erdafitinib with the dosage reduced by 1 dose level
Serum phosphate level is >10.0 mg/dL or significant alteration in baseline renal function or grade 3 hypocalcemia (corrected serum calcium of <7.0–6.0 mg/dL; ionized calcium <0.9–0.8 mmol/L; hospitalization indicated)	Withhold erdafitinib until the serum phosphate level is <5.5 mg/dL (or baseline), renal dysfunction has resolved to G ≤1 or baseline, and hypocalcemia has resolved to G ≤1 or baseline. Monitor serum phosphate, serum creatinine, and serum calcium weekly. Consider adding a phosphate binder as described above Resume erdafitinib with the dosage reduced by 2 dose levels

(continued)

Treatment Modifications (*continued*)

Central Serous Retinopathy/Retinal Pigment Epithelial Detachment (CSR/RPED)

Grade 1 (asymptomatic; clinical or diagnostic observations only)	Withhold erdafitinib and perform serial ophthalmologic exams. If resolution occurs within 4 weeks, resume erdafitinib with the dosage reduced by 1 dose level. Then, if no recurrence for a month after resuming, consider re-escalation
	If stable for 2 consecutive monthly eye exams but not resolved, consider resuming erdafitinib but with the dosage reduced by 1 dose level
Grade 2 (visual acuity 20/40 or better or ≤3 lines of decreased vision from baseline)	Withhold erdafitinib until resolution. If resolution occurs within 4 weeks, may resume erdafitinib with the dosage reduced by 1 dose level
Grade 3 (visual acuity worse than 20/40 or > 3 lines of decreased vision from baseline)	Withhold erdafitinib until resolution. If resolution occurs within 4 weeks, may resume erdafitinib with the dosage reduced by 2 dose levels. If the toxicity recurs, consider permanent discontinuation of erdafitinib
Grade 4 (visual acuity 20/200 or worse in affected eye)	Permanently discontinue erdafitinib

Other Toxicities

Any other G3 toxicity	Withhold erdafitinib until the toxicity resolves to G ≤1 or baseline, then may resume with the dosage reduced by 1 dose level
Any other G4 toxicity	Permanently discontinue erdafitinib

Drug Interactions

Strong CYP2C9 inhibitor	If coadministration of erdafitinib with a strong CYP2C9 or strong CYP3A4 inhibitor cannot be avoided, then monitor closely for erdafitinib adverse reactions and consider dose modification accordingly
Strong CYP3A4 inhibitor	
Strong CYP2C9 inducer	Avoid coadministration of erdafitinib with either strong CYP2C9 inducers or strong CYP3A4 inducers
Strong CYP3A4 inducer	
Moderate CYP2C9 inducer	If possible, consider an alternative medication that is not a moderate CYP2C9 inducer or moderate CYP3A4 inducer
Moderate CYP3A4 inducer	If a moderate CYP2C9 inducer or moderate CYP3A4 inducer must be given from the start of erdafitinib therapy, then administer erdafitinib at the usual recommended dose, initially at 8 mg/day with the potential to increase to 9 mg/day If a moderate CYP2C9 inducer or moderate CYP3A4 inducer is introduced after the initial erdafitinib dose increase period has occurred, then consider increasing the erdafitinib dose to 9 mg/day based on tolerability and serum phosphate levels If the moderate CYP2C9 inducer or moderate CYP3A4 inducer is subsequently discontinued, continue the same dosage of erdafitinib in the absence of toxicity
Medication known to alter serum phosphate levels	Avoid co-administration of serum phosphate level-altering medications with erdafitinib before the initial dose increase period
CYP3A4 substrate with narrow therapeutic index	Avoid concurrent use of a sensitive CYP3A4 substrate with erdafitinib
OCT2 substrate	Consider use of an alternative medication that is not an OCT2 substrate or consider reducing the dose of the OCT2 substrate based on tolerability
P-glycoprotein (P-gp) substrate	If coadministration of a P-gp substrate with erdafitinib is unavoidable, then separate erdafitinib administration by at least 6 hours before or after administration of the P-gp substrate with a narrow therapeutic index

Adverse Events (N = 99)

Grade (%)*	Erdafitinib (N = 99)	
	Grade 1–2	Grade ≥3
Hyperphosphatemia	75	2
Stomatitis	47	10
Diarrhea	46	4
Dry mouth	45	0
Decreased appetite	38	0
Dysgeusia	36	1
Fatigue	30	2
Dry skin	32	0
Alopecia	29	0
Constipation	27	1
Hand-foot syndrome	18	5
Central serous retinopathy†	18	3
Anemia	16	4
Asthenia	13	7
Nausea	19	1
Dry eye	18	1
Onycholysis	16	2
Alanine aminotransferase increased	15	2
Paronychia	14	3
Blurred vision	17	0
Nail dystrophy	10	6

Grade (%)*	Erdafitinib (N = 99)	
	Grade 1–2	Grade ≥3
Urinary tract infection	11	5
Vomiting	11	2
Hyponatremia	1	11
Hematuria	8	2
Dyspnea	6	2
Nail disorder	5	3
Acute kidney injury	4	2
Cataract	4	2
Colitis	3	2
General deterioration in physical health	1	4
Keratitis	2	3
Aphthous ulcer	2	2
Increase in gamma-glutamyltransferase	1	2
Urosepsis	0	3

The table includes adverse events of any cause reported in >15% of patients along with adverse events of grade ≥3 that were reported in >1 patient. No deaths were attributed to study treatment. Treatment discontinuation owing to treatment-emergent adverse events occurred in 13% of patients, including retinal detachment (n = 2), palmar-plantar erythrodysesthesia (n = 2), dry mouth (n = 2), and skin or nail events (n = 2). A dose reduction was required in 55% of patients; the most common reasons for dose reduction were stomatitis (n = 16) and hyperphosphatemia (n = 9)
*According to the National Cancer Institute Common Terminology Criteria for Adverse Events, version 4.0
†Central serous retinopathy was a grouped term including: retinal detachment, vitreous detachment, retinal edema, retinopathy, chorioretinopathy, detachment of retinal pigment epithelium, and detachment of macular retinal pigment epithelium

METASTATIC • SUBSEQUENT THERAPY

BLADDER CANCER REGIMEN: ENFORTUMAB VEDOTIN

Rosenberg JE et al. J Clin Oncol 2019;37:2592–2600
Protocol for: Rosenberg JE et al. J Clin Oncol 2019;37:2592–2600
PADCEV (enfortumab vedotin-ejfv) prescribing information. Bothell, WA: Seattle Genetics, Inc; December 2019

Enfortumab vedotin-ejfv 1.25 mg/kg (maximum dose = 125 mg) per dose; administer intravenously in a volume of 0.9% sodium chloride injection, 5% dextrose injection, or Lactated Ringer's Injection sufficient to produce a concentration within the range 0.3–4 mg/mL over 30 minutes for 3 doses on days 1, 8 and 15, every 28 days, until disease progression (total dose/4-week cycle = 3.75 mg/kg; maximum dose/4-week cycle = 375 mg)

> *Note:* Ensure adequate venous access is present for administration of enfortumab vedotin. Severe extravasation reactions have occurred including bullae, exfoliation, and secondary cellulitis

Dry eye prophylaxis (primary prophylaxis is optional)

Lubricating ophthalmic solution (active and inert ingredients vary by brand); administer 2 drops by intraocular instillation into each eye 4 times per day starting with the first enfortumab vedotin dose

> *Note:* Advise patients to report any new-onset or worsening ocular symptoms and consider ophthalmologic evaluation as clinically indicated. Treatment-related dry eye events occurred in 19% of patients

Supportive Care

Antiemetic prophylaxis
Emetogenic potential is: **MODERATE**
See Chapter 42 for antiemetic recommendations

Hematopoietic growth factor (CSF) prophylaxis
Primary prophylaxis is **NOT** indicated
See Chapter 43 for more information

Antimicrobial prophylaxis
Risk of fever and neutropenia is **LOW**
> *Antimicrobial primary prophylaxis to be considered:*
> • Antibacterial—not indicated
> • Antifungal—not indicated
> • Antiviral— not indicated unless patient previously had an episode of HSV

Patient Population Studied

EV-201 was a global, single-arm, two-cohort, phase 2, multicenter study designed to assess the efficacy and safety of enfortumab vedotin. Cohort 1 enrolled platinum- and anti–PD-1/L1–treated patients with Eastern Cooperative Oncology Group performance status scores of 1 or less. Platinum treatment was defined as platinum-containing chemotherapy in the neoadjuvant and/or adjuvant setting with recurrent or progressive disease within 12 months of completion, or platinum in the locally advanced or metastatic setting

Demographic and Disease Characteristics at Baseline

Characteristic	Patients (N = 125)
Male sex	88 (70)
Age, years	
Median (min, max)	69 (40, 84)
Age group, years	
<75	91 (73)
≥75	34 (27)
Region	
North America	117 (94)
Asia	8 (6)
ECOG performance status	
0	40 (32)
1	85 (68)
Primary tumor location	
Bladder/other	81 (65)
Upper tract*	44 (35)
Histology type	
Urothelial carcinoma only	84 (67)
Urothelial carcinoma with squamous differentiation	15 (12)
Urothelial carcinoma with other histologic variants	26 (21)
Metastasis sites (all had metastatic disease)	
Lymph nodes only	13 (10)
Visceral disease†	112 (90)
Bone	51 (41)
Liver	50 (40)
Lung	53 (42)
No. of prior systemic therapies in locally advanced or metastatic setting‡	
Median (min, max)	3 (1, 6)
≥3	63 (50)

(continued)

Patient Population Studied (*continued*)

Demographic and Disease Characteristics at Baseline

Characteristic	Patients (N = 125)
Best response to PD-1/L1– containing therapy	
Responder	25 (20)
Nonresponder	100 (80)
PD-L1 status by combined positive score§	
<10	78/120 (65
≥10	42/120 (35
Nectin–4 expression level, H-score€	
Median (max, min)	290 (14, 300)

Note: Data are represented as No. (%) unless otherwise indicated
ECOG, Eastern Cooperative Oncology Group; max, maximum; min, minimum; PD-1/L1, programmed death 1 or programmed death ligand 1
*Including renal pelvis, ureter, and kidney
†A patient may have metastatic disease in more than one location
‡Including anti-PD-1/L1–containing therapy in the neoadjuvant/adjuvant setting with progression or recurrence within 3 months after therapy completion, or platinum-based therapy in the neoadjuvant/adjuvant setting with progression or recurrence within 12 months after therapy conclusion
§*Five patients did not have tumor samples evaluable for PD-L1 or nectin–4 expression levels
€Nectin–4 levels were assessed by immunohistochemistry in tumor biopsies. Immunohistochemistry images were scored by a pathologist using the H-score method (H-score = [percentage of strong positive tumor cells 3 3] + [percentage of moderate positive tumor cells 3 2] + [percentage of weak positive tumor cells 3 1]). A score of 0 indicates no expression, and a score of 300 indicates the maximum possible expression with this assay

Treatment Monitoring

1. History and physical exam at each visit, CBC with differential, ALT, AST, total bilirubin, alkaline phosphatase
2. Closely monitor blood glucose levels in patients with, or at risk for, diabetes mellitus or hyperglycemia. If blood glucose is elevated (>250 mg/dL), withhold enfortumab vedotin
3. Monitor patients for symptoms of new or worsening peripheral neuropathy
4. Monitor patients for ocular disorders. Consider artificial tears for prophylaxis of dry eyes and ophthalmologic evaluation if ocular symptoms occur or do not resolve. Consider treatment with ophthalmic topical steroids, if indicated after an ophthalmic exam
5. Monitor patients for skin reactions
6. Monitor the infusion site closely during administration for signs and symptoms of possible extravasation
7. Assess response with imaging initially at eight-week intervals and every 8–12 weeks thereafter

Efficacy

Summary of Responses Per Blinded Independent Central Review

Response	Patients (N = 125)
Objective response rate [95% CI]	55 (44) [35.1–53.2]
Best overall response*	
Complete response	15 (12)
Partial response	40 (32)
Stable disease	35 (28)
Progressive disease	23 (18)
Not evaluable†	12 (10)
Median time to response (range)	1.84 months (1.2–9.2 months)—most responses identified by the first disease assessment
Median duration of response (range)	7.6 months (0.95–11.301; 95% CI, 4.93–7.46)
Duration of response with CR	3.61–11.31 months
Estimated median PFS	5.8 months (95% CI, 4.9–7.5)
Estimated median OS	11.7 months (95% CI, 9.1 to not reached)
ORR in patients with prior response to anti–PD-1/L1 therapy	56%
ORR in patients without a response to anti–PD-1/L1 therapy	41%
ORR with liver metastases	38%
ORR with ≥3 prior lines of therapy	41%

Similar responses were observed in patients with poor prognostic characteristics, including and

Note: Data are presented as No. (%)
CR, complete response; NE, not evaluable; ORR, objective response rate; OS, overall survival; PD, progressive disease; PFS, progression-free survival; PR, partial response; SD, stable disease
*Best overall response according to RECIST v1.1
†Includes 10 patients who did not have any response assessment postbaseline, 1 patient who had uninterpretable postbaseline assessment, and 1 patient whose postbaseline assessment did not meet the minimum interval requirement for stable disease

Treatment Modifications

ENFORTUMAB VEDOTIN

Enfortumab Vedotin Dose Levels

Starting dose	1.25 mg/kg (maximum dose = 125 mg) per dose
Dose level −1	1 mg/kg (maximum dose = 100 mg) per dose
Dose level −2	0.75 mg/kg (maximum dose = 75 mg) per dose
Dose level −3	0.5 mg/kg (maximum dose = 50 mg) per dose

Adverse Event	Dose Modifications
Blood glucose >250 mg/dL*	Withhold enfortumab vedotin until elevated blood glucose has improved to ≤ 250 mg/dL, then resume treatment at the same dose level
First occurrence of G2 peripheral neuropathy	Withhold until G≤1, then resume treatment at the same dose level
Second occurrence of G2 peripheral neuropathy	Withhold until G≤1, then resume treatment with dose reduced by one dose level
G≥3 peripheral neuropathy	Permanently discontinue enfortumab vedotin
G3 skin reactions	Withhold enfortumab vedotin until G≤1, then resume treatment at the same dose level or consider dose reduction by one dose level
Recurrent G3 skin reactions	Permanently discontinue enfortumab vedotin
G4 skin reactions	
Other G3 nonhematologic toxicity	Withhold enfortumab vedotin until G≤1, then resume treatment at the same dose level or consider dose reduction by one dose level
Other G4 nonhematologic toxicity	Permanently discontinue enfortumab vedotin
G3 hematologic toxicity or G2 thrombocytopenia	Withhold enfortumab vedotin until G≤1, then resume treatment at the same dose level or consider dose reduction by one dose level
G4 hematologic toxicity	Withhold enfortumab vedotin until G≤1, then resume treatment with dose reduced by one dose level or discontinue treatment
New onset of ocular disorder	Consider artificial tears for prophylaxis of dry eyes and ophthalmologic evaluation if ocular symptoms occur or do not resolve
Intractable ocular disorders	Consider treatment with ophthalmic topical steroids, if indicated after an ophthalmic exam. Consider dose interruption or dose reduction of enfortumab vedotin for symptomatic ocular disorders
Moderate (Child-Pugh B) or severe (Child-Pugh C) hepatic impairment	Avoid use of enfortumab vedotin
Concomitant use of a strong CYP3A4 inhibitor is unavoidable	Monitor closely for enfortumab vedotin adverse effects

*Patients with baseline hemoglobin A1C ≥8% were excluded

Adverse Events

Summary of Adverse Events in Patients Receiving Enfortumab Vedotin

Variable	Patients (N = 125)	
Any adverse event	125 (100)	
Treatment-related adverse events	117 (94)	
G ≥3 treatment-related adverse events	68 (54)	
Treatment-related serious adverse events	24 (19)	
Treatment-related adverse events resulting in treatment discontinuation	15 (12)	
Treatment-related adverse events leading to death*	0 (0)	
Treatment-related adverse events occurring in ≥20% (preferred term)	Any Grade	G ≥3
Fatigue	62 (50)	7 (6)
Alopecia	61 (49)	0
Decreased appetite	55 (44)	1 (1)
Dysgeusia	50 (40)	0
Peripheral sensory neuropathy	50 (40)	2 (2)
Nausea	49 (39)	3 (2)
Diarrhea	40 (32)	3 (2)
Rash maculopapular	27 (22)	5 (4)
Weight decreased	28 (22)	1 (1)
Dry skin	28 (22)	0

Note: Data are presented as No. (%)
*There were no treatment-related deaths during the 30-day safety reporting period. One death as a result of interstitial lung disease that occurred outside the safety reporting period was reported as treatment related

Selected Laboratory Abnormalities Reported in ≥10% (G2–4) or ≥5% (G3–4) of Patients Treated with Enfortumab Vedotin in EV–201

Adverse Reaction	% G2–4*	% G3–4*
Hematology		
Hemoglobin decreased	34	10
Lymphocytes decreased	32	10
Neutrophils decreased	14	5
Leukocytes decreased	14	4
Chemistry		
Phosphate decreased	34	10
Creatinine increased	20	2
Potassium decreased	19†	1
Lipase increased	14	9
Glucose increased	–‡	8
Sodium decreased	8	8
Urate increased	7	7

*Denominator for each laboratory parameter is based on the number of patients with a baseline and posttreatment laboratory value available for 121 or 122 patients
†Includes grade 1 (potassium 3.0–3.5 mmol/L) through grade 4
‡CTCAE grade 2 is defined as fasting glucose >160–250 mg/dL. Fasting glucose levels were not measured in EV–201. However, 23 (19%) patients had non-fasting glucose >160–250 mg/dL

7. Breast Cancer

Rachel Yung, MD, Nancy E. Davidson, MD, and Jennifer M. Specht, MD

Epidemiology

Incidence: 279,100 (male: 2620; female: 276,480. Estimated new cases for 2020 in the United States)
128.5 per 100,000 females per year
Deaths: Estimated 42,690 in 2020 (male: 520; female: 42,170)
Median age: 62 years

Stage at Presentation
Local: 64.4%
Regional: 27.7%
Distant: 5.7%
Unknown: 2.3%

DeSantis CE et al. CA Cancer J Clin 2019;69:438–451
Siegel R et al. CA Cancer J Clin 2020;70:7–30
Surveillance, Epidemiology and End Results (SEER) Program, available from http://seer.cancer.gov [accessed June 2020]

Pathology

Invasive Carcinoma
1. Ductal   49–75%
2. Lobular   5–16%
3. Medullary   3–9%
4. Mucinous   1–2%
5. Tubular   1–3%

Harris JR et al. Disease of the Breast, 4th ed. Philadelphia: Lippincott Williams & Wilkins; 2010

Work-up

Ductal carcinoma in situ:
1. History and physical
2. Bilateral diagnostic mammogram
3. Pathology review with ER status
4. Consideration of breast MRI (optional)
5. Genetic counseling if patient is high risk for hereditary breast cancer
6. Assess distress and refer to supportive services

Stages I & II invasive breast cancer:
1. History and physical
2. Diagnostic bilateral mammogram
3. Pathology review with ER, PR, and HER2 status
4. Consider breast MRI (optional), with special considerations for mammographically occult tumors, lobular carcinomas, or evaluation of in situ component
5. Genetic counseling if the patient is at high risk for hereditary breast cancer
6. CBC with platelets, LFTs, and alkaline phosphatase, and/or targeted staging imaging if symptoms are present concerning for metastatic disease
7. Pregnancy testing and counseling for fertility concerns if premenopausal
8. Assess distress and refer to supportive services

Stage III invasive breast cancer:
1. History and physical
2. Diagnostic bilateral mammogram
3. Pathology review with ER, PR, and HER2 status
4. Consider breast MRI (optional), with special considerations for mammographically occult tumors, lobular carcinomas or evaluation of in situ component
5. Genetic counseling if the patient is at high risk for hereditary breast cancer
6. CBC with platelets, comprehensive metabolic panel (including LFTs) if symptoms are present concerning for metastatic disease
7. Consider bone scan, abdominal ± pelvis CT or US or MRI, and chest imaging. FDG PET/CT also may be helpful in situations where standard staging studies are equivocal or suspicious
8. Pregnancy testing and counseling for fertility concerns if premenopausal
9. Assess distress and refer to supportive services

(continued)

(continued)

Stage IV:

1. History and physical
2. Diagnostic bilateral mammogram if de novo metastatic disease
3. Determination of tumor ER, PR, and HER2 status on a metastatic biopsy if possible
4. Tumor biomarker testing for FDA-approved targeted therapies
5. CBC with platelets, comprehensive metabolic panel (including LFTs)
6. Diagnostic CT with contrast of chest, abdomen, and pelvis or MRI with contrast.
7. Bone scan to assess for skeletal metastases. FDG PET/CT also may be helpful in situations where standard staging studies are equivocal or suspicious. Brain MRI with contrast if suspicious CNS symptoms
8. Genetic counseling and testing for consideration of FDA-approved targeted therapies
9. Assess distress and refer to supportive services (ie, social work, palliative care)
10. Discuss goals of therapy, adopt shared decision-making, and document course of care

Staging

DEFINITIONS OF AJCC 8th EDITION TNM

Definition of Primary Tumor (T)—Clinical and Pathological

T Category	T Criteria
TX	Primary tumor cannot be assessed
T0	No evidence of primary tumor
Tis (DCIS)*	Ductal carcinoma in situ
Tis (Paget)	Paget disease of the nipple NOT associated with invasive carcinoma and/or carcinoma in situ (DCIS) in the underlying breast parenchyma. Carcinomas in the breast parenchyma associated with Paget disease are categorized based on the size and characteristics of the parenchymal disease, although the presence of Paget disease should still be noted
T1	Tumor ≤20 mm in greatest dimension
T1mi	Tumor ≤1 mm in greatest dimension
T1a	Tumor >1 mm but ≤5 mm in greatest dimension (round any measurement >1.0–1.9 mm to 2 mm).
T1b	Tumor >5 mm but ≤10 mm in greatest dimension
T1c	Tumor >10 mm but ≤20 mm in greatest dimension
T2	Tumor >20 mm but ≤50 mm in greatest dimension
T3	Tumor >50 mm in greatest dimension
T4	Tumor of any size with direct extension to the chest wall and/or to the skin (ulceration or macroscopic nodules); invasion of the dermis alone does not qualify as T4
T4a	Extension to the chest wall; invasion or adherence to pectoralis muscle in the absence of invasion of chest wall structures does not qualify as T4
T4b	Ulceration and/or ipsilateral macroscopic satellite nodules and/or edema (including peau d'orange) of the skin that does not meet the criteria for inflammatory carcinoma
T4c	Both T4a and T4b are present
T4d	Inflammatory carcinoma

*Lobular carcinoma in situ (LCIS) is a benign entity and is removed from TNM staging in the *AJCC Cancer Staging Manual, 8th Edition*

Definition of Regional Lymph Nodes—Clinical (cN)

cN Category	cN Criteria
cNX*	Regional lymph nodes cannot be assessed (eg, previously removed)
cN0	No regional lymph node metastases (by imaging or clinical examination)
cN1	Metastases to movable ipsilateral Level I, II axillary lymph node(s)
cN1mi**	Micrometastases (approximately 200 cells, larger than 0.2 mm, but none larger than 2.0 mm)
cN2	Metastases in ipsilateral Level I, II axillary lymph nodes that are clinically fixed or matted; or in ipsilateral internal mammary nodes in the absence of axillary lymph node metastases
cN2a	Metastases in ipsilateral Level I, II axillary lymph nodes fixed to one another (matted) or to other structures
cN2b	Metastases only in ipsilateral internal mammary nodes in the absence of axillary lymph node metastases
cN3	Metastases in ipsilateral infraclavicular (Level III axillary) lymph node(s) with or without Level I, II axillary lymph node involvement; or in ipsilateral internal mammary lymph node(s) with Level I, II axillary lymph node metastases; or metastases in ipsilateral supraclavicular lymph node(s) with or without axillary or internal mammary lymph node involvement
cN3a	Metastases in ipsilateral infraclavicular lymph node(s)
cN3b	Metastases in ipsilateral internal mammary lymph node(s) and axillary lymph node(s)
cN3c	Metastases in ipsilateral supraclavicular lymph node(s)

(continued)

Staging (continued)

Definition of Regional Lymph Nodes—Pathologic (pN)

pN Category	pN Criteria
pNX	Regional lymph nodes cannot be assessed (eg, not removed for pathologic study or previously removed)
pN0	No regional lymph node metastasis identified or ITCs only
pN0(i+)	ITCs only (malignant cell clusters no larger than 0.2 mm) in regional lymph node(s)
pN0(mol+)	Positive molecular findings by reverse transcriptase polymerase chain reaction (RT-PCR); no ITCs detected
pN1	Micrometastases; or metastases in 1–3 axillary lymph nodes; and/or clinically negative internal mammary nodes with micrometastases or macrometastases by sentinel lymph node biopsy
pN1mi	Micrometastases (approximately 200 cells, larger than 0.2 mm, but none larger than 2.0 mm)
pN1a	Metastases in 1–3 axillary lymph nodes, at least one metastasis larger than 2.0 mm
pN1b	Metastases in ipsilateral internal mammary sentinel nodes, excluding ITCs
pN1c	pN1a and pN1b combined
pN2	Metastases in 4–9 axillary lymph nodes; or positive ipsilateral internal mammary lymph nodes by imaging in the absence of axillary lymph node metastases
pN2a	Metastases in 4–9 axillary lymph nodes (at least one tumor deposit larger than 2.0 mm)
pN2b	metastases in clinically detected internal mammary lymph nodes with or without microscopic confirmation; with pathologically negative axillary nodes
pN3	Metastases in 10 or more axillary lymph nodes; or in infraclavicular (Level III axillary) lymph nodes; or positive ipsilateral internal mammary lymph nodes by imaging in the presence of one or more positive level I, II axillary lymph nodes; or in more than three axillary lymph nodes and micrometastases or macrometastases by sentinel lymph node biopsy in clinically negative ipsilateral internal mammary lymph nodes; or in ipsilateral supraclavicular lymph nodes
pN3a	Metastases in 10 or more axillary lymph nodes (at least one tumor deposit larger than 2.0 mm); or metastases to the infraclavicular (level III axillary lymph) nodes
pN3b	pN1a or pN2a in the presence of cN2b (positive internal mammary nodes by imaging); or pN2a in the presence of pN1b
pN3c	Metastases in ipsilateral supraclavicular lymph nodes

Note: (sn) and (f) suffixes should be added to the N category to denote confirmation of metastasis by sentinel node biopsy or FNA/core needle biopsy respectively, with NO further resection of nodes ITC, refers to Isolated tumor cell clusters

Definition of Regional Lymph Nodes—Clinical (cN) (continued)

Note: (sn) and (f) suffixes should be added to the N category to denote confirmation of metastasis by sentinel node biopsy or fine needle aspiration/core needle biopsy respectively.

*The cNX category is used sparingly in cases where regional lymph nodes have previously been surgically removed or where there is no documentation of physical examination of the axilla

**cN1mi is rarely used but may be appropriate in cases where sentinel node biopsy is performed before tumor resection, most likely to occur in cases treated with neoadjuvant therapy

Definition of Distant Metastasis (M)

M Category	M Criteria
M0	No clinical or radiographic evidence of distant metastases*
cM0(i+)	No clinical or radiographic evidence of distant metastases in the presence of tumor cells or deposits no larger than 0.2 mm detected microscopically or by molecular techniques in circulating blood, bone marrow, or other nonregional nodal tissue in a patient without symptoms or signs of metastases
cM1	Distant metastases detected by clinical and radiographic means
pM1	Any histologically proven metastases in distant organs; or if in non-regional nodes, metastases greater than 0.2 mm

*Note that imaging studies are not required to assign the cM0 category

Staging *(continued)*

AJCC Anatomic Stage Groups

Note: should only be used in regions where biomarker testing for HER2, ER, and PR are unavailable

Stage	T	N	M
Stage 0	Tis	N0	M0
Stage IA	T1	N0	M0
Stage IB	T0	N1mi	M0
Stage IB	T1	N1mi	M0
Stage IIA	T0	N1	M0
Stage IIA	T1	N1	M0
Stage IIA	T2	N0	M0
Stage IIB	T2	N1	M0
Stage IIB	T3	N0	M0
Stage IIIA	T0	N2	M0
Stage IIIA	T1	N2	M0
Stage IIIA	T2	N2	M0
Stage IIIA	T3	N1	M0
Stage IIIA	T3	N2	M0
Stage IIIB	T4	N0	M0
Stage IIIB	T4	N1	M0
Stage IIIB	T4	N2	M0
Stage IIIC	Any T	N3	M0
Stage IV	Any T	Any N	M1

Note:
1. T1 includes T1mi
2. T0 and T1 tumors with nodal micrometastases (N1mi) are staged as Stage IB
3. T2, T3, and T4 tumors with nodal micrometastases (N1mi) are staged using the N1 category
4. M0 includes M0(i+)
5. The designation pM0 is not valid; any M0 is clinical
6. If a patient presents with M1 disease prior to neoadjuvant systemic therapy, the stage is Stage IV and remains Stage IV regardless of response to neoadjuvant therapy.
7. Stage designation may be changed if postsurgical imaging studies reveal the presence of distant *metastases*, provided the studies are performed within 4 months of diagnosis in the absence of *disease progression*, and provided the patient has not received neoadjuvant therapy
8. Staging following neoadjuvant therapy is denoted with a "yc" or "yp" prefix to the T and N classification. There is no anatomic stage group assigned if there is a complete pathologic response (pCR) to neoadjuvant therapy, for example, ypT0ypN0cM0.

(continued)

Staging (continued)

AJCC Clinical Prognostic Stage
Note: Clinical Prognostic Stage applies to all patients with breast cancer for clinical classification and staging.

TNM	Grade	HER2 Status	ER Status	PR Status	Clinical Prognostic Stage Group
Tis N0 M0	Any	Any	Any	Any	0
T1* N0 M0 T0 N1mi M0 T1* N1mi M0	G1	Positive	Positive	Positive	IA
				Negative	IA
			Negative	Positive	IA
				Negative	IA
		Negative	Positive	Positive	IA
				Negative	IA
			Negative	Positive	IA
				Negative	IB
	G2	Positive	Positive	Positive	IA
				Negative	IA
			Negative	Positive	IA
				Negative	IA
		Negative	Positive	Positive	IA
				Negative	IA
			Negative	Positive	IA
				Negative	IB
	G3	Positive	Positive	Positive	IA
				Negative	IA
			Negative	Positive	IA
				Negative	IA
		Negative	Positive	Positive	IA
				Negative	IB
			Negative	Positive	IB
				Negative	IB
T0 N1** M0 T1* N1** M0 T2 N0 M0	G1	Positive	Positive	Positive	IB
				Negative	IIA
			Negative	Positive	IIA
				Negative	IIA
		Negative	Positive	Positive	IB
				Negative	IIA
			Negative	Positive	IIA
				Negative	IIA

(*continued*)

Staging (continued)

TNM	Grade	HER2 Status	ER Status	PR Status	Clinical Prognostic Stage Group
	G2	Positive	Positive	Positive	IB
				Negative	IIA
			Negative	Positive	IIA
				Negative	IIA
		Negative	Positive	Positive	IB
				Negative	IIA
			Negative	Positive	IIA
				Negative	IIB
	G3	Positive	Positive	Positive	IB
				Negative	IIA
			Negative	Positive	IIA
				Negative	IIA
		Negative	Positive	Positive	IIA
				Negative	IIB
			Negative	Positive	IIB
				Negative	IIB
T2 N1*** M0 T3 N0 M0	G1	Positive	Positive	Positive	IB
				Negative	IIA
			Negative	Positive	IIA
				Negative	IIB
		Negative	Positive	Positive	IIA
				Negative	IIB
			Negative	Positive	IIB
				Negative	IIB
	G2	Positive	Positive	Positive	IB
				Negative	IIA
			Negative	Positive	IIA
				Negative	IIB
		Negative	Positive	Positive	IIA
				Negative	IIB
			Negative	Positive	IIB
				Negative	IIIB
	G3	Positive	Positive	Positive	IB
				Negative	IIB
			Negative	Positive	IIB
				Negative	IIB
		Negative	Positive	Positive	IIB
				Negative	IIIA
			Negative	Positive	IIIA
				Negative	IIIB

(continued)

Staging (continued)

TNM	Grade	HER2 Status	ER Status	PR Status	Clinical Prognostic Stage Group
T0 N2 M0 T1* N2 M0 T2 N2 M0 T3 N1*** M0 T3 N2 M0	G1	Positive	Positive	Positive	IIA
				Negative	IIIA
			Negative	Positive	IIIA
				Negative	IIIA
		Negative	Positive	Positive	IIA
				Negative	IIIA
			Negative	Positive	IIIA
				Negative	IIIB
	G2	Positive	Positive	Positive	IIA
				Negative	IIIA
			Negative	Positive	IIIA
				Negative	IIIA
		Negative	Positive	Positive	IIA
				Negative	IIIA
			Negative	Positive	IIIA
				Negative	IIIB
	G3	Positive	Positive	Positive	IIB
				Negative	IIIA
			Negative	Positive	IIIA
				Negative	IIIA
		Negative	Positive	Positive	IIIA
				Negative	IIIB
			Negative	Positive	IIIB
				Negative	IIIC
T4 N0 M0 T4 N1*** M0 T4 N2 M0 Any T N3 M0	G1	Positive	Positive	Positive	IIIA
				Negative	IIIB
			Negative	Positive	IIIB
				Negative	IIIB
		Negative	Positive	Positive	IIIB
				Negative	IIIB
			Negative	Positive	IIIB
				Negative	IIIC

(continued)

Staging (continued)

TNM	Grade	HER2 Status	ER Status	PR Status	Clinical Prognostic Stage Group
	G2	Positive	Positive	Positive	IIIA
				Negative	IIIB
			Negative	Positive	IIIB
				Negative	IIIB
		Negative	Positive	Positive	IIIB
				Negative	IIIB
			Negative	Positive	IIIB
				Negative	IIIC
	G3	Positive	Positive	Positive	IIIB
				Negative	IIIB
			Negative	Positive	IIIB
				Negative	IIIB
		Negative	Positive	Positive	IIIB
				Negative	IIIC
			Negative	Positive	IIIC
				Negative	IIIC
Any T Any N M1	Any	Any	Any	Any	IV

*T1 Includes T1mi

**N1 does not include N1mi. T1 N1mi M0 and T0 N1mi M0 cancers are included for prognostic staging with T1 N0 M0 cancers of the same prognostic factor status

***N1 includes N1mi. T2, T3, and T4 cancers and N1mi are included for prognostic staging with T2 N1, T3 N1, and T4 N1, respectively

Note:

1. Because N1mi categorization requires evaluation of the entire node, and cannot be assigned on the basis of an FNA or core biopsy, N1mi can only be used with Clinical Prognostic Staging when clinical staging is based on a resected lymph node in the absence of resection of the primary cancer, such as the situation where sentinel node biopsy is performed prior to receipt of neoadjuvant chemotherapy or endocrine therapy
2. For cases with lymph node involvement with no evidence of primary tumor (eg, T0 N1, etc.) or with breast ductal carcinoma *in situ* (eg, Tis N1, etc.), the grade, HER2, ER, and PR information from the tumor in the lymph node should be used for assigning stage group
3. For cases where HER2 is determined to be "equivocal" by ISH (FISH or CISH) testing under the 2013 ASCO/CAP HER2 testing guidelines, the HER2 "negative" category should be used for staging in the Clinical Prognostic Stage Group table

The prognostic value of these Prognostic Stage Groups is based on populations of persons with breast cancer that have been offered and mostly treated with appropriate endocrine and/or systemic chemotherapy (including anti-HER2 therapy)

(*continued*)

Staging (continued)

AJCC Pathologic Prognostic Stage
Note: Applies to patients with breast cancer treated with surgery as the initial treatment

TNM	Grade	HER2	ER Status	PR Status	Pathologic Prognostic Stage Group
Tis N0 M0 T1* N0 M0 T0 N1mi M0 T1* N1mi M0	Any	Any	Any	Any	0
	G1	Positive	Positive	Positive	IA
				Negative	IA
			Negative	Positive	IA
				Negative	IA
		Negative	Positive	Positive	IA
				Negative	IA
			Negative	Positive	IA
				Negative	IA
	G2	Positive	Positive	Positive	IA
				Negative	IA
			Negative	Positive	IA
				Negative	IA
		Negative	Positive	Positive	IA
				Negative	IA
			Negative	Positive	IA
				Negative	IB
	G3	Positive	Positive	Positive	IA
				Negative	IA
			Negative	Positive	IA
				Negative	IA
		Negative	Positive	Positive	IA
				Negative	IA
			Negative	Positive	IA
				Negative	IB
T0 N1** M0 T1* N1** M0 T2 N0 M0	G1	Positive	Positive	Positive	IA
				Negative	IB
			Negative	Positive	IB
				Negative	IIA
		Negative	Positive	Positive	IA
				Negative	IB
			Negative	Positive	IB
				Negative	IIA

(continued)

Staging (continued)

TNM	Grade	HER2	ER Status	PR Status	Pathologic Prognostic Stage Group
	G2	Positive	Positive	Positive	IA
				Negative	IB
			Negative	Positive	IB
				Negative	IIA
		Negative	Positive	Positive	IA
				Negative	IIA
			Negative	Positive	IIA
				Negative	IIA
	G3	Positive	Positive	Positive	IA
				Negative	IIA
			Negative	Positive	IIA
				Negative	IIA
		Negative	Positive	Positive	IB
				Negative	IIA
			Negative	Positive	IIA
				Negative	IIA
T2 N1*** M0 T3 N0 M0	G1	Positive	Positive	Positive	IA
				Negative	IIB
			Negative	Positive	IIB
				Negative	IIB
		Negative	Positive	Positive	IA
				Negative	IIB
			Negative	Positive	IIB
				Negative	IIB
	G2	Positive	Positive	Positive	IB
				Negative	IIB
			Negative	Positive	IIB
				Negative	IIB
		Negative	Positive	Positive	IB
				Negative	IIB
			Negative	Positive	IIB
				Negative	IIB
	G3	Positive	Positive	Positive	IB
				Negative	IIB
			Negative	Positive	IIB
				Negative	IIB
		Negative	Positive	Positive	IIA
				Negative	IIB
			Negative	Positive	IIB
				Negative	IIIA

(continued)

Staging (*continued*)

TNM	Grade	HER2	ER Status	PR Status	Pathologic Prognostic Stage Group
T0 N2 M0 T1* N2 M0 T2 N2 M0 T3 N1*** M0 T3 N2 M0	G1	Positive	Positive	Positive	IB
				Negative	IIIA
			Negative	Positive	IIIA
				Negative	IIIA
		Negative	Positive	Positive	IB
				Negative	IIIA
			Negative	Positive	IIIA
				Negative	IIIA
	G2	Positive	Positive	Positive	IB
				Negative	IIIA
			Negative	Positive	IIIA
				Negative	IIIA
		Negative	Positive	Positive	IB
				Negative	IIIA
			Negative	Positive	IIIA
				Negative	IIIB
	G3	Positive	Positive	Positive	IIA
				Negative	IIIA
			Negative	Positive	IIIA
				Negative	IIIA
		Negative	Positive	Positive	IIB
				Negative	IIIA
			Negative	Positive	IIIA
				Negative	*IIIC*
T4 N0 M0 T4 N1*** M0 T4 N2 M0 Any T N3 M0	G1	Positive	Positive	Positive	IIIA
				Negative	IIIB
			Negative	Positive	IIIB
				Negative	IIIB
		Negative	Positive	Positive	IIIA
				Negative	IIIB
			Negative	Positive	IIIB
				Negative	IIIB

(*continued*)

Staging (continued)

TNM	Grade	HER2	ER Status	PR Status	Pathologic Prognostic Stage Group
	G2	Positive	Positive	Positive	IIIA
				Negative	IIIB
			Negative	Positive	IIIB
				Negative	IIIB
		Negative	Positive	Positive	IIIA
				Negative	IIIB
			Negative	Positive	IIIB
				Negative	IIIC
	G3	Positive	Positive	Positive	IIIB
				Negative	IIIB
			Negative	Positive	IIIB
				Negative	IIIB
		Negative	Positive	Positive	IIIB
				Negative	IIIC
			Negative	Positive	IIIC
				Negative	IIIC
Any T Any N M1	Any	Any	Any	Any	IV

*T1 includes T1mi

**N1 does not include N1mi. T1 N1mi M0 and T0 N1mi M0 cancers are included for prognostic staging with T1 N0 M0 cancers of the same prognostic factor status

***N1 includes N1mi. T2, T3, and T4 cancers and N1mi are included for prognostic staging with T2 N1, T3 N1, and T4 N1, respectively

Note:

1. For cases with lymph node involvement with no evidence of primary tumor (eg, T0 N1, etc.) or with breast ductal carcinoma *in situ* (eg, Tis N1, etc.), the grade, HER2, ER and PR information from the tumor in the lymph node should be used for assigning stage group
2. For cases where HER2 is determined to be "equivocal" by ISH (FISH or CISH) testing under the 2013 ASCO/CAP HER2 testing guidelines, HER2 "negative" category should be used for staging in the Pathologic Prognostic Stage Group Table
3. The prognostic value of these Prognostic Stage Groups is based on populations of persons with breast cancer that have been offered and mostly treated with appropriate endocrine and/or systemic chemotherapy (including anti-HER2 therapy)

(*continued*)

Staging (continued)

Genomic Profile for Pathologic Prognostic Staging When OncotypeDx® Score Is Less than 11

TNM	Grade	HER2 Status	ER Status	PR Status	Pathologic Prognostic Stage Group
T1 N0 M0 T2 N0 M0	Any	Negative	Positive	Any	IA

Note:
1. Obtaining genomic profiles is NOT required for assigning Pathologic Prognostic Stage. However genomic profiles may be performed for use in determining appropriate treatment. If the OncotypeDx® test is performed in cases with a T1N0M0 or T2N0M0 cancer that is HER2-negative and ER-positive, and the recurrence score is less than 11, the case should be assigned Pathologic Prognostic Stage Group IA
2. If OncotypeDx® is not performed, or if it is performed and the OncotypeDx® score is not available, or is 11 or greater for patients with T1–2 N0 M0 HER2-negative, ER-positive cancer, then the Prognostic Stage Group is assigned based on the anatomic and biomarker categories shown above
3. OncotypeDx® is the only multigene panel included to classify Pathologic Prognostic Stage because prospective Level I data supports this use for patients with a score less than 11. Future updates to the staging system may include results from other multigene panels to assign cohorts of patients to Prognostic Stage Groups based on the then available evidence. Inclusion or exclusion in this staging table of a genomic profile assay is not an endorsement of any specific assay and should not limit appropriate clinical use of any genomic profile assay based on evidence available at the time of treatment

Amin MB et al, editors. AJCC Cancer Staging Manual. 8th ed. New York: Springer; 2017

5-Year Disease-Specific Survival

AJCC 8th Edition Prognostic Stage	MD Anderson Registry*	California Cancer Registry*
Stage IA	99.6%	99.3%
Stage IB	99.3%	97.5%
Stage IIA	97.9%	94.3%
Stage IIB	97.0%	93.0%
Stage IIIA	95.0%	88.0%
Stage IIIB	93.4%	83.6%
Stage IIIC	78.0%	67.6%
Stage IV	Not applicable	35.5%

*Included 3327 patients with stage I to IIIC breast cancer who underwent surgery as initial intervention at MD Anderson Cancer Center from 2007–2013, with complete vital status data through 31 December 2016. Median follow-up = 5 years
†California Cancer Registry population database (n = 54,727 patients with stage I to IV breast cancer treated between 2005–2009); complete vital status data through 31 December 2014. Median follow-up = 7 years
Weiss A et al. JAMA Oncol 2018;4:203–209

Expert Opinion

Breast cancer is best treated with a multidisciplinary approach with involvement of breast surgery, radiation oncology, imaging expertise, medical oncology, pathology, and other specialists as needed. This is especially important in patients with early-stage breast cancer

Clinical trial participation should be encouraged

Ductal Carcinoma In Situ (DCIS)
Local therapy:
- Surgical management of DCIS is central
- Local treatment options include (a) lumpectomy plus whole breast radiation, (b) lumpectomy with accelerated partial breast irradiation (APBI), (c) lumpectomy without radiation, and (d) mastectomy ± sentinel lymph node biopsy (SLNB) without radiation

Systemic therapy:
- In ER positive DCIS treated surgically with lumpectomy, endocrine therapy decreases risk of ipsilateral local recurrence as well as contralateral risk reduction
- Endocrine therapy does not affect overall survival, and shared decision-making is critical
- Endocrine therapy options are tamoxifen for premenopausal women and aromatase inhibitors or tamoxifen for postmenopausal women

Early-Stage Breast Cancer
Local therapy:
- Local treatment is lumpectomy plus radiation versus mastectomy ± radiation
- In certain circumstances for women age >70 years with ER positive breast cancer taking adjuvant endocrine therapy, radiation post-lumpectomy may safely be omitted
- Axillary nodal status should be assessed by sentinel lymph node biopsy (SLNB) for those with clinical N0 disease or by ultrasound-guided biopsy for those with clinically node-positive disease when neoadjuvant systemic therapy is planned
- Patients with a +SLNB do not need to undergo ALND if they fit criteria for Z11/Amaros
- Post-mastectomy radiation therapy (PMRT) should be considered in those with pretreatment clinical indications (tumor >5 cm, positive axillary nodes, close surgical margins) and less than pCR for those undergoing neoadjuvant therapy

Decisions regarding **adjuvant therapy** *must be individualized, but general guidelines are outlined below:*
Adjuvant Chemotherapy Principles:
- Patients with cancers >1 cm that are ER negative, PR negative, HER2 negative (triple negative) should be considered for multiagent chemotherapy. For patients with triple-negative breast cancer (TNBC) >2 cm or node positive, a regimen including anthracycline and taxane is recommended
- Patients with cancers that are HER2 positive >1 cm should typically be treated with cytotoxic chemotherapy in addition to a HER2-directed agent
- Preoperative treatment of larger triple negative and HER2+ breast cancers is favored since pathologic response at time of surgery can inform recommendations for adjuvant systemic therapy
- Molecular assays (such as the 21- or 70-gene recurrence score) can be incorporated into decision-making regarding adjuvant chemotherapy treatment for patients with ER-positive HER2-negative disease node-negative and limited node-positive (1–3) disease

Adjuvant Endocrine Therapy Principles for Patients with Stage I–III Invasive Disease:
- In patients with ER-positive and/or PR-positive disease, adjuvant endocrine therapy should be recommended, and adherence monitored and encouraged
- In women who are premenopausal/perimenopausal at diagnosis and with disease of high enough risk to warrant adjuvant chemotherapy, ovarian suppression/ablation with aromatase inhibitor or tamoxifen is recommended. For premenopausal women with low-risk hormone receptor–positive disease, tamoxifen is recommended. When patient becomes menopausal, transition to AI can be considered. If patient remains premenopausal after 5 years of tamoxifen, consider an additional 5 years of tamoxifen to total duration of 10 years
- In women who are postmenopausal at diagnosis, an aromatase inhibitor should be used in one of the following adjuvant dosing strategies based on assessment of risk and patient preference:
  - **Upfront** (AI for 5 years)
  - **Sequential** (tamoxifen for 2–3 years followed by an AI to complete 5 years of therapy *or* an AI for 2–3 years followed by tamoxifen to complete 5 years of therapy)
  - **Extended** (tamoxifen for 5 years followed by an AI for 5 years)
- Men with ER positive breast cancer should be treated with adjuvant tamoxifen (if AI must be considered it is recommended to use with a GNRH agonist)
- Extended aromatase inhibitor therapy (>5 years) should be considered for patients with high-risk, node-positive disease
- Neoadjuvant endocrine therapy may be considered for postmenopausal patients with hormone receptor–positive breast cancer
- Consider addition of adjuvant bisphosphonate for post-menopausal women with higher risk breast cancer or low bone mineral density who will be prescribed adjuvant AI

(continued)

Expert Opinion (*continued*)

Locally Advanced (LABC) and Inflammatory Breast Cancer (IBC)
- Treatment of locally advanced or inflammatory breast cancer is best accomplished with a multidisciplinary treatment team
- For patients with locally advanced or inflammatory breast cancer, staging to evaluate for distant metastases is warranted
- Neoadjuvant or pre-operative systemic therapy is the treatment of choice for patients with LABC or IBC
- Neoadjuvant systemic therapy for LABC or IBC should be informed by breast cancer subtype. For patients with hormone receptor–positive, HER2-negative breast cancer, an anthracycline- and taxane-containing regimen is preferred
- Clinical breast exam and/or breast imaging (ultrasound, diagnostic mammogram, or MRI) should be used to evaluate response to neoadjuvant therapy and to inform surgical management
- For patients with IBC, total mastectomy with completion level I/II axillary node dissection is recommended. Post-mastectomy radiation to chest wall and regional nodes also is recommended to optimize local control
- Initial SLNB, rather than upfront ALND, may be performed in selected node-positive patients who receive neoadjuvant therapy and have resolution of clinically positive lymph nodes. Outside of a study, a positive SLNB should be treated with an ALND at the time of publication
- PMRT should be considered in those with pretreatment clinical indications (tumor >5 cm, positive axillary nodes, close surgical margins) and less than pCR for those undergoing neoadjuvant therapy

Metastatic Disease
Chemotherapy: In general, single chemotherapy agents (monotherapy) may be used sequentially. If a rapid clinical response is needed, combination chemotherapy regimens may be used
Endocrine therapy: For patients with ER-positive and/or PR-positive disease without visceral involvement or with low-volume disease, primary endocrine therapy is preferred. CDK4/6 inhibitors in combination with endocrine therapy have demonstrated efficacy with improvement in overall survival and should be considered in first- or second-line setting

	Palbociclib	Ribociclib	Abemaciclib
Use with: AI Fulvestrant Tamoxifen Use alone (monotherapy)	✓ ✓	✓ ✓ ✓	✓ ✓ ✓ ✓
Approved for use in: First-line MBC Second-line MBC	✓ ✓	✓ ✓	✓ ✓
Patient population Postmenopausal Premenopausal	✓ ✓	✓ ✓	✓
Side effects	Neutropenia, fatigue, nausea, alopecia	Neutropenia, fatigue	Diarrhea, neutropenia, nausea

HER2-directed therapy *(IHC 3+ or FISH+):* In first line, trastuzumab and pertuzumab should be used in combination with a taxane for patients with ER- and PR-negative disease given survival benefit. Taxane, pertuzumab, and trastuzumab are often used for patients with hormone receptor–positive, HER2-positive metastatic breast cancer, but endocrine therapy with HER2-targeted agents may also be considered. TDM1 should typically be used as second-line therapy. Third line and beyond includes HER2-directed therapy with chemotherapy or dual HER2-directed agents
Immunotherapy: For patients with metastatic TNBC and evidence of tumor PDL1 expression, nab-paclitaxel with atezolizumab has demonstrated improvement in overall survival and should be considered. Pembrolizumab also may be used for the treatment of patients with metastatic, microsatellite instability-high (MSI-H), or mismatch repair–deficient (dMMR) breast cancer who have progressed following prior treatment and who have no satisfactory alternative treatment options. This is a rapidly evolving field, and participation in available clinical trials is highly recommended
Bone disease present: Use of a bone-stabilizing agent such as denosumab, zoledronic acid, or pamidronate disodium should be added to prevent skeletal-related events
Participation in clinical trials may supplant these recommendations

Gradishar WJ. Ann Oncol 2013;24:2492–2500
Jankowitz RC et al. Breast 2013;22(Suppl 2):S165–S170
Jelovac D, Emens LA. Oncology (Williston Park) 2013;27:166–175

SYSTEMIC ADJUVANT TREATMENT GUIDELINES
Standard Risk Histologies: Ductal, Lobular, Mixed, and Metaplastic

1. **Hormone receptor–positive HER2-negative:**

   Tumor ≤0.5 cm or microinvasive:
   - N0: consider adjuvant endocrine therapy
   - N1mi: Adjuvant endocrine therapy ± adjuvant chemotherapy

   Tumor >0.5 cm and pN0–1:
   - Consider tumor gene expression testing, such as the 21- or 70-gene assay and determine clinical risk by standard prognostic features
   - Assay not done: adjuvant endocrine therapy ± adjuvant chemotherapy
   - For high-risk tumors (by genomic and/or clinical risk), adjuvant chemotherapy in addition to adjuvant endocrine therapy
   - For low-risk tumors (by genomic and/or clinical risk), adjuvant endocrine therapy alone

   Anatomic stage III disease (T3N1 or TxN2–3):
   - Adjuvant chemotherapy followed by endocrine therapy

2. **Hormone receptor–positive HER2-positive pT1, pT2, or pT3 and pN0 or pN1mi:**

   Tumor ≤0.5 cm or microinvasive:
   - N0: consider adjuvant endocrine therapy
   - N1mi: adjuvant endocrine therapy ± adjuvant chemotherapy + trastuzumab (eg, paclitaxel + trastuzumab)

   Tumor 0.6–1.0 cm:
   - N0: consider adjuvant endocrine therapy alone
   - N0 or N1mic: Adjuvant endocrine therapy ± adjuvant chemotherapy and trastuzumab (eg, paclitaxel + trastuzumab)

   Tumor >1.0 cm and N0:
   - Neoadjuvant or adjuvant chemotherapy + trastuzumab ± pertuzumab and adjuvant endocrine therapy

   Node positive:
   - Neoadjuvant chemotherapy + trastuzumab + pertuzumab and adjuvant endocrine therapy
   - For patients treated with neoadjuvant therapy who have residual disease at surgery, we recommend treatment with adjuvant TDM1 or consideration of neratinib with endocrine therapy
   - We recommend a full year of adjuvant HER2-directed therapy

3. **Hormone receptor–negative HER2-positive pT1, pT2, or pT3 and pN0 or pN1mi:**

   Tumor ≤0.5 cm or microinvasive:
   - N0: no adjuvant therapy
   - N1mi: consider adjuvant chemotherapy + trastuzumab

   Tumor 0.6–1.0 cm and N0 or N1mi:
   - Consider adjuvant chemotherapy + trastuzumab (eg, paclitaxel + trastuzumab)

   Tumor >1.0 cm and N0:
   - Neoadjuvant or adjuvant chemotherapy + trastuzumab ± pertuzumab

   Node positive:
   - Neoadjuvant chemotherapy + trastuzumab + pertuzumab
   - For patients treated with neoadjuvant therapy that have residual disease at surgery, we recommend treatment with adjuvant TDM1 or consideration pertuzumab
   - We recommend a full year of HER2-directed therapy

4. **Hormone receptor–negative HER2-negative: pT1, pT2, or pT3 and pN0 or pN1mi:**

   Tumor ≤0.5 cm or microinvasive:
   - N0: no adjuvant therapy
   - N1mi: Consider adjuvant chemotherapy

   Tumor 0.6–1.0 cm:
   - Consider adjuvant chemotherapy

   Tumor >1.0 cm:
   - Neoadjuvant or adjuvant chemotherapy

   Node positive:
   - Neoadjuvant chemotherapy including an anthracycline and taxane unless contraindicated. The addition of carboplatin to neoadjuvant therapy for TNBC patients has been shown to improve rate of pathologic complete response, but improvement in event free and overall survival is less certain
   - Participation in clinical trials is recommended

Favorable Histologies: Tubular, Colloid

1. **ER-positive and/or PR-positive pT1, pT2, or pT3 and pN0 or pN1mi:**

   Tumor <1.0–2.9 cm and N0:
   - No adjuvant therapy

   Tumor ≥3.0 cm and N0:
   - Consider adjuvant endocrine therapy

   Node positive:
   - Adjuvant endocrine therapy
   - Adjuvant endocrine therapy ± adjuvant chemotherapy

2. **ER-negative and PR-negative:**

   Repeat ER and PR status; if truly negative, treat as standard risk breast cancer histology

ADJUVANT OR NEOADJUVANT CHEMOTHERAPY REGIMENS FOR HER2-NEGATIVE BREAST CANCER

Preferred

1. Dose-dense AC (doxorubicin and cyclophosphamide) followed by weekly paclitaxel
2. Dose-dense AC (doxorubicin and cyclophosphamide) followed by paclitaxel every 2 weeks
3. TC (docetaxel and cyclophosphamide)

Other Adjuvant Regimens

1. AC (doxorubicin/cyclophosphamide) followed by docetaxel every 3 weeks
2. FEC (fluorouracil/epirubicin/cyclophosphamide) followed by docetaxel
3. FEC followed by weekly paclitaxel
4. Dose-dense AC (doxorubicin/cyclophosphamide) or AC given every 3 weeks
5. FEC (fluorouracil/epirubicin/cyclophosphamide)
6. CMF (cyclophosphamide/methotrexate/fluorouracil)
7. TAC (docetaxel/doxorubicin/cyclophosphamide)

ADJUVANT OR NEOADJUVANT CHEMOTHERAPY REGIMENS FOR HER2 POSITIVE BREAST CANCER

Preferred:

1. AC (doxorubicin/cyclophosphamide) followed by paclitaxel + trastuzumab +/-pertuzumab*
2. TCH ± P (docetaxel/carboplatin/trastuzumab/±pertuzumab*)
3. TH (paclitaxel/trastuzumab)
   - For patients with residual disease after neoadjuvant therapy, adjuvant TDM1 is indicated
   - For patients with high-risk HER2+ breast cancer, adjuvant neratinib (ER+) and/or pertuzumab may be considered

*Neoadjuvant pertuzumab should be administered to patients receiving neoadjuvant therapy with ≥T2 or ≥N1, HER2-positive, early-stage breast cancer

Other regimens:

1. Docetaxel + trastuzumab ± pertuzumab followed by FEC (fluorouracil/epirubicin/cyclophosphamide)
2. AC (doxorubicin/cyclophosphamide) followed by docetaxel with trastuzumab ± pertuzumab
3. Docetaxel, cyclophosphamide, and trastuzumab

PREFERRED CHEMOTHERAPY FOR METASTATIC BREAST CANCER (MBC)

Chemotherapy

Single Agents

Anthracyclines:

1. Doxorubicin
2. Epirubicin
3. Doxorubicin HCl liposomal injection

Taxanes:

1. Paclitaxel
2. Docetaxel
3. Paclitaxel protein-bound particles for injectable suspension (albumin-bound)

Antimetabolites:

1. Capecitabine
2. Gemcitabine

Microtubule inhibitors:

1. Vinorelbine
2. Eribulin

Other Single Agents

1. Cyclophosphamide
2. Mitoxantrone
3. Cisplatin or carboplatin
4. Etoposide (oral)
5. Ixabepilone

Chemotherapy Combinations

1. FEC (fluorouracil/epirubicin/cyclophosphamide)
2. AC (doxorubicin/cyclophosphamide)
3. CMF (cyclophosphamide/methotrexate/fluorouracil)
4. Docetaxel/capecitabine
5. GT (gemcitabine/paclitaxel)
6. Ixabepilone + capecitabine

(continued)

(*continued*)

Targeted Agents:

1. For patients with germline *BRCA*1/2 mutations, olaparib or talazoparib are recommended

2. For patients with hormone receptor–positive, HER2-negative breast cancer with PIK3CA mutation (detected by molecular panel testing of tumor or blood), alpelisib + fulvestrant is recommended in second line

3. For patients with TNBC and tumor PD-L1 expression, atezolizumab and nab-paclitaxel is preferred in first line

HER2-Directed Therapies:

Preferred First-line Agents for HER2-Positive Disease

1. Pertuzumab + trastuzumab + docetaxel

2. Pertuzumab + trastuzumab + paclitaxel

Other First-line Agents for HER2-Positive Disease
Trastuzumab alone or in combination with:

1. Paclitaxel + carboplatin

2. Paclitaxel

3. Docetaxel

4. Vinorelbine

5. Capecitabine

6. Doxorubicin liposomal (Doxil®)

Preferred Agent for Trastuzumab-Exposed HER2-Positive Disease

1. ado-Trastuzumab emtansine (TDM-1)

2. fam-Trastuzumab deruxtecan-nxki

Other Agents for Trastuzumab-exposed HER2-Positive Disease

1. Lapatinib + capecitabine ± trastuzumab

2. Trastuzumab + capecitabine

3. Trastuzumab + lapatinib

For Patients with HER2-Positive Disease with Brain Metastases

1. Lapatinib + capecitabine

2. TDM1

3. Neratinib + capecitabine

4. "High dose" trastuzumab + pertuzumab

5. Tucatinib + capecitabine + trastuzumab

ADJUVANT • HORMONE-RECEPTOR POSITIVE • PREMENOPAUSAL

BREAST CANCER REGIMEN: EXEMESTANE PLUS OVARIAN SUPPRESSION

Pagani O et al. N Engl J Med 2014;371:107–118
Protocol for: Pagani O et al. N Engl J Med 2014;371:107–118

Triptorelin pamoate injectable suspension 3.75 mg; administer as a single intramuscular injection into either buttock on day 1, every 28 days, for 5 years (total dosage/28-day cycle = 3.75 mg)

Notes:

- Alternate injection site periodically

- After at least 6 months of therapy, may consider bilateral oophorectomy or bilateral ovarian irradiation as an alternative to ongoing treatment with gonadotropin-releasing hormone (GnRH) agonist, if desired

- Goserelin may be considered as an alternative to triptorelin:

    - **Goserelin acetate implant** 3.6 mg; administer as a single subcutaneous injection into the anterior abdominal wall below the navel line on day 1, every 28 days, for 5 years (total dosage/28-day cycle = 3.6 mg), *plus:*

Exemestane 25 mg; administer orally, once daily after a meal, continually for 5 years (total dose/week = 175 mg)

Notes:

- Exemestane should begin between 6 and 8 weeks after the first dose of GnRH agonist if chemotherapy was not administered to allow for suppression of ovarian function, or concurrently with GnRH agonist if chemotherapy is administered

- Exemestane is metabolized by cytochrome P450 (CYP) CYP3A subfamily enzymes. Avoid concurrent use with strong CYP3A4 inducers (eg, rifampin, carbamazepine, phenytoin, phenobarbital, St. John's wort) if possible. If concurrent use with a strong CYP3A4 inducer is required, increase the exemestane dose to 50 mg per day

Supportive Care

Antiemetic prophylaxis
Emetogenic potential is **MINIMAL–LOW**
See Chapter 42 for antiemetic recommendations

Hematopoietic growth factor (CSF) prophylaxis
Primary prophylaxis is **NOT** indicated
See Chapter 43 for more information

Antimicrobial prophylaxis
Risk of fever and neutropenia is **LOW**
   Antimicrobial primary prophylaxis to be considered:
   - Antibacterial—not indicated
   - Antifungal—not indicated
   - Antiviral—not indicated unless patient previously had an episode of HSV

Patient Population Studied

The analysis included data from two phase 3 trials (the Tamoxifen and Exemestane Trial [TEXT] and the Suppression of Ovarian Function Trial [SOFT]) involving a total of 4690 premenopausal women with histologically proven hormone receptor–positive breast cancer. All patients either had undergone total mastectomy with or without subsequent radiotherapy or had undergone breast-conserving surgery with subsequent radiotherapy. All patients in TEXT as well as patients in SOFT who did not undergo chemotherapy (that is, those for whom adjuvant tamoxifen alone was considered suitable) were randomized within 12 weeks after definitive surgery. Patients in SOFT who received adjuvant or neoadjuvant chemotherapy were randomized within 8 months after completion of chemotherapy, upon confirmation of a premenopausal level of estradiol. Patients in TEXT (N = 2672) were randomized to receive either oral exemestane (25 g daily) plus ovarian suppression in the form of triptorelin (3.75 mg intramuscular injection every 28 days) or oral tamoxifen (20 mg daily) plus triptorelin. Patients in TEXT who underwent chemotherapy (which was optional) started it concomitantly with ovarian suppression. In TEXT, oral endocrine therapy was started either after the completion of chemotherapy or, in those who did not receive chemotherapy, 6–8 weeks after the initiation of ovarian suppression. Patients in SOFT (N = 3066) were randomized to receive exemestane plus ovarian suppression (in the form of triptorelin, bilateral oophorectomy, or ovarian irradiation), tamoxifen plus ovarian suppression, or tamoxifen alone (the latter group is not included in this analysis). In SOFT, adjuvant oral endocrine therapy was allowed prior to randomization

Efficacy (N = 4690)

	Exemestane Plus Ovarian Suppression (N = 2346)	Tamoxifen Plus Ovarian Suppression (N = 2344)	
5-year survival free from disease	91.1%	87.3%	HR 0.72, 95% CI 0.60–0.85; P<0.001
Freedom from distant recurrence at 5 years	93.8%	92.0%	HR 0.78; 95% CI 0.62 to 0.97; P = 0.02
Freedom from breast cancer at 5 years	92.8%	88.8%	HR 0.66, 95% CI 0.55–0.80; P<0.001
Overall survival at 5 years	95.9%	96.9%	HR 1.14, 95% CI 0.86–1.51; P = 0.37

Median follow-up 68 months

Therapy Monitoring

1. Assess adherence and persistence to adjuvant therapy at each visit
2. Decreases in bone mineral density may occur albeit to a lower extent with exemestane. Consider bone mineral density monitoring every 24 months
3. Decreases in HDL can occur with exemestane. Consider cholesterol monitoring
4. At baseline, consider pregnancy test in females of reproductive potential. Cases of pregnancy during routine use of GnRH analogues has occurred; therefore discuss the role of effective nonhormone-based contraception

Treatment Modifications

Exemestane Plus Ovarian Suppression

General Dose Adjustment	
If a strong CYP3A inducer must be used	Increase exemestane dose to 50 mg by mouth once daily or transition to an alternative aromatase inhibitor
Vaginal dryness or dyspareunia	Continue exemestane and GnRH analogue at current doses. Treat with vaginal moisturizers and lubricants. Consider low-dose topical estrogen. For persistent bothersome symptoms, consider discontinuation of ovarian suppression and exemestane and instead switch to tamoxifen
Vasomotor symptoms (eg, hot flushes, night sweats)	Continue exemestane and GnRH analogue at current doses. Consider treatment with a selective serotonin reuptake inhibitor (SSRI) or a serotonin and norepinephrine reuptake inhibitor (SNRI) for bothersome symptoms. Primarily nocturnal symptoms may be treated with gabapentin administered at bedtime. For persistent bothersome symptoms, consider discontinuation of ovarian suppression and exemestane and instead switch to tamoxifen

Exemestane
- Dose: 25-mg tablet
- Do not administer to premenopausal women. Do not co-administer with estrogen-containing agents because these could interfere with its pharmacologic action
- Adverse events considered drug related or of indeterminate cause include hot flashes (13%), nausea (9%), fatigue (8%), increased sweating (4%), and increased appetite (3%). Less frequent adverse events of any cause (from 2% to 5%) include fever, generalized weakness, paresthesia, pathologic fracture, bronchitis, sinusitis, rash, itching, urinary tract infection, and lymphedema

Adverse Events (N = 4643)

Grade (%)*	Exemestane Plus Ovarian Suppression (N = 2318)		Tamoxifen Plus Ovarian Suppression (N = 2325)	
	Grade 1–2	Grade 3–4	Grade 1–2	Grade 3–4
Any targeted event	68	31	69	29
Hot flushes	82	10	81	12
Musculoskeletal symptoms	78	11	71	5
Fatigue	58	3	60	3
Insomnia	54	4	54	4
Sweating	55	0	59	0
Vaginal dryness	52	0	47	0
Depression	47	4	46	4
Decreased libido	45	0	41	0
Osteoporosis	38	<1	25	<1
Nausea	30	<1	28	<1
Dyspareunia	28	2	24	1
Hypertension	16	7	15	7
Urinary incontinence	13	<1	18	<1
Injection-site reaction	7	<1	8	<1
Fractures	6	1	4	<1
Allergic reaction or hypersensitivity	4	<1	4	<1
Hyperglycemia†	2	<1	3	<1
Glucose intolerance†	2	<1	2	<1
Thrombosis or embolism	<1	<1	<1	2
CNS hemorrhage	<1	<1	<1	<1
Cardiac ischemia or infarction	<1	<1	<1	<1
CNS cerebrovascular ischemia	<1	<1	<1	<1

*According to the National Cancer Institute Common Terminology Criteria for Adverse Events, version 3.0
†May be an underestimate because the event was added as a targeted adverse event partway through the trials. Targeted adverse events are included in the table. No patients had a targeted grade 5 adverse event. CNS, central nervous system

ADJUVANT • HER2-NEGATIVE

BREAST CANCER REGIMEN: DOCETAXEL + DOXORUBICIN + CYCLOPHOSPHAMIDE (TAC)

Nabholtz JM et al. J Clin Oncol 2001;19:314–321 [Treatment for metastatic disease]
Nabholtz J-M et al. Proc Am Soc Clin Oncol 2002;21:36a [Abstract 141; adjuvant treatment]

Premedication:
Dexamethasone 8 mg/dose; administer orally twice daily for 3 days, starting on the day before docetaxel administration (total dose/cycle = 48 mg)
Hydration with 1000 mL 0.9% sodium chloride injection (0.9% NS); administer intravenously 500 mL before starting cyclophosphamide and 500 mL after completing cyclophosphamide

Doxorubicin HCl 50 mg/m^2; administer by intravenous injection over 3–5 minutes on day 1, every 3 weeks for 6 cycles
(total dosage/cycle = 50 mg/m^2), *followed by:*
Cyclophosphamide 500 mg/m^2; administer intravenously in 100–500 mL 0.9% NS or 5% dextrose injection (D5W), over 15–60 minutes on day 1, every 3 weeks for 6 cycles (total dosage/cycle = 500 mg/m^2), *followed by:*
Docetaxel 75 mg/m^2; administer intravenously in a volume of 0.9% NS or D5W sufficient to produce a docetaxel concentration within the range 0.3–0.74 mg/mL over 60 minutes on day 1, every 3 weeks for 6 cycles (total dosage/cycle = 75 mg/m^2)

Supportive Care
Antiemetic prophylaxis
Emetogenic potential is **HIGH**. *Potential for delayed symptoms*
See Chapter 42 for antiemetic recommendations

Hematopoietic growth factor (CSF) prophylaxis
Primary prophylaxis is indicated with one of the following:
   Filgrastim (G-CSF) 5 mcg/kg per day, by subcutaneous injection, *or*
   Pegfilgrastim (pegylated filgrastim) 6 mg/0.6 mL, by subcutaneous injection for 1 dose
   • Begin use from 24–72 hours after myelosuppressive chemotherapy is completed
   • Continue daily filgrastim until ANC ≥5000/mm^3
See Chapter 43 for more information

Antimicrobial prophylaxis
Risk of fever and neutropenia is **LOW**
   Antimicrobial primary prophylaxis to be considered:
   • Antibacterial—not indicated
   • Antifungal—not indicated
   • Antiviral—not indicated, unless patient previously had an episode of HSV

Steroid-associated gastritis
Add a **proton pump inhibitor** during steroid use to prevent gastritis and duodenitis

Treatment Modifications

Adverse Events	Treatment Modifications
Febrile neutropenia or documented infection after treatment	Reduce docetaxel dosage to 60 mg/m^2 during subsequent cycles
G3 or G4 nausea, vomiting, or diarrhea despite appropriate prophylaxis	Reduce doxorubicin dosage to 40 mg/m^2 during subsequent cycles
First episode of G3 or G4 stomatitis	Reduce doxorubicin dosage to 40 mg/m^2 during subsequent cycles
Second episode of G3 or G4 stomatitis	Reduce docetaxel dosage to 60 mg/m^2 during subsequent cycles
G3 or G4 neuropathy	Discontinue treatment
Other severe adverse events	Hold treatment until toxicity resolves to G ≤1, then resume at decreased dosages appropriate for the toxicity

Dosages reduced for adverse events are not re-escalated

Patient Population Studied

Nabholtz JM et al. J Clin Oncol 2001;19:314–321 [Treatment for metastatic disease]
Nabholtz J-M et al. Proc Am Soc Clin Oncol 2002;21:36a [Abstract 141]

Study of 745 patients with node-positive primary breast cancer treated with adjuvant TAC and 54 patients with metastatic breast cancer and no prior chemotherapy for metastatic disease. All patients were anthracycline-naïve

Toxicity (N = 745)

Nabholtz J-M et al. 2002

Toxicity	Percentage
Febrile neutropenia	24%
G3/4 infection	2.8%
G3/4 asthenia	11%
G3/4 stomatitis	7%
CHF	1.2%

Therapy Monitoring

1. *Before each cycle:* CBC with differential and platelet count, LFTs, and serum electrolytes
2. *Prior to therapy:* Determination of LVEF by echocardiogram or MUGA scan

Efficacy

Nabholtz J-M et al. 2002

	TAC (N = 745)	FAC (N = 746)
Disease-free survival*	82%	74%
Overall survival	TAC demonstrated a reduction in risk of 25% compared with FAC	

*Median follow-up was 33 months

ADJUVANT • HER2-NEGATIVE

BREAST CANCER REGIMEN: DOSE-DENSE DOXORUBICIN + CYCLOPHOSPHAMIDE, THEN PACLITAXEL EVERY 2 WEEKS (DDAC → P)

Citron ML et al. J Clin Oncol 2003;21:1431–1439

Note: Doxorubicin and cyclophosphamide (ddAC) are given in combination, followed sequentially by paclitaxel (P). Both ddAC and P are given for 4 complete cycles

Hydration with 1000 mL 0.9% sodium chloride injection (0.9% NS); administer intravenously 500 mL before starting cyclophosphamide and 500 mL after completing cyclophosphamide

Doxorubicin HCl 60 mg/m^2; administer by intravenous injection over 3–5 minutes on day 1, every 14 days for 4 cycles (total dosage/cycle = 60 mg/m^2)

Cyclophosphamide 600 mg/m^2; administer intravenously in 100–500 mL 0.9% NS or 5% dextrose injection (D5W) over 15–60 minutes on day 1, every 14 days for 4 cycles (total dosage/cycle = 600 mg/m^2)

Filgrastim 5 mcg/kg per day; administer subcutaneously for 7 consecutive days on days 3–9, every 14 days for 4 cycles

• Calculated doses may be rounded by ±10% to use the most economical combination of commercially available products (containing 300 mcg or 480 mcg)

After 4 cycles, doxorubicin + cyclophosphamide are followed by:

Premedication:

Dexamethasone 10 mg/dose; administer orally for 2 doses 12 hours and 6 hours before paclitaxel (total dose/cycle = 20 mg), *or*

Dexamethasone 20 mg; administer intravenously over 10–15 minutes, 30–60 minutes before paclitaxel (total dose/cycle = 20 mg)

Note: Dexamethasone doses may be gradually decreased in the absence of hypersensitivity reactions during repeated paclitaxel treatments

Diphenhydramine 50 mg; administer by intravenous injection 30–60 minutes before paclitaxel

Cimetidine 300 mg (or **ranitidine** 50 mg, **famotidine** 20 mg, or an equivalent histamine receptor [H$_2$]-subtype antagonist); administer intravenously over 15–30 minutes, 30–60 minutes before paclitaxel

Paclitaxel 175 mg/m^2; administer intravenously in a volume of 0.9% NS or D5W sufficient to produce a concentration within the range 0.3–1.2 mg/mL over 3 hours, on day 1, every 14 days for 4 cycles (total dosage/cycle = 175 mg/m^2)

Filgrastim 5 mcg/kg per day; administer subcutaneously for 7 consecutive days on days 3–9, every 14 days for 4 cycles

• Calculated doses may be rounded by ±10% to use the most economical combination of commercially available products (containing 300 mcg or 480 mcg)

Supportive Care with Doxorubicin + Cyclophosphamide (AC) Chemotherapy

Antiemetic prophylaxis

Emetogenic potential is **HIGH**. *Potential for delayed symptoms*

See Chapter 42 for antiemetic recommendations

Hematopoietic growth factor (CSF) prophylaxis

Primary prophylaxis is indicated as described in the regimens

See Chapter 43 for more information

Antimicrobial prophylaxis

Risk of fever and neutropenia is **LOW**

   Antimicrobial primary prophylaxis to be considered:

• Antibacterial—not indicated

• Antifungal—not indicated

• Antiviral—not indicated, unless patient previously had an episode of HSV

Supportive Care with Paclitaxel (P) Chemotherapy

Antiemetic prophylaxis

Emetogenic potential is **LOW**

See Chapter 42 for antiemetic recommendations

Hematopoietic growth factor (CSF) prophylaxis

Primary prophylaxis is indicated as described in the regimens

See Chapter 43 for more information

Antimicrobial prophylaxis

Risk of fever and neutropenia is **LOW**

   Antimicrobial primary prophylaxis to be considered:

• Antibacterial—not indicated

• Antifungal—not indicated

• Antiviral—not indicated, unless patient previously had an episode of HSV

Treatment Modifications

Adverse Events	Treatment Modifications
ANC <1000/mm^3, or platelets <100,000/mm^3 at start of cycle	Delay treatment until ANC ≥1000/mm^3 and platelets ≥100,000/mm^3. If a treatment delay is >3 weeks, consider decreasing implicated drug dosage by 25%
G3/4 nonhematologic toxicity	If adjustment indicated, decrease implicated drug dosage by 25%
G3/4 neuropathy	Discontinue paclitaxel

Patient Population Studied

Women with node-positive operable breast cancer. Chemotherapy was given adjuvantly after recovery from surgery. A total of 2005 females were randomly assigned to receive one of the following regimens: (1) sequential A × 4 → P × 4 → C × 4 with doses every 3 weeks; (2) sequential A × 4 → P × 4 → C × 4 every 2 weeks with filgrastim; (3) concurrent AC × 4 → P × 4 every 3 weeks; or (4) concurrent AC × 4 → P × 4 every 2 weeks with filgrastim

Toxicity

Toxicity	AC → P (N = 495) G3/4	A → P → C (N = 493) G3/4
Hematologic Toxicity		
Leukopenia	6%	<1%
Neutropenia	9%	3%
Thrombocytopenia	<1%	0
Anemia	<1%	<1%
RBC transfusions	13% of cycles	1% of cycles
Nonhematologic Toxicity		
Nausea	8%	7%
Vomiting	6%	4%
Diarrhea	1%	3%
Stomatitis	3%	1%
Cardiac function	<1%	1%
Phlebitis/thrombosis	1%	1%
Sensory	4%	4%
Myalgias/arthralgias	5%	5%
Infection	3%	4%

Efficacy

		Survival* Disease-Free	Overall
Dose-dense regimens (every 2 weeks)	N = 988	82%	92%
Standard 3-week-interval regimens	N = 985	75%	90%

*Median follow-up of 36 months; no difference between sequential and concurrent arms in efficacy

Therapy Monitoring

1. *Before each cycle:* CBC with differential and platelet count, LFTs, and serum electrolytes
2. *Prior to therapy:* Determination of LVEF by echocardiogram or MUGA scan

ADJUVANT • HER2-NEGATIVE
BREAST CANCER REGIMEN: DOXORUBICIN + CYCLOPHOSPHAMIDE, THEN WEEKLY PACLITAXEL (AC → P)

Perez EA et al. J Clin Oncol 2001;19:4216–4223
Seidman AD et al. J Clin Oncol 1998;16:3353–3361
Sparano JA et al. N Engl J Med 2008;358:1663–1671

Hydration with 1000 mL 0.9% sodium chloride injection (0.9% NS); administer intravenously 500 mL before starting cyclophosphamide and 500 mL after completing cyclophosphamide

Doxorubicin HCl 60 mg/m^2; administer by intravenous injection over 3–5 minutes on day 1 every 21 days for 4 cycles (total dosage/cycle = 60 mg/m^2)

Cyclophosphamide 600 mg/m^2; administer intravenously in 100–500 mL 0.9% NS or 5% dextrose injection (D5W) over 30–60 minutes on day 1, every 21 days for 4 cycles (total dosage/cycle = 600 mg/m^2), *followed after 4 cycles by:*

Premedication:
Dexamethasone 10 mg/dose; administer orally for 2 doses at 12 hours and 6 hours before paclitaxel (total dose/cycle = 20 mg), *or*
Dexamethasone 20 mg; administer intravenously over 10–15 minutes, 30–60 minutes before starting paclitaxel (total dose/cycle = 20 mg)
Diphenhydramine 50 mg; administer intravenously 30 minutes prior to starting paclitaxel
Cimetidine 300 mg (or **ranitidine** 50 mg, or **famotidine** 20 mg, or an equivalent histamine receptor [H$_2$]-subtype antagonist); administer intravenously over 15–30 minutes, 30–60 minutes before starting paclitaxel

Paclitaxel 80 mg/m^2 per dose; administer intravenously in a volume of 0.9% NS or D5W sufficient to produce a concentration within the range 0.3–1.2 mg/mL over 60 minutes, weekly for 12 consecutive weeks (total dosage/21-day cycle = 240 mg/m^2)

Supportive Care with Doxorubicin + Cyclophosphamide (AC) Chemotherapy
Antiemetic prophylaxis
*Emetogenic potential is **HIGH**. Potential for delayed symptoms*
See Chapter 42 for antiemetic recommendations

Hematopoietic growth factor (CSF) prophylaxis
Primary prophylaxis may be indicated
See Chapter 43 for more information

Antimicrobial prophylaxis
*Risk of fever and neutropenia is **LOW***
  Antimicrobial primary prophylaxis to be considered:
  • Antibacterial—not indicated
  • Antifungal—not indicated
  • Antiviral—not indicated, unless patient previously had an episode of HSV

Supportive Care with Paclitaxel (P) Chemotherapy
Antiemetic prophylaxis
*Emetogenic potential is **LOW***
See Chapter 42 for antiemetic recommendations

Hematopoietic growth factor (CSF) prophylaxis
*Primary prophylaxis is **NOT** indicated*
See Chapter 43 for more information

Antimicrobial prophylaxis
*Risk of fever and neutropenia is **LOW***
  Antimicrobial primary prophylaxis to be considered:
  • Antibacterial—not indicated
  • Antifungal—not indicated
  • Antiviral—not indicated, unless patient previously had an episode of HSV

Treatment Modifications: AC

Bear HD et al. J Clin Oncol 2003;21:4165–4174
Citron ML et al. J Clin Oncol 2003;21:1431–1439

Adverse Events	Treatment Modifications
Absolute neutrophil count (ANC) <1500/mm³ or platelets <100,000/mm³ at start of cycle*	Delay treatment until ANC ≥1500/mm³ and platelets ≥100,000/mm³. Give filgrastim after chemotherapy during subsequent cycles
First episode of febrile neutropenia	Give filgrastim after chemotherapy during subsequent cycles[†]
Second episode of febrile neutropenia	During subsequent cycles, consider prophylaxis with ciprofloxacin[‡]
Third episode of febrile neutropenia	Decrease both doxorubicin and cyclophosphamide dosages by 25%

*Although an ANC of 1500/mm³ is often identified as a minimum acceptable ANC to safely proceed with treatment, recent data shows that an ANC ≥1000/mm³ is acceptable if filgrastim is given after chemotherapy
[†]Filgrastim 5 mcg/kg per day; administer subcutaneously starting at least 24 hours after completing chemotherapy until ANC >5000/mm³
[‡]Ciprofloxacin 500 mg orally twice daily for 7 consecutive days starting on day 5

Treatment Modifications: Paclitaxel

Adverse Events	Treatment Modifications
ANC ≤800/mm³ or platelets ≤50,000/mm³	Hold treatment until ANC >800/mm³ and platelets >50,000/mm³, then resume with weekly paclitaxel dosage reduced by 10 mg/m²
G2 motor or sensory neuropathies	Reduce weekly paclitaxel dosage by 10 mg/m² without interrupting planned treatment
Other nonhematologic adverse events G2 or G3	Hold treatment until adverse events resolve to G ≤1, then resume with weekly paclitaxel dosage reduced by 10 mg/m²
Patients who cannot tolerate paclitaxel at 60 mg/m² per week	Discontinue treatment
Treatment delay >2 weeks	Decrease weekly paclitaxel dosage by 10 mg/m² or consider discontinuing treatment

Patient Population Studied

Sparano JA. N Engl J Med 2008;258:1663–1671

Study of 4950 patients with operable, hormone receptor–positive adenocarcinoma of the breast with either (a) histologically involved lymph nodes (tumor stage T1, T2, or T3 and nodal stage N1 or N2) or (b) "high-risk, axillary node-negative disease" (T2 or T3, N0) without distant metastases. Of the study patients, 88% were node-positive and 19% HER2neu+. All patients received 4 cycles of intravenous doxorubicin and cyclophosphamide at 3-week intervals and were assigned to intravenous paclitaxel or docetaxel given at 3-week intervals for 4 cycles or at 1-week intervals for 12 cycles. The primary end point was disease-free survival

Efficacy (N = 4950)

Sparano JA. N Engl J Med 2008;258:1663–1671

	Number of Patients	5-Year DFS (%)	Hazard Ratio for DFS*	5-Year OS (%)	Hazard Ratio for OS*
Paclitaxel every 3 weeks	1253	76.9	1	86.5	1
Weekly paclitaxel	1231	81.5	1.27, P = 0.006	89.7	1.32, P = 0.01
Docetaxel every 3 weeks	1236	81.2	1.23, P = 0.020	87.3	1.13, P = 0.25
Weekly docetaxel	1230	77.6	1.09, P = 0.290	86.2	1.02, P = 0.80

DFS, Disease-free survival; OS, overall survival
*Hazard ratio >1 favors the group receiving that therapy

Toxicity of Paclitaxel and Docetaxel

Sparano JA. N Engl J Med 2008;258:1663–1671

Toxicity*	Paclitaxel Every 3 Weeks	Weekly Paclitaxel	Docetaxel Every 3 Weeks	Weekly Docetaxel
	Percentage			
Neutropenia[†]	4	2	46	3
Febrile neutropenia[†]	<1	1	16	1
Infection	3	3	13	4
Stomatitis	<1	0	5	2
Fatigue	2	3	9	11
Myalgia	7	2	6	1
Arthralgia	6	2	6	1
Lacrimation	<1	0	<1	5
G3/4 neuropathy	5	8	4	6
G2/3/4 neuropathy	20	27	16	16

*Tabulation of G3/4 toxic effects and G2/3/4 neuropathies resulting from the taxane component of therapy that occurred in at least 5% of all treated patients
[†]Information on only G4 neutropenia (ANC <500/mm^3) was collected

Therapy Monitoring

1. *Weekly:* CBC with differential and platelet count
2. *Monthly:* LFTs and serum electrolytes
3. *Prior to therapy:* Determination of LVEF by echocardiogram or MUGA scan

ADJUVANT • HER2-NEGATIVE

BREAST CANCER REGIMEN: DOCETAXEL + CYCLOPHOSPHAMIDE (TC) EVERY 3 WEEKS × 4 CYCLES

Jones S et al. J Clin Oncol 2006;24:5381–5387
Jones S et al. J Clin Oncol 2009;27:1177–1183

Hydration with 1000 mL 0.9% sodium chloride injection (0.9% NS); administer intravenously 500 mL before starting cyclophosphamide and 500 mL after completing cyclophosphamide

Premedication:
Dexamethasone 8 mg/dose; administer orally every 12 hours for 3 days starting on the day before docetaxel administration (total dose/cycle = 48 mg)
Docetaxel 75 mg/m²; administer intravenously in a volume of 0.9% NS or 5% dextrose injection (D5W) sufficient to produce a docetaxel concentration within the range 0.3–0.74 mg/mL over 30–60 minutes on day 1 every 21 days for 4 cycles (total dosage/cycle = 75 mg/m²)
Cyclophosphamide 600 mg/m²; administer intravenously in 100–500 mL 0.9% NS or D5W over 30–60 minutes on day 1 every 21 days for 4 cycles (total dosage/cycle = 600 mg/m²)

Supportive Care
Antiemetic prophylaxis
Emetogenic potential is **MODERATE**
See Chapter 42 for antiemetic recommendations

Hematopoietic growth factor (CSF) prophylaxis
Primary prophylaxis is recommended
See Chapter 43 for more information

Antimicrobial prophylaxis
Risk of fever and neutropenia is **LOW**
   Antimicrobial primary prophylaxis to be considered:
   • Antibacterial—not indicated
   • Antifungal—not indicated
   • Antiviral—not indicated, unless patient previously had an episode of HSV

Steroid-associated gastritis
Add a **proton pump inhibitor** during steroid use to prevent gastritis and duodenitis

Efficacy

	7-Year DFS		7-Year OS	
TC × 4 (N = 506)	81%	HR = 0.74 (95% CI, 0.56–0.98) P = 0.033	87%	HR = 0.69 (95% CI, 0.50–0.97) P = 0.032
AC × 4 (N = 510)	75%		82%	

Unplanned, exploratory analyses of disease-free survival hazard ratios (HR) and CI

	Hazard Ratio	95% Confidence Interval (CI)
HER2– (TC = 55; AC = 69)	0.56	0.30–1.05
HER2+ (TC = 28; AC = 18)	0.73	0.32–1.70
ER- and PR– (TC = 136; AC = 158)	0.70	0.44–1.10
ER+ or PR+ (TC = 368; AC = 351)	0.79	0.56–1.13
Age ≥65 (TC = 78; AC = 82)	0.70	0.40–1.24
Age <65 (TC = 428; AC = 428)	0.76	0.55–1.04

AC, doxorubicin + cyclophosphamide; DFS, Disease-free survival; ER, estrogen receptor; OS, overall survival; PR, progesterone receptor; TC, docetaxel + cyclophosphamide

Treatment Modifications

Patients were taken off treatment if administration of any study drug was delayed more than 2 weeks as a result of drug-related toxicities. *No dose reductions were permitted.* No prophylactic growth factors were used and the use of oral prophylactic antibiotics was at the discretion of the treating physician

Patient Population Studied

Phase 3 randomized prospective clinical trial comparing 4 cycles of doxorubicin + cyclophosphamide (AC) with 4 cycles of docetaxel + cyclophosphamide (TC) as adjuvant chemotherapy in 1016 women with operable stage I–III invasive breast cancer. Eligible patients had a Karnofsky performance status of ≥80% and no evidence of metastatic disease. Before treatment, a complete surgical excision of the primary tumor (lumpectomy and axillary dissection or modified radical mastectomy) was performed. Neoadjuvant chemotherapy was *not* permitted. Eligible primary tumor size was ≥1.0 cm and <7.0 cm. Patients were randomly assigned to 4 cycles of either standard-dose AC (60 and 600 mg/m², respectively) or TC (75 and 600 mg/m², respectively) administered on day 1 of each 21-day cycle for 4 cycles as adjuvant treatment after complete surgical excision of the primary tumor. Chemotherapy was administered before radiation therapy (XRT) when XRT was indicated (breast conservation or postoperative XRT for patient with 4 or more involved axillary lymph nodes). On completion of 4 cycles of chemotherapy (±XRT), tamoxifen was administered to all patients with hormone receptor–positive breast cancer for 5 years. The majority (71%) of patients had breast cancer that was estrogen receptor (ER)-positive and/or progesterone receptor (PR)-positive. The number of patients with node-negative disease was balanced between groups (47% TC and 49% AC); 12% of TC and 9% of AC patients had ≥4 positive nodes

Toxicity*

Frequency of Most Common Adverse Events (All Grades)*

	TC Patients (N = 506)				AC Patients (N = 510)			
	Grade (%)				Grade (%)			
	1	2	3	4	1	2	3	4
Hematologic								
Anemia	3	2	<1	<1	4	2	1	<1
Neutropenia	<1	1	10	51	1	2	12	43
Thrombocytopenia	<1	<1	0	<1	<1	<1	1	0
Nonhematologic								
Asthenia	43	32	3	<1	41	31	4	<1
Edema	27	7	<1	0	17	3	<1	<1
Fever	14	5	3	2	11	4	2	<1
Infection	8	4	7	<1	7	5	8	<1
Myalgia	22	10	1	<1	11	5	<1	<1
Nausea	38	13	2	<1	43	32	7	<1
Phlebitis	8	3	<1	0	1	1	0	0
Stomatitis	23	10	<1	<1	29	15	1	1
Vomiting	9	5	<1	<1	21	16	5	<1

AC, doxorubicin and cyclophosphamide; TC, Docetaxel and cyclophosphamide
*NCI-Common Toxicity Criteria v1. Treatment-related toxicities were reported using Coding Symbols for a Thesaurus of Adverse Reaction Terms (COSTART) and summarized by highest grade per patient

Therapy Monitoring

1. *Baseline:* LFTs, serum chemistry, CBC with differential and platelet count
2. *Follow-up:* CBC with differential and platelet count at start of each cycle

ADJUVANT • HER2-NEGATIVE

BREAST CANCER REGIMEN: CYCLOPHOSPHAMIDE + EPIRUBICIN + FLUOROURACIL (FEC) × 4 CYCLES → WEEKLY PACLITAXEL × 8 CYCLES

Martín M et al. J Natl Cancer Inst 2008;100:805–814

FEC × 4 cycles
Hydration with 0.9% sodium chloride injection (0.9% NS); administer intravenously 500 mL before starting cyclophosphamide and 500 mL after completing cyclophosphamide

Fluorouracil 600 mg/m²; administer by intravenous injection over 1–3 minutes on day 1, every 21 days for 4 cycles (total dosage/cycle = 600 mg/m²)

Epirubicin HCl 90 mg/m²; administer by intravenous injection over 3–5 minutes on day 1, every 21 days for 4 cycles (total dosage/cycle = 90 mg/m²)

Cyclophosphamide 600 mg/m²; administer intravenously in 100–500 mL 0.9% NS or 5% dextrose injection (D5W) over 30–60 minutes on day 1, every 21 days for 4 cycles (total dosage/cycle = 600 mg/m²)

Supportive Care
Antiemetic prophylaxis
Emetogenic potential is **HIGH**. *Potential for delayed symptoms*
See Chapter 42 for antiemetic recommendations

Hematopoietic growth factor (CSF) prophylaxis
Primary prophylaxis may be indicated
See Chapter 43 for more information

Antimicrobial prophylaxis
Risk of fever and neutropenia is **LOW**
  Antimicrobial primary prophylaxis to be considered:
  • Antibacterial—not indicated
  • Antifungal—not indicated
  • Antiviral—not indicated, unless patient previously had an episode of HSV

Paclitaxel, weekly × 8 weeks
Follows 3 weeks after completing 4 cycles of FEC

Premedication:
Dexamethasone 10 mg/dose; administer orally or intravenously for 2 doses at 12 hours and 6 hours before paclitaxel, *or*
Dexamethasone 20 mg; administer intravenously 30–60 minutes before paclitaxel (total dose/cycle = 20 mg)
Note: Dexamethasone doses may be gradually decreased in the absence of hypersensitivity reactions during repeated paclitaxel treatments
Diphenhydramine 50 mg; administer by intravenous injection 30–60 minutes before paclitaxel
Cimetidine 300 mg (or **ranitidine** 50 mg, or **famotidine** 20 mg, or an equivalent histamine receptor [H_2]-subtype antagonist); administer intravenously over 15–30 minutes, 30–60 minutes before starting paclitaxel administration

Paclitaxel 100 mg/m²; administer intravenously in a volume of 0.9% NS or D5W sufficient to produce a concentration within the range 0.3–1.2 mg/mL over 60 minutes, once weekly for 8 weeks (total dosage/week = 100 mg/m²)

Supportive Care
Antiemetic prophylaxis
Emetogenic potential is **LOW**
See Chapter 42 for antiemetic recommendations

Hematopoietic growth factor (CSF) prophylaxis
Primary prophylaxis may be indicated
See Chapter 43 for more information

Antimicrobial prophylaxis
Risk of fever and neutropenia is **LOW**
  Antimicrobial primary prophylaxis to be considered:
  • Antibacterial—not indicated
  • Antifungal—not indicated
  • Antiviral—not indicated, unless patient previously had an episode of HSV

(continued)

(continued)

Notes:

On completion of chemotherapy, tamoxifen (20 mg daily; administer orally for 5 years) was mandatory for all patients whose tumors were positive for estrogen receptor, progesterone receptor, or both (according to institutional guidelines). Subsequently an amendment to the study protocol allowed the use of aromatase inhibitors in postmenopausal women

1. Radiotherapy was mandatory after breast-conserving surgery, and was administered after mastectomy according to the guidelines of each participating institution, mostly to women with tumors >5 cm or with ≥4 affected lymph nodes

2. Prophylaxis with filgrastim (granulocyte colony-stimulating factor) was not routine. However, secondary prophylaxis with filgrastim was mandatory among patients who had at least 1 episode of febrile neutropenia or an infection

Treatment Modifications—FEC

Adverse Events	Treatment Modifications
WBC <3500/mm^3 or platelets <100,000/mm^3 on first day of a cycle	Delay treatment for a maximum of 2 weeks until WBC >3500/mm^3 and platelets >100,000/mm^3. Continue at full dosages if counts recover within 2 weeks
If after 2 weeks WBC <3500/mm^3 or platelets <100,000/mm^3 reduce all drugs' dosages as follows:	
WBC 3000–3499/mm^3, or platelets 75,000–99,999/mm^3	Reduce dosages by 25%
WBC 2500–2999/mm^3 and platelets ≥75,000/mm^3	Reduce dosages by 50%
WBC <2500/mm^3, or platelets <75,000/mm^3	Hold treatment
ANC <1500/mm^3, or platelets <100,000/mm^3 at start of cycle	Delay treatment until ANC ≥1500/mm^3 and platelets ≥100,000/mm^3. Give filgrastim* in subsequent cycles
Hematologic recovery >3 weeks	Discontinue treatment
First episode of febrile neutropenia	Give filgrastim* during subsequent cycles
Second episode of febrile neutropenia	During subsequent cycles, consider prophylaxis with ciprofloxacin†
Third episode of febrile neutropenia	Decrease chemotherapy doses by 20% (epirubicin by 20 mg/m^2, fluorouracil and cyclophosphamide by 100 mg/m^2) and administer filgrastim* + ciprofloxacin†
First episode of G4 documented infection	Add filgrastim* and ciprofloxacin† prophylaxis during subsequent cycles
Second episode of G4 documented infection	Decrease chemotherapy doses by 20% (epirubicin by 20 mg/m^2, fluorouracil and cyclophosphamide by 100 mg/m^2) and administer filgrastim* + ciprofloxacin†
Third episode of G4 documented infection	Discontinue chemotherapy
Serum bilirubin levels 2 to 3 mg/dL (34.1 to 51.3 mmol/L)	Reduce epirubicin dose by 50%
Bilirubin levels ≥3 mg/dL (≥51.3 mmol/L)	Discontinue treatment
G3 stomatitis	Reduce epirubicin and fluorouracil dosage by 50% during subsequent cycles
Any other G3 nonhematologic toxicity	Reduce the dosage of all drugs 25%
G4 nonhematologic toxicity	Discontinue chemotherapy

Treatment Modifications—Paclitaxel

Adverse Events	Treatment Modifications
ANC ≤800/mm^3 or platelets ≤50,000/mm^3	Hold treatment until ANC >800/mm^3 and platelets >50,000/mm^3, then resume with weekly paclitaxel dosage reduced by 10 mg/m^2
G2 motor or sensory neuropathies	Reduce weekly paclitaxel dosage by 10 mg/m^2 without interrupting planned treatment
Other nonhematologic adverse events G2 or G3	Hold treatment until adverse events resolve to G ≤1, then resume with weekly paclitaxel dosage reduced by 10 mg/m^2
Patients who cannot tolerate paclitaxel at 60 mg/m^2 per week	Discontinue treatment
Treatment delay >2 weeks	Decrease weekly paclitaxel dosage by 10 mg/m^2 or consider discontinuing treatment

*Filgrastim 5 mcg/kg per day; administer subcutaneously starting at least 24 hours after completing chemotherapy until ANC ≥5000/mm^3

†Ciprofloxacin 500 mg administer orally twice daily for 7 days starting on day 5

Patient Population Studied

Study of 1246 women who had undergone primary curative surgery (ie, mastectomy, tumorectomy, or lumpectomy) with axillary lymph node dissection (in which at least 6 lymph nodes were isolated) for operable unilateral carcinoma of the breast (stage T1–T3) and were found to have node-positive breast cancer. All patients had at least 1 axillary lymph node that was positive for cancer on histologic examination. The margins of resected specimens had to be histologically free of invasive carcinoma and ductal carcinoma in situ. A complete staging work-up was carried out within 16 weeks before registration in the study. Criteria for exclusion included advanced disease (ie, stage T4, N2 or N3, or M1) and motor or sensory neuropathy of NCI Common Toxicity Criteria G2 or more

Efficacy

Analysis of Events in the ITT Population

	FEC (N = 632)		FEC-P (N = 614)	
	No of Pts	%	No of Pts	%
No event	439	69.5	468	76.2
An event	193	30.5	146	23.8
Relapse of breast cancer	174	27.6	113	18.4
Local only, regional only or both	30	4.8	11	1.8
Distant	141	22.3	101	16.4
Local and second primary	1	0.2	0	0
Second primary cancer	16	2.5	23	3.7
Contralateral breast cancer	4	0.6	7	1.1

FEC, Fluorouracil, epirubicin, and cyclophosphamide; FEC-P, FEC + paclitaxel

DFS, RFS, and OS by Kaplan-Meier Method

	FEC	FEC-P	P Value	HR	CI
Unadjusted 5-year DFS	72.1%	78.5%	0.006	0.74	0.60–0.92
Adjusted 5-year DFS*	—	—	0.006	0.77	0.62–0.95
5-Year distant RFS	78.1%	83.8%	0.006	0.70	0.54–0.90
5-Year OS	87.1%	89.9%	0.109	0.78	0.57–1.06

CI, confidence interval; DFS, disease-free survival; FEC, fluorouracil, epirubicin, and cyclophosphamide; FEC-P, FEC + paclitaxel; HR, hazard ratio; RFS, relapse-free survival; OS, overall survival
*Adjusted for lymph node status, age, tumor size, histology, hormone receptor status, and hormonal therapy

Toxicity*

Toxicity	FEC	FEC-P
G3/4 neutropenia	25.5%	19.1%
G3/4 febrile neutropenia	9.5%	5.1%
G3/4 fatigue	2.4%	4.2%
G3/4 nausea	5.9%	5.4%
G3/4 vomiting	9.9%	7.3%
G3/4 stomatitis	4.9%	3.1%
Amenorrhea	58%	65%
G2 alopecia	>90%	>90%
G2 neuropathy	N/A	22.2%
G3 neuropathy	N/A	3.7%
G2 arthralgia/myalgia	N/A	20.6%
G3 arthralgia/myalgia	N/A	2.8%
G2 LV dysfunction	7.2%	7.8%

*Comparison of treatment arms as follows:
FEC, Six 21-day cycles of fluorouracil 600 mg/m², epirubicin 90 mg/m², and cyclophosphamide 600 mg/m²
FEC-P, Four 21-day cycles of the same FEC schedule and, after 3 weeks of no treatment, eight 1-week courses of paclitaxel 100 mg/m²

Therapy Monitoring

1. *Before each cycle:* CBC with differential and platelet count, serum total bilirubin
2. *Before each treatment with paclitaxel:* Neurologic examination
3. *Prior to therapy:* Determination of LVEF by echocardiogram or MUGA scan

ADJUVANT • HER2-NEGATIVE

BREAST CANCER REGIMEN: CYCLOPHOSPHAMIDE + EPIRUBICIN + FLUOROURACIL (FEC) × 3 CYCLES → DOCETAXEL × 3 CYCLES

Roché HJ. Clin Oncol 2006;24:5664–5671

FEC (cyclophosphamide + epirubicin + fluorouracil) × 3 cycles

Hydration before and after cyclophosphamide with 0.9% sodium chloride injection (0.9% NS); administer intravenously 500 mL before starting cyclophosphamide and 500 mL after completing cyclophosphamide

Fluorouracil 500 mg/m²; administer by intravenous injection over 1–3 minutes on day 1, every 21 days for 3 cycles (total dosage/cycle = 500 mg/m²)
Epirubicin HCl 100 mg/m²; administer by intravenous injection over 3–5 minutes on day 1, every 21 days for 3 cycles (total dosage/cycle = 100 mg/m²)
Cyclophosphamide 500 mg/m²; administer intravenously in 100–500 mL 0.9% NS or 5% dextrose injection (D5W) over 30–60 minutes on day 1, every 21 days for 3 cycles (total dosage/cycle = 500 mg/m²)

Supportive Care

Antiemetic prophylaxis
Emetogenic potential is **HIGH**. Potential for delayed symptoms
See Chapter 42 for antiemetic recommendations

Hematopoietic growth factor (CSF) prophylaxis
Primary prophylaxis may be indicated
See Chapter 43 for more information

Antimicrobial prophylaxis
Risk of fever and neutropenia is **LOW**
    Antimicrobial primary prophylaxis to be considered:
- Antibacterial—not indicated
- Antifungal—not indicated
- Antiviral—not indicated, unless patient previously had an episode of HSV

Docetaxel × 3 cycles

Premedication:
Dexamethasone 8 mg/dose; administer orally twice daily for 3 days, starting on the day before docetaxel administration (total dose/cycle = 48 mg)
Docetaxel 100 mg/m²; administer intravenously in a volume of 0.9% NS or D5W sufficient to produce a final docetaxel concentration of 0.3–0.74 mg/mL over 30–60 minutes on day 1, every 21 days for 3 cycles (total dosage/cycle = 100 mg/m²)

Supportive Care

Antiemetic prophylaxis
Emetogenic potential is **LOW**
See Chapter 42 for antiemetic recommendations

Hematopoietic growth factor (CSF) prophylaxis
Primary prophylaxis is indicated with one of the following:
    Filgrastim (G-CSF) 5 mcg/kg per day, by subcutaneous injection, *or*
    Sargramostim (GM-CSF) 250 mcg/m² per day, by subcutaneous injection
    Begin use from 24–72 h after myelosuppressive chemotherapy is completed
See Chapter 43 for more information

Antimicrobial prophylaxis
Risk of fever and neutropenia is **LOW**
    Antimicrobial primary prophylaxis to be considered:
- Antibacterial—not indicated
- Antifungal—not indicated
- Antiviral—not indicated, unless patient previously had an episode of HSV

Treatment Modifications

Adverse Events	Treatment Modifications
WBC <3500/mm³ or platelets <100,000/mm³ on first day of a cycle	Delay treatment for a maximum of 2 weeks until WBC >3500/mm³ and platelets >100,000/mm³. Continue at full dosages if counts recover within 2 weeks
If after 2 weeks WBC <3500/mm³ or platelets <100,000/mm³, reduce all drugs' dosages as follows:	
WBC 3000–3499/mm³, or platelets 75,000–99,999/mm³	Reduce dosages by 25%
WBC 2500–2999/mm³ and platelets ≥75,000/mm³	Reduce dosages by 50%
WBC <2500/mm³, or platelets <75,000/mm³	Hold treatment
ANC <1500/mm³, or platelets <100,000/mm³ at start of cycle	Delay treatment until ANC ≥1500/mm³ and platelets ≥100,000/mm³. Give filgrastim* in subsequent cycles
Hematologic recovery >3 weeks	Discontinue treatment
Second episode of febrile neutropenia	During subsequent cycles, consider prophylaxis with ciprofloxacin†
Third episode of febrile neutropenia	Decrease chemotherapy doses by 20% (epirubicin by 20 mg/m², fluorouracil and cyclophosphamide by 100 mg/m², and docetaxel by 20 mg/m²) and administer filgrastim* + ciprofloxacin†
First episode of G4 documented infection	During subsequent cycles, consider prophylaxis with ciprofloxacin†

(continued)

Efficacy

Analysis of Events in the ITT Population

	FEC (N = 996)		FEC-D (N = 1003)		HR	95% CI	P Value*
	No of Pts	%	No of Pts	%			
First event†	264	26.5	218	21.7	0.80	0.67–0.96	0.012
Relapse of breast cancer	235	23.6	190	18.9	0.78	0.64–0.94	0.010
Local only	40	4	28	2.8	—	—	—
Regional (± local)	15	1.5	12	1.2	—	—	—
Distant (± local or regional)	180	18.1	150	14.9	—	—	—
Contralateral breast cancer	23	2.3	21	2.1	0.80	0.47–1.37	0.43
Any death	135	13.5	100	10.0	0.73	0.56–0.94	0.017
Of breast cancer	123	12.3	89	8.9	—	—	—

FEC, fluorouracil, epirubicin, and cyclophosphamide; FEC-D, fluorouracil, epirubicin, and cyclophosphamide followed by docetaxel; HR, hazard ratio; ITT, intention-to-treat
*Log-rank test adjusted for nodal involvement and age
†First event defined according to the disease-free survival criteria (ie, local relapse, regional relapse, distant relapse, contralateral breast cancer, death of any cause)

Cox Regression Model Analysis for Disease-Free Survival (DFS) in the Intention-to-Treat (ITT) Population

	HR	95% CI	P Value
FEC	1	—	—
FEC-D	0.82	0.69 to 0.99	0.034

DFS and OS by Kaplan-Meier Method

	FEC	FEC-D	P Value
5-Year DFS	73.2%	78.4%	0.012
5-Year OS	86.7%	90.7%	0.017

Treatment Modifications
(continued)

Second episode of G4 documented infection	Decrease chemotherapy doses by 20% (epirubicin by 20 mg/m², fluorouracil and cyclophosphamide by 100 mg/m², and docetaxel by 20 mg/m²) and administer filgrastim* + ciprofloxacin†
Third episode of G4 documented infection	Discontinue chemotherapy
Serum bilirubin levels 2–3 mg/dL (34.1–51.3 mmol/L)	Reduce epirubicin dose by 50%
Bilirubin levels ≥3 mg/dL (≥51.3 mmol/L)	Discontinue treatment
G3 stomatitis	Reduce epirubicin and fluorouracil dosage by 50% during subsequent cycles
G4 nonhematologic toxicity	Discontinue chemotherapy
G2 motor or sensory neuropathies	Reduce docetaxel dosage by 20–50 mg/m²
G3/4 motor or sensory neuropathies	Discontinue docetaxel

*Filgrastim 5 mcg/kg per day; administer subcutaneously starting at least 24 hours after completing chemotherapy until ANC ≥5000/mm³
†Ciprofloxacin 500 mg; administer orally twice daily for 7 days starting on day 5

Patient Population Studied

Study of 1999 patients with operable node-positive breast cancer who were randomly assigned to receive fluorouracil 500 mg/m², epirubicin 100 mg/m², and cyclophosphamide 500 mg/m² (FEC) intravenously on day 1 every 21 days for 6 cycles or the same regimen of FEC for 3 cycles followed by docetaxel 100 mg/m² intravenously on day 1 every 21 days for 3 cycles

Toxicity*

Event	Percent of Patients		P Value
	FEC (N = 995)	FEC-D (N = 1001)	
G3/4 Hematologic			
Neutropenia on day 21	33.6	28.1	0.008
Neutropenia on day 21, cycles 4–6	20.2	10.9	<0.001
Febrile neutropenia	8.4	11.2	0.03
Febrile neutropenia, cycles 4–6	3.7	7.4	0.005
GCSF	27	22.2	0.01
GCSF, cycles 5 and 6	24.8	9.5	<0.001
Infection	1.6	1.6	0.99
Anemia	1.4	0.7	0.12
Thrombocytopenia	0.3	0.4	0.71
Nonhematologic			
G3/4 Nausea-vomiting	20.5	11.2	<0.001
G3/4 Nausea-vomiting, cycles 4–6	11	1.6	<0.001
G3/4 Stomatitis	4.0	5.9	0.054
G3/4 Stomatitis, cycles 4–6	2.3	4.0	0.030
Alopecia grade 3	83.9	82.6	0.40
Edema moderate or severe, cycles 4–6	0.3	4.8	<0.001
Nail disorder moderate or severe, cycles 4–6	1.0	10.3	<0.001
Any cardiac event reported as SAE†	1.3	0.4	0.030

*Toxicity graded according to WHO criteria and serious adverse events (SAEs) defined according to International Conference on Harmonization (ICH) guidelines
†Although rare overall, there were fewer cardiac events after FEC-D (P = 0.03), attributable mainly to the lower anthracycline cumulative dose

Therapy Monitoring

1. *Before each cycle:* CBC with differential and platelet count, serum total bilirubin
2. *Before each cycle with docetaxel:* Neurologic examination
3. *Prior to therapy:* Determination of LVEF by echocardiogram or MUGA scan

ADJUVANT • HER2-NEGATIVE

BREAST CANCER REGIMEN: ADJUVANT CAPECITABINE FOR RESIDUAL INVASIVE CARCINOMA AFTER NEOADJUVANT CHEMOTHERAPY AND SURGERY

Masuda M et al. N Engl J Med 2017;376:2147–2159
Protocol for: Masuda M et al. N Engl J Med 2017;376:2147–2159

The regimen consists of either 6 or 8 cycles of adjuvant capecitabine. When indicated, adjuvant radiation therapy may be administered either before initiation of capecitabine or concurrent with capecitabine. When indicated, adjuvant hormone therapy may be initiated either concurrently with capecitabine or following completion of capecitabine

Capecitabine 1250 mg/m^2 per dose; administer orally twice daily within 30 minutes after a meal for 14 consecutive days (28 doses) on days 1–14, followed by 7 days without treatment, repeated every 21 days, for either 6 or 8 cycles (total dosage/21-day cycle = 35,000 mg/m^2)
Notes:
- Doses are rounded to use combinations of 500-mg and 150-mg tablets that most closely approximate calculated values
- In practice, treatment often is begun with capecitabine 1000 mg/m^2 per dose twice daily for 14 consecutive days on days 1–14, every 21 days, because of a high rate of dose reduction with higher dosages, especially in non-Asian patients or those being treated in Western countries (total dosage/cycle = 28,000 mg/m^2)
- Patients who miss a dose of capecitabine should be instructed to continue with the usual dosing schedule without making up the missed dose and to contact their physician for further instructions
- Patients who take too much (ie, overdose) capecitabine should contact their doctor immediately and present to the emergency department for further care and consideration for timely treatment with the antidote uridine triacetate
- Initial capecitabine dosage should be decreased by 25% in patients with moderate renal impairment (baseline creatinine clearance = 30–50 mL/min [0.5–0.83 mL/s]); ie, a dosage reduction from 1250 mg/m^2 per dose to 950 mg/m^2 per dose, twice daily. Capecitabine use is contraindicated in persons with severe renal impairment (creatinine clearance <30 mL/min [<0.5 mL/s])
- Although food decreases the rate and extent of drug absorption and the time to peak plasma concentration and systemic exposure (AUC) for both capecitabine and fluorouracil, product labeling recommends giving capecitabine within 30 minutes after the end of a meal because established safety and efficacy data are based on administration with food

Supportive Care
Antiemetic prophylaxis
Emetogenic potential is **LOW**
See Chapter 42 for antiemetic recommendations

Hematopoietic growth factor (CSF) prophylaxis
Primary prophylaxis is **NOT** indicated
See Chapter 43 for more information

Antimicrobial prophylaxis
Risk of fever and neutropenia is **LOW**
   Antimicrobial primary prophylaxis to be considered:
   - Antibacterial—not indicated
   - Antifungal—not indicated
   - Antiviral—not indicated, unless patient previously had an episode of HSV

Diarrhea management
Latent or delayed-onset diarrhea:
Loperamide 4 mg orally initially after the first loose or liquid stool, *then*
Loperamide 2 mg orally every 2 hours during waking hours, *plus*
Loperamide 4 mg orally every 4 hours during hours of sleep
- Continue for at least 12 hours after diarrhea resolves
- Recurrent diarrhea after a 12-hour diarrhea-free interval is treated as a new episode
- Rehydrate orally with fluids and electrolytes during a diarrheal episode
- If a patient develops blood or mucus in stool, dehydration, or hemodynamic instability, or if diarrhea persists >48 hours despite loperamide, stop loperamide and evaluate urgently in clinic or hospitalize the patient for IV hydration. Alternatively, a trial of **diphenoxylate hydrochloride** 2.5 mg with **atropine sulfate** 0.025 mg (eg, Lomotil)
- Initial adult dose is 2 tablets 4 times daily until control has been achieved, after which the dose may be reduced to meet individual requirements. Control may often be maintained with as little as 2 tablets daily
- Clinical improvement of acute diarrhea is usually observed within 48 hours. If improvement of chronic diarrhea after treatment with a maximum daily dose of 8 tablets is not observed within 10 days, control is unlikely with further administration

Hand-foot syndrome
For patients who develop a hand-foot syndrome, use topical emollients (eg, Aquaphor), topical or orally administered steroids, antihistamine agents (H$_1$-receptor antagonists), or pyridoxine 50–150 mg/day administered orally

Patient Population Studied

The trial involved 910 patients with HER2-negative residual invasive breast cancer (stage I–IIIB) after neoadjuvant chemotherapy (anthracycline, taxane, or both) and surgery. Eligible patients were aged 20–74 years and had an Eastern Cooperative Oncology Group (ECOG) performance status score ≤1. Patients were randomized to receive standard postsurgical therapy (including endocrine therapy in patients with estrogen receptor–positive disease and radiotherapy if indicated) plus oral capecitabine (1250 mg/m² twice per day on days 1–14 of a 3-week cycle for 6–8 cycles) or standard postsurgical therapy alone

Efficacy (N = 910)

Full Analysis			
	Standard Postsurgical Therapy + Capecitabine (N = 443)	Standard Postsurgical Therapy Alone (N = 444)	Between-group Comparison
3-year survival free from disease	82.8%	73.9%	HR 0.70 (95% CI, 0.53–0.92)
5-year survival free from disease	74.1%	67.6%	
3-year overall survival	94.0%	88.9%	HR 0.59 (95% CI, 0.39–0.90)
5-year overall survival	89.2%	83.6%	

Median follow-up 3.6 years

Triple-negative Subset			
	Standard Postsurgical Therapy + Capecitabine (N = 139)	Standard Postsurgical Therapy Alone (N = 147)	Between-group Comparison
5-year disease-free survival	69.8%	56.1%	HR 0.58; 95% CI, 0.39–0.87
5-year overall survival	78.8%	70.3%	HR 0.52 (95% CI, 0.30–0.90)

Therapy Monitoring

1. During first cycle and in any cycle after a dose adjustment, weekly CBC with differential and platelet count to assess dose
2. Before each cycle: Physical examination, CBC with differential and platelet count, liver function tests, renal function tests
3. Patients receiving concomitant capecitabine and oral coumarin-derivative anticoagulant therapy should have their anticoagulant response (INR or prothrombin time) monitored frequently in order to adjust the anticoagulant dose accordingly
4. Monitor for signs/symptoms of HFS [hand-foot syndrome], SJS/TEN [Stevens-Johnson syndrome and toxic epidermal necrolysis], hydration status, diarrhea, mucositis, and signs of infection

Note: Toxicity in the setting of DPD deficiency occurs early and is characterized by severe mucositis, diarrhea, neutropenia, and neurotoxicity. It occurs in individuals with homozygous or certain compound heterozygous mutations in the DPD gene that result in complete or near complete absence of DPD activity. Discontinue capecitabine permanently. There is insufficient data to recommend a specific dose in patients with partial DPD activity as measured by any specific test

Treatment Modifications

CAPECITABINE

Starting dose	1250 mg/m^2 per dose
Dose level −1	950 mg/m^2 per dose
Dose level −2	625 mg/m^2 per dose

Toxicity	Dose Modification
On day 1 of a cycle: WBC <3000/mm^3, or ANC <1500/mm^3, or platelet count <75,000/ mm^3, or HFS >G1, or AST/ALT >2.5× ULN, or SCr >1.5× ULN, or total bilirubin >1.5× ULN, or diarrhea >G1	Delay start of cycle for up to 3 weeks until WBC ≥3000/mm^3, ANC ≥1500/mm^3, platelet count ≥75,000/mm^3, HFS G ≤1, AST/ALT ≤2.5× ULN, SCr ≤1.5× ULN, total bilirubin ≤1.5× ULN, and diarrhea G ≤1. Upon recovery, resume capecitabine with any applicable dose reductions as described elsewhere in this table. If recovery does not occur within 3 weeks, consider discontinuation of capecitabine
ANC <1000/mm^3 or platelets <50,000/mm^3 during a cycle	Withhold administration of therapy until resolves to ANC ≥1500/mm^3 or baseline and platelets ≥75,000/mm^3. Administer one lower dose level in subsequent cycle(s)
ANC <500/mm^3 or platelets <25,000/mm^3 during cycle (G4 toxicity)	Discontinue permanently OR If physician deems it to be in the patient's best interest to continue, interrupt until resolved to ≤G1, then resume therapy at one lower dose level in subsequent cycle(s)
G2/3/4 diarrhea G2/3/4 mucositis G2/3/4 dehydration G2/3/4 hand-and-foot syndrome HFS or palmar-plantar erythrodysesthesia (PPE) or chemotherapy-induced acral erythema‡	Stop administration of capecitabine; provide supportive care. Do not resume capecitabine until toxicity resolved to ≤G1. If toxicity is G4, discontinue capecitabine. Otherwise, in subsequent cycle(s) administer a lower dose of capecitabine. Note that once the dose has been reduced, it should not be increased at a later time
Stevens-Johnson syndrome and toxic epidermal necrolysis (TEN) (Severe mucocutaneous reactions, some with fatal outcome)	Discontinue treatment permanently
Other nonhematologic toxicities: G1 toxicity	Continue capecitabine without dose reduction
Other nonhematologic toxicities: First* occurrence of G2 toxicity‡	Interrupt capecitabine for up to 3 weeks until toxicity resolves to G ≤1, then reinitiate at the original dose along with prophylactic treatment for the toxicity when feasible. If recovery does not occur within 3 weeks, consider discontinuation of capecitabine
Other nonhematologic toxicities: Second* occurrence of G2 toxicity‡, or first* occurrence of G3 toxicity	Interrupt capecitabine for up to 3 weeks until toxicity resolves to G ≤1, then reinitiate at dose level −1, along with prophylactic treatment for the toxicity when feasible. Do not increase the capecitabine dose in subsequent cycles. If recovery does not occur within 3 weeks, consider discontinuation of capecitabine
Other nonhematologic toxicities: Third* occurrence of G2 toxicity‡, or second* occurrence of G3 toxicity	Interrupt capecitabine for up to 3 weeks until toxicity resolves to G ≤1, then reinitiate at dose level −2, along with prophylactic treatment for the toxicity when feasible. Do not increase the capecitabine dose in subsequent cycles. If recovery does not occur within 3 weeks, consider discontinuation of capecitabine
Other nonhematologic toxicities: Fourth* occurrence of G2 toxicity‡, or third* occurrence of G3 toxicity first* occurrence of G4 toxicity	Discontinue capecitabine unless the treating physician decides that continued administration is beneficial to the patent, in which case capecitabine is interrupted until the toxicity resolves to G ≤1, and then reinitiated at dose level −2 along with prophylactic treatment for the toxicity when feasible. Do not increase the capecitabine dose in subsequent cycles. If recovery does not occur within 3 weeks, consider discontinuation of capecitabine

*Refers to number of occurrences of the same type of toxicity
†Grading of hand-foot syndrome
- G1: Numbness, dysesthesia/paresthesia, tingling, painless swelling or erythema of the hands and/or feet and/or discomfort that does not disrupt normal activities
- G2: Painful erythema and swelling of the hands and/or feet and/or discomfort affecting the patient's activities of daily living
- G3: Moist desquamation, ulceration, blistering or severe pain of the hands and/or feet and/or severe discomfort that causes the patient to be unable to work or perform activities of daily living
‡Excluding alopecia, dysgeusia, anemia which can be managed with transfusions, and other toxicities which do not have a potential to become serious or life-threatening. If a grade 2 toxicity occurs upon completion of the 2-week treatment period but resolves during the 1-week recovery period prior to initiation of the subsequent cycle, then administration can be continued at the same dose
WBC, white blood count; ANC, absolute neutrophil count; HFS, hand-foot syndrome; AST, aspartate aminotransferase; ALT, alanine aminotransferase; ULN, upper limit of normal; CrCl, creatinine clearance; DPD, dihydropyrimidine dehydrogenase

Adverse Events (N = 902)

Grade (%)*	Standard Postsurgical Therapy + Capecitabine (N = 443)		Standard Postsurgical Therapy Alone (N = 459)	
	Grade 1–2	Grade 3–4	Grade 1–2	Grade 3–4
Hand-foot syndrome†	62	11	0	0
Leukopenia	62	2	19	<1
Thrombocytopenia	54	<1	7	0
Anemia	40	0	12	0
Neutropenia	37	6	9	0
Increased alanine aminotransferase level	36	0	9	<1
Increased lactate dehydrogenase level	32	0	8	0
Increased bilirubin level	32	<1	2	<1
Increased aspartate aminotransferase level	28	<1	6	<1
Increased alkaline phosphatase level	26	0	15	<1
Fatigue	24	1	2	0
Nausea	22	0	<1	0
Mucositis or stomatitis	21	<1	<1	0
Diarrhea	19	3	<1	0
Anorexia	16	<1	1	<1
Vomiting	7	<1	<1	<1
Increased creatinine level	5	0	3	0

*According to the National Cancer Institute Common Terminology Criteria for Adverse Events, version 3.0
†Graded from 1 to 3 with higher grades indicating more severe symptoms or disability
Adverse events assessed within 6 months of randomization are included in the table. All serious events resolved and did not result in death

ADJUVANT • HER2-POSITIVE

BREAST CANCER REGIMEN: DOCETAXEL + TRASTUZUMAB FOLLOWED BY CYCLOPHOSPHAMIDE + EPIRUBICIN + FLUOROURACIL (FEC)

Joensuu H et al. N Engl J Med 2006;354:809–820
Joensuu H et al. J Clin Oncol 2009;27:5685–5692

Docetaxel + Trastuzumab: weeks 1 through 9
Trastuzumab 4 mg/kg (loading dose); administer intravenously in 250 mL 0.9% sodium chloride injection (0.9% NS) over at least 90 minutes, 1 day before the first dose of docetaxel is administered (total trastuzumab dosage during the first treatment week = 4 mg/kg), *followed during subsequent weeks by:*
Trastuzumab 2 mg/kg per week; administer intravenously in 250 mL 0.9% NS over 30 minutes, weekly, continually for 8 weeks (total trastuzumab dosage/week during the second to ninth weeks = 2 mg/kg)
Note:
Trastuzumab administration preceded docetaxel administration on days when both drugs were administered.
Trastuzumab administration duration may be decreased from 90 to 30 minutes if administration over longer durations is well tolerated

Premedication:
Dexamethasone 8 mg/dose; administer orally twice daily for 3 days, starting on the day before docetaxel administration (total dose/cycle = 48 mg)

Docetaxel 80 mg/m² or 100 mg/m²; administer by intravenous infusion in a volume of 0.9% NS or 5% dextrose injection (D5W) sufficient to produce a final docetaxel concentration of 0.3–0.74 mg/mL over 60 minutes on day 1, every 21 days for 3 cycles (total dosage/cycle = 80 mg/m² or 100 mg/m²)
Note:
An independent study monitoring committee recommended the docetaxel dosage be reduced because of a high incidence of febrile neutropenia following treatment. Therefore, 41% of patients received docetaxel 100 mg/m² and 59% received docetaxel 80 mg/m² as the starting dose

Supportive Care
Antiemetic prophylaxis
Emetogenic potential is **LOW**
See Chapter 42 for antiemetic recommendations

Hematopoietic growth factor (CSF) prophylaxis
Primary prophylaxis may be indicated
See Chapter 43 for more information

Antimicrobial prophylaxis
Risk of fever and neutropenia is **LOW–INTERMEDIATE**
(risk varies directly with docetaxel dosage)
  Antimicrobial primary prophylaxis to be considered:
  • Antibacterial—consider a fluoroquinolone or no prophylaxis
  • Antifungal—not indicated
  • Antiviral—not indicated, unless patient previously had an episode of HSV

Trastuzumab infusion reactions
• A symptom complex most commonly consisting of chills and/or fever may occur in as many as 40% of patients during the first infusion of trastuzumab. These symptoms occur infrequently with subsequent trastuzumab infusions. Other signs and/or symptoms may include nausea, vomiting, pain (in some cases at tumor sites), rigors, headache, dizziness, dyspnea, hypotension, rash, and asthenia. Although the symptoms are usually mild to moderate in severity, infrequently, trastuzumab may need to be discontinued
• When such a symptom complex is observed, it can be treated with or without reduction in the rate of trastuzumab infusion, and:
  ▪ **Acetaminophen** 650 mg; administer orally
  ▪ **Diphenhydramine** 25–50 mg; administer orally or by intravenous injection, and

(continued)

Treatment Modifications

Adverse Events	Treatment Modifications
WBC <3500/mm³ or platelets <100,000/mm³ on the first day of a cycle	Delay treatment for a maximum of 2 weeks until WBC >3500/mm³ and platelets >100,000/mm³. Continue at full dosages if counts recover within 2 weeks
If after 2 weeks WBC <3500/mm³ or platelets <100,000/mm³, reduce all drug dosages as follows:	
WBC 3000–3499/mm³, or platelets 75,000–99,999/mm³	Reduce dosages by 20%
WBC 2500–2999/mm³ and platelets ≥75,000/mm³	Reduce dosages by 50%
WBC <2500/mm³, or platelets <75,000/mm³	Hold treatment
ANC <1500/mm³, or platelets <100,000/mm³ at start of cycle	Delay treatment until ANC ≥1500/mm³ and platelets ≥100,000/mm³. Give filgrastim* in subsequent cycles
Hematologic recovery >3 weeks	Discontinue treatment
First episode of febrile neutropenia or documented infection after treatment	Filgrastim* prophylaxis administered during subsequent cycles
Second episode of febrile neutropenia or documented infection after treatment	Reduce docetaxel dosage to 60 mg/m² during subsequent cycles; administer filgrastim* and consider prophylaxis with ciprofloxacin†
Third episode of febrile neutropenia or documented infection after treatment	Discontinue chemotherapy
G3/4 stomatitis	Reduce docetaxel dosage to 60 mg/m² during subsequent cycles. Reduce epirubicin and fluorouracil dosage by 50% during subsequent cycles

(continued)

(continued)

- **Meperidine** 12.5–25 mg; administer by intravenous injection every 10 minutes if needed for shaking chills (generally, cumulative doses >50 mg are not needed; use with caution in persons with moderate or more severely impaired renal function)

FEC (cyclophosphamide + epirubicin + fluorouracil): weeks 10 through 18

Hydration with 0.9% sodium chloride injection (0.9% NS); administer intravenously 500 mL before starting cyclophosphamide and 500 mL after completing cyclophosphamide administration

Fluorouracil 600 mg/m²; administer by intravenous injection over 1–3 minutes on day 1, every 21 days for 3 cycles (total dosage/cycle = 600 mg/m²)

Epirubicin HCl 60 mg/m²; administer by intravenous injection over 3–5 minutes on day 1, every 21 days for 3 cycles (total dosage/cycle = 60 mg/m²)

Cyclophosphamide 600 mg/m²; administer intravenously in 100–500 mL 0.9% NS or D5W over 30–60 minutes on day 1, every 21 days for 3 cycles (total dosage/cycle = 600 mg/m²)

Supportive Care

Antiemetic prophylaxis
Emetogenic potential is **HIGH**. *Potential for delayed symptoms*
See Chapter 42 for antiemetic recommendations

Hematopoietic growth factor (CSF) prophylaxis
Primary prophylaxis is **NOT** indicated

Antimicrobial prophylaxis
Risk of fever and neutropenia is **LOW**
  Antimicrobial primary prophylaxis to be considered:
  - Antibacterial—not indicated
  - Antifungal—not indicated
  - Antiviral—not indicated, unless patient previously had an episode of HSV

Efficacy

	Patient Number	Recurrence				Deaths
		Distant	Local or Regional	Contralateral Breast Cancer	Any	
All Study Participants						
Docetaxel/FEC	502	12.2	3.2	1.6	13.3	7.8
Vinorelbine/FEC	507	18.7	5.3	2.6	21.5	10.8
Patients with HER2-positive Cancers						
Docetaxel/FEC/ trastuzumab	54	5.6	3.7	1.9	9.3	7.4
Docetaxel/FEC	58	25.9	10.3	1.7	25.9	17.2
Vinorelbine/ FEC/trastuzumab	61	27.9	8.2	4.9	36.1	13.1
Vinorelbine/FEC	58	25.9	6.9	0	27	19.0

Joensuu H et al. J Clin Oncol 2009;27:5685–5692

Treatment Modifications
(continued)

G3/4 neuropathy	Discontinue treatment
Serum bilirubin levels 2 to 3 mg/dL (34.2 to 51.3 mmol/L)	Reduce epirubicin dosage by 50%
Bilirubin levels ≥3 mg/dL (≥51.3 mmol/L)	Discontinue treatment
Any other G3 nonhematologic toxicity	Hold treatment until toxicity resolves to G ≤1, then resume treatment with dosages of all drugs reduced by 25%
G4 nonhematologic toxicity	Discontinue chemotherapy
LVEF has declined by ≥16 percentage points from baseline, or has declined by 10–15 percentage points from baseline to a value below the lower limit of the normal range OR Symptomatic congestive heart failure	Withhold trastuzumab and repeat LVEF assessment at 4-week intervals until improvement, which may require prolonged interruption. For a persistent decline in LVEF, consider a cardio-oncology consultation and weigh the benefits and risks of continuing trastuzumab in the individual patient

*Filgrastim 5 mcg/kg per day; administer subcutaneously starting at least 24 hours after completing chemotherapy until ANC ≥5000/mm³
†Ciprofloxacin 500 mg; administer orally twice daily for 7 days starting on day 5
Note: Dosages reduced for adverse events are not re-escalated

Patient Population Studied

Joensuu H et al. N Engl J Med 2006;354:809–820

Study of 1010 women with axillary node-positive or high-risk node-negative breast cancer were randomly assigned to receive 3 cycles of docetaxel or vinorelbine, followed in both groups by 3 cycles of fluorouracil, epirubicin, and cyclophosphamide (FEC). Women with HER2-positive cancer (n = 232) were further assigned to either receive or not receive trastuzumab for 9 weeks with docetaxel or vinorelbine. The median follow-up time was 62 months after random assignment

Toxicity

Adverse Event	Docetaxel No Trastuzumab (N = 447)		Docetaxel + Trastuzumab (N = 54)	
	% G1/2	% G3/4	% G1/2	% G3/4
Anemia	66	0.5	63	0
Neutropenia	1.6	98.5	0	100
Thrombocytopenia	3.7	0	0	0
Neutropenic fever	0	23	0	29.6
Infection/no neutropenia	39.2	5	43.1	5.9
Vomiting	10.2	0.5	11.8	0
Stomatitis	71.1	2.7	66	4
Alopecia	98	N/A	100	N/A
Nail problems	55.9	N/A	47.9	N/A
Skin rash	55.6	0.9	60	0
Phlebitis	8.9	0	6	0
Allergic reaction	11.7	2	13.5	5.8
Neuropathy, motor	30.5	1.4	27.5	0
Neuropathy, sensory	49.5	0.2	57.4	0
Edema	61.6	1.6	62	0
Fatigue	83	8.2	76	8
Any adverse effect	100	10	100	100

Joensuu H et al. N Engl J Med 2006;354:809–820

Toxicity: Left Ventricular Ejection Fraction (LVEF) During Follow-up Among Study Participants Who Had Breast Cancer with *HER2/neu* Amplification

Treatment Group	Before Chemotherapy	Last Cycle of Chemotherapy	12 Months > Chemotherapy	36 Months > Chemotherapy
Docetaxel Plus FEC (N = 58)				
Median LVEF (%)	67	64	64	64
Range LVEF (%)	53–83	48–78	45–79	52–76
No. of patients	56	51	49	24
Docetaxel Plus FEC and trastuzumab (N = 54)				
Median LVEF (%)	66	65	66	69
Range LVEF (%)	49–82	51–78	51–83	49–77
No. of patients	50	48	48	30

Joensuu H et al. N Engl J Med 2006;354:809–820

FEC Toxicity (N = 632)*

Toxicity	Percentage of Patients
G3/4 neutropenia	25.5%
G3/4 febrile neutropenia	9.5%
G3/4 fatigue	2.4%
G3/4 nausea	5.9%
G3/4 vomiting	9.9%
G3/4 stomatitis	4.9%
Amenorrhea	58%
G2 alopecia	>90%
G2 neuropathy	N/A
G3 neuropathy	N/A
G2 arthralgia/myalgia	N/A
G3 arthralgia/myalgia	N/A
G2 LV dysfunction	7.2%

*FEC = Six 21-day cycles of fluorouracil 600 mg/m², epirubicin 90 mg/m², and cyclophosphamide 600 mg/m²
Martín M et al. J Natl Cancer Inst 2008;100:805–814

Therapy Monitoring

General:

1. *Before each cycle:* CBC with differential and platelet count, LFTs, serum electrolytes, BUN, and creatinine
2. Conduct thorough cardiac assessment, including history, physical examination, and determination of LVEF by echocardiogram or MUGA scan at baseline immediately prior to initiation of trastuzumab and upon completion of trastuzumab (prior to initiation of epirubicin)
3. Patients should have a pre-treatment LVEF ≥55%
4. Repeat LVEF measurement at 4-week intervals if trastuzumab is withheld for significant left ventricular cardiac dysfunction

FEC Toxicity[*][†] (N = 995)

Event	Percentage of Patients
Neutropenia on day 21	33.6
Neutropenia on day 21, cycles 4–6	20.2
Febrile neutropenia	8.4
Febrile neutropenia, cycles 4–6	3.7
GCSF	27
GCSF, cycles 5 and 6	24.8
Infection	1.6
Anemia	1.4
Thrombocytopenia	0.3
G3/4 nausea-vomiting	20.5
G3/4 nausea-vomiting, cycles 4–6	11
G3/4 stomatitis	4.0
G3/4 stomatitis, cycles 4–6	2.3
Alopecia grade 3	83.9
Edema moderate or severe, cycles 4–6	0.3
Nail disorder moderate or severe, cycles 4–6	1.0
Any cardiac event reported as SAE	1.3

[*]FEC = Three 21-day cycles of fluorouracil 500 mg/m^2, epirubicin 100 mg/m^2, and cyclophosphamide 500 mg/m^2; GCSF, granulocyte-colony stimulating factor
[†]Toxicity graded according to WHO criteria and serious adverse events (SAEs) defined according to International Conference on Harmonization (ICH) guidelines

Roché H. J Clin Oncol 2006;24:5664–5671

ADJUVANT • HER2-POSITIVE

BREAST CANCER REGIMEN: PACLITAXEL + TRASTUZUMAB

Tolaney SM et al. N Engl J Med 2015;372:134–141

The regimen consists of 12 weeks of treatment with weekly paclitaxel and trastuzumab, followed by 40 additional weeks of trastuzumab monotherapy (to complete a total of 1 year of trastuzumab). Patients who underwent segmental mastectomy were required to receive either partial-breast radiation (completed prior to initiation of paclitaxel + trastuzumab) or radiation of the whole breast (which was initiated after completion of paclitaxel treatment and concurrent with trastuzumab monotherapy). Patients with hormone receptor–positive tumors also received adjuvant hormonal therapy initiated after completion of paclitaxel

Schedule for first week of paclitaxel + trastuzumab

Premedications for paclitaxel:
> **Dexamethasone** 10 mg; administer intravenously 30–60 minutes before paclitaxel, *plus:*
> **Diphenhydramine** 50 mg; administer intravenously 30–60 minutes before paclitaxel, *plus:*
> **Cimetidine** 300 mg (or **ranitidine** 50 mg, or **famotidine** 20 mg, or an equivalent histamine receptor [H_2]-subtype antagonist); administer intravenously over 15–30 minutes, 30–60 minutes before paclitaxel

Paclitaxel 80 mg/m²; administer intravenously in a volume of 0.9% sodium chloride injection (0.9% NS) or 5% dextrose injection (D5W) sufficient to produce a concentration within the range 0.3–1.2 mg/mL over 60 minutes (total dosage during the first treatment week = 80 mg/m²)
- *Note:* The study protocol allowed for paclitaxel to be administered either before or after trastuzumab administration during the concomitant phase

Trastuzumab 4 mg/kg (loading dose); administer intravenously in 250 mL 0.9% NS over 90 minutes once (total trastuzumab dosage during the first treatment week = 4 mg/kg)
Note: A syndrome most commonly consisting of chills and/or fever may occur in as many as 40% of patients during the first infusion of trastuzumab. These symptoms occur infrequently with subsequent trastuzumab infusions. Other signs and/or symptoms may include nausea, vomiting, pain (in some cases at tumor sites), rigors, headache, dizziness, dyspnea, hypotension, rash, and asthenia. Although the symptoms are usually mild to moderate in severity, infrequently, trastuzumab may need to be discontinued
- When such a syndrome is observed, it can be treated with or without reduction in the rate of trastuzumab infusion, and:
  - **Acetaminophen** 650 mg; administer orally, *plus:*
  - **Diphenhydramine** 25–50 mg; administer orally or by intravenous injection, *plus:*
  - **Meperidine** 12.5–25 mg; administer by intravenous injection every 10 minutes if needed for shaking chills (generally, cumulative doses >50 mg are not needed; use with caution in persons with moderate or more severely impaired renal function)

Schedule for paclitaxel + trastuzumab during weeks 2 through 12 (initiate 1 week after the initial doses of paclitaxel and trastuzumab):

Premedication for paclitaxel:
> **Dexamethasone** 10 mg; administer intravenously 30–60 minutes before each dose of paclitaxel, *plus:*
> **Diphenhydramine** 50 mg; administer intravenously 30–60 minutes before each dose of paclitaxel, *plus:*
> **Cimetidine** 300 mg (or **ranitidine** 50 mg, or **famotidine** 20 mg, or an equivalent histamine receptor [H_2]-subtype antagonist); administer intravenously over 15–30 minutes, 30–60 minutes before each dose of paclitaxel

Paclitaxel 80 mg/m² per week; administer intravenously in a volume of 0.9% NS or D5W sufficient to produce a concentration within the range 0.3–1.2 mg/mL over 60 minutes, weekly, for 11 weeks (total dosage/week = 80 mg/m²)
- *Note:* the study protocol allowed for paclitaxel to be administered either before or after trastuzumab administration during the concomitant phase

Trastuzumab 2 mg/kg per week; administer intravenously in 250 mL 0.9% NS over 30 minutes, weekly, for 11 weeks (total trastuzumab dosage/week during weeks 2–12 = 2 mg/kg)

(continued)

Patient Population Studied

This multicenter, single-arm study involved 406 patients with node-negative, HER2-positive adenocarcinoma of the breast. Patients with tumor of size >3 cm in the greatest dimension were ineligible. All patients received a loading dose of intravenous trastuzumab (4 mg/kg) on day 1 followed by intravenous trastuzumab (2 mg/kg) and paclitaxel (80 mg/m²) weekly for 12 weeks. Thereafter, patients completed a full year of intravenous trastuzumab treatment (ie, an additional 40 weeks) at either the same weekly dose or at a dose of 6 mg/kg every 3 weeks. Patients who had undergone lumpectomy received either partial-breast radiation before initiation of study treatment or whole-breast radiation after the completion of paclitaxel therapy. Adjuvant hormonal therapy after the completion of paclitaxel therapy was recommended for women with hormone receptor–positive tumors

Efficacy (N = 406)

3-year survival free of invasive disease	98.7% (95% CI 97.6–99.8)
3-year survival free of recurrence	99.2% (95% CI 98.4–100)

Note: Median follow-up was 4.0 years; maximum follow-up was 6.2 years

(continued)

Note: If a patient misses a weekly trastuzumab dose by more than 7 days, a re-loading dose of trastuzumab should be given as trastuzumab 4 mg/kg (loading dose); administer intravenously in 250 mL 0.9% NS over 90 minutes once. This should be followed 7 days later by resumption of 2 mg/kg weekly maintenance doses

Schedule for trastuzumab during weeks 13 through 52 (initiate 1 week after the last dose of combined weekly trastuzumab + paclitaxel):

Trastuzumab 6 mg/kg per dose; administer intravenously in 250 mL 0.9% NS over 30–90 minutes, every 3 weeks for up to 13 cycles not to exceed 52 weeks of total trastuzumab therapy (total trastuzumab dosage/3-week cycle during weeks 13–52 = 6 mg/kg)

Note: If a patient misses a 6-mg/kg trastuzumab dose by more than 7 days, a re-loading dose of trastuzumab should be given as trastuzumab 8 mg/kg (loading dose); administer intravenously in 250 mL 0.9% NS over 90 minutes once. This should be followed 21 days later by resumption of 6-mg/kg maintenance doses repeated every 3 weeks

Supportive Care

Antiemetic prophylaxis
Emetogenic potential on days with paclitaxel is **LOW**
Emetogenic potential on days of trastuzumab monotherapy is **MINIMAL**
See Chapter 42 for antiemetic recommendations

Hematopoietic growth factor (CSF) prophylaxis
Primary prophylaxis is not indicated
See Chapter 43 for more information

Antimicrobial prophylaxis
Risk of fever and neutropenia is **LOW**
   Antimicrobial primary prophylaxis to be considered:
   • Antibacterial—not indicated
   • Antifungal—not indicated
   • Antiviral—not indicated, unless patient previously had an episode of HSV

Therapy Monitoring

1. Before the start of weekly paclitaxel treatment: CBC with differential, serum electrolytes, BUN, creatinine, AST or ALT, and alkaline phosphatase

2. Weekly during paclitaxel treatment: CBC with differential

3. Conduct thorough cardiac assessment, including history, physical examination, and determination of LVEF by echocardiogram or MUGA scan at baseline immediately prior to initiation of trastuzumab and every 3 months during therapy

4. Patients should have a pre-treatment LVEF ≥55%

5. Repeat LVEF measurement at 4-week intervals if trastuzumab is withheld for significant left ventricular cardiac dysfunction

6. Observe closely for hypersensitivity reactions, especially during the first and second infusions

7. Monitor for symptoms of pulmonary toxicity

8. Verify pregnancy status prior to the initiation of therapy. Advise patients of the risks of embryo-fetal death and birth defects and the need for contraception

Treatment Modifications

WEEKLY PACLITAXEL DOSE MODIFICATIONS	
Paclitaxel starting dose	80 mg/m²
Paclitaxel dose level −1	70 mg/m²
Paclitaxel dose level −2	60 mg/m²

Adverse Event	Treatment Modifications
Severe hypersensitivity reaction	Discontinue infusion immediately and administer appropriate support. For hypersensitivity reaction G ≤3, initial management includes temporary discontinuation of infusion for 30 minutes, and administration of additional intravenous antihistamines and glucocorticoids. Upon resolution of symptoms, infusion may be restarted at a slower rate if deemed safe. If G4 hypersensitivity is experienced, stabilize the cardiorespiratory system and use epinephrine as needed, then permanently discontinue paclitaxel*
Febrile neutropenia (ANC <1000/mm³ with temperature >38°C or >100.4°F), or ANC <1000/mm³ for ≥7 days	Reduce paclitaxel dose by one dose level and consider adding filgrastim in subsequent cycles, if applicable
Febrile neutropenia (ANC <1000/mm³ with temperature >38°C or >100.4°F), or ANC <1000/mm³ for ≥7 days despite dose reduction of 10 mg/m²	Administer filgrastim in subsequent cycles. If already administering filgrastim, reduce paclitaxel dose an additional dose level
Platelet nadir <50,000/mm³, or platelets <100,000/mm³ for ≥7 days	Reduce paclitaxel dose by one level
ANC ≤ 800/mm³ or platelets ≤50,000/mm³ at the start of a cycle	Hold treatment until ANC >800/mm³ and platelets >50,000/mm³, then resume with weekly paclitaxel dosage reduced by one dose level
G2 motor or sensory neuropathies	Reduce weekly paclitaxel dosage by one dose level without interrupting planned treatment

(continued)

Treatment Modifications (*continued*)

G3 motor or sensory neuropathies	Withhold paclitaxel until toxicity resolves to G ≤2 then resume with weekly paclitaxel dosage reduced by one dose level
G4 motor or sensory neuropathies	Discontinue paclitaxel
Other nonhematologic adverse events G2/3 (not including alopecia)	Hold treatment until adverse events resolve to <G1, then resume with weekly paclitaxel dosage reduced by one dose level
Patients who cannot tolerate paclitaxel at 60 mg/m² per week	Discontinue paclitaxel
Treatment delay >2 weeks	Decrease weekly paclitaxel dosage by one dose level or consider discontinuing treatment

TRASTUZUMAB

Adverse Event	Dose Modification
Mild or moderate infusion reaction*	Decrease the rate of infusion
Infusion reaction with dyspnea or clinically significant hypotension	Interrupt the infusion. Administer medical therapy as indicated including epinephrine, corticosteroids, diphenhydramine, bronchodilators, and oxygen. Observe patients closely for 60 minutes if the reaction occurs after the first infusion and for 30 minutes if it occurs after subsequent infusions. Prior to resumption of the trastuzumab infusion, pre-medicate with antihistamines and/or corticosteroids *Note:* While some patients tolerate the resumption of trastuzumab infusions, others have recurrent severe infusion reactions despite premedications
Severe or life-threatening infusion reaction (including bronchospasm, anaphylaxis, angioedema, hypoxia, and severe hypotension; usually reported during or immediately following the initial infusion)*	Interrupt the infusion. Administer medical therapy as indicated including epinephrine, corticosteroids, diphenhydramine, bronchodilators, and oxygen. Patients should be evaluated and carefully monitored until complete resolution of signs and symptoms. Discontinue trastuzumab
LVEF has declined by ≥16 percentage points from baseline, or has declined by 10–15 percentage points from baseline to a value below the lower limit of the normal range OR Symptomatic congestive heart failure	Withhold trastuzumab and repeat LVEF assessment at 4-week intervals until improvement, which may require prolonged interruption. For a persistent decline in LVEF, consider a cardio-oncology consultation and weigh the benefits and risks of continuing trastuzumab in the individual patient
Pulmonary toxicity	Discontinue trastuzumab in patients experiencing pulmonary toxicity that is attributable to trastuzumab

*Infusion reactions consist of a symptom complex characterized by fever and chills, and on occasion included nausea, vomiting, pain (in some cases at tumor sites), headache, dizziness, dyspnea, hypotension, rash, and asthenia

Adverse Events (N = 406)

Grade (%)	Grade 2	Grade 3	Grade 4
Fatigue	20	2	0
Diarrhea	12	1	0
Neuropathy	10	3	0
Neutropenia	6	4	<1
Hyperglycemia	9	2	0
Leukopenia	7	2	0
Allergic reaction	7	1	<1
Increased alanine aminotransferase level	6	2	0
Anemia	7	<1	0

The most common adverse events that occurred during the study treatment are shown, although alopecia was expected in the vast majority of patients and so data related to this adverse effect were not collected. During the 12 weeks of combined paclitaxel + trastuzumab therapy, 3.2% patients reported at least one grade 3 neuropathy episode. During the 12-month study protocol, 0.5% patients developed symptomatic congestive heart failure, but recovered after discontinuation of trastuzumab. An additional 3.2% had clinically significant asymptomatic reduction of ejection fraction that resulted in interruption of trastuzumab treatment, but the ejection fraction in all but 0.5% normalized, enabling the 2.7% to complete the trastuzumab treatment. Grade 3 or 4 allergic reaction to the study treatment was experienced by 1.7% of patients and almost all of these patients were unable to complete the protocol. A total of 7.4% patients discontinued the study owing to toxic effects

ADJUVANT • HER2-POSITIVE

BREAST CANCER REGIMEN: DOCETAXEL + CARBOPLATIN + TRASTUZUMAB + PERTUZUMAB (TCHP)

von Minckwitz G et al. N Engl J Med 2017;377:122–131
Protocol for: von Minckwitz G et al. N Engl J Med 2017;377:122–131

The regimen consists of 1 year of adjuvant pertuzumab + trastuzumab therapy given with a standard adjuvant chemotherapy regimen, initiated concurrent with taxane (paclitaxel or docetaxel) therapy. Standard chemotherapy regimens studied included (1) carboplatin + docetaxel x 6 cycles (described here); (2) fluorouracil + epirubicin + cyclophosphamide (FEC) × 3–4 cycles followed by either docetaxel × 4 doses or weekly paclitaxel × 12 doses; and (3) doxorubicin + cyclophosphamide (AC) or epirubicin + cyclophosphamide (EC) × 4 cycles followed by either docetaxel × 4 doses or weekly paclitaxel × 12 doses. Hormonal therapy and/or radiation therapy, when indicated, are initiated after completion of taxane (paclitaxel or docetaxel) therapy and may be given concurrent with trastuzumab + pertuzumab

Docetaxel + carboplatin + trastuzumab + pertuzumab (TCHP)

Trastuzumab every 21 days for 6 cycles:
- *Loading Dose:* **Trastuzumab** 8 mg/kg; administer intravenously in 250 mL 0.9% sodium chloride injection (0.9% NS) over 90 minutes as a loading dose before pertuzumab on day 1, cycle 1 only (total dosage during the first cycle = 8 mg/kg), *followed 3 weeks later by:*
  - *Note:* A syndrome most commonly consisting of chills and/or fever may occur in as many as 40% of patients during the first infusion of trastuzumab. These symptoms occur infrequently with subsequent trastuzumab infusions. Other signs and/or symptoms may include nausea, vomiting, pain (in some cases at tumor sites), rigors, headache, dizziness, dyspnea, hypotension, rash, and asthenia. Although the symptoms are usually mild to moderate in severity, infrequently, trastuzumab may need to be discontinued
  - When such a syndrome is observed, it can be treated with or without reduction in the rate of trastuzumab infusion, and:
    - Acetaminophen 650 mg; administer orally, *plus:*
    - Diphenhydramine 25–50 mg; administer orally or by intravenous injection, *plus:*
    - Meperidine 12.5–25 mg; administer by intravenous injection every 10 minutes if needed for shaking chills (generally, cumulative doses >50 mg are not needed; use with caution in persons with moderate or more severely impaired renal function)
- *Maintenance Doses:* **Trastuzumab** 6 mg/kg; administer intravenously in 250 mL 0.9% NS over 30 minutes before pertuzumab on day 1, every 3 weeks for 5 cycles (total dosage/cycle = 6 mg/kg)
  - *Note:* If a patient misses a 6-mg/kg trastuzumab dose by more than 7 days, a re-loading dose of trastuzumab should be given as trastuzumab 8 mg/kg (loading dose); administer intravenously in 250 mL 0.9% NS over 90 minutes once. This should be followed 21 days later by resumption of 6-mg/kg maintenance doses repeated every 3 weeks

Pertuzumab every 21 days for 6 cycles:
- *Loading Dose:* **Pertuzumab** 840 mg initial (loading) dose; administer intravenously in 250 mL 0.9% NS over 60 minutes as a loading dose after trastuzumab on day 1, cycle 1 only (total dosage during the first cycle = 840 mg), *followed 3 weeks later by:*
- *Maintenance Doses:* **Pertuzumab** 420 mg per dose; administer intravenously in 250 mL 0.9% NS over 30–60 minutes after trastuzumab on day 1, every 3 weeks for 5 cycles (total dose/3-week cycle = 420 mg)
  - *Note:* If a patient misses a 420-mg pertuzumab dose by more than 21 days (ie, ≥6 weeks between two sequential infusions), a re-loading dose of pertuzumab should be given as pertuzumab 840-mg (loading) dose; administer intravenously in 250 mL 0.9% NS over 60 minutes as a loading dose once. This should be followed 21 days later by resumption of 420-mg maintenance doses repeated every 3 weeks

Alternatively, a fixed dose combination product containing pertuzumab, trastuzumab, and hyaluronidase (PHESGO™) for subcutaneous injection may be used instead of intravenous pertuzumab and trastuzumab as follows:
- *Loading Dose:* **Pertuzumab, trastuzumab, and hyaluronidase (PHESGO™) for subcutaneous injection** 1200 mg, 600 mg, and 30,000 units, respectively; administer as a 15 mL subcutaneous injection into the thigh over 8 minutes once on day 1, cycle 1 only (total dosage during the first cycle = 1200 mg pertuzumab, 600 mg trastuzumab, and 30,000 units hyaluronidase), *followed 3 weeks later by:*
- *Maintenance Doses:* **Pertuzumab, trastuzumab, and hyaluronidase (PHESGO™) for subcutaneous injection** 600 mg, 600 mg, and 20,000 units, respectively; administer as a 10 mL subcutaneous injection into the thigh over 5 minutes on day 1, every 3 weeks, for 5 cycles (total dosage/3-week cycle = 600 mg pertuzumab, 600 mg trastuzumab, and 20,000 units hyaluronidase)
  - *Notes:*
    - Alternate the injection site between the left and right thigh, avoiding the last injection site by ≥2.5 cm. Avoid injection into areas that are hard, red, bruised, or tender.
    - Observe patients for at least 30 minutes after the loading dose and for at least 15 minutes after maintenance doses.
    - If a scheduled injection is delayed and the interval between injections is <6 weeks, then administer the maintenance dose. If the interval between injections is ≥6 weeks, then administer a loading dose followed 3 weeks later by resumption of maintenance dosing.

Carboplatin target AUC = 6 mg/mL × min; administer intravenously in 250 mL 5% dextrose injection (D5W) or 0.9% NS over 30–60 minutes after pertuzumab on day 1, every 3 weeks for 6 cycles (total dose/cycle calculated to achieve a target AUC = 6 mg/mL × min), *followed by:*

Prophylaxis for fluid retention and hypersensitivity reactions from docetaxel:
Dexamethasone 8 mg/dose; administer orally twice daily for 3 days, starting on the day before docetaxel administration (total dose/cycle = 48 mg)

(continued)

(*continued*)

Docetaxel 75 mg/m²; administer intravenously in a volume of 0.9% NS or D5W sufficient to produce a final docetaxel concentration of 0.3–0.74 mg/mL over 60 minutes after carboplatin on day 1, every 3 weeks for 6 cycles (total dosage/cycle = 75 mg/m²)

Three weeks after completing combination (TCHP) chemotherapy, continue trastuzumab + pertuzumab to complete a total of 52 weeks of HER2-directed therapy as follows:

Trastuzumab 6 mg/kg; administer intravenously in 250 mL 0.9% NS over 30 minutes before pertuzumab on day 1, every 3 weeks for up to 12 cycles not to exceed 52 weeks of total trastuzumab therapy (total dosage/3-week cycle = 6 mg/kg)
 ▪ *Note:* If a patient misses a 6-mg/kg trastuzumab dose by more than 7 days, a re-loading dose of trastuzumab should be given as trastuzumab 8 mg/kg (loading dose); administer intravenously in 250 mL 0.9% NS over 90 minutes once. This should be followed 21 days later by resumption of 6-mg/kg maintenance doses repeated every 3 weeks

Pertuzumab 420 mg per dose; administer intravenously in 250 mL 0.9% NS over 30–60 minutes after trastuzumab on day 1, every 3 weeks for up to 12 cycles not to exceed 52 weeks of total pertuzumab therapy (total dose/3-week cycle = 420 mg)
 ▪ *Note:* If a patient misses a 420-mg pertuzumab dose by more than 21 days (ie, ≥6 weeks between two sequential infusions), a re-loading dose of pertuzumab should be given as pertuzumab 840-mg (loading) dose; administer intravenously in 250 mL 0.9% NS over 60 minutes as a loading dose once. This should be followed 21 days later by resumption of 420-mg maintenance doses repeated every 3 weeks

Alternatively, a fixed dose combination product containing pertuzumab, trastuzumab, and hyaluronidase (PHESGO™) for subcutaneous injection may be used instead of intravenous pertuzumab and trastuzumab as follows:
• *Maintenance Doses:* **Pertuzumab, trastuzumab, and hyaluronidase (PHESGO™) for subcutaneous injection** 600 mg, 600 mg, and 20,000 units, respectively; administer as a 10 mL subcutaneous injection into the thigh over 5 minutes on day 1, every 3 weeks, for up to 12 cycles not to exceed 52 weeks of total therapy (total dosage/3-week cycle = 600 mg pertuzumab, 600 mg trastuzumab, and 20,000 units hyaluronidase)
  ▪ *Notes:*
   ○ Alternate the injection site between the left and right thigh, avoiding the last injection site by ≥2.5 cm. Avoid injection into areas that are hard, red, bruised, or tender.
   ○ Observe patients for at least 30 minutes after the loading dose and for at least 15 minutes after maintenance doses.
   ○ If a scheduled injection is delayed and the interval between injections is <6 weeks, then administer the maintenance dose. If the interval between injections is ≥6 weeks, then administer a loading dose (as described above) followed 3 weeks later by resumption of maintenance dosing.

Supportive Care
Antiemetic prophylaxis
*Emetogenic potential on days with TCHP combination chemotherapy is **HIGH**. Potential for delayed symptoms*
*Emetogenic potential on days with trastuzumab + pertuzumab (without carboplatin + docetaxel) is **LOW***
See Chapter 42 for antiemetic recommendations

Hematopoietic growth factor (CSF) prophylaxis
Primary prophylaxis may be indicated
See Chapter 43 for more information

Antimicrobial prophylaxis
*Risk of fever and neutropenia is **INTERMEDIATE***
 Antimicrobial primary prophylaxis to be considered:
 • Antibacterial—not indicated
 • Antifungal—not indicated
 • Antiviral—not indicated, unless patient previously had an episode of HSV

Carboplatin dose
Carboplatin dose is based on a formula described by Calvert et al. to achieve a target area under the plasma concentration versus time curve (AUC)

$$\text{Total Carboplatin Dose (mg)} = (\text{target AUC})(\text{GFR} + 25)$$

In practice, creatinine clearance (CrCl) is used in place of glomerular filtration rate (GFR). CrCl can be estimated from the equation of Cockcroft and Gault, thus:

$$\text{For males, CrCl} = \frac{(140 - \text{age[years]} \times (\text{body weight [kg]})}{72 \times (\text{serum creatinine [mg/dL]})}$$

$$\text{For females, CrCl} = \frac{(140 - \text{age[years]} \times (\text{body weight [kg]})}{72 \times (\text{serum creatinine [mg/dL]})} \times 0.85$$

Calvert AH et al. J Clin Oncol 1989;7:1748–1756
Cockcroft DW, Gault MH. Nephron 1976;16:31–41
Jodrell DI et al. J Clin Oncol 1992;10:520–528
Sorensen BT et al. Cancer Chemother Pharmacol 1991;28:397–401

(*continued*)

(*continued*)

Note: On October 8, 2010, the U.S. Food and Drug Administration (FDA) identified a potential safety issue with carboplatin dosing based on recent changes in the measurement of serum creatinine. By the end of 2010, all clinical laboratories in the United States will use the standardized isotope dilution mass spectrometry (IDMS) method to measure serum creatinine, which could result in an overestimation of the GFR in some patients with normal renal function. A carboplatin dose calculated with an IDMS-measured serum creatinine result using the Calvert formula could exceed an expected exposure (AUC) and result in increased drug-related toxicity. Provided actual GFR measurements are made to assess renal function, carboplatin can be safely dosed according to the Calvert formula described in product labeling. If GFR (or creatinine clearance) is estimated based on serum creatinine measurements by the IDMS method, the FDA recommended for patients with normal renal function capping an estimated GFR at 125 mL/min for any targeted AUC value. No greater estimated GFR values should be used.

Diarrhea management
Latent or delayed-onset diarrhea:
Loperamide 4 mg orally initially after the first loose or liquid stool, *then*
Loperamide 2 mg orally every 2 hours during waking hours, *plus*
Loperamide 4 mg orally every 4 hours during hours of sleep
- Continue for at least 12 hours after diarrhea resolves
- Recurrent diarrhea after a 12-hour diarrhea-free interval is treated as a new episode
- Rehydrate orally with fluids and electrolytes during a diarrheal episode
- If a patient develops blood or mucus in stool, dehydration, or hemodynamic instability, or if diarrhea persists >48 hours despite loperamide, stop loperamide and evaluate urgently in clinic or hospitalize the patient for IV hydration
- Alternatively, a trial of **diphenoxylate hydrochloride** 2.5 mg with **atropine sulfate** 0.025 mg (eg, Lomotil)
- Initial adult dose is 2 tablets 4 times daily until control has been achieved, after which the dose may be reduced to meet individual requirements. Control may often be maintained with as little as 2 tablets daily
- Clinical improvement of acute diarrhea is usually observed within 48 hours. If improvement of chronic diarrhea after treatment with a maximum daily dose of 8 tablets is not observed within 10 days, control is unlikely with further administration

Patient Population Studied

This prospective, multicenter, double-blind, randomized, placebo-controlled trial involved 4805 patients with nonmetastatic, adequately excised, invasive HER2-positive breast cancer. Eligible patients had node-positive or high-risk node-negative disease and baseline left ventricular ejection fraction ≥55%. All patients had to receive their first dose of chemotherapy within 8 weeks of definitive breast surgery. All patients received standard adjuvant chemotherapy and intravenous trastuzumab (8-mg/kg loading dose and then 6 mg/kg every 3 weeks for a maximum of 18 weeks). Patients were randomly assigned to also receive intravenously either placebo or pertuzumab (840-mg loading dose and then 420 g every 3 weeks for a maximum of 18 weeks). Patients with hormone receptor–positive disease received standard endocrine therapy from the end of chemotherapy and were supposed to continue with this therapy for at least 5 years. Radiotherapy was administered as clinically indicated after chemotherapy and concurrently with anti-HER2 therapy

Therapy Monitoring

1. Prior to each cycle of TCHP: CBC with differential, serum electrolytes, BUN, creatinine, AST or ALT, and alkaline phosphatase
2. Conduct thorough cardiac assessment, including history, physical examination, and determination of LVEF by echocardiogram or MUGA scan at baseline immediately prior to initiation of trastuzumab and every 3 months during therapy.
3. Patients should have a pre-treatment LVEF ≥55%
4. Repeat LVEF measurement at 4-week intervals if trastuzumab and/or pertuzumab are withheld for significant left ventricular cardiac dysfunction
5. Monitor for symptoms of pulmonary toxicity
6. Verify pregnancy status prior to the initiation of therapy. Advise patients of the risks of embryo-fetal death and birth defects and the need for contraception
7. Avoid using concomitant strong CYP3A4 inhibitors (eg, ketoconazole, itraconazole, clarithromycin, atazanavir, indinavir, nefazodone, nelfinavir, ritonavir, saquinavir, telithromycin, and voriconazole). Consider a 50% docetaxel dose reduction if patients require coadministration of a strong CYP3A4 inhibitor

Efficacy (N = 4804)

Efficacy Variable	Pertuzumab + Trastuzumab + Standard Adjuvant Chemotherapy (N = 2400)	Placebo + Trastuzumab + Standard Adjuvant Chemotherapy (N = 2404)	Hazard Ratio (95% CI) and P Value
Invasive-disease-free survival in the ITT population (n = 2400 in pertuzumab arm and n = 2404 in placebo arm)			
Invasive-disease-free survival events	7.1%	8.7%	0.81 (0.66–1.00); 0.045
3 year invasive-disease-free survival rate	94.1%	93.2%	
Invasive-disease-free survival in patients with node-negative disease (n = 897 in pertuzumab arm and n = 902 in placebo arm)*			
Invasive-disease-free survival events	3.6%	3.2%	1.13 (0.68–1.86); 0.64
Invasive-disease-free survival in patients with node-positive disease (n = 1503 in pertuzumab arm and n = 1502 in placebo arm)*			
Invasive-disease-free survival events	9.2%	12.1%	0.77 (0.62–0.96); 0.02
3 year invasive-disease-free survival rate	92.0%	90.2%	
Invasive-disease-free survival in patients with hormone receptor–negative disease (n = 864 in pertuzumab arm and n = 858 in placebo arm)*			
Invasive-disease-free survival events	8.2%	10.6%	0.76 (0.56–1.04); 0.08
3 year invasive-disease-free survival rate	92.8%	91.2%	
Invasive-disease-free survival in patients with hormone receptor–positive disease (n = 1536 in pertuzumab arm and n = 1546 in placebo arm)*			
Invasive-disease-free survival events	6.5%	7.7%	0.86 (0.66–1.13); 0.28
3 year invasive-disease-free survival rate	94.8%	94.4%	

Note: Median follow-up was 45.4 months
*Exploratory subgroup analyses

Treatment Modifications

DOCETAXEL AND CARBOPLATIN DOSE MODIFICATIONS

Docetaxel starting dose	75 mg/m^2	Carboplatin starting dose	AUC 6
Docetaxel dose level −1	60 mg/m^2	Carboplatin dose level −1	AUC 5
Docetaxel dose level −2	50 mg/m^2	Carboplatin dose level −2	AUC 4
Docetaxel dose level −3	Discontinue docetaxel	Carboplatin dose level −3	Discontinue carboplatin

Adverse Event	Treatment Modifications
Severe hypersensitivity reaction	Discontinue docetaxel or carboplatin infusion immediately and administer appropriate support. For hypersensitivity reaction less G ≤3, initial management includes temporary discontinuation of infusion for 30 minutes, and administration of additional intravenous antihistamines and glucocorticoids. Upon resolution of symptoms, the docetaxel infusion may be restarted at a slower rate if deemed safe. Rechallenge with carboplatin will require institution of a desensitization regimen. If G4 hypersensitivity is experienced, stabilize the cardiorespiratory system and use epinephrine as needed, then permanently discontinue docetaxel or carboplatin.* Rechallenge with carboplatin will require institution of a desensitization regimen
Febrile neutropenia (ANC <1000/mm^3 with temperature >38°C or >100.4°F), or ANC <500/mm^3 for ≥7 days	Withhold treatment until resolution of toxicity. Administer filgrastim in subsequent cycles
Febrile neutropenia (ANC <1000/mm^3 with temperature >38°C or >100.4°F), or ANC <500/mm^3 for ≥7 days despite administration of filgrastim	Reduce docetaxel and carboplatin one dose level; continue filgrastim administration
Platelet nadir <50,000/mm^3, or platelets <100,000/mm^3 for ≥7 days	Reduce docetaxel and carboplatin dose by one level
ANC <1500/mm^3 and/or platelets <100,000/mm^3 at the start of a cycle	Hold treatment until ANC ≥1500/mm^3 and platelets ≥100,000/mm^3, then resume with docetaxel and carboplatin dosage reduced by one dose level

(continued)

Treatment Modifications (continued)

Adverse Event	Treatment Modifications
Day 1 ANC <1500/mm^3 and/or platelet count <100,000/mm^3	Withhold docetaxel and carboplatin until ANC ≥1500/mm^3 and platelet count ≥100,000/mm^3
ANC <1500/mm^3 and/or platelet count <100,000/mm^3 despite a 2-week delay but with ANC >1,000/mm^3 and platelet count >75,000/mm^3	Resume therapy with docetaxel and carboplatin dosages reduced by one dose level. Consider filgrastim
Bilirubin > ULN, or AST/ALT >1.5 × ULN and AP >2.5 × ULN	Withhold docetaxel until bilirubin ≤ ULN or AST/ALT ≤1.5 and AP ≤2.5 × ULN, then resume docetaxel dosage reduced by one dose level
Severe or cumulative cutaneous reactions	Withhold treatment until resolution of toxicity. Reduce docetaxel dosage one dose level
G3/4 stomatitis	
G1 neurotoxicity of any duration (paresthesias/dysesthesias that do not interfere with function)	Continue docetaxel and carboplatin treatment
G2 neurotoxicity of 1–7 days duration (paresthesias/dysesthesias interfering with function, but not activities of daily living)	Continue docetaxel and carboplatin treatment but can delay start for up to 7 days until G ≤1
G2 neurotoxicity of >7 days duration (paresthesias/dysesthesias interfering with function, but not activities of daily living)	Withhold docetaxel and carboplatin until toxicity G ≤1, then resume docetaxel and carboplatin treatment, but reduce dosages by one dose level. If G2 toxicity persists after 3 weeks of delay, discontinue docetaxel and carboplatin*
G3 neurotoxicity of 1–7 days duration (paresthesias/dysesthesias with pain or with function impairment interfering with activities of daily living)	Withhold docetaxel and carboplatin. Resume with docetaxel and carboplatin dosages reduced one dose level when toxicity has resolved to G ≤1
Second episode of G3 neurotoxicity of 1–7 days duration (paresthesias/dysesthesias with pain or with function impairment interfering with activities of daily living)	Discontinue docetaxel and carboplatin*
G3 neurotoxicity of >7 days duration (paresthesias/dysesthesias with pain or with function impairment interfering with activities of daily living)	Discontinue docetaxel and carboplatin*
Persistent paresthesias/dysesthesias that are disabling or life-threatening	Discontinue docetaxel and carboplatin*
G1 musculoskeletal pain not controlled by analgesics of any duration	Continue docetaxel and carboplatin treatment
G2 musculoskeletal pain not controlled by analgesics of 1–7 days duration	
G2 musculoskeletal pain not controlled by analgesics of >7 days duration	Continue docetaxel and carboplatin treatment or withhold docetaxel and carboplatin for persistent G2. When toxicity G ≤1, resume treatment with dosages that are one dose lower. If G2 toxicity persists resulting in a delay of >3 weeks, discontinue docetaxel and carboplatin*
First episode of G3 musculoskeletal pain not controlled by analgesics of 1–7 days duration	Continue docetaxel and carboplatin treatment
Second episode of G3 musculoskeletal pain not controlled by analgesics of 1–7 days duration	Discontinue docetaxel and carboplatin*
First episode of G3 musculoskeletal pain not controlled by analgesics of >7 days duration	Withhold docetaxel and carboplatin. When toxicity G ≤1, resume treatment with dosages that are one dose level lower. If >G2 toxicity persists resulting in a delay of >3 weeks, discontinue docetaxel and carboplatin*
Second episode of G3 musculoskeletal pain not controlled by analgesics of >7 days duration	Discontinue docetaxel and carboplatin*
Docetaxel-related fluid retention	Consider 1- to 5-day treatment with dexamethasone starting one day before docetaxel administration. Consider diuretics for symptomatic relief and to limit the severity of fluid retention
Other G2 nonhematologic adverse event that occurs during a cycle but results in a delay in the start of the next cycle	Hold treatment until adverse events resolve to G ≤1, then resume with docetaxel and/or carboplatin dosages reduced by one dose level

(continued)

Treatment Modifications (*continued*)

Adverse Event	Treatment Modifications
Other G3 nonhematologic adverse event that occurs during a cycle but resolves prior to the start of the next cycle or requires a delay in the start of the next cycle	Hold treatment until adverse events resolve to G ≤1, then resume with docetaxel and/or carboplatin dosages reduced by one dose level
Other G4 nonhematologic adverse event that occurs during a cycle but resolves prior to the start of the next cycle	Hold treatment until adverse events resolve to G ≤1, then resume with docetaxel and/or carboplatin dosages reduced by two dose levels or discontinue docetaxel and carboplatin*
Other G4 nonhematologic adverse event that occurs during a cycle but requires a delay in the start of the next cycle	Discontinue docetaxel and/or carboplatin*
Any treatment delay >3 weeks	Discontinue docetaxel and/or carboplatin*

TRASTUZUMAB AND PERTUZUMAB

Note: Dose reductions are not recommended for trastuzumab or pertuzumab

Adverse Event	Adverse Event
Mild or moderate infusion reaction	Decrease the rate of infusion
Infusion reaction with dyspnea or clinically significant hypotension	Interrupt the infusion. Administer medical therapy as indicated including epinephrine, corticosteroids, diphenhydramine, bronchodilators, and oxygen. Observe patients closely for 60 minutes if the reaction occurs after the first infusion and for 30 minutes if it occurs after subsequent infusions. Prior to resumption of the infusion, premedicate with antihistamines and/or corticosteroids. Note: While some patients tolerate the resumption of infusions, others have recurrent severe infusion reactions despite premedications
Severe or life-threatening infusion reaction (including bronchospasm, anaphylaxis, angioedema, hypoxia, and severe hypotension; usually reported during or immediately following the initial infusion)	Interrupt the infusion reaction. Administer medical therapy as indicated including epinephrine, corticosteroids, diphenhydramine, bronchodilators, and oxygen. Patients should be evaluated and carefully monitored until complete resolution of signs and symptoms. Discontinue pertuzumab and trastuzumab
LVEF has declined by ≥16 percentage points from baseline, or has declined by 10–15 percentage points from baseline to a value below the lower limit of the normal range OR Symptomatic congestive heart failure	Withhold pertuzumab and trastuzumab and repeat LVEF assessment at 4-week intervals until improvement, which may require prolonged interruption. For a persistent decline in LVEF, consider a cardio-oncology consultation and weigh the benefits and risks of continuing pertuzumab and trastuzumab in the individual patient

*If docetaxel and/or carboplatin are discontinued or withheld beyond the time of start of the next cycle, treatment with pertuzumab and trastuzumab may continue

Adverse Events (N = 4769)

Grade ≥3 Adverse Events (%)	Pertuzumab + Trastuzumab + Standard Adjuvant Chemotherapy (N = 2364)	Placebo + Trastuzumab + Standard Adjuvant Chemotherapy (N = 2405)
All	64	57
Neutropenia	16	16
Febrile neutropenia	12	11
Decreased neutrophil count	10	10
Diarrhea	10	4
Anemia	7	5

Toxicities included in the table are grade ≥3 events that occurred in ≥5% of patients in either treatment group. Fatal adverse events occurred in 0.8% of each treatment group. Primary cardiac events occurred in 0.7% of the pertuzumab group and 0.3% of the placebo group. Secondary cardiac events occurred in 2.7% of the pertuzumab group and 2.8% of the placebo group. A total of 7.8% of patients in the pertuzumab group and 6.4% of patients in the placebo group discontinued treatment for safety reasons

ADJUVANT • HER2-POSITIVE

BREAST CANCER REGIMEN: DOCETAXEL + TRASTUZUMAB + PERTUZUMAB (DHP)

von Minckwitz G et al. N Engl J Med 2017;377:122–131
Protocol for: von Minckwitz G et al. N Engl J Med 2017;377:122–131

The regimen consists of 1 year of adjuvant pertuzumab + trastuzumab therapy given with a standard adjuvant chemotherapy regimen, initiated concurrent with taxane (paclitaxel or docetaxel) therapy. Standard chemotherapy regimens studied included (1) carboplatin + docetaxel × 6 cycles; (2) fluorouracil + epirubicin + cyclophosphamide (FEC) × 3–4 cycles followed by either docetaxel × 4 doses or weekly paclitaxel × 12 doses; and (3) doxorubicin + cyclophosphamide (AC) or epirubicin + cyclophosphamide (EC) × 4 cycles followed by either docetaxel × 4 doses or weekly paclitaxel × 12 doses. Hormonal therapy and/or radiation therapy, when indicated, are initiated after completion of taxane (paclitaxel or docetaxel) therapy and may be given concurrent with trastuzumab + pertuzumab. **The below regimen describes the combination of adjuvant docetaxel + trastuzumab + pertuzumab intended to be used after completion of anthracycline-based chemotherapy (ie, FEC × 3–4 cycles or AC x 4 cycles).** Please refer to separate descriptions of FEC and AC regimens

Adjuvant docetaxel + trastuzumab + pertuzumab (initiate after completion of anthracycline-based adjuvant chemotherapy such as fluorouracil + epirubicin + cyclophosphamide [FEC] × 3–4 cycles or doxorubicin + cyclophosphamide [AC] × 4 cycles)

Trastuzumab every 21 days for up to 18 cycles (not to exceed 52 weeks of total trastuzumab therapy):
- *Loading Dose:* **Trastuzumab** 8 mg/kg; administer intravenously in 250 mL 0.9% sodium chloride injection (0.9% NS) over 90 minutes as a loading dose before pertuzumab on day 1, cycle 1 only (total dosage during the first cycle = 8 mg/kg), *followed 3 weeks later by:*
  - ▪ *Note:* A syndrome most commonly consisting of chills and/or fever may occur in as many as 40% of patients during the first infusion of trastuzumab. These symptoms occur infrequently with subsequent trastuzumab infusions. Other signs and/or symptoms may include nausea, vomiting, pain (in some cases at tumor sites), rigors, headache, dizziness, dyspnea, hypotension, rash, and asthenia. Although the symptoms are usually mild to moderate in severity, infrequently, trastuzumab may need to be discontinued
  - ▪ When such a syndrome is observed, it can be treated with or without reduction in the rate of trastuzumab infusion, and:
    - ○ Acetaminophen 650 mg; administer orally, *plus:*
    - ○ Diphenhydramine 25–50 mg; administer orally or by intravenous injection, *plus:*
    - ○ Meperidine 12.5–25 mg; administer by intravenous injection every 10 minutes if needed for shaking chills (generally, cumulative doses >50 mg are not needed; use with caution in persons with moderate or more severely impaired renal function)
- *Maintenance Doses:* **Trastuzumab** 6 mg/kg; administer intravenously in 250 mL 0.9% NS over 30 minutes before pertuzumab on day 1, every 3 weeks for up to 17 cycles not to exceed 52 weeks of total trastuzumab therapy (total dosage/3-week cycle = 6 mg/kg)
  - ▪ *Note:* If a patient misses a 6-mg/kg trastuzumab dose by more than 7 days, a re-loading dose of trastuzumab should be given as trastuzumab 8 mg/kg (loading dose); administer intravenously in 250 mL 0.9% NS over 90 minutes once. This should be followed 21 days later by resumption of 6-mg/kg maintenance doses repeated every 3 weeks

Pertuzumab every 21 days for up to 18 cycles (not to exceed 52 weeks of total pertuzumab therapy):
- *Loading Dose:* **Pertuzumab** 840 mg initial (loading) dose; administer intravenously in 250 mL 0.9% NS over 60 minutes as a loading dose after trastuzumab on day 1, cycle 1 only (total dosage during the first cycle = 840 mg), *followed 3 weeks later by:*
- *Maintenance Doses:* **Pertuzumab** 420 mg per dose; administer intravenously in 250 mL 0.9% NS over 30–60 minutes after trastuzumab on day 1, every 3 weeks for up to 17 cycles not to exceed 52 weeks of total pertuzumab therapy (total dosage/3-week cycle = 420 mg)
  - ▪ *Note:* If a patient misses a 420-mg pertuzumab dose by more than 21 days (ie, ≥6 weeks between two sequential infusions), a re-loading dose of pertuzumab should be given as pertuzumab 840-mg (loading) dose; administer intravenously in 250 mL 0.9% NS over 60 minutes as a loading dose once. This should be followed 21 days later by resumption of 420-mg maintenance doses repeated every 3 weeks

Alternatively, a fixed dose combination product containing pertuzumab, trastuzumab, and hyaluronidase (PHESGO™) for subcutaneous injection may be used instead of intravenous pertuzumab and trastuzumab as follows:
- *Loading Dose:* **Pertuzumab, trastuzumab, and hyaluronidase (PHESGO™) for subcutaneous injection** 1200 mg, 600 mg, and 30,000 units, respectively; administer as a 15 mL subcutaneous injection into the thigh over 8 minutes once on day 1, cycle 1 only (total dosage during the first cycle = 1200 mg pertuzumab, 600 mg trastuzumab, and 30,000 units hyaluronidase), *followed 3 weeks later by:*
- *Maintenance Doses:* **Pertuzumab, trastuzumab, and hyaluronidase (PHESGO™) for subcutaneous injection** 600 mg, 600 mg, and 20,000 units, respectively; administer as a 10 mL subcutaneous injection into the thigh over 5 minutes on day 1, every 3 weeks, for up to 17 cycles not to exceed 52 weeks of total therapy (total dosage/3-week cycle = 600 mg pertuzumab, 600 mg trastuzumab, and 20,000 units hyaluronidase)
  - ▪ *Notes:*
    - ○ Alternate the injection site between the left and right thigh, avoiding the last injection site by ≥2.5 cm. Avoid injection into areas that are hard, red, bruised, or tender.
    - ○ Observe patients for at least 30 minutes after the loading dose and for at least 15 minutes after maintenance doses.
    - ○ If a scheduled injection is delayed and the interval between injections is <6 weeks, then administer the maintenance dose. If the interval between injections is ≥6 weeks, then administer a loading dose followed 3 weeks later by resumption of maintenance dosing.

Prophylaxis for fluid retention and hypersensitivity reactions from docetaxel:

Dexamethasone 8 mg/dose; administer orally twice daily for 3 days, starting on the day before docetaxel administration (total dose/cycle = 48 mg)

(continued)

Docetaxel 75 mg/m^2; administer intravenously in a volume of 0.9% NS or 5% dextrose injection (D5W) sufficient to produce a final docetaxel concentration of 0.3–0.74 mg/mL over 60 minutes after pertuzumab on day 1, every 3 weeks for 4 cycles (total dosage/cycle = 75 mg/m^2)

• *Notes:*
  ▪ Some formulations of docetaxel contain alcohol; use caution or consider using a non–alcohol-containing formulation in patients who are sensitive to alcohol

Supportive Care
Antiemetic prophylaxis
Emetogenic potential on days with docetaxel or pertuzumab is **LOW**
See Chapter 42 for antiemetic recommendations

Hematopoietic growth factor (CSF) prophylaxis
Primary prophylaxis may be indicated (only applies to docetaxel cycles)
See Chapter 43 for more information

Antimicrobial prophylaxis
Risk of fever and neutropenia is **LOW**
  Antimicrobial primary prophylaxis to be considered:
  • Antibacterial—not indicated
  • Antifungal—not indicated
  • Antiviral—not indicated, unless patient previously had an episode of HSV

Diarrhea management
Latent or delayed-onset diarrhea:
Loperamide 4 mg orally initially after the first loose or liquid stool, *then*
Loperamide 2 mg orally every 2 hours during waking hours, *plus*
Loperamide 4 mg orally every 4 hours during hours of sleep
• Continue for at least 12 hours after diarrhea resolves
• Recurrent diarrhea after a 12-hour diarrhea-free interval is treated as a new episode
• Rehydrate orally with fluids and electrolytes during a diarrheal episode
• If a patient develops blood or mucus in stool, dehydration, or hemodynamic instability, or if diarrhea persists >48 hours despite loperamide, stop loperamide and evaluate urgently in clinic or hospitalize the patient for IV hydration
• Alternatively, a trial of **diphenoxylate hydrochloride** 2.5 mg with **atropine sulfate** 0.025 mg (eg, Lomotil)
• Initial adult dose is 2 tablets 4 times daily until control has been achieved, after which the dose may be reduced to meet individual requirements. Control may often be maintained with as little as 2 tablets daily
• Clinical improvement of acute diarrhea is usually observed within 48 hours. If improvement of chronic diarrhea after treatment with a maximum daily dose of 8 tablets is not observed within 10 days, control is unlikely with further administration

Patient Population Studied

This prospective, multicenter, double-blind, randomized, placebo-controlled trial involved 4805 patients with nonmetastatic, adequately excised, invasive HER2-positive breast cancer. Eligible patients had node-positive or high-risk node-negative disease and baseline left ventricular ejection fraction ≥55%. All patients had to receive their first dose of chemotherapy within 8 weeks of definitive breast surgery. All patients received standard adjuvant chemotherapy and intravenous trastuzumab (8-mg/kg loading dose and then 6 mg/kg every 3 weeks for a maximum of 18 weeks). Patients were randomly assigned to also receive intravenously either placebo or pertuzumab (840-mg loading dose and then 420 g every 3 weeks for a maximum of 18 weeks). Patients with hormone receptor–positive disease received standard endocrine therapy from the end of chemotherapy and were supposed to continue with this therapy for at least 5 years. Radiotherapy was administered as clinically indicated after chemotherapy and concurrently with anti-HER2 therapy

Efficacy (N = 4805)

	Pertuzumab + Trastuzumab + Standard Adjuvant Chemotherapy (N = 2400)	Placebo + Trastuzumab + Standard Adjuvant Chemotherapy (N = 2405)	
3-year survival free from invasive disease	94.1%	93.2%	HR 0.81, 95% CI 0.66–1.00; P = 0.045
Overall survival	96.7%	96.3%	HR 0.89, 95% CI 0.66–1.21; P = 0.467

Note: Median follow-up was 45.4 months

Therapy Monitoring

1. Prior to each cycle of docetaxel: CBC with differential, serum electrolytes, BUN, creatinine, AST or ALT, and alkaline phosphatase
2. Conduct thorough cardiac assessment, including history, physical examination, and determination of LVEF by echocardiogram or MUGA scan at baseline immediately prior to initiation of trastuzumab and every 3 months during therapy
3. Patients should have a pre-treatment LVEF ≥55%
4. Repeat LVEF measurement at 4-week intervals if trastuzumab and/or pertuzumab are withheld for significant left ventricular cardiac dysfunction
5. Monitor for symptoms of pulmonary toxicity
6. Verify pregnancy status prior to the initiation of therapy. Advise patients of the risks of embryo-fetal death and birth defects and the need for contraception
7. Avoid using concomitant strong CYP3A4 inhibitors (eg, ketoconazole, itraconazole, clarithromycin, atazanavir, indinavir, nefazodone, nelfinavir, ritonavir, saquinavir, telithromycin, and voriconazole). Consider a 50% docetaxel dose reduction if patients require co-administration of a strong CYP3A4 inhibitor

Treatment Modifications

DOCETAXEL DOSE MODIFICATIONS

Docetaxel starting dose	75 mg/m^2
Docetaxel dose level −1	60 mg/m^2
Docetaxel dose level −2	50 mg/m^2
Docetaxel dose level −3	Discontinue docetaxel

Adverse Event	Treatment Modifications
Severe hypersensitivity reaction	Discontinue infusion immediately and administer appropriate support. For hypersensitivity reaction less G ≤3, initial management includes temporary discontinuation of infusion for 30 minutes, and administration of additional intravenous antihistamines and glucocorticoids. Upon resolution of symptoms, infusion may be restarted at a slower rate if deemed safe. If G4 hypersensitivity is experienced, stabilize the cardiorespiratory system and use epinephrine as needed, then permanently discontinue docetaxel*
Febrile neutropenia (ANC <1000/mm^3 with temperature >38°C or >100.4°F), or ANC <500/mm^3 for ≥7 days	Withhold treatment until resolution of toxicity. Administer filgrastim in subsequent cycles
Febrile neutropenia (ANC <1000/mm^3 with temperature >38°C or >100.4°F), or ANC <500/mm^3 for ≥7 days despite administration of filgrastim	Reduce docetaxel one dose level; continue filgrastim administration
Platelet nadir <50,000/mm^3, or platelets <100,000/mm^3 for ≥7 days	Reduce docetaxel dose by one level
ANC <1500/mm^3 or platelets <100,000/mm^3 at the start of a cycle	Hold treatment until ANC≥1500/mm^3 and platelets ≥100,000/mm^3, then resume with docetaxel dosage reduced by one dose level
Bilirubin > ULN, or AST/ALT >1.5 × ULN and AP >2.5 × ULN	Withhold docetaxel until bilirubin ≤ ULN or AST/ALT ≤1.5 and AP ≤2.5 × ULN, then resume docetaxel dosage reduced by one dose level
Severe or cumulative cutaneous reactions	Withhold treatment until resolution of toxicity. Reduce docetaxel dosage one dose level
G3/4 stomatitis	
G1 neurotoxicity of any duration (paresthesias/dysesthesias that do not interfere with function)	Continue docetaxel treatment
G2 neurotoxicity of 1–7 days duration (paresthesias/dysesthesias interfering with function, but not activities of daily living)	Continue docetaxel treatment but can delay start for up to seven days until G ≤1

(continued)

Treatment Modifications (continued)

Adverse Event	Treatment Modifications
G2 neurotoxicity of >7 days duration (paresthesias/dysesthesias interfering with function, but not activities of daily living)	Withhold docetaxel until toxicity G ≤1, then resume docetaxel treatment, but reduce dose by one dose level. If G2 toxicity persists after 3 weeks of delay, discontinue docetaxel*
G3 neurotoxicity of 1–7 days duration (paresthesias/dysesthesias with pain or with function impairment interfering with activities of daily living)	Withhold docetaxel. Resume with docetaxel dose reduced one dose level when toxicity has resolved to G ≤1
Second episode of G3 neurotoxicity of 1–7 days duration (paresthesias/dysesthesias with pain or with function impairment interfering with activities of daily living)	Discontinue docetaxel*
G3 neurotoxicity of >7 days duration (paresthesias/dysesthesias with pain or with function impairment interfering with activities of daily living)	Discontinue docetaxel*
Persistent paresthesias/dysesthesias that are disabling or life-threatening	Discontinue docetaxel*
G1 musculoskeletal pain not controlled by analgesics of any duration	Continue docetaxel treatment
G2 musculoskeletal pain not controlled by analgesics of 1–7 days duration	
G2 musculoskeletal pain not controlled by analgesics of >7 days duration	Continue docetaxel treatment or withhold docetaxel for persistent G2. When toxicity G ≤1, resume treatment with dose that is one dose lower. If G2 toxicity persists resulting in a delay of >3 weeks, discontinue docetaxel*
First episode of G3 musculoskeletal pain not controlled by analgesics of 1–7 days duration	Continue docetaxel treatment
Second episode of G3 musculoskeletal pain not controlled by analgesics of 1–7 days duration	Discontinue docetaxel*
First episode of G3 musculoskeletal pain not controlled by analgesics of >7 days duration	Withhold docetaxel. When toxicity G ≤1, resume treatment with dose that is one dose level lower. If >G2 toxicity persists resulting in a delay of >3 weeks, discontinue docetaxel*
Second episode of G3 musculoskeletal pain not controlled by analgesics of >7 days duration	Discontinue docetaxel*
Docetaxel-related fluid retention	Consider 1- to 5-day treatment with dexamethasone starting one day before docetaxel administration. Consider diuretics for symptomatic relief and to limit the severity of fluid retention
Other G2 nonhematologic adverse event that occurs during a cycle but results in a delay in the start of the next cycle	Hold treatment until adverse events resolve to G ≤1, then resume with docetaxel dosage reduced by one dose level
Other G3 nonhematologic adverse event that occurs during a cycle but resolves prior to the start of the next cycle or requires a delay in the start of the next cycle	Hold treatment until adverse events resolve to G ≤1, then resume with docetaxel dosage reduced by one dose level
Other G4 nonhematologic adverse event that occurs during a cycle but resolves prior to the start of the next cycle	Hold treatment until adverse events resolve to G ≤1, then resume with docetaxel dosage reduced by two dose levels or discontinue docetaxel*
Other G4 nonhematologic adverse event that occurs during a cycle but requires a delay in the start of the next cycle	Discontinue docetaxel*
Any treatment delay >3 weeks	Discontinue docetaxel*

PERTUZUMAB AND TRASTUZUMAB

Note: Dose reductions are not recommended for trastuzumab or pertuzumab. If the adverse event is clearly attributable to either pertuzumab or trastuzumab, then treatment with the other medication not responsible for the adverse event may be continued without interruption at the discretion of the medically responsible health care provider

(continued)

Treatment Modifications (continued)

Adverse Event	Treatment Modifications
Mild or moderate infusion reaction	Decrease the rate of infusion
Infusion reaction with dyspnea or clinically significant hypotension	Interrupt the infusion. Administer medical therapy as indicated including epinephrine, corticosteroids, diphenhydramine, bronchodilators, and oxygen. Observe patients closely for 60 minutes if the reaction occurs after the first infusion and for 30 minutes if it occurs after subsequent infusions. Prior to resumption of the infusion, premedicate with antihistamines and/or corticosteroids. Note: While some patients tolerate the resumption of infusions, others have recurrent severe infusion reactions despite premedications
Severe or life-threatening infusion reaction (including bronchospasm, anaphylaxis, angioedema, hypoxia, and severe hypotension; usually reported during or immediately following the initial infusion)	Interrupt the infusion. Administer medical therapy as indicated including epinephrine, corticosteroids, diphenhydramine, bronchodilators, and oxygen. Patients should be evaluated and carefully monitored until complete resolution of signs and symptoms. Discontinue the offending agent. If trastuzumab is discontinued, then pertuzumab should also be discontinued
LVEF has declined by ≥16 percentage points from baseline, or has declined by 10–15 percentage points from baseline to a value below the lower limit of the normal range OR Symptomatic congestive heart failure	Withhold pertuzumab and trastuzumab and repeat LVEF assessment at 4-week intervals until improvement, which may require prolonged interruption. For a persistent decline in LVEF, consider a cardio-oncology consultation and weigh the benefits and risks of continuing pertuzumab and trastuzumab in the individual patient

*If docetaxel is discontinued or withheld beyond the time of start of the next cycle, treatment with pertuzumab and trastuzumab may continue

Adverse Events (N = 4769)

Grade ≥3 Adverse Events (%)	Pertuzumab + Trastuzumab + Standard Adjuvant Chemotherapy (N = 2364)	Placebo + Trastuzumab + Standard Adjuvant Chemotherapy (N = 2405)
All	64	57
Neutropenia	16	16
Febrile neutropenia	12	11
Decreased neutrophil count	10	10
Diarrhea	10	4
Anemia	7	5

Toxicities included in the table are grade ≥3 events that occurred in ≥5% of patients in either treatment group. Fatal adverse events occurred in 0.8% of each treatment group. Primary cardiac events occurred in 0.7% of the pertuzumab group and 0.3% of the placebo group. Secondary cardiac events occurred in 2.7% of the pertuzumab group and 2.8% of the placebo group. A total of 7.8% of patients in the pertuzumab group and 6.4% of patients in the placebo group discontinued treatment for safety reasons

ADJUVANT • HER2-POSITIVE

BREAST CANCER REGIMEN: WEEKLY PACLITAXEL + TRASTUZUMAB + PERTUZUMAB

von Minckwitz G et al. N Engl J Med 2017;377:122–131
Protocol for: von Minckwitz G et al. N Engl J Med 2017;377:122–131

The regimen consists of 1 year of adjuvant pertuzumab + trastuzumab therapy given with a standard adjuvant chemotherapy regimen, initiated concurrent with taxane (paclitaxel or docetaxel) therapy. Standard chemotherapy regimens studied included (1) carboplatin + docetaxel × 6 cycles; (2) fluorouracil + epirubicin + cyclophosphamide (FEC) × 3–4 cycles followed by either docetaxel × 4 doses or weekly paclitaxel × 12 doses; and (3) doxorubicin + cyclophosphamide (AC) or epirubicin + cyclophosphamide (EC) × 4 cycles followed by either docetaxel × 4 doses or weekly paclitaxel × 12 doses. Hormonal therapy and/or radiation therapy, when indicated, are initiated after completion of taxane (paclitaxel or docetaxel) therapy and may be given concurrent with trastuzumab + pertuzumab. **The below regimen describes the combination of adjuvant weekly paclitaxel + trastuzumab + pertuzumab intended to be used after completion of anthracycline-based chemotherapy (ie, FEC × 3–4 cycles or AC × 4 cycles).** Please refer to separate descriptions of FEC and AC regimens

Adjuvant weekly paclitaxel + trastuzumab + pertuzumab [initiate after completion of anthracycline-based adjuvant chemotherapy such as fluorouracil + epirubicin + cyclophosphamide (FEC) × 3–4 cycles or doxorubicin + cyclophosphamide (AC) × 4 cycles]

Trastuzumab every 21 days for up to 18 cycles (not to exceed 52 weeks of total trastuzumab therapy):
- *Loading Dose:* **Trastuzumab** 8 mg/kg; administer intravenously in 250 mL 0.9% sodium chloride injection (0.9% NS) over 90 minutes as a loading dose before pertuzumab on day 1, cycle 1 only (total dosage during the first cycle = 8 mg/kg), *followed 3 weeks later by:*
  - *Note:* A syndrome most commonly consisting of chills and/or fever may occur in as many as 40% of patients during the first infusion of trastuzumab. These symptoms occur infrequently with subsequent trastuzumab infusions. Other signs and/or symptoms may include nausea, vomiting, pain (in some cases at tumor sites), rigors, headache, dizziness, dyspnea, hypotension, rash, and asthenia. Although the symptoms are usually mild to moderate in severity, infrequently, trastuzumab may need to be discontinued
  - When such a syndrome is observed, it can be treated with or without reduction in the rate of trastuzumab infusion, and:
    - **Acetaminophen** 650 mg; administer orally, *plus:*
    - **Diphenhydramine** 25–50 mg; administer orally or by intravenous injection, *plus:*
    - **Meperidine** 12.5–25 mg; administer by intravenous injection every 10 minutes if needed for shaking chills (generally, cumulative doses >50 mg are not needed; use with caution in persons with moderate or more severely impaired renal function)
- *Maintenance Doses:* **Trastuzumab** 6 mg/kg; administer intravenously in 250 mL 0.9% NS over 30 minutes before pertuzumab on day 1, every 3 weeks for up to 17 cycles not to exceed 52 weeks of total trastuzumab therapy (total dosage/3-week cycle = 6 mg/kg)
  - *Note:* If a patient misses a 6-mg/kg trastuzumab dose by more than 7 days, a re-loading dose of trastuzumab should be given as trastuzumab 8 mg/kg (loading dose); administer intravenously in 250 mL 0.9% NS over 90 minutes once. This should be followed 21 days later by resumption of 6-mg/kg maintenance doses repeated every 3 weeks

Pertuzumab every 21 days for up to 18 cycles (not to exceed 52 weeks of total pertuzumab therapy):
- *Loading Dose:* **Pertuzumab** 840 mg initial (loading) dose; administer intravenously in 250 mL 0.9% NS over 60 minutes as a loading dose after trastuzumab on day 1, cycle 1 only (total dosage during the first cycle = 840 mg), *followed 3 weeks later by:*
- *Maintenance Doses:* **Pertuzumab** 420 mg per dose; administer intravenously in 250 mL 0.9% NS over 30–60 minutes after trastuzumab on day 1, every 3 weeks for up to 17 cycles not to exceed 52 weeks of total pertuzumab therapy (total dosage/3-week cycle = 420 mg)
  - *Note:* If a patient misses a 420-mg pertuzumab dose by more than 21 days (ie, ≥6 weeks between two sequential infusions), a re-loading dose of pertuzumab should be given as pertuzumab 840-mg (loading) dose; administer intravenously in 250 mL 0.9% NS over 60 minutes as a loading dose once. This should be followed 21 days later by resumption of 420-mg maintenance doses repeated every 3 weeks

Alternatively, a fixed dose combination product containing pertuzumab, trastuzumab, and hyaluronidase (PHESGO™) for subcutaneous injection may be used instead of intravenous pertuzumab and trastuzumab as follows:
- *Loading Dose:* **Pertuzumab, trastuzumab, and hyaluronidase (PHESGO™)** for subcutaneous injection 1200 mg, 600 mg, and 30,000 units, respectively; administer as a 15 mL subcutaneous injection into the thigh over 8 minutes once on day 1, cycle 1 only (total dosage during the first cycle = 1200 mg pertuzumab, 600 mg trastuzumab, and 30,000 units hyaluronidase), *followed 3 weeks later by:*
- *Maintenance Doses:* **Pertuzumab, trastuzumab, and hyaluronidase (PHESGO™)** for subcutaneous injection 600 mg, 600 mg, and 20,000 units, respectively; administer as a 10 mL subcutaneous injection into the thigh over 5 minutes on day 1, every 3 weeks, for up to 17 cycles not to exceed 52 weeks of total therapy (total dosage/3-week cycle = 600 mg pertuzumab, 600 mg trastuzumab, and 20,000 units hyaluronidase)
  - *Notes:*
    - Alternate the injection site between the left and right thigh, avoiding the last injection site by ≥2.5 cm. Avoid injection into areas that are hard, red, bruised, or tender.
    - Observe patients for at least 30 minutes after the loading dose and for at least 15 minutes after maintenance doses.
    - If a scheduled injection is delayed and the interval between injections is <6 weeks, then administer the maintenance dose. If the interval between injections is ≥6 weeks, then administer a loading dose followed 3 weeks later by resumption of maintenance dosing.

(continued)

(continued)

Premedications for paclitaxel:

Dexamethasone 10 mg; administer intravenously 30–60 minutes before each paclitaxel dose

Diphenhydramine 50 mg; administer intravenously 30–60 minutes before each paclitaxel dose

Cimetidine 300 mg (or **ranitidine** 50 mg, or **famotidine** 20 mg, or an equivalent histamine receptor [H_2]-subtype antagonist); administer intravenously over 15–30 minutes, 30–60 minutes before each paclitaxel dose

Paclitaxel 80 mg/m² per dose; administer intravenously in a volume of 0.9% NS or 5% dextrose injection (D5W) sufficient to produce a concentration within the range 0.3–1.2 mg/mL over 60 minutes, on day 1, 8, and 15, every 21 days for 4 cycles (total dosage per week = 80 mg/m²; total dosage per 3-week cycle = 240 mg/m²)

Note: Administer paclitaxel after pertuzumab on days when trastuzumab and pertuzumab are also scheduled

Supportive Care
Antiemetic prophylaxis
Emetogenic potential on days with paclitaxel is **LOW**

Emetogenic potential on days with pertuzumab and trastuzumab (without paclitaxel) is **MINIMAL**

See Chapter 42 for antiemetic recommendations

Hematopoietic growth factor (CSF) prophylaxis
Primary prophylaxis is not indicated

See Chapter 43 for more information

Antimicrobial prophylaxis
Risk of fever and neutropenia is **LOW**

Antimicrobial primary prophylaxis to be considered:

- Antibacterial—not indicated

- Antifungal—not indicated

- Antiviral—not indicated, unless patient previously had an episode of HSV

Diarrhea management
Latent or delayed-onset diarrhea:

Loperamide 4 mg orally initially after the first loose or liquid stool, *then*

Loperamide 2 mg orally every 2 hours during waking hours, *plus*

Loperamide 4 mg orally every 4 hours during hours of sleep

- Continue for at least 12 hours after diarrhea resolves

- Recurrent diarrhea after a 12-hour diarrhea-free interval is treated as a new episode

- Rehydrate orally with fluids and electrolytes during a diarrheal episode

- If a patient develops blood or mucus in stool, dehydration, or hemodynamic instability, or if diarrhea persists >48 hours despite loperamide, stop loperamide and evaluate urgently in clinic or hospitalize the patient for IV hydration

- Alternatively, a trial of **diphenoxylate hydrochloride** 2.5 mg with **atropine sulfate** 0.025 mg (eg, Lomotil)

- Initial adult dose is 2 tablets 4 times daily until control has been achieved, after which the dose may be reduced to meet individual requirements. Control may often be maintained with as little as 2 tablets daily

- Clinical improvement of acute diarrhea is usually observed within 48 hours. If improvement of chronic diarrhea after treatment with a maximum daily dose of 8 tablets is not observed within 10 days, control is unlikely with further administration

Patient Population Studied

This prospective, multicenter, double-blind, randomized, placebo-controlled trial involved 4805 patients with nonmetastatic, adequately excised, invasive HER2-positive breast cancer. Eligible patients had node-positive or high-risk node-negative disease and baseline left ventricular ejection fraction ≥55%. All patients had to receive their first dose of chemotherapy within 8 weeks of definitive breast surgery. All patients received standard adjuvant chemotherapy and intravenous trastuzumab (8-mg/kg loading dose and then 6 mg/kg every 3 weeks for a maximum of 18 weeks). Patients were randomly assigned to also receive intravenously either placebo or pertuzumab (840-mg loading dose and then 420 g every 3 weeks for a maximum of 18 weeks). Patients with hormone receptor–positive disease received standard endocrine therapy from the end of chemotherapy and were supposed to continue with this therapy for at least 5 years. Radiotherapy was administered as clinically indicated after chemotherapy and concurrently with anti-HER2 therapy

Efficacy (N = 4805)

	Pertuzumab + Trastuzumab + Standard Adjuvant Chemotherapy (N = 2400)	Placebo + Trastuzumab + Standard Adjuvant Chemotherapy (N = 2405)	
3-year survival free from invasive disease	94.1%	93.2%	HR 0.81, 95% CI 0.66–1.00; P = 0.045
Overall survival	96.7%	96.3%	HR 0.89, 95% CI 0.66–1.21; P = 0.467

Note: Median follow-up was 45.4 months

Therapy Monitoring

1. Before the start of treatment: CBC with differential, serum electrolytes, BUN, creatinine, AST or ALT, and alkaline phosphatase
2. Once per week during paclitaxel therapy: CBC with differential, serum electrolytes, BUN, creatinine, AST or ALT, and alkaline phosphatase
3. Conduct thorough cardiac assessment, including history, physical examination, and determination of LVEF by echocardiogram or MUGA scan at baseline immediately prior to initiation of trastuzumab and every 3 months during therapy
4. Patients should have a pre-treatment LVEF ≥55%
5. Repeat LVEF measurement at 4-week intervals if trastuzumab and/or pertuzumab are withheld for significant left ventricular cardiac dysfunction
6. Monitor for symptoms of pulmonary toxicity
7. Verify pregnancy status prior to the initiation of therapy. Advise patients of the risks of embryo-fetal death and birth defects and the need for contraception
8. Avoid using concomitant strong CYP3A4 inhibitors (eg, ketoconazole, itraconazole, clarithromycin, atazanavir, indinavir, nefazodone, nelfinavir, ritonavir, saquinavir, telithromycin, and voriconazole). Consider a 50% paclitaxel dose reduction if patients require co-administration of a strong CYP3A4 inhibitor

Treatment Modifications

PACLITAXEL DOSE MODIFICATIONS

Paclitaxel starting dose	80 mg/m^2
Paclitaxel dose level −1	64 mg/m^2
Paclitaxel dose level −2	Discontinue paclitaxel

Adverse Event	Treatment Modifications
Severe hypersensitivity reaction	Discontinue infusion immediately and administer appropriate support. For hypersensitivity reaction G ≤3, initial management includes temporary discontinuation of infusion for 30 minutes, and administration of additional intravenous antihistamines and glucocorticoids. Upon resolution of symptoms, infusion may be restarted at a slower rate if deemed safe. If G4 hypersensitivity is experienced, stabilize the cardiorespiratory system and use epinephrine as needed, then permanently discontinue paclitaxel*
Febrile neutropenia (ANC <1000/mm^3 with temperature >38°C or >100.4°F), or ANC <500/mm^3 for ≥7 days	Withhold treatment until resolution of toxicity. Administer filgrastim in subsequent cycles
Febrile neutropenia (ANC <1000/mm^3 with temperature >38°C or >100.4°F), or ANC <500/mm^3 for ≥7 days despite administration of filgrastim	Reduce paclitaxel one dose level; continue filgrastim administration
Platelet nadir <50,000/mm^3, or platelets <100,000/mm^3 for ≥7 days	Reduce paclitaxel dose by one level
ANC ≤800/mm^3 or platelets ≤50,000/mm^3 at the start of a cycle	Hold treatment until ANC >800/mm^3 and platelets >50,000/mm^3, then resume with paclitaxel dosage reduced by one dose level

(continued)

Treatment Modifications (continued)

Adverse Event	Treatment Modifications
AST/ALT >2 to ≤10 × ULN and bilirubin <2× ULN,	Withhold paclitaxel until AST/ALT <2× ULN then resume with paclitaxel dosage reduced by one dose level
AST/ALT >10 × ULN and/or bilirubin >5× ULN	Discontinue paclitaxel*
G3/4 stomatitis	Withhold treatment until resolution of toxicity. Reduce paclitaxel dosage one dose level
G1 neurotoxicity of any duration (paresthesias/dysesthesias that do not interfere with function)	Continue paclitaxel treatment
G2 neurotoxicity of 1–7 days duration (paresthesias/dysesthesias interfering with function, but not activities of daily living)	Continue paclitaxel treatment but can delay start for up to seven days until G ≤1
G2 neurotoxicity of >7 days duration (paresthesias/dysesthesias interfering with function, but not activities of daily living)	Withhold paclitaxel until toxicity G ≤1, then resume paclitaxel treatment, but reduce dose by one dose level. If G2 toxicity persists after 3 weeks of delay, discontinue paclitaxel*
G3 neurotoxicity of 1–7 days duration (paresthesias/dysesthesias with pain or with function impairment interfering with activities of daily living)	Withhold paclitaxel. Resume with paclitaxel dose reduced one dose level when toxicity has resolved to G ≤1
Second episode of G3 neurotoxicity of 1–7 days duration (paresthesias/dysesthesias with pain or with function impairment interfering with activities of daily living)	Discontinue paclitaxel*
G3 neurotoxicity of >7 days duration (paresthesias/dysesthesias with pain or with function impairment interfering with activities of daily living)	Discontinue paclitaxel*
Persistent paresthesias/dysesthesias that are disabling or life-threatening	Discontinue paclitaxel*
G1 musculoskeletal pain not controlled by analgesics of any duration	Continue paclitaxel treatment
G2 musculoskeletal pain not controlled by analgesics of 1–7 days duration	
G2 musculoskeletal pain not controlled by analgesics of >7 days duration	Continue paclitaxel treatment or withhold paclitaxel for persistent G2. When toxicity G ≤1, resume treatment with dose that is one dose level lower. If G2 toxicity persists resulting in a delay of >3 weeks, discontinue paclitaxel*
First episode of G3 musculoskeletal pain not controlled by analgesics of 1–7 days duration	Continue paclitaxel treatment
Second episode of G3 musculoskeletal pain not controlled by analgesics of 1–7 days duration	Discontinue paclitaxel*
First episode of G3 musculoskeletal pain not controlled by analgesics of >7 days duration	Withhold paclitaxel. When toxicity G ≤1, resume treatment with dose that is one dose lower. If >G2 toxicity persists resulting in a delay of >3 weeks, discontinue paclitaxel*
Second episode of G3 musculoskeletal pain not controlled by analgesics of >7 days duration	Discontinue paclitaxel*
Other G2 nonhematologic adverse event that occurs during a cycle but results in a delay in the start of the next cycle	Hold treatment until adverse events resolve to G ≤1, then resume with paclitaxel dosage reduced by one dose level
Other G3 nonhematologic adverse event that occurs during a cycle but resolves prior to the start of the next cycle or requires a delay in the start of the next cycle	Hold treatment until adverse events resolve to G ≤1, then resume with paclitaxel dosage reduced by one dose level
Other G4 nonhematologic adverse event that occurs during a cycle but resolves prior to the start of the next cycle	Hold treatment until adverse events resolve to G ≤1, then resume with paclitaxel dosage reduced by two dose levels or discontinue paclitaxel*
Other G4 nonhematologic adverse event that occurs during a cycle but requires a delay in the start of the next cycle	Discontinue paclitaxel*
Any treatment delay >3 weeks	Discontinue paclitaxel*

(continued)

Treatment Modifications (*continued*)

PERTUZUMAB AND TRASTUZUMAB

Note: Dose reductions are not recommended for trastuzumab or pertuzumab

Adverse Event	Treatment Modifications
Mild or moderate infusion reaction	Decrease the rate of infusion
Infusion reaction with dyspnea or clinically significant hypotension	Interrupt the infusion. Administer medical therapy as indicated including epinephrine, corticosteroids, diphenhydramine, bronchodilators, and oxygen. Observe patients closely for 60 minutes if the reaction occurs after the first infusion and for 30 minutes if it occurs after subsequent infusions. Prior to resumption of the infusion, premedicate with antihistamines and/or corticosteroids. Note: While some patients tolerate the resumption of infusions, others have recurrent severe infusion reactions despite premedications
Severe or life-threatening infusion reaction (including bronchospasm, anaphylaxis, angioedema, hypoxia, and severe hypotension; usually reported during or immediately following the initial infusion)	Interrupt the infusion. Administer medical therapy as indicated including epinephrine, corticosteroids, diphenhydramine, bronchodilators, and oxygen. Patients should be evaluated and carefully monitored until complete resolution of signs and symptoms. Discontinue the offending agent. If trastuzumab is discontinued, then pertuzumab should also be discontinued
LVEF has declined by ≥16 percentage points from baseline, or has declined by 10–15 percentage points from baseline to a value below the lower limit of the normal range OR Symptomatic congestive heart failure	Withhold pertuzumab and trastuzumab and repeat LVEF assessment at 4-week intervals until improvement, which may require prolonged interruption. For a persistent decline in LVEF, consider a cardio-oncology consultation and weigh the benefits and risks of continuing pertuzumab and trastuzumab in the individual patient

*If paclitaxel is discontinued or withheld beyond the time of start of the next cycle, treatment with pertuzumab and trastuzumab may continue

Adverse Events (N = 4769)

Grade ≥3 Adverse Events (%)	Pertuzumab + Trastuzumab + Standard Adjuvant Chemotherapy (N = 2364)	Placebo + Trastuzumab + Standard Adjuvant Chemotherapy (N = 2405)
All	64	57
Neutropenia	16	16
Febrile neutropenia	12	11
Decreased neutrophil count	10	10
Diarrhea	10	4
Anemia	7	5

Toxicities included in the table are grade ≥3 events that occurred in ≥5% of patients in either treatment group. Fatal adverse events occurred in 0.8% of each treatment group. Primary cardiac events occurred in 0.7% of the pertuzumab group and 0.3% of the placebo group. Secondary cardiac events occurred in 2.7% of the pertuzumab group and 2.8% of the placebo group. A total of 7.8% of patients in the pertuzumab group and 6.4% of patients in the placebo group discontinued treatment for safety reasons

ADJUVANT • HER2-POSITIVE

BREAST CANCER REGIMEN: ADJUVANT ADO-TRASTUZUMAB EMTANSINE (T-DM1) FOR RESIDUAL INVASIVE CARCINOMA AFTER NEOADJUVANT CHEMOTHERAPY + TRASTUZUMAB

von Minckwitz G et al. N Engl J Med 2019;380:617–628
Protocol for: von Minckwitz G et al. N Engl J Med 2019;380:617–628
Supplementary appendix to: von Minckwitz G et al. N Engl J Med 2019;380:617–628

ado-Trastuzumab emtansine 3.6 mg/kg; administer intravenously in 250 mL 0.9% sodium chloride injection on day 1, every 21 days, for 14 cycles (total dosage/3-week cycle = 3.6 mg/kg)

Exposure	Administration Rate	Monitoring
First infusion	Intravenously over 90 minutes	• Patients should be observed closely for infusion-related reactions, especially during the first infusion
Second and subsequent infusions	1. Intravenously over 30 minutes if prior administration was tolerated 2. Subsequent doses may be administered at the rate tolerated during the most recently administered treatment	• Administration should be slowed or interrupted if a patient develops an infusion-related reaction • Permanently discontinue ado-trastuzumab emtansine for life-threatening infusion-related reactions

Notes:
• Administer ado-trastuzumab emtansine through an administration set that contains a sterile, non-pyrogenic, low protein-binding in-line polyethersulfone filter with pore size within the range of 0.2–0.22 μm
• Ado-trastuzumab emtansine should be initiated within 12 weeks following surgery
• Patients who could not tolerate ado-trastuzumab emtansine were allowed, at the investigator's discretion, to complete the remainder of adjuvant therapy with trastuzumab
• Adjuvant endocrine therapy (eg, tamoxifen or an aromatase inhibitor) may be administered concomitantly with ado-trastuzumab emtansine for patients with hormone receptor–positive (ie, estrogen receptor and/or progesterone receptor) disease
• Adjuvant radiation therapy, when indicated, may be given concomitantly with ado-trastuzumab emtansine

Supportive Care
Antiemetic prophylaxis
Emetogenic potential is **LOW**
See Chapter 42 for antiemetic recommendations

Hematopoietic growth factor (CSF) prophylaxis
Primary prophylaxis is not indicated
See Chapter 43 for more information

Antimicrobial prophylaxis
Risk of fever and neutropenia is **LOW**
  Antimicrobial primary prophylaxis to be considered:
  • Antibacterial—not indicated
  • Antifungal—not indicated
  • Antiviral—not indicated, unless patient previously had an episode of HSV

Patient Population Studied

The multicenter, randomized, open-label, phase 3 study involved 1486 patients with HER2-positive early breast cancer (clinical T1–4, N0–3, M0 at presentation; excluding clinical stage T1aN0 and T1bN0) who had undergone taxane-based neoadjuvant chemotherapy including at least 9 weeks of preoperative trastuzumab and who were found to have residual invasive disease in the breast or axillary lymph node surgical specimen. Prior neoadjuvant use of anthracyclines, alkylating agents, and other HER2-targeted agents was also permitted. Patients with gross residual disease after mastectomy, positive margins following breast-conserving surgery, progressive disease during neoadjuvant therapy, or cardiopulmonary dysfunction (including New York Heart Association class II or worse heart failure, or history of left ventricular ejection fraction <40%) were ineligible. Patients were randomized within 12 weeks following surgery 1:1 to fourteen 3-week cycles of either adjuvant ado-trastuzumab emtansine or adjuvant trastuzumab. Patients also received adjuvant radiation therapy and endocrine therapy when indicated

Efficacy (N = 1486)

	ado-Trastuzumab Emtansine (N = 743)	Trastuzumab (N = 743)	
Median invasive disease-free survival*	Not estimable	Not estimable	HR 0.50 (95% CI 0.39–0.64); P<0.001
3-year invasive disease-free survival	88.3%	77.0%	
Median distant recurrence-free survival†	Not estimable	Not estimable	HR 0.50 (95% CI 0.45–0.79)
3-year distant recurrence-free survival	89.7%	83.0%	
Median overall survival	Not estimable	Not estimable	HR 0.70 (95% CI 0.47–1.05) P = 0.08‡

*Invasive disease-free survival was defined as the time from randomization until the date of the first occurrence of one of the following: recurrence of ipsilateral invasive breast tumor, recurrence of ipsilateral locoregional invasive breast cancer, contralateral invasive breast cancer, distant disease recurrence, or death from any cause
†Distant recurrence was defined as evidence of breast cancer in any anatomic site (other than ipsilateral invasive breast tumor or recurrence of locoregional invasive breast cancer) that was either histologically confirmed or clinically diagnosed as recurrent invasive breast cancer
‡Not statistically significant at the time of this prespecified interim analysis based on an alpha level set at 0.000032
Note: Median follow-up was 41.4 months in the ado-trastuzumab emtansine group and 40.9 months in the trastuzumab group

Therapy Monitoring

1) *Prior to each cycle:* CBC with differential and platelet count, serum electrolytes and LFTs
2) *LVEF assessment:* recommended at baseline and repeat serially every 3–4 months for adjuvant treatment

Treatment Modifications

ADO-TRASTUZUMAB EMTANSINE

Starting dose	3.6 mg/kg
Dose level −1	3 mg/kg
Dose level −2	2.4 mg/kg
Dose level −3	Discontinue ado-trastuzumab emtansine*

*If ado-trastuzumab emtansine is discontinued due to toxicity, then consider the appropriateness of completing therapy with trastuzumab (ie, when the toxicity is not related to the trastuzumab component)

Adverse Event	Dose Modification
Hematologic Toxicity	
Day 1 platelet count <75,000/mm³	Withhold ado-trastuzumab emtansine until platelet count recovers to ≥75,000/mm³. Determine if dose reduction is necessary based on nadir platelet count as described below
Platelet count nadir 25,000–50,000/mm³	Withhold ado-trastuzumab emtansine until platelet count recovers to ≥75,000/mm³, then resume treatment at the same dose level
Platelet count nadir <25,000/mm³	Withhold ado-trastuzumab emtansine until platelet count recovers to ≥75,000/mm³, then resume treatment with the dosage reduced by 1 dose level

(continued)

Treatment Modifications (*continued*)

Adverse Event	Dose Modification
Hepatic Toxicity	
AST or ALT >2.5× to ≤5× ULN (G2)	Treat at the same ado-trastuzumab emtansine dose level
AST or ALT >5× to ≤20× ULN (G3)	Withhold ado-trastuzumab emtansine until AST and ALT recover to G ≤2, then resume ado-trastuzumab emtansine with dosage decreased by one dose level
AST or ALT >20× ULN (G4)	Permanently discontinue ado-trastuzumab emtansine. Consider completing therapy with trastuzumab
Total bilirubin >1.5× to ≤3× ULN (G2)	Withhold ado-trastuzumab emtansine until total bilirubin recovers to G ≤1, then resume ado-trastuzumab emtansine at the same dose level
Total bilirubin >3× to ≤10× ULN (G3)	Withhold ado-trastuzumab emtansine until total bilirubin recovers to G ≤1, then resume ado-trastuzumab emtansine with dosage decreased by one dose level
Total bilirubin >10× ULN (G4)	Permanently discontinue ado-trastuzumab emtansine. Consider completing therapy with trastuzumab
AST or ALT >3× ULN and total bilirubin >2× ULN	Permanently discontinue ado-trastuzumab emtansine. Consider completing therapy with trastuzumab
Patient diagnosed with nodular regenerative hepatic hyperplasia	Permanently discontinue ado-trastuzumab emtansine. Consider completing therapy with trastuzumab
Cardiac Toxicity	
Symptomatic CHF	Discontinue ado-trastuzumab emtansine
LVEF <40%	Withhold ado-trastuzumab emtansine. Repeat LVEF assessment within 3 weeks. If LVEF <40% is confirmed, discontinue ado-trastuzumab emtansine
LVEF 40% to ≤45%, and decrease is ≥10% points from baseline measurement	Withhold ado-trastuzumab emtansine. Repeat LVEF assessment within 3 weeks. If LVEF has not recovered to within 10% points from baseline, discontinue ado-trastuzumab emtansine
LVEF 40% to ≤45%, and decrease is <10% points from baseline	Continue ado-trastuzumab emtansine treatment. Repeat LVEF assessment within 3 weeks
LVEF >45%	Continue ado-trastuzumab emtansine at the same dose level
Other Toxicities	
G3/4 peripheral neuropathy	Withhold ado-trastuzumab emtansine until symptoms abate to G ≤2 then resume treatment with ado-trastuzumab emtansine
Patients diagnosed with interstitial lung disease or pneumonitis	Permanently discontinue ado-trastuzumab emtansine
G1/2 infusion-related reaction	Interrupt infusion and provide supportive care as clinically indicated (eg, oxygen supplementation, inhaled beta-agonist, antihistamine, antipyretic, and/or corticosteroid). When symptoms have resolved, resume the infusion at ≤50% of the prior rate and increase by 50% increments every 30 minutes as tolerated until the rate at which the reaction occurred is reached. Administer the next infusion over 90 minutes. Consider premedication with corticosteroid, antihistamine, and antipyretic prior to subsequent infusions
Life-threatening (G ≥3) infusion-related reactions	Permanently discontinue ado-trastuzumab emtansine

Note:
1. Ado-trastuzumab emtansine dosages should not be re-escalated after a dosage reduction is made
2. If a planned dose is delayed or missed, it should be administered as soon as possible. Do not wait until the next planned cycle. The schedule of administration should be adjusted to maintain a 3-week interval between doses.

Adverse Events (N = 1460)

Adverse Event* (%)	ado-Trastuzumab Emtansine (N = 740)	Trastuzumab (N = 720)
Any adverse event	98.8	93.3
Grade ≥3 adverse event	25.7	15.4
Adverse event leading to death†	0.1	0
Serious adverse event	12.7	8.1
Adverse event leading to discontinuation of trial drug‡	18.0	2.1
Decreased platelet count, grade ≥3	5.7	0.3
Hypertension, grade ≥3	2.0	1.2
Radiation-related skin injury, grade ≥3	1.4	1.0
Peripheral sensory neuropathy, grade ≥3	1.4	0
Decreased neutrophil count, grade ≥3	1.2	0.7
Hypokalemia, grade ≥3	1.2	0.1
Fatigue, grade ≥3	1.1	0.1
Anemia, grade ≥3	1.1	0.1

Toxicities included in the table are those which occurred from the first dose of study treatment through 30 days after the final dose of treatment and adverse events with an onset in the follow-up period that was determined to be related to the trial drug. Patients may have had more than one adverse event

*Based on the National Cancer Institute Common Terminology Criteria for Adverse Events (NCI CTCAE) v4.0

†Fatal event due to intracranial hemorrhage after a fall with a platelet count of 55,000/mm³

‡The most common adverse event leading to discontinuation in the trastuzumab group was a decreased ejection fraction (1.4%). The most common adverse events leading to discontinuation in the ado-trastuzumab emtansine group were thrombocytopenia (4.2%), hyperbilirubinemia (2.6%), increased aspartate aminotransferase level (1.6%), increased alanine aminotransferase level (1.5%), peripheral sensory neuropathy (1.5%), and a decreased ejection fraction (1.2%)

ADJUVANT • HER2-POSITIVE

BREAST CANCER REGIMEN: NERATINIB AFTER TRASTUZUMAB-BASED ADJUVANT THERAPY

Martin M et al. Lancet Oncol 2017;18:1688–1700
Chan A et al. Lancet Oncol 2016;17:367–377

The regimen consists of 1 year of continuous treatment with neratinib. Neratinib may be administered concurrent with adjuvant endocrine therapy for patients with hormone receptor–positive breast cancer

Neratinib 240 mg/dose; administer orally once daily, with food, continually on days 1–28, every 28 days, for 12 cycles (total dosage/28-day cycle = 6720 mg)

Notes:
- Patients should be instructed to take prophylactic loperamide during the first 2 cycles (8 weeks) of treatment. During weeks 1–2 of treatment, patients should take loperamide 4 mg orally, three times per day. During weeks 3–8 of treatment, patients should be instructed to take loperamide 4 mg orally, two times per day. Provide patients with instructions to adjust the dose of loperamide to a goal of 1–2 bowel movements per day. During weeks 9–52 of neratinib treatment, patients may take loperamide on an as needed basis (ie, as per diarrhea management section below)
- Patients who delay taking neratinib at a regularly scheduled time should take the next dose at the next regularly scheduled time
- Neratinib tablets should be swallowed whole
  - Neratinib is metabolized by cytochrome P450 (CYP) CYP3A subfamily enzymes. Avoid concurrent use with moderate or strong CYP3A4 inhibitors and moderate or strong CYP3A4 inducers
  - Neratinib is an inhibitor of P-glycoprotein (P-gp). Use caution when co-administering neratinib with P-gp substrates that have narrow therapeutic indices (eg, digoxin and dabigatran)
  - The solubility of neratinib is increased at acidic pH. Thus, gastric acid–reducing medications may interfere with absorption of neratinib and should be avoided when possible
    - Avoid concomitant use of proton pump inhibitors
    - If antacid medications must be used, separate neratinib administration from antacid administration by at least 3 hours
    - If a histamine receptor [H_2]-subtype antagonist must be used, administer neratinib at least 10 hours following a dose of histamine receptor [H_2]-subtype antagonist and at least 2 hours before the next dose of histamine receptor [H_2]-subtype antagonist
- Advise patients to not consume grapefruit and grapefruit juice as they may inhibit CYP3A in the gut wall and increase the bioavailability of neratinib
- Dose adjustment for severe hepatic impairment (Child Pugh-C): reduce each neratinib dose to 80 mg

Supportive Care
Antiemetic prophylaxis
Emetogenic potential is **MINIMAL–LOW**
See Chapter 42 for antiemetic recommendations

Hematopoietic growth factor (CSF) prophylaxis
Primary prophylaxis is **NOT** indicated
See Chapter 43 for more information

Antimicrobial prophylaxis
Risk of fever and neutropenia is **LOW**
  Antimicrobial primary prophylaxis to be considered:
- Antibacterial—not indicated
- Antifungal—not indicated
- Antiviral—not indicated unless patient previously had an episode of HSV

Diarrhea prophylaxis
Diarrhea prophylaxis is recommended during the first 8 weeks of therapy:
  Weeks 1–2: **Loperamide** 4 mg orally, three times per day
  Weeks 3–8: **Loperamide** 4 mg orally, two times per day

Patient Population Studied

This ongoing, randomized, double-blind, placebo-controlled, phase 3 trial involved 2840 patients with stage 1–3c operable HER2-positive breast cancer who had completed neoadjuvant and adjuvant chemotherapy plus trastuzumab within 1 year of randomization and had no evidence of disease recurrence or metastatic disease at the time of enrollment. Eligible patients were aged ≥18 years, had Eastern Cooperative Oncology Group (ECOG) performance status ≤1, and had normal organ function, including normal left ventricular ejection fraction. Patients received oral placebo or neratinib (240 mg) once daily for 1 year

Efficacy (N = 2840)

Martin M et al. Lancet Oncol 2017;18:1688–1700

Intention-to-treat Population

	Neratinib (N = 1420)	Placebo (N = 1420)	
5-year survival free from invasive disease	90.2%	87.7%	HR 0.73, 95% CI 0.57–0.92; P = 0.0083
Incidence of local or regional invasive recurrence	0.8%	2.5%	
Incidence of distant recurrence	6.4%	7.8%	
5-year survival free from disease	89.7%	86.8%	HR 0.71, 95% CI 0.56–0.89; P = 0.0035
5-year survival free from distant disease	91.6%	89.9%	HR 0.78, 95% CI 0.60–1.01; P = 0.065

Hormone Receptor–Positive Population

	Neratinib (N = 816)	Placebo (N = 815)	
Survival free from invasive disease	—	—	HR 0.60, 95% CI 0.43–0.83

Hormone-receptor negative population

	Neratinib (N = 604)	Placebo (N = 605)	
Survival free from invasive disease	—	—	HR 0.95, 95% CI 0.66–1.35

Note: Median duration of treatment was 353 days and 360 days in the neratinib and placebo groups, respectively. Median follow-up was 5.2 years

Therapy Monitoring

1. Monitor CBC with differential and LFTs. Obtain prior to the start of therapy, every 2 weeks for the first 2 months, monthly for the next 2 months, and as clinically indicated
2. Monitor for diarrhea, liver dysfunction, and the use of strong or moderate CYP3A4 inhibitors or inducers
3. Obtain a pregnancy test in females of reproductive potential. Advise females of reproductive potential to use effective contraception

Treatment Modifications

NERATINIB

Starting dose	240 mg by mouth once daily with food
Dose level −1	200 mg by mouth once daily with food
Dose level −2	160 mg by mouth once daily with food
Dose level −3	120 mg by mouth once daily with food

Diarrhea

G1 diarrhea (increase of <4 stools per day over baseline)	• Continue neratinib at the current dose
G2 diarrhea (increase of 4–6 stools per day over baseline) lasting <5 days	• Adjust antidiarrheal treatment • Modify diet • Maintain ~2L of fluid intake/day
G3 diarrhea (increase of ≥7 stools per day over baseline; incontinence; limiting self-care ADLs) lasting ≤2 days	• Once toxicity resolves to G ≤1 or baseline, start loperamide 4 mg with each subsequent neratinib administration

(continued)

Treatment Modifications (continued)

Diarrhea

Any grade diarrhea with complicated features (eg, requiring hospitalization, dehydration, fever, hypotension, renal failure, G3/4 neutropenia)	• Interrupt neratinib • Adjust antidiarrheal treatment • Modify diet • Maintain ~2L of fluid intake/day • If diarrhea resolves to G ≤1 in 1 week or less, then resume neratinib treatment at the same dose. Start loperamide 4 mg with each subsequent neratinib administration • If diarrhea resolves to G ≤1 in longer than 1 week, then resume neratinib treatment at one lower dose level. Start loperamide 4 mg with each subsequent neratinib administration
G2 diarrhea lasting ≥5 days despite optimal medical therapy	
G3 diarrhea lasting >2 days despite optimal medical therapy	
G4 diarrhea (life-threatening consequences; urgent intervention indicated)	Permanently discontinue neratinib
Diarrhea recurs to G ≥2 at a dose of 120 mg per day	Permanently discontinue neratinib

Hepatic Impairment or Hepatotoxicity

Patients with severe hepatic impairment (Child-Pugh class C)	Reduce neratinib starting dose to 80 mg by mouth once daily with food
G3 ALT (>5–20× ULN) or G3 hyperbilirubinemia (>3–10× ULN)	Interrupt neratinib. Evaluate alternative causes. Resume neratinib at the next lower dose level if recovery to G ≤1 toxicity occurs within 3 weeks
Recurrent G3 ALT (>5–20× ULN) or G3 hyperbilirubinemia (>3–10× ULN)	Permanently discontinue neratinib
G4 ALT (>20× ULN) or G4 hyperbilirubinemia (>10× ULN)	Evaluate alternative causes. Permanently discontinue neratinib

Other Toxicities

Any other G3 toxicity	Interrupt neratinib for up to 3 weeks until recovery to G ≤1 or baseline. Then resume neratinib at one lower dose level
Any other G4 toxicity	Permanently discontinue neratinib
Failure to recover to G0–1 from treatment-related toxicity	Permanently discontinue neratinib
Toxicities that result in a treatment delay >3 weeks	
Inability to tolerate 120 mg daily	

Drug Interactions

Strong or moderate CYP3A4 inhibitors	Do not administer neratinib—increase area under the curve (AUC)
Strong or moderate CYP3A4 inducers	Avoid their use—decrease area under the curve (AUC)

Note: Advise patients of potential risk to a fetus and to use effective contraception

ADL, activity of daily living; ALT, alanine aminotransferase; ULN, upper limit of normal

Adverse Events (N = 2816)

Grade (%)*	Neratinib (N = 1408)			Placebo (N = 1408)		
	Grade 1–2	Grade 3	Grade 4	Grade 1–2	Grade 3	Grade 4
Diarrhea	55	40	<1	34	2	0
Nausea	41	2	0	21	<1	0
Fatigue	25	2	0	20	<1	0
Vomiting	23	3	0	8	<1	0
Abdominal pain	22	2	0	10	<1	0
Headache	19	<1	0	19	<1	0
Upper abdominal pain	14	<1	0	7	<1	0
Rash	15	<1	0	7	0	0
Decreased appetite	12	<1	0	3	0	0
Muscle spasms	11	<1	0	3	<1	0
Dizziness	10	<1	0	9	<1	0
Arthralgia	6	<1	0	11	<1	0

*According to the National Cancer Institute Common Terminology Criteria for Adverse Events, version 3.0 Treatment-emergent toxicities for which grade 1–2 adverse events occurred in ≥10% patients in either group are shown; these toxicities were reported in the 2-year follow-up manuscript. No deaths were attributed to study treatment. Treatment discontinuation owing to treatment-emergent adverse events occurred in 28% and 5% of the neratinib and placebo groups, respectively

ADJUVANT • NEOADJUVANT • HER2-POSITIVE

BREAST CANCER REGIMEN: DOCETAXEL + CARBOPLATIN + TRASTUZUMAB (TCH)

Slamon S et al. N Engl J Med 2011;365:1273–1283 [Third interim analysis phase 3 randomized trial comparing doxorubicin and cyclophosphamide followed by docetaxel (AC → T) with doxorubicin and cyclophosphamide followed by docetaxel and trastuzumab (AC → TH) with docetaxel, carboplatin, and trastuzumab (TCH) in HER2neu-positive early breast cancer patients: BCIRG 006 Study]

TCH regimen
Premedication:
Dexamethasone 8 mg/dose; administer orally twice daily for 3 days, starting on the day before docetaxel administration (total dose/cycle = 48 mg)

Docetaxel 75 mg/m²; administer intravenously in a volume of 0.9% sodium chloride injection (0.9% NS) or 5% dextrose injection (D5W) sufficient to produce a final docetaxel concentration of 0.3–0.74 mg/mL over 30–60 minutes on day 1, every 3 weeks for 6 cycles (total dosage/cycle = 75 mg/m²)
Carboplatin target AUC = 6 mg/mL × min; administer intravenously in 250 mL D5W or 0.9% NS over 30–60 minutes on day 1, every 3 weeks for 6 cycles (total dose/cycle calculated to achieve a target AUC = 6 mg/mL × min), *concurrently with:*
Trastuzumab every 21 days for 6 cycles:
  Loading Dose: **Trastuzumab** 8 mg/kg; administer intravenously in 250 mL 0.9% NS over 90 minutes as a loading dose on day 1, cycle 1 only (total dosage during the first cycle = 8 mg/kg), *followed 3 weeks later by:*
  Maintenance Doses: **Trastuzumab** 6 mg/kg; administer intravenously in 250 mL 0.9% NS over 30 minutes on day 1, every 3 weeks for 5 cycles (total dosage/cycle = 6 mg/kg)

Three weeks after completing combination (TCH) chemotherapy:
Trastuzumab 6 mg/kg; administer intravenously in 250 mL 0.9% NS over 30 minutes every 3 weeks for 11 doses (total dosage/3-week cycle = 6 mg/kg)

Supportive Care
Antiemetic prophylaxis
Emetogenic potential on days with TCH combination chemotherapy is **HIGH**. *Potential for delayed symptoms*
Emetogenic potential on days with trastuzumab alone is **LOW**
See Chapter 42 for antiemetic recommendations

Hematopoietic growth factor (CSF) prophylaxis
Primary prophylaxis may be indicated
See Chapter 43 for more information

Antimicrobial prophylaxis
Risk of fever and neutropenia is **LOW**
  Antimicrobial primary prophylaxis to be considered:
  • Antibacterial—not indicated
  • Antifungal—not indicated
  • Antiviral—not indicated, unless patient previously had an episode of HSV

(continued)

Treatment Modifications

Adverse Events	Treatment Modifications
WBC <3500/mm³, or absolute neutrophil count (ANC) <1500/mm³, or platelets <100,000/mm³ on first day of a cycle	Delay treatment for a maximum of 2 weeks until WBC >3500/mm³, ANC >1500/mm³, and platelets >100,000/mm³. Continue at full dosages if counts recover within 2 weeks. Give filgrastim* in subsequent cycles
If after 2 weeks WBC <3500/mm³, ANC <1500/mm³, or platelets <100,000/mm³, reduce all drugs' dosages as follows:	
WBC 3000–3499/mm³, ANC 1000–1500/mm³, or platelets 75,000–99,999/mm³	Reduce dosages by 20%
WBC 2500–2999/mm³, ANC 500–1000/mm³, or platelets ≥ 75,000/mm³	Reduce dosages by 50%
WBC <2500/mm³, ANC <500/mm³, or platelets <75,000/mm³	Hold treatment
Hematologic recovery >3 weeks	Discontinue treatment
First episode of febrile neutropenia or documented infection after treatment	Filgrastim* prophylaxis administered during subsequent cycles
Second episode of febrile neutropenia or documented infection after treatment	Reduce docetaxel dosage to 60 mg/m² during subsequent cycles, administer filgrastim* and consider prophylaxis with ciprofloxacin†
Third episode of febrile neutropenia or documented infection after treatment	Discontinue chemotherapy
G3/4 stomatitis	Reduce docetaxel dosage to 60 mg/m² during subsequent cycles
G3/4 neuropathy	Discontinue treatment

(continued)

Treatment Modifications
(continued)

Other severe adverse events	Hold treatment until toxicity resolves to G ≤1, then resume at decreased dosages appropriate for the toxicity
LVEF has declined by ≥16 percentage points from baseline, or has declined by 10–15 percentage points from baseline to a value below the lower limit of the normal range OR Symptomatic congestive heart failure	Withhold trastuzumab and repeat LVEF assessment at 4-week intervals until improvement, which may require prolonged interruption. For a persistent decline in LVEF, consider a cardio-oncology consultation and weigh the benefits and risks of continuing trastuzumab in the individual patient

*Filgrastim 5 mcg/kg per day; administer subcutaneously starting at least 24 hours after completing chemotherapy until ANC ≥5000/mm³
†Ciprofloxacin 500 mg; administer orally twice daily for 7 days starting on day 5
Note: Dosages reduced for adverse events are not re-escalated

Patient Population Studied

Study of 3222 women with HER2+ by FISH, T1–3, N0/N1, M0 breast cancer (AC → T: 1073; AC→TH: 1074; TCH: 1075). Stratified by nodes and hormonal receptor status

Therapy Monitoring

1. *Before each cycle:* CBC with differential and platelet count, LFTs, serum electrolytes, BUN, and creatinine

2. *Hearing test:* At baseline and as needed

3. Conduct thorough cardiac assessment, including history, physical examination, and determination of LVEF by echocardiogram or MUGA scan at baseline immediately prior to initiation of trastuzumab and every 3 months during therapy

4. Patients should have a pre-treatment LVEF ≥55%

5. Repeat LVEF measurement at 4-week intervals if trastuzumab is withheld for significant left ventricular cardiac dysfunction

(*continued*)

Trastuzumab infusion reactions:
• A symptom complex most commonly consisting of chills and/or fever may occur in as many as 40% of patients during the first infusion of trastuzumab. These symptoms occur infrequently with subsequent trastuzumab infusions. Other signs and/or symptoms may include nausea, vomiting, pain (in some cases at tumor sites), rigors, headache, dizziness, dyspnea, hypotension, rash, and asthenia. Although the symptoms are usually mild to moderate in severity, infrequently, trastuzumab may need to be discontinued
• When such a symptom complex is observed, it can be treated with or without reduction in the rate of trastuzumab infusion, and:
  ▪ **Acetaminophen** 650 mg; administer orally
  ▪ **Diphenhydramine** 25–50 mg; administer orally or by intravenous injection, and
  ▪ **Meperidine** 12.5–25 mg; administer by intravenous injection every 10 minutes if needed for shaking chills (generally, cumulative doses >50 mg are not needed; use with caution in persons with moderate or more severely impaired renal function)

Treatment plan notes:
• One year of trastuzumab therapy = 51 weeks or 17 total doses (6 doses [cycles] with docetaxel and carboplatin and 11 doses [cycles] of single-agent trastuzumab)

Carboplatin dose
Carboplatin dose is based on a formula described by Calvert et al. to achieve a target area under the plasma concentration versus time curve (AUC)

$$\text{Total Carboplatin Dose (mg)} = (\text{target AUC})(\text{GFR} + 25)$$

In practice, creatinine clearance (CrCl) is used in place of glomerular filtration rate (GFR). CrCl can be estimated from the equation of Cockcroft and Gault, thus:

$$\text{For males, CrCl} = \frac{(140 - \text{age[years]}) \times (\text{body weight [kg]})}{72 \times (\text{serum creatinine [mg/dL]})}$$

$$\text{For females, CrCl} = \frac{(140 - \text{age[years]}) \times (\text{body weight [kg]})}{72 \times (\text{serum creatinine [mg/dL]})} \times 0.85$$

Calvert AH et al. J Clin Oncol 1989;7:1748–1756
Cockcroft DW , Gault MH. Nephron 1976;16:31–41
Jodrell DI et al. J Clin Oncol 1992;10:520–528
Sorensen BT et al. Cancer Chemother Pharmacol 1991;28:397–401

Note: On October 8, 2010, the U.S. Food and Drug Administration (FDA) identified a potential safety issue with carboplatin dosing based on recent changes in the measurement of serum creatinine. By the end of 2010, all clinical laboratories in the United States will use the standardized isotope dilution mass spectrometry (IDMS) method to measure serum creatinine, which could result in an overestimation of the GFR in some patients with normal renal function. A carboplatin dose calculated with an IDMS-measured serum creatinine result using the Calvert formula could exceed an expected exposure (AUC) and result in increased drug-related toxicity. Provided actual GFR measurements are made to assess renal function, carboplatin can be safely dosed according to the Calvert formula described in product labeling. If GFR (or creatinine clearance) is estimated based on serum creatinine measurements by the IDMS method, the FDA recommended for patients with normal renal function capping an estimated GFR at 125 mL/min for any targeted AUC value. No greater estimated GFR values should be used.

Note

In the neoadjuvant setting, consider adding Pertuzumab to TCH chemotherapy
Give pertuzumab every 21 days for 6 cycles:

Loading Dose: **Pertuzumab** 840 mg; administer intravenously in 250 mL of 0.9% NS over 90 minutes on day 1 after trastuzumab, cycle 1 only (total dose during the first cycle = 840 mg), *followed 3 weeks later by:*

Maintenance Doses: **Pertuzumab** 420 mg; administer intravenously in 250 mL of 0.9% NS over 30–60 minutes on day 1 after trastuzumab, every 3 weeks for 5 cycles (total dose/cycle = 420 mg)

Schneeweiss A et al. Ann Oncol 2013;24:2278–2284

Efficacy

Third Planned Efficacy Analysis: 65 Months Follow-up*

	AC → T	AC → TH	AC → TH vs AC → T		TCH	TCH vs AC → T		AC → TH vs TCH
			HR	P Value		HR	P Value	P Value
All Patients								
	N = 1073	N = 1074			N = 1075			
DFS	75%	84%	0.64	<0.001	81%	0.75	0.04	0.21
OS	87%	92%	0.63	<0.001	91%	0.77	0.038	0.14
Patients with Negative Lymph Nodes								
	N = 309	N = 310			N = 309			
DFS	85%	93%	0.47	0.003	90%	0.64	0.057	—
OS	93%	97%	0.38	0.02	96%	0.56	0.11	—
Patients with Positive Lymph Nodes								
	N = 764	N = 764			N = 766			
DFS	71%	80%	0.68	0.0003	78%	0.78	0.013	—
Patients with ≥4 Positive Lymph Nodes								
	N = 350	N = 350			N = 352			
DFS	61%	73%	0.66	0.002	72%	0.66	0.002	—

AC → T, doxorubicin (Adriamycin) + cyclophosphamide followed by docetaxel; AC → TH, doxorubicin + cyclophosphamide followed by docetaxel plus trastuzumab (Herceptin) then trastuzumab alone; DFS, disease-free survival; OS, overall survival; TCH, docetaxel plus carboplatin plus concurrent trastuzumab then trastuzumab alone
*DFS and OS values are at 65 months

Toxicity

	AC → T N = 1050		AC → TH N = 1068		TCH N = 1056	
	% All G	% G3/4	% All G	% G3/4	% All G	% G3/4
Nonhematologic Toxicity						
Neuropathy, sensory	48.6		49.7		36.1*	
Neuropathy, motor	5.2		6.3		4.2*	
Nail changes	49.3		43.6		28.7*	
Myalgia	52.8	5.2	55.5	5.2	38.6*	1.8*
Renal failure	0		0		0.1	
G3/4 creatinine	0.6		0.3		0.1	
Arthralgia		3.2		3.3		1.4*
Fatigue		7		7.2		7.2
Hand-foot syndrome		1.9		1.4		0*
Stomatitis		3.5		2.9		1.4*
Diarrhea		3.0		5.6		5.4
Nausea		5.9		5.7		4.8
Vomiting		6.1		6.7		3.5*
Irregular menses		27		24.3		26.5
Hematologic Toxicity						
Neutropenia		63.5		71.6		66.2*
Leucopenia		51.9		60.4		48.4*
Neutropenic infection		9.3		10.9		9.6
Febrile neutropenia		11.5		12.1		11.2
Anemia		2.4		3.1*		5.8
Thrombocytopenia		1.6		2.1*		6.1
Acute leukemia	0.6		0.1		0.1	
Cardiac Toxicity						
G3/4 LV dysfunction (CHF)[†]	7/1050		21/1068		4/1056	
>10% Relative LVEF decline[‡]	11%		19%		9%	

AC → T, doxorubicin (Adriamycin) + cyclophosphamide followed by docetaxel; AC→TH, doxorubicin + cyclophosphamide followed by docetaxel plus trastuzumab (Herceptin) then trastuzumab alone; CHF, congestive heart failure; LV, left ventricular; LVEF, left ventricular ejection fraction; TCH, docetaxel plus carboplatin plus concurrent trastuzumab then trastuzumab alone

*Less statistically significantly events than the comparator groups

[†]AC → T vs AC → TH: P = 0.0121; AC → TH vs TCH: p <0.001; AC → T vs TCH: P = 0.3852

[‡]AC → T vs AC → TH: p <0.001; AC → TH vs TCH: p <0.001; AC → T vs TCH: P = 0.19

ADJUVANT • NEOADJUVANT • HER2-POSITIVE

BREAST CANCER REGIMEN: DOXORUBICIN + CYCLOPHOSPHAMIDE, THEN PACLITAXEL + TRASTUZUMAB, THEN TRASTUZUMAB ALONE (AC × 4 → TH × 12 WEEKS → H × 40 WEEKS)

Romond EH et al. N Engl J Med 2005;353:1673–1684
Seidman AD et al. J Clin Oncol 2001;19:2587–2595

AC (doxorubicin + cyclophosphamide) regimen

Hydration with 0.9% sodium chloride injection (0.9% NS); administer intravenously 500 mL before starting cyclophosphamide and 500 mL after completing cyclophosphamide administration

Doxorubicin HCl 60 mg/m^2; administer by intravenous injection over 3–5 minutes on day 1, every 21 days for 4 cycles (total dosage/cycle = 60 mg/m^2)

Cyclophosphamide 600 mg/m^2; administer intravenously in 100–500 mL 0.9% NS or 5% dextrose injection (D5W) over 15–60 minutes on day 1, every 21 days for 4 cycles (total dosage/cycle = 600 mg/m^2)

Supportive Care

Antiemetic prophylaxis
Emetogenic potential is **HIGH**. *Potential for delayed symptoms*
See Chapter 42 for antiemetic recommendations

Hematopoietic growth factor (CSF) prophylaxis
Primary prophylaxis is **NOT** *indicated*
See Chapter 43 for more information

Antimicrobial prophylaxis
Risk of fever and neutropenia is **LOW**
  Antimicrobial primary prophylaxis to be considered:
  • Antibacterial—not indicated
  • Antifungal—not indicated
  • Antiviral—not indicated, unless patient previously had an episode of HSV

Weekly TH (paclitaxel + trastuzumab) regimen

Schedule for first week of paclitaxel + trastuzumab

Trastuzumab 4 mg/kg (loading dose); administer intravenously in 250 mL 0.9% NS over at least 90 minutes, 1 day before the first dose of paclitaxel is administered (total trastuzumab dosage during the first treatment week = 4 mg/kg), *followed 1 day later by:*

Premedication for paclitaxel:
Dexamethasone 10 mg; administer intravenously 30–60 minutes before paclitaxel (total dose/cycle = 10 mg)
Note: Dexamethasone doses may be gradually reduced in 2- to 4-mg increments if a patient has no hypersensitivity reactions during repeated paclitaxel treatments
Diphenhydramine 50 mg; administer intravenously 30–60 minutes before paclitaxel
Cimetidine 300 mg (or **ranitidine** 50 mg, or **famotidine** 20 mg, or an equivalent histamine receptor [H$_2$]-subtype antagonist); administer intravenously over 15–30 minutes, 30–60 minutes before starting paclitaxel administration

Paclitaxel 80 mg/m^2; administer intravenously in a volume of 0.9% NS or D5W sufficient to produce a concentration within the range 0.3–1.2 mg/mL over 60 minutes (total dosage = 80 mg/m^2)

Paclitaxel + trastuzumab during the second and subsequent weeks
Premedication for paclitaxel:
Dexamethasone 10 mg; administer intravenously 30–60 minutes before paclitaxel
Note: If a patient does not experience any manifestations of hypersensitivity or an allergic reaction after 8 paclitaxel infusions, the **dexamethasone** dose may be reduced as follows:

Weeks 9 and 10:	**Dexamethasone 8 mg IV**
Weeks 11 and 12:	**Dexamethasone 6 mg IV**
Weeks 13 and beyond:	**Dexamethasone 4 mg IV**

Diphenhydramine 50 mg; administer by intravenous injection 30–60 minutes before paclitaxel

Cimetidine 300 mg (or **ranitidine** 50 mg, or **famotidine** 20 mg, or an equivalent histamine receptor [H$_2$]-subtype antagonist); administer intravenously over 15–30 minutes, 30–60 minutes before starting paclitaxel administration

(continued)

(*continued*)

Paclitaxel 80 mg/m² per week; administer intravenously in a volume of 0.9% NS or D5W sufficient to produce a concentration within the range 0.3–1.2 mg/mL over 60 minutes, weekly, for 11 weeks (total dosage/week = 80 mg/m²), *followed immediately afterward by:*

Trastuzumab 2 mg/kg per week; administer intravenously in 250 mL 0.9% NS over 30 minutes, weekly, for 11 weeks (total trastuzumab dosage/week during the second and later weeks = 2 mg/kg)

Note: The duration of trastuzumab administration may be decreased from an initial infusion duration of 90 to 30 minutes if administration over longer durations is well tolerated

Supportive Care
Antiemetic prophylaxis
Emetogenic potential is **LOW**
See Chapter 42 for antiemetic recommendations

Hematopoietic growth factor (CSF) prophylaxis
Primary prophylaxis is NOT indicated
See Chapter 43 for more information

Antimicrobial prophylaxis
Risk of fever and neutropenia is **LOW**
   Antimicrobial primary prophylaxis to be considered:
   • Antibacterial—not indicated
   • Antifungal—not indicated
   • Antiviral—not indicated, unless patient previously had an episode of HSV

Weekly H (*trastuzumab*) regimen
Trastuzumab 2 mg/kg per week; administer intravenously in 250 mL 0.9% NS over 30 minutes, weekly, for 40 weeks (total trastuzumab dosage/week = 2 mg/kg)

Supportive Care
Antiemetic prophylaxis
Emetogenic potential is **MINIMAL**
See Chapter 42 for antiemetic recommendations

Hematopoietic growth factor (CSF) prophylaxis
Primary prophylaxis is **NOT** *indicated*
See Chapter 43 for more information

Antimicrobial prophylaxis
Risk of fever and neutropenia is **LOW**
   Antimicrobial primary prophylaxis to be considered:
   • Antibacterial—not indicated
   • Antifungal—not indicated
   • Antiviral—not indicated, unless patient previously had an episode of HSV

Trastuzumab infusion reactions
• A symptom complex most commonly consisting of chills and/or fever may occur in as many as 40% of patients during the first infusion of trastuzumab. These symptoms occur infrequently with subsequent trastuzumab infusions. Other signs and/or symptoms may include nausea, vomiting, pain (in some cases at tumor sites), rigors, headache, dizziness, dyspnea, hypotension, rash, and asthenia. Although the symptoms are usually mild to moderate in severity, infrequently, trastuzumab may need to be discontinued
• When such a symptom complex is observed, it can be treated with or without reduction in the rate of trastuzumab infusion, and:
   ▪ **Acetaminophen** 650 mg; administer orally
   ▪ **Diphenhydramine** 25–50 mg; administer orally or by intravenous injection, and
   ▪ **Meperidine** 12.5–25 mg; administer by intravenous injection every 10 minutes if needed for shaking chills (generally, cumulative doses >50 mg are not needed; use with caution in persons with moderate or more severely impaired renal function)

Treatment Modifications: Cyclophosphamide + Doxorubicin

Adverse Events	Treatment Modifications
Absolute neutrophil count (ANC) <1500/mm^3, or WBC <3500/mm^3, or platelets <100,000/mm^3 at start of cycle*	Delay treatment for a maximum of 2 weeks until ANC ≥1500/mm^3, WBC ≥3500/mm^3, and platelets ≥100,000/mm^3. Continue at full dosages if counts recover within 2 weeks. Give filgrastim† after chemotherapy during subsequent cycles
If after 2 weeks ANC <1500/mm^3, or WBC <3500/mm^3, or platelets <100,000/mm^3, reduce all drug dosages as follows:	
ANC 1000–1500/mm^3, WBC 3000–3499/mm^3, or platelets 75,000–99,999/mm^3	Reduce cyclophosphamide and doxorubicin dosages by 20%
ANC 500–1000/mm^3, WBC 2500–2999/mm^3, and platelets ≥75,000/mm^3	Reduce cyclophosphamide and doxorubicin dosages by 50%
ANC <500/mm^3, WBC <2500/mm^3, or platelets <75,000/mm^3	Hold treatment
First episode of febrile neutropenia	Give filgrastim† after chemotherapy during subsequent cycles
Second episode of febrile neutropenia	During subsequent cycles, consider prophylaxis with ciprofloxacin‡
Third episode of febrile neutropenia	Decrease both doxorubicin and cyclophosphamide dosages by 25%

*Although an ANC of 1500/mm^3 is often identified as a minimum acceptable ANC to safely proceed with treatment, recent data shows that an ANC ≥1000/mm^3 is acceptable if filgrastim is given after chemotherapy
†Filgrastim 5 mcg/kg per day; administer subcutaneously starting at least 24 hours after completing chemotherapy until ANC ≥5000/mm^3
‡Ciprofloxacin 500 mg; administer orally twice daily for 7 days starting on day 5

Treatment Modifications: Paclitaxel and Trastuzumab

Adverse Events	Adverse Events
ANC ≤800/mm^3, platelets ≤50,000/mm^3, or documented infection	Hold treatment until ANC >1000/mm^3, platelets >100,000/mm^3, and/or infection resolved, then resume with weekly paclitaxel dosage reduced by 10 mg/m^2
G2 motor or sensory neuropathies	Reduce weekly paclitaxel dosage by 10 mg/m^2 without interrupting planned treatment
G2 nonhematologic adverse events (other than sensory or motor neuropathies)	Hold treatment until adverse events resolve to G ≤1, then resume with weekly paclitaxel dosage reduced by 10 mg/m^2
G3 nonhematologic adverse events (other than sensory or motor neuropathies)	Hold treatment until adverse events resolve to G ≤1, then resume with weekly paclitaxel dosage reduced by 20 mg/m^2
Patients who cannot tolerate paclitaxel at 60 mg/m^2 per week	Discontinue treatment
Treatment delay >2 weeks	Decrease weekly paclitaxel dosage by 10 mg/m^2 or consider discontinuing treatment
LVEF has declined by ≥16 percentage points from baseline, or has declined by 10–15 percentage points from baseline to a value below the lower limit of the normal range OR Symptomatic congestive heart failure	Withhold trastuzumab and repeat LVEF assessment at 4-week intervals until improvement, which may require prolonged interruption. For a persistent decline in LVEF, consider a cardio-oncology consultation and weigh the benefits and risks of continuing trastuzumab in the individual patient.

Patient Population Studied

Romond EH et al. J Clin Oncol 2005;16:1673–1684: Report of two trials that treated 1672 women with a regimen of AC followed by paclitaxel with trastuzumab, followed by trastuzumab alone [AC → P + H → H]. Two studies were combined in one analysis: (a) National Surgical Adjuvant Breast and Bowel Project trial B-31 and (b) North Central Cancer Treatment Group trial N9831. Both trials enrolled women with a pathologic diagnosis of adenocarcinoma of the breast with immunohistochemical staining for HER2 protein of 3+ intensity or amplification of the *HER2* gene on fluorescence in situ hybridization. Initially, required patients to have histologically proven, node-positive disease; subsequently, N9831 was amended to include patients with high-risk node-negative disease (defined as a tumor that was more than 2 cm in diameter and positive for estrogen receptors or progesterone receptors or as a tumor that was more than 1 cm in diameter and negative for both estrogen receptors and progesterone receptors). Other requirements included a left ventricular ejection fraction (LVEF) that met or exceeded the lower limit of normal. Complete resection of the primary tumor and axillary-node dissection were required (negative sentinel-node biopsy was allowed in trial N9831). Patients were ineligible if they had one of several cardiac risk factors

Note

In the neoadjuvant setting, consider adding pertuzumab to paclitaxel and trastuzumab
Give pertuzumab every 21 days for 4 cycles:
Loading Dose: **Pertuzumab** 840 mg; administer intravenously in 250 mL of 0.9% NS over 90 minutes on the same day as trastuzumab, but after completing trastuzumab administration (total dose during the first cycle = 840 mg), *followed 3 weeks later by:*
Maintenance Doses: **Pertuzumab** 420 mg; administer intravenously in 250 mL of 0.9% NS over 30–60 minutes after trastuzumab, every 3 weeks for 3 cycles (total dose/3-week cycle = 420 mg)

Schneeweiss A et al. Ann Oncol 2013;24:2278–2284

Efficacy (Combined Analysis of NSABP B-31 and NCCTG N9831)

Romond EH et al. N Engl J Med 2005;353:1673–1684

	AC → PTX N = 1679	AC → P + H → H N = 1672	Hazard Ratio
3-Year DFS	75.4%	87.1%	0.48
4-Year DFS	67.1%	85.3%	
3 Years free of distant recurrence	81.5%	90.4%	0.47
4 Years free of distant recurrence	79.3%	89.7%	
3-Year OS	91.7%	94.3%	0.67
4-Year OS	86.6%	91.4%	
Isolated brain metastases as first event, B-31*	11/872	21/864	
Isolated brain metastases as first event, N9831*	4/807	12/808	
Brain metastases as first/subsequent event, B-31*	35/872	28/864	0.79

AC → PTX, doxorubicin (Adriamycin) + cyclophosphamide followed by paclitaxel; AC → P + H → H, doxorubicin + cyclophosphamide followed by paclitaxel plus trastuzumab (Herceptin) then trastuzumab alone; DFS, disease-free survival; OS, overall survival
*The imbalance in brain metastases as first events can be attributed to earlier failures at other distant sites among patients in the control group

Toxicity

Romond EH et al. N Engl J Med 2005;353:1673–1684

	AC → PTX N = 1679	AC → P + H → H N = 1672
NYHA III/IV CHF* or cardiac death at 3 years, B-31[†]	0.8%[‡]	4.1%[§]
NYHA III/IV CHF* or cardiac death at 3 years, N9831[†]	0	2.9%[ϵ]
Interstitial pneumonitis, B-31		4/864**
Interstitial pneumonitis, N9831		5/808[††]
Other toxicities	Similar CTC v2 toxicities[‡‡]	

AC → PTX, doxorubicin (Adriamycin) + cyclophosphamide followed by paclitaxel; AC → P + H → H, doxorubicin + cyclophosphamide followed by paclitaxel plus trastuzumab (Herceptin) then trastuzumab alone
*New York Heart Association classes III or IV congestive heart failure
[†]Cumulative incidence in patients who remained free of cardiac symptoms during doxorubicin and cyclophosphamide therapy and who had LVEF values that met requirements for the initiation of trastuzumab therapy
[‡]Four patients had congestive heart failure, and 1 died from cardiac causes
[§]Thirty-one patients had congestive heart failure. (Amongst 27 patients followed ≥6 months after onset of CHF, only 1 reported persistent symptoms of CHF)
[ϵ]Twenty patients had congestive heart failure; 1 died of cardiomyopathy
**One died
[††]G3+ pneumonitis or pulmonary infiltrates; 1 died
[‡‡]During treatment with paclitaxel alone or with trastuzumab, there was little imbalance between treatment groups in the incidence of any Common Toxicity Criteria version 2.0

Therapy Monitoring

General:
1. *At intervals:* CBC with differential and platelet count, LFTs, serum electrolytes, BUN, and creatinine
2. Conduct thorough cardiac assessment, including history, physical examination, and determination of LVEF by echocardiogram or MUGA scan at baseline, after completion of doxorubicin and prior to initiation of trastuzumab, and every 3 months during trastuzumab therapy
3. Patients should have a pre-treatment LVEF ≥55%
4. Repeat LVEF measurement at 4-week intervals if trastuzumab is withheld for significant left ventricular cardiac dysfunction

For doxorubicin + cyclophosphamide:
1. *Each cycle:* CBC with differential and platelet count, serum electrolytes, LFTs

For weekly paclitaxel
1. *Every week:* CBC with differential and platelet count
2. *Every 3 to 4 weeks:* LFTs, serum electrolytes, calcium, and magnesium

ADJUVANT • NEOADJUVANT • HER2-POSITIVE

BREAST CANCER REGIMEN: DOXORUBICIN + CYCLOPHOSPHAMIDE (AC) FOLLOWED BY DOCETAXEL WITH TRASTUZUMAB (TH) (AC → TH)

Slamon D. Abstract 62. SABCS 2009
Slamon D et al. N Engl J Med 2011;365:1273–1283 [Third interim analysis phase 3 randomized trial comparing doxorubicin and cyclophosphamide followed by docetaxel (AC → T) with doxorubicin and cyclophosphamide followed by docetaxel and trastuzumab (AC → TH) with docetaxel, carboplatin, and trastuzumab (TCH) in HER2neu-positive early breast cancer patients: BCIRG 006 study]

Hydration with 0.9% sodium chloride injection (0.9% NS); administer 500 mL before starting cyclophosphamide and 500 mL after completing cyclophosphamide administration

Doxorubicin HCl 60 mg/m²; administer by intravenous injection over 3–5 minutes on day 1, every 21 days for 4 cycles (total dosage/cycle = 60 mg/m²)
Cyclophosphamide 600 mg/m²; administer intravenously in 100–500 mL 0.9% NS or 5% dextrose injection (D5W) over 15–60 minutes on day 1, every 21 days for 4 cycles (total dosage/cycle = 600 mg/m²)

Supportive Care
Antiemetic prophylaxis
Emetogenic potential is **HIGH**. Potential for delayed symptoms
See Chapter 42 for antiemetic recommendations

Hematopoietic growth factor (CSF) prophylaxis
Primary prophylaxis is **NOT** indicated
See Chapter 43 for more information

Antimicrobial prophylaxis
Risk of fever and neutropenia is **LOW**
Antimicrobial primary prophylaxis to be considered:
- Antibacterial—not indicated
- Antifungal—not indicated
- Antiviral—not indicated, unless patient previously had an episode of HSV

Followed by:
Trastuzumab every 21 days for 4 cycles,
Loading Dose: **Trastuzumab** 4 mg/kg; administer intravenously in 250 mL 0.9% NS over 90 minutes on day 1 only during the first cycle, *then*
Maintenance Dose: **Trastuzumab** 2 mg/kg per dose; administer intravenously in 250 mL 0.9% NS over 30 minutes, once weekly on days 8 and 15 during cycle 1, and days 1, 8, and 15 during cycles 2–4 (total dosage during the first cycle = 8 mg/kg; total dosage during cycles 2–4 = 6 mg/kg)

Premedication:
Dexamethasone 8 mg/dose; administer orally twice daily for 3 days, starting on the day before docetaxel administration (total dose/cycle = 48 mg)

Docetaxel 100 mg/m²; administer intravenously in a volume of 0.9% NS or D5W sufficient to produce a final docetaxel concentration within the range of 0.3–0.74 mg/mL over 60 minutes on day 1 after trastuzumab, every 21 days for 4 cycles (total dosage/cycle = 100 mg/m²)

Supportive Care
Antiemetic prophylaxis
Emetogenic potential is **LOW**
See Chapter 42 for antiemetic recommendations

Hematopoietic growth factor (CSF) prophylaxis
Primary prophylaxis may be indicated
See Chapter 43 for more information

(continued)

Note

In the neoadjuvant setting, consider adding pertuzumab with docetaxel and trastuzumab chemotherapy
Give Pertuzumab every 21 days for 4 cycles:
Loading dose: **Pertuzumab** 840 mg; administer intravenously in 250 mL of 0.9% NS over 90 minutes on day 1 after trastuzumab, cycle 1 only (total dose during the first cycle = 840 mg), *followed 3 weeks later by:*
Maintenance doses: **Pertuzumab** 420 mg; administer intravenously in 250 mL of 0.9% NS over 30–60 minutes on day 1 after trastuzumab, every 3 weeks for 3 cycles (total dose/cycle = 420 mg)

Schneeweiss A et al. Ann Oncol 2013;24:2278–2284

Treatment Modifications

Adverse Events	Treatment Modifications
WBC <3500/mm³, or absolute neutrophil count (ANC) <1500/mm³, or platelets <100,000/mm³ on first day of a cycle	Delay treatment for a maximum of 2 weeks until WBC >3500/mm³, ANC >1500/mm³, and platelets >100,000/mm³. Continue at full dosages if counts recover within 2 weeks. Give filgrastim* in subsequent cycles

If after 2 weeks, WBC <3500/mm³, ANC <500/mm³, or platelets <100,000/mm³, reduce all drug dosages as follows:

WBC 3000–3499/mm³, ANC 1000–1500/mm³, or platelets 75,000–99,999/mm³	Reduce dosages by 20%
WBC 2500–2999/mm³, ANC 500–1000/mm³, or platelets ≥75,000/mm³	Reduce dosages by 50%
WBC <2500/mm³, ANC <500/mm³, or platelets <75,000/mm³	Hold treatment
Hematologic recovery >3 weeks	Discontinue treatment

(*continued*)

Antimicrobial prophylaxis
Risk of fever and neutropenia is **INTERMEDIATE**
   Antimicrobial primary prophylaxis to be considered:
- Antibacterial—consider a fluoroquinolone or no prophylaxis
- Antifungal—not indicated
- Antiviral—not indicated, unless patient previously had an episode of HSV

Four cycles of trastuzumab and docetaxel are followed by:
Trastuzumab 6 mg/kg; administer intravenously in 250 mL 0.9% NS over 30 minutes on day 1, every 21 days for 9 months to complete 1 year of trastuzumab

Supportive Care
Antiemetic prophylaxis
Emetogenic potential is **LOW**
See Chapter 42 for antiemetic recommendations

Hematopoietic growth factor (CSF) prophylaxis
Primary prophylaxis is **NOT** *indicated*
See Chapter 43 for more information

Antimicrobial prophylaxis
Risk of fever and neutropenia is **LOW**
   Antimicrobial primary prophylaxis to be considered:
- Antibacterial—not indicated
- Antifungal—not indicated
- Antiviral—not indicated, unless patient previously had an episode of HSV

Trastuzumab infusion reactions
- A symptom complex most commonly consisting of chills and/or fever may occur in as many as 40% of patients during the first infusion of trastuzumab. These symptoms occur infrequently with subsequent trastuzumab infusions. Other signs and/or symptoms may include nausea, vomiting, pain (in some cases at tumor sites), rigors, headache, dizziness, dyspnea, hypotension, rash, and asthenia. Although the symptoms are usually mild to moderate in severity, infrequently, trastuzumab may need to be discontinued
- When such a symptom complex is observed, it can be treated with or without reduction in the rate of trastuzumab infusion, and:
  - **Acetaminophen** 650 mg; administer orally
  - **Diphenhydramine** 25–50 mg; administer orally or by intravenous injection, and
  - **Meperidine** 12.5–25 mg; administer by intravenous injection every 10 minutes if needed for shaking chills (generally, cumulative doses >50 mg are not needed; use with caution in persons with moderate or more severely impaired renal function)

Treatment Modifications
(*continued*)

First episode of febrile neutropenia or documented infection after treatment	Filgrastim* prophylaxis administered during subsequent cycles
Second episode of febrile neutropenia or documented infection after treatment	Reduce docetaxel dosage to 60 mg/m² or doxorubicin and cyclophosphamide dosages by 25% during subsequent cycles; administer filgrastim* and consider prophylaxis with ciprofloxacin†
Third episode of febrile neutropenia or documented infection after treatment	Discontinue chemotherapy
G3/4 stomatitis	Reduce docetaxel dosage to 60 mg/m² or doxorubicin dosage by 25% during subsequent cycles
G3/4 neuropathy	Discontinue treatment
Other severe adverse events	Hold treatment until toxicity resolves to G ≤1, then resume at decreased dosages appropriate for the toxicity
LVEF has declined by ≥16 percentage points from baseline, or has declined by 10–15 percentage points from baseline to a value below the lower limit of the normal range OR Symptomatic congestive heart failure	Withhold trastuzumab and repeat LVEF assessment at 4-week intervals until improvement, which may require prolonged interruption. For a persistent decline in LVEF, consider a cardio-oncology consultation and weigh the benefits and risks of continuing trastuzumab in the individual patient.

*Filgrastim 5 mcg/kg per day; administer subcutaneously starting at least 24 hours after completing chemotherapy until ANC ≥5000/mm³
†Ciprofloxacin 500 mg; administer orally twice daily for 7 days starting on day 5
Note: Dosages reduced for adverse events are not re-escalated

Patient Population Studied

Study of 3222 women with HER2+ by FISH, T1–3, N0/N1, M0 breast cancer (AC → T: 1073; AC → TH: 1074; TCH: 1075). Stratified by nodes and hormonal receptor status

Therapy Monitoring

1. *Before each cycle:* CBC with differential and platelet count, LFTs, serum electrolytes, BUN, and creatinine
2. *Hearing test:* At baseline and as needed
3. Conduct thorough cardiac assessment, including history, physical examination, and determination of LVEF by echocardiogram or MUGA scan at baseline, after completion of doxorubicin and prior to initiation of trastuzumab, and every 3 months during trastuzumab therapy

Efficacy

Third Planned Efficacy Analysis: 65 Months Follow-up*

	AC → T	AC → TH	AC → TH vs AC → T		TCH	TCH vs AC → T		AC → TH vs TCH
			HR	*P* Value		HR	P Value	P Value
All Patients								
	N = 1073	N = 1074			N = 1075			
DFS	75%	84%	0.64	<0.001	81%	0.75	0.04	0.21
OS	87%	92%	0.63	<0.001	91%	0.77	0.038	0.14
Patients with Negative Lymph Nodes								
	N = 309	N = 310			N = 309			
DFS	85%	93%	0.47	0.003	90%	0.64	0.057	—
OS	93%	97%	0.38	0.02	96%	0.56	0.11	—
Patients with Positive Lymph Nodes								
	N = 764	N = 764			N = 766			
DFS	71%	80%	0.68	0.0003	78%	0.78	0.013	—
Patients with ≥4 Positive Lymph Nodes								
	N = 350	N = 350			N = 352			
DFS	61%	73%	0.66	0.002	72%	0.66	0.002	—

AC → T, doxorubicin (Adriamycin) + cyclophosphamide followed by docetaxel; AC → TH, doxorubicin + cyclophosphamide followed by docetaxel plus trastuzumab (Herceptin) then trastuzumab alone; DFS, disease-free survival; OS, overall survival; TCH, docetaxel plus carboplatin plus concurrent trastuzumab, then trastuzumab alone
*DFS and OS values are at 65 months

Toxicity

	AC → T N = 1050		AC → TH N = 1068		TCH N = 1056	
	% All G	%G3/4	% All G	% G3/4	% All G	% G3/4
Nonhematologic Toxicity						
Neuropathy, sensory	48.6		49.7		36.1*	
Neuropathy, motor	5.2		6.3		4.2*	
Nail changes	49.3		43.6		28.7*	
Myalgia	52.8	5.2	55.5	5.2	38.6*	1.8*
Renal failure	0		0		0.1	
G3/4 creatinine	0.6		0.3		0.1	
Arthralgia		3.2		3.3		1.4*
Fatigue		7		7.2		7.2
Hand-foot syndrome		1.9		1.4		0*
Stomatitis		3.5		2.9		1.4*
Diarrhea		3.0		5.6		5.4
Nausea		5.9		5.7		4.8
Vomiting		6.1		6.7		3.5*
Irregular menses		27		24.3		26.5
Hematologic Toxicity						
Neutropenia		63.5		71.6		66.2*
Leucopenia		51.9		60.4		48.4*
Neutropenic infection		9.3		10.9		9.6
Febrile neutropenia		11.5		12.1		11.2
Anemia		2.4		3.1*		5.8
Thrombocytopenia		1.6		2.1*		6.1
Acute leukemia	0.6		0.1		0.1	
Cardiac Toxicity						
G3/4 LV dysfunction (CHF)[†]	7/1050		21/1068		4/1056	
>10% Relative LVEF decline[‡]	11%		19%		9%	

AC → T, doxorubicin (Adriamycin) + cyclophosphamide followed by docetaxel; AC → TH, doxorubicin + cyclophosphamide followed by docetaxel plus trastuzumab (Herceptin) then trastuzumab alone; TCH, docetaxel plus carboplatin plus concurrent trastuzumab, then trastuzumab alone; LV, left ventricular; CHF, congestive heart failure; LVEF, left ventricular ejection fraction
*Less statistically significantly events than the comparator groups
[†]AC → T vs AC → TH: P = 0.0121; AC → TH vs TCH: p <0.001; AC → T vs TCH: P = 0.3852
[‡]AC → T vs AC → TH: p <0.001; AC → TH vs TCH: p <0.001; AC → T vs TCH: P = 0.19

NEOADJUVANT • HER2-POSITIVE

BREAST CANCER REGIMEN: NEOADJUVANT FLUOROURACIL + EPIRUBICIN + CYCLOPHOSPHAMIDE (FEC) THEN NEOADJUVANT DOCETAXEL + TRASTUZUMAB + PERTUZUMAB (DHP) THEN ADJUVANT TRASTUZUMAB

Schneeweiss A et al. Ann Oncol 2013;24:2278–2284

The below regimen consists of 3 cycles of neoadjuvant fluorouracil + epirubicin + cyclophosphamide (FEC) followed by 3 cycles of neoadjuvant trastuzumab + pertuzumab + docetaxel followed by adjuvant trastuzumab to complete a total of one year of trastuzumab therapy. Additional adjuvant therapy (eg, radiation, hormone therapy, and/or chemotherapy) should be considered after surgery, as indicated

<u>Neoadjuvant fluorouracil + epirubicin + cyclophosphamide (FEC) × 3 cycles</u>

Hydration before and after cyclophosphamide with 0.9% sodium chloride injection (0.9% NS); administer intravenously 500 mL before starting cyclophosphamide and 500 mL after completing cyclophosphamide

Fluorouracil 500 mg/m^2; administer by intravenous injection over 1–3 minutes on day 1, every 21 days for 3 cycles (total dosage/3-week cycle = 500 mg/m^2)

Epirubicin HCl 100 mg/m^2; administer by intravenous injection over 3–5 minutes on day 1, every 21 days for 3 cycles (total dosage/3-week cycle = 100 mg/m^2)

Cyclophosphamide 600 mg/m^2; administer intravenously in 100–500 mL 0.9% NS or 5% dextrose injection (D5W) over 30–60 minutes on day 1, every 21 days for 3 cycles (total dosage/3-week cycle = 600 mg/m^2)

<u>After completion of neoadjuvant fluorouracil + epirubicin + cyclophosphamide (FEC) × 3 cycles, then administer neoadjuvant docetaxel + trastuzumab + pertuzumab (DHP) × 3 cycles as follows:</u>

Trastuzumab every 21 days for 3 cycles:
- *Loading Dose:* **Trastuzumab** 8 mg/kg; administer intravenously in 250 mL 0.9% NS over 90 minutes as a loading dose before pertuzumab on day 1, cycle 1 only (total dosage during the first cycle = 8 mg/kg), *followed 3 weeks later by:*
  - *Note:* A syndrome most commonly consisting of chills and/or fever may occur in as many as 40% of patients during the first infusion of trastuzumab. These symptoms occur infrequently with subsequent trastuzumab infusions. Other signs and/or symptoms may include nausea, vomiting, pain (in some cases at tumor sites), rigors, headache, dizziness, dyspnea, hypotension, rash, and asthenia. Although the symptoms are usually mild to moderate in severity, infrequently, trastuzumab may need to be discontinued
  - When such a syndrome is observed, it can be treated with or without reduction in the rate of trastuzumab infusion, and:
    - **Acetaminophen** 650 mg; administer orally, *plus:*
    - **Diphenhydramine** 25–50 mg; administer orally or by intravenous injection, *plus:*
    - **Meperidine** 12.5–25 mg; administer by intravenous injection every 10 minutes if needed for shaking chills (generally, cumulative doses >50 mg are not needed; use with caution in persons with moderate or more severely impaired renal function)
- *Maintenance Doses:* **Trastuzumab** 6 mg/kg; administer intravenously in 250 mL 0.9% NS over 30 minutes before pertuzumab on day 1, every 3 weeks for 2 cycles (total dosage/3-week cycle = 6 mg/kg)
  - *Note:* If a patient misses a 6 mg/kg trastuzumab dose by more than 7 days, a re-loading dose of trastuzumab should be given as trastuzumab 8 mg/kg (loading dose); administer intravenously in 250 mL 0.9% NS over 90 minutes once. This should be followed 21 days later by resumption of 6-mg/kg maintenance doses repeated every 3 weeks

Pertuzumab every 21 days for 3 cycles:
- *Loading Dose:* **Pertuzumab** 840 mg initial (loading) dose; administer intravenously in 250 mL 0.9% NS over 60 minutes as a loading dose after trastuzumab on day 1, cycle 1 only (total dosage during the first cycle = 840 mg), *followed 3 weeks later by:*
- *Maintenance Doses:* **Pertuzumab** 420 mg per dose; administer intravenously in 250 mL 0.9% NS over 30–60 minutes after trastuzumab on day 1, every 3 weeks for 2 cycles (total dosage/3-week cycle = 420 mg)
  - *Note:* If a patient misses a 420-mg pertuzumab dose by more than 21 days (ie, ≥6 weeks between two sequential infusions), a re-loading dose of pertuzumab should be given as pertuzumab 840-mg (loading) dose; administer intravenously in 250 mL 0.9% NS over 60 minutes as a loading dose once. This should be followed 21 days later by resumption of 420-mg maintenance doses repeated every 3 weeks

Alternatively, a fixed dose combination product containing pertuzumab, trastuzumab, and hyaluronidase (PHESGO™) for subcutaneous injection may be used instead of intravenous pertuzumab and trastuzumab as follows:
- *Loading Dose:* **Pertuzumab, trastuzumab, and hyaluronidase (PHESGO™) for subcutaneous injection** 1200 mg, 600 mg, and 30,000 units, respectively; administer as a 15 mL subcutaneous injection into the thigh over 8 minutes once on day 1, cycle 1 only (total dosage during the first cycle = 1200 mg pertuzumab, 600 mg trastuzumab, and 30,000 units hyaluronidase), *followed 3 weeks later by:*
- *Maintenance Doses:* **Pertuzumab, trastuzumab, and hyaluronidase (PHESGO™) for subcutaneous injection** 600 mg, 600 mg, and 20,000 units, respectively; administer as a 10 mL subcutaneous injection into the thigh over 5 minutes on day 1, every 3 weeks, for 2 cycles (total dosage/3-week cycle = 600 mg pertuzumab, 600 mg trastuzumab, and 20,000 units hyaluronidase)

(continued)

(continued)

- *Notes:*
  - Alternate the injection site between the left and right thigh, avoiding the last injection site by ≥2.5 cm. Avoid injection into areas that are hard, red, bruised, or tender.
  - Observe patients for at least 30 minutes after the loading dose and for at least 15 minutes after maintenance doses.
  - If a scheduled injection is delayed and the interval between injections is <6 weeks, then administer the maintenance dose. If the interval between injections is ≥6 weeks, then administer a loading dose followed 3 weeks later by resumption of maintenance dosing.

Prophylaxis for fluid retention and hypersensitivity reactions from docetaxel:
Dexamethasone 8 mg/dose; administer orally twice daily for 3 days, starting on the day before docetaxel administration (total dose/cycle = 48 mg)

Docetaxel 75 mg/m²; administer intravenously in a volume of 0.9% NS or D5W sufficient to produce a final docetaxel concentration of 0.3–0.74 mg/mL over 60 minutes after pertuzumab on day 1, every 3 weeks for 3 cycles (total dosage/3-week cycle = 75 mg/m²)

Notes:
- Some formulations of docetaxel contain alcohol; use caution or consider using a non–alcohol-containing formulation in patients who are sensitive to alcohol
- If no dose limiting toxicities are observed after the first docetaxel dose, escalate the docetaxel dose to 100 mg/m² in cycles 2–3 as follows:
  - **Docetaxel** 100 mg/m²; administer intravenously in a volume of 0.9% NS or D5W sufficient to produce a final docetaxel concentration of 0.3–0.74 mg/mL over 60 minutes after pertuzumab on day 1, every 3 weeks for 2 cycles (ie, cycles 2 and 3) (total dosage/cycle during cycles 2 and 3 if dose escalated = 100 mg/m²)

After surgery, continue adjuvant trastuzumab for up to 15 additional cycles (not to exceed 52 weeks of total trastuzumab therapy) as follows:
Trastuzumab every 21 days for up to 15 cycles (not to exceed 52 weeks of total trastuzumab therapy):
- *Loading Dose:* **Trastuzumab** 8 mg/kg; administer intravenously in 250 mL 0.9% NS over 90 minutes as a loading dose on day 1, cycle 1 only (total dosage during the first cycle = 8 mg/kg), *followed 3 weeks later by:*
  - *Note:* A syndrome most commonly consisting of chills and/or fever may occur in as many as 40% of patients during the first infusion of trastuzumab. These symptoms occur infrequently with subsequent trastuzumab infusions. Other signs and/or symptoms may include nausea, vomiting, pain (in some cases at tumor sites), rigors, headache, dizziness, dyspnea, hypotension, rash, and asthenia. Although the symptoms are usually mild to moderate in severity, infrequently, trastuzumab may need to be discontinued
  - When such a syndrome is observed, it can be treated with or without reduction in the rate of trastuzumab infusion, and:
    - **Acetaminophen** 650 mg; administer orally, *plus:*
    - **Diphenhydramine** 25–50 mg; administer orally or by intravenous injection, *plus:*
    - **Meperidine** 12.5–25 mg; administer by intravenous injection every 10 minutes if needed for shaking chills (generally, cumulative doses >50 mg are not needed; use with caution in persons with moderate or more severely impaired renal function)
- *Maintenance Doses:* **Trastuzumab** 6 mg/kg; administer intravenously in 250 mL 0.9% NS over 30 minutes on day 1, every 3 weeks for up to 15 cycles not to exceed 52 weeks of total trastuzumab therapy (total dosage/3-week cycle = 6 mg/kg)
  - *Note:* If a patient misses a 6 mg/kg trastuzumab dose by more than 7 days, a re-loading dose of trastuzumab should be given as trastuzumab 8 mg/kg (loading dose); administer intravenously in 250 mL 0.9% NS over 90 minutes once. This should be followed 21 days later by resumption of 6-mg/kg maintenance doses repeated every 3 weeks

Supportive Care
Antiemetic prophylaxis
Emetogenic potential during neoadjuvant fluorouracil + epirubicin + cyclophosphamide (FEC) is **HIGH.** *Potential for delayed symptoms*
Emetogenic potential during neoadjuvant docetaxel + trastuzumab + pertuzumab (DHP) is **LOW**
Emetogenic potential during adjuvant trastuzumab monotherapy is **MINIMAL**
See Chapter 42 for antiemetic recommendations

Hematopoietic growth factor (CSF) prophylaxis
Primary prophylaxis may be indicated following neoadjuvant fluorouracil + epirubicin + cyclophosphamide (FEC) cycles and/or following neoadjuvant docetaxel + trastuzumab + pertuzumab cycles
See Chapter 43 for more information

Antimicrobial prophylaxis
Risk of fever and neutropenia is **LOW**
Antimicrobial primary prophylaxis to be considered:
- Antibacterial—not indicated
- Antifungal—not indicated

(continued)

(continued)

- Antiviral—not indicated, unless patient previously had an episode of HSV

Diarrhea management
Latent or delayed-onset diarrhea:
  Loperamide 4 mg orally initially after the first loose or liquid stool, *then*
  Loperamide 2 mg orally every 2 hours during waking hours, *plus*
  Loperamide 4 mg orally every 4 hours during hours of sleep
- Continue for at least 12 hours after diarrhea resolves
- Recurrent diarrhea after a 12-hour diarrhea-free interval is treated as a new episode
- Rehydrate orally with fluids and electrolytes during a diarrheal episode
- If a patient develops blood or mucus in stool, dehydration, or hemodynamic instability, or if diarrhea persists >48 hours despite loperamide, stop loperamide and evaluate urgently in clinic or hospitalize the patient for IV hydration
- Alternatively, a trial of **diphenoxylate hydrochloride** 2.5 mg with **atropine sulfate** 0.025 mg (eg, Lomotil)
- Initial adult dose is 2 tablets 4 times daily until control has been achieved, after which the dose may be reduced to meet individual requirements. Control may often be maintained with as little as 2 tablets daily
- Clinical improvement of acute diarrhea is usually observed within 48 hours. If improvement of chronic diarrhea after treatment with a maximum daily dose of 8 tablets is not observed within 10 days, control is unlikely with further administration

Patient Population Studied

The international, multicenter, randomized, open-label, phase 2 trial (TRYPHAENA) involved 225 patients with operable, previously untreated, locally advanced or inflammatory, HER2-positive breast cancer. Eligible patients were aged ≥18 years and had an Eastern Cooperative Oncology Group (ECOG) performance status score ≤1. Patients were randomly assigned to receive six cycles of one of the following treatment combinations every 3 weeks: three cycles of intravenous trastuzumab (initial dose 8 mg/kg and then 6 mg/kg) plus pertuzumab (initial dose 840 mg and then 420 mg) plus 5-fluorouracil (500 mg/m^2) plus epirubicin (100 mg/m^2) plus cyclophosphamide (600 mg/m^2) and then three cycles of intravenous trastuzumab (6 mg/kg) plus pertuzumab (420 mg) plus docetaxel (75 mg/m^2 and then 100 mg/m^2 if tolerated) (group A); three cycles of intravenous 5-fluorouracil (500 mg/m^2) plus epirubicin (100 mg/m^2) plus cyclophosphamide (600 mg/m^2) and then three cycles of intravenous trastuzumab (initial dose 8 mg/kg and then 6 mg/kg) plus pertuzumab (initial dose 840 mg and then 420 mg) plus docetaxel (75 mg/m^2 and then 100 mg/m^2 if tolerated) (group B); or six cycles of intravenous trastuzumab (initial dose 8 mg/kg and then 6 mg/kg) plus pertuzumab (initial dose 840 mg and then 420 mg) plus carboplatin (dose of 6 area under the curve) plus docetaxel (75 mg/m^2) (group C). Patients were scheduled to subsequently undergo surgery and continue trastuzumab to complete 1 year of treatment, and to receive further adjuvant treatment according to local guidelines

Efficacy (N = 225)

	Group A (N = 73)	Group B (N = 75)	Group C (N = 77)
Rate of pathologic complete response in the breast	61.6%	57.3%	66.2%
Rate of clinical complete response	50.7%	28.0%	40.3%

Note: The median time on study, including post-treatment follow-up, was 20–21 months for the three treatment groups. A greater proportion of patients in group C presented with locally advanced disease

Therapy Monitoring

1. Prior to each cycle of DHP and FEC: CBC with differential, serum bilirubin, AST/ALT, alkaline phosphatase, and creatinine
2. Conduct thorough cardiac assessment, including history, physical examination, and determination of LVEF by echocardiogram or MUGA scan at baseline, after completion of epirubicin and immediately prior to initiation of trastuzumab, and then every 3 months during trastuzumab therapy
3. Patients should have a pre-treatment LVEF ≥55%
4. Repeat LVEF measurement at 4-week intervals if trastuzumab and/or pertuzumab are withheld for significant left ventricular cardiac dysfunction
5. Monitor for symptoms of pulmonary toxicity
6. Verify pregnancy status prior to the initiation of therapy. Advise patients of the risks of embryo-fetal death and birth defects and the need for contraception
7. Avoid using concomitant strong CYP3A4 inhibitors (eg, ketoconazole, itraconazole, clarithromycin, atazanavir, indinavir, nefazodone, nelfinavir, ritonavir, saquinavir, telithromycin, and voriconazole). Consider a 50% docetaxel dose reduction if patients require co-administration of a strong CYP3A4 inhibitor

Treatment Modifications

FLUOROURACIL + EPIRUBICIN + CYCLOPHOSPHAMIDE (FEC)

Adverse Event	Treatment Modification
Neutropenia/Thrombocytopenia	
G1 ANC (1500–1999/mm³) or G1 thrombocytopenia (<LLN to 75,000/mm³)	Maintain dose and schedule
G2 ANC (1,000–1499/mm³) or G2 thrombocytopenia (<75,000–50,000/mm³)	Reduce dosages by 15–20%
G3 ANC (500–999/mm³) or G3 thrombocytopenia (<50,000–25,000/mm³)	Hold treatment until toxicity resolves to G ≤2, then reduce dosages by 15–20%
G4 ANC (<500/mm³) or G4 thrombocytopenia (<25,000/mm³)	Hold treatment until toxicity resolves to G ≤2, then reduce dosages by 30–40%
Febrile neutropenia (ANC <1000/mm³ with single temperature >38.3°C [101°F] or a sustained temperature of ≥38°C [100.4°F] for more than 1 hour)	Hold treatment until neutropenia resolves, then reduce dosages by 30–40%. Consider adding filgrastim
Day 1 ANC <1500/mm³ and/or platelet count <100,000/mm³	Withhold therapy until ANC >1500/mm³ and/or platelet count >100,000/mm³
ANC <1500/mm³ and/or platelet count <100,000/mm³ despite a 2-week delay, but with ANC >1000/mm³ and platelet count >75,000/mm³	Resume therapy with fluorouracil, epirubicin, and cyclophosphamide dosage reduced by 30–40%. Consider filgrastim
Diarrhea	
G1 (2–3 stools/day > baseline)	Maintain dose and schedule
G2 (4–6 stools/day > baseline)	Delay until diarrhea resolves to baseline, then reduce dosage of fluorouracil 15–20%
G3 (7–9 stools/day > baseline)	
G4 (≥10 stools/day > baseline)	Delay until diarrhea resolves to baseline, then reduce dosage of fluorouracil by 30–40%
Other Nonhematologic Toxicities	
Bilirubin 1.2 to 3 mg/dL or AST 2–4× ULN	Reduce epirubicin dosage by 50%
Bilirubin >3 mg/dL or AST >4× ULN	Reduce epirubicin dosage by 75%; reduce cyclophosphamide dose by 25%
LVEF is 40%, or is 40% to 45% with a 10% or greater absolute decrease below the pretreatment	Withhold epirubicin and repeat LVEF assessment within approximately 3 weeks. Discontinue epirubicin if the LVEF has not improved or has declined further, unless the benefits for the individual patient outweigh the risks
G2–4 mucositis (moderate pain or ulcer that does not interfere with oral intake; modified diet indicated or worse)	Decrease only fluorouracil by 20%
Any other G1 toxicity	Maintain dose and schedule
Any other G2 toxicity	Hold treatment until toxicity resolves to G ≤1, then reduce dosages by 15–20%
Any other G3 toxicity	Hold treatment until toxicity resolves to G ≤1, then reduce dosages by 15–20%
Any other G4 toxicity	Hold treatment until toxicity resolves to G ≤1, then reduce dosages by 30–50%

Note: Patients who are pregnant or who become pregnant should be apprised of the potential hazard to the fetus; women of childbearing potential should be advised to avoid becoming pregnant during therapy

Treatment Modifications (continued)

DOCETAXEL DOSE MODIFICATIONS

Docetaxel starting dose	75 mg/m²
Docetaxel dose level −1	60 mg/m²
Docetaxel dose level −2	50 mg/m²
Docetaxel dose level −3	Discontinue docetaxel

Adverse Event	Treatment Modifications
Severe hypersensitivity reaction	Discontinue infusion immediately and administer appropriate support. For hypersensitivity reaction less G ≤3, initial management includes temporary discontinuation of infusion for 30 minutes, and administration of additional intravenous antihistamines and glucocorticoids. Upon resolution of symptoms, infusion may be restarted at a slower rate if deemed safe. If G4 hypersensitivity is experienced, stabilize the cardiorespiratory system and use epinephrine as needed, then permanently discontinue docetaxel*
Febrile neutropenia (ANC <1000/mm³ with temperature >38°C or >100.4°F), or ANC <500/mm³ for ≥7 days	Withhold treatment until resolution of toxicity. Administer filgrastim in subsequent cycles
Febrile neutropenia (ANC <1000/mm³ with temperature >38°C or >100.4°F), or ANC <500/mm³ for ≥7 days despite administration of filgrastim	Reduce docetaxel one dose level; continue filgrastim administration
Platelet nadir <50,000/mm³, or platelets <100,000/mm³ for ≥7 days	Reduce docetaxel dose by one level
ANC <1500/mm³ and/or platelets <100,000/mm³ at the start of a cycle	Hold treatment until ANC ≥1500/mm³ and platelets ≥100,000/mm³, then resume with docetaxel dosage reduced by one dose level
Bilirubin > ULN, or AST/ALT >1.5 × ULN and AP >2.5 × ULN	Withhold docetaxel until bilirubin ≤ ULN or AST/ALT ≤1.5 and AP ≤2.5 × ULN, then resume docetaxel dosage reduced by one dose level
Severe or cumulative cutaneous reactions G3/4 stomatitis	Withhold treatment until resolution of toxicity. Reduce docetaxel dosage one dose level
G1 neurotoxicity of any duration (paresthesias/dysesthesias that do not interfere with function)	Continue docetaxel treatment
G2 neurotoxicity of 1–7 days duration (paresthesias/dysesthesias interfering with function, but not activities of daily living)	Continue docetaxel treatment but can delay start for up to seven days until G ≤1
G2 neurotoxicity of >7 days duration (paresthesias/dysesthesias interfering with function, but not activities of daily living)	Withhold docetaxel until toxicity G ≤1, then resume docetaxel treatment, but reduce dose by one dose level. If G2 toxicity persists after 3 weeks of delay, discontinue docetaxel*
G3 neurotoxicity of 1–7 days duration (paresthesias/dysesthesias with pain or with function impairment interfering with activities of daily living)	Withhold docetaxel. Resume with docetaxel dose reduced one dose level when toxicity has resolved to G ≤1
Second episode of G3 neurotoxicity of 1–7 days duration (paresthesias/dysesthesias with pain or with function impairment interfering with activities of daily living)	Discontinue docetaxel*
G3 neurotoxicity of >7 days duration (paresthesias/dysesthesias with pain or with function impairment interfering with activities of daily living)	Discontinue docetaxel*
Persistent paresthesias/dysesthesias that are disabling or life-threatening	Discontinue docetaxel*

(continued)

Treatment Modifications *(continued)*

Adverse Event	Treatment Modifications
G1 musculoskeletal pain not controlled by analgesics of any duration	Continue docetaxel treatment
G2 musculoskeletal pain not controlled by analgesics of 1–7 days duration	
G2 musculoskeletal pain not controlled by analgesics of >7 days duration	Continue docetaxel treatment or withhold docetaxel for persistent G2. When toxicity G ≤1, resume treatment with dose that is one dose lower. If G2 toxicity persists resulting in a delay of >3 weeks, discontinue docetaxel*
First episode of G3 musculoskeletal pain not controlled by analgesics of 1–7 days duration	Continue docetaxel treatment
Second episode of G3 musculoskeletal pain not controlled by analgesics of 1–7 days duration	Discontinue docetaxel*
First episode of G3 musculoskeletal pain not controlled by analgesics of >7 days duration	Withhold docetaxel. When toxicity G ≤1, resume treatment with dose that is one dose lower. If >G2 toxicity persists resulting in a delay of >3 weeks discontinue docetaxel*
Second episode of G3 musculoskeletal pain not controlled by analgesics of >7 days duration	Discontinue docetaxel*
Docetaxel-related fluid retention	Consider 1- to 5-day treatment with dexamethasone starting one day before docetaxel administration. Consider diuretics for symptomatic relief and to limit the severity of fluid retention
Other G2 nonhematologic adverse event that occurs during a cycle but results in a delay in the start of the next cycle	Hold treatment until adverse events resolve to G ≤1, then resume with docetaxel dosage reduced by one dose level
Other G3 nonhematologic adverse event that occurs during a cycle but resolves prior to the start of the next cycle or requires a delay in the start of the next cycle	Hold treatment until adverse events resolve to G ≤1, then resume with docetaxel dosage reduced by one dose level
Other G4 nonhematologic adverse event that occurs during a cycle but resolves prior to the start of the next cycle	Hold treatment until adverse events resolve to G ≤1, then resume with docetaxel dosage reduced by two dose levels or discontinue docetaxel*
Other G4 nonhematologic adverse event that occurs during a cycle but requires a delay in the start of the next cycle	Discontinue docetaxel*
Any treatment delay >3 weeks	

NEOADJUVANT PERTUZUMAB AND TRASTUZUMAB OR ADJUVANT TRASTUZUMAB ALONE

Note: Dose reductions are not recommended for trastuzumab or pertuzumab

Adverse Event	Treatment Modifications
Mild or moderate infusion reaction	Decrease the rate of infusion
Infusion reaction with dyspnea or clinically significant hypotension	Interrupt the infusion. Administer medical therapy as indicated including epinephrine, corticosteroids, diphenhydramine, bronchodilators, and oxygen. Observe patients closely for 60 minutes if the reaction occurs after the first infusion and for 30 minutes if it occurs after subsequent infusions. Prior to resumption of the infusion, premedicate with antihistamines and/or corticosteroids. Note: While some patients tolerate the resumption of infusions, others have recurrent severe infusion reactions despite premedications
Severe or life-threatening infusion reaction (including bronchospasm, anaphylaxis, angioedema, hypoxia, and severe hypotension; usually reported during or immediately following the initial infusion)	Interrupt the infusion reaction. Administer medical therapy as indicated including epinephrine, corticosteroids, diphenhydramine, bronchodilators, and oxygen. Patients should be evaluated and carefully monitored until complete resolution of signs and symptoms. Discontinue pertuzumab and trastuzumab

(continued)

Treatment Modifications (*continued*)

Adverse Event	Treatment Modifications
LVEF has declined by ≥16 percentage points from baseline, or has declined by 10–15 percentage points from baseline to a value below the lower limit of the normal range OR Symptomatic congestive heart failure	Withhold pertuzumab and trastuzumab and repeat LVEF assessment at 4-week intervals until improvement, which may require prolonged interruption. For a persistent decline in LVEF, consider a cardio-oncology consultation and weigh the benefits and risks of continuing pertuzumab and trastuzumab in the individual patient

*If docetaxel is discontinued or withheld beyond the time of start of the next cycle, treatment with pertuzumab and trastuzumab may continue

Adverse Events (N = 223)

Grade 3–5 events* (%)	Group A (N = 72)	Group B (N = 75)	Group C (N = 76)
Neutropenia	47	43	46
Febrile neutropenia	18	9	17
Leukopenia	19	12	12
Diarrhea	4	5	12
Anemia	1	3	17
Thrombocytopenia	0	0	12
Vomiting	0	3	5
Drug hypersensitivity	3	0	3
Fatigue	0	0	4
Increased alanine aminotransferase level	0	0	4

*According to the National Cancer Institute Common Terminology Criteria for Adverse Events, version 3.0
The most common grade 3–4 adverse events that occurred during the neoadjuvant treatment are included in the table. No deaths were reported during the neoadjuvant treatment. The incidences of symptomatic left ventricular systolic dysfunction and significant decline in left ventricular ejection fraction were low in all groups. Grade ≥3 adverse events were rare during adjuvant treatment

NEOADJUVANT • HER2-POSITIVE

BREAST CANCER REGIMEN: NEOADJUVANT DOCETAXEL + CARBOPLATIN + TRASTUZUMAB + PERTUZUMAB (TCHP) THEN ADJUVANT TRASTUZUMAB

Schneeweiss A et al. Ann Oncol 2013;24:2278–2284

The regimen consists of 6 cycles of neoadjuvant docetaxel + carboplatin + trastuzumab + pertuzumab (TCHP) followed by adjuvant trastuzumab to complete a total of 1 year trastuzumab therapy. Additional adjuvant therapy (eg, radiation, hormone therapy, and/or chemotherapy) should be considered after surgery, as indicated

Neoadjuvant docetaxel + carboplatin + trastuzumab + pertuzumab (TCHP)

Trastuzumab every 21 days for 6 cycles:
- *Loading Dose:* **Trastuzumab** 8 mg/kg; administer intravenously in 250 mL 0.9% sodium chloride injection (0.9% NS) over 90 minutes as a loading dose before pertuzumab on day 1, cycle 1 only (total dosage during the first cycle = 8 mg/kg), *followed 3 weeks later by:*
  - *Note:* A syndrome most commonly consisting of chills and/or fever may occur in as many as 40% of patients during the first infusion of trastuzumab. These symptoms occur infrequently with subsequent trastuzumab infusions. Other signs and/or symptoms may include nausea, vomiting, pain (in some cases at tumor sites), rigors, headache, dizziness, dyspnea, hypotension, rash, and asthenia. Although the symptoms are usually mild to moderate in severity, infrequently, trastuzumab may need to be discontinued
  - When such a syndrome is observed, it can be treated with or without reduction in the rate of trastuzumab infusion, and:
    - Acetaminophen 650 mg; administer orally, *plus:*
    - Diphenhydramine 25–50 mg; administer orally or by intravenous injection, *plus:*
    - Meperidine 12.5–25 mg; administer by intravenous injection every 10 minutes if needed for shaking chills (generally, cumulative doses >50 mg are not needed; use with caution in persons with moderate or more severely impaired renal function)
- *Maintenance Doses:* **Trastuzumab** 6 mg/kg; administer intravenously in 250 mL 0.9% NS over 30 minutes before pertuzumab on day 1, every 3 weeks for 5 cycles (total dosage/cycle = 6 mg/kg)
  - *Note:* If a patient misses a 6-mg/kg trastuzumab dose by more than 7 days, a re-loading dose of trastuzumab should be given as trastuzumab 8 mg/kg (loading dose); administer intravenously in 250 mL 0.9% NS over 90 minutes once. This should be followed 21 days later by resumption of 6-mg/kg maintenance doses repeated every 3 weeks

Pertuzumab every 21 days for 6 cycles:
- *Loading Dose:* **Pertuzumab** 840 mg initial (loading) dose; administer intravenously in 250 mL 0.9% NS over 60 minutes as a loading dose after trastuzumab on day 1, cycle 1 only (total dosage during the first cycle = 840 mg), *followed 3 weeks later by:*
- *Maintenance Doses:* **Pertuzumab** 420 mg per dose; administer intravenously in 250 mL 0.9% NS over 30–60 minutes after trastuzumab on day 1, every 3 weeks for 5 cycles (total dose/3-week cycle = 420 mg)
  - *Note:* If a patient misses a 420-mg pertuzumab dose by more than 21 days (ie, ≥6 weeks between two sequential infusions), a re-loading dose of pertuzumab should be given as pertuzumab 840-mg (loading) dose; administer intravenously in 250 mL 0.9% NS over 60 minutes as a loading dose once. This should be followed 21 days later by resumption of 420-mg maintenance doses repeated every 3 weeks

Alternatively, a fixed dose combination product containing pertuzumab, trastuzumab, and hyaluronidase (PHESGO™) for subcutaneous injection may be used instead of intravenous pertuzumab and trastuzumab as follows:
- *Loading Dose:* **Pertuzumab, trastuzumab, and hyaluronidase (PHESGO™) for subcutaneous injection** 1200 mg, 600 mg, and 30,000 units, respectively; administer as a 15 mL subcutaneous injection into the thigh over 8 minutes once on day 1, cycle 1 only (total dosage during the first cycle = 1200 mg pertuzumab, 600 mg trastuzumab, and 30,000 units hyaluronidase), *followed 3 weeks later by:*
- *Maintenance Doses:* **Pertuzumab, trastuzumab, and hyaluronidase (PHESGO™) for subcutaneous injection** 600 mg, 600 mg, and 20,000 units, respectively; administer as a 10 mL subcutaneous injection into the thigh over 5 minutes on day 1, every 3 weeks, for 5 cycles (total dosage/3-week cycle = 600 mg pertuzumab, 600 mg trastuzumab, and 20,000 units hyaluronidase)
  - *Notes:*
    - Alternate the injection site between the left and right thigh, avoiding the last injection site by ≥2.5 cm. Avoid injection into areas that are hard, red, bruised, or tender.
    - Observe patients for at least 30 minutes after the loading dose and for at least 15 minutes after maintenance doses.
    - If a scheduled injection is delayed and the interval between injections is <6 weeks, then administer the maintenance dose. If the interval between injections is ≥6 weeks, then administer a loading dose followed 3 weeks later by resumption of maintenance dosing.

Carboplatin target AUC = 6 mg/mL × min; administer intravenously in 250 mL 5% dextrose injection (D5W) or 0.9% NS over 30–60 minutes after pertuzumab on day 1, every 3 weeks for 6 cycles (total dose/cycle calculated to achieve a target AUC = 6 mg/mL × min), *followed by:*

Prophylaxis for fluid retention and hypersensitivity reactions from docetaxel:
Dexamethasone 8 mg/dose; administer orally twice daily for 3 days, starting on the day before docetaxel administration (total dose/cycle = 48 mg)

Docetaxel 75 mg/m²; administer intravenously in a volume of 0.9% NS or D5W sufficient to produce a final docetaxel concentration of 0.3–0.74 mg/mL over 60 minutes after carboplatin on day 1, every 3 weeks for 6 cycles (total dosage/cycle = 75 mg/m²)

(continued)

(continued)

After surgery, continue adjuvant trastuzumab for up to 12 additional cycles (not to exceed 52 weeks of total trastuzumab therapy) as follows:

Trastuzumab every 21 days for up to 12 cycles (not to exceed 52 weeks of total trastuzumab therapy):

- *Loading Dose:* **Trastuzumab** 8 mg/kg; administer intravenously in 250 mL 0.9% sodium chloride injection (0.9% NS) over 90 minutes as a loading dose on day 1, cycle 1 only (total dosage during the first cycle = 8 mg/kg), *followed 3 weeks later by:*

  - *Note:* A syndrome most commonly consisting of chills and/or fever may occur in as many as 40% of patients during the first infusion of trastuzumab. These symptoms occur infrequently with subsequent trastuzumab infusions. Other signs and/or symptoms may include nausea, vomiting, pain (in some cases at tumor sites), rigors, headache, dizziness, dyspnea, hypotension, rash, and asthenia. Although the symptoms are usually mild to moderate in severity, infrequently, trastuzumab may need to be discontinued

  - When such a syndrome is observed, it can be treated with or without reduction in the rate of trastuzumab infusion, and:
    - Acetaminophen 650 mg; administer orally, *plus:*
    - Diphenhydramine 25–50 mg; administer orally or by intravenous injection, *plus:*
    - Meperidine 12.5–25 mg; administer by intravenous injection every 10 minutes if needed for shaking chills (generally, cumulative doses >50 mg are not needed; use with caution in persons with moderate or more severely impaired renal function)

- *Maintenance Doses:* **Trastuzumab** 6 mg/kg; administer intravenously in 250 mL 0.9% NS over 30 minutes on day 1, every 3 weeks for up to 12 cycles not to exceed 52 weeks of total trastuzumab therapy (total dosage/3-week cycle = 6 mg/kg)

  - *Note:* If a patient misses a 6-mg/kg trastuzumab dose by more than 7 days, a re-loading dose of trastuzumab should be given as trastuzumab 8 mg/kg (loading dose); administer intravenously in 250 mL 0.9% NS over 90 minutes once. This should be followed 21 days later by resumption of 6-mg/kg maintenance doses repeated every 3 weeks

Supportive Care
Antiemetic prophylaxis
Emetogenic potential during neoadjuvant cycles (TCHP) is **HIGH***. Potential for delayed symptoms*
Emetogenic potential during adjuvant cycles (trastuzumab only) is **MINIMAL**
See Chapter 42 for antiemetic recommendations

Hematopoietic growth factor (CSF) prophylaxis
Primary prophylaxis may be indicated during neoadjuvant (TCHP) cycles
See Chapter 43 for more information

Antimicrobial prophylaxis
Risk of fever and neutropenia is **INTERMEDIATE**
Antimicrobial primary prophylaxis to be considered:

- Antibacterial—not indicated
- Antifungal—not indicated
- Antiviral—not indicated, unless patient previously had an episode of HSV

Carboplatin dose
Carboplatin dose is based on a formula described by Calvert et al. to achieve a target area under the plasma concentration versus time curve (AUC)

$$\text{Total Carboplatin Dose (mg)} = (\text{target AUC})(\text{GFR} + 25)$$

In practice, creatinine clearance (CrCl) is used in place of glomerular filtration rate (GFR). CrCl can be estimated from the equation of Cockcroft and Gault, thus:

$$\text{For males, CrCl} = \frac{(140 - \text{age[years]}) \times (\text{body weight [kg]})}{72 \times (\text{serum creatinine [mg/dL]})}$$

$$\text{For females, CrCl} = \frac{(140 - \text{age[years]}) \times (\text{body weight [kg]})}{72 \times (\text{serum creatinine [mg/dL]})} \times 0.85$$

Calvert AH et al. J Clin Oncol 1989;7:1748–1756
Cockcroft DW, Gault MH. Nephron 1976;16:31–41
Jodrell DI et al. J Clin Oncol 1992;10:520–528
Sorensen BT et al. Cancer Chemother Pharmacol 1991;28:397–401

Note: On October 8, 2010, the U.S. Food and Drug Administration (FDA) identified a potential safety issue with carboplatin dosing based on recent changes in the measurement of serum creatinine. By the end of 2010, all clinical laboratories in the United States will use the standardized isotope dilution mass spectrometry (IDMS) method to measure serum creatinine, which could result in an overestimation of the GFR in some patients with normal renal function. A carboplatin dose calculated with an IDMS-measured serum creatinine result using the Calvert formula could exceed an expected exposure (AUC) and result in increased drug-related toxicity. Provided actual GFR measurements are made to assess renal function, carboplatin can be safely dosed according to the Calvert formula described in product labeling. If GFR (or creatinine clearance) is estimated based on serum creatinine measurements by the IDMS method, the FDA recommended for patients with normal renal function capping an estimated GFR at 125 mL/min for any targeted AUC value. No greater estimated GFR values should be used.

(continued)

(continued)

Carboplatin dosing. May 23, 2013. Available from: http://www.fda.gov/AboutFDA/CentersOffices/OfficeofMedicalProductsandTobacco/CDER/ucm228974.htm [accessed February 26, 2014]

Diarrhea management

Latent or delayed-onset diarrhea:

Loperamide 4 mg orally initially after the first loose or liquid stool, *then*

Loperamide 2 mg orally every 2 hours during waking hours, *plus*

Loperamide 4 mg orally every 4 hours during hours of sleep

- Continue for at least 12 hours after diarrhea resolves

- Recurrent diarrhea after a 12-hour diarrhea-free interval is treated as a new episode

- Rehydrate orally with fluids and electrolytes during a diarrheal episode

- If a patient develops blood or mucus in stool, dehydration, or hemodynamic instability, or if diarrhea persists >48 hours despite loperamide, stop loperamide and evaluate urgently in clinic or hospitalize the patient for IV hydration

- Alternatively, a trial of **diphenoxylate hydrochloride** 2.5 mg with **atropine sulfate** 0.025 mg (eg, Lomotil)

- Initial adult dose is 2 tablets 4 times daily until control has been achieved, after which the dose may be reduced to meet individual requirements. Control may often be maintained with as little as 2 tablets daily

- Clinical improvement of acute diarrhea is usually observed within 48 hours. If improvement of chronic diarrhea after treatment with a maximum daily dose of 8 tablets is not observed within 10 days, control is unlikely with further administration

Patient Population Studied

The international, multicenter, randomized, open-label, phase 2 trial (TRYPHAENA) involved 225 patients with operable, previously untreated, locally advanced or inflammatory, HER2-positive breast cancer. Eligible patients were aged ≥18 years and had an Eastern Cooperative Oncology Group (ECOG) performance status score ≤1. Patients were randomly assigned to receive six cycles of one of the following treatment combinations every 3 weeks: three cycles of intravenous trastuzumab (initial dose 8 mg/kg and then 6 mg/kg) plus pertuzumab (initial dose 840 mg and then 420 mg) plus 5-fluorouracil (500 mg/m²) plus epirubicin (100 mg/m²) plus cyclophosphamide (600 mg/m²) and then three cycles of intravenous trastuzumab (6 mg/kg) plus pertuzumab (420 mg) plus docetaxel (75 mg/m² and then 100 mg/m² if tolerated) (group A); three cycles of intravenous 5-fluorouracil (500 mg/m²) plus epirubicin (100 mg/m²) plus cyclophosphamide (600 mg/m²) and then three cycles of intravenous trastuzumab (initial dose 8 mg/kg and then 6 mg/kg) plus pertuzumab (initial dose 840 mg and then 420 mg) plus docetaxel (75 mg/m² and then 100 mg/m² if tolerated) (group B); or six cycles of intravenous trastuzumab (initial dose 8 mg/kg and then 6 mg/kg) plus pertuzumab (initial dose 840 mg and then 420 mg) plus carboplatin (dose of 6 area under the curve) plus docetaxel (75 mg/m²) (group C). Patients were scheduled to subsequently undergo surgery and continue trastuzumab to complete 1 year of treatment, and to receive further adjuvant treatment according to local guidelines

Efficacy (N = 225)

	Group A (N = 73)	Group B (N = 75)	Group C (N = 77)
Rate of pathologic complete response in the breast	61.6%	57.3%	66.2%
Rate of clinical complete response	50.7%	28.0%	40.3%

Note: The median time on study, including post-treatment follow-up, was 20–21 months for the three treatment groups. A greater proportion of patients in group C presented with locally advanced disease

Therapy Monitoring

1. Prior to each cycle of TCHP: CBC with differential, serum electrolytes, BUN, creatinine, AST or ALT, and alkaline phosphatase

2. Conduct thorough cardiac assessment, including history, physical examination, and determination of LVEF by echocardiogram or MUGA scan at baseline immediately prior to initiation of trastuzumab and every 3 months during therapy

3. Patients should have a pre-treatment LVEF ≥55%

4. Repeat LVEF measurement at 4-week intervals if trastuzumab and/or pertuzumab are withheld for significant left ventricular cardiac dysfunction

5. Monitor for symptoms of pulmonary toxicity

6. Verify pregnancy status prior to the initiation of therapy. Advise patients of the risks of embryo-fetal death and birth defects and the need for contraception

7. Avoid using concomitant strong CYP3A4 inhibitors (eg, ketoconazole, itraconazole, clarithromycin, atazanavir, indinavir, nefazodone, nelfinavir, ritonavir, saquinavir, telithromycin, and voriconazole). Consider a 50% docetaxel dose reduction if patients require co-administration of a strong CYP3A4 inhibitor

Treatment Modifications

DOCETAXEL AND CARBOPLATIN DOSE MODIFICATIONS

Docetaxel starting dose	75 mg/m²	Carboplatin starting dose	AUC 6
Docetaxel dose level −1	60 mg/m²	Carboplatin dose level −1	AUC 5
Docetaxel dose level −2	50 mg/m²	Carboplatin dose level −2	AUC 4
Docetaxel dose level −3	Discontinue docetaxel	Carboplatin dose level −3	Discontinue carboplatin

Adverse Event	Treatment Modifications
Severe hypersensitivity reaction	Discontinue docetaxel or carboplatin infusion immediately and administer appropriate support. For hypersensitivity reaction G ≤3, initial management includes temporary discontinuation of infusion for 30 minutes, and administration of additional intravenous antihistamines and glucocorticoids. Upon resolution of symptoms, the docetaxel infusion may be restarted at a slower rate if deemed safe. Rechallenge with carboplatin will require institution of a desensitization regimen. If G4 hypersensitivity is experienced' stabilize the cardiorespiratory system and use epinephrine as needed, then permanently discontinue docetaxel or carboplatin.* Rechallenge with carboplatin will require institution of a desensitization regimen
Febrile neutropenia (ANC <1000/mm³ with temperature >38°C or >100.4°F), or ANC <500/mm³ for ≥7 days	Withhold treatment until resolution of toxicity. Administer filgrastim in subsequent cycles
Febrile neutropenia (ANC <1000/mm³ with temperature >38°C or >100.4°F), or ANC <500/mm³ for ≥7 days despite administration of filgrastim	Reduce docetaxel and carboplatin one dose level; continue filgrastim administration
Platelet nadir <50,000/mm³, or platelets <100,000/mm³ for ≥7 days	Reduce docetaxel and carboplatin dosages by one level
ANC <1500/mm³ and/or platelets <100,000/mm³ at the start of a cycle	Hold treatment until ANC ≥1500/mm³ and platelets ≥100,000/mm³, then resume with docetaxel and carboplatin dosage reduced by one dose level
Day 1 ANC <1500/mm³ and/or platelet count <100,000/mm³	Withhold docetaxel and carboplatin until ANC ≥1500/mm³ and platelet count ≥100,000/mm³
ANC <1500/mm³ and/or platelet count <100,000/mm³ despite a 2-week delay, but with ANC >1000/mm³ and platelet count >75,000/mm³	Resume therapy with docetaxel and carboplatin dosage reduced by one dose level. Consider filgrastim
Bilirubin > ULN, or AST/ALT >1.5 × ULN and AP >2.5 × ULN	Withhold docetaxel until bilirubin ≤ ULN or AST/ALT ≤1.5 and AP ≤2.5 × ULN, then resume docetaxel dosage reduced by one dose level
Severe or cumulative cutaneous reactions G3/4 stomatitis	Withhold treatment until resolution of toxicity. Reduce docetaxel dosage one dose level
G1 neurotoxicity of any duration (paresthesias/dysesthesias that do not interfere with function)	Continue docetaxel and carboplatin treatment
G2 neurotoxicity of 1–7 days duration (paresthesias/dysesthesias interfering with function, but not activities of daily living)	Continue docetaxel and carboplatin treatment but can delay start for up to seven days until G ≤1
G2 neurotoxicity of >7 days duration (paresthesias/dysesthesias interfering with function, but not activities of daily living)	Withhold docetaxel and carboplatin until toxicity G ≤1, then resume docetaxel and carboplatin treatment, but reduce dosages by one dose level. If G2 toxicity persists after 3 weeks of delay, discontinue docetaxel and carboplatin*
G3 neurotoxicity of 1–7 days duration (paresthesias/dysesthesias with pain or with function impairment interfering with activities of daily living)	Withhold docetaxel and carboplatin. Resume with docetaxel and carboplatin dosages reduced one dose level when toxicity has resolved to G ≤1

(continued)

Treatment Modifications (*continued*)

Adverse Event	Treatment Modifications
Second episode of G3 neurotoxicity of 1–7 days duration (paresthesias/dysesthesias with pain or with function impairment interfering with activities of daily living)	Discontinue docetaxel and carboplatin*
G3 neurotoxicity of >7 days duration (paresthesias/dysesthesias with pain or with function impairment interfering with activities of daily living)	Discontinue docetaxel and carboplatin*
Persistent paresthesias/dysesthesias that are disabling or life-threatening	Discontinue docetaxel and carboplatin*
G1 musculoskeletal pain not controlled by analgesics of any duration	Continue docetaxel and carboplatin treatment
G2 musculoskeletal pain not controlled by analgesics of 1–7 days duration	
G2 musculoskeletal pain not controlled by analgesics of >7 days duration	Continue docetaxel and carboplatin treatment or withhold docetaxel and carboplatin for persistent G2. When toxicity G ≤1, resume treatment with dosages that are one dose lower. If G2 toxicity persists resulting in a delay of >3 weeks discontinue docetaxel and carboplatin*
First episode of G3 musculoskeletal pain not controlled by analgesics of 1–7 days duration	Continue docetaxel and carboplatin treatment
Second episode of G3 musculoskeletal pain not controlled by analgesics of 1–7 days duration	Discontinue docetaxel and carboplatin*
First episode of G3 musculoskeletal pain not controlled by analgesics of >7 days duration	Withhold docetaxel and carboplatin. When toxicity G ≤1, resume treatment with dosages that are one dose level lower. If >G2 toxicity persists resulting in a delay of >3 weeks discontinue docetaxel and carboplatin*
Second episode of G3 musculoskeletal pain not controlled by analgesics of >7 days duration	Discontinue docetaxel and carboplatin*
Docetaxel-related fluid retention	Consider 1- to 5-day treatment with dexamethasone starting one day before docetaxel administration. Consider diuretics for symptomatic relief and to limit the severity of fluid retention
Other G2 nonhematologic adverse event that occurs during a cycle but results in a delay in the start of the next cycle	Hold treatment until adverse events resolve to G ≤1, then resume with docetaxel and/or carboplatin dosages reduced by one dose level
Other G3 nonhematologic adverse event that occurs during a cycle but resolves prior to the start of the next cycle or requires a delay in the start of the next cycle	Hold treatment until adverse events resolve to G ≤1, then resume with docetaxel and/or carboplatin dosages reduced by one dose level
Other G4 nonhematologic adverse event that occurs during a cycle but resolves prior to the start of the next cycle	Hold treatment until adverse events resolve to G ≤1, then resume with docetaxel and/or carboplatin dosages reduced by two dose levels or discontinue docetaxel and carboplatin*
Other G4 nonhematologic adverse event that occurs during a cycle but requires a delay in the start of the next cycle	Discontinue docetaxel and/or carboplatin*
Any treatment delay >3 weeks	Discontinue docetaxel and/or carboplatin*

(*continued*)

Treatment Modifications (*continued*)

TRASTUZUMAB AND PERTUZUMAB

Note: Dose reductions are not recommended for trastuzumab or pertuzumab

Adverse Event	Treatment Modifications
Mild or moderate infusion reaction	Decrease the rate of infusion
Infusion reaction with dyspnea or clinically significant hypotension	Interrupt the infusion. Administer medical therapy as indicated including epinephrine, corticosteroids, diphenhydramine, bronchodilators, and oxygen. Observe patients closely for 60 minutes if the reaction occurs after the first infusion and for 30 minutes if it occurs after subsequent infusions. Prior to resumption of the infusion, premedicate with antihistamines and/or corticosteroids. Note: While some patients tolerate the resumption of infusions, others have recurrent severe infusion reactions despite premedications
Severe or life-threatening infusion reaction (including bronchospasm, anaphylaxis, angioedema, hypoxia, and severe hypotension; usually reported during or immediately following the initial infusion)*	Interrupt the infusion reaction. Administer medical therapy as indicated including epinephrine, corticosteroids, diphenhydramine, bronchodilators, and oxygen. Patients should be evaluated and carefully monitored until complete resolution of signs and symptoms. Discontinue pertuzumab and trastuzumab
LVEF has declined by ≥16 percentage points from baseline, or has declined by 10–15 percentage points from baseline to a value below the lower limit of the normal range OR Symptomatic congestive heart failure	Withhold pertuzumab and trastuzumab and repeat LVEF assessment at 4-week intervals until improvement, which may require prolonged interruption. For a persistent decline in LVEF, consider a cardio-oncology consultation and weigh the benefits and risks of continuing pertuzumab and trastuzumab in the individual patient

*If docetaxel and/or carboplatin are discontinued or withheld beyond the time of start of the next cycle, treatment with pertuzumab and trastuzumab may continue

Adverse Events (N = 223)

Grade 3–5 Events* (%)	Group A (N = 72)	Group B (N = 75)	Group C (N = 76)
Neutropenia	47	43	46
Febrile neutropenia	18	9	17
Leukopenia	19	12	12
Diarrhea	4	5	12
Anemia	1	3	17
Thrombocytopenia	0	0	12
Vomiting	0	3	5
Drug hypersensitivity	3	0	3
Fatigue	0	0	4
Increased alanine aminotransferase level	0	0	4

*According to the National Cancer Institute Common Terminology Criteria for Adverse Events, version 3.0
The most common grade 3–4 adverse events that occurred during the neoadjuvant treatment are included in the table. No deaths were reported during the neoadjuvant treatment. The incidences of symptomatic left ventricular systolic dysfunction and significant decline in left ventricular ejection fraction were low in all groups. Grade ≥3 adverse events were rare during adjuvant treatment

NEOADJUVANT • TRIPLE-NEGATIVE
BREAST CANCER REGIMEN: CARBOPLATIN + PACLITAXEL THEN DOSE-DENSE DOXORUBICIN + CYCLOPHOSPHAMIDE

Sikov WM et al. J Clin Oncol 2015;33:13–21

The regimen consists of four cycles of neoadjuvant paclitaxel and carboplatin followed sequentially by 4 cycles of neoadjuvant dose-dense doxorubicin + cyclophosphamide

Neoadjuvant carboplatin + paclitaxel

Premedications for paclitaxel:

Dexamethasone 10 mg; administer intravenously 30–60 minutes before each paclitaxel dose
Diphenhydramine 50 mg; administer intravenously 30–60 minutes before each paclitaxel dose
Cimetidine 300 mg (or **ranitidine** 50 mg, or **famotidine** 20 mg, or an equivalent histamine receptor [H$_2$]-subtype antagonist); administer intravenously over 15–30 minutes, 30–60 minutes before each paclitaxel dose

Paclitaxel 80 mg/m^2 per dose; administer intravenously in a volume of 0.9% sodium chloride injection (0.9% NS) or 5% dextrose injection (D5W) sufficient to produce a concentration within the range 0.3–1.2 mg/mL over 60 minutes, on day 1, 8, and 15, every 21 days for 4 cycles (total dosage per week = 80 mg/m^2; total dosage per 3-week cycle = 240 mg/m^2)
Carboplatin target AUC = 6 mg/mL × min; administer intravenously in 250 mL D5W or 0.9% NS over 30–60 minutes after paclitaxel on day 1, every 3 weeks for 4 cycles (total dose/3-week cycle calculated to achieve a target AUC = 6 mg/mL × min)

After completion of 4 cycles of carboplatin + paclitaxel, then administer 4 cycles of neoadjuvant dose-dense doxorubicin + cyclophosphamide as follows:

Hydration with 1000 mL 0.9% NS; administer intravenously 500 mL before starting cyclophosphamide and 500 mL after completing cyclophosphamide

Doxorubicin HCl 60 mg/m^2; administer by intravenous injection over 3–5 minutes on day 1, every 14 days for 4 cycles (total dosage/14-day cycle = 60 mg/m^2)

Cyclophosphamide 600 mg/m^2; administer intravenously in 100–500 mL 0.9% NS or D5W over 15–60 minutes on day 1, every 14 days for 4 cycles (total dosage/14-day cycle = 600 mg/m^2)
• *Note: hematopoietic growth factor (CSF) support is required with dose-dense doxorubicin + cyclophosphamide. Choose one of the following options:*
  ▪ **Filgrastim** 5 mcg/kg per day; administer subcutaneously for 7 consecutive days on days 3–9, every 14 days for 4 cycles
    ○ Calculated dose may be rounded to use the most economical combination of commercially available products (containing 300 mcg or 480 mcg)
or
  ▪ **Pegfilgrastim** 6 mg; administer subcutaneously once on day 2 (at least 24 hours after completion of chemotherapy), every 14 days for 4 cycles

Supportive Care
Antiemetic prophylaxis
*Emetogenic potential on days with carboplatin is **HIGH**. Potential for delayed symptoms*
*Emetogenic potential on days when only paclitaxel is administered is **LOW***
*Emetogenic potential on days with doxorubicin + cyclophosphamide is **HIGH**. Potential for delayed symptoms*

Hematopoietic growth factor (CSF) prophylaxis
Primary prophylaxis is not indicated during paclitaxel + carboplatin cycles
Primary prophylaxis is required during dose-dense doxorubicin + cyclophosphamide cycles; see above description
See Chapter 43 for more information

Antimicrobial prophylaxis
*Risk of fever and neutropenia is **INTERMEDIATE***
  Antimicrobial primary prophylaxis to be considered:
  • Antibacterial—not indicated
  • Antifungal—not indicated
  • Antiviral—not indicated, unless patient previously had an episode of HSV

(continued)

Patient Population Studied

The randomized, 2×2 factorial, open-label, phase 2 trial (Cancer and Leukemia Group B [CALGB] 40603 trial) involved 433 patients with operable, previously untreated, stage II–III, noninflammatory, invasive, HER2-negative breast cancer with estrogen receptor and progesterone receptor expression ≤10%. All patients were scheduled to receive paclitaxel (80 mg/m^2) once per week for 12 weeks and then doxorubicin (60 mg/m^2) and cyclophosphamide (600 mg/m^2) once every 2 weeks with myeloid growth factor support for four cycles. Starting concurrently with the paclitaxel treatment, patients also received carboplatin (dose of 6 area under the curve) once every 3 weeks for four cycles and/or bevacizumab (10 mg/kg) once every 2 weeks for nine cycles if randomly and independently assigned to receive either/both of those treatments. Patients were scheduled to undergo assessment for eligibility for breast-conserving surgery, followed by surgery, 4–8 weeks after the last dose of chemotherapy (and therefore ≥6 weeks after the last dose of bevacizumab in patients assigned to that treatment). Note that bevacizumab is not approved by the U.S. Food and Drug Administration for the neoadjuvant treatment of breast cancer

(*continued*)

Carboplatin dose

Carboplatin dose is based on a formula described by Calvert et al. to achieve a target area under the plasma concentration versus time curve (AUC)

$$\text{Total carboplatin dose (mg)} = (\text{target AUC})(\text{GFR} + 25)$$

In practice, creatinine clearance (CrCl) is used in place of glomerular filtration rate (GFR). CrCl can be estimated from the equation of Cockcroft and Gault, thus:

$$\text{For males, CrCl} = \frac{(140 - \text{age[years]}) \times (\text{body weight [kg]})}{72 \times (\text{serum creatinine [mg/dL]})}$$

$$\text{For females, CrCl} = \frac{(140 - \text{age[years]}) \times (\text{body weight [kg]})}{72 \times (\text{serum creatinine [mg/dL]})} \times 0.85$$

Calvert AH et al. J Clin Oncol 1989;7:1748–1756
Cockcroft DW, Gault MH. Nephron 1976;16:31–41
Jodrell DI et al. J Clin Oncol 1992;10:520–528
Sorensen BT et al. Cancer Chemother Pharmacol 1991;28:397–401

Note: On October 8, 2010, the U.S. Food and Drug Administration (FDA) identified a potential safety issue with carboplatin dosing based on recent changes in the measurement of serum creatinine. By the end of 2010, all clinical laboratories in the United States will use the standardized isotope dilution mass spectrometry (IDMS) method to measure serum creatinine, which could result in an overestimation of the GFR in some patients with normal renal function. A carboplatin dose calculated with an IDMS-measured serum creatinine result using the Calvert formula could exceed an expected exposure (AUC) and result in increased drug-related toxicity. Provided actual GFR measurements are made to assess renal function, carboplatin can be safely dosed according to the Calvert formula described in product labeling. If GFR (or creatinine clearance) is estimated based on serum creatinine measurements by the IDMS method, the FDA recommended for patients with normal renal function capping an estimated GFR at 125 mL/min for any targeted AUC value. No greater estimated GFR values should be used.

Efficacy (N = 433)

	Paclitaxel then Doxorubicin + Cyclophosphamide (N = 107)	Bevacizumab with Paclitaxel then Doxorubicin + Cyclophosphamide (N = 105)	Carboplatin + Paclitaxel then Doxorubicin + Cyclophosphamide (N = 111)	Bevacizumab with Carboplatin + Paclitaxel then Doxorubicin + Cyclophosphamide (N = 110)
Rate of pathologic complete response in the breast	42%	50%	53%	67%
Rate of pathologic complete response in the breast and absence of any tumor deposit ≥0.2 mm in sampled axillary nodes	39%	43%	49%	60%

	No Carboplatin (± Bevacizumab, with Paclitaxel then Doxorubicin + Cyclophosphamide) (N = 212)	Carboplatin (± Bevacizumab + Paclitaxel then Doxorubicin + Cyclophosphamide) (N = 221)	
Rate of pathologic complete response in the breast	46%	60%	OR 1.76; P = 0.0018
Rate of pathologic complete response in the breast and absence of any tumor deposit ≥0.2 mm in sampled axillary nodes	41%	54%	OR 1.71; P = 0.0029

(*continued*)

Efficacy (N = 433) *(continued)*

	No Bevacizumab (± Carboplatin + Paclitaxel then Doxorubicin + Cyclophosphamide) (N = 218)	Bevacizumab (± Carboplatin + Paclitaxel then Doxorubicin + Cyclophosphamide (N = 215)	
Rate of pathologic complete response in the breast	48%	59%	OR 1.58; P = 0.0089
Rate of pathologic complete response in the breast and absence of any tumor deposit ≥0.2 mm in sampled axillary nodes	44%	52%	OR 1.36; P = 0.0570

Therapy Monitoring

1. Prior to the start of therapy and prior to each dose of carboplatin + paclitaxel or doxorubicin + cyclophosphamide: CBC with differential, serum bilirubin, AST/ALT, and creatinine
2. Prior to the start of therapy perform a thorough cardiac assessment, including history, physical examination, and determination of LVEF by echocardiogram or MUGA scan at baseline prior to initiation of doxorubicin. Reevaluate LVEF during doxorubicin treatment if clinical symptoms of heart failure are present
3. Verify pregnancy status prior to the initiation of therapy. Advise patients of the risks of embryo-fetal death and birth defects and the need for contraception
4. Avoid using concomitant strong CYP3A4 inhibitors (eg, ketoconazole, itraconazole, clarithromycin, atazanavir, indinavir, nefazodone, nelfinavir, ritonavir, saquinavir, telithromycin, and voriconazole). Consider a 50% paclitaxel dose reduction if patients require co-administration of a strong CYP3A4 inhibitor

Treatment Modifications

CARBOPLATIN + PACLITAXEL

Paclitaxel starting dose	80 mg/m²		Carboplatin starting dose AUC 6
Paclitaxel dose level −1	60 mg/m²	Carboplatin dose level −1	AUC 4.5
Paclitaxel dose level −2	40 mg/m²	Carboplatin dose level −2	AUC 3
Paclitaxel dose level −3	Discontinue paclitaxel and proceed to dose-dense AC	Carboplatin dose level −3	Discontinue carboplatin and proceed to dose-dense AC

Adverse Event	Treatment Modifications
Severe hypersensitivity reaction	Discontinue paclitaxel or carboplatin infusion immediately and administer appropriate support. For hypersensitivity reaction less G ≤3, initial management includes temporary discontinuation of infusion for 30 minutes, and administration of additional intravenous antihistamines and glucocorticoids. Upon resolution of symptoms, the paclitaxel infusion may be restarted at a slower rate if deemed safe. Rechallenge with carboplatin will require institution of a desensitization regimen. If G4 hypersensitivity is experienced, stabilize the cardiorespiratory system and use epinephrine as needed, then permanently discontinue paclitaxel or carboplatin. Rechallenge with carboplatin will require institution of a desensitization regimen
Febrile neutropenia (ANC <1000/mm³ with temperature >38°C or >100.4°F), or ANC <500/mm³ for ≥7 days, or ANC <100/mm³ at any time	Withhold treatment until resolution of toxicity. Reduce paclitaxel and carboplatin dosages by one dose level. Administer filgrastim in subsequent cycles

(continued)

Treatment Modifications (*continued*)

Adverse Event	Treatment Modifications
ANC <800/mm³ on day 1, 8, or 15	Omit paclitaxel and do not make up the paclitaxel dose; consider resuming paclitaxel one week later if ANC ≥800/mm³ If ANC <800/mm³ on the day of carboplatin treatment (ie, day 1), then delay carboplatin until ANC ≥800/mm³
If paclitaxel is omitted for 2 consecutive weeks for ANC <800/mm³	Decrease paclitaxel and carboplatin dosages by one dose level for all subsequent doses
If paclitaxel is omitted for 3 consecutive weeks for ANC <800/mm³	Discontinue paclitaxel and carboplatin and begin dose-dense AC when ANC ≥1000/mm³ and platelets ≥75,000/mm³
Platelet nadir <25,000/mm³ at any time	Reduce carboplatin dosage by one level for all subsequent doses
Platelets ≥50,000/mm³ but <75,000/mm³ on day 1 of a cycle	Delay carboplatin until platelets ≥75,000/mm³ and then resume carboplatin at one lower dose level. Administer paclitaxel without delay at the current dose
Platelets <50,000/mm³ on day 1 of a cycle	Delay carboplatin until platelets ≥75,000/mm³ and then resume carboplatin at one lower dose level. Omit paclitaxel and do not make up the paclitaxel dose; consider resuming paclitaxel one week later if platelets ≥50,000/mm³
Platelets <50,000/mm³ on day 8 or 15 of a cycle	Omit paclitaxel and do not make up the paclitaxel dose; consider resuming paclitaxel one week later if platelets ≥50,000/mm³. Reduce all subsequent carboplatin doses by one dose level
Bilirubin >1.5 × ULN, or ALT >5 × ULN	Omit paclitaxel and do not make up the paclitaxel dose; consider resuming paclitaxel at the same dose 1 week later if bilirubin ≤1.5 × ULN and ALT ≤5 × ULN
Treatment is delayed or omitted for 3 consecutive weeks for hepatic dysfunction	Discontinue paclitaxel + carboplatin and proceed to treatment with dose-dense AC when bilirubin ≤1.5 × ULN and ALT ≤2.5 × ULN
G2 neurotoxicity of >7 days duration (paresthesias/dysesthesias interfering with function, but not activities of daily living)	Decrease the dose of paclitaxel by one dose level for all subsequent doses. Continue carboplatin at the same dose
G3 neurotoxicity >7 days duration (paresthesias/dysesthesias with pain or with function impairment interfering with activities of daily living)	Omit paclitaxel and do not make up the paclitaxel dose; consider resuming paclitaxel at one lower dose level if neuropathy improves to G ≤2. Delay the carboplatin dose until neuropathy improves to G ≤2, then resume carboplatin at one lower dose level
G3 neurotoxicity that does not improve within 3 weeks (paresthesias/dysesthesias with pain or with function impairment interfering with activities of daily living)	Discontinue paclitaxel + carboplatin and proceed to treatment with dose-dense AC
Persistent paresthesias/ dysesthesias that are disabling or life-threatening	
Other G2 nonhematologic adverse event that occurs during a cycle but results in a delay in the start of the next cycle	Hold treatment until adverse events resolve to <G1, then resume with paclitaxel and/or carboplatin dosages reduced by one dose level
Other G3 nonhematologic adverse event that occurs during a cycle but resolves prior to the start of the next cycle or requires a delay in the start of the next cycle	
Other G4 nonhematologic adverse event that occurs during a cycle but resolves prior to the start of the next cycle	Hold treatment until adverse events resolve to G <1, then resume with paclitaxel and/or carboplatin dosages reduced by one dose level or discontinue paclitaxel and/or carboplatin
Other G4 nonhematologic adverse event that occurs during a cycle but requires a delay in the start of the next cycle	Discontinue paclitaxel and/or carboplatin
Any treatment delay >3 weeks	

(*continued*)

Treatment Modifications (*continued*)

DOSE-DENSE DOXORUBICIN + CYCLOPHOSPHAMIDE

DOXORUBICIN DOSE LEVELS

Doxorubicin starting dose	60 mg/m²
Doxorubicin dose level −1	50 mg/m²
Doxorubicin dose level −2	40 mg/m²
Doxorubicin dose level −3	Discontinue doxorubicin

CYCLOPHOSPHAMIDE DOSE LEVELS

Cyclophosphamide starting dose	600 mg/m²
Cyclophosphamide dose level −1	500 mg/m²
Cyclophosphamide dose level −2	400 mg/m²
Cyclophosphamide dose level −3	Discontinue cyclophosphamide

Adverse Event	Treatment Modifications
Neutropenia/Thrombocytopenia	
ANC <1000/mm³ or platelets <75,000/mm³ on day 1 of a cycle	Withhold doxorubicin and cyclophosphamide. Repeat CBC with differential weekly and resume treatment when ANC ≥1000/mm³ and platelets ≥75,000/mm³. If therapy is delayed by more than 1 week, then reduce doxorubicin and cyclophosphamide dosages by one dose level dosages and doses should be flipped
Febrile neutropenia (ANC <1000/mm³ with single temperature >38.3°C [101°F] or a sustained temperature of ≥38°C [100.4°F] for more than one hour)	Hold treatment until neutropenia resolves, then reduce dosages of doxorubicin and cyclophosphamide by one dose level
Other nonhematologic toxicities	
Bilirubin 1.2–3.0 mg/dL	Administer 30 mg/m² doxorubicin
Bilirubin 3.1–5 mg/dL	Administer 450 mg/m² cyclophosphamide and 15 mg/m² doxorubicin
Bilirubin >5 mg/dL	Discontinue cyclophosphamide and doxorubicin
LVEF is 40%, or is 40% to 45% with a 10% or greater absolute decrease below the pretreatment	Withhold doxorubicin and repeat LVEF assessment within approximately 4 weeks. Discontinue doxorubicin if the LVEF has not improved or has declined further, unless the benefits for the individual patient outweigh the risks
Any other G1 toxicity	Maintain dose and schedule
Any other G2 toxicity	Hold treatment until toxicity resolves to G ≤1, then reduce dosages of doxorubicin and cyclophosphamide by one dose level
Any other G3 toxicity	Hold treatment until toxicity resolves to G ≤1, then reduce dosages of doxorubicin and cyclophosphamide by one or two dose levels
Any other G4 toxicity	Hold treatment until toxicity resolves to G ≤1, then reduce dosages of doxorubicin and cyclophosphamide by two dose levels

Note: Patients who are pregnant or who become pregnant should be apprised of the potential hazard to the fetus; women of childbearing potential should be advised to avoid becoming pregnant during therapy

Adverse Events (N = 433)

Grade 3–4 Events* (%)	Paclitaxel then Doxorubicin + Cyclophosphamide (N = 107)	Bevacizumab with Paclitaxel then Doxorubicin + Cyclophosphamide (N = 105)	Carboplatin + Paclitaxel then Doxorubicin + Cyclophosphamide (N = 111)	Bevacizumab with Carboplatin + Paclitaxel then Doxorubicin + Cyclophosphamide (N = 110)
Neutropenia	22	27	56	67
Thrombocytopenia	4	3	20	26
Leukopenia	12	13	13	25
Febrile neutropenia	7	9	12	24
Fatigue	10	12	10	20
Pain	3	6	3	11
Nausea	4	4	3	8
Peripheral neuropathy	2	6	7	4
Hypertension	2	12	0	10
Hemoglobin	0	2	4	5
Hypokalemia	3	1	6	2
Vomiting	2	2	2	4
Mucositis	2	0	1	4
Diarrhea	0	3	2	3
Increased alanine aminotransferase level	0	3	0	3

*According to the National Cancer Institute Common Terminology Criteria for Adverse Events, version 4.0

Grade 3–4 Events* (%)	No Carboplatin (± Bevacizumab, with Paclitaxel then Doxorubicin + Cyclophosphamide) (N = 212)	Carboplatin (± Bevacizumab + Paclitaxel then Doxorubicin + Cyclophosphamide (N = 221)
Neutropenia	25	62
Thrombocytopenia	3	23
Leukopenia	13	19
Febrile neutropenia	8	18
Fatigue	11	15
Pain	4	7
Nausea	4	5
Peripheral neuropathy	4	5
Hypertension	7	5
Hemoglobin	1	5
Hypokalemia	2	4
Vomiting	2	3
Mucositis	1	2
Diarrhea	1	2
Increased alanine aminotransferase level	1	1

*According to the National Cancer Institute Common Terminology Criteria for Adverse Events, version 4.0

(*continued*)

Adverse Events (N = 433) (continued)

Grade 3–4 Events* (%)	No Bevacizumab (± Carboplatin + Paclitaxel then Doxorubicin + Cyclophosphamide) (N = 218)	Bevacizumab (± Carboplatin + Paclitaxel then Doxorubicin + Cyclophosphamide) (N = 215)
Neutropenia	39	47
Leukopenia	12	20
Febrile neutropenia	9	16
Fatigue	10	16
Thrombocytopenia	12	15
Hypertension	1	11
Pain	3	8
Nausea	3	6
Peripheral neuropathy	5	5
Hemoglobin	2	4
Vomiting	2	3
Diarrhea	1	3
Increased alanine aminotransferase level	0	3
Mucositis	1	2
Hypokalemia	5	1

*According to the National Cancer Institute Common Terminology Criteria for Adverse Events, version 4.0

HORMONAL THERAPY AGENTS
BREAST CANCER REGIMEN: HORMONAL THERAPY AGENTS

Selective Estrogen Receptor Modulators
Tamoxifen 20 mg daily; administer orally

Selective Estrogen Receptor Downregulator
Fulvestrant 500 mg/treatment; administer by intramuscular injection, 250 mg into each buttock, on days 1, 15, 29, and once monthly thereafter

Aromatase Inhibitors
Anastrozole 1 mg daily; administer orally
Letrozole 2.5 mg daily; administer orally
Exemestane 25 mg daily; administer orally

Progestins
Megestrol Acetate 40 mg 4 times daily; administer orally

LHRH Agonists
Goserelin 3.6 mg implant every 28 days; administer subcutaneously
Goserelin 10.8 mg implant every 3 months; administer subcutaneously

Efficacy

Tamoxifen

Prevention:	50% reduction in breast cancer (invasive and noninvasive) in women at increased risk (5-year risk of 1.66%)
Adjuvant:	50% reduction in recurrence, 28% reduction in mortality
Metastatic:	Response rate 30–70% depending on ER/PR status: ER+/PR+ > ER+/PR− > ER−/PR+

Fulvestrant

Metastatic:	At least equivalent to anastrozole

Anastrozole

Adjuvant:	Superior disease-free survival vs tamoxifen
Metastatic:	Likely superior to tamoxifen

Letrozole

Neoadjuvant:	Superior to tamoxifen
Adjuvant:	Improved DFS when started after 5 years of tamoxifen
Metastatic:	Superior to tamoxifen

Exemestane

Metastatic:	Superior to megestrol acetate

Progestins

Metastatic:	Equivalent to tamoxifen

LHRH Agonists

Adjuvant:	Evidence of efficacy in combination with tamoxifen for premenopausal women
Metastatic:	Evidence of efficacy in combination with tamoxifen for premenopausal women

Baum M et al. Lancet 2002;359:2131–2139
Ellis MJ et al. J Clin Oncol 2001;19:3808–3816
Fisher B et al. J Natl Cancer Inst 1998;90:1371–1388
Goss PE et al. N Engl J Med 2003;349:1793–1802
Kaufmann M et al. J Clin Oncol 2000;18:1399–1411
Klijn JGM et al. J Clin Oncol 2001;19:343–353
Mouridsen H et al. J Clin Oncol 2001;19:2596–2606
Nabholtz JM et al. J Clin Oncol 2000;18:3758–3767
Osborne CK et al. J Clin Oncol 2002;20:3386–3395

Toxicity

Note: Pregnancy is contraindicated with all hormonal therapies

Tamoxifen

	Increase over Placebo Group
Endometrial cancer	1.39 per 1000 women/year
PE*	0.46 per 1000 women/year
DVT†	0.5 per 1000 women/year
CVA‡	0.53 per 1000 women/year
Cataracts	3.1 per 1000 women/year

	Tamoxifen	Placebo
Hot flashes	45.7%	28.7%
Vaginal discharge	29%	13%

Tamoxifen (ATAC DATA)

Hot flashes	39.7%
Vaginal bleeding	8.2%
Endometrial cancer	0.7%
VTE§	3.5%
Fractures	3.7%
Musculoskeletal	21.3%

Fulvestrant

Toxicities similar to anastrozole without musculoskeletal side effects. Injection-site reaction

Anastrozole (ATAC DATA)

Hot flashes	34.3%
Vaginal bleeding	4.5%
Endometrial cancer	0.1%
VTE§	2.1%
Fractures	5.9%
Musculoskeletal	27.8%

(continued)

Therapy Monitoring

Tamoxifen

1. LFTs >1 month, then every 3–6 months
2. Serum chemistries and LFTs every 6 months

Fulvestrant

1. Clinic visit at 1 month
2. Serum chemistries and LFTs every 6 months

Anastrozole

1. Clinic visit at 1 month
2. Bone density scan at baseline and every 6–12 months when used as adjuvant therapy
3. Serum chemistries and LFTs every 6 months

Letrozole

1. Clinic visit at 1 month
2. Bone density scan at baseline and every 6–12 months when used as adjuvant therapy
3. Serum chemistries and LFTs every 6 months

Exemestane

1. Clinic visit at 1 month
2. Bone density scan at baseline and every 6–12 months when used as adjuvant therapy
3. Serum chemistries and LFTs every 6 months

Megestrol

1. Clinic visit, serum chemistries, and LFTs at 1 month then every 3–6 months
2. Monitor adrenal function every 3 months
3. *Note:* Consider replacement (or stress dose) steroids with withdrawal or physiologic stress

LHRH Agonists (Goserelin)

1. Clinic visit at 1 month
2. Serum chemistries and LFTs every 6 months

Toxicity (*continued*)

Letrozole

Toxicities similar to anastrozole

Exemestane

Toxicities similar to anastrozole with weight gain

Megestrol

Weight gain/edema
Hyperglycemia
Sedation
Thromboemboli

Goserelin

Hot flashes	70%
Tumor flare	23%
Nausea	11%
Edema	5%

*Pulmonary embolism
†Deep venous thrombosis
‡Cerebrovascular accident
§Venous thromboembolism

Baum M et al. Lancet 2002;359:2131–2139
Fisher B et al. J Natl Cancer Inst 1998;90:1371–1388
Robertson JFR et al. Cancer 2003;98:229–238
Stuart NSA et al. Eur J Cancer 1996;32A:1888–1892

METASTATIC • HORMONE RECEPTOR-POSITIVE • HER2-NEGATIVE

BREAST CANCER REGIMEN: PALBOCICLIB + LETROZOLE

Finn RS et al. N Engl J Med 2016;375:1925–1936
Supplementary appendix to: Finn RS et al. N Engl J Med 2016;375:1925–1936
Protocol for: Finn RS et al. N Engl J Med 2016;375:1925–1936

Palbociclib 125 mg/dose; administer orally once daily, with food, for 21 consecutive days on days 1–21, followed by 7 days without treatment, repeated every 28 days, until disease progression (total dosage/28-day cycle = 2,625 mg), *plus:*
Notes:
• Patients who delay taking palbociclib at a regularly scheduled time or who vomit after taking a dose of palbociclib should take the next dose at the next regularly scheduled time

• Palbociclib capsules should be swallowed whole

• Palbociclib is metabolized by cytochrome P450 (CYP) CYP3A subfamily enzymes. Avoid concurrent use with strong CYP3A4 inhibitors (eg, clarithromycin, indinavir, itraconazole, ketoconazole, lopinavir/ritonavir, nefazodone, nelfinavir, posaconazole, ritonavir, saquinavir, telaprevir, telithromycin, verapamil, voriconazole) whenever possible. If concurrent use with a strong CYP3A4 inhibitor is required, reduce each palbociclib dose to 75 mg. Avoid concurrent use with moderate CYPA4 inducers (eg, bosentan, efavirenz, etravirine, modafinil, nafcillin) and strong CYP3A4 inducers (eg, rifampin, carbamazepine, phenytoin, phenobarbital, St. John's wort)

• Palbociclib is a time-dependent inhibitor of CYP3A enzymes and thus may alter the metabolism of CYP3A substrates. Use caution when a CYP3A substrate with a narrow therapeutic index is co-prescribed with palbociclib (eg, alfentanil, cyclosporine, tacrolimus, sirolimus, dihydroergotamine, ergotamine, everolimus, fentanyl, pimozide, quinidine)

• Advise patients to not consume grapefruit and grapefruit juice as they may inhibit CYP3A in the gut wall and increase the bioavailability of palbociclib

Letrozole 2.5 mg/dose; administer orally once daily, without regard to food, continually on days 1–28, every 28 days, until disease progression (total dosage/28-day cycle = 70 mg)
Notes:
• Patients who delay taking a letrozole dose at a regularly scheduled time may take the missed dose if the time to the next regularly scheduled dose is >12 hours away

• Dose adjustment for patients with cirrhosis or severe hepatic impairment: 2.5 mg orally every other day

Supportive Care
Antiemetic prophylaxis
Emetogenic potential is **LOW**
See Chapter 42 for antiemetic recommendations

Hematopoietic growth factor (CSF) prophylaxis
Primary prophylaxis is **NOT** indicated
See Chapter 43 for more information

Antimicrobial prophylaxis
Risk of fever and neutropenia is **LOW**
Antimicrobial primary prophylaxis to be considered:
• Antibacterial—not indicated
• Antifungal—not indicated
• Antiviral—not indicated unless patient previously had an episode of HSV

Patient Population Studied

The PALOMA-2 study was a phase 3, double-blinded study that involved 666 postmenopausal women with advanced estrogen receptor–positive, HER2-negative breast cancer who had not received any prior systemic treatment for their advanced disease. Patients were required to have an Eastern Cooperative Oncology Group (ECOG) performance status score ≤2. Patients were randomized 2:1 to receive either the combination of palbociclib + letrozole (n = 444) or placebo + letrozole (n = 222)

Efficacy (N = 666)

	Palbociclib + Letrozole (N = 444)	Placebo + Letrozole (N = 222)	
Median progression-free survival	24.8 months (95% CI, 22.1–NE)	14.5 months (95% CI, 12.9–17.1)	HR 0.58, 95% CI 0.46–0.72; P<0.001
Confirmed objective response rate, all patients*	42.1% (95% CI, 37.5–46.9)	34.7% (95% CI, 28.4–41.3)	P = 0.06
Median duration of response, all patients	22.5 months (95% CI, 19.-28.0)	16.8 months (95% CI, 14.2–28.5)	—
Clinical benefit rate, all patients†	84.9% (95% CI, 81.2–88.1)	70.3% (95% CI, 63.8–76.2)	P<0.001
Confirmed objective response rate, patients with measurable disease*	55.3% (95% CI, 49.9–60.7)	44.4% (95% CI, 36.9–52.2)	P = 0.03
Median duration of response, patients with measurable disease	22.5 months (95% CI, 19.8–28.0)	16.8 months (95% CI, 15.4–28.5)	—
Clinical benefit rate, patients with measurable disease†	84.3% (95% CI, 80.0–88.0)	70.8% (95% CI, 63.3–77.5)	P<0.001

Objective response rate includes patients with either a complete or partial response to treatment
†*Clinical benefit rate* includes patients with either a complete or partial response or stable disease for ≥24 weeks
Note: Median follow-up was 23 months. Follow-up for overall survival is ongoing

Therapy Monitoring

1. Monitor CBC with differential and LFTs. Obtain prior to the start of therapy, every 2 weeks for the first 2 months, monthly for the next 2 months, and as clinically indicated
2. For patients who experience a maximum of G1 or 2 neutropenia in the first 6 cycles, monitor complete blood counts for subsequent cycles every 3 months, prior to the beginning of a cycle and as clinically indicated
3. Decreases in bone mineral density may occur. Consider bone mineral density monitoring
4. Increases in total cholesterol may occur. Consider cholesterol monitoring
5. Obtain a pregnancy test in females of reproductive potential. Advise females of reproductive potential to use effective contraception
6. Response assessment: imaging studies every 3–6 months based on patient and disease characteristics

Treatment Modifications

PALBOCICLIB + LETROZOLE	
PALBOCICLIB	
	Palbociclib
Starting dose	125 mg daily
Dose level −1	100 mg daily
Dose level −2	75 mg daily
Dose level −3	Discontinue therapy

(continued)

Treatment Modifications (continued)

Hematologic Toxicity

G1/2 hematologic toxicity	Observe and continue with administered dose
G3 hematologic toxicity (ANC <1000/mm^3 or platelet <50,000/mm^3)	*Day 1 of ensuing cycle:* Withhold palbociclib. Resume at same dose when ANC ≥1000/mm^3 and platelets ≥50,000/mm^3. Growth factor support is rarely needed *Day 15 of first two cycles:* If G3 on day 15 of a cycle, continue with current dose and repeat CBC on 22nd day of cycle. If G3 finish cycle; if G4 withhold palbociclib. Resume at one dose level lower when ANC >1000/mm^3 and platelets >50,000/mm^3
Prolonged (>1 week) G3 hematologic toxicity (ANC <1000/mm^3 or platelet <50,000/mm^3) or recurrent G3 neutropenia on day 1 of ensuing cycle	Withhold palbociclib. Resume at one lower dose level when ANC >1000/mm^3 and platelets >50,000/mm^3
Grade 3 neutropenia with fever ≥38.5 °C and/or infection	Withhold palbociclib. Resume at one lower dose level when ANC >1000/mm^3 and platelets >50,000/mm^3. Growth factor support is rarely needed
G4 (ANC <500/mm^3 or platelet <25,000/mm^3) or recurrent G3 hematologic toxicity	Withhold palbociclib. Resume at one lower dose level when ANC >1000/mm^3 and platelets >50,000/mm^3. Growth factor support is rarely needed

Hepatotoxicity

G1 AST/ALT elevation (ULN–3× ULN) G2 AST/ALT elevation (>3–5× ULN) WITHOUT increase in total bilirubin above 2× ULN	Observe carefully and continue with administered dose
Persistent or Recurrent G2 AST/ALT elevation or G3 (>5–20× ULN) WITHOUT increase in total bilirubin above 2× ULN	Withhold palbociclib. Resume at one lower dose level when toxicity resolves to ≤G1. Monitor carefully for need of additional reductions
Elevation in AST and/or ALT >3 × ULN WITH total bilirubin >2× ULN, in the absence of cholestasis	Discontinue palbociclib
Grade 4 (>20× ULN)	Discontinue palbociclib

Other Nonhematologic Toxicities

G1/2 nonhematologic toxicity	Observe carefully and continue with administered dose
Persistent or recurrent G ≥3 toxicity that does not resolve with maximal supportive measures within 7 days to baseline or G1	Withhold palbociclib. Resume at one lower dose level when toxicity resolves to ≤G1 or to G ≤2 (if not considered a safety risk for the patient). Monitor carefully for need of additional reductions

General Dose Adjustments

If a strong CYP3A inhibitor must be used (eg, clarithromycin, indinavir, itraconazole, ketoconazole, lopinavir/ritonavir, nefazodone, nelfinavir, posaconazole, ritonavir, saquinavir, telaprevir, telithromycin, and voriconazole, grapefruit, or grapefruit juice)	Begin therapy with 75 mg palbociclib daily. If toxicity occurs then discontinue palbociclib
Strong CYP3A inhibitor is discontinued	Increase the dose of palbociclib to the dose that was used prior to initiation of the strong CYP3A inhibitor after 3–5 half-lives of the inhibitor have transpired
Strong CYP3A inducer (eg, phenytoin, rifampin, carbamazepine, enzalutamide, and St John's wort) is required	May decrease palbociclib plasma concentrations. Avoid concomitant use of strong CYP3A inducers

Note: Advise patients who are to receive palbociclib of potential risk to a fetus and to use effective contraception

LETROZOLE

- Dose: 2.5 mg once daily
- Patients with cirrhosis or severe hepatic impairment: 2.5 mg every other day
- In patients with advanced disease, treatment with letrozole should continue until tumor progression is evident
- The most common adverse events (>20%) are hot flashes, arthralgia; flushing, asthenia, edema, arthralgia, headache, dizziness, hypercholesterolemia, sweating increased, bone pain; and musculoskeletal. These should be managed symptomatically

Adverse Events (N = 666)

Grade (%)*	Palbociclib + Letrozole (N = 444)			Placebo + Letrozole (N = 222)		
	Any Grade	Grade 3	Grade 4	Any Grade	Grade 3	Grade 4
Any adverse event	98.9	62.2	13.5	95.5	22.1	2.3
Neutropenia	79.5	56.1	10.4	6.3	0.9	0.5
Leukopenia	39.0	24.1	0.7	2.3	0	0
Fatigue	37.4	1.8	0	27.5	0.5	0
Nausea	35.1	0.2	0	26.1	1.8	0
Arthralgia	33.3	0.7	0	33.8	0.5	0
Alopecia	32.9	0	0	15.8	0	0
Diarrhea	26.1	1.4	0	19.4	1.4	0
Cough	25.0	0	0	18.9	0	0
Anemia	24.1	5.2	0.2	9.0	1.8	0
Back pain	21.6	1.4	0	21.6	0	0
Headache	21.4	0.2	0	26.1	1.8	0
Hot flush	20.9	0	0	30.6	0	0
Constipation	19.4	0.5	0	15.3	0.5	0
Rash	17.8	0.9	0	11.7	0.5	0
Asthenia	16.9	2.3	0	11.7	0	0
Thrombocytopenia	15.5	1.4	0.2	1.4	0	0
Vomiting	15.5	0.5	0	16.7	1.4	0
Pain in extremity	15.3	0.2	0	17.6	1.4	0
Stomatitis	15.3	0.2	0	5.9	0	0
Decreased appetite	14.9	0.7	0	9.0	0	0
Dyspnea	14.9	1.1	0	13.5	1.4	0
Insomnia	14.9	0	0	11.7	0	0
Dizziness	14.2	0.5	0	14.9	0	0
Nasopharyngitis	14.0	0	0	9.9	0	0
Upper respiratory tract infection	13.3	0	0	11.3	0	0
Dry skin	12.4	0	0	5.9	0	0
Pyrexia	12.4	0	0	8.6	0	0
Myalgia	11.9	0	0	9.0	0	0
Urinary tract infection	11.9	1.1	0	7.7	0	0
Abdominal pain	11.3	0.9	0	5.4	0	0
Peripheral edema	11.3	0	0	6.3	0	0
Dysgeusia	10.1	0	0	5.0	0	0
Dyspepsia	9.2	0	0	12.2	0.5	0
Anxiety	8.1	0	0	11.3	0	0

*According to the National Cancer Institute Common Terminology Criteria for Adverse Events, version 4.0
Adverse events from any cause that were reported in ≥10% of patients in either treatment group are included in the table

METASTATIC • HORMONE RECEPTOR-POSITIVE • HER2-NEGATIVE

BREAST CANCER REGIMEN: PALBOCICLIB + FULVESTRANT

Cristofanilli M et al. Lancet Oncol 2016;17:425–439

Note: The regimen as described below is for postmenopausal women. It may also be used for perimenopausal or premenopausal women if concurrent gonadotropin-releasing hormone (GnRH) agonist (eg, goserelin) is administered starting at least 4 weeks prior to initiation of treatment

Palbociclib 125 mg/dose; administer orally once daily, with food, for 21 consecutive days on days 1–21, followed by 7 days without treatment, every 28 days, until disease progression (total dosage/28-day cycle = 2,625 mg), *plus:*
Notes:
- Patients who delay taking palbociclib at a regularly scheduled time or who vomit after taking a dose of palbociclib should take the next dose at the next regularly scheduled time
- Palbociclib capsules should be swallowed whole
- Palbociclib is metabolized by cytochrome P450 (CYP) CYP3A subfamily enzymes. Avoid concurrent use with strong CYP3A4 inhibitors (eg, clarithromycin, indinavir, itraconazole, ketoconazole, lopinavir/ritonavir, nefazodone, nelfinavir, posaconazole, ritonavir, saquinavir, telaprevir, telithromycin, verapamil, voriconazole) whenever possible. If concurrent use with a strong CYP3A4 inhibitor is required, reduce each palbociclib dose to 75 mg. Avoid concurrent use with moderate CYPA4 inducers (eg, bosentan, efavirenz, etravirine, modafinil, nafcillin) and strong CYP3A4 inducers (eg, rifampin, carbamazepine, phenytoin, phenobarbital, St. John's wort)
- Palbociclib is a time-dependent inhibitor of CYP3A enzymes and thus may alter the metabolism of CYP3A substrates. Use caution when a CYP3A substrate with a narrow therapeutic index is co-prescribed with palbociclib (eg, alfentanil, cyclosporine, tacrolimus, sirolimus, dihydroergotamine, ergotamine, everolimus, fentanyl, pimozide, quinidine)
- Advise patients to not consume grapefruit and grapefruit juice as they may inhibit CYP3A in the gut wall and increase the bioavailability of palbociclib

Fulvestrant 500 mg/treatment; administer by slow intramuscular injection over 1–2 minutes per injection, 250 mg into each buttock, as follows:
   Cycle 1: administer on day 1 and 15 (total dosage/28-day cycle during cycle 1 = 1000 mg)
   Cycle 2 and beyond: administer on day 1 only, every 28 days, until disease progression (total dosage/28-day cycle during cycle ≥2 = 500 mg)
Note: Dose adjustment for moderate hepatic impairment (Child Pugh-B): reduce fulvestrant dose to 250 mg (ie, only one injection) per treatment

Supportive Care
Antiemetic prophylaxis
Emetogenic potential is **LOW**
See Chapter 42 for antiemetic recommendations

Hematopoietic growth factor (CSF) prophylaxis
Primary prophylaxis is **NOT** *indicated*
See Chapter 43 for more information

Antimicrobial prophylaxis
Risk of fever and neutropenia is **LOW**
   Antimicrobial primary prophylaxis to be considered:
   - Antibacterial—not indicated
   - Antifungal—not indicated
   - Antiviral—not indicated unless patient previously had an episode of HSV

Patient Population Studied

The international, multicenter, double-blind, randomized, phase 3 trial (PALOMA-3) involved 521 patients with hormone receptor–positive, HER2-negative metastatic breast cancer that has progressed on previous endocrine therapy. Eligible patients were aged ≥18 years and had an Eastern Cooperative Oncology Group (ECOG) performance status score ≤1. All patients received intramuscular injections of fulvestrant (500 mg) on days 1 and 15 of the first 4-week cycle and then on day 1 of subsequent cycles. Patients were randomly assigned (2:1) to also receive oral palbociclib (125 mg) or matching placebo on days 1–21 of the 4-week cycle. All premenopausal or perimenopausal women also received goserelin at the time of fulvestrant administration. Study treatment continued until disease progression, unacceptable adverse effects, study withdrawal, or death

Efficacy (N = 521)

	Palbociclib + Fulvestrant (N = 347)	Placebo + Fulvestrant (N = 174)	
Median progression-free survival	9.5 months	4.6 months	HR 0.46, 95% CI 0.36–0.59; P<0.0001
Objective response rate*	19%	9%	OR 2.47, 95% CI 1.36–4.91; P = 0.0019
Clinical benefit rate†	67%	40%	OR 3.05, 95% CI 2.07–4.61; P<0.0001

*Objective response rate includes patients with either a complete or partial response to treatment
†Clinical benefit rate includes patients with either a complete or partial response or stable disease for ≥24 weeks
Note: Median follow-up was 8.9 months

Therapy Monitoring

1. Monitor CBC and LFTs. Obtain prior to the start of therapy, every 2 weeks for the first 2 months, monthly for the next 2 months, and as clinically indicated
2. For patients who experience a maximum of Grade 1 or 2 neutropenia in the first 6 cycles, monitor complete blood counts for subsequent cycles every 3 months, prior to the beginning of a cycle and as clinically indicated
3. Monitor patients for signs and symptoms of thrombosis and pulmonary embolism and treat as medically appropriate
4. Response assessment: Imaging studies every 2–3 months

Treatment Modifications

PALBOCICLIB + FULVESTRANT

PALBOCICLIB

	Palbociclib
Starting dose	125 mg daily
Dose level −1	100 mg daily
Dose level −2	75 mg daily
Dose level −3	Discontinue therapy

Hematologic Toxicity

G1/2 hematologic toxicity	Observe and continue with administered dose
G3 hematologic toxicity (ANC <1000/mm³ or platelet <50,000/mm³)	*Day 1 of ensuing cycle:* Withhold palbociclib. Resume at same dose when ANC ≥1000/mm³ and platelets ≥50,000/mm³. Growth factor support is rarely needed. *Day 15 of first two cycles:* If G3 on day 15 of a cycle, continue with current dose and repeat CBC on 22nd day of cycle. If G3 finish cycle; if G4 withhold palbociclib. Resume at one dose level lower when ANC >1000/mm³ and platelets >50,000/mm³
Prolonged (>1 week) G3 hematologic toxicity (ANC <1000/mm³ or platelet <50,000/mm³) or recurrent G3 neutropenia on day 1 of ensuing cycle	Withhold palbociclib. Resume at one lower dose level when ANC >1000/mm³ and platelets >50,000/mm³
Grade 3 neutropenia with fever ≥38.5°C and/or infection	Withhold palbociclib. Resume at one lower dose level when ANC >1000/mm³ and platelets >50,000/mm³. Growth factor support is rarely needed
G4 (ANC <500/mm³ or platelet <25,000/mm³) or recurrent G3 hematologic toxicity	Withhold palbociclib. Resume at one lower dose level when ANC >1000/mm³ and platelets >50,000/mm³. Growth factor support is rarely needed

(continued)

Treatment Modifications (*continued*)

Hepatotoxicity

G1 AST/ALT elevation (ULN–3× ULN) G2 AST/ALT elevation (>3–5× ULN) WITHOUT increase in total bilirubin above 2× ULN	Observe carefully and continue with administered dose
Persistent or recurrent G2 AST/ALT elevation or G3 (>5–20× ULN) WITHOUT increase in total bilirubin above 2× ULN	Withhold palbociclib. Resume at one lower dose level when toxicity resolves to ≤G1. Monitor carefully for need of additional reductions
Elevation in AST and/or ALT >3 × ULN WITH total bilirubin >2× ULN, in the absence of cholestasis	Discontinue palbociclib
Grade 4 (>20.0 × ULN)	Discontinue palbociclib

Other Nonhematologic Toxicities

G1/2 nonhematologic toxicity	Observe carefully and continue with administered dose
Persistent or recurrent G ≥3 toxicity that does not resolve with maximal supportive measures within 7 days to baseline or G1	Withhold palbociclib. Resume at one lower dose level when toxicity resolves to G ≤1 or to G ≤2 (if not considered a safety risk for the patient). Monitor carefully for need of additional reductions

General Dose Adjustments

If a strong CYP3A inhibitor must be used (eg, clarithromycin, indinavir, itraconazole, ketoconazole, lopinavir/ritonavir, nefazodone, nelfinavir, posaconazole, ritonavir, saquinavir, telaprevir, telithromycin, and voriconazole, grapefruit, or grapefruit juice)	Begin therapy with 75 mg palbociclib daily. If toxicity occurs then discontinue palbociclib
Strong CYP3A inhibitor is discontinued	Increase the dose of palbociclib to the dose that was used prior to initiation of the strong CYP3A inhibitor after 3–5 half-lives of the inhibitor have transpired
Strong CYP3A inducer (eg, phenytoin, rifampin, carbamazepine, enzalutamide, and St John's wort) is required	May decrease palbociclib plasma concentrations. Avoid concomitant use of strong CYP3A inducers

Note: Advise patients who are to receive palbociclib of potential risk to a fetus and to use effective contraception

FULVESTRANT

- The recommended dose is 500 mg. A dose of 250 mg is recommended for patients with moderate hepatic impairment (Child-Pugh class B). Fulvestrant has not been evaluated in patients with severe hepatic impairment (Child-Pugh class C)
- Administered IM; use with caution in patients with bleeding diatheses, thrombocytopenia, or anticoagulant use
- The most common, clinically significant adverse events occurring in ≥5% of patients receiving 500 mg fulvestrant were: injection site pain, nausea, bone pain, arthralgia, headache, back pain, fatigue, pain in extremity, hot flash, vomiting, anorexia, asthenia, musculoskeletal pain, cough, dyspnea, and constipation
- There are no known drug-drug interactions

Adverse Events (N = 517)

Grade (%)*	Palbociclib + Fulvestrant (N = 345)		Placebo + Fulvestrant (N = 172)	
	Grade 1–2	Grade 3–4	Grade 1–2	Grade 3–4
Neutropenia	16	65	3	<1
Leukopenia	22	28	3	1
Infections	40	2	27	3
Fatigue	37	2	27	1
Nausea	32	0	27	<1
Anemia	25	3	9	2
Headache	23	<1	19	0
Thrombocytopenia	19	2	0	0
Diarrhea	21	0	18	<1
Constipation	19	0	16	0
Alopecia	17	0	6	0
Vomiting	17	<1	14	<1
Hot flush	15	0	16	<1
Decreased appetite	14	<1	8	<1
Rash	14	<1	5	0
Back pain	14	1	15	2
Cough	15	0	13	0
Arthralgia	14	<1	16	0
Pain in extremity	12	0	10	2
Stomatitis	12	<1	2	0
Dizziness	12	<1	9	0
Dyspnea	11	0	7	1
Pyrexia	11	<1	5	0
Injection-site pain	6	<1	10	0

*According to the National Cancer Institute Common Terminology Criteria for Adverse Events, version 4.0 Toxicities that occurred in ≥10% of patients in any treatment group are included in the table. No treatment-related deaths occurred; in the palbociclib plus fulvestrant group, two patients died as a result of disease progression, one owing to hepatic failure, one as a result of disseminated intravascular coagulation, and one due to deterioration of general physical health. Treatment discontinuation owing to adverse effects occurred in 4% of the palbociclib plus fulvestrant group and 2% of the placebo plus fulvestrant group

METASTATIC • HORMONE RECEPTOR-POSITIVE • HER2-NEGATIVE

BREAST CANCER REGIMEN: RIBOCICLIB + LETROZOLE

Janni W et al. Breast Cancer Res Treat 2018;169:469–479
Hortobagyi GN et al. Ann Oncol 2018;29:1541–1547
Hortobagyi GN et al. N Engl J Med 2016;375:1738–1748

Ribociclib 600 mg/dose; administer orally once daily, without regard to food, for 21 consecutive days on days 1–21, followed by 7 days without treatment, repeated every 28 days, until disease progression (total dosage/28-day cycle = 12,600 mg), *plus:*
Notes:

- Patients who delay taking ribociclib at a regularly scheduled time or who vomit after taking a dose of ribociclib should take the next dose at the next regularly scheduled time
- Ribociclib tablets should be swallowed whole
- Ribociclib is metabolized by cytochrome P450 (CYP) CYP3A subfamily enzymes. Avoid concurrent use with strong CYP3A4 inhibitors (eg, clarithromycin, indinavir, itraconazole, ketoconazole, lopinavir/ritonavir, nefazodone, nelfinavir, posaconazole, ritonavir, saquinavir, telaprevir, telithromycin, verapamil, voriconazole) whenever possible. If concurrent use with a strong CYP3A4 inhibitor is required, reduce each ribociclib dose to 400 mg. Avoid concurrent use with strong CYP3A4 inducers (eg, rifampin, carbamazepine, phenytoin, phenobarbital, St. John's wort)
- Ribociclib is a moderate inhibitor of CYP3A enzymes and thus may alter the metabolism of CYP3A substrates. Use caution when a CYP3A substrate with a narrow therapeutic index is co-prescribed with ribociclib (eg, alfentanil, cyclosporine, tacrolimus, sirolimus, dihydroergotamine, ergotamine, everolimus, fentanyl, pimozide, quinidine)
- Avoid coadministration of ribociclib with other drugs that have the potential to prolong the QTc interval
- Advise patients to not consume grapefruit, grapefruit juice, pomegranates, or pomegranate juice as they may inhibit CYP3A in the gut wall and increase the bioavailability of ribociclib
- Dose adjustment for patients with moderate-severe hepatic impairment (Child-Pugh class B or C): 400 mg orally once daily

Letrozole 2.5 mg/dose; administer orally once daily, without regard to food, continually on days 1–28, every 28 days, until disease progression (total dosage/28-day cycle = 70 mg)
Notes:

- Patients who delay taking a letrozole dose at a regularly scheduled time may take the missed dose if the time to the next regularly scheduled dose is >12 hours away
- Dose adjustment for patients with cirrhosis or severe hepatic impairment: 2.5 mg orally every other day

Supportive Care

Antiemetic prophylaxis
Emetogenic potential is **LOW**
See Chapter 42 for antiemetic recommendations

Hematopoietic growth factor (CSF) prophylaxis
Primary prophylaxis is **NOT** indicated
See Chapter 43 for more information

Antimicrobial prophylaxis
Risk of fever and neutropenia is **LOW**
 Antimicrobial primary prophylaxis to be considered:

- Antibacterial—not indicated
- Antifungal—not indicated
- Antiviral—not indicated unless patient previously had an episode of HSV

Patient Population Studied

The international, randomized, double-blind, placebo-controlled, phase 3 trial (MONALEESA-2) involved 668 postmenopausal women with hormone receptor–positive, HER2-negative, advanced breast cancer who had not received any prior systemic treatment for their advanced disease. Eligible patients had an Eastern Cooperative Oncology Group (ECOG) performance status score ≤1 and had recurrent or metastatic disease. All patients received 4-week cycles of oral letrozole (2.5 mg daily). Patients were randomly assigned to also receive oral ribociclib (600 mg) or placebo on days 1–21 of the 4-week cycle. Study treatment continued until disease progression, unacceptable adverse effects, death, or discontinuation of either of the study drugs for other reasons

Efficacy (N = 668)

	Ribociclib + Letrozole (N = 334)	Placebo + Letrozole (N = 334)	
Median progression-free survival	25.3 months	16.0 months	HR 0.568, 95% CI 0.457–0.704; $P = 9.63 \times 10^{-8}$
Overall response rate*	42.5%	28.7%	$P = 9.18 \times 10^{-5}$
Clinical benefit rate†	79.9%	73.1%	—
Duration of response	26.7 months	18.6 months	—

*Overall response rate includes patients with either a complete or partial response to treatment
†Clinical benefit rate includes patients with either a complete or partial response or stable disease for ≥24 weeks
Note: Median follow-up was 26.4 months

Therapy Monitoring

1. Monitor CBC with differential and LFTs. Obtain prior to the start of therapy, every 2 weeks for the first 2 months, monthly for the next 4 months, and as clinically indicated
2. For patients who experience a maximum of G1 or 2 neutropenia in the first 6 cycles, monitor complete blood counts for subsequent cycles every 3 months, prior to the beginning of a cycle, and as clinically indicated
3. Monitor serum electrolytes (including potassium, calcium, phosphorus, and magnesium). Obtain prior to the start of treatment, monthly for 6 months, and as clinically indicated. Correct any abnormality before starting ribociclib
4. Evaluate ECG for QTc prolongation. Obtain prior to the start of therapy and only initiate treatment if QTc is <450 msec. Repeat ECG at approximately day 14 of the first cycle and at the beginning of cycle 2, then as clinically indicated. *Note:* the goal QTc for subsequent ECGs on treatment is ≤480 msec
5. Decreases in bone mineral density may occur. Consider bone mineral density monitoring
6. Increases in total cholesterol may occur. Consider cholesterol monitoring
7. Obtain a pregnancy test in females of reproductive potential. Advise females of reproductive potential to use effective contraception
8. Response assessment: imaging studies every 3–6 months based on patient and disease characteristics

Treatment Modifications

RIBOCICLIB + LETROZOLE	
Ribociclib	
Starting dose	600 mg/dose
Dose level −1	400 mg/dose
Dose level −2	200 mg/dose
Dose level −3	Discontinue therapy

Hematologic Toxicity

G1/2 neutropenia (ANC 1000/mm³ to < LLN)	Observe and continue with administered dose
G3 neutropenia (ANC 500/mm³ to <1000/mm³)	Withhold ribociclib. Resume at same dose when ANC ≥1000/mm³
Recurrent G3 neutropenia (ANC 500/mm³ to <1000/mm³)	Withhold ribociclib. Resume at one lower dose level when ≥1000/mm³
G3 neutropenic fever (ANC <1000/mm³ with single episode of fever >38.3°C or >38°C sustained for more than one hour and/or concurrent infection)	
G4 neutropenia (ANC <500/mm³)	

(continued)

Treatment Modifications (continued)

Hepatotoxicity

Patients with moderate or severe hepatic impairment (Child-Pugh class B or C)	Reduce ribociclib starting dose to 400 mg by mouth daily for 21 consecutive days followed by 7 days without treatment
Either G1 AST/ALT elevation (ULN–3× ULN), or G2 AST/ALT elevation (>3–5× ULN) with baseline at G2 WITHOUT increase in total bilirubin above 2× ULN	Monitor LFTs frequently and continue with administered dose
G2 AST/ALT elevation (>3–5× ULN) with baseline less than G2 WITHOUT increase in total bilirubin above 2× ULN	Withhold ribociclib. Resume at same dose level when toxicity resolves to ≤ baseline grade. Monitor LFTs frequently
Either recurrent G2 AST/ALT elevation with baseline less than G2, or G3 AST/ALT elevation (>5–20× ULN) WITHOUT increase in total bilirubin above 2× ULN	Withhold ribociclib. Resume at one lower dose level when toxicity resolves to ≤ baseline grade. Monitor LFTs frequently
Either recurrent G3 AST/ALT elevation (>5–20× ULN) despite prior dose reduction, or G4 AST/ALT elevation (>20× ULN) WITHOUT increase in total bilirubin above 2× ULN	Discontinue ribociclib
G ≥2 ALT/AST elevation (>3× ULN) with total bilirubin >2× ULN, in the absence of cholestasis, irrespective of baseline grade	Discontinue ribociclib

QT Prolongation

ECGs with QTcF >480 msec	Withhold ribociclib. Resume at one lower dose level when QTcF resolves to <481 msec. Monitor ECGs frequently If QTcF ≥481 msec recurs, withhold ribociclib. Resume at one lower dose level when QTcF resolves to <481 msec. Monitor ECGs frequently
ECGs with QTcF >500 msec and NOT associated with torsades de pointes, polymorphic ventricular tachycardia, unexplained syncope, or signs/symptoms of serious arrhythmia	Withhold ribociclib. Resume at one lower dose level when QTcF resolves to <481 msec. Monitor ECGs frequently
ECGs with either QTcF >500 msec or >60 msec increase from baseline AND associated with torsades de pointes, polymorphic ventricular tachycardia, unexplained syncope, or signs/symptoms of serious arrhythmia	Permanently discontinue ribociclib

Other Toxicities (Excluding Neutropenia, Hepatotoxicity, and QT Interval Prolongation)

Other G1/2 toxicity	Initiate appropriate therapy if indicated and observe carefully and continue with administered dose
Other G3 toxicity	Withhold ribociclib. Resume at same dose level when toxicity resolves to ≤G1. Monitor carefully for need of additional reductions
Recurrent other G3 toxicity	Withhold ribociclib. Resume at one lower dose level when toxicity resolves to ≤G1. Monitor carefully for need of additional reductions
Other G4 toxicity	Discontinue ribociclib

Renal Impairment

Patients with severe renal impairment (eGFR <30 mL/min/1.73m²)	Reduce ribociclib starting dose to 200 mg by mouth daily for 21 consecutive days followed by 7 days without treatment

General Dose Adjustments

If a strong CYP3A inhibitor must be used	Begin therapy with 400 mg ribociclib by mouth daily for 21 consecutive days followed by 7 days without treatment
Strong CYP3A inhibitor is discontinued	Increase the ribociclib dose to the dose used prior to initiation of the inhibitor, after 5 half-lives of the strong CYP3A inhibitor have transpired

Note: Advise patients of potential risk to a fetus and to use effective contraception

ANC, absolute neutrophil count; LLN, lower limit of normal; LFTs, liver function tests; ECG, electrocardiogram; QTcF, QT interval corrected by Fridericia's formula; eGFR, estimated glomerular filtration rate

(continued)

Treatment Modifications (*continued*)

Letrozole

- Dose: 2.5 mg once daily
- Patients with cirrhosis or severe hepatic impairment: 2.5 mg every other day
- In patients with advanced disease, treatment with letrozole should continue until tumor progression is evident
- The most common adverse events (>20%) were hot flashes, arthralgia; flushing, asthenia, edema, arthralgia, headache, dizziness, hypercholesterolemia, sweating increased, bone pain; and musculoskeletal. These should be managed symptomatically

Adverse Events (N = 664)

Grade (%)*	Ribociclib + Letrozole (N = 334)		Placebo + Letrozole (N = 330)	
	Grade 1–2	Grade 3–4	Grade 1–2	Grade 3–4
Neutropenia	15	62	5	1
Nausea	51	2	30	<1
Fatigue	38	3	32	<1
Diarrhea	36	2	24	<1
Alopecia	34	0	16	0
Vomiting	30	4	16	<1
Arthralgia	32	<1	32	1
Leukopenia	12	21	4	<1
Constipation	27	1	22	0
Headache	27	<1	20	<1
Hot flush	24	<1	25	0
Back pain	21	3	20	<1
Cough	23	0	21	0
Rash	21	1	9	0
Anemia	19	2	5	1
Decreased appetite	19	1	15	<1
Abnormal liver function tests	10	10	4	2

*According to the National Cancer Institute Common Terminology Criteria for Adverse Events, version 4.03
Toxicities that occurred in ≥20% of either treatment group are included in the table. A total of 10 on-treatment deaths were reported: two in each treatment group were a result of underlying breast cancer; in the ribociclib plus letrozole group, an additional two died as a result of acute respiratory failure, one died owing to pneumonia, one experienced sudden death, and one died due to an unknown cause; in the placebo plus letrozole group, an additional patient died due to subdural hematoma. Treatment discontinuation owing to adverse events occurred in 8.1% of the ribociclib plus letrozole group and 2.4% of the placebo plus letrozole group

METASTATIC • HORMONE RECEPTOR-POSITIVE • HER2-NEGATIVE

BREAST CANCER REGIMEN: ABEMACICLIB + NON-STEROIDAL AROMATASE INHIBITOR

Goetz MP et al. J Clin Oncol 2017;35:3638–3646
Protocol for: Goetz MP et al. J Clin Oncol 2017;35:3638–3646
Johnston S et al. NPJ Breast Cancer. 2019;5:5

Abemaciclib 150 mg/dose; administer orally twice daily (approximately every 12 hours), with or without food, continually on days 1–28, every 28 days, until disease progression (total dosage/28-day cycle = 8400 mg), *plus:*
Notes:

- Patients who delay taking abemaciclib at a regularly scheduled time or who vomit after taking a dose of abemaciclib should take the next dose at the next regularly scheduled time

- Abemaciclib tablets should be swallowed whole

- Abemaciclib is metabolized by cytochrome P450 (CYP) CYP3A subfamily enzymes. Avoid concurrent use with ketoconazole, which increased abemaciclib exposure by 16-fold. Avoid concurrent use with other strong CYP3A4 inhibitors whenever possible. If concurrent use with a strong CYP3A4 inhibitor other than ketoconazole is required, reduce each abemaciclib dose by 50%. Avoid concurrent use with strong CYP3A4 inducers (eg, rifampin, carbamazepine, phenytoin, phenobarbital, St. John's wort)

- Advise patients to not consume grapefruit and grapefruit juice as they may inhibit CYP3A in the gut wall and increase the bioavailability of abemaciclib

- Dose adjustment for severe hepatic impairment (Child Pugh-C): reduce the abemaciclib dosing frequency to *once* daily

Choose only *one* of the following non-steroidal aromatase inhibitors:

Letrozole 2.5 mg/dose; administer orally once daily, without regard to food, continually on days 1–28, every 28 days, until disease progression (total dosage/28-day cycle = 70 mg), *or:*
Note:

- Patients who delay taking a letrozole dose at a regularly scheduled time may take the missed dose if the time to the next regularly scheduled dose is >12 hours away

- Dose adjustment for patients with cirrhosis or severe hepatic impairment: 2.5 mg orally every *other* day

Anastrozole 1 mg/dose; administer orally once daily, without regard to food, continually on days 1–28, every 28 days, until disease progression (total dosage/28-day cycle = 28 mg)
Note:

- Patients who delay taking an anastrozole dose at a regularly scheduled time may take the missed dose if the time to the next regularly scheduled dose is >12 hours away

- Dose adjustment for patients with severe hepatic impairment: has not been studied

Supportive Care
Antiemetic prophylaxis
Emetogenic potential is **MINIMAL–LOW**
See Chapter 42 for antiemetic recommendations

Hematopoietic growth factor (CSF) prophylaxis
Primary prophylaxis is **NOT** indicated
See Chapter 43 for more information

Antimicrobial prophylaxis
Risk of fever and neutropenia is **LOW**
   Antimicrobial primary prophylaxis to be considered:
   - Antibacterial—not indicated

   - Antifungal—not indicated

   - Antiviral—not indicated unless patient previously had an episode of HSV

(continued)

Patient Population Studied

The international, multicenter, randomized, double-blind, placebo-controlled, phase 3 trial (MONARCH-3) involved 493 patients with hormone receptor–positive, HER2-negative advanced breast cancer. Eligible patients were aged ≥18 years, had an Eastern Cooperative Oncology Group (ECOG) performance status score ≤1, and had metastatic disease or locoregionally recurrent breast cancer not amenable to surgical resection or curative radiotherapy. Patients who had received any prior systemic therapy for advanced breast cancer were not eligible. All patients received an oral non-steroidal aromatase inhibitor (1 mg anastrozole or 2.5 mg letrozole) daily. Patients were randomly assigned (2:1) to also receive oral abemaciclib (150 mg) or matching placebo twice daily. Study treatment continued until disease progression, unacceptable adverse events, study withdrawal, or death

Therapy Monitoring

1. Monitor CBC and LFTs. Obtain prior to the start of therapy, every 2 weeks for the first 2 months, monthly for the next 2 months, and as clinically indicated

2. Monitor patients for signs and symptoms of thrombosis and pulmonary embolism and treat as medically appropriate

3. Instruct patients at the first sign of loose stools to initiate antidiarrheal therapy, increase oral fluids, and notify their health care provider

4. Response assessment: imaging studies every 3 to 6 month based on patient and disease characteristics

(continued)

Diarrhea management
Latent or delayed-onset diarrhea:
Loperamide 4 mg orally initially after the first loose or liquid stool, *then*
Loperamide 2 mg orally every 2 hours during waking hours, *plus*
Loperamide 4 mg orally every 4 hours during hours of sleep
- Continue for at least 12 hours after diarrhea resolves
- Recurrent diarrhea after a 12-hour diarrhea-free interval is treated as a new episode
- Rehydrate orally with fluids and electrolytes during a diarrheal episode
- If a patient develops blood or mucus in stool, dehydration, or hemodynamic instability, or if diarrhea persists >48 hours despite loperamide, stop loperamide and evaluate urgently in clinic or hospitalize the patient for IV hydration
- Alternatively, a trial of **diphenoxylate hydrochloride** 2.5 mg with **atropine sulfate** 0.025 mg (eg, Lomotil)
- Initial adult dose is 2 tablets 4 times daily until control has been achieved, after which the dose may be reduced to meet individual requirements. Control may often be maintained with as little as 2 tablets daily
- Clinical improvement of acute diarrhea is usually observed within 48 hours. If improvement of chronic diarrhea after treatment with a maximum daily dose of 8 tablets is not observed within 10 days, control is unlikely with further administration

Efficacy (N = 493)

	Abemaciclib + Aromatase Inhibitor (N = 328)	Placebo + Aromatase Inhibitor (N = 165)	
Median progression-free survival	28.18 months	14.76 months	HR 0.540, 95% CI 0.418–0.698; P = 0.000002
Objective response rate*	49.7%	37.0%	P = 0.005
Clinical benefit rate†	78.0%	71.5%	P = 0.101

*Objective response rate includes patients with either a complete or partial response to treatment. There were 9 complete responses (2.7%) in the abemaciclib arm and 1 (0.6%) in the placebo arm
†Clinical benefit rate includes patients with either a complete or partial response or stable disease for ≥6 months
Note: Median follow-up was 26.73 months

Treatment Modifications

ABEMACICLIB + NON-STEROIDAL AROMATASE INHIBITOR

ABEMACICLIB

	Abemaciclib
Starting dose	150 mg twice daily
Dose level −1	100 mg twice daily
Dose level −2	50 mg twice daily
Dose level −3	Discontinue therapy

(continued)

Treatment Modifications (*continued*)

Hematologic Toxicity

G1/2 hematologic toxicity	Observe and continue with administered dose
G3 hematologic toxicity (ANC <1000/mm³ or platelet <50,000/mm³)	Withhold abemaciclib. Resume at same dose when ANC >1000/mm³ and platelets >50,000/mm³. Growth factor support is rarely needed for treatment and should not be used for prevention or to maintain a higher dosing
G4 (ANC <500/mm³ or platelet <25,000/mm³) or recurrent G3 hematologic toxicity	Withhold abemaciclib. Resume at one lower dose level when ANC >1000/mm³ and platelets >50,000/mm³. Growth factor support is rarely needed for treatment and should not be used for prevention or to maintain a higher dosing

Diarrhea

G1 diarrhea (<4 stools/day over baseline)	Observe and continue with administered dose if acceptable to patient and health care provider. Otherwise reduce dose one level
G2 diarrhea (4–6 stools/day over baseline; limiting instrumental ADLs)	Observe and continue with administered dose. However, if toxicity does not resolve to ≤G1 within 24 hours then withhold abemaciclib. Resume the previously administered dose if acceptable to patient and health care provider. Otherwise reduce dose one level
Persistent G2 diarrhea or G2 that recurs after resuming dose that previously resulted in G2 diarrhea	Withhold abemaciclib. Resume at one lower dose level when symptoms resolve to ≤G1
G3/4 diarrhea (≥7 stools/day over baseline limiting self-care ADLs or requiring hospitalization)	Withhold abemaciclib. Resume at one lower dose level when symptoms resolve to ≤G1. Monitor carefully for need of additional reductions

Hepatotoxicity

Patients with severe hepatic impairment (Child Pugh-C)	Administer abemaciclib dose once daily
G1 AST/ALT elevation (ULN–3× ULN) G2 AST/ALT elevation (>3–5× ULN) WITHOUT increase in total bilirubin above 2× ULN	Observe carefully and continue with administered dose
Persistent or Recurrent G2 AST/ALT elevation or G3 (>5–20× ULN) WITHOUT increase in total bilirubin above 2× ULN	Withhold abemaciclib. Resume at one lower dose level when toxicity resolves to ≤G1. Monitor carefully for need of additional reductions
Elevation in AST and/or ALT >3× ULN WITH total bilirubin >2 × ULN, in the absence of cholestasis	Discontinue abemaciclib
Grade 4 (>20.0 × ULN)	Discontinue abemaciclib

Other Nonhematologic Toxicities

G1/2 nonhematologic toxicity	Observe carefully and continue with administered dose
Persistent or recurrent G2 toxicity that does not resolve with maximal supportive measures within 7 days to baseline or G1	Withhold abemaciclib. Resume at one lower dose level when toxicity resolves to ≤G1. Monitor carefully for need of additional reductions
G3/4	Withhold abemaciclib. Resume at one lower dose level when toxicity resolves to ≤G1. Monitor carefully for need of additional reductions. For G4 toxicity, consider discontinuation of abemaciclib

General Dose Adjustments

If systemic treatment with ketoconazole is required	Avoid concomitant use of abemaciclib with ketoconazole
If a strong CYP3A inhibitor other than ketoconazole must be used (eg, clarithromycin, indinavir, itraconazole, lopinavir/ritonavir, nefazodone, nelfinavir, posaconazole, ritonavir, saquinavir, telaprevir, telithromycin, and voriconazole, grapefruit, or grapefruit juice)	Begin therapy with 100 mg abemaciclib twice daily. If toxicity occurs, reduce the dose further to 50 mg twice daily
Strong CYP3A inhibitor is discontinued	Increase the dose of abemaciclib one dose level at a time starting after 3–5 half-lives of the inhibitor have transpired

Note: Advise patients of potential risk to a fetus and to use effective contraception

(*continued*)

Treatment Modifications (continued)

NON-STEROIDAL AROMATASE INHIBITOR

Anastrozole

- Dose: One 1-mg tablet taken once daily
- Use with care in women with pre-existing ischemic heart disease
- Most common side effects (with an incidence of >10%) were: hot flashes, asthenia, arthritis, pain, arthralgia, pharyngitis, hypertension, depression, nausea and vomiting, rash, osteoporosis, fractures, back pain, insomnia, headache, peripheral edema and lymphedema, regardless of causality

Letrozole *(Note: In MONARCH 3, the majority of patients [79.1%] received letrozole)*

- Dose: 2.5 mg once daily
- Patients with cirrhosis or severe hepatic impairment: 2.5 mg every other day
- The most common adverse events (>20%) were hot flashes, arthralgia; flushing, asthenia, edema, arthralgia, headache, dizziness, hypercholesterolemia, sweating increased, bone pain; and musculoskeletal

Adverse Events (N = 488)

Grade (%)*	Abemaciclib + Non-steroidal Aromatase Inhibitor (N = 327)		Placebo + Non-steroidal Aromatase Inhibitor (N = 161)	
	Grade 1–2	Grade 3–4	Grade 1–2	Grade 3–4
Any adverse event	43	55	69	22
Diarrhea	72	9	29	1
Neutropenia	20	21	<1	1
Fatigue	38	2	32	0
Infections and infestations	34	5	25	3
Nausea	38	<1	19	1
Abdominal pain	28	1	11	1
Anemia	23	6	4	1
Vomiting	27	1	10	2
Alopecia	27	—	11	—
Decreased appetite	23	1	9	<1
Leukopenia	13	8	2	<1
Increased blood creatinine level	17	2	4	0
Constipation	15	<1	12	0
Increased alanine aminotransferase level	9	6	5	2
Headache	15	<1	15	0

*According to the National Cancer Institute Common Terminology Criteria for Adverse Events, version 4.0
Treatment-emergent toxicities that occurred in ≥15% of patients in either treatment group are included in the table. Of the abemaciclib plus aromatase inhibitor and placebo plus aromatase inhibitor groups, respectively, 2.4% and 1.2% died due to treatment-related adverse events. Treatment discontinuations owing to adverse events occurred in 19.6% of patients in the abemaciclib plus aromatase inhibitor group and 2.5% of the placebo plus aromatase inhibitor group

Goetz MP et al. J Clin Oncol 2017;35:3638–46

METASTATIC • HORMONE RECEPTOR-POSITIVE • HER2-NEGATIVE

BREAST CANCER REGIMEN: ABEMACICLIB + FULVESTRANT

Sledge GW et al. J Clin Oncol 2017;35:2875–2884
Protocol for: Sledge GW et al. J Clin Oncol 2017;35:2875–2884

Note: The regimen as described below is for postmenopausal women. It may also be used for perimenopausal or premenopausal women if concurrent gonadotropin-releasing hormone (GnRH) agonist (eg, goserelin or leuprolide) is administered starting at least 4 weeks prior to initiation of treatment and given ongoing

Abemaciclib 150 mg/dose; administer orally twice daily (approximately every 12 hours), with or without food, continually on days 1–28, every 28 days, until disease progression (total dosage/28-day cycle = 8400 mg), *plus:*
Notes:
- Patients who delay taking abemaciclib at a regularly scheduled time or who vomit after taking a dose of abemaciclib should take the next dose at the next regularly scheduled time
- Abemaciclib tablets should be swallowed whole
- Abemaciclib is metabolized by cytochrome P450 (CYP) CYP3A subfamily enzymes. Avoid concurrent use with ketoconazole, which increased abemaciclib exposure by 16-fold. Avoid concurrent use with other strong CYP3A4 inhibitors whenever possible. If concurrent use with a strong CYP3A4 inhibitor other than ketoconazole is required, reduce each abemaciclib dose by 50%. Avoid concurrent use with strong CYP3A4 inducers (eg, rifampin, carbamazepine, phenytoin, phenobarbital, St. John's wort)
- Advise patients to not consume grapefruit and grapefruit juice as they may inhibit CYP3A in the gut wall and increase the bioavailability of abemaciclib
- Dose adjustment for severe hepatic impairment (Child Pugh-C): reduce the abemaciclib dosing frequency to *once* daily

Fulvestrant 500 mg/treatment; administer by slow intramuscular injection over 1–2 minutes per injection, 250 mg into each buttock, as follows:
Cycle 1: administer on day 1 and 15 (total dosage/28-day cycle during cycle 1 = 1000 mg)
Cycle 2 and beyond: administer on day 1 only, every 28 days, until disease progression (total dosage/28-day cycle during cycle ≥2 = 500 mg)
Note: Dose adjustment for moderate hepatic impairment (Child Pugh-B): reduce fulvestrant dose to 250 mg (ie, only one injection) per treatment

Supportive Care
Antiemetic prophylaxis
Emetogenic potential is **MINIMAL–LOW**
See Chapter 42 for antiemetic recommendations

Hematopoietic growth factor (CSF) prophylaxis
Primary prophylaxis is **NOT** *indicated*
See Chapter 43 for more information

Antimicrobial prophylaxis
Risk of fever and neutropenia is **LOW**
Antimicrobial primary prophylaxis to be considered:
- Antibacterial—not indicated
- Antifungal—not indicated
- Antiviral—not indicated unless patient previously had an episode of HSV

Diarrhea management
Latent or delayed-onset diarrhea:
Loperamide 4 mg orally initially after the first loose or liquid stool, *then*
Loperamide 2 mg orally every 2 hours during waking hours, *plus*
Loperamide 4 mg orally every 4 hours during hours of sleep
- Continue for at least 12 hours after diarrhea resolves
- Recurrent diarrhea after a 12-hour diarrhea-free interval is treated as a new episode
- Rehydrate orally with fluids and electrolytes during a diarrheal episode
- If a patient develops blood or mucus in stool, dehydration, or hemodynamic instability, or if diarrhea persists >48 hours despite loperamide, stop loperamide and evaluate urgently in clinic or hospitalize the patient for IV hydration
- Alternatively, a trial of **diphenoxylate hydrochloride** 2.5 mg with **atropine sulfate** 0.025 mg (eg, Lomotil)
- Initial adult dose is 2 tablets 4 times daily until control has been achieved, after which the dose may be reduced to meet individual requirements. Control may often be maintained with as little as 2 tablets daily
- Clinical improvement of acute diarrhea is usually observed within 48 hours. If improvement of chronic diarrhea after treatment with a maximum daily dose of 8 tablets is not observed within 10 days, control is unlikely with further administration

Efficacy (N = 669)

	Abemaciclib + Fulvestrant (N = 446)	Placebo + Fulvestrant (N = 223)	
Median progression-free survival	16.4 months	9.3 months	HR 0.553, 95% CI 0.449–0.681; P<0.001
Objective response rate*	35.2%	16.1%	P<0.001
Clinical benefit rate†	72.2%	56.1	P<0.001

*Objective response rate includes patients with either a complete or partial response to treatment. No complete responses were observed
†Clinical benefit rate includes patients with either a complete or partial response or stable disease for ≥6 months
Note: Median follow-up was 19.5 months

Therapy Monitoring

1. Monitor CBC and LFTs. Obtain prior to the start of therapy, every 2 weeks for the first 2 months, monthly for the next 2 months, and as clinically indicated
2. Monitor patients for signs and symptoms of thrombosis and pulmonary embolism and treat as medically appropriate
3. Instruct patients at the first sign of loose stools to initiate antidiarrheal therapy, increase oral fluids, and notify their health care provider
4. Response assessment: Imaging studies every 2–3 months

Patient Population Studied

The international, multicenter, randomized, double-blind, placebo-controlled, phase 3 trial (MONARCH-2) involved 669 patients with hormone receptor–positive, HER2-negative advanced breast cancer that has progressed while or ≤12 months after receiving prior endocrine therapy. Eligible patients were aged ≥18 years and had an Eastern Cooperative Oncology Group (ECOG) performance status score ≤1. Patients who had received more than one prior endocrine therapy or any prior chemotherapy for advanced breast cancer were not eligible. All patients received intramuscular injections of fulvestrant (500 mg) on days 1 and 15 of the first 4-week cycle and then on day 1 of subsequent cycles. Patients were randomly assigned (2:1) to also receive oral abemaciclib (initially 200 mg but reduced to 150 mg) or placebo twice daily. All premenopausal or perimenopausal women also received a gonadotropin-releasing hormone agonist. Study treatment continued until disease progression, study withdrawal, or death

Treatment Modifications

ABEMACICLIB + FULVESTRANT

ABEMACICLIB

	Abemaciclib
Starting dosage	150 mg twice daily
Dosage level −1	100 mg twice daily
Dosage level −2	50 mg twice daily
Dosage level −3	Discontinue therapy

Hematologic Toxicity

G1/2 hematologic toxicity	Observe and continue with administered dose
G3 hematologic toxicity (ANC <1000/mm³ or platelet <50,000/mm³)	Withhold abemaciclib. Resume at same dose when ANC >1000/mm³ and platelets >50,000/mm³. Growth factor support is rarely needed for treatment and should not be used for prevention or to maintain a higher dosing
G4 (ANC <500/mm³ or platelet <25,000/mm³) or recurrent G3 hematologic toxicity	Withhold abemaciclib. Resume at one lower dose level when ANC >1000/mm³ and platelets >50,000/mm³. Growth factor support is rarely needed for treatment and should not be used for prevention or to maintain a higher dosing

Diarrhea

G1 diarrhea (<4 stools/day over baseline)	Observe and continue with administered dose if acceptable to patient and health care provider. Otherwise reduce dose one level

(continued)

Treatment Modifications (continued)

Diarrhea

G2 diarrhea (4–6 stools/day over baseline; limiting instrumental ADLs	Observe and continue with administered dose. However, if toxicity does not resolve to ≤G1 within 24 hours, then withhold abemaciclib. Resume the previously administered dose if acceptable to patient and health care provider. Otherwise reduce dose one level
Persistent G2 diarrhea or G2 that recurs after resuming dose that previously resulted in G2 diarrhea	Withhold abemaciclib. Resume at one lower dose level when symptoms resolve to ≤G1
G3/4 diarrhea (≥7 stools/day over baseline limiting self-care ADLs or requiring hospitalization)	Withhold abemaciclib. Resume at one lower dose level when symptoms resolve to ≤G1. Monitor carefully for need of additional reductions

Hepatotoxicity

Patients with severe hepatic impairment (Child Pugh-C)	Administer abemaciclib dose once daily
G1AST/ALT elevation (ULN–3× ULN) G2 AST/ALT elevation (>3–5× ULN) WITHOUT increase in total bilirubin above 2× ULN	Observe carefully and continue with administered dose
Persistent or recurrent G2 AST/ALT elevation or G3 (>5–20× ULN) WITHOUT increase in total bilirubin above 2× ULN	Withhold abemaciclib. Resume at one lower dose level when toxicity resolves to ≤G1. Monitor carefully for need of additional reductions
Elevation in AST and/or ALT >3× ULN WITH total bilirubin >2 × ULN, in the absence of cholestasis	Discontinue abemaciclib
Grade 4 (>20.0 × ULN)	Discontinue abemaciclib

Other Nonhematologic Toxicities

G1/2 nonhematologic toxicity	Observe carefully and continue with administered dose
Persistent or recurrent G2 toxicity that does not resolve with maximal supportive measures within 7 days to baseline or G1	Withhold abemaciclib. Resume at one lower dose level when toxicity resolves to ≤G1. Monitor carefully for need of additional reductions
G3/4	Withhold abemaciclib. Resume at one lower dose level when toxicity resolves to ≤G1. Monitor carefully for need of additional reductions. For G4 toxicity, consider discontinuation of abemaciclib

General Dose Adjustments

If systemic treatment with ketoconazole is required	Avoid concomitant use of abemaciclib with ketoconazole
If a strong CYP3A inhibitor other than ketoconazole must be used (eg, clarithromycin, indinavir, itraconazole, lopinavir/ritonavir, nefazodone, nelfinavir, posaconazole, ritonavir, saquinavir, telaprevir, telithromycin, and voriconazole, grapefruit, or grapefruit juice)	Begin therapy with 100 mg abemaciclib twice daily. If toxicity occurs, reduce the dose further to 50 mg twice daily
Strong CYP3A inhibitor is discontinued	Increase the dose of abemaciclib one dose level at a time starting after 3–5 half-lives of the inhibitor have transpired

Note: Advise patients who are to receive abemaciclib of potential risk to a fetus and to use effective contraception

FULVESTRANT

- The recommended dose is 500 mg. A dose of 250 mg is recommended for patients with moderate hepatic impairment (Child-Pugh class B). Fulvestrant has not been evaluated in patients with severe hepatic impairment (Child-Pugh class C)
- Administered IM; use with caution in patients with bleeding diatheses, thrombocytopenia, or anticoagulant use
- The most common, clinically significant adverse events occurring in ≥5% of patients receiving 500 mg fulvestrant were: injection site pain, nausea, bone pain, arthralgia, headache, back pain, fatigue, pain in extremity, hot flash, vomiting, anorexia, asthenia, musculoskeletal pain, cough, dyspnea, and constipation
- There are no known drug-drug interactions. Fulvestrant does not significantly inhibit any of the major CYP isoenzymes, and studies indicate therapeutic doses of fulvestrant have no inhibitory effects on CYP 3A4 or alter blood levels of drug metabolized by that enzyme. Dosage adjustment is thus not necessary in patients co-prescribed CYP3A4 inhibitors or inducers

Adverse Events (N = 664)

Grade (%)*	Abemaciclib + Fulvestrant (N = 441)		Placebo + Fulvestrant (N = 223)	
	Grade 1–2	Grade 3–4	Grade 1–2	Grade 3–4
Any	39	60	66	23
Diarrhea	73	13	24	<1
Neutropenia	20	27	2	2
Nausea	42	3	22	<1
Fatigue	37	3	26	<1
Abdominal pain	33	2	15	<1
Anemia	22	7	3	<1
Leukopenia	20	9	2	0
Decreased appetite	25	1	12	<1
Vomiting	25	<1	9	2
Headache	20	<1	15	<1
Dysgeusia	18	—	3	—
Alopecia	16	—	2	—
Thrombocytopenia	12	3	2	<1
Stomatitis	15	<1	10	0
Constipation	13	<1	13	<1
Increased alanine aminotransferase level	9	4	4	2
Cough	13	0	11	0
Pruritus	13	0	6	0
Dizziness	12	<1	6	0
Increased aspartate aminotransferase level	10	2	4	3
Increased blood creatinine level	11	<1	<1	0
Arthralgia	11	<1	14	<1
Peripheral edema	12	0	7	0
Rash	10	1	4	0
Upper respiratory tract infection	11	0	7	<1
Dyspnea	8	3	10	1
Pyrexia	10	<1	5	<1
Muscle weakness	10	<1	6	0
Hot flush	10	0	10	0
Decreased weight	10	<1	2	<1
Back pain	9	<1	12	<1

*According to the National Cancer Institute Common Terminology Criteria for Adverse Events, version 4.0
Treatment-emergent toxicities that occurred in ≥10% of patients in either treatment group are included in the table. Three patients in the abemaciclib plus fulvestrant group died due to treatment-related adverse events: two as a result of sepsis and one as a result of viral pneumonia. Treatment discontinuations owing to adverse events occurred in 15.9% of patients in the abemaciclib plus fulvestrant group and 3.1% of the placebo plus fulvestrant group

METASTATIC • HORMONE RECEPTOR-POSITIVE • HER2-NEGATIVE • PIK3CA-MUTATED
ALPELISIB + FULVESTRANT

André F et al. N Engl J Med. 2019;380:1929–1940
Supplementary appendix to: André F et al. N Engl J Med. 2019;380:1929–1940
Protocol for: André F et al. N Engl J Med. 2019;380:1929–1940
PIQRAY (alpelisib) prescribing information. East Hanover, NJ: Novartis Pharmaceuticals Corporation; revised 2019 May

Fulvestrant 500 mg/treatment; administer by slow intramuscular injection over 1–2 minutes per injection, 250 mg into each buttock, as follows:
   Cycle 1: administer on day 1 and 15 (total dosage/28-day cycle during cycle 1 = 1000 mg)
   Cycle 2 and beyond: administer on day 1 only, every 28 days, until disease progression (total dosage/28-day cycle during cycle ≥2 = 500 mg)
Note: Dose adjustment for moderate hepatic impairment (Child Pugh-B): reduce fulvestrant dose to 250 mg (ie, only one injection) per treatment

Alpelisib 300 mg per dose; administer orally once per day, with food, continually until disease progression (total dosage/week = 2100 mg)
Notes:
- Alpelisib tablets should be swallowed whole. Do not crush, chew, or split tablets
- Patients who delay taking an alpelisib dose at a regularly scheduled time may administer the missed dose with food if within 9 hours of the usual dosing time. If >9 hours, skip the missed dose and resume treatment at the next regularly scheduled time
- Alpelisib primarily undergoes spontaneous and enzymatic hydrolysis and is metabolized to a lesser extent by CYP3A4. Avoid concomitant use with strong CYP3A inducers
- Alpelisib is a substrate for BCRP (ABCG2). If coadministration of alpelisib with a BCRP inhibitor is unavoidable, then monitor closely for alpelisib adverse reactions
- Alpelisib induces CYP2C9 expression. If alpelisib is used concomitantly with a sensitive CYP2C9 substrate, monitor closely for loss of effect of the substrate

Supportive Care
Antiemetic prophylaxis
Emetogenic potential is **MINIMAL–LOW**
See Chapter 42 for antiemetic recommendations

Hematopoietic growth factor (CSF) prophylaxis
Primary prophylaxis is **NOT** *indicated*
See Chapter 43 for more information

Antimicrobial prophylaxis
Risk of fever and neutropenia is **LOW**
   Antimicrobial primary prophylaxis to be considered:
- Antibacterial—not indicated. *Pneumocystis jirovecii* prophylaxis is recommended (eg, cotrimoxazole)
- Antifungal—not indicated
- Antiviral—antiherpes antivirals (eg, acyclovir, famciclovir, valacyclovir). Consider pre-emptive cytomegalovirus (CMV) management in CMV seropositive patients treated with idelalisib

Diarrhea management
Loperamide 4 mg orally initially after the first loose or liquid stool, *then*
Loperamide 2 mg orally every 2 hours during waking hours, *plus*
Loperamide 4 mg orally every 4 hours during hours of sleep
- Continue for at least 12 hours after diarrhea resolves
- Recurrent diarrhea after a 12-hour diarrhea-free interval is treated as a new episode
- Rehydrate orally with fluids and electrolytes during a diarrheal episode
- If a patient develops blood or mucus in stool, dehydration, or hemodynamic instability, or if diarrhea persists >48 hours despite loperamide, stop loperamide and evaluate urgently in clinic or hospitalize the patient for IV hydration
- Alternatively, a trial of **diphenoxylate hydrochloride** 2.5 mg with **atropine sulfate** 0.025 mg (eg, Lomotil)
- Initial adult dose is 2 tablets 4 times daily until control has been achieved, after which the dose may be reduced to meet individual requirements. Control may often be maintained with as little as 2 tablets daily
- Clinical improvement of acute diarrhea is usually observed within 48 hours. If improvement of chronic diarrhea after treatment with a maximum daily dose of 8 tablets is not observed within 10 days, control is unlikely with further administration

Patient Population Studied

SOLAR-1 was a randomized, double-blind, placebo-controlled, international, phase 3 trial that involved 572 adult patients with hormone receptor-positive, HER2-negative, advanced breast cancer that had been previously treated with an aromatase inhibitor. Patients were enrolled into either the *PIK3CA*-mutated cohort (n = 341) or into the *PIK3CA*-wild type cohort (n = 231). Within each cohort, patients were randomized 1:1 to receive either the combination of fulvestrant + alpelisib or fulvestrant + placebo. Male patients and post-menopausal female patients were eligible to participate. Patients were required to have tumor tissue available for analysis of *PIK3CA* mutational status at a central laboratory, to have an Eastern Cooperative Oncology Group performance status of ≤1, and adequate organ function. Patients were excluded if they had received chemotherapy for advanced disease; had received prior fulvestrant; had received an inhibitor of PI3K, AKT, or mTOR; had uncontrolled central nervous system metastases, type 1 diabetes or uncontrolled type 2 diabetes, or if they had current pneumonitis. The primary end point of the study was progression-free survival (PFS) in patients with *PIK3CA*-mutated cancer. Of 341 patients enrolled in the *PIK3CA*-mutated cohort, 52% were in their first line of treatment for advanced disease and 47% were in their second line, 57% had visceral metastases, and 6% had received prior treatment with a CDK4/6 inhibitor

Efficacy (N = 341)

	PIK3CA-Mutated Cohort*		
Efficacy Variable	**Alpelisib + Fulvestrant (n = 169)**	**Placebo + Fulvestrant (n = 172)**	**Between-group Comparison**
Investigator-assessed PFS (Primary End Point) (n = 169 alpelisib arm, n = 172 placebo arm)			
Median PFS—months (95% CI)	11.0 (7.5–14.5)	5.7 (3.7–7.4)	HR 0.65 (95% CI, 0.50–0.85); P<0.0001
Response (n = 169 alpelisib arm, n = 172 placebo arm)[†]			
ORR—n/N (%) [95% CI]	45/169 (26.6) [20.1–34.0]	22/172 (12.8) [8.2–18.7]	—
Clinical benefit[‡]—n/N (%) [95% CI]	104/169 (61.5) [53.8–68.9]	78/172 (45.3) [37.8–53.1]	—
CR—n/N (%)	1/169 (0.6)	2/172 (1.2)	—
PR—n/N (%)	44/169 (26.0)	20/169 (11.6)	—
SD—n/N (%)	58/169 (34.3)	63/172 (36.6)	—
Neither CR nor PD[§]—n/N (%)	38/169 (22.5)	25/172 (14.5)	—
PD—n/N (%)	16/169 (9.5)	53/172 (30.8)	—
Unknown—n/N (%)	12/169 (7.1)	9/172 (5.2)	—

*Refer to the publication for efficacy analyses involving the *PIK3CA*-wild type cohort. Proof-of-concept criteria were not met in this cohort; median (95% CI) PFS was 7.4 months (5.4–9.3) in the alpelisib arm and 5.6 months (3.9–9.1) in the placebo arm (HR, 0.85; 95% CI, 0.58–1.25; posterior probability of true hazard ratio <1.00, 79.4%)
[†]Investigator-assessed per RECIST, v1.1. Refer to the publication for response analyses in the subgroup of patients with measurable disease at baseline (n = 262 in the *PIK3CA*-mutated cohort)
[‡]Defined as CR or PR or SD lasting ≥24 weeks, or the status of having neither a CR nor PD for ≥24 weeks
[§]In this category, the best overall response was evaluated only in patients who had no measurable disease at baseline per RECIST v1.1
PFS, progression-free survival; CI, confidence interval; HR, hazard ratio; ORR, overall response rate; CR, complete response; PR, partial response; SD, stable disease; PD, progressive disease; RECIST, Response Evaluation Criteria In Solid Tumors
Note: At the data cutoff date of 12 June 2018, the median (range) duration of follow-up in the *PIK3CA*-mutated cohort was 20.0 (10.7–33.3) months

Therapy Monitoring

1. *Prior to initiation of therapy and then periodically (as clinically indicated):* fasting plasma glucose and hemoglobin A1c
   a. Optimize blood glucose control prior to therapy
2. Monitor periodically for and advise patients to report signs and symptoms of interstitial lung disease (ILD)/pneumonitis such as cough, dyspnea, fatigue, and rales on chest auscultation. If ILD/pneumonitis is suspected, then evaluate promptly with radiographic imaging (eg, chest x-ray and/or CT scan) and other tests as clinically indicated to rule out neoplastic or infectious etiologies. Consider consultation with a pulmonologist
3. Advise patients to promptly report diarrhea associated with alpelisib therapy and provide instructions for self-management with increased oral fluids and antidiarrheal medication (eg, loperamide), when appropriate. In patients with diarrhea who are at risk for dehydration, monitor BUN, serum creatinine, and electrolytes and consider the need for administration of oral and/or intravenous fluids and electrolytes
4. Monitor periodically for cutaneous reactions related to alpelisib. Advise patients to promptly report new dermatologic symptoms. Consider consultation with a dermatologist

Treatment Modifications

ALPELISIB TREATMENT MODIFICATIONS*

Alpelisib Dose Levels

Starting dose	300 mg orally once daily
Dose level −1	250 mg orally once daily
Dose level −2	200 mg orally once daily
Dose level −3	Discontinue alpelisib

Note: Only 1 dose reduction is permitted for pancreatitis

Hyperglycemia

Adverse Reaction	Treatment Modification
G1 (FPG > ULN—160 mg/dL)	Continue alpelisib at the current dose. Initiate or further intensify antihyperglycemic therapy[†]
G2 (FPG >160—250 mg/dL)	Continue alpelisib at the current dose. Initiate or further intensify antihyperglycemic therapy.[†] If FPG does not decrease to ≤160 mg/dL within 21 days under optimized antihyperglycemic therapy, then reduce the alpelisib dosage by 1 dose level and follow FPG value specific recommendations
G3 (FPG >250–500 mg/dL)	Withhold alpelisib. Initiate or further intensify antihyperglycemic therapy[†] and consider additional antihyperglycemic therapy for 1–2 days until hyperglycemia improves.[‡] Administer IV hydration and consider appropriate treatment (eg, interventions for electrolyte disturbances, DKA, and/or HHNS). If FPG decreases to ≤160 mg/dL within 3 to 5 days under appropriate antihyperglycemic treatment, resume alpelisib at 1 lower dose level. If FPG does not decrease to ≤160 mg/dL within 3 to 5 days under appropriate antihyperglycemic treatment, consultation with a physician with expertise in the treatment of hyperglycemia is recommended. If FPG does not decrease to ≤160 mg/dL within 21 days following appropriate antihyperglycemic treatment, then permanently discontinue alpelisib treatment
G4 (FPG >500 mg/dL)	Withhold alpelisib. Initiate or intensify appropriate antihyperglycemic treatment[†] (administer IV hydration and consider appropriate treatment (eg, interventions for electrolyte disturbances, DKA, and/or HHNS), re-check FPG within 24 hours and as clinically indicated. If FPG decreases to ≤500 mg/dL, follow FPG value specific recommendations for G3. If FPG is confirmed at >500 mg/dL, then permanently discontinue alpelisib

Dermatologic Toxicity

G1 rash (<10% BSA involved)	Continue alpelisib at the same dose. Consider consultation with a dermatologist. Initiate topical corticosteroid treatment. Consider initiating an oral antihistamine to manage symptoms if applicable
G2 rash (10–30% BSA involved)	Continue alpelisib at the same dose. Consider consultation with a dermatologist. Initiate or intensify topical corticosteroid and oral antihistamine treatment. Consider initiating low-dose systemic corticosteroid treatment
G3 rash (eg, severe rash not responsive to medical management or >30% BSA involved)	Withhold alpelisib. Consider consultation with a dermatologist. Initiate or intensify topical/systemic corticosteroid and oral antihistamine treatment. Once improved to G ≤1, resume alpelisib at the same dose level (for first occurrence of rash) or at the next lower dose level (for second occurrence of rash)
G4 rash (eg, severe bullous, blistering, or exfoliating skin conditions; or any % BSA involvement associated with extensive superinfection, with IV antibiotics indicated; life-threatening consequences)	Permanently discontinue alpelisib. Consider consultation with a dermatologist

(continued)

Treatment Modifications (*continued*)

Gastrointestinal and Hepatic Toxicities

G1 diarrhea	Continue alpelisib at the current dose. Initiate appropriate medical therapy and monitor as clinically indicated
G2 diarrhea	Initiate or intensify appropriate medical therapy and monitor as clinically indicated. Withhold alpelisib until recovery to G ≤1, then resume alpelisib at the same dose
G ≥3 diarrhea	Initiate or intensify appropriate medical therapy and monitor as clinically indicated. Withhold alpelisib until recovery to G ≤1, then resume alpelisib with the dosage reduced by 1 dose level
G2 or G3 pancreatitis, first occurrence	Initiate appropriate medical therapy and monitor as clinically indicated. Withhold alpelisib until recovery to G ≤1, then resume alpelisib with the dosage reduced by 1 dose level
G2 or G3 pancreatitis, second occurrence	Permanently discontinue alpelisib
G4 pancreatitis (any occurrence)	Permanently discontinue alpelisib
G2 bilirubin elevation	Withhold alpelisib until recovery to G ≤1. If recovery occurs within 14 days, then resume therapy at the same dose. If recovery occurs after 14 days, then resume therapy with the dosage reduced by 1 dose level
G3 bilirubin elevation	Withhold alpelisib until recovery to G ≤1, then resume alpelisib with the dosage reduced by 1 dose level
G4 bilirubin elevation	Permanently discontinue alpelisib

Other Toxicities

G1 or G2 other toxicities	Continue alpelisib at the same dose. Initiate appropriate medical therapy and monitor as clinically indicated
G3 other toxicities	Withhold alpelisib until recovery to G ≤1, then resume alpelisib with the dosage reduced by 1 dose level
G4 other toxicities	Permanently discontinue alpelisib

*Grading of toxicities for the purpose of adverse reaction management should be as per the National Cancer Institute Common Terminology Criteria for Adverse Events (NCI-CTCAE). For hyperglycemia, utilize NCI-CTCAE v4.03; for all other toxicities, utilize NCI-CTCAE v5.0

†Initiate or intensify antihyperglycemic therapy, including metformin and insulin sensitizers (eg, TZDs or DPP-4 inhibitors). Review respective prescribing information and local diabetes treatment guidelines for dosing and dose titration recommendations. Metformin was recommended in the SOLAR-1 trial with the following guidance: Initiate metformin 500 mg once daily. Based on tolerability, metformin dose may be increased to 500 mg twice daily, followed by 500 mg with breakfast, and 1000 mg with dinner, followed by further increase to 1000 mg twice daily if needed

‡In the SOLAR-1 trial, insulin was used for 1–2 days until resolution of hyperglycemia. However, this may not be necessary in the majority of alpelisib-induced hyperglycemia, given the short half-life (8–9 hours) of alpelisib and the expectation that glucose levels will improve after interruption of alpelisib

FULVESTRANT

- The recommended dose is 500 mg. A dose of 250 mg is recommended for patients with moderate hepatic impairment (Child-Pugh class B). Fulvestrant has not been evaluated in patients with severe hepatic impairment (Child-Pugh class C)
- Administered IM; use with caution in patients with bleeding diatheses, thrombocytopenia, or anticoagulant use
- The most common, clinically significant adverse events occurring in ≥5% of patients receiving 500 mg fulvestrant were: injection site pain, nausea, bone pain, arthralgia, headache, back pain, fatigue, pain in extremity, hot flash, vomiting, anorexia, asthenia, musculoskeletal pain, cough, dyspnea, and constipation
- There are no known drug-drug interactions

Adverse Events (N = 571)

Event Grade* (%)	Alpelisib + Fulvestrant (n = 284)			Placebo + Fulvestrant (n = 287)		
	Any Grade	Grade 3	Grade 4	Any Grade	Grade 3	Grade 4
Any AE	99.3	64.4	11.6	92.0	30.3	5.2
Hyperglycemia[†]	63.7	32.7	3.9	9.8	0.3	0.3
Diarrhea[‡]	57.7	6.7	0	15.7	0.3	0
Nausea[‡]	44.7	2.5	0	22.3	0.3	0
Decreased appetite	35.6	0.7	0	10.5	0.3	0
Rash[§]	35.6	9.9	0	5.9	0.3	0
Vomiting[‡]	27.1	0.7	0	9.8	0.3	0
Weight loss	26.8	3.9	0	2.1	0	0
Stomatitis	24.6	2.5	0	6.3	0	0
Fatigue	24.3	3.5	0	17.1	1.0	0
Asthenia	20.4	1.8	0	12.9	0	0
Alopecia	19.7	0	0	2.4	0	0
Mucosal inflammation	18.3	2.1	0	1.0	0	0
Pruritus	18.0	0.7	0	5.6	0	0
Headache	17.6	0.7	0	13.2	0	0
Dysgeusia	16.5	0	0	3.5	0	0
Arthralgia	11.3	0.4	0	16.4	1.0	0

*Graded per the National Cancer Institute Common Terminology Criteria for Adverse Events version 4.03

[†]AEs related to hyperglycemia (including DM, hyperglycemia, insulin resistance, metabolic syndrome, and others) were reported in 65.8% of patients in the alpelisib arm (G ≥3 in 38.0%) and in 10.5% of patients in the placebo arm (G ≥3 in 0.7%)

[‡]GI toxicities (including N/V/D, and others) were reported in 75.4% of patients in the alpelisib arm (G ≥3 in 8.8%) and in 34.8% of patients in the placebo arm (G ≥3 in 1.0%)

[§]AEs related to rash (including rash, rash follicular, rash generalized, rash maculopapular, and others were reported in 53.9% of patients in the alpelisib arm (G ≥3 in 20.1%) and in 8.4% of patients in the placebo arm (G ≥3 in 0.3%)

Note: AEs included in the table are those that were reported as a single term, at any grade, in ≥15% of patients in either group. Three adverse events of special interest (pancreatitis, severe cutaneous reaction, and pneumonitis) were reported and are not included in the table. Hypersensitivity (as a grouped term) occurred in 16.5% of patients in the alpelisib arm (G ≥3 in 1.8%) and in 4.2% of patients in the placebo arm (grade ≥3 in none) but was not included in the table because no single term was reported in ≥15% of patients

AE, adverse event; DM, diabetes mellitus; GI, gastrointestinal; N/V/D, nausea/vomiting/diarrhea

METASTATIC

BREAST CANCER REGIMEN: DOXORUBICIN, EVERY 3 WEEKS

Chan S et al. J Clin Oncol 1999;17:2341–2354

Doxorubicin 75 mg/m²; administer intravenously over 15–20 min on day 1, every 3 weeks for 7 cycles (total dosage/cycle = 75 mg/m²)

Notes:
- A maximum of 7 cycles was established because of the unacceptable incidence of CHF associated with cumulative doxorubicin dosages >550 mg/m². Continuation of treatment is given on a case-by-case basis
- Doxorubicin use is discontinued for either a decrease in LVEF (cardiac ejection fraction) ≥10% (absolute units) or a LVEF decline to <50%

Supportive Care
Antiemetic prophylaxis
*Emetogenic potential is **HIGH**. Potential for delayed emetic symptoms*
See Chapter 42 for antiemetic recommendations

Hematopoietic growth factor (CSF) prophylaxis
Primary prophylaxis may be indicated
See Chapter 43 for more information

Antimicrobial prophylaxis
*Risk of fever and neutropenia is **LOW***
Antimicrobial primary prophylaxis to be considered:
- Antibacterial—not indicated
- Antifungal—not indicated
- Antiviral—not indicated, unless patient previously had an episode of HSV

Treatment Modifications

Adverse Event	Dose Modification
G4 neutropenia	Administer 75% dosage
ANC <1000/mm³	Delay next cycle until ANC ≥1000/mm³
Platelet count <100,000/mm³	Delay next cycle until platelet count ≥100,000/mm³
G3/4 nonhematologic toxicity	Delay next cycle until nonhematologic toxicities decrease to G ≤1
Bilirubin 1.2–3.0 mg/dL (21–51 µmol/L)	Administer 50% dosage
Bilirubin 3.1–5 mg/dL (53–86 µmol/L)	Administer 25% dosage

Patient Population Studied

Study of 326 patients with MBC randomized to either doxorubicin 75 mg/m² or docetaxel 100 mg/m² every 3 weeks. All patients had previously received alkylating agent chemotherapy (eg, cyclophosphamide, methotrexate, and fluorouracil [CMF], or its variants) either in the adjuvant setting or for advanced disease. Criteria for exclusion included: more than 1 line of chemotherapy for advanced or metastatic disease; previous treatment with anthracyclines, anthracenes, or a taxane; no alkylating agent in last chemotherapeutic regimen

Efficacy* (N = 147)

% Complete response	4.8
% Partial response	28.5

Median time to progression	21 weeks
Median time to treatment failure	18 weeks
Median overall survival	14 months†

*All randomized patients. Evaluated by WHO Criteria
†26% of patients received taxane-containing therapy

Toxicity (N = 193)

Toxicity	Percentage of Patients
Neutropenia, all grades	96.7
G3 neutropenia	11.1
G4 neutropenia	77.8
Febrile neutropenia	12.3
G3/4 infection	4.3
G3/4 anemia	16.1
RBC transfusion	20.9
G4 thrombocytopenia	7.5
>20% LVEF decrease*	31.7
>40% LVEF decrease*	16

*Number of patients assessable for LVEF: 101

Therapy Monitoring

1. CBC with differential and platelet count, and serum LFTs and bilirubin before each treatment. Consider intracycle assessment in early cycles
2. LVEF assessment (MUGA or echocardiography) before starting doxorubicin, after completing 300 mg/m², then before every subsequent treatment

METASTATIC

BREAST CANCER REGIMEN: WEEKLY PACLITAXEL

Perez EA et al. J Clin Oncol 2001;19:4216–4223

Premedication:

Dexamethasone 10 mg/dose; administer orally for 2 doses 12 hours and 6 hours before paclitaxel (total dose/cycle = 20 mg), *or*

Dexamethasone 20 mg; administer intravenously over 10–15 minutes, 30–60 minutes before paclitaxel (total dose/cycle = 20 mg)

Note: Dexamethasone doses may be gradually decreased in the absence of hypersensitivity reactions during repeated paclitaxel treatments

Diphenhydramine 25–50 mg; administer orally 60 minutes before paclitaxel, *or* administer by intravenous injection 30–60 minutes before paclitaxel

Cimetidine 300 mg (or **ranitidine** 150 mg, **famotidine** 20–40 mg, or an equivalent histamine receptor [H_2]-subtype antagonist); administer orally 60 minutes before paclitaxel, *or* cimetidine 300 mg (or ranitidine 50 mg, famotidine 20 mg); administer intravenously over 15–30 minutes, 30–60 minutes before paclitaxel

Paclitaxel 80 mg/m^2 per dose; administer intravenously in a volume of 0.9% sodium chloride injection or 5% dextrose injection sufficient to produce a concentration within the range 0.3–1.2 mg/mL over 60 minutes, weekly for 4 consecutive weeks, every 4 weeks (total dosage/4-week cycle = 320 mg/m^2)

Supportive Care

Antiemetic prophylaxis
Emetogenic potential is **LOW**
See Chapter 42 for antiemetic recommendations

Hematopoietic growth factor (CSF) prophylaxis
Primary prophylaxis is **NOT** indicated
See Chapter 43 for more information

Antimicrobial prophylaxis
Risk of fever and neutropenia is **LOW**
   Antimicrobial primary prophylaxis to be considered:
   • Antibacterial—not indicated
   • Antifungal—not indicated
   • Antiviral—not indicated, unless patient previously had an episode of HSV

Treatment Modifications

Adverse Events	Treatment Modifications
ANC ≤800/mm^3 or platelets ≤50,000/mm^3	Hold treatment until ANC >800/mm^3 and platelets >50,000/mm^3, then resume with weekly paclitaxel dosage reduced by 10 mg/m^2
G2 motor or sensory neuropathies	Reduce weekly paclitaxel dosage by 10 mg/m^2 without interrupting planned treatment
Other nonhematologic adverse events G2 or G3	Hold treatment until adverse events resolve to G ≤1, then resume with weekly paclitaxel dosage reduced by 10 mg/m^2
Patients who cannot tolerate paclitaxel at 60 mg/m^2 per week	Discontinue treatment
Treatment delay >2 weeks	Decrease weekly paclitaxel dosage by 10 mg/m^2 or consider discontinuing treatment

Patient Population Studied

Study of 212 women with metastatic breast cancer who had previously received up to 2 chemotherapy regimens for metastatic disease. Prior taxane treatment was allowed if the administration interval was every 3 weeks or less frequently

Efficacy (N = 177 Evaluable) as Defined

Overall response	21.5%
Partial response	19.2%
Complete response	2.3%
Stable disease	41.8%
Median overall survival (OS)	12.8 months
Median time to progression (TTP)	4.7 months

Toxicity NCI Common Toxicity Criteria Scale (N = 211)

Toxicity	%G1/2	%G3	%G4
Hematologic Toxicity			
Neutropenia	40	10	5
Thrombocytopenia	25	0.5	0.5
Anemia	83	9	0
Febrile neutropenia	0	1	0
Infection	3	0	0
Nonhematologic Toxicity			
Anaphylaxis	1	0.5	0.5
Neuropathy	59	9	0
Arthralgia/myalgia	23	2	0
Asthenia	44	4	0
Edema	16	0.5	0
Nausea	25	1	0
Vomiting	9	1	0
Diarrhea	22	0.5	0
Stomatitis	19	0.5	0
Alopecia	43	0	0
Nail changes	20	0	0
Rash	18	0.5	0

Therapy Monitoring

1. *Before each dose:* CBC with leukocyte differential count and platelet counts
2. *Every third or every fourth cycle during therapy:* LFTs, serum electrolytes

METASTATIC

BREAST CANCER REGIMEN: PACLITAXEL EVERY 3 WEEKS

Nabholtz J-M et al. J Clin Oncol 1996;14:1858–1867

Premedication:
Dexamethasone 10 mg/dose; administer orally for 2 doses 12 hours and 6 hours before paclitaxel (total dose/cycle = 20 mg) *or*
Dexamethasone 20 mg; administer intravenously over 10–15 minutes, 30–60 minutes before paclitaxel (total dose/cycle = 20 mg)
Note: Dexamethasone doses may be gradually decreased in the absence of hypersensitivity reactions during repeated paclitaxel treatments
Diphenhydramine 25–50 mg; administer orally 60 minutes before paclitaxel, *or* administer by intravenous injection 30–60 minutes before paclitaxel
Cimetidine 300 mg (or **ranitidine** 150 mg, **famotidine** 20–40 mg, or an equivalent histamine receptor $[H_2]$-subtype antagonist); administer orally 60 minutes before paclitaxel, *or* cimetidine 300 mg (or ranitidine 50 mg or famotidine 20 mg); administer intravenously over 15–30 minutes, 30–60 minutes before paclitaxel
Paclitaxel 175 mg/m^2; administer intravenously in a volume of 0.9% sodium chloride injection or 5% dextrose injection sufficient to produce a concentration within the range 0.3–1.2 mg/mL over 3 hours on day 1, every 3 weeks (total dosage/cycle = 175 mg/m^2)

Supportive Care
Antiemetic prophylaxis
Emetogenic potential is **LOW**
See Chapter 42 for antiemetic recommendations

Hematopoietic growth factor (CSF) prophylaxis
Primary prophylaxis is **NOT** indicated
See Chapter 43 for more information

Antimicrobial prophylaxis
Risk of fever and neutropenia is **LOW**
  Antimicrobial primary prophylaxis to be considered:
  • Antibacterial—not indicated
  • Antifungal—not indicated
  • Antiviral—not indicated, unless patient previously had an episode of HSV

Treatment Modifications

Adverse Events	Treatment Modifications
WHO G3/4 neutropenia for ≥7 days	Decrease paclitaxel dosage by 25%
Platelet counts ≤100,000/mm^3 for ≥7 days	
Febrile neutropenia, documented infection, or hemorrhage	
WHO G3 mucositis	
WHO G >2 paresthesias	Discontinue therapy
Symptomatic arrhythmia or heart block >1°	
Other major organ toxicities WHO G >2	
Severe hypersensitivity reaction	

Patient Population Studied

Study of 471 women with measurable metastatic breast cancer who had received 1 prior chemotherapy regimen (as adjuvant therapy or for metastatic disease), or 2 prior regimens (1 adjuvant and 1 for metastatic disease)

Efficacy (N = 471)

WHO Criteria

	Paclitaxel Dosage (mg/m^2)	
	175	135
Complete response	5%	2%
Partial response	24%	20%
Stable disease (>4 weeks)	43%	42%
Progressive disease	27%	36%
Median progression-free survival	4.2 months	3.0 months
Median overall survival	11.7 months	10.5 months

Response According to Pretreatment Characteristics

ECOG performance status 0	35% (33/95)	32% (30/93)
ECOG performance status 1	27% (25/91)	15% (15/100)
ECOG performance status 2	19% (7/37)	18% (6/34)
Disease in soft tissue only	50% (19/38)	31% (10/32)
Disease in bone ± soft tissue	37% (10/27)	22% (6/27)
Visceral ± bone ± soft tissue	23% (36/158)	21% (35/168)
Prior adjuvant therapy only	36% (25/69)	29% (20/68)
Prior metastatic therapy only	26% (23/88)	14% (12/87)
Adjuvant and metastatic therapy	26% (17/66)	26% (19/72)

Toxicity (N = 471)

WHO Toxicity Criteria

Toxicity	Paclitaxel Dosage (mg/m²)	
	175	135
Hematologic Toxicity		
G3 or G4 leukopenia	34%	24%
G3 or G4 neutropenia	67%	50%
G3/4 neutropenia for ≥7 days	11%	5%
G3 or G4 thrombocytopenia	3%	2%
G3 or G4 anemia	4%	2%
Febrile neutropenia	4%	2%
Infection any grade	23%	15%
Nonhematologic Toxicity		
Severe hypersensitivity*	—	<1%
Bradycardia <50 BPM	3%	4%
G3 or G4 peripheral neuropathy	7%	3%
G3 arthralgia/myalgia	16%	9%
Edema, any grade	13%	16%
G3 or G4 nausea/vomiting	5%	5%
G3 mucositis	3%	<1%

*Includes any of the following: hypotension requiring vasopressors, angioedema, respiratory distress requiring bronchodilators, or generalized urticarial

Therapy Monitoring

Before each cycle: CBC with differential and platelet count. Consider intracycle monitoring during first few cycles

METASTATIC

BREAST CANCER REGIMEN: WEEKLY DOCETAXEL

Burstein HJ et al. J Clin Oncol 2000;18:1212–1219

Premedication:
Dexamethasone 8 mg/dose; administer orally for 3 doses at approximately 12 hours and 1 hour before docetaxel, and 12 hours after docetaxel administration (total dose/week = 24 mg)
Diphenhydramine 50 mg; administer by intravenous injection 30 minutes before docetaxel
Docetaxel 40 mg/m^2; administer intravenously in a volume of 0.9% sodium chloride injection or 5% dextrose injection sufficient to produce a final docetaxel concentration within the range 0.3–0.74 mg/mL over 60 minutes, every week for 6 consecutive weeks, every 8 weeks (total dosage/8-week cycle = 240 mg/m^2)

Supportive Care
Antiemetic prophylaxis
*Emetogenic potential is **LOW***
See Chapter 42 for antiemetic recommendations

Hematopoietic growth factor (CSF) prophylaxis
*Primary prophylaxis is **NOT** indicated*
See Chapter 43 for more information

Antimicrobial prophylaxis
*Risk of fever and neutropenia is **LOW***
Antimicrobial primary prophylaxis to be considered:
- Antibacterial—not indicated
- Antifungal—not indicated
- Antiviral—not indicated, unless patient previously had an episode of HSV

Treatment Modifications

Adverse Events	Treatment Modifications
G2 neurotoxicity	Decrease docetaxel dosage by 25%*
Febrile neutropenia	
G4 thrombocytopenia	
Any G3 nonhematologic adverse event	
G4 nonhematologic toxicity	Consider discontinuing treatment
ANC <1000/mm^3	Hold treatment until ANC >1000/mm^3, platelets >100,000/mm^3, bilirubin normalizes, and AST <1.5 × ULN. If delay is >3 weeks, consider discontinuing therapy
Platelets <100,000/mm^3	
Bilirubin greater than upper limit of normal (ULN) range	
AST >1.5 ULN	
ANC <1000/mm^3 for >2 weeks	Consider adding filgrastim during subsequent cycles
Patients who miss 1–2 weekly treatments in a cycle, but remain eligible for retreatment	Consider retreatment during week 7 of the affected cycle

*Do not re-escalate dose after a dosage decrease

Patient Population Studied

Study of 29 women with metastatic breast cancer with prior treatment of metastatic disease limited to 1 prior chemotherapy regimen. No limitation on prior hormonal therapy

Efficacy (N = 29)

Partial response	41%
Stable disease ≥6 months	17%

Toxicity (N = 29)

NCI Common Toxicity Criteria Scale		
Toxicity	% G1/2	% G3/4
Hematologic Toxicity		
Neutropenia	28	14
Anemia	86	0
Nonhematologic Toxicity		
Nausea/vomiting	34	3
Gastritis	24	3
Diarrhea	24	3
Stomatitis	17	0
Constipation	3	3
Alopecia	66	0
Fatigue	59	14
Excessive lacrimation	52	0
Fluid retention	45	0
Pleural effusion	31	0
Dysgeusia	24	0
Sensory neuropathy	17	3
Motor neuropathy	3	3
Arthralgia	14	0
Dry mouth	14	0
Phlebitis	14	0
Hypersensitivity	3	0

Therapy Monitoring

1. *Weekly, before each docetaxel dose:* CBC with differential and platelet count
2. *Every other week:* Liver function tests

METASTATIC

BREAST CANCER REGIMEN: DOCETAXEL EVERY 3 WEEKS

Chan S et al. J Clin Oncol 1999;17:2341–2354

Premedication:
Dexamethasone 8 mg/dose; administer orally twice daily for 3 days, starting on the day before docetaxel administration (total dose/cycle = 48 mg)
Docetaxel 100 mg/m²; administer intravenously in a volume of 0.9% sodium chloride injection or 5% dextrose injection sufficient to produce a final docetaxel concentration within the range 0.3–0.74 mg/mL over 60 minutes on day 1, every 3 weeks (total dosage/cycle = 100 mg/m²)

Supportive Care
Antiemetic prophylaxis
Emetogenic potential is **LOW**
See Chapter 42 for antiemetic recommendations

Hematopoietic growth factor (CSF) prophylaxis
Primary prophylaxis is **NOT** *indicated*
See Chapter 43 for more information

Antimicrobial prophylaxis
Risk of fever and neutropenia is **LOW**
Antimicrobial primary prophylaxis to be considered:
- Antibacterial—not indicated
- Antifungal—not indicated
- Antiviral—not indicated, unless patient previously had an episode of HSV

Treatment Modifications

Adverse Events	Treatment Modifications
First episode of hematologic or nonhematologic adverse events G ≥3 other than alopecia and anemia	Reduce docetaxel dosage from 100 mg/m² to 75 mg/m²
Second episode of hematologic or nonhematologic adverse events G3 other than alopecia and anemia	Reduce docetaxel dosage from 75 mg/m² to 55 mg/m²

Patient Population Studied

Study of 159 women with metastatic breast cancer who had previously received chemotherapy containing an alkylating agent in the adjuvant setting or for advanced disease. No prior taxoid treatment. Performance status of at least 60% Karnofsky index

Efficacy (N = 148)

WHO Criteria

	Randomized Patients	Assessable Patients
Overall response	47.8% (95% CI, 40.1–55.5%)	52% (95% CI, 44–60.1%)
Complete response	6.8%	7.4%
Median time to progression	26 weeks	27 weeks
Median time to treatment failure	—	22 weeks
Median overall survival	—	15 months

Toxicity

NCI Common Toxicity Criteria

Toxicity	%G3/4	% Overall
Hematologic Toxicity		
Neutropenia	93.5	97.4
Anemia	4.4	88.6
Thrombocytopenia	1.3	4.4
Febrile neutropenia	—	5.7
Infection	2.5	—
Nonhematologic Toxicity		
Acute		
Nausea	3.1	39.6
Vomiting	3.1	22.6
Stomatitis	5	59.7
Diarrhea	10.7	50.3
Skin toxicity	1.9	37.7
Allergy	2.5	17.6
Chronic		
Alopecia	—	91.2
Asthenia	14.5	59.7
Nail disorder	2.5	44
Neurosensory	5	42.8
Neuromotor	5	18.2
Fluid retention	5	59.7

Therapy Monitoring

1. *Weekly:* CBC with differential and platelet count
2. *Before each docetaxel dose:* CBC with differential and platelet count, LFTs, and serum electrolytes

METASTATIC

BREAST CANCER REGIMEN: ALBUMIN-BOUND PACLITAXEL

Gradishar WJ et al. J Clin Oncol 2009;27:3611–3619

Paclitaxel protein-bound particles for injectable suspension (albumin-bound paclitaxel, nab-paclitaxel) 100 mg/m^2 or 150 mg/m^2 per dose*; administer intravenously (undiluted) for 3 doses on days 1, 8, and 15, every 4 weeks (total dosage/cycle may range from 300–450 mg/m^2, depending on the amount of drug given per dose event)

*Initial Dosages in Patients with Hepatic Impairment			
ALT (SGOT)		Serum Bilirubin	Initial Dosage (% of Planned Dosage)†
<10 × ULN	AND	> ULN to ≤1.25 × ULN	100%
<10 × ULN		1.26–2 × ULN	75%
<10 × ULN		2.01–5 × ULN	50%
>10 × ULN	OR	>5 × ULN	Withhold nab-paclitaxel

ULN, upper limit of normal range
†Extrapolated from product labeling for Abraxane for injectable suspension (paclitaxel protein-bound particles for injectable suspension) (albumin bound), October 2013; Celgene Corporation, Summit, NJ

Supportive Care

Antiemetic prophylaxis
Emetogenic potential is **LOW**
See Chapter 42 for antiemetic recommendations

Hematopoietic growth factor (CSF) prophylaxis
Primary prophylaxis is **NOT** *indicated*
See Chapter 43 for more information

Antimicrobial prophylaxis
Risk of fever and neutropenia is **LOW**
  Antimicrobial primary prophylaxis to be considered:
  • Antibacterial—not indicated
  • Antifungal—not indicated
  • Antiviral—not indicated, unless patient previously had an episode of HSV

Patient Population Studied

Study of 302 patients with stage IV metastatic breast cancer who had not previously received treatment for metastatic disease who were randomly assigned to 1 of 3 treatment regimens with nab-paclitaxel or docetaxel. Prior neoadjuvant or adjuvant chemotherapy was allowed if at least 1 year had elapsed since administration. Forty-three percent of patients had previously received chemotherapy in the adjuvant or neoadjuvant settings, and 10% of patients had grade 1 neuropathy before receiving study therapy

Treatment Modifications

Adverse Event	Treatment Modification
ANC <500/mm^3 for ≥1 week	Withhold nab-paclitaxel until symptoms resolve to G ≤1, then resume at a dosage decreased by 25%
Sensory neuropathy G2	Delay nab-paclitaxel until symptoms resolve to G ≤1, then resume treatment at the same dosage and schedule
Sensory neuropathy G ≥3	Withhold nab-paclitaxel until symptoms resolve to G ≤1, then resume on the same administration schedule with a dosage decreased by 25%. Do not re-escalate nab-paclitaxel dosage during subsequent use
Second recurrence of sensory neuropathy G ≥3 after dosage reduction	Withhold nab-paclitaxel until symptoms resolve to G ≤1, then resume on the same administration schedule with a dosage decreased by an additional 25% (total 50% dosage reduction). Do not re-escalate nab-paclitaxel dosage during subsequent use
Third recurrence of sensory neuropathy G ≥3 after 2 dosage reductions	Discontinue nab-paclitaxel
Severe hypersensitivity reaction	Discontinue nab-paclitaxel
Hypotension, during the 30-minute infusion (may occur in 5% of patients)	Most often occurs without symptoms and requires neither specific therapy nor treatment discontinuation
Bradycardia, during the 30-minute infusion (may occur in <1% of patients)	Most often occurs without symptoms and require neither specific therapy nor treatment discontinuation

Efficacy

RECIST*

	nab-Paclitaxel		
	300 mg/m² Every 3 Weeks	100 mg/m² Weekly*	150 mg/m² Weekly†
Overall response rate	37%	45%	49%
Partial response	36%	45%	49%
Complete response	1%	0	0
Stable disease ≥16 weeks	32%	30%	31%
Median progression-free survival	11 months	12.9 months	12.9 months

*RECIST, Response Evaluation Criteria in Solid Tumors (Therasse P et al. J Natl Cancer Inst 2000;92:205–216)
†Weekly regimens are given for 3 consecutive weeks followed by 1 week without retreatment during a 4-week cycle

Toxicity

NCI Common Terminology Criteria for Adverse Events

Toxicity	300 mg/m² Every 3 Weeks	100 mg/m² Weekly*	150 mg/m² Weekly*
	Percentage of Patients Experiencing Toxicity		
G1/2 neutropenia	49	55	47
G1/2 sensory neuropathy	56	50	54
G1/2 fatigue	31	34	42
G1/2 arthralgia	31	19	35
Alopecia	47	57	53
G3/4 neutropenia	44	25	44
G3/4 sensory neuropathy	17	8	14
G3/4 fatigue	5	0	3
G3/4 arthralgia	1	0	0

*Weekly regimens are given for 3 consecutive weeks followed by 1 week without retreatment during a 4-week cycle

Therapy Monitoring

1. *Before each dose:* CBC with differential count and platelet count, LFTs, and neurologic exam
2. *Weekly:* CBC with differential and platelet count through cell count nadirs, particularly for a 150-mg/m² for 3-weeks-out-of-4-weeks regimen

METASTATIC

BREAST CANCER REGIMEN: CAPECITABINE

Bajetta E et al. J Clin Oncol 2005;23:2155–2161
Blum JL et al. J Clin Oncol 1999;17:485–493
Blum JL et al. Cancer 2001;92:1759–1768
Reichardt P et al. Ann Oncol 2003;14:1227–1233
Xeloda (capecitabine) Tablets, Film Coated for Oral Use Product Label, December 2013. Genentech USA, Inc., South San Francisco, CA

Capecitabine 1250 mg/m^2 per dose; administer orally twice daily within 30 minutes after a meal for 14 consecutive days (28 doses) on days 1–14, every 3 weeks (total dosage/cycle = 35,000 mg/m^2)

Notes:
- Capecitabine is given for 2 consecutive weeks followed by 1 week without treatment
- Doses are rounded to use combinations of 500-mg and 150-mg tablets that most closely approximate calculated values
- In practice, treatment often is begun with capecitabine 1000 mg/m^2 per dose twice daily for 14 consecutive days on days 1–14, every 3 weeks, because of a high rate of dose reduction with higher dosages (total dosage/cycle = 28,000 mg/m^2)
- Initial capecitabine dosage should be decreased by 25% in patients with moderate renal impairment (baseline creatinine clearance = 30–50 mL/min [0.5–0.83 mL/s]); ie, a dosage reduction from 1250 mg/m^2 per dose, to 950 mg/m^2 per dose, twice daily. Capecitabine use is contraindicated in persons with severe renal impairment (creatinine clearance <30 mL/min [<0.5 mL/s])
- Although food decreases the rate and extent of drug absorption and the time to peak plasma concentration and systemic exposure (AUC) for both capecitabine and fluorouracil, product labeling recommends giving capecitabine within 30 minutes after the end of a meal because established safety and efficacy data are based on administration with food

Supportive Care
Antiemetic prophylaxis
Emetogenic potential is **LOW**
See Chapter 42 for antiemetic recommendations

Hematopoietic growth factor (CSF) prophylaxis
Primary prophylaxis is **NOT** indicated
See Chapter 43 for more information

Antimicrobial prophylaxis
Risk of fever and neutropenia is **LOW**
   Antimicrobial primary prophylaxis to be considered:
- Antibacterial—not indicated
- Antifungal—not indicated
- Antiviral—not indicated, unless patient previously had an episode of HSV

Diarrhea management
Latent or delayed-onset diarrhea:
Loperamide 4 mg orally initially after the first loose or liquid stool, *then*
Loperamide 2 mg orally every 2 hours during waking hours, *plus*
Loperamide 4 mg orally every 4 hours during hours of sleep
- Continue for at least 12 hours after diarrhea resolves
- Recurrent diarrhea after a 12-hour diarrhea-free interval is treated as a new episode
- Rehydrate orally with fluids and electrolytes during a diarrheal episode
- If a patient develops blood or mucus in stool, dehydration, or hemodynamic instability, or if diarrhea persists >48 hours despite loperamide, stop loperamide and evaluate urgently in clinic or hospitalize the patient for IV hydration
- Alternatively, a trial of **diphenoxylate hydrochloride** 2.5 mg with **atropine sulfate** 0.025 mg (eg, Lomotil)
- Initial adult dose is 2 tablets 4 times daily until control has been achieved, after which the dose may be reduced to meet individual requirements. Control may often be maintained with as little as 2 tablets daily
- Clinical improvement of acute diarrhea is usually observed within 48 hours. If improvement of chronic diarrhea after treatment with a maximum daily dose of 8 tablets is not observed within 10 days, control is unlikely with further administration

Hand-foot reaction
For patients who develop a hand-foot reaction, use topical emollients (eg, Aquaphor), topical or orally administered steroids, antihistamine agents (H$_1$-receptor antagonists), or pyridoxine 50–150 mg/day administered orally

Treatment Modifications

Adapted from NCI of Canada CTC

Adverse Event	Dose Modification
First G2 toxicity	Hold capecitabine and resume after adverse events resolve to G ≤1. No change in dosage required
Second G2 toxicity	Hold capecitabine and resume after adverse events resolve to G ≤1. Reduce dosage by 25%
Third G2 toxicity	Hold capecitabine and resume after adverse events resolve to G ≤1. Reduce dosage by 50%
Fourth G2 toxicity	Discontinue capecitabine
First G3 toxicity	Hold capecitabine and resume after adverse events resolve to G ≤1. Reduce dosage by 25%
Second G3 toxicity	Hold capecitabine and resume after adverse events resolve to G ≤1. Reduce dosage by 50%
Third G3 toxicity	Discontinue capecitabine
First G4 toxicity	Hold capecitabine and resume after adverse events resolve to G ≤1. Reduce dosage by 50%
Second G4 toxicity	Discontinue capecitabine
Diarrhea, nausea, and vomiting	Treat symptomatically. Resume previous dosage if toxicity is adequately controlled within 2 days after initiation of treatment. If control takes longer, reduce the capecitabine dosage, or if it occurs despite prophylaxis, reduce the capecitabine dosage 25–50%

Patient Population Studied

Study of 75 patients with metastatic breast cancer who developed disease progression during or after taxane-containing chemotherapy (Blum JL et al. Cancer 2001;92:1759–1768)

Toxicity (Adapted from Blum et al, 1999)*

Xeloda (capecitabine) Tablets, Film Coated for Oral Use Product Label, December 2013. Genentech USA, Inc., South San Francisco, CA

Adverse Events	% All Grades	% G3/4
Hematologic Toxicity		
Neutropenia	26	4
Anemia	72	4
Thrombocytopenia	24	4
Lymphopenia	94	59
Nonhematologic Toxicity		
Diarrhea	57	15
Hand-foot syndrome	57	11
Nausea	53	4
Fatigue	41	8
Vomiting	37	4
Dermatitis	37	1
Stomatitis	24	7
Anorexia	23	3
Hyperbilirubinemia	22	11
Paresthesia	21	1
Abdominal pain	20	4
Constipation	15	1
Eye irritation	15	—
Pyrexia	12	1
Dyspepsia	8	—
Nail disorder	7	—
Laboratory Abnormalities		
Hyperbilirubinemia	22	11
Increased alkaline phosphatase	—	3.7

*Twice-daily oral capecitabine at 1255 mg/m² per dose given for 2 treatment weeks, followed by a 1-week rest period and repeated in 3-week cycles (total daily dose = 2510 mg/m²)
Incidence of selected adverse reactions possibly or probably related to treatment in ≥5% of patients participating in a single arm trial in stage IV breast cancer (n = 162)

Efficacy (N = 75)

Blum JL et al. Cancer 2001;92:1759–1768

WHO Criteria	
Intention-to-treat overall response	26%
Intention-to-treat stable disease >6 weeks	31%
Median time to progressive disease	3.2 months (95% CI, 2.3–4.3)
Median time to treatment failure in all patients	3.2 months (95% CI, 2.2–4.4)
Median duration of response in 17 patients with PR	8.3 months (95% CI, 7–9.9)
Median survival in intention-to-treat population	12.2 months (95% CI, 8.0–15.3)
Median survival in 21 patients with stable disease	12.9 months
Median survival in 17 patients with CR/PR	Not reached

Subgroup Analysis	CR/PR
Paclitaxel pretreated	27%
Paclitaxel failed	33%
Paclitaxel resistant	20%
Docetaxel pretreated	28%
Docetaxel failed	38%
Docetaxel resistant	17%

CR, Complete response; PR, partial response

Therapy Monitoring

1. *Before starting each cycle:* CBC with differential and platelet counts. Consider intracycle monitoring in first few cycles
2. *Every other cycle:* Serum electrolytes, serum creatinine and BUN, and LFTs
3. Frequently monitor anticoagulant response (INR or PT) in patients who use coumarin anticoagulants (eg, warfarin) and capecitabine concomitantly, and adjust anticoagulant dose accordingly, or consider alternative anticoagulant agents

METASTATIC

BREAST CANCER REGIMEN: GEMCITABINE

Blackstein M et al. Oncology 2002;62:2–8
Carmichael J et al. J Clin Oncol 1995;13:2731–2736

Gemcitabine 800–1200 mg/m^2 per dose; administer by intravenous infusion in 50–250 mL 0.9% sodium chloride injection (0.9% NS) over 30 minutes on days 1, 8, and 15, every 28 days for up to 8 cycles (total dosage/cycle = 2400–3600 mg/m^2)

Note: Gemcitabine use in patients with concurrent liver metastases or a preexisting history of hepatitis, alcoholism, or liver cirrhosis, may lead to exacerbation of the underlying hepatic insufficiency

Supportive Care

Antiemetic prophylaxis
Emetogenic potential is **LOW**
See Chapter 42 for antiemetic recommendations

Hematopoietic growth factor (CSF) prophylaxis
Primary prophylaxis is **NOT** indicated
See Chapter 43 for more information

Antimicrobial prophylaxis
Risk of fever and neutropenia is **LOW**
  Antimicrobial primary prophylaxis to be considered:
  • Antibacterial—not indicated
  • Antifungal—not indicated
  • Antiviral—not indicated, unless patient previously had an episode of HSV

Treatment Modifications

Adverse Events	Treatment Modifications
ANC 1000–1499/mm^3, WBC 1000–1999/mm^3, or platelets 50,000–99,999/mm^3 on day of treatment	Reduce dosage by 25%
ANC and WBC <1000/mm^3 or platelets <50,000/mm^3 on day of treatment	Hold treatment until ANC and WBC >1000/mm^3, and platelets >50,000/mm^3. Resume treatment with gemcitabine dosage reduced by 50%
ANC and WBC <500/mm^3, or platelets <25,000/mm^3 on day of treatment	Consider discontinuing therapy
WHO G3 nonhematologic adverse events (excluding nausea, vomiting, and alopecia)	Decrease dosage by 50%, or withhold treatment until recovery to G ≤1
WHO G4 nonhematologic adverse events	Hold treatment until resolution to G ≤1 then resume with a 50% dose reduction

Patient Population Studied

Blackstein M et al. Oncology 2002;62:2–8

Study of 39 patients with metastatic breast cancer who had not previously received chemotherapy for metastatic disease

Efficacy (N = 35)

WHO Criteria	
Overall response rate	37.1% (95% CI, 21.5–55.1)
Complete response rate	5.7%
Partial response rate	31.4%
Median time to progression	5.1 months (95% CI, 3.5–5.8)
Median response duration in 13 responders	8.8 months (95% CI, 5.2–12.7)
Median overall survival	21.1 months (95% CI, 11–26.9)
Estimated 1-year survival	65%

Toxicity (N = 39)

Blackstein M et al. Oncology 2002;62:2–8

WHO Criteria		
Toxicity	% G1/2	% G3/4
Hematologic Toxicity		
Anemia	60.6	9.1
Neutropenia*	36.4	30.3
Thrombocytopenia*	25	6.3
Laboratory Abnormalities		
Alkaline phosphatase increase	35.3	0
Alanine aminotransferase increase	58.8	5.9
Bilirubin increase	2.9	2.9
Nonhematologic Toxicity		
Allergic	12.9	0
Cutaneous	30.7	2.6
Diarrhea	23.1	0
Fever	15.4	0
Infection	10.3	2.6
Nausea/vomiting	41.1	10.3
Pulmonary	12.9	5.2
Alopecia	46.2	0

Dose Delivery	
Total cycles completed	211
Median cycles/patient	4 (Range: 0–4)
Dosage reductions	102
Dose omissions	69
Dose delays	5
Median dosage intensity	1053 mg/m^2 per week (range: 400–1212 mg/m^2 week)

*Leukopenia was the most common reason for gemcitabine dosage reductions (78.4%) and omissions (58.0%), while thrombocytopenia resulted in 14% and 13% of reductions and omissions, respectively

Therapy Monitoring

Before starting each treatment: CBC with differential and platelet count, LFTs, serum creatinine and BUN, and serum electrolytes. Consider intracycle assessment in first few cycles

METASTATIC

BREAST CANCER REGIMEN: ERIBULIN MESYLATE

Cortes J et al. J Clin Oncol 2010;28:3922–3928
Cortes J et al. Lancet 2011;377:914–923

Eribulin mesylate 1.4 mg/m^2 per dose*; administer (undiluted) by slow intravenous injection over 2–5 minutes for 2 doses on days 1 and 8, every 21 days (total dosage/cycle = 2.8 mg/m^2)

*Dosage Recommendations for Impaired Liver and Renal Function

Condition	Dosage (Days 1 and 8; 21-day Cycle)
Mild hepatic impairment (Child-Pugh A)	1.1 mg/m^2 per dose (total dosage/cycle = 2.2 mg/m^2)
Moderate hepatic impairment (Child-Pugh B)	0.7 mg/m^2 per dose (total dosage/cycle = 1.4 mg/m^2)
Moderate renal impairment (creatinine clearance: 30–50 mL/min [0.5–0.83 mL/s])	1.1 mg/m^2 per dose (total dosage/cycle = 2.2 mg/m^2)

Supportive Care

Antiemetic prophylaxis
*Emetogenic potential is **LOW***
See Chapter 42 for antiemetic recommendations

Hematopoietic growth factor (CSF) prophylaxis
Primary prophylaxis is **NOT** indicated
See Chapter 43 for more information

Antimicrobial prophylaxis
*Risk of fever and neutropenia is **LOW***
  Antimicrobial primary prophylaxis to be considered:
  • Antibacterial—not indicated
  • Antifungal—not indicated
  • Antiviral—not indicated, unless patient previously had an episode of HSV

Treatment Modifications

Eribulin Mesylate Dosage Levels	
Dosage Level 1	1.4 mg/m^2
Dosage Level −1	1.1 mg/m^2
Dosage Level −2	0.7 mg/m^2

Adverse Events	Treatment Modifications
ANC <1000/mm^3 on cycle days 1 or 8	Hold eribulin mesylate. Administer when ANC >1000/mm^3
Platelet count <75,000/mm^3 on cycle days 1 or 8	Hold eribulin mesylate. Administer when platelet count >75,000/mm^3
Nonhematologic toxicities G ≥3 on cycle days 1 or 8	Hold eribulin mesylate. Administer when toxicities G <2
ANC <1000/mm^3 on cycle day 8 resolved by day 15	Give eribulin mesylate at a dosage decreased by 1 dose level but do not administer less than 0.7 mg/m^2. Initiate a subsequent cycle no sooner than 2 weeks later
Platelet count <75,000/mm^3 on cycle day 8 resolved by day 15	
Nonhematologic toxicities G ≥3 on cycle day 8 resolved by day 15	
ANC <1000/mm^3 on cycle day 8 and still <1000/mm^3 on day 15	Omit day 8 eribulin mesylate dose
Platelet count <75,000/mm^3 on cycle day 8 and still <75,000/mm^3 on day 15	
Nonhematologic toxicities G ≥3 on cycle day 8 and still G ≥3 on day 15	
ANC <500/mm^3 for >7 days	Permanently decrease eribulin mesylate dosage by one dosage level but do not administer <0.7 mg/m^2
ANC <1000/mm^3 with fever or infection	
Platelet count <25,000/mm^3	
Platelet count <50,000/mm^3 requiring transfusion	
Nonhematologic toxicities G ≥3 lasting >7 days	
Omission or delay of a day 8 dose during the previous cycle for toxicity	

Note: After any dosage decrease, do not re-escalate eribulin mesylate dosages during subsequent treatments

Patient Population Studied

Cortes J et al. Lancet 2011;377:914–923
EMBRACE trial (study E7389-G000-305). A phase 3 open-label, multicenter study that enrolled women with locally recurrent or metastatic breast cancer and randomly allocated them (2:1) to eribulin mesylate or treatment of physician's choice (TPC). Patients were previously treated for locally recurrent or metastatic breast cancer (508 eribulin mesylate vs 254 TPC). Patients were heavily pretreated (median of 4 previous chemotherapy regimens); 559 (73%) of 762 patients had received capecitabine previously. No TPC patient received supportive care alone; most (238 [96%] of 247) received chemotherapy, which was most often vinorelbine, gemcitabine, or capecitabine. Overall, 16% (123 of 762 patients) had HER2-positive disease, and 19% (144 patients) had triple-negative disease. The most common metastatic sites were bone and liver; 386 (51%) of 762 patients had metastatic disease involving 3 or more organs. Randomization was stratified by geographical region, previous capecitabine treatment, and human epidermal growth factor receptor 2 status. The primary end point was overall survival in the intention-to-treat population

Efficacy (N = 508)

RECIST

	Independent Review	Investigator Review
Median overall survival	13.1 months	
1-Year survival rates	53.9%	
Median duration of treatment	3.9 months (range: 0.7–16.3)	
Median progression-free survival	3.7 months (95% CI, 3.3–3.9)	3.6 months (95% CI, 3.3–3.7)

Best Overall Tumor Response

Complete response	3 (1%)	1 (<1%)
Partial response	54 (12%)	61 (13%)
Stable disease	208 (44%)	219 (47%)
Progressive disease	190 (41%)	176 (38%)
Not evaluable	12 (3%)	11 (2%)
Unknown	1 (<1%)	0
Objective response rate	57 (12%) (95% CI, 9.4–15.5)	62 (13%) (95% CI, 10.3–16.7)

RECIST, Response Evaluation Criteria in Solid Tumors (Therasse P et al. J Natl Cancer Inst 2000;92:205–216)

Therapy Monitoring

1. ECG at baseline (pretreatment on cycle 1, day 1), prior to treatment on day 8, and prior to all eribulin mesylate treatments in patients with CHF or bradyarrhythmias, and in patients concomitantly using drugs known to prolong the QT/QTc interval. Avoid use in patients with congenital long QT syndrome
2. *Before each dose:* CBC with differential and platelet count, serum sodium, potassium, magnesium, creatinine and BUN, and LFTs. Correct electrolyte abnormalities before commencing treatment
3. *Before each cycle:* Neurologic examination

Toxicity (N = 503)*

NCI-CTCAE

	% All Grades	% G3	% G4
Hematologic			
Neutropenia	52	21	24
Leucopenia	23	12	2
Anemia	19	2	<1
Nonhematologic			
Asthenia/fatigue	54	8	1
Alopecia	45	—	—
Peripheral neuropathy[†]	35	8	<1
Nausea	35	1	0
Constipation	25	1	0
Arthralgia/ myalgia	22	<1	0
Weight loss	21	1	0
Pyrexia	21	<1	0
Anorexia	19	<1	0
Headache	19	<1	0
Diarrhea	18	0	0
Vomiting	18	1	<1
Back pain	16	1	<1
Dyspnea	16	4	0
Cough	14	0	0
Bone pain	12	2	0
Pain in extremity	11	1	0
Mucosal inflammation	9	1	0
Palmar-plantar erythrodysesthesia	1	<1	0

NCI-CTCAE, National Cancer Institute, Common Terminology Criteria for Adverse Events, v.3.0. At: http://ctep.cancer.gov/protocolDevelopment/electronic_applications/ctc.htm [accessed December 7, 2013]
*Dose interruptions, delays, and reductions were undertaken in 28 (6%), 248 (49%), and 145 (29%) of 503 patients, respectively
†Peripheral neuropathy includes neuropathy, peripheral, neuropathy, peripheral motor neuropathy, polyneuropathy, peripheral sensory neuropathy, peripheral sensorimotor neuropathy, demyelinating polyneuropathy, and paresthesia

METASTATIC

BREAST CANCER REGIMEN: DOXORUBICIN + CYCLOPHOSPHAMIDE (AC)

Nabholtz JM et al. J Clin Oncol 2003;21:968–975

Hydration with 1000 mL 0.9% sodium chloride injection (0.9% NS); administer intravenously 500 mL before starting cyclophosphamide and 500 mL after completing cyclophosphamide

Doxorubicin HCl 60 mg/m^2; administer by intravenous injection over 3–5 minutes on day 1, every 21 days, for up to 8 cycles (total dosage/cycle = 60 mg/m^2)

Cyclophosphamide 600 mg/m^2; administer intravenously in 100–500 mL 0.9% NS or 5% dextrose injection over 15–60 minutes on day 1, every 21 days, for up to 8 cycles (total dosage/cycle = 600 mg/m^2)

Supportive Care

Antiemetic prophylaxis
Emetogenic potential is **HIGH**. Potential for delayed symptoms
See Chapter 42 for antiemetic recommendations

Hematopoietic growth factor (CSF) prophylaxis
Primary prophylaxis may be indicated
See Chapter 43 for more information

Antimicrobial prophylaxis
Risk of fever and neutropenia is **LOW**
   Antimicrobial primary prophylaxis to be considered:
   • Antibacterial—not indicated
   • Antifungal—not indicated
   • Antiviral—not indicated, unless patient previously had an episode of HSV

Treatment Modifications

Bear HD et al. J Clin Oncol 2003;21:4165–4174
Citron ML et al. J Clin Oncol 2003;21:1431–1439

Adverse Events	Treatment Modifications
Absolute neutrophil count (ANC) <1500/mm^3 or platelets <100,000/mm^3 at start of cycle*	Delay treatment until ANC ≥1500/mm^3 and platelets ≥100,000/mm^3. Give filgrastim after chemotherapy during subsequent cycles
First episode of febrile neutropenia	Give filgrastim after chemotherapy during subsequent cycles[†]
Second episode of febrile neutropenia	During subsequent cycles, consider prophylaxis with ciprofloxacin[‡]
Third episode of febrile neutropenia	Decrease both doxorubicin and cyclophosphamide dosages by 25%

*Although an ANC of 1500/mm^3 is often identified as a minimum acceptable ANC to safely proceed with treatment, recent data shows that an ANC ≥1000/mm^3 is acceptable if filgrastim is given after chemotherapy
[†]Filgrastim 5 mcg/kg per day; administer subcutaneously starting at least 24 hours after completing chemotherapy until ANC ≥5000/mm^3
[‡]Ciprofloxacin 500 mg orally twice daily for 7 consecutive days starting on day 5

Patient Population Studied

This was a randomized, multicenter, open-label, phase 3 study involving 429 patients with metastatic breast cancer who were randomized to receive doxorubicin + cyclophosphamide (n = 215) or doxorubicin + docetaxel (n = 214). Patients were required to have adequate organ function, a Karnofsky performance status of ≥60%, and a normal left ventricular ejection fraction. Patients who had previously received adjuvant or neoadjuvant non-anthracycline-containing chemotherapy were eligible

Toxicity (n = 210)*

Toxicity	AC (n = 210)
Neutropenia, overall	97%
Neutropenia, G3/4	88%
Febrile neutropenia	10%
Infection, G3/4	2%
Thrombocytopenia, overall	27.6%
Thrombocytopenia, G3/4	9.1%
Septic death	0.5%
Alopecia	93%
Nausea	78%
Vomiting	61%
Stomatitis	49%
Diarrhea	16%
Neurosensory toxicity	7%
Asthenia	49%
Edema	4%
Nail changes	7%
Skin rashes	4%
Allergy	1%
Congestive heart failure, G3/4	4%
LVEF decrease >10 percentage points from baseline and <LLN	18%
LVEF decrease ≥20 percentage points from baseline	13%
LVEF decrease ≥30 percentage points from baseline	6%
Discontinued due to cardiac toxicity	8%

Therapy Monitoring

1. *Before each cycle:* CBC with differential and platelet counts, LFTs, serum electrolytes, BUN, and creatinine
2. *Prior to therapy:* Determination of LVEF by echocardiogram or MUGA scan

Efficacy

Outcome	Doxorubicin + Cyclophosphamide (n = 215)	Doxorubicin + Docetaxel (n = 214)	Between-group Comparison
Median time to progression	31.9 weeks (95% CI, 27.4–36.0)	37.3 weeks (95% CI, 33.4–42.1)	P = 0.014
Median time to treatment failure	23.7 weeks (95% CI, 20.6–26.0)	25.6 weeks (95% CI, 22.3–28.0)	P = 0.048
Median overall survival	21.7 months (95% CI, 19.8–25.2)	22.5 months (95% CI, 19.0–26.4)	P = 0.26
Overall response rate	47%	59%	P = 0.009
Complete response rate	7%	10%	—
Partial response rate	39%	49%	—
No change	33%	24%	—
Progression	15%	10%	—
Not assessable	6%	7%	—

METASTATIC

BREAST CANCER REGIMEN: CYCLOPHOSPHAMIDE + EPIRUBICIN + FLUOROURACIL (FEC 100)

Brufman G et al. Ann Oncol 1997;8:155–162

Fluorouracil 500 mg/m²; administer by intravenous injection over 1–3 minutes on day 1, every 21 days for 6 cycles (total dosage/cycle = 500 mg/m²)

Epirubicin HCl 100 mg/m²; administer by intravenous injection over 3–5 minutes on day 1, every 21 days for 6 cycles (total dosage/cycle = 100 mg/m²)

Hydration with 1000 mL 0.9% sodium chloride injection (0.9% NS); administer intravenously 500 mL before starting cyclophosphamide and 500 mL after completing cyclophosphamide

Cyclophosphamide 500 mg/m²; administer intravenously in 100–500 mL 0.9% NS or 5% dextrose injection over 15–60 minutes on day 1, every 21 days for 6 cycles (total dosage/cycle = 500 mg/m²)

Note: A maximum of 8 total cycles was allowed in case of complete response

Supportive Care
Antiemetic prophylaxis
Emetogenic potential is **HIGH**. *Potential for delayed symptoms*
See Chapter 42 for antiemetic recommendations

Hematopoietic growth factor (CSF) prophylaxis
Primary prophylaxis is indicated with one of the following:

Filgrastim (G-CSF) 5 mcg/kg per day by subcutaneous injection, *or*

Pegfilgrastim (pegylated filgrastim) 6 mg/0.6 mL by subcutaneous injection for 1 dose

- Begin use from 24–72 hours after myelosuppressive chemotherapy is completed
- Continue daily filgrastim until ANC ≥5000/mm³

See Chapter 43 for more information

Antimicrobial prophylaxis
Risk of fever and neutropenia is **LOW**
Antimicrobial primary prophylaxis to be considered:
- Antibacterial—not indicated
- Antifungal—not indicated
- Antiviral—not indicated, unless patient previously had an episode of HSV

Patient Population Studied

This was a multicenter, international, randomized, controlled trial involving 456 patients with metastatic histologically proven breast cancer who received fluorouracil, epirubicin, and cyclophosphamide (FEC) with an epirubicin dose of either 50 mg/m² (FEC50) or 100 mg/m² (FEC100). Patients were required to have measurable disease, a World Health Organization/Eastern Cooperative Oncology Group performance status of ≤2, and normal organ function (including a left ventricular ejection fraction of ≥10% below lowest normal value for the institution). Patients were allowed to have received adjuvant chemotherapy but prior anthracycline exposure was limited to ≤60 mg/m². Prior hormonal therapy was allowed so long as it had been discontinued ≥4 weeks previously without evidence of a withdrawal response

Treatment Modifications

Adverse Events	Treatment Modifications
ANC <1500/mm³, or platelets <100,000/mm³ at start of cycle	Delay treatment until ANC ≥1500/mm³ and platelets ≥100,000/mm³
Hematologic recovery >3 weeks	Discontinue treatment
First episode of febrile neutropenia	During subsequent cycles, consider prophylaxis with ciprofloxacin*
Second episode of febrile neutropenia	Decrease chemotherapy doses by 20% (epirubicin by 20 mg/m², fluorouracil and cyclophosphamide by 100 mg/m²) and administer ciprofloxacin*
First episode of G4 documented infection	Add ciprofloxacin prophylaxis during subsequent cycles*
Second episode of G4 documented infection	Decrease chemotherapy doses by 20% (epirubicin by 20 mg/m², fluorouracil and cyclophosphamide by 100 mg/m²) and administer ciprofloxacin*
Third episode of G4 documented infection	Discontinue chemotherapy
Serum total bilirubin levels 2–3 mg/dL (34.2–51.3 mmol/L)	Reduce epirubicin dose by 50%
Serum bilirubin levels ≥3 mg/dL (≥51.3 mmol/L)	Discontinue treatment

*Ciprofloxacin 500 mg orally twice daily for 7 consecutive days starting on day 5

Efficacy

	FEC 50 (n = 208)*	FEC 100 (n = 182)*	
Overall response	41%	57%	P = 0.003
Complete response	7%	12%	—
Median time to progression	7 months	7.6 months	P = 0.53
Overall survival†	17	18	P = 0.54

FEC 50, fluorouracil + cyclophosphamide + epirubicin 50 mg/m²; FEC 100, fluorouracil + cyclophosphamide + epirubicin 100 mg/m²
*Evaluable patients
†Analysis included all randomized patients (FEC 50, n = 241; FEC 100, n = 212)

Toxicity

Toxicity	FEC 100		FEC 50	
	G1/2	G3/4	G1/2	G3/4
Neutropenia	12%	86%	46%	31%
Thrombocytopenia	18%	6%	4%	2%
Anemia	69%	7%	32%	1%
Nausea/vomiting	64%	30%	65%	26%
Mucositis	30%	10%	12%	0%
Alopecia	23%	72%	38%	56%

Therapy Monitoring

1. *Weekly:* CBC with differential and platelet count
2. *Before each cycle:* CBC with differential and platelet count, LFTs, and serum electrolytes
3. *Prior to therapy:* Determination of LVEF by echocardiogram or MUGA scan

METASTATIC

BREAST CANCER REGIMEN: CYCLOPHOSPHAMIDE + METHOTREXATE + FLUOROURACIL (CMF; ORAL)

De Lena M et al. Cancer 1975;35:1108–1115

Cyclophosphamide 100 mg/m^2 per day; administer orally for 14 consecutive days on days 1–14, every 4 weeks, until disease progression (total dosage/4-week cycle = 1400 mg/m^2)

Note: Encourage patients to supplement their usual oral hydration with (extra) non–alcohol-containing fluids, 1000–2000 mL/day, to take cyclophosphamide doses at the beginning of a waking cycle, and to void urine frequently while taking cyclophosphamide

Methotrexate 40 mg/m^2 per dose; administer by intravenous injection over ≤1 minute for 2 doses on days 1 and 8, every 4 weeks, until disease progression (total dosage/4-week cycle = 80 mg/m^2)

Fluorouracil 600 mg/m^2 per dose; administer by intravenous injection over 1–3 minutes for 2 doses on days 1 and 8, every 4 weeks, until disease progression (total dosage/4-week cycle = 1200 mg/m^2)

Supportive Care

Antiemetic prophylaxis
Emetogenic potential on Days 1–14 is
LOW–MODERATE
See Chapter 42 for antiemetic recommendations

Hematopoietic growth factor (CSF) prophylaxis
Primary prophylaxis is NOT indicated
See Chapter 43 for more information

Antimicrobial prophylaxis
*Risk of fever and neutropenia is **LOW***
Antimicrobial primary prophylaxis to be considered:
- Antibacterial—not indicated
- Antifungal—not indicated
- Antiviral—not indicated, unless patient previously had an episode of HSV

Treatment Modifications

Adverse Events	Treatment Modifications
WBC <3500/mm^3 or platelets <100,000/mm^3 on first day of a cycle	Delay treatment for a maximum of 2 weeks until WBC >3500/mm^3 and platelets >100,000/mm^3. Continue at full dosages if counts recover within 2 weeks
If after 2 weeks WBC <3500/mm^3 or platelets <100,000/mm^3 reduce all drugs' dosages as follows:	
WBC 3000–3499/mm^3, or platelets 75,000–99,999/mm^3	Reduce dosages by 25%
WBC 2500–2999/mm^3 and platelets ≥75,000/mm^3	Reduce dosages by 50%
WBC <2500/mm^3, or platelets <75,000/mm^3	Hold treatment
ANC <1500/mm^3, or platelets <100,000/mm^3 at start of cycle	Delay treatment until ANC ≥1500/mm^3 and platelets ≥100,000/mm^3. Give filgrastim* in subsequent cycles
Hematologic recovery >3 weeks	Discontinue treatment
First episode of febrile neutropenia	Give filgrastim* during subsequent cycles
Second episode of febrile neutropenia	During subsequent cycles, consider prophylaxis with ciprofloxacin†
Third episode of febrile neutropenia	Decrease chemotherapy doses by 20% and administer filgrastim* + ciprofloxacin†
First episode of G4 documented infection	Add filgrastim* and ciprofloxacin† prophylaxis during subsequent cycles
Second episode of G4 documented infection	Decrease chemotherapy doses by 20% and administer filgrastim* + ciprofloxacin†
Third episode of G4 documented infection	Discontinue chemotherapy
G3 stomatitis	Reduce methotrexate and fluorouracil dosage by 50% during subsequent cycles
G4 nonhematologic toxicity	Discontinue chemotherapy

*Filgrastim 5 mcg/kg per day; administer subcutaneously for 8 consecutive days (days 3–10)
†Ciprofloxacin 500 mg orally twice daily for 7 consecutive days starting on day 5

Patient Population Studied

Study of 82 women with advanced breast cancer randomized to receive doxorubicin + vincristine versus cyclophosphamide + methotrexate + fluorouracil (CMF). All patients have a performance status of ≥50, a life expectancy >2 months, and measurable disease (preferably soft tissue involvement)

Toxicity (n = 40)

Toxicity (N = 40)	% of Patients
Grade 1 leukopenia	58%
Grade 2 leukopenia	10%
Grade 1 thrombocytopenia	3%
Grade 2 thrombocytopenia	5%
Loss of hair	53%
Stomatitis	25%
Cystitis	20%
Amenorrhea	3%
No toxicity	7%

Efficacy (n = 40)

Type of Response	Cyclophosphamide + Methotrexate + Fluorouracil (CMF) N = 40
None	2 (5%)
Progression	12 (30%)
Objective improvement	7 (18%)
Partial (≥50%)	15 (30%)
Complete	4 (10%)
Complete + partial	19 (48%)
Total number with response	26 (65%)

Therapy Monitoring

Before each cycle: CBC with differential and platelet counts

METASTATIC

BREAST CANCER REGIMEN: DOCETAXEL + CAPECITABINE

O'Shaughnessy J et al. J Clin Oncol 2002;12:2812–2823

Premedication:

Dexamethasone 8 mg/dose; administer orally twice daily for 3 days, starting on the day before docetaxel administration (total dose/cycle = 48 mg)

Docetaxel 75 mg/m^2; administer intravenously in a volume of 0.9% sodium chloride injection (0.9% NS) or 5% dextrose injection (D5W) sufficient to produce a final docetaxel concentration within the range 0.3–0.74 mg/mL over 60 minutes on day 1, every 3 weeks (total dosage/cycle = 75 mg/m^2)

Capecitabine 1250 mg/m^2 per dose; administer orally twice daily with approximately 200 mL water within 30 minutes after a meal for 14 consecutive days on days 1–14 (28 doses), every 3 weeks (total dosage/cycle = 35,000 mg/m^2)

Notes:
- Capecitabine is given for 2 consecutive weeks followed by 1 week without treatment
- Doses are rounded to use combinations of 500-mg and 150-mg tablets that most closely approximate calculated values
- In practice, treatment often is begun with capecitabine 1000 mg/m^2 per dose twice daily for 14 consecutive days on days 1–14, every 3 weeks, because of a high rate of dose reduction with higher dosages (total dosage/cycle = 28,000 mg/m^2)
- Initial capecitabine dosage should be decreased by 25% in patients with moderate renal impairment (baseline creatinine clearance = 30–50 mL/min [0.5–0.83 mL/s]); ie, a dosage reduction from 1250 mg/m^2 per dose to 950 mg/m^2 per dose, twice daily. Capecitabine use is contraindicated in persons with severe renal impairment (creatinine clearance <30 mL/min [<0.5 mL/s])
- Although food decreases the rate and extent of drug absorption and the time to peak plasma concentration and systemic exposure (AUC) for both capecitabine and fluorouracil, product labeling recommends giving capecitabine within 30 minutes after the end of a meal because established safety and efficacy data are based on administration with food

Supportive Care

Antiemetic prophylaxis
Emetogenic potential is **LOW**
See Chapter 42 for antiemetic recommendations

Hematopoietic growth factor (CSF) prophylaxis
Primary prophylaxis is **NOT** *indicated*
See Chapter 43 for more information

Antimicrobial prophylaxis
Risk of fever and neutropenia is **LOW**
  Antimicrobial primary prophylaxis to be considered:
  - Antibacterial—not indicated
  - Antifungal—not indicated
  - Antiviral—not indicated, unless patient previously had an episode of HSV

Diarrhea management

Latent or delayed-onset diarrhea:
  Loperamide 4 mg orally initially after the first loose or liquid stool, *then*
  Loperamide 2 mg orally every 2 hours during waking hours, *plus*
  Loperamide 4 mg orally every 4 hours during hours of sleep
  - Continue for at least 12 hours after diarrhea resolves
  - Recurrent diarrhea after a 12-hour diarrhea-free interval is treated as a new episode
  - Rehydrate orally with fluids and electrolytes during a diarrheal episode
  - If a patient develops blood or mucus in stool, dehydration, or hemodynamic instability, or if diarrhea persists >48 hours despite loperamide, stop loperamide and evaluate urgently in clinic or hospitalize the patient for IV hydration
  - Alternatively, a trial of **diphenoxylate hydrochloride** 2.5 mg with **atropine sulfate** 0.025 mg (eg, Lomotil)
  - Initial adult dose is 2 tablets 4 times daily until control has been achieved, after which the dose may be reduced to meet individual requirements. Control may often be maintained with as little as 2 tablets daily
  - Clinical improvement of acute diarrhea is usually observed within 48 hours. If improvement of chronic diarrhea after treatment with a maximum daily dose of 8 tablets is not observed within 10 days, control is unlikely with further administration

Hand-foot reaction

For patients who develop a hand-foot reaction, use topical emollients (eg, Aquaphor), topical or orally administered steroids, antihistamine agents (H$_1$-receptor antagonists), or pyridoxine 50–150 mg/day; administer orally

Treatment Modifications

NCI of Canada CTC

Adverse Event	Treatment Modification
First G2*	Withhold chemotherapy until adverse events resolve to G ≤1, then resume
Recurrent G2 (second episode)* or Any G3	Withhold chemotherapy for up to 2 weeks • If adverse events resolve to G ≤1 within 2 weeks, resume treatment with docetaxel and capecitabine dosage decreased by 25% If adverse events do not resolve to G ≤1 within 2 weeks, docetaxel is permanently discontinued, but capecitabine treatment may resume after adverse events resolve to G ≤1 at a dosage decreased by 25%
Recurrent G2 (third episode)* or Recurrent G3 (second episode) or Any G4	Permanently discontinue docetaxel. Withhold capecitabine for up to 2 weeks. If adverse events resolve to G ≤1 within 2 weeks, resume capecitabine treatment at 50% of the previous dosage
Recurrent G2 (fourth episode)* or Recurrent G3 (third episode) or Recurrent G4 (second episode)	Permanently discontinue capecitabine
Patients who continue capecitabine alone without evidence of adverse events G ≥2 during a cycle	Capecitabine dosage may be escalated by 25% greater than the previously administered dose during each subsequent cycle
G3/4 neutropenia	Withhold docetaxel. Resume docetaxel only after ANC ≥1500/mm^3; continue capecitabine treatment without interruption
G3/4 neutropenia + any other G2 clinical adverse event Neutropenia + fever ≥38°C	Discontinue capecitabine. Consider hospitalization for management
ANC <500/mm^3 for >7 days at 75 mg/m^2 docetaxel	Withhold docetaxel until ANC ≥1500/mm^3 and patient is afebrile for ≥48 hours, then resume docetaxel at 55 mg/m^2
ANC <500/mm^3 for >7 days at 55 mg/m^2 docetaxel	Permanently discontinue docetaxel

*Except isolated neutropenia

Efficacy (N = 256)

WHO Criteria		
Response Category	Percentage	95% Confidence Interval
Overall response	42%	36–48%
Complete response	5%	2–8%
Stable disease >6 weeks	38%	32–44%
Median time to progression	6.1 months	5.4–6.5 months
12-Month survival	57%	51–63%
Median survival	14.5 months	12.3–16.3 months

Patient Population Studied

Study of 255 patients with metastatic breast cancer with prior anthracycline, no prior docetaxel, and less than 3 prior chemotherapy regimens

Toxicity (N = 251)

NCI of Canada CTC		
Toxicity	% G3*	% G4*
Hematologic Toxicity		
Neutropenia[†‡]	5	11
Febrile neutropenia[‡§]	3	13
Nonhematologic Toxicity		
Hand-foot syndrome	24	N/A
Stomatitis	17	0.4
Diarrhea	14	0.4
Nausea	6	—
Fatigue/asthenia	8	0.4
Alopecia	6	—
Laboratory Abnormalities[‡]		
Hyperglycemia	13	1
Hyperbilirubinemia	6.8	2
Elevated ALT/AST	1.6	2.8

*National Cancer Institute of Canada common toxicity criteria scale, except hand-foot syndrome
[†]Requiring medical intervention; eg, antibiotics, hematopoietic growth factor support. The overall incidence of G3 or G4 adverse events was greatest during the first treatment cycle (38%)
[‡]Six patients withdrew from further treatment for adverse events, including neutropenia, thrombocytopenia, and increased liver transaminases, each in 1 patient, respectively, and hyperbilirubinemia in 3 patients
[§]The most common cause of hospitalization was febrile neutropenia (12%)
Dose reductions, treatment interruptions:
- 65% of patients required dose reduction of capecitabine alone (4%), docetaxel alone (10%), or both drugs (51%) for adverse events
- Capecitabine treatment interruption was required in 34% of cycles
- Adverse events, either alone or in combination, most frequently leading to capecitabine treatment interruption, included:
  - Hand-foot syndrome (11.1%)
  - Diarrhea (8.5%)
  - Stomatitis (4.6%)

Note: Deaths classified as probably, possibly, or remotely related to study treatment, during or within 28 days after completing study, occurred in 3 patients (1.2%) in association with enterocolitis, sepsis, and pulmonary edema, each in 1 patient

Therapy Monitoring

Start of each cycle: CBC with leukocyte differential count and platelet counts, LFTs, and serum electrolytes. Consider intracycle assessment in first few cycles

METASTATIC

BREAST CANCER REGIMEN: PACLITAXEL AND GEMCITABINE

Albain KS et al. J Clin Oncol 2008;26:3950–3957

Premedication:

Dexamethasone 10 mg/dose; administer orally for 2 doses 12 hours and 6 hours before paclitaxel (total dose/cycle = 20 mg), *or*

Dexamethasone 20 mg; administer intravenously over 10–15 minutes, 30–60 minutes before paclitaxel (total dose/cycle = 20 mg)

Note:

Dexamethasone doses may be gradually decreased in the absence of hypersensitivity reactions during repeated paclitaxel treatments

Diphenhydramine 25–50 mg administer orally 60 minutes before paclitaxel, *or* administer by intravenous injection 30–60 minutes before paclitaxel

Cimetidine 300 mg (or **ranitidine** 150 mg, **famotidine** 20–40 mg, or an equivalent histamine receptor [H_2]-subtype antagonist); administer orally 60 minutes before paclitaxel, *or* cimetidine 300 mg (or ranitidine 50 mg, famotidine 20 mg); administer intravenously over 15–30 minutes, 30–60 minutes before paclitaxel

Paclitaxel 175 mg/m^2; administer intravenously in a volume of 0.9% sodium chloride injection (0.9% NS) or 5% dextrose injection sufficient to produce a concentration within the range 0.3–1.2 mg/mL over 3 hours, on day 1 before gemcitabine, every 21 days (total dosage/cycle = 175 mg/m^2)

Gemcitabine 1250 mg/m^2 per dose; administer intravenously in 50–250 mL 0.9% NS over 30–60 minutes for 2 doses on days 1 and 8, every 21 days (total dosage/cycle = 2500 mg/m^2)

Supportive Care

Antiemetic prophylaxis

Emetogenic potential is **LOW**

See Chapter 42 for antiemetic recommendations

Hematopoietic growth factor (CSF) prophylaxis

Primary prophylaxis is **NOT** indicated

See Chapter 43 for more information

Antimicrobial prophylaxis

Risk of fever and neutropenia is **LOW**

Antimicrobial primary prophylaxis to be considered:

• Antibacterial—not indicated

• Antifungal—not indicated

• Antiviral—not indicated, unless patient previously had an episode of HSV

Patient Population Studied

Women with locally recurrent or metastatic breast carcinoma after 1 neoadjuvant/adjuvant regimen participated in a multicenter, open-label, phase 3 trial, in which 266 patients were randomly assigned to receive gemcitabine + paclitaxel and 263 to receive paclitaxel alone. All patients assigned to a treatment arm were analyzed for efficacy on the basis of intention-to-treat, and all who received at least 1 dose of chemotherapy were evaluated for safety

Efficacy (N = 266)

	% Response or Duration	95% CI
Overall response rate	41.4%	35.4–47.3
Complete responses	7.9%	
Partial response	33.5%	
Overall response rate, nonvisceral sites only	56.9%	
Overall response rate, visceral sites	35.6%	
Duration of response	9.89 months	8.31–11.73
Median time to progression	6.14 months	5.32–6.70
Progression-free survival	5.9 months	
Median overall survival	18.6 months	

Treatment Modifications

Adverse Events	Treatment Modifications
ANC 1000–1499/mm^3 or platelets 50,000–99,999/mm^3 on days 1 or 8	Proceed with treatment, but decrease gemcitabine dosage by 25%
ANC <1000/mm^3 or platelets <50,000/mm^3 on day 1	Withhold treatment until ANC is >1000/mm^3 and platelets >50,000/mm^3, then resume treatment and give filgrastim from day 9 until postnadir ANC >5000/mm^3
ANC <500/mm^3 on day of treatment, febrile neutropenia during cycle, or ANC <500/mm^3 for ≥7 days during cycle	Withhold treatment until ANC is >1000/mm^3, then resume treatment with gemcitabine dosage decreased by 25%, and give filgrastim from day 9 until post-nadir ANC >5000/mm^3
ANC <500/mm^3 on day of treatment (second episode) after decreasing gemcitabine dosage and with filgrastim use	Withhold treatment until ANC is >1000/mm^3, then resume treatment with gemcitabine and paclitaxel dosages decreased by 25%, and give filgrastim from day 9 until postnadir ANC >5000/mm^3
Platelet count <25,000/mm^3 on day of treatment	Withhold treatment until platelet count is >50,000/mm^3, then resume treatment with paclitaxel dosage decreased by 25%
G3 nonhematologic adverse events (excluding nausea, vomiting, and alopecia)	Withhold treatment until adverse events recover to G ≤1, then resume treatment with gemcitabine and paclitaxel dosages decreased by 25%
G4 nonhematologic adverse events	Withhold treatment until adverse events recover to G ≤1, then resume treatment with gemcitabine and paclitaxel dosages decreased by 50%
G >2 paresthesias	Discontinue paclitaxel; consider alternative treatment
Symptomatic arrhythmia or heart block >1°	
Other major organ toxicities G >2	
Severe hypersensitivity reaction	

Toxicity (N = 261)

National Cancer Institute Common Toxicity Criteria, version 2.0

	G2 (%)	% G3	% G4
Hematologic Toxicities*			
Neutropenia	13.4	30.3	17.6
Febrile neutropenia	1.1	4.6	0.4
Thrombocytopenia	1.5	5.7	0.4
Anemia	22.2	5	0.8
Nonhematologic Toxicities			
Alopecia	63.6	13.4	3.8
Fatigue[†]	12.3	6.1	0.8
Sensory neuropathy	18.4	5.3	0.4
Motor neuropathy	6.1	2.3	0.4
Myalgia	16.5	4.2	0
Nausea	19.9	1.1	0
Emesis	13.4	1.9	0
Arthralgia	11.5	2.7	0
Diarrhea	8	3.1	0
Stomatitis/pharyngitis	3.8	1.1	0.4
Dyspnea	3.4	1.5[‡]	0.4[‡]
Bone pain	4.2	1.5	0
Laboratory Abnormalities			
Increased ALT	4.2	5	0
Increased AST	6.5	1.5	0

*Treatment delays were most often related to hematologic toxicities
[†]G3/4 fatigue often not associated with anemia
[‡]Patients who developed G3/4 dyspnea had active disease in the lungs or pleura

Therapy Monitoring

1. *Start of each cycle:* CBC with leukocyte differential count and platelet count, LFTs, neurologic examination
2. *Before gemcitabine:* CBC with leukocyte differential count and platelet count. Consider intracycle monitoring in early cycles

METASTATIC • HER2-POSITIVE • HORMONE RECEPTOR-POSITIVE
BREAST CANCER REGIMEN: LAPATINIB + TRASTUZUMAB + AROMATASE INHIBITOR

Johnston SRD et al. J Clin Oncol 2021;39:79–89
Johnston SRD et al. J Clin Oncol 2018;36:741–748
Protocol for: Johnston SRD et al. J Clin Oncol 2018;36:741–748

Trastuzumab every 21 days until disease progression, *plus:*

- *Loading Dose:* **Trastuzumab** 8 mg/kg; administer intravenously in 250 mL 0.9% sodium chloride injection (0.9% NS) over 90 minutes as a loading dose on day 1, cycle 1 only (total dosage during the first cycle = 8 mg/kg), *followed 3 weeks later by:*

  - *Note:* A syndrome most commonly consisting of chills and/or fever may occur in as many as 40% of patients during the first infusion of trastuzumab. These symptoms occur infrequently with subsequent trastuzumab infusions. Other signs and/or symptoms may include nausea, vomiting, pain (in some cases at tumor sites), rigors, headache, dizziness, dyspnea, hypotension, rash, and asthenia. Although the symptoms are usually mild to moderate in severity, infrequently, trastuzumab may need to be discontinued

  - When such a syndrome is observed, it can be treated with or without reduction in the rate of trastuzumab infusion, and:
    - **Acetaminophen** 650 mg; administer orally, *plus:*
    - **Diphenhydramine** 25–50 mg; administer orally or by intravenous injection, *plus:*
    - **Meperidine** 12.5–25 mg; administer by intravenous injection every 10 minutes if needed for shaking chills (generally, cumulative doses >50 mg are not needed; use with caution in persons with moderate or more severely impaired renal function)

- *Maintenance Doses:* **Trastuzumab** 6 mg/kg; administer intravenously in 250 mL 0.9% NS over 30 minutes on day 1, every 3 weeks until disease progression (total dosage/3-week cycle = 6 mg/kg)

  - *Note:* If a patient misses a 6-mg/kg trastuzumab dose by more than 7 days, a re-loading dose of trastuzumab should be given as **trastuzumab** 8 mg/kg (loading dose); administer intravenously in 250 mL 0.9% NS over 90 minutes once. This should be followed 21 days later by resumption of 6-mg/kg maintenance doses repeated every 3 weeks

Lapatinib 1000 mg/dose; administer orally, once daily either at least one hour before or at least 1 hour after a meal, continually, until disease progression (total dosage/week = 7000 mg), *plus:*
Notes:

- Patients who delay taking lapatinib at a regularly scheduled time should take the next dose at the next regularly scheduled time
- Lapatinib is metabolized by cytochrome P450 (CYP) CYP3A subfamily enzymes. Avoid concurrent use with strong CYP3A4 inhibitors (eg, ketoconazole, itraconazole, clarithromycin, atazanavir, indinavir, nefazodone, nelfinavir, ritonavir, saquinavir, telithromycin, voriconazole) whenever possible. If concurrent use with a strong CYP3A4 inhibitor is required, reduce each lapatinib dose by approximately 65%. If the strong CYP3A4 inhibitor is subsequently discontinued, increase lapatinib to the standard dose after a 1-week washout period. Avoid concurrent use with strong CYP3A4 inducers (eg, phenytoin, carbamazepine, rifampin, rifabutin, rifapentine, phenobarbital, St. John's wort) whenever possible. If concurrent use with a strong CYP3A4 inducer is required, the dose of lapatinib should be titrated gradually from 1000 mg/dose up to 3500 mg/dose based on tolerability. If the strong CYP3A4 inducer is subsequently discontinued, reduce the lapatinib dose back to the standard dosage
- Lapatinib inhibits CYP3A4, CYP2C8 and P-glycoprotein *in vitro*. Use caution and consider dose reduction when narrow-therapeutic index substrates of these enzymes and transport systems (eg, digoxin) are coadministered with lapatinib
- Advise patients to not consume grapefruit and grapefruit juice as they may inhibit CYP3A in the gut wall and increase the bioavailability of lapatinib

Choose only one of the following aromatase inhibitors:

Anastrozole 1 mg/dose; administer orally once daily, without regard to food, continually until disease progression (total dosage/week = 7 mg), *or:*
Notes:
- Patients who delay taking an anastrozole dose at a regularly scheduled time may take the missed dose if the time to the next regularly scheduled dose is >12 hours away

Letrozole 2.5 mg/dose; administer orally once daily, without regard to food, continually until disease progression (total dosage/week = 17.5 mg), *or:*
Notes:
- Patients who delay taking a letrozole dose at a regularly scheduled time may take the missed dose if the time to the next regularly scheduled dose is >12 hours away
- Dose adjustment for patients with cirrhosis or severe hepatic impairment: 2.5 mg orally every *other* day

Exemestane 25 mg/dose; administer orally, once daily after a meal, continually until disease progression (total dosage/week = 175 mg), *or:*
- *Note:* Exemestane is metabolized by cytochrome P450 (CYP) CYP3A subfamily enzymes. Avoid concurrent use with strong CYP3A4 inducers (eg, rifampin, carbamazepine, phenytoin, phenobarbital, St. John's wort) if possible. If concurrent use with a strong CYP3A4 inducer is required, increase the exemestane dose to 50 mg per day

(*continued*)

(continued)

Supportive Care

Antiemetic prophylaxis

Emetogenic potential of lapatinib is **LOW**

Emetogenic potential of trastuzumab is **MINIMAL**

See Chapter 42 for antiemetic recommendations

Hematopoietic growth factor (CSF) prophylaxis

Primary prophylaxis is **NOT** indicated

See Chapter 43 for more information

Antimicrobial prophylaxis

Risk of fever and neutropenia is **LOW**

Antimicrobial primary prophylaxis to be *CONSIDERED*:

- Antibacterial—not indicated

- Antifungal—not indicated

- Antiviral—not indicated unless patient previously had an episode of HSV

Diarrhea management

Latent or delayed-onset diarrhea:

Loperamide 4 mg orally initially after the first loose or liquid stool, *then*

Loperamide 2 mg orally every 2 hours during waking hours, *plus*

Loperamide 4 mg orally every 4 hours during hours of sleep

- Continue for at least 12 hours after diarrhea resolves

- Recurrent diarrhea after a 12-hour diarrhea-free interval is treated as a new episode

- Rehydrate orally with fluids and electrolytes during a diarrheal episode

- If a patient develops blood or mucus in stool, dehydration, or hemodynamic instability, or if diarrhea persists >48 hours despite loperamide, stop loperamide and evaluate urgently in clinic or hospitalize the patient for IV hydration

- Alternatively, a trial of **diphenoxylate hydrochloride** 2.5 mg with **atropine sulfate** 0.025 mg (eg, Lomotil)

- Initial adult dose is 2 tablets 4 times daily until control has been achieved, after which the dose may be reduced to meet individual requirements. Control may often be maintained with as little as 2 tablets daily

- Clinical improvement of acute diarrhea is usually observed within 48 hours. If improvement of chronic diarrhea after treatment with a maximum daily dose of 8 tablets is not observed within 10 days, control is unlikely with further administration

Patient Population Studied

The randomized, open-label, phase 3 trial (ALTERNATIVE) involved 355 postmenopausal women with HER2-positive, hormone receptor–positive, metastatic breast cancer. Eligible patients were aged ≥18 years, had an Eastern Cooperative Oncology Group (ECOG) performance status score ≤1, and had prior treatment with endocrine therapy and disease progression during or after a prior regimen containing trastuzumab plus chemotherapy in the neoadjuvant or first-line metastatic setting. Patients were randomized to receive one of the following treatment strategies: intravenous trastuzumab (first dose 8 mg/kg then 6 mg/kg) every 3 weeks plus oral lapatinib (1000 mg) and oral aromatase inhibitor daily; intravenous trastuzumab (first dose 8 mg/kg then 6 mg/kg) every 3 weeks plus oral aromatase inhibitor daily; or oral lapatinib (1500 mg) and oral aromatase inhibitor daily. The investigators' choices for the aromatase inhibitor were letrozole (2.5 mg), anastrozole (1 mg), or exemestane (25 mg)

Efficacy (N = 355)

	Lapatinib + Trastuzumab + Aromatase Inhibitor (N = 120)	Trastuzumab + Aromatase Inhibitor (N = 117)	Lapatinib + Aromatase Inhibitor (N = 118)
Median progression-free survival	11 months	5.6 months	8.3 months
Overall response rate*	31.7%	13.7%	18.6%
Clinical benefit rate†	40%	30%	34%
Duration of response	14.0 months	8.4 months	11.1 months

*Overall response rate includes patients with either a complete or partial response to treatment

†Clinical benefit rate includes patients with either a complete or partial response or stable disease for ≥6 months

Note: The overall median duration of treatment was 53.6 weeks. The median duration of lapatinib treatment was 35.8 weeks and 24.7 weeks for the triple therapy and double therapy groups, respectively. The median duration of trastuzumab was 36 weeks and 18 weeks for the triple therapy and double therapy groups, respectively

Therapy Monitoring

1. Instruct patients at the first sign of loose stools to initiate antidiarrheal therapy, increase oral fluids, and notify their health care provider

2. Monitor CBC with differential and LFTs prior to the start of therapy, every 4–6 weeks during treatment, and as clinically indicated

3. In patients at risk for QTc prolongation, monitor ECG and electrolytes at baseline and periodically during treatment with lapatinib

4. Conduct thorough cardiac assessment, including history, physical examination, and determination of LVEF by echocardiogram or MUGA scan at baseline immediately prior to initiation of trastuzumab and every 3 months during therapy. In patients with metastatic disease, the frequency of post-baseline cardiac monitoring in asymptomatic patients may be individualized based on the clinical judgment of the medically responsible health care provider

5. Patients should have a pre-treatment LVEF ≥55%

6. Repeat LVEF measurement at 4-week intervals if trastuzumab is withheld for significant left ventricular cardiac dysfunction

7. Monitor for symptoms of pulmonary toxicity (trastuzumab, lapatinib)

8. Avoid using concomitant strong CYP3A4 inhibitors (eg, ketoconazole, itraconazole, clarithromycin, atazanavir, indinavir, nefazodone, nelfinavir, ritonavir, saquinavir, telithromycin, and voriconazole). Consider a lapatinib dose reductions if patients require co-administration of a strong CYP3A4 inhibitor

9. Obtain a pregnancy test in females of reproductive potential. Advise females of reproductive potential to use effective contraception

10. Response assessment: imaging studies every 2–3 months

Treatment Modifications

TRASTUZUMAB	
Adverse Event	**Dose Modification**
Mild or moderate infusion reaction*	Decrease the rate of infusion
Infusion reaction with dyspnea or clinically significant hypotension	Interrupt the infusion. Administer medical therapy as indicated including epinephrine, corticosteroids, diphenhydramine, bronchodilators, and oxygen. Observe patients closely for 60 minutes if the reaction occurs after the first infusion and for 30 minutes if it occurs after subsequent infusions. Prior to resumption of the trastuzumab infusion, premedicate with antihistamines and/or corticosteroids. *Note:* While some patients tolerate the resumption of trastuzumab infusions, others have recurrent severe infusion reactions despite premedications
Severe or life-threatening infusion reaction (including bronchospasm, anaphylaxis, angioedema, hypoxia, and severe hypotension; usually reported during or immediately following the initial infusion)*	Interrupt the infusion. Administer medical therapy as indicated including epinephrine, corticosteroids, diphenhydramine, bronchodilators, and oxygen. Patients should be evaluated and carefully monitored until complete resolution of signs and symptoms. Discontinue trastuzumab
LVEF has declined by ≥16 percentage points from baseline, or has declined by 10–15 percentage points from baseline to a value below the lower limit of the normal range OR Symptomatic congestive heart failure	Withhold trastuzumab and repeat LVEF assessment at 4-week intervals until improvement, which may require prolonged interruption. Discontinue trastuzumab if the LVEF does not improve or if it declines further, unless the benefits for the individual patient outweigh the risks
Pulmonary toxicity	Discontinue trastuzumab in patients experiencing pulmonary toxicity

*Infusion reactions consist of a symptom complex characterized by fever and chills, and on occasion included nausea, vomiting, pain (in some cases at tumor sites), headache, dizziness, dyspnea, hypotension, rash, and asthenia

(continued)

Treatment Modifications (*continued*)

LAPATINIB DOSE MODIFICATIONS

Lapatinib starting dose	1000 mg
Lapatinib dose level −1	750 mg
Lapatinib dose level −2	Discontinue lapatinib
Decreased left ventricular ejection fraction (LVEF) G ≥2 or greater by NCI CTCAE v3 or LVEF < institution's lower limit of normal	Discontinue lapatinib. Resume lapatinib after ≥2 weeks if the LVEF recovers to normal and the patient is asymptomatic
Diarrhea that is G3 or G1/2 with complicating features (moderate to severe abdominal cramping, nausea or vomiting G ≥2, decreased performance status, fever, sepsis, neutropenia, frank bleeding, or dehydration)	Withhold lapatinib. When resolves to G ≤1 resume at one dose lower
G4 diarrhea	Discontinue lapatinib
G3/4 elevation in LFTs	Discontinue lapatinib
Erythema multiforme, Stevens-Johnson syndrome, or toxic epidermal necrolysis (eg, progressive skin rash often with blisters or mucosal lesions) suspected	Discontinue lapatinib
G ≥3 pulmonary symptoms indicative of interstitial lung disease/pneumonitis	Discontinue lapatinib
Other G2 nonhematologic adverse event that occurs during a cycle but results in a delay in the start of the next cycle	Hold treatment until adverse events resolve to G <1, then resume lapatinib with dosage reduced by one dose level
Other G3 nonhematologic adverse event that occurs during a cycle but resolves prior to the start of the next cycle or requires a delay in the start of the next cycle	
Other G4 nonhematologic adverse event that occurs during a cycle but resolves prior to the start of the next cycle	Hold treatment until adverse events resolve to G <1, then resume lapatinib with dosage reduced by one dose level or discontinue
Other G4 nonhematologic adverse event that occurs during a cycle but requires a delay in the start of the next cycle	Discontinue lapatinib
Any treatment delay >3 weeks	Discontinue lapatinib

AROMATASE INHIBITORS

Letrozole (reversible non-steroidal aromatase inhibitor, triazole derivative)

- Dose: 2.5 mg once daily
- Patients with cirrhosis or severe hepatic impairment: 2.5 mg every other day
- In patients with advanced disease, treatment with letrozole should continue until tumor progression is evident
- The most common adverse events (>20%) were hot flashes, arthralgia; flushing, asthenia, edema, arthralgia, headache, dizziness, hypercholesterolemia, sweating increased, bone pain; and musculoskeletal. These should be managed symptomatically

Anastrozole (reversible non-steroidal aromatase inhibitor, triazole derivative)

- Dose: One 1-mg tablet taken once daily
- Use with care in women with pre-existing ischemic heart disease
- Most common side effects (with an incidence of >10%) were: hot flashes, asthenia, arthritis, pain, pharyngitis, hypertension, depression, nausea and vomiting, rash, osteoporosis, fractures, back pain, insomnia, headache, peripheral edema and lymphedema, regardless of causality

Exemestane (irreversible steroidal aromatase inhibitor)

- Dose: 25-mg tablet
- Do not administer to premenopausal women. Do not co-administer with estrogen-containing agents as these could interfere with its pharmacologic action
- Adverse events considered drug related or of indeterminate cause include hot flashes (13%), nausea (9%), fatigue (8%), increased sweating (4%), and increased appetite (3%). Less frequent adverse events of any cause (from 2% to 5%) include fever, generalized weakness, paresthesia, pathologic fracture, bronchitis, sinusitis, rash, itching, urinary tract infection, and lymphedema

Adverse Events (N = 353)

Grade (%)*	Lapatinib + Trastuzumab + Aromatase Inhibitor (N = 118)		Trastuzumab + Aromatase Inhibitor (N = 116)		Lapatinib + Aromatase Inhibitor (N = 119)	
	Grade 1–2	Grade 3–4	Grade 1–2	Grade 3–4	Grade 1–2	Grade 3–4
Any event	58	34	52	22	60	32
Diarrhea	56	13	9	0	45	6
Rash	36	0	2	0	25	3
Paronychia	30	0	0	0	13	2
Nausea	22	0	9	0	20	2
Decreased appetite	18	0	3	0	13	0
Stomatitis	17	0	3	0	12	<1
Arthralgia	12	<1	12	0	14	0
Dermatitis acneiform	13	0	2	0	8	<1
Fatigue	11	<1	10	0	13	2
Alopecia	10	0	2	0	7	0
Vomiting	10	0	0	<1	14	0
Palmar-plantar erythrodysesthesia syndrome	10	0	<1	0	8	<1
Cough	8	0	15	0	8	0
Increased alanine aminotransferase level	7	0	2	4	12	3
Pain in extremity	6	<1	3	0	10	0
Increased aspartate aminotransferase level	0	0	4	4	12	5
Headache	0	0	9	<1	14	2

*According to the National Cancer Institute Common Terminology Criteria for Adverse Events, version 4.0

Toxicities that occurred in ≥10% of patients in any treatment group are included in the table. One death in the lapatinib plus aromatase inhibitor group was due to cardiogenic shock and organ failure. One death in the trastuzumab plus aromatase inhibitor group was due to cardiopulmonary arrest. All other deaths (three in the triple therapy group, three in the trastuzumab plus aromatase inhibitor group, and five in the lapatinib plus aromatase inhibitor group) were due to disease progression. Treatment discontinuation owing to adverse events occurred in 3% of the triple therapy group, 6% of the trastuzumab plus aromatase inhibitor group, and 9% of the lapatinib plus aromatase inhibitor group

METASTATIC • HER2-POSITIVE

BREAST CANCER REGIMEN: TRASTUZUMAB

Esteva FJ et al. J Clin Oncol 2002;20:1800–1808
Leyland-Jones B et al. J Clin Oncol 2003;21:3965–3971
Vogel CL et al. J Clin Oncol 2002;20:719–726

Trastuzumab 4 mg/kg initial (loading) dose; administer intravenously in 250 mL 0.9% sodium chloride injection (0.9% NS), over at least 90 minutes (total initial dosage = 4 mg/kg), *followed at weekly intervals by:*
Trastuzumab 2 mg/kg per dose; administer intravenously in 250 mL 0.9% NS over 30–90 minutes, every week, continually (total dosage/week = 2 mg/kg)
Note: Administration duration may be decreased from 90 to 30 minutes if administration over longer durations is well tolerated
or
Trastuzumab 8 mg/kg initial (loading) dose; administer intravenously in 250 mL 0.9% NS over at least 90 minutes (total initial dosage = 8 mg/kg), *followed 3 weeks later by:*
Trastuzumab 6 mg/kg per dose; administer intravenously in 250 mL 0.9% NS over 30–90 minutes, every 3 weeks, continually (total dosage/3-week cycle = 6 mg/kg)
Note: Administration duration may be decreased from 90 to 30 minutes if administration over longer durations is well tolerated

Supportive Care

Antiemetic prophylaxis
Emetogenic potential is **MINIMAL**
See Chapter 42 for antiemetic recommendations

Hematopoietic growth factor (CSF) prophylaxis
Primary prophylaxis is **NOT** *indicated*
See Chapter 43 for more information

Antimicrobial prophylaxis
Risk of fever and neutropenia is **LOW**
   Antimicrobial primary prophylaxis to be considered:
   • Antibacterial—not indicated
   • Antifungal—not indicated
   • Antiviral—not indicated, unless patient previously had an episode of HSV

Trastuzumab infusion reactions

• A symptom complex most commonly consisting of chills and/or fever may occur in as many as 40% of patients during the first infusion of trastuzumab. These symptoms occur infrequently with subsequent trastuzumab infusions. Other signs and/or symptoms may include nausea, vomiting, pain (in some cases at tumor sites), rigors, headache, dizziness, dyspnea, hypotension, rash, and asthenia. Although the symptoms are usually mild to moderate in severity, infrequently, trastuzumab may need to be discontinued

• When such a symptom complex is observed, it can be treated with or without reduction in the rate of trastuzumab infusion, and:

  ■ **Acetaminophen** 650 mg; administer orally

  ■ **Diphenhydramine** 25–50 mg; administer orally or by intravenous injection, and

  ■ **Meperidine** 12.5–25 mg; administer by intravenous injection every 10 minutes if needed for shaking chills (generally, cumulative doses >50 mg are not needed; use with caution in persons with moderate or more severely impaired renal function)

Patient Population Studied

Vogel CL et al. J Clin Oncol 2002;20:719–726

Study of 84 women with HER2-overexpressing (IHC 3+) metastatic breast cancer with no prior cytotoxic chemotherapy for metastatic disease. Also enrolled were 27 women with HER-2 (IHC 2+) metastatic breast cancer

Treatment Modifications

Adverse Events	Treatment Modifications
LVEF has declined by ≥16 percentage points from baseline, or has declined by 10–15 percentage points from baseline to a value below the lower limit of the normal range OR Symptomatic congestive heart failure	Withhold trastuzumab and repeat LVEF assessment at 4-week intervals until improvement, which may require prolonged interruption. Discontinue trastuzumab if the LVEF does not improve or if it declines further, unless the benefits for the individual patient outweigh the risks

Efficacy (N = 84*)

Vogel CL et al. J Clin Oncol 2002;20:719–726

Overall response[†]	35%*
Complete response[†]	8%*
Clinical benefit[‡]	48%*

*Patients with 3+ HER2 overexpression by IHC
[†]>50% of objective responses lasted >12 months
[‡]CR, PR, MR, or stable disease for >6 months

Toxicity

Seidman A et al. J Clin Oncol 2002;20:1215–1221
Vogel CL et al. J Clin Oncol 2002;20:719–726

NCI-CTC		
Toxicity	**Severity**	
Cardiac Toxicity		
Any	NYHA Classes III/IV	
Cardiac dysfunction	3–7%	2–4%
Noncardiac Toxicity		
	Any	Severe
Pain	59%	8%
Asthenia	53%	7%
Nausea	37%	3%
Fever	36%	2%
Chest pain	25%	3%
Chills	22%	0
Rash	20%	0
Dyspnea	15%	0

Therapy Monitoring

1. Conduct thorough cardiac assessment, including history, physical examination, and determination of LVEF by echocardiogram or MUGA scan at baseline immediately prior to initiation of trastuzumab and every 3 months during therapy. In patients with metastatic disease, the frequency of post-baseline cardiac monitoring in asymptomatic patients may be individualized based on the clinical judgment of the medically responsible health care provider

2. Patients should have a pre-treatment LVEF ≥55%

   Repeat LVEF measurement at 4-week intervals if trastuzumab is withheld for significant left ventricular cardiac dysfunction

METASTATIC • HER2-POSITIVE

BREAST CANCER REGIMEN: DOCETAXEL + TRASTUZUMAB + PERTUZUMAB (DHP)

Baselga J et al. N Engl J Med 2012;366:109–119

Trastuzumab 8 mg/kg initial (loading) dose; administer intravenously in 250 mL 0.9% sodium chloride injection (0.9% NS) over at least 90 minutes (total initial dosage = 8 mg/kg), *followed 3 weeks later by:*
Trastuzumab 6 mg/kg per dose; administer intravenously in 250 mL 0.9% NS over 30–90 minutes, every 3 weeks, continually (total dosage/3-week cycle = 6 mg/kg)
Note: Administration duration may be decreased from 90 to 30 minutes if administration over longer durations is well tolerated

Premedication for docetaxel:
Dexamethasone 8 mg/dose; administer orally every 12 hours for 3 days starting on the day before docetaxel administration (total dose/cycle = 48 mg)
Docetaxel 75 mg/m²; administer intravenously in a volume of 0.9% NS or 5% dextrose injection (D5W) sufficient to produce a docetaxel concentration within the range 0.3–0.74 mg/mL over 60 minutes on day 1, every 3 weeks for at least 6 cycles (total dosage/cycle = 75 mg/m²)

Pertuzumab 840 mg initial (loading) dose; administer intravenously in 250 mL 0.9% NS over 60 minutes (total initial dose = 840 mg), *followed 3 weeks later by:*
Pertuzumab 420 mg per dose; administer intravenously in 250 mL 0.9% NS over 30–60 minutes, every 3 weeks, continually (total dose/3-week cycle = 420 mg)

Note: Treatment continued until disease progression or the development of adverse effects that could not be effectively managed

Alternatively, a fixed dose combination product containing pertuzumab, trastuzumab, and hyaluronidase (PHESGO™) for subcutaneous injection may be used instead of intravenous pertuzumab and trastuzumab as follows:
• *Loading Dose:* **Pertuzumab, trastuzumab, and hyaluronidase (PHESGO™) for subcutaneous injection** 1200 mg, 600 mg, and 30,000 units, respectively; administer as a 15 mL subcutaneous injection into the thigh over 8 minutes once on day 1, cycle 1 only (total dosage during the first cycle = 1200 mg pertuzumab, 600 mg trastuzumab, and 30,000 units hyaluronidase), *followed 3 weeks later by:*
• *Maintenance Doses:* **Pertuzumab, trastuzumab, and hyaluronidase (PHESGO™) for subcutaneous injection** 600 mg, 600 mg, and 20,000 units, respectively; administer as a 10 mL subcutaneous injection into the thigh over 5 minutes on day 1, every 3 weeks, continually (total dosage/3-week cycle = 600 mg pertuzumab, 600 mg trastuzumab, and 20,000 units hyaluronidase)
  ▪ Notes:
    ◦ Alternate the injection site between the left and right thigh, avoiding the last injection site by ≥2.5 cm. Avoid injection into areas that are hard, red, bruised, or tender.
    ◦ Observe patients for at least 30 minutes after the loading dose and for at least 15 minutes after maintenance doses.
    ◦ If a scheduled injection is delayed and the interval between injections is <6 weeks, then administer the maintenance dose. If the interval between injections is ≥6 weeks, then administer a loading dose followed 3 weeks later by resumption of maintenance dosing.

Supportive Care
Antiemetic prophylaxis
Emetogenic potential is **LOW**
See Chapter 42 for antiemetic recommendations

Hematopoietic growth factor (CSF) prophylaxis
Primary prophylaxis may be indicated
See Chapter 43 for more information

(continued)

Patient Population Studied

The Clinical Evaluation of Pertuzumab and Trastuzumab (CLEOPATRA) study was a randomized, double-blind, placebo-controlled, phase 3 trial involving patients with HER2-positive metastatic breast cancer in which the efficacy and safety of pertuzumab versus placebo were evaluated in combination with trastuzumab plus docetaxel as first-line treatment for patients with HER2-positive metastatic breast cancer. Among 808 patients enrolled in the study, 402 were assigned to receive pertuzumab and 406 to receive placebo (control), both in combination with trastuzumab and docetaxel. Eligible patients had locally recurrent, unresectable, or metastatic HER2-positive breast cancer and may have received 1 hormonal treatment for metastatic breast cancer before randomization. Patients may have received adjuvant or neoadjuvant chemotherapy with or without trastuzumab before randomization, with an interval of at least 12 months between completion of the adjuvant or neoadjuvant therapy and the diagnosis of metastatic breast cancer. Median age was 54 years; 78% of patients had visceral involvement, and about 50% of patients had ER-positive and 50% ER-negative disease. Approximately half of the patients had not previously received adjuvant/neoadjuvant chemotherapy, and among them, approximately 10% had received trastuzumab. Patients were stratified according to geographic region (Asia, Europe, North America, or South America) and prior treatment status (prior adjuvant or neoadjuvant chemotherapy vs no prior treatment)

Efficacy

Overall Response, Independent Review		
	Placebo + Trastuzumab + Docetaxel (N = 336)	Pertuzumab + Trastuzumab + Docetaxel (N = 343)
	no. (%)	no. (%)
Objective response	233 (69.3)	275 (80.2)
CR	14 (4.2)	19 (5.5)
PR	219 (65.2)	256 (74.6)
SD	70 (20.8)	50 (14.6)
PD	28 (8.3)	13 (3.8)

(*continued*)

Antimicrobial prophylaxis
Risk of fever and neutropenia is **LOW**
Antimicrobial primary prophylaxis to be considered:
- Antibacterial—not indicated
- Antifungal—not indicated
- Antiviral—not indicated unless patient previously had an episode of HSV

Trastuzumab infusion reactions
- A symptom complex most commonly consisting of chills and/or fever may occur in as many as 40% of patients during the first infusion of trastuzumab. These symptoms occur infrequently with subsequent trastuzumab infusions. Other signs and/or symptoms may include nausea, vomiting, pain (in some cases at tumor sites), rigors, headache, dizziness, dyspnea, hypotension, rash, and asthenia. Although the symptoms are usually mild to moderate in severity, infrequently, trastuzumab may need to be discontinued
- When such a symptom complex is observed, it can be treated with or without reduction in the rate of trastuzumab infusion, and:
  - **Acetaminophen** 650 mg orally
  - **Diphenhydramine** 25–50 mg orally or by intravenous injection, and
  - **Meperidine** 12.5–25 mg by intravenous injection every 10 minutes if needed for shaking chills (generally, cumulative doses >50 mg are not needed; use with caution in persons with moderate or more severely impaired renal function)

Diarrhea management
Latent or delayed-onset diarrhea:
Loperamide 4 mg orally initially after the first loose or liquid stool, *then*
Loperamide 2 mg orally every 2 hours during waking hours, *plus*
Loperamide 4 mg orally every 4 hours during hours of sleep
- Continue for at least 12 hours after diarrhea resolves
- Recurrent diarrhea after a 12-hour diarrhea-free interval is treated as a new episode
- Rehydrate orally with fluids and electrolytes during a diarrheal episode
- If a patient develops blood or mucus in stool, dehydration, or hemodynamic instability, or if diarrhea persists >48 hours despite loperamide, stop loperamide and evaluate urgently in clinic or hospitalize the patient for IV hydration
- Alternatively, a trial of **diphenoxylate hydrochloride** 2.5 mg with **atropine sulfate** 0.025 mg (eg, Lomotil)
- Initial adult dose is 2 tablets 4 times daily until control has been achieved, after which the dose may be reduced to meet individual requirements. Control may often be maintained with as little as 2 tablets daily
- Clinical improvement of acute diarrhea is usually observed within 48 hours. If improvement of chronic diarrhea after treatment with a maximum daily dose of 8 tablets is not observed within 10 days, control is unlikely with further administration

Oral care
Prophylaxis and treatment for mucositis/stomatitis
General advice:
- Encourage patients to maintain intake of nonalcoholic fluids
- Evaluate patients for oral pain and provide analgesic medications
- Consider histamine (H_2-subtype) receptor antagonists (eg, ranitidine, famotidine), or a proton pump inhibitor for epigastric pain

Patients with intact oral mucosa:
- Clean the mouth, tongue, and gums by brushing after every meal and at bedtime with an ultrasoft toothbrush with fluoride toothpaste
- Floss teeth gently every day unless contraindicated. If gums bleed and hurt, avoid bleeding or sore areas, but floss other teeth
- Patients may use saline or commercial bland, nonalcoholic rinses
- Do not use mouthwashes that contain alcohols

If mucositis or stomatitis is present:
- Keep the mouth moist utilizing water, ice chips, sugarless gum, sugar-free hard candies, or a saliva substitute

Therapy Monitoring

1. *Day 1 (Every cycle):* CBC with differential and platelet count and serum electrolytes and LFTs
2. Conduct thorough cardiac assessment, including history, physical examination, and determination of LVEF by echocardiogram or MUGA scan at baseline immediately prior to initiation of trastuzumab and every 3 months during therapy. In patients with metastatic disease, the frequency of post-baseline cardiac monitoring in asymptomatic patients may be individualized based on the clinical judgment of the medically responsible health care provider
3. Patients should have a pre-treatment LVEF ≥55%
4. Repeat LVEF measurement at 4-week intervals if trastuzumab and/or pertuzumab are withheld for significant left ventricular cardiac dysfunction

(*continued*)

(*continued*)

Rinse mouth several times a day to remove debris

- Use a solution of ¼ teaspoon (1.25 g) each of baking soda and table salt (sodium chloride) in 1 quart (~950 mL) of warm water. Follow with a plain water rinse
- Do not use mouthwashes that contain alcohols

Advise patients who develop mucositis to:

- Choose foods that are easy to chew and swallow
- Take small bites of food, chew slowly, and sip liquids with meals
- Encourage soft, moist foods such as cooked cereals, mashed potatoes, and scrambled eggs
- For trouble swallowing, soften food with gravies, sauces, broths, yogurt, or other bland liquids
- Avoid sharp, crunchy foods; hot, spicy, or highly acidic foods (eg, citrus fruits and juices); sugary foods; toothpicks; tobacco products; alcoholic drinks

Toxicity

Adverse Event	Placebo + Trastuzumab + Docetaxel (N = 397)	Pertuzumab + Trastuzumab + Docetaxel (N = 407)
	no. (%)	
Most Common Events, all grades		
Diarrhea	184 (46.3)	272 (66.8)
Alopecia	240 (60.5)	248 (60.9)
Neutropenia	197 (49.6)	215 (52.8)
Nausea	165 (41.6)	172 (42.3)
Fatigue	146 (36.8)	153 (37.6)
Rash	96 (24.2)	137 (33.7)
Decreased appetite	105 (26.4)	119 (29.2)
Mucosal inflammation	79 (19.9)	113 (27.8)
Asthenia	120 (30.2)	106 (26.0)
Peripheral edema	119 (30.0)	94 (23.1)
Constipation	99 (24.9)	61 (15.0)
Dry skin	17 (4.3)	43 (10.6)
Grade ≥3 Events		
Neutropenia	182 (45.8)	199 (48.9)
Febrile neutropenia	30 (7.6)	56 (13.8)
Leukopenia	58 (14.6)	50 (12.3)
Anemia	14 (3.5)	10 (2.5)
Diarrhea	20 (5.0)	32 (7.9)
Peripheral neuropathy	7 (1.8)	11 (2.7)
Asthenia	6 (1.5)	10 (2.5)
Fatigue	13 (3.3)	9 (2.2)
Left ventricular systolic dysfunction	11 (2.8)	5 (1.2)
Dyspnea	8 (2.0)	4 (1.0)

Treatment Modifications

Adverse Event	Dose Modification
Pertuzumab-related infusion reactions	Slow or interrupt pertuzumab infusion. Consider use of supportive medication to treat symptoms (H_1- and H_2-receptor antagonist antihistamines, steroids) if needed. Reinitiate at a slower rate only when symptoms abate
Serious hypersensitivity	Discontinue immediately. Consider permanent discontinuation of pertuzumab
If trastuzumab is withheld	Pertuzumab also should be withheld
LVEF has declined by ≥16 percentage points from baseline, or has declined by 10–15 percentage points from baseline to a value below the lower limit of the normal range OR Symptomatic congestive heart failure	Withhold pertuzumab and trastuzumab and repeat LVEF assessment at 4-week intervals until improvement, which may require prolonged interruption. Discontinue pertuzumab and trastuzumab if the LVEF does not improve or if it declines further, unless the benefits for the individual patient outweigh the risks
Dose modifications for organ dysfunction	
Hepatic impairment	No adjustment needed
Renal impairment	No adjustment needed

Note: Pertuzumab dose reductions are not recommended

METASTATIC • HER2-POSITIVE

BREAST CANCER REGIMEN: DOCETAXEL EVERY 3 WEEKS + WEEKLY TRASTUZUMAB

Marty M et al. J Clin Oncol 2005;23:4265–4274

Premedication:

Dexamethasone 8 mg/dose; administer orally twice daily for 3 days, starting on the day before docetaxel administration (total dose/cycle = 48 mg)

Docetaxel 100 mg/m^2; administer intravenously in a volume of 0.9% sodium chloride injection (0.9% NS) or 5% dextrose injection sufficient to produce a docetaxel concentration within the range 0.3–0.74 mg/mL over 60 minutes on day 1, every 3 weeks for 6 cycles (total dosage/cycle = 100 mg/m^2)

Trastuzumab 4 mg/kg initial (loading) dose; administer intravenously in 250 mL 0.9% NS, over at least 90 minutes (total initial dosage = 4 mg/kg), *followed at weekly intervals by:*
Trastuzumab 2 mg/kg per dose; administer intravenously in 250 mL 0.9% NS over 30–90 minutes, every week, continually until disease progression (total dosage/week = 2 mg/kg)
Notes: Administration duration may be decreased from 90 to 30 minutes if administration over longer durations is well tolerated
Patients who tolerated combination treatment and did not develop disease progression may receive docetaxel for more than 6 cycles

Supportive Care
Antiemetic prophylaxis
Emetogenic potential is LOW
See Chapter 42 for antiemetic recommendations

Hematopoietic growth factor (CSF) prophylaxis
Primary prophylaxis is indicated with one of the following:
  Filgrastim (G-CSF) 5 mcg/kg per day by subcutaneous injection, *or*
  Pegfilgrastim (pegylated filgrastim) 6 mg/0.6 mL by subcutaneous injection for 1 dose
  Begin use from 24–72 hours after myelosuppressive chemotherapy is completed
See Chapter 43 for more information

Antimicrobial prophylaxis
Risk of fever and neutropenia is LOW–INTERMEDIATE
  Antimicrobial primary prophylaxis to be considered:
  • Antibacterial—consider a fluoroquinolone or no prophylaxis
  • Antifungal—not indicated
  • Antiviral—not indicated, unless patient previously had an episode of HSV

Trastuzumab infusion reactions
• A symptom complex most commonly consisting of chills and/or fever may occur in as many as 40% of patients during the first infusion of trastuzumab. These symptoms occur infrequently with subsequent trastuzumab infusions. Other signs and/or symptoms may include nausea, vomiting, pain (in some cases at tumor sites), rigors, headache, dizziness, dyspnea, hypotension, rash, and asthenia. Although the symptoms are usually mild to moderate in severity, infrequently, trastuzumab may need to be discontinued
• When such a symptom complex is observed, it can be treated with or without reduction in the rate of trastuzumab infusion, and:
  ▪ **Acetaminophen** 650 mg; administer orally
  ▪ **Diphenhydramine** 25–50 mg; administer orally or by intravenous injection, and
  ▪ **Meperidine** 12.5–25 mg; administer by intravenous injection every 10 minutes if needed for shaking chills (generally, cumulative doses >50 mg are not needed; use with caution in persons with moderate or more severely impaired renal function)

Treatment Modifications

Adverse Events	Treatment Modifications
LVEF has declined by ≥16 percentage points from baseline, or has declined by 10–15 percentage points from baseline to a value below the lower limit of the normal range OR Symptomatic congestive heart failure	Withhold trastuzumab and repeat LVEF assessment at 4-week intervals until improvement, which may require prolonged interruption. Discontinue trastuzumab if the LVEF does not improve or if it declines further, unless the benefits for the individual patient outweigh the risks
First episode of hematologic or nonhematologic adverse events G ≥3 other than alopecia and anemia	Reduce docetaxel dosage from 100 mg/m^2 to 75 mg/m^2
Second episode of hematologic or nonhematologic adverse events G3 other than alopecia and anemia	Reduce docetaxel dosage from 75 mg/m^2 to 55 mg/m^2

Patient Population Studied

Study of 188 patients with HER2-positive MBC included in an open-label, comparative, randomized, multicenter, multinational trial comparing the efficacy and safety of first-line trastuzumab plus docetaxel vs docetaxel alone

Efficacy (N = 92)

WHO Criteria

Outcome	Percentage or Duration
Overall response rate	61%
Complete response	7%
Partial response	54%
Stable disease	27%
Median duration of response	11.7 months
Median time to progression	11.7 months
Median overall survival*	31.2 months

*Kaplan-Meier estimate

Therapy Monitoring

1. *Start of each cycle:* CBC with leukocyte differential count and platelet counts, LFTs, and serum electrolytes. Consider intracycle assessment in first few cycles

2. Conduct thorough cardiac assessment, including history, physical examination, and determination of LVEF by echocardiogram or MUGA scan at baseline immediately prior to initiation of trastuzumab and every 3 months during therapy. In patients with metastatic disease, the frequency of post-baseline cardiac monitoring in asymptomatic patients may be individualized based on the clinical judgment of the medically responsible health care provider

3. Patients should have a pre-treatment LVEF ≥55%

4. Repeat LVEF measurement at 4-week intervals if trastuzumab is withheld for significant left ventricular cardiac dysfunction

Toxicity (N = 92)

NCI-CTC		
Adverse Events	% Total	% G3/4
Nonhematologic Toxicity		
Alopecia	67	10
Asthenia	45	10
Nausea	45	0
Diarrhea	43	5
Peripheral edema	40	1
Paresthesia	32	0
Vomiting	29	3
Pyrexia	30	1
Constipation	27	2
Myalgia	27	3
Arthralgia	27	4
Rash	24	1
Fatigue	24	3
Mucosal inflammation	23	2
Erythema	23	1
Anorexia	22	2
Headache	21	5
Increased lacrimation	21	1
Epistaxis	20	0
Hematologic Toxicity		
Anemia	—	1
Thrombocytopenia	—	0
Leukopenia	—	20
Neutropenia	—	32
Febrile neutropenia/neutropenic sepsis	—	23

Changes in Left Ventricular Ejection Fraction from Baseline: Worst Value up to 6 Cycles and Overall

	Worse up to Cycle 6	Overall
Increase or no change	41	20
Absolute decrease <15%	48	63
Absolute decrease ≥15%	11	17
Absolute value <40%	1	1

NCI-CTC, National Cancer Institute (USA) Common Toxicity Criteria, version 2.0. At: http://ctep.cancer.gov/protocolDevelopment/electronic_applications/ctc.htm [accessed December 7, 2013]

METASTATIC • HER2-POSITIVE
BREAST CANCER REGIMEN: WEEKLY DOCETAXEL + TRASTUZUMAB

Esteva FJ et al. J Clin Oncol 2002;20:1800–1808

Initial treatment (first cycle):
Trastuzumab 4 mg/kg (loading dose); administer intravenously in 250 mL 0.9% sodium chloride injection (0.9% NS), over at least 90 minutes 1 day before the first dose of docetaxel is administered (total initial dosage = 4 mg/kg)

Premedication for docetaxel:
Dexamethasone 4 mg/dose; administer orally for 3 doses at approximately 12 hours and 1 hour before docetaxel, and 12 hours after docetaxel administration (total dose during week 1 = 12 mg)
Docetaxel 35 mg/m^2; administer intravenously in a volume of 0.9% NS or 5% dextrose injection (D5W), sufficient to produce a final docetaxel concentration within the range 0.3–0.74 mg/mL over 30 minutes, the day after the initial (loading) dose of trastuzumab

Second and subsequent treatments:
Premedication for docetaxel:
Dexamethasone 4 mg/dose; administer orally for 3 doses at approximately 12 hours and 1 hour before docetaxel, and 12 hours after docetaxel administration (total dose during week 1 = 12 mg)
• Initially, dexamethasone is given approximately every 12 hours for 3 doses, starting the evening before docetaxel administration
• If no significant fluid retention or hypersensitivity reactions occur during the first 2 cycles, give dexamethasone 4 mg/dose orally every 12 hours for 2 doses on the day of docetaxel administration, with the first dose given at least 1 hour before docetaxel
• If there is no evidence of fluid retention after a fourth cycle, give a single dose of dexamethasone 4 mg orally just before docetaxel administration

Docetaxel 35 mg/m^2 per dose; administer intravenously in a volume of 0.9% NS or D5W sufficient to produce a final docetaxel concentration within the range 0.3–0.74 mg/mL over 30 minutes, weekly for 3 consecutive weeks (days 1, 8, and 15), every 4 weeks (total dosage/4-week cycle = 105 mg/m^2), *followed by:*
Trastuzumab 2 mg/kg per dose; administer intravenously in 250 mL 0.9% NS over 30–90 minutes, weekly for 3 consecutive weeks (days 1, 8, and 15), every 4 weeks (after an initial 4-mg/kg dose, the total dosage/4-week cycle for the second and subsequent cycles = 6 mg/kg)

Note: Trastuzumab administration duration may be decreased from 90 to 30 minutes if administration over longer durations is well tolerated

Supportive Care
Antiemetic prophylaxis
Emetogenic potential on days with trastuzumab alone is **MINIMAL–LOW**
Emetogenic potential on days with docetaxel is **LOW**
See Chapter 42 for antiemetic recommendations

Hematopoietic growth factor (CSF) prophylaxis
Primary prophylaxis is **NOT** indicated
See Chapter 43 for more information

Antimicrobial prophylaxis
Risk of fever and neutropenia is **LOW**
  Antimicrobial primary prophylaxis to be considered:
  • Antibacterial—not indicated
  • Antifungal—not indicated
  • Antiviral—not indicated, unless patient previously had an episode of HSV

Trastuzumab infusion reactions
• A symptom complex most commonly consisting of chills and/or fever may occur in as many as 40% of patients during the first infusion of trastuzumab. These symptoms occur infrequently with subsequent trastuzumab infusions. Other signs and/or symptoms may include nausea, vomiting, pain (in some cases at tumor sites), rigors, headache, dizziness, dyspnea, hypotension, rash, and asthenia. Although the symptoms are usually mild to moderate in severity, infrequently, trastuzumab may need to be discontinued
• When such a symptom complex is observed, it can be treated with or without reduction in the rate of trastuzumab infusion, and:
  ▪ **Acetaminophen** 650 mg; administer orally
  ▪ **Diphenhydramine** 25–50 mg; administer orally or by intravenous injection, and
  ▪ **Meperidine** 12.5–25 mg; administer by intravenous injection every 10 minutes if needed for shaking chills (generally, cumulative doses >50 mg are not needed; use with caution in persons with moderate or more severely impaired renal function)

Treatment Modifications

Adverse Events	Treatment Modifications*
ANC <500/mm^3	Reduce docetaxel dosage by 5 mg/m^2 per week
Febrile neutropenia	
Platelets <50,000/mm^3	
G2 nonhematologic adverse events	
G3 nonhematologic adverse events (except fatigue)	Reduce docetaxel dosage by 10 mg/m^2 per week
G3 fatigue	Reduce docetaxel dosage by 5 mg/m^2 per week
LVEF has declined by ≥16 percentage points from baseline, or has declined by 10–15 percentage points from baseline to a value below the lower limit of the normal range OR Symptomatic congestive heart failure	Withhold trastuzumab and repeat LVEF assessment at 4-week intervals until improvement, which may require prolonged interruption. Discontinue trastuzumab if the LVEF does not improve or if it declines further, unless the benefits for the individual patient outweigh the risks

*Minimum docetaxel dosage to continue treatment = 20 mg/m^2

Patient Population Studied

Study of 30 women with HER2-overexpressing (FISH+ or IHC 3+) metastatic breast cancer who had not received >3 prior chemotherapy regimens. No limitation on prior hormonal therapy

Efficacy (N = 30)

ECOG Criteria	
Overall response	63% (95% CI, 44–80%)
Complete response	None
Partial response	63%
Minor response	7%
Stable disease >4 months	20%

Toxicity (N = 30)

NCI of Canada CTC			
	G1/2	**G3**	**G4**
Hematologic Toxicity			
Neutropenia	49%	16%	10%
Anemia	56%	0	0
Thrombocytopenia	3%	0	0
Febrile neutropenia	0	3%	0
Nonhematologic Toxicity			
Left ventricle dysfunction	26%	3%	0
Diarrhea	60%	6%	0
Alopecia	80%	NR	NR
Fatigue	62%	20%	0
Excessive lacrimation	93%	0	0
Edema	46%	0	0
Pleural effusion	26%	3%	0
Myalgia	60%	NR	NR
Neuropathy	36%	3%	0
Onycholysis	50%	0	0
Hypersensitivity	0	6%	0

NR, not reported

Therapy Monitoring

1. *Before each docetaxel dose:* CBC with differential and platelet count and LFTs
2. *Every second or third cycle:* Serum electrolytes, calcium, magnesium
3. Conduct thorough cardiac assessment, including history, physical examination, and determination of LVEF by echocardiogram or MUGA scan at baseline immediately prior to initiation of trastuzumab and every 3 months during therapy. In patients with metastatic disease, the frequency of post-baseline cardiac monitoring in asymptomatic patients may be individualized based on the clinical judgment of the medically responsible health care provider
4. Patients should have a pre-treatment LVEF ≥55%
5. Repeat LVEF measurement at 4-week intervals if trastuzumab is withheld for significant left ventricular cardiac dysfunction

METASTATIC • HER2-POSITIVE

BREAST CANCER REGIMEN: TRASTUZUMAB + PACLITAXEL, EVERY 3 WEEKS

Leyland-Jones B et al. J Clin Oncol 2003;21:3965–3971
Slamon DJ et al. N Engl J Med 2001;344:783–792

Initial treatment (first cycle):
Premedication for paclitaxel:
Dexamethasone 20 mg/dose; administer orally for 2 doses at 12 hours and 6 hours before paclitaxel (total dose/cycle = 40 mg)
Diphenhydramine 50 mg; administer by intravenous injection 30–60 minutes before paclitaxel
Cimetidine 300 mg (or **ranitidine** 50 mg, **famotidine** 20 mg, or an equivalent histamine receptor [H$_2$]-subtype antagonist); administer intravenously in 20–50 mL 0.9% sodium chloride injection (0.9% NS) or 5% dextrose injection (D5W) over 15–30 minutes, 30–60 minutes before paclitaxel
Paclitaxel 175 mg/m^2; administer intravenously in a volume of 0.9% NS or D5W sufficient to produce a concentration within the range 0.3–1.2 mg/mL over 3 hours, 24 hours before the first dose of trastuzumab (total dosage = 175 mg/m^2)
Trastuzumab 8 mg/kg (loading dose); administer intravenously in 250 mL 0.9% NS over at least 90 minutes, 24 hours after the initial paclitaxel dose (total initial dosage = 8 mg/kg)

Second and subsequent treatments:
Trastuzumab 6 mg/kg per dose; administer intravenously in 250 mL 0.9% NS over 30–90 minutes, on day 1 before paclitaxel, every 3 weeks (total dosage/cycle = 6 mg/kg)
Note: Trastuzumab administration duration may be decreased from 90 to 30 minutes if administration over longer durations is well tolerated
Premedication for paclitaxel:
Dexamethasone 20 mg/dose; administer orally for 2 doses at 12 hours and 6 hours before paclitaxel (total dose/cycle = 40 mg)
Diphenhydramine 50 mg; administer by intravenous injection 30–60 minutes before paclitaxel
Cimetidine 300 mg (or **ranitidine** 50 mg, **famotidine** 20 mg, or an equivalent histamine receptor [H$_2$]-subtype antagonist); administer intravenously in 20–50 mL 0.9% NS or D5W over 15–30 minutes, 30–60 minutes before paclitaxel
Paclitaxel 175 mg/m^2; administer intravenously in a volume of 0.9% NS or D5W sufficient to produce a concentration within the range 0.3–1.2 mg/mL over 3 hours, on day 1 starting 30 minutes after completing trastuzumab administration, every 3 weeks for a total of 6 cycles (total dosage/cycle = 175 mg/m^2)

Supportive Care
Antiemetic prophylaxis
Emetogenic potential on days with docetaxel is **LOW**
Emetogenic potential on days with trastuzumab alone is **MINIMAL–LOW**
See Chapter 42 for antiemetic recommendations

Hematopoietic growth factor (CSF) prophylaxis
Primary prophylaxis is **NOT** indicated
See Chapter 43 for more information

Antimicrobial prophylaxis
Risk of fever and neutropenia is **LOW**
   Antimicrobial primary prophylaxis to be considered:
 • Antibacterial—not indicated
 • Antifungal—not indicated
 • Antiviral—not indicated, unless patient previously had an episode of HSV

Trastuzumab infusion reactions
• A symptom complex most commonly consisting of chills and/or fever may occur in as many as 40% of patients during the first infusion of trastuzumab. These symptoms occur infrequently with subsequent trastuzumab infusions. Other signs and/or symptoms may include nausea, vomiting, pain (in some cases at tumor sites), rigors, headache, dizziness, dyspnea, hypotension, rash, and asthenia. Although the symptoms are usually mild to moderate in severity, infrequently, trastuzumab may need to be discontinued
• When such a symptom complex is observed, it can be treated with or without reduction in the rate of trastuzumab infusion, and:
  ▪ **Acetaminophen** 650 mg; administer orally
  ▪ **Diphenhydramine** 25–50 mg; administer orally or by intravenous injection, and
  ▪ **Meperidine** 12.5–25 mg; administer by intravenous injection every 10 minutes if needed for shaking chills (generally, cumulative doses >50 mg are not needed; use with caution in persons with moderate or more severely impaired renal function)

Treatment Modifications

Nabholtz J-M et al. J Clin Oncol 1996; 14:1858–1867

Adverse Events	Treatment Modifications
G3/4 ANC for ≥7 days	Reduce paclitaxel dosage by 25%
Any thrombocytopenia for >7 days	
Febrile neutropenia, documented infection, or hemorrhage	
G3 mucositis	
G3/4 neuropathy	Discontinue paclitaxel
Severe hypersensitivity reaction	Discontinue trastuzumab
LVEF has declined by ≥16 percentage points from baseline, or has declined by 10–15 percentage points from baseline to a value below the lower limit of the normal range OR Symptomatic congestive heart failure	Withhold trastuzumab and repeat LVEF assessment at 4-week intervals until improvement, which may require prolonged interruption. Discontinue trastuzumab if the LVEF does not improve or if it declines further, unless the benefits for the individual patient outweigh the risks

Patient Population Studied

Leyland-Jones B et al. J Clin Oncol 2003;21:3965–3971

Study of 92 women with HER2 (IHC 2+, IHC 3+, or FISH+) progressive metastatic breast cancer that had not previously received chemotherapy for metastatic disease

Efficacy (N = 32)

Leyland-Jones B et al. J Clin Oncol 2003;21:3965–3971

WHO Criteria	
Overall response	59%
Complete response	13%
Partial response	47%
Median duration of response	10.5 months

Therapy Monitoring

1. *Every 3 weeks:* CBC with differential and platelet count, LFTs, and serum electrolytes. Consider intracycle assessment in early cycles
2. Conduct thorough cardiac assessment, including history, physical examination, and determination of LVEF by echocardiogram or MUGA scan at baseline immediately prior to initiation of trastuzumab and every 3 months during therapy. In patients with metastatic disease, the frequency of post-baseline cardiac monitoring in asymptomatic patients may be individualized based on the clinical judgment of the medically responsible health care provider
3. Patients should have a pre-treatment LVEF ≥55%
4. Repeat LVEF measurement at 4-week intervals if trastuzumab is withheld for significant left ventricular cardiac dysfunction

Note

Consider adding pertuzumab in combination with trastuzumab + paclitaxel chemotherapy
Loading Dose: **Pertuzumab** 840 mg; administer intravenously in 250 mL of 0.9% NS over 90 minutes after trastuzumab, cycle 1 only (total dose during the first cycle = 840 mg), *followed 3 weeks later by:*
Maintenance Doses: **Pertuzumab** 420 mg; administer intravenously in 250 mL of 0.9% NS over 30–60 minutes on day 1 after trastuzumab, every 3 weeks (total dose/cycle = 420 mg)

Datko F et al. Cancer Res 2012;72(24 Suppl 3) [Cancer Therapy & Research Center-American Association of Cancer Research. 35th annual San Antonio Breast Cancer Symposium; poster P5-18–20]

Toxicity (N = 91)

Slamon DJ et al. N Engl J Med 2001;344:783–792

NCI-CTCv2		
Toxicity	% All	% Severe
Hematologic Toxicity		
Leukopenia	24	6
Anemia	14	1
Infection	46	1
Nonhematologic Toxicity		
Any type		
Abdominal pain	34	3
Asthenia	62	8
Back pain	36	8
Chest pain	30	3
Chills	42	1
Fever	47	2
Headache	36	7
Infection	46	1
Pain	60	10
Cardiac dysfunction	13	2*
Digestive Tract		
Anorexia	24	1
Constipation	25	0
Diarrhea	45	1
Nausea	50	3
Stomatitis	10	0
Vomiting	37	9
Musculoskeletal System		
Arthralgia	37	9
Myalgia	38	7
Nervous System		
Paresthesia	47	2
Respiratory system		
Increased coughing	42	0
Dyspnea not related to heart failure	28	1
Pharyngitis	22	0
Skin		
Alopecia	56	26
Rash	38	1

*New York Heart Association class III or IV

METASTATIC • HER2-POSITIVE

BREAST CANCER REGIMEN: WEEKLY PACLITAXEL + TRASTUZUMAB

Seidman AD et al. J Clin Oncol 2008;26:1642–1649

Initial treatment (first week)

Trastuzumab 4 mg/kg (loading dose); administer intravenously in 250 mL 0.9% sodium chloride injection (0.9% NS) over at least 90 minutes, 1 day before the first dose of paclitaxel is administered (total dosage during the first treatment week = 4 mg/kg)

Premedication for paclitaxel:
Dexamethasone 10 mg; administer intravenously over 10–15 minutes, 30–60 minutes before paclitaxel
Diphenhydramine 50 mg; administer by intravenous injection 30–60 minutes before paclitaxel
Cimetidine 300 mg (or **ranitidine** 50 mg, **famotidine** 20 mg, or an equivalent histamine receptor [H_2]-subtype antagonist); administer in 20–50 mL 0.9% NS or 5% dextrose injection (D5W) over 15–30 minutes, 30–60 minutes before paclitaxel
Paclitaxel 80 mg/m²; administer intravenously in a volume of 0.9% NS or D5W sufficient to produce a concentration within the range 0.3–1.2 mg/mL over 60 minutes (total dosage = 80 mg/m²)

Schedule for second and subsequent weeks
Premedication for paclitaxel:
Dexamethasone 10 mg; administer intravenously over 10–15 minutes, 30–60 minutes before paclitaxel
Note: Dexamethasone doses may be gradually reduced in 2- to 4-mg increments if the patient has no hypersensitivity reactions during repeated paclitaxel treatments
Diphenhydramine 50 mg; administer intravenously per push 30–60 minutes before paclitaxel
Cimetidine 300 mg (or **ranitidine** 50 mg, **famotidine** 20 mg, or an equivalent histamine receptor [H_2]-subtype antagonist); administer in 20–50 mL 0.9% NS or D5W over 15–30 minutes, 30–60 minutes before paclitaxel
Paclitaxel 80 mg/m² per dose; administer intravenously in a volume of 0.9% NS or D5W sufficient to produce a concentration within the range 0.3–1.2 mg/mL over 60 minutes, every week, continually (total dosage/week = 80 mg/m²), *followed by:*
Trastuzumab 2 mg/kg per dose; administer intravenously in 250 mL 0.9% NS over 30–90 minutes, every week, continually (total dosage/week during the second & subsequent weeks = 2 mg/kg)
Note: The duration of trastuzumab administration may be decreased from 90 to 30 minutes if administration over longer durations is well tolerated

Supportive Care
Antiemetic prophylaxis
Emetogenic potential on days with trastuzumab alone is **MINIMAL–LOW**
Emetogenic potential on days with paclitaxel is **LOW**
See Chapter 42 for antiemetic recommendations

Hematopoietic growth factor (CSF) prophylaxis
Primary prophylaxis is **NOT** *indicated*
See Chapter 43 for more information

Antimicrobial prophylaxis
Risk of fever and neutropenia is **LOW**
Antimicrobial primary prophylaxis to be considered:
- Antibacterial—not indicated
- Antifungal—not indicated
- Antiviral—not indicated, unless patient previously had an episode of HSV

Trastuzumab infusion reactions
- A symptom complex most commonly consisting of chills and/or fever may occur in as many as 40% of patients during the first infusion of trastuzumab. These symptoms occur infrequently with subsequent trastuzumab infusions. Other signs and/or symptoms may include nausea, vomiting, pain (in some cases at tumor sites), rigors, headache, dizziness, dyspnea, hypotension, rash, and asthenia. Although the symptoms are usually mild to moderate in severity, infrequently, trastuzumab may need to be discontinued
- When such a symptom complex is observed, it can be treated with or without reduction in the rate of trastuzumab infusion, and:
  - **Acetaminophen** 650 mg; administer orally
  - **Diphenhydramine** 25–50 mg; administer orally or by intravenous injection, and
  - **Meperidine** 12.5–25 mg; administer by intravenous injection every 10 minutes if needed for shaking chills (generally, cumulative doses >50 mg are not needed; use with caution in persons with moderate or more severely impaired renal function)

Treatment Modifications

Adverse Events	Treatment Modifications
ANC <1000/mm³ or platelets <100,000/mm³ on a day of planned treatment	Hold paclitaxel until ANC ≥1000/mm³ and platelets ≥100,000/mm³
If >2 weeks are required for recovery to ANC ≥1000/mm³ and platelets ≥100,000/mm³	Reduce paclitaxel dosage by 20 mg/m²
Platelet nadir count ≤50,000/mm³	
Documented infection	
G2 nonhematologic adverse events	Reduce paclitaxel dosage by 10 mg/m²
G3 nonhematologic adverse events	Hold paclitaxel until toxicity resolves to G ≤2 and reduce paclitaxel dosage by 20 mg/m² during subsequent treatments
LVEF has declined by ≥16 percentage points from baseline, or has declined by 10–15 percentage points from baseline to a value below the lower limit of the normal range OR Symptomatic congestive heart failure	Withhold trastuzumab and repeat LVEF assessment at 4-week intervals until improvement, which may require prolonged interruption. Discontinue trastuzumab if the LVEF does not improve or if it declines further, unless the benefits for the individual patient outweigh the risks

Efficacy

Patients	Paclitaxel Dose Frequency	Response (%)	95% CI	OR	95% CI for OR	P Value
All patients (combined)	3-Weekly Weekly	29 42	25–34 37–47	1.75	1.28–2.37	0.0004
All patients (limited)	3-Weekly Weekly	35 42	28–41 37–47	1.36	0.96–1.23	0.093
HER2-negative (limited)	3-Weekly Weekly	24 42	16–34 34–51	2.29	1.27–4.08	0.0063
HER2-negative (limited)	No trastuzumab Trastuzumab	32 39	23–41 29–48	1.35	0.78–2.34	0.29
HER2-positive (limited)	3-Weekly Weekly	59 55	46–69 45–65	0.99	0.49–1.63	0.71

Toxicity

G3 and G4 Hematologic Toxicity by Paclitaxel Dosing (n = 572)

Measure	Treatment Arm	% G3	% G4
WBC	3-Weekly	8	1
	Weekly	6	2
Platelets	3-Weekly	2	0
	Weekly	1	1
Hemoglobin	3-Weekly	3	0
	Weekly	5	<1
Granulocytes/bands	3-Weekly	10	5
	Weekly	5	3
Lymphocytes	3-Weekly	8	4
	Weekly	15	4

G3 and G4 Hematologic Toxicity by Trastuzumab Use (n = 572)

Measure	Treatment Arm	% G3	% G4
WBC	No trastuzumab	8	3
	Trastuzumab	5	<10
Platelets	No trastuzumab	2	<1
	Trastuzumab	0	<1
Hemoglobin	No trastuzumab	5	0
	Trastuzumab	3	<1
Granulocytes/bands	No trastuzumab	7	6
	Trastuzumab	8	2
Lymphocytes	No trastuzumab	15	6
	Trastuzumab	10	2

G3 and G4 Nonhematologic Toxicity by Paclitaxel Dosing Schedule (n = 572)

Toxicity	Treatment	% G3	% G4
Infection	3-Weekly	4	0
	Weekly	5	1
Diarrhea	3-Weekly	3	0
	Weekly	5	0
Dyspnea	3-Weekly	3	1
	Weekly	5	2
Edema	3-Weekly	1	0
	Weekly	5	1
Neurosensory	3-Weekly	12	0
	Weekly	24	<1
Neuromotor	3-Weekly	4	0
	Weekly	9	0
Malaise/fatigue	3-Weekly	5	0
	Weekly	6	<1
Hyperglycemia	3-Weekly	7	1
	Weekly	4	1

NCI, CTC, National Cancer Institute (USA) Common Toxicity Criteria and Common Terminology Criteria for Adverse Events, all versions. At: http://ctep.cancer.gov/protocolDevelopment/electronic_applications/ctc.htm [accessed December 7, 2013]

Patient Population Studied

Patients were randomly assigned to paclitaxel 175 mg/m^2 every 3 weeks or 80 mg/m^2 weekly. After the first 171 patients, all HER2-positive patients received trastuzumab; HER2 non-overexpressers were randomly assigned to receive or not receive trastuzumab, in addition to paclitaxel. A total of 577 patients were treated on 9840 (limited). An additional 158 patients (158 patients from the 175-mg/m^2 arm of CALGB 9342) were included in analyses, for a total of 735 patients

Therapy Monitoring

1. *Every week:* CBC with differential and platelet count
2. *Every other cycle:* LFTs, serum electrolytes, calcium, and magnesium
3. Conduct thorough cardiac assessment, including history, physical examination, and determination of LVEF by echocardiogram or MUGA scan at baseline immediately prior to initiation of trastuzumab and every 3 months during therapy. In patients with metastatic disease, the frequency of post-baseline cardiac monitoring in asymptomatic patients may be individualized based on the clinical judgment of the medically responsible health care provider
4. Patients should have a pre-treatment LVEF ≥55%
5. Repeat LVEF measurement at 4-week intervals if trastuzumab is withheld for significant left ventricular cardiac dysfunction

Note

Consider adding pertuzumab in combination with trastuzumab + paclitaxel chemotherapy
Loading Dose: **Pertuzumab** 840 mg; administer intravenously in 250 mL of 0.9% NS over 90 minutes after trastuzumab, cycle 1 only (total dose during the first cycle = 840 mg), *followed 3 weeks later by:*
Maintenance Doses: **Pertuzumab** 420 mg; administer intravenously in 250 mL of 0.9% NS over 30–60 minutes on the same day as trastuzumab but after trastuzumab, every 3 weeks (total dose/cycle = 420 mg)

Datko F et al. Cancer Res 2012;72(24 Suppl 3) [Cancer Therapy & Research Center-American Association of Cancer Research. 35th annual San Antonio Breast Cancer Symposium; poster P5-18–20]

METASTATIC • HER2-POSITIVE

BREAST CANCER REGIMEN: ADO-TRASTUZUMAB EMTANSINE
(T-DM1)

Verma S et al. N Engl J Med 2012;367:1783–1791

ado-Trastuzumab emtansine 3.6 mg/kg; administer intravenously in 250 mL 0.9% sodium chloride injection on day 1, every 21 days (total dosage/cycle = 3.6 mg/kg)

Exposure	Administration Rate	Monitoring
First infusion	Intravenously over 90 minutes	• Patients should be observed closely for infusion-related reactions, especially during the first infusion • Administration should be slowed or interrupted if a patient develops an infusion-related reaction • Permanently discontinue ado-trastuzumab for life-threatening infusion-related reactions
Second and subsequent infusions	• Intravenously over 30 minutes if prior administration was tolerated • Subsequent doses may be administered at the rate tolerated during the most recently administered treatment	

Supportive Care
Antiemetic prophylaxis
Emetogenic potential is **LOW**
See Chapter 42 for antiemetic recommendations

Hematopoietic growth factor (CSF) prophylaxis
Primary prophylaxis is **NOT** *indicated*
See Chapter 43 for more information

Antimicrobial prophylaxis
Risk of fever and neutropenia is **LOW**
  Antimicrobial primary prophylaxis to be considered:
  • Antibacterial—not indicated
  • Antifungal—not indicated
  • Antiviral—not indicated, unless patient previously had an episode of HSV

Efficacy

Independent Review

	Lapatinib Plus Capecitabine (N = 389)	ado-Trastuzumab Emtansine (N = 397)	Difference	P Value
	no. (%)	no. (%)		
CR or PR	120 (30.8)	173 (43.6)	12.7 (6.0–19.4)	<0.001
CR	2 (0.5)	4 (1.0%)		
PR	118 (30.3)	169 (42.6)		
Duration of CR or PR (months)				
Median	6.5	12.6		
95% CI	5.5–7.2	8.4–20.8		

Therapy Monitoring

1. *Before each cycle:* CBC with differential and platelet count, serum electrolytes and LFTs
2. Conduct thorough cardiac assessment, including history, physical examination, and determination of LVEF by echocardiogram or MUGA scan at baseline immediately prior to initiation of trastuzumab and every 3 months during therapy and upon completion of ado-trastuzumab emtansine. In patients with metastatic disease, the frequency of post-baseline cardiac monitoring in asymptomatic patients may be individualized based on the clinical judgment of the medically responsible health care provider
3. Patients should have a pre-treatment LVEF ≥55%
4. Repeat LVEF measurement at 4-week intervals if ado-trastuzumab emtansine is withheld for significant left ventricular cardiac dysfunction

Patient Population Studied

The EMILIA study, a randomized phase 3 trial, assessed the efficacy and safety of lapatinib plus capecitabine (496 patients) versus ado-trastuzumab (495 patients) in patients with HER2-positive advanced breast cancer previously treated with trastuzumab and a taxane. In both treatment arms, 61% of patients had previously received anthracycline therapy, 41% endocrine therapy, 84% had received trastuzumab, and 39% >1 prior chemotherapy regimen for locally advanced or metastatic disease

Toxicity

	Lapatinib Plus Capecitabine (N = 488)		ado-Trastuzumab (N = 490)	
	All Grades (%)	G3/4 (%)	All Grades (%)	G3/4 (%)
Diarrhea	389 (79.7)	101 (20.7)	114 (23.3)	8 (1.6)
Palmar-plantar erythrodysesthesia	283 (58.0)	80 (16.4)	6 (1.2)	0
Vomiting	143 (29.3)	22 (4.5)	93 (19.0)	4 (0.8)
Neutropenia	42 (8.6)	21 (4.3)	29 (5.9)	10 (2)
Hypokalemia	42 (8.6)	20 (4.1)	42 (8.6)	11 (2.2)
Fatigue	136 (27.9)	17 (3.5)	172 (35.1)	12 (2.4)
Nausea	218 (44.7)	12 (2.5)	192 (39.2)	4 (0.8)
Mucosal Inflammation	93 (19.1)	11 (2.3)	33 (6.7)	1 (0.2)
Anemia	39 (8.0)	8 (1.6)	51 (10.4)	13 (2.7)
Elevated ALT	43 (8.8)	7 (1.4)	83 (16.9)	14 (2.9)
Elevated AST	46 (9.4)	4 (0.8)	110 (22.4)	21 (4.3)
Thrombocytopenia	12 (2.5)	1 (0.2)	137 (28.0)	63 (12.9)

Treatment Modification for ado-Trastuzumab Emtansine

ado-Trastuzumab Dose Levels	Dosage
Starting dosage	3.6 mg/kg
First dose reduction	3 mg/kg
Second dose reduction	2.4 mg/kg
Requirement for further dose reduction	Discontinue ado-trastuzumab emtansine

Dose delays	If significant related toxicities (other than those described below) have not recovered to G1 or baseline, dose may be delayed for up to 42 days from the last dose. If treatment resumes, it may be at either the same dose level or one dose level lower
Platelet nadir 25,000–50,000/mm³	Withhold ado-trastuzumab emtansine until platelet count recovers to ≥75,000/mm³, then resume treatment at the same dose level
Platelet nadir <25,000/mm³	Withhold ado-trastuzumab emtansine until platelet count recovers to ≥75,000/mm³, then resume treatment with ado-trastuzumab emtansine 3 mg/kg every 3 weeks
AST or ALT >2× to ≤5× ULN (G2)	Treat at the same ado-trastuzumab emtansine dose level
AST or ALT >5× to ≤20× ULN (G3)	Withhold ado-trastuzumab emtansine until AST and ALT recover to G ≤2, then resume ado-trastuzumab emtansine with dosage decreased by one dose level
AST or ALT >20× ULN (G4)	Permanently discontinue ado-trastuzumab emtansine
Total bilirubin >1.5× to ≤3× ULN (G2)	Withhold ado-trastuzumab emtansine until total bilirubin recovers to G ≤1, then resume ado-trastuzumab emtansine at the same dose level
Total bilirubin >3× to ≤10× ULN (G3)	Withhold ado-trastuzumab emtansine until total bilirubin recovers to G ≤1, then resume ado-trastuzumab emtansine with dosage decreased by one dose level

(continued)

Treatment Modification for ado-Trastuzumab Emtansine (*continued*)

Total bilirubin >10× ULN (G4)	Permanently discontinue ado-trastuzumab emtansine
AST or ALT >3× ULN and total bilirubin >2× ULN	Permanently discontinue ado-trastuzumab emtansine
Patients diagnosed with nodular regenerative hepatic hyperplasia	Permanently discontinue ado-trastuzumab emtansine
Symptomatic CHF (G ≥3 left ventricular systolic dysfunction per NCI CTCAE v3.0)	Discontinue ado-trastuzumab emtansine
LVEF <40%	Withhold ado-trastuzumab emtansine. Repeat LVEF assessment within 3 weeks. If LVEF <40% is confirmed, discontinue ado-trastuzumab emtansine
LVEF 40% to ≤45%, and decrease is ≥10% points from baseline measurement	Withhold ado-trastuzumab emtansine. Repeat LVEF assessment within 3 weeks. If LVEF has not recovered to within 10% points from baseline, discontinue ado-trastuzumab emtansine
LVEF 40% to ≤45%, and decrease is <10% points from baseline	Continue ado-trastuzumab emtansine treatment. Repeat LVEF assessment within 3 weeks
LVEF >45%	Continue treatment with ado-trastuzumab emtansine
G3/4 peripheral neuropathy	Withhold ado-trastuzumab emtansine until symptoms abate to G ≤2 then resume treatment with ado-trastuzumab emtansine
Patients diagnosed with interstitial lung disease or pneumonitis	Permanently discontinue ado-trastuzumab emtansine
Life-threatening infusion-related reactions	Permanently discontinue ado-trastuzumab emtansine

Note: ado-trastuzumab emtansine dosages should not be re-escalated after a dosage reduction is made. If a planned dose is delayed or missed, it should be administered as soon as possible: Do not wait until the next planned cycle. The schedule of administration should be adjusted to maintain a 3-week interval between doses

METASTATIC • HER2-POSITIVE
BREAST CANCER REGIMEN: CAPECITABINE + TRASTUZUMAB

Bartsch R et al. J Clin Oncol 2007;25:3853–3858

Trastuzumab 8 mg/kg initial (loading) dose; administer intravenously in 250 mL sodium chloride injection (0.9% NS) over at least 90 minutes (total initial dosage = 8 mg/kg), *followed 3 weeks later by:*

Trastuzumab 6 mg/kg per dose; administer intravenously in 250 mL 0.9% NS over 30–90 minutes, every 3 weeks, continually (total dosage/3-week cycle = 6 mg/kg)

Note: Administration duration may be decreased from 90 to 30 minutes if administration over longer durations is well tolerated

Capecitabine 1250 mg/m^2 per dose; administer orally twice daily within 30 minutes after a meal for 14 consecutive days on days 1–14, every 3 weeks (total dosage/cycle = 35,000 mg/m^2)

Notes:
- Capecitabine is given for 2 consecutive weeks followed by 1 week without treatment
- Doses are rounded to use combinations of 500-mg and 150-mg tablets that most closely approximate calculated values
- In practice, treatment often is begun with capecitabine 1000 mg/m^2 per dose twice daily for 14 consecutive days on days 1–14, every 3 weeks, because of a high rate of dose reduction with higher dosages (total dosage/cycle = 28,000 mg/m^2)
- Initial capecitabine dosage should be decreased by 25% in patients with moderate renal impairment (baseline creatinine clearance = 30–50 mL/min [0.5–0.83 mL/s]); ie, a dosage reduction from 1250 mg/m^2 per dose to 950 mg/m^2 per dose, twice daily. Capecitabine use is contraindicated in persons with severe renal impairment (creatinine clearance <30 mL/min [<0.5 mL/s])
- Although food decreases the rate and extent of drug absorption and the time to peak plasma concentration and systemic exposure (AUC) for both capecitabine and fluorouracil, product labeling recommends giving capecitabine within 30 minutes after the end of a meal because established safety and efficacy data are based on administration with food

Supportive Care
Antiemetic prophylaxis
Emetogenic potential on days with capecitabine is **LOW**
Emetogenic potential on days with trastuzumab alone is **MINIMAL–LOW**
See Chapter 42 for antiemetic recommendations

Hematopoietic growth factor (CSF) prophylaxis
Primary prophylaxis is **NOT** *indicated*
See Chapter 43 for more information

Antimicrobial prophylaxis
Risk of fever and neutropenia is LOW
Antimicrobial primary prophylaxis to be considered:
- Antibacterial—not indicated
- Antifungal—not indicated
- Antiviral—not indicated, unless patient previously had an episode of HSV

Diarrhea management
Latent or delayed-onset diarrhea:
Loperamide 4 mg orally initially after the first loose or liquid stool, *then*
Loperamide 2 mg orally every 2 hours during waking hours, *plus*
Loperamide 4 mg orally every 4 hours during hours of sleep
- Continue for at least 12 hours after diarrhea resolves
- Recurrent diarrhea after a 12-hour diarrhea-free interval is treated as a new episode
- Rehydrate orally with fluids and electrolytes during a diarrheal episode
- If a patient develops blood or mucus in stool, dehydration, or hemodynamic instability, or if diarrhea persists >48 hours despite loperamide, stop loperamide and evaluate urgently in clinic or hospitalize the patient for IV hydration
- Alternatively, a trial of **diphenoxylate hydrochloride** 2.5 mg with **atropine sulfate** 0.025 mg (eg, Lomotil)

(continued)

Treatment Modifications

Dose Adjustments for Capecitabine

Adverse Event	Dose Modification
First G2 toxicity	Hold capecitabine and resume after adverse events resolve to G ≤1. No change in dosage required
Second G2 toxicity	Hold capecitabine and resume after adverse events resolve to G ≤1. Reduce dosage by 25%
Third G2 toxicity	Hold capecitabine and resume after adverse events resolve to G ≤1. Reduce dosage by 50%
Fourth G2 toxicity	Discontinue capecitabine
First G3 toxicity	Hold capecitabine and resume after adverse events resolve to G ≤1. Reduce dosage by 25%
Second G3 toxicity	Hold capecitabine and resume after adverse events resolve to G ≤1. Reduce dosage by 50%
Third G3 toxicity	Discontinue capecitabine
First G4 toxicity	Hold capecitabine and resume after adverse events resolve to G ≤1. Reduce dosage by 50%
Second G4 toxicity	Discontinue capecitabine
LVEF has declined by ≥16 percentage points from baseline, or has declined by 10–15 percentage points from baseline to a value below the lower limit of the normal range OR Symptomatic congestive heart failure	Withhold trastuzumab and repeat LVEF assessment at 4-week intervals until improvement, which may require prolonged interruption. Discontinue trastuzumab if the LVEF does not improve or if it declines further, unless the benefits for the individual patient outweigh the risks

(continued)

- Initial adult dose is 2 tablets 4 times daily until control has been achieved, after which the dose may be reduced to meet individual requirements. Control may often be maintained with as little as 2 tablets daily
- Clinical improvement of acute diarrhea is usually observed within 48 hours. If improvement of chronic diarrhea after treatment with a maximum daily dose of 8 tablets is not observed within 10 days, control is unlikely with further administration

Hand-foot reaction

For patients who develop a hand-foot reaction, use topical emollients (eg, Aquaphor), topical or orally administered steroids, antihistamine agents (H_1-receptor antagonists), or pyridoxine 50–150 mg/day; administer orally

Trastuzumab infusion reactions

- A symptom complex most commonly consisting of chills and/or fever may occur in as many as 40% of patients during the first infusion of trastuzumab. These symptoms occur infrequently with subsequent trastuzumab infusions. Other signs and/or symptoms may include nausea, vomiting, pain (in some cases at tumor sites), rigors, headache, dizziness, dyspnea, hypotension, rash, and asthenia. Although the symptoms are usually mild to moderate in severity, infrequently, trastuzumab may need to be discontinued
- When such a symptom complex is observed, it can be treated with or without reduction in the rate of trastuzumab infusion, and:
  - **Acetaminophen** 650 mg; administer orally
  - **Diphenhydramine** 25–50 mg; administer orally or by intravenous injection, and
  - **Meperidine** 12.5–25 mg; administer by intravenous injection every 10 minutes if needed for shaking chills (generally, cumulative doses >50 mg are not needed; use with caution in persons with moderate or more severely impaired renal function)

Patient Population Studied

Study of 40 patients with advanced breast cancer. All had prior adjuvant or palliative anthracycline and taxane or vinorelbine treatment; further, a minimum of 1 earlier line of trastuzumab-containing therapy for metastatic disease was obligatory

Efficacy

	All Patients (N = 40)	Second Line (N = 21)	> Second Line (N = 19)
	Percentage or Duration		
Overall response rate	20	19	21.1
Complete response	2.5	—	5.3
Partial response	17.5	19	15.8
Stable disease ≥6 months	50	47.6	52.6
Stable disease <6 months	2.5	4.8	—
Progressive disease	27.5	28.6	26.3
Median time to progression	8 months (95% CI: 6.07–9.93)	7 months (95% CI: 2.99–11.01)	8 months (95% CI: 5.94–10.06)
Median overall survival	24 months (95% CI: 20.23–27.77)		

Toxicity

WHO Criteria

Toxicity	% G1	% G2	% G3	% G4
Neutropenia	17.5	15	—	—
Thrombocytopenia	10	—	—	—
Anemia	45	5	—	—
Diarrhea	2.5	20	5	—
Fatigue	—	2.5	—	—
Hand-foot syndrome	10	25	15	—
Nausea/vomiting	5			
Stomatitis	2.5	5	—	—

Therapy Monitoring

1. *Days 1 and 10 of the first cycle:* Complete blood count with differential
2. *Day 1 during consecutive cycles:* Blood count with differential if no G3/G4 hematologic toxicity observed
3. Conduct thorough cardiac assessment, including history, physical examination, and determination of LVEF by echocardiogram or MUGA scan at baseline immediately prior to initiation of trastuzumab and every 3 months during therapy. In patients with metastatic disease, the frequency of post-baseline cardiac monitoring in asymptomatic patients may be individualized based on the clinical judgment of the medically responsible health care provider
4. Patients should have a pre-treatment LVEF ≥55%
5. Repeat LVEF measurement at 4-week intervals if trastuzumab is withheld for significant left ventricular cardiac dysfunction

METASTATIC • HER2-POSITIVE

BREAST CANCER REGIMEN: TUCATINIB + CAPECITABINE + TRASTUZUMAB

Murthy RK et al. N Engl J Med 2020;382:597–609
TUKYSA (tucatinib) prescribing information. Bothell, WA: Seattle Genetics, Inc; revised 2020 April

Tucatinib 300 mg per dose; administer orally twice per day (approximately every 12 hours), with or without food, continually on days 1–21, every 3 weeks, until disease progression (total dosage/3-week cycle = 12,600 mg)
Notes:
- Patients who miss a dose of tucatinib or who vomit after taking a dose should be instructed to take the next dose at the next regularly scheduled time
- Tucatinib tablets should be swallowed whole. Do not crush, chew, split, or dissolve tablets
- Reduce the tucatinib dose to 200 mg orally twice per day in patients with severe (Child-Pugh class C) hepatic impairment
- Tucatinib is metabolized primarily by cytochrome P450 (CYP) CYP2C8 and to a lesser degree by CYP3A
  - Avoid concurrent use with strong CYP3A4 inducers and moderate CYP2C8 inducers
  - If a strong CYP2C8 inhibitor must be administered concurrently, then decrease the tucatinib dosage to 100 mg twice per day and monitor closely for adverse events. If the strong CYP2C8 inhibitor is subsequently discontinued, then increase the tucatinib dose (after 3 plasma half-lives of the inhibitor have transpired) to the dose that was used before starting the inhibitor
- Tucatinib is a strong CYP3A4 inhibitor. Avoid concomitant use with CYP3A4 substrates that have a narrow therapeutic index
- Tucatinib inhibits P-glycoprotein (P-gp). Use caution and consider reducing the dose of P-gp substrates that have a narrow therapeutic index
- Tucatinib inhibits OCT2/MATE1-mediated transport of creatinine which may result in a reduction of renal tubular secretion of creatinine and therefore an increased serum creatinine level which may not represent a decrease in the glomerular filtration rate

Capecitabine 1000 mg/m² per dose; administer orally twice daily within 30 minutes after a meal for 14 consecutive days on days 1–14, followed by 7 days without treatment, every 3 weeks, until disease progression (total dosage/cycle = 28,000 mg/m²)
Notes:
- Doses are rounded to use combinations of 500-mg and 150-mg tablets that most closely approximate calculated values
- Initial capecitabine dosage should be decreased by 25% in patients with moderate renal impairment (baseline creatinine clearance = 30–50 mL/min [0.5–0.83 mL/s]); ie, a dosage reduction from 1000 mg/m² per dose to 750 mg/m² per dose, twice daily. Capecitabine use is contraindicated in persons with severe renal impairment (creatinine clearance <30 mL/min [<0.5 mL/s])
- Although food decreases the rate and extent of drug absorption and the time to peak plasma concentration and systemic exposure (AUC) for both capecitabine and fluorouracil, product labeling recommends giving capecitabine within 30 minutes after the end of a meal because established safety and efficacy data are based on administration with food

Trastuzumab 8 mg/kg initial (loading) dose; administer intravenously in 250 mL sodium chloride injection (0.9% NS) over at least 90 minutes once on day 1 of cycle 1 only (total initial loading dosage = 8 mg/kg), *followed 3 weeks later by:*

Trastuzumab 6 mg/kg per dose; administer intravenously in 250 mL 0.9% NS over 30–90 minutes on day 1, every 3 weeks beginning with cycle 2, until disease progression (total dosage/3-week cycle in cycle 2 and beyond = 6 mg/kg)
Notes:
- Administration duration may be decreased from 90 to 30 minutes if administration over longer durations is well tolerated
- If a patient misses a 6 mg/kg trastuzumab dose by more than 7 days, a re-loading dose of trastuzumab should be given as trastuzumab 8 mg/kg (loading dose); administer intravenously in 250 mL 0.9% NS over 90 minutes once. This should be followed 21 days later by resumption of 6-mg/kg maintenance doses repeated every 3 weeks

Supportive Care
Antiemetic prophylaxis
Emetogenic potential of capecitabine is **MINIMAL–LOW**
Emetogenic potential of tucatinib is **MODERATE–HIGH.** Due to the continuous, twice-daily schedule of tucatinib administration, an individualized approach is recommended to determine if a patient requires prophylactic antiemetic premedication or, more simply, an antiemetic medication administered on an as-needed basis
Emetogenic potential of trastuzumab is **MINIMAL–LOW**
See Chapter 42 for antiemetic recommendations

Hematopoietic growth factor (CSF) prophylaxis
Primary prophylaxis is **NOT** indicated
See Chapter 43 for more information

(continued)

(*continued*)

Antimicrobial prophylaxis
Risk of fever and neutropenia is **LOW**
  Antimicrobial primary prophylaxis to be considered:
  • Antibacterial—not indicated

  • Antifungal—not indicated

  • Antiviral—not indicated, unless patient previously had an episode of HSV

Diarrhea management
  Loperamide 4 mg orally initially after the first loose or liquid stool, *then*
  Loperamide 2 mg orally every 2 hours during waking hours, *plus*
  Loperamide 4 mg orally every 4 hours during hours of sleep
  • Continue for at least 12 hours after diarrhea resolves

  • Recurrent diarrhea after a 12-hour diarrhea-free interval is treated as a new episode

  • Rehydrate orally with fluids and electrolytes during a diarrheal episode

  • If a patient develops blood or mucus in stool, dehydration, or hemodynamic instability, or if diarrhea persists >48 hours despite loperamide, stop loperamide and evaluate urgently in clinic or hospitalize the patient for IV hydration

  • Alternatively, a trial of **diphenoxylate hydrochloride** 2.5 mg with **atropine sulfate** 0.025 mg (eg, Lomotil)

  • Initial adult dose is 2 tablets 4 times daily until control has been achieved, after which the dose may be reduced to meet individual requirements. Control may often be maintained with as little as 2 tablets daily

  • Clinical improvement of acute diarrhea is usually observed within 48 hours. If improvement of chronic diarrhea after treatment with a maximum daily dose of 8 tablets is not observed within 10 days, control is unlikely with further administration

Hand-foot reaction
For patients who develop a hand-foot reaction, use topical emollients (eg, Aquaphor), topical or orally administered steroids, antihistamine agents (H_1-receptor antagonists), or pyridoxine 50–150 mg/day; administer orally

Trastuzumab infusion reactions
• A symptom complex most commonly consisting of chills and/or fever may occur in as many as 40% of patients during the first infusion of trastuzumab. These symptoms occur infrequently with subsequent trastuzumab infusions. Other signs and/or symptoms may include nausea, vomiting, pain (in some cases at tumor sites), rigors, headache, dizziness, dyspnea, hypotension, rash, and asthenia. Although the symptoms are usually mild to moderate in severity, infrequently, trastuzumab may need to be discontinued

• When such a symptom complex is observed, it can be treated with or without reduction in the rate of trastuzumab infusion, and:

  ▪ **Acetaminophen** 650 mg; administer orally

  ▪ **Diphenhydramine** 25–50 mg; administer orally or by intravenous injection, and

  ▪ **Meperidine** 12.5–25 mg; administer by intravenous injection every 10 minutes if needed for shaking chills (generally, cumulative doses >50 mg are not needed; use with caution in persons with moderate or more severely impaired renal function)

Patient Population Studied

The HER2CLIMB study was a phase 2, international, double-blind, placebo-controlled study which randomized patients with HER2-positive advanced breast cancer 2:1 to either tucatinib (n = 320) vs placebo (n = 160), each in combination with trastuzumab and capecitabine. Prior treatment with trastuzumab, pertuzumab, and ado-trastuzumab emtansine was required. The presence of brain metastases were not an exclusion criterion, though symptomatic patients were required to undergo local therapy prior to enrolling. Likewise, patients with brain metastases >2 cm required approval by the medical monitor prior to enrolling. The primary outcome of the study was progression-free survival (PFS) in the first 480 patients enrolled. Secondary outcomes applied to the total population (n = 612 patients) and included overall survival, PFS in patients with brain metastases, confirmed objective response rate, and safety. In the tucatinib arm (n = 410), the median (range) number of prior therapies was 4 (2–14), and 46% of patients had the presence or history of brain metastases at baseline

Efficacy (N = 612)

Efficacy Variable	Tucatinib Arm (n = 410 total population)	Placebo Arm (n = 202 total population)	Between-group Comparison
PFS in Primary End Point Analysis Population (n = 320 tucatinib arm, n = 160 placebo arm)			
Median PFS—months (95% CI)	7.8 (7.5–9.6)	5.6 (4.2–7.1)	HR 0.54 (95% CI, 0.42–0.71); P<0.001*
PFS rate at 1 year—% (95% CI)	33.1 (26.6–39.7)	12.3 (6.0–20.9)	—
OS in the Total Trial Population (n = 410 tucatinib arm, n = 202 placebo arm)			
Median OS—months (95% CI)	21.9 (18.3–31.0)	17.4 (13.6–19.9)	HR 0.66 (95% CI, 0.50–0.88); P = 0.005†
OS rate at 2 years—% (95% CI)	44.9 (36.6–52.8)	26.6 (15.7–38.7)	—
PFS in Patients with Brain Metastases (n = 198 tucatinib arm, n = 93 placebo arm)			
Median PFS—months (95% CI)	7.6 (6.2–9.5)	5.4 (4.1–5.7)	HR 0.48 (95% CI, 0.34–0.69); P<0.001‡
Response§ in Patients with Measurable Disease (n = 340 tucatinib arm, n = 171 placebo arm)			
ORR—n/N (%) [95% CI]	138/340 (40.6) [35.3–46.0]	39/171 (22.8) [16.7–29.8]	P = 0.00008ǀ
CR—n/N (%)	3/340 (0.9)	2/171 (1.2)	—
PR—n/N (%)	135/340 (39.7)	37/171 (21.6)	—
SD—n/N (%)	155/340 (45.6)	100/171 (58.5)	—
PD—n/N (%)	27/340 (7.9)	24/171 (14.0)	—
NE—n/N (%)	0	1/171 (0.6)	—
NA—n/N (%)	20/340 (5.9)	7/171 (4.1)	—

*Two-sided alpha level of 0.05
†Multiplicity-adjusted two-sided alpha level of 0.007 at the first interim analysis
‡Multiplicity-adjusted two-sided alpha level of 0.008 at the first interim analysis
§Blinded independent central review, RECIST v1.1
ǀStratified Cochran-Mantel-Haenszel test
PFS, progression-free survival; CI, confidence interval; HR, hazard ratio; OS, overall survival; ORR, objective response rate; CR, complete response; PR, partial response; SD, stable disease; PD, progressive disease; NE, not evaluable; NA, not available
Note: At the data cutoff date of 4 September 2019, the median follow-up in the total population was 14.0 months

Therapy Monitoring

1. *Prior to therapy in females of reproductive potential:* pregnancy test
2. *Day 1 of each cycle:* CBC with differential, total bilirubin, ALT, AST, BUN, serum creatinine
   a. Consider more frequent monitoring of CBC with differential and liver function tests as clinically indicated
3. *Day 10 of the first cycle:* Complete blood count with differential
4. Observe closely for hypersensitivity reactions, especially during the first and second infusions
5. Conduct thorough cardiac assessment, including history, physical examination, and determination of LVEF by echocardiogram or MUGA scan at baseline immediately prior to initiation of trastuzumab. In patients with metastatic disease, the frequency of post-baseline cardiac monitoring in asymptomatic patients may be individualized based on the clinical judgment of the medically responsible health care provider
   a. Patients should have a pre-treatment LVEF ≥55%
   b. Repeat LVEF measurement at 4-week intervals if trastuzumab is withheld for significant left ventricular cardiac dysfunction
6. *Monitor periodically for symptoms of:* palmar plantar erythrodysesthesia, diarrhea, nausea, vomiting, coronary vasospasm, and stomatitis

Treatment Modifications

TRASTUZUMAB TREATMENT MODIFICATIONS

Adverse Event	Dose Modification
Mild or moderate infusion reaction*	Decrease the rate of infusion
Infusion reaction with dyspnea or clinically significant hypotension	Interrupt the infusion. Administer medical therapy as indicated including epinephrine, corticosteroids, diphenhydramine, bronchodilators, and oxygen. Observe patients closely for 60 minutes if the reaction occurs after the first infusion and for 30 minutes if it occurs after subsequent infusions. Prior to resumption of the trastuzumab infusion, premedicate with antihistamines and/or corticosteroids *Note:* While some patients tolerate the resumption of trastuzumab infusions, others have recurrent severe infusion reactions despite premedications
Severe or life-threatening infusion reaction (including bronchospasm, anaphylaxis, angioedema, hypoxia, and severe hypotension; usually reported during or immediately following the initial infusion)*	Interrupt the infusion. Administer medical therapy as indicated including epinephrine, corticosteroids, diphenhydramine, bronchodilators, and oxygen. Patients should be evaluated and carefully monitored until complete resolution of signs and symptoms. Discontinue trastuzumab
LVEF has declined by ≥16 percentage points from baseline, or has declined by 10–15 percentage points from baseline to a value below the lower limit of the normal range OR Symptomatic congestive heart failure	Withhold trastuzumab and repeat LVEF assessment at 4-week intervals until improvement, which may require prolonged interruption. Discontinue trastuzumab if the LVEF does not improve or if it declines further, unless the benefits for the individual patient outweigh the risks
Pulmonary toxicity	Discontinue trastuzumab in patients experiencing pulmonary toxicity

CAPECITABINE TREATMENT MODIFICATIONS

Adverse Event	Dose Modification
First G2 toxicity	Hold capecitabine and resume after adverse events resolve to G ≤1. No change in dosage required
Second G2 toxicity	Hold capecitabine and resume after adverse events resolve to G ≤1. Reduce dosage by 25%
Third G2 toxicity	Hold capecitabine and resume after adverse events resolve to G ≤1. Reduce dosage by 50%
Fourth G2 toxicity	Discontinue capecitabine
First G3 toxicity	Hold capecitabine and resume after adverse events resolve to G ≤1. Reduce dosage by 25%
Second G3 toxicity	Hold capecitabine and resume after adverse events resolve to G ≤1. Reduce dosage by 50%
Third G3 toxicity	Discontinue capecitabine
First G4 toxicity	Hold capecitabine and resume after adverse events resolve to G ≤1. Reduce dosage by 50%
Second G4 toxicity	Discontinue capecitabine

TUCATINIB TREATMENT MODIFICATIONS

Tucatinib Dose Levels

Starting dose	300 mg orally twice daily
Dose level −1	250 mg orally twice daily
Dose level −2	200 mg orally twice daily
Dose level −3	150 mg orally twice daily
Dose level −4	Discontinue tucatinib

Adverse Event	Dose Modification
	Diarrhea
G3[†] diarrhea without anti-diarrheal treatment	Initiate or optimize appropriate medical therapy. Withhold tucatinib until recovery to G ≤1, then resume tucatinib at the same dose level
G3[†] diarrhea with anti-diarrheal treatment	Initiate or optimize appropriate medical therapy. Withhold tucatinib until recovery to G ≤1, then resume tucatinib with the dosage reduced by 1 dose level
G4[†] diarrhea	Permanently discontinue tucatinib

(*continued*)

Treatment Modifications (*continued*)

Hepatotoxicity

G2 bilirubin (>1.5 to 3× ULN)	Withhold tucatinib until recovery to G ≤1, then resume tucatinib at the same dose level
G3 ALT or AST (>5 to 20× ULN) or G3 bilirubin (>3 to 10× ULN)	Withhold tucatinib until recovery to G ≤1, then resume tucatinib with the dosage reduced by 1 dose level
G4 ALT or AST (>20× ULN) OR G4 bilirubin (>10X× ULN)	Permanently discontinue tucatinib
ALT or AST >3× ULN AND Bilirubin >2× ULN	Permanently discontinue tucatinib

Other Adverse Reactions

G3[†] other adverse reaction	Withhold tucatinib until recovery to G ≤1, then resume tucatinib with the dosage reduced by 1 dose level
G4[†] other adverse reaction	Permanently discontinue tucatinib

*Infusion reactions consist of a symptom complex characterized by fever and chills, and on occasion included nausea, vomiting, pain (in some cases at tumor sites), headache, dizziness, dyspnea, hypotension, rash, and asthenia
[†]Graded according to the National Cancer Institute Common Terminology Criteria for Adverse Events Version 4.03
LVEF, left ventricular ejection fraction; ULN, upper limit of normal; ALT, alanine aminotransferase; AST, aspartate aminotransferase

Toxicity (N = 601)

Event*	Tucatinib Arm (n = 404)		Placebo Arm (n = 197)	
Grade (%)	Grade 1–2	Grade ≥3	Grade 1–2	Grade ≥3
Any adverse event	99.3	55.2	97.0	48.7
Diarrhea	80.9	12.9	53.3	8.6
PPE syndrome	63.4	13.1	52.8	9.1
Nausea	58.4	3.7	43.7	3.0
Fatigue	45.0	4.7	43.1	4.1
Vomiting	35.9	3.0	25.4	3.6
Stomatitis	25.5	2.5	14.2	0.5
Decreased appetite	24.8	0.5	19.8	0
Headache	21.5	0.5	20.3	1.5
AST increased	21.3	4.5	11.2	0.5
ALT increased	20.0	5.4	6.6	0.5

*Adverse events were defined according to the Medical Dictionary for Regulatory Activities, version 22.0 and graded according to the National Cancer Institute Common Terminology Criteria for Adverse Events, version 4.03
Note: Adverse events (AEs) are included in the table if they were reported in ≥20% of patients in the tucatinib arm. AEs led to discontinuation of tucatinib in 5.7% of patients, to discontinuation of placebo in 3.0%, to discontinuation of capecitabine in 9.8% (10.1% in the tucatinib arm and 9.1% in the placebo arm). Serum creatinine increased in 13.9% of the patients in the tucatinib arm and in 1.5% in the placebo arm, presumably due to inhibition of MATE1 and MATE2-K
PPE, palmar-plantar erythrodysesthesia; AST, aspartate aminotransferase; ALT, alanine aminotransferase

METASTATIC • HER2-POSITIVE

BREAST CANCER REGIMEN: FAM-TRASTUZUMAB DERUXTECAN

Modi S et al. N Engl J Med 2020;382:610–621
Protocol for: Modi S et al. N Engl J Med 2020;382:610–621
Supplementary appendix to: Modi S et al. N Engl J Med 2020;382:610–621
ENHURTU (fam-trastuzumab deruxtecan-nxki) prescribing information. Basking Ridge, NJ: Daiichi Sankyo, Inc; 2019 December

fam-Trastuzumab deruxtecan-nxki 5.4 mg/kg; administer intravenously in 100 mL 5% dextrose injection (D5W) on day 1, every 21 days, until disease progression (total dosage/3-week cycle = 5.4 mg/kg)

Exposure	Administration Rate	Monitoring
First infusion	Intravenously over 90 minutes	• Patients should be observed closely for infusion-related reactions, especially during the first infusion • Administration should be slowed or interrupted if a patient develops an infusion-related reaction • Permanently discontinue fam-trastuzumab deruxtecan-nxki for severe infusion-related reactions
Second and subsequent infusions	1. Intravenously over 30 minutes if prior administration was tolerated 2. Subsequent doses may be administered at the rate tolerated during the most recently administered treatment	

Note:
• Prepare fam-trastuzumab deruxtecan-nxki in an infusion bag composed of polyvinyl chloride or polyolefin; protect the infusion bag from light
• Administer fam-trastuzumab deruxtecan-nxki through an administration set composed of either polyolefin or polybutadiene that contains an in-line polyethersulfone or polysulfone filter with pore size of either 0.20 or 0.22 μm

Supportive Care
Antiemetic prophylaxis
Emetogenic potential is **MODERATE**
See Chapter 42 for antiemetic recommendations

Hematopoietic growth factor (CSF) prophylaxis
Primary prophylaxis is **NOT** *indicated*
See Chapter 43 for more information

Antimicrobial prophylaxis
Risk of fever and neutropenia is **LOW**
   Antimicrobial primary prophylaxis to be considered:
   • Antibacterial—not indicated
   • Antifungal—not indicated
   • Antiviral—not indicated, unless patient previously had an episode of HSV

Patient Population Studied

DESTINY-Breast01 was a two-part, open-label, single-group, multicenter, international, phase 2 registration study evaluating trastuzumab deruxtecan in adults with HER2-positive advanced breast cancer who had received prior ado-trastuzumab emtansine. Patients were required to have an Eastern Cooperative Oncology Group performance status of ≤1 and a left ventricular ejection fraction of ≥50%. Patients were excluded if they had untreated or symptomatic brain metastases, a history of interstitial lung disease (ILD)/pneumonitis requiring steroids or current ILD/pneumonitis. Part 1 of the study included a pharmacokinetics stage (dose levels of 5.4 mg/kg [n = 22], 6.4 mg/kg [n = 22], and 7.4 mg/kg [n = 21]) and a dose-finding stage (5.4 mg/kg [n = 28] and 6.4 mg/kg [n = 26]). Part 2 of the study evaluated efficacy and safety of the recommended dose of 5.4 mg/kg (n = 134) in patients who had experienced disease progression during or following prior ado-trastuzumab emtansine (part 2a, n = 130) or who had discontinued ado-trastuzumab due to other reasons (part 2b, n = 4). Among the 184 patients in the primary efficacy population who received the recommended dose of 5.4 mg/kg and who had experienced progression during or following ado-trastuzumab emtansine, the median (range) age was 55 (28–96) years, 23.9% were age ≥65 years, 52.7% had hormone receptor–positive tumors, the median (range) number of previous therapies was 6 (2–27) and included trastuzumab emtansine (100%), trastuzumab (100%), pertuzumab (65.8%), and other anti-HER2 therapies (54.3%)

Efficacy (N =184)

Efficacy Variable	fam-Trastuzumab Deruxtecan (n = 184)*
Confirmed Responses† (n = 184)*	
ORR—% (95% CI)	60.9 (53.4–68.0)
Partial response—%	54.9
Complete response—%	6.0
Median TTR—months (95% CI)	1.6 (1.4–2.6)
Median DOR—months (95% CI)	14.8 (13.8–16.9)
Disease control rate‡—% (95% CI)	97.3 (93.8–99.1)
Clinical benefit rate§—% (95% CI)	76.1 (69.3–82.1)
Progressive disease—%	1.6
Not evaluable—%	1.1
Survival (n = 184)*	
Median PFS—months (95% CI)	16.4 (12.7–NR)
OS at 6 months—% (95% CI)	93.9 (89.3–96.6)
OS at 12 months—% (95% CI)	86.2 (79.8–90.7)
PFS (n = 24 patients with baseline treated and asymptomatic brain metastases)	
Median PFS—months (95% CI)	18.1 (6.7–18.1)

*184 patients who were treated at a dose of 5.4 mg/kg and had experienced disease progression during or after prior ado-trastuzumab emtansine therapy
†Per independent central review using modified Response Evaluation Criteria in Solid Tumors version 1.1
‡Disease control rate included patients with stable disease, partial response, or complete response
§Clinical benefit rate included patients with stable disease lasting ≥6 months, partial response, or complete response
ORR, objective response rate; CI, confidence interval; TTR, time to response; DOR, duration of response; PFS, progression-free survival; NR, not reached; OS, overall survival
Note: The data cutoff date for this analysis was 1 August 2019 at which time the median (range) follow-up was 11.1 (0.7–19.9) months

Therapy Monitoring

1. *Prior to initiation of therapy in females of reproductive potential:* pregnancy test
2. *Before each cycle:* CBC with differential and platelet count
3. Conduct thorough cardiac assessment, including history, physical examination, and determination of LVEF by echocardiogram or MUGA scan at baseline immediately prior to initiation of fam-trastuzumab deruxtecan and then at regular intervals (as clinically indicated) during therapy. In patients with metastatic disease, the frequency of post-baseline cardiac monitoring in asymptomatic patients may be individualized based on the clinical judgment of the medically responsible health care provider
4. Patients should have a pre-treatment LVEF ≥50%
5. Repeat LVEF measurement at 3-week intervals if fam-trastuzumab deruxtecan is withheld for significant left ventricular cardiac dysfunction
6. Monitor periodically for signs and symptoms of interstitial lung disease (ILD)/pneumonitis such as cough, dyspnea, fatigue, and rales on chest auscultation. If ILD/pneumonitis is suspected, then evaluate promptly with radiographic imaging (eg, chest x-ray and/or CT scan) and other tests as clinically indicated. Consider consultation with a pulmonologist

Treatment Modifications

FAM-TRASTUZUMAB DERUXTECAN	
FAM-Trastuzumab Deruxtecan Dose Levels	
Starting dose	5.4 mg/kg
Dose level −1	4.4 mg/kg
Dose level −2	3.2 mg/kg
Dose level −3	Discontinue fam-trastuzumab deruxtecan

Adverse Event	Treatment Modification
	Neutropenia
G3 neutropenia (ANC <1,000/mm³ to 500/mm³)	Withhold fam-trastuzumab deruxtecan until neutrophil count improves to ≥1,000/mm³, then continue at the same dose
G4 neutropenia (ANC <500/mm³)	Withhold fam-trastuzumab deruxtecan until neutrophil count improves to ≥1,000/mm³, then continue with the dosage reduced by 1 dose level
Febrile neutropenia (ANC <1,000/mm³ and temperature >38.3°C or a sustained temperature of ≥38.0°C for more than 1 hour	Withhold fam-trastuzumab deruxtecan until resolution of febrile neutropenia, then continue with the dosage reduced by 1 dose level

(continued)

Treatment Modifications (*continued*)

Pulmonary Toxicity

Patient with cough, dyspnea, fever, and/or any signs or symptoms of new-onset or worsening respiratory dysfunction—ILD/pneumonitis is suspected	Withhold fam-trastuzumab deruxtecan while pulmonary status is clarified. Evaluate promptly with radiographic imaging (eg, chest x-ray and/or CT scan) and other tests as clinically indicated. Consider consultation with a pulmonologist
G1 (asymptomatic) ILD/pneumonitis is confirmed	Consider corticosteroid treatment (eg, ≥0.5 mg/kg/day prednisolone or equivalent initially for 2–4 weeks and then gradually tapered). Withhold fam-trastuzumab deruxtecan until resolution of ILD/pneumonitis to G0, then: If resolves in ≤28 days from the date of onset, then maintain the current dose If resolves in >28 days from the date of onset, then reduce the dosage by 1 dose level
G ≥2 or symptomatic ILD/pneumonitis is confirmed	Administer corticosteroid treatment promptly (eg, ≥1 mg/kg/day prednisolone or equivalent initially and continued until improvement, and then tapered gradually (eg, over 4 weeks). Permanently discontinue fam-trastuzumab deruxtecan

Cardiac Toxicity

Symptomatic CHF	Permanently discontinue fam-trastuzumab deruxtecan
LVEF <40% or absolute decrease from baseline is >20 percentage points	Withhold fam-trastuzumab deruxtecan. Repeat LVEF assessment within 3 weeks. If LVEF <40% or absolute decrease from baseline >20 percentage points is confirmed, then permanently discontinue fam-trastuzumab deruxtecan
LVEF 40% to ≤45%, and decrease is ≥10 and ≤20 percentage points from baseline measurement	Withhold fam-trastuzumab deruxtecan. Repeat LVEF assessment within 3 weeks. If LVEF has not recovered to within 10 percentage points from baseline, then permanently discontinue fam-trastuzumab deruxtecan. If LVEF recovers to within 10 percentage points from baseline, then resume fam-trastuzumab deruxtecan at the same dose
LVEF 40% to ≤45%, and decrease is <10 percentage points from baseline	Continue fam-trastuzumab deruxtecan treatment. Repeat LVEF assessment within 3 weeks
LVEF >45% and decrease is ≥10 and ≤20 percentage points from baseline measurement	Continue fam-trastuzumab deruxtecan at the same dose level

Infusion-Related Reactions

G1/2 infusion-related reaction (infusion interruption indicated but responds promptly to symptomatic treatment [eg, antihistamines, NSAIDs, narcotics, IV fluids]; prophylactic medications indicated for ≤24 hours; or better)	Interrupt infusion and provide supportive care as clinically indicated (eg, oxygen supplementation, inhaled beta-agonist, antihistamine, antipyretic, and/or corticosteroid). When symptoms have resolved, resume the infusion at ≤50% of the prior rate and increase by 50% increments every 30 minutes as tolerated until the rate at which the reaction occurred is reached. Administer the next infusion over 90 minutes. Consider premedication with corticosteroid, antihistamine, and/or antipyretic prior to subsequent infusions
Severe (G ≥3) infusion-related reaction (prolonged [eg, not rapidly responsive to symptomatic medication and/or brief interruption of infusion]; recurrence of symptoms following initial improvement; hospitalization indicated for clinical sequelae; or worse)	Permanently discontinue fam-trastuzumab deruxtecan

Note:
1. fam-Trastuzumab deruxtecan dosages should not be re-escalated after a dosage reduction is made
2. If a planned dose is delayed or missed, it should be administered as soon as possible. Do not wait until the next planned cycle. Administer the infusion at the rate and dose the patient tolerated in the most recent infusion. The schedule of administration should be adjusted to maintain a 3-week interval between doses
3. Grading of toxicities is per the National Cancer Institute Common Terminology Criteria for Adverse Events (NCI CTCAE) version 4.03

Adverse Events (N = 148)

Adverse event* (%)	fam-Trastuzumab Deruxtecan (N = 184)		
	Any Grade	Grade 3	Grade 4
AEs Occurring in >15% of Patients			
Any AE†	99.5	48.4	3.8
Nausea	77.7	7.6	0
Fatigue	49.5	6.0	0
Alopecia	48.4	0.5	0
Vomiting	45.7	4.3	0
Constipation	35.9	0.5	0
Decreased neutrophil count‡	34.8	19.6	1.1
Decreased appetite	31.0	1.6	0
Anemia§	29.9	8.2	0.5
Diarrhea	29.3	2.7	0
Decreased white-cell count‖	21.2	6.0	0.5
Decreased platelet count¶	21.2	3.8	0.5
Headache	19.6	0	0
Cough	19.0	0	0
Abdominal pain**	16.8	1.1	0
Decreased lymphocyte count††	14.1	6.0	0.5
Adverse Events of Special Interest			
ILD‡‡	13.6	0.5	0
Prolonged QT interval	4.9	1.1	0
IRR	2.2	0	0
Decreased LVEF§§	1.6	0.5‖	0

*Based on the National Cancer Institute Common Terminology Criteria for Adverse Events (NCI CTCAE) v4.003
†Includes AEs reported by the investigator of G ≥3 occurring in ≥6% of patients
‡Includes preferred terms neutrophil count decreased and neutropenia
§Includes preferred terms hematocrit decreased, hemoglobin decreased, red-cell count decreased, and anemia
‖Includes preferred terms white-cell count decreased and leukopenia
¶Includes preferred terms platelet count decreased and thrombocytopenia
**Includes preferred terms abdominal discomfort, abdominal pain, abdominal pain lower, and abdominal pain upper
††Includes preferred terms lymphocyte count decreased and lymphopenia
‡‡ILD was determined by an independent adjudication committee. Four patients who had grade 5 events are included in the category of any grade
§§LVEF was measured on echocardiography or multigated acquisition scans every four cycles
‖LVEF was >55% during treatment in this patient
Note: AEs G ≥3 occurred in 57.1% of patients, the most common of which were neutropenia, anemia, nausea, leukopenia, lymphopenia, and fatigue. Neutropenic fever occurred in 1.6% of patients. AEs led to dose interruption in 35.3% of patients, to dose reduction in 23.4%, and to permanent discontinuation in 15.2%. AEs that led to permanent discontinuation in ≥2 patients included pneumonitis (n = 11), and ILD (n = 5). Therapy-related ILD occurred in 25 (13.6%) patients; 10.9% were G1/2, 0.5% were G3, there were no G4 events, and 2.2% (n = 4) were G5. Median (range) time to ILD onset was 193 (42–535) days. At data cutoff, the status of the patients with ILD was: recovered (n = 7), recovery (n = 2), ongoing (n = 10), died (n = 4) and unknown (n = 2). Median (range) duration of ILD was 34 (3–179) days
AE, adverse event; ILD, interstitial lung disease; IRR, infusion-related reaction; LVEF, left ventricular ejection fraction

METASTATIC • TRIPLE-NEGATIVE

BREAST CANCER REGIMEN: SINGLE-AGENT PLATINUM (CARBOPLATIN OR CISPLATIN)

Isakoff SJ et al. J Clin Oncol 2015;33:1902–1909

Select either carboplatin or cisplatin:

Hydration for cisplatin: 0.9% sodium chloride injection (0.9% NS), ≥1000 mL before and after cisplatin; administer intravenously over a minimum of 2–4 hours. Encourage patients to increase oral nonalcoholic fluid intake. Monitor and replace magnesium/electrolytes as needed

Cisplatin 75 mg/m²; administer intravenously in 1000 mL 0.9% NS over 1–2 hours on day 1 every 3 weeks until disease progression (total dosage/cycle = 75 mg/m²)
or
Carboplatin target AUC = 6 mg/mL × min; administer intravenously in 250 mL 5% dextrose injection (D5W) or 0.9% NS over 30–60 minutes on day 1 every 3 weeks until disease progression (total dose/cycle calculated to achieve a target AUC = 6 mg/mL × min)

Carboplatin dose

Carboplatin dose is based on a formula described by Calvert et al. to achieve a target area under the plasma concentration versus time curve (AUC):

$$\text{Total carboplatin dose (mg)} = (\text{target AUC})(\text{GFR} + 25)$$

In practice, creatinine clearance (CrCl) is used in place of glomerular filtration rate (GFR). CrCl can be estimated from the equation of Cockcroft and Gault, thus:

$$\text{For males, CrCl} = \frac{(140 - \text{age[years]}) \times (\text{body weight [kg]})}{72 \times (\text{serum creatinine [mg/dL]})}$$

$$\text{For males, CrCl} = \frac{(140 - \text{age[years]}) \times (\text{body weight [kg]})}{72 \times (\text{serum creatinine [mg/dL]})}$$

Calvert AH et al. J Clin Oncol 1989;7:1748–1756
Cockcroft DW, Gault MH. Nephron 1976;16:31–41
Jodrell DI et al. J Clin Oncol 1992;10:520–528
Sorensen BT et al. Cancer Chemother Pharmacol 1991;28:397–401

Note: On October 8, 2010, the U.S. Food and Drug Administration (FDA) identified a potential safety issue with carboplatin dosing based on recent changes in the measurement of serum creatinine. By the end of 2010, all clinical laboratories in the United States will use the standardized isotope dilution mass spectrometry (IDMS) method to measure serum creatinine, which could result in an overestimation of the GFR in some patients with normal renal function. A carboplatin dose calculated with an IDMS-measured serum creatinine result using the Calvert formula could exceed an expected exposure (AUC) and result in increased drug-related toxicity. Provided actual GFR measurements are made to assess renal function, carboplatin can be safely dosed according to the Calvert formula described in product labeling. If GFR (or creatinine clearance) is estimated based on serum creatinine measurements by the IDMS method, the FDA recommended for patients with normal renal function capping an estimated GFR at 125 mL/min for any targeted AUC value. No greater estimated GFR values should be used.

Supportive Care

Antiemetic prophylaxis
Emetogenic potential: **HIGH**. Potential for delayed symptoms
See Chapter 42 for antiemetic recommendations

Hematopoietic growth factor (CSF) prophylaxis
Primary prophylaxis is not indicated
See Chapter 43 for more information

Antimicrobial prophylaxis
Risk of fever and neutropenia is **LOW**
    Antimicrobial primary prophylaxis to be considered:
    • Antibacterial—not indicated
    • Antifungal—not indicated
    • Antiviral—not indicated, unless patient previously had an episode of HSV

Patient Population Studied

The multicenter, open-label, single-arm, phase 2 trial involved 86 patients with metastatic or locally recurrent, unresectable, triple-negative breast cancer. Eligible patients had an Eastern Cooperative Oncology Group (ECOG) performance status score ≤2 and life expectancy >12 weeks. Patients who had more than one prior cytotoxic chemotherapy treatment for metastatic disease, or had previously undergone cisplatin or carboplatin therapy, were not eligible. Patients received either cisplatin (75 mg/m²) or carboplatin (at dose 6 area under the curve) once every 3 weeks, with treatment chosen at the discretion of the treating physician. After cycle 1, growth factors were permitted and treatment cycles could be extended to 4 weeks, at the discretion of the treating physician. Oral magnesium and potassium supplementation was encouraged. Treatment continued until disease progression, unacceptable adverse effects, or withdrawal of consent

Efficacy (N = 86)

Overall response rate*	25.6%
Median progression-free survival	2.9 months
Median overall survival	11.0 months

*Overall response rate includes patients with either a complete or partial response to treatment
Note: Median follow-up was 49.9 months. Overall response rates did not differ significantly between the patients taking cisplatin and those taking carboplatin (32.6% vs 18.6%; P = 0.22)

Therapy Monitoring

1. Monitor CBC with differential, BUN, creatinine, and electrolytes. Obtain prior to the start of each cycle, and 10–14 days after a dose for the first 2 cycles. For patients who experience any neutropenia or thrombocytopenia in the first 2 cycles, continue monitoring CBC with differential 10–14 days after a dose in subsequent cycles and as clinically indicated

2. Monitor for neuropathy and hearing loss clinically and with ancillary studies as clinically indicated (especially with cisplatin)

3. Response assessment: imaging studies every 6–12 weeks

Treatment Modifications

CISPLATIN

Adverse Event	Treatment Modification
G2 hematologic toxicities (ANC <1500/mm³, hemoglobin <8.5 g/dL, or platelets <75,000/mm³) within 24 hours of scheduled start of a cycle	Delay start of cycle. Resume cisplatin when ANC ≥1500/mm³, hemoglobin ≥8.5 g/dL, and platelets ≥100,000/mm³. If after 3 weeks ANC <1500/mm³, hemoglobin <8.5 g/dL, or platelets <100,000/mm³, then discontinue treatment
G3 hematologic toxicities (ANC <1000/mm³ or platelets count <50,000/mm³) at any time during a cycle	Hold therapy until abnormal value returns to baseline. Then decrease cisplatin dosage by 25% or, if platelet count was acceptable and G3 toxicity was due to low neutrophil count, administer filgrastim support and monitor carefully
G4 hematologic toxicities (ANC <500/mm³ or platelets count <25,000/mm³) at any time during a cycle	Hold therapy until abnormal value returns to baseline. Then decrease cisplatin dosage by 50% or, if platelet count was acceptable and G3 toxicity was due to low neutrophil count, reduce dosage by 25% and administer filgrastim support with careful monitoring
Serum creatinine ≥1.5 mg/dL (≥130 μmol/L) and/or BUN ≥25 mg/dL (≥8.92 mmol/L)	Withhold cisplatin until serum creatinine <1.5 mg/dL (<130 μmol/L) and BUN <25 mg/dL (<8.92 mmol/L). Then consider a decrease in cisplatin dosage by 25%
Peripheral neuropathy of G ≥3	Permanently discontinue cisplatin
Cisplatin induced hearing loss G ≥3	
Occurrence of an adverse event requiring a third dose reduction	
Significant hypersensitivity reaction to cisplatin (hypotension, dyspnea, and angioedema requiring therapy) *Note:* Allergic reaction to cisplatin including anaphylaxis risk is increased in patients previously exposed to platinum therapy	May occur within minutes of administration. Interrupt the infusion in patients with clinically significant infusion reactions. Discontinue therapy or consider desensitization and a rechallenge
Other G ≥3 nonhematologic toxicities (except nausea, vomiting, elevated transaminases, and alopecia)	Delay treatment until toxicity resolves to baseline, then decrease cisplatin dose by 25% from previous dose level

CARBOPLATIN

Starting dose	AUC 6
Dose level −1	AUC 5
Dose level −2	AUC 4

Adverse Event	Treatment Modification
G2 hematologic toxicities (ANC <1500/mm³, hemoglobin <8.5 g/dL, or platelets <75,000/mm³) within 24 hours of scheduled start of a cycle	Delay start of cycle. Resume treatment when ANC ≥1500/mm³, hemoglobin ≥8.5 g/dL, or platelets ≥75,000/mm³. If after 3 weeks ANC <1500/mm³, hemoglobin <8.5 g/dL, or platelets <80,000/mm³, then discontinue treatment
G3 hematologic toxicities (ANC <1,000/mm³ or platelets count <50,000/mm³) at any time during a cycle	Hold therapy until returns to baseline. Then decrease carboplatin dosage by one dose level or, if platelet count was acceptable and G3 toxicity was due to low neutrophil count, administer filgrastim support and monitor carefully
G4 hematologic toxicities (ANC <500/mm³ or platelets count <25,000/mm³) at any time during a cycle	Hold therapy until returns to baseline. Then decrease carboplatin dosage by two dose levels or, if platelet count was acceptable and G3 toxicity was due to low neutrophil count, reduce dosage by one dose level and administer filgrastim support with careful monitoring
Severe (G3/4) nonhematologic toxicities, except nausea/vomiting	Hold or decrease by 50% depending on clinical judgment
Significant hypersensitivity reaction to carboplatin (hypotension, dyspnea, and angioedema requiring therapy) *Note:* Allergic reaction to carboplatin including anaphylaxis risk is increased in patients previously exposed to platinum therapy	May occur within minutes of administration. Interrupt the infusion in patients with clinically significant infusion reactions. Discontinue therapy or consider desensitization and a rechallenge

Adverse Events (N = 86)

Grade (%)*	All patients (N = 86)		Cisplatin (N = 43)		Carboplatin (N =43)	
	Grade 1–2	Grade 3–4	Grade 1–2	Grade 3–4	Grade 1–2	Grade 3–4
Hemoglobin	67	6	79	2	56	9
Fatigue	58	8	56	12	60	5
Hyperglycemia	41	6	44	5	37	7
Neutropenia	35	7	44	5	26	9
Dyspnea	23	6	23	7	23	5
Hyponatremia	13	5	14	7	12	2

*According to the National Cancer Institute Common Terminology Criteria for Adverse Events, version 3.0
Toxicities are included in the table if grade 3–4 events occurred in ≥5% of patients. No treatment-related deaths were reported. Treatment discontinuation owing to treatment-related adverse effects occurred in 10 patients

METASTATIC • TRIPLE-NEGATIVE

BREAST CANCER REGIMEN: ATEZOLIZUMAB + NAB-PACLITAXEL

Schmid P et al. N Engl J Med 2018;379:2108–2121
Protocol for: Schmid P et al. N Engl J Med 2018;379:2108–2121
Supplementary appendix to: Schmid P et al. N Engl J Med 2018;379:2108–2121
Tecentriq (atezolizumab) prescribing information. South San Francisco, CA: Genentech, Inc; revised 2019 March
Abraxane (paclitaxel protein-bound particles for injectable suspension) prescribing information. Summit, NJ: Celgene Corporation; revised 2018 August

Regimen note: The U.S. Food and Drug Administration (FDA) limits approval of this regimen to patients with unresectable locally advanced or metastatic triple-negative breast cancer whose tumors express PD-L1 (PD-L1-stained tumor-infiltrating immune cells of any intensity covering ≥1% of the tumor area), as determined by an FDA-approved test

Atezolizumab 840 mg per dose; administer intravenously in 250 mL 0.9% sodium chloride injection, USP, over 60 minutes, for 2 doses on day 1 and 15, prior to nab-paclitaxel, every 28 days, until disease progression (total dosage/4-week cycle = 1680 mg)
Notes:

- Atezolizumab may be administered through an administration set either with or without a low-protein binding in-line filter with pore size within the range of 0.2–0.22 μm

- If the initial infusion is well tolerated, subsequent administration may be completed over 30 minutes

- Severe infusion-related reactions have occurred in patients in clinical trials of atezolizumab

  - Interrupt or slow the administration rate in patients with mild or moderate infusion-related reactions

  - Permanently discontinue atezolizumab in patients who experience infusion reactions G ≥3

Paclitaxel protein-bound particles for injectable suspension (albumin-bound paclitaxel, nab-paclitaxel) 100 mg/m² per dose; administer intravenously (undiluted) over 30 minutes for 3 doses on days 1, 8, and 15, every 28 days (total dosage/4-week cycle = 300 mg/m²)
  Note: The protocol states that in the absence of disease progression or unacceptable toxicity, a target of 6 cycles of nab-paclitaxel should be administered, with no mandated maximum number of cycles. Patients in the atezolizumab plus nab-paclitaxel arm of the study who had PD-L1-positive tumors received a median of 6 (range, 1–34) cycles of nab-paclitaxel and a median of 7 (range, 1–35) cycles of atezolizumab (Supplementary appendix to Schmid et al, 2018)

Supportive Care
Antiemetic prophylaxis
Emetogenic potential on days with nab-paclitaxel and/or atezolizumab is **LOW**
See Chapter 42 for antiemetic recommendations

Hematopoietic growth factor (CSF) prophylaxis
Primary prophylaxis is **NOT** *indicated*
See Chapter 43 for more information

Antimicrobial prophylaxis
Risk of fever and neutropenia is **LOW**
  Antimicrobial primary prophylaxis to be considered:
  - Antibacterial—not indicated

  - Antifungal—not indicated

  - Antiviral—not indicated, unless patient previously had an episode of HSV

Patient Population Studied

The multicenter, multinational, randomized, placebo-controlled, phase 3 study involved 902 patients with untreated, metastatic or locally advanced unresectable, triple-negative breast cancer. Eligible patients were aged ≥18 years, with an Eastern Cooperative Oncology Group (ECOG) performance status score ≤1, and adequate organ and bone marrow function. Patients with brain metastases were excluded unless they were previously treated, asymptomatic, and not requiring ongoing treatment with dexamethasone. Patients with history of autoimmune disease, history of prior allogeneic transplant, HIV infection, active hepatitis B or C infection, active tuberculosis infection, or those receiving systemic steroids or immunosuppressants were ineligible. Patients were randomized 1:1 to receive albumin-bound paclitaxel plus atezolizumab, or albumin-bound paclitaxel plus placebo, until disease progression. Patients without toxicity or disease progression were targeted to receive at least 6 cycles of albumin-bound paclitaxel, with no limit on the maximum number of allowable cycles. Patients were stratified by prior receipt of taxane therapy in the neoadjuvant or adjuvant setting, presence of liver metastases, and PD-L1 expression on tumor-infiltrating immune cells (expressed as a percentage of tumor area [<1%, PD-L1 negative; ≥1%, PD-L1 positive])

Efficacy (N = 902)

	nab-Paclitaxel + Atezolizumab (N = 451, Intention-to-treat Population; n = 185, PD-L1-positive Subgroup)	nab-Paclitaxel + Placebo (N = 451, Intention-to-treat Population; n = 184, PD-L1-positive Subgroup)	
Median progression-free survival in the intention-to-treat population	7.2 months	5.5 months	HR 0.80 (95% CI 0.69–0.92); P = 0.0025
Median progression-free survival in the PD-L1-positive subgroup	7.5 months	5.0 months	HR 0.62 (95% CI 0.49–0.78); P<0.001
Median overall survival in the intention-to-treat population	21.3 months	17.6 months	HR 0.87 (95% CI 0.69–1.02); P = 0.08
Median overall survival in the PD-L1-positive subgroup	25.0 months	15.5 months	HR 0.62 (95% CI 0.45–0.86)
Objective response rate in the intention-to-treat population*	56%	45.9%	OR 1.52 (95% CI 1.16–1.97); P = 0.002‡
Median duration of response in the intention-to-treat population†	7.4 months	5.6 months	HR 0.78 (95% CI 0.63–0.98)
Objective response rate in the PD-L1-positive subgroup*	58.9%	42.6%	OR 1.96 (95% CI 1.29–2.98); P = 0.002‡
Median duration of response in the PD-L1-positive subgroup†	8.5 months	5.5 months	HR 0.60 (95% CI 0.43–0.86)

**Objective response rate* was evaluated by the investigators according to the Response Evaluation Criteria in Solid Tumors, version 1.1
†Determined for those patients who experienced an objective response
‡Not statistically significant due to alpha level set at 0.001
Note: Median follow-up time was 13.0 months in the nab-paclitaxel plus atezolizumab group and 12.5 months in the nab-paclitaxel plus placebo group. 2.9 months in the intention to treat population 11.9 months in the carfilzomib group and 11.1 months in the bortezomib group

Therapy Monitoring

1. *Prior to each dose of nab-paclitaxel:* CBC with differential and platelet count, liver function tests, neurologic exam
2. *Monitoring for atezolizumab:*
   a. Initially at the time of each atezolizumab dose, and eventually every 6–12 weeks, perform a total body skin examination with attention to ALL mucous membranes as well as a complete review of systems
   b. Monitor patients for signs and symptoms of pneumonitis. Evaluate patients with suspected pneumonitis with chest x-ray, CT, and pulse oximetry. For ≥2 toxicity may include nasal swab, sputum culture and sensitivity, blood culture and sensitivity, and urine culture and sensitivity
   c. Monitor patients for signs and symptoms of colitis. Encourage patients to report diarrhea immediately to any member of the health care team
   d. Draw AST, ALT, and bilirubin prior to each atezolizumab infusion and/or weekly if there are grade 1 liver function test elevations. Note, no intervention is recommended for G1 LFT abnormalities. For ≥2 toxicity work up for other causes of elevated LFTs including viral hepatitis
   e. Use basic metabolic panel (Na, K, CO_2, glucose) and patient history as screening tools for hypophysitis including hypopituitarism and adrenal insufficiency. If in doubt evaluate AM adrenocorticotropic hormone (ACTH) and cortisol levels. Consider ACTH stimulation test for indeterminate results
   f. Test thyroid function at the start of treatment, periodically during atezolizumab treatment, and as indicated based on clinical evaluation and for clinical signs and symptoms of thyroid disorders. Test for TSH and free thyroxine (FT4) every 4–6 weeks as part of routine clinical monitoring on therapy or for case detection in symptomatic patients
   g. Measure glucose at baseline and with each atezolizumab treatment during the first 12 weeks and every 6 weeks thereafter
   h. Obtain a serum creatinine prior to every atezolizumab dose. If creatinine is found to be newly elevated consider holding therapy while other potential causes are evaluated. Note, routine urinalysis is not necessary other than to rule out urinary tract infections, etc
   i. Obtain a complete rheumatologic history and perform an examination of all peripheral joints for tenderness, swelling, and range of motion. Examine the spine. Consider plain x-ray/imaging to exclude metastases and evaluate joint damage (erosions), if appropriate
   j. In patients at high risk for infections and in appropriately selected patients based on an infectious disease evaluation, draw screening laboratories (HIV, hepatitis A and B, and blood QuantiFERON for TB) to prepare patients to start infliximab

Treatment Modifications

NAB-PACLITAXEL DOSE MODIFICATIONS

nab-Paclitaxel Dose Levels

Starting dose	100 mg/m^2
Dose level −1	75 mg/m^2
Dose level −2	50 mg/m^2
Dose level −3	Discontinue nab-paclitaxel*

*If a toxicity is clearly attributable to either nab-paclitaxel or atezolizumab and requires a delay or discontinuation of therapy, then the other medication that is not responsible for the adverse reaction may be continued without interruption, as clinically appropriate

Adverse Reaction	Dose Modification
Hematologic Toxicity	
Day 1 ANC <1500/mm^3	Delay the start of the nab-paclitaxel cycle until ANC ≥1500/mm^3. If a delay of >7 days is required for the initiation of the cycle, then reduce the nab-paclitaxel dosage by 1 dose level
Day 1 platelet count <100,000/mm^3	Delay the start of the nab-paclitaxel cycle until platelet count ≥100,000/mm^3
Day 8 ANC <500/mm^3	Delay the day 8 nab-paclitaxel dose until ANC ≥500/mm^3. If ANC remains <500/mm^3 for >7 days, then reduce subsequent nab-paclitaxel dosages by 1 dose level
Day 8 platelet count <50,000/mm^3	Delay the day 8 nab-paclitaxel dose until platelet count ≥50,000/mm^3, then reduce subsequent nab-paclitaxel dosages by 1 dose level
Day 15 ANC <500/mm^3	Omit the day 15 nab-paclitaxel dose (do not make up) in the current cycle. If ANC remains <500/mm^3 for >7 days, then reduce subsequent nab-paclitaxel dosages by 1 dose level
Day 15 platelet count <50,000/mm^3	Omit the day 15 nab-paclitaxel dose (do not make up) in the current cycle. Reduce the nab-paclitaxel dosage by 1 dose level in subsequent cycles
Nadir ANC <500/mm^3 persisting for >7 days at any time	Reduce the nab-paclitaxel dosage by 1 dose level in subsequent cycles
Neutropenic fever (ANC <500/mm^3 with temperature >38°C)	Reduce the nab-paclitaxel dosage by 1 dose level in subsequent cycles
Neurologic Toxicity	
G3/4 peripheral neuropathy	Withhold nab-paclitaxel until symptoms improve to G ≤1, then reduce the nab-paclitaxel dosage by 1 dose level
Hepatic Toxicity	
AST <10× ULN *and* total bilirubin >ULN to ≤1.25× ULN	Administer nab-paclitaxel without delay at the same dose
AST <10× ULN *and* total bilirubin >1.25× ULN to ≤2× ULN	Withhold nab-paclitaxel until AST <10× ULN *and* bilirubin ≤1.25× ULN, then reduce the nab-paclitaxel dosage by 1 dose level in subsequent cycles. If the toxicity does not resolve within 3 weeks, then discontinue nab-paclitaxel
AST <10× ULN *and* bilirubin >2× ULN to ≤5× ULN	Withhold nab-paclitaxel until AST <10× ULN *and* bilirubin ≤1.25× ULN, then reduce the nab-paclitaxel dosage by 2 dose levels. If the toxicity does not resolve within 3 weeks, then discontinue nab-paclitaxel
AST >10× ULN *or* bilirubin >5× ULN	Discontinue nab-paclitaxel

(continued)

Treatment Modifications (*continued*)

ATEZOLIZUMAB DOSE MODIFICATIONS

*If a toxicity is clearly attributable to either nab-paclitaxel or atezolizumab and requires a delay or discontinuation of therapy, then the other medication that is not responsible for the adverse reaction may be continued without interruption, as clinically appropriate

Adverse Reaction	Grade/Severity	Dose Modification
Colitis	G1	Loperamide 4 mg as starting dose then 2 mg before each meal and after each loose stool until without diarrhea for 12 hours, with maximum of 16 mg loperamide per day. If G1 diarrhea or colitis persists for >14 days, then add prednisolone 0.5–1 mg/kg (non-enteric-coated) or consider oral budesonide 9 mg daily if no bloody diarrhea
	G2/3 diarrhea or colitis	Withhold atezolizumab. Loperamide 4 mg as starting dose then 2 mg before each meal and after each loose stool until without diarrhea for 12 hours, with maximum of 16 mg loperamide per day. Administer oral prednisone/prednisolone at a dose of 0.5–2 mg/kg/day or its equivalent. When improves to G1, begin a slow corticosteroid taper over at least 4 weeks. Resume atezolizumab upon symptom control, or when prednisone/prednisolone daily dose <10 mg
	G4 diarrhea or colitis	Permanently discontinue atezolizumab. Loperamide 4 mg as starting dose then 2 mg before each meal and after each loose stool until without diarrhea for 12 hours, with maximum of 16 mg loperamide per day. Administer 1–2 mg/kg IV (methyl)prednisolone and convert to 0.5–2 mg/kg prednisone/prednisolone orally each day or its equivalent only after a response. Taper over at least 4 weeks when symptoms improve. If does not improve over 72 hours or worsens, perform flexible sigmoidoscopy/colonoscopy to document colitis then begin infliximab 5 mg/kg (if no perforation/sepsis/TB/hepatitis/NYHA III/IV CHF). If no response, add MMF 500–1000 mg twice daily. If worse on MMF, consider addition of tacrolimus or ATG
Pneumonitis	G2	Withhold atezolizumab. Consider pneumocystis prophylaxis depending on the clinical context and cover with empiric antibiotics. Administer oral prednisone/prednisolone at a dose of 1–2 mg/kg/day or its equivalent. When improves to G1, begin a slow corticosteroid taper over at least 4 weeks. If does not respond adequately after 48 hours, then administer 2–4 mg/kg IV (methyl)prednisolone and convert to 0.5–2 mg/kg prednisone/prednisolone orally each day or its equivalent only after a response, followed by a taper over at least 6 weeks when symptoms improve to G1, titrating to symptoms. Resume atezolizumab upon symptom control, or when prednisone/prednisolone daily dose <10 mg
	G3/4	Permanently discontinue atezolizumab. Consider *Pneumocystis* prophylaxis depending on the clinical context; cover with empiric antibiotics. Administer 2–4 mg/kg IV (methyl)prednisolone and convert to 1–2 mg/kg prednisone/prednisolone orally each day or its equivalent only after a response, followed by a taper over at least 8 weeks when symptoms improve to G1, titrating to symptoms. If when initially treated improvement does not occur within 48–72, hours begin infliximab 5 mg/kg (if no perforation/sepsis/TB/hepatitis/NYHA III/IV CHF). If no response to infliximab, add MMF 500–1000 mg twice daily. Consider MMF especially if has concurrent hepatic toxicity
Hepatitis	G2 (AST or ALT >3–5× ULN or total bilirubin >1.5–3× ULN)	Withhold atezolizumab. Administer oral prednisone/prednisolone at a dose of 1–2 mg/kg/day or its equivalent. When improves to G1, begin a slow corticosteroid taper over at least 4 weeks. Resume atezolizumab upon symptom control, or when prednisone/prednisolone daily dose <10 mg
	G3/4 (AST or ALT >5× ULN or total bilirubin >3× ULN)	Permanently discontinue atezolizumab. Administer 1–2 mg/kg IV (methyl)prednisolone and convert to 0.5–2 mg/kg prednisone/prednisolone orally each day or its equivalent only after a response. Taper over at least 6 weeks when symptoms improve. If no response, add MMF 500–1000 mg twice daily. If worse on MMF, consider adding tacrolimus or ATG
Hypophysitis	G2/3 (Moderate symptoms, ie, headache but no visual disturbance or fatigue/mood alteration but hemodynamically stable, no electrolyte disturbance)	Administer analgesia as needed for headache. Withhold atezolizumab. Administer oral prednisone/prednisolone at a dose of 0.5–2 mg/kg/day or its equivalent. When improves to G1, begin a slow corticosteroid taper over at least 4 weeks. If no improvement in 48 hours, administer 1–2 mg/kg IV (methyl)prednisolone and convert to 0.5–2 mg/kg prednisone/prednisolone orally each day or its equivalent only after a response. Taper over at least 4 weeks when symptoms improve to 5 mg prednisone/prednisolone or equivalent; do not stop steroids. Resume atezolizumab upon symptom control, or when prednisone/prednisolone daily dose <10 mg
	G4 (Severe mass effect symptoms, ie, severe headache, any visual disturbance or severe hypoadrenalism, ie, hypotension, severe electrolyte disturbance)	Permanently discontinue atezolizumab. Administer analgesia as needed for headache. Administer 1–2 mg/kg IV (methyl)prednisolone and convert to 0.5–2 mg/kg prednisone/prednisolone orally each day or its equivalent only after a response. Taper over at least 4 weeks when symptoms improve to 5 mg prednisone/prednisolone or equivalent; do not stop steroids

(*continued*)

Treatment Modifications (continued)

Adverse Reaction	Grade/Severity	Dose Modification
Adrenal insufficiency	G2	Withhold atezolizumab. Administer oral prednisone/prednisolone at a dose of 0.5–2 mg/kg/day or its equivalent. When improves to G1, begin a slow corticosteroid taper over at least 4 weeks. Serially assess adrenal function and continue steroids at replacement doses (20–40 mg hydrocortisone daily ~2/3 dose in AM upon awakening and ~1/3 at 4 PM) until recovery of adrenal function is documented. Resume atezolizumab upon symptom control, or when prednisone/prednisolone daily dose <10 mg
	G3/4	Permanently discontinue atezolizumab. Administer oral prednisone/prednisolone at a dose of 0.5–2 mg/kg/day or its equivalent. When improves to G1, begin a slow corticosteroid taper over at least 4 weeks. Serially assess adrenal function and continue steroids at replacement doses (20–40 mg hydrocortisone daily ~2/3 dose in AM upon awakening and ~1/3 at 4 PM) until recovery of adrenal function is documented
Type 1 diabetes mellitus	G3 hyperglycemia	Withhold atezolizumab. Admit to hospital to manage hyperglycemia. Role of corticosteroids in preventing complete loss of insulin producing cells is unknown and not recommended. Resume atezolizumab upon symptom control, or when prednisone/prednisolone daily dose <10 mg
	G4 hyperglycemia	Permanently discontinue atezolizumab. Admit to hospital to manage hyperglycemia. Role of corticosteroids in preventing complete loss of insulin producing cells is unknown and not recommended
Nephritis and renal dysfunction	G2/3 (serum creatinine 1.5–6× ULN)	Withhold atezolizumab. Administer oral prednisone/prednisolone at a dose of 0.5–2 mg/kg/day or its equivalent. When improves to G1, begin a slow corticosteroid taper over at least 4 weeks. If does not respond adequately, then administer 0.5–1 mg/kg IV (methyl)prednisolone and convert to 0.5–2 mg/kg prednisone/prednisolone orally each day or its equivalent only after a response, followed by a taper over at least 4 weeks when improves to G1. Resume atezolizumab upon symptom control, or when prednisone/prednisolone daily dose <10 mg
	G4 (serum creatinine >6× ULN)	Permanently discontinue atezolizumab. Administer 0.5–1 mg/kg IV (methyl)prednisolone and convert to 0.5–2 mg/kg prednisone/prednisolone orally each day or its equivalent only after a response, followed by a taper over at least 4 weeks when improves to G1
Skin	G1/2	Continue atezolizumab. Avoid skin irritants, avoid sun exposure, topical emollients recommended. Topical steroid (mild strength for G1, moderate/potent strength for G2) cream once or twice daily ± oral or topical antihistamines for itching
	G3 rash or suspected SJS or TEN	Withhold atezolizumab. Avoid skin irritants, avoid sun exposure, topical emollients recommended. Administer oral or topical antihistamines for itching. Administer oral prednisone/prednisolone at a dose of 0.5–2 mg/kg or its equivalent daily for 3 days followed by a slow corticosteroid taper over at least 4 weeks when the rash improves to G1. If does not respond adequately, then administer 0.5–1 mg/kg IV (methyl)prednisolone and convert to 0.5–2 mg/kg prednisone/prednisolone orally each day or its equivalent only after a response, followed by a taper over at least 4 weeks when the rash improves to G1. Resume atezolizumab upon symptom control, or when prednisone/prednisolone daily dose <10 mg
	G4 rash or confirmed SJS or TEN	Avoid skin irritants, avoid sun exposure, topical emollients recommended. Administer oral or topical antihistamines for itching. Administer 1–2 mg/kg IV (methyl)prednisolone and convert to oral steroids 0.5–2 mg/kg prednisone/prednisolone each day or its equivalent only after a response. Taper over at least 4 weeks when the rash improves to G1. Permanently discontinue atezolizumab
Encephalitis	Confusion or altered behavior, headaches, alteration in Glasgow Coma Scale, motor or sensory deficits, speech abnormality, may or may not be febrile	Initially withhold atezolizumab, but permanently discontinue atezolizumab if there is no doubt as to diagnosis. Exclude bacterial and ideally viral infections prior to high-dose steroids. Administer oral prednisone/prednisolone at a dose of 0.5–2 mg/kg/day or its equivalent. When symptoms improve, begin a slow corticosteroid taper over at least 4–8 weeks. If symptoms are severe, administer 1–2 mg/kg IV (methyl)prednisolone and convert to 0.5–2 mg/kg prednisone/prednisolone orally each day or its equivalent only after a response. Consider concurrent empiric antiviral (IV acyclovir) and antibacterial therapy
Aseptic meningitis	Headache, photophobia, neck stiffness with fever or may be afebrile, vomiting; normal cognition/cerebral function (distinguishes from encephalitis)	
Other syndromes include neurosarcoidosis, posterior reversible leukoencephalopathy syndrome (PRES), Vogt-Koyanagi-Harada syndrome, demyelination, vasculitic encephalopathy, and generalized seizures		

(continued)

Treatment Modifications (continued)

Adverse Reaction	Grade/Severity	Dose Modification
Transverse myelitis	Acute or subacute neurologic signs/symptoms of motor/sensory/autonomic origin; most have sensory level; often bilateral symptoms	Initially withhold atezolizumab, but permanently discontinue atezolizumab if there is no doubt as to diagnosis. Administer 2 mg/kg IV (methyl)prednisolone or consider 1 g/day and convert to 0.5–2 mg/kg prednisone/prednisolone orally each day or its equivalent only after a response. When symptoms improve begin a slow corticosteroid taper over at least 4–8 weeks. Plasmapheresis may be required if steroids do not bring about improvement
Myocarditis	G3	Permanently discontinue atezolizumab. Administer 2 mg/kg IV (methyl)prednisolone or consider 1 g/day and convert to 0.5–2 mg/kg prednisone/prednisolone orally each day or its equivalent only after a response. When symptoms improve, begin a slow corticosteroid taper over at least 4–8 weeks. If no response, add MMF 500–1000 mg twice daily. If worse on MMF, consider adding tacrolimus
Peripheral neurologic toxicity	Moderate: some interference with ADL, symptoms concerning to patient	Withhold atezolizumab. Initial observation reasonable or initiate prednisone/prednisolone 0.5–1 mg/kg (if progressing, eg, from mild) and/or pregabalin or duloxetine for pain. When symptoms improve begin a slow corticosteroid taper over at least 4 weeks. Resume atezolizumab upon symptom control, or when prednisone/prednisolone daily dose <10 mg
	Severe: limits self-care and aids warranted, life threatening, eg, respiratory problems	Permanently discontinue atezolizumab. Administer 1–2 mg/kg IV (methyl)prednisolone and convert to 0.5–2 mg/kg prednisone/prednisolone orally each day or its equivalent only after a response. Taper over at least 4–8 weeks when symptoms improve to G1
Guillain-Barré syndrome	Progressive symmetrical muscle weakness with absent or reduced tendon reflexes—involves extremities, facial, respiratory and bulbar and oculomotor muscles; dysregulation of autonomic nerves	Permanently discontinue atezolizumab. Use of steroids not recommended in idiopathic Guillain-Barré syndrome; however, a trial of (methyl)prednisolone 1–2 mg/kg is reasonable, converting to 0.5–2 mg/kg prednisone/prednisolone orally each day or its equivalent only after a response. If no improvement or worsening, plasmapheresis or IVIG indicated
Myasthenia gravis	Fluctuating muscle weakness (proximal limb, trunk, ocular, eg, ptosis/diplopia or bulbar) with fatigability, respiratory muscles also may be involved	Permanently discontinue atezolizumab. Administer pyridostigmine at an initial dose of 30 mg three times daily. Administer oral prednisone/prednisolone at a dose of 0.5–2 mg/kg/day or its equivalent or 1–2 mg/kg IV (methyl)prednisolone depending on the severity of symptoms. If begun with IV, convert to 0.5–2 mg/kg prednisone/prednisolone orally each day or its equivalent only after a response. If no improvement or worsening, plasmapheresis or IVIG may be considered. Additional immunosuppressants used in myasthenia gravis include azathioprine, cyclosporine, and mycophenolate. Avoid certain medications, eg, ciprofloxacin, beta-blockers, that may precipitate cholinergic crisis
Other syndromes including motor and sensory peripheral neuropathy, multifocal radicular neuropathy/plexopathy, autonomic neuropathy, phrenic nerve palsy, cranial nerve palsies (eg, facial nerve, optic nerve, hypoglossal nerve)		Permanently discontinue atezolizumab. Administer oral prednisone/prednisolone at a dose of 0.5–2 mg/kg/day or its equivalent or 1–2 mg/kg IV (methyl)prednisolone depending on the severity of symptoms. If begun with IV, convert to 0.5–2 mg/kg prednisone/prednisolone orally each day or its equivalent only after a response
Arthralgia	G1 (Mild pain with inflammation, erythema or joint swelling)	Continue atezolizumab. Administer acetaminophen (paracetamol) and ibuprofen
	G2 (Moderate pain with inflammation, erythema or joint swelling that limits ADLs)	Withhold atezolizumab. Administer higher doses of acetaminophen (paracetamol) and ibuprofen and use diclofenac or naproxen or etoricoxib. If inadequately controlled, consider intra-articular steroid injections for large joints or administer oral prednisone/prednisolone at a dose of 0.5–2 mg/kg/day or its equivalent. When improves to G1, begin a slow corticosteroid taper over at least 4 weeks. If does not respond adequately, then administer 0.5–1 mg/kg IV (methyl)prednisolone and convert to 0.5–2 mg/kg prednisone/prednisolone orally each day or its equivalent only after a response, followed by a taper over at least 4 weeks when improves to G1. Resume atezolizumab upon symptom control, or when prednisone/prednisolone daily dose <10 mg
	G3 (Severe pain; irreversible joint damage; disabling; limits self-care ADL)	Withhold atezolizumab. Administer 0.5–1 mg/kg IV (methyl)prednisolone and convert to 0.5–2 mg/kg prednisone/prednisolone orally each day or its equivalent only after a response, followed by a taper over at least 4 weeks when improves to G1. In severe cases, infliximab or another anti–TNF alpha drug may be required for improvement of arthritis. Resume atezolizumab upon symptom control, or when prednisone/prednisolone daily dose <10 mg

(continued)

Treatment Modifications (*continued*)

Adverse Reaction	Grade/Severity	Dose Modification
Other	First occurrence of other G3	Withhold atezolizumab. Administer oral prednisone/prednisolone at a dose of 0.5–2 mg/kg/day or its equivalent. When improves to G1, begin a slow corticosteroid taper over at least 4 weeks. Resume atezolizumab upon symptom control, or when prednisone/prednisolone daily dose <10 mg
	Recurrence of same G3	Permanently discontinue atezolizumab. Administer 1–2 mg/kg IV (methyl)prednisolone and convert to 0.5–2 mg/kg prednisone/prednisolone orally each day or its equivalent only after a response. Taper over at least 4–8 weeks when symptoms improve to G1
	Life-threatening or G4	
	Requirement for ≥10 mg/day prednisone or equivalent for >12 weeks	Permanently discontinue atezolizumab
	Persistent G2/3 adverse reactions lasting ≥12 weeks	

ADL, activities of daily living; ALT, alanine aminotransferase; AST, aspartate aminotransferase; ATG, anti-thymocyte globulin; SJS, Stevens-Johnson Syndrome; TEN, toxic epidermal necrolysis; ULN, upper limit of normal

Notes on general supportive care:
• Steroid taper in most cases will proceed over a minimum of 1 month but if symptoms improve rapidly a 2-week taper can be considered. If steroids are administered for more than 4 weeks, consider PCP prophylaxis (cotrimoxazole 480 mg twice daily M/W/F or inhaled pentamidine if has cotrimoxazole allergy), regular random blood glucose, vitamin D level and starting calcium/vitamin D supplementation per guidelines

Adverse Events (N = 890)

Grade (%)*	nab-Paclitaxel plus Atezolizumab (N = 452)		nab-Paclitaxel plus Placebo (N = 438)	
	Grade 1–2	Grade 3–4	Grade 1–2	Grade 3–4
Alopecia	55.8	0.7	57.3	0.2
Fatigue	42.7	4.0	41.3	3.4
Nausea	44.9	1.1	36.3	1.8
Diarrhea	31.2	1.3	32.2	2.1
Anemia	24.8	2.9	23.3	3.0
Constipation	24.3	0.7	24.4	0.2
Cough	24.8	0	18.9	0
Headache	22.8	0.4	21.0	0.9
Peripheral neuropathy	16.2	5.5	19.4	2.7
Neutropenia	12.6	8.2	7.1	8.2
Decreased appetite	19.5	0.7	17.4	0.7
Vomiting	18.6	0.9	15.8	1.1
Pyrexia	18.1	0.7	10.7	0
Arthralgia	17.7	0.2	15.8	0.2
Rash	16.8	0.4	16.0	0.5
Dyspnea	15.0	0.9	13.9	0.7
Peripheral sensory neuropathy	13.9	2.0	10.0	1.8

(*continued*)

Treatment Modifications (continued)

Grade (%)*	nab-Paclitaxel plus Atezolizumab (N = 452)		nab-Paclitaxel plus Placebo (N = 438)	
	Grade 1–2	Grade 3–4	Grade 1–2	Grade 3–4
Peripheral edema	14.4	0.2	14.2	1.4
Myalgia	13.7	0.4	14.6	0.7
Back pain	13.9	1.3	12.8	0.5
Dizziness	13.9	0	10.7	0
Dysgeusia	13.7	0	13.7	0
Hypothyroidism	13.7	0	3.4	0
Pruritus	13.7	0	10.3	0
Neutrophil count decreased	8.0	4.6	7.5	3.4
Asthenia	11.9	0.4	10.5	0.9
Urinary tract infection	10.8	0.9	10.0	0.5
Insomnia	11.3	0	11.0	0.7
Pain in extremity	10.4	0.4	9.6	0.2
Nasopharyngitis	10.8	0	8.4	0
Upper respiratory tract infection	9.5	1.1	9.1	0
Increase alanine aminotransferase	8.6	1.8	8.0	1.1
Abdominal pain	9.7	0.4	11.9	0.2
Infusion-related reactions	1.1	0	1.1	0
Immune-related hepatitis (diagnosis)	0.9	1.3	1.4	0.2
Immune-related hepatitis (lab abnormalities)	10.0	3.8	10.5	2.7
Immune-related hypothyroidism	17.3	0	4.3	0
Immune-related hyperthyroidism	4.2	0.2	1.4	0
Immune-related pneumonitis	2.9	0.2	0.2	0
Immune-related meningoencephalitis	1.1	0	0.5	0
Immune-related colitis	0.9	0.2	0.5	0.2
Immune-related adrenal insufficiency	0.7	0.2	0	0
Immune-related pancreatitis	0.2	0.2	0	0
Immune-related diabetes mellitus	0	0.2	0.2	0.2
Immune-related nephritis	0	0.2	0	0
Immune-related rash	33.2	0.9	25.6	0.5

*According to the National Cancer Institute Common Terminology Criteria for Adverse Events, version 4.0
Note: Adverse events occurring in ≥10% in either group (irrespective of treatment attribution) and adverse events of special interest are included in the table. Fatal adverse events occurred in 1.3% of the nab-paclitaxel plus atezolizumab group and in 0.7% of the nab-paclitaxel plus placebo group

METASTATIC • TRIPLE-NEGATIVE

BREAST CANCER REGIMEN: SACITUZUMAB GOVITECAN

Bardia A et al. N Engl J Med 2019;380:741–751
Protocol for: Bardia A et al. N Engl J Med 2019;380:741–751
Supplementary appendix to: Bardia A et al. N Engl J Med 2019;380:741–751
TRODELVY (sacituzumab govitecan-hziy) prescribing information. Morris Plains, NJ: Immunomedics, Inc; revised 2020 April

Premedications for sacituzumab govitecan-hziy:

• *Antiemetics (all cycles):*

▪ Sacituzumab govitecan-hziy is moderately emetogenic; the U.S. Food and Drug Administration (FDA)-approved prescribing information recommends premedication with a two- or three-drug combination regimen (eg, dexamethasone + a 5-HT3 receptor antagonist ± an NK1 receptor antagonist)

• *Infusion reaction prophylaxis (all cycles):*

▪ **Acetaminophen** 650–1000 mg; administer orally 30 minutes prior to sacituzumab govitecan-hziy for 2 doses on days 1 and 8, every 21 days

▪ **Diphenhydramine** 25–50 mg; administer orally or intravenously 30 minutes prior to sacituzumab govitecan-hziy for 2 doses on days 1 and 8, every 21 days

▪ **Ranitidine** 50 mg (or an equivalent histamine receptor [H_2]–subtype antagonist); administer intravenously (or an equivalent dosage, ie, **ranitidine** 150 mg, administered orally) 30 minutes prior to sacituzumab govitecan-hziy for 2 doses on days 1 and 8, every 21 days

• *Prior non-life-threatening hypersensitivity reaction:*

▪ If the patient experienced a prior non-life-threatening hypersensitivity reaction and a corticosteroid was not already being administered for antiemetic purposes, then consider adding:

  ○ **Dexamethasone** 12 mg; administer orally or intravenously 30 minutes prior to sacituzumab govitecan-hziy for 2 doses on days 1 and 8, every 21 days

• *Prior acute cholinergic toxicity:*

▪ If an excessive acute cholinergic response (eg, abdominal cramping, diarrhea, salivation) has occurred with a previous dose, then consider adding:

  ○ **Atropine sulfate** 0.25–1 mg; administer subcutaneously or intravenously 30 minutes prior to sacituzumab govitecan-hziy for 2 doses on days 1 and 8, every 21 days

Sacituzumab govitecan-hziy 10 mg/kg per dose; administer intravenously, in a volume of 0.9% sodium chloride injection (0.9% NS) sufficient to produce a final concentration ranging from 1.1–3.4 mg/mL and not to exceed 500 mL, over 3 hours, for 2 doses on days 1 and 8, every 21 days, until disease progression (total dosage/3-week cycle = 20 mg/kg)

• For patients who have tolerated ≥1 prior infusion over 3 hours, may administer subsequent infusions over 1–2 hours

• Flush the line with 20 mL of 0.9% NS after completion of the sacituzumab govitecan-hziy infusion

• Prepare sacituzumab govitecan-hziy in a bag that is protected from light and that is composed of polypropylene

• For patients who weigh >170 kg, divide the total dose of sacituzumab govitecan-hziy equally between two polypropylene bags each containing 500 mL 0.9% NS and infuse sequentially such that the total volume of 1000 mL is infused over the proper duration of 1–3 hours, depending on dose number and prior infusion reaction history

• Administer sacituzumab govitecan-hziy in a setting with immediate access to emergency equipment and medications for management of severe hypersensitivity reactions

• SN-38 (the cytotoxic component of sacituzumab govitecan-hziy) is known to be metabolized by UGT1A1

▪ Avoid concomitant administration with UGT1A1 inhibitors or inducers

▪ Patients who have reduced UGT1A1 activity (eg, patients who are homozygous or heterozygous for UGT1A1*28) may be at increased risk for toxicity related to sacituzumab govitecan-hziy and should be monitored closely and have doses adjusted as necessary based on treatment tolerance

(continued)

Efficacy (N = 108)

Efficacy Variable	Sacituzumab Govitecan-hziy (N = 108)
Response	
ORR*—n/N (%)	36/108 (33.3)
PR—n/N (%)	33/108 (30.6)
CR—n/N (%)	3/108 (2.8)
Median TTR—months (range)	2.0 (1.6–13.5)
Median DOR—months (95% CI)	7.7 (4.9–10.8)
CBR†—n/N (%)	49/108 (45.4)
Survival	
Median PFS—months (95% CI)	5.5 (4.1–6.3)
Estimated PFS at 6 months—%	41.9
Estimated PFS at 12 months—%	15.1
Median OS—months (95% CI)	13.0 (11.2–13.7)
Estimated OS at 6 months—%	78.5
Estimated OS at 12 months—%	51.3

*Per local review using Response Evaluation Criteria in Solid Tumors version 1.1
†Clinical benefit rate included PR + CR + stable disease lasting ≥6 months
Note: The data cutoff date for this analysis was 1 December 2017 at which time the median follow-up was 9.7 (range, 0.3–36.5) months
ORR, objective response rate; PR, partial response; CR, complete response; TTR, time to response; DOR, duration of response; CBR, clinical benefit rate; PFS, progression-free survival; OS, overall survival

(*continued*)

Supportive Care
Antiemetic prophylaxis
Emetogenic potential is **MODERATE**
See Chapter 42 for antiemetic recommendations

Hematopoietic growth factor (CSF) prophylaxis
Primary prophylaxis is not indicated
Note: The U.S. FDA-approved prescribing information contains a Black Box Warning that states, in part, to consider G-CSF for secondary prophylaxis
See Chapter 43 for more information

Antimicrobial prophylaxis
Risk of fever and neutropenia is **LOW**
  Antimicrobial primary prophylaxis to be considered:
  • Antibacterial—not indicated
  • Antifungal—not indicated
  • Antiviral—not indicated, unless patient previously had an episode of HSV

Acute cholinergic syndrome
Atropine sulfate 0.25–1 mg; administer subcutaneously or intravenously if abdominal cramping or diarrhea develop during or within 1 hour after sacituzumab govitecan-hziy administration
• If symptoms are severe, add as primary prophylaxis 30 minutes before sacituzumab govitecan-hziy during subsequent doses
• Acute cholinergic syndrome may be characterized by: abdominal cramping, diarrhea, diaphoresis, hypotension, flushing, bradycardia, rhinitis, increased salivation, miosis, and lacrimation

Diarrhea management
Latent or delayed-onset diarrhea:
Evaluate for infectious causes of diarrhea and if negative, promptly initiate loperamide as follows:
  Loperamide 4 mg orally initially after the first loose or liquid stool, *then*
  Loperamide 2 mg with every episode of diarrhea for a maximum of 16 mg daily
  • Continue for at least 12 hours after diarrhea resolves
  • Recurrent diarrhea after a 12-hour diarrhea-free interval is treated as a new episode
  • Rehydrate orally with fluids and electrolytes during a diarrheal episode
  • If diarrhea persists >48 hours despite loperamide, stop loperamide and consider evaluation in an ambulatory or hospital setting and treatment with intravenous hydration

Persistent diarrhea requiring hospitalization:
  Octreotide 100–150 mcg subcutaneously 3 times daily. Maximum total daily dose is 1500 mcg

Therapy Monitoring

1. *Prior to initiation of therapy in females of reproductive potential:* pregnancy test
2. *Prior to initiation of therapy, where available:* consider genotyping for UGT1A1; patients who are homozygous or heterozygous for the UGT1A1*28 allele may be at higher risk for toxicity and should be monitored closely
3. *On day 1 and 8 of each cycle:* CBC with differential and platelet count; assess for nausea and vomiting symptoms
4. *Before infusion, during infusion, and for 30 minutes after completion of each infusion:*
   a. Monitor vital signs and for signs and symptoms of an infusion-related reaction or hypersensitivity reaction
   b. Monitor for an acute cholinergic syndrome characterized by abdominal cramping, acute diarrhea, diaphoresis, hypotension, flushing, bradycardia, rhinitis, increased salivation, and lacrimation
5. *Periodically:*
   a. Advise the patient to report late-onset diarrhea. In patients with diarrhea, rule out infectious causes (eg, *Clostridium difficile*) and if negative, administer loperamide. For diarrhea that persists >48 hours or for severe symptoms of any duration, consider assessing the patient in an ambulatory or hospital setting and providing IV hydration and repletion of electrolytes as clinically indicated

Patient Population Studied

The IMMU-132-01 study was a phase 1/2, basket design, open-label, single-arm, multicenter trial that initially involved patients with a variety of solid tumors who had received at least 1 prior treatment for metastatic disease. Based on promising initial results in 69 patients with metastatic triple-negative breast cancer (MTNBC), the protocol was amended to include MTNBC patients who had received ≥2 prior lines of therapy (including a taxane). The analysis published by Bardia et al in 2019 describes results in all patients who received a 10 mg/kg dose as ≥3rd-line therapy (n = 108). Patients were required to have an Eastern Cooperative Oncology Group performance status (ECOG PS) of ≤1. Patients were excluded if they had bulky (>7 cm) disease, brain metastases (unless treated, asymptomatic, and not requiring high dose steroids), or Gilbert disease. The median age of patients included in the analysis was 55 (range, 31–80) years. The majority (76%) were White. All had an ECOG PS of either 0 (28.7%) or 1 (71.3%). Visceral metastases (solid organs not including the brain) were present in 76.9% and brain metastases were present in 2%. The median number of prior anticancer regimens was 3 (range, 2–10)

Treatment Modifications

SACITUZUMAB GOVITECAN-HZIY TREATMENT MODIFICATIONS

Sacituzumab Govitecan-hziy Dose Levels

Starting dose	10 mg/kg
Dose level –1	7.5 mg/kg
Dose level –2	5 mg/kg
Dose level –3	Discontinue sacituzumab govitecan-hziy

Note: Do not re-escalate the sacituzumab govitecan-hziy dose once it has been reduced for an adverse reaction

Adverse Event	Dose Modification		
Infusion-Related Reactions			
G ≤3 infusion-related reaction (prolonged [eg, not rapidly responsive to symptomatic medication and/or brief interruption of infusion]; recurrence of symptoms following initial improvement; hospitalization indicated for clinical sequelae; or less severe)	Slow or interrupt the infusion rate and provide supportive care as clinically indicated (eg, oxygen supplementation, inhaled beta-agonist, antihistamine, antipyretic, and/or corticosteroid). When symptoms have resolved, resume the infusion at ≤50% of the prior rate and increase by 50% increments every 30 minutes as tolerated until the rate at which the reaction occurred is reached. Administer the next infusion over 3 hours with continued premedication consisting of, at minimum, dexamethasone, acetaminophen, diphenhydramine, and an H2-receptor antagonist		
G4 infusion-related reaction (life-threatening consequences; urgent intervention indicated)	Permanently discontinue sacituzumab govitecan-hziy		
Severe Neutropenia			
G4 neutropenia (ANC <500/mm^3) for ≥7 days OR G3 febrile neutropenia (ANC <1,000/mm^3 and temperature ≥38.5°C) OR At time of scheduled treatment, G ≥3 neutropenia (ANC <1000/mm^3) which delays dosing by 2 or 3 weeks for recovery to G ≤1 (ANC ≥1500/mm^3)	*First occurrence*	Reduce the dose by 25% and administer G-CSF	
	Second occurrence	Reduce the dose by 50% and continue G-CSF	
	Third occurrence	Discontinue treatment	
At time of scheduled treatment, G ≥3 neutropenia (ANC <1000/mm^3) which delays dosing beyond 3 weeks for recovery to G ≤1 (ANC ≥1500/mm^3)	Discontinue treatment		
Severe Non-neutropenic Toxicity			
G4 nonhematologic toxicity of any duration OR Any G ≥3 nausea, vomiting, or diarrhea due to treatment that is not controlled with antiemetic and antidiarrheal agents OR Other G ≥3 nonhematologic toxicity persisting >48 hours despite optimal medical management OR At time of scheduled treatment, G ≥3 non-neutropenic hematologic or nonhematologic toxicity that delays dose by 2 or 3 weeks for recovery to G ≤1	*First occurrence*	Reduce the dose by 25%	
	Second occurrence	Reduce the dose by 50%	
	Third occurrence	Discontinue treatment	
At time of scheduled treatment, G ≥3 non-neutropenic hematologic or nonhematologic toxicity that does not recover to G ≤1 within 3 weeks	Discontinue treatment		
Drug Interactions			
Patient is taking a UGT1A1 inducer or UGT1A1 inhibitor	Avoid concomitant use		

Note: Grading of toxicities is per the National Cancer Institute Common Terminology Criteria for Adverse Events (NCI CTCAE) version 4.0
ANC, absolute neutrophil count; G-CSF, granulocyte colony-stimulating factor

Adverse Events (N = 108)

Adverse Event* (%)	Sacituzumab Govitecan-hziy (N = 108)			Adverse Event* (%)	Sacituzumab Govitecan-hziy (N = 108)		
	Any Grade	Grade 3	Grade 4		Any Grade	Grade 3	Grade 4
Any AE	100	66	19	Increased ALT	14	1	0
GI disorders	94	19	0	Decreased weight	14	0	0
Nausea	67	6	0	Increased alkaline phosphatase level	11	2	0
Diarrhea	62	8	0	Increased blood LDH level	10	0	0
Vomiting	49	6	0	Nervous system disorders	55	4	0
Constipation	34	1	0	Headache	21	1	0
Abdominal pain†	25	1	0	Dizziness	20	0	0
Mucositis‡	14	0	0	Neuropathy⁶	19	0	0
General disorders and administration-site conditions	76	9	0	Dysgeusia	11	0	0
Fatigue and asthenia	55	8	0	Infections and infestations	52	10	2
Peripheral edema	16	0	0	Respiratory infection#	21	3	0
Pyrexia	12	0	0	UTI	20	3	0
Blood and lymphatic system disorders	74	23	14	Musculoskeletal and connective-tissue disorders	52	0	0
Neutropenia§	64	26	16	Back pain	22	0	0
Anemia	50	11	0	Arthralgia	16	0	0
Metabolism and nutrition disorders	65	19	2	Pain in extremity	10	0	0
Decreased appetite	30	0	0	Respiratory, thoracic, and mediastinal disorders	51	4	1
Hyperglycemia	24	3	1	Cough and productive cough	19	0	0
Hypomagnesemia	21	1	0	Dyspnea	19	2	1
Hypokalemia	18	2	0	Psychiatric disorders	25	1	0
Hypophosphatemia	15	9	0	Insomnia	14	0	0
Dehydration	13	4	0				
Skin and subcutaneous tissue disorders	61	5	0				
Alopecia	36	0	0				
Rash‖	28	2	0				
Pruritus	16	0	0				
Dry skin	14	1	0				
Abnormal values	57	20	6				
Decreased WBC count	21	8	3				
Prolonged aPTT	14	2	0				
Increased AST	14	1	0				

*Based on the National Cancer Institute Common Terminology Criteria for Adverse Events (NCI CTCAE) v4.0
†Includes abdominal pain, abdominal distension, upper abdominal pain, abdominal discomfort, and abdominal tenderness
‡Includes stomatitis and mucosal inflammation
§Includes neutropenia and decreased neutrophil counts. Febrile neutropenia (FN) of all grades was reported in 10 patients (9%), FN of grade 3 in 7 (%), and FN of grade 4 in 2 (2%)
‖Includes maculopapular rash, generalized rash, dermatitis acneiform, and skin disorder
⁶Includes peripheral neuropathy, paresthesia, peripheral sensory neuropathy, and hypoesthesia
#Includes URTI, viral URTI, influenza, bronchitis, and RSV infection
Note: The table includes adverse events of any grade that occurred in at least 10% of patients. The *Medical Dictionary for Regulatory Activities* system organ class and preferred terms are reported whenever possible
AE, adverse event; GI, gastrointestinal; WBC, white blood cell; aPTT, activated partial thromboplastin time; AST, aspartate aminotransferase; ALT, alanine aminotransferase; LDH, lactate dehydrogenase; UTI, urinary tract infection

METASTATIC • GERMLINE *BRCA* MUTATION • HER2-NEGATIVE
BREAST CANCER REGIMEN: OLAPARIB

Robson M et al. N Engl J Med 2017;377:523–533
Protocol for: Robson M et al. N Engl J Med 2017;377:523–533

Olaparib tablets 300 mg/dose; administer orally twice daily (approximately every 12 hours), without regard to food, continually until disease progression (total dose/week = 4200 mg)

Notes:
- Only prescribe olaparib *tablets* (rather than capsules) for the treatment of metastatic breast cancer, as described by Robson et al. There are marked differences in pharmacokinetics with olaparib tablets versus olaparib capsules; olaparib capsules must not be substituted for olaparib tablets on a mg-per-mg basis
- Patients who delay taking olaparib tablets at a regularly scheduled time or who vomit after taking olaparib tablets should take the next dose at the next regularly scheduled time
- Olaparib is metabolized by cytochrome P450 (CYP) CYP3A subfamily enzymes. Avoid concurrent use with moderate or strong CYP3A4 inhibitors whenever possible. If concurrent use with a *moderate* CYP3A4 inhibitor is required, reduce olaparib dose to 150 mg orally twice daily. If concurrent use with a *strong* CYP3A4 inhibitor is required, reduce olaparib dose to 100 mg orally twice daily. Avoid concurrent use with moderate or strong CYP3A4 inducers (eg, rifampin, carbamazepine, phenytoin, phenobarbital, St. John's wort)
- Advise patients to not consume grapefruit, grapefruit juice, Seville oranges, or Seville orange juice, as they may inhibit CYP3A in the gut wall and increase the bioavailability of olaparib

Supportive Care
Antiemetic prophylaxis
Emetogenic potential is **LOW**
See Chapter 42 for antiemetic recommendations

Hematopoietic growth factor (CSF) prophylaxis
Primary prophylaxis is **NOT** indicated
See Chapter 43 for more information

Antimicrobial prophylaxis
Risk of fever and neutropenia is **LOW**
Antimicrobial primary prophylaxis to be considered:
- Antibacterial—not indicated
- Antifungal—not indicated
- Antiviral—not indicated unless patient previously had an episode of HSV

Patient Population Studied

The international, multicenter, open-label, randomized, controlled, phase 3 trial (OlympiAD) involved 302 patients with HER2-negative metastatic breast cancer with germline *BRCA* mutation. Eligible patients were aged ≥18 years, had previously received no more than two chemotherapy regimens for metastatic disease, and had previously received neoadjuvant or adjuvant therapy for metastatic disease with an anthracycline (unless contraindicated) and a taxane. Patients were randomized (2:1) to receive oral olaparib (300 mg twice daily) or standard therapy. Standard therapy was defined as 21-day cycles involving oral capecitabine (2500 mg/m² daily, divided into two doses) for 14 days, intravenous eribulin mesylate (1.4 mg/m²) on days 1 and 8, or intravenous vinorelbine (30 mg/m²) on days 1 and 8. Treatment continued until disease progression or unacceptable adverse effects

Efficacy (N = 302)

	Olaparib (N = 205)	Standard Therapy (N = 97)	
Median progression-free survival	7.0 months	4.2 months	HR 0.58, 95% CI 0.43–0.80; P<0.001
Median overall survival	19.3 months	19.6 months	HR 0.90, 95% CI 0.63–1.29; P = 0.57

Note: Median follow-up was 14.5 months in the olaparib group and 14.1 months in the standard-therapy group

Therapy Monitoring

1. *Once per week initially then once per month:* CBC with differential and platelet count
2. *Before the start of a cycle:* CBC with differential, serum electrolytes
3. Monitor patients for pneumonitis. Query symptoms of cough, dyspnea, or fever. Obtain radiologic investigations as needed
4. Monitor patients for hematological toxicity at baseline and monthly thereafter. Discontinue if MDS/AML is confirmed
5. *Every 2–3 months:* Imaging to assess response

Treatment Modifications

Olaparib

Note: DO NOT substitute Lynparza (olaparib) tablets (100 mg and 150 mg) with Lynparza (olaparib) capsules (50 mg) on a milligram-to-milligram basis due to differences in the dosing and bioavailability of each formulation

Starting dose	300 mg twice daily in tablet form
Dose level −1	250 mg twice daily in tablet form
Dose level −2	200 mg twice daily in tablet form

Adverse Event	Treatment Modification
Dyspnea, cough, fever, and radiologic abnormalities—pneumonitis is suspected	Interrupt olaparib until pulmonary status clarified
Pneumonitis is confirmed	Discontinue olaparib
Creatinine clearance 31–50 mL/min	Reduce olaparib to 200 mg twice daily
Administration of a moderate CYP3A inhibitor required	Reduce olaparib dose to 150 mg twice daily
Administration of a strong CYP3A inhibitor required	Reduce olaparib dose to 100 mg twice daily
G ≥2 nonhematologic toxicity	Wait for toxicity to resolve to G1, then reduce olaparib one dose level
G ≥2 hematologic toxicity	Wait for toxicity to resolve to G1, then reduce olaparib one dose level
MDS/AML confirmed	Discontinue olaparib

Note: Olaparib can cause fetal harm. Advise females of reproductive potential of the potential risk to a fetus and to use effective contraception

Adverse Events (N = 296)

Grade (%)*	Olaparib (n = 205)		Standard Therapy (n = 91)	
	Grade 1–2	Grade 3–5	Grade 1–2	Grade 3–5
Any adverse event	60	37	46	51
Nausea	58	0	34	1
Anemia	24	16	22	4
Vomiting	30	0	14	1
Fatigue	26	3	22	1
Neutropenia	18	9	23	26
Diarrhea	20	<1	22	0
Headache	19	<1	13	2
Cough	17	0	7	0
Decreased white cell count	13	3	11	10
Decreased appetite	16	0	12	0
Pyrexia	14	0	18	0
Increased alanine aminotransferase level	10	1	16	1
Increased aspartate aminotransferase level	7	2	16	0
Palmar-plantar erythrodysesthesia	<1	0	19	2

*According to the National Cancer Institute Common Terminology Criteria for Adverse Events, version 4.0
Adverse events that occurred in ≥15% patients in either treatment group are shown. Median total treatment duration was 8.2 months in the olaparib group and 3.4 months in the standard-therapy group. One death (owing to sepsis) occurred in the olaparib group and one death (dyspnea, with disease progression as a secondary cause) occurred in the standard-therapy group. Treatment discontinuation owing to an adverse event occurred in 4.9% of the olaparib group and 7.7% of the standard-therapy group

METASTATIC • GERMLINE *BRCA* MUTATION • HER2-NEGATIVE

BREAST CANCER REGIMEN: TALAZOPARIB

Litton JK et al. N Engl J Med 2018;379:753–763
Protocol for: Litton JK et al. N Engl J Med 2018;379:753–763
Supplementary appendix to: Litton JK et al. N Engl J Med 2018;379:753–763
Talzenna (talazoparib) prescribing information. New York, NY: Pfizer Labs; revised 2018 October

Talazoparib 1 mg per dose; administer orally once daily, without regard to food, continually until disease progression (total dose/week = 7 mg)
- Patients who delay taking a talazoparib dose at a regularly scheduled time or who vomit after taking a talazoparib dose should take the next dose at the next regularly scheduled time

- Talazoparib capsules should be swallowed whole. Do not crush, chew, dissolve, or open capsules

  - Starting dose in hepatic impairment: no dose adjustment is recommended in patients with mild hepatic impairment (total bilirubin ≤1× ULN **and aspartate aminotransferase** [AST] >1× ULN, or total bilirubin >1× ULN **and <1.5× ULN with any AST**). No recommendation for dosing can be made for patients with moderate or severe hepatic impairment due to lack of data in these populations

  - Starting dose in renal impairment: reduce the starting talazoparib dose to 0.75 mg by mouth once daily in patients with moderate renal impairment (creatinine clearance ≥30 mL/minute and <60 mL/minute). No recommendation for dosing can be made for patients with severe renal impairment (creatinine clearance <30 mL/minute) or for those undergoing hemodialysis due to lack of data in these populations

- Talazoparib is a substrate of the P-glycoprotein (P-gp) transporter. Concomitant administration of talazoparib with P-gp inhibitors (eg, amiodarone, carvedilol, clarithromycin, itraconazole, and verapamil) increased talazoparib exposure by 45%, resulting in more frequent requirement for dose reduction. Thus, P-gp inhibitors should be avoided with talazoparib if possible. If concomitant use of a P-gp inhibitor with talazoparib is unavoidable, then reduce the talazoparib starting dose to 0.75 mg once daily. If the P-gp inhibitor is subsequently discontinued, then increase the talazoparib dose to the dose used prior to initiation of the P-gp inhibitor once 3–5 half-lives of the P-gp inhibitor have transpired. There are insufficient data on the potential effect of P-gp inducers on talazoparib pharmacokinetics

- Talazoparib is a substrate of the BCRP transporter. There are insufficient data on the potential effect of BCRP inhibitors on talazoparib pharmacokinetics; concomitant use may increase talazoparib exposure

Supportive Care
Antiemetic prophylaxis
Emetogenic potential is **MINIMAL–LOW**
See Chapter 42 for antiemetic recommendations

Hematopoietic growth factor (CSF) prophylaxis
Primary prophylaxis is **NOT** *indicated*
See Chapter 43 for more information

Antimicrobial prophylaxis
Risk of fever and neutropenia is **LOW**
  Antimicrobial primary prophylaxis to be considered:
- Antibacterial—not indicated

- Antifungal—not indicated

- Antiviral—not indicated, unless patient previously had an episode of HSV

Patient Population Studied

The multicenter, randomized, open label, phase 3 study involved 431 patients with metastatic breast cancer and a germline deleterious or suspected deleterious *BRCA*1 or *BRCA*2 mutation as detected with the BRACAnalysis test (Myriad Genetics). Eligible patients were aged ≥18 years, with an Eastern Cooperative Oncology Group (ECOG) performance status score ≤1, had adequate organ and bone marrow function, and were previously treated with a maximum of 3 prior cytotoxic regimens for metastatic disease (including a taxane, anthracycline, or both [if not contraindicated]). Prior platinum-based therapy was allowed if there was at least a 6-month disease-free interval (when administered in the neoadjuvant or adjuvant setting) or in the absence of progressive disease documented during or within 8 weeks following therapy (when used in the metastatic setting). Patients with stable brain metastases were eligible if they had been previously treated and were receiving low-dose or no corticosteroids. Patients were randomized 2:1 to receive either talazoparib or standard single-agent chemotherapy (capecitabine, gemcitabine, eribulin, or vinorelbine) until disease progression, unacceptable toxicity, or withdrawal of consent

Efficacy (N = 431)

	Talazoparib (n = 287)	Standard Single-agent Chemotherapy (n = 144)	
Median progression-free survival	8.6 months	5.6 months	HR 0.54 (95% CI 0.41–0.71); P<0.001
Median overall survival	22.3 months	19.5 months	HR 0.76 (95% CI 0.55–1.06); P = 0.11
Objective response rate*	62.6%	27.2%	P<0.001
Complete response rate*	5.5%	0%	
Median time to response†	2.6 months	1.7 months	
Median duration of response†	5.4 months	3.1 months	
Clinical benefit rate at 24 weeks‡	68.6%	36.1%	P<0.001

*According to Response Evaluation Criteria in Solid Tumors, version 1.1, among patients with measurable disease. Confirmation of complete response or partial response was not required
†Among patients with an objective response
‡Clinical benefit included patients with complete response, partial response, or stable disease
Note: The median duration of follow-up was 11.2 months for progression-free survival

Therapy Monitoring

1. *Every 3–4 weeks:* CBC with differential and platelet count, liver function tests, serum electrolytes, BUN, serum creatinine
2. Myelodysplastic syndrome/acute myeloid leukemia (MDS/AML) has occurred in patients exposed to talazoparib. Monitor patients for hematological toxicity and discontinue if MDS/AML is confirmed
3. Apprise pregnant women of the potential risk to a fetus. Advise females of reproductive potential to use effective contraception during treatment and for at least 7 months after the last dose of talazoparib. Advise male patients with female partners of reproductive potential or who are pregnant to use effective contraception during treatment and for at least 4 months following the last dose of talazoparib
4. Every 2–3 months: imaging to assess response

Treatment Modifications

Talazoparib	
Starting dose	1 mg by mouth once daily
Dose level −1	0.75 mg by mouth once daily
Dose level −2	0.5 mg by mouth once daily
Dose level −3	0.25 mg by mouth once daily
Dose level −4	Discontinue talazoparib

Adverse Event	Treatment Modification
Hematologic Toxicity	
Hemoglobin <8 g/dL	Interrupt talazoparib. Transfuse red blood cells as indicated in accordance with local guidelines. When hemoglobin improves to ≥9 g/dL, resume talazoparib with the dosage reduced by 1 dose level
Platelet count <50,000/mm³	Interrupt talazoparib. Transfuse platelets as indicated in accordance with local guidelines. When the platelet count improves to ≥75,000/mm³, resume talazoparib with the dosage reduced by 1 dose level
ANC <1000/mm³	Interrupt talazoparib until the ANC improves to ≥1500/mm³, then resume talazoparib with the dosage reduced by 1 dose level
MDS/AML confirmed	Discontinue talazoparib

(continued)

Treatment Modifications (*continued*)

Renal Impairment

Moderate renal impairment (creatinine clearance ≥30 mL/minute and <60 mL/minute)	Reduce the starting talazoparib dose to 0.75 mg by mouth once daily
Severe renal impairment (creatinine clearance <30 mL/minute) or undergoing hemodialysis	No recommendation for dosing available due to lack of data in these populations

Drug-Drug Interactions

Concomitant use of a P-gp inhibitor (eg, amiodarone, carvedilol, clarithromycin, itraconazole, and verapamil) is unavoidable	Reduce the talazoparib starting dose to 0.75 mg by mouth once daily. If the P-gp inhibitor is subsequently discontinued, then increase the talazoparib dose to the dose used prior to initiation of the P-gp inhibitor once 3–5 half-lives of the P-gp inhibitor have transpired
Concomitant use of a BCRP inhibitor (eg, cyclosporine, eltrombopag, imatinib, gefitinib, proton pump inhibitors) is unavoidable	Do not modify the talazoparib starting dose. Monitor for the potential for increased frequency and severity of adverse reactions

Other Toxicities

G ≥3 nonhematologic toxicity where prophylaxis is not considered feasible or toxicity persists despite treatment	Interrupt talazoparib until resolution of toxicity to G ≤1 or baseline, then resume talazoparib with the dosage reduced by 1 dose level

ANC, absolute neutrophil count; MDS, myelodysplastic syndrome; AML, acute myelogenous leukemia; P-gp, P-glycoprotein

Talzenna (talazoparib) prescribing information. New York, NY: Pfizer Labs; revised 2018 October

Adverse Events (N = 412)

Grade (%)*	Talazoparib (N = 286)		Physician's Choice (N = 126)	
	Grade 1–2	Grade 3–4	Grade 1–2	Grade 3–4
Anemia	13.6	39.2	13.5	4.8
Neutropenia	13.6	21.0	7.9	34.9
Thrombocytopenia	12.2	14.7	5.6	1.6
Febrile neutropenia	0	0.3	0	0.8
Fatigue	48.6	1.7	39.7	3.2
Nausea	48.3	0.3	45.2	1.6
Headache	30.8	1.7	21.4	0.8
Alopecia	25.2	0	27.8	0
Vomiting	22.4	2.4	21.4	1.6
Diarrhea	21.3	0.7	20.6	5.6
Constipation	21.7	0.3	21.4	0
Decreased appetite	21.0	0.3	21.4	0.8
Back pain	18.5	2.4	14.3	1.6
Dyspnea	15.0	2.4	12.7	2.4
Palmar-plantar erythrodysesthesia	1.0	0.3	19.8	2.4
Pleural effusion	0.3	1.7	4.8	4.0

*According to the National Cancer Institute Common Terminology Criteria for Adverse Events, version 4.03

Note: The table includes all-grade nonhematologic adverse events occurring in ≥20% of patients, grade 3–4 nonhematologic adverse events occurring in ≥2.4% of patients, and hematologic adverse events. No cases of acute myeloid leukemia or myelodysplastic syndrome were reported in the talazoparib group. Adverse events leading to study drug discontinuation occurred in 5.9% of the talazoparib group and 8.7% of the chemotherapy group. Adverse events requiring dose interruption or reduction occurred in 66% of the talazoparib group (most commonly due to hematologic adverse events) and 60% of the chemotherapy group. One patient in each group had a fatal adverse event related to study drug (1 patient due to veno-occlusive disease in the talazoparib group, and 1 patient due to sepsis in the chemotherapy group)

8. Carcinoma of Unknown Primary

David R. Spigel, MD and F. Anthony Greco, MD

Epidemiology

Incidence: Unknown* (Estimated at 30,000–45,000 patients/year)
Median age: Varies by histology (usually sixth decade)
Male to female ratio: M ≅ F

Stage at Presentation
Local/regional: <10%
≥2 sites: >90%

*Due to patient heterogeneity and tumor registry misclassification

American Cancer Society. Cancer Facts & Figures 2013 Greco FA, Hainsworth JD. In: DeVita VT Jr et al, editors. Cancer: Principles & Practice of Oncology, 10th ed. Philadelphia: Wolters Kluwer; 2015:1720–1737
Hainsworth JD et al. J Clin Oncol 1991;9:1931–1938
Hainsworth JD, Greco FA. N Engl J Med 1993;329:257–263

Pathology

Adenocarcinoma (well differentiated or moderately differentiated)	60%
Poorly differentiated carcinoma/ (± features of adenocarcinoma)	29%
Poorly differentiated malignant neoplasm	5%
Squamous carcinoma	5%
Neuroendocrine carcinoma	1%

Greco FA, Hainsworth JD. In: DeVita VT Jr et al, editors. Cancer: Principles & Practice of Oncology, 10th ed. Philadelphia: Wolters Kluwer; 2015:1720–1737Hainsworth JD, Greco FA. N Engl J Med 1993;329:257–263

Work-up

Clinical evaluation
- H&P, including pelvic, breast, and rectal exams
- CBC
- Comprehensive metabolic profile
- Urinalysis
- Occult blood in feces
- Lactate dehydrogenase (LDH)
- Serum human chorionic gonadotropin (HCG)
- Alpha-fetoprotein (AFP)
- Carcinoembryonic antigen (CEA)
- CA 19-9, CA 27–29 (or CA 15-3), CA 125; PSA (men)
- Chest/abdominal/pelvic CT; mammograms (women)

Where appropriate:
- Positron emission tomography (PET)
- Bronchoscopy, and panendoscopy (particularly for squamous carcinomas neck)

Pathologic studies
- Core needle or excisional biopsy preferred over fine-needle aspiration (FNA)/cytology (consider rebiopsy if insufficient material from initial biopsy)
- Immunohistochemistry (IHC) analyses for:
  - CK7

  CK20
  - TTF-1

  CDX-2
  - Other IHC stains depending on results of above listed stains and clinical features
  - Consider gene signature profiling of biopsy specimen for tissue of origin

Where appropriate:
- Electron microscopy
- Cytogenetic analysis
- Molecular profiling of biopsy specimen with next generation sequencing (NGS)

Focused Work-up

Presentation	Men	Women
Head and neck or supraclavicular adenopathy	• ENT exam • Testicular ultrasound	• ENT exam • Mammography, ER/PR • Pathologic evaluation
Axillary adenopathy	• Mammography	• Mammography, ER/PR • (Consider ultrasound or MRI)
Mediastinal involvement	• HCG/AFP	• HCG/AFP • Mammography, ER/PR
Chest (effusion and/or nodules) involvement	• Bronchoscopy	• Mammography, ER/PR • CA 125
Peritoneal involvement	• Chest/abdominal/pelvic CT • PSA	• Intravaginal ultrasound • Mammography, ER/PR • CA 125
Retroperitoneal mass	• Ultrasound • HCG/AFP • Testicular ultrasound	• Chest/abdominal/pelvic CT • Mammography, ER/PR • CA 125
Inguinal adenopathy	• Anoscopy/colonoscopy	• Anoscopy/colonoscopy • Mammography, ER/PR • CA 125
Hepatic involvement	• Colonoscopy • AFP	• Colonoscopy • AFP • Mammography, ER/PR
Skeletal involvement	• Bone scan	• Bone scan • Mammography, ER/PR
Brain involvement		• Mammography, ER/PR

Greco FA, Hainsworth JD. In: DeVita VT Jr et al, editors. Cancer: Principles & Practice of Oncology, 10th ed. Philadelphia: Wolters Kluwer; 2015:1720–1737

Survival

All Patients With First-Line Empiric Chemotherapy
• 1-Year survival: 35–40%
• 2-Year survival: 15–20%
• 3-Year survival: 10–15%
• 5-Year survival: 10%
• 8-Year survival: <10%

Survival varies by histology and clinical subsets

Expert Opinion

General: In the past for most patients who did not fit into a favorable prognostic group and presenting with poor prognostic features and disseminated disease, the prognosis was poor with empiric chemotherapy. However, survival has improved for a minority of patients with otherwise unfavorable prognostic factors. Empiric regimens were the preferred approach in the past and continue to be acceptable alternatives to offer patients; however, emerging data now highly suggest that a more tailored approach to therapy is superior for many patients. With the emergence of modern molecular testing to help define the cancer type and potentially actionable genetic alterations, the focus has shifted from empiric combination chemotherapy to more tailored site-specific therapies. Clinical features, immunohistochemical evaluation, and molecular profiling used together can now identify the cancer type in about 90% of patients. The detailed molecular characterization of these tumors by NGS is also likely to suggest appropriate and perhaps more effective targeted therapies including immunotherapy. Furthermore, as therapies for known primary cancers improve and become more selective based on biomarkers (including genetic findings in the cancer cells), newer therapeutic approaches should be evaluated in the appropriate CUP subsets as well

Recognizing favorable subsets: Most patients with unknown primary cancer have variable clinical and pathologic presentations, making treatment selection somewhat empiric. However, approximately 20% of patients present with recognizable features characteristic of known primary cancers where specific therapies are more established. It is important to recognize these favorable clinical and pathologic subsets when choosing therapy, such as local therapy with curative intent in a patient with isolated neck nodes involved with squamous cell carcinoma or a woman with isolated axillary adenocarcinoma

Empiric therapy: **Cytotoxic chemotherapy combinations may be used, particularly for patients without highly suspected cancer type.** Paclitaxel/carboplatin (± etoposide) and gemcitabine/irinotecan or gemcitabine/platinum are broad-spectrum regimens that can be used in patients who present without characteristic clinical or pathologic features, particularly in patients with adenocarcinomas. The combination of oxaliplatin and capecitabine was found to have modest activity as a salvage treatment for patients with CUP. This regimen should be considered in patients with clinical and pathologic features suggesting a primary site in the gastrointestinal tract

Empiric therapy for unknown primary tumors can also include regimens in the appropriate clinical setting. When one's clinical suspicion is NSCLC, despite the absence of a definitive primary site, paclitaxel/carboplatin + bevacizumab or pemetrexed/platinum regimens are appropriate for a patient who is otherwise eligible. Immunotherapy with immune checkpoint blockers or targeted therapy also should be considered. Likewise, if the clinical impression is of a primary colorectal malignancy, for example in a patient with hepatic metastases and a negative endoscopic evaluation, choosing infusional fluorouracil and oxaliplatin (FOLFOX) + bevacizumab would be a reasonable option, particular in those with IHC staining highly suggesting a lower intestinal primary (CK7−, CK20+, CDX-2+).

Tailoring therapy: Advances in imaging (PET/CT) and in our use of immunohistochemistry (TTF-1, CDX2, CK20, CK7, etc.) have helped expand our ability to identify a primary site at diagnosis. However, none of these tests is absolute, and they still leave clinicians with some degree of uncertainty for some patients when assessing prognosis and selecting treatment. Recently, genomic and proteomic technologies have emerged as additional tools to potentially help identify a tumor's primary origin. These tests analyze which genes are active or inactive in the tumor specimen and compare these genetic signatures with gene profiles from known tumor libraries. Several commercial tests are now available, but they still require additional prospective validation. Encouraging results have been obtained by performing molecular profiling with a reverse transcriptase polymerase chain reaction (RT-PCR) assay (Cancer Type ID; bioTheranostics, Inc., San Diego, CA). The assay can be performed on formalin-fixed paraffin-embedded biopsy specimens. In a blinded study, 15 of the 20 assay predictions (75%) were correct (95% confidence interval, 60–85%), corresponding to the actual latent primary sites identified later after the initial diagnosis of CUP. Moreover, in a large prospective trial 194 patients with CUP received assay-directed site-specific treatment. The median survival was 12.5 months—and longest in tumor types regarded as clinically more responsive (eg, breast, colorectal) when compared with more resistant tumor types (eg, biliary, pancreatic).Others have reported similar findings for retrospective and prospective studies. As these diagnostic tests improve, along with our understanding of molecular targets critical to cancer cell growth, we will be better able to select optimal therapies for our patients with unknown primary cancers. Immunotherapy with immune checkpoint blockers now is standard therapy for several advanced cancers, and patients with CUP who are felt to harbor these cancers should be considered for a therapeutic trial of immunotherapy

Greco FA. Nat Rev Clin Oncol 2017;14:5–6
Greco FA et al. J Natl Cancer Inst 2013;105:782–789
Greco FA et al. Oncologist 2010;15:500–506
Hainsworth JD et al. Am Soc Clin Oncol Educ Book 2018;23:20–25
Hainsworth JD et al. J Clin Oncol 2007;25:1747–1752
Hainsworth JD et al. J Clin Oncol 2013;31:217–223
Moran S et al. Lancet Oncol 2016;17:1386–1395
Varadhachary GR et al. Int J Clin Oncol 2014;19:479–484
Varadhachary GR et al. J Clin Oncol 2008;26:4442–4448
Yoon HH et al. Ann Oncol 2016;27:339–344

FIRST-LINE

CARCINOMA OF UNKNOWN PRIMARY REGIMEN: PACLITAXEL + CARBOPLATIN

Hainsworth JD et al. Cancer 2015;121:1654–1661
Hainsworth JD et al. J Clin Oncol 1997;15:2385–2393

Premedication against hypersensitivity reactions to paclitaxel:
Dexamethasone 10 mg/dose; orally for 2 doses at 12 hours and 6 hours before each paclitaxel dose, *or*
Dexamethasone 20 mg/dose; intravenously over 10–15 minutes, 30–60 minutes before each paclitaxel dose (total dosage/21-day cycle = 20 mg)
Diphenhydramine 50 mg, by intravenous injection 30–60 minutes before each paclitaxel dose
Cimetidine 300 mg (or **ranitidine** 50 mg, **famotidine** 20 mg, or an equivalent histamine [H$_2$]-subtype receptor antagonist) intravenously over 15–30 minutes, 30–60 minutes before each paclitaxel dose

Paclitaxel 175 mg/m^2/dose; administer intravenously diluted in a volume of 0.9% sodium chloride injection (0.9% NS) or 5% dextrose injection (D5W) to a concentration within the range 0.3 to 1.2 mg/mL, over 3 hours, prior to carboplatin on day 1, every 21 days (total dosage/21-day cycle = 175 mg/m^2)

Carboplatin (calculated dose) AUC = 6 mg/mL × min; administer intravenously diluted in 250 mL D5W or 0.9% NS over 30–60 minutes after paclitaxel on day 1, every 21 days (total dosage/21-day cycle calculated to produce an AUC = 6 mg/mL × min)

Supportive Care
Antiemetic prophylaxis
Emetogenic potential on day 1 is **HIGH**. *Potential for delayed symptoms*
See Chapter 42 for antiemetic recommendations

Hematopoietic growth factor (CSF) prophylaxis
Primary prophylaxis is **NOT** *indicated*
See Chapter 43 for more information

Antimicrobial prophylaxis
Risk of fever and neutropenia is **LOW**
  Antimicrobial primary prophylaxis to be considered:
  • Antibacterial—not indicated
  • Antifungal—not indicated
  • Antiviral—not indicated unless patient previously had an episode of HSV

Carboplatin dose is based on a formula described by Calvert et al. to achieve a target area under the plasma concentration versus time curve (AUC)

$$\text{Total carboplatin dose (mg)} = (\text{target AUC}) \times (\text{GFR} + 25)$$

In practice, creatinine clearance (Clcr) is used in place of glomerular filtration rate (GFR). Clcr can be estimated from the equation of Cockcroft and Gault, thus:

$$\text{For males, CrCl} = \frac{(140 - \text{age [years]}) \times (\text{body weight [kg]})}{72 \times (\text{serum creatinine [mg/dL]})}$$

$$\text{For females, CrCl} = \frac{(140 - \text{age [years]}) \times (\text{body weight [kg]})}{72 \times (\text{serum creatinine [mg/dL]})} \times 0.85$$

Note: On October 8, 2010, the U.S. FDA identified a potential safety issue with carboplatin dosing. By the end of 2010, all clinical laboratories in the United States will use the standardized Isotope Dilution Mass Spectrometry (IDMS) method to measure serum creatinine, which could result in an overestimation of the GFR in some patients with normal renal function. A carboplatin dose calculated from an estimated creatinine clearance based on an IDMS-measured serum creatinine could exceed exposure predicted by the Calvert formula and result in increased drug-related toxicity

Provided actual GFR measurements are made to assess renal function, carboplatin can be safely dosed according to the Calvert formula described in product labeling

If GFR (or Clcr) is estimated using serum creatinine measurements by the IDMS method, the FDA recommended for patients with normal renal function limiting estimated GFR (Clcr) to not more than 125 mL/min for any targeted AUC value

Calvert AH et al. J Clin Oncol 1989;7:1748–1756
Cockcroft DW, Gault MH. Nephron 1976;16:31–41
Jodrell DI et al. J Clin Oncol 1992;10:520–528
Sorensen BT et al. Cancer Chemother Pharmacol 1991;28:397–401
U.S. Food and Drug Administration. Carboplatin dosing. May 23, 2013. Available from: http://www.fda.gov/AboutFDA/CentersOffices/OfficeofMedicalProductsandTobacco/CDER/ucm228974.htm [accessed February 26, 2014]

Patient Population Studied

The international, multicenter, randomized, phase 2 trial involved 85 patients with cancer of unknown primary site (CUP) and a histologic diagnosis of adenocarcinoma, poorly differentiated carcinoma, or squamous carcinoma. Eligible patients had Eastern Cooperative Oncology Group performance score ≤2. Patients who had subsets of CUP that had a recognized favorable prognosis with specific treatments, and patients who had previously received systemic treatment for CUP, were not eligible. Patients were randomly assigned to receive paclitaxel and carboplatin with or without belinostat treatment. The efficacy and toxicity data for the control group (that is, those assigned to no belinostat) are provided; these 43 patients had received at least one and up to six 21-day cycles of intravenous paclitaxel (175 mg/m^2 over 1–3 hours on day 1) and carboplatin (area under the concentration time curve of 6 over 30–60 minutes on day 1).

Efficacy (N = 43)

Median progression-free survival	5.3 months
Median overall survival	9.1 months
Objective response rate	21%
Median duration of response	5.3 months

Treatment Modifications

PACLITAXEL AND CARBOPLATIN DOSE MODIFICATIONS

Paclitaxel Dose Levels		Carboplatin Dose Levels	
Paclitaxel starting dose	175 mg/m^2	Carboplatin starting dose	AUC = 6 mg/mL × min
Paclitaxel dose level −1	140 mg/m^2	Carboplatin dose level −1	AUC = 4.5 mg/mL × min
Paclitaxel dose level −2	100 mg/m^2	Carboplatin dose level −2	AUC = 3 mg/mL × min

Adverse Event	Treatment Modification
Hematologic Toxicity	
Day 1: ANC <1500/mm^3 *or* platelets <100,000/mm^3	Delay treatment until ANC ≥1500/mm^3 and platelets ≥100,000/mm^3, then re-treat with paclitaxel and carboplatin doses reduced by one dose level. Consider adding filgrastim in subsequent cycles
Febrile neutropenia (ANC <1000/mm^3 with single temperature >38.3°C [101°F] or a sustained temperature of ≥38°C [100.4°F] for more than 1 hour)	Reduce paclitaxel and carboplatin doses by one dose level and consider adding filgrastim in subsequent cycles, if applicable
Neuropathy	
G2 motor or sensory neuropathies	Reduce paclitaxel dosage by one dose level without interrupting its planned treatment
G3 peripheral neuropathy	Reduce paclitaxel dosage by two dose levels or an additional level if already reduced by one level for G2 toxicity. Continuation of paclitaxel is at the discretion of the medically responsible health care provider
G4 peripheral neuropathy	Discontinue paclitaxel
Hypersensitivity Reactions	
Moderate hypersensitivity during paclitaxel infusion	Patient may be re-treated. Base a decision to re-treat on reaction severity and the medically responsible care provider's judgment
Severe hypersensitivity during paclitaxel infusion	Discontinue paclitaxel
Hypersensitivity reaction to carboplatin including anaphylaxis (risk is increased in patients previously exposed to platinum therapy)	May occur within minutes of administration. Interrupt the infusion in patients with clinically significant infusion reactions. Manage with appropriate supportive therapy including standard epinephrine, corticosteroids, and antihistamines. May consider desensitization for subsequent doses if benefits thought to outweigh risk
Hepatic Impairment	
AST (SGOT) and ALT (SGPT) < 10× ULN and bilirubin between 1.26 to 2× ULN	Reduce starting paclitaxel dosage to 135 mg/m^2. May administer full dose of carboplatin

(continued)

Treatment Modifications (*continued*)

Adverse Event	Treatment Modification
AST (SGOT) and ALT (SGPT) < 10× ULN and bilirubin between 2.01 to 5× ULN	Reduce starting paclitaxel dosage to 90 mg/m². May administer full dose of carboplatin
AST (SGOT) and ALT (SGPT) ≥ 10× ULN or bilirubin >5× ULN	Discontinue paclitaxel. May administer full dose of carboplatin

Other Toxicities

Other reversible G ≥3 toxicities (except nausea, vomiting, elevated transaminases, and alopecia)	Delay treatment until toxicity resolves to baseline or G ≤1, then decrease the dose of the suspected offending medication(s) by one dose level during subsequent cycles

Note: Can cause fetal harm. Advise women of potential risk to the fetus

AUC, area under the curve; ANC, absolute neutrophil count; WBC, white blood cell count; AST, aspartate aminotransferase; ALT, alanine aminotransferase; ULN, upper limit of normal

Hematopoietic growth factors may be used as secondary prophylaxis at the discretion of a treating physician but should not substitute for recommended dose modifications for hematologic toxicities

Hainsworth JD et al. Cancer 2015;121:1654–1661

Hainsworth JD et al. J Clin Oncol 1997;15:2385–2393

Paclitaxel injection, USP prescribing information. Lake Forest, IL: Hospira, Inc; 2012 February

Therapy Monitoring

Prior to each cycle: CBC with differential and platelet count, serum creatinine, BUN, liver function tests

Response evaluation after 2 treatment cycles. If objective response or stable disease with symptomatic improvement recorded, administer 2–4 more cycles for a total of 4–6 cycles

Notes

1. This regimen is easier to administer and less toxic than cisplatin-based regimens
2. Toxicity is primarily myelosuppression

Toxicity (N = 44*)

	Grade 3–4 Event (%)
Fatigue	9
Nausea	9
Pain	7
Thrombocytopenia	7
Anemia	5
Anorexia	5
Neuropathy	5
Neutropenia	5
Vomiting	5
Diarrhea	2
Hypersensitivity reaction	2

*One patient received study treatment but was later identified as being ineligible for the efficacy analysis because of no measurable disease according to RECIST. Treatment-related grade 3–4 toxicities are included in the table. No treatment-related deaths occurred

FIRST-LINE

CARCINOMA OF UNKNOWN PRIMARY REGIMEN: PACLITAXEL + CARBOPLATIN + ETOPOSIDE

Hainsworth JD et al. Cancer 2015;121:1654–1661
Hainsworth JD et al. Cancer J 2010;16:70–75
Hainsworth JD et al. J Clin Oncol 1997;15:2385–2393

Premedication against hypersensitivity reactions to paclitaxel:
Dexamethasone 10 mg/dose; orally for 2 doses at 12 hours and 6 hours before each paclitaxel dose, *or*
Dexamethasone 20 mg/dose; intravenously over 10–15 minutes, 30–60 minutes before each paclitaxel dose (total dosage/21-day cycle = 20 mg)
Diphenhydramine 50 mg, by intravenous injection 30–60 minutes before each paclitaxel dose
Cimetidine 300 mg (or **ranitidine** 50 mg, **famotidine** 20 mg, or an equivalent histamine [H_2]-subtype receptor antagonist) intravenously over 15–30 minutes, 30–60 minutes before each paclitaxel dose

Paclitaxel 200 mg/m^2/dose; administer intravenously diluted in a volume of 0.9% sodium chloride injection (0.9% NS) or 5% dextrose injection (D5W) to a concentration within the range 0.3 to 1.2 mg/mL, over 3 hours, prior to carboplatin on day 1, every 21 days (total dosage/21-day cycle = 200 mg/m^2)

• Or, may administer paclitaxel at a dose of 175 mg/m^2 as described by Hainsworth et al 2015, thus: **paclitaxel** 175 mg/m^2/dose; administer intravenously diluted in a volume of 0.9% NS or D5W to a concentration within the range 0.3–1.2 mg/mL, over 3 hours, prior to carboplatin on day 1, every 21 days (total dosage/cycle = 175 mg/m^2)

Carboplatin (calculated dose) AUC = 6 mg/mL × min; administer intravenously diluted in 250 mL D5W or 0.9% NS over 30–60 minutes after paclitaxel on day 1, every 21 days (total dosage/cycle calculated to produce an AUC = 6 mg/mL × min)

Etoposide 50 mg per dose; administer orally for 5 doses on days 1, 3, 5, 7, and 9, every 21 days, *plus:*
Etoposide 100 mg per dose; administer orally for 5 doses on days 2, 4, 6, 8, and 10, every 21 days (total dosage/21-day cycle = 750 mg)

Supportive Care
Antiemetic prophylaxis
Emetogenic potential on day 1 is **HIGH**. *Potential for delayed symptoms*
Emetogenic potential on days 2 to 10 is **LOW**
See Chapter 42 for antiemetic recommendations

Hematopoietic growth factor (CSF) prophylaxis
Primary prophylaxis is **NOT** *indicated*
See Chapter 43 for more information

Antimicrobial prophylaxis
Risk of fever and neutropenia is **LOW**
Antimicrobial primary prophylaxis to be considered:
• Antibacterial—not indicated
• Antifungal—not indicated
• Antiviral—not indicated unless patient previously had an episode of HSV

Carboplatin dose is based on a formula described by Calvert et al. to achieve a target area under the plasma concentration versus time curve (AUC)

$$\text{Total carboplatin dose (mg)} = (\text{target AUC}) \times (\text{GFR} + 25)$$

In practice, creatinine clearance (Clcr) is used in place of glomerular filtration rate (GFR). Clcr can be estimated from the equation of Cockcroft and Gault, thus:

$$\text{For males, CrCl} = \frac{(140 - \text{age [years]}) \times (\text{body weight [kg]})}{72 \times (\text{serum creatinine [mg/dL]})}$$

$$\text{For females, CrCl} = \frac{(140 - \text{age [years]}) \times (\text{body weight [kg]})}{72 \times (\text{serum creatinine [mg/dL]})} \times 0.85$$

(continued)

Patient Population Studied

The multicenter, randomized, phase 3 trial involved 198 patients with previously untreated cancer of unknown primary site (CUP) and a histologic diagnosis of adenocarcinoma, poorly differentiated adenocarcinoma, poorly differentiated carcinoma, or poorly differentiated squamous carcinoma. Eligible patients had Eastern Cooperative Oncology Group performance score ≤2. Patients with syndromes that had a recognized favorable prognosis with specific treatments were not eligible. Patients were randomly assigned to receive up to six 21-day cycles of intravenous paclitaxel (200 mg/m^2 over 1 hour on day 1), intravenous carboplatin (area under the curve of 6 on day 1), and oral etoposide (50 mg alternating with 100 mg on days 1–10), or intravenous irinotecan (100 mg/m^2 on days 1 and 8) and intravenous gemcitabine (1000 mg/m^2 on days 1 and 8). All patients who had continued response or stable disease after completion of chemotherapy received maintenance therapy with oral gefitinib (250 mg daily) for up to 24 months. The efficacy and toxicity data for the group that received paclitaxel, carboplatin, and etoposide (N = 93) are provided.

(*continued*)

Note: On October 8, 2010, the U.S. FDA identified a potential safety issue with carboplatin dosing. By the end of 2010, all clinical laboratories in the United States will use the standardized Isotope Dilution Mass Spectrometry (IDMS) method to measure serum creatinine, which could result in an overestimation of the GFR in some patients with normal renal function. A carboplatin dose calculated from an estimated creatinine clearance based on an IDMS-measured serum creatinine could exceed exposure predicted by the Calvert formula and result in increased drug-related toxicity

Provided actual GFR measurements are made to assess renal function, carboplatin can be safely dosed according to the Calvert formula described in product labeling

If GFR (or Clcr) is estimated using serum creatinine measurements by the IDMS method, the FDA recommended for patients with normal renal function limiting estimated GFR (Clcr) to not more than 125 mL/min for any targeted AUC value

Calvert AH et al. J Clin Oncol 1989;7:1748–1756
Cockcroft DW, Gault MH. Nephron 1976;16:31–41
Jodrell DI et al. J Clin Oncol 1992;10:520–528
Sorensen BT et al. Cancer Chemother Pharmacol 1991;28:397–401
U.S. Food and Drug Administration. Carboplatin dosing. May 23, 2013. Available from: http://www.fda.gov/AboutFDA/CentersOffices/OfficeofMedicalProductsandTobacco/CDER/ucm228974.htm [accessed February 26, 2014]

Efficacy (N = 93)

Median overall survival	7.4 months
Median progression-free survival	3.3 months
Objective response rate*	18%

*The objective response rate included partial and complete responses; only one complete response was reported
Note: Median follow-up for the whole study (N = 198) was 29 months

Treatment Modifications

PACLITAXEL, CARBOPLATIN, ETOPOSIDE DOSE MODIFICATIONS

Paclitaxel Dose Levels		Carboplatin Dose Levels		Etoposide Dose Levels	
Paclitaxel starting dose	175 or 200 mg/m²	Carboplatin starting dose	AUC = 6 mg/mL × min	Etoposide starting dose	50 mg/dose on days 1, 3, 5, 7, 9, *plus* 100 mg/dose on days 2, 4, 6, 8, 10 (total dosage/21-day cycle = 750 mg)
Paclitaxel dose level −1	140 mg/m²	Carboplatin dose level −1	AUC = 4.5 mg/mL × min	Etoposide dose level −1	50 mg/dose on days 1, 3, 5, 7, *plus* 100 mg/dose on days 2, 4, 6, 8 (total dosage/21-day cycle = 600 mg)
Paclitaxel dose level −2	100 mg/m²	Carboplatin dose level −2	AUC = 3 mg/mL × min	Etoposide dose level −2	50 mg/dose on days 1, 3, 5, *plus* 100 mg/dose on days 2, 4, 6 (total dosage/21-day cycle = 450 mg)

Adverse Event	Treatment Modification
Hematologic Toxicity	
Day 1: ANC <1500/mm³ *or* platelets <75,000/mm³	Delay treatment until ANC >1500/mm³ and platelets >75,000/mm³, then re-treat either without dose reduction or, at the discretion of the medically responsible health care provider, with paclitaxel, carboplatin, and/or etoposide doses reduced by one dose level. Consider adding filgrastim in subsequent cycles
Day 8: WBC <1000/mm³ *or* platelets <75,000/mm³	Omit days 8, 9, and 10 etoposide doses during the current cycle only
Febrile neutropenia (ANC <1000/mm³ with single temperature >38.3°C [101°F] or a sustained temperature of ≥38°C [100.4°F] for more than 1 hour)	Reduce paclitaxel, carboplatin, and etoposide doses by one dose level and consider adding filgrastim in subsequent cycles, if applicable
Neuropathy	
G2 motor or sensory neuropathies	Reduce paclitaxel dosage by one dose level without interrupting its planned treatment
G3 peripheral neuropathy	Reduce paclitaxel dosage by two dose levels or an additional level if already reduced by one level for G2 toxicity. Continuation of paclitaxel is at the discretion of the medically responsible health care provider
G4 peripheral neuropathy	Discontinue paclitaxel

(*continued*)

Treatment Modifications (continued)

Adverse Event	Treatment Modification
Hypersensitivity Reactions	
Moderate hypersensitivity during paclitaxel infusion	Patient may be re-treated. Base a decision to re-treat on reaction severity and the medically responsible care provider's judgment
Severe hypersensitivity during paclitaxel infusion	Discontinue paclitaxel
Hypersensitivity reaction to carboplatin including anaphylaxis (risk is increased in patients previously exposed to platinum therapy)	May occur within minutes of administration. Interrupt the infusion in patients with clinically significant infusion reactions. Manage with appropriate supportive therapy including standard epinephrine, corticosteroids, and antihistamines. May consider desensitization for subsequent doses if benefits thought to outweigh risk
Hepatic Impairment	
AST (SGOT) and ALT (SGPT) < 10× ULN and bilirubin between 1.26 to 2× ULN	Reduce starting paclitaxel dosage to 135 mg/m². May administer full dose of carboplatin. May administer full dose of etoposide in the absence of concurrent renal impairment
AST (SGOT) and ALT (SGPT) < 10× ULN and bilirubin between 2.01 to 5× ULN	Reduce starting paclitaxel dosage to 90 mg/m². May administer full dose of carboplatin. May administer full dose of etoposide in the absence of concurrent renal impairment
AST (SGOT) and ALT (SGPT) ≥ 10× ULN or bilirubin >5× ULN	Discontinue paclitaxel. May administer full dose of carboplatin. May administer full dose of etoposide in the absence of concurrent renal impairment
Other Toxicities	
Other reversible G ≥3 toxicities (except nausea, vomiting, elevated transaminases, and alopecia)	Delay treatment until toxicity resolves to baseline or G ≤1, then decrease the dose of the suspected offending medication(s) by one dose level during subsequent cycles

Note: Can cause fetal harm. Advise women of potential risk to the fetus
AUC, area under the curve; ANC, absolute neutrophil count; WBC, white blood cell count; AST, aspartate aminotransferase; ALT, alanine aminotransferase; ULN, upper limit of normal
Hematopoietic growth factors may be used as secondary prophylaxis at the discretion of a treating physician, but should not substitute for recommended dose modifications for hematologic toxicities
Paclitaxel injection, USP prescribing information. Lake Forest, IL: Hospira, Inc; 2012 February
Hainsworth JD et al. Cancer 2015;121:1654–1661Hainsworth JD et al. Cancer J 2010;16:70–75
Hainsworth JD et al. J Clin Oncol 1997;15:2385–2393

Therapy Monitoring

Prior to each cycle: CBC with differential and platelet count, serum creatinine, BUN, liver function tests
Weekly during therapy: CBC with differential and platelet count
Response evaluation: every 2 cycles

Notes

1. Responses are similar in adenocarcinoma and poorly differentiated carcinoma
2. This regimen is easier to administer and less toxic than cisplatin-based regimens
3. Toxicity is primarily myelosuppression

Toxicity (N = 93)

Grade (%)*	Grade 3	Grade 4
Red blood cell transfusion	24	0
Neutropenia	18	17
Thrombocytopenia	5	3
Anemia	8	1
Fatigue	8	1
Neutropenic fever	9	0
Nausea/vomiting	6	0
Dyspnea	2	1
Anorexia	2	0

Grade (%)*	Grade 3	Grade 4
Hypersensitivity reaction	2	0
Stomatitis/ mucositis	2	0
Arthralgia/myalgia	1	0
Bleeding	1	0
Diarrhea	1	0

*According to the National Cancer Institute Common Toxicity Criteria for Adverse Events, version 3.0. Treatment-related grade 3-4 toxicities are included in the table. A total of 8% of patients did not complete chemotherapy owing to treatment-related toxicity. Two patients (2%) had a treatment-related death

FIRST-LINE

CARCINOMA OF UNKNOWN ORIGIN REGIMEN: GEMCITABINE + IRINOTECAN

Hainsworth JD et al. Cancer J 2010;16:70–75

Gemcitabine 1000 mg/m^2 per dose; administer intravenously in 0.9% sodium chloride injection diluted to a concentration ≥0.1 mg/mL over 30 minutes, for 2 doses on days 1 and 8, every 21 days (total dosage/21-day cycle = 2000 mg/m^2)

Irinotecan 100 mg/m^2 per dose; administer intravenously diluted in a volume of 5% dextrose injection to a concentration within the range of 0.12–2.8 mg/mL over 90 minutes, for 2 doses on days 1 and 8, every 21 days (total dosage/21-day cycle = 200 mg/m^2)

Supportive Care
Antiemetic prophylaxis
Emetogenic potential is **MODERATE**
See Chapter 42 for antiemetic recommendations

Hematopoietic growth factor (CSF) prophylaxis
Primary prophylaxis is **NOT** indicated
See Chapter 43 for more information

Antimicrobial prophylaxis
Risk of fever and neutropenia is **LOW**
   Antimicrobial primary prophylaxis to be considered:
   • Antibacterial—not indicated
   • Antifungal—not indicated
   • Antiviral—not indicated unless patient previously had an episode of HSV

Diarrhea management
Latent or delayed-onset diarrhea:
   Loperamide 4 mg orally initially after the first loose or liquid stool, then
   Loperamide 2 mg orally every 2 hours during waking hours, plus
   Loperamide 4 mg orally every 4 hours during hours of sleep
• Continue for at least 12 hours after diarrhea resolves
• Recurrent diarrhea after a 12-hour diarrhea-free interval is treated as a new episode
• Rehydrate orally with fluids and electrolytes during a diarrheal episode
• If diarrhea persists >48 hours despite loperamide, stop loperamide and hospitalize the patient for IV hydration
Alternatively, a trial of **diphenoxylate hydrochloride** 2.5 mg with **atropine sulfate** 0.025 mg (eg, Lomotil®)
• Initial adult dose is two tablets four times daily until control has been achieved, after which the dose may be reduced to meet individual requirements. Control may often be maintained with as little as two tablets daily
• Clinical improvement of acute diarrhea is usually observed within 48 hours. If improvement of chronic diarrhea after treatment with a maximum daily dose of 8 tablets is not observed within 10 days, control is unlikely with further administration

Persistent diarrhea:
   Octreotide 100–150 mcg subcutaneously 3 times daily. Maximum total daily dose is 1500 mcg

Antibiotic therapy during latent or delayed-onset diarrhea:
   A fluoroquinolone (eg, ciprofloxacin 500 mg orally every 12 hours) if absolute neutrophil count is <500/mm^3, with or without accompanying fever in association with diarrhea
   • Antibiotics should also be administered if patient is hospitalized with prolonged diarrhea and should be continued until diarrhea resolves

Abigerges D et al. J Natl Cancer Inst 1994;86:446–449
*Rothenberg ML et al. J Clin Oncol 2001;19:3801–3807
Wadler S et al. J Clin Oncol 1998;16:3169–3178

Acute cholinergic syndrome
Atropine sulfate 0.25–1 mg; administer subcutaneously or intravenously if abdominal cramping or diarrhea develop during or within 1 hour after irinotecan administration
• If symptoms are severe, add as primary prophylaxis at least 30 minutes before irinotecan during subsequent cycles
For irinotecan, acute cholinergic syndrome may be characterized by abdominal cramping, diarrhea, diaphoresis, hypotension, flushing, bradycardia, rhinitis, increased salivation, miosis, and lacrimation

Patient Population Studied

The multicenter, randomized, phase 3 trial involved 198 patients with previously untreated cancer of unknown primary site (CUP) and a histologic diagnosis of adenocarcinoma, poorly differentiated adenocarcinoma, poorly differentiated carcinoma, or poorly differentiated squamous carcinoma. Eligible patients had Eastern Cooperative Oncology Group performance score ≤2. Patients with syndromes that had a recognized favorable prognosis with specific treatments were not eligible. Patients were randomly assigned to receive 21-day cycles of intravenous paclitaxel (200 mg/m² over 1 hour on day 1), intravenous carboplatin (area under the curve of 6 on day 1), and oral etoposide (50 mg alternating with 100 mg on days 1–10), or intravenous irinotecan (100 mg/m² on days 1 and 8) and intravenous gemcitabine (1000 mg/m² on days 1 and 8). All patients who had continued response or stable disease after completion of chemotherapy received maintenance therapy with oral gefitinib (250 mg daily) for up to 24 months. The efficacy and toxicity data for the group that received irinotecan and gemcitabine (N = 105) are provided.

Efficacy (N = 105)

Median overall survival	8.5 months
Median progression-free survival	5.3 months
Objective response rate*	18%

*The objective response rate included partial and complete responses; however, only partial responses were experienced by patients in this treatment group
Note: Median follow-up for the whole study (N = 198) was 29 months

Treatment Modifications*

GEMCITABINE + IRINOTECAN

Dose Levels

	Gemcitabine	Irinotecan
Starting dose	1000 mg/m²/dose on day 1 and 8	100 mg/m²/dose on day 1 and 8
Dose level −1	750 mg/m²/dose on day 1 and 8	75 mg/m²/dose on day 1 and 8
Dose level −2	500 mg/m²/dose on day 1 and 8	50 mg/m²/dose on day 1 and 8

Adverse Event	Treatment Modification
Hematologic Toxicity	
Day 1 ANC ≥1500/mm³ *and* platelet count ≥100,000/mm³	Do not delay treatment. Administer day 1 gemcitabine and irinotecan at dose level 1
Day 1 ANC ≥1000/mm³ to <1500/mm³ *or* platelet count ≥75,000/mm³ to <100,000/mm³	Do not delay treatment. Administer day 1 gemcitabine and irinotecan at dose level −1
Day 1 ANC <1000/mm³ *or* platelet count <75,000/mm³	Delay treatment at least one week and until ANC ≥1500/mm³ and platelet count ≥100,000/mm³, then administer day 1 gemcitabine and irinotecan at dose level −1. Consider use of hematopoietic growth factor (CSF) prophylaxis in subsequent cycles for dose-limiting neutropenia
Day 8 ANC ≥1500/mm³ *and* platelet count ≥100,000/mm³	Do not delay treatment. Administer day 8 gemcitabine and irinotecan at dose level −1
Day 8 ANC ≥1000/mm³ to <1500/mm³ *or* platelet count ≥75,000/mm³ to <100,000/mm³	Do not delay treatment. Administer day 8 gemcitabine and irinotecan at dose level −1
Day 8 ANC <1000/mm³ *or* platelet count <75,000/mm³	Withhold day 8 gemcitabine and irinotecan. Repeat CBC with differential and platelet count on day 15. If day 15 ANC ≥1500/mm³ and platelet count ≥100,000/mm³, then administer the day 8 treatment on day 15 and schedule the subsequent cycle to begin 7 days later. Consider use of hematopoietic growth factor (CSF) prophylaxis in subsequent cycles for dose-limiting neutropenia
Febrile neutropenia (ANC <1000/mm³ with single temperature >38.3°C [101°F] or a sustained temperature of ≥38°C [100.4°F] for more than 1 hour) during the prior cycle	Administer all subsequent cycles at one lower dose level. Consider use of hematopoietic growth factor (CSF) prophylaxis in subsequent cycles

(continued)

Treatment Modifications (*continued*)

Adverse Event	Treatment Modification
Diarrhea	
G1/2 diarrhea (2–6 stools/day above baseline)	Maintain dose and schedule of gemcitabine and irinotecan. Maximize supportive care
G3 diarrhea (≥7 stools/day above baseline)	Delay gemcitabine and irinotecan until diarrhea resolves to baseline, then reduce dosage of irinotecan by 1 dose level. Maximize supportive care
G4 diarrhea (life-threatening consequences; urgent intervention indicated)	Delay gemcitabine and irinotecan until diarrhea resolves to baseline, then reduce dosage of irinotecan by 2 dosage levels. Maximize supportive care
Hepatic Impairment	
Bilirubin >ULN to ≤2 mg/dL *and* ALT/AST ≤3× ULN in a patient *without* liver metastasis	Reduce irinotecan dosage by one dose level. Do not reduce gemcitabine dosage
Serum bilirubin >2 mg/dL *or* ALT/AST >3× ULN in a patient *without* liver metastasis	Withhold all treatment until bilirubin ≤2 mg/dL and ALT/AST ≤3× ULN
Bilirubin >ULN to ≤2 mg/dL *and* ALT/AST ≤5× ULN in a patient *with* liver metastasis	Reduce irinotecan dosage by one dose level. Do not reduce gemcitabine dosage
Serum bilirubin >2 mg/dL *or* ALT/AST >5× ULN in a patient *with* liver metastasis	Withhold all treatment until bilirubin ≤2 mg/dL and ALT/AST ≤5× ULN
Hypersensitivity Reactions	
Severe hypersensitivity reaction to gemcitabine or irinotecan is noted	Permanently discontinue gemcitabine or irinotecan
Pharmacogenomics Dose Adjustments	
Patient is known to be homozygous for the UGT1A1*28 allele	Consider reducing the starting dosage of irinotecan by 1 dose level
Drug Interactions	
Patient requires treatment with a strong CYP3A4 inducer	Consider substituting the strong CYP3A4 inducer with a non-enzyme inducing therapy ≥2 weeks prior to administration of irinotecan. If coadministration of a strong CYP3A4 inducer with irinotecan is unavoidable, then the appropriate starting dose of irinotecan has not been defined. Monitor closely for loss of irinotecan efficacy
Patient requires treatment with a strong CYP3A4 inhibitor or UGT1A1 inhibitor	Discontinue strong CYP3A4 inhibitors at least 1 week prior to administration of irinotecan. Do not administer strong CYP3A4 or UGT1A1 inhibitors with irinotecan unless there are no therapeutic alternatives, in which case monitor closely for irinotecan toxicity
Other Toxicities	
Unexplained new or worsening dyspnea or evidence of severe pulmonary toxicity	Discontinue gemcitabine and irinotecan immediately and assess for gemcitabine- and/or irinotecan-related pulmonary toxicity
Hemolytic-uremic syndrome (HUS)	Discontinue gemcitabine for HUS or severe renal impairment
Capillary Leak Syndrome	Discontinue gemcitabine
Posterior reversible encephalopathy syndrome (PRES)	Discontinue gemcitabine
Other reversible G ≥3 non-hematologic toxicities (except nausea, vomiting, elevated transaminases, and alopecia)	Delay treatment until toxicity resolves to baseline, then decrease gemcitabine and irinotecan dosages by one dose level from previous dose levels

ANC, absolute neutrophil count; CBC, complete blood count; ULN, upper limit of normal; ALT, alanine aminotransferase; AST, aspartate aminotransferase

Note:
- Patients who are pregnant or who become pregnant should be apprised of the potential hazard to the fetus; women of childbearing potential should be advised to avoid becoming pregnant during therapy
- Gemcitabine may cause severe and life-threatening toxicity when administered during or within 7 days of radiation therapy

Camptosar (irinotecan) prescribing information. New York, NY: Pfizer, Inc; 2014 December

Gemzar (gemcitabine) prescribing information. Indianapolis, IN: Lilly USA, LLC; 2018 November

Hainsworth JD et al. Cancer 2005;104:1992–1997

Hainsworth JD et al. Cancer J 2010;16:70–75

Therapy Monitoring

1. *Day 1 and day 8 of each cycle:* CBC with differential and platelet count, liver function tests, serum electrolytes, BUN, and serum creatinine
2. Pulmonary toxicity and respiratory failure: Discontinue gemcitabine and irinotecan immediately for unexplained new or worsening dyspnea or evidence of severe pulmonary toxicity
3. Gemcitabine has been associated with hemolytic uremic syndrome (HUS). Consider further work-up in patients with evidence of microangiopathic hemolysis and/or renal failure
4. Increased toxicity with infusion time greater than 60 minutes or dosing more frequently than once weekly may occur with gemcitabine; monitor carefully
5. Gemcitabine has been associated with Capillary Leak Syndrome. Monitor weight, volume status, and vital signs
6. Irinotecan has been associated with acute (cholinergic) diarrhea and late-onset diarrhea. Advise patients to promptly report symptoms of diarrhea and provide instructions for self-management
7. Gemcitabine may exacerbate the toxic effects of radiation therapy. Do not administer gemcitabine during or within 7 days of radiation therapy
8. Gemcitabine has been associated with posterior reversible encephalopathy syndrome (PRES). Monitor for a syndrome of headache, altered consciousness, visual disturbances, seizures, and/or hypertension
9. *Response evaluation:* Every 2 cycles

Toxicity (N = 105)

Grade (%)*	Grade 3	Grade 4
Neutropenia	10	1
Red blood cell transfusion	10	0
Diarrhea	6	0
Fatigue	3	1
Nausea/vomiting	4	0
Anemia	3	0
Constipation	3	0
Thrombocytopenia	3	0
Arthralgia/myalgia	2	0
Anorexia	1	0
Bleeding	1	0

*According to the National Cancer Institute Common Toxicity Criteria for Adverse Events, version 3.0 Treatment-related grade 3–4 toxicities are included in the table. A total of 19% of patients did not complete chemotherapy owing to treatment-related toxicity. One patient (1%) had a treatment-related death

SUBSEQUENT THERAPY

CARCINOMA OF UNKNOWN PRIMARY REGIMEN: OXALIPLATIN + CAPECITABINE

Hainsworth JD et al. Cancer 2010;116:2448–2454

Oxaliplatin 130 mg/m^2; administer intravenously in 250–500 mL 5% dextrose injection over 2 hours on day 1, every 21 days (total dosage/cycle = 130 mg/m^2)

Capecitabine 1000 mg/m^2 per dose; administer orally twice daily (approximately every 12 hours) for 28 doses on days 1–14, every 21 days, (total dose/cycle = 28,000 mg/m^2)

Notes:
- Capecitabine is given for 2 consecutive weeks followed by 1 week without treatment
- Doses are rounded to use combinations of 500-mg and 150-mg tablets that most closely approximate calculated values
- Although food decreases the rate and extent of drug absorption and the time to peak plasma concentration and systemic exposure (AUC) for both capecitabine and fluorouracil, product labeling recommends giving capecitabine within 30 minutes after the end of a meal because established safety and efficacy data are based on administration with food

Note: Patients with objective response or stable disease after 2 cycles continued treatment for 6 cycles or until disease progression. Patients who continued to benefit and were tolerating treatment well had the option to receive additional treatment cycles at the discretion of their physician

Note: Leukocyte growth factors are not routinely used during cycle 1 but may be used subsequently as secondary prophylaxis according to standard guidelines

Note: The combination of oxaliplatin and capecitabine has activity as a salvage treatment for patients with CUP. Consider in patients with clinical and pathologic features suggesting a primary site in the gastrointestinal tract

Supportive Care
Antiemetic prophylaxis
Emetogenic potential on day 1 is **MODERATE**
Emetogenic potential on days with capecitabine alone is **LOW**
See Chapter 42 for antiemetic recommendations

Hematopoietic growth factor (CSF) prophylaxis
Primary prophylaxis is NOT indicated
See Chapter 43 for more information

Antimicrobial prophylaxis
Risk of fever and neutropenia is LOW
   Antimicrobial primary prophylaxis to be considered:
- Antibacterial—not indicated
- Antifungal—not indicated
- Antiviral—not indicated, unless patient previously had an episode of HSV

Oral care
Standard prophylaxis and treatment for mucositis/stomatitis

Hand-foot reaction (palmar-plantar erythrodysesthesia, PPE)
For patients who develop a hand-foot reaction, use topical emollients (eg, Aquaphor®), topical or orally administered steroids, antihistamine agents (H$_1$-receptor antagonists), or pyridoxine
   Pyridoxine may provide relief for discomfort/pain associated with PPE, although the mechanism through which this occurs remains unclear
- The suggested pyridoxine starting dose is 50 mg/day, which may be increased to a maximum of 200 mg/day
- Patients who develop G1/2 PPE while receiving doxorubicin HCl liposome injection may receive a fixed daily dose of pyridoxine 200 mg. This may allow for treatment to be completed without dosage reduction, treatment delay, or recurrence of PPE

Treatment Modifications

Adverse Event	Dose Modification
ANC <1500/mm^3 or platelet count <75,000/mm^3 on day 1 of a cycle	Delay treatment for 1 week and remeasure blood counts. If, after a 1-week delay, ANC ≥1500/mm^3 and platelet count ≥75,000/mm^3, decrease dosages of both agents by 25% and resume treatment
ANC <1500/mm^3 or platelet count <75,000/mm^3 after a 1-week delay	Delay treatment for 1 additional week and remeasure blood counts. If, after a second 1-week delay, ANC ≥1500/mm^3 and platelet count ≥75,000/mm^3, decrease dosages of both agents by 25% and resume treatment
ANC <1500/mm^3 or platelet count <75,000/mm^3 after a second 1-week delay	Discontinue therapy
Hospitalization for fever and neutropenia	Continue therapy with dosages of both drugs decreased by 25% in subsequent cycles
Neutropenia and fever during a 14-day course of capecitabine	Discontinue capecitabine for remainder of cycle
G2 peripheral neuropathy	Reduce dose of oxaliplatin by 25% during subsequent cycles
G3/4 peripheral neuropathy	Discontinue oxaliplatin; continue single agent capecitabine if patient is benefiting
Laryngopharyngeal dysesthesia during oxaliplatin administration	Increase duration of subsequent oxaliplatin infusions from 2 to 6 hours
G >1 hand-foot syndrome during or after capecitabine	Discontinue remaining capecitabine doses for ongoing cycle. Delay starting a subsequent cycle of therapy until the hand-foot syndrome recovers to G ≤1. Give capecitabine during subsequent cycles at dosages decreased by 25%

(continued)

Efficacy* (N = 48)

Complete response	0
Partial response	19%
Stable disease at first evaluation[†]	46%
Remission duration in 9 patients who achieved PR	Median 10 months (range: 2–48 months)
Median progression-free survival	3.7 months
Median overall survival[‡]	9.7 months
1 Year PFS	22%

*RECIST criteria (Response Evaluation Criteria in Solid Tumors, Therasse P et al. J Natl Cancer Inst 2000;92:205–216)
[†]8/22 with SD had SD >3 months, and 4/22 had SD >6 months
[‡]28 patients (58%) subsequently received further treatment for CUP

Note: Patients received a median of 12 weeks (4 cycles) of treatment (range: 3–66 weeks). Fifteen patients completed ≥6 cycles with oxaliplatin + capecitabine

Toxicity (N = 48 patients; 209 Treatment Courses)*

	% G3	% G4
Hematologic		
Neutropenia	3 (6%)	—
Thrombocytopenia	4 (8%)	2 (4%)
Anemia	—	1 (2%)
Febrile neutropenia	—	1 (2%)
Nonhematologic		
Nausea/vomiting	24 (50%)	2 (4%)
Dehydration	9 (19%)	—
Diarrhea	2 (4%)	1 (2%)
Peripheral neuropathy	2 (4%)	—
Mucositis	2 (4%)	—
Treatment-related hospitalizations	13 (27%)	
Treatment-related deaths	—	
Treatment discontinued for toxicity	6 (12.5%)	

*NCI CTCAE, National Cancer Institute (USA) Common Terminology Criteria for Adverse Events, version 3. At: http://ctep.cancer.gov/protocolDevelopment/electronic_applications/ctc.htm [accessed December 7, 2013]

Therapy Monitoring

At the beginning of each 21-day cycle, patients seen and examined by physician. Complete blood counts and serum electrolytes, creatinine, LFTs performed. Response assessment every 2 cycles

Treatment Modifications
(continued)

Hand-foot syndrome G >1 after 2 dose reductions, or requiring delay of >2 weeks for symptoms to resolve	Discontinue capecitabine; continue oxaliplatin in patients benefiting from treatment
Other nonhematologic toxicity G >2	Reduce offending agents' dosages by 25% during subsequent courses
Irreversible nonhematologic toxicity, or toxicity that requires treatment delay >2 weeks	Discontinue therapy

Patient Population Studied

Histologically or cytologically confirmed CUP. Eligible tumor histologies included adenocarcinoma, poorly differentiated adenocarcinoma, poorly differentiated carcinoma, squamous carcinoma, and poorly differentiated neuroendocrine carcinoma. Patients were required to have been treated previously with 1 chemotherapy regimen but could not have previously received oxaliplatin, capecitabine, or fluorouracil. Patients may also have had treatment with 1 immunotherapy or targeted therapy regimen

Previous chemotherapy: Taxane/platinum-based: 30 (63%); bevacizumab/erlotinib: 5 (10%); taxane ± bevacizumab: 3 (6%); irinotecan/gemcitabine: 5 (10%); platinum/etoposide: 2 (4%); others (1 regimen each): 3 (6%)—22 of 31 patients had previously received carboplatin or cisplatin

Best response to previous treatment: Complete: 1 (2%); partial: 11 (23%); stable disease or progression: 33 (69%); unknown: 3 (6%)

9. Central Nervous System Cancers

Lyndon Kim, MD, and Howard A. Fine, MD

Epidemiology

Incidence: 23,890 (male: 13,590; female: 10,300. Estimated new cases for 2020 in the United States)
7.5 per 100,000 men vs Male 5.4 per 100,000 women vs Female

Deaths: Estimated 18,020 in 2020 (male: 10,190; Female vs female: 7830)

Median age at diagnosis: 59 years

Male to female ratio: Slight male predominance in the incidence of malignant brain tumors (Male:Female 1.39: 1)

Siegel R et al. CA Cancer J Clin 2020;70:7–30
Surveillance, Epidemiology and End Results (SEER) Program, available from http://seer.cancer.gov [accessed in 2020]

Work-up

1. Neuroimaging study (MRI of the brain preferred over CT)
   No other staging work-up is required except:
2. Primary CNS lymphoma: MRI of spine, lumbar puncture, and ophthalmologic examination
3. Medulloblastoma: MRI of spine and lumbar puncture when safe to do so

Pathology

I. **Neuroepithelial Tumors**
   A. Glial tumors (45–50%)
      a. Diffuse astrocytic tumors (75%)
         1. Diffuse astrocytoma (grade II): 20%
            i. Diffuse astrocytoma, IDH-mutant
               Gemistocytic astrocytoma, IDH-mutant
            ii. Diffuse astrocytoma, IDH-wildtype
         2. Anaplastic astrocytoma (AA grade III): 30%
            i. Anaplastic astrocytoma, IDH-mutant
            ii. Anaplastic astrocytoma, IDH-wildtype
         3. Glioblastoma (GB, grade IV): 50%
            i. Glioblastoma, IDH-wildtype
               Giant cell glioblastoma
               Gliosarcoma: <5% of GB
               Epithelioid glioblastoma
            ii. Glioblastoma, IDH-mutant
         4. Diffuse midline glioma H3 K27M-mutant (grade IV)
      b. Oligodendrogliomas/ oligoastrocytomas (5–10%)
         1. Oligodendroglioma (O, grade II)
            i. Oligodendroglioma, IDH-mutant, 1p19q-codeleted

         2. Anaplastic oligodendroglioma (AO, grade III)
            i. Anaplastic oligodendroglioma, IDH-mutant, 1p19q-codeleted
         3. Oligoastrocytoma (OA, grade II)
            i. Oligoastrocytoma NOS (Most OA will fall into this category if molecular testing for oligodendroglioma and astrocytoma is not diagnostic)
            ii. Oligoastrocytoma (IDH-mutant, 1p19q-codeleted on oligodendroglioma side, IDH-mutant vs wildtype, 1p19q-intact on astrocytoma side)
         4. Anaplastic oligoastrocytoma (AOA grade III)
            i. Anaplastic oligoastrocytoma NOS (Most AOA will fall into this category if molecular testing for oligodendroglioma or astrocytoma is not diagnostic)
            ii. Anaplastic oligoastrocytoma (IDH mutant, 1p19q-codeleted on oligodendroglioma side, IDH-mutant vs wildtype, 1p19q-intact on astrocytoma side)
      c. Other astrocytic tumors (<5%)
         1. Pilocytic astrocytoma (grade I)
         2. Subependymal giant cell astrocytoma (grade I)

         3. Pleomorphic xanthoastrocytoma (grade II)
         4. Anaplastic pleomorphic xanthoastrocytoma (grade III)
      d. Ependymal tumors (5%)
         1. Subependymoma (grade I)
         2. Myxopapillary ependymoma (grade I)
         3. Ependymoma (grade II)
            Papillary ependymoma
            Clear cell ependymoma
            Tanycytic ependymoma
         4. Ependymoma. RELA fusion-positive (grade II or III)
         5. Anaplastic ependymoma (grade III)
   B. Neuronal and mixed glial-neuronal tumors (<1%)
      1. Central neurocytoma (grade II)
      2. Dysembryoplastic neuroepithelial tumor (DNET) (grade I)
      3. Desmoplastic infantile astrocytoma and ganglioglioma (grade I)
      4. Gangliocytoma (grade I)
      5. Ganglioglioma (grade I)
      6. Anaplastic ganglioglioma (grade III)
      7. Dysplastic gangliocytoma of cerebellum (Lhermitte-Duclos disease) (grade I)
      8. Paraganglioma

(continued)

Pathology *(continued)*

C. Nonglial tumors
- a. Embryonal tumors (<5%)
  - 1. Medulloblastoma (grade IV)
    - i. Medulloblastoma, WNT-activated
    - ii. Medulloblastoma, SHH activated and TP53-mutant
      Medulloblastoma, SHH activated and TP53-wildtype
      Medulloblastoma, non-WNT/non-SHH
    - iii. Medulloblastoma group 3
    - iv. Medulloblastoma group 4
  - 2. CNS neuroblastoma (grade IV)
  - 3. Atypical teratoid/rhabdoid tumors (AT/RT) (grade IV)
- b. Choroid plexus tumors (<1%)
  - 1. Choroid plexus papilloma (grade I)
  - 2. Atypical choroid plexus papilloma (grade II)
  - 3. Choroid plexus carcinoma (grade III)
- c. Pineal tumors (<1%)
  - 1. Pineocytoma (grade I)
  - 2. Pineoblastoma (grade IV)

II. **Meningeal Tumors (15–28%)**
1. Meningioma (grade I): (>80–90%)
   - a. Secretory meningioma (grade I)
   - b. Fibrous meningioma (grade I)
   - c. Atypical meningioma (grade II): (10–20%)
   - d. Clear cell meningioma (grade II)
   - e. Chordoid meningioma (grade II)
   - f. Anaplastic (malignant) meningioma (grade III): (2%)
   - g. Papillary meningioma (grade III)
   - h. Rhabdoid meningioma (grade III)

III. **Nerve Sheath Tumors, Cranial and Peripheral Nerves (4–8%)**
1. Schwannoma (grade I)
2. Neurofibroma (grade I)
3. Malignant peripheral nerve sheath tumor (grade II, III, or IV)

IV. **Mesenchymal, Non-meningothelial Tumors**
1. Solitary fibrous tumor/hemangiopericytoma (grade I, II, or III)
   - Grade I
   - Grade II
   - Grade III
2. Hemangioblastoma (grade I)
3. Hemangioma

V. **Primary CNS Lymphoma (PCNSL) (3–5%)**
1. Diffuse large B-cell lymphoma of the CNS
2. Immunodeficiency-associated CNS lymphomas
   - AIDS-related diffuse large B-cell lymphoma
   - EBV-positive diffuse large B-cell lymphoma
   - Lymphomatoid granulomatosis
3. Intravascular large B-cell lymphoma
4. T-cell and NK/T-cell lymphoma of the CNS
5. Anaplastic large cell lymphoma, ALK positive
6. Anaplastic large cell lymphoma, ALK negative
7. MALT lymphoma of the dura

VI. **Germ Cell Tumors (<1%)**
1. Germinoma
2. Embryonal carcinoma
3. York sac tumor
4. Choriocarcinoma
5. Teratoma
6. Teratoma with malignant transformation
7. Mixed germ cell tumor

VII. **Histiocytic Tumors**
1. Langerhans cell histiocytosis
2. Erdheim-Chester disease
3. Juvenile xanthogranuloma
4. Histiocytic sarcoma

VIII. **Melanocytic Tumors**
1. Meningeal melanocytosis
2. Meningeal melanocytoma
3. Meningeal melanoma
4. Meningeal melanomatosis

IX. **Tumors of the sellar region**
1. Craniopharyngioma (grade I)
   - Adamantinomatous craniopharyngioma
   - Papillary craniopharyngioma
2. Granular cell tumor (grade I)
3. Pituicytoma (grade I)
4. Spindle cell oncocytoma (grade I)

X. **Metastatic Tumors**

Adesina AM et al. Histopathology of primary tumors of the central nervous system. In: Prados M (editors). Brain Cancer: American Cancer Society Atlas of Clinical Oncology. Hamilton, Ontario: BC Decker Inc.; 2002:16–47
Greenberg H et al. Brain Tumors. Oxford: Oxford University Press; 1999:1–26
WHO Classification of Tumors. Lyon: IARC Press; 2000:6–7
WHO Classification of Tumors of the Central Nervous System, 2016. Acta Neuropathol 2016;131:803–820

Staging

(TNM staging does not apply to most brain tumors because they rarely metastasize. Embryonal tumors such as medulloblastoma are exceptions to this rule)

	WHO Grade*						
WHO Designation*	Grade	Nuclear Atypia	Mitosis	Endothelial Proliferation	Necrosis	IDH Mutation	MGMT Methylation
Pilocytic astrocytoma	I	-	-	-	-	Not applicable usually - or very low	Not applicable usually low
Diffuse astrocytoma	II	+	Usually -	-	-	+ (65–90%)	Usually + (>80%)
Anaplastic astrocytoma	III	+	+	±	-	Usually + (65–90%)	Usually+ (40–60%)
Glioblastoma	IV	+	+, Active	Usually +	+	Usually - (wildtype)	Usually - (<35%)

*The 2000 WHO grading system stratified previous low-grade astrocytomas (WHO grades I and II) into different subtypes. WHO grade I pilocytic astrocytoma is characteristically well circumscribed, cystic, and localized. WHO grade II diffuse astrocytoma, like WHO grades III and IV, is characteristically infiltrative and progressive. The current 2016 CNS WHO Classification incorporated molecular information (IDH1 and 2, and 1p19q codeletion status) into the diagnosis of brain tumors, most significantly, astrocytomas and oligodendrogliomas, in addition to histology. Several previously known brain tumors, such as oligoastrocytoma and medulloblastoma, were redefined and tumors like gliomatosis cerebri and primitive neuroectodermal tumor were eliminated, while some new ones were added. Most of the oligoastrocytomas that cannot be diagnosed by IDH mutation and 1p19q codeletion status as oligodendroglioma or astrocytoma are now under oligoastrocytoma NOS (not otherwise specified). Unless two distinctively separate oligodendroglioma or astrocytoma are present, the diagnosis of oligoastrocytoma is discouraged

Kleihues P et al. Histological Typing Tumours of the Central Nervous System. 2nd ed. WHO. Berlin: Springer-Verlag; 1993
WHO Classification of Tumors. Lyon: IARC Press; 2000:6–7
WHO Classification of Tumors of the Central Nervous System, 2016. Acta Neuropathol 2016;131:803–820

Prognosis

Median Survival*	
Grade I	>10 years
Grade II	5–8 years
Grade III	3–5 years
Grade IV	1.2–1.5 year

*Because oligodendrogliomas and oligoastrocytomas are uniquely sensitive to both chemotherapy and radiation therapy with better overall survival and prognosis, every effort should be made to look for oligodendroglial cell components, confirmed by the presence of IDH 1 and 2 mutation and 1p19q codeletion, and provide proper treatment options based on the pathology and molecular information

Burger PC et al. Cancer 1985;56:1106–1111
Piepmeier J et al. Neurosurgery 1987;67:177–181

Expert Opinion

In 2016, WHO released an update to its CNS classification with significant changes. The current classification incorporated molecular information, mainly, into the diagnosis of diffusely infiltrating astrocytomas and oligodendrogliomas in addition to histology. For the diagnosis of diffuse astrocytomas, mutation of IDH 1 and 2 (collectively IDH mutation) and negative codeletion of 1p19 are required while both IDH mutation and codeletion of 1p19 are required for the diagnosis of oligodendrogliomas. For example, IDH mutated diffusely infiltrating glioma with astrocytic features without 1p19q codeletion will be diagnosed as astrocytoma. Likewise, IDH mutant tumor that morphologically resembles oligodendroglioma but without 1p19q codeletion will be also diagnosed as astrocytoma, not oligodendroglioma. As stated, IDH1 is a marker of infiltrating gliomas, both astrocytic and oligodendroglial cells. 1p19q codeletion is required for the diagnosis of oligodendrogliomas

IDH1 recognizes only the most common mutation (IDH-R132H) which accounts for about 90% of all glioma-associated IDH mutations. In rare cases, if there is no evidence of immunohistochemical IDH mutation, a mutational analysis is recommended to check other IDH1 and 2 mutation. IDH1 and 2 mutated diffuse astrocytomas have significantly better prognosis than IDH wildtype (non-mutated). MGMT methylated gliomas also have a better tumor response and prognosis than MGMT unmethylated gliomas

Grade I Astrocytoma (Pilocytic Astrocytoma)
Pilocytic astrocytoma is a rare tumor commonly seen in the pediatric or young adult population and in patients with neurofibromatosis type 1 (NF1), Li-Fraumeni syndrome, and tuberous sclerosis. Although WHO grade I and II tumors are grouped together under the category of low-grade gliomas, they are distinctively different. The tumor is slow growing and well circumscribed, and MRI findings reveal a homogenously enhancing lesion with an associated macrocyst commonly seen in the cerebellum, brainstem, and optic pathways. The tumor is often cystic, and, if solid, tends to be well circumscribed. The presence of Rosenthal fibers, which appear as elongated worm-like or corkscrew-like eosinophilic (pink) bundles on H&E stain, helps the diagnosis. IDH is non-mutated (wildtype) or has very low mutation, and the role of MGMT methylation status is not well established compared with other diffusely infiltrating gliomas. The majority of tumors have a unique BRAF-KIAA1549L fusion gene

(*continued*)

Expert Opinion (continued)

1. **Observation following surgery:** Most patients can be cured if tumor can be completely resected by surgery. Following surgery, patients can be simply observed. In patients who had incomplete resection of tumor, the clinical course is often benign and the tumor may remain inactive. Therefore, the role of postoperative radiation therapy in these patients is controversial. For recurrent tumor, re-resection, if possible, or radiation therapy may be offered

Grade II Astrocytomas (Diffuse Astrocytoma)

Diffuse astrocytoma patients can be found in the young adult population. Although considered as a low grade, the prognosis is still not optimal with overall survival of 5-8 years. MRI usually reveals nonenhancing lesion that could be best seen on T2 or FLAIR images. Traditionally, close observation for low-risk patients and radiation therapy for high-risk patients were recommended as standard of care, but with the recent phase 3 clinical trial results revealing significant overall survival benefit of combining radiation and chemotherapy, radiation therapy followed by PCV chemotherapy for high-risk low-grade gliomas is now considered as standard of care as well as for the most low-risk low-grade glioma patients who carry some borderline high risk features,

1. **Observation:** If surgery or radiation therapy is not an option, patients with the following good prognostic factors can be closely monitored with serial scans:

   - Young age (<40 years)
   - Asymptomatic
   - Good performance score (KPS >70)
   - Near or complete resection
   - Small nonenhancing lesion
   - Low Ki67 or MIB-1 proliferative index
   - Presence of IDH1 or IDH2 mutation

   Note: about a third of patients who have nonenhancing lesions may ultimately prove on biopsy to have anaplastic tumors. Thus, close surveillance (particularly early on until the natural course of the diseases becomes apparent) is recommended for all patients with diffuse astrocytomas for whom a watch-and-wait strategy is employed

2. **Treatment:** General indications for treatment include:

   - Older patient (>40 years)
   - Symptomatic
   - Large (>5 cm) or inoperable lesion
   - Enhancement on imaging studies
   - High Ki67 or MIB-1 proliferative index
   - Lack of IDH1 or IDH2 mutation

   a. **Radiation therapy:** Radiation dose for low-grade gliomas is 54 Gy in 27-30 fractions (1.8-2.0 Gy per fraction per day). Patients with the highest risk factor, such as age >40 with unresectable, symptomatic, >5 cm large astrocytomas that cross the midline, should be treated with radiation therapy. However, if radiation therapy was chosen as a treatment option, then chemotherapy with PCV should be added based on the RTOG 9082 clinical trial for low-grade gliomas that randomized PCV chemotherapy after radiation therapy versus radiation therapy alone. Radiation therapy alone is reserved for those who could not tolerate combination radiation therapy or chemotherapy such as PCV or temozolomide.

   Delayed radiation-mediated neurotoxicity remains a concern, although prospective studies suggest it occurs less commonly than was once feared

   Factors that increase the chance of clinically significant delayed radiation-induced neurotoxicity include:

   - Large radiation fields
   - Large fraction dose and total dose
   - Older age
   - Underlying neurodegenerative disease
   - Radiation of temporal and frontal lobes

   For patients considered at significant risk of radiation-induced neurotoxicity, treatment with temozolomide alone is a consideration, although the data suggest that the period of tumor control is generally relatively short

   b. **Chemotherapy:** Chemotherapy with deferred radiation therapy can be considered especially for those patients with large inoperable tumors or whose tumors have mutated IDH1 and IDH2, unable to tolerate radiation therapy or chemoradiation therapy. Temozolomide, an oral agent, has shown efficacy in unirradiated low-grade gliomas especially with mutated IDH and methylated MGMT. It causes no delayed neurotoxicity and can be considered as a treatment option for low-grade gliomas requiring treatment to defer radiation therapy. At a median follow-up of 45.5 months and after the tumors of 246/477 patients had progressed, there was no statistical difference in the primary end point, progression-free survival (PFS). Overall toxicity was mild. Grade 3 hematologic toxicity was observed in 9% of the temozolomide-treated patients. In addition, depending on the circumstances, both active surveillance and PCV or temozolomide alone with deferred radiation therapy could also be considered as an alternative therapy. However, chemotherapy alone with deferred radiation therapy could affect the overall survival when compared with combination chemoradiation

Baumert BG et al. Lancet Oncol 2016;17:1521–1532

(continued)

Expert Opinion (continued)

c. **Chemoradiation therapy:** The timing of adjuvant therapy in low-grade glioma, especially low-risk, has been a controversial topic for decades, but the present data from recent phase 3 clinical trials provide the convincing evidence that, once the decision for adjuvant therapy is made, radiation therapy and PCV should be the treatment of choice. Therefore, radiation therapy followed by PCV chemotherapy is now considered as standard of care for patients with high-risk low-grade gliomas (astrocytomas, oligoastrocytomas, oligodendrogliomas, and neurofibromatosis) and even most of the low-risk low-grade glioma patients who require adjuvant treatment beyond surgery. Recent long-term follow-up results of the phase 3 RTOG 9802* clinical trial revealed a significant survival benefit for patients who were randomized to radiation followed by PCV chemotherapy compared with radiation therapy alone. Median survival time was 13.3 years and 7.8 years, respectively. Additional molecular and genetic studies are ongoing to further identify patients who would most likely benefit from chemotherapy. Patients who are felt to be appropriate candidates for radiation therapy or chemotherapy should be considered for chemoradiation therapy. Combination chemoradiation therapy with temozolomide should be considered for those IDH wildtype grade II or III gliomas, especially those with glioblastoma-like features such as TERTp mutation, trisomy of 7, or 10q loss of heterozygosity. The interim results of the European phase 3 clinical trial for patients with newly diagnosed non 1p19q codeleted anaplastic gliomas suggested a survival benefit of combination chemoradiation followed by monthly temozolomide over radiation therapy alone. The overall survival at 5 years with adjuvant temozolomide was 55.9% compared with 44.1% radiation therapy alone. Although not directly applicable for grade II astrocytoma, this radiation therapy with adjuvant temozolomide approach which is commonly used in the treatment of malignant gliomas is also well adopted for this tumor type. The ongoing CODEL phase 3 trial for 1p,19q codeleted high risk grade II and grade III glioma patients randomized to radiation/temozolomide vs radiation/PCV would provide some comparative insight on how to manage this subgroup of patients. Additional randomized trial for non 1p19q codeleted low grade astrocytoma should be considered.

*A Phase 2 Study of Observation in Favorable Low-Grade Glioma and A Phase 3 Study of Radiation with or without PCV Chemotherapy in Unfavorable Low-Grade Glioma. NCI Press Release February 03, 2014

Fisher BJHC et al. Int J Radiat Oncol Biol Phys 2015;91:497–504

Grade III Astrocytoma (Anaplastic Astrocytoma)

Anaplastic astrocytoma is an aggressive tumor that has overall survival of 3-5 years. MRI often reveals heterogeneous enhancement that is usually intermixed with nonenhancing tumor, although as many as half of all anaplastic astrocytomas may be largely nonenhancing. Mitosis, endothelial proliferation, and atypia can be seen. IDH is usually mutated and MGMT is mostly methylated

1. **Treatment:**

a. **Radiation therapy:** Radiation dose for malignant gliomas is 59.4-60 Gy in 30-33 fractions (1.8-2.0 Gy per fraction per day). Radiation therapy has been the standard of care for anaplastic astrocytoma; however, per recent phase 3 clinical trial results, if radiation therapy is chosen, then it should be combined with chemotherapy as discussed above. Radiation therapy alone could be an option for selected patients who could not tolerate combined radiation therapy and chemotherapy with PCV

b. **Chemotherapy:** The standard of care for anaplastic gliomas had been surgery followed by radiation therapy. However, in patients with newly diagnosed anaplastic gliomas (anaplastic oligodendroglioma, oligoastrocytoma, and astrocytoma), the NOA-04 phase 3 trial compared the efficacy and safety of radiotherapy followed by chemotherapy at progression with the reverse sequence. The results showed comparable results with either initial radiotherapy or initial chemotherapy (Wick et al, 2009). Median TTF (hazard ratio [HR]=1.2; 95% CI, 0.8-1.8), PFS (HR=1.0; 95% CI, 0.7-1.3), and overall survival (HR=1.2; 95% CI, 0.8-1.9) were similar for radiation therapy and procarbazine, lomustine, and vincristine (PCV)/temozolomide. A more recent phase 3 study of elderly patients with anaplastic astrocytoma and glioblastoma patients (NOA-08) randomly assigned patients to receive either chemotherapy (temozolomide) versus radiation therapy as initial treatment. This study showed no difference in time to treatment failure, progression-free survival, or overall survival (median overall survival, 8.6 months [95% CI, 7.3-10.2] in the temozolomide group and 9.6 months [8.2-10.8] in the radiotherapy group [HR=1.09; 95% CI, 0.84-1.42; noninferiority=0.033]), leading the authors to conclude that temozolomide alone is noninferior to radiotherapy alone in the treatment of elderly patients with malignant astrocytoma (Wick et al, 2012).

c. **Chemoradiation Therapy:** Trials of radiation followed by PCV have established the significant benefit of combining PCV chemotherapy after radiation. If possible, all patients who are eligible should be offered radiation therapy followed by PCV

Alternatively, the use of concurrent and postirradiation temozolomide therapy, an approach employed in newly diagnosed glioblastoma, also has become widely accepted for the treatment of other types of malignant gliomas, such as anaplastic astrocytoma. Although popular, the role of combining chemoradiation therapy for grade II or III gliomas has not been fully established yet, but patients with IDH wildtype anaplastic astrocytoma with features of glioblastoma such as TERTp mutation, trisomy 7, or 10q loss of heterozygosity should consider chemoradiation with temozolomide. The interim results of the Concurrent and Adjuvant Temozolomide chemotherapy in Non-1p19q Codeleted Anaplastic Glioma (CATNON) trial suggested a survival benefit of adjuvant temozolomide compared with radiation therapy alone in newly diagnosed non 1p19q codeleted IDH mutant grade III glioma patients and if confirmed on the final analysis, this approach could become another standard treatment option for this subgroup of patients.

Wick W et al. J Clin Oncol 2009;27:5874–5880
Wick W et al. Lancet Oncol 2012;13:707–715
Van Den Vent M et al. J Clin Oncol 2019, Abstact DOI: 10.1200/JCO.2019.37.15_suppl.2000 Journal of Clinical Oncology 37, no. 15_suppl (May 20, 2019) 2000-2000. Second interim and first molecular analysis of the EORTC randomized phase III intergroup CATNON trial on concurrent and adjuvant temozolomide in anaplastic glioma without 1p/19q codeletion.

Grade IV Astrocytomas (Glioblastoma)

Glioblastomas are the most common malignant tumors of the elderly population. The tumor grows rapidly and causes significant morbidity and mortality with an overall survival of 14-18 months. Imaging studies usually reveal a heterogeneously enhancing lesion or lesions with a

(continued)

Expert Opinion (continued)

significant amount of surrounding edema. Increased number of mitosis, endothelial proliferation, atypia, and necrosis are commonly seen. Mostly, MGMT is unmethylated and IDH1 and 2 are wildtype (non-mutant) in de novo, primary glioblastoma (>90%). However, those patients whose tumors have evolved from lower-grade astrocytomas (grade II or III) tend to have mutant IDH1 and 2 and methylated MGMT (secondary glioblastoma). 1p 19q is non-codeleted. ATRX is intact and TP53 is mutated

Glioblastoma can be further divided into classic, proneuronal, and mesenchymal subtypes:

- **Classic subtype:** Enriched in stem cell and cell cycle genes, is common in adults and has the greatest response to aggressive chemo- and radiation therapy. It is characterized by chromosome 7 amplification paired with chromosome 10 loss, lack of TP53 mutation, and EGFR amplification/Notch/SHH signaling.
- **Proneuronal subtype:** Enriched in neurodevelopmental genes, is common in young adults; it corresponds to secondary glioblastoma that has a better outcome than mesenchymal subtype. It is characterized by IDH/TP53 mutations/positivity for the glioma-CpG island methylator phenotype (G-CIMP) - a feature of low grade gliomas - and normal EGFR/PTEN/Notch signaling.
- **Mesenchymal subtype:** enriched in angiogenesis and inflammatory genes, is common in older adults and is associated with worse outcome. It is characterized by EGFR amplification/PTEN loss/NF1mutation/Akt signaling. Although they tend to have poorer prognosis, potentially, they may have favorable outcome to aggressive immunotherapy and chemo- and radiation therapy (Olar A, Aldape KD. J Pathol 2014;232:165–177; Verhaak RGW et al. Cancer Cell 2010;17:98)

Behnan J et al. Brain 2019;142:847–888
Herrlinger U et al. Lancet 2019;393:678–688
Kreisl TN et al. J Clin Oncol 2009;27:740–745
Olar A, Aldape KD. J Pathol 2014;232:165–177
Stupp R et al. N Engl J Med 2005;352:987–996
Verhaak RGW et al. Cancer Cell 2010;17:98
Xiu J et al. Oncotarget 2016;7:21556–21569

1. **Treatment:**

Chemoradiation therapy:

Initial therapy:
- For patients age 18-70 years, combined radiation therapy with low-dose daily temozolomide followed by monthly temozolomide is the standard of care. (Stupp R et al. N Engl J Med 2005;352:987–996)
- Combined radiation therapy with low-dose daily temozolomide followed by monthly temozolomide can be also considered for patients who are older than 70 years with a good performance status
- Alternatively, for patients 70 years or older with a poor performance status, temozolomide or radiation therapy alone can be an option. A 2- or 3-week course of hypofractionated radiation therapy could be an option for patients with poor performance status
- Radiation therapy followed by one of the nitrosoureas (carmustine [BCNU] or lomustine [CCNU]) is an option for those who could not receive temozolomide
- The phase 3 CeReG/NOA-09 clinical trial for newly diagnosed hypermethylated MGMT glioblastoma suggested an overall survival benefit of the combination radiation therapy, lomustine (CCNU), and temozolomide compared with radiation therapy and temozolomide. Median overall survival was 48.1 months for the radiation, lomustine (CCNU), and temozolomide arm compared with 31.4 months in the radiation therapy plus temozolomide arm

Recurrent disease:
- Bevacizumab is the treatment of choice for patients for whom it is not medically or neurologically contraindicated (Kreisl TN et al. J Clin Oncol 2009;27:740–745)
- Reirradiation (with stereotactic radiosurgery or radiotherapy), laser interstitial thermal therapy with biopsy, or tumor treating fields (TTFs, Optune) can be considered
- Re-treatment with a continuous low-dose (metronomic) temozolomide dosing schedule is an option especially for patients who have never been treated with bevacizumab and responded well to their original temozolomide with the last treatment >6 months and whose tumor has a methylated MGMT status (see below)
- Second-line chemotherapeutic agents such as carmustine (BCNU), lomustine (CCNU), or carboplatin also are options
- Recently, the FDA approved pembrolizumab, a PD-1 inhibitor, for any solid organ tumor patients who harbor mismatch repair deficiency (dMMR), which makes it a unique treatment option for those who exhibit dMMR. To further enhance the antitumoral effect of the immune response, combining immunotherapies with dendritic cell vaccines, molecular targeted therapies, oncolytic viral therapies, and CAR-T cells are being actively investigated
- Other vaccine trials (ICT-107, DCVax), virus-based immunotherapy trials such as Toca 511, molecular targeted drugs for malignant gliomas expressing EGFR or EGFRviii (erlotinib, ABT-414), and other immunotherapeutic agents including checkpoint inhibitors (nivolumab: BMS-498 trial) and multikinase inhibitors have been studied with only modest response rates. Other novel innovative therapeutic approaches are desperately needed
- Recently, a multi-platform molecular profiling of 1035 glioblastomas revealed mutations in 39 genes of 48 tested. MGMT methylation was seen in 43%. There was expression of PD-L1 in 19% and PD-1 in 46%, BRCA1 mutation in 5%, and BRCA2 mutation in 7%, making these biomarkers potential targets for immunomodulatory agents and PARP inhibitors, respectively. EGFRvIII was also seen in 19%, confirming

(continued)

Expert Opinion (*continued*)

EGFR as an important therapeutic target. Analysis of 17 metachronous paired tumors showed frequent biomarker changes, including MGMT methylation and EGFR aberrations, indicating the need for a re-biopsy for tumor profiling to direct subsequent therapy. Advances in molecular genetic profiling, proteogenomics, and other new diagnostic technologies will further enhance planning for future personalized biomarker-based clinical trials and identifying effective treatments based on tumor biomarkers (Xiu J et al. Oncotarget 2016;7:21556–21569)

• Participation in a well-designed clinical trial is highly recommended

Diffuse Midline Glioma H3 K27M-mutant (Grade IV)

H3 K27M-mutant diffuse midline glioma is an aggressive tumor that predominantly affects children but can be also seen in adults. The tumor occurs in a midline location such as brainstem but can be also seen in thalamus or spinal cord harboring a K27M mutation in either H3F3A or HIST1H3B/C. This tumor represents the majority of the previously known diffuse intrinsic pontine gliomas. A preliminary data from earlier study and currently ongoing phase 2 clinical trial, targeting H3K27M with ONC201, a highly selective antagonist of dopamine receptor D2, revealed significant tumor response in a number of pediatric and young adult patients. Additional results after the completion of the clinical trial are highly anticipated

Phase 2 Trials of Continuous Low-dose Temozolomide for Patients with Recurrent Malignant Glioma

Reference	N	TMZ Daily Dose, Schedule	ORR (%)	PFS6 (%)	Median OS (Months)
Khan	27	75 mg/m², 42/70 days	14	27	8
Brandes	33	75 mg/m², 21/28 days	9	30	10
Wick	64	150 mg/m², 7/14 days	15	44	9
Perry	33	*Early progression on adjuvant TMZ,* 50 mg/m², 28/28 days	3	27	NA
	27	*Progression on extended TMZ,* 50 mg/m², 28/28 days	0	7	NA
	28	*Rechallenge,* 50 mg/m², 28/28 days	11	36	NA
Kong	38	40–50 m², 28/28 days	5	32	13
Abacioglu	16	100 mg/m², 21/28 days	7	25	7
Verhoeff	15	50 mg/m², 28/28 days + bevacizumab 10 mg/kg q21d	NA	7	4
Desjardins	32	50 mg/m², 28/28 days + bevacizumab 10 mg/kg q14d	28	19	6
Omuro	37	All patients, 50 mg/m², 28/28 days	11	19	7
		Bevacizumab failures, 50 mg/m², 28/28 days	0	11	4
		Bevacizumab naïve, 50 mg/m², 28/28 days	20	26	13

NA, not available; ORR, objective response rate (complete + partial responses); PFS6, progression-free at 6 months; TMZ, temozolomide

Abacioglu U et al. J Neurooncol 2011;103:585–593
Brandes AA et al. Br J Cancer 2006;95:1155–1160
Desjardins A et al. Cancer 2011;118:1302–1312
Khan RB et al. Neuro Oncol 2002;4:39–43
Kong DS et al. Neuro Oncol 2010;12:289–296
Omuro A et al. Neuro Oncol 2013;15:242–250
Perry JR et al. J Clin Oncol 2010;28:2051–2057
Verhoeff JJ et al. Ann Oncol 2010;21:1723–1727
Wick A et al. J Clin Oncol 2007;25:3357–3361

Oligodendroglioma (WHO Grade II)

Oligodendrogliomas are rare tumors that can respond extremely well to radiation and chemotherapy. They appear as "fried egg" round cells under the microscope, and imaging studies that show calcifications can help establish the diagnosis. Per recent 2016 CNS WHO Classification, codeletion of 1p19q and IDH1 and 2 mutation are required to establish the diagnosis and it usually confers a good prognosis. In addition, MGMT is mostly methylated

1. **Observation:** Patients with the following good prognostic factors can be closely monitored with serial scans:
   • Young age (<40 years)
   • Asymptomatic
   • Good performance score (KPS >70)
   • Small non-enhancing lesion
   • Nearly or completely resected tumor
   • Low Ki67 or MIB-1 proliferative index
   • Codeletion of 1p and 19q
   • Presence of IDH1 or IDH2 mutation

(*continued*)

Expert Opinion (*continued*)

2. **Treatment:**

General indications for treatment include:

- Older patient (>40 years)
- Symptomatic
- Poor performance score (<70)
- Large or inoperable, enhancing tumor
- High mitotic proliferative index
- Lack of IDH1 or IDH2 mutation
- Intact 1p and 19q status

   a. **Chemotherapy:** If the tumor cannot be completely resected, radiation therapy or chemotherapy can be considered as oligodendrogliomas can respond to either treatment extremely well. However, because oligodendrogliomas with 1p19q codeletion can be exquisitely sensitive to chemotherapy, temozolomide or PCV can be offered as alternative treatments, especially for young patients with good prognostic features, in order to avoid the potential radiation induced delayed neurotoxicity

   b. **Radiation therapy:** Radiation dose for low-grade gliomas is 54 Gy in 27-30 fractions (1.8-2.0 Gy per fraction per day). Radiation therapy is usually reserved for patients with poor prognostic features, for those who are unable to tolerate chemotherapy, or for chemotherapy-resistant and progressive disease

   c. **Combined chemotherapy and radiation therapy:** The RTOG 9802* phase 2/3 trial for high-risk low-grade gliomas (astrocytomas, oligodendrogliomas, oligoastrocytomas, and neurofibromatosis) revealed a significant long-term survival benefit for patients who were randomized to radiation followed by PCV chemotherapy over radiation therapy alone. Median survival time was 13.3 years for the radiation plus PCV arm and 7.8 years for the radiation alone arm. Based on these findings, this combination therapy is now considered as the standard treatment for high-risk low-grade gliomas especially when oligodendrogliomas are well known to be extremely sensitive to radiation therapy and chemotherapy. Additional molecular and genetic studies from this trial are still ongoing to further identify patients who would most likely benefit from chemotherapy. Patients who are felt to be appropriate candidates for radiation therapy or chemotherapy should be considered for chemoradiation therapy

*A Phase 2 Study of Observation in Favorable Low-Grade Glioma and A Phase 3 Study of Radiation with or without PCV Chemotherapy in Unfavorable Low-Grade Glioma. NCI Press Release February 03, 2014

Anaplastic Oligodendroglioma (WHO Grade III)
Anaplastic oligodendrogliomas, like grade II oligodendrogliomas, can be extremely sensitive to radiation and chemotherapy. Per the recent 2016 CNS WHO classification, co-deletion of 1p 19q is required to establish the diagnosis and it usually confers a good prognosis. In addition, IDH is mutated and MGMT is usually methylated

1. **Treatment:** Combined chemotherapy with PCV and pre- or postradiation therapy is the standard. Radiation therapy alone and chemotherapy alone are reserved for patients who could not tolerate combination therapy

   a. **Chemotherapy:** If the tumor cannot be completely resected, radiation therapy or chemotherapy can be considered as oligodendrogliomas can respond to either treatment extremely well. However, because oligodendrogliomas with 1p19q codeletion can be exquisitely sensitive to chemotherapy, temozolomide or PCV can be offered as alternative treatments, especially for young patients with good prognostic features such as gross total resection, small residual tumor, or IDH mutation, in order to avoid the potential radiation-induced delayed neurotoxicity. PCV is the drug of choice for 1p19q co-deleted anaplastic oligodendrogliomas

   b. **Radiation therapy:** Radiation dose for malignant gliomas is 59.4-60 Gy in 30-33 fractions (1.8-2.0 Gy per fraction per day). Radiation therapy is usually reserved for patients with poor prognostic features, who are unable to tolerate chemotherapy or chemoradiation therapy

   c. **Combined chemotherapy and radiation therapy:** Three recent long-term follow-up results from the phase 3 randomized trials for newly diagnosed anaplastic oligodendrogliomas revealed a significant survival benefit for combination PCV chemotherapy and radiation therapy over radiation therapy alone (van den Bent et al, 2012; Cairncross et al, 2012, Buckner 2014). These trials also validated the role of 1p19q as a predictive biomarker for survival. Therefore, PCV chemotherapy given either pre- or postradiation therapy is now considered as the standard of treatment. However, because PCV chemotherapy compared to temozolomide carries a greater toxicity with a less-favorable dosing schedule and administration, many still debate accepting PCV chemotherapy as standard of care. The role of concurrent radiation-and-postradiation chemotherapy with temozolomide, the standard treatment for glioblastomas, is now commonly adopted for the treatment of other malignant gliomas like anaplastic oligodendrogliomas. However, the survival benefit temozolomide over radiation therapy followed by PCV has not been established yet. A more direct comparison study is being performed with an ongoing CODEL phase 3 trial for newly diagnosed 1p19q co-deleted anaplastic or low-grade glioma patients randomized to radiation therapy followed by PCV or radiation therapy with concurrent and then adjuvant temozolomide

Buckner JC et al. J Clin Oncol 2014;32(15_suppl):2000
Buckner JC et al. N Engl J Med 2016;374:1344–1355
Cairncross GC et al. J Clin Oncol 2013;31:337–343
van den Bent MJ et al. J Clin Oncol 2006;24:2715–2722
van den Bent MJ et al. J Clin Oncol 2012;43:2229
van den Bent et al. J Clin Oncol 2013;31:344–350
van den Bent MJ. Neuro Oncol 2014;16:1570–1574

(*continued*)

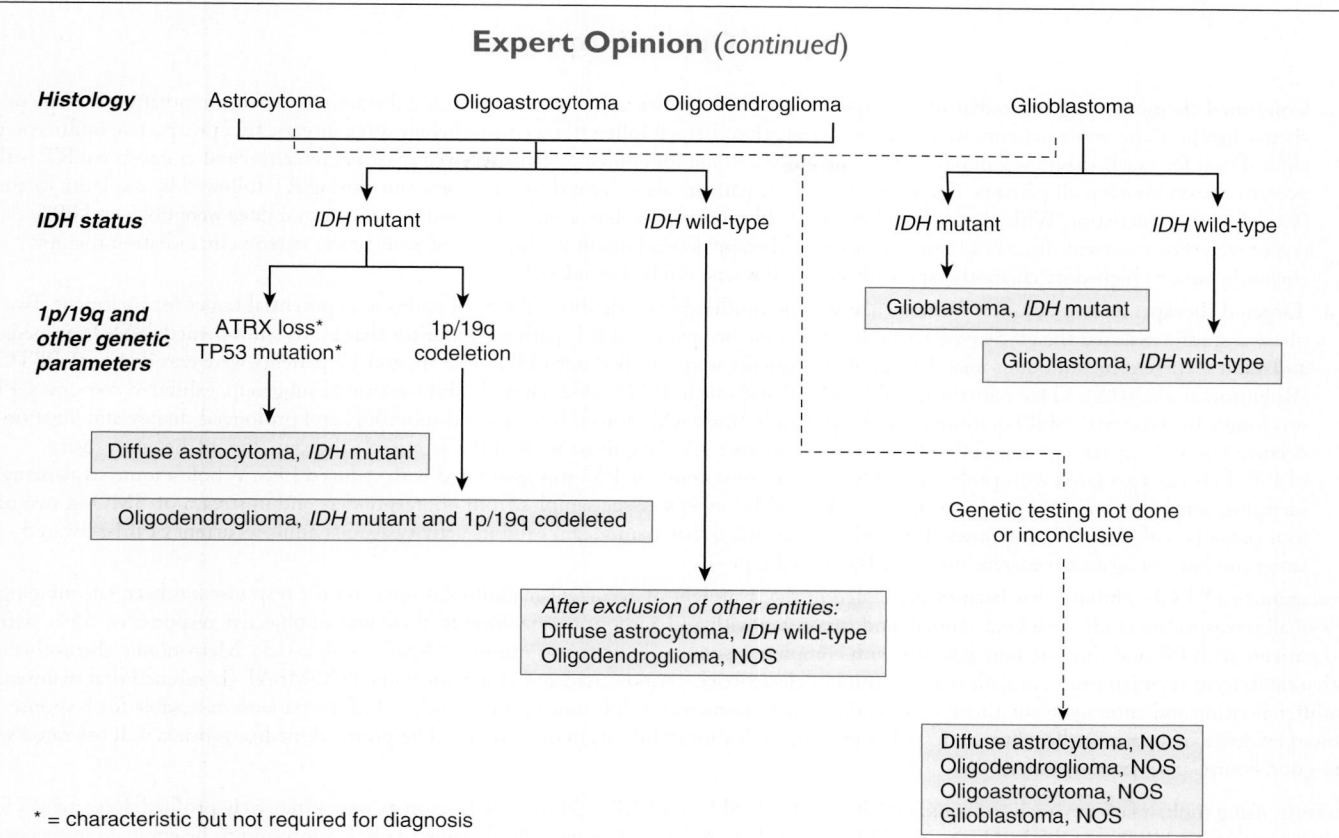

Figure 9-1. A simplified algorithm for classification of the diffuse gliomas based on histological and genetic features (see text and 2016 CNS WHO for details). A caveat to this diagram is that the diagnostic "flow" does not necessarily always proceed from histology first to molecular genetic features next, since molecular signatures can sometimes outweigh histological characteristics in achieving an "integrated" diagnosis. A similar algorithm can be followed for anaplastic level diffuse gliomas.

* Characteristic but not required for diagnosis
Reproduced with permission from Louis DN et al. 2016 World
Health Organization Histological Classification of Tumours of
the Central Nervous System. International Agency for Research

Medulloblastoma

Medulloblastoma usually occurs in children and young adults. The tumor is aggressive in nature and has a high propensity to spread through the cerebrospinal fluid, resulting in distant metastasis within the central nervous system. A thorough staging work-up, including a careful examination of the cerebrospinal fluid and spine, is required. Medulloblastoma usually arises in the posterior fossa causing hydrocephalus and associated obstructive symptoms, including headaches, nausea, vomiting, and gait difficulties requiring urgent ventriculoperitoneal shunt placement to relieve the intracranial pressure. Tumor cells are compactly arranged, small round or ovoid with hyperchromatic nuclei and scant cytoplasm. They lie in small and poorly defined groups or in a pseudorosette pattern

Recent advances in molecular and genetic profiling along with long-established histologic variants have affected the classification of medulloblastoma into four major molecular genetic groups: WNT-activated, SHH-activated, and the numerically designated group 3 and group 4 (WHO CNS tumor classification, 2016) and some of these histological and genetic variants have significant prognostic and therapeutic implications. WNT-activated classic histology cell subgroup is a low-risk tumor with the best prognosis. SHH-activated subgroup is the most common tumor and TP53-wild type could be a potential target for hedgehog pathway inhibitors like vismodegib, a smoothened homologue (SMO) antagonist. A recent clinical trial for recurrent medulloblastoma with vismodegib demonstrated a favorable tumor response in patients with SHH-activated medulloblastoma. On the other hand, SHH-activated, TP53-mutant type is a high-risk tumor with a poor prognosis, and vismodegib was not found to be effective. Non-WNT/non-SHH, group 3 subtype is associated with metastasis and has a poor prognosis. Similarly, non-WNT/non-SHH, group 4 subtype also has a tendency for metastasis and the treatment for these two groups is fairly similar

1. **Treatment:**

   a. **Radiation therapy:** Craniospinal radiation therapy is the standard of care. For patients with low risk who had complete resection or minimal residual disease <1.5 cm without metastases, local radiation to the site of surgical bed and adjacent area is considered adequate. Proton therapy, if available, is becoming more widely used

   b. **Chemotherapy:** Chemotherapy is usually provided after the completion of radiation therapy. When chemotherapy is considered, craniospinal radiation dose can be reduced to minimize the toxicity (Packer et al, 2006). Chemotherapy usually consists of platinum compound, cyclophosphamide, etoposide, vincristine, nitrosourea such as carmustine (BCNU), or lomustine (CCNU).

Expert Opinion (continued)

c. **Combined chemotherapy and radiation therapy:** Due to the high risk of early recurrence and distant metastasis on radiation therapy or chemotherapy alone, most patients are treated with radiation therapy followed by chemotherapy after surgery. In a prospective multicenter clinical trial for newly diagnosed nonmetastatic medulloblastoma for adults, patients received maximal resection and craniospinal RT with posterior fossa boost in all patients. Forty-nine out of 70 patients also received weekly vincristine during RT followed by cisplatin, lomustine (CCNU), and vincristine. With a median follow-up of 44 months, the 4-year event-free and overall survival rates were 68% and 89%, respectively. For recurrent disease, additional radiation therapy depending on the location of recurrence, stereotactic radiation therapy, chemotherapy, or high-dose chemotherapy with stem cell rescue can be considered

d. **Targeted therapy:** Recent advances in molecular genetic profiling have identified the SSH pathway as potential target for treatment. Two phase 2 studies assessed the efficacy of vismodegib, a sonic hedgehog (SHH) pathway inhibitor that binds smoothened (SMO), in pediatric and adult recurrent medulloblastoma. A total of 31 patients were enrolled onto PBTC-025B, and 12 patients were enrolled onto PBTC-32 (Robinson et al, 2015). Three patients in PBTC-025B and one in PBTC-032, all with SHH-activated subgroup, exhibited responses. PFS was longer in those with SHH-activated subgroup than in those with non-SHH-activated subgroup, and prolonged disease stabilization occurred in 41% of patient cases of SHH-activated subgroup. Among those with SHH-activated subgroup, loss of heterozygosity of PTCH1 was associated with prolonged PFS, and diffuse staining of P53 was associated with reduced PFS. Whole-exome sequencing identified mutations in SHH genes downstream from SMO in 4/4 tissue samples from nonresponders and upstream of SMO in two of four patients with favorable responses. The authors concluded that vismodegib exhibits activity against adult recurrent SHH-activated subgroup but not against recurrent non-SHH-activated type

Bevacizumab, a VEGF inhibitor, has been incorporated in the treatment of recurrent medulloblastoma and the response has been encouraging. In a small retrospective study with bevacizumab and irinotecan with and without temozolomide, there was an objective response of 55%, with two patients with PR and three of nine patients with complete response. Toxicity was minimal (Aguila et al, 2013). Metronomic chemotherapy with a multiagent regimen protocol with temozolomide, celecoxib, cis-retinoic acid and etoposide named COMBAT (combined oral maintenance biodifferentiating and antiangiogenic therapy), in children with refractory solid tumors, revealed that 9 of 14 patients assessable for response showed evidence of treatment benefit manifested as prolonged disease stabilization or response. The protocol medication was well tolerated with very good compliance (Sterba et al, 2006)

Recently, using multi-platform analysis including NGS, IHC, FISH, and CISH, 36 medulloblastomas were extensively profiled. Researchers found high expression of MRP1, TUBB3, PTEN, TOP2A, TS, RRM1, and TOP1 in medulloblastoma. TOP1 was found to be enriched in metastatic medulloblastoma relative to posterior fossa cases. HER2, EGFR amplification, and CDK6 amplification were not seen. PD-1 + T cell tumor infiltration was rare. PD-L1 tumor expression was uncommon and TML was low, indicating that immune checkpoint inhibitors as a monotherapy might not be prioritized for therapeutic consideration based on biomarker expression. Potential therapeutic drugs are available for several of the frequently expressed targets, providing a justification for the consideration in future clinical trials (Hashimoto et al, 2018)

Other vaccine immunotherapy and chimeric antigen receptor (CAR) T cells targeting human epidermal growth factor receptor 2 (HER2), which is overexpressed in medulloblastomas, are being investigated

Hashimoto Y et al. J Neurooncol 2018;139:713–720
Packer RJ et al. J Clin Oncol 2006;24:4202–4208
Robinson GW et al. J Clin Oncol 2015;33:2646–2654 [For PBTC–025B; 12 were enrolled onto PBTC–032]
Sterba J et al. Onkologie 2006;29:308–213

Primary Central Nervous System Lymphomas

Primary central nervous system lymphomas are rare non-Hodgkin lymphomas arising within the central nervous system without systemic involvement. They occur mostly in the elderly population and in patients who are immunocompromised. The most common type is diffuse large B-cell lymphoma, and they invariably express CD20. MRI findings usually reveal homogenously enhancing lesion(s) involving periventricle or splenium (butterfly lesion). If a primary central system lymphoma is suspected, a stereotactic biopsy is sufficient to establish the diagnosis as this tumor can be successfully treated with radiation and methotrexate-containing chemotherapy with high cure rates. However, in the presence of significant mass effect, partial or total resection can be considered. As an initial work-up, a thorough examination of eyes and cerebrospinal fluid are required because of the propensity to involve these sites. If a primary central nervous system lymphoma is suspected, the administration of steroids is discouraged as steroids can be oncolytic and could cause a decrease in the size of the tumor, making the diagnosis difficult. Steroids are usually administered after the biopsy or surgery. Recent advances in molecular genetic profiling added a significant improvement in understanding and targeting the key pathways that might further enhance primary CNS lymphoma treatment

1. **Treatment:**

a. **Chemotherapy:** High-dose methotrexate (3.5-8 g/m^2) given alone or as part of multiagent regimen remains the standard therapy (Batchelor et al, 2003). Even at high dose as a single agent the treatment is well tolerated and causes minimal side effects. The complete response and survival rates are found to be comparable or better than radiation therapy. Delayed neurotoxicity commonly seen in long-term survivors of whole-brain radiation therapy is less frequent. Because of high central nervous system penetration of the drug, patients with ocular, cerebrospinal fluid, or leptomeningeal involvement can be safely treated with high-dose methotrexate alone without concurrent radiation or intraocular or intrathecal chemotherapy. CD20-directed rituximab in combination with high-dose methotrexate also is commonly used (Chamberlain and Johnston, 2010). Patients who receive high-dose methotrexate alone can be treated with rituximab as maintenance therapy following high-dose methotrexate. For recurrence, re-treatment with high-dose methotrexate with and without rituximab (Chamberlain and Johnston, 2010), topotecan (Voloschin et al, 2008), high-dose cytarabine, pemetrexed (Raizer), or temozolomide can be considered.

(continued)

Expert Opinion (*continued*)

If chemotherapy is not considered a good option because of the patient's high comorbidities, renal failure, or inability to tolerate chemotherapy, radiation therapy could be considered as an alternative option

In newly diagnosed primary central nervous system lymphoma patients who responded to a chemotherapy trial, a phase 2 study of a methotrexate-based chemotherapy regimen followed by high-dose chemotherapy with autologous stem cell transplantation and reduced-dose whole-brain radiation therapy revealed an encouraging high response rate and survival results that warrant further investigation in a larger phase 3 trial (Colombat et al, 2006)

b. **Radiation therapy:** Radiation therapy was a standard of care in the past, but because of high treatment failure and high incidence of delayed neurotoxicity commonly seen in long-term survivors, this approach is no longer considered as first-line therapy. However, radiation therapy is still considered for patients who have poor performance status and/or are unable to tolerate chemotherapy or for recurrent disease

c. **Chemoradiation therapy:** The recent RTOG 0227 phase I/II clinical trial with methotrexate, rituximab, and temozolomide, followed by whole-brain radiotherapy and postirradiation temozolomide for newly diagnosed primary central nervous system lymphoma (Glass et al, 2016), has revealed a significant improvement in 2-year overall survival of 80.8% and 2-year progression-free survival of 63.6% with a median follow-up of 3.6 years. Low-dose radiation (36 Gy) was provided after methotrexate, rituximab, and temozolomide, and patients were then placed on monthly temozolomide. Cognitive function and quality of life improved or stabilized after therapy

Similarly, recent long-term follow-up results of a phase 2 trial of rituximab and high-dose methotrexate-based multiagent chemotherapy with vincristine and procarbazine (R-MVP) followed by consolidation, reduced-dose radiation therapy, and high-dose cytarabine for newly diagnosed primary central nervous system lymphoma revealed a high rate of response and overall survival with favorable cognitive outcomes compared with historical controls treated with whole-brain radiation therapy alone (Morris et al, 2013). Results showed that 60% achieved a CR after R-MPV and received rdWBRT. The 2-year PFS for this group was 77%; median PFS was 7.7 years. Median overall survival (OS) was not reached (median follow-up for survivors, 5.9 years); 3-year OS was 87%. The overall (n=52) median PFS was 3.3 years, and median OS was 6.6 years. A randomized phase 3 Radiation Therapy Oncology Group trial based on this phase 2 regimen with or without reduced-dose whole-brain radiation therapy was recently closed for enrollment, and the final results are pending

d. **Molecular targeted therapy:** Significant progress has been made in the treatment of PCNSL in recent decades. However, although the response rate and the overall survival have much improved with high-dose methotrexate-based chemotherapy and incorporation of low-dose radiation therapy, the response rate remains 60-80% and once they recur, their prognosis becomes poor despite additional salvage therapy. Increased insight into the pathophysiology of PCNSL has led to the introduction of targeted therapies in the treatment of tumor recurrence. Single agents such as rituximab for CD20-positive disease and temozolomide have been tested in small clinical trials with modest benefits. Ibrutinib is an irreversible selective inhibitor of Bruton tyrosine kinase (BTK) that has shown clinical activity in DLBCL

PCNSL is sensitive to upstream and downstream NF-kB pathway inhibitors such as ibrutinib. A total of 52 patients with recurrent PCNSL or ocular lymphoma were enrolled in the phase 2 trial for recurrent PCNSL, and the first 18 patients had 3 complete and 7 partial responses after 2 months of treatment (Soussain 2019). There was clinical, radiological, and biological activity of ibrutinib in the brain, CSF, spinal cord, and intraocular compartment. The disease control rate was 70% in evaluable patients, and the overall response rate in evaluable patients was 59% which is encouraging. Toxicity was acceptable except in 2 patients who developed pulmonary aspergillosis (one patient recovered; the other patient died). Based on these encouraging results, additional ibrutinib-based clinical trials are being investigated

e. **Immunotherapy:** Immunotherapy with monoclonal antibodies, such as PD-1 or PDL-1 inhibitors (ie, nivolumab and pembrolizumab or avelumab and durvalumab, respectively), may help the body's immune system attack the cancer and may interfere with the ability of tumor cells to grow and spread. PD-1 blockade has shown safety and encouraging results in the treatment of Hodgkin lymphoma patients and is promising in the treatment of non-Hodgkin lymphoma. PD-1/PD-L1 and tumor-infiltrating lymphocytes have been detected in PCNSL. Nivolumab is an anti-PD1 checkpoint inhibitor that has shown encouraging activity in one case report (Nayak et al, 2016). Three out of three patients with recurrent PCNSL showed clinical response and two had radiographic response (1 CR and 1 PR). Combining immunotherapy and ibrutinib and other molecular targeted therapies are currently investigated and, if eligible, a participation in the clinical trial is encouraged

Batchelor TJ et al. Clin Oncol 2003;21:1044–1049
Chamberlain MC, et al Neuro Oncol 2010;2:736–744
Colombat P et al. Bone Marrow Transplant 2006;38:417–420
Morris PG et al. J Clin Oncol 2013;31:3971–3979
Voloschin AD et al. J Neurooncol 2008;86:211–215
Soussain C et al. Eur J Cancer 2019;117:121–130
Nayak L, et al Neurology 2016;86(16_suppl):P6.280

Meningiomas
Meningiomas are rare brain tumors arising from the meninges. They usually affect the elderly population and have a slight female preponderance. Calcifications and bone involvement can be seen on CT scan. MRI scan usually reveals a dural-based homogenously enhancing lesion that has a typical tail sign

Benign Meningiomas (Grade I):
1. **Observation:** Grade I meningiomas are slow-growing benign tumors that have an excellent prognosis with overall survival >10 years. They can be simply followed without any therapeutic intervention
2. **Treatment:**
   a. **Surgery:** If the tumor grows and/or a patient becomes symptomatic, surgery may be indicated

(continued)

Expert Opinion (continued)

Atypical Meningiomas (Grade II)
1. **Observation:** For most atypical meningioma patients, close observation following surgery is usually sufficient if the patient is asymptomatic and the pathology showed a mitotic index <4/10 HPFs
2. **Treatment:**
   a. **Radiation therapy:** Radiation can be considered if the patient is symptomatic and/or the pathology showed a high mitotic index of >4/10 HPFs. Participation in the ongoing NRG Oncology BN-003 clinical trial that randomizes observation versus radiation therapy for atypical meningioma is encouraged

Anaplastic (Malignant) Meningiomas (Grade III):
Malignant meningiomas with anaplastic features such as sarcoma, carcinoma, or melanoma-like histology are a rapidly growing tumor that carries a poor prognosis with overall survival <2-3 years. MRI scan typically reveals a significant vasogenic edema. Octreotide scan or gallium-68 dotatate scan can reveal the presence of octreotide receptors for potential therapeutic targets. Mitotic index is usually high at >20/10 HPFs
1. **Treatment:**
   a. **Surgery followed by radiation therapy:** For newly diagnosed anaplastic meningioma, the standard of care is surgery followed by radiation therapy. For recurrent tumors, surgery, additional radiation therapy, or stereotactic radiation therapy can be considered
   b. **Chemotherapy/immunotherapy/molecular targeted therapy:** Hydroxyurea (Chamberlain et al, 2012) has shown some modest benefits but other chemotherapeutic agents like temozolomide have limited use in the management of recurrent or progressive meningiomas. However, if the tumor reveals MGMT methylation, temozolomide can be considered

Immunomodulating agents, such as interferon α (Chamberlain and Glantz, 2008) and somatostatin analogs for somatostatin receptor–positive tumors (positive octreotide scan) (Chamberlain et al, 2007) have shown some modest responses that can be durable

Hormonal receptors, especially progesterone receptors, are expressed in two-thirds of the meningiomas; this has created a great interest in the potential role of the potent progesterone inhibitor mifepristone, but a large phase 3 clinical trial randomizing mifepristone versus placebo failed to show benefit of mifepristone over placebo

Researchers are currently studying molecularly targeted approaches such as sunitinib (VEGF and VEGFR; Kaley et al, 2015) and everolimus (mTOR) and bevacizumab (VEGF) as single agents or in combination (Shih et al, 2016), and the response has been favorable with improved response rate and progression-free survival. Other molecular targeted agents such as SMO, AKT, and FAK CDK4/6 inhibitors also are being actively investigated

Recently, a phase 2 clinical trial combining sandostatin (octreotide) LAR and everolimus (mTOR inhibitor) for refractory and progressive meningioma (Graillon et al, 2017) was reported. It revealed an encouraging PFS6 of 58.2% and PFS12 of 38%, with a median follow-up of 12.3 months. Pre-therapeutic growth rate was decreased more than 50% in 29 of 35 tumors (18 of 20 patients) during the first 3 months

Bevacizumab, as a single agent or in combination with chemotherapy (Lou et al, 2012), can be safely administered and appears to have encouraging antitumor effects. In a phase 2 trial (Grimm et al, 2015), 40 patients with recurrent meningioma were treated with bevacizumab (15 benign meningioma [BM], 22 atypical meningioma [AM], and 13 malignant meningioma [MM]), and it demonstrated mainly stable disease: 100% BM, 85% AM, and 82% MM. PFS-6, mPFS, and mOS were 87%, 22.5 months, and 35.6 months for BM; 77%, 15.3 months, and not reached for AM; and 46%, 3.7 months, and 12.4 months for MM, respectively. Additional clinical trials to investigate the efficacy and side effects are warranted. A phase 2 trial evaluated the efficacy of everolimus plus bevacizumab in patients with recurrent, progressive meningioma (Shih et al, 2016). The best response of SD was observed in 15 patients (88%), and 6 patients had SD for >12 months. Overall median PFS was 22 months. The median duration of disease stabilization was 10 months

A recent molecular genetic profiling of 115 meningiomas by multi-platform analysis (NGS, FISH, IHC, and CISH) revealed EGFR (93%, n=44), PTEN, BCRP, MRP1, and MGMT (55%, n=97). The most frequent mutation among all grades occurred in the NF2 gene at 85% (11 of 13). Recurring SMO and AKT1 also were occasionally detected. PD-L1 also was expressed in 25% of grade III cases (2 of 8) but not in grade I or II tumors. PD-1+ T cells were present in 46% of meningiomas (24 of 52). TOP2A and TS expression increased with grade. If predicated on tumor expression, therapeutics directed toward NF2 and TOP2A could be considered for most meningioma patients, and tumors that express other biomarkers could be also potential targets for therapeutic approach (Everson et al, 2018) which needs to be further explored in a proper clinical trial setting

In that regard, a multi-institutional, three-arm, phase 2 Alliance clinical trial of SMO (vismodegib), AKT1 (afuresertib), or NF2 (FAK inhibitor, GSK2256098) inhibitors in progressive meningiomas with SMO, AKT1, or NF2 *mutations*, respectively, is open for accrual, and if eligible, participation in the clinical trial is strongly encouraged

Chamberlain M. Neuro Oncol 2012;107:315–321
Chamberlain M, Glantz MJ. Cancer 2008;113:2146–2151
Everson RG et al. J Neurooncol 2018;139:469–478
Graillon T et al. J Clin Oncol 2017; 35(15_suppl):2011
Grimm SA et al. J Clin Oncol 2015;33(15_suppl):2055
Kaley TJ et al. Neuro Oncol 2015;17:116–121
Lou E et al. Neuro Oncol 2012;109:63–70
Shih KC et al. Neuro Oncol 2016;129:281–288

GRADE 2 GLIOMA, NEWLY DIAGNOSED

CNS CANCER REGIMEN: PROCARBAZINE, LOMUSTINE, AND VINCRISTINE AFTER RADIATION

Buckner JC et al. N Engl J Med 2016;374:1344–1355
Protocol for: Buckner JC et al. N Engl J Med 2016;374:1344–1355

Radiation therapy once daily at 1.8 Gy/fraction for 5 days/week for a total of 30 fractions (total dosage = 54 Gy), *followed by:*

Begin chemotherapy after completion of radiation therapy:

Lomustine (CCNU) 110 mg/m^2; administer orally as a single dose, without food, on day 1, every 8 weeks, for 6 cycles (total dosage/8-week cycle = 110 mg/m^2)
Note: to reduce the likelihood of a medication error leading to severe myelosuppression, prescribe, dispense, and administer only enough capsules to supply 1 dose of lomustine. Educate patients that only 1 dose of lomustine is to be taken every 8 weeks and only after documentation of adequate hematologic recovery. (ISMP, 2014. https://www.ismp.org/resources/oral-chemotherapy-we-simply-must-do-better. Accessed June 20, 2018)

Procarbazine 60 mg/m^2/ day; administer orally once daily for 14 consecutive days on days 8–21, every 8 weeks, for 6 cycles (total dosage/8-week cycle = 840 mg/m^2)
Note: because procarbazine is a weak monoamine oxidase inhibitor, one should restrict tyramine-containing foods in patients receiving procarbazine

Vincristine 1.4 mg/m^2 per dose (maximum single dose = 2 mg); administer by intravenous infusion over 15 minutes in 50 mL 0.9% sodium chloride injection (0.9% NS) for 2 doses, on days 8 and 29, every 8 weeks, for 6 cycles (total dosage/8-week cycle = 2.8 mg/m^2, but *not* >4 mg/8-week cycle)

Supportive Care
Antiemetic prophylaxis
Emetogenic potential on day 1 and days 8–21 is **MODERATE–HIGH**
Emetogenic potential on day 29 is **MINIMAL**
See Chapter 42 for antiemetic recommendations

Hematopoietic growth factor (CSF) prophylaxis
Primary prophylaxis is **NOT** *indicated*
See Chapter 43 for more information

Antimicrobial prophylaxis
Risk of fever and neutropenia is **LOW**
  Antimicrobial primary prophylaxis to be considered:
- Antibacterial—not indicated
- Antifungal—not indicated
- Antiviral—not indicated unless patient previously had an episode of HSV

Patient Population Studied

This multicenter, randomized, phase 3 trial (Radiation Therapy Oncology Group [RTOG] 9802) with long-term follow-up involved 251 patients with histologically confirmed grade 2 astrocytoma, oligodendroglioma, or oligoastrocytoma. Eligible patients had a Karnofsky performance status score ≥60, had a neurologic function score ≤3, and had undergone a subtotal resection or biopsy if aged 18–39 years or a biopsy or resection of any of the tumor if aged ≥40 years. Patients who had previously received radiation therapy to the brain or head and neck region, or had received prior chemotherapy for any reason, were not eligible. All patients received 30 fractions of 1.8 Gy radiation (prescribed to the isocenter) over 6 weeks. Patients randomly assigned to also receive chemotherapy subsequently received 6 cycles of lomustine, procarbazine, and vincristine

Efficacy (N = 251)

	Radiation Plus Procarbazine, Lomustine, and Vincristine (N = 125)	Radiation Only (N = 126)	
Median progression-free survival	10.4 years (95% CI 6.1–not reached)	4.0 years (95% CI 3.1–5.5)	HR 0.50; P <0.001
Median overall survival	13.3 years (95% CI 10.6–not reached)	7.8 years (95% CI 6.1–9.8)	HR 0.59; P = 0.003

Note: median follow-up was 11.9 years

Therapy Monitoring

1. *Prior to the start of each cycle:* CBC with differential, platelet count, LFTs, BUN, creatinine, electrolytes; consider baseline pulmonary function testing (PFTs) especially in patients with any pulmonary symptoms

2. *Weekly during PCV chemotherapy:* CBC with differential, platelet count, LFTs, BUN, creatinine, electrolytes. Repeat PFTs if symptoms of potential pulmonary compromise develop. Note, monitor blood counts weekly for 6 weeks after a dose: thrombocytopenia occurs at about 4 weeks postadministration and persists for 1–2 weeks, while leukopenia occurs at 5–6 weeks after a dose and persists for 1–2 weeks

3. *Response assessment:* contrast-enhanced MRI of the brain after completion of radiation therapy, prior to cycle 3, prior to cycle 5, 4 months after completion of PCV chemotherapy, then every 6 months for 2 years, then yearly

Treatment Modifications

RADIATION FOLLOWED BY PROCARBAZINE, LOMUSTINE, AND VINCRISTINE

Starting lomustine dose	110 mg/m^2 as a single dose
Starting procarbazine dose	60 mg/m^2/day for 14 consecutive days
Starting vincristine dose	1.4 mg/m^2 per dose (maximum = 2 mg) × 2 doses days 8 and 29

Adverse Event	Treatment Modifications
Day 1 ANC <1500/mm^3 or platelets <100,000/mm^3	Delay start of cycle until ANC ≥1500/mm^3 and platelets ≥100,000/mm^3. Note that day 8 and day 29 vincristine should not be delayed for hematologic toxicity
Nadir ANC ≥500/mm^3 and platelet count ≥50,000/mm^3	Continue with same dose
Nadir ANC <500/mm^3 or platelet count <50,000/mm^3	Delay therapy until ANC ≥1500/mm^3 and platelets ≥100,000/mm^3. Reduce lomustine and procarbazine dosages by 25–50%. Do not reduce vincristine dose
G ≥2 nonhematologic toxicity that does not recover to G ≤1 within 2 weeks (>8 weeks between cycles) Any G ≥2 nonhematologic toxicity that recurs at the next cycle to G ≥2	Discontinue regimen
G ≥3 nausea or vomiting, persistent despite maximum antiemetic therapy	Reduce doses of lomustine and/or procarbazine by 25% for G3 or 50% for G4 for all subsequent doses
Other G3/4 nonhematologic toxicities	Delay attributable medication(s) until resolution to G ≤1, then reduce dose of attributable medication(s) by 25% for G3 or 50% for G4 toxicity in subsequent doses. For G4 toxicity, consider permanent discontinuation of therapy
Urticarial rash	Discontinue procarbazine unless attributable to another concomitant medication
G ≥2 liver toxicity (AST/ALT >3× ULN) and/or G ≥2 bilirubin (>1.5–3× ULN)	Delay therapy until resolution to G ≤1 (AST/ALT ≤3× ULN; bilirubin ≤1.5× ULN), then reduce lomustine, procarbazine, and vincristine by 25%
Patient concurrently taking drugs known to inhibit drug metabolism by hepatic cytochrome P450 isoenzymes in the CYP 3A subfamily	Adjust vincristine dose
Total serum bilirubin >3 mg/dL: delay vincristine until total bilirubin ≤1.5 mg/dL	Reduce vincristine dose by 50% in all subsequent cycles
Severe abdominal pain or severe jaw pain	Reduce vincristine dose by 50% for all subsequent doses
G ≥3 peripheral neuropathy or G ≥3 motor neuropathy	Discontinue vincristine
Painful paresthesia or peripheral weakness	Discontinue vincristine
SIADH	Reduce vincristine dose or discontinue vincristine
Constipation, abdominal cramps, paralytic ileus	Temporarily discontinue vincristine. Treat symptoms. Resume vincristine when normal bowel function restored. Administer a routine prophylactic regimen against constipation
Creatinine clearance 10–50 mL/min	Reduce lomustine dose by 25%
Creatinine clearance <10 mL/min	Reduce lomustine dose by 50–75%

(continued)

Treatment Modifications (*continued*)

Adverse Event	Treatment Modifications
Any pulmonary symptoms, but with PFT showing DLco ≥ the predicted value	Continue with same lomustine dose
Any pulmonary symptoms, but with PFT showing <60% of the predicted value	Discontinue lomustine
Decreased oxygen saturation at rest (eg, pulse oximeter <88% or Pao$_2$ ≤55 mm Hg)	
Shortness of breath at rest or shortness of breath that limits self-care or ADLs	
Severe cough limiting self-care or ADLs	
Cumulative lomustine dosage >1100 mg/m^2	Discontinue lomustine due to concerns of developing pulmonary fibrosis

Notes:
- Usually no more than a total of 6 cycles (660 mg/m^2) of lomustine is recommended in this regimen. Patients receiving >1100 mg/m^2 cumulative lomustine dosage have a higher risk of developing pulmonary toxicity. Patients with a baseline FVC or DLco <70% are particularly at risk (GLEOSTINE [lomustine] capsules; June 2018 product label. NextSource Biotechnology, LLC, Miami, FL)
- Patients who are pregnant or who become pregnant should be apprised of the potential hazard to the fetus from therapy with lomustine, procarbazine, and vincristine

Adverse Events (N = 251)

Grade (%)	Radiation Plus Procarbazine, Lomustine, and Vincristine (N = 125)		Radiation Only (N = 126)	
	Grade 1/2	Grade 3/4	Grade 1/2	Grade 3/4
Gastrointestinal disorder	76	10	30	2
Blood or bone marrow disorder	25	51	3	<1
Constitutional symptoms	61	9	50	4
Fatigue	58	6	49	3
Nausea	60	2	19	2
Neutropenia	14	44	0	<1
Decreased platelet count	26	18	2	0
Decreased hemoglobin	34	5	2	0
Hepatic disorder	29	4	2	0
Vomiting	30	3	4	2
Anorexia	25	<1	7	0
Constipation	23	0	2	0
Weight loss	19	3	6	<1
Infection	19	2	<1	0
Increased ALT	10	2	0	0
Increased AST	10	<1	0	0
Requirement for packed RBC transfusion	<1	2	0	0
Lymphopenia	2	<1	<1	0
Platelet transfusion	0	<1	0	0
Febrile neutropenia	<1	0	0	0

Note: no Grade 5 events were recorded

ANAPLASTIC OLIGODENDROGLIOMA AND ANAPLASTIC OLIGOASTROCYTOMA, NEWLY DIAGNOSED

CNS CANCER REGIMEN: PROCARBAZINE, LOMUSTINE (CCNU), AND VINCRISTINE (PCV) AFTER RADIATION

van den Bent MJ et al. J Clin Oncol 2013;31:344–350
van den Bent MJ et al. J Clin Oncol 2006;24:2715–2722

PCV chemotherapy started within 4 weeks after the end of RT
Lomustine 110 mg/m^2; administer orally as a single dose on day 1, every 6 weeks for a total of 6 cycles (total dosage/cycle = 110 mg/m^2)

Note: to reduce the likelihood of a medication error leading to severe myelosuppression, prescribe, dispense, and administer only enough capsules to supply one dose of lomustine. Educate patients that only one dose of lomustine is to be taken no more frequently than every 6 weeks and only after documentation of adequate hematologic recovery. (ISMP, 2014. https://www.ismp.org/resources/oral-chemotherapy-we-simply-must-do-better. Accessed June 20, 2018)

Procarbazine 60 mg/m^2 per day; administer orally for 14 consecutive days on days 8–21, every 6 weeks for a total of 6 cycles (total dosage/cycle = 840 mg/m^2)

Note: because procarbazine is a weak monoamine oxidase inhibitor, clinicians should guide patients who receive the drug in limiting their dietary intake of tyramine-containing foods and beverages

Vincristine 1.4 mg/m^2; administer per dose (maximum single dose = 2 mg); administer by intravenous infusion over 15 minutes in 50 mL 0.9% sodium chloride injection for 2 doses, on days 8 and 29, every 6 weeks for a total of 6 cycles (total dosage/cycle = 2.8 mg/m^2; maximum dose/cycle = 4 mg)

Radiotherapy within 6 weeks after surgery. 45 Gy is administered to the planning target volume-1 (PTV-1) in twenty-five 1.8-Gy fractions, 5 days/week over 5 weeks. Thereafter, a boost of 14.4 Gy (up to a cumulative dose of 59.4 Gy) is delivered to the PTV-2 in 8 fractions of 1.8 Gy, 1 fraction per day, 5 fractions per week. PTV-2 is to include the nonenhancing tumor area and/or the enhancing area as visible on the postoperative CT scan with contrast with a 1.5-cm margin; in case of a nonenhancing tumor on CT scan, a postoperative MRI scan with and without gadolinium is recommended to further define the tumor volume

Supportive Care
Antiemetic prophylaxis
Emetogenic potential on day 1 and days 8–21 is **MODERATE–HIGH**
Emetogenic potential on day 29 is **MINIMAL**
See Chapter 42 for antiemetic recommendations

Hematopoietic growth factor (CSF) prophylaxis
Primary prophylaxis is **NOT** *indicated*
See Chapter 43 for more information

Antimicrobial prophylaxis
Risk of fever and neutropenia is **LOW**
  Antimicrobial primary prophylaxis to be considered:
  • Antibacterial—not indicated
  • Antifungal—not indicated
  • Antiviral—not indicated unless patient previously had an episode of HSV

Note: treatment at the time of progression was left to the discretion of local investigators, but the study protocol strongly advised treating physicians to consider (PCV) chemotherapy, especially for patients in the RT-only arm

Patient Population Studied

Patient Characteristic	Radiotherapy Plus PCV (N = 185)	Radiotherapy Only (N = 183)
	Number of Patients (Percentage)	
Age, years: median (range)	48.6 (18.6–68.7)	49.8 (19.2–68.7)
Sex: Male/Female	102/83	110/73
WHO performance status: 0/1/2	155 (84)/30 (16)	153/30/84/16
Previous resection for low-grade tumor: Yes/No	27 (15)/156 (84)	25 (14)/157 (86)

(continued)

Treatment Modifications (continued)

Enhancement of the tumor: Yes/No	144 (78)/33 (18)	140 (77)/29 (16)
Tumor localization: Frontal/Elsewhere	89 (48)/96 (52)	84 (47)/98 (53)
MMSE score: 27–30/<27	116 (63)/46 (25)	14 (62)/53 (29)

Extent of resection*
   Biopsy
   Partial resection
   Total resection
	27 (15)
	 100 (54)
	 58 (31)
		25 (14)
		 83 (45)
		 75 (41)

Pathology
   Oligodendroglioma
   Oligoastrocytoma
   Missing
	139 (75)
	 44 (24)
	 2 (1)
		126 (69)
		 56 (31)
		 1 (1)

1p/19q determined 1p/19q loss 1p loss 19q loss No loss	155 42 (27) 24 (15) 18 (12) 71 (46)	156 36 (23) 24 (15) 20 (13) 76 (49)

*The extent of resection as assessed by the neurosurgeon
MMSE, Mini-Mental State Examination; PCV, procarbazine, lomustine, and vincristine

Efficacy

Median and 5-Year Overall Survival and Progression-Free Survival According to Assigned Treatment in the Various Subgroups

	Overall Survival				Progression-free Survival			
	Median	95% CI	% 5-y	95% CI	Median	95% CI	% 5-y	95% CI
Intent-to-treat Population (N_{RT} = 183; $N_{RT/PCV}$ = 185)								
RT	30.6	21.5–44.5	37.0	30.0–44.0	13.2	9.2–17.9	22	16.0–27.9
RT/PCV	42.3	28.7–62.0	43.4	36.2–50.5	24.3	17.4–40.7	37.5	30.5–44.4
1p/19q Status								
Deleted 1p/19q (N = 80)								
RT	111.8	75.7–134.3	73.0	55.6–84.4	49.9	27.8–101.8	46.0	29.6–60.9
RT/PCV	NR		76.2	60.3–86.4	156.8	68.1–NR	71.4	55.2–82.7
	HR, 0.56 (95% CI, 0.31–1.03); P = 0.0594				HR, 0.42 (95% CI, 0.24 to 0.74); P = 0.002			
Nondeleted 1p/19q (N = 236)								
RT	21.1	17.6–28.7	25.1	17.7–33.0	8.7	7.1–11.7	13.5	8.1–20.3
RT/PCV	25.0	18.0–36.8	31.6	23.3–40.2	14.8	9.9–21.1	25.4	17.8–33.7
	HR, 0.83 (95% CI, 0.62–1.10); P = 0.185				HR, 0.73 (95% CI, 0.56–0.97); P = 0.026			
IDH Status								
Mutated (N = 81)								
RT	64.8	36.9–111.8	52.8	35.5–67.4	36.0	17.2–58.6	33.3	18.8–48.6
RT/PCV	NR		68.2	52.3–79.8	71.2	47.1–NR	59.1	43.2–71.9
Wild type (N = 97)								
RT	14.7	11.9–19.1	16.0	7.5–27.4	6.8	5.4–8.6	4.0	0.74–12.1
RT/PCV	19.0	14.6–30.2	21.3	11.0–33.8	10.0	7.8–18.2	17.0	8.0–29.0

(continued)

Efficacy (continued)

MGMT Promoter							
Methylated (N = 136)							
RT	43.3	21.9–66.2	41.9	29.6–53.8	15.2	8.7–34.5	21.0	11.9–31.8
RT/PCV	70.9	42.0–136.8	54.8	42.7–65.4	55.6	20.4–73.6	48.0	36.2–58.8
Unmethylated (N = 47)							
RT	15.6	11.4–19.1	8.3	1.4–23.3	7.1	4.4–8.7	4.2	0.3–17.6
RT/PCV	16.3	9.1–30.3	17.4	5.4–35.0	9.8	4.6–15.4	17.4	5.4–35.0
Confirmed Anaplastic Oligodendroglial Histology at Central Review (N_{RT} = 126; $N_{RT/PCV}$ = 131)							
RT	28.7	19.3–41.7	33.0	25.0–41.3	10.4	8.4–16.9	17.9	11.8–25.1
RT/PCV	35.0	24.2–56.2	41.5	33.0–49.8	19.1	15.2–40.0	35.4	27.3–43.6
	HR, 0.73 (95% CI, 0.55–0.96)						

*The increase in OS was achieved despite the fact that the median number of PCV cycles was 3, with only 30% of patients completing the intended 6 cycles; most patients who discontinued PCV prematurely did so for (usually asymptomatic) hematologic toxicity or for tumor progression

CI, confidence interval; IDH, isocitrate dehydrogenase; MGMT, O_6-methylguanine-DNA methyltransferase; NR, not reached; PCV, procarbazine, lomustine, and vincristine; RT, radiotherapy

Therapy Monitoring

1. *Weekly:* CBC with differential
2. *Before each treatment:* LFTs
3. *Every 3–4 cycles:* Pulmonary function tests

Treatment Modifications

Adverse Event	Dose Modification
WBC nadir during the prior cycle 2000–3000/mm³, or platelets 25,000–75,000/mm³	Reduce lomustine and procarbazine dosages by 10–25%
WBC nadir during the prior cycle <2000/mm³, or platelets <25,000/mm³	Reduce lomustine and procarbazine dosages by 25–50%
Severe neurotoxicity; eg, painful paresthesia or peripheral weakness	Discontinue vincristine
Cumulative lomustine dosage >1100 mg/m², or worsening forced vital capacity (FVC) or carbon monoxide diffusing capacity (DL_{co})*	Discontinue lomustine

*Usually no more than a total of 6–7 cycles of lomustine (660–770 mg/m²) is recommended. Patients receiving cumulative lomustine dosages >1100 mg/m² are at increased risk for developing pulmonary toxicity. Patients with baseline FVC or DL_{co} <70% are particularly at risk

Adverse Effects

- Most patients who discontinued PCV prematurely did so for (usually asymptomatic) hematologic toxicity or for tumor progression
- A quality-of-life analysis that was part of this study has shown that patients in the RT/PCV arm complained more frequently of nausea/vomiting, loss of appetite, and drowsiness during and shortly after PCV chemotherapy
- However, no long-term effects of PCV chemotherapy on quality of life were identified

G3/4 Toxicity in the Patients Who Started PCV Chemotherapy (N = 161)

Toxicity	Grade 3	Grade 4
	Number of Patients (Percentage)	
WBC count	43 (27)	5 (3)
Neutrophils	39 (24)	13 (8)
Platelets	23 (14)	11 (7)
Hemoglobin	10 (6)	1 (1)
Any hematologic toxicity	51 (32)	23 (14)
Nausea	9 (6)	—
Vomiting	10 (6)	—
Polyneuropathy	3 (2)	—
Allergic skin reactions	2 (1)	—

PCV, procarbazine, lomustine, and vincristine

ANAPLASTIC OLIGODENDROGLIOMA AND ANAPLASTIC OLIGOASTROCYTOMA, NEWLY DIAGNOSED

CNS CANCER REGIMEN: PROCARBAZINE, LOMUSTINE, AND VINCRISTINE BEFORE RADIATION

Cairncross G et al. J Clin Oncol 2006;24:2707–2714
Cairncross G et al. J Clin Oncol 2013;31:337–343
Protocol for: Cairncross G et al. J Clin Oncol 2013;31:337–343

Lomustine (CCNU) 130 mg/m²; administer orally as a single dose, without food, on day 1, every 6 weeks, for 4 cycles (total dosage/6-week cycle = 130 mg/m²)
Note: to reduce the likelihood of a medication error leading to severe myelosuppression, prescribe, dispense, and administer only enough capsules to supply 1 dose of lomustine. Educate patients that only 1 dose of lomustine is to be taken every 6 weeks and only after documentation of adequate hematologic recovery. (ISMP, 2014. https://www.ismp.org/resources/oral-chemotherapy-we-simply-must-do-better. Accessed June 20, 2018)

Procarbazine 75 mg/m²/day; administer orally once daily for 14 consecutive days on days 8–21, every 6 weeks, for 4 cycles (total dosage/6-week cycle = 1050 mg/m²)
Note: because procarbazine is a weak monoamine oxidase inhibitor, one should restrict tyramine-containing foods in patients receiving procarbazine

Vincristine 1.4 mg/m² per dose; administer by intravenous infusion over 15 minutes in 50 mL 0.9% sodium chloride injection (0.9% NS) for 2 doses, on days 8 and 29, every 6 weeks, for 4 cycles (total dosage/6-week cycle = 2.8 mg/m²)
Note: the dose of vincristine is *not* capped in this regimen (Cairncross et al, 2006)

Begin radiation therapy within 6 weeks of the last dose of chemotherapy:

Radiation therapy once daily at 1.8 Gy/fraction for 5 days/week for a total of 33 fractions (total dosage = 59.4 Gy)
Notes:
The first 28 fractions were delivered to the initial target volume
The last 5 fractions were delivered to the boost volume

Supportive Care
Antiemetic prophylaxis
Emetogenic potential on day 1 and days 8–21 is **MODERATE–HIGH**
Emetogenic potential on day 29 is **MINIMAL**
See Chapter 42 for antiemetic recommendations

Hematopoietic growth factor (CSF) prophylaxis
Primary prophylaxis is **NOT** *indicated*
See Chapter 43 for more information

Antimicrobial prophylaxis
Risk of fever and neutropenia is **LOW**
   Antimicrobial primary prophylaxis to be considered:
   • Antibacterial—not indicated
   • Antifungal—not indicated
   • Antiviral—not indicated unless patient previously had an episode of HSV

Patient Population Studied

This multicenter, randomized, phase 3 trial (Radiation Therapy Oncology Group [RTOG] 9402) with long-term follow-up involved 291 patients with anaplastic oligodendroglioma or anaplastic oligoastrocytoma. Eligible patients were aged ≥18 years and had a Karnofsky performance status score ≥60. Patients randomly assigned to receive chemotherapy in addition to radiation received 4 cycles of the following regimen every 6 weeks before radiation: oral lomustine (130 mg/m²) on day 1, oral procarbazine (75 mg/m² daily) on days 8–21, and intravenous vincristine (1.4 mg/m²) on days 8 and 29. Radiation was administered within 6 weeks of the last chemotherapy dose in patients assigned to chemotherapy and within 1 week of randomization in all other patients. All patients received 33 fractions of 1.8 Gy radiation, with 1 fraction administered per day, 5 days per week

Efficacy (N = 291)

	Procarbazine, Lomustine, and Vincristine Plus Radiation (N = 148)	Radiation Only (N = 143)	
Median overall survival	4.6 years	4.7 years	HR 0.79, 95% CI 0.60–1.04; P = 0.1
Median progression-free survival	NR	NR	HR 0.68, 95% CI 0.53–0.88; P = 0.003

Note: median follow-up was 11.3 years. NR, not reported

For patients with codeleted (1p/19q) tumors (N = 126):

	Procarbazine, Lomustine, and Vincristine Plus Radiation (N = 59)	Radiation Only (N = 67)	
Median overall survival	14.7 years	7.3 years	HR 0.59, 95% CI 0.37–0.95; P = 0.03
Median progression-free survival	8.4 years	2.9 years	HR 0.47, 95% CI 0.30–0.72; P < 0.001

For patients with noncodeleted tumors (N = 137):

	Procarbazine, Lomustine, and Vincristine Plus Radiation (N = 76)	Radiation Only (N = 61)	
Median overall survival	2.6 years	2.7 years	HR 0.85, 95% CI 0.58–1.23; P = 0.39
Median progression-free survival	1.2 years	1.0 years	HR 0.81, 95% CI 0.56–1.16; P = 0.24

Therapy Monitoring

1. *Prior to the start of each cycle:* CBC with differential, platelet count, LFTs, BUN, creatinine, electrolytes; consider baseline pulmonary function testing (PFTs) especially in a patient with any pulmonary symptoms
2. *Weekly during PCV chemotherapy:* CBC with differential, platelet count, LFTs, BUN, creatinine, electrolytes. Repeat PFTs if symptoms of potential pulmonary compromise develop. Note, monitor blood counts weekly for 6 weeks after a dose: thrombocytopenia occurs at about 4 weeks postadministration and persists for 1–2 weeks, while leukopenia occurs at 5–6 weeks after a dose and persists for 1–2 weeks
3. *Response assessment:* perform follow-up MRI or CT scans before each cycle and 4–6 weeks after RT; thereafter, perform scans at increasing intervals, and after 5 years, annually, or as needed

Treatment Modifications

PROCARBAZINE, LOMUSTINE, AND VINCRISTINE FOLLOWED BY RADIATION

Starting lomustine dose	130 mg/m² as a single dose
Starting procarbazine dose	75 mg/m²/day for 14 consecutive days
Starting vincristine dose	1.4 mg/m² per dose (no maximum dose) ×2 doses days 8 and 29

Adverse Event	Treatment Modifications
Day 1 ANC <1500/mm³ or platelets <100,000/mm³	Delay start of cycle until ANC ≥1500/mm³ and platelets ≥100,000/mm³. Note that day 8 and day 29 vincristine should not be delayed for hematologic toxicity
Nadir ANC ≥500/mm³ and platelet count ≥50,000/mm³	Continue with same dose
Nadir ANC <500/mm³ or platelet count <50,000/mm³	Delay therapy until ANC ≥1500/mm³ and platelets ≥100,000/mm³. Reduce lomustine and procarbazine dosages by 25–50%. Do not reduce vincristine dose

(continued)

Treatment Modifications (*continued*)

Adverse Event	Treatment Modifications
G ≥2 nonhematologic toxicity that does not recover to G ≤1 within 2 weeks (>8 weeks between cycles)	Discontinue regimen
Any G ≥2 nonhematologic toxicity that recurs at the next cycle to G ≥2	
G ≥3 nausea or vomiting, persistent despite maximum antiemetic therapy	Reduce doses of lomustine and/or procarbazine by 25% for G3 or 50% for G4 for all subsequent doses
Other G3/4 nonhematologic toxicities	Delay attributable medication(s) until resolution to G ≤1, then reduce dose of attributable medication(s) by 25% for G3 or 50% for G4 toxicity in subsequent doses. For G4 toxicity, consider permanent discontinuation of therapy
Urticarial rash	Discontinue procarbazine unless attributable to another concomitant medication
G ≥2 liver toxicity (AST/ALT >3× ULN) and/or G ≥2 bilirubin (>1.5–3× ULN)	Delay therapy until resolution to G ≤1 (AST/ALT ≤3× ULN; bilirubin ≤1.5× ULN), then reduce lomustine, procarbazine, and vincristine by 25%
Patient concurrently taking drugs known to inhibit drug metabolism by hepatic cytochrome P450 isoenzymes in the CYP3A subfamily	Adjust vincristine dose
Total serum bilirubin >3 mg/dL: delay vincristine until total bilirubin ≤1.5 mg/dL	Reduce vincristine dose by 50% in all subsequent cycles
Severe abdominal pain or severe jaw pain	Reduce vincristine dose by 50% for all subsequent doses
G ≥3 peripheral neuropathy or G ≥3 motor neuropathy	Discontinue vincristine
Painful paresthesia or peripheral weakness	Discontinue vincristine
SIADH	Reduce vincristine dose or discontinue vincristine
Constipation, abdominal cramps, paralytic ileus	Temporarily discontinue vincristine. Treat symptoms. Resume vincristine when normal bowel function restored. Administer a routine prophylactic regimen against constipation
Creatinine clearance 10–50 mL/min	Reduce lomustine dose by 25%
Creatinine clearance <10 mL/min	Reduce lomustine dose by 50–75%
Any pulmonary symptoms, but with PFT showing DLco ≥ the predicted value	Continue with same lomustine dose
Any pulmonary symptoms, but with PFT showing <60% of the predicted value	Discontinue lomustine
Decreased oxygen saturation at rest (eg, pulse oximeter <88% or Pao_2 ≤55 mm Hg)	
Shortness of breath at rest or shortness of breath that limits self-care or ADLs	
Severe cough-limiting self-care or ADLs	
Cumulative lomustine dosage >1100 mg/m^2	Discontinue lomustine due to concerns of developing pulmonary fibrosis

Note: usually no more than a total of 4 cycles (520 mg/m^2) of lomustine is recommended in this regimen. Patients receiving >1100 mg/m^2 cumulative lomustine dosage have a higher risk of developing pulmonary toxicity. Patients with a baseline FVC or DLco <70% are particularly at risk (GLEOSTINE [lomustine] capsules; June 2018 product label. NextSource Biotechnology, LLC, Miami, FL).

Adverse Events

Grade 3/4 Toxicities (%)*	Procarbazine, Lomustine, and Vincristine Plus Radiation		Radiation Only
	During Chemotherapy (N = 146)	Within 90 Days of Starting Radiation (N = 141)	Within 90 Days of Starting Radiation (N = 131)
Any hematologic	56	4	0
Neutropenia	42	3	0
Thrombocytopenia	37	2	0
Any neurologic	13	2	1
Any gastrointestinal	9	0	0
Nausea or vomiting	8	0	0
Peripheral neuropathy	8	0	0
Other neurologic	5	1	<1
Anemia	5	0	0
Pulmonary	4	1	0
Dermatologic	4	0	2
Hepatic	4	0	0
Autonomic neuropathy	2	0	0
Other gastrointestinal	2	0	0
Fever†	1	0	0
Ototoxicity	<1	<1	1
Cognitive change	<1	<1	0
Affective disturbance	<1	0	1

*According to the National Cancer Institute Common Terminology Criteria for Adverse Events, version 1
†Fatal in one patient
Note: Grade 3/4 toxicities reported in the short-term follow-up manuscript are shown. Serious late toxicities were uncommon. The long-term follow-up manuscript reported 2 early deaths that were attributed to chemotherapy-induced neutropenia

ANAPLASTIC ASTROCYTOMA, NEWLY DIAGNOSED

CNS CANCER REGIMEN: TEMOZOLOMIDE

Bower M et al. Cancer Chemother Pharmacol 1997;40:484–488
Wick W et al. J Clin Oncol 2009;27:5874–5880
Wick W et al. Lancet Oncol 2012;13:707–715

Cycle 1:
Temozolomide 150 mg/m^2 per day; administer orally for 5 consecutive days, on days 1–5 of a 4-week cycle (total dosage/cycle = 750 mg/m^2)
Cycle 2 and subsequent cycles:
Temozolomide 200 mg/m^2 per day; administer orally for 5 consecutive days, on days 1–5, every 4 weeks (total dosage/cycle = 1000 mg/m^2)

Supportive Care
Antiemetic prophylaxis
Emetogenic potential: **MODERATE**
See Chapter 42 for antiemetic recommendations

Hematopoietic growth factor (CSF) prophylaxis
Primary prophylaxis is **NOT** indicated
See Chapter 43 for more information

Antimicrobial prophylaxis
Risk of fever and neutropenia is **LOW**
   Antimicrobial primary prophylaxis to be considered:
   • Antibacterial—not indicated
   • Antifungal—not indicated
   • Antiviral—not indicated unless patient previously had an episode of HSV

Patient Population Studied

NOA-04 Randomized Phase 3 Trial of Sequential Radiochemotherapy of Anaplastic Glioma with Procarbazine, Lomustine, and Vincristine (PCV) or Temozolomide (TMZ) (n = 318)
Wick W et al. J Clin Oncol 2009;27:5874–5880

A phase 3 trial of 318 patients with newly diagnosed anaplastic gliomas assigned 2:1:1 to receive upfront therapy with conventional radiotherapy (arm A, n = 139), PCV (arm B1, n = 54), or temozolomide (arm B2, n = 53) at diagnosis. Temozolomide was dosed at 200 mg/m^2 per day for 5 days every 4 weeks. After progression or unacceptable toxicity, patients in arm A were then randomized to receive either PCV or temozolomide and patients in arm B1 or B2 underwent radiation therapy

Temozolomide Chemotherapy Alone Versus Radiotherapy Alone for Malignant Astrocytoma in the Elderly: The NOA-08 Randomized Phase 3 Trial (n = 373)
Wick W et al. Lancet Oncol 2012;13:707–715

A randomized phase 3 trial of elderly (age >65 years) patients with anaplastic astrocytoma or glioblastoma and a Karnofsky performance score of ≥60. Patients received either temozolomide 100 mg/m^2/day (7 days on/7 days off schedule) (n = 195) or radiotherapy (n = 178)

Multicenter CRC Phase 2 Trial of Temozolomide in Recurrent or Progressive High-Grade Glioma (n = 103)
Bower M et al. Cancer Chemother Pharmacol 1997;40:484–488

A multicenter phase 2 trial of 103 patients with progressive or recurrent supratentorial high-grade gliomas. Temozolomide was dosed at 150 mg/m^2 for 5 days in cycle 1 and escalated to 200 mg/m^2 beginning in cycle 2 if tolerated

Efficacy

NOA-04 Randomized Phase 3 Trial of Sequential Radiochemotherapy of Anaplastic Glioma with Procarbazine, Lomustine, and Vincristine (PCV) or Temozolomide (TMZ) (n = 318)

Wick W et al. J Clin Oncol 2009;27:5874–5880

TTF, PFS, and OS	Radiotherapy (n = 139)		PCV or TMZ (n = 135)	
	Median	95% CI	Median	95% CI
TTF, months	42.7+		43.8	37.4–NR
Anaplastic astrocytoma	32.0	23.3–NR	29.4	19.0–NR
Anaplastic oligoastrocytoma	54+		54+	
Anaplastic oligodendroglioma	54+		54+	
Treatment failure at 48 months, %	55.5	46.3–64.6	46.4	36.7–56.2
PFS, months	30.6	16.3–42.8	31.9	21.1–37.3
Anaplastic astrocytoma	10.8	8.9–28.3	18.2	12.1–24.2
Anaplastic oligoastrocytoma Anaplastic oligodendroglioma	52.1	36.5–NR	52.7	33.9–NR
OS, months	72.1		82.6	
OS at 48 months, %	72.6	63.8–81.4	64.6	54.6–74.7

NR, not reached; OS, overall survival; PFS, progression-free survival; TTF, time to treatment failure

Temozolomide Chemotherapy Alone Versus Radiotherapy Alone for Malignant Astrocytoma in the Elderly: The NOA-08 Randomized, Phase 3 Trial (n = 373)

Wick W et al. Lancet Oncol 2012;13:707–715

Entire Temozolomide Group[†]	
Overall survival at 6 months	66.7% (95% CI 60.0–73.0)
Overall survival at 1 year	34.4% (95% CI 27.6–41.4)
Median overall survival	8.6 months (95% CI 7.3–10.2)
Event-free survival at 6 months	30.1% (95% CI 23.6–36.6)
Event-free survival at 1 year	12.0% (95% CI 7.9–17.1)
Median event-free survival	3.3 months (95% CI 3.2–4.1)
Patients with Methylated MGMT Promoter	
Median overall survival	NR (95% CI 10.1–NR)[‡]
Median event-free survival	8.4 months (95% CI 5.5–11.7)[§]

*Designed as a noninferiority trial
[†]Values are for ITT (intent-to-treat) population. The noninferiority of temozolomide for overall survival and event-free survival were also confirmed in the per-protocol population
[‡]Compared with 7 months (95% CI 5.7–8.7) for patients with an unmethylated tumor MGMT promoter
[§]Compared with 3.3 months (95% CI 3.0–3.5) for patients with an unmethylated tumor MGMT promoter
95% CI, 95% confidence interval; MGMT, O$_6$-methylguanine-DNA-methyltransferase; NR, not reached

Therapy Monitoring

1. *Weekly:* CBC with differential
2. *Every 4 weeks:* Serum electrolytes, mineral panel, and LFTs

Treatment Modifications

TEMOZOLOMIDE DOSE MODIFICATION

G ≤1 myelosuppression in cycle 1	Escalate temozolomide dosage to 200 mg/m^2 per day, days 1–5
Day 1 ANC <1,500/mm^3 or platelet count <100,000/mm^3	Delay therapy until ANC ≥1500/mm^3 and platelet count ≥100,000/mm^3. Consider dose reduction based on nadir ANC and platelet count as outlined below
Nadir ANC <1000/mm^3 and/or nadir platelet count <50,000/mm^3	Postpone treatment until ANC ≥1500/mm^3 and platelet count ≥100,000/mm^3 and then reduce the temozolomide dosage by 50 mg/m^2/dose
Grade 3 nonhematologic toxicity (except for alopecia, nausea, or vomiting)	Postpone treatment until nonhematologic toxicity Grade ≤1, then reduce the temozolomide dosage by 50 mg/m^2/dose
Recurrent Grade 3 nonhematologic toxicity (except for alopecia, nausea, or vomiting), despite previous dose reduction	Discontinue temozolomide
Grade 4 nonhematologic toxicity	

Efficacy (continued)

Multicenter CRC Phase 2 Trial of Temozolomide in Recurrent or Progressive High-Grade Glioma (n = 103)

Bower M et al. Cancer Chemother Pharmacol 1997;40:484–488

Objective response	11%
Stable disease	47%
Median survival	5.8 months
Progression-free survival at 6 months	22%

Note: the study included 18 patients not evaluable for response

Adverse Events

Phase 3 NOA-04 Study

Toxicity in the First and Recurrence Treatments

Grade 2/3 Adverse Event According to CTCAE	TMZ (N = 108)
Allergic reaction	1 (0.9%)
Alopecia/local skin reaction	0
Cephalgia	1 (0.9%)
Diarrhea	3 (2.8%)
Hematologic (Grades 3 to 4)	6 (5.6%)
Herpes zoster infection	2 (1.8%)
Infection (Grades 2 to 4)	2 (1.8%)
Obstipation	2 (1.8%)
Polyneuropathy	0
Pneumonia	2 (1.8%)
Pneumonitis	0
Tumor bleed, thromboembolic events	3 (2.8%)
Transaminase elevation	2 (1.8%)

CTCAE, National Cancer Institute (USA) Common Terminology Criteria for Adverse Events
Wick W et al. J Clin Oncol 2009;27:5874–5880

Phase 3 NOA-08 Study (n = 195)

	Numbers of Grades 2–4 Adverse Events*		
	Grade 2	Grade 3	Grade 4
Hematologic Toxic Effects			
Neutropenia	56	12	4
Lymphocytopenia	60	44	2
Thrombocytopenia	36	12	2

(continued)

Adverse Events (continued)

Nonhematologic Toxic Effects

Liver enzyme elevation	42	26	4
Infection	54	26	9
Thromboembolic event	16	18	6
Asthenia/fatigue	37	21	3
Nausea/vomiting	32	6	0
Weight loss/inappetence	8	2	0
Neurologic symptoms	73	27	9
Seizures	14	15	2
Cutaneous (dermatitis, allergic rash, alopecia)	15	1	0

Wick W et al. Lancet Oncol 2012;13:707–715

*N = 195 refers to number of patients. However, number of events are total events and if the grade of an adverse event had returned to 1, subsequent events of Grades 2 to 4 were counted as new events, so that a patient could have more than 1 event

Phase 2 CRC Study (n = 101)

% CTC Grade

	None	G1	G2	G3	G4
Hematologic					
Neutropenia	82	6	8	1	4
Thrombocytopenia	53	29	6	6	7
Anemia	64	32	4	0	1
Lymphopenia	12	10	20	43	16
Nonhematologic					
Nausea	40	18	21	22	0
Vomiting	41	8	27	24	1
Constipation	59	13	17	12	0
Mucositis	76	14	8	3	0
Increased ALT	53	36	9	3	0
Increased ALP	75	26	0	0	0
Increased bilirubin	95	0	5	0	1

	None	Mild	Moderate	Severe
Lethargy*	49	5	14	33
Anorexia*	64	17	10	10

Bower M et al. Cancer Chemother Pharmacol 1997;40:484–488

*No CTC grading available. National Cancer Institute (USA) Common Toxicity Criteria (CTC) and Common Terminology Criteria for Adverse Events (CTCAE), all versions. At: http://ctep.cancer.gov/protocolDevelopment/electronic_applications/ctc.htm [accessed December 7, 2013]

ANAPLASTIC ASTROCYTOMA, NEWLY DIAGNOSED

CNS CANCER REGIMEN: RADIATION PLUS EITHER TEMOZOLOMIDE, LOMUSTINE, OR CARMUSTINE

Chang S et al. Neuro Oncol 2017;19:252–258

Radiation therapy once daily at 1.8 Gy/fraction for 5 days/week for a total of 33 fractions (total dosage =59.4 Gy), *plus:*
Notes:
The first 28 fractions were delivered to the initial target volume
The last 5 fractions were delivered to the boost volume

Choose *only one* **of the following chemotherapy regimens:**
Temozolomide 200 mg/m²/day; administer orally once daily for 5 consecutive days, on days 1–5, starting on the first day of radiation therapy, on an empty stomach with water at bedtime, every 4 weeks for 12 cycles (total dosage/4-week cycle = 1000 mg/m²), *or:*
- *Note:* patients who vomit after taking temozolomide should be instructed to take their next dose at the next regularly scheduled time

Lomustine 130 mg/m²; administer orally as a single dose, without food, on day 1, starting on the first day of radiation therapy, every 8 weeks, for 6 cycles (total dosage/8-week cycle = 130 mg/m²), *or:*
- *Note:* to reduce the likelihood of a medication error leading to severe myelosuppression, prescribe, dispense, and administer only enough capsules to supply one dose of lomustine. Educate patients that only one dose of lomustine is to be taken every 8 weeks and only after documentation of adequate hematologic recovery. (ISMP, 2014. https://www.ismp.org/resources/oral-chemotherapy-we-simply-must-do-better. Accessed June 20, 2018)

Carmustine 80 mg/m² per dose; administer intravenously in 100–250 mL 5% dextrose injection (D5W) over at least 60 minutes for 3 consecutive days, on days 1–3, starting on the first day of radiation therapy, every 8 weeks for 6 cycles (total dosage/8-week cycle = 240 mg/m²)

Supportive Care
Antiemetic prophylaxis
Emetogenic potential on days with temozolomide is **MODERATE**
Emetogenic potential on days with lomustine is **MODERATE–HIGH**
Emetogenic potential on days with carmustine is **HIGH**
See Chapter 42 for antiemetic recommendations

Hematopoietic growth factor (CSF) prophylaxis
Primary prophylaxis is **NOT** *indicated*
See Chapter 43 for more information

Antimicrobial prophylaxis
Risk of fever and neutropenia is **LOW**
   Antimicrobial primary prophylaxis to be considered:
- Antibacterial—not indicated; consider *Pneumocystis jirovecii* prophylaxis (eg, cotrimoxazole)
- Antifungal—not indicated
- Antiviral—not indicated unless patient previously had an episode of HSV

Patient Population Studied

This prospective, multicenter, randomized, phase 3 trial (NRG Oncology Radiation Therapy Oncology Group [RTOG] 9813) involved 196 patients with unifocal, newly diagnosed anaplastic astrocytoma or oligoastrocytoma for which the oligodendroglial component was ≤25%. Eligible patients were aged ≥18 years and had a Karnofsky performance status score ≥60. Patients who had prior malignancy within 5 years or who had received prior cranial radiation of chemotherapy were not eligible. All patients received radiation therapy. Patients were randomly assigned to receive temozolomide or a nitrosourea

Efficacy (N = 196)

	Radiation Plus Temozolomide (N = 97)	Radiation Plus Nitrosourea (N = 99)	Hazard Ratio (HR) in Multivariate Analysis
Median overall survival*	3.9 years	3.8 years	HR 0.81, 95% CI 0.57–1.15; P = 0.24
Median progression-free survival	NR	NR	HR 0.70, 95% CI 0.50–0.98; P = 0.039
Time to tumor progression	NR	NR	HR 0.80, 95% CI 0.55–1.16; P = 0.24

*Overall survival was the primary end point
Note: the median follow-up was 3.6 years
NR, not reported

Therapy Monitoring

1. *Prior to day 1 of each cycle:* CBC with differential, platelet count, LFTs, BUN, creatinine, electrolytes
2. *Weekly:* CBC with differential, platelet count (monitor blood counts weekly for 6 weeks after a dose). With the nitrosoureas thrombocytopenia occurs at about 4 weeks postadministration and persists for 1–2 weeks, while leukopenia occurs at 5–6 weeks after a dose and persists for 1–2 weeks
3. *Response assessment:* contrast-enhanced MRI of the brain every 6 weeks for 6 months, then every 12 weeks thereafter

Treatment Modifications

TEMOZOLOMIDE or LOMUSTINE (CCNU) or CARMUSTINE (BCNU)

Adverse Event	Treatment Modification
TEMOZOLOMIDE or LOMUSTINE (CCNU) or CARMUSTINE (BCNU)—DOSE MODIFICATION	
Hematologic Toxicity	
Day 1 WBC <4000/mm^3, ANC <1500/mm^3 or platelets <100,000/mm^3	Delay start of treatment until WBC ≥4000/mm^3, ANC ≥1500/mm^3, and platelets ≥100,000/mm^3
Nadirs during prior cycle: WBC 2000–2999/mm^3; ANC 1000–1500/mm^3; platelets 50,000–75,000/mm^3	Withhold administration of therapy until WBC ≥4000/mm^3, ANC ≥1500/mm^3, and platelets ≥100,000/mm^3. Consider administering 75% of dose taken at the time toxicity occurred in subsequent cycle(s)
Nadirs during prior cycle: WBC <2000/mm^3; ANC <1000/mm^3; platelets <50,000/mm^3	Withhold administration of therapy until WBC ≥4000/mm^3, ANC ≥1500/mm^3, and platelets ≥100,000/mm^3. Administer 50–75% of dose taken at the time toxicity occurred in subsequent cycle(s)
Nadirs during prior cycle: WBC <1000/mm^3, ANC <500/mm^3 or platelets <25,000/mm^3 during cycle (G4 toxicity)	Discontinue permanently *or* if physician deems it to be in the patient's best interest to continue, interrupt until resolved to G ≤1, then resume therapy with dose ≤50% that at the time G4 toxicity occurred
Nonhematologic Toxicity	
Other G1 nonhematologic toxicity	Continue treatment and maintain dose in subsequent cycle
Other G2 nonhematologic toxicity (1st occurrence)	Interrupt until resolved to G ≤1; administer 100% of dose in subsequent cycle
Other G2 nonhematologic toxicity (2nd occurrence)	Interrupt until resolved to G ≤1; administer 75% of initial dose in subsequent cycle. *Note:* once the dose has been reduced, it should not be increased at a later time
Other G2 nonhematologic toxicity (3rd occurrence)	Interrupt until resolved to G ≤1; administer 50% of initial drug dose in subsequent cycle. *Note:* once the dose has been reduced, it should not be increased at a later time
Other G2 nonhematologic toxicity (4th occurrence)	Discontinue treatment permanently
Other G3 nonhematologic toxicity (1st occurrence)	Interrupt until resolved to G ≤1; administer 75% of initial drug dose in subsequent cycle. *Note:* once the dose has been reduced, it should not be increased at a later time

(continued)

Adverse Events (*continued*)

Nonhematologic Toxicity

Other G3 nonhematologic toxicity (2nd occurrence)	Interrupt until resolved to G ≤1; administer 50% of initial drug dose in subsequent cycle. *Note:* once the dose has been reduced, it should not be increased at a later time
Other G3 nonhematologic toxicity (3rd occurrence)	Discontinue treatment permanently
Any other G ≥2 nonhematologic toxicity that does not recover to G ≤1 within 2 weeks	Discontinue chemotherapy
Other G4 nonhematologic toxicity (1st occurrence)	Discontinue permanently *or* if physician deems it to be in the patient's best interest to continue, interrupt until resolved to G ≤1, then resume therapy with dose ≤50% that at the time G4 toxicity occurred. *Note:* once the dose has been reduced, it should not be increased at a later time

TEMOZOLOMIDE DOSE MODIFICATION

Starting temozolomide dose	200 mg/m² days 1–5
Drug-related increase in serum bilirubin to >3× ULN (G3)	Delay therapy until resolution to G ≤1 (AST/ALT ≤3× ULN; bilirubin ≤1.5× ULN). When treatment is resumed administer 50–66% of the dose taken at the time toxicity occurred. If serum bilirubin >10× ULN discontinue therapy. *Note:* once the dose has been reduced, it should not be increased at a later time

Temozolomide dose adjustment for renal impairment: No formal recommendations exist; use with caution
Temozolomide dose adjustments for hepatic impairment:
• Mild to moderate hepatic impairment: no dose reduction necessary
• Severe hepatic impairment: use caution; no data available

LOMUSTINE (CCNU) DOSE MODIFICATIONS

Starting lomustine dose	130 mg/m² as a single dose on day 1
G ≥3 liver toxicity (AST/ALT >5× ULN) and/or G ≥2 bilirubin (>1.5–3× ULN)	Delay therapy until resolution to G ≤1 (AST/ALT ≤3× ULN; bilirubin ≤1.5× ULN). When treatment is resumed, administer lomustine at 70% of the dose taken at the time toxicity occurred
Any pulmonary symptoms, but with PFT showing DLco ≥ the predicted value	Continue with same lomustine dose
Any pulmonary symptoms, but with PFT showing <60% of the predicted value	Discontinue lomustine
Decreased oxygen saturation at rest (eg, pulse oximeter <88% or Pao₂ ≤55 mm Hg) or ADL	
Shortness of breath at rest or shortness of breath that limits self-care or ADL	
Severe cough limiting self-care or ADL	

Notes:
6 × 130 = 780 mg/m² of lomustine is recommended. Patients receiving >1100 mg/m² cumulative lomustine dosage have a higher risk of developing pulmonary toxicity; however, this should not be reached. Patients with a baseline FVC or DLco <70% are particularly at risk (GLEOSTINE [lomustine] capsules; June 2018 product label. NextSource Biotechnology, LLC, Miami, FL)
Lomustine dose adjustment for renal impairment:
• Creatinine clearance 10–50 mL/minute: reduce dose by 25%
• Creatinine clearance <10 mL/minute: reduce dose by 50–75%
Lomustine dose adjustments for hepatic impairment: no formal recommendations exist; use with caution

CARMUSTINE (BCNU) DOSE MODIFCATION

Starting carmustine dose	80 mg/m²/day for 3 consecutive days

Note: 6 × 80 × 3 = 1440 mg/m² *is recommended.* Patients receiving cumulative carmustine dosage >1440 mg/m² are at risk of developing pulmonary fibrosis, or worsening of FVC or DLco

Carmustine dose adjustment for renal impairment: creatinine clearance <10 mL/min: Discontinue carmustine
Carmustine dose adjustments for hepatic impairment: no formal recommendations exist; use with caution

Adverse Events (N = 195)

Grade (%)*	Radiation Plus Temozolomide (N = 96)		Radiation Plus Nitrosourea (N = 99)	
	Grade 1/2	Grade 3–5	Grade 1/2	Grade 3–5
Worst overall toxicity	52	48	24	76
Worst nonhematologic toxicity	68	32	66	34

*According to the National Cancer Institute Common Terminology Criteria for Adverse Events, version 2
Note: the majority of toxicities were related to myelosuppression. Two Grade 5 toxicities were reported for each treatment group: death owing to myocardial ischemia and death owing to neutropenia were reported for the temozolomide group, and death owing to adult respiratory distress syndrome and death owing to pulmonary embolism were reported for the nitrosourea group

GLIOBLASTOMA, NEWLY DIAGNOSED

CNS CANCER REGIMEN: TEMOZOLOMIDE WITH RADIATION THERAPY

Stupp R et al. J Clin Oncol 2002;20:1375–1382
Stupp R et al. N Engl J Med 2005;352:987–996

Temozolomide with radiation therapy:
Temozolomide 75 mg/m^2 per day; administer orally, continually, 7 days/week for 6–7 weeks in a fasting state 1 hour before radiation therapy (RT), and in the morning in a fasting state on days without RT (total dosage/6- to 7-week cycle = 3150–3675 mg/m^2)
Radiation therapy once daily at 2 Gy/fraction for 5 days/week for a total of 60 Gy

Adjuvant temozolomide starting 4 weeks after completing RT:
Temozolomide 200 mg/m^2 per day; administer orally for 5 consecutive days, on days 1–5 every 28 days for up to 6 cycles (total dosage/cycle = 1000 mg/m^2)

Supportive Care
Antiemetic prophylaxis
Emetogenic potential: **MODERATE**
See Chapter 42 for antiemetic recommendations

Hematopoietic growth factor (CSF) prophylaxis
Primary prophylaxis is **NOT** indicated
See Chapter 43 for more information

Antimicrobial prophylaxis
Risk of fever and neutropenia is **LOW**
  Antimicrobial primary prophylaxis to be considered:
  • Antibacterial—not indicated
  • Antifungal—not indicated
  • Antiviral—not indicated unless patient previously had an episode of HSV

Patient Population Studied

A multicenter phase 3 trial of 573 patients with newly diagnosed GBM in which 287 patients received temozolomide with RT

Efficacy (N = 287)

Median Survival	14.6 Months
1-year survival	61.1%
2-year survival	26.5%

Therapy Monitoring

1. *Weekly:* CBC with differential
2. *Every 4 weeks:* Serum electrolytes, chemistry panel, and LFTs

Treatment Modifications

Adverse Event	Dose Modification
WBC <3000/mm^3 or platelets <100,000/mm^3 on day 1 of any cycle	Delay retreatment for 1 week
After a 1-week delay, if WBC <2000/mm^3 or platelets <75,000/mm^3	Reduce temozolomide dosage by 25%
After a 1-week delay, if WBC <1000/mm^3 or platelets <25,000/mm^3	Reduce temozolomide dosage by 50%

Adapted from Stupp R et al. J Clin Oncol 2002;20:375–1382, in which dose modifications were not specified

Adverse Effects (N = 287)

Temozolomide with Radiation Therapy (N = 287)

Toxicity	% CTC Grade	
	G2	G3/G4
Hematologic Toxicity		
Leukopenia	N/A	2
Neutropenia	N/A	4
Thrombocytopenia	N/A	3
Anemia	N/A	<1
Any	N/A	7
Nonhematologic Toxicity		
Fatigue	26	7
Other constitutional symptoms	7	2
Rash/other dermatologic	9	1
Infection	1	3
Vision	14	1
Nausea/vomiting	13	<1

Adjuvant Temozolomide After RT (N = 287)

Toxicity	% CTC Grade	
	G2	G3/4
Hematologic Toxicity		
Leukopenia	N/A	5
Neutropenia	N/A	4
Thrombocytopenia	N/A	11
Anemia	N/A	1
Any	N/A	14
Nonhematologic Toxicity		
Fatigue	25	6
Other constitutional symptoms	4	2
Rash/other dermatologic	5	2
Infection	2	5
Vision	10	<1
Nausea/vomiting	18	1

CTC, National Cancer Institute (USA) Common Toxicity Criteria, version 2.0. At: http://ctep.cancer.gov/protocolDevelopment/electronic_applications/ctc.htm [accessed December 7, 2013]

GLIOBLASTOMA, RECURRENT
CNS CANCER REGIMEN: BEVACIZUMAB ± IRINOTECAN

Kreisl T et al. J Clin Oncol 2009;27:740–745

Initial therapy:
Bevacizumab 10 mg/kg per dose; administer intravenously in 100 mL 0.9% sodium chloride injection, USP (0.9% NS) on days 1 and 15, every 28 days (total dosage/4-week cycle = 20 mg/kg)
- First dose is administered over 90 minutes
- Second dose may be administered over 60 minutes, if the first dose was well tolerated
- Third and subsequent doses may be administered over 30 minutes, if doses administered over 60 minutes were well tolerated

Therapy after documented tumor progression:
Bevacizumab 10 mg/kg per dose; administer intravenously in 100 mL 0.9% NS on days 1 and 15, every 28 days (total dosage/4-week cycle = 20 mg/kg), *plus*
Irinotecan

Patients receiving non–enzyme-inducing antiepileptic drugs (NEIAED) 125 mg/m^2 per dose; administer intravenously over 90 minutes in 250 mL 0.9% NS or 5% dextrose injection, USP (D5W) on days 1 and 15, every 28 days (total dosage/4-week cycle = 250 mg/m^2)

Patients receiving enzyme-inducing antiepileptic drugs (EIAED) 340 mg/m^2 per dose; administer intravenously over 90 minutes in 250 mL 0.9% NS or D5W on days 1 and 15, every 28 days (total dosage/4-week cycle = 680 mg/m^2)

Supportive Care
Antiemetic prophylaxis
Emetogenic potential with bevacizumab alone is **MINIMAL**
Emetogenic potential with bevacizumab + irinotecan is **MODERATE**
See Chapter 42 for antiemetic recommendations

Hematopoietic growth factor (CSF) prophylaxis
Primary prophylaxis is **NOT** indicated
See Chapter 43 for more information

Antimicrobial prophylaxis
Risk of fever and neutropenia is **LOW**
Antimicrobial primary prophylaxis to be considered:
- Antibacterial—not indicated
- Antifungal—not indicated
- Antiviral—not indicated, unless patient previously had an episode of HSV

Acute cholinergic syndrome
Atropine sulfate 0.25–1 mg administer subcutaneously or intravenously if abdominal cramping or diarrhea develop during or within 1 hour after irinotecan administration
- If symptoms are severe, add as primary prophylaxis at least 30 min before irinotecan during subsequent cycles
- For irinotecan, acute cholinergic syndrome may be characterized by abdominal cramping, diarrhea, diaphoresis, hypotension, flushing, bradycardia, rhinitis, increased salivation, meiosis, and lacrimation

Diarrhea management
Latent or delayed-onset diarrhea:
Loperamide 4 mg orally initially after the first loose or liquid stool, *then*
Loperamide 2 mg orally every 2 hours during waking hours, *plus*
Loperamide 4 mg orally every 4 hours during hours of sleep
- Continue for at least 12 hours after diarrhea resolves
- Recurrent diarrhea after a 12-hour diarrhea free interval is treated as a new episode
- Rehydrate orally with fluids and electrolytes during a diarrheal episode
- If a patient develops blood or mucus in stool, dehydration, or hemodynamic instability, or if diarrhea persists >48 hours despite loperamide, stop loperamide and hospitalize the patient for IV hydration

Alternatively, a trial of **diphenoxylate hydrochloride** 2.5 mg **with atropine sulfate** 0.025 mg (eg, Lomotil)
- Initial adult dose is two tablets four times daily until control has been achieved, after which the dose may be reduced to meet individual requirements. Control may often be maintained with as little as two tablets daily
- Clinical improvement of acute diarrhea is usually observed within 48 hours. If improvement of chronic diarrhea after treatment with a maximum daily dose of 8 tablets is not observed within 10 days, control is unlikely with further administration

(continued)

(*continued*)

Persistent diarrhea:
  Octreotide 100–150 mcg subcutaneously 3 times daily. Maximum total daily dose is 1500 mcg
Antibiotic therapy during latent or delayed-onset diarrhea:
  A fluoroquinolone (eg, **ciprofloxacin** 500 mg orally every 12 hours) if absolute neutrophil count <500/mm^3 with or without accompanying fever in association with diarrhea
  • Antibiotics should also be administered if patient is hospitalized with prolonged diarrhea and should be continued until diarrhea resolves

*Rothenberg ML et al. J Clin Oncol 2001;19:3801–3807; Abigerges D et al. J Natl Cancer Inst 1994;86:446–449; Wadler S et al. J Clin Oncol 1998;16:3169–3178

Treatment Modifications: Bevacizumab-Related Adverse Events

Note: there are no recommended dose reductions for the use of bevacizumab. Consequently, bevacizumab use is either temporarily interrupted or discontinued

Adverse Event	Toxicity Grade	Dose Modification/Action to Be Taken
Allergic reactions or acute infusional reactions/cytokine release syndrome	G1–3	Premedications should be given before the next dose, and infusion time may not be shortened for subsequent infusions. For patients with G3 reactions, bevacizumab infusion should be stopped and not restarted on the same day. At a physician's discretion, bevacizumab may be permanently discontinued or reinstituted with premedications and at a rate designed to complete administration over 90 ± 15 minutes. If bevacizumab is reinstituted, the patient should be closely monitored for a duration comparable to or longer than the duration of the previous reactions
	G4	Discontinue bevacizumab
Arterial thrombosis • Cardiac ischemia/infarction • CNS ischemia (TIA, CVA) • Any peripheral or visceral arterial ischemia/thrombosis	G2 (if new or worsened after starting bevacizumab therapy)	Discontinue bevacizumab
	G3/4	Discontinue bevacizumab
Venous thrombosis	G3 or asymptomatic G4	• Hold bevacizumab treatment. If the planned duration of full-dose anticoagulation is <2 weeks, bevacizumab should be withheld until the full-dose anticoagulation period is over. Prophylaxis against pulmonary emboli can be accomplished through placement of an IVC filter • If the planned duration of full-dose anticoagulation is >2 weeks, permanently discontinue bevacizumab • If thromboemboli worsen/recur upon resumption of therapy, discontinue bevacizumab
	G4 (symptomatic)	Discontinue bevacizumab

(*continued*)

Toxicity (N = 48)

Toxicity	% G1	% G2	% G3	% G4
Thromboembolic events			4.2	8.4
Hypertension		8.4	4.2	
Hypophosphatemia		4.2	6.3	
Thrombocytopenia		4.2	2.1	
Hepatic dysfunction			2.1	
Proteinuria	2.1			
Bowel perforation			2.1	

Patient Population Studied

A phase 2 study of 48 patients with recurrent glioblastoma

Efficacy (N = 48)

Partial response	71%
6-month survival rate	57%
6-month progression-free survival	29%
Median overall survival	31 weeks
Median progression-free survival	16 weeks

Note: of 19 patients treated with bevacizumab plus irinotecan at progression, there were no objective radiographic responses

Therapy Monitoring

1. *Every 2 weeks:* CBC with differential, urinalysis for urine protein: creatinine ratio, BP check
2. *Every 4 weeks:* CBC with differential, serum electrolytes, mineral panel, and LFTs

Treatment Modifications:
Bevacizumab-Related Adverse Events (*continued*)

Adverse Event	Toxicity Grade	Dose Modification/Action to Be Taken
Hypertension (treat with antihypertensive medications as needed. The goal of BP control should be consistent with general medical practice)	If BP is controlled medically	Continue bevacizumab
	Persistent or symptomatic HTN	Hold bevacizumab. If treatment is delayed for >4 weeks because of uncontrolled hypertension, discontinue bevacizumab
	G4	Discontinue bevacizumab
Proteinuria (proteinuria should be monitored by urine analysis for urine protein:creatinine [UPC] ratio prior to every dose of bevacizumab)	UPC ratio <3.5	Continue bevacizumab
	UPC ratio ≥3.5	Hold bevacizumab until UPC recovers to <3.5. If therapy is held for >2 months because of proteinuria, discontinue bevacizumab
	G4 or nephrotic syndrome	Discontinue bevacizumab
Wound dehiscence requiring medical or surgical intervention		Discontinue bevacizumab
GI perforation, GI leak, or fistula		Discontinue bevacizumab

GLIOBLASTOMA, RECURRENT

CNS CANCER REGIMEN: LOMUSTINE (CCNU)

Batchelor TT. J Clin Oncol 2013;31:3212–3218

Lomustine 110 mg/m²; administer orally as a single dose on day 1, every 6–8 weeks for a total of 6 cycles (total dosage/cycle = 110 mg/m²)

Note: to reduce the likelihood of a medication error leading to severe myelosuppression, prescribe, dispense, and administer only enough capsules to supply one dose of lomustine. Educate patients that only one dose of lomustine is to be taken no more frequently than ever 6 weeks and only after documentation of adequate hematologic recovery. (ISMP, 2014. https://www.ismp.org/resources/oral-chemotherapy-we-simply-must-do-better. Accessed June 20, 2018)

Supportive Care

Antiemetic prophylaxis

Emetogenic potential on day 1 is
MODERATE–HIGH
See Chapter 42 for antiemetic recommendations

Hematopoietic growth factor (CSF) prophylaxis

*Primary prophylaxis is **NOT** indicated*
See Chapter 43 for more information

Antimicrobial prophylaxis

*Risk of fever and neutropenia is **LOW***
Antimicrobial primary prophylaxis to be considered:
- Antibacterial—not indicated
- Antifungal—not indicated
- Antiviral—not indicated unless patient previously had an episode of HSV

Patient Population Studied

Patients with recurrent glioblastoma, prior treatment with a temozolomide-containing chemotherapy regimen, prior treatment with radiation, Karnofsky performance status (KPS) ≥70, Mini-Mental Status Examination score ≥15, and who had not received any prior anti-VEGF therapy or cranial radiation within 3 months before study entry

Treatment Modifications

Adverse Event	Dose Modification
WBC nadir during the prior cycle 2000–3000/mm³, or platelets 25,000–75,000/mm³	Reduce lomustine dosage by 10–25%
WBC nadir during the prior cycle <2000/mm³, or platelets <25,000/mm³	Reduce lomustine and dosage by 25–50%
Cumulative lomustine dosage >1100 mg/m², or worsening forced vital capacity (FVC) or carbon monoxide diffusing capacity (DLco)*	Discontinue lomustine

Note: usually no more than a total of 6–7 cycles of lomustine (660–770 mg/m²) is recommended. Patients receiving cumulative lomustine dosages >1100 mg/m² are at increased risk for developing pulmonary toxicity. Patients with baseline FVC or DLco<70% are particularly at risk
CCNSB (lomustine) Capsules; May 2013 product label. Next Source Biotechnology, LLC, Miami, FL

Toxicity

Grades 3/4 Adverse Events	Placebo + Lomustine (n = 64)	
	Number	%
Any AE, ≥ Grade 3	39	60.9
Thrombocytopenia	14	22
Neutropenia	2	3.1
Fatigue	6	9.4
Leukopenia	3	4.7
Platelet count decreased	1	1.6
Anemia	0	
Hypertension	0	
ALT increased	0	
GGT increased	2	3.1
WBC decreased	3	4.7
Diarrhea	1	1.6
Pulmonary embolism	4	6.3
Lymphopenia	5	7.8
Convulsion	3	4.7
Intracranial hemorrhage	2	3.1

AE, adverse event; GGT, γ-glutamyltransferase

Efficacy

Best Overall Response	Lomustine + Placebo (n = 56)	
	Number	%
Overall response rate	5	8.9
Complete response (CR)	0	—
Partial response (PR)	5	8.9
Stable disease	23	41.1
Unconfirmed CR	0	—
Unconfirmed PR	2	3.6
PD	16	28.6
Nonevaluable	5	8.9
Median reduction in contrast-enhanced tumor area	+14% increase	
APF6 proportions	25%	
Corticosteroid usage	+5%	
Median progression-free survival	82 days (first quartile = 42 days, third quartile = 168 days)	
Median overall survival	9.8 months	

GLIOBLASTOMA, RECURRENT

CNS CANCER REGIMEN: LOMUSTINE AND BEVACIZUMAB

Taal W et al. Lancet Oncol 2014;15:943–953
Wick W et al. N Engl J Med 2017;377:1954–1963
Protocol for: Wick W et al. N Engl J Med 2017;377:1954–1963 https://www.nejm.org/doi/suppl/10.1056/
NEJMoa1707358/suppl_file/nejmoa1707358_protocol.pdf

Bevacizumab 10 mg/kg per dose; administer intravenously in 100 mL 0.9% sodium chloride injection on days 1, 15, and 29, every 6 weeks until disease progression (total dosage/6-week cycle = 30 mg/kg), *plus:*
Note: bevacizumab administration duration for the initial dose is 90 minutes. If administration is well tolerated, the administration duration may be decreased stepwise during subsequent administrations to 60 minutes and, finally, to a minimum duration of 30 minutes

Lomustine 90 mg/m^2 (maximum dose = 160 mg); administer orally as a single dose, without food, on day 1, every 6 weeks, until disease progression (total dosage/6-week cycle = 90 mg/m^2; maximum dosage/6-week cycle = 160 mg)
Notes:
- In the absence of ≥Grade 2 hematologic toxicity, may increase the lomustine dose to 110 mg/m^2 starting with cycle 2,
  thus:
    - **Lomustine** 110 mg/m^2 (maximum dose = 200 mg); administer orally as a single dose, without food, on day 1, every 6 weeks, until disease progression (total dosage/6-week cycle = 110 mg/m^2; maximum dosage/6-week cycle = 200 mg)
    - To reduce the likelihood of a medication error leading to severe myelosuppression, prescribe, dispense, and administer only enough capsules to supply 1 dose of lomustine. Educate patients that only 1 dose of lomustine is to be taken no more frequently than every 6 weeks and only after documentation of adequate hematologic recovery. (ISMP, 2014. https://www.ismp.org/resources/oral-chemotherapy-we-simply-must-do-better. Accessed June 20, 2018)

Supportive Care
Antiemetic prophylaxis
Emetogenic potential on day 1 is **MODERATE–HIGH**
Emetogenic potential on days 15 and 29 is **MINIMAL**
See Chapter 42 for antiemetic recommendations

Hematopoietic growth factor (CSF) prophylaxis
Primary prophylaxis is **NOT** *indicated*
See Chapter 43 for more information

Antimicrobial prophylaxis
Risk of fever and neutropenia is **LOW**
  Antimicrobial primary prophylaxis to be considered:
  - Antibacterial—not indicated
  - Antifungal—not indicated
  - Antiviral—not indicated unless patient previously had an episode of HSV

Patient Population Studied

A multicenter, randomized, phase 3 trial (European Organisation for Research and Treatment of Cancer [EORTC] 26101) involved 437 patients with progressive glioblastoma after standard chemoradiation. Patients were randomly assigned in a 2:1 ratio to lomustine plus bevacizumab or lomustine alone. Patients in the combination therapy group received lomustine (90 mg/m^2 with maximal dose of 160 mg, but increased to 110 mg/m^2 with maximal dose of 200 mg if no Grade >1 hematologic toxic effects were noted in the first cycle) every 6 weeks plus bevacizumab (10 mg/kg) every 2 weeks. Patients in the monotherapy group received lomustine (110 mg/m^2; maximal dose of 200 mg) every 6 weeks

Therapy Monitoring

1. *Prior to each dose of lomustine:* CBC with differential, platelet count, LFTs, BUN, creatinine, electrolytes
2. Baseline pulmonary function studies with frequent PFTs during treatment
3. *Prior to each dose of bevacizumab:* vital signs, urine dipstick for protein (perform 24-hour urine collection if ≥2+ protein)
4. *Weekly:* CBC with differential, platelet count (monitor blood counts weekly for 6 weeks after a dose). Thrombocytopenia occurs at about 4 weeks postadministration and persists for 1–2 weeks. Leukopenia occurs at 5–6 weeks after a dose and persists for 1–2 weeks
5. *Response assessment:* contrast-enhanced MRI of the brain every 6 weeks for 6 months, then every 12 weeks thereafter

Efficacy (N = 437)

	Lomustine plus Bevacizumab (N = 288)	Lomustine Alone (N = 149)	
Median overall survival	9.1 months	8.6 months	HR 0.95, 95% CI 0.74–1.21; P = 0.65
Median progression-free survival	4.2 months	1.5 months	HR 0.49, 95% CI 0.39–0.61; P <0.001
Objective response rate	41.5%	13.9%	

Treatment Modification

BEVACIZUMAB DOSE MODIFICATIONS

Adverse Event	Treatment Modification
Gastrointestinal perforations (gastrointestinal perforations, fistula formation in the gastrointestinal tract, intra-abdominal abscess), fistula formation involving an internal organ	Discontinue bevacizumab permanently
Serious bleeding	
Wound dehiscence requiring medical intervention	
Nephrotic syndrome	
Hypertensive crisis or hypertensive encephalopathy or reversible posterior leukoencephalopathy syndrome (RPLS)	
Congestive heart failure	
Necrotizing fasciitis	
Severe arterial or venous thromboembolic events	Discontinue bevacizumab permanently; the safety of reinitiating bevacizumab after a thromboembolic event is resolved is not known
Moderate to severe proteinuria	Patients with a ≥2+ urine dipstick reading should undergo further assessment, eg, a 24-hour urine collection. Suspend bevacizumab administration for ≥2 g of proteinuria/24 h and resume when proteinuria is <2 g/24 h
Severe hypertension not controlled with medical management	Hold bevacizumab pending further evaluation and treatment of hypertension
Mild, clinically insignificant infusion reaction	Decrease the rate of infusion
Clinically significant but not severe infusion reaction	Interrupt the infusion in patients with clinically significant infusion reactions and consider resuming at a slower rate following resolution. If decision is made to restart, the infusion may be continued at ≤50% of the rate prior to the reaction and increased in 50% increments every 30 minutes if well tolerated. Infusions may be restarted at the full rate during the next cycle
Severe infusion reaction—hypertension, hypertensive crises associated with neurologic signs and symptoms, wheezing, oxygen desaturation, G3 hypersensitivity, chest pain, headaches, rigors, and diaphoresis	Stop infusion and administer appropriate medical therapy (eg, epinephrine, corticosteroids, intravenous antihistamines, bronchodilators, and/or oxygen). Discontinue bevacizumab
Planned elective surgery	Suspended bevacizumab at least 28 days before elective surgery and do not resume for at least 28 days after surgery or until surgical incision is fully healed
Recent hemoptysis	Do not administer bevacizumab
Evidence of rectosigmoid involvement by pelvic examination or bowel involvement on CT scan or clinical symptoms of bowel obstruction	

LOMUSTINE DOSE MODIFICATIONS

Lomustine dose levels	
Dose level +1	110 mg/m² as a single dose; maximum 200 mg
Starting dose	90 mg/m² as a single dose; maximum 160 mg
Dose level −1	75 mg/m² as a single dose; maximum 130 mg
No G >1 neutropenia and no G >1 thrombocytopenia during cycle 1	Increase lomustine to dose level +1 beginning with cycle 2
Day 1 WBC <4000/mm³ or platelets <100,000/mm³	Delay therapy until WBC ≥4000/mm³ and platelets ≥100,000/mm³

(continued)

Treatment Modification (*continued*)

LOMUSTINE DOSE MODIFICATIONS

Lomustine dose levels

WBC nadir during the prior cycle <2000/mm³, or ANC nadir during the prior cycle <1000/mm³, or platelet nadir during the prior cycle <50,000/mm³	Delay therapy until WBC ≥4000/mm³ and platelets ≥100,000/mm³ if necessary, then reduce lomustine to dose level −1 in subsequent cycle(s)
G ≥3 liver toxicity (AST/ALT >5× ULN) and/or G ≥2 bilirubin (>1.5–3× ULN)	Delay therapy until resolution to G ≤1 (AST/ALT ≤3× ULN; bilirubin ≤1.5× ULN), then reduce lomustine 1 dose level in subsequent cycle(s)
Any G4 nonhematologic toxicity	Discontinue lomustine
G ≥2 nonhematologic toxicity that does not recover to G ≤1 within 2 weeks	
Any G ≥2 nonhematologic toxicity that recurs at the next cycle to G ≥2	
Any pulmonary symptoms, but with PFT showing DLco ≥ predicted value	Continue with same lomustine dose
Any pulmonary symptoms, but with PFT showing <60% of predicted value	Discontinue lomustine
Decreased oxygen saturation at rest (eg, pulse oximeter <88% or Pao₂ ≤55 mm Hg)	
Shortness of breath at rest or shortness of breath that limits self-care or ADL	
Severe cough limiting self-care or ADL	
Cumulative lomustine dosage >1100 mg/m²	Discontinue lomustine due to concerns of developing pulmonary fibrosis
Creatinine clearance 10–50 mL/min	Reduce lomustine dose by 25%
Creatinine clearance <10 mL/min	Reduce lomustine dose by 50–75%

Notes:
- Usually no more than a total of 6–7 cycles (660–770 mg/m²) of lomustine is recommended. Patients receiving >1100 mg/m² cumulative lomustine dosage have a higher risk of developing pulmonary toxicity. Patients with a baseline FVC or DLco <70% are particularly at risk (GLEOSTINE [lomustine] capsules; June 2018 product label. NextSource Biotechnology, LLC, Miami, FL)
- Patients who are pregnant or who become pregnant should be apprised of the potential hazard to the fetus from therapy with lomustine

Adverse Events (N = 430)

Grade 3–5* adverse events were recorded in 63.6% of patients assigned to lomustine plus bevacizumab and in 38.1% of patients assigned to lomustine alone. Grade 3–5 adverse events of special interest were pulmonary embolism (in 5% of the combination therapy group), arterial hypertension (in 24% of the combination therapy group and in <1% of the monotherapy group), and hematologic toxic effects (in 54% of the combination therapy group and in 50% of the monotherapy group). Deaths unrelated to the tumor were noted for 5 patients (2%) assigned to combination therapy (2 from myocardial infarctions, 1 from large-intestine perforation, 1 from sepsis, and 1 from intracranial hemorrhage) and 1 patient (<1%) assigned to monotherapy (as a result of lung infection). Treatment-related adverse events occurred in 85.2% and 53.1% of patients assigned to combination therapy and monotherapy, respectively, and treatment-related serious adverse events occurred in 38.5% and 9.5% of patients, respectively

*According to the National Cancer Institute Common Terminology Criteria for Adverse Events, version 4.0

PRIMARY CNS LYMPHOMA, NEWLY DIAGNOSED

CNS CANCER REGIMEN: HIGH-DOSE METHOTREXATE

Batchelor T et al. J Clin Oncol 2003;21:1044–1049

Induction phase:
Methotrexate every 14 days until complete response (CR) or a maximum of 8 cycles are delivered

Consolidation phase:
For patients achieving a CR during induction, give 2 cycles of methotrexate every 14 days, then give:

Maintenance phase:
Eleven cycles of methotrexate every 28 days

Hydration before, during, and after methotrexate:
Before methotrexate administration:
5% dextrose injection (D5W) or 5% dextrose/0.45% sodium chloride injection (D5W/0.45% NS) with 50–100 mEq sodium bicarbonate injection/L; administer intravenously at 100–150 mL/hour

- Adjust infusion rate to achieve and maintain a urine output ≥100 mL/hour for ≥4 hours before starting methotrexate
- Adjust sodium bicarbonate to produce a urine pH within the range ≥7.0 to ≤8.0 before starting methotrexate

During methotrexate administration:
No additional hydration (see below)

After methotrexate administration:
D5W or D5W/0.45% NS with 50–100 mEq sodium bicarbonate injection/L; administer intravenously at 100–150 mL/hour until serum methotrexate concentration <0.1 μmol/L

- Adjust infusion rate to maintain urine output ≥100 mL/hour
- Adjust sodium bicarbonate to maintain urine pH ≥7.0 to ≤8.0

Methotrexate 8000 mg/m^2 in 500–1000 mL D5W with 50–100 mEq sodium bicarbonate per dose; administer intravenously over 4 hours (total dosage every 14 days [induction and consolidation cycles] and every 28 days [maintenance cycles] = 8000 mg/m^2)
(Add sodium bicarbonate in amounts sufficient to produce a bicarbonate concentration equivalent to fluid used for the same volume of hydration fluid given over a 4-hour period)

Leucovorin calcium 25 mg per dose; administer intravenously every 6 hours for 4 doses, starting 24 hours after methotrexate administration began

Six hours after the last dose of intravenously administered leucovorin, start oral leucovorin or continue with intravenous leucovorin calcium every 6 hours if patient is nauseated or vomiting, otherwise:

Leucovorin calcium 25 mg per dose; administer orally or intravenously every 6 hours until serum methotrexate concentration <0.1 μmol/L

Supportive Care
Antiemetic prophylaxis
Emetogenic potential is **MODERATE**
See Chapter 42 for antiemetic recommendations

Hematopoietic growth factor (CSF) prophylaxis
Primary prophylaxis is **NOT** *indicated*
See Chapter 43 for more information

Antimicrobial prophylaxis
Risk of fever and neutropenia is **LOW**
  Antimicrobial primary prophylaxis to be considered:
  - Antibacterial—not indicated
  - Antifungal—not indicated
  - Antiviral—not indicated, unless patient previously had an episode of HSV

Patient Population Studied

A multicenter phase 2 trial of 25 patients with newly diagnosed non-AIDS-related primary CNS lymphoma (PCNSL). Previous radiation therapy was not allowed

Efficacy (N = 24)

Complete response*	50%
Partial response	21%
Stable disease	4.2%
Median progression-free survival	12.8 months
Median overall survival	>22.8 months

*Median number of cycles to CR = 6

Treatment Modifications

Methotrexate dosage is based on a measured creatinine clearance before treatment commences. For any creatinine clearance <100 mL/min, methotrexate dosage is calculated by multiplying the planned dosage (8000 mg/m^2) by the ratio between the measured creatinine clearance (CrCl) and 100

Example:
For a measured CrCl = 75 mL/min:

$$\frac{75}{100} = 0.75 \ (ie, 75\%)$$

Thus, the adjusted methotrexate dosage is:

8000 mg/m^2 × 0.75 = 6000 mg/m^2

Toxicity

(N = 25 Patients; N = 287 Cycles)

Toxicity	% Patients
G ≥3/4 toxicity	48
No G3/4 toxicity	52
Leukoencephalopathy	—

Batchelor T et al. J Clin Oncol 2003;21:1044–1049

(N = 31 Patients; N = 375 Cycles)*

Toxicity	% Cycles
Leukopenia (<2000 WBC/mm³)	1
Nonoliguric acute renal failure	1
G3 mucositis	2
Leukoencephalopathy	—
Acute cerebral dysfunction	—
Delayed methotrexate clearance†	13

Guha-Thakurta N et al. J Neurooncol 1999;43:259–268

*Treatment:
1. Methotrexate 8000 mg/m² for ≥3 induction cycles
2. Methotrexate 3500–8000 mg/m²/cycle until CR
3. Methotrexate 3500 mg/m²/month for 3 months
4. Methotrexate 3500 mg/m²/3 months indefinitely
Median: 10 cycles/patient (range: 3–30 cycles)

†Risk factors for delayed methotrexate clearance:
1. Cycle intervals <10 days
2. Concurrent SIADH or diabetes insipidus
3. Acute renal failure
4. "Third-space" fluid compartments (eg, effusions)

Therapy Monitoring

Before each treatment cycle:
1. CBC with differential
2. Serum electrolytes
3. LFTs
4. 24-hour urine collection for creatinine clearance

During hospitalization:
1. Check urine output and pH frequently
2. Daily CBC with differential and serum electrolytes
3. Monitor daily methotrexate levels starting the day after methotrexate administration begins and continue until serum methotrexate concentrations are <0.1 μmol/L. In patients with renal impairment or pleural effusion, continue leucovorin and check serum methotrexate concentrations daily until methotrexate is undetectable

Notes

1. The regimen is for the treatment of primary central nervous system lymphoma for which radiation therapy has been deferred
2. In patients with renal impairment or an effusion, consider empirically continuing leucovorin calcium administration until serum methotrexate concentrations become undetectable

PRIMARY CNS LYMPHOMA, NEWLY DIAGNOSED

CNS CANCER REGIMEN: HIGH-DOSE METHOTREXATE AND RITUXIMAB WITH DEFERRED RADIOTHERAPY

Chamberlain MC, Johnson SK. Neuro Oncol 2010;12:736–744

INDUCTION (≥4 BI-WEEKLY CYCLES)
Methotrexate; administer intravenously over 6 hours on day 1, every 2 weeks

Methotrexate Dosage

Estimated or measured creatinine clearance	≥60 mL/minute (≥1 mL/s)	<60 mL/minute (<1 mL/s)
Methotrexate	8000 mg/m² (total dosage/2-week cycle = 8000 mg/m²)	4000 mg/m² (total dosage/2-week cycle = 4000 mg/m²)

Note: for logistical practicality and efficiency, parenteral admixtures containing methotrexate may include a portion or all of the fluid and sodium bicarbonate needed to meet hydration and urinary alkalinization requirements during methotrexate administration

Hydration before, during, and after methotrexate:
Administer intravenously 1500–3000 mL/m² per day. Administer a solution containing a total amount of sodium not greater than 0.9% sodium chloride injection (ie, 154 mEq/1000 mL) by intravenous infusion during methotrexate administration and for at least 24 hours afterward
• Commence fluid administration 2–12 hours before starting methotrexate, depending upon a patient's fluid status
• Urine output should be at least 100 mL/hour before starting methotrexate infusion
• Urine pH should be ≥7.0 but ≤8.0 before, during, and after methotrexate administration
• Maintain hydration at a rate that maintains urine output of at least 100 mL/hours until the serum methotrexate concentration is <0.1 μmol/L
• Adverse effects attributable to methotrexate are related to systemic methotrexate concentrations *and* the duration for which concentrations are maintained

Sodium bicarbonate 50–150 mEq/1000 mL is added to parenteral hydration solutions to maintain urine pH ≥7.0 to ≤8.0

Base Solution Sodium Content	Sodium Bicarbonate Additive	Total Sodium Content
0.45% Sodium chloride injection (0.45% NS)		
77 mEq/L	50–75 mEq	125–152 mEq/L
0.2% Sodium chloride injection (0.2% NS)		
34 mEq/L	100–125 mEq	134–159 mEq/L
5% Dextrose injection (D5W)		
0	125–150 mEq	125–150 mEq/L
D5W/0.45% NS		
77 mEq/L	50–75 mEq	125–152 mEq/L
D5W/0.2% NS		
34 mEq/L	100–125 mEq	134–159 mEq/L

Leucovorin calcium 10 mg/m²; administer intravenously in 25–250 mL 0.9% NS or D5W over 15–30 minutes every 6 hours starting 24 hours after methotrexate administration begins, and continue until serum methotrexate concentrations are ≤0.1 μmol/L, every 2 weeks for a minimum of 4 cycles. When serum methotrexate concentrations are ≤0.1 μmol/L, discontinue intravenous hydration and leucovorin, *then:*
• Give **leucovorin** calcium 25 mg; administer orally every 6 hours for 2 days (8 doses), *and*
• Continue hydration orally with >1500 mL/m² (>50 fluid ounces/m²) for 3 days after intravenous hydration is discontinued

Rituximab 375 mg/m²; administer intravenously in 0.9% NS or D5W diluted to a concentration within the range 1–4 mg/mL between days 7 and 10 every 2 weeks for a minimum of 4 cycles; ie, within a 2-week cycle, during the week when methotrexate is not given (total dosage/2-week cycle = 375 mg/m²)

Notes on rituximab administration:
• Administer initially at a rate of 50 mg/hour. If hypersensitivity or infusion reactions do not occur during the first 30 minutes, increase the rate by 50 mg/hour every 30 minutes as tolerated to a maximum rate of 400 mg/hour
• During subsequent treatments, if previous rituximab administration was well tolerated, start at 100 mg/hour and increase the rate by 100 mg/hour every 30 minutes as tolerated to a maximum rate of 400 mg/hour
• Interrupt rituximab administration for fever, chills, edema, congestion of the head and neck mucosa, hypertension, and other serious adverse events. Resume rituximab administration after adverse events abate

(continued)

(*continued*)

MAINTENANCE (4-WEEK CYCLES)
Methotrexate; administer intravenously over 6 hours on day 1, every 4 weeks

Methotrexate Dosage

Estimated or measured creatinine clearance	≥60 mL/minute (≥1 mL/s)	<60 mL/minute (<1 mL/s)
Methotrexate	8000 mg/m² (Total dosage/4-week cycle = 8000 mg/m²)	4000 mg/m² (Total dosage/4-week cycle = 4000 mg/m²)

Note: for logistical practicality and efficiency, parenteral admixtures containing methotrexate may include a portion or all of the fluid and sodium bicarbonate needed to meet hydration and urinary alkalinization requirements during methotrexate administration

Hydration before, during, and after methotrexate:
Administer intravenously 1500–3000 mL/m² per day. Administer a solution containing a total amount of sodium not greater than 0.9% sodium chloride injection (ie, 154 mEq/1000 mL) by intravenous infusion during methotrexate administration and for at least 24 hours afterward
- Commence fluid administration 2–12 hours before starting methotrexate, depending upon a patient's fluid status
- Urine output should be at least 100 mL/hour before starting methotrexate infusion
- Urine pH should be ≥7.0 but ≤8.0 before, during, and after methotrexate administration
- Maintain hydration at a rate that maintains urine output of at least 100 mL/hour until the serum methotrexate concentration is <0.1 µmol/L
- Adverse effects attributable to methotrexate are related to systemic methotrexate concentrations *and* the duration for which concentrations are maintained

Sodium bicarbonate 50–150 mEq/1000 mL is added to parenteral hydration solutions to maintain urine pH ≥7.0 to ≤8.0

Base Solution Sodium Content	Sodium Bicarbonate Additive	Total Sodium Content
0.45% Sodium Chloride Injection (0.45% NS)		
77 mEq/L	50–75 mEq	125–152 mEq/L
0.2% Sodium Chloride Injection (0.2% NS)		
34 mEq/L	100–125 mEq	134–159 mEq/L
5% Dextrose Injection (D5W)		
0	125–150 mEq	125–150 mEq/L
D5W/0.45% NS		
77 mEq/L	50–75 mEq	125–152 mEq/L
D5W/0.2% NS		
34 mEq/L	100–125 mEq	134–159 mEq/L

Leucovorin calcium 10 mg/m²; administer intravenously in 25–250 mL 0.9% NS or D5W over 15–30 minutes every 6 hours starting 24 hours after methotrexate administration begins, and continue until serum methotrexate concentrations are ≤0.1 µmol/L, every 4 weeks
- When serum methotrexate concentrations are ≤0.1 µmol/L, discontinue intravenous hydration and leucovorin, *then:*
- Give **leucovorin calcium** 25 mg; administer orally every 6 hours for 2 days (8 doses), *and*
- Continue hydration orally with >1500 mL/m² (>50 fluid ounces/m²) for 3 days after intravenous hydration is discontinued

Leucovorin Rescue Guidelines

Clinical Situation	Serum Methotrexate Concentration*	Leucovorin Dosage, Schedule, and Duration
Normal methotrexate elimination	• ≤10 µmol/L at 24 hours, *or* • ≤1 µmol/L at 48 hours, *or* • ≤0.2 µmol/L at 72 hours	• Give leucovorin calcium 10 mg/m² intravenously every 6 hours until serum methotrexate concentrations are <0.1 µmol/L (<1 × 10⁻⁷ mol/L, or <100 nmol/L), then give leucovorin calcium 25 mg orally every 6 hours for 8 doses
Delayed/late methotrexate elimination	• ≥10 µmol/L at 24 hours, *or* • ≥1 µmol/L at 48 hours, *or* • ≥0.1 µmol/L at 72 hours, *or* • ≥0.05 µmol/L at 96 hours, *or* • ≥100% increase in serum creatinine concentration at 24 hours after methotrexate administration	• Give leucovorin calcium 100 mg/m² intravenously every 3 hours • When serum methotrexate concentration results are <0.1 µmol/L the leucovorin dosage may be decreased to 10 mg/m² intravenously given every 3 hours until the serum methotrexate concentration is <0.05 µmol/L or undetectable

*After methotrexate administration is begun
Methotrexate concentration conversions: 1 µmol/L = 10^{-6} mol/L = 1000 nmol/L

Patient Population Studied

Patient Characteristic
N = 40
Forty patients (25 men; 15 women), aged 18–93 years (median: 61.5 years), with newly diagnosed B-cell primary central nervous system lymphoma (PCNSL). Histopathology was determined by stereotactic biopsy in 29 patients, resective surgery in 9 patients, cerebrospinal fluid (CSF) flow cytometry in 1, and vitrectomy in 1 patient

Variables	Number of Patients (Percentage)
Age, Median (range)	61.5 y (18–93 y)
≥50 y/≥70 y	33 (82.5)/17(42.5)
Sex, Male/Female	25 (62.5)/15 (37.5)
Location of tumor	
Frontal	18 (45)
Temporal	3 (7.5)
Parietal	9 (22.5)
Corpus callosum	9 (22.5)
Deep gray nuclei	5 (12.5)
Occipital	2 (5)
Cerebellum	3 (7.5)
Brainstem	1 (2.5)
Subarachnoid/ ventricular	2 (5)
Multilobar	12 (30)
Extent of initial surgery	
Subtotal resection	9 (22.5)
Biopsy	29 (72.5)
Vitrectomy	1 (2.5)
Response to up-front chemotherapy	
Complete response	24 (60)
Partial response	8 (20)
Progressive disease	8 (20)
Progression-free survival to up-front chemotherapy	
Median (range)	21 mo (2–78 mo)

(*continued*)

Efficacy (N = 40)

Following induction with 4–6 cycles of methotrexate/rituximab (N = 40)	
Complete radiographic response	24 (60%)
Partial radiographic response	8 (20%)*
Progressive disease	8 (20%)
Following maintenance methotrexate (N = 40)	
Progression during maintenance	4 (10%)
At conclusion of induction and maintenance methotrexate (N = 28)[†]	
Complete radiographic response	27/28
Partial radiographic response	1/28
Median OS	33.5 months (11–80 months)
Median PFS	21.0 months (95% CI, 13.8–28.2)
Entire cohort (N = 40)	
Median overall survival, entire cohort	29.0 months (95% CI, 19.7–38.3)
Probability of disease-free survival, <50 years	86% (6/7)
Probability of disease-free survival, 50–59 years	33% (4/12)
Probability of disease-free survival, 60–69 years	25% (1/4)
Probability of disease-free survival, >70 years	0 (0/17)

*Six of the 8 patients (75%) with a PR to induction methotrexate/rituximab converted to a complete response with maintenance methotrexate
[†]6–8 months of total therapy

Treatment Monitoring

1. CBC with differential every week
2. Serum creatinine and liver function tests at the beginning of each cycle
3. Serum creatinine levels and serum methotrexate concentrations at 24 hours, 48 hours, and 72 hours after administration of methotrexate began, continuing at least until a serum methotrexate concentration ≤0.1 µmol/L is achieved

Treatment Modifications

Adverse Event	Treatment Modification
G ≥3 hematologic toxicity on day 1 of a cycle or G >1 nonhematologic toxicity on day 1 of a cycle	Withhold treatment until all hematologic toxicity has resolved to G ≤2 and all nonhematologic toxicity has resolved to G ≤1
G ≥4 toxicity ascribed to methotrexate	Reduce the methotrexate dosage by 50%
G ≥3 toxicity ascribed to methotrexate after the dosage has been reduced by 50%	Discontinue methotrexate

Patient Population Studied
(continued)

Variables	Number of Patients (Percentage)
Salvage therapy at recurrence	
Temozolomide	9 (22.5)
Procarbazine, Lomustine (CCNU), Vincristine	5 (12.5)
Methotrexate	1 (2.5)
Whole brain irradiation	8 (20)
Response to salvage therapy	
Complete response	2 (9)
Partial response	12 (67)
Progressive disease	4 (22)
Progression-free survival to salvage therapy	
Median (range)	6 mo (1 – 38+ mo)
Overall survival	
Median (range)	29 mo (6 – 80+ mo)
Alive and disease free	20 (50)
≤50 y of age	7/9 (78)
>50 y of age	8/31 (26)
>60 y of age	0/20 (0)

Toxicity

Toxicity	G2	G3	G4	G5	Total
Anemia	1	2	0	0	3
Fatigue	6	1	0	0	7
Hepatic	2	1	0	0	3
Hyperglycemia	6	2	0	0	8
Neutropenia without fever	1	4	0	0	5
Nausea	2	0	0	0	2
Renal	13	4	2	0	19
Thrombophlebitis	0	2	0	0	2
Totals	31	16	2	0	49

PRIMARY CNS LYMPHOMA, NEWLY DIAGNOSED

CNS CANCER REGIMEN: INDUCTION RITUXIMAB, METHOTREXATE, AND TEMOZOLIMIDE, FOLLOWED BY WHOLE-BRAIN RADIOTHERAPY AND POSTIRRADIATION TEMOZOLOMIDE

Glass J et al. J Clin Oncol 2016;34:1620–1625

Regimen overview: the regimen consists of a single dose of intravenous rituximab 375 mg/m² followed 3 days later by initiation of high-dose methotrexate 3.5 g/m² given every 2 weeks for 5 doses (during weeks 1, 3, 5, 7, and 9) and two 5-day courses of temozolomide 100 mg/m²/day (during weeks 4 and 8). Twice-daily whole-brain radiation therapy is given for a total of 30 fractions (during weeks 11, 12, and 13), followed lastly by ten 5-day courses of single-agent temozolomide maintenance, initiated at 150 mg/m²/day with the first course and then escalated to 200 mg/m²/day for remaining courses, repeated every 4 weeks (during weeks 14, 18, 22, 26, 30, 34, 38, 42, 46, and 50)

Premedications for rituximab:
Acetaminophen 650–1000 mg; administer orally 30–60 minutes before starting rituximab, *plus*
Diphenhydramine 25–50 mg; administer orally or intravenously 30–60 minutes before starting rituximab

Rituximab 375 mg/m²; administer intravenously in 0.9% sodium chloride (0.9% NS) or 5% dextrose injection (D5W) diluted to a concentration within the range 1–4 mg/mL once, 3 days prior to the first (week 1) dose of methotrexate (total dosage = 375 mg/m²)

Notes on rituximab administration:
- Administer initially at a rate of 50 mg/h. If hypersensitivity or infusion reactions do not occur during the first 30 minutes, increase the rate by 50 mg/h every 30 minutes as tolerated to a maximum rate of 400 mg/h
- Interrupt rituximab administration for fever, chills, edema, congestion of the head and neck mucosa, hypertension, and other serious adverse events. Resume rituximab administration after adverse events abate

Hydration before, during, and after each methotrexate administration:
Before each methotrexate administration:
5% D5W or 5% dextrose/0.45% sodium chloride injection (D5W/0.45% NS) with 50–100 mEq sodium bicarbonate injection/L; administer intravenously at 100–150 mL/h
- Adjust infusion rate to achieve and maintain a urine output ≥100 mL/h for ≥4 hours before starting methotrexate
- Adjust sodium bicarbonate content to produce a urine pH within the range ≥7.0 to ≤8.0 before starting methotrexate

During each methotrexate administration:
No additional hydration (see below)

Immediately after each methotrexate administration:
D5W or D5W/0.45% NS with 50–100 mEq sodium bicarbonate injection/L; administer intravenously at 100–150 mL/h until serum methotrexate concentration <0.1 μmol/L
- Adjust infusion rate to maintain urine output ≥100 mL/h
- Adjust sodium bicarbonate content to maintain urine pH ≥7.0 to ≤8.0

Methotrexate 3500 mg/m² in 500 mL D5W or 0.45% NS injection, with 50–100 mEq sodium bicarbonate per dose; administer intravenously over 4 hours, every 14 days for 5 doses during weeks 1, 3, 5, 7, and 9 (total dosage every 14 days = 3500 mg/m²)
Notes:
- Add sodium bicarbonate in amounts sufficient to produce a bicarbonate concentration equivalent to fluid used for the same volume of hydration fluid given over a 4-hour period
- No methotrexate dose reduction is necessary for patients with a creatinine clearance ≥50 mL/min
- Methotrexate should not be administered if creatinine clearance is <50 mL/min
- Avoid nonsteroidal anti-inflammatory drugs (NSAIDs), salicylates, sulfonamides, penicillins, probenecid, and proton pump inhibitors during methotrexate therapy
- Preservative-free formulations of methotrexate injection should be used for high-dose therapy

Leucovorin calcium 25 mg per dose; administer orally or intravenously in 25–250 mL 0.9% NS or D5W over 15–30 minutes every 6 hours, starting 24 hours after each methotrexate administration began, and continue until serum methotrexate concentration <0.1 μmol/L, repeated every 14 days for 5 courses during weeks 1, 3, 5, 7, and 9

When serum methotrexate concentrations are ≤0.1 μmol/L, discontinue intravenous hydration and intravenous leucovorin, *then:*
- Give **leucovorin calcium** 25 mg; administer orally every 6 hours for 2 days (8 doses), *and*
- Continue hydration orally with >1500 mL/m² (>50 fluid ounces/m²) for 3 days after intravenous hydration is discontinued

(continued)

(*continued*)

Leucovorin Rescue Guidelines

Clinical Situation	Serum Methotrexate Concentration*	Leucovorin Dosage, Schedule, and Duration
Normal methotrexate elimination	• ≤10 µmol/L at 24 hours, *or* • ≤1 µmol/L at 48 hours, *or* • ≤0.1 µmol/L at 72 hours	• Give leucovorin calcium 25 mg intravenously every 6 hours until serum methotrexate concentrations are <0.1 µmol/L (<1 × 10^{-7} mol/L, or <100 nmol/L), then give leucovorin calcium 25 mg orally every 6 hours for 2 days (8 doses)
Delayed/late methotrexate elimination	• ≥10 µmol/L at 24 hours, *or* • ≥1 µmol/L at 48 hours, *or* • ≥0.1 µmol/L at 72 hours, *or* • ≥0.05 µmol/L at 96 hours, *or* • ≥100% increase in serum creatinine concentration at 24 hours after methotrexate administration	• Give leucovorin calcium 100 mg/m^2 intravenously every 3 hours • When serum methotrexate concentration results are <0.1 µmol/L, the leucovorin dosage may be decreased to 10 mg/m^2 intravenously given every 3 hours until the serum methotrexate concentration is <0.05 µmol/L or undetectable • *Consider* administration of glucarpidase (if methotrexate concentration is >1 µmol/L in the setting of acute kidney injury)

*After methotrexate administration is begun
Methotrexate concentration conversions: 1 µmol/L = 10^{-6} mol/L = 1000 nmol/L

Temozolomide 100 mg/m^2/day; administer orally once daily for 5 consecutive days, on an empty stomach with water at bedtime, every 4 weeks for 2 cycles during weeks 4 and 8 (total dosage/4-week course = 500 mg/m^2)
• *Note:* patients who vomit after taking temozolomide should be instructed to take their next dose at the next regularly scheduled time

Whole-brain radiation therapy twice daily at 1.2 Gy/fraction for 5 days/week for a total of 30 fractions during weeks 11, 12, and 13 (total dosage = 36 Gy)

Temozolomide; administer orally once daily for 5 consecutive days, on an empty stomach with water at bedtime, every 4 weeks, for 10 cycles during weeks 14, 18, 22, 26, 30, 34, 38, 42, 46, and 50, *as follows:*
• *Week 14*: administer 150 mg/m^2/day (total dosage/4-week course during week 14 = 750 mg/m^2)
• *Weeks 18, 22, 26, 30, 34, 38, 42, 46, and 50*: administer 200 mg/m^2/day (total dosage/4-week course = 1000 mg/m^2)
• *Note:* patients who vomit after taking temozolomide should be instructed to take their next dose at the next regularly scheduled time

Supportive Care
Antiemetic prophylaxis
Emetogenic potential on days with methotrexate or temozolomide is **MODERATE**
Emetogenic potential on day with rituximab is **MINIMIAL**
See Chapter 42 for antiemetic recommendations

Hematopoietic growth factor (CSF) prophylaxis
Primary prophylaxis is **NOT** *indicated*
See Chapter 43 for more information

Antimicrobial prophylaxis
Risk of fever and neutropenia is **LOW**
  Antimicrobial primary prophylaxis to be considered:
• Antibacterial—not indicated; *Pneumocystis jirovecii* prophylaxis is recommended (eg, cotrimoxazole)
• Antifungal—not indicated
• Antiviral— antiherpes antivirals (eg, acyclovir, famciclovir, valacyclovir)

Patient Population Studied

This phase 1/2 trial (Radiation Therapy Oncology Group [RTOG] 0227) involved 53 patients with newly diagnosed primary central nervous system lymphoma (PCNSL). Of the enrolled patients, 12 took part in both the phase 1 and phase 2 portions of the trial and the remainder were enrolled in only the phase 2 portion

Efficacy (N = 53)

2-year overall survival	80.8%
Estimated median overall survival	7.5 years
2-year progression-free survival	63.6%
Estimated median progression-free survival	5.4 years

Note: of the 53 patients initially treated, 45 completed the initial chemotherapy and 42 received the whole-brain radiotherapy. After completion of the initial chemotherapy, 35 patients were assessable for radiographic response. Median follow-up time for eligible living patients was 3.6 years

Therapy Monitoring

1. *Prior to rituximab administration:* Hepatitis B surface antigen, hepatitis B core antibody (total antibody, or IgG only)
2. *Prior to the first dose of methotrexate:* 24-hour urine collection for creatinine clearance, serum creatinine
3. *Prior to each dose of methotrexate:* CBC with differential, platelet count, BUN, serum creatinine, estimated creatinine clearance (Cockroft-Gault method), AST, ALT, total bilirubin, electrolytes, serum bicarbonate, urine output, urine pH, review medication list for potential drug-drug interactions
4. *Following each dose of methotrexate, until methotrexate concentration is <0.1 μmol/L:*

    Daily: methotrexate concentration (draw first sample 24 hours after start of methotrexate infusion and repeat every 24 hours), CBC with differential, platelet count, BUN, serum creatinine, AST, ALT, total bilirubin, weight, fluid balance

    At least every 8 hours during methotrexate administration: urine pH
5. *Prior to each course of temozolomide:* CBC with differential, platelet count, AST, ALT, total bilirubin, urine hCG (women of childbearing potential only)
6. During first cycle and in any cycle after a dose adjustment, weekly CBC with differential and platelet count to assess dose
7. *Response assessment:* at the completion of initial rituximab, methotrexate, temozolomide chemotherapy, after completion of radiation therapy, every 2 months during postradiation temozolomide, at completion of temozolomide, every 3 months from the end of treatment until 2 years since the start of treatment, every 6 months for 3 to 5 years

Treatment Modifications

PRERADIATION [Methotrexate, Rituximab, and Temozolomide]

Methotrexate, Rituximab, and Temozolomide—Hematologic Toxicity

ANC <1000/mm³ or platelet count <70,000/mm³ on weeks 4/8 at start of temozolomide but persisting for <2 weeks	Withhold temozolomide until ANC ≥1000/mm³ and platelet count ≥70,000/mm³. Chemotherapy can then be administered at full dose
ANC <1000/mm³ or platelet count <70,000/mm³ on weeks 4/8 at start of temozolomide but persisting for ≥2 weeks	Withhold treatment until ANC ≥1000/mm³ and platelet count >70,000/mm³. Temozolomide can then be administered but at 25% reduced dose. The dose of methotrexate is not reduced for hematologic toxicity
Recurrence of ANC <1000/mm³ or platelet count <70,000/mm³ on weeks 4/8 at start of temozolomide persisting for ≥2 weeks despite a previous dose reduction	Discontinue temozolomide
ANC <1000/mm³ or platelet count <70,000/mm³ at time of methotrexate administration on weeks 1, 3, 5, 7 and 9	Delay administration of methotrexate until ANC ≥1000/mm³ and platelet count >70,000/mm³. The dose of methotrexate is not reduced for hematologic toxicity
ANC <1000/mm³ at any time during treatment	Administer filgrastim if deemed to be of value

Methotrexate, Rituximab, and Temozolomide—Nonhematologic Toxicity

Serum bilirubin >1.2 mg/dL at time of methotrexate administration on weeks 1, 3, 5, 7, and 9	Delay administration of methotrexate until recovery
ALT >450 U/L at time of methotrexate administration on weeks 1, 3, 5, 7, and 9	
Mucositis with as yet no evidence of healing at time of methotrexate administration on weeks 1, 3, 5, 7, and 9	
G ≥2 nephrotoxicity from methotrexate (serum creatinine >1.5× baseline value, or >1.5× laboratory ULN)	Obtain 24-hour urine collection for CrCl prior to the next dose of methotrexate. The CrCl must be >50 mL/min per 1.73 m² to receive additional methotrexate

(continued)

Treatment Modifications (*continued*)

Methotrexate, Rituximab, and Temozolomide—Rituximab Infusion-Related Toxicity

Onset of infusion-related events (fevers, chills, rigors, edema, congestion of the head and neck mucosa, hypotension) during rituximab infusion	1. Interrupt rituximab infusion 2. For fever, chills: Give additional dose of acetaminophen 650 mg orally and diphenhydramine 25–50 mg by intravenous push 3. For rigors: Give meperidine 12.5–25 mg by intravenous push ± promethazine 12.5–25 mg by intravenous infusion in at least 10 mL 0.9% NS or D5W over 5–15 minutes. If after 15–20 minutes the response to a single dose is considered inadequate, the dose may be repeated 4. After symptoms resolve, resume rituximab infusion at a minimum of 50% reduction in the rate at which the event occurred. If no further infusion-related events, increase the rate by 50 mg/h every 30 minutes, as tolerated, up to a maximum rate of 400 mg/h
Dyspnea or wheezing, without allergic findings (urticaria, or tongue or laryngeal edema) during rituximab infusion	1. Interrupt rituximab infusion immediately 2. Give hydrocortisone 100 mg by intravenous push (or glucocorticoid equivalent) 3. Give an additional dose of diphenhydramine 25–50 mg by intravenous push and an H$_2$-antagonist (ranitidine 50 mg or famotidine 20 mg) by intravenous push 4. After symptoms resolve, resume rituximab infusion at a minimum of 50% reduction in the rate at which the event occurred. If no further infusion-related events, increase the rate by 50 mg/h every 30 minutes, as tolerated, up to a maximum rate of 400 mg/h

Note: medications and equipment for the treatment of hypersensitivity reactions should be available for immediate use in the event of a reaction during rituximab administration (eg, intravenous fluids, epinephrine, antihistamines, glucocorticoids, and oxygen)

POSTRADIATION CHEMOTHERAPY [Temozolomide daily for 5 days every 28 days on weeks 14– 50]

Temozolomide—Hematologic Toxicity

ANC <1000/mm^3 or platelet count <70,000/mm^3 on day of start of a course of temozolomide but persisting for <2 weeks	Withhold treatment until the ANC ≥1000/mm^3 and platelet count >70,000/mm^3. Temozolomide can then be administered at full dose
ANC <1000/mm^3 or platelet count <70,000/mm^3 on day of start of a course of temozolomide but persisting for ≥2 weeks	Withhold treatment until the ANC ≥1000/mm^3 and platelet count >70,000/mm^3. Temozolomide can then be administered but at 25% reduced dose
Recurrence of ANC <1000/mm^3 or platelet count <70,000/mm^3 on day of start of a course of temozolomide persisting for ≥2 weeks despite a previous dose reduction	Discontinue chemotherapy
ANC <1000/mm^3 at any time during treatment	Administer filgrastim if deemed to be of value

Temozolomide—Nonhematologic Toxicity

G1	Continue treatment and maintain dose in subsequent cycle
G2 (1st occurrence)	Interrupt until resolved to G ≤1; administer 100% of original dose in subsequent cycle
G2 (2nd occurrence)	Interrupt until resolved to G ≤1; administer 75–80% of original dose in subsequent cycle. *Note:* once the dose has been reduced, it should not be increased at a later time
G2 (3rd occurrence)	Interrupt until resolved to G ≤1; administer 50% of original dose in subsequent cycle. *Note:* once the dose has been reduced, it should not be increased at a later time
G2 (4th occurrence)	Discontinue treatment permanently
G3 (1st occurrence)	Interrupt until resolved to G ≤1; administer 75–80% of original dose in subsequent cycle. *Note:* once the dose has been reduced, it should not be increased at a later time
G3 (2nd occurrence)	Interrupt until resolved to G ≤1; administer 50% of original dose in subsequent cycle. *Note:* once the dose has been reduced, it should not be increased at a later time
G3 (3rd occurrence)	Discontinue treatment permanently
G4 (1st occurrence)	Discontinue permanently *or* if physician deems it to be in the patient's best interest to continue, interrupt until resolved to G ≤1, then resume therapy with doses ≤50% of that at the time G4 toxicity occurred. *Note:* once the dose has been reduced, it should not be increased at a later time

Adverse Events (N = 53)

Grade (%)*	Chemotherapy-Related Toxicities (Prior to Start of Whole-brain Radiotherapy; N = 53)		Toxicities Related to Chemotherapy and Acute Radiotherapy (After Start of Whole-brain Radiotherapy; N = 42)	
	Grade 3	Grade 4	Grade 3	Grade 4
Hematologic	17	4	2	12
Metabolic	11	0	2	0
Hepatic	11	0	0	0
Neurologic	9	0		
Constitutional	6	2	2	0
Gastrointestinal	2	2	5	0
Pain	4	2	0	0
Renal/genitourinary	6	0	0	0
Cardiovascular	4	0	2	0
Ocular	2	0	2	0
Auditory/hearing	0	0	2	0
Coagulation	0	0	2	0
Dermatologic	0	0	2	0
Febrile neutropenia	2	0	0	0
Musculoskeletal	0	0	0	0

*According to the National Cancer Institute Common Terminology Criteria for Adverse Events, version 2.0

Note: Grade 3 and 4 toxicities defined as being definitely, probably, or possibly related to phase 2 treatment are included. Hematologic toxicities that occurred during radiotherapy were attributed to prior chemotherapy

PRIMARY CNS LYMPHOMA, NEWLY DIAGNOSED

CNS CANCER REGIMEN: RITUXIMAB, METHOTREXATE, PROCARBAZINE, AND VINCRISTINE FOLLOWED BY CONSOLIDATION, REDUCED-DOSE WHOLE-BRAIN RADIOTHERAPY, AND CYTARABINE (R-MPV → RT + C)

Morris PG et al. J Clin Oncol 2013;31:3971–3979
Shah GD et al. J Clin Oncol 2007;25:4730–4735

Induction Chemotherapy: Five 14-Day Cycles

Premedication for rituximab:
Acetaminophen 650–1000 mg orally, *plus*
Diphenhydramine 25–50 mg orally or intravenously, 30–60 minutes before starting rituximab
Rituximab 500 mg/m^2; administer intravenously in 0.9% sodium chloride injection (0.9% NS) or 5% dextrose injection (D5W), USP, diluted to a concentration within the range 1–4 mg/mL on day 1, every 2 weeks, for 5–7 cycles (total dosage/cycle = 500 mg/m^2)

Notes on rituximab administration:
• Administer initially at a rate of 50 mg/h. If hypersensitivity or infusion reactions do not occur during the first 30 minutes, increase the rate by 50 mg/h every 30 minutes as tolerated to a maximum rate of 400 mg/h
• During subsequent treatments, if previous rituximab administration was well tolerated, start at 100 mg/hour and increase by 100 mg/hour every 30 minutes as tolerated to a maximum rate of 400 mg/hour
• Interrupt rituximab administration for fever, chills, edema, congestion of the head and neck mucosa, hypertension, and other serious adverse events. Resume rituximab administration after adverse events abate

Methotrexate 3500 mg/m^2; administer intravenously over 2 hours on day 2, every 2 weeks, for 5–7 cycles (total dosage/cycle *not* including intrathecal therapy = 3500 mg/m^2)
Note: for logistical practicality and efficiency, parenteral admixtures containing methotrexate may include a portion or all of the fluid and sodium bicarbonate needed to meet hydration and urinary alkalinization requirements during methotrexate administration

Hydration before, during, and after methotrexate:
Administer 1500–3000 mL/m^2 per day. Use a solution containing a total amount of sodium not greater than 0.9% sodium chloride injection (ie, ≤154 mEq/1000 mL), by intravenous infusion during methotrexate administration and for at least 24 hours afterward
• Commence fluid administration 2–12 hours before starting methotrexate, depending upon a patient's fluid status
• Urine output should be at least 100 mL/h before starting methotrexate infusion
• Maintain hydration at a rate that maintains urine output of at least 100 mL/h until the serum methotrexate concentration is <0.05 μmol/L
• Adverse effects attributable to methotrexate are related to systemic methotrexate concentrations *and* the duration for which concentrations are maintained

Sodium bicarbonate 50–150 mEq/1000 mL is added to parenteral hydration solutions to maintain urine pH ≥7.0 to ≤8.0

Base Solution Sodium Content	Sodium Bicarbonate Additive	Total Sodium Content
0.45% Sodium Chloride Injection (0.45% NS)		
77 mEq/L	50–75 mEq	125–152 mEq/L
0.2% Sodium Chloride Injection (0.2% NS)		
34 mEq/L	100–125 mEq	134–159 mEq/L
5% Dextrose Injection (D5W)		
0	125–150 mEq	125–150 mEq/L
D5W/0.45% NS		
77 mEq/L	50–75 mEq	125–152 mEq/L
D5W/0.2% NS		
34 mEq/L	100–125 mEq	134–159 mEq/L

Leucovorin calcium 25 mg/m^2; administer intravenously in 25–250 mL 0.9% NS or D5W over 15–30 minutes every 6 hours starting 24 hours after methotrexate administration began, for at least 72 hours (≥12 doses) or until serum methotrexate concentrations are ≤0.05 μmol/L or undetectable, every 2 weeks, for 5–7 cycles

(continued)

(*continued*)

Leucovorin Rescue Guidelines

Clinical Situation	Serum Methotrexate Concentration*	Leucovorin Dosage, Schedule, and Duration
Normal methotrexate elimination	• ≤10 µmol/L at 24 hours, *or* • ≤1 µmol/L at 48 hours, *or* • ≤0.2 µmol/L at 72 hours	• Give leucovorin calcium 25 mg/m² intravenously every 6 hours until serum methotrexate concentrations are <0.1 µmol/L (<1 × 10⁻⁷ mol/L or <100 nmol/L), then give leucovorin calcium 25 mg orally every 6 hours for 8 doses
Delayed/late methotrexate elimination	• ≥10 µmol/L at 24 hours, *or* • ≥1 µmol/L at 48 hours, *or* • ≥0.1 µmol/L at 72 hours, *or* • ≥0.05 µmol/L at 96 hours *or* • ≥100% increase in serum creatinine concentration at 24 hours after methotrexate administration	• Give leucovorin calcium 100 mg/m² intravenously every 3 hours • When serum methotrexate concentration results are <0.1 µmol/L the leucovorin dosage may be decreased to 10 mg/m² intravenously given every 3 hours until the serum methotrexate concentration is <0.05 µmol/L or undetectable

*After methotrexate administration began
Methotrexate concentration conversions: 1 µmol/L = 10^{-6} mol/L = 1000 nmol/L

Vincristine 1.4 mg/m² (maximum dose = 2.8 mg); administer by intravenous infusion over 15 minutes in 50 mL 0.9% NS on day 2, every 2 weeks, for 5–7 cycles (total dosage/cycle = 1.4 mg/m²; maximum dose/cycle = 2.8 mg)

Procarbazine 100 mg/m² per day; administer orally for 7 consecutive days on days 1 through 7, *only* during odd-numbered cycles (cycles 1, 3, 5 ± 7; ie, every 4 weeks) for 3 or 4 cycles (total dosage/cycle = 700 mg/m²)
> *Note:* because procarbazine is a weak monoamine oxidase inhibitor, clinicians should guide patients who receive the drug in limiting their dietary intake of tyramine-containing foods and beverages

For patients with cerebrospinal fluid cytologically positive for lymphoma:
Preservative-free methotrexate 12 mg; administer intrathecally via intraventricular catheter or reservoir (eg, Ommaya) once per cycle between days 5 and 8, every 2 weeks, for 5–7 cycles

Supportive Care
Antiemetic prophylaxis
Emetogenic potential of rituximab on day 1 is **MINIMAL**
Emetogenic potential of procarbazine on days 1-7 during odd-numbered cycles is **MODERATE–HIGH**
Emetogenic potential of methotrexate on day 2 is **MODERATE**
See Chapter 42 for antiemetic recommendations

Hematopoietic growth factor (CSF) prophylaxis
Primary prophylaxis is indicated with:
> **Filgrastim** (G-CSF) 5 mcg/kg per day, by subcutaneous injection
> • Begin use during odd-numbered cycles on day 8 (24 hours after the last dose of procarbazine)
> • Begin use during even-numbered cycles 24 hours after serum methotrexate concentrations are <0.01 µmol/L (<1 × 10⁻⁸ mol/L, <10 nmol/L, or undetectable)
> • Discontinue daily filgrastim use at least 24 hours before resuming myelosuppressive treatment

See Chapter 43 for more information

Antimicrobial prophylaxis
Risk of fever and neutropenia is **INTERMEDIATE**
> Antimicrobial primary prophylaxis to be considered:
> • Antibacterial—consider a fluoroquinolone or no prophylaxis; *Pneumocystis jirovecii* prophylaxis is recommended (eg, cotrimoxazole)
> • Antifungal—recommended; consider use during periods of neutropenia
> • Antiviral—antiherpes antivirals (eg, acyclovir, famciclovir, valacyclovir)

Infusion reactions associated with rituximab
Fevers, chills, and rigors
1. Interrupt rituximab administration for severe symptoms, and give:
> • **Acetaminophen** 650 mg; administer orally for fever. For persistent or recurrent symptoms, repeat administration every 4–6 hours as needed during rituximab administration
> • **Diphenhydramine** 25–50 mg; administer orally or by intravenous injection for pruritus, hypotension, or angioedema. For persistent or recurrent symptoms, repeat administration every 4–6 hours as needed during rituximab administration
> • **Meperidine** 12.5–25 mg; administer by intravenous injection every 10–20 minutes as needed for shaking chills (generally, cumulative doses >100 mg are not needed; use repeated doses with caution in persons with moderate or more severely impaired renal function)

(*continued*)

(continued)

2. If rituximab administration was interrupted, resume infusion at a slower rate than the maximum rate previously attempted. Rate escalation may be reattempted at smaller incremental steps with close monitoring. Do not exceed the maximum recommended rate of 400 mg/hour

Dyspnea or wheezing without allergic findings (urticaria, or tongue or laryngeal edema)
1. Interrupt rituximab administration immediately
2. Give **hydrocortisone** 100 mg; administer by intravenous injection (or an alternative steroid with equivalent glucocorticoid potency)
3. Give a **histamine (H$_2$) receptor antagonist** (ranitidine 50 mg, cimetidine 300 mg, or famotidine 20 mg); administer intravenously over 15–30 minutes
4. After symptoms resolve, resume rituximab administration at 25 mg/hour with close monitoring. Do not increase the administration rate

CONSOLIDATION AFTER RADIOTHERAPY: TWO 28-DAY CYCLES
Cytarabine 3000 mg/m^2 per day (maximum daily dose = 6000 mg); administer intravenously in 25–500 mL 0.9% NS or D5W over 3 hours for 2 days (2 doses), on days 1 and 2, every 28 days (total dosage/cycle = 6000 mg/m^2; maximum dose/cycle = 12,000 mg)

Supportive Care
Antiemetic prophylaxis
Emetogenic potential is **MODERATE**
See Chapter 42 for antiemetic recommendations

Hematopoietic growth factor (CSF) prophylaxis
Primary prophylaxis is indicated with one of the following:
   Filgrastim (G-CSF) 5 mcg/kg per day; administer by subcutaneous injection, *or*
   Pegfilgrastim (pegylated filgrastim) 6 mg/0.6 mL; administer by subcutaneous injection for 1 dose
   • Begin use from 24–72 hours after cytarabine is completed
   • Continue daily filgrastim use until ANC ≥10,000/mm^3 on two measurements separated temporally by ≥12 hours
   • Discontinue daily filgrastim use at least 24 hours before administering myelosuppressive treatment. Do not administer pegfilgrastim within 14 days before resuming myelosuppressive treatment
See Chapter 43 for more information

Antimicrobial prophylaxis
Risk of fever and neutropenia is **INTERMEDIATE**
   Antimicrobial primary prophylaxis to be considered:
   • Antibacterial—consider a fluoroquinolone or no prophylaxis; *Pneumocystis jirovecii* prophylaxis is recommended (eg, cotrimoxazole)
   • Antifungal—recommended; consider use during periods of neutropenia
   • Antiviral—antiherpes antivirals (eg, acyclovir, famciclovir, valacyclovir)

Keratitis prophylaxis
Steroid ophthalmic drops (prednisolone 1% or dexamethasone 0.1%): administer 2 drops by intraocular instillation into each eye every 6 hours starting prior to the first cytarabine dose and continuing until 48 hours after high-dose cytarabine is completed

Patients with CSF evidence of malignancy received 12 mg of intra-Ommaya methotrexate between cycles

Response Assessment After Five Induction Chemotherapy Cycles*

Assessment	Plan
Complete response (CR)	Reduced-dose whole-brain radiotherapy (rdWBRT) (23.40 Gy in 1.8-Gy fractions × 13 fractions) 3–5 weeks after chemotherapy completion. Opposed lateral radiation fields were used to include the whole brain down to the level of C2 (so-called German helmet shape) and excluded the anterior two-thirds of the orbit
Partial response (PR)	Two additional cycles of R-MPV, and, if a CR was achieved, rdWBRT was given as previously described. Otherwise, a standard dose of WBRT (45 Gy in 25 fractions) was offered
Stable or progressive disease	Standard WBRT. Patients with ocular involvement were irradiated without orbital shielding to the full dose of 23.40 Gy (patients in CR) or to a dose of 36 Gy (patients with less than a CR)

*Response was assessed using International PCNSL Collaborative Group criteria, based on imaging, corticosteroid use, and CSF cytology and slit-lamp examination in case of CSF or ocular involvement

Patient Population Studied

Clinical Characteristics (N = 30)

Characteristic	
Age (years), median/range	57 (30–76)
Sex, Male/Female	17/13
Karnofsky performance score, median/range	70 (50–90)
Positive CSF	6
Ocular involvement	3

Therapy Monitoring

1. *Weekly:* CBC with differential
2. *Before each treatment:* serum creatinine and liver function tests
3. *Every 3–4 cycles:* pulmonary function test

Treatment Modifications

Adverse Event	Dose Modification
WBC nadir during the previous cycle 2000–3000/mm³, or platelets 25,000–75,000/mm³	Reduce procarbazine dosage by 10–25%
WBC nadir during the previous cycle <2000/mm³, or platelets <25,000/mm³	Reduce procarbazine dosage by 25–50%
Severe neurotoxicity; eg, painful paresthesia or peripheral weakness	Discontinue vincristine
Leucovorin doses	See leucovorin guidelines

Efficacy

Time Point	Complete Response Number (Percentage)	Partial Response Number (Percentage)	Overall Response Number (Percentage)
After ≥5 cycles	12 (44%)	13 (59%)	25 (93%)
After all cycles	21 (78%)	4 (15%)	25 (93%)

R-MPV, rituximab, methotrexate, procarbazine, and vincristine

Efficacy*

Reduced-dose Whole-brain Radiotherapy (rdWBRT) (N = 31)

Median PFS[†]	7.7 years	
Median OS[†]	Not reached	
Median PFS <60 years[†]	Not reached	P = 0.02
Median PFS ≥60 years[†]	4.4 years	
Median OS <60 years[†]	Not reached	P = 0.17
Median OS ≥60 years[†]	Not reached	
1-year PFS	84% (95% CI, 71–97)	
2-year PFS	77% (95% CI, 63–92)	
3-year PFS	71% (95% CI, 55–87)	
1-year OS	94% (95% CI, 85–100)	
2-year OS	90% (95% CI, 80–100)	
3-year OS	87% (95% CI, 75–99)	
5-year OS	80% (95% CI, 66–94)	
1-year PFS patients <60 years	94% (95% CI, 82–100)	
2-year PFS patients <60 years	94% (95% CI, 82–100)	
3-year PFS patients <60 years	88% (95% CI, 71–100)	
1-year PFS patients ≥60 years	73% (95% CI, 51–96)	
2-year PFS patients ≥60 years	60% (95% CI, 35–85)	
3-year PFS patients ≥60 years	53% (95% CI, 28–79)	

Entire Cohort (N = 52)

Median PFS[‡]	3.3 years	
Median OS[‡]	6.6 years	
Median PFS <60 years[‡]	7.7 years	P = 0.09
Median PFS ≥60 years[‡]	1.4 years	
Median OS <60 years[‡]	Not reached	P = 0.14
Median OS ≥60 years[‡]	5.5 years	

(continued)

Toxicity (N = 52)*

Acute renal failure	3%
Septic shock	2%
Fatal febrile neutropenia >2 cycles	2%
G4/5 neutropenia[†]	13%
G3 anemia	10%
G3 thrombocytopenia	27%
G3 lymphopenia	40%
G3 neutropenia	20%

*Median number of R-MPV (rituximab, methotrexate, procarbazine, and vincristine) cycles received was 5 (range: 0–7)
[†]Includes 2 of the first 5 treated patients; the protocol was amended to require prophylactic filgrastim

Toxicity

Exploratory Neuropsychological and Imaging Correlates (N = 12 treated with rdWBRT)

- *At baseline:* cognitive impairment present in several domains
- *After induction chemotherapy:* significant improvement in executive (P <0.01) and verbal memory (P <0.05)
- *During follow-up:* no evidence of significant cognitive decline except for motor speed (P <0.05)
- *During follow-up:* no evidence of depressed mood, and self-reported quality of life remained stable during the follow-up period
- *At baseline:* 5/12 patients had G ≥2 white matter disease
- *After induction chemotherapy:* 1/12 patients had G ≥2 white matter disease
- *At 4-year evaluation:* 5/12 patients had G2 and 2/12 patients had G3 white matter disease
- *During follow-up:* no patient developed Fazekas scores of 4 or 5

Efficacy* (continued)

Entire Cohort (N = 52)

1-year PFS	65% (95% CI, 52–78)
2-year PFS	57% (95% CI, 44–71)
3-year PFS	51% (95% CI, 38–65)
1-year OS	85% (95% CI, 75–94)
2-year OS	81% (95% CI, 70–91)
3-year OS	77% (95% CI, 65–88)
5-year OS	70% (95% CI, 57–83)
1-year PFS patients <60 years	68% (95% CI, 50–86)
2-year PFS patients <60 years	64% (95% CI, 45–83)
3-year PFS patients <60 years	64% (95% CI, 45–83)
1-year PFS patients ≥60 years	63% (95% CI, 45–81)
2-year PFS patients ≥60 years	47% (95% CI, 28–66)
3-year PFS patients ≥60 years	38% (95% CI, 19–57)

*The favorable regimen performance in patients expected to have a poor prognosis (elderly and low KPS) abrogated the predictive value of the Memorial Sloan Kettering Cancer Center RPA class, and no differences were seen in PFS or OS according to methotrexate pharmacokinetic parameters
[†]Median follow-up of 5.9 years for survivors
[‡]Median follow-up of 5.6 years for survivors

PRIMARY CNS LYMPHOMA, RECURRENT

CNS CANCER REGIMEN: PEMETREXED

Raizer JJ et al. Cancer 2012;118:3743–3748

Folic acid 350–1000 mcg daily; administer orally, beginning 1–3 weeks before chemotherapy and continuing throughout treatment with pemetrexed and for 21 days after the last pemetrexed dose, *and*

Cyanocobalamin (vitamin B$_{12}$) 1000 mcg; administer intramuscularly every 9 weeks, beginning 1–3 weeks before chemotherapy and continuing throughout treatment with pemetrexed, *and*

Dexamethasone 4 mg; administer intravenously or orally twice daily for 3 consecutive days, starting the day before each pemetrexed administration to decrease the risk of severe skin rash associated with pemetrexed

Pemetrexed 900 mg/m^2; administer intravenously in 100 mL 0.9% sodium chloride injection (0.9% NS) over 10 minutes for 2 doses on day 1 and day 22, repeated every 42 days until disease progression (total dosage/6-week cycle = 1800 mg/m^2)
Note: patients continued pemetrexed until disease progression. If a complete response (CR) was achieved, pemetrexed was discontinued after administration of 1 additional cycle (ie, 2 doses) post-documentation of CR

Supportive Care
Antiemetic prophylaxis
Emetogenic potential is **LOW**
See Chapter 42 for antiemetic recommendations

Hematopoietic growth factor (CSF) prophylaxis
Primary prophylaxis is **NOT** *indicated*
See Chapter 43 for more information

Antimicrobial prophylaxis
Risk of fever and neutropenia is **LOW**
  Antimicrobial primary prophylaxis to be considered:
  • Antibacterial—*Pneumocystis jirovecii* prophylaxis is recommended (eg, cotrimoxazole)
  • Antifungal—not indicated
  • Antiviral—not indicated unless patient previously had an episode of HSV

Steroid-associated gastritis
Add a proton pump inhibitor or H$_2$-receptor antagonist during dexamethasone use to prevent gastritis and duodenitis

Patient Population Studied

This study involved 11 patients with refractory or relapsed primary central nervous system lymphoma (PCNSL). Eligible patients were aged >18 years, had a Karnofsky performance status score ≥60, and had to have undertaken at least 1 prior failed chemotherapy regimen

Therapy Monitoring

1. *Prior to each dose of pemetrexed:* CBC with differential, platelet count, liver function tests, BUN/serum creatinine, electrolytes,
2. *Weekly during treatment:* CBC with differential, platelet count
3. *Response assessment:* clinical examination prior to each dose of pemetrexed, contrast-enhanced MRI of brain at baseline and then repeated approximately every 6–9 weeks

Efficacy (N = 11)

Median progression-free survival	5.7 months
Progression-free survival at 6 months	45%
Progression-free survival at 12 months	27%
Median overall survival	10.1 months
Overall survival at 12 months	45%
Overall response rate*	55%
Disease control rate†	91%

*Overall response rate includes patients with either a complete or partial response to treatment. A complete response was observed in 36% of patients
†Disease control rate includes patients with a complete or partial response to treatment or stable disease
Note: median follow-up was 10.1 months

Treatment Modifications

PEMETREXED	
Adverse Event	**Treatment Modification**
Delay cycle until ANC is >1500/mm^3 and platelet count >100,000/mm^3	
ANC nadir <500/mm^3 + platelet nadir ≥50,000/mm^3	Delay therapy up to 21 days until ANC >1500/mm^3 and platelet count >100,000/mm^3, then reduce pemetrexed dose by 25% for subsequent cycles
Platelet nadir <50,000/mm^3 without bleeding + any ANC nadir	
Platelet nadir <50,000/mm^3 with bleeding + any ANC nadir	Delay therapy up to 21 days until ANC>1500/mm^3 and platelet count >100,000/mm^3, then reduce dose by 50% for subsequent cycles
G3 toxicity other than mucositis or elevated transaminases	Delay start of pemetrexed for up to 21 days until G ≤1 or returns to baseline, then reduce dose by 25% for subsequent cycles
G4 toxicity other than mucositis	
Any grade diarrhea requiring hospitalization or G ≥3 diarrhea	
G ≥3 mucositis	Delay start of pemetrexed for up to 21 days until G ≤1 or returns to baseline, then reduce dose by 50% for subsequent cycles
ALT and AST >1.5× ULN in a patient without liver metastasis	Withhold pemetrexed until ALT and AST ≤1.5× ULN
ALT and AST >2.5× ULN in a patient *with liver metastasis* with alkaline phosphatase >2.5× ULN	Withhold pemetrexed until ALT and AST ≤2.5× ULN and alkaline phosphatase ≤2.5× ULN
Severe hypersensitivity reaction to pemetrexed	Permanently discontinue pemetrexed
Third occurrence of an adverse event requiring a dose reduction	
G ≥3 neurotoxicity	
Creatinine clearance <45 mL/min	Delay pemetrexed until creatinine clearance is ≥45 mL/min

Note: delays of ≤42 days are permitted for recovery from pemetrexed-related toxicities

Adverse Events (N = 11)

Grade (%)	Grade 1	Grade 2	Grade 3	Grade 4	Grade 5
Thrombocytopenia	0	18	27	18	0
Leukopenia	0	18	27	9	0
Infection	0	9	18	0	18
Anemia	9	9	18	9	0
Fatigue	27	9	9	0	0
Increased ALT or AST	0	18	9	0	0
Stomatitis	9	9	0	0	0
Cellulitis	0	9	0	0	0
Neuropathy	0	9	0	0	0
Skin rash	0	9	0	0	0
Weight loss	0	9	0	0	0
Diarrhea	9	0	0	0	0
Fever	9	0	0	0	0
Lymphocytosis	9	0	0	0	0
Nausea	9	0	0	0	0

Note: four patients discontinued treatment because of toxicities: 2 owing to pneumonia, 1 owing to cellulitis, and 1 owing to clinical decline in the setting of Grade 2 thrombocytopenia. One patient died of unknown cause

PRIMARY CNS LYMPHOMA, RECURRENT

CNS CANCER REGIMEN: HIGH-DOSE CYTARABINE

Chamberlain MC. J Neurooncol 2016;126:545–550

Cytarabine 3000 mg/m² per dose; administer intravenously in 100–1000 mL 0.9% sodium chloride injection or 5% dextrose injection over 3 hours, every 12 hours for 4 doses (2 doses/day) on days 1 and 2, every 28 days, until disease progression (total dosage/cycle = 12,000 mg/m²)

Note:

- Patients with renal dysfunction and/or elderly patients are at increased risk of high-dose cytarabine-induced cerebellar toxicity; consider initiating treatment at a reduced dose. Dose reduction recommendations vary; one commonly cited reference (Kintzel PE, Dorr RT. Cancer Treat Rev 1995;21:33–64) suggests:
  - Creatinine clearance 46–60 mL/min: Reduce dose to 1800 mg/m² per dose
  - Creatinine clearance 31–45 mL/min: Reduce dose to 1500 mg/m² per dose
  - Creatinine clearance <30 mL/min: Consider use of alternative drug

Supportive Care

Antiemetic prophylaxis
Emetogenic potential is **MODERATE**
See Chapter 42 for antiemetic recommendations

Hematopoietic growth factor (CSF) prophylaxis
Primary prophylaxis is indicated with one of the following:
Filgrastim (G-CSF) 5 mcg/kg/day, by subcutaneous injection, or
Pegfilgrastim (pegylated filgrastim) 6 mg/0.6 mL, by subcutaneous injection for 1 dose
- Begin use from 24–72 hours after myelosuppressive chemotherapy is completed
- Continue daily filgrastim use until ANC ≥5000/mm³ after the leukocyte nadir
- Discontinue daily filgrastim use at least 24 hours before administering myelosuppressive treatment. Do not administer pegfilgrastim within 14 days before administering myelosuppressive treatment

See Chapter 43 for more information

Antimicrobial prophylaxis
Risk of fever and neutropenia is **HIGH**
Antimicrobial primary prophylaxis is recommended:
- Antibacterial—consider fluoroquinolone prophylaxis during periods of neutropenia
- Antifungal—fluconazole is recommended during periods of neutropenia
- Antiviral—antiherpes antivirals (eg, acyclovir, famciclovir, valacyclovir)

Keratitis prophylaxis
Steroid ophthalmic drops (prednisolone 1% or dexamethasone 0.1%); administer 2 drops by intraocular instillation into each eye every 6 hours starting prior to the first cytarabine dose and continuing until 48 hours after high-dose cytarabine is completed

Efficacy (N = 14)

Median progression-free survival	3 months
6-month progression-free survival	0%
Median overall survival	12 months

Therapy Monitoring

1. CBC with differential and platelet counts and comprehensive metabolic panel daily during chemotherapy
2. *Outpatient monitoring post-chemotherapy:* CBC with differential, platelets, and comprehensive metabolic panel, 2–3 times weekly until counts recover
3. Monitor for signs of cerebellar toxicity (nystagmus, dysmetria, and ataxia) before each dose of cytarabine
4. Patients who receive high-dose cytarabine need to be closely monitored for changes in renal function. Renal dysfunction is highly correlated with an increased risk of cerebellar toxicity
5. *Response assessment:* contrast-enhanced MRI of the brain prior to each cycle of chemotherapy

Patient Population Studied

A retrospective review was performed for 14 patients with recurrent primary central nervous system lymphoma (PCNSL) after having failed first-line treatment (high-dose methotrexate plus rituximab) and second-line therapy (first salvage; temozolomide in 5 patients, high-dose methotrexate plus rituximab in 5 patients, and procarbazine plus lomustine plus vincristine in 4 patients). All patients received high-dose cytarabine

Treatment Modifications

HIGH-DOSE CYTARABINE

Adverse Event	Treatment Modification
Fever, myalgia, bone pain, occasionally chest pain, maculopapular rash, conjunctivitis and malaise, 6–12 hours following drug administration (cytarabine or Ara-C syndrome).	Corticosteroids are beneficial in treating or preventing this syndrome. If the symptoms are deemed treatable, continue therapy with cytarabine and pretreat with corticosteroids
Neurologic (cerebellar) toxicity	Hold cytarabine. Patients who develop CNS symptoms should not receive subsequent high-dose cytarabine.
ANC <1000/mm^3 or platelet count <50,000/mm^3	Consider suspending or modifying doses/schedule. *Note:* ANC and platelet count may continue to fall after the drug is stopped and reach lowest values after drug-free intervals of 12–24 days. When definite signs of marrow recovery appear, restart therapy

Adverse Events (N = 14)

Grade (%)*	Grade 1/2	Grade 3	Grade 4
Neutropenia	43	36	21
Anemia	29	57	14
Lymphopenia	43	43	14
Mucositis	43	43	14
Thrombocytopenia	21	71	7
Fatigue	43	50	7
Neutropenic fever	14	29	7
Conjunctivitis	36	21	0
Nausea	43	14	0
Infection without neutropenia	7	14	0
Encephalopathy	14	7	0

*According to the National Cancer Institute Common Terminology Criteria for Adverse Events
Note: no treatment-related deaths were recorded and no patient discontinued therapy because of toxicity

PRIMARY CNS LYMPHOMA, RECURRENT
CNS CANCER REGIMEN: IBRUTINIB

Soussain C et al. Eur J Can 2019;117:121–130

Ibrutinib 560 mg/dose; administer orally, once daily with a glass of water, without regard to food, continually until disease progression (total dose/week = 3920 mg)

Notes:

- Administration with food increases ibrutinib exposure approximately 2-fold compared with administration after overnight fasting. The U.S. Food and Drug Administration–approved prescribing information does not make specific recommendations regarding administration of ibrutinib with regard to food (Imbruvica [ibrutinib] prescribing information. Sunnyvale, CA: Pharmacyclics LLC; Revised August 2018). Others have also concluded that no food restrictions are needed given the relative safety profile of ibrutinib and because repeated drug intake in fasted conditions is unlikely (de Jong J et al. Cancer Chemother Pharmacol 2015;75:907–916)

- Ibrutinib capsules should be swallowed whole; do not break, open, or chew capsules. Ibrutinib tablets should be swallowed whole; do not cut, crush, or chew tablets

- Patients who delay taking ibrutinib at a regularly scheduled time may administer the missed dose as soon as possible on the same day, and then resume the normal schedule the following day. Do not administer an extra dose of ibrutinib to make up for a missed dose

- Ibrutinib is metabolized predominantly by CYP3A. Refer to treatment modification section for initial dose adjustment recommendations for patients requiring concurrent treatment with moderate or strong CYP3A inhibitors. Avoid concomitant use of ibrutinib with strong CYP3A inducers

- Advise patients to not consume grapefruit products or Seville oranges as they may inhibit CYP3A in the gut wall and increase the bioavailability of ibrutinib

- Serious bleeding events, some fatal, have been reported in patients treated with ibrutinib. Grade ≥3 bleeding events were reported to occur in 3% of patients exposed to ibrutinib. All-grade bleeding (including bruising and petechia) occurred in approximately 44% of patients. Ibrutinib may exacerbate the risk of bleeding when administered concurrently with anticoagulant and/or antiplatelet drugs; use caution and monitor closely for bleeding with concomitant use. Consider the risks and benefits of interrupting ibrutinib treatment at least 3–7 days prior to and following elective surgery depending on the risk of bleeding and type of surgery

- Reduce the ibrutinib starting dose to 140 mg dose, administered orally once daily for mild (Child-Pugh class A) hepatic impairment. Reduce the ibrutinib starting dose to 70 mg dose, administered orally once daily for moderate (Child-Pugh class B) hepatic impairment. Avoid ibrutinib in patients with severe (Child-Pugh class C) hepatic impairment

Supportive Care
Antiemetic prophylaxis
Emetogenic potential is **LOW**
See Chapter 42 for antiemetic recommendations

Hematopoietic growth factor (CSF) prophylaxis
Primary prophylaxis is **NOT** *indicated*
See Chapter 43 for more information

Antimicrobial prophylaxis
Risk of fever and neutropenia is **LOW**
Antimicrobial primary prophylaxis to be considered:
- Antibacterial—not indicated. Consider prophylaxis for *P. jirovecii* (eg, cotrimoxazole)
- Antifungal—not indicated
- Antiviral— not indicated unless patient previously had an episode of HSV

Patient Population Studied

The iLOC study was an open-label, prospective, multicenter, phase 2 trial intended to assess the tolerance and efficacy of ibrutinib monotherapy (28-day cycles) in relapsed or refractory primary central nervous system lymphomas (PCNSL). This study involved 52 adult immunocompetent patients with relapsed or refractory PCNSL or primary vitreoretinal lymphoma. Patients were eligible if they had an Eastern Cooperative Oncology Group performance status of <2 and had received prior therapy with high-dose methotrexate

Efficacy (N = 52)

Therapeutic Response (after 2 Cycles of Treatment), n = 52

Patient Group	Response, n (%)					
	CR + uCR	PR	ORR	SD	DC	PD
Intent-to-treat population, n = 52	10 (19)	17 (33)	27 (52)	5 (10)	32 (62)	20 (38)
Population evaluable for response, n = 44*	10 (23)	16 (36)	26 (59)	5 (11)	31 (70)	13 (30)
Brain lesion at inclusion, n = 30	3 (10)	11 (37)	14 (47)	3 (10)	17 (57)	13 (43)
No brain lesion at inclusion, n = 14	7 (50)	5 (36)	12 (86)	2 (14)	14 (100)	0

Overall Response Rate and Disease Control Rate (After Multiple Cycles), n = 44 evaluable patients*

	After Cycle 4	After Cycle 6	After Cycle 9	After Cycle 12
ORR, %	39	27	29	25
DCR, %	39	32	32	27
Patients not reaching the time point, n	19	28	27	32

Median Survival[†], n = 44

Median progression-free survival, months	4.8 months (95% CI 2.8–12.7)
Median overall survival, months	19.2 months (95% CI 7.2–NR)

Median Survival[†] (intent-to-treat population), n = 52

Median progression-free survival, months	3.3 months (95% CI 2.0–6.4)
Median overall survival, months	14.4 months (95% CI 4.2–21.2)

CR, complete response; uCR, unconfirmed CR; PR, partial response; SD, stable disease; DC, disease control; PD, progressive disease; CI, confidence interval; NR, not reached
*44 patients were evaluable for response having received 90% of the planned dose of ibrutinib during the first month of treatment
[†]The median follow-up period was 25.7 months

Therapy Monitoring

1. *Prior to initiation of ibrutinib:* CBC with differential, serum bilirubin, ALT or AST, alkaline phosphatase
2. *At least monthly:* CBC with differential
3. *Periodically:* monitor for signs and symptoms of cardiac arrhythmias (eg, atrial fibrillation and atrial flutter) and check electrocardiogram if present, signs and symptoms of bleeding (especially if concomitant antiplatelet or anticoagulant medication[s] used), signs and symptoms of infection (including progressive multifocal leukoencephalopathy), blood pressure, presence of second primary malignancies, and diarrhea

Treatment Modifications

IBRUTINIB	
Starting dose	560 mg by mouth once a day
Adverse Event	**Treatment Modification**
Drug Interactions	
Treatment with a moderate CYP3A inhibitor is required	Reduce ibrutinib starting dose to 280 mg by mouth once daily during concomitant therapy
Treatment with voriconazole 200 mg by mouth twice a day is required, *or:* Treatment with posaconazole suspension 100 mg by mouth once daily is required, *or:* Treatment with posaconazole suspension 100–200 mg by mouth twice a day is required	Reduce ibrutinib starting dose to 140 mg by mouth once daily during concomitant therapy

(continued)

Treatment Modifications (*continued*)

Drug Interactions

Treatment with posaconazole suspension 200 mg by mouth three times a day is required, *or:* Treatment with posaconazole suspension 400 mg by mouth twice a day is required, *or:* Treatment with posaconazole 300 mg intravenously once a day is required, *or:* Treatment with posaconazole delayed-release tablets 300 mg by mouth once a day is required	Reduce ibrutinib starting dose to 70 mg by mouth once daily during concomitant therapy
Treatment with other strong CYP3A inhibitors besides those listed above is required	Avoid concomitant use of ibrutinib with other strong CYP3A inhibitors besides those listed above If the other strong CYP3A inhibitor is to be used short-term (eg, ≤7 days) then interrupt ibrutinib therapy during use of the strong CYP3A inhibitor
Treatment with a strong CYP3A inducer is required	Avoid concomitant use of ibrutinib with strong CYP3A inducers
Treatment with antiplatelet and/or anticoagulant medications is required	Bleeding risk may be increased. Monitor closely for signs and symptoms of bleeding

Hypertension

Hypertension	Adjust existing antihypertensive medications and/or initiate antihypertensive treatment as appropriate

Hepatic Impairment

Child-Pugh class A hepatic impairment	Reduce ibrutinib starting dose to 140 mg by mouth once a day
Child-Pugh class B hepatic impairment	Reduce ibrutinib starting dose to 70 mg by mouth once a day
Child-Pugh class C hepatic impairment	Avoid ibrutinib use

Other Toxicities

Surgical procedure is required during treatment with ibrutinib	Consider benefit-risk of withholding ibrutinib for at least 3–7 days prior to and following surgery depending on the type of surgery and the risk of bleeding
First occurrence of G ≥3 nonhematologic toxicity, G ≥3 neutropenia with infection or fever, or G4 hematologic toxicity	Interrupt ibrutinib until resolution to G1 or baseline, then resume ibrutinib at the same dose (eg, 560 mg by mouth once a day). Consider use of G-CSF for G4 neutropenia lasting >7 days or for life-threatening neutropenic complications
Second occurrence of G ≥3 nonhematologic toxicity, G ≥3 neutropenia with infection or fever, or G4 hematologic toxicity	Interrupt ibrutinib until resolution to G1 or baseline, then resume ibrutinib at 420 mg by mouth once a day. Consider use of G-CSF for G4 neutropenia lasting > 7 days or for life-threatening neutropenic complications
Third occurrence of G ≥3 nonhematologic toxicity, G ≥3 neutropenia with infection or fever, or G4 hematologic toxicity	Interrupt ibrutinib until resolution to G1 or baseline, then resume ibrutinib at 280 mg by mouth once a day. Consider use of G-CSF for G4 neutropenia lasting > 7 days or for life-threatening neutropenic complications
Fourth occurrence of G ≥3 nonhematologic toxicity, G ≥3 neutropenia with infection or fever, or G4 hematologic toxicity	Discontinue ibrutinib

G-CSF, granulocyte colony stimulating factor
Imbruvica (ibrutinib) prescribing information. Sunnyvale, CA: Pharmacyclics LLC; Revised August 2018

Adverse Events (N = 52)

Grade (%)	Grade 1	Grade 2	Grade 3	Grade 4	Grade 5
Bronchopulmonary aspergillosis	0	2	0	0	2
Erysipelas	0	2	2	0	0
Pneumonia	0	0	2	0	0
Cerebral hemorrhage	2	2	0	0	0
Atrial fibrillation	0	2	2	0	0
Diarrhea	2	2	0	0	0
Mouth ulceration	2	0	0	0	0
Asthenia	0	2	0	0	0
Pyrexia	0	0	2	0	0
Blue toe syndrome	0	2	0	0	0
Hematoma	2	0	0	0	0
Neutropenia	0	0	0	4	0
Febrile neutropenia	0	0	2	0	0
Leukopenia	0	0	2	0	0
Hyphema	0	2	2	0	0
Muscle spasms	0	4	0	0	0
Alanine aminotransferase increased	0	0	2	2	0
Gamma-glutamyl transferase increased	0	0	2	2	0

PRIMARY CNS LYMPHOMA, RECURRENT

CNS CANCER REGIMEN: NIVOLUMAB

Nayak L et al. Blood 2017;129:3071–3073
OPDIVO (nivolumab) prescribing information.
Princeton, NJ: Bristol-Myers Squibb Company; Revised September 2019

Note that U.S. Food and Drug Administration (FDA)-approved nivolumab regimens include fixed doses of nivolumab and allow for a shortened infusion duration of 30 minutes, consistent with the regimens approved on 5 March 2018, thus:

Nivolumab 240 mg; administer intravenously over 30 minutes in a volume of 0.9% NS or D5W, not to exceed 160 mL and sufficient to produce a nivolumab concentration within the range 1–10 mg/mL, every 2 weeks until disease progression (total dosage/2-week cycle = 240 mg)

- Administer nivolumab through an administration set that contains a sterile, non-pyrogenic, low protein-binding in-line filter with pore size within the range of 0.2–1.2 μm
- Nivolumab can cause severe infusion-related reactions

OR

Nivolumab 480 mg; administer intravenously over 30 minutes in a volume of 0.9% NS or D5W not to exceed 160 mL and sufficient to produce a nivolumab concentration within the range 1–10 mg/mL, every 4 weeks until disease progression (total dosage/4-week cycle = 480 mg)

- Administer nivolumab through an administration set that contains a sterile, non-pyrogenic, low protein-binding in-line filter with pore size within the range of 0.2–1.2 μm
- Nivolumab can cause severe infusion-related reactions

Supportive Care

Antiemetic prophylaxis
Emetogenic potential with nivolumab is **MINIMAL**
See Chapter 42 for antiemetic recommendations

Hematopoietic growth factor (CSF) prophylaxis
Primary prophylaxis is **NOT** *indicated*
See Chapter 43 for more information

Antimicrobial prophylaxis
Risk of fever and neutropenia is **LOW**
  Antimicrobial primary prophylaxis to be considered:
  - Antibacterial—not indicated
  - Antifungal—not indicated
  - Antiviral—not indicated unless patient previously had an episode of HSV

Patient Population Studied

This case series describes a consecutive series of 5 patients from 3 institutions who received nivolumab for recurrent/refractory primary CNS lymphoma (n = 4) and CNS recurrence of primary testicular lymphoma (n = 1) and who had at least 13 months of follow-up. The median age was 64 years (range 54–85 years) and the median Karnofsky performance status (KPS) was 70% (range 40–80%). These patients had received standard-of-care regimens and had no other options available before starting nivolumab therapy. In addition to nivolumab, several patients also received a variety of adjunctive therapies, including rituximab in 1 patient, radiation immediately prior to nivolumab initiation in 2 patients, and corticosteroids in 1 patient which were discontinued within 1 month

Efficacy (N = 5)

All 5 patients had clinical and radiographic responses to therapy, with 4 of 5 patients achieving complete responses. In addition, 4 patients who were symptomatic before initiating nivolumab experienced complete or near-complete resolution of neurologic symptoms after treatment. All 5 patients were alive at the median follow-up point of 17 months. Additionally, 3 patients remained progression-free at 13+ and 17+ months following initiation of nivolumab

Therapy Monitoring

1. Initially at the time of each dose, and eventually every 6–12 weeks, perform a total body skin examination with attention to ALL mucous membranes as well as a complete review of systems
2. Monitor patients for signs and symptoms of pneumonitis. Evaluate patients with suspected pneumonitis with chest x-ray, CT, and pulse oximetry. For ≥2 toxicity, may include nasal swab, sputum culture and sensitivity, blood culture and sensitivity, and urine culture and sensitivity
3. Monitor patients for signs and symptoms of colitis. Encourage patients to report diarrhea immediately to any member of the health care team
4. Draw AST, ALT, and bilirubin prior to each infusion and/or weekly if there are Grade 1 liver function test elevations. Note, no treatment is recommended for G1 LFT abnormalities. For ≥2 toxicity, work up for other causes of elevated LFTs including viral hepatitis
5. Use basic metabolic panel (Na, K, CO_2, glucose) and patient history as screening tools for hypophysitis including hypopituitarism and adrenal insufficiency. If in doubt, evaluate AM adrenocorticotropic hormone (ACTH) and cortisol levels. Consider ACTH stimulation test for indeterminate results
6. Assess thyroid function at the start of treatment, periodically during treatment, and as indicated based on clinical evaluation) and for clinical signs and symptoms of thyroid disorders. Test for TSH and free thyroxine (FT4) every 4 to 6 weeks as part of routine clinical monitoring of therapy or for case detection in symptomatic patients
7. Measure glucose at baseline and with each treatment during the first 12 weeks and every 6 weeks thereafter
8. Obtain a serum creatinine prior to every dose. If creatinine is found to be newly elevated, consider holding therapy while other potential causes are evaluated. Note, routine urinalysis is not necessary other than to rule out urinary tract infections, etc
9. Obtain a complete rheumatologic history and perform an examination of all peripheral joints for tenderness, swelling, and range of motion. Examine the spine. Consider plain x-ray/imaging to exclude metastases and evaluate joint damage (erosions), if appropriate
10. In patients at high risk for infections and in appropriately selected patients based on an infectious disease evaluation, draw screening laboratories (HIV, hepatitis A and B, and blood QuantiFERON for TB) to prepare patients to start infliximab

Treatment Modifications

RECOMMENDED DOSE MODIFICATIONS FOR NIVOLUMAB

Adverse Event	Grade/Severity	Treatment Modification
Infusion reaction	Clinically significant but not severe infusion reaction	Interrupt the infusion in patients with clinically significant infusion reactions and consider resuming at a slower rate following resolution. If decision is made to restart, begin at ≤50% of the rate prior to the reaction and increase in 50% increments every 30 minutes if well tolerated. Infusions may be restarted at the full rate during the next cycle
	G3/4 (severe infusion reaction—pyrexia, chills, flushing, hypotension, dyspnea, wheezing, back pain, abdominal pain, and urticaria). Not rapidly responsive to brief interruption of infusion	Stop infusion and administer appropriate medical therapy (eg, epinephrine, corticosteroids, intravenous antihistamines, bronchodilators and/or oxygen). Discontinue nivolumab
Colitis	G1	Loperamide 4 mg as starting dose then 2mg before each meal and after each loose stool until without diarrhea for 12 hours, with maximum of 16 mg loperamide per day. If G1 diarrhea or colitis persists >14 days, then add prednisolone 0.5–1 mg/kg (non-enteric-coated) or consider oral budesonide 9 mg daily if no bloody diarrhea
	G2/3 diarrhea or colitis	Withhold nivolumab. Loperamide 4 mg as starting dose then 2mg before each meal and after each loose stool until without diarrhea for 12 hours, with maximum of 16 mg loperamide per day. Administer oral prednisone/prednisolone at a dose of 0.5 to 2 mg/kg/day or its equivalent. When improves to G1, begin a slow corticosteroid taper over at least 4 weeks. Resume nivolumab upon symptom control, or when prednisone/prednisolone daily dose <10 mg
	G4 diarrhea or colitis	Permanently discontinue nivolumab. Loperamide 4 mg as starting dose then 2 mg before each meal and after each loose stool until without diarrhea for 12 hours, with maximum of 16 mg loperamide per day. Administer 1–2 mg/kg IV (methyl)prednisolone and convert to 0.5–2 mg/kg prednisone/prednisolone orally each day or its equivalent only after a response. Taper over at least 4 weeks when symptoms improve. If does not improve over 72 hours or worsens, perform flexible sigmoidoscopy/colonoscopy to document colitis then begin infliximab 5 mg/kg (if no perforation/sepsis/TB/hepatitis/NYHA III/IV CHF). If no response, add MMF 500–1000 mg twice daily. If worse on MMF, consider addition of tacrolimus or ATG
Pneumonitis	G2	Withhold nivolumab. Consider pneumocystis prophylaxis depending on the clinical context and coverage with empiric antibiotics. Administer oral prednisone/prednisolone at a dose of 1–2 mg/kg/day or its equivalent. When improves to G1, begin a slow corticosteroid taper over at least 4 weeks. If does not respond adequately after 48 hours, then administer 2–4 mg/kg IV (methyl)prednisolone and convert to 0.5–2 mg/kg prednisone/prednisolone orally each day or its equivalent only after a response, followed by a taper over at least 6 weeks when symptoms improve to G1, titrating to symptoms. Resume nivolumab upon symptom control, or when prednisone/prednisolone daily dose <10 mg
	G3/4	Permanently discontinue nivolumab. Consider pneumocystis prophylaxis depending on the clinical context; cover with empiric antibiotics. Administer 2–4 mg/kg IV (methyl)prednisolone and convert to 1–2 mg/kg prednisone/prednisolone orally each day or its equivalent only after a response, followed by a taper over at least 8 weeks when symptoms improve to G1, titrating to symptoms. If when initially treated improvement does not occur within 48–72 hours, begin infliximab 5 mg/kg (if no perforation/sepsis/TB/hepatitis/NYHA III/IV CHF). If no response to infliximab, add MMF 500–1000 mg twice daily. Consider MMF especially if has concurrent hepatic toxicity
Hepatitis	G2 (AST or ALT >3–5× ULN or total bilirubin >1.5–3× ULN)	Withhold nivolumab. Administer oral prednisone/prednisolone at a dose of 1 to 2 mg/kg/day or its equivalent. When improves to G1, begin a slow corticosteroid taper over at least 4 weeks. Resume nivolumab upon symptom control, or when prednisone/prednisolone daily dose <10 mg
	G3/4 (AST or ALT >5× ULN or total bilirubin >3× ULN)	Permanently discontinue nivolumab. Administer 1–2 mg/kg IV (methyl)prednisolone and convert to 0.5–2 mg/kg prednisone/prednisolone orally each day or its equivalent only after a response. Taper over at least 6 weeks when symptoms improve. If no response, add MMF 500–1000 mg twice daily. If worse on MMF, consider adding tacrolimus or ATG

(continued)

Treatment Modifications (*continued*)

RECOMMENDED DOSE MODIFICATIONS FOR NIVOLUMAB

Adverse Event	Grade/Severity	Treatment Modification
Hypophysitis	G2/3 (moderate symptoms, ie, headache but no visual disturbance or fatigue/mood alteration but hemodynamically stable, no electrolyte disturbance)	Administer analgesia as needed for headache. Withhold nivolumab. Administer oral prednisone/prednisolone at a dose of 0.5 to 2 mg/kg/day or its equivalent. When improves to G1, begin a slow corticosteroid taper over at least 4 weeks. If no improvement in 48 hours, administer 1–2 mg/kg IV (methyl)prednisolone and convert to 0.5–2 mg/kg prednisone/prednisolone orally each day or its equivalent only after a response. Taper over at least 4 weeks when symptoms improve to 5 mg prednisone/prednisolone or equivalent; do not stop steroids. Resume nivolumab upon symptom control, or when prednisone/prednisolone daily dose <10 mg
	G4 (severe mass effect symptoms, ie, severe headache, any visual disturbance or severe hypoadrenalism, ie, hypotension, severe electrolyte disturbance)	Permanently discontinue nivolumab. Administer analgesia as needed for headache. Administer 1–2 mg/kg IV (methyl)prednisolone and convert to 0.5–2 mg/kg prednisone/prednisolone orally each day or its equivalent only after a response. Taper over at least 4 weeks when symptoms improve to 5 mg prednisone/prednisolone or equivalent; do not stop steroids
Adrenal insufficiency	G2	Withhold nivolumab. Administer oral prednisone/prednisolone at a dose of 0.5 to 2 mg/kg/day or its equivalent. When improves to G1, begin a slow corticosteroid taper over at least 4 weeks. Serially assess adrenal function and continue steroids at replacement doses (20–40 mg hydrocortisone daily ~2/3 dose in AM upon awakening and ~1/3 at 4 PM) until recovery of adrenal function is documented. Resume nivolumab upon symptom control, or when prednisone/prednisolone daily dose <10 mg
	G3/4	Permanently discontinue nivolumab. Administer oral prednisone/prednisolone at a dose of 0.5 to 2 mg/kg/day or its equivalent. When improves to G1, begin a slow corticosteroid taper over at least 4 weeks. Serially assess adrenal function and continue steroids at replacement doses (20–40 mg hydrocortisone daily ~2/3 dose in AM upon awakening and ~1/3 at 4 PM) until recovery of adrenal function is documented
Type 1 diabetes mellitus	G3 hyperglycemia	Withhold nivolumab. Admit to hospital to manage hyperglycemia. Role of corticosteroids in preventing complete loss of insulin-producing cells is unknown and not recommended. Resume nivolumab upon symptom control, or when prednisone/prednisolone daily dose <10 mg
	G4 hyperglycemia	Permanently discontinue nivolumab. Admit to hospital to manage hyperglycemia. Role of corticosteroids in preventing complete loss of insulin-producing cells is unknown and not recommended.
Nephritis and renal dysfunction	G2/3 (serum creatinine 1.5–6× ULN)	Withhold nivolumab. Administer oral prednisone/prednisolone at a dose of 0.5 to 2 mg/kg/day or its equivalent. When improves to G1, begin a slow corticosteroid taper over at least 4 weeks. If does not respond adequately, then administer 0.5–1 mg/kg IV (methyl)prednisolone and convert to 0.5–2 mg/kg prednisone/prednisolone orally each day or its equivalent only after a response, followed by a taper over at least 4 weeks when improves to G1. Resume nivolumab upon symptom control, or when prednisone/prednisolone daily dose <10 mg
	G4 (serum creatinine >6× ULN)	Permanently discontinue nivolumab. Administer 0.5–1 mg/kg IV (methyl)prednisolone and convert to 0.5–2 mg/kg prednisone/prednisolone orally each day or its equivalent only after a response, followed by a taper over at least 4 weeks when improves to G1
Skin	G1/2	Continue nivolumab. Avoid skin irritants, avoid sun exposure, topical emollients recommended. Topical steroid (mild strength for G1, moderate/potent strength for G2) cream once or twice daily ± oral or topical antihistamines for itching.
	G3 rash or suspected SJS or TEN	Withhold nivolumab. Avoid skin irritants, avoid sun exposure, topical emollients recommended. Administer oral or topical antihistamines for itching. Administer oral prednisone/prednisolone at a dose of 0.5–2 mg/kg or its equivalent daily for 3 days followed by a slow corticosteroid taper over at least 4 weeks when the rash improves to G1. If does not respond adequately, then administer 0.5–1 mg/kg IV (methyl)prednisolone and convert to 0.5–2 mg/kg prednisone/prednisolone orally each day or its equivalent only after a response, followed by a taper over at least 4 weeks when the rash improves to G1. Resume nivolumab upon symptom control, or when prednisone/prednisolone daily dose <10 mg
	G4 rash or confirmed SJS or TEN	Avoid skin irritants, avoid sun exposure, topical emollients recommended. Administer oral or topical antihistamines for itching. Administer 1–2 mg/kg IV (methyl)prednisolone and convert to oral steroids 0.5–2 mg/kg prednisone/prednisolone each day or its equivalent only after a response. Taper over at least 4 weeks when the rash improves to G1. Permanently discontinue nivolumab

(*continued*)

Treatment Modifications (*continued*)

RECOMMENDED DOSE MODIFICATIONS FOR NIVOLUMAB

Adverse Event	Grade/Severity	Treatment Modification
Encephalitis	Confusion or altered behavior, headaches, alteration in Glasgow Coma Scale, motor or sensory deficits, speech abnormality, may or may not be febrile	Initially withhold nivolumab, but permanently discontinue nivolumab if there is no doubt as to diagnosis. Exclude bacterial and ideally viral infections prior to high-dose steroids. Administer oral prednisone/prednisolone at a dose of 0.5–2 mg/kg/day or its equivalent. When symptoms improve, begin a slow corticosteroid taper over at least 4–8 weeks. If symptoms are severe, administer 1–2 mg/kg IV (methyl)prednisolone and convert to 0.5–2 mg/kg prednisone/prednisolone orally each day or its equivalent only after a response. Consider concurrent empiric antiviral (IV acyclovir) and antibacterial therapy
Aseptic meningitis	Headache, photophobia, neck stiffness with fever or may be afebrile, vomiting; normal cognition/cerebral function (distinguishes from encephalitis)	
Other syndromes include neurosarcoidosis, posterior reversible leukoencephalopathy syndrome (PRES), Vogt-Harada-Koyanagi syndrome, demyelination, vasculitic encephalopathy, and generalized seizures		
Transverse myelitis	Acute or subacute neurologic signs/symptoms of motor/sensory/autonomic origin; most have sensory level; often bilateral symptoms	Initially withhold nivolumab, but permanently discontinue nivolumab if there is no doubt as to diagnosis. Administer 2 mg/kg IV (methyl)prednisolone or consider 1 g/day and convert to 0.5–2 mg/kg prednisone/prednisolone orally each day or its equivalent only after a response. When symptoms improve, begin a slow corticosteroid taper over at least 4–8 weeks. Plasmapheresis may be required if steroids do not bring about improvement
Myocarditis	G3	Permanently discontinue nivolumab. Administer 2 mg/kg IV (methyl)prednisolone or consider 1 g/day and convert to 0.5–2 mg/kg prednisone/prednisolone orally each day or its equivalent only after a response. When symptoms improve, begin a slow corticosteroid taper over at least 4–8 weeks. If no response, add MMF 500–1000 mg twice daily. If worse on MMF, consider adding tacrolimus
Peripheral neurologic toxicity	Moderate: some interference with ADL, symptoms concerning to patient	Withhold nivolumab. Initial observation reasonable or initiate prednisone/prednisolone 0.5–1 mg/kg (if progressing, eg, from mild) and/or pregabalin or duloxetine for pain. When symptoms improve, begin a slow corticosteroid taper over at least 4 weeks. Resume nivolumab upon symptom control, or when prednisone/prednisolone daily dose <10 mg
	Severe: limits self-care and aids warranted, life-threatening, eg, respiratory problems	Permanently discontinue nivolumab. Administer 1–2 mg/kg IV (methyl)prednisolone and convert to 0.5–2 mg/kg prednisone/prednisolone orally each day or its equivalent only after a response. Taper over at least 4–8 weeks when symptoms improve to G1
Guillain-Barré syndrome	Progressive symmetrical muscle weakness with absent or reduced tendon reflexes—involves extremities, facial, respiratory, and bulbar and oculomotor muscles; dysregulation of autonomic nerves	Permanently discontinue nivolumab. Use of steroids not recommended in idiopathic Guillain-Barré syndrome; however, a trial of (methyl)prednisolone 1–2 mg/kg is reasonable, converting to 0.5–2 mg/kg prednisone/prednisolone orally each day or its equivalent only after a response. If no improvement or worsening, plasmapheresis or IVIG indicated
Myasthenia gravis	Fluctuating muscle weakness (proximal limb, trunk, ocular, eg, ptosis/diplopia or bulbar) with fatigability; respiratory muscles may also be involved	Permanently discontinue nivolumab. Administer pyridostigmine at an initial dose of 30 mg three times daily. Administer oral prednisone/prednisolone at a dose of 0.5 to 2 mg/kg/day or its equivalent or 1–2 mg/kg IV (methyl)prednisolone depending on the severity of symptoms. If begin with IV, convert to 0.5–2 mg/kg prednisone/prednisolone orally each day or its equivalent only after a response. If no improvement or worsening, plasmapheresis or IVIG may be considered. Additional immunosuppressants used in myasthenia gravis include azathioprine, cyclosporine, and mycophenolate. Avoid certain medications, eg, ciprofloxacin, beta-blockers, that may precipitate cholinergic crisis
Other syndromes including motor and sensory peripheral neuropathy, multifocal radicular neuropathy/plexopathy, autonomic neuropathy, phrenic nerve palsy, cranial nerve palsies (eg, facial nerve, optic nerve, hypoglossal nerve)		Permanently discontinue nivolumab. Administer oral prednisone/prednisolone at a dose of 0.5 to 2 mg/kg/day or its equivalent or 1–2 mg/kg IV (methyl)prednisolone depending on the severity of symptoms. If begin with IV, convert to 0.5–2 mg/kg prednisone/prednisolone orally each day or its equivalent only after a response

(*continued*)

Treatment Modifications (*continued*)

RECOMMENDED DOSE MODIFICATIONS FOR NIVOLUMAB

Adverse Event	Grade/Severity	Treatment Modification
Arthralgia	G1 (mild pain with inflammation, erythema, or joint swelling)	Continue nivolumab. Administer acetaminophen (paracetamol) and ibuprofen
	G2 (Moderate pain with inflammation, erythema, or joint swelling that limits ADLs)	Withhold nivolumab. Administer higher doses of acetaminophen (paracetamol) and ibuprofen and use diclofenac or naproxen or etoricoxib. If inadequately controlled, consider intra-articular steroid injections for large joints or administer oral prednisone/prednisolone at a dose of 0.5 to 2 mg/kg/day or its equivalent. When improves to G1, begin a slow corticosteroid taper over at least 4 weeks. If does not respond adequately, then administer 0.5–1 mg/kg IV (methyl) prednisolone and convert to 0.5–2 mg/kg prednisone/prednisolone orally each day or its equivalent only after a response, followed by a taper over at least 4 weeks when improves to G1. Resume nivolumab upon symptom control, or when prednisone/prednisolone daily dose <10 mg
	G3 (severe pain; irreversible joint damage; disabling; limits self-care ADL)	Withhold nivolumab. Administer 0.5–1 mg/kg IV (methyl)prednisolone and convert to 0.5–2 mg/kg prednisone/prednisolone orally each day or its equivalent only after a response, followed by a taper over at least 4 weeks when improves to G1. In severe cases, infliximab or another anti–TNF-alpha drug may be required for improvement of arthritis. Resume nivolumab upon symptom control, or when prednisone/prednisolone daily dose <10 mg
Other	First occurrence of other G3	Withhold nivolumab. Administer oral prednisone/prednisolone at a dose of 0.5 to 2 mg/kg/day or its equivalent. When improves to G1, begin a slow corticosteroid taper over at least 4 weeks. Resume nivolumab upon symptom control, or when prednisone/prednisolone daily dose <10 mg
	Recurrence of same G3	Permanently discontinue nivolumab. Administer 1–2 mg/kg IV (methyl)prednisolone and convert to 0.5–2 mg/kg prednisone/prednisolone orally each day or its equivalent only after a response. Taper over at least 4–8 weeks when symptoms improve to G1
	Life-threatening or G4	
	Requirement for ≥10 mg/day prednisone or equivalent for >12 weeks	Permanently discontinue nivolumab
	Persistent G2/3 adverse reactions lasting ≥12 weeks	

ADL, activities of daily living; ALT, alanine aminotransferase; AST, aspartate aminotransferase; ATG, anti-thymocyte globulin; SJS, Stevens-Johnson Syndrome; TEN, toxic epidermal necrolysis; ULN, upper limit of normal

Notes on general supportive care:
• Steroid taper in most cases will proceed over a minimum of one month but if symptoms improve rapidly, a two-week taper can be considered. If steroids are administered for more than 4 weeks, consider PCP prophylaxis (cotrimoxazole 480 mg twice daily M/W/F or inhaled pentamidine if has cotrimoxazole allergy), regular random blood glucose, VitD level, and starting calcium/VitD supplementation as per guidelines

Adverse Events (N = 5)

Two patients experienced Grade 2 toxicities associated with nivolumab (pruritis in 1 patient and fatigue in another). One patient developed worsening renal insufficiency (Grade 4), requiring discontinuation of nivolumab after 3 doses

MENINGIOMA, RECURRENT
CNS CANCER REGIMEN: LONG-ACTING OCTREOTIDE ACETATE

Chamberlain MC et al. Neurology 2007;69:969–973

Octreotide acetate for injectable suspension 30 mg per dose; administer by intramuscular injection (intragluteally) every 4 weeks (total dose/cycle = 30 mg)

Note: if after 2 cycles of therapy a patient has achieved stable disease or a better response and has tolerated a 30-mg dose, the dose of long-acting octreotide acetate may be increased to 40 mg every 4 weeks for the third and subsequent cycles of therapy (total dose/cycle = 40 mg)

Note: for patients not previously treated with subcutaneously administered octreotide acetate, it is recommended to start with the administration of subcutaneous octreotide at a dosage of 0.1 mg 3 times daily for a short period (approximately 2 weeks) to assess the response and systemic tolerability of octreotide before initiating the treatment with long-acting octreotide acetate

Note: limited published data indicate somatostatin analogs might decrease the metabolic clearance of compounds known to be metabolized by cytochrome P450. Use with caution drugs mainly metabolized by CYP3A4 and which have a low therapeutic index (eg, quinidine, terfenadine)

Supportive Care
Antiemetic prophylaxis
Emetogenic potential is **MINIMAL**
See Chapter 42 for antiemetic recommendations

Hematopoietic growth factor (CSF) prophylaxis
Primary prophylaxis is **NOT** indicated
See Chapter 43 for more information

Antimicrobial prophylaxis
Risk of fever and neutropenia is **LOW**
Antimicrobial primary prophylaxis to be considered:
- Antibacterial—*Pneumocystis jirovecii* prophylaxis is recommended (eg, cotrimoxazole)
- Antifungal—not indicated
- Antiviral—not indicated unless patient previously had an episode of HSV

Patient Characteristics and Individual Efficacy

Age/Gender	PATH	LOC	SUR	RT, Gy	SUR	EBRT	SRT	CHEMORx	KPS	#Cy	RESP	OS
M/62	I/Yes	LF LFP RCS	No	No	No	No	15	Celebrex (SD)	90	11	PR/12*	12*
M/83	III/Yes	LF LT Falx SS	STR	No	No	No	No	No	80	15	PR/15*	15*
F/41	I/No	CS LSW	STR	54	X2	No	18	TAM 30 (SD) HU 4.5 (PD)	90	8	PR/8	20+
M/67	III/No	BF	GTR	55	X2	No	No	No	60	8	SD/8*	8*
F/65	III/No	LTP	STR	58.4	X2	No	12.9	TMZ + erlotinib2 (PD)	70	2	PD/2	10
F/68	II/No	RSW	STR	58.4	X1	No	No	αIFN 12 (SD)	90	6	PR/6	11+
F/26	III/Yes	RT RF Spine CSF	GTR	59.4	X4	No	12	HU 2 (PD) TMZ 2 (PD)	60	2	PD/2	3
F/45	I/No	RSB RSF CbPA	STR	No	No	No	18	No	80	5	SD/5*	5*

(continued)

Patient Characteristics and Individual Efficacy (continued)

Age/Gender	PATH	LOC	SUR	RT, Gy	SUR	EBRT	SRT	CHEMORx	KPS	#Cy	RESP	OS
F/52	I/No	LS LCS	No	No	No	No	No	HU 3 (PD)	90	6	SD/20	20+
F/87	II/Yes	RF	STR	No	X1	61	No	No	70	3	PD/3	4
F/51	I/No	LF	GTR	54	No	No	No	HU 3 (PD)	80	3	PD/3	8+†
M/61	I/No	RF RP	GTR	No	X2	54	18	HU 3 (PD)	60	3	PD/3	7+†
F/51	III/No	RF	STR	54	X1	No	18	Thal 13 (SD) HU 3 (PD)	50	6	PD/3	7+†
F/84	II/No	RCS	Bx	No	No	No	No	HU 3 (PD)	80	5	SD/5*	5*
FX/74	I/No	LSW	GTR	No	No	54	No	HU 3 (PD)	80	3	PD/3	4
M/72	I/No	LCS	Bx	54	No	No	No	HU 6 (PD)	70	6	PR/6	7+

Column descriptions (in left-to-right order): Age/Gender (in years); PATH, histology, WHO grade/multifocal; LOC, tumor location; surgery; RT, radiotherapy; Gy, Gray; EBRT, SUR (assuming surgery); external beam radiotherapy; SRT, stereotactic radiotherapy; CHEMORx, chemotherapy, number of cycles* (best response); KPS, Karnofsky performance status; #Cy, number of cycles (cycle defined as 4 weeks); RESP, response assessment/duration in months; OS, overall survival

LOC (tumor location) (order of appearance): LF, left frontal; LFP, left frontoparietal; RCS, right cavernous sinus; LT, left temporal; SS, sphenoid sinus; CS, cavernous sinus; LSW, left sphenoid wing; BF, bifrontal; LTP, left temporoparietal; RSW, right sphenoid wing; RT, right temporal; RF, right frontal, RSB, right skull; base; CbA, cerebellopontine angle; LS, left sphenoid; LCS, left cavernous sinus

Other (alphabetically): αIFN, interferon alfa; Bx, biopsy; CR, complete response; GTR, gross total resection; HU, hydroxyurea; NE, nonevaluable; PD, progressive disease; PR, partial response; SD, stable disease; STR, subtotal resection; TAM, tamoxifen; Thal, thalidomide; TMZ, temozolomide

*Alive on octreotide acetate
†Alive

Efficacy

Partial response	4/16
Stable disease	5/16
Progressive disease	7/16
6-month progression-free survival	44% (7/16)
Median duration of response	5.0 months (range: 2–20+ months)
Median overall survival	7.5 months (range: 3–20+ months)

Treatment Modifications

Adverse Event	Treatment Modification
Asymptomatic gallstones	Continue long-acting octreotide acetate depending on reassessment of the benefit-to-risk ratio. Either way, no action is required except to continue monitoring with increased frequency if treatment with long-acting octreotide acetate is continued
Symptomatic gallstones	Long-acting octreotide acetate may be either stopped or continued, depending on reassessment of the benefit-to-risk ratio. Either way, the gallstones should be treated like any other symptomatic gallstones

Treatment/Therapy Monitoring

1. Ultrasound examination of the gallbladder prior to commencing octreotide treatment and at approximately 6-month intervals throughout treatment
2. Monitor vitamin B_{12} levels in patients who have a history of vitamin B_{12} deprivation

Toxicity

Adverse Drug Reactions Reported in Clinical Studies

Gastrointestinal Disorders

Very common	Diarrhea, abdominal pain, nausea, constipation, flatulence
Common	Dyspepsia, vomiting, abdominal bloating, steatorrhea, loose stools, discoloration of feces

Nervous System Disorders

Very common	Headache
Common	Dizziness

Endocrine Disorders

Common	Hypothyroidism, thyroid dysfunction (eg, decreased TSH, decreased total T_4, and decreased free T_4)

Hepatobiliary Disorders

Very common	Cholelithiasis
Common	Cholecystitis, biliary sludge, hyperbilirubinemia

Metabolism and Nutrition Disorders*

Very common	Hyperglycemia
Common	Hypoglycemia, impaired glucose tolerance, anorexia
Uncommon	Dehydration

General Disorders and Administration Site Reactions

Very common	Localized pain at injection site

Laboratory Investigations

Common	Elevated transaminase levels
Uncommon	Depressed vitamin B_{12} levels and abnormal Schilling tests

Skin and Subcutaneous Tissue Disorders

Common	Pruritus, rash, alopecia

Respiratory Disorders

Common	Dyspnea

Cardiac Disorders

Common	Bradycardia
Uncommon	Tachycardia

Very common: ≥1/10; Common: ≥1/100, <1/10; Uncommon: ≥1/1000, <1/100
*Note: because of its inhibitory action on growth hormone, glucagon, and insulin release, long-acting somatostatin may affect glucose regulation. Postprandial glucose tolerance may be impaired. In some instances, a state of persistent hyperglycemia may be induced as a result of chronic administration

MENINGIOMA, RECURRENT

CNS CANCER REGIMEN: BEVACIZUMAB

Grimm SA et al. J Clin Oncol 2015;33(15_suppl):2055

Bevacizumab 10 mg/kg; administer intravenously in 100 mL 0.9% sodium chloride injection, every 2 weeks, until disease progression (total dosage/2-week cycle = 10 mg/kg)

Notes:

- Bevacizumab administration duration for the initial dose is 90 minutes. If administration is well tolerated, the administration duration may be decreased stepwise during subsequent administrations to 60 minutes and, finally, to a minimum duration of 30 minutes

- The protocol allowed stable patients to switch to an every-3-week schedule of bevacizumab after 6 months of therapy as follows:

  - **Bevacizumab** 15 mg/kg; administer intravenously in 100 mL 0.9% sodium chloride injection, every 3 weeks, until disease progression (total dosage/3-week cycle = 15 mg/kg)

    ○ *Note:* bevacizumab administration duration for the initial dose is 90 minutes. If administration is well tolerated, the administration duration may be decreased stepwise during subsequent administrations to 60 minutes and, finally, to a minimum duration of 30 minutes

Supportive Care

Antiemetic prophylaxis
Emetogenic potential is **MINIMAL**
See Chapter 42 for antiemetic recommendations

Hematopoietic growth factor (G-CSF) prophylaxis
Primary prophylaxis is **NOT** *indicated*
See Chapter 43 for more information

Antimicrobial prophylaxis
Risk of fever and neutropenia is **LOW**
  Antimicrobial primary prophylaxis to be considered:
  - *Antibacterial—not indicated*
  - *Antifungal—not indicated*
  - *Antiviral—not indicated unless patient previously had an episode of HSV*

Patient Population Studied

This open-label, non-randomized, phase 2 trial included 40 total adult patients with progressive benign (n = 15), atypical (n = 22), or malignant meningioma (n = 13) and evaluated treatment with bevacizumab. Patients were eligible for the trial if they had histologically proven recurrent or progressive intracranial meningioma (including benign, atypical, or malignant meningioma in patients with or without neurofibromatosis type 1 or 2) or if they had histologically proven intracranial hemangiopericytoma, hemangioblastoma (with or without metastatic disease), acoustic neuroma, or intracranial schwannoma. Unequivocal evidence of tumor progression by MRI was required. Patients may have had recent resection of recurrent tumor so long as at least 4 weeks had passed and there was residual evaluable disease. Prior radiation therapy was allowed if more than 8 weeks prior to registration. Prior systemic therapy had to have been completed >4 weeks (cytotoxic chemotherapy) or >2 weeks (biologic therapy) before registration. Additionally, a Karnofsky performance status ≥ 60% and adequate organ function were required. Notable exclusion criteria included prior therapy with VEGF inhibitors; life expectancy of <12 weeks; history of stroke, myocardial infarction, coagulopathy, bleeding diathesis, bowel perforation, major surgery within 28 days; or minor surgery within 7 days of start of treatment

Therapy Monitoring

1. Observe closely for hypersensitivity reactions, especially during the first and second bevacizumab infusions
2. Vital signs (including blood pressure measurement) prior to each cycle or more frequently as indicated during treatment
3. Assess proteinuria by urine dipstick and/or urinary protein creatinine ratio prior to each cycle. Patients with a ≥2+ urine dipstick reading should undergo further assessment with a 24-hour urine collection

Efficacy (N = 40)*

Efficacy Variable	Bevacizumab (N = 40)*
Response in progressive benign meningioma patients (n = 15)	
PR—%	0
SD—%	100
PD—%	0
Response in atypical meningioma patients (n = 22)	
PR—%	5
SD—%	85
PD—%	10
Response in malignant meningioma patients (n = 13)	
PR—%	0
SD—%	82
PD—%	18
Survival in progressive benign meningioma patients (n = 15)	
PFS at 6 months—%	87
Median PFS—months	22.5
Median OS—months	35.6
Response in atypical meningioma patients (n = 22)	
PFS at 6 months—%	77
Median PFS—months	15.3
Median OS—months	NR
Response in malignant meningioma patients (n = 13)	
PFS at 6 months—%	46
Median PFS—months	3.7
Median OS—months	12.4

*The authors reported that 40 patients were treated and note that there were 15 patients with benign progressive meningioma, 22 with atypical meningioma, and 13 with malignant meningioma, which totals 50 patients. Percentages are reproduced as reported in the abstract

NR, not reached; PFS, progression-free survival; OS, overall survival; PR, partial response; SD, stable disease; PD, progressive disease
Note: all data in the table were reported in Grimm et al, 2015. Median Karnofsky performance status was 80, and median age was 54 years

Treatment Modifications

BEVACIZUMAB DOSE MODIFICATIONS

Adverse Event	Treatment Modification
Gastrointestinal perforations (gastrointestinal perforations, fistula formation in the gastrointestinal tract, intra-abdominal abscess), fistula formation involving an internal organ	Discontinue bevacizumab permanently
Serious bleeding	
Wound dehiscence requiring medical intervention	
Nephrotic syndrome	
Hypertensive crisis or hypertensive encephalopathy or reversible posterior leukoencephalopathy syndrome (RPLS)	
Congestive heart failure	
Necrotizing fasciitis	
Severe arterial or venous thromboembolic events	Discontinue bevacizumab permanently; the safety of reinitiating bevacizumab after a thromboembolic event is resolved is not known
Moderate to severe proteinuria	Patients with a ≥2+ dipstick reading should undergo further assessment, eg, 24-hour urine collection. Suspend bevacizumab administration for ≥2 g proteinuria/24 h and resume when proteinuria is <2 g/24 h
Severe hypertension not controlled with medical management	Hold bevacizumab pending further evaluation and treatment of hypertension
Mild, clinically insignificant infusion reaction	Decrease the rate of infusion
Clinically significant but not severe infusion reaction	Interrupt the infusion and consider resuming at a slower rate following resolution. If decision is made to restart, the infusion may be continued at ≤50% of the rate prior to the reaction and increased in 50% increments every 30 minutes if well tolerated. Infusions may be restarted at the full rate during the next cycle
Severe infusion reaction (hypertension, hypertensive crises associated with neurologic signs and symptoms, wheezing, oxygen desaturation, G3 hypersensitivity, chest pain, headaches, rigors, and diaphoresis)	Stop infusion and administer appropriate medical therapy (eg, epinephrine, corticosteroids, intravenous antihistamines, bronchodilators, and/or oxygen). Discontinue bevacizumab
Planned elective surgery	Suspend bevacizumab at least 28 days before elective surgery and do not resume for at least 28 days after surgery or until surgical incision is fully healed
Recent hemoptysis	Do not administer bevacizumab
Evidence of rectosigmoid involvement by pelvic examination or bowel involvement on CT scan or clinical symptoms of bowel obstruction	

Adverse Events (N = 40)

Event	Bevacizumab (N = 40)*	
Grade (N)*	Grade 3	Grade 4
Hypertension	10	0
Proteinuria	2	0
Hyponatremia	2	0
Fatigue	1	0
Bruising	1	0
Nausea/vomiting	1	0
Epistaxis	1	0
Pancreatitis	1	0
Perianal infection	1	0
Ataxia	1	0
Thrombus/embolism	1	0
Anemia	0	1
Wound infection	0	1
Elevated lipase	0	1
Weakness	0	1

*The abstract does not explicitly indicate whether the numbers reported for adverse events represent numbers of patients or percentages of patients; for purposes of this table it has been assumed that the authors intended the numbers to represent the numbers of patients
The authors note that toxicity was minimal and expected for bevacizumab

MENINGIOMA, RECURRENT

CNS CANCER REGIMEN: BEVACIZUMAB + EVEROLIMUS

Shih KC et al. J Neurooncol 2016;129:281–288

Bevacizumab 10 mg/kg; administer intravenously in 100 mL 0.9% sodium chloride injection, every 2 weeks, until disease progression (total dosage/2-week cycle = 10 mg/kg), *plus:*
- *Note:* bevacizumab administration duration for the initial dose is 90 minutes. If administration is well tolerated, the administration duration may be decreased stepwise during subsequent administrations to 60 minutes and, finally, to a minimum duration of 30 minutes

Everolimus 10 mg/dose; administer orally, once daily either consistently with food or without food, continually until disease progression (total dosage/week = 70 mg)
Notes:
- Patients who delay taking everolimus at a regularly scheduled time should be instructed to administer the missed dose if the delay is ≤6 hours following the normal time of administration. If the delay is >6 hours, take the next dose at the next regularly scheduled time
- Everolimus is a substrate for cytochrome P450 (CYP) CYP3A subfamily enzymes and P-glycoprotein (P-gp). Avoid everolimus use with a concomitant P-gp inhibitor and strong CYP3A4 inhibitor. If everolimus must be used with a concomitant P-gp inhibitor and moderate CYP3A4 inhibitor, reduce the dose of everolimus. Avoid concomitant use of St. John's Wort. If concurrent use with a P-gp and strong CYP3A4 inducer is required, consider doubling the everolimus dose
- Advise patients to not consume grapefruit and grapefruit juice as they may inhibit CYP3A in the gut wall and increase the bioavailability of everolimus
- Everolimus undergoes extensive hepatic metabolism. Reduce the everolimus dose in patients with mild (Child-Pugh class A) hepatic dysfunction by 25%, moderate (Child-Pugh class B) hepatic dysfunction by 50%, and severe (Child-Pugh class C) hepatic dysfunction by 75% (if benefits outweigh risks)

Supportive Care
Antiemetic prophylaxis
Emetogenic potential of bevacizumab is **MINIMAL**
Emetogenic potential of everolimus is **MINIMAL–LOW**
See Chapter 42 for antiemetic recommendations

Hematopoietic growth factor (G-CSF) prophylaxis
Primary prophylaxis is **NOT** indicated
See Chapter 43 for more information

Antimicrobial prophylaxis
Risk of fever and neutropenia is **LOW**
  Antimicrobial primary prophylaxis to be considered:
  - Antibacterial—not indicated
  - Antifungal—not indicated
  - Antiviral—not indicated unless patient previously had an episode of HSV

Prophylaxis and treatment for mucositis/stomatitis
  General advice:
  - Dexamethasone alcohol-free mouthwash used concomitantly with everolimus decreases the incidence of stomatitis (Rugo HS et al. Lancet Oncol 2017;18:654–662):
    - **Dexamethasone 0.5 mg/5mL alcohol-free oral solution** 10 mL/dose; swish for 2 minutes and then expectorate four times per day during treatment with everolimus
  - Encourage patients to maintain intake of nonalcoholic fluids
  - Evaluate patients for oral pain and provide analgesic medications
  - Consider histamine (H_2-subtype) receptor antagonists (eg, **ranitidine**, **famotidine**), or a proton pump inhibitor for epigastric pain
  Patients with intact oral mucosa:
  - Clean the mouth, tongue, and gums by brushing after every meal and at bedtime with an ultra-soft toothbrush with fluoride toothpaste
  - Floss teeth gently every day unless contraindicated. If gums bleed and hurt, avoid bleeding or sore areas, but floss other teeth

(continued)

Efficacy (N = 17)

Efficacy Variable	Bevacizumab + Everolimus (N = 17)*
Survival in all patients (n = 16)*	
Median PFS—months (95% CI)	22.0 (4.5–26.8)
PFS rate at 6 months—%	69
PFS rate at 12 months—%	57
PFS rate at 18 months—%	57
Median OS—months (95% CI)	23.85 (9.0–33.1)
OS rate at 18 months—%	69
PFS in patients with WHO grade I (benign) tumors (n = 4)	
Median PFS—months (95% CI)	17.58 (0.91–26.4)
PFS in patients with WHO grade II or III (atypical or malignant) tumors (n = 12)	
Median PFS—months (95% CI)	22.05 (4.27–23.85)
Tumor response in all patients (n = 17)*	
CR rate—n/N (%)	0/17 (0)
PR rate—n/N (%)	0/17 (0)
SD rate—n/N (%)	15/17 (88)*
PD rate—n/N (%)	1/17 (6)
Not evaluable rate—n/N (%)*	1/17 (6)
Median duration of SD—months (range)	10 (2–29)

*A total of 18 patients were enrolled in the study, but 1 patient had no evidence of disease on a pre-treatment MRI and was thus not treated or included in the analyses. Additionally, 1 patient died due to disease after one 28-day cycle of treatment and was not evaluated for tumor response or PFS. Note that the tumor response data table in the paper reported data from a total of 17 patients, 1 of which was not evaluable. The table was re-created here for consistency, but the SD rate of *evaluable patients only* would be 15/16 = 94%
Note: the study was closed early due to slow accrual and never reached the projected enrollment of 41 patients. Treatment response was evaluated by MRI using the MacDonald criteria. PFS and OS were estimated using Kaplan-Meier methods. Median follow-up for PFS was 20 months (range, 4–31)
CI, confidence interval; PFS, progression-free survival; OS, overall survival; CR, complete response; PR, partial response; SD, stable disease; PD, progressive disease

(continued)

- Patients may use saline or commercial bland, nonalcoholic rinses
  - Do not use mouthwashes that contain alcohols

If mucositis or stomatitis is present:
- Keep the mouth moist utilizing water, ice chips, sugarless gum, sugar-free hard candies, or a saliva substitute
- Rinse mouth several times a day to remove debris
  - Use a solution of ¼ teaspoon (1.25 g) each of baking soda and table salt (**sodium chloride**) in 1 quart (~950 mL) of warm water. Follow with a plain water rinse
  - Do not use mouthwashes that contain alcohols

Diarrhea management
Loperamide 4 mg orally initially after the first loose or liquid stool, *then*
Loperamide 2 mg orally every 2 hours during waking hours, *plus*
Loperamide 4 mg orally every 4 hours during hours of sleep
- Continue for at least 12 hours after diarrhea resolves
- Recurrent diarrhea after a 12-hour diarrhea-free interval is treated as a new episode
- Rehydrate orally with fluids and electrolytes during a diarrheal episode
- If a patient develops blood or mucus in stool, dehydration, or hemodynamic instability, or if diarrhea persists >48 hours despite loperamide, stop loperamide and evaluate urgently in clinic or hospitalize the patient for IV hydration
- Alternatively, a trial of **diphenoxylate hydrochloride** 2.5 mg with **atropine sulfate** 0.025 mg (eg, Lomotil)
- Initial adult dose is 2 tablets 4 times daily until control has been achieved, after which the dose may be reduced to meet individual requirements. Control may often be maintained with as little as 2 tablets daily
- Clinical improvement of acute diarrhea is usually observed within 48 hours. If improvement of chronic diarrhea after treatment with a maximum daily dose of 8 tablets is not observed within 10 days, control is unlikely with further administration

Patient Population Studied

NCT00972335 was an open-label, non-controlled phase 2 trial included 17 adult patients with progressive or refractory meningioma and evaluated treatment with bevacizumab plus everolimus. Patients were eligible if they had symptomatic WHO grade I, II, or III progressive or refractory meningioma for which they had undergone surgical resection (if possible) or definitive radiotherapy for unresectable or recurrent disease, and for which they had received ≤ 1 systemic therapy. Patients were also required to have measurable disease, an ECOG performance status of 0–2, a life expectancy of ≥12 weeks, adequate organ function, and the ability to swallow and retain whole pills. Patients were excluded if they had received prior treatment with bevacizumab, other anti-angiogenic drugs, or mTOR inhibitors; if they had evidence of bleeding diathesis or significant coagulopathy (without therapeutic anticoagulation); myocardial infarction, unstable angina, or stroke/TIA within 6 months of beginning treatment; cardiac arrythmia requiring medication; if they were undergoing chronic systemic treatment with immunosuppressive drugs; if they had HIV; or if they were using CYP3A4 inhibitors or inducers

Therapy Monitoring

Bevacizumab:
1. Observe closely for hypersensitivity reactions, especially during the first and second bevacizumab infusions
2. Vital signs (including blood pressure measurement) prior to each cycle or more frequently as indicated during treatment
3. Assess proteinuria by urine dipstick and/or urinary protein creatinine ratio prior to each cycle. Patients with a ≥2+ urine dipstick reading should undergo further assessment with a 24-hour urine collection

Everolimus:
1. Baseline and periodically:
   a. CBC with differential and platelet count, ALT, AST, bilirubin, alkaline phosphatase, BUN, and serum creatinine
   b. Fasting serum glucose and lipid panel. When possible, achieve optimal glucose and lipid control prior to initiation of everolimus
   c. Monitor for symptoms of pulmonary toxicity, infection, and stomatitis
2. Everolimus may impair wound healing; use caution and strongly consider withholding therapy in the peri-surgical period.
3. Advise patients to avoid live vaccines and close contact with those who have received live vaccines
4. Complete treatment of any pre-existing invasive fungal infections prior to initiating everolimus

Treatment Modifications

BEVACIZUMAB DOSE MODIFICATIONS

Adverse Event	Treatment Modification
Gastrointestinal perforations (gastrointestinal perforations, fistula formation in the gastrointestinal tract, intra-abdominal abscess), fistula formation involving an internal organ	Discontinue bevacizumab permanently
Serious bleeding	
Wound dehiscence requiring medical intervention	
Nephrotic syndrome	
Hypertensive crisis or hypertensive encephalopathy or reversible posterior leukoencephalopathy syndrome (RPLS)	
Congestive heart failure	
Necrotizing fasciitis	
Severe arterial or venous thromboembolic events	Discontinue bevacizumab permanently; the safety of reinitiating bevacizumab after a thromboembolic event is resolved is not known
Moderate to severe proteinuria	Patients with a ≥2+ dipstick reading should undergo further assessment, eg, 24-hour urine collection. Suspend bevacizumab administration for ≥2 g proteinuria/24 h and resume when proteinuria is <2 g/24 h
Severe hypertension not controlled with medical management	Hold bevacizumab pending further evaluation and treatment of hypertension
Mild, clinically insignificant infusion reaction	Decrease the rate of infusion
Clinically significant but not severe infusion reaction	Interrupt the infusion and consider resuming at a slower rate following resolution. If decision is made to restart, the infusion may be continued at ≤50% of the rate prior to the reaction and increased in 50% increments every 30 minutes if well tolerated. Infusions may be restarted at the full rate during the next cycle
Severe infusion reaction (hypertension, hypertensive crises associated with neurologic signs and symptoms, wheezing, oxygen desaturation, G3 hypersensitivity, chest pain, headaches, rigors, and diaphoresis)	Stop infusion and administer appropriate medical therapy (eg, epinephrine, corticosteroids, intravenous antihistamines, bronchodilators, and/or oxygen). Discontinue bevacizumab
Planned elective surgery	Suspend bevacizumab at least 28 days before elective surgery and do not resume for at least 28 days after surgery or until surgical incision is fully healed
Recent hemoptysis	Do not administer bevacizumab
Evidence of rectosigmoid involvement by pelvic examination or bowel involvement on CT scan or clinical symptoms of bowel obstruction	

EVEROLIMUS DOSE MODIFICATIONS

Starting dose level	10 mg orally once daily
Dose level −1	5 mg orally once daily
Dose level −2	5 mg orally once every *other* day
Dose level −3	Discontinue everolimus

Adverse Event	Dose Modification
Radiologic changes suggestive of noninfectious pneumonitis with few or no symptoms	Can continue everolimus therapy without dose alteration but with careful monitoring
Radiologic changes suggestive of noninfectious pneumonitis with moderate symptoms	Withhold everolimus until symptoms improve. Consider using corticosteroids. If symptoms improve, consider reintroducing everolimus one dose lower with careful continued monitoring

(continued)

Treatment Modifications (*continued*)

Adverse Event	Dose Modification
Radiologic changes suggestive of noninfectious pneumonitis with severe symptoms	Discontinue everolimus. Consider using corticosteroids
Diagnosis of a medically significant infection	Withhold everolimus and institute appropriate treatment promptly. Consider discontinuing everolimus
Diagnosis of invasive systemic fungal infection	Discontinue everolimus and treat with appropriate antifungal therapy
G1/2 stomatitis	Withhold everolimus and administer topical treatments (avoid alcohol- or peroxide-containing mouthwashes as they may exacerbate the condition). Do not use antifungal agents unless fungal infection has been diagnosed. If symptoms improve to <G1, everolimus treatment may begin with either the same dose or one dose level lower
G3 stomatitis	Withhold everolimus and administer topical treatments (avoid alcohol- or peroxide-containing mouthwashes as they may exacerbate the condition). Do not use antifungal agents unless fungal infection has been diagnosed. If symptoms improve to <G1, everolimus treatment may begin with one dose level lower
G4 stomatitis	Discontinue everolimus
G3 elevated blood glucose or G3 hyperlipidemia	Withhold everolimus until improvement to G ≤2, then resume everolimus at 1 lower dose level
G4 elevated blood glucose or G4 hyperlipidemia	Consider permanently discontinuing everolimus
G2 thrombocytopenia	Withhold everolimus until improvement to G ≤1, then resume at the same dose
G3/4 thrombocytopenia	Withhold everolimus until improvement to G ≤1, then resume everolimus with the dosage reduced by 1 dose level
G3 neutropenia	Withhold everolimus until improvement to G ≤2, then resume at the same dose
G4 neutropenia	Withhold everolimus until improvement to G ≤2, then resume everolimus with the dosage reduced by 1 dose level
G3 febrile neutropenia	Withhold everolimus until ANC improves to G ≤2 and no fever, then resume everolimus with the dosage reduced by 1 dose level
G4 febrile neutropenia	Permanently discontinue everolimus
Other intolerable G2 nonhematologic toxicities	Withhold everolimus until improvement to G ≤1, then resume at the same dose. If the same G2 nonhematologic toxicity recurs, withhold everolimus until improvement to G ≤1 and then resume everolimus with the dosage reduced by 1 dose level
Other G3 nonhematologic toxicities	Withhold everolimus until improvement to G ≤1, then consider resuming everolimus with the dosage reduced by 1 dose level. If the same G3 nonhematologic toxicity recurs, then permanently discontinue everolimus
Other G4 nonhematologic toxicities	Permanently discontinue everolimus

Adapted in part from AFINITOR (everolimus) prescribing information. East Hanover, NJ: Novartis Pharmaceuticals Corporation; Revised January 2020

Adverse Events (N = 17)

Event Grade (%)	Bevacizumab + Everolimus (n = 17)		
	Grade 1	Grade 2	Grade 3
Thrombocytopenia	41	12	6
Anemia	29	6	0
Leukopenia	12	0	0
Neutropenia	6	6	0
Hypercholesterolemia	24	24	6*
Mucositis	29	24	0
Fatigue	35	6	6
Proteinuria	0	24	12
Hypertriglyceridemia	18	12	6*
Rash/desquamation	12	18	6
Diarrhea	24	6	6
Hypertension	6	18	6
Limb edema	6	24	0
Vomiting	12	6	6
Anorexia	18	6	0
Nausea	18	6	0
Hyperglycemia	6	12	0
Oral cavity pain	6	12	0
Epistaxis	12	6	0
Headache	12	6	0
Arthralgia	12	6	0

*These patients (1 per adverse event) met inclusion criteria for cholesterol and triglycerides levels on enrollment, but had elevated cholesterol levels at baseline

Adverse events included in the table were treatment-related adverse events graded according to the National Cancer Institute Common Terminology Criteria for Adverse Events (NCI-CTC AE) v3 in all patients who received treatment. No Grade 4 or 5 events were reported. Treatment discontinuation due to toxicity occurred in 4 patients, for reasons of Grade 3 colitis, Grade 3 chronic thrombotic microangiopathy/Grade 3 proteinuria, Grade 2 proteinuria/nephrotic syndrome, and Grade 3 thrombocytopenia (n = 1 each). Other reasons for treatment discontinuation included disease progression (n = 6), intercurrent illness (n = 2), patient request (n = 2), and death due to disease, investigator discretion, and patient withdrawal of consent (n = 1 each)

MEDULLOBLASTOMA, NEWLY DIAGNOSED

CNS CANCER REGIMEN: CRANIOSPINAL CHEMORADIOTHERAPY FOLLOWED BY ADJUVANT CISPLATIN + VINCRISTINE + LOMUSTINE

Friedrich C et al. Eur J Cancer 2013;49:893–903
Packer RJ et al. J Clin Oncol 2006;24:4202–4208
Packer RJ et al. J Neurosurg 1994;81:690–698

Chemoradiotherapy:

Craniospinal radiation therapy once daily at 1.8 Gy/fraction for 5 days/week for a total of 13 fractions (total dosage of craniospinal radiation = 23.4 Gy), *followed by:*

Notes:

- The whole brain treatment volume extends to the entire frontal lobe and cribriform plate region

- The spinal treatment volume extends laterally to cover the recesses of the vertebral bodies with at least 1 cm margin on either side and inferiorly 1–2 cm below the termination of the thecal sac

- The duration of craniospinal radiation therapy is not to exceed 20 days

Posterior fossa boost radiation therapy once daily at 1.8 Gy/fraction for 5 days/week for a total of 18 fractions [total dosage of posterior fossa boost radiation = 32.4 Gy; total dosage of all radiation therapy (craniospinal + posterior fossa boost) = 55.8 Gy]

Notes:

- The boost volume includes the entire posterior fossa with a 1-cm margin around the tentorium. The study protocol originally administered boost radiotherapy by parallel opposing fields, but later allowed conformal radiation therapy techniques

- The total duration of radiation therapy, including craniospinal radiation and posterior fossa radiation boost, is not to exceed 51 days

Vincristine 1.5 mg/m^2 (maximum dose = 2 mg) per dose; administer by intravenous infusion over 15 minutes in 50 mL 0.9% sodium chloride injection (0.9% NS) every 7 days during radiation therapy until either completion of radiation therapy or for up to 8 doses, whichever comes first (total dosage/week during radiation therapy = 1.5 mg/m^2; total maximum dosage/week during radiation therapy = 2 mg)

- *Note:* adult patients are at higher risk for vincristine neurotoxicity; monitor closely during therapy. Consider dose modification or omission of vincristine during radiotherapy in adult patients

Adjuvant chemotherapy (begin 6 weeks after completion of radiation therapy):

Lomustine 75 mg/m^2; administer orally as a single dose, without food, on day 1, every 6 weeks, for 8 cycles (total dosage/6-week cycle = 75 mg/m^2), *plus:*

- *Note:* to reduce the likelihood of a medication error leading to severe myelosuppression, prescribe, dispense, and administer only enough capsules to supply one dose of lomustine. Educate patients that only one dose of lomustine is to be taken every 6 weeks and only after documentation of adequate hematologic recovery (ISMP, 2014. https://www.ismp.org/resources/oral-chemotherapy-we-simply-must-do-better. Accessed June 20, 2018)

Hydration before cisplatin: ≥1000 mL 0.9% NS; intravenously over a minimum of 1 hour before commencing cisplatin administration

Cisplatin 75 mg/m^2; administer intravenously, diluted in 100–250 mL 0.9% NS over 6 hours on day 2, every 6 weeks, for 8 cycles (total dosage/6-week cycle = 75 mg/m^2), *plus:*

Hydration after cisplatin: Administer by intravenous infusion ≥1000 mL 0.9% NS over a minimum of 1 hour. Encourage patients to increase oral intake of non-alcoholic fluids, and provide electrolyte replacement as needed (potassium, magnesium, sodium)

Vincristine 1.5 mg/m^2 (maximum dose = 2 mg) per dose; administer by intravenous infusion over 15 minutes in 50 mL 0.9% NS for 3 doses on days 2, 8, and 15, every 6 weeks, for 8 cycles (total dosage/6-week cycle = 4.5 mg/m^2; total maximum dosage/6-week cycle = 6 mg)

Supportive Care

Antiemetic prophylaxis

Emetogenic potential of vincristine during radiotherapy is **MINIMAL**

Emetogenic potential on day 1 of adjuvant chemotherapy is **MODERATE TO HIGH**

Emetogenic potential on day 2 of adjuvant chemotherapy is **HIGH**. *Potential for delayed symptoms*

Emetogenic potential on days 8 and 15 of adjuvant chemotherapy is **MINIMAL**

See Chapter 42 for antiemetic recommendations

Hematopoietic growth factor (CSF) prophylaxis

Primary prophylaxis is **NOT** *indicated*

See Chapter 43 for more information

Antimicrobial prophylaxis

Risk of fever and neutropenia is **LOW**

Antimicrobial primary prophylaxis to be considered:

- Antibacterial—not indicated

- Antifungal—not indicated

- Antiviral—not indicated unless patient previously had an episode of HSV

Patient Population Studied

This randomized phase 3 trial included 379 mostly pediatric patients with non-disseminated medulloblastoma and compared treatment with lomustine plus cisplatin plus vincristine (n = 193) to cyclophosphamide plus cisplatin plus vincristine (n = 186). Patients were eligible for the trial if they had histologically confirmed posterior fossa medulloblastoma, if they were between 3–21 years old at diagnosis, if they had no evidence of disseminated disease on MRI of the full brain and spine pre- or postoperatively or on cytologic examination of lumbar CSF (between surgery and radiation therapy), if they had <1.5 cm³ of residual tumor volume on neuroimaging within 21 days postoperatively, and if they had adequate organ function. Patients with brainstem involvement could partake. Patients were excluded from the trial if they had received any previous chemotherapy or radiotherapy (other than corticosteroids)

Efficacy (N = 379)

Efficacy Variable	Lomustine + Cisplatin + Vincristine (N = 193)	Cyclophosphamide + Cisplatin + Vincristine (N = 186)
Survival by treatment group (n = 379 total; n per group as in the column headers)		
EFS rate at 5 years—% ± SE	82 ± 2.8	80 ± 3.1
OS rate at 5 years—% ± SE*	87 ± 2.6	85 ± 2.8
Survival in entire cohort (n = 379)		
EFS rate at 5 years—% ± SE	81 ± 2.1	
OS rate at 5 years—% ± SE*	86 ± 1.9	
Survival in patients with excessive anaplasia (n = 48)†		
EFS rate at 5 years—% ± SE	73 ± 6.4‡	
OS rate at 5 years—% ± SE*	75 ± 6.4ᶜ	
Survival in patients without excessive anaplasia (n = 279 total)†		
EFS rate at 5 years—% ± SE	83 ± 2.3‡	
OS rate at 5 years—% ± SE*	89 ± 1.9ᶜ	

*OS is reported as an actuarial survival probability
†Central pathologic review was performed on 358 of 421 samples by neuropathologists in which they evaluated tumors for evidence of excessive focal or diffuse anaplasia. There was no difference in EFS between focal and diffuse severe anaplasia, nor were there any differences in patterns of failure or relapse between anaplastic and non-anaplastic tumors
‡P = 0.087 for the comparison of patients with vs without excessive anaplasia
ᶜP = 0.005 for the comparison of patients with vs without excessive anaplasia
Note: of 421 patients enrolled in the study, 42 patients were excluded from analysis after central review of imaging found that they met exclusion criteria, including postoperative residual disease >1.5 cm³ (15 patients), metastatic disease (15 patients), ineligible pathology (4), incomplete staging (4), and others. The remaining 379 analyzed patients included 66 patients who had no clear evidence of excess residual or metastatic disease, but whose studies were incompletely evaluable due to poor quality or incomplete submissions. Randomization was stratified by age and brainstem involvement. All analyses were performed in the intention-to-treat population. EFS and OS were assessed by institutional review. Analysis found a significant effect of assessability (comparing fully assessable patients to those who were incompletely assessable, those who were ineligible due to unequivocal excess residual, and those with disseminated disease) on 5-year EFS (log-rank P <0.005), with 5-year EFS of 36% in patients with disseminated disease and 83% in those who were fully assessable. The median follow-up time was just over 5 years, with all patients having been followed for ≥3 years
SE, standard error; EFS, event-free survival; OS, overall survival

Therapy Monitoring

1. *Prior to the start of each adjuvant chemotherapy cycle:* CBC with differential and platelet count, BUN, serum creatinine, potassium, magnesium, liver function tests (ALT, AST, total bilirubin, direct bilirubin, alkaline phosphate); consider baseline pulmonary function testing (PFTs) especially in patients with any pulmonary symptoms
2. *Weekly during adjuvant chemotherapy:* CBC with differential and platelet count, BUN, serum creatinine, potassium, magnesium, liver function tests (ALT, AST, total bilirubin, direct bilirubin, alkaline phosphate); repeat PFTs if symptoms of potential pulmonary compromise develop
3. *Vincristine toxicity:* perform a neurologic exam prior to each dose

Treatment Modifications

CISPLATIN + VINCRISTINE + LOMUSTINE

Adverse Event	Treatment Modifications
Day 1 ANC <750/mm^3 or platelets <75,000/mm^3	Delay start of cycle until ANC ≥750/mm^3 and platelets ≥75,000/mm^3. Note that day 8 and day 15 vincristine should not be delayed for hematologic toxicity
Patient concurrently taking drugs known to inhibit drug metabolism by hepatic cytochrome P450 isoenzymes in the CYP 3A subfamily	Adjust vincristine dose
Total serum bilirubin 1.5–3 mg/dL	Reduce vincristine dose by 50%
Total serum bilirubin >3 mg/dL	Withhold vincristine
Severe abdominal pain or severe jaw pain	Reduce vincristine dose by 50% for all subsequent doses
G ≥3 peripheral neuropathy or G ≥3 motor neuropathy	Withhold vincristine until symptoms have resolved to G ≤1, then resume at full dosage. If symptoms recur to G ≥3, then again withhold vincristine until resolution to G ≤1 and either reduce subsequent vincristine doses by 50% or discontinue vincristine.
SIADH	Reduce vincristine dose or discontinue vincristine
Constipation, abdominal cramps, paralytic ileus	Temporarily discontinue vincristine. Treat symptoms. Resume vincristine at full dose when normal bowel function restored. Administer a routine prophylactic regimen against constipation
Creatinine clearance <50% of baseline value	Withhold cisplatin until improvement in creatinine clearance to ≥50% of baseline value, then reduce subsequent cisplatin doses by 50%
Creatinine clearance ≥50% but <75% of baseline value	Reduce cisplatin dose by 50%
Cisplatin induced hearing loss G ≥3	Permanently discontinue cisplatin
Significant hypersensitivity reaction to cisplatin (hypotension, dyspnea, and angioedema requiring therapy) *Note:* allergic reaction to cisplatin including anaphylaxis risk is increased in patients previously exposed to platinum therapy	May occur within minutes of administration. Interrupt the infusion in patients with clinically significant infusion reactions. Discontinue therapy or can consider desensitization and a rechallenge
Any pulmonary symptoms, but with PFT showing DLco ≥ the predicted value	Continue with same lomustine dose
Any pulmonary symptoms, but with PFT showing <60% of the predicted value	Discontinue lomustine
Decreased oxygen saturation at rest (eg, pulse oximeter <88% or Pao$_2$ ≤55 mm Hg)	
Shortness of breath at rest or shortness of breath that limits self-care or ADLs	
Severe cough limiting self-care or ADLs	
Cumulative lomustine dosage >1100 mg/m^2	Discontinue lomustine due to concerns of developing pulmonary fibrosis

Notes:
- Usually no more than a total of 8 cycles (600 mg/m^2) of lomustine is recommended in this regimen. Patients receiving >1100 mg/m^2 cumulative lomustine dosage have a higher risk of developing pulmonary toxicity. Patients with a baseline FVC or DLco <70% are particularly at risk (GLEOSTINE [lomustine] capsules; June 2018 product label. NextSource Biotechnology, LLC, Miami, FL)

Adverse Events (N = 379)

Event Category	Lomustine + Cisplatin + Vincristine (N = 193)		Cyclophosphamide + Cisplatin + Vincristine (N = 186)	
Grade (%)	Grade 3 or 4	Grade 4	Grade 3 or 4	Grade 4
Hematologic	97	82*	98	90*
Hepatic	12	1.7	11	2.2
Renal	9	1.1	5	0
Pulmonary	3.4	1.6	2.2	1.6
Nervous system	51	5.4	46	3.8
Hearing	28	5.8	23	6.7
Electrolytes	6.2†	1.7	12†	3.9
Infection	18*	1.6‡	30*	6.9‡
Performance score reduction	21†	4.9	14†	4.8

*P <0.01 for the comparison between treatment regimens
†P <0.1 for the comparison between treatment regimens
‡ P <0.05 for the comparison between treatment regimens
This table includes the cumulative rate of adverse events over the full course of therapy. No deaths were reported due to adverse events of therapy

Secondary malignant neoplasms in the lomustine + cisplatin + vincristine group

Event	Month
Myelodysplastic syndrome	76
Pilocytic astrocytoma	77
T-cell acute lymphoblastic leukemia	38
Basal cell carcinoma	56

Secondary malignant neoplasms in the cyclophosphamide + cisplatin + vincristine group

Event	Month
Malignant glioma (cerebellar)	62
Glioblastoma (temporal)	63
Glioblastoma (cerebellar)	44

MEDULLOBLASTOMA, NEWLY DIAGNOSED

CNS CANCER REGIMEN: CRANIOSPINAL CHEMORADIOTHERAPY FOLLOWED BY ADJUVANT CISPLATIN + VINCRISTINE + CYCLOPHOSPHAMIDE

Friedrich C et al. Eur J Cancer 2013;49:893–903
Packer RJ et al. J Clin Oncol 2006;24:4202–4208
Packer RJ et al. J Neurosurg 1994;81:690–698

Chemoradiotherapy:

Craniospinal radiation therapy once daily at 1.8 Gy/fraction for 5 days/week for a total of 13 fractions (total dosage of craniospinal radiation = 23.4 Gy), *followed by:*

Notes:
- The whole brain treatment volume extends to the entire frontal lobe and cribriform plate region
- The spinal treatment volume extends laterally to cover the recesses of the vertebral bodies with at least 1 cm margin on either side and inferiorly 1–2 cm below the termination of the thecal sac
- The duration of craniospinal radiation therapy is not to exceed 20 days

Posterior fossa boost radiation therapy once daily at 1.8 Gy/fraction for 5 days/week for a total of 18 fractions [total dosage of posterior fossa boost radiation = 32.4 Gy; total dosage of all radiation therapy (craniospinal + posterior fossa boost) = 55.8 Gy]

Notes:
- The boost volume includes the entire posterior fossa with a 1 cm margin around the tentorium. The study protocol originally administered boost radiotherapy by parallel opposing fields, but later allowed conformal radiation therapy techniques
- The total duration of radiation therapy, including craniospinal radiation and posterior fossa radiation boost, is not to exceed 51 days

Vincristine 1.5 mg/m² (maximum dose = 2 mg) per dose; administer by intravenous infusion over 15 minutes in 50 mL 0.9% sodium chloride injection (0.9% NS) every 7 days during radiation therapy until either completion of radiation therapy or for up to 8 doses, whichever comes first (total dosage/week during radiation therapy = 1.5 mg/m²; total maximum dosage/week during radiation therapy = 2 mg)
- *Note:* adult patients are at higher risk for vincristine neurotoxicity; monitor closely during therapy. Consider dose modification or omission of vincristine during radiotherapy in adult patients

Adjuvant chemotherapy (begin 6 weeks after completion of radiation therapy):

Hydration before cisplatin: ≥1000 mL 0.9% NS; intravenously over a minimum of 1 hour before commencing cisplatin administration on day 1

Cisplatin 75 mg/m²; administer intravenously, diluted in 100–250 mL 0.9% NS over 1–6 hours on day 1, every 6 weeks, for 8 cycles (total dosage/6-week cycle = 75 mg/m²), *plus:*

Hydration after cisplatin: Administer by intravenous infusion ≥1000 mL 0.9% NS over a minimum of 1 hour on day 1. Encourage patients to increase oral intake of non-alcoholic fluids, and provide electrolyte replacement as needed (potassium, magnesium, sodium)

Vincristine 1.5 mg/m² (maximum dose = 2 mg) per dose; administer by intravenous infusion over 15 minutes in 50 mL 0.9% NS for 3 doses on days 1, 8, and 15, every 6 weeks, for 8 cycles (total dosage/6-week cycle = 4.5 mg/m²; total maximum dosage/6-week cycle = 6 mg)
- *Note:* Packer RJ et al administered vincristine on days 2, 8, and 15; however, for convenience the schedule has been modified above to days 1, 8, and 15

Intravenous hydration before cyclophosphamide administration:
0.9% NS 500–1000 mL; administer over at least 1 hour on days 22 and 23

Cyclophosphamide 1000 mg/m² per dose; administer intravenously in 25–250 mL 0.9% NS or **5% dextrose injection** over 60 minutes, for 2 doses given on days 22 and 23, every 6 weeks, for 8 cycles (total dosage/6-week cycle = 2000 mg/m²)

(continued)

Patient Population Studied

This randomized phase 3 trial included 379 mostly pediatric patients with non-disseminated medulloblastoma and compared treatment with lomustine plus cisplatin plus vincristine (n = 193) to cyclophosphamide plus cisplatin plus vincristine (n = 186). Patients were eligible for the trial if they had histologically confirmed posterior fossa medulloblastoma, if they were between 3–21 years old at diagnosis, if they had no evidence of disseminated disease on MRI of the full brain and spine pre- or postoperatively or on cytologic examination of lumbar CSF (between surgery and radiation therapy), if they had <1.5 cm³ of residual tumor volume on neuroimaging within 21 days postoperatively, and if they had adequate organ function. Patients with brainstem involvement could partake. Patients were excluded from the trial if they had received any previous chemotherapy or radiotherapy (other than corticosteroids)

Therapy Monitoring

1. *Prior to the start of each adjuvant chemotherapy cycle:* CBC with differential and platelet count, BUN, serum creatinine, potassium, magnesium, liver function tests (ALT, AST, total bilirubin, direct bilirubin, alkaline phosphate)

2. *Weekly during adjuvant chemotherapy:* CBC with differential and platelet count, BUN, serum creatinine, potassium, magnesium, liver function tests (ALT, AST, total bilirubin, direct bilirubin, alkaline phosphate)

3. *Vincristine toxicity:* Perform a neurologic exam prior to each dose

(continued)

Intravenous hydration after cyclophosphamide administration:
0.9% NS 500–1000 mL; administer over at least 1 hour on days 22 and 23

Supportive Care
Antiemetic prophylaxis
Emetogenic potential of vincristine during radiotherapy is **MINIMAL**
Emetogenic potential on day 1 of adjuvant chemotherapy is **HIGH**. *Potential for delayed symptoms*
Emetogenic potential on days 8 and 15 of adjuvant chemotherapy is **MINIMAL**
Emetogenic potential on days 22 and 23 of adjuvant chemotherapy is **MODERATE**
See Chapter 42 for antiemetic recommendations

Hematopoietic growth factor (CSF) prophylaxis
Primary prophylaxis is **NOT** *indicated*
See Chapter 43 for more information

Antimicrobial prophylaxis
Risk of fever and neutropenia is **LOW**
  Antimicrobial primary prophylaxis to be considered:
  • Antibacterial—not indicated
  • Antifungal—not indicated
  • Antiviral—not indicated unless patient previously had an episode of HSV

Efficacy (N = 379)

Efficacy Variable	Lomustine + Cisplatin + Vincristine (N = 193)	Cyclophosphamide + Cisplatin + Vincristine (N = 186)
Survival by treatment group (n = 379 total; n per group as in the column headers)		
EFS rate at 5 years—% ± SE	82 ± 2.8	80 ± 3.1
OS rate at 5 years—% ± SE*	87 ± 2.6	85 ± 2.8
Survival in entire cohort (n = 379)		
EFS rate at 5 years—% ± SE	81 ± 2.1	
OS rate at 5 years—% ± SE*	86 ± 1.9	
Survival in patients with excessive anaplasia (n = 48)[†]		
EFS rate at 5 years—% ± SE	73 ± 6.4[‡]	
OS rate at 5 years—% ± SE*	75 ± 6.4[ϲ]	
Survival in patients without excessive anaplasia (n = 279 total)[†]		
EFS rate at 5 years—% ± SE	83 ± 2.3[‡]	
OS rate at 5 years—% ± SE*	89 ± 1.9[ϲ]	

*OS is reported as an actuarial survival probability
[†]Central pathologic review was performed on 358 of 421 samples by neuropathologists in which they evaluated tumors for evidence of excessive focal or diffuse anaplasia. There was no difference in EFS between focal and diffuse severe anaplasia, nor were there any differences in patterns of failure or relapse between anaplastic and non-anaplastic tumors
[‡]$P = 0.087$ for the comparison of patients with vs without excessive anaplasia
[ϲ]$P = 0.005$ for the comparison of patients with vs without excessive anaplasia
Note: of 421 patients enrolled in the study, 42 patients were excluded from analysis after central review of imaging found that they met exclusion criteria, including postoperative residual disease > 1.5 cm^3 (15 patients), metastatic disease (15 patients), ineligible pathology (4), incomplete staging (4), and others. The remaining 379 analyzed patients included 66 patients who had no clear evidence of excess residual or metastatic disease, but whose studies were incompletely evaluable due to poor quality or incomplete submissions. Randomization was stratified by age and brainstem involvement. All analyses were performed in the intention-to-treat population. EFS and OS were assessed by institutional review. Analysis found a significant effect of assessability (comparing fully assessable patients to those who were incompletely assessable, those who were ineligible due to unequivocal excess residual, and those with disseminated disease) on 5-year EFS (log-rank P <0.005), with 5-year EFS of 36% in patients with disseminated disease and 83% in those who were fully assessable. The median follow-up time was just over 5 years, with all patients having been followed for ≥3 years
SE, standard error; EFS, event-free survival; OS, overall survival

Treatment Modifications

CISPLATIN + VINCRISTINE + CYCLOPHOSPHAMIDE

Adverse Event	Treatment Modifications
Day 1 ANC <1000/mm^3 or platelets <100,000/mm^3	Delay start of cycle until ANC ≥1000/mm^3 and platelets ≥100,000/mm^3. Note that day 8 and day 15 vincristine should not be delayed for hematologic toxicity
Patient concurrently taking drugs known to inhibit drug metabolism by hepatic cytochrome P450 isoenzymes in the CYP 3A subfamily	Adjust vincristine dose
Total serum bilirubin 1.5–3 mg/dL	Reduce vincristine dose by 50%
Total serum bilirubin >3 mg/dL	Withhold vincristine
Severe abdominal pain or severe jaw pain	Reduce vincristine dose by 50% for all subsequent doses
G ≥3 peripheral neuropathy or G ≥3 motor neuropathy	Withhold vincristine until symptoms have resolved to G ≤1, then resume at full dosage. If symptoms recur to G ≥3, then again withhold vincristine until resolution to G ≤1 and either reduce subsequent vincristine doses by 50% or discontinue vincristine
SIADH	Reduce vincristine dose or discontinue vincristine
Constipation, abdominal cramps, paralytic ileus	Temporarily discontinue vincristine. Treat symptoms. Resume vincristine at full dose when normal bowel function restored. Administer a routine prophylactic regimen against constipation
Creatinine clearance <50% of baseline value	Withhold cisplatin until improvement in creatinine clearance to ≥50% of baseline value, then reduce subsequent cisplatin doses by 50%
Creatinine clearance ≥50% but <75% of baseline value	Reduce cisplatin dose by 50%
Cisplatin induced hearing loss G ≥3	Permanently discontinue cisplatin
Significant hypersensitivity reaction to cisplatin (hypotension, dyspnea, and angioedema requiring therapy) *Note:* allergic reaction to cisplatin including anaphylaxis risk is increased in patients previously exposed to platinum therapy	May occur within minutes of administration. Interrupt the infusion in patients with clinically significant infusion reactions. Discontinue therapy or can consider desensitization and a rechallenge

Adverse Events (N = 379)

Event category	Lomustine + Cisplatin + Vincristine (N = 193)		Cyclophosphamide + Cisplatin + Vincristine (N = 186)	
Grade (%)	Grade 3 or 4	Grade 4	Grade 3 or 4	Grade 4
Hematologic	97	82*	98	90*
Hepatic	12	1.7	11	2.2
Renal	9	1.1	5	0
Pulmonary	3.4	1.6	2.2	1.6
Nervous system	51	5.4	46	3.8
Hearing	28	5.8	23	6.7
Electrolytes	6.2†	1.7	12†	3.9
Infection	18*	1.6‡	30*	6.9‡
Performance score reduction	21†	4.9	14†	4.8

*P <0.01 for the comparison between treatment regimens
†P <0.1 for the comparison between treatment regimens
‡P <0.05 for the comparison between treatment regimens
This table includes the cumulative rate of adverse events over the full course of therapy. No deaths were reported due to adverse events of therapy

Secondary malignant neoplasms in the lomustine + cisplatin + vincristine group

Event	Month
Myelodysplastic syndrome	76
Pilocytic astrocytoma	77
T-cell acute lymphoblastic leukemia	38
Basal cell carcinoma	56

Secondary malignant neoplasms in the cyclophosphamide + cisplatin + vincristine group

Event	Month
Malignant glioma (cerebellar)	62
Glioblastoma (temporal)	63
Glioblastoma (cerebellar)	44

MEDULLOBLASTOMA, NEWLY DIAGNOSED

CNS CANCER REGIMEN: CRANIOSPINAL CHEMORADIOTHERAPY FOLLOWED BY ADJUVANT CISPLATIN + LOMUSTINE + VINCRISTINE + CYCLOPHOSPHAMIDE (COG ACNS0331)

Michalski JM et al. Int J Radiat Oncol Biol Phys 2016;96:937–938
Protocol for ACNS0331, version date 9/28/12, available at: https://www.skion.nl/workspace/uploads/ACNS0331DOC-versie–28092012_1.pdf [accessed 11 July 2020]

Chemoradiotherapy (begin within 31 days of definitive surgery):
Craniospinal radiation therapy once daily at 1.8 Gy/fraction for 5 days/week for a total of 13 fractions (total dosage of craniospinal radiation = 23.4 Gy), *followed by:*

Involved field boost radiation therapy once daily at 1.8 Gy/fraction for 5 days/week for a total of 17 fractions (total dosage of involved field boost radiation therapy = 30.6 Gy; cumulative dosage to the boost volume [craniospinal + involved field boost radiation] = 54 Gy)

Vincristine 1.5 mg/m² (maximum dose = 2 mg) per dose; administer by intravenous infusion over 15 minutes in 50 mL 0.9% sodium chloride injection (0.9% NS) every 7 days, starting 1 week after initiation of craniospinal radiation therapy, for 6 doses during weeks 2 through 7 of radiation therapy (total dosage/week during radiation therapy = 1.5 mg/m²; total maximum dosage/week during radiation therapy = 2 mg)
• *Note:* adult patients are at higher risk for vincristine neurotoxicity; monitor closely during therapy. Consider dose modification or omission of vincristine during radiotherapy in adult patients

Maintenance chemotherapy (begin 4 weeks after completion of radiation therapy; a total of 9 cycles of chemotherapy are administered comprising "A" and "B" cycles administered in the following sequence: AABAABAAB):

"A" cycles (to be administered in cycles 1, 2, 4, 5, 7, and 8; "A" cycle length = 6 weeks)

Hydration before cisplatin: ≥1000 mL 0.9% NS; intravenously over a minimum of 1 hour before commencing cisplatin administration

Cisplatin 75 mg/m²; administer intravenously, diluted in 100–250 mL 0.9% NS over 6 hours on day 1, for 6 cycles during cycles 1, 2, 4, 5, 7, and 8 (total dosage/6-week "A" cycle = 75 mg/m²), *plus:*

Hydration after cisplatin: Administer by intravenous infusion ≥1000 mL 0.9% NS over a minimum of 1 hour. Encourage patients to increase oral intake of non-alcoholic fluids, and provide electrolyte replacement as needed (potassium, magnesium, sodium)

Lomustine 75 mg/m²; administer orally as a single dose, without food, on day 1, for 6 cycles during cycles 1, 2, 4, 5, 7, and 8 (total dosage/6-week "A" cycle = 75 mg/m²), *plus:*
• *Note:* to reduce the likelihood of a medication error leading to severe myelosuppression, prescribe, dispense, and administer only enough capsules to supply one dose of lomustine. Educate patients that only one dose of lomustine is to be taken no more frequently than every 6 weeks and only after documentation of adequate hematologic recovery. (ISMP, 2014. https://www.ismp.org/resources/oral-chemotherapy-we-simply-must-do-better. Accessed June 20, 2018)

Vincristine 1.5 mg/m² (maximum dose = 2 mg) per dose; administer by intravenous infusion over 15 minutes in 50 mL 0.9% NS for 3 doses on days 1, 8, and 15, **for 6 cycles during cycles 1, 2, 4, 5, 7, and 8** (total dosage/6-week "A" cycle = 4.5 mg/m²; total maximum dosage/6-week "A" cycle = 6 mg)

"B" cycles (to be administered in cycles 3, 6, and 9; "B" cycle length = 4 weeks)

Intravenous hydration before cyclophosphamide administration:
0.9% NS 500–1000 mL; administer over at least 1 hour on days 1 and 2

Cyclophosphamide 1000 mg/m² per dose; administer intravenously in 25–250 mL 0.9% NS or **5% dextrose injection** (D5W) over 60 minutes, for 2 doses given on days 1 and 2, for 3 cycles **during cycles 3, 6, and 9** (total dosage/4-week "B" cycle = 2000 mg/m²)

Intravenous hydration after cyclophosphamide administration:
0.9% NS 500–1000 mL; administer over at least 1 hour on days 1 and 2

Mesna 360 mg/m² per dose; administer intravenously, diluted with 0.9% NS or D5W to a concentration within the range of 1–20 mg/mL, over 15 minutes just prior to the start of each cyclophosphamide infusion and repeated at hours 4 and 8 after the start of each cyclophosphamide infusion on days 1 and 2, for 3 cycles during cycles 3, 6, and 9 (total dosage/4-week "B" cycle = 2160 mg)

Vincristine 1.5 mg/m² (maximum dose = 2 mg) per dose; administer by intravenous infusion over 15 minutes in 50 mL 0.9% NS for 2 doses on days 1 and 8, for 3 **cycles during cycles 3, 6, and 9** (total dosage/4-week "B" cycle = 3 mg/m²; total maximum dosage/4-week "B" cycle = 4 mg)

Supportive Care
Antiemetic prophylaxis
*Emetogenic potential of vincristine during radiotherapy is **MINIMAL***
*Emetogenic potential on day 1 of "A" cycles is **HIGH**. Potential for delayed symptoms*
*Emetogenic potential on days 8 and 15 of "A" cycles is **MINIMAL***
*Emetogenic potential on days 1 and 2 of "B" cycles is **MODERATE***
*Emetogenic potential on day 8 of "B" cycles is **MINIMAL***
See Chapter 42 for antiemetic recommendations

(continued)

(continued)

Hematopoietic growth factor (CSF) prophylaxis
*Primary prophylaxis is **NOT** indicated*
See Chapter 43 for more information

Antimicrobial prophylaxis
*Risk of fever and neutropenia is **LOW***
Antimicrobial primary prophylaxis to be considered:
- Antibacterial—not indicated
- Antifungal—not indicated
- Antiviral—not indicated unless patient previously had an episode of HSV

Patient Population Studied

COG ACNS0331 was a randomized, comparative, open-label, phase 3 trial that included 464 pediatric patients with average-risk medulloblastoma. All eligible patients (n = 464) were randomized to receive either a radiation boost to the posterior fossa (standard volume, n = 237) or involved field radiation therapy (IFRT, experimental reduced volume, n = 227). Further, patients aged 3–7 years old (n = 226) were additionally randomized to receive either standard dose craniospinal irradiation (23.4 Gy, n = 110) or reduced dose craniospinal irradiation (18 Gy, n = 116). All patients received maintenance treatment with cisplatin, cyclophosphamide, lomustine, and vincristine. Patients were eligible if they were age 3–21 years; if they had histologically confirmed posterior fossa medulloblastoma with average-risk disease; minimum volume, non-disseminated disease (defined as residual tumor size of ≤1.5 cm^2 on MRI within 21 days of surgery and lack of metastatic disease in the head, spine, or CSF); a Karnofsky performance status of 50–100% in those > 16 years old or a Lansky performance status of 30–100% in those ≤16 years old; and adequate organ function. Patients were excluded if they had received any prior chemotherapy, corticosteroid therapy, or radiation therapy

Efficacy (N = 464)

Efficacy Variable	PFRT + Either Standard-Dose CSI or Low-Dose CSI* (n = 237)	IFRT + Either Standard-Dose CSI or Low-Dose CSI* (n = 227)	Standard-Dose CSI + Either PFRT or IFRT* in Patients Age 3–7 (n = 110)	Low-Dose CSI + Either PFRT or IFRT* in Patients Age 3–7 (n = 116)
Survival in entire cohort comparing IFRT to PFRT regardless of CSI dose (n = 464)				
EFS rate at 5 years—%	80.8 ± 3.0[†]	82.2 ± 2.9[†]	N/A	N/A
OS rate at 5 years—%	85.2 ± 2.6	84.1 ± 2.8	N/A	N/A
Survival in patients age 3–7 comparing low dose CSI to standard dose CSI dose regardless of boost volume (PFRT or IFRT) (n = 226)				
EFS rate at 5 years—%	N/A	N/A	82.6 ± 4.2[‡]	72.1 ± 4.8[‡]
OS rate at 5 years—%	N/A	N/A	85.9 ± 3.8	78.1 ± 4.4
Local treatment failure in entire cohort comparing IFRT to PFRT regardless of CSI dose (n = 464)				
Local failure rate at 5 years—%	3.7 ± 1.3[ϵ]	1.9 ± 0.1[ϵ]	N/A	N/A
Isolated distant treatment failure in patients age 3–7 comparing low dose CSI to standard dose CSI dose regardless of boost volume (PFRT or IFRT) (n = 226)				
Isolated distant failure rate at 5 years—%	N/A	N/A	8.2 ± 2.8[□]	12.8 ± 3.2[□]

*All patients received chemotherapy with cisplatin + lomustine + vincristine + cyclophosphamide
[†]Between-group differences comparing PFRT and IFRT were analyzed for noninferiority by comparing a one-sided 1-β confidence interval for the hazard ratio with a prespecified noninferiority margin of 1.6. The upper limit of the 94% confidence interval of the hazard ratio comparing EFS between treatments was 1.3, which was less than the prespecified margin of 1.6 and the authors concluded that IFRT was noninferior to PFRT
[‡]Between-group differences comparing standard and low dose CSI were analyzed for noninferiority by comparing a one-sided 1-β confidence interval for the hazard ratio with a prespecified noninferiority margin of 1.6. The upper limit of the 80% confidence interval of the hazard ratio comparing EFS between treatments was 1.9, which was more than the prespecified margin of 1.6 and the authors concluded that noninferiority of low dose CSI to standard dose CSI was not established
[ϵ]P = 0.178. 64% of posterior fossa failures included neuraxis failure. No IFRT patients had an isolated posterior fossa failure outside the boost volume
[□]P = 0.115
Note: of 549 patients enrolled, only 464 were considered eligible and without anaplasia or excessive residual disease as assessed by central review. All analyses were performed in the intention to treat population. EFS and OS rates were estimated using the Kaplan-Meier method. The analysis of the between-group difference in standard vs low dose CSI was stratified by receipt of PFRT or IFRT, and the analysis of the between-group difference in PFRT vs IFRT was stratified by CSI dose received. Median follow-up time for EFS was 6.6 years
Abbreviations: PFRT, posterior fossa radiation therapy; IFRT, involved-field radiation therapy; CSI, craniospinal irradiation; EFS, event-free survival; OS, overall survival

Therapy Monitoring

1. *Prior to the start of each maintenance chemotherapy cycle:* CBC with differential and platelet count, BUN, serum creatinine, potassium, magnesium, liver function tests (ALT, AST, total bilirubin, direct bilirubin, alkaline phosphate); consider baseline pulmonary function testing (PFTs) especially in patients with any pulmonary symptoms

2. *Weekly during maintenance chemotherapy:* CBC with differential and platelet count, BUN, serum creatinine, potassium, magnesium, liver function tests (ALT, AST, total bilirubin, direct bilirubin, alkaline phosphate); repeat PFTs if symptoms of potential pulmonary compromise develop

3. *Vincristine toxicity:* Perform a neurologic exam prior to each dose

Treatment Modifications

CISPLATIN + LOMUSTINE + VINCRISTINE (A CYCLES) AND CYCLOPHOSPHAMIDE + VINCRISTINE (B CYCLES)

Adverse Event	Treatment Modifications
Day 1 ANC ≥1000/mm^3 and platelet count ≥75,000/mm^3 and patient is due for either an "A" cycle or a "B" cycle	Proceed with cycle at the same dosage
Day 1 platelet count <75,000/mm^3 and patient is due for an "A" cycle	Delay start of cycle until platelet count ≥75,000/mm^3, then proceed with the dose of lomustine reduced to 38 mg/m^2 and with the doses of cisplatin and vincristine unchanged. Refer to treatment modifications below based on ANC if more stringent
Day 1 ANC <750/mm^3 and patient is due for an "A" cycle	Delay start of cycle until ANC ≥750/mm^3, then proceed with the dose of lomustine reduced to 20 mg/m^2 and with the doses of cisplatin and vincristine unchanged. If there is a ≥2 week delay in treatment due to neutropenia, then add G-CSF in subsequent cycles
Day 1 ANC 750–999/mm^3 and patient is due for an "A" cycle	Proceed without delay but with the dose of lomustine reduced to 38 mg/m^2 and with the doses of cisplatin and vincristine unchanged
Day 1 platelet count <75,000/mm^3 and patient is due for a "B" cycle	Delay start of cycle until platelet count ≥75,000/mm^3, then proceed with the dose of cyclophosphamide reduced to 750 mg/m^2 per dose and with the dose of vincristine unchanged. Reduce each mesna dose by 25% accordingly. Refer to treatment modifications below based on ANC if more stringent
Day 1 ANC <750/mm^3 and patient is due for a "B" cycle	Delay start of cycle until ANC ≥750/mm^3, then proceed with the dose of cyclophosphamide reduced to 500 mg/m^2 per dose and with the dose of vincristine unchanged. Reduce each mesna dose by 50% accordingly. If there is a ≥2 week delay in treatment due to neutropenia, then add G-CSF in subsequent cycles
Day 1 ANC 750–999/mm^3 and patient is due for a "B" cycle	Proceed without delay but with the dose of cyclophosphamide reduced to 750 mg/m^2 per dose and with the dose of vincristine unchanged. Reduce each mesna dose by 25% accordingly
Patient concurrently taking drugs known to inhibit drug metabolism by hepatic cytochrome P450 isoenzymes in the CYP 3A subfamily	Adjust vincristine dose
Direct bilirubin 1.5–1.9 mg/dL and total serum bilirubin ≤1.9 mg/dL	Reduce vincristine dose by 50%
Total serum bilirubin >1.9 mg/dL	Withhold vincristine
G ≥3 peripheral neuropathy or G ≥3 motor neuropathy	Withhold vincristine until symptoms have resolved to G ≤1, then resume at full dosage. If symptoms recur to G ≥3, then again withhold vincristine until resolution to G ≤1 and either reduce subsequent vincristine doses by 50% or discontinue vincristine
SIADH	Reduce vincristine dose or discontinue vincristine
Constipation, abdominal cramps, paralytic ileus	Temporarily discontinue vincristine. Treat symptoms. Resume vincristine at full dose when normal bowel function restored. Administer a routine prophylactic regimen against constipation
Creatinine clearance <50% of baseline value	Withhold cisplatin until improvement in creatinine clearance to ≥50% of baseline value, then reduce subsequent cisplatin doses by 50%

(continued)

Treatment Modifications (*continued*)

Creatinine clearance ≥50% but <75% of baseline value	Reduce cisplatin dose by 50%
Cisplatin induced hearing loss G ≥3	Permanently discontinue cisplatin
Significant hypersensitivity reaction to cisplatin (hypotension, dyspnea, and angioedema requiring therapy) *Note:* allergic reaction to cisplatin including anaphylaxis risk is increased in patients previously exposed to platinum therapy	May occur within minutes of administration. Interrupt the infusion in patients with clinically significant infusion reactions. Discontinue therapy or can consider desensitization and a rechallenge
Any pulmonary symptoms, but with PFT showing DLco ≥ the predicted value	Continue with same lomustine dose
Any pulmonary symptoms, but with PFT showing <60% of the predicted value	Discontinue lomustine
Decreased oxygen saturation at rest (eg, pulse oximeter <88% or Pao_2 ≤55 mm Hg)	
Shortness of breath at rest or shortness of breath that limits self-care or ADLs	
Severe cough limiting self-care or ADLs	
Cumulative lomustine dosage >1100 mg/m^2	Discontinue lomustine due to concerns of developing pulmonary fibrosis

Notes:
- Usually no more than a total of 6 cycles (450 mg/m^2) of lomustine is recommended in this regimen. Patients receiving >1100 mg/m^2 cumulative lomustine dosage have a higher risk of developing pulmonary toxicity. Patients with a baseline FVC or DLco <70% are particularly at risk (GLEOSTINE [lomustine] capsules; June 2018 product label. NextSource Biotechnology, LLC, Miami, FL)

Adverse Events

Ten patients developed secondary malignancies during the study; no additional information available from the abstract.

Michalski JM et al. Int J Radiat Oncol Biol Phys 2016;96:937–938

10. Cervical Cancer

Peter G. Rose, MD

Epidemiology

Incidence: 13,800 (Estimated new cases for 2020 in the United States)

7.3 per 100,000 women per year

Deaths: Estimated 4290 in 2020

Median age: 50 years

Stage at Presentation	
Localized:	44%
Regional:	36%
Distant:	15%
Unstaged:	4%

Siegel R et al. CA Cancer J Clin 2020;70:7-30
Surveillance, Epidemiology and End Results (SEER) Program, available from http://seer.cancer.gov [accessed June 2020]

Work-up

Stage IA/stage IB1:	• H&P
	• CBC with platelet count, LFTs, BUN, creatinine
	• Cervical biopsy (pathologic review)
	• Cone biopsy as indicated
	• Chest x-ray, intravenous pyelogram, for IB1 MRI ± PET
Stage IB2 or greater:	• Consider examination under anesthesia
Stages III/IV:	• Consider cystoscopy/proctoscopy

Pathology

Squamous cell carcinomas • Large cell, keratinizing • Large cell, nonkeratinizing • Small cell (not neuroendocrine) • Verrucous carcinoma	75–80%
Adenocarcinomas **HPV associated** Usual endocervical (villoglandular and micropapillary variants) Mucinous Intestinal Signet ring Adenosquamous (Invasive stratified mucin-producing carcinoma variant) **Non-HPV associated*** Gastric Clear cell Endometrioid Mesonephric	23%
Glassy cell carcinoma	Rare
Neuroendocrine small cell carcinoma	Rare

* NonHPV Associated adenocarcinomas more often have lymphovascular invasion and lymph node metastases and are associated with worse survival

Hunter RD in: Souhami RL et al editors. Oxford Textbook of Oncology, 2nd ed., New York, Oxford University Press 2002:1835-1837

Stolnicu S, et al. Virchows Archiv 2019; 475:537-49.

Histologic Grade

Gx	Cannot be assessed
G1	Well differentiated
G2	Moderately differentiated
G3	Poorly differentiated
G4	Undifferentiated

Staging

FIGO Stage (2018)

I	Cervical carcinoma is strictly confined to uterus (extension to corpus should be disregarded)
IA	Invasive carcinoma diagnosed only by microscopy, with maximum depth of invasion <5 mm*
IA1	Measured stromal invasion <3 mm in depth
IA2	Measured stromal invasion ≥3 mm and <5 mm in depth
IB	Invasive carcinoma with measured deepest invasion ≥5 mm (greater than stage IA), lesion limited to the cervix uteri†
IB1	Invasive carcinoma ≥5 mm depth of stromal invasion and <2 cm in greatest dimension
IB2	Invasive carcinoma ≥2 cm and <4 cm in greatest dimension
IB3	Invasive carcinoma ≥4 cm in greatest dimension
II	The carcinoma invades beyond the uterus, but has not extended onto the lower third of the vagina or to the pelvic wall
IIA	Involvement limited to the upper two-thirds of the vagina without parametrial involvement
IIA1	Invasive carcinoma <4 cm in greatest dimension
IIA2	Invasive carcinoma ≥4 cm in greatest dimension
IIB	With parametrial involvement but not up to the pelvic wall
III	The carcinoma involves the lower third of the vagina and/or extends to the pelvic wall and/or causes hydronephrosis or non-functioning kidney and/or involves pelvic and/or paraaortic lymph nodes‡
IIIA	Carcinoma involves the lower third of the vagina, with no extension to the pelvic wall
IIIB	Extension to the pelvic wall and/or hydronephrosis or non-functioning kidney (unless known to be due to another cause)
IIIC	Involvement of pelvic and/or paraaortic lymph nodes, irrespective of tumor size and extent (with r and p notations)‡
IIIC1	Pelvic lymph node metastasis only
IIIC2	Paraaortic lymph node metastasis
IV	The carcinoma has extended beyond the true pelvis or has involved (biopsy proven) the mucosa of the bladder or rectum. A bullous edema, as such, does not permit a case to be allotted to stage IV
IVA	Spread of the growth to adjacent organs
IVB	Spread to distant organs

*Imaging and pathology can be used, when available, to supplement clinical findings with respect to tumor size and extent, in all stages
†The involvement of vascular/lymphatic spaces does not change the staging. The lateral extent of the lesion is no longer considered
‡Adding notation of r (imaging) and p (pathology) to indicate the findings that are used to allocate the case to stage IIIC. For example, if imaging indicates pelvic lymph node metastasis, the stage allocation would be stage IIIC1r and, if confirmed by pathologic findings, it would be stage IIIc1p. The type of imaging modality or pathology technique used should always be documented. When in doubt, the lower staging should be assigned

Bhatla N et al. Int J Gynecol Obstet 2019;145:129–135

Overall 5-Year Survival Relative to FIGO* Disease Stage

Stage	% Survival
IA1	94.6
IA2	92.6
IB1	97.0
IB2	92.1
IB3	83.1
IIA	76
IIB	73.3
IIIA	50.5
IIIB	46.4
IVA	29.6
IVB	22

*International Federation of Gynecology and Obstetrics

Expert Opinion

1. The use of concurrent chemotherapy and radiation has reduced the overall mortality rate of locally advanced cervical cancer by nearly 50%

2. Concurrent chemoradiation should be given to women with high-risk local disease or regionally advanced disease

3. Dose adjustments for nephrotoxicity are presented as specified in the original trials. In a patient with creatinine clearance of <60 cc per minute would recommend replacing cisplatin with carboplatin at an AUC of 2

4. In cervical cancer, survival rates and rates of local control appear to correlate with radiation dose and the time of administration. Better results are achieved with higher radiation doses and shorter periods of administration

5. Chemotherapy agents with single-agent activity include:
   - **Cisplatin:** Considered the most active drug with response rates of 20–30%. In combination with paclitaxel, cisplatin (at a dosage of 50 mg/m^2) remains the platinum compound of choice in chemotherapy-naïve patients despite less toxicity with carboplatin based on a randomized trial. Japanese GOG 0505 (Kitagawa R et al. J Clin Oncol 2015;33:2129–2135)
   - **Paclitaxel:** 17% response rate in GOG trial (McGuire WP et al. J Clin Oncol 1996;14:792–795)
   - **Vinorelbine:** 18% response rate in patients with recurrent/metastatic carcinoma of the cervix (Morris M et al. J Clin Oncol 1998;16:1094–1098; Lacava JA et al. J Clin Oncol 1997;15:604–609); and 45% response rate in patients with previously untreated, locally advanced cervical cancer (Lhommé C et al. Eur J Cancer 2000;36:194–199)
   - **Toptecan:** 18.6% response rate in advanced, recurrent, or persistent squamous cell carcinoma of the uterine cervix (Muderspach LI et al. Gynecol Oncol 2001;81:213–215)
   - **Gemcitabine:** 11–18% response rate in patients with advanced disease (Goedhals L et al. Proc Am Soc Clin Oncol 1996;15:296 [abstract 819]; Hansen HH. Ann Oncol 1996;7(Suppl 1):29 [abstract 058])
   - **Irinotecan:** 13.3% response rate in patients with recurrent squamous carcinoma of the cervix (Look KY et al. Gynecol Oncol 1998;70:334–338)
   - **Ifosfamide:** Active in patients who have not received prior chemotherapy with response rates of 16–40% (Coleman RE et al. Cancer Chemother Pharmacol 1986;18:280–283; Meanwell CA et al. Cancer Treat Rep 1986;70:727–730; Sutton GP et al. Am J Obstet 1993;168:805–807)
   - **Nab paclitaxel:** It is also well-tolerated in women who have experienced a paclitaxel-associated hypersensitivity reaction (Maurer K et al. J Gynecol Oncol 2017;28:e38)

6. Platinum combinations yield high response rates, particularly in patients with no prior radiation therapy

7. Two randomized trials have shown improvement in progression-free survival (Long HJ III et al. J Clin Oncol 2005;26:4626–4633; Moore DH et al. J Clin Oncol 2004;22:3113–3119), with one trial demonstrating an improvement in survival for combinations (Long HJ III et al. J Clin Oncol 2005;26:4626–4633)

8. The GOG completed a randomized phase 3 trial of 4 cisplatin (CIS)-containing doublet combinations in stage IVB, recurrent or persistent cervical carcinoma. The study demonstrated that in patients with stage IVB, recurrent or persistent cancer, the combination of paclitaxel 135 mg/m^2 over 24 hours with cisplatin 50 mg/m^2 was superior to combinations of vinorelbine 30 mg/m^2, or gemcitabine 1000 mg/m^2, or topotecan 0.75 mg/m^2 with cisplatin 50 mg

9. In view of the fact that most patients currently receive cisplatin-based chemoradiation, a subsequent trial GOG 240 compared the combination of paclitaxel with cisplatin versus paclitaxel and topotecan. The study had a secondary randomization to bevacizumab. The trial demonstrated that despite prior platinum exposure during chemoradiation, patients who received the combination of paclitaxel with cisplatin had a higher response rate and progression-free survival but no improvement in overall survival when compared to patients who received paclitaxel and topotecan. Patients who received bevacizumab had a statistically improved survival by 3.7 months. There were increased toxicities including gastrointestinal and genitourinary fistula, hypertension greater than grade 2, neutropenia greater than grade 4, and thromboembolism

10. Risk factors for poorer survival include black race, performance status = 1, pelvic disease, prior cisplatin, and progression-free interval <1 year. The addition of bevacizumab resulted in improved outcomes for patients with 2–3 risk factors (HR PFS 0.69, HR OS 0.67) and for patients with 4–5 risk factors (HR PFS 0.51, HR OS 0.54), but not for patients with 0–1 risk factors. Tewari et al. Clin Cancer Res 2015;21:5480–7. Since the addition of bevacizumab increased toxicities, it should be avoided for patients with 0–1 risk factor.

11. The combination of carboplatin and paclitaxel was compared to cisplatin and paclitaxel in a randomized trial. Both were equally effective in patients who had previously received platinum compounds during radiation, but the combination of cisplatin and paclitaxel was superior for patients who are chemotherapy naïve (Kitagawa R et al. J Clin Oncol 2015;33:2129–2135)

CONCOMITANT CHEMORADIATION

CERVICAL CANCER REGIMEN: CONCURRENT RADIATION THERAPY + CHEMOTHERAPY/WEEKLY CISPLATIN

Keys HM et al. N Engl J Med 1999;340:1154–1161
Rose PG et al. N Engl J Med 1999;340:1144–1153

Note: Chemotherapy is given concomitantly with radiation therapy

Cisplatin 40 mg/m^2 per dose (maximum weekly dose 70 mg); administer intravenously in 50–250 mL 0.9% sodium chloride injection (0.9% NS) over 60 minutes weekly for 6 doses during weeks 1–6 (days 1, 8, 15, 22, 29, and 36) starting 4 hours before radiation therapy (total dosage/week = 40 mg/m^2)

Optional hydration with cisplatin: ≥500 mL 0.9% NS; administer intravenously at ≥100 mL/hour before and after cisplatin administration. Also, encourage patients to increase oral intake of nonalcoholic fluids and provide electrolyte replacement as needed (potassium, magnesium, sodium)

Supportive Care
Antiemetic prophylaxis
Emetogenic potential is **HIGH**. Potential for delayed symptoms
See Chapter 42 for antiemetic recommendations

Hematopoietic growth factor (CSF) prophylaxis
Primary prophylaxis is **NOT** indicated
See Chapter 43 for more information

Antimicrobial prophylaxis
Risk of fever and neutropenia is **LOW**
   Antimicrobial primary prophylaxis to be considered:
- Antibacterial—not indicated
- Antifungal—not indicated
- Antiviral—not indicated unless patient previously had an episode of HSV

Treatment Modifications

Adverse Event	Dose Modification
WBC <2000/mm^3	Delay radiation therapy for up to 1 week until WBC >2000/mm^3
Radiation-related gastrointestinal or genitourinary toxicity	Delay radiation therapy for up to 1 week until symptoms resolve
WBC <2500/mm^3 or platelet count <50,000/mm^3	Hold cisplatin until WBC >2500/mm^3 and platelet >50,000/mm^3
G2 neurotoxicity	Reduce cisplatin dosage to 30 mg/m^2 per dose or substitute Carboplatin AUC of 2
G ≥3 neurotoxicity	Discontinue cisplatin
Serum creatinine ≥2 mg/dL (≥177 μmol/L)	Reduce cisplatin dosage to 30 mg/m^2 per dose
Serum creatinine ≥2 mg/dL (≥177 μmol/L) despite reduction of cisplatin dosage to 30 mg/m^2	Discontinue cisplatin and substitute carboplatin dosed to achieve a target AUC of 2 mg/mL × min

Patient Population Studied

Women with untreated invasive squamous cell carcinoma, adenosquamous carcinoma, or adenocarcinoma of the cervix of International Federation of Gynecology and Obstetrics stage IB3 (limited to cervix ≥4 cm), stage IIB (localized disease with parametrial involvement), stage III (extension of tumor to the pelvic wall), or stage IVA (involvement of the bladder and rectal mucosa). Patients with disease outside the pelvis and those with metastases to paraaortic lymph nodes or intraperitoneal disease were not eligible

Therapy Monitoring

Every week: CBC with differential, serum magnesium, BUN, and creatinine

Toxicity (N = 176)

	% G1	% G2	% G3	% G4
Hematologic				
Leukopenia	17	26	21	2
Thrombocytopenia	15	4	2	0
Other hematologic	13	27	10	5
Nonhematologic				
Gastrointestinal	32	28	8	4
Genitourinary	11	6	3	2
Cutaneous	7	6	1	1
Neurologic	6	8	1	0
Pulmonary	0	1	0	0
Cardiovascular	0	0	0	0
Fever	2	4	0	0
Fatigue	5	3	0	0
Pain	2	2	0	0
Weight loss	2	2	1	0
Hypomagnesemia	3	2	2	1
Other*	5	2	1	2

NCI Common Toxicity Criteria (version not specified). All versions available at: http://ctep.cancer.gov/protocolDevelopment/electronic_applications/ctc.htm [accessed December 7, 2013]
*Includes G3 renal abnormalities (serum creatinine 3.1–6 times institutional upper limit of normal), G3 electrolyte imbalance, G3 dehydration, G3 hepatic infection, G4 lymphopenia, G4 vaginal necrosis, G4 edema, and G4 renal abnormalities (serum creatinine >6 times institutional upper limit of normal)

G1, minimal; G2, mild; G3, moderate; G4, severe
Rose PG et al. N Engl J Med 1999;340:1144–1153

Notes

1. Number of cycles of chemotherapy:

No. of Cycles	% of Patients
0	0.6
1	1.1
2	1.1
3	4
4	10.2
5	33.5
≥6	49.4

2. Radiation therapy (RT) administered:

Percentage of patients who received ≥85% of prescribed RT to both points A and B	90%
Median delay in patients receiving ≥85% of prescribed RT	8 days
Median duration of treatment	9 weeks

3. The rate of local recurrences was significantly lower than the comparison arm with hydroxyurea, whereas the rate of distant recurrences, especially in the lungs, was only slightly less. These results suggest that the principal effect of cisplatin is radiosensitization

Efficacy (N = 176)

	%	P Value*
Probability of progression-free survival at 48 months	62	0.001
Probability of survival at 48 months	66.5	0.004
Progression-free survival at 24 months	67[†]	—
Local progression	19[†]	—
Lung metastases	20[†]	—

*Compared with control group (RT + hydroxyurea)
[†]In control group (RT + hydroxyurea), progression-free survival at 24 months = 47%, local progression = 30%, and lung metastases = 10%

Rose PG et al. N Engl J Med 1999;340:1144–1153

ADVANCED/RECURRENT • FIRST-LINE

CERVICAL CANCER REGIMEN: CISPLATIN + PACLITAXEL

Moore DH et al. J Clin Oncol 2004;22:3113–3119 (GOG 169, 204)

Premedication for paclitaxel:

Dexamethasone 20 mg/dose; administer orally or intravenously for 2 doses at 12 hours and 6 hours before paclitaxel

Note: If patient has no acute toxicities to paclitaxel, the dexamethasone doses at 12 hours and 6 hours before paclitaxel may eventually be omitted

Diphenhydramine 50 mg; administer intravenously 30 minutes before paclitaxel

Cimetidine 300 mg, *or* **ranitidine** 50 mg, *or* **famotidine** 20 mg; administer intravenously over 5–20 minutes, 30 minutes before paclitaxel

Paclitaxel 135 mg/m^2; administer by continuous intravenous infusion in a volume of 0.9% sodium chloride injection (0.9% NS) or 5% dextrose injection (D5W) sufficient to produce a concentration within the range 0.3–1.2 mg/mL over 24 hours on day 1, every 3 weeks for 6 cycles (total dosage/cycle = 135 mg/m^2)

Hydration before and after cisplatin:
≥1000 mL 0.45% sodium chloride injection; administer intravenously over a minimum of 2–4 hours. Encourage patients to increase oral intake of nonalcoholic fluids, and provide electrolyte replacement as needed (potassium, magnesium, sodium)

Cisplatin 50 mg/m^2; administer intravenously in 50–250 mL 0.9% NS at a rate of 1 mg/min on day 2 after completing paclitaxel administration, every 3 weeks for 6 cycles (total dosage/cycle = 50 mg/m^2)

Note: Begin cisplatin within 4 hours after completing paclitaxel administration

Supportive Care
Antiemetic prophylaxis
Emetogenic potential during paclitaxel administration is **LOW**
Emetogenic potential on day 2 is **HIGH**. *Potential for delayed symptoms*
See Chapter 42 for antiemetic recommendations

Hematopoietic growth factor (CSF) prophylaxis
Primary prophylaxis may be indicated
See Chapter 43 for more information

Antimicrobial prophylaxis
Risk of fever and neutropenia is **LOW**
   Antimicrobial primary prophylaxis to be considered:
   • Antibacterial—not indicated
   • Antifungal—not indicated
   • Antiviral—not indicated unless patient previously had an episode of HSV

Treatment Modifications

Cisplatin Dose Levels	
Initial dosage	50 mg/m^2
Dose level −1	37.5 mg/m^2
Dose level −2	25 mg/m^2
Paclitaxel Dose Levels	
Initial dosage	135 mg/m^2
Dose level −1	110 mg/m^2
Dose level −2	90 mg/m^2

(continued)

Patient Population Studied

A study of women with advanced (stage IVB), recurrent, or persistent squamous cell carcinoma of the uterine cervix, 24% of whom had received prior chemotherapy and radiation

Efficacy (N = 130)

Complete response	15%
Partial response	21%
Overall response rate (ORR)	36%
ORR, prior chemoradiotherapy (n = 31)	32%
ORR, no prior chemoradiotherapy (n = 99)	37%
Progression-free survival	4.8 months
Progression-free survival, no prior therapy	4.9 months
Median survival	9.7 months
Median survival, no prior therapy	9.9 months

Toxicity (N = 129)

	% G1	% G2	% G3	% G4
Hematologic				
Leukopenia	12.4	22.5	35.7	17
Granulocytopenia	7.8	7.8	20.9	45.7
Thrombocytopenia	30.2	3.1	1.6	2.3
Anemia	10.9	31	22.5	5.4
Nonhematologic				
Nausea/vomiting	29.5	20.9	9.3	0.8
Other gastrointestinal	14	9.3	6.2	0.8
Cardiac	1.6	1.6	1.6	0
Neurologic	19.4	13.2	3.1	0
Fever	1.6	13.2	0	0.8
Dermatologic	2.3	1.6	1.6	0.8
Alopecia	11.6	52.7	0	0
Genitourinary	6.2	10.9	0.8	0
Renal	4.7	7	2.3	0

Treatment Modifications (*continued*)

Adverse Event	Dose Modification
Day 1 ANC <1500/mm³ *or* platelet count <100,000/mm³	Hold chemotherapy until ANC ≥1500/mm³ *and* platelet count ≥100,000/mm³
ANC <1500/mm³ *or* platelet count <100,000/mm³ persists ≥2 weeks beyond the scheduled start of cycle	Discontinue therapy
G4 thrombocytopenia	Reduce paclitaxel dosage by 1 level; continue with same cisplatin dosage
G3/4 ANC with fever*	
G3/4 ANC with fever despite paclitaxel dosage reduction by 1 dose level	Administer filgrastim with all subsequent courses
G3/4 ANC with fever despite paclitaxel dose reduction and filgrastim	Reduce paclitaxel dosage by 1 level or 20%; continue with same cisplatin dosage
G2 peripheral neuropathy	Reduce paclitaxel dosage by 2 dose levels
G3/4 peripheral neuropathy	Hold paclitaxel until neuropathy G ≤1; then reduce paclitaxel dosage by 2 dose levels. If G3/4 toxicity persists >2 weeks beyond scheduled start of next cycle, discontinue paclitaxel
G2 hepatic toxicity	Hold paclitaxel until toxicity G ≤1; then reduce paclitaxel dosage by 1 dose level
G3/4 hepatic toxicity	Hold paclitaxel until toxicity G ≤1; then reduce paclitaxel dosage by 1–2 dose levels. If G3/4 toxicity persists >2 weeks beyond scheduled start of cycle, discontinue paclitaxel
G2/3/4 nephrotoxicity	Hold cisplatin until serum creatinine ≤1.5 mg/dL (≤133 µmol/L); then resume treatment
	Discontinue cisplatin if creatinine >1.5 mg/dL (>133 µmol/L) >2 weeks beyond scheduled start of next cycle
G2 peripheral neuropathy or ototoxicity†	Reduce cisplatin dosage by 2 dose levels
G3/4 peripheral neuropathy or ototoxicity	Hold cisplatin until neuropathy G ≤1 then reduce cisplatin dosage by 2 dose levels. If G3/4 toxicity persists >2 weeks beyond scheduled start of next cycle, discontinue cisplatin
G4 gastrointestinal toxicity	Continue cisplatin at same dosage
Second event of G4 gastrointestinal toxicity	Reduce cisplatin dosage by 1 dose level

*Use filgrastim if thought beneficial
†G2 Ototoxicity consists of tinnitus and symptomatic hearing loss

Note: Management of paclitaxel hypersensitivity reaction:
1. Discontinue infusion
2. Wait for symptoms to resolve
3. If symptoms were not life-threatening, repeat premedications (dexamethasone, diphenhydramine, and cimetidine or ranitidine or famotidine) in preparation for restarting infusion
4. Administer 1 mL of the original paclitaxel solution diluted in 100 mL of the same base solution over 1 hour, then
5. Administer 5 mL of the original paclitaxel solution diluted in 100 mL of the same base solution over 1 hour, then
6. Administer 10 mL of the original paclitaxel solution diluted in 100 mL of the same base solution over 1 hour, then
7. Administer the remaining original solution at the original infusion rate

Therapy Monitoring

1. *Every 15 minutes for the first hour of the paclitaxel infusion:* Vital signs including blood pressure, respiratory rate, and temperature
2. *Once per week:* CBC with differential
3. *Before the start of a cycle:* CBC with differential, serum calcium, magnesium, potassium, bilirubin, and creatinine

ADVANCED/RECURRENT • FIRST-LINE

CERVICAL CANCER REGIMEN: PACLITAXEL + CARBOPLATIN

Kitagawa R et al. J Clin Oncol 2015;33:2129–2135

Paclitaxel premedications:

Dexamethasone 10 mg/dose; orally for 2 doses at 12 hours and 6 hours before each paclitaxel dose, *or*

Dexamethasone 20 mg/dose; intravenously over 10–15 minutes, 30–60 minutes before each paclitaxel dose (total dose/cycle = 20 mg)

Diphenhydramine 50 mg, by intravenous injection 30–60 minutes before each paclitaxel dose

Cimetidine 300 mg (or **ranitidine** 50 mg, **famotidine** 20 mg, or an equivalent histamine [H_2]-subtype receptor antagonist) intravenously over 15–30 minutes, 30–60 minutes before each paclitaxel dose

Paclitaxel 175 mg/m²; administer intravenously, diluted in a volume of 0.9% sodium chloride injection (0.9% NS) or 5% dextrose injection (D5W) sufficient to produce a concentration within the range 0.3–1.2 mg/mL, over 3 hours on day 1, prior to carboplatin, every 21 days for up to 6 cycles (total dosage/cycle = 175 mg/m²)

Carboplatin target AUC = 5 mg/mL × min; administer intravenously in 250 mL D5W or 0.9% NS over 60 minutes after paclitaxel on day 1, every 21 days for up to 6 cycles (total dose/cycle calculated to achieve a target AUC = 5 mg/mL × min)

Supportive Care

Antiemetic prophylaxis

Emetogenic potential is **HIGH**. *Potential for delayed symptoms*

Hematopoietic growth factor (CSF) prophylaxis

*Primary prophylaxis is **NOT** indicated*

See Chapter 43 for more information

Antimicrobial prophylaxis

*Risk of fever and neutropenia is **LOW***

  Antimicrobial primary prophylaxis to be considered:

  • Antibacterial—not indicated

  • Antifungal—not indicated

  • Antiviral—not indicated, unless patient previously had an episode of HSV

Carboplatin dose

Carboplatin dose is based on a formula described by Calvert et al. to achieve a target area under the plasma concentration versus time curve (AUC)

$$\text{Total carboplatin dose (mg)} = (\text{target AUC}) \times (\text{GFR} + 25)$$

In practice, creatinine clearance (CrCl) is used in place of glomerular filtration rate (GFR). CrCl can be estimated from the equation of Cockcroft and Gault, thus:

$$\text{For males, CrCl} = \frac{(140 - \text{age [years]}) \times (\text{body weight [kg]})}{72 \times (\text{serum creatinine [mg/dL]})}$$

$$\text{For females, CrCl} = \frac{(140 - \text{age [years]}) \times (\text{body weight [kg]})}{72 \times (\text{serum creatinine [mg/dL]})} \times 0.85$$

Calvert AH et al. J Clin Oncol 1989;7:1748–1756
Cockcroft DW , Gault MH. Nephron 1976;16:31–41
Jodrell DI et al. J Clin Oncol 1992;10:520–528
Sorensen BT et al. Cancer Chemother Pharmacol 1991;28:397–401

Note: On October 8, 2010, the U.S. Food and Drug Administration (FDA) identified a potential safety issue with carboplatin dosing based on recent changes in the measurement of serum creatinine. By the end of 2010, all clinical laboratories in the United States will use the standardized isotope dilution mass spectrometry (IDMS) method to measure serum creatinine, which could result in an overestimation of the GFR in some patients with normal renal function. A carboplatin dose calculated with an IDMS-measured serum creatinine result using the Calvert formula could exceed an expected exposure (AUC) and result in increased drug-related toxicity. Provided actual GFR measurements are made to assess renal function, carboplatin can be safely dosed according to the Calvert formula described in product labeling. If GFR (or creatinine clearance) is estimated based on serum creatinine measurements by the IDMS method, the FDA recommended for patients with normal renal function capping an estimated GFR at 125 mL/min for any targeted AUC value. No greater estimated GFR values should be used per U.S. FDA.

Carboplatin dosing. May 23, 2013. Available from: http://www.fda.gov/AboutFDA/CentersOffices/OfficeofMedicalProductsandTobacco/CDER/ucm228974.htm [accessed February 26, 2014]

Patient Population Studied

This multicenter, randomized, open-label, phase 3 trial involved 253 patients with histologically confirmed, primary stage IVB or first or second recurrent carcinoma of the uterine cervix not amenable to curative surgery or radiotherapy. Eligible patients were aged 20–75 years, with an Eastern Cooperative Oncology Group (ECOG) performance status score ≤2, and had no more than 1 prior platinum-based chemotherapy, including concurrent chemoradiotherapy, and no prior chemotherapy with taxanes. Patients were randomized (1:1) to receive 21-day cycles of either paclitaxel (175 mg/m^2 intravenously over 3 h on day 1) and carboplatin (area under the curve of 5 mg/mL/min intravenously over 1 h on day 1, immediately after paclitaxel administration, and with a maximum dose of 1000 mg) or paclitaxel (135 mg/m^2 intravenously over 24 h on day 1) and cisplatin (50 mg/m^2 intravenously on day 2) for a maximum of 6 cycles or until disease progression or unacceptable toxicity

Efficacy (N = 253)

	Paclitaxel + Carboplatin (N = 126)	Paclitaxel + Cisplatin (N = 127)	
Median overall survival	17.5 months	18.3 months	HR 0.994, 90% CI 0.789–1.253; P = 0.032
Median progression-free survival	6.2 months	6.9 months	HR 1.041, 90% CI 0.803–1.351; P = 0.053

Note: Median duration of follow-up was 17.6 months

Therapy Monitoring

1. Before therapy: History and physical exam, CBC with differential, renal and liver function tests, serum electrolytes
2. Prior to each cycle: CBC with differential, serum electrolytes, BUN, serum creatinine, serum bilirubin, AST, and ALT
3. CBC with differential initially also at day 10–14
4. Observe closely for hypersensitivity reactions, especially during the first and second infusions
5. Every 2–3 months: CT scans to assess response

Treatment Modifications

PACLITAXEL AND CARBOPLATIN DOSE MODIFICATIONS

Paclitaxel Dose Levels		Carboplatin Dose Levels	
Paclitaxel starting dose	175 mg/m^2	Carboplatin starting dose	AUC = 5 mg/mL × min
Paclitaxel dose level −1	140 mg/m^2	Carboplatin dose level −1	AUC = 4 mg/mL × min
Paclitaxel dose level −2	120 mg/m^2	Carboplatin dose level −2	AUC = 3 mg/mL × min

Adverse Event	Treatment Modifications
G ≥3 hematologic toxicities (ANC <1000/mm^3; platelet count <50,000/mm^3)	Interrupt therapy until returns to baseline. Then decrease drug dosages by one dose level
Febrile neutropenia (ANC <1000/mm^3 with temperature >38°C or >100.4°F)	Reduce paclitaxel and carboplatin by one dose level and consider adding filgrastim in subsequent cycles, if applicable
Febrile neutropenia (ANC <1000/mm^3 with temperature >38°C or >100.4°F) despite dose reduction of paclitaxel and carboplatin	Administer filgrastim in subsequent cycles. If already administering filgrastim, reduce paclitaxel and carboplatin doses an additional one dose level
G2 motor or sensory neuropathies	Reduce paclitaxel dosage by one dose level without interrupting its planned treatment
G3 peripheral neuropathy	Reduce paclitaxel dosage by two dose levels or an additional level if already reduced by one level for G2 toxicity. Continuation of paclitaxel is at the discretion of the medically responsible care provider
G4 peripheral neuropathy	Discontinue paclitaxel
Moderate hypersensitivity during paclitaxel infusion	Patient may be retreated. Base a decision to re-treat on reaction severity and the medically responsible care provider's judgment

(continued)

Treatment Modifications (*continued*)

Adverse Event	Treatment Modifications
Severe hypersensitivity during paclitaxel infusion	Discontinue paclitaxel
G ≥2 arthralgias/myalgias	Add dexamethasone as secondary prophylaxis
G3 arthralgia/myalgia despite dexamethasone prophylaxis	Reduce paclitaxel dosage by one dose level
AST (SGOT) and ALT (SGPT) < 10× ULN and bilirubin between 1.26 to 2× ULN	Reduce starting paclitaxel dosage to 135 mg/m^2
AST (SGOT) and ALT (SGPT) < 10× ULN and bilirubin between 2.01 to 5× ULN	Reduce starting paclitaxel dosage to 90 mg/m^2
AST (SGOT) and ALT (SGPT) ≥ 10× ULN or bilirubin >5× ULN	Discontinue paclitaxel
Hypersensitivity reaction to carboplatin including anaphylaxis (risk is increased in patients previously exposed to platinum therapy)	May occur within minutes of administration. Interrupt the infusion in patients with clinically significant infusion reactions. Manage with appropriate supportive therapy including standard epinephrine, corticosteroids, and antihistamines. May consider desensitization for subsequent doses if benefits thought to outweigh risk
Other G ≥3 nonhematologic toxicities (except nausea, vomiting, elevated transaminases, and alopecia)	Delay treatment until toxicity resolves to baseline, then decrease both drug dosages by one dose level from previous dose levels
Treatment delay >2 weeks	Decrease dosage by one dose level for each drug or consider discontinuing treatment

Note: Can cause fetal harm. Advise women of potential risk to the fetus

Adverse Events (N = 251)

Grade 3–4 (%)*	Paclitaxel + Carboplatin (N = 126)	Paclitaxel + Cisplatin (N = 125)
Neutropenia	76	85
Anemia	44	31
Thrombocytopenia	25	3
Fatigue	8	4
Febrile neutropenia	7	16
Infection	5	5
Sensory neuropathy	5	0
Nausea/vomiting	3	6
Creatinine	0	2

*According to the National Cancer Institute Common Terminology Criteria for Adverse Events, version 3.0
Note: Grade 3–4 treatment-related toxicities that occurred in >5% of either group, or were of special interest, are included in the table. Treatment discontinuation owing to adverse events occurred in 9.5% and 11.8% of the paclitaxel + carboplatin and paclitaxel + cisplatin groups, respectively. One patient in the paclitaxel + carboplatin group died owing to interstitial pneumonitis related to protocol treatment

ADVANCED/RECURRENT • FIRST-LINE

CERVICAL CANCER REGIMEN: CISPLATIN + TOPOTECAN

Long HJ III et al. J Clin Oncol 2005;23:4626–4633 (GOG 179, 204)

Topotecan HCl 0.75 mg/m² per day; administer intravenously in 50–250 mL 0.9% sodium chloride injection (0.9% NS) or 5% dextrose injection (D5W) over 30 minutes for 3 consecutive days on days 1–3, every 21 days (total dosage/cycle = 2.25 mg/m²)

Hydration before and after cisplatin: ≥1000 mL 0.45% sodium chloride injection; administer intravenously over a minimum of 2–4 hours. Encourage patients to increase oral intake of nonalcoholic fluids, and provide electrolyte replacement as needed (potassium, magnesium, sodium)

Cisplatin 50 mg/m²; administer intravenously in 50–250 mL 0.9% NS at 1 mg/min on day 1, every 21 days (total dosage/cycle = 50 mg/m²)

Note: Administer cisplatin within 4 hours after completing topotecan administration

Supportive Care
Antiemetic prophylaxis
*Emetogenic potential on day 1 is **HIGH**. Potential for delayed symptoms*
*Emetogenic potential on days 2 and 3 is **LOW***
See Chapter 42 for antiemetic recommendations

*Hematopoietic growth factor (**CSF**) prophylaxis*
Primary prophylaxis may be indicated
See Chapter 43 for more information

Antimicrobial prophylaxis
*Risk of fever and neutropenia is **LOW***
   Antimicrobial primary prophylaxis to be considered:
- Antibacterial—not indicated
- Antifungal—not indicated
- Antiviral—not indicated unless patient previously had an episode of HSV

Patient Population Studied

A study of women with advanced (stage IVB), recurrent or persistent carcinoma of the uterine cervix, who were unsuitable candidates for curative treatment with surgery and/or radiation therapy. Histologic types included squamous, adenosquamous, and adenocarcinoma. Prior cisplatin therapy was allowed

Treatment Modifications

Cisplatin Dose Levels	
Initial dosage	50 mg/m²
Dose level −1	37.5 mg/m²
Dose level −2	25 mg/m²

Topotecan Dose Levels	
Initial dosage	0.75 mg/m² per d × 3 d
Dose level −1	0.6 mg/m² per d × 3 d
Dose level −2	0.45 mg/m² per d × 3 d

Topotecan Dosage Modifications	
Total Bilirubin (mg/dL)	% Starting Topotecan Dosage
≤2.0 (≤34.2 μmol/L)	100
2.1–3.0 (35.9–51.3 μmol/L)	50
>3.0 (>51.3 μmol/L)	25

(continued)

Treatment Modifications (*continued*)

Adverse Event	Dose Modification
Day 1 ANC <1500/mm³ *or* platelet count <100,000/mm³	Hold chemotherapy until ANC ≥1500/mm³ *and* platelet count ≥100,000/mm³
G4 thrombocytopenia	Reduce topotecan dosage 1 level; continue with same cisplatin dosage
G3/4 ANC with fever	
G3/4 ANC with fever despite 1 dose level reduction	Administer filgrastim with all subsequent courses
G2/3/4 nephrotoxicity	Hold cisplatin until serum creatinine ≤1.5 mg/dL (≤133 µmol/L); then resume treatment. If creatinine >1.5 mg/dL >2 weeks beyond scheduled start of next cycle, discontinue cisplatin
G2 peripheral neuropathy or ototoxicity*	Reduce cisplatin dosage by 2 levels
G3/4 peripheral neuropathy or ototoxicity	Hold cisplatin until neuropathy G ≤1; then reduce cisplatin dosage by 2 levels. If G3/4 toxicity persists >2 weeks beyond scheduled start of next cycle, discontinue cisplatin
G4 gastrointestinal toxicity	Continue cisplatin at same dosage
Second event of G4 gastrointestinal toxicity	Reduce cisplatin dosage by 1 level
G2/3 mucositis or diarrhea	Reduce topotecan dosage by 1 level
G4 mucositis or diarrhea	Reduce topotecan dosage by 1–2 levels
Recurrent mucositis or diarrhea despite dosage reduction or persistence of mucositis/diarrhea >2 weeks beyond scheduled start of next cycle	Discontinue topotecan

*G2 ototoxicity consists of tinnitus and symptomatic hearing loss

Toxicity (N = 147)

	% G3	% G4
Hematologic		
Leukopenia	39.4	23.8
Granulocytopenia	24.5	45.6
Thrombocytopenia	24.5	6.8
Anemia	40	6.1
Other hematologic	11.6	2.7
Nonhematologic		
Infection	14.2	3.4
Renal	6.1	6.1
Nausea	12.2	1.4
Emesis	13.6	1.4
Other gastrointestinal	10.9	2.7
Metabolic	8.8	4.8
Neuropathy	0.7	—
Other neurologic	2	0.7
Cardiovascular	4.8	4.1
Pulmonary	2.7	—
Pain	19	2
Constitutional	7.5	—
Hemorrhage	5.4	0.7
Hepatic	3.4	1.4

NCI, CTC, National Cancer Institute (USA) Common Toxicity Criteria, version 2.0. At: http://ctep.cancer.gov/protocolDevelopment/electronic_applications/ctc.htm [accessed December 7, 2013]

Efficacy (N = 147)

Complete response	10%
Partial response	16%
Stable disease	45%
Median progression-free survival	4.6 months
Median survival	9.4 months

Gynecologic Oncology Group Criteria

Therapy Monitoring

1. *Once per week:* CBC with differential
2. *Before the start of a cycle:* CBC with differential, serum calcium, magnesium, potassium, bilirubin, and creatinine

ADVANCED/RECURRENT • FIRST-LINE
CERVICAL CANCER REGIMEN: CISPLATIN + GEMCITABINE

Burnett AF et al. Gynecol Oncol 2000;76:63–66 (GOG 204)

Gemcitabine 1250 mg/m^2 per dose; administer intravenously diluted to a concentration ≥0.1 mg/mL in 0.9% sodium chloride injection (0.9% NS) over 30 minutes for 2 doses on days 1 and 8, every 21 days (total dosage/cycle = 2500 mg/m^2)

Note: After gemcitabine administration, flush the patient's vascular access device with 75–125 mL of 0.9% NS

Hydration before and after cisplatin: ≥1000 mL 0.45% sodium chloride injection; administer by intravenous infusion over a minimum of 2–4 hours. Encourage patients to increase oral intake of nonalcoholic fluids, and provide electrolyte replacement as needed (potassium, magnesium, sodium)

Cisplatin 50 mg/m^2; administer intravenously in 50–250 mL 0.9% NS over 60 minutes on day 1 after completing gemcitabine administration, every 21 days (total dosage/cycle = 50 mg/m^2)

Note: Administer cisplatin on day 1 within 4 hours after completing gemcitabine

Supportive Care
Antiemetic prophylaxis
*Emetogenic potential on day 1 is **HIGH**. Potential for delayed symptoms*
*Emetogenic potential on day 8 is **LOW***
See Chapter 42 for antiemetic recommendations

Hematopoietic growth factor (CSF) prophylaxis
*Primary prophylaxis is **NOT** indicated*
See Chapter 43 for more information

Antimicrobial prophylaxis
*Risk of fever and neutropenia is **LOW***
   Antimicrobial primary prophylaxis to be considered:
- Antibacterial—not indicated
- Antifungal—not indicated
- Antiviral—not indicated unless patient previously had an episode of HSV

Treatment Modifications

Cisplatin Dose Levels	
Initial dosage	50 mg/m^2
Dose level −1	37.5 mg/m^2
Dose level −2	25 mg/m^2

Gemcitabine Dose Levels	
Initial dosage	1250 mg/m^2
Dose level −1	1000 mg/m^2
Dose level −2	800 mg/m^2

Gemcitabine Dosage Modification	
Total Bilirubin (mg/dL)	% of Starting Gemcitabine Dosage
≤2.0 (≤34.2 µmol/L)	100
2.1–3.0 (35.9–51.3 µmol/L)	50
>3.0 (>51.3 µmol/L)	25

Note: Gemcitabine dose reductions at any time after day 1 of cycle 1 will be continued throughout the rest of the study

(continued)

Patient Population Studied

Phase 2 trial in patients with advanced, persistent, or recurrent squamous cell carcinoma of the cervix

Treatment Modifications (*continued*)

Adverse Event	Dose Modification
Day 1 ANC <1500/mm^3 *or* platelet count <100,000/mm^3	Hold chemotherapy until ANC ≥1500/mm^3 *and* platelet count ≥100,000/mm^3
ANC <1500/mm^3 *or* platelet count <100,000/mm^3 that persists ≥3 weeks beyond the scheduled start of cycle	Discontinue therapy
>2-week delay until ANC ≥1500/mm^3 *and* platelet count ≥100,000/mm^3	Reduce gemcitabine by 1 dose level
Day 8 ANC ≥1500/mm^3 *or* platelet count ≥100,000/mm^3	Administer day 1 gemcitabine dosage on day 8
Day 8 ANC 1000–1499/mm^3 *or* platelet count 75,000–99,000/mm^3	Reduce gemcitabine on day 8 by 1 dose level from day 1 level
Day 8 ANC <1500/mm^3 *or* platelet count <100,000/mm^3	Withhold day 8 gemcitabine dose; reduce gemcitabine dosage by 1 dose level in ensuing cycles on day 8
G4 thrombocytopenia	Reduce gemcitabine by 1 dose level; continue with same cisplatin dosage
G3/4 ANC with fever*	Reduce gemcitabine dosage by 1 dose level; continue with same cisplatin dosage
G3/4 ANC with fever despite 1 dose level reduction	Administer filgrastim with all subsequent courses
G3/4 ANC with fever despite gemcitabine dose reduction and filgrastim	Reduce gemcitabine dosage by 1 dose level or 20%; continue with same cisplatin dosage
G1 mucositis or diarrhea	Hold gemcitabine until toxicity resolves; then resume with same dosage
G2/3 mucositis or diarrhea	Hold gemcitabine until toxicity G ≤1; reduce subsequent dosages by 1 dose level
Mucositis or diarrhea that is G4 or that persists >2 weeks, or repeated episodes of persistent toxicity G ≥2	Hold gemcitabine until toxicity G ≤1; consider discontinuing gemcitabine
G2/3/4 nephrotoxicity	Hold cisplatin until serum creatinine ≤1.5 mg/dL (≤133 µmol/L) then resume treatment. If creatinine >1.5 mg/dL >2 weeks beyond scheduled start of next cycle, discontinue cisplatin
G2 peripheral neuropathy or ototoxicity†	Reduce cisplatin dosage by 2 dose levels
G3/4 peripheral neuropathy or ototoxicity	Hold cisplatin and gemcitabine until neuropathy G ≤1 then reduce cisplatin dosage by 2 dose levels. If G3/4 toxicity persists >2 weeks beyond scheduled start of next cycle, discontinue cisplatin
G4 gastrointestinal toxicity	Continue cisplatin at same dosage
Second event of G4 gastrointestinal toxicity	Reduce cisplatin dosage by 1 dose level

*Use filgrastim if thought beneficial
†G2 ototoxicity consists of tinnitus and symptomatic hearing loss. If neurotoxicity occurs, it will most likely be cisplatin-related

Efficacy (N = 17)

Complete response	5.9%
Partial response*	35.3%
Median survival patients with response	12 months
Median survival patients without response	7 months

*Six patients; three had received prior radiation therapy
GOG Response Criteria

Toxicity (N = 82 cycles)

	% G3	% G4
Hematologic		
Neutropenia	7.3	2.4
Anemia	1.2	1.2
Median leukocyte nadir	3145/mm^3	
Median platelet nadir	174,000/mm^3	
Nonhematologic		
Gastrointestinal	2.4	0

Therapy Monitoring

1. *Once per week:* CBC with differential
2. *Before the start of a cycle:* CBC with differential, serum calcium, magnesium, potassium, bilirubin, and creatinine

ADVANCED/RECURRENT • FIRST-LINE

CERVICAL CANCER REGIMEN: PACLITAXEL + TOPOTECAN ± BEVACIZUMAB

Tewari KS et al. N Engl J Med 2014;370:734–737
Supplementary appendix to: Tewari KS et al. N Engl J Med 2014;370:734–737
Protocol for: Tewari KS et al. N Engl J Med 2014;370:734–737
Tiersten AD et al. Gynecol Oncol 2004;92:635–638

Paclitaxel Premedications
Dexamethasone 10 mg per dose; administer orally for 2 doses at 12 hours and 6 hours before each paclitaxel dose, *or*
Dexamethasone 20 mg per dose; administer intravenously over 10–15 minutes, 30–60 minutes before each paclitaxel dose (total dose/cycle = 20 mg)
Diphenhydramine 50 mg, administer by intravenous injection 30–60 minutes before each paclitaxel dose
Cimetidine 300 mg (or **ranitidine** 50 mg, **famotidine** 20 mg, or an equivalent histamine [H_2]-subtype receptor antagonist) administer intravenously over 15–30 minutes, 30–60 minutes before each paclitaxel dose

Paclitaxel 175 mg/m²; administer intravenously, diluted in a volume of 0.9% sodium chloride injection (0.9% NS) or 5% dextrose injection (D5W) sufficient to produce a concentration within the range of 0.3–1.2 mg/mL, over 3 hours on day 1, prior to topotecan, every 21 days until disease progression or complete response (total dosage/cycle = 175 mg/m²)

Topotecan 0.75 mg/m² per dose; administer intravenously, diluted in 50–250 mL 0.9% NS or D5W over 30 minutes for 3 consecutive days, on days 1–3, every 21 days until disease progression or complete response (total dosage/cycle = 2.25 mg/m²)

Bevacizumab 15 mg/kg; administer intravenously, diluted in 100 mL 0.9% NS over 30–90 minutes on day 1, every 21 days until disease progression or complete response (total dosage/cycle = 15 mg/kg)

Notes about bevacizumab administration: The duration of administration for the initial dose is 90 minutes. If administration is well tolerated, the administration duration may be decreased stepwise during subsequent administrations to 60 minutes and, finally, to a minimum duration of 30 minutes

Supportive Care
Antiemetic prophylaxis
Emetogenic potential on days 1–3 is **LOW**
See Chapter 42 for antiemetic recommendations

Hematopoietic growth factor (CSF) prophylaxis
Primary prophylaxis is **NOT** *indicated*
See Chapter 43 for more information

Antimicrobial prophylaxis
Risk of fever and neutropenia is **LOW**
 Antimicrobial primary prophylaxis to be considered:
 • Antibacterial—not indicated
 • Antifungal—not indicated
 • Antiviral—not indicated, unless patient previously had an episode of HSV

Patient Population Studied

This international, multicenter, randomized, phase 3 trial involved 452 patients with metastatic, persistent, or recurrent cervical carcinoma. Eligible patients had a Gynecologic Oncology Group (GOG) performance status score ≤1. Patients with recurrent disease who were candidates for curative therapy by means of pelvic exenteration were ineligible. Patients were randomly assigned to one of four 21-day cycle intravenous regimens: (1) cisplatin (50 mg/m²) plus paclitaxel (135 mg/m² over 24 hours, or 175 mg/m² over 3 hours); (2) cisplatin (50 mg/m²) plus paclitaxel (135 mg/m² over 24 hours, or 175 mg/m² over 3 hours) plus bevacizumab (15 mg/kg); (3) topotecan (0.75 mg/m² per day on days 1–3) plus paclitaxel (175 mg/m² over 3 hours on day 1); or (4) topotecan (0.75 mg/m² per day on days 1–3) plus paclitaxel (175 mg/m² over 3 hours on day 1) plus bevacizumab (15 mg/kg on day 1)

Efficacy (N = 452)

	Topotecan + Paclitaxel (± Bevacizumab) (N = 223)	Cisplatin + Paclitaxel (± Bevacizumab) (N = 229)	
Median overall survival	12.5 months	15 months	HR 1.20, 99% CI 0.82–1.76; P = 0.88
Median progression-free survival	5.7 months	7.6 months	HR 1.39, 99% CI 1.09–1.77; P = 0.008
Overall response rate*	37%	47%	

*Overall response rate includes patients with either a complete or a partial response to treatment. Data shown for analysis made at median duration of follow-up was 20.8 months

Note: Median duration of follow-up at the interim analysis (shown for overall survival and progression-free survival) was 12.5 months

Therapy Monitoring

1. Before therapy: History and physical examination, CBC with differential, renal and liver function tests, serum electrolytes
2. Prior to each cycle: CBC with differential, serum electrolytes, BUN, serum creatinine, serum bilirubin, AST, and ALT
3. CBC with differential initially and also at days 10–14
4. Observe closely for hypersensitivity reactions, especially during the first and second infusions of paclitaxel and bevacizumab
5. Blood pressure before every infusion of bevacizumab and every 2 weeks, or more frequently, as indicated during treatment
6. Prior to each bevacizumab infusion: Assess proteinuria by urine dipstick and/or urinary protein creatinine ratio. Patients with a urine dipstick reading ≥2+ should undergo further assessment with 24-hour urine collection
7. Every 2–3 months: CT scans to assess response

Treatment Modifications

BEVACIZUMAB DOSAGE MODIFICATIONS

Adverse Event	Treatment Modification
Treatment delay of >3 weeks or patient whose G3 toxicity recurs after resumption of therapy	Discontinue bevacizumab permanently
G4 nonhematologic toxicity	
Gastrointestinal perforations (gastrointestinal perforations, fistula formation in the gastrointestinal tract, intra-abdominal abscess), fistula formation involving an internal organ	Discontinue bevacizumab permanently. Continue chemotherapy after toxicity has resolved
Wound dehiscence requiring medical intervention	
Nephrotic syndrome	
Hypertensive crisis or hypertensive encephalopathy or reversible posterior leukoencephalopathy syndrome (RPLS)	
Congestive heart failure	
Necrotizing fasciitis	
Serious bleeding defined as G ≥2 pulmonary or CNS hemorrhage	Discontinue bevacizumab permanently. Continue chemotherapy after toxicity has resolved
G3 hemorrhage (any site) in patient receiving full-dose anticoagulation	Discontinue bevacizumab permanently. Continue chemotherapy after toxicity has resolved

(*continued*)

Treatment Modifications (*continued*)

Adverse Event	Treatment Modification
G3 hemorrhage in sites other than pulmonary or CNS	Withhold bevacizumab and chemotherapy until (1) bleeding has resolved, and (2) hemoglobin level is stable. Resume bevacizumab and chemotherapy after toxicity has resolved provided (1) evaluation does not uncover a bleeding diathesis that would increase the risk of continuing therapy, and (2) there is no anatomic or pathologic condition that can increase the risk of hemorrhage recurrence
Recurrence of any G3 hemorrhage	Discontinue bevacizumab permanently. Continue chemotherapy
Patients with any grade arterial thromboembolic events (including cerebrovascular ischemia, cardiac ischemia/infarction, peripheral or visceral arterial ischemia)	Discontinue bevacizumab permanently. Continue chemotherapy after toxicity has resolved
Symptomatic G4 venous thrombosis	Discontinue bevacizumab permanently. Continue chemotherapy after toxicity has resolved
Asymptomatic G4 or any G3 venous thrombosis with planned duration of full-dose anticoagulation ≤2 weeks	Withhold bevacizumab until the full-dose anticoagulation period is over, then resume bevacizumab and chemotherapy
Asymptomatic G4 or any G3 venous thrombosis with planned duration of full-dose anticoagulation >2 weeks	Withhold bevacizumab initially as patient is assessed. Bevacizumab may then be resumed during the period of full-dose anticoagulation if *all* of the following criteria are met: (1) must have an in-range INR (usually between 2 and 3) on a stable dose of warfarin (or other anticoagulant) or on stable dose of heparin prior to restarting bevacizumab treatment; (2) there is no evidence of a pathologic condition that carries high risk of bleeding (eg, tumor involving major vessels); (3) the patient has not had hemorrhagic events while receiving bevacizumab; and (4) the patient is benefiting from the bevacizumab therapy (no evidence of disease progression)
G3/4 coagulopathy	Withhold bevacizumab until PT/PTT resolves to G1. For patients with PT/INR > therapeutic range while on therapeutic warfarin, hold bevacizumab until PT/INR is within the therapeutic range
Moderate to severe proteinuria	Patients with a urine dipstick reading ≥2+ should undergo further assessment, eg, 24-hour urine collection. Suspend bevacizumab administration for ≥2 g of proteinuria/24 h and resume when proteinuria is <2 g/24 h
G4 proteinuria or nephrotic syndrome	Discontinue bevacizumab permanently. Continue chemotherapy after toxicity has resolved
For hypertension (systolic >150 mm Hg or diastolic >100 mm Hg) not controlled by medical management or symptomatic hypertension	Hold bevacizumab pending further evaluation and treatment of hypertension. Medication classes used for management of patients with G3 hypertension receiving bevacizumab include angiotensin-converting enzyme inhibitors, diuretics, and calcium channel blockers. The goal for blood pressure control should be consistent with general medical practice guidelines. For controlled hypertension, defined as systolic ≤150 mm Hg and diastolic ≤90 mm Hg, continue bevacizumab therapy
Treatment is delayed for > 4 weeks due to uncontrolled hypertension	Discontinue bevacizumab
Mild, clinically insignificant infusion reaction	Decrease the rate of infusion
Clinically significant but not severe infusion reaction	Interrupt the infusion in patients with clinically significant infusion reactions and consider resuming at a slower rate following resolution. If decision is made to restart, the infusion may be continued at ≤50% of the rate prior to the reaction and increased in 50% increments every 30 minutes if well tolerated. Infusions may be restarted at the full rate during the next cycle
Severe infusion reaction—hypertension, hypertensive crises associated with neurologic signs and symptoms, wheezing, oxygen desaturation, G3 hypersensitivity, chest pain, headaches, rigors, and diaphoresis	Stop infusion and administer appropriate medical therapy (eg, epinephrine, corticosteroids, intravenous antihistamines, bronchodilators, and/or oxygen). Discontinue bevacizumab

(continued)

Treatment Modifications (*continued*)

Adverse Event	Treatment Modification
Planned elective surgery	Suspend bevacizumab at least 28 days before elective surgery and do not resume for at least 28 days after surgery or until surgical incision is fully healed
Recent hemoptysis	Do not administer bevacizumab
Evidence of recto-sigmoid involvement by pelvic examination or bowel involvement on CT scan or clinical symptoms of bowel obstruction	
Reversible posterior leukoencephalopathy syndrome (RPLS)	Withhold bevacizumab pending work-up and management, including control of blood pressure. Discontinue bevacizumab upon confirming the diagnosis of RPLS. *Note:* the diagnosis of RPLS should be made with MRI and its complete resolution confirmed with MRI. Resumption of bevacizumab may be considered in patients who have had documented benefit from bevacizumab, provided that RPLS was mild and has completely resolved clinically and radiographically within 2–4 weeks
Platelet count <50,000/mm³	Withhold bevacizumab until platelet count >75,000/mm³. If platelet count of <50,000/mm³ persists for >3 weeks, discontinue bevacizumab; continue chemotherapy only to the extent felt safe
G3 hematologic toxicities (ANC <1000/mm³; platelet count <50,000/mm³)	Hold bevacizumab as chemotherapy is held
G4 hematologic toxicities (thrombocytopenia) (ANC <500/mm³; platelet count <25,000/mm³)	

PACLITAXEL AND TOPOTECAN DOSAGE MODIFICATIONS

Paclitaxel Dose Levels		Topotecan Dose Levels	
Paclitaxel starting dose	175 mg/m²	Starting dose	0.75 mg/m² for 3 consecutive days
Paclitaxel dose level −1	140 mg/m²	Dose level −1	0.6 mg/m² for 3 consecutive days
Paclitaxel dose level −2	105 mg/m²	Dose level −2	0.45 mg/m² for 3 consecutive days

Adverse Event	Treatment Modifications
ANC ≤1500/mm³ or platelets ≤100,000/mm³ at the start of a cycle	Hold all therapy (paclitaxel, topotecan, and bevacizumab) until ANC >1500/mm³ and platelets >100,000/mm³. See below for recommended paclitaxel and topotecan dosage reductions based on nadir ANC and platelet counts
G4 thrombocytopenia (platelet count <25,000/mm³) of any duration	Reduce both topotecan and paclitaxel dosages by 1 dose level
G4 neutropenia (ANC <500/mm³) lasting >7 days	Reduce both topotecan and paclitaxel dosages by 1 dose level
Febrile neutropenia (ANC <1000/mm³ with temperature >38°C or >100.4°F), or ANC <500/mm³ for ≥7 days	Reduce both topotecan and paclitaxel dosages by 1 dose level and consider adding filgrastim in subsequent cycles
Recurrence of febrile neutropenia (ANC <1000/mm³ with temperature >38°C or >100.4°F), or ANC <500/mm³ for ≥7 days despite prior dose reduction of topotecan and paclitaxel	Administer filgrastim in subsequent cycles and continue topotecan and paclitaxel at the same dosages. If already administering filgrastim, then reduce both the topotecan and paclitaxel dosages by an additional 1 dose level
G2 motor or sensory neuropathies	Reduce the paclitaxel dosage by 2 dose levels without interrupting planned treatment. Do not reduce the topotecan dose
G ≥3 peripheral neuropathy	Interrupt therapy with paclitaxel until peripheral neuropathy improves to G ≤1, then reduce the paclitaxel dosage by 2 dose levels. Do not reduce the topotecan dose

(*continued*)

Treatment Modifications (*continued*)

PACLITAXEL AND TOPOTECAN DOSAGE MODIFICATIONS

Paclitaxel Dose Levels	Topotecan Dose Levels
Moderate hypersensitivity during paclitaxel infusion	Patient may be re-treated with paclitaxel. Base a decision to re-treat on reaction severity and the medically responsible care provider's judgment
Severe hypersensitivity during paclitaxel infusion	Discontinue therapy
G ≥2 arthralgias/myalgias	Add dexamethasone as secondary prophylaxis
G3 arthralgia/myalgia despite dexamethasone prophylaxis	Reduce paclitaxel dosage 1 dose level
G ≥2 AST (SGOT) or ALT (SGPT), or G ≥2 bilirubin	Interrupt paclitaxel until improvement to G ≤1, then reduce the paclitaxel dosage by 1 dose level. See below for topotecan dosing in the setting of hyperbilirubinemia
Total bilirubin between 2.1 and 3.0 mg/dL	Reduce the topotecan dosage by 50% without interrupting planned treatment. See above for paclitaxel dosing in the setting of hepatic impairment
Total bilirubin between 2.1 and 3.0 mg/dL	Reduce the topotecan dosage by 75% without interrupting planned treatment. See above for paclitaxel dosing in the setting of hepatic impairment
G2/3 mucositis or diarrhea	Reduce topotecan dosage by 1 level. Do not reduce paclitaxel dose
G4 mucositis or diarrhea	Reduce topotecan dosage by 1 or 2 levels or consider discontinuing topotecan. Do not reduce paclitaxel dose
Recurrent mucositis or diarrhea despite dosage reduction or persistence of mucositis/diarrhea >2 weeks beyond scheduled start of next cycle	Discontinue topotecan
Pulmonary symptoms indicative of interstitial lung disease (eg, cough, fever, dyspnea, and/or hypoxia)	Discontinue topotecan and evaluate. If a new diagnosis of interstitial lung disease is confirmed, discontinue topotecan
Other G ≥3 nonhematologic toxicities (except nausea, vomiting, elevated transaminases and alopecia)	Delay treatment until toxicity resolves to baseline, then decrease topotecan and paclitaxel dosages by 1 dose level from previous levels
Treatment delay >2 weeks	Decrease topotecan and paclitaxel dosages by 1 dose level, or consider discontinuing treatment

Adverse Events (N = 439)

Seven patients in the topotecan group died from a treatment-related cause (4 owing to infection with G4 neutropenia, 1 owing to infection with unknown absolute neutrophil count, 1 owing to gastrointestinal perforation, and 1 owing to adult respiratory distress syndrome) compared with 1 patient in the cisplatin group (owing to infection with G4 neutropenia)

ADVANCED/RECURRENT • FIRST-LINE

CERVICAL CANCER REGIMEN: PACLITAXEL + CISPLATIN + BEVACIZUMAB

Tewari KS et al. N Engl J Med 2014;370:734–737
Supplementary appendix to: Tewari KS et al. N Engl J Med 2014;370:734–737
Protocol for: Tewari KS et al. N Engl J Med 2014;370:734–737

Paclitaxel premedications:

Dexamethasone 10 mg/dose; orally for 2 doses at 12 hours and 6 hours before each paclitaxel dose, or

Dexamethasone 20 mg/dose; intravenously over 10–15 minutes, 30–60 minutes before each paclitaxel dose (total dosage/21-day cycle = 20 mg)

Diphenhydramine 50 mg, by intravenous injection 30–60 minutes before each paclitaxel dose

Cimetidine 300 mg (or **ranitidine** 50 mg, **famotidine** 20 mg, or an equivalent histamine [H_2]-subtype receptor antagonist) intravenously over 15–30 minutes, 30–60 minutes before each paclitaxel dose

Paclitaxel 175 mg/m²; administer intravenously, diluted in a volume of 0.9% sodium chloride injection (0.9% NS) or 5% dextrose injection (D5W) sufficient to produce a concentration within the range 0.3–1.2 mg/mL, over 3 hours on day 1, prior to cisplatin, every 21 days until disease progression or complete response (total dosage/21-day cycle = 175 mg/m²)

Hydration before cisplatin: 1000 mL 0.9% NS; intravenously over a minimum of 1 hour before commencing cisplatin administration

Cisplatin 50 mg/m²; administer intravenously, diluted in 100–500 mL 0.9% NS over 30–90 minutes on day 1, after completion of paclitaxel, every 21 days until disease progression or complete response (total dosage/21-day cycle = 50 mg/m²)

Hydration after cisplatin: Administer by intravenous infusion ≥1000 mL 0.9% NS over a minimum of 2 hours. Encourage patients to increase oral intake of nonalcoholic fluids, and provide electrolyte replacement as needed (potassium, magnesium, sodium)

Bevacizumab 15 mg/kg; intravenously, diluted in 100 mL 0.9% NS over 30–90 minutes on day 1, every 21 days until disease progression or complete response (total dosage/21-day cycle = 15 mg/kg)

Notes about bevacizumab administration: The duration of administration for the initial dose is 90 minutes. If administration is well tolerated, the administration duration may be decreased stepwise during subsequent administrations to 60 minutes and, finally, to a minimum duration of 30 minutes

Treatment notes: the protocol allowed various dosing and schedules of paclitaxel + cisplatin + bevacizumab; the above described dosing and schedule was chosen based on superior convenience

Supportive Care

Antiemetic prophylaxis
Emetogenic potential on a treatment day with cisplatin is **HIGH**. *Potential for delayed emetic symptoms*
See Chapter 42 for antiemetic recommendations

Hematopoietic growth factor (CSF) prophylaxis
Primary prophylaxis is **NOT** *indicated*
See Chapter 43 for more information

Antimicrobial prophylaxis
Risk of fever and neutropenia is **LOW**
   Antimicrobial primary prophylaxis to be considered:
- Antibacterial—not indicated
- Antifungal—not indicated
- Antiviral—not indicated, unless patient previously had an episode of HSV

Patient Population Studied

This international, multicenter, randomized, phase 3 trial involved 452 patients with metastatic, persistent, or recurrent cervical carcinoma. Eligible patients had a Gynecologic Oncology Group (GOG) performance status score ≤1. Patients with recurrent disease who were candidates for curative therapy by means of pelvic exenteration were ineligible. Patients were randomly assigned to one of four 21-day cycle intravenous regimens: (1) cisplatin (50 mg/m²) plus paclitaxel (135 mg/m² over 24 hours, or 175 mg/m² over 3 hours), (2) cisplatin (50 mg/m²) plus paclitaxel (135 mg/m² over 24 hours, or 175 mg/m² over 3 hours) plus bevacizumab (15 mg/kg), (3) topotecan (0.75 mg/m²/day on days 1–3) plus paclitaxel (175mg/m² over 3 hours on day 1), or (4) topotecan (0.75 mg/m²/day on days 1–3) plus paclitaxel (175mg/m² over 3 hours on day 1) plus bevacizumab (15 mg/kg on day 1)

Efficacy (N = 229 or 452)

	Cisplatin + Paclitaxel + Bevacizumab (N = 115)	Cisplatin + Paclitaxel (N = 114)	
Median overall survival	17.5 months	14.3 months	HR 0.68, 95% CI 0.48–0.97; P = 0.04
Overall response rate*	50%	45%	P = 0.51

	Cisplatin or Topotecan + Paclitaxel + Bevacizumab (N = 227)	Cisplatin or Topotecan + Paclitaxel (N = 225)	
Median overall survival	17.0 months	13.3 months	HR 0.71, 95% CI 0.54–0.95; P = 0.004
Median progression-free survival	8.2 months	5.9 months	HR 0.67, 95% CI 0.54–0.82; P = 0.002
Overall response rate*	48%	36%	P = 0.008

*Overall response rate includes patients with either a complete or partial response to treatment
Note: Median duration of follow-up was 20.8 months

Therapy Monitoring

1. Before therapy: History and physical exam, CBC with differential, renal and liver function tests, serum electrolytes
2. Prior to each cycle: CBC with differential, serum electrolytes, BUN, serum creatinine, serum bilirubin, AST, and ALT
3. CBC with differential initially also at day 10–14
4. Observe closely for hypersensitivity reactions, especially during the first and second infusions
5. Blood pressure before every infusion of bevacizumab and every two weeks or more frequently as indicated during treatment
6. Before every infusion of bevacizumab: assess proteinuria by urine dipstick and/or urinary protein creatinine ratio. Patients with a ≥2+ urine dipstick reading should undergo further assessment with a 24-hour urine collection
7. Every 2–3 months: CT scans to assess response

Treatment Modifications

BEVACIZUMAB DOSE MODIFICATIONS

Adverse Event	Treatment Modification
Treatment delay of more than three weeks or whose G3 toxicity recurs after resumption of therapy	Discontinue bevacizumab permanently
G4 nonhematologic toxicity	
Gastrointestinal perforations (gastrointestinal perforations, fistula formation in the gastrointestinal tract, intra-abdominal abscess), fistula formation involving an internal organ	Discontinue bevacizumab permanently. Continue chemotherapy after toxicity has resolved
Wound dehiscence requiring medical intervention	
Nephrotic syndrome	
Hypertensive crisis or hypertensive encephalopathy or reversible posterior leukoencephalopathy syndrome (RPLS)	
Congestive heart failure	
Necrotizing fasciitis	
Serious bleeding defined as G ≥2 pulmonary or CNS hemorrhage	Discontinue bevacizumab permanently. Continue chemotherapy after toxicity has resolved

(continued)

Treatment Modifications (continued)

Adverse Event	Treatment Modification
G3 hemorrhage (any site) in patient receiving full dose anti-coagulation	Discontinue bevacizumab permanently. Continue chemotherapy after toxicity has resolved
G3 hemorrhage in sites other than pulmonary or CNS	Withhold bevacizumab and chemotherapy until (1) bleeding has resolved and (2) hemoglobin level is stable. Resume bevacizumab and chemotherapy after toxicity has resolved provided (1) evaluation does not uncover a bleeding diathesis that would increase the risk of continuing therapy and (2) there is no anatomic or pathologic condition that can increase the risk of hemorrhage recurrence
Recurrence of any G3 hemorrhage	Discontinue bevacizumab permanently. Continue chemotherapy
Patients with any grade arterial thromboembolic events (including cerebrovascular ischemia, cardiac ischemia/infarction, peripheral or visceral arterial ischemia)	Discontinue bevacizumab permanently. Continue chemotherapy after toxicity has resolved
Symptomatic G4 venous thrombosis	Discontinue bevacizumab permanently. Continue chemotherapy after toxicity has resolved
Asymptomatic G4 or any G3 venous thrombosis with planned duration of full-dose anticoagulation ≤2 weeks	Withhold bevacizumab until the full-dose anticoagulation period is over, then resume bevacizumab and chemotherapy
Asymptomatic G4 or any G3 venous thrombosis with planned duration of full-dose anticoagulation >2 weeks	Withhold bevacizumab initially as patient is assessed. Bevacizumab may then be resumed during the period of full-dose anticoagulation if ALL of the following criteria are met: (1) must have an in-range INR (usually between 2 and 3) on a stable dose of warfarin (or other anticoagulant) or on stable dose of heparin prior to restarting bevacizumab treatment; (2) there is no evidence of a pathologic condition that carries high risk of bleeding (eg, tumor involving major vessels); (3) the patient has not had hemorrhagic events while receiving bevacizumab; and (4) the patient is benefiting from the bevacizumab therapy (no evidence of disease progression)
G3/4 coagulopathy	Withhold bevacizumab until PT/PTT resolves to G1. For patients with PT/INR > therapeutic range while on therapeutic warfarin, hold bevacizumab until PT/INR is within the therapeutic range
Moderate to severe proteinuria	Patients with a 2+ or greater urine dipstick reading should undergo further assessment, eg, a 24-h urine collection. Suspend bevacizumab administration for ≥2 grams of proteinuria/24 h and resume when proteinuria is <2 grams/24 h
G4 proteinuria or nephrotic syndrome	Discontinue bevacizumab permanently. Continue chemotherapy after toxicity has resolved
For hypertension (systolic >150 mmHg or diastolic >100 mmHg) not controlled by medical management or symptomatic hypertension	Hold bevacizumab pending further evaluation and treatment of hypertension. Medication classes used for management of patients with G3 hypertension receiving bevacizumab include angiotensin-converting enzyme inhibitors, diuretics, and calcium channel blockers. The goal for blood pressure control should be consistent with general medical practice guidelines. For controlled hypertension, defined as systolic ≤150 mmHg and diastolic ≤90 mmHg, continue bevacizumab therapy
Treatment is delayed for >4 weeks due to uncontrolled hypertension	Discontinue bevacizumab
Mild, clinically insignificant infusion reaction	Decrease the rate of infusion
Clinically significant but not severe infusion reaction	Interrupt the infusion in patients with clinically significant infusion reactions and consider resuming at a slower rate following resolution. If decision is made to restart, the infusion may be continued at ≤50% of the rate prior to the reaction and increased in 50% increments every 30 minutes if well tolerated. Infusions may be restarted at the full rate during the next cycle
Severe infusion reaction—hypertension, hypertensive crises associated with neurologic signs and symptoms, wheezing, oxygen desaturation, G3 hypersensitivity, chest pain, headaches, rigors, and diaphoresis	Stop infusion and administer appropriate medical therapy (eg, epinephrine, corticosteroids, intravenous antihistamines, bronchodilators and/or oxygen). Discontinue bevacizumab
Planned elective surgery	Suspend bevacizumab at least 28 days before elective surgery and do not resume for at least 28 days after surgery or until surgical incision is fully healed

(continued)

Treatment Modifications (*continued*)

Adverse Event	Treatment Modification
Recent hemoptysis	Do not administer bevacizumab
Evidence of recto-sigmoid involvement by pelvic examination or bowel involvement on CT scan or clinical symptoms of bowel obstruction	
Reversible posterior leukoencephalopathy syndrome (RPLS)	Withhold bevacizumab pending work-up and management, including control of blood pressure. Discontinue bevacizumab upon confirming the diagnosis of RPLS. *Note:* The diagnosis of RPLS should be made with MRI and its complete resolution confirmed with MRI. *Note:* Resumption of bevacizumab may be considered in patients who have had documented benefit from bevacizumab, provided that RPLS was mild and has completely resolved clinically and radiographically within 2–4 weeks
Platelet count <50,000/mm³	Withhold bevacizumab until platelet count >75,000/mm³. If platelet count of <50,000/mm³ persists for >3 weeks, discontinue bevacizumab; continue chemotherapy only to the extent felt safe
G3 hematologic toxicities (ANC <1000/mm³; platelet count <50,000/mm³)	Hold bevacizumab as chemotherapy is held
G4 hematologic toxicities (thrombocytopenia) (ANC <500/mm³; platelet count <25,000/mm³)	

PACLITAXEL AND CISPLATIN DOSE MODIFICATIONS

Paclitaxel Dose Levels		Cisplatin Dose Levels	
Paclitaxel starting dose	175 mg/m²	Cisplatin starting dose	50 mg/m²
Paclitaxel dose level −1	140 mg/m²	Cisplatin dose level −1	37.5 mg/m²
Paclitaxel dose level −2	105 mg/m²	Cisplatin dose level −2	25 mg/m²

Adverse Event	Treatment Modifications
ANC ≤1500/mm³ or platelets ≤100,000/mm³ at the start of a cycle	Hold all therapy (cisplatin, paclitaxel, and bevacizumab) until ANC >1500/mm³ and platelets >100,000/mm³. See below for recommended paclitaxel dose reductions based on nadir ANC and platelet counts
G4 thrombocytopenia (platelet count <25,000/mm³) of any duration	Reduce paclitaxel dose by one dose level. Do not reduce the cisplatin dose
G4 neutropenia (ANC <500/mm²) lasting >7 days	Reduce paclitaxel dose by one dose level. Do not reduce the cisplatin dose
Febrile neutropenia (ANC <1000/mm³ with temperature >38°C or >100.4°F), or ANC <500/mm³ for ≥7 days	Reduce paclitaxel dosage by one dose level and consider adding filgrastim in subsequent cycles. Do not reduce the cisplatin dose
Recurrence of febrile neutropenia (ANC <1000/mm³ with temperature >38°C or >100.4°F), or ANC <500/mm³ for ≥7 days despite prior dose reduction of paclitaxel	Administer filgrastim in subsequent cycles and continue paclitaxel at the same dose. If already administering filgrastim, then reduce paclitaxel dose by an additional one dose level. Do not reduce the cisplatin dose
G2 motor or sensory neuropathies	Reduce both paclitaxel and cisplatin dosages by two dose levels without interrupting planned treatment
G ≥3 peripheral neuropathy	Interrupt therapy with paclitaxel and cisplatin until peripheral neuropathy improves to G ≤1, then reduce both paclitaxel and cisplatin dosages by two dose levels
Moderate hypersensitivity during paclitaxel infusion	Patient may be re-treated with paclitaxel. Base a decision to re-treat on reaction severity and the medically responsible care provider's judgment
Severe hypersensitivity during paclitaxel infusion	Discontinue paclitaxel

(*continued*)

Treatment Modifications (continued)

Adverse Event	Treatment Modifications
G ≥2 arthralgias/myalgias	Add dexamethasone as secondary prophylaxis
G3 arthralgia/myalgia despite dexamethasone prophylaxis	Reduce paclitaxel dosage one dose level
G ≥2 AST (SGOT) or ALT (SGPT), or G ≥2 bilirubin	Interrupt paclitaxel until improvement to G ≤1, then reduce paclitaxel dosage by one dose level. Continue cisplatin at the same dose
G2 ototoxicity (tinnitus, hearing loss)	Reduce cisplatin dosage by two dose levels without interrupting planned treatment. Do not reduce the paclitaxel dose
G ≥3 ototoxicity (tinnitus, hearing loss)	Interrupt therapy with cisplatin until ototoxicity improves to G ≤1, then reduce the cisplatin dosage by two dose levels. Do not reduce the paclitaxel dose
Severe hypersensitivity reaction to cisplatin is noted	Permanently discontinue cisplatin. May consider cisplatin desensitization if benefit thought to outweigh risk
Serum creatinine ≥1.5 mg/dL (≥130 μmol/L)	Withhold cisplatin until serum creatinine <1.5 mg/dL (<130 μmol/L), then decrease cisplatin dosage by one dose level; if already reduced, then reduce again
Other G ≥3 nonhematologic toxicities (except nausea, vomiting, elevated transaminases, and alopecia)	Delay all treatment until toxicity resolves to baseline, then decrease cisplatin and paclitaxel dosages by one dose level from previous dose levels
Treatment delay >2 weeks	Decrease dosage by one dose level for cisplatin and paclitaxel, or consider discontinuing treatment

Adverse Events (N = 439)

	Cisplatin or Topotecan + Paclitaxel + Bevacizumab (N = 220)	Cisplatin or/ Topotecan + Paclitaxel (N = 219)	
Grade ≥2 gastrointestinal events, excluding fistulas	52	44	OR 1.38, 95% CI 0.93–2.04; P = 0.10
Grade ≥4 neutropenia	35	26	OR 1.56, 95% CI 1.02–2.40; P = 0.04
Grade ≥2 pain	32	28	OR 1.21, 95% CI 0.79–1.85; P = 0.41
Grade ≥2 hypertension	25	2	OR 17.50, 95% CI 6.23–67.50; *P* <0.001
Grade ≥3 thromboembolism	8	1	OR 6.42, 95% CI 1.83–34.4; P = 0.001
Grade ≥3 fistula	6	<1	OR 13.69, 95% CI 2.01–584.00; P = 0.002
Grade ≥3 febrile neutropenia	5	5	OR 1.00, 95% CI 0.40–2.48; P = 1.00
Grade ≥3 genitourinary bleeding	3	<1	OR 6.11, 95% CI 0.73–282.00; P = 0.12
Grade ≥3 gastrointestinal bleeding	2	<1	OR 4.04, 95% CI 0.39–200.00; P = 0.37
Grade ≥3 proteinuria	2	0	P = 0.12
Grade ≥3 central nervous system bleeding	0	0	NA

Note: Selected toxicities are included in the table. Toxicities were graded according to the National Cancer Institute Common Terminology Criteria for Adverse Events, version 4.0. Four patients in the bevacizumab group died from a treatment-related cause (three owing to infection with grade 4 neutropenia and one owing to infection with unknown absolute neutrophil count) compared with four patients who did not receive bevacizumab (two owing to infection with grade 4 neutropenia, one owing to gastrointestinal perforation, and one owing to adult respiratory distress syndrome) compared with one patient in the cisplatin group (owing to infection with grade 4 neutropenia)

ADVANCED/RECURRENT • SUBSEQUENT THERAPY

CERVICAL CANCER REGIMEN: PEMBROLIZUMAB

Chung HC et al. J Clin Oncol 2019;37:1470–1478
Protocol for: Chung HC et al. J Clin Oncol 2019;37:1470–1478

Pembrolizumab 200 mg; administer intravenously over 30 minutes in a volume of 0.9% sodium chloride injection (0.9% NS) or 5% dextrose injection (D5W) sufficient to produce a pembrolizumab concentration within the range 1–10 mg/mL every 3 weeks for up to 24 months (total dose/3-week cycle = 200 mg), *or:*

Alternative pembrolizumab dose and schedule as per the U.S. FDA regimens approved on April 28, 2020:

Pembrolizumab 400 mg; administer intravenously over 30 minutes in a volume of 0.9% NS or D5W sufficient to produce a pembrolizumab concentration within the range 1–10 mg/mL every 6 weeks for up to 24 months (total dose/6-week cycle = 400 mg)

- Administer pembrolizumab with an administration set that contains a sterile, non-pyrogenic, low protein-binding in-line or add-on filter with pore size within the range of 0.2–5 μm
- Pembrolizumab can cause severe or life-threatening infusion-related reactions, including hypersensitivity and anaphylaxis
- The U.S. Food and Drug Administration approved indication for pembrolizumab as subsequent therapy for recurrent or metastatic cervical cancer is limited to patients with PD-L1 expressing tumors (combined positive score [CPS] ≥1). CPS is calculated as the number of PD-L1 staining cells (including tumor cells, lymphocytes, and macrophages/histocytes) divided by the total number of viable tumor cells, multiplied by 100

Supportive Care

Antiemetic prophylaxis
Emetogenic potential is **MINIMAL**
See Chapter 42 for antiemetic recommendations

Hematopoietic growth factor (CSF) prophylaxis
Primary prophylaxis is **NOT** *indicated*
See Chapter 43 for more information

Antimicrobial prophylaxis
Risk of fever and neutropenia is **LOW**
  Antimicrobial primary prophylaxis to be considered:
  - Antibacterial—not indicated
  - Antifungal—not indicated
  - Antiviral—not indicated unless patient previously had an episode of HSV

Patient Population Studied

KEYNOTE–158 was an international, open-label, multicohort, phase 2 study of single-agent pembrolizumab in multiple advanced solid tumors progressing after standard systemic therapy. Cohort E included 98 adult patients with histologically or cytologically confirmed advanced cervical cancer who had disease progression during or intolerance to at least 1 prior line of standard treatment. PD-L1 combined positive score (CPS) was ≥1 in 82/98 patients (83.7%). Patients were required to have an Eastern Cooperative Oncology Group (ECOG) performance status of 0–1, adequate organ function, and measurable disease. Tumors were assessed for PD-L1 expression but patients could be enrolled irrespective of expression status. Patients were excluded if they had active central nervous system metastases, had active autoimmune disease requiring recent immunosuppressive therapy within the prior 2 years, or had a history of pneumonitis requiring steroids or current pneumonitis

Efficacy

| Antitumor Activity | Total Population (N = 98)* | PD-L1-Positive Population [CPS ≥1] | | PD-L1-Negative (N = 15) |
		Total (N = 82)	Previously Treated (N = 77)†	
ORR	12 (12.2)	12 (14.6)	11 (14.3)	0 (0.0)
95% CI	6.5–20.4	7.8–24.2	7.4–24.1	0.0–21.8
DCR	30 (30.6)	27 (32.9)	24 (31.2)	3 (20.0)
95% CI	21.7–40.7	22.9–44.2	21.2–42.7	4.3–48.1

(continued)

Efficacy (continued)

Antitumor Activity	Total Population (N = 98)*	PD-L1-Positive Population [CPS ≥1]		PD-L1-Negative (N = 15)
		Total (N = 82)	Previously Treated (N = 77)†	
Best overall response				
CR	3 (3.1)	3 (3.7)	2 (2.6)	0 (0.0)
PR	9 (9.2)	9 (11.0)	9 (11.7)	0 (0.0)
SD	18 (18.4)	15 (18.3)	13 (16.9)	3 (20.0)
Progressive disease	55 (56.1)	44 (53.7)	42 (54.5)	10 (66.7)
Not evaluable‡	5 (5.1)	4 (4.9)	4 (5.2)	1 (6.7)
Not assessable§	8 (8.2)	7 (8.5)	7 (9.1)	1 (6.7)
Time to response, months‖				
Median (range)	2.1 (1.6–4.1)	2.1 (1.6–4.1)	2.2 (1.6–4.1)	
Duration of response, months‖ϵ				
Median (range)	NR (≥3.7 to ≥18.6)	NR (≥3.7 to ≥18.6)	NR (≥4.1 to ≥18.6)	

Note: Data are presented as No. (%) unless otherwise indicated

Abbreviations: PD-L1, programmed death ligand 1; CPS, combined positive score; ORR, objective response rate; CI, confidence interval; DCR, disease control rate; CR, complete response; PR, partial response; SD, stable disease; NR, not reached

*Includes 1 patient who had disease not evaluable for PD-L1 expression
†Patients who had received one or more line of chemotherapy for recurrent or metastatic disease
‡Patients who had one or more postbaseline tumor assessment, none of which were evaluable
§Patients who had no postbaseline tumor assessment because of death, withdrawal of consent, loss to follow-up, or start of new anticancer therapy
‖Evaluated in patients who had a CR or PR (n = 12 for total population, n = 12 for PD-L1–positive population)
ϵEstimated using Kaplan-Meier method

Therapy Monitoring

- Initially at the time of each dose, and eventually every 6–12 weeks, perform a total body skin examination with attention to ALL mucous membranes as well as a complete review of systems
- Monitor patients for signs and symptoms of pneumonitis. Evaluate patients with suspected pneumonitis with chest x-ray, CT, and pulse oximetry. For ≥2 toxicity, may include nasal swab, sputum culture and sensitivity, blood culture and sensitivity, and urine culture and sensitivity
- Monitor patients for signs and symptoms of colitis. Encourage patients to report diarrhea immediately to any member of the health care team
- Draw AST, ALT, and bilirubin prior to each infusion and/or weekly if there are grade 1 liver function test elevations. Note, no treatment is recommended for G1 LFT abnormalities. For ≥2 toxicity, work up for other causes of elevated LFTs including viral hepatitis
- Use basic metabolic panel (Na, K, CO_2, glucose) and patient history as screening tools for hypophysitis including hypopituitarism and adrenal insufficiency. If in doubt, evaluate AM adrenocorticotropic hormone (ACTH) and cortisol levels. Consider ACTH stimulation test for indeterminate results
- Assess thyroid function at the start of treatment, periodically during treatment, and as indicated based on clinical evaluation, and for clinical signs and symptoms of thyroid disorders. Test for TSH and free thyroxine (FT4) every 4 to 6 weeks as part of routine clinical monitoring on therapy or for case detection in symptomatic patients
- Measure glucose at baseline and with each treatment during the first 12 weeks and every 6 weeks thereafter
- Obtain a serum creatinine prior to every dose. If creatinine is found to be newly elevated, consider holding therapy while other potential causes are evaluated. Note, routine urinalysis is not necessary other than to rule out urinary tract infections, etc.
- Obtain a complete rheumatologic history and perform an examination of all peripheral joints for tenderness, swelling, and range of motion. Examine the spine. Consider plain x-ray/imaging to exclude metastases and evaluate joint damage (erosions), if appropriate
- In patients at high risk for infections and in appropriately selected patients based on an infectious disease evaluation, draw screening laboratories (HIV, hepatitis A and B, and blood QuantiFERON for TB) to prepare patients to start infliximab
- Response evaluation: Every 2–4 months

Treatment Modifications

RECOMMENDED DOSE MODIFICATIONS FOR PEMBROLIZUMAB

Adverse Event	Grade/Severity	Treatment Modification
Infusion reaction	Clinically significant but not severe infusion reaction	Interrupt the infusion in patients with clinically significant infusion reactions and consider resuming at a slower rate following resolution. If decision is made to restart, begin at ≤50% of the rate prior to the reaction and increase in 50% increments every 30 minutes if well tolerated. Infusions may be restarted at the full rate during the next cycle
	G3/4 (severe infusion reaction— pyrexia, chills, flushing, hypotension, dyspnea, wheezing, back pain, abdominal pain, and urticaria). Not rapidly responsive to brief interruption of infusion	Stop infusion and administer appropriate medical therapy (eg, epinephrine, corticosteroids, intravenous antihistamines, bronchodilators and/or oxygen). Discontinue pembrolizumab
Colitis	G1	Loperamide 4 mg as starting dose then 2mg before each meal and after each loose stool until without diarrhea for 12 hours, with maximum of 16 mg loperamide per day. If G1 diarrhea or colitis persists >14 days, then add prednisolone 0.5–1 mg/kg (non-enteric coated) or consider oral budesonide 9 mg daily if no bloody diarrhea
	G2/3 diarrhea or colitis	Withhold pembrolizumab. Loperamide 4 mg as starting dose then 2mg before each meal and after each loose stool until without diarrhea for 12 hours, with maximum of 16 mg loperamide per day. Administer oral prednisone/prednisolone at a dose of 0.5–2 mg/kg/day or its equivalent. When improves to G1, begin a slow corticosteroid taper over at least 4 weeks. Resume pembrolizumab upon symptom control, or when prednisone/prednisolone daily dose <10 mg
	G4 diarrhea or colitis	Permanently discontinue pembrolizumab. Loperamide 4 mg as starting dose then 2 mg before each meal and after each loose stool until without diarrhea for 12 hours, with maximum of 16 mg loperamide per day. Administer 1–2 mg/kg IV (methyl) prednisolone and convert to 0.5–2 mg/kg prednisone/prednisolone orally each day or its equivalent only after a response. Taper over at least 4 weeks when symptoms improve. If does not improve over 72 hours or worsens, perform flexible sigmoidoscopy/ colonoscopy to document colitis then begin infliximab 5 mg/kg (if no perforation/ sepsis/TB/hepatitis/NYHA III/IV CHF). If no response add mycophenolate mofetil (MMF) 500–1000 mg twice daily. If worse on MMF, consider addition of tacrolimus or anti-thymocyte globulin (ATG)
Pneumonitis	G2	Withhold pembrolizumab. Consider pneumocystis prophylaxis depending on the clinical context and coverage with empiric antibiotics. Administer oral prednisone/prednisolone at a dose of 1–2 mg/kg/day or its equivalent. When improves to G1, begin a slow corticosteroid taper over at least 4 weeks. If does not respond adequately after 48 hours, then administer 2–4 mg/kg IV (methyl)prednisolone and convert to 0.5–2 mg/kg prednisone/prednisolone orally each day or its equivalent only after a response, followed by a taper over at least 6 weeks when symptoms improve to G1, titrating to symptoms. Resume pembrolizumab upon symptom control, or when prednisone/prednisolone daily dose <10 mg
	G3/4	Permanently discontinue pembrolizumab. Consider pneumocystis prophylaxis depending on the clinical context; cover with empiric antibiotics. Administer 2–4 mg/kg IV (methyl)prednisolone and convert to 1–2 mg/kg prednisone/prednisolone orally each day or its equivalent only after a response, followed by a taper over at least 8 weeks when symptoms improve to G1, titrating to symptoms. If when initially treated improvement does not occur within 48–72 hours, begin infliximab 5 mg/kg (if no perforation/ sepsis/TB/hepatitis/NYHA III/IV CHF). If no response to infliximab, add mycophenolate mofetil (MMF) 500–1000 mg twice daily. Consider MMF especially if has concurrent hepatic toxicity
Hepatitis	G2 (AST or ALT >3–5× ULN or total bilirubin >1.5–3× ULN)	Withhold pembrolizumab. Administer oral prednisone/prednisolone at a dose of 1 to 2 mg/kg/day or its equivalent. When improves to G1, begin a slow corticosteroid taper over at least 4 weeks. Resume pembrolizumab upon symptom control, or when prednisone/prednisolone daily dose <10 mg

(continued)

Treatment Modifications (*continued*)

Adverse Event	Grade/Severity	Treatment Modification
	G3/4 (AST or ALT >5× ULN or total bilirubin >3× ULN)	Permanently discontinue pembrolizumab. Administer 1–2 mg/kg IV (methyl) prednisolone and convert to 0.5–2 mg/kg prednisone/prednisolone orally each day or its equivalent only after a response. Taper over at least 6 weeks when symptoms improve. If no response, add MMF 500–1000 mg twice daily. If worse on MMF, consider adding tacrolimus or ATG
Hypophysitis	G2/3 (moderate symptoms, ie, headache but no visual disturbance or fatigue/mood alteration but hemodynamically stable, no electrolyte disturbance)	Administer analgesia as needed for headache. Withhold pembrolizumab. Administer oral prednisone/prednisolone at a dose of 0.5–2 mg/kg/day or its equivalent. When improves to G1, begin a slow corticosteroid taper over at least 4 weeks. If no improvement in 48 hours, administer 1–2 mg/kg IV (methyl)prednisolone and convert to 0.5–2 mg/kg prednisone/prednisolone orally each day or its equivalent only after a response. Taper over at least 4 weeks when symptoms improve to 5 mg prednisone/prednisolone or equivalent; do not stop steroids. Resume pembrolizumab upon symptom control, or when prednisone/prednisolone daily dose <10 mg
	G4 (severe mass effect symptoms, ie, severe headache, any visual disturbance or severe hypoadrenalism, ie, hypotension, severe electrolyte disturbance)	Permanently discontinue pembrolizumab. Administer analgesia as needed for headache. Administer 1–2 mg/kg IV (methyl)prednisolone and convert to 0.5–2 mg/kg prednisone/prednisolone orally each day or its equivalent only after a response. Taper over at least 4 weeks when symptoms improve to 5 mg prednisone/prednisolone or equivalent; do not stop steroids
Adrenal insufficiency	G2	Withhold pembrolizumab. Administer oral prednisone/prednisolone at a dose of 0.5–2 mg/kg/day or its equivalent. When improves to G1, begin a slow corticosteroid taper over at least 4 weeks. Serially assess adrenal function and continue steroids at replacement doses (20–40 mg hydrocortisone daily ~2/3 dose in AM upon awakening and ~1/3 at 4 PM) until recovery of adrenal function is documented. Resume pembrolizumab upon symptom control, or when prednisone/prednisolone daily dose <10 mg
	G3/4	Permanently discontinue pembrolizumab. Administer oral prednisone/prednisolone at a dose of 0.5–2 mg/kg/day or its equivalent. When improves to G1, begin a slow corticosteroid taper over at least 4 weeks. Serially assess adrenal function and continue steroids at replacement doses (20–40 mg hydrocortisone daily ~2/3 dose in AM upon awakening and ~1/3 at 4 PM) until recovery of adrenal function is documented
Type 1 diabetes mellitus	G3 hyperglycemia	Withhold pembrolizumab. Admit to hospital to manage hyperglycemia. Role of corticosteroids in preventing complete loss of insulin-producing cells is unknown and not recommended. Resume pembrolizumab upon symptom control, or when prednisone/prednisolone daily dose <10 mg
	G4 hyperglycemia	Permanently discontinue pembrolizumab. Admit to hospital to manage hyperglycemia. Role of corticosteroids in preventing complete loss of insulin-producing cells is unknown and not recommended
Nephritis and renal dysfunction	G2/3 (serum creatinine 1.5–6× ULN)	Withhold pembrolizumab. Administer oral prednisone/prednisolone at a dose of 0.5–2 mg/kg/day or its equivalent. When improves to G1, begin a slow corticosteroid taper over at least 4 weeks. If does not respond adequately, then administer 0.5–1 mg/kg IV (methyl)prednisolone and convert to 0.5–2 mg/kg prednisone/prednisolone orally each day or its equivalent only after a response, followed by a taper over at least 4 weeks when improves to G1. Resume pembrolizumab upon symptom control, or when prednisone/prednisolone daily dose <10 mg
	G4 (serum creatinine >6× ULN)	Permanently discontinue pembrolizumab. Administer 0.5–1 mg/kg IV (methyl) prednisolone and convert to 0.5–2 mg/kg prednisone/prednisolone orally each day or its equivalent only after a response, followed by a taper over at least 4 weeks when improves to G1
Skin	G1/2	Continue pembrolizumab. Avoid skin irritants, avoid sun exposure, topical emollients recommended. Topical steroid (mild strength for G1, moderate/potent strength for G2) cream once or twice daily ± oral or topical antihistamines for itching

(*continued*)

Treatment Modifications (*continued*)

Adverse Event	Grade/Severity	Treatment Modification
	G3 rash or suspected SJS or TEN	Withhold pembrolizumab. Avoid skin irritants, avoid sun exposure, topical emollients recommended. Administer oral or topical antihistamines for itching. Administer oral prednisone/prednisolone at a dose of 0.5–2 mg/kg or its equivalent daily for 3 days followed by a slow corticosteroid taper over at least 4 weeks when the rash improves to G1. If does not respond adequately, then administer 0.5–1 mg/kg IV (methyl) prednisolone and convert to 0.5–2 mg/kg prednisone/prednisolone orally each day or its equivalent only after a response, followed by a taper over at least 4 weeks when the rash improves to G1. Resume pembrolizumab upon symptom control, or when prednisone/prednisolone daily dose <10 mg
	G4 rash or confirmed SJS or TEN	Avoid skin irritants, avoid sun exposure, topical emollients recommended. Administer oral or topical antihistamines for itching. Administer 1–2 mg/kg IV (methyl) prednisolone and convert to oral steroids 0.5–2 mg/kg prednisone/prednisolone each day or its equivalent only after a response. Taper over at least 4 weeks when the rash improves to G1. Permanently discontinue pembrolizumab
Encephalitis	Confusion or altered behavior, headaches, alteration in Glasgow Coma Scale, motor or sensory deficits, speech abnormality, may or may not be febrile	Initially withhold pembrolizumab, but permanently discontinue pembrolizumab if there is no doubt as to diagnosis. Exclude bacterial and ideally viral infections prior to high-dose steroids. Administer oral prednisone/prednisolone at a dose of 0.5–2 mg/kg/day or its equivalent. When symptoms improve, begin a slow corticosteroid taper over at least 4–8 weeks. If symptoms are severe, administer 1–2 mg/kg IV (methyl) prednisolone and convert to 0.5–2 mg/kg prednisone/prednisolone orally each day or its equivalent only after a response. Consider concurrent empiric antiviral (IV acyclovir) and antibacterial therapy
Aseptic meningitis	Headache, photophobia, neck stiffness with fever or may be afebrile, vomiting; normal cognition/cerebral function (distinguishes from encephalitis)	
Other syndromes include neurosarcoidosis, posterior reversible leukoencephalopathy syndrome (PRES), Vogt-Koyanagi-Harada syndrome, demyelination, vasculitic encephalopathy, and generalized seizures		
Transverse myelitis	Acute or subacute neurologic signs/symptoms of motor/sensory/autonomic origin; most have sensory level; often bilateral symptoms	Initially withhold pembrolizumab, but permanently discontinue pembrolizumab if there is no doubt as to diagnosis. Administer 2 mg/kg IV (methyl)prednisolone or consider 1 g/day and convert to 0.5–2 mg/kg prednisone/prednisolone orally each day or its equivalent only after a response. When symptoms improve, begin a slow corticosteroid taper over at least 4–8 weeks. Plasmapheresis may be required if steroids do not bring about improvement
Myocarditis	G3	Permanently discontinue pembrolizumab. Administer 2 mg/kg IV (methyl)prednisolone or consider 1 g/day and convert to 0.5–2 mg/kg prednisone/prednisolone orally each day or its equivalent only after a response. When symptoms improve, begin a slow corticosteroid taper over at least 4–8 weeks. If no response, add MMF 500–1000 mg twice daily. If worse on MMF, consider adding tacrolimus
Peripheral neurologic toxicity	Moderate: some interference with ADL, symptoms concerning to patient	Withhold pembrolizumab. Initial observation reasonable or initiate prednisone/prednisolone 0.5–1 mg/kg (if progressing, eg, from mild) and/or pregabalin or duloxetine for pain. When symptoms improve, begin a slow corticosteroid taper over at least 4 weeks. Resume pembrolizumab upon symptom control, or when prednisone/prednisolone daily dose <10 mg
	Severe: limits self-care and aids warranted, life threatening, eg, respiratory problems	Permanently discontinue pembrolizumab. Administer 1–2 mg/kg IV (methyl) prednisolone and convert to 0.5–2 mg/kg prednisone/prednisolone orally each day or its equivalent only after a response. Taper over at least 4–8 weeks when symptoms improve to G1
Guillain-Barré syndrome	Progressive symmetrical muscle weakness with absent or reduced tendon reflexes—involves extremities and facial, respiratory, and bulbar and oculomotor muscles; dysregulation of autonomic nerves	Permanently discontinue pembrolizumab. Use of steroids not recommended in idiopathic Guillain-Barré syndrome; however, a trial of (methyl)prednisolone 1–2 mg/kg is reasonable, converting to 0.5–2 mg/kg prednisone/prednisolone orally each day or its equivalent only after a response. If no improvement or worsening, plasmapheresis or IVIG indicated

(continued)

Treatment Modifications (continued)

Adverse Event	Grade/Severity	Treatment Modification
Myasthenia gravis	Fluctuating muscle weakness (proximal limb, trunk, ocular, eg, ptosis/diplopia or bulbar) with fatigability, respiratory muscles may also be involved	Permanently discontinue pembrolizumab. Administer pyridostigmine at an initial dose of 30 mg three times daily. Administer oral prednisone/prednisolone at a dose of 0.5–2 mg/kg/day or its equivalent or 1–2 mg/kg IV (methyl)prednisolone depending on the severity of symptoms. If begin with IV, convert to 0.5–2 mg/kg prednisone/prednisolone orally each day or its equivalent only after a response. If no improvement or worsening, plasmapheresis or IVIG may be considered. Additional immunosuppressants used in myasthenia gravis include azathioprine, cyclosporine, and mycophenolate. Avoid certain medications, eg, ciprofloxacin, beta-blockers, that may precipitate cholinergic crisis
Other syndromes including motor and sensory peripheral neuropathy, multifocal radicular neuropathy/plexopathy, autonomic neuropathy, phrenic nerve palsy, cranial nerve palsies (eg, facial nerve, optic nerve, hypoglossal nerve)		Permanently discontinue pembrolizumab. Administer oral prednisone/prednisolone at a dose of 0.5–2 mg/kg/day or its equivalent or 1–2 mg/kg IV (methyl)prednisolone depending on the severity of symptoms. If begin with IV, convert to 0.5–2 mg/kg prednisone/prednisolone orally each day or its equivalent only after a response
Arthralgia	G1 (mild pain with inflammation, erythema or joint swelling)	Continue pembrolizumab. Administer acetaminophen (paracetamol) and ibuprofen
	G2 (moderate pain with inflammation, erythema, or joint swelling that limits ADLs)	Withhold pembrolizumab. Administer higher doses of acetaminophen (paracetamol) and ibuprofen and use diclofenac or naproxen or etoricoxib. If inadequately controlled, consider intra-articular steroid injections for large joints or administer oral prednisone/prednisolone at a dose of 0.5–2 mg/kg/day or its equivalent. When improves to G1, begin a slow corticosteroid taper over at least 4 weeks. If does not respond adequately, then administer 0.5–1 mg/kg IV (methyl)prednisolone and convert to 0.5–2 mg/kg prednisone/prednisolone orally each day or its equivalent only after a response, followed by a taper over at least 4 weeks when improves to G1. Resume pembrolizumab upon symptom control, or when prednisone/prednisolone daily dose <10 mg
	G3 (severe pain; irreversible joint damage; disabling; limits self-care ADL)	Withhold pembrolizumab. Administer 0.5–1 mg/kg IV (methyl)prednisolone and convert to 0.5–2 mg/kg prednisone/prednisolone orally each day or its equivalent only after a response, followed by a taper over at least 4 weeks when improves to G1. In severe cases, infliximab or another anti-TNF alpha drug may be required for improvement of arthritis. Resume pembrolizumab upon symptom control, or when prednisone/prednisolone daily dose <10 mg
Other	First occurrence of other G3	Withhold pembrolizumab. Administer oral prednisone/prednisolone at a dose of 0.5–2 mg/kg/day or its equivalent. When improves to G1, begin a slow corticosteroid taper over at least 4 weeks. Resume pembrolizumab upon symptom control, or when prednisone/prednisolone daily dose <10 mg
	Recurrence of same G3	Permanently discontinue pembrolizumab. Administer 1–2 mg/kg IV (methyl)prednisolone and convert to 0.5–2 mg/kg prednisone/prednisolone orally each day or its equivalent only after a response. Taper over at least 4–8 weeks when symptoms improve to G1
	Life-threatening or G4	
	Requirement for ≥10 mg/day prednisone or equivalent for >12 weeks	Permanently discontinue pembrolizumab
	Persistent G2/3 adverse reactions lasting ≥12 weeks	

ADL, activities of daily living; ALT, alanine aminotransferase; AST, aspartate aminotransferase; ATG, anti-thymocyte globulin; SJS, Stevens-Johnson Syndrome; TEN, toxic epidermal necrolysis; ULN, upper limit of normal.

Notes on general supportive care:
- Steroid taper in most cases will proceed over a minimum of 1 month, but if symptoms improve rapidly, a 2-week taper can be considered. If steroids are administered for more than 4 weeks, consider PCP prophylaxis (cotrimoxazole 480 mg twice daily M/W/F or inhaled pentamidine if cotrimoxazole allergy), regular random blood glucose, VitD level and starting calcium/VitD supplementation as per guidelines

Notes on pregnancy and breastfeeding:
- Pembrolizumab can cause fetal harm. If used during pregnancy, or if the patient becomes pregnant during treatment, apprise the patient of the potential hazard to a fetus. Females of reproductive potential should use highly effective contraception during treatment and for 4 months after the last dose of pembrolizumab
- It is not known whether pembrolizumab is excreted in human milk. Therefore, it is recommended that women discontinue nursing during treatment with and for 4 months after the final dose of pembrolizumab

Adverse Events (N = 98)

Grade (%)	Pembrolizumab (N = 98)	
	Grade 1–2	Grade 3–4
Treatment-related adverse events of any grade*		
Any*	53	12
Hypothyroidism*	10	0
Decreased appetite*	9	0
Fatigue*	9	0
Diarrhea*	7	1
AST increased*	5	2
Asthenia*	6	1
Pyrexia*	6	1
Hyperthyroidism*	7	0
Arthralgia*	5	1
Nausea*	6	0
Pruritus*	6	0
Rash*	6	0
Vomiting*	6	0
Abdominal pain*	5	0
ALT increased*	0	3
Immune-mediated adverse events and infusion reactions[†]		
Hypothyroidism[†]	11	0
Hyperthyroidism[†]	9	0
Infusion-related reaction[†]	3	0
Colitis[†]	2	0
Hepatitis[†]	0	2
Severe skin reactions[†]	0	2
Adrenal insufficiency[†]	0	1
Myositis[†]	1	0
Pneumonitis[†]	1	0
Uveitis[†]	1	0

*Includes treatment-related adverse events of any grade that occurred in ≥5 patients or of grade 3–4 that occurred in ≥2 patients
[†]Occurring in ≥1 patient; immune-mediated events were based on a list of terms specified by the sponsor and were considered regardless of attribution to the treatment or immune relatedness as determined by the investigator; related terms were included

11. Chronic Lymphocytic Leukemia

Dhaval Mehta, MD, and Kanti Rai, MD

Epidemiology

Incidence:	21,040 (male: 12,930; female: 8110. Estimated new cases for 2020 in the United States). 191,000 (worldwide). Incidence rates: 6.0 and 3.3 cases per 100,000 population per year among men and women respectively
Deaths:	4060 (male: 2330; female: 1730. Estimated deaths for 2020 in the United States). Estimated 61,000 per year worldwide
Median age:	70 years
Male to female ratio:	1.3:1

Stage at Presentation (Rai):

Stage 0:	31%
Stage I/II:	59%
Stages III/IV:	10%

Global Burden of Disease Cancer Collaboration et al. JAMA Oncol 2017:3:524–548

Siegel R et al. CA Cancer J Clin 2020;70:7–30

Surveillance, Epidemiology and End Results (SEER) Program, available from http://seer.cancer.gov (accessed in 2020)

Work-up

Essential

1. Medical history and PE: attention to node-bearing areas, including the Waldeyer ring, and to size of liver and spleen
2. Performance status
3. B-symptoms
4. Laboratory work-up: CBC with differential, LDH, comprehensive metabolic panel

Useful in certain circumstances

1. Quantitative immunoglobulins
2. β_2-Microglobulin
3. Reticulocyte count, haptoglobin, direct Coombs test
4. Uric acid
5. Chest, abdomen, and pelvis CT scans with contrast of diagnostic quality prior to initiation of therapy
6. Hepatitis B testing if CD20 monoclonal antibody contemplated
7. Pregnancy testing in women of child-bearing age (if chemotherapy planned)
8. Unilateral bone marrow biopsy + aspirate at initiation of therapy
9. MUGA scan/echocardiogram if anthracycline-based regimen is indicated
10. PET/CT scan to direct nodal biopsy, if histologic transformation is suspected
11. Discussion of sperm banking and fertility issues

Informative for prognostic and/or therapy determination

1. CpG-stimulated metaphase karyotype
2. FISH analysis to detect: +12, del(11q), del(13q), del(17p)
3. TP53 sequencing
4. Molecular analysis to detect immunoglobulin heavy-chain variable gene (IGHV) mutation status

Diagnosis

NCI working group diagnostic criteria

1. Absolute lymphocytosis in the peripheral blood with a count of $\geq 5 \times 10^9$ B lymphocytes and cells morphologically mature in appearance
2. The clonality of the B cells must be confirmed by flow cytometry
3. The monoclonal B-cell lymphocytes express low levels of surface immunoglobulins, simultaneously with CD5, CD23, CD19, and CD20

Hallek M et al. Blood 2008;111:5446–5456

Prognosis

Unfavorable risk factors

1. Advanced clinical stage
2. Rapid lymphocyte doubling time (<6 months)
3. TP53 mutation by DNA sequencing, and/or del(17p)
4. Unmutated IGHV genes (≤2 % mutation)
5. Diffuse bone marrow lymphocytic involvement
6. del(11q) by interphase (FISH) cytogenetics (normal karyotype and trisomy 12 have an intermediate prognosis, while 13q deletion has a good prognosis)*
7. Complex karyotype (≥3 unrelated) on conventional karyotyping
8. CD38 (>30%), ZAP-70 expression (>20%), CD49d (>30%) measured via flow cytometry

*Döehner H et al. N Engl J Med 2000;343:1910–1916

Staging and Survival

Kay NE et al. Hematology Am Soc Hematol Educ Program 2002:193–213

Rai	Lymphocytosis	Lymph Node Enlargement	Spleen/Liver Enlargement	Hemoglobin <11 g/dL	Platelets <100,000/mm³	Survival (Years)
0	Yes	No	No	No	No	>13
I	Yes	Yes	No	No	No	8
II	Yes	±	Yes	No	No	6
III	Yes	±	±	Yes*	No	4
IV	Yes	±	±	±	Yes*	2

*Not immune-related

Expert Opinion

Chronic lymphocytic leukemia (CLL) is one of the most common leukemias in the Western world, characterized by progressive proliferation of functionally incompetent lymphocytes, which are monoclonal in origin. The diagnosis requires a count of >5000 circulating CLL type cells per cubic millimeter. CLL is an extremely heterogenous disease, while there had been a general belief that CLL is an indolent disease associated with a prolonged life span (10–20 years) and the eventual cause of death may be unrelated to CLL. However, this observation is true for <30 percent of all CLL cases. Some patients die rapidly, within 2–3 years from diagnosis, from complications or causes directly related to CLL. Other patients live for 5–10 years with an initial course that is relatively benign followed by a terminal phase lasting 1–2 years. The diagnosis of CLL does not imply the need for immediate treatment; rather, a number of iWCLL indications justify the need for patient-specific therapy

Hallek M et al. Blood 2018;131:2745–2760

Treatment by stage:

- Asymptomatic early stage disease (Rai 0, Binet A) should be monitored without therapy rather than active immediate treatment
- Intermediate (stages I and II) and high risk (stages III and IV) according to the Rai classification or at Binet stage B or C usually benefit from the initiation of treatment. Some of these patients (in particular, Rai intermediate risk or Binet stage B) can be monitored without therapy until they have evidence for progressive or symptomatic disease

Indications for treatment include:

- Evidence of progressive marrow failure as manifested by the development or worsening of anemia (hemoglobin <11 g/dL) and/or thrombocytopenia (platelets <100 × 10⁹/L)
- Constitutional symptoms: Any one of the following disease-related symptoms must be present:
  a. Unintentional weight loss ≥10% within the previous 6 months
  b. Significant fatigue; that is, Eastern Cooperative Oncology Group performance status 2 or worse (cannot work or unable to perform usual activities)

(continued)

(*continued*)

   c. Fevers >100.5°F (>38.0°C) for ≥2 weeks without other evidence of infection

   d. Night sweats for more than 1 month without evidence of infection

- Massive, progressive, or symptomatic splenomegaly
- Massive, progressive, or symptomatic lymphadenopathy
- Autoimmune anemia and/or thrombocytopenia that is poorly responsive to corticosteroids or other second-line treatments (splenectomy, intravenous immunoglobulin, and/or immunosuppressive agents, rituximab)
- Rapidly increasing lymphocytosis with an increase of >50% over 2 months or lymphocyte doubling time of <6 months

Note: Recurrent bacterial infections are common in patients with CLL, but we do not view this as a reason to treat the underlying CLL unless any of the above mentioned criteria for initiating therapy exist. We would first attempt therapy with intravenous gamma globulin (IVIG) monthly for the prevention of recurrent bacterial infections. If IVIG is not successful in preventing recurrent bacterial infections, then we would initiate therapy

Isolated hypogammaglobulinemia or monoclonal paraproteinemia do not constitute a basis for initiating therapy. Patients with CLL may present with a markedly elevated leukocyte count; however, the symptoms associated with leukocyte aggregates that develop in patients with acute leukemia rarely occur in patients with CLL. Therefore, the absolute lymphocyte count should not be used as the sole indicator for initiating treatment

Therapy: There are multiple treatment options available for patients with CLL and most have not been directly compared. Hence, there is not one treatment that is considered the "standard of care" for all patients. The choice of therapy depends upon patient characteristics including age, performance status, comorbidities, compliance, and the expected goals of care based upon disease risk factors. Once a patient meets iWCLL guidelines for treatment, we recommend checking del(17p)/TP53 mutation and IgVH mutation testing before consideration of various therapeutic approaches

A) If del(17p)/TP53 mutation-positive, patients will benefit from targeted therapy such as BTK inhibitors (such as ibrutinib, ibrutinib + rituximab, acalabrutinib) or BCL-2 inhibitors (such as venetoclax ± obinutuzumab) rather than chemoimmunotherapy approaches. Among the targeted agents, we have the longest efficacy and safety data for ibrutinib, although patients with a history of atrial fibrillation, significant hepatic impairment (Child-Pugh class B/C), severe bleeding, or current anticoagulant use remain at high risk for ibrutinib-related complications. Initial reports suggest venetoclax-based regimens can achieve MRD-negativity in the majority of patients whereas ibrutinib rarely achieves MRD-negativity

B) If negative for del(17p)/TP53 mutation, and IgVH unmutated, patients are likely to benefit from targeted therapy (such as ibrutinib, ibrutinib + rituximab, venetoclax + obinutuzumab)

C) If negative for del(17p)/TP53 mutation and IgVH mutated, then we recommend treatment based on patients' performance status, age, fitness, preference for definite vs indefinite treatment, and patients' compliance and preferences. For these populations, apart from targeted therapies as discussed above (ibrutinib or venetoclax-based regimens) which remain options, chemoimmunotherapy regimens such as FCR (younger patients), BR (older patients), and chlorambucil + obinutuzumab (older unfit patients) can be considered as they do provide treatment-free intervals with reasonable efficacy data

D) Patients with CLL are not cured with conventional therapy. While most patients will have an initial complete or partial response to treatment, all will relapse eventually. Asymptomatic relapse does not necessarily require immediate treatment but should be followed closely for the development of active disease. Targeted agents (eg, Bruton's tyrosine kinase [BTK] inhibitors, PI3-kinase inhibitors, BCL2 inhibitors, and novel antibodies) and other investigational therapies (eg, chimeric antigen receptor T cells) are changing the landscape of treatment options for relapsed or refractory disease. Allogenic HCT is reserved only for fit patients with relapsed disease

E) The CLL treatment landscape has changed tremendously over the last 5–10 years, and several cooperative group–led clinical trials are underway to define the optimal duration of treatment for newer targeted therapies as well as to understand resistance mechanisms leading to progression. Clinical trial participation is strongly encouraged for all patients to advance further treatment modalities

Abrisqueta P et al. Blood 2009;114:4916–4921
Badoux X et al. Blood 2011;117:3016–3024
Badoux XC et al. Blood 2011;118:Abstract 98
Chowdhury O et al. Br J Haematol;155:519–521
Coiffier B et al. Blood 2008;111:1094
Delgado J et al. Blood 2009;114:2581–2588
Döhner H et al. N Engl J Med 2000;343:1910–1916
Fischer K et al. J Clin Oncol 2012;30:3209–3216
Hallek M et al. Blood 2018;131:2745–2760
Hallek M et al. Lancet 2010;376:1164–1174
Knauf WU et al. J Clin Oncol 2009;27:4378
Moreton P et al. J Clin Oncol 2005;23:2971–2979
Rai KR et al. N Engl J Med 2000;343:1750–1757
Rai KR, Stilgenbauer S. www.uptodate.com/contents/overview-of-the-treatment-of-chronic-lymphocytic-leukemia. (Accessed June 2020)
Samaniego F et al. Blood 2008;112–309
Wierda WG et al. J Clin Oncol 2010;28:1749

FIRST-LINE

CHRONIC LYMPHOCYTIC LEUKEMIA REGIMEN: IBRUTINIB

Woyach JA et al. N Engl J Med 2018;379:2517–2528
Protocol for: Woyach JA et al. N Engl J Med 2018;379:2517–2528
Supplementary appendix to: Woyach JA et al. N Engl J Med 2018;379:2517–2528
IMBRUVICA (ibrutinib) prescribing information. Sunnyvale, CA: Pharmacyclics LLC; revised 2019 July

Ibrutinib 420 mg/dose; administer orally, once daily with a glass of water, without regard to food, continually until disease progression (total dose/week = 2940 mg)

Notes:
- Administration with food increases ibrutinib exposure approximately two-fold compared with administration after overnight fasting. Clinical studies instructed that ibrutinib be taken at least 30 minutes before eating or at least 2 hours after a meal at approximately the same time each day (Protocol for: Woyach JA et al. N Engl J Med 2018;379:2517–2528). However, the U.S. Food and Drug Administration–approved prescribing information does not make specific recommendations regarding administration of ibrutinib with regard to food. (Imbruvica [ibrutinib] prescribing information. Sunnyvale, CA: Pharmacyclics LLC; revised 2018 August). Others have also concluded that no food restrictions are needed given the relative safety profile of ibrutinib and because repeated drug intake in fasted conditions is unlikely (de Jong J et al. Cancer Chemother Pharmacol 2015;75:907–916)
- Ibrutinib capsules should be swallowed whole; do not break, open, or chew capsules. Ibrutinib tablets should be swallowed whole; do not cut, crush, or chew tablets
- Patients who delay taking ibrutinib at a regularly scheduled time may administer the missed dose as soon as possible on the same day, and then resume the normal schedule the following day. Do not administer an extra dose of ibrutinib to make up for a missed dose
- Ibrutinib is metabolized predominantly by CYP3A. Refer to treatment modification section for initial dose adjustment recommendations for patients requiring concurrent treatment with moderate or strong CYP3A inhibitors. Avoid concomitant use of ibrutinib with strong CYP3A inducers
- Advise patients to not consume grapefruit products or Seville oranges as they may inhibit CYP3A in the gut wall and increase the bioavailability of ibrutinib
- Serious bleeding events, some fatal, have been reported in patients treated with ibrutinib. Grade ≥3 bleeding events were reported to occur in 3% of patients. All-grade bleeding (including bruising and petechia) occurred in approximately 44% of patients. Ibrutinib may exacerbate the risk of bleeding when administered concurrently with anticoagulant and/or antiplatelet drugs; use caution and monitor closely for bleeding with concomitant use. Consider the risks and benefits of interrupting ibrutinib treatment at least 3–7 days prior to and following elective surgery depending on the risk of bleeding and type of surgery
- After initiation of ibrutinib, lymphocytosis occurs commonly and should not be considered as an indicator of disease progression. An absolute lymphocyte count (ALC) above 5000/mcL together with a ≥50% increase from baseline occurred in two-thirds of patients in CLL studies. Lymphocytosis occurs during the first month of therapy and resolves by a median of 14 weeks
- Reduce the ibrutinib starting dose to 140 mg, administered orally once daily for mild (Child-Pugh class A) hepatic impairment. Reduce the ibrutinib starting dose to 70 mg, administered orally once daily for moderate (Child-Pugh class C) hepatic impairment. Avoid ibrutinib in patients with severe (Child-Pugh class C) hepatic impairment
- Tumor lysis syndrome may rarely occur with ibrutinib therapy. Consider appropriate monitoring and precautions (eg, anti-hyperuricemic therapy, hydration) in patients with high baseline risk (eg, high tumor burden, renal impairment)

Supportive Care
Antiemetic prophylaxis
Emetogenic potential is **MINIMAL–LOW**
See Chapter 42 for antiemetic recommendations

Hematopoietic growth factor (CSF) prophylaxis
Primary prophylaxis is **NOT** indicated
See Chapter 43 for more information

Antimicrobial prophylaxis
Risk of fever and neutropenia is **LOW**
    Antimicrobial primary prophylaxis to be considered:
- Antibacterial—not indicated. Consider prophylaxis for *P. jirovecii* (eg, cotrimoxazole)
- Antifungal—not indicated
- Antiviral—antiherpes antivirals (eg, acyclovir, famciclovir, valacyclovir)

Patient Population Studied

This multicenter, cooperative-group, randomized, controlled, open-label, phase 3 trial included 547 adults (≥65 years old) with chronic lymphocytic leukemia (CLL) who were randomized to receive ibrutinib alone, ibrutinib plus rituximab, or bendamustine plus rituximab. Patients were included if they had an indication for treatment according to IWCLL 2008 criteria, had an intermediate- or high-risk Rai stage, had an Eastern Cooperative Oncology Group (ECOG) performance score of 0–2, and if they had normal organ function. Patients were ineligible if they had undergone major surgery within 10 days or minor surgery within 7 days; if they were previously treated for CLL (other than with palliative steroids or rituximab for autoimmune complications); if they had active hepatitis B or history of cardiovascular disease; or if they were receiving treatment with anticoagulation (heparin or warfarin), >20 mg prednisone (or equivalent) daily, intravenous antibiotics, or strong CYP3A4/5 inhibitors/inducers

Efficacy (N = 524)

	Ibrutinib Alone (n = 178)	Ibrutinib + Rituximab (n = 170)	Bendamustine + Rituximab (BR) (n = 176)	
Median progression-free survival	NR	NR	43 Months (95% CI, 38–NR)	
Estimated progression-free survival, 2 years*	87% (95% CI, 81–92)	88% (95% CI, 81–92)	74% (95% CI, 66–80)	HR 0.39 (95% CI, 0.26–0.58); P<0.001 for ibrutinib vs BR HR 0.38 (95% CI, 0.25–0.59); P<0.001 for ibrutinib + rituximab vs BR HR 1.00 (95% CI, 0.62–1.62); P = 0.49 for ibrutinib + rituximab vs ibrutinib
Estimated overall survival, 2 years[†]	90% (95% CI, 85–94)	94% (95% CI, 89–97)	95% (95% CI, 91–98)	P≥0.65 for all pairwise comparisons
Overall response rate[†‡]	93% (95% CI, 88–96)	94% (95% CI, 89–97)	81% (95% CI, 75–87)	
Complete response rate[†‡]	7% (95% CI, 4–12)	12% (95% CI, 8–18)	26% (95% CI, 20–33)	
Undetectable minimal residual disease rate[†ϵ]	1% (95% CI, <1–3)	4% (95% CI, 2–8)	8% (95% CI, 5–13)	

HR, hazard ratio; CI, confidence interval
*Log-rank P value is reported from one-sided analysis with an α of 0.025 from the per-protocol analysis. The same conclusions were made with an intention-to-treat analysis of the data
[†]Intention-to-treat analysis with two-sided P value reported, if one was reported. N = 182 for ibrutinib alone and ibrutinib + rituximab and 183 for bendamustine + rituximab
[‡]Response determined by CT and physical examination
[ϵ]Based on a flow-based assay at cycle 9

Therapy Monitoring

1. *Prior to initiation of ibrutinib:* CBC with differential, serum bilirubin, ALT or AST, alkaline phosphatase, potassium, calcium, phosphorus, LDH, uric acid, and serum creatinine
2. *At least monthly:* CBC with differential
3. *Periodically:* monitor for signs and symptoms of cardiac arrhythmias (eg, atrial fibrillation and atrial flutter) and check electrocardiogram if present, signs and symptoms of bleeding (especially if concomitant antiplatelet or anticoagulant medication[s] are used), signs and symptoms of infection (including progressive multifocal leukoencephalopathy), blood pressure, presence of second primary malignancies, and diarrhea
4. *During initiation of therapy in patients with high tumor burden or renal dysfunction:* monitor for tumor lysis syndrome (potassium, calcium, phosphorus, LDH, uric acid, and serum creatinine)
5. *Response assessment every 1–3 months:* physical examination, CBC with differential, CT scans (in select patients for evaluation of adenopathy). Note that lymphocytosis occurs commonly following initiation of ibrutinib and should not be considered as an indicator of disease progression

Treatment Modifications

Ibrutinib for Chronic Lymphocytic Leukemia

Starting dose: 420 mg by mouth once a day

Adverse Event	Treatment Modification
Treatment with a moderate CYP3A inhibitor is required	Reduce ibrutinib starting dose to 280 mg by mouth once daily during concomitant therapy
Treatment with voriconazole 200 mg by mouth twice a day is required, *or:* Treatment with posaconazole suspension 100 mg by mouth once daily is required, *or:* Treatment with posaconazole suspension 100–200 mg by mouth twice a day is required	Reduce ibrutinib starting dose to 140 mg by mouth once daily during concomitant therapy
Treatment with posaconazole suspension 200 mg by mouth three times a day is required, *or:* Treatment with posaconazole suspension 400 mg by mouth twice a day is required, *or:* Treatment with posaconazole 300 mg intravenously once a day is required, *or:* Treatment with posaconazole delayed-release tablets 300 mg by mouth once a day is required	Reduce ibrutinib starting dose to 70 mg by mouth once daily during concomitant therapy
Treatment with other strong CYP3A inhibitors besides those listed above is required	Avoid concomitant use of ibrutinib with other strong CYP3A inhibitors besides those listed above. If the other strong CYP3A inhibitor is to be used short-term (eg, ≤7 days), then interrupt ibrutinib therapy during use of the strong CYP3A inhibitor
Treatment with a strong CYP3A inducer is required	Avoid concomitant use of ibrutinib with strong CYP3A inducers
Treatment with antiplatelet and/or anticoagulant medications is required	Bleeding risk may be increased. Monitor closely for signs and symptoms of bleeding
Child-Pugh class A hepatic impairment	Reduce ibrutinib starting dose to 140 mg by mouth once a day
Child-Pugh class B hepatic impairment	Reduce ibrutinib starting dose to 70 mg by mouth once a day
Child-Pugh class C hepatic impairment	Avoid ibrutinib use
Surgical procedure is required during treatment with ibrutinib	Consider benefit-risk of withholding ibrutinib for at least 3–7 days prior to and following surgery depending on the type of surgery and the risk of bleeding
Hypertension	Adjust existing anti-hypertensive medications and/or initiate anti-hypertensive treatment as appropriate
First occurrence of G ≥3 non-hematologic toxicity, G ≥3 neutropenia with infection or fever, or G4 hematologic toxicity	Interrupt ibrutinib until resolution to G1 or baseline, then resume ibrutinib at the same dose (eg, 420 mg by mouth once a day). Consider use of G-CSF for G4 neutropenia lasting > 7 days or for life-threatening neutropenic complications
Second occurrence of G ≥3 nonhematologic toxicity, G ≥3 neutropenia with infection or fever, or G4 hematologic toxicity	Interrupt ibrutinib until resolution to G1 or baseline, then resume ibrutinib at 280 mg by mouth once a day. Consider use of G-CSF for G4 neutropenia lasting >7 days or for life-threatening neutropenic complications
Third occurrence of G ≥3 nonhematologic toxicity, G ≥3 neutropenia with infection or fever, or G4 hematologic toxicity	Interrupt ibrutinib until resolution to G1 or baseline, then resume ibrutinib at 140 mg by mouth once a day. Consider use of G-CSF for G4 neutropenia lasting >7 days or for life-threatening neutropenic complications
Fourth occurrence of G ≥3 nonhematologic toxicity, G ≥3 neutropenia with infection or fever, or G4 hematologic toxicity	Discontinue ibrutinib

G-CSF, granulocyte colony stimulating factor
Imbruvica (ibrutinib) prescribing information. Sunnyvale, CA: Pharmacyclics LLC; revised 2018 August

Adverse Events (N = 537)

Event	Ibrutinib Alone (n = 180)			Ibrutinib + Rituximab (n = 181)			Bendamustine + Rituximab (n = 176)		
	Grade 3 (%)	Grade 4 (%)	Grade 5 (%)	Grade 3 (%)	Grade 4 (%)	Grade 5 (%)	Grade 3 (%)	Grade 4 (%)	Grade 5 (%)
Any hematologic	33	8	NR	27	12	NR	35	26	NR
Anemia	11	1	NR	6	0	NR	12	0	NR
Decreased neutrophil count	8	7	NA	11	10	NA	22	18	NA
Decreased platelet count	5	2	NA	4	1	NA	9	6	NA
Any nonhematologic	54	7	13	55	7	12	43	11	9
Bleeding	1	1	0	2	1	1	0	0	0
Infection	16	3	1	15	4	1	10	3	2
Febrile neutropenia	2	NR	NR	1	NR	NR	7	NR	NR
Atrial fibrillation	8	1	NR	6	0	NR	3	0	NR
Hypertension	29	0	NR	33	1	NR	14	1	NR
Secondary cancer	5	1	2	7	1	1	3	0	1
Unexplained or unwitnessed death	NA	NA	4	NA	NA	2	NA	NA	1
Abdominal infection	1	NR	NR	1	NR	NR	0	NR	NR
Respiratory tract infection	6	NR	1	9	NR	0	8	NR	0
CNS infection	1	1	0	1	0	0	0	0	1
Sepsis	NR	3	1	NR	4	1	NR	3	1
UTI	2	NR	NR	3	NR	NR	2	NR	NR

NR, not reported; NA, not applicable; CNS, central nervous system; UTI, urinary tract infection

Adverse events were reported regardless of attribution and if they occurred during treatment or follow-up, but not those that occurred after crossover. Data were included only for patients who received the treatment delineated. Death occurred during treatment or within 30 days of discontinuation in 7% of patients in the ibrutinib and ibrutinib + rituximab groups and 1% of patients in the bendamustine + rituximab group. Richter's transformation occurred in 2 patients in the ibrutinib + rituximab group and in 1 patient in the bendamustine + rituximab group

FIRST-LINE

CHRONIC LYMPHOCYTIC LEUKEMIA REGIMEN: IBRUTINIB + RITUXIMAB

Shanafelt TD et al. N Engl J Med 2019;381:432–443
Protocol for: Shanafelt TD et al. N Engl J Med 2019;381:432–443
Supplementary appendix to: Shanafelt TD et al. N Engl J Med 2019;381:432–443
IMBRUVICA (ibrutinib) prescribing information. Sunnyvale, CA: Pharmacyclics LLC; revised 2019 July

Ibrutinib 420 mg/dose; administer orally, once daily with a glass of water, without regard to food, continually on days 1–28, beginning with cycle 1, every 28 days, until disease progression (total dosage/28-day cycle = 11,760 mg)

Notes:

- Administration with food increases ibrutinib exposure approximately 2-fold compared with administration after overnight fasting. Clinical studies instructed that ibrutinib be taken at least 30 minutes before eating or at least 2 hours after a meal at approximately the same time each day (Protocol for: Shanafelt TD et al. N Engl J Med 2019; 381:432–443). However, the U.S. Food and Drug Administration–approved prescribing information does not make specific recommendations regarding administration of ibrutinib with regard to food. (IMBRUVICA [ibrutinib] prescribing information. Sunnyvale, CA: Pharmacyclics LLC; Revised 2019 July). Others also have concluded that no food restrictions are needed given the relative safety profile of ibrutinib and because repeated drug intake in fasted conditions is unlikely (de Jong J et al. Cancer Chemother Pharmacol 2015;75:907–916)

- Ibrutinib capsules should be swallowed whole; do not break, open, or chew capsules. Ibrutinib tablets should be swallowed whole; do not cut, crush, or chew tablets

- Patients who delay taking ibrutinib at a regularly scheduled time may administer the missed dose as soon as possible on the same day, and then resume the normal schedule the following day. Do not administer an extra dose of ibrutinib to make up for a missed dose

- Ibrutinib is metabolized predominantly by CYP3A. Refer to treatment modification section for initial dose adjustment recommendations for patients requiring concurrent treatment with moderate or strong CYP3A inhibitors. Avoid concomitant use of ibrutinib with strong CYP3A inducers

- Advise patients to not consume grapefruit products or Seville oranges as they may inhibit CYP3A in the gut wall and increase the bioavailability of ibrutinib

- Serious bleeding events, some fatal, have been reported in patients treated with ibrutinib. Grade ≥3 bleeding events were reported to occur in 3% of patients. All-grade bleeding (including bruising and petechia) occurred in approximately 44% of patients. Ibrutinib may exacerbate the risk of bleeding when administered concurrently with anticoagulant and/or antiplatelet drugs; use caution and monitor closely for bleeding with concomitant use. Consider the risks and benefits of interrupting ibrutinib treatment at least 3–7 days prior to and following elective surgery depending on the risk of bleeding and type of surgery

- After initiation of ibrutinib, lymphocytosis occurs commonly and should not be considered as an indicator of disease progression. An absolute lymphocyte count (ALC) >5000/mcL together with a ≥50% increase from baseline occurred in two-thirds of patients in CLL studies. Lymphocytosis occurs during the first month of therapy and resolves by a median of 14 weeks

- Reduce the ibrutinib starting dose to 140 mg, administered orally once daily for mild (Child-Pugh class A) hepatic impairment. Reduce the ibrutinib starting dose to 70 mg, administered orally once daily for moderate (Child-Pugh class C) hepatic impairment. Avoid ibrutinib in patients with severe (Child-Pugh class C) hepatic impairment

- Tumor lysis syndrome may rarely occur with ibrutinib therapy. Consider appropriate monitoring and precautions (eg, anti-hyperuricemic therapy, hydration) in patients with high baseline risk (eg, high tumor burden, renal impairment)

Rituximab to be administered as follows:

Cycle*	Day	Rituximab Dose	Rituximab Administration[†‡]
2	1	50 mg/m^2	Administer intravenously in 0.9% NS or D5W, diluted to a concentration within the range 1–4 mg/mL, over 4 hours. Do not escalate the rate
2	2	325 mg/m^2	Administer intravenously in 0.9% NS or D5W, diluted to a concentration within the range 1–4 mg/mL. Infuse initially at 50 mg/hour. If hypersensitivity or infusion reactions do not occur during the first 30 minutes, increase the rate by 50 mg/hour every 30 minutes as tolerated to a maximum rate of 400 mg/hour. During subsequent treatments, if previous rituximab administration was well tolerated, start at 100 mg/hour and increase by 100 mg/hour every 30 minutes as tolerated to a maximum rate of 400 mg/hour
3, 4, 5, 6, and 7	1	500 mg/m^2	

0.9% NS, 0.9% sodium chloride; D5W, 5% dextrose injection

Note: Rituximab begins with cycle 2

*Cycle length is 28 days

[†]*Premedications for rituximab*

- **Acetaminophen** 650–1000 mg; administer orally 30–60 minutes before each rituximab dose, *plus*
- **Diphenhydramine** 25–50 mg; administer orally or intravenously 30–60 minutes before each rituximab dose

[‡]Interrupt rituximab administration for fever, chills, edema, congestion of the head and neck mucosa, hypertension, and other serious adverse events. Resume rituximab administration after adverse events abate

(continued)

(*continued*)

Supportive Care

Antiemetic prophylaxis

Emetogenic potential of ibrutinib is **MINIMAL–LOW**

Emetogenic potential of rituximab is **MINIMAL**

See Chapter 42 for antiemetic recommendations

Hematopoietic growth factor (CSF) prophylaxis

Primary prophylaxis is **NOT** *indicated*

See Chapter 43 for more information

Antimicrobial prophylaxis

Risk of fever and neutropenia is **LOW**

   Antimicrobial primary prophylaxis to be considered:

- Antibacterial—not indicated. Consider prophylaxis for *P. jirovecii* (eg, cotrimoxazole)
- Antifungal—not indicated
- Antiviral—antiherpes antivirals (eg, acyclovir, famciclovir, valacyclovir)

Patient Population Studied

This multicenter, open-label, randomized, phase 3 trial involved 529 adults with previously untreated chronic lymphocytic leukemia (CLL) or small lymphocytic lymphoma (SLL). Eligible patients were 70 years of age or younger and were deemed appropriate candidates for treatment by the criteria set forth by the International Workshop on Chronic Lymphocytic Leukemia 2008 guidelines. Patients were excluded if they had a chromosome 17p13 deletion (due to known poor response to the control arm of fludarabine + cyclophosphamide + rituximab) or if they required therapy with a strong CYP3A4 inhibitor or anticoagulation with warfarin. Randomization was stratified based on age (<60 years vs 60–70 years old), Eastern Cooperative Oncology Group (ECOG) performance status (0 or 1 vs ≥2), Rai stage (0 to II [low/intermediate risk] vs III or IV [high risk]), and the presence or absence of chromosome 11q22.3 deletion. Patients were randomly assigned 2:1 to receive ibrutinib-rituximab or chemoimmunotherapy (fludarabine + cyclophosphamide + rituximab)

Efficacy (N = 529)

Endpoint	Ibrutinib + Rituximab (N = 354)	Fludarabine-Cyclophosphamide-Rituximab (FCR) (N = 175)	Between-Group Comparison
Progression-free survival at 3 years among all patients*	89.4% (95% CI 86.0–93.0)	72.9% (95% CI 65.3–81.3)	HR 0.35 (95% CI 0.22–0.56) $P<0.001$
Overall survival at 3 years among all patients[†]	98.8% (95% CI 97.6–100)	91.5% (95% CI 86.2–97.0)	HR 0.17 (95% CI 0.05–0.54) $P<0.001$
Progression-free survival at 3 years among patients known to have IGHV-unmutated CLL (n = 210 ibrutinib-rituximab; n = 71 FCR)	90.7%	62.5%	HR 0.26 (95% CI 0.14–0.50)
Progression-free survival at 3 years among patients known to have IGHV-mutated CLL[‡] (n = 70 ibrutinib-rituximab; n = 44 FCR)	87.7%	88.0%	HR 0.44 (95% CI 0.14–1.36); P = 0.0708
Overall response, determined by physical exam[§]	95.8% (95% CI 93.1–97.6)	81.1% (95% CI 74.5–86.6)	—
Complete response, with or without WBC count normalization (including CT scan and bone marrow results)[§]	17.2% (95% CI 13.4–21.6)	30.3% (95% CI 23.6–37.7)	—
Negative for minimal residual disease in peripheral blood at 12 months (n = 276 ibrutinib-rituximab; n = 103 FCR)	8.3% (95% CI 5.4–12.2)	59.2% (95% CI 49.1–68.8)	—

HR, hazard ratio; WBC, white blood cell

*Progression-free survival defined as the time from randomization to documented progression of CLL or death without documented progression. The median follow-up time was 33.6 months

Therapy Monitoring

1. *Prior to treatment initiation:* CBC with differential, serum bilirubin, ALT or AST, alkaline phosphatase, potassium, calcium, phosphorus, LDH, uric acid, serum creatinine, and hepatitis B core antibody (IgG or total) and hepatitis B core antigen

2. *During each rituximab infusion and for at least 1 hour after infusion completion:* signs and symptoms of infusion-related reaction, vital signs at least every 30 minutes

3. *At least monthly:* CBC with differential

4. *Periodically:* monitor for signs and symptoms of cardiac arrhythmias (eg, atrial fibrillation and atrial flutter) and check electrocardiogram if present, signs and symptoms of bleeding (especially if concomitant antiplatelet or anticoagulant medication[s] used), signs and symptoms of infection (including progressive multifocal leukoencephalopathy), blood pressure, presence of second primary malignancies, and diarrhea

5. *During initiation of therapy in patients with high tumor burden or renal dysfunction:* monitor for tumor lysis syndrome (potassium, calcium, phosphorus, LDH, uric acid, and serum creatinine)

6. *Response assessment every 1–3 months:* physical examination, CBC with differential, CT scans (in select patients for evaluation of adenopathy). Note that lymphocytosis occurs commonly following initiation of ibrutinib and should not be considered as an indicator of disease progression

Treatment Modifications

Ibrutinib for Chronic Lymphocytic Leukemia	
Starting dose: 420 mg by mouth once a day	
Adverse Event	**Treatment Modification**
Treatment with a moderate CYP3A inhibitor is required	Reduce ibrutinib starting dose to 280 mg by mouth once daily during concomitant therapy
Treatment with voriconazole 200 mg by mouth twice a day is required, or: Treatment with posaconazole suspension 100 mg by mouth once daily is required, or: Treatment with posaconazole suspension 100–200 mg by mouth twice a day is required	Reduce ibrutinib starting dose to 140 mg by mouth once daily during concomitant therapy
Treatment with posaconazole suspension 200 mg by mouth three times a day is required, or: Treatment with posaconazole suspension 400 mg by mouth twice a day is required, or: Treatment with posaconazole 300 mg intravenously once a day is required, or: Treatment with posaconazole delayed-release tablets 300 mg by mouth once a day is required	Reduce ibrutinib starting dose to 70 mg by mouth once daily during concomitant therapy
Treatment with other strong CYP3A inhibitors besides those listed above is required	Avoid concomitant use of ibrutinib with other strong CYP3A inhibitors besides those listed above If the other strong CYP3A inhibitor is to be used short-term (eg, ≤7 days), then interrupt ibrutinib therapy during use of the strong CYP3A inhibitor
Treatment with a strong CYP3A inducer is required	Avoid concomitant use of ibrutinib with strong CYP3A inducers
Treatment with antiplatelet and/or anticoagulant medications is required	Bleeding risk may be increased. Monitor closely for signs and symptoms of bleeding
Child-Pugh class A hepatic impairment	Reduce ibrutinib starting dose to 140 mg by mouth once a day
Child-Pugh class B hepatic impairment	Reduce ibrutinib starting dose to 70 mg by mouth once a day
Child-Pugh class C hepatic impairment	Avoid ibrutinib use
Surgical procedure is required during treatment with ibrutinib	Consider benefit-risk of withholding ibrutinib for at least 3–7 days prior to and following surgery depending on the type of surgery and the risk of bleeding
Hypertension	Adjust existing anti-hypertensive medications and/or initiate anti-hypertensive treatment as appropriate

(continued)

Treatment Modifications (*continued*)

Adverse Event	Treatment Modification
First occurrence of G ≥3 nonhematologic toxicity, G ≥3 neutropenia with infection or fever, or G4 hematologic toxicity	Interrupt ibrutinib until resolution to G1 or baseline, then resume ibrutinib at the same dose (eg, 420 mg by mouth once a day). Consider use of G-CSF for G4 neutropenia lasting > 7 days or for life-threatening neutropenic complications
Second occurrence of G ≥3 nonhematologic toxicity, G ≥3 neutropenia with infection or fever, or G4 hematologic toxicity	Interrupt ibrutinib until resolution to G1 or baseline, then resume ibrutinib at 280 mg by mouth once a day. Consider use of G-CSF for G4 neutropenia lasting > 7 days or for life-threatening neutropenic complications
Third occurrence of G ≥3 nonhematologic toxicity, G ≥3 neutropenia with infection or fever, or G4 hematologic toxicity	Interrupt ibrutinib until resolution to G1 or baseline, then resume ibrutinib at 140 mg by mouth once a day. Consider use of G-CSF for G4 neutropenia lasting > 7 days or for life-threatening neutropenic complications
Fourth occurrence of G ≥3 nonhematologic toxicity, G ≥3 neutropenia with infection or fever, or G4 hematologic toxicity	Discontinue ibrutinib

G-CSF, granulocyte colony stimulating factor
Imbruvica (ibrutinib) prescribing information. Sunnyvale, CA: Pharmacyclics LLC; revised 2018 August

RITUXIMAB

Rituximab Infusion-Related Toxicities

Onset of infusion-related events (fevers, chills, rigors, edema, congestion of the head and neck mucosa, hypotension)
1. Interrupt rituximab infusion
2. For fever, chills: Give additional dose of **acetaminophen** 650 mg orally and **diphenhydramine** 25–50 mg by intravenous push
3. For rigors: Give **meperidine** 12.5–25 mg by intravenous push ± **promethazine** 12.5–25 mg by intravenous infusion in at least 10 mL 0.9% NS or D5W over 5–15 minutes. If after 15–20 minutes the response to a single dose is considered inadequate, the dose may be repeated
4. After symptoms resolve, resume rituximab infusion at a minimum of 50% reduction in the rate at which the event occurred. If no further infusion-related events, increase the rate by 50 mg/hour every 30 minutes, as tolerated, up to a maximum rate of 400 mg/hour

Dyspnea or wheezing, without allergic findings (urticaria, or tongue or laryngeal edema)
1. Interrupt rituximab infusion immediately
2. Give **hydrocortisone** 100 mg by intravenous push (or glucocorticoid equivalent)
3. Give an additional dose of **diphenhydramine** 25–50 mg by intravenous push and a histamine H2-antagonist (**ranitidine** 50 mg or **famotidine** 20 mg) by intravenous push
4. After symptoms resolve, resume rituximab infusion at a minimum of 50% reduction in the rate at which the event occurred. If no further infusion-related events, increase the rate by 50 mg/hour every 30 minutes, as tolerated, up to a maximum rate of 400 mg/hour

Note: Medications and equipment for the treatment of hypersensitivity reactions should be available for immediate use in the event of a reaction during administration (eg, intravenous fluids, epinephrine, antihistamines, glucocorticoids, oxygen)

Adverse Events* (N = 510)

Event	Ibrutinib + Rituximab (n = 352)			Fludarabine-Cyclophosphamide-Rituximab (n = 158)		
	Grade 3 (%)	Grade 4 (%)	Grade 5 (%)	Grade 3 (%)	Grade 4 (%)	Grade 5 (%)
Anemia	4.8	0	0	10.8	3.8	0
Hemolysis	0.6	0	0	1.9	0.6	0
Leukocytosis	17.3	0.3	0	7.6	0	0

(*continued*)

Adverse Events* (N = 510) (continued)

Event	Ibrutinib + Rituximab (n = 352)			Fludarabine-Cyclophosphamide-Rituximab (n = 158)		
	Grade 3 (%)	Grade 4 (%)	Grade 5 (%)	Grade 3 (%)	Grade 4 (%)	Grade 5 (%)
Lymphocyte count decreased	2.8	0	0	27.2	20.3	0
Lymphocyte count increased	21.9	0	0	7.6	0	0
Neutropenia	10.8	14.8	0	22.2	22.8	0
Thrombocytopenia	2.6	1.7	0	10.1	5.1	0
Infection†	8	1.1	0.3	5.7	3.2	0.6
Febrile neutropenia	2.3	0	0	13.3	2.5	0
Increased ALT	1.7	0.6	0	0.6	0	0
Increased AST	2.6	0	0	1.3	0	0
Hyperglycemia	3.4	0.6	0	5.1	0	0
Hyponatremia	3.1	0	0	1.9	0	0
Atrial fibrillation	2.6	0.6	0	0.6	0.6	0
Hypertension	18.5	0.3	0	8.2	0	0
Fatigue	2	0	0	2.5	0	0
Maculopapular rash	3.1	0	0	5.1	0	0
Diarrhea	4.3	0	0	1.3	0	0

ALT, alanine aminotransferase; AST, aspartate aminotransferase
*Adverse event data include all adverse events of Grade 3 or higher that occurred in >2% of patients who started the assigned treatment in either group
†Events described as infection included sepsis, sinusitis, skin infection, upper respiratory infection, urinary tract infection, infectious enterocolitis, lung infection, penile infection, scrotal infection, soft-tissue infection, lymph gland infection, tooth infection, kidney infection, and catheter-associated infection

FIRST-LINE

CHRONIC LYMPHOCYTIC LEUKEMIA REGIMEN: VENETOCLAX + OBINUTUZUMAB

Fischer K et al. N Engl J Med 2019;380:2225–2236
Protocol for: Fischer K et al. N Engl J Med 2019;380:2225–2236
Supplementary appendix to: Fischer K et al. N Engl J Med 2019;380:2225–2236
VENCLEXTA (venetoclax) prescribing information. North Chicago, IL: AbbVie, Inc; revised 2019 July
GAZYVA (obinutuzumab) prescribing information. South San Francisco, CA: Genentech, Inc; revised 2017 November

The regimen consists of obinutuzumab administered for six cycles on an every-28-day schedule (cycle 1, day 1 = 100 mg; cycle 1, day 2 = 900 mg; cycles 2–6, day 1 = 1000 mg/dose). Beginning on cycle 1, day 22, venetoclax is administered as a 5-week ramp-up to a target dose of 400 mg orally once daily taken continuously through the end of cycle 12.

Premedications for obinutuzumab

- **Acetaminophen** 650–1000 mg; administer orally at least 30 minutes prior to every dose of obinutuzumab
- **Diphenhydramine** 50 mg; administer orally or intravenously at least 30 minutes prior to obinutuzumab
  - Required for cycle 1, day 1 and cycle 1, day 2 infusions
  - Required for subsequent infusions only if the previous infusion was complicated by a Grade 1–3 infusion-related reaction
- Corticosteroid premedication is required for cycle 1, day 1 and cycle 1, day 2 infusions. For subsequent infusions, administer corticosteroid premedication only if the absolute lymphocyte count is >25 × 10^9/L OR if the previous dose was complicated by a Grade 3 infusion-related reaction. Choose only ONE of the following options, when indicated:
  - **Dexamethasone** 20 mg; administer intravenously at least 1 hour prior to obinutuzumab, *or:*
  - **Methylprednisolone** 80 mg; administer intravenously at least 1 hour prior to obinutuzumab

Prophylaxis for tumor lysis syndrome is recommended for high-risk patients (eg, high tumor burden, absolute lymphocyte count >25 × 10^9/L, bulky lymphadenopathy, or renal impairment):

- **Hydration;** encourage oral hydration (eg, ≥3 L/day) starting 1–2 days prior to the first obinutuzumab dose. Consider administering additional *intravenous* hydration prior to the infusion if needed. Continue hydration prior to subsequent obinutuzumab infusions if needed
- **Allopurinol** 300 mg per dose; administer orally twice per day starting 12–24 hours prior to the first obinutuzumab infusion. Continue prophylaxis prior to subsequent obinutuzumab infusions if needed
  - Reduce allopurinol dose to 300 mg by mouth once daily for patients with renal impairment

Obinutuzumab; administer intravenously diluted in 0.9% sodium chloride (0.9% NS) injection to a final concentration ranging from 0.4 mg/mL to 4 mg/mL, for 6 cycles (see table below for dose, dilution, infusion rate, and schedule information)

Notes:

- Hepatitis B virus (HBV) reactivation, in some cases resulting in fulminant hepatitis, hepatic failure, and death, can occur in patients receiving CD20-directed cytolytic antibodies, including obinutuzumab. Screen all patients for HBV infection before treatment initiation. Monitor HBV-positive patients during and after treatment with obinutuzumab and consider antiviral prophylaxis. Discontinue obinutuzumab and concomitant medications in the event of HBV reactivation
- Obinutuzumab can cause severe and life-threatening infusion reactions. Symptoms may include hypotension, tachycardia, dyspnea, and respiratory symptoms (eg, bronchospasm, larynx and throat irritation, wheezing, laryngeal edema). Other common symptoms include nausea, vomiting, diarrhea, hypertension, flushing, headache, pyrexia, and chills
  - *Two-thirds of patients experienced a reaction to the first 1000 mg infused of obinutuzumab. Infusion reactions can also occur with subsequent infusions*
- Hypotension may occur as an infusion reaction. Consider withholding antihypertensive treatments for 12 hours prior to and during each obinutuzumab infusion, and for the first hour after administration until blood pressure is stable

(continued)

(continued)

Cycle and Day*	Obinutuzumab Dose	Volume of 0.9% NS for Dilution	Obinutuzumab Administration	Total Dose per 28-day Cycle
Cycle 1, Day 1	100 mg	100 mL	Infuse over 4 hours at 25 mg/hour. Do not increase infusion rate	Cycle 1 = 3000 mg
Cycle 1, Day 2	900 mg	250 mL	If no infusion reaction occurred during the previous dose, begin infusion at 50 mg/hour and increase by 50 mg/hour every 30 minutes to a maximum rate of 400 mg/hour. If an infusion reaction occurred during the previous dose, begin infusion at 25 mg/hour and increase by 50 mg/hour every 30 minutes to a maximum rate of 400 mg/hour	
Cycle 1, Day 8	1000 mg	250 mL	If no infusion reaction occurred during the previous dose and the final infusion rate was ≥100 mg/hour, start at 100 mg/hour and increase by 100 mg/hour every 30 minutes to a maximum rate of 400 mg/hour. If an infusion reaction occurred during the previous dose, begin infusion at 50 mg/hour and increase by 50 mg/hour every 30 minutes to a maximum rate of 400 mg/hour	
Cycle 1, Day 15	1000 mg	250 mL		
Cycle 2–6, Day 1 only	1000 mg	250 mL		Cycles 2–6 = 1000 mg

*Cycle length = 28 days

Venetoclax; administer orally once daily with 240 mL water within 30 minutes of completion of a meal (preferably breakfast) continuously through cycle 12 or until disease progression, whichever occurs first (see table below for dosing schedule)

Standard 5-Week Dose Escalation Schedule*

Week of Treatment	Venetoclax Dose per Day	Total Venetoclax Dosage per Week
Week 1	20 mg	140 mg
Week 2	50 mg	350 mg
Week 3	100 mg	700 mg
Week 4	200 mg	1400 mg
Week 5 and beyond	400 mg	2800 mg

***Advise patients to keep the medication in its original packaging during the first 4 weeks of therapy**
Venclexta (venetoclax tablets) prescribing information. North Chicago, IL: AbbVie Inc; 2018 November

Notes:
• Venetoclax tablets should be swallowed whole. Do not chew, crush, or break venetoclax tablets
• Patients who delay taking venetoclax at a regularly scheduled time may administer the missed dose within 30 minutes of completion of a meal if within 8 hours of the usual dosing time. If >8 hours, skip the missed dose and resume treatment at the next regularly scheduled time. Patients who vomit after a dose of venetoclax should not repeat the dose but rather take the next dose at the next regularly scheduled time
• Venetoclax is a substrate of cytochrome P450 (CYP) CYP3A subfamily enzymes, P-glycoprotein (P-gp), and BCRP. Venetoclax is a weak inhibitor of CYP2C8, CYP2C9, and UGT1A1 in vitro but due to high protein binding is predicted to cause clinically insignificant inhibition of these enzymes in vivo. Venetoclax is a P-gp and BCRP inhibitor and weak OATP1B1 inhibitor in vitro
  ▪ Avoid concurrent use with strong or moderate CYP3A inducers at all times
  ▪ Avoid concurrent use with strong CYP3A4 inhibitors throughout the venetoclax dose escalation period
    ○ For patients who have completed venetoclax dose-escalation and are maintained on a steady dose of venetoclax, reduce the venetoclax dose to 100 mg if concomitant use of a strong CYP3A inhibitor is unavoidable and monitor closely for side effects. If the strong CYP3A inhibitor is subsequently discontinued, resume the venetoclax dose that was administered prior to introduction of the inhibitor 2–3 days after discontinuation of the inhibitor
    ○ For patients who have completed venetoclax dose-escalation and are maintained on a steady dose of venetoclax, reduce the venetoclax dose to 70 mg if concomitant use of posaconazole is unavoidable and monitor closely for side effects. If posaconazole is subsequently discontinued, resume the venetoclax dose that was administered prior to introduction of posaconazole 2–3 days after discontinuation of posaconazole
  ▪ Reduce the venetoclax dose by ≥50% if concomitant use of a moderate CYP3A4 inhibitor or P-gp inhibitor is unavoidable and monitor closely for side effects. If the moderate CYP3A4 inhibitor is subsequently discontinued, resume the venetoclax dose that was administered prior to introduction of the inhibitor 2–3 days after discontinuation of the inhibitor

(continued)

(*continued*)

- Advise patients to not consume grapefruit products, Seville oranges, or starfruit as they may inhibit CYP3A in the gut wall and increase the bioavailability of venetoclax

- Coadministration of venetoclax with warfarin caused increased exposure to *R*-warfarin and *S*-warfarin. Monitor the international normalized ratio closely in patients coadministered warfarin

- Venetoclax inhibits P-gp. Concomitant use of narrow therapeutic index P-gp substrates (eg, digoxin, everolimus, sirolimus) should be avoided when possible. If use of a P-gp substrate is unavoidable, then administer the P-gp substrate ≥6 hours before venetoclax

- Venetoclax can cause rapid death of leukemic cells leading to rapid onset of tumor lysis syndrome (TLS) during the dose escalation period in some patients. In clinical trials of venetoclax, fatal cases of tumor lysis syndrome have occurred which led to the development of a step-wise dose escalation approach to initiation of venetoclax. Assess tumor burden (eg, CT scan, absolute lymphocyte count) and TLS laboratory measurements (eg, potassium, uric acid, phosphorus, calcium, creatinine, lactate dehydrogenase) and correct any abnormalities prior to initiation of venetoclax. Based on the tumor burden and baseline renal function assessments, determine the risk of TLS in order to guide decisions regarding optimal setting of therapy initiation (inpatient vs outpatient), hydration requirements, and frequency of TLS laboratory monitoring according to the table below

TLS Risk Assessment and Supportive Care

Tumor Burden		Prophylaxis*		Blood Chemistry† Monitoring
		Hydration	Anti-hyperuricemic therapy	Setting and frequency of assessment
Low	All LN < 5 cm AND ALC <25 × 10⁹/L	Oral (1.5–2 L/day)	Allopurinol	Outpatient: • For the first dose of 20 mg and 50 mg; pre-dose, 6–8 hours, 24 hours • For subsequent ramp-up doses; pre-dose‡
Medium	Any LN 5–10 cm OR ALC ≥25 × 10⁹/L	Oral (1.5–2 L/day) and consider additional intravenous	Allopurinol	Outpatient: • For the first dose of 20 mg and 50 mg; pre-dose, 6–8 hours, 24 hours (for patients with CrCl <80 mL/min consider hospitalization with frequent laboratory monitoring as described below for high-risk patients) • For subsequent ramp-up doses; pre-dose‡
High	Any LN ≥10 cm OR ALC ≥25 × 10⁹/L AND Any LN ≥5 cm	Oral (1.5–2 L/day) and intravenous (150–200 mL/hour as tolerated)	Allopurinol; consider rasburicase if baseline uric acid is elevated	In hospital: • For the first dose of 20 mg and 50 mg; pre-dose, 4, 8, 12, and 24 hours Outpatient: • For subsequent ramp-up doses; pre-dose, 6–8 hours, 24 hours

TLS, tumor lysis syndrome; LN, lymph node; ALC, absolute lymphocyte count; CrCl, creatinine clearance

*Initiate a xanthine oxidase inhibitor (eg, allopurinol) 2–3 days prior to initiation of venetoclax. Continue the xanthine oxidase inhibitor for up to 5 weeks depending upon ongoing risk of TLS. Encourage oral hydration (1.5–2 L/day) starting 2 days before and on the day of the first venetoclax dose and each dose escalation

†Blood chemistries = potassium, uric acid, phosphorus, calcium, serum creatinine (evaluate in real time)

‡For patients at continued risk of TLS, monitor chemistries at 6–8 hours and at 24 hours at each subsequent outpatient ramp-up dose

Venclexta (venetoclax tablets) prescribing information. North Chicago, IL: AbbVie Inc; 2018 November

Supportive Care

Antiemetic prophylaxis
Emetogenic potential (all days) is **MINIMAL–LOW**
See Chapter 42 for antiemetic recommendations

Hematopoietic growth factor (CSF) prophylaxis
Primary prophylaxis is **NOT** indicated
See Chapter 43 for more information

Antimicrobial prophylaxis
Risk of fever and neutropenia is **LOW**
Antimicrobial primary prophylaxis to be considered:
- Antibacterial—consider prophylaxis with a fluoroquinolone during periods of prolonged neutropenia only (eg, <500/mm³ for ≥7 days) until ANC recovery. *Pneumocystis jirovecii* prophylaxis is recommended (eg, cotrimoxazole)
- Antifungal—not indicated
- Antiviral—antiherpes antivirals (eg, acyclovir, famciclovir, valacyclovir)

Patient Population Studied

This randomized, multinational, multicenter, open-label, active-controlled, phase 3 trial involved 432 adult patients who had previously untreated CD20+ chronic lymphocytic leukemia (CLL) and were determined to require treatment (Binet stage C or symptomatic disease). Eligibility was determined based on the presence of coexisting conditions, with a total score of >6 on the Cumulative Illness Rating Scale (range 0–56, higher score indicating greater impairment of organ systems) or a creatinine clearance of <70 mL/min. Patients with known central nervous system involvement or transformation of CLL to aggressive non-Hodgkin lymphoma were excluded. Patients were randomly assigned to receive combination therapy with venetoclax and obinutuzumab or chlorambucil and obinutuzumab

Efficacy (N = 432)

End Point	Venetoclax + Obinutuzumab (n = 216)	Chlorambucil + Obinutuzumab (n = 216)	Between-Group Comparison
Progression-free survival events*	30 events	77 events	HR 0.35 95% CI 0.23–0.53 P<0.001
Progression-free survival at 24 months	88.2% 95% CI, 83.7–92.6%	64.1% 95% CI, 57.4–70.8%	
Negative for minimal residual disease in peripheral blood at 3 months†	75.5%	32.5%	P<0.001
Negative for minimal residual disease in bone marrow at 3 months†	56.9%	17.1%	P<0.001
Patients with any response to treatment	84.7%	71.3%	P<0.001
Patients with complete response to treatment‡	49.5%	23.1%	P<0.001
Median overall survival§	NR	NR	

HR, hazard ratio, CI, confidence interval; NR, not reached
*Progression-free survival defined as the time from randomization to the first occurrence of progression, relapse, or death from any cause. Events referred to disease progression or death. After a median follow-up of 28.1 months, in the venetoclax-obinutuzumab group there were 14 events of disease progression and 16 deaths. In the chlorambucil-obinutuzumab group there were 69 events of disease progression and 8 deaths
†Minimal residual disease negativity was consistently more common across all subgroups
‡The percentages of patients with complete response and minimal residual disease negativity in peripheral blood or bone marrow were significantly higher with venetoclax-obinutuzumab than with chlorambucil-obinutuzumab
§The median follow-up time was 28.1 months. Overall survival did not differ significantly between the groups for the complete observation period. All-cause mortality was 9.3% in the venetoclax-obinutuzumab compared with 7.9% in the chlorambucil-obinutuzumab group

Therapy Monitoring

1. *Prior to initiation of venetoclax:*
   a. Assess tumor burden (CBC with differential, CT scan) and baseline chemistries (potassium, uric acid, phosphorus, calcium, serum creatinine, LDH) to determine the risk for tumor lysis syndrome (TLS). Decisions regarding treatment setting (inpatient vs outpatient) and frequency of laboratory monitoring depend upon TLS risk assessment (see above table)
   b. Verify adherence to the prescribed xanthine oxidase inhibitor regimen (eg, allopurinol) to begin 2–3 days prior to venetoclax initiation
   c. Screen for the presence of drug-drug interactions involving venetoclax
   d. Prescribe the appropriate combination of venetoclax tablet strengths (available in 10-mg, 50-mg, and 100-mg tablets) in sufficient quantities to accommodate the planned venetoclax dose-escalation and maintenance dosing schedule
2. *Tumor lysis syndrome monitoring during venetoclax ramp-up:* monitor potassium, uric acid, phosphorus, calcium, and serum creatinine at the frequency described in the above table corresponding to the patient's risk for tumor lysis syndrome
3. *Periodically throughout venetoclax treatment:* CBC with differential
4. *Prior to initiation of rituximab:* hepatitis B core antibody (IgG or total) and hepatitis B core antigen
5. *Response assessment every 2–3 months:* physical examination, CBC with differential, CT scans (in select patients for evaluation of adenopathy)

Treatment Modifications

VENETOCLAX AND OBINUTUZUMAB

Dose at Interruption	Restart Dose*†
400 mg	300 mg
300 mg	200 mg
200 mg	100 mg
100 mg	50 mg‡
50 mg	20 mg‡
20 mg	10 mg‡

*If patients interrupt venetoclax for >1 week during the 5-week ramp-up period or interrupt venetoclax for >2 weeks during maintenance therapy, reassess the risk of TLS to determine if reinitiation with a reduced dose of venetoclax is necessary
†During the venetoclax ramp-up phase, continue the reduced venetoclax dose for 1 week before further dose escalation
‡Consider discontinuing venetoclax for patients who require dose reductions to <100 mg for >2 weeks

Tumor Lysis Syndrome

Adverse Event	Treatment Modification
Prior to initiation of venetoclax: • Potassium, phosphorus, or uric acid >ULN • Corrected calcium <LLN • Serum creatinine ≥25% above baseline value	Correct pre-existing tumor lysis syndrome abnormalities prior to initiation of venetoclax
Laboratory TLS Blood chemistry (potassium, phosphorus, uric acid, calcium, serum creatinine) suggestive of TLS *without* clinical sequelae	Withhold venetoclax until resolution. Correct laboratory abnormalities and increase frequency of monitoring If abnormalities resolve within 48 hours, resume venetoclax at the same dose. If resolution requires >48 hours, then resume venetoclax at a reduced dose
Clinical TLS Blood chemistry (potassium, phosphorus, uric acid, calcium, serum creatinine) suggestive of TLS *with* clinical sequelae (eg, serum creatinine ≥1.5× ULN, cardiac arrhythmia, seizure, sudden cardiac death)	Correct laboratory abnormalities and increase frequency of monitoring Withhold venetoclax until resolution and then resume venetoclax at a reduced dose
Potassium > ULN in the setting of TLS	Withhold venetoclax until resolution. Increase frequency of monitoring. If resolution occurs within 24–48 hours of the last dose, resume venetoclax at the same dose. If resolution requires >48 hours, then resume at a reduced dose Perform STAT ECG and begin telemetry. Consider the following interventions: • Sodium polystyrene sulfonate 15 g by mouth once • Furosemide 20 mg IV push once • Insulin 10 units IV push once plus 25 g of 50% dextrose IV push once (may omit glucose if serum glucose is ≥250 mg/dL) • If there is ECG evidence of life-threatening arrhythmia, then administer calcium gluconate 1000 mg in 100 mL D5W IV over 30 minutes once • Consult nephrology for consideration of dialysis for severe, refractory, or rapidly worsening hyperkalemia, especially in the setting of concomitant AKI
Uric acid ≥8.0 mg/dL in the setting of TLS	Withhold venetoclax until resolution. Increase frequency of monitoring. If resolution occurs within 24–48 hours of the last dose, resume venetoclax at the same dose. If resolution requires >48 hours, then resume at a reduced dose Consider a single dose of rasburicase 3–6 mg (fixed dose) IV over 30 minutes. Optimize the dose of xanthine oxidase inhibitor (eg, allopurinol) and the rate of IV hydration, as tolerated

(continued)

Treatment Modifications (*continued*)

Adverse Event	Treatment Modification
Phosphorus ≥5.0 mg/dL in the setting of TLS	Withhold venetoclax until resolution. Increase frequency of monitoring. If resolution occurs within 24–48 hours of the last dose, resume venetoclax at the same dose. If resolution requires >48 hours, then resume at a reduced dose
	Administer a phosphate binder (eg, aluminum hydroxide, calcium carbonate, sevelamer carbonate, or lanthanum carbonate) with meals. Place patient on a low-phosphate diet. Optimize the rate of IV hydration, as tolerated. Consult nephrology for consideration of hemodialysis, especially if phosphorus ≥10 mg/dL or with concomitant AKI
Serum creatinine increases ≥25% from baseline in the setting of TLS	Withhold venetoclax until resolution. Increase frequency of monitoring. If resolution occurs within 24–48 hours of the last dose, resume venetoclax at the same dose. If resolution requires >48 hours, then resume at a reduced dose
	Start or increase rate of IV hydration. For severe AKI, consider nephrology consultation
Corrected calcium ≤7.0 mg/dL and patient is symptomatic (eg, muscle cramps, hypotension, tetany, cardiac arrhythmias) in the setting of TLS	Withhold venetoclax until resolution. Increase frequency of monitoring. If resolution occurs within 24–48 hours of the last dose, resume venetoclax at the same dose. If resolution requires >48 hours, then resume at a reduced dose
	Perform STAT ECG and begin telemetry. Administer calcium gluconate 1000 mg in 100 mL D5W IV over 30 minutes once
Hematologic Toxicities	
G ≥3 neutropenia (ANC <1000/mm³)	Withhold venetoclax (and obinutuzumab if neutropenia occurs during cycles 1–6) for at least 1 week. G-CSF may be administered with venetoclax if indicated to reduce the risk of infection associated with neutropenia. When ANC improves to ≥1000/mm³ and platelets are ≥75,000/mm³, then resume venetoclax with the dosage reduced by 1 dose level and resume obinutuzumab (if applicable) at the same dose
G4 thrombocytopenia (platelet count <25,000/mm³) and/or symptomatic bleeding, first occurrence	Withhold venetoclax (and obinutuzumab if event occurs during cycles 1–6). Transfuse platelets as clinically indicated per institutional standards. When platelet count improves to ≥50,000/mm³ without transfusion support for 5 days, resume venetoclax and obinutuzumab at the same dose
G4 thrombocytopenia (platelet count <25,000/mm³) and/or symptomatic bleeding, recurrent	Withhold venetoclax (and obinutuzumab if event occurs during cycles 1–6). Transfuse platelets as clinically indicated per institutional standards. When platelet count improves to ≥50,000/mm³ without transfusion support for 5 days, resume venetoclax with the dosage reduced by 1 dose level and resume obinutuzumab at the same dose
Drug-Drug Interactions	
Concomitant therapy with a strong or moderate CYP3A inducer is required	Do not administer a strong or moderate CYP3A inducer with venetoclax
Concomitant therapy with a strong CYP3A4 inhibitor is required during the venetoclax 5-week ramp-up period	Do not administer a strong CYP3A4 inhibitor during the venetoclax ramp-up period
Concomitant therapy with a strong CYP3A4 inhibitor is required in a patient taking a steady daily dosage of venetoclax (after ramp-up phase)	Consider alternative medications. If the strong CYP3A4 inhibitor is unavoidable, then reduce the venetoclax dose to 100 mg
Concomitant therapy with posaconazole is required in a patient taking a steady daily dosage of venetoclax (after ramp-up phase)	Consider alternative medications. If posaconazole is unavoidable, then reduce the venetoclax dose to 70 mg
Concomitant therapy with a moderate CYP3A4 inhibitor or P-gp inhibitor is required (any phase of treatment)	Consider alternative medications. If the moderate CYP3A4 inhibitor or P-gp inhibitor is unavoidable, then reduce the venetoclax dose by at least 50%
Concomitant strong or moderate CYP3A4 inhibitor, posaconazole, or P-gp inhibitor is subsequently discontinued	Resume the venetoclax dosage that was used prior to concomitant use of a strong or moderate CYP3A4 inhibitor, posaconazole, or P-gp inhibitor 2–3 days after discontinuation of the inhibitor
Concomitant therapy with warfarin is required	Monitor international normalized ratio frequently

(continued)

Treatment Modifications (continued)

Adverse Event	Treatment Modification
Concomitant therapy with a P-gp substrate is required	Consider alternative medications. If concomitant use is unavoidable, administer the P-gp substrate at least 6 hours before the administration of venetoclax

Other Toxicities

Other G3/4 nonhematologic toxicity attributable to venetoclax, first occurrence	Withhold venetoclax until resolution to G ≤1 or baseline, then resume venetoclax at the same dose
Other G3/4 nonhematologic toxicity attributable to venetoclax, second and subsequent occurrences	Withhold venetoclax until resolution to G ≤1 or baseline, then resume venetoclax at a lower dose. At the discretion of the medically responsible health care provider, a larger dose reduction than that described above may be considered depending on the severity of the toxicity
Immunization with a live attenuated vaccine is indicated prior to, during, or after therapy with venetoclax and obinutuzumab	Do not administer live attenuated vaccines prior to, during, or after treatment with venetoclax and obinutuzumab until B-cell recovery occurs

TLS, tumor lysis syndrome; ULN, upper limit of normal; LLN, lower limit of normal; ECG, electrocardiogram; IV, intravenous; AKI, acute kidney injury; ANC, absolute neutrophil count; G-CSF, granulocyte-colony stimulating factor; P-gp, P-glycoprotein

OBINUTUZUMAB

Obinutuzumab Infusion-Related Toxicities

G ≤2 obinutuzumab infusion-related reaction	1. Interrupt obinutuzumab infusion or reduce infusion rate by at least 50% 2. For fever, chills: Give additional dose of **acetaminophen** 650 mg orally and **diphenhydramine** 25–50 mg by intravenous push 3. For dyspnea/wheezing: Give additional dose of **diphenhydramine** 25–50 mg by intravenous push. Give a histamine H2-antagonist (**ranitidine** 50 mg or **famotidine** 20 mg) by intravenous push. Give **hydrocortisone** 100 mg (or glucocorticoid equivalent) by intravenous push 4. For rigors: Give **meperidine** 12.5–25 mg by intravenous push ± **promethazine** 12.5–25 mg by intravenous infusion in at least 10 mL 0.9% NS or D5W over 5–15 minutes. If after 15–20 minutes the response to a single dose is considered inadequate, the dose may be repeated 5. After symptoms resolve, continue or resume obinutuzumab infusion at a minimum of 50% reduction in the rate at which the event occurred. If no further infusion-related events, increase the infusion rate at the increments and intervals as appropriate for the treatment cycle dose. Note, for CLL patients only, the cycle 1, day 1 infusion rate may be increased back up to 25 mg/hour after 1 hour but not increased further. 6. Refer to the "premedications for obinutuzumab" section within the regimen description to determine appropriate premedications for the subsequent cycle
G3 obinutuzumab infusion-related reaction, first occurrence	1. Interrupt obinutuzumab infusion 2. For fever, chills: Give additional dose of **acetaminophen** 650 mg orally and **diphenhydramine** 25–50 mg by intravenous push 3. For dyspnea/wheezing: Give additional dose of **diphenhydramine** 25–50 mg by intravenous push. Give a histamine H2-antagonist (**ranitidine** 50 mg or **famotidine** 20 mg) by intravenous push. Give **hydrocortisone** 100 mg (or glucocorticoid equivalent) by intravenous push 4. For rigors: Give **meperidine** 12.5–25 mg by intravenous push ± **promethazine** 12.5–25 mg by intravenous infusion in at least 10 mL 0.9% NS or D5W over 5–15 minutes. If after 15–20 minutes the response to a single dose is considered inadequate, the dose may be repeated 5. After symptoms resolve, resume obinutuzumab infusion at a minimum of 50% reduction in the rate at which the event occurred. If no further infusion-related events, increase the infusion rate at the increments and intervals as appropriate for the treatment cycle dose. Note, for CLL patients only, the cycle 1, day 1 infusion rate may be increased back up to 25 mg/hour after 1 hour but not increased further. If G3 infusion-related reaction recurs during rechallenge, then permanently discontinue obinutuzumab 6. Refer to the "premedications for obinutuzumab" section within the regimen description to determine appropriate premedications for the subsequent cycle

(continued)

Treatment Modifications (continued)

Obinutuzumab Infusion-Related Toxicities

G3 obinutuzumab infusion-related reaction, recurrent (following rechallenge on the same day of treatment)	Permanently discontinue obinutuzumab and provide supportive care
G4 obinutuzumab infusion-related reaction	Permanently discontinue obinutuzumab and provide supportive care
Serum sickness or hypersensitivity reaction	Permanently discontinue obinutuzumab and provide supportive care

Note: Medications and equipment for the treatment of hypersensitivity reactions should be available for immediate use in the event of a reaction during administration (eg, intravenous fluids, epinephrine, antihistamines, glucocorticoids, and oxygen)

Protocol for: Fischer K et al. N Engl J Med 2019;380:2225–2236
VENCLEXTA (venetoclax) prescribing information. North Chicago, IL: AbbVie, Inc; revised 2019 July
GAZYVA (obinutuzumab) prescribing information. South San Francisco, CA: Genentech, Inc; revised 2017 November

Adverse Events (N = 426)

Event	Venetoclax + Obinutuzumab (N = 212)		Chlorambucil + Obinutuzumab (N = 214)	
	Grade 1–2 (%)	Grade 3–5 (%)	Grade 1–2 (%)	Grade 3–5 (%)
Neutropenia	4	56	10	52
Anemia	9	8	13	7
Thrombocytopenia	40	28	23	56
Diarrhea	24	4	14	1
Nausea	19	0	21	1
Constipation	13	0	9	0
Fatigue	19	2	22	1
Upper respiratory tract infection	16	1	16	1
Blood creatinine increased	74	6	72	2
Hypocalcemia	58	9	54	4
Hyperkalemia	37	4	32	3
Hyperuricemia	0	38	0	38

Fatal adverse reactions that occurred in the absence of disease progression and within 28 days of the last study treatment were reported in 4 patients (2%) in the venetoclax-obinutuzumab group, most often from infection. In the venetoclax-obinutuzumab group, adverse reactions led to treatment discontinuation in 16% of patients, dose reduction in 21%, and dose interruption in 74% of patients. Other noteworthy adverse events in the obinutuzumab-venetoclax group include all-grade febrile neutropenia (6%), all-grade pneumonia (9%), all-grade urinary tract infection (6%), all-grade sepsis (4%), all-grade tumor lysis syndrome (1%), Grade 4 neutropenia (32%), Grade 4 thrombocytopenia (8%), Grade 4 hypocalcemia (8%), Grade 4 hyperuricemia (7%), Grade 4 increase in blood creatinine (3%), Grade 4 hypercalcemia (3%), and Grade 2 hypokalemia (2%)
*Neutropenia led to dose interruption of venetoclax-obinutuzumab in 41% of patients, dose reduction in 13%, and discontinuation in 2%

VENCLEXTA (venetoclax) prescribing information. North Chicago, IL: AbbVie, Inc; revised 2019 July

FIRST-LINE

CHRONIC LYMPHOCYTIC LEUKEMIA REGIMEN: FLUDARABINE + CYCLOPHOSPHAMIDE + RITUXIMAB (FCR)

Fischer K et al. Blood 2016;127:208–215
Supplement to: Fischer K et al. Blood 2016;127:208–215
Hallek M et al. Lancet 2010;376:1164–1174
Supplementary appendix to: Hallek M et al. Lancet 2010;376:1164–1174

Consider prophylaxis against tumor lysis syndrome in high-risk patients (eg, high tumor burden)—cycle 1:

Allopurinol 300 mg/day; administer orally or intravenously for 7 consecutive days, days 1–7 of cycle 1 only in patients at high risk for tumor lysis syndrome

Premedications for rituximab
Acetaminophen 650–1000 mg; administer orally 30–60 minutes before each rituximab dose, *plus*
Diphenhydramine 25–50 mg; administer orally or intravenously 30–60 minutes before each rituximab dose

4-Week Cycles

Cycle 1	Cycles 2–6
Rituximab 375 mg/m²; administer intravenously for 1 dose on the day prior to fludarabine + cyclophosphamide initiation (ie, day 0) during cycle 1 only (total dosage during cycle 1 = 375 mg/m²)	**Rituximab** 500 mg/m² per dose; administer intravenously on day 1, every 28 days, for 5 cycles (total dosage/28-day cycle during cycles 2–6 = 500 mg/m²)

Rituximab is diluted in 0.9% sodium chloride injection (0.9% NS) or 5% dextrose injection (D5W) to a concentration within the range 1–4 mg/mL

Rituximab administration:

- Infuse initially at 50 mg/hour. If hypersensitivity or infusion reactions do not occur during the first 30 minutes, increase the rate by 50 mg/hour every 30 minutes as tolerated to a maximum rate of 400 mg/hour. During subsequent treatments if previous rituximab administration was well tolerated, start at 100 mg/hour and increase by 100 mg/hour every 30 minutes as tolerated to a maximum rate of 400 mg/hour
- Interrupt rituximab administration for fever, chills, edema, congestion of the head and neck mucosa, hypertension, and other serious adverse events. Resume rituximab administration after adverse events abate

Cycles 1–6

Cyclophosphamide 250 mg/m² per day; administer intravenously in 100 mL 0.9% NS or D5W over 30 minutes daily for 3 consecutive days on days 1–3, every 28 days for 6 cycles (total dosage/28-day cycle = 750 mg/m²)

Fludarabine 25 mg/m² per day; administer intravenously in 100–125 mL 0.9% NS or D5W over 30 minutes daily for 3 consecutive days on days 1–3, every 28 days for 6 cycles (total dosage/28-day cycle = 75 mg/m²)

Treatment notes:
- Cyclophosphamide and fludarabine administration begin 1 day after completing rituximab administration only during the first cycle
- During cycles 2–6, the day on which rituximab is given (day 1) and the first day on which cyclophosphamide and fludarabine are administered coincide
- Fludarabine dose adjustments in renal impairment:
  - *Creatinine clearance (CrCl) 50–79 mL/minute:* fludarabine 20 mg/m² per day on days 1–3
  - *CrCl 30–49 mL/minute:* fludarabine 15 mg/m² per day on days 1–3
  - *CrCl <30 mL/minute:* do not administer fludarabine

Supportive Care
Antiemetic prophylaxis
Emetogenic potential on Cycle 1, Day 0 is **MINIMAL**
Emetogenic potential on Cycles 1–6, Days 1–3 is **MODERATE**
See Chapter 42 for antiemetic recommendations

Hematopoietic growth factor (CSF) prophylaxis
Primary prophylaxis is indicated with one of the following:
Filgrastim (G-CSF) 5 mcg/kg per day by subcutaneous injection, *or*
Pegfilgrastim (pegylated filgrastim) 6 mg/0.6 mL by subcutaneous injection for 1 dose
- Begin use 24–72 hours after myelosuppressive chemotherapy is completed

See Chapter 43 for more information

(continued)

(continued)

Antimicrobial prophylaxis
Risk of fever and neutropenia is **INTERMEDIATE**
   Antimicrobial primary prophylaxis to be considered:
- Antibacterial—consider a fluoroquinolone or no prophylaxis; *P. jirovecii* prophylaxis is recommended (eg, cotrimoxazole)
- Antifungal—consider use during periods of prolonged neutropenia
- Antiviral—antiherpes antivirals (eg, acyclovir, famciclovir, valacyclovir)

Patient Population Studied

The prospective, international, multicenter, randomized, open-label, phase 3 trial (CLL8) involved 817 treatment-naïve patients with immunophenotypically confirmed CLL with Binet stage C, or Binet stage A or B with confirmed active disease. Eligible patients had Eastern Cooperative Oncology Group performance status score ≤1, low comorbidity, and creatine clearance ≥70 mL/min. Patients with clinically apparent autoimmune cytopenia or active second malignancy were ineligible. Patients were randomly assigned to receive six 28-day cycles of intravenous fludarabine (25 mg/m^2 per day on days 1–3) and cyclophosphamide (250 mg/m^2 per day on days 1–3) with or without rituximab (375 mg/m^2 1 day before the first treatment cycle and then 500 mg/m^2 on day 1 of subsequent treatment cycles)

Efficacy (N = 817)

	Fludarabine + Cyclophosphamide + Rituximab (n = 408)	Fludarabine + Cyclophosphamide (n = 409)	
Median progression-free survival	56.8 months	32.9 months	HR 0.59, 95% CI 0.50–0.69; P<0.001
Median overall survival	Not reached	86.0 months	HR 0.68, 95% CI 0.54–0.89; P = 0.001

Note: Median duration of follow-up was 5.9 years

Therapy Monitoring

1. *Prior to treatment initiation:* CBC with differential, chemistries (potassium, uric acid, phosphorus, calcium, serum creatinine, LDH), serum bilirubin, ALT or AST, hepatitis B core antibody (IgG or total) and hepatitis B core antigen, urine pregnancy test (women of child-bearing potentially only)
2. *Prior to each cycle:* CBC with differential, chemistries (potassium, uric acid, phosphorus, calcium, serum creatinine, LDH), serum bilirubin, ALT or AST
3. *Weekly during treatment:* CBC with differential
4. *During each rituximab infusion and for at least 1 hour after infusion completion:* signs and symptoms of infusion-related reaction, vital signs every 30 minutes
5. *In patients at high risk for tumor lysis syndrome (eg, high tumor burden, renal dysfunction, rapidly increasing absolute lymphocyte count, markedly elevated LDH, baseline abnormalities in laboratory indices of tumor lysis syndrome [potassium, phosphate, uric acid, calcium, serum creatinine]):* consider frequent monitoring of laboratory indices of tumor lysis syndrome, intravenous hydration, and prophylaxis with a xanthine oxidase inhibitor (eg, allopurinol) during the first cycle
6. *Monitor periodically for:*
   a. Signs and symptoms of infection (including progressive multifocal leukoencephalopathy)
   b. Signs and symptoms of hemorrhagic cystitis
7. *Response assessment every 2–3 months:* physical examination, CBC with differential, CT scans (in select patients for evaluation of adenopathy)

Treatment Modifications

FLUDARABINE + CYCLOPHOSPHAMIDE

Dose Levels

	Fludarabine	Cyclophosphamide
Starting dose	25 mg/m^2/dose on days 1–3	250 mg/m^2/dose on days 1–3
Dose level –1	20 mg/m^2/dose on days 1–3	200 mg/m^2/dose on days 1–3
Dose level –2	15 mg/m^2/dose on days 1–3	150 mg/m^2/dose on days 1–3

Note: Rituximab dose is not reduced

Infectious Complications

Active infection	Interrupt fludarabine, cyclophosphamide, and rituximab until resolution of infection, then resume treatment at either the same dose, or reduced by one dose level, depending on the severity of infection. Do not reduce the rituximab dose
New or changes in pre-existing neurologic symptoms (eg, confusion, dizziness, loss of balance, vision problems, aphasia, ambulation issues): PML suspected	Interrupt fludarabine, cyclophosphamide, and rituximab until central nervous system status clarified. Work-up may include (but is not limited to) consultation with a neurologist, brain MRI, and LP
PML is confirmed	Discontinue fludarabine, cyclophosphamide, and rituximab
HBV reactivation	Discontinue fludarabine, cyclophosphamide, and rituximab. Institute appropriate treatment for HBV. Upon resolution of HBV reactivation, resumption of fludarabine, cyclophosphamide, and rituximab should be discussed with a physician with expertise in management of HBV

Hematologic Toxicity

Initial and recurrent episodes of any of the following: G3 neutropenia (ANC ≥500/mm^3 to <1000/mm^3) or G4 neutropenia (ANC <500/mm^3) or Platelet count <80,000/mm^3	Delay fludarabine, cyclophosphamide, and rituximab until improvement to G ≤2 neutropenia and platelet count ≥80,000/mm^3 (or recovery to baseline levels). Consider increasing the frequency of CBC with differential monitoring
	In the setting of a rapid decrease in hemoglobin, consider the possibility of fludarabine-induced or auto-immune hemolytic anemia and perform appropriate laboratory work-up (eg, LDH, total bilirubin, direct bilirubin, haptoglobin, reticulocyte count, Coombs test)
	Consider transfusion of platelets or red blood cells, or treatment with G-CSF (if not already being given prophylactically), as indicated. For G4 neutropenia persisting for >1 week, consider prophylaxis with antibiotic (eg, ciprofloxacin), antiviral (eg, acyclovir), and antifungal (eg, fluconazole) until improvement of neutropenia to G ≤3. For G ≥3 thrombocytopenia, consider holding concomitant antiplatelet and anticoagulation medications, if applicable
	Upon recovery, decrease fludarabine and cyclophosphamide by one dose level. Do not reduce the dose of rituximab
Fludarabine-induced hemolytic anemia suspected or confirmed	Permanently discontinue fludarabine. May continue cyclophosphamide and rituximab at the same dose at the discretion of the medically responsible health care provider

Renal Insufficiency*

CrCl >70 mL/minute	No dose reductions are necessary
CrCl 50–70 mL/minute*	Reduce fludarabine dose to 20 mg/m^2/dose. No dose reduction necessary for cyclophosphamide or rituximab
CrCl 30–49 mL/minute*	Reduce fludarabine dose to 15 mg/m^2/dose. No dose reduction necessary for cyclophosphamide or rituximab
CrCl <30 mL/minute*	Fludarabine use is not recommended. No dose reduction necessary for cyclophosphamide or rituximab

(continued)

Treatment Modifications (*continued*)

Drug-Drug Interactions

Patient requires concomitant therapy with antihypertensive medication(s)	On days of rituximab treatment, and especially with the initial dose, weigh the risk versus benefit of delaying administration of the antihypertensive medication(s) until after completion of the rituximab infusion due to the potential risk of rituximab infusion-related hypotension
Live attenuated vaccine is indicated during or after rituximab administration	Avoid administration of a live attenuated vaccine during rituximab therapy and following therapy until adequate B-cell recovery has occurred

*In the studies conducted by Fischer et al and Hallek et al, patients with a baseline CrCl <70 mL/minute were excluded. Consider regimen other than FCR for patients with renal insufficiency

PML, progressive multifocal leukoencephalopathy; MRI, magnetic resonance imaging; LP, lumbar puncture; HBV, hepatitis B virus; ANC, absolute neutrophil count; CBC, complete blood count; LDH, lactate dehydrogenase; G-CSF, granulocyte-colony stimulating factor; CrCl, creatinine clearance

Fludarabine phosphate injection prescribing information. Princeton, NJ: Sandoz; 2010 December

RITUXIMAB

Rituximab Infusion-Related Toxicities

Onset of infusion-related events (fevers, chills, rigors, edema, congestion of the head and neck mucosa, hypotension)
1. Interrupt rituximab infusion
2. For fever, chills: Give additional dose of **acetaminophen** 650 mg orally and **diphenhydramine** 25–50 mg by intravenous push
3. For rigors: Give **meperidine** 12.5–25 mg by intravenous push ± **promethazine** 12.5–25 mg by intravenous infusion in at least 10 mL 0.9% NS or D5W over 5–15 minutes. If after 15–20 minutes the response to a single dose is considered inadequate, the dose may be repeated
4. After symptoms resolve, resume rituximab infusion at a minimum of 50% reduction in the rate at which the event occurred. If no further infusion-related events, increase the rate by 50 mg/hour every 30 minutes, as tolerated, up to a maximum rate of 400 mg/hour

Dyspnea or wheezing, without allergic findings (urticaria, or tongue or laryngeal edema)
1. Interrupt rituximab infusion immediately
2. Give **hydrocortisone** 100 mg by intravenous push (or glucocorticoid equivalent)
3. Give an additional dose of **diphenhydramine** 25–50 mg by intravenous push and a histamine H2-antagonist (**ranitidine** 50 mg or **famotidine** 20 mg) by intravenous push
4. After symptoms resolve, resume rituximab infusion at a minimum of 50% reduction in the rate at which the event occurred. If no further infusion-related events, increase the rate by 50 mg/hour every 30 minutes, as tolerated, up to a maximum rate of 400 mg/hour

Note: Medications and equipment for the treatment of hypersensitivity reactions should be available for immediate use in the event of a reaction during administration (eg, intravenous fluids, epinephrine, antihistamines, glucocorticoids, oxygen)

Adverse Events (N = 800)

Grade 3–4* events during treatment (data from Hallek M et al. Lancet 2010;376:1164–1174):

Event	Event Percentage: Fludarabine + Cyclophosphamide + Rituximab (n = 404)	Event Percentage: Fludarabine + Cyclophosphamide (n = 396)	
Hematologic toxicity	56	40	P<0.0001
Neutropenia	34	21	P<0.0001
Infections, total	25	21	P = 0.18
Leukocytopenia	24	12	P<0.0001
Infections, not specified	21	17	P = 0.19
Thrombocytopenia	7	11	P = 0.07
Anemia	5	7	P = 0.42

(*continued*)

Adverse Events (N = 800) (continued)

Event	Event Percentage: Fludarabine + Cyclophosphamide + Rituximab (n = 404)	Event Percentage: Fludarabine + Cyclophosphamide (n = 396)	
Viral infection	4	4	P = 0.95
Bacterial infection	3	1	P = 0.14
Autoimmune hemolytic anemia	<1	1	P = 0.69
Fungal infection	<1	<1	P = 0.33
Tumor lysis syndrome	<1	<1	P = 0.55
Cytokine release syndrome	<1	0	P = 0.32
Parasitic infection	<1	0	P = 0.32

*According to the National Cancer Institute Common Toxicity Criteria, version 2

Note: Treatment-related deaths occurred in 2% and 3%, respectively, of the patients who were and were not assigned to receive rituximab

Long-term safety events (data from Fischer K et al. Blood 2016;127:208–215)

Event	Event Percentage: Fludarabine + Cyclophosphamide + Rituximab (n = 404)	Event Percentage: Fludarabine + Cyclophosphamide (n = 396)
Prolonged neutropenia, 2 months after the end of treatment	17	9
Prolonged neutropenia, 12 months after the end of treatment	4	4
Solid tumor	6	7
Richter's transformation	3	6
Hematologic neoplasia	3	3
Basalioma, squamous cell	2	3

FIRST-LINE

CHRONIC LYMPHOCYTIC LEUKEMIA REGIMEN: BENDAMUSTINE + RITUXIMAB (BR)

Eichhorst B et al. Lancet Oncol 2016;17:928–942
Supplementary appendix to: Eichhorst B et al. Lancet Oncol 2016;17:928–942

Premedications for rituximab
Acetaminophen 650–1000 mg; administer orally 30–60 minutes before each rituximab dose, *plus*
Diphenhydramine 25–50 mg; administer orally or intravenously 30–60 minutes before each rituximab dose

4-Week Cycles	
Cycle 1	Cycles 2–6
Rituximab 375 mg/m²; administer intravenously for 1 dose on the day prior to bendamustine initiation (ie, day 0) during cycle 1 only (total dosage during cycle 1 = 375 mg/m²)	**Rituximab** 500 mg/m² per dose; administer intravenously on day 1, every 28 days, for 5 cycles (total dosage/28-day cycle during cycles 2–6 = 500 mg/m²)

Rituximab is diluted in 0.9% sodium chloride injection (0.9% NS) or 5% dextrose injection (D5W) to a concentration within the range 1–4 mg/mL

Rituximab administration:

- Infuse initially at 50 mg/hour. If hypersensitivity or infusion reactions do not occur during the first 30 minutes, increase the rate by 50 mg/hour every 30 minutes as tolerated to a maximum rate of 400 mg/hour. During subsequent treatments if previous rituximab administration was well tolerated, start at 100 mg/hour and increase by 100 mg/hour every 30 minutes as tolerated to a maximum rate of 400 mg/hour
- Interrupt rituximab administration for fever, chills, edema, congestion of the head and neck mucosa, hypertension, and other serious adverse events. Resume rituximab administration after adverse events abate

Premedications for bendamustine HCl: premedications are not necessary for primary prophylaxis of infusion-related reactions. In the event of a non-severe infusion-related reaction, consider adding a histamine receptor (H_1)-subtype antagonist (eg, **diphenhydramine** 25–50 mg intravenously or orally), an antipyretic (eg, **acetaminophen** 650–1000 mg orally), and a corticosteroid (eg, **methylprednisolone** 100 mg intravenously) administered 30 minutes prior to bendamustine HCl administration in subsequent cycles

Bendamustine HCl 90 mg/m² per dose; administer intravenously in a volume of 0.9% sodium chloride injection (0.9% NS) sufficient to produce a concentration with the range 0.2–0.6 mg/mL over 30–60 minutes, on 2 consecutive days, days 1 and 2, every 28 days for 6 cycles (total dosage/28-day cycle = 180 mg/m²)

Notes:

- Bendamustine HCl can cause severe infusion-related reactions
  - For Grade 1–2 infusion-related reactions, consider rechallenge with the addition of antihistamine, antipyretic, and corticosteroid premedications (as described in the above premedication section)
  - For Grade 3 infusion-related reactions, consider permanent discontinuation versus rechallenge with the addition of antihistamine, antipyretic, and corticosteroid premedications (as described in the above premedication section) after weighing risks and benefits
  - For Grade 4 infusion-related reactions, permanently discontinue bendamustine HCl
- Coadministration of strong CYP1A2 inhibitors (eg, ciprofloxacin, fluvoxamine) may increase exposure to bendamustine HCl and decrease exposure to its active metabolites. Concomitant CYP1A2 inducers (eg, omeprazole, cigarette smoking) may decrease exposure to bendamustine HCl and increase exposure to its active metabolites. Use caution, or select an alternative therapy, when coadministration of bendamustine HCl with strong CYP1A2 inhibitors or inducers is unavoidable
- Bendamustine HCl formulations may vary by country; consult local regulatory-approved labeling for guidance. For example, in the United States, the Food and Drug Administration approved Bendeka under Section 505(b)(2) of the Federal Food, Drug, and Cosmetic Act on 7 December 2015. The Bendeka product labeling contains specific dilution and administration instructions, *thus:*

  Bendamustine HCl (Bendeka, where available) 90 mg/m² per dose; administer intravenously in a volume of 0.9% NS or 5% dextrose injection (D5W) sufficient to produce a concentration with the range 1.85–5.6 mg/mL, over 10 minutes, on 2 consecutive days, days 1 and 2, every 28 days for 6 cycles (total dosage/cycle = 180 mg/m²)

Supportive Care
Antiemetic prophylaxis
Emetogenic potential on days with bendamustine is **MODERATE**
Emetogenic potential on day with rituximab ONLY (ie, cycle 1, day 0) is **MINIMAL**
See Chapter 42 for antiemetic recommendations

(continued)

(continued)

Hematopoietic growth factor (CSF) prophylaxis
Primary prophylaxis **MAY** be indicated
See Chapter 43 for more information

Antimicrobial prophylaxis
Risk of fever and neutropenia is **INTERMEDIATE**
  Antimicrobial primary prophylaxis to be considered:
  • Antibacterial—consider a fluoroquinolone or no prophylaxis; *P. jirovecii* prophylaxis is recommended (eg, cotrimoxazole)
  • Antifungal—consider use during periods of prolonged neutropenia
  • Antiviral—antiherpes antivirals (eg, acyclovir, famciclovir, valacyclovir)

Patient Population Studied

The international, multicenter, randomized, open-label, phase 3, non-inferiority trial (CLL10) involved 561 treatment-naïve patients with advanced CLL (Binet stage C), or confirmed active disease, who required treatment according to the International Workshop on Chronic Lymphocytic Leukemia criteria. Eligible patients had Eastern Cooperative Oncology Group performance status score ≤2, low comorbidity, and creatine clearance ≥70 mL/min. Patients with del(17p) as detected by fluorescence in-situ hybridization, impaired renal function other than that caused by abdominal lymph node mass, Richter transformation, or active second malignancy requiring treatment were ineligible. Patients were randomly assigned to receive six 28-day cycles of intravenous fludarabine (25 mg/m² per day on days 1–3), cyclophosphamide (250 mg/m² per day on days 1–3), and rituximab (375 mg/m² 1 day before the first treatment cycle and then 500 mg/m² on day 1 of subsequent treatment cycles), or bendamustine (90 mg/m² per day on days 1 and 2) and rituximab (375 mg/m² 1 day before the first treatment cycle and then 500 mg/m² on day 1 of subsequent treatment cycles)

Efficacy (N = 561)

	Bendamustine + Rituximab (n = 279)	Fludarabine + Cyclophosphamide + Rituximab (n = 282)	
Median progression-free survival	41.7 months	55.2 months	HR 1.643; 90.4% CI 1.308–2.064; P = 0.003
Overall survival at 3 years	92%	91%	HR 1.034; 95% CI 0.620–1.724; P = 0.897
Overall response rate*	96%	95%	P = 1.0

*Overall response rate included patients with complete remission, complete remission with incomplete marrow recovery, or partial remission

Note: Median duration of follow-up was 37.1 months

Therapy Monitoring

1. *Prior to treatment initiation:* CBC with differential, chemistries (potassium, uric acid, phosphorus, calcium, serum creatinine, LDH), serum bilirubin, ALT or AST, hepatitis B core antibody (IgG or total) and hepatitis B core antigen, urine pregnancy test (women of child-bearing potentially only)
2. *Prior to each cycle:* CBC with differential, chemistries (potassium, uric acid, phosphorus, calcium, serum creatinine, LDH), serum bilirubin, ALT or AST
3. *Weekly during treatment:* CBC with differential
4. *During each rituximab infusion and for at least 1 hour after infusion completion:* signs and symptoms of infusion-related reaction, vital signs every 30 minutes
5. *In patients at high risk for tumor lysis syndrome (eg, high tumor burden, renal dysfunction, rapidly increasing absolute lymphocyte count, markedly elevated LDH, baseline abnormalities in laboratory indices of tumor lysis syndrome [potassium, phosphate, uric acid, calcium, serum creatinine]):* consider frequent monitoring of laboratory indices of tumor lysis syndrome, intravenous hydration, and prophylaxis with a xanthine oxidase inhibitor (eg, allopurinol) during the first cycle
6. *Monitor periodically for:*
   a. Signs and symptoms of infection (including progressive multifocal leukoencephalopathy)
   b. Signs and symptoms of dermatologic toxicity
7. *Response assessment every 2–3 months:* physical examination, CBC with differential, CT scans (in select patients for evaluation of adenopathy)

Treatment Modifications

Bendamustine Dose Modifications

Starting dose	90 mg/m² per dose on days 1 and 2
Dose level −1	70 mg/m² per dose on days 1 and 2
Dose level −2	50 mg/m² per dose on days 1 and 2
Dose level −3	Discontinue bendamustine

Note: Rituximab dose is not reduced

Hematologic Toxicity

Day 1 platelet count less than 75,000/mm³ or day 1 ANC <1000/mm³	Delay start of cycle until platelet count ≥75,000/mm³ and ANC ≥1000/mm³ or until recovery to near baseline values, then reduce by 1 dose level for subsequent cycles. Consider G-CSF use in subsequent cycles for dose-limiting neutropenia
G4 hematologic toxicity occurring in the previous cycle	Delay start of cycle until platelet count ≥75,000/mcL and ANC ≥1000/mcL or until recovery to near baseline values, then reduce by 1 dose level for subsequent cycles. Consider G-CSF use in subsequent cycles for dose-limiting neutropenia or severe neutropenic complications

Infectious Complications

Active infection	Interrupt bendamustine and rituximab until resolution of infection, then resume treatment at either the same dose, or reduced by one dose level, depending on the severity of infection
New or changes in pre-existing neurologic symptoms (eg, confusion, dizziness, loss of balance, vision problems, aphasia, ambulation issues): PML suspected	Interrupt bendamustine and rituximab until central nervous system status clarified. Work-up may include (but is not limited to) consultation with a neurologist, brain MRI, and LP
PML is confirmed	Discontinue bendamustine and rituximab
HBV reactivation	Discontinue bendamustine and rituximab. Institute appropriate treatment for HBV. Upon resolution of HBV reactivation, resumption of bendamustine and rituximab should be discussed with a physician with expertise in management of HBV

Drug-Drug Interactions

Patient requires concomitant therapy with antihypertensive medication(s)	On days of rituximab treatment, and especially with the initial dose, weigh the risk versus benefit of delaying administration of the antihypertensive medication(s) until after completion of the rituximab infusion due to the potential risk of rituximab infusion-related hypotension
Live attenuated vaccine is indicated during or after rituximab administration	Avoid administration of a live attenuated vaccine during rituximab therapy and following therapy until adequate B-cell recovery has occurred
Patient requires concomitant therapy with a CYP1A2 inhibitor (eg, fluvoxamine, ciprofloxacin)	Consider alternative treatment instead of the CYP1A2 inhibitor. If the CYP1A2 inhibitor cannot be avoided, use caution and monitor carefully for bendamustine adverse effects
Patient requires concomitant therapy with a CYP1A2 inducer (eg, omeprazole), or patient is a smoker	Consider alternative treatment instead of the CYP1A2 inducer. Recommend cessation of smoking, if applicable. If the CYP1A2 inducer cannot be avoided, use caution and monitor carefully for reduced bendamustine efficacy

Other Toxicities

G ≥2 nonhematologic toxicity during the prior cycle	Delay start of cycle until nonhematologic toxicity resolves to G ≤1 or baseline, then reduce by 1 dose level for subsequent cycles

(continued)

Treatment Modifications (continued)

RITUXIMAB

Rituximab Infusion-Related Toxicities

Onset of infusion-related events (fevers, chills, rigors, edema, congestion of the head and neck mucosa, hypotension)
1. Interrupt rituximab infusion
2. For fever, chills: Give additional dose of **acetaminophen** 650 mg orally and **diphenhydramine** 25–50 mg by intravenous push
3. For rigors: Give **meperidine** 12.5–25 mg by intravenous push ± **promethazine** 12.5–25 mg by intravenous infusion in at least 10 mL 0.9% NS or D5W over 5–15 minutes. If after 15–20 minutes the response to a single dose is considered inadequate, the dose may be repeated
4. After symptoms resolve, resume rituximab infusion at a minimum of 50% reduction in the rate at which the event occurred. If no further infusion-related events, increase the rate by 50 mg/hour every 30 minutes, as tolerated, up to a maximum rate of 400 mg/hour

Dyspnea or wheezing, without allergic findings (urticaria, or tongue or laryngeal edema)
1. Interrupt rituximab infusion immediately
2. Give **hydrocortisone** 100 mg by intravenous push (or glucocorticoid equivalent)
3. Give an additional dose of **diphenhydramine** 25–50 mg by intravenous push and a histamine H2-antagonist (**ranitidine** 50 mg or **famotidine** 20 mg) by intravenous push
4. After symptoms resolve, resume rituximab infusion at a minimum of 50% reduction in the rate at which the event occurred. If no further infusion-related events, increase the rate by 50 mg/hour every 30 minutes, as tolerated, up to a maximum rate of 400 mg/hour

Note: Medications and equipment for the treatment of hypersensitivity reactions should be available for immediate use in the event of a reaction during administration (eg, intravenous fluids, epinephrine, antihistamines, glucocorticoids, oxygen)

Adverse Events (N = 557)

Event	Event Percentage:* Bendamustine + Rituximab (n = 278)		Event Percentage:* Fludarabine + Cyclophosphamide + Rituximab (n = 279)	
	Grade 1–2	Grade 3–5	Grade 1–2	Grade 3–5
Hematologic toxic events	1	68	1	91
Infections, total	41	27	37	40
Infection with unspecified pathogen	44	15	42	25
Neutropenia	<1	59	<1	84
Leukocytopenia	<1	49	<1	80
Viral infection	15	4	18	9
Thrombocytopenia	4	14	3	22
Allergic conditions	4	10	3	5
Pneumonia	5	9	4	12
Cardiac and pulmonary disorders	4	9	4	9
Skin reactions	9	4	8	3
Other	6	6	9	4
Gastrointestinal disorders	5	6	7	8
Anemia	<1	10	1	14
Neurologic and psychiatric disorders	5	4	4	4

(continued)

Adverse Events (N = 557) *(continued)*

Event	Event Percentage:* Bendamustine + Rituximab (n = 278)		Event Percentage:* Fludarabine + Cyclophosphamide + Rituximab (n = 279)	
	Grade 1–2	Grade 3–5	Grade 1–2	Grade 3–5
Pyrexia	5	2	6	<1
Laboratory abnormalities	2	3	2	3
Trauma and orthopedic problems	2	3	2	3
Secondary neoplasia	<1	4	<1	7
Bacterial infection	2	2	2	2
Arthritis and arthralgia	3	<1	3	<1
Sepsis	0	2	0	3
Fungal infection	2	0	2	1
Renal disorders	1	<1	1	3
Urticaria	<1	1	<1	0
Fatigue	1	<1	2	<1

*According to the National Cancer Institute Common Terminology Criteria for Adverse Events, version 3
Note: Adverse events that occurred during the whole study period are included. A total of 13% of the bendamustine + rituximab group and 23% of the fludarabine + cyclophosphamide + rituximab group discontinued study treatment owing to toxic effects (P = 0.003). Deaths related to treatment were reported for 2% of the bendamustine + rituximab group and 5% of the fludarabine + cyclophosphamide + rituximab group

FIRST-LINE

CHRONIC LYMPHOCYTIC LEUKEMIA REGIMEN: FLUDARABINE + RITUXIMAB

Byrd JC et al. Blood 2003;101:6–14
Woyach JA et al. J Clin Oncol 2011;29:1349–1355

Premedication:
Allopurinol 300 mg/day; administer orally for 14 consecutive days on days 1–14
Acetaminophen 650 mg; administer orally 30 minutes before rituximab
Diphenhydramine 25–50 mg; administer by intravenous injection 30 minutes before rituximab

Fludarabine 25 mg/m^2 per day; administer by intravenous infusion in 100–125 mL 5% dextrose injection (D5W) or 0.9% sodium chloride injection (0.9% NS) over 20–30 minutes for 5 consecutive day on days 1–5, every 28 days for 6 cycles (total dosage/cycle = 125 mg/m^2)

Cycle 1: Rituximab 375 mg/m^2 per dose; administer by intravenous infusion in a volume of D5W or 0.9% NS sufficient to produce a concentration within the range 1–4 mg/mL for 2 doses on days 1 and 4 (total dosage/cycle 1 = 750 mg/m^2)

Cycles 2–6: Rituximab 375 mg/m^2; administer by intravenous infusion in a volume of D5W or 0.9% NS sufficient to produce a concentration within the range 1–4 mg/mL on day 1, every 28 days for 5 cycles (total dosage/cycle = 375 mg/m^2)

Supportive Care
Antiemetic prophylaxis
Emetogenic potential is **MINIMAL**
See Chapter 42 for antiemetic recommendations

Hematopoietic growth factor (CSF) prophylaxis
Primary prophylaxis may be indicated
See Chapter 43 for more information

Antimicrobial prophylaxis
Risk of fever and neutropenia is **INTERMEDIATE**
Antimicrobial primary prophylaxis to be considered:

- Antibacterial—consider a fluoroquinolone or no prophylaxis; *P. jirovecii* prophylaxis is recommended (eg, cotrimoxazole)

- Antifungal—consider concomitant use with cotrimoxazole, during periods of neutropenia

- Antiviral—antiherpes antivirals (eg, acyclovir, famciclovir, valacyclovir)

Nonhematologic Toxicity (NCI CTC)

Toxicity	% G1/2	% G3/4
Nausea	48	0
Vomiting	16	0
Myalgias	28	0
Fatigue/malaise	62	0
Dyspnea/hypoxemia*	12	14
Hypotension*	10	6
Fever*	32	0
Chills/rigors*	36	0
G3/4 pulmonary toxicity	3 cases	
Thrombocytopenic purpura	1 case	
Pure red cell aplasia	1 case	

*Infusion-related toxicities occurred in 100% of patients during the first administration of rituximab. Usually G1/2, although 20% experienced G3/4. Only 2 patients (4%) experienced infusion-related adverse events during a second administration

Patient Population Studied

Study of 104 previously untreated patients with symptomatic CLL

Efficacy (N = 104)

Overall response rate	84%
Complete response rate	38%
Estimated 5-year progression-free survival	28%
Median overall survival	85 months

Adverse Events (N = 51)

Hematologic Toxicity (Modified NCI Criteria for CLL)

Toxicity	% G1/2	% G3/4
Neutropenia	8	76
Thrombocytopenia	47	20
Anemia	65	4
Infection	43	20

Treatment Modifications

Adverse Event	Treatment Modification
Fludarabine-Related Toxicities	
G3 neutropenia, thrombocytopenia, or anemia	Delay treatment until recovery to within 20% of baseline, then resume treatment with dosage of fludarabine reduced by 25%
G4 neutropenia, thrombocytopenia, or anemia	Delay treatment until recovery to within 20% of baseline, then resume treatment with dosage of fludarabine reduced by 50%
Infection without G3/4 neutropenia	Hold treatment until infection resolves, then restart at the same dosages
Evidence of autoimmune hemolytic anemia or thrombocytopenia	Replace rituximab and fludarabine with alternative treatment as appropriate
Grade ≥2 nonhematologic adverse events attributable to fludarabine, except nausea, vomiting, fatigue, diarrhea, infusion-related fever, or chills	Reduce fludarabine dosage by 50%
G3/4, or irreversible G2 nonhematologic toxicity	Reduce fludarabine dosage by 50%, or consider withdrawing fludarabine

RITUXIMAB

Rituximab Infusion-Related Toxicities

Onset of infusion-related events (fevers, chills, rigors, edema, congestion of the head and neck mucosa, hypotension)
1. Interrupt rituximab infusion
2. For fever, chills: Give additional dose of **acetaminophen** 650 mg orally and **diphenhydramine** 25–50 mg by intravenous push
3. For rigors: Give **meperidine** 12.5–25 mg by intravenous push ± **promethazine** 12.5–25 mg by intravenous infusion in at least 10 mL 0.9% NS or D5W over 5–15 minutes. If after 15–20 minutes the response to a single dose is considered inadequate, the dose may be repeated
4. After symptoms resolve, resume rituximab infusion at a minimum of 50% reduction in the rate at which the event occurred. If no further infusion-related events, increase the rate by 50 mg/hour every 30 minutes, as tolerated, up to a maximum rate of 400 mg/hour

Dyspnea or wheezing, without allergic findings (urticaria, or tongue or laryngeal edema)
1. Interrupt rituximab infusion immediately
2. Give **hydrocortisone** 100 mg by intravenous push (or glucocorticoid equivalent)
3. Give an additional dose of **diphenhydramine** 25–50 mg by intravenous push and a histamine H2-antagonist (**ranitidine** 50 mg or **famotidine** 20 mg) by intravenous push
4. After symptoms resolve, resume rituximab infusion at a minimum of 50% reduction in the rate at which the event occurred. If no further infusion-related events, increase the rate by 50 mg/hour every 30 minutes, as tolerated, up to a maximum rate of 400 mg/hour

Note: Medications and equipment for the treatment of hypersensitivity reactions should be available for immediate use in the event of a reaction during administration (eg, intravenous fluids, epinephrine, antihistamines, glucocorticoids, oxygen)

Therapy Monitoring

1. *Prior to treatment initiation:* CBC with differential, chemistries (potassium, uric acid, phosphorus, calcium, serum creatinine, LDH), serum bilirubin, ALT or AST, hepatitis B core antibody (IgG or total) and hepatitis B core antigen, urine pregnancy test (women of child-bearing potentially only)
2. *Prior to each cycle:* CBC with differential, chemistries (potassium, uric acid, phosphorus, calcium, serum creatinine, LDH), serum bilirubin, ALT or AST
3. *Weekly during treatment:* CBC with differential
4. *During each rituximab infusion and for at least 1 hour after infusion completion:* signs and symptoms of infusion-related reaction, vital signs every 30 minutes
5. *In patients at high risk for tumor lysis syndrome (eg, high tumor burden, renal dysfunction, rapidly increasing absolute lymphocyte count, markedly elevated LDH, baseline abnormalities in laboratory indices of tumor lysis syndrome [potassium, phosphate, uric acid, calcium, serum creatinine]):* consider frequent monitoring of laboratory indices of tumor lysis syndrome, intravenous hydration, and prophylaxis with a xanthine oxidase inhibitor (eg, allopurinol) during the first cycle
6. *Monitor periodically for:*
   a. Signs and symptoms of infection (including progressive multifocal leukoencephalopathy)
   b. Signs and symptoms of dermatologic toxicity
7. *Response assessment every 2–3 months:* physical examination, CBC with differential, CT scans (in select patients for evaluation of adenopathy)

Note

Recommended as initial therapy for patients with CLL. This regimen is increasingly used in combination with cyclophosphamide

SUBSEQUENT THERAPY
CHRONIC LYMPHOCYTIC LEUKEMIA REGIMEN: VENETOCLAX

Davids M et al. Clin Lymphoma Myeloma Leuk 2017;17(Suppl 2):S302
Jones JA et al. Lancet Oncol 2018;19:65–75
Supplementary appendix to: Jones JA et al. Lancet Oncol 2018;19:65–75
Venclexta (venetoclax tablets) prescribing information. North Chicago, IL: AbbVie Inc; 2018 November

Venetoclax; administer orally once daily with 240 mL water within 30 minutes of completion of a meal (preferably breakfast) continuously for up to 2 years or until disease progression (see tables below for dosing schedule, choose either the Standard 5-Week Dose Escalation Schedule OR the Accelerated 3-Week Dose Escalation Schedule)

Standard 5-Week Dose Escalation Schedule*

Week of Treatment	Venetoclax Dose per Day	Total Venetoclax Dosage per Week
Week 1	20 mg	140 mg
Week 2	50 mg	350 mg
Week 3	100 mg	700 mg
Week 4	200 mg	1400 mg
Week 5 and beyond†	400 mg	2800 mg

*The standard 5-week dose escalation schedule is approved by the U.S. Food and Drug Administration and is appropriate for the majority of patients initiating treatment with venetoclax. Advise patients to keep the medication in its original packaging during the first 4 weeks of therapy

†If no response is achieved by week 12, consider increasing the venetoclax dose to 600 mg orally once daily (total venetoclax dosage/week = 4200 mg) per Jones et al. Follow high-risk tumor lysis syndrome precautions (eg, IV hydration, allopurinol ± rasburicase) as outlined in the table below and admit the patient to the hospital for frequent laboratory monitoring (pre-dose, 4, 8, 12, and 24 hours) if electing to escalate to 600 mg

Venclexta (venetoclax tablets) prescribing information. North Chicago, IL: AbbVie Inc; 2018 November

Accelerated 3-Week Dose Escalation Schedule*

Week and Day of Treatment	Venetoclax Dose per day	Total Venetoclax Dosage per Week
Week 1 Day 1	20 mg	Week 1: 520 mg
Week 1 Days 2 and 3	50 mg	
Week 1 Days 4, 5, 6, and 7	100 mg	
Week 2	200 mg	Week 2: 1400 mg
Week 3 and beyond	400 mg	Week 3 and beyond: 2800 mg

*Patients with high tumor burden (any lymph node ≥10 cm OR any lymph node ≥5 cm AND absolute lymphocyte count ≥25 × 10⁹/L) who were experiencing symptomatic rapid disease progression following treatment with a B-cell receptor pathway inhibitor were allowed to be treated according to an accelerated 3-week dose escalation schedule. Note that this schedule is not approved by the U.S. Food and Drug Administration and is considered to be "off-label"

†If no response is achieved by week 12, consider increasing the venetoclax dose to 600 mg orally once daily (total venetoclax dosage/week = 4200 mg) per Jones et al. Follow high-risk tumor lysis syndrome precautions (eg, IV hydration, allopurinol ± rasburicase) as outlined in the table below and admit the patient to the hospital for frequent laboratory monitoring (pre-dose, 4, 8, 12, and 24 hours) if electing to escalate to 600 mg

Davids M et al. Clin Lymphoma Myeloma Leuk 2017;17(Suppl 2):S302
Jones JA et al. Lancet Oncol 2018;19:65–75
Supplementary appendix to: Jones JA et al. Lancet Oncol 2018;19:65–75

Notes:
• Venetoclax tablets should be swallowed whole. Do not chew, crush, or break venetoclax tablets.
• Patients who delay taking venetoclax at a regularly scheduled time may administer the missed dose within 30 minutes of completion of a meal if within 8 hours of the usual dosing time. If >8 hours, skip the missed dose and resume treatment at the next regularly scheduled time. Patients who vomit after a dose of venetoclax should not repeat the dose but rather take the next dose at the next regularly scheduled time

(continued)

(*continued*)

- Venetoclax is a substrate of cytochrome P450 (CYP) CYP3A subfamily enzymes, P-glycoprotein (P-gp), and BCRP. Venetoclax is a weak inhibitor of CYP2C8, CYP2C9, and UGT1A1 in vitro but due to high protein binding is predicted to cause clinically insignificant inhibition of these enzymes in vivo. Venetoclax is a P-gp and BCRP inhibitor and weak OATP1B1 inhibitor in vitro
  - Avoid concurrent use with strong or moderate CYP3A inducers at all times
  - Avoid concurrent use with strong CYP3A4 inhibitors throughout the venetoclax dose escalation period.
    - For patients who have completed venetoclax dose-escalation and are maintained on a steady dose of venetoclax, reduce the venetoclax dose to 100 mg if concomitant use of a strong CYP3A inhibitor is unavoidable and monitor closely for side effects. If the strong CYP3A inhibitor is subsequently discontinued, resume the venetoclax dose that was administered prior to introduction of the inhibitor 2–3 days after discontinuation of the inhibitor
    - For patients who have completed venetoclax dose-escalation and are maintained on a steady dose of venetoclax, reduce the venetoclax dose to 70 mg if concomitant use of posaconazole is unavoidable and monitor closely for side effects. If posaconazole is subsequently discontinued, resume the venetoclax dose that was administered prior to introduction of posaconazole 2–3 days after discontinuation of posaconazole
  - Reduce the venetoclax dose by ≥50% if concomitant use of a moderate CYP3A4 inhibitor or P-gp inhibitor is unavoidable and monitor closely for side effects. If the moderate CYP3A4 inhibitor is subsequently discontinued, resume the venetoclax dose that was administered prior to introduction of the inhibitor 2–3 days after discontinuation of the inhibitor
  - Advise patients to not consume grapefruit products, Seville oranges, or starfruit as they may inhibit CYP3A in the gut wall and increase the bioavailability of venetoclax
  - Coadministration of venetoclax with warfarin caused increased exposure to *R*-warfarin and *S*-warfarin. Monitor the international normalized ratio closely in patients coadministered warfarin
  - Venetoclax inhibits P-gp. Concomitant use of narrow therapeutic index P-gp substrates (eg, digoxin, everolimus, sirolimus) should be avoided when possible. If use of a P-gp substrate is unavoidable, then administer the P-gp substrate ≥6 hours before venetoclax
- Venetoclax can cause rapid death of leukemic cells leading to rapid onset of tumor lysis syndrome (TLS) during the dose escalation period in some patients. In clinical trials of venetoclax, fatal cases of tumor lysis syndrome have occurred which led to the development of a step-wise dose escalation approach to initiation of venetoclax. Assess tumor burden (eg, CT scan, absolute lymphocyte count) and TLS laboratory measurements (eg, potassium, uric acid, phosphorus, calcium, creatinine, lactate dehydrogenase) and correct any abnormalities prior to initiation of venetoclax. Based on the tumor burden and baseline renal function assessments, determine the risk of TLS in order to guide decisions regarding optimal setting of therapy initiation (inpatient vs outpatient), hydration requirements, and frequency of TLS laboratory monitoring according to the table below

TLS Risk Assessment and Supportive Care				
		Prophylaxis*		Blood Chemistry† Monitoring
Tumor Burden		Hydration	Anti-hyperuricemic therapy	Setting and frequency of assessment
Low	All LN < 5 cm AND ALC <25 × 10⁹/L	Oral (1.5–2 L/day)	Allopurinol	Outpatient: • For the first dose of 20 mg and 50 mg; pre-dose, 6–8 hours, 24 hours • For subsequent ramp-up doses; pre-dose‡
Medium	Any LN 5 –10 cm OR ALC ≥25 × 10⁹/L	Oral (1.5–2 L/day) and consider additional intravenous	Allopurinol	Outpatient: • For the first dose of 20 mg and 50 mg; pre-dose, 6–8 hours, 24 hours (for patients with CrCl <80 mL/min consider hospitalization with frequent laboratory monitoring as described below for high-risk patients) • For subsequent ramp-up doses; pre-dose‡
High (standard 5-week dose escalation)	Any LN ≥10 cm OR ALC ≥25 × 10⁹/L AND Any LN ≥5 cm	Oral (1.5–2 L/day) and intravenous (150–200 mL/hour as tolerated)	Allopurinol; consider rasburicase if baseline uric acid is elevated	In hospital: • For the first dose of 20 mg and 50 mg; pre-dose, 4, 8, 12, and 24 hours Outpatient: • For subsequent ramp-up doses; pre-dose, 6–8 hours, 24 hours

(*continued*)

(continued)

		TLS Risk Assessment and Supportive Care		
		Prophylaxis*		Blood Chemistry† Monitoring
Tumor Burden		Hydration	Anti-hyperuricemic therapy	Setting and frequency of assessment
High (accelerated 3-week dose escalation)	Any LN ≥10 cm OR ALC ≥25 × 10⁹/L AND Any LN ≥5 cm	Oral (1.5–2 L/day) and intravenous (150–200 mL/hour as tolerated)	Allopurinol; consider rasburicase if baseline uric acid is elevated	In hospital: • Hospitalize patients prior to initiation of venetoclax and through at least 24 hours after reaching the 200-mg dose (ie, until week 2, day 2) provided that there is no evidence of clinical or laboratory TLS. Rehospitalize patients the evening prior to dose escalation to the 400-mg dose (ie, rehospitalize on the evening of week 2, day 7) and until 24 hours following administration of the 400-mg dose (ie, until week 3 day 2) provided that there is no evidence of clinical or laboratory TLS • During all days of hospitalization during accelerated 3-week dose escalation; pre-dose, 4, 8, 12, and 24 hours

TLS, tumor lysis syndrome; LN, lymph node; ALC, absolute lymphocyte count; CrCl, creatinine clearance

*Initiate a xanthine oxidase inhibitor (eg, allopurinol) 2–3 days prior to initiation of venetoclax. Continue the xanthine oxidase inhibitor for up to 5 weeks depending upon ongoing risk of TLS. Encourage oral hydration (1.5–2 L/day) starting 2 days before and on the day of the first venetoclax dose and each dose escalation

†Blood chemistries = potassium, uric acid, phosphorus, calcium, serum creatinine (evaluate in real time)

‡For patients at continued risk of TLS, monitor chemistries at 6–8 hours and at 24 hours at each subsequent outpatient ramp-up dose

Davids M et al. Clin Lymphoma Myeloma Leuk 2017;17(Suppl 2):S302
Jones JA et al. Lancet Oncol 2018;19:65–75
Supplementary appendix to: Jones JA et al. Lancet Oncol 2018;19:65–75
Venclexta (venetoclax tablets) prescribing information. North Chicago, IL: AbbVie Inc; 2018 November

Supportive Care
Antiemetic prophylaxis
Emetogenic potential is **MINIMAL–LOW**
See Chapter 42 for antiemetic recommendations

Hematopoietic growth factor (CSF) prophylaxis
Primary prophylaxis may be indicated
See Chapter 43 for more information

Antimicrobial prophylaxis
Risk of fever and neutropenia is **LOW**
Antimicrobial primary prophylaxis to be considered:
• Antibacterial—consider prophylaxis with a fluoroquinolone during periods of prolonged neutropenia only (eg, <500/mm³ for ≥7 days) until ANC recovery
• Antifungal— not indicated
• Antiviral—antiherpes antivirals (eg, acyclovir, famciclovir, valacyclovir)

Patient Population Studied

The multicenter, non-randomized, open-label, phase 2 trial involved 127 patients with relapsed or refractory CLL. Eligible patients were aged ≥18 years, had an Eastern Cooperative Oncology Group performance status score ≤2, and had previously received B-cell receptor inhibitor therapy, with ibrutinib or idelalisib being their last such therapy. Patients with Richter's transformation, active and uncontrolled autoimmune cytopenias, unresolved toxicity from previous therapy, or a history of allogeneic stem-cell transplantation within 1 year of study entry were ineligible. All patients received oral venetoclax (20 mg once daily for 1 week, followed by weekly ramp-up to 50 mg, 100 mg, and 200 mg daily, up to a final dose of 400 mg daily by week 5) for up to 2 years. After the response assessment at week 12, dose escalation to 600 mg was allowed in the expansion cohort if the patient had not responded to treatment

Efficacy (N = 91 Patients Who Had Received Ibrutinib Before Enrollment: 43 in Main Cohort and 48 in Expansion Cohort)

Overall response rate*	65%
Median progression-free survival	24.7 months

*Overall response rate included patients with complete response (including with incomplete bone marrow recovery), nodular partial response, or partial response at 24 weeks in the main cohort and 36 weeks in the expansion cohort

Note: Median duration of follow-up was 14 months (19 months for the main cohort and 12 months for the expansion cohort)

Therapy Monitoring

1. *Prior to initiation of venetoclax:*
   a. Assess tumor burden (CBC with differential, CT scan) and baseline chemistries (potassium, uric acid, phosphorus, calcium, serum creatinine, LDH) to determine the risk for tumor lysis syndrome (TLS). Decisions regarding treatment setting (inpatient vs outpatient) and frequency of laboratory monitoring depend upon TLS risk assessment (see above table)
   b. Verify adherence to the prescribed xanthine oxidase inhibitor regimen (eg, allopurinol) to begin 2–3 days prior to venetoclax initiation
   c. Screen for the presence of drug-drug interactions involving venetoclax
   d. Prescribe the appropriate combination of venetoclax tablet strengths (available in 10-mg, 50-mg, and 100-mg tablets) in sufficient quantities to accommodate the planned venetoclax dose-escalation and maintenance dosing schedule
2. *Tumor lysis syndrome monitoring during venetoclax ramp-up:* monitor potassium, uric acid, phosphorus, calcium, and serum creatinine at the frequency described in the above table corresponding to the patient's risk for tumor lysis syndrome
3. *Periodically throughout treatment:* CBC with differential
4. *Response assessment every 2–3 months:* physical examination, CBC with differential, CT scans (in select patients for evaluation of adenopathy)

Treatment Modifications

VENETOCLAX

Dose at Interruption	Restart Dose*†
400 mg	300 mg
300 mg	200 mg
200 mg	100 mg
100 mg	50 mg‡
50 mg	20 mg‡
20 mg	10 mg‡

*If patients interrupt venetoclax for >1 week during the 5-week ramp-up period or interrupt venetoclax for >2 weeks during maintenance therapy, reassess the risk of TLS to determine if reinitiation with a reduced dose of venetoclax is necessary
†During the venetoclax ramp-up phase, continue the reduced venetoclax dose for 1 week before further dose escalation
‡Consider discontinuing venetoclax for patients who require dose reductions to <100 mg for >2 weeks

Tumor Lysis Syndrome

Adverse Event	Treatment Modification
Prior to initiation of venetoclax: • Potassium, phosphorus, or uric acid > ULN • Corrected calcium < LLN • Serum creatinine ≥25% above baseline value	Correct pre-existing tumor lysis syndrome abnormalities prior to initiation of venetoclax
Laboratory TLS Blood chemistry (potassium, phosphorus, uric acid, calcium, serum creatinine) suggestive of TLS *without* clinical sequelae	Withhold venetoclax until resolution. Correct laboratory abnormalities and increase frequency of monitoring If abnormalities resolve within 48 hours, resume venetoclax at the same dose. If resolution requires >48 hours, then resume venetoclax at a reduced dose

(continued)

Treatment Modifications (*continued*)

Adverse Event	Treatment Modification
Clinical TLS Blood chemistry (potassium, phosphorus, uric acid, calcium, serum creatinine) suggestive of TLS *with* clinical sequelae (eg, serum creatinine ≥1.5× ULN, cardiac arrhythmia, seizure, sudden cardiac death)	Correct laboratory abnormalities and increase frequency of monitoring Withhold venetoclax until resolution and then resume venetoclax at a reduced dose
Potassium > ULN in the setting of TLS	Withhold venetoclax until resolution. Increase frequency of monitoring. If resolution occurs within 24–48 hours of the last dose, resume venetoclax at the same dose. If resolution requires >48 hours, then resume at a reduced dose Perform STAT ECG and begin telemetry. Consider the following interventions: • Sodium polystyrene sulfonate 15 g by mouth once • Furosemide 20 mg IV push once • Insulin 10 units IV push once plus 25 g of 50% dextrose IV push once (may omit glucose if serum glucose is ≥250 mg/dL) • If there is ECG evidence of life-threatening arrhythmia, then administer calcium gluconate 1000 mg in 100 mL D5W IV over 30 minutes once • Consult nephrology for consideration of dialysis for severe, refractory, or rapidly worsening hyperkalemia, especially in the setting of concomitant AKI
Uric acid ≥8.0 mg/dL in the setting of TLS	Withhold venetoclax until resolution. Increase frequency of monitoring. If resolution occurs within 24–48 hours of the last dose, resume venetoclax at the same dose. If resolution requires >48 hours, then resume at a reduced dose Consider a single dose of rasburicase 3–6 mg (fixed dose) IV over 30 minutes. Optimize the dose of xanthine oxidase inhibitor (eg, allopurinol) and the rate of IV hydration, as tolerated
Phosphorus ≥5.0 mg/dL in the setting of TLS	Withhold venetoclax until resolution. Increase frequency of monitoring. If resolution occurs within 24–48 hours of the last dose, resume venetoclax at the same dose. If resolution requires >48 hours, then resume at a reduced dose Administer a phosphate binder (eg, aluminum hydroxide, calcium carbonate, sevelamer carbonate, or lanthanum carbonate) with meals. Place patient on a low-phosphate diet. Optimize the rate of IV hydration, as tolerated. Consult nephrology for consideration of hemodialysis, especially if phosphorus ≥10 mg/dL or with concomitant AKI
Serum creatinine increases ≥25% from baseline in the setting of TLS	Withhold venetoclax until resolution. Increase frequency of monitoring. If resolution occurs within 24–48 hours of the last dose, resume venetoclax at the same dose. If resolution requires >48 hours, then resume at a reduced dose Start or increase rate of IV hydration. For severe AKI, consider nephrology consultation
Corrected calcium ≤7.0 mg/dL and patient is symptomatic (eg, muscle cramps, hypotension, tetany, cardiac arrhythmias) in the setting of TLS	Withhold venetoclax until resolution. Increase frequency of monitoring. If resolution occurs within 24–48 hours of the last dose, resume venetoclax at the same dose. If resolution requires >48 hours, then resume at a reduced dose Perform STAT ECG and begin telemetry. Administer calcium gluconate 1000 mg in 100 mL D5W IV over 30 minutes once
Hematologic Toxicities	
G3 neutropenia (ANC ≥500/mm^3 and <1000/mm^3) with infection or fever; or G4 neutropenia (ANC <500/mm^3); or G4 thrombocytopenia (platelet count <25,000/mm^3), first occurrence	Withhold venetoclax until resolution to G ≤1 or baseline, then resume venetoclax at the same dose G-CSF may be administered with venetoclax if indicated to reduce the risk of infection associated with neutropenia
G3 neutropenia (ANC ≥500/mm^3 and <1000/mm^3) with infection or fever; or G4 neutropenia (ANC <500/mm^3); or G4 thrombocytopenia (platelet count <25,000/mm^3), second and subsequent occurrences	Withhold venetoclax until resolution to G ≤1 or baseline, then resume venetoclax at a reduced dose. At the discretion of the medically responsible health care provider, a larger dose reduction than that described above may be considered depending on the severity of the toxicity G-CSF may be administered with venetoclax if indicated to reduce the risk of infection associated with neutropenia

(*continued*)

Treatment Modifications (*continued*)

Adverse Event	Treatment Modification
Drug-Drug Interactions	
Concomitant therapy with a strong or moderate CYP3A inducer is required	Do not administer a strong or moderate CYP3A inducer with venetoclax
Concomitant therapy with a strong CYP3A4 inhibitor is required during the venetoclax 5-week ramp-up period	Do not administer a strong CYP3A4 inhibitor during the venetoclax ramp-up period
Concomitant therapy with a strong CYP3A4 inhibitor is required in a patient taking a steady daily dosage of venetoclax (after ramp-up phase)	Consider alternative medications. If the strong CYP3A4 inhibitor is unavoidable, then reduce the venetoclax dose to 100 mg
Concomitant therapy with posaconazole is required in a patient taking a steady daily dosage of venetoclax (after ramp-up phase)	Consider alternative medications. If posaconazole is unavoidable, then reduce the venetoclax dose to 70 mg
Concomitant therapy with a moderate CYP3A4 inhibitor or P-gp inhibitor is required (any phase of treatment)	Consider alternative medications. If the moderate CYP3A4 inhibitor or P-gp inhibitor is unavoidable, then reduce the venetoclax dose by at least 50%
Concomitant strong or moderate CYP3A4 inhibitor, posaconazole, or P-gp inhibitor is subsequently discontinued	Resume the venetoclax dosage that was used prior to concomitant use of a strong or moderate CYP3A4 inhibitor, posaconazole, or P-gp inhibitor 2–3 days after discontinuation of the inhibitor
Concomitant therapy with warfarin is required	Monitor international normalized ratio frequently
Concomitant therapy with a P-gp substrate is required	Consider alternative medications. If concomitant use is unavoidable, administer the P-gp substrate at least 6 hours before the administration of venetoclax
Suboptimal Response to Venetoclax	
No response to venetoclax by week 12	Consider increasing the venetoclax dose to 600 mg orally once daily (total venetoclax dosage/week = 4200 mg) per Jones et al. Follow high-risk tumor lysis syndrome precautions (eg, IV hydration, allopurinol ± rasburicase) as outlined in the table above and admit the patient to the hospital for frequent laboratory monitoring (pre-dose, 4, 8, 12, and 24 hours) if electing to escalate to 600 mg
Other Toxicities	
Other G3/4 nonhematologic toxicity, first occurrence	Withhold venetoclax until resolution to G ≤1 or baseline, then resume venetoclax at the same dose
Other G3/4 nonhematologic toxicity, second and subsequent occurrences	Withhold venetoclax until resolution to G ≤1 or baseline, then resume venetoclax at a lower dose. At the discretion of the medically responsible health care provider, a larger dose reduction than that described above may be considered depending on the severity of the toxicity
Immunization with a live attenuated vaccine is indicated prior to, during, or after therapy with venetoclax	Do not administer live attenuated vaccines prior to, during, or after treatment with venetoclax until B-cell recovery occurs
Venetoclax may cause fetal harm. Advise females of reproductive potential of the potential risk to a fetus and to use effective contraception during treatment	

TLS, tumor lysis syndrome; ULN, upper limit of normal; LLN, lower limit of normal; ECG, electrocardiogram; IV, intravenous; AKI, acute kidney injury; ANC, absolute neutrophil count; G-CSF, granulocyte-colony stimulating factor; P-gp, P-glycoprotein

Adverse Events (N = 91 Patients Who Had Received Ibrutinib Before Enrollment: 43 in Main Cohort and 48 in Expansion Cohort)

Event	Grade 1–2 (%)	Grade 3–5 (%)	Event	Grade 1–2 (%)	Grade 3–5 (%)
Neutropenia	11	51	Bruising	17	0
Nausea	56	1	Hypoalbuminemia	14	2
Anemia	24	29	Increased alanine aminotransferase level	12	3
Diarrhea	45	7	Dyspnea	13	2
Thrombocytopenia	19	29	Hyperkalemia	14	1
Fatigue	36	7	Febrile neutropenia	0	13
Decreased white blood cell count	16	19	Increased blood bilirubin level	12	1
Cough	26	0	Dizziness	13	0
Upper respiratory tract infection	26	0	Extremity pain	13	0
Decreased lymphocyte count	10	15	Hyperuricemia	13	0
Hypocalcemia	20	3	Hypertension	5	7
Vomiting	22	1	Chills	11	1
Peripheral edema	23	0	Hyperphosphatemia	12	0
Hypokalemia	16	5	Oropharyngeal pain	12	0
Abdominal pain	17	4	Rash	12	0
Headache	20	1	Pneumonia	4	7
Constipation	21	0	Hyperglycemia	5	5
Increased aspartate aminotransferase level	18	2			
Pyrexia	19	1			
Hyponatremia	12	7			
Hypophosphatemia	5	13			
Arthralgia	18	0			
Back pain	18	0			

*According to the National Cancer Institute Common Terminology Criteria for Adverse Events, version 4.0

Note: Safety was monitored for 30 days after treatment. Treatment-emergent toxicities are included if Grade 1–2 adverse events occurred in ≥10% of patients or Grade ≥3 adverse events occurred in ≥5% of patients. A total of 7% discontinued treatment owing to adverse events. No treatment-related deaths occurred, although six deaths due to adverse events occurred within 30 days of the last dose of venetoclax (from *Corynebacterium* sepsis, possible cytokine release syndrome on subsequent therapy, mechanical asphyxia, multi-organ failure, septic shock, and for an unknown reason)

SUBSEQUENT THERAPY
CHRONIC LYMPHOCYTIC LEUKEMIA REGIMEN: VENETOCLAX + RITUXIMAB

Seymour JF et al. N Engl J Med 2018;378:1107–1120
Supplementary appendix to: Seymour JF et al. N Engl J Med 2018;378:1107–1120
Seymour JF et al. Lancet Oncol 2017;18:230–240
Supplementary appendix to: Seymour JF et al. Lancet Oncol 2017;18:230–240
Venclexta (venetoclax tablets) prescribing information. North Chicago, IL: AbbVie Inc; 2018 November

The regimen consists of venetoclax administered as a 5-week ramp-up to a target dose of 400 mg orally once daily. After 7 doses of venetoclax 400 mg have been administered, rituximab is added to the regimen administered for six cycles on an every-28-day schedule (cycle 1 = 375 mg/m^2/dose, cycles 2–6 = 500 mg/m^2/dose). Venetoclax is then continued for a maximum of 2 years from the first cycle of rituximab, or until disease progression, whichever comes first.

Venetoclax; administer orally once daily with 240 mL water within 30 minutes of completion of a meal (preferably breakfast) continuously for up to 2 years from the initial rituximab dose or until disease progression (see table below for dosing schedule)

Standard 5-Week Dose Escalation Schedule*		
Week of Treatment	Venetoclax Dose per Day	Total Venetoclax Dosage per Week
Week 1	20 mg	140 mg
Week 2	50 mg	350 mg
Week 3	100 mg	700 mg
Week 4	200 mg	1400 mg
Week 5 and beyond	400 mg	2800 mg

*Advise patients to keep the medication in its original packaging during the first 4 weeks of therapy

Venclexta (venetoclax tablets) prescribing information. North Chicago, IL: AbbVie Inc; 2018 November

Notes:
- Venetoclax tablets should be swallowed whole. Do not chew, crush, or break venetoclax tablets
- Patients who delay taking venetoclax at a regularly scheduled time may administer the missed dose within 30 minutes of completion of a meal if within 8 hours of the usual dosing time. If >8 hours, skip the missed dose and resume treatment at the next regularly scheduled time. Patients who vomit after a dose of venetoclax should not repeat the dose but rather take the next dose at the next regularly scheduled time
- Venetoclax is a substrate of cytochrome P450 (CYP) CYP3A subfamily enzymes, P-glycoprotein (P-gp), and BCRP. Venetoclax is a weak inhibitor of CYP2C8, CYP2C9, and UGT1A1 in vitro but due to high protein binding is predicted to cause clinically insignificant inhibition of these enzymes in vivo. Venetoclax is a P-gp and BCRP inhibitor and weak OATP1B1 inhibitor in vitro
  - Avoid concurrent use with strong or moderate CYP3A inducers at all times
  - Avoid concurrent use with strong CYP3A4 inhibitors throughout the venetoclax dose escalation period
    - For patients who have completed venetoclax dose-escalation and are maintained on a steady dose of venetoclax, reduce the venetoclax dose to 100 mg if concomitant use of a strong CYP3A inhibitor is unavoidable and monitor closely for side effects. If the strong CYP3A inhibitor is subsequently discontinued, resume the venetoclax dose that was administered prior to introduction of the inhibitor 2–3 days after discontinuation of the inhibitor
    - For patients who have completed venetoclax dose-escalation and are maintained on a steady dose of venetoclax, reduce the venetoclax dose to 70 mg if concomitant use of posaconazole is unavoidable and monitor closely for side effects. If posaconazole is subsequently discontinued, resume the venetoclax dose that was administered prior to introduction of posaconazole 2–3 days after discontinuation of posaconazole
  - Reduce the venetoclax dose by ≥50% if concomitant use of a moderate CYP3A4 inhibitor or P-gp inhibitor is unavoidable and monitor closely for side effects. If the moderate CYP3A4 inhibitor is subsequently discontinued, resume the venetoclax dose that was administered prior to introduction of the inhibitor 2–3 days after discontinuation of the inhibitor
  - Advise patients to not consume grapefruit products, Seville oranges, or starfruit as they may inhibit CYP3A in the gut wall and increase the bioavailability of venetoclax
  - Coadministration of venetoclax with warfarin caused increased exposure to *R*-warfarin and *S*-warfarin. Monitor the international normalized ratio closely in patients coadministered warfarin
  - Venetoclax inhibits P-gp. Concomitant use of narrow therapeutic index P-gp substrates (eg, digoxin, everolimus, sirolimus) should be avoided when possible. If use of a P-gp substrate is unavoidable, then administer the P-gp substrate ≥6 hours before venetoclax

(continued)

(continued)

- Venetoclax can cause rapid death of leukemic cells leading to rapid onset of tumor lysis syndrome (TLS) during the dose escalation period in some patients. In clinical trials of venetoclax, fatal cases of tumor lysis syndrome have occurred which led to the development of a step-wise dose escalation approach to initiation of venetoclax. Assess tumor burden (eg, CT scan, absolute lymphocyte count) and TLS laboratory measurements (eg, potassium, uric acid, phosphorus, calcium, creatinine, lactate dehydrogenase) and correct any abnormalities prior to initiation of venetoclax. Based on the tumor burden and baseline renal function assessments, determine the risk of TLS in order to guide decisions regarding optimal setting of therapy initiation (inpatient vs outpatient), hydration requirements, and frequency of TLS laboratory monitoring according to the table below

TLS Risk Assessment and Supportive Care

Tumor Burden		Prophylaxis*		Blood Chemistry† Monitoring
		Hydration	Anti-hyperuricemic therapy	Setting and frequency of assessment
Low	All LN < 5 cm AND ALC <25 × 10⁹/L	Oral (1.5–2 L/day)	Allopurinol	Outpatient: • For the first dose of 20 mg and 50 mg; pre-dose, 6–8 hours, 24 hours • For subsequent ramp-up doses; pre-dose‡
Medium	Any LN 5–10 cm OR ALC ≥25 × 10⁹/L	Oral (1.5–2 L/day) and consider additional intravenous	Allopurinol	Outpatient: • For the first dose of 20 mg and 50 mg; pre-dose, 6–8 hours, 24 hours (for patients with CrCl <80 mL/min consider hospitalization with frequent laboratory monitoring as described below for high-risk patients) • For subsequent ramp-up doses; pre-dose‡
High	Any LN ≥10 cm OR ALC ≥25 × 10⁹/L AND Any LN ≥5 cm	Oral (1.5–2 L/day) and intravenous (150–200 mL/hour as tolerated)	Allopurinol; consider rasburicase if baseline uric acid is elevated	In hospital: • For the first dose of 20 mg and 50 mg; pre-dose, 4, 8, 12, and 24 hours Outpatient: • For subsequent ramp-up doses; pre-dose, 6–8 hours, 24 hours

TLS, tumor lysis syndrome; LN, lymph node; ALC, absolute lymphocyte count; CrCl, creatinine clearance

*Initiate a xanthine oxidase inhibitor (eg, allopurinol) 2–3 days prior to initiation of venetoclax. Continue the xanthine oxidase inhibitor for up to 5 weeks depending upon ongoing risk of TLS. Encourage oral hydration (1.5–2 L/day) starting 2 days before and on the day of the first venetoclax dose and each dose escalation

†Blood chemistries = potassium, uric acid, phosphorus, calcium, serum creatinine (evaluate in real-time)

‡For patients at continued risk of TLS, monitor chemistries at 6–8 hours and at 24 hours at each subsequent outpatient ramp-up dose

Venclexta (venetoclax tablets) prescribing information. North Chicago, IL: AbbVie Inc; 2018 November

Note: A total of 6 rituximab infusions are administered *beginning after completion of the 5-week venetoclax ramp-up* (ie, start rituximab at week 6 of venetoclax therapy) according to the below schedule:

Premedications for rituximab
Acetaminophen 650–1000 mg; administer orally 30–60 minutes before each rituximab dose, *plus*
Diphenhydramine 25–50 mg; administer orally or intravenously 30–60 minutes before each rituximab dose

Rituximab 375 mg/m²; administer intravenously in 0.9% sodium chloride injection (0.9% NS) or 5% dextrose injection (D5W), diluted to a concentration within the range 1–4 mg/mL, for 1 dose during week 6 of venetoclax therapy (total dosage of initial rituximab dose = 375 mg/m²), *followed in four weeks by:*

Rituximab 500 mg/m² per dose; administer intravenously in 0.9% NS or D5W, diluted to a concentration within the range 1–4 mg/mL, on day 1, every 28 days, for 5 doses (total dosage/28-day cycle = 500 mg/m²)

Rituximab administration:
- Infuse initially at 50 mg/hour. If hypersensitivity or infusion reactions do not occur during the first 30 minutes, increase the rate by 50 mg/hour every 30 minutes as tolerated to a maximum rate of 400 mg/hour. During subsequent treatments, if previous rituximab administration was well tolerated, start at 100 mg/hour and increase by 100 mg/hour every 30 minutes as tolerated to a maximum rate of 400 mg/hour
- Interrupt rituximab administration for fever, chills, edema, congestion of the head and neck mucosa, hypertension, and other serious adverse events. Resume rituximab administration after adverse events abate

(continued)

(continued)

Supportive Care

Antiemetic prophylaxis
Emetogenic potential (all days) is **MINIMAL–LOW**
See Chapter 42 for antiemetic recommendations

Hematopoietic growth factor (CSF) prophylaxis
Primary prophylaxis is **NOT** *indicated*
See Chapter 43 for more information

Antimicrobial prophylaxis
Risk of fever and neutropenia is **LOW**
    Antimicrobial primary prophylaxis to be considered:
- Antibacterial—consider prophylaxis with a fluoroquinolone during periods of prolonged neutropenia only (eg, <500/mm^3 for ≥7 days) until ANC recovery. *Pneumocystis jirovecii* prophylaxis is recommended (eg, cotrimoxazole)
- Antifungal—not indicated
- Antiviral—antiherpes antivirals (eg, acyclovir, famciclovir, valacyclovir)

Patient Population Studied

The international, multicenter, randomized, open-label, phase 3 trial (MURANO) involved 389 patients with relapsed or refractory CLL that required therapy. Eligible patients were aged ≥18 years, had an Eastern Cooperative Oncology Group performance status score ≤1, and had received 1–3 previous treatments, including at least 1 treatment that involved chemotherapy. Patients were randomly assigned (1:1) to receive oral venetoclax (administered initially at a dose of 20 mg daily and gradually increased to the target dose of 400 g daily over a 5-week schedule of gradual dose escalation; administered at 400 mg daily thereafter for 2 years) and intravenous rituximab therapy (started after the patient reached the target venetoclax dose of 400 mg daily; initial dose 375 mg/m², followed by 500 mg/m² every 28 days for a total of six infusions) or six 28-day cycles of intravenous bendamustine (70 mg/m² on days 1 and 2) and rituximab (375 mg/m² on day 1 of cycle 1, followed by 500 mg/m² on day 1 of subsequent cycles)

Efficacy (N = 389)

	Venetoclax + Rituximab (n = 194)	Bendamustine + Rituximab (n = 195)	
Progression-free survival at 2 years	84.9%	36.3%	HR 0.17; 95% CI 0.11–0.25; P<0.001
Overall survival at 2 years	91.9%	86.6%	HR 0.48; 95% CI 0.25–0.90
Overall response rate*	92.3%	72.3%	

*Overall response rate included patients with complete response, complete response with incomplete hematologic recovery, nodular partial response, or partial response, as assessed by the independent review committee

Note: Median duration of follow-up was 23.8 months. Median progression-free survival had not been reached in the venetoclax group, and median overall survival had not been reached in either group

Therapy Monitoring

1. *Prior to initiation of venetoclax:*
   a. Assess tumor burden (CBC with differential, CT scan) and baseline chemistries (potassium, uric acid, phosphorus, calcium, serum creatinine, LDH) to determine the risk for tumor lysis syndrome (TLS). Decisions regarding treatment setting (inpatient vs outpatient) and frequency of laboratory monitoring depend upon TLS risk assessment (see above table)
   b. Verify adherence to the prescribed xanthine oxidase inhibitor regimen (eg, allopurinol) to begin 2–3 days prior to venetoclax initiation
   c. Screen for the presence of drug-drug interactions involving venetoclax
   d. Prescribe the appropriate combination of venetoclax tablet strengths (available in 10-mg, 50-mg, and 100-mg tablets) in sufficient quantities to accommodate the planned venetoclax dose-escalation and maintenance dosing schedule
2. *Tumor lysis syndrome monitoring during venetoclax ramp-up:* monitor potassium, uric acid, phosphorus, calcium, and serum creatinine at the frequency described in the above table corresponding to the patient's risk for tumor lysis syndrome
3. *Periodically throughout venetoclax treatment:* CBC with differential
4. *Prior to initiation of rituximab:* hepatitis B core antibody (IgG or total) and hepatitis B core antigen
5. *Response assessment every 2–3 months:* physical examination, CBC with differential, CT scans (in select patients for evaluation of adenopathy)

Treatment Modifications

VENETOCLAX

Dose at Interruption	Restart Dose*†
400 mg	300 mg
300 mg	200 mg
200 mg	100 mg
100 mg	50 mg‡
50 mg	20 mg‡
20 mg	10 mg‡

*If patients interrupt venetoclax for >1 week during the 5-week ramp-up period or interrupt venetoclax for >2 weeks during maintenance therapy, reassess the risk of TLS to determine if reinitiation with a reduced dose of venetoclax is necessary
†During the venetoclax ramp-up phase, continue the reduced venetoclax dose for 1 week before further dose escalation
‡Consider discontinuing venetoclax for patients who require dose reductions to <100 mg for > 2 weeks

Tumor Lysis Syndrome

Adverse Event	Treatment Modification
Prior to initiation of venetoclax: • Potassium, phosphorus, or uric acid > ULN • Corrected calcium < LLN • Serum creatinine ≥25% above baseline value	Correct pre-existing tumor lysis syndrome abnormalities prior to initiation of venetoclax
Laboratory TLS Blood chemistry (potassium, phosphorus, uric acid, calcium, serum creatinine) suggestive of TLS *without* clinical sequelae	Withhold venetoclax until resolution. Correct laboratory abnormalities and increase frequency of monitoring If abnormalities resolve within 48 hours, resume venetoclax at the same dose. If resolution requires >48 hours, then resume venetoclax at a reduced dose
Clinical TLS Blood chemistry (potassium, phosphorus, uric acid, calcium, serum creatinine) suggestive of TLS *with* clinical sequelae (eg, serum creatinine ≥1.5× ULN, cardiac arrhythmia, seizure, sudden cardiac death)	Correct laboratory abnormalities and increase frequency of monitoring Withhold venetoclax until resolution and then resume venetoclax at a reduced dose
Potassium > ULN in the setting of TLS	Withhold venetoclax until resolution. Increase frequency of monitoring. If resolution occurs within 24–48 hours of the last dose, resume venetoclax at the dose. If resolution requires >48 hours, then resume at a reduced dose Perform STAT ECG and begin telemetry. Consider the following interventions: • Sodium polystyrene sulfonate 15 g by mouth once • Furosemide 20 mg IV push once • Insulin 10 units IV push once plus 25 g of 50% dextrose IV push once (may omit glucose if serum glucose is ≥250 mg/dL) • If there is ECG evidence of life-threatening arrhythmia, then administer calcium gluconate 1000 mg in 100 mL D5W IV over 30 minutes once • Consult nephrology for consideration of dialysis for severe, refractory, or rapidly worsening hyperkalemia, especially in the setting of concomitant AKI
Uric acid ≥8.0 mg/dL in the setting of TLS	Withhold venetoclax until resolution. Increase frequency of monitoring. If resolution occurs within 24–48 hours of the last dose, resume venetoclax at the same dose. If resolution requires >48 hours, then resume at a reduced dose Consider a single dose of rasburicase 3–6 mg (fixed dose) IV over 30 minutes. Optimize the dose of xanthine oxidase inhibitor (eg, allopurinol) and the rate of IV hydration, as tolerated

(continued)

Treatment Modifications (*continued*)

Adverse Event	Treatment Modification
Phosphorus ≥5.0 mg/dL in the setting of TLS	Withhold venetoclax until resolution. Increase frequency of monitoring. If resolution occurs within 24–48 hours of the last dose, resume venetoclax at the same dose. If resolution requires >48 hours, then resume at a reduced dose Administer a phosphate binder (eg, aluminum hydroxide, calcium carbonate, sevelamer carbonate, or lanthanum carbonate) with meals. Place patient on a low-phosphate diet. Optimize the rate of IV hydration, as tolerated. Consult nephrology for consideration of hemodialysis, especially if phosphorus ≥10 mg/dL or with concomitant AKI
Serum creatinine increases ≥25% from baseline in the setting of TLS	Withhold venetoclax until resolution. Increase frequency of monitoring. If resolution occurs within 24–48 hours of the last dose, resume venetoclax at the same dose. If resolution requires >48 hours, then resume at a reduced dose Start or increase rate of IV hydration. For severe AKI, consider nephrology consultation
Corrected calcium ≤7.0 mg/dL and patient is symptomatic (eg, muscle cramps, hypotension, tetany, cardiac arrhythmias) in the setting of TLS	Withhold venetoclax until resolution. Increase frequency of monitoring. If resolution occurs within 24–48 hours of the last dose, resume venetoclax at the same dose. If resolution requires >48 hours, then resume at a reduced dose Perform STAT ECG and begin telemetry. Administer calcium gluconate 1000 mg in 100 mL D5W IV over 30 minutes once
Hematologic Toxicities	
G3 neutropenia (ANC ≥500/mm^3 and <1000/mm^3) with infection or fever; or G4 neutropenia (ANC <500/mm^3); or G4 thrombocytopenia (platelet count <25,000/mm^3), first occurrence	Withhold venetoclax until resolution to G ≤1 or baseline, then resume venetoclax at the same dose G-CSF may be administered with venetoclax if indicated to reduce the risk of infection associated with neutropenia
G3 neutropenia (ANC ≥500/mm^3 and <1000/mm^3) with infection or fever; or G4 neutropenia (ANC <500/mm^3); or G4 thrombocytopenia (platelet count <25,000/mm^3), second and subsequent occurrences	Withhold venetoclax until resolution to G ≤1 or baseline, then resume venetoclax at a reduced dose. At the discretion of the medically responsible health care provider, a larger dose reduction than that described above may be considered depending on the severity of the toxicity G-CSF may be administered with venetoclax if indicated to reduce the risk of infection associated with neutropenia
Drug-Drug Interactions	
Concomitant therapy with a strong or moderate CYP3A inducer is required	Do not administer a strong or moderate CYP3A inducer with venetoclax
Concomitant therapy with a strong CYP3A4 inhibitor is required during the venetoclax 5-week ramp-up period	Do not administer a strong CYP3A4 inhibitor during the venetoclax ramp-up period
Concomitant therapy with a strong CYP3A4 inhibitor is required in a patient taking a steady daily dosage of venetoclax (after ramp-up phase)	Consider alternative medications. If the strong CYP3A4 inhibitor is unavoidable, then reduce the venetoclax dose to 100 mg
Concomitant therapy with posaconazole is required in a patient taking a steady daily dosage of venetoclax (after ramp-up phase)	Consider alternative medications. If posaconazole is unavoidable, then reduce the venetoclax dose to 70 mg
Concomitant therapy with a moderate CYP3A4 inhibitor or P-gp inhibitor is required (any phase of treatment)	Consider alternative medications. If the moderate CYP3A4 inhibitor or P-gp inhibitor is unavoidable, then reduce the venetoclax dose by at least 50%
Concomitant strong or moderate CYP3A4 inhibitor, posaconazole, or P-gp inhibitor is subsequently discontinued	Resume the venetoclax dosage that was used prior to concomitant use of a strong or moderate CYP3A4 inhibitor, posaconazole, or P-gp inhibitor 2–3 days after discontinuation of the inhibitor
Concomitant therapy with warfarin is required	Monitor international normalized ratio frequently
Concomitant therapy with a P-gp substrate is required	Consider alternative medications. If concomitant use is unavoidable, administer the P-gp substrate at least 6 hours before the administration of venetoclax

(*continued*)

Treatment Modifications (continued)

Adverse Event	Treatment Modification
Other Toxicities	
Other G3/4 nonhematologic toxicity, first occurrence	Withhold venetoclax until resolution to G ≤1 or baseline, then resume venetoclax at the same dose
Other G3/4 nonhematologic toxicity, second and subsequent occurrences	Withhold venetoclax until resolution to G ≤1 or baseline, then resume venetoclax at a lower dose. At the discretion of the medically responsible health care provider, a larger dose reduction than that described above may be considered depending on the severity of the toxicity
Immunization with a live attenuated vaccine is indicated prior to, during, or after therapy with venetoclax	Do not administer live attenuated vaccines prior to, during, or after treatment with venetoclax until B-cell recovery occurs

Venetoclax may cause fetal harm. Advise females of reproductive potential of the potential risk to a fetus and to use effective contraception during treatment

TLS, tumor lysis syndrome; ULN, upper limit of normal; LLN, lower limit of normal; ECG, electrocardiogram; IV, intravenous; AKI, acute kidney injury; ANC, absolute neutrophil count; G-CSF, granulocyte-colony stimulating factor; P-gp, P-glycoprotein

RITUXIMAB

Rituximab Infusion-Related Toxicities

Onset of infusion-related events (fevers, chills, rigors, edema, congestion of the head and neck mucosa, hypotension)
1. Interrupt rituximab infusion
2. For fever, chills: Give additional dose of **acetaminophen** 650 mg orally and **diphenhydramine** 25–50 mg by intravenous push
3. For rigors: Give **meperidine** 12.5–25 mg by intravenous push ± **promethazine** 12.5–25 mg by intravenous infusion in at least 10 mL 0.9% NS or D5W over 5–15 minutes. If after 15–20 minutes the response to a single dose is considered inadequate, the dose may be repeated
4. After symptoms resolve, resume rituximab infusion at a minimum of 50% reduction in the rate at which the event occurred. If no further infusion-related events, increase the rate by 50 mg/hour every 30 minutes, as tolerated, up to a maximum rate of 400 mg/hour

Dyspnea or wheezing, without allergic findings (urticaria, or tongue or laryngeal edema)
1. Interrupt rituximab infusion immediately
2. Give **hydrocortisone** 100 mg by intravenous push (or glucocorticoid equivalent)
3. Give an additional dose of **diphenhydramine** 25–50 mg by intravenous push and a histamine H2-antagonist (**ranitidine** 50 mg or **famotidine** 20 mg) by intravenous push
4. After symptoms resolve, resume rituximab infusion at a minimum of 50% reduction in the rate at which the event occurred. If no further infusion-related events, increase the rate by 50 mg/hour every 30 minutes, as tolerated, up to a maximum rate of 400 mg/hour

Note: Medications and equipment for the treatment of hypersensitivity reactions should be available for immediate use in the event of a reaction during administration (eg, intravenous fluids, epinephrine, antihistamines, glucocorticoids, oxygen)

Adverse Events (N = 382)

Event	All-Grade Adverse Events (%)	
	Venetoclax + Rituximab (n = 194)	Bendamustine + Rituximab (n = 188)
Neutropenia	61	44
Diarrhea	40	16
Upper respiratory tract infection	22	15
Nausea	21	34
Fatigue	18	21

(continued)

Adverse Events (N = 382) *(continued)*

Event	All-Grade Adverse Events (%)	
	Venetoclax + Rituximab (n = 194)	Bendamustine + Rituximab (n = 188)
Cough	18	16
Anemia	15	23
Pyrexia	15	20
Constipation	14	21
Thrombocytopenia	13	22
Headache	11	10
Insomnia	11	6
Nasopharyngitis	11	5
Bronchitis	10	7
Pneumonia	9	12
Infusion-related reaction	8	24
Vomiting	8	12
Rash	7	13
Febrile neutropenia	4	10

Note: Toxicities are included if adverse events occurred in ≥10% of patients in either group, regardless of relationship to study drug. Deaths were reported in 5% and 6% of the venetoclax + rituximab and bendamustine + rituximab groups, respectively

Event	Grade 3–4 Adverse Events (%)	
	Venetoclax + Rituximab (N = 194)	Bendamustine + Rituximab (N = 188)
Neutropenia	58	39
Infections and infestations	18	22
Anemia	11	14
Thrombocytopenia	6	10
Pneumonia	5	8
Febrile neutropenia	4	10
Tumor lysis syndrome	3	1
Hypogammaglobulinemia	2	0
Hyperglycemia	2	0
Infusion-related reaction	2	5
Hypotension	0	3

Note: Toxicities are included if a ≥2% difference in incidence of Grade 3–4 adverse events occurred between the groups

SUBSEQUENT THERAPY
CHRONIC LYMPHOCYTIC LEUKEMIA REGIMEN: IDELALISIB + RITUXIMAB

Coutré SE et al. Leuk Lymphoma 2015;56:2779–2786
Furman RR et al. N Engl J Med 2014;370:997–1007
Supplementary appendix to: Furman RR et al. N Engl J Med 2014;370:997–1007
Protocol for: Furman RR et al. N Engl J Med 2014;370:997–1007
Zydelig (idelalisib) prescribing information. Foster City, CA: Gilead Sciences, Inc; 2018 October

Idelalisib 150 mg per dose; administer orally twice per day, without regard to food, continually until disease progression (total dosage/week = 2100 mg)

Notes:
- Idelalisib tablets should be swallowed whole
- Patients who delay taking an idelalisib dose at a regularly scheduled time may administer the missed dose if within 6 hours of the usual dosing time. If >6 hours, skip the missed dose and resume treatment at the next regularly scheduled time
- Idelalisib is metabolized by aldehyde oxidase and CYP3A (major routes) and by UGT1A4 (minor route). If concomitant use with a strong CY3A inhibitor is unavoidable, monitor closely for idelalisib side effects. Avoid concomitant use with strong CYP3A inducers
- Idelalisib was shown in vitro to inhibit CYP2C8, CYP2C19, UGT1A1 and to induce CYP2B6. Idelalisib increased the mean C_{max} of midazolam (a sensitive CYP3A substrate) by 2.4-fold and the mean area under the curve of midazolam by 5.4-fold. Thus, avoid concomitant use with sensitive CYP3A substrates

Note: A total of 8 rituximab infusions are administered according to the below schedule (first dose of rituximab to be administered on the same day as idelalisib initiation):

Premedications for rituximab
Acetaminophen 650–1000 mg; administer orally 30–60 minutes before each rituximab dose, *plus*
Diphenhydramine 25–50 mg; administer orally or intravenously 30–60 minutes before each rituximab dose

Rituximab 375 mg/m²; administer intravenously in 0.9% sodium chloride injection (0.9% NS) or 5% dextrose injection (D5W), diluted to a concentration within the range 1–4 mg/mL, for 1 dose on the day of idelalisib initiation (total dosage of initial rituximab dose = 375 mg/m²), *followed in two weeks by:*

Rituximab 500 mg/m² per dose; administer intravenously in 0.9% NS or D5W, diluted to a concentration within the range 1–4 mg/mL, every 2 weeks for 4 doses (total dosage/2-week cycle = 500 mg/m²), *followed in 4 weeks by:*

Rituximab 500 mg/m² per dose; administer intravenously in 0.9% NS or D5W, diluted to a concentration within the range 1–4 mg/mL, every 4 weeks for 3 doses (total dosage/4-week cycle = 500 mg/m²)

Rituximab administration:
- Infuse initially at 50 mg/hour. If hypersensitivity or infusion reactions do not occur during the first 30 minutes, increase the rate by 50 mg/hour every 30 minutes as tolerated to a maximum rate of 400 mg/hour. During subsequent treatments if previous rituximab administration was well tolerated, start at 100 mg/hour and increase by 100 mg/hour every 30 minutes as tolerated to a maximum rate of 400 mg/hour
- Interrupt rituximab administration for fever, chills, edema, congestion of the head and neck mucosa, hypertension, and other serious adverse events. Resume rituximab administration after adverse events abate

Supportive Care
Antiemetic prophylaxis
*Emetogenic potential on days of idelalisib ± rituximab is **LOW***
See Chapter 42 for antiemetic recommendations

Hematopoietic growth factor (CSF) prophylaxis
*Primary prophylaxis is **NOT** indicated*
See Chapter 43 for more information

Antimicrobial prophylaxis
*Risk of fever and neutropenia is **LOW***
  Antimicrobial primary prophylaxis to be considered:
- Antibacterial—not indicated. *Pneumocystis jirovecii* prophylaxis is recommended (eg, cotrimoxazole)
- Antifungal—not indicated
- Antiviral—antiherpes antivirals (eg, acyclovir, famciclovir, valacyclovir). Consider pre-emptive cytomegalovirus (CMV) management in CMV seropositive patients treated with idelalisib

Patient Population Studied

The international, multicenter, randomized, double-blind, placebo-controlled, phase 3 trial involved 220 patients with relapsed CLL and coexisting conditions. Eligible patients had previous treatment that included either a CD20 antibody-based regimen or at least two cytotoxic regimens, had CLL that had progressed within 24 months after their last treatment, and had a Cumulative Illness Rating Scale score >6, estimated creatinine clearance <60 mL/min, or severe neutropenia or thrombocytopenia as a result of cumulative myelotoxicity from previous therapies. Patients were randomly assigned to receive intravenous rituximab (initial dose 375 mg/m^2, followed by 500 mg/m^2 every 2 weeks for four doses and then every 4 weeks for three doses) with either oral idelalisib (150 mg twice daily) or placebo

Efficacy (N = 220)

	Rituximab + Idelalisib (n = 110)	Rituximab + Placebo (n = 110)	
Progression-free survival at 24 weeks	93%	46%	HR 0.15, 95% CI 0.08–0.28; unadjusted P<0.001
Overall survival at 12 months	92%	80%	HR 0.28, 95% CI 0.09–0.86; P = 0.02
Overall response rate*	81%	13%	OR 29.92; P<0.001

*Overall response rate included patients with complete or partial response; however, all observed responses were partial

Note: Median duration of treatment was 3.8 months in the rituximab + idelalisib group and 2.9 months in the rituximab + placebo group; the study was terminated early owing to a recommendation by the data and safety monitoring board. At the time the study was terminated, median progression-free survival had not yet been reached in the rituximab + idelalisib group, and median overall survival had not been reached in either treatment group

Therapy Monitoring

1. *Prior to initiation of idelalisib:* CBC with differential, chemistries (potassium, uric acid, phosphorus, calcium, serum creatinine, LDH), liver function tests (serum bilirubin, ALT, AST, alkaline phosphatase), urine pregnancy test (women of child-bearing potentially only)

2. *Prior to initiation of rituximab:* hepatitis B core antibody (IgG or total) and hepatitis B core antigen

3. *During treatment with idelalisib:*
   a. Monitor liver function tests (ALT, AST, and serum bilirubin) in all patients at least every 2 weeks for the first 3 months of treatment, then at least every 4 weeks for the next 3 months, then at least every 1–3 months thereafter. Monitor at least weekly if ALT or AST increases to >5× ULN or if bilirubin increases to >1.5× ULN until resolution to ≤1× ULN
   b. Monitor CBC with differential at least every 2 weeks for the first 6 months of therapy, and at least weekly while absolute neutrophil count is <1000/mm^3 or platelet count is <50,000/mm^3
   c. Monitor periodically for:
      i. Signs and symptoms of diarrhea/colitis. Median time to onset of any grade diarrhea/colitis was 1.9 (range, 0–29.8) months across trials. Median time to onset of Grade 1 or 2 diarrhea/colitis was 1.5 (range, 0–15.2) months. Median time to onset of Grade 3 or 4 diarrhea/colitis was 7.1 (range, 0.5–29.8) months
      ii. Signs and symptoms of intestinal perforation
      iii. Signs and symptoms of dermatologic toxicity or hypersensitivity reactions
      iv. Signs and symptoms of pneumonitis
      v. Signs and symptoms of infection (including sepsis, pneumonia, *Pneumocystis jiroveci* pneumonia, and cytomegalovirus)

4. *Response assessment every 2–3 months:* physical examination, CBC with differential, CT scans (in select patients for evaluation of adenopathy)

Treatment Modifications

IDELALISIB	
Starting dose	150 mg by mouth twice a day
Dose level −1	100 mg by mouth twice a day

Pulmonary Toxicity	
Dyspnea, cough, fever, hypoxia (decline by ≥5% O₂ saturation), and/or radiologic abnormalities: pneumonitis is suspected	Interrupt idelalisib until pulmonary status clarified. Perform extensive evaluations for infectious etiology, including testing for PJP
Symptomatic pneumonitis or organizing pneumonia (any grade) is confirmed	Discontinue idelalisib and initiate appropriate treatment with corticosteroids

Infectious Complications	
G ≥3 sepsis or pneumonia	Interrupt idelalisib until resolution of infection, then resume at the same dose
CMV infection (any grade) or CMV viremia	Interrupt idelalisib until viremia and/or infection has resolved. Upon resolution, idelalisib may be resumed at the same dose; if resumed then monitor blood CMV PCR or pp65 antigen detection at least monthly during ongoing treatment
PJP infection is suspected	Interrupt idelalisib during workup for suspected PJP infection
PJP infection is confirmed	Permanently discontinue idelalisib

Gastrointestinal Toxicity	
G1 diarrhea (increase of <4 stools per day over baseline) or Early-onset (≤8 weeks), G2 diarrhea (increase of 4–6 stools per day over baseline)	Continue idelalisib at the current dose without interruption. Discontinue other medications that may cause diarrhea, if applicable. Rule out infectious causes of diarrhea (eg, *Clostridium difficile*, *Salmonella*, *Escherichia coli*, *Campylobacter*). Consider colonoscopy in atypical cases (eg, bloody diarrhea), or for refractory diarrhea. Early-onset uncomplicated diarrhea (Grade 1 and sometimes Grade 2) is often self-limiting and may occasionally respond to antimotility agents (eg, loperamide) and dietary modification (avoidance of lactose, alcohol, and high-osmolar supplements; increase in oral clear liquids; consumption of frequent small, bland meals, etc) Monitor at least weekly until resolution (median time to resolution in trials ranged from 1 week to 1 month) and then resume normal diet See below for early-onset G2 diarrhea that does not respond to antimotility agents
Late-onset (>8 weeks), G2 diarrhea (increase of 4–6 stools per day over baseline) or Early-onset (>8 weeks), G2 diarrhea (increase of 4–6 stools per day over baseline) unresponsive to antimotility agents or G3 diarrhea (increase of ≥7 stools per day over baseline, or requiring hospitalization) or G4 diarrhea (life-threatening consequences; urgent intervention indicated)	Interrupt idelalisib. Determine the need for hospitalization and/or IV hydration. Discontinue other medications that may cause diarrhea, if applicable. Rule out infectious causes of diarrhea (eg, *Clostridium difficile*, *Salmonella*, *Escherichia coli*, *Campylobacter*). Consider colonoscopy in atypical cases (eg, bloody diarrhea), or for refractory diarrhea. Diarrhea responds poorly to antimotility (eg, loperamide) agents. Implement dietary modification (avoidance of lactose, alcohol, and high-osmolar supplements; increase in oral clear liquids; consumption of frequent small, bland meals, etc) After ruling out infectious diarrhea, consider treatment with budesonide 9 mg by mouth once daily until resolution to G ≤1, followed by taper. Alternatively, systemic corticosteroids (initial dose = prednisolone 1 mg/kg or equivalent) may be administered until resolution to G ≤1, followed by taper Monitor at least weekly until resolution (median time to resolution in trials ranged from 1 week to 1 month) and then resume normal diet In cases of G2 or G3 diarrhea, upon resolution to G ≤1 then consider resumption of idelalisib, per clinical judgement, at dose level −1 with or without concomitant budesonide prophylaxis In cases of G4 diarrhea, permanently discontinue idelalisib
Intestinal perforation	Permanently discontinue idelalisib

(continued)

Treatment Modifications (continued)

Hematologic Toxicity

G3 neutropenia (ANC ≥500/mm³ to <1000/mm³)	Continue idelalisib at the current dose without interruption. Monitor ANC at least once per week
G4 neutropenia (ANC <500/mm³)	Interrupt idelalisib. Monitor ANC at least once per week until ANC ≥500/mm³, then resume idelalisib at dose level −1
G3 thrombocytopenia (platelet count ≥25,000/mm³ to <50,000/mm³)	Continue idelalisib at the current dose without interruption. Monitor platelet count at least once per week
G4 thrombocytopenia (platelet count <25,000/mm³)	Interrupt idelalisib. Monitor platelet count at least once per week until platelet count ≥25,000/mm³, then resume idelalisib at dose level −1

Hepatic Toxicity

G2 elevation in ALT or AST (ALT or AST >3 to ≤5× ULN) or G2 elevation in bilirubin (bilirubin >1.5 to ≤3× ULN)	Continue idelalisib at the current dose without interruption Monitor liver function tests at least weekly until resolution to ≤1× ULN, then resume normal frequency of monitoring
G3 elevation in ALT or AST (ALT or AST >5 to ≤20× ULN) or G3 elevation in bilirubin (bilirubin >3 to ≤10× ULN)	Interrupt idelalisib. Monitor liver function tests at least weekly until resolution to ≤1× ULN, then may resume idelalisib at dose level −1
G4 elevation in ALT or AST (ALT or AST >20× ULN) or G4 elevation in bilirubin (bilirubin >10× ULN)	Permanently discontinue idelalisib

Dermatologic and Immunologic Toxicities

SJS or TEN is suspected	Interrupt idelalisib until dermatologic status is clarified
SJS or TEN is confirmed	Permanently discontinue idelalisib
Other G ≥3 cutaneous reaction	Permanently discontinue idelalisib
Severe allergic reaction or anaphylactic reaction	Permanently discontinue idelalisib

Drug-Drug Interactions

Concomitant therapy with a strong CYP3A inhibitor is required	Consider alternative medication. If the strong CYP3A inhibitor is unavoidable, then monitor patients more frequently for idelalisib adverse reactions
Concomitant therapy with a strong CYP3A inducer is required	Do not administer a strong CYP3A inducer with idelalisib
Concomitant therapy with a CYP3A substrate with a narrow therapeutic index is required	Do not administer idelalisib with sensitive CYP3A substrates
Concomitant therapy with other hepatotoxic medications or medications which cause diarrhea	Avoid coadministration of idelalisib with other medications which are hepatotoxic or which cause diarrhea
Patient requires concomitant therapy with antihypertensive medication(s)	On days of rituximab treatment, and especially with the initial dose, weigh the risk versus benefit of delaying administration of the antihypertensive medication(s) until after completion of the rituximab infusion due to the potential risk of rituximab infusion-related hypotension
Live attenuated vaccine is indicated during or after rituximab administration	Avoid administration of a live attenuated vaccine during rituximab therapy and following therapy until adequate B-cell recovery has occurred

(continued)

Treatment Modifications (continued)

Other Toxicities

Other severe or life-threatening toxicity, first occurrence	Interrupt idelalisib until resolution of toxicity. Upon resolution, consider resuming idelalisib at dose level −1, per the discretion of the medically responsible health care provider
Other severe or life-threatening toxicity, second occurrence	Permanently discontinue idelalisib

Coutré SE et al. Leuk Lymphoma 2015;56:2779–2786
Zydelig (idelalisib) prescribing information. Foster City, CA: Gilead Sciences, Inc; 2018 October

PJP, *Pneumocystis jirovecii* pneumonia; CMV, cytomegalovirus; PCR, polymerase chain reaction; ANC, absolute neutrophil count; ALT, alanine aminotransferase; AST, aspartate aminotransferase; ULN, upper limit of normal; SJS, Stevens-Johnson syndrome; TEN, toxic epidermal necrolysis

RITUXIMAB

Rituximab Infusion-Related Toxicities

Onset of infusion-related events (fevers, chills, rigors, edema, congestion of the head and neck mucosa, hypotension)
1. Interrupt rituximab infusion
2. For fever, chills: Give additional dose of **acetaminophen** 650 mg orally and **diphenhydramine** 25–50 mg by intravenous push
3. For rigors: Give **meperidine** 12.5–25 mg by intravenous push ± **promethazine** 12.5–25 mg by intravenous infusion in at least 10 mL 0.9% NS or D5W over 5–15 minutes. If after 15–20 minutes the response to a single dose is considered inadequate, the dose may be repeated
4. After symptoms resolve, resume rituximab infusion at a minimum of 50% reduction in the rate at which the event occurred. If no further infusion-related events, increase the rate by 50 mg/hour every 30 minutes, as tolerated, up to a maximum rate of 400 mg/hour

Dyspnea or wheezing, without allergic findings (urticaria, or tongue or laryngeal edema)
1. Interrupt rituximab infusion immediately
2. Give **hydrocortisone** 100 mg by intravenous push (or glucocorticoid equivalent)
3. Give an additional dose of **diphenhydramine** 25–50 mg by intravenous push and a histamine H2-antagonist (**ranitidine** 50 mg or **famotidine** 20 mg) by intravenous push
4. After symptoms resolve, resume rituximab infusion at a minimum of 50% reduction in the rate at which the event occurred. If no further infusion-related events, increase the rate by 50 mg/hour every 30 minutes, as tolerated, up to a maximum rate of 400 mg/hour

Note: Medications and equipment for the treatment of hypersensitivity reactions should be available for immediate use in the event of a reaction during administration (eg, intravenous fluids, epinephrine, antihistamines, glucocorticoids, oxygen)

Adverse Events (N = 217)

Event	Rituximab + Idelalisib (n = 110)		Rituximab + Placebo (n = 107)	
	Grade 1–2 (%)	Grade ≥3 (%)	Grade 1–2 (%)	Grade ≥3 (%)
Any adverse event	35	56	47	48
Neutropenia	27	34	26	22
Increased alanine aminotransferase or aspartate aminotransferase level	29	5	18	<1
Pyrexia	26	3	17	<1
Anemia	20	5	16	14
Fatigue	21	3	25	2
Nausea	24	0	21	0
Chills	20	2	16	0
Diarrhea	15	4	14	0

(continued)

Adverse Events (N = 217) *(continued)*

Event	Rituximab + Idelalisib (n = 110)		Rituximab + Placebo (n = 107)	
	Grade 1–2 (%)	Grade ≥3 (%)	Grade 1–2 (%)	Grade ≥3 (%)
Thrombocytopenia	7	10	10	16
Infusion-related reaction	15	0	24	4
Cough	15	0	23	2
Constipation	12	0	11	0
Decreased appetite	12	0	7	<1
Vomiting	12	0	7	0
Dyspnea	9	2	16	3
Night sweats	10	0	7	0
Rash	8	2	6	0

*According to the National Cancer Institute Common Terminology Criteria for Adverse Events, version 4.03

Note: Toxicities that occurred in ≥10% of either treatment group during treatment are included

Event	Serious Adverse Event (%)	
	Rituximab + Idelalisib (N = 110)	Rituximab + Placebo (N = 107)
Any serious adverse event	40	35
Pneumonia	6	8
Pyrexia	6	3
Febrile neutropenia	5	6
Sepsis	4	3
Pneumonitis	4	<1
Diarrhea	3	<1
Neutropenia	3	<1
Pneumocystis jirovecii pneumonia	3	<1
Neutropenic sepsis	3	0
Dyspnea	<1	4
Cellulitis	<1	3

Note: Serious toxicities that occurred in ≥3 patients in either treatment group are included

SUBSEQUENT THERAPY

CHRONIC LYMPHOCYTIC LEUKEMIA REGIMEN: ACALABRUTINIB

Byrd JC et al. N Engl J Med 2016;374:323–332
Protocol for: Byrd JC et al. N Engl J Med 2016;374:323–332
Supplementary appendix to: Byrd JC et al. N Engl J Med 2016;374:323–332

Acalabrutinib 100 mg per dose; administer orally with water twice per day (approximately every 12 hours), without regard to food, continuously until disease progression (total dosage/week = 1400 mg)

Notes:
- Acalabrutinib capsules should be swallowed whole. Do not break, open, or chew capsules
- Patients who delay taking acalabrutinib at a regularly scheduled time may administer the missed dose if within 3 hours of the usual dosing time. If >3 hours, skip the missed dose and resume treatment at the next regularly scheduled time
- Acalabrutinib is metabolized predominantly by CYP3A. Avoid concomitant use with strong CYP3A inhibitors. If a strong CYP3A inhibitor must be used short-term (eg, ≤7 days), interrupt acalabrutinib treatment during treatment with the inhibitor. If concomitant use of a moderate CYP3A inhibitor is unavoidable, then reduce the acalabrutinib dose to 100 mg by mouth once daily. If concomitant use of a strong CYP3A inducer is unavoidable, increase the acalabrutinib dose to 200 mg by mouth twice a day
- Among patients with hematologic malignancies treated with acalabrutinib, skin cancer was diagnosed as a secondary primary malignancy in 7% of patients. Thus, counsel patients to apply sunscreen and avoid prolonged sun exposure during treatment with acalabrutinib
- The solubility of acalabrutinib is increased at acidic pH. Thus, gastric acid–reducing medications may interfere with absorption of acalabrutinib and should be avoided when possible
  - A 5-day course of omeprazole reduced acalabrutinib area under the curve (AUC) by 43%. Since proton pump inhibitors (PPIs) have long-lasting effects on gastric pH, avoid concomitant use of PPIs with acalabrutinib
  - A 1000-mg dose of calcium carbonate coadministered with acalabrutinib reduced acalabrutinib AUC by 53%. Thus, if antacid medications are required, separate acalabrutinib administration from antacid administration by ≥2 hours
  - If a histamine receptor (H2)-subtype antagonist must be used, administer acalabrutinib at least 10 hours following a dose of histamine receptor (H2)-subtype antagonist and at least 2 hours before the next dose of histamine receptor (H2)-subtype antagonist
- Serious bleeding events, some fatal, have been reported in patients with hematologic malignancies treated with acalabrutinib. Grade ≥3 bleeding events were reported to occur in 2% of patients. All-grade bleeding (including bruising and petechia) occurred in approximately 50% of patients. Acalabrutinib may exacerbate the risk of bleeding when administered concurrently with anticoagulant and/or antiplatelet drugs; use caution and monitor closely for bleeding with concomitant use. Consider the risks and benefits of interrupting acalabrutinib treatment 3–7 days prior to and following elective surgery depending on the risk of bleeding and type of surgery
- Hepatitis B virus (HBV) reactivation has been reported in patients treated with acalabrutinib. Monitor HBV positive patients during and after treatment with acalabrutinib and consider antiviral prophylaxis

Supportive Care
Antiemetic prophylaxis
Emetogenic potential is **MINIMAL–LOW**
See Chapter 42 for antiemetic recommendations

Hematopoietic growth factor (CSF) prophylaxis
Primary prophylaxis is **NOT** indicated
See Chapter 43 for more information

Antimicrobial prophylaxis
Risk of fever and neutropenia is **LOW**
  Antimicrobial primary prophylaxis to be considered:
  - Antibacterial—not indicated
  - Antifungal—not indicated
  - Antiviral—antiherpes antivirals (eg, acyclovir, famciclovir, valacyclovir)

Patient Population Studied

The international, multicenter, uncontrolled, phase 1–2 study involved 61 patients with relapsed CLL. Eligible patients had Eastern Cooperative Oncology Group performance status score ≤2. Patients with any cancer that limited life expectancy to <2 years, who needed warfarin therapy, had active gastrointestinal inflammation or malabsorption, or were using medications associated with torsades des pointes, high-grade atrioventricular block, or a corrected QT interval ≥480 ms, were ineligible. In the phase 1, dose-escalation part of the study, patients were successively enrolled in cohorts that were to receive oral acalabrutinib at a dose of 100 mg, 175 mg, 250 mg, or 400 mg once daily. In phase 2, patients received oral acalabrutinib 100 mg twice daily

Efficacy (N = 60)

Overall response rate*	95%

*Overall response rate included patients with complete or partial response (with or without lymphocytosis); however, no complete response was noted

Note: Median duration of follow-up was 14.3 months

Therapy Monitoring

1. *Prior to initiation of acalabrutinib:* hepatitis B core antibody (IgG or total), hepatitis B surface antigen
2. *Monthly:* CBC with differential
3. *Periodically:* monitor for atrial fibrillation and atrial flutter, signs and symptoms of bleeding (especially if concomitant antiplatelet or anticoagulant medication[s] are used), signs and symptoms of infection, presence of second primary malignancies (including skin cancer and other carcinomas)
4. *Response assessment every 1–3 months:* physical examination, CBC with differential, CT scans (in select patients for evaluation of adenopathy)

Treatment Modifications

ACALABRUTINIB

Starting dose	100 mg by mouth twice a day
Dose level −1	100 mg by mouth daily

Hematologic and Nonhematologic Toxicities

Adverse Event	Treatment Modification	
Occurrence of any of the following: • G3 thrombocytopenia (platelet count ≥25,000/mm³ and <50,000/mm³) with bleeding OR • G4 thrombocytopenia (platelet count <25,000/mm³) OR • G4 neutropenia (ANC <500/mm³) lasting >7 days OR • G ≥3 nonhematologic toxicity	First occurrence	Interrupt acalabrutinib. Once toxicity resolves to G ≤1 or baseline, then resume acalabrutinib without dose reduction
	Second occurrence	Interrupt acalabrutinib. Once toxicity resolves to G ≤1 or baseline, then resume acalabrutinib without dose reduction
	Third occurrence	Interrupt acalabrutinib. Once toxicity resolves to G ≤1 or baseline, then resume acalabrutinib at a reduced dose of 100 mg by mouth once daily
	Fourth occurrence	Discontinue acalabrutinib

Drug-Drug Interactions

Concomitant therapy with a strong CYP3A inhibitor is required	Avoid coadministration of a strong CYP3A inhibitor with acalabrutinib. If the strong CYP3A inhibitor is to be used short-term, then interrupt acalabrutinib therapy
Concomitant therapy with a moderate CYP3A inhibitor is required	Reduce the acalabrutinib dose to 100 mg by mouth once daily. If the moderate CYP3A inhibitor is subsequently discontinued, then increase the acalabrutinib dose back to the dose that was used prior to initiation of the inhibitor
Concomitant therapy with a strong CYP3A inducer is required	Consider use of an alternative medication. If concurrent use of a strong CYP3A inducer with acalabrutinib is unavoidable, then increase the acalabrutinib dose to 200 mg by mouth twice daily. If the strong CYP3A inducer is subsequently discontinued, then reduce the acalabrutinib dose back to the dose that was used prior to initiation of the inducer
Concomitant therapy with a proton pump inhibitor is required	Avoid coadministration of a proton pump inhibitor with acalabrutinib
Concomitant therapy with an H2-receptor antagonist is required	Administer acalabrutinib 2 hours before administration of a H2-receptor antagonist
Concomitant therapy with an antacid is required	Separate administration of acalabrutinib from administration of antacid medication by at least 2 hours
Concomitant therapy with antiplatelet medication(s) or anticoagulants is required	The risk of bleeding with acalabrutinib may be further increased. Monitor closely for signs of bleeding

Treatment Modifications (continued)

Other	
Planned elective surgery	Consider the benefit-risk of withholding acalabrutinib for 3–7 days pre- and post-surgery depending upon the type of surgery, risk of bleeding, and status of SLL/CLL
Severe liver dysfunction (total bilirubin between 3–10× ULN and any AST) or Child-Pugh class C liver dysfunction	Acalabrutinib pharmacokinetics have not been evaluated in patients with severe liver dysfunction, therefore no dose recommendation can be made

ANC, absolute neutrophil count; ULN, upper limit of normal; AST, aspartate aminotransferase; SLL, small lymphocytic lymphoma; CLL, chronic lymphocytic leukemia

Adverse Events (N = 61)

Event	Grade 1–2 (%)*	Grade 3–4 (%)*
Headache	43	0
Diarrhea	38	2
Increased weight	25	2
Pyrexia	20	3
Upper respiratory tract infection	23	0
Fatigue	18	3
Peripheral edema	21	0
Hypertension	13	7
Nausea	20	0
Contusion	18	0
Arthralgia	15	2
Petechiae	16	0
Decreased weight	16	0

*According to the National Cancer Institute Common Terminology Criteria for Adverse Events, version 4.03

Note: Toxicities that occurred in ≥15% of patients are included, regardless of cause. One Grade 5 event (pneumonia) was reported

SUBSEQUENT THERAPY
CHRONIC LYMPHOCYTIC LEUKEMIA REGIMEN: IBRUTINIB

Brown JR et al. Leukemia 2018;32:83–91
Byrd JC et al. N Engl J Med 2014;371:213–223
Supplementary appendix to: Byrd JC et al. N Engl J Med 2014;371:213–223
Protocol for: Byrd JC et al. N Engl J Med 2014;371:213–223
Imbruvica (ibrutinib) prescribing information. Sunnyvale, CA: Pharmacyclics LLC; revised 2018 August

Ibrutinib 420 mg/dose; administer orally, once daily with a glass of water, without regard to food, continually until disease progression (total dose/week = 2940 mg)

Notes:

- Administration with food increases ibrutinib exposure approximately 2-fold compared with administration after overnight fasting. Clinical studies instructed that ibrutinib be taken at least 30 minutes before eating or at least 2 hours after a meal at approximately the same time each day (Protocol for: Byrd JC et al. N Engl J Med 2014;371:213–223). However, the U.S. Food and Drug Administration–approved prescribing information does not make specific recommendations regarding administration of ibrutinib with regard to food. (Imbruvica [ibrutinib] prescribing information. Sunnyvale, CA: Pharmacyclics LLC; revised 2018 August). Others also have concluded that no food restrictions are needed given the relative safety profile of ibrutinib and because repeated drug intake in fasted conditions is unlikely (de Jong J et al. Cancer Chemother Pharmacol 2015;75:907–916)

- Ibrutinib capsules should be swallowed whole; do not break, open, or chew capsules. Ibrutinib tablets should be swallowed whole; do not cut, crush, or chew tablets

- Patients who delay taking ibrutinib at a regularly scheduled time may administer the missed dose as soon as possible on the same day, and then resume the normal schedule the following day. Do not administer an extra dose of ibrutinib to make up for a missed dose

- Ibrutinib is metabolized predominantly by CYP3A. Refer to treatment modification section for initial dose adjustment recommendations for patients requiring concurrent treatment with moderate or strong CYP3A inhibitors. Avoid concomitant use of ibrutinib with strong CYP3A inducers

- Advise patients to not consume grapefruit products or Seville oranges as they may inhibit CYP3A in the gut wall and increase the bioavailability of ibrutinib

- Serious bleeding events, some fatal, have been reported in patients treated with ibrutinib. Grade ≥3 bleeding events were reported to occur in 3% of patients. All-grade bleeding (including bruising and petechia) occurred in approximately 44% of patients. Ibrutinib may exacerbate the risk of bleeding when administered concurrently with anticoagulant and/or antiplatelet drugs; use caution and monitor closely for bleeding with concomitant use. Consider the risks and benefits of interrupting ibrutinib treatment at least 3–7 days prior to and following elective surgery depending on the risk of bleeding and type of surgery

- After initiation of ibrutinib, lymphocytosis occurs commonly and should not be considered as an indicator of disease progression. An absolute lymphocyte count (ALC) >5000/mcL together with a ≥50% increase from baseline occurred in two-thirds of patients in CLL studies. Lymphocytosis occurs during the first month of therapy and resolves by a median of 14 weeks

- Reduce the ibrutinib starting dose to 140 mg, administered orally once daily for mild (Child-Pugh class A) hepatic impairment. Reduce the ibrutinib starting dose to 70 mg, administered orally once daily for moderate (Child-Pugh class C) hepatic impairment. Avoid ibrutinib in patients with severe (Child-Pugh class C) hepatic impairment

- Tumor lysis syndrome may rarely occur with ibrutinib therapy. Consider appropriate monitoring and precautions (eg, anti-hyperuricemic therapy, hydration) in patients with high baseline risk (eg, high tumor burden, renal impairment)

Supportive Care
Antiemetic prophylaxis
Emetogenic potential is **MINIMAL TO LOW**
See Chapter 42 for antiemetic recommendations

Hematopoietic growth factor (CSF) prophylaxis
Primary prophylaxis is **NOT** indicated
See Chapter 43 for more information

Antimicrobial prophylaxis
Risk of fever and neutropenia is **LOW**
   Antimicrobial primary prophylaxis to be considered:
   - Antibacterial—not indicated. Consider prophylaxis for *P. jirovecii* (eg, cotrimoxazole)
   - Antifungal—not indicated
   - Antiviral—antiherpes antivirals (eg, acyclovir, famciclovir, valacyclovir)

Patient Population Studied

The international, multicenter, randomized, open-label, phase 3 trial (RESONATE) involved 391 patients with relapsed/refractory CLL and high-risk prognostic factors. Eligible patients had Eastern Cooperative Oncology Group performance score <2, had received at least one previous therapy, and were considered inappropriate candidates for purine analogue treatment because they had a short progression-free interval after chemoimmunotherapy, they had coexisting illnesses, were aged ≥70 years, or had a chromosome 17p13.1 deletion. Patients requiring warfarin or strong CYP3A4/5 inhibitors were ineligible. Patients were randomly assigned (1:1) to receive either oral ibrutinib (420 mg daily) until disease progression or unacceptable toxicity or intravenous ofatumumab for up to 24 weeks (initial dose at week 1: 300 mg, followed by 2000 mg weekly for 7 weeks and then every 4 weeks for 16 weeks)

Efficacy (N = 391)

	Ibrutinib (n = 195)	Ofatumumab (n = 196)	
Median progression-free survival	Not reached	8.1 months	HR 0.106, 95% CI 0.075–0.151; P<0.0001
Overall response rate*	90%	25%	P<0.0001

*Overall response rate included patients with complete response (with complete or incomplete hematopoietic recovery) or partial remission (with or without lymphocytosis)

Notes: Median duration of follow-up was 19 months (maximum 26 months on study)

Therapy Monitoring

1. *Prior to initiation of ibrutinib:* CBC with differential, serum bilirubin, ALT or AST, alkaline phosphatase, potassium, calcium, phosphorus, LDH, uric acid, and serum creatinine
2. *At least monthly:* CBC with differential
3. *Periodically:* monitor for signs and symptoms of cardiac arrhythmias (eg, atrial fibrillation and atrial flutter) and check electrocardiogram if present, signs and symptoms of bleeding (especially if concomitant antiplatelet or anticoagulant medication[s] are used), signs and symptoms of infection (including progressive multifocal leukoencephalopathy), blood pressure, presence of second primary malignancies, and diarrhea
4. *During initiation of therapy in patients with high tumor burden or renal dysfunction:* monitor for tumor lysis syndrome (potassium, calcium, phosphorus, LDH, uric acid, and serum creatinine)
5. *Response assessment every 1–3 months:* physical examination, CBC with differential, CT scans (in select patients for evaluation of adenopathy). Note that lymphocytosis occurs commonly following initiation of ibrutinib and should not be considered as an indicator of disease progression

Treatment Modifications

Ibrutinib for Chronic Lymphocytic Leukemia	
Starting dose: 420 mg by mouth once a day	
Adverse Event	**Treatment Modification**
Treatment with a moderate CYP3A inhibitor is required	Reduce ibrutinib starting dose to 280 mg by mouth once daily during concomitant therapy
Treatment with voriconazole 200 mg by mouth twice a day is required, *or:* Treatment with posaconazole suspension 100 mg by mouth once daily is required, *or:* Treatment with posaconazole suspension 100–200 mg by mouth twice a day is required	Reduce ibrutinib starting dose to 140 mg by mouth once daily during concomitant therapy
Treatment with posaconazole suspension 200 mg by mouth three times a day is required, *or:* Treatment with posaconazole suspension 400 mg by mouth twice a day is required, *or:* Treatment with posaconazole 300 mg intravenously once a day is required, *or:* Treatment with posaconazole delayed-release tablets 300 mg by mouth once a day is required	Reduce ibrutinib starting dose to 70 mg by mouth once daily during concomitant therapy

(continued)

Treatment Modifications (*continued*)

Adverse Event	Treatment Modification
Treatment with other strong CYP3A inhibitors besides those listed above is required	Avoid concomitant use of ibrutinib with other strong CYP3A inhibitors besides those listed above If the other strong CYP3A inhibitor is to be used short-term (eg, ≤7 days), then interrupt ibrutinib therapy during use of the strong CYP3A inhibitor
Treatment with a strong CYP3A inducer is required	Avoid concomitant use of ibrutinib with strong CYP3A inducers
Treatment with antiplatelet and/or anticoagulant medications is required	Bleeding risk may be increased. Monitor closely for signs and symptoms of bleeding
Child-Pugh class A hepatic impairment	Reduce ibrutinib starting dose to 140 mg by mouth once a day
Child-Pugh class B hepatic impairment	Reduce ibrutinib starting dose to 70 mg by mouth once a day
Child-Pugh class C hepatic impairment	Avoid ibrutinib use
Surgical procedure is required during treatment with ibrutinib	Consider benefit-risk of withholding ibrutinib for at least 3–7 days prior to and following surgery depending on the type of surgery and the risk of bleeding
Hypertension	Adjust existing anti-hypertensive medications and/or initiate anti-hypertensive treatment as appropriate
First occurrence of G ≥3 nonhematologic toxicity, G ≥3 neutropenia with infection or fever, or G4 hematologic toxicity	Interrupt ibrutinib until resolution to G1 or baseline, then resume ibrutinib at the same dose (eg, 420 mg by mouth once a day). Consider use of G-CSF for G4 neutropenia lasting >7 days or for life-threatening neutropenic complications
Second occurrence of G ≥3 nonhematologic toxicity, G ≥3 neutropenia with infection or fever, or G4 hematologic toxicity	Interrupt ibrutinib until resolution to G1 or baseline, then resume ibrutinib at 280 mg by mouth once a day. Consider use of G-CSF for G4 neutropenia lasting >7 days or for life-threatening neutropenic complications
Third occurrence of G ≥3 nonhematologic toxicity, G ≥3 neutropenia with infection or fever, or G4 hematologic toxicity	Interrupt ibrutinib until resolution to G1 or baseline, then resume ibrutinib at 140 mg by mouth once a day. Consider use of G-CSF for G4 neutropenia lasting >7 days or for life-threatening neutropenic complications
Fourth occurrence of G ≥3 nonhematologic toxicity, G ≥3 neutropenia with infection or fever, or G4 hematologic toxicity	Discontinue ibrutinib

G-CSF, granulocyte colony stimulating factor
Note: Ibrutinib can cause fetal harm. Advise females of reproductive potential of the potential risk to a fetus and to use effective contraception and avoid becoming pregnant while taking ibrutinib and for 1 month after cessation of treatment

Imbruvica (ibrutinib) prescribing information. Sunnyvale, CA: Pharmacyclics LLC; revised 2018 August

Adverse Events (N = 195)

Event	Ibrutinib (N = 195)		
	Grade 1–2 (%)*	Grade 3–4 (%)*	Grade 5 (%)*
Diarrhea	49	5	0
Fatigue	31	4	0
Nausea	30	2	0
Pyrexia	28	2	0
Cough	26	<1	0
Neutropenia	6	19	0
Anemia	19	6	0
Upper respiratory tract infection	25	<1	0
Peripheral edema	19	0	0
Sinusitis	18	<1	0
Arthralgia	17	2	0
Muscle spasms	18	<1	0
Constipation	18	0	0
Pneumonia	5	10	2
Thrombocytopenia	11	6	0
Headache	15	2	0
Vomiting	17	0	0

*According to the National Cancer Institute Common Terminology Criteria for Adverse Events, version 4.0

Note: The most common adverse events are included (for median follow-up 19 months). A total of 13 patients discontinued treatment owing to adverse events. Deaths were reported for 10 patients (4 owing to pneumonia, 2 to sepsis, 1 to neutropenic sepsis, 1 to cardiac arrest, 1 to gastrointestinal carcinoma, and 1 sudden death); none of the Grade 5 infections was considered related to study treatment

12. Chronic Myeloid Leukemia

Michael W.N. Deininger, MD, PhD, Diana Brewer, PA, and Brian J. Druker, MD

Epidemiology

Incidence: Estimated new cases for 2019 in the United States: 8990 (male: 5250; female: 3740)

Deaths: Estimated 1140 in 2019 (male: 660; female: 480)

Median age: 65 years

Phase at Presentation
Chronic phase: 85–90%
Accelerated phase and blast crisis: 10–15%

Cervantes F et al. Haematologica 1999;84:324–327
O'Brien SG et al. N Engl J Med 2003;348:994–1004
Siegel R et al. CA Cancer J Clin 2019;69:7–34
Surveillance, Epidemiology and End Results (SEER) Program, available from http://seer.cancer.gov (accessed in 2019)

Pathology

Peripheral blood findings at diagnosis: median (range)

1. WBC: 174,000/mm^3 (15–850/mm^3)
2. Hemoglobin: 10.3 g/dL (4.9–16.6 g/dL)
3. Platelet count: 430,000/mm^3 (17–3182/mm^3)
4. Left-shifted white cell differential, basophilia, and eosinophilia
5. Blasts: <15%—chronic phase

Bone marrow findings at diagnosis

1. Increased cellularity
2. Increased myeloid-to-erythroid ratio with full myeloid maturation
3. Blasts <15%—chronic phase
4. Basophilia
5. Megakaryocyte hyperplasia
6. Reticulin fibrosis

Cytogenetics and molecular diagnostics

1. Philadelphia (Ph) chromosome including variant translocations (90%)
2. BCR-ABL translocation by FISH (95%)*
3. BCR-ABL transcripts by RT-PCR (95%)*
4. Chromosomal abnormalities in addition to the Ph chromosome (clonal evolution)
   - Rare in chronic phase at diagnosis, common in accelerated and blast phase
   - Major route abnormalities: trisomy 8, trisomy 19, second Ph and isochromosome 17
   - Minor route abnormalities: all others except loss of Y chromosome
   - Major route abnormalities at diagnosis in chronic phase are associated with shorter progression-free and overall survival with imatinib
   - Some minor route abnormalities such as deletion 7 and 3q26.2 abnormalities also carry a poor prognosis
   - Newly acquired chromosomal abnormalities on therapy define progression to accelerated phase

*Approximately 5% of patients with morphologically and clinically typical CML are negative for BCR-ABL by FISH and RT-PCR; these patients do not have CML but constitute a heterogeneous group including atypical CML, chronic neutrophilic leukemia, and non-classifiable myeloproliferative neoplasms. They do not respond to imatinib or other tyrosine kinase inhibitors. The data given here do not apply to this group of patients

Deininger MWN. Semin Hematol 2003;40(2 Suppl 2):50–55
Johansson B et al. Acta Haematol 2002;107:76–94
Mitelman F. Leuk Lymphoma 1993;11(Suppl 1):11–15
Savage DG et al. Br J Haematol 1997;96:111–116
Thiele J et al. Leuk Lymphoma 2000;36:295–308
Fabarius A et al. Blood 2011;118;6760–6768
Wang W et al. Blood 2016;127:2742–2750
Deininger et al. Nat Rev Cancer 2017;17:425–440

Work-up

History and physical examination

1. Spleen size by palpation (cm below left costal margin)
2. Sites of extramedullary involvement other than hepatosplenomegaly

Laboratory studies

1. CBC and leukocyte differential, complete metabolic panel, phosphorus, magnesium, uric acid, and LDH
2. HLA typing for patients who are candidates for allogeneic hematopoietic cell transplantation
3. Bone marrow aspirate and biopsy (bone marrow cytogenetics can detect chromosomal abnormalities other than Ph chromosome that are not detectable using peripheral blood)
4. Baseline BCR-ABL1 transcript levels by quantitative reverse transcriptase polymerase reaction (QPCR) before initiation of treatment
5. If collection of bone marrow is not feasible, fluorescence in situ hybridization (FISH) on a peripheral blood specimen with dual probes for *BCR* and *ABL1* genes
6. Hepatitis panel as postmarketing data has shown reactivation in hepatitis following initiation of therapy with tyrosine kinase inhibitors; Hep B surface antigen (HBsAg), hepatitis B surface antibody (HBsAb), hepatitis B core antibody (anti-HBc), IgM anti-HBc, IgG anti-HBc
7. Baseline ECG
8. Baseline lipid panel, HgbA1c and ankle brachial index (ABI) in patients considered for second- or third-generation TKIs
9. Consider baseline cardiac ultrasound for patients with high cardiovascular risk

Additional considerations

1. Thoroughly review past medical and family history and comorbidities
2. Consider toxicity profile for TKI treatment selection
3. Consider multidisciplinary approach, including cardiology consult, and ensure close collaboration with primary care providers
4. Provide patient education; review treatment-related side effects and common management, drug/drug interactions, optimization of overall health with a focus on reducing metabolic and cardiovascular risks (encourage lifestyle modifications; smoking cessation, healthy diet, and exercise)
5. Emphasize importance of strict adherence to therapy and monitoring
6. Discuss contraceptives and family planning as appropriate

Classification of Disease: Phases of Disease

Chronic phase	Bone marrow and peripheral blood blasts <15% Peripheral blood promyelocytes and blasts combined <30% Peripheral blood basophils <20% Platelets >100,000/mm³
Accelerated phase	Bone marrow and peripheral blood blasts 15–30% Peripheral blood promyelocytes + blasts ≥30% (but blasts alone <30%) Peripheral blood basophils ≥20% Platelets ≤100,000/mm³ (unless related to therapy)
Blast crisis	Bone marrow or peripheral blood blasts ≥30% Flow cytometry to determine cell lineage: Myeloid immunophenotype: MPO-positive Lymphoid immunophenotype: TdT-positive

Cytogenetic abnormalities in addition to the Philadelphia chromosome (typically, isochromosome 17, trisomy 8, trisomy 19, second Ph chromosome), even in the absence of other defining criteria, indicate accelerated phase if they occur on therapy, and high risk if they occur at diagnosis. Adverse prognostic significance is best documented for isochromosome 17 and 3q26.2 abnormalities

Fabarius A et al. Blood 2011;118:6760–6768
Johansson B et al. Acta Haematol 2002;107:76–94
Talpaz M et al. Blood 2002;99:1928–1937
Wang W et al. Blood 2016;127:2742–2750

CML Risk Stratification

Calculation of Relative Risk

Adapted from Hasford J et al. Blood 2011;118:686–692

Study		Calculation	Risk Definition by Calculation
Sokal et al, 1984		Exp 0.0116 × (age − 43.4)	Low risk: <0.8
	+	0.0345 × (spleen − 7.51)	Intermediate risk: 0.8–1.2
	+	0.188 × ([platelet count ÷ 700]² − 0.563)	High risk: >1.2
	+	0.0887 × (myeloblasts − 2.10)	
Euro Hasford et al, 1998		0.666 when age ≥50 years	Low risk: ≤780
	+	(0.042 × spleen)	Intermediate risk: 781–1480
	+	1.0956 when platelet count >1500 × 10⁹ L	High risk: >1480
	+	(0.0584 × myeloblast)	
	+	0.20399 when basophils >3%	
	+	(0.0413 × eosinophils) × 100	

(continued)

CML Risk Stratification *(continued)*

Study		Calculation	Risk Definition by Calculation
ELTS Pfirrmann et al, 2016	+ + +	$0.0025 \times$ (age in completed years/10)^3 $0.0615 \times$ spleen size below costal margin $0.1052 \times$ blasts in peripheral blood $0.4104 \times$ (platelet count/1000)$^{-0.5}$	Low risk: ≤1.5680
			Intermediate risk: >1.5680 but ≤2.2185 High risk: >2.2185

Calculation of the risk requires use of clinical and hematologic data at diagnosis, prior to any treatment:
- Age is given in years
- Spleen is given in centimeters below the costal margin (maximum distance)
- Myeloblasts, eosinophils, and basophils are given in percentage of peripheral blood differential

Relative risk for the Sokal calculation is expressed as exponential of the total; that for the Hasford calculation is expressed as the total × 1000

To calculate Sokal and Euro risk score, go to:
www.leukemia-net.org/content/leukemias/cml/euro__and_sokal_score/index_eng.html
To calculate ELTS risk score, go to:
www.leukemia-net.org/content/leukemias/cml/elts_score/index_eng.html

Hasford J et al. J Natl Cancer Inst 1998;90:850–858
Pfirrmann M et al. Leukemia 2016;30:48–56
Sokal JE et al. Blood 1984;63:789–799

Approximate relationship between response, the putative number of leukemic cells, and the level of BCR-ABL transcripts
Adapted from Baccarani M et al. Blood 2006;108:1809–1820

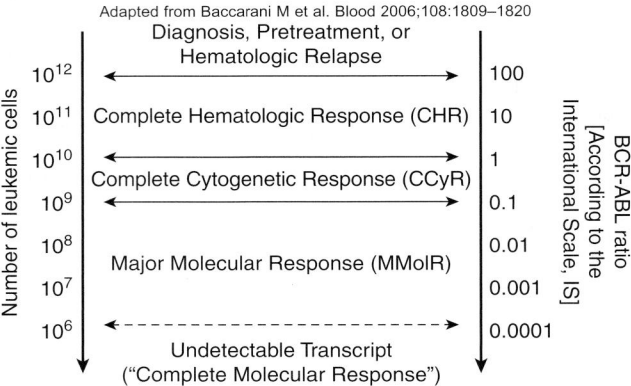

Response Definitions and Monitoring
Adapted from Baccarani M et al. Blood 2013;122:872–884

	Complete Hematologic Response (CHR)*	Cytogenetic Response (CyR)†	Molecular Response (MolR)‡

Definitions	• Normalization of blood counts:
	  ▪ Platelet count <450,000/mm^3
	  ▪ WBC <10,000/mm^3;
	  ▪ Differential without immature granulocytes and <5% basophils
	• Spleen not palpable
	  ▪ Disappearance of CML symptoms
		• Percentage of 20 marrow metaphases with Ph detected by karyotyping:
		  ▪ Complete (CCyR)* = 0%
		  ▪ Partial/Major (MCyR) = 1–35%
		  ▪ Minor CyR = 36–65%
		  ▪ Minimal CyR = 66–95%
		  ▪ None = >95%
			• Major molecular response (MMolR)* = ≥3-log$_{10}$ reduction in *BCR-ABL1* transcripts (≤0.10% IS)
			• Deep molecular response (DMR) = ≥4-log$_{10}$ reduction in *BCR-ABL1* transcripts (≤0.01% IS)§
			• "Complete (CMR, CMolR)" = transcript not detectable§

Monitoring	• Check CBC every 2 weeks until CHR achieved and confirmed • Once CHR achieved, check CBC every 3 months unless otherwise required	• Check CyR at 3, 6, 12 months and then at least every 6 months until CCyR achieved and confirmed • Once CCyR achieved, check every 12 months	• Check every 3 months • Perform mutational analysis in case of treatment failure, suboptimal response, or >5-fold increase in transcript level

*Complete HR, complete CCyR, and major MolR should be confirmed on at least 2 occasions
†CyR is evaluated by karyotyping of at least 20 marrow metaphases. FISH of peripheral blood cells should be used only if marrow metaphases cannot be obtained
‡MolR is assessed on peripheral white blood cells. Following quantitative real time PCR (qRT-PCR) analysis, the BCR-ABL1/control gene transcript ratio is determined using the International Scale (IS) standardized baseline. The international scale for measuring MolR is that proposed by Hughes T et al. Blood 2006;108:28–37
§There is no universal definition of complete molecular response (CMR, CMolR), as negativity of a test result is a function of the test sensitivity as well as of the sample quality. It is best practice to indicate test sensitivity and avoid the term CMR

(continued)

CML Risk Stratification (continued)

Recommendations for Cytogenetic and Molecular Monitoring
Adapted from Baccarani M et al. Blood 2013;122:872–884

At diagnosis	Chromosome banding analysis (CBA) of marrow cell metaphases
	FISH in case of Ph negativity to identify variant or cryptic translocations
	Qualitative PCR (identification of transcript type)
During treatment	Quantitative real-time PCR (RQ-PCR) for the determination of *BCR-ABL1* transcripts level on the international scale, to be performed every 3 months until MMR (BCR-ABL ≤0.1%, or MR$^{3.0}$) has been achieved, then every 3–6 months *and/or*
	Karyotyping of marrow cell metaphases (at least 20) to be performed at 3, 6, and 12 months until a CCyR has been achieved, then every 12 months. If adequate molecular monitoring is performed, karyotyping during follow-up is optional. In patients with atypical BCR-ABL1 transcripts who cannot be monitored by standard RQ-qPCR, FISH on white blood cells can replace karyotyping once CCyR has been documented
Failure, progression	RQ-PCR, mutational analysis, and CBA of marrow cell metaphases. Immunophenotyping in BP
Warning	Molecular and cytogenetic tests to be performed more frequently. CBA of marrow cell metaphases recommended in case of myelodysplasia or CCA/Ph⁻ with chromosome 7 involvement

CCA/Ph⁻ clonal chromosome abnormalities in Ph⁻ cells; FISH, fluorescence in situ hybridization
Note: The response can be assessed either with RQ-PCR or with cytogenetics, depending on the local laboratory facilities, but RQ-PCR is preferred if there is access to high-quality testing with results expressed on the international scale. Karyotyping and mutational analysis by conventional Sanger sequencing or next generation sequencing (NGS) are indicated in case of progression or failure. Bone marrow karyotyping is also indicated if myelodysplastic features (unexpected leucopenia, thrombocytopenia, or anemia) develop

Treatment Options Based on BCR-ABL1 Mutation Profile

Mutation	TKI Sensitive/Treatment Recommendation
Y253H, E255K/V, or F359V/C/I	Dasatinib
F317L/V/I/C, T315A, or V299L	Nilotinib
E255K/V, F317L/V/I/C, F359 V/C/I, T315A, or Y253H	Bosutinib
T315I	Ponatinib

Baccarani M et al. Blood 2013;122:872–884
Cortes JE et al. J Clin Oncol 2016;34;2333–2340
Soverini S et al. Blood 2011;118:1208–1215

Early Treatment Response Milestones to TKIs as First-Line Treatment
Per NCCN Guidelines Version 3.2020

Time	TKI-resistant Disease*	Possible TKI Resistance†	TKI-sensitive Disease
Diagnosis/baseline	NA	High risk *or* CCA/Ph⁺, major route‡	NA
3 months on TKI treatment		BCR-ABL1 >10%	BCR-ABL1 >1%–10% or BCR-ABL1 ≤1%
6 months on TKI treatment	BCR-ABL1 >10%		BCR-ABL1 >1%–10% or BCR-ABL1 ≤1%
12 months on TKI treatment	BCR-ABL1 >10%	BCR-ABL1 >1–10%	BCR-ABL1 ≤0.1%

(*continued*)

Treatment Options Based on BCR-ABL1 Mutation Profile (continued)

Time	TKI-resistant Disease*	Possible TKI Resistance†	TKI-sensitive Disease
Then, and at any time	Loss of CHR Loss of CCyR Confirmed loss of MMR§ New mutation CCA/Ph+	CCA/Ph− (−7 or 7q−)	BCR-ABL1 ≤0.1%

Radich JP. J Natl Compr Canc Netw 2018;16:1108–1135

CCA, clonal chromosomal abnormalities; CCyR, complete cytogenetic response, Philadelphia chromosome (Ph) not detected by karyotyping in 20/20 marrow metaphases; CHR, complete hematologic response; CyR, cytogenetic response; NA, not applicable

*Failure implies patient should be moved to other treatments when available
†Possible TKI resistance implies that the characteristics of the disease and the response to treatment require more frequent monitoring to permit timely changes in therapy in case of treatment failure
‡Major route abnormalities include +8, +der(22)t(9;22)(q34;q11), ider(22)(q10) t(9;22)(q34,q11), isochromosome(17)(q10), and trisomy 19. Note that several minor route abnormalities such as inv(3)(q21q26), t(3;3)(q21;q26) and −7 are associated with inferior outcomes
§To be confirmed on 2 occasions, at least 1 of which with BCR-ABL ≥1%

Clinical Considerations for Transition to Second-Line Treatment
Per NCCN Guidelines Version 3.2020

	Clinical Considerations	Second-line Treatment
TKI-resistant disease*	Evaluate patient compliance and drug interactions Consider mutational analysis	Switch to alternate TKI and evaluate for allogeneic HCT
Possible TKI resistance†	Evaluate patient compliance and drug interactions Consider mutational analysis Consider bone marrow cytogenetic analysis to assess from MCyR at 3 months or CCyR at 12 months	Switch to alternate TKI or continue same TKI (other than imatinib) or increase imatinib dose to a max of 800 mg and consider evaluation for allogeneic HCT
TKI-sensitive disease	Monitor response and side effects	Continue same TKI

Radich JP. J Natl Compr Canc Netw 2018;16:1108–1135

Nuances

1. Consider adherence to therapy (either patient compliance and/or treatment interruptions based on adverse events) when evaluating disease status and treatment response
2. Use clinical judgment when evaluating treatment response: Consider the overall decline in BCR-ABL1 transcripts from baseline; both the degree and rate of change over time and its relation to the expected treatment milestones to guide decision-making on whether to continue same TKI versus switching therapy

Definitions of the Response to Second-Line Therapy in Case of Failure of Imatinib
Adapted from Baccarani M et al. Blood 2013;122:872–884

	Failure	Warning	Optimal
Diagnosis/baseline	NA	No CHR or loss of CHR on imatinib *or* Lack of CyR to first-line TKI *or* High risk	NA
3 months on TKI treatment	No CHR *or* Ph+ >95% *or* New mutations	BCR-ABL1 >10% *and/or* Ph+ 65–95%	BCR-ABL1 ≤10% *and/or* Ph+ <65%
6 months on TKI treatment	BCR-ABL1 >10% *and/or* Ph+ >65% *and/or* New mutations	Ph+ 35–65%	BCR-ABL1 ≤10% *and/or* Ph+ <35%

(continued)

Nuances *(continued)*

	Failure	Warning	Optimal
12 months on TKI treatment	BCR-ABL1 >10% *and/or* Ph+ >35% *and/or* New mutations	BCR-ABL1 1–10% *and/or* Ph+ 1–35%	BCR-ABL1 <1% *and/or* Ph+ 0
Then, and at any time	Loss of CHR *or* Loss of CCyR or PCyR New mutations Confirmed loss of MMR* CCA/Ph+	CCA/Ph− (−7 or 7q−) *or* BCR-ABL1 >0.1%	BCR-ABL1 ≤0.1%

CCA/Ph+, clonal chromosome abnormalities in Ph+ cells; CCA/Ph−, clonal chromosome abnormalities in Ph− cells; MMR, BCR-ABL1 ≥0.1% = MR3.0 or better; NA, not applicable
*In 2 consecutive tests, in which 1 notes a BCR-ABL transcript level ≥1%

Rates of CCyR and MMR

Adapted from Mealing S et al. Exp Hematol Oncol 2013;2:5

Percentage with Complete Cytogenic Response (CCyR)

	Dasatinib			Nilotinib 600 mg			Nilotinib 800 mg			Imatinib 400 mg			Imatinib 800 mg			Bosutinib 400 mg		
Time (months)	6	12	18	6	12	18	6	12	18	6	12	18	6	12	18	6	12	18
Study																		
DASISION	73	85	85*							59	73	82*						
ENESTnd				67	63	85	80	78	82	45	65	74						
Baccarani et al										50	58		52	64	74			
German CML IV										22	50	67	34	63				
Cortes et al										45	66		57	70				
ISTAHIT										20	82		44	69				
SPIRIT										50	58		69	65				
S0325 Intergroup†											67			85				
BFORE											66						77	

(continued)

Nuances *(continued)*

	Dasatinib	Nilotinib 600 mg	Nilotinib 800 mg	Imatinib 400 mg	Imatinib 800 mg	Bosutinib 400 mg
Percentage with Major Molecular Response (MMR) at 12 Months						
Baccarani et al.				33	40	
DASISION	46			28		
ENESTnd		44	43	22		
German CML IV				31	55	
Cortes et al.				40	46	
SPIRIT				38	49	
S0325 Intergroup†				36	53	
BFORE				37		47

*24 months
†Based on blood specimens collected 295–406 days after randomization. (If a patient's molecular response was tested more than once during that interval, only the result obtained closest to day 365 was included in this analysis)
Baccarani M et al. Blood 2009;113:4497–4504
Cotes JE et al. J Clin Oncol 2010;28:424–430
Cortes JE et al. J Clin Oncol 2018;36:231–237 (BFORE)
Deininger MW et al. Br J Hematol 2014;164:223–232 (S0325 Intergroup)
Hehlmann R et al. J Clin Oncol 2011;29;1634–1642

Hehlmann R et al. J Clin Oncol 2014; 32, 415–423 (CML IV)
Hughes TP et al. Blood 2014;123;1353–1360 (ENESTnd)
Kantarjian HM et al. Blood 2012;119:1123–1129 (DASISION)
Kantarjian HM et al. N Engl J Med 2010;362:2260–2270 (DASISION)
Larson RA et al. Leukemia 2012:26:2197–2203 (ENESTnd)
Petzer AL et al. Haematologica 2010;95:908–913 (ISTAHIT)
Preudhomme C et al. N Engl J Med 2010;363:2511–2521 (SPIRIT)
Saglio G et al. N Engl J Med 2010;362:2251–2259 (ENESTnd)

Expert Opinion

FDA-Approved Indications and Usage

1. Imatinib is approved for:
   • Newly diagnosed adult and pediatric patients with CML* in chronic phase
   • Patients with CML in blast crisis (BC), in accelerated phase (AP), or in chronic phase (CP) after failure of interferon α therapy
   • Adult patients with relapsed or refractory Philadelphia chromosome-positive acute lymphoblastic leukemia (Ph+ ALL)
   • Pediatric patients with Ph+ ALL in combination with chemotherapy

2. Dasatinib is approved for:
   • Newly diagnosed adult and pediatric patients *(1 year of age or older)* with CML in chronic phase
   • Adults with chronic-, accelerated-, or myeloid or lymphoid blast-phase CML with resistance or intolerance to prior therapy that included imatinib
   • Adults with Ph+ ALL with resistance or intolerance to prior therapy

3. Nilotinib is approved for:
   • Newly diagnosed adults with CML in chronic phase
   • Adults with chronic- or accelerated-phase CML with resistance or intolerance to prior therapy that included imatinib
   • First- and second-line TKI in pediatric patients *(1 year of age or older)* with CML in chronic phase

4. Bosutinib is approved for:
   • Newly diagnosed adult patients with CML in chronic phase
   • Adult patients with chronic-, accelerated-, or blast-phase CML with resistance or intolerance to prior therapy

5. Ponatinib is approved for:
   • T315I-positive CML (chronic phase, accelerated phase, or blast phase) or T315I-positive Ph+ ALL
   • Chronic-phase, accelerated-phase, or blast-phase CML or Ph+ ALL for whom no other tyrosine kinase inhibitor therapy is indicated

6. Omacetaxine mepesuccinate is approved for:
   • Adult patients with chronic- or accelerated-phase CML with resistance and/or intolerance to two or more tyrosine kinase inhibitors

*According to the WHO, chronic myeloid leukemia (CML) is defined by the presence of the Ph chromosome or the *BCR-ABL1* fusion gene in the context of a myeloproliferative neoplasm. Therefore "Ph chromosome–positive" is redundant

(continued)

Expert Opinion (*continued*)

Treatment options:

1. In the opinion of some experts, imatinib remains the standard drug therapy regimen for the initial treatment of all phases of CML. This is based on its overall efficacy and long-term safety profile. In the opinion of others, nilotinib, dasatinib, and bosutinib represent better first-line options than imatinib due to faster and deeper molecular responses. The latter are a prerequisite for a trial of treatment-free remission (TFR). There is universal agreement that the availability of four first-line therapies provides clinicians with a range of options for managing intolerance and resistance

2. Although imatinib is a highly effective therapy, it has limitations: with 8 years of follow-up, 16% of IRIS patients discontinued treatment for insufficient efficacy and 6% for adverse events. These outcomes led to clinical trials that tested whether first-line use of more potent tyrosine kinase inhibitors, such as dasatinib, nilotinib, and bosutinib, may reduce the rate of failures. Promising results in single-arm studies with dasatinib, nilotinib, and bosutinib led to randomized trials comparing dasatinib to imatinib (Dasatinib versus Imatinib Study in Treatment-Naïve CML Patients [DASISION] study), nilotinib to imatinib (Evaluating Nilotinib Efficacy and Safety in Clinical Trials of Newly Diagnosed Ph-positive CML Patients [ENESTnd] study), and bosutinib to imatinib (Bosutinib Trial in First-Line Chronic Myelogenous Leukemia Treatment [BFORE] study). All studies found newer agents superior to imatinib with respect to:
   - Complete cytogenetic responses (CCyR)
   - Major molecular responses (MMR), and
   - Deep molecular responses (DMR)

   These observations led to their approval for first-line therapy of CML-CP

3. Dasatinib, nilotinib, and bosutinib provide several advantages
   - Response milestones are achieved sooner and in a greater proportion of patients
   - Progression to advanced disease is reduced (statistically significant only for nilotinib)

   However, the numeric advantages are slight, overall survival is not significantly different, and some late side effects have been observed for the second-generation inhibitors (nilotinib: peripheral occlusive arterial disease, and other cardiovascular adverse events; dasatinib: pulmonary hypertension)
   - Second-generation TKIs should be considered in patients with high Sokal or ELTS scores and patients in whom treatment-free remission is a critical goal of therapy, eg, women who desire to become pregnant. Imatinib is a safe choice in older patients with high cardiovascular risk
   - More general recommendations will require long-term follow-up of large populations

4. In aggregate dasatinib, bosutinib, and nilotinib control BCR-ABL1 mutations that confer resistance to imatinib, with the exception of the T315I mutation. However, activity against individual mutants can vary, and the choice between dasatinib, bosutinib, and nilotinib can be partially rationalized based on *BCR-ABL1* genotype (kinase domain mutation analysis) and patient history (risk of adverse events). However, the three second-generation TKIs have not been compared in a prospective study

5. The most problematic point mutation is the BCR-ABL^{T315I} "gatekeeper" mutation. BCR-ABL^{T315I} is insensitive to imatinib, dasatinib, nilotinib, and bosutinib

6. Ponatinib has in vitro activity against BCR-ABL1^{T315I} and other resistant mutants. However, certain T315I-inclusive compound mutants exhibit high-level resistance. Ponatinib has demonstrated considerable clinical activity in patients with and without BCR-ABL^{T315I}, especially in the chronic phase of CML, but cardiovascular safety concerns prevent its use in second-line therapy, except in the case of BCR-ABL^{T315I}

7. Interferon α or peginterferon α-2b may be considered in exceptional cases, in particular during pregnancy given the teratogenicity of TKIs. However interferon α is generally ineffective in patients with disease resistant to tyrosine kinase inhibitors

8. Hydroxyurea is used for lowering excessively high white blood cell counts and in the case of clinical signs/symptoms of leukostasis, if the diagnosis is uncertain, and in the case of intolerance or resistance to tyrosine kinase inhibitors. Hydroxyurea is considered a palliative regimen, as it does not usually induce lasting responses

9. Although the Sokal score was developed in patients treated with chemotherapy, it also predicts the likelihood of achieving a complete cytogenetic response to imatinib (91% vs 84% vs 69% at 48 months for low-, intermediate-, and high-risk patients, respectively). Complete cytogenetic response is associated with a favorable outcome

10. The definitions of disease phases given above were used in the clinical trials of imatinib that led to regulatory approval. They are widely used, but alternative definitions also exist

11. AML- or ALL-type chemotherapy is indicated for TKI-resistant CML in myeloid and lymphoid blast crisis, respectively. No data from controlled trials are available to demonstrate superiority of one regimen over another. All efforts should be made to proceed to allogeneic hematopoietic cell transplantation as soon as possible. Complete hematologic remission is achieved in 40–60% of patients

Cortes J et al. Am J Hematol 2013;88:350–354
Cortes J et al. Blood 2012;120:2573–2580
Cortes JE et al. J Clin Oncol. 2018 Jan 20;36:231–237
Cortes JE et al. N Engl J Med 2012;367:2075–2088
Derderian PM et al. Am J Med 1993;94:69–74
Druker BJ et al. N Engl J Med 2006;355:2408–2417
Jabbour E et al. Blood 2011;117:1822–1827
Jabbour E et al. Blood 2011;118:4541–4546
Kantarjian H et al. N Engl J Med 2006;354:2542–2551

Kantarjian HM et al. Am J Med 1987;83:445–454
Kantarjian HM et al. Blood 2012;119:1123–1129
Kantarjian HM et al. Lancet Oncol 2011;12:841–851
Kantarjian HM et al. N Engl J Med 2010;362:2260–2270
Khoury HJ et al. Blood 2012;119:3403–3412
Michallet M et al. Leukemia 2004:18;309–315
Saglio G et al. N Engl J Med 2010;362:2251–2259
Talpaz M et al. N Engl J Med 2006;354:2531–2541

(*continued*)

Expert Opinion (continued)

Treatment-Free Remission (TFR): Guidance

Treatment-Free Remission Clinical Trials
Adapted from Saußele S et al. Leukemia 2016;30:1638–1647

Study	Number	Treatment Before Discontinuation	Response Required for Discontinuation	Definition of Relapse	TFR % (Median Follow-up Time)
			Trials of imatinib discontinuation		
STIM1	100	IFN then imatinib for ≥3 years	CMR for ≥2 years	Loss of MMR or ≥1-log increase in Bcr/Abl	40% (95% CI 29–47) at 24 months and 38% at 60 months
STIM2	200	Imatinib for ≥3 years	As for STIM	Loss of MMR or ≥1-log increase in Bcr/Abl	Preliminary results 46% (95% CI 38–56) at 24 months
ALLG CML8	40	Imatinib for ≥3 years	UMRD ≥ 2 years	Loss of MMR or confirmed loss of MR4.5	47% at 24 months
According to STIM	80	Imatinib for ≥3 years	As for STIM; confirmed CMR with occasional weakly positive samples also were considered eligible	Loss of MMR	64% (95% CI 54–75) at 2 years
EURO-SKI	755	Imatinib, nilotinib, and dasatinib	MR4 for ≥1 year; TKI for >3 years	Loss of MMR	50% at 24 months
ISAV	112	Imatinib	Undetectable PCR (3 PCRs)	Loss of MMR	52% at 36 months
DESTINY	168	Imatinib, nilotinib, and dasatinib	MR4 and stable response under half standard dose for 12 months	Loss of MMR	72% at 36 months
			Trials of nilotinib/dasatinib discontinuation		
STOP 2G-TKI pilot	60	Nilotinib or dasatinib	CMR for median 29 months (range, 21–39)	Loss of MMR	63% at 12 months and 53% at 48 months
ENESTFreedom	190	Nilotinib front line	MR4.5 for ≥1 year	Loss of MMR	49% at 96 weeks
ENESTop	163	Second-line nilotinib (≥3 years total; ≥2 years NIL)	MR4.5 for ≥1 year	Confirmed loss of MR4 or any loss of MMR	50% at 96 weeks
ENESTPath	1058	Imatinib (<2 years) and nilotinib	MR4.5 for ≥1 year vs MR4.5 for ≥2 years randomized	Confirmed loss of MR4 or any loss of MMR	In progress
ENESTGoal	300	Imatinib (≥1 years) without MMR followed by nilotinib	MR4.5 for ≥ 1 year	Confirmed loss of MR4 or any loss of MMR	In progress
DADI trial (dasatinib discontinuation)	88 (63 discontinued)	Dasatinib consolidation for 1 year within trial	Deep molecular response, definition unclear	Loss of deep molecular response at any assessment	48% at 24 months
DASFREE dasatinib functional cure CA180–406 Study	~74	≥2 years dasatinib treatment	MR4.5 for ≥ 1year	Loss of MMR	46% at 24 months

(continued)

Expert Opinion (continued)

Trials of nilotinib/dasatinib discontinuation					
CML V (TIGER) Nilotinib ± PEG-IFN	650	Nilotinib (3 years) vs nilotinib + PEG-IFN (2 years)	MR4 for ≥1 year + PEG IFN maintenance	Loss of MMR	In progress

ALLG, Australasian Leukemia & Lymphoma Group; CI, confidence interval; CML, chronic myeloid leukemia; CMR, complete molecular response; Destiny, De-escalation and stopping treatment of imatinib, nilotinib or dasatinib in CML; ENEST, nilotinib treatment-free remission studies; EURO-SKI, Europe stops tyrosine kinase inhibitor trial; 2G-TKI, second-generation TKIs; IFN, interferon; MMR, major molecular response; MR4, MR4.5 molecular response level corresponding to a 4- or 4.5-log reduction from the standardized baseline, respectively; PEG, polyethylene glycol; STIM, stop imatinib trial; TFR, treatment-free remission; TKI, tyrosine kinase inhibitor; UMRD, undetectable minimal residual disease

Note: Multiple clinical trials have noted ~40% of patients who have stable deep molecular response remain in treatment-free remission (TFR) after stopping first-line treatment (per table)

Clark RE et al. Lancet Haematol 2017;4:e310–e316 (DESTINY)
Etienne G at al. J Clin Oncol 2017;35:298–305 (STIM1)
Hochhaus A et al. Leukemia 2017;31:1525–1531 (ENESTFreedom)
Imagawa J et al. Lancet Haematol 2015;2:e528–e535 (DADI)
Mahon FX et al. Lancet Oncol 2010;11:1029–1035 (STIM1)
Mori S et al. Am J Hematol 2015;90:910–914 (ISAV)
Nakamae H et al. Haematologica 2017;102:77 (DADI)
Nicolini FE et al. Blood 2013;122:abstract 654 (STIM2)
Rousselot P et al. J Clin Oncol 2014;32:424–430 (ASTIM)
Rea D et al. Blood 2017;129:846–854 (STOP 2G)
Ross DM et al. Blood 2013;122:515–522 (TWISTER)
Ross DM et al. J Cancer Res Clin Oncol 2018;144:945–954 (ENESTop)
Saußele S et al. Lancet 2018;19:747–757 (EURO-SKI)
Saußele S et al. Leukemia 2016;30:1638–1647
Shah NP et al. Leuk Lymphoma 2020;61:650–659 (DASFREE)
NCCN guidelines on treatment-free remission
Lee S-E et al. Haematologica 2016;101:717–723 (TKI Withdrawal Syndrome)
Radich JP et al. J Natl Compr Canc Netw 2018;16:1108–1135

Eligibility for TKI Discontinuation

1. Age ≥18 years
2. Chronic phase CML with no prior history of accelerated or blast phase CML
3. On approved TKI therapy for at least 3 years*
4. Prior evidence of quantifiable BCR-ABL transcript
5. Stable molecular response (MR4; BCR-ABL1 ≤0.01% IS) for ≥2 years, as documented on at least 4 tests, performed at least 3 months apart
6. Access to a reliable qPCR test with a sensitivity of detection of at least MR4.5 (BCR-ABL 1 ≤0.0032% IS) and that provides results within 2 weeks

Additional Considerations

1. Consider consultation with a CML specialist to review appropriateness for TKI discontinuation. It is recommended to have a thorough discussion of the potential risks versus benefits of treatment discontinuation, review TKI withdrawal syndrome (footnote below), and devise plan for strict adherence to close monitoring as well as threshold to resume therapy in the event of disease progression (defined as loss of MMR, >0.1% IS)

Monitoring after TKI Discontinuation

1. Molecular monitoring every 4 weeks for the first year following, then every 6 weeks for the second year, and every 12 weeks thereafter (indefinitely*)—recommended for patients who remain in MMR (MR3; BCR-ABL1 ≤0.1% IS) after discontinuation of TKI therapy

*Although the majority of patients who experience disease recurrence tend to do so within the first 6 months following discontinuation, recurrence can occur at any time, in some instances even years later

Treatment Reinitiation

1. Prompt reinitiation of TKI within 4 weeks of loss of MMR with molecular monitoring every 4 weeks until MMR is re-established, then transition to monitoring every 12 weeks thereafter. The majority of patients are anticipated to regain their response with previous TKI
2. For those patients who fail to achieve MMR after 3 months of TKI resumption, BCR-ABL1 kinase domain mutational analysis should be performed and monthly molecular monitoring should be continued for another 6 months

Note: Consensus from the National Comprehensive Cancer Network acknowledges that the feasibility of TFR following discontinuation of bosutinib or ponatinib has not yet been evaluated in clinical studies. However, it is assumed that response rates will be similar irrespective of the TKI in patients eligible to discontinue therapy having achieved and maintained a durable and deep molecular response >2 years. TKI withdrawal syndrome can and does occur in ~10–30% of patients following discontinuation. Often these symptoms are mild to moderate but can vary in severity, with typical duration of symptoms lasting weeks to several months, most often with complete resolution by 1 year following discontinuation. Symptoms commonly experienced are either aggravation or new development of musculoskeletal pain and/or pruritis and rash. These myalgias and arthralgias can often be effectively treated with over-the-counter anti-inflammatories and analgesics and/or antihistamines

INITIAL THERAPY

CHRONIC MYELOID LEUKEMIA REGIMEN: IMATINIB (FIRST-GENERATION TKI)

Deininger MWN et al. J Clin Oncol 2003;21:1637–1647

Chronic phase CML:
Initial dose:
Imatinib 400 mg/day; administer orally, continually, with the largest meal of the day (total dose/week = 2800 mg)
Dose escalation:
Escalate to **Imatinib** 600 mg/day; administer orally, continually, with the largest meal of the day (total dose/week = 4200 mg), if:
1. BCR-ABL1 >10% response at 3 months, *or*
2. BCR-ABL1 >1%–10% at 12 months

Accelerated and blast phase CML:
Initial dose:
Imatinib 600 mg/day; administer orally, continually, with the largest meal of the day

Supportive Care
Antiemetic prophylaxis
Emetogenic potential is **MINIMAL–LOW**
See Chapter 42 for antiemetic recommendations

Hematopoietic growth factor (G-CSF) prophylaxis
Primary prophylaxis is **NOT** indicated
See Chapter 43 for more information

Antimicrobial prophylaxis
Risk of fever and neutropenia is **LOW**
   Antimicrobial primary prophylaxis to be considered:
   • Antibacterial—not indicated
   • Antifungal—not indicated
   • Antiviral—not indicated, unless patient previously had an episode of HSV

Patient Population Studied

Study of 553 patients with newly diagnosed CML in chronic phase

Efficacy (Chronic Phase, N = 553)*

Complete hematologic response	98%
Complete cytogenetic response	87%
Partial cytogenetic response (1–35% Ph⁺ metaphases)	5%
Freedom from progression to accelerated phase or blast crisis	93%

*Projected rates at 60 months
Druker BJ et al. N Engl J Med 2006;355:2408–2417

Therapy Monitoring

1. *CBC:* Weekly; every 2 weeks after achievement of complete hematologic response; every 4–6 weeks after achievement of a complete cytogenetic response
2. *Blood chemistry:* Weekly; every 4–8 weeks after achievement of complete hematologic response
3. *Quantitative RT-PCR for BCR-ABL from peripheral blood:* Every 3 months until MMR has been achieved, then every 3–6 months
4. *Bone marrow cytogenetics:* Every 3 months until complete cytogenetic response, then at 12- to 24-month intervals (only if no access to reliable qPCR testing or in case of atypical transcripts not measurable by standard qPCR assays)
5. *FISH (peripheral blood):* In case of atypical transcripts, once CCyR has been achieved

Treatment Modifications

Hematologic Toxicity (No Modifications for Anemia)

G1/2	No dose modifications
G3	Hold imatinib until toxicity resolves to Grade 1*, then restart at 400 mg/day
Recurrent G3	Hold imatinib until toxicity resolves to Grade 1, then restart at 300 mg/day
G4	Withhold imatinib until toxicity resolves to Grade 1, then restart at 300 mg/day
Recurrent G4	Hold imatinib until toxicity resolves to Grade 1, then restart at 300 mg/day†

Nonhematologic Toxicity

G1	No dose modifications
G2/3	Hold imatinib until toxicity resolves to Grade 1, then restart at 400 mg/day
Recurrent G2/3	Hold imatinib until toxicity resolves to Grade 1, then restart at 300 mg/day
G4	Hold imatinib until toxicity resolves to Grade 1, then restart at 300 mg/day
Recurrent G4	Discontinue imatinib

*Consider filgrastim for persistent neutropenia
†No dose reduction to <300 mg/day
Deininger MWN et al. J Clin Oncol 2003;21:1637–1647

Toxicity (In >10% of patients, N = 553)

Toxicity	% G1/2	% G3/4
Hematologic AE		
Thrombocytopenia	48.8	7.8
Neutropenia	46.5	14.3
Anemia	41.5	3.1
Nonhematologic AE		
Superficial edema	54.6	0.9
Nausea	43	0.7
Increased liver transaminases	38.1	5.1
Muscle cramps	37	1.3
Musculoskeletal pain	33.8	2.7
Rash	31.9	2.0
Fatigue	33.4	1.1
Diarrhea	31	1.8
Headache	30.8	0.4
Joint pain	25.9	2.4
Abdominal pain	24.6	2.4
Nasopharyngitis	22.0	—
Myalgia	19.9	1.5
Hemorrhage	20.2	0.7
Vomiting	15.4	1.5
Dyspepsia	16.2	—
Pharyngolaryngeal pain	15.8	0.2
Cough	14.3	0.2
Dizziness	13.6	0.9
Upper respiratory infection	14.3	0.2
Weight gain	12.5	0.9
Pyrexia	12.4	0.7
Insomnia	12.2	—

O'Brien SG et al. N Engl J Med 2003;348:994–1004

Notes

Consider testing plasma imatinib concentrations in patients with suboptimal response, as imatinib levels >1000 ng/mL are associated with higher likelihood of achieving MMR

In patients who develop disease progression while receiving imatinib, reevaluate the option of allogeneic stem cell transplantation and determine eligibility for clinical trial as an alternative switching to alternate TKI

Guilhot F et al. Haematologica 2012;97:731–738
Larson RA et al. Blood 2008;111:4022–4028

INITIAL THERAPY

CHRONIC MYELOID LEUKEMIA REGIMEN: DASATINIB (SECOND-GENERATION TKI)

Kantarjian HM et al. N Engl J Med 2010;362:2260–2270

Chronic phase CML:
Initial dose:
Dasatinib 100 mg/day; administer orally, continually, with or without a meal (total dose/week = 700 mg)
Dose escalation:
Escalate to **dasatinib** 140 mg/day; administer orally, continually, with or without a meal in case of insufficient response (total dose/week = 980 mg)

Accelerated phase and blast crisis CML:
Initial dose:
Dasatinib 140 mg/day; administer orally, continually, with or without meal (total dose/week = 980 mg)

Dose escalation:
Escalate to **dasatinib** 180 mg/day; administer orally, continually, with or without a meal in case of insufficient response (total dose/week = 1260 mg)

Supportive Care
Antiemetic prophylaxis
Emetogenic potential is **MINIMAL–LOW**
See Chapter 42 for antiemetic recommendations

Hematopoietic growth factor (G-CSF) prophylaxis
Primary prophylaxis is **NOT** *indicated*
See Chapter 43 for more information

Antimicrobial prophylaxis
Risk of fever and neutropenia is **LOW**
Antimicrobial primary prophylaxis to be considered:
- Antibacterial—not indicated
- Antifungal—not indicated
- Antiviral—not indicated, unless patient previously had an episode of HSV

Patient Population Studied

Study of patients with newly diagnosed CML in chronic phase treated with dasatinib 100 mg daily (n = 259) compared with imatinib 400 mg daily (n = 260) for frontline treatment by the DASISION trial

Efficacy (Chronic Phase, N = 259)

Confirmed complete cytogenetic response by 12 months	77%
Complete cytogenetic response by 12 months	83%
Major molecular response at any time	52%
Major molecular response by 12 months	46%

Note: Of the 547 patients evaluated for eligibility, 28 were not randomly assigned to a study treatment: 20 patients no longer met the inclusion criteria, 3 refused to participate, and 5 had other reasons. Data for the 519 patients who were randomly assigned (259 in the dasatinib group and 260 in the imatinib group) were included in the analysis of efficacy, and data for 258 in the dasatinib group and 258 in the imatinib group were included in the analysis of safety

Kantarjian HM et al. N Engl J Med 2010;362:2260–2270

Therapy Monitoring

1. *CBC:* Weekly; every 2 weeks after achievement of complete hematologic response; every 4–6 weeks after achievement of a complete cytogenetic response
2. *Blood chemistry:* Weekly; every 4–8 weeks after achievement of complete hematologic response
3. *Quantitative RT-PCR for BCR-ABL from peripheral blood:* Every 3 months until MMR has been achieved, then every 3–6 months
4. *Bone marrow cytogenetics:* Every 3 months until complete cytogenetic response, then at 12- to 24-month intervals (only if no access to reliable qPCR testing or in case of atypical transcripts not measurable by standard qPCR assays)
5. *FISH (peripheral blood):* In case of atypical transcripts, once CCyR has been achieved
6. *ECG and ECHO:* then annually; sooner if indicated

Toxicity (In >10% of Patients, N = 258)

Toxicity	% All Grades	% G3/4
Hematologic AE		
Anemia	90	10
Neutropenia	65	21
Thrombocytopenia	70	19
Nonhematologic AE		
Fluid retention	19	1
Superficial edema	9	0
Pleural effusion	10	0
Fluid retention "other"	5	1
Headache	12	0
Diarrhea	17	<1
Fatigue	8	<1
Nausea	8	0
Vomiting	5	0
Rash	11	0
Myalgia	6	0
Muscle inflammation	4	0
Musculoskeletal pain	11	0

Kantarjian HM et al. N Engl J Med 2010;362:2260–2270

Treatment Modifications

Notes

Hematologic Toxicity: Chronic Phase (No Modifications for Anemia)

G1/2	No dose modifications
ANC <500/mm^3*	Hold dasatinib until ANC ≥1000/mm^3 Recovery within 7 days: resume at 100 mg/day Recovery within >7 days or first recurrence: resume at 80 mg/day Second recurrence: discontinue
Platelet count <50,000/mm^3	Hold dasatinib until platelet count is ≥50,000/mm^3 Recovery within ≤7 days: resume at 100 mg/day Recovery within >7 days or first recurrence: resume at 80 mg/day Second recurrence: discontinue drug
Platelet count <25,000/mm^3	Hold dasatinib until platelet count is ≥50,000/mm^3 and resume at 80 mg/day First recurrence: Hold dasatinib until platelet count is ≥50,000/mm^3 and resume at 80 mg/day Second recurrence: discontinue drug

Hematologic Toxicity: Accelerated or Blastic Phase

G1–3	No dose modifications
G4–first occurrence	If cytopenia is unrelated to leukemia (bone marrow assessment), hold dasatinib until recovery to platelet count ≥20,000/mm^3 and ANC ≥1000/mm^3 and resume at 140 mg/day†
G4–second occurrence	Hold dasatinib until recovery to platelet count ≥20,000/mm^3 and ANC ≥1000/mm^3, and resume at 100 mg/day
G4–third occurrence	Hold dasatinib until recovery to platelet count ≥20,000/mm^3 and ANC ≥1000/mm^3, and resume at 80 mg/day

Nonhematologic Toxicity

G1	No dose modifications
G2/3	Hold dasatinib until toxicity resolves to Grade 1, then restart at 100 mg/day
Recurrent G2/3	Hold dasatinib until toxicity resolves to Grade 1, then restart at 80 mg/day
G4	Hold dasatinib until toxicity resolves to Grade 1, then restart at 80 mg/day
Recurrent G4	Discontinue dasatinib

*Consider filgrastim for persistent neutropenia; consider eltrombopag for persistent thrombocytopenia
†Consider dose escalation to 80 mg/day in case of leukemia-related cytopenia
packageinserts.bms.com/pi/pi_sprycel.pdf (accessed December 2011)

Notes

Fluid retention events (ascites, edema, pleural and pericardial effusion): consider diuretics and supportive care

For pleural/pericardial effusion: in addition to diuretics and dose interruption, consider short course of steroids (prednisone)

Evaluate for pulmonary arterial hypertension (PAH) in case of unexplained dyspnea or chest pain (~3% PAH incidence vs 0% with imatinib, DASSION trial)

In patients who develop disease progression while receiving dasatinib, re-evaluate the option of allogeneic stem cell transplantation and determine eligibility for clinical trial as an alternative to switching to alternate TKI

INITIAL THERAPY

CHRONIC MYELOID LEUKEMIA REGIMEN: NILOTINIB (SECOND-GENERATION TKI)

Saglio G et al. N Engl J Med 2010;362:2251–2259

Chronic phase CML:
Nilotinib 300 mg; administer orally twice daily, continually, at least 2 hours after the last and 1 hour before the next meal

Accelerated phase CML:
Nilotinib 400 mg; administer orally twice daily, continually, at least 2 hours after the last and 1 hour before the next meal

Note: Dose escalation is not indicated

Supportive Care
Antiemetic prophylaxis
Emetogenic potential is **MINIMAL–LOW**
See Chapter 42 for antiemetic recommendations

*Hematopoietic growth factor (**G-CSF**) prophylaxis*
Primary prophylaxis is **NOT** indicated
See Chapter 43 for more information

Antimicrobial prophylaxis
Risk of fever and neutropenia is **LOW**
  Antimicrobial primary prophylaxis to be considered:
  • Antibacterial—not indicated
  • Antifungal—not indicated
  • Antiviral—not indicated, unless patient previously had an episode of HSV

Patient Population Studied

Study of patients with newly diagnosed CML in chronic phase treated with either nilotinib 300 mg BID (n = 282) versus nilotinib 400 mg BID (n = 281) compared to imatinib (n = 283) for frontline treatment by the ENESTnd trial

Efficacy
(Chronic Phase, N = 563)

	Nilotinib 300 mg BID	Nilotinib 400 mg BID
Complete cytogenetic response by 6 months	67%	80%
Complete cytogenetic response by 12 months	63%	78%
Major molecular response by 12 months	44%	43%

Saglio G et al. N Engl J Med 2010;362:2251–2259

Therapy Monitoring

1. *CBC:* Weekly; every 2 weeks after achievement of complete hematologic response; every 4–6 weeks after achievement of a complete cytogenetic response

2. *Blood chemistry:* Weekly; every 4–8 weeks after achievement of complete hematologic response

3. *Quantitative RT-PCR for BCR-ABL from peripheral blood:* Every 3 months until MMR has been achieved, then every 3–6 months

4. *Bone marrow cytogenetics:* Every 3 months until complete cytogenetic response, then at 12- to 24-month intervals (only if no access to reliable qPCR testing or in case of atypical transcripts not measurable by standard qPCR assays)

5. *FISH (peripheral blood):* In case of atypical transcripts, once CCyR has been achieved

6. *ECG and ECHO:* then annually; sooner if indicated; repeat ECG 1 week after initiation on therapy and subsequent resumption of therapy following any treatment interruption or dose escalation

Treatment Modifications

Hematologic Toxicity (No Modifications for Anemia)

G1/2	No dose modifications
G3/4	Hold nilotinib until toxicity resolves to Grade 2. Recovery within 2 weeks: restart at 400 mg twice daily. Recovery within >2 weeks: restart at 400 mg/day

Nonhematologic Toxicity (Noncardiac)

G1/2	No dose modifications
G3/4	Hold nilotinib until toxicity resolves to Grade 1, then restart at 400 mg/day. If tolerated, consider re-escalation to 400 mg twice daily

QT Prolongation

QTcF >480 ms	Hold nilotinib and correct any hypokalemia and/or hypomagnesemia. QTcF <450 ms and within 20 ms of baseline within 2 weeks: resume at 400 mg twice daily. QTcF 450–480 ms: resume at 400 mg/day; if recurrence of QTcF >480 ms, discontinue nilotinib

www.novartis.us/sites/www.novartis.us/files/tasigna.pdf (accessed, December 2011)

Toxicity (In >10% of Patients Treated with 300 mg [n = 279] vs 400 mg [n = 277])

Toxicity	Nilotinib 300 mg BID n = 279	Nilotinib 400 mg BID n = 277	Nilotinib 300 mg BID n = 279	Nilotinib 400 mg BID n = 277
	% All Grades		% G3/4	
Hematologic AE				
Thrombocytopenia	48 vs 49%		10 vs 12%	
Anemia	38 vs 38%		3 vs 3%	
Neutropenia	43 vs 38%		12 vs 10%	
Nonhematologic AE				
Rash	31 vs 36%		<1 vs 3%	
Alopecia	8 vs 13%		0 vs 0%	
Pruritus	15 vs 13%		<1 vs <1%	
Headache	14 vs 21%		1 vs 1%	
Fatigue	11 vs 9%		0 vs 1%	
Diarrhea	8 vs 6%		1 vs 0%	
Vomiting	5 vs 9 %		0 vs 1%	
Nausea	11 vs 19%		<1 vs 1%	
Muscle spasm	7 vs 6%		0 vs 1%	
Myalgia	10 vs 10%		<1 vs 0%	
Peripheral edema	5 vs 5%		0 vs 0%	
Eyelid edema	1 vs 2%		0 vs <1%	
Periorbital edema	<1 vs 1%		0 vs 0%	

Saglio G et al. N Engl J Med 2010;362:2251–2259

Notes

Correct hypokalemia and hypophosphatemia before initiating nilotinib therapy and monitor serum electrolytes during nilotinib treatment

Monitor ECG for QT prolongation at baseline, within 7 days after initiating therapy or when changing the dose, and periodically thereafter

Use the Fridericia correction of the QT interval (QTcF) for all calculations

Monitor and minimize cardiovascular risk factors (HbA1c; lipid panel, blood pressure); annual ankle-brachial index (ABI) testing is recommended

In patients who develop disease progression while receiving nilotinib, reevaluate the option of allogeneic stem cell transplantation and determine eligibility for clinical trial as an alternative to switching to alternate TKI

INITIAL THERAPY

CHRONIC MYELOID LEUKEMIA REGIMEN: BOSUTINIB (SECOND-GENERATION TKI)

Cortes JE et al. J Clin Oncol 2018;36:231–237

Newly diagnosed chronic phase CML:
Bosutinib 400 mg/day; administer orally with food, continually

Accelerated or blast-phase CML with resistance or intolerance to prior therapy:
Bosutinib 500 mg/day; administer orally with food, continually

Notes:

1. If a dose is missed by more than 12 hours, the patient should skip the dose and resume taking the usual prescribed dose on the following day

2. Consider dose escalations to 500 mg or 600 mg once daily with food in patients who do not reach complete hematologic response (CHR) by week 8 or a complete cytogenetic response (CCyR) by week 12, and who did not have G ≥3 adverse reactions

3. *Use in case of hepatic impairment:* In patients with pre-existing mild, moderate, and severe hepatic impairment (Child-Pugh classes A, B, and C, respectively), the recommended dose of bosutinib is 200 mg daily. A daily dose of 200 mg in patients with hepatic impairment is predicted to result in systemic exposure (area under the concentration curve; AUC) similar to the AUC seen in patients with normal hepatic function receiving 500 mg daily. However, there are no clinical data for efficacy at the dose of 200 mg once daily in patients with hepatic impairment and CML

Supportive Care

Antiemetic prophylaxis
Emetogenic potential is **MINIMAL–LOW**
See Chapter 42 for antiemetic recommendations

Hematopoietic growth factor (G-CSF) prophylaxis
Primary prophylaxis is **NOT** indicated
See Chapter 43 for more information

Antimicrobial prophylaxis
Risk of fever and neutropenia is **LOW**
  Antimicrobial primary prophylaxis to be considered:
  • Antibacterial—not indicated
  • Antifungal—not indicated
  • Antiviral—not indicated, unless patient previously had an episode of HSV

Patient Population Studied

Study of patients with newly diagnosed CML in chronic phase treated with bosutinib 400 mg daily (n = 246) compared with imatinib 400 mg daily (n = 241) for frontline treatment by the BFORE trial

Efficacy (Chronic Phase, N = 268)

Major molecular response at 12 months	47%
Complete cytogenetic response by 12 months	77%

Cortes JE et al. J Clin Oncol 2018;36:231–237

Treatment Monitoring

1. *CBC:* Weekly; every 2 weeks after achievement of complete hematologic response; every 4–6 weeks after achievement of a complete cytogenetic response

2. *Blood chemistry:* Weekly; every 4–8 weeks after achievement of complete hematologic response

3. *Quantitative RT-PCR for BCR-ABL from peripheral blood:* Every 3 months until MMR has been achieved, then every 3–6 months

4. *Bone marrow cytogenetics:* Every 3 months until complete cytogenetic response, then at 12- to 24-month intervals (only if no access to reliable qPCR testing or in case of atypical transcripts not measurable by standard qPCR assays)

5. *FISH (peripheral blood):* In case of atypical transcripts, once CCyR has been achieved

6. *ECG and ECHO:* then annually; sooner if indicated

Treatment Modifications

Adverse Event	Treatment Modification
AST/ALT >5× ULN	Withhold bosutinib until AST/ALT ≤2.5 × ULN, then resume use at 400 mg once daily
AST/ALT >5× ULN >4 weeks	Discontinue bosutinib
AST/ALT ≤3× ULN concurrently with bilirubin elevations >2× ULN and alkaline phosphatase <2× ULN (Hy's law case definition)	Discontinue bosutinib
G3/4 diarrhea (≥7 stools/day over baseline/ pretreatment)	Withhold bosutinib until recovery to G ≤1 and resume at 400 mg once daily
Other G3/4 nonhematologic toxicity	Withhold bosutinib until recovery to G ≤1, then resume use at 400 mg once daily. If clinically appropriate, consider re-escalating the dose of bosutinib to 500 mg once daily
First episode of ANC <1000 × 10^6/L or platelets <50,000 × 10^6/L with recovery in <2 weeks	Withhold bosutinib until ANC ≥1000 × 10^6/L and platelets ≥50,000 × 10^6/L. Resume treatment with bosutinib at the same dose
Second episode of ANC <1000 × 10^6/L or platelets <50,000 × 10^6/L with recovery in <2 weeks	Withhold bosutinib until ANC ≥1000 × 10^6/L and platelets ≥50,000 × 10^6/L then resume bosutinib at a dose 100 mg less than the dose previously administered
ANC <1000 × 10^6/L or platelets <50,000 × 10^6/L with recovery in <2 weeks	Withhold bosutinib until ANC ≥1000 × 10^6/L and platelets ≥50,000 × 10^6/L, then resume bosutinib use at a dose 100 mg less than the dose previously administered
Fluid retention (pericardial effusion, pleural effusion, pulmonary edema, and/or peripheral edema)	Monitor and manage patients using standards of care. Interrupt, decrease the dose, or discontinue bosutinib as necessary

Adverse Events

Newly diagnosed patients with chronic phase CML

Cortes JE et al. J Clin Oncol 2018;36:231–237

Grade (%)*	Bosutinib N = 268	
	Grade 1/2	Grade 3–5
Gastrointestinal	71	11
Diarrhea	62	8
Nausea	35	0
Vomiting	17	1
Abdominal pain	16	2
Hematologic AEs	29	16
Thrombocytopenia	21	14
Anemia	15	3
Neutropenia	4	7
Leukopenia	4	1
Musculoskeletal	28	2
Muscle spasms	2	0
Arthralgia	10	1
Myalgia	3	<1
Pain in extremity	4	<1
Infections	41	3
Upper respiratory tract infection	8	<1
Liver function	16	24
ALT increased	12	19
AST increased	13	10
Fatigue	19	<1
Rash	19	<1

Grade (%)*	Bosutinib N = 268	
	Grade 1/2	Grade 3–5
Headache	18	1
Lipase increased	4	10
Pyrexia	12	1
Peripheral edema	4	0
Asthenia	11	0
Periorbital edema	1	0
Decreased appetite	10	<1
ALT increased	40	23
AST increased	37	12
Increased amylase	23	2
Decreased calcium	24	1
Increased creatine kinase	27	1
Increased creatinine[‡]	93	0
Increased glucose	44	2
Decreased potassium	6	1
Increased lipase	26	13
Decreased phosphate	39	4
Decreased hemoglobin[§]	80	7
Decreased ANC	31	9
Decreased platelets	53	14
Decreased leukocytes	44	6

Notes

Consider slow upward dose titration to improve tolerability with treatment initiation on bosutinib; 100 mg/day × 1 week, then increase by 100 mg/day per week until reaching desired dose

Transaminitis (increase in AST and/or ALT) occurs in ~20% patients. In patients with pre-existing mild, moderate, and severe hepatic impairment, the recommended dose of bosutinib is 200 mg daily

In patients who develop disease progression while receiving bosutinib, the option of allogeneic stem cell transplantation should be reevaluated as well as eligibility for clinical trial in addition to consideration for switching to alternate TKI

SUBSEQUENT THERAPY

CHRONIC MYELOID LEUKEMIA REGIMEN: PONATINIB (ICLUSIG; THIRD-GENERATION TKI)

Cortes JE et al. N Engl J Med 2012;367:2075–2088
Cortes JE et al. Blood 2018;132:393–404

PACE was a single-arm, open-label, international, multicenter, phase 2 trial in adult patients with CML or Ph⁺ ALL who were resistant or intolerant to dasatinib or nilotinib, or who had the T315I mutation regardless of prior TKI use (N = 449; n = 270 CP-CML, n = 85 APCML, n = 62 BPCML, n = 32 Ph⁺ ALL). Five-year results reflect data analysis as of 6 February 2017, with median follow-up of 37.3 months for all patients and 56.8 months (range, 0.1–73.1 months) for CP-CML patients

Chronic-, accelerated-, or blast-phase CML: patients for whom no other TKI therapy is indicated or who have the T315I mutation
Chronic-phase CML:
Ponatinib hydrochloride 30 mg/day; administer orally with or without food, continually for 28 consecutive days, on days 1–28, every 4 weeks (total dose/28-day cycle = 840 mg). Consider dose modification in older patient population, especially patients with increased cardiovascular risk and based on response and tolerance

Accelerated- and blast-phase CML:
Ponatinib hydrochloride 45 mg/day; administer orally with or without food, continually for 28 consecutive days, on days 1–28, every 4 weeks (total dose/28-day cycle = 1260 mg)

Notes:
- On the basis of safety, pharmacokinetic, and pharmacodynamic data, 45 mg of ponatinib was determined to be the maximum tolerated dose
- The optimal dose of ponatinib has not been identified. In clinical trials, the starting dose of ponatinib was 45 mg administered orally once daily. However, 59% of the patients required dose reductions to 30 mg or 15 mg once daily during the course of therapy
- More safety information will become available when an ongoing trial (OPTIC) is completed

Notes:
- Consider starting patients on 30 mg once daily. Although the starting dose according to package insert is 45 mg once daily, it is common to start patients on 30 mg once daily for better tolerability
- Consider reducing the dose of ponatinib for CP CML and AP CML patients who have achieved a major cytogenetic response
- Reduce to 15 mg once daily when administering ponatinib with strong CYP3A subfamily inhibitors

Supportive Care
Antiemetic prophylaxis
Emetogenic potential is **MINIMAL**
See Chapter 42 for antiemetic recommendations

Hematopoietic growth factor (G-CSF) prophylaxis
Primary prophylaxis is **NOT** indicated
See Chapter 43 for more information

Antimicrobial prophylaxis
Risk of fever and neutropenia is **LOW**
   Antimicrobial primary prophylaxis to be considered:
- Antibacterial—not indicated
- Antifungal—not indicated
- Antiviral—not indicated unless patient previously had an episode of HSV

Patient Population Studied

Patients with a diagnosis of CML whose disease had relapsed or was resistant to standard care, or for which no standard care was available or acceptable. Ph-positive disease was classified and characterized as relapsed or refractory disease on the basis of standard criteria. In addition, patients were required to have an Eastern Cooperative Oncology Group performance status of 2 or lower

Study of patients with CML in chronic phase or Philadelphia chromosome–positive ALL resistant or intolerant to dasatinib or nilotinib or with T315I mutation treated by ponatinib on the phase 2 PACE trial (N = 449)

N = 449	Resistant or intolerant to dasatinib or nilotinib (n = 203) vs T315I mutation regardless of prior TKI use (n = 64)			
	Chronic Phase (n = 270)	Accelerated Phase (n = 85)	Blast Phase (n = 62)	Ph⁺ ALL (n = 32)

Efficacy (Chronic Phase, N = 267)

Major molecular response at any time during the 5-year study	40%
4.0-log molecular response	30%
4.5-log molecular response	24%
Complete cytogenetic response at any time during the 5-year study	54%
Major cytogenetic response at any time during the 5-year study	60%

Median follow-up was 37.3 months for all patients and 56.8 months (range, 0.1–73.1 months) for CP-CML patients

	Accelerated Phase (n = 85)	Blast Phase (n = 62)	Ph+ ALL (n = 32)
MaCHR	61%	31%	41%
CHR	55%	21%	34%
MCyR	49%	23%	47%
CCyR	31%	18%	NA
MMR	22%	NA	NA

Cortes JE et al. Blood 2018;132:393–404

Treatment Monitoring

1. *CBC:* Weekly; during the first 3 cycles after starting ponatinib, and every second week during subsequent cycles thereafter
2. *Blood chemistry including pancreatic enzymes:* at baseline and weekly during the first 2 cycles, then every second week during subsequent cycles
3. *Quantitative RT-PCR for BCR-ABL1 from peripheral blood:* Every 3 months
4. *Bone marrow cytogenetics:* Every 3 months until complete cytogenetic response, then at 12- to 24-month intervals (only if no access to reliable qPCR testing or in case of atypical transcripts not measurable by standard qPCR assays)
5. *FISH (peripheral blood):* In case of atypical transcripts, once CCyR has been achieved
6. *ECG and ECHO:* then annually; sooner if indicated
7. Optimization and reduction of CV risk factors

Note: Monitor patients with accelerated or blast phase more frequently as clinically indicated

Treatment Modifications

Adverse Event	Treatment Modification
First arterial thrombotic event	Interrupt and consider discontinuation of ponatinib
Second arterial thrombotic event	Discontinue ponatinib
First episode of G3/4 hepatotoxicity	Interrupt and then reduce or discontinue ponatinib
Second episode of G3/4 hepatotoxicity	Discontinue ponatinib
First occurrence of ANC <1 × 10^9/L or platelet <50 × 10^9/L	Interrupt ponatinib and resume initial 45-mg dose after recovery to ANC ≥1.5 × 10^9/L and platelet ≥75 × 10^9/L
Second occurrence of ANC <1 × 10^9/L or platelet <50 × 10^9/L	Interrupt ponatinib and resume at 30 mg after recovery to ANC ≥1.5 × 10^9/L and platelet ≥75 × 10^9/L
Third occurrence of ANC <1 × 10^9/L or platelet <50 × 10^9/L	Interrupt ponatinib and resume at 15 mg after recovery to ANC ≥1.5 × 10^9/L and platelet ≥75 × 10^9/L
Elevation of liver transaminase >3 × ULN (G ≥2) at a ponatinib dose of 45 mg	Discontinue ponatinib and monitor hepatic function. Resume ponatinib at 30 mg after recovery to G ≤1 (<3 × ULN)
Elevation of liver transaminase >3 × ULN (G ≥2) at a ponatinib dose of 30 mg	Discontinue ponatinib and monitor hepatic function. Resume ponatinib at 15 mg after recovery to G ≤1 (<3 × ULN)
Elevation of liver transaminase >3 × ULN (G ≥2) at a ponatinib dose of 15 mg	Discontinue ponatinib
Elevation of liver transaminase >3 × ULN (G ≥2) concurrent with an elevation of bilirubin >2 × ULN and alkaline phosphatase <2 × ULN	Discontinue ponatinib
Asymptomatic G1/2 elevation of serum lipase	Consider interruption or dose reduction of ponatinib

(continued)

Treatment Modifications (*continued*)

Adverse Event	Treatment Modification
Asymptomatic G3/4 elevation of lipase (>2 × ULN) or asymptomatic radiologic pancreatitis (G2 pancreatitis) at a ponatinib dose of 45 mg	Interrupt ponatinib and resume at 30 mg after recovery to G ≤1 (<1.5 × ULN)
Asymptomatic G3/4 elevation of lipase (>2 × ULN) or asymptomatic radiologic pancreatitis (G2 pancreatitis) at a ponatinib dose of 30 mg	Interrupt ponatinib and resume at 15 mg after recovery to G ≤1 (<1.5 × ULN)
Asymptomatic G3/4 elevation of lipase (>2 × ULN) or asymptomatic radiologic pancreatitis (G2 pancreatitis) at a ponatinib dose of 15 mg	Discontinue ponatinib
Symptomatic G3 pancreatitis at a ponatinib dose of 45 mg	Interrupt ponatinib and resume at 30 mg after complete resolution of symptoms and after recovery of lipase elevation to G ≤1
Symptomatic G3 pancreatitis at a ponatinib dose of 30 mg	Interrupt ponatinib and resume at 15 mg after complete resolution of symptoms and after recovery of lipase elevation to G ≤1
Symptomatic G3 pancreatitis at a ponatinib dose of 15 mg	Discontinue ponatinib
G4 pancreatitis	Discontinue ponatinib

Notes:
Arterial thrombosis: Cardiovascular, cerebrovascular, and peripheral vascular thrombosis, including fatal myocardial infarction and stroke, have occurred in ponatinib-treated patients. In clinical trials, serious arterial thrombosis occurred in 8% of ponatinib-treated patients. Interrupt and consider discontinuation of ponatinib in patients who develop arterial thrombotic events
Hepatic toxicity: Hepatotoxicity, liver failure, and death have occurred in ponatinib-treated patients. Monitor hepatic function prior to and during treatment. Interrupt and then reduce or discontinue ponatinib for hepatotoxicity

Toxicity (In >20% of Patients, N = 449)

N = 449	Resistant or intolerant to dasatinib or nilotinib (n = 203) or T315I mutation regardless of prior TKI use (n = 64)			
	Chronic Phase (n = 270)	Accelerated Phase (n = 85)	Blast Phase (n = 62)	Ph⁺ ALL (n = 32)

	Any Grade	Grade 3/4	Any Grade	Grade 3/4	Any Grade	Grade 3/4	Any Grade	Grade 3/4
	CP-CML n = 270		AP-CML n = 85		BP-CML n = 62		Ph⁺ ALL n = 32	
Nonhematologic AE								
Arthralgia	33 vs 3%		34 vs 2%		19 vs 0%		13 vs 0%	
Increased lipase	27 vs 13%		15 vs 13%		15 vs 13%		9 vs 6%	
Fatigue	30 vs 2%		38 vs 5%		26 vs 5%		28 vs 0%	
Rash*	47 vs 4%		38 vs 5%		35 vs 5%		22 vs 3%	
Dry skin	42 vs 3%		32 vs 1%		26 vs 2%		25 vs 0%	
Pyrexia	26 vs 1%		40 vs 7%		37 vs 3%		25 vs 0%	
Diarrhea	20 vs ≤1%		29 vs 2%		24 vs 3%		13 vs 3%	
Vomiting	19 vs 1%		27 vs 0%		27 vs 2%		25 vs 0%	
Constipation	41 vs 3%		29 vs 2%		27 vs 0%		53 vs 3%	
Nausea	29 vs ≤1%		32 vs 0%		34 vs 2%		22 vs 0%	
Headache	43 vs 3%		31 vs 1%		31 vs 3%		25 vs 0%	
Hypertension†	37 vs 14%		26 vs 11%		21 vs 8%		25 vs 9%	

(*continued*)

Toxicity (In >20% of Patients, N = 449) *(continued)*

	Any Grade	Grade 3/4	Any Grade	Grade 3/4	Any Grade	Grade 3/4	Any Grade	Grade 3/4
	CP-CML n = 270		AP-CML n = 85		BP-CML n = 62		Ph⁺ ALL n = 32	
Nonhematologic AE								
Myalgia	24 vs 1%		21 vs 0%		18 vs 0%		6 vs 0%	
Pain in extremity	24 vs 3%		20 vs 0%		13 vs 0%		13 vs 0%	
Abdominal pain	46 vs 10%		42 vs 8%		34 vs 8%		31 vs 6%	
Hematologic AE								
Thrombocytopenia	46 vs 35%		53 vs 44%		37 vs 35%		22 vs 19%	
Neutropenia	20 vs 17%		37 vs 37%		35 vs 29%		25 vs 22%	
Anemia	20 vs 10%		37 vs 22%		34 vs 32%		25 vs 19%	

*Combines the terms erythematous, macular, and popular rash
†At baseline, 379 of 449 patients (84%) had elevated blood pressure (212 of 449 [47%] had blood pressure ≥140/90 mmHg); 307 of 449 patients (68%) experienced any increase from baseline in blood pressure on study

Notes:
Patients on ponatinib are at significant risk of vascular occlusive events and hypertension. Minimizing risk factors, careful monitoring, and prompt management of adverse events are mandatory. Risks and benefits of ponatinib must be weighed carefully and discussed with patients, depending on cardiovascular risk profile and disease risk. The U.S. Food and Drug Administration (FDA) and the European Medicines Agency have published warnings and recommendations regarding the use of ponatinib. The FDA has determined vascular occlusion events in the phase 2 (PACE) study as shown below. Careful cardiovascular monitoring is part of the ongoing OPTIC trial that compares 45 vs 30 vs 15 mg ponatinib daily and will clarify the incidence of cardiovascular toxicity according to dose and with stringent pre-specified criteria

Vascular Occlusion Incidence in Ponatinib-Treated Patients in Phase 2 Trial According to Risk Categories

	Prior History of Ischemia, Hypertension, Diabetes, or Hyperlipidemia	No History of Ischemia, Hypertension, Diabetes, or Hyperlipidemia
Age: 49 or younger	18% (6/33)	12% (13/112)
Age: 50 to 74 years	33% (50/152)	18% (20/114)
Age: 75 and older	56% (14/25)	46% (6/13)
All age groups	33% (70/210)	16% (39/239)
Total	24% (109/449)	

- All BCR-ABL1 TKIs, with the exception of imatinib, increase cardiovascular risk
- Monitoring recommendations are available from several publications, including Moslehi JJ, Deininger M. J Clin Oncol 2015;33:4210–4218

(continued)

Toxicity (In >20% of Patients, N = 449) (*continued*)

Provisional recommendations for cardiovascular/cardiometabolic follow-up of patients on BCR-ABL1 TKIs (adapted from Moslehi JJ, Deininger M. J Clin Oncol 2015;33:4210–4218)

		Imatinib	Nilotinib	Dasatinib	Bosutinib	Ponatinib
Baseline	Clinical cardiovascular assessment, including BP	Follow good clinical practice	REC	REC	REC	REC
	Fasting glucose		REC	ACI	ACI	REC
	Fasting lipid panel		REC	ACI	ACI	REC
	Echocardiogram		ACI	ACI	ACI	ACI
	ECG		REC*	REC	ACI	ACI
	Ankle-brachial index		REC	ACI	ACI	REC
1-month follow-up	Clinical cardiovascular assessment		REC	REC	ACI	REC
	Blood pressure check		ACI	ACI	ACI	REC
3- to 6-month follow-up	Clinical cardiovascular assessment		REC	REC	REC	REC
	Blood pressure check		REC	ACI	ACI	REC
	Fasting glucose		REC	ACI	ACI	ACI
	Fasting lipid panel		REC	ACI	ACI	REC
	Echocardiogram		ACI*	ACI	ACI	ACI
	ECG		ACI*	ACI	ACI	ACI
	Ankle-brachial index		REC	ACI	ACI	REC

ACI, as clinically indicated; REC, recommended
*ECG prior to starting, after 7 days after starting and after each dose change (package insert)

Note: Practice guidelines regarding prevention of cardiovascular toxicity should be followed, including tobacco cessation counseling. In symptomatic patients or those with high cardiovascular risk, consider referral to cardiologist

SUBSEQUENT THERAPY

CHRONIC MYELOID LEUKEMIA REGIMEN: OMACETAXINE MEPESUCCINATE

Cortes J et al. Am J Hematol 2013;88:350–354
Cortes J et al. Blood 2012;120:2573–2580

Chronic- or accelerated-phase chronic CML with resistance and/or intolerance to 2 or more tyrosine kinase inhibitors (TKIs):

Omacetaxine mepesuccinate 1.25 mg/m^2 per dose by subcutaneous injection:
Induction regimen schedule
Doses are given twice daily for 14 consecutive days, on days 1–14, every 28 days until patients achieve a hematologic response (total dosage/28-day cycle = 35 mg/m^2)

Maintenance regimen schedule
Doses are given twice daily for 7 consecutive days, on days 1–7, every 28 days for as long as patients experience clinical benefit from treatment (total dosage/28-day cycle = 17.5 mg/m^2)

Supportive Care
Antiemetic prophylaxis
*Emetogenic potential is **LOW***
See Chapter 42 for antiemetic recommendations

*Hematopoietic growth factor (**G-CSF**) prophylaxis*
Primary prophylaxis may be indicated
See Chapter 43 for more information

Antimicrobial prophylaxis
*Risk of fever and neutropenia is **LOW***
  Antimicrobial primary prophylaxis to be considered:
  • Antibacterial—not indicated
  • Antifungal—not indicated
  • Antiviral—not indicated unless patient previously had an episode of HSV

Patient Population Studied

The efficacy of omacetaxine mepesuccinate was evaluated using a combined cohort of adult patients with CML from two trials. The combined cohort consisted of patients who had received two or more approved TKIs and had, at a minimum, documented evidence of resistance or intolerance to dasatinib and/or nilotinib. Resistance was defined as one of the following: no complete hematologic response (CHR) by 12 weeks (whether lost or never achieved); or no cytogenetic response by 24 weeks (ie, 100% Ph$^+$) (whether lost or never achieved); or no major cytogenetic response (MCyR) by 52 weeks (ie, ≥35% Ph$^+$) (whether lost or never achieved); or progressive leukocytosis. Intolerance was defined as 1 of the following: (1) G3/4 nonhematologic toxicity that did not resolve with adequate intervention; (2) G4 hematologic toxicity lasting more than 7 days; or (3) any G ≥2 toxicity unacceptable to the patient. Patients with NYHA class III or IV heart disease, active ischemia, or other uncontrolled cardiac conditions were excluded

A total of 76 patients with chronic-phase CML were included in the efficacy analysis. The demographics were as follows: median age 59 years, and 30% were 65 years of age or older. All had previously received two or more TKIs, including imatinib. Thirty-six patients (47%) had failed treatment with imatinib, dasatinib, and nilotinib. Most patients had also received prior non-TKI treatments, most commonly hydroxyurea (54%), interferon (30%), and/or cytarabine (29%)

Efficacy

The accelerated FDA approval was based on combined data from two open-label single-arm trials enrolling patients with CML in chronic phase (CML-CP) or in accelerated phase (CML-AP). The efficacy population included 76 patients with CML-CP who had received two or more prior TKIs, including imatinib

Efficacy Results for Patients with CP CML

The efficacy end point was based on MCyR

	Patients (N = 76)
Primary response—MCyR	
Total with MCyR, n (%)	14 (18.4)
95% confidence interval	(10.5–29)
Cytogenetic response, n (%)	
Confirmed complete	6 (7.9)
Confirmed partial	3 (3.9)
Mean time to MCyR onset (n = 14)	3.5 months
Median duration of MCyR (n = 14)	12.5 months (Kaplan-Meier estimate)

Cytogenetic response evaluation is based on standard cytogenetic analysis (at least 20 metaphases)
Complete: no Ph$^+$ cells; partial: >0 to 35% Ph$^+$ cells

Treatment Monitoring

1. *CBC:* Weekly during induction and initial maintenance cycles

2. After initial maintenance cycles, monitor CBCs every 2 weeks, or as clinically indicated

3. *Blood chemistry:* particularly monitor blood glucose concentrations frequently especially in patients with diabetes or risk factors for diabetes

4. *Quantitative RT-PCR for BCR-ABL from peripheral blood or bone marrow:* Every 3–6 months

5. *Bone marrow cytogenetics:* Every 3 months until complete cytogenetic response, then at 12- to 24-month intervals (only if no access to reliable qPCR testing or in case of atypical transcripts not measurable by standard qPCR assays)

Treatment Modifications

G4 neutropenia (ANC <0.5 × 10⁹/L) or G3 thrombocytopenia (<50 × 10⁹/L) during a cycle	Delay start of next cycle until ANC ≥1 × 10⁹/L and platelet count ≥50 × 10⁹/L. Also, for the next cycle, reduce the number of dosing days by 2 days (eg, to 12 or 5 days)
G3/4 Nonhematologic toxicity	Interrupt and/or delay omacetaxine mepesuccinate until toxicity is G ≤1. Also, for the next cycle, reduce the number of dosing days by 2 days (eg, to 12 or 5 days)
G2 AE unresponsive to supportive care	Interrupt treatment until G ≤1, then resume omacetaxine mepesuccinate at full dose
G ≥3 AE unresponsive to supportive care	Interrupt treatment until G ≤1 then resume omacetaxine mepesuccinate, reducing the number of treatment days by 2 in subsequent cycles

Toxicity

Adverse Reactions Occurring in at Least 10% of Patients (Chronic Myeloid Leukemia—Chronic Phase)

Adverse Reaction	Number (%) of Patients (N = 108)	
	All Reactions	G3/4 Reactions
Patients with ≥1 commonly occurring adverse reaction	107 (99)	94 (87)
Blood and lymphatic system disorders		
Thrombocytopenia	80 (74)	72 (67)
Anemia	66 (61)	39 (36)
Neutropenia	54 (50)	49 (45)
Lymphopenia	18 (17)	17 (16)
Bone marrow failure	11 (10)	11 (10)
Febrile neutropenia	11 (10)	11 (10)
Gastrointestinal disorders		
Diarrhea	45 (42)	1 (1)
Nausea	35 (32)	1 (1)
Constipation	16 (15)	0
Abdominal pain, upper	15 (14)	0
Vomiting	13 (12)	0
General disorders and administration-site conditions		
Fatigue	28 (26)	5 (5)
Pyrexia	26 (24)	1 (1)
Asthenia	25 (23)	1 (1)
Edema peripheral	14 (13)	0
Infusion and injection site–related reactions	37 (34)	0
Infections and infestations		
Bacterial, viral, fungal, and nonspecified infections	50 (46)	12 (11)
Musculoskeletal and connective tissue disorders		
Arthralgia	20 (19)	1 (1)
Pain in extremity	14 (13)	1 (1)
Back pain	12 (11)	2 (2)
Nervous system disorders		
Headache	20 (19)	1 (1)
Psychiatric disorders		
Insomnia	11 (10)	0
Respiratory, thoracic, and mediastinal disorders		
Cough	17 (16)	1 (1)
Epistaxis	16 (15)	1 (1)
Skin and subcutaneous tissue disorders		
Alopecia	16 (15)	0
Rash	11 (10)	0

Note: Safety data were evaluated in 163 patients, including 108 patients with CML-CP and 55 patients with CML-AP who received at least 1 dose of omacetaxine mepesuccinate and an additional 4 patients with CML-CP from another open-label, single-arm trial. Ten deaths were reported within 30 days after the last omacetaxine mepesuccinate dose. Four of these were attributed to progressive disease, 4 to cerebral hemorrhage, 1 to multiorgan failure, and 1 to unknown causes

SUBSEQUENT THERAPY

CHRONIC MYELOID LEUKEMIA REGIMEN: HYDROXYUREA

Hehlmann R et al. Blood 1994;84:4064–4077

Starting dose: **Hydroxyurea** 40 mg/kg; administer orally after meals, continually, as a single daily dose or divided into 2 doses (total dosage/week (initially) = 280 mg/kg)

1. Optimal dose is determined **empirically**, with very frequent monitoring of CBC (eg, every 3 days)

2. A dose of 1000–2000 mg/day is frequently sufficient for patients with WBC <100,000/mm^3. With higher WBCs and a need to rapidly lower WBC, hydroxyurea 6000–8000 mg/day may be required initially

3. Total daily dose depends on disease activity and is extremely variable (range: hydroxyurea 500–15,000 mg/day)

4. Therapeutic goal is normalization of the WBC (target: 5000–10,000/mm^3). This may require significantly higher or lower doses than the initial dose. If response is insufficient, aggressiveness of dose escalation must match aggressiveness of the disease. Frequent monitoring of WBC is mandatory during changes to the regimen

   a. Slowly rising WBC or failure to achieve therapeutic target: increase total daily hydroxyurea dose 25–50%, assess effect after 5–7 days before further escalation

   b. Rapidly rising WBC: increase total daily hydroxyurea dose by 50–100%, assess effect of dose increase for 3 days before further dose escalation

5. Very high doses carry a risk of prolonged aplasia

Supportive Care
Antiemetic prophylaxis
Emetogenic potential is **MINIMAL–LOW**
See Chapter 42 for antiemetic recommendations

Hematopoietic growth factor (G-CSF) prophylaxis
Primary prophylaxis is **NOT** *indicated*
See Chapter 43 for more information

Antimicrobial prophylaxis
Risk of fever and neutropenia is **LOW**
Antimicrobial primary prophylaxis to be considered:
- Antibacterial—not indicated
- Antifungal—not indicated
- Antiviral—not indicated, unless patient previously had an episode of HSV

Patient Population Studied

Study of 194 patients with newly diagnosed CML in chronic phase

Efficacy (N = 194)

5-year survival: 45%

Therapy Monitoring

1. *CBC:* Initially, at least weekly, then every 2–4 weeks after achieving stable blood counts
2. *Blood chemistry profile:* Every 6 months

Treatment Modifications

Hematologic Toxicity	
G1	No dose modifications. G1 WBC or ANC are acceptable or even desirable
G2 or G3	Hold hydroxyurea until toxicity resolves to G1, then restart at 75% of initial dose
Recurrent G2/3	Hold hydroxyurea until toxicity resolves to G1, then restart at 50% of initial dose
G4	Hold hydroxyurea until toxicity resolves to G1, then restart at 25% of initial dose
Recurrent G4	Hold hydroxyurea until toxicity resolves to G1, then restart at 50% of the previous dose

Nonhematologic Toxicity	
G1	No dose modifications
G2/3	Hold hydroxyurea until toxicity resolves to G1, then restart at initial dose
Recurrent G2/3	Hold hydroxyurea until toxicity resolves to G1, then restart at 75% of initial dose
G4	Hold hydroxyurea until toxicity resolves to G1, then restart at 50% of dose previously administered
Recurrent G4	Discontinue hydroxyurea

Toxicity

Hematologic side effects
1. Neutropenia and anemia are common, whereas thrombocytopenia is rare*
2. Cytopenias are usually rapidly reversible (within 3–4 days)
3. High doses and/or failure to interrupt treatment despite cytopenia may result in prolonged aplasia

Relatively common nonhematologic side effects
1. Gastrointestinal symptoms (stomatitis, anorexia, nausea, vomiting, diarrhea)
2. Acute skin reactions (rash, ulceration, dermatomyositis-like changes, erythema)

Rare, nonhematologic side effects
1. Chronic skin reactions (hyperpigmentation, atrophy of skin and nails, skin cancer, alopecia)
2. Headache, drowsiness, convulsions
3. Fever, chills, asthenia
4. Renal and hepatic impairment

Important note: A comprehensive and detailed analysis of nonhematologic toxicity from a controlled trial is not available

Notes

Hydroxyurea is the drug of choice when a rapid reduction of the white cell count is clinically mandated but the diagnosis of BCR-ABL-positive CML has not been established

Hydroxyurea may be indicated in cases of TKI intolerance or resistance

SUBSEQUENT THERAPY

CHRONIC MYELOID LEUKEMIA REGIMEN: INTERFERON

Baccarani M et al. Blood 2002;99:1527–1535
Hehlmann R et al. Blood 1994;84:4064–4077
Michallet M et al. Leukemia 2004:18;309–315

Premedication:
Acetaminophen 500–650 mg/dose; administer orally, every 4–6 hours as needed

Target dose of interferon α:
Interferon α-2a 5 million IU/m² per day; administer subcutaneously, continually (preferably at bedtime) (total dosage/week = 35 million IU/m²)

or

Interferon α-2b 5 million IU/m² per day; administer subcutaneously, continually (preferably at bedtime) (total dosage/week = 35 million IU/m²)

Typical dose of interferon α:
5 million IU/m² per day. To increase tolerability, interferon α should be started at low doses (eg, 1.5 million IU/m² per day) with gradual increases over several weeks until the target dose is achieved

Alternative formulation, polyethylene glycol–modified rINF-α2b (peginterferon α-2b): approved for the treatment of hepatitis C and adjuvant treatment for melanoma but may be considered off label for CML

Typical dose of peginterferon α-2b:
1.5 mcg/kg/week; administered subcutaneously, intramuscularly, or intravenously. The volume of peginterferon α-2b to be injected depends on the strength of peginterferon α-2b and the patient's body weight. In a phase 1 study, 6-mcg/kg/week dosing was considered a safe alternative to patients with CML who failed interferon α

Talpaz M, et al. Blood 2001; 2001:98;1708–1713

Supportive Care
Antiemetic prophylaxis
Emetogenic potential is **MINIMAL–LOW**
See Chapter 42 for antiemetic recommendations

Hematopoietic growth factor (G-CSF) prophylaxis
Primary prophylaxis is **NOT** indicated
See Chapter 43 for more information

Antimicrobial prophylaxis
Risk of fever and neutropenia is **LOW**
  Antimicrobial primary prophylaxis to be considered:
  • Antibacterial—not indicated
  • Antifungal—not indicated
  • Antiviral—not indicated, unless patient previously had an episode of HSV

Patient Population Studied

Patients with newly diagnosed CML in chronic phase treated with interferon α: n = 263

Baccarani M et al. Blood 2002;99:1527–1535

Efficacy (N = 263)

Complete or partial hematologic response	74%
Complete cytogenetic response	7.6%
Partial cytogenetic response	10.3%
5-year survival	65%

Baccarani M et al. Blood 2002;99:1527–1535

Therapy Monitoring

1. *CBC:* Weekly; every 3–4 weeks after achievement of complete hematologic response, if counts are stable; every 4–6 weeks after achievement of complete cytogenetic response
2. *Blood chemistry:* Twice weekly; every 4–6 weeks after achievement of complete hematologic response
3. *Quantitative RT-PCR for BCR-ABL from peripheral blood or bone marrow:* Every 3–6 months
4. *Bone marrow cytogenetics:* Every 3 months until complete cytogenetic response, then at 12- to 24-month intervals (only if no access to reliable qPCR testing or in case of atypical transcripts not measurable by standard qPCR assays)
5. *FISH (peripheral blood):* In case of atypical transcripts, once CCyR has been achieved

Treatment Modifications

The practical management of patients receiving interferon α is complex. The simplified dose modification schema shown below is only a minimal guideline

Nonhematologic Toxicity

G1	No dose reduction
G2	Reduce interferon α dosage by 25%
G3/4	Stop interferon α. Restart at 50% of the previously administered dose after toxicity resolves. If resumption is tolerated, increase to 75% of the dose that produced G3/4 toxicity

Hematologic Toxicity

G1/2	No dose reduction
G3	Reduce interferon α dosage in 25% decrements until abates to Grade <3
G4	Stop interferon α. Restart at a dosage decreased by 50% when toxicity resolves; increase dosage to 75% of the dose that produced G4 toxicity if tolerated

Modified from O'Brien S et al. Leuk Lymphoma 1996;23:247–252

Toxicity

Toxicity	% (All Grades)
Fever	92
Asthenia or fatigue	88
Myalgia	68
Chills	63
Anorexia	48
Arthralgia/bone pain	47
Headache	44
Nausea, vomiting	37
Diarrhea	37
Depression	28
Cough	19
Hair changes	18
Skin rashes	18
Decreased mental status	16

(continued)

Efficacy (N = 344)

	Pegylated rIFN-a2b n = 171	rIFN-a2b n = 173
Complete cytogenetic response at 12 months	8%	8%
Partial cytogenetic response	15%	20%
Major cytogenetic response (total)	23%	28%
Complete cytogenetic response at or beyond 12 months	10%	10%

Michallet M et al. Leukemia 2004:18;309–315

Therapy Monitoring:

1. *CBC:* Weekly; every 2–4 weeks after achievement of complete hematologic response, if counts are stable; every 4–6 weeks after achievement of complete cytogenetic response
2. *Blood chemistry:* Twice weekly; every 4–6 weeks after achievement of complete hematologic response
3. *Quantitative RT-PCR for BCR-ABL from peripheral blood or bone marrow:* Every 3–6 months
4. *Bone marrow cytogenetics:* Every 3 months until complete cytogenetic response, then at 12- to 24-month intervals (only if no access to reliable qPCR testing or in case of atypical transcripts not measurable by standard qPCR assays)
5. *FISH (peripheral blood):* In case of atypical transcripts, once CCyR has been achieved

Toxicity (*continued*)

Toxicity	% (All Grades)
Sweating	15
Dizziness	11
Sleep disturbances	11
Paresthesia	8
Dyspnea	8
Cardiac dysrhythmia	7
Involuntary movements	7
Dry skin	7
Pruritus	7
Visual disturbances	6

Roferon-A (interferon alfa–2a, recombinant) product label. Nutley, NJ: Hoffmann-La Roche Inc., 2004

Patient Population Studied

Patients with newly diagnosed CML in chronic phase treated with interferon α vs pegylated interferon α: n = 173 and n =171, respectively

Treatment Modifications

The practical management of patients receiving pegylated interferon α-2b

Hematologic Toxicity	Reduce Dose	Discontinue Therapy
WBC	1.0 to <1.5 × 109/L	<1.0 × 109/L
Neutrophils	0.5 to <0.75 × 109/L	<0.5 × 109/L
Platelets	25 to <50 × 109/L (adults)	<25 × 109/L (adults)
Hemoglobin in patients without history of cardiac disease	N/A	<8.5 g/dL
Hemoglobin in patients with history of cardiac disease	≥2-g/dL decrease in hemoglobin during any 4-week period during treatment	<8.5 g/dL or <12 g/dL after 4 weeks of dose reduction

*Refer to full prescribing information for complete details as well as for the guidelines for modification or discontinuation of pegylated interferon α and for scheduling visits for patients with depression

Toxicity

Toxicity	Pegylated rIFN-α2b	rIFN-α2b	Pegylated rIFN-a2b	rIFN-α2b
	% (All Grades)		% (Grade 3/4)	
Nonhematologic AE				
Fever	82%	77%	15%	13%
Headache	78%	75%	9%	6%
Rigors	69%	63%	3%	5%
Anorexia	67%	58%	5%	8%
Fatigue	61%	63%	12%	13%
Myalgia	61%	63%	3%	6%
Nausea	64%	60%	4%	5%
Diarrhea	61%	51%	6%	5%
Arthralgia	54%	49%	8%	6%
Asthenia	56%	46%	6%	8%
Musculoskeletal pain	48%	48%	10%	6%
Back pain	46%	47%	6%	5%
Weight decrease	49%	40%	5%	9%
Depression	37%	31%	8%	6%
Hepatic enzymes increased	8%	7%	5%	6%
Hematologic AE				
Thrombocytopenia	25%	27%	12%	14%
Leukopenia	11%	11%	4%	6%
Neutropenia	8%	8%	4%	5%

WARNING: RISK OF SERIOUS DISORDERS. See full prescribing information for complete boxed warning.
• May cause or aggravate fatal or life-threatening neuropsychiatric, autoimmune, ischemic, and infectious disorders. Monitor closely and withdraw therapy with persistently severe or worsening signs or symptoms of the above disorders

Notes

Interferon α is reserved for patients who are intolerant of imatinib, nilotinib, and dasatinib. Patients whose disease is resistant to these drugs usually do not respond to interferon α. An alternative, polyethylene glycol–modified rIFN-α-2b, is a novel formulation with a longer half-life that allows for weekly dosing and has a similar safety and efficacy profile

There is general consensus recommending against the use of TKIs during pregnancy due to the risk of teratogenicity with malformations, spontaneous abortion, or fetal growth retardation. Interferon α is a safe alternative treatment option during pregnancy particularly in the first and second trimesters, where the risk of TKI-related teratogenicity is highest, and can serve as a useful treatment option during pregnancy when TKIs are contraindicated

Pavlovsky C et al. Case Rep Hematol 2012;2012:624590
Balsat M et al. Eur J Haematol 2018;101:774–780

13. Colorectal Cancer

Jennifer M. Duff, MD, Jason Starr, DO, and Carmen Joseph Allegra, MD

Epidemiology

Incidence

Colorectal (CRC) cancer:	145,600 estimated new cases in 2019: 101,420 colon cancer and 44,180 rectal cancer
Deaths:	51,020 estimated in 2019
Median age at diagnosis:	67 years
Lifetime risk of developing CRC:	4.2 percent of men and women will be diagnosed in their lifetime. CRC is more common in men compared with women, and in those of African-American descent

Surveillance, Epidemiology and End Results (SEER) Program, available from http://seer.cancer.gov [accessed 2019]
https://www.cancer.net/cancer-types/colorectal-cancer/statistics [accessed 2019]

Colorectal Cancer Subsites

Proximal colon:	41%
Distal Colon:	22%
Rectum:	28%
Other:	8%

Staging Distribution: Colon

Local:	38%
Regional:	35%
Distant:	23%

Staging Distribution: Rectum

Local:	41%
Regional:	34%
Distant:	19%

Howlader N et al, editors. SEER Cancer Statistics Review, 1975–2016. Bethesda, MD: National Cancer Institute; 2019
Siegel RL et al. Colorectal Cancer Statistics, 2017. CA Cancer J Clin 2017;67:177–193

Five-year Survival

Colorectal Cancer: Five-year Relative Survival by Stage at Diagnosis

Localized (cancer confined to primary site)	90%
Regional (cancer spread to regional lymph nodes)	72%
Distant (cancer metastasized)	14%

https://seer.cancer.gov/statfacts/html/colorect.html#survival [accessed 2020]

Amin MB et al, editors. AJCC Cancer Staging Manual 8th Ed. New York: Springer; 2017

Work-up

Colon and Rectal Cancer Appropriate for Resection	H&P, CBC, serum electrolytes, LFTs, serum creatinine, BUN, and CEA. Full colonoscopy, CT scan of thorax and abdomen, and pelvis with IV and oral contrast, pathology review *Rectal lesions:* pelvic MRI with contrast or endoscopic ultrasound PET scans are not routinely performed, used to clarify findings from a contrasted CT scan or if the patient has a contraindication to receiving contrast MSI or MMR testing should be performed in all patients with a personal history of colon cancer to evaluate for the risk of Lynch syndrome and provide prognostic value in stage II CRC
Stage IV	As above plus extended RAS analysis and BRAF V600E mutation testing

https://www.nccn.org/professionals/physician_gls/pdf/rectal_blocks.pdf [accessed March 2017]

Pathology

World Health Organization Classification
1. Adenocarcinoma (>90%)
2. Mucinous adenocarcinoma
3. Adenosquamous carcinoma
4. Small cell carcinoma
5. Medullary carcinoma
6. Signet ring adenocarcinoma
7. Squamous cell carcinoma
8. Undifferentiated

Skibber JM et al. Cancer of the colon. In: DeVita VT Jr et al. editors. Cancer: Principles & Practice of Oncology, 10th ed. Philadelphia: Wolters Kluwer; 2015:1216–1270

Expert Opinion

Stage II colon cancer:

- Given the relatively low risk for recurrence for most patients with stage II colon cancer, the routine use of adjuvant chemotherapy for medically fit patients with stage II colon cancer is not recommended. The QUASAR trial is the largest study comprising stage II CRC patients that showed a statistical benefit for using adjuvant fluorouracil (5FU)/leucovorin (LV)
- Most experts recommend that adjuvant chemotherapy be considered for patients with high-risk stage II disease.
- Those considered at higher risk for recurrence include patients with:
  - Inadequately sampled nodes (less than 12)
  - T4 lesions
  - Localized perforation
  - Poorly differentiated histology (excluding MSI-high tumors)
  - Lymphatic/vascular invasion
  - Perineural invasion
  - Bowel obstruction
- Defective mismatch repair proteins (dMMR) leading to MMR deficiency and microsatellite instability (MSI-H) are found in 15–20% of colon cancers. This deficiency is associated with a low risk of recurrence and an important factor when considering adjuvant chemotherapy for stage II patients. Adjuvant chemotherapy is not recommended in low-risk, MSI-H disease
- Oxaliplatin's role in stage II colon cancer is a topic of debate. A post-hoc analysis of the MOSAIC trial showed no difference in DFS at 6 years with the use of FOLFOX (fluorouracil, leucovorin, oxaliplatin) versus 5FU/LV in DFS with the addition of oxaliplatin although the power to detect a difference if one existed was small due to the relatively small number of patients treated. For patients being considered for adjuvant therapy, experts suggest treating low-risk stage II disease with 5FU/LV or capecitabine alone, and 5FU/LV, capecitabine, or oxaliplatin-based adjuvant therapy (FOLFOX, CAPOX, FLOX) for high-risk disease

Stage III colon cancer:

- Systemic combined chemotherapy is the principal adjuvant therapy for stage III colon cancer
- Combinations include oxaliplatin with bolus or infusional 5FU/LV
- The addition of oxaliplatin to leucovorin modulated 5FU has shown improved disease-free survival (DFS) and overall survival compared with 5FU/LV and is considered the standard
- Similar improvements in DFS have been demonstrated when either oxaliplatin is added to weekly bolus 5FU/LV (FLOX regimen) or infusional 5FU (FOLFOX regimen)
- mFOLFOX-6 is more commonly used compared to FOLFOX-4 for convenience as it eliminates the day 2 bolus 5FU
- Capecitabine can be used in place of bolus or infusional 5FU
- Trials testing the benefit of irinotecan, bevacizumab, and cetuximab have all been negative in the adjuvant setting
- Standard adjuvant therapy is prescribed for 6 months with either XELOX or FOLFOX. A shorter duration of chemotherapy was recently analyzed in the IDEA trial, suggesting that 3 months of oxaliplatin-based combination therapy may be noninferior to 6 months of treatment in a subset of stage III colon cancer patients. The trial reports that 3-year disease free survival (DFS) was slightly shorter with 3 months of adjuvant chemotherapy compared to 6 months for the entire cohort. However, for the subset of patients with lower-risk stage III disease, defined as spread within 1–3 lymph nodes and not T4, 3 months of chemotherapy produced similar benefit compared to 6 months, particularly with the use of CAPOX. Although this noninferiority study did not meet its primary end point, the findings should be considered for select patients with resected stage III colon cancer

Stage IV colon and rectal cancer:

- The choice of therapy is based on consideration of
  - The type and timing of the prior therapy that has been administered
  - The differing toxicity profiles of the constituent drugs
  - RAS mutational status and molecular profiling
  - The possibility of resection of metastases

(continued)

Staging

Primary Tumor (T)

TX	Primary tumor cannot be assessed
T0	No evidence of primary tumor
Tis	Carcinoma in situ: intraepithelial or invasion of lamina propria*
T1	Tumor invades submucosa
T2	Tumor invades muscularis propria
T3	Tumor invades through the muscularis propria into pericolorectal tissues
T4a	Tumor penetrates to the surface of the visceral peritoneum
T4b	Tumor directly invades or is adherent to other organs or structures†

*Tis includes cancer cells confined within the glandular basement membrane (intraepithelial) or mucosal lamina propria (intramucosal) with no extension through the muscularis mucosae into the submucosa
†Direct invasion in T4 includes invasion of other organs or other segments of the colorectum as a result of direct extension through the serosa, as confirmed on microscopic examination (for example, invasion of the sigmoid colon by a carcinoma of the cecum) or, for cancers in a retro-peritoneal or subperitoneal location, direct invasion of other organs or structures by virtue of extension beyond the muscularis propria (ie, respectively, a tumor on the posterior wall of the descending colon invading the left kidney or lateral abdominal wall; or a mid or distal rectal cancer with invasion of prostate, seminal vesicles, cervix, or vagina)

Regional Lymph Node (N)

NX	Regional lymph nodes cannot be assessed
N0	No regional lymph node metastasis
N1	Metastasis in one to three regional lymph nodes
N1a	Metastasis in one regional lymph node
N1b	Metastasis in two to three regional lymph nodes
N1c	Tumor deposit(s) in the subserosa, mesentery, or nonperitonealized pericolic or perirectal tissues without regional nodal metastasis
N2	Metastasis in four or more regional lymph nodes
N2a	Metastasis in four to six regional lymph nodes
N2b	Metastasis in seven or more regional lymph nodes

Expert Opinion (continued)

- Approximately 35% of patients have stage IV disease at presentation and 20–50% with stage II or III disease progress to stage IV
- Patients can be classified as potentially curable or noncurable
- Up to 60% of patients presenting with liver metastases who underwent a surgical resection were alive at 5 years in a report from Memorial Sloan-Kettering Cancer Center (MSKCC)
- Patients with untreated metastatic disease may be treated initially with FOLFOX (or XELOX) or FOLFIRI plus a biologic including vascular endothelial growth factor (VEGF) inhibitor, bevacizumab, or if RAS wild-type epidermal growth factor receptor (EGFR) inhibitors, cetuximab or panitumumab. The phase 3 CALGB/SWOG 80405 study provides the strongest available evidence for primary tumor location being a predictive marker for response to therapy. It reports that in RAS wild-type tumors, those with right-sided tumors had better overall survival using bevacizumab in first-line treatment compared to cetuximab. Left-sided tumors had better survival utilizing cetuximab in first-line treatment compared to bevacizumab. Expert panels recommend consideration of first-line EGFR inhibitors in RAS wild-type tumors that originated in the left side of the colon. The median survival approaching 2.5 years for patients with metastatic colorectal cancer treated initially with multi-agent therapy sets a benchmark
- Unfortunately, patients whose cancers harbor a BRAF mutation have a particularly poor outcome regardless of chemotherapeutic intervention
- Patients with progressive disease who have received fluorouracil-based therapy may be treated with chemotherapy consisting of FOLFIRI, irinotecan, or FOLFOX (or XELOX) in addition to continuation of anti-VEGF therapy or the addition of anti-EGFR therapy for those patients whose cancers do not contain a mutation in KRAS or NRAS. If the tumor is MSI-H, then use of the immune checkpoint inhibitors (pembrolizumab or nivolumab) can be considered for second-line treatment and beyond
- The oral anti-VEGF protein kinase inhibitor regorafenib and an oral combination of a nucleoside analog with a thymidine phosphorylase inhibitor, trifluridine/tipiracil (TAS102), have activity in patients with disease that is refractory to the above listed agents

Rectal cancer:
- Preoperative chemoradiotherapy and postoperative chemoradiotherapy yield similar DFS and OS for patients with full-thickness muscularis involvement (T3), adjacent structure invasion (T4), and/or regional node involvement (N1/N2)
- Preoperative chemoradiotherapy, generally favored as a sphincter-sparing operation, is more likely to be technically feasible when compared to an initial surgical approach
- Adjuvant chemotherapy is offered to patients who have undergone preoperative chemoradiotherapy
- Adjuvant chemotherapy for stages II and III is firmly established, albeit in the pre-neoadjuvant era. It remains the standard of care in the United States
- Induction chemotherapy prior to chemoradiotherapy can also be considered. Advantages to this approach may be a higher rate of completion of systemic therapy to address micrometastatic disease

Guidelines for molecular analysis of colorectal cancers and significance of cell free DNA (cfDNA)
- Patients with a personal history of colorectal cancer of any stage should have MMR or MSI testing performed on the tumor to identify Lynch syndrome
- MSI-H or MMR deficiency in low-risk stage II disease likely has a good prognosis and does not benefit from 5FU-based adjuvant chemotherapy
- BRAF V600E analysis should be performed in MMR deficient tumors with loss of MLH1 to evaluate for Lynch syndrome. If identified, this strongly suggests sporadic loss of MLH1 due to hypermethylation
- When anti-EGFR therapy is being considered, the tumor sample must be analyzed for extended RAS mutational status. This testing includes KRAS and NRAS exon 2, 3, and 4
- BRAF V600E mutational analysis should be performed for prognostic stratification in metastatic disease. Identification of BRAF V600E makes response to anti-EGFR therapy unlikely

(continued)

Staging (continued)

Distant Metastasis (M)

M0	No distant metastasis
M1	Distant metastasis
M1a	Metastasis confined to one organ or site (eg, liver, lung, ovary, nonregional node) without peritoneal metastasis
M1b	Metastases in more than one organ/site without peritoneal metastasis
M1c	Metastasis to the peritoneal surface is identified alone or with other site or organ metastasis

Anatomic Stage/Prognostic Groups

Stage	T	N	M
0	Tis	N0	M0
I	T1	N0	M0
	T2	N0	M0
IIA	T3	N0	M0
IIB	T4a	N0	M0
IIC	T4b	N0	M0
IIIA	T1–2	N1/N1c	M0
	T1	N2a	M0
IIIB	T3–T4a	N1/N1c	M0
	T2–T3	N2a	M0
	T1–T2	N2b	M0
IIIC	T4a	N2a	M0
	T3–T4a	N2b	M0
	T4b	N1-N2	M0
IVA	Any T	Any N	M1a
IVB	Any T	Any N	M1b
IVC	Any T	Any N	M1c

Amin MB et al, editors. AJCC Cancer Staging Manual. 8th ed. New York: Springer; 2017

Expert Opinion (*continued*)

• Retrospective studies suggest that the presence of cfDNA after resection of local and locally advanced colon cancer is strongly associated with recurrence risk. The clinical utility of cfDNA is still under study

Alberts SR et al. JAMA 2012;307:1383–1393
Allegra CJ et al. J Clin Oncol 2013;31:359–364
André T et al. J Clin Oncol 2009;27:3109–3116
Bertagnolli MM et al. J Clin Oncol 2011;29:3153–3162
Cassidy J et al. J Clin Oncol 2008;26:2006–2012
Fong Y et al. Ann Surg 1999;230:309–321
Grothey A et al. Lancet 2013;381:303–312
Haller DG et al. J Clin Oncol 2011;29:1465–1471
Hurwitz H et al. N Engl J Med 2004;350:2335–2342
Quasar Collaborative Group, Gray R et al. Lancet 2007;370:2020–2029
Saltz LB et al. J Clin Oncol 2007;25:3456–3461
Sauer R et al. N Engl J Med 2004;351:1731–1740
Sepulveda AR et al. J Clin Oncol 2017;35:1453–1486
Seymour MT et al. Lancet 2007;370:143–152
Shi Q et al. J Clin Oncol 2017;35:abstr LBA1
Spindler KG et al. Oncologist 2017;22:1049–1055
Van Cutsem E et al. J Clin Oncol 2011;29:2011–2019
https://www.nccn.org/professionals/physician_gls/pdf/rectal_blocks.pdf [accessed March 2017]

ADJUVANT

COLORECTAL CANCER REGIMEN: LEUCOVORIN + INFUSIONAL FLUOROURACIL + OXALIPLATIN (MODIFIED FOLFOX6)

André T et al. N Engl J Med 2004;350:2343–2351
Hochster HS et al. J Clin Oncol 2008;26:3523–3529
Tournigand C et al. J Clin Oncol 2004;22:229–237

mFOLFOX–6: 12 CYCLES (André et al) OF ADJUVANT THERAPY

Note: see separate LEUCOVORIN + INFUSIONAL FLUOROURACIL + OXALIPLATIN (FOLFOX) regimen description for use in metastatic disease

Oxaliplatin 85 mg/m^2; administer intravenously over 2 hours in 500 mL 5% dextrose injection (D5W) on day 1, every 2 weeks, concurrently with leucovorin (or levoleucovorin) administration, for 12 cycles (total dosage/cycle = 85 mg/m^2), *plus:*

Either: **(racemic) leucovorin calcium** 400 mg/m^2 *or* **levoleucovorin calcium** 200 mg/m^2; administer intravenously over 2 hours in 25–500 mL D5W on day 1, every 2 weeks, concurrently with oxaliplatin, for 12 cycles (total dosage/cycle for racemic leucovorin = 400 mg/m^2, for levoleucovorin = 200 mg/m^2), *followed by:*

> *Note:* Although Hochster et al report a 350-mg fixed dose of racemic leucovorin with modified FOLFOX6, many institutions prefer to use the body surface area–based dose of racemic leucovorin, 400 mg/m^2, or levoleucovorin, 200 mg/m^2, reported in the original FOLFOX6 regimen by Tournigand et al

Fluorouracil 400 mg/m^2; administer by intravenous injection over 1–2 minutes after leucovorin (or levoleucovorin) on day 1, every 2 weeks, for 12 cycles, *followed by:*

Fluorouracil 2400 mg/m^2; administer by continuous intravenous infusion over 46 hours in 100–1000 mL 0.9% sodium chloride injection (0.9% NS) or D5W, starting on day 1 every 2 weeks, for 12 cycles (total fluorouracil dosage/cycle = 2800 mg/m^2)
> *Note:* The fluorouracil bolus dose (400 mg/m^2) can be omitted for better hematologic tolerance

> *Note:* Oxaliplatin must not be mixed with sodium chloride injection. Therefore, when leucovorin and oxaliplatin are given concurrently via the same administration set tubing, both drugs must be administered in D5W

Supportive Care
Antiemetic prophylaxis
Emetogenic potential on day 1 is **MODERATE**
Emetogenic potential on day 2 is **LOW**
See Chapter 42 for antiemetic recommendations

Hematopoietic growth factor (G-CSF) prophylaxis
Primary prophylaxis is **NOT** *indicated*
See Chapter 43 for more information

Antimicrobial prophylaxis
Risk of fever and neutropenia is **LOW**
> *Antimicrobial primary prophylaxis to be considered:*
> • Antibacterial—not indicated
> • Antifungal—not indicated
> • Antiviral—not indicated unless patient previously had an episode of HSV

Diarrhea management
Latent or delayed-onset diarrhea*:
> **Loperamide** 4 mg orally initially after the first loose or liquid stool, *then* 2-4 mg orally every 2-4 hours or **diphenoxylate hydrochloride** 2.5 mg **with atropine sulfate** 0.025 mg (e.g., Lomotil®)

Persistent diarrhea
> **Octreotide** 100–150 mcg subcutaneously 3 times daily. Maximum total daily dose is 1500 mcg
Antibiotic therapy during latent or delayed-onset diarrhea:
> A fluoroquinolone (eg, **ciprofloxacin** 500 mg orally every 12 hours) if absolute neutrophil count <500/mm^3 with or without accompanying fever in association with diarrhea
> • Antibiotics should also be administered if patient is hospitalized with prolonged diarrhea and should be continued until diarrhea resolves

Oral care
Standard prophylaxis and treatment for mucositis/stomatitis

*Abergerges D et al. J Natl Cancer Inst 1994;86:446–449

Patient Population Studied

A multicenter, randomized, phase 3 study involved 2246 patients who had undergone complete resection of histologically proven stage II/III colon cancer. Eligible patients were aged 18–75 years and had a Karnofsky performance status score ≥60 and a carcinoembryonic antigen level <10 ng/mL. Patients who had received previous chemotherapy, immunotherapy, or radiotherapy were not eligible. Patients were randomly assigned (1:1) to receive fluorouracil + leucovorin with or without oxaliplatin.

Efficacy (N = 2246)

Disease-free survival at 3 years	78.2% with fluorouracil + leucovorin + oxaliplatin 72.9% fluorouracil + leucovorin only P = 0.002
Overall survival at 3 years	87.7% with fluorouracil + leucovorin + oxaliplatin 86.6% fluorouracil + leucovorin only

Therapy Monitoring

1. *Before each cycle:* H&P, CBC with differential, LFTs, and CEA if being used to monitor disease
2. *Every 2–3 months:* CT scans to assess response in patients presenting with advanced colorectal cancer

Treatment Modifications

Treatment Modifications (mFOLFOX–6)

Adverse Event	Treatment Modification
Day 1 persistent nonhematologic toxicity G ≥2	Delay start of next cycle until the severity of all toxicities are G ≤1; omit fluorouracil by intravenous bolus injection in subsequent cycles
Day 1 ANC ≤1500/mm³ *or* platelet count ≤100,000/mm³	Delay start of next cycle until ANC >1500/mm³ *and* platelet count >100,000/mm³; omit fluorouracil by intravenous bolus injection in subsequent cycles
G4 neutropenia (<500/mm³), G3/4 thrombocytopenia (<50,000/mm³) or G4 diarrhea (life-threatening; urgent intervention required)	Reduce oxaliplatin dosage to 75 mg/m² and omit fluorouracil by intravenous bolus injection in subsequent cycles
G ≥3 non-neurologic toxicity	Reduce infusional fluorouracil dosage to 2000 mg/m²
G2 paresthesia (persistent paresthesia or dysesthesia, moderate in nature without functional impairment other than limiting instrumental ADLs)	Reduce oxaliplatin dosage to 75 mg/m²
Persistent G2 paresthesia/dysesthesia	Discontinue oxaliplatin
Persistent painful paresthesia or G3 neuropathy (persistent paresthesia or dysesthesia with persistent functional impairment limiting self-care and ADLs)	Discontinue oxaliplatin

ADLs, activities of daily living; ANC, absolute neutrophil count
Tournigand C et al. J Clin Oncol 2004;22:229–237

Adverse Events (N = 2219)

Grade (%)*	Fluorouracil + Leucovorin + Oxaliplatin			Fluorouracil + Leucovorin Only			P Value	
	Grade 1/2	Grade 3	Grade 4	Grade 1/2	Grade 3	Grade 4	All Grades	Grades 3–4
Nonhematologic Adverse Events								
Paresthesia	80	12	—	15	<1	–	<0.001	0.001
Nausea	68	5	<1	59	2	<1	<0.001	<0.001
Diarrhea	46	8	3	42	5	2	<0.001	<0.001
Vomiting	41	5	<1	23	<1	<1	<0.001	<0.001
Stomatitis	39	3	0	37	2	<1	0.34	0.41
Skin (including hand-foot syndrome)	30	1	<1	33	2	<1	0.05	0.67
Alopecia	30	—	—	28	—	—	0.28	—
Allergic reaction	7	2	<1	2	<1	<1	<0.001	<0.001
Hematologic Adverse Events								
Neutropenia	38	29	12	35	4	1	<0.001	<0.001
Neutropenia with fever or infection	0	1	<1	0	<1	<1	<0.001	<0.001
Thrombocytopenia	76	2	<1	19	<1	<1	<0.001	0.001
Anemia	75	<1	<1	67	<1	0	<0.001	0.09
Thrombosis or phlebitis	5	1	<1	5	2	<1	0.48	0.29

*According to the National Cancer Institute Common Toxicity Criteria for Adverse Events, version 1

ADJUVANT

COLORECTAL CANCER: CAPECITABINE + OXALIPLATIN (XELOX)

Haller DG et al. J Clin Oncol 2011;29:1465–1471

Note: See XELOX ± bevacizumab regimen specifically for use in metastatic disease

Oxaliplatin 130 mg/m²; administer intravenously in 250–500 mL 5% dextrose injection over 2 hours on day 1, every 3 weeks, for 8 cycles (total dosage/cycle = 130 mg/m²), *plus*
Capecitabine 1000 mg/m² per dose; administer orally twice daily (approximately every 12 hours, within 30 minutes after a meal) for 14 consecutive days, on days 1–14 (28 doses), every 3 weeks for 8 cycles (total dosage/cycle = 28,000 mg/m²)

Note: Capecitabine monotherapy was continued in patients who refused or discontinued oxaliplatin because of toxicity
XELOX was compared to 2 fluorouracil and leucovorin (folinic acid) (FU/FA) regimens given either for 6 cycles over 24 weeks or 4 cycles over 32 weeks (Haller DG et al. J Clin Oncol 2005;23:8671–8678)

Supportive Care
Antiemetic prophylaxis
Emetogenic potential on day 1 is **MODERATE**
Emetogenic potential on days with capecitabine alone is **MINIMAL–LOW**
See Chapter 42 for antiemetic recommendations

Hematopoietic growth factor (G-CSF) prophylaxis
Primary prophylaxis may be indicated
See Chapter 43 for more information

Antimicrobial prophylaxis
Risk of fever and neutropenia is **LOW**
  Antimicrobial primary prophylaxis to be considered:
  • Antibacterial—not indicated
  • Antifungal—not indicated
  • Antiviral—not indicated, unless patient previously had an episode of HSV

Hand-foot reaction (palmar-plantar erythrodysesthesia, PPE)
For patients who develop a hand-foot reaction, use topical emollients (eg, Aquaphor®), topical or orally administered steroids, antihistamine agents (H₁-receptor antagonists), or pyridoxine
  • Pyridoxine may provide relief for discomfort/pain associated with PPE, although the mechanism through which this occurs remains unclear
  • The suggested pyridoxine starting dose is 50 mg/day, which may be increased to a maximum of 200 mg/day

Diarrhea management
Latent or delayed-onset diarrhea*:
Loperamide 4 mg orally initially after the first loose or liquid stool, *then* 2-4 mg orally every 2-4 hours or **diphenoxylate hydrochloride** 2.5 mg **with atropine sulfate** 0.025 mg (e.g., Lomotil®)

*Abigerges D et al. J Natl Cancer Inst 1994; 86:446–449
Rothenberg ML et al. J Clin Oncol 2001; 19:3801–3807
Wadler S et al. J Clin Oncol 1998; 16:3169–3178

Oral care
Standard prophylaxis and treatment for mucositis/stomatitis

Treatment Modifications

Adverse Event	Dose Modification
ANC nadir <1000/mm³ *or* platelet nadir <50,000/mm³ after treatment	Delay treatment until ANC is ≥1000/mm³ *and* platelet count is ≥50,000/mm³, then decrease oxaliplatin dosage by 25%, and decrease daily capecitabine dosages by 50% during subsequent cycles.* Alternatively, consider using hematopoietic growth factors
Persistent G1/G2 neuropathy	Delay oxaliplatin 1 week. After toxicity resolves, resume oxaliplatin at a dosage decreased to 100 mg/m² during subsequent cycles
"Transient" G3/4 neuropathy (7–14 days)	Hold oxaliplatin. After toxicity resolves, resume oxaliplatin at a dosage decreased to 100 mg/m² during subsequent cycles
Persistent G3/4 neuropathy	Discontinue oxaliplatin
G3/4 diarrhea or stomatitis despite capecitabine dose reductions	Reduce oxaliplatin dosage to 100 mg/m²
G3/4 nonhematologic adverse events other than renal function and neurotoxicity	Reduce oxaliplatin and capecitabine dosages by 25% during subsequent cycles
G2 stomatitis, diarrhea, or nausea	Hold capecitabine; resume capecitabine at full dosage after resolution of toxicity
Second episode of G2 stomatitis, diarrhea, or nausea	Hold capecitabine; resume capecitabine with dosage reduced by 25% after toxicity resolves
Third episode of G2 stomatitis, diarrhea, or nausea	Hold capecitabine; resume capecitabine with dosage reduced by 50% after toxicity resolves
Fourth episode of G2 stomatitis, diarrhea, or nausea	Discontinue capecitabine

(continued)

Efficacy

The authors concluded "The addition of oxaliplatin to capecitabine improves DFS in patients with stage III colon cancer. XELOX is an additional adjuvant treatment option for these patients."

	XELOX	FU/FA
3-year DFS	70.9% (95% CI, 67.9–73.9)	66.5% (95% CI, 63.4–69.6)
4-year DFS	68.4% (95% CI, 65.3–71.4)	62.3% (95% CI, 59.1–65.5)
5-year DFS	66.1% (95% CI, 62.9–69.4)	59.8% (95% CI, 56.4–63.1)
3-year RFS	72.1	67.5
4-year RFS	69.7% (95% CI, 66.7–72.8)	63.3% (95% CI, 60.1–66.5)
5-year RFS	67.8% (95% CI, 64.6–71.0)	60.9% (95% CI, 57.6–64.2)
OS*	79.1	76.1
	(HR, 0.87; 95% CI, 0.72–1.05; P = 0.1486)	
5-year OS	77.6% (95% CI, 74.7–80.3)	74.2% (95% CI, 71.3–77.2)

DFS, disease-free survival; FU/FA, fluorouracil/folinic acid (leucovorin); OS, overall survival; RFS, relapse-free survival; XELOX, capecitabine plus oxaliplatin
*After median follow-up of 57.0 months

Efficacy (Intention to Treat)

End Point	Follow-Up (months)	Number of Patients	Number of Patients with Event	Hazard Ratio (95% CI)	P (Log-Rank Test)
DFS	55.0				
XELOX	—	944	295	0.80 (0.69–0.93)	0.0045
FU/FA	—	942	353		
RFS	55.0				
XELOX	—	944	278	0.78 (0.67–0.92)	0.0024
FU/FA	—	942	340		
OS	57.0				
XELOX	—	944	197	0.87 (0.72–1.05)	0.1486
FU/FA	—	942	225		

DFS, disease-free survival; FU/FA, fluorouracil/folinic acid (leucovorin); OS, overall survival; RFS, relapse-free survival; XELOX, capecitabine plus oxaliplatin

Treatment Modifications
(continued)

Adverse Event	Dose Modification
G3 stomatitis, diarrhea, or nausea	Hold capecitabine. If G3 toxicity is adequately controlled within 2 days, resume capecitabine at full dosage when toxicity abates to G ≤1. If G3 toxicity takes >2 days to be controlled, resume capecitabine with dosage reduced by 25% after toxicity abates to G ≤1
Second episode of G3 stomatitis, diarrhea, or nausea	Hold capecitabine. If G3 toxicity is controlled adequately within 2 days, then resume capecitabine with dosage reduced by 50% after toxicity abates to G ≤1
Third episode of G3 stomatitis, diarrhea, or nausea	Discontinue capecitabine
G4 stomatitis, diarrhea, or nausea	Discontinue capecitabine. Resume capecitabine with dosage reduced by 50% after toxicity resolves
G1 capecitabine-associated PPE[†]	Begin pyridoxine 50 mg orally 3 times daily and continue capecitabine without dose modification
G2 capecitabine-associated PPE[†]	Begin pyridoxine 50 mg orally 3 times daily and withhold capecitabine. Resume capecitabine with dosage reduced by 15% after toxicity resolves
G3 capecitabine-associated PPE[†]	Begin pyridoxine 50 mg orally 3 times daily and withhold capecitabine. Resume capecitabine with dosage reduced by 30% after toxicity resolves
Recurrent G3 capecitabine-associated PPE[†]	Begin pyridoxine 50 mg orally 3 times daily and withhold capecitabine. Resume capecitabine with dosage reduced by 50% after toxicity resolves

*Treatment delays for unresolved adverse events of >3 weeks duration warrant discontinuation of treatment
[†]PPE, palmar-plantar erythrodysesthesia (hand-foot syndrome)

Patient Population Studied

Patients with histologically confirmed stage III colon carcinoma (T1–4/N1–2/M0), defined as a tumor located ≥15 cm from the anal verge or above the peritoneal reflection. Surgery with curative intent was performed in all patients ≤8 weeks before random assignment, by which time full recovery from surgery was required

Patient Characteristic (n = 944)

	Percentage of Patients
Age—median (range)	61 years (22–83 years)
Sex —male/female	54%/46%
ECOG performance status 0 1	 74% 25%
Primary tumor classification T1–2 T3 T4 TX	 11% 74% 15% <1%
Regional lymph nodes classification N0 N1 N2	 <1% 65% 35%
Histologic appearance Well differentiated Moderately differentiated Poorly differentiated Undetermined/unknown/data missing	 11% 70% 15% 4

Efficacy—Multivariate Analysis

Variable	DFS HR (95% CI)	P	OS HR (95% CI)	P
Stratification				
Treatment (XELOX vs FU/FA)	0.78 (0.67–0.92)	0.0022	0.88 (0.72–1.06)	0.1836
Lymph nodes (≤3 vs >3)	0.55 (0.43–0.70)	<0.001	0.48 (0.35–0.64)	<0.001
Baseline CEA (normal vs abnormal)	0.41 (0.32–0.52)	<0.001	0.41 (0.31–0.54)	<0.001
Region by lymph node interaction	0.98 (0.95–1.01)	0.1597	0.98 (0.95–1.01)	0.2231
Prognostic				
Sex (male vs female)	1.13 (0.96–1.32)	0.1321	1.18 (0.97–1.44)	0.0919
Age (10-year intervals)*	1.07 (0.99–1.15)	0.0819	1.17 (1.06–1.28)	0.0016
Time from surgery to randomization (10-day intervals)*	1.09 (1.01–1.17)	0.0254	1.10 (1.00–1.21)	0.0395

CEA, carcinoembryonic antigen; CI, confidence interval; DFS, disease-free survival; HR, hazard ratio; FU/FA, fluorouracil/folinic acid (leucovorin); OS, overall survival; XELOX, capecitabine plus oxaliplatin
*Continuous variable: increase in hazard ratio represents risk increase per pre-defined increment

Treatment Monitoring

1. Before starting treatment: History and physical examination, ECG, CEA determination, CBC with differential, and serum chemistries
2. During treatment: CBC with differential and serum chemistries before each treatment cycle
3. Tumor assessments: Abdominal computed tomography, magnetic resonance imaging, or ultrasound, at baseline, every 6 months for the first 4 years, and annually thereafter. CEA levels every 3 months for the first 3 years and every 6 months thereafter

Toxicity

Most Common Treatment-Related AEs

Schmoll H-J et al. J Clin Oncol 2007;25:102–109

	XELOX (n = 938)		FU/LV (n = 926)	
	Percent of Patients		Percent of Patients	
	All Grades (≥20%)*	Grade 3/4 (≥5%)*	All Grades (≥20%)*	Grade 3/4 (≥5%)*
Patients with at least 1 AE	98%	55%	94%	47%
Neurosensory toxicity	78%	11%	7%	<1%
Nausea	66%	5%	57%	4%
Diarrhea	60%	19%	72%	20%
Vomiting	43%	6%	25%	3%
Fatigue	35%	N/R	34%	N/R
Hand-foot syndrome	29%	5%	10%	<1%
Neutropenia	27%	9%	28%	16%
Thrombocytopenia	N/R	5%	N/R	<1%
Anorexia	24%	N/R	18%	N/R
Stomatitis	21%	<1%	51%	9%
Abdominal pain	17%	2%	18%	2%
Alopecia	4%	N/R	20%	N/R
Dehydration	N/R	3%	N/R	3%
Hypokalemia	N/R	2%	N/R	2%
Febrile neutropenia	N/R	<1%	N/R	4%

AE, adverse event; FU/LV, fluorouracil/leucovorin; N/R, not reported; XELOX, capecitabine and oxaliplatin
*Reported if any grade of AE occurred in >20% or G3/4 occurred in >5% of patients in either treatment arm with some exceptions

Analysis of Safety by Age

Schmoll H-J et al. J Clin Oncol 2007;25:102–109

	XELOX		FU/LV	
	Age of Patients			
Patient Condition and Event	<65 Years (n = 583)	≥65 Years (n = 355)	<65 Years (n = 544)	≥65 Years (n = 382)
	%	%	%	%
Patients with AEs	99%	99%	95%	96%
Patients with grade 3/4 AEs	57%	65%	52%	53%
Patients with grade 4 AEs	5%	10%	10%	12%
Patients with serious AEs	17%	30%	23%	26%
Grade 3/4 events				
Diarrhea	17%	23%	20%	21%
Vomiting	7%	6%	3%	3%
Nausea	5%	6%	4%	5%
Dehydration	2%	7%	3%	3%
Stomatitis	<1%	1%	9%	9%
Neutropenia/ granulocytopenia	9%	8%	17%	15%
Febrile neutropenia	<1%	<1%	4%	5%
Infections/ infestations	2%	5%	4%	5%
Hand-foot syndrome	6%	4%	<1%	<1%
Neurosensory toxicity	12%	10%	<1%	—
Cardiac disorders	1%	2%	1%	2%
Venous thromboembolic events	1%	3%	3%	2%
Patients withdrawn due to AEs	16%	30%	8%	9%

AE, adverse event; FU/LV, fluorouracil/leucovorin; XELOX, capecitabine and oxaliplatin

ADJUVANT
COLORECTAL CANCER REGIMEN: CAPECITABINE

Twelves C et al. N Engl J Med 2005;352:2696–2704

Capecitabine 1250 mg/m² per dose; administer orally with water within 30 minutes after a meal twice daily for 28 doses on days 1–14, every 3 weeks, for 8 cycles (total dosage/cycle = 35,000 mg/m²)

Notes:
- Capecitabine is given for 2 consecutive weeks followed by 1 week without treatment
- Doses are rounded down to approximate a calculated dose using combinations of 500-mg and 150-mg tablets
- In practice, treatment often is begun with capecitabine 1000 mg/m² per dose twice daily for 28 doses on days 1–14 (total dosage/cycle = 28,000 mg/m²), especially in North American patients. Dosage may be increased during subsequent cycles if initial treatment at a lesser dosage is tolerated

Supportive Care
Antiemetic prophylaxis
Emetogenic potential is **LOW**
See Chapter 42 for antiemetic recommendations

Hematopoietic growth factor (G-CSF) prophylaxis
Primary prophylaxis is **NOT** *indicated*
See Chapter 43 for more information

Antimicrobial prophylaxis
Risk of fever and neutropenia is **LOW**
  Antimicrobial primary prophylaxis to be considered:
- Antibacterial—not indicated
- Antifungal—not indicated
- Antiviral—not indicated unless patient previously had an episode of HSV

Diarrhea management
Latent or delayed-onset diarrhea*:
  Loperamide 4 mg orally initially after the first loose or liquid stool, *then*
  Loperamide 2 mg orally every 2 hours during waking hours, *plus*
  Loperamide 4 mg orally every 4 hours during hours of sleep
- Continue for at least 12 hours after diarrhea resolves
- Recurrent diarrhea after a 12-hour diarrhea-free interval is treated as a new episode
- Rehydrate orally with fluids and electrolytes during a diarrheal episode
- If diarrhea persists >48 hours despite loperamide, stop loperamide and hospitalize the patient for IV hydration

Persistent diarrhea:
  Octreotide 100–150 mcg subcutaneously 3 times daily. Maximum total daily dose is 1500 mcg

Antibiotic therapy during latent or delayed-onset diarrhea:
  A fluoroquinolone (eg, **ciprofloxacin** 500 mg orally every 12 hours) if absolute neutrophil count is <500/mm³ with or without accompanying fever in association with diarrhea
- Antibiotics should also be administered if patient is hospitalized with prolonged diarrhea and should be continued until diarrhea resolves

*Abigerges D et al. J Natl Cancer Inst 1994;86:446–449
Rothenberg ML et al. J Clin Oncol 2001;19:3801–3807
Wadler S et al. J Clin Oncol 1998;16:3169–3178

Oral care
Standard prophylaxis and treatment for mucositis/stomatitis

Hand-foot reaction (palmar-plantar erythrodysesthesia, PPE)
For patients who develop a hand-foot reaction, use topical emollients (eg, Aquaphor®), topical or orally administered steroids, antihistamine agents (H_1-receptor antagonists), or pyridoxine
- Pyridoxine may provide relief for discomfort/pain associated with PPE although the mechanism through which this occurs remains unclear
- The suggested pyridoxine starting dose is 50 mg/day, which may be increased to a maximum of 200 mg/day

Patient Population Studied

Patients receiving adjuvant therapy for histologically confirmed stage III colon cancer. Patients were randomized to receive capecitabine or leucovorin/bolus fluorouracil

Efficacy (N = 1987)

	Capecitabine	Fluorouracil + Leucovorin	Hazard Ratio	P Value for Equivalence*	P Value for Superiority*
DFS	65.3%	61.3%	HR 0.87 (95% CI, 0.75–1.00)	<0.001†	0.05
RFS	67.7%	63.2%	HR 0.86 (95% CI, 0.74–0.99)	—	0.04
OS	80%	76.9%	HR 0.84 (95% CI, 0.69–1.01)	<0.001‡	0.07

Data presented are with a median follow-up of 3.8 years
DFS, disease-free survival; RFS, relapse-free survival; OS, overall survival
*P values for equivalence are one-sided; P values for superiority were calculated by Wald chi-square test
†Upper limit of hazard ratio met the pre-specified noninferiority margin of 1.20
‡Upper limit of hazard ratio met the pre-specified noninferiority margin of 1.25

Therapy Monitoring

1. *Before each cycle:* H&P, CBC with differential, CEA, serum electrolytes, creatinine, BUN, and LFTs

Treatment Modifications

Adverse Event	Dose Modification
First occurrence of a G2 toxicity	No dose reduction*
Second occurrence of a given G2 toxicity	Reduce dosage by 25%*
First occurrence of a G3 toxicity	
Third occurrence of a given G2 toxicity	Reduce dosage by 50%*
Second occurrence of a given G3 toxicity	
Any G4 toxicity	
Fourth occurrence of a given G2 toxicity	Discontinue capecitabine
Third occurrence of a given G3 toxicity	
Second occurrence of a given G4 toxicity	
Both G4 hematologic and G4 nonhematologic toxicity	

*Interrupt capecitabine treatment until toxicity resolves to G ≤1
National Cancer Institute of Canada Common Toxicity Criteria

Toxicity (N = 995)

	% All Grades	% Grade 3–4
Diarrhea	46	11
Nausea or vomiting	36	3
Stomatitis	22	2
Hand-foot syndrome	60	17
Fatigue or asthenia	23	1
Abdominal pain	10	2
Alopecia	6	0
Lethargy	10	<1
Anorexia	9	<1
Neutropenia	32	2
Hyperbilirubinemia	50	20

The table includes treatment-related adverse events reported in ≥10% of patients in either arm included in the safety population

METASTATIC • FIRST-LINE

COLORECTAL CANCER REGIMEN: LEUCOVORIN + INFUSIONAL FLUOROURACIL + OXALIPLATIN (FOLFOX)

André T et al. N Engl J Med 2004;350:2343–2351
Cheeseman SL et al. Br J Cancer 2002;87:393–399
de Gramont A et al. J Clin Oncol 2000;18:2938–2947
Rothenberg ML et al. J Clin Oncol 2003;21:2059–2069
Tournigand C et al. J Clin Oncol 2004;22:229–237

FOLFOX–4 (de Gramont et al, Rothenberg et al, André et al):
Oxaliplatin 85 mg/m² administer intravenously over 2 hours in 250 mL 5% dextrose injection (D5W) on day 1, every 2 weeks, concurrently with leucovorin administration (total dosage/cycle = 85 mg/m²)

Note: Oxaliplatin must not be mixed with sodium chloride injection. Therefore, when leucovorin and oxaliplatin are given concurrently via the same administration set tubing, both drugs must be administered in D5W

Leucovorin calcium 200 mg/m² per day; administer intravenously over 2 hours in 25–500 mL D5W for 2 consecutive days, on days 1 and 2, every 2 weeks (total dosage/cycle = 400 mg/m²) *followed by:*
Fluorouracil 400 mg/m² per day; administer by intravenous injection over 1–4 minutes after leucovorin for 2 consecutive days, on days 1 and 2, every 2 weeks, *followed by:*
Fluorouracil 600 mg/m² per day; administer by continuous intravenous infusion over 22 hours in 100–1000 mL 0.9% sodium chloride injection (0.9% NS) or D5W for 2 consecutive days, on days 1 and 2, every 2 weeks (total dosage/cycle = 2000 mg/m²)
or

mFOLFOX–6 (Tournigand et al, Cheeseman et al)
Oxaliplatin 85 mg/m²; administer intravenously over 2 hours in 500 mL D5W on day 1, every 2 weeks, concurrently with leucovorin administration (total dosage/cycle = 85 mg/m²)

Note: Oxaliplatin must not be mixed with sodium chloride injection. Therefore, when leucovorin and oxaliplatin are given concurrently via the same administration set tubing, both drugs must be administered in D5W
Either: **(racemic) leucovorin calcium** 400 mg/m² *or* **levoleucovorin calcium** 200 mg/m²; administer intravenously over 2 hours in 25–500 mL 0.9% NS or D5W on day 1, every 2 weeks (total dosage/cycle for racemic leucovorin = 400 mg/m², for levoleucovorin = 200 mg/m²), *followed by:*

Fluorouracil 400 mg/m²; administer by intravenous injection over 1–2 minutes after leucovorin on day 1, every 2 weeks, *followed by:*
Fluorouracil 2400 mg/m²; administer by continuous intravenous infusion over 46 hours in 100–1000 mL 0.9% NS or D5W, starting on day 1 every 2 weeks (total dosage/cycle = 2800 mg/m²)
• Infusional fluorouracil dosage may be increased to 3000 mg/m² by continuous intravenous infusion over 46 hours, starting on cycle 3, day 1, and repeated every 2 weeks in patients who do not develop adverse effects G >1 during the first 2 cycles (total dosage/cycle = 3400 mg/m²)
Note: The fluorouracil loading dose (400 mg/m²) can be omitted for better hematologic tolerance

Supportive Care
Antiemetic prophylaxis
Emetogenic potential on day 1 is **MODERATE**
Emetogenic potential on day 2 is **LOW to MODERATE**
See Chapter 42 for antiemetic recommendations

Hematopoietic growth factor (G-CSF) prophylaxis
Primary prophylaxis is **NOT** *indicated*
See Chapter 43 for more information

Antimicrobial prophylaxis
Risk of fever and neutropenia is **LOW**
  Antimicrobial primary prophylaxis to be considered:
  • Antibacterial—not indicated
  • Antifungal—not indicated
  • Antiviral—not indicated unless patient previously had an episode of HSV

(continued)

Patient Population Studied

Patients with previously untreated advanced colorectal cancer

Treatment Modifications (FOLFOX–4)

Adverse Event	Dose Modification
Any G2/3/4 nonhematologic toxicity	Delay start of next cycle until the severity of all toxicities are G ≤1 and decrease fluorouracil loading dosage from 400 mg/m² to 300 mg/m²
ANC ≤1500/mm³ or platelet count ≤100,000/mm³	Delay start of next cycle until ANC >1500/mm³ *and* platelet count >100,000/mm³
G3/4 nonneurologic	Reduce fluorouracil and oxaliplatin dosages by 20%
G3/4 ANC	Reduce oxaliplatin dosage by 20%
Persistent (≥14 days) paresthesias	Reduce oxaliplatin dosage by 20%
Temporary (7–14 days) painful paresthesias	
Temporary (7–14 days) functional impairment	
Persistent (≥14 days) painful paresthesias	Discontinue oxaliplatin
Persistent (≥14 days) functional impairment	

de Gramont A et al. J Clin Oncol 2000;18:2938–2947

(*continued*)

Diarrhea management

Latent or delayed-onset diarrhea*:
   Loperamide 4 mg orally initially after the first loose or liquid stool, *then*
   Loperamide 2 mg orally every 2 hours during waking hours, *plus*
   Loperamide 4 mg orally every 4 hours during hours of sleep
   • Continue for at least 12 hours after diarrhea resolves
   • Recurrent diarrhea after a 12-hour diarrhea-free interval is treated as a new episode
   • Rehydrate orally with fluids and electrolytes during a diarrheal episode
   • If diarrhea persists >48 hours despite loperamide, stop loperamide and hospitalize the patient for IV hydration

Persistent diarrhea:
   Octreotide 100–150 mcg subcutaneously 3 times daily. Maximum total daily dose is 1500 mcg

Antibiotic therapy during latent or delayed-onset diarrhea:
   A fluoroquinolone (eg, **ciprofloxacin** 500 mg orally every 12 hours) if absolute neutrophil count <500/mm^3 with or without accompanying fever in association with diarrhea
   • Antibiotics should also be administered if patient is hospitalized with prolonged diarrhea and should be continued until diarrhea resolves

*Abigerges D et al. J Natl Cancer Inst 1994;86:446–449
Rothenberg ML et al. J Clin Oncol 2001;19:3801–3807
Wadler S et al. J Clin Oncol 1998;16:3169–3178

Oral care
Standard prophylaxis and treatment for mucositis/stomatitis

Toxicity (N = 209) (FOLFOX–4)

	% G1	% G2	% G3	% G4
Nonhematologic				
Nausea	44	22.5	5.7	NA
Vomiting	24	24.4	4.3	1.5
Diarrhea	30.6	16.3	8.6	3.3
Mucositis	24.9	12.9	5.3	0.5
Cutaneous	19.6	9.1	0	0
Alopecia	15.8	1.9	NA	NA
Neurologic	20.6	29.2	18.2	NA
Hematologic				
Neutropenia	14.3	14.3	29.7	12
Thrombocytopenia	62.2	11.5	2	0.5
Anemia	59.8	23.5	3.3	0

de Gramont A et al. J Clin Oncol 2000;18:2938–2947

Treatment Modifications (FOLFOX–6)

Adverse Event	Dose Modification
ANC ≤1500/mm^3 or platelet count ≤100,000/mm^3 or persistent nonhematologic toxicity G ≥2	Delay start of next cycle until ANC >1500/mm^3 and platelet count >100,000/mm^3; omit fluorouracil by intravenous injection
G ≥3 toxicity	Reduce fluorouracil dosage to 2000 mg/m^2
G4 ANC, G3/4 thrombocytopenia or G4 diarrhea	Reduce oxaliplatin dosage to 75 mg/m^2
G2 paresthesias (persistent paresthesia or dysesthesia without functional impairment)	Reduce oxaliplatin dosage to 75 mg/m^2
Persistent G2/3 paresthesia/dysesthesia	Discontinue oxaliplatin
Persistent painful paresthesia or G3 neurotoxicity (persistent paresthesia or dysesthesia with persistent functional impairment)	Discontinue oxaliplatin

Tournigand C et al. J Clin Oncol 2004;22:229–237

Toxicity (N = 110) (FOLFOX–6)

	% G1	% G2	% G3	% G4
Nonhematologic				
Nausea	39	25	3	0
Vomiting	22	17	3	0
Diarrhea	28	13	9	2
Mucositis	35	10	1	0
Cutaneous	17	5	2	0
Alopecia	19	9	NA	NA
Neurologic*	26	37	34	NA
Fatigue	17	15	3	0
Hematologic				
Neutropenia	18	20	31	13
Thrombocytopenia	57	21	5	0
Anemia	39	12	3	0

*Neurotoxicity scale:
G1 = Short-lasting paresthesia with complete regression by next cycle
G2 = Persistent paresthesia or dysesthesia without functional impairment
G3 = Persistent functional impairment

Tournigand C et al. J Clin Oncol 2004;22:229–237

Efficacy (N = 210)

Intent-to-Treat Analysis

Objective response	50%
Complete response	1.4%
Partial response	48.6%
Stable disease	31.9%
Progressive disease	10%
Median survival	16.2 months

de Gramont A et al. J Clin Oncol 2000;18:2938–2947
WHO Criteria

Therapy Monitoring

1. *Before each cycle:* H&P, CBC with differential, CEA serum electrolytes, and LFTs
2. *Every 2–3 months:* CT scans to assess response in patients presenting with advanced colorectal cancer

METASTATIC • FIRST-LINE
COLORECTAL CANCER REGIMEN: MODIFIED FOLFOX6 ± BEVACIZUMAB

Venook AP et al. JAMA 2017;317:2392–2401
Venook AP et al. J Clin Oncol 2016;34(suppl):abstract 3504

Bevacizumab 5 mg/kg; administer intravenously in 100 mL 0.9% sodium chloride injection (0.9% NS), every 2 weeks, until disease progression (total dosage/2-week cycle = 5 mg/kg), *followed by:*

Oxaliplatin 85 mg/m²; administer intravenously over 2 hours in 500 mL 5% dextrose injection (D5W) on day 1, every 2 weeks, concurrently with leucovorin (or levoleucovorin) administration, until disease progression (total dosage/cycle = 85 mg/m²), *plus:*

Leucovorin calcium 400 mg/m²; administer intravenously over 2 hours in 25–500 mL D5W on day 1, every 2 weeks, concurrently with oxaliplatin, until disease progression (total dosage/2-week cycle = 400 mg/m²), *followed by:*

Fluorouracil 400 mg/m²; administer by intravenous injection over 1–2 minutes after leucovorin on day 1, every 2 weeks, until disease progression, *followed by:*

Fluorouracil 2400 mg/m²; administer by continuous intravenous infusion over 46 hours in 100–1000 mL 0.9% sodium chloride injection (0.9% NS) or D5W, starting on day 1 every 2 weeks, until disease progression (total fluorouracil dosage/cycle = 2800 mg/m²)

Notes:
• The fluorouracil bolus dose (400 mg/m²) can be omitted for better hematologic tolerance
• Oxaliplatin must not be mixed with sodium chloride injection. Therefore, when leucovorin and oxaliplatin are given concurrently via the same administration set tubing, both drugs must be administered in D5W
• Bevacizumab administration duration for the initial dose is 90 minutes. If administration is well tolerated, the administration duration may be decreased stepwise during subsequent administrations to 60 minutes and, finally, to a minimum duration of 30 minutes

Supportive Care
Antiemetic prophylaxis
Emetogenic potential on day 1 is **MODERATE**
Emetogenic potential on day 2 is **LOW**
See Chapter 42 for antiemetic recommendations

Hematopoietic growth factor (G-CSF) prophylaxis
Primary prophylaxis is **NOT** *indicated*
See Chapter 43 for more information

Antimicrobial prophylaxis
Risk of fever and neutropenia is **LOW**
  Antimicrobial primary prophylaxis to be considered:
  • Antibacterial—not indicated
  • Antifungal—not indicated
  • Antiviral—not indicated unless patient previously had an episode of HSV

Diarrhea management
Latent or delayed-onset diarrhea*:
Loperamide 4 mg orally initially after the first loose or liquid stool, *then*
Loperamide 2 mg orally every 2 hours during waking hours, *plus*
Loperamide 4 mg orally every 4 hours during hours of sleep
• Continue for at least 12 hours after diarrhea resolves
• Recurrent diarrhea after a 12-hour diarrhea-free interval is treated as a new episode
• Rehydrate orally with fluids and electrolytes during a diarrheal episode
• If a patient develops blood or mucus in stool, dehydration, or hemodynamic instability, or if diarrhea persists >48 hours despite loperamide, stop loperamide and hospitalize the patient for intravenous hydration
  Alternatively, a trial of **diphenoxylate hydrochloride** 2.5 mg with **atropine sulfate** 0.025 mg (eg, Lomotil)
• Initial adult dose is 2 tablets 4 times daily until control has been achieved, after which the dose may be reduced to meet individual requirements. Control may often be maintained with as little as 2 tablets daily
• Clinical improvement of acute diarrhea is usually observed within 48 hours. If improvement of chronic diarrhea after treatment with a maximum daily dose of 8 tablets is not observed within 10 days, control is unlikely with further administration

*Abigerges D et al. J Natl Cancer Inst 1994; 86:446–449
Rothenberg ML et al. J Clin Oncol 2001; 19:3801–3807
Wadler S et al. J Clin Oncol 1998; 16:3169–3178

(continued)

(*continued*)

Persistent diarrhea:
   Octreotide 100–150 mcg subcutaneously 3 times daily. Maximum total daily dose is 1500 mcg
Antibiotic therapy during latent or delayed-onset diarrhea:
   A fluoroquinolone (eg, **ciprofloxacin** 500 mg orally every 12 hours) if absolute neutrophil count <500/mm³ with or without accompanying fever in association with diarrhea
   • Antibiotics should also be administered if patient is hospitalized with prolonged diarrhea and should be continued until diarrhea resolves

Oral care
Standard prophylaxis and treatment for mucositis/stomatitis

Patient Population Studied

CALGB/SWOG 80405 was a cooperative group, multicenter, multinational, randomized clinical trial involving 1137 adult patients with pathologically confirmed untreated locally advanced or metastatic colorectal cancer. Patients were required to have an Eastern Cooperative Oncology Group (ECOG) performance status of 0 or 1, adequate organ function, and, according to a protocol amendment, KRAS wild-type (codons 12 and 13) disease. The choice of therapy with mFOLFOX6 or FOLFIRI was per patient and physician discretion before enrollment. From November 2005 to September 2009, patients were randomized 1:1:1 to receive cetuximab, bevacizumab, or the combination of cetuximab and bevacizumab in addition to the chosen chemotherapy regimen. The arm containing the combination of both cetuximab and bevacizumab was subsequently discontinued by protocol amendment and thereafter patients were randomized 1:1 to receive either cetuximab or bevacizumab

Efficacy (N = 1137)

	mFOLFOX–6/FOLFIRI + Bevacizumab (N = 559 with KRAS Wild-Type Disease)	mFOLFOX–6/FOLFIRI + Cetuximab (N = 578 with KRAS Wild-Type Disease)	
Median OS*	29.0 months	30.0 months	HR 0.88 (95% CI, 0.77–1.01); P = 0.08
Median PFS*	10.6 months	10.5 months	HR 0.95 (95% CI, 0.84–1.08); P = 0.45
Response rate*	55.2%	59.6%	P = 0.13

Median follow-up was 47.4 months (range, 0.0–110.7 months)
OS, overall survival; PFS, progression-free survival
*Analysis restricted to KRAS wild-type population

	Median Overall Survival		
	Right-sided Primary Tumor Location*	Left-sided Primary Tumor Location†	
mFOLFOX–6/FOLFIRI + cetuximab (N = 578)	16.4 months	37.5 months	HR 1.97 (95% CI, 1.56–2.48)
mFOLFOX–6/FOLFIRI + bevacizumab (N = 559)	24.5 months	32.1 months	HR 1.26 (95% CI, 1.00–1.58)

*Right side was defined as extending from the cecum to the hepatic flexure
†Left side was defined as extending from the splenic flexure to the rectum
In KRAS wild-type patients with left-sided primary tumor location, cetuximab-based chemotherapy was superior to bevacizumab-based chemotherapy (P = 0.04). In KRAS wild-type patients with right-sided primary tumors, bevacizumab-based chemotherapy was superior to cetuximab-based chemotherapy (P = 0.03)
Venook AP et al. J Clin Oncol 2016;34(suppl):abstract 3504

Therapy Monitoring

1. *Before each cycle:* H&P, CBC with differential, serum bilirubin, AST or ALT, alkaline phosphatase, serum creatinine, BUN, and CEA if being used to monitor disease
2. Observe closely for hypersensitivity reactions, especially during the first and second bevacizumab infusions
3. Blood pressure every 2 weeks or more frequently as indicated during treatment
4. Assess proteinuria by urine dipstick and/or urinary protein creatinine ratio prior to each cycle. Patients with a ≥2+ urine dipstick reading should undergo further assessment with a 24-hour urine collection
5. Every 2–3 months: CT scans to assess response

Treatment Modifications

BEVACIZUMAB DOSE MODIFICATIONS

Adverse Event	Treatment Modification
Gastrointestinal perforations (gastrointestinal perforations, fistula formation in the gastrointestinal tract, intra-abdominal abscess), fistula formation involving an internal organ	Discontinue bevacizumab permanently
Serious bleeding	
Wound dehiscence requiring medical intervention	
Nephrotic syndrome	
Hypertensive crisis or hypertensive encephalopathy or reversible posterior leukoencephalopathy syndrome (RPLS)	
Congestive heart failure	
Necrotizing fasciitis	
Severe arterial or venous thromboembolic events	Discontinue bevacizumab permanently; the safety of reinitiating bevacizumab after a thromboembolic event is resolved is not known
Moderate to severe proteinuria	Patients with a ≥2+ dipstick reading should undergo further assessment, eg, 24-hour urine collection. Suspend bevacizumab administration for ≥2 g proteinuria/24 h and resume when proteinuria is <2 g/24 h
Severe hypertension not controlled with medical management	Hold bevacizumab pending further evaluation and treatment of hypertension
Mild, clinically insignificant infusion reaction	Decrease the rate of infusion
Clinically significant but not severe infusion reaction	Interrupt the infusion and consider resuming at a slower rate following resolution. If decision is made to restart, the infusion may be continued at ≤50% of the rate prior to the reaction and increased in 50% increments every 30 minutes if well tolerated. Infusions may be restarted at the full rate during the next cycle
Severe infusion reaction (hypertension, hypertensive crises associated with neurologic signs and symptoms, wheezing, oxygen desaturation, G3 hypersensitivity, chest pain, headaches, rigors, and diaphoresis)	Stop infusion and administer appropriate medical therapy (eg, epinephrine, corticosteroids, intravenous antihistamines, bronchodilators and/or oxygen). Discontinue bevacizumab
Planned elective surgery	Suspend bevacizumab at least 28 days before elective surgery and do not resume for at least 28 days after surgery or until surgical incision is fully healed
Recent hemoptysis	Do not administer bevacizumab
Evidence of rectosigmoid involvement by pelvic examination or bowel involvement on CT scan or clinical symptoms of bowel obstruction	

(continued)

Treatment Modifications (*continued*)

mFOLFOX 6 DOSE MODIFICATIONS

Adverse Event	Treatment Modification
Day 1 persistent nonhematologic toxicity G ≥2	Delay start of next cycle until the severity of all toxicities are G ≤1; omit fluorouracil by intravenous bolus injection in subsequent cycles
Day 1 ANC ≤1500/mm³ *or* platelet count ≤100,000/mm³	Delay start of next cycle until ANC >1500/mm³ *and* platelet count >100,000/mm³; omit fluorouracil by intravenous bolus injection in subsequent cycles
G4 neutropenia (<500/mm³), G3/4 thrombocytopenia (<50,000/mm³) or G4 diarrhea (life-threatening; urgent intervention required)	Reduce oxaliplatin dosage to 75 mg/m² and omit fluorouracil by intravenous bolus injection in subsequent cycles
G ≥3 non-neurologic toxicity	Reduce infusional fluorouracil dosage to 2000 mg/m²
G2 paresthesia (persistent paresthesia or dysesthesia, moderate in nature without functional impairment other than limiting instrumental ADLs)	Reduce oxaliplatin dosage to 75 mg/m²
Persistent G2 paresthesia/dysesthesia	Discontinue oxaliplatin
Persistent painful paresthesia or G3 neuropathy (persistent paresthesia or dysesthesia with persistent functional impairment limiting self-care and ADLs)	Discontinue oxaliplatin

ADLs, activities of daily living; ANC, absolute neutrophil count
Tournigand C et al. J Clin Oncol 2004;22:229–237

Adverse Events (N = 1092)

	mFOLFOX/FOLFIRI + Bevacizumab (n = 539)		mFOLFOX/FOLFIRI + Cetuximab (n = 553)	
	Grade 3	Grade 4	Grade 3	Grade 4
Blood or bone marrow adverse events	23	6	25	7
Fatigue	7	1	9	1
Diarrhea	8	<1	11	0
Sensory neuropathy	13	1	13	0

Included in the table are grade ≥3 adverse events at least possibly related to treatment and occurring in at least 10% of patients in either treatment group
Deaths at least possibly related to protocol therapy occurred in 8 patients in the bevacizumab group and in 7 patients in the cetuximab group.
The authors note that grade 1–2 rash predominated in the cetuximab arm and grade 1–2 hypertension predominated in the bevacizumab arm

METASTATIC • FIRST-LINE
COLORECTAL CANCER: CAPECITABINE + OXALIPLATIN (XELOX) ± BEVACIZUMAB

Cassidy J et al. J Clin Oncol 2008;26:2006–2012
Saltz LB et al. J Clin Oncol 2008;26:2013–2019

Oxaliplatin 130 mg/m^2; administer intravenously in 250–500 mL 5% dextrose injection over 2 hours on day 1, every 21 days, until disease progression (total dosage/3-week cycle = 130 mg/m^2)

Capecitabine 1000 mg/m^2 per dose; administer orally twice daily (approximately every 12 hours, within 30 minutes after a meal) for 14 consecutive days, on days 1–14 (28 doses), every 21 days, until disease progression (total dosage/3-week cycle = 28,000 mg/m^2)

The above regimen (XELOX) may be given with or without bevacizumab as described below:

> **Bevacizumab** 7.5 mg/kg; administer intravenously in 100 mL 0.9% sodium chloride injection (0.9% NS) every 3 weeks, until disease progression (total dosage/3-week cycle = 7.5 mg/kg)
>
> *Note:* Bevacizumab administration duration for the initial dose is 90 minutes. If administration is well tolerated, the administration duration may be decreased stepwise during subsequent administrations to 60 minutes and, finally, to a minimum duration of 30 minutes

Supportive Care
Antiemetic prophylaxis
Emetogenic potential on day 1 is **MODERATE**
Emetogenic potential on days with capecitabine alone is **MINIMAL–LOW**
See Chapter 42 for antiemetic recommendations

Hematopoietic growth factor (G-CSF) prophylaxis
Primary prophylaxis may be indicated
See Chapter 43 for more information

Antimicrobial prophylaxis
Risk of fever and neutropenia is **LOW**
> *Antimicrobial primary prophylaxis to be considered:*
> - Antibacterial—not indicated
> - Antifungal—not indicated
> - Antiviral—not indicated, unless patient previously had an episode of HSV

Hand-foot reaction (palmar-plantar erythrodysesthesia, PPE)
For patients who develop a hand-foot reaction, use topical emollients (eg, Aquaphor®), topical or orally administered steroids, antihistamine agents (H$_1$-receptor antagonists), or pyridoxine
> - Pyridoxine may provide relief for discomfort/pain associated with PPE, although the mechanism through which this occurs remains unclear
> - The suggested pyridoxine starting dose is 50 mg/day, which may be increased to a maximum of 200 mg/day

Diarrhea management
Latent or delayed-onset diarrhea:*
> **Loperamide** 4 mg orally initially after the first loose or liquid stool, *then* 2-4 mg orally every 2-4 hours or **diphenoxylate hydrochloride** 2.5 mg **with atropine sulfate** 0.025 mg (e.g., Lomotil®)

*Abigerges D et al. J Natl Cancer Inst 1994; 86:446–449
Rothenberg ML et al. J Clin Oncol 2001; 19:3801–3807
Wadler S et al. J Clin Oncol 1998; 16:3169–3178

Oral care
Standard prophylaxis and treatment for mucositis/stomatitis

Patient Population Studied

The multinational, multicenter, randomized, double-blind (with respect to bevacizumab vs. placebo), 2 × 2 factorial design trial involved 2034 patients with histologically confirmed unresectable metastatic colorectal cancer who had not received prior systemic therapy for metastatic disease. The study was originally a randomized two-arm study comparing XELOX and FOLFOX4, but it was amended to a 2 × 2 factorial design to assess the effect of bevacizumab. Patients were required to have an Eastern Cooperative Oncology Group (ECOG) performance status of 0 or 1 and adequate organ function. Patients were excluded if they had received prior oxaliplatin or bevacizumab; had clinically significant cardiovascular disease; had clinically detectable ascites; were treated with full-dose anticoagulation; had central nervous system metastases; had a severe nonhealing wound, ulcer, or fracture; had a known bleeding disorder or coagulopathy; or had proteinuria ≥500 mg/24 hours. Patients were randomly assigned to either capecitabine + oxaliplatin (XELOX) ± bevacizumab or to fluorouracil/folinic acid + oxaliplatin (FOLFOX–4) ± bevacizumab after stratification by region, ECOG performance status, presence of liver metastases, alkaline phosphatase, and number of metastatic sites

Efficacy

	FOLFOX4 + Placebo/ Bevacizumab (n = 1017)	XELOX + Placebo/ Bevacizumab (n = 1017)	
Median progression-free survival	8.5 months	8.0 months	HR 1.04 (97.5% CI, 0.93–1.16)*
Median overall survival	19.6 months	19.8 months	HR 0.99 (97.5% CI, 0.88–1.12)
Overall response rate (investigator-assessed)	48%	47%	OR 0.94 (97.5% CI, 0.77–1.15)†
Median duration of response	7.6 months	7.5 months	HR 1.00 (97.5% CI, 0.85–1.18)

*Non-inferiority was concluded if the upper limit of the 97.5% CI was below the non-inferiority margin of 1.23
†Non-inferiority was concluded if the lower limit of the 97.5% CI was above the non-inferiority margin of 0.66

	XELOX/FOLFOX4 + Placebo (n = 701)	XELOX/FOLFOX4 + Bevacizumab (n = 699)	
Median progression-free survival	8.0 months	9.4 months	HR 0.83 (97.5% CI, 0.72–0.95); P = 0.0023
Median overall survival	19.9 months	21.3 months	HR 0.89 (97.5% CI, 0.76–1.03); P = 0.0769
Overall response rate (investigator-assessed)	49%	47%	OR 0.90 (97.5% CI, 0.71–1.14)†; P = 0.31
Median duration of response	7.4 months	8.45 months	HR 0.82 (97.5% CI, 0.66–1.01); P = 0.0307

Therapy Monitoring

1. Prior to each cycle of capecitabine + oxaliplatin: CBC with differential, serum bilirubin, AST or ALT, alkaline phosphatase, serum creatinine, CEA if being used to follow disease. Assessment for peripheral neuropathy

2. If bevacizumab is included in the treatment regimen:

   a. Observe closely for hypersensitivity reactions, especially during the first and second bevacizumab infusions

   b. Blood pressure every 2 weeks or more frequently as indicated during treatment (if bevacizumab is given)

   c. Assess proteinuria by urine dipstick and/or urinary protein creatinine ratio prior to each cycle. Patients with a ≥2+ urine dipstick reading should undergo further assessment with a 24-hour urine collection

3. Every 2–3 months: CT scans to assess response

Treatment Modifications

BEVACIZUMAB DOSE MODIFICATIONS

Adverse Event	Treatment Modification
Gastrointestinal perforations (gastrointestinal perforations, fistula formation in the gastrointestinal tract, intra-abdominal abscess), fistula formation involving an internal organ	Discontinue bevacizumab permanently
Serious bleeding	
Wound dehiscence requiring medical intervention	
Nephrotic syndrome	
Hypertensive crisis or hypertensive encephalopathy or reversible posterior leukoencephalopathy syndrome (RPLS)	
Congestive heart failure	
Necrotizing fasciitis	
Severe arterial or venous thromboembolic events	Discontinue bevacizumab permanently; the safety of reinitiating bevacizumab after a thromboembolic event is resolved is not known
Moderate to severe proteinuria	Patients with a ≥2+ dipstick reading should undergo further assessment, eg, 24-hour urine collection. Suspend bevacizumab administration for ≥2 g proteinuria/24 h and resume when proteinuria is <2 g/24 h

(continued)

Treatment Modifications (continued)

Adverse Event	Treatment Modification
Severe hypertension not controlled with medical management	Hold bevacizumab pending further evaluation and treatment of hypertension
Mild, clinically insignificant infusion reaction	Decrease the rate of infusion
Clinically significant but not severe infusion reaction	Interrupt the infusion and consider resuming at a slower rate following resolution. If decision is made to restart, the infusion may be continued at ≤50% of the rate prior to the reaction and increased in 50% increments every 30 minutes if well tolerated. Infusions may be restarted at the full rate during the next cycle
Severe infusion reaction (hypertension, hypertensive crises associated with neurologic signs and symptoms, wheezing, oxygen desaturation, G3 hypersensitivity, chest pain, headaches, rigors, and diaphoresis)	Stop infusion and administer appropriate medical therapy (eg, epinephrine, corticosteroids, intravenous antihistamines, bronchodilators and/or oxygen). Discontinue bevacizumab
Planned elective surgery	Suspend bevacizumab at least 28 days before elective surgery and do not resume for at least 28 days after surgery or until surgical incision is fully healed
Recent hemoptysis	Do not administer bevacizumab
Evidence of rectosigmoid involvement by pelvic examination or bowel involvement on CT scan or clinical symptoms of bowel obstruction	

CAPECITABINE + OXALIPLATIN DOSE MODIFICATIONS

ANC nadir <1000/mm³ *or* platelet nadir <50,000/mm³ after treatment	Delay treatment until ANC is ≥1000/mm³ *and* platelet count is ≥50,000/mm³, then decrease oxaliplatin dosage by 25%, and decrease daily capecitabine dosages by 50% during subsequent cycles.* Alternatively, consider using hematopoietic growth factors
Persistent G1/G2 neuropathy	Delay oxaliplatin 1 week. After toxicity resolves, resume oxaliplatin at a dosage decreased to 100 mg/m² during subsequent cycles
"Transient" G3/4 neuropathy (7–14 days)	Hold oxaliplatin. After toxicity resolves, resume oxaliplatin at a dosage decreased to 100 mg/m² during subsequent cycles
Persistent G3/4 neuropathy	Discontinue oxaliplatin
G3/4 diarrhea or stomatitis despite capecitabine dose reductions	Reduce oxaliplatin dosage to 100 mg/m²
G3/4 nonhematologic adverse events other than renal dysfunction and neurotoxicity	Reduce oxaliplatin and capecitabine dosages by 25% during subsequent cycles
G2 stomatitis, diarrhea, or nausea	Hold capecitabine; resume capecitabine at full dosage after resolution of toxicity
Second episode of G2 stomatitis, diarrhea, or nausea	Hold capecitabine; resume capecitabine with dosage reduced by 25% after toxicity resolves
Third episode of G2 stomatitis, diarrhea, or nausea	Hold capecitabine; resume capecitabine with dosage reduced by 50% after toxicity resolves
Fourth episode of G2 stomatitis, diarrhea, or nausea	Discontinue capecitabine
G3 stomatitis, diarrhea, or nausea	Hold capecitabine. If G3 toxicity is adequately controlled within 2 days, resume capecitabine at full dosage when toxicity abates to G ≤1. If G3 toxicity takes >2 days to be controlled, resume capecitabine with dosage reduced by 25% after toxicity abates to G ≤1
Second episode of G3 stomatitis, diarrhea, or nausea	Hold capecitabine. If G3 toxicity is controlled adequately within 2 days, then resume capecitabine with dosage reduced by 50% after toxicity abates to G ≤1
Third episode of G3 stomatitis, diarrhea, or nausea	Discontinue capecitabine
G4 stomatitis, diarrhea, or nausea	Discontinue capecitabine. Resume capecitabine with dosage reduced by 50% after toxicity resolves
G1 capecitabine-associated PPE[†]	Begin pyridoxine 50 mg orally 3 times daily and continue capecitabine without dose modification
G2 capecitabine-associated PPE[†]	Begin pyridoxine 50 mg orally 3 times daily and withhold capecitabine. Resume capecitabine with dosage reduced by 15% after toxicity resolves
G3 capecitabine-associated PPE[†]	Begin pyridoxine 50 mg orally 3 times daily and withhold capecitabine. Resume capecitabine with dosage reduced by 30% after toxicity resolves
Recurrent G3 capecitabine-associated PPE[†]	Begin pyridoxine 50 mg orally 3 times daily and withhold capecitabine. Resume capecitabine with dosage reduced by 50% after toxicity resolves

*Treatment delays for unresolved adverse events of >3 weeks duration warrant discontinuation of treatment
[†]PPE, palmar-plantar erythrodysesthesia (hand-foot syndrome)

Adverse Events

Grade (%)*	FOLFOX4 Alone or FOLFOX + Placebo (n = 649)		XELOX Alone or XELOX + Placebo (n = 655)	
	Grade 1/2	Grade 3/4	Grade 1/2	Grade 3/4
Nausea	59	5	58	5
Diarrhea	49	11	45	20
Neutropenia	15	43	20	7
Fatigue	37	8	33	5
Vomiting	35	4	38	5
Paresthesia	34	4	32	5
Stomatitis	35	2	20	1
Anorexia	25	3	25	2
Hand-foot syndrome	9	1	24	6
Constipation	25	2	22	1
Pyrexia	25	1	18	1
Abdominal pain	23	4	21	5
Thrombocytopenia	20	3	15	7
Peripheral neuropathy	16	4	16	4
Asthenia	17	4	15	4

Included in the table are adverse events occurring in >20% of patients (treatment-related and unrelated). Patients who received bevacizumab were not included in this table

Grade (%)	FOLFOX4/XELOX + Placebo (n = 675)	Bevacizumab + FOLFOX4/ XELOX (n = 694)
	Grade 3/4	Grade 3/4
Venous thromboembolism	5	8
Hypertension	1	4
Bleeding	1	2
Arterial thromboembolic events*	1	2
Gastrointestinal perforations	<1	1
Wound healing complications	<1	<1
Fistula/intra-abdominal abscess	0	1
Proteinuria	0	1

Only adverse events of special interest to bevacizumab are included in the table
*Also includes ischemic cardiac events

METASTATIC • FIRST-LINE
COLORECTAL CANCER REGIMEN: CETUXIMAB + FOLFOX4

Bokemeyer C et al. J Clin Oncol 2009;27:663–671
Cunningham D et al. N Engl J Med 2004;351:337–345
de Gramont A et al. J Clin Oncol 2000;18:2938–2947

Warning:

1. Severe infusion reactions occurred with the administration of cetuximab in approximately 3% of patients (17/633), rarely with fatal outcome (<1 in 1000)

2. Approximately 90% of severe infusion reactions are associated with the first infusion of cetuximab despite the use of prophylactic antihistamines

3. Infusion reactions are characterized by the rapid onset of airway obstruction (bronchospasm, stridor, hoarseness), urticaria, and/or hypotension

4. Caution must be exercised with every cetuximab infusion, as there were patients who experienced their first severe infusion reaction during later infusions

5. Provocative test doses do not reliably predict hypersensitivity reactions to cetuximab administration and are not recommended

Mild to moderate infusion reactions

• Interrupt or slow the cetuximab infusion rate

• Permanently decrease the administration rate by 50%

• Give antihistamine prophylaxis before repeated treatments

Severe reactions

• Immediately interrupt cetuximab therapy

• Administer epinephrine, glucocorticoids, intravenous antihistamines, bronchodilators, and oxygen as needed

• Permanently discontinue further treatment

Cetuximab premedication:
Diphenhydramine 50 mg by intravenous injection before cetuximab administration (other H_1-receptor antagonists may be substituted)

Initial cetuximab dose:
Cetuximab 400 mg/m^2; administer intravenously over 120 minutes (maximum infusion rate = 5 mL/min [10 mg/min]) as a single dose (total initial dosage = 400 mg/m^2)

Maintenance cetuximab doses:
Cetuximab 250 mg/m^2; administer intravenously over 60 minutes (maximum infusion rate = 5 mL/min [10 mg/min]) every week (total weekly dosage = 250 mg/m^2)

Notes:

• Cetuximab is intended for direct administration and should not be diluted

• Maximum infusion rate = 5 mL (10 mg)/min (300 mL/h, or 600 mg/h)

• Administer cetuximab through a low protein-binding inline filter with pore size = 0.22 μm

• Use 0.9% sodium chloride injection to flush vascular access devices after administration is completed

FOLFOX–4 (de Gramont A et al.):
Oxaliplatin 85 mg/m^2; administer intravenously in 250 mL 5% dextrose injection (D5W) over 2 hours concurrently with leucovorin administration, on day 1 every 2 weeks (total dosage/cycle = 85 mg/m^2)
Note: Oxaliplatin must not be mixed with sodium chloride injection. Therefore, when leucovorin and oxaliplatin are given concurrently via a Y-connector, both drugs must be administered in D5W
Leucovorin calcium 200 mg/m^2 per dose; administer intravenously in 25–500 mL D5W over 2 hours on 2 consecutive days, on days 1 and 2, every 2 weeks (total dosage/cycle = 400 mg/m^2), *followed by:*
Fluorouracil 400 mg/m^2 per dose; administer by intravenous injection over 1–2 minutes after leucovorin on 2 consecutive days, on days 1 and 2, every 2 weeks, *followed by:*
Fluorouracil 600 mg/m^2 per dose; administer by continuous intravenous infusion in 100–1000 mL 0.9% sodium chloride injection (0.9% NS) or D5W over 22 hours on 2 consecutive days, on days 1 and 2, every 2 weeks (total dosage/cycle = 2000 mg/m^2)
Note: **Fluorouracil** boluses (400 mg/m^2 by intravenous injection) may be omitted for better hematologic tolerance

Supportive Care
Antiemetic prophylaxis
Emetogenic potential on days with cetuximab is **MINIMAL**
Emetogenic potential on days with oxaliplatin is **MODERATE**
Emetogenic potential on days with fluorouracil and leucovorin alone is **LOW**
See Chapter 42 for antiemetic recommendations

(continued)

(continued)

Hematopoietic growth factor (G-CSF) prophylaxis
Primary prophylaxis may be indicated
See Chapter 43 for more information

Antimicrobial prophylaxis
*Risk of fever and neutropenia is **LOW***
   Antimicrobial primary prophylaxis to be considered:
- Antibacterial—not indicated
- Antifungal—not indicated
- Antiviral—not indicated unless patient previously had an episode of HSV

Diarrhea management
Latent or delayed-onset diarrhea*:
  Loperamide 4 mg orally initially after the first loose or liquid stool, *then*
  Loperamide 2 mg orally every 2 hours during waking hours, *plus*
  Loperamide 4 mg orally every 4 hours during hours of sleep
- Continue for at least 12 hours after diarrhea resolves
- Recurrent diarrhea after a 12-hour diarrhea-free interval is treated as a new episode
- Rehydrate orally with fluids and electrolytes during a diarrheal episode
- If a patient develops blood or mucus in stool, dehydration, or hemodynamic instability, or if diarrhea persists >48 hours despite loperamide, stop loperamide and hospitalize the patient for IV hydration

Alternatively, a trial of **diphenoxylate hydrochloride** 2.5 mg with **atropine sulfate** 0.025 mg (eg, Lomotil)
- Initial adult dose is 2 tablets 4 times daily until control has been achieved, after which the dose may be reduced to meet individual requirements. Control may often be maintained with as little as 2 tablets daily
- Clinical improvement of acute diarrhea is usually observed within 48 hours. If improvement of chronic diarrhea after treatment with a maximum daily dose of 8 tablets is not observed within 10 days, control is unlikely with further administration

Persistent diarrhea:
  Octreotide 100–150 mcg subcutaneously 3 times daily. Maximum total daily dose is 1500 mcg
Antibiotic therapy during latent or delayed-onset diarrhea:
  A fluoroquinolone (eg, **ciprofloxacin** 500 mg orally every 12 hours) if absolute neutrophil count <500/mm^3 with or without accompanying fever in association with diarrhea
- Antibiotics should also be administered if patient is hospitalized with prolonged diarrhea and should be continued until diarrhea resolves

*Abigerges D et al. J Natl Cancer Inst 1994;86:446–449
Rothenberg ML et al. J Clin Oncol 2001;19:3801–3807
Wadler S et al. J Clin Oncol 1998;16:3169–3178

Hand-foot reaction (palmar-plantar erythrodysesthesia, PPE)
For patients who develop a hand-foot reaction, use topical emollients (eg, Aquaphor®), topical or orally administered steroids, antihistamine agents (H$_1$-receptor antagonists), or pyridoxine
- Pyridoxine may provide relief for discomfort/pain associated with PPE although the mechanism through which this occurs remains unclear
- The suggested pyridoxine starting dose is 50 mg/day, which may be increased to a maximum of 200 mg/day

Patient Population Studied

463 patients with histologically confirmed, first occurrence of a nonresectable, EGFR-expressing metastatic colorectal cancer (mCRC) with a life expectancy of >12 weeks; an Eastern Cooperative Oncology Group Performance Status (ECOG-PS) >2. Patients were ineligible if they had a history of previous exposure to EGFR-targeted therapy or previous chemotherapy (except adjuvant treatment) for mCRC

Efficacy*

	ITT (N = 337)		KRAS WT (N = 134)		KRAS MT (N = 99)	
	F	F + C	F	F + C	F	F + C
Complete response (%)	0.6	1	1	3	2	0
Partial response (%)	35	44	36	57	45	33
Progression-free survival (months)	7.2	7.2	7.2	7.7	8.6	5.5
Percent progression-free at 3 months	85	83	78	93	87	78
Percent progression-free at 6 months	59	53	54	66	69	39
Percent progression-free at 9 months	34	34	27	47	42	20
Percent progression-free at 12 months	12	24	13	30	14	6

C, Cetuximab; F, FOLFOX–4 (oxaliplatin, leucovorin, and fluorouracil); ITT, intention to treat; MT, mutant; WT, wild type
*Modified WHO criteria

Therapy Monitoring

1. *Before each cycle:* H&P, CBC with differential, CEA if initially elevated, serum electrolytes, serum magnesium, and LFTs
2. *Every 2–3 months:* CT scans to assess response in patients presenting with advanced colorectal cancer

Treatment Modifications

ERBITUX (Cetuximab) product label, August 2013. Manufactured by ImClone Systems Incorporated, Branchburg, NJ. Distributed and marketed by Bristol-Myers Squibb Company, Princeton, NJ, and Eli Lilly and Company, Indianapolis, IN

Cetuximab Infusion Reactions

Mild/moderate (G1/2)	Permanently decrease administration rates by 50%
Severe (G3/4)	Immediately and permanently discontinue

Cetuximab Dermatologic Toxicity—Severe (G3/4)

Occurrence	Cetuximab	Improvement	Cetuximab Dosage
First	Delay infusion 1–2 weeks	Yes	Continue at 250 mg/m^2
		No	Discontinue
Second	Delay infusion 1–2 weeks	Yes	Decrease to 200 mg/m^2
		No	Discontinue
Third	Delay infusion 1–2 weeks	Yes	Decrease to 150 mg/m^2
		No	Discontinue
Fourth	Discontinue		

Information from the product label: www.erbitux.com [accessed October 15, 2013]

(*continued*)

Treatment Modifications (continued)

Fluorouracil and Oxaliplatin

Any G2/3/4 nonhematologic toxicity	Delay start of next cycle until the severity of all toxicities is G ≤1
ANC ≤1500/mm³ or platelet count ≤100,000/mm³	Delay start of next cycle until ANC >1500/mm³ and platelet count >100,000/mm³
G3/4 Nonneurologic	Reduce fluorouracil and oxaliplatin dosages by 20%
G3/4 ANC	Reduce oxaliplatin dosage by 20%
Persistent (≥14 days) paresthesias	Reduce oxaliplatin dosage by 20%
Temporary (7–14 days) painful paresthesias	
Temporary (7–14 days) functional impairment	
Persistent (≥14 days) painful paresthesias	Discontinue oxaliplatin
Persistent (≥14 days) functional impairment	

Adapted in part from de Gramont A et al. J Clin Oncol 2000;18:2938–2947

Relevant G3/4 Adverse Events Occurring in ≥3% of Patients*

G3/4 Adverse Event	FOLFOX4	Cetuximab + FOLFOX4
Any G3/4 event	70	78
Neutropenia	34	30
Rash[†]	0.6	11
Diarrhea[†]	7	8
Leukopenia	6	7
Thrombocytopenia	2	4
Fatigue[†]	3	4
Palmar-plantar erythrodysesthesia (PPE)[†]	0.6	4
Peripheral sensory neuropathy[†]	7	4
Anemia[†]	2	4
Composite Categories		
Skin reactions[†‡]	0.6	18
Infusion-related reactions[§]	2	5

*National Cancer Institute (USA) Common Toxicity Criteria, version 2.0. At: http://ctep.cancer.gov/protocolDevelopment/electronic_applications/ctc.htm [accessed October 11, 2013]

[†]No G4 adverse events

[‡]The special adverse event category skin reactions included the following Medical Dictionary for Regulatory Activities 8.1 terms: acne, acne pustular, cellulitis, dermatitis acneiform, dry skin, erysipelas, erythema, face edema, folliculitis, growth of eyelashes, hair growth abnormal, hypertrichosis, nail bed infection, nail bed inflammation, nail disorder, nail infection, paronychia, pruritus, rash, rash erythematous, rash follicular, rash generalized, rash macular, rash maculopapular, rash popular, rash pruritic, rash pustular, skin exfoliation, skin hyperpigmentation, skin necrosis, staphylococcal scalded skin syndrome, telangiectasia, wound necrosis, xerosis

[§]The special adverse event category infusion-related reactions included the following Medical Dictionary for Regulatory Activities 8.1 terms: acute respiratory failure, apnea, asthma, bronchial obstruction, bronchospasm, cyanosis, dyspnea, dyspnea at rest, dyspnea exacerbated, dyspnea exertional, hypoxia, orthopnea, respiratory distress, respiratory failure, chills, hyperpyrexia, pyrexia, acute myocardial infarction, angina pectoris, blood pressure decreased, cardiac failure, cardiopulmonary failure, clonus, convulsion, epilepsy, hypotension, infusion-related reaction, loss of consciousness, myocardial infarction, myocardial ischemia, shock, sudden death, and syncope, occurring on the first day of treatment; and anaphylactic reaction, anaphylactic shock, anaphylactoid reaction, anaphylactoid shock, drug hypersensitivity, and hypersensitivity, occurring at any time during treatment

Note: The median duration of cetuximab treatment was 24 weeks, with 84% of patients having a relative dose intensity (RDI) of ≥80%. Similar numbers of patients in both arms had RDIs of ≥80% for oxaliplatin (75% and 80% of patients receiving cetuximab plus FOLFOX–4 and FOLFOX–4, respectively) and FU (67% and 70% of patients, respectively). Reductions and delays in cetuximab dosing were primarily because of skin reactions, and delays in chemotherapy dosing were because of hematologic, GI, or neurologic reactions

METASTATIC • FIRST-LINE

COLORECTAL CANCER REGIMEN: PANITUMUMAB + MODIFIED FOLFOX6

Cheeseman SL et al. Br J Cancer 2002;87:393–399
de Gramont A et al. J Clin Oncol 2000;18:2938–2947
Douillard J-Y et al. J Clin Oncol 2010;28:4697–4705

Panitumumab 6 mg/kg; administer intravenously in 0.9% sodium chloride injection (100 mL for doses ≤1000 mg; 150 mL for doses >1000 mg; product concentration should be <10 mg/mL) over 60–90 minutes on day 1 before mFOLFOX6 chemotherapy, every 2 weeks (total dosage/cycle = 6 mg/kg)

Notes:
- Severe infusion reactions occur in approximately 1% of patients (anaphylactic reactions, bronchospasm, fever, chills, and hypotension). Dose adjustment or discontinuation of panitumumab is warranted depending on the severity of the reaction
- Panitumumab should always be administered by a rate-controlling device via a low-protein-binding 0.22-μm inline filter
- Flush line before and after panitumumab with 0.9% sodium chloride injection
- Doses ≤1000 mg should be administered over 60 minutes; >1000 mg should be administered over 90 minutes
- If tolerated, subsequent infusions may be administered over 30 minutes
- The routine use of an antihistamine prior to panitumumab administration is not recommended by the manufacturer; however, doing so may prevent infusion reactions

mFOLFOX–6 (Cheeseman et al):
Oxaliplatin 85 mg/m^2; administer intravenously in 250 mL 5% dextrose injection (D5W) over 2 hours concurrently with leucovorin administration, on day 1, every 2 weeks (total dosage/cycle = 85 mg/m^2)

Note: Oxaliplatin must not be mixed with sodium chloride injection. Therefore, when leucovorin and oxaliplatin are given concurrently via a Y-connector, both drugs must be administered in D5W
Leucovorin calcium 400 mg/m^2 per dose; administer intravenously in 25–500 mL D5W over 2 hours on day 1, every 2 weeks (total dosage/cycle = 400 mg/m^2), *followed by:*
Fluorouracil 400 mg/m^2 per dose; administer by intravenous injection over 1–2 minutes after leucovorin on day 1, every 2 weeks, *followed by:*
Fluorouracil 2400 mg/m^2 per dose; administer by continuous intravenous infusion in 100–1000 mL 0.9% sodium chloride injection or D5W over 46 hours every 2 weeks (total dosage/cycle = 2800 mg/m^2)

Note: **Fluorouracil** boluses (400 mg/m^2 by intravenous injection) may be omitted for better hematologic tolerance

Supportive Care
Antiemetic prophylaxis
Emetogenic potential on day 1 is **MODERATE**
Emetogenic potential on day 2 is **LOW**
See Chapter 42 for antiemetic recommendations

Hematopoietic growth factor (G-CSF) prophylaxis
Primary prophylaxis is **NOT** indicated
See Chapter 43 for more information

Antimicrobial prophylaxis
Risk of fever and neutropenia is **LOW**
   Antimicrobial primary prophylaxis to be considered:
- Antibacterial—not indicated
- Antifungal—not indicated
- Antiviral—not indicated unless patient previously had an episode of HSV

(continued)

Patient Population Studied

An open-label, multicenter, phase 3 trial comparing the efficacy of panitumumab-FOLFOX-4 with FOLFOX-4 alone in patients with *previously untreated* metastatic colorectal cancer (mCRC) according to tumor KRAS status. Patients with Eastern Cooperative Oncology Group Performance Status 0 or 1 versus 2 were randomly assigned (1:1) to receive either panitumumab-FOLFOX-4 or FOLFOX-4. The primary objective of the study was to assess the treatment effect on progression-free survival (PFS) of the addition of panitumumab to FOLFOX-4 as initial therapy for mCRC in patients with wild-type (WT) KRAS tumors and also in patients with mutant (MT) KRAS tumors. The study was amended to compare PFS (primary end point) and overall survival (secondary end point) according to KRAS status before any efficacy analyses

Treatment Modifications

Adverse Event	Dose Modification
G1/2 infusion reaction to panitumumab	Decrease infusion rate by 50% for duration of infusion
G3/4 infusion reaction to panitumumab	Immediately and permanently discontinue infusion
G3/4 or intolerable dermatologic reaction to panitumumab	Withhold panitumumab. If toxicity improves to G ≤2 and patient symptomatically improves after withholding no more than 2 doses, resume treatment at 50% of original dose. If toxicity does not improve to G ≤2 within 1 month, permanently discontinue panitumumab. *Note:* **If toxicities do not recur**, subsequent doses of panitumumab may be increased by increments of 25% of original dose until a 6-mg/kg dose is achieved
Recurrence of G3/4 or intolerable dermatologic reaction to panitumumab	Permanently discontinue infusion

(continued)

(continued)

Diarrhea management
Latent or delayed-onset diarrhea*:
  Loperamide 4 mg orally initially after the first loose or liquid stool, *then*
  Loperamide 2 mg orally every 2 hours during waking hours, *plus*
  Loperamide 4 mg orally every 4 hours during hours of sleep
- Continue for at least 12 hours after diarrhea resolves
- Recurrent diarrhea after a 12-hour diarrhea-free interval is treated as a new episode
- Rehydrate orally with fluids and electrolytes during a diarrheal episode
- If diarrhea persists >48 hours despite loperamide, stop loperamide and hospitalize the patient for IV hydration

Persistent diarrhea:
  Octreotide 100–150 mcg subcutaneously 3 times daily. Maximum total daily dose is 1500 mcg
Antibiotic therapy during latent or delayed-onset diarrhea:
  A fluoroquinolone (eg, **ciprofloxacin** 500 mg orally every 12 hours) if absolute neutrophil count <500/mm^3 with or without accompanying fever in association with diarrhea
- Antibiotics should also be administered if patient is hospitalized with prolonged diarrhea and should be continued until diarrhea resolves

*Abigerges D et al. J Natl Cancer Inst 1994;86:446–449
Rothenberg ML et al. J Clin Oncol 2001;19:3801–3807
Wadler S et al. J Clin Oncol 1998;16:3169–3178

Oral care
Standard prophylaxis and treatment for mucositis/stomatitis

Efficacy (N = 649)*

	Wild-Type KRAS		Mutant KRAS	
	FOLFOX4 (N = 190)	FOLFOX4 + Panitumumab (N = 165)	FOLFOX4 (N = 142)	FOLFOX4 + Panitumumab (N = 152)
Progression-free survival	8 months	9.6 months	8.8 months	7.3 months
Overall survival	19.7 months	23.9 months	19.3 months	15.5 months
Overall response rate	48%	55%	40%	40%

*RECIST (Response Evaluation Criteria in Solid Tumors. Therasse P et al. J Natl Cancer Inst 2000;92:205–216)
Note: Metastasectomy of any site was attempted in 10.5% of patients treated with panitumumab-FOLFOX-4 and 9.4% of patients treated with FOLFOX-4 with WT KRAS status; complete resections were achieved in 8.3% and 7.0% of patients, respectively

Note: Treatment-emergent binding antipanitumumab antibodies were detected in 14 (3.0%) of 470 patients who received panitumumab. Neutralizing antibodies were detected in postdose samples from 2 (0.4%) of 470 patients

Treatment Modifications
(continued)

Adverse Event	Dose Modification
Any G2/3/4 nonhematologic toxicity	Delay start of next cycle until the severity of all toxicities is G ≤1
ANC ≤1500/mm^3 or platelet count ≤100,000/mm^3	Delay start of next cycle until ANC >1500/mm^3 and platelet count >100,000/mm^3
G3/4 Nonneurologic	Reduce fluorouracil and oxaliplatin dosages by 20%
G3/4 ANC	Reduce oxaliplatin dosage by 20%
Persistent (≥14 days) paresthesias	Reduce oxaliplatin dosage by 20%
Temporary (7–14 days) painful paresthesias	
Temporary (7–14 days) functional impairment	
Persistent (≥14 days) painful paresthesias	Discontinue oxaliplatin
Persistent (≥14 days) functional impairment	

Adapted in part from de Gramont A et al. J Clin Oncol 2000;18:2938–2947

Toxicity* (N = 539)

	% G3/4
Any G3/4 event	82
Neutropenia	40.2
Skin toxicity	33.8
Diarrhea	18.9
Neurologic toxicities	16.3
Hypokalemia	9.5
Fatigue	8.5
Mucositis	7.4
Hypomagnesemia	6.1
Pulmonary embolism	3
Paronychia	2.8
Febrile neutropenia	2.8
Panitumumab infusion-related reaction‡	<1

*NCI Common Terminology Criteria for Adverse Events, v3. At: http://ctep.cancer.gov/protocolDevelopment/electronic_applications/ctc.htm [accessed October 11, 2013]
†Includes patients with wild-type (WT) KRAS and mutant (MT) KRAS who were treated with panitumumab
‡Grade 3 panitumumab-related infusion reactions occurred in 2 patients; both patients received additional panitumumab treatment after premedication

Therapy Monitoring

1. *Before each cycle:* H&P, CBC with differential, CEA if initially elevated, serum electrolytes, serum magnesium, and LFTs
2. *Every 2–3 months:* CT scans to assess response in patients presenting with advanced colorectal cancer

METASTATIC • FIRST-LINE

COLORECTAL CANCER REGIMEN: LEUCOVORIN + INFUSIONAL FLUOROURACIL + IRINOTECAN (FOLFIRI)

Douillard JY et al. Lancet 2000;355:1041–1047
Tournigand C et al. J Clin Oncol 2004;22:229–237

Common to both alternative regimens (Douillard et al and Tournigand et al):
Irinotecan 180 mg/m²; administer intravenously over 90 minutes in 500 mL 5% dextrose injection (D5W) on day 1, every 2 weeks (total dosage/cycle = 180 mg/m²), *plus one of the following alternative regimens:*

Douillard et al. Lancet 2000;355:1041–1047

(Racemic) leucovorin calcium 200 mg/m² per day; administer intravenously over 1 hour in 25–500 mL 0.9% sodium chloride injection (0.9% NS) or D5W for 2 consecutive days, on days 1 and 2, every 2 weeks (total dosage/cycle = 400 mg/m²) *followed by:*
Fluorouracil 400 mg/m² per day; administer by intravenous injection over 1–2 minutes after leucovorin for 2 consecutive days, on days 1 and 2, every 2 weeks, *followed by:*
Fluorouracil 600 mg/m² per day; administer by continuous intravenous infusion over 22 hours in 100–1000 mL 0.9% NS or D5W for 2 consecutive days, on days 1 and 2, every 2 weeks (total dosage/cycle = 2000 mg/m²)
or

Tournigand et al. J Clin Oncol 2004;22:229–237

Either: **(racemic) leucovorin calcium** 400 mg/m² *or* **levoleucovorin calcium** 200 mg/m²; administer intravenously over 2 hours in 25–500 mL 0.9% NS or D5W on day 1, every 2 weeks (total dosage/cycle for racemic leucovorin = 400 mg/m², for levoleucovorin = 200 mg/m²), *followed by:*
Fluorouracil 400 mg/m²; administer by intravenous injection over 1–2 minutes after leucovorin on day 1, every 2 weeks, *followed by:*
Fluorouracil 2400 mg/m²; administer by continuous intravenous infusion over 46 hours in 100–1000 mL 0.9% NS or D5W, starting on day 1 every 2 weeks (total dosage/cycle = 2800 mg/m²)
• Infusional fluorouracil dosage may be increased to 3000 mg/m² by continuous intravenous infusion over 46 hours, starting on cycle 3, day 1, and repeated every 2 weeks in patients who do not develop adverse effects G >1 during the first 2 cycles (total dosage/cycle = 3400 mg/m²)

Supportive Care
Antiemetic prophylaxis
Emetogenic potential on day 1 is **MODERATE**
Emetogenic potential on day 2 is **LOW**
See Chapter 42 for antiemetic recommendations

Hematopoietic growth factor (G-CSF) prophylaxis
Primary prophylaxis is **NOT** *indicated*
See Chapter 43 for more information

Antimicrobial prophylaxis
Risk of fever and neutropenia is **LOW**
   Antimicrobial primary prophylaxis to be considered:
   • Antibacterial—not indicated
   • Antifungal—not indicated
   • Antiviral—not indicated unless patient previously had an episode of HSV

Acute cholinergic syndrome
Atropine sulfate 0.25–1 mg administer subcutaneously or intravenously if abdominal cramping or diarrhea develop during or within 1 hour after irinotecan administration
• If symptoms are severe, add as primary prophylaxis at least 30 min before irinotecan during subsequent cycles
• For irinotecan, acute cholinergic syndrome may be characterized by: abdominal cramping, diarrhea, diaphoresis, hypotension, flushing, bradycardia, rhinitis, increased salivation, miosis, and lacrimation

Diarrhea management
Latent or delayed-onset diarrhea*:
   Loperamide 4 mg orally initially after the first loose or liquid stool, *then*

(continued)

Treatment Modifications

Camptosar, irinotecan hydrochloride injection product label. New York: Pharmacia & Upjohn; July 2005

	Dosage Levels		
	Initial	−1	−2
Irinotecan	180 mg/m²	150 mg/m²	120 mg/m²
Leucovorin	Racemic leucovorin calcium 400 mg/m² or levoleucovorin calcium 200 mg/m²		
Bolus fluorouracil	400 mg/m²	300 mg/m²	
Infusional fluorouracil	600 mg/m²	480 mg/m²	360 mg/m²
Infusional fluorouracil	2400 mg/m²	2000 mg/m²	1800 mg/m²

Notes:
• Dose modifications are based on the National Cancer Institute (USA) Common Toxicity Criteria. At: http://ctep.cancer.gov/protocolDevelopment/electronic_applications/ctc.htm [accessed October 11, 2013]
• Before beginning a treatment cycle, patients should have baseline bowel function (similar to that before the start of treatment) without antidiarrheal therapy for 24 hours, ANC ≥1500/mm³, and platelet count ≥100,000/mm³
• Treatment should be delayed 1–2 weeks to allow for recovery from treatment-related toxicities. If a patient has not recovered after 2 weeks, consider stopping therapy
If toxicity occurs despite 2 dose reductions (ie, on level −2), discontinue therapy

Toxicity	Modifications for Irinotecan and Fluorouracil
Neutropenia/Thrombocytopenia	
G1 ANC (1500–1999/mm³) or G1 thrombocytopenia	Maintain dose and schedule
G2 ANC (1000–1499/mm³) or G2 thrombocytopenia	Reduce dosages by 1 dosage level
G3 ANC (500–999/mm³) or G3 thrombocytopenia	Hold treatment until toxicity resolves to G ≤2, then reduce dosages by 1 dosage level

(continued)

(continued)

Loperamide 2 mg orally every 2 hours during waking hours, *plus*
Loperamide 4 mg orally every 4 hours during hours of sleep
- Continue for at least 12 hours after diarrhea resolves
- Recurrent diarrhea after a 12-hour diarrhea-free interval is treated as a new episode
- Rehydrate orally with fluids and electrolytes during a diarrheal episode
- If diarrhea persists >48 hours despite loperamide, stop loperamide and hospitalize the patient for IV hydration

Persistent diarrhea:
Octreotide 100–150 mcg subcutaneously 3 times daily. Maximum total daily dose is 1500 mcg

Antibiotic therapy during latent or delayed-onset diarrhea:
A fluoroquinolone (eg, **ciprofloxacin** 500 mg orally every 12 hours) if absolute neutrophil count is <500/mm^3 with or without accompanying fever in association with diarrhea
- Antibiotics should also be administered if patient is hospitalized with prolonged diarrhea and should be continued until diarrhea resolves

*Abigerges D et al. J Natl Cancer Inst 1994;86:446–449
Rothenberg ML et al. J Clin Oncol 2001;19:3801–3807
Wadler S et al. J Clin Oncol 1998;16:3169–3178

Oral care
Standard prophylaxis and treatment for mucositis/stomatitis

Hand-foot reaction (palmar-plantar erythrodysesthesia, PPE)
For patients who develop a hand-foot reaction, use topical emollients (eg, Aquaphor®), topical or orally administered steroids, antihistamine agents (H$_1$-receptor antagonists), or pyridoxine
- Pyridoxine may provide relief for discomfort/pain associated with PPE although the mechanism through which this occurs remains unclear
- The suggested pyridoxine starting dose is 50 mg/day, which may be increased to a maximum of 200 mg/day

Therapy Monitoring

1. *Before each cycle:* H&P, CBC with differential, CEA serum electrolytes, and LFTs
2. *Every 2–3 months:* CT scans to assess response

Patient Population Studied

A study of 199 patients with previously untreated advanced colorectal cancer

Efficacy (N* = 169/198)

Confirmed overall response	40.8% (34.8%)†
Complete response	3.6% (3.0%)
Partial response	37.3% (31.8%)
Median time to progression	6.7 months
Median survival	17.4 months

*Evaluable = 169 patients; intention-to-treat = 198 patients. Both totals include patients receiving weekly and 2-weekly regimens
†Percent of evaluable patients (percent of intention-to-treat patients)

Douillard JY et al. Lancet 2000;355:1041–1047

Treatment Modifications
(continued)

Toxicity	Modifications for Irinotecan and Fluorouracil
Neutropenia/Thrombocytopenia	
G4 ANC (<500/mm^3) or G4 thrombocytopenia	Hold treatment until toxicity resolves to G ≤2, then reduce dosages by 2 dosage levels
Febrile neutropenia	Hold treatment until neutropenia resolves, then reduce dosages by 2 dosage levels
Diarrhea	
G1 (2–3 stools/day > baseline)	Maintain dose and schedule
G2 (4–6 stools/day > baseline)	Delay until diarrhea resolves to baseline, then reduce dosage by 1 dosage level
G3 (7–9 stools/day > baseline)	Delay until diarrhea resolves to baseline, then reduce dosage by 1 dosage level
G4 (≥10 stools/day > baseline)	Delay until diarrhea resolves to baseline, then reduce dosage by 2 dosage levels
Other Nonhematologic Toxicities	
Any G1 toxicity	Maintain dose and schedule
Any G2 toxicity	Hold treatment until toxicity resolves to G ≤1, then reduce dosage by 1 dosage level
Any G3 toxicity	Hold treatment until toxicity resolves to G ≤1, then reduce dosage by 1 dosage level
Any G4 toxicity	Hold treatment until toxicity resolves to G ≤1, then reduce dosage by 2 dosage levels
G2–4 mucositis	Decrease only fluorouracil by 20%

André T et al. Eur J Cancer 1999;35:1343–1347
Douillard JY et al. Lancet 2000;355:1041–1047
Tournigand C et al. J Clin Oncol 2004;22:229–237

Toxicity (N = 54)

	% All G	% G3/4
Nonhematologic		
Diarrhea	68.3	13.1
Nausea	58.6	2.1
Alopecia	56.6	—
Asthenia	44.8	6.2
Vomiting	41.4	2.8
Mucositis	38.6	4.1
Cholinergic syndrome	28.3	1.4
Anorexia	17.2	2.1
Pain other than abdominal	9.7	0.7
Nonabdominal pain	8.3	—
Hand-foot syndrome	9	0.7
Hematologic		
Anemia	97.2	2.1
Neutropenia	82.5	46.2
Fever with G3/4 neutropenia	—	3.4
Infection with G3/4 neutropenia	—	2.1

Douillard JY et al. Lancet 2000;355:1041–1047

METASTATIC • FIRST-LINE
COLORECTAL CANCER REGIMEN: FOLFIRI + BEVACIZUMAB

Heinemann V et al. Lancet Oncol 2014;15:1065–1075
Venook AP et al. JAMA 2017;317:2392–2401
Venook AP et al. J Clin Oncol 2016;34(suppl):abstract 3504

Bevacizumab 5 mg/kg; administer intravenously in 100 mL 0.9% sodium chloride injection (0.9% NS), every 2 weeks, until disease progression (total dosage/2-week cycle = 5 mg/kg), *followed by:*

Irinotecan 180 mg/m²; administer intravenously over 90 minutes in 500 mL 5% dextrose injection (D5W) on day 1, every 2 weeks, until disease progression (total dosage/2-week cycle = 180 mg/m²), *plus:*

Either: **(racemic) leucovorin calcium** 400 mg/m² *or* **levoleucovorin calcium** 200 mg/m²; administer intravenously over 2 hours in 25–500 mL 0.9% NS or D5W on day 1, every 2 weeks, until disease progression (total dosage/2-week cycle for racemic leucovorin = 400 mg/m², for levoleucovorin = 200 mg/m²), *followed by:*

Fluorouracil 400 mg/m²; administer by intravenous injection over 1–2 minutes after leucovorin on day 1, every 2 weeks, until disease progression, *followed by:*

Fluorouracil 2400 mg/m²; administer by continuous intravenous infusion over 46 hours in 100–1000 mL 0.9% NS or D5W, starting on day 1, every 2 weeks, until disease progression (total fluorouracil dosage/2-week cycle = 2800 mg/m²)

Note: Bevacizumab administration duration for the initial dose is 90 minutes. If administration is well tolerated, the administration duration may be decreased stepwise during subsequent administrations to 60 minutes and, finally, to a minimum duration of 30 minutes

Supportive Care

Antiemetic prophylaxis
Emetogenic potential on day 1 is **MODERATE**
Emetogenic potential on day 2 is **LOW**
See Chapter 42 for antiemetic recommendations

Hematopoietic growth factor (G-CSF) prophylaxis
Primary prophylaxis is **NOT** indicated
See Chapter 43 for more information

Antimicrobial prophylaxis
Risk of fever and neutropenia is **LOW**
  Antimicrobial primary prophylaxis to be considered:
- Antibacterial—not indicated
- Antifungal—not indicated
- Antiviral—not indicated unless patient previously had an episode of HSV

Acute cholinergic syndrome
Atropine sulfate 0.25–1 mg subcutaneously or intravenously if abdominal cramping or diarrhea develop during or within 1 hour after irinotecan administration
- If symptoms are severe, add as primary prophylaxis at least 30 minutes before irinotecan during subsequent cycles
- For irinotecan, acute cholinergic syndrome may be characterized by abdominal cramping, diarrhea, diaphoresis, hypotension, flushing, bradycardia, rhinitis, increased salivation, miosis, and lacrimation

Diarrhea management
Latent or delayed-onset diarrhea*:
  Loperamide 4 mg orally initially after the first loose or liquid stool, *then*
  Loperamide 2 mg orally every 2 hours during waking hours, *plus*
  Loperamide 4 mg orally every 4 hours during hours of sleep
- Continue for at least 12 hours after diarrhea resolves
- Recurrent diarrhea after a 12-hour diarrhea-free interval is treated as a new episode
- Rehydrate orally with fluids and electrolytes during a diarrheal episode
- If a patient develops blood or mucus in stool, dehydration, or hemodynamic instability, or if diarrhea persists >48 hours despite loperamide, stop loperamide and hospitalize the patient for intravenous hydration

  Alternatively, a trial of **diphenoxylate hydrochloride** 2.5 mg with **atropine sulfate** 0.025 mg (eg, Lomotil)
- Initial adult dose is 2 tablets 4 times daily until control has been achieved, after which the dose may be reduced to meet individual requirements. Control may often be maintained with as little as 2 tablets daily
- Clinical improvement of acute diarrhea is usually observed within 48 hours. If improvement of chronic diarrhea after treatment with a maximum daily dose of 8 tablets is not observed within 10 days, control is unlikely with further administration

(continued)

(*continued*)

Persistent diarrhea:
  Octreotide 100–150 mcg subcutaneously 3 times daily. Maximum total daily dose is 1500 mcg
Antibiotic therapy during latent or delayed-onset diarrhea:
  A fluoroquinolone (eg, **ciprofloxacin** 500 mg orally every 12 hours) if absolute neutrophil count <500/mm³ with or without accompanying fever in association with diarrhea
  • Antibiotics should also be administered if patient is hospitalized with prolonged diarrhea and should be continued until diarrhea resolves

*Abigerges D et al. J Natl Cancer Inst 1994; 86:446–449
Rothenberg ML et al. J Clin Oncol 2001; 19:3801–3807
Wadler S et al. J Clin Oncol 1998; 16:3169–3178

Patient Population Studied

FIRE-3 was a phase 3, open-label, multinational, randomized, controlled clinical trial involving 592 adult patients in Germany and Austria with histologically confirmed, untreated, stage IV colorectal adenocarcinoma. A protocol amendment required patients to have KRAS exon 2 wild type tumors. Patients were required to have an Eastern Cooperative Oncology Group (ECOG) performance status of 0 or 2 and adequate organ function. Prior treatment with adjuvant chemotherapy was allowed if it was completed ≥6 months before enrollment. Patients were excluded if they had brain metastases; clinically significant coronary heart disease; a myocardial infarction within the past 12 months; a risk of uncontrolled arrhythmia; an acute or subacute intestinal obstruction; a history of chronic inflammatory bowel disease; symptomatic peritoneal carcinomatosis; serious non-healing wounds, ulcers, or fractures; uncontrolled hypertension; nephrotic syndrome; an arterial thromboembolism or severe hemorrhage in the past 6 months; a bleeding diathesis or thrombotic tendency; a known dihydropyrimidine dehydrogenase deficiency; Gilbert syndrome; or if they were receiving therapeutic anticoagulation treatment. Patients were randomized 1:1 to receive either FOLFIRI + cetuximab or FOLFIRI + bevacizumab.

Efficacy (N = 592)

	FOLFIRI + Cetuximab (n = 297 in Intention-to-Treat Population)	FOLFIRI + Bevacizumab (n = 295 in Intention-to-Treat Population)	
Objective response rate	62%	58%	OR 1.18 (95% CI, 0.85–1.64); P = 0.18
Median progression-free survival	10.0 months (95% CI, 8.8–10.8)	10.3 months (95% CI, 9.8–11.3)	HR 1.06 (95% CI, 0.88–1.26); P = 0.55
Median overall survival	28.7 months (95% CI, 24.0–36.6)	25.0 months (95% CI, 22.7–27.6)	HR 0.77 (95% CI, 0.62–0.96); P = 0.017

Median follow-up was 33.0 months (interquartile range, 19.0–55.4)
OR, odds ratio; CI, confidence interval; HR, hazard ratio

Therapy Monitoring

1. *Before each cycle:* H&P, CBC with differential, serum bilirubin, AST or ALT, alkaline phosphatase, serum creatinine, BUN, and CEA if being used to monitor disease
2. Observe closely for hypersensitivity reactions, especially during the first and second bevacizumab infusions
3. Blood pressure every 2 weeks or more frequently as indicated during treatment
4. Assess proteinuria by urine dipstick and/or urinary protein creatinine ratio prior to each cycle. Patients with a ≥2+ urine dipstick reading should undergo further assessment with a 24-hour urine collection
5. Every 2–3 months: CT scans to assess response

Treatment Modifications

BEVACIZUMAB DOSE MODIFICATIONS

Adverse Event	Treatment Modification
Gastrointestinal perforations (gastrointestinal perforations, fistula formation in the gastrointestinal tract, intra-abdominal abscess), fistula formation involving an internal organ	Discontinue bevacizumab permanently
Serious bleeding	
Wound dehiscence requiring medical intervention	
Nephrotic syndrome	
Hypertensive crisis or hypertensive encephalopathy or reversible posterior leukoencephalopathy syndrome (RPLS)	
Congestive heart failure	
Necrotizing fasciitis	
Severe arterial or venous thromboembolic events	Discontinue bevacizumab permanently; the safety of reinitiating bevacizumab after a thromboembolic event is resolved is not known
Moderate to severe proteinuria	Patients with a ≥2+ dipstick reading should undergo further assessment, eg, 24-hour urine collection. Suspend bevacizumab administration for ≥2 g proteinuria/24 h and resume when proteinuria is <2 g/24 h
Severe hypertension not controlled with medical management	Hold bevacizumab pending further evaluation and treatment of hypertension
Mild, clinically insignificant infusion reaction	Decrease the rate of infusion
Clinically significant but not severe infusion reaction	Interrupt the infusion and consider resuming at a slower rate following resolution. If decision is made to restart, the infusion may be continued at ≤50% of the rate prior to the reaction and increased in 50% increments every 30 minutes if well tolerated. Infusions may be restarted at the full rate during the next cycle
Severe infusion reaction (hypertension, hypertensive crises associated with neurologic signs and symptoms, wheezing, oxygen desaturation, G3 hypersensitivity, chest pain, headaches, rigors, and diaphoresis)	Stop infusion and administer appropriate medical therapy (eg, epinephrine, corticosteroids, intravenous antihistamines, bronchodilators and/or oxygen). Discontinue bevacizumab
Planned elective surgery	Suspend bevacizumab at least 28 days before elective surgery and do not resume for at least 28 days after surgery or until surgical incision is fully healed
Recent hemoptysis	Do not administer bevacizumab
Evidence of rectosigmoid involvement by pelvic examination or bowel involvement on CT scan or clinical symptoms of bowel obstruction	

FOLFIRI DOSE MOFICIATIONS

	Dosage Levels		
	Initial	Dose level −1	Dose level −2
Irinotecan	180 mg/m²	150 mg/m²	120 mg/m²
Leucovorin	Racemic leucovorin 400 mg/m² or levoleucovorin 200 mg/m²		
Fluorouracil injection (bolus)	400 mg/m²	320 mg/m²	240 mg/m²
Fluorouracil infusion	2400 mg/m²	2000 mg/m²	1600 mg/m²

Notes:
- Dose modifications are based on the National Cancer Institute (USA) Common Toxicity Criteria. At: http://ctep.cancer.gov/protocolDevelopment/electronic_applications/ctc.htm [accessed October 11, 2013]
- Before beginning a treatment cycle, patients should have baseline bowel (similar to that before start of treatment) function without antidiarrheal therapy for 24 hours, ANC ≥1500/mm³, and platelet count ≥100,000/mm³
- Treatment should be delayed 1–2 weeks to allow for recovery from treatment-related toxicities
- If a patient has not recovered after 2 weeks, consider stopping therapy. If toxicity occurs despite 2 dose reductions (ie, on level −2), discontinue therapy

(continued)

Treatment Modifications (*continued*)

Adverse Event	Treatment Modification for Irinotecan and Fluorouracil
G1 neutropenia (ANC 1500–1999/mm^3) or G1 thrombocytopenia (75,000/mm^3 to less than normal limits)	Maintain dose and schedule
G2 neutropenia (ANC 1000–1499/mm^3) or G2 thrombocytopenia (≥50,000 to <75,000/mm^3)	Reduce dosage by 1 dosage level
G3 neutropenia (ANC 500–999/mm^3) or G3 thrombocytopenia (≥10,000 to <50,000/mm^3)	Hold treatment until toxicity resolves to G ≤2, then reduce dosage by 1 dosage level
G4 neutropenia (ANC <500/mm^3) or G4 thrombocytopenia (<10,000/mm^3)	Hold treatment until toxicity resolves to G ≤2, then reduce dosage by 2 dosage levels
Febrile neutropenia	Hold treatment until neutropenia resolves, then reduce dosage by 2 dosage levels
Diarrhea	
G1 (2–3 stools/day > baseline)	Maintain dose and schedule
G2 (4–6 stools/day > baseline)	Delay until diarrhea resolves to baseline then reduce dosage by 1 dosage level
G3 (7–9 stools/day > baseline)	Delay until diarrhea resolves to baseline then reduce dosage by 1 dosage level
G4 (≥10 stools/day > baseline)	Delay until diarrhea resolves to baseline then reduce dosage by 2 dosage levels
Other Nonhematologic Toxicities	
Any G1 toxicity	Maintain dose and schedule
Any G2 toxicity	Hold treatment until toxicity resolves to G ≤1, then reduce dosage by 1 dosage level
Any G3 toxicity	Hold treatment until toxicity resolves to G ≤1, then reduce dosage by 1 dosage level
Any G4 toxicity	Hold treatment until toxicity resolves to G ≤1, then reduce dosage by 2 dosage levels
G2–4 mucositis	Decrease only fluorouracil by 20%

André T et al. Eur J Cancer 1999;35:1343–1347
Camptosar, irinotecan hydrochloride injection product label. New York: Pharmacia & Upjohn; July 2005
Douillard JY et al. Lancet 2000;355:1041–1047
Tournigand C et al. J Clin Oncol 2004;22:229–237

Adverse Events (N = 592)

	FOLFIRI + Cetuximab (n = 297)		FOLFIRI + Bevacizumab (n = 295)	
	Grade 1–2	Grade 3–5	Grade 1–2	Grade 3–5
Hematologic toxicity	63	25	69	21
Skin reaction	61	26	42	2
Acneiform rash	61	17	8	0
Liver toxicity	60	7	55	6
Fatigue	49	1	54	1
Diarrhea	46	11	49	14
Nausea	45	3	58	5
Pain	45	5	51	7
Stomatitis	38	4	41	4
Infection	38	8	40	8
Hypocalcemia	33	2	17	2
Hypomagnesemia	31	4	14	1
Paronychia	31	6	9	0
Alopecia	30	1	36	2
Hypokalemia	29	7	16	3
Desquamation	29	7	11	1
Obstipation	25	1	23	1
Hand-foot syndrome	23	3	14	1
Vomiting	22	2	29	3
Polyneuropathy	21	0	22	<1
Bleeding/hemorrhage	21	1	28	<1
Edema	16	1	9	<1
Hypertonia	15	6	32	7
Fever (without ANC <1000)	14	1	14	<1
Nephrotoxicity	13	1	19	1
Decreased appetite	13	1	13	1
Weight decreased	10	1	12	<1
Thrombosis (any)	3	6	5	6
Thromboembolic event	2	5	1	6
Infusional-related allergic reaction	4	4	<1	0
Infection with neutropenia	1	2	3	3
Dyspnea	6	2	6	1
Abscesses fistulae	1	<1	4	1
Dizziness	10	<1	11	0
Hyperkalemia	4	<1	6	1
Weight increased	2	<1	4	1
Mental disorder	8	0	7	1

Included in the table are adverse events (all-grade) which occurred in at least 5% of patients in either arm. Adverse events were classified and graded according to the National Cancer Institute Common Terminology Criteria for Adverse Events, version 3.0

METASTATIC • FIRST-LINE

COLORECTAL CANCER REGIMEN: CETUXIMAB + FOLFIRI

Van Cutsem E et al. N Engl J Med 2009;360:1408–1417

Warning:

1. Severe infusion reactions occurred with the administration of cetuximab in approximately 3% (17/633) of patients, rarely with fatal outcome (<1 in 1000)

2. Approximately 90% of severe infusion reactions are associated with the first infusion of cetuximab despite the use of prophylactic antihistamines

3. Infusion reactions are characterized by the rapid onset of airway obstruction (bronchospasm, stridor, hoarseness), urticaria, and/or hypotension

4. Caution must be exercised with every cetuximab infusion, as there were patients who experienced their first severe infusion reaction during later infusions

5. Provocative test doses do not reliably predict hypersensitivity reactions to cetuximab administration and are not recommended

Mild to moderate infusion reactions
• Interrupt or slow the cetuximab infusion rate
• Permanently decrease the administration rate by 50%
• Give antihistamine prophylaxis before repeated treatments

Severe reactions
• Immediately interrupt cetuximab therapy
• Administer epinephrine, glucocorticoids, intravenous antihistamines, bronchodilators, and oxygen as needed
• Permanently discontinue further treatment

Cetuximab premedication:
Diphenhydramine 50 mg; administer by intravenous injection before cetuximab administration (other H_1-receptor antagonists may be substituted)

Initial cetuximab dose:
Cetuximab 400 mg/m^2; administer intravenously over 120 minutes (maximum infusion rate = 5 mL/min [10 mg/min]) as a single dose (total initial dosage = 400 mg/m^2)

Maintenance cetuximab doses:
Cetuximab 250 mg/m^2; administer intravenously over 60 minutes (maximum infusion rate = 5 mL/min [10 mg/min]) every week (total weekly dosage = 250 mg/m^2)

Notes:
• Cetuximab is intended for direct administration and should not be diluted
• Maximum infusion rate = 5 mL (10 mg)/min (300 mL/h, *or* 600 mg/h)
• Administer cetuximab through a low protein-binding inline filter with pore size = 0.22 μm
• Use 0.9% sodium chloride injection to flush vascular access devices after administration is completed

Irinotecan 180 mg/m^2; administer intravenously over 90 minutes in 500 mL 5% dextrose injection (D5W) on day 1, every 2 weeks (total dosage/cycle = 180 mg/m^2), *plus:*
Either: (**racemic**) **leucovorin calcium** 400 mg/m^2 *or* **levoleucovorin calcium** 200 mg/m^2; administer intravenously over 2 hours in 25–500 mL 0.9% sodium chloride injection (0.9% NS) or D5W on day 1, every 2 weeks (total dosage/cycle for racemic leucovorin = 400 mg/m^2, for levoleucovorin = 200 mg/m^2), *followed by:*
Fluorouracil 400 mg/m^2; administer by intravenous injection over 1–2 minutes after leucovorin on day 1, every 2 weeks, *followed by:*
Fluorouracil 2400 mg/m^2; administer by continuous intravenous infusion over 46 hours in 100–1000 mL 0.9% NS or D5W, starting on day 1, every 2 weeks (total dosage/cycle = 2800 mg/m^2)

(continued)

Patient Population Studied

An open-label, multicenter study, comparing 14-day cycles of cetuximab plus FOLFIRI and FOLFIRI alone, randomized and treated 1198 patients. The primary end point was progression-free survival time. Inclusion criteria included histologically confirmed adenocarcinoma of the colon or rectum, first occurrence of metastatic disease that could not be resected for curative purposes, immunohistochemical evidence of tumor EGFR expression, and Eastern Cooperative Oncology Group (ECOG) performance status score of 2 or less. Exclusion criteria were previous exposure to an anti-EGFR therapy or irinotecan-based chemotherapy, previous chemotherapy for metastatic colorectal cancer, adjuvant treatment that was terminated 6 months or less before the start of treatment on trial

Efficacy (N = 1198)

	FOLFIRI (n = 599)	**FOLFIRI + Cetuximab** (n = 599)
Median progression-free survival	8 months	8.9 months
Median overall survival	18.6 months	19.9 months
Complete response	0.3%	0.5%
Partial response	38.4%	46.4%

Therapy Monitoring

1. *Before each cycle:* H&P, CBC with differential, CEA if initially elevated, serum electrolytes, serum magnesium, and LFTs

2. *Every 2–3 months:* CT scans to assess response in patients presenting with advanced colorectal cancer

(continued)

Supportive Care
Antiemetic prophylaxis
Emetogenic potential on day 1 is **MODERATE**
Emetogenic potential on day 2 is **LOW**
See Chapter 42 for antiemetic recommendations

Hematopoietic growth factor (G-CSF) prophylaxis
Primary prophylaxis is **NOT** *indicated*
See Chapter 43 for more information

Antimicrobial prophylaxis
Risk of fever and neutropenia is **LOW**
   Antimicrobial primary prophylaxis to be considered:
   • Antibacterial—not indicated
   • Antifungal—not indicated
   • Antiviral—not indicated unless patient previously had an episode of HSV

Acute cholinergic syndrome
Atropine sulfate 0.25–1 mg subcutaneously or intravenously if abdominal cramping or diarrhea develop during or within 1 hour after irinotecan administration
• If symptoms are severe, add as primary prophylaxis at least 30 minutes before irinotecan during subsequent cycles
• For irinotecan, acute cholinergic syndrome may be characterized by abdominal cramping, diarrhea, diaphoresis, hypotension, flushing, bradycardia, rhinitis, increased salivation, miosis, and lacrimation

Diarrhea management
Latent or delayed-onset diarrhea*:
   Loperamide 4 mg orally initially after the first loose or liquid stool, *then*
   Loperamide 2 mg orally every 2 hours during waking hours, *plus*
   Loperamide 4 mg orally every 4 hours during hours of sleep
   • Continue for at least 12 hours after diarrhea resolves
   • Recurrent diarrhea after a 12-hour diarrhea-free interval is treated as a new episode
   • Rehydrate orally with fluids and electrolytes during a diarrheal episode
   • If diarrhea persists >48 hours despite loperamide, stop loperamide and hospitalize the patient for IV hydration

Persistent diarrhea:
   Octreotide 100–150 mcg subcutaneously 3 times daily. Maximum total daily dose is 1500 mcg
Antibiotic therapy during latent or delayed-onset diarrhea:
   A fluoroquinolone (eg, **ciprofloxacin** 500 mg orally every 12 hours) if absolute neutrophil count <500/mm^3 with or without accompanying fever in association with diarrhea
   • Antibiotics should also be administered if patient is hospitalized with prolonged diarrhea and should be continued until diarrhea resolves

*Abigerges D et al. J Natl Cancer Inst 1994;86:446–449
Rothenberg ML et al. J Clin Oncol 2001;19:3801–3807
Wadler S et al. J Clin Oncol 1998;16:3169–3178

Hand-foot reaction (palmar-plantar erythrodysesthesia, PPE)
For patients who develop a hand-foot reaction, use topical emollients (eg, Aquaphor®), topical or orally administered steroids, antihistamine agents (H$_1$-receptor antagonists), or pyridoxine
   • Pyridoxine may provide relief for discomfort/pain associated with PPE although the mechanism through which this occurs remains unclear
   • The suggested pyridoxine starting dose is 50 mg/day, which may be increased to a maximum of 200 mg/day

Treatment Modifications

ERBITUX (cetuximab) injection, for intravenous infusion, product label, August 2013

Cetuximab Infusion Reactions

Mild/moderate (G1/2)	Permanently decrease administration rates by 50%
Severe (G3/4)	Immediately and permanently discontinue

Cetuximab Dermatologic Toxicity—Severe (G3/4)

Occurrence	Cetuximab	Improvement	Cetuximab Dosage
First	Delay infusion 1–2 weeks	Yes	Continue at 250 mg/m²
		No	Discontinue
Second	Delay infusion 1–2 weeks	Yes	Decrease to 200 mg/m²
		No	Discontinue
Third	Delay infusion 1–2 weeks	Yes	Decrease to 150 mg/m²
		No	Discontinue
Fourth	Discontinue		

Information from the product label: www.erbitux.com [accessed April 23, 2013]

Irinotecan and Fluorouracil

	Dosage Levels		
	Initial	−1	−2
Irinotecan	180 mg/m²	150 mg/m²	120 mg/m²
Leucovorin	Racemic leucovorin calcium 400 mg/m² *or* levoleucovorin calcium 200 mg/m²		
Fluorouracil injection	400 mg/m²	320 mg/m²	240 mg/m²
Infusional fluorouracil	2400 mg/m²	2000 mg/m²	1600 mg/m²

Notes:
- Dose modifications are based on the National Cancer Institute (USA) Common Toxicity Criteria. At: http://ctep.cancer.gov/protocolDevelopment/electronic_applications/ctc.htm [accessed October 11, 2013]
- Before beginning a treatment cycle, patients should have baseline bowel function (similar to that before start of treatment) without antidiarrheal therapy for 24 hours, ANC ≥1500/mm³, and platelet count ≥100,000/mm³
- Treatment should be delayed 1–2 weeks to allow for recovery from treatment-related toxicities
- If a patient has not recovered after 2 weeks, consider stopping therapy. If toxicity occurs despite 2 dose reductions (ie, on level −2), discontinue therapy
- Patients with prolonged, severe myelosuppression should be considered for UGT1A1*28 testing.

Toxicity	Modifications for Irinotecan and Fluorouracil
Neutropenia/Thrombocytopenia	
G1 ANC (1500–1999/mm³) or G1 thrombocytopenia (75,000/mm³ to less than normal limits)	Maintain dose and schedule
G2 ANC (1000–1499/mm³) or G2 thrombocytopenia (≥50,000 to <75,000/mm³)	Reduce dosage by 1 dosage level
G3 ANC (500–999/mm³) or G3 thrombocytopenia (≥10,000 to <50,000/mm³)	Hold treatment until toxicity resolves to G ≤2, then reduce dosage by 1 dosage level
G4 ANC (<500/mm³) or G4 thrombocytopenia (<10,000/mm³)	Hold treatment until toxicity resolves to G ≤2, then reduce dosage by 2 dosage levels
Febrile neutropenia	Hold treatment until neutropenia resolves, then reduce dosage by 2 dosage levels

(*continued*)

Treatment Modifications (*continued*)

Diarrhea	
G1 (2–3 stools/day > baseline)	Maintain dose and schedule
G2 (4–6 stools/day > baseline)	Delay until diarrhea resolves to baseline then reduce dosage by 1 dosage level
G3 (7–9 stools/day > baseline)	Delay until diarrhea resolves to baseline then reduce dosage by 1 dosage level
G4 (≥10 stools/day > baseline)	Delay until diarrhea resolves to baseline then reduce dosage by 2 dosage levels
Other Nonhematologic Toxicities	
Any G1 toxicity	Maintain dose and schedule
Any G2 toxicity	Hold treatment until toxicity resolves to G ≤1, then reduce dosage by 1 dosage level
Any G3 toxicity	Hold treatment until toxicity resolves to G ≤1, then reduce dosage by 1 dosage level
Any G4 toxicity	Hold treatment until toxicity resolves to G ≤1, then reduce dosage by 2 dosage levels
G2–4 mucositis	Decrease only fluorouracil by 20%

André T et al. Eur J Cancer 1999;35:1343–1347
Camptosar, irinotecan hydrochloride injection product label. New York: Pharmacia & Upjohn; July 2005
Douillard JY et al. Lancet 2000;355:1041–1047
Tournigand C et al. J Clin Oncol 2004;22:229–237

Most Common G3/4 Adverse Events and Special Adverse Event Categories in the Safety Population, According to Treatment Group

MedDRA Preferred Term*	FOLFIRI (N = 602)	FOLFIRI + Cetuximab (N = 600)	P Value
Any	61	79.3	<0.001
Neutropenia[†]	24.6	28.2	0.16
Leukopenia	5.1	7.2	0.15
Diarrhea	10.5	15.7	0.008
Fatigue	4.7	5.3	0.59
Rash	0	8.2	<0.001
Dermatitis acneiform	0	5.3	<0.001
Vomiting	5	4.7	0.80
Special Adverse Events			
Skin reactions			
All	0.2	19.7	<0.001
Acne-like rash	0	16.2	<0.001
Infusion-related reaction	0	2.5	<0.001

*Among the Medical Dictionary for Regulatory Activities (MedDRA, version 10.0) preferred terms, no grade 4 reactions were reported for dermatitis acneiform, acne-like rash, or all skin reactions
[†]Grade 3 or 4 febrile neutropenia was reported in 18 of the 600 patients (3.0%) receiving cetuximab plus FOLFIRI and in 13 of the 602 patients (2.2%) receiving FOLFIRI alone

METASTATIC • FIRST-LINE
COLORECTAL CANCER REGIMEN: PANITUMUMAB + FOLFIRI

Douillard JY et al. Lancet 2000;355:1041–1047
Peeters M et al. J Clin Oncol 2010;28:4706–4713
Tournigand C et al. J Clin Oncol 2004;22:229–237

Panitumumab 6 mg/kg; administer intravenously in 0.9% sodium chloride injection (100 mL for doses ≤1000 mg; 150 mL for doses >1000 mg; product concentration should be <10 mg/mL) over 60–90 minutes on day 1 before FOLFIRI chemotherapy, every 2 weeks (total dosage/cycle = 6 mg/kg)

Notes:
- Severe infusion reactions occur in approximately 1% of patients (anaphylactic reactions, bronchospasm, fever, chills, and hypotension). Dose adjustment or discontinuation of panitumumab is warranted depending on the severity of the reaction
- Panitumumab should always be administered by a rate-controlling device via a low-protein-binding 0.22-μm inline filter
- Flush line before and after panitumumab with 0.9% sodium chloride injection
- Doses ≤1000 mg should be administered over 60 minutes; >1000 mg should be administered over 90 minutes
- If tolerated, subsequent infusions may be administered over 30 minutes
- The routine use of an antihistamine prior to panitumumab administration is not recommended by the manufacturer; however, doing so may prevent infusion reactions

Irinotecan 180 mg/m^2; administer intravenously over 90 minutes in 500 mL 5% dextrose injection (D5W) on day 1, every 2 weeks (total dosage/cycle = 180 mg/m^2), *plus:*
Either: (**racemic**) **leucovorin calcium** 400 mg/m^2 *or* **levoleucovorin calcium** 200 mg/m^2; administer intravenously over 2 hours in 25–500 mL 0.9% sodium chloride injection (0.9% NS) or D5W on day 1, every 2 weeks (total dosage/cycle for racemic leucovorin = 400 mg/m^2, for levoleucovorin = 200 mg/m^2), *followed by:*
Fluorouracil 400 mg/m^2; administer by intravenous injection over 1–2 minutes after leucovorin on day 1, every 2 weeks, *followed by:*
Fluorouracil 2400 mg/m^2; administer by continuous intravenous infusion over 46 hours in 100–1000 mL 0.9% NS or D5W, starting on day 1, every 2 weeks (total dosage/cycle = 2800 mg/m^2)

Supportive Care
Antiemetic prophylaxis
Emetogenic potential on day 1 is **MODERATE**
Emetogenic potential on day 2 is **LOW**
See Chapter 42 for antiemetic recommendations

Hematopoietic growth factor (G-CSF) prophylaxis
Primary prophylaxis is **NOT** *indicated*
See Chapter 43 for more information

Antimicrobial prophylaxis
Risk of fever and neutropenia is **LOW**
   Antimicrobial primary prophylaxis to be considered:
   - Antibacterial—not indicated
   - Antifungal—not indicated
   - Antiviral—not indicated unless patient previously had an episode of HSV

Acute cholinergic syndrome
Atropine sulfate 0.25–1 mg subcutaneously or intravenously if abdominal cramping or diarrhea develop during or within 1 hour after irinotecan administration
- If symptoms are severe, add as primary prophylaxis at least 30 minutes before irinotecan during subsequent cycles
- For irinotecan, acute cholinergic syndrome may be characterized by abdominal cramping, diarrhea, diaphoresis, hypotension, flushing, bradycardia, rhinitis, increased salivation, miosis, and lacrimation

Diarrhea management
Latent or delayed-onset diarrhea:
   Loperamide 4 mg orally initially after the first loose or liquid stool, *then*
   Loperamide 2 mg orally every 2 hours during waking hours, *plus*
   Loperamide 4 mg orally every 4 hours during hours of sleep
   - Continue for at least 12 hours after diarrhea resolves
   - Recurrent diarrhea after a 12-hour diarrhea-free interval is treated as a new episode

(continued)

(continued)

- Rehydrate orally with fluids and electrolytes during a diarrheal episode
- If diarrhea persists >48 hours despite loperamide, stop loperamide and hospitalize the patient for IV hydration

*Abigerges D et al. J Natl Cancer Inst 1994;86:446–449
Rothenberg ML et al. J Clin Oncol 2001;19:3801–3807
Wadler S et al. J Clin Oncol 1998;16:3169–3178

Persistent diarrhea:
   Octreotide 100–150 mcg subcutaneously 3 times daily. Maximum total daily dose is 1500 mcg
Antibiotic therapy during latent or delayed-onset diarrhea:
   A fluoroquinolone (eg, **ciprofloxacin** 500 mg orally every 12 hours) if absolute neutrophil count <500/mm^3 with or without accompanying fever in association with diarrhea
   - Antibiotics should also be administered if patient is hospitalized with prolonged diarrhea and should be continued until diarrhea resolves

Oral care
Standard prophylaxis and treatment for mucositis/stomatitis

Treatment Modifications

Adverse Event	Dose Modification
G1/2 infusion reaction to panitumumab	Decrease infusion rate by 50% for duration of infusion
G3/4 infusion reaction to panitumumab	Immediately and permanently discontinue infusion
G3/4 or intolerable dermatologic reaction to panitumumab	Withhold panitumumab. If toxicity improves to G ≤2 and patient symptomatically improves after withholding no more than 2 doses, resume treatment at 50% of the original dose. If toxicity does not improve to G ≤2 within 1 month, permanently discontinue panitumumab *Note:* **If toxicities do not recur**, subsequent doses of panitumumab may be increased by increments of 25% of original dose until a 6-mg/kg dose is achieved
Recurrence of G3/4 or intolerable dermatologic reaction to panitumumab	Permanently discontinue panitumumab
Any G2/3/4 nonhematologic toxicity	Delay start of next cycle until the severity of all toxicities is G ≤1
ANC ≤1500/mm^3 or platelet count ≤100,000/mm^3	Delay start of next cycle until ANC >1500/mm^3 and platelet count >100,000/mm^3

Dosage Levels			
	Initial	−1	−2
Irinotecan	180 mg/m^2	150 mg/m^2	120 mg/m^2
Leucovorin	Racemic leucovorin calcium 400 mg/m^2 or levoleucovorin calcium 200 mg/m^2		
Fluorouracil injection	400 mg/m^2	320 mg/m^2	240 mg/m^2
Infusional fluorouracil	2400 mg/m^2	2000 mg/m^2	1600 mg/m^2

Notes:
- Dose modifications are based on the National Cancer Institute (USA) Common Toxicity Criteria. At: http://ctep.cancer.gov/protocolDevelopment/electronic_applications/ctc.htm [accessed October 11, 2013]
- Before beginning a treatment cycle, patients should have baseline bowel function (similar to that before start of treatment) without antidiarrheal therapy for 24 hours, ANC ≥1500/mm^3, and platelet count ≥100,000/mm^3
- Treatment should be delayed 1–2 weeks to allow for recovery from treatment-related toxicities
- If a patient has not recovered after 2 weeks, consider stopping therapy
- If toxicity occurs despite 2 dose reductions (ie, on level −2), discontinue therapy

(continued)

Treatment Modifications (*continued*)

Toxicity	Modifications for Irinotecan and Fluorouracil
Neutropenia/Thrombocytopenia	
G1 ANC (1500–1999/mm^3) or G1 thrombocytopenia (75,000/mm^3 to less than normal limits)	Maintain dose and schedule
G2 ANC (1000–1499/mm^3) or G2 thrombocytopenia (≥50,000 to <75,000/mm^3)	Reduce dosage by 1 dosage level
G3 ANC (500–999/mm^3) or G3 thrombocytopenia (≥10,000 to <50,000/mm^3)	Hold treatment until toxicity resolves to G ≤2, then reduce dosage by 1 dosage level
G4 ANC (<500/mm^3) or G4 thrombocytopenia (<10,000/mm^3)	Hold treatment until toxicity resolves to G ≤2, then reduce dosage by 2 dosage levels
Febrile neutropenia	Hold treatment until neutropenia resolves, then reduce dosage by 2 dosage levels
Diarrhea	
G1 (2–3 stools/day > baseline)	Maintain dose and schedule
G2 (4–6 stools/day > baseline)	Delay until diarrhea resolves to baseline then reduce dosage by 1 dosage level
G3 (7–9 stools/day > baseline)	Delay until diarrhea resolves to baseline then reduce dosage by 1 dosage level
G4 (≥10 stools/day > baseline)	Delay until diarrhea resolves to baseline then reduce dosage by 2 dosage levels
Other Nonhematologic Toxicities	
Any G1 toxicity	Maintain dose and schedule
Any G2 toxicity	Hold treatment until toxicity resolves to G ≤1, then reduce dosage by 1 dosage level
Any G3 toxicity	Hold treatment until toxicity resolves to G ≤1, then reduce dosage by 1 dosage level
Any G4 toxicity	Hold treatment until toxicity resolves to G ≤1, then reduce dosage by 2 dosage levels
G2–4 mucositis	Decrease only fluorouracil by 20%

André T et al. Eur J Cancer 1999;35:1343–1347
Camptosar, irinotecan hydrochloride injection product label. New York: Pharmacia & Upjohn; July 2005
Douillard JY et al. Lancet 2000;355:1041–1047
Tournigand C et al. J Clin Oncol 2004;22:229–237

Efficacy (N = 1083)*

	Wild-Type (WT) KRAS		Mutant (MT) KRAS	
	FOLFIRI (n = 294)	FOLFIRI + Panitumumab (n = 303)	FOLFIRI (n = 248)	FOLFIRI + Panitumumab (n = 238)
Progression-free survival	3.9 months	5.9 months	4.9 months	5.0 months
Overall survival	12.5 months	14.5 months	11.1 months	11.8 months
Overall response rate	10%	35%	14%	13%

*RECIST (Response Evaluation Criteria in Solid Tumors. Therasse P et al. J Natl Cancer Inst 2000;92:205–216)

Patient Population Studied

A study of 1186 patients with Eastern Cooperative Oncology Group (ECOG) Performance Status of 0, 1, or 2 and a diagnosis of adenocarcinoma of the colon or rectum. *Only one prior chemotherapy regimen for metastatic colorectal cancer (mCRC) consisting of first-line fluoropyrimidine-based chemotherapy was allowed.* Patients were excluded if they previously received irinotecan or anti-EGFR therapy. Radiographically confirmed disease progression must have occurred during or within 6 months after first-line chemotherapy

Toxicity* (N = 539†)

	% G3/4
Any G3/4 event	68.6
Skin toxicity	34.5
Neutropenia	16.9
Diarrhea	13.5
Mucositis	8.3
Hypokalemia	5.4
Pulmonary embolism	4.1
Hypomagnesemia	3.7
Dehydration	3.3
Paronychia	2.8
Febrile neutropenia	1.7
Panitumumab infusion-related reaction‡	<1

*NCI CTCAE, National Cancer Institute (USA) Common Terminology Criteria for Adverse Events, version 3. At: http://ctep.cancer.gov/protocolDevelopment/electronic_applications/ctc.htm [accessed December 7, 2013]
†Includes patients with WT KRAS and MT KRAS who were treated with panitumumab
‡Grade 3 panitumumab-related infusion reactions occurred in 2 patients; these patients did not receive additional panitumumab treatment

Therapy Monitoring

1. *Before each cycle:* H&P, CBC with differential, CEA if initially elevated, serum electrolytes, serum magnesium, and LFTs
2. *Every 2–3 months:* CT scans to assess response in patients presenting with advanced colorectal cancer

METASTATIC

COLORECTAL CANCER REGIMEN: MODIFIED DE GRAMONT 5-FLUOROURACIL+LEUCOVORIN

Braun MS et al. Br J Cancer 2003;89:1155–1158
Cheeseman SL et al. Br J Cancer 2002;87:393–399

Modified de Gramont (MdG); (Cheeseman et al):

Note: **Although the Modified de Gramont (leucovorin + fluorouracil) regimen was evaluated in patients with advanced colorectal cancer, it may also be used in practice for adjuvant therapy (12 cycles) as an alternative to mFOLFOX6 in patients for whom the addition of oxaliplatin is either contraindicated or is unlikely to provide benefit**

Either: **(racemic) leucovorin calcium** 350 mg (fixed dose) *or* **levoleucovorin calcium** 175 mg (fixed dose); administer intravenously over 2 hours in 25–500 mL 0.9% sodium chloride injection (0.9% NS) or 5% dextrose injection (D5W) on day 1, every 2 weeks (total dosage/cycle for racemic leucovorin = 350 mg, for levoleucovorin = 175 mg), *followed by:*
Note: Although Cheeseman et al report a 350-mg fixed dose of racemic leucovorin with the modified de Gramont regimen, many institutions instead prefer to use the body surface area–based dose of racemic leucovorin, 400 mg/m^2, or levoleucovorin, 200 mg/m^2, as reported in the FOLFOX6 regimen (Tournigand C et al. J Clin Oncol 2004;22:229–237)

Fluorouracil 400 mg/m^2; administer by intravenous injection over 5 minutes after leucovorin on day 1, every 2 weeks, *followed by:*
Fluorouracil 2400 mg/m^2; administer by continuous intravenous infusion over 46 hours in 100–1000 mL 0.9% NS or D5W, starting on day 1 every 2 weeks (total fluorouracil dosage/cycle = 2800 mg/m^2)
Note: Although Cheeseman et al report that the maximum tolerated dose of fluorouracil infusion was 2800 mg/m^2 over 46 hours, most institutions prefer to use a dose of 2400 mg/m^2 as indicated above.

Supportive Care
Antiemetic prophylaxis
Emetogenic potential on day 1 and day 2 is **LOW**
See Chapter 42 for antiemetic recommendations

Hematopoietic growth factor (CSF) prophylaxis
Primary prophylaxis is **NOT** *indicated*
See Chapter 43 for more information

Antimicrobial prophylaxis
Risk of fever and neutropenia is **LOW**
  Antimicrobial primary prophylaxis to be CONSIDERED:
  • Antibacterial—not indicated
  • Antifungal—not indicated
  • Antiviral—not indicated unless patient previously had an episode of HSV

Diarrhea management
Latent or delayed-onset diarrhea*:
  Loperamide 4 mg orally initially after the first loose or liquid stool, *then*
  Loperamide 2 mg orally every 2 hours during waking hours, *plus*
  Loperamide 4 mg orally every 4 hours during hours of sleep
  • Continue for at least 12 hours after diarrhea resolves
  • Recurrent diarrhea after a 12-hour diarrhea-free interval is treated as a new episode
  • Rehydrate orally with fluids and electrolytes during a diarrheal episode
  • If a patient develops blood or mucus in stool, dehydration, or hemodynamic instability, or if diarrhea persists >48 hours despite loperamide, stop loperamide and hospitalize the patient for intravenous hydration

(continued)

Patient Population Studied

This was a prospective, multicenter, phase 1/2 study involving patients with metastatic colorectal cancer. Patients were not excluded if they had received prior chemotherapy for metastatic disease. Forty-six patients received the modified de Gramont regimen (leucovorin plus fluorouracil); the first 32 patients were enrolled in a dose-escalation phase to determine the optimal dose of 46-hour continuous infusion fluorouracil and received starting doses of 2000 mg/m^2, 2400 mg/m^2, 2800 mg/m^2, or 3200 mg/m^2. Following this, the 2800 mg/m^2 dose level was expanded to enroll an additional 14 patients

Efficacy (N = 22)

Median failure-free survival	9.3 months
Median overall survival	16.8 months
Complete or partial response rate*	36%

*Response rate was assessed by the investigator using World Health Organization criteria for 22 patients with measurable disease who received MdG at fluorouracil 400 mg/m^2 bolus plus fluorouracil 2800 mg/m^2 46-hour infusion as first-line therapy

Therapy Monitoring

1. *Before each cycle:* H&P, CBC with differential, LFTs, and CEA if being used to monitor disease
2. *Every 2–3 months:* CT scans to assess response in patients presenting with advanced colorectal cancer

(continued)

Alternatively, a trial of **diphenoxylate hydrochloride** 2.5 mg with **atropine sulfate** 0.025 mg (eg, Lomotil)
- Initial adult dose is 2 tablets 4 times daily until control has been achieved, after which the dose may be reduced to meet individual requirements. Control may often be maintained with as little as 2 tablets daily
- Clinical improvement of acute diarrhea is usually observed within 48 hours. If improvement of chronic diarrhea after treatment with a maximum daily dose of 8 tablets is not observed within 10 days, control is unlikely with further administration

*Abigerges D et al. J Natl Cancer Inst 1994; 86:446–449
Rothenberg ML et al. J Clin Oncol 2001; 19:3801–3807
Wadler S et al. J Clin Oncol 1998; 16:3169–3178

Persistent diarrhea:
Octreotide 100–150 mcg subcutaneously 3 times daily. Maximum total daily dose is 1500 mcg
Antibiotic therapy during latent or delayed-onset diarrhea:
A fluoroquinolone (eg, **ciprofloxacin** 500 mg orally every 12 hours) if absolute neutrophil count <500/mm^3 with or without accompanying fever in association with diarrhea
- Antibiotics should also be administered if patient is hospitalized with prolonged diarrhea and should be continued until diarrhea resolves

Oral care
Standard prophylaxis and treatment for mucositis/stomatitis

Treatment Modifications

Modified de Gramont
(5-Fluorouracil + Leucovorin)
Treatment Modifications

Adverse Event	Treatment Modification
Day 1 persistent nonhematologic toxicity G ≥2	Delay start of next cycle until the severity of all toxicities is G ≤1 and omit fluorouracil by intravenous bolus injection. If a 2-week delay or two separate delays of 1 week are required, reduce subsequent chemotherapy doses (fluorouracil infusion but not leucovorin) by 20%
Day 1 ANC ≤1500/mm^3 *or* platelet count ≤100,000/mm^3	Delay start of next cycle until ANC >1500/mm^3 *and* platelet count >100,000/mm^3; omit fluorouracil by intravenous bolus injection. If a 2-week delay or two separate delays of 1 week are required, reduce subsequent chemotherapy doses (fluorouracil infusion, but not leucovorin) by 20%
G4 neutropenia (<500/mm^3), G3/4 thrombocytopenia (<50,000/mm^3) or G4 diarrhea (life-threatening; urgent intervention required)	Omit fluorouracil by intravenous bolus injection in subsequent cycles
G ≥3 non-neurologic toxicity	Reduce infusional fluorouracil dosage to 2000 mg/m^2

Note: Do not adjust leucovorin for toxicity
Tournigand C et al. J Clin Oncol 2004;22:229–237

Adverse Events (N = 33 patients)

Grade* (%)	Grade 2	Grade 3/4
Nonhematologic Adverse Events		
Nausea or vomiting	13%	13%
Mucositis	3%	0%
Diarrhea	7%	0%
Hand-foot syndrome	3%	7%
Lethargy	13%	13%
Infection	10%	7%
Hematologic Adverse Events		
Leukopenia or neutropenia	0%	3%
Thrombocytopenia	0%	0%

*According to the National Cancer Institute Common Terminology Criteria for Adverse Events, version 2
Note: The 7% of patients with G3/4 infection also includes two patients who experienced grade 5 (fatal) infections

METASTATIC

COLORECTAL CANCER REGIMEN: CAPECITABINE

Van Cutsem E et al. J Clin Oncol 2001;19:4097–4106

Capecitabine 1250 mg/m^2 per dose; administer orally with water within 30 minutes after a meal twice daily for 28 doses on days 1–14, every 3 weeks (total dosage/3-week cycle = 35,000 mg/m^2)

Notes:
Capecitabine is given for 2 consecutive weeks followed by 1 week without treatment
Doses are rounded down to approximate a calculated dose using combinations of 500-mg and 150-mg tablets
In practice, treatment often is begun with capecitabine 1000 mg/m^2 per dose twice daily for 28 doses on days 1–14 (total dosage/cycle = 28,000 mg/m^2). Dosage may be increased during subsequent cycles if initial treatment at a lesser dosage is tolerated

Supportive Care
Antiemetic prophylaxis
*Emetogenic potential is **LOW***
See Chapter 42 for antiemetic recommendations

*Hematopoietic growth factor (**G-CSF**) prophylaxis*
*Primary prophylaxis is **NOT** indicated*
See Chapter 43 for more information

Antimicrobial prophylaxis
*Risk of fever and neutropenia is **LOW***
  Antimicrobial primary prophylaxis to be considered:
  • Antibacterial—not indicated
  • Antifungal—not indicated
  • Antiviral—not indicated unless patient previously had an episode of HSV

Diarrhea management
Latent or delayed-onset diarrhea*:
  Loperamide 4 mg orally initially after the first loose or liquid stool, *then*
  Loperamide 2 mg orally every 2 hours during waking hours, *plus*
  Loperamide 4 mg orally every 4 hours during hours of sleep
  • Continue for at least 12 hours after diarrhea resolves
  • Recurrent diarrhea after a 12-hour diarrhea-free interval is treated as a new episode
  • Rehydrate orally with fluids and electrolytes during a diarrheal episode
  • If diarrhea persists >48 hours despite loperamide, stop loperamide and hospitalize the patient for IV hydration

Persistent diarrhea:
  Octreotide 100–150 mcg subcutaneously 3 times daily. Maximum total daily dose is 1500 mcg
Antibiotic therapy during latent or delayed-onset diarrhea:
  A fluoroquinolone (eg, **ciprofloxacin** 500 mg orally every 12 hours) if absolute neutrophil count is <500/mm^3 with or without accompanying fever in association with diarrhea
  • Antibiotics should also be administered if patient is hospitalized with prolonged diarrhea and should be continued until diarrhea resolves

*Abigerges D et al. J Natl Cancer Inst 1994;86:446–449
Rothenberg ML et al. J Clin Oncol 2001;19:3801–3807
Wadler S et al. J Clin Oncol 1998;16:3169–3178

Oral care
Standard prophylaxis and treatment for mucositis/stomatitis

Hand-foot reaction (palmar-plantar erythrodysesthesia, PPE)
For patients who develop a hand-foot reaction, use topical emollients (eg, Aquaphor®), topical or orally administered steroids, antihistamine agents (H$_1$-receptor antagonists), or pyridoxine
  • Pyridoxine may provide relief for discomfort/pain associated with PPE although the mechanism through which this occurs remains unclear
  • The suggested pyridoxine starting dose is 50 mg/day, which may be increased to a maximum of 200 mg/day

Patient Population Studied

Patients receiving first-line treatment for metastatic colorectal cancer. For advanced disease, this regimen should be considered for special cases; eg, elderly patients

Efficacy (N = 301)

Complete response	0.3%
Partial response	18.6%
Stable disease	56.8%
Mean duration of response	7.2 months
Median time to progression	5.2 months
Median survival	13.2 months

Van Cutsem E et al. J Clin Oncol 2001;19:4097–4106

Treatment Modifications

Adverse Event	Dose Modification
First occurrence of a G2 toxicity	No dose reduction*
Second occurrence of a given G2 toxicity	Reduce dosage by 25%*
First occurrence of a G3 toxicity	
Third occurrence of a given G2 toxicity	Reduce dosage by 50%*
Second occurrence of a given G3 toxicity	
Any G4 toxicity	
Fourth occurrence of a given G2 toxicity	Discontinue capecitabine
Third occurrence of a given G3 toxicity	
Second occurrence of a given G4 toxicity	
Both G4 hematologic and G4 nonhematologic toxicity	

*Interrupt capecitabine treatment until is toxicity resolves to G ≤1
National Cancer Institute of Canada Common Toxicity Criteria

Toxicity (N = 297)

	% All G	% G3	% G4
Nonhematologic			
Diarrhea	50.2	9.4	1.3
Hand-foot syndrome	48	16.2	0
Nausea	37.7	—	—
Stomatitis	21.9	1	0.3
Vomiting	18.5	—	—
Fatigue	10	—	—
Increased bilirubin*,†	—	23.6	4.7
Hematologic			
Anemia	—	2.7	0
Neutropenia	—	0	2
Thrombocytopenia	—	0.7	0.3

*G3 and G4 correspond to G2 and G3 in updated National Cancer Institute of Canada Common Toxicity Criteria
†Eight (10%) patients with G3/4 hyperbilirubinemia also had G3 abnormalities in ALT or AST

Van Cutsem E et al. J Clin Oncol 2001;19:4097–4106

Therapy Monitoring

1. *Before each cycle:* H&P, CBC with differential, CEA, serum electrolytes, creatinine, BUN, and LFTs
2. *Every 2–3 months:* CT scans to assess cancer status in patients presenting with advanced colorectal cancer

METASTATIC • FIRST-LINE

COLORECTAL CANCER REGIMEN: BOLUS FLUOROURACIL + LEUCOVORIN (ROSWELL PARK REGIMEN)

Haller DG et al. J Clin Oncol 2005;23:8671–8678
Petrelli N et al. J Clin Oncol 1989;7:1419–1426
Wolmark N et al. J Clin Oncol 1999;17:3553–3559

Leucovorin calcium 500 mg/m^2; administer intravenously in 250 mL 0.9% sodium chloride injection (0.9% NS) over 2 hours once per week for 6 consecutive weeks (weeks 1–6), every 8 weeks (total dosage/8-week cycle = 3000 mg/m^2)

Fluorouracil 500 mg/m^2; administer by intravenous injection over 1–2 minutes, starting 1 hour after leucovorin once per week for 6 consecutive weeks (weeks 1–6), every 8 weeks (total dosage/8-week cycle = 3000 mg/m^2)

Supportive Care
Antiemetic prophylaxis
Emetogenic potential is **LOW**
See Chapter 42 for antiemetic recommendations

Hematopoietic growth factor (G-CSF) prophylaxis
Primary prophylaxis is **NOT** *indicated*
See Chapter 43 for more information

Antimicrobial prophylaxis
Risk of fever and neutropenia is **LOW**
  Antimicrobial primary prophylaxis to be considered:
  • Antibacterial—not indicated
  • Antifungal—not indicated
  • Antiviral—not indicated unless patient previously had an episode of HSV

Diarrhea management
Latent or delayed-onset diarrhea*:
  Loperamide 4 mg orally initially after the first loose or liquid stool, *then*
  Loperamide 2 mg orally every 2 hours during waking hours, *plus*
  Loperamide 4 mg orally every 4 hours during hours of sleep
  • Continue for at least 12 hours after diarrhea resolves
  • Recurrent diarrhea after a 12-hour diarrhea-free interval is treated as a new episode
  • Rehydrate orally with fluids and electrolytes during a diarrheal episode
  • If diarrhea persists >48 hours despite loperamide, stop loperamide and hospitalize the patient for IV hydration

Persistent diarrhea:
  Octreotide 100–150 mcg subcutaneously 3 times daily. Maximum total daily dose is 1500 mcg

Antibiotic therapy during latent or delayed-onset diarrhea:
  A fluoroquinolone (eg, **ciprofloxacin** 500 mg orally every 12 hours) if absolute neutrophil count is <500/mm^3 with or without accompanying fever in association with diarrhea
  • Antibiotics should also be administered if patient is hospitalized with prolonged diarrhea and should be continued until diarrhea resolves

*Abigerges D et al. J Natl Cancer Inst 1994;86:446–449
Rothenberg ML et al. J Clin Oncol 2001;19:3801–3807
Wadler S et al. J Clin Oncol 1998;16:3169–3178

Oral care
Standard prophylaxis and treatment for mucositis/stomatitis

Patient Population Studied

This was a prospective randomized study involving 343 patients with histologically confirmed unresectable metastatic or recurrent colorectal carcinoma who had not received prior systemic chemotherapy or radiation treatment. Patients were required to have an Eastern Cooperative Oncology Group performance status of ≤2 and have adequate organ function.

Efficacy (N = 343)

	5FU + High-Dose Leucovorin
Response rate	30.3%
Median overall survival	55 weeks

5FU, fluorouracil; DFS, disease-free survival
*Comparison between fluorouracil + high dose leucovorin versus fluorouracil alone
†Comparison between fluorouracil + high dose leucovorin versus fluorouracil + low-dose leucovorin

Therapy Monitoring

1. *Before each cycle:* H&P, CBC with differential, CEA, serum electrolytes, creatinine, BUN, and LFTs

Treatment Modifications

Adverse Event	Dose Modification*
Any G1 toxicity	Maintain dose
Any G2 toxicity	Hold treatment until toxicity resolves to G ≤1. If toxicity occurs after the fourth weekly dose, stop until the next cycle; then resume at same dosage. If diarrhea occurs, reduce fluorouracil to 400 mg/m² per dose
Any G3/4 toxicity	Hold treatment until toxicity resolves to G ≤1. If toxicity occurs after the fourth weekly dose, stop until next cycle; then resume with fluorouracil 400 mg/m² per dose. If diarrhea occurs, reduce fluorouracil to 350 mg/m² per dose
Further toxicity	Reduce fluorouracil to 300 mg/m² per dose. If diarrhea occurs, reduce fluorouracil to 250 mg/m² dose

*Leucovorin dosage remains constant at 500 mg/m² per dose
Adapted from NSABP C–07 protocol
Wolmark N et al. Proc Am Soc Clin Oncol 2005;23:246S (abstract 3500)

Adverse Events (n = 109)

Toxicity	%G1–2	%G3–5
Nausea	53	10
Diarrhea	48	25
Skin	21	4
Mucositis	32	4
Anemia	46	2
Leukopenia	39	8
Thrombocytopenia	15	3

The table includes toxicities observed in the fluorouracil + high-dose leucovorin arm
Wolmark N et al. J Clin Oncol 1999;17:3553–3539

METASTATIC • SUBSEQUENT THERAPY

COLORECTAL CANCER REGIMEN: BEVACIZUMAB + FOLFIRI OR FOLFOX4 AFTER FIRST PROGRESSION ON BEVACIZUMAB

Bevacizumab 5 mg/kg; administer intravenously in 100 mL 0.9% sodium chloride injection (0.9% NS) every 2 weeks (total dosage/cycle = 5 mg/kg)

Note: Administration duration for the initial dose is 90 minutes. If administration is well tolerated, the administration duration may be decreased stepwise during subsequent administrations to 60 minutes and, finally, to a minimum duration of 30 minutes

FOLFIRI (*Tournigand C et al. J Clin Oncol 2004;22:229–237*):

Irinotecan 180 mg/m^2; administer intravenously over 90 minutes in 500 mL 5% dextrose injection (D5W) on day 1, every 2 weeks (total dosage/cycle = 180 mg/m^2), *plus:*
Either: (**racemic**) **leucovorin calcium** 400 mg/m^2 *or* **levoleucovorin calcium** 200 mg/m^2; administer intravenously over 2 hours in 25–500 mL 0.9% NS or D5W on day 1, every 2 weeks (total dosage/cycle for racemic leucovorin = 400 mg/m^2, for levoleucovorin = 200 mg/m^2), *followed by:*
Fluorouracil 400 mg/m^2; administer by intravenous injection over 1–2 minutes after leucovorin on day 1, every 2 weeks, *followed by:*
Fluorouracil 2400 mg/m^2; administer by continuous intravenous infusion over 46 hours in 100–1000 mL 0.9% NS or D5W, starting on day 1, every 2 weeks (total dosage/cycle = 2800 mg/m^2)

Supportive Care
Antiemetic prophylaxis
Emetogenic potential on day 1 is **MODERATE**
Emetogenic potential on day 2 is **LOW**
See Chapter 42 for antiemetic recommendations

Hematopoietic growth factor (G-CSF) prophylaxis
Primary prophylaxis is **NOT** *indicated*
See Chapter 43 for more information

Antimicrobial prophylaxis
Risk of fever and neutropenia is **LOW**
Antimicrobial primary prophylaxis to be considered:
- Antibacterial—not indicated
- Antifungal—not indicated
- Antiviral—not indicated unless patient previously had an episode of HSV

Acute cholinergic syndrome
Atropine sulfate 0.25–1 mg subcutaneously or intravenously if abdominal cramping or diarrhea develop during or within 1 hour after irinotecan administration
- If symptoms are severe, add as primary prophylaxis at least 30 minutes before irinotecan during subsequent cycles
- For irinotecan, acute cholinergic syndrome may be characterized by: abdominal cramping, diarrhea, diaphoresis, hypotension, flushing, bradycardia, rhinitis, increased salivation, miosis, and lacrimation

Diarrhea management
Latent or delayed-onset diarrhea*:
Loperamide 4 mg orally initially after the first loose or liquid stool, *then*
Loperamide 2 mg orally every 2 hours during waking hours, *plus*
Loperamide 4 mg orally every 4 hours during hours of sleep
- Continue for at least 12 hours after diarrhea resolves
- Recurrent diarrhea after a 12-hour diarrhea-free interval is treated as a new episode
- Rehydrate orally with fluids and electrolytes during a diarrheal episode
- If diarrhea persists >48 hours despite loperamide, stop loperamide and hospitalize the patient for IV hydration

Persistent diarrhea:
Octreotide 100–150 mcg subcutaneously 3 times daily. Maximum total daily dose is 1500 mcg
Antibiotic therapy during latent or delayed-onset diarrhea:
A fluoroquinolone (eg, **ciprofloxacin** 500 mg orally every 12 hours) if absolute neutrophil count <500/mm^3 with or without accompanying fever in association with diarrhea
- Antibiotics should also be administered if patient is hospitalized with prolonged diarrhea and should be continued until diarrhea resolves

*Abigerges D et al. J Natl Cancer Inst 1994;86:446–449
Rothenberg ML et al. J Clin Oncol 2001;19:3801–3807
Wadler S et al. J Clin Oncol 1998;16:3169–3178

(*continued*)

(*continued*)

BEVACIZUMAB + mFOLFOX6

Bevacizumab 5 mg/kg; administer intravenously in 100 mL 0.9% sodium chloride injection (0.9% NS) every 2 weeks (total dosage/cycle = 15 mg/kg)

Note: Administration duration for the initial dose is 90 minutes. If administration is well tolerated, the administration duration may be decreased stepwise during subsequent administrations to 60 minutes and, finally, to a minimum duration of 30 minutes

mFOLFOX6 (*Cheeseman SL. Br J Cancer. 2002;87:393–399*): **Oxaliplatin** 85 mg/m^2; administer intravenously in 250 mL 5% dextrose injection (D5W) over 2 hours concurrently with leucovorin administration, on day 1, every 2 weeks (total dosage/cycle = 85 mg/m^2)

Note: Oxaliplatin must not be mixed with sodium chloride injection. Therefore, when leucovorin and oxaliplatin are given concurrently via a Y-connector, both drugs must be administered in D5W

Leucovorin calcium 400 mg/m^2 per dose; administer intravenously in 25–500 mL D5W over 2 hours on day 1, every 2 weeks (total dosage/cycle = 400 mg/m^2), *followed by:*
Fluorouracil 400 mg/m^2 per dose; administer by intravenous injection over 1–2 minutes after leucovorin on day 1, every 2 weeks, *followed by:*
Fluorouracil 2400 mg/m^2 per dose; administer by continuous intravenous infusion in 100–1000 mL 0.9% NS or D5W over 46 hours every 2 weeks (total dosage/cycle = 2800 mg/m^2)

Note: **Fluorouracil** boluses (400 mg/m^2 by intravenous injection) may be omitted for better hematologic tolerance

Supportive Care
Antiemetic prophylaxis
Emetogenic potential on day 1 is **MODERATE**
Emetogenic potential on day 2 is **LOW**
See Chapter 42 for antiemetic recommendations

Hematopoietic growth factor (G-CSF) prophylaxis
Primary prophylaxis may be indicated
See Chapter 43 for more information

Antimicrobial prophylaxis
Risk of fever and neutropenia is **LOW**
  Antimicrobial primary prophylaxis to be considered:
  • Antibacterial—not indicated
  • Antifungal—not indicated
  • Antiviral—not indicated unless patient previously had an episode of HSV

Diarrhea management
Latent or delayed-onset diarrhea*:
  Loperamide 4 mg orally initially after the first loose or liquid stool, *then*
  Loperamide 2 mg orally every 2 hours during waking hours, *plus*
  Loperamide 4 mg orally every 4 hours during hours of sleep
  • Continue for at least 12 hours after diarrhea resolves
  • Recurrent diarrhea after a 12-hour diarrhea-free interval is treated as a new episode
  • Rehydrate orally with fluids and electrolytes during a diarrheal episode
  • If a patient develops blood or mucus in stool, dehydration, or hemodynamic instability, or if diarrhea persists >48 hours despite loperamide, stop loperamide and hospitalize the patient for IV hydration
  Alternatively, a trial of **diphenoxylate hydrochloride** 2.5 mg with **atropine sulfate** 0.025 mg (eg, Lomotil)
  • Initial adult dose is 2 tablets 4 times daily until control has been achieved, after which the dose may be reduced to meet individual requirements. Control may often be maintained with as little as 2 tablets daily
  • Clinical improvement of acute diarrhea is usually observed within 48 hours. If improvement of chronic diarrhea after treatment with a maximum daily dose of 8 tablets is not observed within 10 days, control is unlikely with further administration

Persistent diarrhea:
  Octreotide 100–150 mcg subcutaneously 3 times daily. Maximum total daily dose is 1500 mcg
Antibiotic therapy during latent or delayed-onset diarrhea:
  A fluoroquinolone (eg, **ciprofloxacin** 500 mg orally every 12 hours) if absolute neutrophil count <500/mm^3 with or without accompanying fever in association with diarrhea
  • Antibiotics should also be administered if patient is hospitalized with prolonged diarrhea and should be continued until diarrhea resolves

*Abigerges D et al. J Natl Cancer Inst 1994;86:446–449
Rothenberg ML et al. J Clin Oncol 2001;19:3801–3807
Wadler S et al. J Clin Oncol 1998;16:3169–3178

Oral care
Standard prophylaxis and treatment for mucositis/stomatitis

Treatment Modifications

Fluorouracil and Oxaliplatin

Any G2/3/4 nonhematologic toxicity	Delay start of next cycle until the severity of all toxicities is G ≤1
ANC ≤1500/mm³ or platelet count ≤100,000/mm³	Delay start of next cycle until ANC >1500/mm³ and platelet count >100,000/mm³
G3/4 Nonneurologic	Reduce fluorouracil and oxaliplatin dosages by 20%
G3/4 ANC	Reduce oxaliplatin dosage by 20%
Persistent (≥14 days) paresthesias	Reduce oxaliplatin dosage by 20%
Temporary (7–14 days) painful paresthesias	
Temporary (7–14 days) functional impairment	
Persistent (≥14 days) painful paresthesias	Discontinue oxaliplatin
Persistent (≥14 days) functional impairment	

Adapted in part from de Gramont A et al. J Clin Oncol 2000;18:2938–2947

Irinotecan and Fluorouracil

	Dosage Levels		
	Initial	**−1**	**−2**
Irinotecan	180 mg/m²	150 mg/m²	120 mg/m²
Leucovorin	Racemic leucovorin calcium 400 mg/m² or levoleucovorin calcium 200 mg/m²		
Fluorouracil injection	400 mg/m²	320 mg/m²	240 mg/m²
Infusional fluorouracil	2400 mg/m²	2000 mg/m²	1600 mg/m²

Notes:
- Dose modifications are based on the National Cancer Institute (USA) Common Toxicity Criteria. At: http://ctep.cancer.gov/protocolDevelopment/electronic_applications/ctc.htm [accessed October 11, 2013]
- Before beginning a treatment cycle, patients should have baseline bowel (similar to that before start of treatment) function without antidiarrheal therapy for 24 hours, ANC ≥1500/mm³, and platelet count ≥100,000/mm³
- Treatment should be delayed 1–2 weeks to allow for recovery from treatment-related toxicities
- If a patient has not recovered after 2 weeks, consider stopping therapy. If toxicity occurs despite 2 dose reductions (ie, on level −2), discontinue therapy

Toxicity	Modifications for Irinotecan and Fluorouracil
Neutropenia/Thrombocytopenia	
G1 ANC (1500–1999/mm³) or G1 thrombocytopenia (75,000/mm³ to less than normal limits)	Maintain dose and schedule
G2 ANC (1000–1499/mm³) or G2 thrombocytopenia (≥50,000 to <75,000/mm³)	Reduce dosage by 1 dosage level
G3 ANC (500–999/mm³) or G3 thrombocytopenia (≥10,000 to <50,000/mm³)	Hold treatment until toxicity resolves to G ≤2, then reduce dosage by 1 dosage level
G4 ANC (<500/mm³) or G4 thrombocytopenia (<10,000/mm³)	Hold treatment until toxicity resolves to G ≤2, then reduce dosage by 2 dosage levels
Febrile neutropenia	Hold treatment until neutropenia resolves, then reduce dosage by 2 dosage levels

(continued)

Treatment Modifications (*continued*)

Diarrhea

G1 (2–3 stools/day > baseline)	Maintain dose and schedule
G2 (4–6 stools/day > baseline)	Delay until diarrhea resolves to baseline then reduce dosage by 1 dosage level
G3 (7–9 stools/day > baseline)	Delay until diarrhea resolves to baseline then reduce dosage by 1 dosage level
G4 (≥10 stools/day > baseline)	Delay until diarrhea resolves to baseline then reduce dosage by 2 dosage levels

Other Nonhematologic Toxicities

Any G1 toxicity	Maintain dose and schedule
Any G2 toxicity	Hold treatment until toxicity resolves to G ≤1, then reduce dosage by 1 dosage level
Any G3 toxicity	Hold treatment until toxicity resolves to G ≤1, then reduce dosage by 1 dosage level
Any G4 toxicity	Hold treatment until toxicity resolves to G ≤1, then reduce dosage by 2 dosage levels
G2–4 mucositis	Decrease only fluorouracil by 20%

André T et al. Eur J Cancer 1999;35:1343–1347
Camptosar, irinotecan hydrochloride injection product label. New York: Pharmacia & Upjohn; July 2005
Douillard JY et al. Lancet 2000;355:1041–1047
Tournigand C et al. J Clin Oncol 2004;22:229–237

Efficacy

Tumor Response by RECIST*

	Bevacizumab + Chemotherapy (n = 404)	Chemotherapy Alone (n = 406)
Complete response	1 (<1%)	2 (<1%)
Partial response	21 (5%)	14 (3%)
Stable disease	253 (63%)	204 (50%)
Progressive disease	87 (22%)	142 (35%)
Missing/not assessable	42 (10%)	44 (11%)

Data are number (%)
*Includes only those patients with one or more measurable lesion at baseline. (RECIST, Response Evaluation Criteria in Solid Tumors. Therasse P et al. J Natl Cancer Inst 2000;92:205–216)

Response Durations

	Bevacizumab + Chemotherapy (n = 404)	Chemotherapy Alone (n = 406)
Median follow-up (months)	11.1 (6.4–15.6)	9.6 (IQR 5.4–13.9)
Median overall survival (months)	11.2 (95% CI 10.4–12.2)	9.8 (95% CI 8.9–10.7)
	HR 0.81 (95% CI 0.69–0.94); P = 0.0062	
Median progression-free survival (months)	5.7 (5.2–6.2)	4.1 (95% CI 3.7–4.4)
	HR 0.68 (95% CI 0.59–0.78); P <0.0001	

Efficacy (continued)

	Bevacizumab + Chemotherapy (n = 404)	Chemotherapy Alone (n = 406)
Median overall survival from start of first-line treatment* (months)	23.9 (95% CI 22.2–25.7)	22.5 (21.4–24.5)
	HR 0.90 (95% CI 0.77–1.05); P = 0.17	
Median overall treatment exposure (months)	4.2 (IQR 2.0–7.2)	3.2 months (1.7–5.2)
Treatment duration with bevacizumab (months)	3.9 (1.8–6.9)	N/A
Exploratory Subgroup Analysis According to KRAS Status (n = 616)		
Progression-free survival KRAS wild type	HR 0.61, 95% CI 0.49–0.77; P <0.0001[†]	
Progression-free survival KRAS mutant	HR 0.70, 95% CI 0.56–0.89; P = 0.003[†]	
Overall survival KRAS wild type	HR 0.69, 95% CI 0.53–0.90; P = 0.005[†‡]	
Overall survival KRAS mutant	HR 0.92, 95% CI 0.71–1.18; P = 0.50[‡]	

*Retrospectively documented
[†]Better outcome with bevacizumab
[‡]Treatment by KRAS status interaction test was negative for both progression-free survival (P = 0.4436) and overall survival (P = 0.1266), indicating there is no evidence treatment effect is dependent on KRAS mutational status

Patient Population Studied

Prospective, randomized, open-label, phase 3 study that enrolled patients if they had: (a) histologically confirmed, measurable metastatic colorectal cancer; (b) Eastern Cooperative Oncology Group (ECOG) performance status 0–2; (c) tumor disease according to RECIST criteria evaluated by investigator up to 4 weeks prior to start of study treatment; (d) previous treatment with bevacizumab plus standard first-line chemotherapy including a fluoropyrimidine plus either oxaliplatin or irinotecan; and (e) they were not candidates for primary metastasectomy. Patients were excluded if they: (a) had a diagnosis of progressive disease for more than 3 months after the last bevacizumab administration; (b) had first-line progression-free survival of less than 3 months; and (c) were given less than 3 months (consecutive) of first-line bevacizumab

Toxicity

Incidence of Grades 3–5 Adverse Events Occurring in ≥ 2% of Patients Given Chemotherapy with or Without Bevacizumab After Disease Progression Following First-Line Bevacizumab-Based Treatment (Safety Population*)

	Bevacizumab + Chemotherapy (n = 401)	Chemotherapy Alone (n = 409)
Neutropenia	65 (16%)	52 (13%)
Leucopenia	16 (4%)	12 (3%)
Asthenia	23 (6%)	17 (4%)
Fatigue	14 (3%)	10 (2%)
Diarrhea	40 (10%)	34 (8%)
Vomiting	14 (3%)	13 (3%)
Nausea	13 (3%)	11 (3%)
Decreased appetite	5 (1%)	9 (2%)
Mucosal inflammation	13 (3%)	4 (1%)
Abdominal pain	15 (4%)	12 (3%)
Polyneuropathy	12 (3%)	6 (1%)
Peripheral neuropathy	5 (1%)	10 (2%)
Hypokalemia	9 (2%)	8 (2%)
Dyspnea	6 (1%)	12 (3%)
Pulmonary embolism	10 (2%)	8 (2%)
Hypertension	7 (2%)	5 (1%)
Bleeding or hemorrhage	8 (2%)	1 (<1%)
Venous thromboembolic events	19 (5%)	12 (3%)
Gastrointestinal perforation	7 (2%)	3 (<1%)
Subileus	8 (2%)	2 (<1%)
Patients who discontinued any treatment because of adverse events	63 (16%)[†]	36 (9%)

*The safety population = 810 patients given ≥1 dose of study drug, including 407 patients in the chemotherapy group and 403 in the chemotherapy plus bevacizumab group. Two patients assigned to chemotherapy plus bevacizumab were not given bevacizumab and, for the safety analyses, were assigned to the chemotherapy group
[†]A total of 53 (13%) patients discontinued chemotherapy only or both bevacizumab and chemotherapy and 10 (2%) discontinued bevacizumab

METASTATIC • SUBSEQUENT THERAPY
COLORECTAL CANCER REGIMEN: INFUSIONAL FLUOROURACIL

Hansen RM et al. J Natl Cancer Inst 1996;88:668–674

Fluorouracil 300 mg/m^2 per day; administer by continuous intravenous infusion in 50–1000 mL 0.9% sodium chloride injection or 5% dextrose injection (total dosage/week = 2100 mg/m^2). Treatment is continued indefinitely until toxicity/disease progression

Supportive Care
Antiemetic prophylaxis
Emetogenic potential is **LOW**
See Chapter 42 for antiemetic recommendations

Hematopoietic growth factor (G-CSF) prophylaxis
Primary prophylaxis is **NOT** *indicated*
See Chapter 43 for more information

Antimicrobial prophylaxis
Risk of fever and neutropenia is **LOW**
  Antimicrobial primary prophylaxis to be considered:
- Antibacterial—not indicated
- Antifungal—not indicated
- Antiviral—not indicated unless patient previously had an episode of HSV

Diarrhea management
Latent or delayed-onset diarrhea*:
  Loperamide 4 mg orally initially after the first loose or liquid stool, *then*
  Loperamide 2 mg orally every 2 hours during waking hours, *plus*
  Loperamide 4 mg orally every 4 hours during hours of sleep
- Continue for at least 12 hours after diarrhea resolves
- Recurrent diarrhea after a 12-hour diarrhea-free interval is treated as a new episode
- Rehydrate orally with fluids and electrolytes during a diarrheal episode
- If diarrhea persists >48 hours despite loperamide, stop loperamide and hospitalize the patient for IV hydration

Persistent diarrhea:
  Octreotide 100–150 mcg subcutaneously 3 times daily. Maximum total daily dose is 1500 mcg
Antibiotic therapy during latent or delayed-onset diarrhea:
  A fluoroquinolone (eg, **ciprofloxacin** 500 mg orally every 12 hours) if absolute neutrophil count is <500/mm^3 with or without accompanying fever in association with diarrhea
- Antibiotics should also be administered if patient is hospitalized with prolonged diarrhea and should be continued until diarrhea resolves

*Abigerges D et al. J Natl Cancer Inst 1994;86:446–449
Rothenberg ML et al. J Clin Oncol 2001;19:3801–3807
Wadler S et al. J Clin Oncol 1998;16:3169–3178

Oral care
Standard prophylaxis and treatment for mucositis/stomatitis

Hand-foot reaction (palmar-plantar erythrodysesthesia, PPE)
For patients who develop a hand-foot reaction, use topical emollients (eg, Aquaphor®), topical or orally administered steroids, antihistamine agents (H$_1$-receptor antagonists), or pyridoxine
- Pyridoxine may provide relief for discomfort/pain associated with PPE although the mechanism through which this occurs remains unclear
- The suggested pyridoxine starting dose is 50 mg/day, which may be increased to a maximum of 200 mg/day

Patient Population Studied

A study of 159 patients with previously untreated metastatic adenocarcinoma of the colon or rectum

Toxicity (N = 159)

Requiring Treatment Interruption

G2 stomatitis	35%
G3 stomatitis	5%
G2/3 hand-foot syndrome	36%
G3 vomiting and diarrhea	3%
G3/4 hematologic	6%
All toxicities	
None	2%
Mild	15%
Moderate	52%
Severe	27%
Life-threatening	4%
Lethal	1%

Treatment Modifications

Adverse Event	Dose Modification
G2 nonhematologic toxicity	Reduce fluorouracil dosage by 50 mg/m^2 per day
G3 nonhematologic toxicity	Reduce fluorouracil dosage by 100 mg/m^2 per day
Hematologic toxicity	No modifications

Therapy Monitoring

1. *Before each cycle:* H&P, CBC with differential, CEA serum electrolytes, and LFTs
2. *Weekly:* CBC with differential count
3. *Every 2–3 months:* CT scans to assess response

Efficacy (N = 159)

Overall response	28%
Complete response	5%
Median survival	13 months

METASTATIC • SUBSEQUENT THERAPY
COLORECTAL CANCER REGIMEN: TRIFLURIDINE/TIPIRACIL (TAS–102)

Mayer RJ et al. N Engl J Med 2015;372:1909–1919

Trifluridine/tipiracil 35 mg/m²/dose (dose based on trifluridine component, maximum dose = 80 mg); administer orally twice per day, with a glass of water within 1 hour of completion of the morning and evening meals, on days 1–5 and days 8–12; repeated every 28 days until disease progression (total dose of trifluridine per 28-day cycle = 700 mg/m²; total maximum dose of trifluridine per 28-day cycle = 1600 mg)

Notes:
• Round each dose to the nearest 5 mg (maximum dose = 80 mg) and administer a combination of 15 mg and/or 20 mg tablets (trifluridine component) as necessary to provide the calculated dose
• Patients who delay taking a trifluridine/tipiracil dose at a regularly scheduled time or who vomit after taking a dose of trifluridine/tipiracil should take the next dose at the next regularly scheduled time

Supportive Care
Antiemetic prophylaxis
Emetogenic potential is **MODERATE**
See Chapter 42 for antiemetic recommendations

Hematopoietic growth factor (CSF) prophylaxis
Primary prophylaxis is **NOT** *indicated*
See Chapter 43 for more information

Antimicrobial prophylaxis
Risk of fever and neutropenia is **LOW**
  Antimicrobial primary prophylaxis to be considered:
  • Antibacterial—not indicated
  • Antifungal—not indicated
  • Antiviral—not indicated unless patient previously had an episode of HSV

Diarrhea management
Latent or delayed-onset diarrhea*:
  Loperamide 4 mg orally initially after the first loose or liquid stool, *then*
  Loperamide 2 mg orally every 2 hours during waking hours, *plus*
  Loperamide 4 mg orally every 4 hours during hours of sleep
  • Continue for at least 12 hours after diarrhea resolves
  • Recurrent diarrhea after a 12-hour diarrhea-free interval is treated as a new episode
  • Rehydrate orally with fluids and electrolytes during a diarrheal episode
  • If a patient develops blood or mucus in stool, dehydration, or hemodynamic instability, or if diarrhea persists >48 hours despite loperamide, stop loperamide and hospitalize the patient for intravenous hydration
  Alternatively, a trial of **diphenoxylate hydrochloride** 2.5 mg with **atropine sulfate** 0.025 mg (eg, Lomotil)
  • Initial adult dose is 2 tablets 4 times daily until control has been achieved, after which the dose may be reduced to meet individual requirements. Control may often be maintained with as little as 2 tablets daily
  • Clinical improvement of acute diarrhea is usually observed within 48 hours. If improvement of chronic diarrhea after treatment with a maximum daily dose of 8 tablets is not observed within 10 days, control is unlikely with further administration

Persistent diarrhea:
  Octreotide 100–150 mcg subcutaneously 3 times daily. Maximum total daily dose is 1500 mcg
Antibiotic therapy during latent or delayed-onset diarrhea:
  A fluoroquinolone (eg, **ciprofloxacin** 500 mg orally every 12 hours) if absolute neutrophil count <500/mm³ with or without accompanying fever in association with diarrhea
  • Antibiotics should also be administered if patient is hospitalized with prolonged diarrhea and should be continued until diarrhea resolves

*Abergerges D et al. J Natl Cancer Inst 1994;86:446–449

Patient Population Studied

A multicenter, randomized, double-blind, phase 3 trial involved 800 patients with biopsy-documented adenocarcinoma of the colon or rectum. Eligible patients were aged ≥18 years, with ECOG (Eastern Cooperative Oncology Group) performance status ≤1, had previously received ≥2 regimens of standard chemotherapies, and had either experienced tumor progression within 3 months after last administration of chemotherapy or had clinically significant adverse events from standard chemotherapies that precluded readministration of those therapies. Patients who had not previously received chemotherapy with a fluoropyrimidine, oxaliplatin, irinotecan, bevacizumab and (in those with KRAS wild-type tumors) either cetuximab or panitumumab were not eligible. Patients were randomly assigned (2:1) to receive trifluridine + tipiracil (TAS–102) or placebo

Efficacy (N = 800)

Median overall survival	7.1 months vs. 5.3 months with placebo HR 0.68, 95% CI 0.58–0.81, P<0.001
Median progression-free survival	2.0 months vs. 1.7 months with placebo HR 0.48, 95% CI 0.41–0.57, P<0.001
Complete or partial response*	1.6% vs 0.4% with placebo; P = 0.29
Disease control*†	44% vs 16% with placebo; P<0.001

*Tumor response was assessed in 760 patients
†Disease control was defined as complete or partial response or stable disease at least 6 weeks after randomization

Therapy Monitoring

1. CBC with differential at a minimum prior to and on day 15 of each cycle. CBC as often as weekly early on in treatment to assess if dose is appropriate
2. Serum bilirubin, AST or ALT, and alkaline phosphatase prior to each cycle; CEA if being used to follow disease
3. Every 2–3 months: CT scans to assess response

Treatment Modifications

TRIFLURIDINE AND TIPIRACIL (TAS–102)

Dose Levels

Starting dose	35 mg/m²/dose (maximum dose = 80 mg) twice daily on days 1–5 and days 8–12 of each 28-day cycle
Dose Level −1	30 mg/m²/dose (maximum dose = 70 mg) twice daily on days 1–5 and days 8–12 of each 28-day cycle
Dose Level −2	25 mg/m²/dose (maximum dose = 60 mg) twice daily on days 1–5 and days 8–12 of each 28-day cycle
Dose Level −3	20 mg/m²/dose (maximum dose = 50 mg) twice daily on days 1–5 and days 8–12 of each 28-day cycle

Alternately find trifluridine and tipiracil dosage calculator at: https://www.lonsurfhcp.com/dosing/dosage-calculator [accessed July 29, 2018]

Adverse Event	Treatment Modification
If at start of new cycle ANC <1,500/mm³; febrile neutropenia; platelets < 75,000/mm³; G3/4 nonhematologic adverse reactions	Withhold the start of trifluridine/tipiracil until ANC ≥1500/mm³; febrile neutropenia is resolved; platelets ≥75,000/mm³; G3/4 nonhematologic adverse reactions have resolved to G0/1 and resume with previous dose
Uncomplicated G4 neutropenia (<1000/mm³) that has recovered to ≥1500/mm³ or G4 thrombocytopenia (<25,000/mm³) that has recovered to ≥75,000/mm³ but that did not delay start of cycle by >1 week	Resume trifluridine/tipiracil at previous dose
Febrile neutropenia	After recovery, resume trifluridine/tipiracil, reducing dose by 5 mg/m²/dose. Do not escalate trifluridine/tipiracil dose after it has been reduced
Uncomplicated G4 neutropenia (<1000/mm³) that has recovered to ≥1500/mm³ or G4 thrombocytopenia (<25,000/mm³) that has recovered to ≥75,000/mm³ but that delayed start of cycle by >1 week	
Nonhematologic G3/4 adverse reactions (except for G3 nausea and/or vomiting controlled by antiemetic therapy or G3 diarrhea responsive to antidiarrheal medication)	
If within a treatment cycle ANC <500/mm³; febrile neutropenia; platelets <50,000/mm³; G3/4 nonhematologic adverse reactions	Withhold trifluridine/tipiracil until ANC ≥500/mm³; febrile neutropenia is resolved; platelets ≥50,000/mm³; G3/4 nonhematologic adverse reactions have resolved to G0/1
Mild hepatic impairment (total bilirubin <1.5′ ULN and normal transaminases)	No adjustment to the starting dose of trifluridine/tipiracil is recommended
Baseline moderate or severe hepatic impairment (total bilirubin >1.5′ ULN and any AST elevation)	Do not initiate trifluridine/tipiracil
Moderate renal impairment (creatinine clearance =30–59 mL/min)	May require dose modifications for increased toxicity
Severe fatigue	Reduce trifluridine/tipiracil dose by 5 mg/m²
G≥2 nausea/vomiting	Institute antiemetic therapy; after resolution of symptoms, resume trifluridine/tipiracil at the dose being used

Note: Trifluridine/tipiracil can cause fetal harm when administered to a pregnant woman. Advise pregnant women of the potential risk to the fetus. Advise females of reproductive potential to use effective contraception during treatment

Adverse Events (N = 798)

Grade (%)*	Trifluridine + Tipiracil (TAS–102)		Placebo	
	Grade 1/2	Grade ≥3	Grade 1/2	Grade ≥3
Any event	29	69	42	52
Nonhematologic Adverse Events				
Nausea	47	2	23	1
Decreased appetite	35	4	25	5
Increase in alkaline phosphatase level	31	8	34	11
Increase in total bilirubin	27	9	15	12
Fatigue	31	4	18	6
Diarrhea	29	3	12	<1
Increase in AST level	25	4	29	6
Vomiting	26	2	14	<1
Increase in ALT level	22	2	23	4
Abdominal pain	19	2	15	4
Fever	17	1	14	<1
Asthenia	15	3	8	3
Increase in creatinine level	13	<1	11	<1
Stomatitis†	8	<1	6	0
Hand-foot syndrome	2	0	2	0
Cardiac ischemia	<1	<1	0	<1
Hematologic Adverse Events				
Leukopenia	56	21	5	0
Anemia	58	18	30	3
Neutropenia	29	38	<1	0
Febrile neutropenia†	0	4	0	0
Thrombocytopenia	37	5	8	<1

*According to the National Cancer Institute Common Terminology Criteria for Adverse Events, version 4.03
†Denotes those events of special interest for fluoropyrimidine treatment
Note: Toxicities are included in the table if all-grade events occurred in ≥10% of patients in the TAS–102 group and occurred more frequently in that group than in the controls, or were of special interest

METASTATIC • SUBSEQUENT THERAPY

COLORECTAL CANCER REGIMEN: PANITUMUMAB + BEST SUPPORTIVE CARE

Van Cutsem E et al. J Clin Oncol 2007;25:1658–1664

Panitumumab 6 mg/kg; administer intravenously in 0.9% sodium chloride injection (100 mL for doses ≤1000 mg; 150 mL for doses >1000 mg; product concentration should be <10 mg/mL) over 60–90 minutes on day 1, every 2 weeks (total dosage/cycle = 6 mg/kg)

Notes:
- Severe infusion reactions occur in approximately 1% of patients (anaphylactic reactions, bronchospasm, fever, chills, and hypotension). Dose adjustment or discontinuation of panitumumab is warranted depending on the severity of the reaction
- Panitumumab should always be administered by a rate-controlling device via a low-protein-binding 0.22-μm inline filter
- Flush line before and after panitumumab with 0.9% sodium chloride injection
- Doses ≤1000 mg should be administered over 60 minutes; >1000 mg should be administered over 90 minutes
  - If tolerated, second and subsequent infusions may be administered over 30 minutes
- The routine use of an antihistamine prior to panitumumab administration is not recommended by the manufacturer; however, doing so may prevent infusion reactions

Supportive Care

Antiemetic prophylaxis
Emetogenic potential is **MINIMAL** to **LOW**
See Chapter 42 for antiemetic recommendations

Hematopoietic growth factor (G-CSF) prophylaxis
Primary prophylaxis is **NOT** indicated
See Chapter 43 for more information

Antimicrobial prophylaxis
Risk of fever and neutropenia is **LOW**
  Antimicrobial primary prophylaxis to be considered:
- Antibacterial—not indicated
- Antifungal—not indicated
- Antiviral—not indicated unless patient previously had an episode of HSV

Diarrhea management
Loperamide 4 mg; administer orally initially after the first loose or liquid stool, *then*
Loperamide 2 mg; administer orally every 2 hours during waking hours, *plus*
Loperamide 4 mg; administer orally every 4 hours during hours of sleep
- Continue for at least 12 hours after diarrhea resolves
- Recurrent diarrhea after a 12-hour diarrhea-free interval is treated as a new episode
- Rehydrate orally with fluids and electrolytes during a diarrheal episode
- If a patient develops blood or mucus in stool, dehydration, or hemodynamic instability, or if diarrhea persists >48 hours despite loperamide, stop loperamide and hospitalize the patient for IV hydration

Alternatively, a trial of **diphenoxylate hydrochloride** 2.5 mg with **atropine sulfate** 0.025 mg (eg, Lomotil®)
- Initial adult dose is two tablets four times daily until control has been achieved, after which the dose may be reduced to meet individual requirements. Control may often be maintained with as little as two tablets daily
- Clinical improvement of acute diarrhea is usually observed within 48 hours. If improvement of chronic diarrhea after treatment with a maximum daily dose of 8 tablets is not observed within 10 days, control is unlikely with further administration

Persistent diarrhea:
Octreotide acetate (solution) 100–150 mcg; administer subcutaneously 3 times daily. Maximum total daily dose is 1500 mcg
Antibiotic therapy during latent or delayed-onset diarrhea:
A fluoroquinolone (eg, **ciprofloxacin** 500 mg orally every 12 hours) if absolute neutrophil count <500/mm^3 with or without accompanying fever in association with diarrhea
- Antibiotics should also be administered if patient is hospitalized with prolonged diarrhea and should be continued until diarrhea resolves

Toxicities (N = 463)

	Panitumumab + BSC		BSC	
	% All Grades	% G3/4	% All Grades	% G3/4
Patients with at least 1 adverse event	100%	34.5	86	19.2
Erythema	64	5	1	0
Dermatitis acneiform	62	7	1	0
Pruritus	57	2	2	0
Skin exfoliation	24	2	0	0
Fatigue	24	4	15	3
Paronychia	24	1	0	0
Abdominal pain	23	7	17	4.7
Anorexia	22	3.5	18	2
Nausea	22	1	15	0
Diarrhea	21	1	11	0
Rash	20	1	1	0
Skin fissures	20	1	0	0
Constipation	19	3	9	1
Vomiting	18	2	12	1
Dyspnea	14	4.8	13	3
Pyrexia	14	0	12	2
Asthenia	14	3	12	2
Cough	14	0	7	0
Back pain	10	2	7	0
Edema peripheral	10	1	6	0
General physical health deterioration	10	7	3	2.1

Note: In the panitumumab group, 36% of patients had declines in blood magnesium levels versus 1% in the BSC group. Grade 3 or 4 hypomagnesemia occurred in 3% of patients and required magnesium supplementation

Patient Population Studied

A study of 463 patients with pathologic diagnosis of metastatic colorectal adenocarcinoma and radiologic documentation of disease progression during or within 6 months following the last administration of fluoropyrimidine, irinotecan, and oxaliplatin. A total of 231 patients were assigned to receive panitumumab + best supportive care (BSC) versus 232 patients assigned to BSC alone. To ensure adequate exposure to prior chemotherapy, average dose-intensity of irinotecan (>65 mg/m^2 per week) and of oxaliplatin (>30 mg/m^2 per week) were required. Other key eligibility criteria included: Eastern Cooperative Oncology Group (ECOG) performance status score of 0–2, 2, or 3 prior chemotherapy regimens for metastatic colorectal cancer, and 1% or more EGFR-positive membrane staining in evaluated tumor cells (primary or metastatic) by immunohistochemistry

Efficacy* (N = 463)

	Panitumumab + BSC (N = 231)	BSC (N = 232)
Median progression-free survival[†]	8 weeks	7.3 weeks
Mean progression-free survival (SE)[†]	13.8 (0.8) weeks	8.5 (0.5) weeks
Progression-free survival at week 8[†]	49%	30%
Overall survival	No significant difference observed between groups (HR,1.00; 95% CI, 0.82–1.22; P = 0.81)	
Overall response rate[‡]	10%	0%

*Assessed by modified RECIST criteria at weeks 8, 12, 16, 24, 32, 40, and 48, and every 3 months thereafter until disease progression (Response Evaluation Criteria in Solid Tumors. Therasse P et al. J Natl Cancer Inst 2000;92:205–216)
[†]Patients receiving panitumumab had a 46% decrease in the relative progression rate compared with patients receiving BSC (HR, 0.54; 95% CI, 0.44–0.66), and a 95% CI for the difference in PFS rates favored panitumumab at all scheduled assessments from weeks 8–32; SE = standard error
[‡]Median time to response was 7.9 (range, 6.7–15.6) weeks and median duration of response was 17.0 (range, 7.9–76.7) weeks; all responses were partial responses

Treatment Modifications

Adverse Event	Dose Modification
G1/2 infusion reaction to panitumumab	Decrease infusion rate by 50% for duration of infusion
G3/4 infusion reaction to panitumumab	Immediately and permanently discontinue infusion
G3/4 or intolerable dermatologic reaction to panitumumab	Withhold panitumumab. If toxicity improves to G ≤2 and patient symptomatically improves after withholding no more than 2 doses, resume treatment at 50% of the original dose. If toxicity does not improve to G ≤2 within 1 month, permanently discontinue panitumumab *Note:* **If toxicities do not recur**, subsequent doses of panitumumab may be increased by increments of 25% of original dose until a 6-mg/kg dose is achieved
Recurrence of G3/4 or intolerable dermatologic reaction to panitumumab	Permanently discontinue infusion
Any G2/3/4 nonhematologic toxicity	Delay start of next cycle until the severity of all toxicities is G ≤1
ANC ≤1500/mm^3 or platelet count ≤100,000/mm^3	Delay start of next cycle until ANC >1500/mm^3 and platelet count >100,000/mm^3

Therapy Monitoring

1. *Before each cycle:* H&P, CBC with differential, CEA if initially elevated, serum electrolytes, serum magnesium, and LFTs
2. *Every 2–3 months:* CT scans to assess response in patients presenting with advanced colorectal cancer

METASTATIC • SUBSEQUENT THERAPY
COLORECTAL CANCER REGIMEN: NIVOLUMAB

Overman MJ et al. Lancet Oncol 2017;18:1182–1191
Waterhouse D et al. Cancer Chemother Pharmacol 2018;81:679–686
Zhao X et al. Ann Oncol 2017;28:2002–2008

Adult patients and pediatric patients weighing ≥40 kg:

Nivolumab 240 mg; administer intravenously over 30 minutes in a volume of 0.9% Sodium Chloride (0.9% NS) or 5% dextrose injection (D5W), not to exceed 160 mL and sufficient to produce a nivolumab concentration within the range 1–10 mg/mL, every 2 weeks until disease progression (total dosage/2-week cycle = 240 mg)
or
Nivolumab 480 mg; administer intravenously over 30 minutes in a volume of 0.9% NS or D5W not to exceed 160 mL and sufficient to produce a nivolumab concentration within the range 1–10 mg/mL, every 4 weeks until disease progression (total dosage/4-week cycle = 480 mg)

Pediatric patients weighing <40 kg:
Nivolumab 3 mg/kg; administer intravenously over 30–60 minutes in a volume of 0.9% NS or D5W , not to exceed 160 mL and sufficient to produce a nivolumab concentration within the range 1–10 mg/mL, every 2 weeks (total dosage/2-week course = 3 mg/kg)

Notes:
- Administer nivolumab through an administration set that contains a sterile, nonpyrogenic, low protein-binding in-line filter with pore size within the range of 0.2–1.2 μm
- Nivolumab can cause severe infusion-related reactions
  - Interrupt or slow the administration rate in patients with mild or moderate infusion-related reactions
  - Discontinue nivolumab in patients who experience severe or life-threatening infusion-related reactions
- Eligibility for treatment with nivolumab requires a patient's colorectal cancer to be identified as microsatellite instability-high (MSI-H) or mismatch repair deficient (dMMR)

Supportive Care
Antiemetic prophylaxis
Emetogenic potential is **MINIMAL**
See Chapter 42 for antiemetic recommendations

Hematopoietic growth factor (CSF) prophylaxis
Primary prophylaxis is **NOT** indicated
See Chapter 43 for more information

Antimicrobial prophylaxis
Risk of fever and neutropenia is **LOW**
   Antimicrobial primary prophylaxis to be considered:
- Antibacterial—not indicated
- Antifungal—not indicated
- Antiviral—not indicated unless patient previously had an episode of HSV

Patient Population Studied

A multicenter, open-label, phase 2 study involved 74 patients with histologically confirmed recurrent or metastatic dMMR or MSI-H colorectal cancer. Eligible patients were aged ≥18 years and had ECOG (Eastern Cooperative Oncology Group) performance status ≤1, measurable disease, and progression on or after, or intolerance of, at least 1 previous line of treatment, including a fluoropyrimidine and oxaliplatin or irinotecan. Patients who had refused chemotherapy were also eligible. Patients received intravenous nivolumab (3 mg/kg) every 2 weeks

Efficacy (N = 74)

Objective response*	31.1%
Rate of complete response	0
Median progression-free survival	14.3 months
Overall survival at 12 months	73%

Note: Median follow-up was 12.0 months
*As assessed by the investigator according to RECIST criteria; the primary end point

Therapy Monitoring

1. CBC with differential at a minimum once per cycle, but initially also at day 10–14
2. Every 2–3 months: CT scans to assess response
3. Observe closely for hypersensitivity reactions, especially during the first and second infusions
4. Draw AST, ALT, and bilirubin prior to each infusion and/or weekly if there are G1 LFT elevations. Note, no treatment is recommended for G1 LFT abnormalities. For G ≥2 toxicity, implement work-up for other causes of elevated LFTs, including viral hepatitis
5. Measure glucose at baseline and with each treatment during the first 12 weeks and every 6 weeks thereafter
6. Obtain a serum creatinine level prior to every dose. If creatinine is found to be newly elevated, consider holding therapy while other potential causes are evaluated. Note: Routine urinalysis is not necessary other than to rule out urinary tract infections
7. Use basic metabolic panel (Na, K, CO_2, glucose) and patient history as screening tools for hypophysitis including hypopituitarism and adrenal insufficiency. If in doubt evaluate morning adrenocorticotropic hormone (ACTH) and cortisol levels. Consider ACTH stimulation test for indeterminate results

(continued)

Therapy Monitoring (*continued*)

8. Assess thyroid function at the start of treatment, periodically during treatment, and as indicated based on clinical evaluation) and for clinical signs and symptoms of thyroid disorders. Test for TSH and free thyroxine (FT^4) every 4–6 weeks as part of routine clinical monitoring of therapy or for case detection in symptomatic patients

9. Obtain CEA if being used to follow disease

10. Initially at the time of each dose, and eventually every 6–12 weeks, perform a total body skin examination with attention to all mucous membranes as well as a complete review of systems

11. Monitor patients for signs and symptoms of pneumonitis. Evaluate patients with suspected pneumonitis with chest x-ray, CT scan, and pulse oximetry. For G ≥2 toxicity, may include nasal swab, sputum culture and sensitivity, blood culture and sensitivity, and urine culture and sensitivity

12. Monitor patients for signs and symptoms of colitis. Encourage patients to report diarrhea immediately to any member of the health care team

13. Obtain a complete rheumatologic history and perform an examination of all peripheral joints for tenderness, swelling, and range of motion. Examine the spine. Consider plain x-ray/imaging to exclude metastases and evaluate joint damage (erosions), if appropriate

14. In patients at high risk for infections and in appropriately selected patients, based on an infectious disease evaluation, draw screening laboratories (HIV, hepatitis A and B, and blood QuantiFERON for TB) to prepare patients to start infliximab

Treatment Modifications

RECOMMENDED DOSE MODIFICATIONS FOR NIVOLUMAB

Adverse Event	Grade/Severity	Treatment Modification
Colitis	G1	Loperamide 4 mg as starting dose then 2 mg before each meal and after each loose stool until without diarrhea for 12 hours, with maximum of 16 mg loperamide per day. If G1 diarrhea or colitis persists for >14 days, then add prednisolone 0.5–1 mg/kg (non-enteric coated) or consider oral budesonide 9 mg daily if no bloody diarrhea
	G2/3 diarrhea or colitis	Withhold nivolumab. Loperamide 4 mg as starting dose then 2 mg before each meal and after each loose stool until without diarrhea for 12 hours, with maximum of 16 mg loperamide per day. Administer oral prednisone/prednisolone at a dose of 0.5–2 mg/kg/day or its equivalent. When symptoms improve to G1, begin a slow corticosteroid taper over at least 4 weeks. Resume nivolumab upon symptom control, or when prednisone/prednisolone daily dose <10 mg
	G4 diarrhea or colitis	Permanently discontinue nivolumab. Loperamide 4 mg as starting dose then 2 mg before each meal and after each loose stool until without diarrhea for 12 hours, with maximum of 16 mg loperamide per day. Administer 1–2 mg/kg intravenous (methyl)prednisolone and convert to 0.5–2 mg/kg prednisone/prednisolone orally each day or its equivalent only after a response. Taper over at least 4 weeks when symptoms improve. If symptoms do not improve over 72 hours or worsen, perform flexible sigmoidoscopy/colonoscopy to document colitis then begin infliximab 5 mg/kg (if no perforation, sepsis, TB, hepatitis, NYHA III/IV CHF). If no response, add MMF 500–1000 mg twice daily. If worse on MMF, consider addition of tacrolimus or ATG
Pneumonitis	G2	Withhold nivolumab. Consider pneumocystis prophylaxis depending on the clinical context and coverage with empiric antibiotics. Administer oral prednisone/prednisolone at a dose of 1–2 mg/kg/day or its equivalent. When symptoms improve to G1, begin a slow corticosteroid taper over at least 4 weeks. If response is not adequate after 48 hours, then administer 2–4 mg/kg intravenous (methyl)prednisolone and convert to 0.5–2 mg/kg prednisone/prednisolone orally each day or its equivalent only after a response, followed by a taper over at least 6 weeks when symptoms improve to G1, titrating to symptoms. Resume nivolumab upon symptom control, or when prednisone/prednisolone daily dose <10 mg
	G3/4	Permanently discontinue nivolumab. Consider pneumocystis prophylaxis depending on the clinical context; cover with empiric antibiotics. Administer 2–4 mg/kg intravenous (methyl)prednisolone and convert to 1–2 mg/kg prednisone/prednisolone orally each day or its equivalent only after a response, followed by a taper over at least 8 weeks when symptoms improve to G1, titrating to symptoms. If, when initially treated, improvement does not occur within 48–72 hours, begin infliximab 5 mg/kg (if no perforation, sepsis, TB, hepatitis, NYHA III/IV CHF). If no response to infliximab, add MMF 500–1000 mg twice daily. Consider MMF especially if concurrent hepatic toxicity

(*continued*)

Treatment Modifications (*continued*)

RECOMMENDED DOSE MODIFICATIONS FOR NIVOLUMAB

Adverse Event	Grade/Severity	Treatment Modification
Hepatitis	G2 (AST or ALT >3–5′ ULN or total bilirubin >1.5–3′ ULN)	Withhold nivolumab. Administer oral prednisone/prednisolone at a dose of 1–2 mg/kg/day or its equivalent. When symptoms improve to G1, begin a slow corticosteroid taper over at least 4 weeks. Resume nivolumab upon symptom control, or when prednisone/prednisolone daily dose <10 mg
	G3/4 (AST or ALT >5′ ULN or total bilirubin >3′ ULN)	Permanently discontinue nivolumab. Administer 1–2 mg/kg intravenous (methyl)prednisolone and convert to 0.5–2 mg/kg prednisone/prednisolone orally each day or its equivalent only after a response. Taper over at least 6 weeks when symptoms improve. If no response, add MMF 500–1000 mg twice daily. If worse on MMF, consider adding tacrolimus or ATG
Hypophysitis	G2/3 (moderate symptoms, ie, headache but no visual disturbance, or fatigue/mood alteration but hemodynamically stable, no electrolyte disturbance)	Administer analgesia as needed for headache. Withhold nivolumab. Administer oral prednisone/prednisolone at a dose of 0.5–2 mg/kg/day or its equivalent. When improves to G1, begin a slow corticosteroid taper over at least 4 weeks. If no improvement in 48 hours, administer 1–2 mg/kg intravenous (methyl)prednisolone and convert to 0.5–2 mg/kg prednisone/prednisolone orally each day or its equivalent only after a response. Taper over at least 4 weeks when symptoms improve to 5 mg prednisone/prednisolone or equivalent; do not stop steroids. Resume nivolumab upon symptom control, or when prednisone/prednisolone daily dose <10 mg
	G4 (severe mass effect symptoms, ie, severe headache, any visual disturbance, or severe hypoadrenalism, ie, hypotension, severe electrolyte disturbance)	Permanently discontinue nivolumab. Administer analgesia as needed for headache. Administer 1–2 mg/kg intravenous (methyl)prednisolone and convert to 0.5–2 mg/kg prednisone/prednisolone orally each day or its equivalent only after a response. Taper over at least 4 weeks when symptoms improve to 5 mg prednisone/prednisolone or equivalent; do not stop steroids
Adrenal insufficiency	G2	Withhold nivolumab. Administer oral prednisone/prednisolone at a dose of 0.5–2 mg/kg/day or its equivalent. When symptoms improve to G1, begin a slow corticosteroid taper over at least 4 weeks. Serially assess adrenal function and continue steroids at replacement doses (20–40 mg hydrocortisone daily ~2/3 dose in morning upon awakening and ~1/3 at 4 PM) until recovery of adrenal function is documented. Resume nivolumab upon symptom control, or when prednisone/prednisolone daily dose <10 mg
	G3/4	Permanently discontinue nivolumab. Administer oral prednisone/prednisolone at a dose of 0.5–2 mg/kg/day or its equivalent. When symptoms improve to G1, begin a slow corticosteroid taper over at least 4 weeks. Serially assess adrenal function and continue steroids at replacement doses (20–40 mg hydrocortisone daily ~2/3 dose in morning upon awakening and ~1/3 at 4 PM) until recovery of adrenal function is documented
Type 1 diabetes mellitus	G3 hyperglycemia	Withhold nivolumab. Admit to hospital to manage hyperglycemia. Role of corticosteroids in preventing complete loss of insulin-producing cells is unknown and not recommended. Resume nivolumab upon symptom control, or when prednisone/prednisolone daily dose <10 mg
	G4 hyperglycemia	Permanently discontinue nivolumab. Admit to hospital to manage hyperglycemia. Role of corticosteroids in preventing complete loss of insulin-producing cells is unknown and not recommended
Nephritis and renal dysfunction	G2/3 (serum creatinine 1.5–6′ ULN)	Withhold nivolumab. Administer oral prednisone/prednisolone at a dose of 0.5–2 mg/kg/day or its equivalent. When symptoms improve to G1, begin a slow corticosteroid taper over at least 4 weeks. If response is not adequate, then administer 0.5–1 mg/kg intravenous (methyl)prednisolone and convert to 0.5–2 mg/kg prednisone/prednisolone orally each day or its equivalent only after a response, followed by a taper over at least 4 weeks when symptoms improve to G1. Resume nivolumab upon symptom control, or when prednisone/prednisolone daily dose <10 mg
	G4 (serum creatinine >6′ ULN)	Permanently discontinue nivolumab. Administer 0.5–1 mg/kg intravenous (methyl)prednisolone and convert to 0.5–2 mg/kg prednisone/prednisolone orally each day or its equivalent only after a response, followed by a taper over at least 4 weeks when symptoms improve to G1

(*continued*)

Treatment Modifications (*continued*)

RECOMMENDED DOSE MODIFICATIONS FOR NIVOLUMAB

Adverse Event	Grade/Severity	Treatment Modification
Skin	G1/2	Continue nivolumab. Avoid skin irritants, avoid sun exposure; topical emollients recommended. Topical steroid (mild strength for G1, moderate/potent strength for G2) cream once or twice daily ± oral or topical antihistamines for itching
	G3 rash or suspected SJS or TEN	Withhold nivolumab. Avoid skin irritants, avoid sun exposure, topical emollients recommended. Administer oral or topical antihistamines for itching. Administer oral prednisone/prednisolone at a dose of 0.5–2 mg/kg or its equivalent daily for 3 days followed by a slow corticosteroid taper over at least 4 weeks when the rash improves to G1. If response is not adequate, then administer 0.5–1 mg/kg intravenous (methyl)prednisolone and convert to 0.5–2 mg/kg prednisone/prednisolone orally each day or its equivalent only after a response, followed by a taper over at least 4 weeks when the rash improves to G1. Resume nivolumab upon symptom control, or when prednisone/prednisolone daily dose <10 mg
	G4 rash or confirmed SJS or TEN	Avoid skin irritants, avoid sun exposure; topical emollients recommended. Administer oral or topical antihistamines for itching. Administer 1–2 mg/kg intravenous (methyl)prednisolone and convert to oral steroids 0.5–2 mg/kg prednisone/prednisolone each day or its equivalent only after a response. Taper over at least 4 weeks when the rash improves to G1. Permanently discontinue nivolumab
Encephalitis	Confusion or altered behavior, headaches, alteration in Glasgow Coma Scale, motor or sensory deficits, speech abnormality, may or may not be febrile	Initially withhold nivolumab, but permanently discontinue nivolumab if there is no doubt as to diagnosis. Exclude bacterial and ideally viral infections prior to high-dose steroids. Administer oral prednisone/prednisolone at a dose of 0.5–2 mg/kg/day or its equivalent. When symptoms improve, begin a slow corticosteroid taper over at least 4–8 weeks. If symptoms are severe, administer 1–2 mg/kg intravenous (methyl)prednisolone and convert to 0.5–2 mg/kg prednisone/prednisolone orally each day or its equivalent only after a response. Consider concurrent empiric antiviral (intravenous acyclovir) and antibacterial therapy
Aseptic meningitis	Headache, photophobia, neck stiffness with fever, or may be afebrile, vomiting; normal cognition/cerebral function (distinguishes from encephalitis)	
Other syndromes include neurosarcoidosis, posterior reversible leukoencephalopathy syndrome (PRES), Vogt-Koyanagi-Harada syndrome, demyelination, vasculitic encephalopathy, and generalized seizures		
Transverse myelitis	Acute or subacute neurologic signs/symptoms of motor, sensory, or autonomic origin; most have sensory level; often bilateral symptoms	Initially withhold nivolumab, but permanently discontinue nivolumab if there is no doubt as to diagnosis. Administer 2 mg/kg intravenous (methyl)prednisolone or consider 1 g/day and convert to 0.5–2 mg/kg prednisone/prednisolone orally each day or its equivalent only after a response. When symptoms improve, begin a slow corticosteroid taper over at least 4–8 weeks. Plasmapheresis may be required if steroids do not bring about improvement
Myocarditis	G3	Permanently discontinue nivolumab. Administer 2 mg/kg intravenous (methyl)prednisolone or consider 1 g/day and convert to 0.5–2 mg/kg prednisone/prednisolone orally each day or its equivalent only after a response. When symptoms improve, begin a slow corticosteroid taper over at least 4–8 weeks. If no response, add MMF 500–1000 mg twice daily. If worse on MMF, consider adding tacrolimus
Peripheral neurologic toxicity	Moderate: some interference with ADLs, symptoms concerning to patient	Withhold nivolumab. Initial observation reasonable or initiate prednisone/prednisolone 0.5–1 mg/kg (if progressing, eg, from mild) and/or pregabalin or duloxetine for pain. When symptoms improve, begin a slow corticosteroid taper over at least 4 weeks. Resume nivolumab upon symptom control, or when prednisone/prednisolone daily dose <10 mg
	Severe: limits self-care and aids warranted, life threatening, eg, respiratory problems	Permanently discontinue nivolumab. Administer 1–2 mg/kg intravenous (methyl)prednisolone and convert to 0.5–2 mg/kg prednisone/prednisolone orally each day or its equivalent only after a response. Taper over at least 4–8 weeks when symptoms improve to G1
Guillain-Barré syndrome	Progressive symmetrical muscle weakness with absent or reduced tendon reflexes—involves extremities, facial, respiratory, bulbar, and oculomotor muscles; dysregulation of autonomic nerves	Permanently discontinue nivolumab. Use of steroids not recommended in idiopathic Guillain-Barré syndrome; however, a trial of (methyl)prednisolone 1–2 mg/kg is reasonable, converting to 0.5–2 mg/kg prednisone/prednisolone orally each day or its equivalent only after a response. If no improvement or worsening, plasmapheresis or IVIG indicated

(*continued*)

Treatment Modifications (*continued*)

RECOMMENDED DOSE MODIFICATIONS FOR NIVOLUMAB

Adverse Event	Grade/Severity	Treatment Modification
Myasthenia gravis	Fluctuating muscle weakness (proximal limb, trunk, ocular, eg, ptosis/diplopia or bulbar) with fatigability, respiratory muscles may also be involved	Permanently discontinue nivolumab. Administer pyridostigmine at an initial dose of 30 mg 3 times daily. Administer oral prednisone/prednisolone at a dose of 0.5–2 mg/kg/day or its equivalent or 1–2 mg/kg intravenous (methyl)prednisolone depending on the severity of symptoms. If treatment begins with intravenous drug, convert to 0.5–2 mg/kg prednisone/prednisolone orally each day or its equivalent only after a response. If no improvement or worsening, plasmapheresis or IVIG may be considered. Additional immunosuppressants used in myasthenia gravis include azathioprine, cyclosporine, and mycophenolate. Avoid certain medications (eg, ciprofloxacin, beta-blockers) that may precipitate cholinergic crisis
Other syndromes, including motor and sensory peripheral neuropathy, multifocal radicular neuropathy/plexopathy, autonomic neuropathy, phrenic nerve palsy, cranial nerve palsies (eg, facial nerve, optic nerve, hypoglossal nerve)		Permanently discontinue nivolumab. Administer oral prednisone/prednisolone at a dose of 0.5–2 mg/kg/day or its equivalent or 1–2 mg/kg intravenous (methyl)prednisolone depending on the severity of symptoms. If treatment begins with intravenous drug, convert to 0.5–2 mg/kg prednisone/prednisolone orally each day or its equivalent only after a response
Arthralgia	G1 (mild pain with inflammation, erythema or joint swelling)	Continue nivolumab. Administer acetaminophen (paracetamol) and ibuprofen
	G2 (moderate pain with inflammation, erythema or joint swelling that limits ADLs)	Withhold nivolumab. Administer higher doses of acetaminophen (paracetamol) and ibuprofen and use diclofenac or naproxen or etoricoxib. If inadequately controlled, consider intra-articular steroid injections for large joints or administer oral prednisone/prednisolone at a dose of 0.5–2 mg/kg/day or its equivalent. When symptoms improve to G1, begin a slow corticosteroid taper over at least 4 weeks. If response is not adequate, then administer 0.5–1 mg/kg intravenous (methyl)prednisolone and convert to 0.5–2 mg/kg prednisone/prednisolone orally each day or its equivalent only after a response, followed by a taper over at least 4 weeks when symptoms improve to G1. Resume nivolumab upon symptom control, or when prednisone/prednisolone daily dose <10 mg
	G3 (severe pain; irreversible joint damage; disabling; limits self-care ADLs)	Withhold nivolumab. Administer 0.5–1 mg/kg intravenous (methyl)prednisolone and convert to 0.5–2 mg/kg prednisone/prednisolone orally each day or its equivalent only after a response, followed by a taper over at least 4 weeks when symptoms improve to G1. In severe cases, infliximab or another anti–TNF-alpha drug may be required for improvement of arthritis. Resume nivolumab upon symptom control, or when prednisone/prednisolone daily dose <10 mg
Other	First occurrence of other G3	Withhold nivolumab. Administer oral prednisone/prednisolone at a dose of 0.5–2 mg/kg/day or its equivalent. When symptoms improve to G1, begin a slow corticosteroid taper over at least 4 weeks. Resume nivolumab upon symptom control, or when prednisone/prednisolone daily dose <10 mg
	Recurrence of same G3	Permanently discontinue nivolumab. Administer 1–2 mg/kg intravenous (methyl)prednisolone and convert to 0.5–2 mg/kg prednisone/prednisolone orally each day or its equivalent only after a response. Taper over at least 4–8 weeks when symptoms improve to G1
	Life-threatening or G4	
	Requirement for ≥10 mg/day prednisone or equivalent for >12 weeks	Permanently discontinue nivolumab
	Persistent G2/3 adverse reactions lasting ≥12 weeks	

ADL, activities of daily living; ALT, alanine aminotransferase; AST, aspartate aminotransferase; ATG, anti-thymocyte globulin; CHF, congestive heart failure; IVIG, intravenous immunoglobulin; MMF, mycophenolate mofetil; NYHA, New York Heart Association; SJS, Stevens-Johnson syndrome; TB, tuberculosis; TEN, toxic epidermal necrolysis; TNF, tumor necrosis factor; ULN, upper limit of normal

Notes on general supportive care:

Steroid taper in most cases will proceed over a minimum of 1 month but if symptoms improve rapidly, a 2-week taper can be considered. If steroids are administered for more than 4 weeks, consider PCP prophylaxis (cotrimoxazole 480 mg twice daily M/W/F or inhaled pentamidine if cotrimoxazole allergy), regular random blood glucose, vitamin D level, and starting calcium/vitamin D supplementation as per guidelines

Notes on pregnancy and breastfeeding:

Nivolumab can cause fetal harm. If used during pregnancy, or if the patient becomes pregnant during treatment, apprise the patient of the potential hazard to a fetus. Females of reproductive potential should use highly effective contraception during treatment and for 5 months after the last dose of nivolumab

It is not known whether nivolumab is excreted in human milk. Therefore, it is recommended that women discontinue nursing during treatment with nivolumab

Adverse Events (N = 74)

Grade (%)*	Grade 1/2	Grade 3/4
Any event	49	20
Fatigue	22	1
Diarrhea	20	1
Pruritus	14	0
Increased lipase	4	8
Rash	11	0
Hypothyroidism	10	0
Nausea	10	0
Asthenia	7	0
Increased AST	7	0
Increased amylase	3	3
Maculopapular rash	5	1
Increased ALT	4	1
Arthralgia	5	0
Dry skin	5	0
Pyrexia	5	0
Stomatitis	3	1
Abdominal pain	1	1
Decreased lymphocyte count	1	1
Increased creatinine	1	1
Acute kidney injury	0	1
Adrenal insufficiency	0	1
Colitis	0	1
Esophagitis	0	1
Gastritis	0	1
Increased GGT	0	1
Pain	0	1

*According to the National Cancer Institute Common Terminology Criteria for Adverse Events, version 4.03
Note: Treatment-related toxicities are included in the table if grade 1/2 events occurred in ≥10% of patients or if any grade 3/4 events occurred. No treatment-related deaths were recorded. In total, 70% of patients experienced a treatment-related adverse event. Six patients discontinued treatment because of treatment-related adverse effects

METASTATIC • SUBSEQUENT THERAPY
COLORECTAL CANCER REGIMEN: PEMBROLIZUMAB

Diaz LA et al. J Clin Oncol 2017;35(suppl):abstr 3071
Freshwater T et al. J Immunother Cancer 2017;5:43
Le DT et al. J Clin Oncol 2016;34(suppl):abstr TPS787
Le DT et al. J Clin Oncol 2018;36(suppl):abstr 3514
Le DT et al. N Engl J Med 2015;372:2509–2520

Pembrolizumab 200 mg; administer intravenously over 30 minutes in a volume of 0.9% sodium chloride injection (0.9% NS) or 5% dextrose injection (D5W), sufficient to produce a pembrolizumab concentration within the range 1–10 mg/mL every 3 weeks for up to 35 cycles (total dose/3-week cycle = 200 mg)
- Administer pembrolizumab with an administration set that contains a sterile, nonpyrogenic, low protein-binding in-line or add-on filter with pore size within the range of 0.2–5 μm

Alternative pembrolizumab dose and schedule as per the U.S. FDA regimens approved on April 28, 2020:
Pembrolizumab 400 mg; administer intravenously over 30 minutes in a volume of 0.9% NS or D5W sufficient to produce a pembrolizumab concentration within the range 1–10 mg/mL every 6 weeks, for a maximum of 2 years of therapy (total dose/6-week cycle = 400 mg)

Notes:
- Pembrolizumab can cause severe or life-threatening infusion-related reactions, including hypersensitivity and anaphylaxis
  - Monitor patients for signs and symptoms of infusion-related reactions including rigors, chills, wheezing, pruritus, flushing, rash, hypotension, hypoxemia, and fever
  - For severe or life-threatening infusion-related reactions (G3 or G4, respectively), stop administration and permanently discontinue pembrolizumab
- Eligibility for treatment with pembrolizumab requires a patient's colorectal cancer to be identified as microsatellite instability-high (MSI-H) or mismatch repair deficient (dMMR)
- The U.S. FDA-approved dose of pembrolizumab for *pediatric* patients with MSI-H or dMMR solid tumors, including colorectal cancer, is 2 mg/kg (maximum dose = 200 mg) intravenously over 30 minutes every 3 weeks, thus, *for pediatric patients:*

  Pembrolizumab 2 mg/kg (maximum dose = 200 mg); administer intravenously over 30 minutes in a volume of 0.9% NS or D5W, sufficient to produce a pembrolizumab concentration within the range 1–10 mg/mL every 3 weeks for up to 35 cycles (total dose/3-week cycle = 2 mg/kg; maximum dose/3-week cycle = 200 mg)
  - Administer pembrolizumab with an administration set that contains a sterile, nonpyrogenic, low protein-binding in-line or add-on filter with pore size within the range of 0.2–5 μm

Supportive Care
Antiemetic prophylaxis
Emetogenic potential is **MINIMAL**
See Chapter 42 for antiemetic recommendations

Hematopoietic growth factor (CSF) prophylaxis
Primary prophylaxis is **NOT** *indicated*
See Chapter 43 for more information

Antimicrobial prophylaxis
Risk of fever and neutropenia is **LOW**
  Antimicrobial primary prophylaxis to be considered:
  - Antibacterial—not indicated
  - Antifungal—not indicated
  - Antiviral—not indicated, unless patient previously had an episode of HSV

Patient Population Studied

A multicenter, phase 2 study involved 41 patients with treatment-refractory progressive metastatic cancer; of these participants, 11 had mismatch repair-deficient (dMMR) colorectal cancer, 21 had mismatch repair-proficient (pMMR) colorectal cancer, and 9 had dMMR noncolorectal cancer. All patients received the study drug, pembrolizumab

Efficacy (N = 41)

	dMMR Colorectal Cancer	pMMR Colorectal Cancer	dMMR Noncolorectal Cancer
Immune-related objective response	40%	0%	71%
Immune-related progression-free survival at 20 weeks	78%	11%	67%
Median progression-free survival	Not reached	2.2 months	5.4 months
Median overall survival	Not reached	5.0 months	Not reached

Note: Median follow-up was 36 weeks for patients with dMMR colorectal cancer, 20 weeks for patients with pMMR colorectal cancer, and 21 weeks for patients with dMMR non-colorectal cancer

Therapy Monitoring

1. CBC with differential at a minimum once per cycle, but initially also at day 10–14

2. Every 2–3 months: CT scans to assess response

3. Observe closely for hypersensitivity reactions, especially during the first and second infusions

4. Draw AST, ALT, and bilirubin prior to each infusion and/or weekly if there are G1 LFT elevations. Note, no treatment is recommended for G1 LFT abnormalities. For G ≥2 toxicity, implement work-up for other causes of elevated LFTs, including viral hepatitis

5. Measure glucose at baseline and with each treatment during the first 12 weeks and every 6 weeks thereafter

6. Obtain a serum creatinine level prior to every dose. If creatinine is found to be newly elevated, consider holding therapy while other potential causes are evaluated. Note, routine urinalysis is not necessary other than to rule out urinary tract infections

7. Use basic metabolic panel (Na, K, CO_2, glucose) and patient history as screening tools for hypophysitis including hypopituitarism and adrenal insufficiency. If in doubt evaluate morning adrenocorticotropic hormone (ACTH) and cortisol levels. Consider ACTH stimulation test for indeterminate results

8. Assess thyroid function at the start of treatment, periodically during treatment, and as indicated based on clinical evaluation, and for clinical signs and symptoms of thyroid disorders. Test for TSH and free thyroxine (FT_4) every 4–6 weeks as part of routine clinical monitoring of therapy or for case detection in symptomatic patients

9. Obtain CEA if being used to follow disease

10. Initially at the time of each dose, and eventually every 6–12 weeks, perform a total body skin examination with attention to all mucous membranes as well as a complete review of systems

11. Monitor patients for signs and symptoms of pneumonitis. Evaluate patients with suspected pneumonitis with chest x-ray, CT scan, and pulse oximetry. For G ≥2 toxicity, may include nasal swab, sputum culture and sensitivity, blood culture and sensitivity, and urine culture and sensitivity

12. Monitor patients for signs and symptoms of colitis. Encourage patients to report diarrhea immediately to any member of the health care team

13. Obtain a complete rheumatologic history and perform an examination of all peripheral joints for tenderness, swelling, and range of motion. Examine the spine. Consider plain x-ray/imaging to exclude metastases and evaluate joint damage (erosions), if appropriate

14. In patients at high risk for infections and in appropriately selected patients, based on an infectious disease evaluation, draw screening laboratories (HIV, hepatitis A and B, and blood QuantiFERON for TB) to prepare patients to start infliximab

Treatment Modifications

RECOMMENDED DOSE MODIFICATIONS FOR PEMBROLIZUMAB

Adverse Event	Grade/Severity	Treatment Modification
Colitis	G1	Loperamide 4 mg as starting dose then 2 mg before each meal and after each loose stool until without diarrhea for 12 hours, with maximum of 16 mg loperamide per day. If G1 diarrhea or colitis persists for >14 days, then add prednisolone 0.5–1 mg/kg (non-enteric coated) or consider oral budesonide 9 mg daily if no bloody diarrhea
	G2/3 diarrhea or colitis	Withhold pembrolizumab. Loperamide 4 mg as starting dose then 2 mg before each meal and after each loose stool until without diarrhea for 12 hours, with maximum of 16 mg loperamide per day. Administer oral prednisone/prednisolone at a dose of 0.5–2 mg/kg/day or its equivalent. When symptoms improve to G1, begin a slow corticosteroid taper over at least 4 weeks. Resume pembrolizumab upon symptom control, or when prednisone/prednisolone daily dose <10 mg
	G4 diarrhea or colitis	Permanently discontinue pembrolizumab. Loperamide 4 mg as starting dose then 2 mg before each meal and after each loose stool until without diarrhea for 12 hours, with maximum of 16 mg loperamide per day. Administer 1–2 mg/kg intravenous (methyl)prednisolone and convert to 0.5–2 mg/kg prednisone/prednisolone orally each day or its equivalent only after a response. Taper over at least 4 weeks when symptoms improve. If symptoms do not improve over 72 hours or worsen, perform flexible sigmoidoscopy/colonoscopy to document colitis then begin infliximab 5 mg/kg (if no perforation, sepsis, TB, hepatitis, NYHA III/IV CHF). If no response, add MMF 500–1000 mg twice daily. If worse on MMF, consider addition of tacrolimus or ATG
Pneumonitis	G2	Withhold pembrolizumab. Consider pneumocystis prophylaxis depending on the clinical context and coverage with empiric antibiotics. Administer oral prednisone/prednisolone at a dose of 1–2 mg/kg/day or its equivalent. When symptoms improve to G1, begin a slow corticosteroid taper over at least 4 weeks. If response is not adequate after 48 hours, then administer 2–4 mg/kg intravenous (methyl)prednisolone and convert to 0.5–2 mg/kg prednisone/prednisolone orally each day or its equivalent only after a response, followed by a taper over at least 6 weeks when symptoms improve to G1, titrating to symptoms. Resume pembrolizumab upon symptom control, or when prednisone/prednisolone daily dose <10 mg
	G3/4	Permanently discontinue pembrolizumab. Consider pneumocystis prophylaxis depending on the clinical context; cover with empiric antibiotics. Administer 2–4 mg/kg intravenous (methyl)prednisolone and convert to 1–2 mg/kg prednisone/prednisolone orally each day or its equivalent only after a response, followed by a taper over at least 8 weeks when symptoms improve to G1, titrating to symptoms. If, when initially treated, improvement does not occur within 48–72 hours, begin infliximab 5 mg/kg (if no perforation, sepsis, TB, hepatitis, NYHA III/IV CHF). If no response to infliximab, add MMF 500–1000 mg twice daily. Consider MMF especially if has concurrent hepatic toxicity
Hepatitis	G2 (AST or ALT >3–5′ ULN or total bilirubin >1.5–3′ ULN)	Withhold pembrolizumab. Administer oral prednisone/prednisolone at a dose of 1–2 mg/kg/day or its equivalent. When symptoms improve to G1, begin a slow corticosteroid taper over at least 4 weeks. Resume pembrolizumab upon symptom control, or when prednisone/prednisolone daily dose <10 mg
	G3/4 (AST or ALT >5′ ULN or total bilirubin >3′ ULN)	Permanently discontinue pembrolizumab. Administer 1–2 mg/kg intravenous (methyl)prednisolone and convert to 0.5–2 mg/kg prednisone/prednisolone orally each day or its equivalent only after a response. Taper over at least 6 weeks when symptoms improve. If no response, add MMF 500–1000 mg twice daily. If worse on MMF, consider adding tacrolimus or ATG
Hypophysitis	G2/3 (moderate symptoms, ie, headache but no visual disturbance, or fatigue/mood alteration but hemodynamically stable, no electrolyte disturbance)	Administer analgesia as needed for headache. Withhold pembrolizumab. Administer oral prednisone/prednisolone at a dose of 0.5–2 mg/kg/day or its equivalent. When symptoms improve to G1, begin a slow corticosteroid taper over at least 4 weeks. If no improvement in 48 hours, administer 1–2 mg/kg intravenous (methyl)prednisolone and convert to 0.5–2 mg/kg prednisone/prednisolone orally each day or its equivalent only after a response. Taper over at least 4 weeks when symptoms improve to 5 mg prednisone/prednisolone or equivalent; do not stop steroids. Resume pembrolizumab upon symptom control, or when prednisone/prednisolone daily dose <10 mg
	G4 (severe mass effect symptoms, ie, severe headache, any visual disturbance, or severe hypoadrenalism, ie, hypotension, severe electrolyte disturbance)	Permanently discontinue pembrolizumab. Administer analgesia as needed for headache. Administer 1–2 mg/kg intravenous (methyl)prednisolone and convert to 0.5–2 mg/kg prednisone/prednisolone orally each day or its equivalent only after a response. Taper over at least 4 weeks when symptoms improve to 5 mg prednisone/prednisolone or equivalent; do not stop steroids

(*continued*)

Treatment Modifications (*continued*)

RECOMMENDED DOSE MODIFICATIONS FOR PEMBROLIZUMAB		
Adverse Event	**Grade/Severity**	**Treatment Modification**
Adrenal insufficiency	G2	Withhold pembrolizumab. Administer oral prednisone/prednisolone at a dose of 0.5–2 mg/kg/day or its equivalent. When symptoms improve to G1, begin a slow corticosteroid taper over at least 4 weeks. Serially assess adrenal function and continue steroids at replacement doses (20–40 mg hydrocortisone daily ~2/3 dose in morning upon awakening and ~1/3 at 4 PM) until recovery of adrenal function is documented. Resume pembrolizumab upon symptom control, or when prednisone/prednisolone daily dose <10 mg
	G3/4	Permanently discontinue pembrolizumab. Administer oral prednisone/prednisolone at a dose of 0.5–2 mg/kg/day or its equivalent. When symptoms improve to G1, begin a slow corticosteroid taper over at least 4 weeks. Serially assess adrenal function and continue steroids at replacement doses (20–40 mg hydrocortisone daily ~2/3 dose in morning upon awakening and ~1/3 at 4 PM) until recovery of adrenal function is documented
Type 1 diabetes mellitus	G3 hyperglycemia	Withhold pembrolizumab. Admit to hospital to manage hyperglycemia. Role of corticosteroids in preventing complete loss of insulin-producing cells is unknown and not recommended. Resume pembrolizumab upon symptom control, or when prednisone/prednisolone daily dose <10 mg
	G4 hyperglycemia	Permanently discontinue pembrolizumab. Admit to hospital to manage hyperglycemia. Role of corticosteroids in preventing complete loss of insulin-producing cells is unknown and not recommended.
Nephritis and renal dysfunction	G2/3 (serum creatinine 1.5–6′ ULN)	Withhold pembrolizumab. Administer oral prednisone/prednisolone at a dose of 0.5–2 mg/kg/day or its equivalent. When symptoms improve to G1, begin a slow corticosteroid taper over at least 4 weeks. If response is not adequate, then administer 0.5–1 mg/kg intravenous (methyl)prednisolone and convert to 0.5–2 mg/kg prednisone/prednisolone orally each day or its equivalent only after a response, followed by a taper over at least 4 weeks when symptoms improve to G1. Resume pembrolizumab upon symptom control, or when prednisone/prednisolone daily dose <10 mg
	G4 (serum creatinine >6′ ULN)	Permanently discontinue pembrolizumab. Administer 0.5–1 mg/kg intravenous (methyl)prednisolone and convert to 0.5–2 mg/kg prednisone/prednisolone orally each day or its equivalent only after a response, followed by a taper over at least 4 weeks when symptoms improve to G1
Skin	G1/2	Continue pembrolizumab. Avoid skin irritants, avoid sun exposure; topical emollients recommended. Topical steroid (mild strength for G1, moderate/potent strength for G2) cream once or twice daily ± oral or topical antihistamines for itching
	G3 rash or suspected SJS or TEN	Withhold pembrolizumab. Avoid skin irritants, avoid sun exposure; topical emollients recommended. Administer oral or topical antihistamines for itching. Administer oral prednisone/prednisolone at a dose of 0.5–2 mg/kg or its equivalent daily for 3 days followed by a slow corticosteroid taper over at least 4 weeks when the rash improves to G1. If rash does not respond adequately, then administer 0.5–1 mg/kg intravenous (methyl)prednisolone and convert to 0.5–2 mg/kg prednisone/prednisolone orally each day or its equivalent only after a response, followed by a taper over at least 4 weeks when the rash improves to G1. Resume pembrolizumab upon symptom control, or when prednisone/prednisolone daily dose <10 mg
	G4 rash or confirmed SJS or TEN	Avoid skin irritants, avoid sun exposure; topical emollients recommended. Administer oral or topical antihistamines for itching. Administer 1–2 mg/kg intravenous (methyl)prednisolone and convert to oral steroids 0.5–2 mg/kg prednisone/prednisolone each day or its equivalent only after a response. Taper over at least 4 weeks when the rash improves to G1. Permanently discontinue pembrolizumab

(*continued*)

Treatment Modifications (*continued*)

RECOMMENDED DOSE MODIFICATIONS FOR PEMBROLIZUMAB

Adverse Event	Grade/Severity	Treatment Modification
Encephalitis	Confusion or altered behavior, headaches, alteration in Glasgow Coma Scale, motor or sensory deficits, speech abnormality, may or may not be febrile	Initially withhold pembrolizumab, but permanently discontinue pembrolizumab if there is no doubt as to diagnosis. Exclude bacterial and ideally viral infections prior to high-dose steroids. Administer oral prednisone/prednisolone at a dose of 0.5–2 mg/kg/day or its equivalent. When symptoms improve, begin a slow corticosteroid taper over at least 4–8 weeks. If symptoms are severe, administer 1–2 mg/kg intravenous (methyl)prednisolone and convert to 0.5–2 mg/kg prednisone/prednisolone orally each day or its equivalent only after a response. Consider concurrent empiric antiviral (intravenous acyclovir) and antibacterial therapy
Aseptic meningitis	Headache, photophobia, neck stiffness with fever, or may be afebrile, vomiting; normal cognition/cerebral function (distinguishes from encephalitis)	
Other syndromes include neurosarcoidosis, posterior reversible leukoencephalopathy syndrome (PRES), Vogt-Koyanagi-Harada syndrome, demyelination, vasculitic encephalopathy, and generalized seizures		
Transverse myelitis	Acute or subacute neurologic signs/symptoms of motor, sensory, or autonomic origin; most have sensory level; often bilateral symptoms	Initially withhold pembrolizumab, but permanently discontinue pembrolizumab if there is no doubt as to diagnosis. Administer 2 mg/kg intravenous (methyl)prednisolone or consider 1 g/day and convert to 0.5–2 mg/kg prednisone/prednisolone orally each day or its equivalent only after a response. When symptoms improve, begin a slow corticosteroid taper over at least 4–8 weeks. Plasmapheresis may be required if steroids do not bring about improvement
Myocarditis	G3	Permanently discontinue pembrolizumab. Administer 2 mg/kg intravenous (methyl)prednisolone or consider 1 g/day and convert to 0.5–2 mg/kg prednisone/prednisolone orally each day or its equivalent only after a response. When symptoms improve, begin a slow corticosteroid taper over at least 4–8 weeks. If no response, add MMF 500–1000 mg twice daily. If worse on MMF, consider adding tacrolimus
Peripheral neurologic toxicity	Moderate: some interference with ADLs, symptoms concerning to patient	Withhold pembrolizumab. Initial observation reasonable or initiate prednisone/prednisolone 0.5–1 mg/kg (if progressing, eg, from mild) and/or pregabalin or duloxetine for pain. When symptoms improve, begin a slow corticosteroid taper over at least 4 weeks. Resume pembrolizumab upon symptom control, or when prednisone/prednisolone daily dose <10 mg
	Severe: limits self-care and aids warranted, life-threatening, eg, respiratory problems	Permanently discontinue pembrolizumab. Administer 1–2 mg/kg intravenous (methyl)prednisolone and convert to 0.5–2 mg/kg prednisone/prednisolone orally each day or its equivalent only after a response. When improved to Grade 0-1, taper over at least 4–8 weeks
Guillain-Barré syndrome	Progressive symmetrical muscle weakness with absent or reduced tendon reflexes—involves extremities, facial, respiratory, bulbar, and oculomotor muscles; dysregulation of autonomic nerves	Permanently discontinue pembrolizumab. Use of steroids not recommended in idiopathic Guillain-Barré syndrome; however, a trial of (methyl)prednisolone 1–2 mg/kg is reasonable, converting to 0.5–2 mg/kg prednisone/prednisolone orally each day or its equivalent only after a response. If no improvement or worsening, plasmapheresis or IVIG indicated
Myasthenia gravis	Fluctuating muscle weakness (proximal limb, trunk, ocular, eg, ptosis/diplopia or bulbar) with fatigability; respiratory muscles may also be involved	Permanently discontinue pembrolizumab. Administer pyridostigmine at an initial dose of 30 mg 3 times daily. Administer oral prednisone/prednisolone at a dose of 0.5–2 mg/kg/day or its equivalent or 1–2 mg/kg intravenous (methyl)prednisolone depending on the severity of symptoms. If treatment begins with intravenous drug, convert to 0.5–2 mg/kg prednisone/prednisolone orally each day or its equivalent only after a response. If no improvement or worsening, plasmapheresis or IVIG may be considered. Additional immunosuppressants used in myasthenia gravis include azathioprine, cyclosporine, and mycophenolate. Avoid certain medications (eg, ciprofloxacin, beta-blockers) that may precipitate cholinergic crisis
Other syndromes, including motor and sensory peripheral neuropathy, multifocal radicular neuropathy/plexopathy, autonomic neuropathy, phrenic nerve palsy, cranial nerve palsies (eg, facial nerve, optic nerve, hypoglossal nerve)		Permanently discontinue pembrolizumab. Administer oral prednisone/prednisolone at a dose of 0.5–2 mg/kg/day or its equivalent or 1–2 mg/kg intravenous (methyl)prednisolone depending on the severity of symptoms. If treatment begins with intravenous drug, convert to 0.5–2 mg/kg prednisone/prednisolone orally each day or its equivalent only after a response

(*continued*)

Treatment Modifications (*continued*)

RECOMMENDED DOSE MODIFICATIONS FOR PEMBROLIZUMAB

Adverse Event	Grade/Severity	Treatment Modification
Arthralgia	G1 (mild pain with inflammation, erythema, or joint swelling)	Continue pembrolizumab. Administer acetaminophen (paracetamol) and ibuprofen
	G2 (moderate pain with inflammation, erythema, or joint swelling that limits ADLs)	Withhold pembrolizumab. Administer higher doses of acetaminophen (paracetamol) and ibuprofen and use diclofenac or naproxen or etoricoxib. If inadequately controlled, consider intra-articular steroid injections for large joints or administer oral prednisone/prednisolone at a dose of 0.5–2 mg/kg/day or its equivalent. When symptoms improve to G1, begin a slow corticosteroid taper over at least 4 weeks. If response is not adequate, then administer 0.5–1 mg/kg intravenous (methyl)prednisolone and convert to 0.5–2 mg/kg prednisone/prednisolone orally each day or its equivalent only after a response, followed by a taper over at least 4 weeks when improves to G1. Resume pembrolizumab upon symptom control, or when prednisone/prednisolone daily dose <10 mg
	G3 (severe pain; irreversible joint damage; disabling; limits self-care ADLs)	Withhold pembrolizumab. Administer 0.5–1 mg/kg intravenous (methyl)prednisolone and convert to 0.5–2 mg/kg prednisone/prednisolone orally each day or its equivalent only after a response, followed by a taper over at least 4 weeks when symptoms improve to G1. In severe cases, infliximab or another anti–TNF-alpha drug may be required for improvement of arthritis. Resume pembrolizumab upon symptom control, or when prednisone/prednisolone daily dose <10 mg
Other	First occurrence of other G3	Withhold pembrolizumab. Administer oral prednisone/prednisolone at a dose of 0.5–2 mg/kg/day or its equivalent. When symptoms improve to G1, begin a slow corticosteroid taper over at least 4 weeks. Resume pembrolizumab upon symptom control, or when prednisone/prednisolone daily dose <10 mg
	Recurrence of same G3	Permanently discontinue pembrolizumab. Administer 1–2 mg/kg intravenous (methyl)prednisolone and convert to 0.5–2 mg/kg prednisone/prednisolone orally each day or its equivalent only after a response. Taper over at least 4–8 weeks when symptoms improve to G1
	Life-threatening or G4	
	Requirement for ≥10 mg/day prednisone or equivalent for >12 weeks	Permanently discontinue pembrolizumab
	Persistent G2/3 adverse reactions lasting ≥12 weeks	

ADL, activities of daily living; ALT, alanine aminotransferase; AST, aspartate aminotransferase; ATG, anti-thymocyte globulin; CHF, congestive heart failure; IVIG, intravenous immunoglobulin; MMF, mycophenolate mofetil; NYHA, New York Heart Association; SJS, Stevens-Johnson syndrome; TB, tuberculosis; TEN, toxic epidermal necrolysis; TNF, tumor necrosis factor; ULN, upper limit of normal

Notes on general supportive care:

Steroid taper in most cases will proceed over a minimum of 1 month but if symptoms improve rapidly, a 2-week taper can be considered. If steroids are administered for more than 4 weeks, consider PCP prophylaxis (cotrimoxazole 480 mg twice daily M/W/F or inhaled pentamidine if cotrimoxazole allergy), regular random blood glucose, vitamin D level, and starting calcium/vitamin D supplementation as per guidelines

Notes on pregnancy and breastfeeding:

Pembrolizumab can cause fetal harm. If used during pregnancy, or if the patient becomes pregnant during treatment, apprise the patient of the potential hazard to a fetus. Females of reproductive potential should use highly effective contraception during treatment and for 4 months after the last dose of pembrolizumab

It is not known whether pembrolizumab is excreted in human milk. Therefore, it is recommended that women discontinue nursing during treatment with and for 4 months after the final dose of pembrolizumab

Adverse Events (N = 41)

Grade (%)*	Grade 1/2	Grade 3/4
Any event	56	41
Pain	34	0
Fatigue	32	0
Allergic rhinitis	29	0
Diarrhea	20	5
Rash or pruritus	24	0
Abdominal pain	24	0
Lymphopenia	0	20
Constipation	20	0
Anemia	2	17
Headache	17	0
Arthralgia	17	0
Myalgia	15	0
Dyspnea	15	0
Pancreatitis (asymptomatic)	15	0
Cold intolerance	15	0
Fever	12	0
Nausea	12	0
Dry mouth	12	0
Dry skin	12	0
Hypoalbuminemia	0	10
Thyroiditis, hypothyroidism, or hypophysitis	10	0
Sinus tachycardia	10	0
Anorexia	10	0
Dizziness	10	0
Cough	10	0
Edema	10	0
Hyponatremia	0	7
Bowel obstruction	0	7
Elevated ALT	2	5
Insomnia	7	0
Upper respiratory infection	7	0

*According to the National Cancer Institute Common Terminology Criteria for Adverse Events, version 4.0
Note: Toxicities are included in the table if all-grade events occurred in >5% of patients

RECTAL CANCER • ADJUVANT • CHEMORADIOTHERAPY

COLORECTAL CANCER REGIMEN: FLUOROURACIL + RADIATION

O'Connell MJ et al. N Engl J Med 1994;331:502–507

Chemotherapy Before or After Radiation
Fluorouracil + calcium leucovorin (Roswell Park, Mayo Clinic, or infusional fluorouracil) or FOLFOX
Note: Systemic chemotherapy is usually administered 4 weeks before or after surgery or chemoradiotherapy

Radiation + Chemotherapy

Fluorouracil 225 mg/m^2 per day; administer by continuous intravenous infusion over 24 hours in 50–1000 mL 0.9% sodium chloride injection or 5% dextrose injection, daily throughout radiation therapy (total dosage/week = 1575 mg/m^2)

Radiation therapy 180 cGy per fraction for 25 fractions (total dose = 4500 cGy), directed at the initial pelvic field, followed by a minimum boost of 540 cGy, to the entire tumor bed, the immediately adjacent lymph nodes, and 2 cm of adjacent tissues (the perineum was excluded after it had received 4500 cGy in patients with abdominoperineal resection). A second boost of 360 cGy was allowed to a smaller field in patients with good to excellent displacement of the small bowel out of the field

Supportive Care
Antiemetic prophylaxis
Emetogenic potential is **LOW**
See Chapter 42 for antiemetic recommendations

Hematopoietic growth factor (G-CSF) prophylaxis
Primary prophylaxis is **NOT** indicated
See Chapter 43 for more information

Antimicrobial prophylaxis
Risk of fever and neutropenia is **LOW**
  Antimicrobial primary prophylaxis to be considered:
  • Antibacterial—not indicated
  • Antifungal—not indicated
  • Antiviral—not indicated unless patient previously had an episode of HSV

Oral care
Standard prophylaxis and treatment for mucositis/stomatitis

Hand-foot reaction (palmar-plantar erythrodysesthesia, PPE)
For patients who develop a hand-foot reaction, use topical emollients (eg, Aquaphor®), topical or orally administered steroids, antihistamine agents (H$_1$-receptor antagonists), or pyridoxine
  • Pyridoxine may provide relief for discomfort/pain associated with PPE although the mechanism through which this occurs remains unclear
  • The suggested pyridoxine starting dose is 50 mg/day, which may be increased to a maximum of 200 mg/day

Patient Population Studied

A study of patients with surgically resected stage II or III rectal cancer with the inferior edge of tumor at or below the level of sacral promontory or within 12 cm of the anal verge

Efficacy (N = 328)

Bolus fluorouracil for 2 cycles ± semustine before and after RT with fluorouracil by continuous infusion during radiation

4-year relapse-free survival	63%
4-year overall survival	70%

O'Connell MJ et al. N Engl J Med 1994;331:502–507

Treatment Modifications

Adverse Event	Dose Modification
G ≥3 gastrointestinal toxicity	Interrupt radiation treatments. Resume when the toxicities decrease to G ≤2
G ≥3 hematologic toxicity	
G ≥3 gastrointestinal toxicity	Interrupt fluorouracil infusion. Resume when the toxicities decrease to G ≤2
G ≥3 hematologic toxicity	

Therapy Monitoring

1. *Before each cycle and weekly during RT:* H&P, CBC with differential, serum electrolytes, BUN, creatinine, and LFTs
2. *Every 2–3 months:* CT scans to assess response

RECTAL CANCER • ADJUVANT • CHEMORADIOTHERAPY
COLORECTAL CANCER: CHEMORADIOTHERAPY WITH CAPECITABINE

Hofheinz R-D et al. Lancet Oncol 2012;13:579–588

Adjuvant Therapy
Before radiation therapy:
Capecitabine 1250 mg/m^2 per dose; administer orally twice daily (approximately every 12 hours, within 30 minutes after a meal) for 14 consecutive days, on days 1–14 (28 doses), every 21 days (weeks 1 and 4), for 2 cycles (total dosage/cycle = 35,000 mg/m^2)

Throughout radiation therapy:
Capecitabine 825 mg/m^2 per dose; administer orally twice daily (approximately every 12 hours, within 30 minutes after a meal) continually throughout and coincident with the duration of radiation therapy (weeks 8 through 12 or 13; total dosage/week = 11,550 mg/m^2), *plus:*
Radiotherapy to a total dose of 50.4 Gy delivered in conventional daily 1.8-Gy fractions on 5 days per week, over 5–6 weeks

Notes:
• Radiotherapy and capecitabine are started on the same day and capecitabine is stopped on the last day of radiotherapy
• Three-dimensional conformal techniques with high-energy photons (6–25 MeV) and belly boards were used. The clinical target volume included the entire macroscopic tumor with a minimum margin of 5 cm, the mesorectum (plus 1.0- to 1.5-cm margin lateral to the pelvic brim), and the iliac and presacral lymph nodes up to the L5–S1 junction (or L4–L5 junction in the case of extensive lymph-node involvement)

After radiation therapy:
Capecitabine 1250 mg/m^2 per dose; administer orally twice daily (approximately every 12 hours, within 30 minutes after a meal) for 14 consecutive days, on days 1–14 (28 doses) every 21 days (weeks 15, 18, and 21), for 3 cycles (total dosage/cycle = 35,000 mg/m^2)

Notes:
• Phenytoin and coumarin-derivative anticoagulant doses may need to be reduced when either drug is administered concomitantly with capecitabine. In patients receiving concomitant capecitabine and oral coumarin-derivative anticoagulant therapy, the INR or prothrombin time should be monitored frequently in order to adjust the anticoagulant dose

Supportive Care
Antiemetic prophylaxis
Emetogenic potential with capecitabine alone is **MINIMAL–LOW**
Emetogenic potential during chemoradiotherapy is at least **LOW**
See Chapter 42 for antiemetic recommendations

Hematopoietic growth factor (G-CSF) prophylaxis
Primary prophylaxis is **NOT** *indicated*
See Chapter 43 for more information

Antimicrobial prophylaxis
Risk of fever and neutropenia is **LOW**
   Antimicrobial primary prophylaxis to be considered:
   • Antibacterial—not indicated
   • Antifungal—not indicated
   • Antiviral—not indicated, unless patient previously had an episode of HSV

Hand-foot reaction (palmar-plantar erythrodysesthesia, PPE)
For patients who develop a hand-foot reaction, use topical emollients (eg, Aquaphor®), topical or orally administered steroids, antihistamine agents (H$_1$-receptor antagonists), or pyridoxine
   • Pyridoxine may provide relief for discomfort/pain associated with PPE although the mechanism through which this occurs remains unclear
   • The suggested pyridoxine starting dose is 50 mg/day, which may be increased to a maximum of 200 mg/day

Diarrhea management
   Loperamide 4 mg; administer orally initially after the first loose or liquid stool, *then*
   Loperamide 2 mg; administer orally every 2 hours during waking hours, *plus*
   Loperamide 4 mg; administer orally every 4 hours during hours of sleep
   • Continue for at least 12 hours after diarrhea resolves
   • Recurrent diarrhea after a 12-hour diarrhea-free interval is treated as a new episode
   • Rehydrate orally with fluids and electrolytes during a diarrheal episode
   • If a patient develops blood or mucus in stool, dehydration, or hemodynamic instability, or if diarrhea persists >48 hours despite loperamide, stop loperamide and hospitalize the patient for IV hydration

(*continued*)

(continued)

Alternatively, a trial of **diphenoxylate hydrochloride** 2.5 mg with **atropine sulfate** 0.025 mg (eg, Lomotil®)
- Initial adult dose is 2 tablets 4 times daily until control has been achieved, after which the dose may be reduced to meet individual requirements. Control may often be maintained with as little as 2 tablets daily
- Clinical improvement of acute diarrhea is usually observed within 48 hours. If improvement of chronic diarrhea after treatment with a maximum daily dose of 8 tablets is not observed within 10 days, control is unlikely with further administration

Rothenberg ML et al. J Clin Oncol 2001;19:3801–3807
Wadler S et al. J Clin Oncol 1998;16:3169–3178

Oral care
Standard prophylaxis and treatment for mucositis/stomatitis

Treatment Modifications

Adverse Event	Dose Modification
G1 toxicity	Continue capecitabine and maintain dose level
First episode of G2 toxicity	Interrupt capecitabine treatment until adverse effects abate to G ≤1. Then, administer same dose in the next cycle
Second episode of G2 toxicity	Interrupt capecitabine treatment until adverse effects abate to G ≤1. Then, administer 75% dose in the next cycle
Third episode of G2 toxicity	Interrupt capecitabine treatment until adverse effects abate to G ≤1. Then, administer 50% dose in the next cycle
Fourth episode of G2 toxicity	Discontinue therapy
First episode of G3 toxicity	Interrupt capecitabine treatment until adverse effects abate to G ≤1. Then, administer 75% dose in the next cycle
Second episode of G3 toxicity	Interrupt capecitabine treatment until adverse effects abate to G ≤1. Then, administer 50% dose in the next cycle
Third episode of G3 toxicity	Discontinue therapy
First episode of G4 toxicity	Discontinue capecitabine treatment unless continued therapy deemed to be in the patient's best interest. In the latter case, interrupt treatment until adverse effects abate to G ≤1. Then, administer 50% dose in the next cycle

Patient Population Studied

A noninferiority, phase 3 trial comparing fluorouracil with capecitabine for perioperative treatment of patients with locally advanced rectal cancer. Patients had histologically confirmed adenocarcinoma of the rectum (defined as a distal tumor border <16 cm from the anal verge, measured by rigid rectoscopy), with no evidence of distant metastases (identified by abdominal ultrasound or CT scan and chest radiograph)

Adjuvant cohort: Had undergone R0 resection (ie, leaving no residual tumor) for pT3–4 N_{any} or $pT_{any} N_{positive}$ nonmetastatic rectal cancer. TME was mandatory for tumors in the lower two-thirds of the rectum, with PME being permitted for those in the upper third, provided a distal margin of at least 5 cm without coning was observed

Neoadjuvant cohort: Had to have a clinical cT3–4 N_{any} or $cT_{any} N_{positive}$ tumor staged by endoscopic ultrasound, provided the lower border of the tumor was 0–16 cm from the anal verge (measured by rigid rectoscopy) and the primary tumor was deemed R0 resectable by TME or PME on the basis of clinical assessment (pelvic CT or MRI were done at the discretion of the local investigators)

Patient Characteristics (N = 197 Treated with Capecitabine)

Age (Range)	65 Years (30–85 Years)
Sex: male-to-female ratio	129 (65%)/68 (35%)
WHO status	
0	120 (61%)
1	60 (30%)
2	3 (2%)
Missing data	14 (7%)
Tumor category*	
T1 or T2	29 (15%)
T3	150 (76%)
T4	15 (8%)
Missing data	3 (2%)
Nodal category*	
Node negative	78 (40%)
Node positive	112 (57%)
Missing data	7 (4%)

*Clinical or pathologic category

Treatment Monitoring

1. *Before starting:* History and physical examination, CEA determination, CBC with differential and serum chemistries
2. *During treatment:* CBC with differential and serum chemistries before each treatment cycle
3. *Tumor assessments:* Abdominal computed tomography, magnetic resonance imaging, or ultrasound, at baseline, every 6 months initially, and annually thereafter. CEA levels every 3 months initially and every 6 months thereafter

Efficacy*

	Capecitabine (n = 197)	Fluorouracil (n = 195)	P
Site of Recurrence			
Local	12 (6%)	14 (7%)	0.67[†]
Distant	37 (19%)	54 (28%)	0.04[†]
Deaths			
Total	38 (19%)	55 (28%)	0.04[†]
Disease-related	26 (13%)	37 (19%)	
Other causes	12 (6%)	15 (8%)	
Unknown	0	3 (2%)	

*Data are cumulative number of events (%)
[†]χ^2 test

Toxicity*[†]

	Capecitabine (n = 197)			Fluorouracil (n = 195)			
	G1/2	G3/4	Total	G1/2	G3/4	Total	P[‡]
Laboratory							
Lowered hemoglobin	58	0	62	49	2	52	0.29
Lowered leucocytes	47	3	50	50	16	68	0.04
Lowered platelets	23	0	23	29	1	32	0.18
Raised creatinine	5	0	5	2	0	2	0.26
Raised bilirubin	6	1	8	1	1	2	0.06
Gastrointestinal							
Nausea	33	2	36	30	0	32	0.63
Vomiting	11	1	14	8	1	9	0.30
Diarrhea	83	17	104	76	4	85	0.07
Mucositis	11	1	12	15	2	17	0.32
Stomatitis	8	0	8	11	0	12	0.35
Abdominal pain	19	1	23	11	0	14	0.13
Proctitis	26	1	31	9	1	10	<0.001
Other							
Fatigue	50	0	55	27	2	29	0.002
Anorexia	13	0	13	5	1	6	0.10
Alopecia	4	0	4	11	0	11	0.06
Hand-foot skin reaction	56	4	62	3	0	3	<0.001
Radiation dermatitis	22	2	29	32	1	35	0.39

*Data are number of patients or P value
[†]National Cancer Institute (USA) Common Toxicity Criteria, version 2.0. At: http://ctep.cancer.gov/protocolDevelopment/electronic_applications/ctc.htm [accessed December 7, 2013]
[‡]χ^2

14. Endometrial Cancer

Don S. Dizon, MD, FACP, FASCO

Epidemiology

Incidence:	61,880 (2019 U.S. estimate)
	27.5 per 100,000 women per year
Deaths:	12,160 (2019 U.S. estimate)
Median age at diagnosis:	63 years

Siegel RL et al. CA Cancer J Clin 2019;69:7–34
Surveillance, Epidemiology and End Results (SEER) Program, available from http://seer.cancer.gov [accessed December 12, 2019]

Pathology

Endometrioid	75–80%
Serous	~10%
Clear cell	<5%
Mucinous	1%
Squamous	<1%
Mixed	10%
Carcinosarcoma	<5%

Rare subtypes:
  Neuroendocrine carcinoma
  Dedifferentiated carcinoma
	<1%

WHO Classification of tumors of the female reproductive organs (Kurman, Carcangiu, Herrington, Young (Eds). World Health Organization, 2014

Diagnosis

Abnormal uterine bleeding	Endometrial curettage
	Endometrial biopsy
No abnormal uterine bleeding, but other symptoms present*	Endometrial curettage and biopsy
	Consider biopsy if distant disease suspected

*Patients may present with nonspecific symptoms, including abdominal bloating, pain, or distention as well as constitutional symptoms

Staging and treatment evaluation

All Patients	Physical exam, including pelvic examination
	Assessment of hereditary risk
	CBC with platelet count Chemistry panel
	Consider CA–125 measurement
High-risk histologies (serous or clear cell cancer), suspected advanced disease, or confirmed stages III/IV	CT chest/abdomen/ pelvis, MRI pelvis, or other imaging (eg, PET scan)

Staging

Staging outlined below is for uterine carcinomas and carcinosarcomas only.

FIGO Stage	TNM	Primary Tumor (T)
	TX	Primary tumor cannot be assessed
	T0	No evidence of primary tumor
I	T1	Tumor confined to corpus uteri (includes endocervical gland involvement)
IA	T1a	Tumor limited to endometrium or invades less than one-half of the myometrium
IB	T1b	Tumor invades one-half or more of the myometrium
II	T2	Tumor invades stromal connective tissue of the cervix but does not extend beyond uterus. Does NOT include endocervical glandular involvement
III	T3	Tumor involves serosa, adnexa, vagina, or parametrium
IIIA	T3a	Tumor involves serosa and/or adnexa (direct extension or metastasis)
IIIB	T3b	Vaginal involvement (direct extension or metastasis) or parametrial involvement
IVA	T4	Tumor invades bladder mucosa and/or bowel mucosa (bullous edema is not sufficient to classify a tumor as T4)

FIGO Stage	TNM Category	Regional Lymph Nodes (N)
	NX	Regional lymph nodes cannot be assessed
	N0	No regional lymph node metastasis
	N0 (i+)	Isolated tumor cells in regional lymph node(s) ≤0.2 mm
IIIC1	N1	Regional lymph node metastasis to pelvic lymph nodes
IIIC1	N1mi	Regional lymph node metastasis (>0.2 mm but ≤2.0 mm in diameter) to pelvic lymph nodes
IIIC1	N1a	Regional lymph node metastasis (>2.0 mm in diameter) to pelvic lymph nodes
IIIC2	N2	Regional lymph node metastasis to para-aortic lymph nodes, with or without positive pelvic lymph nodes
IIIC2	N2mi	Regional lymph node metastasis (>0.2 mm but ≤2.0 mm in diameter) to para-aortic lymph nodes, with or without positive pelvic nodes
IIIC2	N2a	Regional lymph node metastasis (>2.0 mm in diameter) to para-aortic lymph nodes, with or without positive pelvic nodes

Note: suffix (sn) is added to the N category when metastasis is identified only by sentinel lymph node biopsy

AJCC Stage Group	T	N	M
Stage I	T1	N0	M0
Stage IA	T1a	N0	M0
Stage IB	T1b	N0	M0
Stage II	T2	N0	M0
Stage III	T3	N0	M0
Stage IIIA	T3a	N0	M0
Stage IIIB	T3b	N0	M0
Stage IIIC1	T1-T3	N1/ N1mi/ N1a	M0
Stage IIIC2	T1-T3	N2/ N2mi/ N2a	M0
Stage IVA	T4	Any N	M0
Stage IVB	Any T	Any N	M1

Amin MB et al, editors. AJCC Cancer Staging Manual. 8th ed. New York: Springer; 2017

Histologic Grade (G)

GX	Grade cannot be assessed
G1	Well differentiated
G2	Moderately differentiated
G3	Poorly differentiated or undifferentiated

Overall 5-Year Survival: Relative to FIGO Disease Stage

FIGO Stage	% Survival at 5 years
Ia	88
Ib	75
II	69
IIIA	58
IIIB	50
IIIC	47
IVA	17
IVB	15

American Cancer Society. Survival Rates for Endometrial Cancer. https://www.cancer.org/cancer/endometrial-cancer/detection-diagnosis-staging/survival-rates.html [accessed March 28, 2018]

FIGO Stage	TNM Category	Distant Metastasis (M)
	M0	No distant metastasis (no pathologic M0; use clinical M to complete stage group)
IVB	MI	Distant metastasis (includes metastasis to inguinal lymph nodes, intraperitoneal disease, lung, liver, or bone). (It excludes metastasis to pelvic or para-aortic lymph nodes, vagina, uterine serosa, or adnexa)

AJCC 8th Edition Prognostic Stage Groups

Expert Opinion

The vast majority of patients with endometrial cancer will present with early-stage disease, and in these patients surgical resection is often curative. However, a not insignificant proportion of women who undergo surgical treatment for endometrial cancer will face a high risk of recurrence. Indeed, as noted above, women with stage II or higher disease have a substantially lower likelihood of surviving their disease at 5 years compared to women with uterine-confined disease. As a result, adjuvant treatment is often recommended. In addition, patients with serous or clear cell adenocarcinoma often face a higher risk of recurrence compared to those women with endometrioid cancers and are often recommended to proceed with adjuvant treatment.

The National Comprehensive Cancer Network (NCCN) has endorsed multiple options for this indication, including radiation therapy (RT) alone, combined-modality treatment (chemotherapy followed by RT in most cases), or even observation. For the most part, however, these patients are often referred for adjuvant chemotherapy, which is supported by a 2014 meta-analysis by Galaal et al. reporting that compared to RT alone, chemotherapy reduced the risk of recurrence by 20% (RR 0.79, 95% CI 0.68–0.93). Despite this, several phase 3 trials were reported in 2017, raising the question of what is the most appropriate treatment of this disease.

The Post-Operative Radiation Therapy in Endometrial Cancer 3 (PORTEC–3) trial enrolled more than 600 women with high-risk endometrial cancer and randomly assigned them to whole pelvic RT or to an investigational regimen consisting of cisplatin during RT followed by 4 cycles of carboplatin and paclitaxel. In this trial, high risk was defined as stage I grade 3 endometrioid tumors associated with deep myometrial invasion or lymphovascular invasion; serous or clear carcinoma (any stage), or stage II–III disease (all histologies). There was no statistically significant benefit to the multimodal investigational treatment when compared to pelvic RT alone in terms of either 5-year failure-free or overall survival. Multimodal treatment was associated with significant toxicities, which persisted out to 24 months, including a higher frequency of grade 3 or worse adverse events during treatment (60% vs. 12% with pelvic RT alone, P<0.0001) and neuropathy at 3 years (8% vs. 1%, respectively, P<0.0001). Despite the overall negative results, a preplanned subset analysis suggested that women with stage III disease did benefit from multimodal therapy in terms of 5-year failure-free survival (69% vs. 58%, respectively, HR 0.66, 95% CI 0.45–0.97). Although not significant, there was a trend toward improved 5-year OS as well (79% vs. 70%, respectively, HR 0.69, 95% CI 0.44–1.09). These data suggest that RT alone might be sufficient treatment in the adjuvant setting for women with endometrial cancer, with the addition of chemotherapy reserved for women with stage III disease.

In the Gynecologic Oncology Group (GOG) 258 trial, more than 700 women were randomly assigned to chemoradiation (cisplatin plus RT) followed by 4 cycles of carboplatin and paclitaxel versus adjuvant chemotherapy (carboplatin and paclitaxel for 6 cycles). Eligibility for this trial included stage III endometrial cancer (all histologies) or early-stage serous or clear cell carcinoma. Similar to PORTEC–3, there was no benefit in recurrence-free survival associated with multimodal treatment compared to adjuvant chemotherapy alone (HR 0.90, 95% CI 0.71–1.10). The intervention was associated with significant reductions in vaginal recurrence (3% vs. 7% with RT alone, HR 0.36, 95% CI 0.16–0.82) and pelvic/para-aortic recurrence rates (10% vs. 21%, HR 0.43, 95% CI 0.28–0.66), but there was no difference in the rate of distant recurrences (28% vs 21%, HR 1.36, 95% CI 1.0–1.86). These data suggest that chemotherapy should remain the standard treatment, particularly for women with advanced endometrial cancer (>90% of the study population).

For women with early-stage endometrial cancer at sufficiently increased risk of recurrence, GOG 249 evaluated combined modality treatment (vaginal brachytherapy plus 3 cycles of carboplatin and paclitaxel) versus pelvic RT. Approximately 75% of these patients had stage I disease and 15% had a serous carcinoma. There was no recurrence-free (HR 0.92, 95% CI 0.69–1.22) or overall survival (HR 1.04, 95% CI 0.71–1.52) advantage associated with combined modality treatment in this population. However, compared to pelvic RT, a substantially larger proportion of patients treated with RT plus chemotherapy experienced serious (grade 3 or greater) toxicity (64% vs. 11%, respectively). Therefore, for women with early-stage disease, these results suggest that RT alone is sufficient treatment.

For women who present with recurrent or metastatic disease, randomized trials support the role of chemotherapy. The Gynecologic Oncology Group (GOG) 177 trial established doxorubicin + cisplatin followed by paclitaxel (TAP) as the standard for systemic treatment of stage III–IV and recurrent endometrial cancer. However, TAP was associated with substantially more toxicity compared with the comparator arm, doxorubicin + cisplatin (AP). Grade 2/3 neurotoxicity occurred in 39% of patients who received TAP compared with 5% of those given AP, and 24% of patients who received TAP discontinued treatment because of toxicities compared with 9% of patients who received AP. As a result, TAP often was not utilized. GOG 209 was subsequently developed to test carboplatin and paclitaxel against TAP as an alternative combination. In this trial of 1300 women with advanced or recurrent endometrial cancer, patients were randomly assigned to receive either:

- TAP: Doxorubicin 45 mg/m^2 + cisplatin 50 mg/m^2 (day 1), followed by paclitaxel 160 mg/m^2 (day 2) every 21 days with hematopoietic growth factor support for a maximum of 7 cycles, *or*
- TC: Paclitaxel 175 mg/m^2 + carboplatin AUC = 6 mg/mL/min (day 1) every 21 days for a maximum of 7 cycles
  - Paclitaxel 135 mg/m^2 and carboplatin AUC = 5 mg/mL/min were given to women with a history of pelvic/spine irradiation

Fleming GF et al. J Clin Oncol 2004;22:2159–2166

Designed as a noninferiority trial, the study had two primary objectives:

1. Determine whether TC was therapeutically equivalent (noninferior) to TAP with respect to overall survival
2. Determine whether TC has a more favorable toxicity profile

A test for homogeneity suggested a consistent effect of treatment with TC across all prespecified subgroups. At interim analysis, the authors concluded: "TC is not inferior to TAP in terms of PFS and OS.… Overall, the toxicity profile favors TC. Thus, TC as prescribed in this study is an acceptable backbone for further trials in combination with 'targeted' therapies."

GOG 209 Interim Analysis

Miller D et al. Gynecol Oncol 2012;125:771

	TAP	TC	
Interim Efficacy Analysis			
PFS	14 months	14 months	HR = 1.03
OS	38 months	32 months	HR = 1.01
Safety/Tolerability			
Discontinued therapy for toxicity*	17.6%	11.9%	
Neutropenia and fever	7%	6%	P = 0.01
G1 sensory neuropathy	26%	19%	P<0.01
G3/4 thrombocytopenia	22.8%	12.8%	P<0.001
G3/4 neutropenia	52.1%	79.7%	P<0.001
G3/4 other hematologic	30.6%	21.2%	P<0.001
G3/4 nausea	8.9%	5.6%	P = 0.024
G3/4 vomiting	7.0%	3.5%	P = 0.006
G3/4 diarrhea	5.7%	2.0%	P<0.001
G3/4 stomatitis	1.3%	0.2%	P = 0.019
G3/4 creatinine elevation	1.9%	0.6%	P = 0.044

TAP, doxorubicin + cisplatin, followed by paclitaxel with growth factor support; TC, paclitaxel + carboplatin
*About two-thirds of patients in each group completed seven planned cycles, and another 10% completed six cycles. The most common reason for discontinuation was completion of protocol specified therapy

Beyond chemotherapy, endocrine treatment remains a viable option for women with advanced or recurrent disease. Agents such as medroxyprogesterone acetate, tamoxifen, and the aromatase inhibitors all have been used with clinical benefit for women with this disease, and activity has not been limited to women whose disease is hormone receptor–positive. As an example, a phase 2 trial that included 66 women with recurrent disease evaluated tamoxifen alternating with megestrol acetate at 3-week intervals. The overall response rate was 27% among 56 eligible patients, with responses noted in women with grade 1 (38%), grade 2 (24%), and grade 3 (22%) tumors. Finally, at the 2018 Society of Gynecologic Oncologists meeting, the results of GOG307 were presented. This randomized phase 2 trial enrolled 74 previously treated patients and randomly assigned them to letrozole (2.5 mg) plus everolimus (10 mg) (EL) or to alternating medroxyprogesterone acetate (200 mg) with tamoxifen (20 mg). While the response rate of both combinations was similar in the intent-to-treat analysis (24% vs. 22%, respectively), among patients who were chemotherapy naïve, EL was associated with an improvement in the response rate (53% vs. 43%).

For women with mismatch repair–deficient, metastatic endometrial cancer, the immune checkpoint inhibitor pembrolizumab can be used based on the tissue agnostic indication approved by the FDA. However, the combination of pembrolizumab and lenvatinib was shown to have anti-tumor activity in a phase 2 trial that enrolled women with metastatic endometrial cancer unselected for mismatch repair deficiency (Makker V et al. Lancet Oncol 2019; 20:711–718). The overall response rate to the combination was almost 40% at week 24. Despite this activity, treatment was shown to be notably toxic with 30% experiencing serious toxicity, including grade 3 diarrhea and grade 3 hypertension in 34% and 8%, respectively.

Summary:

1. For most women with endometrial cancer, surgery remains the mainstay of treatment. Most women deemed to be at high risk for relapse based on stage or histology should be offered adjuvant therapy. There is still considerable debate regarding standard treatment in this situation but for women with early-stage high-risk disease (eg, stage I serous carcinoma), adjuvant pelvic RT alone is a reasonable alternative to three cycles of chemotherapy (with vaginal brachytherapy). For women with more advanced disease, adjuvant chemotherapy consisting of carboplatin and paclitaxel is the mainstay of treatment

2. Patients unable to receive combination chemotherapy (eg, secondary to clinically relevant pre-existing comorbidity) may be treated with one of several previously noted cytotoxic agents with known biological activity in metastatic endometrial cancer

3. Endocrine therapy remains a viable option for women with recurrent, advanced, or metastatic endometrial cancer

de Boer SM et al. Lancet Oncol. 2018 Mar;19(3):295–309
Fiorica JV et al. Gynecol Oncol. 2004 Jan;92(1):10–4
Galaal K et al. Cochrane Database Syst Rev 2014;2014(5):CD010681
Matei D et al. N Engl J Med 2019;380:2317–2326
NCCN Clinical Practice Guidelines in Oncology: Uterine Neoplasms (version 1.2018), available from https://www.nccn.org/professionals/physician_gls/PDF/uterine.pdf [accessed 2018]
Randall M et al. J Clin Oncol 2019;37:1810–1818
Slomovitz BM et al. Gynecol Oncol 2018;149:2

ADJUVANT

ENDOMETRIAL CANCER REGIMEN: CISPLATIN WITH CONCURRENT PELVIC RADIATION THERAPY FOLLOWED BY CARBOPLATIN + PACLITAXEL

de Boer SM et al. Lancet Oncol 2018;19(3):295–309

The regimen is initiated within 4–6 weeks (but not more than 8 weeks) following surgery (total abdominal hysterectomy or laparoscopic hysterectomy plus bilateral salpingo-oophorectomy, with or without lymphadenectomy). The regimen consists of 27 once-daily fractions (Monday through Friday) of pelvic radiation therapy during weeks 1, 2, 3, 4, 5, and 6, and 2 doses of cisplatin given concurrently with radiation therapy during week 1 and week 4. Three weeks after completion of radiation therapy (and at least 28 days following the last cisplatin dose), adjuvant chemotherapy consisting of 4 cycles of carboplatin + paclitaxel is initiated.

Cisplatin with concurrent pelvic radiation therapy (initiate within 4–6 weeks [maximum of 8 weeks] following surgery)

Pelvic radiation therapy once daily at 1.8 Gy/fraction for 5 days/week for a total of 27 fractions during weeks 1, 2, 3, 4, 5, and 6 (total dosage = 48.6 Gy)

Notes:
- A reduced total dosage of 45 Gy was allowed for some sites participating in the study when it was consistent with standard practice, *thus, alternatively may consider*: **Pelvic radiation therapy** once daily at 1.8 Gy/fraction for 5 days/week for a total of 25 fractions during weeks 1, 2, 3, 4, and 5 (total dosage = 45 Gy)
- A brachytherapy boost was given to the vaginal vault in cases of cervical involvement (glandular, stromal, or both).

Hydration before cisplatin: ≥1000 mL 0.9% sodium chloride injection (0.9% NS); administer intravenously over a minimum of 2–4 hours

Cisplatin 50 mg/m² per dose; administer intravenously in 50–500 mL 0.9% NS over 60 minutes for 2 doses on day 1 (during week 1 of radiation therapy) and day 29 (during week 4 of radiation therapy) (total cisplatin dosage during radiation therapy = 100 mg/m²)

Hydration after cisplatin: ≥1000 mL 0.9% NS; administer intravenously over a minimum of 2–4 hours. Encourage patients to increase oral intake of nonalcoholic fluids. Monitor serum electrolytes and replace as needed (potassium, magnesium, sodium)

Supportive Care
Antiemetic prophylaxis
Emetogenic potential is **HIGH**. *Potential for delayed symptoms*
See Chapter 42 for antiemetic recommendations

Hematopoietic growth factor (CSF) prophylaxis
Primary prophylaxis is **NOT** *indicated*
See Chapter 43 for more information

Antimicrobial prophylaxis
Risk of fever and neutropenia is **LOW**
    Antimicrobial primary prophylaxis to be CONSIDERED:
- Antibacterial—not indicated
- Antifungal—not indicated
- Antiviral—not indicated unless patient previously had an episode of HSV

Adjuvant carboplatin and paclitaxel (initiate 3 weeks after completion of radiation therapy and at least 28 days following the last dose of cisplatin)

Premedication for paclitaxel:
    Dexamethasone 10 mg/dose; administer orally for 2 doses 12 hours and 6 hours before each paclitaxel dose, *or:*
    Dexamethasone 20 mg/dose; administer intravenously over 10–15 minutes, 30–60 minutes before each paclitaxel dose, *plus:*
    Diphenhydramine 50 mg; administer by intravenous injection 30 minutes before each paclitaxel dose, *plus:*
    Cimetidine 300 mg (or **ranitidine** 50 mg, **famotidine** 20 mg, or an equivalent histamine receptor (H₂ subtype)–antagonist); administer intravenously over 15–30 minutes, 30–60 minutes before each paclitaxel dose

Paclitaxel 175 mg/m²; administer intravenously in a volume of 0.9% NS or 5% dextrose injection (D5W) sufficient to produce a concentration within the range 0.3–1.2 mg/mL over 3 hours, before carboplatin on day 1, every 3 weeks for 4 cycles (total dosage/cycle = 175 mg/m²)

Carboplatin (calculated dose) AUC = 5 mg/mL × min; administer intravenously in 250 mL 0.9% NS or D5W over 60 minutes, after completing paclitaxel on day 1, every 3 weeks for 4 cycles (total dosage/cycle calculated to produce a target AUC = 6 mg/mL × min)

(continued)

(continued)

Treatment plan notes:

Carboplatin dose

Carboplatin dose is based on a formula described by Calvert et al. to achieve a target area under the plasma concentration versus time curve (AUC):

$$\text{Total Carboplatin Dose (mg)} = (\text{target AUC}) \times (\text{GFR} + 25)$$

In practice, creatinine clearance (CrCl) is used in place of glomerular filtration rate (GFR). CrCl can be estimated from the equation of Cockcroft and Gault, thus:

$$\text{For males}, \text{CrCl} = \frac{(140 - \text{age}[y]) \times (\text{body weight } [\text{kg}])}{72 \times (\text{serum creatinine } [\text{mg/dL}])}$$

$$\text{For females}, \text{CrCl} = \frac{(140 - \text{age}[y]) \times (\text{body weight } [\text{kg}])}{72 \times (\text{serum creatinine } [\text{mg/dL}])} \times 0.85$$

Calvert AH et al. J Clin Oncol 1989;7:1748–1756
Cockcroft DW, Gault MH. Nephron 1976;16:31–41
Jodrell DI et al. J Clin Oncol 1992;10:520–528
Sørensen BT et al. Cancer Chemother Pharmacol 1991;28:397–401

Note: On October 8, 2010, the U.S. Food and Drug Administration (FDA) identified a potential safety issue with carboplatin dosing based on recent changes in the measurement of serum creatinine. By the end of 2010, all clinical laboratories in the USA will use the standardized Isotope Dilution Mass Spectrometry (IDMS) method to measure serum creatinine, which could result in an overestimation of the GFR in some patients with normal renal function. A carboplatin dose calculated with an IDMS-measured serum creatinine result using the Calvert formula could exceed an expected exposure (AUC) and result in increased drug-related toxicity.

Provided actual GFR measurements are made to assess renal function, carboplatin can be safely dosed according to the Calvert formula described in product labeling

If GFR (or creatinine clearance) is estimated based on serum creatinine measurements by the IDMS method, the FDA recommended for patients with normal renal function capping an estimated GFR at 125 mL/min for any targeted AUC value. No greater estimated GFR values should be used.

U.S. FDA. Carboplatin dosing [online] updated 27 Nov. 2015. Available at: http://wayback.archive-it.org/7993/20170113081146/http://www.fda.gov/AboutFDA/CentersOffices/OfficeofMedicalProductsandTobacco/CDER/ucm228974.htm [accessed 4 Jan. 2018]

Supportive Care
Antiemetic prophylaxis
Emetogenic potential is **HIGH**. *Potential for delayed symptoms.*
See Chapter 42 for antiemetic recommendations

Hematopoietic growth factor (CSF) prophylaxis
Primary prophylaxis is **NOT** *indicated*
See Chapter 43 for more information

Antimicrobial prophylaxis
Risk of fever and neutropenia is **LOW**
  Antimicrobial primary prophylaxis to be CONSIDERED:
  • Antibacterial—not indicated
  • Antifungal—not indicated
  • Antiviral—not indicated unless patient previously had an episode of HSV

Patient Population Studied

This international, randomized, open-label, phase 3 trial (PORTEC–3) involved 660 patients with high-risk endometrial cancer. Eligible patients were aged ≥18 years and had WHO performance score 0–2. Patients were randomly assigned (1:1) to receive radiotherapy (48.6 Gy in 1.8-Gy fractions given on 5 days per week) or chemoradiotherapy (2 cycles of intravenous cisplatin 50 mg/m² given in the first and fourth week of radiotherapy, followed by 4 cycles of intravenous carboplatin AUC5 and paclitaxel 175 mg/m² at 21-day intervals). Treatment was recommended to start within 4–6 weeks, and no later than 8 weeks, after surgery.

Efficacy (N = 660)

	Chemoradiotherapy (N = 330)	Radiotherapy (N = 330)	
Overall survival at 5 years	81.8%	76.7%	Unadjusted HR 0.81 (95% CI 0.58–1.13); P = 0.213 HR adjusted for stratification factors HR 0.76 (95% CI 0.54–1.06); P = 0.109
Failure-free survival* at 5 years	75.5%	68.6%	Unadjusted HR 0.76 (95% CI 0.57–1.02); P = 0.067 HR adjusted for stratification factors HR 0.71 (95% CI 0.53–0.95); P = 0.022

*Failure-free survival was defined as no relapse or death related to endometrial cancer or treatment
Note: Median duration of follow-up was 60.2 months

Therapy Monitoring

1. Before each cycle of chemotherapy: History and physical examination. CBC with differential; renal and liver function tests; serum electrolytes
2. Monitor renal function prior to initiation and during therapy
3. CBC with differential every 2 weeks

Treatment Modifications

CISPLATIN DOSE MODIFICATIONS

Starting dose	Cisplatin 50 mg/m^2 IV
Dose level −1	Cisplatin 40 mg/m^2 IV

Adverse Event	Treatment Modification
ANC <1500/mm^3 or platelets <100,000/mm^3 on day of cisplatin treatment	Delay cisplatin administration by 1 week and until ANC recovery to ≥1500/mm^3 and platelet recovery to ≥100,000/mm^3 and then proceed at the full dose
G ≥2 peripheral neuropathy	Discontinue cisplatin
G ≥2 tinnitus or hearing loss	Discontinue cisplatin
Severe hypersensitivity reaction to cisplatin is noted	May occur within minutes of administration. Interrupt the infusion in patients with clinically significant infusion reactions. Manage with appropriate supportive therapy, including standard epinephrine, corticosteroids, and antihistamines. May consider desensitization for subsequent doses if benefits thought to outweigh risk. Note that the requirement for desensitization if further therapy is contemplated applies to both cisplatin and carboplatin
Serum creatinine ≥1.5 mg/dL (≥130 μmol/L)	Delay cisplatin administration by 1 week and until serum creatinine <1.5 mg/dL (<130 μmol/L), then decrease cisplatin dosage by 1 dose level
Other G ≥3 nonhematologic toxicities (except nausea, vomiting, elevated transaminases, and alopecia)	Delay cisplatin administration by 1 week and until toxicity resolves to baseline, then decrease cisplatin dose by 1 dose level
Cisplatin treatment delay >1 week	Discontinue cisplatin

PACLITAXEL AND CARBOPLATIN DOSE MODIFICATIONS

Paclitaxel Dose Levels		Carboplatin Dose Levels	
Paclitaxel starting dose	175 mg/m^2	Carboplatin starting dose	AUC = 5 mg/mL × min
Paclitaxel dose level −1	140 mg/m^2	Carboplatin dose level −1	AUC = 4 mg/mL × min
Paclitaxel dose level −2	120 mg/m^2	Carboplatin dose level −2	AUC = 3 mg/mL × min

(continued)

Treatment Modifications (*continued*)

Adverse Event	Treatment Modification
G ≥3 hematologic toxicities (ANC <1000/mm³; platelet count <50,000/mm³)	Interrupt therapy until value returns to baseline. Then decrease drug dosages by 1 dose level
Febrile neutropenia (ANC <1000/mm³ with temperature >38°C or >100.4°F)	Reduce paclitaxel and carboplatin by 1 dose level and consider adding filgrastim in subsequent cycles, if applicable
Febrile neutropenia (ANC <1000/mm³ with temperature >38°C or >100.4°F) despite dosage reduction of paclitaxel and carboplatin	Administer filgrastim in subsequent cycles. If already administering filgrastim, reduce paclitaxel and carboplatin dosages by 1 additional dose level
G2 motor or sensory neuropathies	Reduce paclitaxel dosage by 1 dose level without interrupting its planned treatment
G3 peripheral neuropathy	Reduce paclitaxel dosage by 2 dose levels or an additional level if already reduced by 1 level for G2 toxicity. Continuation of paclitaxel is at the discretion of the medically responsible care provider
G4 peripheral neuropathy	Discontinue paclitaxel
Moderate hypersensitivity during paclitaxel infusion	Patient may be re-treated. Base a decision to re-treat on reaction severity and the medically responsible care provider's judgment
Severe hypersensitivity during paclitaxel infusion	Discontinue paclitaxel
G ≥2 arthralgias/myalgias	Add dexamethasone as secondary prophylaxis
G3 arthralgia/myalgia despite dexamethasone prophylaxis	Reduce paclitaxel dosage by 1 dose level
AST and ALT <10× ULN and bilirubin between 1.26 and 2× ULN	Reduce starting paclitaxel dosage to 135 mg/m²
AST and ALT <10× ULN and bilirubin between 2.01 and 5× ULN	Reduce starting paclitaxel dosage to 90 mg/m²
AST and ALT ≥10× ULN or bilirubin >5× ULN	Discontinue paclitaxel
Hypersensitivity reaction to carboplatin, including anaphylaxis (risk is increased in patients previously exposed to platinum therapy)	May occur within minutes of administration. Interrupt the infusion in patients with clinically significant infusion reactions. Manage with appropriate supportive therapy, including standard epinephrine, corticosteroids, and antihistamines. May consider desensitization for subsequent doses if benefits thought to outweigh risk
Other G ≥3 nonhematologic toxicities (except nausea, vomiting, elevated transaminases, and alopecia)	Delay treatment until toxicity resolves to baseline, then decrease both drug dosages by 1 dose level from previous levels
Treatment delay >2 weeks	Decrease dosage by 1 dose level for each drug or consider discontinuing treatment

ANC, absolute neutrophil count; ADL, activity of daily living; AST, aspartate aminotransferase; ALT, alanine aminotransferase; ULN, upper limit of normal

Adverse Events (N = 660)

Grade (%)*	Chemoradiotherapy (N = 330)		Radiotherapy (N = 330)	
	Grade 2	Grade 3–4	Grade 2	Grade 3–4
Any hematologic	30	45	6	5
Any gastrointestinal	44	14	24	5
Alopecia	57	—	<1	—
Leukocytes	30	23	<1	<1
Lymphocytes	15	33	5	5
Diarrhea	32	11	21	4
Any pain	31	9	7	1
Hemoglobin	32	8	0	0
Neutrophils	19	20	<1	<1
Any neuropathy	25	7	<1	0
Sensory neuropathy	24	7	0	0
Nausea	21	3	7	<1
Fatigue	21	3	2	0
Joint pain	16	3	<1	0
Muscle pain	16	3	<1	0
Platelets	7	5	0	0
Vomiting	9	2	3	0
Constipation	10	<1	2	0
Infection without neutropenia	6	4	<1	<1
Anorexia	9	<1	3	1
Allergy	7	2	<1	0
Hypertension	6	2	4	<1
Genitourinary: frequency or urgency	7	<1	3	<1
Pelvic, back, or limb pain	3	3	1	0
Pulmonary: dyspnea	4	2	<1	0
Dermatitis	5	<1	2	<1
Metabolic or laboratory	5	<1	<1	0
Motor neuropathy	4	1	<1	0
Auditory or hearing	4	<1	<1	<1
Infection with neutropenia	<1	2	0	0
Febrile neutropenia	—	3	—	<1
Thrombosis or embolism	<1	1	0	0

*According to the National Cancer Institute Common Terminology Criteria for Adverse Events, version 3.0
Note: Adverse events that occurred during treatment in ≥5% of patients or were significantly different between the two patient groups are included in the table. No treatment-related deaths were reported

METASTATIC

ENDOMETRIAL CANCER REGIMEN: PACLITAXEL + CARBOPLATIN (TC)

Sorbe B et al. Int J Gynecol Cancer 2008;18:803–808

Premedication for paclitaxel:

Dexamethasone 20 mg per dose; administer orally or intravenously in 10–50 mL 0.9% sodium chloride injection (0.9% NS) or 5% dextrose injection (D5W) for 2 doses, 12–14 hours and 6–7 hours before starting paclitaxel

Diphenhydramine 50 mg, by intravenous injection 30 minutes before starting paclitaxel

Cimetidine 300 mg (or **ranitidine** 50 mg, **famotidine** 20 mg, or an equivalent histamine receptor (H2 subtype)–antagonist; administer intravenously over 15–30 minutes, 30 minutes before starting paclitaxel

Paclitaxel 175 mg/m^2; administer intravenously in a volume of 0.9% NS or D5W sufficient to produce a solution with concentration within the range 0.3–1.2 mg/mL over 3 hours on day 1 every 3 weeks (total dosage/cycle = 175 mg/m^2)

Carboplatin* AUC = 5 mg/mL × min; administer intravenously in 50–150 mL D5W over 60 minutes, on day 1, every 3 weeks (total dosage/cycle calculated to produce an AUC = 6 mg/mL × min) (see equation below)

*Carboplatin dose is based on Calvert et al.'s formula to achieve a target area under the plasma concentration versus time curve (AUC) [AUC units = mg/mL × min]

$$\text{Total Carboplatin dose (mg)} = (\text{target AUC}) \times (\text{GFR} + 25)$$

In practice, creatinine clearance (CrCl) is used in place of glomerular filtration rate (GFR). CrCl can be calculated from the equation of Cockcroft and Gault:

$$\text{For males, CrCl} = \frac{(140 - \text{age[years]}) \times (\text{body weight [kg]})}{72 \times (\text{serum creatinine [mg/dL]})}$$

$$\text{For females, CrCl} = \frac{(140 - \text{age[years]}) \times (\text{body weight [kg]})}{72 \times (\text{serum creatinine [mg/dL]})} \times 0.85$$

Note: On October 8, 2010, the U.S. Food and Drug Administration (FDA) identified a potential safety issue with carboplatin dosing based on recent changes in the measurement of serum creatinine. By the end of 2010, all clinical laboratories in the USA will use the standardized Isotope Dilution Mass Spectrometry (IDMS) method to measure serum creatinine, which could result in an overestimation of the GFR in some patients with normal renal function. A carboplatin dose calculated with an IDMS-measured serum creatinine result using the Calvert formula could exceed an expected exposure (AUC) and result in increased drug-related toxicity

Provided actual GFR measurements are made to assess renal function, carboplatin can be safely dosed according to the Calvert formula described in product labeling

If GFR (or creatinine clearance) is estimated based on serum creatinine measurements by the IDMS method, the FDA recommended for patients with normal renal function capping an estimated GFR at 125 mL/min for any targeted AUC value. No greater estimated GFR values should be used

U.S. FDA. Carboplatin dosing. [online] May 23, 2013. Available from: http://www.fda.gov/AboutFDA/CentersOffices/OfficeofMedicalProductsandTobacco/CDER/ucm228974.htm [accessed February 26, 2014]

Calvert AH et al. J Clin Oncol 1989;7:1748–1756
Cockcroft DW, Gault MH. Nephron 1976;16:31–41
Jodrell DI et al. J Clin Oncol 1992;10:520–528
Sørensen BT et al. Cancer Chemother Pharmacol 1991;28:397–401

(continued)

Patient Population Studied

A prospective, phase 2, multicenter study evaluating carboplatin and paclitaxel in the treatment of patients with primary advanced or recurrent endometrial carcinoma. Sixty-six patients were enrolled: 18 with primary advanced tumors and 48 with recurrences. All histologic types and tumor grades were allowed

Efficacy (N = 66)

Complete response	29%
Partial response	38%
Median progression-free survival	14 months
3-year progression-free survival	18.2%
5-year progression-free survival	12.5%
Median overall survival	26 months
3-year overall survival	33.3%
5-year overall survival	20.3%

Primary Advanced Cases (N = 18)

Complete response	50%
Partial response	33%
Median progression-free survival	14 months
Median survival	19 months

Recurrent Cases (N = 48)

Complete response	21%
Partial response	40%
Median progression-free survival	14 months
Median survival	27 months

Assessment: Clinical examination, gynecologic examination under anesthesia, transvaginal and transabdominal ultrasound, and computerized tomography were used in the evaluation of the tumor status. WHO response criteria were used to evaluate tumor

Note: Prior radiotherapy was not associated with response rate (P = 0.565), PFS rate (P = 0.420), or OS rate (P = 0.637) in this study

(continued)

Supportive Care

Antiemetic prophylaxis
*Emetogenic potential: **HIGH**. Potential for delayed symptoms*
See Chapter 42 for antiemetic recommendations

Hematopoietic growth factor (CSF) prophylaxis
Primary prophylaxis may be indicated
See Chapter 43 for more information

Antimicrobial prophylaxis
*Risk of fever and neutropenia is **LOW***
   Antimicrobial primary prophylaxis to be considered:
   • Antibacterial—not indicated
   • Antifungal—not indicated
   • Antiviral—not indicated unless patient previously had an episode of HSV

Toxicity (N = 66)

Adverse Events	% of Patients			
	Grade (%)			
	1	2	3	4
Hematologic				
Anemia	40.9	43.9	—	—
Neutropenia*	25.8	15.2	4.5	3.0
Thrombocytopenia	47	3.0	1.5	3.0
Nonhematologic				
Infection/fever	—	—	—	—
Renal	42.2	—	—	—
Cardiac	7.6	—	—	—
Neurologic†	37.9	31.8	13.6	—
Nausea/vomiting	39.4	16.7	4.5	1.5

*In 6 cases (9.1%), chemotherapy was stopped because of this toxicity
†In 13 cases (19.7%), therapy was prematurely stopped because of this toxicity
In 2 cases, allergic reactions prohibited completion of therapy
NCI CTC, National Cancer Institute (USA) Common Toxicity Criteria, version 2.0. At: http://ctep.cancer.gov/ protocolDevelopment/electronic_applications/ctc.htm [accessed December 7, 2013]

Therapy Monitoring

1. Physical examination, CBC, and serum creatinine before each chemotherapy cycle
2. Efficacy assessment every 2–3 cycles

Treatment Modifications

Adverse Event	Dose Modification
At start of a cycle ANC ≤1000/mm³ or platelet count ≤100,000/mm³	Delay start of cycle up to 2 weeks until ANC >1000/mm³ *and* platelet count >100,000/mm³
ANC ≤1000/mm³ or platelet count ≤100,000/mm³ for more than 2 weeks but less than 3 weeks after scheduled start of next cycle	Reduce paclitaxel and carboplatin dosages by 20% (140 mg/m² and AUC = 4, respectively)
At start of a cycle ANC ≤1000/mm³ or platelet count ≤100,000/mm³ despite dose reduction	Delay start of cycle up to 2 weeks until ANC >1000/mm³ *and* platelet count >100,000/mm³, then administer filgrastim or pegfilgrastim after completing chemotherapy without changing chemotherapy dosages
Serum creatinine >2 mg/dL (>177 µmol/L) or G ≥3 peripheral neuropathy	Delay start of cycle up to 2 weeks; if serum creatinine does not decrease to ≤2 mg/dL (≤177 µmol/L) or G peripheral neuropathy within that 2-week period, discontinue therapy

METASTATIC

ENDOMETRIAL CANCER REGIMEN: PEMBROLIZUMAB + LENVATINIB

Makker V et al. Ann Oncol 2019;30(suppl_5):v403–v434
Makker V et al. Lancet Oncol 2019;20:711–718
Supplementary appendix to: Makker V et al. Lancet Oncol 2019;20:711–718
KEYTRUDA (pembrolizumab) prescribing information. Whitehouse Station, NJ: Merck & Co.; revised 2019 September
Lenvima (lenvatinib) prescribing information. Woodcliff Lake, NJ: Eisai Inc; revised 2019 September

Pembrolizumab 200 mg; administer intravenously over 30 minutes in a volume of 0.9% sodium chloride injection or 5% dextrose injection sufficient to produce a pembrolizumab concentration within the range 1–10 mg/mL every 3 weeks for up to 24 months (total dose/3-week cycle = 200 mg)

Alternative pembrolizumab dose and schedule as per the U.S. FDA regimens approved on April 28, 2020:

Pembrolizumab 400 mg; administer intravenously over 30 minutes in a volume of 0.9% NS or D5W sufficient to produce a pembrolizumab concentration within the range 1–10 mg/mL every 6 weeks for up to 24 months (total dose/6-week cycle = 400 mg)
- Administer pembrolizumab with an administration set that contains a sterile, non-pyrogenic, low-protein-binding in-line or add-on filter with pore size within the range of 0.2–5 μm
- Pembrolizumab can cause severe or life-threatening infusion-related reactions, including hypersensitivity and anaphylaxis

Lenvatinib 20 mg per dose; administer orally once daily, without regard to food, continuously until disease progression (total dosage/week = 140 mg)
- Lenvatinib capsules should ideally be swallowed whole. Patients who have difficulty swallowing whole lenvatinib capsules may instead place the appropriate combination of whole capsules necessary to administer the required dose in 15 mL of water or apple juice in a glass container for at least 10 minutes. After 10 minutes, the contents of the glass container should be stirred for at least 3 minutes and then the resulting mixture should be swallowed orally. After drinking, rinse the glass container with an additional 15 mL of water or apple juice and swallow the liquid to ensure complete administration of the lenvatinib dose
- A missed dose of lenvatinib may be taken up to 12 hours before a subsequently scheduled dose
- Reduce the lenvatinib starting dose to 10 mg per dose, administered orally once daily for severe (Child-Pugh class C) hepatic impairment
- Reduce the lenvatinib starting dose to 10 mg per dose, administered orally once daily for severe (creatinine clearance <30 mL/minute) renal impairment
- Patients with pre-existing hypertension should have blood pressure adequately controlled (blood pressure ≤150/90 mm Hg) prior to initiation of treatment with lenvatinib

Supportive Care
Antiemetic prophylaxis
Emetogenic potential of lenvatinib is **MODERATE to HIGH**
Emetogenic potential of pembrolizumab is **MINIMAL**
See Chapter 42 for antiemetic recommendations

Hematopoietic growth factor (CSF) prophylaxis
Primary prophylaxis is **NOT** *indicated*
See Chapter 43 for more information

Antimicrobial prophylaxis
Risk of fever and neutropenia is **LOW**
   Antimicrobial primary prophylaxis to be considered:
- Antibacterial—not indicated
- Antifungal—not indicated
- Antiviral—not indicated unless patient previously had an episode of HSV

Patient Population Studied

This was a phase 1b/2, open-label, single-arm, multicenter study involving 108 adult patients with pathologically confirmed metastatic endometrial cancer. Patients could have received between 0–2 prior systemic regimens. Patients were required to have an Eastern Cooperative Oncology Group (ECOG) performance status of ≤2, measurable disease according to immune-related Response Evaluation Criteria In Solid Tumors (irRECIST), a life expectancy of ≥12 weeks, adequate blood pressure control, and adequate organ function. Patients who had received prior lenvatinib, anti–PD-1 drugs, or anti–PD-L-1 drugs were excluded.

Efficacy (N = 108)

Investigator Assessment per irRECIST	Pembrolizumab + Lenvatinib		
	Total (N = 108)	Not MSI-H or dMMR (n = 94)	MSI-H/dMMR
ORR_{WK24}	38.0% (95% CI, 28.8–47.8)	36.2% (95% CI, 26.5–46.7)	63.6% (95% CI, 30.8–89.1)
ORR	38.9% (95% CI, 29.7–48.7)	37.2% (95% CI, 27.5–47.8)	63.6% (95% CI, 30.8–89.1)
Complete response	7.4%	7.3%	9.1%
Partial response	31.5%	29.8%	54.5%
Median duration of response	21.2 months (95% CI, 7.6–NR)	NE months (95% CI, 7.4–NR)	21.2 months (95% CI, 7.3–NR)
Median progression-free survival	7.4 months (95% CI, 5.3–8.7)	7.4 months (95% CI, 5.0–7.6)	18.9 months (95% CI, 4.0–NR)
Median overall survival	16.7 months (95% CI, 15.0–NR)	16.4 (95% CI, 13.5–25.9)	NR (7.4–NR)
Time to response, mean (SD)	2.6 months (1.6)	2.5 months (1.5)	2.9 (1.8)

irRECIST, immune-related Response Evaluation Criteria In Solid Tumors; MSI-H, microsatellite instability-high; dMMR, mismatch repair deficient; ORR_{WK24}, objective response rate at week 24; ORR, objective response rate; NR, not reached; NE, not estimable

Efficacy data are from the final analysis with a data cutoff, January 10, 2019

Makker V et al. Ann Oncol 2019;30(suppl_5):v403–v434

Therapy Monitoring

1. Lenvatinib:
   a. Check ALT, AST, bilirubin, and alkaline phosphatase at baseline, every 2 weeks for 2 months, and then at least monthly thereafter
   b. Check BUN and serum creatinine at baseline and then periodically
   c. Check serum calcium at baseline and at least monthly
   d. Check TSK and free thyroxine (FT4) every 4–6 weeks as outlined below for pembrolizumab
   e. Monitor urine dipstick for protein at baseline and then periodically during treatment. If 2+, then perform a 24-hour urine collection for protein
   f. Monitor blood pressure at baseline, after 1 week, every 2 weeks for 2 months, and then at least monthly thereafter
   g. Check an electrocardiogram (ECG) at baseline and periodically in patients at increased risk for QT prolongation (eg, congenital long QT syndrome, heart failure, bradyarrhythmias, or in patients taking concomitant medications known to prolong the QT interval)
   h. Monitor periodically for signs and symptoms of cardiac dysfunction, arterial thrombosis, reversible posterior leukoencephalopathy syndrome (RPLS), fistula formation, gastrointestinal perforation, and wound-healing complications
2. Pembrolizumab:
   a. Initially at the time of each dose, and eventually every 6–12 weeks, perform a total body skin examination with attention to ALL mucous membranes as well as a complete review of systems
   b. Monitor patients for signs and symptoms of pneumonitis. Evaluate patients with suspected pneumonitis with chest x-ray, CT, and pulse oximetry. For ≥2 toxicity, may include nasal swab, sputum culture and sensitivity, blood culture and sensitivity, and urine culture and sensitivity
   c. Monitor patients for signs and symptoms of colitis. Encourage patients to report diarrhea immediately to any member of the health care team

(continued)

Toxicity (N = 53)

	% of Patients	
	Grade (%)	
Adverse Events	1–2	3
Any treatment-related adverse event	25	68
Serious treatment-related adverse event	4	25
Fatigue	49	6
Hypothyroidism	47	0
Diarrhea	43	8
Decreased appetite	40	0
Nausea	38	0
Stomatitis	34	0
Weight loss	28	0
Arthralgia	26	0
Palmar-plantar erythrodysesthesia syndrome	26	6
Hypertension	25	34
Vomiting	25	0
Headache	23	0

(continued)

Toxicity (N = 53) (continued)

Adverse Events	% of Patients Grade (%)	
	1–2	3
Dry mouth	17	0
Dry skin	13	0
Abdominal pain	11	0
Constipation	11	0
Increased aspartate aminotransferase	8	2
Anemia	6	2
Hyponatremia	4	4
Increased lipase	4	2
Increased alanine aminotransferase	4	2
Prolonged QT interval	4	2
Hypokalemia	2	2
Acute kidney injury	0	4
Pulmonary embolism	0	4
Syncope	0	4
Adrenal insufficiency	0	2
Cardiac failure	0	2
Colitis	0	2
Dysarthria	0	2
Hypertensive encephalopathy	0	2
Ischemic colitis	0	2
Neutropenia	0	2
Pancreatitis	0	2
Retinal vein occlusion	0	2
Small intestinal obstruction	0	2
Upper abdominal pain	0	2

Adverse events included in the table are grade 1–2 treatment-related adverse events with an incidence of ≥10% and all grade 3. There were no grade 4 treatment-related adverse events. There was 1 grade 5 treatment-related adverse event (intracranial hemorrhage). Grading is per the National Cancer Institute Common Terminology Criteria for Adverse Events (version 4.03). Data cutoff for adverse events was November 1, 2017
Makker V et al. Lancet Oncol 2019;20:711–718

Therapy Monitoring (continued)

d. Draw AST, ALT, and bilirubin prior to each infusion and/or weekly if there are grade 1 liver function test elevations. Note, no treatment is recommended for G1 LFT abnormalities. For ≥2 toxicity, work up for other causes of elevated LFTs including viral hepatitis

e. Use basic metabolic panel (Na, K, CO2, glucose) and patient history as screening tools for hypophysitis including hypopituitarism and adrenal insufficiency. If in doubt, evaluate AM adrenocorticotropic hormone (ACTH) and cortisol levels. Consider ACTH stimulation test for indeterminate results

f. Assess thyroid function at the start of treatment, periodically during treatment, and as indicated based on clinical evaluation, and for clinical signs and symptoms of thyroid disorders. Test for TSH and free thyroxine (FT4) every 4–6 weeks as part of routine clinical monitoring of therapy or for case detection in symptomatic patients

g. Measure glucose at baseline and with each treatment during the first 12 weeks and every 6 weeks thereafter

h. Obtain a serum creatinine prior to every dose. If creatinine is found to be newly elevated, consider holding therapy while other potential causes are evaluated. Note, routine urinalysis is not necessary other than to rule out urinary tract infections, etc

i. Obtain a complete rheumatologic history and perform an examination of all peripheral joints for tenderness, swelling, and range of motion. Examine the spine. Consider plain x-ray/imaging to exclude metastases and evaluate joint damage (erosions), if appropriate

j. In patients at high risk for infections and in appropriately selected patients based on an infectious disease evaluation, draw screening laboratories (HIV, hepatitis A and B, and blood QuantiFERON for TB) to prepare patients to start infliximab

Treatment Modifications

RECOMMENDED DOSE MODIFICATIONS FOR LENVATINIB

Starting dose	20 mg by mouth once daily
Dose Level −1	14 mg by mouth once daily
Dose Level −2	10 mg by mouth once daily
Dose Level −3	Discontinue lenvatinib

Lenvatinib Dose Modification—Cardiovascular Toxicity

Adverse Event	Treatment Modification
Either of the following: • G2 hypertension (SBP 140–159 mm Hg or DBP 90–99 mm Hg) • G3 hypertension (SBP ≥160 mm Hg or DBP ≥100 mm Hg) on suboptimal antihypertensive therapy	Continue lenvatinib at the same dose and optimize antihypertensive therapy. Monitor blood pressure frequently
G3 hypertension (SBP ≥160 mm Hg or DBP ≥100 mm Hg) persistent despite optimal antihypertensive therapy	Withhold lenvatinib until hypertension controlled to G ≤2, then resume lenvatinib at one lower dose level. Monitor blood pressure frequently
G4 hypertension (life-threatening consequences [eg, malignant hypertension, transient or permanent neurologic deficit, hypertensive crisis]; urgent intervention indicated)	Permanently discontinue lenvatinib
G3 cardiac dysfunction	Withhold lenvatinib until cardiac dysfunction improves to G ≤1 or baseline, then resume lenvatinib at one lower dose level or discontinue lenvatinib depending upon the severity and persistence of cardiac dysfunction
G4 cardiac dysfunction	Permanently discontinue lenvatinib
QTc prolongation (>500 ms, or >60 ms increase from baseline)	Withhold lenvatinib until QTc improves to ≤480 ms or baseline, then resume at one lower dose level. Correct hypomagnesemia and/or hypokalemia if applicable
Arterial thromboembolic event	Permanently discontinue lenvatinib

Lenvatinib Dose Modification—Gastrointestinal Toxicity

Gastrointestinal perforation	Permanently discontinue lenvatinib
G3/4 fistula formation	Permanently discontinue lenvatinib
Either of the following: • G1 diarrhea • G2 diarrhea lasting ≤2 weeks	Continue current lenvatinib dose and optimize antidiarrheal medications
Any of the following: • G2 diarrhea lasting >2 weeks • G3 diarrhea • G4 diarrhea developing in a patient not receiving an optimal antidiarrheal regimen	Withhold lenvatinib until diarrhea resolves to ≤G1 or baseline, then resume lenvatinib at 1 lower dose level. Antidiarrheal treatment for symptoms may continue indefinitely as a preventive measure
Recurrent or persistent G4 diarrhea in a patient receiving an optimal antidiarrheal regimen	Permanently discontinue lenvatinib

Lenvatinib Dose Modification—Hepatic Toxicity and Hepatic Impairment

G3/4 hepatotoxicity (ALT/AST >5× ULN, bilirubin >3× ULN)	Withhold lenvatinib until hepatotoxicity improves to G ≤1, then resume lenvatinib at one lower dose level or discontinue lenvatinib depending upon the severity and persistence of hepatotoxicity
Hepatic failure	Permanently discontinue lenvatinib
Severe hepatic impairment (Child-Pugh class C)	Reduce initial lenvatinib dose to 10 mg orally once daily

(continued)

Treatment Modifications (continued)

Lenvatinib Dose Modification—Renal Toxicity and Renal Impairment

G3/4 AKI (SCr >3× baseline or >4 mg/dL; hospitalization indicated; life-threatening consequences; dialysis indicated)	Initiate prompt evaluation and correction of dehydration if applicable. Withhold lenvatinib until toxicity improves to G ≤1 or baseline, then resume at one lower dose level or discontinue lenvatinib depending upon the severity and persistence of renal impairment
Severe renal impairment (CrCl <30 mL/min*)	Reduce initial lenvatinib dose to 10 mg orally once daily
Urine dipstick proteinuria ≥2+	Continue lenvatinib at current dose and obtain a 24-hour urine protein
Proteinuria ≥2 grams in 24 hours	Withhold lenvatinib until <2 grams of proteinuria per 24 hours, then resume lenvatinib at one lower dose level
Nephrotic syndrome	Permanently discontinue lenvatinib

Lenvatinib Dose Modification—Other Toxicities

RPLS	Withhold lenvatinib until fully resolved, then resume at a reduced dose or discontinue depending on severity and persistence of neurologic symptoms
Planned elective surgery	Withhold lenvatinib for at least 6 days prior to scheduled surgery. Resume lenvatinib after surgery based on clinical assessment of adequate wound healing
Patient with wound healing complications	Permanently discontinue lenvatinib
Other toxicities (eg, hand-foot skin reaction, rash, nausea/vomiting, stomatitis, hemorrhage) • Other persistent/intolerable G2 toxicities • Other G3 toxicities	Withhold lenvatinib until toxicity improves to G ≤1 or baseline, then resume lenvatinib at one lower dose level
G4 laboratory abnormality	Withhold lenvatinib until toxicity improves to G ≤1 or baseline, then resume lenvatinib at one lower dose level
Other G4 toxicity	Permanently discontinue lenvatinib

*CrCl calculated using the Cockcroft-Gault equation using actual body weight
SBP, systolic blood pressure; DBP, diastolic blood pressure; ALT, alanine aminotransferase; AST, aspartate aminotransferase; AKI, acute kidney injury; SCr, serum creatinine; CrCl, creatinine clearance; RPLS, reversible posterior leukoencephalopathy syndrome
Lenvima (lenvatinib) prescribing information. Woodcliff Lake, NJ: Eisai Inc; revised 2019 September

RECOMMENDED DOSE MODIFICATIONS FOR PEMBROLIZUMAB

Adverse Event	Grade/Severity	Treatment Modification
Infusion reaction	Clinically significant but not severe infusion reaction	Interrupt the infusion in patients with clinically significant infusion reactions and consider resuming at a slower rate following resolution. If decision is made to restart, begin at 50% of the rate prior to the reaction and increase in 50% increments every 30 minutes if well tolerated. Infusions may be restarted at the full rate during the next cycle
	G3/4 (severe infusion reaction—pyrexia, chills, flushing, hypotension, dyspnea, wheezing, back pain, abdominal pain, and urticaria). Not rapidly responsive to brief interruption of infusion	Stop infusion and administer appropriate medical therapy (eg, epinephrine, corticosteroids, intravenous antihistamines, bronchodilators, and/or oxygen). Discontinue pembrolizumab

(continued)

Treatment Modifications (*continued*)

RECOMMENDED DOSE MODIFICATIONS FOR PEMBROLIZUMAB

Adverse Event	Grade/Severity	Treatment Modification
Colitis	G1	Loperamide 4 mg as starting dose then 2 mg before each meal and after each loose stool until without diarrhea for 12 hours, with maximum of 16 mg loperamide per day. If G1 diarrhea or colitis persists >14 days, then add prednisolone 0.5–1 mg/kg (non-enteric-coated) or consider oral budesonide 9 mg daily if no bloody diarrhea
	G2/3 diarrhea or colitis	Withhold pembrolizumab. Loperamide 4 mg as starting dose then 2 mg before each meal and after each loose stool until without diarrhea for 12 hours, with maximum of 16 mg loperamide per day. Administer oral prednisone/prednisolone at a dose of 0.5–2 mg/kg/day or its equivalent. When symptoms improve to G1, begin a slow corticosteroid taper over at least 4 weeks. Resume pembrolizumab upon symptom control, or when prednisone/prednisolone daily dose <10 mg
	G4 diarrhea or colitis	Permanently discontinue pembrolizumab. Loperamide 4 mg as starting dose then 2 mg before each meal and after each loose stool until without diarrhea for 12 hours, with maximum of 16 mg loperamide per day. Administer 1–2 mg/kg IV (methyl)prednisolone and convert to 0.5–2 mg/kg prednisone/prednisolone orally each day or its equivalent only after a response. Taper over at least 4 weeks when symptoms improve. If does not improve over 72 hours or worsens, perform flexible sigmoidoscopy/colonoscopy to document colitis then begin infliximab 5 mg/kg (if no perforation/sepsis/TB/hepatitis/NYHA III/IV CHF). If no response, add MMF 500–1000 mg twice daily. If worse on MMF, consider addition of tacrolimus or ATG
Pneumonitis	G2	Withhold pembrolizumab. Consider pneumocystis prophylaxis depending on the clinical context and coverage with empiric antibiotics. Administer oral prednisone/prednisolone at a dose of 1–2 mg/kg/day or its equivalent. When symptoms improve to G1, begin a slow corticosteroid taper over at least 4 weeks. If does not respond adequately after 48 hours, then administer 2–4 mg/kg IV (methyl)prednisolone and convert to 0.5–2 mg/kg prednisone/prednisolone orally each day or its equivalent only after a response, followed by a taper over at least 6 weeks when symptoms improve to G1, titrating to symptoms. Resume pembrolizumab upon symptom control, or when prednisone/prednisolone daily dose <10 mg
	G3/4	Permanently discontinue pembrolizumab. Consider pneumocystis prophylaxis depending on the clinical context; cover with empiric antibiotics. Administer 2–4 mg/kg IV (methyl)prednisolone and convert to 1–2 mg/kg prednisone/prednisolone orally each day or its equivalent only after a response, followed by a taper over at least 8 weeks when symptoms improve to G1, titrating to symptoms. If, when initially treated improvement does not occur within 48–72 hours, begin infliximab 5 mg/kg (if no perforation/sepsis/TB/hepatitis/NYHA III/IV CHF). If no response to infliximab, add MMF 500–1000 mg twice daily. Consider MMF especially if has concurrent hepatic toxicity
Hepatitis	G2 (AST or ALT >3–5× ULN or total bilirubin >1.5–3× ULN)	Withhold pembrolizumab. Administer oral prednisone/prednisolone at a dose of 1 to 2 mg/kg/day or its equivalent. When symptoms improve to G1, begin a slow corticosteroid taper over at least 4 weeks. Resume pembrolizumab upon symptom control, or when prednisone/prednisolone daily dose <10 mg
	G3/4 (AST or ALT >5× ULN or total bilirubin >3× ULN)	Permanently discontinue pembrolizumab. Administer 1–2 mg/kg IV (methyl)prednisolone and convert to 0.5–2 mg/kg prednisone/prednisolone orally each day or its equivalent only after a response. Taper over at least 6 weeks when symptoms improve. If no response, add MMF 500–1000 mg twice daily. If worse on MMF, consider adding tacrolimus or ATG
Hypophysitis	G2/3 (Moderate symptoms, ie, headache but no visual disturbance or fatigue/mood alteration but hemodynamically stable, no electrolyte disturbance)	Administer analgesia as needed for headache. Withhold pembrolizumab. Administer oral prednisone/prednisolone at a dose of 0.5–2 mg/kg/day or its equivalent. When symptoms improve to G1, begin a slow corticosteroid taper over at least 4 weeks. If no improvement in 48 hours, administer 1–2 mg/kg IV (methyl)prednisolone and convert to 0.5–2 mg/kg prednisone/prednisolone orally each day or its equivalent only after a response. Taper over at least 4 weeks when symptoms improve to 5 mg prednisone/prednisolone or equivalent; do not stop steroids. Resume pembrolizumab upon symptom control, or when prednisone/prednisolone daily dose <10 mg
	G4 (Severe mass effect symptoms, ie, severe headache, any visual disturbance or severe hypoadrenalism, ie, hypotension, severe electrolyte disturbance)	Permanently discontinue pembrolizumab. Administer analgesia as needed for headache. Administer 1–2 mg/kg IV (methyl)prednisolone and convert to 0.5–2 mg/kg prednisone/prednisolone orally each day or its equivalent only after a response. Taper over at least 4 weeks when symptoms improve to 5 mg prednisone/prednisolone or equivalent; do not stop steroids

(*continued*)

Treatment Modifications (*continued*)

RECOMMENDED DOSE MODIFICATIONS FOR PEMBROLIZUMAB

Adverse Event	Grade/Severity	Treatment Modification
Adrenal insufficiency	G2	Withhold pembrolizumab. Administer oral prednisone/prednisolone at a dose of 0.5–2 mg/kg/day or its equivalent. When symptoms improve to G1, begin a slow corticosteroid taper over at least 4 weeks. Serially assess adrenal function and continue steroids at replacement doses (20–40 mg hydrocortisone daily ~2/3 dose in AM upon awakening and ~1/3 at 4 PM) until recovery of adrenal function is documented. Resume pembrolizumab upon symptom control, or when prednisone/prednisolone daily dose <10 mg
	G3/4	Permanently discontinue pembrolizumab. Administer oral prednisone/prednisolone at a dose of 0.5–2 mg/kg/day or its equivalent. When symptoms improve to G1, begin a slow corticosteroid taper over at least 4 weeks. Serially assess adrenal function and continue steroids at replacement doses (20–40 mg hydrocortisone daily ~2/3 dose in AM upon awakening and ~1/3 at 4 PM) until recovery of adrenal function is documented
Type 1 diabetes mellitus	G3 hyperglycemia	Withhold pembrolizumab. Admit to hospital to manage hyperglycemia. Role of corticosteroids in preventing complete loss of insulin-producing cells is unknown and not recommended. Resume pembrolizumab upon symptom control, or when prednisone/prednisolone daily dose <10 mg
	G4 hyperglycemia	Permanently discontinue pembrolizumab. Admit to hospital to manage hyperglycemia. Role of corticosteroids in preventing complete loss of insulin-producing cells is unknown and not recommended
Nephritis and renal dysfunction	G2/3 (serum creatinine 1.5–6× ULN)	Withhold pembrolizumab. Administer oral prednisone/prednisolone at a dose of 0.5–2 mg/kg/day or its equivalent. When symptoms improve to G1, begin a slow corticosteroid taper over at least 4 weeks. If does not respond adequately, then administer 0.5–1 mg/kg IV (methyl)prednisolone and convert to 0.5–2 mg/kg prednisone/prednisolone orally each day or its equivalent only after a response, followed by a taper over at least 4 weeks when symptoms improve to G1. Resume pembrolizumab upon symptom control, or when prednisone/prednisolone daily dose <10 mg
	G4 (serum creatinine >6× ULN)	Permanently discontinue pembrolizumab. Administer 0.5–1 mg/kg IV (methyl)prednisolone and convert to 0.5–2 mg/kg prednisone/prednisolone orally each day or its equivalent only after a response, followed by a taper over at least 4 weeks when symptoms improve to G1
Skin	G1/2	Continue pembrolizumab. Avoid skin irritants, avoid sun exposure, topical emollients recommended. Topical steroid (mild strength for G1, moderate/potent strength for G2) cream once or twice daily ± oral or topical antihistamines for itching
	G3 rash or suspected SJS or TEN	Withhold pembrolizumab. Avoid skin irritants, avoid sun exposure, topical emollients recommended. Administer oral or topical antihistamines for itching. Administer oral prednisone/prednisolone at a dose of 0.5–2 mg/kg or its equivalent daily for 3 days followed by a slow corticosteroid taper over at least 4 weeks when the rash improves to G1. If does not respond adequately, then administer 0.5–1 mg/kg IV (methyl)prednisolone and convert to 0.5–2 mg/kg prednisone/prednisolone orally each day or its equivalent only after a response, followed by a taper over at least 4 weeks when the rash improves to G1. Resume pembrolizumab upon symptom control, or when prednisone/prednisolone daily dose <10 mg
	G4 rash or confirmed SJS or TEN	Avoid skin irritants, avoid sun exposure, topical emollients recommended. Administer oral or topical antihistamines for itching. Administer 1–2 mg/kg IV (methyl)prednisolone and convert to oral steroids 0.5–2 mg/kg prednisone/prednisolone each day or its equivalent only after a response. Taper over at least 4 weeks when the rash improves to G1. Permanently discontinue pembrolizumab

(*continued*)

Treatment Modifications (continued)

RECOMMENDED DOSE MODIFICATIONS FOR PEMBROLIZUMAB

Adverse Event	Grade/Severity	Treatment Modification
Encephalitis	Confusion or altered behavior, headaches, alteration in Glasgow Coma Scale, motor or sensory deficits, speech abnormality, may or may not be febrile	Initially withhold pembrolizumab, but permanently discontinue pembrolizumab if there is no doubt as to diagnosis. Exclude bacterial and ideally viral infections prior to high-dose steroids. Administer oral prednisone/prednisolone at a dose of 0.5–2 mg/kg/day or its equivalent. When symptoms improve, begin a slow corticosteroid taper over at least 4–8 weeks. If symptoms are severe, administer 1–2 mg/kg IV (methyl)prednisolone and convert to 0.5–2 mg/kg prednisone/prednisolone orally each day or its equivalent only after a response. Consider concurrent empiric antiviral (IV acyclovir) and antibacterial therapy
Aseptic meningitis	Headache, photophobia, neck stiffness with fever or may be afebrile, vomiting; normal cognition/cerebral function (distinguishes from encephalitis)	
Other syndromes include neurosarcoidosis, posterior reversible leukoencephalopathy syndrome (PRES), Vogt-Koyanagi-Harada syndrome, demyelination, vasculitic encephalopathy, and generalized seizures		
Transverse myelitis	Acute or subacute neurologic signs/symptoms of motor/sensory/autonomic origin; most have sensory level; often bilateral symptoms	Initially withhold pembrolizumab, but permanently discontinue pembrolizumab if there is no doubt as to diagnosis. Administer 2 mg/kg IV (methyl)prednisolone or consider 1 g/day and convert to 0.5–2 mg/kg prednisone/prednisolone orally each day or its equivalent only after a response. When symptoms improve, begin a slow corticosteroid taper over at least 4–8 weeks. Plasmapheresis may be required if steroids do not bring about improvement
Myocarditis	G3	Permanently discontinue pembrolizumab. Administer 2 mg/kg IV (methyl)prednisolone or consider 1 g/day and convert to 0.5–2 mg/kg prednisone/prednisolone orally each day or its equivalent only after a response. When symptoms improve, begin a slow corticosteroid taper over at least 4–8 weeks. If no response, add MMF 500–1000 mg twice daily. If worse on MMF, consider adding tacrolimus
Peripheral neurologic toxicity	Moderate: some interference with ADL, symptoms concerning to patient	Withhold pembrolizumab. Initial observation reasonable or initiate prednisone/prednisolone 0.5–1 mg/kg (if progressing, eg, from mild) and/or pregabalin or duloxetine for pain. When symptoms improve, begin a slow corticosteroid taper over at least 4 weeks. Resume pembrolizumab upon symptom control, or when prednisone/prednisolone daily dose <10 mg
	Severe: limits self-care and aids warranted, life threatening, eg, respiratory problems	Permanently discontinue pembrolizumab. Administer 1–2 mg/kg IV (methyl)prednisolone and convert to 0.5–2 mg/kg prednisone/prednisolone orally each day or its equivalent only after a response. Taper over at least 4–8 weeks when symptoms improve to G1
Guillain-Barré syndrome	Progressive symmetrical muscle weakness with absent or reduced tendon reflexes—involves extremities, facial, respiratory, and bulbar and oculomotor muscles; dysregulation of autonomic nerves	Permanently discontinue pembrolizumab. Use of steroids not recommended in idiopathic Guillain-Barré syndrome; however, a trial of (methyl)prednisolone 1–2 mg/kg is reasonable, converting to 0.5–2 mg/kg prednisone/prednisolone orally each day or its equivalent only after a response. If no improvement or worsening, plasmapheresis or IVIG indicated
Myasthenia gravis	Fluctuating muscle weakness (proximal limb, trunk, ocular, eg, ptosis/diplopia or bulbar) with fatigability, respiratory muscles may also be involved	Permanently discontinue pembrolizumab. Administer pyridostigmine at an initial dose of 30 mg three times daily. Administer oral prednisone/prednisolone at a dose of 0.5–2 mg/kg/day or its equivalent or 1–2 mg/kg IV (methyl)prednisolone depending on the severity of symptoms. If begin with IV, convert to 0.5–2 mg/kg prednisone/prednisolone orally each day or its equivalent only after a response. If no improvement or worsening, plasmapheresis or IVIG may be considered. Additional immunosuppressants used in myasthenia gravis include azathioprine, cyclosporine, and mycophenolate. Avoid certain medications, eg, ciprofloxacin, beta-blockers, that may precipitate cholinergic crisis
Other syndromes including motor and sensory peripheral neuropathy, multifocal radicular neuropathy/plexopathy, autonomic neuropathy, phrenic nerve palsy, cranial nerve palsies (eg, facial nerve, optic nerve, hypoglossal nerve)		Permanently discontinue pembrolizumab. Administer oral prednisone/prednisolone at a dose of 0.5–2 mg/kg/day or its equivalent or 1–2 mg/kg IV (methyl)prednisolone depending on the severity of symptoms. If begin with IV, convert to 0.5–2 mg/kg prednisone/prednisolone orally each day or its equivalent only after a response

(continued)

Treatment Modifications (*continued*)

RECOMMENDED DOSE MODIFICATIONS FOR PEMBROLIZUMAB

Adverse Event	Grade/Severity	Treatment Modification
Arthralgia	G1 (mild pain with inflammation, erythema, or joint swelling)	Continue pembrolizumab. Administer acetaminophen (paracetamol) and ibuprofen
	G2 (moderate pain with inflammation, erythema, or joint swelling that limits ADLs)	Withhold pembrolizumab. Administer higher doses of acetaminophen (paracetamol) and ibuprofen and use diclofenac or naproxen or etoricoxib. If inadequately controlled, consider intra-articular steroid injections for large joints or administer oral prednisone/prednisolone at a dose of 0.5–2 mg/kg/day or its equivalent. When symptoms improve to G1, begin a slow corticosteroid taper over at least 4 weeks. If does not respond adequately, then administer 0.5–1 mg/kg IV (methyl)prednisolone and convert to 0.5–2 mg/kg prednisone/prednisolone orally each day or its equivalent only after a response, followed by a taper over at least 4 weeks when symptoms improve to G1. Resume pembrolizumab upon symptom control, or when prednisone/prednisolone daily dose <10 mg
	G3 (severe pain; irreversible joint damage; disabling; limits self-care ADL)	Withhold pembrolizumab. Administer 0.5–1 mg/kg IV (methyl)prednisolone and convert to 0.5–2 mg/kg prednisone/prednisolone orally each day or its equivalent only after a response, followed by a taper over at least 4 weeks when symptoms improve to G1. In severe cases, infliximab or another anti–TNF-alpha drug may be required for improvement of arthritis. Resume pembrolizumab upon symptom control, or when prednisone/prednisolone daily dose <10 mg
Other	First occurrence of other G3	Withhold pembrolizumab. Administer oral prednisone/prednisolone at a dose of 0.5–2 mg/kg/day or its equivalent. When symptoms improve to G1, begin a slow corticosteroid taper over at least 4 weeks. Resume pembrolizumab upon symptom control, or when prednisone/prednisolone daily dose <10 mg
	Recurrence of same G3	Permanently discontinue pembrolizumab. Administer 1–2 mg/kg IV (methyl)prednisolone and convert to 0.5–2 mg/kg prednisone/prednisolone orally each day or its equivalent only after a response. Taper over at least 4–8 weeks when symptoms improve to G1
	Life-threatening or G4	
	Requirement for ≥10 mg/day prednisone or equivalent for >12 weeks	Permanently discontinue pembrolizumab
	Persistent G2/3 adverse reactions lasting ≥12 weeks	

ADL, activities of daily living; ALT, alanine aminotransferase; AST, aspartate aminotransferase; ATG, anti-thymocyte globulin; SJS, Stevens-Johnson Syndrome; TEN, toxic epidermal necrolysis; ULN, upper limit of normal

Notes on general supportive care:
- Steroid taper in most cases will proceed over a minimum of 1 month but if symptoms improve rapidly, a 2-week taper can be considered. If steroids are administered for more than 4 weeks, consider PCP prophylaxis (cotrimoxazole 480 mg twice daily M/W/F or inhaled pentamidine if has cotrimoxazole allergy), regular random blood glucose, VitD level, and starting calcium/VitD supplementation per guidelines

15. Esophageal Cancer

Sunnie Kim, MD and John Marshall, MD

Epidemiology

Incidence:	16,940 (male: 13,360; female: 3580. Estimated new cases for 2017 in the United States)
	8.1 per 100,000 male, 1.8 per 100,000 female
Deaths:	Estimated 15,690 in 2014 (male: 12,720; female: 2970)
Median age at diagnosis*:	67 years
Male to female ratio[†]:	3:1 for squamous cell carcinoma and 7.5:1 for adenocarcinoma
Stage at presentation:	Locoregional disease: 52%
	Distant metastasis: 48%

*Zhang Y. World J Gastroenterol 2013;19:5598–5606
[†]Mathieu LN. Dis Esophagus 2014;27:757–763
Siegel R et al. CA Cancer J Clin 2017;67:7–30
Surveillance, Epidemiology and End Results (SEER) Program, available from http://seer.cancer.gov [accessed 2017]

Pathology

Upper to midthoracic esophagus:	Predominantly squamous cell carcinoma
Distal esophagus and GE junction:	Predominantly adenocarcinoma
Other rare pathology:	Basaloid-squamous carcinoma (1.9%)* or small cell carcinomas

Especially in white men, the incidence of adenocarcinoma of the gastroesophageal junction (GEJ) has risen significantly in the United States, whereas that of squamous cell carcinoma has slightly decreased. In the 1960s, squamous cell cancer accounted for 90% or more of esophageal cancer. Data from 1996 suggested that they occur with equal frequency, and by 2004 the trend had changed further. This is thought to be related to increase in body mass index and Barrett esophagus.

*Abe K et al. Am J Surg Pathol 1996;20:453–461
Brown LM et al. J Natl Cancer Inst 2008;100:1184–1187
Daly JM et al. Cancer 1996;78:1820–1828

Work-up

1. H&P, esophagogastroduodenoscopy with biopsy, CBC, serum electrolytes, BUN, creatinine, LFTs and mineral panel, CT scan of chest and abdomen ± pelvis (if clinically indicated)

2. In patients with locoregional cancer with no evidence of M1 disease, a PET scan and endoscopic ultrasound (EUS) should be performed

3. For locoregional cancer at or above the carina, a bronchoscopy must be considered

4. In selected patients with local-regional GE junction cancer, a laparoscopic staging of the peritoneal cavity may be warranted

5. In addition, for patients with locoregional cancer (stages I–III), a multidisciplinary evaluation is required, including nutritional assessment. The need for supplementation depends on the severity of dysphagia and the overall nutritional status (>10% weight loss). Enteral nutritional support is preferred (PEG is avoided if surgery is a consideration)

6. If metastatic disease is documented or suspected, MSI or MMR deficiency should be tested. For metastatic adenocarcinoma, PD-L1 and HER2 expression should be tested

NCCN. Guidelines for Patients: Esophageal and Esophagogastric Junction Cancers. Version 4.2017

Staging

Primary Tumor (T)

TX	Primary tumor cannot be assessed
T0	No evidence of primary tumor
Tis	High-grade dysplasia
T1	Tumor invades lamina propria, muscularis mucosae, or submucosa
T1a	Tumor invades lamina propria or muscularis mucosae
T1b	Tumor invades submucosa

(continued)

Staging Groupings for Esophageal Adenocarcinoma

Stage	T	N	M	G
0	Tis (HGD*)	0	0	1
IA	1	0	0	1–2
IB	1	0	0	3
	2	0	0	1–2
IIA	2	0	0	3
IIB	3	0	0	Any
	1–2	1	0	Any

(continued)

Staging (continued)

Primary Tumor (T) (continued)

T2	Tumor invades muscularis propria
T3	Tumor invades adventitia
T4a	Resectable cancer invades adjacent structures such as pleura, pericardium, diaphragm
T4b	Unresectable cancer invades adjacent structures such as aorta, vertebral body, trachea

Regional Lymph Nodes (N) (Any Periesophageal Lymph Node from Cervical Nodes to Celiac Nodes)

NX	Regional lymph nodes cannot be assessed
N0	No regional lymph node metastases
N1	1–2 positive regional lymph nodes
N2	3–6 positive regional lymph nodes
N3	≥7 positive regional lymph nodes

Metastases

M0	No distant metastases
M1	Distant metastases

Grade

1	Well-differentiated
2	Moderately differentiated
3	Poorly differentiated
4	Undifferentiated

Cancer Location

Upper thoracic	20–25 cm from incisors
Middle thoracic	>25–30 cm from incisors
Lower thoracic	>30–40 cm from incisors
Esophagogastric junction	The Siewert classification described categories of esophageal cancer based on location. Type I: Located between 5 and 1 cm proximal to the anatomic Z-line Type II: Located between 1 cm proximal and 2 cm distal to the Z-line Type III: Located between 2 and 5 cm distal to Z-line Siewert type I tumors often arise from Barrett esophagus due to gastroesophageal reflux, while type III tumors have shared risk factors with more distal gastric adenocarcinomas

Staging Groupings for Esophageal Adenocarcinoma (continued)

Stage	T	N	M	G
IIIA	1–2	2	0	Any
	3	1	0	Any
	4a	0	0	Any
IIIB	3	2	0	Any
IIIC	4a	1–2	0	Any
	4b	Any	0	Any
	Any	3	0	Any
IV	Any	Any	1	Any

*High-grade dysplasia

Staging Groupings for Esophageal Squamous Cell Carcinoma

Stage	T	N	M	G	Location
0	is (HGD*)	0	0	1	Any
IA	1	0	0	1	Any
IB	1	0	0	2–3	Any
	2–3	0	0	1	Lower
IIA	2–3	0	0	1	Upper/middle
	2–3	0	0	2–3	Lower
IIB	2–3	0	0	2–3	Upper/middle
	1–2	1	0	Any	Any
IIIA	1–2	2	0	Any	Any
	3	1	0	Any	Any
	4a	0	0	Any	Any
IIIB	3	2	0	Any	Any
IIIC	4a	1–2	0	Any	Any
	4b	Any	0	Any	Any
	Any	3	0	Any	Any
IV	Any	Any	1	Any	Any

*High-grade dysplasia
Amin MB et al. editors. AJCC Cancer Staging Manual. 8th ed. New York: Springer; 2017

Five-Year Survival Adenocarcinoma

Stage 0	≈82
Stage IA	≈77
Stage IB	≈63
Stage IIA	≈50
Stage IIB	≈40
Stage IIIA	≈25
Stage IIIB	≈18
Stage IIIC	≈14

Rice TW et al. Ann Surg Oncol 2010;17:1721–1724

Five-Year Survival Squamous Cell Carcinoma

Stage 0	≈71
Stage IA	≈71
Stage IB	≈61
Stage IIA	≈53
Stage IIB	≈41
Stage IIIA	≈25
Stage IIIB	≈18
Stage IIIC	≈14

Rice TW et al. Ann Surg Oncol 2010;17:1721–1724

Expert Opinion

Management of localized/locally advanced disease:
A distinction must be made between the treatment of localized/locally advanced *esophageal squamous cell carcinoma* and *esophageal adenocarcinoma*

Squamous cell carcinoma:
- Treatment should be surgery or concurrent chemoradiotherapy followed by surgery
- The role of surgery in patients who have a complete endoscopic response to chemoradiotherapy is unclear

Adenocarcinoma:
- Treatment should be multimodality with surgery
  - Preoperative radiation with concurrent chemotherapy, followed by surgery (preferred for esophageal cancer)
  - Perioperative chemotherapy (FLOT4: Al-Batran SE et al. Ann Oncol 2017;28(suppl_5):v605–v649 and MAGIC: Cunningham D et al. N Engl J Med 2006;355:11–20). Studies evaluated both gastric and GEJ adenocarcinomas
  - Postoperative chemotherapy and radiation (INT 116: Macdonald JS et al. N Engl J Med 2001;345:725–730). Study evaluated both gastric and GEJ adenocarcinomas

Chemotherapy:
Squamous cell carcinoma:
- No single standard chemotherapy regimen
  - Active agents include fluoropyrimidines, platinums, taxanes, and irinotecan
  - Immunotherapy with checkpoint inhibitors targeting PD-1/PD-L1 is under investigation

Adenocarcinoma:
- Tend to be grouped with gastric and gastroesophageal adenocarcinomas
- Locally advanced disease
  - Preoperative chemoradiotherapy regimens: fluoropyrimidines, platinums, and taxanes are active agents
  - Perioperative chemotherapy regimens: 5-FU, oxaliplatin, and docetaxel combination regimen (FLOT) is the new standard of care over epirubicin, cisplatin, and 5-FU (ECF)
- Metastatic disease
  - Combination chemotherapy with platinum and fluoropyrimidine is the standard. In patients with good functional status, modified docetaxel, cisplatin, fluoropyrimidine (mDCF) can be used, which showed improved efficacy and less toxicity than DCF (Shah MA et al. J Clin Oncol 2015;33:3874–387)
- **Targeted therapies** against HER2 and VEGFR2
  - **Trastuzumab:** The ToGA study (Bang Y-J et al. Lancet 2010;376:687–697) showed that the addition of trastuzumab to cisplatin and fluoropyrimidine combination improved survival in metastatic HER2-positive gastric and gastroesophageal adenocarcinomas. The role of continued HER2-directed therapy after progression on first-line therapy is under investigation
  - **Ramucirumab:** The REGARD study (Fuchs CS et al. Lancet 2014;383:31–39) showed that ramucirumab (a monoclonal antibody VEGFR-2 antagonist) compared to placebo prolonged survival in patients with advanced gastric or GEJ cancers progressing after first-line chemotherapy. The RAINBOW study (Wilke H et al. Lancet Oncol 2014;15:1224–1235) showed that combination ramucirumab and paclitaxel improved survival compared to placebo plus paclitaxel in previously treated gastric or GEJ cancers. Combination ramucirumab and paclitaxel is the standard for second-line treatment for patients with advanced GEJ adenocarcinomas
- Immunotherapy with checkpoint inhibitors targeting PD-1
  - Pembrolizumab, which targets PD-1, is approved for use in GEJ adenocarcinomas that are PD-L1–positive in patients who have received two or more lines of prior systemic therapies including a fluoropyrimidine- and platinum-containing regimen or are MSI-H/MMR-deficient (Le DT et al. N Engl J Med 2015;372:2509–2520)

Palliative approaches include:
- Stents
- Photodynamic therapy
- Radiation
- Chemotherapy

Locoregional cancer defined as:
- Potentially resectable, or
- Unresectable, which includes T4 lesion, supraclavicular adenopathy, and celiac nodal metastasis in patients with upper or mid-thoracic esophageal cancer

PREOPERATIVE CHEMORADIOTHERAPY

ESOPHAGEAL CANCER REGIMEN: FLUOROURACIL + CISPLATIN + RADIATION

Tepper J et al. J Clin Oncol 2008;26:1086–1092

Note: The regimen consists of preoperative chemoradiotherapy (cisplatin and fluorouracil) followed by surgery performed between 3–8 weeks after completion of radiation therapy in patients who remained operable candidates based on restaging

Hydration before cisplatin: 1000 mL 0.9% sodium chloride (0.9% NS); intravenously over a minimum of 1 hour before commencing cisplatin administration

Cisplatin 100 mg/m^2/dose; administer intravenously in 100–500 mL of 0.9% NS over 30–90 minutes for a total of 2 doses, prior to commencement of fluorouracil infusion, on days 1 and 29 (total dosage during chemoradiation therapy = 200 mg/m^2)

Hydration after cisplatin: Administer by intravenous infusion ≥1000 mL 0.9% NS over a minimum of 2 hours. Encourage patients to increase oral intake of nonalcoholic fluids, and provide electrolyte replacement as needed (potassium, magnesium, sodium)

Fluorouracil 1000 mg/m^2 per day; administer by continuous intravenous infusion in 500–1000 mL 0.9% NS or 5% dextrose injection (D5W) over 24 hours for 4 consecutive days on days 1–4 and repeated for an additional 4 consecutive days on days 29–32 (total dosage during chemoradiation therapy = 8000 mg/m^2)

Radiation 1.8 Gy/day for 5 days/week
Starts concurrently (within 24 hours) of chemotherapy
Planned cumulative dose = 50.4 Gy (duration of planned treatment is 5 weeks, 3 days)
The final 5.4-Gy treatment is given as a boost

Supportive Care

Antiemetic prophylaxis
*Emetogenic potential on days with cisplatin is **HIGH**. Potential for delayed symptoms*
*Emetogenic potential on days with fluorouracil alone is **LOW***
*Emetogenic potential of radiation therapy to the upper abdomen is **MODERATE***
See Chapter 42 for antiemetic recommendations

Hematopoietic growth factor (CSF) prophylaxis
*Primary prophylaxis is **NOT** indicated*
See Chapter 43 for more information

Antimicrobial prophylaxis
*Risk of fever and neutropenia is **LOW***
   Antimicrobial primary prophylaxis to be considered:
   • Antibacterial—not indicated
   • Antifungal—not indicated
   • Antiviral—not indicated unless patient previously had an episode of HSV

Patient Population Studied

The phase 3 trial (CALGB 9781) involved 56 patients with histologically documented, untreated squamous cell carcinoma or adenocarcinoma of the thoracic esophagus (below 20 cm) or gastro-esophageal junction and with <2 cm distal spread into the gastric cardia. The investigators had planned to include 475 patients, but the study was closed early due to poor accrual. Eligible patients had tumors that were considered surgically resectable (T1–3, NX), including regional thoracic lymph node (N1) metastases. Patients with evidence of distant metastatic disease, who had previously received chemotherapy or radiation therapy for this tumor, or who had previously had any radiation therapy that would overlap with radiation fields required for this malignancy, were ineligible. Patients were randomly assigned to receive preoperative chemoradiotherapy followed by surgery or surgery alone. Preoperative chemotherapy included a bolus intravenous infusion of cisplatin (100 mg/m^2) over 30 minutes on day 1 followed by a continuous intravenous infusion of fluorouracil (1000 mg/m^2/day) over 96 h through to day 4, and the same bolus intravenous infusion of cisplatin (100 mg/m^2) over 30 minutes on day 29 followed by a continuous intravenous infusion of fluorouracil (1000 mg/m^2/day) over 96 h through to day 32. Radiotherapy (1.8 Gy/5 days/week for 5.5 weeks; total 50.4 Gy) was scheduled to begin within 24 h of the start of chemotherapy. Surgery was due to be performed 3–8 weeks after completion of chemoradiotherapy or within 6 weeks of randomization in patients assigned to undergo only surgery

Efficacy (N = 56)

	Trimodality Therapy (N = 30)	Surgery Alone (N = 26)
Median overall survival	4.48 years	1.79 years
Median progression-free survival	3.47 years	1.01 years

Note: Median duration of follow-up was 6 years

Therapy Monitoring

1. *Before therapy:* History and physical exam. CBC with differential, renal and liver function tests, serum electrolytes
2. Monitor renal function prior to initiation and during therapy
3. CBC with differential every 2 weeks
4. Within 4 weeks after completion of radiation therapy, restage with a CT of the chest and abdomen and repeat esophagogastroduodenoscopy. Patients with progressive or unresectable disease are not offered surgery

Treatment Modifications

CISPLATIN + 5-FLUOROURACIL

The goal of therapy is to administer the second cycle on time and to avoid treatment delays if possible

Adverse Event	Treatment Modification
G >3 hematologic toxicities (ANC <1000/mm^3; platelet count <50,000/mm^3)	Delay dose until ANC is >1,500/mm^3 and platelet count >100,000/mm^3
Febrile neutropenia (ANC <1000/mm^3 with single temperature >38.3°C [101°F] or a sustained temperature of ≥38°C [100.4°F] for more than 1 hour)	Hold treatment until neutropenia resolves
Serum creatinine ≥1.5 mg/dL (≥130 μmol/L) and/or BUN ≥25 mg/dL (≥8.92 mmol/L)	Withhold cisplatin until serum creatinine <1.5 mg/dL (<130 μmol/L) and BUN <25 mg/dL (<8.92 mmol/L)
Peripheral neuropathy G ≥3	Discontinue cisplatin. G4 discontinue permanently; G3 may reinstitute if toxicity resolves within 2–3 weeks to G ≤1
Cisplatin induced hearing loss G ≥3	
G1 diarrhea (2–3 stools/day > baseline)	Maintain dose and schedule
G2 diarrhea (4–6 stools/day > baseline)	Delay until diarrhea resolves to baseline, then reduce dosage of fluorouracil by 15–20%
G3 diarrhea (7–9 stools/day > baseline)	
G4 diarrhea (≥10 stools/day > baseline)	Delay until diarrhea resolves to baseline, then reduce dosage of fluorouracil by 30–40%
Other G ≥3 nonhematologic toxicities (except nausea, vomiting, elevated transaminases, and alopecia)	Delay treatment until toxicity resolves to baseline

Adverse Events (N = 28 Patients Who Underwent Trimodality Therapy)

Grade (%)*	Grade 3	Grade 4	Grade 5
Lymphocytes	8	38	0
Esophagitis/dysphagia	27	15	0
White blood cells	25	11	0
Infection	30	0	4
Granulocytes/bands	15	12	0
Pain	16	8	0
Other gastrointestinal	14	5	0
Hemoglobin	11	4	0
Platelets	7	4	0
Nausea	11	0	0
Weight loss	11	0	0
Dysrhythmias	8	0	0

*According to the CALGB Expanded Common Toxicity Criteria
Note: Toxicities are included in the table if grade ≥3 toxicities occurred in ≥10% of the patients receiving trimodality therapy. In total, 57% of patients who received the preoperative chemoradiotherapy experienced at least one grade ≥3 hematologic toxicity. One patient died as a result of treatment-related toxicity (infection)

PREOPERATIVE CHEMORADIOTHERAPY

ESOPHAGEAL CANCER REGIMEN: OXALIPLATIN + PROTRACTED INFUSION FLUOROURACIL AND EXTERNAL BEAM RADIATION THERAPY (EBRT) PRIOR TO SURGERY

Leichman L et al. Proc Am Soc Clin Oncol 2009;27:205s [abstract 4513]

Neoadjuvant combined modality therapy:
Oxaliplatin 85 mg/m^2 per dose; administer intravenously in 250–500 mL 5% dextrose injection (D5W) over 2 hours for 3 doses on days 1, 15, and 29 (total dosage/course = 255 mg/m^2)
Protracted infusion fluorouracil 180 mg/m^2 per day; administer by continuous intravenous infusion in 50–1000 mL 0.9% sodium chloride injection (0.9% NS) or D5W over 24 hours for 35 consecutive days, days 8–43 (total dosage/35-day course = 6300 mg/m^2)
External beam radiation therapy 180 cGy/day starting day 8, on 5 days/week for 25 fractions, to a total dose of 4500 cGy

Esophagectomy:
Two to 4 weeks after completing neoadjuvant combined modality therapy
Adjuvant chemotherapy (optional after recovery from surgery):
Oxaliplatin 85 mg/m^2 per dose; administer intravenously in 250–500 mL D5W over 2 hours for 3 doses on days 1, 15, and 29 (total dosage/course = 255 mg/m^2)
Protracted infusion fluorouracil 180 mg/m^2 per day; administer by continuous intravenous infusion in 50–1000 mL 0.9% NS or D5W over 24 hours for 35 consecutive days, days 8–43 (total dosage/35-day course = 6300 mg/m^2)
Note: Postoperative chemotherapy was not given to all patients; it was not given to patients with pathologic complete response. In the study reported, <50% received postoperative chemotherapy. The investigators recommended completing *all* therapy before surgery

Supportive Care
Antiemetic prophylaxis
*Emetogenic potential on days with oxaliplatin is **MODERATE**, on days with fluorouracil without EBRT is **LOW**, and on days with fluorouracil + EBRT is **LOW–MODERATE***
See Chapter 42 for antiemetic recommendations

Hematopoietic growth factor (CSF) prophylaxis
*Primary prophylaxis is **NOT** indicated*
See Chapter 43 for more information

Antimicrobial prophylaxis
*Risk of fever and neutropenia is **LOW***
   Antimicrobial primary prophylaxis to be considered:
   • Antibacterial—not indicated
   • Antifungal—not indicated
   • Antiviral—not indicated unless patient previously had an episode of HSV

Patient Population Studied

Clinical stage II/III esophageal adenocarcinoma, Zubrod PS ≤2, and tumor <2 cm into the gastric cardia

Treatment Modifications

Adverse Event	Dose Modifications*
Inadequate hematologic recovery at time of oxaliplatin administration (absolute neutrophil count <1500/mm^3 or platelet count <10,0000/mm^3)	Delay therapy 1 week
Persistent G2 or any G3 neuropathy	Reduced oxaliplatin dosage by 25%

Adverse Event (N = 90)

Toxicity Grade (G)	Percentage of Patients
Any G3 toxicity	43%
Any G4 toxicity	18%
Any G gastrointestinal toxicity	39%
Any G flu-like/fatigue	22%
Any G pulmonary toxicity	17%
Any G hematologic toxicity	16%
Any G mucositis toxicity	14%
Any G neurologic toxicity	3%
Death due to protocol*	4.5%

*Two a result of neoadjuvant combined modality therapy, two to surgery

Efficacy (N = 90)

Patients undergoing surgery	77 (86%)
Pathologic complete response	30 (33%)
Cancer in situ or T1N0M0	9 (10%)

Therapy Monitoring

1. Complete blood counts with differential leukocyte counts at least weekly
2. LFTs, serum BUN, and creatinine before each chemotherapy administration
3. Assessment of response after neoadjuvant combined modality therapy and after surgery

PREOPERATIVE CHEMORADIOTHERAPY

ESOPHAGEAL CANCER REGIMEN: CARBOPLATIN + PACLITAXEL + CONCURRENT RADIOTHERAPY

van Hagen P et al. N Engl J Med 2012;366:2074–2084

Hypersensitivity prophylaxis before paclitaxel:

Dexamethasone 20 mg per dose; administer orally for 2 doses: the first dose between 12 and 14 hours before starting paclitaxel, and a second dose 6–7 hours before starting paclitaxel

• Alternatively, give **dexamethasone** 10 mg; administer intravenously 30 minutes before starting paclitaxel

Diphenhydramine 50 mg; administer by intravenous injection 30 minutes before starting paclitaxel

Cimetidine 300 mg (or **ranitidine** 50 mg, **famotidine** 20 mg, or an equivalent histamine receptor (H2 subtype)–antagonist); administer intravenously over 15–30 minutes, 30-60 minutes before starting paclitaxel

Paclitaxel 50 mg/m² per dose; administer intravenously diluted in 0.9% NS or D5W to a concentration within the range 0.3–1.2 mg/mL over 60 minutes before carboplatin for 5 doses on days 1, 8, 15, 22, and 29 (total dosage/course = 250 mg/m²), *with:*

Carboplatin AUC = 2 mg/mL × min per dose; administer intravenously diluted in 0.9% NS or D5W to a concentration >0.5 mg/mL over 60 minutes after paclitaxel for 5 doses on days 1, 8, 15, 22, and 29 (total course includes 5 doses each calculated to produce an AUC = 2 mg/mL × min)

Radiation Therapy

External beam radiation, using 3D conformal radiation technique

Fractionation Schedule

Administer a total dose of 41.4 Gy in 23 fractions of 1.8 Gy, 5 fractions per week, starting the first day of the first cycle of chemotherapy

Position of the Patient

Supine position. Assess reproducibility by orthogonal laser

Definitions of Target Volumes and Critical Structures

Define gross tumor volume (GTV) as the primary tumor and any enlarged regional lymph nodes, and draw on each relevant CT slice. Use available information including physical examination, endoscopy, EUS, and CT-thorax/abdomen to determine the GTV. The planning target volume (PTV) should provide a proximal and distal margin of 4 cm. In case of tumor extension into the stomach, use a distal margin of 3 cm. Provide a 2-cm radial margin around the GTV to include the area of subclinical involvement around the GTV and to compensate for tumor motion and setup variations. Contour both lungs. Contour the heart on all slices; include the infundibulum of the right ventricle and the apex of both atria in its cranial border and exclude the great vessels as much as possible. Define the caudal border as the lowest part of the left ventricle's inferior wall that is distinguishable from the liver. Contour the spinal canal to represent the spinal cord

Simulation Procedure

Prior to the start of the irradiation, make a planning CT scan from the cricoid to L1 vertebra with a slice thickness of 5 mm, with the patient in treatment position. Determine the isocenter at the planning CT

Radiation Technique

Use a multiple-field technique. Give treatment with a combination of anterior/posterior, oblique, or lateral field. Use customized blocks or a multileaf collimator to shape the treatment fields. Have all patients undergo 3D planning. Use beam's eye view (BEV) to ensure optimal target volume coverage and optimal normal tissue sparing. Choose the most appropriate technical solutions (eg, beam quality, field arrangement, conformal therapy planning) as long as they comply with ICRU 50/62 safety margins and homogeneity requirements

Normal Tissue Tolerance

Obtain dose-volume-histograms (DVHs) of both lungs, the heart, and spinal cord for all patients. Use DVHs primarily to document normal tissue damage. Use DVHs to help select the most appropriate treatment plan. Minimize the risks for severe pneumonitis for patients by the use of BEV planning and field-shaping (with optimal sparing of both lungs). Do not exceed spinal cord tolerance (50 Gy)

(continued)

Dose Modification

Adverse Event	Treatment Modification
WBC <1000/mm³ and/or platelets <50,000/mm³ on days 8, 15, 22, and 29	Delay chemotherapy by 1 week until WBC count is >1000/mm³ and platelet count is >50,000/mm³
Febrile neutropenia (ANC <500/mm³ and fever >38.5°C [≤101.3°F])	Hold chemotherapy
Severe bleeding requiring ≥2 platelet transfusions	Hold chemotherapy
Hypersensitivity: Mild symptoms (eg flushing, rash, pruritus)	Complete paclitaxel infusion. Supervise at bedside. No treatment required
Hypersensitivity: Moderate symptoms (eg rash, flushing, mild dyspnea, chest discomfort, mild hypotension)	Stop paclitaxel infusion, give IV antihistamine (clemastine 2 mg or diphenhydramine 50 mg IV, or equivalent antihistamine) and dexamethasone (10 mg IV). After symptoms abate, resume paclitaxel infusion at a rate of 20 mL/hour for 15 minutes, then 50 mL/hour for 15 minutes. Then, if symptoms of hypersensitivity do not recur, at full dose rate until infusion is completed
Hypersensitivity: Severe symptoms (one or more of the following): respiratory distress requiring treatment, generalized urticaria, angioedema, hypotension requiring therapy	Stop paclitaxel infusion, give IV antihistamine and steroid as above. Add epinephrine or bronchodilators if indicated, discontinue therapy
Creatinine ≤1.5 × the upper limit of normal on the day of retreatment	Continue therapy

(continued)

(*continued*)

External Beam Equipment

Use megavoltage equipment with photon energies ≥6 MV. Use a multileaf collimator or individually shaped blocks to shape the irradiation portal according to the planning target volume

Dose Specification

Specify the prescription dose at the ICRU 50/62 reference point, which will be the isocenter for most patients. Ensure the daily prescription dose will be 1.8 Gy at the ICRU reference point and ensure the 95% isodose encompasses the entire planning target volume (PTV). Do not exceed the prescription dose by >7% (ICRU 50/62 guidelines) at the maximum to the PTV. Use tissue density inhomogeneity correction

Treatment Verification

Obtain portal images during the first fraction of all fields. On indication repeat portal images

Note: The median time between the end of chemoradiotherapy and surgery was 6.6 weeks (inter quartile range: 5.7–7.9)

Supportive Care

Antiemetic prophylaxis

Emetogenic potential is **HIGH** on days with chemotherapy with potential for delayed symptoms

Emetogenic potential with radiation therapy alone is **LOW–MODERATE**

See Chapter 42 for antiemetic recommendations

Hematopoietic growth factor (CSF) prophylaxis

Primary prophylaxis is **NOT** indicated

See Chapter 43 for more information

Antimicrobial prophylaxis

Risk of fever and neutropenia is **LOW**

   Antimicrobial primary prophylaxis to be considered:

   • Antibacterial—not indicated

   • Antifungal—not indicated

   • Antiviral—not indicated unless patient previously had an episode of HSV

Efficacy

	Chemoradiotherapy + Surgery (N = 161)	Surgery Alone (N = 161)	P
R0 resection achieved	148 (92%)	111 (69%)	<0.001
Median number of lymph nodes resected	15	18	0.77
≥1 positive lymph node in resection specimen	50 (31%)	120 (75%)	<0.001
Median disease-free survival	Not reached	24.2 months	<0.001 HR, 0.498 95% CI 0.357–0.693
Median overall survival (ITT)	49.4 months	24.0 months	0.003 HR, 0.657 95% CI 0.495–0.871
1-year overall survival rate	82%	70%	HR, 0.665 95% CI 0.500–0.884
2-year overall survival rate	67%	50%	
3-year overall survival rate	58%	44%	
5-year overall survival rate	47%	34%	

Dose Modification (*continued*)

Adverse Event	Treatment Modification
Creatinine is >1.5 × the upper limit of normal	Establish IV hydration the evening preceding treatment at a flow rate sufficient to correct volume deficits and produce a urine flow ≥50 mL/hour. Repeat serum creatinine measurement in the morning. If repeated serum creatinine result is ≤1.5 × the upper limit of normal, proceed with treatment. Stop chemotherapy if the repeated serum creatinine result is >1.5 × the upper limit of normal
Mucositis with oral ulcers or protracted vomiting despite antiemetic premedication	Delay chemotherapy 1 week
G ≤2 neurotoxicity	Continue therapy
G >2 neurotoxicity	Discontinue chemotherapy
Asymptomatic bradycardia or isolated and asymptomatic ventricular extrasystoles	Continue therapy under continuous cardiac monitoring
First-degree AV block	Continue therapy under continuous cardiac monitoring
Symptomatic arrhythmia or AV block (except first degree) or other heart blocks	Continue therapy under continuous cardiac monitoring. Stop paclitaxel, manage arrhythmia according to standard practice until patient goes off protocol
G4 radiation induced esophagitis	Hold both chemotherapy and radiotherapy until the esophagitis is G ≤3

Toxicity

Adverse Events During Neoadjuvant Chemoradiotherapy and After Surgery*		
Event	Chemoradiotherapy and Surgery (N = 171)	Surgery Alone (N = 186)
Postoperative Events		
Event	Number of Patients (%)†	
Pulmonary complications‡	78/168 (46)	82/186 (44)
Cardiac complications§	36/168 (21)	31/186 (17)
Chylothorax	17/168 (10)	11/186 (6)
Mediastinitis	5/168 (3)	12/186 (6)
Anastomotic leakage	36/161 (22)	48/161 (30)
Death		
In hospital	6/168 (4)	8/186 (4)
After 30 days	4/168 (2)	5/186 (3)
Events During Chemoradiotherapy		
Event	Number of Patients (%)	
	Any Grade	Grade ≥3
Anorexia	51 (30)	9 (5)
Alopecia	25 (15)	—
Constipation	47 (27)	1 (1)
Diarrhea	30 (18)	2 (1)
Esophageal perforation	1 (1)	1 (1)
Esophagitis	32 (19)	2 (1)
Fatigue	115 (67)	5 (3)
Nausea	91 (53)	2 (1)
Neurotoxic effects	25 (15)	—
Vomiting	43 (25)	1 (1)
Leukopenia	103 (60)	11 (6)
Neutropenia	16 (9)	4 (2)
Thrombocytopenia	92 (54)	1 (1)

*Adverse events according to NCI CTCAE, National Cancer Institute (USA) Common Terminology Criteria for Adverse Events, version 3. At: http://ctep.cancer.gov/protocolDevelopment/electronic_applications/ctc.htm [accessed December 7, 2013]

†168/171 patients treated with chemoradiotherapy underwent surgery

‡Includes pneumonia (isolation of pathogen from sputum culture and a new or progressive infiltrate on CXR), serious atelectasis (lobar collapse on chest radiograph), pneumothorax (collection of air, requiring drainage), pleural effusion (collection of fluid, requiring drainage), pulmonary embolus (detected on spiral CT or V/Q mismatch on scintigraphy), and acute respiratory failure (partial pressure of arterial oxygen <60 mm Hg while breathing ambient air)

§Including arrhythmia (any change in rhythm requiring treatment), myocardial infarction, and left ventricular failure (marked pulmonary edema on CXR)

Patient Population Studied

Patients with histologically confirmed, potentially curable squamous cell carcinoma, adenocarcinoma, or large-cell undifferentiated carcinoma of the esophagus or esophagogastric junction (ie, tumors involving both the cardia and the esophagus on endoscopy) were eligible for inclusion in the study. The upper border of the tumor had to be ≥3 cm below the upper esophageal sphincter. Patients who had proximal gastric tumors with minimal invasion of the esophagus were excluded. The length and width of the tumor could not exceed 8 cm and 5 cm, respectively. Only patients with tumors of clinical stage T1N1 or T2–3N0–1 and no clinical evidence of metastatic spread (M0), according to the International Union against Cancer tumor–node–metastasis (TNM) classification, were enrolled. Eligible patients had a World Health Organization performance status score ≤2 and had lost ≤10% of body weight

Treatment Monitoring

1. Tumor assessment every 2 cycles
2. CBC with differential and serum creatinine: weekly while receiving chemotherapy; and at completion of chemoradiotherapy
3. During the first year after treatment completed, see patients every 3 months. In the second year, every 6 months, and then at the end of each year until 5 years after treatment

METASTATIC • FIRST-LINE
ESOPHAGEAL CANCER: CISPLATIN + CAPECITABINE

Kang Y-K et al. Ann Oncol 2009;20:666–673

Hydration before cisplatin: 1000 mL 0.9% sodium chloride injection (0.9% NS); administer intravenously over a minimum of 1 hour before commencing cisplatin administration
Cisplatin 80 mg/m²; administer intravenously in 50–500 mL 0.9% NS over 2 hours on day 1, every 3 weeks (total dosage/cycle = 80 mg/m²)
Hydration after cisplatin: ≥1000 mL 0.9% NS; administer intravenously over a minimum of 2 hours. Monitor and replace magnesium and other electrolytes as needed. Encourage patients to increase their intake of nonalcoholic fluids
Capecitabine 1000 mg/m² per dose; administer orally twice daily with water within 30 minutes after a meal for 14 consecutive days (28 doses) on days 1–14, every 3 weeks (total dosage/cycle = 28,000 mg/m²)

Supportive Care
Antiemetic prophylaxis
Emetogenic potential on day 1 is **HIGH**. *Potential for delayed symptoms*
Emetogenic potential with capecitabine alone is **MINIMAL–LOW**
See Chapter 42 for antiemetic recommendations

Hematopoietic growth factor (CSF) prophylaxis
Primary prophylaxis may be indicated
See Chapter 43 for more information

Antimicrobial prophylaxis
Risk of fever and neutropenia is **LOW**
  Antimicrobial primary prophylaxis to be considered:
- Antibacterial—not indicated
- Antifungal—not indicated
- Antiviral—not indicated unless patient previously had an episode of HSV

Oral care
Risk of mucositis/stomatitis is **HIGH**
  General advice:
- Encourage patients to maintain intake of nonalcoholic fluids
- Evaluate patients for oral pain and provide analgesic medications
- Consider histamine (H₂-subtype) receptor antagonists (eg, ranitidine, famotidine), or a proton pump inhibitor for epigastric pain
- Probiotics containing *Lactobacillus* sp. may be beneficial in preventing diarrhea
  Patients with intact oral mucosa:
- Clean the mouth, tongue, and gums by brushing after every meal and at bedtime with an ultrasoft toothbrush with fluoride toothpaste
- Floss teeth gently every day unless contraindicated. If gums bleed and hurt, avoid bleeding or sore areas, but floss other teeth
- Patients may use saline or commercial bland, nonalcoholic rinses
  - Do not use mouthwashes that contain alcohols
  If mucositis or stomatitis is present:
- Keep the mouth moist utilizing water, ice chips, sugarless gum, sugar-free hard candies, or a saliva substitute
- Rinse mouth several times a day to remove debris
  - Use a solution of ¼ teaspoon (1.25 g) each of baking soda and table salt (sodium chloride) in 1 quart (~950 mL) of warm water. Follow with a plain-water rinse
  - Do not use mouthwashes that contain alcohols
- Foam-tipped swabs (eg, Toothettes) are useful in moisturizing oral mucosa, but ineffective for cleansing teeth and removing plaque
- Advise patients who develop mucositis to:
  - Choose foods that are easy to chew and swallow
  - Take small bites of food, chew slowly, and sip liquids with meals
  - Encourage soft, moist foods such as cooked cereals, mashed potatoes, and scrambled eggs
  - For trouble swallowing, soften food with gravies, sauces, broths, yogurt, or other bland liquids
  - Avoid sharp, crunchy foods; hot, spicy, or highly acidic foods (eg, citrus fruits and juices); sugary foods; toothpicks; tobacco products; alcoholic drinks

Treatment Modifications

Adverse Event	Dose Modification
ANC nadir <1000/mm^3 *or* platelet nadir <50,000/mm^3 after treatment	Delay treatment until ANC ≥1000/mm^3 *and* platelet ≥50,000/mm^3, then decrease cisplatin dosage by 25%, and decrease daily capecitabine dosages by 50% during subsequent cycles*. Alternatively, consider using hematopoietic growth factors
Serum creatinine >1.5 mg/dL (>133 μmol/L), but <3 mg/dL (<265 μmol/L) *or* creatinine clearance >40 mL/min but <60 mL/min (>0.66 mL/s, but <1 mL/s)	Delay treatment until serum creatinine ≤1.5 mg/dL (≤133 μmol/L), then decrease cisplatin dosage by 50%*
Serum creatinine >3 mg/dL (>265 μmol/L) *or* creatinine clearance <40 mL/min (<0.66 mL/s)	Stop cisplatin
Persistent G2 neuropathy	Hold cisplatin until toxicity resolves to G ≤1; reduce dose by 25% for subsequent cycles
Transient G3/4 neuropathy (duration 7–14 days)	Hold cisplatin. Resume cisplatin after toxicity resolves with dosage reduced by 25% for subsequent cycles
Persistent G3/4 neuropathy	Discontinue cisplatin
G3/4 nonhematologic adverse events other than renal function and neurotoxicity	Reduce cisplatin and capecitabine dosages by 25% for subsequent cycles
G2 stomatitis, diarrhea, or nausea	Hold capecitabine; resume capecitabine at full dosage after resolution of toxicity
Second episode of G2 stomatitis, diarrhea, or nausea	Hold capecitabine; resume capecitabine with dosage reduced by 25% after resolution of toxicity
Third episode of G2 stomatitis, diarrhea, or nausea	Hold capecitabine; resume capecitabine with dosage reduced by 50% after resolution of toxicity
Fourth episode of G2 stomatitis, diarrhea, or nausea	Discontinue capecitabine
G3 stomatitis, diarrhea, or nausea, first episode	Hold capecitabine; if G3 toxicity is adequately controlled within 2 days, resume capecitabine at full dosage when toxicity resolves to G ≤1. If G3 toxicity takes >2 days to be controlled, resume capecitabine with dosage reduced by 25% after toxicity resolves to G ≤1
Second episode of G3 stomatitis, diarrhea, or nausea	Hold capecitabine; if G3 toxicity is controlled adequately within 2 days, then resume capecitabine with dosage reduced by 50% after toxicity resolves to G ≤1
Third episode of G3 stomatitis, diarrhea, or nausea	Discontinue capecitabine
G4 stomatitis, diarrhea, or nausea	Withhold capecitabine. Resume capecitabine with dosage reduced by 50% after toxicity resolves
G1 capecitabine-associated PPE[†]	Begin pyridoxine 50 mg orally 3 times daily and continue capecitabine without dose modification
G2 capecitabine-associated PPE[†]	Begin pyridoxine 50 mg orally 3 times daily and withhold capecitabine. Resume capecitabine with dosage reduced by 15% after toxicity resolves
G3 capecitabine-associated PPE[†]	Begin pyridoxine 50 mg orally 3 times daily and withhold capecitabine. Resume capecitabine with dosage reduced by 30% after toxicity resolves
Recurrent G3 capecitabine-associated PPE[†]	Begin pyridoxine 50 mg orally 3 times daily and withhold capecitabine. Resume capecitabine with dosage reduced by 50% after toxicity resolves

*Treatment delays for unresolved adverse events of >3 weeks duration warrant discontinuation of treatment
[†]PPE, Palmar-plantar erythrodysesthesia (hand-foot syndrome)

Efficacy

	Capecitabine + Cisplatin	Fluorouracil + Cisplatin	Hazard Ratio (95% CI)	P Value
Median progression-free survival	5.6 months	5.0 months	0.81 (0.63–1.04)	<0.001*
Median overall survival	10.5 months	9.3 months	0.85 (0.64–1.13)	0.008*
Objective response rate	46 (38–55)[†]	32 (24–41)[†]	1.80 (1.11–2.94)[‡]	0.020
Complete response	2%	3%	—	—
Partial response	44%	29%	—	—
Mean time to response	3.7 months	3.8 months	1.61 (1.10–2.35)	0.015
Median duration of response	7.6 months	6.2 months	0.88 (0.56–1.36)	0.554

*For noninferiority versus 1.25
[†]95% CI in parentheses
[‡]Odds ratio (95% CI)

Patient Population Studied

Patients with histologically confirmed measurable advanced gastric cancer, a Karnofsky performance status of 70 or more, no previous chemotherapy other than neoadjuvant or adjuvant regimens, no radiotherapy to target lesions, and adequate hepatic, cardiac, and renal function, the latter defined as an estimated creatinine clearance ≥ 60 mL/min estimated with the Cockcroft and Gault formula

Treatment Monitoring

1. Tumor assessment every 2 cycles
2. CBC with differential before the start of a new cycle

Toxicity

Treatment-Related Adverse Events (in >15% of Patients) by NCI-CTC*

	No. (%) of Patients							
	Capecitabine + Cisplatin (n = 156)				Fluorouracil + Cisplatin (n = 155)			
Adverse Event	G1	G2	G3	G4	G1	G2	G3	G4
Nausea	49 (31)	35 (22)	3 (2)	—	44 (28)	37 (24)	4 (3)	—
Vomiting	32 (21)	33 (21)	10 (6)	1 (<1)	31 (20)	47 (30)	13 (8)	—
Diarrhea	9 (6)	14 (9)	7 (4)	1 (<1)	11 (7)	6 (4)	6 (4)	1 (<1)
Stomatitis	11 (7)	4 (3)	3 (2)	—	15 (10)	16 (10)	10 (6)	—
Neutropenia	2 (1)	24 (15)	22 (14)	3 (2)	2 (1)	15 (10)	23 (15)	6 (4)
Leucopenia	3 (2)	15 (10)	4 (3)	—	4 (3)	16 (10)	4 (3)	2 (1)
Anorexia	23 (15)	18 (12)	3 (2)	—	23 (15)	19 (12)	1 (<1)	—
Fatigue	15 (10)	8 (5)	1 (<1)	—	11 (7)	3 (2)	1 (<1)	—
Asthenia	10 (6)	9 (6)	3 (2)	—	14 (9)	12 (8)	1 (<1)	—
Hand-foot syndrome	20 (13)	8 (5)	6 (4)	—	5 (3)	1 (<1)	—	—

*NCI, CTC, National Cancer Institute (USA) Common Toxicity Criteria, version 2.0. At: http://ctep.cancer.gov/protocolDevelopment/electronic_applications/ctc.htm [accessed December 7, 2013]

METASTATIC • FIRST-LINE

ESOPHAGEAL CANCER REGIMEN: OXALIPLATIN + FLUOROURACIL + LEUCOVORIN (FOLFOX)

Mauer AM et al. Ann Oncol 2005;16:1320–1325

Oxaliplatin 85 mg/m²; administer intravenously in 250–500 mL 5% dextrose injection (D5W) over 2 hours on day 1, every 14 days (total dosage/cycle = 85 mg/m²)
Leucovorin 500 mg/m² per day; administer by intravenous infusion in 10–500 mL 0.9% sodium chloride injection (0.9% NS) or D5W over 2 hours for 2 doses on days 1 and 2, every 14 days (total dosage/cycle = 1000 mg/m²); *followed each day by:*
Fluorouracil 400 mg/m² per day; administer by intravenous push or infusion in 10–100 mL 0.9% NS or D5W over 2–15 minutes for 2 doses on days 1 and 2, every 14 days; *followed immediately afterward by:*
Fluorouracil 600 mg/m² per day; administer by continuous intravenous infusion over 22 hours in 50–1000 mL 0.9% NS or D5W for 2 doses on days 1 and 2, every 14 days (total dosage/cycle = 2000 mg/m²)

Note:

• Patients were counseled to avoid exposure to cold liquids or air because the acute neurotoxicity encountered with oxaliplatin appears to be exacerbated by exposure to cold

Supportive Care
Antiemetic prophylaxis
Emetogenic potential on day 1 is **HIGH**
Emetogenic potential on day 2 is **LOW**
See Chapter 42 for antiemetic recommendations

Hematopoietic growth factor (CSF) prophylaxis
Primary prophylaxis is **NOT** indicated
See Chapter 43 for more information

Antimicrobial prophylaxis
Risk of fever and neutropenia is **LOW**
   Antimicrobial primary prophylaxis to be considered:
   • Antibacterial—not indicated
   • Antifungal—not indicated
   • Antiviral—not indicated unless patient previously had an episode of HSV

Oral care
• Encourage patients to maintain intake of nonalcoholic fluids

If mucositis or stomatitis is present:
• Rinse mouth several times a day with ¼ teaspoon (1.25 g) each of baking soda and table salt in 1 quart of warm water. Follow with a plain water rinse
   ▪ Do not use mouthwashes that contain alcohols

Diarrhea management
Latent or delayed-onset diarrhea*:
   Loperamide 4 mg; administer orally initially after the first loose or liquid stool, then
   Loperamide 2 mg every 2 hours while awake; every 4 hours during sleep
   Alternatively, a trial of **diphenoxylate hydrochloride** 2.5 mg with **atropine sulfate** 0.025 mg (eg, Lomotil) two tablets four times daily until control has been achieved.

Persistent diarrhea:
Octreotide acetate (solution) 100–150 mcg; administer subcutaneously 3 times daily.

Antibiotic therapy during latent or delayed-onset diarrhea:
A fluoroquinolone (eg, **ciprofloxacin** 500 mg orally every 12 hours) if absolute neutrophil count <500/mm³

*Abigerges D et al. J Natl Cancer Inst 1994;86:446–449
Rothenberg ML et al. J Clin Oncol 2001;19:3801–3807
Wadler S et al. J Clin Oncol 1998;16:3169–3178

Patient Population Studied

Recurrent or metastatic cancer of the esophagus or gastric cardia. Prior treatment with a single chemotherapy regimen and radiotherapy allowed. Eastern Cooperative Oncology Group (ECOG) performance status of 0, 1, or 2. Laboratory measures required at study entry: creatinine ≤1.5 times the institutional upper limit of normal or creatinine clearance ≥50 mL/min; bilirubin ≤1.5 mg/dL; and glutamic–oxaloacetic transaminase <2 times the institutional limit of normal

Adverse Events (N = 35)

Hematologic Toxicity					
Toxicity Grade	**G1**	**G2**	**G3**	**G4**	**G5**
Leukopenia	6	14	7	1	0
Neutropenia	2	3	12	10	1
Thrombocytopenia	14	2	2	1	0
Anemia	17	9	3	0	0

Nonhematologic Toxicity					
Toxicity Grade	**G1**	**G2**	**G3**	**G4**	**G5**
Fatigue	14	15	2	1	—
Vomiting	9	7	1	0	—
Stomatitis	5	4	0	0	–
Anorexia	13	5	2	0	—
Diarrhea	6	3	4	0	—
Laryngodysesthesia	0	0	0	0	—
Neuropathy, motor	3	0	0	0	—
Neuropathy, sensory	13	8	1	0	—
Respiratory	0	4	1	0	—
Infection	1	1	1	0	—
Creatinine elevation	0	0	0	1*	—

*Reversible renal insufficiency secondary to oxaliplatin-induced hemolysis
NCI CTC, National Cancer Institute (USA) Common Toxicity Criteria, version 2.0. At: http://ctep.cancer.gov/protocolDevelopment/electronic_applications/ctc.htm [accessed December 7, 2013]

Therapy Monitoring

1. Complete blood counts with differential leukocyte counts at least weekly
2. LFTs, serum BUN, and creatinine before each cycle of chemotherapy
3. Assessment of response after every 4 cycles of therapy

Treatment Modifications

Adverse Event	Dose Modifications*
Inadequate hematologic recovery by day 15 (ANC <1500/mm^3 *or* platelet count <100,000/mm^3)	Delay therapy 1 week
G4 neutropenia or thrombocytopenia	Reduce oxaliplatin and fluorouracil dosages 25% in subsequent cycle
G3/4 stomatitis or diarrhea	Reduce oxaliplatin and fluorouracil dosages by 25% in the subsequent cycle after recovery to baseline
Persistent G2 or any G3 neuropathy	Reduce oxaliplatin dosages by 25%
Febrile or prolonged neutropenia	Administer prophylactic granulocyte colony stimulating factor in subsequent cycles

*Based on the worst toxicity observed during the previous course

Efficacy (N = 35)

	Number (%)
Complete response	1 (2.5%)
Partial response	13 (37%)
Overall RR, all patients[†]	40% (95% CI, 24–57%)
Overall RR, chemotherapy-naïve patients	45% (95% CI, 27–64%)
Overall RR, previously treated patients	0 (95% CI, 0–53%)
Stable disease (≥4 cycles of chemotherapy)	10 (29%)
Progressive disease	10 (29%)
Not evaluated	1 (2.5%)
Median PFS, all patients	4.6 months (95% CI, 2.2–6.8)
Median PFS, chemotherapy-naïve patients	4.9 months[‡]
Median PFS, previously treated patients	1.7 months[‡]
1-year PFS probability	0.15
Median OS, all patients	7.1 months (95% CI, 5.9–10.9)
Median OS, chemotherapy-naïve patients	7.6 months[§]
Median OS, previously treated patients	2.1 months[§]
1-year survival probability	0.31 (95% CI, 0.17–0.47)
2-year survival probability	0.11

*WHO Criteria
[†]Histology of responding patients: adenocarcinoma (13) adenosquamous (1)
[‡]P = 0.0009; log-rank test
[§]P = 0.011; log-rank test

METASTATIC • FIRST-LINE

ESOPHAGEAL CANCER REGIMEN: CISPLATIN + CAPECITABINE ± TRASTUZUMAB

Bang Y-J et al. Lancet 2010;376:687–697

Hydration with cisplatin: ≥1000 mL 0.9% sodium chloride injection (0.9% NS); administer intravenously at ≥100 mL/hour before and after cisplatin administration. Also, encourage patients to increase oral intake of nonalcoholic fluids. Monitor serum electrolytes and replace as needed (potassium, magnesium, sodium)

Cisplatin 80 mg/m^2; administer intravenously in 100–250 mL 0.9% NS over 60 minutes on day 1, every 3 weeks, for 6 cycles (total dosage/cycle = 80 mg/m^2)

Capecitabine 1000 mg/m^2 per dose; administer orally twice daily (approximately every 12 hours) with water within 30 minutes after a meal for 28 doses on days 1–14, every 3 weeks, for 6 cycles (total dosage/cycle = 28,000 mg/m^2)

Trastuzumab

- **Initial dose:** Trastuzumab 8 mg/kg; administer intravenously in 250 mL 0.9% NS over 90 minutes (total dosage during cycle 1 = 8 mg/kg), *followed after 3 weeks by:*
- **Subsequent doses:** Trastuzumab 6 mg/kg per dose; administer intravenously in 250 mL 0.9% NS over 30–90 minutes (total dosage/cycle = 6 mg/kg)

Notes: Trastuzumab treatment continues every 3 weeks until disease progression, unacceptable toxicities, or patient withdrawal

An optimal sequence for drug administration is suggested by experimental evidence, but has not been proved in clinical trials (Li X-L. Cancer Invest 2010;28:1038–1047)

Supportive Care

Antiemetic prophylaxis

Emetogenic potential on day 1 is **HIGH**

Emetogenic potential on days with capecitabine alone is **LOW**

See Chapter 42 for antiemetic recommendations

Hematopoietic growth factor (CSF) prophylaxis

Primary prophylaxis is **NOT** indicated

See Chapter 43 for more information

Antimicrobial prophylaxis

Risk of fever and neutropenia is **LOW**

Antimicrobial primary prophylaxis to be considered:

- Antibacterial—not indicated
- Antifungal—not indicated
- Antiviral—not indicated unless patient previously had an episode of HSV

Trastuzumab infusion reactions:

- A symptom complex most commonly consisting of chills and/or fever may occur in as many as 40% of patients during the first infusion of trastuzumab. These symptoms occur infrequently with subsequent trastuzumab infusions. Other signs and/or symptoms may include nausea, vomiting, pain (in some cases at tumor sites), rigors, headache, dizziness, dyspnea, hypotension, rash, and asthenia. Although the symptoms are usually mild to moderate in severity, infrequently, trastuzumab may need to be discontinued
- When such a symptom complex is observed, it can be treated with or without reduction in the rate of trastuzumab infusion, and:
  - **Acetaminophen** 650 mg; administer orally
  - **Diphenhydramine** 25–50 mg administer orally or by intravenous injection, and
  - **Meperidine** 12.5–25 mg; administer by intravenous injection every 10 minutes if needed for shaking chills (generally, cumulative doses >50 mg are not needed; use with caution in persons with moderate or more severely impaired renal function)

Treatment plan notes:

- LVEF assessment (MUGA or echocardiography) every 3 months in patients receiving trastuzumab

(*continued*)

Patient Population Studied

Patients with measurable or nonmeasurable histologically confirmed inoperable locally advanced, recurrent, or metastatic adenocarcinoma of the stomach or gastroesophageal junction with defined HER2+ status who had not previously received treatment for metastatic disease. New immunohistochemistry scoring criteria (Hofmann M et al. Histopathology 2008;52:797–805) determined eligibility. Patients whose tumor samples scored 3+ on immunohistochemical staining for HER2 or if samples were FISH positive (HER2:CEP17 ratio ≥2) were eligible to participate

Therapy Monitoring

1. LVEF assessments at baseline and at least every 12 weeks
2. Complete blood counts and leukocyte differential counts at least weekly
3. LFTs, serum BUN, and creatinine before each cycle of chemotherapy
4. Assessment of response every 6 weeks

(continued)

Hand-foot reaction (palmar-plantar erythrodysesthesia, PPE)
Use topical emollients (eg, Aquaphor), topical or orally administered steroids, antihistamines, or pyridoxine 50–200 mg/day

Diarrhea management
Latent or delayed onset-diarrhea:
Loperamide 4 mg; administer orally initially after the first loose or liquid stool, *then*
Loperamide 2 mg every 2 hours while awake; every 4 hours during sleep
Alternatively, a trial of **diphenoxylate hydrochloride** 2.5 mg with **atropine sulfate** 0.025 mg (eg, Lomotil) two tablets four times daily until control achieved

Persistent diarrhea:
Octreotide acetate (solution) 100–150 mcg; administer subcutaneously 3 times daily

Antibiotic therapy during latent or delayed-onset diarrhea:
A fluoroquinolone (eg, **ciprofloxacin** 500 mg orally every 12 hours) if absolute neutrophil count <500/mm³

*Abigerges D et al. J Natl Cancer Inst 1994;86:446–449
Rothenberg ML et al. J Clin Oncol 2001;19:3801–3807
Wadler S et al. J Clin Oncol 1998;16:3169–3178

Oral care
Encourage patients to maintain intake of nonalcoholic fluids

If mucositis or stomatitis is present:
• Rinse mouth several times a day with ¼ teaspoon (1.25 g) each of baking soda and table salt in 1 quart of warm water. Follow with a plain water rinse
  ▪ Do not use mouthwashes that contain alcohols

Treatment Modifications

Adverse Event	Dose Modifications*
Inadequate hematologic recovery by day 21 (absolute neutrophil count <1500/mm³ *or* platelet count <100,000/mm³)	Delay cisplatin and capecitabine for 1 week or until myelosuppression resolves
Recurrent treatment delay because of myelosuppression	Delay cisplatin and capecitabine for 1 week *or* until myelosuppression resolves, *then* decrease cisplatin and capecitabine dosage by 25% during subsequent treatments
Capecitabine	
G2 stomatitis, diarrhea, or nausea	Hold capecitabine; resume capecitabine at full dose after resolution of toxicity
Second episode of G2 stomatitis, diarrhea, or nausea	Hold capecitabine; resume capecitabine with dosage reduced by 25% after resolution of toxicity
Third episode of G2 stomatitis, diarrhea, or nausea	Hold capecitabine; resume capecitabine with dosage reduced by 50% after resolution of toxicity
Fourth episode of G2 stomatitis, diarrhea, or nausea	Discontinue capecitabine
G3 stomatitis, diarrhea, or nausea	Hold capecitabine; if G3 toxicity is adequately controlled within 2 days, then on resolution of toxicity to G ≤2, resume capecitabine at full dosage. If G3 toxicity takes >2 days to be controlled, then on resolution of toxicity to G ≤2, resume capecitabine with dosage decreased by 25%
Second episode of G3 stomatitis, diarrhea, or nausea	Hold capecitabine; if G3 toxicity is adequately controlled within 2 days, then on resolution of toxicity to G ≤2, resume capecitabine with dosage reduced by 50%
Third episode of G3 stomatitis, diarrhea, or nausea	Discontinue capecitabine
G4 stomatitis, diarrhea, or nausea	Discontinue capecitabine or on resolution of toxicity resume capecitabine with dosage reduced by 50%
G1 capecitabine-associated plantar-palmar erythema (PPE)	Begin pyridoxine 50 mg 3 times daily and continue capecitabine without dose modification

(continued)

Treatment Modifications (continued)

Capecitabine

G2 capecitabine-associated PPE	Begin pyridoxine 50 mg 3 times daily; withhold capecitabine until symptoms resolve, then resume capecitabine with dosage reduced by 15%
G3 capecitabine-associated PPE	Begin pyridoxine 50 mg 3 times daily; withhold capecitabine until symptoms resolve, then resume capecitabine with dosage reduced by 30%
Recurrent G3 capecitabine-associated PPE	Begin pyridoxine 50 mg 3 times daily; withhold capecitabine until symptoms resolve, then resume capecitabine with dosage reduced by 50%

Cisplatin

Reduction in creatinine clearance* to ≤60% of on study value	Delay therapy 1 week. If creatinine clearance does not recover to pretreatment values, then consider reducing cisplatin dose
Creatinine clearance* 40–60 mL/min (0.66–1 mL/s)	Consider reducing cisplatin so that dose in milligrams equals the creatinine clearance* value in mL/min[†]
Creatinine clearance* <40 mL/min (<0.66 mL/s)	Hold cisplatin
Clinically significant ototoxicity	Discontinue cisplatin
Persistent (>14 days) peripheral neuropathy without functional impairment	Decrease cisplatin dose by 50%
Clinically significant sensory loss—persistent (>14 days) peripheral neuropathy with functional impairment	Discontinue cisplatin

Trastuzumab

Trastuzumab toxicity was managed by treatment interruptions

*Creatinine clearance used as a measure of glomerular filtration rate
[†]This also applies to patients with creatinine clearance (GFR) of 40–60 mL/min at the outset of treatment

Efficacy

	Chemotherapy + Trastuzumab (n = 294)	Chemotherapy Alone (n = 290)
Median overall survival	13.8 months (95% CI, 12–16)	11.1 months (95% CI, 10–13)
Median PFS	6.7 months (95% CI, 6–8)*	5.5 months (95% CI, 5–6)[†]
Duration of response	6.9 months (95% CI, 6–8)*	4.8 months (95% CI, 4–6)[†]
Overall tumor response rate	139 (47%)	100 (35%)
CR	16 (5%)	7 (2%)
PR	123 (42%)	93 (32%)

*N = 139
[†]N = 100

Post-hoc exploratory analysis

	High HER2 Expression (IHC 2+ and FISH+ or IHC 3+)		Low HER2 Expression (IHC 0 or 1+ and FISH+)	
	Chemotherapy + Trastuzumab	Chemotherapy Alone	Chemotherapy + Trastuzumab	Chemotherapy Alone
Hazard ratio	0.65 (95% CI, 0.51–0.83)		1.07 (95% CI, 0.70–1.62)	
Median OS	16.0 months	11.8 months	10 months	8.7 months

IHC, HER2 immunohistochemistry
There was evidence of a significant interaction test (P = 0.036) between treatment and the two HER2 subgroups (high HER2 expression vs. low HER2 expression)

Adverse Events

NCI-CTCAE, National Cancer Institute (USA) Common Terminology Criteria for Adverse Events, version 3.0 and serious adverse events according to International Conference on Harmonisation guidelines. Available at: http://ctep.cancer.gov/protocolDevelopment/electronic_applications/ctc.htm [accessed December 7, 2013]

Adverse events of all grades (>5%) and G3/4 (≥1%) plus adverse events of any grade with ≤5% difference between groups

	Trastuzumab + Chemotherapy (N = 294)		Chemotherapy Alone (N = 290)	
	All Grades	G3/4	All Grades	G3/4
Any adverse event	292 (99%)	201 (68%)	284 (98%)	198 (68%)
Gastrointestinal Disorders				
Nausea	197 (67%)	22 (7%)	184 (63%)	21 (7%)
Vomiting	147 (50%)	18 (6%)	134 (46%)	22 (8%)
Diarrhea	109 (37%)	27 (9%)	80 (28%)	11 (4%)
Constipation	75 (26%)	2 (1%)	93 (32%)	5 (2%)
Stomatitis	72 (24%)	2 (1%)	43 (15%)	6 (2%)
Abdominal pain	66 (22%)	7 (2%)	56 (19%)	5 (2%)
Dysphagia	19 (6%)	7 (2%)	10 (3%)	1 (<1%)
Blood and Lymphatic System Disorders				
Neutropenia	157 (53%)	79 (27%)	165 (57%)	88 (30%)
Anemia	81 (28%)	36 (12%)	61 (21%)	30 (10%)
Thrombocytopenia	47 (16%)	14 (5%)	33 (11%)	8 (3%)
Febrile neutropenia	15 (5%)	15 (5%)	8 (3%)	8 (3%)
General, Metabolic, and Other Disorders				
Anorexia	135 (46%)	19 (6%)	133 (46%)	18 (6%)
Fatigue	102 (35%)	12 (4%)	82 (28%)	7 (2%)
Hand-foot syndrome	75 (26%)	4 (1%)	64 (22%)	5 (2%)
Weight decreased	69 (23%)	6 (2%)	40 (14%)	7 (2%)
Asthenia	55 (19%)	14 (5%)	53 (18%)	10 (3%)
Fever	54 (18%)	3 (1%)	36 (12%)	0
Renal impairment	47 (16%)	2 (1%)	39 (13%)	3 (1%)
Mucosal inflammation	37 (13%)	6 (2%)	18 (6%)	2 (1%)
Nasopharyngitis	37 (13%)	0	17 (6%)	0
Chills	23 (8%)	1 (<1%)	0	0
Hypokalemia	22 (7%)	13 (4%)	13 (4%)	7 (2%)
Dehydration	18 (6%)	7 (2%)	16 (6%)	5 (2%)
Dyspnea	9 (3%)	1 (<1%)	16 (6%)	5 (2%)

Serious Adverse Events

	Trastuzumab + Chemotherapy (N = 294)	Chemotherapy Alone (N = 290)
Serious adverse events	95 (32%)	81 (28%)
Adverse events leading to dose modifications or treatment interruption	246 (84%)	237 (82%)
60-day mortality	15 deaths (5%)	20 deaths (7%)
Treatment-related mortality	10 deaths (3%)	3 deaths (1%)
Severe infusion reactions (G ≥3; eg, allergic reaction or hypersensitivity, chills, arthralgia, dyspnea)	17 (6%)	NR
Cardiac adverse events	17 (6%)	18 (6%)
G3/4	4 patients, 9 events	9 patients, 9 events
Cardiac dysfunction (LVEF decrease ≥10%, or decrease to absolute LVEF <50%)	11 (5%)*	2 (1%)†

*N = 237
†N = 187

METASTATIC • SUBSEQUENT THERAPY
ESOPHAGEAL CANCER REGIMEN: RAMUCIRUMAB + PACLITAXEL

FDA and EMA prescribing information
Wilke H et al. Lancet Oncol 2014;15:1224–1235
Supplement to: Wilke H et al. Lancet Oncol 2014;15:1224–1235

Prophylaxis for infusion-related reaction from ramucirumab:
   Diphenhydramine 50 mg; administer intravenously, 30–60 minutes before each
   ramucirumab dose (note diphenhydramine is also indicated for prophylaxis with paclitaxel,
   as described below), *plus*
   Acetaminophen 650 –1000 mg; administer orally, 30–60 minutes before ramucirumab
   (only if history of grade 1–2 infusion reaction), *plus*
   Dexamethasone 8 mg; administer orally or intravenously, 30–60 minutes before
   ramucirumab (only if history of grade 1–2 infusion reaction; note dexamethasone is also
   indicated for prophylaxis with paclitaxel as described below)

Ramucirumab 8 mg/kg/dose; administer intravenously in 250 mL of 0.9% sodium
chloride injection (0.9% NS) over 1 hour for 2 doses on days 1 and 15, prior to paclitaxel,
every 28 days, until disease progression (total dosage/28-day cycle = 16 mg/kg)

• Administration of ramucirumab with an administration set that contains a low-protein-
  binding in-line or add-on filter with pore size of 0.22 μm is recommended
• Flush the line with 0.9% NS following completion of the ramucirumab infusion

Prophylaxis for infusion-related reaction from paclitaxel:
   Diphenhydramine 50 mg; administer intravenously 30–60 minutes before each paclitaxel
   dose (note diphenhydramine is also indicated for prophylaxis with ramucirumab as described
   above), *plus:*
   Dexamethasone 10 mg; administer intravenously 30–60 minutes before each paclitaxel dose,
   plus:
   Cimetidine 300 mg (or **ranitidine** 50 mg, or **famotidine** 20 mg, or an equivalent
   histamine receptor [H$_2$]-subtype antagonist); administer intravenously over 15–30 minutes,
   30–60 minutes before each paclitaxel dose

Paclitaxel 80 mg/m^2/dose; administer intravenously in a volume of 0.9% NS or 5% dextrose
injection (D5W) sufficient to produce a concentration within the range 0.3–1.2 mg/mL over
1 hour for 3 doses on day 1, 8, and 15, every 28 days, until disease progression (total
dosage/28-day cycle = 240 mg/m^2)

• *Note:* Administer paclitaxel after ramucirumab on days when both medications are scheduled

Supportive Care
Antiemetic prophylaxis
Emetogenic potential on days 1, 8, and 15 is **LOW**
See Chapter 39 for antiemetic recommendations

Hematopoietic growth factor (CSF) prophylaxis
Primary prophylaxis is **NOT** *indicated*
See Chapter 43 for more information

Antimicrobial prophylaxis
Risk of fever and neutropenia is **LOW**
   Antimicrobial primary prophylaxis to be considered:
   • Antibacterial—not indicated
   • Antifungal—not indicated
   • Antiviral—not indicated unless patient previously had an episode of HSV

Patient Population Studied

The international, multicenter, randomized, placebo-controlled, double-blind, phase 3 trial (RAINBOW) involved 665 patients with metastatic or non-resectable, locally advanced gastric or gastroesophageal junction adenocarcinoma and disease progression on or within 4 months after first-line chemotherapy (platinum and fluoropyrimidine doublet with or without anthracycline). Eligible patients were aged ≥18 years and had Eastern Cooperative Oncology Group (ECOG) performance status score ≤1. Patients with squamous or undifferentiated gastric cancer; gastrointestinal perforation, fistulae, or any arterial thromboembolic event within 6 months before randomization; any significant bleeding or any significant venous thromboembolism within 3 months before randomization; or poorly controlled hypertension were ineligible. Patients were randomly assigned (1:1) to receive 28-day cycles of intravenous ramucirumab (8 mg/kg on days 1 and 15) and paclitaxel (80 mg/m^2 on days 1, 8, and 15) or placebo (on days 1 and 15) and paclitaxel (80 mg/m^2 on days 1, 8, and 15)

Efficacy (N = 665)

	Ramucirumab and Paclitaxel (n = 330)	Placebo and Paclitaxel (n = 335)	
Median overall survival	9.6 months	7.4 months	HR 0.807, 95% CI 0.678–0.962; P = 0.017
Median progression-free survival	4.4 months	2.9 months	HR 0.635, 95% CI 0.536–0.752; P<0.0001
Objective response rate*	28%	16%	P = 0.0001
Disease control rate†	80%	64%	P<0.0001

Objective response rate included patients with complete or partial response, as assessed by investigators according to RECIST version 1.1
†*Disease control rate* included complete response, partial response, or stable disease
Note: Median duration of follow-up was 7.9 months

Therapy Monitoring

1. *Before the start of a cycle:* CBC with differential, serum electrolytes, BUN, creatinine, bilirubin, AST or ALT, and alkaline phosphatase
2. *Once per week:* CBC with differential and platelet count
3. Blood pressure every 2 weeks or more frequently as indicated during treatment
4. *Prior to each dose of ramucirumab:* Assess proteinuria by urine dipstick and/or urinary protein creatinine ratio. Patients with a ≥2+ urine dipstick reading should undergo further assessment with a 24-hour urine collection
5. Observe closely for hypersensitivity reactions, especially during the first and second infusions
6. *Every 2–3 months:* Imaging to assess response

Treatment Modifications

RAMUCIRUMAB DOSE MODIFICATIONS

Starting dose	8 mg/kg
Dose level −1	6 mg/kg
Dose level −2	5 mg/kg

Adverse Event	Treatment Modification
G1/2 infusion-related reaction	Stop ramucirumab. Administer dexamethasone intravenously at commonly used antiemetic doses of 8–20 mg (or equivalent) and acetaminophen, then resume infusion at 50% of previous rate. Use the 50% infusion rate for all subsequent administrations
Prior G1/2 infusion-related reaction	Pre-medicate with dexamethasone intravenously at commonly used antiemetic doses of 8–20 mg (or equivalent), acetaminophen, and diphenhydramine 50 mg intravenously prior to each subsequent ramucirumab infusion
G3/4 infusion-related reaction	Permanently discontinue ramucirumab
G3/4 hypertension (SBP ≥160 mm Hg or DBP ≥100 mm Hg; medical intervention indicated; >1 drug or more intensive therapy than previously used indicated; or worse)	Interrupt ramucirumab until controlled with medical management then resume ramucirumab; if unable to control with medical management, discontinue ramucirumab
Reversible posterior leukoencephalopathy syndrome (RPLS)	Permanently discontinue ramucirumab

(continued)

Adverse Events (N = 656)

Grade (%)*	Ramucirumab and Paclitaxel (n = 327)		Placebo and Paclitaxel (n = 329)	
	Grade 1–2	Grade ≥3	Grade 1–2	Grade ≥3
Fatigue	45	12	38	5
Neutropenia	14	41	12	19
Neuropathy	38	8	32	5
Decreased appetite	37	3	28	4
Abdominal pain	30	6	26	3
Nausea	33	2	30	2
Anemia	26	9	26	10
Leukopenia	17	17	14	7
Alopecia	33	0	38	<1
Diarrhea	29	4	22	2
Epistaxis	31	0	7	0
Vomiting	24	3	17	4
Peripheral edema	24	2	13	<1

(continued)

Treatment Modifications (continued)

Urine protein ≥2 g/24 hours	Interrupt ramucirumab. Reinitiate treatment reduced by one dose level once the urine protein level returns to <2 g/24 hours
Reoccurrence of urine protein ≥2 g/24 hours	Interrupt ramucirumab. Reinitiate treatment reduced by one dose level once the urine protein level returns to <2 g/24 hours
Urine protein >3 g/24 hours or nephrotic syndrome	Permanently discontinue ramucirumab
Anticipated wound healing	Stop ramucirumab ≥4 weeks prior to a scheduled surgery until wound is fully healed; discontinue ramucirumab if patient develops wound healing complications
G3/4 bleeding, arterial thromboembolic event, gastrointestinal perforation	Permanently discontinue ramucirumab
G3/4 fatigue/asthenia	Interrupt ramucirumab. Reinstitute treatment at a reduced dose once toxicity is G1
G3/4 stomatitis/mucosal inflammation	

WEEKLY PACLITAXEL DOSE MODIFICATIONS

Paclitaxel starting dose	80 mg/m²
Paclitaxel dose level −1	70 mg/m²
Paclitaxel dose level −2	60 mg/m²

Adverse Event	Treatment Modifications
Febrile neutropenia (ANC <1000/mm³ with temperature >38°C or >100.4°F), or ANC <1000/mm³ for ≥7 days	Reduce paclitaxel dose by 10 mg/m² and consider adding filgrastim in subsequent cycles, if applicable
Febrile neutropenia (ANC <1000/mm³ with temperature >38°C or >100.4°F), or ANC <1000/mm³ for ≥7 days despite dose reduction of 10 mg/m²	Administer filgrastim in subsequent cycles. If already administering filgrastim, reduce paclitaxel dose an additional 10 mg/m²
Platelet nadir <50,000/mm³, or platelets <100,000/mm³ for ≥7 days	Reduce paclitaxel dose by one level
ANC <800/mm³ or platelets <50,000/mm³ at the start of a cycle	Hold treatment until ANC >800/mm³ and platelets >50,000/mm³, then resume with weekly paclitaxel dosage reduced by 10 mg/m²
G2 motor or sensory neuropathies	Reduce weekly paclitaxel dosage by 10 mg/m² without interrupting planned treatment
Other nonhematologic adverse events G2/3	Hold treatment until adverse events resolve to <G1, then resume with weekly paclitaxel dosage reduced by 10 mg/m²
Patients who cannot tolerate paclitaxel at 60 mg/m² per week	Discontinue treatment
Treatment delay >2 weeks	Decrease weekly paclitaxel dosage by 10 mg/m² or consider discontinuing treatment

Adverse Events (N = 656) (continued)

Grade (%)*	Ramucirumab and Paclitaxel (n = 327)		Placebo and Paclitaxel (n = 329)	
	Grade 1–2	Grade ≥3	Grade 1-2	Grade ≥3
Constipation	21	0	21	<1
Stomatitis	19	<1	7	<1
Pyrexia	17	<1	11	<1
Proteinuria	15	1	6	0
Malignant neoplasm progression	2	14	<1	18
Weight decreased	12	2	14	1
Thrombocytopenia	12	2	4	2
Rash	13	0	9	0
Dyspnea	10	2	9	<1
Cough	12	0	8	0
Back pain	11	1	11	2
Hypoalbuminemia	10	1	4	<1
Ascites	6	4	4	4
Myalgia	10	0	10	<1
Headache	10	0	6	<1

*According to the National Cancer Institute Common Terminology Criteria for Adverse Events, version 4.02
Note: Treatment-emergent toxicities that occurred in ≥10% of patients in the ramucirumab plus paclitaxel group are included in the table, irrespective of causality. Treatment-emergent adverse events leading to death occurred in 12% of the ramucirumab plus paclitaxel group and 16% of the placebo plus paclitaxel group; in each group, 2% of patients experienced an adverse event leading to death with a causal relation to any study drug

METASTATIC • SUBSEQUENT THERAPY

ESOPHAGEAL CANCER REGIMEN: PEMBROLIZUMAB

Fuchs CS et al. JAMA Oncol 2018;4:e180013
Supplement 1 to: Fuchs CS et al. JAMA Oncol 2018;4:e180013
Supplement 2 to: Fuchs CS et al. JAMA Oncol 2018;4:e180013
Shah MA et al. J Clin Oncol 2019;37:4010

- **Pembrolizumab** 200 mg; administer intravenously over 30 minutes in a volume of 0.9% sodium chloride injection (0.9% NS) or 5% dextrose injection (D5W) sufficient to produce a pembrolizumab concentration within the range 1–10 mg/mL every 3 weeks until disease progression for up to 24 months (total dosage/3-week cycle = 200 mg)
- Alternative pembrolizumab dose and schedule as per the U.S. FDA regimens approved on April 28, 2020:
- **Pembrolizumab** 400 mg; administer intravenously over 30 minutes in a volume of 0.9% NS or D5W sufficient to produce a pembrolizumab concentration within the range 1–10 mg/mL every 6 weeks for up to 24 months (total dose/6-week cycle = 400 mg)
- Administer pembrolizumab with an administration set that contains a sterile, nonpyrogenic, low-protein-binding in-line or add-on filter with pore size within the range of 0.2–5 μm

Pembrolizumab can cause severe or life-threatening infusion-related reactions, including hypersensitivity and anaphylaxis

Patients who achieved a confirmed complete response after receiving at least 8 cycles of pembrolizumab could discontinue treatment after receiving 2 doses beyond the determination of complete response

Supportive Care
Antiemetic prophylaxis
Emetogenic potential is **MINIMAL**
See Chapter 42 for antiemetic recommendations

Hematopoietic growth factor (CSF) prophylaxis
Primary prophylaxis is **NOT** *indicated*
See Chapter 43 for more information

(continued)

Patient Population Studied

Cohort 1 of the international, multicenter, open-label, single-arm, multicohort (3-cohort), phase 2 trial (KEYNOTE–059) involved 259 patients with histologically or cytologically confirmed recurrent or metastatic gastric or gastroesophageal junction adenocarcinoma (only Siewert types II and III) incurable by locally approved therapies. Eligible patients were aged ≥18 years, had disease progression after 2 or more prior chemotherapy regimens that included a fluoropyrimidine and a platinum doublet, had human epidermal growth factor receptor 2/neu-negative disease (or human epidermal growth factor receptor 2/neu-positive disease if previously treated with trastuzumab), had Eastern Cooperative Oncology Group (ECOG) performance score status ≤1, and had life expectancy ≥3 months. Patients received pembrolizumab monotherapy infusion (200 mg over 30 minutes) on day 1 of every 3-week cycle for up to 35 cycles

The phase 3 KEYNOTE–181 study compared pembrolizumab versus chemo as second-line therapy for patients with advanced SCC and ACC of the esophagus. Patients were randomized to pembrolizumab 200 mg on day 1 of every 3-week cycle for up to 2 years versus investigator choice of chemotherapy (paclitaxel, docetaxel, or irinotecan). In CPS PD-L1 ≥10 for SCC, median OS was 10.3 months versus 6.7 months, leading to FDA approval for pembrolizumab in advanced CPS ≥10 SCC with disease progression after ≥1 line of systemic therapy

Efficacy (N = 259)

Objective response rate*	11.6%
Duration of response	8.4 months
Disease control rate†	27.0%
Median progression-free survival	2.0 months
Median overall survival	5.6 months

Objective response rate was the primary efficacy end point and included patients with complete or partial response, as per RECIST version 1.1 by central review
†*Disease control rate* included complete response, partial response, or stable disease for ≥2 months
Note: Median duration of follow-up was 5.8 months. In total, 2.3% experienced a complete response

Therapy Monitoring

1. Initially at the time of each dose, and eventually every 6–12 weeks, perform a total body skin examination with attention to *all* mucous membranes as well as a complete review of systems
2. Monitor patients for signs and symptoms of pneumonitis. Evaluate patients with suspected pneumonitis with chest x-ray, CT scan, and pulse oximetry. For toxicity G ≥2, may include nasal swab, sputum culture and sensitivity, blood culture and sensitivity, and urine culture and sensitivity
3. Monitor patients for signs and symptoms of colitis. Encourage patients to report diarrhea immediately to any member of the healthcare team
4. Draw AST, ALT, and bilirubin prior to each infusion and/or weekly if there are G1 LFT elevations. *Note:* No treatment is recommended for G1 LFT abnormalities. For toxicity G ≥2, work up for other causes of elevated LFTs, including viral hepatitis
5. Use basic metabolic panel (Na, K, CO_2, glucose) and patient history as screening tools for hypophysitis, including hypopituitarism and adrenal insufficiency. If in doubt, evaluate morning adrenocorticotropic hormone (ACTH) and cortisol levels. Consider ACTH stimulation test for indeterminate results
6. Assess thyroid function at the start of treatment, periodically during treatment, and as indicated based on clinical evaluation, and for clinical signs and symptoms of thyroid disorders. Test for TSH and free thyroxine (FT4) every 4–6 weeks as part of routine clinical monitoring on therapy or for case detection in symptomatic patients
7. Measure glucose at baseline and with each treatment during the first 12 weeks and every 6 weeks thereafter

(continued)

(continued)

Antimicrobial prophylaxis
Risk of fever and neutropenia is **LOW**
Antimicrobial primary prophylaxis to be considered:
- Antibacterial—not indicated
- Antifungal—not indicated
- Antiviral—not indicated unless patient previously had an episode of HSV

Therapy Monitoring *(continued)*

8. Obtain a serum creatinine level prior to every dose. If creatinine is found to be newly elevated, consider holding therapy while other potential causes are evaluated. *Note:* Routine urinalysis is not necessary other than to rule out urinary tract infections, etc

9. Obtain a complete rheumatologic history and perform an examination of all peripheral joints for tenderness, swelling, and range of motion. Examine the spine. Consider plain x-ray/imaging to exclude metastases and evaluate joint damage (erosions), if appropriate

10. In patients at high risk for infections and in appropriately selected patients based on an infectious disease evaluation, draw screening laboratories (HIV, hepatitis A and B, and blood QuantiFERON for TB) to prepare patients to start infliximab

11. Response evaluation: Every 2–4 months

Treatment Modifications

RECOMMENDED DOSAGE MODIFICATIONS FOR PEMBROLIZUMAB

Adverse Event	Grade/Severity	Treatment Modification
Infusion reaction	Clinically significant but not severe infusion reaction	Interrupt the infusion in patients with clinically significant infusion reactions and consider resuming at a slower rate following resolution. If decision is made to restart, begin at ≤50% of the rate prior to the reaction and increase in 50% increments every 30 minutes if well tolerated. Infusions may be restarted at the full rate during the next cycle
	G3/4 (severe infusion reaction—pyrexia, chills, flushing, hypotension, dyspnea, wheezing, back pain, abdominal pain, and urticaria). Not rapidly responsive to brief interruption of infusion	Stop infusion and administer appropriate medical therapy (eg, epinephrine, corticosteroids, intravenous antihistamines, bronchodilators, and/or oxygen). Discontinue pembrolizumab
Colitis	G1	Loperamide 4 mg as starting dose, then 2 mg before each meal and after each loose stool until without diarrhea for 12 hours, with maximum of 16 mg loperamide per day. If G1 diarrhea or colitis persists >14 days, add prednisolone 0.5–1 mg/kg (non-enteric-coated) or consider oral budesonide 9 mg daily if no bloody diarrhea
	G2/3 diarrhea or colitis	Withhold pembrolizumab. Loperamide 4 mg as starting dose, then 2 mg before each meal and after each loose stool until without diarrhea for 12 hours, with maximum of 16 mg loperamide per day. Administer oral prednisone/prednisolone at a dose of 0.5–2 mg/kg per day or its equivalent. When symptoms improve to G1, begin a slow corticosteroid taper over at least 4 weeks. Resume pembrolizumab upon symptom control, or when prednisone/prednisolone daily dosage <10 mg
	G4 diarrhea or colitis	Permanently discontinue pembrolizumab. Loperamide 4 mg as starting dose, then 2 mg before each meal and after each loose stool until without diarrhea for 12 hours, with maximum of 16 mg loperamide per day. Administer 1–2 mg/kg intravenous (methyl)prednisolone and convert to 0.5–2 mg/kg prednisone/prednisolone orally each day or its equivalent only after a response. Taper over at least 4 weeks when symptoms improve. If symptoms do not improve over 72 hours or worsen, perform flexible sigmoidoscopy/colonoscopy to document colitis, then begin infliximab 5 mg/kg (if no perforation, sepsis, TB, hepatitis, NYHA III/IV CHF). If no response, add MMF 500–1000 mg twice daily. If worse on MMF, consider addition of tacrolimus or ATG

(continued)

Treatment Modifications (*continued*)

RECOMMENDED DOSAGE MODIFICATIONS FOR PEMBROLIZUMAB

Adverse Event	Grade/Severity	Treatment Modification
Pneumonitis	G2	Withhold pembrolizumab. Consider pneumocystis prophylaxis depending on the clinical context and coverage with empiric antibiotics. Administer oral prednisone/prednisolone at a dose of 1–2 mg/kg per day or its equivalent. When symptoms improve to G1, begin a slow corticosteroid taper over at least 4 weeks. If response is not adequate after 48 hours, administer 2–4 mg/kg intravenous (methyl)prednisolone and convert to 0.5–2 mg/kg prednisone/prednisolone orally each day or its equivalent only after a response, followed by a taper over at least 6 weeks when symptoms improve to G1, titrating to symptoms. Resume pembrolizumab upon symptom control, or when prednisone/prednisolone daily dosage <10 mg
	G3/4	Permanently discontinue pembrolizumab. Consider pneumocystis prophylaxis depending on the clinical context; cover with empiric antibiotics. Administer 2–4 mg/kg intravenous (methyl)prednisolone and convert to 1–2 mg/kg prednisone/prednisolone orally each day or its equivalent only after a response, followed by a taper over at least 8 weeks when symptoms improve to G1, titrating to symptoms. If, when initially treated, improvement does not occur within 48–72 hours, begin infliximab 5 mg/kg (if no perforation, sepsis, TB, hepatitis, NYHA III/IV CHF). If no response to infliximab, add MMF 500–1000 mg twice daily. Consider MMF especially if concurrent hepatic toxicity
Hepatitis	G2 (AST or ALT >3–5× ULN or total bilirubin >1.5–3× ULN)	Withhold pembrolizumab. Administer oral prednisone/prednisolone at a dose of 1–2 mg/kg per day or its equivalent. When symptoms improve to G1, begin a slow corticosteroid taper over at least 4 weeks. Resume pembrolizumab upon symptom control, or when prednisone/prednisolone daily dosage <10 mg
	G3/4 (AST or ALT >5× ULN or total bilirubin >3× ULN)	Permanently discontinue pembrolizumab. Administer 1–2 mg/kg intravenous (methyl)prednisolone and convert to 0.5–2 mg/kg prednisone/prednisolone orally each day or its equivalent only after a response. Taper over at least 6 weeks when symptoms improve. If no response, add MMF 500–1000 mg twice daily. If worse on MMF, consider adding tacrolimus or ATG
Hypophysitis	G2/3 (moderate symptoms, ie, headache but no visual disturbance or fatigue/mood alteration but hemodynamically stable, no electrolyte disturbance)	Administer analgesia as needed for headache. Withhold pembrolizumab. Administer oral prednisone/prednisolone at a dosage of 0.5–2 mg/kg per day or its equivalent. When symptoms improve to G1, begin a slow corticosteroid taper over at least 4 weeks. If no improvement in 48 hours, administer 1–2 mg/kg intravenous (methyl)prednisolone and convert to 0.5–2 mg/kg prednisone/prednisolone orally each day or its equivalent only after a response. Taper over at least 4 weeks when symptoms improve to 5 mg prednisone/prednisolone or equivalent; do not stop steroids. Resume pembrolizumab upon symptom control, or when prednisone/prednisolone daily dosage <10 mg
	G4 (severe mass effect symptoms, ie, severe headache, any visual disturbance or severe hypoadrenalism, ie, hypotension, severe electrolyte disturbance)	Permanently discontinue pembrolizumab. Administer analgesia as needed for headache. Administer 1–2 mg/kg intravenous (methyl)prednisolone and convert to 0.5–2 mg/kg prednisone/prednisolone orally each day or its equivalent only after a response. Taper over at least 4 weeks when symptoms improve to 5 mg prednisone/prednisolone or equivalent; do not stop steroids
Adrenal insufficiency	G2	Withhold pembrolizumab. Administer oral prednisone/prednisolone at a dosage of 0.5–2 mg/kg per day or its equivalent. When symptoms improve to G1, begin a slow corticosteroid taper over at least 4 weeks. Serially assess adrenal function and continue steroids at replacement doses (20–40 mg hydrocortisone daily ~2/3 dose in morning upon awakening and ~1/3 at 4 PM) until recovery of adrenal function is documented. Resume pembrolizumab upon symptom control, or when prednisone/prednisolone daily dosage <10 mg
	G3/4	Permanently discontinue pembrolizumab. Administer oral prednisone/prednisolone at a dosage of 0.5–2 mg/kg per day or its equivalent. When symptoms improve to G1, begin a slow corticosteroid taper over at least 4 weeks. Serially assess adrenal function and continue steroids at replacement doses (20–40 mg hydrocortisone daily ~2/3 dose in morning upon awakening and ~1/3 at 4 PM) until recovery of adrenal function is documented

(*continued*)

Treatment Modifications (continued)

RECOMMENDED DOSAGE MODIFICATIONS FOR PEMBROLIZUMAB

Adverse Event	Grade/Severity	Treatment Modification
Type 1 diabetes mellitus	G3 hyperglycemia	Withhold pembrolizumab. Admit to hospital to manage hyperglycemia. Role of corticosteroids in preventing complete loss of insulin-producing cells is unknown and use is not recommended. Resume pembrolizumab upon symptom control, or when prednisone/prednisolone daily dosage <10 mg
	G4 hyperglycemia	Permanently discontinue pembrolizumab. Admit to hospital to manage hyperglycemia. Role of corticosteroids in preventing complete loss of insulin-producing cells is unknown and use is not recommended
Nephritis and renal dysfunction	G2/3 (serum creatinine 1.5–6× ULN)	Withhold pembrolizumab. Administer oral prednisone/prednisolone at a dose of 0.5–2 mg/kg per day or its equivalent. When symptoms improve to G1, begin a slow corticosteroid taper over at least 4 weeks. If response is not adequate, administer 0.5–1 mg/kg intravenous (methyl)prednisolone and convert to 0.5–2 mg/kg prednisone/prednisolone orally each day or its equivalent only after a response, followed by a taper over at least 4 weeks when symptoms improve to G1. Resume pembrolizumab upon symptom control, or when prednisone/prednisolone daily dosage <10 mg
	G4 (serum creatinine >6× ULN)	Permanently discontinue pembrolizumab. Administer 0.5–1 mg/kg intravenous (methyl)prednisolone and convert to 0.5–2 mg/kg prednisone/prednisolone orally each day or its equivalent only after a response, followed by a taper over at least 4 weeks when symptoms improve to G1
Skin	G1/2	Continue pembrolizumab. Avoid skin irritants, avoid sun exposure; topical emollients recommended. Topical steroid (mild strength for G1, moderate/potent strength for G2) cream once or twice daily ± oral or topical antihistamines for itching
	G3 rash or suspected SJS or TEN	Withhold pembrolizumab. Avoid skin irritants, avoid sun exposure; topical emollients recommended. Administer oral or topical antihistamines for itching. Administer oral prednisone/prednisolone at a dose of 0.5–2 mg/kg or its equivalent daily for 3 days followed by a slow corticosteroid taper over at least 4 weeks when the rash improves to G1. If rash does not respond adequately, administer 0.5–1 mg/kg intravenous (methyl)prednisolone and convert to 0.5–2 mg/kg prednisone/prednisolone orally each day or its equivalent only after a response, followed by a taper over at least 4 weeks when the rash improves to G1. Resume pembrolizumab upon symptom control, or when prednisone/prednisolone daily dosage <10 mg
	G4 rash or confirmed SJS or TEN	Avoid skin irritants, avoid sun exposure; topical emollients recommended. Administer oral or topical antihistamines for itching. Administer 1–2 mg/kg intravenous (methyl)prednisolone and convert to oral steroids 0.5–2 mg/kg prednisone/prednisolone each day or its equivalent only after a response. Taper over at least 4 weeks when the rash improves to G1. Permanently discontinue pembrolizumab
Encephalitis	Confusion or altered behavior, headaches, alteration in Glasgow Coma Scale, motor or sensory deficits, speech abnormality; may or may not be febrile	Initially withhold pembrolizumab, but permanently discontinue pembrolizumab if there is no doubt as to diagnosis. Exclude bacterial and ideally viral infections prior to high-dose steroids. Administer oral prednisone/prednisolone at a dosage of 0.5–2 mg/kg per day or its equivalent. When symptoms improve, begin a slow corticosteroid taper over at least 4–8 weeks. If symptoms are severe, administer 1–2 mg/kg intravenous (methyl)prednisolone and convert to 0.5–2 mg/kg prednisone/prednisolone orally each day or its equivalent only after a response. Consider concurrent empiric antiviral (intravenous acyclovir) and antibacterial therapy
Aseptic meningitis	Headache, photophobia, neck stiffness with fever, or may be afebrile, vomiting; normal cognition/cerebral function (distinguishes from encephalitis)	
Other syndromes include neurosarcoidosis, posterior reversible leukoencephalopathy syndrome (PRES), Vogt-Harada-Koyanagi syndrome, demyelination, vasculitic encephalopathy, and generalized seizures		
Transverse myelitis	Acute or subacute neurologic signs/symptoms of motor, sensory, autonomic origin; most have sensory level; often bilateral symptoms	Initially withhold pembrolizumab, but permanently discontinue pembrolizumab if there is no doubt as to diagnosis. Administer 2 mg/kg intravenous (methyl)prednisolone or consider 1 g/day and convert to 0.5–2 mg/kg prednisone/prednisolone orally each day or its equivalent only after a response. When symptoms improve, begin a slow corticosteroid taper over at least 4–8 weeks. Plasmapheresis may be required if steroids do not bring about improvement

(continued)

Treatment Modifications (*continued*)

RECOMMENDED DOSAGE MODIFICATIONS FOR PEMBROLIZUMAB

Adverse Event	Grade/Severity	Treatment Modification
Myocarditis	G3	Permanently discontinue pembrolizumab. Administer 2 mg/kg intravenous (methyl) prednisolone or consider 1 g/day and convert to 0.5–2 mg/kg prednisone/prednisolone orally each day or its equivalent only after a response. When symptoms improve, begin a slow corticosteroid taper over at least 4–8 weeks. If no response, add MMF 500–1000 mg twice daily. If worse on MMF, consider adding tacrolimus
Peripheral neurologic toxicity	Moderate: some interference with ADL, symptoms concerning to patient	Withhold pembrolizumab. Initial observation reasonable or initiate prednisone/prednisolone 0.5–1 mg/kg (if progressing, eg, from mild) and/or pregabalin or duloxetine for pain. When symptoms improve, begin a slow corticosteroid taper over at least 4 weeks. Resume pembrolizumab upon symptom control, or when prednisone/prednisolone daily dosage <10 mg
	Severe: limits self-care and aids warranted, life-threatening, eg, respiratory problems	Permanently discontinue pembrolizumab. Administer 1–2 mg/kg intravenous (methyl) prednisolone and convert to 0.5–2 mg/kg prednisone/prednisolone orally each day or its equivalent only after a response. Taper over at least 4–8 weeks when symptoms improve to G1
Guillain-Barré syndrome	Progressive symmetrical muscle weakness with absent or reduced tendon reflexes—involves extremities; facial, respiratory, and bulbar and oculomotor muscles; dysregulation of autonomic nerves	Permanently discontinue pembrolizumab. Use of steroids not recommended in idiopathic Guillain-Barré syndrome; however, a trial of (methyl)prednisolone 1–2 mg/kg is reasonable, converting to 0.5–2 mg/kg prednisone/prednisolone orally each day or its equivalent only after a response. If no improvement or worsening, plasmapheresis or IVIG is indicated
Myasthenia gravis	Fluctuating muscle weakness (proximal limb, trunk, ocular, eg, ptosis/diplopia or bulbar) with fatigability; respiratory muscles may also be involved	Permanently discontinue pembrolizumab. Administer pyridostigmine at an initial dose of 30 mg 3 times daily. Administer oral prednisone/prednisolone at a dosage of 0.5–2 mg/kg per day or its equivalent or 1–2 mg/kg intravenous (methyl)prednisolone, depending on the severity of symptoms. If treatment begins with intravenous drug, convert to 0.5–2 mg/kg prednisone/prednisolone orally each day or its equivalent only after a response. If no improvement or worsening, plasmapheresis or IVIG may be considered. Additional immunosuppressants used in myasthenia gravis include azathioprine, cyclosporine, and mycophenolate. Avoid certain medications, e.g. ciprofloxacin, beta blockers, that may precipitate cholinergic crisis
Other syndromes, including motor and sensory peripheral neuropathy, multifocal radicular neuropathy/plexopathy, autonomic neuropathy, phrenic nerve palsy, cranial nerve palsies (eg, facial nerve, optic nerve, hypoglossal nerve)		Permanently discontinue pembrolizumab. Administer oral prednisone/prednisolone at a dosage of 0.5–2 mg/kg per day or its equivalent or 1–2 mg/kg intravenous (methyl)prednisolone, depending on the severity of symptoms. If treatment begins with intravenous drug, convert to 0.5–2 mg/kg prednisone/prednisolone orally each day or its equivalent only after a response
Arthralgia	G1 (mild pain with inflammation, erythema, or joint swelling)	Continue pembrolizumab. Administer acetaminophen (paracetamol) and ibuprofen
	G2 (moderate pain with inflammation, erythema, or joint swelling that limits ADLs)	Withhold pembrolizumab. Administer higher doses of acetaminophen (paracetamol) and ibuprofen and use diclofenac or naproxen or etoricoxib. If inadequately controlled, consider intra-articular steroid injections for large joints or administer oral prednisone/prednisolone at a dosage of 0.5–2 mg/kg per day or its equivalent. When symptoms improve to G1, begin a slow corticosteroid taper over at least 4 weeks. If response is not adequate, administer 0.5–1 mg/kg intravenous (methyl)prednisolone and convert to 0.5–2 mg/kg prednisone/prednisolone orally each day or its equivalent only after a response, followed by a taper over at least 4 weeks when symptoms improve to G1. Resume pembrolizumab upon symptom control, or when prednisone/prednisolone daily dosage <10 mg
	G3 (severe pain; irreversible joint damage; disabling; limits self-care ADLs)	Withhold pembrolizumab. Administer 0.5–1 mg/kg intravenous (methyl)prednisolone and convert to 0.5–2 mg/kg prednisone/prednisolone orally each day or its equivalent only after a response, followed by a taper over at least 4 weeks when symptoms improve to G1. In severe cases, infliximab or another anti–TNF-alpha drug may be required for improvement of arthritis. Resume pembrolizumab upon symptom control, or when prednisone/prednisolone daily dosage <10 mg

(*continued*)

Treatment Modifications (continued)

RECOMMENDED DOSAGE MODIFICATIONS FOR PEMBROLIZUMAB

Adverse Event	Grade/Severity	Treatment Modification
Other	First occurrence of other G3	Withhold pembrolizumab. Administer oral prednisone/prednisolone at a dosage of 0.5–2 mg/kg per day or its equivalent. When symptoms improve to G1, begin a slow corticosteroid taper over at least 4 weeks. Resume pembrolizumab upon symptom control, or when prednisone/prednisolone daily dosage <10 mg
	Recurrence of same G3	Permanently discontinue pembrolizumab. Administer 1–2 mg/kg intravenous (methyl) prednisolone and convert to 0.5–2 mg/kg prednisone/prednisolone orally each day or its equivalent only after a response. Taper over at least 4–8 weeks when symptoms improve to G1
	Life-threatening or G4	
	Requirement for ≥10 mg/day prednisone or equivalent for >12 weeks	Permanently discontinue pembrolizumab
	Persistent G2/3 adverse reactions lasting ≥12 weeks	

ADL, activities of daily living; ALT, alanine aminotransferase; AST, aspartate aminotransferase; ATG, anti-thymocyte globulin; NYHA, New York Heart Association; SJS, Stevens-Johnson syndrome; TEN, toxic epidermal necrolysis; ULN, upper limit of normal

Notes on general supportive care:

- Steroid taper in most cases will proceed over a minimum of 1 month, but if symptoms improve rapidly, a 2-week taper can be considered. If steroids are administered for more than 4 weeks, consider PCP prophylaxis (cotrimoxazole 480 mg twice daily M/W/F or inhaled pentamidine if cotrimoxazole allergy), regular random blood glucose, vitamin D level, and starting calcium/vitamin D supplementation per guidelines

Notes on pregnancy and breastfeeding:

- Pembrolizumab can cause fetal harm. If used during pregnancy, or if the patient becomes pregnant during treatment, apprise the patient of the potential hazard to a fetus. Females of reproductive potential should use highly effective contraception during treatment and for 4 months after the last dose of pembrolizumab
- It is not known whether pembrolizumab is excreted in human milk. Therefore, it is recommended that women discontinue nursing during treatment with and for 4 months after the final dose of pembrolizumab

Adverse Events (N = 259)

Grade (%)*	Grade 1/2	Grade 3	Grade 4/5
Fatigue	17	2	0
Pruritus	9	0	0
Rash	8	<1	0
Hypothyroidism	7	<1	0
Decreased appetite	7	0	0
Anemia	4	3	0
Nausea	6	<1	0
Diarrhea	5	1	0
Arthralgia	5	<1	0

*According to the National Cancer Institute Common Terminology Criteria for Adverse Events, version 4.0
Note: Treatment-related toxicities that occurred in ≥5% are included in the table. In total, 60.2% of patients experienced at least 1 treatment-related toxicity of any grade and 17.8% of patients experienced at least 1 G ≥3 treatment-related toxicity. Treatment discontinuation owing to treatment-related adverse events was reported for 0.8%. Deaths considered by the investigator to have been related to treatment were reported for 0.8% (1 death as a result of acute kidney injury and 1 as a result of pleural effusion)

16. Gastric Cancer

Jonas W. Feilchenfeldt, MD, and Manish A. Shah, MD

Epidemiology

Incidence: 27,600 estimated new cases for 2020 in United States
Male: 16,980; Female: 10,620
9.3 per 100,000 male, 5.3 per 100,000 female (2016 figures)
The incidence of gastric cancer varies with different geographic regions
Deaths: Estimated 11,010 in 2020 (male: 6650; female: 4360)
Median age: 68 years
Male to female ratio: ~2:1

Stage at Presentation

Localized	28%
Regional	26%
Distant	36%
Unknown	10%

Kamangar F et al. J Clin Oncol 2006;24:2137–2150
Siegel R et al. CA Cancer J Clin 2020;70:7–30
Surveillance, Epidemiology and End Results (SEER) Program, available from http://seer.cancer.gov [accessed in 2020]

Work-up

1. Multidisciplinary evaluation
2. History and physical examination
3. CBC and chemistry profile
4. CT abdomen with contrast; CT/ultrasound pelvis in women
5. Chest imaging*
6. Esophagogastroduodenoscopy (EGD)
7. PET-CT or PET scan (optional)
8. Endoscopic ultrasound (EUS) (optional)
9. *Helicobacter pylori* test[†] (optional)

*A combined CT scan of chest and abdomen is a pragmatic option
[†]Chey WD et al. Am J Gastroenterol 2007;102:1808–1825

Locoregional (stages cT1b–cT4a; cM0):
Laparoscopy is performed to evaluate for peritoneal spread when considering chemoradiation or surgery.
Laparoscopy is not indicated if a palliative resection is planned. Laparoscopy allows patients to be categorized into one of the following groups:
1. Medically fit (medically able to tolerate major abdominal surgery), potentially resectable
2. Medically fit (medically able to tolerate major abdominal surgery), unresectable
3. Medically unfit

Stage IV (cT4b; cM1):
1. No further work-up necessary
Note: PET-CT may have a role for monitoring chemotherapy response

Pathology

Stemmermann GN et al. Gastric cancer: pathology. In: Kelsen DP et al (editors). Gastrointestinal Oncology: Principles and Practice. Baltimore, MD: Lippincott Williams & Wilkins, 2008:257–274

Borrmann Classification
Based on gross appearance
Any of the 4 types may coexist
Type I:	Polypoid
Type II:	Fungating
Type III:	Ulcerated
Type IV:	Infiltrative

Lauren Classification
Pattern of local invasion based on histologic features
1. Intestinal: composed of cohesive neoplastic cells that form glands and tubular structures
2. Diffuse: scattered neoplastic cells that invade individually with minimal intercellular cohesion
3. Unclassified

World Health Organization Classification
1. Intraepithelial neoplasia—adenoma
2. Carcinoma
3. Adenocarcinoma (intestinal type, diffuse type)
4. Papillary adenocarcinoma
5. Tubular adenocarcinoma
6. Mucinous adenocarcinoma
7. Signet ring cell carcinoma
8. Adenosquamous carcinoma
9. Squamous cell carcinoma
10. Undifferentiated carcinoma
11. Others

Staging

Primary Tumor (T)

TX	Primary tumor cannot be assessed
T0	No evidence of primary tumor
Tis	Carcinoma in situ: intraepithelial tumor without invasion of the lamina propria, high-grade dysplasia
T1	Tumor invades lamina propria, muscularis mucosae, or submucosa
T1a	Tumor invades lamina propria or muscularis mucosae
T1b	Tumor invades submucosa
T2	Tumor invades muscularis propria*
T3	Tumor penetrates subserosal connective tissue without invasion of visceral peritoneum or adjacent structures†‡
T4	Tumor invades serosa (visceral peritoneum) or adjacent structures†‡
T4a	Tumor invades serosa (visceral peritoneum)
T4b	Tumor invades adjacent structures/organs

*A tumor may penetrate the muscularis propria with extension into the gastrocolic or gastrohepatic ligaments, or into the greater or lesser omentum, without perforation of the visceral peritoneum covering these structures. In this case, the tumor is classified T3. If there is perforation of the visceral peritoneum covering the gastric ligaments or the omentum, the tumor should be classified T4

†The adjacent structures of the stomach include the spleen, transverse colon, liver, diaphragm, pancreas, abdominal wall, adrenal gland, kidney, small intestine, and retroperitoneum

‡Intramural extension to the duodenum or esophagus is not considered invasion of an adjacent structure, but is classified using the depth of the greatest invasion in any of these sites

Regional Lymph Nodes (N)

NX	Regional lymph node(s) cannot be assessed
N0	No regional lymph node metastasis
N1	Metastasis in 1 to 2 regional lymph nodes
N2	Metastasis in 3 to 6 regional lymph nodes
N3	Metastasis in 7 or more regional lymph nodes
N3a	Metastasis in 7 to 15 regional lymph nodes
N3b	Metastasis in 16 or more regional lymph nodes

Distant Metastasis (M)

M0	No distant metastasis
M1	Distant metastasis

AJCC 8th Edition Prognostic Stage Groups: Clinical (cTNM)

Group	T	N	M
0	Tis	N0	M0
I	T1	N0	M0
I	T2	N0	M0
IIA	T1	N1	M0
	T1	N2	M0
	T1	N3	M0
	T2	N1	M0
	T2	N2	M0
	T2	N3	M0
IIB	T3	N0	M0
	T4a	N0	M0
III	T3	N1	M0
	T3	N2	M0
	T3	N3	M0
	T4a	N1	M0
	T4a	N2	M0
	T4a	N3	M0
IVA	T4b	Any N	M0
IVB	Any T	Any N	M1

AJCC 8th Edition Prognostic Stage Groups: Pathological (pTNM)

Group	T	N	M
0	Tis	N0	M0
IA	T1	N0	M0
IB	T2	N0	M0
	T1	N1	M0
IIA	T3	N0	M0
	T2	N1	M0
	T1	N2	M0
IIB	T4a	N0	M0
	T3	N1	M0
	T2	N2	M0
	T1	N3a	M0
IIIA	T4b	N0	M0
	T4a	N2	M0
	T4a	N1	M0
	T3	N2	M0
	T2	N3a	M0
IIIB	T4b	N2	M0
	T4b	N1	M0
	T4a	N3a	M0
	T3	N3a	M0
	T2	N3b	M0
	T1	N3b	M0
IIIC	T4b	N3b	M0
	T4b	N3a	M0
	T4a	N3b	M0
	T3	N3b	M0
IV	Any T	Any N	M1

AJCC 8th Edition Prognostic Stage Groups: Post-Neoadjuvant Therapy (ypTNM)

Group	T	N	M
I	T1	N0	M0
	T2	N0	M0
	T1	N1	M0
II	T3	N0	M0
	T2	N1	M0
	T1	N2	M0
	T4a	N0	M0
	T3	N1	M0
	T2	N2	M0
	T1	N3	M0
III	T4a	N1	M0
	T3	N2	M0
	T2	N3	M0
	T4b	N0	M0
	T4b	N1	M0
	T4a	N2	M0
	T3	N3	M0
	T4b	N2	M0
	T4b	N3	M0
	T4a	N3	M0
IV	Any T	Any N	M1

AJCC 8TH EDITION STAGING
Amin MB et al (editors). AJCC Cancer Staging Manual. 8th ed. New York: Springer; 2017

Treatment and Survival by Stage

Stage	Treatment	5-Year Survival Rate
Stage 0 (in situ)	Surgery	>90%
Stage IA	Surgery	60–80%
Stage IB	Surgery ± adjuvant therapy	50–60%
Stage II	Surgery + adjuvant therapy	30–50%
Stage IIIA	Surgery + adjuvant therapy	~20% (distal tumors)
Stage IIIB	Surgery + adjuvant therapy	~10%
Stage IV	Palliative chemotherapy, radiation therapy	~5%

Expert Opinion

1. Diffuse gastric histology and peritoneal spread may adversely affect the motility of the gastrointestinal tract. Consider promotility agents

2. Common sites of metastatic spread: *Lymphatic:* M1 lymph nodes include para-aortic nodes. Supradiaphragmatic and mediastinal nodes may also be involved. Rare involvement of the left supraclavicular nodes occurs via the thoracic duct. *Blood-borne hematogenous:* Distant metastases to the liver, lungs, bone, and skin. Either hematogenous spread or neoplastic seeding of the peritoneum, mesentery, and omentum can result in massive bilateral involvement of the ovaries (Krukenberg tumor)

3. For locally advanced, nonmetastatic disease, several studies demonstrate benefit with adjuvant therapy:
   - Perioperative chemotherapy
   - Postoperative chemoradiation
   - Postoperative chemotherapy (preferred in Asia)

4. All tumors should be examined for HER2 status. HER2-positive patients should receive cisplatin/capecitabine- and trastuzumab-based therapy

5. In second line, either single-agent docetaxel or single-agent irinotecan can be administered

Bonin SR et al. Gastric cancer. In: Pazdur R et al (editors). Cancer Management: A Multidisciplinary Approach, 7th ed. The Oncology Group, 2003:259–270
D'Angelica M et al. Ann Surg 2004;240:808–816

6. **New tool for treatment monitoring: 18-fluorodeoxyglucose-PET**
   a. Although no data exist to routinely perform a PET-CT for staging purposes, the MUNICON trial points to a role of PET in predicting response to treatment in localized disease
   b. The trial included 119 patients with locally advanced adenocarcinoma of the esophagogastric junction who underwent staging with PET prior to initiating treatment. PET was repeated after 2 weeks of chemotherapy. Tumors with a decrease of 35% of standard uptake values (SUVs) were considered "responders." Difference of overall survival between responders and nonresponders was significant at censured follow-up of 2.3 years

Lordick F et al. Lancet Oncol 2007;8:797–805

7. A study reporting poor prognostic factors in locally advanced and metastatic esophagogastric cancer analyzed prognostic factors based on three randomized trials (N = 1080)

Ross P et al. J Clin Oncol 2002;20:1996–2004
Tebbutt NC et al. Ann Oncol 2002;13:1568–1575
Webb A et al. J Clin Oncol 1997;15:261–267

(continued)

Expert Opinion (continued)

Multivariate Baseline Prognostic Model and Logistic Regression Model for Tumor Response to Chemotherapy
Chau I et al. J Clin Oncol 2004;22:2395–2403

Multivariate Baseline Prognostic Model

Factors	Hazard Ratio	99% CI	P Value
Performance status 2–3	1.575	1.251–1.981	<0.0001
Liver metastasis	1.409	1.139–1.743	<0.0001
Peritoneal metastasis	1.329	1.013–1.743	0.007
Alkaline phosphatase ≥100 units/L	1.412	1.136–1.755	<0.0001

Multivariate Logistic Regression Model for Tumor Response to Chemotherapy

Factors	Risk Ratio	99% CI	P Value
Performance Status 2–3	0.469	0.280–0.787	<0.001
Peritoneal metastasis	0.475	0.254–0.889	0.002
Alkaline phosphatase ≥100 units/L	0.655	0.433–0.992	0.009

Surgical Options
Resectable Tumors
1. Tis or T1* limited to mucosa (T1a)
   - Gastrectomy (endoscopic resection in experienced centers)
2. T1b-T3[†]
   - Distal gastrectomy
   - Subtotal gastrectomy (preferred for distal gastric cancers)
   - Total gastrectomy

   Notes:
   - Gastric resection should encompass the regional lymph nodes (D1), with a desired goal of removing/examining ≥15 lymph nodes[‡,§]
   - Consider placing a feeding jejunostomy tube especially if postoperative chemoradiation appears a likely recommendation

Criteria of unresectability
Locoregionally advanced
1. Level 3 or 4 lymph node highly suspicious on imaging or confirmed by biopsy
2. Invasion or encasement of major vascular structures
3. Distant metastasis or peritoneal seeding (including positive peritoneal cytology)

*Soetikno R et al. J Clin Oncol 2005;23:4490–4498
[†]Ito H et al. J Am Coll Surg 2004;199:880–886
[‡]Hartgrink HH et al. J Clin Oncol 2004;22:2069–2077
[§]Schwarz RE et al. Ann Surg Oncol 2007;14:317–328

LOCOREGIONAL DISEASE • PERIOPERATIVE

GASTRIC CANCER REGIMEN: FLUOROURACIL + LEUCOVORIN + OXALIPLATIN + DOCETAXEL (FLOT)

Al-Batran SE et al. Lancet 2019;393:1948–1957
Supplementary appendix to: Al-Batran SE et al. Lancet 2019;393:1948–1957

Premedication for docetaxel:
Dexamethasone 8 mg/dose; administer orally twice daily for 3 days, starting on the day before docetaxel administration (total dose/cycle = 48 mg)

Docetaxel 50 mg/m^2; administer intravenously diluted in a volume of 0.9% sodium chloride injection (0.9% NS) or 5% dextrose injection (D5W) sufficient to produce a docetaxel concentration within the range 0.3–0.74 mg/mL over 60 minutes on day 1, every 14 days, for a total of 8 cycles (4 preoperative cycles and 4 postoperative cycles) (total dosage/2-week cycle = 50 mg/m^2)

Oxaliplatin 85 mg/m^2; administer intravenously over 2 hours in 500 mL D5W on day 1, every 2 weeks, concurrently with leucovorin administration, for a total of 8 cycles (4 preoperative cycles and 4 postoperative cycles) (total dosage/2-week cycle = 85 mg/m^2), *plus:*

Leucovorin calcium 200 mg/m^2; administer intravenously over 60 minutes in 250 mL D5W on day 1 during the last hour of the oxaliplatin infusion, every 14 days, for a total of 8 cycles (4 preoperative cycles and 4 postoperative cycles) (total dosage/2-week cycle = 200 mg/m^2), *followed by:*
Fluorouracil 2600 mg/m^2; administer by continuous intravenous infusion in 50–1000 mL 0.9% NS or D5W over 24 hours on day 1 only, every 14 days, for a total of 8 cycles (4 preoperative cycles and 4 postoperative cycles) (total dosage/2-week cycle = 2600 mg/m^2)
Note: Oxaliplatin must not be mixed with sodium chloride injection. Therefore, when leucovorin and oxaliplatin are given concurrently via the same administration set tubing, both drugs must be administered in D5W

Supportive Care
Antiemetic prophylaxis
Emetogenic potential on day 1 is **MODERATE**.
See Chapter 42 for antiemetic recommendations

Hematopoietic growth factor (CSF) prophylaxis
Primary prophylaxis is **NOT** *indicated*
See Chapter 43 for more information

Antimicrobial prophylaxis
Risk of fever and neutropenia is **LOW**
Antimicrobial primary prophylaxis to be considered:
- Antibacterial—not indicated
- Antifungal—not indicated
- Antiviral—not indicated unless patient previously had an episode of HSV

Diarrhea management
Latent or delayed-onset diarrhea*:
Loperamide 4 mg orally initially after the first loose or liquid stool, *then* 2–4 mg orally every 2–4 hours or **diphenoxylate hydrochloride** 2.5 mg **with atropine sulfate** 0.025 mg (eg, Lomotil), 2 tablets orally four times per day

*Abigerges D et al. J Natl Cancer Inst 1994;86:446–449
Rothenberg ML et al. J Clin Oncol 2001;19:3801–3807
Wadler S et al. J Clin Oncol 1998;16:3169–3178

Oral care
Standard prophylaxis and treatment for mucositis/stomatitis

Patient Population Studied

This multicenter, randomized, open-label, active controlled, phase 3 trial included 716 adult German patients with locally advanced gastric cancer who were randomized to receive either perioperative 5-fluorouracil, leucovorin, oxaliplatin, and docetaxel (FLOT) or perioperative cisplatin plus epirubicin and either 5-fluorouracil or capecitabine (ECF/ECX). Patients were eligible if they had histologically proven, resectable, gastric or gastro-esophageal junction adenocarcinomas of clinical stage ≥cT2, nodal positive disease (cN+), or both, with no evidence of distant metastases. Patients were also required to have normal cardiac, renal, and hepatic function; an Eastern Cooperative Oncology Group (ECOG) performance status of ≤ 2; no prior gastric cancer resection; and prior cytostatic chemotherapy

Efficacy (N = 716)

	FLOT (N = 360)	ECF/ECX (N = 356)	
Underwent R0 resection	85%	78%	P = 0.0162
Median overall survival*	50 months (95% CI, 38.33–NR)	35 months (95% CI, 27.35–46.26)	HR 0.77 (95% CI, 0.63–0.94); P = 0.012
Median disease-free survival*	30 months‡	18 months‡	HR 0.75 (95% CI, 0.62–0.91); P = 0.0036
Estimated overall survival, 2 years	68% (95% CI, 63–73)	59% (95% CI, 53–64)	
Estimated overall survival, 3 years	57% (95% CI, 52–62)	48% (95% CI, 43–54)	
Estimated overall survival, 5 years	45% (95% CI, 38–51)	36% (95% CI, 30–42)	

HR, hazard ratio; CI, confidence interval; NR, not reached
Note that the primary end point was changed from disease-free survival to overall survival during the study at the request of the independent scientific committee of the German Cancer Aid, but that both end points were reached
*In the intention-to-treat population. Log-rank P value is reported

Therapy Monitoring

1. *Before each cycle:* Interval medical history with emphasis on clinical toxicities, physical examination, weight, performance status, CBC with differential, blood urea nitrogen, serum creatinine, and LFTs
2. Perform restaging by means of computed CT or MRI and endoscopy before surgery
3. Schedule surgery for 4 weeks after the last dose of preoperative chemotherapy. Study protocol required transthoracic esophagectomy (Ivor-Lewis procedure) with resection of the proximal stomach and 2-field (mediastinal and abdominal) lymphadenectomy for type 1 gastroesophageal junction cancers and gastrectomy with transhiatal distal esophagectomy plus D2 lymphadenectomy for types 2 and 3 gastro-esophageal junction cancers. For gastric tumors, total or subtotal distal gastrectomy with D2 lymphadenectomy was performed
4. *Response evaluation:* Clinical follow-up at 3-month intervals for 2 years, then at 6-month intervals for 3 years, and yearly thereafter. Follow-up consists of physical examination, CBC, liver function tests, and CT as clinically indicated

Treatment Modification

Adverse Event	Dose Modification
Leukocytes $<3.0 \times 10^9/L$*; platelets $<100 \times 10^9/L$; or any nonhematologic toxicity G ≥2	• Use supportive care as indicated, including growth factors† • Do not start a new cycle until leukocytes $≥3.0 \times 10^9/L$*; platelets $≥100 \times 10^9/L$; and any nonhematologic toxicity G <2 in the absence of fever or a relevant infection
Febrile neutropenia despite the use of G-CSF	• Reduce dosage of oxaliplatin by 25% to 64 mg/m² • Reduce dosage of docetaxel by 25% to 37.5 mg/m²
Thrombocytopenia causing bleeding	
Any other hematologic DLT	
Second occurrence of febrile neutropenia despite the use of G-CSF and despite a 25% dose reduction of oxaliplatin and docetaxel	• Reduce dosage of oxaliplatin an additional 25% to 43 mg/m², a dose that is 50% of the original dose • Reduce dosage of docetaxel an additional 25% to 25 mg/m², a dose that is 50% of the original dose
Second occurrence of thrombocytopenia causing bleeding despite a 25% dose reduction of oxaliplatin and docetaxel	
Second occurrence of any other hematologic DLT despite a 25% dose reduction of oxaliplatin and docetaxel	
Third occurrence of febrile neutropenia despite the use of G-CSF and despite a 50% dose reduction of oxaliplatin and docetaxel	Discontinue oxaliplatin and docetaxel
Third occurrence of thrombocytopenia causing bleeding despite a 50% dose reduction of oxaliplatin and docetaxel	
Third occurrence of any other hematologic DLT despite a 50% dose reduction of oxaliplatin and docetaxel	

(continued)

Treatment Modification (*continued*)

Adverse Event	Dose Modification
Creatinine clearance <40 mL/min but >30 mL/min	Administer hyperhydration for 48 hours and repeat creatinine clearance. If repeat creatinine clearance is >40 mL/min, do not alter oxaliplatin dose. If creatinine clearance is still 30–40 mL/min, reduce oxaliplatin dose to 64 mg/m^2 or 75% of the initial dose
Creatinine clearance of <30 mL/min	Discontinue oxaliplatin treatment. 5-FU and docetaxel administration can be continued
First occurrence of G ≥3 nonhematologic toxicity, and select G2 toxicities of concern to the physician	Reduce the dose of the chemotherapeutic agent most likely responsible for the observed toxicity to 75% of the initial dose (for all further cycles)—64 mg/m^2 for oxaliplatin, 37.5 mg/m^2 for docetaxel, and 1950 mg/m^2 for 5-FU
Second occurrence of G ≥3 nonhematologic toxicity, and select G2 toxicities of concern to the physician despite a 25% dose reduction of the suspected agent	Reduce the dose of the chemotherapeutic agent most likely responsible for the observed toxicity an additional 25% to 50% of the initial dose (for all further cycles)—43 mg/m^2 for oxaliplatin; 25 mg/m^2 for docetaxel and 1300 mg/m^2 for 5-FU
Third occurrence of G ≥3 nonhematologic toxicity, and select G2 toxicities of concern to the physician despite a 50% dose reduction of the suspected agent	Discontinue the relevant drug(s) or discontinue all therapy

Dose adjustments for oxaliplatin neurotoxicity

Neurotoxicity	7 days	>7 and <14 days	Present Between Cycle
Cold-induced dysesthesia	No change	No change	No change
Paresthesia	No change	No change	Reduce dose to 43 mg/m^2 on d1
Paresthesia with pain	No change	Reduce dose to 75% of starting dose or 64 mg/m^2 on d1	Stop oxaliplatin[‡] continue docetaxel/5-FU/LV
Paresthesia with functional impairment	No change	Reduce dose to 50% of starting dose or 43 mg/m^2 on d1	Stop oxaliplatin[‡] continue docetaxel/5-FU/LV

*Neutrophil count is not relevant. Make decisions based on leukocyte count, provided the patient has no infection, fever, or other side effects that are possibly neutropenia-related
[†]Granulocyte colony-stimulating factor (GCSF) is not used as primary prophylaxis but can be added if needed
[‡]Usually, discontinuation will be permanent. However, consider resumption of oxaliplatin if complete recovery from the related symptoms occurs and if the treating physician decides that this is in the best interest of the patient and if the toxicity is not expected to reoccur

Adverse Events (N = 708)

Event	FLOT (N = 354)		ECF/ECX (N = 354)	
Grade (%)	Grade 1 or 2	Grade 3 or 4	Grade 1 or 2	Grade 3 or 4
Diarrhea	52	10	29	4
Vomiting	32	2	29	8
Nausea	60	7	61	16
Constipation	21	1	24	<1
Stomatitis or mucositis	28	1	30	3
Leukopenia	51	27	49	21
Neutropenia	24	51	26	39
Anemia	80	3	80	6
Thrombocytopenia	39	2	35	3
Serum AST elevation	33	1	12	<1
Serum ALT elevation	36	2	16	<1
Fever	22	1	8	1
Peripheral neuropathy	64	7	34	2
Pain	47	6	48	4
Alopecia	62	N/A	62	N/A
Renal	11	0	28	<1
Infections	17	18	18	9
Thromboembolic	4	3	9	6
Toxic death*	4	3	9	6

*Defined as chemotherapy-related toxicity resulting in death
Adverse events are included in the table if they were reported in ≥20% of the patients at Grade 1 or 2 or ≥ 5% of patients at Grade 3 or 4. These data include all patients who were randomized and who received treatment (per protocol population). Febrile neutropenia was reported in 2 patients in the ECF/ECX group and 7 patients in the FLOT group. The rate of serious adverse events related to treatment was similar between FLOT (27%) and ECF/ECX (27%) groups. Grade 3 or 4 nausea was less common in the FLOT group than in the ECF/ECX group, most likely due to the less emetogenic nature of oxaliplatin vs cisplatin. Note that, for the FLOT group, more patients started postoperative therapy and toxicity was evaluated every 2 weeks, whereas toxicity was evaluated every 3 weeks for the ECF/ECX group, possibly increasing the rates of adverse events in the FLOT group. Median follow-up for both groups was 43 months

LOCOREGIONAL DISEASE • PERIOPERATIVE

GASTRIC CANCER REGIMEN: CAPECITABINE + OXALIPLATIN (CAPOX)

Kim GM et al. Eur J Cancer 2012;48(4):518–526

Note: this perioperative regimen is used in clinical practice as described below based on an extrapolation of evidence in patients with advanced gastric cancer

Oxaliplatin 130 mg/m^2; administer intravenously in 250–500 mL 5% dextrose injection over 2 hours on day 1, every 21 days, for a total of 6 planned cycles (3 preoperative and 3 postoperative) (total dosage/3-week cycle = 130 mg/m^2)

Capecitabine 1000 mg/m^2 per dose; administer orally twice daily (approximately every 12 hours, within 30 minutes after a meal) for 14 consecutive days, on days 1–14 (28 doses), followed by 7 days without therapy, every 21 days, for a total of 6 planned cycles (3 preoperative and 3 postoperative) (total dosage/3-week cycle = 28,000 mg/m^2)

Supportive Care

Antiemetic prophylaxis

Emetogenic potential on day 1 is **MODERATE**

Emetogenic potential on days with capecitabine alone is **MINIMAL–LOW**

See Chapter 42 for antiemetic recommendations

Hematopoietic growth factor (G-CSF) prophylaxis

Primary prophylaxis is **NOT** *indicated*

See Chapter 43 for more information

Antimicrobial prophylaxis

Risk of fever and neutropenia is **LOW**

   Antimicrobial primary prophylaxis to be considered:

- Antibacterial—not indicated

- Antifungal—not indicated

- Antiviral—not indicated, unless patient previously had an episode of HSV

Hand-foot reaction (palmar-plantar erythrodysesthesia, PPE)

- For patients who develop a hand-foot reaction, use topical emollients (eg, Aquaphor), topical or orally administered steroids, antihistamine agents (H$_1$-receptor antagonists), or pyridoxine

- **Pyridoxine** may provide relief for discomfort/pain associated with PPE although the mechanism through which this occurs remains unclear

- The suggested **pyridoxine** starting dose is **50 mg/day**, which may be increased to a maximum of 200 mg/day

Diarrhea management

Latent or delayed-onset diarrhea*:

Loperamide 4 mg orally initially after the first loose or liquid stool, *then* 2–4 mg orally every 2–4 hours or **diphenoxylate hydrochloride** 2.5 mg with **atropine sulfate** 0.025 mg (eg, Lomotil) 2 tablets orally four times per day

*Abigerges D et al. J Natl Cancer Inst 1994;86:446–449
Rothenberg ML et al. J Clin Oncol 2001;19:3801–3807
Wadler S et al. J Clin Oncol 1998;16:3169–3178

Oral care

Standard prophylaxis and treatment for mucositis/stomatitis

Patient Population Studied

This perioperative regimen is used in clinical practice based on an extrapolation of evidence from a randomized, phase 2 trial that included 129 patients with advanced gastric cancer and compared treatment with S-1 plus oxaliplatin (SOX) or capecitabine plus oxaliplatin (CAPOX). Patients were eligible if they had histologically confirmed metastatic or recurrent gastric adenocarcinoma with measurable or evaluable lesions, if they had never received previous chemotherapy (except for adjuvant or preoperative chemotherapy more than 6 months before enrollment that didn't include S-1, capecitabine, or oxaliplatin), and if they had an ECOG performance score of 0–2 and adequate organ function. Patients were excluded if they had brain metastases, neuropathy of grade >2, or uncontrolled comorbid conditions

Efficacy (N = 129)

	S–1 + Oxaliplatin (SOX) (N = 65)	Capecitabine + Oxaliplatin (CAPOX) (N = 64)	
Median time to progression*†	6.2 months (95% CI, 4.92–7.48)	7.2 months (95% CI, 5.87–8.54)	HR 1.06 (95% CI, 0.72–1.57); P = 0.767
Median overall survival*†	12.4 months (95% CI, 8.796–16.01)	13.3 months (95% CI, 10.26–16.34)	HR 1.08 (95% CI, 0.74–1.58); P = 0.686
Estimated survival rate, 12 months*	52%	59%	—
Complete response rate‡	0%	2%	—
Partial response rate‡	40%	42%	—
Stable disease rate‡	51%	40%	—
Progressive disease rate‡	7%	16%	—
Overall objective response rate‡	40% (95% CI, 26–54)	44% (95% CI, 29–60)	—
Disease control rate‡	91%	84%	—

HR, hazard ratio; CI, confidence interval

*Time to progression and overall survival were analyzed in a modified intention-to-treat population that included all patients who ever received a dose of a trial drug. Of 130 patients enrolled in the study, 129 received a dose of trial drug and were thus included in the analysis

†P values were calculated using the log-rank test

‡Response rates were graded according to RECIST v1.0 criteria and were generated from a modified intention-to-treat population that included only patients who received at least one dose of trial drug and who had measurable lesions. This population included 53 patients in the SOX group and 45 patients in the CAPOX group

All data included in this table were reported in the paper titled *A randomized phase II trial of S-1-oxaliplatin versus capecitabine–oxaliplatin in advanced gastric cancer*. Data in this paper were generated with a median follow-up time of 13 months (no range or group breakdown reported)

Therapy Monitoring

1. *Before each cycle:* Interval medical history with emphasis on clinical toxicities, physical examination, weight, performance status, CBC with differential, blood urea nitrogen, serum creatinine, and LFTs
2. Perform restaging by means of computed CT or MRI and endoscopy before surgery
3. *Response evaluation:* Clinical follow-up at 3-month intervals for 2 years, then at 6-month intervals for 3 years, and yearly thereafter. Follow-up consists of physical examination, CBC, liver function tests, and CT as clinically indicated

CAPECITABINE AND OXALIPLATIN DOSE MODIFICATIONS

	Capecitabine Dose	Oxaliplatin Dose
Starting dose	1000 mg/m² /dose twice per day	130 mg/m²
Dose level −1	750 mg/m² /dose twice per day	100 mg/m²
Dose level −2	500 mg/m² /dose twice per day	70 mg/m²

Adverse Event	Treatment Modification
Symptomatic toxicity, ANC <1500/mm³ or platelet count <75,000/mm³	Delay treatment up to 3 weeks. If after 3 weeks symptomatic toxicity has not improved, ANC is still <1500/mm³, or platelet count still <75,000/mm³, then discontinue treatment
G4 ANC (<500/mm³), G4 thrombocytopenia (<25,000/mm³), or febrile neutropenia with ANC <1000/mm³ + a single temperature of >38.3°C (101°F) or a sustained temperature of 38°C (100.4°F) for more than 1 hour or G3 nausea/vomiting, diarrhea, or stomatitis	Delay treatment until ANC is ≥1500/mm³ *and* platelet count is ≥75,000/mm³, then reduce the doses of oxaliplatin and capecitabine by one dose level beginning with the next cycle. Consider using hematopoietic growth factors. *Note:* Treatment delays for unresolved adverse events of >3 weeks duration warrant discontinuation of treatment
G2/3 hand-foot syndrome or palmar-plantar erythrodysesthesia or chemotherapy-induced acral erythema* G2/3 diarrhea, stomatitis, nausea, or dehydration	Withhold capecitabine; provide supportive care. Do not resume capecitabine until toxicity resolved to G ≤1. In subsequent cycle(s), *permanently* reduce the capecitabine dosage by 1 dose level

(continued)

Therapy Monitoring (continued)

Second episode of G2/3 diarrhea, stomatitis, nausea, or dehydration	Hold capecitabine; resume capecitabine with dosage reduced by one dose level after toxicity resolves
G4 diarrhea, stomatitis, nausea, or dehydration	Permanently discontinue capecitabine
Stevens-Johnson syndrome and toxic epidermal necrolysis (severe mucocutaneous reactions, some with fatal outcome)	
Capecitabine-induced coronary vasospasm/cardiac ischemia	
G3/4 diarrhea or stomatitis despite capecitabine dose reductions	Reduce oxaliplatin dosage by one dose level
Creatinine clearance 30–50 mL/minute	Reduce the capecitabine dosage by 1 dose level
Creatinine clearance <30 mL/minute	Withhold capecitabine
Persistent G1/G2 neuropathy	Delay oxaliplatin 1 week. After toxicity resolves, resume oxaliplatin at a dosage decreased by one dose level during subsequent cycles
"Transient" G3/4 neuropathy (7–14 days)	Hold oxaliplatin. After toxicity resolves, resume oxaliplatin at a dosage decreased by one dose level during subsequent cycles
Persistent G3/4 neuropathy	Discontinue oxaliplatin
Other G3/4 nonhematologic adverse events	Reduce oxaliplatin and capecitabine dosages by one dose level during subsequent cycles

ANC, absolute neutrophil count; CBC, complete blood count
Grading of hand-foot syndrome is as follows:
- G1: Numbness, dysesthesia/paresthesia, tingling, painless swelling or erythema of the hands and/or feet and/or discomfort which does not disrupt normal activities
- G2: Painful erythema and swelling of the hands and/or feet and/or discomfort affecting the patient's activities of daily living
- G3: Moist desquamation, ulceration, blistering, or severe pain of the hands and/or feet and/or severe discomfort that causes the patient to be unable to work or perform activities of daily living

Adverse Events (N = 129)

Event	S–1 + Oxaliplatin (SOX) (N = 65)		Capecitabine + Oxaliplatin (CAPOX) (N = 64)	
	Grade (%)			
	Grade 1 or 2	Grade 3–4	Grade 1 or 2	Grade 3–4
Neutropenia	48	9	44	19
Leukopenia	45	8	50	3
Anemia	78	12	89	3
Thrombocytopenia	49	15	52	14
Asthenia	40	2	42	8
Anorexia	49	3	47	3
Nausea	45	3	38	5
Vomiting	40	2	30	3
Diarrhea	26	5	30	5
Neuropathy	38	3	44	5
Hand-foot syndrome	3	0	23	2
Infection	11	9	8	6

Data were included from the modified intention-to-treat population, which includes only patients who received at least one dose of trial drug. Adverse events were graded according to National Cancer Institute Common Terminology Criteria for Adverse Events (NCI-CTCAE) version 3.0. The only adverse event with a statistically significant difference in incidence was all-grade hand-foot syndrome (P <0.001). There was no difference in overall incidence of Grade 3 or 4 adverse events between groups. Febrile neutropenia occurred in 1 patient in each arm. There were no treatment-related deaths in either group in this study

LOCOREGIONAL DISEASE • PERIOPERATIVE

GASTRIC CANCER REGIMEN: FLUOROURACIL + LEUCOVORIN + OXALIPLATIN (FOLFOX)

Enzinger P et al. J Clin Oncol 2016;34(23):2736–2742

Note: This perioperative regimen is used in clinical practice as described below based on an extrapolation of evidence in patients with advanced gastric cancer

Oxaliplatin 85 mg/m^2; administer intravenously over 2 hours in 500 mL 5% dextrose injection (D5W) on day 1, every 2 weeks, concurrently with leucovorin administration, for a total of 6 planned cycles (3 preoperative and 3 postoperative) (total dosage/cycle = 85 mg/m^2), *plus:*
Leucovorin calcium 400 mg/m^2; administer intravenously over 2 hours in 25–500 mL D5W on day 1, every 2 weeks, concurrently with oxaliplatin, for a total of 6 planned cycles (3 preoperative and 3 postoperative) (total dosage/cycle = 400 mg/m^2), *followed by:*
Fluorouracil 400 mg/m^2; administer by intravenous injection over 1–2 minutes after leucovorin on day 1, every 2 weeks, for a total of 6 planned cycles (3 preoperative and 3 postoperative), *followed by:*
Fluorouracil 2400 mg/m^2; administer by continuous intravenous infusion over 46 hours in 100–1000 mL 0.9% sodium chloride injection (0.9% NS) or D5W, starting on day 1 every 2 weeks, for a total of 6 planned cycles (3 preoperative and 3 postoperative) (total fluorouracil dosage/cycle = 2800 mg/m^2)
Note: The fluorouracil bolus dose (400 mg/m^2) can be omitted for better hematologic tolerance
Note: Oxaliplatin must not be mixed with sodium chloride injection. Therefore, when leucovorin and oxaliplatin are given concurrently via the same administration set tubing, both drugs must be administered in D5W

Supportive Care
Antiemetic prophylaxis
Emetogenic potential on day 1 is **MODERATE**
Emetogenic potential on day 2 is **LOW**
See Chapter 42 for antiemetic recommendations

Hematopoietic growth factor (G-CSF) prophylaxis
Primary prophylaxis is **NOT** *indicated*
See Chapter 43 for more information

Antimicrobial prophylaxis
Risk of fever and neutropenia is **LOW**
Antimicrobial primary prophylaxis to be considered:
- *Antibacterial—not indicated*
- *Antifungal—not indicated*
- *Antiviral—not indicated unless patient previously had an episode of HSV*

Diarrhea management
Latent or delayed-onset diarrhea*:
Loperamide 4 mg orally initially after the first loose or liquid stool, *then* 2–4 mg orally every 2–4 hours or **diphenoxylate hydrochloride** 2.5 mg with **atropine sulfate** 0.025 mg (eg, Lomotil) 2 tablets orally four times per day

*Abigerges D et al. J Natl Cancer Inst 1994;86:446–449
Rothenberg ML et al. J Clin Oncol 2001;19:3801–3807
Wadler S et al. J Clin Oncol 1998;16:3169–3178

Oral care
Standard prophylaxis and treatment for mucositis/stomatitis

Patient Population Studied

This perioperative regimen is used in clinical practice as described above based on an extrapolation of evidence from a randomized phase 2 trial that enrolled 245 adult patients with metastatic esophageal or gastroesophageal junction (GEJ) cancer and compared treatment with cetuximab plus either ECF (epirubicin, cisplatin, and fluorouracil) or IC (irinotecan and cisplatin) or FOLFOX (oxaliplatin, leucovorin, fluorouracil). Patients were eligible if they had metastatic adenocarcinoma or squamous cell carcinoma of the esophagus or GEJ (type I or II by Siewert classification) with measurable disease according to RECIST v1.0, and if they had an ECOG performance status of 0 to 2. Patients were excluded from the trial if they had received previous chemotherapy, radiotherapy, or anti-EGFR therapy. Note that this study was completed before the publication of two randomized studies that showed **no benefit** with the addition of EGFR-directed monoclonal antibodies to chemotherapy in patients with advanced esophagogastric cancer (Waddell T et al. Lancet Oncol 2013;14:481–489 and Lordick F et al. Lancet Oncol 2013;14:490–499). Therefore, in clinical practice, cetuximab is omitted from this regimen

Efficacy (N = 245)

	Epirubicin + Cisplatin + Fluorouracil (ECF) + Cetuximab (N = 82)	Irinotecan + Cisplatin (IC) + Cetuximab (N = 83)	Leucovorin + Fluorouracil + Oxaliplatin (FOLFOX) + Cetuximab (N = 80)	
Complete response rate*	1.5%	1.4%	3.0%	
Partial response rate*	58.7%	43.6%	50.0%	
Stable disease rate*	22.2%	32.4%	27.2%	
Progressive disease rate*	7.9%	15.5%	12.1%	
Objective response rate*	60.3% (95% CI, 47.2–72.4)	45.1% (95% CI, 33.2–57.3)	53.0% (95% CI, 42.5–68.1)	P <0.001 for each treatment group compared with null hypothesis
Response duration*	7.1 months (range, 1.1–65.8)	6.5 months (range, 0.5–26.5)	6.6 months (range, 2.4–60.1)	
Median overall survival rate[†]	11.6 months (95% CI, 8.1–13.4 months)	8.6 months (95% CI, 6.0–12.4 months)	11.8 months (95% CI, 8.8–13.9 months)	No significant pairwise comparisons
Median progression-free survival[†]	7.1 months (95% CI, 4.5–8.4)	4.9 months (95% CI, 3.9–6.0)	6.8 months (95% CI, 5.4–8.1%)	No significant pairwise comparisons
Median time to treatment failure[†]	5.6 months (95% CI, 3.9–7.2)	4.3 months (95% CI, 3.6–5.5)	6.7 months (95% CI, 4.8–7.4)	P = 0.012 for comparison of IC+C with FOLFOX+C; no other pairwise comparisons significant

HR, hazard ratio; CI, confidence interval

Response data (including duration of response) included only adenocarcinoma patients who received ≥1 cycle of chemotherapy (n = 200). Time to event data included all patients who received ≥1 cycle of chemotherapy (n = 213)

*Response rate graded according to RECIST v1.0 criteria

[†]Comparisons were unplanned

Therapy Monitoring

1. *Before each cycle:* H&P, CBC with differential, serum bilirubin, AST, ALT, and alkaline phosphatase, CEA if initially elevated, serum electrolytes and serum magnesium
2. Perform restaging by means of computed CT or MRI and endoscopy before surgery
3. *Response evaluation:* Clinical follow-up at 3-month intervals for 2 years, then at 6-month intervals for 3 years, and yearly thereafter. Follow-up consists of physical examination, CBC, liver function tests, and CT as clinically indicated

Treatment Modifications

Adverse Event	Dose Modification
Any G2/3/4 nonhematologic toxicity	Delay start of next cycle until the severity of all toxicities are G ≤1
ANC ≤1500/mm³ or platelet count ≤100,000/mm³	Delay start of next cycle until ANC >1500/mm³ and platelet count >100,000/mm³
G3/4 Nonneurologic toxicity	Reduce fluorouracil and oxaliplatin dosages by 20%
G3/4 neutropenia	Reduce oxaliplatin dosage by 20%
Persistent (≥14 days) paresthesias	Reduce oxaliplatin dosage by 20%
Temporary (7–14 days) painful paresthesias	
Temporary (7–14 days) functional impairment	
Persistent (≥14 days) painful paresthesias	Discontinue oxaliplatin
Persistent (≥14 days) functional impairment	

Adapted in part from de Gramont A et al. J Clin Oncol 2000;18:2938–2947

Adverse Events (N = 213)

Event	Epirubicin + Cisplatin + Fluorouracil (ECF) (N = 67)	Irinotecan + Cisplatin (IC) (N = 73)	Leucovorin + Fluorouracil + Oxaliplatin (FOLFOX) (N = 73)
		Cetuximab +	
Treatment modifications	91%	85%	73%
		P = 0.013	
Treatment discontinued due to adverse events	19%	26%	11%
		P = 0.17	
Treatment-related death	6.0%	8.2%	2.7%
Grade (%)	Grade 3–5	Grade 3–5	Grade 3–5
All Hematologic	53	59	46
		P = 0.32	
Neutropenia	49	51	43
Leukocytopenia	13	22	16
Anemia	7	13	7
Thrombocytopenia	4	8	3
Lymphopenia	7	11	3
All Nonhematologic	73	77	66
Constitutional symptoms	13	21	16
Dermatologic	17	11	22
Gastrointestinal	31	41 ($\uparrow$P = 0.04)	22
Infection	12	7	7
Metabolic	18	34 ($\uparrow$P = 0.09)	26
Neurologic	15	3 ($\downarrow$P = 0.02)	16
Pain	8	3	3
Pulmonary	4	3	0
Vascular	7	9	4
Death (not CTCAE defined)	4	0	0

Adverse events were included if they were reported by patients who received any trial drug, if they were of Grade 3–5, and if they were at least possibly related to treatment according to CTCAE version 3 criteria. 58% of treated patients stopped treatment because of disease progression, 13% due to adverse effects, and 11% due to withdrawal of consent

LOCOREGIONAL DISEASE • PERIOPERATIVE

GASTRIC CANCER REGIMEN: CISPLATIN + FLUOROURACIL (CF)

Ychou M et al. J Clin Oncol 2011;29:1715–1721
Protocol for: Ychou M et al. J Clin Oncol 2011;29:1715–1721
Supplementary appendix to: Ychou M et al. J Clin Oncol 2011;29:1715–1721

Fluorouracil 800 mg/m^2 per day; administer by continuous intravenous infusion in 50–1000 mL 0.9% sodium chloride injection (0.9% NS) or 5% dextrose injection (D5W) over 24 hours for 5 consecutive days, on days 1–5, every 28 days, for a total of 6 cycles (2–3 preoperative cycles and 3–4 post-operative cycles) (total dosage/cycle = 4000 mg/m^2)

Hydration before cisplatin: ≥1000 mL 0.9% NS; administer intravenously over a minimum of 3 hours
Cisplatin 100 mg/m^2; administer intravenously in 100–500 mL of 0.9% NS over 1 hour on day 1, every 28 days, for a total of 6 cycles (2–3 preoperative cycles and 3–4 post-operative cycles) (total dosage/cycle = 100 mg/m^2)
Hydration after cisplatin: ≥1000 mL 0.9% NS; administer intravenously over a minimum of 3 hours. Encourage increased oral fluid intake. Goal is to achieve a urine output of ≥100 mL/hour. Monitor and replace magnesium and other electrolytes as needed

Supportive Care
Antiemetic prophylaxis
*Emetogenic potential on day 1 is **HIGH**. Potential for delayed emetic symptoms*
*Emetogenic potential on days 2–5 is **LOW***
See Chapter 42 for antiemetic recommendations

Hematopoietic growth factor (CSF) prophylaxis
*Primary prophylaxis is **NOT** indicated*
See Chapter 43 for more information

Antimicrobial prophylaxis
*Risk of fever and neutropenia is **LOW***
   Antimicrobial primary prophylaxis to be considered:
   • Antibacterial—not indicated
   • Antifungal—not indicated
   • Antiviral—not indicated unless patient previously had an episode of HSV

Diarrhea management
Latent or delayed-onset diarrhea*:
Loperamide 4 mg orally initially after the first loose or liquid stool, *then* 2–4 mg orally every 2–4 hours or **diphenoxylate hydrochloride** 2.5 mg with **atropine sulfate** 0.025 mg (eg, Lomotil) 2 tablets orally four times per day

*Abigerges D et al. J Natl Cancer Inst 1994;86:446–449
Rothenberg ML et al. J Clin Oncol 2001;19:3801–3807
Wadler S et al. J Clin Oncol 1998;16:3169–3178

Oral care
Standard prophylaxis and treatment for mucositis/stomatitis

Patient Population Studied

This international, open-label, randomized phase 3 trial involved 224 adult patients with histologically proven adenocarcinoma of the lower third of the esophagus, gastroesophageal junction, or stomach that was judged suitable for curative resection. Patients were required to have a WHO performance status of 0 or 1. Eligible patients were randomly assigned to either perioperative chemotherapy followed by surgical resection (CS group) or surgical resection alone (S group)

Efficacy (N = 224)

Endpoint	Chemotherapy + Surgery (N = 113)	Surgical Resection Alone (N = 111)	Between-Group Comparison
5-year overall survival rate*	38% (95% CI 29–47%)	24% (95% CI 17–33%)	HR 0.69 (95% CI 0.50–0.95) P = 0.02
5-year disease-free survival rate	34% (95% CI 26–44%)	19% (95% CI 13–28%)	HR 0.65 (95% CI 0.48–0.89) P = 0.003
Patients with locoregional recurrence only	14 patients (12%)	9 patients (8%)	—
Patients with distant recurrence only	35 patients (30%)	42 patients (38%)	—
Patients with both locoregional and distant recurrence	14 patients (12%)	20 patients (18%)	—

HR, hazard ratio, CI, confidence interval
*In the multivariable analysis, two significant prognostic factors for overall survival were the administration of preoperative chemotherapy (P = 0.01) and tumor site (P <0.01). No statistically significant variation of chemotherapy effect according to tumor site was observed

Therapy Monitoring

1. *Before each cycle:* History and physical examination, BUN, serum creatinine, electrolytes, serum bilirubin, AST, ALT, and alkaline phosphatase
2. *Weekly:* CBC with differential, BUN, serum creatinine, electrolytes
3. Perform restaging by means of computed CT or MRI and endoscopy before surgery
4. *Response evaluation:* Clinical follow-up at 3-month intervals for 2 years, then at 6-month intervals for 3 years, and yearly thereafter. Follow-up consists of physical examination, CBC, liver function tests, and CT as clinically indicated

Treatment Modifications

CISPLATIN + 5-FLUOROURACIL

ANC nadir <1000/mm^3 *or* platelet nadir <50,000/mm^3 after treatment	Delay treatment until ANC is ≥1000/mm^3 *and* platelet count is ≥50,000/mm^3, then decrease cisplatin and 5-fluorouracil dosages by 25%. Alternatively, consider using hematopoietic growth factors
Recurrent treatment delay because of myelosuppression	Delay therapy for 1 week, or until myelosuppression resolves, then decrease cisplatin and 5-fluorouracil dosages by 25% during subsequent treatments
Sepsis during an episode of neutropenia	
Reduction in creatinine clearance* to 60% of on-study value	Delay therapy 1 week. If creatinine clearance does not recover to pretreatment values, then consider reducing cisplatin dose
Creatinine clearance* 40–60 mL/min (0.66–1 mL/s)	Consider reducing cisplatin so that dose in milligrams equals the creatinine clearance* value in mL/min (mL/s × 1/0.0166)†
Creatinine clearance* <40 mL/min (<0.66 mL/s)	Hold cisplatin
Clinically significant ototoxicity	Discontinue cisplatin
Persistent (>14 days) peripheral neuropathy without functional impairment	Decrease cisplatin dosage by 50%
Clinically significant sensory loss—persistent (>14 days) peripheral neuropathy with functional impairment	Discontinue cisplatin
G ≥3 nausea, vomiting	Decrease cisplatin dosage by 25%
G2 stomatitis or diarrhea	Hold 5-fluorouracil; resume 5-fluorouracil at full dosage after resolution of toxicity

(continued)

Treatment Modifications (*continued*)

Second episode of G2 stomatitis or diarrhea	Hold 5-fluorouracil; resume 5-fluorouracil with dosage reduced to 75% of the starting dose after toxicity resolves
Third episode of G2 stomatitis or diarrhea	Hold 5-fluorouracil; resume 5-fluorouracil with dosage reduced to 50% of the starting dose after toxicity resolves
Fourth episode of G2 stomatitis or diarrhea	Discontinue 5-fluorouracil
G3 stomatitis or diarrhea	Hold 5-fluorouracil. If G3 toxicity is adequately controlled within 2 days, resume 5-fluorouracil at full dosage when toxicity abates to G ≤1. If G3 toxicity takes >2 days to be controlled, resume 5-fluorouracil with dosage reduced to 75% of the starting dose after toxicity abates to G ≤1
Second episode of G3 stomatitis or diarrhea	Hold 5-fluorouracil. If G3 toxicity is controlled adequately within 2 days, then resume 5-fluorouracil with dosage reduced to 50% of the starting dose after toxicity abates to G ≤1
Third episode of G3 stomatitis or diarrhea	Discontinue 5-fluorouracil
G4 stomatitis or diarrhea	Discontinue 5-fluorouracil

Note: Treatment delays for unresolved adverse events of >3 weeks' duration warrant discontinuation of treatment
*Creatinine clearance is used as a measure of glomerular filtration rate
†This also applies to patients with creatinine clearance (GFR) of 40–60 mL/min at the outset of treatment

Adverse Events (N = 109)

	WHO Grade 3–4 Toxicity, % Chemotherapy + Surgery (N = 109)
Neutropenia	20.2
Leukopenia	5.5
Thrombocytopenia	5.5
Nausea/vomiting	9.2
Cardiotoxicity	3.7
Mucositis	3.7
Diarrhea	1.8
Neurotoxicity	0.9
Nephrotoxicity*	0.9
Fever	0.9
Ototoxicity	0.9
Other	4.6

*One patient died from acute renal failure considered to be related to the study drugs

LOCOREGIONAL DISEASE • ADJUVANT

GASTRIC CANCER REGIMEN: FLUOROURACIL + LEUCOVORIN + RADIATION

Macdonald JS et al. N Engl J Med 2001;345:725–730

Following curative surgery, patients receive 5 cycles of chemotherapy and concomitant radiotherapy spanning cycles 2 and 3 (based on a regimen described by Poon MA et al. J Clin Oncol 1989;7:1407–1418)

Cycle 1, neoadjuvant chemotherapy only:
Leucovorin 20 mg/m^2 per day; administer intravenously in 25–100 mL of 0.9% sodium chloride injection (0.9% NS) or 5% dextrose injection (D5W) over 5–15 minutes for 5 consecutive days on days 1–5 (total dosage/cycle = 100 mg/m^2)
Fluorouracil 425 mg/m^2 per day; administer intravenously in 25–100 mL 0.9% NS or D5W over 5–30 minutes after leucovorin for 5 consecutive days on days 1–5 (total dosage/cycle = 2125 mg/m^2)

Cycles 2 and 3, chemotherapy plus radiation:
Starts 28 days after the start of cycle 1 (ie, day 29)
Leucovorin 20 mg/m^2 per day; administer intravenously in 25–100 mL of 0.9% NS or D5W over 5–15 minutes for 4 consecutive days on days 1–4 during the first week of radiation therapy (total dosage during the first week of combined chemoradiation = 80 mg/m^2)
Fluorouracil 400 mg/m^2 per day; administer intravenously in 25–100 mL of 0.9% NS or D5W over 5–30 minutes after leucovorin for 4 consecutive days on days 1–4 during the first week of radiation therapy (total dosage during first week of combined chemoradiation = 1600 mg/m^2)
Radiation 180 cGy/day for 5 days/week for 5 consecutive weeks (total dose 4500 cGy in twenty-five 180-cGy fractions)
• Radiation fields must be evaluated carefully
• One-third of patients require field adjustments (INT-0116 study)
Leucovorin 20 mg/m^2 per day; administer intravenously in 25–100 mL of 0.9% NS or D5W over 5–15 minutes for 3 consecutive days on days 3–5 during the fifth week of radiation therapy (total dosage during the fifth week of combined chemoradiation = 60 mg/m^2)
Fluorouracil 400 mg/m^2 per day; administer intravenously in 25–100 mL of 0.9% NS or D5W over 5–30 minutes after leucovorin for 3 consecutive days on days 3–5 during the fifth week of radiation therapy (total dosage during the fifth week of combined chemoradiation = 1200 mg/m^2)

Cycles 4 and 5, chemotherapy only:
Starts 1 month after completing radiation therapy
Leucovorin 20 mg/m^2 per day; administer intravenously in 25–100 mL of 0.9% NS or D5W over 5–15 minutes on days 1–5, every 4 weeks for 2 cycles (total dosage/cycle = 100 mg/m^2)
Fluorouracil 425 mg/m^2 per day; administer intravenously in 25–100 mL of 0.9% NS or D5W over 5–30 minutes after leucovorin on days 1–5 every 4 weeks, for 2 cycles (total dosage/cycle = 2125 mg/m^2)

Supportive Care
Antiemetic prophylaxis
Emetogenic potential is **LOW** for chemotherapy alone
Emetogenic potential is at least **MODERATE** during chemoradiation
See Chapter 42 for antiemetic recommendations

Hematopoietic growth factor (CSF) prophylaxis
Primary prophylaxis is **NOT** indicated
See Chapter 43 for more information

Antimicrobial prophylaxis
Risk of fever and neutropenia is **LOW**
  Antimicrobial primary prophylaxis to be considered:
  • Antibacterial—not indicated
  • Antifungal—not indicated
  • Antiviral—not indicated unless patient previously had an episode of HSV

Oral care
Standard prophylaxis and treatment for mucositis/stomatitis

Patient Population Studied

A study of 556 evaluable patients with stage IB-IV M0 gastric cancer who had undergone curative surgery were randomly assigned to receive adjuvant chemoradiation or observation alone. **Patients had completely recovered from resection and were no longer losing weight**

Efficacy (N = 281)[*]

Median overall survival	36 months
3-year disease-free survival	48%
Median relapse free survival	30 months
Local recurrence	19%
Regional relapse[†]	65%
Distant relapses	33%

*Intention-to-treat analysis
[†]Typically, abdominal carcinomatosis

Cessation of Chemoradiotherapy (N = 281)

Reason	No. of Patients (%)
Protocol treatment completed	181 (64)
Toxic effects	49 (17)
Patient declined further treatment	23 (8)
Progression of disease	13 (5)
Death	3 (1)
Other	12 (4)

Therapy Monitoring

1. *Prior to each cycle:* Interval history with emphasis on clinical toxicities, physical examination, CBC with differential, serum creatinine, and LFTs
2. *Response evaluation:* Clinical follow-up at 3-month intervals for 2 years, then at 6-month intervals for 3 years, and yearly thereafter. Follow-up consists of physical examination, CBC, liver function tests, chest radiography, and CT as clinically indicated

(continued)

(*continued*)

Hand-foot reaction (palmar-plantar erythrodysesthesia, PPE)
- For patients who develop a hand-foot reaction, use topical emollients (eg, Aquaphor), topical or orally administered steroids, antihistamine agents (H_1-receptor antagonists), or pyridoxine
- **Pyridoxine** may provide relief for discomfort/pain associated with PPE although the mechanism through which this occurs remains unclear
- The suggested **pyridoxine** starting dose is 50 mg/day, which may be increased to a maximum of 200 mg/day

Treatment Modifications

Dose modification as clinically indicated based on the most significant toxicity
Recommendations apply to all 5 chemotherapy cycles

Starting dose	Fluorouracil 425 mg/m^2 (without radiation) or 400 mg/m^2 (with radiation)
Dosage level −1	Fluorouracil 350 mg/m^2
Dosage level −2	Fluorouracil 300 mg/m^2

Adverse Event	Dose Modification
Myelosuppression/ thrombocytopenia	Consider reducing chemotherapy doses during subsequent cycles
G2 stomatitis, diarrhea, or nausea	Hold 5-fluorouracil; resume 5-fluorouracil at full dosage after resolution of toxicity
Second episode of G2 stomatitis, diarrhea, or nausea	Hold 5-fluorouracil; resume 5-fluorouracil with dosage reduced by one dosage level after toxicity resolves
Third episode of G2 stomatitis, diarrhea, or nausea	Hold 5-fluorouracil; resume 5-fluorouracil with dosage reduced by one additional dosage level after toxicity resolves
Fourth episode of G2 stomatitis, diarrhea, or nausea	Discontinue 5-fluorouracil
G3 stomatitis, diarrhea, or nausea	Hold 5-fluorouracil. If G3 toxicity is adequately controlled within 2 days, resume 5-fluorouracil at full dosage when toxicity abates to G ≤1. If G3 toxicity takes >2 days to be controlled, resume 5-fluorouracil with dosage reduced by one dosage level after toxicity abates to G ≤1
Second episode of G3 stomatitis, diarrhea, or nausea	Hold 5-fluorouracil. If G3 toxicity is controlled adequately within 2 days, then resume 5-fluorouracil with dosage reduced by one additional dosage level after toxicity abates to G ≤1
Third episode of G3 stomatitis, diarrhea, or nausea	Discontinue 5-fluorouracil
G4 stomatitis, diarrhea, or nausea	Discontinue 5-fluorouracil. Resume 5-fluorouracil with dosage reduced by 50% after toxicity resolves
G1 capecitabine-associated PPE[†]	Begin pyridoxine 50 mg orally 3 times daily and continue 5-flurouracil without dose modification
G2 capecitabine-associated PPE[†]	Begin pyridoxine 50 mg orally 3 times daily and withhold capecitabine. Resume 5-fluorouracil with dosage reduced by 15% after toxicity resolves
G3 capecitabine-associated PPE[†]	Begin pyridoxine 50 mg orally 3 times daily and withhold capecitabine. Resume 5-fluorouracil with dosage reduced by 30% after toxicity resolves
Recurrent G3 capecitabine-associated PPE[†]	Begin pyridoxine 50 mg orally 3 times daily and withhold capecitabine. Resume 5-fluorouracil with dosage reduced by 50% after toxicity resolves

Toxicity (N = 273)

Event	Toxicity Grade ≥3 No. of Patients (%)
Hematologic	148 (54)
Gastrointestinal	89 (33)
Influenza-like symptoms	25 (9)
Infection	16 (6)
Neurologic	12 (4)
Cardiovascular	11 (4)
Pain	9 (3)
Metabolic	5 (2)
Hepatic	4 (1)
Lung-related	3 (1)
Death*	3 (1)

*One patient died from a cardiac event, one from pulmonary fibrosis, and one from sepsis complicating myelosuppression

LOCOREGIONAL DISEASE • ADJUVANT

GASTRIC CANCER REGIMEN: CAPECITABINE AND OXALIPLATIN AFTER D2 GASTRECTOMY

Bang Y-J et al. Lancet 2012;379:315–321

Capecitabine 1000 mg/m² per dose; administer orally twice daily for 14 consecutive days, on days 1–14, every 3 weeks for 8 cycles (total dosage/cycle = 28,000 mg/m²), *plus:*
Oxaliplatin 130 mg/m²; administer intravenously in 250–500 mL 5% dextrose injection over 2 hours on day 1, every 3 weeks, for 8 cycles (total dosage/cycle = 130 mg/m²)

Supportive Care

Antiemetic prophylaxis
Emetogenic potential on Day 1 is **MODERATE**
Emetogenic potential on days with capecitabine alone is **MINIMAL–LOW**
See Chapter 42 for antiemetic recommendations

Hematopoietic growth factor (CSF) prophylaxis
Primary prophylaxis may be indicated
See Chapter 43 for more information

Antimicrobial prophylaxis
Risk of fever and neutropenia is **LOW**
  Antimicrobial primary prophylaxis to be considered:
  • Antibacterial—not indicated
  • Antifungal—not indicated
  • Antiviral—not indicated, unless patient previously had an episode of HSV

Diarrhea management
Latent or delayed-onset diarrhea*:
Loperamide 4 mg orally initially after the first loose or liquid stool, *then* 2–4 mg orally every 2–4 hours or **diphenoxylate hydrochloride** 2.5 mg with **atropine sulfate** 0.025 mg (eg, Lomotil) 2 tablets orally four times per day

*Abigerges D et al. J Natl Cancer Inst 1994;86:446–449
Rothenberg ML et al. J Clin Oncol 2001;19:3801–3807
Wadler S et al. J Clin Oncol 1998;16:3169–3178

Oral care
Standard prophylaxis and treatment for mucositis/stomatitis

Hand-foot reaction (palmar-plantar erythrodysesthesia, PPE)
• For patients who develop a hand-foot reaction, use topical emollients (eg, Aquaphor), topical or orally administered steroids, antihistamine agents (H_1-receptor antagonists), or pyridoxine
• **Pyridoxine** may provide relief for discomfort/pain associated with PPE although the mechanism through which this occurs remains unclear
• The suggested **pyridoxine** starting dose is 50 mg/day, which may be increased to a maximum of 200 mg/day

Patient Population Studied

Patients with histologically confirmed gastric adenocarcinoma without evidence of metastatic disease. Only patients whose tumors were American Joint Committee on Cancer/Union Internationale Contre le Cancer (AJCC/UICC) stage II (T2N1, T1N2, T3N0), IIIA (T3N1, T2N2, T4N0), or IIIB (T3N2) were eligible. All patients had curative D2 gastrectomy and achieved R0 resection ≤6 weeks before randomization. At least 15 lymph nodes were examined. All surgeons were experienced (>50 procedures per year), and standard operating procedures were predefined

Patient Characteristics (N = 520)

Age (years)	56.1 (11.1)
Men	373 (72%)
Karnofsky performance status 90–100	90%
Time since surgery (months)	1.14 (0.17)
AJCC/UICC stage	
IB	1 (<1%)
II	253 (49%)
IIIA	193 (37%)
IIIB	73 (14%)
IV	0
Tumor stage	
T1	8 (2%)
T2	282 (54%)
T3	227 (44%)
T4	3 (1%)
Tumor location	
Antrum (lower third)	237 (46%)
Body (middle third)	166 (32%)
Body and antrum	31 (6%)
Fundus (upper third)	46 (9%)
Fundus and body	10 (2%)
Gastro-esophageal junction	15 (3%)
Whole gastric	6 (1%)
Other (multiple localizations)	9 (2%)
Lymph nodes examined	45.0 (17.4)
Nodal status	
N0	47 (9%)
N1	313 (60%)
N2	160 (31%)

Data are mean (SD), n (%), or median (interquartile range)
AJCC/UICC, American Joint Cancer Committee/Union Internationale Contre le Cancer

Efficacy

(Study Compared Adjuvant CAPE-OX After Surgery vs Surgery Only)

	Surgery Only (N = 515)	Surgery + CAPE-OX (N = 520)
Relapsed, developed a new gastric cancer, or died by time of data cutoff	163 (32%)	106 (20%)
3-year disease-free survival (DFS)	59% (95% CI, 53–64)	74% (95% CI, 69–79)
	HR 0.56, 95% CI 0.44–0.72; P <0.0001	
3-year DFS, stage II	71% (95% CI, 64–78)	85% (95% CI, 79–90)
3-year DFS, stage IIIa	51% (95% CI, 42–60)	66% (95% CI, 57–75)
3-year DFS stage IIIb	33% (95% CI, 15–51)	61% (95% CI, 48–73)
Deaths by time of data cutoff	85 (17%)	65 (13%)
3-year overall survival	78% (95% CI, 74–83)	83% (95% CI, 79–87)
	HR 0.72, 95% CI 0.52–1.00; P = 0.0493	
Recurrence or new gastric cancer	155 (30%)	96 (18%)
Peritoneal recurrence	56 (11%)	47 (9%)
Locoregional recurrence	44 (8.5%)	21 (4%)
Recurrence at distant sites	78 (15%)	49 (9.4%)

CAPE-OX, capecitabine and oxaliplatin

Treatment Monitoring

Before each cycle: Physical examination with attention to clinical toxicities, CBC with differential, serum creatinine, serum magnesium, and LFTs

Treatment Modifications

Adverse Event	Dose Modification
ANC nadir <1000/mm^3 *or* platelet nadir <50,000/mm^3 after treatment	Delay treatment until ANC ≥1000/mm^3 *and* platelet ≥50,000/mm^3, then decrease oxaliplatin dosage by 25%, and decrease daily capecitabine dosages by 50% during subsequent cycles*. Alternately consider using hematopoietic growth factors
Persistent G1/G2 neuropathy	Delay oxaliplatin 1 week. Resume oxaliplatin after toxicity resolves at a dosage decreased to 100 mg/m^2 during subsequent cycles
"Transient" G3/4 neuropathy (7–14 days duration)	Hold oxaliplatin. Resume oxaliplatin after toxicity resolves at a dosage decreased to 100 mg/m^2 during subsequent cycles
Persistent G3/4 neuropathy	Discontinue oxaliplatin
G3/4 diarrhea or stomatitis despite capecitabine dose reductions	Reduce oxaliplatin dosage to 100 mg/m^2
G3/4 nonhematologic adverse events other than renal function and neurotoxicity	Reduce cisplatin and capecitabine dosages by 25% for subsequent cycles
G2 stomatitis, diarrhea, or nausea	Hold capecitabine; resume capecitabine at full dosage after resolution of toxicity
Second episode of G2 stomatitis, diarrhea, or nausea	Hold capecitabine; resume capecitabine with dosage reduced by 25% after resolution of toxicity
Third episode of G2 stomatitis, diarrhea, or nausea	Hold capecitabine; resume capecitabine with dosage reduced by 50% after resolution of toxicity
Fourth episode of G2 stomatitis, diarrhea, or nausea	Discontinue capecitabine

(continued)

Treatment Modifications (*continued*)

Adverse Event	Dose Modification
G3 stomatitis, diarrhea, or nausea	Hold capecitabine. If G3 toxicity is adequately controlled within 2 days, resume capecitabine at full dosage when toxicity resolves to G ≤1. If G3 toxicity takes >2 days to be controlled, resume capecitabine with dosage reduced by 25% after toxicity resolves to G ≤1
Second episode of G3 stomatitis, diarrhea, or nausea	Hold capecitabine; if G3 toxicity is controlled adequately within 2 days, then resume capecitabine with dosage reduced by 50% after toxicity resolves to G ≤1
Third episode of G3 stomatitis, diarrhea, or nausea	Discontinue capecitabine
G4 stomatitis, diarrhea, or nausea	Withhold capecitabine. Resume capecitabine with dosage reduced by 50% after toxicity resolves
G1 capecitabine-associated PPE[†]	Begin pyridoxine 50 mg orally 3 times daily and continue capecitabine without dose modification
G2 capecitabine-associated PPE[†]	Begin pyridoxine 50 mg orally 3 times daily and withhold capecitabine. Resume capecitabine with dosage reduced by 15% after toxicity resolves
G3 capecitabine-associated PPE[†]	Begin pyridoxine 50 mg orally 3 times daily and withhold capecitabine. Resume capecitabine with dosage reduced by 30% after toxicity resolves
Recurrent G3 capecitabine-associated PPE[†]	Continue pyridoxine 50 mg orally 3 times daily and withhold capecitabine. Resume capecitabine with dosage reduced by 50% after toxicity resolves

*Treatment delays for unresolved adverse events of >3 weeks' duration warrant discontinuation of treatment
[†]PPE, palmar-plantar erythrodysesthesia (hand-foot syndrome)

Toxicity

Adverse events reported by ≥10% of patients (safety population*)
Capecitabine and Oxaliplatin (N = 496)

	All Grades	Grades 3/4
Patients with ≥1 adverse event	490 (99%)	279 (56%)
Nausea	326 (66%)	39 (8%)
Neutropenia	300 (60%)	107 (22%)
Decreased appetite	294 (59%)	23 (5%)
Peripheral neuropathy	277 (56%)	12 (2%)
Diarrhea	236 (48%)	9 (2%)
Vomiting	191 (39%)	37 (7%)
Fatigue	156 (31%)	23 (5%)
Thrombocytopenia	130 (26%)	40 (8%)
Hand–foot syndrome	93 (19%)	5 (1%)
Asthenia	87 (18%)	10 (2%)
Abdominal pain	85 (17%)	8 (2%)
Constipation	63 (13%)	1 (<1%)
Dizziness	64 (13%)	3 (<1%)
Stomatitis, all	59 (12%)	3 (<1%)
Weight decreased	59 (12%)	1 (<1%)
Peripheral sensory neuropathy	50 (10%)	3 (<1%)

Data are n (%)
*Patients who received ≥1 dose of capecitabine or oxaliplatin

METASTATIC DISEASE • FIRST-LINE
GASTRIC CANCER REGIMEN: FLUOROURACIL + LEUCOVORIN + OXALIPLATIN (FOLFOX) ± TRASTUZUMAB

Bang YJ et al. Lancet 2010;376(9742):687–697
Enzinger P et al. J Clin Oncol 2016;34(23):2736–2742
HERCEPTIN (trastuzumab) for injection prescribing information. South San Francisco, CA: Genentech, Inc; updated November 2018

Oxaliplatin 85 mg/m²; administer intravenously over 2 hours in 500 mL 5% dextrose injection (D5W) on day 1, every 2 weeks, concurrently with leucovorin administration, until disease progression (total dosage/cycle = 85 mg/m²), *plus:*
Leucovorin calcium 400 mg/m²; administer intravenously over 2 hours in 25–500 mL D5W on day 1, every 2 weeks, concurrently with oxaliplatin, until disease progression (total dosage/cycle = 400 mg/m²), *followed by:*
Fluorouracil 400 mg/m²; administer by intravenous injection over 1–2 minutes after leucovorin on day 1, every 2 weeks, until disease progression, *followed by:*
Fluorouracil 2400 mg/m²; administer by continuous intravenous infusion over 46 hours in 100–1000 mL 0.9% sodium chloride injection (0.9% NS) or D5W, starting on day 1 every 2 weeks, until disease progression (total fluorouracil dosage/cycle = 2800 mg/m²)
Note: The fluorouracil bolus dose (400 mg/m²) can be omitted for better hematologic tolerance
Note: Oxaliplatin must not be mixed with sodium chloride injection. Therefore, when leucovorin and oxaliplatin are given concurrently via the same administration set tubing, both drugs must be administered in D5W

The above regimen (FOLFOX) may be given with trastuzumab for HER2-positive patients as described below:
Loading Dose: **Trastuzumab** 6 mg/kg; administer intravenously in 250 mL 0.9% NS over 90 minutes as a loading dose on day 1, cycle 1 only (total dosage during the first cycle = 6 mg/kg), *followed 2 weeks later by:*
Maintenance Doses: **Trastuzumab** 4 mg/kg; administer intravenously in 250 mL 0.9% NS over 30 minutes on day 1, every 14 days, until disease progression (total dosage during each maintenance cycle = 4 mg/kg)

Note: Assess left ventricular ejection fraction (LVEF) prior to initiating trastuzumab and at regular intervals during treatment

Supportive Care
Antiemetic prophylaxis
Emetogenic potential on day 1 is **MODERATE**
Emetogenic potential on day 2 is **LOW**
See Chapter 42 for antiemetic recommendations

Hematopoietic growth factor (G-CSF) prophylaxis
Primary prophylaxis is **NOT** *indicated*
See Chapter 43 for more information

Antimicrobial prophylaxis
Risk of fever and neutropenia is **LOW**
  Antimicrobial primary prophylaxis to be considered:
  • *Antibacterial—not indicated*
  • *Antifungal—not indicated*
  • *Antiviral—not indicated unless patient previously had an episode of HSV*

Diarrhea management
Latent or delayed-onset diarrhea*:
Loperamide 4 mg orally initially after the first loose or liquid stool, *then* 2–4 mg orally every 2–4 hours or **diphenoxylate hydrochloride** 2.5 mg with **atropine sulfate** 0.025 mg (eg, Lomotil) 2 tablets orally four times per day

*Abigerges D et al. J Natl Cancer Inst 1994;86:446–449
Rothenberg ML et al. J Clin Oncol 2001;19:3801–3807
Wadler S et al. J Clin Oncol 1998;16:3169–3178

Oral care
Standard prophylaxis and treatment for mucositis/stomatitis

Patient Population Studied

This perioperative regimen is used in clinical practice as described above based on an extrapolation of evidence from a randomized phase 2 trial that enrolled 245 adult patients with metastatic esophageal or gastroesophageal junction (GEJ) cancer and compared treatment with cetuximab plus ECF (epirubicin, cisplatin, and fluorouracil) or IC (irinotecan and cisplatin) or FOLFOX (oxaliplatin, leucovorin, fluorouracil). Patients were eligible if they had metastatic adenocarcinoma or squamous cell carcinoma of the esophagus or GEJ (type I or II by Siewert classification) with measurable disease according to RECIST v1.0, and if they had an ECOG performance status of 0 to 2. Patients were excluded from the trial if they had received previous chemotherapy, radiotherapy, or anti-EGFR therapy, Note that this study was completed before the publication of two randomized studies which showed **no benefit** with the addition of EGFR-directed monoclonal antibodies to chemotherapy in patients with advanced esophagogastric cancer (Waddell T et al. Lancet Oncol 2013;14:481–489 and Lordick F et al. Lancet Oncol 2013;14:490–499). Therefore, in clinical practice, cetuximab is omitted from this regimen

Efficacy (N = 245)

	Cetuximab +			
	Epirubicin + Cisplatin + Fluorouracil (ECF) (N = 82)	Irinotecan + Cisplatin (IC) (N = 83)	Leucovorin + Fluorouracil + Oxaliplatin (FOLFOX) (N = 80)	
Complete response rate*	1.5%	1.4%	3.0%	
Partial response rate*	58.7%	43.6%	50.0%	
Stable disease rate*	22.2%	32.4%	27.2%	
Progressive disease rate*	7.9%	15.5%	12.1%	
Objective response rate*	60.3% (95% CI, 47.2–72.4)	45.1% (95% CI, 33.2–57.3)	53.0% (95% CI, 42.5–68.1)	P <0.001 for each treatment group compared to null hypothesis
Response duration*	7.1 months (range, 1.1–65.8)	6.5 months (range, 0.5–26.5)	6.6 months (range, 2.4–60.1)	
Median overall survival rate$^{\epsilon}$	11.6 months (95% CI, 8.1–13.4 months)	8.6 months (95% CI, 6.0–12.4 months)	11.8 months (95% CI, 8.8–13.9 months)	No significant pairwise comparisons
Median progression-free survival$^{\epsilon}$	7.1 months (95% CI, 4.5–8.4)	4.9 months (95% CI, 3.9–6.0)	6.8 months (95% CI, 5.4–8.1%)	No significant pairwise comparisons
Median time to treatment failure$^{\epsilon}$	5.6 months (95% CI, 3.9–7.2)	4.3 months (95% CI, 3.6–5.5)	6.7 months (95% CI, 4.8–7.4)	P = 0.012 for comparison of IC+C with FOLFOX+C; no other pairwise comparisons significant

HR, hazard ratio; CI, confidence interval
Response data (including duration of response) included only adenocarcinoma patients who received ≥1 cycle of chemotherapy (n = 200). Time to event data included all patients who received ≥1 cycle of chemotherapy (n = 213)
*Response rate graded according to RECIST v1.0 criteria.
$^{\epsilon}$Comparisons were unplanned

Therapy Monitoring

1. *Before each cycle:* History and physical examination with attention to neurologic exam
2. CBC with differential at a minimum once per cycle, but initially also at day 10–14
3. Serum bilirubin, AST, ALT, and alkaline phosphatase prior to each cycle
4. CA 19–9 and/or CEA prior to each cycle if detectable and being used to monitor disease
5. *Every 2–3 months:* CT scans to assess response

Treatment Modifications

Treatment Modifications—TRASTUZUMAB

Adverse Event	Dose Modification
Mild or moderate infusion reaction*	Decrease the rate of infusion
Infusion reaction with dyspnea or clinically significant hypotension	Interrupt the infusion reaction. Administer medical therapy as indicated including epinephrine, corticosteroids, diphenhydramine, bronchodilators, and oxygen. Observe patients closely for 60 minutes if the reaction occurs after the first infusion and for 30 minutes if it occurs after subsequent infusions. Prior to resumption of the trastuzumab infusion, premedicate with antihistamines and/or corticosteroids. *Note:* While some patients tolerate the resumption of trastuzumab infusions, others have recurrent severe infusion reactions despite premedications
Severe or life-threatening infusion reaction (includes bronchospasm, anaphylaxis, angioedema, hypoxia, and severe hypotension, usually reported during or immediately following the initial infusion)*	Interrupt the infusion reaction. Administer medical therapy as indicated including epinephrine, corticosteroids, diphenhydramine, bronchodilators, and oxygen. Patients should be evaluated and carefully monitored until complete resolution of signs and symptoms. Discontinue trastuzumab

(continued)

Treatment Modifications (continued)

Adverse Event	Dose Modification
≥16% absolute decrease in LVEF from pre-treatment values	Withhold trastuzumab dosing for at least 4–8 weeks. Resume trastuzumab if, within 4–8 weeks, the LVEF returns to normal limits and the absolute decrease from baseline is ≤15%
LVEF below institutional limits of normal and ≥10% absolute decrease in LVEF from pre-treatment values	
Persistent (>8 weeks) LVEF decline or suspension of trastuzumab dosing on ≥3 occasions for cardiomyopathy	Permanently discontinue trastuzumab
Pulmonary toxicity	Discontinue trastuzumab in patients experiencing pulmonary toxicity

*Infusion reactions consist of a symptom complex characterized by fever and chills, and on occasion included nausea, vomiting, pain (in some cases at tumor sites), headache, dizziness, dyspnea, hypotension, rash, and asthenia

Treatment Modifications—FOLFOX

Adverse Event	Treatment Modification

Notes:
- Before beginning treatment cycle, patients should have baseline bowel function similar to that before the start of treatment, without antidiarrheal therapy for 24 hours, ANC ≥1500/mm³, and platelet count ≥100,000/mm³
- Treatment should be delayed 1–2 weeks to allow for recovery from treatment-related toxicities. If toxicities have not resolved after 2 weeks, consider stopping therapy
- Dose modifications are based on the National Cancer Institute (USA) Common Toxicity Criteria V5.0. At: http://ctep.cancer.gov/protocolDevelopment/electronic_applications/ctc.htm

Neutropenia/Thrombocytopenia

G1 ANC (1500–1999/mm³) or G1 thrombocytopenia (<LLN–75,000/mm³)	Maintain dose and schedule
G2 ANC (1000–1499/mm³) or G2 thrombocytopenia (<75,000–50,000/mm³)	Reduce oxaliplatin dosage to 70 mg/m² and fluorouracil by intravenous bolus injection to 300 mg/m²
G3 ANC (500–999/mm³) or G3 thrombocytopenia (<50,000–25,000/mm³)	Hold treatment until toxicity resolves to G ≤2, then reduce oxaliplatin dosage to 70 mg/m² and omit fluorouracil by intravenous bolus injection in subsequent cycles
G4 ANC (<500/mm³) or G4 thrombocytopenia (<25,000/mm³)	Hold treatment until toxicity resolves to G ≤2, then reduce oxaliplatin dosage to 60–70 mg/m², reduce infusional fluorouracil to 2000 mg/m², and omit fluorouracil by intravenous bolus injection in subsequent cycles
Febrile neutropenia (ANC <1000/mm³ with single temperature >38.3°C [101°F] or a sustained temperature of ≥38°C [100.4°F] for more than one hour)	Hold treatment until neutropenia resolves, then reduce oxaliplatin dosage to 60–70 mg/m², reduce infusional fluorouracil to 2000 mg/m², and omit fluorouracil by intravenous bolus injection in subsequent cycles
Day 1 ANC ≤1500/mm³ or platelet count ≤100,000/mm³	Delay start of next cycle until ANC >1500/mm³ and platelet count >100,000/mm³; omit fluorouracil by intravenous bolus injection in subsequent cycles

Diarrhea

Notes: Before beginning a treatment cycle, patients should have baseline bowel function (similar to that before the start of treatment) without antidiarrheal therapy for 24 hours

G1 (2–3 stools/day > baseline)	Maintain dose and schedule
G2 (4–6 stools/day > baseline)	Delay until diarrhea resolves to baseline, then reduce oxaliplatin dosage to 70 mg/m² and fluorouracil by intravenous bolus injection to 300 mg/m²
G3 (7–9 stools/day > baseline)	Delay until diarrhea resolves to baseline, then reduce oxaliplatin dosage to 60–70 mg/m², infusional fluorouracil to 1600–2000 mg/m², and omit fluorouracil by intravenous bolus injection
G4 (≥10 stools/day > baseline; life-threatening; urgent intervention required)	Delay until diarrhea resolves to baseline, then reduce oxaliplatin dosage to 60 mg/m², infusional fluorouracil to 1600 mg/m², and omit fluorouracil by intravenous bolus injection

(continued)

Treatment Modifications (*continued*)

Other Nonhematologic Toxicities	
Day 1 persistent nonhematologic toxicity G ≥2	Delay start of next cycle until the severity of all toxicities are G ≤1; omit fluorouracil by intravenous bolus injection in subsequent cycles
G ≥3 non-neurologic toxicity	Reduce infusional fluorouracil dosage to 2000 mg/m²
G2 paresthesia (persistent paresthesia or dysesthesia, moderate in nature without functional impairment other than limiting instrumental ADL)	Reduce oxaliplatin dosage to 60–70 mg/m²
Persistent G2 paresthesia/dysesthesia	Discontinue oxaliplatin
Persistent painful paresthesia or G3 neuropathy (persistent paresthesia or dysesthesia with persistent functional impairment limiting self-care and ADL)	

Adapted from Tournigand C et al. J Clin Oncol 2004;22:229–237

Adverse Events (N = 213)

Event	Cetuximab +		
	Epirubicin + Cisplatin + Fluorouracil (ECF) (N = 67)	Irinotecan + Cisplatin (IC) (N = 73)	Leucovorin + Fluorouracil + Oxaliplatin (FOLFOX) (N = 73)
Treatment modifications	91%	85%	73%
	P = 0.013		
Treatment discontinued due to adverse events	19%	26%	11%
	P = 0.17		
Treatment-related death	6.0%	8.2%	2.7%
Grade (%)	Grade 3–5	Grade 3–5	Grade 3–5
All Hematologic	53	59	46
	P = 0.32		
Neutropenia	49	51	43
Leukocytopenia	13	22	16
Anemia	7	13	7
Thrombocytopenia	4	8	3
Lymphopenia	7	11	3
All Nonhematologic	73	77	66
Constitutional symptoms	13	21	16
Dermatologic	17	11	22
Gastrointestinal	31	41 (↑P = 0.04)	22
Infection	12	7	7
Metabolic	18	34 (↑P = 0.09)	26
Neurologic	15	3 (↓P = 0.02)	16
Pain	8	3	3
Pulmonary	4	3	0
Vascular	7	9	4
Death (not CTCAE defined)	4	0	0

Adverse events were included if they were reported by patients who received any trial drug, if they were of Grade 3–5, and if they were at least possibly related to treatment according to CTCAE version 3 criteria. 58% of treated patients stopped treatment because of disease progression, 13% due to adverse effects, and 11% due to withdrawal of consent

METASTATIC DISEASE • FIRST-LINE

GASTRIC CANCER REGIMEN: CAPECITABINE + OXALIPLATIN (CAPOX) ± TRASTUZUMAB

Bang YJ et al. Lancet 2010;376(9742):687–697
Kim GM et al. Eur J Cancer 2012;48(4):518–526
HERCEPTIN (trastuzumab) for injection prescribing information. South San Francisco, CA: Genentech, Inc; updated November 2018

Oxaliplatin 130 mg/m^2; administer intravenously in 250–500 mL 5% dextrose injection over 2 hours on day 1, every 21 days, until disease progression (total dosage/3-week cycle = 130 mg/m^2)

Capecitabine 1000 mg/m^2 per dose; administer orally twice daily (approximately every 12 hours, within 30 minutes after a meal) for 14 consecutive days, on days 1–14 (28 doses), every 21 days, until disease progression (total dosage/3-week cycle = 28,000 mg/m^2)

The above regimen (CAPOX) may be given with trastuzumab for HER2-positive patients as described below:

Loading Dose: **Trastuzumab** 8 mg/kg; administer intravenously in 250 mL 0.9% NS over 90 minutes as a loading dose on day 1, cycle 1 only (total dosage during the first cycle = 8 mg/kg), *followed 3 weeks later by:*

Maintenance Doses: **Trastuzumab** 6 mg/kg; administer intravenously in 250 mL 0.9% NS over 30 minutes on day 1, every 21 days, until disease progression (total dosage during each maintenance cycle = 6 mg/kg)

Note: Assess left ventricular ejection fraction (LVEF) prior to initiating trastuzumab and at regular intervals during treatment

Supportive Care
Antiemetic prophylaxis
Emetogenic potential on day 1 is **MODERATE**
Emetogenic potential on days with capecitabine alone is **MINIMAL–LOW**
See Chapter 42 for antiemetic recommendations

Hematopoietic growth factor (G-CSF) prophylaxis
Primary prophylaxis is **NOT** indicated
See Chapter 43 for more information

Antimicrobial prophylaxis
Risk of fever and neutropenia is **LOW**
   Antimicrobial primary prophylaxis to be considered:
   • Antibacterial—not indicated
   • Antifungal—not indicated
   • Antiviral—not indicated, unless patient previously had an episode of HSV

Hand-foot reaction (palmar-plantar erythrodysesthesia, PPE)
• For patients who develop a hand-foot reaction, use topical emollients (eg, Aquaphor), topical or orally administered steroids, antihistamine agents (H$_1$-receptor antagonists), or pyridoxine
• **Pyridoxine** may provide relief for discomfort/pain associated with PPE although the mechanism through which this occurs remains unclear
• The suggested **pyridoxine** starting dose is 50 mg/day, which may be increased to a maximum of 200 mg/day

Diarrhea management
Latent or delayed-onset diarrhea:
Loperamide 4 mg orally initially after the first loose or liquid stool, *then* 2–4 mg orally every 2–4 hours or **diphenoxylate hydrochloride** 2.5 mg with **atropine sulfate** 0.025 mg (eg, Lomotil) 2 tablets orally four times per day

*Abigerges D et al. J Natl Cancer Inst 1994;86:446–449
Rothenberg ML et al. J Clin Oncol 2001;19:3801–3807
Wadler S et al. J Clin Oncol 1998;16:3169–3178

Oral care
Standard prophylaxis and treatment for mucositis/stomatitis

Patient Population Studied

Based in part on a randomized, phase 2 trial included 129 patients with advanced gastric cancer and compared treatment with S-1 plus oxaliplatin (SOX) or capecitabine plus oxaliplatin (CAPOX). Patients were eligible if they had histologically confirmed metastatic or recurrent gastric adenocarcinoma with measurable or evaluable lesions, if they had never received previous chemotherapy (except for adjuvant or preoperative chemotherapy more than 6 months before enrollment that didn't include S-1, capecitabine, or oxaliplatin), if they had an ECOG performance score of 0–2, and adequate organ function. Patients were excluded if they had brain metastases, neuropathy of grade >2, or uncontrolled comorbid conditions

Efficacy (N = 129)

	S–1 + Oxaliplatin (SOX) (N = 65)	Capecitabine + Oxaliplatin (CAPOX) (N = 64)	
Median time to progression†	6.2 months (95% CI, 4.92–7.48)	7.2 months (95% CI, 5.87–8.54)	HR 1.06 (95% CI, 0.72–1.57); P = 0.767
Median overall survival†	12.4 months (95% CI, 8.796–16.01)	13.3 months (95% CI, 10.26–16.34)	HR 1.08 (95% CI, 0.74–1.58); P = 0.686
Estimated survival rate, 12 months	52%	59%	
Complete response rate‡	0%	2%	
Partial response rate‡	40%	42%	
Stable disease rate‡	51%	40%	
Progressive disease rate‡	7%	16%	
Overall objective response rate‡	40% (95% CI, 26–54)	44% (95% CI, 29–60)	
Disease control rate‡	91%	84%	

HR, hazard ratio; CI, confidence interval
†P Values were calculated using the log-rank test
‡Response rates were graded according to RECIST v1.0 criteria and were generated from a modified intention-to-treat population which included only patients who received at least one dose of trial drug and who had measurable lesions. This population included 53 patients in the SOX group and 45 patients in the CAPOX group

Therapy Monitoring

1. *Prior to each cycle of capecitabine + oxaliplatin:* CBC with differential, serum bilirubin, AST or ALT, alkaline phosphatase, serum creatinine. Assessment for peripheral neuropathy
2. *Every 2–3 months:* CT scans to assess response

Treatment Modifications

Treatment Modifications—TRASTUZUMAB	
Adverse Event	**Dose Modification**
Mild or moderate infusion reaction*	Decrease the rate of infusion
Infusion reaction with dyspnea or clinically significant hypotension	Interrupt the infusion reaction. Administer medical therapy as indicated including epinephrine, corticosteroids, diphenhydramine, bronchodilators, and oxygen. Observe patients closely for 60 minutes if the reaction occurs after the first infusion and for 30 minutes if it occurs after subsequent infusions. Prior to resumption of the trastuzumab infusion, premedicate with antihistamines and/or corticosteroids *Note:* While some patients tolerate the resumption of trastuzumab infusions, others have recurrent severe infusion reactions despite premedications
Severe or life-threatening infusion reaction (includes bronchospasm, anaphylaxis, angioedema, hypoxia, and severe hypotension, usually reported during or immediately following the initial infusion)*	Interrupt the infusion reaction. Administer medical therapy as indicated including epinephrine, corticosteroids, diphenhydramine, bronchodilators, and oxygen. Patients should be evaluated and carefully monitored until complete resolution of signs and symptoms. Discontinue trastuzumab
≥16% absolute decrease in LVEF from pre-treatment values	Withhold trastuzumab dosing for at least 4–8 weeks. Resume trastuzumab if, within 4–8 weeks, the LVEF returns to normal limits and the absolute decrease from baseline is ≤15%
LVEF below institutional limits of normal and ≥10% absolute decrease in LVEF from pre-treatment values	
Persistent (>8 weeks) LVEF decline or suspension of trastuzumab dosing on ≥3 occasions for cardiomyopathy	Permanently discontinue trastuzumab
Pulmonary toxicity	Discontinue trastuzumab in patients experiencing pulmonary toxicity

*Infusion reactions consist of a symptom complex characterized by fever and chills, and on occasion included nausea, vomiting, pain (in some cases at tumor sites), headache, dizziness, dyspnea, hypotension, rash, and asthenia

Treatment Modifications (continued)

CAPECITABINE AND OXALIPLATIN DOSE MODIFICATIONS

	Capecitabine dose	Oxaliplatin dose
Starting dose	1000 mg/m^2/dose twice per day	130 mg/m^2
Dose level −1	750 mg/m^2/dose twice per day	100 mg/m^2
Dose level −2	500 mg/m^2/dose twice per day	70 mg/m^2

Adverse Event	Treatment Modification
Symptomatic toxicity, ANC <1500/mm^3, or platelet count <75,000/mm^3	Delay treatment up to 3 weeks. If after 3 weeks symptomatic toxicity has not improved, ANC is still <1500/mm^3, or platelet count still <75,000/mm^3, then discontinue treatment
G4 ANC (<500/mm^3), G4 thrombocytopenia (<25,000/mm^3), or febrile neutropenia with ANC <1000/mm^3 + a single temperature of >38.3°C (101°F) or a sustained temperature of 38°C (100.4°F) for more than one hour or G3 nausea/vomiting, diarrhea, or stomatitis	Delay treatment until ANC is ≥1500/mm^3 *and* platelet count is ≥75,000/mm^3, then reduce the doses of oxaliplatin and capecitabine by one dose level beginning with the next cycle. Consider using hematopoietic growth factors. *Note:* Treatment delays for unresolved adverse events of >3 weeks' duration warrant discontinuation of treatment
G2/3 hand-foot syndrome or palmar-plantar erythrodysesthesia or chemotherapy-induced acral erythema*	Withhold capecitabine; provide supportive care. Do not resume capecitabine until toxicity resolved to G ≤1. In subsequent cycle(s), *permanently* reduce the capecitabine dosage by 1 dose level
G2/3 diarrhea, stomatitis, nausea, or dehydration	
Second episode of G2/3 diarrhea, stomatitis, nausea, or dehydration	Hold capecitabine; resume capecitabine with dosage reduced by one dose level after toxicity resolves
G4 diarrhea, stomatitis, nausea, or dehydration	Permanently discontinue capecitabine
Stevens-Johnson syndrome and toxic epidermal necrolysis (severe mucocutaneous reactions, some with fatal outcome)	
Capecitabine-induced coronary vasospasm/cardiac ischemia	
G3/4 diarrhea or stomatitis despite capecitabine dose reductions	Reduce oxaliplatin dosage by one dose level
Creatinine clearance 30–50 mL/minute	Reduce the capecitabine dosage by 1 dose level
Creatinine clearance <30 mL/minute	Withhold capecitabine
Persistent G1/G2 neuropathy	Delay oxaliplatin 1 week. After toxicity resolves, resume oxaliplatin at a dosage decreased by one dose level during subsequent cycles
"Transient" G3/4 neuropathy (7–14 days)	Hold oxaliplatin. After toxicity resolves, resume oxaliplatin at a dosage decreased by one dose level during subsequent cycles
Persistent G3/4 neuropathy	Discontinue oxaliplatin
Other G3/4 nonhematologic adverse events	Reduce oxaliplatin and capecitabine dosages by one dose level during subsequent cycles

ANC, absolute neutrophil count; CBC, complete blood count
Grading of hand-foot syndrome is as follows:
• G1: Numbness, dysesthesia/paresthesia, tingling, painless swelling, or erythema of the hands and/or feet and/or discomfort which does not disrupt normal activities
• G2: Painful erythema and swelling of the hands and/or feet and/or discomfort affecting the patient's activities of daily living
• G3: Moist desquamation, ulceration, blistering, or severe pain of the hands and/or feet and/or severe discomfort that causes the patient to be unable to work or perform activities of daily living

Adverse Events

Event	S–1 + Oxaliplatin (SOX) (N = 65)		Capecitabine + Oxaliplatin (CAPOX) (N = 64)	
Grade (%)	Grade 1/2	Grade 3/4	Grade 1/2	Grade 3/4
Neutropenia	48	9	44	19
Leukopenia	45	8	50	3
Anemia	78	12	89	3
Thrombocytopenia	49	15	52	14
Asthenia	40	2	42	8
Anorexia	49	3	47	3
Nausea	45	3	38	5
Vomiting	40	2	30	3
Diarrhea	26	5	30	5
Neuropathy	38	3	44	5
Hand-foot syndrome*	3	0	23	2
Infection	11	9	8	6

Data were included from the modified intention-to-treat population, which includes only patients who received at least one dose of trial drug. Adverse events were graded according to National Cancer Institute Common Terminology Criteria for Adverse Events (NCI-CTCAE) version 3.0
*Only adverse event with a statistically significant difference in incidence (P <0.001)

METASTATIC DISEASE • FIRST-LINE

GASTRIC CANCER REGIMEN: CISPLATIN + EITHER FLUOROURACIL (CF) OR CAPECITABINE (CX) ± TRASTUZUMAB

Bang YJ et al. Lancet 2010;376:687–697
Kang YK et al. Ann Oncol 2009;20:666–673
Supplementary webappendix to: Bang YJ et al. Lancet 2010;376:687–697

Either:
Capecitabine 1000 mg/m² per dose; administer orally twice daily for 14 consecutive days, on days 1–14 (28 doses), followed by 7 days without treatment, every 3 weeks (total dosage/cycle = 28,000 mg/m²)
Or:
Fluorouracil 800 mg/m² per day; administer by continuous intravenous infusion in 50–1000 mL 0.9% sodium chloride injection (0.9% NS) or 5% dextrose injection over 24 hours for 5 consecutive days, on days 1–5, every 3 weeks (total dosage/cycle = 4000 mg/m²)
With:
Hydration before cisplatin: 1000 mL 0.9% NS; administer intravenously over a minimum of 1 hour before commencing cisplatin administration
(optional) **Mannitol** 12.5–25 g; administer by intravenous injection or intravenous infusion over 5–15 minutes before starting cisplatin
• Mannitol may be given to patients who have received adequate hydration. Continued hydration is essential to ensure diuresis
• Mannitol may be prepared as an admixture (in the same container) with cisplatin

Cisplatin 80 mg/m²; administer intravenously in 50–500 mL 0.9% NS over 2 hours on day 1, every 3 weeks (total dosage/cycle = 80 mg/m²)
Hydration after cisplatin: ≥1000 mL 0.9% NS; administer intravenously over a minimum of 2 hours. Monitor and replace magnesium and other electrolytes as needed. Encourage patients to increase their intake of nonalcoholic fluids

Regimen notes:
• Regarding duration of therapy, in the study by Kang et al, cisplatin and fluorouracil/capecitabine were administered until disease progression, lack of clinical benefit, or intolerable toxicity. In the study by Bang et al, which evaluated the same regimens either alone or with trastuzumab, cytotoxic chemotherapy was given for a maximum of 6 cycles and trastuzumab was continued until disease progression or unacceptable toxicity

The above regimens (cisplatin + fluorouracil or capecitabine) may be given with trastuzumab for HER2-positive patients as described below:
• *Loading Dose:* **Trastuzumab** 8 mg/kg; administer intravenously in 250 mL 0.9% NS over 90 minutes as a loading dose on day 1, cycle 1 only (total dosage during the first cycle = 8 mg/kg), *followed 3 weeks later by:*
• *Maintenance Doses:* **Trastuzumab** 6 mg/kg; administer intravenously in 250 mL 0.9% NS over 30 minutes on day 1, every 21 days, until disease progression (total dosage during each maintenance cycle = 6 mg/kg)
Note: Assess left ventricular ejection fraction (LVEF) prior to initiating trastuzumab and at regular intervals during treatment

Supportive Care
Antiemetic prophylaxis
Emetogenic potential on days with cisplatin is **HIGH**. *Potential for delayed emetic symptoms*
Emetogenic potential on days with capecitabine or fluorouracil is **LOW**
Emetogenic potential on days with trastuzumab alone is **MINIMAL**
See Chapter 42 for antiemetic recommendations

Hematopoietic growth factor (CSF) prophylaxis
Primary prophylaxis is **NOT** *indicated*
See Chapter 43 for more information

Antimicrobial prophylaxis
Risk of fever and neutropenia is **LOW**
　Antimicrobial primary prophylaxis to be considered:
• Antibacterial—not indicated
• Antifungal—not indicated
• Antiviral—not indicated, unless patient previously had an episode of HSV

Diarrhea management
Latent or delayed-onset diarrhea*:
Loperamide 4 mg orally initially after the first loose or liquid stool, *then* 2–4 mg orally every 2–4 hours or **diphenoxylate hydrochloride** 2.5 mg with **atropine sulfate** 0.025 mg (eg, Lomotil) 2 tablets orally four times per day

*Abigerges D et al. J Natl Cancer Inst 1994;86:446–449
Rothenberg ML et al. J Clin Oncol 2001;19:3801–3807
Wadler S et al. J Clin Oncol 1998;16:3169–3178

Oral care
Standard prophylaxis and treatment for mucositis/stomatitis

(continued)

(*continued*)

Hand-foot reaction (palmar-plantar erythrodysesthesia, PPE)
- For patients who develop a hand-foot reaction, use topical emollients (eg, Aquaphor), topical or orally administered steroids, antihistamine agents (H_1-receptor antagonists), or pyridoxine
- **Pyridoxine** may provide relief for discomfort/pain associated with PPE although the mechanism through which this occurs remains unclear
- The suggested **pyridoxine** starting dose is 50 mg/day, which may be increased to a maximum of 200 mg/day

Patient Population Studied

Kang YK et al. Ann Oncol 2009;20:666–673
This international, multicenter, randomized, open-label, phase 3 trial involved 316 adult patients, age 18–75 years, with histologically confirmed advanced gastric cancer. Participants were eligible if they had Karnofsky performance status of ≥70: and had not received previous chemotherapy (except neoadjuvant or adjuvant regimens)

Bang YJ et al. Lancet 2010;376:687–697
This international, multicenter, open-label, phase 3 randomized controlled trial involved 594 adult patients with gastric or gastroesophageal junction cancer. Patients were eligible for inclusion if they had histologically confirmed inoperable locally advanced, recurrent, or metastatic adenocarcinoma of the stomach or gastroesophageal junction. Additionally, eligible patients had tumors that showed overexpression of human epidermal growth factor receptor 2 (HER2) protein. Participants were excluded if they had previous chemotherapy for metastatic disease, congestive heart failure or baseline left ventricular ejection fraction <50%, transmural myocardial infarction, uncontrolled hypertension (systolic blood pressure >180 mmHg or diastolic blood pressure >100 mmHg), or active gastrointestinal bleeding

Efficacy

Kang YK et al. Ann Oncol 2009;20:666–673

End Point	Cisplatin + Capecitabine (N = 139)	Cisplatin + 5-Fluorouracil (N = 137)	Between-Group Comparison
Median progression-free survival	5.6 months (95% CI 4.9–7.3)	5.0 months (95% CI 4.2–6.3)	HR 0.81 (95% CI 0.63–1.04) P <0.001*
Median overall survival	10.5 (95% CI 9.3–11.2)	9.3 (95% CI 7.4–10.6)	HR 0.85 (95% CI 0.64–1.13) P = 0.008*
Overall response rate	46% (95% CI 38–55)	32% (95% CI 24–41)	OR 1.80 (95% CI 1.11–2.94) P = 0.020
Patients with complete response	2%	3%	—
Patients with partial response	44%	29%	—
Mean time to response	3.7 months	3.8 months	HR 1.61 (95% CI 1.10–2.35) P = 0.015
Median duration of response	7.6 months	6.2 months	HR 0.88 (95% CI 0.56–1.36) P = 0.554

HR, hazard ratio, CI, confidence interval; OR, odds ratio
*P value for noninferiority versus 1.25. The upper limit of the two-sided 95% CI for the hazard ratio did not exceed the prespecified noninferiority margin of 1.25

Efficacy

Bang YJ et al. Lancet 2010;376:687–697

End Point	Trastuzumab + Chemotherapy (Cisplatin + Capecitabine or Fluorouracil) (N = 294)	Chemotherapy Alone (Cisplatin + Capecitabine or Fluorouracil) (N = 290)	Between-Group Comparison
Median overall survival	13.8 months (95% CI 12–16)	11.1 months (95% CI 10–13)	HR 0.74 (95% CI 0.60–0.91) P = 0.0046
Median progression-free survival	6.7 months (95% CI 6–8)	5.5 months (95% CI 5–6)	HR 0.71 (95% CI 0.59–0.85) P = 0.0002
Time to progression	7.1 months (95% CI 6–8)	5.6 months (95% CI 5–6)	HR 0.70 (95% CI 0.58–0.85) P = 0.0003
Duration of response	6.9 months (95% CI 6–8)*	4.8 months (95% CI 4–6)†	HR 0.54 (95% CI 0.40–0.73) P <0.0001

(*continued*)

Efficacy (continued)

End Point	Trastuzumab + Chemotherapy (Cisplatin + Capecitabine or Fluorouracil) (N = 294)	Chemotherapy Alone (Cisplatin + Capecitabine or Fluorouracil) (N = 290)	Between-Group Comparison
Overall tumor response rate	47%	35%	OR 1.70 (95% CI 1.22–2.38) P = 0.0017
Patients with complete response	5%	2%	OR 2.33 (95% CI 0.94–5.74) P = 0.0599
Patients with partial response	42%	32%	OR 1.52 (95% CI 1.09–2.14) P = 0.0145

HR, hazard ratio, CI, confidence interval; OR, odds ratio
*For the analysis of duration of response, N = 139 in the trastuzumab + chemotherapy group
†For the analysis of duration of response, N = 100 in the chemotherapy alone group

Therapy Monitoring

1. *Before each cycle:* History and physical examination, BUN, serum creatinine, electrolytes, serum bilirubin, AST, ALT, and alkaline phosphatase
2. *Weekly:* CBC with differential, BUN, serum creatinine, electrolytes
3. *Every 2–3 months:* CT scans to assess response

Treatment Modifications

Treatment Modifications—TRASTUZUMAB

Adverse Event	Dose Modification
Mild or moderate infusion reaction*	Decrease the rate of infusion
Infusion reaction with dyspnea or clinically significant hypotension	Interrupt the infusion reaction. Administer medical therapy as indicated including epinephrine, corticosteroids, diphenhydramine, bronchodilators, and oxygen. Observe patients closely for 60 minutes if the reaction occurs after the first infusion and for 30 minutes if it occurs after subsequent infusions. Prior to resumption of the trastuzumab infusion, premedicate with antihistamines and/or corticosteroids. *Note:* While some patients tolerate the resumption of trastuzumab infusions, others have recurrent severe infusion reactions despite premedications
Severe or life-threatening infusion reaction (includes bronchospasm, anaphylaxis, angioedema, hypoxia, and severe hypotension, usually reported during or immediately following the initial infusion)*	Interrupt the infusion reaction. Administer medical therapy as indicated including epinephrine, corticosteroids, diphenhydramine, bronchodilators, and oxygen. Patients should be evaluated and carefully monitored until complete resolution of signs and symptoms. Discontinue trastuzumab
≥16% absolute decrease in LVEF from pre-treatment values	Withhold trastuzumab dosing for at least 4–8 weeks. Resume trastuzumab if, within 4–8 weeks, the LVEF returns to normal limits and the absolute decrease from baseline is ≤15%
LVEF below institutional limits of normal and ≥10% absolute decrease in LVEF from pre-treatment values	
Persistent (>8 weeks) LVEF decline or suspension of trastuzumab dosing on ≥3 occasions for cardiomyopathy	Permanently discontinue trastuzumab
Pulmonary toxicity	Discontinue trastuzumab in patients experiencing pulmonary toxicity

*Infusion reactions consist of a symptom complex characterized by fever and chills, and on occasion included nausea, vomiting, pain (in some cases at tumor sites), headache, dizziness, dyspnea, hypotension, rash, and asthenia

(continued)

Treatment Modifications (*continued*)

Treatment Modifications—CAPECITABINE/5-FLUOROURACIL + CISPLATIN	
ANC nadir <1000/mm³ *or* platelet nadir <50,000/mm³ after treatment	Delay treatment until ANC is ≥1000/mm³ *and* platelet count is ≥50,000/mm³, then decrease cisplatin and 5-fluorouracil dosages by 25%, or if using capecitabine, decrease daily capecitabine dosages by 50% during subsequent cycles*. Alternatively, consider using hematopoietic growth factors
Recurrent treatment delay because of myelosuppression	Delay therapy for 1 week, or until myelosuppression resolves, then decrease cisplatin and 5-fluorouracil dosages by 25% during subsequent treatments or if using capecitabine, decrease daily capecitabine dosages by 50% during subsequent cycles*
Sepsis during an episode of neutropenia	
Reduction in creatinine clearance* to 60% of on-study value	Delay therapy 1 week. If creatinine clearance does not recover to pretreatment values, then consider reducing cisplatin dose
Creatinine clearance* 40–60 mL/min (0.66–1 mL/s)	Consider reducing cisplatin so that dose in milligrams equals the creatinine clearance* value in mL/min (mL/s × 1/0.0166)† If the patient is receiving capecitabine and the creatinine clearance is <50 mL/min, then reduce the capecitabine dosage by 1 dose level
Creatinine clearance* <40 mL/min (<0.66 mL/s)	Hold cisplatin If the patient is receiving capecitabine and the creatinine clearance is 30–40 mL/min, then reduce the capecitabine dosage by 1 dose level; if the creatinine clearance is <30 mL/min, then withhold capecitabine
Clinically significant ototoxicity	Discontinue cisplatin
Persistent (>14 days) peripheral neuropathy without functional impairment	Decrease cisplatin dosage by 50%
Clinically significant sensory loss—persistent (>14 days) peripheral neuropathy with functional impairment	Discontinue cisplatin
G3 nausea, vomiting	Decrease cisplatin dosage by 25%
G2 stomatitis or diarrhea	Hold capecitabine/5-fluorouracil; resume capecitabine/5-fluorouracil at full dosage after resolution of toxicity
Second episode of G2 stomatitis or diarrhea	Hold capecitabine/5-fluorouracil; resume capecitabine/5-fluorouracil with dosage reduced by 25% after toxicity resolves
Third episode of G2 stomatitis or diarrhea	Hold capecitabine/5-fluorouracil; resume capecitabine/5-fluorouracil with dosage reduced by 50% after toxicity resolves
Fourth episode of G2 stomatitis or diarrhea	Discontinue capecitabine/5-fluorouracil
G3 stomatitis or diarrhea	Hold capecitabine/5-fluorouracil. If G3 toxicity is adequately controlled within 2 days, resume capecitabine/5-fluorouracil at full dosage when toxicity abates to G ≤1. If G3 toxicity takes >2 days to be controlled, resume capecitabine/5-fluorouracil with dosage reduced by 25% after toxicity abates to G ≤1
Second episode of G3 stomatitis or diarrhea	Hold capecitabine/5-fluorouracil. If G3 toxicity is controlled adequately within 2 days, then resume capecitabine/5-fluorouracil with dosage reduced by 50% after toxicity abates to G ≤1
Third episode of G3 stomatitis or diarrhea	Discontinue capecitabine/5-fluorouracil
G4 stomatitis or diarrhea	Discontinue capecitabine/5-fluorouracil. Resume capecitabine/5-fluorouracil with dosage reduced by 50% after toxicity resolves
G1 capecitabine-associated PPE†	Begin pyridoxine 50 mg orally 3 times daily and continue capecitabine without dose modification
G2 capecitabine-associated PPE†	Begin pyridoxine 50 mg orally 3 times daily and withhold capecitabine. Resume capecitabine with dosage reduced by 15% after toxicity resolves
G3 capecitabine-associated PPE†	Begin pyridoxine 50 mg orally 3 times daily and withhold capecitabine. Resume capecitabine with dosage reduced by 30% after toxicity resolves
Recurrent G3 capecitabine-associated PPE†	Begin pyridoxine 50 mg orally 3 times daily and withhold capecitabine. Resume capecitabine with dosage reduced by 50% after toxicity resolves

Adverse Events

Kang YK et al. Ann Oncol 2009;20:666–673

Grade (%)	Cisplatin + Capecitabine (N = 156)		Cisplatin + 5-Fluorouracil (N = 155)	
	Grade 1–2	Grade 3–4	Grade 1–2	Grade 3–4
Nausea	53	2	52	3
Vomiting	42	7	50	8
Diarrhea	15	5	11	5
Stomatitis	10	2	20	6
Neutropenia	16	16	11	19
Leukopenia	12	3	13	4
Anorexia	27	2	27	<1
Fatigue	15	<1	9	<1
Asthenia	12	2	17	<1
Hand-foot syndrome*	18	4	4	0

*Hand-foot syndrome was more frequent in the cisplatin + capecitabine group than the cisplatin + 5-fluorouracil group, but it led to treatment discontinuation in one patient

Adverse Events

Bang YJ et al. Lancet 2010;376:687–697

Grade (%)	Trastuzumab + Chemotherapy (Cisplatin + Capecitabine or Fluorouracil) (N = 294)		Chemotherapy Alone (Cisplatin + Capecitabine or Fluorouracil) (N = 290)	
	Grade 1–2	Grade 3–4	Grade 1–2	Grade 3–4
Nausea	60	7	56	7
Vomiting	44	6	38	8
Diarrhea	28	9	24	4
Constipation	25	1	30	2
Stomatitis	23	1	13	2
Abdominal pain	20	2	17	2
Dysphagia	4	2	3	<1
Neutropenia	26	27	27	30
Anemia	16	12	11	10
Thrombocytopenia	11	5	8	3
Febrile neutropenia	0	5	0	3
Anorexia	40	6	40	6
Fatigue	31	4	26	2
Hand-foot syndrome	25	1	20	2
Weight decreased	21	2	12	2
Asthenia	14	5	15	3
Pyrexia	17	1	12	0
Renal impairment	15	1	12	1
Mucosal inflammation	11	2	5	1
Nasopharyngitis	13	0	6	0
Chills	8	<1	0	0
Hypokalemia	3	4	2	2
Dehydration	4	2	4	2
Dyspnea	3	<1	4	2

METASTATIC DISEASE • FIRST-LINE

GASTRIC CANCER REGIMEN: FLUOROURACIL + LEUCOVORIN + IRINOTECAN (FOLFIRI) ± TRASTUZUMAB

Bang YJ et al. Lancet 2010;376(9742):687–697
Guimbaud R et al. J Clin Oncol 2014;32:3520–3526
Protocol for: Guimbaud R et al. J Clin Oncol 2014;32:3520–3526
Supplementary appendix to: Guimbaud R et al. J Clin Oncol 2014;32:3520–3526
HERCEPTIN (trastuzumab) for injection prescribing information. South San Francisco, CA: Genentech, Inc; updated November 2018

Irinotecan 180 mg/m²; administer intravenously over 90 minutes in 500 mL 5% dextrose injection (D5W) on day 1, every 2 weeks, until disease progression (total dosage/cycle = 180 mg/m²), *plus:*

Leucovorin calcium 400 mg/m²; administer intravenously over 2 hours in 25–500 mL 0.9% sodium chloride (0.9% NS) or D5W on day 1, every 2 weeks, until disease progression (total dosage/cycle = 400 mg/m², *followed by:*

Fluorouracil 400 mg/m²; administer by intravenous injection over 2–4 minutes after leucovorin on day 1, every 2 weeks, until disease progression, *followed by:*

Fluorouracil 2400 mg/m²; administer by continuous intravenous infusion over 46 hours in 100–1000 mL 0.9% NS or D5W, starting on day 1, every 2 weeks, until disease progression (total dosage/cycle = 2800 mg/m²)

The above regimen (FOLFIRI) may be given with trastuzumab for HER2-positive patients as described below:
- *Loading Dose:* **Trastuzumab** 6 mg/kg; administer intravenously in 250 mL 0.9% NS over 90 minutes as a loading dose on day 1, cycle 1 only (total dosage during the first cycle = 6 mg/kg), *followed 2 weeks later by:*
- *Maintenance Doses:* **Trastuzumab** 4 mg/kg; administer intravenously in 250 mL 0.9% NS over 30 minutes on day 1, every 14 days, until disease progression (total dosage during each maintenance cycle = 4 mg/kg)

Note: Assess left ventricular ejection fraction (LVEF) prior to initiating trastuzumab and at regular intervals during treatment

Supportive Care
Antiemetic prophylaxis
Emetogenic potential on day 1 is **MODERATE**
Emetogenic potential on day 2 is **LOW**
See Chapter 42 for antiemetic recommendations

Hematopoietic growth factor (CSF) prophylaxis
Primary prophylaxis is **NOT** indicated
See Chapter 43 for more information

Antimicrobial prophylaxis
Risk of fever and neutropenia is **LOW**
   Antimicrobial primary prophylaxis to be considered:
   - *Antibacterial—not indicated*
   - *Antifungal—not indicated*
   - *Antiviral—not indicated unless patient previously had an episode of HSV*

Acute cholinergic syndrome
Atropine sulfate 0.25–1 mg; administer subcutaneously or intravenously if abdominal cramping or diarrhea develop during or within 1 hour after irinotecan administration
- If symptoms are severe, add as primary prophylaxis at least 30 min before irinotecan during subsequent cycles
- For irinotecan, acute cholinergic syndrome may be characterized by: abdominal cramping, diarrhea, diaphoresis, hypotension, flushing, bradycardia, rhinitis, increased salivation, miosis, and lacrimation

Diarrhea management
Latent or delayed-onset diarrhea*:
Loperamide 4 mg orally initially after the first loose or liquid stool, *then* 2–4 mg orally every 2–4 hours or **diphenoxylate hydrochloride** 2.5 mg with **atropine sulfate** 0.025 mg (eg, Lomotil) 2 tablets orally four times per day

*Abigerges D et al. J Natl Cancer Inst 1994;86:446–449
Rothenberg ML et al. J Clin Oncol 2001;19:3801–3807
Wadler S et al. J Clin Oncol 1998;16:3169–3178

Oral care
Standard prophylaxis and treatment for mucositis/stomatitis

Patient Population Studied

This international, prospective, open, randomized, phase 3 study enrolled 416 patients with histologically confirmed, unresectable, locally advanced or metastatic gastric or esophagogastric junction adenocarcinoma. Participants were eligible if they had WHO performance score of ≤2, no previous palliative chemotherapy (≥6 months from adjuvant chemotherapy was allowed), ≥3 weeks from previous radiotherapy. The second-line treatment was prespecified, with second-line FOLFIRI for patients originally in the ECX arm and second-line ECX for patients in the FOLFIRI arm

Efficacy (N = 416)

End Point	Epirubicin + Cisplatin + Capecitabine (ECX) (N = 209)	Fluorouracil + Leucovorin + Irinotecan (FOLFIRI) (N = 207)	Between-Group Comparison
Median time to treatment failure*	3.24 months (95% CI 3.48–4.65)	5.08 months (95% CI 4.53–5.68)	HR 0.77 (95% CI 0.63–0.93) P = 0.008
Median progression-free survival	5.29 months (95% CI 4.53–6.31)	5.75 months (95% CI 5.19–6.74)	HR 0.99 (95% CI 0.81–1.21) P = 0.96
Median overall survival	9.49 months (95% CI 8.77–11.14)	9.72 months (95% CI 8.54–11.27)	HR 1.01, (95% CI 0.82–1.24) P = 0.95
ORR to first-line treatment[†]	39.2%	37.8%	—
ORR to second-line treatment[‡]	13.7%	10.1%	—
Reasons for treatment discontinuation			
Disease progression	48%	62%	—
Toxicity	14.5%	3.9%	—
Patient request	9.8%	6.4%	—
Change in general status	15%	15%	—
Death	6.5%	10%	—

HR, hazard ratio, CI, confidence interval; OR, odds ratio; ORR, objective response rate

[†]The objective response rate to first-line treatment was determined in 189 patients in the ECX group and 198 patients in the FOLFIRI arm

[‡]The objective response rate was also determined for second-line treatment. Study participants were able to receive second-line treatment, as predetermined in the study protocol. Patients in the ECX group received the FOLFIRI regimen as second-line treatment and patients in the FOLFIRI group received ECX as second-line treatment

Therapy Monitoring

1. *Before each cycle:* History and physical examination
2. CBC with differential at a minimum once per cycle, but initially also at day 10–14
3. Serum bilirubin, AST, ALT, and alkaline phosphatase prior to each cycle
4. CA 19-9 and/or CEA prior to each cycle if detectable and being used to monitor disease
5. *Every 2–3 months:* CT scans to assess response

Treatment Modifications

FOLFIRI DOSE MODIFICATIONS

	Initial Dose Level	Dose Level −1	Dose Level −2
Irinotecan	180 mg/m²	150 mg/m²	120 mg/m²
Leucovorin	Racemic leucovorin calcium 400 mg/m² or levoleucovorin calcium 200 mg/m²	Omit	
Bolus fluorouracil	400 mg/m²	300 mg/m²	Omit
Infusional fluorouracil	2400 mg/m²	2000 mg/m²	1600 mg/m²

Note:
• Before beginning a treatment cycle, patients should have baseline bowel function (similar to that before the start of treatment) without antidiarrheal therapy for 24 hours, ANC ≥1500/mm³, and platelet count ≥100,000/mm³. Treatment should be delayed 1–2 weeks to allow for recovery from treatment-related toxicities. If toxicities have not resolved after 2 weeks, consider stopping therapy. If toxicity occurs despite 2 dose reductions (ie, on dose level −2), discontinue therapy. Dose modifications are based on the National Cancer Institute (USA) Common Toxicity Criteria V5.0. At: http://ctep.cancer.gov/protocolDevelopment/electronic_applications/ctc.htm

(continued)

Treatment Modifications (*continued*)

Adverse Event	Treatment Modification for Irinotecan and Fluorouracil
Neutropenia/Thrombocytopenia	
G1 ANC (1500–1999/mm³) or G1 thrombocytopenia (<LLN—75,000/mm³)	Maintain dose and schedule
G2 ANC (1000–1499/mm³) or G2 thrombocytopenia (<75,000—50,000/mm³)	Reduce dosages by 1 dosage level
G3 ANC (500–999/mm³) or G3 thrombocytopenia (<50,000—25,000/mm³)	Hold treatment until toxicity resolves to G ≤2, then reduce dosages by 1 dosage level
G4 ANC (<500/mm³) or G4 thrombocytopenia (<25,000/mm³)	Hold treatment until toxicity resolves to G ≤2, then reduce dosages by 2 dosage levels
Febrile neutropenia (ANC <1000/mm³ with single temperature >38.3°C [101°F] or a sustained temperature of ≥38°C [100.4°F] for more than 1 hour)	Hold treatment until neutropenia resolves, then reduce dosages by 2 dosage levels
Diarrhea	
G1 (2–3 stools/day > baseline)	Maintain dose and schedule
G2 (4–6 stools/day > baseline)	Delay until diarrhea resolves to baseline, then reduce dosage by 1 dosage level
G3 (7–9 stools/day > baseline)	Delay until diarrhea resolves to baseline, then reduce dosage by 1 or 2 dosage levels
G4 (≥10 stools/day > baseline)	Delay until diarrhea resolves to baseline, then reduce dosage by 2 dosage levels
Other Nonhematologic Toxicities	
G2–4 mucositis (moderate pain or ulcer that does not interfere with oral intake; modified diet indicated or worse)	Decrease only fluorouracil by 20%
Any G1 toxicity	Maintain dose and schedule
Any G2 toxicity	Hold treatment until toxicity resolves to G ≤1, then reduce dosage by 1 dosage level
Any G3 toxicity	Hold treatment until toxicity resolves to G ≤1, then reduce dosage by 1 or 2 dosage levels
Any G4 toxicity	Hold treatment until toxicity resolves to G ≤1, then reduce dosage by 2 dosage levels

ANC, absolute neutrophil count; LLN, lower limit of normal

Note:
- No dose adjustment is recommended for patients with renal impairment
- Irinotecan dose adjustments for hepatic impairment:
  - *Bilirubin >ULN to ≤2 mg/dL:* consider reducing initial irinotecan dose by one dose level
  - *Bilirubin >2 mg/dL:* irinotecan use is not recommended
- Fluorouracil dose adjustments for hepatic impairment:
  - *Bilirubin >5 mg/dL:* fluorouracil use is not recommended

Neuzillet C et al. World J Gastroenterol 2012;18:4533–4541
Camptosar, irinotecan hydrochloride injection product label, July 2005. New York, NY: Pharmacia & Upjohn Company, Division of Pfizer, Inc.; 2005

Treatment Modifications—TRASTUZUMAB

Adverse Event	Dose Modification
Mild or moderate infusion reaction*	Decrease the rate of infusion
Infusion reaction with dyspnea or clinically significant hypotension	Interrupt the infusion reaction. Administer medical therapy as indicated including epinephrine, corticosteroids, diphenhydramine, bronchodilators, and oxygen. Observe patients closely for 60 minutes if the reaction occurs after the first infusion and for 30 minutes if it occurs after subsequent infusions. Prior to resumption of the trastuzumab infusion, premedicate with antihistamines and/or corticosteroids. *Note:* While some patients tolerate the resumption of trastuzumab infusions, others have recurrent severe infusion reactions despite premedications

(*continued*)

Treatment Modifications (continued)

Adverse Event	Dose Modification
Severe or life-threatening infusion reaction (includes bronchospasm, anaphylaxis, angioedema, hypoxia, and severe hypotension, usually reported during or immediately following the initial infusion)*	Interrupt the infusion reaction. Administer medical therapy as indicated including epinephrine, corticosteroids, diphenhydramine, bronchodilators, and oxygen. Patients should be evaluated and carefully monitored until complete resolution of signs and symptoms. Discontinue trastuzumab
≥16% absolute decrease in LVEF from pre-treatment values	Withhold trastuzumab dosing for at least 4–8 weeks. Resume trastuzumab if, within 4–8 weeks, the LVEF returns to normal limits and the absolute decrease from baseline is ≤15%
LVEF below institutional limits of normal and ≥10% absolute decrease in LVEF from pre-treatment values	
Persistent (>8 weeks) LVEF decline or suspension of trastuzumab dosing on ≥3 occasions for cardiomyopathy	Permanently discontinue trastuzumab
Pulmonary toxicity	Discontinue trastuzumab in patients experiencing pulmonary toxicity

*Infusion reactions consist of a symptom complex characterized by fever and chills, and on occasion included nausea, vomiting, pain (in some cases at tumor sites), headache, dizziness, dyspnea, hypotension, rash, and asthenia

Adverse Events

Grade (%)	Epirubicin + Cisplatin + Capecitabine (ECX)		Fluorouracil + Leucovorin + Irinotecan (FOLFIRI)	
	Grade 1–2	Grade 3–4	Grade 1–2	Grade 3–4
First-Line Treatment	N = 200		N = 203	
Nonhematologic	42.5%	53.5%	44.3%	53.2%
Hematologic	30.0%	64.5%	59.1%	38.4%
Overall	12.5%	83.5%	28.6%	69.0%
Deaths*	7		5	
Second-Line Treatment	N = 101		N = 81	
Nonhematologic	49.5%	46.5%	44.4%	54.3%
Hematologic	52.5%	43.6%	54.3%	43.2%
Overall	28.7%	67.3%	27.2%	71.6%
Deaths*	2		2	

*Deaths were related to hematologic toxicities (6 deaths), global deterioration of the patient (5 deaths), sudden death and/or stroke (3 deaths), acute renal failure (1 death), and digestive toxicity (1 death)

METASTATIC DISEASE • FIRST-LINE

GASTRIC CANCER REGIMEN: MODIFIED DOCETAXEL + CISPLATIN + FLUOROURACIL (MDCF) ± TRASTUZUMAB

Bang YJ et al. Lancet 2010;376(9742):687–697
Mondaca S et al. Gastric Cancer 2019;22(2):355–362
Shah MA et al. J Clin Oncol 2015;33(33):3874–3879
HERCEPTIN (trastuzumab) for injection prescribing information. South San Francisco, CA: Genentech, Inc; updated November 2018

Premedication for docetaxel:
Dexamethasone 8 mg/dose; administer orally twice daily for 3 days, starting on the day before docetaxel administration (total dose/cycle = 48 mg)
Docetaxel 40 mg/m^2; administer intravenously diluted in a volume of 0.9% sodium chloride injection (0.9% NS) or 5% dextrose injection (D5W) sufficient to produce a docetaxel concentration within the range 0.3–0.74 mg/mL over 60 minutes on day 1, every 14 days, until disease progression (total dosage/2-week cycle = 40 mg/m^2)

Hydration before cisplatin: ≥500 mL 0.9% NS; administer intravenously over a minimum of 1 hour
Cisplatin 40 mg/m^2; administer intravenously in 100–250 mL 0.9% NS over 30 minutes on day 1, every 14 days, until disease progression (total dosage/2-week cycle = 40 mg/m^2)
Hydration after cisplatin: ≥500 mL 0.9% NS; administer intravenously over a minimum of 1 hour. Encourage increased oral intake of nonalcoholic fluids. Goal is to achieve a urine output of ≥100 mL/hour. Monitor and replace magnesium and other electrolytes as needed

Leucovorin calcium 400 mg/m^2; administer intravenously over 30 minutes in 25–500 mL D5W on day 1, every 14 days, until disease progression (total dosage/2-week cycle = 400 mg/m^2), *followed by:*
Fluorouracil 400 mg/m^2; administer by intravenous injection over 1–2 minutes after leucovorin on day 1, every 2 weeks, until disease progression, *followed by:*
Fluorouracil 1000 mg/m^2 per day; administer by continuous intravenous infusion in 50–1000 mL 0.9% NS or D5W over 24 hours for 2 consecutive days, on days 1–2, every 14 days, until disease progression (total dosage/2-week cycle = 2400 mg/m^2)
Regimen notes:
• In the clinical trial (Shah et al, 2015), cisplatin was administered on day 2 or day 3; but, for practical reasons, many institutions prefer to administer on day 1 as outlined above
• The clinical trial (Shah et al, 2015) protocol allowed discontinuation of cisplatin, docetaxel, and/or fluorouracil after 6 months of therapy for cumulative toxicity and permitted continued less-intensive maintenance therapy with the remaining agent(s)

The above regimen (modified DCF) may be given with trastuzumab for HER2-positive patients as described below:
– *Loading Dose:* **Trastuzumab** 6 mg/kg; administer intravenously in 250 mL 0.9% NS over 90 minutes as a loading dose on day 1, cycle 1 only (total dosage during the first cycle = 6 mg/kg), *followed 2 weeks later by:*
– *Maintenance Doses:* **Trastuzumab** 4 mg/kg; administer intravenously in 250 mL 0.9% NS over 30 minutes on day 1, every 14 days, until disease progression (total dosage during each maintenance cycle = 4 mg/kg)
Note: Assess left ventricular ejection fraction (LVEF) prior to initiating trastuzumab and at regular intervals during treatment

Supportive Care
Antiemetic prophylaxis
Emetogenic potential on day 1 is **HIGH**. *Potential for delayed emetic symptoms*
Emetogenic potential on day 2 is **LOW**
See Chapter 42 for antiemetic recommendations

Hematopoietic growth factor (CSF) prophylaxis
Primary prophylaxis is **NOT** *indicated*
See Chapter 43 for more information

(*continued*)

Patient Population Studied

Shah MA et al. J Clin Oncol 2015;33(33):3874–3879
This randomized, phase 2 trial included 85 adult patients with metastatic gastric or gastroesophageal junction (GEJ) adenocarcinoma and compared treatment with modified docetaxel + cisplatin + fluorouracil (mDCF) to parent DCF + G-CSF. Patients were eligible if they had pathologically confirmed gastric or GEJ cancer without previous treatment for metastatic disease, histologic or imaging-based confirmation of metastasis, radiographically evaluable disease (by RECIST v1.0 criteria), a Karnofsky performance status ≥70% (ECOG performance status <2), and adequate organ function. Patients were excluded if they had previously received chemotherapy or chemoradiotherapy <6 months before registration, if they had ever received cisplatin or docetaxel as part of adjuvant therapy, if they had received chemotherapy for incurable gastric or GEJ adenocarcinoma, brain or CNS metastasis, significant cardiovascular disease, clinically significant hearing loss or tinnitus, or if they had another malignancy within the past 3 years (excluding basal cell carcinoma of skin, cervical carcinoma in situ, or nonmetastatic prostate cancer). HER2 status was not a variable in this paper and no information on its presence in the enrolled patients was included

Mondaca S et al. Gastric Cancer 2019;22(2):355–362
This single-arm, multicenter, phase 2 trial included 26 adult patients with HER2-positive metastatic gastric or gastroesophageal junction (GEJ) adenocarcinoma who were treated with a modified docetaxel + cisplatin + fluorouracil + trastuzumab (mDCF + T) regimen. Patients were eligible if they had pathologically confirmed metastatic gastric or GEJ adenocarcinoma without previous treatment for metastatic or unresectable disease, radiographically evaluable disease (by RECIST v1.0 criteria), HER2-positive disease (defined as IHC staining intensity of 3+ on a scale from 0 to 3+ or IHC 2+ with ERBB2 amplification confirmed by FISH), a Karnofsky performance status ≥70% (ECOG performance status <2), and adequate organ function. Patients were excluded if they had previously received adjuvant or perioperative docetaxel or cisplatin, brain or CNS metastasis, significant cardiovascular disease, or clinically significant hearing loss or tinnitus, or if they had another malignancy within the past 3 years (excluding basal cell carcinoma of skin, cervical carcinoma in situ, or nonmetastatic prostate cancer)

(*continued*)

Antimicrobial prophylaxis
Risk of fever and neutropenia is **LOW**
Antimicrobial primary prophylaxis to be considered:

- Antibacterial—not indicated
- Antifungal—not indicated
- Antiviral—not indicated unless patient previously had an episode of HSV

Diarrhea management
Latent or delayed-onset diarrhea:
Loperamide 4 mg orally initially after the first loose or liquid stool, *then* 2–4 mg orally every 2–4 hours or **diphenoxylate hydrochloride** 2.5 mg with **atropine sulfate** 0.025 mg (eg, Lomotil) 2 tablets orally four times per day

*Abigerges D et al. J Natl Cancer Inst 1994;86:446–449
Rothenberg ML et al. J Clin Oncol 2001;19:3801–3807
Wadler S et al. J Clin Oncol 1998;16:3169–3178

Oral care
Standard prophylaxis and treatment for mucositis/stomatitis

Efficacy (N = 85)

Shah MA et al. J Clin Oncol 2015;33(33):3874–3879

	Modified Docetaxel + Cisplatin + Fluorouracil (mDCF) (N = 54)	Parent Docetaxel + Cisplatin + Fluorouracil + Growth Factor (DCF + G-CSF) (N = 31)	
Median progression-free survival*	9.7 months (95% CI, 5.8–11.6)	6.5 months (95% CI, 3.9–9.4)	HR not reported; P = 0.2; no significant difference between gastric cancer types (P = 0.4)
Progression-free survival, 6 months	63%	53%	
6-month therapeutic failure-free survival	56%	51%	
Median overall survival*	18.8 months (95% CI, 14.9–24.5)	12.6 months (95% CI, 6.7–16)	HR not reported; P = 0.007
Overall survival, 12 months	63%	55%	
Overall survival, 24 months	30%	12%	
Objective response rate (complete + partial response)†	49%	33%	HR not reported; P = 0.2

HR, hazard ratio; CI, confidence interval
*Statistical analysis of differences between treatments in median progression-free survival and median overall survival rates were performed using the permutation log-rank test
†P Value was calculated using Fischer's exact test

Efficacy (N = 26)

Mondaca S et al. Gastric Cancer 2019;22(2):355–362

Modified Docetaxel + Cisplatin + Fluorouracil + Trastuzumab (mDCF + T) (N = 26)	
Median progression-free survival*	13 months (95% CI, 6.4–20.7)
Progression-free survival, 6 months*	73% (95% CI, 51–86)
Median overall survival*	24.9 months (95% CI, 14.4–42.5)
Overall survival, 12 months*	73%
Overall survival, 24 months*	56%
Objective response rate	65% (95% CI, 46–80)
Complete response	4% (Duration, 77 months)
Partial response	62% (Duration, 19 months)
Stable disease	23% (Duration, 6 months)
Disease progression	4%

HR, hazard ratio; CI, confidence interval
*Progression-free survival and overall survival were estimated using the Kaplan-Meier method
RECIST v1.0 criteria were used to grade tumors for response rate determination and progression-free survival

Therapy Monitoring

1. *Before each cycle:* History and physical examination with attention to neurotoxicity, CBC with differential, serum electrolytes, magnesium, calcium, creatinine, BUN, and serum bilirubin, AST, ALT, and alkaline phosphatase prior to each cycle
2. CA 19–9 and/or CEA prior to each cycle if detectable and being used to monitor disease
3. *Day 8 (at least initially):* CBC with differential, serum electrolytes, magnesium, calcium, creatinine, BUN
4. *Every 2–3 months:* CT scans to assess response

Treatment Modifications

Treatment Modifications—TRASTUZUMAB

Adverse Event	Dose Modification
Mild or moderate infusion reaction*	Decrease the rate of infusion
Infusion reaction with dyspnea or clinically significant hypotension	Interrupt the infusion reaction. Administer medical therapy as indicated including epinephrine, corticosteroids, diphenhydramine, bronchodilators, and oxygen. Observe patients closely for 60 minutes if the reaction occurs after the first infusion and for 30 minutes if it occurs after subsequent infusions. Prior to resumption of the trastuzumab infusion, premedicate with antihistamines and/or corticosteroids. *Note:* While some patients tolerate the resumption of trastuzumab infusions, others have recurrent severe infusion reactions despite premedications
Severe or life-threatening infusion reaction (includes bronchospasm, anaphylaxis, angioedema, hypoxia, and severe hypotension, usually reported during or immediately following the initial infusion)*	Interrupt the infusion reaction. Administer medical therapy as indicated including epinephrine, corticosteroids, diphenhydramine, bronchodilators, and oxygen. Patients should be evaluated and carefully monitored until complete resolution of signs and symptoms. Discontinue trastuzumab
≥16% absolute decrease in LVEF from pre-treatment values	Withhold trastuzumab dosing for at least 4–8 weeks. Resume trastuzumab if, within 4–8 weeks, the LVEF returns to normal limits and the absolute decrease from baseline is ≤15%
LVEF below institutional limits of normal and ≥10% absolute decrease in LVEF from pre-treatment values	
Persistent (>8 weeks) LVEF decline or suspension of trastuzumab dosing on ≥3 occasions for cardiomyopathy	Permanently discontinue trastuzumab
Pulmonary toxicity	Discontinue trastuzumab in patients experiencing pulmonary toxicity

*Infusion reactions consist of a symptom complex characterized by fever and chills, and on occasion included nausea, vomiting, pain (in some cases at tumor sites), headache, dizziness, dyspnea, hypotension, rash, and asthenia

Treatment Modifications—DOCETAXEL + CISPLATIN + 5-FLUOROURACIL (DCF)

ANC nadir <1000/mm^3 or platelet nadir <50,000/mm^3 after treatment	Delay treatment until ANC is ≥1000/mm^3 and platelet count is ≥50,000/mm^3, then cisplatin, 5-fluorouracil, and docetaxel dosages by 20–25%. Alternatively, consider using hematopoietic growth factors*
Recurrent treatment delay because of myelosuppression	Delay therapy for 1 week, or until myelosuppression resolves, then decrease cisplatin, 5-fluorouracil, and docetaxel dosages by 20–25% during subsequent treatments*
Sepsis during an episode of neutropenia	
Reduction in creatinine clearance* to 60% of on-study value	Delay therapy 1 week. If creatinine clearance does not recover to pretreatment values, then consider reducing cisplatin dose
Creatinine clearance* 40–60 mL/min (0.66–1 mL/s)	Consider reducing cisplatin so that dose in milligrams equals the creatinine clearance* value in mL/min (mL/s × 1/0.0166)†
Creatinine clearance* <40 mL/min (<0.66 mL/s)	Hold cisplatin
Clinically significant ototoxicity	Discontinue cisplatin
Persistent (>14 days) peripheral neuropathy without functional impairment	Decrease cisplatin and docetaxel dosages by 50%
Clinically significant sensory loss—persistent (>14 days) peripheral neuropathy with functional impairment	Discontinue cisplatin and docetaxel
G3 nausea, vomiting	Decrease cisplatin dosage by 25%
G2 stomatitis or diarrhea	Hold 5-fluorouracil; resume 5-fluorouracil at full dosage after resolution of toxicity
Second episode of G2 stomatitis or diarrhea	Hold 5-fluorouracil; resume 5-fluorouracil with dosage reduced by 25% after toxicity resolves
Third episode of G2 stomatitis or diarrhea	Hold 5-fluorouracil; resume 5-fluorouracil with dosage reduced by 50% after toxicity resolves
Fourth episode of G2 stomatitis or diarrhea	Discontinue 5-fluorouracil

(*continued*)

Treatment Modifications (*continued*)

Treatment Modifications—DOCETAXEL + CISPLATIN + 5-FLUOROURACIL (DCF)

G3 stomatitis or diarrhea	Hold 5-fluorouracil. If G3 toxicity is adequately controlled within 2 days, resume 5-fluorouracil at full dosage when toxicity abates to G ≤1. If G3 toxicity takes >2 days to be controlled, resume 5-fluorouracil with dosage reduced by 25% after toxicity abates to G ≤1
Second episode of G3 stomatitis or diarrhea	Hold 5-fluorouracil. If G3 toxicity is controlled adequately within 2 days, then resume 5-fluorouracil with dosage reduced by 50% after toxicity abates to G ≤1
Third episode of G3 stomatitis or diarrhea	Discontinue 5-fluorouracil
G4 stomatitis or diarrhea	Discontinue 5-fluorouracil. Resume 5-fluorouracil with dosage reduced by 50% after toxicity resolves

*Treatment delays for unresolved adverse events of >3 weeks' duration warrant discontinuation of treatment
*Creatinine clearance is used as a measure of glomerular filtration rate
†This also applies to patients with GFR of 40–60 mL/min at the outset of treatment

Adverse Events (n = 85)

Shah MA et al. J Clin Oncol 2015;33(33):3874–3879

Event	Modified Docetaxel + Cisplatin + Fluorouracil (mDCF) (N = 54)		Parent Docetaxel + Cisplatin + Fluorouracil + Growth Factors (DCF + G-CSF) (N = 31)*	
Any Grade 3/4 event	76%		90%	
Any Grade 3/4 hematologic event	59%		61%	
Any Grade 3/4 nonhematologic event	46%		74%	
Any Grade 3/4 event in first 3 months	54%		71%	
Hospitalization in first 3 months	22%		53%	
Hospitalized for febrile neutropenia	33%		31%	
Hospitalized for febrile GI toxicity	25%		44%	
Grade (%)	Grade 2	Grade 3/4	Grade 2	Grade 3/4
Allergy or hypersensitivity	7	6	0	0
Anorexia	15	0	6	13
Dysgeusia	9	0	3	0
Nausea	19	2	29	23
Vomiting	6	2	26	19
Dehydration	6	6	13	10
Diarrhea	11	6	26	3
Mucositis	13	0	42	13
Fatigue	41	11	55	13
Neuropathy	24	4	13	13
Alopecia	17	0	10	0
Hypomagnesemia	19	2	23	13
Hypophosphatemia	6	13	6	32
Hypokalemia	2	9	10	13
Thromboembolism	4	20	13	19
Hemorrhage	0	0	0	3

(*continued*)

Adverse Events (n = 85) (continued)

Grade (%)	Grade 2	Grade 3/4	Grade 2	Grade 3/4
GI perforation	0	0	0	3
AST or ALT elevation	0	3	3	0
Hemoglobin	56	11	45	39
Thrombocytopenia	19	4	8	3
Leukopenia	35	44	23	48
Neutropenia (without fever)	17	56	13	45
Febrile neutropenia	0	9	0	16

Adverse events were graded according to National Cancer Institute Common Terminology Criteria for Adverse Events (NCI-CTCAE) version 3.0
*As delineated by a prespecified rule, the DCF + G-CSF arm was closed after 31 patients were enrolled due to excessive toxicity within the first 3 months

Adverse Events (n = 26)

Mondaca S et al. Gastric Cancer 2019;22(2):355–362

Event	Modified Docetaxel + Cisplatin + Fluorouracil + Trastuzumab (mDCF + T) (N = 26)	
Grade (%)	Grade 1/2	Grade 3/4
Fatigue	27	23
Hypophosphatemia	0	15
Hypokalemia	8	12
Hyponatremia	19	4
Hyperglycemia	23	4
Hypersensitivity reaction	19	12
Dehydration	8	12
Diarrhea	31	8
GI hemorrhage	0	8
Anorexia	8	4
Hyperbilirubinemia	8	4
Hypoalbuminemia	4	4
Epiphora	23	4
Nausea	38	4
Syncope	0	4
Thromboembolism	4	4
Neutropenia	19	42
Lymphopenia	0	31
Anemia	38	27
Thrombocytopenia	46	4

• Adverse events were graded according to National Cancer Institute Common Terminology Criteria for Adverse Events (NCI-CTCAE) version 3.0
• Study was closed before reaching the estimated sample size due to slow accrual
• Three patients (~12%) discontinued treatment due to toxicity, two of which reported G3 GI bleeding and one of which reported persistent G2 anorexia
• There were no deaths that were considered drug-related

METASTATIC DISEASE • SECOND-LINE

GASTRIC CANCER REGIMEN: RAMUCIRUMAB + PACLITAXEL

Wilke H et al. Lancet Oncol 2014;15(11):1224–1235
Supplementary appendix to: Wilke H et al. Lancet Oncol 2014;15(11):1224–1235
CYRAMZA (ramucirumab) prescribing information. Indianapolis, IN: Eli Lilly and Company; revised November 2019

Prophylaxis for infusion-related reaction from ramucirumab:
Diphenhydramine 25–50 mg; administer intravenously, 30–60 minutes before starting ramucirumab, *plus*
Acetaminophen 650–1000 mg; administer orally, 30–60 minutes before starting ramucirumab (only if history of Grade 1–2 infusion reaction), *plus*
Dexamethasone 8 mg; administer orally or intravenously, 30–60 minutes before starting ramucirumab (only if history of Grade 1–2 infusion reaction)
Ramucirumab 8 mg/kg; administer intravenously in 250 mL of 0.9% sodium chloride injection (0.9% NS) over 1 hour, prior to paclitaxel administration, for 2 doses on day 1 and day 15, every 28 days, until disease progression (total dosage/4-week cycle = 16 mg/kg)
- Ramucirumab should be administered through an administration set with a low-protein-binding in-line filter with pore size of 0.22 μm
- Flush the line with 0.9% NS at the end of the infusion
- If the first infusion is tolerated, all subsequent ramucirumab infusions may be administered over 30 minutes
- Ramucirumab can cause severe infusion-related reactions
  - Reduce the ramucirumab infusion rate by 50% for Grade 1 or Grade 2 infusion reactions and add acetaminophen and dexamethasone to infusion-related reaction prophylaxis regimen, as described above, in subsequent cycles
  - Permanently discontinue ramucirumab for Grade 3 or Grade 4 infusion-related reactions

Premedication for paclitaxel:
Dexamethasone 16 mg; administer intravenously over 10–15 minutes, 30 minutes before starting paclitaxel (total dose/cycle = 16 mg)
- *Note:* in the absence of hypersensitivity reaction following the initial paclitaxel infusion, the dexamethasone dose may be reduced for subsequent paclitaxel infusions (eg, dexamethasone 8 mg prior to the second paclitaxel dose, and dexamethasone 4 mg prior to the third and subsequent paclitaxel doses)
Diphenhydramine 25–50 mg; administer intravenously 30 minutes prior to starting paclitaxel
- *Note:* on days when the patient is receiving ramucirumab, a single dose of diphenhydramine may be given as premedication for both ramucirumab and paclitaxel
Cimetidine 300 mg (or **ranitidine** 50 mg, or **famotidine** 20 mg, or an equivalent histamine receptor (H_2)-subtype antagonist); administer intravenously over 15–30 minutes, 30 minutes before starting paclitaxel

Paclitaxel 80 mg/m² per dose; administer intravenously in a volume of 0.9% NS or D5W sufficient to produce a concentration within the range 0.3–1.2 mg/mL over 60 minutes, for 3 doses on day 1, day 8, and day 15, every 28 days (total dosage/28-day cycle = 240 mg/m²)

Supportive Care
Antiemetic prophylaxis
Emetogenic potential is **LOW**
See Chapter 42 for antiemetic recommendations

Hematopoietic growth factor (CSF) prophylaxis
Primary prophylaxis is **NOT** indicated
See Chapter 43 for more information

Antimicrobial prophylaxis
Risk of fever and neutropenia is **LOW**
  Antimicrobial primary prophylaxis to be considered:
  - *Antibacterial—not indicated*
  - *Antifungal—not indicated*
  - *Antiviral—not indicated unless patient previously had an episode of HSV*

Patient Population Studied

The RAINBOW study was a randomized, placebo-controlled, double-blind, phase 3 trial that included 665 adult patients with previously treated advanced gastric or gastroesophageal junction (GEJ) adenocarcinoma and compared treatment with paclitaxel plus either placebo or ramucirumab. Patients were eligible if they had metastatic or nonresectable, locally advanced gastric or GEJ cancer, documented objective radiologic or clinical disease progression during or within 4 months of the last dose of first-line platinum and fluoropyrimidine doublet with or without anthracycline, and an Eastern Cooperative Oncology Group (ECOG) performance score of 0 or 1. Patients were excluded if they had GI perforation, fistulae, or arterial thromboembolic events within 6 months or any significant GI bleeding or any significant venous thromboembolism within 3 months of randomization, or if they had poorly controlled hypertension

Efficacy (N = 6650)

	Ramucirumab + Paclitaxel (N = 330)	Placebo + Paclitaxel (N = 335)	
Median overall survival	9.6 months (95% CI, 8.5–10.8)	7.4 months (95% CI, 6.3–8.4)	Stratified HR 0.807 (95% CI, 0.678–0.962); P = 0.017 Preplanned multivariable analysis: HR 0.745 (95% CI, 0.626–0.888); P = 0.0010
Overall survival, 6 months	72% (95% CI, 66–76)	57% (95% CI, 51–62)	
Overall survival, 12 months	40% (95% CI, 35–45)	30% (95% CI, 25–35)	
Median progression-free survival	4.4 months (95% CI, 4.2–5.3)	2.9 months (95% CI, 2.8–3.0)	HR 0.635 (95% CI, 0.536–0.752); P <0.0001 Preplanned multivariate analysis: HR 0.599 (95% CI, 0.506–0.708); P <0.0001
Progression-free survival, 6 months	36% (95% CI, 31–41)	17% (95% CI, 13–22)	
Progression-free survival, 9 months	22% (95% CI, 17–27)	10% (95% CI, 7–14)	
Objective response rate[†]	28% (95% CI, 23–33)	16% (95% CI, 13–20)	P = 0.0001
Disease control rate[†]	80% (95% CI, 75–84)	64% (95% CI, 58–69)	P <0.0001
Median duration of response	4.4 months (IQR, 2.8–7.5)	2.8 months (IQR, 1.4–4.4)	
Complete response rate	<1%	<1%	
Partial response rate	27%	16%	
Stable disease	52%	47%	
Progressive disease	13%	25%	

HR, hazard ratio; CI, confidence interval; IQR, interquartile range

Therapy Monitoring

1. *Before the start of a cycle:* CBC with differential, BUN, creatinine, serum bilirubin, AST or ALT, and alkaline phosphatase
2. *Once per week:* CBC with differential and platelet count
3. Observe closely for hypersensitivity reactions, especially during the first and second ramucirumab infusions
4. Blood pressure every 2 weeks or more frequently as indicated during treatment
5. Assess proteinuria by urine dipstick and/or urinary protein creatinine ratio prior to each cycle. Patients with a ≥2+ urine dipstick reading should undergo further assessment with a 24-hour urine collection
6. Thyroid function at outset and every 3 months while on therapy
7. *Every 2–3 months:* Imaging to assess response

Treatment Modification

RAMUCIRUMAB DOSE MODIFICATIONS

Starting dose	8 mg/kg
Dose level −1	6 mg/kg
Dose level −2	5 mg/kg

Adverse Event	Treatment Modification
G1/2 infusion-related	Stop ramucirumab. Administer dexamethasone intravenously at commonly used antiemetic doses of 8–20 mg (or equivalent) and acetaminophen, then resume infusion at 50% of previous rate. Use the 50% infusion rate for all subsequent administrations
Prior G1/2 infusion-related reaction	Premedicate with dexamethasone intravenously at commonly used antiemetic doses of 8–20 mg (or equivalent) and acetaminophen prior to each ramucirumab infusion. Can also use diphenhydramine 25–50 mg intravenously
G3/4 infusion-related reaction	Permanently discontinue ramucirumab
G3/4 hypertension (SBP ≥160 mm Hg or DBP ≥100 mm Hg; medical intervention indicated; >1 drug or more intensive therapy than previously used indicated; or worse)	Interrupt ramucirumab until controlled with medical management then resume ramucirumab; if unable to control with medical management discontinue ramucirumab
Reversible posterior leukoencephalopathy syndrome (RPLS)	Permanently discontinue ramucirumab
Urine protein ≥2 g/24 hours	Interrupt ramucirumab. Reinitiate treatment at a reduced dose once the urine protein level returns to <2 g/24 hours
Reoccurrence of urine protein ≥2 g/24 hours	Interrupt ramucirumab and reduce the dose once the urine protein level returns to <2 g/24 hours
Urine protein >3 g/24 hours or nephrotic syndrome	Permanently discontinue ramucirumab
Anticipated wound healing	Stop ramucirumab prior to a scheduled surgery until wound is fully healed; discontinue ramucirumab if patient develops wound-healing complications
G3/4 bleeding, arterial thromboembolic event, gastrointestinal perforation	Permanently discontinue ramucirumab
G3/4 fatigue/asthenia	Interrupt ramucirumab. Reinstitute treatment at a reduced dose once toxicity is G1
G3/4 stomatitis/mucosal inflammation	

PACLITAXEL DOSE MODIFICATIONS

Paclitaxel starting dose	80 mg/m^2
Paclitaxel dose level −1	70 mg/m^2
Paclitaxel dose level −2	60 mg/m^2

Adverse Event	Treatment Modifications
Febrile neutropenia (ANC <1000/mm^3 with temperature >38°C or >100.4°F), or ANC <1000/mm^3 for ≥7 days	Reduce paclitaxel dose by one dose level and consider adding filgrastim in subsequent cycles, if applicable
Febrile neutropenia (ANC <1000/mm^3 with temperature >38°C or >100.4°F), or ANC <1000/mm^3 for ≥7 days despite dose reduction of 10 mg/m^2	Administer filgrastim in subsequent cycles. If already administering filgrastim, reduce paclitaxel dose an additional dose level
Platelet nadir <50,000/mm^3, or platelets <100,000/mm^3 for ≥7 days	Reduce paclitaxel dose by one level
Day 1 ANC <1,500/mm^3 and/or platelet count <100,000/mm^3	Withhold paclitaxel until ANC >1500/mm^3 and/or platelet count <100,000/mm^3

(*continued*)

Treatment Modification (*continued*)

ANC <1500/mm³ and/or platelet count <100,000/mm³ despite a 2-week delay, but with ANC >1000/mm³ and platelet count >75,000/mm³	Resume therapy with paclitaxel dosage reduced by one dose level. Consider filgrastim
G2 motor or sensory neuropathies	Reduce weekly paclitaxel dosage by one dose level without interrupting planned treatment
G3 motor or sensory neuropathies	Withhold paclitaxel until toxicity resolves to G ≤2, then resume with weekly paclitaxel dosage reduced by one dose level
G4 motor or sensory neuropathies	Discontinue paclitaxel
Other nonhematologic adverse events G2/3	Hold treatment until adverse events resolve to <G1, then resume with weekly paclitaxel dosage reduced by one dose level
Patients who cannot tolerate paclitaxel at 60 mg/m² per week	Discontinue paclitaxel
Treatment delay >2 weeks	Decrease weekly paclitaxel dosage by one dose level or consider discontinuing treatment

Adverse Events

Event	Ramucirumab + Paclitaxel (N = 327)	Placebo + Paclitaxel (N = 329)
Dose reduction of ramucirumab	5%	1%
Disease progression as reason for treatment discontinuation	72%	76%
Treatment discontinued due to adverse events	12%	11%
Serious adverse events	47%	42%
Treatment-emergent adverse events leading to death	12%	16%

Grade (%)	Grade 1–2	Grade 3–5	Grade 1–2	Grade 3–5
Any treatment-emergent adverse event	17	82	35	63
Fatigue*	45	12	38	5
Neuropathy*	38	8	32	5
Decreased appetite	37	3	28	4
Abdominal pain*	30	6	26	3
Nausea	33	2	30	2
Alopecia	33	0	38	<1
Diarrhea	29	4	22	2
Epistaxis	31	0	7	0
Vomiting	24	3	17	4
Peripheral edema	24	2	13	<1
Hypertension	10	14	2	2
Constipation	21	0	21	<1
Stomatitis	19	<1	7	<1
Pyrexia	17	<1	11	<1

(*continued*)

Adverse Events (continued)

Grade (%)	Grade 1–2	Grade 3–5	Grade 1–2	Grade 3–5
Proteinuria	15	1	6	0
Malignant neoplasm progression	2	14	<1	18
Weight decreased	12	2	14	1
Dyspnea	10	2	9	<1
Rash*	13	0	9	0
Cough	12	0	8	0
Back pain	11	1	11	2
Hypoalbuminemia*	10	1	4	<1
Myalgia	10	0	10	<1
Ascites	6	4	4	4
Headache	10	0	6	<1
Neutropenia*	14	41	12	19
Anemia*	26	9	26	10
Leukopenia*	17	17	14	7
Thrombocytopenia*	12	2	4	2

*Consolidated adverse event category with synonymous MEdDRA-preferred terms
Adverse events were included in the table if they were deemed treatment-emergent, irrespective of causality, and if they were reported in ≥10% of patients in the ramucirumab + paclitaxel group

Adverse Events of Special Interest

Event Grade (%)	Ramucirumab + Paclitaxel (N = 327)		Placebo + Paclitaxel (N = 329)	
	Grade 1–2	Grade 3–5	Grade 1–2	Grade 3–5
Bleeding or hemorrhage	38	4	16	2
Proteinuria	16	1	6	0
Liver injury or failure	12	5	9	4
Hypertension	10	15	3	3
Gastrointestinal hemorrhage*	6	4	5	2
Infusion-related reaction	5	<1	4	0
Renal failure	5	2	3	<1
Congestive heart failure	2	<1	<1	<1
Venous thromboembolic events	2	2	2	3
Arterial thromboembolic events	<1	<1	<1	<1
Gastrointestinal perforation	0	1	<1	0

*Events pooled as gastrointestinal hemorrhage are also pooled as bleeding or hemorrhage

METASTATIC DISEASE • SECOND-LINE

GASTRIC CANCER REGIMEN: PACLITAXEL

Hironaka S et al. J Clin Oncol 2013;31:4438–4444
Protocol for: Hironaka S et al. J Clin Oncol 2013;31:4438–4444

Premedication for paclitaxel:
Dexamethasone 16 mg; administer intravenously over 10–15 minutes, 30 minutes before starting paclitaxel (total dose/cycle = 16 mg)
Note: in the absence of hypersensitivity reaction following the initial paclitaxel infusion, the dexamethasone dose may be reduced for subsequent paclitaxel infusions (eg, dexamethasone 8 mg prior to the second paclitaxel dose, and dexamethasone 4 mg prior to the third and subsequent paclitaxel doses)
Diphenhydramine 25–50 mg; administer intravenously 30 minutes prior to starting paclitaxel
Cimetidine 300 mg (or **ranitidine** 50 mg, or **famotidine** 20 mg, or an equivalent histamine receptor (H_2)-subtype antagonist); administer intravenously over 15–30 minutes, 30 minutes before starting paclitaxel

Paclitaxel 80 mg/m^2 per dose; administer intravenously in a volume of 0.9% NS or D5W sufficient to produce a concentration within the range 0.3–1.2 mg/mL over 60 minutes, for 3 doses on day 1, day 8, and day 15, every 28 days (total dosage/28-day cycle = 240 mg/m^2)

Supportive Care
Antiemetic prophylaxis
*Emetogenic potential is **LOW***
See Chapter 42 for antiemetic recommendations

Hematopoietic growth factor (CSF) prophylaxis
*Primary prophylaxis is **NOT** indicated*
See Chapter 43 for more information

Antimicrobial prophylaxis
*Risk of fever and neutropenia is **LOW***
  Antimicrobial primary prophylaxis to be considered:
  • *Antibacterial—not indicated*
  • *Antifungal—not indicated*
  • *Antiviral—not indicated unless patient previously had an episode of HSV*

Patient Population Studied

WJOG 4007 was a prospective, multicenter, randomized, open-label, parallel-group, phase 3 trial conducted in Japan that involved 223 patients with histologically confirmed metastatic or recurrent gastric adenocarcinoma. Inclusion criteria included Eastern Cooperative Oncology Group performance status of 0 to 2, disease progression during or within 1 month after receiving the final dose of first-line chemotherapy with fluoropyrimidine plus platinum, and no severe peritoneal metastasis. Patients who experienced disease progression during treatment or within 6 months after treatment completion with adjuvant or neoadjuvant chemotherapy (fluoropyridine plus platinum) also were eligible

Therapy Monitoring

1. *Before the start of a cycle:* CBC with differential, BUN, creatinine, serum bilirubin, AST or ALT, and alkaline phosphatase
2. *Once per week:* CBC with differential and platelet count
3. Observe closely for hypersensitivity reactions, especially during the first and second paclitaxel infusions
4. *Every 2–3 months:* Imaging to assess response

Efficacy (N = 219)

Endpoint	Paclitaxel (N = 108)	Irinotecan (N = 111)	Between-Group Comparison
Median overall survival	9.5 months (95% CI 8.4–10.7)	8.4 months (95% CI 7.6–9.8)	HR 1.13 (95% CI 0.86–1.49) P = 0.38*
Median progression-free survival	3.6 months (95% CI 3.3–3.8)	2.3 months (95% CI 2.2–3.1)	HR 1.14 (95% CI 0.88–1.49) P = 0.33*
Response rate	19/91 (20.9%)	12/88 (13.6%)	P = 0.24†

HR, hazard ratio, CI, confidence interval
After a median follow-up period of 17.6 months, there were 203 (92.7%) deaths reported in the study cohort
*Two-sided log-rank P value
†Fisher's exact P value

PACLITAXEL DOSE MODIFICATIONS

Paclitaxel starting dose	80 mg/m^2
Paclitaxel dose level −1	70 mg/m^2
Paclitaxel dose level −2	60 mg/m^2

Adverse Event	Treatment Modifications
Febrile neutropenia (ANC <1000/mm^3 with temperature >38°C or >100.4°F), or ANC <1000/mm^3 for ≥7 days	Reduce paclitaxel dose by one dose level and consider adding filgrastim in subsequent cycles, if applicable
Febrile neutropenia (ANC <1000/mm^3 with temperature >38°C or >100.4°F), or ANC <1000/mm^3 for ≥7 days despite dose reduction of 10 mg/m^2	Administer filgrastim in subsequent cycles. If already administering filgrastim, reduce paclitaxel dose an additional dose level
Platelet nadir <50,000/mm^3, or platelets <100,000/mm^3 for ≥7 days	Reduce paclitaxel dose by one level
Day 1 ANC <1,500/mm^3 and/or platelet count <100,00/mm^3	Withhold paclitaxel until ANC >1500/mm^3 and/or platelet count <100,00/mm^3

(continued)

Efficacy (N = 219) *(continued)*

Adverse Event	Treatment Modifications
ANC <1,500/mm³ and/or platelet count <100,00/mm³ despite a 2-week delay, but with ANC >1000/mm³ and platelet count >75,000/mm³	Resume therapy with paclitaxel dosage reduced by one dose level. Consider filgrastim
G2 motor or sensory neuropathies	Reduce weekly paclitaxel dosage by one dose level without interrupting planned treatment
G3 motor or sensory neuropathies	Withhold paclitaxel until toxicity resolves to G ≤2 then resume with weekly paclitaxel dosage reduced by one dose level
G4 motor or sensory neuropathies	Discontinue paclitaxel
Other nonhematologic adverse events G2/3	Hold treatment until adverse events resolve to <G1, then resume with weekly paclitaxel dosage reduced by one dose level
Patients who cannot tolerate paclitaxel at 60 mg/m² per week	Discontinue paclitaxel
Treatment delay >2 weeks	Decrease weekly paclitaxel dosage by one dose level or consider discontinuing treatment

Adverse Events

Grade (%)	Paclitaxel (N = 108)		Irinotecan (N = 110)	
	Grade 1–2	Grade 3–4	Grade 1–2	Grade 3–4
Leukopenia	61	20.4	50.3	19.1
Neutropenia	50	28.7	30.9	39.1
Anemia	42.6	21.3	46.4	30
Thrombocytopenia	4.7	0.9	11.8	1.8
Febrile neutropenia	0	2.8	0	9.1
Nausea	28.7	1.9	51	4.5
Vomiting	17.6	2.8	35.5	0.9
Anorexia	38.9	7.4	52.8	17.3
Diarrhea	18.5	0.9	40	4.5
Sensory neuropathy	50	7.4	1.8	0
Bilirubin	6.5	2.8	15.5	3.6
AST	25.9	3.7	30	8.2
ALT	19.4	2.8	34.6	2.7
Hyponatremia	15.7	3.7	16.3	15.5
Treatment-related death*	0	0	0	1.8

*Treatment-related death occurred in 2 patients in the irinotecan group. Cause of death = gastric perforation in one patient and pneumonia in the other

METASTATIC DISEASE • SECOND-LINE

GASTRIC CANCER REGIMEN: IRINOTECAN

Kang JH et al. J Clin Oncol 2012;30:1513–1518

Irinotecan 150 mg/m²; administer intravenously in 500 mL D5W over 90 minutes on day 1, every 2 weeks (total dosage/cycle = 150 mg/m²)

Supportive Care
Antiemetic prophylaxis
Emetogenic potential is **MODERATE**
See Chapter 42 for antiemetic recommendations

Hematopoietic growth factor (CSF) prophylaxis
Primary prophylaxis may be indicated
See Chapter 43 for more information

Antimicrobial prophylaxis
Risk of fever and neutropenia is **LOW**
  Antimicrobial primary prophylaxis to be considered:
  • Antibacterial—not indicated
  • Antifungal—not indicated
  • Antiviral—not indicated, unless patient previously had an episode of HSV

Acute cholinergic syndrome
Atropine sulfate 0.25–1 mg; administer subcutaneously or intravenously if abdominal cramping or diarrhea develops during or within 1 hour after irinotecan administration
• If symptoms are severe, add as primary prophylaxis at least 30 min before irinotecan during subsequent cycles
• For irinotecan, acute cholinergic syndrome may be characterized by abdominal cramping, diarrhea, diaphoresis, hypotension, flushing, bradycardia, rhinitis, increased salivation, miosis, and lacrimation

Diarrhea management
Latent or delayed-onset diarrhea*:
Loperamide 4 mg orally initially after the first loose or liquid stool, *then* 2–4 mg orally every 2–4 hours or **diphenoxylate hydrochloride** 2.5 mg with **atropine sulfate** 0.025 mg (eg, Lomotil) 2 tablets orally four times per day

*Abigerges D et al. J Natl Cancer Inst 1994;86:446–449
Rothenberg ML et al. J Clin Oncol 2001;19:3801–3807
Wadler S et al. J Clin Oncol 1998;16:3169–3178

Oral care
Standard prophylaxis and treatment for mucositis/stomatitis

Efficacy

	Docetaxel N = 66*; 42†	Irinotecan N = 60*; 50†	BSC N = 62	
Partial response	7/42	5/50	—	—
Stable disease	18/42	21/50	—	—
Median duration of therapy (95% CI)	4.4 months (3.8–4.9)	4.2 months (3.4–5.0)	—	—
Median overall survival (95% CI)	5.3 months (4.1–6.5)		3.8 months (3.1–4.5)	HR = 0.657 (0.485–0.891) One-sided P = 0.007
Median overall survival (95% CI)	5.2 months (3.8–6.6)	6.5 months (4.5–8.5)	—	Two-sided P = 0.116

BSC, best supportive care; CI, confidence interval; HR, hazard ratio
*Number of patients treated with docetaxel or irinotecan or given BSC
†Number of patients who had measurable disease

Univariate Analyses for Survival

Clinical Parameter	HR	95% CI	P Value
Age			
≤ Median (56 years)	1	—	0.686
> Median	1.063	0.789–1.433	
Sex			
Male	1	—	0.267
Female	0.831	0.599–1.152	
Number of prior chemotherapy regimens			
1	1	—	<0.001
2	2.044	1.440–2.901	
Response to prior therapy			
No	1	—	0.123
Yes	0.784	0.576–1.068	
ECOG performance status			
0	1	—	<0.001
1	2.022	1.494–2.736	
Number of metastatic sites			
1	1	—	0.173
≥2	1.239	0.911–1.686	
Interval from last therapy, months			
<3	1	—	0.030
≥3	0.682	0.483–0.964	

HR, hazard ratio

Patient Population Studied

Patients with histologically confirmed advanced gastric cancer who had not received benefit after one or two chemotherapy regimens for metastatic disease consisting of either fluoropyrimidine- or platinum-based chemotherapy, or a fluoropyrimidine and platinum combination. Exclusion criteria included more than two prior chemotherapy regimens or prior exposure to both taxanes and irinotecan

Patient Characteristics (N = 133)

Characteristic	Number (%)
Age, years—median (range)	56 (31–83)
Sex—male/female	93 (70%)/40 (30%)
Number of prior chemotherapy regimens	
1	100 (75%)
2	33 (25%)
Prior surgery	29 (22%)
Prior adjuvant treatment	20 (15%)
Response to prior chemotherapy	
No	79 (59%)
Yes	54 (41%)
ECOG performance status	
0	72 (54%)
1	61 (46%)
Number of metastatic sites	
1	42 (32%)
≥2	91 (68%)
Involved sites	
Peritoneum	56 (42%)
Liver	30 (23%)
Lymph node	50 (38%)
Lung	12 (9%)
Bone	10 (8%)
Interval from last chemotherapy	
<3	101 months
≥3	32 months

Treatment Monitoring

1. CBC with differential, serum electrolytes, magnesium and calcium, BUN, creatinine, and liver function tests before the start of a new cycle
2. Tumor assessment every two cycles

Treatment Modifications

Irinotecan Dosage Levels

Initial	Level −1	Level −2
150 mg/m²	120 mg/m²	90 mg/m²

Notes:
- Dose modifications are based on National Cancer Institute (USA) Common Terminology Criteria for Adverse Events, version 3.0
- Before beginning a treatment cycle, patients should have baseline bowel function without antidiarrheal therapy for 24 hours, ANC ≥1500/mm³, and platelet count ≥100,000/mm³
- Treatment should be delayed 1–2 weeks to allow for recovery from treatment-related toxicities
- If a patient has not recovered after 2 weeks, consider stopping therapy. If toxicity occurs despite 2 dose reductions (ie, on level −2), discontinue therapy

Adverse Event	Dose Modifications
Neutropenia/Thrombocytopenia	
G1 ANC (1500–1999/mm³) or G1 thrombocytopenia (75,000/mm³ to less than normal limits)	Maintain dose and schedule
G2 ANC (1000–1499/mm³) or G2 thrombocytopenia (≥50,000 to <75,000/mm³)	Reduce dosage by 1 dosage level
G3 ANC (500–999/mm³) or G3 thrombocytopenia (≥10,000 to <50,000/mm³)	Hold treatment until toxicity resolves to G ≤2, then reduce dosage by 1 dosage level
G4 ANC (<500/mm³) or G4 thrombocytopenia (<10,000/mm³)	Hold treatment until toxicity resolves to G ≤2, then reduce dosage by 1 dosage level
Febrile neutropenia	Hold treatment until neutropenia resolves, then reduce dosage by 2 dosage levels
Diarrhea	
G1 (2–3 stools/day greater than baseline)	Maintain dose and schedule
G2 or G3 (4–9 stools/day greater than baseline)	Delay until diarrhea resolves to baseline, then reduce dosage by 1 dosage level
G4 (≥10 stools/day greater than baseline)	Delay until diarrhea resolves to baseline, then reduce dosage by 2 dosage levels
Other Nonhematologic Toxicities	
Any G1 toxicity	Maintain dose and schedule
Any G2 or G3 toxicity	Hold treatment until toxicity resolves to G ≤2, then reduce dosage by 1 dosage level
Any G4 toxicity	Hold treatment until toxicity resolves to G ≤2, then reduce dosage by 2 dosage level. If resolution of symptoms does not occur then discontinue irinotecan

André T et al. Eur J Cancer 1999;35:1343–1347
Camptosar, irinotecan hydrochloride injection product label, July 2005. New York, NY: Pharmacia & Upjohn Company, Division of Pfizer, Inc; 2005
Douillard JY et al. Lancet 2000;355:1041–1047
Tournigand C et al. J Clin Oncol 2004;22:229–237

Toxicity

Adverse Event	Docetaxel (N = 66)		Irinotecan (N = 60)		Best Supportive Care (N = 62)	
	% All G	% G3/4	% All G	% G3/4	% All G	% G3/4
Neutropenia	62%	15%	58%	18%	13%	2%
Anemia	76%	30%	77%	32%	61%	23%
Thrombocytopenia	24%	2%	22%	3%	5%	0%
Fatigue	38%	26%	22%	10%	40%	27%
Anorexia	17%	6%	33%	5%	47%	10%
Nausea	21%	5%	32%	3%	32%	6%
Diarrhea	14%	3%	15%	8%	18%	5%
Stomatitis	15%	3%	18%	5%	5%	2%

METASTATIC DISEASE • THIRD-LINE

GASTRIC CANCER REGIMEN: PEMBROLIZUMAB

Fuchs CS et al. JAMA Oncol 2018;4(5):e180013
Protocol for: Fuchs CS et al. JAMA Oncol 2018;4(5):e180013
Supplementary online content for: Fuchs CS et al. JAMA Oncol 2018;4(5):e180013
KEYTRUDA (pembrolizumab) injection prescribing information. Whitehouse Station, NJ: Merck & Co., Inc; updated January 2020

Note: The U.S. Food and Drug Administration–approved indication for pembrolizumab as first-line therapy for metastatic gastric cancer is limited to patients with PD-L1 expressing tumors (Combined Positive Score [CPS] ≥1) with disease progression on or after ≥2 prior lines of therapy including fluoropyrimidine- and platinum-containing chemotherapy and, if appropriate, HER2/neu-targeted therapy. CPS is calculated as the number of PD-L1-staining cells (including tumor cells, lymphocytes, and macrophages) divided by the total number of viable tumor cells, multiplied by 100

Pembrolizumab 200 mg; administer intravenously over 30 minutes in a volume of 0.9% sodium chloride injection (0.9% NS) or 5% dextrose injection (D5W) sufficient to produce a pembrolizumab concentration within the range 1–10 mg/mL every 3 weeks for up to 24 months (total dose/3-week cycle = 200 mg), *or:*

Pembrolizumab 400 mg; administer intravenously over 30 minutes in a volume of 0.9% NS D5W sufficient to produce a pembrolizumab concentration within the range 1–10 mg/mL every 6 weeks for up to 24 months (total dose/6-week cycle = 400 mg)
- Administer pembrolizumab with an administration set that contains a sterile, non-pyrogenic, low-protein-binding in-line or add-on filter with pore size within the range of 0.2–5 μm
- Pembrolizumab can cause severe or life-threatening infusion-related reactions, including hypersensitivity and anaphylaxis

Supportive Care
Antiemetic prophylaxis
Emetogenic potential is **MINIMAL**
See Chapter 42 for antiemetic recommendations

Hematopoietic growth factor (CSF) prophylaxis
Primary prophylaxis is **NOT** indicated
See Chapter 43 for more information

Antimicrobial prophylaxis
Risk of fever and neutropenia is **LOW**
   Antimicrobial primary prophylaxis to be considered:
   - Antibacterial—not indicated
   - Antifungal—not indicated
   - Antiviral—not indicated unless patient previously had an episode of HSV

Patient Population Studied

KEYNOTE-059 was a single-arm, open-label, global, multicohort, phase 2 trial that included 259 adult patients with advanced gastric or gastroesophageal junction (GEJ) cancer who had failed to benefit from 2 or more prior chemotherapy regimens and assessed treatment with pembrolizumab monotherapy. Patients were eligible if they had histologically or cytologically confirmed recurrent or metastatic gastric or GEJ adenocarcinoma (only Siewert types II and III) incurable by approved therapies, if they had measurable disease (according to RECIST v1.1), if they had disease progression after ≥2 previous chemotherapy regimens that included a fluoropyrimidine and a platinum doublet (as adjuvant treatment or for metastatic disease; perioperative, neoadjuvant, or adjuvant regimens were not considered previous regimens unless the patient's disease progressed during or within 6 months after adjuvant therapy), if they had HER2/neu-negative (or HER2/neu-positive if previously treated with trastuzumab) disease, and if they had an Eastern Cooperative Oncology Group performance status of ≤1. Patients were excluded from the study if they had clinical evidence of ascites, severe autoimmune disease that required systemic treatment in the previous 2 years or a diagnosis of immunodeficiency, a history of or active non-infectious pneumonitis, or active infection requiring systemic therapy

Therapy Monitoring

1. Initially at the time of each dose, and eventually every 6–12 weeks, perform a total body skin examination with attention to *all* mucous membranes as well as a complete review of systems

2. Monitor patients for signs and symptoms of pneumonitis. Evaluate patients with suspected pneumonitis with chest x-ray, CT, and pulse oximetry. For ≥2 toxicity, may include nasal swab, sputum culture and sensitivity, blood culture and sensitivity, and urine culture and sensitivity

3. Monitor patients for signs and symptoms of colitis. Encourage patients to report diarrhea immediately to any member of the health care team

4. Draw AST, ALT, and bilirubin prior to each infusion and/or weekly if there are Grade 1 liver function test elevations. Note, no treatment is recommended for G1 LFT abnormalities. For ≥2 toxicity, work up for other causes of elevated LFTs including viral hepatitis

5. Use basic metabolic panel (Na, K, CO_2, glucose) and patient history as screening tools for hypophysitis including hypopituitarism and adrenal insufficiency. If in doubt, evaluate AM adrenocorticotropic hormone (ACTH) and cortisol levels. Consider ACTH stimulation test for indeterminate results

6. Assess thyroid function at the start of treatment, periodically during treatment, and, as indicated, based on clinical evaluation and for clinical signs and symptoms of thyroid disorders. Test for TSH and free thyroxine (FT4) every 4 to 6 weeks as part of routine clinical monitoring on therapy or for case detection in symptomatic patients

7. Measure glucose at baseline and with each treatment during the first 12 weeks and every 6 weeks thereafter

8. Obtain a serum creatinine prior to every dose. If creatinine is found to be newly elevated, consider holding therapy while other potential causes are evaluated. Note that routine urinalysis is not necessary other than to rule out urinary tract infections, etc

9. Obtain a complete rheumatologic history and perform an examination of all peripheral joints for tenderness, swelling, and range of motion. Examine the spine. Consider plain x-ray/imaging to exclude metastases and evaluate joint damage (erosions), if appropriate

(continued)

Efficacy (N = 259)

Pembrolizumab Monotherapy (N = 259)

Objective response rate (CR + PR)	11.6% (95% CI, 8.0–16.1)
Disease control rate (CR + PR + stable disease ≥2 months)	27.0% (95% CI, 21.7–32.9)
Complete response rate	2.3% (95% CI, 0.9–5.0)
Partial response rate	9.3% (95% CI, 6.0–13.5)
Stable disease rate	16.2% (95% CI, 11.9–21.3)
Progressive disease rate	56.0% (95% CI, 49.7–62.1)
Median duration of response*	8.4 months (range, 1.6+–17.3+)
Median time to objective response	2.1 months (range, 1.7–6.6)
Patients with reduction in measurable tumor size†	42.6%
Median progression-free survival	2.0 months (95% CI, 2.0–2.1)
Progression-free survival, 6 months	14.1% (95% CI, 10.1–18.7)
Median overall survival	5.6 months (95% CI, 4.3–6.9)
Overall survival, 6 months	46.5% (95% CI, 40.2–52.6)
Overall survival, 12 months	23.4% (95% CI, 17.6–29.7)

Among 148 Patients with PD-L1-positive Tumors‡

Objective response rate (CR + PR)	15.5% (95% CI, 10.1–22.4)
Complete response rate (CR + PR)	2.0% (95% CI, 0.4–5.8)
Median duration of response	16.3 months (range, 1.6+–17.3+)
ORR with pembrolizumab as third-line treatment	22.7% (95% CI, 13.8–33.8)
CR with pembrolizumab as third-line treatment	2.7% (95% CI, 0.3–9.3)
Median duration of response with pembrolizumab as third-line treatment	8.1 months (1.6+–17.3+)

Among 109 Patients with PD-L1-negative Tumors‡

Objective response rate (CR + PR)	6.4% (95% CI, 2.6–12.8)
Complete response rate (CR + PR)	2.8% (95% CI, 0.6–7.8)
Median duration of response	6.9 months (range, 2.4–7.0+)
ORR with pembrolizumab as third-line treatment	8.6% (95% CI, 2.9–19)
CR with pembrolizumab as third-line treatment	3.4% (95% CI, 0.4–11.9)
Median duration of response with pembrolizumab as third-line treatment	6.9 months (4.4+–7.0+)

Among 7 Patients with High Microsatellite Instability Samples (MSI)ᶜ

Objective response rate	57.1% (95% CI, 18.4–90.1)

Among 167 Patients Without High MSIᶜ

Objective response rate	9.0% (95% CI, 5.1–14.4)

HR, hazard ratio; CI, confidence interval
*+ indicates no progressive disease at the last assessment
†Among the 223 patients who had 1 or more post-baseline radiologic imaging evaluations
‡Tumors were considered PD-L1-positive if the combined positive score (percentage of positive cells in the sample) was ≥1%
ᶜPatient samples were considered high MSI if ≥2 of 5 mononucleotide repeat markers (NR21, NR24, BAT25, BAT26, and MONO27) were changed compared with normal controls. Of 259 patients enrolled, 174 patients had samples assessed for MSI and 7 were determined to be high-MSI samples

Therapy Monitoring
(continued)

10. In patients at high risk for infections and in appropriately selected patients based on an infectious disease evaluation, draw screening laboratories (HIV, hepatitis A and B, and blood QuantiFERON for TB) to prepare patients to start infliximab
11. *Response evaluation:* Every 2 to 4 months

Treatment Modifications

RECOMMENDED DOSE MODIFICATIONS FOR PEMBROLIZUMAB

Adverse Event	Grade/Severity	Treatment Modification
Infusion reaction	Clinically significant but not severe infusion reaction	Interrupt the infusion in patients with clinically significant infusion reactions and consider resuming at a slower rate following resolution. If decision is made to restart, begin at ≤50% of the rate prior to the reaction and increase in 50% increments every 30 minutes if well tolerated. Infusions may be restarted at the full rate during the next cycle
	G3/4 (severe infusion reaction—pyrexia, chills, flushing, hypotension, dyspnea, wheezing, back pain, abdominal pain, and urticaria). Not rapidly responsive to brief interruption of infusion	Stop infusion and administer appropriate medical therapy (eg, epinephrine, corticosteroids, intravenous antihistamines, bronchodilators, and/or oxygen). Discontinue pembrolizumab
Colitis	G1	Loperamide 4 mg as starting dose then 2 mg before each meal and after each loose stool until without diarrhea for 12 hours, with maximum of 16 mg loperamide per day. If G1 diarrhea or colitis persists >14 days, then add prednisolone 0.5–1 mg/kg (non-enteric-coated) or consider oral budesonide 9 mg daily if no bloody diarrhea
	G2/3 diarrhea or colitis	Withhold pembrolizumab. Loperamide 4 mg as starting dose then 2 mg before each meal and after each loose stool until without diarrhea for 12 hours, with maximum of 16 mg loperamide per day. Administer oral prednisone/prednisolone at a dose of 0.5 to 2 mg/kg/day or its equivalent. When improves to G1, begin a slow corticosteroid taper over at least 4 weeks. Resume pembrolizumab upon symptom control, or when prednisone/prednisolone daily dose <10 mg
	G4 diarrhea or colitis	Permanently discontinue pembrolizumab. Loperamide 4 mg as starting dose then 2 mg before each meal and after each loose stool until without diarrhea for 12 hours, with maximum of 16 mg loperamide per day. Administer 1–2 mg/kg IV (methyl)prednisolone and convert to 0.5–2 mg/kg prednisone/prednisolone orally each day or its equivalent only after a response. Taper over at least 4 weeks when symptoms improve. If does not improve over 72 hours or worsens, perform flexible sigmoidoscopy/colonoscopy to document colitis then begin infliximab 5 mg/kg (if no perforation/sepsis/TB/hepatitis/NYHA III/IV CHF). If no response, add MMF 500–1000 mg twice daily. If worse on MMF, consider addition of tacrolimus or ATG
Pneumonitis	G2	Withhold pembrolizumab. Consider pneumocystis prophylaxis depending on the clinical context and coverage with empiric antibiotics. Administer oral prednisone/prednisolone at a dose of 1–2 mg/kg/day or its equivalent. When improves to G1, begin a slow corticosteroid taper over at least 4 weeks. If does not respond adequately after 48 hours, then administer 2–4 mg/kg IV (methyl)prednisolone and convert to 0.5–2 mg/kg prednisone/prednisolone orally each day or its equivalent only after a response, followed by a taper over at least 6 weeks when symptoms improve to G1, titrating to symptoms. Resume pembrolizumab upon symptom control, or when prednisone/prednisolone daily dose <10 mg
	G3/4	Permanently discontinue pembrolizumab. Consider pneumocystis prophylaxis depending on the clinical context; cover with empiric antibiotics. Administer 2–4 mg/kg IV (methyl)prednisolone and convert to 1–2 mg/kg prednisone/prednisolone orally each day or its equivalent only after a response, followed by a taper over at least 8 weeks when symptoms improve to G1, titrating to symptoms. If when initially treated improvement does not occur within 48–72 hours, begin infliximab 5 mg/kg (if no perforation/sepsis/TB/hepatitis/NYHA III/IV CHF). If no response to infliximab, add MMF 500–1000 mg twice daily. Consider MMF especially if has concurrent hepatic toxicity
Hepatitis	G2 (AST or ALT >3–5× ULN or total bilirubin >1.5–3× ULN)	Withhold pembrolizumab. Administer oral prednisone/prednisolone at a dose of 1 to 2 mg/kg/day or its equivalent. When improves to G1, begin a slow corticosteroid taper over at least 4 weeks. Resume pembrolizumab upon symptom control, or when prednisone/prednisolone daily dose <10 mg
	G3/4 (AST or ALT >5× ULN or total bilirubin >3× ULN)	Permanently discontinue pembrolizumab. Administer 1–2 mg/kg IV (methyl)prednisolone and convert to 0.5–2 mg/kg prednisone/prednisolone orally each day or its equivalent only after a response. Taper over at least 6 weeks when symptoms improve. If no response, add MMF 500–1000 mg twice daily. If worse on MMF, consider adding tacrolimus or ATG

(continued)

Treatment Modifications (*continued*)

Hypophysitis	G2/3 (moderate symptoms, ie, headache but no visual disturbance or fatigue/mood alteration but hemodynamically stable, no electrolyte disturbance)	Administer analgesia as needed for headache. Withhold pembrolizumab. Administer oral prednisone/prednisolone at a dose of 0.5 to 2 mg/kg/day or its equivalent. When improves to G1, begin a slow corticosteroid taper over at least 4 weeks. If no improvement in 48 hours, administer 1–2 mg/kg IV (methyl)prednisolone and convert to 0.5–2 mg/kg prednisone/prednisolone orally each day or its equivalent only after a response. Taper over at least 4 weeks when symptoms improve to 5 mg prednisone/prednisolone or equivalent; do not stop steroids. Resume pembrolizumab upon symptom control, or when prednisone/prednisolone daily dose <10 mg
	G4 (severe mass effect symptoms, ie, severe headache, any visual disturbance or severe hypoadrenalism, ie, hypotension, severe electrolyte disturbance)	Permanently discontinue pembrolizumab. Administer analgesia as needed for headache. Administer 1–2 mg/kg IV (methyl)prednisolone and convert to 0.5–2 mg/kg prednisone/prednisolone orally each day or its equivalent only after a response. Taper over at least 4 weeks when symptoms improve to 5 mg prednisone/prednisolone or equivalent; do not stop steroids
Adrenal insufficiency	G2	Withhold pembrolizumab. Administer oral prednisone/prednisolone at a dose of 0.5 to 2 mg/kg/day or its equivalent. When improves to G1, begin a slow corticosteroid taper over at least 4 weeks. Serially assess adrenal function and continue steroids at replacement doses (20–40 mg hydrocortisone daily ~2/3 dose in AM upon awakening and ~1/3 at 4 PM) until recovery of adrenal function is documented. Resume pembrolizumab upon symptom control, or when prednisone/prednisolone daily dose <10 mg
	G3/4	Permanently discontinue pembrolizumab. Administer oral prednisone/prednisolone at a dose of 0.5 to 2 mg/kg/day or its equivalent. When improves to G1, begin a slow corticosteroid taper over at least 4 weeks. Serially assess adrenal function and continue steroids at replacement doses (20–40 mg hydrocortisone daily ~2/3 dose in AM upon awakening and ~1/3 at 4 PM) until recovery of adrenal function is documented
Type 1 diabetes mellitus	G3 hyperglycemia	Withhold pembrolizumab. Admit to hospital to manage hyperglycemia. Role of corticosteroids in preventing complete loss of insulin-producing cells is unknown and not recommended. Resume pembrolizumab upon symptom control, or when prednisone/prednisolone daily dose <10 mg
	G4 hyperglycemia	Permanently discontinue pembrolizumab. Admit to hospital to manage hyperglycemia. Role of corticosteroids in preventing complete loss of insulin-producing cells is unknown and not recommended
Nephritis and renal dysfunction	G2/3 (serum creatinine 1.5–6× ULN)	Withhold pembrolizumab. Administer oral prednisone/prednisolone at a dose of 0.5 to 2 mg/kg/day or its equivalent. When improves to G1, begin a slow corticosteroid taper over at least 4 weeks. If does not respond adequately, then administer 0.5–1 mg/kg IV (methyl)prednisolone and convert to 0.5–2 mg/kg prednisone/prednisolone orally each day or its equivalent only after a response, followed by a taper over at least 4 weeks when improves to G1. Resume pembrolizumab upon symptom control, or when prednisone/prednisolone daily dose <10 mg
	G4 (serum creatinine >6× ULN)	Permanently discontinue pembrolizumab. Administer 0.5–1 mg/kg IV (methyl)prednisolone and convert to 0.5–2 mg/kg prednisone/prednisolone orally each day or its equivalent only after a response, followed by a taper over at least 4 weeks when improves to G1
Skin	G1/2	Continue pembrolizumab. Avoid skin irritants, avoid sun exposure, topical emollients recommended. Topical steroid (mild strength for G1, moderate/potent strength for G2) cream once or twice daily ± oral or topical antihistamines for itching
	G3 rash or suspected SJS or TEN	Withhold pembrolizumab. Avoid skin irritants, avoid sun exposure, topical emollients recommended. Administer oral or topical antihistamines for itching. Administer oral prednisone/prednisolone at a dose of 0.5–2 mg/kg or its equivalent daily for 3 days followed by a slow corticosteroid taper over at least 4 weeks when the rash improves to G1. If does not respond adequately, then administer 0.5–1 mg/kg IV (methyl)prednisolone and convert to 0.5–2 mg/kg prednisone/prednisolone orally each day or its equivalent only after a response, followed by a taper over at least 4 weeks when the rash improves to G1. Resume pembrolizumab upon symptom control, or when prednisone/prednisolone daily dose <10 mg
	G4 rash or confirmed SJS or TEN	Avoid skin irritants, avoid sun exposure, topical emollients recommended. Administer oral or topical antihistamines for itching. Administer 1–2 mg/kg IV (methyl)prednisolone and convert to oral steroids 0.5–2 mg/kg prednisone/prednisolone each day or its equivalent only after a response. Taper over at least 4 weeks when the rash improves to G1. Permanently discontinue pembrolizumab

(*continued*)

Treatment Modifications (*continued*)

Encephalitis	Confusion or altered behavior, headaches, alteration in Glasgow Coma Scale, motor or sensory deficits, speech abnormality, may or may not be febrile	Initially withhold pembrolizumab, but permanently discontinue pembrolizumab if there is no doubt as to diagnosis. Exclude bacterial and ideally viral infections prior to high-dose steroids. Administer oral prednisone/prednisolone at a dose of 0.5–2 mg/kg/day or its equivalent. When symptoms improve, begin a slow corticosteroid taper over at least 4–8 weeks. If symptoms are severe, administer 1–2 mg/kg IV (methyl)prednisolone and convert to 0.5–2 mg/kg prednisone/prednisolone orally each day or its equivalent only after a response. Consider concurrent empiric antiviral (IV acyclovir) and antibacterial therapy
Aseptic meningitis	Headache, photophobia, neck stiffness with fever or may be afebrile, vomiting; normal cognition/cerebral function (distinguishes from encephalitis)	
Other syndromes include neurosarcoidosis, posterior reversible leukoencephalopathy syndrome (PRES), Vogt-Koyanagi-Harada syndrome, demyelination, vasculitic encephalopathy, and generalized seizures		
Transverse myelitis	Acute or subacute neurological signs/symptoms of motor/sensory/autonomic origin; most have sensory level; often bilateral symptoms	Initially withhold pembrolizumab, but permanently discontinue pembrolizumab if there is no doubt as to diagnosis. Administer 2 mg/kg IV (methyl)prednisolone or consider 1 g/day and convert to 0.5–2 mg/kg prednisone/prednisolone orally each day or its equivalent only after a response. When symptoms improve, begin a slow corticosteroid taper over at least 4–8 weeks. Plasmapheresis may be required if steroids do not bring about improvement
Myocarditis	G3	Permanently discontinue pembrolizumab. Administer 2 mg/kg IV (methyl)prednisolone or consider 1 g/day and convert to 0.5–2 mg/kg prednisone/prednisolone orally each day or its equivalent only after a response. When symptoms improve, begin a slow corticosteroid taper over at least 4–8 weeks. If no response, add MMF 500–1000 mg twice daily. If worse on MMF, consider adding tacrolimus
Peripheral neurologic toxicity	Moderate: some interference with ADL, symptoms concerning to patient	Withhold pembrolizumab. Initial observation reasonable or initiate prednisone/prednisolone 0.5–1 mg/kg (if progressing, eg, from mild) and/or pregabalin or duloxetine for pain. When symptoms improve, begin a slow corticosteroid taper over at least 4 weeks. Resume pembrolizumab upon symptom control, or when prednisone/prednisolone daily dose <10 mg
	Severe: limits self-care and aids warranted, life-threatening, eg, respiratory problems	Permanently discontinue pembrolizumab. Administer 1–2 mg/kg IV (methyl)prednisolone and convert to 0.5–2 mg/kg prednisone/prednisolone orally each day or its equivalent only after a response. Taper over at least 4–8 weeks when symptoms improve to G1
Guillain-Barré syndrome	Progressive symmetrical muscle weakness with absent or reduced tendon reflexes—involves extremities, facial, respiratory, and bulbar and oculomotor muscles; dysregulation of autonomic nerves	Permanently discontinue pembrolizumab. Use of steroids not recommended in idiopathic Guillain-Barré syndrome; however, a trial of (methyl)prednisolone 1–2 mg/kg is reasonable, converting to 0.5–2 mg/kg prednisone/prednisolone orally each day or its equivalent only after a response. If no improvement or worsening, plasmapheresis or IVIG indicated
Myasthenia gravis	Fluctuating muscle weakness (proximal limb, trunk, ocular, eg, ptosis/diplopia or bulbar) with fatigability, respiratory muscles also may be involved	Permanently discontinue pembrolizumab. Administer pyridostigmine at an initial dose of 30 mg three times daily. Administer oral prednisone/prednisolone at a dose of 0.5 to 2 mg/kg/day or its equivalent or 1–2 mg/kg IV (methyl)prednisolone depending on the severity of symptoms. If begin with IV, convert to 0.5–2 mg/kg prednisone/prednisolone orally each day or its equivalent only after a response. If no improvement or worsening, plasmapheresis or IVIG may be considered. Additional immunosuppressants used in myasthenia gravis include azathioprine, cyclosporine, and mycophenolate. Avoid certain medications, eg, ciprofloxacin, beta-blockers, that may precipitate cholinergic crisis
Other syndromes including motor and sensory peripheral neuropathy, multifocal radicular neuropathy/plexopathy, autonomic neuropathy, phrenic nerve palsy, cranial nerve palsies (eg, facial nerve, optic nerve, hypoglossal nerve)		Permanently discontinue pembrolizumab. Administer oral prednisone/prednisolone at a dose of 0.5 to 2 mg/kg/day or its equivalent or 1–2 mg/kg IV (methyl)prednisolone depending on the severity of symptoms. If begin with IV, convert to 0.5–2 mg/kg prednisone/prednisolone orally each day or its equivalent only after a response

(*continued*)

Treatment Modifications (*continued*)

Arthralgia	G1 (mild pain with inflammation, erythema, or joint swelling)	Continue pembrolizumab. Administer acetaminophen (paracetamol) and ibuprofen
	G2 (moderate pain with inflammation, erythema, or joint swelling that limits ADLs)	Withhold pembrolizumab. Administer higher doses of acetaminophen (paracetamol) and ibuprofen and use diclofenac or naproxen or etoricoxib. If inadequately controlled, consider intra-articular steroid injections for large joints or administer oral prednisone/prednisolone at a dose of 0.5 to 2 mg/kg/day or its equivalent. When improves to G1, begin a slow corticosteroid taper over at least 4 weeks. If does not respond adequately, then administer 0.5–1 mg/kg IV (methyl)prednisolone and convert to 0.5–2 mg/kg prednisone/prednisolone orally each day or its equivalent only after a response, followed by a taper over at least 4 weeks when improves to G1. Resume pembrolizumab upon symptom control, or when prednisone/prednisolone daily dose <10 mg
	G3 (severe pain; irreversible joint damage; disabling; limits self-care ADL)	Withhold pembrolizumab. Administer 0.5–1 mg/kg IV (methyl)prednisolone and convert to 0.5–2 mg/kg prednisone/prednisolone orally each day or its equivalent only after a response, followed by a taper over at least 4 weeks when improves to G1. In severe cases, infliximab or another anti–TNF-alpha drug may be required for improvement of arthritis. Resume pembrolizumab upon symptom control, or when prednisone/prednisolone daily dose <10 mg
Other	First occurrence of other G3	Withhold pembrolizumab. Administer oral prednisone/prednisolone at a dose of 0.5 to 2 mg/kg/day or its equivalent. When improves to G1, begin a slow corticosteroid taper over at least 4 weeks. Resume pembrolizumab upon symptom control, or when prednisone/prednisolone daily dose <10 mg
	Recurrence of same G3	Permanently discontinue pembrolizumab. Administer 1–2 mg/kg IV (methyl)prednisolone and convert to 0.5–2 mg/kg prednisone/prednisolone orally each day or its equivalent only after a response. Taper over at least 4–8 weeks when symptoms improve to G1
	Life-threatening or G4	
	Requirement for ≥10 mg/day prednisone or equivalent for >12 weeks	Permanently discontinue pembrolizumab
	Persistent G2/3 adverse reactions lasting ≥12 weeks	

ADL, activities of daily living; ALT, alanine aminotransferase; AST, aspartate aminotransferase; ATG, anti-thymocyte globulin; SJS, Stevens-Johnson Syndrome; TEN, toxic epidermal necrolysis; ULN, upper limit of normal

Notes on general supportive care:
- Steroid taper in most cases will proceed over a minimum of one month but if symptoms improve rapidly, a two-week taper can be considered. If steroids are administered for more than 4 weeks, consider PCP prophylaxis (cotrimoxazole 480 mg twice daily M/W/F or inhaled pentamidine if has cotrimoxazole allergy), regular random blood glucose, VitD level and starting calcium/VitD supplementation as per guidelines

Adverse Events (N = 259)

Pembrolizumab Monotherapy (N = 259)	
All-cause, any grade adverse events	95.8%
1 or more Grade 3–5 adverse events	61.4%
≥1 treatment-related adverse events of any grade	60.2%
≥1 G3–5 treatment-related adverse event	17.8%
Treatment discontinuation due to treatment-related adverse event	0.8%
≥1 immune-related adverse events of any grade	17.8%
G3/4 immune-mediated events (none fatal)	4.6%

Grade (%)	Any Grade	Grade 3
Fatigue	49 (18.9%)	6 (2.3%)
Pruritis	23 (8.9%)	0
Rash	22 (8.5%)	2 (0.8%)
Hypothyroidism	20 (7.7%)	1 (0.4%)
Decreased appetite	19 (7.3%)	0
Anemia	18 (6.9%)	7 (2.7%)
Nausea	18 (6.9%)	2 (0.8%)
Diarrhea	17 (6.6%)	3 (1.2%)
Arthralgia	15 (5.8%)	1 (0.4%)

Note that the table includes treatment-related adverse events that occurred in ≥5% of patients. There were no treatment-related Grade 4–5 events. However, there were two Grade 5 events (acute kidney injury and pleural effusion) that were considered related to pembrolizumab by the investigators. The most common reasons for discontinuation were disease progression (64.9%), death (10.0%), and adverse events (7.7%)

17. Gestational Trophoblastic Neoplasia

John R. Lurain, MD

Epidemiology

Gestational trophoblastic disease (GTD) is a spectrum of inter-related abnormal proliferations of the placental trophoblast, encompassing benign hydatidiform mole (complete and partial) as well as malignant gestational trophoblastic neoplasia (GTN), which includes invasive mole (IM), choriocarcinoma (CC), placental site trophoblastic tumor (PSTT), and epithelioid trophoblastic tumor (ETT)

Complete Hydatidiform Mole (CHM)
- Incidence: 1 in 1000–2000 pregnancies in the United States and Europe, but higher in Asia and Latin America
- Risk Factors: extremes of reproductive age (<20 and >40), prior molar pregnancy
- GTN: develops in about 15–20% (12–18% IM and 2–3% CC) after molar evacuation

Partial Hydatidiform Mole (PHM)
- Incidence: 3 in 1000 pregnancies
- Risk Factors: possible history of irregular menses and prolonged oral contraceptive use
- GTN: develops in 1–5% after molar evacuation (almost all IM)

Choriocarcinoma
- Incidence: 1 in 40,000 pregnancies
- Risk Factors: history of complete hydatidiform mole (1000× more likely to arise from a CHM, although one-half of cases develop from other pregnancy events)
- Common sites of metastasis: lungs (80%), brain (10%), liver (10%), vagina (~5%)

PSTT/ETT
- Incidence: <0.2% of all cases of GTD
- Risk Factors: insufficient data exist to adequately characterize any risk factors; however, 95% develop following a term pregnancy or nonmolar abortion and may present many months or years later

Lurain JR. Am J Obstet Gynecol 2010;203:531–539

Clinicopathology

Disease	Pathologic Features	Clinical Factors
Complete mole	• Diploid (46,XX, rarely 46,XY) • Absent fetus/embryo • Diffuse swelling of villi • Diffuse trophoblastic hyperplasia	• Vaginal bleeding • Large for dates uterine size • Bilateral theca-lutein cysts • Medical complications • hCG often >100,000 mIU/mL • 15–20% postmolar GTN
Partial mole	• Triploid • Abnormal fetus/embryo • Focal swelling of villi • Focal trophoblastic hyperplasia	• Pre-D&C diagnosis usually incomplete or missed abortion • Medical complications rare • hCG rarely >100,000 mIU/mL • <5% postmolar GTN
Invasive mole	• Swollen villi • Hyperplastic trophoblast • Myometrial invasion	• Irregular postmolar vaginal bleeding • Persistent hCG elevation • Most often diagnosed clinically rather than pathologically • 15% metastatic—lung/vagina
Choriocarcinoma	• Abnormal trophoblastic hyperplasia • Absent villi • Hemorrhage • Necrosis	• Irregular vaginal bleeding after any pregnancy event • hCG elevation • Symptoms associated with vascular spread to distant sites
PSTT	• Intermediate trophoblastic hyperplasia • Absent villi • Less hemorrhage and necrosis • Vascular and lymphatic invasion • Tumor cells stain positive for hPL	• Enlarged uterus • Total hCG low • Free beta subunit of hCG elevated • Relatively chemoresistant • Mainly surgical treatment
ETT	• Chorionic-type intermediate trophoblast • Extensive necrosis • Rare hemorrhage • Tumor cells stain positive for p63	• Enlarged uterus; cervical tumor • Metastases with associated symptoms • No or very low elevation of hCG • Relatively chemoresistant

hCG, human chorionic gonadotropin; hPL, human placental lactogen; PSTT, placental site trophoblastic tumor; ETT, epithelioid trophoblastic tumor
Modified from Lurain JR. Am J Obstet Gynecol 2010;203:531–539

Staging

FIGO Anatomic Staging System for GTN

Stage	Extent of GTN
I	Confined to the uterus
II	Extends outside the uterus but is limited to the genital structures (adnexa, vagina, broad ligament)
III	Extends to the lungs, with or without known genital tract involvement
IV	All other metastatic sites

FIGO (Modified WHO) Prognostic Scoring System for GTN

Note: This scoring system does not apply to patients with placental site or epithelioid trophoblastic tumors

Prognostic Factor	0	1	2	4
Age (years)	≤39	>39	—	—
Antecedent pregnancy	Hydatidiform mole	Abortion	Term pregnancy	—
Interval from index pregnancy	<4 months	4–6 months	7–12 months	>12 months
Pretreatment hCG level (IU/L)	<1000	1000–10,000	>10,000–100,000	>100,000
Largest tumor size including uterus	—	3–4 cm	≥5 cm	—
Sites of metastases	Lung*	Spleen, kidney	GI tract	Brain, liver
Number of metastases identified*	0	1–4	5–8	>8
Previous ineffective chemotherapy	—	—	Single drug	≥2 drugs

*Chest x-ray is used to count the number of metastases for risk score assessment

Note: Total score for a patient is obtained by adding individual scores for each prognostic factor

Total Score	Risk
0–6	Low risk
≥7	High risk

Both FIGO Anatomic Staging and Prognostic Scoring System should be used. By convention, the FIGO stage is depicted by a Roman numeral and is followed by the prognostic score depicted by an Arabic numeral. The two values are separated by a colon (eg, III:9)

Kohorn EI. Int J Gynecol Cancer 2001;11:73–77
Ngan HYS et al. Int J Gynaecol Obstet 2018;143:79–85

Work-up

Once a diagnosis of GTN has been made, it is necessary to determine the extent of disease

Once the initial work-up is completed, patients are categorized according to FIGO risk group, as above

1. H&P
2. Serum hCG

Note: For staging purposes, the hCG level that is important is that obtained immediately before instituting treatment and not the hCG obtained at the time of the previous molar evacuation

3. CBC, LFT, serum electrolytes, BUN, creatinine, PTT, and PT
4. Chest x-ray
5. CT of chest, abdomen, and pelvis
6. MRI brain (especially in patients with lung lesions. Asymptomatic patients with a normal chest x-ray are unlikely to have brain metastasis)
7. TSH, T_4 (elevations of thyroid tests are not common in patients with GTN but can occur mostly in association with hydatidiform mole)

Lurain JR. Am J Obstet Gynecol 2011;204:11–18

Survival

GTN can be cured predictably even in the presence of widespread metastases. Overall survival is >95%, with survival rates approaching 100% for stage I and stages II/III with score <7 and 80–90% for stage IV or score ≥7 disease

Expert Opinion

Nonmetastatic GTN

1. Patients with nonmetastatic GTN (FIGO stage I) should be treated with single-agent methotrexate or dactinomycin chemotherapy. Several different outpatient chemotherapy protocols have been used, yielding excellent and fairly comparable results. Hysterectomy may be used as part of primary therapy in patients who no longer desire to preserve fertility

2. Cure is anticipated in 100% of patients with nonmetastatic GTN. Approximately 80% of patients will be cured by the initial single-agent chemotherapy regimen. Most of the remaining patients will be placed into permanent remission with an alternate single agent. Multiagent chemotherapy is needed in <10%, and hysterectomy is required in <5% of patients to achieve cure

    a. Methotrexate given intravenously for 5 days every 2 weeks (Chapman-Davis E et al. Gynecol Oncol 2012;125:572–575) results in the highest primary remission rate of approximately 90%

    b. Methotrexate + leucovorin (folinic acid) given over 8 days every 2 weeks[†,‡,§] is reported to have decreased toxicity (especially stomatitis), but is associated with a more frequent need for a change in chemotherapy (20–25%) to achieve remission

    c. Methotrexate 30–50 mg/m^2 by intramuscular injection once weekly or methotrexate 300 mg/m^2 by intravenous infusion in 25–1000 mL 0.9% NS or D5W over 12 hours followed by leucovorin 15 mg/dose by intramuscular injection or orally every 12 hours for 4 doses starting 24 hours after beginning the methotrexate. These two treatment protocols are NOT recommended because of the lower primary remission rates of 53–70% and the more frequent need for multiagent chemotherapy to achieve remission

    d. Dactinomycin given intravenously at a flat dose of 0.5 mg daily for 5 days every 2 weeks[**] or 1.25 mg/m^2 (max 2 mg) once every 2 weeks[††] are acceptable alternatives to methotrexate

    - Dactinomycin generally causes more nausea and alopecia than methotrexate and produces vesicant injury if extravasation into perivascular tissues occurs. Therefore, dactinomycin is most often used as secondary therapy in the presence of methotrexate resistance or as primary therapy when patients have hepatic or renal compromise or effusions contraindicating the use of methotrexate

Low-Risk Metastatic GTN

1. Patients categorized as having low-risk metastatic GTN (FIGO stages II and III, score <7) can usually be treated successfully with sequential single-agent chemotherapy (Chapman-Davis E et al. Gynecol Oncol 2012;125:572–575), with:

    - A 5-day methotrexate or dactinomycin regimen[¶]
    - An 8-day methotrexate and leucovorin regimen

2. When resistance to sequential single-agent chemotherapy develops, multiagent chemotherapy as for high-risk disease should be given. Hysterectomy may become necessary to eradicate persistent, chemotherapy-resistant disease in the uterus, or it may be performed as adjuvant treatment coincident with the initiation of chemotherapy to shorten the duration of treatment if fertility preservation is not desired

3. Cure rate for low-risk metastatic GTN approaches 100%. Because approximately 30–50% of patients in this category develop resistance to the first chemotherapeutic agent, it is important to carefully monitor patients for evidence of drug resistance so that a change in chemotherapy can be made at the earliest possible time. Eventually, 5–15% of patients treated with sequential single-agent chemotherapy will require multiagent chemotherapy or surgery to achieve remission

High-Risk Metastatic GTN

1. Patients with high-risk metastatic GTN (FIGO stage IV or score ≥7) should be treated initially with multiagent chemotherapy with or without adjuvant surgery or radiation therapy. The EMA/CO protocol, or some variation of it, is currently the treatment of choice for high-risk metastatic GTN because of low toxicity allowing adherence to treatment schedule and relatively high complete response rates of 70–80%[‡‡,§§]

2. Patients with widely metastatic disease as evidenced by very high FIGO scores (>12) are at significant risk for pulmonary, intraperitoneal, and intracranial hemorrhage leading to early death after commencement of chemotherapy. These patients may benefit from low-dose induction chemotherapy with etoposide 100 mg/m^2 and cisplatin 20 mg/m^2 days 1 and 2 every 7 days for 1–3 courses prior to starting standard EMA/CO (Alifrangis et al, 2013)

3. When central nervous system metastases are present, whole-brain irradiation (3000 cGy in 200-cGy fractions), intrathecal methotrexate, or stereotactic irradiation in selected patients, is usually given simultaneously with the initiation of systemic chemotherapy. During radiotherapy, the methotrexate infusion dosage in the EMA/CO protocol is increased to 1000 mg/m^2 and 30 mg of leucovorin is given every 12 hours for 3 days starting 32 hours after the methotrexate infusion begins. Reported cure rates with brain metastases are 50–80%, depending on patient symptoms as well as number, size, and location of brain lesions (Savage et al, 2015)

4. Adjuvant surgical procedures, especially hysterectomy and pulmonary resection for chemotherapy-resistant disease, as well as procedures to control hemorrhage, are important components in the management of high-risk GTN. Almost 50% of high-risk patients treated with EMA/CO will require one or more operations in order to effect cure

(continued)

Expert Opinion (continued)

5. Cure rates for high-risk metastatic GTN of 80–90% are now achievable with intensive multimodality treatment with EMA/CO chemotherapy, along with adjuvant radiotherapy or surgery when indicated. Approximately 30% of high-risk patients will fail to achieve a complete response from first-line therapy or relapse from remission. Salvage therapy with platinum-containing drug combinations, such as:

> Etoposide + cisplatin/etoposide + methotrexate + dactinomycin (EP/EMA),
>
> Bleomycin + etoposide + cisplatin (BEP),
>
> Etoposide + ifosfamide + cisplatin (VIP) or ifosfamide + carboplatin + etoposide (ICE), and
>
> Paclitaxel + cisplatin alternating with paclitaxel + etoposide (TP/TE),

often in conjunction with surgical resection of sites of persistent tumor, will result in cure of most of these high-risk patients with resistant disease (Lurain et al 2012; Abu-Rustum et al 2019)

Intermediate Trophoblastic Tumor: Placental Site Trophoblastic Tumor (PSTT) and Epithelioid Trophoblastic Tumor (ETT)

1. Because of the relative resistance of PSTT and ETT to chemotherapy and the risk of lymphatic spread, hysterectomy and lymph node dissection is the recommended treatment

2. Patients with metastatic disease and patients with nonmetastatic disease with poor prognostic factors, including long interval between last pregnancy and diagnosis (>2 years), deep myometrial invasion, tumor necrosis, and mitotic count > 5/10 HPFs, should receive chemotherapy with a platinum-containing regimen, such as EP/EMA or TP/TE. Excision of metastatic disease should also be undertaken, when possible

3. The survival rate is approximately 100% for nonmetastatic disease and 50–60% for metastatic disease (Horowitz et al Gynecol Oncol 2017 and Froeling et al 2019)

*Lawrie TA et al. Cochrane Database Syst Rev 2016;6:CD007102
†McNeish IA et al. J Clin Oncol 2002;20:1838–1844
‡Sita-Lumsden A et al. Br J Cancer 2012;107:1810–1814
§Growden WB et al. Gynecol Oncol 2009;112:353–357
¶Osborne RJ et al. J Clin Oncol 2011;29:825–831
**Osathanondh R et al. Cancer 1975;36:863–866
††Petrilli ES et al. Cancer 1987;60:2173–2176
‡‡Lurain JR et al. J Reprod Med 2010;55:199–207
§§Lurain JR, Schink JC. J Reprod Med 2012;57:219–224

Abu-Rustum NR et al. J Natl Compr Canc Netw 2019;17:1374–1391
Alifrangis C et al. J Clin Oncol 2013;31:280–286
Froeling FEM et al. Br J Cancer 2019;120:587–594
Horowitz NS et al. Gynecol Oncol 2017;144:208–214
Savage P et al. Gynecol Oncol 2015;137:73–76

FIRST-LINE • NONMETASTATIC • LOW-RISK METASTATIC

GESTATIONAL TROPHOBLASTIC NEOPLASIA REGIMEN: METHOTREXATE

Chapman-Davis E et al. Gynecol Oncol 2012;125:572–575
Lurain JR, Elfstrand EP. Am J Obstet Gynecol 1995;172:574–579
Roberts JP, Lurain JR. Am J Obstet Gynecol 1996;174:1917–1924

Methotrexate 0.4 mg/kg (maximum daily dose = 25 mg) per day; administer by intravenous injection daily for 5 consecutive days on days 1–5, every 2 weeks (total dosage/14-day cycle = 2 mg/kg, maximum dose/14-day cycle = 125 mg)

Recommendations:

1. Administer treatment courses as often as toxicity permits, usually every 14 days
2. Encourage increased oral fluid intake or, if NPO, give parenteral hydration
3. Avoid drugs that can alter methotrexate elimination, such as non-steroidal anti-inflammatory drugs, omeprazole (and possibly other proton pump inhibitors), penicillins, probenecid, and salicylates
4. Administer two additional cycles after the first normal hCG level

Note: Determination of GFR before treatment does not predict for methotrexate clearance and potential toxicity, but serum creatinine that is within normal limits and a GFR >60 mL/min are generally accepted as adequate renal function

Supportive Care
Antiemetic prophylaxis
Emetogenic potential on days 1–5: **MINIMAL**
See Chapter 42 for antiemetic recommendations

Hematopoietic growth factor (CSF) prophylaxis
Primary prophylaxis is **NOT** *indicated*
See Chapter 43 for more information

Antimicrobial prophylaxis
Risk of fever and neutropenia is **LOW**

Oral care
Prophylaxis and treatment for mucositis/stomatitis
  General advice:
  • Encourage patients to maintain intake of nonalcoholic fluids

  If mucositis or stomatitis is present:
  • Rinse mouth several times a day to remove debris
    ■ Use a solution of ¼ teaspoon (1.25 g) each of baking soda and table salt (sodium chloride) in 1 quart (~950 mL) of warm water. Follow with a plain water rinse
    ■ Do not use mouthwashes that contain alcohols

Treatment Modifications

Adverse Event	Dose Modification
G ≤1 toxicity	Continue therapy if easy to manage
G2 toxicity	Consider a 20% reduction in methotrexate dosage
G ≥3 toxicity	Discontinue methotrexate and institute other therapy

Patient Population Studied

Retrospective review of 253 patients with nonmetastatic gestational trophoblastic tumors (invasive mole [209] or choriocarcinoma [44]) treated from 1962 to 1990. Antecedent pregnancy was hydatidiform mole (230), abortion (16), and term or preterm delivery (7). A mean of 4.7 courses (range, 1–7) of single-agent methotrexate was administered

Efficacy (N = 253)

Treatment	% Complete Response
Methotrexate alone	89.3*
Methotrexate + dactinomycin	8.7
Multiagent chemotherapy or surgery	2.0
Survival	100

*Six patients (2.4%) had a relapse 1–9 months after achieving a complete response. All were placed into a permanent remission with additional chemotherapy

Toxicity (N = 253)

Stomatitis	G3 (16 patients) mild to moderate (many)
Conjunctivitis	3 patients
Pleuritic/peritoneal pain	3 patients
Hair loss	None
Nausea/vomiting	Not common
Toxicity requiring dose reduction	11 patients (4.3%)
Toxicity requiring change in therapy*	12 patients (4.7%)

*Reasons: G3 stomatitis (5), rash and stomatitis (4); prolonged neutropenia (2), elevated LFTs (1)

Therapy Monitoring

1. *Every other week:* PE, CBC with differential, serum electrolytes, LFTs, serum creatinine, BUN, and hCG
2. *Methotrexate levels:* Not routinely performed
3. *Complete remission:* Three consecutive weekly hCG levels within normal range
4. *Resistance to treatment:* hCG plateau over two consecutive treatments or an hCG rise after any treatment
5. *Following remission:* hCG levels are obtained monthly for 12 months, and every 3 months during the second year

FIRST LINE • NONMETASTATIC • LOW-RISK METASTATIC

GESTATIONAL TROPHOBLASTIC NEOPLASIA REGIMEN: METHOTREXATE WITH LEUCOVORIN

Bagshawe KD et al. Br J Obstet Gynaecol 1989;96:795–802
Berkowitz RS et al. Gynecol Oncol 1986;23:111–118
McNeish IA et al. J Clin Oncol 2002;20:1838–1844
Sita-Lumsden A et al. Br J Cancer 2012;107:1810–1814

Methotrexate 1 mg/kg (maximum daily dose = 50 mg) per dose; administer by intramuscular injection for 4 doses on days 1, 3, 5, and 7, every 2 weeks (total dosage/14-day cycle = 4 mg/kg, or a maximum total dose of 200 mg)

Leucovorin calcium 0.1 mg/kg or 15 mg fixed dose; administer orally or by intramuscular injection for 4 doses on days 2, 4, 6, and 8, at 30 hours after each dose of methotrexate, every 2 weeks (total dosage/cycle = 0.4 mg/kg or 60 mg)

Notes:

1. Administer treatment courses as often as toxicity permits after a minimum rest period of 7 days (usually every 14 days)

2. Encourage increased oral fluid intake or, if NPO, give parenteral hydration

3. Avoid drugs that can alter methotrexate elimination, such as non-steroidal anti-inflammatory drugs, omeprazole (and possibly other proton pump inhibitors), penicillins, probenecid, and salicylates

4. Administer two additional cycles after the first normal hCG level

Supportive Care

Antiemetic prophylaxis
Emetogenic potential on days 1, 3, 5, and 7: **MINIMAL**
See Chapter 42 for antiemetic recommendations

Hematopoietic growth factor (CSF) prophylaxis
Primary prophylaxis is **NOT** indicated
See Chapter 43 for more information

Antimicrobial prophylaxis
Risk of fever and neutropenia is **LOW**
   Antimicrobial primary prophylaxis to be considered:
   • Antibacterial—not indicated
   • Antifungal—not indicated
   • Antiviral—not indicated unless patient previously had an episode of HSV

Treatment Modifications

Adverse Event	Dose Modification
G ≤1 toxicity	Continue therapy if easy to manage
G2 toxicity including LFTs	Consider a 20% reduction in methotrexate dosage
G ≥3 toxicity including LFTs	Discontinue methotrexate and institute other therapy

Patient Population Studied

Patients with low-risk GTN

Efficacy (N = 348)

Outcome	% of Patients
Changed treatment for drug resistance	20
Relapsed	4
Survival	347/348 (99.75)

One death attributed to concurrent non-Hodgkin lymphoma
Bagshawe KD et al. Br J Obstet Gynaecol 1989;96:795–802

Toxicity (N = 185)

Toxicity	% of Patients
Hepatotoxicity; normalized in 1 week	14.1
Granulocytopenia without infection or need for antibiotics	5.9; no secondary infections
Thrombocytopenia without need for platelets	1.6; without infections
Pleuritic chest pain	3.1
Nausea/vomiting	1; requiring intravenous therapy
Alopecia	0
Toxicity requiring change in therapy*	6

Bagshawe KD et al. Br J Obstet Gynaecol 1989;96:795–802
Berkowitz RS et al. Gynecol Oncol 1986;23:111–118

Therapy Monitoring

1. *Every other week:* PE, CBC with differential, serum electrolytes, LFTs, serum creatinine, BUN, and hCG

2. *Methotrexate levels:* Not routinely performed

3. *Complete remission:* Three consecutive weekly hCG levels within normal range

4. *Resistance to treatment:* hCG plateau over two consecutive treatments or hCG rise after any treatment

5. *Following remission:* hCG levels are obtained monthly for 12 months and every 3 months during the second year

FIRST LINE • NONMETASTATIC • LOW-RISK METASTATIC

GESTATIONAL TROPHOBLASTIC NEOPLASIA REGIMEN: DACTINOMYCIN

Osathanondh R et al. Cancer 1975;36:863–866
Petrilli ES et al. Cancer 1987;60:2173–2176

Dactinomycin 12 mcg/kg or fixed dose 0.5 mg per day; administer by intravenous injection over 1–2 minutes for 5 consecutive days on days 1–5, every 2 weeks (total dosage/cycle = 60 mcg/kg or 2.5 mg)
Osathanondh R et al. Cancer 1975;36:863–866

Notes:

1. Therapy was reinstituted only when and if the human chorionic gonadotropin (hCG) level reached a plateau for 2 consecutive weeks, or again increased
2. Patients who did not respond after 2 consecutive cycles were classified as having resistant disease

Alternate regimen:
Dactinomycin 1.25 mg/m^2 (max 2 mg); administer by intravenous injection over 1–2 minutes, on day 1 every 2 weeks (total dosage/cycle = 1.25 mg/m^2)

Petrilli ES et al. Cancer 1987;60:2173–2176

Note: This is an acceptable regimen for the treatment of nonmetastatic postmolar GTN, but should be used with caution for metastatic disease, known choriocarcinoma, or as secondary therapy to treat methotrexate-resistant disease where the 5-day regimen is more appropriate (Lurain JR et al. J Reprod Med 2012;57:283–287; Prouvot C et al. Int J Gynecol Cancer 2018;28:1038–1044)

Supportive Care
Antiemetic prophylaxis—first regimen
Emetogenic potential on days 1–5: **MODERATE**

Antiemetic prophylaxis—alternate regimen
Emetogenic potential: **MODERATE**
See Chapter 42 for antiemetic recommendations

Hematopoietic growth factor (CSF) prophylaxis
Primary prophylaxis is **NOT** *indicated*
See Chapter 43 for more information

Antimicrobial prophylaxis
Risk of fever and neutropenia is **LOW**
  Antimicrobial primary prophylaxis to be considered:
  • Antibacterial—not indicated
  • Antifungal—not indicated
  • Antiviral—not indicated unless patient previously had an episode of HSV

Treatment Modifications

Adverse Event	Dose Modification
WBC <3000/mm^3	Hold dactinomycin until WBC >3000/mm^3
ANC <1500/mm^3	Hold dactinomycin until ANC >1500/mm^3
Platelet count <100,000/mm^3	Hold dactinomycin until platelet >100,000/mm^3
Hepatotoxicity before or during treatment (LFTs ≥3× ULN)	Hold dactinomycin until LFTs ≤1.5× ULN
Increasing hCG level	Discontinue dactinomycin
Plateau in hCG levels after 2 cycles of dactinomycin	Discontinue dactinomycin

Patient Population Studied

A study of 70 patients (previously untreated) with nonmetastatic (31) and metastatic (39) gestational trophoblastic disease accrued from 1965 to 1973

Efficacy (N = 70*)

	Nonmetastatic GTN (N = 31)			Metastatic GTN (N = 39)		
	Non-CC	CC	Total	Non-CC	CC	Total
CR[†]	93%	100%	94%	76%	56%	67%

*CC = choriocarcinoma
[†]CR (complete response) = hCG in normal range for 3 consecutive weeks off therapy

Toxicity (N = 32)

Goldstein DP et al. Obstet Gynecol 1972;39:341–345

Toxicity	% of Patients
Hematologic	
WBC <2500/mm^3	25
ANC <1500/mm^3	38
Platelets <100,000/mm^3	16
Nonhematologic	
SGOT (AST) >50 units/L	22
Nausea and vomiting	66
Stomatitis	38
Skin rash	34
Alopecia	44

Therapy Monitoring

1. *Every other week:* PE, CBC with differential, serum electrolytes, LFTs, serum creatinine, BUN, and hCG
2. *Complete remission:* Three consecutive weekly hCG levels within normal range
3. *Resistance to treatment:* hCG plateau over two consecutive treatments or a hCG rise after any treatment
4. *Following remission:* hCG levels are obtained monthly for 12 months and every 3 months during the second year

Notes:

1. In current practice, dactinomycin is most frequently used as secondary therapy after the development of methotrexate resistance, rather than as primary therapy, because it causes more nausea and alopecia and is more expensive than methotrexate, and produces local tissue injury if extravasation occurs while administered
2. Dactinomycin is appropriate as primary therapy for patients with liver or renal disease or with large effusions that are relative contraindications to methotrexate

FIRST-LINE • HIGH-RISK METASTATIC

GESTATIONAL TROPHOBLASTIC NEOPLASIA REGIMEN: ETOPOSIDE + METHOTREXATE + DACTINOMYCIN + CYCLOPHOSPHAMIDE + VINCRISTINE (EMA/CO)

Bower M et al. J Clin Oncol 1997;15:2636–2643
Escobar PF et al. Gynecol Oncol 2003;91:552–557
Kim SJ et al. Gynecol Oncol 1998;71:247–253
Lu W-G et al. Int J Gynecol Cancer 2008;18:357–362
Turan T et al. Int J Gynecol Cancer 2006;16:1432–1438

EMA component (days 1–3):

Dactinomycin 0.5 mg (fixed dose) per day; administer by intravenous injection over 1–2 minutes for 2 consecutive days on days 1 and 2, every 2 weeks (total dose/cycle = 1 mg)

Etoposide 100 mg/m² per day; administer intravenously diluted in 0.9% sodium chloride injection (0.9% NS) to a concentration within the range of 0.2–0.4 mg/mL over 60 minutes for 2 consecutive days on days 1 and 2, every 2 weeks (total dosage/cycle = 200 mg/m²)

Methotrexate 100 mg/m²; administer intravenously by injection or in 25 mL 0.9% NS or 5% dextrose injection (D5W) over 5 minutes, given on day 1, *followed immediately afterward by:*

Methotrexate 200 mg/m²; administer intravenously in ≥1000 mL 0.9% NS over 12 hours on day 1, every 2 weeks (total dosage/cycle = 300 mg/m²)
Note: See dose adjustment for patients with documented CNS metastases, below

Leucovorin calcium 15 mg; administer orally or by intramuscular injection every 12 hours for 4 doses on days 2 and 3, beginning 24 hours after the start of methotrexate infusion, every 2 weeks (total dose/cycle = 60 mg). *Note:* See dose adjustment for CNS metastases below

CO component (day 8):

Vincristine 1 mg/m² (maximum dose, 2 mg); administer by intravenous infusion over 15 minutes in 50 mL 0.9% NS, given on day 8, every 2 weeks (total dosage/cycle = 1 mg/m²; maximum dose/cycle = 2 mg)

Cyclophosphamide 600 mg/m²; administer intravenously in 250 mL 0.9% NS over 30 minutes, given on day 8, every 2 weeks (total dosage/cycle = 600 mg/m²)

CNS treatment for patients with documented brain metastases:

3000-cGy whole-brain radiation; administer in fifteen 200-cGy fractions given 5 times per week for 3 weeks

Dexamethasone as needed, 4 mg; administer orally every 6 hours while radiation is administered, tapering over 2–4 weeks after the completion of radiation

Alternative approach: Surgical excision, stereotactic radiation, or intrathecal methotrexate

Methotrexate 1000 mg/m²; administer by continuous intravenous infusion over 24 hours in 1000 mL 0.9% NS on day 1, every 2 weeks (total dosage/cycle = 1000 mg/m²)

Leucovorin calcium 30 mg; administer orally, intramuscularly, or intravenously every 12 hours for 6 doses on days 2–4, beginning 32 hours after the start of methotrexate infusion, every 2 weeks (total dose/cycle = 180 mg)

Note: During CNS therapy, the methotrexate regimen given during the *EMA component* is replaced with **methotrexate** 1000 mg/m² by continuous intravenous infusion over 24 hours *for 2–3 cycles,* and the leucovorin calcium dose is increased to 30 mg/dose

Encourage increased oral fluid intake or, if NPO, give parenteral hydration

Duration of therapy:

Repeat EMA alternating weekly with CO to serologic remission (serum hCG <5 IU/L), then administer for an additional 4–8 weeks (2–4 cycles) of therapy. In the report by Escobar et al of 45 high-risk GTT patients, 4–7 cycles were administered with a mean of 5.5 cycles

Supportive Care
Antiemetic prophylaxis—EMA/CO
Emetogenic potential on days 1 and 2: **MODERATE–HIGH**

Antiemetic prophylaxis—during methotrexate for CNS treatment
Emetogenic potential: **MODERATE**
See Chapter 42 for antiemetic recommendations

Hematopoietic growth factor (CSF) prophylaxis
Primary prophylaxis is **NOT** indicated
Secondary prophylaxis **IS** indicated
See Chapter 43 for more information

Antimicrobial prophylaxis
Risk of fever and neutropenia is **LOW**
  Antimicrobial primary prophylaxis to be considered:
  • Antibacterial—not indicated
  • Antifungal—not indicated
  • Antiviral—not indicated unless patient previously had an episode of HSV

Treatment Modifications

Adverse Event	Dose Modification
WBC <3000/mm^3, platelets <100,000/mm^3, or liver transaminases >1.5× ULN	Hold therapy until WBC ≥3000/mm^3, platelets ≥100,000/mm^3, and liver transaminases ≤1.5× ULN
More than 1 treatment delay for WBC <3000/mm^3	Administer filgrastim 300 mcg/day subcutaneously on days 9–14 of all subsequent cycles
Hgb <10 g/dL	Transfuse as needed and administer erythropoietin
Peripheral neuropathy G >2	Discontinue vincristine

Patient Population Studied

Women with high-risk GTN. Almost one-half had received prior chemotherapy

Efficacy (N = 272)

Bower M et al. J Clin Oncol 1997;15:2636–2643

All Patients		Prior Therapy	
		No	Yes
Complete response	78.3%*	78%	79%
Progressive disease	17.2%†	14%	21%
Early deaths	4%	8%	—
Cumulative overall 5-year survival rate	86%		
Disease-specific 5-year survival rate	88%		

*Sixteen of 213 patients suffered relapse after attaining a complete response
†Forty-seven patients developed resistance to EMA/CO. Sixteen of 21 (76%) patients without prior therapy and 17 of 26 (65%) patients with prior therapy underwent successful salvage treatment and were alive and in remission at the time of publication

Efficacy (N = 45)

Escobar PF et al. Gynecol Oncol 2003;91:552–557

All Patients		Prior Therapy	
		No	Yes
Initial complete response	71%	76%	65%
Successful salvage therapy	20%*	—	—
Died of disease	9%	—	—
Survival†	91%	92%	90%

*All achieved remission with cisplatin-based therapy
†Median follow-up 36 months

Toxicity (N = 257 cycle)

Escobar PF et al. Gynecol Oncol 2003;91:552–557

	% Cycles		
	G1	G2	G3
Anemia	0.8	8.5	5.8
Neutropenia	6.6	5.4	1.6
Thrombocytopenia	1.6	—	—
Alopecia	All patients		

Gastrointestinal toxicity (nausea, vomiting, diarrhea, and stomatitis) occurred in some patients but was G3 requiring hospitalization in only 1 patient
The EMA-CO chemotherapy regimen produced no life-threatening toxicity, caused grade 3–4 hematologic toxicity in 1.6% of cycles, and was associated with neutropenia necessitating a 1-week delay in treatment in only 13.5% of cycles

Toxicity (N = 272 patients)

Bower M et al. J Clin Oncol 1997;15:2636–2643

Two cases of AML FAB subtypes M1 and M5

Therapy Monitoring

1. *Every other week*: PE, CBC with differential, serum electrolytes, LFTs, serum creatinine, BUN, and hCG
2. *Methotrexate levels*: Not routinely performed
3. *Complete remission*: Three consecutive weekly hCG levels within normal range
4. *Resistance to treatment*: hCG plateau over two consecutive treatments or a hCG rise after any treatment
5. *Following remission*: hCG levels are obtained monthly for 12 months and every 3 months during the second year

REFRACTORY • HIGH-RISK METASTATIC • PSTT/ETT FIRST-LINE

GESTATIONAL TROPHOBLASTIC NEOPLASIA REGIMEN: EP/EMA (ETOPOSIDE + CISPLATIN/ETOPOSIDE + METHOTREXATE + DACTINOMYCIN)

Lurain JR et al. J Reprod Med 2012;57:219–224
Lurain JR et al. J Reprod Med 2010;55:199–207
Mao Y et al. Int J Gynaecol Obstet 2007;98:44–47
Newlands ES et al. J Clin Oncol 2000;18:854–859

EP component (day 1)
Etoposide 150 mg/m²; administer intravenously diluted in 0.9% sodium chloride injection (0.9% NS) or 5% dextrose injection (D5W) to a concentration within the range of 0.2–0.4 mg/mL over 60 minutes, on day 1, every 2 weeks
Cisplatin 25 mg/m²; administer intravenously in 1000 mL 0.9% NS over 4 hours every 4 hours for 3 doses (total duration of continuous infusion is 12 hours) on day 1, every 2 weeks (total dosage/2-week cycle = 75 mg/m²)
Hydration after cisplatin: Encourage increased oral intake of nonalcoholic fluids if possible. Monitor and replace magnesium, potassium, and other electrolytes as needed

EMA component (days 8–10)
Dactinomycin 0.5 mg (fixed dose); administer by intravenous injection over 1–2 minutes, on day 8 every 2 weeks (total dose/2-week cycle = 0.5 mg)
Etoposide 100 mg/m²; administer intravenously in 0.9% NS or D5W to a concentration within the range of 0.2–0.4 mg/mL over 60 minutes, on day 8, every 2 weeks (total dosage/2-week cycle = 250 mg/m² [sum of EP + EMA regimens])
Methotrexate 100 mg/m²; administer intravenously by injection or in 25 mL 0.9% NS or D5W over 5 minutes, given on day 8, *followed immediately afterward by* **methotrexate** 200 mg/m²; administer intravenously in ≥1000 mL 0.9% NS over 12 hours on day 8 every 2 weeks (total dosage/2-week cycle = 300 mg/m²)
Leucovorin calcium 15 mg; administer orally, intravenously, or by intramuscular injection every 12 hours for 4 doses on days 9 and 10, beginning 24 hours after the start of methotrexate infusion, every 2 weeks (total dose/cycle = 60 mg)

Recommendations:
1. EP and EMA components of treatment are alternated at weekly intervals
2. Encourage increased oral fluid intake or, if NPO, give parenteral hydration
3. Avoid concomitant use of drugs that can alter methotrexate elimination, such as non-steroidal anti-inflammatory drugs, omeprazole (and perhaps other proton pump inhibitors), penicillins, probenecid, and salicylates

Supportive Care
Antiemetic prophylaxis—EP regimen
Emetogenic potential: **HIGH**. Potential for delayed symptoms

Antiemetic prophylaxis—EMA regimen
Emetogenic potential: **MODERATE**
See Chapter 42 for antiemetic recommendations

Hematopoietic growth factor (CSF) prophylaxis
Primary prophylaxis is indicated:
Filgrastim (G-CSF) 300 mcg per day by subcutaneous injection days 9–14
• Begin use on day 9 (24 hours after myelosuppressive chemotherapy is completed)
• Discontinue use at least 24 hours before myelosuppressive treatment resumes
See Chapter 43 for more information

Antimicrobial prophylaxis
Risk of fever and neutropenia is **LOW**
Antimicrobial primary prophylaxis to be considered:
• Antibacterial—not indicated
• Antifungal—not indicated
• Antiviral—not indicated unless patient previously had an episode of HSV

Treatment Modifications

Adverse Event	Dose Modification
WBC count <2000/mm³, *and* platelet count <75,000/mm³	Hold therapy until WBC count ≥2000/mm³ *and* platelet count ≥75,000/mm³
Serum creatinine >1.5× ULN	Measure or estimate creatinine clearance (CrCl) and reduce cisplatin dose by the same percentage as the reduction in CrCl from baseline
G ≥2 mucositis	Double the dose of leucovorin and double the duration of administration (8 doses) before considering methotrexate dose reduction
Any treatment delay for WBC count <2000/mm³	Administer filgrastim 300 mcg/day, subcutaneously on days 9–14 of all subsequent cycles

Patient Population Studied

A study of 42 women with high-risk GTN refractory to or relapsing after EMA/CO chemotherapy. Patients either (1) had improvement while receiving EMA/CO but a persistently low hCG level or (2) developed a re-elevation of hCG after having a complete response to prior treatment with EMA/CO

Efficacy

Response	Alive in Remission
hCG Plateau on EMA/CO* (n = 22)	
—	21 (95%)
Resistant to or Relapsed After EMA/CO† (n = 12)	
12 (100%)	9 (75%)
Placental Site Trophoblastic Tumor (n = 8)	
—	4 (50%)

*hCG sufficiently close to normal range, but not possible to evaluate response
†>1-log decline in hCG

Surgical Procedures in Patients Receiving EP/EMA

	Effect on hCG Response		
Operation	Decreased	None	Not Assessed
Hysterectomy	2	4	4
Thoracotomy	1	3	5
Craniotomy	2	0	1
Total	5 (23%)	7 (32%)	10 (45%)

Toxicity*

	% G3	% G4
Hematologic (n = 25)		
Anemia	20	—
Leukopenia	48	20
Thrombocytopenia	24	16

Ten patients (40%) had multiple G3/4 toxicities

	% G3	% G4
Nonhematologic (n = 22)		
Elevated BUN	32%	9%

*Complete results on patients treated before 1988 were no longer available. In the 42 patients:
• Treatment delays because of myelosuppression were observed in 37 of 42 patients (88%)
• Dose reductions were required in 16 of 42 patients (38%)
• Filgrastim was administered to 13 of 42 patients (31%)

NCI, CTC, National Cancer Institute (USA) Common Toxicity Criteria, version 2.0. At: http://ctep.cancer.gov/protocolDevelopment/electronic_applications/ctc.htm

Therapy Monitoring

1. *Every week:* PE, CBC with differential, serum electrolytes, LFTs, serum creatinine, BUN, and hCG
2. *Methotrexate levels:* Not routinely performed
3. *Complete remission:* Three consecutive weekly hCG levels within normal range
4. *Resistance to treatment:* hCG plateau over two consecutive treatments or a hCG rise after any treatment
5. *Following remission:* hCG levels are obtained monthly for 12 months, and every 3 months during the second year

REFRACTORY • HIGH-RISK METASTATIC • PSTT/ETT FIRST-LINE

GESTATIONAL TROPHOBLASTIC NEOPLASIA REGIMEN: (TP/TE) PACLITAXEL + CISPLATIN/PACLITAXEL + ETOPOSIDE

Wang J et al. Ann Oncol 2008;19:1578–1583

Day 1: TP component
Primary prophylaxis against hypersensitivity reactions to paclitaxel:
Dexamethasone 20 mg/dose; administer orally for 2 doses every 6 hours, starting approximately 12 hours before paclitaxel administration begins
Cimetidine 300 mg (or equivalent histaminergic receptor [H_2 subtype] antagonist); administer intravenously over 15–30 minutes + **diphenhydramine** 25–50 mg (or equivalent H_1 receptor antagonist); administer intravenously 30–60 minutes before starting paclitaxel administration
Paclitaxel 135 mg/m²; administer intravenously in a volume of 0.9% sodium chloride injection (0.9% NS) or 5% dextrose injection (D5W) sufficient to produce a solution with concentration within the range 0.3–1.2 mg/mL over 3 hours (total dosage/cycle for TP + TE = 270 mg/m²)

Hydration before cisplatin: Administer intravenously ≥1000 mL 0.9% NS over a minimum of 2–4 hours
Cisplatin 60–75 mg/m² with 12.5 g **mannitol**; administer intravenously in 1000 mL 0.9% NS after paclitaxel over 2–3 hours (total dosage/cycle = 60–75 mg/m²)
Hydration after cisplatin: Administer intravenously ≥1000 mL 0.9% NS over a minimum of 2–4 hours. Also encourage increased oral intake of nonalcoholic fluids. Monitor and replace magnesium and other electrolytes as needed

Day 15: TE component
Primary prophylaxis against hypersensitivity reactions to paclitaxel:
Dexamethasone 20 mg/dose; administer orally for 2 doses every 6 hours, starting approximately 12 hours before paclitaxel administration begins
Cimetidine 300 mg (or equivalent H_2 receptor antagonist); administer intravenously over 15–30 minutes + **diphenhydramine** 25–50 mg (or equivalent H_1 receptor antagonist); administer intravenously 30–60 minutes before starting paclitaxel administration
Paclitaxel 135 mg/m²; administer intravenously in a volume of 0.9% NS or D5W sufficient to produce a solution with concentration within the range 0.3–1.2 mg/mL over 3 hours, *followed by:*
Etoposide 150 mg/m²; administer intravenously diluted in 0.9% NS to a concentration within the range of 0.2–0.4 mg/mL over at least 60 minutes (total dosage/cycle = 150 mg/m²)

Supportive Care
Antiemetic prophylaxis
Emetogenic potential on day 1: **HIGH**. *Potential for delayed symptoms after cisplatin*
Emetogenic potential on day 15: **LOW**
See Chapter 42 for antiemetic recommendations

Hematopoietic growth factor (CSF) prophylaxis
Primary prophylaxis is indicated:
   Pegfilgrastim 6 mg by subcutaneous injection days 2 and 16 of each cycle
See Chapter 43 for more information

Antimicrobial prophylaxis
Risk of fever and neutropenia is **LOW**
   Antimicrobial primary prophylaxis to be considered:
   • Antibacterial—not indicated
   • Antifungal—not indicated
   • Antiviral—not indicated unless patient previously had an episode of HSV

Recommendations:
1. TP and TE components of treatment are alternated at 2-week intervals
2. Encourage increased oral fluid intake or, if NPO, give parenteral hydration
3. *Duration of therapy:* Repeat TP alternating with TE to serologic remission (serum hCG <5 IU/L), then administer for an additional 8–16 weeks (2–4 cycles) of therapy

Treatment Modifications

Adverse Event	Dose Modification
WBC count <3000/mm³ *and* platelet count <100,000/mm³	Hold therapy until WBC count ≥3000/mm³ *and* platelet count ≥100,000/mm³
Serum creatinine >1.5 mg/dL (>133 μmol/L)	Measure or estimate creatinine clearance (CrCl) and reduce cisplatin dose by the same percentage as the reduction in CrCl from baseline
Platelet nadir <50,000/mm³	Decrease doses of all drugs by 20%
Peripheral neuropathy G >2	Discontinue therapy or possibly substitute docetaxel 60 mg/m² for paclitaxel

Patient Population Studied

A trial in which 24 women with relapsed/refractory GTN or placental site trophoblastic tumor (PSTT) were treated with TP/TE: 16 had failed to benefit from previous chemotherapy, including 6 who had received cisplatin-containing regimens and 8 who had prior treatment-induced toxic effects

Efficacy (N = 24)

Category	Complete Response	Partial Response	Alive in Remission
Relapsed disease (N = 16)	3 (19%)	5 (31%)*	7 (44%)*
Prior treatment toxic (N = 8)[†]	2 (25%)	2 (25%)[§]	6 (75%)[‡]
Total (N = 24)	5 (21%)	7 (29%)	13 (54%)

*Median follow-up = 25 months; 4 patients with PR entered remission/cured with subsequent surgery and/or chemotherapy
[†]Four not assessable for response because hCG already normal or close to normal at start
[‡]Median follow-up = 19 months
[§]Two patients (1 PR and 1 not assessable for response) entered remission/cured with subsequent surgery and/or chemotherapy

Toxicity (N = 24)

	% G1	% G2	% G3	% G4
Neutropenia	—	—	42	
Thrombocytopenia	—	—	13	
Anemia	8		—	—
Neuropathy	17	—	4	—
Nausea	13	—	—	—

Therapy Monitoring

1. *Every other week:* Physical examination, CBC with differential, serum electrolytes, LFTs, serum creatinine, BUN, and hCG
2. *Complete remission:* Three consecutive weekly hCG levels within normal range
3. *Resistance to treatment:* hCG plateau over two consecutive treatments or a hCG rise after any treatment
4. *Following remission:* hCG levels are obtained monthly for 12 months and every 3 months during the second year

18. Hairy Cell Leukemia

Maximilian Stahl, MD and Martin S. Tallman, MD

Epidemiology

Incidence: 2% of all leukemia (approximately 600–800 new patients per year in the United States)

Median age: 52 years

Male to female ratio: Approximately 4:1

Bernstein L et al. Cancer Res 1990;50:3605–3609
Staines A, Cartwright RA. Br J Haematol 1993;85:714–717

Pathology

Peripheral blood findings at diagnosis

1. Pancytopenia: 50%
2. "Leukemic" phase with a WBC >1000/mm³: 10–20%
3. Monocytopenia
4. Hairy cells identified in most patients, but the number is usually low and may be difficult to identify in the peripheral blood because of low numbers and staining technique

Bone marrow findings at diagnosis

1. Hypercellularity
2. Hairy cell infiltration: diffuse, patchy, or interstitial
   a. Diffuse infiltration: Often results in complete effacement of bone marrow
   b. Patchy infiltration: Subtle small clusters of hairy cells present focally or throughout the bone marrow
   c. Interstitial infiltration: Hairy cells do not form well-defined discreet aggregates, but merge almost imperceptibly with surrounding normal hematopoietic tissue
3. Hairy cell nuclei are usually round, oval, or indented, and are widely separated from each other by abundant clear or lightly eosinophilic cytoplasm. Rarely, hairy cells can be convoluted or spindle shaped
4. Extravasated blood cells create blood lakes in the bone marrow similar to those observed in the spleen
5. Mast cells are often numerous
6. Reticulin stain of the bone marrow almost always shows moderate to marked increase in reticulin fibers
7. Approximately 10–20% of patients show a hypocellular bone marrow

Immunophenotyping, cytogenetics, and molecular diagnostic studies

1. *Cytochemical studies:* Tartrate-resistant acid phosphatase (**TRAP**) stain. However, TRAP is not specific for HCL
2. *Hairy cell immunophenotype:* CD19(+), CD20(+), CD22(+), CD79B(+), CD5(−), CD10(−), CD11C(+), CD25 Sub(+), FMC(+), CD103(+), CD45(+)
3. *Clonal cytogenetics:* Abnormalities in approximately two-thirds of patients. Chromosomes 1, 2, 5, 6, 11, 14, 19, and 20 are most frequently involved. Chromosome 5 is altered in approximately 40%, most commonly as a trisomy 5, pericentric inversion, and interstitial deletions involving band 5q13. However, the identification of cytogenetic abnormalities in a patient with a definite diagnosis of HCL is usually not important as it does not influence, as far as is currently determined, prognosis or therapy

Work-up

1. H&P
2. CBC with differential, serum electrolytes, BUN, creatinine, LFTs, and uric acid
3. Bone marrow aspirate and biopsy for tartrate-resistant acid phosphatase (TRAP) (although TRAP is not required for the diagnosis, has been largely abandoned, and has been supplanted by immunophenotyping) and morphologic review; immunophenotyping by flow cytometry with B cell–associated antibodies, including CD20, CD79A, or DBA.44

Tallman MS et al. Hairy cell leukemia. In: Hoffman (editor). Hematology: Basic Principles and Practice, 3rd ed. Philadelphia, Churchill Livingstone, 2000:1363–1372

(*continued*)

(continued)

Bartl R et al. Am J Clin Pathol 1983;79:531–545
Brunning RD et al. Atlas of Tumor Pathology, 3rd Series, Fascicle 9. Washington DC, AFIP, 1994; pp 277–278
Burke JS et al. Am J Clin Pathol 1978;70:876–884
Burke JS et al. Semin Oncol 1984;11:334–346
Cornfield DB et al. Am J Hematol 2001;67:223–226
Ellison DJ et al. Blood 1994;84:4310–4315
Flandrin G et al. Semin Oncol 1984;11(4 Suppl 2):458–471
Golomb HM et al. Ann Intern Med 1978;89(Part 1):677–683
Haglund U et al. Blood 1994;83:2637–2645
Hakimian D et al. Blood 1993;82:1798–1802
Hanson CA et al. Am J Surg Pathol 1989;13:671–679
Hounieu H et al. Am J Clin Pathol 1992;98:26–33
Katayama I. Hematol Oncol Clin North Am 1988;2:585–602
Kluin-Nelemans HC et al. Blood 1994;84:3134–3141
Kroft SH et al. Blood Rev 1995;9:234–250
Lee WM, Beckstead JH. Cancer 1982;50:2207–2210
Robbins BA et al. Blood 1993;82:1277–1287
Sausville JE et al. Am J Clin Pathol 2003;119:213–217
Turner A, Kjeldsberg CR. Medicine (Baltimore) 1978;57:477–499
Wheaton S et al. Blood 1996;87:1556–1560
Yam LT et al. N Engl J Med 1971;284:357–360

Prognosis

Therapy with purine analogs: pentostatin (2'-deoxycoformycin) or cladribine (2-chlorodeoxyadenosine)

Complete remission	70–90%
Peripheral remission	10–20%
No response	5–10%
Relapse rate	5–25%
Estimated 5-year survival rate	85–90%
5- to 10-year survival rate	80–90%

Catovsky D et al. Leuk Lymphoma 1994;14:109–113
Dearden CE et al. Br J Haematol 1999;106:515–519
Flinn IW et al. Blood 2000;96:2981–2986
Goodman GR et al. J Clin Oncol 2003;21:891–896
Grever M et al. J Clin Oncol 1995;13:974–982
Hoffman MA et al. J Clin Oncol 1997;15:1138–1142
Jehn U et al. Ann Hematol 1999;78:139–144
Kraut EH et al. Blood 1994;84:4061–4063
Saven A et al. Blood 1998;92:1918–1926
Tallman MS et al. Blood 1992;80:2203–2209
Tallman MS et al. Blood 1996;88:1954–1959

Differential Diagnosis

Other small B-cell lymphoproliferative disorders associated with splenomegaly:
1. Prolymphocytic leukemia
   a. Marked elevation in the WBC
   b. Characteristic morphology of the prolymphocytes
   c. Different immunophenotypic profile
2. Splenic marginal zone lymphoma (splenic lymphoma with villous lymphocytes)
   a. Cells do not usually exhibit TRAP positivity
   b. Bone marrow infiltrates are demarcated sharply
   c. Different immunophenotypic profile; CD103(−)
3. HCL variant
   a. Morphologic features between hairy cells and prolymphocytes
   b. Usually associated with leukocytosis/lack of monocytopenia
   c. Absence of CD25 expression
4. Systemic mastocytosis
   a. Mast cells are negative for B-cell markers, and positive for tryptase

Catovsky D et al. Semin Oncol 1984;11:362–369
Cawley JC et al. Leuk Res 1980;4:547–559
de Totero D et al. Blood 1993;82:528–535
Galton DA et al. Br J Haematol 1974;27:7–23
Horny HP et al. Am J Clin Pathol 1988;89:335–340
Isaacson PG et al. Blood 1994;84:3828–3834
Kroft SH et al. Blood Rev 1995;9:234–250
Matutes E et al. Blood 1994;83:1558–1562
Matutes E et al. Leukemia 2001;15:184–186
Melo JV et al. Br J Haematol 1986;63:377–387
Melo JV et al. Br J Haematol 1987;65:23–29
Mulligan SP et al. Br J Haematol 1991;78:206–209
Sainati L et al. Blood 1990;76:157–162
Troussard X et al. Br J Haematol 1996;93:731–736

Expert Opinion

- A diagnosis of HCL by itself is not necessarily an indication to initiate treatment. If a patient is maintaining safe peripheral blood counts, the conservative approach is to "watch and wait" until counts decrease
- Treatment is indicated when a patient has developed life-threatening cytopenias (absolute neutrophil count <1000/mm^3, hemoglobin <11 g/dL, or platelet count <100,000/mm^3), or in the presence of symptomatic splenomegaly or constitutional symptoms attributable to the disease
- There is no clear advantage to either purine analog as initial treatment for patients with previously untreated HCL with respect to long-term outcome. The ease of administration of cladribine, which requires only a single course of therapy, may offer some advantages over pentostatin
- Patients should be followed closely during treatment and for several months after completion of therapy, with special attention to appropriate surveillance and treatment for infection resulting from myelosuppression. An improvement in peripheral blood counts after purine nucleoside analog treatment may require weeks and sometimes months. Bone marrow biopsy to confirm a complete response is usually performed 3 months after cladribine. However, if the peripheral blood counts return to normal, splenomegaly resolves and the patient is asymptomatic, one can argue not to carry out another bone marrow biopsy as the results will likely not influence further therapy. Even if the marrow demonstrates a small amount of HCL, further therapy is not indicated outside the context of a clinical trial exploring the potential benefits of additional therapy for residual disease
- For patients who do not respond to initial therapy with a purine analog, the suggested therapeutic option is treatment with a different purine analog. However, the lack of excellent response to one purine analog is exceedingly uncommon and would prompt a reevaluation of the diagnosis
- If relapse is suspected, the bone marrow should be reexamined before restarting therapy. In patients who achieved an initial, durable complete response to a purine analog lasting longer than 1–2 years, a reasonable course of action would be to re-treat the patient with either the same agent or an alternative purine analog. If there was an initial remission of short duration (eg, <1 year), a repeated course of the original therapy is unlikely to result in a second remission of equivalent or longer duration. Re-treatment with a second cycle of cladribine or pentostatin leads to a second complete remission in up to 70% of patients
- The anti-CD20 antibody rituximab has been evaluated in patients with relapsed/refractory HCL and should be considered in patients who are not eligible to enroll in a clinical trial. Rituximab following cladribine has been reported to be very effective in previously untreated patients and has been also used in relapsed and refractory disease. In the previously untreated setting, it is not clear whether such a combination improves overall survival compared with cladribine alone. While some clinicians recommend this regimen, it has not clearly been established as a new standard of care. Such a combination may be highly effective in patients with hairy cell leukemia variant
- Clinical trials using the truncated *Pseudomonas* exotoxin-linked recombinant anti-CD22 antibody (BL22) have shown high response rates in patients with previously treated HCL
- Although not yet approved by the FDA, clinical trials using the BRAF inhibitor vemurafenib have resulted in high response rates in patients with purine analog–refractory or relapsed *BRAF* V600E–mutated classic HCL
- Patients with HCL are often at an increased risk of bacterial, viral, and fungal infections due to neutropenia due to their disease, which is further aggravated by the immunosuppressive effect of purine analog–based therapy. However, evidence for the use of specific prevention strategies has not been validated in clinical trials, and practice patterns vary among groups. In our practice we use antiherpes antivirals (acyclovir) during the entire disease course, antibacterial (fluoroquinolone) and antifungal prophylaxis during neutropenia, and anti-PJP prophylaxis during treatment with rituximab

Estey EH et al. Blood 1992;79:882–887
Grever MR. Blood 2010;115:21–28
Grever M, Abdel-Wahab O. Blood 2017;129:553–560
Kreitman RJ et al. J Clin Oncol 2009;27:2983–2990
Kreitman RJ et al. N Engl J Med 2001;345:241–247
Saven A et al. Blood 1998;92:1918–1926
Tallman MS et al. Blood 1992;80:2203–2209
Tallman MS, Polliack A. Leuk Lymphoma 2009;50(Suppl 1):2–7
Tiacci E et al. N Engl J Med 2015;373(18):1733–1747

FIRST-LINE • RELAPSE AFTER INITIAL DURABLE COMPLETE RESPONSE TO PURINE ANALOG

HAIRY CELL LEUKEMIA REGIMEN: CLADRIBINE + RITUXIMAB

Ravandi F et al. Blood. 2011;118(14):3818–3823

Cladribine 5.6 mg/m² per dose; administer intravenously, diluted in 100–500 mL 0.9% sodium chloride (0.9% NS), over 2 hours daily for 5 consecutive days to complete a single course of therapy (total dosage = 28 mg/m²), *followed by:*

Initiate rituximab approximately 4 weeks after initiation of cladribine as follows:

Premedications for rituximab
Acetaminophen 650–1000 mg; administer orally 30–60 minutes before each rituximab dose, every 7 days for 8 cycles, *plus*
Diphenhydramine 25–50 mg; administer orally or intravenously 30–60 minutes before each rituximab dose, every 7 days for 8 cycles

Rituximab 375 mg/m²; administer intravenously in 0.9% sodium chloride injection (0.9% NS) or 5% dextrose injection (D5W), diluted to a concentration within the range 1–4 mg/mL, on day 1, every 7 days for 8 cycles (total dosage/1-week cycle = 375 mg/m²)

Rituximab administration:
• Infuse initially at 50 mg/hour. If hypersensitivity or infusion reactions do not occur during the first 30 minutes, increase the rate by 50 mg/hour every 30 minutes as tolerated to a maximum rate of 400 mg/hour. During subsequent treatments if previous rituximab administration was well tolerated, start at 100 mg/hour and increase by 100 mg/hour every 30 minutes as tolerated to a maximum rate of 400 mg/hour
• Interrupt rituximab administration for fever, chills, edema, congestion of the head and neck mucosa, hypertension, and other serious adverse events. Resume rituximab administration after adverse events abate

Supportive Care
Antiemetic prophylaxis
Emetogenic potential is **MINIMAL**
See Chapter 42 for antiemetic recommendations

Hematopoietic growth factor (CSF) prophylaxis
Primary prophylaxis is not indicated
See Chapter 43 for more information

Antimicrobial prophylaxis
Risk of fever and neutropenia is **INTERMEDIATE**
  Antimicrobial primary prophylaxis to be considered:
  • Antibacterial—consider a fluoroquinolone or no prophylaxis; *P. jirovecii* prophylaxis is recommended (eg, cotrimoxazole)
  • Antifungal—consider use during periods of prolonged neutropenia
  • Antiviral—antiherpes antivirals (eg, acyclovir, famciclovir, valacyclovir)

Optional: **Allopurinol** 300 mg/day; administer orally, beginning on the first day of cladribine administration and continue for 2 weeks. Tumor lysis is uncommon, and allopurinol need not be routinely administered. In addition, cutaneous disorders have occasionally been reported when cladribine is used with allopurinol

Patient Population Studied

The phase 2 study cohort involved 36 previously untreated patients with hairy cell leukemia, including five with the variant form. Eligible patients had a new diagnosis of hairy cell leukemia with active disease, Eastern Cooperative Oncology Group performance score ≤2, and adequate organ function. Active disease was defined as ≥1 of the following: (1) hemoglobin <10 g/dL or transfusions of ≥2 units of packed red blood cells per month, absolute neutrophil count <1500/mm³, platelet count <100,000/mm³, or >25% decline from baseline over 3 months in 1 or more cell lines; (2) circulating hairy cells at least 1000/mm³ or extramedullary hairy cell leukemia; and (3) recurrent infections, progressive decline in performance status, or symptomatic splenomegaly. Patients with known infection with HIV, or hepatitis B or C, were not eligible. Patients received daily intravenous cladribine (5.6 mg/m² over 2 hours) for 5 days and then, approximately 28 days after the initiation of cladribine, eight weekly doses of rituximab (375 mg/m²/dose)

Efficacy (N = 36)

Complete response rate	100%
Relapse rate*	3%

*Over a median follow-up of 25 months; the one patient who relapsed had the variant form of hairy cell leukemia

Therapy Monitoring

1. *Every other day during the week in which cladribine is administered:* CBC with differential and platelet count, potassium, calcium, phosphorus, uric acid, LDH, serum creatinine, blood urea nitrogen, liver function tests. Monitor for presence of rash and fevers
2. *Prior to initiation of rituximab:* hepatitis B core antibody (IgG or total) and hepatitis B surface antigen
3. *Weekly starting the week after cladribine completion and until rituximab completion:* CBC with differential and platelet count
4. *Response assessment 2–3 months after completion of therapy:* bone marrow aspirate and biopsy
5. *Long-term follow-up:* CBC with differential and platelet count every 3–6 months for 2 years, then every 6 months for 3 years

Treatment Modifications

CLADRIBINE + RITUXIMAB

Renal Impairment

Estimated creatinine clearance 10–50 mL/minute	Reduce the cladribine dose by 25%. Do not adjust the rituximab dose
Estimated creatinine clearance <10 mL/minute	Reduce the cladribine dose by 50%. Do not adjust the rituximab dose

RITUXIMAB

Rituximab Infusion-Related Toxicities

Onset of infusion-related events (fevers, chills, rigors, edema, congestion of the head and neck mucosa, hypotension)
1. Interrupt rituximab infusion
2. For fever, chills: Give additional dose of **acetaminophen** 650 mg orally and diphenhydramine 25–50 mg by intravenous push
3. For rigors: Give **meperidine** 12.5–25 mg by intravenous push ± **promethazine** 12.5–25 mg by intravenous infusion in at least 10 mL 0.9% NS or D5W over 5–15 minutes. If after 15–20 minutes the response to a single dose is considered inadequate, the dose may be repeated
4. After symptoms resolve, resume rituximab infusion at a minimum of 50% reduction in the rate at which the event occurred. If no further infusion-related events, increase the rate by 50 mg/hour every 30 minutes, as tolerated, up to a maximum rate of 400 mg/hour

Dyspnea or wheezing, without allergic findings (urticaria, or tongue or laryngeal edema)
1. Interrupt rituximab infusion immediately
2. Give **hydrocortisone** 100 mg by intravenous push (or glucocorticoid equivalent)
3. Give an additional dose of **diphenhydramine** 25–50 mg by intravenous push and a histamine H2-antagonist (**ranitidine** 50 mg or **famotidine** 20 mg) by intravenous push
4. After symptoms resolve, resume rituximab infusion at a minimum of 50% reduction in the rate at which the event occurred. If no further infusion-related events, increase the rate by 50 mg/hour every 30 minutes, as tolerated, up to a maximum rate of 400 mg/hour

Note: Medications and equipment for the treatment of hypersensitivity reactions should be available for immediate use in the event of a reaction during administration (eg, intravenous fluids, epinephrine, antihistamines, glucocorticoids, and oxygen)

Adverse Events (N = 36)

No Grade 3 or 4 nonhematologic therapy-related toxicities were reported. Reversible Grade 3 or 4 infections (such as neutropenic fever, cellulitis, and herpes zoster dermatitis) that were possibly related to therapy were reported for 33% of patients. The following Grade 1 and 2 adverse events also were recorded: fatigue, fever, nausea, rash, weight gain, and weight loss

FIRST-LINE • RELAPSE AFTER INITIAL DURABLE COMPLETE RESPONSE TO PURINE ANALOG

HAIRY CELL LEUKEMIA REGIMEN: CLADRIBINE (2-CHLORO–2'-DEOXYADENOSINE, 2-CDA)

Chacko J et al. Br J Haematol 1999;105:1145–1146
Cheson BD et al. J Clin Oncol 1998;16:3007–3015
Lauria F et al. Blood 1997;89:1838–1839
Robak T et al. Leuk Lymphoma 1996;22:107–111
Tallman MS et al. Blood 1992;80:2203–2209
Tallman MS et al. Blood 1996;88:1954–1959

Cladribine 0.1 mg/kg per day; administer by continuous intravenous infusion in 100–500 mL 0.9% sodium chloride injection, (0.9% NS), over 24 hours for 7 consecutive days (total dosage/cycle = 0.7 mg/kg)

or

Cladribine 0.14 mg/kg per day; administer intravenously in 100–500 mL of 0.9% NS over 2 hours for 5 consecutive days (total dosage/cycle = 0.7 mg/kg)

or

Cladribine 0.15 mg/kg per dose; administer intravenously in 100–500 mL 0.9% NS over 3 hours once weekly for 6 consecutive weeks (total dosage/cycle = 0.9 mg/kg)

Chacko J et al. Br J Haematol 1999;105:1145–1146
Lauria F et al. Blood 1997;89:1838–1839

Supportive Care
Antiemetic prophylaxis
See Chapter 42 for antiemetic recommendations
Emetogenic potential is **MINIMAL**
See Chapter 42 for antiemetic recommendations

Hematopoietic growth factor (CSF) prophylaxis
Primary prophylaxis is not indicated

Antimicrobial prophylaxis
Risk of fever and neutropenia is **INTERMEDIATE**
- Antibacterial—consider a fluoroquinolone or no prophylaxis; *P. jirovecii* prophylaxis is recommended (eg, cotrimoxazole)
- Antifungal—consider use during neutropenia
- Antiviral—antiherpes antivirals (eg, acyclovir) as patients may develop herpes viral infections as a result of their underlying disease even without the influence of purine analog therapy

Optional: **Allopurinol** 300 mg/day; administer orally, beginning on the first day of cladribine administration and continue for 2 weeks. Tumor lysis is uncommon and allopurinol need not be routinely administered. In addition, cutaneous disorders have occasionally been reported when cladribine is used with allopurinol

Therapy Monitoring

1. *Every other day for the week of therapy, then weekly for the next 7 weeks:* CBC and serum electrolytes, BUN, creatinine, LFTs, and uric acid
2. *Three months after the completion of therapy:* Bone marrow aspirate and biopsy
3. *Long-term follow-up:* CBC every 3–6 months for 2 years, and then every 6 months for 3 years

Treatment Modifications

Cladribine Dose	No Modification
Platelet count <15,000/mm^3	Administer platelets
Symptomatic anemia or hemoglobin <7 g/dL	Administer packed red blood cells

Patient Population Studied

Patients with newly diagnosed as well as relapsed and refractory disease

Efficacy

Complete remission rate	75–90%
Partial remission rate	5–20%
Relapse rate	5–50%

Toxicity (N = 895)

Cheson BD et al. J Clin Oncol 1998;16:3007–3015

	% G1	% G2	% G3	% G4
All Toxicities				
Maximum grade	21	20	22	6
Nonhematologic Toxicities				
Maximum grade	14	18	17	4
Hemorrhage	2	2	0.6	0.6
Nausea/vomiting	14	4	0.5	0.3
Infection	1	13	13	3
Pulmonary	3	2	0.7	0.7
Skin	8	5	4	0.5
Neurologic Toxicities				
Maximum grade	18	6	1	0.1
Motor	8	3	1	0
Headache	11	2	0.3	0
Constipation	5	1	0	0.1

Hematologic Toxicities

ANC <1000/mm³ or >50% decrease from baseline, or platelet count <100,000/mm³ or >50% decrease from baseline*	66%
Fever >38.3°C (101°F)*	48%
Peripheral vein chemical phlebitis*	12%

*Tallman MS et al. Blood 1992;80:2203–2209 (N = 26)

Notes

Cladribine may be administered to patients with relapsed or refractory disease

FIRST-LINE • RELAPSE AFTER INITIAL DURABLE COMPLETE RESPONSE TO PURINE ANALOG

HAIRY CELL LEUKEMIA REGIMEN: PENTOSTATIN (2'-DEOXYCOFORMYCIN, DCF)

Grever M et al. J Clin Oncol 1995;13:974–982

Hydration: 5% Dextrose/0.9% sodium chloride injection or 5% dextrose/0.45% sodium chloride injection; administer intravenously 1000 mL before and at least 500 mL after pentostatin administration

Pentostatin 4 mg/m²; administer intravenously over 20–30 minutes in 25–50 mL 0.9% sodium chloride injection (0.9% NS) or 5% dextrose injection (D5W) every 2 weeks until complete remission (total dosage per 2-week course = 4 mg/m²)

then

Pentostatin 4 mg/m²; administer intravenously over 20–30 minutes in 25–50 mL 0.9% NS or D5W every 2 weeks for 2 courses (total dosage per 2-week course = 4 mg/m²)

Supportive Care
Antiemetic prophylaxis
Emetogenic potential is **MINIMAL**
See Chapter 42 for antiemetic recommendations

Hematopoietic growth factor (CSF) prophylaxis
Primary prophylaxis should be considered in patients with:
ANC <500/mm³ or in patients with history of recurrent episodes of fever and neutropenia
　Pegfilgrastim (pegylated filgrastim) 6 mg/0.6 mL by subcutaneous injection for 1 dose
　• Begin use from 24–72 hours after myelosuppressive chemotherapy is completed

Antimicrobial prophylaxis
Risk of fever and neutropenia is **INTERMEDIATE**
　• Antibacterial—consider a fluoroquinolone or no prophylaxis; *P. jirovecii* prophylaxis is recommended (eg, cotrimoxazole)
　• Antifungal—no prophylaxis
　• Antiviral—antiherpes antivirals (eg, acyclovir) as patients may develop herpes viral infections as a result of their underlying disease even without the influence of purine analog therapy

Allopurinol: Tumor lysis is uncommon and allopurinol need not be routinely administered

Treatment Modifications

Toxicity	Treatment Modification
Serum creatinine >20% over baseline	Hold pentostatin until serum creatinine returns to baseline or creatinine clearance on a 24-hour urine collection is >50 mL/min (>0.83 mL/s)
New or suspected infection	Hold pentostatin until successful therapy being administered
G2 nonhematologic toxicity	Reduce pentostatin by 33% after toxicity G ≤1
G3 nonhematologic toxicity	Reduce pentostatin by 50% after toxicity G ≤1
G4 nonhematologic toxicity	Discontinue pentostatin

Therapy Monitoring

1. *Two to 3 times per week during therapy:* CBC and serum electrolytes, BUN, creatinine, LFTs, and uric acid
2. *Three months after the completion of therapy:* bone marrow aspirate and biopsy
3. *Long-term follow-up:* CBC every 3–6 months for 2 years, and then every 6 months for 3 years

Patient Population Studied

Study of 154 patients with previously untreated hairy cell leukemia

Efficacy

Complete remission rate	70–80%
Partial remission rate	5–20%
Relapse rate	10–25%

Toxicity (N = 154)

Toxicity	% G3	% G4
Allergy/rash	2.6	0
Nausea/vomiting/anorexia	12	0
Chills/fever	1.3	0
Diarrhea	1.3	0
Neurologic	0.7	0
Hepatic	0.7	0
Renal	0.7	0
Anemia	0.7	0
Granulocytopenia (G4)	5.2	14
Thrombocytopenia	2.6	0
Suspected infection during induction	53%	
Systemic antibiotics during induction	27%	

SECOND-LINE

HAIRY CELL LEUKEMIA REGIMEN: MOXETUMOMAB PASUDOTOX-TDFK

Kreitman RJ et al. Leukemia 2018;32(8):1768–1777
Supplementary appendix to: Kreitman RJ et al. Leukemia 2018;32(8):1768–1777
Kreitman RJ et al. Blood 2018;131(21):2331–2334
Supplementary materials to: Kreitman RJ et al. Blood 2018;131(21):2331–2334
Kreitman RJ et al. J Clin Oncol 2012;30(15):1822–1828
Lumoxiti (moxetumomab pasudotox-tdfk) prescribing information. Wilmington, DE: Astrazeneca Pharmaceuticals, LP; revised 2018 September

Moxetumomab pasudotox-tdfk premedications:

Diphenhydramine 25–50 mg; administer orally or by intravenous injection (or **hydroxyzine** 25 mg administered orally) 30–90 minutes before each moxetumomab pasudotox-tdfk infusion on days 1, 3, and 5, every 28 days for up to 6 cycles, *plus:*

Famotidine 20 mg; administer orally or by intravenous injection (or **ranitidine** 150 mg administered orally, or **ranitidine** 50 mg administered by intravenous injection, or **cimetidine** 300 mg administered orally or by intravenous injection) 30–90 minutes before each moxetumomab pasudotox-tdfk infusion on days 1, 3, and 5, every 28 days for up to 6 cycles, *plus:*

Acetaminophen 650–1000 mg; administer orally or by intravenous injection 30–90 minutes before each moxetumomab pasudotox-tdfk infusion on days 1, 3, and 5, every 28 days for up to 6 cycles

If history of prior severe infusion-related reaction, then add:
   Dexamethasone 10–20 mg; administer orally or by intravenous injection 30–90 minutes before each moxetumomab pasudotox-tdfk infusion (only if history of prior severe infusion-related reaction) on days 1, 3, and 5, every 28 days for up to 6 cycles

Hydration prior to moxetumomab pasudotox-tdfk:
   0.9% sodium chloride injection (0.9% NS) 1000 mL (or 500 mL if weight <50 kg); administer intravenously over 2–4 hours prior to each moxetumomab pasudotox-tdfk infusion on days 1, 3, and 5, every 28 days for up to 6 cycles

Moxetumomab pasudotox-tdfk 0.04 mg/kg per dose; administer intravenously, diluted in 50 mL 0.9% NS containing 1 mL of solution stabilizer, over 30 minutes for 3 doses on days 1, 3, and 5, every 28 days for up to 6 cycles or until complete response (total dosage/28-day cycle = 0.12 mg/kg)

Post-moxetumomab pasudotox-tdfk infusion medications:
   Diphenhydramine 25–50 mg; administer orally (or **hydroxyzine** 25 mg orally) every 6 hours for 24 hours following each infusion of moxetumomab pasudotox-tdfk on days 1, 3, and 5, every 28 days for up to 6 cycles
   Famotidine 20 mg; administer orally every 12 hours (or **ranitidine** 150 mg orally every 12 hours, or **cimetidine** 300 mg orally every 6 hours) for 24 hours following each infusion of moxetumomab pasudotox-tdfk on days 1, 3, and 5, every 28 days for up to 6 cycles
   Acetaminophen 650–1000 mg; administer orally every 6 hours for 24 hours following each infusion of moxetumomab pasudotox-tdfk on days 1, 3, and 5, every 28 days for up to 6 cycles
   Dexamethasone 4 mg; administer orally twice per day for 24 hours following each infusion of moxetumomab pasudotox-tdfk on days 1, 3, and 5, every 28 days for up to 6 cycles

Thrombotic microangiopathy prophylaxis following moxetumomab pasudotox-tdfk infusion (consider in patients with platelet count ≥100,000/mm³):
   Aspirin 75–100 mg; administer orally once daily on days 1–8, every 28 days for up to 6 cycles

Hydration after moxetumomab pasudotox-tdfk
   0.9% NS 1000 mL (or 500 mL if weight <50 kg); administer intravenously over 2–4 hours after each moxetumomab pasudotox-tdfk infusion. Advise patient to consume up to 3000 mL (2000 mL if weight <50 kg) of oral fluids per 24 hours on days 1–8, every 28 days for up to 6 cycles

(continued)

Patient Population Studied

The international, multicenter, single-arm, open-label study involved 80 patients with histologically confirmed relapsed/refractory hairy cell leukemia who had previously received at least two systemic therapies, including at least one purine nucleoside analog. Eligible patients had an Eastern Cooperative Oncology Group performance score ≤2 and adequate hepatic and renal function. All patients received intravenous moxetumomab pasudotox (0.04 mg/kg over 30 minutes) on days 1, 3, and 5 of a 28-day cycle for a maximum of six cycles

Efficacy (N = 80)

Durable complete response rate*	30%
Objective response rate	75%
Complete response rate	41%

*Complete response with maintenance of hematologic remission for >180 days
Note: The median duration of follow-up was 16.7 months

Therapy Monitoring

1. *Prior to each infusion:* physical examination, vital signs, weight, fluid balance, CBC with differential and platelet count, serum creatinine, blood urea nitrogen, estimated creatinine clearance, serum electrolytes (sodium, potassium, chloride, bicarbonate, phosphate, calcium, magnesium), total bilirubin, direct bilirubin, ALT or AST, serum albumin, alkaline phosphatase, lactate dehydrogenase

2. *During each infusion on days 1, 3, and 5 of each cycle:* monitor vital signs every 30 minutes during the moxetumomab pasudotox-tdfk infusion and for 1 hour following completion of the infusion

3. *On approximately day 8 and day 15 of each cycle:* CBC with differential and platelet count, serum creatinine, blood urea nitrogen, serum electrolytes (sodium, potassium, chloride, bicarbonate, phosphate, calcium, magnesium), total bilirubin, direct bilirubin, ALT or AST, serum albumin, alkaline phosphatase, lactate dehydrogenase

(continued)

(continued)

Notes:
- After each moxetumomab pasudotox-tdfk infusion, flush the intravenous administration line with a volume of 0.9% NS adequate to clear the priming volume of the tubing. Infuse the 0.9% NS flush at the same rate as the moxetumomab pasudotox-tdfk infusion
- Do not administer moxetumomab pasudotox-tdfk in patients with severe renal impairment (creatinine clearance ≤29 mL/minute)
- Changes in dose due to fluctuations in weight should be made between cycles only when a change in weight of >10% is observed from the baseline weight used to calculate the first dose of cycle 1. Do not change the dose within a particular cycle

Supportive Care
Antiemetic prophylaxis
Emetogenic potential is **MINIMAL-LOW**
See Chapter 42 for antiemetic recommendations

Hematopoietic growth factor (CSF) prophylaxis
Primary prophylaxis is **NOT** *indicated*
See Chapter 43 for more information

Antimicrobial prophylaxis
Risk of fever and neutropenia is **LOW**
  Antimicrobial primary prophylaxis to be considered:
  - Antibacterial—not indicated
  - Antifungal—not indicated
  - Antiviral—antiherpes antivirals (eg, acyclovir, famciclovir, valacyclovir)

Treatment Modifications

MOXETUMOMAB PASUDOTOX-TDFK

Capillary Leak Syndrome

Patient meets both of the following criteria: • Weight increased by an absolute value of 2.5 kg or by ≥5% relative to the baseline weight measured on day 1 of the current cycle • Patient is hypotensive Capillary leak syndrome is suspected	• Interrupt moxetumomab pasudotox-tdfk during assessment • Promptly assess for peripheral edema, hypoalbuminemia, and respiratory symptoms (including dyspnea and cough). If capillary leak syndrome is suspected, then assess oxygen saturation and examine the patient for evidence of pulmonary edema and/or serosal effusions (and consider appropriate radiologic imaging as clinically indicated) • If G ≤1 capillary leak syndrome is confirmed, may resume moxetumomab pasudotox-tdfk and monitor closely for worsening signs, symptoms, and laboratory evidence of capillary leak syndrome
G2 capillary leak syndrome (symptomatic; medical intervention indicated) is confirmed	• Interrupt moxetumomab pasudotox-tdfk • Consider the need for hospitalization. Provide appropriate supportive measures including treatment with oral or intravenous corticosteroids and monitor weight, albumin levels, and blood pressure until resolution • Upon resolution of symptoms, may resume moxetumomab pasudotox at the same dose

(continued)

Therapy Monitoring
(continued)

4. *Periodically or as clinically indicated:* signs and symptoms of capillary leak syndrome, signs and symptoms of hemolytic uremic syndrome, peripheral smear review (if hemolytic uremic syndrome suspected), signs and symptoms of thrombosis, fluid balance, vital signs, weight

5. *Response assessment:*
   a. *Prior to each 28-day cycle of moxetumomab pasudotox-tdfk:* physical examination (assessment for splenomegaly and lymphadenopathy), CBC with differential and platelet count
   b. *Upon documentation of hematologic remission (hemoglobin >11 g/dL [without transfusion], platelets >100,000/mm³, and absolute neutrophil count >1500/mm³):* consider CT scans, bone marrow biopsy, and/or flow cytometry (on peripheral blood and/or marrow aspirate) as indicated to document response

6. *Long-term follow-up:* CBC with differential and platelet count every 3–6 months for 2 years, then every 6 months for 3 years

Treatment Modifications (continued)

MOXETUMOMAB PASUDOTOX-TDFK

Capillary Leak Syndrome

G3 capillary leak syndrome (severe symptoms; medical intervention indicated)	• Permanently discontinue moxetumomab pasudotox-tdfk • Consider the need for hospitalization. Provide appropriate supportive measures including treatment with oral or intravenous corticosteroids and monitor weight, albumin levels, and blood pressure until resolution
G4 capillary leak syndrome (life-threatening consequences; urgent intervention indicated)	

Hemolytic Uremic Syndrome

Worsening anemia, thrombocytopenia, and renal function—hemolytic uremic syndrome is suspected	• Interrupt moxetumomab pasudotox-tdfk during assessment • Promptly check blood lactate dehydrogenase, indirect bilirubin, and blood smear schistocytes for evidence of hemolysis • If hemolytic uremic syndrome is ruled out, may continue moxetumomab pasudotox-tdfk at the same dose if no other dose-limiting toxicities are present
Hemolytic uremic syndrome is confirmed (any grade)	• Permanently discontinue moxetumomab pasudotox-tdfk • Consider the need for hospitalization. Treat with appropriate supportive measures and fluid replacement. Monitor blood chemistry, complete blood count with differential and platelet count, and renal function until resolution. *Note:* plasma exchange was not necessary during clinical trials of moxetumomab pasudotox

Renal Impairment and Renal Toxicity

Baseline estimated creatinine clearance is ≤29 mL/minute	Avoid use of moxetumomab pasudotox-tdfk
G ≥2 increase in serum creatinine (>1.5× baseline or ULN) in patients with baseline serum creatinine ≤ULN	Delay moxetumomab pasudotox-tdfk dosing until recovery to G ≤1, then continue at the same dose
G ≥3 increase in serum creatinine (>3× baseline or ULN) in patients with baseline serum creatinine elevation of G1 (>1 to ≤1.5× ULN) or G2 (>1.5 to ≤3× ULN)	Delay moxetumomab pasudotox-tdfk dosing until recovery to ≤ baseline grade, then continue at the same dose

Infusion-Related Reaction

Severe infusion-related reaction	• Interrupt the moxetumomab pasudotox-tdfk infusion until resolution of symptoms. Institute appropriate medical management • Administer a corticosteroid (eg, dexamethasone 10–20 mg administered orally or intravenously) 30 minutes prior to resuming moxetumomab pasudotox-tdfk infusion and prior to all subsequent moxetumomab pasudotox-tdfk infusions as described in the therapy administration section

Adverse Events (N = 80)

Grade (%)*	Grade 1–2	Grade 3–4
Edema, peripheral	39	0
Nausea	33	3
Fatigue	34	0
Headache	33	0
Pyrexia	30	1
Hypophosphatemia	14	10
Hypocalcemia	24	0
Constipation	23	0
Anemia	11	10
Increased alanine aminotransferase	20	1
Diarrhea	21	0
Decreased lymphocyte count	0	20
Hypoalbuminemia	20	0
Hypokalemia	14	3
Hypertension	8	8
Decreased platelet count	5	6
Hyponatremia	9	3
Decreased white blood cell count	1	9
Capillary leak syndrome	6	3
Upper respiratory infection	6	3
Decreased neutrophil count	1	6
Hemolytic uremic syndrome	3	5
Febrile neutropenia	1	5
Neutropenia	0	5
Hypoxia	3	3
Acute kidney injury	1	3
Lung infection	1	3
Erysipelas	0	3

*According to the National Cancer Institute Common Toxicity Criteria for Adverse Events, version 4.03 Toxicities of any grade that occurred in ≥20% of patients or of Grade 3–4 that occurred in ≥2.5% of patients are included in the table. Three patients died, but none of the deaths was considered related to treatment

SECOND-LINE

HAIRY CELL LEUKEMIA REGIMEN: RITUXIMAB

Hagberg H, Lundholm L. Br J Haematol 2001;115:609–611
Lauria F et al. Haematologica 2001;86:1046–1050
Nieva J et al. Blood 2003;102:810–813

Premedication:
1. **Acetaminophen** 650–1000 mg; administer orally, 30–60 minutes before rituximab
2. **Diphenhydramine** 25–50 mg; administer orally or by intravenous injection 30–60 minutes before rituximab

Rituximab 375 mg/m² per week; administer intravenously in 0.9% sodium chloride injection (0.9% NS) or 5% dextrose injection (D5W) diluted to a concentration within the range of 1–4 mg/mL for 4 consecutive weeks (total dosage per 4-week course = 1500 mg/m²)

or

Rituximab 375 mg/m² per week; administer intravenously in 0.9% NS or D5W diluted to a concentration within the range of 1–4 mg/mL for 8 consecutive weeks with an additional 4 weekly doses (maximum of 12 doses) if a patient does not achieve a complete remission, but shows signs of continual improvement (total dosage per 8-week and 12-week courses = 3000 mg/m² and 4500 mg/m², respectively)

Thomas DA et al. Blood 2003;102:3906–3911

Rituximab infusion rates:
First dose: Start at an initial rate of 50 mg/hour. If hypersensitivity or infusion reactions do not occur during the first 30 minutes, increase the rate by 50 mg/hour every 30 minutes, to a maximum rate of 400 mg/hour
Subsequent doses: If previous administration was well tolerated, start at 100 mg/hour, and, if tolerated, increase by 100 mg/hour every 30 minutes, to a maximum rate of 400 mg/hour

Supportive Care
Antiemetic prophylaxis
Emetogenic potential is **MINIMAL**
See Chapter 42 for antiemetic recommendations

Hematopoietic growth factor (CSF) prophylaxis
Primary prophylaxis is **NOT** indicated
See Chapter 43 for more information

Antimicrobial prophylaxis
Risk of fever and neutropenia is **LOW**
   Antimicrobial primary prophylaxis to be considered:
   • Antibacterial—*P. jirovecii* prophylaxis is recommended (eg, cotrimoxazole)
   • Antifungal—not indicated
   • Antiviral—not indicated, unless patient previously had an episode of HSV

Optional: **Allopurinol** 300 mg/day; administer orally, beginning on the first day of rituximab administration and continuing for 2 weeks. Tumor lysis is uncommon and allopurinol need not be routinely administered

Patient Population Studied

Relapsed or refractory HCL

Efficacy

Thomas DA et al. Blood 2003;102:3906–3911

Overall response rate	80%
Complete response rate	53%
Partial response rate	27%*
No response	20%

*Includes 2 additional patients who achieved complete remission by hematologic parameters but had residual marrow disease (1–5% hairy cells)
Duration of response: With median follow-up of 32 months, 5 of 12 patients had progression of disease at 8, 12, 18, 23, and 39 months from the start of therapy

Toxicity (N = 15)

Thomas DA et al. Blood 2003;102:3906–3911

Toxicity	No. of Patients	G	Dose No.
Fever and chills	9	1	1
Nausea and vomiting	4	1	1, 2
Hypotension*	1	1	1
Palpitations*	1	2	1, 2
Shortness of breath*	1	2	1
Myalgia	1	3	All 8
Fatigue	2	1, 2	1, 2
Back pain	1	1	1
Rash	1	1	1
Infection	0	—	—

*Infusional events associated with the first dose. Rapid resolution occurred with temporary cessation of the infusion

Therapy Monitoring

1. *Weekly prior to each dose of rituximab:* CBC
2. *One to 3 months after the completion of therapy:* bone marrow aspirate and biopsy with immunophenotyping
3. *Long-term follow-up:* CBC every 3–6 months for 2 years, and then every 6 months for 3 years

Treatment Modifications

Fever, chills, hypotension, and other toxicities:
Slow or interrupt rituximab administration

Severe hypersensitivity reactions:
1. Interrupt administration
2. **Diphenhydramine** 25–50 mg; administration by intravenous injection is recommended
3. Additional treatment with diphenhydramine, bronchodilators, intravenous hydrocortisone, and/or intravenous hydration may be indicated
4. Resume infusion at a 50% reduction in rate when symptoms have completely resolved
5. Medications for the treatment of hypersensitivity reactions should be available for immediate use in the event of a reaction during administration (eg, intravenous fluids, epinephrine, antihistamines, glucocorticoids, O_2)
6. In many cases, the infusion can be resumed at a 50% reduction in rate when symptoms have completely resolved

Notes

1. Patients requiring close monitoring during first and all subsequent infusions include those with preexisting cardiac and pulmonary conditions, prior clinically significant cardiopulmonary adverse events, or circulating malignant cells >25,000/mm^3 with or without evidence of high tumor burden
2. No clear benefit of 12 doses versus 4 doses

SECOND-LINE

HAIRY CELL LEUKEMIA REGIMEN: VEMURAFENIB

Tiacci E et al. N Engl J Med 2015;373:1733–1747
Protocol for: Tiacci E et al. N Engl J Med 2015;373:1733–1747
Supplementary appendix to: Tiacci E et al. N Engl J Med 2015;373:1733–1747

Vemurafenib 960 mg per dose; administer orally, twice daily without regard to food (total dose/week = 13,440 mg)
Notes:
- Confirm presence of the *BRAF* V600E mutation prior to initiation of therapy
- The optimal duration of therapy is unknown. In the Italian phase 2 study, vemurafenib was administered for a median of 16 weeks; in the U.S. phase 2 study, vemurafenib was administered for a median 18 weeks
- The chapter authors' practice is to treat patients with vemurafenib for 3 months and then assess response to therapy. If a complete remission (CR) without presence of minimal residual disease (MRD) is achieved, then therapy is stopped. If patients achieve a CR but have evidence of MRD or have evidence of persistent disease, treatment is continued for another 3 months and then response is reassessed at 6 months. If there is still evidence of disease at that point, therapy is continued for another 3 months and then stopped

Supportive Care
Antiemetic prophylaxis
*Emetogenic potential is **MINIMAL–LOW***
See Chapter 42 for antiemetic recommendations

Hematopoietic growth factor (CSF) prophylaxis
Primary prophylaxis is **NOT** indicated
See Chapter 43 for more information

Antimicrobial prophylaxis
Risk of fever and neutropenia is **LOW**
  Antimicrobial primary prophylaxis to be considered:
- Antibacterial—not indicated
- Antifungal—not indicated
- Antiviral—antiherpes antivirals (eg, acyclovir, famciclovir, valacyclovir)

Patient Population Studied

Vemurafenib was studied in separate U.S.-based and Italy-based phase 2 trials, which were published jointly. The patient population for both trials were patients with classical hairy cell leukemia, who relapsed after or were refractory to treatment with purine analogs. The phase 2 studies in the U.S. and Italy involved 26 and 28 patients, respectively. Eligible patients were required to have a hemoglobin level of <11g/dL (Italian study)/10g/dL (U.S. study), an absolute neutrophil count of <1500/mm³ (Italian study)/1000/mm³ (U.S. study), or a platelet count of <100,000/mm³ (both studies) and were required to have a *BRAF* V600E mutation. Patients with a previous malignancy within the past 2 years were excluded except for patients with treated and controlled squamous cell carcinoma of the skin or carcinoma in situ of the cervix or melanoma carrying a *BRAF* V600E mutation. Patients received vemurafenib orally at a dose of 960 mg twice per day. In the Italian trial, patients received vemurafenib for a minimum of 8 weeks and if they did not achieve a complete response, for a maximum of 16 weeks. In the U.S. study, patients received vemurafenib for 12 weeks and if there was presence of residual disease, they could receive up to 12 additional weeks. At the time of data cut-off, in the Italian study, vemurafenib was administered for a median of 16 weeks and in the U.S. study vemurafenib was administered for a median of 18 weeks

Efficacy (N = 54)

	Italian Trial (N = 28)	U.S. Trial (N = 26)
Overall response rate	96%	100%
Complete response rate	35%	42%

Note: In the Italian study, the median relapse-free survival was 9 months. In the U.S. trial, the cumulative incidence of relapse at 1 year was 27%

Therapy Monitoring

1. *Clinic visits:* should occur weekly for the first month and then monthly thereafter. A thorough skin and head and neck examination to monitor for squamous cell carcinoma should be conducted prior to the start of treatment and at least every 2 months while on therapy and continuing for 6 months after discontinuation of vemurafenib
2. *CBC with differential and platelet count:* weekly for the first month then monthly during active treatment
3. *Liver function tests:* evaluate prior to initiation of therapy and then monthly during treatment, or more frequently if clinically indicated
4. *Serum creatinine:* monitor at baseline and then periodically during treatment
5. *Electrocardiogram and electrolytes (eg, potassium, magnesium, and calcium):* monitor on day 1 prior to the first dose of vemurafenib and after 2 weeks of treatment and then every month for the next 3 months followed by monitoring every 3 months thereafter
6. *Long-term follow-up:* CBC with differential and platelet count every 3–6 months for 2 years, then every 6 months for 3 years

Treatment Modifications

VEMURAFENIB DOSE MODIFICATIONS

Dose level 1 (starting dose)	960 mg twice daily
Dose level −1	720 mg twice daily
Dose level −2	480 mg twice daily
Dose level −3	Discontinue vemurafenib

Note: Re-escalation of the vemurafenib dosage after dose reduction is not recommended

Adverse Reaction	Therapy Modification
Cutaneous squamous cell carcinoma (SCC)	Do not interrupt therapy or modify the dose of vemurafenib. Manage the SCC lesion(s) by excision
Severe hypersensitivity or cutaneous reaction (eg, anaphylaxis, generalized rash and erythema, drug reaction with eosinophilia and systemic symptoms [DRESS] syndrome, Stevens-Johnson syndrome/toxic epidermal necrolysis)	Permanently discontinue vemurafenib
QTc >500 ms or increase in baseline by >60 ms	Withhold vemurafenib. Evaluate electrolytes (potassium, magnesium, and calcium) and replete if necessary. Upon improvement of QTc to ≤500 ms, resume vemurafenib with the dosage reduced by 1 dose level. If the QTc does not improve to ≤500 ms and remains >60 ms above baseline despite correction and control of risk factors (eg, electrolyte abnormalities, congestive heart failure, bradyarrhythmias), then permanently discontinue vemurafenib
Uveitis	In clinical trials of vemurafenib with melanoma, uveitis occurred in 2.1% of patients. Consider managing with steroid and mydriatic ophthalmic drops
Other Grade 1 or tolerable Grade 2 toxicities	Do not modify the vemurafenib dose
Other intolerable Grade 2 toxicities or Grade 3 toxicities	For symptomatic drug reactions (eg, arthralgia, fatigue, rash, photosensitivity), consider withholding vemurafenib until improvement to G ≤1, then resume vemurafenib and consider reducing the dosage by 1 dose level. Arthralgia is common and can be first managed with prednisone 5–10 mg daily before dose reduction is attempted
Other Grade 4 toxicities	Discontinue permanently or withhold therapy until G ≤1 and then resume vemurafenib with the dosage reduced by 2 dose levels

Adverse Events (N = 54)

Serious Adverse Event (%)	Italian Trial (N = 28)			U.S. Trial (N = 26)		
	Grade 2	Grade 3	Total	Grade 2	Grade 3	Total
Arthralgia or arthritis	36	7	43	31	0	31
Rash or erythema	39	7	46	42	19	62
Cutaneous basal-cell carcinoma	7*	0	7	4	0	4
Cutaneous superficial melanoma	0	4	4	0	0	0
Cutaneous squamous cell carcinoma	0	0	0	12†	0	12
Skin papilloma	7	0	7	0	0	0
Photosensitivity reaction	7	0	7	0	8	8
Hyperkeratosis	11	0	11	0	0	0
Panniculitis	7	0	7	0	0	0
Pancreatitis	4‡	7	11	0	0	0
Increased pancreatic enzymes	4	4	7	0	0	0
Hyperbilirubinemia	7	4	11	12	0	12
Any increased aminotransferase	4	0	4	12	4	15
Increased alkaline phosphatase	0	0	0	0	8	8
Pain in the hands or feet	7	0	7	8	0	8
Headache	4	0	4	0	0	0
Increased blood creatinine	7	0	7	4	0	4
Seborrheic keratosis	7	0	7	0	0	0
Asthenia	4	0	4	0	8	8
Musculoskeletal pain	4	0	4	0	0	0
Abdominal pain	4	0	4	0	0	0
Pyrexia	0	0	0	0	4	4
Nausea	0	0	0	4	0	4
Alopecia	0	0	0	4	0	4

Adverse events were included in the table if they occurred in at least 1 patient in either trial and were considered to be drug-related. There were no Grade 4 events reported in either study. All cutaneous tumors that developed in the study were managed by simple excision
*Two basal cell carcinomas developed in one patient. The other patient had a history of basal cell carcinoma
†All three patients had a history of squamous cell carcinoma
‡The patient with a Grade 2 pancreatitis in the Italian trial had elevated pancreatic enzyme(s) but did not have clinical symptoms or radiologic abnormalities associated with pancreatitis

19. Head and Neck Cancers

Pol Specenier, MD, PhD and JB Vermorken, MD, PhD

Epidemiology

Incidence: Estimated new cases for 2019 in the United States
Tongue: 17,060 (male, 12,550; female, 4510)
Mouth: 14,310 (male, 8430; female, 5880)
Pharynx; 17,870 (male, 14,450; female, 3420)
Other oral cavity: 3760 (male, 2710; female, 1050)
Larynx: 12,410, (male, 9860; female, 2550)

Deaths: Estimated deaths in 2019 in the United States
Tongue: 3020 (male, 2220; female, 800)
Mouth: 2740 (male, 1800; female, 940)
Pharynx: 3450 (male, 2660; female, 790)
Other oral: 1650 (male, 1290; female, 360)
Larynx: 3760 (male, 3010; female, 750)

Median age: Oral cavity and pharynx 63 years
Tongue 63 years
Larynx 65 years
Male to female ratio: 2.76:1

Siegel R et al. CA Cancer J Clin 2019;69:7–34
Surveillance, Epidemiology and End Results (SEER) Program, available from http://seer.cancer.gov [accessed October 2019]

Pathology

1. Squamous carcinomas (90%)
2. Lymphomas
3. Salivary gland tumors (adenocarcinoma, adenoid cystic carcinoma, mucoepidermoid carcinoma)
4. Sarcomas
5. Melanomas

Work-up

1. History and physical examination
2. ENT examination
3. Laryngoscopy with biopsy of suspicious lesions
4. CT and/or MRI of the head and neck
5. X-ray or CT of chest (to rule out metastatic disease or second primary tumor)
6. Needle biopsy of lymph node not associated with obvious primary tumor
7. PET (CT) in locally advanced disease

Organ Site–Specific Work-up

1. Ethmoid sinus: H&P, CT and/or MRI, CXR, pathology review if diagnosis with incomplete excision
2. Maxillary sinus: H&P, head and neck CT with contrast ± MRI, CXR, dental/prosthetic consultation as indicated
3. Salivary glands: H&P, CT/MRI, CXR, pathology review
4. Lip, oral cavity: H&P, CT/MRI, panorex, biopsy, preanesthesia studies, dental evaluation
5. Hypopharynx: H&P, biopsy, CXR or chest CT, CT with contrast or MRI of primary and neck, examination under anesthesia with laryngoscopy/esophagoscopy, preanesthesia studies, dental evaluation, multidisciplinary consultation as indicated
6. Glottic larynx: Same work-up as for hypopharynx + CT scan with contrast and thin cuts of the larynx or MRI of primary, speech and swallowing studies

Staging

Primary Tumor (T)

- Differs for each site
- For larynx and hypopharynx cancers, vocal cord paralysis indicates at least T3
- Local invasion of adjacent structures indicates T4

Clinical Regional Lymph Node (N) Definitions for Cancers of the Oral Cavity, Major Salivary Glands, Paranasal Sinuses, Nasal Cavity, Oropharynx (p16[−]), Hypopharynx, and Larynx

NX	Regional lymph nodes cannot be assessed
N0	No regional lymph node metastasis
N1	Metastasis in a single ipsilateral lymph node, 3 cm or less in greatest dimension and ENE(−)
N2	Metastasis in a single ipsilateral lymph node, larger than 3 cm but not larger than 6 cm in greatest dimension and ENE(−), or in multiple ipsilateral lymph nodes, none larger than 6 cm in greatest dimension and ENE(−), or in bilateral or contralateral lymph nodes, none larger than 6 cm in greatest dimension and ENE(−)
N2a	Metastasis in a single ipsilateral lymph node, larger than 3 cm but not larger than 6 cm in greatest dimension and ENE(−)
N2b	Metastasis in multiple ipsilateral lymph nodes, none larger than 6 cm in greatest dimension and ENE(−)
N2c	Metastasis in bilateral or contralateral lymph nodes, none more than 6 cm in greatest dimension and ENE(−)
N3	Metastasis in a lymph node, more than 6 cm in greatest dimension and ENE(−), or in any lymph node(s) with clinically overt ENE(+)
N3a	Metastasis in a lymph node, larger than 6 cm in greatest dimension and ENE(−)
N3b	Metastasis in any lymph node(s) with clinically overt ENE(+)

Note: A "U" designation is used for any N category to indicate metastasis above the lower border of the cricoid and a "L" designation may be used for any N category to indicate metastasis below the lower border of the cricoid

Clinical Regional Lymph Node (N) Definitions for HPV-related (p16[+]) Squamous Cell Carcinoma of the Oropharynx

NX	Regional lymph nodes cannot be assessed
N0	No regional lymph node metastasis
N1	One or more ipsilateral lymph nodes, none larger than 6 cm
N2	Contralateral or bilateral lymph nodes, none larger than 6 cm
N3	Lymph node(s) larger than 6 cm

Clinical Regional Lymph Node (N) Definitions for Epithelial Tumors of the Nasopharynx

NX	Regional lymph nodes cannot be assessed
N0	No regional lymph node metastasis
N1	Unilateral metastasis in cervical lymph node(s) and/or unilateral or bilateral metastasis in retropharyngeal lymph node(s), 6 cm or smaller in greatest dimension, above the caudal border of cricoid cartilage
N2	Bilateral metastasis in cervical lymph node(s), 6 cm or smaller in greatest dimension, above the caudal border of cricoid cartilage
N3	Unilateral or bilateral metastasis in cervical lymph node(s), larger than 6 cm in greatest dimension, and/or extension below the caudal border of cricoid cartilage

Distant Metastasis (M)

M0	No distant metastasis
M1	Distant metastasis

Staging Groups for Cancers of Oral Cavity, Oropharynx (p16[−]), Hypopharynx, Larynx, Major Salivary Glands, Nasal Cavity, and Paranasal Sinuses*

	T (Primary)	N	M
Stage 0	Tis	N0	M0
Stage I	T1	N0	M0
Stage II	T2	N0	M0
Stage III†	T3	N0	M0
	T1	N1	M0
	T2	N1	M0
	T3	N1	M0
Stage IVA‡	T4a	N0	M0
	T4a	N1	M0
	T1	N2	M0
	T2	N2	M0
	T3	N2	M0
	T4a	N2	M0
Stage IVB	T4b	Any N	M0
	Any T	N3	M0
Stage IVC	Any T	Any N	M1

*The same for all primary sites, *except* cancers of the nasopharynx and HPV-related (p16[+]) squamous cell carcinoma of the oropharynx
†Patients with cancer of the major salivary glands with T0, N1, M0 disease are also classified as stage III
‡Patients with cancer of the major salivary glands with T0, N2, M0 disease are also classified as stage IVA

Staging (continued)

Staging Groups for HPV-related (p16[+]) Squamous Cell Carcinoma of the Oropharynx

	T (Primary)	N	M
Stage I	T0	N0	M0
	T1	N0	M0
	T2	N0	M0
	T0	N1	M0
	T1	N1	M0
	T2	N1	M0
Stage II	T0	N2	M0
	T1	N2	M0
	T2	N2	M0
	T3	N0	M0
	T3	N1	M0
	T3	N2	M0
Stage III	T0	N3	M0
	T1	N3	M0
	T2	N3	M0
	T3	N3	M0
	T4	N0	M0
	T4	N1	M0
	T4	N2	M0
	T4	N3	M0
Stage IV	Any T	Any M	M1

Staging Groups for Epithelial Tumors of the Nasopharynx

	T (Primary)	N	M
Stage 0	Tis	N0	M0
Stage I	T1	N0	M0
Stage II	T0	N1	M0
	T1	N1	M0
	T2	N0	M0
	T2	N1	M0
Stage III	T0	N2	M0
	T1	N2	M0
	T2	N2	M0
	T3	N0	M0
	T3	N1	M0
	T3	N2	M0
Stage IVA	T4	N0	M0
	T4	N1	M0
	T4	N2	M0
	Any T	N3	M0
Stage IVB	Any T	Any M	M1

Amin MB et al, editors. AJCC Cancer Staging Manual. 8th ed. New York: Springer; 2017

Larynx: 5-Year Relative Survival by Stage at Diagnosis for All Races, Both Sexes

Stage at Diagnosis	5-Year Relative Survival (%)
Localized (confined to primary site)	76.1
Regional (spread to regional lymph nodes)	42.8
Distant (cancer has metastasized)	35.3

Surveillance, Epidemiology and End Results (SEER) Program, available from http://seer.cancer.gov [accessed 3 October 2019]

Oral Cavity and Pharynx: 5-Year Relative Survival by Stage at Diagnosis for All Races, Both Sexes

Stage at Diagnosis	5-Year Relative Survival (%)
Localized (confined to primary site)	84.4
Regional (spread to regional lymph nodes)	66.0
Distant (cancer has metastasized)	39.1

Surveillance, Epidemiology and End Results (SEER) Program, available from http://seer.cancer.gov [accessed 3 October 2019]

Tongue: 5-Year Relative Survival by Stage at Diagnosis for All Races, Both Sexes

Stage at Diagnosis	5-Year Relative Survival (%)
Localized (confined to primary site)	81.3
Regional (spread to regional lymph nodes)	67.8
Distant (cancer has metastasized)	39

Surveillance, Epidemiology and End Results (SEER) Program, available from http://seer.cancer.gov [accessed 3 October 2019]

Expert Opinion
Treatment

General: All patients should have access to a *multidisciplinary team* with expertise in all aspects of care for patients with head and neck cancer including:
1. Head and neck surgery
2. Radiation oncology
3. Medical oncology
4. Reconstructive surgery
5. Dentistry
6. Speech and swallowing therapy
7. Diagnostic radiology
8. Pathology
9. Nutrition support
10. Social work

Smoking cessation counseling is indicated

Resectable versus unresectable disease: The tumor is considered unresectable when a team of surgeons with particular expertise in head and neck cancer has serious doubts about the ability to remove the gross tumor with a reasonable likelihood of local control, even with the addition of adjuvant chemoradiation

Postoperative chemoradiation: Postoperative cisplatin-based chemoradiation using *cisplatin 100 mg/m² every 3 weeks* is superior to irradiation alone in patients with adverse risk factors in the resection specimen. Postoperative chemoradiation is:
1. Indicated in patients with extracapsular nodal spread and/or positive surgical margins
2. To be considered in patients with:
   - pT3 or pT4 primary
   - N2 or N3 nodal disease
   - Perineural invasion
   - Vascular tumor embolism

Postoperative chemoradiation should be started within 6 weeks after surgery, but note that combined-modality treatment is associated with a substantial increase in adverse effects

Organ preservation: In some patients with resectable disease, a combination of chemotherapy and definitive irradiation can spare a functional organ without sacrificing the probability of cure. Each patient should be evaluated by the multidisciplinary team in order to offer to a patient the best options

Definitive nonsurgical treatment for patients with unresectable disease or as organ preservation:
- *Concurrent chemoradiation using cisplatin 100 mg/m² every 3 weeks for 3 doses should still be considered the standard regimen*
- Cetuximab with irradiation can be used in patients who cannot tolerate cisplatin-based chemotherapy
- PET-CT imaging 12 weeks after the end of chemoradiation may help to select patients with initial N2 or N3 disease who achieved a complete response from combined modality treatment for whom elective neck dissection is unnecessary
- *Salvage surgery* is indicated in patients with residual tumor at the *primary site* whenever the disease is resectable at that time
- *Neck dissection* is indicated in cases of residual *disease in the neck*

Considerations in patients undergoing chemoradiation:
1. All patients for whom chemoradiation is planned should be evaluated and treated by a dentist before the start of treatment
2. Follow patients closely during chemoradiation with special attention to:
   - Hydration
   - Nutritional status
   - Electrolyte balance
3. Tube feeding is indicated in cases of a 10% decrease of body weight. Some centers prefer prophylactic tube feeding before the start of chemoradiation
4. Swallowing exercises during and after treatment are strongly advocated in order to diminish the risk of permanent disturbance of oral food intake
5. Adequate analgesic therapy often including opioids may be required

(continued)

(continued)

Induction chemotherapy:

1. **TPF (docetaxel + cisplatin + fluorouracil)** *is to be considered the current standard induction chemotherapy regimen in cases where induction chemotherapy is considered appropriate*

2. Induction chemotherapy reduces the risk of distant metastases but should not be considered standard treatment pending the results of ongoing randomized phase 3 trials

3. Induction chemotherapy may be an option for specific patient categories

Recurrent/metastatic disease: Active single agents include:

1. Cisplatin
2. Carboplatin
3. Paclitaxel
4. Docetaxel
5. Fluorouracil
6. Methotrexate
7. Ifosfamide
8. Bleomycin
9. Cetuximab
10. Pembrolizumab
11. Nivolumab

Consideration in recurrent/metastatic disease:

1. Response rates with single cytotoxic agents range from 15% to 30% in nonrandomized trials

2. In randomized comparisons *platinum-based combination chemotherapy regimens (in particular cisplatin plus infusional fluorouracil) induce higher response rates than single-agent chemotherapy but at the cost of increased toxicity*

3. Pembrolizumab with chemotherapy improved overall survival versus cetuximab with chemotherapy in patients with a combined positive score (CPS) $\geq$1. Pembrolizumab monotherapy improved overall survival when compared to cetuximab with chemotherapy. Pembrolizumab either as a single agent or in combination with chemotherapy can be considered the new standard of care in patients with a CPS $\geq$1. The choice between pembrolizumab monotherapy and the combination with chemotherapy should be based on factors including the need of a (rapid) tumor response and the level of CPS

4. The addition of cetuximab to cisplatin and fluorouracil improves survival without a significant increase in serious toxicities. *The combination of cisplatin + fluorouracil + cetuximab, therefore, is still the preferred regimen in patients with a CPS <1 who are most likely to benefit from combination chemotherapy*

5. Single-agent chemotherapy is still an option in patients with a decreased performance status or in a frail condition:
   - Weekly methotrexate is the best-studied regimen for that indication
   - (Weekly) taxanes and cetuximab may be adequate alternatives

6. Nivolumab and pembrolizumab prolong survival when compared to investigator's choice therapy (single-agent docetaxel, cetuximab, or methotrexate) in patients who fail platin-based chemo(radio)therapy, and represent the new standard of care in patients who did not previously receive an immune checkpoint inhibitor

7. Selected patients with a locoregional relapse may be salvaged by surgery or re-irradiation
   - Metastatic disease outside the head/neck area is present in only 10% at presentation, but 20% of those treated for cure with surgery and/or radiation or with chemoradiation develop metastatic disease outside the locoregional area, commonly concurrent with a locoregional recurrence
   - Patients cured of the initial tumor have a 2–6% per year incidence of second primary tumors, commonly diagnosed in the upper aerodigestive tract

Note regarding thyroid function: Patients who received thyroid gland irradiation are prone to the development of hypothyroidism. Thyroid-stimulating hormone should be followed every 6–12 months for the lifetime of affected patients

Bernier J et al. Head Neck 2005;27:843–850
Bernier J et al. N Engl J Med 2004;350:1945–1952
Burtness B et al. Lancet 2019;394:1915–1928
Cohen EEW et al. Lancet 2019;393:156–167
Ferris RL et al. N Engl J Med 2016;375:1856–1867
Forastiere AA et al. N Engl J Med 2003;349:2091–2098
Haddad RI, Shin DM. N Engl J Med 2008;359:1143–1154
Lefebvre JL. Lancet Oncol 2006;7:745–755
Posner MR et al. N Engl J Med 2007;357:1705–1715
Vermorken JB, Specenier P. Ann Oncol 2010;21(suppl 7):vii252–vii261
Vermorken JB et al. Cancer 2008;112:2710–2719
Vermorken JB et al. N Engl J Med 2007;357:1695–1704
Vermorken JB et al. N Engl J Med 2008;359:1116–1127

CONCOMITANT CHEMORADIATION

HEAD AND NECK CANCER REGIMEN: CISPLATIN WITH RADIATION THERAPY

Adelstein DJ et al. J Clin Oncol 2003;21:92–98
Forastiere AA et al. N Engl J Med 2003;349:2091–2098

Pretreatment: Consider dental evaluation, percutaneous feeding tube, and nutrition evaluation
Hydration before, during, and after cisplatin administration ± mannitol:
* *Pre-cisplatin hydration* with 1000 mL 0.9% sodium chloride injection (0.9% NS); administer with potassium and magnesium supplementation as needed based on pretreatment laboratory results
* *Mannitol diuresis:* May be given to patients who have received adequate hydration. A dose of **mannitol 12.5–25 g** may be administered by intravenous injection or a short infusion before or during cisplatin administration, or prepared as an admixture with cisplatin. Continued intravenous hydration is essential
* *Continued mannitol diuresis:* In an inpatient or day-hospital setting, one may administer additional mannitol in the form of an intravenous infusion: **mannitol 10–40 g;** administer intravenously over 1–4 hours. This can be done either during or immediately after cisplatin, but requires maintenance of adequate intravenously administered fluids during and for hours after mannitol administration
* *Post-cisplatin hydration* with ≥1000 mL 0.9% NS; administer with potassium and magnesium supplementation as needed based on measured values

Cisplatin 100 mg/m²; administer intravenously in 50–1000 mL 0.9% NS over 60 minutes on day 1, every 3 weeks for 3 cycles during radiation (total dosage/cycle = 100 mg/m²)
Radiation therapy at least 70 Gy to primary site and clinically positive nodes given in daily (Monday–Friday) fractions of 2 Gy/day over 7 weeks; at least 50 Gy to entire neck

Supportive Care
Antiemetic prophylaxis
Emetogenic potential on day 1 is **HIGH**. *Potential for delayed symptoms*
See Chapter 42 for antiemetic recommendations

Hematopoietic growth factor (CSF) prophylaxis
Primary prophylaxis is **NOT** *indicated*
See Chapter 43 for more information

Antimicrobial prophylaxis
Risk of fever and neutropenia is **LOW**
   Antimicrobial primary prophylaxis to be considered:
* Antibacterial—not indicated
* Antifungal—not indicated
* Antiviral—not indicated unless patient previously had an episode of HSV

Oral care (mucositis prophylaxis and management)
Risk of mucositis/stomatitis is HIGH
   General advice:
* Encourage patients to maintain intake of nonalcoholic fluids
* Evaluate patients for oral pain and provide analgesic medications
* Consider histamine (H₂-subtype) receptor antagonists (eg, ranitidine, famotidine), or a proton pump inhibitor for epigastric pain
* *Lactobacillus* sp.–containing probiotics may be beneficial in preventing diarrhea
   Patients with intact oral mucosa:
* Clean the mouth, tongue, and gums by brushing after every meal and at bedtime with an ultra-soft toothbrush with fluoride toothpaste
* Floss teeth gently every day unless contraindicated. If gums bleed and hurt, avoid bleeding or sore areas, but floss other teeth
* Patients may use saline or commercial bland, nonalcoholic rinses
   ▪ Do not use mouthwashes that contain alcohols

(continued)

Treatment Modifications

Adverse Event	Dose Modification*
Creatinine clearance <50 mL/min (<0.83 mL/s)	Ineligible for therapy
Day 1, 22, or 43 ANC <1500/mm³ or platelets <100,000/mm³	Delay cisplatin until ANC >1500/mm³ *and* platelets >100,000/mm³, for up to 3 weeks. Discontinue cisplatin if recovery has not occurred after a 3-week delay
ANC nadir <500/mm³	Reduce cisplatin dosage to 75 mg/m²
Platelet nadir <25,000/mm³	
G1 neurotoxicity or ototoxicity	
Serum creatinine 1.5–2.0 mg/dL (133–177 µmol/L)	Hold cisplatin†, then reduce dosage to 75 mg/m²
ANC nadir <500/mm³ with a cisplatin dosage of 75 mg/m²	Reduce cisplatin dosage to 50 mg/m²
Platelet nadir <25,000/mm³ with a cisplatin dosage of 75 mg/m²	
G2 neurotoxicity or ototoxicity	
Serum creatinine 2.1–3.0 mg/dL (186–265 µmol/L)	Hold cisplatin†, then reduce dosage to 50 mg/m²
ANC nadir <500/mm³ with a cisplatin dosage of 50 mg/m²	Discontinue cisplatin
Platelet nadir <25,000/mm³ with a cisplatin dosage of 50 mg/m²	
Serum creatinine >3.0 mg/dL (>265µmol/L)	
G3/4 neurotoxicity or ototoxicity	

*The use of colony-stimulating factors is discouraged
†Hold cisplatin dosage until serum creatinine <1.5 mg/dL (<133 µmol/L) or within 0.2 mg/dL (17.7 µmol/L) of baseline

(continued)

If mucositis or stomatitis is present:

- Keep the mouth moist utilizing water, ice chips, sugarless gum, sugar-free hard candies, or a saliva substitute
- Rinse mouth several times a day to remove debris
  - Use a solution of ¼ teaspoon (1.25 g) each of baking soda and table salt (sodium chloride) in 1 quart (~950 mL) of warm water. Follow with a plain water rinse
  - Do not use mouthwashes that contain alcohols
- Foam-tipped swabs (eg, Toothettes) are useful in moisturizing oral mucosa, but ineffective for cleansing teeth and removing plaque
- Advise patients who develop mucositis to:
  - Choose foods that are easy to chew and swallow
  - Take small bites of food, chew slowly, and sip liquids with meals
  - Encourage soft, moist foods such as cooked cereals, mashed potatoes, and scrambled eggs
  - For trouble swallowing, soften food with gravies, sauces, broths, yogurt, or other bland liquids
  - Avoid sharp, crunchy foods; hot, spicy, or highly acidic foods (eg, citrus fruits and juices); sugary foods; toothpicks; tobacco products; alcoholic drinks

Efficacy

Larynx Preservation Regimen (N = 172)*

Complete response	90.6%
Laryngeal preservation at median 3.8 years follow-up	84%
2-year estimated overall survival	74%
2-year estimated laryngectomy-free survival[†]	66%
2-year estimated disease-free survival	61%
5-year estimated overall survival	54%
5-year estimated laryngectomy-free survival[†]	45%
5-year estimated disease-free survival	36%
Percentage receiving >95% of planned RT dose	91%
Moderate[‡] or worse speech impairment at 2 year[§]	11%
Moderate[‡] or worse speech impairment at 1 year[§]	6%
Able to swallow only soft foods or liquids at 1 year	23%
Able to swallow only soft foods or liquids at 2 years	15%
Unable to swallow at 1 year	3%

*Forastiere AA et al. N Engl J Med 2003;349:2091–2098
[†]Composite end point on which the sample size of the trial was predicated. Either laryngectomy or death from any cause constituted treatment failure
[‡]Difficulty in pronouncing some words and being understood on the telephone
[§]*Note:* Information on speech and swallowing was available from only 78% of patients who were disease-free and had an intact larynx

Patient Population Studied

Organ preservation: Patients with previously untreated stage III or stage IV squamous cell carcinoma of the glottic or supraglottic larynx, the surgical treatment of which would require total laryngectomy. The disease had to be considered curable with surgery and postoperative radiation therapy. Karnofsky performance status (PS) at least 60%; adequate organ function; creatinine clearance at least 50 mL/min (≥0.83 mL/s)
Unresectable: Patients with stage III/IV unresectable squamous cancer excluding nasopharyngeal cancer, or cancers of the paranasal sinuses or parotid glands. ECOG PS 0–1, adequate organ function

Efficacy

Patients with Unresectable Squamous Cell Head and Neck Cancer (N = 87)*

Complete response	40.2%
3-year overall survival	37%
Median survival	19.1 months
3-year disease-specific survival	51%
Compliance	85.1%
Distant metastasis as first site of recurrence	21.8%

*Adelstein DJ et al. J Clin Oncol 2003;21:92–98

Toxicity (N = 266)

Organ Preservation (n = 171); Unresectable (n = 95)

	% G3–5 Toxicity	
Toxicity	Organ Preservation	Unresectable
Hematologic	47	42
Leukopenia		18
Anemia		3
Thrombocytopenia		
Mucosal	43	45
Pharyngeal/esophageal	35	—
Nausea or vomiting	20	16
Laryngeal	18	—
Dermatologic*	7	7
Infection	4	—
Renal/genitourinary	4	8
Neurologic	5	—
Other (not specified)	40	—
G5 toxicity	5	4

*Within radiation field

Therapy Monitoring

1. *Before cisplatin and weekly after treatment:* CBC with differential, serum electrolytes, calcium, and magnesium
2. *Weekly follow-up recommended during therapy:* Attention to signs and symptoms of dehydration as supplemental hydration and nutritional support often are required
3. *Every 4–6 months:* Thyroid function studies

CONCOMITANT CHEMORADIATION

HEAD AND NECK CANCER REGIMEN: CISPLATIN ALONE *OR* CISPLATIN + FLUOROURACIL WITH RADIATION THERAPY

Adelstein DJ et al. J Clin Oncol 2003;21:92–98

Pretreatment: Consider dental evaluation, percutaneous feeding tube, and nutrition evaluation

Hydration before, during, and after cisplatin administration ± mannitol:

- *Pre-cisplatin hydration* with 1000 mL 0.9% sodium chloride injection (0.9% NS); administer intravenously with potassium and magnesium supplementation as needed based on pretreatment laboratory results
- *Mannitol diuresis:* May be given to patients who have received adequate hydration. A dose of **mannitol** 12.5–25 g may be administered by intravenous injection or a short infusion before or during cisplatin administration, or prepared as an admixture with cisplatin. Continued intravenous hydration is essential
- *Continued mannitol diuresis:* In an inpatient or day-hospital setting, one may administer additional mannitol in the form of an intravenous infusion: **mannitol** 10–40 g; administer intravenously over 1–4 hours. This can be done either during or immediately after cisplatin, but requires maintenance of adequate intravenously administered fluids during and for hours after mannitol administration
- *Post-cisplatin hydration* with ≥1000 mL 0.9% NS; administer intravenously with potassium and magnesium supplementation as needed based on measured values

Cisplatin 100 mg/m^2; administer intravenously in 50–1000 mL 0.9% NS over 60 minutes on day 1, every 3 weeks for 3 cycles during radiation (total dosage/cycle = 100 mg/m^2)

Radiation therapy administered to a total dose of 70 Gy given continually in single, daily, 2-Gy fractions over 7 weeks

Supportive Care

Antiemetic prophylaxis

Emetogenic potential on day 1 is **HIGH**. *Potential for delayed symptoms*

See Chapter 42 for antiemetic recommendations

Hematopoietic growth factor (CSF) prophylaxis

Primary prophylaxis is **NOT** *indicated*

See Chapter 43 for more information

Antimicrobial prophylaxis

Risk of fever and neutropenia is **LOW**

   Antimicrobial primary prophylaxis to be considered:

- Antibacterial—not indicated
- Antifungal—not indicated
- Antiviral—not indicated unless patient previously had an episode of HSV

Or

Cisplatin 75 mg/m^2; administer intravenously in 50–1000 mL 0.9% NS over 60 minutes on day 1, every 4 weeks for 3 cycles during radiation (total dosage/cycle = 75 mg/m^2), *followed by:*

Fluorouracil 1000 mg/m^2 per day; administer in 50–1000 mL 0.9% NS or D5W by continuous intravenous infusion over 24 hours for 4 consecutive days, on days 1–4, every 4 weeks for 3 cycles during radiation (total dosage/cycle = 4000 mg/m^2)

Concurrent radiation therapy, at a rate of 2 Gy/day, split as follows:

- *First chemotherapy cycle:* A total of 30 Gy administered as 15 daily fractions of 2 Gy/fraction, 5 days/week, starting on day 1 of cycle 1
- *Third chemotherapy cycle:* A total of 30–40 Gy administered as 15–20 daily fractions of 2 Gy/fraction, 5 days/week, starting on day 1 of cycle 3
- Administer 30–40 Gy for a total dose of 60–70 Gy depending on response

(continued)

Patient Population Studied

A study of 295 patients with a histologically confirmed diagnosis of squamous cell or undifferentiated stage III or IV, nonmetastatic, carcinoma of the head and neck, excluding tumors originating in the nasopharynx, paranasal sinus, or parotid gland. Unresectability was predefined for each tumor site as follows:

- *Hypopharynx:* tumor extension across the midline of the posterior pharyngeal wall or fixed to the cervical spine
- *Larynx:* direct extension into surrounding muscle or skin or >3 cm subglottic extension
- *Oral cavity:* functional reconstruction not possible
- *Base of tongue:* extension into the root of tongue or refusal of total glossectomy
- *Tonsil:* extension into the pterygoid region as manifested by clinical trismus or demonstrated radiographically, or tumor extension across the midline of the pharyngeal wall or direct invasion into the soft tissue of the neck

Adequate organ function and an ECOG performance score ≤1 were required

Efficacy

	Cisplatin + Radiation N = 95	Cisplatin + Fluorouracil + Radiation N = 94
Complete response rate	40.2%	49.4%*
Estimated 3-year survival	37%	27%
Median overall survival, months	19.1	13.8
Disease-specific survival rates	51%	41%

*Includes patients undergoing mid-course surgical resection

(*continued*)

Note: The radiation therapy break is planned to allow for the possibility of surgical resection in patients whose disease is rendered resectable after the first 2 courses of chemotherapy and the first 30 Gy of radiation. Patients who do not achieve a complete response after the first 2 courses of chemotherapy and the first 30 Gy of radiation, or whose disease remains unresectable, complete chemoradiation without surgery.

As a result of the break, almost 7 additional weeks were required to complete treatment

Supportive Care
Antiemetic prophylaxis
Emetogenic potential on day 1 is **HIGH**. Potential for delayed symptoms
Emetogenic potential on days with fluorouracil ± RT is **LOW–MODERATE**
See Chapter 42 for antiemetic recommendations

Hematopoietic growth factor (CSF) prophylaxis
Primary prophylaxis is **NOT** indicated
See Chapter 43 for more information

Antimicrobial prophylaxis
Risk of fever and neutropenia is **LOW**
  Antimicrobial primary prophylaxis to be considered:
  • Antibacterial—not indicated
  • Antifungal—not indicated
  • Antiviral—not indicated unless patient previously had an episode of HSV

Oral care (mucositis prophylaxis and management)
Risk of mucositis/stomatitis is **HIGH**
  General advice:
  • Encourage patients to maintain intake of nonalcoholic fluids
  • Evaluate patients for oral pain and provide analgesic medications
  • Consider histamine (H$_2$-subtype) receptor antagonists (eg, ranitidine, famotidine), or a proton pump inhibitor for epigastric pain
  • *Lactobacillus* sp.–containing probiotics may be beneficial in preventing diarrhea
  Patients with intact oral mucosa:
  • Clean the mouth, tongue, and gums by brushing after every meal and at bedtime with an ultra-soft toothbrush with fluoride toothpaste
  • Floss teeth gently every day unless contraindicated. If gums bleed and hurt, avoid bleeding or sore areas, but floss other teeth
  • Patients may use saline or commercial bland, nonalcoholic rinses
    ▪ Do not use mouthwashes that contain alcohols
  If mucositis or stomatitis is present:
  • Keep the mouth moist utilizing water, ice chips, sugarless gum, sugar-free hard candies, or a saliva substitute
  • Rinse mouth several times a day to remove debris
    ▪ Use a solution of ¼ teaspoon (1.25 g) each of baking soda and table salt (sodium chloride) in 1 quart (~950 mL) of warm water. Follow with a plain water rinse
    ▪ Do not use mouthwashes that contain alcohols
  • Foam-tipped swabs (eg, Toothettes) are useful in moisturizing oral mucosa, but ineffective for cleansing teeth and removing plaque
  • Advise patients who develop mucositis to:
    ▪ Choose foods that are easy to chew and swallow
    ▪ Take small bites of food, chew slowly, and sip liquids with meals
    ▪ Encourage soft, moist foods such as cooked cereals, mashed potatoes, and scrambled eggs
    ▪ For trouble swallowing, soften food with gravies, sauces, broths, yogurt, or other bland liquids
    ▪ Avoid sharp, crunchy foods; hot, spicy, or highly acidic foods (eg, citrus fruits and juices); sugary foods; toothpicks; tobacco products; alcoholic drinks

G3–5 Toxicity

	Cisplatin + Radiation N = 95	Cisplatin + Fluorouracil + Radiation N = 94	P Value
Nausea/vomiting	15	8	
Mucositis/dysphagia	43	44	
Leukopenia	40	29	<0.001
Thrombocytopenia	3	3	
Anemia	17	18	
Renal	8	0	0.01
Skin	7	2	
Feeding tube	49	48	
Toxic death	4	2	
All G3–5	85	72	0.02
Treatment regimen compliance*	85.1%	73%	0.05

*As measured by treatment completion

Therapy Monitoring

1. *Day 1 of each cycle:* Medical history and physical exam, CBC with differential, LFTs, electrolytes, BUN, and creatinine
2. *Diagnostic imaging:* At treatment completion and 3 months later

Dose Modification

Note: It is anticipated that radiation therapy will continue despite the development of significant mucositis and/or myelosuppression

Adverse Event	Dose Modification
G3/4 hematologic toxicity	Hold chemotherapy for up to 3 weeks until toxicity resolves to G ≤1. If toxicity has not resolved to G ≤1 within 3 weeks, do not administer next cycle
G3/4 nonhematologic toxicity other than alopecia, fatigue, malaise, and nail changes (exceptions: neurotoxicity, ototoxicity, and mucositis as detailed below)	
G3/4 neurotoxicity or ototoxicity	Discontinue chemotherapy
G4 mucositis	

CONCOMITANT CHEMORADIATION
HEAD AND NECK CANCER REGIMEN: CISPLATIN + PACLITAXEL WITH RADIATION THERAPY

Garden AS et al. J Clin Oncol 2004;22:2856–2864

Pretreatment: Consider dental evaluation, percutaneous feeding tube, and nutrition evaluation

Premedication:

Dexamethasone 8–20 mg; administer by intravenous injection or short intravenous infusion 30 minutes before paclitaxel

Diphenhydramine 50 mg; administer by intravenous injection 30–60 minutes before paclitaxel

Cimetidine 300 mg (or **ranitidine** 50 mg, **famotidine** 20 mg, or an equivalent histamine receptor (H2 subtype)–antagonist); administer intravenously over 15–30 minutes, 30-60 minutes before paclitaxel

Paclitaxel 30 mg/m² per dose; administer intravenously in a volume of 0.9% sodium chloride injection (0.9% NS), or 5% dextrose injection (D5W) sufficient to produce a concentration within the range 0.3–1.2 mg/mL over 3–24 hours weekly, on day 1, for 7 consecutive weeks (total dosage/7-week cycle = 210 mg/m²)

Optional: **Dexamethasone** 4 mg; administer orally every 6 hours for 4 doses following paclitaxel with glucose monitoring if indicated

Cisplatin 20 mg/m² per dose; administer intravenously in 100–1000 mL 0.9% NS over 15–60 minutes weekly on day 2, for 7 consecutive weeks (total dosage/7-week cycle = 140 mg/m²)

Radiation at least 70 Gy to primary site and clinically positive nodes given in daily (Monday–Friday) fractions of 2 Gy/day over 7 weeks

Supportive Care

Antiemetic prophylaxis

Emetogenic potential on days with paclitaxel is **LOW**

Emetogenic potential on days with cisplatin is **HIGH**

See Chapter 42 for antiemetic recommendations

Hematopoietic growth factor (CSF) prophylaxis

Primary prophylaxis is **NOT** indicated

See Chapter 43 for more information

Antimicrobial prophylaxis

Risk of fever and neutropenia is **LOW**

   Antimicrobial primary prophylaxis to be considered:

- Antibacterial—not indicated

- Antifungal—consider use during neutropenia and for anticipated mucositis

- Antiviral—not indicated unless patient previously had an episode of HSV

Oral care (mucositis prophylaxis and management)

Risk of mucositis/stomatitis is **MODERATE**

   General advice:

- Encourage patients to maintain intake of nonalcoholic fluids

- Evaluate patients for oral pain and provide analgesic medications

- Consider histamine (H$_2$-subtype) receptor antagonists (eg, ranitidine, famotidine), or a proton pump inhibitor for epigastric pain

- *Lactobacillus* sp.–containing probiotics may be beneficial in preventing diarrhea

   Patients with intact oral mucosa:

- Clean the mouth, tongue, and gums by brushing after every meal and at bedtime with an ultra-soft toothbrush with fluoride toothpaste

- Floss teeth gently every day unless contraindicated. If gums bleed and hurt, avoid bleeding or sore areas, but floss other teeth

- Patients may use saline or commercial bland, nonalcoholic rinses
  - Do not use mouthwashes that contain alcohols

   If mucositis or stomatitis is present:

- Keep the mouth moist utilizing water, ice chips, sugarless gum, sugar-free hard candies, or a saliva substitute

- Rinse mouth several times a day to remove debris
  - Use a solution of ¼ teaspoon (1.25 g) each of baking soda and table salt (sodium chloride) in 1 quart (~950 mL) of warm water. Follow with a plain water rinse
  - Do not use mouthwashes that contain alcohols

- Foam-tipped swabs (eg, Toothettes) are useful in moisturizing oral mucosa, but ineffective for cleansing teeth and removing plaque

- Advise patients who develop mucositis to:
  - Choose foods that are easy to chew and swallow
  - Take small bites of food, chew slowly, and sip liquids with meals
  - Encourage soft, moist foods such as cooked cereals, mashed potatoes, and scrambled eggs
  - For trouble swallowing, soften food with gravies, sauces, broths, yogurt, or other bland liquids
  - Avoid sharp, crunchy foods; hot, spicy, or highly acidic foods (eg, citrus fruits and juices); sugary foods; toothpicks; tobacco products; alcoholic drinks

Patient Population Studied

A study of 77 patients with stage III or stage IV M0 squamous cancer of oral cavity, oropharynx, or hypopharynx, previously untreated, assigned to 1 of 3 arms in a randomized phase 2 RTOG trial. ECOG PS at least 70% and adequate organ function are required

Efficacy (N = 77)

Complete response	82%
Estimated 2-year disease-free survival	51.3%
Estimated 2-year overall survival	66.6%

Toxicity (N = 77)

	% G3/4
Nonhematologic	84
Hematologic	39
Mucositis	10 (G4)
Skin	3 (G4)
% Late Grade 4 Toxicities* (N = 72)	
Bone	4.2
Mucous membrane	1.4
Pharynx and esophagus	1.4
Larynx	1.4
Spinal cord	1.4
Skin	0
Subcutaneous tissue	0

*No grade 5 toxicities

Therapy Monitoring

1. *Weekly:* CBC with differential, serum electrolytes, calcium, and magnesium. Weekly follow-up recommended during therapy with attention to signs and symptoms of dehydration because supplemental hydration and nutritional support are often required
2. *Every 4–6 months:* Thyroid function studies

Treatment Modifications

Adverse Event	Dose Modification
Creatinine clearance <50 mL/min (<0.83 mL/s)	Ineligible for therapy
ANC <1000/mm^3 *or* platelets <75,000/mm^3 at the time of chemotherapy administration	Delay chemotherapy until ANC >1000/mm^3 *and* platelets >75,000/mm^3. Discontinue chemotherapy if recovery has not occurred after a 3-week delay
Serum creatinine >1.5 mg/dL (>133μmol/L) or 20% higher than baseline value if baseline was >1.5 mg/dL	Hold cisplatin dosage until serum creatinine <1.5 mg/dL (<133 μmol/L) or within 0.2 mg/dL (17.7 mol/L) of baseline
G2 neurotoxicity or ototoxicity	Hold cisplatin and paclitaxel until neurotoxicity resolves to G ≤1
G3/4 neurotoxicity or ototoxicity	Discontinue chemotherapy

CONCOMITANT CHEMORADIATION

HEAD AND NECK CANCER REGIMEN: CARBOPLATIN + FLUOROURACIL WITH RADIATION THERAPY

Calais G et al. J Natl Cancer Inst 1999;91:2081–2086

Pretreatment: Consider dental evaluation, percutaneous feeding tube, and nutrition evaluation
Carboplatin 70 mg/m² per day; administer intravenously in 50–100 mL 5% dextrose injection (D5W) or 0.9% sodium chloride injection (0.9% NS) over 15–30 minutes for 4 consecutive days, given on days 1–4, every 3 weeks (total dosage/cycle = 280 mg/m²)
Fluorouracil 600 mg/m² per day; administer by continuous intravenous infusion in 50–1000 mL 0.9% NS or D5W over 24 hours for 4 consecutive days, given on days 1–4, every 3 weeks (total dosage/cycle = 2400 mg/m²)
Radiation 2 Gy/day, 5 fractions per week to tumor and clinically positive nodes to a total dose of 70 Gy

Supportive Care
Antiemetic prophylaxis
Emetogenic potential is **MODERATE**
See Chapter 42 for antiemetic recommendations

Hematopoietic growth factor (CSF) prophylaxis
Primary prophylaxis is **NOT** indicated
See Chapter 43 for more information

Antimicrobial prophylaxis
Risk of fever and neutropenia is **LOW**
  Antimicrobial primary prophylaxis to be considered:
  • Antibacterial—not indicated
  • Antifungal—not indicated
  • Antiviral—not indicated unless patient previously had an episode of HSV

Diarrhea management
Latent or delayed-onset diarrhea*:
  Loperamide 4 mg orally initially after the first loose or liquid stool, *then*
  Loperamide 2 mg orally every 2 hours during waking hours, *plus*
  Loperamide 4 mg orally every 4 hours during hours of sleep
  • Continue for at least 12 hours after diarrhea resolves
  • Recurrent diarrhea after a 12-hour diarrhea-free interval is treated as a new episode
  • Rehydrate orally with fluids and electrolytes during a diarrheal episode
  • If diarrhea persists >48 hours despite loperamide, stop loperamide and hospitalize the patient for IV hydration
Persistent diarrhea:
  Octreotide 100–150 mcg subcutaneously 3 times daily. Maximum total daily dose is 1500 mcg
Antibiotic therapy during latent or delayed-onset diarrhea:
• A fluoroquinolone (eg, **ciprofloxacin** 500 mg orally every 12 hours) if absolute neutrophil count <500/mm³ with or without accompanying fever in association with diarrhea
• Antibiotics should also be administered if patient is hospitalized with prolonged diarrhea and should be continued until diarrhea resolves

*Rothenberg ML et al. J Clin Oncol 2001;19:3801–3807
Abigerges D et al. J Natl Cancer Inst 1994;86:446–449
Wadler S et al. J Clin Oncol 1998;16:3169–3178

Oral care
Risk of mucositis/stomatitis is HIGH
  General advice:
  • Encourage patients to maintain intake of nonalcoholic fluids
  • Evaluate patients for oral pain and provide analgesic medications
  • Consider histamine (H₂-subtype) receptor antagonists (eg, ranitidine, famotidine), or a proton pump inhibitor for epigastric pain
  • *Lactobacillus* sp.–containing probiotics may be beneficial in preventing diarrhea

(continued)

Patient Population Studied

A study of 109 patients with previously untreated stage III or stage IV squamous cell carcinoma of the oropharynx without evidence of distant metastases. Patients were assigned to the chemoradiation arm of a randomized phase 3 trial with Karnofsky PS at least 60% and adequate organ function

Efficacy (N = 109)

Locoregional control	66%
3-year overall survival	51%
3-year disease-free survival	42%
Median survival	29.2 months

Toxicity (N = 109)

	% of Patients
Acute Nonhematologic Toxicity	
G3/4 mucositis	71
Erythema/pruritis/dry desquamation	44
Moist desquamation	23
Weight loss >10% body mass	14
Need for feeding tube	36
G5 toxicities	0.9
Acute Hematologic Toxicity	
G3/4 neutropenia	4
G3/4 thrombocytopenia	6
G3/4 anemia	3
Late Toxicities	
G3/4 xerostomia	10
Severe cervical fibrosis	12

(*continued*)

Patients with intact oral mucosa:
- Clean the mouth, tongue, and gums by brushing after every meal and at bedtime with an ultra-soft toothbrush with fluoride toothpaste
- Floss teeth gently every day unless contraindicated. If gums bleed and hurt, avoid bleeding or sore areas, but floss other teeth
- Patients may use saline or commercial bland, nonalcoholic rinses
  - Do not use mouthwashes that contain alcohols

If mucositis or stomatitis is present:
- Keep the mouth moist utilizing water, ice chips, sugarless gum, sugar-free hard candies, or a saliva substitute
- Rinse mouth several times a day to remove debris
  - Use a solution of ¼ teaspoon (1.25 g) each of baking soda and table salt (sodium chloride) in 1 quart (~950 mL) of warm water. Follow with a plain water rinse
  - Do not use mouthwashes that contain alcohols
- Foam-tipped swabs (eg, Toothettes) are useful in moisturizing oral mucosa, but ineffective for cleansing teeth and removing plaque
- Advise patients who develop mucositis to:
  - Choose foods that are easy to chew and swallow
  - Take small bites of food, chew slowly, and sip liquids with meals
  - Encourage soft, moist foods such as cooked cereals, mashed potatoes, and scrambled eggs
  - For trouble swallowing, soften food with gravies, sauces, broths, yogurt, or other bland liquids
  - Avoid sharp, crunchy foods; hot, spicy, or highly acidic foods (eg, citrus fruits and juices); sugary foods; toothpicks; tobacco products; alcoholic drinks

Therapy Monitoring

1. *Weekly:* CBC with differential, serum electrolytes, calcium, and magnesium. Weekly follow-up recommended during therapy with attention to signs and symptoms of dehydration because supplemental hydration and nutritional support are often required
2. *Every 4–6 months:* Thyroid function studies

Treatment Modifications

Adverse Event	Dose Modification
Creatinine clearance <50 mL/min (<0.83 mL/s)	Ineligible for therapy
ANC <1000/mm^3 *or* platelets <75,000/mm^3 at time of chemotherapy administration	Delay chemotherapy until ANC >1000/mm^3 *and* platelets >75,000/mm^3
G ≥2 neurotoxicity	Hold carboplatin until neurotoxicity resolves to G ≤1
G3/4 neurotoxicity	Discontinue carboplatin
G ≥2 diarrhea (4–6 stools/day > baseline)	Delay until diarrhea resolves to baseline
G ≥2 mucositis	Delay chemotherapy until toxicity resolves to G ≤1
G ≥2 nonhematologic toxicity	

CONCOMITANT CHEMORADIATION
HEAD AND NECK CANCER REGIMEN: CISPLATIN WITH RADIATION THERAPY

Forastiere AA et al. N Engl J Med 2003;349:2091–2098

Pretreatment: Consider dental evaluation, percutaneous feeding tube, and nutrition evaluation

Chemoradiation

Hydration before, during, and after cisplatin administration ± mannitol:
- *Pre-cisplatin hydration* with 1000 mL 0.9% sodium chloride injection (0.9% NS); administer intravenously with potassium and magnesium supplementation as needed based on pretreatment laboratory results
- *Mannitol diuresis:* May be given to patients who have received adequate hydration. A dose of **mannitol** 12.5–25 g may be administered by intravenous injection or a short infusion before or during cisplatin administration, or prepared as an admixture with cisplatin. Continued intravenous hydration is essential
- *Continued mannitol diuresis:* In an inpatient or day-hospital setting, one may administer additional mannitol in the form of an intravenous infusion: **mannitol** 10–40 g; administer intravenously over 1–4 hours. This can be done either during or immediately after cisplatin, but requires maintenance of adequate intravenously administered fluids during and for hours after mannitol administration
- *Post-cisplatin hydration* with ≥1000 mL 0.9% NS; administer intravenously with potassium and magnesium supplementation as needed based on measured values

Cisplatin 100 mg/m^2; administer intravenously in 50–1000 mL 0.9% NS over 60 minutes on day 1, every 3 weeks for 3 cycles during radiation (total dosage/cycle = 100 mg/m^2)
Radiotherapy 70 Gy given in 35 fractions of 2 Gy/fraction over 7 weeks to the primary tumor and clinically positive nodes; 50 Gy in fractions of 2 Gy to the entire neck

Supportive Care
Antiemetic prophylaxis
Emetogenic potential on days with cisplatin is **HIGH**. *Potential for delayed symptoms*
See Chapter 42 for antiemetic recommendations

Hematopoietic growth factor (CSF) prophylaxis
Primary prophylaxis is **NOT** *indicated*
See Chapter 43 for more information

Antimicrobial prophylaxis
Risk of fever and neutropenia is **LOW**
  Antimicrobial primary prophylaxis to be considered:
  - Antibacterial—not indicated
  - Antifungal—not indicated
  - Antiviral—not indicated unless patient previously had an episode of HSV

Oral care
Risk of mucositis/stomatitis is **HIGH**
  General advice:
  - Encourage patients to maintain intake of nonalcoholic fluids
  - Evaluate patients for oral pain and provide analgesic medications
  - Consider histamine (H$_2$-subtype) receptor antagonists (eg, ranitidine, famotidine), or a proton pump inhibitor for epigastric pain
  - *Lactobacillus* sp.–containing probiotics may be beneficial in preventing diarrhea

  Patients with intact oral mucosa:
  - Clean the mouth, tongue, and gums by brushing after every meal and at bedtime with an ultra-soft toothbrush with fluoride toothpaste
  - Floss teeth gently every day unless contraindicated. If gums bleed and hurt, avoid bleeding or sore areas, but floss other teeth
  - Patients may use saline or commercial bland, nonalcoholic rinses
    - Do not use mouthwashes that contain alcohols

  If mucositis or stomatitis is present:
  - Keep the mouth moist utilizing water, ice chips, sugarless gum, sugar-free hard candies, or a saliva substitute
  - Rinse mouth several times a day to remove debris
    - Use a solution of ¼ teaspoon (1.25 g) each of baking soda and table salt (sodium chloride) in 1 quart (~950 mL) of warm water. Follow with a plain water rinse
    - Do not use mouthwashes that contain alcohols

(continued)

(continued)

- Foam-tipped swabs (eg, Toothettes) are useful in moisturizing oral mucosa, but ineffective for cleansing teeth and removing plaque
- Advise patients who develop mucositis to:
  - Choose foods that are easy to chew and swallow
  - Take small bites of food, chew slowly, and sip liquids with meals
  - Encourage soft, moist foods such as cooked cereals, mashed potatoes, and scrambled eggs
  - For trouble swallowing, soften food with gravies, sauces, broths, yogurt, or other bland liquids
  - Avoid sharp, crunchy foods; hot, spicy, or highly acidic foods (eg, citrus fruits and juices); sugary foods; toothpicks; tobacco products; alcoholic drinks

Induction Chemotherapy Followed by Radiotherapy

Cisplatin 100 mg/m²; administer intravenously in 50–1000 mL 0.9% NS over 60 minutes on day 1, every 3 weeks for 3 cycles (total dosage/cycle = 100 mg/m²), *followed by:*
Fluorouracil 1000 mg/m² per day; administer in 50–1000 mL 0.9% NS or D5W by continuous intravenous infusion over 24 hours for 5 consecutive days on days 1–5, every 3 weeks for 3 cycles (total dosage/cycle = 5000 mg/m²)
After 2 cycles of cisplatin + fluorouracil, evaluate extent of response and disease status in the neck with indirect laryngoscopy and CT imaging of the neck
- If evaluation reveals a complete or partial response of the primary tumor and no sign of progression in the neck, a third course of cisplatin plus fluorouracil is given, followed by radiotherapy
- If evaluation reveals less than partial response of the primary tumor or with progression in the neck, laryngectomy followed by adjuvant radiotherapy is recommended
Radiotherapy, 70 Gy given in 35 fractions of 2 Gy/fraction over 7 weeks to the primary tumor and clinically positive nodes; 50 Gy in fractions of 2 Gy to the entire neck

Surgery
Patients with either a single lymph node ≥3 cm or with multiple lymph node metastases on initial clinical staging of the neck should undergo neck dissection 8 weeks after completing radiotherapy. Laryngectomy should be performed in patients who had histologically proven persistent or recurrent carcinoma after the completion of treatment, or who had an inadequate response after 2 courses of induction chemotherapy

Supportive Care
Antiemetic prophylaxis
Emetogenic potential on days with cisplatin is **HIGH**. *Potential for delayed symptoms*
Emetogenic potential on days with fluorouracil alone is **LOW**
See Chapter 42 for antiemetic recommendations

Hematopoietic growth factor (CSF) prophylaxis
Primary prophylaxis is **NOT** *indicated*
See Chapter 43 for more information

Antimicrobial prophylaxis
Risk of fever and neutropenia is **LOW**
  Antimicrobial primary prophylaxis to be considered:
- Antibacterial—not indicated
- Antifungal—not indicated
- Antiviral—not indicated unless patient previously had an episode of HSV

Oral care
Risk of mucositis/stomatitis is **HIGH**
  General advice:
- Encourage patients to maintain intake of nonalcoholic fluids
- Evaluate patients for oral pain and provide analgesic medications
- Consider histamine (H₂-subtype) receptor antagonists (eg, ranitidine, famotidine), or a proton pump inhibitor for epigastric pain
- *Lactobacillus* sp.—containing probiotics may be beneficial in preventing diarrhea
  Patients with intact oral mucosa:
- Clean the mouth, tongue, and gums by brushing after every meal and at bedtime with an ultra-soft toothbrush with fluoride toothpaste
- Floss teeth gently every day unless contraindicated. If gums bleed and hurt, avoid bleeding or sore areas, but floss other teeth
- Patients may use saline or commercial bland, nonalcoholic rinses
  - Do not use mouthwashes that contain alcohols

(continued)

(*continued*)

If mucositis or stomatitis is present:
- Keep the mouth moist utilizing water, ice chips, sugarless gum, sugar-free hard candies, or a saliva substitute
- Rinse mouth several times a day to remove debris
  - Use a solution of ¼ teaspoon (1.25 g) each of baking soda and table salt (sodium chloride) in 1 quart (~950 mL) of warm water. Follow with a plain water rinse
  - Do not use mouthwashes that contain alcohols
- Foam-tipped swabs (eg, Toothettes) are useful in moisturizing oral mucosa, but ineffective for cleansing teeth and removing plaque
- Advise patients who develop mucositis to:
  - Choose foods that are easy to chew and swallow
  - Take small bites of food, chew slowly, and sip liquids with meals
  - Encourage soft, moist foods such as cooked cereals, mashed potatoes, and scrambled eggs
  - For trouble swallowing, soften food with gravies, sauces, broths, yogurt, or other bland liquids
  - Avoid sharp, crunchy foods; hot, spicy, or highly acidic foods (eg, citrus fruits and juices); sugary foods; toothpicks; tobacco products; alcoholic drinks

Patient Population Studied

A study of 547 patients with biopsy-proven, previously untreated, stage III or IV squamous cell carcinoma of the larynx for whom surgical treatment would require total laryngectomy. Excluded were patients with large T4 tumors, defined as tumors penetrating through the cartilage or extending >1 cm into the base of tongue, and patients with a stage T1 primary tumor. Karnofsky performance score of ≥60 and adequate organ function were required

Efficacy

	Induction Chemotherapy (Cisplatin + Fluorouracil) → RT (N = 168)	Radiotherapy Alone (N = 156)	Chemoradiation (Cisplatin + RT) (N = 171)
Larynx Preservation Rate			
At 2 years	84%	67%	72%
Estimated Laryngectomy-free Survival			
At 2 years	59%	53%	66%
At 5 years	43%	38%	45%
Estimated Overall Survival			
At 2 years	76%	75%	74%
At 5 years	55%	56%	54%
Estimated Disease-free Survival			
At 2 years	52%	44%	61%
At 5 years	38%	27%	36%

Toxicity

	G3/4 Toxicity					
	Induction Chemotherapy (Cisplatin + Fluorouracil) → RT (N = 168)		Radiotherapy Alone (N = 156)		Chemoradiation (Cisplatin + RT) (N = 171)	
	% G3	% G4	% G3	% G4	% G3	% G4
Hematologic	26	26	8	6.5	37	10
Infection	2.5	2.5	1	—	4	—
Mucositis	16	4	23	1	37	5
Pharyngeal/esophageal	—	—	19	—	35	—
Laryngeal	—	—	13	0.5	17	1
Radiation dermatitis	—	—	10	—	6	1
Nausea/vomiting	12	2	—	—	16	1
Renal/genitourinary	2	—	1	—	3.5	0.5
Neurologic	2.5	0.5	—	—	5	0.5
Other	12	4	10	1	34	6.5
Overall maximal	37	29	42	8	58	19

Note: Deaths caused by treatment occurred in 3% of the group assigned to induction cisplatin plus fluorouracil followed by radiotherapy, 3% of the group assigned to RT alone, and 5% percent of the group assigned to radiotherapy with concurrent cisplatin

Therapy Monitoring

1. *Day 1 of each cycle:* Medical history and physical exam, CBC with differential, LFTs, electrolytes, BUN, and creatinine
2. *Posttreatment reevaluation:* 8 weeks after the completion of therapy by examination of the head and neck and CT imaging. If persistent disease is suspected, perform the examination while the patient is under anesthesia so that direct laryngoscopy can be performed
3. *Scheduled follow-up visits:* Complete examination of the head and neck, with evaluation for late toxicity

Dose Modification

Note: It is anticipated that radiation therapy will continue despite the development of significant mucositis and/or myelosuppression

Adverse Event	Dose Modification
G3/4 hematologic toxicity	Hold chemotherapy up to 3 weeks until toxicity resolves to G ≤1. If toxicity has not resolved to G ≤1 within 3 weeks, do not administer next cycle
G3/4 nonhematologic toxicity other than alopecia, fatigue, malaise, and nail changes (exceptions: neurotoxicity, ototoxicity, and mucositis as detailed below)	
G3/4 neurotoxicity or ototoxicity	Discontinue chemotherapy
G4 mucositis	

CONCOMITANT CHEMORADIATION

HEAD AND NECK CANCER REGIMEN: CETUXIMAB + RADIATION

Bonner JA et al. N Engl J Med 2006;354:567–578

Pretreatment: Consider dental evaluation, percutaneous feeding tube, and nutrition evaluation
Premedication:

Diphenhydramine 50 mg (or an equivalent [H$_1$] antihistamine); administer by intravenous injection or as a short infusion 30 minutes prior to cetuximab administration
Note: Severe infusion reactions can occur with the administration of cetuximab. Approximately 90% of severe reactions were associated with the first infusion despite the use of prophylactic antihistamines

Initial dose:

Cetuximab 400 mg/m^2; administer intravenously over 120 minutes (maximum infusion rate = 5 mL [10 mg] per min) 1 week prior to radiation therapy

Maintenance doses:

Cetuximab 250 mg/m^2 per dose; administer intravenously over 60 minutes (maximum infusion rate = 5 mL [10 mg] per min), weekly ± **radiation**
Note: If administering radiation, administer cetuximab weekly for the duration of radiation

Radiation Regimens Used in the Randomized Trial

Regimen	Total Radiation Dose	Once-Daily Fractions	Twice-Daily Fractions
Once daily	70.0 Gy 35 fractions	2.0 Gy/fraction 5 fractions/week 7 weeks	Not applicable
Twice daily	72.0–76.8 Gy 60–64 fractions	Not applicable	1.2 Gy/fraction; 10 fractions/week for 6.0–6.5 weeks
Concomitant boost	72.0 Gy 42 fractions	32.4 Gy 1.8 Gy/fraction 5 fractions/week for 3.6 weeks	*Morning dose:* 21.6 Gy; 1.8 Gy/fraction; 5 fractions/week; 2.4 weeks *Afternoon dose:* 18.0 Gy; 1.5 Gy/fraction; 5 fractions/week; 2.4 weeks

Supportive Care
Antiemetic prophylaxis
Emetogenic potential with cetuximab is **MINIMAL**
See Chapter 42 for antiemetic recommendations

Hematopoietic growth factor (CSF) prophylaxis
Primary prophylaxis is **NOT** *indicated*
See Chapter 43 for more information

Antimicrobial prophylaxis
Risk of fever and neutropenia is **LOW**
  Antimicrobial primary prophylaxis to be considered:
  • Antibacterial—not indicated
  • Antifungal—not indicated
  • Antiviral—not indicated unless patient previously had an episode of HSV

Oral care
Risk of mucositis/stomatitis is **HIGH**
  General advice:
  • Encourage patients to maintain intake of nonalcoholic fluids
  • Evaluate patients for oral pain and provide analgesic medications
  • Consider histamine (H$_2$-subtype) receptor antagonists (eg, ranitidine, famotidine), or a proton pump inhibitor for epigastric pain
  • *Lactobacillus* sp.–containing probiotics may be beneficial in preventing diarrhea

(continued)

Patient Population Studied

A study of 424 patients with stage III or IV nonmetastatic measurable squamous cell carcinoma of the oropharynx, hypopharynx, or larynx who were randomly assigned to receive high-dose radiotherapy alone (n = 213) or high-dose radiotherapy plus cetuximab (n = 211)

Efficacy (N = 211)

	Radiotherapy Alone (n = 213)	Radiotherapy Plus Cetuximab (n = 211)
Locoregional Control		
Median duration (months)	14.9	24.4
Median Duration of Locoregional Control According to Site (Months)		
Oropharynx	23	49
Larynx	11.9	12.9
Hypopharynx	10.3	12.5
Median Duration of Locoregional Control According to Stage		
Stage III	16.2	38.9
Stage IV	13.5	20.9
Progression-Free Survival		
Median duration (months)	12.4	17.1
Rate at 2 years (%)	37	46
Overall Survival (OS)		
Median duration (months)	29.3	49
Median Duration of OS According to Site		
Oropharynx	30.3	>66
Larynx	31.6	32.8
Hypopharynx	13.5	13.7

(continued)

(continued)

Patients with intact oral mucosa:
- Clean the mouth, tongue, and gums by brushing after every meal and at bedtime with an ultra-soft toothbrush with fluoride toothpaste
- Floss teeth gently every day unless contraindicated. If gums bleed and hurt, avoid bleeding or sore areas, but floss other teeth
- Patients may use saline or commercial bland, nonalcoholic rinses
  - Do not use mouthwashes that contain alcohols

If mucositis or stomatitis is present:
- Keep the mouth moist utilizing water, ice chips, sugarless gum, sugar-free hard candies, or a saliva substitute
- Rinse mouth several times a day to remove debris
  - Use a solution of ¼ teaspoon (1.25 g) each of baking soda and table salt (sodium chloride) in 1 quart (~950 mL) of warm water. Follow with a plain water rinse
  - Do not use mouthwashes that contain alcohols
- Foam-tipped swabs (eg, Toothettes) are useful in moisturizing oral mucosa, but ineffective for cleansing teeth and removing plaque
- Advise patients who develop mucositis to:
  - Choose foods that are easy to chew and swallow
  - Take small bites of food, chew slowly, and sip liquids with meals
  - Encourage soft, moist foods such as cooked cereals, mashed potatoes, and scrambled eggs
  - For trouble swallowing, soften food with gravies, sauces, broths, yogurt, or other bland liquids
  - Avoid sharp, crunchy foods; hot, spicy, or highly acidic foods (eg, citrus fruits and juices); sugary foods; toothpicks; tobacco products; alcoholic drinks

Efficacy (N = 211) *(continued)*

Median Duration of OS According to Stage

Stage III	42.9	55.2
Stage IV	24.2	47.4

Median Duration of OS According to Radiotherapy Regimen (Months)

Once daily	15.3	18.9
Twice daily	53.3	58.9
Concomitant boost	31	>66

Toxicity (N = 208)

Adverse Event	Radiotherapy Alone (N = 212)		Radiotherapy Plus Cetuximab (N = 208)	
	% All Grades	% G3–5	% All Grades	% G3–5
Mucositis	94	52	93	56
Acneiform rash*	10	1	87	17
Radiation dermatitis	90	18	86	23
Weight loss	72	7	84	11
Xerostomia	71	3	72	5
Dysphagia	63	30	65	26
Asthenia	49	5	56	4
Nausea	37	2	49	2
Constipation	30	5	35	5
Taste perversion	28	0	29	0
Vomiting	23	4	29	2
Pain	28	7	28	6
Anorexia	23	2	27	2
Fever	13	1	26	1
Pharyngitis	19	4	26	3

Toxicity (N = 208) *(continued)*

Adverse Event	Radiotherapy Alone (N = 212)		Radiotherapy Plus Cetuximab (N = 208)	
	% All Grades	% G3–5	% All Grades	% G3–5
Dehydration	19	8	25	6
Oral candidiasis	22	0	20	0
Coughing	19	0	20	<1
Voice alteration	22	0	19	2
Diarrhea	13	1	19	2
Headache	8	<1	19	<1
Pruritus	4	0	16	0
Infusion reaction*	2	0	15	3
Insomnia	14	0	15	0
Dyspepsia	9	1	14	0
Increased sputum	15	1	13	<1
Infection	9	1	13	1
Anxiety	9	1	11	<1
Chills	5	0	11	0
Anemia	13	6	3	1

*With the exception of acneiform rash and infusion-related events, the incidence rates of G3–5 reactions were similar in the 2 treatment groups

Note: Four patients discontinued cetuximab because of hypersensitivity reactions after the test dose or first dose

Dose Modification

Infusion Reaction

Severity	Cetuximab Dosage
G1/2	Reduce dosage by 50%
G3/4	Discontinue cetuximab

Severe Acneiform Rash*

Improvement		Subsequent Treatment Modifications by Outcome	
		No Improvement	
First occurrence	Delay cetuximab treatment for 1–2 weeks	Resume with cetuximab 250 mg/m² weekly	Discontinue cetuximab
Second occurrence		Resume with cetuximab 200 mg/m² weekly	
Third occurrence		Resume with cetuximab 150 mg/m² weekly	
Fourth occurrence		Discontinue cetuximab	

*In patients with mild and moderate skin toxicity, treatment should continue without dose modification

Therapy Monitoring

Weekly: CBC with differential, serum electrolytes, calcium, and magnesium weekly during radiation

Notes

Indications:
• Cetuximab, in combination with radiation therapy, is indicated for the treatment of locally or regional advanced squamous cell carcinoma of the head and neck

Bonner JA et al. N Engl J Med 2006;354:567–578

• Cetuximab as a single agent is indicated for the treatment of patients with recurrent or metastatic squamous cell carcinoma of the head and neck after prior platinum-based therapy has failed

Trigo J et al. Proc Am Soc Clin Oncol 2004;23:488s [abstract 5502]

• Evaluated the efficacy of cetuximab monotherapy in 103 patients with platinum-refractory, recurrent, or metastatic squamous cell carcinoma of the head and neck in a multicenter phase 2 study. An initial dose of cetuximab 400 mg/m² was followed by cetuximab 250 mg/m² weekly, until disease progression, with an option to switch to cetuximab plus the same platinum agent on which patients' disease had previously progressed after disease progression occurred with cetuximab monotherapy. Drug-related adverse events in >10% of patients included skin rash/acne 80% (1% G3), fatigue 24% (4% G3), fever/chills 19% (2% G3), nail changes 15% (all G1/2), and nausea 13% (1% G3). There was 1 treatment-related death as a result of a hypersensitivity reaction in a patient for whom mechanical ventilation was not suitable. Preliminary efficacy data were as follows: 5 CR, 12 PR, 38 SD, 47 PD, and 1 not assessable, for an overall objective response rate of 16.5% (95% CI, 9.9–25.1%). The disease control rate was 53.4% (95% CI, 43.3–63.3%). Median TTP and median survival were 85 days and 175 days, respectively

LOCALLY ADVANCED • INDUCTION CHEMOTHERAPY FOLLOWED BY CHEMORADIATION

HEAD AND NECK CANCER REGIMEN: DOCETAXEL + CISPLATIN + FLUOROURACIL (TPF) *OR* CISPLATIN + FLUOROURACIL (PF) FOLLOWED BY RADIATION THERAPY

Posner MR et al. N Engl J Med 2007;357:1705–1715

Pretreatment: Consider dental evaluation, percutaneous feeding tube, and nutrition evaluation

Induction Chemotherapy (Three Cycles of TPF or PF)

Hydration before, during, and after cisplatin administration ± mannitol:
- *Pre-cisplatin hydration* with 1000 mL 0.9% sodium chloride injection (0.9% NS); administer intravenously with potassium and magnesium supplementation as needed based on pretreatment laboratory results
- *Mannitol diuresis:* May be given to patients who have received adequate hydration. A dose of **mannitol** 12.5–25 g may be administered by intravenous injection or a short intravenous infusion before or during cisplatin administration, or prepared as an admixture with cisplatin. Continued intravenous hydration is essential
- *Continued mannitol diuresis:* In an inpatient or day-hospital setting, one may administer additional mannitol in the form of an intravenous infusion: **mannitol** 10–40 g; administer intravenously over 1–4 hours. This can be done either during or immediately after cisplatin, but requires maintenance of adequate intravenously administered fluids during and for hours after mannitol administration
- *Post-cisplatin hydration* with ≥1000 mL 0.9% NS; administer intravenously with potassium and magnesium supplementation as needed based on measured values

TPF induction chemotherapy:
Dexamethasone 8 mg/dose; administer orally or intravenously twice daily for 6 doses starting the day before docetaxel administration (total dose/cycle = 48 mg) as prophylaxis against docetaxel-related hypersensitivity reactions, skin toxic effects, and fluid retention
Docetaxel 75 mg/m²; administer intravenously in a volume of 0.9% NS or 5% dextrose injection (D5W) sufficient to produce a docetaxel concentration within the range 0.3–0.74 mg/mL over 60 minutes on day 1, every 21 days for 3 cycles (total dosage/cycle = 75 mg/m²), *followed by:*
Cisplatin 100 mg/m²; administer intravenously in 50–1000 mL 0.9% NS over 0.5–3 hours on day 1, every 21 days for 3 cycles (total dosage/cycle = 100 mg/m²), *followed by:*
Fluorouracil 1000 mg/m² per day; administer in 50–1000 mL 0.9% NS or D5W by continuous intravenous infusion over 24 hours for 4 consecutive days, on days 1–4, every 21 days for 3 cycles (total dosage/cycle = 4000 mg/m²)
Prophylactic antibiotics days 5–14

Or

PF induction chemotherapy:
Cisplatin 100 mg/m²; administer intravenously in 50–1000 mL 0.9% NS over 0.5–3 hours on day 1, every 21 days for 3 cycles (total dosage/cycle = 100 mg/m²), *followed by*
Fluorouracil 1000 mg/m² per day; administer intravenously in 50–1000 mL 0.9% NS or D5W by continuous infusion over 24 hours for 5 consecutive days, days 1–5, every 21 days for 3 cycles (total dosage/cycle = 5000 mg/m²)

Note: Induction chemotherapy is discontinued in case of (a) disease progression; (b) a reduction in tumor after 2 cycles <25% (WHO) or <30% (RECIST); or (c) unacceptable toxicity

Supportive Care for Patients Receiving Either TPF or PF Chemotherapies
Antiemetic prophylaxis
Emetogenic potential on day 1 is **HIGH**. *Potential for delayed symptoms*
Emetogenic potential on days with fluorouracil alone is **LOW**
See Chapter 42 for antiemetic recommendations

Diarrhea management
Latent or delayed-onset diarrhea*:
Loperamide 4 mg orally initially after the first loose or liquid stool, *then*
Loperamide 2 mg orally every 2 hours during waking hours, *plus*
Loperamide 4 mg orally every 4 hours during hours of sleep
- Continue for at least 12 hours after diarrhea resolves
- Recurrent diarrhea after a 12-hour diarrhea-free interval is treated as a new episode
- Rehydrate orally with fluids and electrolytes during a diarrheal episode
- If a patient develops blood or mucus in stool, dehydration, or hemodynamic instability, or if diarrhea persists >48 hours despite loperamide, stop loperamide and hospitalize the patient for IV hydration

(continued)

(*continued*)

Persistent diarrhea:
   Octreotide 100–150 mcg subcutaneously 3 times daily. Maximum total daily dose is 1500 mcg
Antibiotic therapy during latent or delayed-onset diarrhea:
• A fluoroquinolone (eg, **ciprofloxacin** 500 mg orally every 12 hours) if absolute neutrophil count <500/mm^3 with or without accompanying fever in association with diarrhea
• Antibiotics should also be administered if patient is hospitalized with prolonged diarrhea and should be continued until diarrhea resolves

*Rothenberg ML et al. J Clin Oncol 2001;19:3801–3807
Abigerges D et al. J Natl Cancer Inst 1994;86:446–449
Wadler S et al. J Clin Oncol 1998;16:3169–3178

Oral care
*Risk of mucositis/stomatitis is **HIGH***
   General advice:
   • Encourage patients to maintain intake of nonalcoholic fluids
   • Evaluate patients for oral pain and provide analgesic medications
   • Consider histamine (H$_2$-subtype) receptor antagonists (eg, ranitidine, famotidine), or a proton pump inhibitor for epigastric pain
   • *Lactobacillus* sp.–containing probiotics may be beneficial in preventing diarrhea

   Patients with intact oral mucosa:
   • Clean the mouth, tongue, and gums by brushing after every meal and at bedtime with an ultra-soft toothbrush with fluoride toothpaste
   • Floss teeth gently every day unless contraindicated. If gums bleed and hurt, avoid bleeding or sore areas, but floss other teeth
   • Patients may use saline or commercial bland, nonalcoholic rinses
      ▪ Do not use mouthwashes that contain alcohols

   If mucositis or stomatitis is present:
   • Keep the mouth moist utilizing water, ice chips, sugarless gum, sugar-free hard candies, or a saliva substitute
   • Rinse mouth several times a day to remove debris
      ▪ Use a solution of ¼ teaspoon (1.25 g) each of baking soda and table salt (sodium chloride) in 1 quart (~950 mL) of warm water. Follow with a plain water rinse
      ▪ Do not use mouthwashes that contain alcohols
   • Foam-tipped swabs (eg, Toothettes) are useful in moisturizing oral mucosa, but ineffective for cleansing teeth and removing plaque
   • Advise patients who develop mucositis to:
      ▪ Choose foods that are easy to chew and swallow
      ▪ Take small bites of food, chew slowly, and sip liquids with meals
      ▪ Encourage soft, moist foods such as cooked cereals, mashed potatoes, and scrambled eggs
      ▪ For trouble swallowing, soften food with gravies, sauces, broths, yogurt, or other bland liquids
      ▪ Avoid sharp, crunchy foods; hot, spicy, or highly acidic foods (eg, citrus fruits and juices); sugary foods; toothpicks; tobacco products; alcoholic drinks

For Patients Who Receive TPF Chemotherapy
Hematopoietic growth factor (CSF) prophylaxis
*Primary prophylaxis is indicated with **1** of the following:*
   Filgrastim (G-CSF) 5 mcg/kg per day by subcutaneous injection, *or*
   Pegfilgrastim (pegylated filgrastim) 6 mg/0.6 mL by subcutaneous injection for 1 dose
   • Begin use from 24–72 hours after myelosuppressive chemotherapy is completed
See Chapter 43 for more information

Antimicrobial prophylaxis
*Risk of fever and neutropenia is **INTERMEDIATE***
   Antimicrobial primary prophylaxis to be considered:
   • Antibacterial—consider a fluoroquinolone or no prophylaxis
      ▪ Posner et al gave antibiotic prophylaxis to patients who received the TPF regimen for 10 days starting on cycle day 5. Choice of antibiotics was not specified
   • Antifungal—consider use during neutropenia and for anticipated mucositis
   • Antiviral—antiherpes antivirals (eg, acyclovir)

For Patients Who Receive PF Chemotherapy
Hematopoietic growth factor (CSF) prophylaxis
*Primary prophylaxis is **NOT** indicated*
See Chapter 43 for more information

(*continued*)

(*continued*)

Antimicrobial prophylaxis
Risk of fever and neutropenia is **LOW**
   Antimicrobial primary prophylaxis to be considered:
   • Antibacterial—not indicated
      ▪ Posner et al gave antibiotic prophylaxis only to patients who received the TPF regimen: patients who received the PF regimen did not receive antimicrobial primary prophylaxis
   • Antifungal—not indicated
   • Antiviral—not indicated unless patient previously had an episode of HSV

- - -

Chemoradiation

(Follows Induction Chemotherapy)

Seven weeks of chemoradiation: Starting between days 22 and 56 of induction chemotherapy cycle 3 (3–8 weeks after the start of cycle 3 of induction chemotherapy)

Radiotherapy:
70–74 Gy to primary tumor in 5 daily fractions/week of 2 Gy/fraction
At least 50 Gy to uninvolved lymph nodes
At least 60–74 Gy to involved lymph nodes
Concurrent chemotherapy:
Carboplatin* (calculated dose) AUC = 1.5 mg/mL · min per dose; administer intravenously diluted to concentrations as low as 0.5 mg/mL with either D5W or 0.9% NS over 1 hour, once weekly for up to 7 doses during the course of radiotherapy (total dose/week calculated to produce a target AUC = 1.5 mg/mL × min)

*Carboplatin dose is based on a formula described by Calvert et al. to achieve a target area under the plasma concentration versus time curve (AUC)

$$\text{Total Carboplatin Dose (mg)} = (\text{target AUC}) \times (\text{GFR} + 25)$$

In practice, creatinine clearance (CrCl) is used in place of glomerular filtration rate (GFR). CrCl can be estimated from the equation of Cockcroft and Gault, thus:

$$\text{For males, CrCl} = \frac{(140 - \text{age[years]}) \times (\text{body weight [kg]})}{72 \times (\text{serum creatinine [mg/dL]})}$$

$$\text{For females, CrCl} = \frac{(140 - \text{age[years]}) \times (\text{body weight [kg]})}{72 \times (\text{serum creatinine [mg/dL]})} \times 0.85$$

Calvert AH et al. J Clin Oncol 1989;7:1748–1756
Cockcroft DW , Gault MH. Nephron 1976;16:31–41
Jodrell DI et al. J Clin Oncol 1992;10:520–528
Sorensen BT et al. Cancer Chemother Pharmacol 1991;28:397–401

Note: On October 8, 2010, the U.S. FDA identified a potential safety issue with carboplatin dosing based on recent changes in the measurement of serum creatinine. By the end of 2010, all clinical laboratories in the United States were required to use the standardized Isotope Dilution Mass Spectrometry (IDMS) method to measure serum creatinine, which can result in an overestimation of the GFR in some patients with normal renal function. A carboplatin dose calculated with an IDMS-measured serum creatinine result using the Calvert formula can exceed an expected exposure (AUC) and result in increased drug-related toxicity
• Provided actual GFR measurements are made to assess renal function, carboplatin can be safely dosed according to the Calvert formula described in product labeling
• If GFR (or creatinine clearance) is estimated based on serum creatinine measurements by the IDMS method, the FDA recommended for patients with normal renal function capping an estimated GFR at 125 mL/min for any targeted AUC value. No greater estimated GFR values should be used
U.S. FDA. Carboplatin dosing. [online] Available from: http://www.fda.gov/AboutFDA/CentersOffices/OfficeofMedicalProductsandTobacco/CDER/ucm228974.htm [accessed February 26, 2014]

Supportive Care
Antiemetic prophylaxis
Emetogenic potential on days when carboplatin is administered is **MODERATE**
See Chapter 42 for antiemetic recommendations

(*continued*)

(*continued*)

Hematopoietic growth factor (CSF) prophylaxis
Primary prophylaxis is **NOT** indicated
See Chapter 43 for more information

Antimicrobial prophylaxis
Risk of fever and neutropenia is **LOW**
   Antimicrobial primary prophylaxis to be considered:
   • Antibacterial—not indicated
   • Antifungal—not indicated
   • Antiviral—not indicated unless patient previously had an episode of HSV

Surgery
(Elective Neck Dissection)
Elective neck dissection 6–12 weeks after end of chemoradiation for patients with initial N2 disease and a partial response to induction chemotherapy, N3 disease, or residual disease after chemoradiation

Patient Population Studied

A study of 539 patients with measurable, nonmetastatic, stage III or IV, histologically proven, previously untreated squamous cell carcinoma of the oral cavity, larynx, oropharynx, or hypopharynx with a tumor deemed to be unresectable (because of tumor fixation, involvement of the nasopharynx, or fixed lymph nodes), or of low surgical curability on basis of advanced tumor stage (3 or 4) or regional node stage (2–3, except T1N2), or if a patient was a candidate for organ preservation. WHO performance status 0 or 1. Adequate organ function and age ≥18 years

Efficacy*

	TPF† (N = 255)	PF† (N = 246)	Hazard Ratio or P Value
ORR after induction chemotherapy	72%	64%	$P = 0.07$
CR rate after induction chemotherapy	17%	15%	$P = 0.66$
Median PFS, months	36	13	0.71 (0.56–0.90)
Estimated 2-year PFS	53%	42%	$P = 0.01$
Estimated 3-year PFS	49%	37%	—
Median OS, months	71	30	0.7 (0.54–0.90)
Estimated 2-year OS	67%	55%	—
Estimated 3-year OS	62%	48%	$P = 0.002$
Median OS resectable tumors, months	NR	42	$P = 0.007$
Median OS unresectable tumors, months	40	21	$P = 0.06$
Loco-regional failure	30%	38%	$P = 0.04$

CR, complete response; ORR, overall response rate; OS, overall survival; PFS, progression-free survival
*WHO Criteria
†TPF, docetaxel + cisplatin + fluorouracil; PF, cisplatin + fluorouracil

Toxicity

	TPF*	PF*
Adverse Events During Induction Chemotherapy	% G3/4 (N = 251)	% G3/4 (N = 243)
Anemia	12	9
Thrombocytopenia	4	11
Neutropenia	83	56
Febrile neutropenia	12	7
Neutropenia and infection	12	8
Mucositis	21	27
Esophagitis, dysphagia, or odynophagia	13	9
Anorexia	12	12
Nausea	14	14
Vomiting	8	10
Diarrhea	7	3
Infection	6	5
Lethargy	5	10
Adverse Events During Chemoradiation	% G3/4 N = 202	% G3/4 N = 184
Mucositis	37	38
Esophagitis, dysphagia, or odynophagia	23	24
Anorexia	11	15
Nausea	6	6
Vomiting	3	5
Diarrhea	0	2
Infection	9	7
Lethargy	6	6

*TPF, docetaxel + cisplatin + 5-fluorouracil; PF, cisplatin + 5-fluorouracil

Therapy Monitoring

1. *Pretreatment evaluation:* Medical history and tumor assessment by clinical evaluation and imaging studies
2. *Toxicity assessment:* Weekly during treatment with chemotherapy
3. *Tumor assessment:* After cycles 2 and 3; then, 6–12 weeks after chemoradiation

Dose Modification

Adverse Event	Dose Modifications
G3/4 hematologic toxicity	Hold chemotherapy up to 2 weeks until toxicity resolves to G ≤1. If toxicity does not resolve to G ≤1 within 2 weeks, then discontinue therapy
G3/4 nonhematologic toxicity other than alopecia, fatigue, malaise, and nail changes (exceptions: neurotoxicity, ototoxicity, and mucositis as detailed below)	Hold chemotherapy up to 2 weeks until toxicity resolves to G ≤1. If toxicity does not resolve to G ≤1 within 2 weeks, then discontinue therapy
G3/4 neurotoxicity or ototoxicity	Discontinue therapy
G4 mucositis and diarrhea	Discontinue therapy
Febrile neutropenia or infection	Administer filgrastim during subsequent cycles
Delay in ANC recovery beyond day 28	
G4 neutropenia ≥7 days	
ANC <2000/mm³; platelet count <100,000/mm³; or hemoglobin <10 g/dL)	Withhold start of RT
Incomplete resolution of mucositis	

LOCALLY ADVANCED • INDUCTION CHEMOTHERAPY FOLLOWED BY RADIOTHERAPY

HEAD AND NECK CANCER REGIMEN: DOCETAXEL + CISPLATIN + FLUOROURACIL (TPF) *OR* CISPLATIN + FLUOROURACIL (PF) FOLLOWED BY RADIATION THERAPY

Vermorken JB et al. N Engl J Med 2007;357:1695–1704

Pretreatment: Consider dental evaluation, percutaneous feeding tube, and nutrition evaluation

Induction Chemotherapy—Three Cycles of TPF or PF

Hydration before, during, and after cisplatin administration ± mannitol:
- *Pre-cisplatin hydration* with 1000 mL 0.9% sodium chloride injection (0.9% NS); administer intravenously with potassium and magnesium supplementation as needed based on pretreatment laboratory results
- *Mannitol diuresis:* May be given to patients who have received adequate hydration. A dose of **mannitol** 12.5–25 g may be administered by intravenous injection or a short infusion before or during cisplatin administration, or prepared as an admixture with cisplatin. Continued intravenous hydration is essential
- *Continued mannitol diuresis:* In an inpatient or day-hospital setting, one may administer additional mannitol in the form of an intravenous infusion: **mannitol** 10–40 g; administer intravenously over 1–4 hours. This can be done either during or immediately after cisplatin, but requires maintenance of adequate intravenously administered fluids during and for hours after mannitol administration
- *Post-cisplatin hydration* with ≥1000 mL 0.9% NS; administer intravenously with potassium and magnesium supplementation as needed based on measured values

Docetaxel + Cisplatin + Fluorouracil (TPF)

Premedication:
Dexamethasone 8 mg/dose; administer orally or intravenously twice daily for 6 doses starting the day before docetaxel administration (total dose/cycle = 48 mg)
- As prophylaxis against docetaxel-related hypersensitivity reactions, skin toxic effects, and fluid retention

Induction chemotherapy:
Docetaxel 75 mg/m^2; administer intravenously in a volume of 0.9% NS or 5% dextrose injection (D5W) sufficient to produce a docetaxel concentration within the range 0.3–0.74 mg/mL over 60 minutes on day 1, every 3 weeks for up to 4 cycles (total dosage/cycle = 75 mg/m^2), *followed by:*
Cisplatin 75 mg/m^2; administer intravenously in 50–1000 mL 0.9% NS over 60 minutes on day 1, every 3 weeks for up to 4 cycles (total dosage/cycle = 75 mg/m^2), *followed by:*
Fluorouracil 750 mg/m^2 per day; administer in 50–1000 mL 0.9% NS or D5W by continuous intravenous infusion over 24 hours for 5 consecutive days, on days 1–5, every 3 weeks for up to 4 cycles (total dosage/cycle = 3750 mg/m^2)

or

Cisplatin + Fluorouracil (PF)

Induction chemotherapy:
Cisplatin 100 mg/m^2; administer intravenously in 50–1000 mL 0.9% NS over 60 minutes on day 1, every 3 weeks for up to 4 cycles (total dosage/cycle = 100 mg/m^2), *followed by:*
Fluorouracil 1000 mg/m^2 per day; administer in 50–1000 mL 0.9% NS or D5W by continuous intravenous infusion over 24 hours for 5 consecutive days, on days 1–5, every 3 weeks for up to 4 cycles (total dosage/cycle = 5000 mg/m^2)

Patient Population Studied

A study of 358 patients with measurable, nonmetastatic stage III or IV, histologically or cytologically proven, previously untreated squamous cell carcinoma of the oral cavity, larynx, oropharynx, or hypopharynx, with a tumor considered to be unresectable by a multidisciplinary team. WHO performance status 0 or 1, adequate organ function, and age 18–70 years

Efficacy

	TPF* (N = 181)	PF* (N = 177)
Median progression-free survival, months	11	8.2
Estimated 3-year progression-free survival	17%	14%
Median overall survival, months	18.8	14.5
Estimated 3-year overall survival	37%	26%
Overall response rate after induction chemotherapy	68%	54%
Complete response rate after induction chemotherapy	8.5%	6.6%

*TPF, Docetaxel + cisplatin + fluorouracil; PF, cisplatin + fluorouracil

(continued)

Supportive Care for Patients Receiving Either TPF or PF Chemotherapies

Antiemetic prophylaxis
Emetogenic potential on day 1 is **HIGH**. *Potential for delayed symptoms*
Emetogenic potential on days with fluorouracil alone is **LOW**
See Chapter 42 for antiemetic recommendations

Diarrhea management
Latent or delayed-onset diarrhea*:
    Loperamide 4 mg orally initially after the first loose or liquid stool, *then*
    Loperamide 2 mg orally every 2 hours during waking hours, *plus*
    Loperamide 4 mg orally every 4 hours during hours of sleep
- Continue for at least 12 hours after diarrhea resolves
- Recurrent diarrhea after a 12-hour diarrhea-free interval is treated as a new episode
- Rehydrate orally with fluids and electrolytes during a diarrheal episode
- If a patient develops blood or mucus in stool, dehydration, or hemodynamic instability, or if diarrhea persists >48 hours despite loperamide, stop loperamide and hospitalize the patient for IV hydration

Persistent diarrhea:
    Octreotide 100–150 mcg subcutaneously 3 times daily. Maximum total daily dose is 1500 mcg

Antibiotic therapy during latent or delayed-onset diarrhea:
    A fluoroquinolone (eg, **ciprofloxacin** 500 mg orally every 12 hours) if absolute neutrophil count <500/mm^3 with or without accompanying fever in association with diarrhea
- Antibiotics should also be administered if patient is hospitalized with prolonged diarrhea and should be continued until diarrhea resolves

*Rothenberg ML et al. J Clin Oncol 2001;19:3801–3807
Abigerges D et al. J Natl Cancer Inst 1994;86:446–449
Wadler S et al. J Clin Oncol 1998;16:3169–3178

Oral care
Risk of mucositis/stomatitis is **HIGH**
  General advice:
- Encourage patients to maintain intake of nonalcoholic fluids
- Evaluate patients for oral pain and provide analgesic medications
- Consider histamine (H$_2$-subtype) receptor antagonists (eg, ranitidine, famotidine), or a proton pump inhibitor for epigastric pain
- *Lactobacillus* sp.—containing probiotics may be beneficial in preventing diarrhea

  Patients with intact oral mucosa:
- Clean the mouth, tongue, and gums by brushing after every meal and at bedtime with an ultra-soft toothbrush with fluoride toothpaste
- Floss teeth gently every day unless contraindicated. If gums bleed and hurt, avoid bleeding or sore areas, but floss other teeth
- Patients may use saline or commercial bland, nonalcoholic rinses
  - Do not use mouthwashes that contain alcohols

If mucositis or stomatitis is present:
- Keep the mouth moist utilizing water, ice chips, sugarless gum, sugar-free hard candies, or a saliva substitute
- Rinse mouth several times a day to remove debris
  - Use a solution of ¼ teaspoon (1.25 g) each of baking soda and table salt (sodium chloride) in 1 quart (~950 mL) of warm water. Follow with a plain water rinse
  - Do not use mouthwashes that contain alcohols
- Foam-tipped swabs (eg, Toothettes) are useful in moisturizing oral mucosa, but ineffective for cleansing teeth and removing plaque

(continued)

Toxicity

Adverse Events During Induction Chemotherapy	TPF* % G3/4 N = 179	PF* % G3/4 N = 173
Anemia	9.2	12.8
Thrombocytopenia	5.2	17.9
Neutropenia	76.9	52.5
Leukopenia	41.6	22.9
Febrile neutropenia	5.2	2.8
Infection	6.9	6.1
Alopecia	11.6	0
Stomatitis	4.6	11.2
Esophagitis, dysphagia, or odynophagia	0.6	0
Anorexia	0.6	3.4
Nausea	0.6	6.7
Vomiting	0.6	4.5
Diarrhea	2.9	3.4
Constipation	0	0.6
Lethargy	2.9	1.7
Weight loss	0	0.6
Gastrointestinal pain	0	0.6
Neurotoxicity	0.6	0.6
Hearing loss	0	2.8
Local toxic effect	0.6	0.6
Toxic deaths	2.3	5.5

*TPF, docetaxel + cisplatin + fluorouracil; PF, cisplatin + fluorouracil

Therapy Monitoring

1. *Day 1 of each cycle:* Medical history and physical exam, CBC with differential, LFTs, electrolytes, BUN, and creatinine
2. *At end of cycles 2 and 4:* Diagnostic imaging

(*continued*)

- Advise patients who develop mucositis to:
  - Choose foods that are easy to chew and swallow
  - Take small bites of food, chew slowly, and sip liquids with meals
  - Encourage soft, moist foods such as cooked cereals, mashed potatoes, and scrambled eggs
  - For trouble swallowing, soften food with gravies, sauces, broths, yogurt, or other bland liquids
  - Avoid sharp, crunchy foods; hot, spicy, or highly acidic foods (eg, citrus fruits and juices); sugary foods; toothpicks; tobacco products; alcoholic drinks

For Patients Who Receive TPF Chemotherapy
Hematopoietic growth factor (CSF) prophylaxis
Primary prophylaxis may be indicated.
- Particularly in patients who do not receive antibiotic prophylaxis
See Chapter 43 for more information

Antimicrobial prophylaxis
Risk of fever and neutropenia is **INTERMEDIATE**
  Antimicrobial primary prophylaxis to be considered:
- Antibacterial—consider a fluoroquinolone or no prophylaxis
  - Vermorken et al gave antibiotic prophylaxis to patients who received the TPF regimen from cycle days 5–15
- Antifungal—consider use during neutropenia and for anticipated mucositis
- Antiviral—not indicated unless patient previously had an episode of HSV

For Patients Who Receive PF Chemotherapy
Hematopoietic growth factor (CSF) prophylaxis
Primary prophylaxis is **NOT** *indicated*
See Chapter 43 for more information

Antimicrobial prophylaxis
Risk of fever and neutropenia is **LOW**
  Antimicrobial primary prophylaxis to be considered:
- Antibacterial—not indicated
  - Vermorken et al gave antibiotic prophylaxis only to patients who received the TPF regimen
- Antifungal—not indicated
- Antiviral—not indicated unless patient previously had an episode of HSV

Radiotherapy
Starting within 4–7 weeks after completion of chemotherapy
- Conventional fractionation (66–70 Gy) *or*
- Accelerated irradiation (70 Gy]) *or*
- Hyperfractionated irradiation (74 Gy)

Surgery
Elective neck dissection can be considered before radiotherapy and again 3 months after the completion of radiotherapy

Dose Modification

Adverse Event	Dose Modification
G3/4 hematologic toxicity	Hold chemotherapy up to 2 weeks until toxicity resolves to G ≤1. If toxicity has not resolved to G ≤1 within 2 weeks, discontinue therapy
G3/4 nonhematologic toxicity other than alopecia, fatigue, malaise, and nail changes (exceptions: neurotoxicity, ototoxicity and mucositis as detailed below)	
G3/4 neurotoxicity or ototoxicity	Discontinue therapy
G4 mucositis and diarrhea	
Febrile neutropenia or infection	Administer filgrastim in subsequent cycles
Delay in ANC recovery beyond day 28	
G4 neutropenia ≥7 days	
ANC <2000/mm³, platelet count <100,000/mm³, or hemoglobin <10 g/dL	Withhold start of RT
Incomplete resolution of mucositis	

POSTOPERATIVE CHEMORADIATION

HEAD AND NECK CANCER REGIMEN: POSTOPERATIVE CHEMORADIATION WITH CISPLATIN

Bernier J et al. N Engl J Med 2004;350:1945–1952
Cooper JS et al. N Engl J Med 2004;350:1937–1944

Pretreatment: Consider dental evaluation, percutaneous feeding tube, and nutrition evaluation

Chemoradiation

Note: Among high-risk patients with resected head and neck cancer, the chemoradiation therapy regimen described significantly improved the rates of local and regional control and disease-free survival. However, compared to RT alone, chemoradiation is associated with a substantial increase in adverse effects

Hydration before, during, and after cisplatin administration ± mannitol:

- *Pre-cisplatin hydration* with 1000 mL 0.9% sodium chloride injection (0.9% NS); administer intravenously with potassium and magnesium supplementation as needed based on pretreatment laboratory results

- *Mannitol diuresis:* May be given to patients who have received adequate hydration. A dose of **mannitol** 12.5–25 g may be administered by intravenous injection or a short infusion before or during cisplatin administration, or prepared as an admixture with cisplatin. Continued intravenous hydration is essential

- *Continued mannitol diuresis:* In an inpatient or day-hospital setting, one may administer additional mannitol in the form of an intravenous infusion: **mannitol** 10–40 g; administer intravenously over 1–4 hours. This can be done either during or immediately after cisplatin, but requires maintenance of adequate intravenously administered fluids during and for hours after mannitol administration

- *Post-cisplatin hydration* with ≥1000 mL 0.9% NS; administer intravenously with potassium and magnesium supplementation as needed based on measured values

Cisplatin 100 mg/m²; administer intravenously in 50–1000 mL 0.9% NS over 60 minutes on day 1, every 3 weeks for 3 cycles during radiation (total dosage/cycle = 100 mg/m²)
Radiotherapy 60–66 Gy in 30–33 fractions of 2 Gy/fraction given continually over 6–6.6 weeks

Supportive Care
Antiemetic prophylaxis
Emetogenic potential on days with cisplatin is **HIGH**. *Potential for delayed symptoms*
See Chapter 42 for antiemetic recommendations

Hematopoietic growth factor (CSF) prophylaxis
Primary prophylaxis is **NOT** *indicated*
See Chapter 43 for more information

Antimicrobial prophylaxis
Risk of fever and neutropenia is **LOW**
  Antimicrobial primary prophylaxis to be considered:
  - Antibacterial—not indicated
  - Antifungal—not indicated
  - Antiviral—not indicated unless patient previously had an episode of HSV

Diarrhea management
Latent or delayed-onset diarrhea*:
  Loperamide 4 mg orally initially after the first loose or liquid stool, *then*
  Loperamide 2 mg orally every 2 hours during waking hours, *plus*
  Loperamide 4 mg orally every 4 hours during hours of sleep
  - Continue for at least 12 hours after diarrhea resolves
  - Recurrent diarrhea after a 12-hour diarrhea-free interval is treated as a new episode
  - Rehydrate orally with fluids and electrolytes during a diarrheal episode
  - If a patient develops blood or mucus in stool, dehydration, or hemodynamic instability, or if diarrhea persists >48 hours despite loperamide, stop loperamide and hospitalize the patient for IV hydration

(continued)

Patient Population Studied

EORTC 22931
A study of 334 patients with previously untreated, histologically proven, squamous cell carcinoma of the oral cavity, oropharynx, hypopharynx, or larynx with (a) tumor stage pT3 or pT4 and any nodal stage except T3N0 of the larynx with negative resection margins, (b) N2/N3 disease, (c) T1/2N1/N2 disease with extranodal spread, (d) positive section margins, (e) perineural involvement, (f) vascular involvement, or (g) oral cavity or oropharyngeal tumors with involvement of lymph nodes at levels IV or V. Adequate organ function, WHO performance status of 0–2, and age ≥18 years
RTOG 9501/Intergroup
A study of 459 patients with squamous cell carcinoma of the oral cavity, oropharynx, larynx, or hypopharynx, who underwent macroscopically complete resection but had at least 1 high-risk characteristic defined as (a) invasion of at least 2 lymph nodes, (b) extracapsular extension of nodal disease, or (c) microscopically involved mucosal margins of resection. Adequate organ function and Karnofsky performance status of ≥60 were required

Therapy Monitoring

1. *Day 1 of each cisplatin treatment:* Medical history and physical exam, CBC with differential, LFTs, electrolytes, BUN, and creatinine
2. *Posttreatment reevaluation:* 8 weeks after the completion of therapy by examination of the head and neck and CT imaging. If persistent disease is suspected, perform the examination while the patient is under anesthesia so that direct laryngoscopy can be performed
3. *Scheduled follow-up visits:* Complete examination of the head and neck, with evaluation for late toxicity

(*continued*)

Persistent diarrhea:
Octreotide 100–150 mcg subcutaneously 3 times daily. Maximum total daily dose is 1500 mcg

Antibiotic therapy during latent or delayed-onset diarrhea:
A fluoroquinolone (eg, **ciprofloxacin** 500 mg orally every 12 hours) if absolute neutrophil count <500/mm^3 with or without accompanying fever in association with diarrhea
- Antibiotics should also be administered if patient is hospitalized with prolonged diarrhea and should be continued until diarrhea resolves

*Rothenberg ML et al. J Clin Oncol 2001;19:3801–3807
Abigerges D et al. J Natl Cancer Inst 1994;86:446–449
Wadler S et al. J Clin Oncol 1998;16:3169–3178

Oral care
Risk of mucositis/stomatitis is **HIGH**
General advice:
- Encourage patients to maintain intake of nonalcoholic fluids
- Evaluate patients for oral pain and provide analgesic medications
- Consider histamine (H$_2$-subtype) receptor antagonists (eg, ranitidine, famotidine), or a proton pump inhibitor for epigastric pain
- *Lactobacillus* sp.—containing probiotics may be beneficial in preventing diarrhea

Patients with intact oral mucosa:
- Clean the mouth, tongue, and gums by brushing after every meal and at bedtime with an ultra-soft toothbrush with fluoride toothpaste
- Floss teeth gently every day unless contraindicated. If gums bleed and hurt, avoid bleeding or sore areas, but floss other teeth
- Patients may use saline or commercial bland, nonalcoholic rinses
  - Do not use mouthwashes that contain alcohols

If mucositis or stomatitis is present:
- Keep the mouth moist utilizing water, ice chips, sugarless gum, sugar-free hard candies, or a saliva substitute
- Rinse mouth several times a day to remove debris
  - Use a solution of ¼ teaspoon (1.25 g) each of baking soda and table salt (sodium chloride) in 1 quart (~950 mL) of warm water. Follow with a plain water rinse
  - Do not use mouthwashes that contain alcohols
- Foam-tipped swabs (eg, Toothettes) are useful in moisturizing oral mucosa, but ineffective for cleansing teeth and removing plaque
- Advise patients who develop mucositis to:
  - Choose foods that are easy to chew and swallow
  - Take small bites of food, chew slowly, and sip liquids with meals
  - Encourage soft, moist foods such as cooked cereals, mashed potatoes, and scrambled eggs
  - For trouble swallowing, soften food with gravies, sauces, broths, yogurt, or other bland liquids
  - Avoid sharp, crunchy foods; hot, spicy, or highly acidic foods (eg, citrus fruits and juices); sugary foods; toothpicks; tobacco products; alcoholic drinks

Dose Modification

Note: Continuity of radiotherapy should be maintained if at all possible. Keep to a minimum interruptions resulting from treatment-related adverse effects

Adverse Event	Dose Modification
On day 12 of any cycle, ANC <1000/mm^3 *or* platelet count <75,000/mm^3	Hold cisplatin until ANC >1000/mm^3 *and* platelet count >75,000/mm^3
G1/2 neurotoxicity	Reduce cisplatin dosage to 60 mg/m^2
G3/4 neurotoxicity or ototoxicity	Discontinue cisplatin
Creatinine clearance 40–50 mL/min (0.66–0.83 mL/s)	Reduce cisplatin dosage to 75 mg/m^2
Creatinine clearance <40 mL/min (<0.66 mL/s)	Discontinue cisplatin

POSTOPERATIVE CHEMORADIATION

HEAD AND NECK CANCER REGIMEN: POSTOPERATIVE CHEMORADIATION WITH CISPLATIN + FLUOROURACIL

Fietkau R et al. Proc Am Soc Clin Oncol 2006;24(18S, Part 1 of 2):281s (abstract 5507)

Chemoradiation

Hydration before, during, and after cisplatin administration:
- *Pre-cisplatin hydration* with 500–1000 mL 0.9% sodium chloride injection (0.9% NS); administer intravenously with potassium and magnesium supplementation as needed based on pretreatment laboratory results
- *Post-cisplatin hydration* with 500–1000 mL 0.9% NS; administer intravenously with potassium and magnesium supplementation as needed based on measured values

Cisplatin 20 mg/m^2 per day; administer intravenously in 50–1000 mL 0.9% NS over 60 minutes for 5 consecutive days, on days 1–5, every 4 weeks for 2 cycles during radiation (total dosage/cycle = 100 mg/m^2), *and*

Fluorouracil 600 mg/m^2 per day; administer in 50–1000 mL 0.9% NS or D5W by continuous intravenous infusion over 24 hours for 5 consecutive days, on days 1–5, every 4 weeks for 2 cycles during radiation (total dosage/cycle = 3000 mg/m^2)

Radiotherapy (50 Gy in case of pN0, 56 Gy in case of pN+ without extracapsular spread, 64 Gy in case of pN+ with extracapsular spread)

Supportive Care
Antiemetic prophylaxis
Emetogenic potential on days with cisplatin is **HIGH**. Potential for delayed symptoms
Emetogenic potential on days with fluorouracil alone is **LOW**
See Chapter 42 for antiemetic recommendations

Hematopoietic growth factor (CSF) prophylaxis
Primary prophylaxis is **NOT** indicated
See Chapter 43 for more information

Antimicrobial prophylaxis
Risk of fever and neutropenia is **LOW**
  Antimicrobial primary prophylaxis to be considered:
  - Antibacterial—not indicated
  - Antifungal—not indicated
  - Antiviral—not indicated unless patient previously had an episode of HSV

Diarrhea management
Latent or delayed-onset diarrhea*:
Loperamide 4 mg orally initially after the first loose or liquid stool, *then*
Loperamide 2 mg orally every 2 hours during waking hours, *plus*
Loperamide 4 mg orally every 4 hours during hours of sleep
- Continue for at least 12 hours after diarrhea resolves
- Recurrent diarrhea after a 12-hour diarrhea-free interval is treated as a new episode
- Rehydrate orally with fluids and electrolytes during a diarrheal episode
- If a patient develops blood or mucus in stool, dehydration, or hemodynamic instability, or if diarrhea persists >48 hours despite loperamide, stop loperamide and hospitalize the patient for IV hydration

Persistent diarrhea:
Octreotide 100–150 mcg subcutaneously 3 times daily. Maximum total daily dose is 1500 mcg
Antibiotic therapy during latent or delayed-onset diarrhea:
A fluoroquinolone (eg, **ciprofloxacin** 500 mg orally every 12 hours) if absolute neutrophil count <500/mm^3 with or without accompanying fever in association with diarrhea
- Antibiotics should also be administered if patient is hospitalized with prolonged diarrhea and should be continued until diarrhea resolves

Oral care
Risk of mucositis/stomatitis is **HIGH**
  General advice:
  - Encourage patients to maintain intake of nonalcoholic fluids
  - Evaluate patients for oral pain and provide analgesic medications
  - Consider histamine (H$_2$-subtype) receptor antagonists (eg, ranitidine, famotidine), or a proton pump inhibitor for epigastric pain
  - *Lactobacillus* sp.–containing probiotics may be beneficial in preventing diarrhea

(continued)

(continued)

Patients with intact oral mucosa:
- Clean the mouth, tongue, and gums by brushing after every meal and at bedtime with an ultra-soft toothbrush with fluoride toothpaste
- Floss teeth gently every day unless contraindicated. If gums bleed and hurt, avoid bleeding or sore areas, but floss other teeth
- Patients may use saline or commercial bland, nonalcoholic rinses
  - Do not use mouthwashes that contain alcohols

If mucositis or stomatitis is present:
- Keep the mouth moist utilizing water, ice chips, sugarless gum, sugar-free hard candies, or a saliva substitute
- Rinse mouth several times a day to remove debris
  - Use a solution of ¼ teaspoon (1.25 g) each of baking soda and table salt (sodium chloride) in 1 quart (~950 mL) of warm water. Follow with a plain water rinse
  - Do not use mouthwashes that contain alcohols
- Foam-tipped swabs (eg, Toothettes) are useful in moisturizing oral mucosa, but ineffective for cleansing teeth and removing plaque
- Advise patients who develop mucositis to:
  - Choose foods that are easy to chew and swallow
  - Take small bites of food, chew slowly, and sip liquids with meals
  - Encourage soft, moist foods such as cooked cereals, mashed potatoes, and scrambled eggs
  - For trouble swallowing, soften food with gravies, sauces, broths, yogurt, or other bland liquids
  - Avoid sharp, crunchy foods; hot, spicy, or highly acidic foods (eg, citrus fruits and juices); sugary foods; toothpicks; tobacco products; alcoholic drinks

Patient Population Studied

A study of 440 patients with pTR1, PT4, or ≥3 positive lymph nodes, or extracapsular spread and no macroscopic residual tumor

Efficacy

	Radiotherapy	Chemoradiation
5-year locoregional control	61.9%	83.3%
5-year rate free of distant metastases	68%	70%
5-year disease survival	50.1%	62.4%
5-year survival	48.6%	58.1%

G3/4 Toxicity (%)

Adverse Event	Radiotherapy	Chemoradiation
Mucositis	12.6	20.8
Dermatitis	8.9	13.1
Leukopenia	0	4.4
Thrombocytopenia	0	1.7
Serum creatinine >1.5× upper limit of normal range	1.2	6.4
Infections	6.9	8.8

Therapy Monitoring

1. *Days 1 and 29:* Medical history and physical exam, CBC with differential, LFTs, electrolytes, BUN, and creatinine
2. *Posttreatment reevaluation:* 8 weeks after the completion of therapy by examination of the head and neck and CT imaging. If persistent disease is suspected, perform the examination while the patient is under anesthesia so that direct laryngoscopy can be performed
3. *Scheduled follow-up visits:* Complete examination of the head and neck, with evaluation for late toxicity

Dose Modification

Note: Continuity of radiotherapy should be maintained if at all possible. Keep to a minimum interruptions resulting from treatment-related adverse effects

Adverse Event	Dose Modification
G3/4 hematologic toxicity attributable to chemotherapy	Hold chemotherapy
G3/4 nonhematologic toxicity other than alopecia, fatigue, malaise, and nail changes attributable to chemotherapy (exception: mucositis as detailed below)	
G4 mucositis	Discontinue therapy

METASTATIC • PD-L1 CPS ≥ 1%

HEAD AND NECK CANCER REGIMEN: PEMBROLIZUMAB

Rischin D et al. J Clin Oncol 2019;37(15_suppl):6000
Burtness B et al. Ann Oncol 2018;29(8_suppl):LBA8_PR
KEYTRUDA (pembrolizumab) prescribing information. Whitehouse Station, NJ: Merck & Co., Inc; revised 2019 September

Pembrolizumab 200 mg; administer intravenously over 30 minutes in a volume of 0.9% sodium chloride injection (0.9% NS) or 5% dextrose injection (D5W) every 3 weeks for up to 24 months (total dose/3-week cycle = 200 mg)

Alternative pembrolizumab dose and schedule as per the U.S. FDA regimens approved on April 28, 2020:

Pembrolizumab 400 mg; administer intravenously over 30 minutes in a volume of 0.9% NS or D5W sufficient to produce a pembrolizumab concentration within the range 1–10 mg/mL every 6 weeks for up to 24 months (total dose/6-week cycle = 400 mg)

- Administer pembrolizumab with an administration set that contains a sterile, non-pyrogenic, low-protein-binding in-line or add-on filter with pore size within the range of 0.2–5 µm
- Pembrolizumab can cause severe or life-threatening infusion-related reactions, including hypersensitivity and anaphylaxis
- The U.S. Food and Drug Administration approved indication for pembrolizumab as first-line therapy for metastatic head and neck squamous cell carcinoma is limited to patients with PD-L1 expressing tumors (combined positive score [CPS] ≥1 as determined by an FDA-approved test). CPS is calculated as the number of PD-L1 staining cells (including tumor cells, lymphocytes, and macrophages) divided by the total number of viable tumor cells, multiplied by 100

Supportive Care

Antiemetic prophylaxis
Emetogenic potential is **MINIMAL**
See Chapter 42 for antiemetic recommendations

Hematopoietic growth factor (CSF) prophylaxis
Primary prophylaxis is **NOT** indicated
See Chapter 43 for more information

Antimicrobial prophylaxis
Risk of fever and neutropenia is **LOW**
  Antimicrobial primary prophylaxis to be considered:
- Antibacterial—not indicated
- Antifungal—not indicated
- Antiviral—not indicated unless patient previously had an episode of HSV

Patient Population Studied

This was a multicenter, open-label, randomized, active-controlled trial involving 882 patients with untreated recurrent or metastatic head and neck squamous cell carcinoma not amenable to curable local treatment. Patients who had active autoimmune disease requiring recent immunosuppressive therapy were excluded. Patients were randomized 1:1:1 to single-agent pembrolizumab, pembrolizumab + chemotherapy (6 cycles of cisplatin or carboplatin and fluorouracil), or cetuximab + chemotherapy, HPV status based on p16 immunohistochemistry, and Eastern Cooperative Group performance status (0 vs 1)

Efficacy (N = 601)

	Pembrolizumab n = 301 Total Population n = 133 with PD-L1 CPS ≥20 n = 257 with PD-L1 CPS ≥1	Cetuximab + Cisplatin + Fluorouracil n = 300 Total Population n = 122 with PD-L1 CPS ≥20 n = 255 with PD-L1 CPS ≥1	
Median overall survival (PD-L1 CPS ≥20)*	14.9 months	10.7 months	HR 0.61 (95% CI, 0.45–0.83), P = 0.0007
Median overall survival (PD-L1 CPS ≥1)*	12.3 months	10.3 months	HR 0.78 (95% CI, 0.64–0.96), P = 0.0086
Median overall survival (total population)†	11.5 months	10.7 months	HR 0.83 (95% CI, 0.70–0.99); P = 0.0199‡
Overall response rate and duration of response (DOR) (PD-L1 CPS ≥20)	23% Median DOR = 20.9 months	36% Median DOR = 4.2 months	—
Overall response rate and DOR (PD-L1 CPS ≥1)*	19% Median DOR = 20.9 months	35% Median DOR = 4.5 months	—
Overall response rate and DOR (total population)†	16.9% Median DOR = 22.6 months	36% Median DOR = 4.5 months	—

*Data from interim analysis with data cutoff of 13 June 2018 after a minimum follow-up of approximately 17 months (Burtness et al, 2018)
†Data from final analysis with data cutoff of 25 Feb 2019, approximately 25 months after the last patient was randomized (Rischin et al, 2019)
‡Demonstrated non-inferiority but did not meet criteria for superiority

Adverse Events (N = 601)

Note: All-cause grade 3–5 adverse events occurred in 54.7% of patients in the pembrolizumab arm compared to 83.3% of patients in the cetuximab + chemotherapy arm

Pembrolizumab group (n = 246)	Any Grade	Grade 3–5
Treatment-related event* (%)		
Any event	63	13
Event leading to treatment discontinuation	6	5
Event leading to death	2	2
Event occurring in 10% or more of patients in either group		
Hypothyroidism	13	<1
Fatigue	13	2
Diarrhea	8	2
Rash	8	<1
Asthenia	7	<1
Anemia	7	<1
Nausea	5	0
Mucosal inflammation	4	<1
Stomatitis	2	<1
Neutrophil count decreased	1	<1
Alopecia	<1	0
Event of interest†		
Any	26	4
Hypothyroidism	15	<1
Pneumonitis	4	1
Infusion-related reaction	3	<1
Severe skin reaction	3	2
Hyperthyroidism	2	0
Colitis	1	0
Guillain-Barré syndrome	1	<1
Hepatitis	1	<1

The median duration of treatment in this population was 2.8 months (IQR 1.2–6.8) for pembrolizumab

*Events were attributed to treatment by the investigator and are listed as indicated by the investigator on the case report form

†Events of interest are those with an immune-related cause and are considered regardless of attribution to study treatment by the investigator. In addition to the specific preferred terms listed, related terms were also included. Data are number of patients with at least one event (% of patients)

Therapy Monitoring

1. Initially at the time of each dose, and eventually every 6–12 weeks, perform a total body skin examination with attention to all mucous membranes as well as a complete review of systems

2. Monitor patients for signs and symptoms of pneumonitis. Evaluate patients with suspected pneumonitis with chest x-ray, CT, and pulse oximetry. For ≥2 toxicity may include nasal swab, and sputum culture and sensitivity

3. Monitor patients for signs and symptoms of colitis. Encourage patients to report diarrhea immediately

4. AST, ALT, and bilirubin prior to each infusion for first 12 weeks and then every 6–12 weeks or weekly if there are grade 1 liver function test elevations. Note, no treatment is recommended for G1 LFT abnormalities. For G≥2 toxicity, work up for other causes of elevated LFTs including viral hepatitis

5. Use basic metabolic panel (Na, K, CO_2, glucose) and patient history as screening tools for hypophysitis including hypopituitarism and adrenal insufficiency. If in doubt, evaluate AM adrenocorticotropic hormone (ACTH) and cortisol levels. Consider ACTH stimulation test for indeterminate results

6. Assess thyroid function at the start of treatment, and periodically during treatment. Test for TSH and free thyroxine (FT4) every 3–24 weeks as part of routine clinical monitoring of therapy or for case detection in symptomatic patients

7. Measure glucose at baseline and with each treatment during the first 12 weeks and every 6–12 weeks thereafter

8. Obtain a serum creatinine prior to every dose during the first 12 weeks and then every other or every third or fourth dose. If creatinine is newly elevated, consider holding therapy while other potential causes are evaluated. Note, routine urinalysis is not necessary other than to rule out urinary tract infections, etc

9. Obtain a complete rheumatologic history and perform an examination of the spine and all peripheral joints for tenderness, swelling, and range of motion

10. In patients at high risk of infections and in appropriately selected patients based on an infectious disease evaluation, draw screening laboratories (HIV, hepatitis A and B, and blood QuantiFERON for TB) to prepare patients to start infliximab

11. Response evaluation: Every 12–24 weeks

Treatment Modifications

RECOMMENDED DOSE MODIFICATIONS FOR PEMBROLIZUMAB

Adverse Event	Grade/Severity	Treatment Modification
Infusion reaction	Clinically significant but not severe infusion reaction	Interrupt the infusion in patients with clinically significant infusion reactions and consider resuming at a slower rate following resolution. If decision is made to restart, begin at ≤50% of the rate prior to the reaction and increase in 50% increments every 30 minutes if well tolerated. Infusions may be restarted at the full rate during the next cycle
	G3/4 (severe infusion reaction—pyrexia, chills, flushing, hypotension, dyspnea, wheezing, back pain, abdominal pain, and urticaria). Not rapidly responsive to brief interruption of infusion	Stop infusion and administer appropriate medical therapy (eg, epinephrine, corticosteroids, intravenous antihistamines, bronchodilators, and/or oxygen). Discontinue pembrolizumab
Colitis	G1	Loperamide 4 mg as starting dose then 2 mg before each meal and after each loose stool until without diarrhea for 12 hours, with maximum of 16 mg loperamide per day. If G1 diarrhea or colitis persists >14 days, then add prednisolone 0.5–1 mg/kg (non-enteric-coated) or consider oral budesonide 9 mg daily if no bloody diarrhea
	G2/3 diarrhea or colitis	Withhold pembrolizumab. Loperamide 4 mg as starting dose then 2 mg before each meal and after each loose stool until without diarrhea for 12 hours, with maximum of 16 mg loperamide per day. Administer oral prednisone/prednisolone at a dose of 0.5–2 mg/kg/day or its equivalent. When improves to G1, begin a slow corticosteroid taper over at least 4 weeks. Resume pembrolizumab upon symptom control, or when prednisone/prednisolone daily dose <10 mg
	G4 diarrhea or colitis	Permanently discontinue pembrolizumab. Loperamide 4 mg as starting dose then 2 mg before each meal and after each loose stool until without diarrhea for 12 hours, with maximum of 16 mg loperamide per day. Administer 1–2 mg/kg IV (methyl)prednisolone and convert to 0.5–2 mg/kg prednisone/prednisolone orally each day or its equivalent only after a response. Taper over at least 4 weeks when symptoms improve. If does not improve over 72 hours or worsens, perform flexible sigmoidoscopy/colonoscopy to document colitis then begin infliximab 5 mg/kg (if no perforation/sepsis/TB/hepatitis/NYHA III/IV CHF). If no response, add MMF 500–1000 mg twice daily. If worse on MMF, consider addition of tacrolimus or ATG
Pneumonitis	G2	Withhold pembrolizumab. Consider pneumocystis prophylaxis depending on the clinical context and coverage with empiric antibiotics. Administer oral prednisone/prednisolone at a dose of 1–2 mg/kg/day or its equivalent. When improves to G1, begin a slow corticosteroid taper over at least 4 weeks. If does not respond adequately after 48 hours, then administer 2–4 mg/kg IV (methyl)prednisolone and convert to 0.5–2 mg/kg prednisone/prednisolone orally each day or its equivalent only after a response, followed by a taper over at least 6 weeks when symptoms improve to G1, titrating to symptoms. Resume pembrolizumab upon symptom control, or when prednisone/prednisolone daily dose <10 mg
	G3/4	Permanently discontinue pembrolizumab. Consider pneumocystis prophylaxis depending on the clinical context; cover with empiric antibiotics. Administer 2–4 mg/kg IV (methyl)prednisolone and convert to 1–2 mg/kg prednisone/prednisolone orally each day or its equivalent only after a response, followed by a taper over at least 8 weeks when symptoms improve to G1, titrating to symptoms. If, when initially treated, improvement does not occur within 48–72 hours, begin infliximab 5 mg/kg (if no perforation/sepsis/TB/hepatitis/NYHA III/IV CHF). If no response to infliximab, add MMF 500–1000 mg twice daily. Consider MMF especially if has concurrent hepatic toxicity
Hepatitis	G2 (AST or ALT >3–5× ULN or total bilirubin >1.5–3× ULN)	Withhold pembrolizumab. Administer oral prednisone/prednisolone at a dose of 1–2 mg/kg/day or its equivalent. When improves to G1, begin a slow corticosteroid taper over at least 4 weeks. Resume pembrolizumab upon symptom control, or when prednisone/prednisolone daily dose <10 mg
	G3/4 (AST or ALT >5× ULN or total bilirubin >3× ULN)	Permanently discontinue pembrolizumab. Administer 1–2 mg/kg IV (methyl)prednisolone and convert to 0.5–2 mg/kg prednisone/prednisolone orally each day or its equivalent only after a response. Taper over at least 6 weeks when symptoms improve. If no response, add MMF 500–1000 mg twice daily. If worse on MMF, consider adding tacrolimus or ATG

(continued)

Treatment Modifications (*continued*)

RECOMMENDED DOSE MODIFICATIONS FOR PEMBROLIZUMAB

Adverse Event	Grade/Severity	Treatment Modification
Hypophysitis	G2/3 (moderate symptoms, ie, headache but no visual disturbance or fatigue/mood alteration but hemodynamically stable, no electrolyte disturbance)	Administer analgesia as needed for headache. Withhold pembrolizumab. Administer oral prednisone/prednisolone at a dose of 0.5–2 mg/kg/day or its equivalent. When improves to G1, begin a slow corticosteroid taper over at least 4 weeks. If no improvement in 48 hours, administer 1–2 mg/kg IV (methyl)prednisolone and convert to 0.5–2 mg/kg prednisone/prednisolone orally each day or its equivalent only after a response. Taper over at least 4 weeks when symptoms improve to 5 mg prednisone/prednisolone or equivalent; do not stop steroids. Resume pembrolizumab upon symptom control, or when prednisone/prednisolone daily dose <10 mg
	G4 (severe mass effect symptoms, ie, severe headache, any visual disturbance or severe hypoadrenalism, ie, hypotension, severe electrolyte disturbance)	Permanently discontinue pembrolizumab. Administer analgesia as needed for headache. Administer 1–2 mg/kg IV (methyl)prednisolone and convert to 0.5–2 mg/kg prednisone/prednisolone orally each day or its equivalent only after a response. Taper over at least 4 weeks when symptoms improve to 5 mg prednisone/prednisolone or equivalent; do not stop steroids
Adrenal insufficiency	G2	Withhold pembrolizumab. Administer oral prednisone/prednisolone at a dose of 0.5–2 mg/kg/day or its equivalent. When improves to G1, begin a slow corticosteroid taper over at least 4 weeks. Serially assess adrenal function and continue steroids at replacement doses (20–40 mg hydrocortisone daily ~2/3 dose in AM upon awakening and ~1/3 at 4 PM) until recovery of adrenal function is documented. Resume pembrolizumab upon symptom control, or when prednisone/prednisolone daily dose <10 mg
	G3/4	Permanently discontinue pembrolizumab. Administer oral prednisone/prednisolone at a dose of 0.5–2 mg/kg/day or its equivalent. When improves to G1, begin a slow corticosteroid taper over at least 4 weeks. Serially assess adrenal function and continue steroids at replacement doses (20–40 mg hydrocortisone daily ~2/3 dose in AM upon awakening and ~1/3 at 4 PM) until recovery of adrenal function is documented
Type 1 diabetes mellitus	G3 hyperglycemia	Withhold pembrolizumab. Admit to hospital to manage hyperglycemia. Role of corticosteroids in preventing complete loss of insulin-producing cells is unknown and not recommended. Resume pembrolizumab upon symptom control, or when prednisone/prednisolone daily dose <10 mg
	G4 hyperglycemia	Permanently discontinue pembrolizumab. Admit to hospital to manage hyperglycemia. Role of corticosteroids in preventing complete loss of insulin-producing cells is unknown and not recommended.
Nephritis and renal dysfunction	G2/3 (serum creatinine 1.5–6X ULN)	Withhold pembrolizumab. Administer oral prednisone/prednisolone at a dose of 0.5–2 mg/kg/day or its equivalent. When improves to G1, begin a slow corticosteroid taper over at least 4 weeks. If does not respond adequately, then administer 0.5–1 mg/kg IV (methyl)prednisolone and convert to 0.5–2 mg/kg prednisone/prednisolone orally each day or its equivalent only after a response, followed by a taper over at least 4 weeks when improves to G1. Resume pembrolizumab upon symptom control, or when prednisone/prednisolone daily dose <10 mg
	G4 (serum creatinine >6X ULN)	Permanently discontinue pembrolizumab. Administer 0.5–1 mg/kg IV (methyl)prednisolone and convert to 0.5–2 mg/kg prednisone/prednisolone orally each day or its equivalent only after a response, followed by a taper over at least 4 weeks when improves to G1
Skin	G1/2	Continue pembrolizumab. Avoid skin irritants, avoid sun exposure, topical emollients recommended. Topical steroid (mild strength for G1, moderate/potent strength for G2) cream once or twice daily ± oral or topical antihistamines for itching
	G3 rash or suspected SJS or TEN	Withhold pembrolizumab. Avoid skin irritants, avoid sun exposure, topical emollients recommended. Administer oral or topical antihistamines for itching. Administer oral prednisone/prednisolone at a dose of 0.5–2 mg/kg or its equivalent daily for 3 days followed by a slow corticosteroid taper over at least 4 weeks when the rash improves to G1. If does not respond adequately, then administer 0.5–1 mg/kg IV (methyl)prednisolone and convert to 0.5–2 mg/kg prednisone/prednisolone orally each day or its equivalent only after a response, followed by a taper over at least 4 weeks when the rash improves to G1. Resume pembrolizumab upon symptom control, or when prednisone/prednisolone daily dose <10 mg
	G4 rash or confirmed SJS or TEN	Avoid skin irritants, avoid sun exposure, topical emollients recommended. Administer oral or topical antihistamines for itching. Administer 1–2 mg/kg IV (methyl)prednisolone and convert to oral steroids 0.5–2 mg/kg prednisone/prednisolone each day or its equivalent only after a response. Taper over at least 4 weeks when the rash improves to G1. Permanently discontinue pembrolizumab

(*continued*)

Treatment Modifications (*continued*)

RECOMMENDED DOSE MODIFICATIONS FOR PEMBROLIZUMAB

Adverse Event	Grade/Severity	Treatment Modification
Encephalitis	Confusion or altered behavior, headaches, alteration in Glasgow Coma Scale, motor or sensory deficits, speech abnormality, may or may not be febrile	Initially withhold pembrolizumab, but permanently discontinue pembrolizumab if there is no doubt as to diagnosis. Exclude bacterial and ideally viral infections prior to high-dose steroids. Administer oral prednisone/prednisolone at a dose of 0.5–2 mg/kg/day or its equivalent. When symptoms improve, begin a slow corticosteroid taper over at least 4–8 weeks. If symptoms are severe, administer 1–2 mg/kg IV (methyl)prednisolone and convert to 0.5–2 mg/kg prednisone/prednisolone orally each day or its equivalent only after a response. Consider concurrent empiric antiviral (IV acyclovir) and antibacterial therapy
Aseptic meningitis	Headache, photophobia, neck stiffness with fever or may be afebrile, vomiting; normal cognition/cerebral function (distinguishes from encephalitis)	
Other syndromes include neurosarcoidosis, posterior reversible leukoencephalopathy syndrome (PRES), Vogt-Koyanagi-Harada syndrome, demyelination, vasculitic encephalopathy, and generalized seizures		
Transverse myelitis	Acute or subacute neurologic signs/symptoms of motor/sensory/autonomic origin; most have sensory level; often bilateral symptoms	Initially withhold pembrolizumab, but permanently discontinue pembrolizumab if there is no doubt as to diagnosis. Administer 2 mg/kg IV (methyl)prednisolone or consider 1 g/day and convert to 0.5–2 mg/kg prednisone/prednisolone orally each day or its equivalent only after a response. When symptoms improve, begin a slow corticosteroid taper over at least 4–8 weeks. Plasmapheresis may be required if steroids do not bring about improvement
Myocarditis	G3	Permanently discontinue pembrolizumab. Administer 2 mg/kg IV (methyl)prednisolone or consider 1 g/day and convert to 0.5–2 mg/kg prednisone/prednisolone orally each day or its equivalent only after a response. When symptoms improve, begin a slow corticosteroid taper over at least 4–8 weeks. If no response, add MMF 500–1000 mg twice daily. If worse on MMF, consider adding tacrolimus
Peripheral neurologic toxicity	Moderate: some interference with ADL, symptoms concerning to patient	Withhold pembrolizumab. Initial observation reasonable or initiate prednisone/prednisolone 0.5–1 mg/kg (if progressing, eg, from mild) and/or pregabalin or duloxetine for pain. When symptoms improve, begin a slow corticosteroid taper over at least 4 weeks. Resume pembrolizumab upon symptom control, or when prednisone/prednisolone daily dose <10 mg
	Severe: limits self-care and aids warranted, life threatening, eg, respiratory problems	Permanently discontinue pembrolizumab. Administer 1–2 mg/kg IV (methyl)prednisolone and convert to 0.5–2 mg/kg prednisone/prednisolone orally each day or its equivalent only after a response. Taper over at least 4–8 weeks when symptoms improve to G1
Guillain-Barré syndrome	Progressive symmetrical muscle weakness with absent or reduced tendon reflexes—involves extremities, facial, respiratory, and bulbar and oculomotor muscles; dysregulation of autonomic nerves	Permanently discontinue pembrolizumab. Use of steroids not recommended in idiopathic Guillain-Barré syndrome; however, a trial of (methyl)prednisolone 1–2 mg/kg is reasonable, converting to 0.5–2 mg/kg prednisone/prednisolone orally each day or its equivalent only after a response. If no improvement or worsening, plasmapheresis or IVIG indicated
Myasthenia gravis	Fluctuating muscle weakness (proximal limb, trunk, ocular, eg, ptosis/diplopia or bulbar) with fatigability, respiratory muscles may also be involved	Permanently discontinue pembrolizumab. Administer pyridostigmine at an initial dose of 30 mg three times daily. Administer oral prednisone/prednisolone at a dose of 0.5–2 mg/kg/day or its equivalent or 1–2 mg/kg IV (methyl)prednisolone depending on the severity of symptoms. If begin with IV, convert to 0.5–2 mg/kg prednisone/prednisolone orally each day or its equivalent only after a response. If no improvement or worsening, plasmapheresis or IVIG may be considered. Additional immunosuppressants used in myasthenia gravis include azathioprine, cyclosporine, and mycophenolate. Avoid certain medications, eg, ciprofloxacin, beta-blockers, that may precipitate cholinergic crisis
Other syndromes including motor and sensory peripheral neuropathy, multifocal radicular neuropathy/plexopathy, autonomic neuropathy, phrenic nerve palsy, cranial nerve palsies (eg, facial nerve, optic nerve, hypoglossal nerve)		Permanently discontinue pembrolizumab. Administer oral prednisone/prednisolone at a dose of 0.5–2 mg/kg/day or its equivalent or 1–2 mg/kg IV (methyl)prednisolone depending on the severity of symptoms. If begin with IV, convert to 0.5–2 mg/kg prednisone/prednisolone orally each day or its equivalent only after a response

(*continued*)

Treatment Modifications (*continued*)

RECOMMENDED DOSE MODIFICATIONS FOR PEMBROLIZUMAB

Adverse Event	Grade/Severity	Treatment Modification
Arthralgia	G1 (mild pain with inflammation, erythema, or joint swelling)	Continue pembrolizumab. Administer acetaminophen (paracetamol) and ibuprofen
	G2 (moderate pain with inflammation, erythema, or joint swelling that limits ADL)	Withhold pembrolizumab. Administer higher doses of acetaminophen (paracetamol) and ibuprofen and use diclofenac or naproxen or etoricoxib. If inadequately controlled, consider intra-articular steroid injections for large joints or administer oral prednisone/prednisolone at a dose of 0.5–2 mg/kg/day or its equivalent. When improves to G1, begin a slow corticosteroid taper over at least 4 weeks. If does not respond adequately, then administer 0.5–1 mg/kg IV (methyl)prednisolone and convert to 0.5–2 mg/kg prednisone/prednisolone orally each day or its equivalent only after a response, followed by a taper over at least 4 weeks when improves to G1. Resume pembrolizumab upon symptom control, or when prednisone/prednisolone daily dose <10 mg
	G3 (severe pain; irreversible joint damage; disabling; limits self-care ADL)	Withhold pembrolizumab. Administer 0.5–1 mg/kg IV (methyl)prednisolone and convert to 0.5–2 mg/kg prednisone/prednisolone orally each day or its equivalent only after a response, followed by a taper over at least 4 weeks when improves to G1. In severe cases, infliximab or another anti–TNF-alpha drug may be required for improvement of arthritis. Resume pembrolizumab upon symptom control, or when prednisone/prednisolone daily dose <10 mg
Other	First occurrence of other G3	Withhold pembrolizumab. Administer oral prednisone/prednisolone at a dose of 0.5–2 mg/kg/day or its equivalent. When improves to G1, begin a slow corticosteroid taper over at least 4 weeks. Resume pembrolizumab upon symptom control, or when prednisone/prednisolone daily dose <10 mg
	Recurrence of same G3	Permanently discontinue pembrolizumab. Administer 1–2 mg/kg IV (methyl)prednisolone and convert to 0.5–2 mg/kg prednisone/prednisolone orally each day or its equivalent only after a response. Taper over at least 4–8 weeks when symptoms improve to G1
	Life-threatening or G4	
	Requirement for ≥10 mg/day prednisone or equivalent for >12 weeks	Permanently discontinue pembrolizumab
	Persistent G2/3 adverse reactions lasting ≥12 weeks	

ADL, activities of daily living; ALT, alanine aminotransferase; AST, aspartate aminotransferase; ATG, anti-thymocyte globulin; SJS, Stevens-Johnson Syndrome; TEN, toxic epidermal necrolysis; ULN, upper limit of normal

Notes on general supportive care: Steroid taper in most cases will proceed over a minimum of 1 month but if symptoms improve rapidly, a 2-week taper can be considered. If steroids are administered for more than 4 weeks, consider PCP prophylaxis (cotrimoxazole 480 mg twice daily M/W/F or inhaled pentamidine if has cotrimoxazole allergy), regular random blood glucose, VitD level, and starting calcium/VitD supplementation per guidelines

METASTATIC

HEAD AND NECK CANCER REGIMEN: PEMBROLIZUMAB + PLATINUM (CISPLATIN OR CARBOPLATIN) + FLUOROURACIL

Rischin D et al. J Clin Oncol 2019;37(15_suppl):6000
Burtness B et al. Ann Oncol 2018;29(8_suppl):LBA8_PR
KEYTRUDA (pembrolizumab) prescribing information. Whitehouse Station, NJ: Merck & Co., Inc; revised 2019 September

Pembrolizumab 200 mg; administer intravenously over 30 minutes in a volume of 0.9% sodium chloride injection (0.9% NS) or 5% dextrose injection (D5W) on day 1, every 21 days, for up to 24 months (total dose/3-week cycle = 200 mg)
Alternative pembrolizumab dose and schedule as per the U.S. FDA regimens approved on April 28, 2020:

Pembrolizumab 400 mg; administer intravenously over 30 minutes in a volume of 0.9% NS or D5W sufficient to produce a pembrolizumab concentration within the range 1–10 mg/mL every 6 weeks for up to 24 months (total dose/6-week cycle = 400 mg)
- Administer pembrolizumab with an administration set that contains a sterile, non-pyrogenic, low-protein-binding in-line or add-on filter with pore size within the range of 0.2–5 µm
- Pembrolizumab can cause severe or life-threatening infusion-related reactions, including hypersensitivity and anaphylaxis

Hydration before, during, and after cisplatin administration:
- *Pre-cisplatin hydration* with 1000 mL 0.9% sodium chloride injection (0.9% NS); administer intravenously with potassium and magnesium supplementation as needed based on pretreatment laboratory results
- Post-cisplatin hydration with ≥1000 mL 0.9% NS; administer intravenously with potassium and magnesium supplementation as needed based on measured values

Cisplatin 100 mg/m²; administer intravenously in 25–250 mL of 0.9% NS over 15–30 minutes, given on day 1, every 21 days, for 6 cycles (total dosage/3-week cycle = 100 mg/m²)
Note: May substitute carboplatin for cisplatin at the discretion of the treating physician. If electing to substitute with carboplatin, then pre- and post-hydration is not necessary. Thus:
Carboplatin target AUC = 5 mg/mL × min; administer intravenously in 250 mL D5W or 0.9% NS over 60 minutes on day 1, every 21 days, for 6 cycles (total dose/3-week cycle calculated to achieve a target AUC = 5 mg/mL × min)

Fluorouracil 1000 mg/m² per day; administer by continuous intravenous infusion in 100–1000 mL 0.9% NS or 5% dextrose injection over 24 hours for 4 consecutive days (96-hour infusion), given on days 1–4, every 21 days, for 6 cycles (total dosage/3-week cycle = 4000 mg/m²)

Carboplatin dose
Carboplatin dose is based on a formula described by Calvert et al. to achieve a target area under the plasma concentration versus time curve (AUC)

$$\text{Total carboplatin dose (mg)} = (\text{target AUC})(\text{GFR} + 25)$$

In practice, creatinine clearance (CrCl) is used in place of glomerular filtration rate (GFR). CrCl can be estimated from the equation of Cockcroft and Gault, thus:

$$\text{For males}, \text{CrCl} = \frac{(140 - \text{age}[\text{years}]) \times (\text{body weight }[\text{kg}])}{72 \times (\text{serum creatinine }[\text{mg/dL}])}$$

$$\text{For females}, \text{CrCl} = \frac{(140 - \text{age}[\text{years}]) \times (\text{body weight }[\text{kg}])}{72 \times (\text{serum creatinine }[\text{mg/dL}])} \times 0.85$$

Calvert AH et al. J Clin Oncol 1989;7:1748–1756
Cockcroft DW, Gault MH. Nephron 1976;16:31–41
Jodrell DI et al. J Clin Oncol 1992;10:520–528
Sorensen BT et al. Cancer Chemother Pharmacol 1991;28:397–401

(continued)

Patient Population Studied

This was a multicenter, open-label, randomized, active-controlled trial involving 882 patients with untreated recurrent or metastatic head and neck squamous cell carcinoma not amenable to curable local treatment. Patients who had active autoimmune disease requiring recent immunosuppressive therapy were excluded. Patients were randomized 1:1:1 to single-agent pembrolizumab, pembrolizumab + chemotherapy (6 cycles of cisplatin or carboplatin and fluorouracil), or cetuximab + chemotherapy after stratification based on tumor PD-L1 expression (TPS ≥50% vs <50%), HPV status based on p16 immunohistochemistry, and Eastern Cooperative Group performance status (0 vs 1)

Adverse Events (N = 882)

All-cause grade 3–5 adverse events occurred in 85.1% of patients in the pembrolizumab + chemotherapy arm compared to 83.3% of patients in the cetuximab + chemotherapy arm

Therapy Monitoring

Monitoring during six cycles of chemotherapy (cisplatin/carboplatin + fluorouracil):
  a. *Before each chemotherapy cycle:* physical exam, CBC with differential, LFTs, serum creatinine, serum electrolytes, calcium, and magnesium
  b. *One week after treatment:* serum creatinine, serum electrolytes, calcium, and magnesium
  c. *Weekly follow-up recommending during at least the first cycle:* attention to signs and symptoms of dehydration as supplemental hydration is often required

Monitoring throughout therapy with pembrolizumab:
  1. Initially at the time of each dose, and eventually every 6–12 weeks, perform a total body skin examination with attention to all mucous membranes as well as a complete review of systems
  2. Monitor patients for signs and symptoms of pneumonitis. Evaluate patients with suspected pneumonitis with chest x-ray, CT, and pulse oximetry. For ≥2 toxicity may include nasal swab, and sputum culture and sensitivity

(continued)

(continued)

Note: On October 8, 2010, the U.S. Food and Drug Administration (FDA) identified a potential safety issue with carboplatin dosing based on recent changes in the measurement of serum creatinine. By the end of 2010, all clinical laboratories in the United States will use the standardized isotope dilution mass spectrometry (IDMS) method to measure serum creatinine, which could result in an overestimation of the GFR in some patients with normal renal function. A carboplatin dose calculated with an IDMS-measured serum creatinine result using the Calvert formula could exceed an expected exposure (AUC) and result in increased drug-related toxicity. Provided actual GFR measurements are made to assess renal function, carboplatin can be safely dosed according to the Calvert formula described in product labeling. If GFR (or creatinine clearance) is estimated based on serum creatinine measurements by the IDMS method, the FDA recommended for patients with normal renal function capping an estimated GFR at 125 mL/min for any targeted AUC value. No greater estimated GFR values should be used per U.S. FDA.

   Carboplatin dosing. May 23, 2013. Available from: http://www.fda.gov/AboutFDA/CentersOffices/OfficeofMedicalProductsandTobacco/CDER/ucm228974.htm [accessed February 26, 2014]

Supportive Care
Antiemetic prophylaxis
Emetogenic potential on days with cisplatin or carboplatin is **HIGH**. *Potential for delayed symptoms*
Emetogenic potential on days with fluorouracil alone is **LOW**
Emetogenic potential on days with pembrolizumab alone is **MINIMAL**
See Chapter 42 for antiemetic recommendations

Hematopoietic growth factor (CSF) prophylaxis
Primary prophylaxis is **NOT** *indicated*
See Chapter 43 for more information

Antimicrobial prophylaxis
Risk of fever and neutropenia is **LOW**
   Antimicrobial primary prophylaxis to be considered:
   • Antibacterial—not indicated
   • Antifungal—not indicated
   • Antiviral—not indicated unless patient previously had an episode of HSV

Diarrhea management
Latent or delayed-onset diarrhea during cisplatin/carboplatin + fluorouracil therapy (below is for management of chemotherapy-induced diarrhea and is not appropriate for immune-mediated colitis related to pembrolizumab)*:
   Loperamide 4 mg orally initially after the first loose or liquid stool, *then*
   Loperamide 2 mg orally every 2 hours during waking hours, *plus*
   Loperamide 4 mg orally every 4 hours during hours of sleep
   • Continue for at least 12 hours after diarrhea resolves
   • Recurrent diarrhea after a 12-hour diarrhea-free interval is treated as a new episode
   • Rehydrate orally with fluids and electrolytes during a diarrheal episode
   • If a patient develops blood or mucus in stool, dehydration, or hemodynamic instability, or if diarrhea persists >48 hours despite loperamide, stop loperamide and hospitalize the patient for IV hydration
Persistent diarrhea:
   Octreotide 100–150 mcg subcutaneously 3 times daily. Maximum total daily dose is 1500 mcg
Antibiotic therapy during latent or delayed-onset diarrhea:
• A fluoroquinolone (eg, **ciprofloxacin** 500 mg orally every 12 hours) if absolute neutrophil count <500/mm³ with or without accompanying fever in association with diarrhea
• Antibiotics should also be administered if patient is hospitalized with prolonged diarrhea and should be continued until diarrhea resolves

*Rothenberg ML et al. J Clin Oncol 2001;19:3801–3807
Abigerges D et al. J Natl Cancer Inst 1994;86:446–449
Wadler S et al. J Clin Oncol 1998;16:3169–3178

(continued)

Therapy Monitoring
(continued)

3. Monitor patients for signs and symptoms of colitis. Encourage patients to report diarrhea immediately

4. AST, ALT, and bilirubin prior to each infusion for first 12 weeks and then every 6–12 weeks or weekly if there are grade 1 liver function test elevations. Note, no treatment is recommended for G1 LFT abnormalities. For G ≥2 toxicity, work up for other causes of elevated LFTs including viral hepatitis

5. Use basic metabolic panel (Na, K, CO_2, glucose) and patient history as screening tools for hypophysitis including hypopituitarism and adrenal insufficiency. If in doubt, evaluate AM adrenocorticotropic hormone (ACTH) and cortisol levels. Consider ACTH stimulation test for indeterminate results

6. Assess thyroid function at the start of treatment, and periodically during treatment. Test for TSH and free thyroxine (FT4) every 3–24 weeks as part of routine clinical monitoring of therapy or for case detection in symptomatic patients

7. Measure glucose at baseline and with each treatment during the first 12 weeks and every 6–12 weeks thereafter

8. Obtain a serum creatinine prior to every dose during the first 12 weeks and then every other or every third or fourth dose. If creatinine is newly elevated, consider holding therapy while other potential causes are evaluated. Note, routine urinalysis is not necessary other than to rule out urinary tract infections, etc

9. Obtain a complete rheumatologic history and perform an examination of the spine and all peripheral joints for tenderness, swelling, and range of motion

10. In patients at high risk of infections and in appropriately selected patients based on an infectious disease evaluation, draw screening laboratories (HIV, hepatitis A and B, and blood QuantiFERON for TB) to prepare patients to start infliximab

11. Response evaluation: Every 12–24 weeks

(continued)

Oral care (mucositis prophylaxis and management)

General advice:

- Encourage patients to maintain intake of nonalcoholic fluids
- Evaluate patients for oral pain and provide analgesic medications
- Consider histamine (H_2-subtype) receptor antagonists (eg, ranitidine, famotidine), or a proton pump inhibitor for epigastric pain
- *Lactobacillus* sp.–containing probiotics may be beneficial in preventing diarrhea

Patients with intact oral mucosa:

- Clean the mouth, tongue, and gums by brushing after every meal and at bedtime with an ultra-soft toothbrush with fluoride toothpaste
- Floss teeth gently every day unless contraindicated. If gums bleed and hurt, avoid bleeding or sore areas, but floss other teeth
- Patients may use saline or commercial bland, nonalcoholic rinses
  - Do not use mouthwashes that contain alcohols

If mucositis or stomatitis is present:

- Keep the mouth moist utilizing water, ice chips, sugarless gum, sugar-free hard candies, or a saliva substitute
- Rinse mouth several times a day to remove debris
  - Use a solution of ¼ teaspoon (1.25 g) each of baking soda and table salt (sodium chloride) in 1 quart (~950 mL) of warm water. Follow with a plain water rinse
  - Do not use mouthwashes that contain alcohols
- Foam-tipped swabs (eg, Toothettes) are useful in moisturizing oral mucosa, but ineffective for cleansing teeth and removing plaque
- Advise patients who develop mucositis to:
  - Choose foods that are easy to chew and swallow
  - Take small bites of food, chew slowly, and sip liquids with meals
  - Encourage soft, moist foods such as cooked cereals, mashed potatoes, and scrambled eggs
  - For trouble swallowing, soften food with gravies, sauces, broths, yogurt, or other bland liquids
  - Avoid sharp, crunchy foods; hot, spicy, or highly acidic foods (eg, citrus fruits and juices); sugary foods; toothpicks; tobacco products; alcoholic drinks

Efficacy (N = 559)

	Pembrolizumab + Cisplatin/ Carboplatin + Fluorouracil n = 281 Total Population n = 126 with PD-L1 CPS ≥20 n = 242 with PD-L1 CPS ≥1	Cetuximab + Cisplatin/ Carboplatin + Fluorouracil n = 278 Total Population n = 110 with PD-L1 CPS ≥20 n = 235 with PD-L1 CPS ≥1	
Median overall survival (PD-L1 CPS ≥20)*	14.7 months	11.0 months	HR 0.60 (95% CI, 0.45–0.82), P = 0.0004
Median overall survival (PD-L1 CPS ≥1)*	13.6 months	10.4 months	HR 0.65 (95% CI, 0.53–0.80), P<0.0001
Median overall survival (total population)†	13.0 months	10.7 months	HR 0.77 (95% CI, 0.63–0.93), P = 0.0034
Overall response rate and duration of response (DOR) (PD-L1 CPS ≥20)*	42.9% Median DOR = 7.1 months	38.2% Median DOR = 4.2 months	—
Overall response rate and DOR (PD-L1 CPS ≥1)*	36.4% Median DOR = 6.7 months	35.7% Median DOR = 4.3 months	—
Overall response rate and DOR (total population)†	36% Median DOR = 6.7 months	36% Median DOR = 4.3 months	—

*Data from final analysis with data cutoff of 25 February 2019, approximately 25 months after the last patient was randomized (Rischin et al, 2019)

†Data from interim analysis with data cutoff of 13 June 2018 after a minimum follow-up of approximately 17 months (Burtness et al, 2018)

Treatment Modifications

RECOMMENDED DOSE MODIFICATIONS FOR CARBOPLATIN/CISPLATIN + FLUOROURACIL

	Cisplatin	Carboplatin	Fluorouracil
Starting Dose	100 mg/m² on day 1	AUC 5 mg/mL × min	1000 mg/m²/day on days 1–4

Note: Patients will receive either cisplatin or carboplatin (not both) in any given cycle

Adverse Event	Treatment Modification
G ≥2 mucositis or G ≥2 palmar-plantar erythrodysesthesia	Reduce the fluorouracil dosage by 20–25%. Do not modify the cisplatin/carboplatin dose
G ≥3 diarrhea (≥7 stools/day above baseline)	Consider a diagnosis of immune-mediated colitis as described below in the pembrolizumab section and complete work-up/treatment as clinically appropriate. If diarrhea is attributable to fluorouracil, then hold fluorouracil until diarrhea resolves to baseline, then reduce the fluorouracil dosage by 25% in subsequent cycles
G3 thrombocytopenia (platelet count <50,000/mm³ and ≥25,000/mm³) or G3 neutropenia (ANC <1000/mm³ and ≥500/mm³)	Reduce the cisplatin dosage by 25% or the carboplatin dosage to AUC 4.5 and then 4.0. Do not change the fluorouracil dosage
G4 thrombocytopenia (platelet count <25,000/mm³) or G4 neutropenia (ANC <500/mm³)	Reduce the cisplatin or carboplatin dosage by 50%. Do not change the fluorouracil dosage. Consider adding G-CSF in subsequent cycles for persistent (>1 week) G4 neutropenia or in case of prior neutropenic fever
Creatinine clearance <50 mL/min	Do not administer cisplatin. Consider substituting carboplatin for cisplatin. Do not modify the fluorouracil dosage
Serum creatinine >1.5 mg/dL and ≤2 mg/dL, or serum creatinine ≥20% higher than baseline if baseline value is >1.5 mg/dL	Delay therapy with cisplatin + fluorouracil until serum creatinine <1.5 mg/dL (<133 µmol/L) or within 0.2 mg/dL (17.7 µmol/L) of baseline, then proceed with the cisplatin dosage reduced by 25% (peak serum creatinine 1.5–2 mg/dL). Alternatively, substitute carboplatin for cisplatin in subsequent cycles.
Serum creatinine >2 mg/dL	Discontinue cisplatin, substituting carboplatin for cisplatin in subsequent cycles
G2 neurotoxicity or ototoxicity	Hold cisplatin until neurotoxicity or ototoxicity resolves to ≤G1, or substitute carboplatin in subsequent cycles
G ≥3 neurotoxicity or ototoxicity	Permanently discontinue cisplatin. Consider substituting carboplatin for cisplatin in subsequent cycles

RECOMMENDED DOSE MODIFICATIONS FOR PEMBROLIZUMAB

Adverse Event	Grade/Severity	Treatment Modification
Infusion reaction	Clinically significant but not severe infusion reaction	Interrupt the infusion in patients with clinically significant infusion reactions and consider resuming at a slower rate following resolution. If decision is made to restart, begin at ≤50% of the rate prior to the reaction and increase in 50% increments every 30 minutes if well tolerated. Infusions may be restarted at the full rate during the next cycle
	G3/4 (severe infusion reaction—pyrexia, chills, flushing, hypotension, dyspnea, wheezing, back pain, abdominal pain, and urticaria). Not rapidly responsive to brief interruption of infusion	Stop infusion and administer appropriate medical therapy (eg, epinephrine, corticosteroids, intravenous antihistamines, bronchodilators, and/or oxygen). Discontinue pembrolizumab

(*continued*)

Treatment Modifications (*continued*)

RECOMMENDED DOSE MODIFICATIONS FOR PEMBROLIZUMAB

Adverse Event	Grade/Severity	Treatment Modification
Colitis	G1	Loperamide 4 mg as starting dose then 2 mg before each meal and after each loose stool until without diarrhea for 12 hours, with maximum of 16 mg loperamide per day. If G1 diarrhea or colitis persists >14 days, then add prednisolone 0.5–1 mg/kg (non-enteric-coated) or consider oral budesonide 9 mg daily if no bloody diarrhea
	G2/3 diarrhea or colitis	Withhold pembrolizumab. Loperamide 4 mg as starting dose then 2 mg before each meal and after each loose stool until without diarrhea for 12 hours, with maximum of 16 mg loperamide per day. Administer oral prednisone/prednisolone at a dose of 0.5–2 mg/kg/day or its equivalent. When improves to G1, begin a slow corticosteroid taper over at least 4 weeks. Resume pembrolizumab upon symptom control, or when prednisone/prednisolone daily dose <10 mg
	G4 diarrhea or colitis	Permanently discontinue pembrolizumab. Loperamide 4 mg as starting dose then 2 mg before each meal and after each loose stool until without diarrhea for 12 hours, with maximum of 16 mg loperamide per day. Administer 1–2 mg/kg IV (methyl)prednisolone and convert to 0.5–2 mg/kg prednisone/prednisolone orally each day or its equivalent only after a response. Taper over at least 4 weeks when symptoms improve. If does not improve over 72 hours or worsens, perform flexible sigmoidoscopy/colonoscopy to document colitis then begin infliximab 5 mg/kg (if no perforation/sepsis/TB/hepatitis/NYHA III/IV CHF). If no response, add MMF 500–1000 mg twice daily. If worse on MMF, consider addition of tacrolimus or ATG
Pneumonitis	G2	Withhold pembrolizumab. Consider pneumocystis prophylaxis depending on the clinical context and coverage with empiric antibiotics. Administer oral prednisone/prednisolone at a dose of 1–2 mg/kg/day or its equivalent. When improves to G1, begin a slow corticosteroid taper over at least 4 weeks. If does not respond adequately after 48 hours, then administer 2–4 mg/kg IV (methyl)prednisolone and convert to 0.5–2 mg/kg prednisone/prednisolone orally each day or its equivalent only after a response, followed by a taper over at least 6 weeks when symptoms improve to G1, titrating to symptoms. Resume pembrolizumab upon symptom control, or when prednisone/prednisolone daily dose <10 mg
	G3/4	Permanently discontinue pembrolizumab. Consider pneumocystis prophylaxis depending on the clinical context; cover with empiric antibiotics. Administer 2–4 mg/kg IV (methyl)prednisolone and convert to 1–2 mg/kg prednisone/prednisolone orally each day or its equivalent only after a response, followed by a taper over at least 8 weeks when symptoms improve to G1, titrating to symptoms. If, when initially treated, improvement does not occur within 48–72 hours, begin infliximab 5 mg/kg (if no perforation/sepsis/TB/hepatitis/NYHA III/IV CHF). If no response to infliximab, add MMF 500–1000 mg twice daily. Consider MMF especially if has concurrent hepatic toxicity
Hepatitis	G2 (AST or ALT >3–5× ULN or total bilirubin >1.5–3X ULN)	Withhold pembrolizumab. Administer oral prednisone/prednisolone at a dose of 1–2 mg/kg/day or its equivalent. When improves to G1, begin a slow corticosteroid taper over at least 4 weeks. Resume pembrolizumab upon symptom control, or when prednisone/prednisolone daily dose <10 mg
	G3/4 (AST or ALT >5× ULN or total bilirubin >3X ULN)	Permanently discontinue pembrolizumab. Administer 1–2 mg/kg IV (methyl)prednisolone and convert to 0.5–2 mg/kg prednisone/prednisolone orally each day or its equivalent only after a response. Taper over at least 6 weeks when symptoms improve. If no response, add MMF 500–1000 mg twice daily. If worse on MMF, consider adding tacrolimus or ATG
Hypophysitis	G2/3 (moderate symptoms, ie, headache but no visual disturbance or fatigue/mood alteration but hemodynamically stable, no electrolyte disturbance)	Administer analgesia as needed for headache. Withhold pembrolizumab. Administer oral prednisone/prednisolone at a dose of 0.5–2 mg/kg/day or its equivalent. When improves to G1, begin a slow corticosteroid taper over at least 4 weeks. If no improvement in 48 hours, administer 1–2 mg/kg IV (methyl)prednisolone and convert to 0.5–2 mg/kg prednisone/prednisolone orally each day or its equivalent only after a response. Taper over at least 4 weeks when symptoms improve to 5 mg prednisone/prednisolone or equivalent; do not stop steroids. Resume pembrolizumab upon symptom control, or when prednisone/prednisolone daily dose <10 mg
	G4 (severe mass effect symptoms, ie, severe headache, any visual disturbance or severe hypoadrenalism, ie, hypotension, severe electrolyte disturbance)	Permanently discontinue pembrolizumab. Administer analgesia as needed for headache. Administer 1–2 mg/kg IV (methyl)prednisolone and convert to 0.5–2 mg/kg prednisone/prednisolone orally each day or its equivalent only after a response. Taper over at least 4 weeks when symptoms improve to 5 mg prednisone/prednisolone or equivalent; do not stop steroids

(*continued*)

Treatment Modifications (*continued*)

RECOMMENDED DOSE MODIFICATIONS FOR PEMBROLIZUMAB

Adverse Event	Grade/Severity	Treatment Modification
Adrenal Insufficiency	G2	Withhold pembrolizumab. Administer oral prednisone/prednisolone at a dose of 0.5–2 mg/kg/day or its equivalent. When improves to G1, begin a slow corticosteroid taper over at least 4 weeks. Serially assess adrenal function and continue steroids at replacement doses (20–40 mg hydrocortisone daily ~2/3 dose in AM upon awakening and ~1/3 at 4 PM) until recovery of adrenal function is documented. Resume pembrolizumab upon symptom control, or when prednisone/prednisolone daily dose <10 mg
	G3/4	Permanently discontinue pembrolizumab. Administer oral prednisone/prednisolone at a dose of 0.5–2 mg/kg/day or its equivalent. When improves to G1, begin a slow corticosteroid taper over at least 4 weeks. Serially assess adrenal function and continue steroids at replacement doses (20–40 mg hydrocortisone daily ~2/3 dose in AM upon awakening and ~1/3 at 4 PM) until recovery of adrenal function is documented
Type 1 diabetes mellitus	G3 hyperglycemia	Withhold pembrolizumab. Admit to hospital to manage hyperglycemia. Role of corticosteroids in preventing complete loss of insulin-producing cells is unknown and not recommended. Resume pembrolizumab upon symptom control, or when prednisone/prednisolone daily dose <10 mg
	G4 hyperglycemia	Permanently discontinue pembrolizumab. Admit to hospital to manage hyperglycemia. Role of corticosteroids in preventing complete loss of insulin-producing cells is unknown and not recommended.
Nephritis and renal dysfunction	G2/3 (serum creatinine 1.5–6× ULN)	Withhold pembrolizumab. Administer oral prednisone/prednisolone at a dose of 0.5–2 mg/kg/day or its equivalent. When improves to G1, begin a slow corticosteroid taper over at least 4 weeks. If does not respond adequately, then administer 0.5–1 mg/kg IV (methyl)prednisolone and convert to 0.5–2 mg/kg prednisone/prednisolone orally each day or its equivalent only after a response, followed by a taper over at least 4 weeks when improves to G1. Resume pembrolizumab upon symptom control, or when prednisone/prednisolone daily dose <10 mg
	G4 (serum creatinine >6× ULN)	Permanently discontinue pembrolizumab. Administer 0.5–1 mg/kg IV (methyl)prednisolone and convert to 0.5–2 mg/kg prednisone/prednisolone orally each day or its equivalent only after a response, followed by a taper over at least 4 weeks when improves to G1
Skin	G1/2	Continue pembrolizumab. Avoid skin irritants, avoid sun exposure, topical emollients recommended. Topical steroid (mild strength for G1, moderate/potent strength for G2) cream once or twice daily ± oral or topical antihistamines for itching
	G3 rash or suspected SJS or TEN	Withhold pembrolizumab. Avoid skin irritants, avoid sun exposure, topical emollients recommended. Administer oral or topical antihistamines for itching. Administer oral prednisone/prednisolone at a dose of 0.5–2 mg/kg or its equivalent daily for 3 days followed by a slow corticosteroid taper over at least 4 weeks when the rash improves to G1. If does not respond adequately, then administer 0.5 –1 mg/kg IV (methyl)prednisolone and convert to 0.5–2 mg/kg prednisone/prednisolone orally each day or its equivalent only after a response, followed by a taper over at least 4 weeks when the rash improves to G1. Resume pembrolizumab upon symptom control, or when prednisone/prednisolone daily dose <10 mg
	G4 rash or confirmed SJS or TEN	Avoid skin irritants, avoid sun exposure, topical emollients recommended. Administer oral or topical antihistamines for itching. Administer 1–2 mg/kg IV (methyl)prednisolone and convert to oral steroids 0.5–2 mg/kg prednisone/prednisolone each day or its equivalent only after a response. Taper over at least 4 weeks when the rash improves to G1. Permanently discontinue pembrolizumab

(*continued*)

Treatment Modifications (continued)

RECOMMENDED DOSE MODIFICATIONS FOR PEMBROLIZUMAB

Adverse Event	Grade/Severity	Treatment Modification
Encephalitis	Confusion or altered behavior, headaches, alteration in Glasgow Coma Scale, motor or sensory deficits, speech abnormality, may or may not be febrile	Initially withhold pembrolizumab, but permanently discontinue pembrolizumab if there is no doubt as to diagnosis. Exclude bacterial and ideally viral infections prior to high-dose steroids. Administer oral prednisone/prednisolone at a dose of 0.5–2 mg/kg/day or its equivalent. When symptoms improve, begin a slow corticosteroid taper over at least 4–8 weeks. If symptoms are severe, administer 1–2 mg/kg IV (methyl)prednisolone and convert to 0.5–2 mg/kg prednisone/prednisolone orally each day or its equivalent only after a response. Consider concurrent empiric antiviral (IV acyclovir) and antibacterial therapy
Aseptic meningitis	Headache, photophobia, neck stiffness with fever or may be afebrile, vomiting; normal cognition/cerebral function (distinguishes from encephalitis)	
Other syndromes include neurosarcoidosis, posterior reversible leukoencephalopathy syndrome (PRES), Vogt-Koyanagi-Harada syndrome, demyelination, vasculitic encephalopathy, and generalized seizures		
Transverse myelitis	Acute or subacute neurologic signs/symptoms of motor/sensory/autonomic origin; most have sensory level; often bilateral symptoms	Initially withhold pembrolizumab, but permanently discontinue pembrolizumab if there is no doubt as to diagnosis. Administer 2 mg/kg IV (methyl)prednisolone or consider 1 g/day and convert to 0.5–2 mg/kg prednisone/prednisolone orally each day or its equivalent only after a response. When symptoms improve, begin a slow corticosteroid taper over at least 4–8 weeks. Plasmapheresis may be required if steroids do not bring about improvement
Myocarditis	G3	Permanently discontinue pembrolizumab. Administer 2 mg/kg IV (methyl)prednisolone or consider 1 g/day and convert to 0.5–2 mg/kg prednisone/prednisolone orally each day or its equivalent only after a response. When symptoms improve, begin a slow corticosteroid taper over at least 4–8 weeks. If no response, add MMF 500–1000 mg twice daily. If worse on MMF, consider adding tacrolimus
Peripheral neurologic toxicity	Moderate: some interference with ADL, symptoms concerning to patient	Withhold pembrolizumab. Initial observation reasonable or initiate prednisone/prednisolone 0.5–1 mg/kg (if progressing, eg, from mild) and/or pregabalin or duloxetine for pain. When symptoms improve, begin a slow corticosteroid taper over at least 4 weeks. Resume pembrolizumab upon symptom control, or when prednisone/prednisolone daily dose <10 mg
	Severe: limits self-care and aids warranted, life threatening, eg, respiratory problems	Permanently discontinue pembrolizumab. Administer 1–2 mg/kg IV (methyl)prednisolone and convert to 0.5–2 mg/kg prednisone/prednisolone orally each day or its equivalent only after a response. Taper over at least 4–8 weeks when symptoms improve to G1
Guillain-Barré syndrome	Progressive symmetrical muscle weakness with absent or reduced tendon reflexes—involves extremities, facial, respiratory, and bulbar and oculomotor muscles; dysregulation of autonomic nerves	Permanently discontinue pembrolizumab. Use of steroids not recommended in idiopathic Guillain-Barré syndrome; however, a trial of (methyl)prednisolone 1–2 mg/kg is reasonable, converting to 0.5–2 mg/kg prednisone/prednisolone orally each day or its equivalent only after a response. If no improvement or worsening, plasmapheresis or IVIG indicated
Myasthenia gravis	Fluctuating muscle weakness (proximal limb, trunk, ocular, eg, ptosis/diplopia or bulbar) with fatigability, respiratory muscles may also be involved	Permanently discontinue pembrolizumab. Administer pyridostigmine at an initial dose of 30 mg three times daily. Administer oral prednisone/prednisolone at a dose of 0.5–2 mg/kg/day or its equivalent or 1–2 mg/kg IV (methyl)prednisolone depending on the severity of symptoms. If begin with IV, convert to 0.5–2 mg/kg prednisone/prednisolone orally each day or its equivalent only after a response. If no improvement or worsening, plasmapheresis or IVIG may be considered. Additional immunosuppressants used in myasthenia gravis include azathioprine, cyclosporine, and mycophenolate. Avoid certain medications, eg, ciprofloxacin, beta-blockers, that may precipitate cholinergic crisis

(continued)

Treatment Modifications (*continued*)

RECOMMENDED DOSE MODIFICATIONS FOR PEMBROLIZUMAB

Adverse Event	Grade/Severity	Treatment Modification
Other syndromes including motor and sensory peripheral neuropathy, multifocal radicular neuropathy/plexopathy, autonomic neuropathy, phrenic nerve palsy, cranial nerve palsies (eg, facial nerve, optic nerve, hypoglossal nerve)		Permanently discontinue pembrolizumab. Administer oral prednisone/prednisolone at a dose of 0.5–2 mg/kg/day or its equivalent or 1–2 mg/kg IV (methyl)prednisolone depending on the severity of symptoms. If begin with IV, convert to 0.5–2 mg/kg prednisone/prednisolone orally each day or its equivalent only after a response
Arthralgia	G1 (mild pain with inflammation, erythema, or joint swelling)	Continue pembrolizumab. Administer acetaminophen (paracetamol) and ibuprofen
	G2 (moderate pain with inflammation, erythema, or joint swelling that limits ADL)	Withhold pembrolizumab. Administer higher doses of acetaminophen (paracetamol) and ibuprofen and use diclofenac or naproxen or etoricoxib. If inadequately controlled, consider intra-articular steroid injections for large joints or administer oral prednisone/prednisolone at a dose of 0.5–2 mg/kg/day or its equivalent. When improves to G1, begin a slow corticosteroid taper over at least 4 weeks. If does not respond adequately, then administer 0.5–1 mg/kg IV (methyl)prednisolone and convert to 0.5–2 mg/kg prednisone/prednisolone orally each day or its equivalent only after a response, followed by a taper over at least 4 weeks when improves to G1. Resume pembrolizumab upon symptom control, or when prednisone/prednisolone daily dose <10 mg
	G3 (severe pain; irreversible joint damage; disabling; limits self-care ADL)	Withhold pembrolizumab. Administer 0.5–1 mg/kg IV (methyl)prednisolone and convert to 0.5–2 mg/kg prednisone/prednisolone orally each day or its equivalent only after a response, followed by a taper over at least 4 weeks when improves to G1. In severe cases, infliximab or another anti–TNF-alpha drug may be required for improvement of arthritis. Resume pembrolizumab upon symptom control, or when prednisone/prednisolone daily dose <10 mg
Other	First occurrence of other G3	Withhold pembrolizumab. Administer oral prednisone/prednisolone at a dose of 0.5–2 mg/kg/day or its equivalent. When improves to G1, begin a slow corticosteroid taper over at least 4 weeks. Resume pembrolizumab upon symptom control, or when prednisone/prednisolone daily dose <10 mg
	Recurrence of same G3	Permanently discontinue pembrolizumab. Administer 1–2 mg/kg IV (methyl)prednisolone and convert to 0.5–2 mg/kg prednisone/prednisolone orally each day or its equivalent only after a response. Taper over at least 4–8 weeks when symptoms improve to G1
	Life-threatening or G4	
	Requirement for ≥10 mg/day prednisone or equivalent for >12 weeks	Permanently discontinue pembrolizumab
	Persistent G2/3 adverse reactions lasting ≥12 weeks	

ADL, activities of daily living; ALT, alanine aminotransferase; AST, aspartate aminotransferase; ATG, anti-thymocyte globulin; SJS, Stevens-Johnson Syndrome; TEN, toxic epidermal necrolysis; ULN, upper limit of normal

Notes on general supportive care:
- Steroid taper in most cases will proceed over a minimum of 1 month but if symptoms improve rapidly, a 2-week taper can be considered. If steroids are administered for more than 4 weeks, consider PCP prophylaxis (cotrimoxazole 480 mg twice daily M/W/F or inhaled pentamidine if has cotrimoxazole allergy), regular random blood glucose, VitD level, and starting calcium/VitD supplementation per guidelines

METASTATIC

HEAD AND NECK CANCER REGIMEN: CISPLATIN + FLUOROURACIL

(See also Methotrexate and Carboplatin + Fluorouracil)
Forastiere AA et al. J Clin Oncol 1992;10:1245–1251
Note: These 3 regimens were compared in a randomized trial. The Efficacy and Toxicity tables provide the comparative data

Hydration before, during, and after cisplatin administration ± mannitol:

• *Pre-cisplatin hydration* with 1000 mL 0.9% sodium chloride injection (0.9% NS); administer intravenously with potassium and magnesium supplementation as needed based on pretreatment laboratory results

• *Mannitol diuresis:* May be given to patients who have received adequate hydration. A dose of **mannitol** 12.5–25 g may be administered by intravenous injection or a short infusion before or during cisplatin administration, or prepared as an admixture with cisplatin. Continued intravenous hydration is essential

• *Continued mannitol diuresis:* In an inpatient or day-hospital setting, one may administer additional mannitol in the form of an intravenous infusion: **mannitol** 10–40 g; administer intravenously over 1–4 hours. This can be done either during or immediately after cisplatin, but requires maintenance of adequate intravenously administered fluids during and for hours after mannitol administration

• Post-cisplatin hydration with ≥1000 mL 0.9% NS; administer intravenously with potassium and magnesium supplementation as needed based on measured values

Cisplatin 100 mg/m^2; administer intravenously in 25–250 mL of 0.9% NS over 15–30 minutes, given on day 1 every 21 days (total dosage/cycle = 100 mg/m^2)
Fluorouracil 1000 mg/m^2 per day; administer by continuous intravenous infusion in 100–1000 mL 0.9% NS or 5% dextrose injection over 24 hours for 4 consecutive days (96-hour infusion), given on days 1–4 every 21 days (total dosage/cycle = 4000 mg/m^2)

Supportive Care
Antiemetic prophylaxis
*Emetogenic potential on days with cisplatin is **HIGH**. Potential for delayed symptoms*
*Emetogenic potential on days with fluorouracil alone is **LOW***
See Chapter 42 for antiemetic recommendations

Hematopoietic growth factor (CSF) prophylaxis
*Primary prophylaxis is **NOT** indicated*
See Chapter 43 for more information

Antimicrobial prophylaxis
*Risk of fever and neutropenia is **LOW***
   Antimicrobial primary prophylaxis to be considered:

   • Antibacterial—not indicated

   • Antifungal—not indicated

   • Antiviral—not indicated unless patient previously had an episode of HSV

Diarrhea management
Latent or delayed-onset diarrhea*:
   Loperamide 4 mg orally initially after the first loose or liquid stool, *then*
   Loperamide 2 mg orally every 2 hours during waking hours, *plus*
   Loperamide 4 mg orally every 4 hours during hours of sleep
   • Continue for at least 12 hours after diarrhea resolves

   • Recurrent diarrhea after a 12-hour diarrhea-free interval is treated as a new episode

   • Rehydrate orally with fluids and electrolytes during a diarrheal episode

   • If a patient develops blood or mucus in stool, dehydration, or hemodynamic instability, or if diarrhea persists >48 hours despite loperamide, stop loperamide and hospitalize the patient for IV hydration
Persistent diarrhea:
   Octreotide 100–150 mcg subcutaneously 3 times daily. Maximum total daily dose is 1500 mcg
Antibiotic therapy during latent or delayed-onset diarrhea:
   • A fluoroquinolone (eg, **ciprofloxacin** 500 mg orally every 12 hours) if absolute neutrophil count <500/mm^3 with or without accompanying fever in association with diarrhea

   • Antibiotics should also be administered if patient is hospitalized with prolonged diarrhea and should be continued until diarrhea resolves

*Rothenberg ML et al. J Clin Oncol 2001;19:3801–3807
Abigerges D et al. J Natl Cancer Inst 1994;86:446–449
Wadler S et al. J Clin Oncol 1998;16:3169–3178

(continued)

(*continued*)

Oral care (mucositis prophylaxis and management)

General advice:

- Encourage patients to maintain intake of nonalcoholic fluids
- Evaluate patients for oral pain and provide analgesic medications
- Consider histamine (H_2-subtype) receptor antagonists (eg, ranitidine, famotidine), or a proton pump inhibitor for epigastric pain
- *Lactobacillus* sp.–containing probiotics may be beneficial in preventing diarrhea

Patients with intact oral mucosa:

- Clean the mouth, tongue, and gums by brushing after every meal and at bedtime with an ultra-soft toothbrush with fluoride toothpaste
- Floss teeth gently every day unless contraindicated. If gums bleed and hurt, avoid bleeding or sore areas, but floss other teeth
- Patients may use saline or commercial bland, nonalcoholic rinses
  - Do not use mouthwashes that contain alcohols

If mucositis or stomatitis is present:

- Keep the mouth moist utilizing water, ice chips, sugarless gum, sugar-free hard candies, or a saliva substitute
- Rinse mouth several times a day to remove debris
  - Use a solution of ¼ teaspoon (1.25 g) each of baking soda and table salt (sodium chloride) in 1 quart (~950 mL) of warm water. Follow with a plain water rinse
  - Do not use mouthwashes that contain alcohols
- Foam-tipped swabs (eg, Toothettes) are useful in moisturizing oral mucosa, but ineffective for cleansing teeth and removing plaque
- Advise patients who develop mucositis to:
  - Choose foods that are easy to chew and swallow
  - Take small bites of food, chew slowly, and sip liquids with meals
  - Encourage soft, moist foods such as cooked cereals, mashed potatoes, and scrambled eggs
  - For trouble swallowing, soften food with gravies, sauces, broths, yogurt, or other bland liquids
  - Avoid sharp, crunchy foods; hot, spicy, or highly acidic foods (eg, citrus fruits and juices); sugary foods; toothpicks; tobacco products; alcoholic drinks

Patient Population Studied

A randomized comparison of 3 treatments: (a) single-agent methotrexate; (b) cisplatin plus fluorouracil; and (c) carboplatin plus fluorouracil. The study enrolled 277 patients with recurrent and metastatic squamous cell carcinoma of the head and neck. The primary objective was to compare separately the response rates of each regimen. Eligible patients had histologically proven squamous cell carcinoma of the head and neck that was either recurrent after attempted cure with surgery and radiation therapy or newly diagnosed disease with distant metastases. Patients with recurrent disease had not previously received chemotherapy for treatment of the recurrence, although they could have received induction chemotherapy ≥6 months before study entry. All patients were required to have measurable disease; a life expectancy of at least 12 weeks; a performance status of 0, 1, or 2 on the SWOG criteria; and a 24-hour creatinine clearance >50 mL/min (>0.83 mL/s)

Therapy Monitoring

1. *Before each cycle:* PE, CBC, LFTs, serum electrolytes, calcium, and magnesium
2. *One week after treatment:* Serum electrolytes, calcium, and magnesium
3. *Weekly follow-up recommended during at least the first cycle:* Attention to signs and symptoms of dehydration as supplemental hydration is often required

Efficacy*

	Methotrexate (n = 87)	Cisplatin + Fluorouracil (n = 85)	Carboplatin + Fluorouracil (n = 86)
Complete response	2	6	2
Partial response	8	26	19
Stable disease/no response	50	37	42
Increasing disease	32	16	25
Assumed no response[†]	8	15	12

*WHO Criteria
[†]Early death or not assessable

Toxicity*

	Methotrexate (n = 87)		Cisplatin + Fluorouracil (n = 85)		Carboplatin + Fluorouracil (n = 86)	
	% G1/2	% G3/4	% G1/2	% G3/4	% G1/2	% G3/4
Hematologic Toxicity						
Anemia	25.3	3.4	55.3	4.7	41.9	14
Granulocytopenia	8	6.9	31.8	8.2	20.9	2.3
Leukopenia	28.7	16.1	42.4	30.6	50	11.6
Thrombocytopenia	9.2	5.7	12.9	5.9	18.6	12.8
Nonhematologic Toxicity						
Diarrhea	3	0	12	2	6	2
Stomatitis	34	10	19	14	28	15
Nausea/vomiting†	38	8	68	8	48	6
Peripheral neuropathy	0	0	5	1	2	0
Ototoxicity	2	0	8	4	2	0
Renal	3	3	18	9	1	1
% G5 toxicity	1.1		1.1		1.2	

*SWOG Criteria
†Lower rates are expected with current antiemetics

Treatment Modifications

Adverse Event	Dose Modification
G ≥2 Mucosal or skin toxicity	Reduce fluorouracil dosage by 20%
G ≥2 Diarrhea (4–6 stools/day > baseline)	Hold fluorouracil until diarrhea resolves to baseline
G3 myelosuppression	Reduce cisplatin dosage by 25%. Do not change fluorouracil dosage
G4 myelosuppression	Reduce cisplatin dosage by 40%. Do not change fluorouracil dosage
Creatinine clearance <50 mL/min (<0.83 mL/s)	Do not administer therapy
Serum creatinine >1.5 mg/dL (>133 μmol/L) or 20% higher than baseline if >1.5 mg/dL (>133 μmol/L)	Hold cisplatin dose until serum creatinine <1.5 mg/dL (<133 μmol/L) or within 0.2 mg/dL (17.7 μmol/L) of baseline
Serum creatinine 1.5–2.0 mg/dL (133–177 μmol/L) immediately before a cycle	Hold cisplatin*, then reduce cisplatin dosage by 25% during subsequent cycles
Serum creatinine 2.1–3.0 mg/dL (186–265μmol/L) immediately before a cycle	Hold cisplatin*, then reduce cisplatin dosage by 50% during subsequent cycles
Serum creatinine >3.0 mg/dL (>265μmol/L) immediately before a cycle	Hold cisplatin
G2 neurotoxicity or ototoxicity	Hold cisplatin until neurotoxicity resolves to G ≤1
G3/4 neurotoxicity or ototoxicity	Discontinue chemotherapy

*Hold cisplatin until serum creatinine <1.5 mg/dL (<133 μmol/L), or within 0.2 mg/dL (17.7 μmol/L) of baseline

METASTATIC
HEAD AND NECK CANCER REGIMEN: CARBOPLATIN + FLUOROURACIL

(See also Methotrexate and Cisplatin + Fluorouracil)
Forastiere AA et al. J Clin Oncol 1992;10:1245–1251
Note: These 3 regimens were compared in a randomized trial. The Efficacy and Toxicity tables provide the comparative data

Carboplatin 300 mg/m²; administer intravenously in 50–500 mL 5% dextrose injection (D5W) or 0.9% sodium chloride injection (0.9% NS) over at least 15 minutes, given on day 1, every 28 days (total dosage/cycle = 300 mg/m²)
Fluorouracil 1000 mg/m² per day; administer by continuous intravenous infusion in 100–1000 mL 0.9% NS or D5W over 24 hours for 4 consecutive days (96-hour infusion), given on days 1–4, every 28 days (total dosage/cycle = 4000 mg/m²)

Supportive Care
Antiemetic prophylaxis
Emetogenic potential on days with carboplatin is **HIGH**. *Potential for delayed symptoms*
Emetogenic potential on days with fluorouracil alone is **LOW**
See Chapter 42 for antiemetic recommendations

Hematopoietic growth factor (CSF) prophylaxis
Primary prophylaxis is **NOT** *indicated*
See Chapter 43 for more information

Antimicrobial prophylaxis
Risk of fever and neutropenia is **LOW**
Antimicrobial primary prophylaxis to be considered:
- Antibacterial—not indicated
- Antifungal—not indicated
- Antiviral—not indicated unless patient previously had an episode of HSV

Diarrhea management
Latent or delayed-onset diarrhea*:
Loperamide 4 mg orally initially after the first loose or liquid stool, *then*
Loperamide 2 mg orally every 2 hours during waking hours, *plus*
Loperamide 4 mg orally every 4 hours during hours of sleep
- Continue for at least 12 hours after diarrhea resolves
- Recurrent diarrhea after a 12-hour diarrhea-free interval is treated as a new episode
- Rehydrate orally with fluids and electrolytes during a diarrheal episode
- If a patient develops blood or mucus in stool, dehydration, or hemodynamic instability, or if diarrhea persists >48 hours despite loperamide, stop loperamide and hospitalize the patient for IV hydration

Persistent diarrhea:
Octreotide 100–150 mcg subcutaneously 3 times daily. Maximum total daily dose is 1500 mcg
Antibiotic therapy during latent or delayed-onset diarrhea:
- A fluoroquinolone (eg, **ciprofloxacin** 500 mg orally every 12 hours) if absolute neutrophil count <500/mm³ with or without accompanying fever in association with diarrhea
- Antibiotics should also be administered if patient is hospitalized with prolonged diarrhea and should be continued until diarrhea resolves

*Rothenberg ML et al. J Clin Oncol 2001;19:3801–3807
Abigerges D et al. J Natl Cancer Inst 1994;86:446–449
Wadler S et al. J Clin Oncol 1998;16:3169–3178

Oral care (mucositis prophylaxis and management)
General advice:
- Encourage patients to maintain intake of nonalcoholic fluids
- Evaluate patients for oral pain and provide analgesic medications
- Consider histamine (H₂-subtype) receptor antagonists (eg, ranitidine, famotidine), or a proton pump inhibitor for epigastric pain
- *Lactobacillus* sp.—containing probiotics may be beneficial in preventing diarrhea
Patients with intact oral mucosa:
- Clean the mouth, tongue, and gums by brushing after every meal and at bedtime with an ultra-soft toothbrush with fluoride toothpaste
- Floss teeth gently every day unless contraindicated. If gums bleed and hurt, avoid bleeding or sore areas, but floss other teeth
- Patients may use saline or commercial bland, nonalcoholic rinses
  - Do not use mouthwashes that contain alcohols

(continued)

(*continued*)

If mucositis or stomatitis is present:
- Keep the mouth moist utilizing water, ice chips, sugarless gum, sugar-free hard candies, or a saliva substitute
- Rinse mouth several times a day to remove debris
  - Use a solution of ¼ teaspoon (1.25 g) each of baking soda and table salt (sodium chloride) in 1 quart (~950 mL) of warm water. Follow with a plain water rinse
  - Do not use mouthwashes that contain alcohols
- Foam-tipped swabs (eg, Toothettes) are useful in moisturizing oral mucosa, but ineffective for cleansing teeth and removing plaque
- Advise patients who develop mucositis to:
  - Choose foods that are easy to chew and swallow
  - Take small bites of food, chew slowly, and sip liquids with meals
  - Encourage soft, moist foods such as cooked cereals, mashed potatoes, and scrambled eggs
  - For trouble swallowing, soften food with gravies, sauces, broths, yogurt, or other bland liquids
  - Avoid sharp, crunchy foods; hot, spicy, or highly acidic foods (eg, citrus fruits and juices); sugary foods; toothpicks; tobacco products; alcoholic drinks

Patient Population Studied

A randomized comparison of 3 treatments: (a) single-agent methotrexate, (b) cisplatin plus fluorouracil, and (c) carboplatin plus fluorouracil. The study enrolled 277 patients with recurrent and metastatic squamous cell carcinoma of the head and neck. The primary objective was to compare separately the response rates of each regimen. Eligible patients had histologically proven squamous cell carcinoma of the head and neck that was either recurrent after attempted cure with surgery and radiation therapy or newly diagnosed disease with distant metastases. Patients with recurrent disease had not previously received chemotherapy for treatment of the recurrence, although they could have received induction chemotherapy ≥6 months before study entry. All patients were required to have measurable disease; a life expectancy of at least 12 weeks; a performance status of 0, 1, or 2 on the SWOG criteria; and a 24-hour creatinine clearance >50 mL/min (>0.83 mL/s)

Efficacy[*]

	Methotrexate (n = 87)	Cisplatin + Fluorouracil (n = 85)	Carboplatin + Fluorouracil (n = 86)
Complete response	2	6	2
Partial response	8	26	19
Stable disease/no response	50	37	42
Increasing disease	32	16	25
Assumed no response[†]	8	15	12

[*]WHO criteria
[†]Early death or not assessable

Toxicity*

	Methotrexate (n = 87)		Cisplatin + Fluorouracil (n = 85)		Carboplatin + Fluorouracil (n = 86)	
	% G1/2	% G3/4	% G1/2	% G3/4	% G1/2	% G3/4
Hematologic Toxicity						
Anemia	25.3	3.4	55.3	4.7	41.9	14
Granulocytopenia	8	6.9	31.8	8.2	20.9	2.3
Leukopenia	28.7	16.1	42.4	30.6	50	11.6
Thrombocytopenia	9.2	5.7	12.9	5.9	18.6	12.8
Nonhematologic Toxicity						
Diarrhea	3	0	12	2	6	2
Stomatitis	34	10	19	14	28	15
Nausea/vomiting†	38	8	68	8	48	6
Peripheral neuropathy	0	0	5	1	2	0
Ototoxicity	2	0	8	4	2	0
Renal	3	3	18	9	1	1
% G5 toxicity	1.1		1.1		1.2	

*SWOG Criteria
†Lower rates are expected with current antiemetics

Therapy Monitoring

1. *Weekly:* PE, CBC, serum electrolytes, LFTs calcium, and magnesium
2. *Weekly follow-up recommended during at least the first cycle:* Attention to signs and symptoms of dehydration as supplemental hydration is often required

Treatment Modifications

Adverse Event	Dose Modification
G ≥2 mucosal or skin toxicity	Reduce fluorouracil dosage by 20%
G ≥2 diarrhea (4–6 stools/day ≤ baseline)	Hold fluorouracil until diarrhea resolves
G3/4 toxicity myelosuppression	Reduce carboplatin dosage by 20%. Do not change fluorouracil dosage
G0/1 myelosuppression	Increase carboplatin dosage by 20% to 360 mg/m^2 on the same administration schedule

METASTATIC

HEAD AND NECK CANCER REGIMEN: CISPLATIN *OR* CARBOPLATIN WITH FLUOROURACIL + CETUXIMAB

Vermorken JB et al. N Engl J Med 2008;359:1116–1127

Cetuximab premedication:
Diphenhydramine 50 mg; administer by intravenous injection or infusion before cetuximab administration (other H_1-receptor antagonists may be substituted)

Initial cetuximab dose:
Cetuximab 400 mg/m²; administer intravenously over 120 minutes (maximum infusion rate = 5 mL [10 mg] per min) as a single loading dose (total initial dosage = 400 mg/m²)

Maintenance cetuximab doses:
Cetuximab 250 mg/m² per dose; administer intravenously over 60 minutes (maximum infusion rate = 5 mL [10 mg] per min) every week (total weekly dosage = 250 mg/m²)

Notes:
Cetuximab is intended for direct administration and should not be diluted
Maximum infusion rate = 5 mL (10 mg)/min
Administer cetuximab through a low-protein-binding in-line filter with pore size = 0.22 μm
Use 0.9% sodium chloride injection to flush vascular access devices after administration is completed
One hour after completing cetuximab administration, either cisplatin *or* carboplatin is given

Cisplatin-Containing Regimen

Hydration before, during, and after cisplatin administration ± mannitol:
- *Pre-cisplatin hydration* with 1000 mL 0.9% sodium chloride injection (0.9% NS); administer intravenously with potassium and magnesium supplementation as needed based on pretreatment laboratory results
- *Mannitol diuresis:* May be given to patients who have received adequate hydration. A dose of **mannitol** 12.5–25 g may be administered by intravenous injection or a short infusion before or during cisplatin administration, or prepared as an admixture with cisplatin. Continued intravenous hydration is essential
- *Continued mannitol diuresis:* In an inpatient or day-hospital setting, one may administer additional mannitol in the form of an intravenous infusion: **mannitol** 10–40 g; administer intravenously over 1–4 hours. This can be done either during or immediately after cisplatin, but requires maintenance of adequate intravenously administered fluids during and for hours after mannitol administration
- *Post-cisplatin hydration* with ≥1000 mL 0.9% NS; administer intravenously with potassium and magnesium supplementation as needed based on measured values

Cisplatin 100 mg/m²; administer intravenously in 50–1000 mL 0.9% NS over 60 minutes on day 1, every 3 weeks (total dosage/cycle = 100 mg/m²), *followed by:*

Fluorouracil 1000 mg/m² per day; administer in 50–1000 mL 0.9% NS or D5W by continuous intravenous infusion over 24 hours for 4 consecutive days, on days 1–4, every 3 weeks (total dosage/cycle = 4000 mg/m²)

Carboplatin-Containing Regimen

Carboplatin* (calculated dose) AUC = 5 mg/mL × min per dose; administer by intravenous infusion diluted to concentrations as low as 0.5 mg/mL with either D5W or 0.9% NS over 1 hour, on day 1, every 3 weeks (total dose/cycle calculated to produce a target AUC = 5 mg/mL × min), *followed by:*

Fluorouracil 1000 mg/m² per day; administer in 50–1000 mL 0.9% NS or D5W by continuous intravenous infusion over 24 hours for 4 consecutive days, on days 1–4, every 3 weeks for 4 cycles (total dosage/cycle = 4000 mg/m²)

*Carboplatin dose is based on a formula described by Calvert et al. to achieve a target area under the plasma concentration versus time curve (AUC)

$$\text{Total Carboplatin Dose (mg)} = (\text{target AUC}) \times (\text{GFR} + 25)$$

In practice, creatinine clearance (CrCl) is used in place of glomerular filtration rate (GFR). CrCl can be estimated from the equation of Cockcroft and Gault, thus:

$$\text{For males, CrCl} = \frac{(140 - \text{age[years]}) \times (\text{body weight [kg]})}{72 \times (\text{serum creatinine [mg/dL]})}$$

$$\text{For females, CrCl} = \frac{(140 - \text{age[years]}) \times (\text{body weight [kg]})}{72 \times (\text{serum creatinine [mg/dL]})} \times 0.85$$

(*continued*)

(*continued*)

Calvert AH et al. J Clin Oncol 1989;7:1748–1756
Cockcroft DW , Gault MH. Nephron 1976;16:31–41
Jodrell DI et al. J Clin Oncol 1992;10:520–528
Sorensen BT et al. Cancer Chemother Pharmacol 1991;28:397–401

Note: On October 8, 2010, the U.S. FDA identified a potential safety issue with carboplatin dosing based on recent changes in the measurement of serum creatinine. By the end of 2010, all clinical laboratories in the United States were required to use the standardized Isotope Dilution Mass Spectrometry (IDMS) method to measure serum creatinine, which can result in an overestimation of the GFR in some patients with normal renal function. A carboplatin dose calculated with an IDMS-measured serum creatinine result using the Calvert formula can exceed an expected exposure (AUC) and result in increased drug-related toxicity

- Provided actual GFR measurements are made to assess renal function, carboplatin can be safely dosed according to the Calvert formula described in product labeling
- If GFR (or creatinine clearance) is estimated based on serum creatinine measurements by the IDMS method, the FDA recommends, for patients with normal renal function, capping an estimated GFR at 125 mL/min for any targeted AUC value. No greater estimated GFR values should be used

U.S. FDA. Carboplatin dosing. [online] October 8, 2010. Available from: http://www.fda.gov/AboutFDA/CentersOffices/OfficeofMedicalProductsandTobacco/CDER/ucm228974.htm [accessed February 26, 2014]

Treatment duration:
Until evidence of disease progression or unacceptable toxicity for a maximum of 6 cycles of chemotherapy. Cetuximab may be continued as a single agent until unacceptable toxicity or disease progression

Supportive Care
Antiemetic prophylaxis
Emetogenic potential on days with cetuximab alone is **MINIMAL**
Emetogenic potential on days with cisplatin or carboplatin is **HIGH**. *Potential for delayed symptoms*
Emetogenic potential on days with fluorouracil alone is **LOW**
See Chapter 42 for antiemetic recommendations

Hematopoietic growth factor (CSF) prophylaxis
Primary prophylaxis is **NOT** indicated
See Chapter 43 for more information

Antimicrobial prophylaxis
Risk of fever and neutropenia is **LOW**
  Antimicrobial primary prophylaxis to be considered:
  - Antibacterial—not indicated
  - Antifungal—not indicated
  - Antiviral—not indicated unless patient previously had an episode of HSV

Diarrhea management
Latent or delayed-onset diarrhea*:
  Loperamide 4 mg orally initially after the first loose or liquid stool, *then*
  Loperamide 2 mg orally every 2 hours during waking hours, *plus*
  Loperamide 4 mg orally every 4 hours during hours of sleep
  - Continue for at least 12 hours after diarrhea resolves
  - Recurrent diarrhea after a 12-hour diarrhea-free interval is treated as a new episode
  - Rehydrate orally with fluids and electrolytes during a diarrheal episode
  - If a patient develops blood or mucus in stool, dehydration, or hemodynamic instability, or if diarrhea persists >48 hours despite loperamide, stop loperamide and hospitalize the patient for IV hydration

Alternatively, a trial of **diphenoxylate hydrochloride** 2.5 mg with **atropine sulfate** 0.025 mg (eg, Lomotil)
  - Initial adult dose is two tablets four times daily until control has been achieved, after which the dose may be reduced to meet individual requirements. Control may often be maintained with as little as two tablets daily
  - Clinical improvement of acute diarrhea is usually observed within 48 hours. If improvement of chronic diarrhea after treatment with a maximum daily dose of 8 tablets is not observed within 10 days, control is unlikely with further administration

Persistent diarrhea:
  Octreotide 100 –150 mcg subcutaneously 3 times daily. Maximum total daily dose is 1500 mcg
Antibiotic therapy during latent or delayed-onset diarrhea:
  A fluoroquinolone (eg, **ciprofloxacin** 500 mg orally every 12 hours) if absolute neutrophil count <500/mm^3 with or without accompanying fever in association with diarrhea
  - Antibiotics should also be administered if patient is hospitalized with prolonged diarrhea and should be continued until diarrhea resolves

(*continued*)

(*continued*)

*Rothenberg ML et al. J Clin Oncol 2001;19:3801–3807
Abigerges D et al. J Natl Cancer Inst 1994;86:446–449
Wadler S et al. J Clin Oncol 1998;16:3169–3178

Oral care

Risk of mucositis/stomatitis is **HIGH**

General advice:

- Encourage patients to maintain intake of nonalcoholic fluids
- Evaluate patients for oral pain and provide analgesic medications
- Consider histamine (H_2-subtype) receptor antagonists (eg, ranitidine, famotidine), or a proton pump inhibitor for epigastric pain
- *Lactobacillus* sp.—containing probiotics may be beneficial in preventing diarrhea

Patients with intact oral mucosa:

- Clean the mouth, tongue, and gums by brushing after every meal and at bedtime with an ultra-soft toothbrush with fluoride toothpaste
- Floss teeth gently every day unless contraindicated. If gums bleed and hurt, avoid bleeding or sore areas, but floss other teeth
- Patients may use saline or commercial bland, nonalcoholic rinses
  - Do not use mouthwashes that contain alcohols

If mucositis or stomatitis is present:

- Keep the mouth moist utilizing water, ice chips, sugarless gum, sugar-free hard candies, or a saliva substitute
- Rinse mouth several times a day to remove debris
  - Use a solution of ¼ teaspoon (1.25 g) each of baking soda and table salt (sodium chloride) in 1 quart (~950 mL) of warm water. Follow with a plain water rinse
  - Do not use mouthwashes that contain alcohols
- Foam-tipped swabs (eg, Toothettes) are useful in moisturizing oral mucosa, but ineffective for cleansing teeth and removing plaque
- Advise patients who develop mucositis to:
  - Choose foods that are easy to chew and swallow
  - Take small bites of food, chew slowly, and sip liquids with meals
  - Encourage soft, moist foods such as cooked cereals, mashed potatoes, and scrambled eggs
  - For trouble swallowing, soften food with gravies, sauces, broths, yogurt, or other bland liquids
  - Avoid sharp, crunchy foods; hot, spicy, or highly acidic foods (eg, citrus fruits and juices); sugary foods; toothpicks; tobacco products; alcoholic drinks

Patient Population Studied

A study of 442 patients with measurable histologically or cytologically confirmed recurrent and/or metastatic squamous cell carcinoma of the head and neck (except nasopharyngeal carcinoma) that was not curable with surgery or radiation. Prior chemotherapy for recurrent disease was not allowed. Prior chemotherapy delivered as part of initial curative therapy was allowed provided it was completed at least 6 months before study entry. Age ≥18 years, adequate organ function, and Karnofsky performance status of ≥70 were required

Efficacy

(PF Comparator = The Same Chemotherapy Without Cetuximab)*			
	PFC[†] (n = 222)	PF[†] (n = 220)	Hazard Ratio (P Value)
Median overall survival, months	10.1	7.4	0.8 (0.04)
Median progression-free survival, months	5.6	3.3	0.54 (<0.001)
Median time to treatment failure, months	4.8	3	0.59 (<0.001)
Median duration of response, months	5.6	4.7	0.76 (0.21)
	PFC (n = 222)	PF (n = 220)	Odds Ratio (P Value)
Overall response rate	36%	20%	2.23 (<0.001)

*WHO
[†]PFC, Cisplatin or carboplatin with fluorouracil + cetuximab; PF, cisplatin or carboplatin with + fluorouracil

Toxicity

Adverse Event	PFC[†] % G3/4 (n = 219)	PF[†] % G3/4 (n = 215)
	(PF Comparator = The Same Chemotherapy Without Cetuximab)*	
Anemia	13	19
Thrombocytopenia	11	11
Neutropenia	22	23
Leukopenia	9	9
Febrile neutropenia	5	5
Sepsis	4	<1
Skin reactions	9	<1
Pneumonia	4	2
Dyspnea	4	8
Respiratory failure	<1	2
Anorexia	5	1
Vomiting	5	3
Asthenia	5	6
Decreased performance status	1	2
Tumor hemorrhage	1	3
Cardiac events	7	4
Hypomagnesemia	5	1
Hypocalcemia	4	1
Hypokalemia	7	5

*NCI, CTC, National Cancer Institute (USA) Common Toxicity Criteria and Common Terminology Criteria for Adverse Events, all versions. Available at: http://ctep.cancer.gov/protocolDevelopment/electronic_applications/ctc.htm [accessed December 7, 2013]
[†]PFC, Cisplatin or carboplatin with fluorouracil + cetuximab; PF, cisplatin or carboplatin with fluorouracil

Therapy Monitoring

1. *Pretreatment evaluation:* Medical history and tumor assessment by clinical evaluation and imaging studies
2. *Response evaluation:* Every 2 cycles

Treatment Modifications

Adverse Event	Dose Modification
First occurrence G3 skin toxicity	Hold cetuximab up to 2 weeks
Second occurrence G3 skin toxicity	Reduce cetuximab dosage to 200 mg/m²
Third occurrence G3 skin toxicity	Reduce cetuximab dosage to 150 mg/m²
Fourth occurrence G3 skin toxicity	Discontinue cetuximab
G ≥2 mucosal or skin toxicity	Reduce fluorouracil dosage 20%
G ≥2 diarrhea (4–6 stools/day greater than baseline)	Hold fluorouracil until diarrhea resolves to baseline
Creatinine clearance ≤50 mL/min (≤0.83 mL/s)	Replace cisplatin with carboplatin AUC = 5 mg/mL × min
G3 myelosuppression	Reduce cisplatin dosage by 25% or carboplatin dosage by 20%. Do not change fluorouracil dosage
G4 myelosuppression	Reduce cisplatin dosage by 40% or carboplatin dosage by 20%. Do not change fluorouracil dosage
Creatinine clearance <50 mL/min (<0.83 mL/s)	Do not administer therapy
Serum creatinine >1.5 mg/dL (>133 μmol/L) or 20% higher than baseline if baseline was >1.5 mg/dL	Hold cisplatin dosage until serum creatinine <1.5 mg/dL (<133 μmol/L) or within 0.2 mg/dL (17.7 μmol/L) of baseline
Serum creatinine 1.5–2.0 mg/dL (133–177 μmol/L) immediately before a cycle	Hold cisplatin,* then reduce cisplatin dosage by 25% during subsequent cycles
Serum creatinine 2.1–3.0 mg/dL (186–265 μmol/L) immediately before a cycle	Hold cisplatin*, then reduce cisplatin dosage by 50% during subsequent cycles
Serum creatinine >3.0 mg/dL immediately before a cycle	Hold cisplatin
G2 neurotoxicity or ototoxicity	Hold cisplatin until neurotoxicity resolves to G ≤1
G3/4 neurotoxicity or ototoxicity	Discontinue chemotherapy
G ≥3 nausea/vomiting despite use of a serotonin (5-HT₃) receptor antagonist + dexamethasone + aprepitant, consistent with published guidelines (see Chapter 43)	Reduce cisplatin dosage or carboplatin dose, or discontinue the platinating agent

*Hold cisplatin until serum creatinine <1.5 mg/dL (<133 μmol/L) or within 0.2 mg/dL (17.7 μmol/L) of baseline

METASTATIC

HEAD AND NECK CANCER REGIMEN: CISPLATIN + PACLITAXEL *OR* CISPLATIN + FLUOROURACIL

Gibson MK et al. J Clin Oncol 2005;23:3562–3567

CISPLATIN + PACLITAXEL

Premedication for paclitaxel
Dexamethasone 20 mg/dose; administer orally or intravenously for 2 doses at 12–14 hours and 6–7 hours before starting paclitaxel (total dose/cycle = 40 mg), *or*
Dexamethasone 20 mg; administer intravenously 30 minutes before administering paclitaxel (total dose/cycle = 20 mg)
plus
Diphenhydramine 50 mg; administer intravenously 30 minutes before administering paclitaxel
Cimetidine 300 mg (*or* **ranitidine** 50 mg *or* **famotidine** 20 mg *or* an equivalent histamine receptor [H$_2$]-subtype antagonist); administer intravenously in 20–50 mL 0.9% sodium chloride injection (0.9% NS) or 5% dextrose injection (D5W) over 15–20 minutes, 30 minutes before administering paclitaxel

Hydration before, during, and after cisplatin administration ± mannitol:
• *Pre-cisplatin hydration* with 1000 mL 0.9% NS; administer intravenously with potassium and magnesium supplementation as needed based on pretreatment laboratory results
• *Mannitol diuresis:* May be given to patients who have received adequate hydration. A dose of **mannitol** 12.5–25 g may be administered by intravenous injection or a short infusion before or during cisplatin administration, or prepared as an admixture with cisplatin. Continued intravenous hydration is essential
• *Continued mannitol diuresis:* In an inpatient or day-hospital setting, one may administer additional mannitol in the form of an intravenous infusion: **mannitol** 10–40 g; administer intravenously over 1–4 hours. This can be done either during or immediately after cisplatin, but requires maintenance of adequate intravenously administered fluids during and for hours after mannitol administration
• *Post-cisplatin hydration* with ≥1000 mL 0.9% NS; administer intravenously with potassium and magnesium supplementation as needed based on measured values

Paclitaxel 175 mg/mg; administer intravenously in a volume of 0.9% NS or D5W sufficient to produce a concentration within the range 0.3–1.2 mg/mL over 3 hours on day 1, every 21 days (total dosage/cycle = 175 mg/m^2), *followed by:*
Cisplatin 75 mg/m^2; administer intravenously in 50–1000 mL 0.9% NS over 60 minutes on day 1, every 21 days (total dosage/cycle = 75 mg/m^2)

Notes: Treatment is continued for at least 6 cycles in patients who continue to respond

Carboplatin (target AUC = 6 mg/mL × min) may be substituted for cisplatin in patients who develop G ≥2 neuropathy or renal impairment (creatinine clearance <50 mL/min [<0.83 mL/s])

Supportive Care
Antiemetic prophylaxis
*Emetogenic potential on day 1 is **HIGH**. Potential for delayed symptoms*
See Chapter 42 for antiemetic recommendations

Hematopoietic growth factor (CSF) prophylaxis
*Primary prophylaxis is **NOT** indicated*
See Chapter 43 for more information

Antimicrobial prophylaxis
*Risk of fever and neutropenia is **LOW***
  Antimicrobial primary prophylaxis to be considered:
  • Antibacterial—not indicated
  • Antifungal—not indicated
  • Antiviral—not indicated unless patient previously had an episode of HSV

(*continued*)

Patient Population Studied

A study of 218 patients with measurable or assessable histologically confirmed squamous cell carcinoma of the head and neck (excluding nasopharyngeal carcinoma) not curable with surgery or radiation. Prior chemotherapy for recurrent disease was not allowed. Prior chemotherapy delivered as part of initial curative therapy was allowed; treatment with paclitaxel or fluorouracil had to be completed more than 12 months before study entry, and treatment with cisplatin had to be completed more than 6 months before study entry. Age ≥18 years, adequate organ function, and ECOG performance status ≤1 were required

Efficacy

	Cisplatin + Fluorouracil	Cisplatin + Paclitaxel
Complete response	6.7%	7%
Partial response	23.1%	19%
Stable disease	55.8%	54%
Progressive disease	3.8%	6%
Not assessable	10.6%	14%

	Cisplatin + Fluorouracil	Cisplatin + Paclitaxel
Median overall survival, months	8.7	8.1
1-year survival	41.4%	32.4%

(continued)

CISPLATIN + FLUOROURACIL

Hydration before, during, and after cisplatin administration ± mannitol:

- *Pre-cisplatin hydration* with 1000 mL 0.9% sodium chloride injection (0.9% NS); administer intravenously with potassium and magnesium supplementation as needed based on pretreatment laboratory results

- *Mannitol diuresis:* May be given to patients who have received adequate hydration. A dose of **mannitol 12.5–25 g** may be administered by intravenous injection or a short infusion before or during cisplatin administration, or prepared as an admixture with cisplatin. Continued intravenous hydration is essential

- *Continued mannitol diuresis:* In an inpatient or day-hospital setting, one may administer additional mannitol in the form of an intravenous infusion: **mannitol 10–40 g**; administer intravenously over 1–4 hours. This can be done either during or immediately after cisplatin, but requires maintenance of adequate intravenously administered fluids during and for hours after mannitol administration

- *Post-cisplatin hydration* with ≥1000 mL 0.9% NS; administer intravenously with potassium and magnesium supplementation as needed based on measured values

Cisplatin 100 mg/m²; administer intravenously in 50–1000 mL 0.9% NS over 60 minutes on day 1, every 21 days (total dosage/cycle = 100 mg/m²)
Fluorouracil 1000 mg/m² per day; administer in 50–1000 mL 0.9% NS or 5% dextrose injection by continuous intravenous infusion over 24 hours for 4 consecutive days, on days 1–4, every 21 days (total dosage/cycle = 4000 mg/m²)

Notes: Treatment is continued for at least 6 cycles in patients who continue to respond. Carboplatin (target AUC = 6 mg/mL × min) may be substituted for cisplatin in patients who develop G ≥2 neuropathy or renal impairment (creatinine clearance <50 mL/min [<0.83 mL/s])

Supportive Care
Antiemetic prophylaxis
Emetogenic potential on days with cisplatin or carboplatin is **HIGH**. *Potential for delayed symptoms*
Emetogenic potential on days with fluorouracil alone is **LOW**
See Chapter 42 for antiemetic recommendations

Hematopoietic growth factor (CSF) prophylaxis
Primary prophylaxis may be indicated
See Chapter 43 for more information

Antimicrobial prophylaxis
Risk of fever and neutropenia is **LOW**
  Antimicrobial primary prophylaxis to be considered:
  - Antibacterial—consider a fluoroquinolone or no prophylaxis
  - Antifungal—not indicated
  - Antiviral—not indicated unless patient previously had an episode of HSV

Diarrhea management
Latent or delayed-onset diarrhea:
  Loperamide 4 mg orally initially after the first loose or liquid stool, *then*
  Loperamide 2 mg orally every 2 hours during waking hours, *plus*
  Loperamide 4 mg orally every 4 hours during hours of sleep
- Continue for at least 12 hours after diarrhea resolves
- Recurrent diarrhea after a 12-hour diarrhea-free interval is treated as a new episode
- Rehydrate orally with fluids and electrolytes during a diarrheal episode
- If a patient develops blood or mucus in stool, dehydration, or hemodynamic instability, or if diarrhea persists >48 hours despite loperamide, stop loperamide and hospitalize the patient for IV hydration

(continued)

Toxicity

Adverse Event	Cisplatin + Fluorouracil % G3–5 n = 106	Cisplatin + Paclitaxel % G3–5 n = 108
Anemia	33	13
Thrombocytopenia	23	4
Neutropenia	67	55
Leukopenia	63	35
Infection	21	13*
Genitourinary	3	1
Stomatitis	31	0
Mucositis	1	0
Diarrhea	6	1
Nausea	19	18
Vomiting	18	10
Fatigue	9	7
Decreased performance status	1	2
Hemorrhage	2†	1†
Cardiac	3†	4
Metabolic	15	10
Dehydration	5	4
Liver	1	3
Hypotension	2	5
Neurosensory	4	5
Neuromotor	3	4
Toxic deaths	7	5

*Includes 4% G5 toxicities
†Includes 1% G5 toxicities

Therapy Monitoring

1. *Pretreatment evaluation:* Medical history and tumor assessment by clinical evaluation and imaging studies
2. *Response evaluation:* Every 2 cycles

(*continued*)

Persistent diarrhea:
Octreotide 100–150 mcg subcutaneously 3 times daily. Maximum total daily dose is 1500 mcg

Antibiotic therapy during latent or delayed-onset diarrhea:
A fluoroquinolone (eg, **ciprofloxacin** 500 mg orally every 12 hours) if absolute neutrophil count <500/mm^3 with or without accompanying fever in association with diarrhea
- Antibiotics should also be administered if patient is hospitalized with prolonged diarrhea and should be continued until diarrhea resolves

*Rothenberg ML et al. J Clin Oncol 2001;19:3801–3807
Abigerges D et al. J Natl Cancer Inst 1994;86:446–449
Wadler S et al. J Clin Oncol 1998;16:3169–3178

Oral care
Risk of mucositis/stomatitis is **HIGH**
  General advice:
- Encourage patients to maintain intake of nonalcoholic fluids
- Evaluate patients for oral pain and provide analgesic medications
- Consider histamine (H$_2$-subtype) receptor antagonists (eg, ranitidine, famotidine), or a proton pump inhibitor for epigastric pain
- *Lactobacillus* sp.–containing probiotics may be beneficial in preventing diarrhea

  Patients with intact oral mucosa:
- Clean the mouth, tongue, and gums by brushing after every meal and at bedtime with an ultra-soft toothbrush with fluoride toothpaste
- Floss teeth gently every day unless contraindicated. If gums bleed and hurt, avoid bleeding or sore areas, but floss other teeth
- Patients may use saline or commercial bland, nonalcoholic rinses
  - Do not use mouthwashes that contain alcohols

  If mucositis or stomatitis is present:
- Keep the mouth moist utilizing water, ice chips, sugarless gum, sugar-free hard candies, or a saliva substitute
- Rinse mouth several times a day to remove debris
  - Use a solution of ¼ teaspoon (1.25 g) each of baking soda and table salt (sodium chloride) in 1 quart (~950 mL) of warm water. Follow with a plain water rinse
  - Do not use mouthwashes that contain alcohols
- Foam-tipped swabs (eg, Toothettes) are useful in moisturizing oral mucosa, but ineffective for cleansing teeth and removing plaque
- Advise patients who develop mucositis to:
  - Choose foods that are easy to chew and swallow
  - Take small bites of food, chew slowly, and sip liquids with meals
  - Encourage soft, moist foods such as cooked cereals, mashed potatoes, and scrambled eggs
  - For trouble swallowing, soften food with gravies, sauces, broths, yogurt, or other bland liquids
  - Avoid sharp, crunchy foods; hot, spicy, or highly acidic foods (eg, citrus fruits and juices); sugary foods; toothpicks; tobacco products; alcoholic drinks

Dose Modifications

Adverse Event	Dose Modification
G4 toxicity	Withhold treatment until G ≤1
G2 hepatic toxicity	Withhold treatment until G ≤1
G3 hepatic toxicity	Withhold treatment until G ≤1, then reduce paclitaxel dosage by 20%
Neutrophil count <1500/mm^3	Withhold treatment until ANC is ≥1500/mm^3
Platelet count <100,000/mm^3	Withhold treatment until platelet count is ≥100,000/mm^3
Nadir thrombocytopenia G4	Reduce dosages of all agents by 20%
G4 neutropenia ≥5 days	Reduce dosages of all agents by 20%
Febrile neutropenia requiring hospitalization and antibiotics	Reduce dosages of all agents by 20%
G ≥2 mucosal or skin toxicity	Reduce fluorouracil dosage by 20%
G3 mucositis	Reduce paclitaxel and fluorouracil dosages by 20%
G ≥2 diarrhea (4–6 stools/day greater than baseline)	Hold fluorouracil until diarrhea resolves to baseline
Creatinine clearance ≤50 mL/min (≤0.83 mL/s)	Replace cisplatin with carboplatin AUC = 6 mg/mL × min
G2 neuropathy	Replace cisplatin with carboplatin AUC = 6 mg/mL × min; do not alter paclitaxel dosage
G2 neuropathy lasting ≥1 cycle after substituting carboplatin for cisplatin	Reduce paclitaxel dosages by 20%
G3 neuropathy	Discontinue therapy

METASTATIC

HEAD AND NECK CANCER REGIMEN: PACLITAXEL + CARBOPLATIN

Pivot X et al. Oncology 2001;60:66–71

Premedication:
Prednisone 60 mg; administer orally twice daily for a total of 4 doses, starting the day before chemotherapy (total dose/cycle = 240 mg), *or*
Dexamethasone 20 mg/dose; administer orally for 2 doses at 12–14 hours and 6–7 hours before starting paclitaxel administration (total dose/cycle = 40 mg), *or*
Dexamethasone 20 mg; administer intravenously 30 minutes before starting paclitaxel administration (total dose/cycle = 20 mg)
Cimetidine 300 mg (*or* **ranitidine** 50 mg *or* **famotidine** 20 mg or an equivalent histamine receptor [H2]-subtype antagonist); administer intravenously over 15–30 minutes, 30–60 minutes before paclitaxel
Diphenhydramine 50 mg; administer by intravenous injection, 30–60 minutes before paclitaxel
Paclitaxel 175 mg/m^2; administer by intravenous infusion in a volume of 0.9% NS or D5W sufficient to produce a concentration within the range 0.3–1.2 mg/mL over 3 hours on day 1, every 21 days (total dosage/cycle = 175 mg/m^2), *followed by:*
Carboplatin (calculated dose) AUC = 6 mg/mL × min; administer by intravenous infusion in 500 mL of 0.9% NS over 2 hours on day 1, every 21 days (total dosage/cycle calculated to produce an AUC of 6 mg/mL × min)

An equation for calculating carboplatin doses developed by Chatelut et al accounts for inter-individual carboplatin clearance (CL) based on patient-specific factors for weight, age, and sex (Chatelut E et al. J Natl Cancer Inst 1995;87:573–580):

$$CL\ (females) = (0.134 \times wt) + \frac{[(218 \times wt) \times (1 - 0.00457 \times age) \times 0.686]}{serum\ creatinine}$$

$$CL\ (males) = (0.134 \times wt) + \frac{[(218 \times wt) \times (1 - 0.00457 \times age)]}{serum\ creatinine}$$

Weight is expressed in kilogram units, age in years, serum creatinine in micromoles/L (micromoles/L = mg/dL × 88.4), and the value for sex is 0 (zero) for males and 1 (one) for females

A carboplatin dose (in milligrams) is calculated from a target area under the plasma concentration versus time curve (AUC) and a value for carboplatin clearance (CL) appropriate for a female or male patient:

$$Carboplatin\ dose\ (mg) = CL\ (mL/min) \times AUC\ (mg \cdot min/mL)$$

Supportive Care
Antiemetic prophylaxis
Emetogenic potential is **HIGH**. *Potential for delayed symptoms*
See Chapter 42 for antiemetic recommendations

Hematopoietic growth factor (CSF) prophylaxis
Primary prophylaxis is indicated with one of the following:
Filgrastim (G-CSF) 5 mcg/kg per day, by subcutaneous injection, *or*
Pegfilgrastim (pegylated filgrastim) 6 mg/0.6 mL, by subcutaneous injection for one dose
• Begin use from 24–72 h after myelosuppressive chemotherapy is completed
• Continue daily filgrastim use until ANC ≥10,000/mm^3 on two measurements separated temporally by ≥12 hours
• Discontinue daily filgrastim use at least 24 hours before administering myelosuppressive treatment. Do not administer pegfilgrastim within 14 days before administering myelosuppressive treatment
See Chapter 43 for more information

(continued)

Patient Population Studied

A study of 27 patients with unresectable recurrent disease or distant metastatic disease. Previous radiation treatment and concomitant or induction chemoradiation were allowed. ECOG performance status 0–2 and adequate organ function were required, including creatinine clearance ≥45 mL/min (≥0.75 mL/s)

Efficacy (N = 27)

Complete response	7.4%
Partial response	22.2%
Stable disease	11.1%
Median duration of response	4.4 months
Median survival	7.2 months
SWOG Criteria	

Toxicity (N = 27)

	% G2	% G3/4
Hematologic		
Anemia	40.7	11.1
Neutropenia	14.8	62.9
Febrile neutropenia	—	18.5
Thrombocytopenia	11.1	14.8
Nonhematologic		
Alopecia	29.6	44.4
Neurotoxicity (neuropathy)	11.1	7.4
Mucositis	11.1	7.4
Nausea/vomiting	7.4	7.4
Cardiotoxicity	—	3.7
G5 toxicity	3.7%*	

*One patient with neutropenia and sepsis
National Cancer Institute Common Toxicity Criteria

(*continued*)

Antimicrobial prophylaxis

Risk of fever and neutropenia is **INTERMEDIATE**

Antimicrobial primary prophylaxis to be considered:

- Antibacterial—consider a fluoroquinolone or no prophylaxis
- Antifungal—consider concomitant use of cotrimoxazole during periods of neutropenia, and in anticipation of mucositis
- Antiviral—not indicated, unless patient previously had an episode of HSV

Oral care

Risk of mucositis/stomatitis is **MODERATE**

General advice:

- Encourage patients to maintain intake of nonalcoholic fluids
- Evaluate patients for oral pain and provide analgesic medications
- Consider histamine (H$_2$-subtype) receptor antagonists (eg, ranitidine, famotidine), or a proton pump inhibitor for epigastric pain
- *Lactobacillus* sp.—containing probiotics may be beneficial in preventing diarrhea

Patients with intact oral mucosa:

- Clean the mouth, tongue, and gums by brushing after every meal and at bedtime with an ultra-soft toothbrush with fluoride toothpaste
- Floss teeth gently every day unless contraindicated. If gums bleed and hurt, avoid bleeding or sore areas, but floss other teeth
- Patients may use saline or commercial bland, nonalcoholic rinses
  - Do not use mouthwashes that contain alcohols

If mucositis or stomatitis is present:

- Keep the mouth moist utilizing water, ice chips, sugarless gum, sugar-free hard candies, or a saliva substitute
- Rinse mouth several times a day to remove debris
  - Use a solution of ¼ teaspoon (1.25 g) each of baking soda and table salt (sodium chloride) in 1 quart (~950 mL) of warm water. Follow with a plain water rinse
  - Do not use mouthwashes that contain alcohols
- Foam-tipped swabs (eg, Toothettes) are useful in moisturizing oral mucosa, but ineffective for cleansing teeth and removing plaque
- Advise patients who develop mucositis to:
  - Choose foods that are easy to chew and swallow
  - Take small bites of food, chew slowly, and sip liquids with meals
  - Encourage soft, moist foods such as cooked cereals, mashed potatoes, and scrambled eggs
  - For trouble swallowing, soften food with gravies, sauces, broths, yogurt, or other bland liquids
  - Avoid sharp, crunchy foods; hot, spicy, or highly acidic foods (eg, citrus fruits and juices); sugary foods; toothpicks; tobacco products; alcoholic drinks

Therapy Monitoring

1. *Before each cycle:* CBC with differential, serum electrolytes, calcium, magnesium, and LFTs
2. *Weekly:* CBC with differential

Treatment Modifications

Adverse Event	Dose Modification
G3/4 mucositis	Reduce paclitaxel dosage by 20%
G3 thrombocytopenia	Reduce paclitaxel dosage by 20%
G4 thrombocytopenia	Reduce paclitaxel dosage by 50%
G4 neutropenia >5 days	Reduce paclitaxel dosage by 20%
ANC <1500/mm^3 or platelets <100,000/ mm^3 at the time of chemotherapy administration	Delay chemotherapy until ANC >1500/ mm^3 *and* platelets >100,000/ mm^3. Discontinue chemotherapy if recovery has not occurred after a 2-week delay
Creatinine clearance (CrCl) <45 mL/min (<0.75 mL/s)	Delay treatment until CrCl >45 mL/ min (>0.75 mL/s). Discontinue therapy if has not recovered by 6 weeks
G2 neurotoxicity	Hold paclitaxel until neurotoxicity resolves to G ≤1
G3/4 neurotoxicity	Discontinue chemotherapy

METASTATIC

HEAD AND NECK CANCER REGIMEN: DOCETAXEL + CISPLATIN

Glisson BS et al. J Clin Oncol 2002;20:1593–1599

Premedication:
Dexamethasone 8 mg; administer orally or intravenously twice daily for 3 days starting the day before docetaxel infusion (total dose/cycle = 48 mg)

Hydration before, during, and after cisplatin administration ± mannitol:
- *Pre-cisplatin hydration* with 1000 mL 0.9% sodium chloride injection (0.9% NS); administer intravenously with potassium and magnesium supplementation as needed based on pretreatment laboratory results
- *Mannitol diuresis:* May be given to patients who have received adequate hydration. A dose of **mannitol** 12.5–25 g may be administered by intravenous injection or a short infusion before or during cisplatin administration, or prepared as an admixture with cisplatin. Continued intravenous hydration is essential
- *Continued mannitol diuresis:* In an inpatient or day-hospital setting, one may administer additional mannitol in the form of an intravenous infusion: **mannitol** 10–40 g; administer intravenously over 1–4 hours. This can be done either during or immediately after cisplatin, but requires maintenance of adequate intravenously administered fluids during and for hours after mannitol administration
- *Post-cisplatin hydration* with ≥1000 mL 0.9% NS; administer intravenously with potassium and magnesium supplementation as needed based on measured values

Docetaxel 75 mg/m²; administer intravenously diluted in a volume of 0.9% NS or 5% dextrose injection sufficient to produce a docetaxel concentration within the range 0.3–0.74 mg/mL over 60 minutes, on day 1, every 21 days (total dosage/cycle = 75 mg/m²), followed by
Cisplatin 75 mg/m²; administer intravenously in 25–250 mL 0.9% NS over 30 minutes on day 1, every 21 days (total dosage/cycle = 75 mg/m²)

Supportive Care
Antiemetic prophylaxis
Emetogenic potential is **HIGH**. Potential for delayed symptoms
See Chapter 42 for antiemetic recommendations

Hematopoietic growth factor (CSF) prophylaxis
Primary prophylaxis is **NOT** indicated
See Chapter 43 for more information

Antimicrobial prophylaxis
Risk of fever and neutropenia is **LOW**
  Antimicrobial primary prophylaxis to be considered:
  - Antibacterial—not indicated
  - Antifungal—not indicated
  - Antiviral—not indicated unless patient previously had an episode of HSV

Oral care (mucositis prophylaxis and management)
Risk of mucositis/stomatitis is **LOW–MODERATE**
  General advice:
  - Encourage patients to maintain intake of nonalcoholic fluids
  - Evaluate patients for oral pain and provide analgesic medications
  - Consider histamine (H₂-subtype) receptor antagonists (eg, ranitidine, famotidine), or a proton pump inhibitor for epigastric pain
  - *Lactobacillus* sp.–containing probiotics may be beneficial in preventing diarrhea
  Patients with intact oral mucosa:
  - Clean the mouth, tongue, and gums by brushing after every meal and at bedtime with an ultra-soft toothbrush with fluoride toothpaste
  - Floss teeth gently every day unless contraindicated. If gums bleed and hurt, avoid bleeding or sore areas, but floss other teeth
  - Patients may use saline or commercial bland, nonalcoholic rinses
    - Do not use mouthwashes that contain alcohols

(continued)

A study of 36 patients with recurrent disease or disease deemed incurable, who had not previously received chemotherapy for recurrent disease and had never received a taxane, were entered in a multicenter phase 2 trial. Performance status ECOG 0–1 and adequate organ function were required, including creatinine clearance ≥50 mL/min (≥0.83 mL/s)

Efficacy (N = 36)

Complete response	6%
Partial response	34%
Stable disease	34%
Median duration of response	4.9 months
Median time to response	5 weeks
Median time to treatment failure	3 months
Median survival	9.6 months
1-year survival	28%
2-year survival	19%

(*continued*)

If mucositis or stomatitis is present:
- Keep the mouth moist utilizing water, ice chips, sugarless gum, sugar-free hard candies, or a saliva substitute
- Rinse mouth several times a day to remove debris
  - Use a solution of ¼ teaspoon (1.25 g) each of baking soda and table salt (sodium chloride) in 1 quart (~950 mL) of warm water. Follow with a plain water rinse
  - Do not use mouthwashes that contain alcohols
- Foam-tipped swabs (eg, Toothettes) are useful in moisturizing oral mucosa, but ineffective for cleansing teeth and removing plaque
- Advise patients who develop mucositis to:
  - Choose foods that are easy to chew and swallow
  - Take small bites of food, chew slowly, and sip liquids with meals
  - Encourage soft, moist foods such as cooked cereals, mashed potatoes, and scrambled eggs
  - For trouble swallowing, soften food with gravies, sauces, broths, yogurt, or other bland liquids
  - Avoid sharp, crunchy foods; hot, spicy, or highly acidic foods (eg, citrus fruits and juices); sugary foods; toothpicks; tobacco products; alcoholic drinks

Treatment Modifications

Adverse Event	Dose Modification
ANC <1500/mm^3 *or* platelets <100,000/mm^3 at the time of chemotherapy administration	Delay chemotherapy until ANC >1500/mm^3 *and* platelets >100,000/mm^3. Discontinue if recovery has not occurred after a 3-week delay
Creatinine clearance <50 mL/min (<0.83 mL/s)	Do not administer therapy
Serum creatinine >1.5 mg/dL (>133 µmol/L) *or* 20% higher than baseline value if baseline was >1.5 mg/dL (>133 µmol/L)	Hold cisplatin until serum creatinine <1.5 mg/dL (<133 µmol/L) *or* within 0.2 mg/dL (17.7 µmol/L) of baseline
Serum creatinine 1.5–2.0 mg/dL (133–177 µmol/L) immediately before a cycle	Hold cisplatin*, then reduce cisplatin dosage by 25% during subsequent cycles
Serum creatinine 2.1–3.0 mg/dL (186–265 µmol/L) immediately before a cycle	Hold cisplatin*, then reduce cisplatin dosage by 50% during subsequent cycles
Serum creatinine >3.0 mg/dL (>265 µmol/L) immediately before a cycle	Hold cisplatin
G2 neurotoxicity or ototoxicity	Hold cisplatin until neurotoxicity resolves to G ≤1
G3/4 neurotoxicity or ototoxicity	Discontinue chemotherapy

*Hold cisplatin until serum creatinine <1.5 mg/dL (<133 µmol/L) or within 0.2 mg/dL (17.7 µmol/L) of baseline

Toxicity (N = 35/36)

	% G1/2	% G3/4
Hematologic (N = 35)		
Neutropenia	NR	80
Thrombocytopenia	NR	3
Anemia	NR	14
Nonhematologic (N = 36)		
Nausea	56	11
Asthenia	53	25
Stomatitis	44	3
Vomiting	41	8
Neurosensory	39	3
Diarrhea	38	6
Infection	27	17
Skin	19	0
Neurosensory, hearing	17	0
Pulmonary	14	8
Allergy	14	8
Neuromotor	14	3
Hypotension	14	0
G5 toxicity	2.8%	

NR, Not reported
National Cancer Institute Common Toxicity Criteria

Therapy Monitoring

1. *Weekly:* CBC with differential
2. *Before each cycle:* Serum electrolytes, creatinine, calcium, magnesium, LFTs, and urinalysis
3. *During dexamethasone:* monitor glucose if indicated

METASTATIC

HEAD AND NECK CANCER REGIMEN: CISPLATIN

Jacobs C et al. J Clin Oncol 1992;10:257–263

Hydration before, during, and after cisplatin administration ± mannitol:

- *Pre-cisplatin hydration* with 1000 mL 0.9% sodium chloride injection (0.9% NS); administer intravenously with potassium and magnesium supplementation as needed based on pretreatment laboratory results

- *Mannitol diuresis:* May be given to patients who have received adequate hydration. A dose of **mannitol** 12.5–25 g may be administered by intravenous injection or a short infusion before or during cisplatin administration, or prepared as an admixture with cisplatin. Continued intravenous hydration is essential

- *Continued mannitol diuresis:* In an inpatient or day-hospital setting, one may administer additional mannitol in the form of an intravenous infusion: **mannitol** 10–40 g; administer intravenously over 1–4 hours. This can be done either during or immediately after cisplatin, but requires maintenance of adequate intravenously administered fluids during and for hours after mannitol administration

- *Post-cisplatin hydration* with ≥1000 mL 0.9% NS; administer intravenously with potassium and magnesium supplementation as needed based on measured values

Cisplatin 100 mg/m²; administer intravenously in 25–250 mL of 0.9% NS over 15–20 minutes every 21 days (total dosage/cycle = 100 mg/m²)

Supportive Care
Antiemetic prophylaxis
Emetogenic potential is **HIGH**. *Potential for delayed symptoms*
See Chapter 42 for antiemetic recommendations

Hematopoietic growth factor (CSF) prophylaxis
Primary prophylaxis is **NOT** *indicated*
See Chapter 43 for more information

Antimicrobial prophylaxis
Risk of fever and neutropenia is **LOW**
  Antimicrobial primary prophylaxis to be considered:
- Antibacterial—not indicated
- Antifungal—consider use during neutropenia and for anticipated mucositis
- Antiviral—not indicated unless patient previously had an episode of HSV

Patient Population Studied

A study of 84 patients with unresectable recurrent disease or newly diagnosed distant metastatic disease who had received no prior chemotherapy, who were randomized to the cisplatin alone arm of a 3-arm phase 3 randomized trial. WHO performance status <4 and good organ function were required. Thirty-six percent had performance status of 2 or 3.

Efficacy (N = 83)

Complete response	3.6%
Partial response	13.3%
Median duration of response	2 months
Median survival	5.7 months

Toxicity (N = 83)

	% G1/2	% G3/4
Hematologic		
Neutropenia	35	1
Thrombocytopenia	11	1
Anemia (Hgb <8 g/dL)	NR	11
Nonhematologic		
Vomiting	54	18
Diarrhea	17	0
Mucositis	3	2
Ototoxicity	3	1
Magnesium <1.5 mg/dL		22%
Creatinine >2 mg/dL (>177 µmol/L)		14%
G >1 cardiovascular toxicity		5%
Alopecia		4%

Therapy Monitoring

1. *Weekly:* CBC with differential
2. *Before each cycle:* serum electrolytes, creatinine, calcium, magnesium, and liver function tests

Treatment Modifications

Adverse Event	Dose Modification
Creatinine clearance <50 mL/min (<0.83 mL/s)	Ineligible for therapy
Day 1 ANC <1500/mm³ *or* platelets <100,000/mm³	Delay cisplatin until ANC >1500/mm³ *and* platelets >100,000/mm³ for up to 3 weeks. Discontinue cisplatin if recovery has not occurred after a 3-week delay
ANC nadir <500/mm³	Reduce dosage to 75 mg/m²
Platelet nadir <25,000/mm³	
G1 neurotoxicity or ototoxicity	
Serum creatinine 1.5–2.0 mg/dL (133–177 µmol/L)	Hold cisplatin until serum creatinine <1.5 mg/dL (<133 µmol/L) or within 0.2 mg/dL (17.7 µmol/L) of baseline, then reduce dosage to 75 mg/m²
ANC nadir <500/mm³ with a cisplatin dosage of 75 mg/m²	Reduce dosage to 50 mg/m²
Platelet nadir <25,000/mm³ with a cisplatin dosage of 75 mg/m²	
G2 neurotoxicity or ototoxicity	
Serum creatinine 2.1–3.0 mg/dL (186–265 µmol/L)	Hold cisplatin until serum creatinine <1.5 mg/dL (<133 µmol/L) or within 0.2 mg/dL (17.7 µmol/L) of baseline, then reduce cisplatin dosage to 50 mg/m²
ANC nadir <500/mm³ with a cisplatin dosage of 50 mg/m²	Discontinue cisplatin
Platelet nadir <25,000/mm³ with a cisplatin dosage of 50 mg/m²	
Serum creatinine >3.0 mg/dL (>265 µmol/L)	
G3/4 neurotoxicity or ototoxicity	

METASTATIC
HEAD AND NECK CANCER REGIMEN: DOCETAXEL

Catimel G et al. Ann Oncol 1994;5:533–537

Premedication:
Dexamethasone 8 mg; administer orally twice daily for 3 days (6 doses), starting the day before docetaxel administration (total dose/cycle = 48 mg)
Docetaxel 100 mg/m²; administer intravenously after dilution in a volume of 0.9% sodium chloride injection or 5% dextrose injection sufficient to produce a final docetaxel concentration within the range 0.3–0.74 mg/mL over 60 minutes every 21 days (total dosage/cycle = 100 mg/m²)

Supportive Care
Antiemetic prophylaxis
Emetogenic potential is **LOW**
See Chapter 42 for antiemetic recommendations

Hematopoietic growth factor (CSF) prophylaxis
Primary prophylaxis is **NOT** *indicated*
See Chapter 43 for more information

Antimicrobial prophylaxis
Risk of fever and neutropenia is **LOW**
   Antimicrobial primary prophylaxis to be considered:
   • Antibacterial—not indicated
   • Antifungal—consider use during neutropenia and for anticipated mucositis
   • Antiviral—not indicated unless patient previously had an episode of HSV

Oral care (mucositis prophylaxis and management)
Risk of mucositis/stomatitis is **MODERATE**
   General advice:
   • Encourage patients to maintain intake of nonalcoholic fluids
   • Evaluate patients for oral pain and provide analgesic medications
   • Consider histamine (H₂-subtype) receptor antagonists (eg, ranitidine, famotidine), or a proton pump inhibitor for epigastric pain
   • *Lactobacillus* sp.–containing probiotics may be beneficial in preventing diarrhea
   Patients with intact oral mucosa:
   • Clean the mouth, tongue, and gums by brushing after every meal and at bedtime with an ultra-soft toothbrush with fluoride toothpaste
   • Floss teeth gently every day unless contraindicated. If gums bleed and hurt, avoid bleeding or sore areas, but floss other teeth
   • Patients may use saline or commercial bland, nonalcoholic rinses
      ▪ Do not use mouthwashes that contain alcohols
   If mucositis or stomatitis is present:
   • Keep the mouth moist utilizing water, ice chips, sugarless gum, sugar-free hard candies, or a saliva substitute
   • Rinse mouth several times a day to remove debris
      ▪ Use a solution of ¼ teaspoon (1.25 g) each of baking soda and table salt (sodium chloride) in 1 quart (~950 mL) of warm water. Follow with a plain water rinse
      ▪ Do not use mouthwashes that contain alcohols
   • Foam-tipped swabs (eg, Toothettes) are useful in moisturizing oral mucosa, but ineffective for cleansing teeth and removing plaque
   • Advise patients who develop mucositis to:
      ▪ Choose foods that are easy to chew and swallow
      ▪ Take small bites of food, chew slowly, and sip liquids with meals
      ▪ Encourage soft, moist foods such as cooked cereals, mashed potatoes, and scrambled eggs
      ▪ For trouble swallowing, soften food with gravies, sauces, broths, yogurt, or other bland liquids
      ▪ Avoid sharp, crunchy foods; hot, spicy, or highly acidic foods (eg, citrus fruits and juices); sugary foods; toothpicks; tobacco products; alcoholic drinks

Patient Population Studied

A trial of 40 patients with unresectable recurrent disease following attempted cure with surgery and/or radiation therapy (may have received neoadjuvant chemotherapy) or newly diagnosed with distant metastases treated in a phase 2 trial. Performance status WHO ≤2, age <75 years, and adequate organ function were required

Efficacy (N = 37)

Complete response	5.4%
Partial response	27%
Stable disease	35%
Median duration of response	6.5 months

Toxicity (N = 39 Patients/166 Cycles)

	G1/2 (% Cycles)	G3/4 (% Cycles)
Hematologic		
Leukopenia	23 (43)	74 (48)
Neutropenia	5 (20)	87 (61)
Anemia	74 (61)	5 (1)
Thrombocytopenia	13 (5)	0 (0)
Nonhematologic		
Skin toxicity	46	7.5
Asthenia	46	23
Peripheral neuropathy	41	—
Nausea	33	2.5
Edema	30.7	—
Vomiting	28.5	2.5
Stomatitis	25.6	13
Diarrhea	25.6	2.5
Phlebitis	23	—
Hypersensitivity	20.5	2.5
Myalgia	13	—

Therapy Monitoring

1. *Weekly:* CBC with differential
2. *During dexamethasone:* monitor glucose if indicated

Treatment Modifications

Adverse Event	Dose Modification
G ≥2 cutaneous toxicity without recovery to G ≤1 at time of retreatment	Reduce docetaxel dosage 25%
G ≥2 peripheral neuropathy without recovery to G ≤1 at time of retreatment	
G4 granulocytopenia lasting more than 7 days or associated with fever >38.5°C (>101.3°F)	
G3/4 nonhematologic toxicity	

METASTATIC • PLATINUM-REFRACTORY

HEAD AND NECK CANCER REGIMEN: PEMBROLIZUMAB

Chow LQM et al. J Clin Oncol 2016;34:3838–3845
Protocol for: Chow LQM et al. J Clin Oncol 2016;34:3838–3845
Cohen EEW et al. Lancet 2019;393:156–167
Supplementary appendix to: Cohen EEW et al. Lancet 2019;393:156–167
Seiwert TY et al. Lancet Oncol 2016;17:956–965
Supplementary appendix to: Seiwert TY et al. Lancet Oncol 2016;17:956–965
KEYTRUDA (pembrolizumab) prescribing information. Whitehouse Station, NJ: Merck & Co., Inc; revised 2019 September

Pembrolizumab 200 mg; administer intravenously over 30 minutes in a volume of 0.9% sodium chloride injection (0.9% NS) or 5% dextrose injection (D5W) sufficient to produce a pembrolizumab concentration within the range 1–10 mg/mL every 21 days for up to 24 months (total dose/3-week cycle = 200 mg)

Alternative pembrolizumab dose and schedule as per the U.S. FDA regimens approved on April 28, 2020:

Pembrolizumab 400 mg; administer intravenously over 30 minutes in a volume of 0.9% NS or D5W sufficient to produce a pembrolizumab concentration within the range 1–10 mg/mL every 6 weeks for up to 24 months (total dose/6-week cycle = 400 mg)

- Administer pembrolizumab with an administration set that contains a sterile, non-pyrogenic, low-protein-binding in-line or add-on filter with pore size within the range of 0.2–5 μm
- Pembrolizumab can cause severe or life-threatening infusion-related reactions, including hypersensitivity and anaphylaxis

Supportive Care
Antiemetic prophylaxis
Emetogenic potential is **MINIMAL**
See Chapter 42 for antiemetic recommendations

Hematopoietic growth factor (CSF) prophylaxis
Primary prophylaxis is **NOT** indicated
See Chapter 43 for more information

Antimicrobial prophylaxis
Risk of fever and neutropenia is **LOW**
  Antimicrobial primary prophylaxis to be considered:
  - Antibacterial—not indicated
  - Antifungal—not indicated
  - Antiviral—not indicated unless patient previously had an episode of HSV

Patient Population Studied

KEYNOTE–040 was an international, multicenter, open-label, randomized, active-controlled, phase 3 trial involving 495 adult patients who met the following eligibility criteria: had squamous cell carcinoma of the head and neck deemed incurable by local therapies; had progressive disease during or following platinum-based therapy for recurrent and/or metastatic disease, or experienced recurrence or progression within 3–6 months following prior multimodal platinum-based therapy for locally advanced disease; had undergone ≤2 prior lines of therapy for recurrent or metastatic disease; had known human papilloma virus (HPV) p16 status for oropharyngeal cancer; had known programmed death ligand 1 (PD-L1) expression status; and had an Eastern Cooperative Oncology Group (ECOG) performance status of 0 or 1. Patients were randomized 1:1 to single-agent pembrolizumab or investigator's choice of standard therapy (docetaxel, methotrexate, or cetuximab) after stratification based on ECOG performance status, p16 status, and PD-L1 proportion score (≥50% vs <50%).

Efficacy (N = 495)

	Pembrolizumab n = 247 in ITT Population n = 196 with PD-L1 CPS ≥1	Standard of Care (Methotrexate, Docetaxel, or Cetuximab) n = 248 in ITT Population n = 191 with PD-L1 CPS ≥1	
Median overall survival (ITT population)	8.4 months	6.9 months	HR 0.80 (95% CI, 0.65–0.98), nominal P = 0.0161
Median overall survival (PD-L1 CPS ≥1%)	8.7 months	7.1 months	HR 0.74 (95% CI, 0.58–0.93), nominal P = 0.0049
Overall response rate* and duration of response (DOR)† (ITT population)	14.6% Median DOR = 18.4 months	10.1% Median DOR = 5.0 months	—

Data reported are from the final analysis conducted with a data cutoff date of 15 May 2017 after a median follow-up of 7.5 months and after 388 total deaths
ITT, intention to treat; CPS, combined proportion score (calculated as the number of PD-L1-staining cells [including tumor cells, lymphocytes, and macrophages] divided by the total number of viable tumor cells, multiplied by 100)
*Includes confirmed and unconfirmed objective responses according to Response Evaluation Criteria in Solid Tumors (RECIST) version 1.1
†Duration of response (DOR) reported only for patients with a confirmed objective response

Therapy Monitoring

- Initially at the time of each dose, and eventually every 6–12 weeks, perform a total body skin examination with attention to all mucous membranes as well as a complete review of systems
- Monitor patients for signs and symptoms of pneumonitis. Evaluate patients with suspected pneumonitis with chest x-ray, CT, and pulse oximetry. For ≥2 toxicity, may include nasal swab, and sputum culture and sensitivity
- Monitor patients for signs and symptoms of colitis. Encourage patients to report diarrhea immediately
- AST, ALT, and bilirubin prior to each infusion for first 12 weeks and then every 6–12 weeks or weekly if there are grade 1 liver function test elevations. Note, no treatment is recommended for G1 LFT abnormalities. For G ≥2 toxicity, work up for other causes of elevated LFTs including viral hepatitis
- Use basic metabolic panel (Na, K, CO_2, glucose) and patient history as screening tools for hypophysitis including hypopituitarism and adrenal insufficiency. If in doubt, evaluate AM adrenocorticotropic hormone (ACTH) and cortisol levels. Consider ACTH stimulation test for indeterminate results
- Assess thyroid function at the start of treatment, and periodically during treatment. Test for TSH and free thyroxine (FT4) every 3–24 weeks as part of routine clinical monitoring on therapy or for case detection in symptomatic patients
- Measure glucose at baseline and with each treatment during the first 12 weeks and every 6–12 weeks thereafter
- Obtain a serum creatinine prior to every dose during the first 12 weeks and then every other or every third or fourth dose. If creatinine is newly elevated, consider holding therapy while other potential causes are evaluated. Note, routine urinalysis is not necessary other than to rule out urinary tract infections, etc
- Obtain a complete rheumatologic history and perform an examination of the spine and all peripheral joints for tenderness, swelling, and range of motion
- In patients at high risk of infections and in appropriately selected patients based on an infectious disease evaluation, draw screening laboratories (HIV, hepatitis A and B, and blood QuantiFERON for TB) to prepare patients to start infliximab
- Response evaluation: Every 12–24 weeks

Adverse Events (N = 480)

Grade (%)	Pembrolizumab (n = 246)		Standard of Care (Methotrexate, Docetaxel, or Cetuximab) (n = 234)	
	Grade 1–2	Grade 3–5	Grade 1–2	Grade 3–5
Hypothyroidism	13	<1	1	0
Fatigue	11	2	18	1
Diarrhea	7	2	10	<1
Rash	7	<1	14	<1
Asthenia	7	<1	10	2
Anemia	7	<1	10	4
Nausea	5	0	12	<1
Mucosal inflammation	3	<1	11	2
Stomatitis	2	<1	7	5
Neutrophil count decreased	1	<1	2	9
Alopecia	<1	0	11	0
Hypothyroidism*	15	<1	4	0
Pneumonitis*	3	1	0	1
Infusion-related reaction*	3	<1	3	<1
Severe skin reaction*	1	2	1	3
Hyperthyroidism*	2	0	<1	0
Colitis*	1	0	<1	0
Guillain-Barré syndrome*	<1	<1	0	0
Hepatitis*	<1	<1	0	0

Note: Toxicities were included in the table if they occurred in at least 10% of patients in either group (all grade) or they were deemed to be of special interest. Grading of adverse events was according to the National Cancer Institute Common Terminology Criteria for Adverse Events, version 4.0. There were four grade 5 adverse events reported in the pembrolizumab arm and two grade 5 events reported in the standard of care arm. Adverse events leading to discontinuation of protocol therapy occurred in 6% of patients in the pembrolizumab arm and in 5% of patients in the standard of care arm. Any grade 3–5 event occurred in 13% of patients in the pembrolizumab arm versus 36% of patients in the standard of care arm

*Adverse event deemed to be of special interest. These events are included due to possible immune-mediated mechanism and are included irrespective of investigator-reported attribution.

Treatment Modifications

RECOMMENDED DOSE MODIFICATIONS FOR PEMBROLIZUMAB

Adverse Event	Grade/Severity	Treatment Modification
Infusion reaction	Clinically significant but not severe infusion reaction	Interrupt the infusion in patients with clinically significant infusion reactions and consider resuming at a slower rate following resolution. If decision is made to restart, begin at ≤50% of the rate prior to the reaction and increase in 50% increments every 30 minutes if well tolerated. Infusions may be restarted at the full rate during the next cycle
	G3/4 (severe infusion reaction—pyrexia, chills, flushing, hypotension, dyspnea, wheezing, back pain, abdominal pain, and urticaria). Not rapidly responsive to brief interruption of infusion	Stop infusion and administer appropriate medical therapy (eg, epinephrine, corticosteroids, intravenous antihistamines, bronchodilators, and/or oxygen). Discontinue pembrolizumab
Colitis	G1	Loperamide 4 mg as starting dose then 2 mg before each meal and after each loose stool until without diarrhea for 12 hours, with maximum of 16 mg loperamide per day. If G1 diarrhea or colitis persists >14 days, then add prednisolone 0.5–1 mg/kg (non-enteric-coated) or consider oral budesonide 9 mg daily if no bloody diarrhea
	G2/3 diarrhea or colitis	Withhold pembrolizumab. Loperamide 4 mg as starting dose then 2 mg before each meal and after each loose stool until without diarrhea for 12 hours, with maximum of 16 mg loperamide per day. Administer oral prednisone/prednisolone at a dose of 0.5–2 mg/kg/day or its equivalent. When improves to G1, begin a slow corticosteroid taper over at least 4 weeks. Resume pembrolizumab upon symptom control, or when prednisone/prednisolone daily dose <10 mg
	G4 diarrhea or colitis	Permanently discontinue pembrolizumab. Loperamide 4 mg as starting dose then 2 mg before each meal and after each loose stool until without diarrhea for 12 hours, with maximum of 16 mg loperamide per day. Administer 1–2 mg/kg IV (methyl)prednisolone and convert to 0.5–2 mg/kg prednisone/prednisolone orally each day or its equivalent only after a response. Taper over at least 4 weeks when symptoms improve. If does not improve over 72 hours or worsens, perform flexible sigmoidoscopy/colonoscopy to document colitis then begin infliximab 5 mg/kg (if no perforation/sepsis/TB/hepatitis/NYHA III/IV CHF). If no response, add MMF 500–1000 mg twice daily. If worse on MMF, consider addition of tacrolimus or ATG
Pneumonitis	G2	Withhold pembrolizumab. Consider pneumocystis prophylaxis depending on the clinical context and coverage with empiric antibiotics. Administer oral prednisone/prednisolone at a dose of 1–2 mg/kg/day or its equivalent. When improves to G1, begin a slow corticosteroid taper over at least 4 weeks. If does not respond adequately after 48 hours, then administer 2–4 mg/kg IV (methyl)prednisolone and convert to 0.5–2 mg/kg prednisone/prednisolone orally each day or its equivalent only after a response, followed by a taper over at least 6 weeks when symptoms improve to G1, titrating to symptoms. Resume pembrolizumab upon symptom control, or when prednisone/prednisolone daily dose <10 mg
	G3/4	Permanently discontinue pembrolizumab. Consider pneumocystis prophylaxis depending on the clinical context; cover with empiric antibiotics. Administer 2–4 mg/kg IV (methyl)prednisolone and convert to 1–2 mg/kg prednisone/prednisolone orally each day or its equivalent only after a response, followed by a taper over at least 8 weeks when symptoms improve to G1, titrating to symptoms. If when initially treated, improvement does not occur within 48–72 hours, begin infliximab 5 mg/kg (if no perforation/sepsis/TB/hepatitis/NYHA III/IV CHF). If, no response to infliximab, add MMF 500–1000 mg twice daily. Consider MMF especially if has concurrent hepatic toxicity
Hepatitis	G2 (AST or ALT >3–5× ULN or total bilirubin >1.5–3× ULN)	Withhold pembrolizumab. Administer oral prednisone/prednisolone at a dose of 1–2 mg/kg/day or its equivalent. When improves to G1, begin a slow corticosteroid taper over at least 4 weeks. Resume pembrolizumab upon symptom control, or when prednisone/prednisolone daily dose <10 mg
	G3/4 (AST or ALT >5× ULN or total bilirubin >3× ULN)	Permanently discontinue pembrolizumab. Administer 1–2 mg/kg IV (methyl)prednisolone and convert to 0.5–2 mg/kg prednisone/prednisolone orally each day or its equivalent only after a response. Taper over at least 6 weeks when symptoms improve. If no response, add MMF 500–1000 mg twice daily. If worse on MMF, consider adding tacrolimus or ATG

(continued)

Treatment Modifications (continued)

RECOMMENDED DOSE MODIFICATIONS FOR PEMBROLIZUMAB

Adverse Event	Grade/Severity	Treatment Modification
Hypophysitis	G2/3 (moderate symptoms, ie, headache but no visual disturbance or fatigue/mood alteration but hemodynamically stable, no electrolyte disturbance)	Administer analgesia as needed for headache. Withhold pembrolizumab. Administer oral prednisone/prednisolone at a dose of 0.5–2 mg/kg/day or its equivalent. When improves to G1, begin a slow corticosteroid taper over at least 4 weeks. If no improvement in 48 hours, administer 1–2 mg/kg IV (methyl)prednisolone and convert to 0.5–2 mg/kg prednisone/prednisolone orally each day or its equivalent only after a response. Taper over at least 4 weeks when symptoms improve to 5 mg prednisone/prednisolone or equivalent; do not stop steroids. Resume pembrolizumab upon symptom control, or when prednisone/prednisolone daily dose <10 mg
	G4 (severe mass effect symptoms, ie, severe headache, any visual disturbance or severe hypoadrenalism, ie, hypotension, severe electrolyte disturbance)	Permanently discontinue pembrolizumab. Administer analgesia as needed for headache. Administer 1–2 mg/kg IV (methyl)prednisolone and convert to 0.5–2 mg/kg prednisone/prednisolone orally each day or its equivalent only after a response. Taper over at least 4 weeks when symptoms improve to 5 mg prednisone/prednisolone or equivalent; do not stop steroids
Adrenal insufficiency	G2	Withhold pembrolizumab. Administer oral prednisone/prednisolone at a dose of 0.5–2 mg/kg/day or its equivalent. When improves to G1, begin a slow corticosteroid taper over at least 4 weeks. Serially assess adrenal function and continue steroids at replacement doses (20–40 mg hydrocortisone daily ~2/3 dose in AM upon awakening and ~1/3 at 4 PM) until recovery of adrenal function is documented. Resume pembrolizumab upon symptom control, or when prednisone/prednisolone daily dose <10 mg
	G3/4	Permanently discontinue pembrolizumab. Administer oral prednisone/prednisolone at a dose of 0.5–2 mg/kg/day or its equivalent. When improves to G1, begin a slow corticosteroid taper over at least 4 weeks. Serially assess adrenal function and continue steroids at replacement doses (20–40 mg hydrocortisone daily ~2/3 dose in AM upon awakening and ~1/3 at 4 PM) until recovery of adrenal function is documented
Type 1 diabetes mellitus	G3 hyperglycemia	Withhold pembrolizumab. Admit to hospital to manage hyperglycemia. Role of corticosteroids in preventing complete loss of insulin-producing cells is unknown and not recommended. Resume pembrolizumab upon symptom control, or when prednisone/prednisolone daily dose <10 mg
	G4 hyperglycemia	Permanently discontinue pembrolizumab. Admit to hospital to manage hyperglycemia. Role of corticosteroids in preventing complete loss of insulin-producing cells is unknown and not recommended
Nephritis and renal dysfunction	G2/3 (serum creatinine 1.5–6× ULN)	Withhold pembrolizumab. Administer oral prednisone/prednisolone at a dose of 0.5–2 mg/kg/day or its equivalent. When improves to G1, begin a slow corticosteroid taper over at least 4 weeks. If does not respond adequately, then administer 0.5–1 mg/kg IV (methyl)prednisolone and convert to 0.5–2 mg/kg prednisone/prednisolone orally each day or its equivalent only after a response, followed by a taper over at least 4 weeks when improves to G1. Resume pembrolizumab upon symptom control, or when prednisone/prednisolone daily dose <10 mg
	G4 (serum creatinine >6× ULN)	Permanently discontinue pembrolizumab. Administer 0.5–1 mg/kg IV (methyl)prednisolone and convert to 0.5–2 mg/kg prednisone/prednisolone orally each day or its equivalent only after a response, followed by a taper over at least 4 weeks when improves to G1

(continued)

Treatment Modifications (*continued*)

RECOMMENDED DOSE MODIFICATIONS FOR PEMBROLIZUMAB

Adverse Event	Grade/Severity	Treatment Modification
Skin	G1/2	Continue pembrolizumab. Avoid skin irritants, avoid sun exposure, topical emollients recommended. Topical steroid (mild strength for G1, moderate/potent strength for G2) cream once or twice daily ± oral or topical antihistamines for itching
	G3 rash or suspected SJS or TEN	Withhold pembrolizumab. Avoid skin irritants, avoid sun exposure, topical emollients recommended. Administer oral or topical antihistamines for itching. Administer oral prednisone/prednisolone at a dose of 0.5–2 mg/kg or its equivalent daily for 3 days followed by a slow corticosteroid taper over at least 4 weeks when the rash improves to G1. If does not respond adequately, then administer 0.5 –1 mg/kg IV (methyl)prednisolone and convert to 0.5–2 mg/kg prednisone/prednisolone orally each day or its equivalent only after a response, followed by a taper over at least 4 weeks when the rash improves to G1. Resume pembrolizumab upon symptom control, or when prednisone/prednisolone daily dose <10 mg
	G4 rash or confirmed SJS or TEN	Avoid skin irritants, avoid sun exposure, topical emollients recommended. Administer oral or topical antihistamines for itching. Administer 1–2 mg/kg IV (methyl)prednisolone and convert to oral steroids 0.5–2 mg/kg prednisone/prednisolone each day or its equivalent only after a response. Taper over at least 4 weeks when the rash improves to G1. Permanently discontinue pembrolizumab
Encephalitis	Confusion or altered behavior, headaches, alteration in Glasgow Coma Scale, motor or sensory deficits, speech abnormality, may or may not be febrile	Initially withhold pembrolizumab, but permanently discontinue pembrolizumab if there is no doubt as to diagnosis. Exclude bacterial and ideally viral infections prior to high-dose steroids. Administer oral prednisone/prednisolone at a dose of 0.5–2 mg/kg/day or its equivalent. When symptoms improve, begin a slow corticosteroid taper over at least 4–8 weeks. If symptoms are severe, administer 1–2 mg/kg IV (methyl)prednisolone and convert to 0.5–2 mg/kg prednisone/prednisolone orally each day or its equivalent only after a response. Consider concurrent empiric antiviral (IV acyclovir) and antibacterial therapy
Aseptic meningitis	Headache, photophobia, neck stiffness with fever or may be afebrile, vomiting; normal cognition/cerebral function (distinguishes from encephalitis)	
Other syndromes include neurosarcoidosis, posterior reversible leukoencephalopathy syndrome (PRES), Vogt-Koyanagi-Harada syndrome, demyelination, vasculitic encephalopathy, and generalized seizures		
Transverse myelitis	Acute or subacute neurologic signs/symptoms of motor/sensory/autonomic origin; most have sensory level; often bilateral symptoms	Initially withhold pembrolizumab, but permanently discontinue pembrolizumab if there is no doubt as to diagnosis. Administer 2 mg/kg IV (methyl)prednisolone or consider 1 g/day and convert to 0.5–2 mg/kg prednisone/prednisolone orally each day or its equivalent only after a response. When symptoms improve, begin a slow corticosteroid taper over at least 4–8 weeks. Plasmapheresis may be required if steroids do not bring about improvement
Myocarditis	G3	Permanently discontinue pembrolizumab. Administer 2 mg/kg IV (methyl)prednisolone or consider 1 g/day and convert to 0.5–2 mg/kg prednisone/prednisolone orally each day or its equivalent only after a response. When symptoms improve, begin a slow corticosteroid taper over at least 4–8 weeks. If no response, add MMF 500–1000 mg twice daily. If worse on MMF, consider adding tacrolimus
Peripheral neurologic toxicity	Moderate: some interference with ADL, symptoms concerning to patient	Withhold pembrolizumab. Initial observation reasonable or initiate prednisone/prednisolone 0.5–1 mg/kg (if progressing, eg, from mild) and/or pregabalin or duloxetine for pain. When symptoms improve, begin a slow corticosteroid taper over at least 4 weeks. Resume pembrolizumab upon symptom control, or when prednisone/prednisolone daily dose <10 mg
	Severe: limits self-care and aids warranted, life threatening, eg, respiratory problems	Permanently discontinue pembrolizumab. Administer 1–2 mg/kg IV (methyl)prednisolone and convert to 0.5–2 mg/kg prednisone/prednisolone each day or its equivalent only after a response. Taper over at least 4–8 weeks when symptoms improve to G1

(*continued*)

Treatment Modifications (continued)

RECOMMENDED DOSE MODIFICATIONS FOR PEMBROLIZUMAB

Adverse Event	Grade/Severity	Treatment Modification
Guillain-Barré syndrome	Progressive symmetrical muscle weakness with absent or reduced tendon reflexes—involves extremities, facial, respiratory, and bulbar and oculomotor muscles; dysregulation of autonomic nerves	Permanently discontinue pembrolizumab. Use of steroids not recommended in idiopathic Guillain-Barré syndrome; however, a trial of (methyl)prednisolone 1–2 mg/kg is reasonable, converting to 0.5–2 mg/kg prednisone/prednisolone orally each day or its equivalent only after a response. If no improvement or worsening, plasmapheresis or IVIG indicated
Myasthenia gravis	Fluctuating muscle weakness (proximal limb, trunk, ocular, eg, ptosis/diplopia or bulbar) with fatigability, respiratory muscles may also be involved	Permanently discontinue pembrolizumab. Administer pyridostigmine at an initial dose of 30 mg three times daily. Administer oral prednisone/prednisolone at a dose of 0.5–2 mg/kg/day or its equivalent or 1–2 mg/kg IV (methyl)prednisolone depending on the severity of symptoms. If begin with IV, convert to 0.5–2 mg/kg prednisone/prednisolone orally each day or its equivalent only after a response. If no improvement or worsening, plasmapheresis or IVIG may be considered. Additional immunosuppressants used in myasthenia gravis include azathioprine, cyclosporine, and mycophenolate. Avoid certain medications, eg, ciprofloxacin, beta-blockers, that may precipitate cholinergic crisis
Other syndromes including motor and sensory peripheral neuropathy, multifocal radicular neuropathy/plexopathy, autonomic neuropathy, phrenic nerve palsy, cranial nerve palsies (eg, facial nerve, optic nerve, hypoglossal nerve)		Permanently discontinue pembrolizumab. Administer oral prednisone/prednisolone at a dose of 0.5–2 mg/kg/day or its equivalent or 1–2 mg/kg IV (methyl)prednisolone depending on the severity of symptoms. If begin with IV, convert to 0.5–2 mg/kg prednisone/prednisolone orally each day or its equivalent only after a response
Arthralgia	G1 (mild pain with inflammation, erythema or joint swelling)	Continue pembrolizumab. Administer acetaminophen (paracetamol) and ibuprofen
	G2 (moderate pain with inflammation, erythema, or joint swelling that limits ADL)	Withhold pembrolizumab. Administer higher doses of acetaminophen (paracetamol) and ibuprofen and use diclofenac or naproxen or etoricoxib. If inadequately controlled, consider intra-articular steroid injections for large joints or administer oral prednisone/prednisolone at a dose of 0.5–2 mg/kg/day or its equivalent. When improves to G1, begin a slow corticosteroid taper over at least 4 weeks. If does not respond adequately, then administer 0.5–1 mg/kg IV (methyl)prednisolone and convert to 0.5–2 mg/kg prednisone/prednisolone orally each day or its equivalent only after a response, followed by a taper over at least 4 weeks when improves to G1. Resume pembrolizumab upon symptom control, or when prednisone/prednisolone daily dose <10 mg
	G3 (severe pain; irreversible joint damage; disabling; limits self-care ADL)	Withhold pembrolizumab. Administer 0.5–1 mg/kg IV (methyl)prednisolone and convert to 0.5–2 mg/kg prednisone/prednisolone orally each day or its equivalent only after a response, followed by a taper over at least 4 weeks when improves to G1. In severe cases, infliximab or another anti–TNF-alpha drug may be required for improvement of arthritis. Resume pembrolizumab upon symptom control, or when prednisone/prednisolone daily dose <10 mg
Other	First occurrence of other G3	Withhold pembrolizumab. Administer oral prednisone/prednisolone at a dose of 0.5–2 mg/kg/day or its equivalent. When improves to G1, begin a slow corticosteroid taper over at least 4 weeks. Resume pembrolizumab upon symptom control, or when prednisone/prednisolone daily dose <10 mg
	Recurrence of same G3	Permanently discontinue pembrolizumab. Administer 1–2 mg/kg IV (methyl)prednisolone and convert to 0.5–2 mg/kg prednisone/prednisolone orally each day or its equivalent only after a response. Taper over at least 4–8 weeks when symptoms improve to G1
	Requirement for ≥10 mg/day prednisone or equivalent for >12 weeks	Permanently discontinue pembrolizumab
	Persistent G2/3 adverse reactions lasting ≥12 weeks	

ADL, activities of daily living; ALT, alanine aminotransferase; AST, aspartate aminotransferase; ATG, anti-thymocyte globulin; SJS, Stevens-Johnson Syndrome; TEN, toxic epidermal necrolysis; ULN, upper limit of normal

Notes on general supportive care:
Steroid taper in most cases will proceed over a minimum of 1 month but if symptoms improve rapidly, a 2-week taper can be considered. If steroids are administered for more than 4 weeks, consider PCP prophylaxis (cotrimoxazole 480 mg twice daily M/W/F or inhaled pentamidine if has cotrimoxazole allergy), regular random blood glucose, VitD level, and starting calcium/VitD supplementation per guidelines

METASTATIC • PLATINUM-REFRACTORY

HEAD AND NECK CANCER REGIMEN: NIVOLUMAB

Ferris RL et al. N Engl J Med 2016;375:1856–1867
Supplementary appendix to: Ferris RL et al. N Engl J Med 2016;375:1856–1867
Protocol for: Ferris RL et al. N Engl J Med 2016;375:1856–1867
OPDIVO (nivolumab) prescribing information. Princeton, NJ: Bristol-Myers Squibb Company; revised 2019 September

The U.S. Food and Drug Administration (FDA)-approved regimens for recurrent or metastatic squamous cell carcinoma of the head and neck include fixed doses of nivolumab and allows for a shortened infusion duration of 30 minutes, consistent with the regimens approved on March 5, 2018, thus:

Nivolumab 240 mg; administer intravenously over 30 minutes in a volume of 0.9% sodium chloride injection (0.9% NS) or 5% dextrose injection (D5W), not to exceed 160 mL and sufficient to produce a nivolumab concentration within the range 1–10 mg/mL, every 2 weeks until disease progression (total dosage/2-week course = 240 mg)

- Administer nivolumab through an administration set that contains a sterile, non-pyrogenic, low-protein-binding in-line filter with pore size within the range of 0.2–1.2 μm.
- Nivolumab can cause severe infusion-related reactions

OR

Nivolumab 480 mg; administer intravenously over 30 minutes in a volume of 0.9% NS or D5W not to exceed 160 mL and sufficient to produce a nivolumab concentration within the range 1–10 mg/mL, every 4 weeks until disease progression (total dosage/4-week course = 480 mg)

- Administer nivolumab through an administration set that contains a sterile, non-pyrogenic, low-protein-binding in-line filter with pore size within the range of 0.2–1.2 μm.
- Nivolumab can cause severe infusion-related reactions

Supportive Care

Antiemetic prophylaxis
Emetogenic potential with nivolumab is **MINIMAL**
See Chapter 42 for antiemetic recommendations

Hematopoietic growth factor (CSF) prophylaxis
Primary prophylaxis is **NOT** indicated
See Chapter 43 for more information

Antimicrobial prophylaxis
Risk of fever and neutropenia is **LOW**
　Antimicrobial primary prophylaxis to be considered:
- Antibacterial—not indicated
- Antifungal—not indicated
- Antiviral—not indicated unless patient previously had an episode of HSV

Patient Population Studied

CheckMate 141 was an international, multicenter, open-label, randomized, active-controlled phase 3 trial involving 361 adult patients who met the following eligibility criteria: had histologically confirmed, recurrent and/or metastatic squamous cell carcinoma of the head and neck deemed incurable by local therapies; had progressive disease within 6 months of platinum-based therapy administered as adjuvant therapy or for primary or recurrent disease; had an Eastern Cooperative Oncology Group (ECOG) performance status of 0 or 1; and had adequate organ function. Patients were excluded if they required immunosuppressive therapy; had an autoimmune disease, systemic immunosuppression, or known human immunodeficiency virus or hepatitis B or C virus infection; or if they had brain metastases. Patients were randomized 2:1 to single-agent nivolumab 2 mg/kg IV every 3 weeks until disease progression or investigator's choice of standard therapy (docetaxel, methotrexate, or cetuximab) after stratification based on prior receipt of cetuximab therapy

Therapy Monitoring

- Initially at the time of each dose, and eventually every 6–12 weeks, perform a total body skin examination with attention to all mucous membranes as well as a complete review of systems
- Monitor patients for signs and symptoms of pneumonitis. Evaluate patients with suspected pneumonitis with chest x-ray, CT, and pulse oximetry. For ≥2 toxicity, may include nasal swab, and sputum culture and sensitivity
- Monitor patients for signs and symptoms of colitis. Encourage patients to report diarrhea immediately
- AST, ALT, and bilirubin prior to each infusion for first 12 weeks and then every 6–12 weeks or weekly if there are grade 1 liver function test elevations. Note, no treatment is recommended for G1 LFT abnormalities. For G ≥2 toxicity, work up for other causes of elevated LFTs including viral hepatitis
- Use basic metabolic panel (Na, K, CO_2, glucose) and patient history as screening tools for hypophysitis including hypopituitarism and adrenal insufficiency. If in doubt, evaluate AM adrenocorticotropic hormone (ACTH) and cortisol levels. Consider ACTH stimulation test for indeterminate results
- Assess thyroid function at the start of treatment, and periodically during treatment. Test for TSH and free thyroxine (FT4) every 3–24 weeks as part of routine clinical monitoring of therapy or for case detection in symptomatic patients
- Measure glucose at baseline and with each treatment during the first 12 weeks and every 6–12 weeks thereafter
- Obtain a serum creatinine prior to every dose during the first 12 weeks and then every other or every third or fourth dose. If creatinine is newly elevated, consider holding therapy while other potential causes are evaluated. Note, routine urinalysis is not necessary other than to rule out urinary tract infections, etc
- Obtain a complete rheumatologic history and perform an examination of the spine and all peripheral joints for tenderness, swelling, and range of motion
- In patients at high risk of infections and in appropriately selected patients based on an infectious disease evaluation, draw screening laboratories (HIV, hepatitis A and B, and blood QuantiFERON for TB) to prepare patients to start infliximab
- Response evaluation: Every 12–24 weeks

Efficacy (N = 361)

	Nivolumab n = 240 (ITT Population) n = 88 (PD-L1 ≥1%)	Standard of Care (Methotrexate, Docetaxel, or Cetuximab) n = 121 (ITT Population) n = 61 (PD-L1 ≥1%)	
Median overall survival (ITT population)	7.5 months	5.1 months	HR 0.70 (97.73% CI, 0.51–0.96), P = 0.01
Overall survival at 1 year	36.0%; 95% CI, 28.5–43.4	16.6%; 95% CI, 8.6–26.8	—
Median overall survival (PD-L1 ≥1%)*	8.7 months	4.6 months	HR 0.55 (95% CI, 0.36–0.83)
Median overall survival (PD-L1 <1%)*	5.7 months	5.8 months	HR 0.89 (95% CI, 0.54–1.45)
p16 positive	9.1 months	4.4 months	HR 56 (95% CI. 0.32–0.99)
p16 negative	7.5 months	5.8 months	HR 0.73 (95% CI, 0.42–1.25)
Overall response rate (ITT population)	13.3%	5.8%	—
Rate of progression-free survival	2.0 months	2.3 months	HR, 0.89; 95% CI, 0.70 to 1.13; P = 0.32

Survival data are from the planned interim analysis conducted with a data cutoff date of 18 December 2015 after a median follow-up of 5.1 months and after 218 total deaths. Overall response rate data are based on a database lock occurring on 5 May 2016

ITT, intention to treat

*Exploratory analysis. HR for death in the analysis of OS in the subgroups of patients with PD-L1 expression levels of 5% or more and of 10% or more were similar to those among patients with PD-L1 expression levels of 1% or more

Adverse Events (N = 347)

Grade (%)	Nivolumab (n = 236)		Standard of Care (Methotrexate, Docetaxel, or Cetuximab) (n = 111)	
	Grade 1/2	Grade 3/4	Grade 1/2	Grade 3/4
Fatigue	12	2	14	3
Nausea	8	0	20	1
Rash	8	0	4	1
Decreased appetite	7	0	7	0
Pruritus	7	0	0	0
Diarrhea	7	0	12	2
Anemia	4	1	12	5
Asthenia	4	<1	13	2
Vomiting	3	0	7	0
Dry skin	3	0	9	0
Stomatitis	2	<1	6	3
Weight loss	2	0	5	0
Mucosal inflammation	1	0	11	2
Peripheral neuropathy	<1	0	6	0
Alopecia	0	0	10	3
Neutropenia	0	0	1	7

Note: Treatment-emergent adverse events were included in the table if they occurred in at least 5% of patients in either group (all grade). Grading of adverse events was according to the National Cancer Institute Common Terminology Criteria for Adverse Events, version 4. There were two grade 5 adverse events reported in the nivolumab arm (n = 1 pneumonitis and n = 1 hypercalcemia) and one grade 5 event reported in the standard of care arm (n = 1 lung infection). Any grade 3–4 event occurred in 13.1% of patients in the nivolumab arm versus 35.1% of patients in the standard of care arm

Treatment Modifications

RECOMMENDED DOSE MODIFICATIONS FOR NIVOLUMAB

Adverse Event	Grade/Severity	Treatment Modification
Infusion reaction	Clinically significant but not severe infusion reaction	Interrupt the infusion in patients with clinically significant infusion reactions and consider resuming at a slower rate following resolution. If decision is made to restart, begin at ≤50% of the rate prior to the reaction and increase in 50% increments every 30 minutes if well tolerated. Infusions may be restarted at the full rate during the next cycle
	G3/4 (severe infusion reaction—pyrexia, chills, flushing, hypotension, dyspnea, wheezing, back pain, abdominal pain, and urticaria). Not rapidly responsive to brief interruption of infusion	Stop infusion and administer appropriate medical therapy (eg, epinephrine, corticosteroids, intravenous antihistamines, bronchodilators, and/or oxygen). Discontinue nivolumab
Colitis	G1	Loperamide 4 mg as starting dose then 2 mg before each meal and after each loose stool until without diarrhea for 12 hours, with maximum of 16 mg loperamide per day. If G1 diarrhea or colitis persists >14 days, then add prednisolone 0.5–1 mg/kg (non-enteric-coated) or consider oral budesonide 9 mg daily if no bloody diarrhea
	G2/3 diarrhea or colitis	Withhold nivolumab. Loperamide 4 mg as starting dose then 2 mg before each meal and after each loose stool until without diarrhea for 12 hours, with maximum of 16 mg loperamide per day. Administer oral prednisone/prednisolone at a dose of 0.5–2 mg/kg/day or its equivalent. When improves to G1, begin a slow corticosteroid taper over at least 4 weeks. Resume nivolumab upon symptom control, or when prednisone/prednisolone daily dose <10 mg
	G4 diarrhea or colitis	Permanently discontinue nivolumab. Loperamide 4 mg as starting dose then 2 mg before each meal and after each loose stool until without diarrhea for 12 hours, with maximum of 16 mg loperamide per day. Administer 1–2 mg/kg IV (methyl)prednisolone and convert to 0.5–2 mg/kg prednisone/prednisolone orally each day or its equivalent only after a response. Taper over at least 4 weeks when symptoms improve. If does not improve over 72 hours or worsens, perform flexible sigmoidoscopy/colonoscopy to document colitis then begin infliximab 5 mg/kg (if no perforation/sepsis/TB/hepatitis/NYHA III/IV CHF). If no response, add MMF 500–1000 mg twice daily. If worse on MMF, consider addition of tacrolimus or ATG
Pneumonitis	G2	Withhold nivolumab. Consider pneumocystis prophylaxis depending on the clinical context and coverage with empiric antibiotics. Administer oral prednisone/prednisolone at a dose of 1–2 mg/kg/day or its equivalent. When improves to G1, begin a slow corticosteroid taper over at least 4 weeks. If does not respond adequately after 48 hours, then administer 2–4 mg/kg IV (methyl)prednisolone and convert to 0.5–2 mg/kg prednisone/prednisolone orally each day or its equivalent only after a response, followed by a taper over at least 6 weeks when symptoms improve to G1, titrating to symptoms. Resume nivolumab upon symptom control, or when prednisone/prednisolone daily dose <10 mg
	G3/4	Permanently discontinue nivolumab. Consider pneumocystis prophylaxis depending on the clinical context; cover with empiric antibiotics. Administer 2–4 mg/kg IV (methyl)prednisolone and convert to 1–2 mg/kg prednisone/prednisolone orally each day or its equivalent only after a response, followed by a taper over at least 8 weeks when symptoms improve to G1, titrating to symptoms. If, when initially treated, improvement does not occur within 48–72 hours, begin infliximab 5 mg/kg (if no perforation/sepsis/TB/hepatitis/NYHA III/IV CHF). If no response to infliximab, add MMF 500–1000 mg twice daily. Consider MMF especially if has concurrent hepatic toxicity

(continued)

Treatment Modifications (*continued*)

RECOMMENDED DOSE MODIFICATIONS FOR NIVOLUMAB

Adverse Event	Grade/Severity	Treatment Modification
Hepatitis	G2 (AST or ALT >3–5× ULN or total bilirubin >1.5–3× ULN)	Withhold nivolumab. Administer oral prednisone/prednisolone at a dose of 1–2 mg/kg/day or its equivalent. When improves to G1, begin a slow corticosteroid taper over at least 4 weeks. Resume nivolumab upon symptom control, or when prednisone/prednisolone daily dose <10 mg
	G3/4 (AST or ALT >5× ULN or total bilirubin >3× ULN)	Permanently discontinue nivolumab. Administer 1–2 mg/kg IV (methyl)prednisolone and convert to 0.5–2 mg/kg prednisone/prednisolone orally each day or its equivalent only after a response. Taper over at least 6 weeks when symptoms improve. If no response, add MMF 500–1000 mg twice daily. If worse on MMF, consider adding tacrolimus or ATG
Hypophysitis	G2/3 (moderate symptoms, ie, headache but no visual disturbance or fatigue/mood alteration but hemodynamically stable, no electrolyte disturbance)	Administer analgesia as needed for headache. Withhold nivolumab. Administer oral prednisone/prednisolone at a dose of 0.5–2 mg/kg/day or its equivalent. When improves to G1, begin a slow corticosteroid taper over at least 4 weeks. If no improvement in 48 hours, administer 1–2 mg/kg IV (methyl)prednisolone and convert to 0.5–2 mg/kg prednisone/prednisolone orally each day or its equivalent only after a response. Taper over at least 4 weeks when symptoms improve to 5 mg prednisone/prednisolone or equivalent; do not stop steroids. Resume nivolumab upon symptom control, or when prednisone/prednisolone daily dose <10 mg
	G4 (severe mass effect symptoms, ie, severe headache, any visual disturbance or severe hypoadrenalism, ie, hypotension, severe electrolyte disturbance)	Permanently discontinue nivolumab. Administer analgesia as needed for headache. Administer 1–2 mg/kg IV (methyl)prednisolone and convert to 0.5–2 mg/kg prednisone/prednisolone orally each day or its equivalent only after a response. Taper over at least 4 weeks when symptoms improve to 5 mg prednisone/prednisolone or equivalent; do not stop steroids
Adrenal insufficiency	G2	Withhold nivolumab. Administer oral prednisone/prednisolone at a dose of 0.5–2 mg/kg/day or its equivalent. When improves to G1, begin a slow corticosteroid taper over at least 4 weeks. Serially assess adrenal function and continue steroids at replacement doses (20–40 mg hydrocortisone daily ~2/3 dose in AM upon awakening and ~1/3 at 4 PM) until recovery of adrenal function is documented. Resume nivolumab upon symptom control, or when prednisone/prednisolone daily dose <10 mg
	G3/4	Permanently discontinue nivolumab. Administer oral prednisone/prednisolone at a dose of 0.5–2 mg/kg/day or its equivalent. When improves to G1, begin a slow corticosteroid taper over at least 4 weeks. Serially assess adrenal function and continue steroids at replacement doses (20–40 mg hydrocortisone daily ~2/3 dose in AM upon awakening and ~1/3 at 4 PM) until recovery of adrenal function is documented
Type 1 diabetes mellitus	G3 hyperglycemia	Withhold nivolumab. Admit to hospital to manage hyperglycemia. Role of corticosteroids in preventing complete loss of insulin-producing cells is unknown and not recommended. Resume nivolumab upon symptom control, or when prednisone/prednisolone daily dose <10 mg
	G4 hyperglycemia	Permanently discontinue nivolumab. Admit to hospital to manage hyperglycemia. Role of corticosteroids in preventing complete loss of insulin-producing cells is unknown and not recommended
Nephritis and renal dysfunction	G2/3 (serum creatinine 1.5–6× ULN)	Withhold nivolumab. Administer oral prednisone/prednisolone at a dose of 0.5–2 mg/kg/day or its equivalent. When improves to G1, begin a slow corticosteroid taper over at least 4 weeks. If does not respond adequately, then administer 0.5–1 mg/kg IV (methyl)prednisolone and convert to 0.5–2 mg/kg prednisone/prednisolone orally each day or its equivalent only after a response, followed by a taper over at least 4 weeks when improves to G1. Resume nivolumab upon symptom control, or when prednisone/prednisolone daily dose <10 mg
	G4 (serum creatinine >6× ULN)	Permanently discontinue nivolumab. Administer 0.5–1 mg/kg IV (methyl)prednisolone and convert to 0.5–2 mg/kg prednisone/prednisolone orally each day or its equivalent only after a response, followed by a taper over at least 4 weeks when improves to G1

(*continued*)

Treatment Modifications (*continued*)

RECOMMENDED DOSE MODIFICATIONS FOR NIVOLUMAB

Adverse Event	Grade/Severity	Treatment Modification
Skin	G1/2	Continue nivolumab. Avoid skin irritants, avoid sun exposure, topical emollients recommended. Topical steroid (mild strength for G1, moderate/potent strength for G2) cream once or twice daily ± oral or topical antihistamines for itching
	G3 rash or suspected SJS or TEN	Withhold nivolumab. Avoid skin irritants, avoid sun exposure, topical emollients recommended. Administer oral or topical antihistamines for itching. Administer oral prednisone/prednisolone at a dose of 0.5–2 mg/kg or its equivalent daily for 3 days followed by a slow corticosteroid taper over at least 4 weeks when the rash improves to G1. If does not respond adequately, then administer 0.5–1 mg/kg IV (methyl)prednisolone and convert to 0.5–2 mg/kg prednisone/prednisolone orally each day or its equivalent only after a response, followed by a taper over at least 4 weeks when the rash improves to G1. Resume nivolumab upon symptom control, or when prednisone/prednisolone daily dose <10 mg
	G4 rash or confirmed SJS or TEN	Avoid skin irritants, avoid sun exposure, topical emollients recommended. Administer oral or topical antihistamines for itching. Administer 1–2 mg/kg IV (methyl)prednisolone and convert to oral steroids 0.5–2 mg/kg prednisone/prednisolone each day or its equivalent only after a response. Taper over at least 4 weeks when the rash improves to G1. Permanently discontinue nivolumab
Encephalitis	Confusion or altered behavior, headaches, alteration in Glasgow Coma Scale, motor or sensory deficits, speech abnormality, may or may not be febrile	Initially withhold nivolumab, but permanently discontinue nivolumab if there is no doubt as to diagnosis. Exclude bacterial and ideally viral infections prior to high-dose steroids. Administer oral prednisone/prednisolone at a dose of 0.5–2 mg/kg/day or its equivalent. When symptoms improve, begin a slow corticosteroid taper over at least 4–8 weeks. If symptoms are severe, administer 1–2 mg/kg IV (methyl)prednisolone and convert to 0.5–2 mg/kg prednisone/prednisolone orally each day or its equivalent only after a response. Consider concurrent empiric antiviral (IV acyclovir) and antibacterial therapy
Aseptic meningitis	Headache, photophobia, neck stiffness with fever or may be afebrile, vomiting; normal cognition/cerebral function (distinguishes from encephalitis)	
Other syndromes include neurosarcoidosis, posterior reversible leukoencephalopathy syndrome (PRES), Vogt-Koyanagi-Harada syndrome, demyelination, vasculitic encephalopathy, and generalized seizures		
Transverse myelitis	Acute or subacute neurologic signs/symptoms of motor/sensory/autonomic origin; most have sensory level; often bilateral symptoms	Initially withhold nivolumab, but permanently discontinue nivolumab if there is no doubt as to diagnosis. Administer 2 mg/kg IV (methyl)prednisolone or consider 1 g/day and convert to 0.5–2 mg/kg prednisone/prednisolone orally each day or its equivalent only after a response. When symptoms improve, begin a slow corticosteroid taper over at least 4–8 weeks. Plasmapheresis may be required if steroids do not bring about improvement
Myocarditis	G3	Permanently discontinue nivolumab. Administer 2 mg/kg IV (methyl)prednisolone or consider 1 g/day and convert to 0.5–2 mg/kg prednisone/prednisolone orally each day or its equivalent only after a response. When symptoms improve, begin a slow corticosteroid taper over at least 4–8 weeks. If no response, add MMF 500–1000 mg twice daily. If worse on MMF, consider adding tacrolimus
Peripheral neurologic toxicity	Moderate: some interference with ADL, symptoms concerning to patient	Withhold nivolumab. Initial observation reasonable or initiate prednisone/prednisolone 0.5–1 mg/kg (if progressing, eg, from mild) and/or pregabalin or duloxetine for pain. When symptoms improve, begin a slow corticosteroid taper over at least 4 weeks. Resume nivolumab upon symptom control, or when prednisone/prednisolone daily dose <10 mg
	Severe: limits self-care and aids warranted, life threatening, eg, respiratory problems	Permanently discontinue nivolumab. Administer 1–2 mg/kg IV (methyl)prednisolone and convert to 0.5–2 mg/kg prednisone/prednisolone orally each day or its equivalent only after a response. Taper over at least 4–8 weeks when symptoms improve to G1

(*continued*)

Treatment Modifications (continued)

RECOMMENDED DOSE MODIFICATIONS FOR NIVOLUMAB

Adverse Event	Grade/Severity	Treatment Modification
Guillain-Barré syndrome	Progressive symmetrical muscle weakness with absent or reduced tendon reflexes—involves extremities, facial, respiratory, and bulbar and oculomotor muscles; dysregulation of autonomic nerves	Permanently discontinue nivolumab. Use of steroids not recommended in idiopathic Guillain-Barré syndrome; however, a trial of (methyl)prednisolone 1–2 mg/kg is reasonable, converting to 0.5–2 mg/kg prednisone/prednisolone orally each day or its equivalent only after a response. If no improvement or worsening, plasmapheresis or IVIG indicated
Myasthenia gravis	Fluctuating muscle weakness (proximal limb, trunk, ocular, eg, ptosis/diplopia or bulbar) with fatigability, respiratory muscles may also be involved	Permanently discontinue nivolumab. Administer pyridostigmine at an initial dose of 30 mg three times daily. Administer oral prednisone/prednisolone at a dose of 0.5–2 mg/kg/day or its equivalent or 1–2 mg/kg IV (methyl)prednisolone depending on the severity of symptoms. If begin with IV, convert to 0.5–2 mg/kg prednisone/prednisolone orally each day or its equivalent only after a response. If no improvement or worsening, plasmapheresis or IVIG may be considered. Additional immunosuppressants used in myasthenia gravis include azathioprine, cyclosporine, and mycophenolate. Avoid certain medications, eg, ciprofloxacin, beta-blockers, that may precipitate cholinergic crisis
Other syndromes including motor and sensory peripheral neuropathy, multifocal radicular neuropathy/plexopathy, autonomic neuropathy, phrenic nerve palsy, cranial nerve palsies (eg, facial nerve, optic nerve, hypoglossal nerve)		Permanently discontinue nivolumab. Administer oral prednisone/prednisolone at a dose of 0.5–2 mg/kg/day or its equivalent or 1–2 mg/kg IV (methyl)prednisolone depending on the severity of symptoms. If begin with IV, convert to 0.5–2 mg/kg prednisone/prednisolone orally each day or its equivalent only after a response
Arthralgia	G1 (mild pain with inflammation, erythema or joint swelling)	Continue nivolumab. Administer acetaminophen (paracetamol) and ibuprofen
	G2 (moderate pain with inflammation, erythema, or joint swelling that limits ADL)	Withhold nivolumab. Administer higher doses of acetaminophen (paracetamol) and ibuprofen and use diclofenac or naproxen or etoricoxib. If inadequately controlled, consider intra-articular steroid injections for large joints or administer oral prednisone/prednisolone at a dose of 0.5–2 mg/kg/day or its equivalent. When improves to G1, begin a slow corticosteroid taper over at least 4 weeks. If does not respond adequately, then administer 0.5–1 mg/kg IV (methyl)prednisolone and convert to 0.5–2 mg/kg prednisone/prednisolone orally each day or its equivalent only after a response, followed by a taper over at least 4 weeks when improves to G1. Resume nivolumab upon symptom control, or when prednisone/prednisolone daily dose <10 mg
	G3 (severe pain; irreversible joint damage; disabling; limits self-care ADL)	Withhold nivolumab. Administer 0.5–1 mg/kg IV (methyl)prednisolone and convert to 0.5–2 mg/kg prednisone/prednisolone orally each day or its equivalent only after a response, followed by a taper over at least 4 weeks when improves to G1. In severe cases, infliximab or another anti–TNF-alpha drug may be required for improvement of arthritis. Resume nivolumab upon symptom control, or when prednisone/prednisolone daily dose <10 mg
Other	First occurrence of other G3	Withhold nivolumab. Administer oral prednisone/prednisolone at a dose of 0.5–2 mg/kg/day or its equivalent. When improves to G1, begin a slow corticosteroid taper over at least 4 weeks. Resume nivolumab upon symptom control, or when prednisone/prednisolone daily dose <10 mg
	Recurrence of same G3	Permanently discontinue nivolumab. Administer 1–2 mg/kg IV (methyl)prednisolone and convert to 0.5–2 mg/kg prednisone/prednisolone orally each day or its equivalent only after a response. Taper over at least 4–8 weeks when symptoms improve to G1
	Life-threatening or G4	
	Requirement for ≥10 mg/day prednisone or equivalent for >12 weeks	Permanently discontinue nivolumab
	Persistent G2/3 adverse reactions lasting ≥12 weeks	

ADL, activities of daily living; ALT, alanine aminotransferase; AST, aspartate aminotransferase; ATG, anti-thymocyte globulin; SJS, Stevens-Johnson Syndrome; TEN, toxic epidermal necrolysis; ULN, upper limit of normal

Notes on general supportive care: Steroid taper in most cases will proceed over a minimum of 1 month but if symptoms improve rapidly a 2-week taper can be considered. If steroids are administered for more than 4 weeks, consider PCP prophylaxis (cotrimoxazole 480 mg twice daily M/W/F or inhaled pentamidine if has cotrimoxazole allergy), regular random blood glucose, VitD level, and starting calcium/VitD supplementation per guidelines

METASTATIC • PLATINUM-REFRACTORY

HEAD AND NECK CANCER REGIMEN: CETUXIMAB

Vermorken JB et al. J Clin Oncol 2007;25:2171–2177

Cetuximab premedication:
Diphenhydramine 50 mg; administer by intravenous injection or infusion before cetuximab administration (other H_1-receptor antagonists may be substituted)

Initial cetuximab dose:
Cetuximab 400 mg/m²; administer intravenously over 120 minutes (maximum infusion rate = 5 mL [10 mg] per min) as a single loading dose (total initial dosage = 400 mg/m²)

Maintenance cetuximab doses:
Cetuximab 250 mg/m² per dose; administer intravenously over 60 minutes (maximum infusion rate = 5 mL [10 mg] per min) every week, continually (total weekly dosage = 250 mg/m²)

Notes:
• Cetuximab is intended for direct administration and should not be diluted
• Maximum infusion rate = 5 mL (10 mg)/min
• Administer cetuximab through a low-protein-binding in-line filter with pore size = 0.22 µm
• Use 0.9% sodium chloride injection to flush vascular access devices after administration is completed

Note: Continue cetuximab single-agent therapy for at least 6 weeks. If tumors appear to respond to treatment and disease stability (SD) is attained, treatment may be continued until progressive disease (PD), clinical deterioration, or unacceptable adverse events are observed

Supportive Care

Antiemetic prophylaxis
Emetogenic potential is **MINIMAL**
See Chapter 42 for antiemetic recommendations

Hematopoietic growth factor (CSF) prophylaxis
Primary prophylaxis is **NOT** *indicated*
See Chapter 43 for more information

Antimicrobial prophylaxis
Risk of fever and neutropenia is **LOW**
Antimicrobial primary prophylaxis to be considered:
  • Antibacterial—not indicated
  • Antifungal—not indicated
  • Antiviral—not indicated unless patient previously had an episode of HSV

Patient Population Studied

A study of 103 patients with measurable metastatic and/or recurrent histologically proven squamous cell carcinoma of the head and neck with documented disease progression within 30 days after a minimum of 2 cycles and a maximum of 6 cycles of chemotherapy: cisplatin-based (≥60 mg/m² per cycle) or carboplatin-based (≥300 mg/m², or dose based on target AUC ≥4 mg/mL × min per cycle). Adequate organ function, a Karnofsky performance status ≥60, and age ≥18 years were required

Efficacy (N = 103)

Overall response rate	0
Complete response rate	13%
Stable disease	33%
Progressive disease	37%
Disease not assessable	18%
Median time to progression	70 days
Median overall survival	178 days

Toxicity (N = 103)*

Adverse Event	% All Grades	% G3/4
Rash	49	1
Acne	26	0
Asthenia	24	4
Nail disorder	16	0
Dry skin	14	0
Fever	14	1
Nausea	13	1
Vomiting	11	2
Dyspnea	5	4
Infusion-related reactions	6	1
Treatment-related death	1 Patient	

*Common Toxicity Criteria, version 2.0, (U.S.) National Cancer Institute

Therapy Monitoring

1. *Pretreatment evaluation:* Medical history and tumor assessment by clinical evaluation and imaging studies
2. *Response evaluation:* Every 6 weeks

Dose Modifications

Adverse Event	Treatment Modifications
Progressive disease, clinical deterioration, or unacceptable toxicity	Discontinue treatment
First occurrence G3 skin toxicity	Hold cetuximab up to 2 weeks
Second occurrence G3 skin toxicity	Reduce cetuximab dosage to 200 mg/m²
Third occurrence G3 skin toxicity	Reduce cetuximab dosage to 150 mg/m²
Fourth occurrence G3 skin toxicity	Discontinue cetuximab

METASTATIC

HEAD AND NECK CANCER (NASOPHARYNGEAL CARCINOMA) REGIMEN: GEMCITABINE + CISPLATIN

Zhang L et al. Lancet 2016;388:1883–1892
Supplementary appendix to: Zhang L et al. Lancet 2016;388:1883–1892

Gemcitabine 1000 mg/m² per dose; administer intravenously in 50–250 mL 0.9% NS over 30 minutes, on days 1 and 8, every 3 weeks for up to 6 cycles (total dosage/3-week cycle = 2000 mg/m²), *followed by:*

Hydration before cisplatin: 0.9% sodium chloride (0.9% NS), ≥1000 mL; intravenously over a minimum of 1 hour before commencing cisplatin administration
Cisplatin 80 mg/m²; administer intravenously in 1000 mL 0.9% NS over 4 hours, following gemcitabine administration, on day 1 every 3 weeks for up to 6 cycles (total dosage/3-week cycle = 80 mg/m²)
Hydration after cisplatin: Administer by intravenous infusion ≥1000 mL 0.9% NS over a minimum of 2 hours. Encourage patients to increase oral intake of non-alcoholic fluids, and provide electrolyte replacement as needed (potassium, magnesium, sodium)

Supportive Care
Antiemetic prophylaxis
Emetogenic potential on day 1 is **HIGH***. Potential for delayed symptoms*
Emetogenic potential on day 8 is **LOW**
See Chapter 42 for antiemetic recommendations

Hematopoietic growth factor (CSF) prophylaxis
Primary prophylaxis is **NOT** indicated
See Chapter 43 for more information

Antimicrobial prophylaxis
Risk of fever and neutropenia is LOW
   Antimicrobial primary prophylaxis to be considered:
   • Antibacterial—not indicated
   • Antifungal—not indicated
   • Antiviral—not indicated unless patient previously had an episode of HSV

Patient Population Studied

The multicenter, open-label, randomized, phase 3 trial performed in China included 362 patients with histologically or cytologically confirmed incurable nasopharyngeal carcinoma. Eligible patients had either primary metastatic disease or developed recurrent disease after radiation therapy (either local or distant recurrence) and had not received prior systemic chemotherapy for advanced disease. Eligible patients were aged >18 years, with an Eastern Cooperative Oncology Group (ECOG) performance status score ≤1, had a life expectancy ≥12 weeks, and had adequate organ function. Patients were randomized to receive gemcitabine plus cisplatin or to receive fluorouracil plus cisplatin

Efficacy (N = 362)

	Gemcitabine + Cisplatin (n = 181)	Fluorouracil + Cisplatin (n = 181)	
Estimated median progression-free survival*	7.0 months (95% CI, 6.3–7.6)	5.6 months (95% CI, 4.9–6.2)	HR 0.55, 95% CI 0.44–0.68; P<0.0001
Estimated median overall survival†	29.1 months (95% CI, 18.7–39.5)	20.9 months (95% CI, 16.0–25.8)	HR 0.62, 95% CI 0.45–0.84; P = 0.0025
Objective response rate*	64%	42%	RR 1.5, 95% CI 1.2–1.9; P<0.0001

*Median follow-up for progression-free survival was 19.4 months (IQR, 12.1–35.6)
†Median follow-up for overall survival was 22.0 months (IQR, 13.0–33.5)
*Objective response rate is the percentage of patients who experienced a partial or complete response according to RECIST version 1.1 evaluated by an independent image committee. In this study, 8% of patients in the gemcitabine + cisplatin arm experienced a complete response compared to 3% of patients in the fluorouracil + cisplatin arm

Adverse Events (N = 353)

	Gemcitabine + Cisplatin (n = 180)		Fluorouracil + Cisplatin (n = 173)	
	Grade 1/2	Grade 3/4	Grade 1/2	Grade 3/4
Leukopenia	46	29	61	9
Neutropenia	43	23	52	13
Anemia	73	4	71	1
Thrombocytopenia	18	13	9	2
ALT increased	19	2	19	1
AST increased	14	2	15	1
Mucosal inflammation	1	0	20	14
Fatigue	11	1	12	1
Weight loss	22	1	20	0
Decreased appetite	21	2	31	4
Nausea	21	2	29	2
Vomiting	8	2	13	1

*According to the National Cancer Institute Common Terminology Criteria for Adverse Events, version 3.0
Note: The safety analysis included all patients who received at least one dose of study drug. No grade 5 drug-related adverse events were reported in the study. Three percent of patients in the gemcitabine + cisplatin group discontinued therapy due to drug-related adverse events versus 8% in the fluorouracil + cisplatin group

Therapy Monitoring

1. *Before therapy:* History and physical exam. CBC with differential, renal and liver function tests, serum electrolytes
2. Monitor hepatic function prior to initiation and during therapy with gemcitabine
3. Pulmonary toxicity and respiratory failure: Discontinue gemcitabine immediately for unexplained new or worsening dyspnea or evidence of severe pulmonary toxicity
4. Monitor renal function and electrolytes prior to initiation and during therapy with cisplatin and gemcitabine, including hemolytic-uremic syndrome (HUS) secondary to gemcitabine
5. Increased toxicity with infusion time >30 minutes or dosing more frequently than once weekly may occur with gemcitabine; monitor carefully

Treatment Modifications

CISPLATIN + GEMCITABINE

Dose Levels

	Gemcitabine	Cisplatin
Starting dose	1000 mg/m²/dose on day 1 and 8	80 mg/m² on day 1
Dose level −1	800 mg/m²/dose on day 1 and 8	64 mg/m² on day 1
Dose level −2	600 mg/m²/dose on day 1 and 8	48 mg/m² on day 1
Dose level −3	Discontinue gemcitabine and cisplatin	

Delay initiation of cycle until ANC is >1500/mm³ and platelet count >100,000/mm³
*Cisplatin dose was also adjusted for patients based on creatinine clearance estimated prior to each cycle by the Cockcroft-Gault formula

Adverse Event	Treatment Modification
G3/4 hematologic toxicities (ANC <1000/mm³; platelet count <50,000/mm³) occurring in the prior cycle	Hold all therapy until returns to baseline. Then decrease the gemcitabine dosage by one dose level. Do not modify the cisplatin dose. Consider use of hematopoietic growth factor (CSF) prophylaxis in subsequent cycles for dose-limiting neutropenia
Day 8 ANC 1000–1499/mm³ and/or platelet count 75,000–99,999/mm³	Administer 50% of day 1 gemcitabine dose
Day 8 ANC <1000/mm³ and/or platelet count <75,000/mm³	Withhold day 8 gemcitabine dose. Consider use of hematopoietic growth factor (CSF) prophylaxis in subsequent cycles for dose-limiting neutropenia
Creatinine clearance (by Cockcroft-Gault method) estimated prior to the current cycle of chemotherapy is ≥60 mL/minute	Administer full dose cisplatin
Creatinine clearance (by Cockcroft-Gault method) estimated prior to the current cycle of chemotherapy is ≥41 mL/minute and <60 mL/minute	Administer a dose of cisplatin (mg/m²) equivalent to the creatinine clearance (mL/minute). For example, if the estimated creatinine clearance is 45 mL/minute, then administer cisplatin at a dose of 45 mg/m²
Creatinine clearance (by Cockcroft-Gault method) estimated prior to the current cycle of chemotherapy is <41 mL/minute	Omit cisplatin in the current cycle of chemotherapy. Proceed with gemcitabine. If creatinine clearance improves to ≥41 mL/minute, then consider resuming cisplatin in subsequent cycles
G ≥2 diarrhea	Hold chemotherapy until toxicity resolves to grade <2, then decrease gemcitabine one dose level
G3/4 mucositis	Decrease gemcitabine dosage by two dose levels
ALT and AST >1.5× ULN in a patient without liver metastasis	Withhold gemcitabine until ALT and AST ≤1.5× ULN
ALT and AST >2.5× ULN in a patient with liver metastasis with alkaline phosphatase >2.5× ULN	Withhold gemcitabine until ALT and AST ≤2.5× ULN and alkaline phosphatase ≤2.5× ULN

(continued)

Treatment Modifications (*continued*)

Adverse Event	Treatment Modification
Peripheral neuropathy G ≥3	G4 discontinue cisplatin permanently; G3 may reinstitute if toxicity resolves within 2–3 weeks to ≤G1
Cisplatin induced hearing loss G ≥3	
Severe hypersensitivity reaction to gemcitabine or cisplatin is noted	Permanently discontinue gemcitabine or cisplatin
Other G ≥3 nonhematologic toxicities (except nausea, vomiting, elevated transaminases and alopecia)	Delay treatment until toxicity resolves to baseline, then decrease the attributable drug dosage(s) by 1 dose level from previous dose level(s)
Unexplained new or worsening dyspnea or evidence of severe pulmonary toxicity	Discontinue gemcitabine immediately and assess for gemcitabine pulmonary toxicity
Hemolytic-uremic syndrome (HUS)	Discontinue gemcitabine for HUS or severe renal impairment
Capillary leak syndrome	Discontinue gemcitabine
Posterior reversible encephalopathy syndrome (PRES)	Discontinue gemcitabine

20. Hepatocellular Carcinoma

Tim Greten, MD, PhD and Cecilia Monge, MD

Epidemiology

Incidence (worldwide)*: 841,080 cases per year
13.9 cases per 100,000 men
4.9 cases per 100,000 women
Deaths (worldwide): 781,631 per year, 5-year OS 18%
Median age: 50–60 years
Male to female ratio: 3.7: 2.5

https://seer.cancer.gov/report_to_nation/infographics/trends_incidence.html

Stage at Presentation

Stage A:	35%
Stage B:	25%
Stage C:	10%
Stage D:	30%

Work-up

History and clinical examination
- **Risk factors for chronic liver disease:** intravenous drug abuse, alcohol intake, metabolic syndrome (obesity, diabetes, arterial hypertension)
- **Symptoms and signs of chronic liver disease:** jaundice, ascites, encephalopathy, bleeding, splenomegaly
- **Performance status and nutritional state**

Laboratory analysis
- **Etiology of liver disease:** HBV (HBsAg, anti-HBc), HCV (anti-HCV), iron status, autoimmune disease, liver function: prothrombin time, albumin, bilirubin
- **Complete blood cell count including platelets**
- **Tumor marker:** serum alpha fetoprotein (AFP)

Assessment of portal hypertension
- **Upper endoscopy:** varices and/or hypertensive gastropathy

Imaging studies
- **Liver dynamic (multiple phase) MRI or CT** for diagnosis and evaluation of tumor extent; number and size of nodules, vascular invasion, extrahepatic spread
- **CT of the chest, abdomen, and pelvis** to rule out extrahepatic spread
- **Imaging performed, interpreted, and reported through the CT MRI Liver Imaging Reporting and Data System (CT/MRI LI-RADS)**— an imaging-based diagnostic system used in patients at high risk of hepatocellular carcinoma (HCC). It assigns each liver abnormality a category that reflects the probability of the finding representing a benign cause, HCC, or other malignancy (see below)

Tumor biopsy
- **Nodules with non-diagnostic imaging**
- **Required to diagnose HCC in non-cirrhotic liver**

Vogel A et al. Ann Oncol 2018;29(Suppl 4):iv238–iv255

Diagnostic Criteria for HCC: CT/MRI LI-RADS
- Diagnosis of HCC can be established based on imaging (without biopsy confirmation) in patients who have cirrhosis
- Criteria on multiphase imaging to enable noninvasive diagnosis of HCC: nodule ≥1 cm, arterial phase hyperenhancement, and depending on size, a combination of washout in the venous or delayed phase, threshold growth, and capsule appearance
- If criteria not met, liver biopsy should be considered
- AFP and other serum biomarkers have a minor role in the diagnosis of HCC
- At-risk patients with abnormal surveillance results or a clinical suspicion of HCC should undergo multiphase CT or MRI for diagnostic testing

(continued)

Work-up (*continued*)

- **LI-RADS system** designates lesions to category codes according to the probability of being benign, HCC, or other hepatic malignant neoplasm (cholangiocarcinoma or combined) (Figure 1)
- The probability of HCC associated with each LI-RADS category guides management
- LI-RADS 1 and LI-RADS 2:
  - Definitely benign (cysts and typical hemangiomas) and probably benign (atypical hemangiomas and focal parenchymal abnormalities) lesions, respectively
  - LI-RADS 1 lesions have an average probability of HCC of 0%
  - LI-RADS 2 lesions have an average probability of HCC of 11%
- LI-RADS 3:
  - Low probability of HCC (vascular pseudo-lesions and small HCCs, distinctive solid nodule with only some imaging features consistent with HCC diagnosis)
  - Average probability of HCC of 33%
  - Followed prospectively, 6–15% are diagnosed as HCC or other malignancy at 24 months
- LI-RADS 4:
  - Probable HCC (≥2-cm encapsulated lesion with arterial phase hyper-enhancement, but without "washout," or ≥2-cm lesion that enhances to the same degree as liver in the arterial phase, but is hypo-enhanced in the post-arterial phases (differential diagnosis includes dysplastic nodule, benign entities, rarely non-HCC malignant neoplasms)
  - Average probability of HCC of 80%
  - Followed prospectively, 46–68% are diagnosed as HCC or other malignancy at 24 months
- LI-RADS 5:
  - Average probability of HCC of 96% or higher and indicates definite HCC

Abd Alkhalik Basha et al. Clin Radiol 2017;72:901.e1–901.e11
Kim Y-Y et al. Eur Radiol 2018;28:2038–2046
Lee SE et al. Eur Radiol 2018;28:1551–1559
Roberts LR et al. Hepatology 2018;67:401–421

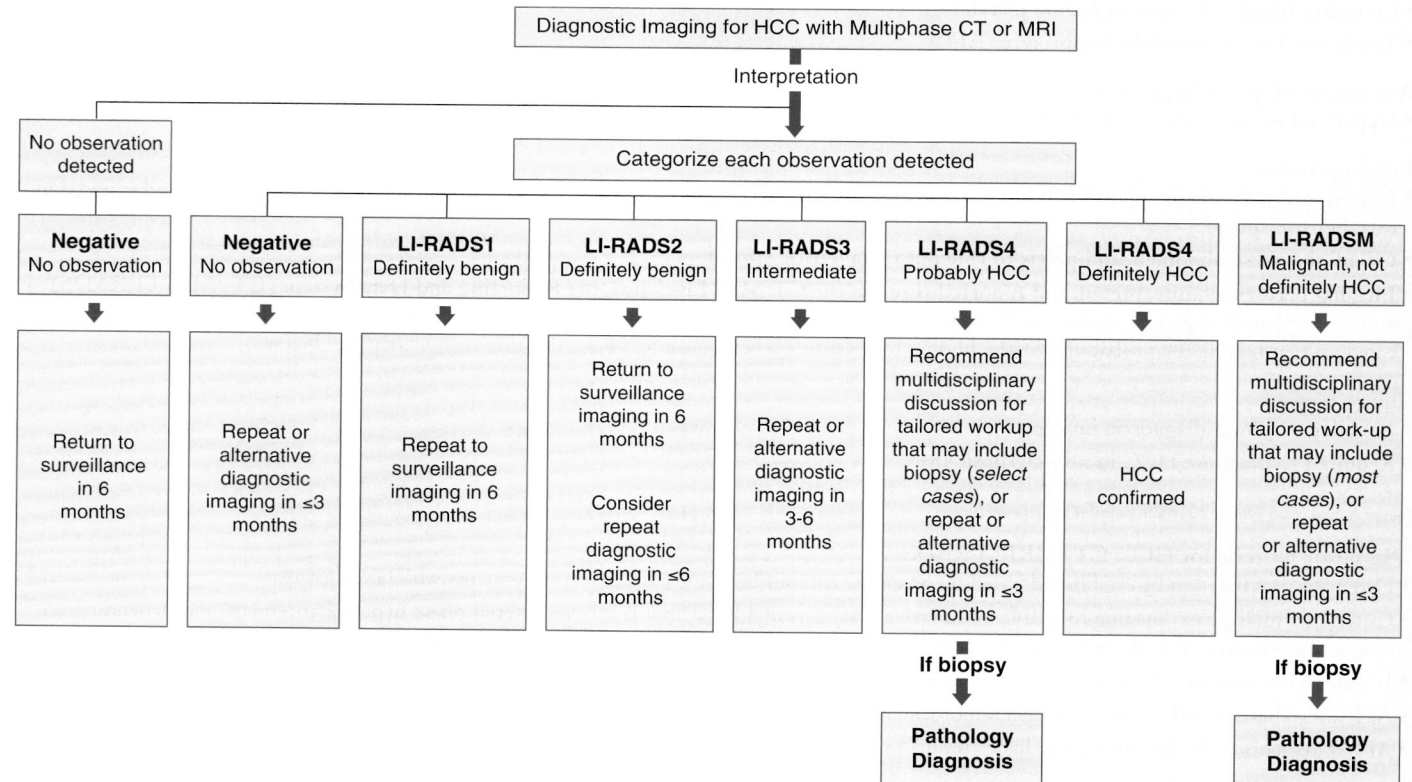

Figure 1. American Association for the Study of Liver Diseases (AASLD) Diagnostic Algorithm

Adapted from Marrero JA et al. Hepatology 2018;68:723–750

(*continued*)

Work-up (continued)

HCC Pathology
- **Well differentiated:** thin plates (1–3 hepatocytes thick), small cells, abnormal reticulin network; increased nuclear density, minimal nuclear atypia, pseudo-glands—fatty change and pseudo-glands; may resemble hepatocyte adenoma; common pattern for small hepatocellular carcinoma
- **Moderately differentiated:** trabecular pattern with 4+ cells thick; tumor cells are larger than in well-differentiated HCC with more eosinophilic cytoplasm, distinct nucleoli, pseudo-glands, bile, and tumor giant cells; most common pattern in advanced HCC
- **Poorly differentiated:** tumor cells are large with hyperchromatic nuclei in compact growth pattern, rare trabeculae; prominent pleomorphism, possibly some spindle cell or small cell areas
- **Others:**
  - **Combined hepatocellular cholangiocarcinoma:** rare (<1%) HCC; cholangiocarcinoma and hepatocellular carcinoma combined
  - **Steatohepatitic HCC:** associated with metabolic syndrome (nonalcoholic fatty liver disease); more fibrosis and more steatosis than that seen in classic HCC; hepatocyte ballooning, Mallory-Denk bodies, inflammation, and pericellular fibrosis
  - **Diffuse cirrhosis-like HCC:** rare HCC (case reports only); extensive and diffuse involvement by small cirrhosis-like nodules that evade radiographic detection

Jain D. Hepatocellular carcinoma—general. www.pathologyoutlines.com. Accessed May 26, 2020
Jain D. Liver & intrahepatic bile ducts tumor. www.pathologyoutlines.com/topic/livertumorHCC.html. Accessed May 26, 2020

Staging

Primary Tumor (T)

TX	Primary tumor cannot be assessed
T0	No evidence of primary tumor
T1	Solitary tumor ≤ 2 cm, or > 2 cm without vascular invasion
T1a	Solitary tumor ≤2 cm in greatest dimension with or without vascular invasion
T1b	Solitary tumor >2 cm in greatest dimension without vascular invasion
T2	Solitary tumor >2 cm with vascular invasion, or multiple tumors, none >5 cm in greatest dimension
T3	Multiple tumors, at least one of which is >5 cm in greatest dimension
T4	Single tumor or multiple tumors of any size involving a major branch of the portal vein or hepatic vein, or tumor(s) with direct invasion of adjacent organs (including the diaphragm) other than the gallbladder or with perforation of visceral peritoneum

Regional Lymph Nodes (N)

NX	Regional lymph nodes cannot be assessed
N0	No regional lymph node metastasis
N1	Regional lymph node metastasis

Distant Metastasis (M)

M0	No distant metastasis (no pathologic M0; use clinical M to complete stage group)
M1	Distant metastasis

Staging

	T	N	M
IA	T1a	N0	M0
IB	T1b	N0	M0
II	T2	N0	M0
IIIA	T3	N0	M0
IIIB	T4	N0	M0
IVA	any T	N1	M0
IVB	any T	any N	M1

Brierley JD, Gospodarowicz MK, Wittekind C (editors). IUCC TNM Classification of Malignant Tumours, 8th edition. Oxford: John Wiley & Sons Inc; 2016
Vogel A et al. Ann Oncol 2018;29(Suppl 4):iv238–iv255

Staging (continued)

Child-Pugh Classification

Measure	Score		
	1 Point	**2 Points**	**3 Points**
Ascites	Absent	Slight	Moderate
Serum bilirubin	<2.0 mg/dL (<34.2 mmol/L)	2.0–3.0 mg/dL (34.2–51.3 mmol/L)	>3.0 mg/dL (>51.3 mmol/L)
Serum albumin	>3.5 g/dL	2.8–3.5 g/dL	<2.8 g/dL
Prothrombin time (seconds prolonged)	<4	4–6	>6
Encephalopathy grade	None	1–2	3–4

Child-Pugh Score

Child-Pugh A	5 or 6 points
Child-Pugh B	7–9 points
Child-Pugh C	>9 points

- Within Child-Pugh A group: measurement of the albumin-bilirubin (ALBI) score predicts prognosis: good prognosis (ALBI 1) and poor prognosis (ALBI 2), with median survival of 26 and 14 months, respectively
- Platelet count >150 × 10^9 cells/L and a non-invasive liver stiffness measurement <20 kPa excludes significant portal hypertension
- Esophageal varices and/or splenomegaly with platelet counts of >150 × 10^9 cells/L suggests portal hypertension (can be measured invasively as appropriate)

Augustin S et al. Hepatology 2017;66:1980–1988
Johnson PJ et al. J Clin Oncol 2015;33:550–558

Survival (BCLC Staging)

Stage	3-Year Survival
Stage 0–A	40–70%
Stage B	50%
Stage C	10%
Stage D	0

Llovet JM et al. J Natl Cancer Inst 2008; 100:698–711

Barcelona Clinic Liver Cancer (BCLC) Classification

	Tumor Status	Child-Pugh Classification	Performance Status
Stage 0—Very Early Stage	Single HCC <2 cm; carcinoma in situ	A	0
Stage A—Early Stage	Single HCC or 3 nodules <3 cm	A–B	0
Stage B—Intermediate Stage	Large/multinodular. Without vascular invasion or extrahepatic spread	A–B	0
Stage C—Advanced Stage	Any size with vascular invasion or extrahepatic spread (N1M1)	A–B	1–2
Stage D—Terminal Stage	Any size	C	3–4

Llovet Jm Et Al. J Natl Cancer Inst 2008;100:698–711

Expert Opinion

TREATMENT ACCORDING TO STAGE

1. **Stage 0–A:** Resection, liver transplant, or ablation
2. **Stage B:** Chemoembolization or other locoregional treatment options
3. **Stage C:** Bevacizumab and atezolizumab, sorafenib, lenvatinib, regorafenib, ramucirumab, cabozantinib, nivolumab, pembrolizumab, nivolumab in combination with ipilimumab
4. **Stage D:** Rest supportive care

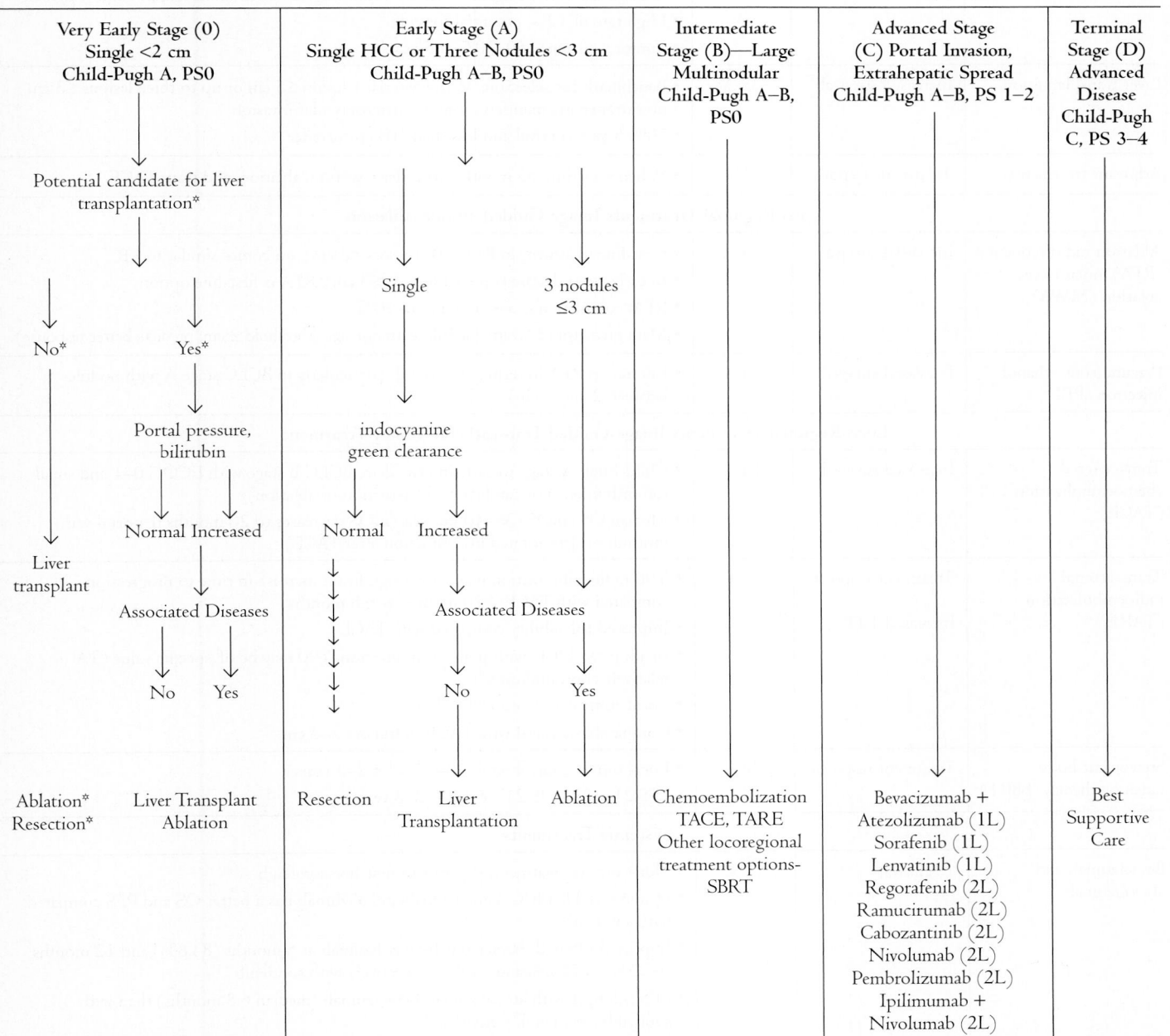

*Very early-stage (BCLC0) patients are considered for resection only if transplant not available. If transplant not an option, ablation first-line option and surgery justified only in patients with contraindication to ablation or in whom ablation fails. If patient eligible for transplant, then strategy of transplantation depending on risk of recurrence per tumor pathology favors resection as the first-line approach. Analysis of resected tumor would distinguish BCLC0 with marginal risk of recurrence (no need to transplant) and more advanced disease with microscopic vascular invasion or satellites that favor transplant because of high risk of recurrence

(*continued*)

Expert Opinion (*continued*)

Therapeutic Strategies/Options

Procedure/Treatment	Benefit	Level of Evidence	Comments
Surgical Treatments			
Surgical resection	Increased survival	3ii A	• Mainstay indication for single tumors with well-reserved liver function • Suitable for Child-Pugh A, possibly Child-Pugh B, contraindicated in Child-Pugh C • High rate of CRs; potential for cure • Tumor recurrence 50–70% at 5 years
Liver transplantation	Increased survival	3ii A	• Benchmark for selection: Milan criteria: 1 lesion ≤5 cm or up to three lesions ≤3 cm, no extrahepatic manifestations, no macrovascular invasion • 70% 5-year survival and less than 10% recurrence
Adjuvant treatments	Treatment response	3 Diii	• When wait time >3 months: consider resection, ablation, and trans TACE
Loco-Regional Treatments Image-Guided Tumor Ablation			
Ablation radiofrequency (RFA), microwave ablation (MWA)	Increased survival	3ii A	• First-line treatment in BCLC 0 (tumors <2 cm); outcomes similar to LR • In early-stage disease (up to 3 lesions ≤3 cm), RFA is first-line option • RFA: complete response rate in 70–90% • Main predictor of treatment failure: tumor size (threshold 2 cm; predicts better response)
Percutaneous ethanol injection (PEI)	Increased survival	3ii A	• Inferior to RFA in terms of survival (particularly in BCLC stage A with nodules between 2 and 4 cm)
Loco-Regional Treatments Image-Guided Transcatheter Tumor Treatment			
Trans-arterial chemoembolization (TACE)	Increased survival	1ii A	• Child-Pugh A stage to early intermediate BCLC B stage with ECOG 0–1 and small tumor burden (not candidates for resection or ablation) • Median OS (mOS) 35–40 months (mOS decreases to 20 months if portal vein invasion or deteriorated liver function after TACE)
Trans-arterial radioembolization (TARE)	Treatment response Increased TTP	2i A	• Y90 radioembolization may have a significant increase in time to progression compared with TACE: >26 months vs 6.8 months • Improved tolerability compared with TACE • In advanced HCC with portal vein invasion, Y90 may be of specific value (TACE relatively contraindicated) • Local control at 2 years 61–81% • Comparable survival with TACE in tumors 3–8 cm
Stereotactic body radiation therapy (SBRT)	Treatment response	2i A	• Local tumor control rates: 68–95% (at 2–3 years) • PFS 21–48%, OS 21–69% (at 2–3 years)
Systemic Treatments			
Bevacizumab and atezolizumab	↑ Survival	1ii A	• Non-curative treatment, superior to first-line sorafenib • In unresectable HCC, bevacizumab-atezolizumab has a better OS and PFS compared with sorafenib • Improved OS with bevacizumab-atezolizumab at 6 months (84.8%) and 12 months (67.2%) vs 72.2% and 54.6% respectively with sorafenib • PFS is longer with atezolizumab-bevacizumab (median 6.8 months) than with sorafenib (median 4.3 months) • Most common Grade 3 or 4 AEs: hypertension, AST increase, ALT increase, fatigue, proteinuria, diarrhea, decreased appetite, pyrexia
Sorafenib	↑ Survival	1i A	• Non-curative treatment that improves survival • First-line in advanced HCC results in an improved OS in Child-Pugh A vs placebo • Benefit in subgroups including macroscopic vascular invasion or extrahepatic spread • Most common Grade 3 AEs: palmar-plantar erythrodysesthesia, diarrhea, hypertension, abdominal pain, hypophosphatemia, thrombocytopenia

(*continued*)

Expert Opinion (*continued*)

Procedure/Treatment	Benefit	Level of Evidence	Comments
Lenvatinib	Noninferior to sorafenib	1ii A	• Noninferior to sorafenib as far as OS benefit versus in first-line setting • PFS of 7.4 months vs 3.7 months with sorafenib • ORR of 24% vs 9% with sorafenib • Lenvatinib has not been studied in patients with 50% or more liver invasion, main portal vein invasion, or invasion of the bile duct • Dosed by weight • Most common AEs: hypertension, diarrhea, decreased appetite, weight loss
Regorafenib	↑ Survival	1ii D	• Treatment of advanced HCC after progressed on and tolerated a minimum dose of sorafenib • Improves OS in the second-line setting (10.6 months vs 7.8 months with placebo), non-curative • Most common Grade 3–4 AEs: hypertension, palmar-plantar erythrodysesthesia, fatigue, diarrhea
Ramucirumab	↑ Survival	1i A	• Treatment of patients with AFP ≥400 ng/mL • Indicated after treatment with sorafenib • Improvement in OS of 8.5 months vs 7.3 months with placebo • Grade 3–4 AEs: hypertension, hyponatremia, increased AST
Cabozantinib	↑ Survival	1ii A	• Indicated in patients previously treated with sorafenib and with disease progression after at least one systemic treatment for HCC, may have received up to two previous systemic regimens for advanced HCC • Improvement in median OS of 10.2 months vs 8.0 months with placebo, non-curative • Most common high-grade AEs: palmar-plantar erythrodysesthesia, hypertension, increased AST, fatigue, diarrhea
Nivolumab	No survival benefit	1ii A	• Treatment of advanced HCC previously treated with sorafenib • Durable ORR of 14%, median duration of response 17 months • Median OS as second-line therapy:15.6 months, non-curative • Well tolerated • In front-line setting vs sorafenib did not show increase in OS (phase 3 study)
Pembrolizumab	No survival benefit	1i A	• Treatment of advanced HCC previously treated with sorafenib • Overall durable response rate of 17%, PFS 4.9 months, non-curative treatment • Well tolerated
Ipilimumab and nivolumab	↑ Survival	1ii A	• Treatment of advanced HCC after failure of sorafenib treatment • Objective response 31%, median duration of response 17 months • Most common AEs: fatigue, diarrhea, rash, pruritus, nausea, musculoskeletal pain, pyrexia, cough, decreased appetite, vomiting, abdominal pain, dyspnea, upper respiratory tract infection, arthralgia, headache, hypothyroidism, decreased weight, dizziness • More than 50% of patients may require systemic steroids to manage AEs

Evidence-based classification adapted from the National Cancer Institute
1 = Randomized controlled trial or meta-analysis (1i = double-blinded, 1ii = non-blinded); 2 = non-randomized controlled trial; 3 = case series (3i = population-based, 3ii = non-population-based, consecutive, 3iii = non-population-based, non-consecutive); A = survival end point; B = cause-specific mortality; C = quality of life; D = indirect surrogates (Di = disease-free survival, Dii = progression-free survival, Diii = tumor response)

Surgical Resection
• Liver resection (LR) is mainstay for single tumors with adequate liver function reserve (R0 resection with sufficient liver reserve in remnant)
• Suitable for Child-Pugh A, possibly Child-Pugh B
• Contraindicated in Child-Pugh C
• Anatomic resection vs non-anatomic wedge resection is subject of debate
• Tumor recurrence observed in 50–70% of cases within 5 years; intrahepatic recurrence often in the first 2 years or new HCC usually occurring beyond 2 years

(*continued*)

Expert Opinion (continued)

- Early recurrence: microvascular invasion, poor histologic differentiation, and multifocal disease are predictors
- Late recurrence: dependent on carcinogenic effect of underlying liver disease
- No effective neo-adjuvant or adjuvant treatment options to reduce risk of recurrence

Berzigotti A et al. Hepatology 2015;61:526–536
Cucchetti A et al. Ann Surg 2009;250:922–928
Fancellu A et al. J Surg Res 2011;171:e33–e45

Liver Transplantation
- Possibility of cure of the tumor and underlying liver disease
- Benchmark for the selection of patients is the Milan criteria: one lesion ≤5 cm, alternatively up to three lesions ≤3 cm, no extrahepatic manifestations, no evidence of macrovascular invasion
- 70% 5-year survival and <10% recurrence expected in patients who fit Milan criteria
- Low availability of liver allografts is a major limitation; long waiting times are associated with disease progression
- When wait time for transplant >3 months, resection ablation and trans-arterial chemoembolization (TACE) should be considered
- No role for systemic chemotherapy prior to transplant

European Association for the Study of the Liver. J Hepatol 2018;69:182–236

Percutaneous Ablation
- Potential curative therapy
- Techniques include percutaneous ethanol injection (PEI), radiofrequency ablation (RFA), microwave ablation (MWA)
- Applicability dependent on tumor size (<3–4 cm), number of tumors (up to 3 tumors), and location (accessibility with CT, MRI, or US guidance)
- RFA: recommended as first-line treatment in early stages of disease (HCC <2 cm); outcomes similar to LR
- Complete response rate after RFA is 70–90% (with up to two procedures)
- Overall survival after RFA is 60 months; recurrence rate is 40–68% at 5 years
- Several randomized controlled trials (RCTs) have confirmed the superiority of RFA over ethanol injection in terms of survival, particularly in BCLC stage A with nodules between 2 and 4 cm
- Stereotactic RFA has technological advantages to conventional RFA and improved outcomes (97% complete pathologic response in nodules >3 cm)
- Effectiveness limited by:
  - Tumor size: not recommended for lesions >5 cm
  - Tumor location: avoid in tumors located in the vicinity of the gallbladder, liver hilum, intestine, or major blood vessels
- Predictors of survival: tumor size, multinodularity, Child-Pugh class, serum AFP level
- RFA is associated with lower complication rates than resection

Bale R et al. Hepatology 2019;70:840–850
Casadei Gardini A et al. Onco Targets Ther 2018;11:6555–6567
Doyle A et al. J Hepatol 2019;70:866–873
Hermida M et al. Cancers (Basel) 2020;12:313
Izumi N et al. J Clin Oncol 2019;37:4002

Chemoembolization (TACE) and other loco-regional therapies
Trans-arterial chemoembolization (TACE)
- TACE prolongs OS in Child-Pugh A or B, intermediate-stage disease BCLC B (liver-confined multinodular disease), ECOG 0–1, small tumor burden (not candidates for resection or ablation) in the absence of portal vein invasion
- Median OS (mOS) of 35–40 months (mOS decreases to 20 months if portal vein invasion or deteriorated liver function after TACE)
- The hepatoma arterial-embolization prognostic (HAP) score defines four prognostic groups; HAP A has an expected OS of 33 months and HAP D an OS of 12 months
- Options include lipiodol-based TACE, doxorubicin-eluting bead (DEB)-TACE
- Conventional TACE (cTACE) and DEB-TACE have similar survival; DEB-TACE is associated with fewer side effects
- Optimal duration and frequency of TACE is not defined
- TACE should not be combined with systemic agents outside of clinical trials

Golfieri R et al. Br J Cancer 2014;111:255–264
Ikeda M et al. J Gastroenterol 2018;53:281–290
Kudo M et al. Lancet Gastroenterol Hepatol 2018;3:37–46
Meyer T et al. Lancet Gastroenterol Hepatol 2017;2:565–575
Waked I et al. J Clin Oncol 2016;34:2046
Yu SC et al. Radiology 2014;270:607–620

(continued)

Expert Opinion (*continued*)

Trans-arterial radioembolization (TARE, also called selective internal radiation therapy or SIRT)
- Similar survival and local tumor control between TACE and TARE in tumors 3–8 cm (phase 2 study)
- TARE has a longer PFS than TACE (> 6 months vs 6.8 months, phase 2 study)
- Downstaging of the tumor is more likely with TARE than with TACE (58% vs 31%)
- Radioembolization with ^{90}Y for advanced HCC compares favorably with other approved therapies for unresectable HCC (retrospective and cohort studies)
- Radioembolization with ^{90}Y has advantages relative to TACE in patients with unresectable HCC, with increased time to progression, improved tolerability, and fewer adverse events (retrospective studies)
- A survival benefit relative to TACE has not been demonstrated
- In advanced HCC with portal vein invasion, ^{90}Y radioembolization may be of specific value (TACE relatively contraindicated)
- Phase 3 study results pending for TARE

Galle PR et al. Hepatology 2018;67:358–380
Mosconi C et al. J Hepatol 2018;69:259–260
Sapir E et al. Int J Radiat Oncol Biol Phys 2018;100:122–130
Shen PC et al. Int J Radiat Oncol Biol Phys 2019;105:307–318

Stereotactic body radiation therapy (SBRT)
- Total doses range from 24 to 60 Gy over three to six fractions
- Local tumor control rate: 68–95% at 2–3 years
- PFS 21–48% and OS rates 21–69% at 2–3 years due to out-of-field progression in untreated liver

Chow PKH et al. J Clin Oncol 2018;36(19):1913–1921
Jang WI et al. Cancer 2020;126(2):363
Ricke J et al. J Hepatol 2019;71(6):1164–1174
Rim CH et al. Radiother Oncol 2019;131:135–144

Systemic Treatment
First-line setting: Bevacizumab + atezolizumab, lenvatinib, sorafenib
Subsequent therapy: Regorafenib, ramucirumab, cabozantinib
Systemic immune therapy: Nivolumab, pembrolizumab, nivolumab + ipilimumab

Bevacizumab and atezolizumab
- In unresectable HCC, bevacizumab-atezolizumab has a better OS and PFS compared with sorafenib
- Improved OS with bevacizumab-atezolizumab at 6 months (84.8%) and 12 months (67.2%) versus 72.2% and 54.6% respectively with sorafenib
- Progression-free survival is longer with atezolizumab-bevacizumab (median 6.8 months, 54.5%) than with sorafenib (median 4.3 months, 37.2%)
- The most common Grade 3 or 4 adverse events (AE) with the combination are hypertension (15 %), aspartate aminotransferase increase (7%), alanine amino transferase increase (4%), fatigue (2%), proteinuria (3%), diarrhea (2%), decreased appetite (1%), pyrexia (1%)

Finn RS et al. N Engl J Med 2020;382:1894–1905

Sorafenib
- First-line treatment in advanced HCC results in an increase in OS in Child-Pugh A versus placebo (10.7 vs 7.9 months)
- Subgroups including macroscopic vascular invasion or extrahepatic spread show an important benefit
- Most common Grade 3 AEs include palmar-plantar erythrodysesthesia (8%), diarrhea (8%), hypertension (2%), abdominal pain (2%), hypophosphatemia (11%), thrombocytopenia (4%)

Llovet JM et al. N Engl J Med 2008;359:378–390

Lenvatinib
- Lenvatinib is noninferior to sorafenib as far as OS benefit in the first-line setting
- PFS with lenvatinib is 7.4 months vs 3.7 months with sorafenib
- The objective response rate with lenvatinib is 24% vs 9% with sorafenib
- Lenvatinib has not been studied in patients with 50% or more liver invasion, main portal vein invasion, or invasion of the bile duct
- Lenvatinib is dosed by weight (<60 kg; 8 mg/day, ≥60 kg; 12 mg/day)
- Most common any grade AEs; hypertension (42%), diarrhea (39%), decreased appetite (34%), weight loss (31%)

Kudo M et al. Lancet 2018;391:1163–1173

(*continued*)

Expert Opinion (continued)

Subsequent therapies:

Regorafenib
- Treatment of advanced HCC after progression on and having tolerated a minimum dose of sorafenib (≥400 mg/day for ≥20 of last 28 days of treatment)
- Improves OS in the second-line setting (10.6 months with regorafenib vs 7.8 months with placebo)
- Most common Grade 3 or 4 AEs: hypertension (15%), palmar-plantar erythrodysesthesia (13%), fatigue (9%), diarrhea (3%)

Bruix J et al. Lancet 2017;389:56–66

Cabozantinib:
- Indicated in patients previously treated with sorafenib and with disease progression after at least one systemic treatment for HCC (may have received up to two previous systemic regimens)
- Improvement in median OS: 10.2 months with cabozantinib versus 8.0 months with placebo
- The most common high-grade AEs were palmar-plantar erythrodysesthesia (17%), hypertension (16%), increased aspartate aminotransferase (AST) level (12%), fatigue (10%), diarrhea (10%)

Abou-Alfa GK et al. N Engl J Med 2018;379:54–63

Ramucirumab
- Indicated after treatment with sorafenib with baseline AFP concentrations ≥400 ng/dL
- Improvement in OS of 8.5 months with ramucirumab vs 7.3 months for placebo
- Grade 3–4 AEs: hypertension (13%), hyponatremia (6%), increased AST (3%)

Zhu AX et al. Lancet Oncol 2019;20:282–296

Systemic Treatments
Immunotherapy: Nivolumab, Pembrolizumab, Ipilimumab and Nivolumab

Nivolumab
- Treatment of advanced HCC previously treated with sorafenib
- Durable objective response rate (ORR) of 14%, median duration of response 17 months (phase 1/2 study with or without previous exposure to sorafenib)
- Median OS as second-line therapy: 15.6 months
- Well-tolerated, side-effect profile similar to that seen in other diseases including pruritus, rash, diarrhea, decreased appetite, rash, AST/ALT, and lipase increase
- Nivolumab in the front-line setting versus sorafenib did not achieve statistical significance for OS (phase 3 study)

El-Khoueiry AB et al. Lancet 2017;389:2492–2502
Yau T PJ et al. Ann Oncol 2019;30:851–934

Pembrolizumab
- Treatment of advanced HCC previously treated with sorafenib
- Overall durable response rate of 17%, PFS of 4.9 months
- Tolerable side-effect profile, similar to safety profile in other diseases
- Pembrolizumab in the second-line setting (after progression on sorafenib) in advanced HCC compared with placebo did not meet statistical significance (phase 3 study)
- Well-tolerated, side-effect profile similar to that seen in other diseases treated with pembrolizumab including AST, ALT, and bilirubin increase, fatigue, pruritus, decreased appetite, diarrhea, abdominal pain, nausea, rash, cough, dyspnea

Zhu AX et al. J Clin Oncol 2020;38:193–202

Nivolumab and Ipilimumab
- Treatment of advanced HCC after failure of sorafenib treatment
- ORR 31%, median duration of response 17 months; disease control rate 49% and 24-month OS rate 40%
- 37% of patients had Grade 3/4 AEs, most common: fatigue, diarrhea, rash, pruritus, nausea, musculoskeletal pain, pyrexia, cough, decreased appetite, vomiting, abdominal pain, dyspnea, upper respiratory tract infection, arthralgia, headache, hypothyroidism, decreased weight, dizziness
- More than 50% of patients may require systemic steroids to manage AEs

Yau T et al. J Clin Oncol 2019;37:4012–4012

LOCOREGIONAL THERAPY

HEPATOCELLULAR CARCINOMA REGIMEN: CHEMOEMBOLIZATION WITH DOXORUBICIN

Llovet JM et al. Lancet 2002;359:1734–1739

Doxorubicin dose adjusted to serum bilirubin concentration (see table below) prepared as an emulsion with 10 mL of ethiodized oil injection administered intra-arterially followed by mechanical obstruction achieved by intra-arterial injection of gelatin sponge fragments suspended in radiologic contrast media until flow stagnation occurred. Chemoembolization was performed at baseline, repeated 2 months and 6 months later, and then every 6 months until disease progression observed

Notes:
• Doxorubicin dosage was based on serum total bilirubin concentration:

Total Bilirubin		Doxorubicin Dosage
(μmol/L)	(mg/dL)	
<25.6	<1.5	75 mg/m^2
25.6–51.3	1.5–3	50 mg/m^2
51.3–85.5	3–5	25 mg/m^2

• Extrahepatic arterial supply of HCC is important. See section on extrahepatic collateral vessels supplying hepatocellular carcinomas (Kim HC et al. Radiographics 2005;25[Suppl 1]:S25–S39)
• The mean numbers of treatment sessions were 3.08 (95% CI 2.4–3.5; range 0–7) for embolization and 2.8 (2.3–3.2; 1–8) for chemoembolization (P = 0.5)

General Guidelines

Prior to embolization:
• **Hydration**
  ▪ Start intravenous **hydration** with 0.9% sodium chloride injection (0.9% NS)
  ▪ Continuous 0.9% NS 100 mL/h beginning a minimum of 6 hours prior to procedure
• **Antibiotic prophylaxis** not always required but may be considered with the first doses given before embolization:
  ▪ **Metronidazole** 500 mg; administer intravenously prior to procedure followed by 500 mg every 12 hours × 3 doses, *plus*
  ▪ **Cefazolin** 1000 mg; administer intravenously prior to procedure followed by **cefazolin** 500 mg; administer intravenously every 8 hours × 5 doses
• **Antiemetic primary prophylaxis:** Give a serotonin receptor (5HT$_3$)-antagonist plus a high-potency glucocorticoid
  Give a serotonin receptor (5HT$_3$) antagonist plus a high-potency glucocorticoid
  ▪ **Ondansetron** 16 mg; administer intravenously or 24 mg orally, *plus*
  ▪ **Dexamethasone** 10–12 mg; administer intravenously or orally 30–60 minutes before the procedure

Post-embolization syndrome:
• The triad of abdominal pain, vomiting, and fever that frequently occurs 24–72 hours after chemoembolization is commonly referred to as post-embolization syndrome
• Post-embolization syndrome uniformly responds to supportive care including analgesics and antiemetics
• Use care administering acetaminophen (paracetamol) and non-steroidal anti-inflammatory drugs in patients with liver cirrhosis

After embolization:
• Continue intravenous **hydration** with 0.9% NS or another clinically appropriate fluid until patient resumes adequate oral fluid intake
• Provide **analgesic support** with parenterally administered opioid medications (**morphine, hydromorphone, fentanyl**) after chemoembolization until patient is able to continue analgesic treatment with oral products
• Continue **antiemetic prophylaxis** with a 5HT$_3$ antagonist plus a high-potency glucocorticoid:
  ▪ **Ondansetron** 8 mg; administer intravenously or orally every 8 hours, *plus*
  ▪ **Dexamethasone** 8 mg; administer intravenously or orally every 8 hours for 2–3 days
• **Filgrastim** (G-CSF) 5 mcg/kg per day; administer by subcutaneous injection
  ▪ May be used for patients who develop an ANC <500/mm^3, neutropenia and fever, or documented infections during neutropenia
  ▪ Discontinue filgrastim at least 24 hours before a chemoembolization procedure

Treatment Modifications

Doxorubicin dosage modifications were based on serum total bilirubin concentrations before treatment

Patient Population Studied

A total of 903 patients were screened and 791 excluded due to early HCC, advanced liver disease, vascular invasion, extrahepatic spread, and end-stage cancer. A total of 112 patients with intermediate BCLC stage (stage B or C) were randomized to conservative treatment (n = 35), embolization (n = 37), or chemoembolization (n = 40)

Patient Characteristics			
	Embolization (n = 37)	Chemoembolization (n = 40)	Control (n = 35)
Demography			
Age, years*	64 (62–67)	63 (61–66)	66 (64–68)
M/F	30/17 (81%/19%)	32/8 (80%/20%)	23/12 (66%/34%)
Cause of cirrhosis			
Hepatitis C virus	30 (81%)	33 (82%)	32 (91%)
Hepatitis B virus	2 (5%)	4 (10%)	1 (3%)
Alcohol	4 (11%)	3 (8%)	1 (3%)
Other	1 (3%)	—	1 (3%)
Tumor-related symptoms			
Ascites	9 (24%)	6 (15%)	11 (31%)
Abdominal pain	7 (19%)	3 (8%)	3 (9%)
Constitutional syndrome	1 (3%)	1 (2%)	4 (11%)
Biochemistry			
Serum bilirubin (mmol/L)*	22.2 (18.8–27.4)	20.5 (18.8–23.9)	25.6 (22.2–29.1)
Prothrombin activity (%)*	81 (75–87)	82 (77–87)	77 (71–83)
Serum albumin (g/L)*	35 (33–37)	35 (33–37)	35 (33–37)
γ-glutamyltranspeptidase*,‡	113 (70–156)	112 (85–139)	101 (66–137)
Alkaline phosphatase*,‡	233 (203–263)	220 (182–258)	257 (202–311)
Distribution of α-fetoprotein concentrations			
<10 mg/L	15	15	11
10–100 mg/L	9	18	16
>100 mg/L	13	7	8
Tumor stage			
Solitary (66%)†	9 (24%)	13 (32%)	8 (23%)
Multinodular	27 (73%)	26 (65%)	27 (77%)
Two nodules	6	7	8
More than two nodules	21	19	19
Diffuse	1 (3%)	1 (3%)	—
Disease characteristics			
Diameter main nodule (mm)*	52 (46–60)	49 (40–58)	44 (39–49)
Bilobar disease	18 (49%)	19 (47%)	18 (51%)

(continued)

Patient Population Studied (*continued*)

Patient Characteristics			
	Embolization (n = 37)	Chemoembolization (n = 40)	Control (n = 35)
Child-Pugh class A/B	27/10	31/9	21/14
Okuda stage I/II	24/13	27/13	22/13
BCLC stage B/C	28/9	35/5	27/8
Performance status			
0	28	35	27
1	7	4	4
2	2	1	4

Data are numbers of patients unless otherwise indicated
*Mean (95% CI)
†Solitary tumors with or without satellites
‡IU/L

Efficacy

1. Chemoembolization-induced objective responses sustained for at least 6 months in 35% (14) of cases, and was associated with a significantly lower rate of portal vein invasion than conservative treatment
2. Probability of portal vein invasion reduced from 58% in control to 17% in patients with chemoembolization
3. Survival probabilities at 1 year and 2 years were 75% and 50% for embolization, and 82% and 63% for chemoembolization
4. Patients who achieved objective responses sustained for at least 6 months had probabilities of survival at 1, 2, and 3 years of 96%, 77%, and 47%, respectively ($P = 0.002$ compared with patients with treatment failure, and $P = 0.006$ vs control group)
5. Treatment allocation was the sole baseline variable independently related to survival (odds ratio 0.45 [95% CI 0.25–0.81], $P = 0.02$) in the Cox regression model. Inclusion of treatment response identified this variable as an independent predictor (odds ratio 0.59 [0.44–0.81], $P = 0.0007$) together with constitutional syndrome (0.46 [0.25–0.86], $P = 0.04$)
6. There were no differences in intention-to-treat survival between nonresponders and the control group (1-year survival 65% vs 63%; 2-year survival 41% vs 26%; $P = 0.3$)

	Embolization (n = 37)	Chemoembolization (n = 40)*	Control (n = 35)*
Mean follow-up, month	21.7	21.2	14.5
Mean follow-up, 95% CI	17.5–26.0	17.3–25.1	10.6–18.4
Probability of survival at 1 year	75%	82%	63%
Probability of survival at 2 years	50%	63%	27%
Probability of survival at 3 years	29%	29%	17%
Mean survival, months	25.3	28.7	17.9
Mean survival, 95% CI	20.3–30.2	23.6–33.7	13.1–22.7
Assessment of Response in 102 Patients Who Survived for at Least 5 Months			
Objective responses	16†	14†	
Probability of portal-vein invasion at 2 years	—	17%	58%
		$P = 0.005$	

*Survival was significantly better in the chemoembolization group than in the control group ($P = 0.009$)
†Embolization vs control, $P = 0.001$; chemoembolization vs control, $P = 0.004$

(*continued*)

Efficacy (continued)

Causes of Death

	Embolization (n = 37)	Chemoembolization (n = 40)	Control (n = 35)	Total (n = 112)
Deaths	25 (67%)	21 (52%)	25 (71%)	71 (63%)
Cause of Death				
Tumor progression	20	14	23	57
Hepatic failure with SD*	4	5	2	11
Other	1[†]	2[‡]	0	3

*SD, stable disease
[†]Neoplasm of lung
[‡]Neoplasm of tongue and treatment-related death (septic shock)

Reasons for Treatment Discontinuation Among Patients Who Received Embolization*

	Embolization (n = 37)	Chemoembolization (n = 40)	Both Groups (n = 77)
Reason			
Tumor progression (portal thrombosis, extrahepatic spread, or performance status >2)	15	9	24
Liver failure without tumor progression	3	2	5
Technical problems (arterial hepatic obstruction, collateral blood flow, low ejection fraction)	3	8	11
Adverse events (leukopenia, ischemic biliary stricture, transient ischemic attack, allergic dermatitis)	1	4	5
Patient's decision	2	4	6
Death on treatment	4	3	7
Other (lung cancer, percutaneous ethanol injection)	2	0	2
Treatment discontinuation	29 (78%)	31 (77%)	60 (78%)
Active treatment at end of follow-up	8 (22%)	9 (23%)	17 (22%)

*There were no significant differences between groups

Toxicity (N = 40)

Adverse Event	Number of Patients
Cholecystitis	2
Leukopenia	2
Ischemic biliary stricture	1
Hepatic infarction	1
Spontaneous bacterial peritonitis	1
Bacteremia	1

Adverse Event	Number of Patients
Septic shock	1
Allergic dermatitis	1
Severe alopecia	1

Other complications associated with TACE procedures in general:
• Hepatic artery occlusion: 4%
• Damage to the hepatic artery: pseudoaneurysm (rare), occlusion, and dissection
• Treatment was discontinued in 60 (78%) patients

Therapy Monitoring

1. *Days 7 and 14 after TACE and then monthly:* CBC and LFTs
2. Response assessment using computed tomography (CT) every 3 months

LOCOGREGIONAL THERAPY

HEPATOCELLULAR CARCINOMA REGIMEN: CHEMOEMBOLIZATION WITH CISPLATIN

Lo C-M et al. Hepatology 2002;35:1164–1171

Chemoembolization: cisplatin (1 mg/mL) emulsified with ethiodized oil injection in equivalent volumes (1:1)
- Administer cisplatin intra-arterially via the left or right hepatic artery as appropriate for tumor vascularization. If selective catheterization is not possible, the cisplatin emulsion is injected into the hepatic artery, distal to the gastroduodenal artery
- The emulsion is injected slowly under fluoroscopic monitoring to a maximum volume of 60 mL ($\leq$30 mg cisplatin) at a controlled rate to prevent retrograde flow, followed by mechanical obstruction achieved by intra-arterial injection of gelatin sponge pellets 1 mm in diameter mixed with gentamicin 40 mg
- Chemoembolization is repeated every 2–3 months until comorbid pathologies, adverse events, or disease progression is observed

Notes:
- Extrahepatic arterial supply of HCC is important. See section on extrahepatic collateral vessels supplying hepatocellular carcinomas (Kim HC et al. Radiographics 2005;25[Suppl 1]:S25–S39)
- Forty patients assigned to the chemoembolization group received a total of 192 courses of chemoembolization, with each patient receiving a median of 4.5 courses (range, 1–15). Ninety-four courses (49%) of the chemoembolization were performed by selective injection into the right or left hepatic artery. The median volume of cisplatin-ethiodized oil emulsion injected in 1 course was 20 mL (range, 2–60), and the dosage was significantly related to the tumor size ($r = 0.70$; $P <0.001$)
- Two patients were scheduled for continuation of chemoembolization as of the date of the latest follow-up. The remaining 38 patients had treatment stopped because of progressive disease (12 patients), death (7 patients), poor liver function (6 patients), adverse effects (6 patients), patient refusal (3 patients), arteriovenous shunting (2 patients), and hepatic artery thrombosis (2 patients)
- The most common clinical adverse effect was a self-limiting syndrome consisting of fever, abdominal pain, and vomiting. The median hospital stay for each course of treatment was 2 days (range, 1–21)

General Guidelines

Prior to embolization:
- **Hydration**
  - Start intravenous **hydration** with 0.9% sodium chloride injection (0.9% NS)
  - Continuous 0.9% NS 100 mL/h beginning a minimum of 6 hours prior to procedure
- **Antibiotic prophylaxis** not always required but may be considered with the first doses given before embolization:
  - **Metronidazole** 500 mg; administer intravenously prior to procedure followed by **Metronidazole** 500 mg; administer intravenously every 12 hours × 3 doses, *plus*
  - **Cefazolin** 1000 mg; administer intravenously prior to procedure followed by **cefazolin** 500 mg; administer intravenously every 8 hours × 5 doses
- **Antiemetic primary prophylaxis** Give a serotonin receptor ($5HT_3$) antagonist plus a high-potency glucocorticoid
  - **Ondansetron** 16 mg; administer intravenously or 24 mg orally, *plus*
  - **Dexamethasone** 10–12 mg; administer intravenously or orally 30–60 minutes before the procedure

Post-embolization syndrome:
- The triad of abdominal pain, vomiting, and fever that frequently occurs 24–72 hours after chemoembolization is commonly referred to as post-embolization syndrome
- Post-embolization syndrome uniformly responds to supportive care including analgesics and antiemetics
- Use care administering acetaminophen (paracetamol) and nonsteroidal anti-inflammatory drugs in patients with liver cirrhosis

After embolization:
- Continue intravenous **hydration** with 0.9% NS or another clinically appropriate fluid until patient resumes adequate oral fluid intake
- Provide **analgesic support** with parenterally administered opioid medications (**morphine, hydromorphone, fentanyl**) after chemoembolization until patient is able to continue analgesic treatment with oral products
- Continue **antiemetic prophylaxis** with a $5HT_3$ antagonist plus a high-potency glucocorticoid:
  - **Ondansetron** 8 mg; administer intravenously or orally every 8 hours, *plus*
  - **Dexamethasone** 8 mg; administer intravenously or orally every 8 hours for 2–3 days
- **Filgrastim** (G-CSF) 5 mcg/kg per day; administer by subcutaneous injection
  - May be used for patients who develop an ANC <500/mm^3, neutropenia and fever, or documented infections during neutropenia
  - Discontinue filgrastim at least 24 hours before a chemoembolization procedure

Treatment Modifications

Withhold or discontinue
chemoembolization for:
• Hepatic artery thrombosis
• Main portal vein thrombosis
• Arteriovenous shunting
• Hepatic encephalopathy
• Ascites not controlled by diuretics
• Variceal bleeding within the last 3 months
• Serum total bilirubin >50 μmol/L
  (>2.9 mg/dL)
• Serum albumin <28 g/L (<2.8 g/dL)
• Prothrombin time 4 seconds > control

Patient Population Studied

A study of 80 patients with Okuda stage I–II HCC and no contraindications for
chemoembolization; 40 assigned to chemoembolization and 39 assigned to control

Baseline Characteristics of the Study Patients According to the Treatment Group

	Chemoembolization (n = 40)	Control (n = 39)
Age (years)*	62 (53–69)	63 (53–70)
Sex (men/women)	36/4	34/5
Serum hepatitis B surface antigen (positive/negative)	34/6	29/10
Serum creatinine, μmol/L*	92 (82–102)	87 (78–98)
Serum total bilirubin, μmol/L*	14 (10–21)	13 (11–23)
Serum albumin, g/L*	38 (32–42)	37 (33–40)
Serum alanine aminotransferase, U/L*	51 (38–83)	53 (35–88)
Prothrombin time, s*	11.5 (10.9–12.4)	11.5 (10.8–12.5)
Serum α-fetoprotein, ng/mL*	505 (55–5, 874)	500 (58–24, 458)
Serum α-fetoprotein (ng/mL; <20/20–500/>500)	6/14/20	8/12/19
Indocyanine green retention at 15 minutes (%)*	24 (6–33)	18 (6–38)
ECOG performance status rating (0/1/2/3)	20/16/3/1	14/19/4/2
Presenting symptom (asymptomatic/symptomatic)	12/28	10/29
Diameter of largest tumor mass, cm*	7 (4–14)	7 (5–11)
Number of tumors (solitary/multinodular)	17/23	15/24
Portal vein obstruction (right/left/main)†	6/3/0	7/5/0
Okuda stage (I/II)	19/21	18/21

Note: P >0.05 for all variables when the two groups are compared
*Values are medians, with interquartile ranges shown in parentheses
†Assessed by computed tomography

Efficacy

Patients with Measurable Disease*

	Chemoembolization (N = 28)	Control (N = 18)
Objective response	39%	6%
	P = 0.014	
Complete response	(0)	(0)
Major responses	11/28 (39.3)	1 (5.55%)
Minor responses	6/28 (21.4%)	2 (11.1%)
Stabilization	7/28 (25%)	6 (33.3%)
Progression	4/28 (14.3%)	9 (50%)

(continued)

Efficacy (continued)

Patients with Measurable AFP[†]

	Chemoembolization (N = 29)	Control (N = 21)
Objective response in α-FP	21/29 (72.4%)	2/21 (9.5%)
	P <0.001	
Complete response in α-FP	9/29 (31%)	0/21 (0)
Major responses α-FP	12/29 (41.4%)	2/21 (9.5%)
Minor responses in α-FP	0/29 (0)	0/21 (0)
Stabilization of α-FP	1/29 (3.4%)	1/21 (4.8%)
Progression of α-FP	7/29 (24.1%)	18/21 (85.7%)

All Patients

	Chemoembolization	Control
1-year survival	57%[‡]	32%[‡]
2-year survival	31%[‡]	11%[‡]
3-year survival	26%[*,‡]	3%[‡]

*Patients who survived more than 3 months and had a measurable tumor on computed tomographic scan
[†]Patients with a baseline serum α-fetoprotein level >20 ng/mL who survived more than 3 months
[‡]Relative risk of death in the chemoembolization group was 0.50; 95% CI, 0.31–0.81; P <0.005

Univariate Analysis of Prognostic Variables for Survival

		Probability of Survival (%)			
Characteristics	Number of Patients	12 Months	24 Months	36 Months	P Value
Study treatment					
Chemoembolization	40	57	31	26	0.002
Control	39	32	11	3	
Sex					
Men	70	44	20	15	NS (0.720)
Women	9	56	33	11	
Age (years)					
≤60	34	35	15	12	NS (0.274)
>60	45	52	26	17	
ECOG performance status rating					
0	34	43	18	9	NS (0.384)
1–3	45	46	23	19	
Presenting symptom					
Asymptomatic	22	77	43	29	0.004
Symptomatic	57	33	13	9	
Tumor size (cm)					
≤5	26	65	39	27	0.019
>5	50	37	13	9	

(continued)

Efficacy (continued)

Characteristics	Number of Patients	Probability of Survival (%)			P Value
		12 Months	24 Months	36 Months	
Tumor number					
Single	32	55	29	16	NS (0.225)
Multiple	47	39	16	14	
Unilobar portal vein obstruction					
Negative	58	60	27	18	<0.001
Positive	21	5	5	5	
Okuda stage					
I	37	61	35	23	0.003
II	42	31	10	7	
Serum albumin (g/L)					
≤37	40	44	16	10	NS (0.341)
>37	39	46	27	19	
Serum bilirubin (μmol/L)					
≤14	41	41	23	18	NS (0.967)
>14	38	49	19	11	
% indocyanine green retention at 15 minutes					
≤20	38	39	20	17	NS (0.635)
>20	41	50	23	13	
α-fetoprotein (ng/mL)					
≤500	40	54	32	19	NS (0.059)
>500	39	36	10	10	

Comparison of Survival Between the Chemoembolization and Control Groups Stratified by Baseline Prognostic Variables*

	Chemoembolization	Control	P Value
Presenting symptom			
Asymptomatic	25.4 (17.5)	16.6 (2.5)	0.039
Symptomatic	11.2 (2.6)	5.2 (1.4)	0.019
Unilobar portal vein obstruction			
Negative	18.0 (3.5)	9.2 (5.6)	0.008
Positive	5.1 (2.2)	2.6 (2.3)	NS (0.406)
Tumor size (cm)			
≤5	29.8 (12.2)	11.5 (3.0)	0.003
>5	11.2 (1.8)	5.3 (1.4)	NS (0.115)
Okuda stage			
I	25.4 (9.1)	11.5 (5.8)	0.016
II	9.2 (4.1)	5.2 (1.5)	0.040

*Values are median survival times in months with standard errors in parentheses

(continued)

Efficacy (continued)

Comparison of Liver Function as Assessed by the Serum Bilirubin Level, Serum Albumin Level, and Indocyanine Green Retention Rate at 15 Minutes

	Chemoembolization Group		Control Group		
	Number of Patients	Median (Interquartile Range)	Number of Patients	Median (Interquartile Range)	P Value
Bilirubin (μmol/L)					
3 months	34	15 (10–31)	24	21 (14–42)	0.038
6 months	24	14 (11–24)	13	17 (10–28)	0.987
9 months	19	16 (10–20)	7	18 (12–32)	0.385
12 months	17	13 (9–23)	9	15 (11–30)	0.517
Albumin (g/L)					
3 months	34	36 (31–40)	24	32 (26–37)	0.073
6 months	24	35 (31–39)	13	35 (28–38)	0.425
9 months	19	35 (31–37)	7	33 (28–36)	0.223
12 months	17	33 (31–39)	9	34 (27–39)	0.499
Indocyanine green retention at 15 minutes (%)					
3 months	32	25 (14–43)	25	36 (20–52)	0.169
6 months	25	25 (18–38)	13	26 (17–51)	0.433
9 months	22	25 (20–34)	10	28 (15–48)	0.405
12 months	17	26 (13–34)	9	32 (22–47)	0.146

Toxicity

(N = 40 Patients/192 Courses)

	Number of Cycles (%)
Fevers ≥38°C (≥100.4°F)*	63 (32.8)
Abdominal pain*	50 (26%)
Vomiting*	32 (16.7%)
Ascites	10 (5.2%)
Gastrointestinal bleeding	8 (4.2%)
Bleeding at femoral puncture	3 (1.6%)
Encephalopathy	3 (1.6%)
Ruptured tumor	2 (1%)
Pleural effusion	2 (1%)
Liver abscess	1 (0.5%)
Hematuria	1 (0.5%)
Hypotension	1 (0.5%)
Bradycardia	1 (0.5%)

*The most common clinical adverse effect was a self-limiting syndrome consisting of fever, abdominal pain, and vomiting. The median hospital stay for each course of treatment was 2 days (range, 1–21)

Therapy Monitoring

1. *Days 7 and 14 after TACE and then monthly:* CBC and LFTs
2. Response assessment using computed tomography (CT) every 3 months

LOCOREGIONAL THERAPY

HEPATOCELLULAR CARCINOMA REGIMEN: DEB-TACE—TRANSARTERIAL CHEMOEMBOLIZATION (TACE) USING DRUG-ELUTING BEADS (DEB)

Lammer J et al. Cardiovasc Intervent Radiol 2010; 33:41–52

Transarterial chemoembolization using drug-eluting beads (DEB), an embolizing device that slowly releases chemotherapy to decrease systemic toxicity

Pretreatment approach:
• A baseline angiography of the celiac trunk, superior mesenteric artery, and hepatic artery is performed using a peripheral arterial approach
• Antibiotic prophylaxis is not required but may be considered

Note: Extrahepatic arterial supply of HCC is important. See section on extra-hepatic collateral vessels supplying hepatocellular carcinomas (Kim HC, Chung JW, Lee W, Jae HJ, Park JH. Radiographics 2005;25[Suppl 1]:S25–S39)

Drug-eluting beads (DEB) (Boston Scientific Corporation, USA) with a diameter ranging between 300 and 700 μm are loaded with **doxorubicin** and mixed with an equal volume of contrast media. Additional unloaded spheres are used to complete the embolization procedure

Doxorubicin 150 mg (bilirubin <1.5 mg/dL; <25.7 μmol/L)

Loading process to obtain a final loading dose of 150 mg doxorubicin per two 2-mL vials of beads:
• Begin about 2 hours before the TACE is planned
• Reconstitute a vial containing doxorubicin 50 mg with 2 mL of sterile water for injection. Mix well to obtain a clear red doxorubicin solution with concentration = 25 mg/mL
• Remove as much of the solution as possible from a vial of beads using a syringe with a small-gauge needle
• Using a syringe and needle, add 2 mL of reconstituted doxorubicin solution directly to the vial of beads
• Agitate the beads in the doxorubicin solution occasionally to encourage mixing. The dark red color of the suspension should become slightly pink and the beads, which are initially blue, should become red, indicating that doxorubicin has been loaded into the beads *Note:* Although the solution retains a red color, the doxorubicin will be loaded. Loading will take a minimum of 20 minutes for the smallest beads and up to 120 minutes for the largest beads
• Prior to use, transfer the beads loaded with doxorubicin to a syringe and add an equal volume of non-ionic contrast media. Invert the syringe gently to obtain an even suspension of beads

Note: Beads should be loaded only with doxorubicin HCl; liposomal formulations of doxorubicin are not suitable for loading into beads. A dose of up to 37.5 mg doxorubicin per mL of beads can be loaded. The maximum recommended total dose of doxorubicin per procedure is 150 mg. Beads loaded with doxorubicin may be stored for up to 24 hours at 2°–8°C (35.6°–46.4°F) in the presence or absence of non-ionic contrast media. Two hours of dwell time for 500–700 μmol DEB has been reported to allow for loading of more than 90% of 100 mg doxorubicin in the beads (Lewis AL et al. J Vasc Interv Radiol 2006;17:1335–1343)

TACE Procedure:
• The vascular network associated with the lesion is carefully evaluated using high-resolution imaging prior to beginning the embolization procedure
• **Highly selective catheterization** is performed with a 3-French microcatheter in order to obtain complete obstruction of the nourishing arteries and avoid damage to non-tumoral liver
• Beads are available in a range of sizes and care should be taken to choose the appropriate size of the bead that best matches the pathology (ie, vascular target/vessel size) and provides the desired clinical outcome
• A delivery catheter is chosen based on the size of the target vessel. Beads can tolerate temporary compression of 20–30% in order to facilitate passage through a delivery catheter
• The delivery catheter is introduced into the target vessel according to standard techniques. The catheter tip is positioned as close as possible to the treatment site to avoid inadvertent occlusion of normal vessels
• Because the beads are not radiopaque, monitoring the embolization under fluoroscopic visualization necessitates adding contrast medium to the DEB suspension
• Care should be taken to ensure proper suspension of the beads in the contrast medium to enhance distribution during injection
• Beads are drawn into a syringe and slowly injected
• After completion of the treatment, the catheter is removed while maintaining gentle suction so as not to dislodge beads still within the catheter lumen
• The embolization end point will be to achieve complete occlusion of the neovascularity, avoiding, however, complete stasis in the afferent artery, which could lead to endothelial damage and subsequent thrombosis precluding future treatments

Note: Treatment is given at 2-month intervals, with a maximum of three chemoembolizations (at baseline, 2 months, and 4 months) with a 6-month follow-up

(continued)

General Guidelines

Prior to embolization:

- **Hydration**
  - Start intravenous **hydration** with 0.9% sodium chloride injection (0.9% NS)
  - Continuous 0.9% NS 100 mL/h beginning a minimum of 6 hours prior to procedure
- **Antibiotic prophylaxis** not always required but may be considered with the first doses given before embolization:
  - **Metronidazole** 500 mg; administer intravenously prior to the procedure followed by **Metronidazole** 500 mg; administer intravenously every 12 hours × 3 doses, *plus*
  - **Cefazolin** 1000 mg; administer intravenously prior to the procedure followed by **Cefazolin** 500 mg; administer intravenously every 8 hours × 5 doses
- **Antiemetic primary prophylaxis:** Give a serotonin receptor ($5HT_3$)-antagonist plus a high-potency glucocorticoid
  - **Ondansetron** 16 mg; administer intravenously *or* 24 mg orally, *plus*
  - **Dexamethasone** 10–12 mg; administer intravenously or orally 30–60 minutes before the procedure

Post-embolization syndrome:

- The triad of abdominal pain, vomiting, and fever that frequently occurs 24–72 hours after chemoembolization is commonly referred to as post-embolization syndrome
- Post-embolization syndrome uniformly responds to supportive care including analgesics and antiemetics
- Use care administering acetaminophen (paracetamol) and nonsteroidal anti-inflammatory drugs in patients with liver cirrhosis

After embolization:

- Continue intravenous **hydration** with 0.9% NS or another clinically appropriate fluid until patient resumes adequate oral fluid intake
- Provide **analgesic support** with parenterally administered opioid medications (**morphine, hydromorphone, fentanyl**) after chemoembolization until the patient is able to continue analgesic treatment with oral products
- Continue **antiemetic prophylaxis** with a $5HT_3$-antagonist plus a high-potency glucocorticoid:
  - **Ondansetron** 8 mg; administer intravenously or orally every 8 hours, *plus*
  - **Dexamethasone** 8 mg; administer intravenously or orally every 8 hours for 2–3 days
- **Filgrastim** (G-CSF) 5 mcg/kg per day; administer by subcutaneous injection
  - May be used for patients who develop an ANC <500/mm^3, neutropenia and fever, or documented infections during neutropenia
  - Discontinue filgrastim at least 24 hours before a chemoembolization procedure

Efficacy

Response Rates

Tumor Response Rate at 6 Months	DC Bead (N = 93)*	cTACE (N = 108)*
Objective response	48/93 (51.6%)	47/108 (43.5%)
	One-sided P = 0.11[†]	
Complete response	25/93 (26.9%)	24/108 (22.2%)
Partial response	23/93 (24.7%)	23/108 (21.3%)
Stable disease	11/93 (11.8%)	9/108 (8.3%)
Disease control rate	59/93 (63.4%)	56/108 (51.9%)
	Two-sided P = 0.11	
Progressive disease	30/93 (32.3%)	44/108 (40.7%)
Advanced-disease patients[‡]		
Objective response, advanced disease[‡]	32/61 (52.4%)	25/72 (34.7)
	Chi-square P = 0.038	

(continued)

Patient Population Studied

A trial in which 212 patients with Child-Pugh A/B cirrhosis (76% male, 59% HCV) with HCC unsuitable for resection without portal invasion or extrahepatic spread and less than 50% liver involvement received chemoembolization with doxorubicin-loaded DEB at doses adjusted for bilirubin and body surface (range, 47–150 mg). Patients were excluded if they had another primary tumor, advanced liver disease (bilirubin levels >3 mg/dL, AST or ALT >5 × upper limit of normal or >250 U/L), advanced tumoral disease (vascular invasion or extrahepatic spread, or diffuse HCC, defined as >50% liver involvement), or contraindications for doxorubicin administration. In this international, multicenter, prospective, randomized single-blind, phase 2 study, patients were randomized to receive doxorubicin with DEB or conventional TACE defined as 50–75 mg/m^2 doxorubicin emulsified in ethiodized oil followed by particle embolization with an embolic agent of choice

Efficacy (continued)

Tumor Response Rate at 6 Months	DC Bead (N = 93)*	cTACE (N = 108)*
Complete response, advanced disease‡	15/61 (24.5%)	10/72 (13.9%)
	Chi-square P = 0.091	
Disease control rate, advanced disease‡	38/61 (63.5%)	32/72 (44.4%)
	Chi-square P = 0.026	
Disease control rate, Child-Pugh B	21/33 (63%)	13/41 (32%)
Disease control rate, ECOG 1	19/30 (63%)	21/66 (32%)
Disease control rate, bilobar	51/86 (59%)	46/94 (49%)
Disease control rate, recurrent disease	17/23 (73%)	13/24 (54%)

*Four DC Bead patients and eight cTACE patients withdrew prior to the first MRI scan. Reasons for these withdrawals were AEs (four DC Bead and four cTACE), withdrawn consent (two cTACE), and post-consent ineligibility (two cTACE)

†The hypothesis of superiority was not met. The difference between groups in favor of DC Bead was 8.1% (two-sided 95% repeated confidence interval [RCI], −4.8 to 22.6%)

‡Advanced disease = 67% of patients with Child-Pugh B, ECOG 1, bilobar or recurrent disease

Toxicity

Incidence of Serious Adverse Events* within 30 Days of a Procedure Analysis by Stratification (Safety Population)

	Number of Patients/Total (%) Number of Events	
	DC Bead (N = 93)	cTACE (N = 108)
Treatment-related SAEs within 30 days of a procedure (primary safety end point)	19 (20.4%) 28 events	21 (19.4%) 24 events
	P = 0.86	
	Number of Patients/Total (%)	
Stratification factor	DC Bead (N = 93)	cTACE (N = 108)
All patients	22/93 (23.7)	32/108 (29.6)
Child-Pugh A	19/77 (24.7)	26/89 (29.2)
Child-Pugh B	3/16 (18.8)	6/19 (31.6)
ECOG 0	17/74 (23.0)	23/80 (28.8)
ECOG 1	5/19 (26.3)	9/28 (32.1)
Unilobar	12/52 (23.1)	18/63 (28.6)
Bilobar	10/41 (24.4)	14/45 (31.1)
No prior curative treatments	19/82 (23.2)	28/95 (29.5)
Recurrent disease	3/11 (27.3)	4/13 (30.8)

*Note: Serious adverse events were defined as events: (1) resulting in death; (2) that were immediately life-threatening; (3) resulting in permanent or significant disability/incapacity; (4) requiring or extending inpatient hospitalization; or (5) congenital anomaly/birth defects. Analysis of treatment groups overall: chi-square test P = 0.34; difference in incidence rates, −6.0%; 95% CI, −18.2 to 6.2

(continued)

Toxicity (continued)

Effects of Systemic Doxorubicin

Events/SWOG Toxicity Grade	DC Bead (N = 93)		cTACE (N = 108)	
	Number of Events	Number of Patients	Number of Events	Number of Patients
All doxorubicin-related events	12	11 (11.8%)	40	28 (25.9%)
	Incidence = −14.1%; 95% CI, −24.7% to −3.5%; P = 0.012			
Alopecia	1	1 (1%)	23	22 (20.4%)
Grade 1	1		12	
Grade 2	0		11	
Marrow suppression	5	5 (5.4%)	8	6 (5.6%)
Grade 1	2		1	
Grade 2	2		1	
Grade 3	1		4	
Grade 4	0		2	
Mucositis	4	4 (4.3%)	7	6 (5.6%)
Grade 1	4		5	
Grade 2	0		1	
Grade 3	0		1	
Skin discoloration	2	2 (2.2%)	2	2 (1.9%)
Grade 1	1		0	
Grade 2	1		2	
Post-embolization syndrome	35	23 (24.7%)	43	28 (25.9%)

Therapy Monitoring

1. *Days 7 and 14 after TACE and then monthly:* CBC and LFTs
2. Response assessment using computed tomography (CT) every 3 months

UNRESECTABLE DISEASE • FIRST-LINE

HEPATOCELLULAR CARCINOMA REGIMEN: ATEZOLIZUMAB + BEVACIZUMAB

Finn RS et al. N Engl J Med 2020;382:1894–1905

Atezolizumab 1200 mg; administer intravenously in 250 mL 0.9% sodium chloride injection, USP, over 60 minutes, every 3 weeks, until disease progression (total dose/3-week cycle = 1200 mg)

Notes:
- Atezolizumab may be administered through an administration set either with or without a low-protein-binding in-line filter with pore size within the range of 0.2–0.22 μm
- If the initial infusion is well tolerated, subsequent administration may be completed over 30 minutes
  - Interrupt or slow the administration rate in patients with mild or moderate infusion-related reactions
  - Permanently discontinue atezolizumab in patients who experience infusion reactions G ≥3

Bevacizumab 15 mg/kg; administer intravenously in 100 mL 0.9% sodium chloride injection, every 3 weeks, until disease progression (total dosage/3-week cycle = 15 mg/kg)

Note:
- Bevacizumab administration duration for the initial dose is 90 minutes. If administration is well tolerated, the administration duration may be decreased stepwise during subsequent administrations to 60 minutes and, finally, to a minimum duration of 30 minutes

Supportive Care
Antiemetic prophylaxis
Emetogenic potential is **MINIMAL**
See Chapter 42 for antiemetic recommendations

Hematopoietic growth factor (G-CSF) prophylaxis
Primary prophylaxis is **NOT** *indicated*
See Chapter 43 for more information

Antimicrobial prophylaxis
Risk of fever and neutropenia is **LOW**
  Antimicrobial primary prophylaxis to be considered:
- Antibacterial—not indicated
- Antifungal—not indicated
- Antiviral—not indicated unless patient previously had an episode of HSV

Treatment Modifications

ATEZOLIZUMAB DOSE MODIFICATIONS

Adverse Reaction	Grade/Severity	Dose Modification
Colitis	G1	Loperamide 4 mg as starting dose then 2 mg before each meal and after each loose stool until without diarrhea for 12 hours, with maximum of 16 mg loperamide per day. If G1 diarrhea or colitis persists for >14 days, then add prednisolone 0.5–1 mg/kg (non-enteric-coated) or consider oral budesonide 9 mg daily if no bloody diarrhea
	G2/3 diarrhea or colitis	Withhold atezolizumab. Loperamide 4 mg as starting dose then 2 mg before each meal and after each loose stool until without diarrhea for 12 hours, with maximum of 16 mg loperamide per day. Administer oral prednisone/prednisolone at a dose of 0.5 to 2 mg/kg/day or its equivalent. When improves to G1, begin a slow corticosteroid taper over at least 4 weeks. Resume atezolizumab upon symptom control, or when prednisone/prednisolone daily dose <10 mg

(continued)

Treatment Modifications (*continued*)

Adverse Reaction	Grade/Severity	Dose Modification
	G4 diarrhea or colitis	Permanently discontinue atezolizumab. Loperamide 4 mg as starting dose then 2 mg before each meal and after each loose stool until without diarrhea for 12 hours, with maximum of 16 mg loperamide per day. Administer 1–2 mg/kg IV (methyl)prednisolone and convert to 0.5–2 mg/kg prednisone/prednisolone orally each day or its equivalent only after a response. Taper over at least 4 weeks when symptoms improve. If does not improve over 72 hours or worsens, perform flexible sigmoidoscopy/colonoscopy to document colitis then begin infliximab 5 mg/kg (if no perforation/sepsis/TB/hepatitis/NYHA III/IV CHF). If no response, add MMF 500–1000 mg twice daily. If worse on MMF, consider addition of tacrolimus or ATG
Pneumonitis	G2	Withhold atezolizumab. Consider pneumocystis prophylaxis depending on the clinical context and cover with empiric antibiotics. Administer oral prednisone/prednisolone at a dose of 1–2 mg/kg/day or its equivalent. When improves to G1, begin a slow corticosteroid taper over at least 4 weeks. If does not respond adequately after 48 hours, then administer 2–4 mg/kg IV (methyl)prednisolone and convert to 0.5–2 mg/kg prednisone/prednisolone orally each day or its equivalent only after a response, followed by a taper over at least 6 weeks when symptoms improve to G1, titrating to symptoms. Resume atezolizumab upon symptom control, or when prednisone/prednisolone daily dose <10 mg
	G3/4	Permanently discontinue atezolizumab. Consider pneumocystis prophylaxis depending on the clinical context; cover with empiric antibiotics. Administer 2–4 mg/kg IV (methyl)prednisolone and convert to 1–2 mg/kg prednisone/prednisolone orally each day or its equivalent only after a response, followed by a taper over at least 8 weeks when symptoms improve to G1, titrating to symptoms. If, when initially treated improvement does not occur within 48–72 hours, begin infliximab 5 mg/kg (if no perforation/sepsis/TB/hepatitis/NYHA III/IV CHF). If no response to infliximab, add MMF 500–1000 mg twice daily. Consider MMF especially if has concurrent hepatic toxicity
Hepatitis	G2 (AST or ALT >3–5× ULN or total bilirubin >1.5–3× ULN)	Withhold atezolizumab. Administer oral prednisone/prednisolone at a dose of 1 to 2 mg/kg/day or its equivalent. When improves to G1, begin a slow corticosteroid taper over at least 4 weeks. Resume atezolizumab upon symptom control, or when prednisone/prednisolone daily dose <10 mg
	G3/4 (AST or ALT >5× ULN or total bilirubin >3× ULN)	Permanently discontinue atezolizumab. Administer 1–2 mg/kg IV (methyl)prednisolone and convert to 0.5–2 mg/kg prednisone/prednisolone orally each day or its equivalent only after a response. Taper over at least 6 weeks when symptoms improve. If no response, add MMF 500–1000 mg twice daily. If worse on MMF, consider adding tacrolimus or ATG
Hypophysitis	G2/3 (moderate symptoms, ie, headache but no visual disturbance or fatigue/mood alteration but hemodynamically stable, no electrolyte disturbance)	Administer analgesia as needed for headache. Withhold atezolizumab. Administer oral prednisone/prednisolone at a dose of 0.5 to 2 mg/kg/day or its equivalent. When improves to G1, begin a slow corticosteroid taper over at least 4 weeks. If no improvement in 48 hours, administer 1–2 mg/kg IV (methyl)prednisolone and convert to 0.5–2 mg/kg prednisone/prednisolone orally each day or its equivalent only after a response. Taper over at least 4 weeks when symptoms improve to 5 mg prednisone/prednisolone or equivalent; do not stop steroids. Resume atezolizumab upon symptom control, or when prednisone/prednisolone daily dose <10 mg
	G4 (severe mass effect symptoms, ie, severe headache, any visual disturbance or severe hypoadrenalism, ie, hypotension, severe electrolyte disturbance)	Permanently discontinue atezolizumab. Administer analgesia as needed for headache. Administer 1–2 mg/kg IV (methyl)prednisolone and convert to 0.5–2 mg/kg prednisone/prednisolone orally each day or its equivalent only after a response. Taper over at least 4 weeks when symptoms improve to 5 mg prednisone/prednisolone or equivalent; do not stop steroids
Adrenal insufficiency	G2	Withhold atezolizumab. Administer oral prednisone/prednisolone at a dose of 0.5 to 2 mg/kg/day or its equivalent. When improves to G1, begin a slow corticosteroid taper over at least 4 weeks. Serially assess adrenal function and continue steroids at replacement doses (20–40 mg hydrocortisone daily ~2/3 dose in AM upon awakening and ~1/3 at 4 PM) until recovery of adrenal function is documented. Resume atezolizumab upon symptom control, or when prednisone/prednisolone daily dose <10 mg

(continued)

Treatment Modifications (*continued*)

Adverse Reaction	Grade/Severity	Dose Modification
	G3/4	Permanently discontinue atezolizumab. Administer oral prednisone/prednisolone at a dose of 0.5 to 2 mg/kg/day or its equivalent. When improves to G1, begin a slow corticosteroid taper over at least 4 weeks. Serially assess adrenal function and continue steroids at replacement doses (20–40 mg hydrocortisone daily ~2/3 dose in AM upon awakening and ~1/3 at 4 PM) until recovery of adrenal function is documented
Type 1 diabetes mellitus	G3 hyperglycemia	Withhold atezolizumab. Admit to hospital to manage hyperglycemia. Role of corticosteroids in preventing complete loss of insulin-producing cells is unknown and not recommended. Resume atezolizumab upon symptom control, or when prednisone/prednisolone daily dose <10 mg
	G4 hyperglycemia	Permanently discontinue atezolizumab. Admit to hospital to manage hyperglycemia. Role of corticosteroids in preventing complete loss of insulin-producing cells is unknown and not recommended
Nephritis and renal dysfunction	G2/3 (serum creatinine 1.5–6× ULN)	Withhold atezolizumab. Administer oral prednisone/prednisolone at a dose of 0.5 to 2 mg/kg/day or its equivalent. When improves to G1, begin a slow corticosteroid taper over at least 4 weeks. If does not respond adequately, then administer 0.5–1 mg/kg IV (methyl) prednisolone and convert to 0.5–2 mg/kg prednisone/prednisolone orally each day or its equivalent only after a response, followed by a taper over at least 4 weeks when improves to G1. Resume atezolizumab upon symptom control, or when prednisone/prednisolone daily dose <10 mg
	G4 (serum creatinine >6× ULN)	Permanently discontinue atezolizumab. Administer 0.5–1 mg/kg IV (methyl)prednisolone and convert to 0.5–2 mg/kg prednisone/prednisolone orally each day or its equivalent only after a response, followed by a taper over at least 4 weeks when improves to G1
Skin	G1/2	Continue atezolizumab. Avoid skin irritants, avoid sun exposure, topical emollients recommended. Topical steroid (mild strength for G1, moderate/potent strength for G2) cream once or twice daily ± oral or topical antihistamines for itching
	G3 rash or suspected SJS or TEN	Withhold atezolizumab. Avoid skin irritants, avoid sun exposure, topical emollients recommended. Administer oral or topical antihistamines for itching. Administer oral prednisone/prednisolone at a dose of 0.5–2 mg/kg or its equivalent daily for 3 days followed by a slow corticosteroid taper over at least 4 weeks when the rash improves to G1. If does not respond adequately, then administer 0.5 –1 mg/kg IV (methyl)prednisolone and convert to 0.5–2 mg/kg prednisone/prednisolone orally each day or its equivalent only after a response, followed by a taper over at least 4 weeks when the rash improves to G1. Resume atezolizumab upon symptom control, or when prednisone/prednisolone daily dose <10 mg
	G4 rash or confirmed SJS or TEN	Avoid skin irritants, avoid sun exposure, topical emollients recommended. Administer oral or topical antihistamines for itching. Administer 1–2 mg/kg IV (methyl)prednisolone and convert to oral steroids 0.5–2 mg/kg prednisone/prednisolone each day or its equivalent only after a response. Taper over at least 4 weeks when the rash improves to G1. Permanently discontinue atezolizumab
Encephalitis	Confusion or altered behavior, headaches, alteration in Glasgow Coma Scale, motor or sensory deficits, speech abnormality, may or may not be febrile	Initially withhold atezolizumab, but permanently discontinue atezolizumab if there is no doubt as to diagnosis. Exclude bacterial and ideally viral infections prior to high-dose steroids. Administer oral prednisone/prednisolone at a dose of 0.5–2 mg/kg/day or its equivalent. When symptoms improve, begin a slow corticosteroid taper over at least 4–8 weeks. If symptoms are severe, administer 1–2 mg/kg IV (methyl)prednisolone and convert to 0.5–2 mg/kg prednisone/prednisolone orally each day or its equivalent only after a response. Consider concurrent empiric antiviral (IV acyclovir) and antibacterial therapy
Aseptic meningitis	Headache, photophobia, neck stiffness with fever or may be afebrile, vomiting; normal cognition/cerebral function (distinguishes from encephalitis)	

(*continued*)

Treatment Modifications (*continued*)

Adverse Reaction	Grade/Severity	Dose Modification
Other syndromes include neurosarcoidosis, posterior reversible leukoencephalopathy syndrome (PRES), Vogt-Koyanagi-Harada syndrome, demyelination, vasculitic encephalopathy, and generalized seizures		
Transverse myelitis	Acute or subacute neurologic signs/symptoms of motor/sensory/autonomic origin; most have sensory level; often bilateral symptoms	Initially withhold atezolizumab, but permanently discontinue atezolizumab if there is no doubt as to diagnosis. Administer 2 mg/kg IV (methyl)prednisolone or consider 1 g/day and convert to 0.5–2 mg/kg prednisone/prednisolone orally each day or its equivalent only after a response. When symptoms improve, begin a slow corticosteroid taper over at least 4–8 weeks. Plasmapheresis may be required if steroids do not bring about improvement
Myocarditis	G3	Permanently discontinue atezolizumab. Administer 2 mg/kg IV (methyl)prednisolone or consider 1 g/day and convert to 0.5–2 mg/kg prednisone/prednisolone orally each day or its equivalent only after a response. When symptoms improve, begin a slow corticosteroid taper over at least 4–8 weeks. If no response, add MMF 500–1000 mg twice daily. If worse on MMF, consider adding tacrolimus
Peripheral neurologic toxicity	Moderate: some interference with ADL, symptoms concerning to patient	Withhold atezolizumab. Initial observation reasonable or initiate prednisone/prednisolone 0.5–1 mg/kg (if progressing, eg, from mild) and/or pregabalin or duloxetine for pain. When symptoms improve, begin a slow corticosteroid taper over at least 4 weeks. Resume atezolizumab upon symptom control, or when prednisone/prednisolone daily dose <10 mg
	Severe: limits self-care and aids warranted, life-threatening, eg, respiratory problems	Permanently discontinue atezolizumab. Administer 1–2 mg/kg IV (methyl)prednisolone and convert to 0.5–2 mg/kg prednisone/prednisolone orally each day or its equivalent only after a response. Taper over at least 4–8 weeks when symptoms improve to G1
Guillain-Barré syndrome	Progressive symmetrical muscle weakness with absent or reduced tendon reflexes—involves extremities; facial, respiratory, bulbar, and oculomotor muscles; dysregulation of autonomic nerves	Permanently discontinue atezolizumab. Use of steroids not recommended in idiopathic Guillain-Barré syndrome; however, a trial of (methyl)prednisolone 1–2 mg/kg is reasonable, converting to 0.5–2 mg/kg prednisone/prednisolone orally each day or its equivalent only after a response. If no improvement or worsening, plasmapheresis or IVIG indicated
Myasthenia gravis	Fluctuating muscle weakness (proximal limb, trunk, ocular, eg, ptosis/diplopia or bulbar) with fatigability; respiratory muscles also may be involved	Permanently discontinue atezolizumab. Administer pyridostigmine at an initial dose of 30 mg three times daily. Administer oral prednisone/prednisolone at a dose of 0.5 to 2 mg/kg/day or its equivalent or 1–2 mg/kg IV (methyl)prednisolone depending on the severity of symptoms. If begin with IV, convert to 0.5–2 mg/kg prednisone/prednisolone orally each day or its equivalent only after a response. If no improvement or worsening, plasmapheresis or IVIG may be considered. Additional immunosuppressants used in myasthenia gravis include azathioprine, cyclosporine, and mycophenolate. Avoid certain medications, eg, ciprofloxacin, beta-blockers, that may precipitate cholinergic crisis
Other syndromes including motor and sensory peripheral neuropathy, multifocal radicular neuropathy/plexopathy, autonomic neuropathy, phrenic nerve palsy, cranial nerve palsies (eg, facial nerve, optic nerve, hypoglossal nerve)		Permanently discontinue atezolizumab. Administer oral prednisone/prednisolone at a dose of 0.5 to 2 mg/kg/day or its equivalent or 1–2 mg/kg IV (methyl)prednisolone depending on the severity of symptoms. If begin with IV, convert to 0.5–2 mg/kg prednisone/prednisolone orally each day or its equivalent only after a response
Arthralgia	G1 (mild pain with inflammation, erythema, or joint swelling)	Continue atezolizumab. Administer acetaminophen (paracetamol) and ibuprofen
	G2 (moderate pain with inflammation, erythema, or joint swelling that limits ADLs)	Withhold atezolizumab. Administer higher doses of acetaminophen (paracetamol) and ibuprofen and use diclofenac or naproxen or etoricoxib. If inadequately controlled, consider intra-articular steroid injections for large joints or administer oral prednisone/prednisolone at a dose of 0.5 to 2 mg/kg/day or its equivalent. When improves to G1, begin a slow corticosteroid taper over at least 4 weeks. If does not respond adequately, then administer 0.5–1 mg/kg IV (methyl)prednisolone and convert to 0.5–2 mg/kg prednisone/prednisolone orally each day or its equivalent only after a response, followed by a taper over at least 4 weeks when improves to G1. Resume atezolizumab upon symptom control, or when prednisone/prednisolone daily dose <10 mg

(*continued*)

Treatment Modifications (*continued*)

Adverse Reaction	Grade/Severity	Dose Modification
	G3 (severe pain; irreversible joint damage; disabling; limits self-care ADL)	Withhold atezolizumab. Administer 0.5–1 mg/kg IV (methyl)prednisolone and convert to 0.5–2 mg/kg prednisone/prednisolone orally each day or its equivalent only after a response, followed by a taper over at least 4 weeks when improves to G1. In severe cases, infliximab or another anti–TNF-alpha drug may be required for improvement of arthritis. Resume atezolizumab upon symptom control, or when prednisone/prednisolone daily dose <10 mg
Other	First occurrence of other G3	Withhold atezolizumab. Administer oral prednisone/prednisolone at a dose of 0.5 to 2 mg/kg/day or its equivalent. When improves to G1, begin a slow corticosteroid taper over at least 4 weeks. Resume atezolizumab upon symptom control, or when prednisone/prednisolone daily dose <10 mg
	Recurrence of same G3	Permanently discontinue atezolizumab. Administer 1–2 mg/kg IV (methyl)prednisolone and convert to 0.5–2 mg/kg prednisone/prednisolone orally each day or its equivalent only after a response. Taper over at least 4–8 weeks when symptoms improve to G1
	Life-threatening or G4	
	Requirement for ≥10 mg/day prednisone or equivalent for >12 weeks	Permanently discontinue atezolizumab
	Persistent G2/3 adverse reactions lasting ≥12 weeks	

ADL, activities of daily living; ALT, alanine aminotransferase; AST, aspartate aminotransferase; ATG, anti-thymocyte globulin; SJS, Stevens-Johnson Syndrome; TEN, toxic epidermal necrolysis; ULN, upper limit of normal

Notes on general supportive care:
- Steroid taper in most cases will proceed over a minimum of 1 month but if symptoms improve rapidly, a 2-week taper can be considered. If steroids are administered for more than 4 weeks, consider PCP prophylaxis (cotrimoxazole 480 mg twice daily M/W/F or inhaled pentamidine if has cotrimoxazole allergy), regular random blood glucose, VitD level, and starting calcium/VitD supplementation per guidelines

BEVACIZUMAB DOSE MODIFICATIONS

Adverse Event	Treatment Modification
Gastrointestinal perforations (gastrointestinal perforations, fistula formation in the gastrointestinal tract, intra-abdominal abscess), fistula formation involving an internal organ	Discontinue bevacizumab permanently
Serious bleeding	
Wound dehiscence requiring medical intervention	
Nephrotic syndrome	
Hypertensive crisis or hypertensive encephalopathy or reversible posterior leukoencephalopathy syndrome (RPLS)	
Congestive heart failure	
Necrotizing fasciitis	
Severe arterial or venous thromboembolic events	Discontinue bevacizumab permanently; the safety of reinitiating bevacizumab after a thromboembolic event is resolved is not known
Moderate to severe proteinuria	Patients with a ≥2+ dipstick reading should undergo further assessment, eg, 24-hour urine collection. Suspend bevacizumab administration for ≥2 g proteinuria/24 h and resume when proteinuria is <2 g/24 h
Severe hypertension not controlled with medical management	Hold bevacizumab pending further evaluation and treatment of hypertension
Mild, clinically insignificant infusion reaction	Decrease the rate of infusion

(*continued*)

Treatment Modifications (*continued*)

Adverse Event	Treatment Modification
Clinically significant but not severe infusion reaction	Interrupt the infusion and consider resuming at a slower rate following resolution. If decision is made to restart, the infusion may be continued at ≤50% of the rate prior to the reaction and increased in 50% increments every 30 minutes if well tolerated. Infusions may be restarted at the full rate during the next cycle
Severe infusion reaction (hypertension, hypertensive crises associated with neurologic signs and symptoms, wheezing, oxygen desaturation, G3 hypersensitivity, chest pain, headaches, rigors, and diaphoresis)	Stop infusion and administer appropriate medical therapy (eg, epinephrine, corticosteroids, intravenous antihistamines, bronchodilators, and/or oxygen). Discontinue bevacizumab
Planned elective surgery	Suspend bevacizumab at least 28 days before elective surgery and do not resume for at least 28 days after surgery or until surgical incision is fully healed
Recent hemoptysis	Do not administer bevacizumab
Evidence of rectosigmoid involvement by pelvic examination or bowel involvement on CT scan or clinical symptoms of bowel obstruction	

Patient Population Studied

IMbrave 150 was a phase 3 randomized, controlled study involving 501 patients with locally advanced metastatic or unresectable hepatocellular carcinoma (or both). Eligible patients had not previously received systemic therapy for liver cancer and had measurable disease that was not amenable to curative or locoregional therapies or that had progressed thereafter. Among key exclusion criteria were a history of autoimmune disease, coinfection with hepatitis B or hepatitis C virus, and untreated or incompletely treated esophageal or gastric varices (assessed with esophagogastroduodenoscopy and treated according to local clinical practice) with bleeding or high risk of bleeding.

Patients were randomly assigned 2:1 to receive the combination of atezolizumab plus bevacizumab or to receive sorafenib

Patient Characteristics at Baseline*		
Variable	Atezolizumab-Bevacizumab (n = 336)	Sorafenib (n = 165)
Median age (IQR)—years	64 (56–71)	66 (59–71)
Male sex—no. (%) 277 (82) 137 (83)		
Geographic region—no. (%)		
Asia, excluding Japan	133 (40)	68 (41)
Rest of the world[†]	203 (60)	97 (59)
ECOG performance status score—no. (%)[‡]		
0	209 (62)	103 (62)
1	127 (38)	62 (38)
Child-Pugh classification—no./total no. (%)[§]		
A5	239/333 (72)	121/165 (73)
A6	94/333 (28)	44/165 (27)
Barcelona Clinic liver cancer stage—no. (%)[€]		
A	8 (2)	6 (4)
B	52 (15)	26 (16)
C	276 (82)	133 (81)

(*continued*)

Patient Population Studied (continued)

Patient Characteristics at Baseline*

Variable	Atezolizumab-Bevacizumab (n = 336)	Sorafenib (n = 165)
Alpha-fetoprotein ≥400 ng/mL—no. (%) 126 (38) 61 (37)		
Presence of macrovascular invasion, extrahepatic spread, or both—no. (%)	258 (77)	120 (73)
Macrovascular invasion	129 (38)	71 (43)
Extrahepatic spread	212 (63)	93 (56)
Varices—no. (%)		
Present at baseline	88 (26)	43 (26)
Treated at baseline	36 (11)	23 (14)
Cause of hepatocellular carcinoma—no. (%)		
Hepatitis B	164 (49)	76 (46)
Hepatitis C	72 (21)	36 (22)
Nonviral		100 (30)	53 (32)
Prior local therapy for hepatocellular carcinoma—no. (%)	161 (48)	85 (52)

Efficacy

Primary Efficacy Outcomes

	Atezolizumab + Bevacizumab (N = 326)	Sorafenib (N = 158)	
Survival at 6 months	84.8% (95% CI, 80.9–88.7)	72.2% (95% CI, 65.1–79.4)	—
Survival at 12 months	67.2% (95% CI, 61.3–73.1)	54.6% (95% CI, 45.2–64.0)	—
Deaths	96 (28.6%)	65 (39.4%)	HR, 0.58; 95% CI 0.42 to 0.79; P <0.001
Disease progression or death	197 (58.6%)	109 (66.1%)	—
Median PFS (months)	6.8 (95% CI, 5.7–8.3)	4.3 (95% CI, 4.0–5.6)	Stratified HR for progression or death, 0.59; 95% CI, 0.47 to 0.76; P <0.001
PFS at 6 months	54.5%	37.2%	

Secondary Efficacy Outcomes*

Variable	RECIST 1.1			HCC-Specific mRECIST		
	Atezolizumab + Bevacizumab (N = 326)	Sorafenib (N = 159)	Difference (P Value)†	Atezolizumab + Bevacizumab (N = 32)	Sorafenib (N = 158)	Difference (P Value)†
Confirmed objective response—no. (% [95% CI])‡	89 (27.3 [22.5–32.5])	19 (11.9 [7.4–18.0])	15.4 (<0.001)	108 (33.2 [28.1–38.6])	21 (13.3 [8.4–19.6])	19.9 (<0.001)
Complete response—no. (%)	18 (5.5)	0	—	33 (10.2)	3 (1.9)	—
Partial response—no. (%)	71 (21.8)	19 (11.9)		75 (23.1)	18 (11.4)	

(continued)

Efficacy (continued)

Variable	RECIST 1.1			HCC-Specific mRECIST		
	Atezolizumab + Bevacizumab (N = 326)	Sorafenib (N = 159)	Difference (P Value)[†]	Atezolizumab + Bevacizumab (N = 32)	Sorafenib (N = 158)	Difference (P Value)[†]
Stable disease—no. (%)	151 (46.3)	69 (43.4)		127 (39.1)	66 (41.8)	
Disease control rate—no. (%)[#]	240 (73.6)	88 (55.3)		235 (72.3)	87 (55.1)	
Progressive disease—no. (%)	64 (19.6)	39 (24.5)		66 (20.3)	40 (25.3)	
Could not be evaluated—no. (%)	8 (2.5)	14 (8.8)		10 (3.1)	14 (8.9)	
Data missing—no. (%)	14 (4.3)	18 (11.3)		14 (4.3)	17 (10.8)	
Ongoing objective response at data cutoff—no./total no. (%)	77/89 (86.5)	13/19 (68.4)		84/108 (77.8)	13/21 (61.9)	

OS, overall survival; PFS, progression-free survival; HR, hazard ratio; CI, confidence interval

*Included are patients who presented with measurable disease according to the Response Evaluation Criteria in Solid Tumors, version 1.1 (RECIST 1.1), and according to hepatocellular carcinoma (HCC)-specific modified RECIST (mRECIST), as assessed at an independent review facility. CI denotes confidence interval

[†]The difference is the between-group difference (atezolizumab-bevacizumab minus sorafenib) in the percentage of patients with confirmed response, expressed in percentage points. The P Value was derived from a Cochran-Mantel-Haenszel test. Randomization, which was performed through an interactive voice-response or Web-response system, included as stratification factors geographic region (Asia excluding Japan vs the rest of the world), alpha-fetoprotein level (<400 ng/mL vs ≥400 ng/mL) at baseline, and macrovascular invasion, extrahepatic spread, or both (yes vs no)

[‡]Confirmed objective response was defined as a response (complete or partial) seen at two consecutive tumor assessments at least 28 days apart

[§]The control rate is the sum of complete response, partial response, and stable disease

Adverse Events

Adverse Events from Any Cause

Variable	Atezolizumab + Bevacizumab (N = 329)	Sorafenib (N = 156)
	Number (%)	
Patients with an adverse event from any cause	323 (98.2)	154 (98.7)
Grade 3 or 4 event*	186 (56.5)	86 (55.1)
Grade 5 event[†]	15 (4.6)	9 (5.8)
Serious adverse event	125 (38.0)	48 (30.8)
Adverse event leading to withdrawal from any trial drug	51 (15.5)	16 (10.3)
Withdrawal from atezolizumab-bevacizumab	23 (7.0)	—
Adverse event leading to dose modification or interruption of any trial drug	163 (49.5)	95 (60.9)
Dose interruption of any trial treatment	163 (49.5)	64 (41.0)
Dose modification of sorafenib	—	58 (37.2)

*Numbers represent the highest grades assigned

[†]Grade 5 events in the atezolizumab-bevacizumab group included gastrointestinal hemorrhage (in 3 patients), pneumonia (in 2 patients), empyema, gastric ulcer perforation, abnormal hepatic function, liver injury, multiple-organ dysfunction syndrome, esophageal varices hemorrhage, subarachnoid hemorrhage, respiratory distress, sepsis, and cardiac arrest (in 1 patient each); Grade 5 events in the sorafenib group included death (in 2 patients), hepatic cirrhosis (in 2 patients), cardiac arrest, cardiac failure, general physical health deterioration, hepatitis E, and peritoneal hemorrhage (in 1 patient each)

Therapy Monitoring

Bevacizumab:

1. Observe closely for hypersensitivity reactions, especially during the first and second bevacizumab infusions
2. Vital signs (including blood pressure measurement) prior to each cycle or more frequently as indicated during treatment
3. Assess proteinuria by urine dipstick and/or urinary protein creatinine ratio prior to each cycle. Patients with a ≥2+ urine dipstick reading should undergo further assessment with a 24-hour urine collection

Atezolizumab:

1. Initially at the time of each atezolizumab dose, and eventually every 6–12 weeks, perform a total-body skin examination with attention to *all* mucous membranes as well as a complete review of systems
2. Monitor patients for signs and symptoms of pneumonitis. Evaluate patients with suspected pneumonitis with chest x-ray, CT, and pulse oximetry. For ≥2 toxicity, may include nasal swab, sputum culture and sensitivity, blood culture and sensitivity, and urine culture and sensitivity

(continued)

(continued)

Therapy Monitoring
(continued)

3. Monitor patients for signs and symptoms of colitis. Encourage patients to report diarrhea immediately to any member of the health care team

4. Draw AST, ALT, and bilirubin prior to each atezolizumab infusion and/or weekly if there are Grade 1 liver function test elevations. Note, no intervention is recommended for G1 LFT abnormalities. For ≥2 toxicity, work up for other causes of elevated LFTs including viral hepatitis

5. Use basic metabolic panel (Na, K, CO$_2$, glucose) and patient history as screening tools for hypophysitis including hypopituitarism and adrenal insufficiency. If in doubt, evaluate AM adrenocorticotropic hormone (ACTH) and cortisol levels. Consider ACTH stimulation test for indeterminate results

6. Assess thyroid function at the start of treatment, periodically during atezolizumab treatment, and as indicated based on clinical evaluation, and for clinical signs and symptoms of thyroid disorders. Test for TSH and free thyroxine (FT4) every 4 to 6 weeks as part of routine clinical monitoring of therapy or for case detection in symptomatic patients

7. Measure glucose at baseline and with each atezolizumab treatment during the first 12 weeks and every 6 weeks thereafter

8. Obtain a serum creatinine prior to every atezolizumab dose. If creatinine is found to be newly elevated, consider holding therapy while other potential causes are evaluated. Note, routine urinalysis is not necessary other than to rule out urinary tract infections, etc.

9. Obtain a complete rheumatologic history and perform an examination of all peripheral joints for tenderness, swelling, and range of motion. Examine the spine. Consider plain x-ray/imaging to exclude metastases and evaluate joint damage (erosions), if appropriate

10. In patients at high risk for infections and in appropriately selected patients based on an infectious disease evaluation, draw screening laboratories (HIV, hepatitis A and B, and blood QuantiFERON for TB) to prepare patients to start infliximab

Adverse Events (continued)

Adverse Events with an Incidence of More Than 10% in Either Group

Event	Sorafenib (N = 156)		Atezolizumab + Bevacizumab (N = 329)	
	Any Grade	Grade 3/4	Any Grade	Grade 3/4
	Number (%)			
Hypertension	98 (29.8)	50 (15.2)	38 (24.4)	19 (12.2)
Fatigue	67 (20.4)	8 (2.4)	29 (18.6)	5 (3.2)
Proteinuria	66 (20.1)	10 (3.0)	11 (7.1)	1 (0.6)
Aspartate aminotransferase increase	64 (19.5)	23 (7.0)	26 (16.7)	8 (5.1)
Pruritus	64 (19.5)	0	15 (9.6)	0
Diarrhea	62 (18.8)	6 (1.8)	77 (49.4)	8 (5.1)
Decreased appetite	58 (17.6)	4 (1.2)	38 (24.4)	6 (3.8)
Pyrexia	59 (17.9)	4 (1.2)	15 (9.6)	2 (1.3)
Alanine aminotransferase increase	46 (14.0)	12 (3.6)	14 (9.0)	2 (1.3)
Constipation	44 (13.4)	0	22 (14.1)	0
Blood bilirubin increase	43 (13.1)	8 (2.4)	22 (14.1)	10 (6.4)
Rash	41 (12.5)	0	27 (17.3)	4 (2.6)
Abdominal pain	40 (12.2)	4 (1.2)	27 (17.3)	4 (2.6)
Nausea	40 (12.2)	1 (0.3)	25 (16.0)	1 (0.6)
Cough	39 (11.9)	0	15 (9.6)	1 (0.6)
Infusion-related reaction	37 (11.2)	8 (2.4)	0	0
Weight decrease	37 (11.2)	0	15 (9.6)	1 (0.6)
Platelet count decrease	35 (10.6)	11 (3.3)	18 (11.5)	2 (1.3)
Epistaxis	34 (10.3)	0	7 (4.5)	1 (0.6)
Asthenia	22 (6.7)	1 (0.3)	21 (13.5)	4 (2.6)
Alopecia	4 (1.2)	0	22 (14.1)	0
PPES	3 (0.9)	0	75 (48.1)	13 (8.3)

PPES, palmar-plantar erythrodysesthesia syndrome

UNRESECTABLE DISEASE • FIRST-LINE
HEPATOCELLULAR CARCINOMA REGIMEN: SORAFENIB

Cheng A-L et al. Lancet Oncol 2009;10:25–34
Llovet JM et al. N Engl J Med 2008;359:378–390

Sorafenib 400 mg per dose (2 × 200 mg); administer orally, twice daily, continually (total dose/week = 5600 mg)

Supportive Care
Antiemetic prophylaxis
Emetogenic potential: **LOW**
See Chapter 42 for antiemetic recommendations

Hematopoietic growth factor (CSF) prophylaxis
Primary prophylaxis is **NOT** *indicated*
See Chapter 43 for more information

Antimicrobial prophylaxis
Risk of fever and neutropenia is **LOW**
Antimicrobial primary prophylaxis to be considered:
- Antibacterial—not indicated
- Antifungal—not indicated
- Antiviral—not indicated, unless patient previously had an episode of HSV

Diarrhea management
Latent or delayed-onset diarrhea*:
   Loperamide 4 mg orally initially after the first loose or liquid stool, *then* 2–4 mg orally every 2–4 hours or **diphenoxylate hydrochloride** 2.5 mg with **atropine sulfate** 0.025 mg (eg, Lomotil)

*Abigerges D et al. J Natl Cancer Inst 1994;86:446–449
Rothenberg ML et al. J Clin Oncol 2001;19:3801–3807
Wadler S et al. J Clin Oncol 1998;16:3169–3178

Dose Modifications

Dose Levels	
Starting dose level	400 mg twice per day
Dose level −1	400 mg daily or 200 mg twice per day
Dose level −2	200 mg daily or 400 mg every other day

Adverse Event	Dose Modification
Cardiovascular toxicity	
G ≥2 cardiac ischemia and/or infarction	Permanently discontinue sorafenib
G3 congestive heart failure	Interrupt until G ≤1; resume treatment with dose decrease one dose level. If no recovery after 30-day interruption, discontinue treatment unless the patient is deriving clinical benefit. If two dose reductions are insufficient, discontinue treatment
G4 congestive heart failure	Permanently discontinue
G 2 hemorrhage requiring medical intervention	Permanently discontinue sorafenib
G2 hypertension (asymptomatic and diastolic pressure 90–99 mm Hg)	Treat with antihypertensive therapy. Continue dosing as scheduled and closely monitor blood pressure

(*continued*)

Dose Modifications (continued)

Adverse Event	Dose Modification
G2 hypertension (symptomatic/persistent) *or* G2 symptomatic increase by >20 mm Hg (diastolic) or >140/90 mm Hg if previously within normal limits *or* G3	Interrupt treatment and treat with antihypertensives until symptoms resolve and diastolic blood pressure <90 mm Hg. When resuming treatment, reduce dose one dose level. If needed, reduce another dose level. If two dose reductions are insufficient, discontinue treatment
G4 hypertension	Permanently discontinue sorafenib
Any grade gastrointestinal perforation	Permanently discontinue sorafenib
QT prolongation: QTc >500 ms or an increase from baseline of 60 ms	Interrupt. Correct electrolyte abnormalities (magnesium, potassium, calcium). Monitor electrolytes and electrocardiograms. Use medical judgement before restarting
Hepatic Toxicity	
Severe drug-induced liver injury: >G3 ALT in the absence of another cause; AST/ALT >3× ULN with bilirubin >2× ULN in the absence of another cause	Permanently discontinue sorafenib
Any grade alkaline phosphatase increase in the absence of known bone pathology and G ≥2 or worse bilirubin increase	
INR ≥1.5, ascites, and/or encephalopathy in the absence of underlying cirrhosis or other organ failure considered to be due to severe drug-induced liver	
Nonhematologic toxicity	
G2 nonhematologic toxicity	Treat on time. Decrease dose one dose level. If two dose reductions are insufficient, discontinue treatment
First occurrence G3 nonhematologic toxicity	Interrupt until G ≤2, then resume with dose decreased one dose level. If two dose reductions are insufficient, discontinue treatment
G3 nonhematologic toxicity without improvement within 7 days	Interrupt until G ≤2, then resume with dose decreased two dose levels. If two dose reductions are insufficient, discontinue treatment
Second or third occurrence of G3 nonhematologic toxicity	Interrupt until G ≤2, then resume with dose decreased two dose levels. If two dose reductions are insufficient, discontinue treatment
Fourth occurrence of G3 nonhematologic toxicity or G4 nonhematologic toxicity	Permanently discontinue sorafenib
Dermatologic toxicity	
First occurrence of G2 dermatologic toxicity (painful erythema and swelling of the hands or feet and/or discomfort affecting the patient's normal activities)	Continue treatment with sorafenib and consider topical therapy for symptomatic relief. If no improvement within 7 days, interrupt sorafenib treatment until toxicity resolves to G0/1
First occurrence of G2 dermatologic toxicity (painful erythema and swelling of the hands or feet and/or discomfort affecting the patient's normal activities) without improvement within 7 days at the reduced dose	Interrupt sorafenib treatment until toxicity resolves to G0/1. Then resume treatment with the sorafenib dose decreased by one dose level (400 mg daily or 400 mg every other day)
Second and third occurrence of G2 dermatologic toxicity (painful erythema and swelling of the hands or feet and/or discomfort affecting the patient's normal activities)	
Fourth occurrence of G2 dermatologic toxicity	Discontinue sorafenib treatment
First occurrence of G3 dermatologic toxicity (moist desquamation, ulceration, blistering, or severe pain of the hands or feet, resulting in inability to work or perform activities of daily living)	Interrupt sorafenib treatment until toxicity resolves to G0/1. Then resume treatment with the sorafenib dose decreased by one dose level (400 mg daily or 400 mg every other day)

(continued)

Dose Modifications (*continued*)

Adverse Event	Dose Modification
Second occurrence of G3 dermatologic toxicity (moist desquamation, ulceration, blistering, or severe pain of the hands or feet, resulting in inability to work or perform activities of daily living)	Interrupt sorafenib treatment until toxicity resolves to G0/1. Then resume treatment with the sorafenib dose decreased by one dose level
Third occurrence of G3 dermatologic toxicity	Discontinue sorafenib treatment

Note on dermatologic toxicity: Following improvement of G2/3 dermatologic toxicity to G0/1 after at least 28 days of treatment on a reduced dose of sorafenib, the dose of sorafenib may be increased one dose level from the reduced dose. Approximately 50% of patients requiring a dose reduction for dermatologic toxicity are expected to meet these criteria for resumption of the higher dose, and roughly 50% of patients resuming the previous dose are expected to tolerate the higher dose (that is, maintain the higher dose level without recurrent G2 or higher dermatologic toxicity)

Patient Population Studied

Llovet JM et al. N Engl J Med 2008; 359:378–390

Multicenter, phase 3, double-blind, placebo-controlled trial. In all, 602 patients with advanced hepatocellular carcinoma who had not previously received systemic treatment were randomly assigned to receive either sorafenib (n = 299) or placebo (n = 303). The study population consisted of patients with advanced-stage hepatocellular carcinoma. Patients were classified as having advanced disease if they were not eligible or had disease progression after surgical or locoregional therapies. Eligibility criteria also included (1) Eastern Cooperative Oncology Group performance status score ≤2; (2) Child-Pugh liver function class A; (3) prothrombin time international normalized ratio ≤2.3 or prothrombin time ≤6 s greater than control; (4) albumin ≥2.8 g/dL; (5) total bilirubin ≤3 mg/dL (≤51.3 μmol/L); and (6) alanine aminotransferase and aspartate aminotransferase ≤5 times the upper limit of normal

Cheng A-L et al. Lancet Oncol 2009;10:25–34

Patients with advanced (unresectable or metastatic) hepatocellular carcinoma who had not received previous systemic therapy were eligible for this trial. Eligibility criteria also included ECOG PS of 0/1/2; Child-Pugh liver function class A; and a life expectancy ≥12 weeks; albumin concentration of at least 28 g/L; total bilirubin concentration of 51.3 μmol/L or less; alanine aminotransferase concentration of ≤5 times the upper limit of normal. Patients who had received previous local therapy, such as surgery, radiotherapy, hepatic arterial embolization, chemoembolization, radiofrequency ablation, percutaneous injection, or cryoablation, were eligible for enrollment in the study, provided that either the target lesion increased in size by 25% or more, or the target lesion had not been treated with local therapy. Furthermore, the local therapy must have been stopped at least 4 weeks before study entry. Patients with recurrent disease after previous resection were considered eligible for the study. Exclusion criteria included previous or concomitant systemic therapy (including new, molecularly targeted therapies)

Demographic and Baseline Characteristics of the Patients (Intention-to-Treat Population)*

Loved JM et al. N Engl J Med 2008; 359:378–390

Variable	Sorafenib (N = 299)	Placebo (N = 303)
Age, years	64.9 ± 11.2	66.3 ± 10.2
Sex, no. (%) male/female	260 (87)/39 (13)	264 (87)/39 (13)
Region, no. (%)		
Europe and Australasia	263 (88)	263 (87)
North America	27 (9)	29 (10)
Central and South America	9 (3)	11 (4)
Cause of disease, no. (%)		
Hepatitis C only	87 (29)	82 (27)
Alcohol only	79 (26)	80 (26)
Hepatitis B only	56 (19)	55 (18)

(*continued*)

Patient Population Studied (*continued*)

Variable	Sorafenib (N = 299)	Placebo (N = 303)
Unknown	49 (16)	56 (19)
Other	28 (9)	29 (10)
ECOG performance status, 0/1/2 no. (%)	161(54)/114(38)/24(8)	164(54)/117(39)/22(7)
BCLC stage, B (intermediate)/C (advanced) no. (%)	54(18)/244(82)[‡]	51(17)/252(83)
Macroscopic vascular invasion, no. (%)	108 (36)	123 (41)
Extrahepatic spread, no. (%)	159 (53)	150 (50)
Lymph nodes, no. (%)	89 (30)	65 (21)
Lung, no. (%)	67 (22)	58 (19)
Macroscopic vascular invasion, extrahepatic spread, or both, absent/present, no. (%)	90 (30)/209 (70)	91 (30)/212 (70)
Child-Pugh class, A/B, no. (%)	284 (95)/14 (5)	297 (98)/6 (2)
Biochemical analysis		
Albumin, g/dL, median (range)	3.9 (2.7–5.3)	4.0 (2.5–5.1)
Total bilirubin, mg/dL, median (range)[†]	07. (0.1–16.4)	0.7 (0.2–6.1)
Alpha-fetoprotein, ng/mL—median (range)	44.3 ($0–208 \times 10^4$)	99.0 ($0–5 \times 10^5$)
Previous therapy, no. (%)[§]		
Surgical resection	57 (19)	62 (20)
Locoregional therapy		
Trans-arterial chemoembolization	86 (29)	90 (30)
Percutaneous ethanol injection	28 (9)	20 (7)
Radiofrequency ablation	17 (6)	12 (4)
Radiotherapy	13 (4)	15 (5)
Systemic anticancer therapy		
Hormonal therapy	7 (2)	8 (3)
Cytotoxic chemotherapy	1 (<1)	1 (<1)
Concomitant systemic antiviral therapy, no. (%)	6 (2)	2 (1)

*Plus–minus values are means ± SD. None of the differences between the two study groups was significant (P ≥0.05)

[†]To convert the values for bilirubin to micromoles per liter, multiply by 17.1

[‡]One patient in the sorafenib group had a BCLC score of D and a Child-Pugh class of C

[§]Patients may have received more than one type of therapy. There was no significant difference between groups in the number of patients who had received previous palliative or curative therapy or previous adjuvant or neoadjuvant therapy (P ≥0.05)

[¶]Radiotherapy was applied to extrahepatic metastatic lesions in all patients except five in the sorafenib group and three in the placebo group

Efficacy

Llovet JM et al. N Engl J Med 2008;359:378–390

Outcome	Sorafenib	Placebo	HR/P Value
Median overall survival, months (95% CI)	10.7 months (9.4–13.3)	7.9 months (6.8–9.1)	0.69 (0.55–0.87) <0.001
1-year survival rate	44%	33%	0.009
Time to symptomatic progression*, median (95% CI)	4.1 months (3.5–4.8)	4.9 months (4.2–6.3)	1.08 (0.88–1.31) 0.77
Time to radiologic progression, median (95% CI)	5.5 months (4.1–6.9)	2.8 months (2.7–3.9)	0.58 (0.45–0.74) <0.001
Level of Response[†]			
Complete response	0	0	NA
Partial response	2%	1%	0.05
Stable disease	71%	67%	0.17
Disease control rate[‡]	43%	32%	0

*Symptomatic progression was defined as a decrease of 4 or more points from the baseline score on the Functional Assessment of Cancer Therapy–Hepatobiliary Symptom Index 8 (FHSI8), deterioration to a score of 4 in Eastern Cooperative Group performance status, or death, whichever occurred first
[†]Response was measured according to RECIST
[‡]Percentage of patients with CR/PR/SD according to RECIST maintained for 28 days

Cheng A-L et al. Lancet Oncol 2009;10:25–34

	Sorafenib Group (n = 150)	Placebo Group (n = 76)
Complete response	0 (0)	0 (0)
Partial response	5 (3.3)	1 (1.3)
Stable disease	81 (54.0)	21 (27.6)
Progressive disease	46 (30.7)	41 (54.0)
Not assessable	18 (12.0)	13 (17.1)
DCR*, n (%; 95% CI)	53 (35.3; 27.7–43.6)	12 (15.8; 8.4–26.0)
Median overall survival	6.5 months (95% CI, 5.56–7.56)	4.2 months (95% CI, 3.75–5.46)
	HR 0.68 (95% CI, 0.50–0.93); P = 0.014	
6-month overall survival	53.3%	36.7%
Median time to progression	2.8 months (95% CI, 2.63–3.58)	1.4 months (95% CI, 1.35–1.55)
	HR 0.57 (95% CI, 0.42–0.79); P = 0.0005	
TTSP as assessed by the FHSI–8[†]	3.5 months (95% CI, 2.80–4.24)	3.4 months (95% CI, 2.40–4.08)
	HR 0.90 (95% CI 0.67–1.22); P = 0.50	

*DCR (disease control rate) = proportion of patients who had the best response of complete response, partial response, or stable disease, maintained ≥4 weeks
[†]Time to symptomatic progression was defined as deterioration to ECOG PS 4 status or a change from baseline score on the 8-item, symptom-focused Functional Assessment of Cancer Therapy–Hepatobiliary Symptom Index (FHSI–8) questionnaire, associated with a deterioration of symptoms

Toxicity

Incidence of Drug-Related Adverse Events (Safety Population)*

Llovet JM et al. N Engl J Med 2008;359:378–390

Adverse Event	Sorafenib (n = 297)			Placebo (n = 302)			P Value	
	Any G	G3	G4	Any G	G3	G4	Any G	G3/4
	Percentage							
Overall incidence	80			52				
Constitutional symptoms								
Fatigue	22	3	1	'6	3	<1	0.07	1.00
Weight loss	9	2	0	1	0	0	<0.001	0.03
Dermatologic events								
Alopecia	14	0	0	2	0	0	<0.001	NA
Dry skin	8	0	0	4	0	0	0.04	NA
Hand–foot skin reaction	21	8	0	3	<1	0	<0.001	<0.001
Pruritus	8	0	0	7	<1	0	0.65	1.0
Rash or desquamation	16	1	0	11	0	0	0.12	0.12
Other	5	1	0	1	0	0	<0.001	0.12
Gastrointestinal events								
Anorexia	14	<1	0	3	1	0	<0.001	1.00
Diarrhea	39	8	0	11	2	0	<0.001	<0.001
Nausea	11	<1	0	8	1	0	0.16	0.62
Vomiting	5	1	0	3	1	0	0.14	0.68
Voice changes	6	0	0	1	0	0	<0.001	NA
Hypertension	5	2	0	2	1	0	0.05	0.28
Liver dysfunction	<1	<1	0	0	0	0	0.50	0.50
Abdominal pain not otherwise specified	8	2	0	3	1	0	0.007	0.17
Bleeding	7	1	0	4	1	<1	0.07	1.00

	Sorafenib (n = 297)	Placebo (n = 302)
Rate of discontinuation	38%	37%
Dose reductions due to adverse events‡	26%	7%
Dose interruptions due to adverse events	44%	30%

NA, not applicable

*Listed are adverse events, as defined by the National Cancer Institute Common Terminology Criteria (version 3.0), that occurred in at least 5% of patients in either study group

†The most frequent adverse events leading to discontinuation of sorafenib were gastrointestinal events (6%), fatigue (5%), and liver dysfunction (5%). Drug-related adverse events leading to permanent treatment discontinuation occurred in 34 patients in the sorafenib group (11%) and 15 patients in the placebo group (5%)

‡The most frequent adverse events leading to dose reductions of sorafenib were diarrhea (8%), hand-foot skin reaction (5%), and rash or desquamation (3%)

Toxicity (*continued*)

Drug-related Adverse Events, Dose Reductions, and Discontinuations

Cheng A-L et al. Lancet Oncol 2009;10:25–34

	Sorafenib Group (n = 149)		Placebo Group (n = 75)	
	All	Grade 3/4	All	Grade 3/4
Drug-related, n (%)*				
HFSR	67 (45.0)	16 (10.7)	2 (2.7)	0 (0)
Diarrhea	38 (25.5)	9 (6.0)	4 (5.3)	0 (0)
Alopecia	37 (24.8)	—	1 (1.3)	—
Fatigue	30 (20.1)	5 (3.4)	6 (8.0)	1 (1.3)
Rash/desquamation	30 (20.1)	1 (0.7)	5 (6.7)	0 (0)
Hypertension	28 (18.8)	3 (2.0)	1 (1.3)	0 (0)
Anorexia	19 (12.8)	0 (0)	2 (2.7)	0 (0)
Nausea	17 (11.4)	1 (0.7)	8 (10.7)	1 (1.3)
Dose reduction, n (%)†	46 (30.9)		2 (2.7)	
HFSR	17 (11.4)	—	0 (0)	—
Diarrhea	11 (7.4)	—	0 (0)	—
Discontinuation, n (%)‡	29 (19.5)		10 (13.3)	
Hemorrhage, upper GI	4 (2.7)	—	3 (4.0)	—
Ascites	4 (2.7)	—	2 (2.7)	—
Fatigue	4 (2.7)	—	0 (0)	—
Liver dysfunction	1 (0.7)	—	2 (2.7)	

HFSR, hand-foot skin reaction; GI, gastrointestinal tract
*Drug-related adverse events in ≥10% of patients in any study group
†Adverse events causing dose reduction ≥5% of patients in any study group
‡Adverse events causing discontinuation ≥2.5% of patients in any study group

Therapy Monitoring

At screening and every 6 weeks: Tumor measurements by computed tomography or magnetic resonance imaging

UNRESECTABLE DISEASE • FIRST-LINE
HEPATOCELLULAR CARCINOMA REGIMEN: LENVATINIB

Kudo M et al. Lancet Oncol 2018;391:1163–1173
Supplementary appendix to: Kudo M et al. Lancet Oncol 2018;391:1163–1173

LENVIMA (lenvatinib) prescribing information. Woodcliff Lake, NJ: Eisai Inc; revised February 2020

For patients with actual body weight ≥60 kg:
Lenvatinib 12 mg per dose; administer orally once daily, without regard to food, continuously until disease progression (total dosage/week = 84 mg)

For patients with actual body weight <60 kg:
Lenvatinib 8 mg per dose; administer orally once daily, without regard to food, continuously until disease progression (total dosage/week = 56 mg)

Notes:
- Lenvatinib capsules should ideally be swallowed whole. Patients who have difficulty swallowing whole lenvatinib capsules may instead place the appropriate combination of whole capsules necessary to administer the required dose in 15 mL of water or apple juice in a glass container for at least 10 minutes. After 10 minutes, the contents of the glass container should be stirred for at least 3 minutes and then the resulting mixture should be swallowed orally. After drinking, rinse the glass container with an additional 15 mL of water or apple juice and swallow the liquid to ensure complete administration of the lenvatinib dose
- A missed dose of lenvatinib may be taken up to 12 hours before a subsequently scheduled dose
- For hepatocellular carcinoma patients who have severe hepatic impairment (Child-Pugh class C), there are insufficient data to recommend a dose of lenvatinib
- For hepatocellular carcinoma patients who have severe renal impairment (CrCl 15–29 mL/min) or end-stage renal disease, there is insufficient data to recommend a dose of lenvatinib
- Patients with pre-existing hypertension should have blood pressure adequately controlled (blood pressure ≤150/90 mm Hg) prior to initiation of treatment with lenvatinib

Supportive Care
Antiemetic prophylaxis
Emetogenic potential is **MODERATE TO HIGH**
See Chapter 42 for antiemetic recommendations

Hematopoietic growth factor (CSF) prophylaxis
Primary prophylaxis is **NOT** indicated
See Chapter 43 for more information

Antimicrobial prophylaxis
Risk of fever and neutropenia is **LOW**
   Antimicrobial primary prophylaxis to be considered:
   - Antibacterial—not indicated
   - Antifungal—not indicated
   - Antiviral—not indicated unless patient previously had an episode of HSV

Diarrhea management
Latent or delayed-onset diarrhea:
   Loperamide 4 mg orally initially after the first loose or liquid stool, *then* 2–4 mg orally every 2–4 hours or **diphenoxylate hydrochloride** 2.5 mg with **atropine sulfate** 0.025 mg (eg, Lomotil)

*Abigerges D et al. J Natl Cancer Inst 1994;86:446–449
Rothenberg ML et al. J Clin Oncol 2001;19:3801–3807
Wadler S et al. J Clin Oncol 1998;16:3169–3178

Treatment Modifications

RECOMMENDED DOSE MODIFICATIONS FOR LENVATINIB

Dose Levels for Lenvatinib

	Actual Weight ≥60 kg	Actual Weight <60 kg
Starting dose	12 by mouth once daily	8 by mouth once daily
Dose level −1	8 by mouth once daily	4 by mouth once daily
Dose level −2	4 by mouth once daily	4 by mouth every other day
Dose level −3	4 by mouth every other day	Discontinue
Dose level −4	Discontinue	

Cardiovascular Toxicity

Adverse Event	Treatment Modification
Either of the following: • G2 hypertension (SBP 140–159 mm Hg or DBP 90–99 mm Hg) • G3 hypertension (SBP ≥160 mm Hg or DBP ≥100 mm Hg) on suboptimal antihypertensive therapy	Continue lenvatinib at the same dose and optimize antihypertensive therapy. Monitor blood pressure frequently
Persistent G3 hypertension (SBP ≥160 mm Hg or DBP ≥100 mm Hg) despite optimal antihypertensive therapy	Withhold lenvatinib until hypertension controlled to G ≤2, then resume lenvatinib at one lower dose level. Monitor blood pressure frequently
G4 hypertension (life-threatening consequences [eg, malignant hypertension, transient or permanent neurologic deficit, hypertensive crisis]; urgent intervention indicated)	Permanently discontinue lenvatinib
G3 cardiac dysfunction	Withhold lenvatinib until cardiac dysfunction improves to G ≤1 or baseline, then resume lenvatinib at one lower dose level or discontinue lenvatinib depending upon the severity and persistence of cardiac dysfunction
G4 cardiac dysfunction	Permanently discontinue lenvatinib
QTc prolongation (>500 ms, or >60-ms increase from baseline)	Withhold lenvatinib until QTc improves to ≤480 ms or baseline, then resume at one lower dose level. Correct hypomagnesemia and/or hypokalemia if applicable
Arterial thromboembolic event	Permanently discontinue lenvatinib

Gastrointestinal Toxicity

Gastrointestinal perforation	Permanently discontinue lenvatinib
G3/4 fistula formation	Permanently discontinue lenvatinib
Either of the following: • G1 diarrhea • G2 diarrhea lasting ≤2 weeks	Continue current lenvatinib dose and optimize antidiarrheal medications
Any of the following: • G2 diarrhea lasting >2 weeks • G3 diarrhea • G4 diarrhea developing in a patient not receiving an optimal antidiarrheal regimen	Withhold lenvatinib until diarrhea resolves to ≤G1 or baseline, then resume lenvatinib at 1 lower dose level. Antidiarrheal treatment for symptoms may continue indefinitely as a preventive measure
Recurrent or persistent G4 diarrhea in a patient receiving an optimal antidiarrheal regimen	Permanently discontinue lenvatinib

Hepatic Toxicity and Hepatic Impairment

G3/4 hepatotoxicity (ALT/AST >5× ULN, bilirubin >3× ULN)	Withhold lenvatinib until hepatotoxicity improves to G ≤1, then resume lenvatinib at one lower dose level or discontinue lenvatinib depending upon the severity and persistence of hepatotoxicity

(continued)

Treatment Modifications (*continued*)

Adverse Event	Treatment Modification
Hepatic failure	Permanently discontinue lenvatinib

Renal Toxicity and Renal Impairment

Adverse Event	Treatment Modification
G3/4 AKI (SCr >3× baseline or >4 mg/dL; hospitalization indicated; life-threatening consequences; dialysis indicated)	Initiate prompt evaluation and correction of dehydration if applicable. Withhold lenvatinib until toxicity improves to G ≤1 or baseline, then resume at one lower dose level or discontinue lenvatinib depending upon the severity and persistence of renal impairment
Urine dipstick proteinuria ≥2+	Continue lenvatinib at current dose and obtain a 24-hour urine protein
Proteinuria ≥2 g in 24 hours	Withhold lenvatinib until <2 grams of proteinuria per 24 hours, then resume lenvatinib at one lower dose level
Nephrotic syndrome	Permanently discontinue lenvatinib

Other Toxicities

Adverse Event	Treatment Modification
RPLS	Withhold lenvatinib until fully resolved, then resume at a reduced dose or discontinue depending on severity and persistence of neurologic symptoms
Planned elective surgery	Withhold lenvatinib for at least 7 days prior to scheduled surgery. Resume lenvatinib after surgery based on clinical assessment of adequate wound healing
Patient with wound-healing complications	Permanently discontinue lenvatinib
Other toxicities (eg, hand-foot skin reaction, rash, nausea/vomiting, stomatitis, hemorrhage, etc) • Other persistent/intolerable G2 toxicities • Other G3 toxicities	Withhold lenvatinib until toxicity improves to G ≤1 or baseline, then resume lenvatinib at one lower dose level
G4 laboratory abnormality	Withhold lenvatinib until toxicity improves to G ≤1 or baseline, then resume lenvatinib at one lower dose level
Other G4 toxicity	Permanently discontinue lenvatinib

*CrCl calculated using the Cockcroft-Gault equation using actual body weight
SBP, systolic blood pressure; DBP, diastolic blood pressure; ALT, alanine aminotransferase; AST, aspartate aminotransferase; AKI, acute kidney injury; SCr, serum creatinine; CrCl, creatinine clearance; RPLS, reversible posterior leukoencephalopathy syndrome
LENVIMA (lenvatinib) prescribing information. Woodcliff Lake, NJ: Eisai Inc; revised February 2020

Patient Population Studied

The REFLECT study was an international, multicenter, phase 3, open-label, randomized, controlled, noninferiority trial that compared lenvatinib versus sorafenib as first-line treatment in 954 patients with unresectable hepatocellular carcinoma. Patients were additionally required to have ≥1 measurable target lesion, have disease categorized as Barcelona Clinic Liver Cancer stage B or C, meet criteria for Child-Pugh class A, have an Eastern Cooperative Oncology Group performance status (ECOG PS) of ≤1, have a blood pressure ≤150/90 mm Hg, have adequate liver function (albumin ≥2.8 g/dL, bilirubin ≤3.0 mg/dL, and aspartate aminotransferase, alkaline phosphatase, and alanine aminotransferase ≤5 times the upper limit of normal), and have adequate organ function. Patients were excluded if they had ≥50% liver occupation by tumor, obvious invasion of the bile duct, or main portal vein invasion

Efficacy (N = 954)

Efficacy Variable	Lenvatinib (N = 478)	Sorafenib (N = 476)	Between-group Comparison
Outcomes*	Months (95% CI)		
Median OS	13.6 (95% CI, 12.1–14.9)	12.3 (95% CI, 10.4–13.9)	HR 0.92 (95% CI, 0.79–1.06)†
Median PFS—months (95% CI)	7.4 (95% CI, 6.9–8.8)	3.7 (95% CI, 3.6–4.6)	HR 0.66 (95% CI, 0.57–0.77), P <0.0001
Median TTP—months (95% CI)	8.9 (95% CI, 7.4–9.2)	3.7 (95% CI, 3.6–5.4)	HR 0.63 (95% CI, 0.53–0.73), P <0.0001
Response	n/N (%) [95% CI]		
Objective response	115/478 (24.1) [20.2–27.9]	44/476 (9.2) [6.6–11.8]	OR 3.13 (95% CI, 2.15–4.56), P <0.0001
Complete response	6/478 (1)	2/476 (<1)	—
Partial response	109/478 (23)	42/476 (9)	—
Stable disease	246/478 (51)	244/476 (51)	—
Stable disease lasting ≥23 weeks	167/478 (35)	139/476 (29)	—
Progressive disease	71/478 (15)	147/476 (31)	—
Unknown or not evaluable	46/478 (10)	41/476 (9)	—
DCR	361/478 (75.5) [71.7–79.4]	288/476 (60.5) [56.1–64.9]	—

*Per investigator review according to modified Response Evaluation Criteria in Solid Tumors (mRECIST) criteria. Refer to Kudo M et al. Lancet 2018;391:1163–1173 for post-hoc analyses based on masked independent imaging review according to modified RECIST and according to RECIST 1.1
†Met criteria for noninferiority of lenvatinib, but not superiority
OS, overall survival; CI, confidence interval; HR, hazard ratio; PFS, progression-free survival; TTP, time to progression; OR, odds ratio; DCR, disease control rate (complete response + partial response + stable disease)
Note: Efficacy end points were assessed in the intention-to-treat population. At the primary analysis data cutoff date of 13 November 2016, the median follow-up time was 27.7 months (IQR, 23.3–32.8) in the lenvatinib group and 27.2 months (IQR, 22.6–31.3) in the sorafenib group. At data cutoff, 701 deaths had occurred

Adverse Events (N = 951)

Adverse Event (AE)	Lenvatinib (N = 476)	Sorafenib (N = 475)
Total treatment-emergent AE	99%	99%
Total treatment-related treatment-emergent AE	94%	95%
Treatment-emergent AE of G ≥3	75%	67%
Treatment-related treatment-emergent AE of G ≥3	57%	49%

Treatment-emergent adverse events occurring in ≥15% of patients in either treatment group

Grade (%)*	% Any Grade	% G ≥3	% Any Grade	% G ≥3
Palmar-plantar erythrodysesthesia	27	3	52	11
Diarrhea	39	4	46	4
Hypertension	42	23	30	14
Decreased appetite	34	5	27	1
Fatigue	30	4	25	4
Alopecia	3	0	25	0

(*continued*)

Adverse Events (N = 951) *(continued)*

Adverse Event (AE)	Lenvatinib (N = 476)		Sorafenib (N = 475)	
Proteinuria	25	6	11	2
Dysphonia	24	<1	12	0
Nausea	20	1	14	1
Abdominal pain	17	2	18	3
Decreased platelet count	18	5	12	3
Elevated aspartate aminotransferase	14	5	17	8
Hypothyroidism	16	0	2	0
Vomiting	16	1	8	1
Constipation	16	1	11	0
Rash	10	0	16	<1
Increased blood bilirubin	15	7	13	5

*Graded accorded to the National Cancer Institute Common Terminology Criteria for Adverse Events (NCI CTCAE) version 4.0
Note: The safety population included all patients who received at least 1 dose of study drug

Therapy Monitoring

1. Check ALT, AST, bilirubin, and alkaline phosphatase at baseline, every 2 weeks for 2 months, and then at least monthly thereafter
2. Check BUN and serum creatinine at baseline and then periodically
3. Check serum calcium at baseline and at least monthly
4. Check TSH and free thyroxine (FT4) every 4–6 weeks
5. Monitor urine dipstick for protein at baseline and then periodically during treatment. If 2+, then perform a 24-hour urine collection for protein.
6. Monitor blood pressure at baseline, after 1 week, every 2 weeks for 2 months, and then at least monthly thereafter
7. Check an electrocardiogram (ECG) at baseline and periodically in patients at increased risk for QT prolongation (eg, congenital long QT syndrome, heart failure, bradyarrhythmias, or in patients taking concomitant medications known to prolong the QT interval)
8. Monitor periodically for signs and symptoms of cardiac dysfunction, arterial thrombosis, reversible posterior leukoencephalopathy syndrome (RPLS), fistula formation, gastrointestinal perforation, and wound-healing complications

UNRESECTABLE DISEASE • SUBSEQUENT THERAPY
HEPATOCELLULAR CARCINOMA REGIMEN: RAMUCIRUMAB

Zhu AX et al. Lancet Oncol 2019;20:282–296
Supplementary appendix to: Zhu AX et al. Lancet Oncol 2019;20:282–296
CYRAMZA (ramucirumab) prescribing information. Indianapolis, IN: Eli Lilly and Company; revised November 2019

Prophylaxis for infusion-related reaction from ramucirumab:

> **Diphenhydramine** 25–50 mg; administer intravenously, 30–60 minutes before starting ramucirumab, *plus*

> **Acetaminophen** 650–1000 mg; administer orally, 30–60 minutes before starting ramucirumab (only if history of Grade 1–2 infusion reaction), *plus*

> **Dexamethasone** 8 mg; administer orally or intravenously, 30–60 minutes before starting ramucirumab (only if history of Grade 1–2 infusion reaction)

Ramucirumab 8 mg/kg; administer intravenously in 250 mL of 0.9% sodium chloride injection (0.9% NS) over 1 hour on day 1, every 2 weeks, until disease progression (total dosage/2-week cycle = 8 mg/kg)

- Ramucirumab should be administered through an administration set with a low-protein-binding in-line filter with pore size of 0.22 μm

- Flush the line with 0.9% NS at the end of the infusion

- If the first infusion is tolerated, all subsequent ramucirumab infusions may be administered over 30 minutes

- Ramucirumab can cause severe infusion-related reactions

  - Reduce the ramucirumab infusion rate by 50% for Grade 1 or Grade 2 infusion reactions and add acetaminophen and dexamethasone to infusion-related reaction prophylaxis regimen, as described above, in subsequent cycles

  - Permanently discontinue ramucirumab for Grade 3 or Grade 4 infusion-related reactions

Supportive Care
Antiemetic prophylaxis
Emetogenic potential is **MINIMAL**
See Chapter 42 for antiemetic recommendations

Hematopoietic growth factor (CSF) prophylaxis
Primary prophylaxis is **NOT** *indicated*
See Chapter 43 for more information

Antimicrobial prophylaxis
Risk of fever and neutropenia is **LOW**
> *Antimicrobial primary prophylaxis to be considered:*

- Antibacterial—not indicated

- Antifungal—not indicated

- Antiviral—not indicated unless patient previously had an episode of HSV

Treatment Modifications

RAMUCIRUMAB TREATMENT MODIFICATIONS

Ramucirumab Dose Levels	
Starting dose	8 mg/kg
Dose level −1	6 mg/kg
Dose level −2	5 mg/kg

Adverse Reaction	**Dose Modification**
Proteinuria	
Urine protein ≥2 g/24 hours	Interrupt ramucirumab. Resume ramucirumab treatment at 6 mg/kg once the urine protein level returns to <2 g/24 hours
Reoccurrence of urine protein ≥2 g/24 hours on a dose of 6 mg/kg	Interrupt ramucirumab. Resume ramucirumab treatment at 5 mg/kg once the urine protein level returns to <2 g/24 hours

(continued)

Treatment Modifications (continued)

Adverse Reaction	Dose Modification
Reoccurrence of urine protein ≥2 g/24 hours on a dose of 5 mg/kg	Permanently discontinue ramucirumab
Urine protein >3 g/24 hours or nephrotic syndrome	
Infusion-related Reactions	
G1/2 infusion-related reaction	Stop ramucirumab. Administer dexamethasone intravenously at commonly used antiemetic doses of 8–20 mg (or equivalent) and acetaminophen, then resume infusion at 50% of previous rate. Use the 50% infusion rate for all subsequent administrations
Prior G1/2 infusion-related reaction	Premedicate with dexamethasone intravenously at commonly used antiemetic doses of 8–20 mg (or equivalent) and acetaminophen prior to each ramucirumab infusion. Continue diphenhydramine 25–50 mg intravenously
G3/4 infusion-related reaction	Permanently discontinue ramucirumab

Hypertension	
G3/4 hypertension	Interrupt ramucirumab until symptoms controlled with medical management; consider dose reduction.
Recurrent G3/4 hypertension unable to be controlled with medical management	Permanently discontinue ramucirumab

Other Adverse Events	
Posterior reversible leukoencephalopathy syndrome (PRES)	Permanently discontinue ramucirumab
G3/4 bleeding	
Arterial thromboembolic event	
Gastrointestinal perforation	
Anticipated wound healing	Stop ramucirumab ≥4 weeks prior to a scheduled surgery and until wound is fully healed; discontinue ramucirumab if patient develops wound-healing complications
G3/4 fatigue/asthenia	Interrupt ramucirumab. Reinstitute treatment at a reduced dose once toxicity is G1
G3/4 stomatitis/mucosal inflammation	

Patient Population Studied

The REACH-2 study was a randomized, double-blind, placebo-controlled, international, multicenter, phase 3 study comparing ramucirumab (n = 197) to placebo (n = 95) in patients with hepatocellular carcinoma that had been previously treated with first-line sorafenib. Additionally, patients were required to have ≥1 measurable lesion, to have disease classified as Barcelona Clinic Liver Cancer stage B or C, to meet criteria for Child-Pugh A liver function, to not be candidates for locoregional therapies, to have an α-fetoprotein level of ≥400 ng/mL, and to have an Eastern Cooperative Oncology Group performance status of ≤1. Noteworthy exclusion criteria included uncontrolled arterial hypertension, a history of or current hepatic encephalopathy, prior liver transplantation, and gastroesophageal varices requiring endoscopic treatment

Efficacy (N = 292)

Efficacy Variable	Ramucirumab (N = 197)	Placebo (N = 95)	Between-group Comparison
Outcomes*	Months (95% CI)		
Median overall survival	8.5 (95% CI, 7.0–10.6)	7.3 (95% CI, 5.4–9.1)	HR 0.710 (95% CI, 0.531–0.949), P = 0.0199[†]
Median progression-free survival	2.8 (95% CI, 2.8–8.4)	1.6 (95% CI, 1.5–2.7)	HR 0.452 (95% CI, 0.339–0.603), P <0.0001[†]
Median time to (radiographic) progression	3.0 (95% CI, 2.8–4.2)	1.6 (95% CI, 1.5–2.7)	HR 0.427 (95% CI, 0.313–0.582), P <0.0001[†]
Response			
Best overall response*	n/N (%) [95% CI]		
Complete response	0	0	—
Partial response	9/197 (4.6)	1/95 (1.1)	—
Stable disease	109/197 (55.3)	36/95 (37.9)	—
Progressive disease	66/197 (33.5)	48/95 (50.5)	—
Not evaluable	13/197 (6.6)	10/95 (10.5)	—
Overall response rate (CR + PR)	9/197 (4.6) [1.7–7.5]	1/95 (1.1) [0.0–3.1]	P = 0.1697[‡]
Disease control rate (ORR + SD)	118/197 (59.9) [53.1–66.7]	37/95 (38.9) [29.1–48.8]	P = 0.0006[‡]

*Based on RECIST version 1.1 criteria assessed by local investigators
[†]Two-sided P Values were log-rank stratified by geographical region, macrovascular invasion, and ECOG PS
[‡]P Value calculated by exact Cochran-Mantel-Haenszel test stratified by randomization strata
CI, confidence interval; HR, hazard ratio; RECIST, Response Evaluation Criteria in Solid Tumors; ECOG PS, Eastern Cooperative Oncology Group Performance Status
Note: Efficacy end points were assessed in the intention-to-treat population. At the data cutoff date of 15 March 2018, the median follow-up time was 7.6 months (IQR, 4.0–12.5) and 221 deaths had occurred

Adverse Events (N = 292)

	Treatment-emergent Adverse Events Occurring in ≥10% of Patients in Either Arm						Treatment-emergent Adverse Events Occurring in ≥10% of Patients in Either Arm, Treatment-related					
	Ramucirumab (N = 197)			Placebo (N = 95)			Ramucirumab (N = 197)			Placebo (N = 95)		
Grade (%)*	G1–2	G3	G4	G1–2	G3	G4	G1–2	G3	G4	G1–2	G3	G4
Fatigue	24	4	NA	14	3	NA	13	1	NA	5	0	NA
Peripheral edema	24	2	0	14	0	0	7	1	0	5	0	0
Decreased appetite	22	2	0	19	1	0	11	0	0	4	0	0
Abdominal pain	18	2	NA	11	2	NA	3	1	NA	3	0	NA
Nausea	19	0	NA	12	0	NA	12	0	NA	2	0	NA
Diarrhea	16	0	0	14	1	0	7	0	0	4	1	0
Headache	14	0	NA	4	1	NA	5	0	NA	0	0	NA
Constipation	13	1	0	19	1	0	1	1	0	3	0	0
Insomnia	11	0	NA	5	1	NA	1	0	NA	0	0	NA
Pyrexia	10	0	0	3	0	0	1	0	0	1	0	0
Vomiting	10	0	0	7	0	0	3	0	0	1	0	0

*Graded according to the National Cancer Institute Common Terminology Criteria for Adverse Events (NCI CTCAE) v4.0
Note: No Grade 5 events were reported in the above categories

Adverse Events (N = 292)

Adverse Event	Treatment-emergent Adverse Events of Special Interest						Treatment-emergent, Treatment-related Adverse Events of Special Interest					
	Ramucirumab (N = 197)			Placebo (N = 95)			Ramucirumab (N = 197)			Placebo (N = 95)		
Grade (%)*	G1–2	G3	G4	G1–2	G3	G4	G1–2	G3	G4	G1–2	G3	G4
Bleeding or hemorrhage event	19	5	1	9	2	1	10	1	0	4	0	1
Epistaxis	13	1	0	3	0	0	7	0	0	2	0	0
GI hemorrhage event	3	4	0	3	2	0	1	0	0	0	0	0
Hepatic hemorrhage event	0	0	1	0	0	0	0	0	0	0	0	0
Pulmonary hemorrhage event	2	1	0	1	0	0	0	0	0	0	0	0
Hypertension	12	13	0	7	5	0	9	8	0	4	2	0
Proteinuria	18	2	0	4	0	0	12	2	0	3	0	0
Arterial thromboembolic event	1	0	1	0	0	0	1	0	1	0	0	0
VTE event	1	0	0	1	1	0	1	0	0	1	0	0
GI perforation	0	1	0	0	2	0	0	1	0	0	0	0
CHF	0	0	0	0	1	0	0	0	0	0	0	0
Fistula	1	0	0	0	0	0	0	0	0	0	0	0
Liver injury or failure	21	14	2	14	15	1	6	2	0	2	0	0
Ascites	14	4	0	5	2	0	2	1	0	1	0	0
HE	1	3	1	0	0	0	1	1	0	0	0	0
IRR	9	0	0	3	0	0	7	0	0	2	0	0

*Graded according to the National Cancer Institute Common Terminology Criteria for Adverse Events (NCI CTCAE) v4.0
Note: Treatment-emergent Grade 5 events included arterial thromboembolic event (ramucirumab, n = 2; placebo, n = 1); CHF (ramucirumab, n = 2); liver injury or failure (ramucirumab, n = 4); ascites (ramucirumab, n = 1). Treatment-emergent, treatment-related Grade 5 events included arterial thromboembolic event (ramucirumab, n = 1); liver injury or failure (ramucirumab, n = 3)
GI, gastrointestinal; VTE, venous thromboembolism; CHF, congestive heart failure; HE, hepatic encephalopathy; IRR, infusion-related reaction

Therapy Monitoring

1. Observe closely for hypersensitivity reactions, especially during the first and second ramucirumab infusions
2. Check blood pressure every 2 weeks or more frequently as indicated during treatment
3. Assess proteinuria by urine dipstick and/or urinary protein creatinine ratio at baseline and every 2 cycles. If protein ≥2+, then collect a 24-hour urine for protein measurement
4. Assess thyroid function at outset and every 3 months while on therapy
5. Monitor for and advise patients to report signs and/or symptoms of bleeding, arterial thromboembolic events, gastrointestinal perforation, impaired wound healing, and posterior reversible encephalopathy syndrome

UNRESECTABLE DISEASE • SUBSEQUENT THERAPY
HEPATOCELLULAR CARCINOMA REGIMEN: CABOZANTINIB

Abou-Alfa GK et al. N Engl J Med 2018;379:54–63
Protocol for: Abou-Alfa GK et al. N Engl J Med 2018;379:54–63
Supplementary appendix to: Abou-Alfa GK et al. N Engl J Med 2018;379:54–63
CABOMETYX (cabozantinib) prescribing information. Alameda, CA: Exelixis, Inc; revised January 2020

Cabozantinib tablets 60 mg dose; administer orally at least 2 hours after or at least 1 hour before eating food, once daily, continually, until disease progression (total dose/week = 420 mg)

Notes:
- Tablets are swallowed whole. Do not crush cabozantinib tablets
- Do not substitute cabozantinib tablets (CABOMETYX) with cabozantinib capsules (COMETRIQ)
- Do not take a missed dose within 12 hours of the next scheduled dose
- In light of the fact that 62% of patients starting at the 60-mg dose had a subsequent dose reduction and 16% discontinued the medication because of adverse effects, clinicians are advised to consider the following:
- *Patients taking CYP3A4 inhibitors*
  - Avoid use of concomitant strong CYP3A4 inhibitors (eg, atazanavir, clarithromycin, indinavir, itraconazole, ketoconazole, nefazodone, nelfinavir, ritonavir, saquinavir, telithromycin, voriconazole)
  - For patients who require treatment with a strong CYP3A4 inhibitor, reduce the daily cabozantinib dose by 20 mg. Resume the dose that was used prior to initiating the CYP3A4 inhibitor 2 to 3 days after discontinuing a strong inhibitor
- *Patients taking strong CYP3A4 inducers*
  - Avoid use of strong CYP3A4 inducers (eg, carbamazepine, phenobarbital, phenytoin, rifabutin, rifampin, rifapentine) concomitantly with cabozantinib if alternative therapy is available
  - Inform patients not to ingest foods or nutritional supplements (eg, St. John's Wort (*Hypericum perforatum*) known to induce cytochrome P450 activity
  - For patients who require treatment with a strong CYP3A4 inducer, increase the daily cabozantinib dose by 20 mg *only if tolerability on the dose without the inducer has been convincingly demonstrated*. Resume the dose that was used prior to initiating a CYP3A4 inducer 2 to 3 days after discontinuing a strong inducer. The daily cabozantinib dose should not exceed 80 mg
- *Patients with hepatic impairment*
  - In patients with moderate hepatic impairment (Child-Pugh class B), reduce the starting dose of cabozantinib to 40 mg once daily
  - Avoid use of cabozantinib in patients with severe hepatic impairment (Child-Pugh class C)

Supportive Care
Antiemetic prophylaxis
Emetogenic potential is **MINIMAL–LOW**
See Chapter 42 for antiemetic recommendations

Hematopoietic growth factor (CSF) prophylaxis
Primary prophylaxis is **NOT** *indicated*
See Chapter 43 for more information

Antimicrobial prophylaxis
Risk of fever and neutropenia is **LOW**
Antimicrobial primary prophylaxis to be considered:

Diarrhea management
Latent or delayed-onset diarrhea*:
Loperamide 4 mg orally initially after the first loose or liquid stool, *then* 2–4 mg orally every 2–4 hours or **diphenoxylate hydrochloride** 2.5 mg with **atropine sulfate** 0.025 mg (eg, Lomotil)

*Abigerges D et al. J Natl Cancer Inst 1994;86:446–449
Rothenberg ML et al. J Clin Oncol 2001;19:3801–3807

Hand-foot reaction (palmar-plantar erythrodysesthesia, PPE)
Use topical emollients (eg, Aquaphor), topical or orally administered steroids, antihistamines, or pyridoxine 50 to 200 mg/day

Treatment Modifications

RECOMMENDED DOSE MODIFICATIONS FOR CABOZANTINIB

Cabozantinib Dose Levels	
Starting dose (level 1)	60 mg orally once daily
Dose level −1	40 mg orally once daily
Dose level −2	20 mg orally once daily
Dose level −3	Consider discontinuing cabozantinib or consider resuming at 20 mg orally once daily, if tolerable, at the discretion of the medically responsible health care provider

Adverse Event	Treatment Modification
G ≥3 hemorrhage	Permanently discontinue cabozantinib
Development of a gastrointestinal perforation or Grade 4 fistula	
Acute MI	
Serious arterial or VTE event requiring medical intervention	
Any hypertension	Treat as needed with standard antihypertensive therapy
Persistent hypertension despite use of maximal antihypertensive medications	Withhold cabozantinib until blood pressure is adequately controlled, then resume cabozantinib with the dosage reduced by 1 dosage level
Evidence of hypertensive crisis or severe hypertension that cannot be controlled with antihypertensive therapy	Discontinue cabozantinib
Intolerable Grade 2 diarrhea	Optimize antidiarrheal regimen. Withhold cabozantinib until improvement to G ≤1, then resume cabozantinib with the dosage reduced by 1 dose level
Grade ≥3 diarrhea not manageable with standard antidiarrheal treatments	
Intolerable Grade 2 palmar-plantar erythrodysesthesia syndrome (skin changes [eg, peeling, blisters, bleeding, edema, or hyperkeratosis] with pain; limiting instrumental ADL)	Withhold cabozantinib until improvement to G ≤1, then resume cabozantinib with the dosage reduced by 1 dose level
Grade 3 palmar-plantar erythrodysesthesia syndrome (severe skin changes [e.g., peeling, blisters, bleeding, edema, or hyperkeratosis] with pain; limiting self-care ADL)	
Patient requires dental surgery or an invasive dental procedure	If possible, withhold cabozantinib for ≥3 weeks prior to the procedure to reduce risk of osteonecrosis of the jaw and poor wound healing
Osteonecrosis of the jaw	Withhold cabozantinib until complete resolution, then reduce the cabozantinib dosage by 1 dose level
Patient requires elective surgery	If possible, withhold cabozantinib for ≥3 weeks prior to elective surgery and for ≥2 weeks after major surgery and until adequate wound healing, whichever is longer
RPLS is suspected (symptoms of headache, seizure, lethargy, confusion, blindness, and/or other visual and neurologic disturbances along with hypertension of any severity)	Withhold cabozantinib until clarification of the patient's neurologic status (ie, with an emergent brain MRI) has occurred
RPLS is confirmed	Discontinue cabozantinib. The safety of reinitiating cabozantinib in a patient who has experienced RPLS is unknown
Urine dipstick >1+ for protein	Continue cabozantinib at the same dose pending results of a 24-hour urine protein

(continued)

Treatment Modifications (*continued*)

Adverse Event	Treatment Modification
Urine protein ≥3 g/24 hours	Withhold cabozantinib until urine protein is <3 g/24 hours, then resume cabozantinib at 1 lower dose level. Consider increasing the frequency of urine protein monitoring upon resumption of cabozantinib
Nephrotic syndrome	Discontinue cabozantinib treatment
Other Adverse Reactions	
Other intolerable Grade 2 adverse reactions	Withhold cabozantinib until improvement to G ≤1 or baseline, then reduce the cabozantinib dosage by 1 dose level
Other G ≥3 adverse reactions	
Hepatic Impairment	
Moderate hepatic impairment (Child-Pugh class B)	Decrease the starting dose of cabozantinib to 40 mg once daily
Drug Interactions	
Patient requires concomitant use of a strong CYP3A4 inhibitor (eg, atazanavir, clarithromycin, indinavir, itraconazole, ketoconazole, nefazodone, nelfinavir, ritonavir, saquinavir, telithromycin, voriconazole)	Reduce the daily cabozantinib dose by 20 mg. Resume the dose that was used prior to initiating the CYP3A4 inhibitor 2 to 3 days after discontinuing a strong inhibitor
Patient requires concomitant use of a strong CYP3A4 inducer (eg, carbamazepine, phenobarbital, phenytoin, rifabutin, rifampin, rifapentine, St. John's Wort)	Increase the daily cabozantinib dose by 20 mg only if tolerability on the dose without the inducer has been convincingly demonstrated. Resume the dose that was used prior to initiating a CYP3A4 inducer 2 to 3 days after discontinuing a strong inducer. The daily cabozantinib dose should not exceed 80 mg

MI, myocardial infarction; VTE, venous thromboembolic event; RPLS, reversible posterior leukoencephalopathy syndrome; UPCR, urine protein to creatinine ratio; MRI, magnetic resonance imaging; ADL, activities of daily living

Patient Population Studied

The CELESTIAL study was a phase 3, double-blind, randomized, placebo-controlled trial that involved 707 adult patients with advanced hepatocellular carcinoma that was not amenable to curative treatment. Eligible patients were previously treated with sorafenib and had experienced disease progression after at least 1 systemic treatment, although up to 2 prior systemic therapies were allowed. Participants had an Eastern Cooperative Oncology Group (ECOG) performance status score of ≤1, Child-Pugh class A liver function, and adequate hematologic and renal function. Patients were excluded if they had received prior treatment with cabozantinib or uncontrolled clinically significant illness. Participants were randomly assigned in a 2:1 ratio to receive cabozantinib or matching placebo

Efficacy (N = 707)

Efficacy Variable	Cabozantinib (N = 470)	Placebo (N = 237)	Between-group Comparison
	Months (95% CI)		
Median overall survival	10.2 (9.1–12.0)	8.0 (6.8–9.4)	HR 0.76 (95% CI, 0.63–0.92); P = 0.005
Median progression-free survival*	5.2 (4.0–5.5)	1.9 (1.9–1.9)	HR 0.44 (95% CI 0.36–0.52); P <0.001
Response to therapy			
Objective response rate*	4%	<1%	P = 0.009
Disease control rate†	64%	33%	—

OS, overall survival; CI, confidence interval; HR, hazard ratio
*Per RECIST version 1.1
†Defined as partial response + stable disease
Note: The median duration of therapy 3.8 months in the cabozantinib group and 2.0 months in the placebo group. The data cutoff date for this second interim analysis was 1 June 2017

Therapy Monitoring

1. *Prior to initiation of cabozantinib:* CBC with differential and platelet count, vital signs, liver function tests, serum electrolytes, oral examination
   a. Control hypertension prior to initiation of cabozantinib
2. *Monitor regularly for:*
   a. Hypertension
   b. Signs and symptoms of bleeding. Avoid initiation of cabozantinib in patients with a recent history of hemorrhage (eg, hemoptysis, hematemesis, or melena)
   c. Signs and symptoms of fistulas and perforations, including abscess and sepsis
   d. Diarrhea
   e. Spot urine for protein measurement every 4–8 weeks (if spot urine dipstick >1+ for protein, perform a 24-hour urine protein)
   f. Signs and symptoms of osteonecrosis of the jaw (jaw pain, osteomyelitis, osteitis, bone erosion, tooth or periodontal infection, toothache, gingival ulceration or erosion, persistent jaw pain or slow healing of the mouth or jaw after dental surgery)
      i. Perform an oral examination prior to initiation of cabozantinib and periodically during treatment
      ii. Advise patients regarding good oral hygiene practices
      iii. Withhold cabozantinib for ≥3 weeks prior to scheduled dental surgery or invasive dental procedures, if possible
      iv. Withhold cabozantinib for development of osteonecrosis of the jaw until complete resolution
3. Withhold cabozantinib for ≥3 weeks prior to elective surgery (including dental surgery) and for ≥2 weeks after major surgery and until adequate wound healing, whichever is longer

Adverse Events (N = 704)

Grade* (%)	Cabozantinib (N = 467)		Placebo (N = 237)	
	Grade 1–2	Grade 3–4	Grade 1–2	Grade 3–4
Diarrhea	43	11	17	2
Decreased appetite	42	6	17	<1
Palmar-plantar erythrodysesthesia	29	17	5	0
Fatigue	35	10	26	4
Nausea	29	2	16	2
Hypertension	12	17	4	2
Vomiting	25	<1	9	3
Increased AST	10	12	4	7
Asthenia	14	8	6	2
Dysphonia	18	1	2	0
Constipation	18	<1	19	0
Abdominal pain	16	2	21	4
Weight loss	16	1	6	0
Increased ALT	12	5	3	2
Mucosal inflammation	12	2	1	<1
Pyrexia	14	0	9	<1
Upper abdominal pain	12	1	13	0
Cough	12	<1	11	0
Peripheral edema	12	1	13	1
Stomatitis	11	2	2	0
Dyspnea	9	3	9	<1
Rash	11	<1	5	<1
Ascites	7	5	8	5
Dysgeusia	12	0	2	0
Hypoalbuminemia	11	<1	5	0
Headache	10	<1	6	<1
Thrombocytopenia	8	3	<1	0
Insomnia	9	<1	7	0
Dizziness	9	<1	6	0
Dyspepsia	10	0	3	0
Anemia	5	5	3	5
Back pain	9	1	9	<1
Increased serum bilirubin	7	3	5	2
Decreased platelet count	6	4	2	1

*Per National Cancer Institute
Common Terminology Criteria for Adverse Events (NCI CTCAE) v4.0
AST, aspartate aminotransferase; ALT, alanine aminotransferase
Note: Adverse events are included in the table, regardless of causality, if they occurred in ≥10% of patients in either group. There were six Grade 5 adverse events in the cabozantinib group (one event each of hepatic failure, broncho-esophageal fistula, portal vein thrombosis, upper gastrointestinal hemorrhage, pulmonary embolism, and hepatorenal syndrome). There was one Grade 5 event in the placebo group (hepatic failure)

UNRESECTABLE DISEASE • SUBSEQUENT THERAPY
HEPATOCELLULAR CARCINOMA REGIMEN: NIVOLUMAB

El-Khoueiry AB et al. Lancet 2017;389:2492–2502
Supplementary appendix to: El-Khoueiry AB et al. Lancet 2017;389:2492–2502
OPDIVO (nivolumab) prescribing information. Princeton, NJ: Bristol-Myers Squibb Company; revised September 2019

Note that the U.S. Food and Drug Administration (FDA)-approved regimens for hepatocellular carcinoma include fixed doses of nivolumab and allow for a shortened infusion duration of 30 minutes, consistent with the regimens approved on 5 March 2018

Nivolumab 240 mg; administer intravenously over 30 minutes in a volume of 0.9% NS or D5W, not to exceed 160 mL and sufficient to produce a nivolumab concentration within the range 1–10 mg/mL, every 2 weeks until disease progression (total dosage/2-week cycle = 240 mg)
- Administer nivolumab through an administration set that contains a sterile, non-pyrogenic, low-protein-binding in-line filter with pore size within the range of 0.2–1.2 μm
- Nivolumab can cause severe infusion-related reactions

or

Nivolumab 480 mg; administer intravenously over 30 minutes in a volume of 0.9% NS or D5W not to exceed 160 mL and sufficient to produce a nivolumab concentration within the range 1–10 mg/mL, every 4 weeks until disease progression (total dosage/4-week cycle = 480 mg)
- Administer nivolumab through an administration set that contains a sterile, non-pyrogenic, low-protein-binding in-line filter with pore size within the range of 0.2–1.2 μm
- Nivolumab can cause severe infusion-related reactions

Supportive Care
Antiemetic prophylaxis
Emetogenic potential with nivolumab is **MINIMAL**
See Chapter 42 for antiemetic recommendations

Hematopoietic growth factor (CSF) prophylaxis
Primary prophylaxis is **NOT** *indicated*
See Chapter 43 for more information

Antimicrobial prophylaxis
Risk of fever and neutropenia is **LOW**
   Antimicrobial primary prophylaxis to be considered:
- Antibacterial—not indicated
- Antifungal—not indicated
- Antiviral—not indicated unless patient previously had an episode of HSV

Treatment Modifications

RECOMMENDED DOSE MODIFICATIONS FOR NIVOLUMAB

Adverse Event	Grade/Severity	Treatment Modification
Infusion reaction	Clinically significant but not severe infusion reaction	Interrupt the infusion in patients with clinically significant infusion reactions and consider resuming at a slower rate following resolution. If decision is made to restart, begin at ≤50% of the rate prior to the reaction and increase in 50% increments every 30 minutes if well tolerated. Infusions may be restarted at the full rate during the next cycle
	G3/4 (severe infusion reaction—pyrexia, chills, flushing, hypotension, dyspnea, wheezing, back pain, abdominal pain, and urticaria). Not rapidly responsive to brief interruption of infusion	Stop infusion and administer appropriate medical therapy (eg, epinephrine, corticosteroids, intravenous antihistamines, bronchodilators, and/or oxygen). Discontinue nivolumab

(continued)

Treatment Modifications (*continued*)

Adverse Event	Grade/Severity	Treatment Modification
Colitis	G1	Loperamide 4 mg as starting dose then 2 mg before each meal and after each loose stool until without diarrhea for 12 hours, with maximum of 16 mg loperamide per day. If G1 diarrhea or colitis persists >14 days, then add prednisolone 0.5–1 mg/kg (non-enteric-coated) or consider oral budesonide 9 mg daily if no bloody diarrhea
	G2/3 diarrhea or colitis	Withhold nivolumab. Loperamide 4 mg as starting dose then 2 mg before each meal and after each loose stool until without diarrhea for 12 hours, with maximum of 16 mg loperamide per day. Administer oral prednisone/prednisolone at a dose of 0.5 to 2 mg/kg/day or its equivalent. When improves to G1, begin a slow corticosteroid taper over at least 4 weeks. Resume nivolumab upon symptom control, or when prednisone/prednisolone daily dose <10 mg
	G4 diarrhea or colitis	Permanently discontinue nivolumab. Loperamide 4 mg as starting dose then 2 mg before each meal and after each loose stool until without diarrhea for 12 hours, with maximum of 16 mg loperamide per day. Administer 1–2 mg/kg IV (methyl)prednisolone and convert to 0.5–2 mg/kg prednisone/prednisolone orally each day or its equivalent only after a response. Taper over at least 4 weeks when symptoms improve. If does not improve over 72 hours or worsens, perform flexible sigmoidoscopy/colonoscopy to document colitis then begin infliximab 5 mg/kg (if no perforation/sepsis/TB/hepatitis/NYHA III/IV CHF). If no response, add MMF 500–1000 mg twice daily. If worse on MMF, consider addition of tacrolimus or ATG
Pneumonitis	G2	Withhold nivolumab. Consider pneumocystis prophylaxis depending on the clinical context and coverage with empiric antibiotics. Administer oral prednisone/prednisolone at a dose of 1–2 mg/kg/day or its equivalent. When improves to G1, begin a slow corticosteroid taper over at least 4 weeks. If does not respond adequately after 48 hours, then administer 2–4 mg/kg IV (methyl)prednisolone and convert to 0.5–2 mg/kg prednisone/prednisolone orally each day or its equivalent only after a response, followed by a taper over at least 6 weeks when symptoms improve to G1, titrating to symptoms. Resume nivolumab upon symptom control, or when prednisone/prednisolone daily dose <10 mg
	G3/4	Permanently discontinue nivolumab. Consider pneumocystis prophylaxis depending on the clinical context; cover with empiric antibiotics. Administer 2–4 mg/kg IV (methyl)prednisolone and convert to 1–2 mg/kg prednisone/prednisolone orally each day or its equivalent only after a response, followed by a taper over at least 8 weeks when symptoms improve to G1, titrating to symptoms. If, when initially treated, improvement does not occur within 48–72 hours, begin infliximab 5 mg/kg (if no perforation/sepsis/TB/hepatitis/NYHA III/IV CHF). If no response to infliximab, add MMF 500–1000 mg twice daily. Consider MMF especially if has concurrent hepatic toxicity
Hepatitis	G2 (AST or ALT >3–5× ULN or total bilirubin >1.5–3× ULN)	Withhold nivolumab. Administer oral prednisone/prednisolone at a dose of 1 to 2 mg/kg/day or its equivalent. When improves to G1, begin a slow corticosteroid taper over at least 4 weeks. Resume nivolumab upon symptom control, or when prednisone/prednisolone daily dose <10 mg
	G3/4 (AST or ALT >5× ULN or total bilirubin >3× ULN)	Permanently discontinue nivolumab. Administer 1–2 mg/kg IV (methyl)prednisolone and convert to 0.5–2 mg/kg prednisone/prednisolone orally each day or its equivalent only after a response. Taper over at least 6 weeks when symptoms improve. If no response, add MMF 500–1000 mg twice daily. If worse on MMF, consider adding tacrolimus or ATG

(*continued*)

Treatment Modifications (continued)

Adverse Event	Grade/Severity	Treatment Modification
Hypophysitis	G2/3 (moderate symptoms, ie, headache but no visual disturbance or fatigue/mood alteration but hemodynamically stable, no electrolyte disturbance)	Administer analgesia as needed for headache. Withhold nivolumab. Administer oral prednisone/prednisolone at a dose of 0.5 to 2 mg/kg/day or its equivalent. When improves to G1, begin a slow corticosteroid taper over at least 4 weeks. If no improvement in 48 hours, administer 1–2 mg/kg IV (methyl)prednisolone and convert to 0.5–2 mg/kg prednisone/prednisolone orally each day or its equivalent only after a response. Taper over at least 4 weeks when symptoms improve to 5 mg prednisone/prednisolone or equivalent; do not stop steroids. Resume nivolumab upon symptom control, or when prednisone/prednisolone daily dose <10 mg
	G4 (severe mass effect symptoms, ie, severe headache, any visual disturbance or severe hypoadrenalism, ie, hypotension, severe electrolyte disturbance)	Permanently discontinue nivolumab. Administer analgesia as needed for headache. Administer 1–2 mg/kg IV (methyl)prednisolone and convert to 0.5–2 mg/kg prednisone/prednisolone orally each day or its equivalent only after a response. Taper over at least 4 weeks when symptoms improve to 5 mg prednisone/prednisolone or equivalent; do not stop steroids
Adrenal insufficiency	G2	Withhold nivolumab. Administer oral prednisone/prednisolone at a dose of 0.5 to 2 mg/kg/day or its equivalent. When improves to G1, begin a slow corticosteroid taper over at least 4 weeks. Serially assess adrenal function and continue steroids at replacement doses (20–40 mg hydrocortisone daily ~2/3 dose in AM upon awakening and ~1/3 at 4 PM) until recovery of adrenal function is documented. Resume nivolumab upon symptom control, or when prednisone/prednisolone daily dose <10 mg
	G3/4	Permanently discontinue nivolumab. Administer oral prednisone/prednisolone at a dose of 0.5 to 2 mg/kg/day or its equivalent. When improves to G1, begin a slow corticosteroid taper over at least 4 weeks. Serially assess adrenal function and continue steroids at replacement doses (20–40 mg hydrocortisone daily ~2/3 dose in AM upon awakening and ~1/3 at 4 PM) until recovery of adrenal function is documented
Type 1 diabetes mellitus	G3 hyperglycemia	Withhold nivolumab. Admit to hospital to manage hyperglycemia. Role of corticosteroids in preventing complete loss of insulin-producing cells is unknown and not recommended. Resume nivolumab upon symptom control, or when prednisone/prednisolone daily dose <10 mg
	G4 hyperglycemia	Permanently discontinue nivolumab. Admit to hospital to manage hyperglycemia. Role of corticosteroids in preventing complete loss of insulin-producing cells is unknown and not recommended
Nephritis and renal dysfunction	G2/3 (serum creatinine 1.5–6× ULN)	Withhold nivolumab. Administer oral prednisone/prednisolone at a dose of 0.5 to 2 mg/kg/day or its equivalent. When improves to G1, begin a slow corticosteroid taper over at least 4 weeks. If does not respond adequately, then administer 0.5–1 mg/kg IV (methyl)prednisolone and convert to 0.5–2 mg/kg prednisone/prednisolone orally each day or its equivalent only after a response, followed by a taper over at least 4 weeks when improves to G1. Resume nivolumab upon symptom control, or when prednisone/prednisolone daily dose <10 mg
	G4 (serum creatinine >6× ULN)	Permanently discontinue nivolumab. Administer 0.5–1 mg/kg IV (methyl)prednisolone and convert to 0.5–2 mg/kg prednisone/prednisolone orally each day or its equivalent only after a response, followed by a taper over at least 4 weeks when improves to G1
Skin	G1/2	Continue nivolumab. Avoid skin irritants, avoid sun exposure, topical emollients recommended. Topical steroid (mild strength for G1, moderate/potent strength for G2) cream once or twice daily ± oral or topical antihistamines for itching

(continued)

Treatment Modifications (continued)

Adverse Event	Grade/Severity	Treatment Modification
	G3 rash or suspected SJS or TEN	Withhold nivolumab. Avoid skin irritants, avoid sun exposure, topical emollients recommended. Administer oral or topical antihistamines for itching. Administer oral prednisone/prednisolone at a dose of 0.5–2 mg/kg or its equivalent daily for 3 days followed by a slow corticosteroid taper over at least 4 weeks when the rash improves to G1. If does not respond adequately, then administer 0.5–1 mg/kg IV (methyl)prednisolone and convert to 0.5–2 mg/kg prednisone/prednisolone orally each day or its equivalent only after a response, followed by a taper over at least 4 weeks when the rash improves to G1. Resume nivolumab upon symptom control, or when prednisone/prednisolone daily dose <10 mg
	G4 rash or confirmed SJS or TEN	Avoid skin irritants, avoid sun exposure, topical emollients recommended. Administer oral or topical antihistamines for itching. Administer 1–2 mg/kg IV (methyl)prednisolone and convert to oral steroids 0.5–2 mg/kg prednisone/prednisolone each day or its equivalent only after a response. Taper over at least 4 weeks when the rash improves to G1. Permanently discontinue nivolumab
Encephalitis	Confusion or altered behavior, headaches, alteration in Glasgow Coma Scale, motor or sensory deficits, speech abnormality, may or may not be febrile	Initially withhold nivolumab, but permanently discontinue nivolumab if there is no doubt as to diagnosis. Exclude bacterial and ideally viral infections prior to high-dose steroids. Administer oral prednisone/prednisolone at a dose of 0.5–2 mg/kg/day or its equivalent. When symptoms improve, begin a slow corticosteroid taper over at least 4–8 weeks. If symptoms are severe, administer 1–2 mg/kg IV (methyl)prednisolone and convert to 0.5–2 mg/kg prednisone/prednisolone orally each day or its equivalent only after a response. Consider concurrent empiric antiviral (IV acyclovir) and antibacterial therapy
Aseptic meningitis	Headache, photophobia, neck stiffness with fever or may be afebrile, vomiting; normal cognition/cerebral function (distinguishes from encephalitis)	
Other syndromes include neurosarcoidosis, posterior reversible leukoencephalopathy syndrome (PRES), Vogt-Koyanagi-Harada syndrome, demyelination, vasculitic encephalopathy, and generalized seizures		
Transverse myelitis	Acute or subacute neurologic signs/symptoms of motor/sensory/autonomic origin; most have sensory level; often bilateral symptoms	Initially withhold nivolumab, but permanently discontinue nivolumab if there is no doubt as to diagnosis. Administer 2 mg/kg IV (methyl)prednisolone or consider 1 g/day and convert to 0.5–2 mg/kg prednisone/prednisolone orally each day or its equivalent only after a response. When symptoms improve, begin a slow corticosteroid taper over at least 4–8 weeks. Plasmapheresis may be required if steroids do not bring about improvement
Myocarditis	G3	Permanently discontinue nivolumab. Administer 2 mg/kg IV (methyl)prednisolone or consider 1 g/day and convert to 0.5–2 mg/kg prednisone/prednisolone orally each day or its equivalent only after a response. When symptoms improve, begin a slow corticosteroid taper over at least 4–8 weeks. If no response, add MMF 500–1000 mg twice daily. If worse on MMF, consider adding tacrolimus
Peripheral neurologic toxicity	Moderate: some interference with ADL, symptoms concerning to patient	Withhold nivolumab. Initial observation reasonable or initiate prednisone/prednisolone 0.5–1 mg/kg (if progressing, eg, from mild) and/or pregabalin or duloxetine for pain. When symptoms improve, begin a slow corticosteroid taper over at least 4 weeks. Resume nivolumab upon symptom control, or when prednisone/prednisolone daily dose <10 mg
	Severe: limits self-care and aids warranted, life-threatening, eg, respiratory problems	Permanently discontinue nivolumab. Administer 1–2 mg/kg IV (methyl)prednisolone and convert to 0.5–2 mg/kg prednisone/prednisolone orally each day or its equivalent only after a response. Taper over at least 4–8 weeks when symptoms improve to G1
Guillain-Barré syndrome	Progressive symmetrical muscle weakness with absent or reduced tendon reflexes—involves extremities; facial, respiratory, bulbar, and oculomotor muscles; dysregulation of autonomic nerves	Permanently discontinue nivolumab. Use of steroids not recommended in idiopathic Guillain-Barré syndrome; however, a trial of (methyl)prednisolone 1–2 mg/kg is reasonable, converting to 0.5–2 mg/kg prednisone/prednisolone orally each day or its equivalent only after a response. If no improvement or worsening, plasmapheresis or IVIG indicated

(continued)

Treatment Modifications (*continued*)

Adverse Event	Grade/Severity	Treatment Modification
Myasthenia gravis	Fluctuating muscle weakness (proximal limb, trunk, ocular, eg, ptosis/diplopia or bulbar) with fatigability; respiratory muscles may also be involved	Permanently discontinue nivolumab. Administer pyridostigmine at an initial dose of 30 mg three times daily. Administer oral prednisone/prednisolone at a dose of 0.5 to 2 mg/kg/day or its equivalent or 1–2 mg/kg IV (methyl)prednisolone depending on the severity of symptoms. If begin with IV, convert to 0.5–2 mg/kg prednisone/prednisolone orally each day or its equivalent only after a response. If no improvement or worsening, plasmapheresis or IVIG may be considered. Additional immunosuppressants used in myasthenia gravis include azathioprine, cyclosporine, and mycophenolate. Avoid certain medications, eg, ciprofloxacin, beta-blockers, that may precipitate cholinergic crisis
	Other syndromes including motor and sensory peripheral neuropathy, multifocal radicular neuropathy/plexopathy, autonomic neuropathy, phrenic nerve palsy, cranial nerve palsies (eg, facial nerve, optic nerve, hypoglossal nerve)	Permanently discontinue nivolumab. Administer oral prednisone/prednisolone at a dose of 0.5 to 2 mg/kg/day or its equivalent or 1–2 mg/kg IV (methyl)prednisolone depending on the severity of symptoms. If begin with IV, convert to 0.5–2 mg/kg prednisone/prednisolone orally each day or its equivalent only after a response
Arthralgia	G1 (mild pain with inflammation, erythema, or joint swelling)	Continue nivolumab. Administer acetaminophen (paracetamol) and ibuprofen
	G2 (moderate pain with inflammation, erythema or joint swelling that limits ADLs)	Withhold nivolumab. Administer higher doses of acetaminophen (paracetamol) and ibuprofen and use diclofenac or naproxen or etoricoxib. If inadequately controlled, consider intra-articular steroid injections for large joints or administer oral prednisone/prednisolone at a dose of 0.5 to 2 mg/kg/day or its equivalent. When improves to G1, begin a slow corticosteroid taper over at least 4 weeks. If does not respond adequately, then administer 0.5–1 mg/kg IV (methyl)prednisolone and convert to 0.5–2 mg/kg prednisone/prednisolone orally each day or its equivalent only after a response, followed by a taper over at least 4 weeks when improves to G1. Resume nivolumab upon symptom control, or when prednisone/prednisolone daily dose <10 mg
	G3 (severe pain; irreversible joint damage; disabling; limits self-care ADL)	Withhold nivolumab. Administer 0.5–1 mg/kg IV (methyl)prednisolone and convert to 0.5–2 mg/kg prednisone/prednisolone orally each day or its equivalent only after a response, followed by a taper over at least 4 weeks when improves to G1. In severe cases, infliximab or another anti–TNF-alpha drug may be required for improvement of arthritis. Resume nivolumab upon symptom control, or when prednisone/prednisolone daily dose <10 mg
Other	First occurrence of other G3	Withhold nivolumab. Administer oral prednisone/prednisolone at a dose of 0.5 to 2 mg/kg/day or its equivalent. When improves to G1, begin a slow corticosteroid taper over at least 4 weeks. Resume nivolumab upon symptom control, or when prednisone/prednisolone daily dose <10 mg
	Recurrence of same G3	Permanently discontinue nivolumab. Administer 1–2 mg/kg IV (methyl)prednisolone and convert to 0.5–2 mg/kg prednisone/prednisolone orally each day or its equivalent only after a response. Taper over at least 4–8 weeks when symptoms improve to G1
	Life-threatening or G4	
	Requirement for ≥10 mg/day prednisone or equivalent for >12 weeks	Permanently discontinue nivolumab
	Persistent G2/3 adverse reactions lasting ≥12 weeks	

ADL, activities of daily living; ALT, alanine aminotransferase; AST, aspartate aminotransferase; ATG, anti-thymocyte globulin; SJS, Stevens-Johnson Syndrome; TEN, toxic epidermal necrolysis; ULN, upper limit of normal

Notes on general supportive care:
• Steroid taper in most cases will proceed over a minimum of 1 month but if symptoms improve rapidly, a 2-week taper can be considered. If steroids are administered for more than 4 weeks, consider PCP prophylaxis (cotrimoxazole 480 mg twice daily M/W/F or inhaled pentamidine if has cotrimoxazole allergy), regular random blood glucose, VitD level, and starting calcium/VitD supplementation per guidelines

Patient Population Studied

The CheckMate 040 study was a multicenter, international, non-comparative, open-label, phase 1/2 study evaluating nivolumab in patients with advanced hepatocellular carcinoma (with or without viral hepatitis). Patients in the dose-escalation phase and those in the dose-expansion phase who had viral hepatitis were required to have been previously treated with ≥1 line of therapy, including sorafenib. The dose expansion phase included 4 cohorts: sorafenib untreated or intolerant without viral hepatitis, sorafenib progressor without viral hepatitis, HCV infected, and HBV infected. The dose escalation phase included 48 patients and the dose expansion phase included 214 patients. Patients were required to have a Child-Pugh score of either ≤7 (dose-escalation phase) or ≤6 (dose-expansion phase), to not be candidates for curative resection or locoregional therapies, and to have an Eastern Cooperative Oncology Group performance status of ≤1. Patients with HBV were required to be taking effective antiviral therapy and to have a viral load <100 IU/mL. Patients who had previously received checkpoint inhibitor therapy were excluded. There was no maximum tolerated dose reached in the dose-escalation phase (doses ranged from 0.1 mg/kg to 10 mg/kg); the dose-expansion group was treated with a dose of 3 mg/kg every 2 weeks

Efficacy (N = 214, Expansion Phase of Trial)

Efficacy Variable	Uninfected, Untreated, or Intolerant (n = 56)	Uninfected Progressor (n = 57)	HCV Infected (n = 50)	HBV Infected (n = 51)	All Patients (n = 214)
Overall Survival (OS) and Progression-free Survival (PFS) *					
Median OS, months (95% CI)	NR	13.2 (8.6–NE)	NR	NR	NR
OS at 6 months, percentage (95% CI)	89 (77–95)	75 (62–85)	85 (72–93)	84 (71–92)	83 (78–88)
OS at 9 months, percentage (95% CI)	82 (68–90)	63 (49–74)	81 (66–90)	70 (55–81)	74 (67–79)
Median PFS, months (95% CI)	5.4 (3.9–8.5)	4.0 (2.6–6.7)	4.0 (2.6–5.7)	4.0 (1.3–4.1)	4.0 (2.9–5.4)
Response					
Best overall response*	n/N (%)				
Complete response (CR)	0/56	2/57 (4)	0/50	1/51 (2)	3/214 (1)
Partial response (PR)	13/56 (23)	10/57 (18)	10/50 (20)	6/51 (12)	39/214 (18)
Stable disease (SD)	29/56 (52)	23/57 (40)	23/50 (46)	21/51 (41)	96/214 (45)
Progressive disease (PD)	13/56 (23)	18/57 (32)	14/50 (28)	23/51 (45)	68/214 (32)
Not evaluable (NE)	1/56 (2)	4/57 (7)	3/50 (6)	0/51	8/214 (4)
	n/N (%) [95% CI]				
Objective response rate (ORR = CR + PR)	13/56 (23) [13–36]	12/57 (21) [11–34]	10/50 (20) [10–34]	7/51 (14) [6–26]	42/214 (20) [15–26]
Disease control rate (DCR = ORR + SD)	42/56 (75) [62–86]	35/57 (61) [48–74]	33/50 (66) [51–79]	28/51 (55) [40–69]	138/214 (64) [58–71]
Median DOR, months (95% CI)	8.4 (8.3–NE)	NR	9.9 (4.5–9.9)	NR	9.9 (8.3–NE)

*Based on RECIST version 1.1 criteria assessed by local investigators
HCV, hepatitis C virus; HBV, hepatitis B virus; CI, confidence interval; NR, not reported; NE, not estimable; DOR, duration of response
Note: Efficacy parameters included in the table are for patients in the dose-expansion phase (n = 214). In the dose-escalation phase, the ORR was 15% (95% CI, 6–28) with 3 patients achieving a CR and 4 patients achieving a PR, the DCR was 58% (95% CI, 43–72), the median time to progression was 3.4 months (95% CI, 1.6–6.9), the median DOR was 17 months (95% CI, 6–24), median OS was 15.0 months (95% CI, 9.6–20.2). Uninfected refers to not infected with hepatitis B or C. Intolerant refers to patients who were unable to tolerate sorafenib. The data cutoff date for this analysis was 8 August 2016

Adverse Events (N = 48, Dose Escalation Phase of Trial)

Grade (%)*	3 mg/kg (N = 10)		All Patients in All Levels of Dose Escalation Phase (N = 48)	
	Any Grade	Grade 3–4	Any Grade	Grade 3–4
Treatment-related serious AEs	0	0	3 (6%)	2 (4%)

(continued)

Adverse Events (N = 48, Dose Escalation Phase of Trial) *(continued)*

Grade (%)*	Any Grade	Grade 3–4	Any Grade	Grade 3–4
AEs leading to discontinuation	1 (10%)	1 (10%)	3 (6%)	3 (6%)
Treatment-related deaths	0	0	0	0
Patients with a treatment-related AE	9 (90%)	2 (20%)	40 (83%)	12 (25%)
Treatment-related AEs Reported in ≥5% of All Patients, Any Grade				
Rash	2 (20%)	0	11 (23%)	0
Pruritus	1 (10%)	0	9 (19%)	0
Diarrhea	1 (10%)	0	5 (10%)	0
Decreased appetite	0	0	5 (10%)	0
Fatigue	0	0	4 (8%)	1 (2%)
Asthenia	1 (10%)	0	3 (6%)	0
Weight decreased	0	0	3 (6%)	0
Nausea	1 (10%)	0	3 (6%)	0
Dry mouth	0	0	3 (6%)	0
AST increase	1 (10%)	1 (10%)	10 (21%)	5 (10%)
ALT increase	2 (20%)	1 (10%)	7 (15%)	3 (6%)
Lipase increase	2 (20%)	1 (10%)	10 (21%)	6 (13%)
Amylase increase	2 (20%)	1 (10%)	9 (19%)	2 (4%)
Anemia	0	0	4 (8%)	1 (2%)
Hypoalbuminemia	0	0	3 (6%)	0
Hyponatremia	0	0	3 (6%)	0

*Adverse events were graded according to the National Cancer Institute Common Terminology Criteria for Adverse Events (NCI CTCAE) v4.03
Note: The table includes data from patients enrolled in the expansion cohort
AE, adverse event; AST, aspartate aminotransferase; ALT, alanine aminotransferase

Therapy Monitoring

1. Initially at the time of each dose, and eventually every 6–12 weeks, perform a total-body skin examination with attention to *all* mucous membranes as well as a complete review of systems
2. Monitor patients for signs and symptoms of pneumonitis. Evaluate patients with suspected pneumonitis with chest x-ray, CT, and pulse oximetry. For ≥2 toxicity, may include nasal swab, sputum culture and sensitivity, blood culture and sensitivity, and urine culture and sensitivity
3. Monitor patients for signs and symptoms of colitis. Encourage patients to report diarrhea immediately to any member of the health care team
4. Draw AST, ALT, and bilirubin prior to each infusion and/or weekly if there are Grade 1 liver function test elevations. Note, no treatment is recommended for G1 LFT abnormalities. For ≥2 toxicity, work up for other causes of elevated LFTs including viral hepatitis
5. Use basic metabolic panel (Na, K, CO2, glucose) and patient history as screening tools for hypophysitis including hypopituitarism and adrenal insufficiency. If in doubt, evaluate AM adrenocorticotropic hormone (ACTH) and cortisol levels. Consider ACTH stimulation test for indeterminate results
6. Assess thyroid function at the start of treatment, periodically during treatment, and as indicated based on clinical evaluation, and for clinical signs and symptoms of thyroid disorders. Test for TSH and free thyroxine (FT4) every 4 to 6 weeks as part of routine clinical monitoring of therapy or for case detection in symptomatic patients
7. Measure glucose at baseline and with each treatment during the first 12 weeks and every 6 weeks thereafter
8. Obtain a serum creatinine prior to every dose. If creatinine is found to be newly elevated, consider holding therapy while other potential causes are evaluated. Note, routine urinalysis is not necessary other than to rule out urinary tract infections, etc
9. Obtain a complete rheumatologic history and perform an examination of all peripheral joints for tenderness, swelling, and range of motion. Examine the spine. Consider plain x-ray/imaging to exclude metastases and evaluate joint damage (erosions), if appropriate
10. In patients at high risk for infections and in appropriately selected patients based on an infectious disease evaluation, draw screening laboratories (HIV, hepatitis A and B, and blood QuantiFERON for TB) to prepare patients to start infliximab

UNRESECTABLE DISEASE • SUBSEQUENT THERAPY

HEPATOCELLULAR CARCINOMA REGIMEN: PEMBROLIZUMAB

Zhu AX et al. Lancet Oncol 2018;19:940–952
Supplementary appendix to: Zhu AX et al. Lancet Oncol 2018;19:940–952
KEYTRUDA (pembrolizumab) injection prescribing information. Whitehouse Station, NJ: Merck & Co., Inc; updated January 2020

Pembrolizumab 200 mg; administer intravenously over 30 minutes in a volume of 0.9% sodium chloride injection (0.9% NS) or 5% dextrose injection (D5W) sufficient to produce a pembrolizumab concentration within the range 1–10 mg/mL every 3 weeks for up to 24 months (total dose/3-week cycle = 200 mg)

Alternative pembrolizumab dose and schedule as per the U.S. FDA regimens approved on April 28, 2020:

Pembrolizumab 400 mg; administer intravenously over 30 minutes in a volume of 0.9% NS or D5W sufficient to produce a pembrolizumab concentration within the range 1–10 mg/mL every 6 weeks for up to 24 months (total dose/6-week cycle = 400 mg)

- Administer pembrolizumab with an administration set that contains a sterile, non-pyrogenic, low-protein-binding in-line or add-on filter with pore size within the range of 0.2–5 μm
- Pembrolizumab can cause severe or life-threatening infusion-related reactions, including hypersensitivity and anaphylaxis

Supportive Care
Antiemetic prophylaxis
Emetogenic potential is **MINIMAL**
See Chapter 42 for antiemetic recommendations

Hematopoietic growth factor (CSF) prophylaxis
Primary prophylaxis is **NOT** indicated
See Chapter 43 for more information

Antimicrobial prophylaxis
Risk of fever and neutropenia is **LOW**
  Antimicrobial primary prophylaxis to be considered:
  - Antibacterial—not indicated
  - Antifungal—not indicated

- Antiviral—not indicated unless patient previously had an episode of HSV

Treatment Modifications

RECOMMENDED DOSE MODIFICATIONS FOR PEMBROLIZUMAB

Adverse Event	Grade/Severity	Treatment Modification
Infusion reaction	Clinically significant but not severe infusion reaction	Interrupt the infusion in patients with clinically significant infusion reactions and consider resuming at a slower rate following resolution. If decision is made to restart, begin at ≤50% of the rate prior to the reaction and increase in 50% increments every 30 minutes if well tolerated. Infusions may be restarted at the full rate during the next cycle
	G3/4 (severe infusion reaction—pyrexia, chills, flushing, hypotension, dyspnea, wheezing, back pain, abdominal pain, and urticaria). Not rapidly responsive to brief interruption of infusion	Stop infusion and administer appropriate medical therapy (eg, epinephrine, corticosteroids, intravenous antihistamines, bronchodilators, and/or oxygen). Discontinue pembrolizumab
Colitis	G1	Loperamide 4 mg as starting dose then 2 mg before each meal and after each loose stool until without diarrhea for 12 hours, with maximum of 16 mg loperamide per day. If G1 diarrhea or colitis persists >14 days, then add prednisolone 0.5–1 mg/kg (non-enteric-coated) or consider oral budesonide 9 mg daily if no bloody diarrhea
	G2/3 diarrhea or colitis	Withhold pembrolizumab. Loperamide 4 mg as starting dose then 2 mg before each meal and after each loose stool until without diarrhea for 12 hours, with maximum of 16 mg loperamide per day. Administer oral prednisone/prednisolone at a dose of 0.5 to 2 mg/kg/day or its equivalent. When improves to G1, begin a slow corticosteroid taper over at least 4 weeks. Resume pembrolizumab upon symptom control, or when prednisone/prednisolone daily dose <10 mg

(continued)

Treatment Modifications (*continued*)

Adverse Event	Grade/Severity	Treatment Modification
	G4 diarrhea or colitis	Permanently discontinue pembrolizumab. Loperamide 4 mg as starting dose then 2 mg before each meal and after each loose stool until without diarrhea for 12 hours, with maximum of 16 mg loperamide per day. Administer 1–2 mg/kg IV (methyl) prednisolone and convert to 0.5–2 mg/kg prednisone/prednisolone orally each day or its equivalent only after a response. Taper over at least 4 weeks when symptoms improve. If does not improve over 72 hours or worsens, perform flexible sigmoidoscopy/colonoscopy to document colitis then begin infliximab 5 mg/kg (if no perforation/sepsis/TB/hepatitis/NYHA III/IV CHF). If no response, add MMF 500–1000 mg twice daily. If worse on MMF, consider addition of tacrolimus or ATG
Pneumonitis	G2	Withhold pembrolizumab. Consider pneumocystis prophylaxis depending on the clinical context and coverage with empiric antibiotics. Administer oral prednisone/prednisolone at a dose of 1–2 mg/kg/day or its equivalent. When improves to G1, begin a slow corticosteroid taper over at least 4 weeks. If does not respond adequately after 48 hours, then administer 2–4 mg/kg IV (methyl)prednisolone and convert to 0.5–2 mg/kg prednisone/prednisolone orally each day or its equivalent only after a response, followed by a taper over at least 6 weeks when symptoms improve to G1, titrating to symptoms. Resume pembrolizumab upon symptom control, or when prednisone/prednisolone daily dose <10 mg
	G3/4	Permanently discontinue pembrolizumab. Consider pneumocystis prophylaxis depending on the clinical context; cover with empiric antibiotics. Administer 2–4 mg/kg IV (methyl)prednisolone and convert to 1–2 mg/kg prednisone/prednisolone orally each day or its equivalent only after a response, followed by a taper over at least 8 weeks when symptoms improve to G1, titrating to symptoms. If, when initially treated, improvement does not occur within 48–72 hours, begin infliximab 5 mg/kg (if no perforation/sepsis/TB/hepatitis/NYHA III/IV CHF). If no response to infliximab, add MMF 500–1000 mg twice daily. Consider MMF especially if has concurrent hepatic toxicity
Hepatitis	G2 (AST or ALT >3–5× ULN or total bilirubin >1.5–3× ULN)	Withhold pembrolizumab. Administer oral prednisone/prednisolone at a dose of 1 to 2 mg/kg/day or its equivalent. When improves to G1, begin a slow corticosteroid taper over at least 4 weeks. Resume pembrolizumab upon symptom control, or when prednisone/prednisolone daily dose <10 mg
	G3/4 (AST or ALT >5× ULN or total bilirubin >3× ULN)	Permanently discontinue pembrolizumab. Administer 1–2 mg/kg IV (methyl) prednisolone and convert to 0.5–2 mg/kg prednisone/prednisolone orally each day or its equivalent only after a response. Taper over at least 6 weeks when symptoms improve. If no response, add MMF 500–1000 mg twice daily. If worse on MMF, consider adding tacrolimus or ATG
Hypophysitis	G2/3 (moderate symptoms, ie, headache but no visual disturbance or fatigue/mood alteration but hemodynamically stable, no electrolyte disturbance)	Administer analgesia as needed for headache. Withhold pembrolizumab. Administer oral prednisone/prednisolone at a dose of 0.5 to 2 mg/kg/day or its equivalent. When improves to G1, begin a slow corticosteroid taper over at least 4 weeks. If no improvement in 48 hours, administer 1–2 mg/kg IV (methyl)prednisolone and convert to 0.5–2 mg/kg prednisone/prednisolone orally each day or its equivalent only after a response. Taper over at least 4 weeks when symptoms improve to 5 mg prednisone/prednisolone or equivalent; do not stop steroids. Resume pembrolizumab upon symptom control, or when prednisone/prednisolone daily dose <10 mg
	G4 (severe mass effect symptoms, ie, severe headache, any visual disturbance or severe hypoadrenalism, ie, hypotension, severe electrolyte disturbance)	Permanently discontinue pembrolizumab. Administer analgesia as needed for headache. Administer 1–2 mg/kg IV (methyl)prednisolone and convert to 0.5–2 mg/kg prednisone/prednisolone orally each day or its equivalent only after a response. Taper over at least 4 weeks when symptoms improve to 5 mg prednisone/prednisolone or equivalent; do not stop steroids
Adrenal insufficiency	G2	Withhold pembrolizumab. Administer oral prednisone/prednisolone at a dose of 0.5 to 2 mg/kg/day or its equivalent. When improves to G1, begin a slow corticosteroid taper over at least 4 weeks. Serially assess adrenal function and continue steroids at replacement doses (20–40 mg hydrocortisone daily ~2/3 dose in AM upon awakening and ~1/3 at 4 PM) until recovery of adrenal function is documented. Resume pembrolizumab upon symptom control, or when prednisone/prednisolone daily dose <10 mg

(*continued*)

Treatment Modifications (continued)

Adverse Event	Grade/Severity	Treatment Modification
	G3/4	Permanently discontinue pembrolizumab. Administer oral prednisone/prednisolone at a dose of 0.5 to 2 mg/kg/day or its equivalent. When improves to G1, begin a slow corticosteroid taper over at least 4 weeks. Serially assess adrenal function and continue steroids at replacement doses (20–40 mg hydrocortisone daily ~2/3 dose in AM upon awakening and ~1/3 at 4 PM) until recovery of adrenal function is documented
Type 1 diabetes mellitus	G3 hyperglycemia	Withhold pembrolizumab. Admit to hospital to manage hyperglycemia. Role of corticosteroids in preventing complete loss of insulin-producing cells is unknown and not recommended. Resume pembrolizumab upon symptom control, or when prednisone/prednisolone daily dose <10 mg
	G4 hyperglycemia	Permanently discontinue pembrolizumab. Admit to hospital to manage hyperglycemia. Role of corticosteroids in preventing complete loss of insulin-producing cells is unknown and not recommended
Nephritis and renal dysfunction	G2/3 (serum creatinine 1.5–6× ULN)	Withhold pembrolizumab. Administer oral prednisone/prednisolone at a dose of 0.5 to 2 mg/kg/day or its equivalent. When improves to G1, begin a slow corticosteroid taper over at least 4 weeks. If does not respond adequately, then administer 0.5–1 mg/kg IV (methyl)prednisolone and convert to 0.5–2 mg/kg prednisone/prednisolone orally each day or its equivalent only after a response, followed by a taper over at least 4 weeks when improves to G1. Resume pembrolizumab upon symptom control, or when prednisone/prednisolone daily dose <10 mg
	G4 (serum creatinine >6× ULN)	Permanently discontinue pembrolizumab. Administer 0.5–1 mg/kg IV (methyl)prednisolone and convert to 0.5–2 mg/kg prednisone/prednisolone orally each day or its equivalent only after a response, followed by a taper over at least 4 weeks when improves to G1
Skin	G1/2	Continue pembrolizumab. Avoid skin irritants, avoid sun exposure, topical emollients recommended. Topical steroid (mild strength for G1, moderate/potent strength for G2) cream once or twice daily ± oral or topical antihistamines for itching
	G3 rash or suspected SJS or TEN	Withhold pembrolizumab. Avoid skin irritants, avoid sun exposure, topical emollients recommended. Administer oral or topical antihistamines for itching. Administer oral prednisone/prednisolone at a dose of 0.5–2 mg/kg or its equivalent daily for 3 days followed by a slow corticosteroid taper over at least 4 weeks when the rash improves to G1. If does not respond adequately, then administer 0.5–1 mg/kg IV (methyl)prednisolone and convert to 0.5–2 mg/kg prednisone/prednisolone orally each day or its equivalent only after a response, followed by a taper over at least 4 weeks when the rash improves to G1. Resume pembrolizumab upon symptom control, or when prednisone/prednisolone daily dose <10 mg
	G4 rash or confirmed SJS or TEN	Avoid skin irritants, avoid sun exposure, topical emollients recommended. Administer oral or topical antihistamines for itching. Administer 1–2 mg/kg IV (methyl)prednisolone and convert to oral steroids 0.5–2 mg/kg prednisone/prednisolone each day or its equivalent only after a response. Taper over at least 4 weeks when the rash improves to G1. Permanently discontinue pembrolizumab
Encephalitis	Confusion or altered behavior, headaches, alteration in Glasgow Coma Scale, motor or sensory deficits, speech abnormality, may or may not be febrile	Initially withhold pembrolizumab, but permanently discontinue pembrolizumab if there is no doubt as to diagnosis. Exclude bacterial and ideally viral infections prior to high-dose steroids. Administer oral prednisone/prednisolone at a dose of 0.5–2 mg/kg/day or its equivalent. When symptoms improve, begin a slow corticosteroid taper over at least 4–8 weeks. If symptoms are severe, administer 1–2 mg/kg IV (methyl)prednisolone and convert to 0.5–2 mg/kg prednisone/prednisolone orally each day or its equivalent only after a response. Consider concurrent empiric antiviral (IV acyclovir) and antibacterial therapy
Aseptic meningitis	Headache, photophobia, neck stiffness with fever or may be afebrile, vomiting; normal cognition/cerebral function (distinguishes from encephalitis)	
	Other syndromes include neurosarcoidosis, posterior reversible leukoencephalopathy syndrome (PRES), Vogt-Koyanagi-Harada syndrome, demyelination, vasculitic encephalopathy, and generalized seizures	
Transverse myelitis	Acute or subacute neurologic signs/symptoms of motor/sensory/autonomic origin; most have sensory level; often bilateral symptoms	Initially withhold pembrolizumab, but permanently discontinue pembrolizumab if there is no doubt as to diagnosis. Administer 2 mg/kg IV (methyl)prednisolone or consider 1 g/day and convert to 0.5–2 mg/kg prednisone/prednisolone orally each day or its equivalent only after a response. When symptoms improve, begin a slow corticosteroid taper over at least 4–8 weeks. Plasmapheresis may be required if steroids do not bring about improvement

(continued)

Treatment Modifications (*continued*)

Adverse Event	Grade/Severity	Treatment Modification
Myocarditis	G3	Permanently discontinue pembrolizumab. Administer 2 mg/kg IV (methyl)prednisolone or consider 1 g/day and convert to 0.5–2 mg/kg prednisone/prednisolone orally each day or its equivalent only after a response. When symptoms improve, begin a slow corticosteroid taper over at least 4–8 weeks. If no response, add MMF 500–1000 mg twice daily. If worse on MMF, consider adding tacrolimus
Peripheral neurologic toxicity	Moderate: some interference with ADL, symptoms concerning to patient	Withhold pembrolizumab. Initial observation reasonable or initiate prednisone/prednisolone 0.5–1 mg/kg (if progressing, eg, from mild) and/or pregabalin or duloxetine for pain. When symptoms improve, begin a slow corticosteroid taper over at least 4 weeks. Resume pembrolizumab upon symptom control, or when prednisone/prednisolone daily dose <10 mg
	Severe: limits self-care and aids warranted, life-threatening, eg, respiratory problems	Permanently discontinue pembrolizumab. Administer 1–2 mg/kg IV (methyl)prednisolone and convert to 0.5–2 mg/kg prednisone/prednisolone orally each day or its equivalent only after a response. Taper over at least 4–8 weeks when symptoms improve to G1
Guillain-Barré syndrome	Progressive symmetrical muscle weakness with absent or reduced tendon reflexes—involves extremities; facial, respiratory, bulbar, and oculomotor muscles; dysregulation of autonomic nerves	Permanently discontinue pembrolizumab. Use of steroids not recommended in idiopathic Guillain-Barré syndrome; however, a trial of (methyl)prednisolone 1–2 mg/kg is reasonable, converting to 0.5–2 mg/kg prednisone/prednisolone orally each day or its equivalent only after a response. If no improvement or worsening, plasmapheresis or IVIG indicated
Myasthenia gravis	Fluctuating muscle weakness (proximal limb, trunk, ocular, eg, ptosis/diplopia or bulbar) with fatigability; respiratory muscles may also be involved	Permanently discontinue pembrolizumab. Administer pyridostigmine at an initial dose of 30 mg three times daily. Administer oral prednisone/prednisolone at a dose of 0.5 to 2 mg/kg/day or its equivalent or 1–2 mg/kg IV (methyl)prednisolone depending on the severity of symptoms. If begin with IV, convert to 0.5–2 mg/kg prednisone/prednisolone orally each day or its equivalent only after a response. If no improvement or worsening, plasmapheresis or IVIG may be considered. Additional immunosuppressants used in myasthenia gravis include azathioprine, cyclosporine, and mycophenolate. Avoid certain medications, eg, ciprofloxacin, beta-blockers, that may precipitate cholinergic crisis
Other syndromes including motor and sensory peripheral neuropathy, multifocal radicular neuropathy/plexopathy, autonomic neuropathy, phrenic nerve palsy, cranial nerve palsies (eg, facial nerve, optic nerve, hypoglossal nerve)		Permanently discontinue pembrolizumab. Administer oral prednisone/prednisolone at a dose of 0.5 to 2 mg/kg/day or its equivalent or 1–2 mg/kg IV (methyl)prednisolone depending on the severity of symptoms. If begin with IV, convert to 0.5–2 mg/kg prednisone/prednisolone orally each day or its equivalent only after a response
Arthralgia	G1 (mild pain with inflammation, erythema, or joint swelling)	Continue pembrolizumab. Administer acetaminophen (paracetamol) and ibuprofen
	G2 (moderate pain with inflammation, erythema, or joint swelling that limits ADLs)	Withhold pembrolizumab. Administer higher doses of acetaminophen (paracetamol) and ibuprofen and use diclofenac or naproxen or etoricoxib. If inadequately controlled, consider intra-articular steroid injections for large joints or administer oral prednisone/prednisolone at a dose of 0.5 to 2 mg/kg/day or its equivalent. When improves to G1, begin a slow corticosteroid taper over at least 4 weeks. If does not respond adequately, then administer 0.5–1 mg/kg IV (methyl)prednisolone and convert to 0.5–2 mg/kg prednisone/prednisolone orally each day or its equivalent only after a response, followed by a taper over at least 4 weeks when improves to G1. Resume pembrolizumab upon symptom control, or when prednisone/prednisolone daily dose <10 mg
	G3 (severe pain; irreversible joint damage; disabling; limits self-care ADL)	Withhold pembrolizumab. Administer 0.5–1 mg/kg IV (methyl)prednisolone and convert to 0.5–2 mg/kg prednisone/prednisolone orally each day or its equivalent only after a response, followed by a taper over at least 4 weeks when improves to G1. In severe cases, infliximab or another anti–TNF-alpha drug may be required for improvement of arthritis. Resume pembrolizumab upon symptom control, or when prednisone/prednisolone daily dose <10 mg
Other	First occurrence of other G3	Withhold pembrolizumab. Administer oral prednisone/prednisolone at a dose of 0.5 to 2 mg/kg/day or its equivalent. When improves to G1, begin a slow corticosteroid taper over at least 4 weeks. Resume pembrolizumab upon symptom control, or when prednisone/prednisolone daily dose <10 mg
	Recurrence of same G3	Permanently discontinue pembrolizumab. Administer 1–2 mg/kg IV (methyl)prednisolone and convert to 0.5–2 mg/kg prednisone/prednisolone orally each day or its equivalent only after a response. Taper over at least 4–8 weeks when symptoms improve to G1
	Life-threatening or G4	

(*continued*)

Treatment Modifications (continued)

Adverse Event	Grade/Severity	Treatment Modification
	Requirement for ≥10 mg/day prednisone or equivalent for >12 weeks	Permanently discontinue pembrolizumab
	Persistent G2/3 adverse reactions lasting ≥12 weeks	

ADL, activities of daily living; ALT, alanine aminotransferase; AST, aspartate aminotransferase; ATG, anti-thymocyte globulin; SJS, Stevens-Johnson Syndrome; TEN, toxic epidermal necrolysis; ULN, upper limit of normal

Notes on general supportive care:
- Steroid taper in most cases will proceed over a minimum of 1 month but if symptoms improve rapidly, a 2-week taper can be considered. If steroids are administered for more than 4 weeks, consider PCP prophylaxis (cotrimoxazole 480 mg twice daily M/W/F or inhaled pentamidine if has cotrimoxazole allergy), regular random blood glucose, VitD level, and starting calcium/VitD supplementation per guidelines

Patient Population Studied

The KEYNOTE–224 trial was a non-randomized, open-label, phase 2 trial that included 104 adults with advanced hepatocellular carcinoma (HCC) previously treated with sorafenib and evaluated treatment with pembrolizumab. Patients were eligible for the trial if they had histologically or cytologically confirmed HCC, if they had documented radiographic progression after treatment with sorafenib or were intolerant to sorafenib, if they had Barcelona Clinical Liver Cancer Stage C or B disease that was not amenable to, or was refractory after, locoregional therapy or to a curative treatment approach, and if they had at least one measurable lesion, an ECOG performance status of ≤ 1, a predicted life expectancy of > 3 months, adequate organ function, and Child-Pugh class A liver disease. Patients were permitted to have chronic hepatitis C infection (treated or untreated) and were permitted to have hepatitis B infection if they were treated with antiviral therapy and had a viral load of <100 IU/mL. Selected exclusion criteria included CNS metastases, prior immunotherapy (anti-PD-1, anti-PD-L1, anti-PD-L2), prior systemic therapy for advanced HCC other than sorafenib, active autoimmune disease, a diagnosis of immunodeficiency, or systemic steroid therapy or other immunosuppressive therapy within 7 days of the first pembrolizumab dose

Efficacy (N = 104)

Efficacy Variable	Pembrolizumab (N = 104)
Response (n = 104)*	**n/N (%) [95% CI]**
Objective response rate	18/104 (17) [11–26]
Complete response	1/104 (<1)
Partial response	17/104 (16)
Stable disease	46/104 (44)
Progressive disease	34/104 (33)
Not assessable*	6/104 (6)
Disease control rate*	64/104 (62) [52–71]
Median time to response, months (IQR)	2.1 (2.1–4.1)
Median duration of response, months (range)	NR (3.1–14.6+*)
Duration of response of ≥9 months*	77%
Survival (n = 104)	
Median progression-free survival, months (95% CI)	4.9 (3.4–7.2)
PFS rate at 12 months, n/N (%) [95% CI]	29/104 (28) [19–37]
Median time to progression, months (95% CI)	4.9 (3.9–8.0)
Median overall survival, months (95% CI)	12.9 (9.7–15.5)
Overall survival rate at 12 months, n/N (%) (95% CI)	56/104 (54) [44–63]

*Not assessable means that patients had a baseline assessment, but no post-baseline assessment by the data cutoff date, including cases of discontinuation or death before the post-baseline scan. Disease control rate includes patients with CR, PR, or SD for ≥6 weeks. The + sign in DOR indicates that the patient with this DOR had no progressive disease at the time of the last assessment. DOR of ≥9 months was assessed in patients with a confirmed CR or PR as their best response and was derived using Kaplan-Meier methods for censored data. An exploratory analysis of response using irRECIST (immune-related RECIST) and mRECIST (modified RECIST) criteria generated similar results as the primary analysis using RECIST v1.1 criteria
CI, confidence interval; NR, not reached
Note: Of 105 patients enrolled, 104 received treatment (1 patient was enrolled in error and not treated) and were included in the analyses. Of these patients, 20% had discontinued sorafenib due to intolerance and 80% discontinued sorafenib due to disease progression. PFS and response were assessed by central imaging review according to RECIST v1.1 criteria. At a data cutoff date of 13 Feb 2018, the median follow-up time was 12.3 months (IQR, 7.6–15.1)

Adverse Events (N = 104)

Treatment-Related Adverse Events

Event	Pembrolizumab (N = 104)	
Grade* (%)	Grade 1–2	Grade 3–5†
Fatigue	17	4
Pruritis	12	0
Diarrhea	11	0
Rash	10	0
Nausea	8	0
Asthenia	7	0
Increased aspartate aminotransferase	7	7
Decreased appetite	6	<1
Myalgia	6	<1
Hypothyroidism	6	0
Increased alanine aminotransferase	5	4
Arthralgia	5	0
Maculopapular rash	5	0
Hyperbilirubinemia	3	2
Dyspnea	4	<1
Anemia	2	<1
Adrenal insufficiency	<1	2
Cardiac failure	0	<1
Diabetic metabolic decompensation	0	<1
Increased gamma-glutamyltransferase	0	<1
Hepatic vein thrombosis	0	<1
Gastric ulcer	0	<1
Hyperlipasemia	0	<1
Iron deficiency anemia	0	<1
Cholestatic jaundice	0	<1
Lichenoid keratosis	0	<1
Lung infection	0	<1
Mucosal inflammation	0	<1
Type 1 diabetes mellitus	0	<1
Generalized rash	0	<1
Vena cava thrombosis	0	<1
Ulcerative esophagitis	0	<1

(continued)

Therapy Monitoring

1. Initially at the time of each dose, and eventually every 6–12 weeks, perform a total-body skin examination with attention to *all* mucous membranes as well as a complete review of systems

2. Monitor patients for signs and symptoms of pneumonitis. Evaluate patients with suspected pneumonitis with chest x-ray, CT, and pulse oximetry. For ≥2 toxicity, may include nasal swab, sputum culture and sensitivity, blood culture and sensitivity, and urine culture and sensitivity

3. Monitor patients for signs and symptoms of colitis. Encourage patients to report diarrhea immediately to any member of the health care team

4. Draw AST, ALT, and bilirubin prior to each infusion and/or weekly if there are Grade 1 liver function test elevations. Note, no treatment is recommended for G1 LFT abnormalities. For ≥2 toxicity, work up for other causes of elevated LFTs including viral hepatitis

5. Use basic metabolic panel (Na, K, CO_2, glucose) and patient history as screening tools for hypophysitis including hypopituitarism and adrenal insufficiency. If in doubt, evaluate AM adrenocorticotropic hormone (ACTH) and cortisol levels. Consider ACTH stimulation test for indeterminate results

6. Assess thyroid function at the start of treatment, periodically during treatment, and as indicated based on clinical evaluation, and for clinical signs and symptoms of thyroid disorders. Test for TSH and free thyroxine (FT4) every 4 to 6 weeks as part of routine clinical monitoring of therapy or for case detection in symptomatic patients

7. Measure glucose at baseline and with each treatment during the first 12 weeks and every 6 weeks thereafter

8. Obtain a serum creatinine prior to every dose. If creatinine is found to be newly elevated, consider holding therapy while other potential causes are evaluated. Note, routine urinalysis is not necessary other than to rule out urinary tract infections, etc

(continued)

Therapy Monitoring
(continued)

9. Obtain a complete rheumatologic history and perform an examination of all peripheral joints for tenderness, swelling, and range of motion. Examine the spine. Consider plain x-ray/imaging to exclude metastases and evaluate joint damage (erosions), if appropriate

10. In patients at high risk for infections and in appropriately selected patients based on an infectious disease evaluation, draw screening laboratories (HIV, hepatitis A and B, and blood QuantiFERON for TB) to prepare patients to start infliximab

Adverse Events (N = 104) *(continued)*

*Graded according to the National Cancer Institute Common Terminology Criteria for Adverse Events (NCI CTCAE) v4.0
†There was 1 treatment-related G4 event (hyperbilirubinemia) and 1 treatment-related G5 event (ulcerative esophagitis); the remainder of the adverse events in this column were Grade 3
Note: Treatment-related adverse events (AEs) were included in the table if they were reported in ≥10% of patients (G1–2) or in ≥1 patient (G3–5). Dose interruption due to AEs occurred in 25%, with the most common reasons being increased aspartate aminotransferase (AST) (4%) or alanine aminotransferase (ALT) (3%), hypothyroidism (2%), and rash (2%). Treatment-related AEs were reported in 73% of subjects (47% of Grade 1–2, 26% of Grade 3–5). Severe treatment-related AEs were reported in 15% of subjects, the most frequent of which were increased AST (4%), increased ALT (2%), and adrenal insufficiency (2%). Study treatment discontinuation due to AEs occurred in 5% of subjects (1 patient each of adrenal insufficiency, increased AST and ALT, elevated bilirubin, cholestatic jaundice, and ulcerative esophagitis)

Immune-mediated Adverse Events of Any Attribution

Event	Pembrolizumab (N = 104)	
Grade (%)	Grade 1–2	Grade 3
At least 1 event	11	4
Hypothyroidism	8	0
Adrenal insufficiency	<1	2
Thyroiditis	2	0
Severe skin reaction	0	<1
Autoimmune colitis	<1	0
Colitis	<1	0
Hyperthyroidism	<1	0
Type 1 diabetes mellitus	0	<1
At least 1 immune-mediated hepatic event*	0	3

*Based on sponsor assessment. Includes 3 events initially reported as increased aspartate and alanine aminotransferases, which were determined to be immune-mediated hepatitis by the sponsor
Note: Immune-mediated adverse events of any attribution were included in the table in order of decreasing frequency. Adverse events were assessed and graded as described in the table footnote above. There were no reports of Grade 4 or 5 immune-mediated adverse events. There were no reported cases of flares of hepatitis B or C virus

UNRESECTABLE DISEASE • SUBSEQUENT THERAPY
HEPATOCELLULAR CARCINOMA REGIMEN: NIVOLUMAB + IPILIMUMAB

Yau T et al. J Clin Oncol 2019;37(suppl 15):4012
OPDIVO (nivolumab) prescribing information. Princeton, NJ: Bristol-Myers Squibb Company; revised March 2020
YERVOY (ipilimumab) prescribing information. Princeton, NJ: Bristol-Myers Squibb Company; revised March 2020

Induction phase (concurrent treatment with nivolumab and ipilimumab):

Nivolumab 1 mg/kg; administer intravenously over 30 minutes in a volume of 0.9% sodium chloride injection (0.9% NS) or 5% dextrose injection (D5W) not to exceed 160 mL and sufficient to produce a nivolumab concentration within the range 1–10 mg/mL on day 1, every 3 weeks for a maximum of 4 doses (total dosage/3-week cycle = 1 mg/kg)

- Administer nivolumab through an administration set that contains a sterile, non-pyrogenic, low-protein-binding in-line filter with pore size within the range of 0.2–1.2 μm.

- Nivolumab can cause severe infusion-related reactions

followed on the same day by:

Ipilimumab 3 mg/kg; administer intravenously over 30 minutes in a volume of 0.9% NS or D5W sufficient to produce an ipilimumab concentration within the range 1–2 mg/mL on day 1, every 3 weeks for a maximum of 4 doses (total dose/3-week cycle = 3 mg/kg)

- Administer ipilimumab through an administration set containing a sterile, non-pyrogenic, low-protein-binding in-line filter

Maintenance phase (single-agent nivolumab):

Note that the U.S. Food and Drug Administration (FDA)-approved maintenance regimens for hepatocellular carcinoma approved on March 10, 2020, include an option for a 240-mg fixed dose administered every 2 weeks and an option for a 480-mg fixed dose administered every 4 weeks; fixed dosing of nivolumab may only be used *after completion* of concurrent treatment with nivolumab and ipilimumab, thus:

Nivolumab 240 mg; administer intravenously over 30 minutes in a volume of 0.9% NS or D5W, not to exceed 160 mL and sufficient to produce a nivolumab concentration within the range 1–10 mg/mL, every 2 weeks until disease progression (total dosage/2-week cycle = 240 mg)

- Administer nivolumab through an administration set that contains a sterile, non-pyrogenic, low-protein-binding in-line filter with pore size within the range of 0.2–1.2 μm

- Nivolumab can cause severe infusion-related reactions

or

Nivolumab 480 mg; administer intravenously over 30 minutes in a volume of 0.9% NS or D5W not to exceed 160 mL and sufficient to produce a nivolumab concentration within the range 1–10 mg/mL, every 4 weeks until disease progression (total dosage/4-week cycle = 480 mg)

- Administer nivolumab through an administration set that contains a sterile, non-pyrogenic, low-protein-binding in-line filter with pore size within the range of 0.2–1.2 μm.

- Nivolumab can cause severe infusion-related reactions

Supportive Care
Antiemetic prophylaxis
Emetogenic potential with nivolumab ± ipilimumab is **MINIMAL**
See Chapter 42 for antiemetic recommendations

Hematopoietic growth factor (CSF) prophylaxis
Primary prophylaxis is **NOT** *indicated*
See Chapter 43 for more information

Antimicrobial prophylaxis
Risk of fever and neutropenia is **LOW**
Antimicrobial primary prophylaxis to be considered:
- Antibacterial—not indicated
- Antifungal—not indicated
- Antiviral—not indicated unless patient previously had an episode of HSV

Treatment Modifications

RECOMMENDED DOSE MODIFICATIONS FOR NIVOLUMAB AND IPILIMUMAB

Adverse Event	Grade/Severity	Treatment Modification
Infusion reaction	Clinically significant but not severe infusion reaction	Interrupt the infusion in patients with clinically significant infusion reactions and consider resuming at a slower rate following resolution. If decision is made to restart, begin at ≤50% of the rate prior to the reaction and increase in 50% increments every 30 minutes if well tolerated. Infusions may be restarted at the full rate during the next cycle
	G3/4 (severe infusion reaction—pyrexia, chills, flushing, hypotension, dyspnea, wheezing, back pain, abdominal pain, and urticaria). Not rapidly responsive to brief interruption of infusion	Stop infusion and administer appropriate medical therapy (eg, epinephrine, corticosteroids, intravenous antihistamines, bronchodilators, and/or oxygen). Discontinue nivolumab and ipilimumab
Colitis	G1	Loperamide 4 mg as starting dose then 2 mg before each meal and after each loose stool until without diarrhea for 12 hours, with maximum of 16 mg loperamide per day. If G1 diarrhea or colitis persists >14 days, then add prednisolone 0.5–1 mg/kg (non-enteric-coated) or consider oral budesonide 9 mg daily if no bloody diarrhea
	G2/3 diarrhea or colitis	Withhold nivolumab and ipilimumab. Loperamide 4 mg as starting dose then 2 mg before each meal and after each loose stool until without diarrhea for 12 hours, with maximum of 16 mg loperamide per day. Administer oral prednisone/prednisolone at a dose of 0.5–2 mg/kg/day or its equivalent. When improves to G1, begin a slow corticosteroid taper over at least 4 weeks. Resume nivolumab and ipilimumab upon symptom control, or when prednisone/prednisolone daily dose <10 mg
	G4 diarrhea or colitis	Permanently discontinue nivolumab and ipilimumab. Loperamide 4 mg as starting dose then 2 mg before each meal and after each loose stool until without diarrhea for 12 hours, with maximum of 16 mg loperamide per day. Administer 1–2 mg/kg intravenously (methyl)prednisolone and convert to 0.5–2 mg/kg prednisone/prednisolone orally each day or its equivalent only after a response. Taper over at least 4 weeks when symptoms improve. If does not improve over 72 hours or worsens, perform flexible sigmoidoscopy/colonoscopy to document colitis then begin infliximab 5 mg/kg (if no perforation/sepsis/TB/hepatitis/NYHA III/IV CHF). If no response, add MMF 500–1000 mg twice daily. If worse on MMF, consider addition of tacrolimus or ATG
Pneumonitis	G2	Withhold nivolumab and ipilimumab. Consider pneumocystis prophylaxis depending on the clinical context and coverage with empiric antibiotics. Administer oral prednisone/prednisolone at a dose of 1–2 mg/kg/day or its equivalent. When improves to G1, begin a slow corticosteroid taper over at least 4 weeks. If does not respond adequately after 48 hours, then administer 2–4 mg/kg intravenously (methyl)prednisolone and convert to 0.5–2 mg/kg prednisone/prednisolone orally each day or its equivalent only after a response, followed by a taper over at least 6 weeks when symptoms improve to G1, titrating to symptoms. Resume nivolumab and ipilimumab upon symptom control, or when prednisone/prednisolone daily dose <10 mg
	G3/4	Permanently discontinue nivolumab and ipilimumab. Consider pneumocystis prophylaxis depending on the clinical context; cover with empiric antibiotics. Administer 2–4 mg/kg intravenously (methyl)prednisolone and convert to 1–2 mg/kg prednisone/prednisolone orally each day or its equivalent only after a response, followed by a taper over at least 8 weeks when symptoms improve to G1, titrating to symptoms. If, when initially treated, improvement does not occur within 48–72 hours, begin infliximab 5 mg/kg (if no perforation/sepsis/TB/hepatitis/NYHA III/IV CHF). If no response to infliximab, add MMF 500–1000 mg twice daily. Consider MMF especially if has concurrent hepatic toxicity

(continued)

Treatment Modifications (*continued*)

Adverse Event	Grade/Severity	Treatment Modification
Hepatitis	G2 (AST or ALT >3–5× ULN or total bilirubin >1.5–3× ULN)	Withhold nivolumab and ipilimumab. Administer oral prednisone/prednisolone at a dose of 1–2 mg/kg/day or its equivalent. When improves to G1, begin a slow corticosteroid taper over at least 4 weeks. Resume nivolumab and ipilimumab upon symptom control, or when prednisone/prednisolone daily dose <10 mg
	G3/4 (AST or ALT >5× ULN or total bilirubin >3× ULN)	Permanently discontinue nivolumab and ipilimumab. Administer 1–2 mg/kg intravenously (methyl)prednisolone and convert to 0.5–2 mg/kg prednisone/prednisolone orally each day or its equivalent only after a response. Taper over at least 6 weeks when symptoms improve. If no response, add MMF 500–1000 mg twice daily. If worse on MMF, consider adding tacrolimus or ATG
Hypophysitis	G2/3 (moderate symptoms, ie, headache but no visual disturbance or fatigue/mood alteration but hemodynamically stable, no electrolyte disturbance)	Administer analgesia as needed for headache. Withhold nivolumab and ipilimumab. Administer oral prednisone/prednisolone at a dose of 0.5–2 mg/kg/day or its equivalent. When improves to G1, begin a slow corticosteroid taper over at least 4 weeks. If no improvement in 48 hours, administer 1–2 mg/kg intravenously (methyl)prednisolone and convert to 0.5–2 mg/kg prednisone/prednisolone orally each day or its equivalent only after a response. Taper over at least 4 weeks when symptoms improve to 5 mg prednisone/prednisolone or equivalent; do not stop steroids. Resume nivolumab and ipilimumab upon symptom control, or when prednisone/prednisolone daily dose <10 mg
	G4 (severe mass effect symptoms, ie, severe headache, any visual disturbance or severe hypoadrenalism, ie, hypotension, severe electrolyte disturbance)	Permanently discontinue nivolumab and ipilimumab. Administer analgesia as needed for headache. Administer 1–2 mg/kg intravenously (methyl)prednisolone and convert to 0.5–2 mg/kg prednisone/prednisolone orally each day or its equivalent only after a response. Taper over at least 4 weeks when symptoms improve to 5 mg prednisone/prednisolone or equivalent; do not stop steroids
Adrenal insufficiency	G2	Withhold nivolumab and ipilimumab. Administer oral prednisone/prednisolone at a dose of 0.5–2 mg/kg/day or its equivalent. When improves to G1, begin a slow corticosteroid taper over at least 4 weeks. Serially assess adrenal function and continue steroids at replacement doses (20–40 mg hydrocortisone daily ~2/3 dose in AM upon awakening and ~1/3 at 4 PM) until recovery of adrenal function is documented. Resume nivolumab and ipilimumab upon symptom control, or when prednisone/prednisolone daily dose <10 mg
	G3/4	Permanently discontinue nivolumab and ipilimumab. Administer oral prednisone/prednisolone at a dose of 0.5–2 mg/kg/day or its equivalent. When improves to G1, begin a slow corticosteroid taper over at least 4 weeks. Serially assess adrenal function and continue steroids at replacement doses (20–40 mg hydrocortisone daily ~2/3 dose in AM upon awakening and ~1/3 at 4 PM) until recovery of adrenal function is documented
Type 1 diabetes mellitus	G3 hyperglycemia	Withhold nivolumab and ipilimumab. Admit to hospital to manage hyperglycemia. Role of corticosteroids in preventing complete loss of insulin-producing cells is unknown and not recommended. Resume nivolumab and ipilimumab upon symptom control, or when prednisone/prednisolone daily dose <10 mg
	G4 hyperglycemia	Permanently discontinue nivolumab and ipilimumab. Admit to hospital to manage hyperglycemia. Role of corticosteroids in preventing complete loss of insulin-producing cells is unknown and not recommended

(*continued*)

Treatment Modifications (continued)

Adverse Event	Grade/Severity	Treatment Modification
Nephritis and renal dysfunction	G2/3 (serum creatinine 1.5–6× ULN)	Withhold nivolumab and ipilimumab. Administer oral prednisone/prednisolone at a dose of 0.5–2 mg/kg/day or its equivalent. When improves to G1, begin a slow corticosteroid taper over at least 4 weeks. If does not respond adequately, then administer 0.5–1 mg/kg intravenously (methyl)prednisolone and convert to 0.5–2 mg/kg prednisone/prednisolone orally each day or its equivalent only after a response, followed by a taper over at least 4 weeks when improves to G1. Resume nivolumab and ipilimumab upon symptom control, or when prednisone/prednisolone daily dose <10 mg
	G4 (serum creatinine >6× ULN)	Permanently discontinue nivolumab and ipilimumab. Administer 0.5–1 mg/kg intravenously (methyl)prednisolone and convert to 0.5–2 mg/kg prednisone/prednisolone orally each day or its equivalent only after a response, followed by a taper over at least 4 weeks when improves to G1
Skin	G1/2	Continue nivolumab and ipilimumab. Avoid skin irritants, avoid sun exposure, topical emollients recommended. Topical steroid (mild strength for G1, moderate/potent strength for G2) cream once or twice daily ± oral or topical antihistamines for itching
	G3 rash or suspected SJS or TEN	Withhold nivolumab and ipilimumab. Avoid skin irritants, avoid sun exposure, topical emollients recommended. Administer oral or topical antihistamines for itching. Administer oral prednisone/prednisolone at a dose of 0.5–2 mg/kg or its equivalent daily for 3 days followed by a slow corticosteroid taper over at least 4 weeks when the rash improves to G1. If does not respond adequately, then administer 0.5–1 mg/kg intravenously (methyl)prednisolone and convert to 0.5–2 mg/kg prednisone/prednisolone orally each day or its equivalent only after a response, followed by a taper over at least 4 weeks when the rash improves to G1. Resume nivolumab and ipilimumab upon symptom control, or when prednisone/prednisolone daily dose <10 mg
	G4 rash or confirmed SJS or TEN	Avoid skin irritants, avoid sun exposure, topical emollients recommended. Administer oral or topical antihistamines for itching. Administer 1–2 mg/kg intravenously (methyl)prednisolone and convert to oral steroids 0.5–2 mg/kg prednisone/prednisolone each day or its equivalent only after a response. Taper over at least 4 weeks when the rash improves to G1. Permanently discontinue nivolumab and ipilimumab
Encephalitis	Confusion or altered behavior, headaches, alteration in Glasgow Coma Scale, motor or sensory deficits, speech abnormality, may or may not be febrile	Initially withhold nivolumab and ipilimumab, but permanently discontinue nivolumab and ipilimumab if there is no doubt as to diagnosis. Exclude bacterial and ideally viral infections prior to high-dose steroids. Administer oral prednisone/prednisolone at a dose of 0.5–2 mg/kg/day or its equivalent. When symptoms improve, begin a slow corticosteroid taper over at least 4–8 weeks. If symptoms are severe, administer 1–2 mg/kg intravenously (methyl)prednisolone and convert to 0.5–2 mg/kg prednisone/prednisolone orally each day or its equivalent only after a response. Consider concurrent empiric antiviral (intravenous acyclovir) and antibacterial therapy
Aseptic meningitis	Headache, photophobia, neck stiffness with fever or may be afebrile, vomiting; normal cognition/cerebral function (distinguishes from encephalitis)	
Other syndromes include neurosarcoidosis, posterior reversible leukoencephalopathy syndrome (PRES), Vogt-Koyanagi-Harada syndrome, demyelination, vasculitic encephalopathy, and generalized seizures		
Transverse myelitis	Acute or subacute neurologic signs/symptoms of motor/sensory/autonomic origin; most have sensory level; often bilateral symptoms	Initially withhold nivolumab and ipilimumab, but permanently discontinue nivolumab and ipilimumab if there is no doubt as to diagnosis. Administer 2 mg/kg intravenously (methyl)prednisolone or consider 1 g/day and convert to 0.5–2 mg/kg prednisone/prednisolone orally each day or its equivalent only after a response. When symptoms improve, begin a slow corticosteroid taper over at least 4–8 weeks. Plasmapheresis may be required if steroids do not bring about improvement

(continued)

Treatment Modifications (continued)

Adverse Event	Grade/Severity	Treatment Modification
Myocarditis	G3	Permanently discontinue nivolumab and ipilimumab. Administer 2 mg/kg intravenously (methyl)prednisolone or consider 1 g/day and convert to 0.5–2 mg/kg prednisone/prednisolone orally each day or its equivalent only after a response. When symptoms improve, begin a slow corticosteroid taper over at least 4–8 weeks. If no response, add MMF 500–1000 mg twice daily. If worse on MMF, consider adding tacrolimus
Peripheral neurologic toxicity	Moderate: some interference with ADL, symptoms concerning to patient	Withhold nivolumab and ipilimumab. Initial observation reasonable or initiate prednisone/prednisolone 0.5–1 mg/kg (if progressing, eg, from mild) and/or pregabalin or duloxetine for pain. When symptoms improve, begin a slow corticosteroid taper over at least 4 weeks. Resume nivolumab and ipilimumab upon symptom control, or when prednisone/prednisolone daily dose <10 mg
	Severe: limits self-care and aids warranted, life-threatening, eg, respiratory problems	Permanently discontinue nivolumab and ipilimumab. Administer 1–2 mg/kg intravenously (methyl)prednisolone and convert to 0.5–2 mg/kg prednisone/prednisolone orally each day or its equivalent only after a response. Taper over at least 4–8 weeks when symptoms improve to G1
Guillain-Barré syndrome	Progressive symmetrical muscle weakness with absent or reduced tendon reflexes—involves extremities; facial, respiratory, bulbar, and oculomotor muscles; dysregulation of autonomic nerves	Permanently discontinue nivolumab and ipilimumab. Use of steroids not recommended in idiopathic Guillain-Barré syndrome; however, a trial of (methyl)prednisolone 1–2 mg/kg is reasonable, converting to 0.5–2 mg/kg prednisone/prednisolone orally each day or its equivalent only after a response. If no improvement or worsening, plasmapheresis or IVIG indicated
Myasthenia gravis	Fluctuating muscle weakness (proximal limb, trunk, ocular, eg, ptosis/diplopia or bulbar) with fatigability; respiratory muscles also may be involved	Permanently discontinue nivolumab and ipilimumab. Administer pyridostigmine at an initial dose of 30 mg three times daily. Administer oral prednisone/prednisolone at a dose of 0.5–2 mg/kg/day or its equivalent or 1–2 mg/kg intravenously (methyl)prednisolone depending on the severity of symptoms. If begin with intravenous, convert to 0.5–2 mg/kg prednisone/prednisolone orally each day or its equivalent only after a response. If no improvement or worsening, plasmapheresis or IVIG may be considered. Additional immunosuppressants used in myasthenia gravis include azathioprine, cyclosporine, and mycophenolate. Avoid certain medications, eg, ciprofloxacin, beta-blockers, that may precipitate cholinergic crisis
Other syndromes including motor and sensory peripheral neuropathy, multifocal radicular neuropathy/plexopathy, autonomic neuropathy, phrenic nerve palsy, cranial nerve palsies (eg, facial nerve, optic nerve, hypoglossal nerve)		Permanently discontinue nivolumab and ipilimumab. Administer oral prednisone/prednisolone at a dose of 0.5–2 mg/kg/day or its equivalent or 1–2 mg/kg intravenously (methyl)prednisolone depending on the severity of symptoms. If begin with intravenous, convert to 0.5–2 mg/kg prednisone/prednisolone orally each day or its equivalent only after a response
Arthralgia	G1 (mild pain with inflammation, erythema or joint swelling)	Continue nivolumab and ipilimumab. Administer acetaminophen (paracetamol) and ibuprofen
	G2 (moderate pain with inflammation, erythema or joint swelling that limits ADLs)	Withhold nivolumab and ipilimumab. Administer higher doses of acetaminophen (paracetamol) and ibuprofen and use diclofenac or naproxen or etoricoxib. If inadequately controlled, consider intra-articular steroid injections for large joints or administer oral prednisone/prednisolone at a dose of 0.5–2 mg/kg/day or its equivalent. When improves to G1, begin a slow corticosteroid taper over at least 4 weeks. If does not respond adequately, then administer 0.5–1 mg/kg intravenously (methyl)prednisolone and convert to 0.5–2 mg/kg prednisone/prednisolone orally each day or its equivalent only after a response, followed by a taper over at least 4 weeks when improves to G1. Resume nivolumab and ipilimumab upon symptom control, or when prednisone/prednisolone daily dose <10 mg

(continued)

Treatment Modifications (continued)

Adverse Event	Grade/Severity	Treatment Modification
	G3 (severe pain; irreversible joint damage; disabling; limits self-care ADL)	Withhold nivolumab and ipilimumab. Administer 0.5–1 mg/kg intravenously (methyl)prednisolone and convert to 0.5–2 mg/kg prednisone/prednisolone orally each day or its equivalent only after a response, followed by a taper over at least 4 weeks when improves to G1. In severe cases, infliximab or another anti–TNF-alpha drug may be required for improvement of arthritis. Resume nivolumab and ipilimumab upon symptom control, or when prednisone/prednisolone daily dose <10 mg
Other	First occurrence of other G3	Withhold nivolumab and ipilimumab. Administer oral prednisone/prednisolone at a dose of 0.5–2 mg/kg/day or its equivalent. When improves to G1, begin a slow corticosteroid taper over at least 4 weeks. Resume nivolumab and ipilimumab upon symptom control, or when prednisone/prednisolone daily dose <10 mg
	Recurrence of same G3	Permanently discontinue nivolumab and ipilimumab. Administer 1–2 mg/kg intravenously (methyl)prednisolone and convert to 0.5–2 mg/kg prednisone/prednisolone orally each day or its equivalent only after a response. Taper over at least 4–8 weeks when symptoms improve to G1
	Life-threatening or G4	
	Requirement for ≥10 mg/day prednisone or equivalent for >12 weeks	Permanently discontinue nivolumab and ipilimumab
	Persistent G2/3 adverse reactions lasting ≥12 weeks	

ADL, activities of daily living; ALT, alanine aminotransferase; AST, aspartate aminotransferase; ATG, anti-thymocyte globulin; SJS, Stevens-Johnson Syndrome; TEN, toxic epidermal necrolysis; ULN, upper limit of normal

Notes on general supportive care:
- Steroid taper in most cases will proceed over a minimum of 1 month but if symptoms improve rapidly, a 2-week taper can be considered. If steroids are administered for more than 4 weeks, consider PCP prophylaxis (cotrimoxazole 480 mg twice daily M/W/F or inhaled pentamidine if has cotrimoxazole allergy), regular random blood glucose, VitD level, and starting calcium/VitD supplementation per guidelines

Patient Population Studied

CheckMate 040 was a multicenter, multiple cohort, open-label trial evaluating nivolumab alone or in combination with other agents in patients with histologically confirmed advanced hepatocellular carcinoma who had progressed on or were intolerant to sorafenib. Patients were required to have Child-Pugh class A cirrhosis and were excluded if they had an active autoimmune disease, brain metastasis, a history of hepatic encephalopathy, clinically significant ascites, human immunodeficiency virus infection, or active infection with hepatitis B (HBV) virus and either hepatitis C (HCV) virus or hepatitis D virus (although patients with only active HBV or HCV infection were allowed to enroll). Arm A (n = 50) evaluated the administration of four 3-week cycles of induction therapy with the combination of ipilimumab 3 mg/kg plus nivolumab 1 mg/kg followed by maintenance therapy with single-agent nivolumab 240 mg administered every 2 weeks

Efficacy (N = 50)

Efficacy Variable	Nivolumab 1 mg/kg + Ipilimumab 3 mg/kg (N = 50)
Response*	**n/N (%)**
Objective response rate	16/50 (32)
Complete response	4/50 (8)
Partial response	12/50 (24)
Stable disease	9/50 (18)
Progressive disease	20/50 (40)
Disease control rate, % (95% CI)	54 (39–68)
Survival	
Median overall survival, months (95% CI)	23 (9–NA)
OS rate at 12 months, % (95% CI)	61 (46–73)
OS rate at 24 months, % (95% CI)	48 (34–61)

*Blinded independent central review per Response Evaluation Criteria in Solid Tumors (RECIST) v1.1
CI, confidence interval; NA, not available
Note: Data cutoff for this analysis was 25 Sep 2018
Yau T et al. J Clin Oncol 2019;37(suppl 15):4012

Adverse Events (N = 49)

Event	Nivolumab + Ipilimumab (N = 49)	
Grade (%)	All Grades	Grades 3–4
Adverse Reactions Occurring in ≥10% of Patients		
Rash	53	8
Pruritus	53	4
Musculoskeletal pain	41	2
Arthralgia	10	0
Diarrhea	39	4
Abdominal pain	22	6
Nausea	20	0
Ascites	14	6
Constipation	14	0
Dry mouth	12	0
Dyspepsia	12	2
Vomiting	12	2
Stomatitis	10	0
Cough	37	0
Dyspnea	14	0
Pneumonitis	10	2
Decreased appetite	35	2
Fatigue	27	2
Pyrexia	27	0
Malaise	18	2
Edema	16	2
Influenza-like illness	14	0
Chills	10	0
Headache	22	0
Dizziness	20	0
Hypothyroidism	20	0
Adrenal insufficiency	18	4
Weight decreased	20	0
Insomnia	18	0
Anemia	10	4
Influenza	10	2
Hypotension	10	0

(continued)

Therapy Monitoring

1. Monitor patients for signs and symptoms of infusion-related reactions including pyrexia, chills, flushing, hypotension, dyspnea, wheezing, back pain, abdominal pain, and urticaria

2. Initially at the time of each dose, and eventually every 6–12 weeks, perform a total-body skin examination with attention to *all* mucous membranes as well as a complete review of systems

3. Monitor patients for signs and symptoms of pneumonitis. Evaluate patients with suspected pneumonitis with chest x-ray, CT, and pulse oximetry. For ≥2 toxicity, may include nasal swab, sputum culture and sensitivity, blood culture and sensitivity, and urine culture and sensitivity

4. Monitor patients for signs and symptoms of colitis. Encourage patients to report diarrhea immediately to any member of the health care team

5. Draw AST, ALT, and bilirubin prior to each infusion and/or weekly if there are Grade 1 liver function test elevations. Note, no treatment is recommended for G1 LFT abnormalities. For ≥2 toxicity, work up for other causes of elevated LFTs including viral hepatitis

6. Use basic metabolic panel (Na, K, CO_2, glucose) and patient history as screening tools for hypophysitis including hypopituitarism and adrenal insufficiency. If in doubt, evaluate AM adrenocorticotropic hormone (ACTH) and cortisol levels. Consider ACTH stimulation test for indeterminate results

7. Assess thyroid function at the start of treatment, periodically during treatment, and as indicated based on clinical evaluation, and for clinical signs and symptoms of thyroid disorders. Test for TSH and free thyroxine (FT4) every 4–6 weeks as part of routine clinical monitoring of therapy or for case detection in symptomatic patients

8. Measure glucose at baseline and with each treatment during the first 12 weeks and every 6 weeks thereafter

9. Obtain a serum creatinine prior to every dose. If creatinine is found to be newly elevated, consider holding therapy while other potential causes are evaluated. Note, routine urinalysis is not necessary other than to rule out urinary tract infections, etc

(continued)

Therapy Monitoring
(continued)

10. Obtain a complete rheumatologic history and perform an examination of all peripheral joints for tenderness, swelling, and range of motion. Examine the spine. Consider plain x-ray/imaging to exclude metastases and evaluate joint damage (erosions), if appropriate

11. In patients at high risk for infections and in appropriately selected patients based on an infectious disease evaluation, draw screening laboratories (HIV, hepatitis A and B, and blood QuantiFERON for TB) to prepare patients to start infliximab

Adverse Events (N = 49) (continued)

Event	Nivolumab + Ipilimumab (N = 49)	
Grade (%)	All Grades	Grades 3–4
Select Laboratory Abnormalities Worsening from Baseline with ≥10% Incidence		
Lymphopenia	53	13
Anemia	43	4.3
Neutropenia	43	9
Leukopenia	40	2.1
Thrombocytopenia	34	4.3
Increased AST	66	40
Increased ALT	66	21
Increased bilirubin	55	11
Increased lipase	51	26
Hyponatremia	49	32
Hypocalcemia	47	0
Increased alkaline phosphatase	40	4.3
Increased amylase	38	15
Hypokalemia	23	4.3
Hyperkalemia	23	4.3
Increased creatinine	21	0
Hypomagnesemia	11	0

Note: other select clinically important adverse reactions reported in <10% of patients included hyperglycemia (8%), colitis (4%), and increased blood creatine phosphokinase (2%)

YERVOY (ipilimumab) prescribing information. Princeton, NJ: Bristol-Myers Squibb Company; revised March 2020

21. HIV-Related Malignancies

Kathryn Lurain, MD, MPH, Robert Yarchoan, MD, and Thomas S. Uldrick, MD, MS

HIV increases the risk of several cancers, including Kaposi sarcoma, aggressive B-cell non-Hodgkin lymphomas, classical Hodgkin lymphoma, HPV-associated cancers (eg, cervical, anal), lung cancer, and oropharyngeal cancer. As people with HIV are aging, incidental cancers also occur in this patient population. Oncologists should be aware of the principles of treating cancer in people living with HIV. Treating these patients requires a multidisciplinary approach that takes into account potential drug-drug interactions and appropriate supportive care. Antiretroviral therapy is almost always indicated, and prophylaxis against opportunistic infections is sometimes required. In general, cancers in people living with HIV should be treated in the same manner as HIV-negative patients, and HIV alone should not be used as a reason to offer less aggressive cancer therapy. Treatments for Kaposi sarcoma, Kaposi sarcoma herpesvirus-associated multicentric Castleman disease, and HIV-related lymphomas are discussed in detail in this chapter. ART is an essential part of the treatment of HIV, regardless of CD4+ T cell count, to reduce the morbidity and mortality of HIV infection. ART may be sufficient in treating many cases of HIV-KS. Guidelines for the use of antiretroviral therapy can be found at www.aidsinfo.nih.gov (U.S. Department of Health and Human Services).

Kaposi Sarcoma (KS)

Epidemiology of KS

Population	Incidence/100,000
United States, overall population, male	1.1*
United States, overall population, female	0.1
HIV-infected in United States in era of effective combination HIV therapy	168
Africa, male	39.3
Africa, female	21.8
HIV-infected in East Africa in era of effective combination HIV therapy	321

*Risk of KS is 4.5 times greater in African-American men than white men in the United States
Howlader N et al. SEER Cancer Statistics Review 1975–2014. Available at seer.cancer.gov [accessed June 2020]
Semeera A et al. Cancer Med 2016;5:1914–1928
Yanik EL et al. J Clin Oncol 2016;34:3276–3283

Pathology

1. All KS is caused by Kaposi sarcoma herpesvirus (KSHV), also called human herpesvirus 8 (HHV-8), a gamma-herpesvirus first identified in 1994
2. Pathology shows a highly vascular tumor with spindle-shaped cells that stain positive for KSHV latency-associated nuclear antigen (LANA)

Moore PS, Chang Y. N Engl J Med 1995;332:1181–1185

Work-up

1. Biopsy to confirm diagnosis
2. HIV serology, HIV viral load, and CD4+ T cell count
3. Assessment of tumor extent:
   - Physical examination of the skin, oral mucosa, and lymph nodes
   - CBC with differential, chemistry panel
   - Chest x-ray
   - Chest CT scan not routinely indicated unless x-ray is abnormal or patient reports respiratory symptoms
   - Fecal occult blood testing and endoscopic evaluation if positive or patient reports gastrointestinal symptoms

Staging (ACTG TIS Staging for Kaposi sarcoma herpesvirus)

Good Risk (0)	Poor Risk (1)
Tumor (T)	
Confined to skin and/or lymph nodes	Tumor-associated edema, infection, or ulceration Extensive/nodular oral KS Gastrointestinal KS KS in other nonnodal viscera
Immune System (I)	
CD4 cells >150/mm^3	CD4 cells <150/mm^3
Systemic Illness (S)	
• No history of opportunistic infection • No B symptoms present • Performance status >70 (Karnofsky scale)	• History of opportunistic infections • B symptoms present >2 weeks ■ (Fevers, night sweats, weight loss >10% of body weight) • Performance status <70 (Karnofsky scale) • Other HIV-related illness (eg, neurologic disease, lymphoma)
Good Risk Disease: T_0S_0, T_1S_0, T_0S_1	Poor Risk Disease: T_1S_1

Staging example:

A patient with KS restricted to the skin and a history of *Pneumocystis jirovecii* (formerly *P. carinii*) pneumonia would be T_0S_1

Notes:

1. In the ART era, baseline immune status (I) is relatively less important prognostically; however, patients with CD4+ T cell counts <100 cells/mm^3 remain at high risk for poor outcomes

2. In the ART era, poor prognosis is T_1S_1. All other stages are considered good prognosis

3. Pulmonary involvement portends the worst survival independent of tumor extension or systemic illness

4. Patients with KS may develop a KSHV-associated inflammatory cytokine syndrome (KICS), which is in part related to interleukin 6. The syndrome includes a constellation of symptoms (edema, respiratory symptoms, gastrointestinal symptoms, fevers), laboratory abnormalities (anemia, hypoalbuminemia, thrombocytopenia), evidence of inflammation (elevated c-reactive protein), and elevated KSHV viral load in blood or effusions. It is associated with a poor prognosis

Krown SE et al. J Clin Oncol 1997;15:3085–3092
Nasti G et al. J Clin Oncol 2003;21:2876–2882
Polizzotto MN et al. Clin Infect Dis 2016;62:730–738

Survival of HIV-Associated KS

Stage	3-Year Survival (%)
$T_0 S_0$	88
$T_1 S_0$	80
$T_0 S_1$	81
$T_1 S_1$	53

Nasti G et al. J Clin Oncol 2003;21:2876–2882

Expert Opinion

Kaposi sarcoma, as an HIV-presenting manifestation in ART-naïve patients, responds to ART in most cases with limited disease. Approximately 20–30% of patients with more advanced disease will have tumor regression with ART alone, but it may take 6–12 months or longer to see tumor regression. Not all patients have adequate disease control with ART despite an undetectable HIV viral load. KS-specific systemic therapy is generally required for extensive cutaneous lesions, tumor-associated edema, visceral disease, disease causing pain or ulcerations, or lesions on cosmetically sensitive areas, such as the face. Around 10% of patients experience progression of KS with the initiation of ART. This is referred to as KS immune reconstitution inflammatory syndrome (KS-IRIS) and is often an indication for systemic KS-directed therapy in addition to ART. KS may require urgent KS-specific systemic therapy if it is associated with excessive bleeding, lung compromise, locally problematic lesions (for example compromising the airways), or rapidly progressive cutaneous disease. Although some are FDA-approved, local therapies, such as radiation, intralesional chemotherapy, and surgery, are generally not useful in treating KS and should be used only to rapidly treat life-threatening lesions such as obstructive lesions involving the upper airway or urethra. Liposomal doxorubicin is usually the first-line choice for systemic treatment in addition to ART. It was compared with paclitaxel in a randomized clinical trial that showed similar efficacy between the two agents; however, paclitaxel had a higher rate of Grade 3 and 4 hematologic toxicities and sensory neuropathy. Therefore, paclitaxel is generally considered second-line therapy in patients who do not respond to liposomal doxorubicin or as first-line in areas where it is unavailable. The immune modulatory derivative of thalidomide, pomalidomide, showed good activity in a phase 2 trial and is now approved by the Food and Drug Administration for first-line treatment of HIV-associated KS that has not responded to ART. Immune modulatory therapy using interferon has some activity, especially in patients with higher CD4+ T cell counts; however, it is no longer used due to its side-effect profile and more effective available therapies. Systemic steroids may exacerbate KS and should be avoided when possible. Patients with KS not associated with HIV also may require systemic therapy, and the indications for treatment are similar to that of patients with HIV on effective ART

Cianfrocca M et al. Cancer 2010;116:3969–3977
Polizzotto MN et al. J Clin Oncol 2016;34:4125–4131

FIRST-LINE • SYSTEMIC

HIV-RELATED KAPOSI SARCOMA REGIMEN: DOXORUBICIN HCL LIPOSOME INJECTION (LIPOSOMAL DOXORUBICIN)

Cianfrocca M. Cancer 2010;116:3969–3977
Northfelt DW et al. J Clin Oncol 1998;16:2445–2451

Important to administer ART to all patients with HIV

Doxorubicin HCl liposome injection 20 mg/m^2; administer intravenously in 250 mL 5% dextrose injection over 60 minutes every 3 weeks (total dosage/cycle = 20 mg/m^2)

Premedication: Generally not required

Supportive Care
Antiemetic prophylaxis
Emetogenic potential: **LOW**
See Chapter 42 for antiemetic recommendations

Hematopoietic growth factor (CSF) prophylaxis
Secondary prophylaxis, if indicated with one of the following:
   Filgrastim (G-CSF) 5 mcg/kg per day by subcutaneous injection, *or*
   Pegfilgrastim (pegylated filgrastim) 6 mg/0.6 mL by subcutaneous injection for one dose
   • Begin use from 24–72 hours after myelosuppressive chemotherapy is completed
   • Most patients do not require growth factor support
See Chapter 43 for more information

Antimicrobial prophylaxis
Risk of fever and neutropenia is **LOW**
   Antimicrobial primary prophylaxis to be considered:
   • Antibacterial—not indicated
   • Antifungal—not indicated
   • Antiviral—not indicated unless patient previously had an episode of HSV
• Opportunistic infection prophylaxis, based on CD4+ T cell count

Hand-foot reaction (palmar-plantar erythrodysesthesia, PPE)
For patients who develop a hand-foot reaction, use topical emollients (eg, Aquaphor), topical or orally administered steroids, antihistamine agents (H$_1$-receptor antagonists), or pyridoxine. Pyridoxine may provide relief for discomfort/pain associated with PPE, although the mechanism through which this occurs remains unclear
   • The suggested pyridoxine starting dose is 50 mg/day, which may be increased to a maximum of 200 mg/day
   • Patients who develop G1/2 PPE while receiving doxorubicin HCl liposome injection may receive a fixed daily dose of pyridoxine 200 mg. This may allow for treatment to be completed without dosage reduction, treatment delay, or recurrence of PPE.

Oral care
Prophylaxis and treatment for mucositis/stomatitis
   General advice:
   • Evaluate patients for oral pain, oral KS, mucositis, and oral candidiasis
   • Consider histamine (H$_2$-subtype) receptor antagonists (eg, ranitidine, famotidine), or a proton pump inhibitor for epigastric pain
   Patients with intact oral mucosa:
   • Clean the mouth, tongue, and gums by brushing with an ultra-soft toothbrush with fluoride toothpaste
   • Patients may use saline or commercial bland, nonalcoholic rinses
   If mucositis or stomatitis is present:
   • Treat oral candidiasis if present using oral nystatin or fluconazole 100 mg daily for 7–14 days
   • Keep the mouth moist utilizing water, ice chips, sugarless gum, sugar-free hard candies, or a saliva substitute
   • Rinse mouth several times a day to remove debris
       ▪ Use a solution of ¼ teaspoon (1.25 g) each of baking soda and table salt (sodium chloride) in 1 quart (~950 mL) of warm water. Follow with a plain water rinse
       ▪ Do not use mouthwashes that contain alcohol
   • Advise patients who develop mucositis to:
       ▪ Choose foods that are easy to chew and swallow
       ▪ Take small bites of food, chew slowly, and sip liquids with meals

Patient Population Studied

In a trial of 258 patients pre-ART with advanced HIV-associated KS, patients were randomly assigned to either pegylated-liposomal doxorubicin 20 mg/m^2 or a doxorubicin, bleomycin, and vincristine (ABV) regimen. Both regimens were administered every 14 days for 6 cycles. A randomized controlled trial of 73 patients performed in the ART era compared pegylated-liposomal doxorubicin 20 mg/m^2 or paclitaxel 100 mg/m^2 every 14 days. The median number of cycles was 8. These studies were not limited to treatment-naïve patients, and improved response rates may be feasible in the first-line setting

Efficacy* (N = 133)

	Pre-ART era	ART Era
Complete response	1%	5%
Partial response	45%	41%
• Flattening of lesions	37%	—
• Decreased sum of products of largest perpendicular diameters	6%	—
• Reduced number and flattening of lesions	1%	—
• Reduced size and flattening of lesions	1%	—
Median time to progression	4.1 months	12.2 months
Median survival	5.3 months	Not reached

*Modified AIDS Clinical Trials Group

Treatment Modifications

Adverse Event	Dose Modification
Grade (G) 3 toxicity other than granulocytopenia	Delay treatment for up to 14 days
ANC <750/mm^3 on cycle day 1	Delay treatment until ANC recovers, G-CSF is indicated to support administration of therapy
Palmar-plantar erythrodysesthesia	Delay treatment. May require dosage reductions

Although Doxil (doxorubicin HCl liposome injection) product labeling indicates dose modifications for increased bilirubin, some protease inhibitors (eg, indinavir, atazanavir) cause a mild hyperbilirubinemia, in which cases dose adjustment may not be necessary

Notes

1. In ART era, 2-year overall survival after with liposomal doxorubicin is >75%
2. Chronic therapy may be required; patients responding to ART may have long-term progression-free survival and require fewer (eg, 4–6) cycles of chemotherapy

Toxicity (N = 133; 37)*,†

	Pre-ART % G3/4	ART Era % G3/4
At least one G3/4 toxicity	92	65
Hematologic		
Leukopenia‡	36	35
ANC <500/mm^3	6	—
Febrile with ANC <500/mm^3	0	2
Febrile neutropenia	—	7
Anemia	9.8	11
Thrombocytopenia	3	7
Septic episodes	6	11
Nonhematologic		
Nausea or vomiting	15	5
Mucositis/stomatitis	5	0
Peripheral neuropathy	6	2
Alopecia	1	—
Palmar-plantar erythrodysesthesia	4	2
Infusion-related reactions§	4.5	—
Cardiac ejection fraction decreased	2 patients	0
≥20% from baseline (n = 47)ᵉ	—	—

*WHO Criteria
†Percentage of patients experiencing G3/4 toxicity
‡44% received G-CSF or GM-CSF in Norfelt study
§Flushing, chest pain, dyspnea, difficulty swallowing, hypotension, back pain
ᵉOne death because of cardiomyopathy

Therapy Monitoring

1. *Before therapy:* CBC with differential, LFTs, BUN and serum creatinine, and cardiac ejection fraction
2. *Before each cycle:* CBC with differential, LFTs, BUN, serum creatinine, and response assessment
3. *Cumulative daunorubicin or doxorubicin dosage ≥500 mg/m^2:* Ejection fraction

FIRST-LINE • SYSTEMIC

HIV-RELATED KAPOSI SARCOMA REGIMEN: PACLITAXEL

Cianfrocca M. Cancer 2010;116:3969–3977
Gill PS et al. J Clin Oncol 1999;17:1876–1883
Welles L et al. J Clin Oncol 1998;16:1112–1121

Important to administer ART to all patients

Premedication: Primary prophylaxis against hypersensitivity reactions from paclitaxel:

Dexamethasone 20 mg; administer intravenously prior to paclitaxel (reduce to 8 mg if no hypersensitivity reactions occur during cycle 1), *plus:*

Diphenhydramine 50 mg; administer by intravenous injection 30 minutes before paclitaxel, *and:*

Ranitidine 50 mg or an equivalent dose of an alternative histamine (H_2) receptor antagonist; administer intravenously in 25–100 mL 0.9% sodium chloride injection (0.9% NS) or 5% dextrose injection (D5W) over 5–30 minutes, 30 minutes before paclitaxel

Paclitaxel 135 mg/m²; administer intravenously, in a volume of 0.9% NS or D5W sufficient to produce a concentration within the range of 0.3–1.2 mg/mL, over 3 hours every 21 days (total dosage/cycle = 135 mg/m²)

or

Premedication: Primary prophylaxis against hypersensitivity reactions from paclitaxel:

Dexamethasone 10 mg/dose for 2 doses; administer orally, 14 and 7 hours prior to paclitaxel, *plus*

Diphenhydramine 50 mg; administer by intravenous injection 30 minutes before paclitaxel, *and:*

Ranitidine 50 mg; administer intravenously in 25–100 mL 0.9% sodium chloride injection or 5% dextrose injection over 5–30 minutes, 30 minutes before paclitaxel

Paclitaxel 100 mg/m²; administer intravenously in a volume of 0.9% NS or D5W sufficient to produce a concentration within the range of 0.3–1.2 mg/mL, over 3 hours every 14–21 days (total dosage/cycle = 100 mg/m²)

Supportive Care

Antiemetic prophylaxis

Emetogenic potential: **MINIMAL**

See Chapter 42 for antiemetic recommendations

Hematopoietic growth factor (CSF) prophylaxis

Secondary prophylaxis, if indicated, with one of the following:

Filgrastim (G-CSF) 5 mcg/kg per day by subcutaneous injection, *or*

Pegfilgrastim (pegylated filgrastim) 6 mg/0.6 mL by subcutaneous injection for 1 dose

- Begin use from 24–72 hours after myelosuppressive chemotherapy is completed
- Most patients do not require growth factor support

See Chapter 43 for more information

Antimicrobial prophylaxis

Risk of fever and neutropenia is **LOW**

Antimicrobial primary prophylaxis to be considered:

- Antibacterial—not indicated
- Antifungal—not indicated
- Antiviral—not indicated, unless patient previously had an episode of herpes simplex virus
- Opportunistic infection prophylaxis, based on CD4+

Oral care

Prophylaxis and treatment for mucositis/stomatitis

General advice:

- Evaluate patients for oral pain, oral KS, mucositis, and oral candidiasis
- Consider histamine (H_2-subtype) receptor antagonists (eg, ranitidine, famotidine), or a proton pump inhibitor for epigastric pain

Patients with intact oral mucosa:

- Clean the mouth, tongue, and gums by brushing with an ultra-soft toothbrush with fluoride toothpaste
- Patients may use saline or commercial bland, non-alcoholic rinses

If mucositis or stomatitis is present:

- Treat oral candidiasis if present using oral nystatin or fluconazole 100 mg daily for 7–14 days
- Keep the mouth moist utilizing water, ice chips, sugarless gum, sugar-free hard candies, or a saliva substitute
- Rinse mouth several times a day to remove debris
  - Use a solution of ¼ teaspoon (1.25 g) each of baking soda and table salt (sodium chloride) in 1 quart (~950 mL) of warm water. Follow with a plain water rinse
  - Do not use mouthwashes that contain alcohol

(continued)

(*continued*)

- Advise patients who develop mucositis to:
  - Choose foods that are easy to chew and swallow
  - Take small bites of food, chew slowly, and sip liquids with meals

Efficacy

	Pre-ART era		ART era
	Welles et al	**Gill et al**	**Cianfrocca et al**
Paclitaxel dose	135 mg/m² every 3 weeks	100 mg/m² every 2 weeks	100 mg/m² every 2 weeks
Objective response rate (PR + CR)	71%	59%	55%
Median progression free survival	7.4 months	—	17.5 months
Median overall survival	13.9 months	15.4 months	53.6 months

Treatment Modifications

Adverse Event	Dose Modification
G4 hematologic toxicity	Decrease paclitaxel dosage by 25%

Saville MW et al. Lancet 1995;346:26–28

Cycle, day 1 ANC <1000/mm³, or platelet count <50,000/mm³	Delay treatment until ANC >1000/mm³, and platelet count >50,000/mm³
ANC <500/mm³ for 7 days	Reduce paclitaxel dosage by 20%
G1/2 peripheral neuropathy*	Reduce paclitaxel dosage by 20%
G3/4 peripheral neuropathy*	Discontinue therapy
Total bilirubin >3.0 mg/dL (>51.3 µmol/L)	Delay treatment until bilirubin <3.0 mg/dL (<51.3 µmol/L), then reduce dosage by 20%
Liver transaminases >5 times the upper limit of normal range	Delay treatment until liver transaminases <3 times the upper limit of normal, then reduce dosage by 20%

*Increased neuropathy reported when using stavudine

Gill PS et al. J Clin Oncol 1999;17:1876–1883

Patient Population Studied

Data from phase 2 trials with advanced KS in treated pre-ART, as well as a randomized controlled trial of 73 patients performed in the ART era, compared pegylated-liposomal doxorubicin 20 mg/m² or paclitaxel 100 mg/m² every 14 days. The median number of cycles was 8. Differences in response rates may be due in part to differences in proportion of treatment-naïve patients in a given study

Toxicity

	Pre-ART era		ART era
	%G1/2*	%G3/4	%G3/4
Hematologic			
Neutropenia†	33	61	37
Anemia	45	27	5
Thrombocytopenia	25	6	3
Nonhematologic			
Alopecia	78	9	—
Fatigue	50	25	5
Rash ± pruritus	9	0	2
Myalgia	21	16	2
Nausea/vomiting	57	13	2
Diarrhea	57	16	0
Neuropathy	45	2	2
Mucositis	18	2	2
Elevated AST	35	5	2

*Includes patients with unknown grades

Cianfrocca M. Cancer 2010;116:3969–3977
Gill PS et al. J Clin Oncol 1999;17:1876–1883
Welles L et al. J Clin Oncol 1998;16:1112–1121

Therapy Monitoring

Before each cycle: CBC with differential, LFTs, BUN, serum creatinine, and physical examination with careful attention to peripheral nerves

Notes

1. Chronic therapy may be required

SUBSEQUENT THERAPY • SYSTEMIC
HIV-RELATED KAPOSI SARCOMA REGIMEN: POMALIDOMIDE

Polizzotto MN et al. J Clin Oncol 2016;34:4125–4131

Pomalidomide 5 mg/dose; administer orally, once daily, without regard to food, for 21 consecutive days on days 1–21, followed by 7 days without treatment, every 28 days until complete response, progressive disease, unacceptable side effects, or for a maximum of 12 months (total dose/4-week cycle = 105 mg)

Notes:

- Patients who delay taking pomalidomide at a regularly scheduled time may take a missed dose if the interval remaining before the next regularly scheduled dose is ≥12 hours

- Do not break, chew, or open pomalidomide capsules

- Women of childbearing potential must not become pregnant while taking pomalidomide, and for at least 4 weeks following the last dose, due to the risk of severe birth defects. Either abstinence from heterosexual contact must be practiced, or at least 2 forms of reliable birth control must be utilized

- Men taking pomalidomide must wear a synthetic or latex condom during sexual contact with a woman of childbearing potential, and must avoid sperm donation during pomalidomide therapy and for at least 4 weeks after discontinuation

- Pomalidomide exposure is reduced in smokers; encourage patients to quit smoking during pomalidomide treatment

- If possible, avoid concomitant use of strong CYP1A2 inhibitors (eg, fluvoxamine, ciprofloxacin). If patients must receive a strong CYP1A2 inhibitor concomitantly, reduce the pomalidomide dose by approximately 50%. If coadministration of the strong inhibitor is discontinued, the pomalidomide dose should be returned to the dose used prior to initiation of a strong CYP1A2 inhibitor

Supportive Care
Antiemetic prophylaxis
Emetogenic potential is **MINIMAL**
See Chapter 39 for antiemetic recommendations

Hematopoietic growth factor (CSF) prophylaxis
Primary prophylaxis is **NOT** indicated
See Chapter 43 for more information

Antimicrobial prophylaxis
Risk of fever and neutropenia is **LOW**
  Antimicrobial primary prophylaxis to be considered:
  - Opportunistic infection prophylaxis, based on CD4+ T cell count (aidsinfo.nih.gov/contentfiles/lvguidelines/adult_oi.pdf [accessed 1 June 2018])
  - Antibacterial—*Pneumocystis jirovecii* prophylaxis may be recommended (eg, cotrimoxazole), depending on CD4 count as per HIV guidelines
  - Antifungal—not indicated
  - Antiviral— not indicated

Thromboprophylaxis
  Aspirin 81–325 mg daily is indicated

Patient Population Studied

The single-center phase 1/2 study included 15 HIV-positive patients with pathologically confirmed, symptomatic KS. Eligible patients had an Eastern Cooperative Oncology Group (ECOG) performance status score ≤2 and life expectancy ≥6 months, had at least five evaluable cutaneous lesions, and had to have been receiving ART with controlled HIV viral load for ≥2 months with progressive KS or ≥3 months without regression. Patients with symptomatic visceral KS, concurrent malignancies not in remission for ≥1 year, previous thromboembolic disease, or procoagulant disorders were not eligible. All patients received oral pomalidomide (5 mg) once daily for days 1–21 of a 28-day cycle and aspirin (81 mg) once daily. Pomalidomide was continued for up to 12 months, or until complete response, progressive disease, unacceptable adverse events, non-adherence, or patient withdrawal of consent.

Efficacy (N = 15)

Overall response rate*	60%
Median time to response	8 weeks (95% CI 4–32)

*Overall response rate is the percentage of patients who experienced a partial or complete response to the study drug

Therapy Monitoring

1. *Before the start of therapy:* CBC with differential, LFTs, BUN, serum creatinine, KSHV viral load
2. *Before each cycle:* CBC with differential, LFTs, BUN, serum creatinine, and response assessment
3. Deep venous thrombosis (DVT) and pulmonary embolism (PE) occur in patients with multiple myeloma treated with pomalidomide. Monitor for DVT and PE
4. *Response assessment:* Cutaneous KS measurement every 1–3 months. Imaging every 1–3 months if visceral KS

Treatment Modifications

POMALIDOMIDE

Note: Because of the embryo-fetal risk, pomalidomide is available only through a restricted program under a Risk Evaluation and Mitigation Strategy (REMS) called "POMALYST REMS"

Adverse Event	Treatment Modification
First occurrence of ANC <500/mm^3 and/or platelet count between 25,000/mm^3 and 50,000/mm^3 at start of a new cycle	Withhold start of cycle until ANC ≥500/mm^3, and platelet count ≥50,000/mm^3, then resume pomalidomide at the same dose
Recurrence of ANC <500/mm^3 or platelet count between 25,000/mm^3 and 50,000/mm^3 at start of a subsequent cycle	Withhold start of cycle until ANC ≥500/mm^3, and platelet count ≥50,000/mm^3 and then resume pomalidomide reduced by 1 mg/dose
Febrile neutropenia (fever ≥38.5°C and ANC <500/mm^3) or severe infection during a cycle	Withhold pomalidomide. When ANC ≥500/mm^3 and infection adequately controlled, resume pomalidomide reduced by 2 mg/dose
Platelet count <25,000/mm^3 at start of a new cycle	Withhold start of cycle until ANC ≥500/mm^3, and platelet count ≥50,000/mm^3, then resume pomalidomide reduced by 1 mg/dose
Any recurrence of platelet count <25,000/mm^3 at start of a subsequent cycle	Withhold start of cycle until ANC ≥500/mm^3, and platelet count ≥50,000/mm^3, then resume pomalidomide reduced by 1 mg/dose
ANC <500/mm^3 or platelet count <25,000/mm^3 occurring *within* a pomalidomide cycle	Hold pomalidomide until ANC >500/mm^3 and platelet count >50,000/mm^3, then resume pomalidomide reduced by 1 mg/dose
ANC <500/mm^3 or platelet count <25,000/mm^3 at any time while on a pomalidomide dose of 1 mg daily	Discontinue pomalidomide
Any other G3/4 adverse event at start of a new cycle or at any time during a cycle	Withhold pomalidomide and restart treatment reduced by 1 mg/dose less than the previous dose when toxicity has resolved to ≤G2 at the physician's discretion
Patients considered to be at higher risk of deep venous thrombosis (DVT) or pulmonary embolism (PE)	Consider anti-coagulation prophylaxis after an assessment of each patient's underlying risk factors

Note: Pomalidomide is a thalidomide analogue and is contraindicated in pregnancy. Thalidomide is a known human teratogen that causes severe life-threatening birth defects. For females of reproductive potential exclude pregnancy before start of treatment and prevent pregnancy during treatment by the use of two reliable methods of contraception

Adverse Events (N = 22; 15 with HIV and 7 without HIV)

Grade (%)*	Grade 1	Grade 2	Grade 3	Grade 4
Neutropenia	59	77	45	9
Rash	64	23	0	0
Constipation	73	5	0	0
Anemia	50	9	0	0
Thrombocytopenia	59	0	0	0
Fatigue	41	9	0	0
Lymphocytopenia	45	5	0	0
Elevated alanine aminotransferase level	32	0	0	0
Edema	9	5	5	0

Grade (%)*	Grade 1	Grade 2	Grade 3	Grade 4
Hypothyroidism	5	14	0	0
Infection	0	9	5	0
Fever	9	5	0	0
Impaired concentration	14	0	0	0
Anxiety	0	5	0	0
Depression	0	5	0	0

*According to the National Cancer Institute Common Terminology Criteria for Adverse Events, version 4.0

Note: Toxicities are included in the table if the events were grade ≥2 and were deemed to be possibly related to the study treatment, or if the possibly-treatment-related events were Grade 1 and occurred in ≥10% of cycles

Kaposi Sarcoma Herpesvirus-Associated Multicentric Castleman Disease (KSHV-MCD)

This is a rare, polyclonal B-cell lymphoproliferative disorder caused by KSHV with flares of inflammatory symptoms, edema, cytopenias, hypoalbuminemia, lymphadenopathy, and splenomegaly. Symptoms are caused by excess inflammatory cytokines, especially human interleukin 6 (IL-6) and interleukin 10 (IL-10) along with viral interleukin 6 (vIL-6). KSHV-associated multicentric Castleman disease is most frequent in people living with HIV but people infected with KSHV, such as men who have sex with men or people living in areas of the world with high KSHV seroprevalence, also are at risk.

Epidemiology

- Approximately 4.3 cases per 10,000 person-years in HIV-positive patients. Incidence may be increasing in ART era
- Often occurs in patients with controlled HIV and preserved CD4+ T cell counts
- Likely underdiagnosed in sub-Saharan Africa where seroprevalence of KSHV is 40–80% in adults
- Patients often have concurrent Kaposi sarcoma and are at high risk of developing non-Hodgkin lymphoma
- Survival <2 years without treatment

Bower M et al. J Clin Oncol 2011;29:2481–2486
Gao SJ et al. Nat Med 1996;2:925–928
Powles T et al. Ann Oncol 2009;20:775–779

Pathology

1. Kaposi sarcoma herpesvirus (KSHV), a gamma-herpesvirus, is the causative agent
2. Pathology shows polyclonal proliferation of KSHV-infected plasmablasts in the mantle zone of KSHV-MCD-involved lymph node follicles
3. KSHV-infected plasmablasts stain positive for KSHV-associated latent nuclear antigen 1 (LANA-1) and often for vIL-6. Some also express other KSHV lytic genes
4. KSHV-infected plasmablasts have a polyclonal pattern of Ig gene rearrangement and express λ light chain–restricted IgM. KS is often seen in the same lymph node

Dupin N et al. Blood 2000;95:1406–1412
Wang HW et al. Semin Diagn Pathol 2016;33:294–306

Work-up

1. Clinical suspicion in patients with fatigue, fevers, night sweats, weight loss, volume overload, rashes, and nonspecific neurologic, sinus, respiratory, and gastrointestinal symptoms, as well as unexplained cytopenias and hypoalbuminemia, especially if they have other KSHV-associated disease (eg, KS). Symptoms may be intermittent
2. Complete blood count with differential, chemistries, albumin, immunoglobulins, C-reactive protein, HIV antibody (if HIV status unknown), HIV viral load, CD4+ T cell count, KSHV viral load
3. Lymph node biopsy (excisional preferred)
4. CT scans of neck, chest, abdomen, and pelvis ± ^{18}FDG PET
5. Skin biopsy if cutaneous KS is suspected
6. All effusions should be sampled and undergo cytopathologic review to rule out concurrent primary effusion lymphoma

Definition of MCD Flare

Fever

At least 3 of the following:
  Peripheral lymphadenopathy
  Enlarged spleen
  Edema
  Pleural effusion
  Ascites
  Cough
  Nasal obstruction
  Xerostomia
  Rash
  Central neurologic symptoms
  Jaundice
  Autoimmune hemolytic anemia

Increased C-reactive protein >20 mg/L

Gérard L et al. J Clin Oncol 2007;25:3350–3356

(*continued*)

Work-up (continued)

NCI KSHV-MCD Modified Clinical Benefit Criteria

Eight Indicator Abnormalities Assessed in Responses

Symptoms
Fevers (includes chills and rigors)
Fatigue (includes lethargy)
Gastrointestinal (includes nausea and anorexia)
Respiratory (includes airway hyperreactivity and cough)

Laboratory abnormalities
Elevated C-reactive protein
Thrombocytopenia
Anemia
Hypoalbuminemia

Note: Assessment of disease activity and treatment response based on assessment of indicator clinical abnormalities that are probably or definitely attributable to KSHV-MCD at each evaluation

Uldrick TS et al. Blood 2014;124:3544–3552

Expert Opinion

KSHV-MCD requires a high level of suspicion on the part of the clinician, as symptoms may overlap with the symptoms of uncontrolled HIV infection, Hodgkin lymphoma, or non-Hodgkin lymphoma. Patients with KSHV-MCD should receive individualized treatment based upon symptoms and laboratory abnormalities. Patients should not be treated based upon radiographic abnormalities alone. For mild disease, weekly rituximab is recommended. In more severe disease or in patients with concurrent KS, rituximab plus liposomal doxorubicin should be considered. Treatment should be continued until resolution of symptoms and improvement in the following laboratory abnormalities: hemoglobin, platelets, albumin, and CRP. If possible, monitoring KSHV viral load is helpful in following patients. There is no role for maintenance therapy in KSHV-MCD. A combination of high-dose zidovudine plus valganciclovir also can have activity but is associated with more relapses and is not frequently utilized

Duration of therapy also should be symptom-based. There are no consensus guidelines for treatment response in KSHV-MCD. The CastlemaB trial defined criteria for an MCD attack warranting treatment as the presence of fever, elevated CRP, and presence of three clinical symptoms. The National Cancer Institute (NCI) criteria for treatment include at least one clinical symptom; the presence of anemia, thrombocytopenia, or hypoalbuminemia; and an elevated CRP. Treatment is continued until resolution of clinical symptoms and significant improvement in marker laboratory abnormalities

FIRST-LINE*

HIV-RELATED KAPOSI SARCOMA HERPESVIRUS-ASSOCIATED MULTICENTRIC CASTLEMAN DISEASE (KSHV-MCD) REGIMEN: RITUXIMAB

Bower M et al. Ann Intern Med 2007;147:836–839
Gérard L et al. J Clin Oncol 2007;25:3350–3356

Important to administer ART to all HIV-positive patients

Premedications for rituximab

Acetaminophen 650–1000 mg; administer orally 30–60 minutes before starting rituximab, *plus:*

Diphenhydramine 25–50 mg; administer orally or intravenously 30–60 minutes before starting rituximab

Rituximab 375 mg/m^2 per dose; administer intravenously in 0.9% sodium chloride injection (0.9% NS) or 5% dextrose injection (D5W), diluted to a concentration within the range 1–4 mg/mL, once weekly for 4 weeks (total dosage/4-week course = 1500 mg/m^2)

Rituximab administration:

- Infuse initially at 50 mg/hour. If hypersensitivity or infusion reactions do not occur during the first 30 minutes, increase the rate by 50 mg/hour every 30 minutes as tolerated to a maximum rate of 400 mg/hour. During subsequent treatments if previous rituximab administration was well tolerated, start at 100 mg/hour and increase by 100 mg/hour every 30 minutes as tolerated to a maximum rate of 400 mg/hour

- Infusion reactions are common during the first administration. Management includes interruption of rituximab administration for fever, chills, edema, congestion of the head and neck mucosa, hypertension, and other serious adverse events. Resume rituximab administration after adverse events abate. (See Treatment Modifications table)

Supportive Care

Antiemetic prophylaxis
Emetogenic potential: **MINIMAL**
See Chapter 39 for antiemetic recommendations

Hematopoietic growth factor (CSF) prophylaxis
Primary prophylaxis is **NOT** *indicated*
See Chapter 43 for more information

Antimicrobial prophylaxis
Risk of fever and neutropenia is **LOW**
  Antimicrobial primary prophylaxis to be considered:
  - Opportunistic infection prophylaxis, based on CD4+ T cell count (aidsinfo.nih.gov/contentfiles/lvguidelines/adult_oi.pdf [accessed 1 June 2018])

  - Antibacterial—not indicated

  - Antifungal—not indicated

  - Antiviral—not indicated unless patient previously had an episode of HSV

Risk of reactivation of viral hepatitis with rituximab administration

- All patients should be tested for active or previous exposure to hepatitis B and C prior to receiving rituximab.

- Providers should ensure patients with active previous exposure to hepatitis B or C are receiving appropriate prophylaxis or treatment prior to initiation of rituximab

- Carriers of hepatitis B receiving rituximab should be on antiretroviral therapy with an NRTI base containing two agents with activity against HBV

Patient Population Studied

The prospective, multicenter, open-label, phase 2 trial by Gérard et al (ARNS 117 CastlemaB trial) involved 24 patients with HIV-associated, biopsy-proven, multicentric Castleman disease who had discontinued chemotherapy. Eligible patients were aged ≥18 years, were infected with HIV, had been treated by combination antiretroviral therapy during the previous 3 months, had been treated with chemotherapy for ≥3 months with clinical response, and had experienced at least one recurrence of multicentric Castleman disease attack after attempt to discontinue chemotherapy. Patients received four weekly intravenous infusions of rituximab (375 mg/m^2).

The multicenter, non-randomized, open-label, single-group, phase 2 trial by Bower et al involved 21 patients with previously untreated, HIV-associated, biopsy-proven, multicentric Castleman disease without microlymphoma. Patients received four weekly intravenous infusions of rituximab (375 mg/m^2). This regimen should be avoided in patients with active Kaposi sarcoma, as this may worsen with administration of rituximab alone.

Efficacy

Gérard et al Trial (N = 24)

Rate of sustained remission* at day 60	22/24 (92%)
Rate of sustained remission persistence at day 365	17/22 (77%)
Estimated event-free survival at 1 year	71%
Estimated disease-free survival at 1 year	77%
Estimated overall survival at 1 year	92%
Occurrence of lymphoma at 1 year	0%

*Sustained remission was defined as the absence of multicentric Castleman disease relapse off chemotherapy

Bower et al Trial (N = 21)

Rate of remission of symptoms	95%
Rate of complete response	29%
Rate of partial response	67%
Relapse-free survival at 2 years	79%
Overall survival at 2 years	95%

Note: Median duration of follow-up was 12 months. One patient died before completion of rituximab therapy as a result of progressive disease

Therapy Monitoring

1. *Before therapy:* CBC with differential, CD4+ T cell count, LFTs, BUN, serum creatinine, KSHV viral load, hepatitis B and C serologies, C-reactive protein
2. *After Treatment:* CBC with differential, CD4+ T cell count, LFTs, BUN, serum creatinine, KSHV viral load, C-reactive protein. Monitor every 1–3 months during the first year

Treatment Modifications

RITUXIMAB

Rituximab Infusion-Related Toxicities

Onset of infusion-related events (fevers, chills, rigors, edema, congestion of the head and neck mucosa, hypotension)
1. Interrupt rituximab infusion
2. For fever, chills: Give additional dose of acetaminophen 650 mg orally and diphenhydramine 25–50 mg by intravenous push
3. For rigors: Give meperidine 12.5–25 mg by intravenous push ± promethazine 12.5–25 mg by intravenous infusion in at least 10 mL 0.9% NS or D5W over 5–15 minutes. If after 15–20 minutes the response to a single dose is considered inadequate, the dose may be repeated
4. After symptoms resolve, resume rituximab infusion at a minimum of 50% reduction in the rate at which the event occurred. If no further infusion-related events, increase the rate by 50 mg/hour every 30 minutes, as tolerated, up to a maximum rate of 400 mg/hour

Dyspnea or wheezing, without allergic findings (urticaria, or tongue or laryngeal edema)
1. Interrupt rituximab infusion immediately
2. Give **hydrocortisone** 100 mg by intravenous push (or glucocorticoid equivalent)
3. Give an additional dose of **diphenhydramine** 25–50 mg by intravenous push and a histamine H2-antagonist (**ranitidine** 50 mg or **famotidine** 20 mg) by intravenous push
4. After symptoms resolve, resume rituximab infusion at a minimum of 50% reduction in the rate at which the event occurred. If no further infusion-related events, increase the rate by 50 mg/hour every 30 minutes, as tolerated, up to a maximum rate of 400 mg/hour

Note: Medications and equipment for the treatment of hypersensitivity reactions should be available for immediate use in the event of a reaction during administration (eg, intravenous fluids, epinephrine, antihistamines, glucocorticoids, oxygen)

Adverse Events

Gérard et al trial (N = 24)
Adverse events were graded according to the Agence National de Recherche sur le Sida et les Hépatites Virales toxicity grading system (www.anrs.fr/). Treatment-related adverse events occurred in nine (38%) patients, generally within 24 hours after the first infusion. The most common events during therapy were chills, fever, headache, pruritus, rash, dizziness, and hypotension; all were mild to moderate in severity and resolved after rituximab infusion was slowed or stopped. Serum sickness occurred in one patient after the second rituximab infusion. Grade 3-4 neutropenia was observed in 3 (13%) patients. During the time between day 60 and day 365, 17 (71%) patients experienced mild-to-moderate infections. During the study, Kaposi sarcoma flares occurred in 8 of 12 patients (67%) who had reported Kaposi sarcoma (either in complete remission or stable) at study entry

Bower et al trial (N = 21)
Adverse events were graded according to the National Cancer Institute Common Terminology Criteria for Adverse Events, version 3.0. No Grade 3–4 toxicities were recorded with rituximab therapy, but Kaposi sarcoma progression occurred during rituximab therapy in 4 of 11 patients (36%) who had cutaneous Kaposi sarcoma at diagnosis

FIRST-LINE

HIV-RELATED KAPOSI SARCOMA HERPESVIRUS-ASSOCIATED MULTICENTRIC CASTLEMAN DISEASE (KSHV-MCD) REGIMEN: RITUXIMAB + LIPOSOMAL DOXORUBICIN

Uldrick TS et al. Blood 2014;124:3544–3552

The regimen consists of cycles of rituximab and doxorubicin HCl liposome injection administered every 3 weeks for up to 2 cycles beyond resolution of KSHV-MCD-related symptoms along with improvement in associated biochemical abnormalities. In the study published by Uldrick et al, a median of 4 (range, 3–9) cycles were administered. Following completion of rituximab and doxorubicin HCl liposome injection, patients were prescribed consolidation with either interferon alpha or valganciclovir plus zidovudine, continued for 6–12 months as tolerated. However, subsequent studies have provided evidence that further therapy in KSHV-MCD is not required due to the low rate of relapse after treatment with rituximab-based therapy and the high success rate of re-treatment (Pria AD et al. Blood 2017;129:2143–2147)

Important to administer ART to all HIV-positive patients

Premedications for rituximab
Acetaminophen 650–1000 mg; administer orally 30–60 minutes before starting rituximab, *plus*
Diphenhydramine 25–50 mg; administer orally or intravenously 30–60 minutes before starting rituximab

Rituximab 375 mg/m²; administer intravenously in 0.9% sodium chloride injection (0.9% NS) or 5% dextrose injection (D5W), diluted to a concentration within the range 1–4 mg/mL on day 1, every 21 days (total dosage/cycle = 375 mg/m²)

Rituximab administration:
- Infuse initially at 50 mg/hour. If hypersensitivity or infusion reactions do not occur during the first 30 minutes, increase the rate by 50 mg/hour every 30 minutes as tolerated to a maximum rate of 400 mg/hour. During subsequent treatments if previous rituximab administration was well tolerated, start at 100 mg/hour and increase by 100 mg/hour every 30 minutes as tolerated to a maximum rate of 400 mg/hour
- Interrupt rituximab administration for fever, chills, edema, congestion of the head and neck mucosa, hypertension, and other serious adverse events. Resume rituximab administration after adverse events abate

Premedication for doxorubicin HCl liposome injection: Generally not required
Doxorubicin HCl liposome injection (pegylated liposomal doxorubicin) 20 mg/m²; administer intravenously in 250 mL D5W over 60 minutes on day 1, every 3 weeks (total dosage/cycle = 20 mg/m²)

Note: Doxorubicin HCl liposome injection can cause severe infusion reactions.
- Temporarily stop the infusion for any grade infusion-related reaction until resolution
- For mild to moderate infusion reactions, resume doxorubicin HCl liposome injection infusion at a reduced rate
- Permanently discontinue doxorubicin HCl liposome injection in the event of a serious or life-threatening infusion-related reaction

Supportive Care
Antiemetic prophylaxis
Emetogenic potential: **LOW**
See Chapter 39 for antiemetic recommendations

Hematopoietic growth factor (CSF) prophylaxis
Primary prophylaxis is **NOT** indicated
See Chapter 43 for more information

Antimicrobial prophylaxis
Risk of fever and neutropenia is **LOW**
  Antimicrobial primary prophylaxis to be considered:
- Opportunistic infection prophylaxis, based on CD4+ T cell count (aidsinfo.nih.gov/contentfiles/lvguidelines/adult_oi.pdf [accessed 1 June 2018])
- Antibacterial—not indicated
- Antifungal—not indicated
- Antiviral—not indicated unless patient previously had an episode of HSV

Risk of reactivation of viral hepatitis with rituximab administration
- All patients should be tested for active or previous exposure to hepatitis B and C prior to receiving rituximab
- Providers should ensure patients with active previous exposure to hepatitis B or C are receiving appropriate prophylaxis or treatment prior to initiation of rituximab
- Carriers of hepatitis B receiving rituximab should be on antiretroviral therapy with an NRTI base containing two agents with activity against HBV

(continued)

(continued)

Hand-foot reaction (palmar-plantar erythrodysesthesia, PPE)
For patients who develop a hand-foot reaction, use topical emollients (eg, Aquaphor), topical or orally administered steroids, antihistamine agents (H_1-receptor antagonists), or pyridoxine. Pyridoxine may provide relief for discomfort/pain associated with PPE, although the mechanism through which this occurs remains unclear

• The suggested pyridoxine starting dose is 50 mg/day, which may be increased to a maximum of 200 mg/day
• Patients who develop G1/2 PPE while receiving doxorubicin HCl liposome injection may receive a fixed daily dose of pyridoxine 200 mg. This may allow for treatment to be completed without dosage reduction, treatment delay, or recurrence of PPE

Oral care
Prophylaxis and treatment for mucositis/stomatitis
  General advice:
  • Encourage patients to maintain intake of nonalcoholic fluids
  • Evaluate patients for oral pain and provide analgesic medications
  • Consider histamine (H_2-subtype) receptor antagonists (eg, ranitidine, famotidine), or a proton pump inhibitor for epigastric pain
  • *Lactobacillus* sp.—containing probiotics may be beneficial in preventing diarrhea

  Patients with intact oral mucosa:
  • Clean the mouth, tongue, and gums by brushing after every meal and at bedtime with an ultra-soft toothbrush with fluoride toothpaste
  • Floss teeth gently every day unless contraindicated. If gums bleed and hurt, avoid bleeding or sore areas, but floss other teeth
  • Patients may use saline or commercial bland, nonalcoholic rinses
    ▪ Do not use mouthwashes that contain alcohol

  If mucositis or stomatitis is present:
  • Keep the mouth moist utilizing water, ice chips, sugarless gum, sugar-free hard candies, or a saliva substitute
  • Rinse mouth several times a day to remove debris
    ▪ Use a solution of ¼ teaspoon (1.25 g) each of baking soda and table salt (sodium chloride) in 1 quart (~950 mL) of warm water. Follow with a plain water rinse
    ▪ Do not use mouthwashes that contain alcohol
  • Foam-tipped swabs (eg, Toothettes) are useful in moisturizing oral mucosa, but ineffective for cleansing teeth and removing plaque
  • Advise patients who develop mucositis to:
    ▪ Choose foods that are easy to chew and swallow
    ▪ Take small bites of food, chew slowly, and sip liquids with meals
    ▪ Encourage soft, moist foods such as cooked cereals, mashed potatoes, and scrambled eggs
    ▪ For trouble swallowing, soften food with gravies, sauces, broths, yogurt, or other bland liquids
    ▪ Avoid sharp, crunchy foods; hot, spicy, or highly acidic foods (eg, citrus fruits and juices); sugary foods; toothpicks; tobacco products; alcoholic drinks

Patient Population Studied

The pilot study included 17 HIV-positive patients with pathologically confirmed KSHV-MCD and concurrent symptomatic KS, progression through virus-activated cytotoxic therapy, or disease severe enough to warrant immunochemotherapy. All patients received intravenous rituximab (375 mg/m^2) and liposomal doxorubicin (20 mg/m^2) every 3 weeks. All patients also received ART. Patients received up to two cycles beyond resolution of symptoms attributable to KSHV-MCD and marked improvement in biochemical abnormalities. Patients received consolidation therapy (interferon α or azidothymidine and valganciclovir) after the study protocol for 6–12 months

Efficacy (N = 17)

Clinical complete response rate	88%
Major clinical response rate*	94%
Biochemical complete response rate	76%
Major biochemical response rate†	88%
Event-free survival at 3 years	69%
Overall survival at 3 years	81%

*Major clinical response rate is the percentage of patients who experienced a clinical complete response to the study drug or symptom-free disease
†Major biochemical response rate is the percentage of patients who experienced a biochemical partial or complete response to the study drug
Note: The median duration of potential follow-up (including consolidation therapy) was 58 months

Therapy Monitoring

1. *Before therapy:* CBC with differential, LFTs, BUN, serum creatinine, KSHV viral load, hepatitis B and C serologies, and left ventricular ejection fraction (LVEF)
2. In addition to baseline monitoring, evaluate LVEF during liposomal doxorubicin treatment if clinical symptoms of heart failure are present
3. *Before each cycle:* CBC with differential, LFTs, BUN, serum creatinine, and response assessment
4. *After treatment:* CBC with differential, LFTs, BUN, serum creatinine, and KSHV viral load. Monitor every 1–3 months based on response to treatment

Treatment Modifications

RITUXIMAB + LIPOSOMAL DOXORUBICIN

RITUXIMAB

Rituximab Infusion-Related Toxicities

Onset of infusion-related events (fevers, chills, rigors, edema, congestion of the head and neck mucosa, hypotension)

1. Interrupt rituximab infusion
2. For fever, chills: Give additional dose of acetaminophen 650 mg orally and diphenhydramine 25–50 mg by intravenous push
3. For rigors: Give meperidine 12.5–25 mg by intravenous push ± promethazine 12.5–25 mg by intravenous infusion in at least 10 mL 0.9% NS or D5W over 5–15 minutes. If after 15–20 minutes the response to a single dose is considered inadequate, the dose may be repeated
4. After symptoms resolve, resume rituximab infusion at a minimum of 50% reduction in the rate at which the event occurred. If no further infusion-related events, increase the rate by 50 mg/hour every 30 minutes, as tolerated, up to a maximum rate of 400 mg/hour

Dyspnea or wheezing, without allergic findings (urticaria, or tongue or laryngeal edema)

1. Interrupt rituximab infusion immediately
2. Give **hydrocortisone** 100 mg by intravenous push (or glucocorticoid equivalent)
3. Give an additional dose of **diphenhydramine** 25–50 mg by intravenous push and a histamine H2-antagonist (**ranitidine** 50 mg or **famotidine** 20 mg) by intravenous push
4. After symptoms resolve, resume rituximab infusion at a minimum of 50% reduction in the rate at which the event occurred. If no further infusion-related events, increase the rate by 50 mg/hour every 30 minutes, as tolerated, up to a maximum rate of 400 mg/hour

Note: Medications and equipment for the treatment of hypersensitivity reactions should be available for immediate use in the event of a reaction during administration (eg, intravenous fluids, epinephrine, antihistamines, glucocorticoids, and oxygen)

Liposomal Doxorubicin

Adverse Event	Treatment Modification
Signs or symptoms of extravasation	Liposomal doxorubicin should be considered an irritant and precautions should be taken to avoid extravasation. Immediately terminate the infusion and restart in another vein. Apply ice over the site of extravasation for approximately 30 minutes
Febrile neutropenia (ANC <1000/mm^3 with temperature >38°C or >100.4°F), or ANC <1000/mm^3 for ≥7 days	Reduce liposomal doxorubicin dose by 25% and consider adding filgrastim in subsequent cycles, if applicable
Febrile neutropenia (ANC <1000/mm^3 with temperature >38°C or >100.4°F), or ANC <1000/mm^3 for ≥7 days despite one dose reduction	Administer filgrastim in subsequent cycles. If already administering filgrastim, reduce liposomal doxorubicin dose by one level
G1 ANC/platelet count (ANC 1500–1,900/mm^3; platelet count 75,000–150,000/mm^3)	Resume treatment with no dose reduction
G2 ANC/platelet count (ANC 1000–1500/mm^3 and platelet count 50,000–<75,000/mm^3)	Wait until ANC ≥1500 and platelets ≥75,000; redose with no dose reduction
G3 ANC/platelet count (ANC 500–999 and platelet count 25,000–<50,000)	Wait until ANC ≥1500 and platelets ≥75,000; redose with no dose reduction
G4 ANC/platelet count (ANC <500 and platelet count <25,000)	Wait until ANC ≥1500 and platelets ≥75,000; redose at 25% dose reduction or continue full dose with cytokine support
G1 hand-foot syndrome (HFS) (mild erythema, swelling, or desquamation not interfering with daily activities)	Redose unless patient has experienced previous G3/4 HFS. If so, delay up to 2 weeks and decrease dose by 25%. Return to original dose interval
G2 hand-foot syndrome (HFS) (erythema, desquamation, or swelling interfering with, but not precluding, normal physical activities; small blisters or ulcerations <2 cm in diameter)	Delay dosing up to 2 weeks or until resolved to G0/1. If after 2 weeks there is no resolution, liposomal doxorubicin should be discontinued. If resolved to G0/1 within 2 weeks, and there are no prior G3/4 HFS, continue treatment at previous dose and return to original dose interval. If patient experienced previous G3/4 toxicity, continue treatment with a 25% dose reduction and return to original dose interval

(continued)

Treatment Modifications (*continued*)

Adverse Event	Treatment Modification
G3 hand-foot syndrome (HFS) (blistering, ulceration, or swelling interfering with walking or normal daily activities; cannot wear regular clothing)	Delay dosing up to 2 weeks or until resolved to G0/1. Decrease dose by 25% and return to original dose interval. If after 2 weeks there is no resolution, liposomal doxorubicin should be discontinued
G4 hand-foot syndrome (HFS) (diffuse or local process causing infectious complications, or a bed-ridden state or hospitalization)	Delay dosing up to 2 weeks or until resolved to G0/1. Decrease dose by 25% and return to original dose interval. If after 2 weeks there is no resolution, liposomal doxorubicin should be discontinued
G1 stomatitis (painless ulcers, erythema, or mild soreness)	Redose unless patient has experienced previous Grade 3 or 4 toxicity. If so, delay up to 2 weeks and decrease dose by 25%. Return to original dose interval
G2 stomatitis (painful erythema, edema, or ulcers, but can eat)	Delay dosing up to 2 weeks or until resolved to G0/1. If after 2 weeks there is no resolution, liposomal doxorubicin should be discontinued. If resolved to G0/1 within 2 weeks and there was no prior G3/4 stomatitis, continue treatment at previous dose and return to original dose interval. If patient experienced previous G3/4 toxicity, continue treatment with a 25% dose reduction and return to original dose interval
G3 stomatitis (painful erythema, edema, or ulcers, and cannot eat)	Delay dosing up to 2 weeks or until resolved to G0/1. Decrease dose by 25% and return to original dose interval. If after 2 weeks there is no resolution, liposomal doxorubicin should be discontinued
G4 stomatitis (requires parenteral or enteral support)	Delay dosing up to 2 weeks or until resolved to G0/1. Decrease dose by 25% and return to liposomal doxorubicin original dose interval. If after 2 weeks there is no resolution, liposomal doxorubicin should be discontinued
Serum bilirubin 1.2–3.0 mg/dL	Reduce liposomal doxorubicin dose by 25%
Serum bilirubin >3 mg/dL	Reduce liposomal doxorubicin dose by 50%
Any other G3/4 nonhematologic drug-related toxicity	Do not dose until recovered to G <2 and reduce dose by 25% for all subsequent cycles
Any other G3/4 nonhematologic drug-related toxicity despite reduced dose	Do not dose until recovered to G <2 and reduce dose by an additional 25% for all subsequent cycles

Note: The liposomal doxorubicin package insert states the following: Cardiac function should be carefully monitored in patients treated with liposomal doxorubicin via endomyocardial biopsy, echocardiography, or multigated radionuclide scans. If these test results indicate possible cardiac injury associated with liposomal doxorubicin therapy, the benefit of continued therapy must be carefully weighed against the risk of myocardial injury

Adverse Events (N = 17)

Grade (%)*	Grade 2	Grade 3	Grade 4
Neutropenia	35	18	6
Fever/infusion reaction	35	18	0
Anemia	24	6	6
Fatigue	12	6	0
Anorexia	12	0	0
CD4 lymphopenia	0	6	0
Bone pain	6	0	0

Grade (%)*	Grade 2	Grade 3	Grade 4
Gastroesophageal reflux	6	0	0
Headache	6	0	0
Rash	6	0	0
Stomatitis	6	0	0

*According to the National Cancer Institute Common Terminology Criteria for Adverse Events, version 3.0

Note: Toxicities are included in the table if the events were grade ≥2 and were deemed to be possibly related to the rituximab + liposomal doxorubicin treatment (not the consolidation therapy)

HIV-Related Lymphomas

Epidemiology

Incidence
- 201 cases/100,000 person-years in HIV-positive individuals in the ART era
- The cumulative incidence of non-Hodgkin lymphoma in people with HIV in the U.S. in the ART era is estimated to be 4.5%

Stage at presentation
- More than 60% have advanced stage III–IV disease with B-cell symptoms
- Extranodal involvement is common

Besson C et al. Blood 2001;98:2339–2344

Pathology

Several aggressive B-cell lymphomas are considered AIDS-defining. Distribution of histologic subtypes tracks with CD4+ T cell count and has been influenced by ART-induced immune preservation. With ART, fewer immunoblastic EBV+ subtypes are seen. AIDS-related non-Hodgkin lymphomas include the following histologies:

1. Diffuse large B-cell lymphoma (DLBCL):
   - Centroblastic: 20–30% Epstein-Barr virus (EBV)+
   - Immunoblastic: 80% EBV+
2. Primary central nervous system lymphoma: 100% EBV+
3. Burkitt lymphoma: 30% EBV+
4. Primary effusion lymphoma: 100% KSHV associated, 80% also EBV+
5. Plasmablastic lymphoma: 100% EBV+; majority also have c-myc rearrangements

Jaffe ES et al. World Health Organization Classification of Tumors: Pathology & Genetics: Tumors of Haematopoietic and Lymphoid Tissues. Lyon, France: IARC Press; 2001:351

Staging

Ann Arbor Staging System for Lymphomas

Stage	Description
I	Single lymph node region
IE	Single extralymphatic organ or site
II	Two or more lymph node regions on the same side of the diaphragm
IIE	Single extranodal site + adjacent nodes
III	Nodal regions on both sides of the diaphragm (III)
IIIE	Nodal regions on both sides of the diaphragm + single extranodal site
IIIS	Nodal regions on both sides of the diaphragm + involvement of spleen
IIISE	Nodal regions on both sides of the diaphragm + single extranodal site + involvement of spleen
IV	Diffuse or disseminated involvement of one or more extralymphatic organs Bone marrow involvement Liver involvement Brain involvement

Absence of associated symptoms is designated A
Presence of symptoms is designated B. B symptoms include unexplained fevers, >10% unexplained weight loss, night sweats

Work-up

1. Assessment of hematologic and biochemical parameters
2. CT scans of chest, abdomen, and pelvis
3. ^{18}FDG-PET scan
4. MRI brain if neurologic symptoms
5. Lumbar puncture for CSF cytology and cell count; flow cytometry if available
6. HIV viral load and CD4 cell count
7. Bone marrow biopsy often not needed based on FDG-PET findings

If primary brain lymphoma is suspected:
1. Brain biopsy is the gold standard
2. Must exclude peripheral disease
3. Slit-lamp exam of optic nerve
4. CSF evaluation for leptomeningeal disease
5. Minimally invasive diagnosis combining ^{18}FDG-PET (or SPECT) with assessment of EBV presence in the CSF by polymerase chain reaction can be used in some cases rather than biopsy
   - If both tests are positive: near 100% positive predictive value for primary brain lymphoma
   - If both tests are negative: near 100% negative predictive value for brain lymphoma
   - If these tests are discordant: biopsy is required to establish the diagnosis

Antinori A et al. J Clin Oncol 1999;17:554–560
Levine AM. Semin Oncol 1990;17:104–112

Survival

Overall survival has improved since the advent of ART:

1. *Diffuse large B-cell lymphoma (DLCBL) and Burkitt Lymphoma*
   - Pre-ART 4–18 months
   - With appropriate therapy and ART, 2 year overall survival 60–90%
2. *PEL*: Median overall survival 22 months, 47% 3-year survival
3. *Plasmablastic lymphoma:* 43% 2-year survival
4. Tumor histology is the primary predictor of response to treatment and overall survival

Besson C et al. Blood 2001;98:2339–2344
Castillo J et al. Am J Hematol 2008;83:804–809
Lurain K et al. Blood 2019; 133:1753–1761

Expert Opinion

Treatment should be based on histology. A pooled analysis of trials in HIV-associated diffuse large B cell lymphoma showed R-EPOCH had improved overall survival compared with R-CHOP. Outcomes with R-CHOP are poor for Burkitt lymphoma and plasmablastic lymphoma, and EPOCH-based therapy is preferred. Concurrent ART with chemotherapy is the standard of care, but initiation of ART should not delay definitive lymphoma treatment. ART regimens containing ritonavir or cobicistat are contraindicated with EPOCH and CHOP, but integrase inhibitor-based regimens are generally safe to administer with these regimens without increased toxicity or dose delay. For patients not on ART or those requiring a change in ART to prevent drug-drug interactions, a reasonable approach is to initiate ART after administration of first cycle of chemotherapy is completed. A small prospective study of AIDS-related primary CNS lymphoma showed high-dose methotrexate and rituximab in combination with ART was safe and showed a 67% 5-year overall survival rate, even in high-risk patients. Expedient diagnosis and curative-intent therapy are crucial in this disease.

Lurain K et al. Blood 2020

FIRST-LINE

HIV-RELATED LYMPHOMA REGIMEN: DOSE-ADJUSTED ETOPOSIDE + PREDNISONE + VINCRISTINE + CYCLOPHOSPHAMIDE + DOXORUBICIN + RITUXIMAB (DA-EPOCH-R)

Barta SK et al. Cancer 2012;118:3977–3983
Bartlett NL et al. J Clin Oncol 2019;37:1790–1799
Protocol for: Bartlett NL et al. J Clin Oncol 2019;37:1790–1799
Data Supplement to: Bartlett NL et al. J Clin Oncol 2019;37:1790–1799
Sparano JA et al. Blood 2010;115:3008–3016

Important Note:
• ART should be continued in patients already on a stable regimen or initiated in patients with newly diagnosed HIV

Premedications for rituximab
Acetaminophen 650–1000 mg; administer orally 30–60 minutes before starting rituximab on day 1, every 21 days, for up to 6 cycles, *plus*
Diphenhydramine 25–50 mg; administer orally or intravenously 30–60 minutes before starting rituximab on day 1, every 21 days, for up to 6 cycles

Rituximab 375 mg/m^2; administer intravenously in 0.9% sodium chloride injection (0.9% NS) or 5% dextrose injection (D5W), diluted to a concentration within the range 1–4 mg/mL, on day 1, every 21 days, for up to 6 cycles (total dosage/3-week cycle = 375 mg/m^2)

Rituximab administration:
• Infuse initially at 50 mg/hour. If hypersensitivity or infusion reactions do not occur during the first 30 minutes, increase the rate by 50 mg/hour every 30 minutes as tolerated to a maximum rate of 400 mg/hour. During subsequent treatments if previous rituximab administration was well tolerated, start at 100 mg/hour and increase by 100 mg/hour every 30 minutes as tolerated to a maximum rate of 400 mg/hour
• Interrupt rituximab administration for fever, chills, edema, congestion of the head and neck mucosa, hypertension, and other serious adverse events. Resume rituximab administration after adverse events abate

Etoposide 50 mg/m^2 per day; administer by continuous intravenous infusion over 24 hours,* for 4 consecutive days, on days 1–4, every 21 days, for up to 6 cycles (total dosage/cycle = 200 mg/m^2) (see therapy modifications section for dosage specifications)

Doxorubicin 10 mg/m^2 per day; administer by continuous intravenous infusion over 24 hours,* for 4 consecutive days, on days 1–4, every 21 days, for up to 6 cycles (total dosage/cycle = 40 mg/m^2) (see therapy modifications section for dosage specifications)

Vincristine 0.4 mg/m^2 per day; administer by continuous intravenous infusion over 24 hours,* for 4 consecutive days, on days 1–4, every 21 days, for up to 6 cycles (total dosage/cycle = 1.6 mg/m^2)
*See Special Instructions below for preparing a 3-in-1 admixture with etoposide, doxorubicin, and vincristine

Prednisone 60 mg/m^2 per dose; administer orally, twice daily for 5 consecutive days, on days 1–5 (10 doses), every 21 days, for up to 6 cycles (total dosage/cycle = 600 mg/m^2)
• The first prednisone dose should be given at least 1 hour before rituximab administration begins
• Patients who were unable to ingest oral medications may receive a parenterally administered steroid at a glucocorticoid equivalent dosage for the same number of doses on the same administration schedule (eg, methylprednisolone 48 mg/m^2 per dose)

Cyclophosphamide 750 mg/m^2; administer intravenously in 100 mL 0.9% NS or D5W over 30 minutes on day 5 (after completing infusional etoposide + doxorubicin + vincristine), every 21 days, for up to 6 cycles (total dosage/cycle = 750 mg/m^2) (see therapy modifications section for dosage specifications)

Supportive Care
Antiemetic prophylaxis
Emetogenic potential on Days 1–5 is **MODERATE**
See Chapter 39 for antiemetic recommendations

Hematopoietic growth factor (CSF) prophylaxis
Primary prophylaxis is indicated with one of the following:
  Filgrastim (G-CSF) 5 mcg/kg per day, by subcutaneous injection, *or:*
  Pegfilgrastim (pegylated filgrastim) 6 mg/0.6 mL, by subcutaneous injection for one dose
• Begin use from 24–72 h after myelosuppressive chemotherapy is completed
• Continue daily filgrastim use until ANC ≥5000/mm^3 after the leukocyte nadir
• Discontinue daily filgrastim use at least 24 hours before administering myelosuppressive treatment. Do not administer pegfilgrastim within 14 days before administering myelosuppressive treatment
See Chapter 43 for more information

Antimicrobial prophylaxis
Risk of fever and neutropenia is **INTERMEDIATE**
  Antimicrobial primary prophylaxis to be considered:
• Opportunistic infection prophylaxis, based on CD4+ T cell count (aidsinfo.nih.gov/contentfiles/lvguidelines/adult_oi.pdf [accessed 1 June 2018])

(continued)

(continued)

- Antibacterial—consider a fluoroquinolone during periods of neutropenia, or no prophylaxis; *P. jirovecii* prophylaxis is recommended (eg, cotrimoxazole)
- Antifungal—consider concomitant use of fluconazole during periods of neutropenia, and in anticipation of mucositis
- Antiviral—anti-herpes antivirals (eg, acyclovir, famciclovir, valacyclovir)

Risk of reactivation of viral hepatitis with rituximab administration

- All patients should be tested for active or previous exposure to hepatitis B and C prior to receiving rituximab
- Providers should ensure patients with active previous exposure to hepatitis B or C are receiving appropriate prophylaxis or treatment prior to initiation of rituximab
- Carriers of hepatitis B receiving rituximab should be on antiretroviral therapy with an NRTI base containing two agents with activity against HBV

Oral care

Prophylaxis and treatment for mucositis/stomatitis

General advice:

- Encourage patients to maintain intake of nonalcoholic fluids
- Evaluate patients for oral pain and provide analgesic medications
- Consider histamine (H$_2$-subtype) receptor antagonists (eg, ranitidine, famotidine), or a proton pump inhibitor for epigastric pain
- *Lactobacillus* sp.–containing probiotics may be beneficial in preventing diarrhea

Patients with intact oral mucosa:

- Clean the mouth, tongue, and gums by brushing after every meal and at bedtime with an ultra-soft toothbrush with fluoride toothpaste
- Floss teeth gently every day unless contraindicated. If gums bleed and hurt, avoid bleeding or sore areas, but floss other teeth
- Patients may use saline or commercial bland, nonalcoholic rinses
  - Do not use mouthwashes that contain alcohol

If mucositis or stomatitis is present:

- Keep the mouth moist utilizing water, ice chips, sugarless gum, sugar-free hard candies, or a saliva substitute
- Rinse mouth several times a day to remove debris
  - Use a solution of ¼ teaspoon (1.25 g) each of baking soda and table salt (sodium chloride) in 1 quart (~950 mL) of warm water. Follow with a plain water rinse
  - Do not use mouthwashes that contain alcohol
- Foam-tipped swabs (eg, Toothettes) are useful in moisturizing oral mucosa, but ineffective for cleansing teeth and removing plaque
- Advise patients who develop mucositis to:
  - Choose foods that are easy to chew and swallow
  - Take small bites of food, chew slowly, and sip liquids with meals
  - Encourage soft, moist foods such as cooked cereals, mashed potatoes, and scrambled eggs
  - For trouble swallowing, soften food with gravies, sauces, broths, yogurt, or other bland liquids
  - Avoid sharp, crunchy foods; hot, spicy, or highly acidic foods (eg, citrus fruits and juices); sugary foods; toothpicks; tobacco products; alcoholic drinks

Additional prophylaxis

Add a **proton pump inhibitor** during prednisone use to prevent gastritis and duodenitis

Give **stool softeners and/or laxatives** during and after vincristine administration

Suggested CNS therapy

Suggested CNS prophylaxis for patients with Burkitt Lymphoma:

Methotrexate 12 mg per dose; administer intrathecally in a volume of **preservative-free** 0.9% NS equivalent to the amount of cerebrospinal fluid removed via lumbar puncture on days 1 and 5, every 21 days, during cycles 3, 4, 5, and 6 only (total dosage/3-week cycle in cycles 3–6 = 24 mg)

Suggested CNS prophylaxis for patients with Diffuse Large B-cell Lymphoma:

Methotrexate 12 mg per dose; administer intrathecally in a volume of **preservative-free** 0.9% NS equivalent to the amount of cerebrospinal fluid removed via lumbar puncture on day 1, every 21 days, during cycles 3, 4, 5, and 6 only (total dosage/3-week cycle in cycles 3–6 = 12 mg)

Suggested CNS treatment (confirmed CNS disease):

Induction: **Methotrexate** 12 mg per dose; administered intrathecally (or 6 mg per dose; if administered via Ommaya reservoir) in a volume of **preservative-free** 0.9% NS equivalent to the amount of cerebrospinal fluid removed, twice weekly for 4 weeks starting on day 1 of cycle 1 (total dose/week via lumbar puncture = 24 mg; total dose/week via Ommaya reservoir = 12 mg), *followed by:*

(continued)

(*continued*)

Consolidation: **Methotrexate** 12 mg per dose; administered intrathecally (or 6 mg per dose; if administered via Ommaya reservoir) in a volume of **preservative-free** 0.9% NS equivalent to the amount of cerebrospinal fluid removed, once weekly for 6 weeks (total dose/week via lumbar puncture = 12 mg; total dose/week via Ommaya reservoir = 6 mg), *followed by:*

Maintenance: **Methotrexate** 12 mg per dose; administered intrathecally (or 6 mg per dose; if administered via Ommaya reservoir) in a volume of **preservative-free** 0.9% NS equivalent to the amount of cerebrospinal fluid removed, once monthly for 4 months (total dose/month via lumbar puncture = 12 mg; total dose/month via Ommaya reservoir = 6 mg)

*General instructions:
To prepare a 3-in-1 admixture with etoposide + doxorubicin + vincristine, dilute all three drug products in 0.9% NS as follows:

Total Dose of Etoposide	Volume of 0.9% NS
≤130 mg	500 mL
>130 mg	1000 mL

Etoposide (base) + doxorubicin + vincristine 3-in-1 admixtures:
Etoposide 50 mg/m^2, doxorubicin hydrochloride 10 mg/m^2, and vincristine sulfate 0.4 mg/m^2 admixtures diluted in 0.9% NS to produce a final etoposide concentration <250 mcg/mL, in polyolefin-lined infusion bags are stable and compatible for 72 hours at 23°–25°C (73.4°–77°F), and at 31°–33°C (87.8°–91.4°F) when protected from exposure to light

Wolfe JL et al. Am J Health Syst Pharm 1999;56:985–989

Etoposide phosphate + doxorubicin + vincristine 3-in-1 admixtures:
Etoposide phosphate, doxorubicin hydrochloride, and vincristine sulfate admixtures diluted in 0.9% NS, to produce a final etoposide concentration <250 mcg/mL in polyolefin-lined infusion bags are stable and compatible for up to 124 hours at 2°–6°C (35.6°–42.8°F) and 35°–40°C (95°–104°F) in the dark and under fluorescent light. In admixtures stored at 35°–40°C (95°–104°F) and exposed to light, the initial drug concentrations decreased slightly but remain within acceptable concentrations

Yuan P et al. Am J Health Syst Pharm 2001;58:594–598

A 3-in-1 admixture does not prevent microbial growth after exposure to bacterial and fungal contamination. With respect to product sterility, expiration dating should be determined by the aseptic techniques used in preparation and local and national guidelines

Patient Population Studied

Sparano JA et al. Rituximab plus concurrent infusional EPOCH chemotherapy is highly effective in HIV-associated B-cell non-Hodgkin lymphoma. Blood 2010;115:3008–3016

AMC034 was a randomized phase 2 trial conducted by the AIDS Malignancy Consortium (AMC) that involved 110 HIV-infected adult patients who were allocated to receive either EPOCH given concurrently with rituximab (n = 54), or EPOCH followed by sequential administration of weekly rituximab (n = 56). Patients were accrued between 2002 and 2006 and were included if they had previously untreated histologically or cytologically confirmed aggressive CD20+ B-cell non-Hodgkin lymphoma. Eligible histologies included diffuse large B-cell lymphoma, Burkitt/Burkitt-like lymphoma, or other aggressive lymphomas associated with HIV infection. Patients were required to have stage II–IV disease or stage I disease with an elevated serum LDH, an Eastern Cooperative Oncology Group performance status of ≤2, adequate hematologic parameters (ANC >1000/mm^3 and platelets >75,000/mm^3 unless due to bone marrow involvement), and adequate organ function (serum creatinine <2 mg/dL, bilirubin <2 mg/dL, ALT and AST <7× upper limit of normal). Patients were excluded if they had lymphoma involving the parenchymal brain or spinal cord, or if they had an acute HIV-associated opportunistic infection requiring treatment. EPOCH was continued for two cycles beyond complete remission, for a minimum of four and a maximum of six cycles. The use of ART was left to the discretion of the treating physician

Barta SK et al. Pooled analysis of AIDS Malignancy Consortium trials evaluating rituximab plus CHOP or infusional EPOCH chemotherapy in HIV-associated non-Hodgkin lymphoma. Cancer 2012;118:3977–3983
A pooled analysis of two AMC trials was conducted with the concurrent R-EPOCH arm (n = 51) from AMC034 and the R-CHOP arm (n = 99) of AMC010. Comparative efficacy data in this regimen overview will be presented from the pooled analysis (Barta et al, 2012)

Note that we chapter authors prefer to administer a more contemporary version of the DA-EPOCH-R regimen to patients with HIV-related lymphoma, such as that described in the Intergroup Trial Alliance/CALGB 50303 study (Bartlett et al, 2019)

Barta SK et al. Cancer 2012;118:3977–3983
Bartlett NL et al. J Clin Oncol 2019;37:1790–1799
Sparano JA et al. Blood 2010;115:3008–3016

Efficacy

Sparano JA et al. Rituximab plus concurrent infusional EPOCH chemotherapy is highly effective in HIV-associated B-cell non-Hodgkin lymphoma. Blood 2010;115:3008–3016

Efficacy Variable	Result in Concurrent R-EPOCH Arm
Response rate in all patients treated with concurrent R-EPOCH (n = 48)	
CR	35/48 (73%)
PR	7/48 (15%)
Survival in all patients treated with concurrent R-EPOCH (n = 48)	
1-year PFS	78%
2-year PFS	66%
2-year OS	70%
CR rate in diffuse large B-cell lymphoma patients treated with concurrent R-EPOCH (n = 35)	
CR	25/35 (71%)
CR rate in Burkitt-like lymphoma and other aggressive subtype patients treated with concurrent R-EPOCH (n = 16)	
CR	10/16 (63%)

CR, complete response; PR, partial response; PFS, progression-free survival; OS, overall survival

Median follow-up in all treated patients was 30 months (range, 0–68 months)

Barta SK et al. Pooled analysis of AIDS Malignancy Consortium trials evaluating rituximab plus CHOP or infusional EPOCH chemotherapy in HIV-associated non-Hodgkin lymphoma. Cancer 2012;118:3977–3983

Efficacy Variable	P Value
Survival in all patients (R-EPOCH, n = 51) vs R-CHOP (n = 99)	
Event-free survival	P<0.001 in favor of R-EPOCH
Overall survival	P<0.01 in favor of R-EPOCH
Survival in low-risk IPI score patients (R-EPOCH, n = 16) vs R-CHOP (n = 41)	
Event-free survival	P=0.06 in favor of R-EPOCH
Overall survival	P<0.05 in favor of R-EPOCH
Survival high-risk IPI score patients (R-EPOCH, n = 35) vs R-CHOP (n = 58)	
Event-free survival	P<0.01 in favor of R-EPOCH
Overall survival	P<0.01 in favor of R-EPOCH

Multivariable Analysis Assessing the Outcomes Complete Response, Event-Free Survival, and Overall Survival Adjusted for Other Prognostic Covariates in All Patients (R-EPOCH, n = 51; R-CHOP, n = 99)

Covariate	Complete Response	Event-free Survival	Overall Survival
Age-adjusted IPI: low risk vs high risk	OR 4.60 (95% CI, 1.97–10.72); P<0.001	HR 0.32 (95% CI, 0.17–0.57); P<0.001	HR 0.28 (95% CI, 0.14–0.55); P<0.001
Baseline CD4 count: ≥100/mm^3 vs <100/mm^3	OR 2.69 (95% CI, 1.25–5.76); P = 0.01	HR 0.42 (95% CI, 0.26–0.69); P<0.001	HR 0.38 (95% CI, 0.22–0.64); P<0.001
Treatment: R-EPOCH vs R-CHOP	OR 1.92 (95% CI, 0.86–4.22); P = 0.11	HR 0.40 (95% CI, 0.23–0.69); P<0.001	HR 0.37 (95% CI, 0.20–0.68); P<0.01

(continued)

Efficacy (continued)

Outcomes of Patients with Diffuse Large B-cell Lymphoma

Covariate	Complete Response	Event-free Survival	Overall Survival
Treatment: R-EPOCH (n = 35) vs R-CHOP (n = 80)	OR 1.92 (95% CI, 0.86–4.25)	HR 0.40 (95% CI, 0.23–0.69)	HR 0.37 (95% CI, 0.20–0.68)

Therapy Monitoring

1. *Before therapy:* CBC with differential, LFTs, BUN, serum creatinine, hepatitis B and C serologies, tumor lysis labs (ie, potassium, phosphate, uric acid, LDH, calcium), and left ventricular ejection fraction (LVEF)
2. Evaluate LVEF during doxorubicin treatment if clinical symptoms of heart failure are present
3. *Day 1 each cycle:* CBC with differential count, LFTs, BUN, and serum creatinine
4. *Twice-weekly during chemotherapy (at least 3 days apart):* CBC with differential
5. *With each cycle and every 3 months thereafter:* CD4+ cell count and viral load (modify prophylaxis for opportunistic infections based upon CD4+ cell count)

Note: Carriers of hepatitis B receiving rituximab should be on antiretroviral therapy with an NRTI base containing two agents with activity against HBV

Treatment Modifications

DOSE-ADJUSTED EPOCH-R (DA-EPOCH-R)

Drug	Dose Level								
	−3	−2	−1	1 (Starting Dose)	2	3	4	5	6
Prednisone (mg/m^2/dose)	60	60	60	60	60	60	60	60	60
Vincristine (mg/m^2/day)	0.4	0.4	0.4	0.4	0.4	0.4	0.4	0.4	0.4
Doxorubicin (mg/m^2/day)	10	10	10	10	12	14.4	17.3	20.7	24.8
Etoposide (mg/m^2/day)	50	50	50	50	60	72	86.4	103.7	124.4
Cyclophosphamide (mg/m^2)	384	480	600	750	900	1080	1296	1555	1866
Rituximab (mg/m^2)	375	375	375	375	375	375	375	375	375

Dose Modification of Doxorubicin, Etoposide, and Cyclophosphamide Based on Twice-Weekly ANC and Platelet Measurements

Note: ANC and platelets should be measured twice per week (3–4 days apart, eg, every Monday and Thursday) beginning 3–4 days after completion of chemotherapy. Dose adjustments for hematologic toxicity apply only to etoposide, doxorubicin, and cyclophosphamide. Only cyclophosphamide is reduced in dose levels −1 through −3

ANC <1000/mm^3 or platelets <100,000/mm^3 on day 1	Delay the cycle until recovery of ANC >1000/mm^3 or platelets >100,00/mm^3
Previous cycle ANC >500/mm^3 on all measurements AND platelet nadir ≥25,000/ mm^{3*}	Increase etoposide, doxorubicin, and cyclophosphamide dosages by 1 dose level
Previous cycle ANC <500/mm^3 on 1 or 2 measurements (3–4 days apart) AND platelet nadir ≥25,000/ mm^{3*}	Maintain the same dose level of etoposide, doxorubicin, and cyclophosphamide
Previous cycle ANC <500/mm^3 on ≥3 measurements (3–4 days apart) OR platelet nadir <25,000/ mm^{3*}	Decrease etoposide, doxorubicin, and cyclophosphamide dosages by 1 dose level

(continued)

Treatment Modifications *(continued)*

Neuropathy

G2 motor neuropathy	Decrease vincristine dose 25%†
G3 sensory neuropathy	Decrease vincristine dose 25%†
G3 motor neuropathy	Decrease vincristine 50%†
G4 neuropathy (any)	Discontinue vincristine, continue other agents†
Ileus or constipation requiring hospitalization	Optimize the prophylactic bowel regimen. Consider reducing the dose of vincristine in the next cycle by 25%. If the ileus or constipation do not recur, then re-escalate the vincristine dose to the full dose in subsequent cycles

Hyperbilirubinemia Secondary to Lymphoma

Total bilirubin >1.5 mg/dL, but <3 mg/dL	Decrease the vincristine dosage by 25%‡ Do not reduce the doxorubicin dosage
Total bilirubin ≥3.0 mg/dL, but ≤7 mg/dL	Reduce the vincristine dosage by 50%‡ Do not reduce the doxorubicin dosage
Total bilirubin >7 mg/dL	Reduce vincristine dosage by 50%‡ Omit doxorubicin until bilirubin improves to ≤7 mg/dL

*ANC and platelet nadir measurements are based on twice-weekly CBC with differential only
†Vincristine dosage is increased to 100% if neuropathy resolves to G1
‡The vincristine dose may be re-escalated as hyperbilirubinemia improves
Protocol for: Bartlett NL et al. J Clin Oncol 2019;37:1790–1799

RITUXIMAB

Rituximab Infusion-Related Toxicities

Onset of infusion-related events (fevers, chills, rigors, edema, congestion of the head and neck mucosa, hypotension)
1. Interrupt rituximab infusion
2. For fever, chills: Give additional dose of acetaminophen 650 mg orally and diphenhydramine 25–50 mg by intravenous push
3. For rigors: Give meperidine 12.5–25 mg by intravenous push ± promethazine 12.5–25 mg by intravenous infusion in at least 10 mL 0.9% NS or D5W over 5–15 minutes. If after 15–20 minutes the response to a single dose is considered inadequate, the dose may be repeated
4. After symptoms resolve, resume rituximab infusion at a minimum of 50% reduction in the rate at which the event occurred. If no further infusion-related events, increase the rate by 50 mg/hour every 30 minutes, as tolerated, up to a maximum rate of 400 mg/hour

Dyspnea or wheezing, without allergic findings (urticaria, or tongue or laryngeal edema)
1. Interrupt rituximab infusion immediately
2. Give **hydrocortisone** 100 mg by intravenous push (or glucocorticoid equivalent)
3. Give an additional dose of **diphenhydramine** 25–50 mg by intravenous push and a histamine H2-antagonist (**ranitidine** 50 mg or **famotidine** 20 mg) by intravenous push
4. After symptoms resolve, resume rituximab infusion at a minimum of 50% reduction in the rate at which the event occurred. If no further infusion-related events, increase the rate by 50 mg/hour every 30 minutes, as tolerated, up to a maximum rate of 400 mg/hour

---

Note: Medications and equipment for the treatment of hypersensitivity reactions should be available for immediate use in the event of a reaction during administration (eg, intravenous fluids, epinephrine, antihistamines, glucocorticoids, oxygen)

Adverse Events

Barta SK et al. Pooled analysis of AIDS Malignancy Consortium trials evaluating rituximab plus CHOP or infusional EPOCH chemotherapy in HIV-associated non-Hodgkin lymphoma. Cancer 2012;118:3977–3983

Risk of Treatment-Associated Death		
Stratification	R-EPOCH (AMC034)	R-CHOP (AMC010)
All patients	5/51 (9%)	13/99 (13%)
Patients with CD4 <50/mm^3	3/8 (38%)	8/22 (36%)
Patients with CD4 ≥50/mm^3	2/43 (5%)	5/77 (6%)

Sparano JA et al. Rituximab plus concurrent infusional EPOCH chemotherapy is highly effective in HIV-associated B-cell non-Hodgkin lymphoma. Blood 2010;115:3008–3016

	Concurrent R-EPOCH (n = 51)
Grade (%)*	Grade 3–4
Neutropenia	43
Anemia	22
Thrombocytopenia	8
Febrile neutropenia	16
Infection	27
Neuropathy	0
Mucositis	2

FIRST-LINE

HIV-RELATED DIFFUSE LARGE B-CELL LYMPHOMA REGIMEN: CYCLOPHOSPHAMIDE + DOXORUBICIN + VINCRISTINE + PREDNISONE (CHOP) ± RITUXIMAB (CHOP ± RITUXIMAB)

Kaplan DL et al. Blood 2005;106:1538–1543

Rituximab premedication
Acetaminophen 650 mg; administer orally 30 minutes before rituximab
Diphenhydramine 50 mg; administer by intravenous injection 30 minutes before rituximab
Rituximab 375 mg/m²; administer intravenously in 0.9% sodium chloride injection (0.9% NS) or 5% dextrose injection (D5W), diluted to a concentration within the range 1–4 mg/mL, on day 1, every 21 days, for a maximum of 6 cycles (total dosage/cycle = 375 mg/m²)

Note: Caution is advised particularly if a patient's CD4+ cell count is <50/mm³

Notes on rituximab administration:
- Infuse initially at 50 mg/hour. If hypersensitivity or infusion reactions do not occur during the first 30 minutes, increase the rate by 50 mg/hour every 30 minutes as tolerated to a maximum rate of 400 mg/hour. During subsequent treatments, if previous rituximab administration was well tolerated, start at 100 mg/hour and increase by 100 mg/hour every 30 minutes as tolerated to a maximum rate of 400 mg/hour
- Interrupt rituximab administration for fever, chills, edema, congestion of the head and neck mucosa, hypertension, and other serious adverse events. Resume rituximab administration after adverse events abate

Cyclophosphamide 750 mg/m²; administer intravenously in 100 mL of 0.9% NS or D5W over 30 minutes, on day 1, every 21 days (total dosage/cycle = 750 mg/m²)
Doxorubicin 50 mg/m²; administer by slow intravenous injection over 3–5 minutes, on day 1, every 21 days (total dosage/cycle = 50 mg/m²)
Vincristine 1.4 mg/m² (maximum dose = 2 mg); administer by intravenous infusion over 15 minutes in 50 mL 0.9% NS on day 1, every 21 days (total dosage/cycle = 1.4 mg/m²; maximum dosage/cycle = 2 mg)
Prednisone 100 mg/day; administer orally for 5 consecutive days, on days 1–5, every 21 days (total dose/cycle = 500 mg)

Supportive Care
Antiemetic prophylaxis
Emetogenic potential: **HIGH.** *Potential for delayed symptoms*
See Chapter 42 for antiemetic recommendations

Hematopoietic growth factor (CSF) prophylaxis
Primary prophylaxis is indicated with one of the following:
   Filgrastim (G-CSF) 5 mcg/kg per day; administer by subcutaneous injection, *or*
   Pegfilgrastim (pegylated filgrastim) 6 mg/0.6 mL; administer by subcutaneous injection for 1 dose
- Begin use from 24–72 hours after myelosuppressive chemotherapy is completed
See Chapter 43 for more information

Antimicrobial prophylaxis
Risk of fever and neutropenia is **INTERMEDIATE**
   Antimicrobial primary prophylaxis to be considered:
- Antibacterial
  - Consider a fluoroquinolone during expected periods of neutropenia, or no prophylaxis
- Opportunistic infection prophylaxis, based on CD4+ (See above)
- Antifungal—not indicated
- Antiviral—not indicated, unless patient previously had an episode of herpes simplex virus infection

Additional prophylaxis
Add a **proton pump inhibitor** during prednisone use to prevent gastritis and duodenitis
Give **stool softeners** and/or laxatives during and after vincristine administration

Patient Population Studied

A 2:1 randomization trial with 95 patients randomized to the CHOP-rituximab arm and 47 patients to the CHOP arm. The study included DLBCL, Burkitt Lymphoma, primary effusion lymphoma, and other unspecified high-grade CD20 + lymphomas. Median CD4+ lymphocyte count was 133 cells/mm³; 79% of patients had stage III/IV disease

Efficacy (N = 47)

Complete response	50%
Median progression-free survival	11 months
Median overall survival	33 months

Treatment Modifications

CYCLOPHOSPHAMIDE + DOXORUBICIN + VINCRISTINE + PREDNISONE DOSE MODIFICATIONS

	Cyclophosphamide Dose Levels	Doxorubicin Dose Levels	Vincristine Dose Levels	Prednisone Dose Levels
Starting dose	750 mg/m^2	50 mg/m^2	1.4 mg/m^2 (max dose of 2 mg)	100 mg
Dose level −1	562.5 mg/m^2	37.5 mg/m^2	1.05 mg/m^2 (max dose of 1.5 mg)	80 mg
Dose level −2	375 mg/m^2	25 mg/m^2	0.7 mg/m^2 (max dose of 1 mg)	60 mg

Hematologic Toxicity

Day 1 platelet count <100,000/mm^3 or ANC <1500/mm^3	Delay start of cycle until platelet count ≥100,000/mm^3 and ANC ≥1500/mm^3, or until recovery to near baseline value, then continue at the same doses
G4 neutropenia (ANC <500/mm^3) during the prior cycle given *without* growth factor (filgrastim, pegfilgrastim) prophylaxis	Administer filgrastim or pegfilgrastim during all subsequent cycles and continue the same doses
Febrile neutropenia (ANC <1000/mm^3 with temperature >38°C or >100.4°F) during the prior cycle given *without* growth factor (filgrastim, pegfilgrastim) prophylaxis	
Febrile neutropenia (ANC <1000/mm^3 with temperature >38°C or >100.4°F) during the prior cycle given *with* growth factor (filgrastim, pegfilgrastim) prophylaxis	Reduce the dose of cyclophosphamide and doxorubicin by 1 dose level for subsequent cycles. Do not change the prednisone or vincristine dose
G ≥3 thrombocytopenia (platelets <50,000/mm^3) during the prior cycle	

Gastrointestinal Toxicities

G ≥3 ileus (severely altered GI function; TPN indicated; tube placement indicated)	Withhold all chemotherapy until resolution of ileus and constipation, then reduce the next dose of vincristine by one dose level with an optimal prophylactic bowel regimen. Do not change the cyclophosphamide, doxorubicin, or prednisone doses
G ≥3 constipation (obstipation with manual evacuation indicated; limiting self-care ADL)	If symptoms do not recur at the reduced vincristine dose, then the vincristine dose may be re-escalated on subsequent cycles with an appropriate prophylactic bowel regimen

Neurologic Toxicities

G3 peripheral sensory neuropathy (severe symptoms; limiting self-care ADL)	Proceed with treatment and reduce the dose of vincristine by one dose level. Do not change the cyclophosphamide, doxorubicin, or prednisone doses
G2 peripheral motor neuropathy (moderate symptoms; limiting instrumental ADL)	If symptoms improve, then the vincristine dose may be re-escalated on subsequent cycles
G3 peripheral motor neuropathy (severe symptoms; limiting self-care ADL)	Proceed with treatment and reduce the dose of vincristine by two dose levels. Do not change the cyclophosphamide, doxorubicin, or prednisone doses
	If symptoms improve, then the vincristine dose may be re-escalated on subsequent cycles
G4 peripheral sensory neuropathy (life-threatening symptoms; urgent intervention indicated)	Discontinue vincristine
G4 peripheral motor neuropathy (life-threatening consequences; urgent intervention indicated)	Do not change the cyclophosphamide, doxorubicin, or prednisone doses
G ≥2 mood alteration (moderate mood alteration) or confusion (moderate disorientation; limiting instrumental ADL)	Withhold prednisone until symptoms return to baseline. Resume prednisone reduced by one dose level. If symptoms persist, reduce by another dose level. Do not change the cyclophosphamide, doxorubicin, or vincristine doses

(continued)

Treatment Modifications (*continued*)

Hepatic Impairment

Serum bilirubin 1.2 to 3 mg/dL	Decrease the doxorubicin dose by 50%
	Additionally, if the bilirubin is 1.5 to 3 mg/dL, then decrease the vincristine dose by 50%
Serum bilirubin 3.1 to 5 mg/dL	Decrease the doxorubicin by 75%
	Do not administer vincristine
Serum bilirubin >5 mg/dL	Do not administer doxorubicin or vincristine

Drug Interactions

Patient requires concomitant therapy with antihypertensive medication(s)	On days of rituximab treatment, and especially with the initial dose, weigh the risk versus benefit of delaying administration of the antihypertensive medication(s) until after completion of the rituximab infusion due to the potential risk of rituximab infusion-related hypotension
Patient requires concomitant therapy with a strong CYP3A4 inhibitor	Patient may have earlier onset of neuromuscular side effects of vincristine. If concomitant use of the strong CYP3A4 inhibitor cannot be avoided, consider dose reduction of vincristine and increased monitoring for toxicity

Other Toxicities

G ≥3 hyperglycemia (insulin therapy initiated; hospitalization indicated)	Withhold prednisone until blood glucose is ≤250 mg/dL. Treat with insulin or other hypoglycemic agents as clinically appropriate and then resume prednisone at the same dose. If hyperglycemia is uncontrolled despite above measures, decrease prednisone by one dose level
LVEF is 40%, or is 40% to 45% with a 10% or greater absolute decrease below the pre-treatment	Withhold doxorubicin and repeat LVEF assessment within approximately 4 weeks. Discontinue doxorubicin if the LVEF has not improved or has declined further, unless the benefits for the individual patient outweigh the risks

RITUXIMAB

Rituximab Infusion-Related Toxicities

Onset of infusion-related events (fevers, chills, rigors, edema, congestion of the head and neck mucosa, hypotension)
1. Interrupt rituximab infusion
2. For fever, chills: Give additional dose of acetaminophen 650 mg orally and diphenhydramine 25–50 mg by intravenous push
3. For rigors: Give meperidine 12.5–25 mg by intravenous push ± promethazine 12.5–25 mg by intravenous infusion in at least 10 mL 0.9% NS or D5W over 5–15 minutes. If after 15–20 minutes the response to a single dose is considered inadequate, the dose may be repeated
4. After symptoms resolve, resume rituximab infusion at a minimum of 50% reduction in the rate at which the event occurred. If no further infusion-related events, increase the rate by 50 mg/hour every 30 minutes, as tolerated, up to a maximum rate of 400 mg/hour

Dyspnea or wheezing, without allergic findings (urticaria, or tongue or laryngeal edema)
1. Interrupt rituximab infusion immediately
2. Give hydrocortisone 100 mg by intravenous push (or glucocorticoid equivalent)
3. Give an additional dose of diphenhydramine 25–50 mg by intravenous push and a histamine H2-antagonist (**ranitidine** 50 mg or **famotidine** 20 mg) by intravenous push
4. After symptoms resolve, resume rituximab infusion at a minimum of 50% reduction in the rate at which the event occurred. If no further infusion-related events, increase the rate by 50 mg/hour every 30 minutes, as tolerated, up to a maximum rate of 400 mg/hour

Note: Medications and equipment for the treatment of hypersensitivity reactions should be available for immediate use in the event of a reaction during administration (eg, intravenous fluids, epinephrine, antihistamines, glucocorticoids, and oxygen)

Toxicity* (N = 47)

	% Patients
G3/4 neutropenia	17
G3/4 anemia	8
Fever and ANC <100/mm^3	8.5
G3/4 infusion reaction	2
G3/4 AST elevation	11
Death caused by infection	2

*National Cancer Institute (USA) Common Toxicity Criteria, version 2.0. Available at: http://ctep.cancer.gov/protocolDevelopment/electronic_applications/ctc.htm [accessed December 7, 2013]

Therapy Monitoring

1. *Before therapy:* CBC with differential, LFTs, BUN, serum creatinine, hepatitis B and C serologies, tumor lysis labs (ie, potassium, phosphate, uric acid, LDH, calcium), and left ventricular ejection fraction (LVEF)
2. *Day 1 of each cycle:* CBC with differential count, LFTs, BUN, serum creatinine
3. *Twice-weekly during chemotherapy:* CBC with differential
4. Evaluate LVEF during doxorubicin treatment if clinical symptoms of heart failure are present
5. *Every 2 cycles:* Tumor restaging

Note

Carriers of hepatitis B receiving rituximab should be on antiretroviral therapy with an NRTI base containing two agents with activity against HBV

22. Hodgkin Lymphoma

Michael Fuchs, MD and Volker Diehl, MD

Epidemiology

Incidence: 8110 Estimated new cases for 2019 in the United States; 3.0 per 100,000 males; 2.3 per 100,000 females
Deaths: Estimated 1000 in 2019
Median age: 39 years
Male to female ratio: 1.3:1

Surveillance, Epidemiology and End Results (SEER) Program, available from http://seer.cancer.gov [accessed in 2019]

Pathology

Since 1944, several classifications have been proposed for Hodgkin lymphoma (HL). Currently, the World Health Organization (WHO) Classification of Hematologic Malignancies is used:

1. Lymphocyte predominant, nodular (NLPHL) (5%)
2. Classic
   a. Lymphocyte-rich (LRCHL) (5%)
   b. Nodular sclerosis (NSHL) (60–80%)
   c. Mixed cellularity (MCHL) (15–30%)
   d. Lymphocyte depleted (LDHL) (1%)
   e. Unclassifiable (<1%)

Swerdlow SH et al (editors). WHO classification of tumours of haematopoietic and lymphoid tissues. In: Bosman FT, Jaffe ES, Lakhani SR, Ohgaki H (editors). World Health Organization Classification of Tumours. Lyon, France: IARC; 2008

Swerdlow SH et al. Blood 2016;127:2375–2390

Work-up

1. History and physical exam
2. Laboratory tests: CBC with differential, ESR, electrolytes, albumin, liver function tests, mineral panel, LDH
3. HIV and hepatitis B and C serologies as clinically indicated
4. Chest x-ray (PA and lateral)
5. CT scan of chest, abdomen, and pelvis (and neck in selected cases)
6. Positron emission tomography (PET) scan
7. Bone marrow aspirate and biopsy
8. Pulmonary function tests
9. Echocardiogram or MUGA scan to determine cardiac ejection fraction
10. Excisional lymph node biopsy to completely assess lymph node architecture is required at initial diagnosis. Fine-needle aspiration biopsy alone is not desirable for the initial diagnosis of lymphoma
11. Fertility counseling, if appropriate

Five-Year Survival Rate

NLPHL	90% (10 years)
Classic HL	70–80%

Jaffe ES et al. (editors). World Health Organization Classification of Tumours. Pathology and Genetics of Tumours of Haematopoietic and Lymphoid Tissues. Lyon, France: IARC Press; 2001

Staging

Ann Arbor Staging Classification for Hodgkin and Non-Hodgkin Lymphomas

Stage	Description
I	Involvement of a single lymph node region (I) or involvement of a single extralymphatic organ or site (IE)
II	Involvement of 2 or more lymph node regions or lymphatic structures on the same side of the diaphragm alone (II) or with involvement of limited, contiguous extralymphatic organ or tissue (IIE)
III	Involvement of lymph node regions on both sides of the diaphragm (III), which may include the spleen (IIIS), or limited, contiguous extralymphatic organ or site (IIIE), or both (IIIES)
IV	Diffuse or disseminated foci of involvement of one or more extralymphatic organs or tissues with or without associated lymphatic involvement

Abbreviations

A	Asymptomatic
B	Unexplained persistent or recurrent fever with temperature higher than 38°C (100.4°F) or recurrent drenching night sweats within 1 month or unexplained loss of >10% body weight within 6 months
E	Limited direct extension into extralymphatic organ from adjacent lymph node

Carbone PP et al. Cancer Res 1971;31:1860–1861

Criteria that predict an unfavorable prognosis in *limited-stage HL* differ among study groups

Patients with one or more of these factors are considered to have an unfavorable prognosis

Factor	EORTC	GHSG	NCIC	Stanford
Age (years)	≥50	—	≥40	—
Histology	—	—	MC/LD	—
ESR/B-symptoms	≥30 mm with any B ≥50 mm without B	≥30 mm with any B ≥50 mm without B	≥50 mm or any B	Any B
Mediastinal mass	MTR ≥0.35	MMR >0.33	10 cm or MMR >0.33	MMR >0.33
Number of nodal sites	≥4	≥3	≥4	—
E-lesions	—	Present	—	—

EORTC, European Organization for Research and Treatment of Cancer; GHSG, German Hodgkin Lymphoma Study Group; NCIC, National Cancer Institute of Canada

For patients with *advanced-stage HL*, the German Hodgkin Lymphoma Study Group (*GHSG*) has developed the following prognostic score model:

Number of Factors	Percentage of the Population	Estimated Freedom from Disease Progression at 5 Years
0	7%	84%
1	22%	77%
2	29%	67%
3	23%	60%
4	12%	51%
5+	7%	42%

Factors: Stage IV; male sex; age >45 years; hemoglobin <10.5 g/dL; WBC ≥15,000/mm^3; lymphocytes <8% or <600/mm^3; albumin <4 g/dL
Hasenclever D, Diehl V. N Engl J Med 1998;339:1506–1514

Expert Opinion

The treatment of adult patients with HL should be stage adapted with respect to age and additional factors such as comorbidities

1. **Patients with early favorable-stage HL**
   - Combined modality treatment with a chemotherapy regimen such as ABVD followed by involved-field radiotherapy (IF-RT) is considered the treatment of choice[*,†] with a 5-year event-free survival rate (EFS) of 98% (data from the H8F trial of the EORTC)

2. **Patients with Stage IA nodular lymphocyte predominant Hodgkin Lymphoma (NLPHL)**
   - Local radiotherapy is widely accepted as the standard treatment due to the excellent prognosis of this subgroup of patients[‡]

3. **Patients with early unfavorable (intermediate)-stage HL**
   - Combined modality treatment, for example, 4–6 cycles of ABVD followed by IF-RT[§]
   - Despite excellent initial remission rates, approximately 15% of patients relapse within 5 years. Thus, an intensification of chemotherapy might improve results. Several ongoing studies are addressing this issue

4. **Patients with advanced-stage HL**
   - *Low-risk patients:* IPS <3 risk factors → FDG-PET might help to identify patients for whom 6–8 cycles of ABVD ± IF-RT are sufficient to achieve a cure
   - *High-risk patients:* IPS >3 risk factors → intensive chemotherapy such as dose-escalated BEACOPP is the treatment of choice.[€] For patients with advanced HL, 6 cycles of BEACOPP escalated are no longer standard of care. The final analysis of the GHSG HD18 trial has shown tailoring therapy by FDG-PET after 2 cycles (PET–2) represents the optimal treatment. Patients with negative PET–2 can be treated with 4 cycles of BEACOPP escalated only. Patients with positive PET–2 should be treated with 6 cycles of BEACOPP escalated
   - The impact of radiotherapy after effective chemotherapy if a CR is achieved is doubtful. Therefore, radiotherapy should be restricted to patients in whom FDG-PET scan demonstrates positive lesions after the end of chemotherapy

5. The following protocols may be considered in the management of patients with Hodgkin lymphoma:

   First-line protocols for newly diagnosed Hodgkin lymphoma
   1. ABVD
   2. A+AVD
   3. Stanford V
   4. BEACOPP

Salvage/induction protocols
1. DHAP
2. ICE
3. IGEV
4. GVD
5. Dexa-BEAM
6. IVE

High-dose/conditioning protocols
1. BEAM
2. CBV

Consolidation after autologous stem cell transplant
1. Brentuximab vedotin

Palliative protocols (regimens/drugs)
1. Brentuximab vedotin
2. Gemcitabine
3. Vinorelbine
4. Bendamustine
5. Nivolumab
6. Pembrolizumab

*Two large randomized clinical trials were published demonstrating an increased risk of relapse if RT was omitted in patients who are PET negative after end of chemotherapy. Thus, omitting radiotherapy cannot be recommended

†Patients older than 60 years of age should not receive dose-escalated BEACOPP because of an increased rate of toxicity. These patients should be treated with 6–8 cycles of ABVD followed by radiotherapy in case of residual lymphomas

‡HL patients who relapse or do not respond to primary treatment require an adequate salvage therapy. For most of them, high-dose chemotherapy (HDCT) followed by autologous stem cell transplantation (ASCT) is the treatment of choice. The best regimen for reinduction therapy has not yet been defined

§Patients with contraindications to undergo ASCT or with multiple relapses should either receive a classic palliative treatment with drugs such as gemcitabine or vinorelbine, or be enrolled in clinical trials evaluating novel approaches

€ASCT still has to be regarded as an experimental approach, as it is associated with high relapse and mortality rates. It should be considered only for patients younger than 30 years of age who are in a good general condition

Bonadonna G et al. J Clin Oncol 2004;22:2835–2841
Diehl V et al. N Engl J Med 2003;348:2386–2395
Engert A et al J Clin Oncol 2003;21:3601–3608
Nogova L et al. Ann Oncol 2005;16:1683–1687
Noordijk EM et al. J Clin Oncol 2006;24:3128–3135

INDUCTION • FIRST-LINE

HODGKIN LYMPHOMA REGIMEN: DOXORUBICIN (ADRIAMYCIN), BLEOMYCIN, VINBLASTINE, DACARBAZINE (ABVD)

Canellos GP et al. N Engl J Med 1992;327:1478–1484
Duggan DB et al. J Clin Oncol 2003;21:607–614
Hoskins PJ et al. J Clin Oncol 2009;27:5390–5396

Doxorubicin 25 mg/m^2 per dose; administer by intravenous injection over 3–5 minutes for 2 doses on days 1 and 15, every 28 days (total dosage/cycle = 50 mg/m^2)

Bleomycin 10 units/m^2 per dose; administer intravenously by slow injection over 10 minutes for 2 doses on days 1 and 15, every 28 days (total dosage/cycle = 20 units/m^2)

Vinblastine 6 mg/m^2 per dose; administer by intravenous injection over 1–2 minutes for 2 doses on days 1 and 15, every 28 days (total dosage/cycle = 12 mg/m^2)

• In accordance with recommendations from the Institute for Safe Medication Practices and in order to avoid inadvertent fatal intrathecal administration, some institutions further dilute vinblastine sulfate in 50 mL of 0.9% sodium chloride injection (0.9% NS) or 5% dextrose injection (D5W) and infuse each dose intravenously over 20 minutes. This method of administration is particularly suited for patients with a central venous access device since slow administration through a peripheral vein can lead to phlebitis.

Dacarbazine 375 mg/m^2 per dose; administer intravenously in 100–250 mL 0.9% NS or D5W over 15–30 minutes for 2 doses on days 1 and 15, every 28 days (total dosage/cycle = 750 mg/m^2)

Note: There is evidence that ABVD can be given without any dose modification on time irrespective of the peripheral blood count (Evens AM et al. Br J Haematol 2007;137:545–552)

Supportive Care
Antiemetic prophylaxis
Emetogenic potential on Days 1 and 15 is **HIGH**
See Chapter 42 for antiemetic recommendations

Hematopoietic growth factor (CSF) prophylaxis
Primary prophylaxis is indicated with:
   Filgrastim (G-CSF) 5 mcg/kg per day, by subcutaneous injection
   • Begin use 24–72 h after myelosuppressive chemotherapy is completed
   • G-CSF use with bleomycin-containing regimens for Hodgkin disease has been associated with an increased rate of pulmonary toxicity
See Chapter 43 for more information

Antimicrobial prophylaxis
Risk of fever and neutropenia is **LOW**
   Antimicrobial primary prophylaxis to be considered:
   • Antibacterial—*Pneumocystis jirovecii* prophylaxis is recommended (eg, cotrimoxazole)

Patient Population Studied

Hoskins PJ et al. J Clin Oncol 2009;27:5390–5396

Multicenter, prospective, randomized controlled trial compared the efficacy and toxicity of 2 chemotherapy regimens, ABVD and Stanford V, in advanced Hodgkin lymphoma

Baseline Demographic and Clinical Characteristics

Characteristic	Treatment Arm		Total (N = 520) Number (%)
	ABVD (n = 261) Number (%)	Stanford V (n = 259) Number (%)	
Age, median (range)	35 years (18–60)	34 years (18–67)	35 years (18–67)
Male sex	154 (59%)	154 (59%)	308 (59%)
Stage			
I to II	119 (46%)	134 (52%)	253 (49%)
III	81 (31%)	72 (28%)	153 (29%)

(continued)

Patient Population Studied (continued)

Characteristic	Treatment Arm		Total (N = 520) Number (%)
	ABVD (n = 261) Number (%)	Stanford V (n = 259) Number (%)	
IV	61 (23%)	53 (20%)	114 (22%)
"B" symptoms present	184 (73%)	185 (75%)	369 (74%)
Bulky disease present	94 (41%)	93 (42%)	187 (41%)
Hasenclever score			
0–1	77 (31%)	90 (36%)	167 (34%)
2–3	136 (55%)	122 (50%)	258 (52%)
4–7	33 (13%)	36 (15%)	69 (14%)
Unknown	15	11	26
Histology			
LP	2 (1%)	6 (3%)	8 (2%)
MC	21 (10%)	20 (10%)	41 (10%)
NS	190 (88%)	178 (86%)	368 (87%)
Other	3 (1%)	3 (1%)	6 (1%)
Not reviewed	45	52	97

LP, lymphocyte predominant; MC, mixed cellularity; NS nodular sclerosing

Treatment Modifications

Adverse Event*	Dose Modification
WBC 3999–3000/mm^3 or platelet count 129,000–100,000/mm^3	Reduce doxorubicin and vinblastine dosages by 50%[†]
WBC 2999–2000/mm^3 or platelet count 99,000–80,000/mm^3	Reduce dacarbazine dosage by 50%. Reduce doxorubicin and vinblastine dosages by 75%[†]
WBC 1999–1500/mm^3 or platelet count 79,000–50,000/mm^3	Reduce dacarbazine dosage by 75%. Hold doxorubicin and vinblastine[†]
WBC <1500/mm^3 or platelet count <50,000/ mm^3	Hold doxorubicin, vinblastine, and dacarbazine[†]
Clinical or radiologic evidence of pulmonary fibrosis or DLCO <50% pretreatment value	Discontinue bleomycin
Moderate to severe renal function impairment (creatinine clearance <50 mL/min [<0.83 mL/s])	Discontinue bleomycin until creatinine clearance improves to ≥50 mL/min

*Refers to values on days 1 or 15
[†]There is evidence that ABVD can be given without any dose modification on time irrespective of the peripheral blood count (Evens AM et al. Br J Haematol 2007;137:545–552)

Therapy Monitoring

1. *Semiweekly and before each cycle:* CBC with differential
2. *Before each cycle:* Physical exam, chest x-ray
3. *After second and each subsequent cycle:* DLCO
4. *Response evaluation:* CT of chest, abdomen, and pelvis every 2 cycles starting after cycle 4. FDG-PET scan at conclusion of therapy to document extent of remission. Bone marrow biopsy (if disease existed before therapy) performed 1 month after completing the sixth cycle

Efficacy

Response	Treatment Arm		Total Number (%)
	ABVD Number (%)	Stanford V Number (%)	
At completion of chemotherapy			
CR	89 (38%)	62 (27%)	151 (33%)
Cru	39 (17%)	21 (9%)	60 (13%)
PR	88 (38%)	133 (58%)	221 (48%)
SD	7 (3%)	7 (3%)	14 (3%)
PD/relapse	9 (4%)	5 (2%)	14 (3%)
Death	1	0	1 (0%)
Unknown	19	20	39
Total	252	248	500
CR/CRu rate*	128/233 (55%)	83/228 (36%)	P<0.0001
At treatment completion			
ORR	228 (92%)	218 (91%)	
CR	113 (46%)	104 (44%)	217 (45%)
CRu	52 (21%)	33 (14%)	85 (17%)
PR	63 (25%)	81 (34%)	144 (30%)
SD	6 (2%)	6 (2%)	12 (2%)
PD/relapse	12 (5%)	15 (6%)	27 (6%)
Death	2 (1%)	0	2 (0)
Unknown	4	9	13
Total	252	248	500
CR/CRu rate†	165/248 (67%)	137/239 (57%)	P = 0.036
Estimated 5-year PFS	76%	74%	
5-year OS rates	90%	92%	HR 0.76, 95% CI 0.41−1.38; P = 0.37

CR, complete response rate; CRu, complete remission unconfirmed; ORR, overall response rate = CR + Cru + PR; PFS, progression-free survival; PR, partial response rate
Note: Treatment completion indicates completion of chemotherapy and radiotherapy

Hoskins PJ et al. J Clin Oncol 2009;27:5390–5396

Toxicity

ABVD

Toxicity	Number of Patients (%)
During initial treatment (N = 412)	
Pulmonary*	101 (24.5%)
Cardiac*	27 (6.6)
Hematologic†	262 (63.6%)
Anorexia†	1 (0.2%)
Fatigue†	7 (1.7%)
Hypotension†	0
After completion of treatment (N = 300)	
Pulmonary*	25 (8.3%)
Cardiac*	10 (3.3%)
Hematologic†	15 (5%)

*G ≥2 dyspnea, partial pressure of oxygen/carbon dioxide, diffusing capacity for carbon monoxide, fibrosis, acute respiratory distress syndrome, noninfectious pneumonitis, cardiac function, or arrhythmia, all of which would result in dose modification or elimination of doxorubicin or bleomycin
†Maximum toxicity G ≥3, severe, life-threatening, or fatal
Note: There were 9 deaths during initial therapy

Duggan DB et al. J Clin Oncol 2003;21:607–614

INDUCTION • FIRST-LINE

HODGKIN LYMPHOMA REGIMEN: BRENTUXIMAB VEDOTIN + DOXORUBICIN + VINBLASTINE + DACARBAZINE (A+AVD)

Connors JM et al. N Engl J Med 2018;378:331–344
Supplementary appendix to: Connors JM et al. N Engl J Med 2018;378:331–344
Protocol for: Connors JM et al. N Engl J Med 2018;378:331–344

Doxorubicin HCl 25 mg/m^2 per dose; administer by intravenous injection over 3–5 minutes for 2 doses on days 1 and 15, every 28 days (total dosage/28-day cycle = 50 mg/m^2)

Vinblastine sulfate 6 mg/m^2 per dose; administer by intravenous injection over 1–2 minutes for 2 doses on days 1 and 15, every 28 days (total dosage/28-day cycle = 12 mg/m^2)
• In accordance with recommendations from the Institute for Safe Medication Practices and in order to avoid inadvertent fatal intrathecal administration, some institutions further dilute vinblastine sulfate in 50 mL of 0.9% sodium chloride injection (0.9% NS) or 5% dextrose injection (D5W) and infuse each dose intravenously over 20 minutes. This method of administration is particularly suited for patients with a central venous access device since slow administration through a peripheral vein can lead to phlebitis. See Chapter 40 for more information. https://www.ismp.org/sites/default/files/attachments/2017-12/TMSBP-for-Hospitalsv2.pdf [accessed September 2, 2018]

Dacarbazine 375 mg/m^2 per dose; administer intravenously in 100–250 mL 0.9% NS or D5W over 15–30 minutes for 2 doses on days 1 and 15, every 28 days, for 6 cycles (total dosage/28-day cycle = 750 mg/m^2)

Brentuximab vedotin 1.2 mg/kg (maximum dose = 120 mg); administer intravenously in a volume of 0.9% NS or D5W sufficient to produce a concentration with the range 0.4–1.8 mg/mL (minimum volume, 100 mL) over 30 minutes for 2 doses, within one hour of completion of dacarbazine, on days 1 and 15, every 28 days for 6 cycles (total dosage/28-day cycle = 2.4 mg/kg; maximum dose/28-day cycle = 240 mg)

Notes:
• The dose for patients whose body weight is >100 kg should be calculated based on a weight of 100 kg
• Brentuximab vedotin can cause severe or life-threatening infusion-related reactions, including hypersensitivity and anaphylaxis
• Monomethyl auristatin E, the cytotoxic component of brentuximab vedotin, is a substrate of CYP3A4/5 and P-glycoprotein (P-gp). Use caution and monitor closely for brentuximab vedotin side effects when coadministering brentuximab vedotin with strong CYP3A4 inhibitors or P-gp inhibitors

Supportive Care
Antiemetic prophylaxis
Emetogenic potential on Days 1 and 15 is **HIGH**
See Chapter 42 for antiemetic recommendations

Hematopoietic growth factor (CSF) prophylaxis
Primary prophylaxis is indicated with one of the following:
  Filgrastim (G-CSF) 5 mcg/kg per day, by subcutaneous injection, *or*
  • Begin use from 24–72 h after myelosuppressive chemotherapy is completed
  • Continue daily filgrastim use until ANC ≥5000/mm^3 after the leukocyte nadir
  • Discontinue daily filgrastim use at least 24 hours before administering myelosuppressive treatment
  Pegfilgrastim (pegylated filgrastim) 6 mg/0.6 mL, by subcutaneous injection for 2 doses per 28-day cycle (eg, on days 2 and 16)
  • Administer between 24–72 h after myelosuppressive chemotherapy is completed
  • Do not administer pegfilgrastim within 14 days before administering myelosuppressive treatment

See Chapter 43 for more information

(continued)

Patient Population Studied

The international, multicenter, randomized, open-label, phase 3 trial (ECHELON–1) involved 1334 patients with histologically confirmed, advanced, classic Hodgkin lymphoma. Eligible patients were aged ≥18 years, with an Eastern Cooperative Oncology Group (ECOG) performance status score ≤2. Patients with nodular lymphocyte-predominant Hodgkin lymphoma were ineligible. Patients were randomized (1:1) to receive intravenous A + AVD (1.2 mg/kg brentuximab vedotin, 25 mg/m^2 doxorubicin, 6 mg/m^2 vinblastine, and 375 mg/m^2 dacarbazine) or ABVD (25 mg/m^2 doxorubicin, 10 units/m^2 bleomycin, 6 mg/m^2 vinblastine, and 375 mg/m^2 dacarbazine) on days 1 and 15 of each 28-day cycle for up to 6 cycles

Efficacy (N = 1334)

	A + AVD (N = 664)	ABVD (N = 670)	
2-year modified progression-free survival*	82.1%	77.2%	HR 0.77, 95% CI 0.60–0.98; P = 0.04

*Modified progression-free survival (the primary efficacy end point) is time to disease progression, death, or modified progression (that is, evidence of noncomplete response after completion of front-line therapy, followed by subsequent anticancer therapy)
Note: Median follow-up time was 24.6 months. An interim analysis of overall survival (a secondary end point) showed no significant difference between the treatment groups

(continued)

Antimicrobial prophylaxis
Risk of fever and neutropenia is **HIGH**
Antimicrobial primary prophylaxis to be considered:
- Antibacterial—consider a fluoroquinolone during periods of neutropenia, or no prophylaxis
- Antifungal—consider concomitant use of fluconazole during periods of neutropenia, and in anticipation of mucositis
- Antiviral—antiherpes antivirals (eg, acyclovir, famciclovir, valacyclovir)

Therapy Monitoring

1. *Prior to initiation of therapy:* CBC with differential and platelet count, serum electrolytes, liver function tests, serum creatinine, BUN, physical exam, urine pregnancy test (women of child-bearing potential only)
2. *In patients at high risk for tumor lysis syndrome (eg, high tumor burden, renal dysfunction, rapidly progressing disease, markedly elevated LDH, baseline abnormalities in laboratory indices of tumor lysis syndrome [potassium, phosphate, uric acid, calcium, serum creatinine]):* consider frequent monitoring of laboratory indices of tumor lysis syndrome, intravenous hydration, and prophylaxis with a xanthine oxidase inhibitor (eg, allopurinol) during cycle 1
3. *During each brentuximab vedotin infusion:* signs and symptoms of infusion-related reaction, vital signs every 30 minutes
4. *On day 1 and 15 of each cycle:* CBC with differential and platelet count, serum electrolytes, liver function tests, serum creatinine, BUN
   a. In patients with compromised bone marrow function or past G ≥3 myelosuppression, consider more frequent monitoring of CBC with differential and platelet count within each cycle
5. *Periodically assess for:* peripheral neuropathy, pulmonary toxicity, severe dermatologic toxicity, gastrointestinal toxicity, infection, and progressive multifocal leukoencephalopathy
6. *Response evaluation:* physical exam prior to each cycle, CT scan with contrast and/or PET scan after cycle 2 and after completion of therapy

Treatment Modifications

BRENTUXIMAB VEDOTIN + DOXORUBICIN + VINBLASTINE + DACARBAZINE (A + AVD)

	Brentuximab Vedotin	Doxorubicin	Vinblastine	Dacarbazine
Starting dose	1.2 mg/kg (maximum dose = 120 mg) per dose	25 mg/m² per dose	6 mg/m² per dose	375 mg/m² per dose
Dose level −1	0.9 mg/kg (maximum dose = 90 mg) per dose	18.75 mg/m² per dose	4.5 mg/m² per dose	280 mg/m² per dose

Adverse Event	Dose Modification
General Dose Modification	
Patient weight >100 kg	Use a maximum weight of 100 kg for calculation of the brentuximab vedotin dose. Follow institutional standards and clinical practice guidelines for calculation of doxorubicin, vinblastine, and dacarbazine doses
Hematologic Adverse Events	
Day 1 or Day 15 platelet count <50,000/mm³ or ANC <1000/mm³	If the patient is not already receiving primary prophylaxis with G-CSF, then add G-CSF with subsequent cycles
	Consider platelet transfusion per institutional guidelines
	The U.S. FDA prescribing information for brentuximab vedotin recommends proceeding with brentuximab vedotin therapy without delay and without dose reduction in case of G3/4 thrombocytopenia and/or G3/4 neutropenia and refers to the U.S. FDA prescribing information for doxorubicin, vinblastine, and dacarbazine for instructions for dose modification and/or delay for these agents. However, these documents provide vague recommendations for dose reduction and delay for hematologic toxicity
	There is evidence to support treating patients receiving a similar regimen, ABVD, at full doses irrespective of neutrophil counts measured on the day of treatment (Evens AM et al. Br J Haematol 2007;137:545–552); however the safety of extrapolating that approach to patients receiving A + AVD is unknown
	In general, maintenance of maximal dose intensity should be the goal of therapy when feasible

(continued)

Treatment Modifications (*continued*)

Hematologic Adverse Events

Therapy modification data from the ECHELON–1 trial in North American patients is presented in the table below for reference

Taken together, the medically responsible health care provider may use discretion for dose reduction, delay, or discontinuation of doxorubicin, vinblastine, and/or dacarbazine for G3/4 neutropenia or G3/4 thrombocytopenia occurring on the day of scheduled treatment for individual patients

Dose modification, delay, or discontinuation of study drug for any reason in North American patients enrolled into the A + AVD arm (n = 249) of the ECHELON–1 study

	BV	Dox	Vinblastine	DTIC
Dose reduced	32%	4%	10%	4%
Dose held	11%	<1%	2%	0
Dose delay	35%	37%	37%	35%
Discontinue	6%	6%	7%	6%

BV, brentuximab vedotin; dox, doxorubicin; DTIC, dacarbazine
Ramchandren R et al. Clin Cancer Res 2019;25:1718–1726

Hepatic Impairment

Patient with mild hepatic impairment (Child-Pugh class A)	Reduce the brentuximab vedotin dose to 0.9 mg/kg (maximum dose = 90 mg) every 2 weeks. See bilirubin criteria to determine if doxorubicin and/or vinblastine dose modification is necessary
Patient with moderate to severe hepatic impairment (Child-Pugh class B or C)	Avoid use of brentuximab vedotin. See bilirubin criteria to determine if doxorubicin and/or vinblastine dose modification is necessary
Serum bilirubin >3 mg/dL	Reduce the dose of vinblastine by 50% Reduce the dose of doxorubicin by 75% if serum bilirubin is >3 but ≤5 mg/dL Omit doxorubicin if serum bilirubin is >5 mg/dL See Child-Pugh criteria to determine if brentuximab vedotin dose modification is necessary

Renal Impairment

Mild renal impairment (CrCl 46–60 mL/min)	Consider reducing the dacarbazine dosage by 20% Do not modify the brentuximab vedotin, doxorubicin, or vinblastine dosages
Moderate renal impairment (CrCl 30–45 mL/min)	Consider reducing the dacarbazine dosage by 25% Do not modify the brentuximab vedotin, doxorubicin, or vinblastine dosages
Severe renal impairment (CrCl <30 mL/min)	Avoid use of brentuximab vedotin Consider reducing the dacarbazine dosage by 30% Do not modify the doxorubicin or vinblastine dosages

Infusion-Related Reaction and Anaphylactic Reaction Adverse Events

Infusion-related reaction during brentuximab vedotin administration	Interrupt infusion and initiate appropriate medical management. For subsequent cycles, premedicate with acetaminophen, antihistamine, and corticosteroids Continue doxorubicin, vinblastine, and dacarbazine at the same dose
Anaphylactic reaction during brentuximab vedotin administration	Permanently discontinue brentuximab vedotin. Continue doxorubicin, vinblastine, and dacarbazine at the same dose
Anaphylactic reaction during dacarbazine administration	Permanently discontinue dacarbazine. Continue brentuximab vedotin, doxorubicin, and vinblastine at the same dose

(*continued*)

Treatment Modifications (*continued*)

Neuropathy Adverse Events

New or worsening G2 neuropathy	Reduce brentuximab vedotin dosage by 1 dose level. Continue doxorubicin, vinblastine, and dacarbazine at the same dose
New or worsening G3 neuropathy	Withhold brentuximab vedotin until improvement to G ≤2 or baseline, then resume at dose level −1 Consider reducing the dose of vinblastine by 1 dose level Continue doxorubicin and dacarbazine at the same dose
G4 neuropathy	Permanently discontinue brentuximab vedotin At the discretion of the medically responsible health care provider, consider either reducing the dose of vinblastine by 1 dose level or permanently discontinuing vinblastine Continue doxorubicin and dacarbazine at the same dose

Pulmonary Adverse Events

New or worsening pulmonary symptoms	Delay brentuximab vedotin and all therapy during evaluation and until symptomatic improvement Upon improvement, depending on the severity of symptoms and results of diagnostic evaluation, consider permanently discontinuing brentuximab vedotin, reducing the brentuximab vedotin dosage to dose level −1, or continuing the same brentuximab vedotin dosage Doxorubicin, vinblastine, and dacarbazine may be continued at full dose upon symptomatic improvement

Severe Dermatologic Adverse Events

SJS or TEN	Permanently discontinue brentuximab vedotin. Upon recovery, continue doxorubicin, vinblastine, and dacarbazine at the same dose

Opportunistic Infection Adverse Events

PML suspected (eg, new neurologic deficit[s])	Delay all therapy during evaluation
PML confirmed	Permanently discontinue brentuximab vedotin. The safety of resuming chemotherapy (doxorubicin, vinblastine, and dacarbazine) in patients following recovery from PML has not been determined

Other Nonhematologic Adverse Events

LVEF is <40%, or is 40% to 45% with a 10% or greater absolute decrease below the pre-treatment	Withhold doxorubicin and repeat LVEF assessment within approximately 4 weeks. Discontinue doxorubicin if the LVEF has not improved or has declined further, unless the benefits for the individual patient outweigh the risks Continue brentuximab vedotin, vinblastine, and dacarbazine at the same dose
Other nonhematologic G3 adverse event (excluding electrolyte abnormalities)	Delay brentuximab vedotin, doxorubicin, vinblastine, and dacarbazine until adverse event resolves to G ≤2 or baseline, then resume treatment at the same doses
Other nonhematologic G4 adverse event (excluding electrolyte abnormalities)	Delay brentuximab vedotin, doxorubicin, vinblastine, and dacarbazine until adverse event resolves to G ≤2 or baseline At the discretion of the medically responsible health care provider, resume treatment at the same doses, or reduce the dosage of the attributable agent(s) by at least 1 dosage level, or discontinue the attributable agent(s)

ANC, absolute neutrophil count; G-CSF, granulocyte-colony stimulating factor; U.S. FDA, United States Food and Drug Administration; ABVD, doxorubicin + bleomycin + vinblastine + dacarbazine; CrCl, creatinine clearance; SJS, Stevens-Johnson Syndrome; TEN, toxic epidermal necrolysis; PML, progressive multifocal leukoencephalopathy; LVEF, left ventricular ejection fraction

Connors JM et al. N Engl J Med 2018;378:331–344
Evens AM et al. Br J Haematol 2007;137:545–552
Ramchandren R et al. Clin Cancer Res 2019;25:1718–1726
Adcetris (brentuximab vedotin) prescribing information. Bothell, WA: Seattle Genetics, Inc; revised 2018 November

Adverse Events (N = 1321)

Grade (%)*	A + AVD (n = 662)		ABVD (n = 659)	
	Grade 1–2	Grade ≥3	Grade 1–2	Grade ≥3
Neutropenia	4	54	5	39
Nausea	50	3	55	1
Constipation	40	2	36	<1
Vomiting	29	3	26	1
Fatigue	29	3	31	1
Peripheral sensory neuropathy	24	5	16	<1
Diarrhea	24	3	18	<1
Pyrexia	24	3	20	2
Peripheral neuropathy	22	4	12	<1
Alopecia	26	<1	22	0
Weight decreased	21	<1	6	<1
Abdominal pain	18	3	9	<1
Anemia	13	8	6	4
Stomatitis	19	2	15	<1
Febrile neutropenia	0	19	0	8
Bone pain	18	<1	10	<1
Insomnia	18	<1	12	<1
Decreased appetite	17	<1	11	<1
Cough	15	0	19	0
Headache	14	<1	14	<1
Arthralgia	13	<1	12	0
Neutrophil count decreased	<1	13	2	10
Dyspepsia	13	<1	11	0
Paresthesia	13	0	11	0
Back pain	12	<1	7	0
Dyspnea	11	1	17	2
Myalgia	12	<1	10	<1
Pain in extremity	12	<1	10	<1
Oropharyngeal pain	11	<1	8	<1
Upper respiratory tract infection	10	<1	10	<1
Alanine aminotransferase increased	7	3	4	<1

*According to the National Cancer Institute Common Terminology Criteria for Adverse Events, version 4.03
Note: Toxicities that occurred in ≥10% of the A + AVD group are included in the table. Treatment discontinuation owing to adverse events occurred in 13% and 16%, respectively, of the A + AVD and ABVD groups. During treatment, nine deaths occurred in the A + AVD group (seven associated with neutropenia and two owing to myocardial infarction) and 13 deaths occurred in the ABVD group (11 due to or associated with pulmonary-related toxicity, one owing to cardiopulmonary failure, and one with unknown cause)

INDUCTION • FIRST-LINE

HODGKIN LYMPHOMA REGIMEN: BLEOMYCIN, ETOPOSIDE, BEACOPP (ADRIAMYCIN), CYCLOPHOSPHAMIDE, VINCRISTINE (ONCOVIN), PROCARBAZINE, PREDNISONE (BEACOPP)

Diehl V et al. J Clin Oncol 1998;16:3810–3821.
Erratum in: N Engl J Med 2005;353:744
Diehl V et al. N Engl J Med 2003;348:2386–2395

BEACOPP

Doxorubicin 25 mg/m^2; administer by intravenous injection over 3–5 minutes on day 1, every 21 days (total dosage/cycle = 25 mg/m^2)

Cyclophosphamide 650 mg/m^2; administer intravenously in 25–250 mL 0.9% sodium chloride injection (0.9% NS) or 5% dextrose injection (D5W) over 10–30 minutes on day 1, every 21 days (total dosage/cycle = 650 mg/m^2)

Etoposide 100 mg/m^2 per day; administer intravenously, diluted in 0.9% NS or D5W to a concentration within the range 0.2–0.4 mg/mL over 1 hour for 3 consecutive days, on days 1, 2, and 3, every 21 days (total dosage/cycle = 300 mg/m^2)

Procarbazine 100 mg/m^2 per day; administer orally for 7 consecutive days on days 1–7, every 21 days (total dosage/cycle = 700 mg/m^2)

Prednisone 40 mg/m^2 per day; administer orally for 14 consecutive days on days 1–14, every 21 days (total dosage/cycle = 560 mg/m^2)

Bleomycin 10 units/m^2; administer by slow intravenous injection over 10 minutes on day 8, every 21 days (total dosage/cycle = 10 units/m^2)

Vincristine 1.4 mg/m^2 (maximum single dose = 2 mg); administer by intravenous infusion over 15 minutes in 50 mL 0.9% NS on day 8, every 21 days (total dosage/cycle = 1.4 mg/m^2; maximum dose/cycle = 2 mg)

Dose-Escalated BEACOPP

Doxorubicin 35 mg/m^2; administer by intravenous injection over 3–5 minutes on day 1, every 21 days (total dosage/cycle = 35 mg/m^2)

Cyclophosphamide 1250 mg/m^2; administer intravenously in 100–1000 mL 0.9% NS or D5W over 10–30 minutes on day 1, every 21 days (total dosage/cycle = 1250 mg/m^2)

Etoposide 200 mg/m^2 per day; administer intravenously, diluted in 0.9% NS or D5W to a concentration within the range 0.2–0.4 mg/mL, over 1 hour for 3 consecutive days, on days 1, 2, and 3, every 21 days (total dosage/cycle = 600 mg/m^2)

Procarbazine 100 mg/m^2 per day; administer orally for 7 consecutive days on days 1–7, every 21 days (total dosage/cycle = 700 mg/m^2)

Prednisone 40 mg/m^2 per day; administer orally for 14 consecutive days on days 1–14, every 21 days (total dosage/cycle = 560 mg/m^2)

Bleomycin 10 units/m^2; administer by slow intravenous injection over 10 minutes on day 8, every 21 days (total dosage/cycle = 10 units/m^2)

Vincristine 1.4 mg/m^2 (maximum single dose = 2 mg); administer by intravenous infusion over 15 minutes in 50 mL 0.9% NS on day 8, every 21 days (total dosage/cycle = 1.4 mg/m^2; maximum dose/cycle = 2 mg)

Special instructions:
Procarbazine is a weak monoamine oxidase inhibitor. Concurrent use of sympathomimetic or tricyclic antidepressant drugs and ingestion of tyramine-rich foods may produce severe hypertensive episodes in a patient receiving procarbazine

Anonymous. Med Lett Drugs Ther 1989;31:11–12
Da Prada M et al. J Neural Transm Suppl 1988;26:31–56
McCabe BJ. J Am Diet Assoc 1986;86:1059–1064

Supportive Care
Antiemetic prophylaxis
Emetogenic potential on Day 1 is **HIGH**
Emetogenic potential on Days 2–7 is **MODERATE**
Emetogenic potential on Day 8 is **MINIMAL**
See Chapter 42 for antiemetic recommendations

Treatment Modifications

Adverse Event	Dose Modification
BEACOPP and Dose-Escalated BEACOPP	
WBC <2500/mm^3 or platelet count <80,000/mm^3	Delay cycle until WBC >2500/mm^3 and platelet count >80,000/mm^3; if delayed >2 weeks, reduce dosage of doxorubicin, cyclophosphamide, etoposide, and procarbazine by 25%
Clinical or radiologic evidence of pulmonary fibrosis or DLCO <50% pretreatment value	Discontinue bleomycin
Moderate to severe impairment renal function (creatinine clearance <50 mL/min [<0.83 mL/s])	Discontinue bleomycin until creatinine clearance improves to ≥50 mL/min (≥0.83 mL/s)
Dose-Escalated BEACOPP	
Any G4 toxicity or a 2-week postponement in start of next cycle per above guidelines	Stepwise reduction of cyclophosphamide and etoposide dosages by 25% of the difference between the escalated dosage and standard BEACOPP; immediate reduction to standard BEACOPP dosages if G4 toxicity occurs in 2 successive cycles

(continued)

(*continued*)

Hematopoietic growth factor (CSF) prophylaxis
Primary prophylaxis is indicated with:

Filgrastim (G-CSF) 300 mcg/day (patients with body weight <75 kg) or 480 mcg/day (body weight ≥75 kg) by subcutaneous injection starting on day 8 and continuing until WBC ≥1000/mm³ on 3 consecutive days
- G-CSF use with bleomycin-containing regimens for Hodgkin disease has been associated with an increased rate of pulmonary toxicity

See Chapter 43 for more information

Antimicrobial prophylaxis
Risk of fever and neutropenia is **INTERMEDIATE**
Antimicrobial primary prophylaxis to be considered:
- Antibacterial—consider a fluoroquinolone or no prophylaxis; *P. jirovecii* prophylaxis is recommended (eg, cotrimoxazole)
- Antifungal—consider use during neutropenia and for anticipated mucositis
- Antiviral—antiherpes antivirals (eg, acyclovir)

Steroid-associated gastritis
Add a **proton pump inhibitor** concurrent with steroid use to prevent gastritis and duodenitis

Patient Population Studied

Phase 3 multicenter trial of 935 patients with advanced-stage HL, ages 16–65 years. Patients were randomized to receive 8 cycles of BEACOPP or dose-escalated BEACOPP. An additional 260 patients were randomized to standard treatment with COPP/ABVD. This arm was prematurely closed because of the superiority of the BEACOPP arms in terms of FFTF. Radiation therapy was planned to sites of initial bulky disease (>5 cm)

Therapy Monitoring

1. *Weekly:* CBC with differential
2. *Before each cycle:* PE, CBC with differential, BUN, creatinine, LFTs, and LDH
3. *After the second and each subsequent cycle:* DLCO
4. *Response evaluation after completion of therapy:* CT of chest, abdomen, and pelvis every 2 cycles starting after cycle 4. FDG-PET scan at conclusion of therapy to document extent of remission. Bone marrow biopsy (if disease existed before therapy) performed 1 month after completing the sixth cycle

Notes

1. Approximately 70% of all patients received radiation therapy after chemotherapy had been completed. However, subsequent studies have demonstrated that the percentage of patients that require radiation can be decreased. The final analysis from the HD15 trial showed that only 11% of patients require additional radiotherapy. RT can be restricted to patients who continue to have areas that are positive by PET scan after the completion of chemotherapy (Engert et al. Lancet 2012;379:1791–1799)
2. Patients older than 60 years of age should not receive dose-escalated BEACOPP because of an increased rate of toxicity

Efficacy (N = 323)

	BEACOPP	Dose-Escalated BEACOPP
Complete remission	88%	96%
Early progression	8%	2%
FFTF at 5 years	76%	87%
OS at 5 years	88%	91%

Toxicity (N = 1140; 854 Cycles)

Toxicity	% G3/4	
	BEACOPP	Dose-Escalated BEACOPP
Leukopenia	73%	98%
Thrombocytopenia	9%	70%
Anemia	17%	66%
Infection	16%	22%
Nausea	12%	20%
Mucositis	2%	8%
Respiratory tract effects	5%	4%

INDUCTION • SALVAGE

HODGKIN LYMPHOMA REGIMEN: DEXAMETHASONE + CYTARABINE (ARA-C) + CISPLATIN (DHAP)

Josting A et al. Ann Oncol 2002;13:1628–1635

Hydration: Administer 0.9% sodium chloride injection (0.9% NS); administer by continuous intravenous infusion at 200–250 mL/h starting 6 hours before cisplatin. Monitor and replace magnesium and other electrolytes as needed

Dexamethasone 40 mg/day; administer intravenously in 10–100 mL 0.9% NS or 5% dextrose injection (D5W) over 15–30 minutes for 4 consecutive days on days 1–4, every 14 days (total dose/cycle = 160 mg)

Cisplatin 100 mg/m^2; administer by continuous intravenous infusion over 24 hours in 100–1000 mL 0.9% NS on day 1, every 14 days (total dosage/cycle = 100 mg/m^2)

Cytarabine 2000 mg/m^2 per dose; administer intravenously in 25–250 mL 0.9% NS or D5W over 3 hours every 12 hours for 2 doses on day 2, every 14 days (total dosage/cycle = 4000 mg/m^2)

Supportive Care

Glucocorticoid eye drops; for example, **dexamethasone sodium phosphate** 0.1% ophthalmic drops; administer 2 drops by instillation into both eyes every 6 hours starting just before cytarabine administration begins, and continuing for 2 days after the last dose of cytarabine

• Steroid eye drops are given to prevent and mitigate conjunctivitis associated with cytarabine excretion in tears

Antiemetic prophylaxis
Emetogenic potential on day 1 is **HIGH**
Emetogenic potential on day 2 is **MODERATE–HIGH**
See Chapter 42 for antiemetic recommendations

Hematopoietic growth factor (CSF) prophylaxis
Primary prophylaxis is indicated with:
   Filgrastim (G-CSF) 5 mcg/kg per day by subcutaneous injection starting 24 hours after the last dose of cytarabine, and continuing until WBC ≥2500/mm^3 for 3 consecutive days
See Chapter 43 for more information

Antimicrobial prophylaxis
Risk of fever and neutropenia is **LOW**
   Antimicrobial primary prophylaxis to be considered:
   • Antibacterial—*P. jirovecii* prophylaxis is recommended (eg, cotrimoxazole)
   • Antifungal—not indicated
   • Antiviral—not indicated unless patient previously had an episode of HSV

Efficacy

	Complete Response	Partial Response	Treatment Failure
All patients	21%	67%	12%
Late relapse	26%	65%	9%
Early relapse	17%	76%	7%
Multiple relapse	23%	69%	8%
Progressive disease	12%	53%	35%

Note: Using the chi-square test for independence, remission status (relapsed HL vs progressive HL) and stage at relapse (Stages I/II vs Stages III/IV) were significant factors for response to DHAP

Treatment Modifications

Adverse Event	Dose Modification
ANC <2500/mm^3 or platelets <80,000/mm^3	Delay start of cycle 2 until ANC >2500/mm^3 and platelets >80,000/mm^3

Otherwise, no treatment modifications specified as part of this tumor-reducing program before autologous stem cell transplantation

Patient Population Studied

Phase 2 multicenter trial, 102 patients with refractory or relapsed HL; age range: 21–64 years. Eleven patients had received COPP/ABVD, ABVD, BEACOPP, or similar regimens as frontline chemotherapy

Definitions	
Primary progressive or refractory	Disease progression during first-line chemotherapy, or only transient response (CR or PR lasting ≤90 days) after induction treatment
Progressive disease	(a) ≥5% increase from nadir in the sum of the products of the greatest perpendicular diameters of any previously identified abnormal lymph node for partial responders or nonresponders; (b) appearance of any new lesion during or ≤90 days after the end of therapy
Relapsed HD	Complete disappearance of all detectable clinical and radiographic evidence of disease and disappearance of all disease-related symptoms if present before therapy for ≥3 months
Early relapse	CR lasting ≥3 months to 12 months
CR in late relapses	CR must last ≥12 months

Toxicity

Toxicity	Number of Courses = 201	
	WHO G3	WHO G4
Leukocytopenia*	50 (25%)	86 (43%)
Thrombocytopenia†	42 (21%)	97 (48%)‡
Anemia§	33 (16%)	1 (0.5%)
Mucositis	0 (0)	0 (0)
Infection€	2 (1%)	0 (0)
Nausea/vomiting	49 (24%)	3 (2%)
Renal	0 (0)	0 (0)
Neurotoxicity	1 (0.5%)	0 (0)
Ototoxicity	2 (1%)	0 (0)

*Duration of WHO Grade 3 leukocytopenia: median 1.1 days (range: 0–6 days)
†Mean number of platelet transfusions: 0.4 (range: 0–4) transfusions
‡Duration of WHO Grade 4 thrombocytopenia: median 1.4 days (range: 0–11 days)
§Mean number of red blood cell units transfused: 0.5 (range: 0–4) units
€Days with fever ≥38°C (≥100.4°F): 0.3 days (range: 0–8 days); neither severe infections nor treatment-related deaths occurred

Therapy Monitoring

1. *Semiweekly and before each cycle:* CBC with differential
2. *Before each cycle:* Physical exam
3. *Response evaluation:* CT of all initially involved sites. Bone marrow biopsy if BM involvement before start of therapy

Notes

1. Stem cell mobilization for autologous stem cell transplantation was performed after the first and, if necessary, the second cycle
2. High-dose chemotherapy and autologous stem cell transplantation was performed after 2 cycles, if patients achieved at least partial remission

INDUCTION • SALVAGE

HODGKIN LYMPHOMA REGIMEN: IFOSFAMIDE + CARBOPLATIN + ETOPOSIDE (ICE)

Moskowitz CH et al. Blood 2001;97:616–623

Etoposide 100 mg/m^2 per day; administer intravenously, diluted in 0.9% sodium chloride injection (0.9% NS) to a concentration within the range of 0.2–0.4 mg/mL, over 60 minutes for 3 consecutive days, on days 1–3, every 2 weeks (total dosage/cycle = 300 mg/m^2)

Carboplatin (calculated dose) AUC = 5 mg/mL × min* (maximum absolute dose/cycle = 800 mg); administer intravenously in 100–500 mL 5% dextrose injection (D5W) or 0.9% NS over 15–30 minutes on day 2, every 2 weeks (total dosage/cycle calculated to produce an AUC = 5 mg/mL × min; maximum absolute dose/cycle = 800 mg)

Ifosfamide 5000 mg/m^2; administer intravenously in 0.9% NS or D5W to a concentration within the range of 0.6–20 mg/mL, prepared as an admixture (in the same container) with **mesna** 5000 mg/m^2; administer by continuous intravenous infusion over 24 hours on day 2, every 2 weeks (total dosage/cycle for ifosfamide = 5000 mg/m^2 and for mesna = 5000 mg/m^2)

*Carboplatin dose is based on Calvert et al's formula to achieve a target area under the plasma concentration versus time curve (AUC) (AUC units = mg/mL × min)

$$\text{Total Carboplatin Dose (mg)} = (\text{Target AUC}) \times (\text{GFR} + 25)$$

In practice, creatinine clearance (CrCl) is used in place of glomerular filtration rate (GFR). CrCl can be calculated from the equation of Cockcroft and Gault:

$$\text{For males, CrCl} = \frac{(140 - \text{age [years]}) \times (\text{body weight [kg]})}{72 \times (\text{serum creatinine [mg/dL]})}$$

$$\text{For females, CrCl} = \frac{(140 - \text{age [years]}) \times (\text{body weight [kg]})}{72 \times (\text{serum creatinine [mg/dL]})} \times 0.85$$

Calvert AH et al. J Clin Oncol 1989;7:1748–1756
Cockcroft DW, Gault MH. Nephron 1976;16:31–41
Jodrell DI et al. J Clin Oncol 1992;10:520–528
Sorensen BT et al. Cancer Chemother Pharmacol 1991;28:397–401

Note: A carboplatin dose calculated with an IDMS-measured serum creatinine result using the Calvert formula could exceed an expected exposure (AUC) and result in increased drug-related toxicity. The FDA recommends capping an estimated GFR at 125 mL/min for any targeted AUC value. No greater estimated GFR values should be used (online) May 23, 2013. Available from: http://www.fda.gov/AboutFDA/CentersOffices/OfficeofMedicalProductsandTobacco/CDER/ucm228974.htm [accessed February 26, 2014]

Supportive Care
Antiemetic prophylaxis
Emetogenic potential on days 1 and 3 is **LOW**
Emetogenic potential on day 2 is **MODERATE–HIGH**
See Chapter 42 for antiemetic recommendations

Hematopoietic growth factor (CSF) prophylaxis
Primary prophylaxis is indicated with:
Filgrastim (G-CSF) 5 mcg/kg per day by subcutaneous injection on days 5–12 (except during peripheral blood progenitor cells mobilization)

Antimicrobial prophylaxis
Risk of fever and neutropenia is **INTERMEDIATE**
Antimicrobial primary prophylaxis to be considered:
- Antibacterial—consider a fluoroquinolone or no prophylaxis; *P. jirovecii* prophylaxis is recommended (eg, cotrimoxazole)
- Antifungal—consider use during neutropenia and for anticipated mucositis
- Antiviral—antiherpes antivirals (eg, acyclovir)

(continued)

Treatment Modifications

Adverse Event	Dose Modification
ANC <1000/mm^3 or platelet count <50,000/mm^3	Delay next cycle until ANC ≥1000/mm^3 and platelet count ≥50,000/mm^3

Patient Population Studied

Phase 2 single-center trial of 65 patients with relapsed or primary refractory HL after chemotherapy/combined modality therapy; age range: 12–59 years

Efficacy

	Percent of Patients Receiving ICE	Event-Free at a Median Follow-up of 43 Months
Complete response	26	82%*
Partial response	58	59%*
Minor response	3	
Progressive disease	12	Median survival = 5 months

*P = 0.10

(*continued*)

Accelerated fractionation involved-field radiotherapy (IFRT):
- Of the 57 patients with chemosensitive disease, 41 received IFRT
- Administered to patients who had nodal sites of disease that measured ≥5 cm prior to the start of ICE chemotherapy or who had residual disease after receiving ICE chemotherapy
- IFRT started within 2 weeks after successful collection of stem cells
- IFRT dose was 18,000–36,000 cGy administered in ten to twenty 180-cGy fractions twice daily (minimal 7-hour interval between fractions) within a period of 5–10 days

Notes:
- Patients who underwent prior radiotherapy to a dose above standard tolerance for a specific site had reduced-dose IFRT or no radiotherapy

Therapy Monitoring

1. *Semi-weekly and before each cycle:* CBC with differential
2. *Before each cycle:* Physical exam
3. *Response evaluation:* CT of all initially involved sites. Bone marrow biopsy if BM involvement before start of therapy

Notes

1. Stem cell mobilization for autologous stem cell transplantation was performed after the second cycle of ICE using filgrastim (10 mcg/kg per day) beginning on day 5, and continuing until the completion of leukapheresis. Leukapheresis was initiated when the white blood cell count was >5000/mm^3
2. Patients who achieved CR, PR, or a minor response received high-dose chemotherapy and autologous stem cell transplantation

Toxicity

Toxicity	Number of Patients
Gram-negative sepsis and neutropenia	1
Pneumonitis and death from aspiration pneumonia and acute respiratory distress syndrome*,†	1
Marantic endocarditis with cerebral emboli and subsequent multisystem organ failure*,†	1
Upper airway bleeding from a tracheal tear that resolved spontaneously†	1
ICE administration delayed beyond planned 14-day interval	40 (62%)
Scheduling difficulty	21 (32%)
Thrombocytopenia	17 (26%)
Infection	2 (3%)
Median Dose Intensities	
Ifosfamide	2187 mg/m^2 per week (87.5%)
Carboplatin	AUC 2.187 mg/mL × min per week (87.5%)
Etoposide	43.5 mg/m^2 per week (87.5%)

*No evidence of HL at time of death
†Toxicity not thought to be caused by chemotherapy

INDUCTION • SALVAGE

LYMPOMA, HODGKIN REGIMEN: IFOSFAMIDE + GEMCITABINE + VINORELBINE (IGEV)

Santoro A et al. Haematologica 2007;92:35–41

Hyperhydration during ifosfamide:
Administer 2000 mL 0.9% sodium chloride injection (0.9% NS) per day by intravenous infusion concurrently with ifosfamide administration, for 4 consecutive days, on days 1–4, every 3 weeks
- If feasible, continue maintenance intravenous hydration during intervals between ifosfamide administration. Encourage oral fluid ingestion. Monitor daily weight, or if implemented in an inpatient setting, monitor fluid input and output. Replace electrolytes as medically appropriate

Ifosfamide 2000 mg/m^2 per day; administer intravenously, diluted in 0.9% NS or 5% dextrose injection (D5W) to a concentration within the range of 0.6–20 mg/mL, over 2 hours for 4 consecutive days, on days 1–4, every 3 weeks (total dosage/cycle = 8000 mg/m^2)

Mesna 2600 mg/m^2 per day; administer intravenously for 4 consecutive days, on days 1–4, every 3 weeks (total dosage/cycle = 10,400 mg/m^2)
- Mesna utilization strategies include:
  1. Mesna 2600 mg/m^2 per day; administer by continuous intravenous infusion in 50–1000 mL 0.9% NS or D5W over 12 hours starting simultaneously with ifosfamide
  2. Mesna 650 mg/m^2 per dose; administer intravenously in 25–100 mL 0.9% NS or D5W over 15–30 minutes every 3 hours for 4 doses each day. The first dose is given when ifosfamide commences (ie, hours 0, 3, 6, and 9)
  3. Mesna 650 mg/m^2; administer intravenously in 25–100 mL 0.9% NS or D5W over 15–30 minutes coincident with the start of ifosfamide administration (hour 0), then mesna 800 mg orally every 3–4 hours for an additional 3 doses (every 3 hours: at hours 3, 6, and 9; every 4 hours: at hours 4, 8, and 12; the regimen results in a different total mesna dose/cycle)

Gemcitabine 800 mg/m^2 per dose; administer intravenously, diluted in 0.9% NS to a concentration as low as 0.1 mg/mL over 30 minutes, for 2 doses on days 1 and 4, every 3 weeks (total dosage/cycle = 1600 mg/m^2), *followed by:*

Vinorelbine 20 mg/m^2; administer intravenously, diluted in 0.9% NS or D5W to a concentration between 1.5 and 3 mg/mL, over 6–10 minutes, on day 1, every 3 weeks (total dosage/cycle = 20 mg/m^2)

Prednisolone 100 mg/day; administer orally, or by intravenous injection or intravenous infusion over 10–30 minutes for 4 consecutive days, on days 1–4, every 3 weeks (total dose/cycle = 400 mg)
- Alternatively, give **prednisone** orally at the same dose and administration schedule, and for the same duration

Supportive Care
Antiemetic prophylaxis
Emetogenic potential on days 1–4 is **MODERATE**
See Chapter 42 for antiemetic recommendations

Hematopoietic growth factor (CSF) prophylaxis
Primary prophylaxis is indicated with:
Filgrastim (G-CSF) 5 mcg/kg per day, by subcutaneous injection on days 7–12, or until apheresis in the course of mobilization commences

Antimicrobial prophylaxis
Risk of fever and neutropenia is **INTERMEDIATE**
Antimicrobial primary prophylaxis to be considered:
- Antibacterial—consider a fluoroquinolone or no prophylaxis; *P. jirovecii* prophylaxis is recommended (eg, cotrimoxazole)
- Antifungal—consider use during neutropenia and for anticipated mucositis
- Antiviral—antiherpes antivirals (eg, acyclovir)

Treatment Modifications

None specified as part of this regimen often used as a preparative regimen

Patient Population Studied

Phase 2 multicenter trial; 91 patients with refractory or relapsed HL; age range: 17–59 years. Nodular sclerosis was the most frequent histologic subtype (74.7%). A high percentage of patients had B symptoms (59.3%), extranodal involvement (47.2%), more than 3 involved sites (45.1%), and/or bulky disease (45.1%)

Efficacy

Response	Proportion
CR	54%
PR	27%
PD	10%

Response Rate According to Disease Status

	CR	PR	IF
Refractory	33.3%	27.8%	38.9%
Relapse	67.3%	27.3%	5.4%

Response Rate According to Prior RT

Prior radiotherapy	60%	30.9%	9.1%
No prior radiotherapy	44.4%	22.2%	33.3%

CR, Complete response; PR, partial response; IF, induction failure

Note:
- Stem cell mobilization was performed at various time points (66% after cycle 3)
- High-dose chemotherapy and autologous stem cell transplantation was performed after 4 IGEV cycles
- Overall, 64 of 74 (86%) patients in complete or partial remission after IGEV proceeded to single (29 cases) or tandem (35 cases) high-dose chemotherapy with PBSC support

Toxicity

Delayed cycles		4.2%
Cycles with dose reductions		8.6%
Cycles with infection		3.5%
Toxicity	**G3**	**G4**
Hematologic Toxicity		
Neutropenia	22.7%	5.7%
Thrombocytopenia	15.3%	4.8%
Anemia	16.6%	1.6%
Nonhematologic Toxicity		
Mucositis	1.9%	0.3%
Nausea	3.2%	0
Cystitis	0.3%	0

Therapy Monitoring

1. *Semi-weekly and before each cycle:* CBC with differential
2. *Before each cycle:* Physical exam
3. *Response evaluation:* CT of all initially involved sites. Bone marrow biopsy if BM involvement before start of therapy

INDUCTION • SALVAGE

HODGKIN LYMPHOMA REGIMEN: HIGH-DOSE IFOSFAMIDE, ETOPOSIDE AND EPIRUBICIN (IVE)

Proctor SJ et al. Ann Oncol 2003;14:i47–i50

Anticonvulsant prophylaxis:
Phenytoin 300 mg/day; administer orally for 6 consecutive days, from day –1 (1 day before chemotherapy begins) through day 5, every 21 days (total dose/cycle = 1800 mg)
Epirubicin 50 mg/m^2; administer by intravenous injection over 3–5 minutes on day 1, every 21 days, for a maximum of 3 cycles (total dosage/cycle = 50 mg/m^2)
Etoposide 200 mg/m^2 per day; administer intravenously, diluted in 0.9% sodium chloride injection (0.9% NS) to a concentration within the range of 0.2–0.4 mg/mL, over 2 hours for 3 consecutive days, days 1–3, every 21 days, for a maximum of 3 cycles (total dosage/cycle = 600 mg/m^2)
Ifosfamide 3000 mg/m^2 per day; administer intravenously, diluted in 0.9% NS or 5% dextrose injection (D5W) to a concentration within the range 0.6 to 20 mg/mL, over 22 hours on 3 consecutive days, days 1–3, every 21 days for a maximum of 3 cycles (total dosage/cycle = 9000 mg/m^2)
Mesna 1800 mg/m^2; administer intravenously in 10–50 mL 0.9% NS or D5W over 15 minutes on day 1 just before starting ifosfamide administration, every 21 days, then:
Mesna 3000 mg/m^2 per day; administer intravenously, diluted in 25–1000 mL 0.9% NS or D5W over 22 hours, for 3 consecutive days, days 1–3, every 21 days, for a maximum of 3 cycles (total dosage/cycle = 9000 mg/m^2), *followed on day 3 by*
Mesna 1636 mg/m^2; administer intravenously in 50–1000 mL 0.9% NS or D5W over 12 hours on day 3, after ifosfamide administration is completed, every 21 days (total mesna dosage/cycle = 12,436 mg/m^2)
- Mesna administered by prolonged infusion over 22 hours at the same time as ifosfamide may be prepared conveniently as an admixture (in the same container) with ifosfamide
- Proctor et al did not identify the amount of mesna they gave after ifosfamide administration was completed. The amount of mesna identified for administration on day 3 after ifosfamide administration is completed is calculated from the amount of mesna given within a 12-hour interval during continuous ifosfamide administration over 22 hours

Note: Hematopoietic growth factor support is not routinely given as primary prophylaxis

Supportive Care
Antiemetic prophylaxis
Emetogenic potential on day 1 is **HIGH**
Emetogenic potential on days 2 and 3 is **MODERATE**
See Chapter 42 for antiemetic recommendations

Hematopoietic growth factor (CSF) prophylaxis
Primary prophylaxis may be indicated
See Chapter 43 for more information

Antimicrobial prophylaxis
Risk of fever and neutropenia is **INTERMEDIATE**
  Antimicrobial primary prophylaxis to be considered:
  - Antibacterial—consider a fluoroquinolone or no prophylaxis; *P. jirovecii* prophylaxis is recommended (eg, cotrimoxazole)
  - Antifungal—consider use during neutropenia
  - Antiviral—antiherpes antivirals (eg, acyclovir)

Patient Population Studied

Phase 2 multicenter trial, 51 patients with refractory or relapsed HL, ages 16–53 years. The majority of patients were treated following a first relapse. Disease histologies included lymphocyte predominant (n = 4), mixed cellularity (n = 8), and nodular sclerosing subtypes (n = 39)

Treatment Modifications

None specified as part of this regimen. Often used as a preparative regimen for hematopoietic stem cell transplantation

Efficacy

Response	Percentage of Patients
Complete response	61
Partial response	22
SD or progression	16

Overall Survival According to Response to Prior Therapy

<PR to primary therapy	8 months
PR to primary therapy	24 months
CR to primary therapy; first relapse	Not reached
CR to primary therapy; second relapse	46 months
CR to primary therapy; second relapse	18 months

Toxicity

Toxicity	Frequency
G4 hematologic toxicity	100% of patients
G3 infections	10% of all courses
Neurotoxicity	2% of patients
Treatment-related deaths	0

Therapy Monitoring

1. *Semi-weekly and before each cycle:* CBC with differential
2. *Before each cycle:* Physical exam
3. *Response evaluation after 3 cycles:* CT scan, and bone marrow biopsy if BM involvement before start of therapy

Notes

Often used as a preparative regimen; 61% of the patients proceeded to high-dose chemotherapy and autologous stem cell transplantation

CONSOLIDATION AFTER AUTOLOGOUS HEMATOPOIETIC STEM CELL TRANSPLANT

HODGKIN LYMPHOMA REGIMEN: BRENTUXIMAB VEDOTIN

Moskowitz CH et al. Lancet 2015;385(9980):1853–1862
Supplementary appendix to: Moskowitz CH et al. Lancet 2015;385(9980):1853–1862

Start brentuximab vedotin between 30 and 45 days after autologous hematopoietic stem cell transplant (auto-HSCT) or upon recovery from auto-HSCT:

Brentuximab vedotin 1.8 mg/kg (maximum dose = 180 mg); administer intravenously in a volume of 0.9% sodium chloride injection or 5% dextrose injection sufficient to produce a concentration with the range 0.4–1.8 mg/mL (minimum volume, 100 mL) over 30 minutes on day 1, every 3 weeks for up to 16 doses (total dosage/cycle = 1.8 mg/kg; maximum dose/cycle = 180 mg)

Notes:
- The dose for patients whose body weight is >100 kg should be calculated based on a weight of 100 kg
- Brentuximab vedotin can cause severe or life-threatening infusion-related reactions, including hypersensitivity and anaphylaxis
- Monomethyl auristatin E, the cytotoxic component of brentuximab vedotin, is a substrate of CYP3A4/5 and P-glycoprotein (P-gp). Use caution and monitor closely for brentuximab vedotin side effects when coadministering brentuximab vedotin with strong CYP3A4 inhibitors or P-gp inhibitors.

Supportive Care
Antiemetic prophylaxis
Emetogenic potential is **LOW**
See Chapter 42 for antiemetic recommendations

Hematopoietic growth factor (CSF) prophylaxis
Primary prophylaxis is **NOT** indicated
See Chapter 43 for more information

Antimicrobial prophylaxis
Risk of fever and neutropenia is **LOW**
   Antimicrobial primary prophylaxis to be considered:
   - Antibacterial—not indicated
   - Antifungal—not indicated
   - Antiviral—antiherpes antivirals (eg, acyclovir, famciclovir, valacyclovir)

Patient Population Studied

The international, multicenter, randomized, double-blind, placebo-controlled, phase 3 trial (AETHERA) involved 329 patients with histologically confirmed, classic Hodgkin lymphoma who had undergone high-dose therapy and autologous stem-cell transplantation. Eligible patients were aged ≥18 years and had primary refractory Hodgkin lymphoma (failure to achieve complete remission), relapsed Hodgkin lymphoma with an initial remission duration <12 months), and/or extranodal involvement at the start of pre-transplantation salvage chemotherapy. Eligible patients also had to have had complete remission, partial remission, or stable disease after pre-transplantation salvage chemotherapy. Patients who had previously received brentuximab vedotin were ineligible. Patients were randomized (1:1) to receive intravenous brentuximab vedotin (1.8 mg/kg) or placebo administered over 30 minutes on day 1 of every 21-day cycle for up to 16 cycles.

Efficacy (N = 329)

	Brentuximab Vedotin (n = 165)	Placebo (n = 164)	
Median progression-free survival	42.9 months	24.1 months	HR 0.57, 95% CI 0.40–0.81; P = 0.0013

Note: Median follow-up time was 30 months. An interim analysis of overall survival (a secondary end point) showed no significant difference between the treatment groups

Therapy Monitoring

1. *Prior to initiation of therapy:* CBC with differential and platelet count, serum electrolytes, liver function tests, serum creatinine, BUN, pregnancy test (women of child-bearing potential only)
2. *During each brentuximab vedotin infusion:* signs and symptoms of infusion-related reaction, vital signs every 30 minutes
3. *Prior to each cycle:* CBC with differential and platelet count, serum electrolytes, liver function tests, serum creatinine, BUN
   a. In patients with compromised bone marrow function or past G ≥3 myelosuppression, consider more frequent monitoring of CBC with differential and platelet count within each cycle
4. *Periodically assess for:* peripheral neuropathy, pulmonary toxicity, severe dermatologic toxicity, gastrointestinal toxicity, infection, and progressive multifocal leukoencephalopathy

Treatment Modifications

BRENTUXIMAB VEDOTIN

Starting dose	1.8 mg/kg (maximum dose = 180 mg) every 3 weeks
Dose Level −1	1.2 mg/kg (maximum dose = 120 mg) every 3 weeks

Adverse Event	Dose Modification
General Dose Modification	
Patient weight >100 kg	Use a maximum weight of 100 kg for calculation of the brentuximab vedotin dose
Hepatic Impairment	
Patient with mild hepatic impairment (Child-Pugh class A)	Reduce dose to 1.2 mg/kg (maximum dose = 120 mg) every 3 weeks
Infusion-Related Reaction and Anaphylactic Reaction Adverse Events	
Infusion-related reaction	Interrupt infusion and initiate appropriate medical management. For subsequent cycles, premedicate with acetaminophen, antihistamine, and corticosteroids
Anaphylactic reaction	Permanently discontinue brentuximab vedotin
Neuropathy Adverse Events	
New or worsening G2/3 neuropathy	Delay brentuximab vedotin until improvement to G ≤1 or baseline, then resume at dose level −1
G4 neuropathy	Permanently discontinue brentuximab vedotin
Hematologic Adverse Events	
G3/4 neutropenia	Delay brentuximab vedotin until improvement to G ≤2. Consider G-CSF prophylaxis during subsequent cycles
Recurrent G4 neutropenia despite use of prophylactic G-CSF	Delay brentuximab vedotin until improvement to G ≤2. Continue G-CSF prophylaxis during subsequent cycles and either reduce brentuximab vedotin to dose level −1 or permanently discontinue brentuximab vedotin
G3 thrombocytopenia First occurrence of G4 thrombocytopenia	Delay brentuximab vedotin until improvement to G ≤2, then resume treatment at the same dose
Second occurrence of G4 thrombocytopenia	Delay brentuximab vedotin until improvement to G ≤2, then resume treatment at dose level −1
Pulmonary Adverse Events	
New or worsening pulmonary symptoms	Delay brentuximab vedotin during evaluation and until symptomatic improvement. Upon improvement, depending on the severity of symptoms and results of diagnostic evaluation, consider permanently discontinuing brentuximab vedotin, reducing to dose level −1, or continuing the same dose
Severe Dermatologic Adverse Events	
SJS or TEN	Permanently discontinue brentuximab vedotin
Opportunistic Infection Adverse Events	
PML suspected (eg, new neurologic deficit[s])	Delay brentuximab vedotin during evaluation
PML confirmed	Permanently discontinue brentuximab vedotin
Other Nonhematologic Adverse Events	
Other nonhematologic G3 adverse event (excluding electrolyte abnormalities)	Delay brentuximab vedotin until adverse event resolves to G ≤1 or baseline, then resume treatment at the same dose
Other nonhematologic G4 adverse event (excluding electrolyte abnormalities)	Delay brentuximab vedotin until adverse event resolves to G ≤1 or baseline, then resume treatment at dose level −1

G-CSF, granulocyte-colony stimulating factor; SJS, Stevens-Johnson Syndrome; TEN, toxic epidermal necrolysis; PML, progressive multifocal leukoencephalopathy

Adcetris (brentuximab vedotin) prescribing information. Bothell, WA: Seattle Genetics, Inc; revised 2018 March
Supplementary appendix to: Moskowitz CH et al. Lancet 2015;385(9980):1853–1862

Adverse Events (N = 327)

Grade (%)*	Brentuximab Vedotin (N = 167)		Placebo (N = 160)	
	Grade 1–2	Grade ≥3	Grade 1–2	Grade ≥3
Peripheral sensory neuropathy	46	10	14	1
Neutropenia	5	29	2	10
Upper respiratory tract infection	26	0	22	1
Fatigue	22	2	16	3
Peripheral motor neuropathy	17	6	1	<1
Nausea	19	3	8	0
Cough	21	0	16	0
Diarrhea	18	2	9	<1
Pyrexia	17	2	16	0
Weight decreased	19	<1	6	0
Arthralgia	17	<1	9	0
Vomiting	14	2	7	0
Abdominal pain	12	2	3	0
Constipation	10	2	3	0
Dyspnea	13	0	6	<1
Decreased appetite	11	<1	6	0
Pruritus	11	<1	8	0
Headache	10	2	8	<1
Muscle spasms	11	0	6	0
Myalgia	10	<1	4	0
Chills	10	0	5	0
Paresthesia	8	2	1	0

*According to the National Cancer Institute Common Terminology Criteria for Adverse Events, version 4

Note: Treatment-emergent toxicities are included in the table if all-grade toxicities occurred in ≥10% or Grade ≥3 toxicities occurred in ≥5% of the brentuximab vedotin group. Treatment discontinuation owing to adverse events occurred in 33% and 6%, respectively, of the brentuximab vedotin and placebo groups. In the brentuximab vedotin group, one patient died within 30 days of treatment from treatment-related acute respiratory distress syndrome associated with pneumonitis and another patient died at day 40 from acute respiratory distress syndrome after an episode of treatment-related acute pancreatitis that had resolved at the time of death

SUBSEQUENT THERAPY

HODGKIN LYMPHOMA REGIMEN: BRENTUXIMAB VEDOTIN

Younes A et al. J Clin Oncol 2012;30:2183–2189

Brentuximab vedotin 1.8 mg/kg (maximum dose = 180 mg); administer intravenously in a volume of 0.9% sodium chloride injection or 5% dextrose injection sufficient to produce a concentration with the range 0.4–1.8 mg/mL (minimum volume, 100 mL) over 30 minutes on day 1, every 3 weeks for up to 16 doses (total dosage/cycle = 1.8 mg/kg; maximum dose/cycle = 180 mg)

Notes:
- The dose for patients whose body weight is >100 kg should be calculated based on a weight of 100 kg
- Brentuximab vedotin can cause severe or life-threatening infusion-related reactions, including hypersensitivity and anaphylaxis
- Monomethyl auristatin E, the cytotoxic component of brentuximab vedotin, is a substrate of CYP3A4/5 and P-glycoprotein (P-gp). Use caution and monitor closely for brentuximab vedotin side effects when coadministering brentuximab vedotin with strong CYP3A4 inhibitors or P-gp inhibitors.

Supportive Care
Antiemetic prophylaxis
Emetogenic potential is LOW
See Chapter 42 for antiemetic recommendations

Hematopoietic growth factor (CSF) prophylaxis
Primary prophylaxis MAY be indicated with one of the following:
  Filgrastim (G-CSF) 5 mcg/kg per day, by subcutaneous injection, *or*
  Pegfilgrastim (pegylated filgrastim) 6 mg/0.6 mL, by subcutaneous injection for 1 dose
- Begin use from 24–72 hours after myelosuppressive chemotherapy is completed
- Continue daily filgrastim use until ANC ≥10,000/mm^3 on 2 measurements separated temporally by ≥12 hours
- Discontinue daily filgrastim use at least 24 hours before administering myelosuppressive treatment. Do not administer pegfilgrastim within 14 days before administering myelosuppressive treatment
See Chapter 43 for more information

Antimicrobial prophylaxis
Risk of fever and neutropenia is LOW
  Antimicrobial primary prophylaxis to be considered:
- Antibacterial—not indicated
- Antifungal—not indicated
- Antiviral—not indicated unless patient previously had an episode of HSV

Treatment Modifications

BRENTUXIMAB VEDOTIN

Starting dose	1.8 mg/kg (maximum dose = 180 mg) every 3 weeks
Dose Level −1	1.2 mg/kg (maximum dose = 120 mg) every 3 weeks

Adverse Event	Dose Modification
	General Dose Modification
Patient weight >100 kg	Use a maximum weight of 100 kg for calculation of the brentuximab vedotin dose

(continued)

Patient Population Studied

Patients with relapsed or refractory HL after high-dose chemotherapy and auto-SCT with histologically documented CD30-positive Hodgkin Reed-Sternberg cells. Patients could not have previously received allogeneic stem-cell transplantation (SCT).

Demographics and Baseline Clinical Characteristics

Demographic or Clinical Characteristic	Patients	
	Number	**Percentage**
Age, median (range)	31 years (15–77 years)	
Sex, male-to-female ratio	48/54	47/53
Race		
Asian	7	7
Black or African American	5	5
White	89	87
Other	1	1
ECOG performance status		
0	42	41
1	60	59
Baseline "B" symptoms	35	34
Bone marrow involvement	8	8
Prior radiation	67	66
Prior chemotherapy regimens, median (range)	3.5 (1–13)	
Primary refractory disease*	72	71
Disease status relative to most recent prior therapy†		
Relapsed†	59	58
Refractory†	43	42
Best response with most recent systemic regimen		
Complete response	12	12

(continued)

Treatment Modifications (continued)

Hepatic Impairment

Patient with mild hepatic impairment (Child-Pugh class A)	Reduce dose to 1.2 mg/kg (maximum dose = 120 mg) every 3 weeks

Infusion-Related Reaction and Anaphylactic Reaction Adverse Events

Infusion-related reaction	Interrupt infusion and initiate appropriate medical management. For subsequent cycles, premedicate with acetaminophen, antihistamine, and corticosteroids
Anaphylactic reaction	Permanently discontinue brentuximab vedotin

Neuropathy Adverse Events

New or worsening G2/3 neuropathy	Delay brentuximab vedotin until improvement to G ≤1 or baseline, then resume at dose level −1
G4 neuropathy	Permanently discontinue brentuximab vedotin

Hematologic Adverse Events

G3/4 neutropenia	Delay brentuximab vedotin until improvement to G ≤2. Consider G-CSF prophylaxis during subsequent cycles
Recurrent G4 neutropenia despite use of prophylactic G-CSF	Delay brentuximab vedotin until improvement to G ≤2. Continue G-CSF prophylaxis during subsequent cycles and either reduce brentuximab vedotin to dose level −1 or permanently discontinue brentuximab vedotin
G3 thrombocytopenia First occurrence of G4 thrombocytopenia	Delay brentuximab vedotin until improvement to G ≤2, then resume treatment at the same dose
Second occurrence of G4 thrombocytopenia	Delay brentuximab vedotin until improvement to G ≤2, then resume treatment at dose level −1

Pulmonary Adverse Events

New or worsening pulmonary symptoms	Delay brentuximab vedotin during evaluation and until symptomatic improvement. Upon improvement, depending on the severity of symptoms and results of diagnostic evaluation, consider permanently discontinuing brentuximab vedotin, reducing to dose level −1, or continuing the same dose

Severe Dermatologic Adverse Events

SJS or TEN	Permanently discontinue brentuximab vedotin

Opportunistic Infection Adverse Events

PML suspected (eg, new neurologic deficit[s])	Delay brentuximab vedotin during evaluation
PML confirmed	Permanently discontinue brentuximab vedotin

Other Nonhematologic Adverse Events

Other nonhematologic G3 adverse event (excluding electrolyte abnormalities)	Delay brentuximab vedotin until adverse event resolves to G ≤1 or baseline, then resume treatment at the same dose
Other nonhematologic G4 adverse event (excluding electrolyte abnormalities)	Delay brentuximab vedotin until adverse event resolves to G ≤1 or baseline, then resume treatment at dose level −1

G-CSF, granulocyte-colony stimulating factor; SJS, Stevens-Johnson Syndrome; TEN, toxic epidermal necrolysis; PML, progressive multifocal leukoencephalopathy

Adcetris (brentuximab vedotin) prescribing information. Bothell, WA: Seattle Genetics, Inc; revised 2018 March
Supplementary appendix to: Moskowitz CH et al. Lancet 2015;385(9980):1853–1862

Patient Population Studied
(continued)

Demographic or Clinical Characteristic	Patients	
	Number	Percentage
Partial response	35	34
Stable disease	23	23
Progressive disease	26	25
Unknown/other	6	6
Number of prior auto-SCT		
1	91	89
2	11	11
Months from auto-SCT to first posttransplantation relapse‡	6.7 (0–131)	
Months from initial diagnosis to first dose of study drug‡	39.9 (11.8–219.7)	

auto-SCT, autologous stem-cell transplantation; ECOG, Eastern Cooperative Oncology Group
*Primary refractory disease = failure to obtain a CR with front-line therapy or relapse within 3 months of front-line therapy
†Relapsed indicates best response of CR or PR to most recent prior therapy, and refractory indicates best response of SD or PD to most recent prior therapy
‡Median (range)

Efficacy (N = 102)

	Patients	
	Number	Percentage
Objective response	76	75
Complete remission	35	34
Partial remission	41	40
Stable disease	22	22
Progressive disease	3	3
Not evaluable	1	1

	Median (95% CI)
Duration of objective response, months	6.7 (3.6–14.8)
Duration of response for patients with CR, months	20.5 (10.8–NE)
Progression-free survival, months	5.6 (5.0–9.0)
Overall survival, months	22.4 (21.7–NE)

NE, not estimable

Toxicity

Drug-Related Adverse Events Reported by > 10% of Patients and G3/4 Incidence of These Events Regardless of Relationship to Brentuximab Vedotin

	Events Related to Brentuximab Vedotin (Any G)		Any G3 Events		Any G4 Events	
	Patients					
Adverse Event	Number	Percent	Number	%	Number	%
Peripheral sensory neuropathy	43	42	8	8	0	0
Nausea	36	35	0	0	0	0
Fatigue	35	34	2	2	0	0
Neutropenia	19	19	14	14	6	6
Diarrhea	18	18	1	1	0	0
Pyrexia	14	14	2	2	0	0
Vomiting	13	13	0	0	0	0
Arthralgia	12	12	0	0	0	0
Pruritus	12	12	0	0	0	0
Myalgia	11	11	0	0	0	0
Peripheral motor neuropathy	11	11	1	1	0	0
Alopecia	10	10	0	0	0	0

Therapy Monitoring

1. *Prior to initiation of therapy:* CBC with differential and platelet count, serum electrolytes, liver function tests, serum creatinine, BUN, pregnancy test (women of child-bearing potential only)

2. *During each brentuximab vedotin infusion:* signs and symptoms of infusion-related reaction, vital signs every 30 minutes

3. *Prior to each cycle:* CBC with differential and platelet count, serum electrolytes, liver function tests, serum creatinine, BUN

   a. In patients with compromised bone marrow function or past G ≥3 myelosuppression, consider more frequent monitoring of CBC with differential and platelet count within each cycle

4. *Periodically assess for:* peripheral neuropathy, pulmonary toxicity, severe dermatologic toxicity, gastrointestinal toxicity, infection, and progressive multifocal leukoencephalopathy

SUBSEQUENT THERAPY

HODGKIN LYMPHOMA REGIMEN: NIVOLUMAB

Younes A et al. Lancet Oncol 2016;17:1283–1294

Nivolumab 3 mg/kg; administer intravenously over 30–60 minutes in a volume of 0.9% sodium chloride injection (0.9% NS) or 5% dextrose injection, USP, not to exceed 160 mL and sufficient to produce a nivolumab concentration within the range 1–10 mg/mL, every 2 weeks (total dosage/2-week course = 3 mg/kg)

- Administer nivolumab through an administration set that contains a sterile, non-pyrogenic, low-protein-binding in-line filter with pore size within the range of 0.2–1.2 μm

Notes:

- Nivolumab can cause severe infusion-related reactions

  - Interrupt or slow the administration rate in patients with mild or moderate infusion-related reactions

  - Discontinue nivolumab in patients who experience severe or life-threatening infusion-related reactions

- Patients who require systemic corticosteroids must be on a dose of ≤10 mg daily prednisone (or equivalent) before initiating treatment with nivolumab

- The U.S. Food and Drug Administration (FDA)-approved regimen for Hodgkin lymphoma includes fixed doses of nivolumab and allows for a shortened infusion duration of 30 minutes, consistent with the regimens approved on 5 March 2018, thus:

Nivolumab 240 mg; administer intravenously over 30–60 minutes in a volume of 0.9% sodium chloride injection (0.9% NS) or 5% dextrose injection, USP, not to exceed 160 mL and sufficient to produce a nivolumab concentration within the range 1–10 mg/mL, every 2 weeks (total dosage/2-week course = 240 mg)

  - Administer nivolumab through an administration set that contains a sterile, nonpyrogenic, low-protein-binding in-line filter with pore size within the range of 0.2–1.2 μm

OR

Nivolumab 480 mg; administer intravenously over 30–60 minutes in a volume of 0.9% sodium chloride injection (0.9% NS) or 5% dextrose injection, USP, not to exceed 160 mL and sufficient to produce a nivolumab concentration within the range 1–10 mg/mL, every 4 weeks (total dosage/4-week course = 480 mg)

  - Administer nivolumab through an administration set that contains a sterile, nonpyrogenic, low-protein-binding in-line filter with pore size within the range of 0.2–1.2 μm

Supportive Care

Antiemetic prophylaxis

Emetogenic potential is **MINIMAL**

See Chapter 39 for antiemetic recommendations

Hematopoietic growth factor (CSF) prophylaxis

Primary prophylaxis is **NOT** *indicated*

See Chapter 43 for more information

Antimicrobial prophylaxis

Risk of fever and neutropenia is **LOW**

Antimicrobial primary prophylaxis to be considered:

- Antibacterial—not indicated

- Antifungal—not indicated

- Antiviral—not indicated unless patient previously had an episode of HSV

Patient Population Studied

The multicenter, noncomparative, single-arm, phase 2 study involved 80 patients with recurrent classic Hodgkin lymphoma who had failed to respond to autologous stem cell transplantation and had either failed to respond to, or relapsed after, subsequent brentuximab vedotin treatment. Eligible patients were aged ≥18 years, with an Eastern Cooperative Oncology Group (ECOG) performance status score ≤1. All patients received 3 mg/kg nivolumab intravenously over 1 hour every 2 weeks until disease progression, death, unacceptable toxicity, withdrawal of consent, or study end

Efficacy (N = 80)

Objective response rate*	66.3%
Median duration of objective response	7.8 months
Proportion of patients who achieved complete remission	9%
Proportion of patients who achieved partial remission	58%
Progression-free survival at 6 months	76.9%
Overall survival at 6 months	98.7%

*Objective response rate (the primary outcome) is the percentage of patients who experienced a best overall response of partial or complete remission, per the revised International Working Group criteria for Malignant Lymphoma (2007 criteria). Best overall response was defined as best response between the first dose and progression or subsequent therapy, whichever occurred first

Note: All efficacy end points listed above were assessed by an independent radiological review committee. Median follow-up time was 8.9 months

Therapy Monitoring

1. Initially at the time of each dose, and eventually every 6–12 weeks, perform a total body skin examination with attention to ALL mucous membranes as well as a complete review of systems
2. Monitor patients for signs and symptoms of pneumonitis. Evaluate patients with suspected pneumonitis with chest x-ray, CT, and pulse oximetry. For ≥2 toxicity, may include nasal swab, sputum culture and sensitivity, blood culture and sensitivity, and urine culture and sensitivity
3. Monitor patients for signs and symptoms of colitis. Encourage patients to report diarrhea immediately to any member of the health care team
4. Draw AST, ALT, and bilirubin prior to each infusion and/or weekly if there are Grade 1 liver function test elevations. Note, no treatment is recommended for G1 LFT abnormalities. For ≥2 toxicity, work up for other causes of elevated LFTs including viral hepatitis
5. Use basic metabolic panel (Na, K, CO_2, glucose) and patient history as screening tools for hypophysitis including hypopituitarism and adrenal insufficiency. If in doubt, evaluate AM adrenocorticotropic hormone (ACTH) and cortisol levels. Consider ACTH stimulation test for indeterminate results
6. Assess thyroid function at the start of treatment, periodically during treatment, and as indicated based on clinical evaluation and for clinical signs and symptoms of thyroid disorders. Test for TSH and free thyroxine (FT4) every 4–6 weeks as part of routine clinical monitoring of therapy or for case detection in symptomatic patients
7. Measure glucose at baseline and with each treatment during the first 12 weeks and every 6 weeks thereafter
8. Obtain a serum creatinine prior to every dose. If creatinine is found to be newly elevated, consider holding therapy while other potential causes are evaluated. Note, routine urinalysis is not necessary other than to rule out urinary tract infections, etc
9. Obtain a complete rheumatologic history and perform an examination of all peripheral joints for tenderness, swelling, and range of motion. Examine the spine. Consider plain x-ray/imaging to exclude metastases and evaluate joint damage (erosions), if appropriate
10. In patients at high risk for infections and in appropriately selected patients based on an infectious disease evaluation, draw screening laboratories (HIV, hepatitis A and B, and blood QuantiFERON for TB) to prepare patients to start infliximab
11. *Response assessment:* CT scan every 3 months during year 1, every 4 months during year 2, then every 6 months thereafter while on therapy. Consider PET scan to confirm complete response or progressive disease as clinically indicated

Treatment Modifications

Adverse Reaction	Grade/Severity	Dose Modification
Colitis	G1	Loperamide 4 mg as starting dose then 2 mg before each meal and after each loose stool until without diarrhea for 12 hours, with maximum of 16 mg loperamide per day. If G1 diarrhea or colitis persists for >14 days, then add prednisolone 0.5–1 mg/kg (non-enteric coated) or consider oral budesonide 9 mg daily if no bloody diarrhea
	G2/3 diarrhea or colitis	Withhold nivolumab. Loperamide 4 mg as starting dose then 2 mg before each meal and after each loose stool until without diarrhea for 12 hours, with maximum of 16 mg loperamide per day. Administer oral prednisone/prednisolone at a dose of 0.5 to 2 mg/kg/day or its equivalent. When improves to G1, begin a slow corticosteroid taper over at least 4 weeks. Resume nivolumab upon symptom control, or when prednisone/prednisolone daily dose <10 mg
	G4 diarrhea or colitis	Permanently discontinue nivolumab. Loperamide 4 mg as starting dose then 2 mg before each meal and after each loose stool until without diarrhea for 12 hours, with maximum of 16 mg loperamide per day. Administer 1–2 mg/kg intravenous (methyl)prednisolone and convert to 0.5–2 mg/kg prednisone/prednisolone orally each day or its equivalent only after a response. Taper over at least 4 weeks when symptoms improve. If does not improve over 72 hours or worsens, perform flexible sigmoidoscopy/colonoscopy to document colitis then begin infliximab 5 mg/kg (if no perforation/sepsis/TB/hepatitis/NYHA III/IV CHF). If no response, add MMF 500–1000 mg twice daily. If worse on MMF, consider addition of tacrolimus or ATG
Pneumonitis	G2	Withhold nivolumab. Consider *Pneumocystis* prophylaxis depending on the clinical context and cover with empiric antibiotics. Administer oral prednisone/prednisolone at a dose of 1–2 mg/kg/day or its equivalent. When improves to G1, begin a slow corticosteroid taper over at least 4 weeks. If does not respond adequately after 48 hours, then administer 2–4 mg/kg intravenous (methyl)prednisolone and convert to 0.5–2 mg/kg prednisone/prednisolone orally each day or its equivalent only after a response, followed by a taper over at least 6 weeks when symptoms improve to G1, titrating to symptoms. Resume nivolumab upon symptom control, or when prednisone/prednisolone daily dose <10 mg

(continued)

Treatment Modifications (continued)

Adverse Reaction	Grade/Severity	Dose Modification
	G3/4	Permanently discontinue nivolumab. Consider *Pneumocystis* prophylaxis depending on the clinical context; cover with empiric antibiotics. Administer 2–4 mg/kg intravenous (methyl)prednisolone and convert to 1–2 mg/kg prednisone/prednisolone orally each day or its equivalent only after a response, followed by a taper over at least 8 weeks when symptoms improve to G1, titrating to symptoms. If when initially treated improvement does not occur within 48–72 hours, begin infliximab 5 mg/kg (if no perforation/sepsis/TB/hepatitis/NYHA III/IV CHF). If no response to infliximab, add MMF 500–1000 mg twice daily. Consider MMF especially if has concurrent hepatic toxicity
Hepatitis	G2 (AST or ALT >3–5× ULN or total bilirubin >1.5–3× ULN)	Withhold nivolumab. Administer oral prednisone/prednisolone at a dose of 1–2 mg/kg/day or its equivalent. When improves to G1, begin a slow corticosteroid taper over at least 4 weeks. Resume nivolumab upon symptom control, or when prednisone/prednisolone daily dose <10 mg
	G3/4 (AST or ALT >5× ULN or total bilirubin >3× ULN)	Permanently discontinue nivolumab. Administer 1–2 mg/kg intravenous (methyl)prednisolone and convert to 0.5–2 mg/kg prednisone/prednisolone orally each day or its equivalent only after a response. Taper over at least 6 weeks when symptoms improve. If no response, add MMF 500–1000 mg twice daily. If worse on MMF, consider adding tacrolimus or ATG
Hypophysitis	G2/3 (moderate symptoms, ie, headache but no visual disturbance or fatigue/mood alteration but hemodynamically stable, no electrolyte disturbance)	Administer analgesia as needed for headache. Withhold nivolumab. Administer oral prednisone/prednisolone at a dose of 0.5–2 mg/kg/day or its equivalent. When improves to G1, begin a slow corticosteroid taper over at least 4 weeks. If no improvement in 48 hours, administer 1–2 mg/kg intravenous (methyl)prednisolone and convert to 0.5–2 mg/kg prednisone/prednisolone orally each day or its equivalent only after a response. Taper over at least 4 weeks when symptoms improve to 5 mg prednisone/prednisolone or equivalent; do not stop steroids. Resume nivolumab upon symptom control, or when prednisone/prednisolone daily dose <10 mg
	G4 (severe mass effect symptoms, ie, severe headache, any visual disturbance or severe hypoadrenalism, ie, hypotension, severe electrolyte disturbance)	Permanently discontinue nivolumab. Administer analgesia as needed for headache. Administer 1–2 mg/kg intravenous (methyl)prednisolone and convert to 0.5–2 mg/kg prednisone/prednisolone orally each day or its equivalent only after a response. Taper over at least 4 weeks when symptoms improve to 5 mg prednisone/prednisolone or equivalent; do not stop steroids
Adrenal insufficiency	G2	Withhold nivolumab. Administer oral prednisone/prednisolone at a dose of 0.5–2 mg/kg/day or its equivalent. When improves to G1, begin a slow corticosteroid taper over at least 4 weeks. Serially assess adrenal function and continue steroids at replacement doses (20–40 mg hydrocortisone daily ~2/3 dose in AM upon awakening and ~1/3 at 4 PM) until recovery of adrenal function is documented. Resume nivolumab upon symptom control, or when prednisone/prednisolone daily dose <10 mg
	G3/4	Permanently discontinue nivolumab. Administer oral prednisone/prednisolone at a dose of 0.5–2 mg/kg/day or its equivalent. When improves to G1, begin a slow corticosteroid taper over at least 4 weeks. Serially assess adrenal function and continue steroids at replacement doses (20–40 mg hydrocortisone daily ~2/3 dose in AM upon awakening and ~1/3 at 4 PM) until recovery of adrenal function is documented
Type 1 diabetes mellitus	G3 hyperglycemia	Withhold nivolumab. Admit to hospital to manage hyperglycemia. Role of corticosteroids in preventing complete loss of insulin-producing cells is unknown and not recommended. Resume nivolumab upon symptom control, or when prednisone/prednisolone daily dose <10 mg
	G4 hyperglycemia	Permanently discontinue nivolumab. Admit to hospital to manage hyperglycemia. Role of corticosteroids in preventing complete loss of insulin-producing cells is unknown and not recommended
Nephritis and renal dysfunction	G2/3 (serum creatinine 1.5–6× ULN)	Withhold nivolumab. Administer oral prednisone/prednisolone at a dose of 0.5–2 mg/kg/day or its equivalent. When improves to G1, begin a slow corticosteroid taper over at least 4 weeks. If does not respond adequately, then administer 0.5–1 mg/kg intravenous (methyl)prednisolone and convert to 0.5–2 mg/kg prednisone/prednisolone orally each day or its equivalent only after a response, followed by a taper over at least 4 weeks when improves to G1. Resume nivolumab upon symptom control, or when prednisone/prednisolone daily dose <10 mg
	G4 (serum creatinine >6× ULN)	Permanently discontinue nivolumab. Administer 0.5–1 mg/kg intravenous (methyl)prednisolone and convert to 0.5–2 mg/kg prednisone/prednisolone orally each day or its equivalent only after a response, followed by a taper over at least 4 weeks when improves to G1

(continued)

Treatment Modifications (continued)

Adverse Reaction	Grade/Severity	Dose Modification
Skin	G1/2	Continue nivolumab. Avoid skin irritants, avoid sun exposure, topical emollients recommended. Topical steroid (mild strength for G1, moderate/potent strength for G2) cream once or twice daily ± oral or topical antihistamines for itching
	G3 rash or suspected SJS or TEN	Withhold nivolumab. Avoid skin irritants, avoid sun exposure, topical emollients recommended. Administer oral or topical antihistamines for itching. Administer oral prednisone/prednisolone at a dose of 0.5–2 mg/kg or its equivalent daily for 3 days followed by a slow corticosteroid taper over at least 4 weeks when the rash improves to G1. If does not respond adequately, then administer 0.5–1 mg/kg intravenous (methyl)prednisolone and convert to 0.5–2 mg/kg prednisone/prednisolone orally each day or its equivalent only after a response, followed by a taper over at least 4 weeks when the rash improves to G1. Resume nivolumab upon symptom control, or when prednisone/prednisolone daily dose <10 mg
	G4 rash or confirmed SJS or TEN	Avoid skin irritants, avoid sun exposure, topical emollients recommended. Administer oral or topical antihistamines for itching. Administer 1–2 mg/kg intravenous (methyl)prednisolone and convert to oral steroids 0.5–2 mg/kg prednisone/prednisolone each day or its equivalent only after a response. Taper over at least 4 weeks when the rash improves to G1. Permanently discontinue nivolumab
Encephalitis	Confusion or altered behavior, headaches, alteration in Glasgow Coma Scale, motor or sensory deficits, speech abnormality, may or may not be febrile	Initially withhold nivolumab, but permanently discontinue nivolumab if there is no doubt as to diagnosis. Exclude bacterial and ideally viral infections prior to high-dose steroids. Administer oral prednisone/prednisolone at a dose of 0.5–2 mg/kg/day or its equivalent. When symptoms improve, begin a slow corticosteroid taper over at least 4–8 weeks. If symptoms are severe, administer 1–2 mg/kg intravenous (methyl)prednisolone and convert to 0.5–2 mg/kg prednisone/prednisolone orally each day or its equivalent only after a response. Consider concurrent empiric antiviral (intravenous acyclovir) and antibacterial therapy
Aseptic meningitis	Headache, photophobia, neck stiffness with fever or may be afebrile, vomiting; normal cognition/cerebral function (distinguishes from encephalitis)	
Other syndromes include neurosarcoidosis, posterior reversible leukoencephalopathy syndrome (PRES), Vogt-Koyanagi-Harada syndrome, demyelination, vasculitic encephalopathy, and generalized seizures		
Transverse myelitis	Acute or subacute neurologic signs/symptoms of motor/sensory/autonomic origin; most have sensory level; often bilateral symptoms	Initially withhold nivolumab, but permanently discontinue nivolumab if there is no doubt as to diagnosis. Administer 2 mg/kg intravenous (methyl)prednisolone or consider 1 g/day and convert to 0.5–2 mg/kg prednisone/prednisolone orally each day or its equivalent only after a response. When symptoms improve, begin a slow corticosteroid taper over at least 4–8 weeks. Plasmapheresis may be required if steroids do not bring about improvement
Myocarditis	G3	Permanently discontinue nivolumab. Administer 2 mg/kg intravenous (methyl)prednisolone or consider 1 g/day and convert to 0.5–2 mg/kg prednisone/prednisolone orally each day or its equivalent only after a response. When symptoms improve, begin a slow corticosteroid taper over at least 4–8 weeks. If no response, add MMF 500–1000 mg twice daily. If worse on MMF, consider adding tacrolimus
Peripheral neurologic toxicity	Moderate: some interference with ADL, symptoms concerning to patient	Withhold nivolumab. Initial observation reasonable or initiate prednisone/prednisolone 0.5–1 mg/kg (if progressing, eg, from mild) and/or pregabalin or duloxetine for pain. When symptoms improve, begin a slow corticosteroid taper over at least 4 weeks. Resume nivolumab upon symptom control, or when prednisone/prednisolone daily dose <10 mg
	Severe: limits self-care and aids warranted, life-threatening, eg, respiratory problems	Permanently discontinue nivolumab. Administer 1–2 mg/kg intravenous (methyl)prednisolone and convert to 0.5–2 mg/kg prednisone/prednisolone orally each day or its equivalent only after a response. Taper over at least 4–8 weeks when symptoms improve to G1

(continued)

Treatment Modifications (continued)

Adverse Reaction	Grade/Severity	Dose Modification
Guillain-Barré syndrome	Progressive symmetrical muscle weakness with absent or reduced tendon reflexes—involves extremities, facial, respiratory, and bulbar and oculomotor muscles; dysregulation of autonomic nerves	Permanently discontinue nivolumab. Use of steroids not recommended in idiopathic Guillain-Barré syndrome; however, a trial of (methyl)prednisolone 1–2 mg/kg is reasonable, converting to 0.5–2 mg/kg prednisone/prednisolone orally each day or its equivalent only after a response. If no improvement or worsening, plasmapheresis or IVIG indicated
Myasthenia gravis	Fluctuating muscle weakness (proximal limb, trunk, ocular, eg, ptosis/diplopia or bulbar) with fatigability, respiratory muscles may also be involved	Permanently discontinue nivolumab. Administer pyridostigmine at an initial dose of 30 mg three times daily. Administer oral prednisone/prednisolone at a dose of 0.5–2 mg/kg/day or its equivalent or 1–2 mg/kg intravenous (methyl)prednisolone depending on the severity of symptoms. If begin with IV, convert to 0.5–2 mg/kg prednisone/prednisolone orally each day or its equivalent only after a response. If no improvement or worsening, plasmapheresis or IVIG may be considered. Additional immunosuppressants used in myasthenia gravis include azathioprine, cyclosporine, and mycophenolate. Avoid certain medications, eg, ciprofloxacin, beta-blockers, that may precipitate cholinergic crisis
Other syndromes including motor and sensory peripheral neuropathy, multifocal radicular neuropathy/plexopathy, autonomic neuropathy, phrenic nerve palsy, cranial nerve palsies (eg, facial nerve, optic nerve, hypoglossal nerve)		Permanently discontinue nivolumab. Administer oral prednisone/prednisolone at a dose of 0.5–2 mg/kg/day or its equivalent or 1–2 mg/kg intravenous (methyl)prednisolone depending on the severity of symptoms. If begin with IV, convert to 0.5–2 mg/kg prednisone/prednisolone orally each day or its equivalent only after a response
Arthralgia	G1 (mild pain with inflammation, erythema, or joint swelling)	Continue nivolumab. Administer acetaminophen (paracetamol) and ibuprofen
	G2 (moderate pain with inflammation, erythema, or joint swelling that limits ADLs)	Withhold nivolumab. Administer higher doses of acetaminophen (paracetamol) and ibuprofen and use diclofenac or naproxen or etoricoxib. If inadequately controlled, consider intra-articular steroid injections for large joints or administer oral prednisone/prednisolone at a dose of 0.5–2 mg/kg/day or its equivalent. When improves to G1, begin a slow corticosteroid taper over at least 4 weeks. If does not respond adequately, then administer 0.5–1 mg/kg intravenous (methyl)prednisolone and convert to 0.5–2 mg/kg prednisone/prednisolone orally each day or its equivalent only after a response, followed by a taper over at least 4 weeks when improves to G1. Resume nivolumab upon symptom control, or when prednisone/prednisolone daily dose <10 mg
	G3 (severe pain; irreversible joint damage; disabling; limits self-care ADL)	Withhold nivolumab. Administer 0.5–1 mg/kg intravenous (methyl)prednisolone and convert to 0.5–2 mg/kg prednisone/prednisolone orally each day or its equivalent only after a response, followed by a taper over at least 4 weeks when improves to G1. In severe cases, infliximab or another anti–TNF-alpha drug may be required for improvement of arthritis. Resume nivolumab upon symptom control, or when prednisone/prednisolone daily dose <10 mg
Other	First occurrence of other G3	Withhold nivolumab. Administer oral prednisone/prednisolone at a dose of 0.5–2 mg/kg/day or its equivalent. When improves to G1, begin a slow corticosteroid taper over at least 4 weeks. Resume nivolumab upon symptom control, or when prednisone/prednisolone daily dose <10 mg
	Recurrence of same G3	Permanently discontinue nivolumab. Administer 1–2 mg/kg intravenous (methyl)prednisolone and convert to 0.5–2 mg/kg prednisone/prednisolone orally each day or its equivalent only after a response. Taper over at least 4–8 weeks when symptoms improve to G1
	Life-threatening or G4	
	Requirement for ≥10 mg/day prednisone or equivalent for >12 weeks	Permanently discontinue nivolumab
	Persistent G2/3 adverse reactions lasting ≥12 weeks	

ADL, activities of daily living; ALT, alanine aminotransferase; AST, aspartate aminotransferase; ATG, anti-thymocyte globulin; SJS, Stevens-Johnson Syndrome; TEN, toxic epidermal necrolysis; ULN, upper limit of normal

Notes on general supportive care:
• Steroid taper in most cases will proceed over a minimum of 1 month but if symptoms improve rapidly, a 2-week taper can be considered. If steroids are administered for more than 4 weeks, consider PCP prophylaxis (cotrimoxazole 480 mg twice daily M/W/F or inhaled pentamidine if has cotrimoxazole allergy), regular random blood glucose, VitD level and starting calcium/VitD supplementation per guidelines

Adverse Events (N = 80)

Grade (%)*	Grade 1–2	Grade 3	Grade 4
Fatigue	25	0	0
Infusion-related reaction	20	0	0
Rash	15	1	0
Pyrexia	14	0	0
Arthralgia	14	0	0
Nausea	13	0	0
Diarrhea	10	0	0
Pruritus	10	0	0
Increased lipase	3	3	3
Neutropenia	4	5	0
Abdominal pain	5	3	0
Vomiting	8	0	0
Myalgia	8	0	0
Increased amylase	3	3	0
Increased aspartate aminotransferase	3	3	0
Constipation	6	0	0
Hyperglycemia	5	0	0

*According to the National Cancer Institute Common Terminology Criteria for Adverse Events, version 4.0
Note: Toxicities included in the table are those deemed to have been related to treatment and to have occurred in ≥5% of patients. No treatment-related deaths occurred

SUBSEQUENT THERAPY

HODGKIN LYMPHOMA
REGIMEN: PEMBROLIZUMAB

Chen R et al. J Clin Oncol 2017;35:2125–2132

Pembrolizumab 200 mg; administer intravenously over 30 minutes in a volume of 0.9% sodium chloride injection (0.9%NS) or 5% dextrose injection (D5W), USP, sufficient to produce a pembrolizumab concentration within the range 1–10 mg/mL every 3 weeks for up to 24 months (total dose/3-week cycle = 200 mg)

Alternative pembrolizumab dose and schedule as per the U.S. FDA regimens approved on April 28, 2020:

Pembrolizumab 400 mg; administer intravenously over 30 minutes in a volume of 0.9% NS or D5W sufficient to produce a pembrolizumab concentration within the range 1–10 mg/mL every 6 weeks for up to 24 months (total dose/6-week cycle = 400 mg)
- Administer pembrolizumab with an administration set that contains a sterile, nonpyrogenic, low-protein-binding in-line or add-on filter with pore size within the range of 0.2–5 μm

Treatment notes:
- The U.S. Food and Drug Administration (FDA)-approved dose of pembrolizumab for *pediatric* patients with classic Hodgkin lymphoma is 2 mg/kg (up to a maximum of 200 mg) intravenously over 30 minutes every 3 weeks for up to 24 months.
- Pembrolizumab can cause severe or life-threatening infusion-related reactions, including hypersensitivity and anaphylaxis
  - Monitor patients for signs and symptoms of infusion-related reactions including rigors, chills, wheezing, pruritus, flushing, rash, hypotension, hypoxemia, and fever
  - For severe or life-threatening infusion-related reactions (G3 or G4, respectively), stop administration and permanently discontinue pembrolizumab

Supportive Care
Antiemetic prophylaxis
Emetogenic potential is **MINIMAL**
See Chapter 42 for antiemetic recommendations

Hematopoietic growth factor (CSF) prophylaxis
Primary prophylaxis is **NOT** *indicated*
See Chapter 43 for more information

(continued)

Patient Population Studied

The multicenter, single-arm, phase 2 KEYNOTE–087 study involved 210 patients with relapsed or refractory classic Hodgkin lymphoma. Eligible patients were aged ≥18 years, with an Eastern Cooperative Oncology Group (ECOG) performance status score ≤1. Patients were divided into three cohorts on the basis of lymphoma progression after (1) autologous stem cell transplantation and subsequent brentuximab vedotin treatment; (2) salvage chemotherapy and brentuximab vedotin treatment; and (3) autologous stem cell transplantation but no subsequent brentuximab vedotin treatment. All patients received 200 mg pembrolizumab intravenously every 3 weeks until disease progression, intolerable toxicity, investigator decision, a maximum of 24 months, or after at least 6 months of therapy if they had attained complete remission and had received at least 2 doses since complete remission was attained

Efficacy (N = 210)

	All Patients	Cohort 1 (n= 69)	Cohort 2 (n = 81)	Cohort 3 (n = 60)
Overall response rate*	69.0%	73.9%	64.2%	70.0%
Proportion of patients who achieved complete remission	22.4%	21.7%	24.7%	20.0%
Progression-free survival at 6 months	72.4%			
Overall survival at 6 months	99.5%			

*Overall response rate (the primary efficacy end point) is the percentage of patients who experienced a partial or complete response, per the Revised Response Criteria for Malignant Lymphomas
Note: All efficacy end points listed above, except overall survival, were assessed by a blinded independent central review. Median exposure to pembrolizumab was 8.3 months and median follow-up time was 10.1 months

Therapy Monitoring

1. Initially at the time of each dose, and eventually every 6–12 weeks, perform a total body skin examination with attention to ALL mucous membranes as well as a complete review of systems
2. Monitor patients for signs and symptoms of pneumonitis. Evaluate patients with suspected pneumonitis with chest x-ray, CT, and pulse oximetry. For ≥2 toxicity, may include nasal swab, sputum culture and sensitivity, blood culture and sensitivity, and urine culture and sensitivity
3. Monitor patients for signs and symptoms of colitis. Encourage patients to report diarrhea immediately to any member of the health care team
4. Draw AST, ALT, and bilirubin prior to each infusion and/or weekly if there are Grade 1 liver function test elevations. Note, no treatment is recommended for G1 LFT abnormalities. For ≥2 toxicity, work up for other causes of elevated LFTs including viral hepatitis
5. Use basic metabolic panel (Na, K, CO_2, glucose) and patient history as screening tools for hypophysitis including hypopituitarism and adrenal insufficiency. If in doubt, evaluate AM adrenocorticotropic hormone (ACTH) and cortisol levels. Consider ACTH stimulation test for indeterminate results
6. Assess thyroid function at the start of treatment, periodically during treatment, and as indicated based on clinical evaluation and for clinical signs and symptoms of thyroid disorders. Test for TSH and free thyroxine (FT4) every 4–6 weeks as part of routine clinical monitoring of therapy or for case detection in symptomatic patients
7. Measure glucose at baseline and with each treatment during the first 12 weeks and every 6 weeks thereafter

(continued)

(continued)

Antimicrobial prophylaxis
Risk of fever and neutropenia is **LOW**
Antimicrobial primary prophylaxis to be considered:
- Antibacterial—not indicated
- Antifungal—not indicated
- Antiviral—not indicated, unless patient previously had an episode of HSV

(continued)

8. Obtain a serum creatinine prior to every dose. If creatinine is found to be newly elevated, consider holding therapy while other potential causes are evaluated. Note, routine urinalysis is not necessary other than to rule out urinary tract infections, etc

9. Obtain a complete rheumatologic history and perform an examination of all peripheral joints for tenderness, swelling, and range of motion. Examine the spine. Consider plain x-ray/imaging to exclude metastases and evaluate joint damage (erosions), if appropriate

10. In patients at high risk for infections and in appropriately selected patients based on an infectious disease evaluation, draw screening laboratories (HIV, hepatitis A and B, and blood QuantiFERON for TB) to prepare patients to start infliximab

11. *Response assessment:* CT scan every 3 months during therapy. Consider PET scan to confirm complete response or progressive disease as clinically indicated

Treatment Modifications

Adverse Reaction	Grade/Severity	Dose Modification
Colitis	G1	Loperamide 4 mg as starting dose then 2 mg before each meal and after each loose stool until without diarrhea for 12 hours, with maximum of 16 mg loperamide per day. If G1 diarrhea or colitis persists for >14 days, then add prednisolone 0.5–1 mg/kg (non-enteric coated) or consider oral budesonide 9 mg daily if no bloody diarrhea
	G2/3 diarrhea or colitis	Withhold pembrolizumab. Loperamide 4 mg as starting dose then 2 mg before each meal and after each loose stool until without diarrhea for 12 hours, with maximum of 16 mg loperamide per day. Administer oral prednisone/prednisolone at a dose of 0.5–2 mg/kg/day or its equivalent. When improves to G1, begin a slow corticosteroid taper over at least 4 weeks. Resume pembrolizumab upon symptom control, or when prednisone/prednisolone daily dose <10 mg
	G4 diarrhea or colitis	Permanently discontinue pembrolizumab. Loperamide 4 mg as starting dose then 2 mg before each meal and after each loose stool until without diarrhea for 12 hours, with maximum of 16 mg loperamide per day. Administer 1–2 mg/kg intravenous (methyl)prednisolone and convert to 0.5–2 mg/kg prednisone/prednisolone orally each day or its equivalent only after a response. Taper over at least 4 weeks when symptoms improve. If does not improve over 72 hours or worsens, perform flexible sigmoidoscopy/colonoscopy to document colitis then begin infliximab 5 mg/kg (if no perforation/sepsis/TB/hepatitis/NYHA III/IV CHF). If no response, add MMF 500–1000 mg twice daily. If worse on MMF, consider addition of tacrolimus or ATG
Pneumonitis	G2	Withhold pembrolizumab. Consider *Pneumocystis* prophylaxis depending on the clinical context and coverage with empiric antibiotics. Administer oral prednisone/prednisolone at a dose of 1–2 mg/kg/day or its equivalent. When improves to G1, begin a slow corticosteroid taper over at least 4 weeks. If does not respond adequately after 48 hours, then administer 2–4 mg/kg intravenous (methyl)prednisolone and convert to 0.5–2 mg/kg prednisone/prednisolone orally each day or its equivalent only after a response, followed by a taper over at least 6 weeks when symptoms improve to G1, titrating to symptoms. Resume pembrolizumab upon symptom control, or when prednisone/prednisolone daily dose <10 mg
	G3/4	Permanently discontinue pembrolizumab. Consider *Pneumocystis* prophylaxis depending on the clinical context; cover with empiric antibiotics. Administer 2–4 mg/kg intravenous (methyl)prednisolone and convert to 1–2 mg/kg prednisone/prednisolone orally each day or its equivalent only after a response, followed by a taper over at least 8 weeks when symptoms improve to G1, titrating to symptoms. If when initially treated improvement does not occur within 48–72 hours, begin infliximab 5 mg/kg (if no perforation/sepsis/TB/hepatitis/NYHA III/IV CHF). If no response to infliximab, add MMF 500–1000 mg twice daily. Consider MMF especially if has concurrent hepatic toxicity
Hepatitis	G2 (AST or ALT >3–5× ULN or total bilirubin >1.5–3× ULN)	Withhold pembrolizumab. Administer oral prednisone/prednisolone at a dose of 1–2 mg/kg/day or its equivalent. When improves to G1, begin a slow corticosteroid taper over at least 4 weeks. Resume pembrolizumab upon symptom control, or when prednisone/prednisolone daily dose <10 mg
	G3/4 (AST or ALT >5× ULN or total bilirubin >3× ULN)	Permanently discontinue pembrolizumab. Administer 1–2 mg/kg intravenous (methyl)prednisolone and convert to 0.5–2 mg/kg prednisone/prednisolone orally each day or its equivalent only after a response. Taper over at least 6 weeks when symptoms improve. If no response, add MMF 500–1000 mg twice daily. If worse on MMF, consider adding tacrolimus or ATG

(continued)

Treatment Modifications (continued)

Adverse Reaction	Grade/Severity	Dose Modification
Hypophysitis	G2/3 (moderate symptoms, ie, headache but no visual disturbance or fatigue/mood alteration but hemodynamically stable, no electrolyte disturbance)	Administer analgesia as needed for headache. Withhold pembrolizumab. Administer oral prednisone/prednisolone at a dose of 0.5 to 2 mg/kg/day or its equivalent. When improves to G1, begin a slow corticosteroid taper over at least 4 weeks. If no improvement in 48 hours, administer 1–2 mg/kg intravenous (methyl)prednisolone and convert to 0.5–2 mg/kg prednisone/prednisolone orally each day or its equivalent only after a response. Taper over at least 4 weeks when symptoms improve to 5 mg prednisone/prednisolone or equivalent; do not stop steroids. Resume pembrolizumab upon symptom control, or when prednisone/prednisolone daily dose <10 mg
	G4 (severe mass effect symptoms, ie, severe headache, any visual disturbance or severe hypoadrenalism, ie, hypotension, severe electrolyte disturbance)	Permanently discontinue pembrolizumab. Administer analgesia as needed for headache. Administer 1–2 mg/kg intravenous (methyl)prednisolone and convert to 0.5–2 mg/kg prednisone/prednisolone orally each day or its equivalent only after a response. Taper over at least 4 weeks when symptoms improve to 5 mg prednisone/prednisolone or equivalent; do not stop steroids
Adrenal insufficiency	G2	Withhold pembrolizumab. Administer oral prednisone/prednisolone at a dose of 0.5–2 mg/kg/day or its equivalent. When improves to G1, begin a slow corticosteroid taper over at least 4 weeks. Serially assess adrenal function and continue steroids at replacement doses (20–40 mg hydrocortisone daily ~2/3 dose in AM upon awakening and ~1/3 at 4 PM) until recovery of adrenal function is documented. Resume pembrolizumab upon symptom control, or when prednisone/prednisolone daily dose <10 mg
	G3/4	Permanently discontinue pembrolizumab. Administer oral prednisone/prednisolone at a dose of 0.5–2 mg/kg/day or its equivalent. When improves to G1, begin a slow corticosteroid taper over at least 4 weeks. Serially assess adrenal function and continue steroids at replacement doses (20–40 mg hydrocortisone daily ~2/3 dose in AM upon awakening and ~1/3 at 4 PM) until recovery of adrenal function is documented
Type 1 diabetes mellitus	G3 hyperglycemia	Withhold pembrolizumab. Admit to hospital to manage hyperglycemia. Role of corticosteroids in preventing complete loss of insulin-producing cells is unknown and not recommended. Resume pembrolizumab upon symptom control, or when prednisone/prednisolone daily dose <10 mg
	G4 hyperglycemia	Permanently discontinue pembrolizumab. Admit to hospital to manage hyperglycemia. Role of corticosteroids in preventing complete loss of insulin-producing cells is unknown and not recommended
Nephritis and renal dysfunction	G2/3 (serum creatinine 1.5–6× ULN)	Withhold pembrolizumab. Administer oral prednisone/prednisolone at a dose of 0.5–2 mg/kg/day or its equivalent. When improves to G1, begin a slow corticosteroid taper over at least 4 weeks. If does not respond adequately, then administer 0.5–1 mg/kg intravenous (methyl)prednisolone and convert to 0.5–2 mg/kg prednisone/prednisolone orally each day or its equivalent only after a response, followed by a taper over at least 4 weeks when improves to G1. Resume pembrolizumab upon symptom control, or when prednisone/prednisolone daily dose <10 mg
	G4 (serum creatinine >6× ULN)	Permanently discontinue pembrolizumab. Administer 0.5–1 mg/kg intravenous (methyl)prednisolone and convert to 0.5–2 mg/kg prednisone/prednisolone orally each day or its equivalent only after a response, followed by a taper over at least 4 weeks when improves to G1
Skin	G1/2	Continue pembrolizumab. Avoid skin irritants, avoid sun exposure, topical emollients recommended. Topical steroid (mild strength for G1, moderate/potent strength for G2) cream once or twice daily ± oral or topical antihistamines for itching
	G3 rash or suspected SJS or TEN	Withhold pembrolizumab. Avoid skin irritants, avoid sun exposure, topical emollients recommended. Administer oral or topical antihistamines for itching. Administer oral prednisone/prednisolone at a dose of 0.5–2 mg/kg or its equivalent daily for 3 days followed by a slow corticosteroid taper over at least 4 weeks when the rash improves to G1. If does not respond adequately, then administer 0.5–1 mg/kg intravenous (methyl)prednisolone and convert to 0.5–2 mg/kg prednisone/prednisolone orally each day or its equivalent only after a response, followed by a taper over at least 4 weeks when the rash improves to G1. Resume pembrolizumab upon symptom control, or when prednisone/prednisolone daily dose <10 mg

(continued)

Treatment Modifications (continued)

Adverse Reaction	Grade/Severity	Dose Modification
	G4 rash or confirmed SJS or TEN	Avoid skin irritants, avoid sun exposure, topical emollients recommended. Administer oral or topical antihistamines for itching. Administer 1–2 mg/kg intravenous (methyl)prednisolone and convert to oral steroids 0.5–2 mg/kg prednisone/prednisolone each day or its equivalent only after a response. Taper over at least 4 weeks when the rash improves to G1. Permanently discontinue pembrolizumab
Encephalitis	Confusion or altered behavior, headaches, alteration in Glasgow Coma Scale, motor or sensory deficits, speech abnormality, may or may not be febrile	Initially withhold pembrolizumab, but permanently discontinue pembrolizumab if there is no doubt as to diagnosis. Exclude bacterial and ideally viral infections prior to high-dose steroids. Administer oral prednisone/prednisolone at a dose of 0.5–2 mg/kg/day or its equivalent. When symptoms improve, begin a slow corticosteroid taper over at least 4–8 weeks. If symptoms are severe, administer 1–2 mg/kg intravenous (methyl)prednisolone and convert to 0.5–2 mg/kg prednisone/prednisolone orally each day or its equivalent only after a response. Consider concurrent empiric antiviral (intravenous acyclovir) and antibacterial therapy
Aseptic meningitis	Headache, photophobia, neck stiffness with fever or may be afebrile, vomiting; normal cognition/cerebral function (distinguishes from encephalitis)	
Other syndromes include neurosarcoidosis, posterior reversible leukoencephalopathy syndrome (PRES), Vogt-Koyanagi-Harada syndrome, demyelination, vasculitic encephalopathy, and generalized seizures		
Transverse myelitis	Acute or subacute neurologic signs/symptoms of motor/sensory/autonomic origin; most have sensory level; often bilateral symptoms	Initially withhold pembrolizumab, but permanently discontinue pembrolizumab if there is no doubt as to diagnosis. Administer 2 mg/kg intravenous (methyl)prednisolone or consider 1 g/day and convert to 0.5–2 mg/kg prednisone/prednisolone orally each day or its equivalent only after a response. When symptoms improve, begin a slow corticosteroid taper over at least 4–8 weeks. Plasmapheresis may be required if steroids do not bring about improvement
Myocarditis	G3	Permanently discontinue pembrolizumab. Administer 2 mg/kg intravenous (methyl)prednisolone or consider 1 g/day and convert to 0.5–2 mg/kg prednisone/prednisolone orally each day or its equivalent only after a response. When symptoms improve, begin a slow corticosteroid taper over at least 4–8 weeks. If no response, add MMF 500–1000 mg twice daily. If worse on MMF, consider adding tacrolimus
Peripheral neurologic toxicity	Moderate: some interference with ADL, symptoms concerning to patient	Withhold pembrolizumab. Initial observation reasonable or initiate prednisone/prednisolone 0.5–1 mg/kg (if progressing, eg, from mild) and/or pregabalin or duloxetine for pain. When symptoms improve, begin a slow corticosteroid taper over at least 4 weeks. Resume pembrolizumab upon symptom control, or when prednisone/prednisolone daily dose <10 mg
	Severe: limits self-care and aids warranted, life-threatening, eg, respiratory problems	Permanently discontinue pembrolizumab. Administer 1–2 mg/kg intravenous (methyl)prednisolone and convert to 0.5–2 mg/kg prednisone/prednisolone orally each day or its equivalent only after a response. Taper over at least 4–8 weeks when symptoms improve to G1
Guillain-Barré syndrome	Progressive symmetrical muscle weakness with absent or reduced tendon reflexes—involves extremities, facial, respiratory, and bulbar and oculomotor muscles; dysregulation of autonomic nerves	Permanently discontinue pembrolizumab. Use of steroids not recommended in idiopathic Guillain-Barré syndrome; however, a trial of (methyl)prednisolone 1–2 mg/kg is reasonable, converting to 0.5–2 mg/kg prednisone/prednisolone orally each day or its equivalent only after a response. If no improvement or worsening, plasmapheresis or IVIG indicated

(continued)

Treatment Modifications (*continued*)

Adverse Reaction	Grade/Severity	Dose Modification
Myasthenia gravis	Fluctuating muscle weakness (proximal limb, trunk, ocular, eg, ptosis/diplopia or bulbar) with fatigability, respiratory muscles may also be involved	Permanently discontinue pembrolizumab. Administer pyridostigmine at an initial dose of 30 mg three times daily. Administer oral prednisone/prednisolone at a dose of 0.5–2 mg/kg/day or its equivalent or 1–2 mg/kg intravenous (methyl)prednisolone depending on the severity of symptoms. If begin with IV, convert to 0.5–2 mg/kg prednisone/prednisolone orally each day or its equivalent only after a response. If no improvement or worsening, plasmapheresis or IVIG may be considered. Additional immunosuppressants used in myasthenia gravis include azathioprine, cyclosporine, and mycophenolate. Avoid certain medications, eg, ciprofloxacin, beta-blockers, that may precipitate cholinergic crisis
Other syndromes including motor and sensory peripheral neuropathy, multifocal radicular neuropathy/plexopathy, autonomic neuropathy, phrenic nerve palsy, cranial nerve palsies (eg, facial nerve, optic nerve, hypoglossal nerve)		Permanently discontinue pembrolizumab. Administer oral prednisone/prednisolone at a dose of 0.5–2 mg/kg/day or its equivalent or 1–2 mg/kg intravenous (methyl)prednisolone depending on the severity of symptoms. If begin with IV, convert to 0.5–2 mg/kg prednisone/prednisolone orally each day or its equivalent only after a response
Arthralgia	G1 (mild pain with inflammation, erythema or joint swelling)	Continue pembrolizumab. Administer acetaminophen (paracetamol) and ibuprofen
	G2 (moderate pain with inflammation, erythema, or joint swelling that limits ADLs)	Withhold pembrolizumab. Administer higher doses of acetaminophen (paracetamol) and ibuprofen and use diclofenac or naproxen or etoricoxib. If inadequately controlled, consider intra-articular steroid injections for large joints or administer oral prednisone/prednisolone at a dose of 0.5–2 mg/kg/day or its equivalent. When improves to G1, begin a slow corticosteroid taper over at least 4 weeks. If does not respond adequately, then administer 0.5–1 mg/kg intravenous (methyl)prednisolone and convert to 0.5–2 mg/kg prednisone/prednisolone orally each day or its equivalent only after a response, followed by a taper over at least 4 weeks when improves to G1. Resume pembrolizumab upon symptom control, or when prednisone/prednisolone daily dose <10 mg
	G3 (severe pain; irreversible joint damage; disabling; limits self-care ADL)	Withhold pembrolizumab. Administer 0.5–1 mg/kg intravenous (methyl)prednisolone and convert to 0.5–2 mg/kg prednisone/prednisolone orally each day or its equivalent only after a response, followed by a taper over at least 4 weeks when improves to G1. In severe cases, infliximab or another anti–TNF-alpha drug may be required for improvement of arthritis. Resume pembrolizumab upon symptom control, or when prednisone/prednisolone daily dose <10 mg
Other	First occurrence of other G3	Withhold pembrolizumab. Administer oral prednisone/prednisolone at a dose of 0.5–2 mg/kg/day or its equivalent. When improves to G1, begin a slow corticosteroid taper over at least 4 weeks. Resume pembrolizumab upon symptom control, or when prednisone/prednisolone daily dose <10 mg
	Recurrence of same G3	Permanently discontinue pembrolizumab. Administer 1–2 mg/kg intravenous (methyl)prednisolone and convert to 0.5–2 mg/kg prednisone/prednisolone orally each day or its equivalent only after a response. Taper over at least 4–8 weeks when symptoms improve to G1
	Life-threatening or G4	
	Requirement for ≥10 mg/day prednisone or equivalent for >12 weeks	Permanently discontinue pembrolizumab
	Persistent G2/3 adverse reactions lasting ≥12 weeks	

ADL, activities of daily living; ALT, alanine aminotransferase; AST, aspartate aminotransferase; ATG, anti-thymocyte globulin; SJS, Stevens-Johnson Syndrome; TEN, toxic epidermal necrolysis; ULN, upper limit of normal

Notes on general supportive care:
- Steroid taper in most cases will proceed over a minimum of one month but if symptoms improve rapidly a two-week taper can be considered. If steroids are administered for more than 4 weeks, consider PCP prophylaxis (cotrimoxazole 480 mg twice daily M/W/F or inhaled pentamidine if has cotrimoxazole allergy), regular random blood glucose, VitD level and starting calcium/VitD supplementation per guidelines

Notes on pregnancy and breast feeding:
- Pembrolizumab can cause fetal harm. If used during pregnancy, or if the patient becomes pregnant during treatment, apprise the patient of the potential hazard to a fetus. Females of reproductive potential should use highly effective contraception during treatment and for 4 months after the last dose of pembrolizumab
- It is not known whether pembrolizumab is excreted in human milk. Therefore, it is recommended that women discontinue nursing during treatment with and for 4 months after the final dose of pembrolizumab

Adverse Events (N = 210)

Grade (%)*	Grade 1–2	Grade 3	Grade 4
Hypothyroidism	12	<1	0
Pyrexia	10	<1	0
Fatigue	9	<1	0
Rash	8	0	0
Diarrhea	6	1	0
Cough	5	<1	0
Headache	6	0	0
Nausea	6	0	0
Neutropenia	3	2	0

*According to the National Cancer Institute Common Terminology Criteria for Adverse Events, version 4.0
Note: Toxicities included in the table are those deemed to have been related to treatment and to have occurred in ≥5% of patients. No treatment-related deaths occurred

23. Lung Cancer

Enriqueta Felip, MD, PhD and Rafael Rosell, MD

Epidemiology

Incidence: 228,150 (male: 116,440; female: 111,710. Estimated new cases for 2019 in the United States)
228,820 (male: 116,300; female: 112,520) in 2020
54.9 per 100,000 male and female per year (63.0 per 100,000 men, 48.9 per 100,000 women)

Deaths: Estimated 142,670 in 2019 (male: 76,650; female: 66,020)

Median age: 70 years

Stage at Presentation

Localized (confined to primary site): 20.1%
Regional (spread to regional lymph nodes): 21.9%
Distant (cancer has metastasized): 51.4%

Siegel R et al. CA Cancer J Clin 2019;69:7–34
Surveillance, Epidemiology and End Results (SEER) Program, available from http://seer.cancer.gov (accessed in 2019)

Pathology

Lung cancer is divided into two major classes:

1. Non–small cell lung cancer (NSCLC):   80–85%
   - Squamous cell carcinoma
   - Adenocarcinoma
   - Large-cell carcinoma
2. Small cell lung cancer (SCLC)   15–20%

Brambilla E et al. Eur Respir J 2001;18:1059–1068

Non–Small Cell Lung Cancer (NSCLC)

Work-up

1. History and physical examination including performance status and weight loss
2. Chest x-ray, PA and lateral
3. CT scan of chest and upper abdomen including adrenals
4. CBC, serum electrolytes, BUN, creatinine, calcium, magnesium, and LFTs
5. CT scan and/or MRI of brain if neurologic history or examination is abnormal
6. Bone scan if there is bone pain, elevated calcium level, or elevated alkaline phosphatase level
7. Assessment of perioperative risks for potential candidates for surgery, including pulmonary function tests (PFTs)

Stages I–II	a. Bronchoscopy
	b. FDG-PET scan
Stages IIIA–IIIB	a. Bronchoscopy
	b. FDG-PET scan
	c. MRI of the chest in superior sulcus tumors
	d. MRI of brain
	e. Bone scan
	f. Mediastinal lymph node biopsy if CT scan shows nodes >1 cm
	Invasive tests: Mediastinoscopy, thoracoscopy, transbronchial needle aspiration, and endoscopic ultrasound and needle aspiration
Stage IV	Biopsy for otherwise potentially resectable patient with isolated adrenal mass or liver lesion

Staging

Primary Tumor (T)

TX	Primary tumor cannot be assessed
T0	No evidence of primary tumor
Tis	Carcinoma in situ
T1	Tumor ≤3 cm in greatest dimension, surrounded by lung or visceral pleura, without bronchoscopic evidence of invasion more proximal than the lobar bronchus (ie, not in the main bronchus)[1]
T1mi	Minimally invasive adenocarcinoma[2]
T1a	Tumor ≤1 in greatest dimension[1]
T1b	Tumor >1 cm but not >2 cm in greatest dimension[1]
T1c	Tumor >2 cm but not >3 cm in greatest dimension[1]
T2	Tumor >3 cm but not >5 cm in greatest dimension or tumor with any of the following features[3] Involves main bronchus regardless of distance to the carina, but without involving the carina Invades visceral pleura Associated with atelectasis or obstructive pneumonitis that extends to the hilar region, either involving part of the lung or the entire lung
T2a	Tumor >3 cm but not >4 cm in greatest dimension
T2b	Tumor >4 cm but not >5 cm in greatest dimension
T3	Tumor >5 cm but not >7 cm in greatest dimension or one that directly invades any of the following: chest wall (including superior sulcus tumors), phrenic nerve, parietal pericardium; or tumor in the main bronchus (<2 cm distal to the carina* but without involvement of the carina; or associated separate tumor nodule(s) in the same lobe as the primary
T4	Tumors >7 cm or one that invades any of the following: diaphragm, mediastinum, heart, great vessels, trachea, recurrent laryngeal nerve, esophagus, vertebral body, carina, separate tumor nodule(s) in a different ipsilateral lobe to that of the primary

Distant Metastases (M)

M0	No distant metastasis
M1	Distant metastasis
M1a	Separate tumor nodule(s) in a contralateral lobe; tumor with pleural or pericardial nodules or malignant pleural or pericardial effusion[4]
M1b	Single extrathoracic metastasis in a single organ[5]
M1c	Multiple extrathoracic metastases in one or several organs

Regional Lymph Nodes (N)

NX	Regional lymph nodes cannot be assessed
N0	No regional lymph node metastasis
N1	Metastasis in ipsilateral peribronchial and/or ipsilateral hilar lymph nodes and intrapulmonary nodes, including involvement by direct extension
N2	Metastasis in ipsilateral mediastinal and/or subcarinal lymph node(s)
N3	Metastasis in contralateral mediastinal, contralateral hilar, ipsilateral or contralateral scalene, or supraclavicular lymph node(s)

(continued)

Staging Groups

Group	T	N	M
Occult carcinoma	TX	N0	M0
0	Tis	N0	M0
IA1	T1mi	N0	M0
	T1a	N0	M0
IA2	T1b	N0	M0
IA3	T1c	N0	M0
IB	T2a	N0	M0
IIA	T2b	N0	M0
IIB	T1a	N1	M0
	T1b	N1	M0
	T1c	N1	M0
	T2a	N1	M0
	T2b	N1	M0
	T3	N0	M0
IIIA	T1a	N2	M0
	T1b	N2	M0
	T1c	N2	M0
	T2a	N2	M0
	T2b	N2	M0
	T3	N1	M0
	T4	N0	M0
	T4	N1	M0
IIIB	T1a	N3	M0
	T1b	N3	M0
	T1c	N3	M0
	T2a	N3	M0
	T2b	N3	M0
	T3	N2	M0
	T4	N2	M0
IIIC	T3	N3	M0
	T4	N3	M0

(continued)

(continued)

1. The uncommon superficial spreading tumor of any size with its invasive component limited to the bronchial wall, which may extend proximal to the main bronchus, is also classified as T1a.
2. Solitary adenocarcinoma (≤3 cm), with a predominantly lepidic pattern and ≤5 mm invasion in greatest dimension in any one focus.
3. T2 tumors with these features are classified T2a if 4 cm or less, or if size cannot be determined and T2b if greater than 4 cm but not larger than 5 cm.
4. Most pleural (pericardial) effusions with lung cancer are due to tumor. In a few patients, however, multiple microscopic examinations of pleural (pericardial) fluid are negative for tumor, and the fluid is non-bloody and is not an exudate. Where these elements and clinical judgment dictate that the effusion is not related to the tumor, the effusion should be excluded as a staging descriptor.
5. This includes involvement of a single distant (nonregional) node.

International Association for the Study of Lung Cancer, 8th ed.

(continued)

Group	T	N	M
IVA	Any T	Any N	M1a
	Any T	Any N	M1b
IVB	Any T	Any N	M1c

International Association for the Study of Lung Cancer, 8th ed.

5-Year Relative Survival Rates

Stage IA1	92%
Stage IA2	83%
Stage IA3	77%
Stage IB	68%
Stage IIA	60%
Stage IIB	53%
Stage IIIA	36%
Stage IIIB	26%
Stage IIIC	13%
Stage IVA	10%
Stage IVB	0%

Goldstraw P et al. J Thorac Oncol 2016;11(1):39–51.

Expert Opinion

1. Surgery is the standard treatment in stage I–II disease. Radiation therapy should be considered in medically inoperable stage I–II disease (inadequate pulmonary function tests or comorbid diseases). SART is recommended for medically inoperable NSCLC patients with node-negative tumors ≤5cm.
2. Four cycles of adjuvant cisplatin-based chemotherapy (a doublet combination) is recommended in patients with pathologic stages II–III. Cisplatin-based chemotherapy may be considered in selected patients with N0 disease and tumor size >4 cm.
3. Preoperative chemotherapy or definitive concurrent chemoradiation is the treatment of choice for resectable stage IIIA disease. Platinum-based chemotherapy and thoracic radiation therapy is the standard treatment for unresectable stage III. Concurrent chemoradiation appears to be better than sequential chemoradiation. In patients with unresectable disease with SD or PR after concurrent chemoradiation, consolidation durvalumab should be considered.
4. Platinum-based chemotherapy prolongs survival, improves symptom control, and yields superior quality of life in stage IV disease.
5. For stage IV, ECOG PS 0–1 NSCLC patients without driver mutations whose tumors express PD-L1 at levels of 50% or greater, 1L pembrolizumab or chemotherapy + immunotherapy (± bevacizumab in non-squamous histology) is recommended in the absence of contraindications to use immunotherapy. For patients with low (TPS<50%) or unknown PD-L1 expression, chemotherapy + immunotherapy should be considered (± bevacizumab in non-squamous histology).
6. In patients with metastatic non-SCC and SCC who have not received prior immunotherapy, and with no contraindications, 2L single-agent pembrolizumab (PD-L1 TPS≥1%), nivolumab, or atezolizumab is recommended.
7. Gefitinib, erlotinib, afatinib, and osimertinib are options available for 1L treatment of patients whose tumors harbor EGFR mutation.

(continued)

Expert Opinion (*continued*)

8. Crizotinib, ceritinib, alectinib, and brigatinib are available options for 1L treatment of patients with ALK rearrangements. Alectinib and brigatinib have shown a significant improvement in PFS versus crizotinib.

9. Lorlatinib has shown activity in patients who have progressed on next-generation ALK TKI.

Hanna N et al. J Clin Oncol. 2017;35(30):3484–3515 (erratum in: J Clin Oncol. 2018;36:304)
Kalemkerian GP et al. J Clin Oncol. 2018;36(9):911–919
Kris MG et al. J Clin Oncol. 2017;35(25):2960–2974.
Planchard D et al. Ann Oncol. 2019;30(5):863–870
Schneider BJ et al. J Clin Oncol. 2018;36(7):710–719

STAGE III NSCLC • CONSOLIDATION AFTER CHEMORADIATION
LUNG CANCER REGIMEN: DURVALUMAB

Antonia SJ et al. N Engl J Med 2017;377(20):1919–1929
Protocol for: Antonia SJ et al. N Engl J Med 2017;377(20):1919–1929
Supplementary appendix to: Antonia SJ et al. N Engl J Med 2017;377(20):1919–1929
Supplementary appendix to: Antonia SJ et al. N Engl J Med 2018;379(24):2342–2350
IMFINZI (durvalumab) injection solution prescribing information. Wilmington, DE: AstraZeneca Pharmaceuticals LP; updated 2019 August

Durvalumab 10 mg/kg; administer intravenously over 60 minutes in a volume of 0.9% sodium chloride injection (0.9% NS) or 5% dextrose injection (D5W) sufficient to produce a durvalumab concentration within the range 1–15 mg/mL, every 2 weeks, until disease progression or a maximum of 12 months (total dosage/2-week course = 10 mg/kg)

Alternative regimen for patients with body weight ≥ 30 kg:
Durvalumab 1500 mg fixed dose; administer intravenously over 60 minutes in a volume of 0.9% NS or D5W sufficient to produce a durvalumab concentration within the range 1–15 mg/mL, every 4 weeks, until disease progression or a maximum of 12 months (total dosage/4-week course = 1500 mg)

Notes:
- Administer durvalumab with an administration set that contains a sterile, nonpyrogenic, low-protein-binding in-line filter with pore size of 0.2–0.22 μm
- Durvalumab can cause severe or life-threatening infusion-related reactions
  - Monitor patients for signs and symptoms of infusion-related reactions
    - During clinical development, urticaria was reported to have developed within 48 hours after durvalumab administration
  - Interrupt or slow the administration rate for mild (G1) or moderate (G2) infusion-related reactions
  - STOP administration and permanently discontinue durvalumab for severe (G3) and life-threatening (G4) infusion-related reactions

Supportive Care
Antiemetic prophylaxis
Emetogenic potential is **MINIMAL**
See Chapter 42 for antiemetic recommendations

Hematopoietic growth factor (CSF) prophylaxis
Primary prophylaxis is **NOT** indicated
See Chapter 43 for more information

Antimicrobial prophylaxis
Risk of fever and neutropenia is **LOW**

Antimicrobial primary prophylaxis to be considered:
- Antibacterial—not indicated
- Antifungal—not indicated
- Antiviral—not indicated, unless patient previously had an episode of HSV

Patient Population Studied

This randomized, double-blind, placebo-controlled, phase 3 trial included 713 adult patients with unresectable non–small cell lung cancer (NSCLC) and compared durvalumab to placebo as consolidation therapy after chemoradiotherapy. Patients were included if they had histologically or cytologically documented unresectable, stage III, locally advanced NSCLC and if they had completed two or more cycles of platinum-based chemotherapy (containing etoposide, vinblastine, vinorelbine, paclitaxel, docetaxel, or pemetrexed) with concomitant definitive radiation therapy (54–66 Gy) where the mean dose to the lung was <20 Gy, the V20 (volume of lung parenchyma that received ≥20 Gy) was <35%, or both. Patients also had to experience no disease progression after this treatment, they had to have a WHO performance status of 0 or 1, they had to have a life expectancy of >12 weeks, and they had to have received their last radiation dose 1–42 days before randomization. Patients were excluded if they had ever received anti-PD-L1 or anti-PD-1 antibodies; if they had received immunotherapy or an investigational drug within 4 weeks before the first dose of durvalumab (6 weeks for monoclonal antibodies); if they had an autoimmune disease within the previous 2 years; if they had a history of primary immunodeficiency, concurrent illness, or infection; or if there were unresolved toxic effects or pneumonitis of Grade ≥2 from previous chemoradiotherapy.

Efficacy (N = 713)

	Durvalumab (n = 476)	Placebo (n = 237)	
Median progression-free survival[*†‡]	17.2 months (95% CI, 13.1–23.9)	5.6 months (95% CI, 4.6–7.7)	HR 0.51 (95% CI, 0.41–0.63)
Estimated progression-free survival, 12 months[*]	55.7% (95% CI, 50.9–60.2)	34.4% (95% CI, 28.2–40.7)	
Estimated progression-free survival, 18 months[*]	49.5% (95% CI, 44.6–54.2)	26.7% (95% CI, 20.9–32.9)	
Median overall survival (months)[‡]	NR (95% CI, 34.7-NR)	28.7 (95% CI, 22.9-NR)	HR 0.68 (99.73% CI, 0.47–0.997); P=0.0025
Overall survival rate, 12 months	83.1% (95% CI, 79.4–86.2)	75.3% (95% CI, 69.2–80.4)	
Overall survival rate, 24 months[‡]	66.3% (95% CI, 61.7–70.4)	55.6% (95% CI, 48.9–61.8)	P=0.005
Median time to death or distant metastasis[†‡]	28.3 months (95% CI, 24.0–34.9)	16.2 months (95% CI, 12.5–21.1)	HR 0.53 (95% CI, 0.41–0.68)
Objective response rate[ϵ]	30.0% (95% CI, 25.79–34.53)	17.8% (95% CI, 12.95–23.65)	P<0.001
Complete response rate[ϵ]	1.8%	0.5%	

HR, hazard ratio; CI, confidence interval; NR, not reached
Data are reported from the updated final overall survival analysis (Antonia SJ et al. N Engl J Med 2018;379:2342–2350) with clarifications below. Median follow-up time was 25.2 months (range 0.2–43.1)
[*]Based on RECIST v1.1 criteria
[†]The interim analysis, with a median follow-up time of 14.5 months, reported a P value of <0.001 for this comparison
[‡]Log-rank P value of intention-to-treat analysis is reported, stratified according to age, sex, and smoking history using a two-sided analysis with a significance level of 2.5%
[ϵ]Estimated with the Clopper-Pearson method and compared with the Fisher's exact test, when compared. The interim analysis reported a risk ratio of 1.78 (95% CI, 1.27–2.51)

Therapy Monitoring

1. Monitor patients for signs and symptoms of infusion-related reactions, including pyrexia, chills, flushing, hypotension, dyspnea, wheezing, back pain, abdominal pain, and urticaria

2. Initially at the time of each dose, and eventually every 6–12 weeks, perform a total-body skin examination with attention to *all* mucous membranes as well as a complete review of systems

3. Monitor patients for signs and symptoms of pneumonitis. Evaluate patients with suspected pneumonitis with chest x-ray, CT scan, and pulse oximetry. For toxicity ≥2, may include nasal swab, sputum culture and sensitivity, blood culture and sensitivity, and urine culture and sensitivity

4. Monitor patients for signs and symptoms of colitis. Encourage patients to report diarrhea immediately to any member of the healthcare team

5. Draw AST, ALT, and bilirubin prior to each infusion and/or weekly if there are G1 LFT elevations. *Note:* no treatment is recommended for G1 LFT abnormalities. For toxicity ≥2, work up for other causes of elevated LFTs, including viral hepatitis

6. Use basic metabolic panel (Na, K, CO_2, glucose) and patient history as screening tools for hypophysitis, including hypopituitarism and adrenal insufficiency. If in doubt, evaluate morning adrenocorticotropic hormone (ACTH) and cortisol levels. Consider ACTH stimulation test for indeterminate results

7. Assess thyroid function at the start of treatment, periodically during treatment, and as indicated based on clinical evaluation, and for clinical signs and symptoms of thyroid disorders. Test for TSH and free thyroxine (FT4) every 4–6 weeks as part of routine clinical monitoring of therapy or for case detection in symptomatic patients

8. Measure glucose at baseline and with each treatment during the first 12 weeks and every 6 weeks thereafter

9. Obtain a serum creatinine level prior to every dose. If creatinine is found to be newly elevated, consider holding therapy while other potential causes are evaluated. *Note:* routine urinalysis is not necessary other than to rule out urinary tract infections, etc

10. Obtain a complete rheumatologic history and perform an examination of all peripheral joints for tenderness, swelling, and range of motion. Examine the spine. Consider plain x-ray/imaging to exclude metastases and evaluate joint damage (erosions), if appropriate

11. In patients at high risk for infections and in appropriately selected patients based on an infectious disease evaluation, draw screening laboratories (HIV, hepatitis A and B, and blood QuantiFERON for TB) to prepare patients to start infliximab

Treatment Modifications

RECOMMENDED DOSE MODIFICATIONS FOR DURVALUMAB

Adverse Event	Grade/Severity	Treatment Modification
Infusion reaction	Clinically significant but not severe infusion reaction	Interrupt the infusion in patients with clinically significant infusion reactions and consider resuming at a slower rate following resolution. If decision is made to restart, begin at ≤50% of the rate prior to the reaction and increase in 50% increments every 30 minutes if well tolerated. Infusions may be restarted at the full rate during the next cycle
	G3/4 (severe infusion reaction—pyrexia, chills, flushing, hypotension, dyspnea, wheezing, back pain, abdominal pain, and urticaria). Not rapidly responsive to brief interruption of infusion	Stop infusion and administer appropriate medical therapy (eg, epinephrine, corticosteroids, intravenous antihistamines, bronchodilators, and/or oxygen). Discontinue durvalumab
Infection	Severe or life-threatening	Withhold durvalumab
Colitis	G1	Loperamide 4 mg as starting dose, then 2 mg before each meal and after each loose stool until without diarrhea for 12 hours, with maximum of 16 mg loperamide per day. If G1 diarrhea or colitis persists >14 days, add prednisolone 0.5–1 mg/kg (non-enteric-coated) or consider oral budesonide 9 mg daily if no bloody diarrhea
	G2/3 diarrhea or colitis	Withhold durvalumab. Loperamide 4 mg as starting dose, then 2 mg before each meal and after each loose stool until without diarrhea for 12 hours, with maximum of 16 mg loperamide per day. Administer oral prednisone/prednisolone at a dose of 0.5–2 mg/kg/day or its equivalent. When symptoms improve to G1, begin a slow corticosteroid taper over at least 4 weeks. Resume durvalumab upon symptom control, or when prednisone/prednisolone daily dose <10 mg
	G4 diarrhea or colitis	Permanently discontinue durvalumab. Loperamide 4 mg as starting dose, then 2 mg before each meal and after each loose stool until without diarrhea for 12 hours, with maximum of 16 mg loperamide per day. Administer 1–2 mg/kg intravenous (methyl)prednisolone and convert to 0.5–2 mg/kg prednisone/prednisolone orally each day or its equivalent only after a response. Taper over at least 4 weeks when symptoms improve. If symptoms do not improve over 72 hours or worsen, perform flexible sigmoidoscopy/colonoscopy to document colitis, then begin infliximab 5 mg/kg (if no perforation, sepsis, TB, hepatitis, NYHA III/IV CHF). If no response, add MMF 500–1000 mg twice daily. If worse on MMF, consider addition of tacrolimus or ATG
Pneumonitis	G2	Withhold durvalumab. Start pneumocystis prophylaxis (while patient is receiving a glucocorticoid dose equivalent to ≥20 mg of prednisone daily for 4 weeks or longer) and coverage with empiric antibiotics. Administer oral prednisone/prednisolone at a dose of 1–2 mg/kg/day or its equivalent. When symptoms improve to G1, begin a slow corticosteroid taper over at least 4 weeks. If response is not adequate after 48 hours, administer 2–4 mg/kg intravenous (methyl)prednisolone and convert to 0.5–2 mg/kg prednisone/prednisolone orally each day or its equivalent only after a response, followed by a taper over at least 6 weeks when symptoms improve to G1, titrating to symptoms. Resume durvalumab upon symptom control, or when prednisone/prednisolone daily dose <10 mg
	G3/4	Permanently discontinue durvalumab. Start pneumocystis prophylaxis (while patient is receiving a glucocorticoid dose equivalent to ≥20 mg of prednisone daily for 4 weeks or longer); cover with empiric antibiotics. Administer 2–4 mg/kg intravenous (methyl)prednisolone and convert to 1–2 mg/kg prednisone/prednisolone orally each day or its equivalent only after a response, followed by a taper over at least 8 weeks when symptoms improve to G1, titrating to symptoms. If, when initially treated, improvement does not occur within 48–72 hours, begin infliximab 5 mg/kg (if no perforation, sepsis, TB, hepatitis, NYHA III/IV CHF). If no response to infliximab, add MMF 500–1000 mg twice daily. Consider MMF, especially if concurrent hepatic toxicity

(continued)

Treatment Modifications (*continued*)

RECOMMENDED DOSE MODIFICATIONS FOR DURVALUMAB

Adverse Event	Grade/Severity	Treatment Modification
Hepatitis	G2 (AST or ALT >3–5× ULN or total bilirubin >1.5–3× ULN)	Withhold durvalumab. Administer oral prednisone/prednisolone at a dosage of 1–2 mg/kg/day or its equivalent. When symptoms improve to G1, begin a slow corticosteroid taper over at least 4 weeks. Resume durvalumab upon symptom control, or when prednisone/prednisolone daily dose <10 mg
	G3/4 (AST or ALT >5× ULN or total bilirubin >3× ULN)	Permanently discontinue durvalumab. Administer 1–2 mg/kg intravenous (methyl) prednisolone and convert to 0.5–2 mg/kg prednisone/prednisolone orally each day or its equivalent only after a response. Taper over at least 6 weeks when symptoms improve. If no response, add MMF 500–1000 mg twice daily. If worse on MMF, consider adding tacrolimus or ATG
Hypophysitis	G2/3 (moderate symptoms, ie, headache but no visual disturbance or fatigue/mood alteration but hemodynamically stable, no electrolyte disturbance)	Administer analgesia as needed for headache. Withhold durvalumab. Administer oral prednisone/prednisolone at a dosage of 0.5–2 mg/kg/day or its equivalent. When symptoms improve to G1, begin a slow corticosteroid taper over at least 4 weeks. If no improvement in 48 hours, administer 1–2 mg/kg intravenous (methyl) prednisolone and convert to 0.5–2 mg/kg prednisone/prednisolone orally each day or its equivalent only after a response. Taper over at least 4 weeks when symptoms improve to 5 mg prednisone/prednisolone or equivalent; do not stop steroids. Resume durvalumab upon symptom control, or when prednisone/prednisolone daily dose <10 mg
	G4 (severe mass effect symptoms, ie, severe headache, any visual disturbance or severe hypoadrenalism, ie, hypotension, severe electrolyte disturbance)	Permanently discontinue durvalumab. Administer analgesia as needed for headache. Administer 1–2 mg/kg intravenous (methyl)prednisolone and convert to 0.5–2 mg/kg prednisone/prednisolone orally each day or its equivalent only after a response. Taper over at least 4 weeks when symptoms improve to 5 mg prednisone/prednisolone or equivalent; do not stop steroids
Adrenal insufficiency	G2	Withhold durvalumab. Administer oral prednisone/prednisolone at a dose of 0.5–2 mg/kg/day or its equivalent. When symptoms improve to G1, begin a slow corticosteroid taper over at least 4 weeks. Serially assess adrenal function and continue steroids at replacement doses (20–40 mg hydrocortisone daily ~2/3 dose in morning upon awakening and ~1/3 at 4:00 pm) until recovery of adrenal function is documented. Resume durvalumab upon symptom control, or when prednisone/prednisolone daily dose <10 mg
	G3/4	Permanently discontinue durvalumab. Administer oral prednisone/prednisolone at a dose of 0.5–2 mg/kg/day or its equivalent. When symptoms improve to G1, begin a slow corticosteroid taper over at least 4 weeks. Serially assess adrenal function and continue steroids at replacement doses (20–40 mg hydrocortisone daily ~2/3 dose in morning upon awakening and ~1/3 at 4:00 PM) until recovery of adrenal function is documented
Type 1 diabetes mellitus	G3 hyperglycemia	Withhold durvalumab. Admit to hospital to manage hyperglycemia. Role of corticosteroids in preventing complete loss of insulin-producing cells is unknown, and use is not recommended. Resume durvalumab upon symptom control, or when prednisone/prednisolone daily dose <10 mg
	G4 hyperglycemia	Permanently discontinue durvalumab. Admit to hospital to manage hyperglycemia. Role of corticosteroids in preventing complete loss of insulin-producing cells is unknown, and use is not recommended

(*continued*)

Treatment Modifications (*continued*)

RECOMMENDED DOSE MODIFICATIONS FOR DURVALUMAB

Adverse Event	Grade/Severity	Treatment Modification
Nephritis and renal dysfunction	G2/3 (serum creatinine 1.5–6× ULN)	Withhold durvalumab. Administer oral prednisone/prednisolone at a dose of 0.5–2 mg/kg/day or its equivalent. When symptoms improve to G1, begin a slow corticosteroid taper over at least 4 weeks. If response is not adequate, administer 0.5–1 mg/kg intravenous (methyl)prednisolone and convert to 0.5–2 mg/kg prednisone/prednisolone orally each day or its equivalent only after a response, followed by a taper over at least 4 weeks when symptoms improve to G1. Resume durvalumab upon symptom control, or when prednisone/prednisolone daily dose <10 mg
	G4 (serum creatinine >6× ULN)	Permanently discontinue durvalumab. Administer 0.5–1 mg/kg intravenous (methyl)prednisolone and convert to 0.5–2 mg/kg prednisone/prednisolone orally each day or its equivalent only after a response, followed by a taper over at least 4 weeks when symptoms improve to G1
Skin	G1/2	Continue durvalumab. Avoid skin irritants and sun exposure; topical emollients recommended. Topical steroid (mild strength for G1, moderate/potent strength for G2) cream once or twice daily ± oral or topical antihistamines for itching
	G3 rash or suspected SJS or TEN	Withhold durvalumab. Avoid skin irritants and sun exposure; topical emollients recommended. Administer oral or topical antihistamines for itching. Administer oral prednisone/prednisolone at a dosage of 0.5–2 mg/kg or its equivalent daily for 3 days followed by a slow corticosteroid taper over at least 4 weeks when the rash improves to G1. If rash does not respond adequately, then administer 0.5–1 mg/kg intravenous (methyl)prednisolone and convert to 0.5–2 mg/kg prednisone/prednisolone orally each day or its equivalent only after a response, followed by a taper over at least 4 weeks when the rash improves to G1. Resume durvalumab upon symptom control, or when prednisone/prednisolone daily dose <10 mg
	G4 rash or confirmed SJS or TEN	Avoid skin irritants and sun exposure; topical emollients recommended. Administer oral or topical antihistamines for itching. Administer 1–2 mg/kg intravenous (methyl)prednisolone and convert to oral steroids 0.5–2 mg/kg prednisone/prednisolone each day or its equivalent only after a response. Taper over at least 4 weeks when the rash improves to G1. Permanently discontinue durvalumab
Encephalitis	Confusion or altered behavior, headaches, alteration in Glasgow Coma Scale, motor or sensory deficits, speech abnormality; may or may not be febrile	Initially withhold durvalumab, but permanently discontinue durvalumab if there is no doubt as to diagnosis. Exclude bacterial and ideally viral infections prior to high-dose steroids. Administer 1–2 mg/kg intravenous (methyl)prednisolone for 5 days or oral prednisone/prednisolone at a dosage of 0.5–2 mg/kg/day or its equivalent. When symptoms improve, begin a slow corticosteroid taper over at least 4–8 weeks. If symptoms are severe, administer 1–2 mg/kg intravenous (methyl)prednisolone and convert to 0.5–2 mg/kg prednisone/prednisolone orally each day or its equivalent only after a response. Consider concurrent empiric antiviral (intravenous acyclovir) and antibacterial therapy
Aseptic meningitis	Headache, photophobia, neck stiffness with fever or may be afebrile, vomiting; normal cognition/cerebral function (distinguishes from encephalitis)	
Other syndromes include neurosarcoidosis, posterior reversible leukoencephalopathy syndrome (PRES), Vogt-Koyanagi-Harada syndrome, demyelination, vasculitic encephalopathy, and generalized seizures		
Transverse myelitis	Acute or subacute neurologic signs/symptoms of motor, sensory, autonomic origin; most have sensory level; often bilateral symptoms	Initially withhold durvalumab, but permanently discontinue durvalumab if there is no doubt as to diagnosis. Administer 2 mg/kg intravenous (methyl)prednisolone or consider 1 g/day and convert to 0.5–2 mg/kg prednisone/prednisolone orally each day or its equivalent only after a response. When symptoms improve, begin a slow corticosteroid taper over at least 4–8 weeks. Plasmapheresis may be required if steroids do not bring about improvement

(*continued*)

Treatment Modifications (*continued*)

RECOMMENDED DOSE MODIFICATIONS FOR DURVALUMAB

Adverse Event	Grade/Severity	Treatment Modification
Myocarditis	G3	Permanently discontinue durvalumab. Administer 2 mg/kg intravenous (methyl) prednisolone or consider 1 g/day and convert to 0.5–2 mg/kg prednisone/prednisolone orally each day or its equivalent only after a response. When symptoms improve, begin a slow corticosteroid taper over at least 4–8 weeks. If no response, add MMF 500–1000 mg twice daily. If worse on MMF, consider adding tacrolimus
Peripheral neurologic toxicity	Moderate: some interference with ADL, symptoms concerning to patient	Withhold durvalumab. Initial observation reasonable or initiate prednisone/prednisolone 0.5–1 mg/kg (if progressing, eg, from mild) and/or pregabalin or duloxetine for pain. When symptoms improve, begin a slow corticosteroid taper over at least 4 weeks. Resume durvalumab upon symptom control, or when prednisone/prednisolone daily dose <10 mg
	Severe: limits self-care and aids warranted, life-threatening, eg, respiratory problems	Permanently discontinue durvalumab. Administer 1–2 mg/kg intravenous (methyl) prednisolone and convert to 0.5–2 mg/kg prednisone/prednisolone orally each day or its equivalent only after a response. Taper over at least 4–8 weeks when symptoms improve to G1
Guillain-Barré syndrome	Progressive symmetrical muscle weakness with absent or reduced tendon reflexes—involves extremities; facial, respiratory, and bulbar and oculomotor muscles; dysregulation of autonomic nerves	Permanently discontinue durvalumab. Use of steroids not recommended in idiopathic Guillain-Barré syndrome; however, a trial of (methyl)prednisolone 1–2 mg/kg is reasonable, converting to 0.5–2 mg/kg prednisone/prednisolone orally each day or its equivalent only after a response. If no improvement or worsening, plasmapheresis or IVIG indicated
Myasthenia gravis	Fluctuating muscle weakness (proximal limb, trunk, ocular, eg, ptosis/diplopia or bulbar) with fatigability; respiratory muscles may also be involved	Permanently discontinue durvalumab. Administer pyridostigmine at an initial dose of 30 mg 3 times daily. Administer oral prednisone/prednisolone at a dose of 0.5–2 mg/kg/day or its equivalent or 1–2 mg/kg intravenous (methyl)prednisolone, depending on the severity of symptoms. If treatment begins with intravenous drug, convert to 0.5–2 mg/kg prednisone/prednisolone orally each day or its equivalent only after a response. If no improvement or worsening, plasmapheresis or IVIG may be considered. Additional immunosuppressants used in myasthenia gravis include azathioprine, cyclosporine, and mycophenolate. Avoid certain medications, eg, ciprofloxacin, beta-blockers, that may precipitate cholinergic crisis
Other syndromes, including motor and sensory peripheral neuropathy, multifocal radicular neuropathy/plexopathy, autonomic neuropathy, phrenic nerve palsy, cranial nerve palsies (eg, facial nerve, optic nerve, hypoglossal nerve)		Permanently discontinue durvalumab. Administer oral prednisone/prednisolone at a dose of 0.5–2 mg/kg/day or its equivalent or 1–2 mg/kg intravenous (methyl) prednisolone, depending on the severity of symptoms. If treatment begins with intravenous drug, convert to 0.5–2 mg/kg prednisone/prednisolone orally each day or its equivalent only after a response
Arthralgia	G1 (mild pain with inflammation, erythema, or joint swelling)	Continue durvalumab. Administer acetaminophen (paracetamol) and ibuprofen
	G2 (moderate pain with inflammation, erythema, or joint swelling that limits ADLs)	Withhold durvalumab. Administer higher doses of acetaminophen (paracetamol) and ibuprofen, and use diclofenac or naproxen or etoricoxib. If inadequately controlled, consider intra-articular steroid injections for large joints or administer oral prednisone/prednisolone at a dosage of 0.5–2 mg/kg/day or its equivalent. When symptoms improve to G1, begin a slow corticosteroid taper over at least 4 weeks. If response is not adequate, administer 0.5–1 mg/kg intravenous (methyl) prednisolone and convert to 0.5–2 mg/kg prednisone/prednisolone orally each day or its equivalent only after a response, followed by a taper over at least 4 weeks when symptoms improve to G1. Resume durvalumab upon symptom control, or when prednisone/prednisolone daily dose <10 mg
	G3 (severe pain; irreversible joint damage; disabling; limits self-care ADLs)	Withhold durvalumab. Administer 0.5–1 mg/kg intravenous (methyl)prednisolone and convert to 0.5–2 mg/kg prednisone/prednisolone orally each day or its equivalent only after a response, followed by a taper over at least 4 weeks when symptoms improve to G1. In severe cases, infliximab or another anti–TNF alpha drug may be required for improvement of arthritis. Resume durvalumab upon symptom control, or when prednisone/prednisolone daily dose <10 mg

(*continued*)

Treatment Modifications (*continued*)

RECOMMENDED DOSE MODIFICATIONS FOR DURVALUMAB

Adverse Event	Grade/Severity	Treatment Modification
Other	First occurrence of other G3	Withhold durvalumab. Administer oral prednisone/prednisolone at a dosage of 0.5–2 mg/kg/day or its equivalent. When symptoms improve to G1, begin a slow corticosteroid taper over at least 4 weeks. Resume durvalumab upon symptom control, or when prednisone/prednisolone daily dose <10 mg
	Recurrence of same G3	Permanently discontinue durvalumab. Administer 1–2 mg/kg intravenous (methyl) prednisolone and convert to 0.5–2 mg/kg prednisone/prednisolone orally each day or its equivalent only after a response. Taper over at least 4–8 weeks when symptoms improve to G1
	Life-threatening or G4	
	Requirement for ≥10 mg/day prednisone or equivalent for >12 weeks	Permanently discontinue durvalumab
	Persistent G2/3 adverse reactions lasting ≥12 weeks	

ADL, activities of daily living; ALT, alanine aminotransferase; AST, aspartate aminotransferase; ATG, anti-thymocyte globulin; IVIG, intravenous immunoglobulin; MMF, mycophenolate mofetil; NYHA, New York Heart Association; SJS, Stevens-Johnson syndrome; TEN, toxic epidermal necrolysis; ULN, upper limit of normal

Notes on general supportive care:

Steroid taper in most cases will proceed over a minimum of 1 month, but if symptoms improve rapidly, a 2-week taper can be considered. If steroids are administered for more than 4 weeks, administer PCP prophylaxis (cotrimoxazole 480 mg twice daily M/W/F or inhaled pentamidine if cotrimoxazole allergy), regular random blood glucose, vitamin D level, and starting calcium/vitamin D supplementation per guidelines

Adverse Events (N = 709)

Event		Durvalumab (n = 475)		Placebo (n = 234)	
Grade (%)		Grade 1 or 2	Grade 3 or 4	Grade 1 or 2	Grade 3 or 4
Cough		35	<1	25	<1
Fatigue		24	<1	19	1
Dyspnea		21	1	21	3
Radiation pneumonitis		19	1	15	<1
Diarrhea		18	<1	18	1
Pyrexia		15	<1	9	0
Nausea		14	0	13	0
Decreased appetite		14	<1	12	<1
Pneumonia		9	4	3	4
Pneumonitis		10	2	5	2
Arthralgia		12	0	11	0
Upper respiratory tract infection		12	<1	10	0
Pruritis		12	0	5	0

(*continued*)

Adverse Events (N = 709) (continued)

Event	Durvalumab (n = 475)		Placebo (n = 234)	
Grade (%)	Grade 1 or 2	Grade 3 or 4	Grade 1 or 2	Grade 3 or 4
Rash	12	<1	8	0
Constipation	12	<1	9	0
Hypothyroidism	11	<1	2	0
Headache	11	<1	8	<1
Asthenia	10	<1	13	<1
Back pain	10	<1	11	<1
Musculoskeletal pain	8	<1	10	<1
Anemia	5	3	8	3

Supplementary appendix to: Antonia SJ et al. N Engl J Med 2018;379(24):2342–2350

Adverse events were included in the table if they were reported in ≥10% of patients in either treatment group in the as-treated population. Adverse events were graded according to the CTCAE v4.03. Patients with multiple adverse events are counted once at the maximum reported grade. Grade 5 events occurred in 4.4% of patients who received durvalumab and 6.0% of patients who received placebo. Discontinuation due to adverse events occurred in 15.4% of durvalumab-treated patients and 9.8% of placebo-treated patients, with the most frequent being pneumonitis (4.8% of durvalumab-treated patients and 2.6% of placebo-treated patients), followed by radiation pneumonitis (1.3% each) and pneumonia (1.1% and 1.3%, respectively).

ADVANCED SQUAMOUS
NSCLC • FIRST-LINE

LUNG CANCER REGIMEN: PEMBROLIZUMAB + PACLITAXEL/NAB-PACLITAXEL + CARBOPLATIN

KEYTRUDA (pembrolizumab) prescribing information. Whitehouse Station, NJ: Merck & Co.; revised 2019 September
Paz-Ares L et al. N Engl J Med 2018;379:2040–2051
Protocol for: Paz-Ares L et al. N Engl J Med 2018;379:2040–2051
Supplementary appendix to: Paz-Ares L et al. N Engl J Med 2018;379:2040–2051

The regimen consists of four cycles of induction therapy consisting of pembrolizumab, either paclitaxel or nab-paclitaxel, and carboplatin, followed by maintenance therapy with single-agent pembrolizumab until disease progression or for a maximum of 2 years of therapy (inclusive of induction therapy).

Induction phase

Pembrolizumab 200 mg; administer intravenously over 30 minutes in a volume of 0.9% sodium chloride injection (0.9% NS) or 5% dextrose injection (D5W) sufficient to produce a pembrolizumab concentration within the range 1–10 mg/mL on day 1, prior to paclitaxel or nab-paclitaxel, every 21 days, for 4 induction cycles (total dose/3-week induction cycle = 200 mg)
- Administer pembrolizumab with an administration set that contains a sterile, non-pyrogenic, low protein-binding in-line or add-on filter with pore size within the range of 0.2–5.0μm
- Pembrolizumab can cause severe or life-threatening infusion-related reactions, including hypersensitivity and anaphylaxis

Choose ONE of the following formulations of paclitaxel:
Paclitaxel protein-bound particles for injectable suspension (nab-paclitaxel) 100 mg/m^2 per dose intravenously once weekly for 3 doses on days 1, 8, and 15, every 21 days, for 4 induction cycles (total dosage/3-week induction cycle = 300 mg/m^2), *or:*
  Paclitaxel premedications:
  Dexamethasone 10 mg/dose; orally for 2 doses at 12 hours and 6 hours before each paclitaxel dose, *or*
  Dexamethasone 20 mg/dose; intravenously over 10–15 minutes, 30–60 minutes before each paclitaxel dose (total dose/cycle = 20 mg)
  Diphenhydramine 50 mg, by intravenous injection 30–60 minutes before each paclitaxel dose
  Cimetidine 300 mg (or **ranitidine** 50 mg, **famotidine** 20 mg, or an equivalent histamine [H$_2$]-subtype receptor antagonist) intravenously over 15–30 minutes, 30–60 minutes before each paclitaxel dose

Paclitaxel 200 mg/m^2; administer intravenously, diluted in a volume of 0.9% NS or D5W sufficient to produce a concentration within the range 0.3–1.2 mg/mL, over 3 hours on day 1, prior to carboplatin, every 21 days, for 4 induction cycles (total dosage/3-week induction cycle = 200 mg/m^2)

Carboplatin target AUC = 6 mg/mL × min; administer intravenously in 250 mL D5W or 0.9% NS over 15–30 minutes on day 1, after paclitaxel or nab-paclitaxel, every 21 days, for 4 induction cycles (total dosage/3-week induction cycle calculated to achieve a target AUC = 6 mg/mL × min)

Supportive Care (Induction Therapy Phase)
Antiemetic prophylaxis
Emetogenic potential on day 1 is **HIGH**. *Potential for delayed symptoms*
Emetogenic potential on days 8 and 15 (if nab-paclitaxel chosen instead of paclitaxel) is **LOW**
See Chapter 42 for antiemetic recommendations

Hematopoietic growth factor (CSF) prophylaxis
Primary prophylaxis is **NOT** *indicated*
See Chapter 43 for more information

Antimicrobial prophylaxis
Risk of fever and neutropenia is LOW
Antimicrobial primary prophylaxis to be considered:
- Antibacterial—not indicated
- Antifungal—not indicated
- Antiviral—not indicated unless patient previously had an episode of HSV

Carboplatin dose
Carboplatin dose is based on a formula described by Calvert et al. to achieve a target area under the plasma concentration versus time curve (AUC)

$$\text{Total carboplatin dose (mg)} = (\text{target AUC})(\text{GFR} + 25)$$

(continued)

(*continued*)

In practice, creatinine clearance (CrCl) is used in place of glomerular filtration rate (GFR). CrCl can be estimated from the equation of Cockcroft and Gault, thus:

$$\text{For males, Clcr} = \frac{(140 - \text{age[years]}) \times (\text{body weight [kg]})}{72 \times (\text{serum creatinine [mg/dl]})}$$

$$\text{For females, Clcr} = \frac{(140 - \text{age[years]}) \times (\text{body weight [kg]})}{72 \times (\text{serum creatinine [mg/dl]})}$$

Calvert AH et al. J Clin Oncol 1989;7:1748–1756
Cockcroft DW, Gault MH. Nephron 1976;16:31–41
Jodrell DI et al. J Clin Oncol 1992;10:520–528
Sorensen BT et al. Cancer Chemother Pharmacol 1991;28:397–401

Maintenance phase
Pembrolizumab 200 mg; administer intravenously over 30 minutes in a volume of 0.9% NS or D5W sufficient to produce a pembrolizumab concentration within the range 1–10 mg/mL on day 1, every 21 days, until disease progression and for a maximum of 2 years of therapy (inclusive of induction therapy) (total dosage/3-week maintenance cycle = 200 mg)
- Administer pembrolizumab with an administration set that contains a sterile, non-pyrogenic, low-protein-binding in-line or add-on filter with pore size within the range of 0.2–5.0μm
- Pembrolizumab can cause severe or life-threatening infusion-related reactions, including hypersensitivity and anaphylaxis

Alternative pembrolizumab dose and schedule as per the U.S. FDA regimens approved on April 28, 2020:

Pembrolizumab 400 mg; administer intravenously over 30 minutes in a volume of 0.9% NS or D5W sufficient to produce a pembrolizumab concentration within the range 1–10 mg/mL every 6 weeks, until disease progression and for a maximum of 2 years of therapy (inclusive of induction therapy) (total dose/6-week cycle = 400 mg)

Supportive care (maintenance therapy phase)
Antiemetic prophylaxis
Emetogenic potential is **MINIMAL**
See Chapter 42 for antiemetic recommendations

Hematopoietic growth factor (CSF) prophylaxis
Primary prophylaxis is **NOT** indicated
See Chapter 43 for more information

Antimicrobial prophylaxis
Risk of fever and neutropenia is **LOW**
   Antimicrobial primary prophylaxis to be considered:
   - Antibacterial—not indicated
   - Antifungal—not indicated
   - Antiviral—not indicated unless patient previously had an episode of HSV

Patient Population Studied

This double-blind, randomized, phase 3 trial involved 559 adult patients with pathologically confirmed stage IV squamous non–small cell lung cancer who had received no previous systemic treatment for metastatic disease. Eligible patients had an Eastern Cooperative Oncology Group (ECOG) performance status of 0 or 1 and had at least one measurable lesion according to the Response Evaluation Criteria in Solid Tumors (RECIST) version 1.1. A tumor sample was required to determine PD-L1 status. Patients were excluded if they had symptomatic central nervous system metastases, a history of noninfectious pneumonitis that required glucocorticoid use, or an active autoimmune disease, or if they were receiving systemic immunosuppressive treatment. Patients were randomized 1:1 to receive pembrolizumab or saline placebo, with all patients also receiving carboplatin and either paclitaxel or nanoparticle albumin-bound [nab]-paclitaxel for the first four cycles.

Efficacy (N = 559)

End Point	Pembrolizumab + Paclitaxel/ nab-Paclitaxel + Carboplatin (n = 278)	Placebo + Paclitaxel/ nab-Paclitaxel + Carboplatin (n = 281)	Between-Group Comparison
Median overall survival	15.9 months (95% CI 13.2–NR)	11.3 months (95% CI 9.5–14.8)	HR 0.64 (95% CI 0.49–0.85) P<0.001
Median progression-free survival*	6.4 months (95% CI 6.2–8.3)	4.8 months (95% CI 4.3–5.7)	HR 0.56 (95% CI 0.45–0.70) P<0.001
Response rate[†]	57.9% (95% CI 51.9–63.8)	38.4% (95% CI 32.7–44.4)	—
Median time to response	1.4 months	1.4 months	—
Median duration of response[‡]	7.7 months (range 1.1+ to 14.7+)	4.8 months (range 1.3+ to 15.8+)	—

NR, not reached; HR, hazard ratio, CI, confidence interval
*A total of 349 events of disease progression or death occurred in the intention-to-treat population, as assessed by means of blind, independent central radiologic review
[†]Response was assessed by means of blind, independent central radiologic review
[‡]Plus sign (+) indicates ongoing response at the time of data cutoff

Therapy Monitoring

1. *Before therapy:* history and physical exam, CBC with differential, renal and liver function tests, serum electrolytes
2. *Prior to each cycle:* CBC with differential, serum electrolytes, BUN, serum creatinine, serum bilirubin, AST, and ALT. For G ≥2 LFT elevations, work up for other causes of elevated LFTs including viral hepatitis
3. CBC with differential initially also at day 10–14
4. Observe closely for hypersensitivity reactions, especially during the first and second paclitaxel and pembrolizumab infusions
5. Initially at the time of each pembrolizumab dose, and eventually every 6–12 weeks, perform a total-body skin examination with attention to ALL mucous membranes as well as a complete review of systems
6. Monitor patients for signs and symptoms of pneumonitis. Evaluate patients with suspected pneumonitis with chest x-ray, CT, and pulse oximetry. For G ≥2 toxicity, may include nasal swab, sputum culture and sensitivity, blood culture and sensitivity, and urine culture and sensitivity
7. Monitor patients for signs and symptoms of colitis. Encourage patients to report diarrhea immediately to any member of the health care team
8. Use basic metabolic panel (Na, K, CO_2, glucose) and patient history as screening tools for hypophysitis including hypopituitarism and adrenal insufficiency. If in doubt, evaluate AM adrenocorticotropic hormone (ACTH) and cortisol levels. Consider ACTH stimulation test for indeterminate results
9. Assess thyroid function at the start of treatment, periodically during treatment, and as indicated based on clinical evaluation, and for clinical signs and symptoms of thyroid disorders. Test for TSH and free thyroxine (FT4) every 4–6 weeks as part of routine clinical monitoring of therapy or for case detection in symptomatic patients
10. Measure glucose at baseline and with each treatment during the first 12 weeks and every 6 weeks thereafter
11. Obtain a complete rheumatologic history and perform an examination of all peripheral joints for tenderness, swelling, and range of motion. Examine the spine. Consider plain x-ray/imaging to exclude metastases and evaluate joint damage (erosions), if appropriate
12. In patients at high risk for infections and in appropriately selected patients based on an infectious disease evaluation, draw screening laboratories (HIV, hepatitis A and B, and blood QuantiFERON for TB) to prepare patients to start infliximab
13. *Every 2–3 months:* CT scans to assess response

Treatment Modifications

DOSE MODIFICATION FOR PEMBROLIZUMAB + PACLITAXEL OR NAB-PACLITAXEL + CARBOPLATIN

Notes:
- Toxicity needs to resolve to Grade ≤1 or baseline prior to resuming a given therapy
- Chemotherapy may be interrupted for a maximum of 6 weeks; pembrolizumab may be interrupted for a maximum of 12 weeks
- If a dose is reduced for toxicity with any agent, do not re-escalate the dose
- If there occur several toxicities and there are conflicting recommendations, then follow the most conservative dose adjustment
- Reduction of one chemotherapy agent and not the other agent is appropriate if the toxicity is clearly related to only one of the treatments
- If the toxicity is related to the combination of both chemotherapy agents, both drugs should be reduced
- If the toxicity is related to the combination of three agents, all three agents should be reduced (if applicable), interrupted, or discontinued according to the recommended dose modifications
- Chemotherapy may be discontinued with continuation of pembrolizumab alone
- Interrupt or discontinue pembrolizumab and continue on chemotherapy alone if appropriate

Dose Levels (DLs)

	Dose Level 0	Dose Level −1	Dose Level −2	Dose Level −3
Carboplatin	AUC 6 on day 1 Maximum dose = 900 mg	AUC 4.5 Maximum dose = 675 mg	AUC 3 Maximum dose = 450 mg	Discontinue
Paclitaxel	200 mg/m² day 1	150 mg/m² day 1	120 mg/m² day 1	Discontinue
nab-Paclitaxel	100 mg/m² days 1, 8 and 15	75 mg/m² days 1, 8 and 15	60 mg/m² days 1, 8 and 15	Discontinue
Pembrolizumab	200 mg fixed dose; the dose should not be reduced, only discontinued			

RECOMMENDED DOSE MODIFICATIONS FOR CARBOPLATIN AND PACLITAXEL OR NANOPARTICLE ALBUMIN-BOUND PACLITAXEL

	Carboplatin	Paclitaxel	*nab*-Paclitaxel
Hematologic Toxicity			
Platelets ≥50,000/mm³ AND ANC ≥500/mm³	No dose reduction	No dose reduction	No dose reduction
Platelets ≥50,000/mm³ AND ANC <500/mm³	DL −1	DL −1	DL −1
Platelets <50,000/mm³ without bleeding AND ANY ANC	DL −1	DL −1	DL −1
Platelets <50,000/mm³ with Grade ≥2 bleeding AND ANY ANC	DL −2	DL −2	DL −2
Any platelet count AND ANC <1000/mm³ + fever ≥38.5°C (101°F)	DL −1	DL −1	DL −1
Non-hematologic Toxicity			
G3/4 nausea or vomiting	DL 0	DL 0	DL 0
G3/4 diarrhea	DL 0	DL −1	DL −1
G3/4 mucositis	DL 0	DL −2	DL 0
G2 motor or sensory neuropathies including peripheral neuropathy or ototoxicity (tinnitus and symptomatic hearing loss)	DL 0	DL −2	DL −2
G3/4 neurotoxicity—peripheral neuropathy or ototoxicity (tinnitus and symptomatic hearing loss)	DL −1	Discontinue	Discontinue

(continued)

Treatment Modifications (*continued*)

Non-hematologic Toxicity

Moderate hypersensitivity during paclitaxel or nab-paclitaxel infusion	DL 0	Patient may be re-treated. Base a decision to re-treat on reaction severity and the medically responsible care provider's judgment	
Severe hypersensitivity during paclitaxel or nab-paclitaxel infusion	DL 0	Discontinue therapy	
Loss of vision for light or colors	Discontinue carboplatin; if recovers, consider resumption at a lower DL	DL 0	DL 0
G≥2 AST (SGOT) or ALT (SGPT), or G ≥3 bilirubin	DL −1	Discontinue	Discontinue
G4 transaminase elevation	Discontinue	Discontinue	Discontinue
Creatinine clearance 41–59 mL/min	For an AUC of 4.5, administer no more carboplatin than 4.5 × (GFR + 25)	DL 0	DL 0
Creatinine clearance 16–40 mL/min			
Allergic reaction to carboplatin including anaphylaxis (risk increased in patients previously exposed to platinum therapy)	May occur within minutes of administration. Interrupt the infusion in patients with clinically significant infusion reactions. May also consider desensitization	DL 0	DL 0
Significant hypersensitivity reaction to carboplatin (hypotension, dyspnea, and angioedema requiring therapy)	Discontinue carboplatin. Can consider desensitization	DL 0	DL 0
Other non-hematologic G2/3/4 adverse events (except nausea, vomiting, elevated transaminases, and alopecia)	Withhold treatment until adverse events resolve to <G1, then resume with dose of attributable medication(s) reduced by one DL		
Second occurrence of other non-hematologic G2/3/4 adverse events (except nausea, vomiting, elevated transaminases, and alopecia)	Withhold treatment until adverse events resolve to <G1, then resume with dose of attributable medication(s) reduced by one DL or discontinue the attributable medication(s)		
Treatment delay >2 weeks	Decrease dosage by one dose level for each drug or consider discontinuing treatment		

RECOMMENDED DOSE MODIFICATIONS FOR PEMBROLIZUMAB

Adverse reaction	Grade/Severity	Dose Modification
Colitis	G1	Loperamide 4 mg as starting dose then 2 mg before each meal and after each loose stool until without diarrhea for 12 hours, with maximum of 16 mg loperamide per day. If G1 diarrhea or colitis persists >14 days, then add prednisolone 0.5–1 mg/kg (non-enteric-coated) or consider oral budesonide 9 mg daily if no bloody diarrhea
	G2/3 diarrhea or colitis	Withhold pembrolizumab. Loperamide 4 mg as starting dose then 2 mg before each meal and after each loose stool until without diarrhea for 12 hours, with maximum of 16 mg loperamide per day. Administer oral prednisone/prednisolone at a dose of 0.5–2.0 mg/kg/day or its equivalent. When improves to G1, begin a slow corticosteroid taper over at least 4 weeks. Resume pembrolizumab upon symptom control, or when prednisone/prednisolone daily dose <10 mg
	G4 diarrhea or colitis	Permanently discontinue pembrolizumab. Loperamide 4 mg as starting dose then 2 mg before each meal and after each loose stool until without diarrhea for 12 hours, with maximum of 16 mg loperamide per day. Administer 1–2 mg/kg IV (methyl) prednisolone and convert to 0.5–2.0 mg/kg prednisone/prednisolone orally each day or its equivalent only after a response. Taper over at least 4 weeks when symptoms improve. If does not improve over 72 hours or worsens, perform flexible sigmoidoscopy/colonoscopy to document colitis then begin infliximab 5 mg/kg (if no perforation/sepsis/TB/hepatitis/NYHA III/IV CHF). If no response, add MMF 500–1000 mg twice daily. If worse on MMF, consider addition of tacrolimus or ATG

(*continued*)

Treatment Modifications (*continued*)

Adverse reaction	Grade/Severity	Dose Modification
Pneumonitis	G2	Withhold pembrolizumab. Consider *Pneumocystis* prophylaxis depending on the clinical context and coverage with empiric antibiotics. Administer oral prednisone/prednisolone at a dose of 1–2 mg/kg/day or its equivalent. When improves to G1, begin a slow corticosteroid taper over at least 4 weeks. If does not respond adequately after 48 hours, then administer 2–4 mg/kg IV (methyl)prednisolone and convert to 0.5–2.0 mg/kg prednisone/prednisolone orally each day or its equivalent only after a response, followed by a taper over at least 6 weeks when symptoms improve to G1, titrating to symptoms. Resume pembrolizumab upon symptom control, or when prednisone/prednisolone daily dose <10 mg
	G3/4	Permanently discontinue pembrolizumab. Consider *PNEUMOCYSTIS* prophylaxis depending on the clinical context; cover with empiric antibiotics. Administer 2–4 mg/kg IV (methyl)prednisolone and convert to 1–2 mg/kg prednisone/prednisolone orally each day or its equivalent only after a response, followed by a taper over at least 8 weeks when symptoms improve to G1, titrating to symptoms. If when initially treated improvement does not occur within 48–72 hours, begin infliximab 5 mg/kg (if no perforation/sepsis/TB/hepatitis/NYHA III/IV CHF). If no response to infliximab, add MMF 500–1000 mg twice daily. Consider MMF especially if has concurrent hepatic toxicity
Hepatitis	G2 (AST or ALT >3–5× ULN or total bilirubin >1.5-3× ULN)	Withhold pembrolizumab. Administer oral prednisone/prednisolone at a dose of 1–2 mg/kg/day or its equivalent. When improves to G1, begin a slow corticosteroid taper over at least 4 weeks. Resume pembrolizumab upon symptom control, or when prednisone/prednisolone daily dose <10 mg
	G3/4 (AST or ALT >5× ULN or total bilirubin >3× ULN)	Permanently discontinue pembrolizumab. Administer 1–2 mg/kg IV (methyl) prednisolone and convert to 0.5–2.0 mg/kg prednisone/prednisolone orally each day or its equivalent only after a response. Taper over at least 6 weeks when symptoms improve. If no response, add MMF 500–1000 mg twice daily. If worse on MMF, consider adding tacrolimus or ATG
Hypophysitis	G2/3 (moderate symptoms, ie, headache but no visual disturbance or fatigue/mood alteration but hemodynamically stable, no electrolyte disturbance)	Administer analgesia as needed for headache. Withhold pembrolizumab. Administer oral prednisone/prednisolone at a dose of 0.5–2.0 mg/kg/day or its equivalent. When improves to G1, begin a slow corticosteroid taper over at least 4 weeks. If no improvement in 48 hours, administer 1–2 mg/kg IV (methyl)prednisolone and convert to 0.5–2.0 mg/kg prednisone/prednisolone orally each day or its equivalent only after a response. Taper over at least 4 weeks when symptoms improve to 5 mg prednisone/prednisolone or equivalent; do not stop steroids. Resume pembrolizumab upon symptom control, or when prednisone/prednisolone daily dose <10 mg
	G4 (severe mass effect symptoms, ie, severe headache, any visual disturbance or severe hypoadrenalism, ie, hypotension, severe electrolyte disturbance)	Permanently discontinue pembrolizumab. Administer analgesia as needed for headache. Administer 1–2 mg/kg IV (methyl)prednisolone and convert to 0.5–2.0 mg/kg prednisone/prednisolone orally each day or its equivalent only after a response. Taper over at least 4 weeks when symptoms improve to 5 mg prednisone/prednisolone or equivalent; do not stop steroids
Adrenal insufficiency	G2	Withhold pembrolizumab. Administer oral prednisone/prednisolone at a dose of 0.5–2.0 mg/kg/day or its equivalent. When improves to G1, begin a slow corticosteroid taper over at least 4 weeks. Serially assess adrenal function and continue steroids at replacement doses (20–40 mg hydrocortisone daily ~2/3 dose in AM upon awakening and ~1/3 at 4:00 PM) until recovery of adrenal function is documented. Resume pembrolizumab upon symptom control, or when prednisone/prednisolone daily dose <10 mg
	G3/4	Permanently discontinue pembrolizumab. Administer oral prednisone/prednisolone at a dose of 0.5–2.0 mg/kg/day or its equivalent. When improves to G1, begin a slow corticosteroid taper over at least 4 weeks. Serially assess adrenal function and continue steroids at replacement doses (20–40 mg hydrocortisone daily ~2/3 dose in AM upon awakening and ~1/3 at 4:00 PM) until recovery of adrenal function is documented

(*continued*)

Treatment Modifications (continued)

Adverse reaction	Grade/Severity	Dose Modification
Type 1 diabetes mellitus	G3 hyperglycemia	Withhold pembrolizumab. Admit to hospital to manage hyperglycemia. Role of corticosteroids in preventing complete loss of insulin-producing cells is unknown and not recommended. Resume pembrolizumab upon symptom control, or when prednisone/prednisolone daily dose <10 mg
	G4 hyperglycemia	Permanently discontinue pembrolizumab. Admit to hospital to manage hyperglycemia. Role of corticosteroids in preventing complete loss of insulin-producing cells is unknown and not recommended
Nephritis and renal dysfunction	G2/3 (serum creatinine 1.5–6× ULN)	Withhold pembrolizumab. Administer oral prednisone/prednisolone at a dose of 0.5–2.0 mg/kg/day or its equivalent. When improves to G1, begin a slow corticosteroid taper over at least 4 weeks. If does not respond adequately, then administer 0.5–1 mg/kg IV (methyl)prednisolone and convert to 0.5–2.0 mg/kg prednisone/prednisolone orally each day or its equivalent only after a response, followed by a taper over at least 4 weeks when improves to G1. Resume pembrolizumab upon symptom control, or when prednisone/prednisolone daily dose <10 mg
	G4 (serum creatinine >6× ULN)	Permanently discontinue pembrolizumab. Administer 0.5–1 mg/kg IV (methyl)prednisolone and convert to 0.5–2.0 mg/kg prednisone/prednisolone orally each day or its equivalent only after a response, followed by a taper over at least 4 weeks when improves to G1
Skin	G1/2	Continue pembrolizumab. Avoid skin irritants, avoid sun exposure, topical emollients recommended. Topical steroid (mild strength for G1, moderate/potent strength for G2) cream once or twice daily ± oral or topical antihistamines for itching
	G3 rash or suspected SJS or TEN	Withhold pembrolizumab. Avoid skin irritants, avoid sun exposure, topical emollients recommended. Administer oral or topical antihistamines for itching. Administer oral prednisone/prednisolone at a dose of 0.5–2.0 mg/kg or its equivalent daily for 3 days followed by a slow corticosteroid taper over at least 4 weeks when the rash improves to G1. If does not respond adequately, then administer 0.5–1 mg/kg IV (methyl)prednisolone and convert to 0.5–2.0 mg/kg prednisone/prednisolone orally each day or its equivalent only after a response, followed by a taper over at least 4 weeks when the rash improves to G1. Resume pembrolizumab upon symptom control, or when prednisone/prednisolone daily dose <10 mg
	G4 rash or confirmed SJS or TEN	Avoid skin irritants, avoid sun exposure, topical emollients recommended. Administer oral or topical antihistamines for itching. Administer 1–2 mg/kg IV (methyl)prednisolone and convert to oral steroids 0.5–2.0 mg/kg prednisone/prednisolone each day or its equivalent only after a response. Taper over at least 4 weeks when the rash improves to G1. Permanently discontinue pembrolizumab
Encephalitis	Confusion or altered behavior, headaches, alteration in Glasgow Coma Scale, motor or sensory deficits, speech abnormality, may or may not be febrile	Initially withhold pembrolizumab, but permanently discontinue pembrolizumab if there is no doubt as to diagnosis. Exclude bacterial and ideally viral infections prior to high-dose steroids. Administer oral prednisone/prednisolone at a dose of 0.5–2.0 mg/kg/day or its equivalent. When symptoms improve, begin a slow corticosteroid taper over at least 4–8 weeks. If symptoms are severe, administer 1–2 mg/kg IV (methyl)prednisolone and convert to 0.5–2.0 mg/kg prednisone/prednisolone orally each day or its equivalent only after a response. Consider concurrent empiric antiviral (IV acyclovir) and antibacterial therapy
Aseptic meningitis	Headache, photophobia, neck stiffness with fever or may be afebrile, vomiting; normal cognition/cerebral function (distinguishes from encephalitis)	
Other syndromes include neurosarcoidosis, posterior reversible leukoencephalopathy syndrome (PRES), Vogt-Koyanagi-Harada syndrome, demyelination, vasculitic encephalopathy, and generalized seizures		
Transverse myelitis	Acute or subacute neurologic signs/symptoms of motor/sensory/autonomic origin; most have sensory level; often bilateral symptoms	Initially withhold pembrolizumab, but permanently discontinue pembrolizumab if there is no doubt as to diagnosis. Administer 2 mg/kg IV (methyl)prednisolone or consider 1 g/day and convert to 0.5–2.0 mg/kg prednisone/prednisolone orally each day or its equivalent only after a response. When symptoms improve, begin a slow corticosteroid taper over at least 4–8 weeks. Plasmapheresis may be required if steroids do not bring about improvement

(continued)

Treatment Modifications (*continued*)

Adverse reaction	Grade/Severity	Dose Modification
Myocarditis	G3	Permanently discontinue pembrolizumab. Administer 2 mg/kg IV (methyl) prednisolone or consider 1 g/day and convert to 0.5–2.0 mg/kg prednisone/prednisolone orally each day or its equivalent only after a response. When symptoms improve, begin a slow corticosteroid taper over at least 4–8 weeks. If no response, add MMF 500–1000 mg twice daily. If worse on MMF, consider adding tacrolimus
Peripheral neurologic toxicity	Moderate: some interference with ADL, symptoms concerning to patient	Withhold pembrolizumab. Initial observation reasonable or initiate prednisone/prednisolone 0.5–1 mg/kg (if progressing, eg, from mild) and/or pregabalin or duloxetine for pain. When symptoms improve, begin a slow corticosteroid taper over at least 4 weeks. Resume pembrolizumab upon symptom control, or when prednisone/prednisolone daily dose <10 mg
	Severe: limits self-care and aids warranted, life-threatening, eg, respiratory problems	Permanently discontinue pembrolizumab. Administer 1–2 mg/kg IV (methyl) prednisolone and convert to 0.5–2.0 mg/kg prednisone/prednisolone orally each day or its equivalent only after a response. Taper over at least 4–8 weeks when symptoms improve to G1
Guillain-Barré syndrome	Progressive symmetrical muscle weakness with absent or reduced tendon reflexes—involves extremities, facial, respiratory, and bulbar and oculomotor muscles; dysregulation of autonomic nerves	Permanently discontinue pembrolizumab. Use of steroids not recommended in idiopathic Guillain-Barré syndrome; however, a trial of (methyl)prednisolone 1–2 mg/kg is reasonable, converting to 0.5–2.0 mg/kg prednisone/prednisolone orally each day or its equivalent only after a response. If no improvement or worsening, plasmapheresis or IVIG indicated
Myasthenia gravis	Fluctuating muscle weakness (proximal limb, trunk, ocular, eg, ptosis/diplopia or bulbar) with fatigability, respiratory muscles also may be involved	Permanently discontinue pembrolizumab. Administer pyridostigmine at an initial dose of 30 mg three times daily. Administer oral prednisone/prednisolone at a dose of 0.5–2.0 mg/kg/day or its equivalent or 1–2 mg/kg IV (methyl) prednisolone depending on the severity of symptoms. If begin with IV, convert to 0.5–2.0 mg/kg prednisone/prednisolone orally each day or its equivalent only after a response. If no improvement or worsening, plasmapheresis or IVIG may be considered. Additional immunosuppressants used in myasthenia gravis include azathioprine, cyclosporine, and mycophenolate. Avoid certain medications, eg, ciprofloxacin, beta-blockers, that may precipitate cholinergic crisis
Other syndromes including motor and sensory peripheral neuropathy, multifocal radicular neuropathy/plexopathy, autonomic neuropathy, phrenic nerve palsy, cranial nerve palsies (eg, facial nerve, optic nerve, hypoglossal nerve)		Permanently discontinue pembrolizumab. Administer oral prednisone/prednisolone at a dose of 0.5–2.0 mg/kg/day or its equivalent or 1–2 mg/kg IV (methyl) prednisolone depending on the severity of symptoms. If begin with IV, convert to 0.5–2.0 mg/kg prednisone/prednisolone orally each day or its equivalent only after a response
Arthralgia	G1 (mild pain with inflammation, erythema or joint swelling)	Continue pembrolizumab. Administer acetaminophen (paracetamol) and ibuprofen
	G2 (moderate pain with inflammation, erythema, or joint swelling that limits ADLs)	Withhold pembrolizumab. Administer higher doses of acetaminophen (paracetamol) and ibuprofen, and use diclofenac or naproxen or etoricoxib. If inadequately controlled, consider intra-articular steroid injections for large joints or administer oral prednisone/prednisolone at a dose of 0.5–2.0 mg/kg/day or its equivalent. When improves to G1, begin a slow corticosteroid taper over at least 4 weeks. If does not respond adequately, then administer 0.5–1 mg/kg IV (methyl) prednisolone and convert to 0.5–2.0 mg/kg prednisone/prednisolone orally each day or its equivalent only after a response, followed by a taper over at least 4 weeks when improves to G1. Resume pembrolizumab upon symptom control, or when prednisone/prednisolone daily dose <10 mg
	G3 (severe pain; irreversible joint damage; disabling; limits self-care ADL)	Withhold pembrolizumab. Administer 0.5–1 mg/kg IV (methyl)prednisolone and convert to 0.5–2.0 mg/kg prednisone/prednisolone orally each day or its equivalent only after a response, followed by a taper over at least 4 weeks when improves to G1. In severe cases, infliximab or another anti–TNF alpha drug may be required for improvement of arthritis. Resume pembrolizumab upon symptom control, or when prednisone/prednisolone daily dose <10 mg

(*continued*)

Treatment Modifications (*continued*)

Adverse reaction	Grade/Severity	Dose Modification
Other	First occurrence of other G3	Withhold pembrolizumab. Administer oral prednisone/prednisolone at a dose of 0.5–2.0 mg/kg/day or its equivalent. When improves to G1, begin a slow corticosteroid taper over at least 4 weeks. Resume pembrolizumab upon symptom control, or when prednisone/prednisolone daily dose <10 mg
	Recurrence of same G3	Permanently discontinue pembrolizumab. Administer 1–2 mg/kg IV (methyl) prednisolone and convert to 0.5–2.0 mg/kg prednisone/prednisolone orally each day or its equivalent only after a response. Taper over at least 4–8 weeks when symptoms improve to G1
	Life-threatening or G4	
	Requirement for ≥10 mg/day prednisone or equivalent for >12 weeks	Permanently discontinue pembrolizumab
	Persistent G2/3 adverse reactions lasting ≥12 weeks	

ADL, activities of daily living; ALT, alanine aminotransferase; AST, aspartate aminotransferase; ATG, anti-thymocyte globulin; SJS, Stevens-Johnson Syndrome; TEN, toxic epidermal necrolysis; ULN, upper limit of normal

Notes on general supportive care:
- Steroid taper in most cases will proceed over a minimum of 1 month, but if symptoms improve rapidly, a 2-week taper can be considered. If steroids are administered for more than 4 weeks, consider PCP prophylaxis (cotrimoxazole 480 mg twice daily M/W/F or inhaled pentamidine if has cotrimoxazole allergy), regular random blood glucose, vitamin D level and starting calcium/vitamin D supplementation per guidelines

Notes on pregnancy and breastfeeding:
- Pembrolizumab can cause fetal harm. If used during pregnancy, or if the patient becomes pregnant during treatment, apprise the patient of the potential hazard to a fetus. Females of reproductive potential should use highly effective contraception during treatment and for 4 months after the last dose of pembrolizumab
- It is not known whether pembrolizumab is excreted in human milk. Therefore, it is recommended that women discontinue nursing during treatment with and for 4 months after the final dose of pembrolizumab

Adverse Events (N = 558)

Grade (%)	Pembrolizumab Combination (n = 278)		Placebo Combination (n = 280)	
	Grade 1–2	Grade 3–5	Grade 1–2	Grade 3–5
Events occurring in ≥15% of patients in either treatment group*				
Anemia	37.7	15.5	31.4	20.4
Alopecia	45.6	0.4	35.3	1.1
Neutropenia	15.1	22.7	8.3	24.6
Nausea	34.5	1.1	30.7	1.4
Thrombocytopenia	23.8	6.8	17.1	6.4
Diarrhea	25.9	4.0	21.1	2.1
Decreased appetite	22.3	2.2	27.5	1.8
Constipation	22.3	0.7	20.7	1.1
Fatigue	19.5	3.2	21.8	3.9
Asthenia	19.4	2.2	17.5	3.6
Arthralgia	19.1	1.4	13.6	0.7
Peripheral neuropathy	19.4	1.1	15.4	0.7

(*continued*)

Adverse Events (N = 558) *(continued)*

Grade (%)	Pembrolizumab Combination (n = 278)		Placebo Combination (n = 280)	
	Grade 1–2	Grade 3–5	Grade 1–2	Grade 3–5
Vomiting	15.8	0.4	9.7	2.1
Cough	12.6	0.7	15.7	1.1
Dyspnea	11.5	1.4	15	1.1
Adverse events of interest in the as-treated population[†]				
Hypothyroidism	7.5	0.4	1.8	0
Hyperthyroidism	6.8	0.4	0.7	0
Pneumonitis	4.0	2.5[‡]	1.0	1.1[‡]
Infusion reaction	1.5	1.4	1.7	0.4
Colitis	0.3	2.2	0.3	1.1
Hepatitis	0	1.8	0	0
Severe skin reaction	0.7	1.1	0	0.4
Hypophysitis	0.4	0.7	0	0
Thyroiditis	0.7	0.4	0	0
Nephritis	0	0.7	0	0.7

*Adverse event data reported in the as-treated population for all adverse events that occurred during the trial period or within 30 days (or within 90 days for serious events). Adverse events that occurred during crossover from the placebo-combination to pembrolizumab monotherapy were excluded. The as-treated population included all patients who underwent randomization and received at least one dose of the assigned combination treatment

†Adverse events of interest are infusion reactions and events with an immune-related cause; they are considered regardless of whether the investigator attributed the event to a trial regimen or considered the event to be immune-related

‡Includes 1 patient (0.4%) in each treatment group who had Grade 5 (fatal) pneumonitis

ADVANCED NON-SQUAMOUS NSCLC • FIRST-LINE
LUNG CANCER REGIMEN: PEMBROLIZUMAB + CISPLATIN/CARBOPLATIN + PEMETREXED

Gadgeel SM et al. J Clin Oncol 2019;37(15_suppl):9013–9013
Gandhi L et al. N Engl J Med 2018;378(22):2078–2092
Protocol for: Gandhi L et al. N Engl J Med 2018;378(22):2078–2092
Supplemental appendix to: Gandhi L et al. N Engl J Med 2018;378(22):2078–2092
KEYTRUDA (pembrolizumab) injection prescribing information. Whitehouse Station, NJ: Merck & Co., Inc; updated 2019 September

The regimen consists of four 3-week cycles of induction therapy consisting of pembrolizumab, pemetrexed, and either cisplatin or carboplatin, followed by maintenance therapy with pembrolizumab (given until disease progression and for a maximum of 24 months of therapy, inclusive of induction therapy) and pemetrexed (given until disease progression)

Induction therapy
Ancillary medications:

Folic acid 350–1000 mcg daily; administer orally, beginning 1–3 weeks before chemotherapy and continuing throughout treatment with pemetrexed and for 21 days after the last pemetrexed dose, *and*

Cyanocobalamin (vitamin B$_{12}$) 1000 mcg; administer intramuscularly every 9 weeks, beginning 1–3 weeks before chemotherapy and continuing throughout treatment with pemetrexed, *and*

Dexamethasone 4 mg; administer intravenously or orally twice daily for 3 consecutive days, starting the day before each pemetrexed administration to decrease the risk of severe skin rash associated with pemetrexed

Pembrolizumab 200 mg; administer intravenously over 30 minutes in a volume of 0.9% sodium chloride injection (0.9% NS) or 5% dextrose injection (D5W) sufficient to produce a pembrolizumab concentration within the range 1–10 mg/mL, on day 1, before pemetrexed, every 21 days, for 4 induction cycles (total dose/3-week induction cycle = 200 mg), *followed by:*
- Administer pembrolizumab with an administration set that contains a sterile, non-pyrogenic, low-protein-binding in-line or add-on filter with pore size within the range of 0.2–5.0μm
- Pembrolizumab can cause severe or life-threatening infusion-related reactions, including hypersensitivity and anaphylaxis
- A 400-mg Q6W dosing regimen for pembrolizumab offers an alternative. This dosing regimen received accelerated approval based on pharmacokinetic data, the relationship of exposure to efficacy, and the relationship of exposure to safety. Continued approval for this dosing may be contingent upon verification and description of clinical benefit in the confirmatory trials.

Pemetrexed 500 mg/m^2; administer intravenously in 100 mL 0.9% NS over 10 minutes on day 1, after pembrolizumab, every 21 days, for 4 induction cycles (total dosage/3-week induction cycle = 500 mg/m^2), *followed by:*

Choose one of the following platinum agents (either carboplatin or cisplatin):

Carboplatin target AUC = 5 mg/mL × min; administer intravenously in 250 mL D5W or 0.9% NS over 15–60 minutes on day 1, every 21 days, for 4 induction cycles (total dose/3-week cycle calculated to achieve a target AUC = 5 mg/mL × min)

OR

Hydration before cisplatin: ≥1000 mL 0.9% NS; intravenously over a minimum of 1 hour before commencing cisplatin administration
Cisplatin 75 mg/m^2; administer intravenously, diluted in 100–250 mL 0.9% NS over 60 minutes on day 1, every 21 days, for 4 induction cycles (total dosage/3-week induction cycle = 75 mg/m^2)
Hydration after cisplatin: Administer by intravenous infusion ≥1000 mL 0.9% NS over a minimum of 2 hours. Encourage patients to increase oral intake of nonalcoholic fluids, and provide electrolyte replacement as needed (potassium, magnesium, sodium)

Supportive Care (Induction Therapy Phase)
Antiemetic prophylaxis
Emetogenic potential is **HIGH.** *Potential for delayed symptoms*
See Chapter 42 for antiemetic recommendations

Hematopoietic growth factor (CSF) prophylaxis
Primary prophylaxis is **NOT** *indicated*
See Chapter 43 for more information

Antimicrobial prophylaxis
Risk of fever and neutropenia is LOW
Antimicrobial primary prophylaxis to be considered:
- Antibacterial—not indicated
- Antifungal—not indicated
- Antiviral—not indicated unless patient previously had an episode of HSV

Carboplatin dose
Carboplatin dose is based on a formula described by Calvert et al. to achieve a target area under the plasma concentration versus time curve (AUC)

$$\text{Total carboplatin dose (mg)} = (\text{target AUC})(\text{GFR} + 25)$$

(continued)

(continued)

In practice, creatinine clearance (CrCl) is used in place of glomerular filtration rate (GFR). CrCl can be estimated from the equation of Cockcroft and Gault, thus:

$$\text{For males, Clcr} = \frac{(140 - \text{age[years]}) \times (\text{body weight [kg]})}{72 \times (\text{serum creatinine [mg/dl]})}$$

$$\text{For females, Clcr} = \frac{(140 - \text{age[years]}) \times (\text{body weight [kg]})}{72 \times (\text{serum creatinine [mg/dl]})} \times 0.85$$

Calvert AH et al. J Clin Oncol 1989;7:1748–1756
Cockcroft DW, Gault MH. Nephron 1976;16:31–41
Jodrell DI et al. J Clin Oncol 1992;10:520–528
Sorensen BT et al. Cancer Chemother Pharmacol 1991;28:397–401

Maintenance therapy
Ancillary medications:

Folic acid 350–1000 mcg daily; administer orally, beginning 1–3 weeks before chemotherapy and continuing throughout treatment with pemetrexed and for 21 days after the last pemetrexed dose, *and*

Cyanocobalamin (vitamin B$_{12}$) 1000 mcg; administer intramuscularly every 9 weeks, beginning 1–3 weeks before chemotherapy and continuing throughout treatment with pemetrexed, *and*

Dexamethasone 4 mg; administer intravenously or orally twice daily for 3 consecutive days, starting the day before each pemetrexed administration to decrease the risk of severe skin rash associated with pemetrexed

Pembrolizumab 200 mg; administer intravenously over 30 minutes in a volume of 0.9% NS or D5W sufficient to produce a pembrolizumab concentration within the range 1–10 mg/mL, on day 1, before pemetrexed, every 21 days, until disease progression and for a maximum of 2 years of therapy (inclusive of induction therapy) (total dose/3-week maintenance cycle = 200 mg), *followed by:*
• Administer pembrolizumab with an administration set that contains a sterile, non-pyrogenic, low-protein-binding in-line or add-on filter with pore size within the range of 0.2–5.0μm
• Pembrolizumab can cause severe or life-threatening infusion-related reactions, including hypersensitivity and anaphylaxis

Alternative pembrolizumab dose and schedule as per the U.S. FDA regimens approved on April 28, 2020:

Pembrolizumab 400 mg; administer intravenously over 30 minutes in a volume of 0.9% NS or D5W sufficient to produce a pembrolizumab concentration within the range 1–10 mg/mL every 6 weeks, until disease progression and for a maximum of 2 years of therapy (inclusive of induction therapy) (total dose/6-week cycle = 400 mg)

Pemetrexed 500 mg/m^2; administer intravenously in 100 mL 0.9% sodium chloride (0.9% NS) over 10-minutes on day 1, after pembrolizumab, every 21 days, until disease progression (total dosage/3-week maintenance cycle = 500 mg/m^2)

Supportive Care (Maintenance Therapy Phase)
Antiemetic prophylaxis
Emetogenic potential is **LOW**
See Chapter 42 for antiemetic recommendations

Hematopoietic growth factor (CSF) prophylaxis
Primary prophylaxis is **NOT** *indicated*
See Chapter 43 for more information

Antimicrobial prophylaxis
Risk of fever and neutropenia is LOW
Antimicrobial primary prophylaxis to be considered:
• Antibacterial—not indicated
• Antifungal—not indicated
• Antiviral—not indicated unless patient previously had an episode of HSV

Patient Population Studied

KEYNOTE-189 was a randomized, double-blind, placebo-controlled, phase 3, international trial that included 616 adult patients and compared treatment with pemetrexed plus a platinum-based chemotherapy drug plus either pembrolizumab or placebo, followed by pemetrexed plus either pembrolizumab or placebo as maintenance therapy. Patients were eligible if they had histologically or cytologically confirmed stage IV non-squamous, non–small cell lung cancer (NSCLC) without sensitizing EGFR or ALK mutations, if they had received no previous systemic treatment for metastatic disease, if they had an Eastern Cooperative Oncology Group (ECOG) performance score of 0 or 1, if they had at least one measurable lesion according to RECIST v1.1 criteria, if they had a life expectancy ≥3 months, if they had adequate organ function, and if they had provided a tumor sample for assessment of PD-L1 status. Patients were excluded from the trial if they had symptomatic CNS metastases, major surgery <3 weeks previously, a history of noninfectious pneumonitis requiring glucocorticoids, active autoimmune disease, if they were receiving systemic immunosuppressive treatment, if they would be expected to require other antineoplastic agents during the trial, or if they had received >30 Gy of radiotherapy to the lung in the previous 6 months (due to the increased risk of pneumonitis with pembrolizumab).

Data included herein are obtained from the initial publication and a subsequent updated abstract (J Clin Oncol 2019;37[15]:9013).

Efficacy (N = 616)

	Cisplatin/Carboplatin + Pemetrexed + Pembrolizumab (n = 410)	Cisplatin/ Carboplatin + Pemetrexed + Placebo (n = 206)	
Median overall survival*†	22.0 months	10.7 months	HR 0.56 (95% CI, 0.45–0.70); P<0.00001
Overall survival in PD-L1 TPS ≥50%*† (n = 202)	NR	NR	HR 0.59 (95% CI, 0.39–0.88)
Overall survival in PD-L1 TPS 1–49%*† (n = 186)	NR	NR	HR 0.62 (95% CI, 0.42–0.92)
Overall survival in PD-L1 TPS <1%*† (n =190)	NR	NR	HR 0.52 (95% CI, 0.36–0.74)
Median PFS2*†‡	17.0 months	9.0 months	HR 0.49 (95% CI, 0.40–0.59); P<0.00001
Median overall survival†	NR	11.3 months (95% CI, 8.7–15.1)	HR 0.49 (95% CI, 0.38–0.64); P<0.001
Estimated overall survival rate (12 months)	69.2% (95% CI, 64.1–73.8)	49.4% (95% CI, 42.1–56.2)	
Median progression-free survival†	8.8 months (95% CI, 7.6–9.2)	4.9 months (95% CI, 4.7–5.5)	HR 0.52 (95% CI, 0.43–0.64); P<0.001
Estimated progression-free survival rate (12 months)	34.1% (95% CI, 28.8–39.5)	17.3% (95% CI, 12.0–23.5)	
Objective response rate (IRC-assessed)§	47.6% (95% CI, 42.6–52.5)	18.9% (95% CI, 13.8–25.0)	Estimated treatment difference 28.6 (95% CI, 21.1–35.4); P<0.0001
Disease control rate	84.6%	70.4%	
Median duration of response¶	11.2 months (range, 1.1+ to 18.0+)	7.8 months (range, 2.1+ to 16.4+)	

HR, hazard ratio; CI, confidence interval; IRC, independent review committee; NR, not reached

*Data from the update paper (abstract only) titled "KEYNOTE-189: Updated OS and progression after the next line of therapy (PFS2) with pembrolizumab (pembro) plus chemo with pemetrexed and platinum vs placebo plus chemo for metastatic non-squamous NSCLC" with a median overall follow-up time of 18.7 months (no range or breakdown by group reported)

†Analyzed with a stratified log-rank test. HRs and 95% CIs were analyzed with the stratified Cox proportional-hazards model and Efron's method for handling tied events to evaluate treatment differences

‡PFS2 defined as time from randomization to disease progression per investigator after start of second-line therapy or death, whichever occurred first

§Differences in response rate were calculated with the stratified method of Miettinen and Nurminen

¶Plus signs indicate that there was no progressive disease at the time of last assessment

All data are from the paper titled "Pembrolizumab plus Chemotherapy in Metastatic Non–Small-Cell Lung Cancer" unless noted. Data in this paper were generated with a median follow-up time of 10.5 months (range, 0.2 to 20.4), the mean (± SD) duration of treatment was 7.4 ± 4.7 months in the pembrolizumab group and 5.4 ± 4.3 months in the placebo group. Tumor response was graded according to RECIST v1.1 criteria. All end points were analyzed in the intention-to-treat population

Therapy Monitoring

1. *Before therapy:* history and physical exam, CBC with differential, renal and liver function tests, serum electrolytes

2. *Prior to each cycle:* CBC with differential, serum electrolytes, BUN, serum creatinine, serum bilirubin, AST, and ALT. For G ≥2 LFT elevations, work up for other causes of elevated LFTs including viral hepatitis

3. CBC with differential initially also at day 10–14

4. Observe closely for hypersensitivity reactions, especially during the first and second pembrolizumab infusions

5. Initially at the time of each pembrolizumab dose, and eventually every 6–12 weeks, perform a total-body skin examination with attention to ALL mucous membranes as well as a complete review of systems

6. Monitor patients for signs and symptoms of pneumonitis. Evaluate patients with suspected pneumonitis with chest x-ray, CT, and pulse oximetry. For G ≥2 toxicity, may include nasal swab, sputum culture and sensitivity, blood culture and sensitivity, and urine culture and sensitivity

7. Monitor patients for signs and symptoms of colitis. Encourage patients to report diarrhea immediately to any member of the health care team

8. Use basic metabolic panel (Na, K, CO_2, glucose) and patient history as screening tools for hypophysitis including hypopituitarism and adrenal insufficiency. If in doubt, evaluate AM adrenocorticotropic hormone (ACTH) and cortisol levels. Consider ACTH stimulation test for indeterminate results

9. Assess thyroid function at the start of treatment, periodically during treatment, and as indicated based on clinical evaluation, and for clinical signs and symptoms of thyroid disorders. Test for TSH and free thyroxine (FT4) every 4–6 weeks as part of routine clinical monitoring of therapy or for case detection in symptomatic patients

10. Measure glucose at baseline and with each treatment during the first 12 weeks and every 6 weeks thereafter

11. Obtain a complete rheumatologic history and perform an examination of all peripheral joints for tenderness, swelling, and range of motion. Examine the spine. Consider plain x-ray/imaging to exclude metastases and evaluate joint damage (erosions), if appropriate

12. In patients at high risk for infections and in appropriately selected patients based on an infectious disease evaluation, draw screening laboratories (HIV, hepatitis A and B, and blood QuantiFERON for TB) to prepare patients to start infliximab

13. *Every 2–3 months:* CT scans to assess response

Treatment Modification

DOSE MODIFICATION FOR CARBOPLATIN/CISPLATIN + PEMETREXED + PEMBROLIZUMAB

Notes:
- Toxicity needs to resolve to Grade ≤1 or baseline prior to resuming a given therapy
- Chemotherapy may be interrupted for a maximum of 6 weeks; pembrolizumab may be interrupted for a maximum of 12 weeks
- If a dose is reduced for toxicity with any agent, do not re-escalate the dose
- If there occur several toxicities and there are conflicting recommendations, then follow the most conservative dose adjustment
- Reduction of one chemotherapy agent and not the other agent is appropriate if the toxicity is clearly related to only one of the treatments
- If the toxicity is related to the combination of both chemotherapy agents, both drugs should be reduced
- If the toxicity is related to the combination of three agents, all three agents should be reduced (if applicable), interrupted, or discontinued according to the recommended dose modifications
- Chemotherapy may be discontinued with continuation of pembrolizumab alone
- Interrupt or discontinue pembrolizumab and continue on chemotherapy alone if appropriate

Dose Levels (DLs)

	Dose Level 0	Dose Level −1	Dose Level −2	Dose Level −3
Cisplatin	75 mg/m²	56 mg/m²	38 mg/m²	Discontinue
Carboplatin	AUC 5 Maximum dose = 750 mg	AUC 3.75 Maximum dose = 562.5 mg	AUC 2.5 Maximum dose = 375 mg	Discontinue
Pemetrexed	500 mg/m²	375 mg/m²	250 mg/m²	Discontinue
Pembrolizumab	200-mg fixed dose; the dose should not be reduced only discontinued			

(*continued*)

Treatment Modification (*continued*)

RECOMMENDED DOSE MODIFICATIONS FOR PEMETREXED, CISPLATIN, AND CARBOPLATIN

	Pemetrexed	Carboplatin	Cisplatin
Hematologic Toxicity			
Platelets ≥50,000/mm³ AND ANC ≥500/mm³	No dose reduction	No dose reduction	No dose reduction
Platelets ≥50,000/mm³ AND ANC <500/mm³	DL −1	DL −1	DL −1
Platelets <50,000/mm³ without bleeding AND ANY ANC	DL −1	DL −1	DL −1
Platelets <50,000/mm³ with Grade ≥2 bleeding AND ANY ANC	DL −2	DL −2	DL −2
Any platelet count AND ANC <1000/mm³ + fever ≥38.5°C (101°F)	DL −1	DL −1	DL −1
Non-hematologic Toxicity			
G3/4 nausea or vomiting	DL 0	DL 0	DL 0
G3/4 diarrhea	DL −1	DL 0	DL −1
G3/4 mucositis	DL −2	DL−0	DL 0
G2 neurotoxicity—peripheral neuropathy or ototoxicity (tinnitus and symptomatic hearing loss)	DL 0	DL 0	DL −2
G3/4 neurotoxicity—peripheral neuropathy or ototoxicity (tinnitus and symptomatic hearing loss)	DL −1	DL −1	Discontinue
Loss of vision for light or colors	DL 0	Discontinue carboplatin; if recovers, consider resumption at a lower DL	DL 0
G3 transaminase elevation	DL −1	DL −1	DL −1
G4 transaminase elevation	Discontinue	Discontinue	Discontinue
Serum creatinine ≥1.5 mg/dL (≥130 μmol/L) on day of treatment	DL 0	DL 0	Ensure patient is adequately hydrated. Hold cisplatin until serum creatinine ≤1.5 mg/dL (≤130 μmol/L) and BUN <25 mg/dL (<8.92 mmol/L). If creatinine >1.5 mg/dL and/or BUN ≥25 mg/dL (≥8.92 mmol/L) >2 weeks beyond scheduled start of next cycle, discontinue cisplatin
Other G3/4 non-hematologic toxicity	Delay attributable medication(s) until resolution to G ≤1, then reduce dose of attributable medication(s) by one DL		
Creatinine clearance 41–59 mL/min	DL 0	For an AUC of 4, administer no more carboplatin than 4 × (GFR + 25)	DL −1
Creatinine clearance 16–40 mL/min			Discontinue cisplatin and consider using carboplatin instead
Allergic reaction to cisplatin or carboplatin including anaphylaxis (risk increased in patients previously exposed to platinum therapy)	DL 0	May occur within minutes of administration. Interrupt the infusion in patients with clinically significant infusion reactions. May also consider desensitization	

(*continued*)

Treatment Modification (*continued*)

RECOMMENDED DOSE MODIFICATIONS FOR PEMBROLIZUMAB

Adverse Reaction	Grade/Severity	Dose Modification
Colitis	G1	Loperamide 4 mg as starting dose then 2 mg before each meal and after each loose stool until without diarrhea for 12 hours, with maximum of 16 mg loperamide per day. If G1 diarrhea or colitis persists >14 days, then add prednisolone 0.5–1 mg/kg (non-enteric-coated) or consider oral budesonide 9 mg daily if no bloody diarrhea
	G2/3 diarrhea or colitis	Withhold pembrolizumab. Loperamide 4 mg as starting dose then 2 mg before each meal and after each loose stool until without diarrhea for 12 hours, with maximum of 16 mg loperamide per day. Administer oral prednisone/prednisolone at a dose of 0.5–2.0 mg/kg/day or its equivalent. When improves to G1, begin a slow corticosteroid taper over at least 4 weeks. Resume pembrolizumab upon symptom control, or when prednisone/prednisolone daily dose <10 mg
	G4 diarrhea or colitis	Permanently discontinue pembrolizumab. Loperamide 4 mg as starting dose then 2 mg before each meal and after each loose stool until without diarrhea for 12 hours, with maximum of 16 mg loperamide per day. Administer 1–2 mg/kg IV (methyl)prednisolone and convert to 0.5–2.0 mg/kg prednisone/prednisolone orally each day or its equivalent only after a response. Taper over at least 4 weeks when symptoms improve. If does not improve over 72 hours or worsens, perform flexible sigmoidoscopy/ colonoscopy to document colitis then begin infliximab 5 mg/kg (if no perforation/sepsis/TB/hepatitis/NYHA III/IV CHF). If no response, add MMF 500–1000 mg twice daily. If worse on MMF, consider addition of tacrolimus or ATG
Pneumonitis	G2	Withhold pembrolizumab. Consider pneumocystis prophylaxis depending on the clinical context and coverage with empiric antibiotics. Administer oral prednisone/prednisolone at a dose of 1–2 mg/kg/day or its equivalent. When improves to G1, begin a slow corticosteroid taper over at least 4 weeks. If does not respond adequately after 48 hours, then administer 2–4 mg/kg IV (methyl)prednisolone and convert to 0.5–2.0 mg/kg prednisone/prednisolone orally each day or its equivalent only after a response, followed by a taper over at least 6 weeks when symptoms improve to G1, titrating to symptoms. Resume pembrolizumab upon symptom control, or when prednisone/prednisolone daily dose <10 mg
	G3/4	Permanently discontinue pembrolizumab. Consider pneumocystis prophylaxis depending on the clinical context; cover with empiric antibiotics. Administer 2–4 mg/kg IV (methyl)prednisolone and convert to 1–2 mg/kg prednisone/prednisolone orally each day or its equivalent only after a response, followed by a taper over at least 8 weeks when symptoms improve to G1, titrating to symptoms. If when initially treated improvement does not occur within 48–72 hours, begin infliximab 5 mg/kg (if no perforation/sepsis/TB/hepatitis/NYHA III/IV CHF). If no response to infliximab, add MMF 500–1000 mg twice daily. Consider MMF especially if has concurrent hepatic toxicity
Hepatitis	G2 (AST or ALT >3–5× ULN or total bilirubin >1.5-3× ULN)	Withhold pembrolizumab. Administer oral prednisone/prednisolone at a dose of 1–2 mg/kg/day or its equivalent. When improves to G1, begin a slow corticosteroid taper over at least 4 weeks. Resume pembrolizumab upon symptom control, or when prednisone/prednisolone daily dose <10 mg
	G3/4 (AST or ALT >5× ULN or total bilirubin >3× ULN)	Permanently discontinue pembrolizumab. Administer 1–2 mg/kg IV (methyl)prednisolone and convert to 0.5–2.0 mg/kg prednisone/ prednisolone orally each day or its equivalent only after a response. Taper over at least 6 weeks when symptoms improve. If no response, add MMF 500–1000 mg twice daily. If worse on MMF, consider adding tacrolimus or ATG

(continued)

Treatment Modification (continued)

Adverse Reaction	Grade/Severity	Dose Modification
Hypophysitis	G2/3 (moderate symptoms, ie, headache but no visual disturbance or fatigue/mood alteration but hemodynamically stable, no electrolyte disturbance)	Administer analgesia as needed for headache. Withhold pembrolizumab. Administer oral prednisone/prednisolone at a dose of 0.5–2.0 mg/kg/day or its equivalent. When improves to G1, begin a slow corticosteroid taper over at least 4 weeks. If no improvement in 48 hours, administer 1–2 mg/kg IV (methyl)prednisolone and convert to 0.5–2.0 mg/kg prednisone/prednisolone orally each day or its equivalent only after a response. Taper over at least 4 weeks when symptoms improve to 5 mg prednisone/prednisolone or equivalent; do not stop steroids. Resume pembrolizumab upon symptom control, or when prednisone/prednisolone daily dose <10 mg
	G4 (severe mass effect symptoms, ie, severe headache, any visual disturbance or severe hypoadrenalism, ie, hypotension, severe electrolyte disturbance)	Permanently discontinue pembrolizumab. Administer analgesia as needed for headache. Administer 1–2 mg/kg IV (methyl)prednisolone and convert to 0.5–2.0 mg/kg prednisone/prednisolone orally each day or its equivalent only after a response. Taper over at least 4 weeks when symptoms improve to 5 mg prednisone/prednisolone or equivalent; do not stop steroids
Adrenal insufficiency	G2	Withhold pembrolizumab. Administer oral prednisone/prednisolone at a dose of 0.5–2.0 mg/kg/day or its equivalent. When improves to G1, begin a slow corticosteroid taper over at least 4 weeks. Serially assess adrenal function and continue steroids at replacement doses (20–40 mg hydrocortisone daily ~2/3 dose in AM upon awakening and ~1/3 at 4:00 PM) until recovery of adrenal function is documented. Resume pembrolizumab upon symptom control, or when prednisone/prednisolone daily dose <10 mg
	G3/4	Permanently discontinue pembrolizumab. Administer oral prednisone/prednisolone at a dose of 0.5–2.0 mg/kg/day or its equivalent. When improves to G1, begin a slow corticosteroid taper over at least 4 weeks. Serially assess adrenal function and continue steroids at replacement doses (20–40 mg hydrocortisone daily ~2/3 dose in AM upon awakening and ~1/3 at 4:00 PM) until recovery of adrenal function is documented
Type 1 diabetes mellitus	G3 hyperglycemia	Withhold pembrolizumab. Admit to hospital to manage hyperglycemia. Role of corticosteroids in preventing complete loss of insulin-producing cells is unknown and not recommended. Resume pembrolizumab upon symptom control, or when prednisone/prednisolone daily dose <10 mg
	G4 hyperglycemia	Permanently discontinue pembrolizumab. Admit to hospital to manage hyperglycemia. Role of corticosteroids in preventing complete loss of insulin-producing cells is unknown and not recommended
Nephritis and renal dysfunction	G2/3 (serum creatinine 1.5–6× ULN)	Withhold pembrolizumab. Administer oral prednisone/prednisolone at a dose of 0.5–2.0 mg/kg/day or its equivalent. When improves to G1, begin a slow corticosteroid taper over at least 4 weeks. If does not respond adequately, then administer 0.5–1 mg/kg IV (methyl)prednisolone and convert to 0.5–2.0 mg/kg prednisone/prednisolone orally each day or its equivalent only after a response, followed by a taper over at least 4 weeks when improves to G1. Resume pembrolizumab upon symptom control, or when prednisone/prednisolone daily dose <10 mg
	G4 (serum creatinine >6× ULN)	Permanently discontinue pembrolizumab. Administer 0.5–1 mg/kg IV (methyl)prednisolone and convert to 0.5–2.0 mg/kg prednisone/prednisolone orally each day or its equivalent only after a response, followed by a taper over at least 4 weeks when improves to G1

(continued)

Treatment Modification (continued)

Adverse Reaction	Grade/Severity	Dose Modification
Skin	G1/2	Continue pembrolizumab. Avoid skin irritants, avoid sun exposure, topical emollients recommended. Topical steroid (mild strength for G1, moderate/potent strength for G2) cream once or twice daily ± oral or topical antihistamines for itching
	G3 rash or suspected SJS or TEN	Withhold pembrolizumab. Avoid skin irritants, avoid sun exposure, topical emollients recommended. Administer oral or topical antihistamines for itching. Administer oral prednisone/prednisolone at a dose of 0.5–2.0 mg/kg or its equivalent daily for 3 days followed by a slow corticosteroid taper over at least 4 weeks when the rash improves to G1. If does not respond adequately, then administer 0.5–1 mg/kg IV (methyl)prednisolone and convert to 0.5–2.0 mg/kg prednisone/prednisolone orally each day or its equivalent only after a response, followed by a taper over at least 4 weeks when the rash improves to G1. Resume pembrolizumab upon symptom control, or when prednisone/prednisolone daily dose <10 mg
	G4 rash or confirmed SJS or TEN	Avoid skin irritants, avoid sun exposure, topical emollients recommended. Administer oral or topical antihistamines for itching. Administer 1–2 mg/kg IV (methyl)prednisolone and convert to oral steroids 0.5–2.0 mg/kg prednisone/prednisolone each day or its equivalent only after a response. Taper over at least 4 weeks when the rash improves to G1. Permanently discontinue pembrolizumab
Encephalitis	Confusion or altered behavior, headaches, alteration in Glasgow Coma Scale, motor or sensory deficits, speech abnormality, may or may not be febrile	Initially withhold pembrolizumab, but permanently discontinue pembrolizumab if there is no doubt as to diagnosis. Exclude bacterial and ideally viral infections prior to high-dose steroids. Administer oral prednisone/prednisolone at a dose of 0.5–2.0 mg/kg/day or its equivalent. When symptoms improve, begin a slow corticosteroid taper over at least 4–8 weeks. If symptoms are severe, administer 1–2 mg/kg IV (methyl)prednisolone and convert to 0.5–2.0 mg/kg prednisone/prednisolone orally each day or its equivalent only after a response. Consider concurrent empiric antiviral (IV acyclovir) and antibacterial therapy
Aseptic meningitis	Headache, photophobia, neck stiffness with fever or may be afebrile, vomiting; normal cognition/cerebral function (distinguishes from encephalitis)	
Other syndromes include neurosarcoidosis, posterior reversible leukoencephalopathy syndrome (PRES), Vogt-Koyanagi-Harada syndrome, demyelination, vasculitic encephalopathy, and generalized seizures		
Transverse myelitis	Acute or subacute neurologic signs/symptoms of motor/sensory/autonomic origin; most have sensory level; often bilateral symptoms	Initially withhold pembrolizumab, but permanently discontinue pembrolizumab if there is no doubt as to diagnosis. Administer 2 mg/kg IV (methyl)prednisolone or consider 1 g/day and convert to 0.5–2.0 mg/kg prednisone/prednisolone orally each day or its equivalent only after a response. When symptoms improve, begin a slow corticosteroid taper over at least 4–8 weeks. Plasmapheresis may be required if steroids do not bring about improvement
Myocarditis	G3	Permanently discontinue pembrolizumab. Administer 2 mg/kg IV (methyl)prednisolone or consider 1 g/day and convert to 0.5–2.0 mg/kg prednisone/prednisolone orally each day or its equivalent only after a response. When symptoms improve, begin a slow corticosteroid taper over at least 4–8 weeks. If no response, add MMF 500–1000 mg twice daily. If worse on MMF, consider adding tacrolimus

(continued)

Treatment Modification (continued)

Adverse Reaction	Grade/Severity	Dose Modification
Peripheral neurologic toxicity	Moderate: some interference with ADL, symptoms concerning to patient	Withhold pembrolizumab. Initial observation reasonable or initiate prednisone/prednisolone 0.5–1 mg/kg (if progressing, eg, from mild) and/or pregabalin or duloxetine for pain. When symptoms improve, begin a slow corticosteroid taper over at least 4 weeks. Resume pembrolizumab upon symptom control, or when prednisone/prednisolone daily dose <10 mg
	Severe: limits self-care and aids warranted, life-threatening, eg, respiratory problems	Permanently discontinue pembrolizumab. Administer 1–2 mg/kg IV (methyl)prednisolone and convert to 0.5–2.0 mg/kg prednisone/prednisolone orally each day or its equivalent only after a response. Taper over at least 4–8 weeks when symptoms improve to G1
Guillain-Barré syndrome	Progressive symmetrical muscle weakness with absent or reduced tendon reflexes—involves extremities, facial, respiratory, and bulbar and oculomotor muscles; dysregulation of autonomic nerves	Permanently discontinue pembrolizumab. Use of steroids not recommended in idiopathic Guillain-Barré syndrome; however, a trial of (methyl)prednisolone 1–2 mg/kg is reasonable, converting to 0.5–2.0 mg/kg prednisone/prednisolone orally each day or its equivalent only after a response. If no improvement or worsening, plasmapheresis or IVIG indicated
Myasthenia gravis	Fluctuating muscle weakness (proximal limb, trunk, ocular, eg, ptosis/diplopia or bulbar) with fatigability, respiratory muscles may also be involved	Permanently discontinue pembrolizumab. Administer pyridostigmine at an initial dose of 30 mg three times daily. Administer oral prednisone/prednisolone at a dose of 0.5–2.0 mg/kg/day or its equivalent or 1–2 mg/kg IV (methyl)prednisolone depending on the severity of symptoms. If begin with IV, convert to 0.5–2.0 mg/kg prednisone/prednisolone orally each day or its equivalent only after a response. If no improvement or worsening, plasmapheresis or IVIG may be considered. Additional immunosuppressants used in myasthenia gravis include azathioprine, cyclosporine, and mycophenolate. Avoid certain medications, eg, ciprofloxacin, beta-blockers, that may precipitate cholinergic crisis
Other syndromes including motor and sensory peripheral neuropathy, multifocal radicular neuropathy/plexopathy, autonomic neuropathy, phrenic nerve palsy, cranial nerve palsies (eg, facial nerve, optic nerve, hypoglossal nerve)		Permanently discontinue pembrolizumab. Administer oral prednisone/prednisolone at a dose of 0.5–2.0 mg/kg/day or its equivalent or 1–2 mg/kg IV (methyl)prednisolone depending on the severity of symptoms. If begin with IV, convert to 0.5–2.0 mg/kg prednisone/prednisolone orally each day or its equivalent only after a response
Arthralgia	G1 (mild pain with inflammation, erythema, or joint swelling)	Continue pembrolizumab. Administer acetaminophen (paracetamol) and ibuprofen
	G2 (moderate pain with inflammation, erythema, or joint swelling that limits ADLs)	Withhold pembrolizumab. Administer higher doses of acetaminophen (paracetamol) and ibuprofen, and use diclofenac or naproxen or etoricoxib. If inadequately controlled, consider intra-articular steroid injections for large joints or administer oral prednisone/prednisolone at a dose of 0.5–2.0 mg/kg/day or its equivalent. When improves to G1, begin a slow corticosteroid taper over at least 4 weeks. If does not respond adequately, then administer 0.5–1 mg/kg IV (methyl)prednisolone and convert to 0.5–2.0 mg/kg prednisone/prednisolone orally each day or its equivalent only after a response, followed by a taper over at least 4 weeks when improves to G1. Resume pembrolizumab upon symptom control, or when prednisone/prednisolone daily dose <10 mg
	G3 (severe pain; irreversible joint damage; disabling; limits self-care ADL)	Withhold pembrolizumab. Administer 0.5–1 mg/kg IV (methyl)prednisolone and convert to 0.5–2.0 mg/kg prednisone/prednisolone orally each day or its equivalent only after a response, followed by a taper over at least 4 weeks when improves to G1. In severe cases, infliximab or another anti–TNF alpha drug may be required for improvement of arthritis. Resume pembrolizumab upon symptom control, or when prednisone/prednisolone daily dose <10 mg

(continued)

Treatment Modification (*continued*)

Adverse Reaction	Grade/Severity	Dose Modification
Other	First occurrence of other G3	Withhold pembrolizumab. Administer oral prednisone/prednisolone at a dose of 0.5–2.0 mg/kg/day or its equivalent. When improves to G1, begin a slow corticosteroid taper over at least 4 weeks. Resume pembrolizumab upon symptom control, or when prednisone/prednisolone daily dose <10 mg
	Recurrence of same G3	Permanently discontinue pembrolizumab. Administer 1–2 mg/kg IV (methyl)prednisolone and convert to 0.5–2.0 mg/kg prednisone/prednisolone orally each day or its equivalent only after a response. Taper over at least 4–8 weeks when symptoms improve to G1
	Life-threatening or G4	
	Requirement for ≥10 mg/day prednisone or equivalent for >12 weeks	Permanently discontinue pembrolizumab
	Persistent G2/3 adverse reactions lasting ≥12 weeks	

ADL, activities of daily living; ALT, alanine aminotransferase; AST, aspartate aminotransferase; ATG, anti-thymocyte globulin; SJS, Stevens-Johnson Syndrome; TEN, toxic epidermal necrolysis; ULN, upper limit of normal

Notes on general supportive care:
- Steroid taper in most cases will proceed over a minimum of 1 month, but if symptoms improve rapidly, a 2-week taper can be considered. If steroids are administered for more than 4 weeks, consider PCP prophylaxis (cotrimoxazole 480 mg twice daily M/W/F or inhaled pentamidine if has cotrimoxazole allergy), regular random blood glucose, vitamin D level and starting calcium/vitamin D supplementation per guidelines

Notes on pregnancy and breastfeeding:
- Pembrolizumab can cause fetal harm. If used during pregnancy, or if the patient becomes pregnant during treatment, apprise the patient of the potential hazard to a fetus. Females of reproductive potential should use highly effective contraception during treatment and for 4 months after the last dose of pembrolizumab
- It is not known whether pembrolizumab is excreted in human milk. Therefore, it is recommended that women discontinue nursing during treatment with and for 4 months after the final dose of pembrolizumab

Adverse Events (N = 607)

Event	Cisplatin/Carboplatin + Pemetrexed + Pembrolizumab (n = 405)		Cisplatin/Carboplatin + Pemetrexed + Placebo (n = 202)	
Grade (%)	Grade 1 or 2	Grade 3–5	Grade 1 or 2	Grade 3–5
Any event	33	67	33	66
Event leading to discontinuation of all treatment*	2	12	<1	7
Event leading to discontinuation of any treatment component*	8	20	4	11
Discontinuation of pembrolizumab or placebo	4	16	2	8
Discontinuation of pemetrexed	6	17	3	8
Discontinuation of platinum-based drug	<1	7	<1	5
Event leading to death	0	7	0	6

(*continued*)

Adverse Events (N = 607) *(continued)*

Event	Cisplatin/Carboplatin + Pemetrexed + Pembrolizumab (n = 405)		Cisplatin/Carboplatin + Pemetrexed + Placebo (n = 202)	
Grade (%)	Grade 1 or 2	Grade 3–5	Grade 1 or 2	Grade 3–5
Events occurring in ≥15% of patients in either group				
Nausea	52	3	49	3
Anemia	30	16	31	15
Fatigue	35	6	36	2
Constipation	34	<1	31	<1
Diarrhea	26	5	18	3
Decreased appetite	27	1	30	<1
Neutropenia	11	16	12	12
Vomiting	20	4	20	3
Cough	21	0	28	0
Dyspnea	18	4	20	5
Asthenia	14	6	21	3
Rash	19	2	10	1
Pyrexia	19	<1	15	0
Peripheral edema	19	<1	13	0
Thrombocytopenia	10	8	7	7
Increased lacrimation	17	0	11	0

Adverse events of any cause and regardless of attribution to treatment by the investigator that occurred during the trial period or 30 days after (90 days for serious events) were included in the table if they were reported by ≥15% of patients in either group except for events related to discontinuation or death. Adverse events were assessed in the as-treated population. Median time on treatment was 7.4 ± 4.7 months for the pembrolizumab group and 5.4 ± 4.3 months for the placebo group. Adverse events reported by patients who crossed over from placebo to pembrolizumab group were not included in the table
*These categories include discontinuation of all drugs in combination (pemetrexed, platinum-based drug, pembrolizumab, or placebo) or any drug of the combination, respectively

Event of Special Interest	Cisplatin/Carboplatin + Pemetrexed + Pembrolizumab 200 mg (n = 405)		Cisplatin/Carboplatin + Pemetrexed + Placebo (n = 202)	
Grade (%)	Grade 1 or 2	Grade 3–5	Grade 1 or 2	Grade 3–5
Any event	14	9	7	4
Hypothyroidism	6	<1	2	0
Pneumonitis	2	3	<1	2
Hyperthyroidism	4	0	3	0
Infusion reaction	2	<1	<1	0

(continued)

Adverse Events (N = 607) *(continued)*

Event of Special Interest	Cisplatin/Carboplatin + Pemetrexed + Pembrolizumab 200 mg (n = 405)		Cisplatin/Carboplatin + Pemetrexed + Placebo (n = 202)	
Grade (%)	Grade 1 or 2	Grade 3–5	Grade 1 or 2	Grade 3–5
Colitis	1	<1	0	0
Severe skin reaction	0	2	<1	2
Nephritis	<1	1	0	0
Hepatitis	<1	<1	0	0
Hypophysitis	<1	0	0	0
Pancreatitis	<1	<1	0	0
Adrenal insufficiency	0	<1	0	<1
Myositis	<1	0	0	0
Thyroiditis	<1	0	0	0
Type 1 diabetes mellitus	0	<1	0	0

Adverse events of special interest (immune-related) were included in the table in descending order regardless of attribution to treatment by the investigators. Adverse events were assessed in the as-treated population. Median time on treatment was 7.4 ± 4.7 months for the pembrolizumab group and 5.4 ± 4.3 months for the placebo group. Adverse events reported by patients who crossed over from placebo to pembrolizumab group were not included in the table. Three events in this table, all pneumonitis, led to death in the pembrolizumab group

ADVANCED NON-SQUAMOUS NSCLC • FIRST-LINE
LUNG CANCER REGIMEN: ATEZOLIZUMAB + BEVACIZUMAB + CARBOPLATIN + PACLITAXEL (ABCP)

Socinski MA et al. N Engl J Med 2018;378:2288–301
Protocol for: Socinski MA et al. N Engl J Med 2018;378:2288–301
Supplementary appendix to: Socinski MA et al. N Engl J Med 2018;378:2288–301
TECENTRIQ (atezolizumab) prescribing information. South San Francisco, CA: Genentech, Inc; revised 2019 May

The regimen consists of either four or six 3-week cycles of induction therapy consisting of atezolizumab, bevacizumab, carboplatin, and paclitaxel (ABCP), followed by maintenance therapy with atezolizumab and bevacizumab given until disease progression. Maintenance therapy cycles are 3 weeks in length when both atezolizumab and bevacizumab are given; however, if bevacizumab is discontinued, then single-agent atezolizumab maintenance therapy may be given as 840 mg every 2 weeks, 1200 mg every 3 weeks, or 1680 mg every 4 weeks.

Induction phase

Atezolizumab 1200 mg per dose; administer intravenously in 250 mL 0.9% sodium chloride injection, USP (0.9% NS) over 60 minutes on day 1, prior to bevacizumab, every 21 days, for 4 or 6 induction cycles (total dosage/3-week cycle = 1200 mg)

Notes:
- Atezolizumab may be administered through an administration set either with or without a low-protein-binding in-line filter with pore size within the range of 0.2–0.22μm. Infusion bag may be composed of polyvinyl chloride (PVC), polyethylene (PE), or polyolefin (PO).
- If the initial infusion is well tolerated, subsequent administration may be completed over 30 minutes
- Severe infusion-related reactions have occurred in patients in clinical trials of atezolizumab
  - Interrupt or slow the administration rate in patients with mild or moderate infusion-related reactions
  - Permanently discontinue atezolizumab in patients who experience infusion reactions Grade ≥3

Bevacizumab 15 mg/kg; intravenously, diluted in 100 mL 0.9% NS over 30–90 minutes on day 1, prior to paclitaxel, every 21 days, for 4 or 6 induction cycles (total dosage/3-week cycle = 15 mg/kg)
- *Notes about bevacizumab administration:* the duration of administration for the initial dose is 90 minutes. If administration is well tolerated, the administration duration may be decreased stepwise during subsequent administrations to 60 minutes and, finally, to a minimum duration of 30 minutes

Paclitaxel premedications:
Dexamethasone 10 mg/dose; orally for 2 doses at 12 hours and 6 hours before each paclitaxel dose, *or*
Dexamethasone 20 mg/dose; intravenously over 10–15 minutes, 30–60 minutes before each paclitaxel dose (total dose/cycle = 20 mg)
Diphenhydramine 50 mg, by intravenous injection 30–60 minutes before each paclitaxel dose
Cimetidine 300 mg (or **ranitidine** 50 mg, **famotidine** 20 mg, or an equivalent histamine [H_2]-subtype receptor antagonist) intravenously over 15–30 minutes, 30–60 minutes before each paclitaxel dose

Paclitaxel 200 mg/m²; administer intravenously, diluted in a volume of 0.9% NS or 5% dextrose injection (D5W) sufficient to produce a concentration within the range 0.3–1.2 mg/mL, over 3 hours on day 1, prior to carboplatin, every 21 days, for 4 or 6 induction cycles (total dosage/3-week cycle in non-Asian patients = 200 mg/m²)
- *Note:* the independent Data Monitoring Committee for IMpower150 noted a higher level of hematologic toxicities in patients from Asian countries and recommended a starting paclitaxel dose of 175 mg/m² in patients of Asian race/ethnicity. Thus, for patients of Asian race/ethnicity, consider:
  - **Paclitaxel** 175 mg/m²; administer intravenously, diluted in a volume of 0.9% NS or D5W sufficient to produce a concentration within the range 0.3–1.2 mg/mL, over 3 hours on day 1, prior to carboplatin, every 21 days, for 4 or 6 induction cycles (total dosage/3-week cycle in Asian patients = 175 mg/m²)

Carboplatin target AUC = 6 mg/mL × min; administer intravenously in 250 mL D5W or 0.9% NS over 15–30 minutes on day 1, after paclitaxel, every 21 days, for 4 or 6 induction cycles (total dosage/3-week cycle calculated to achieve a target AUC = 6 mg/mL × min)

Supportive Care (Induction Therapy)
Antiemetic prophylaxis
Emetogenic potential is **HIGH**. *Potential for delayed symptoms*
See Chapter 42 for antiemetic recommendations

Hematopoietic growth factor (CSF) prophylaxis (induction therapy)
Primary prophylaxis is **NOT** *indicated*
See Chapter 43 for more information

Antimicrobial prophylaxis (induction therapy)
Risk of fever and neutropenia is LOW
Antimicrobial primary prophylaxis to be considered:
- Antibacterial—not indicated
- Antifungal—not indicated
- Antiviral—not indicated unless patient previously had an episode of HSV

(continued)

(*continued*)

Carboplatin dose
Carboplatin dose is based on a formula described by Calvert et al. to achieve a target area under the plasma concentration versus time curve (AUC)

$$\text{Total carboplatin dose (mg)} = (\text{target AUC})(\text{GFR} + 25)$$

In practice, creatinine clearance (CrCl) is used in place of glomerular filtration rate (GFR). CrCl can be estimated from the equation of Cockcroft and Gault, thus:

$$\text{For males, Clcr} = \frac{(140 - \text{age[years]}) \times (\text{body weight [kg]})}{72 \times (\text{serum creatinine [mg/dl]})}$$

$$\text{For females, Clcr} = \frac{(140 - \text{age[years]}) \times (\text{body weight [kg]})}{72 \times (\text{serum creatinine [mg/dl]})} \times 0.85$$

Calvert AH et al. J Clin Oncol 1989;7:1748–1756
Cockcroft DW, Gault MH. Nephron 1976;16:31–41
Jodrell DI et al. J Clin Oncol 1992;10:520–528
Sorensen BT et al. Cancer Chemother Pharmacol 1991;28:397–401

Maintenance phase
    Atezolizumab 1200 mg per dose; administer intravenously in 250 mL 0.9% NS over 60 minutes on day 1, before bevacizumab, every 21 days, until disease progression (total dosage/3-week cycle = 1200 mg)
    • Atezolizumab may be administered through an administration set either with or without a low-protein-binding in-line filter with pore size within the range of 0.2–0.22μm. Infusion bag may be composed of polyvinyl chloride (PVC), polyethylene (PE), or polyolefin (PO).
    • If the initial infusion is well tolerated, subsequent administration may be completed over 30 minutes
    • Severe infusion-related reactions have occurred in patients in clinical trials of atezolizumab
        ■ Interrupt or slow the administration rate in patients with mild or moderate infusion-related reactions
        ■ Permanently discontinue atezolizumab in patients who experience infusion reactions Grade ≥3
    • If bevacizumab is discontinued and continued maintenance treatment with single-agent atezolizumab is indicated, then any of the following 3 dosing schedules may be chosen:
        ■ **Atezolizumab** 840 mg per dose; administer intravenously in 250 mL 0.9% sodium chloride injection, USP (0.9% NS) over 60 minutes on day 1, every 14 days, until disease progression (total dosage/2-week cycle = 840 mg), *or:*
        ■ **Atezolizumab** 1200 mg per dose; administer intravenously in 250 mL 0.9% NS over 60 minutes on day 1, every 21 days, until disease progression (total dosage/3-week cycle = 1200 mg), *or:*
        ■ **Atezolizumab** 1680 mg per dose; administer intravenously in 250 mL 0.9% NS over 60 minutes on day 1, every 28 days, until disease progression (total dosage/4-week cycle = 1680 mg)
Bevacizumab 15 mg/kg; intravenously, diluted in 100 mL 0.9% NS over 30–90 minutes on day 1, after atezolizumab, every 21 days, until disease progression (total dosage/3-week cycle = 15 mg/kg)
    • *Notes about bevacizumab administration:* The duration of administration for the initial dose is 90 minutes. If administration is well tolerated, the administration duration may be decreased stepwise during subsequent administrations to 60 minutes and, finally, to a minimum duration of 30 minutes

Supportive Care (Maintenance Therapy)
Antiemetic prophylaxis
Emetogenic potential is **MINIMAL**
See Chapter 42 for antiemetic recommendations

Hematopoietic growth factor (CSF) prophylaxis (maintenance therapy)
Primary prophylaxis is **NOT** *indicated*
See Chapter 43 for more information

Antimicrobial prophylaxis (maintenance therapy)
Risk of fever and neutropenia is LOW
    Antimicrobial primary prophylaxis to be considered:
    • Antibacterial—not indicated
    • Antifungal—not indicated
    • Antiviral—not indicated unless patient previously had an episode of HSV

Patient Population Studied

This international, open-label, randomized, phase 3 study involved adult patients with stage IV or recurrent metastatic non-squamous non–small cell lung cancer for which they had not previously received chemotherapy. Eligible patients had a baseline Eastern Cooperative Oncology Group (ECOG) performance status of 0 or 1 and tumor tissue available for biomarker testing. Patients with any PD-L1 immunohistochemistry status were eligible. Patients with *EGFR* or *ALK* mutations were eligible if they had experienced disease progression or unacceptable side effects from treatment with at least one approved tyrosine kinase inhibitor. Patients were excluded if they had untreated central nervous system metastases, if they had an autoimmune disease, or if they had received previous immunotherapy or anti-CTLA-4 therapy within 6 weeks of randomization. Patients who had received adjuvant or neoadjuvant chemotherapy were eligible if the last treatment was ≥6 months before randomization. Patients were randomized in a 1:1:1 ratio to receive atezolizumab + carboplatin + paclitaxel (ACP group), atezolizumab + bevacizumab + carboplatin + paclitaxel (ABCP group), or bevacizumab + carboplatin + paclitaxel (BCP group). Randomization was stratified according to sex, presence or absence of liver metastases at baseline, and PD-L1 tumor expression. The wild-type genotype (WT) population contained 356 patients assigned to the ABCP group and 336 patients assigned to the BCP group. The ABCP group was compared to the BCP group before comparison of the ACP and BCP groups. The referenced publication only presents data for the comparison of ABCP vs. BCP.

Efficacy (N = 684)

End Point	ABCP Group (n = 353)	BCP Group (n = 331)	Between-Group Comparison
Median progression-free survival in WT population*	8.3 months (95% CI 7.7–9.8)	6.8 months (95% CI 6.0–7.1)	HR 0.62 (95% CI 0.52–0.74) P<0.001
Progression-free survival rate in WT population at 6 months	66.9% (95% CI 61.9–71.8)	56.1% (95% CI 50.7–61.5)	
Progression-free survival rate in WT population at 12 months	36.5% (95% CI 31.2–41.9)	18.0% (95% CI 13.4–22.6)	
Median overall survival in WT population	19.2 months (95% CI 17.0–23.8)	14.7 months (95% CI 13.3–16.9)	HR 0.78 (95% CI 0.64–0.96) P=0.02
Overall survival rate in WT population at 12 months	67.3% (95% CI 62.4–72.2)	60.6% (95% CI 55.3–65.9)	
Overall survival rate in WT population at 24 months	43.4% (95% CI 36.9–49.9)	33.7% (95% CI 27.4–40.0)	
Objective response rate in WT population	63.5% (95% CI, 58.2–68.5)	48.0% (95% CI, 42.5–53.6)	-
Complete response rate in WT population	3.7% (95% CI, 2.0–6.2)	1.2% (95% CI, 0.3–3.1)	
Partial response rate in WT population	59.8% (95% CI, 54.5–64.9)	46.8% (95% CI, 41.4–52.4)	
Stable disease rate in WT population	21.5% (95% CI, 17.6–26.5)	34.7% (95% CI, 29.6–40.1)	
Median (range) duration of response in WT population	11.2 (0.5 to 24.9+)	5.7 (0.0+ to 22.1)	
Patients with ongoing response at the data-cutoff date	46.2%	23.5%	

WT, wild-type (ie, ALK and EGFR wild-type); HR, hazard ratio, CI, confidence interval
*At the time of data cutoff (September 15, 2017), the medium duration of follow-up was 15.4 months in the ABCP group and 15.5 months in the BCP group

Therapy Monitoring

1. *Before therapy:* history and physical exam, CBC with differential, renal and liver function tests, serum electrolytes

2. *Prior to each cycle:* CBC with differential, serum electrolytes, BUN, serum creatinine, serum bilirubin, AST, and ALT. For G ≥2 LFT elevations, work up for other causes of elevated LFTs including viral hepatitis

3. CBC with differential initially also at day 10–14

4. Blood pressure before every infusion of bevacizumab and every 2 weeks or more frequently as indicated during treatment

5. Assess proteinuria by urine dipstick and/or urinary protein creatinine ratio. Patients with a ≥2+ urine dipstick reading should undergo further assessment with a 24-hour urine collection

6. Observe closely for hypersensitivity reactions, especially during the first and second bevacizumab and atezolizumab infusions

7. Initially at the time of each atezolizumab dose, and eventually every 6–12 weeks, perform a total-body skin examination with attention to ALL mucous membranes as well as a complete review of systems

8. Monitor patients for signs and symptoms of pneumonitis. Evaluate patients with suspected pneumonitis with chest x-ray, CT, and pulse oximetry. For ≥2 toxicity, may include nasal swab, sputum culture and sensitivity, blood culture and sensitivity, and urine culture and sensitivity

9. Monitor patients for signs and symptoms of colitis. Encourage patients to report diarrhea immediately to any member of the health care team

10. Use basic metabolic panel (Na, K, CO_2, glucose) and patient history as screening tools for hypophysitis including hypopituitarism and adrenal insufficiency. If in doubt, evaluate AM adrenocorticotropic hormone (ACTH) and cortisol levels. Consider ACTH stimulation test for indeterminate results

11. Assess thyroid function at the start of treatment, periodically during treatment, and as indicated based on clinical evaluation, and for clinical signs and symptoms of thyroid disorders. Test for TSH and free thyroxine (FT4) every 4–6 weeks as part of routine clinical monitoring of therapy or for case detection in symptomatic patients

12. Measure glucose at baseline and with each treatment during the first 12 weeks and every 6 weeks thereafter

13. Obtain a complete rheumatologic history and perform an examination of all peripheral joints for tenderness, swelling, and range of motion. Examine the spine. Consider plain x-ray/imaging to exclude metastases and evaluate joint damage (erosions), if appropriate

14. In patients at high risk for infections and in appropriately selected patients based on an infectious disease evaluation, draw screening laboratories (HIV, hepatitis A and B, and blood QuantiFERON for TB) to prepare patients to start infliximab

15. *Every 2–3 months:* CT scans to assess response

Treatment Modifications

DOSE MODIFICATIONS FOR ATEZOLIZUMAB + BEVACIZUMAB + CARBOPLATIN + PACLITAXEL

Notes:

• When several toxicities with different grades of severity occur at the same time, the dose modifications should be according to the highest grade observed

• If a toxicity is considered to be due solely to one component of the treatment (ie, atezolizumab, bevacizumab, carboplatin, or paclitaxel) and the dose of that component is delayed or modified in accordance with the guidelines below, other components may be administered if there is no contraindication

• When treatment is temporarily interrupted because of toxicity caused by bevacizumab, atezolizumab, carboplatin, and/or paclitaxel (if applicable), the treatment cycles will be restarted such that the atezolizumab and bevacizumab (if applicable) infusions remain synchronized and aligned with the chemotherapy schedule

• If a toxicity is considered to be due solely to one chemotherapy drug, the dose of the other chemotherapy drug does not require modification

• If it is anticipated that chemotherapy will be delayed by ≥2 weeks, then atezolizumab/bevacizumab should be given without the chemotherapy if there is no contraindication

• Do not reduce the bevacizumab dose. If adverse events occur that necessitate holding bevacizumab, the dose will remain unchanged once treatment resumes

• Temporarily suspend bevacizumab if a patient experiences a serious adverse event or a G3/4 non-serious adverse event assessed as related to bevacizumab. If the event resolves to G≤1, bevacizumab may be restarted at the same dose level

• The appropriate interval between the last dose of bevacizumab and major surgery is unknown. Because bevacizumab has a half-life of approximately 21 days, elective surgery should be delayed whenever possible, but if necessary, bevacizumab should be held for ≥28 days prior to the procedure. Re-initiation of bevacizumab following surgery should not occur for ≥28 days and until wounds have fully healed

• At the start of each cycle, the ANC must be ≥1500/mm³ and the platelet count must be ≥100,000/mm³. Treatment may be delayed for up to 42 days from the last dose to allow sufficient time for recovery

• Growth factors may be used in lieu of a dose reduction for neutropenic fever or Grade 4 neutropenia in accordance with ASCO and NCCN guidelines. Upon recovery, dose adjustments at the start of a subsequent cycle will be based on the lowest platelet and neutrophil values from the previous cycle

(continued)

Treatment Modifications *(continued)*

RECOMMENDED DOSE MODIFICATIONS FOR CARBOPLATIN + PACLITAXEL

	Carboplatin	Paclitaxel
Hematologic Toxicity		
First episode of febrile neutropenia and ANC <1500/mm^3 on day 1 of next cycle	Withhold chemotherapy up to 3 weeks until ANC ≥1500/mm^3. When toxicity resolves, resume carboplatin at AUC 4.5. *Note:* if after 3 weeks ANC is not ≥1500/mm^3, can delay start of cycle further, discontinue chemotherapy, or resume carboplatin at AUC 4.5. However, if chemotherapy is held longer than 42 days from the last dose, all study treatment should be discontinued	Withhold chemotherapy up to 3 weeks until ANC ≥1500/mm^3. When toxicity resolves, resume paclitaxel at 150 mg/m^2. *Note:* if after 3 weeks ANC is not ≥1500/mm^3, can delay start of cycle further, discontinue chemotherapy, or resume paclitaxel at 150 mg/m^2. However, if chemotherapy is held longer than 42 days from the last dose, all study treatment should be discontinued
First episode of febrile neutropenia and ANC ≥1500/mm^3 on day 1 of next cycle	Carboplatin AUC 4.5	Paclitaxel 150 mg/m^2
First episode of thrombocytopenia with platelet count <100,000 on day 1 of next cycle AND platelet count nadir of 25,000/mm^3 or <50,000/mm^3 with bleeding or requiring transfusion	Withhold chemotherapy up to 3 weeks until platelet count ≥100,000/mm^3. When toxicity resolves, resume carboplatin at AUC 4.5. *Note:* if after 3 weeks platelet count is not ≥100,000/mm^3, can delay start of cycle further, discontinue chemotherapy, or resume carboplatin at AUC 4.5. However, if chemotherapy is held longer than 42 days from the last dose, all study treatment should be discontinued	Withhold chemotherapy up to 3 weeks until platelet count ≥100,000/mm^3. When toxicity resolves, resume paclitaxel at 150 mg/m^2. *Note:* if after 3 weeks platelet count is not ≥100,000/mm^3, can delay start of cycle further, discontinue chemotherapy, or resume paclitaxel at 150 mg/m^2. However, if chemotherapy is held longer than 42 days from the last dose, all study treatment should be discontinued
First episode of thrombocytopenia with platelet count ≥100,000 on day 1 of next cycle and platelet count nadir of 25,000/mm^3 or <50,000/mm^3 with bleeding or requiring transfusion	Carboplatin AUC 4.5	Paclitaxel 150 mg/m^2
Second episode of febrile neutropenia and ANC <1500/mm^3 on day 1 of next cycle	Withhold chemotherapy up to 3 weeks until ANC ≥1500/mm^3. When toxicity resolves, resume carboplatin at AUC 3.5 or according to physician judgment and local standard practice. *Note:* if after 3 weeks ANC is not ≥1500/mm^3, can delay start of cycle further, discontinue chemotherapy, or resume carboplatin at AUC 3.5. However, if chemotherapy is held longer than 42 days from the last dose, all study treatment should be discontinued	Withhold chemotherapy up to 3 weeks until ANC ≥1500/mm^3. When toxicity resolves, resume paclitaxel at 120 mg/m^2. *Note:* if after 3 weeks ANC is not ≥1500/mm^3, can delay start of cycle further, discontinue chemotherapy, or resume paclitaxel at 120 mg/m^2. However, if chemotherapy is held longer than 42 days from the last dose, all study treatment should be discontinued
Second episode of febrile neutropenia and ANC ≥1500/mm^3 on day 1 of next cycle	Carboplatin AUC 3.5 or according to physician judgment and local standard practice	Paclitaxel 120 mg/m^2

(continued)

Treatment Modifications (*continued*)

	Carboplatin	Paclitaxel
Hematologic Toxicity		
Second episode of thrombocytopenia with platelet count <100,000 on day 1 of next cycle AND platelet count nadir of 25,000/mm³ or <50,000/mm³ with bleeding or requiring transfusion	Withhold chemotherapy up to 3 weeks until platelet count ≥100,000/mm³. When toxicity resolves, resume carboplatin at AUC 3.5 or according to physician judgment and local standard practice. *Note:* if after 3 weeks platelet count is not ≥100,000/mm³, can delay start of cycle further, discontinue chemotherapy, or resume carboplatin at AUC 3.5. However, if chemotherapy is held longer than 42 days from the last dose, all study treatment should be discontinued	Withhold chemotherapy up to 3 weeks until platelet count ≥100,000/mm³. When toxicity resolves, resume paclitaxel at 120 mg/m². *Note:* if after 3 weeks platelet count is not ≥100,000/mm³, can delay start of cycle further, discontinue chemotherapy, or resume paclitaxel at 120 mg/m². However, if chemotherapy is held longer than 42 days from the last dose, all study treatment should be discontinued
Second episode of thrombocytopenia with platelet count ≥100,000 on day 1 of next cycle and platelet count nadir of 25,000/mm³ or <50,000/mm³ with bleeding or requiring transfusion	Carboplatin AUC 3.5 or according to physician judgment and local standard practice	Paclitaxel 120 mg/m²
Third episode of febrile neutropenia	Discontinue chemotherapy	
Third episode of platelet count nadir of 25,000/mm³ or <50,000/mm³ with bleeding or requiring transfusion	Discontinue chemotherapy	
Non-hematologic Toxicity		
G3/4 nausea or vomiting	Withhold carboplatin and paclitaxel until toxicity resolves to G ≤ 1. When toxicity resolves, resume carboplatin and paclitaxel at 75% of previous dose. If tolerated, increase the carboplatin and paclitaxel dose back to 100% as soon as possible	
G3/4 diarrhea	Withhold carboplatin and paclitaxel until toxicity resolves to G ≤ 1. When toxicity resolves, resume carboplatin and paclitaxel at 75% of previous dose	
G3/4 mucositis	Withhold carboplatin and paclitaxel until toxicity resolves to G ≤ 1. When toxicity resolves, resume carboplatin and paclitaxel at 75% of previous dose	
Any mucositis on day 1 of a cycle	Withhold carboplatin and paclitaxel. Reduce dose to 75% of the previous dose and administer when the oral mucositis is completely resolved. If the oral mucositis/stomatitis has not cleared in 3 weeks, discontinue chemotherapy	
Acute G3 oral mucositis at any time	Reduce carboplatin and paclitaxel to 75% of the previous and administer when the oral mucositis is completely cleared. This is a permanent dose reduction	
SGOT (AST) <10× ULN AND serum bilirubin ≤1.25× ULN	N/A	No change in paclitaxel dose
SGOT (AST) <10× ULN AND serum bilirubin 1.26–2.0× ULN	N/A	Withhold treatment. Reduce dose to 75% of the previous dose and administer when toxicity completely resolved
SGOT (AST) <10× ULN AND serum bilirubin 2.01–5.0× ULN	N/A	Withhold treatment. Reduce dose to 50% of the previous dose and administer when toxicity completely resolved
SGOT (AST) >10× ULN OR serum bilirubin >5 ULN	N/A	Discontinue paclitaxel
Asymptomatic bradycardia	N/A	No change in paclitaxel dose
Symptomatic arrhythmia during infusion	N/A	Stop paclitaxel infusion, and manage arrhythmia according to standard practice. Paclitaxel treatment will be discontinued
Chest pain and/or symptomatic hypotension (<90/60 mmHg or requires fluid replacement)	N/A	Stop paclitaxel infusion. Perform an ECG. Give IV diphenhydramine and dexamethasone if hypersensitivity is considered. Also consider epinephrine or bronchodilators if chest pain is not thought to be cardiac. Discontinue paclitaxel treatment and provide cardiovascular support as appropriate

(*continued*)

Treatment Modifications (*continued*)

	Carboplatin	Paclitaxel
Non-hematologic Toxicity		
G2 neurotoxicity—peripheral neuropathy or ototoxicity (tinnitus and symptomatic hearing loss)	N/A	Withhold treatment. Reduce dose by 25% of the previous dose and administer when toxicity recovers to G ≤ 1
G3/4 neurotoxicity—peripheral neuropathy or ototoxicity (tinnitus and symptomatic hearing loss)	N/A	Withhold treatment. Reduce dose by 50% of the previous dose and administer when toxicity resolves to G ≤ 1
Allergic reaction/hypersensitivity to paclitaxel—mild symptoms	N/A	Complete paclitaxel infusion. Supervise at bedside. No treatment required
Allergic reaction/hypersensitivity to paclitaxel—moderate symptoms	N/A	Stop paclitaxel infusion. Give 25–50 mg diphenhydramine IV and 10 mg dexamethasone IV. Resume paclitaxel infusion after symptoms resolve at a 20 mL/hour for 15 minutes, then 40 mL/hour for 15 minutes, then if no further symptoms, at full-dose rate until infusion is complete. If symptoms recur, stop infusion and discontinue paclitaxel
Allergic reaction/hypersensitivity to paclitaxel—severe life-threatening symptoms	N/A	Stop paclitaxel infusion. Give 25–50 mg diphenhydramine IV and 10 mg dexamethasone IV. Add epinephrine or bronchodilators if indicated. Discontinue paclitaxel
Loss of vision for light or colors	Discontinue carboplatin; if recovers, consider resumption at a lower dose	N/A
Other G1/2 non-hematologic toxicity	Withhold carboplatin and/or paclitaxel until the patient recovers completely or to G1 toxicity. Resume treatment at the previous dose. Monitor carefully for recurrence of toxicity. If G1/2 toxicity recurs, then resume treatment at 75% dose (permanent dose reduction)	
Other G3/4 non-hematologic toxicity	Withhold carboplatin and/or paclitaxel until the patient recovers completely or to G1 toxicity. For G3 toxicities, resume treatment at 75% dose (permanent dose reduction). For G4 toxicities, resume treatment at 50% of dose (permanent dose reduction). If recovery to G1 toxicity does not occur within 3 weeks, discontinue chemotherapy	
Creatinine clearance 41–59 mL/min	For an AUC of 4.5, administer no more carboplatin than $4.5 \times (GFR + 25)$	
Creatinine clearance 16–40 mL/min		
Allergic reaction to carboplatin including anaphylaxis (risk increased in patients previously exposed to platinum therapy)	May occur within minutes of administration. Interrupt the infusion in patients with clinically significant infusion reactions. May also consider desensitization	

RECOMMENDED DOSE MODIFICATIONS FOR BEVACIZUMAB

Treatment delay of more than three-weeks or whose G3 toxicity recurs after resumption of therapy	Discontinue bevacizumab permanently. Continue chemotherapy after toxicity has resolved
G4 non-hematologic toxicity	
Gastrointestinal perforations, any grade	Discontinue bevacizumab permanently. Continue chemotherapy after toxicity has resolved
Intra-abdominal abscess	
Fistula formation involving any internal organ, any grade	
Wound dehiscence requiring medical intervention, any grade	
Necrotizing fasciitis	
Administration of bevacizumab is delayed due to toxicity for >42 days beyond when the next dose should have been given	
G1 hypertension (asymptomatic, transient [<24 hr] blood pressure increase by >20 mmHg [diastolic] or to >150/100 mmHg if previously within normal limits)	Do not alter the bevacizumab dose

(*continued*)

Treatment Modifications (*continued*)

RECOMMENDED DOSE MODIFICATIONS FOR BEVACIZUMAB

G2 hypertension (recurrent or persistent [>24 hr] or symptomatic increase by >20 mmHg [diastolic] or to >150/100 mmHg if previously within normal limits)	Hold bevacizumab. Start antihypertensive therapy. Once blood pressure is <150/100 mmHg, may continue bevacizumab therapy. Medication classes used for management of patients with hypertension receiving bevacizumab include angiotensin-converting enzyme inhibitors, diuretics, and calcium channel blockers. The goal for blood pressure control should be consistent with general medical practice guidelines. For controlled hypertension, defined as systolic ≤150 mmHg and diastolic ≤90 mmHg, continue bevacizumab therapy
G3 hypertension—requires more than one antihypertensive drug or more intensive therapy than previously	If not controlled to 150/90 mmHg with medication, discontinue bevacizumab
G4 hypertension (including hypertensive encephalopathy)	Discontinue bevacizumab
G1 pulmonary or brain or spinal cord hemorrhage	Hold bevacizumab until (1) the bleeding has resolved and hemoglobin is stable; (2) there is no bleeding diathesis that would increase the risk of continued bevacizumab therapy; (3) there is no anatomic or pathologic condition that significantly increases the risk of hemorrhage recurrence with re-initiation of bevacizumab
G3 non-pulmonary or non-brain or non-spinal cord hemorrhage	
Serious bleeding defined as G ≥2 pulmonary or brain or spinal cord hemorrhage	Discontinue bevacizumab permanently. Continue chemotherapy after toxicity has resolved
G3 hemorrhage in sites other than pulmonary or brain or spinal cord	Withhold bevacizumab until (1) bleeding has resolved and (2) hemoglobin level is stable. Resume chemotherapy after toxicity has resolved provided (1) evaluation does not uncover a bleeding diathesis that would increase the risk of continuing therapy and (2) there is no anatomical or pathologic condition that can increase the risk of hemorrhage recurrence
Recurrence of any G3 hemorrhage	Discontinue bevacizumab permanently. Continue chemotherapy after toxicity has resolved
G3 hemorrhage in patient receiving full dose anti-coagulation	
Any grade arterial thromboembolic events (including cerebrovascular ischemia, cardiac ischemia/infarction, peripheral or visceral arterial ischemia)	Discontinue bevacizumab permanently. Continue chemotherapy after toxicity has resolved
Symptomatic G4 venous thrombosis	Discontinue bevacizumab permanently. Continue chemotherapy after toxicity has resolved
Asymptomatic G4 or any G3 venous thrombosis with planned duration of full-dose anticoagulation ≤2 weeks	Withhold bevacizumab until the full-dose anticoagulation period is over, then resume bevacizumab and chemotherapy
Asymptomatic G4 or any G3 venous thrombosis with planned duration of full-dose anticoagulation >2 weeks	Withhold bevacizumab initially as patient is assessed. Bevacizumab may then be resumed during the period of full-dose anticoagulation if ALL of the following criteria are met: (1) must have an in-range INR (usually between 2 and 3) on a stable dose of warfarin (or other anticoagulant) or on stable dose of heparin prior to restarting bevacizumab treatment; (2) there is no evidence of a pathological condition that carries high risk of bleeding (eg, tumor involving major vessels); (3) the patient has not had hemorrhagic events while receiving bevacizumab; and (4) the patient is benefiting from the bevacizumab therapy (no evidence of disease progression)
G3/4 coagulopathy	Withhold bevacizumab until PT/PTT resolves to G1. For patients with PT/INR > therapeutic range while on therapeutic warfarin, hold bevacizumab until PT/INR is within the therapeutic range
G1/2 left ventricular dysfunction	Continue with bevacizumab
G3 left ventricular dysfunction	Withhold bevacizumab until toxicity resolves to G ≤ 1
G4 left ventricular dysfunction	Discontinue bevacizumab
Moderate to severe proteinuria	Patients with a 2+ or greater urine dipstick reading should undergo further assessment, eg, a 24-hour urine collection. Suspend bevacizumab administration for ≥2 grams of proteinuria/24 h and resume when proteinuria is <2 grams/24 h
G4 proteinuria or nephrotic syndrome	Discontinue bevacizumab permanently. Continue chemotherapy after toxicity has resolved
Mild, clinically insignificant infusion reaction	Decrease the rate of infusion

(*continued*)

Treatment Modifications (continued)

RECOMMENDED DOSE MODIFICATIONS FOR BEVACIZUMAB

Clinically significant but not severe infusion reaction	Interrupt the infusion in patients with clinically significant infusion reactions and consider resuming at a slower rate following resolution. If decision is made to restart, the infusion may be continued at ≤50% of the rate prior to the reaction and increased in 50% increments every 30 minutes if well tolerated. Infusions may be restarted at the full rate during the next cycle
NCI CTCAE G3/4 allergic reaction/hypersensitivity, adult respiratory distress syndrome, or bronchospasm (regardless of grade) will be discontinued from bevacizumab treatment	Stop infusion and administer appropriate medical therapy (eg, epinephrine, corticosteroids, intravenous antihistamines, bronchodilators, and/or oxygen). Discontinue bevacizumab
Planned elective surgery	Suspend bevacizumab at least 28 days before elective surgery and do not resume for at least 28 days after surgery or until surgical incision is fully healed
Evidence of recto-sigmoid involvement by pelvic examination or bowel involvement on CT scan or clinical symptoms of bowel obstruction	Do not administer bevacizumab
Reversible posterior leukoencephalopathy syndrome (RPLS)	Withhold bevacizumab pending work-up and management, including control of blood pressure. Discontinue bevacizumab upon confirming the diagnosis of RPLS *Note:* the diagnosis of RPLS should be made with MRI and its complete resolution confirmed with MRI *Note:* resumption of bevacizumab may be considered in patients who have had documented benefit from bevacizumab, provided that RPLS was mild and has completely resolved clinically and radiographically within 2–4 weeks
Platelet count <50,000/mm³	Withhold bevacizumab until platelet count >75,000/mm³. If platelet count of <50,000/mm³ persists for >3 weeks, discontinue bevacizumab; continue chemotherapy only to the extent felt safe
G3 hematologic toxicities (ANC <1000/mm³; platelet count <50,000/mm³)	Hold bevacizumab as chemotherapy is held
G4 hematologic toxicities (thrombocytopenia) (ANC <500/mm³; platelet count <25,000/mm³)	

RECOMMENDED DOSE MODIFICATIONS FOR ATEZOLIZUMAB

Adverse Reaction	Grade/Severity	Dose Modification
Colitis	G1	Loperamide 4 mg as starting dose then 2 mg before each meal and after each loose stool until without diarrhea for 12 hours, with maximum of 16 mg loperamide per day. If G1 diarrhea or colitis persists >14 days, then add prednisolone 0.5–1 mg/kg (non-enteric-coated) or consider oral budesonide 9 mg daily if no bloody diarrhea
	G2/3 diarrhea or colitis	Withhold atezolizumab. Loperamide 4 mg as starting dose then 2 mg before each meal and after each loose stool until without diarrhea for 12 hours, with maximum of 16 mg loperamide per day. Administer oral prednisone/prednisolone at a dose of 0.5–2.0 mg/kg/day or its equivalent. When improves to G1, begin a slow corticosteroid taper over at least 4 weeks. Resume atezolizumab upon symptom control, or when prednisone/prednisolone daily dose <10 mg
	G4 diarrhea or colitis	Permanently discontinue atezolizumab. Loperamide 4 mg as starting dose then 2 mg before each meal and after each loose stool until without diarrhea for 12 hours, with maximum of 16 mg loperamide per day. Administer 1–2 mg/kg IV (methyl) prednisolone and convert to 0.5–2.0 mg/kg prednisone/prednisolone orally each day or its equivalent only after a response. Taper over at least 4 weeks when symptoms improve. If does not improve over 72 hours or worsens, perform flexible sigmoidoscopy/colonoscopy to document colitis then begin infliximab 5 mg/kg (if no perforation/sepsis/TB/hepatitis/NYHA III/IV CHF). If no response, add MMF 500–1000 mg twice daily. If worse on MMF, consider addition of tacrolimus or ATG

(continued)

Treatment Modifications (*continued*)

Adverse Reaction	Grade/Severity	Dose Modification
Pneumonitis	G2	Withhold atezolizumab. Consider pneumocystis prophylaxis depending on the clinical context and coverage with empiric antibiotics. Administer oral prednisone/prednisolone at a dose of 1–2 mg/kg/day or its equivalent. When improves to G1, begin a slow corticosteroid taper over at least 4 weeks. If does not respond adequately after 48 hours, then administer 2–4 mg/kg IV (methyl)prednisolone and convert to 0.5–2.0 mg/kg prednisone/prednisolone orally each day or its equivalent only after a response, followed by a taper over at least 6 weeks when symptoms improve to G1, titrating to symptoms. Resume atezolizumab upon symptom control, or when prednisone/prednisolone daily dose <10 mg
	G3/4	Permanently discontinue atezolizumab. Consider pneumocystis prophylaxis depending on the clinical context; cover with empiric antibiotics. Administer 2–4 mg/kg IV (methyl)prednisolone and convert to 1–2 mg/kg prednisone/prednisolone orally each day or its equivalent only after a response, followed by a taper over at least 8 weeks when symptoms improve to G1, titrating to symptoms. If when initially treated improvement does not occur within 48–72 hours, begin infliximab 5 mg/kg (if no perforation/sepsis/TB/hepatitis/NYHA III/IV CHF). If no response to infliximab, add MMF 500–1000 mg twice daily. Consider MMF especially if has concurrent hepatic toxicity
Hepatitis	G2 (AST or ALT >3–5× ULN or total bilirubin >1.5-3× ULN)	Withhold atezolizumab. Administer oral prednisone/prednisolone at a dose of 1–2 mg/kg/day or its equivalent. When improves to G1, begin a slow corticosteroid taper over at least 4 weeks. Resume atezolizumab upon symptom control, or when prednisone/prednisolone daily dose <10 mg
	G3/4 (AST or ALT >5× ULN or total bilirubin >3× ULN)	Permanently discontinue atezolizumab. Administer 1–2 mg/kg IV (methyl)prednisolone and convert to 0.5–2.0 mg/kg prednisone/prednisolone orally each day or its equivalent only after a response. Taper over at least 6 weeks when symptoms improve. If no response, add MMF 500–1000 mg twice daily. If worse on MMF, consider adding tacrolimus or ATG
Hypophysitis	G2/3 (moderate symptoms, ie, headache but no visual disturbance or fatigue/mood alteration but hemodynamically stable, no electrolyte disturbance)	Administer analgesia as needed for headache. Withhold atezolizumab. Administer oral prednisone/prednisolone at a dose of 0.5–2.0 mg/kg/day or its equivalent. When improves to G1, begin a slow corticosteroid taper over at least 4 weeks. If no improvement in 48 hours, administer 1–2 mg/kg IV (methyl)prednisolone and convert to 0.5–2.0 mg/kg prednisone/prednisolone orally each day or its equivalent only after a response. Taper over at least 4 weeks when symptoms improve to 5 mg prednisone/prednisolone or equivalent; do not stop steroids. Resume atezolizumab upon symptom control, or when prednisone/prednisolone daily dose <10 mg
	G4 (severe mass effect symptoms, ie, severe headache, any visual disturbance or severe hypoadrenalism, ie, hypotension, severe electrolyte disturbance)	Permanently discontinue atezolizumab. Administer analgesia as needed for headache. Administer 1–2 mg/kg IV (methyl)prednisolone and convert to 0.5–2.0 mg/kg prednisone/prednisolone orally each day or its equivalent only after a response. Taper over at least 4 weeks when symptoms improve to 5 mg prednisone/prednisolone or equivalent; do not stop steroids

(*continued*)

Treatment Modifications (*continued*)

Adverse Reaction	Grade/Severity	Dose Modification
Adrenal insufficiency	G2	Withhold atezolizumab. Administer oral prednisone/ prednisolone at a dose of 0.5–2.0 mg/kg/day or its equivalent. When improves to G1, begin a slow corticosteroid taper over at least 4 weeks. Serially assess adrenal function and continue steroids at replacement doses (20–40 mg hydrocortisone daily ~2/3 dose in AM upon awakening and ~1/3 at 4:00 PM) until recovery of adrenal function is documented. Resume atezolizumab upon symptom control, or when prednisone/prednisolone daily dose <10 mg
	G3/4	Permanently discontinue atezolizumab. Administer oral prednisone/prednisolone at a dose of 0.5–2.0 mg/kg/ day or its equivalent. When improves to G1, begin a slow corticosteroid taper over at least 4 weeks. Serially assess adrenal function and continue steroids at replacement doses (20–40 mg hydrocortisone daily ~2/3 dose in AM upon awakening and ~1/3 at 4:00 PM) until recovery of adrenal function is documented
Type 1 diabetes mellitus	G3 hyperglycemia	Withhold atezolizumab. Admit to hospital to manage hyperglycemia. Role of corticosteroids in preventing complete loss of insulin-producing cells is unknown and not recommended. Resume atezolizumab upon symptom control, or when prednisone/prednisolone daily dose <10 mg
	G4 hyperglycemia	Permanently discontinue atezolizumab. Admit to hospital to manage hyperglycemia. Role of corticosteroids in preventing complete loss of insulin-producing cells is unknown and not recommended
Nephritis and renal dysfunction	G2/3 (serum creatinine 1.5–6× ULN)	Withhold atezolizumab. Administer oral prednisone/ prednisolone at a dose of 0.5–2.0 mg/kg/day or its equivalent. When improves to G1, begin a slow corticosteroid taper over at least 4 weeks. If does not respond adequately, then administer 0.5–1 mg/kg IV (methyl)prednisolone and convert to 0.5–2.0 mg/kg prednisone/prednisolone orally each day or its equivalent only after a response, followed by a taper over at least 4 weeks when improves to G1. Resume atezolizumab upon symptom control, or when prednisone/prednisolone daily dose <10 mg
	G4 (serum creatinine >6× ULN)	Permanently discontinue atezolizumab. Administer 0.5–1 mg/kg IV (methyl)prednisolone and convert to 0.5–2.0 mg/ kg prednisone/prednisolone orally each day or its equivalent only after a response, followed by a taper over at least 4 weeks when improves to G1

(*continued*)

Treatment Modifications (*continued*)

Adverse Reaction	Grade/Severity	Dose Modification
Skin	G1/2	Continue atezolizumab. Avoid skin irritants, avoid sun exposure, topical emollients recommended. Topical steroid (mild strength for G1, moderate/potent strength for G2) cream once or twice daily ± oral or topical antihistamines for itching
	G3 rash or suspected SJS or TEN	Withhold atezolizumab. Avoid skin irritants, avoid sun exposure, topical emollients recommended. Administer oral or topical antihistamines for itching. Administer oral prednisone/prednisolone at a dose of 0.5–2.0 mg/kg or its equivalent daily for 3 days followed by a slow corticosteroid taper over at least 4 weeks when the rash improves to G1. If does not respond adequately, then administer 0.5–1 mg/kg IV (methyl)prednisolone and convert to 0.5–2.0 mg/kg prednisone/prednisolone orally each day or its equivalent only after a response, followed by a taper over at least 4 weeks when the rash improves to G1. Resume atezolizumab upon symptom control, or when prednisone/prednisolone daily dose <10 mg
	G4 rash or confirmed SJS or TEN	Avoid skin irritants, avoid sun exposure, topical emollients recommended. Administer oral or topical antihistamines for itching. Administer 1–2 mg/kg IV (methyl)prednisolone and convert to oral steroids 0.5–2.0 mg/kg prednisone/prednisolone each day or its equivalent only after a response. Taper over at least 4 weeks when the rash improves to G1. Permanently discontinue atezolizumab
Encephalitis	Confusion or altered behavior, headaches, alteration in Glasgow Coma Scale, motor or sensory deficits, speech abnormality, may or may not be febrile	Initially withhold atezolizumab, but permanently discontinue atezolizumab if there is no doubt as to diagnosis. Exclude bacterial and ideally viral infections prior to high-dose steroids. Administer oral prednisone/prednisolone at a dose of 0.5–2.0 mg/kg/day or its equivalent. When symptoms improve, begin a slow corticosteroid taper over at least 4–8 weeks. If symptoms are severe, administer 1–2 mg/kg IV (methyl)prednisolone and convert to 0.5–2.0 mg/kg prednisone/prednisolone orally each day or its equivalent only after a response. Consider concurrent empiric antiviral (IV acyclovir) and antibacterial therapy
Aseptic meningitis	Headache, photophobia, neck stiffness with fever or may be afebrile, vomiting; normal cognition/cerebral function (distinguishes from encephalitis)	
Other syndromes include neurosarcoidosis, posterior reversible leukoencephalopathy syndrome (PRES), Vogt-Koyanagi-Harada syndrome, demyelination, vasculitic encephalopathy, and generalized seizures		
Transverse myelitis	Acute or subacute neurologic signs/symptoms of motor/sensory/autonomic origin; most have sensory level; often bilateral symptoms	Initially withhold atezolizumab, but permanently discontinue atezolizumab if there is no doubt as to diagnosis. Administer 2 mg/kg IV (methyl)prednisolone or consider 1 g/day and convert to 0.5–2.0 mg/kg prednisone/prednisolone orally each day or its equivalent only after a response. When symptoms improve, begin a slow corticosteroid taper over at least 4–8 weeks. Plasmapheresis may be required if steroids do not bring about improvement
Myocarditis	G3	Permanently discontinue atezolizumab. Administer 2 mg/kg IV (methyl)prednisolone or consider 1 g/day and convert to 0.5–2.0 mg/kg prednisone/prednisolone orally each day or its equivalent only after a response. When symptoms improve, begin a slow corticosteroid taper over at least 4–8 weeks. If no response, add MMF 500–1000 mg twice daily. If worse on MMF, consider adding tacrolimus

(continued)

Treatment Modifications (continued)

Adverse Reaction	Grade/Severity	Dose Modification
Peripheral neurologic toxicity	Moderate: some interference with ADL, symptoms concerning to patient	Withhold atezolizumab. Initial observation reasonable or initiate prednisone/prednisolone 0.5–1 mg/kg (if progressing, eg, from mild) and/or pregabalin or duloxetine for pain. When symptoms improve begin a slow corticosteroid taper over at least 4 weeks. Resume atezolizumab upon symptom control, or when prednisone/prednisolone daily dose <10 mg
	Severe: limits self-care and aids warranted, life-threatening, eg, respiratory problems	Permanently discontinue atezolizumab. Administer 1–2 mg/kg IV (methyl)prednisolone and convert to 0.5–2.0 mg/kg prednisone/prednisolone orally each day or its equivalent only after a response. Taper over at least 4–8 weeks when symptoms improve to G1
Guillain-Barré syndrome	Progressive symmetrical muscle weakness with absent or reduced tendon reflexes—involves extremities, facial, respiratory, and bulbar and oculomotor muscles; dysregulation of autonomic nerves	Permanently discontinue atezolizumab. Use of steroids not recommended in idiopathic Guillain-Barré syndrome; however, a trial of (methyl)prednisolone 1–2 mg/kg is reasonable, converting to 0.5–2.0 mg/kg prednisone/prednisolone orally each day or its equivalent only after a response. If no improvement or worsening, plasmapheresis or IVIG indicated
Myasthenia gravis	Fluctuating muscle weakness (proximal limb, trunk, ocular, eg, ptosis/diplopia or bulbar) with fatigability, respiratory muscles may also be involved	Permanently discontinue atezolizumab. Administer pyridostigmine at an initial dose of 30 mg three times daily. Administer oral prednisone/prednisolone at a dose of 0.5–2.0 mg/kg/day or its equivalent or 1–2 mg/kg IV (methyl)prednisolone depending on the severity of symptoms. If begin with IV, convert to 0.5–2.0 mg/kg prednisone/prednisolone orally each day or its equivalent only after a response. If no improvement or worsening, plasmapheresis or IVIG may be considered. Additional immunosuppressants used in myasthenia gravis include azathioprine, cyclosporine, and mycophenolate. Avoid certain medications, eg, ciprofloxacin, beta-blockers, that may precipitate cholinergic crisis
Other syndromes including motor and sensory peripheral neuropathy, multifocal radicular neuropathy/plexopathy, autonomic neuropathy, phrenic nerve palsy, cranial nerve palsies (eg, facial nerve, optic nerve, hypoglossal nerve)		Permanently discontinue atezolizumab. Administer oral prednisone/prednisolone at a dose of 0.5–2.0 mg/kg/day or its equivalent or 1–2 mg/kg IV (methyl)prednisolone depending on the severity of symptoms. If begin with IV, convert to 0.5–2.0 mg/kg prednisone/prednisolone orally each day or its equivalent only after a response
Arthralgia	G1 (mild pain with inflammation, erythema, or joint swelling)	Continue atezolizumab. Administer acetaminophen (paracetamol) and ibuprofen
	G2 (moderate pain with inflammation, erythema, or joint swelling that limits ADLs)	Withhold atezolizumab. Administer higher doses of acetaminophen (paracetamol) and ibuprofen, and use diclofenac or naproxen or etoricoxib. If inadequately controlled, consider intra-articular steroid injections for large joints or administer oral prednisone/prednisolone at a dose of 0.5–2.0 mg/kg/day or its equivalent. When improves to G1, begin a slow corticosteroid taper over at least 4 weeks. If does not respond adequately, then administer 0.5–1 mg/kg IV (methyl)prednisolone and convert to 0.5–2.0 mg/kg prednisone/prednisolone orally each day or its equivalent only after a response, followed by a taper over at least 4 weeks when improves to G1. Resume atezolizumab upon symptom control, or when prednisone/prednisolone daily dose <10 mg
	G3 (severe pain; irreversible joint damage; disabling; limits self-care ADL)	Withhold atezolizumab. Administer 0.5–1 mg/kg IV (methyl)prednisolone and convert to 0.5–2.0 mg/kg prednisone/prednisolone orally each day or its equivalent only after a response, followed by a taper over at least 4 weeks when improves to G1. In severe cases, infliximab or another anti–TNF alpha drug may be required for improvement of arthritis. Resume atezolizumab upon symptom control, or when prednisone/prednisolone daily dose <10 mg

(continued)

Treatment Modifications (*continued*)

Adverse Reaction	Grade/Severity	Dose Modification
Other	First occurrence of other G3	Withhold atezolizumab. Administer oral prednisone/prednisolone at a dose of 0.5–2.0 mg/kg/day or its equivalent. When improves to G1, begin a slow corticosteroid taper over at least 4 weeks. Resume atezolizumab upon symptom control, or when prednisone/prednisolone daily dose <10 mg
	Recurrence of same G3	Permanently discontinue atezolizumab. Administer 1–2 mg/kg IV (methyl)prednisolone and convert to 0.5–2.0 mg/kg prednisone/prednisolone orally each day or its equivalent only after a response. Taper over at least 4–8 weeks when symptoms improve to G1
	Life-threatening or G4	
	Requirement for ≥10 mg/day prednisone or equivalent for >12 weeks	Permanently discontinue atezolizumab
	Persistent G2/3 adverse reactions lasting ≥12 weeks	

ADL, activities of daily living; ALT, alanine aminotransferase; AST, aspartate aminotransferase; ATG, anti-thymocyte globulin; SJS, Stevens-Johnson Syndrome; TEN, toxic epidermal necrolysis; ULN, upper limit of normal

Notes on general supportive care:
• Steroid taper in most cases will proceed over a minimum of 1 month, but if symptoms improve rapidly, a 2-week taper can be considered. If steroids are administered for more than 4 weeks, consider PCP prophylaxis (cotrimoxazole 480 mg twice daily M/W/F or inhaled pentamidine if has cotrimoxazole allergy), regular random blood glucose, vitamin D level and starting calcium/vitamin D supplementation per guidelines

Notes on pregnancy and breastfeeding:
• Atezolizumab can cause fetal harm. If used during pregnancy, or if the patient becomes pregnant during treatment, apprise the patient of the potential hazard to a fetus. Females of reproductive potential should use highly effective contraception during treatment and for 4 months after the last dose of atezolizumab
• It is not known whether atezolizumab is excreted in human milk. Therefore, it is recommended that women discontinue nursing during treatment with and for 4 months after the final dose of atezolizumab

Adverse Events (N = 787)

Grade (%)	ABCP Group (n = 393)		BCP Group (n = 394)	
	Grade 1–2	Grade 3–4	Grade 1–2	Grade 3–4
Alopecia	46.6	0	43.9	0
Peripheral neuropathy	35.9	2.8	28.7	2.3
Nausea	30.3	3.8	25.6	2.0
Fatigue	22.4	3.3	20.1	2.5
Anemia	17.8	6.1	18.0	5.8
Decreased appetite	19.6	2.5	14.2	0.8
Diarrhea	17.8	2.8	14.7	0.5
Neutropenia	4.6	13.7	6.1	11.2
Hypertension	12.7	6.4	10.7	6.3
Arthralgia	16.0	0.8	14.0	1.0
Constipation	16.5	0	11.4	0

(continued)

Adverse Events (N = 787) (*continued*)

Grade (%)	ABCP Group (n = 393)		BCP Group (n = 394)	
	Grade 1–2	Grade 3–4	Grade 1–2	Grade 3–4
Asthenia	13.2	1.3	13.5	2.8
Epistaxis	12.7	1.0	17.3	0
Vomiting	12.7	1.5	12.9	1.3
Decreased platelet count	8.7	5.1	8.9	2.3
Myalgia	12.0	.5	11.7	0.3
Thrombocytopenia	9.2	4.1	7.1	4.3
Proteinuria	10.4	2.5	9.4	2.8
Decreased neutrophil count	3.6	8.7	2.5	6.3
Rash	12.0	1.3	5.1	0
Stomatitis	10.9	1.0	5.1	0.3
Paresthesia	10.7	0	9.1	0.3
Febrile neutropenia*	0.5	9.2	0	5.8

Adverse event data were reported for the intent-to-treat population for treatment-related adverse events with an incidence of ³10%. For Grade 3–4 events, treatment-related adverse events with an incidence of 5% or higher were listed

The incidence of Grade 5 treatment-related adverse events was 2.8% in the ABCP group and 2.3% in the BCP group

*Not included in these figures are 3 patients (0.8%) in the ABCP group and 0 patients in the BCP group who experienced Grade 5 febrile neutropenia

ADVANCED NON-SQUAMOUS NSCLC • FIRST-LINE
LUNG CANCER REGIMEN: PACLITAXEL + CARBOPLATIN + BEVACIZUMAB

Johnson DH et al. J Clin Oncol 2004;22:2184–2191
Sandler AB et al. N Engl J Med 2006;355:2542–2550

Premedication (primary prophylaxis against hypersensitivity reactions from paclitaxel):
Dexamethasone 20 mg/dose for 2 doses; administer orally the evening before and the morning of chemotherapy prior to paclitaxel, *plus:*
Diphenhydramine 50 mg; administer by intravenous injection 30 minutes before paclitaxel, *and:*
Ranitidine 50 mg or **cimetidine** 300 mg; administer intravenously in 25–100 mL 0.9% sodium chloride injection (0.9% NS) or 5% dextrose injection (D5W) over 5–30 minutes, 30 minutes before paclitaxel
Paclitaxel 200 mg/m²; administer intravenously in a volume of 0.9% NS or D5W sufficient to produce a solution with concentration within the range 0.3–1.2 mg/mL over 3 hours on day 1, every 3 weeks (total dosage/cycle = 200 mg/m²)

Carboplatin (calculated dose) AUC = 6 mg/mL × min; administer intravenously diluted in D5W or 0.9% NS to a concentration as low as 0.5 mg/mL over 15–30 minutes on day 1, 60 minutes after completing paclitaxel, every 3 weeks (total dosage/cycle calculated to produce an AUC = 6 mg/mL × min) (see equation below)

Bevacizumab 15 mg/kg; administer intravenously in 100 mL 0.9% NS every 3 weeks on day 1, (total dosage/cycle = 15 mg/kg)

Note: administration duration for the initial bevacizumab dose is 90 minutes. If administration is well tolerated, the administration duration may be decreased stepwise during subsequent administrations to 60 minutes and, finally, to a minimum duration of 30 minutes

Supportive Care
Antiemetic prophylaxis
Emetogenic potential: **HIGH**. *Potential for delayed symptoms*
See Chapter 42 for antiemetic recommendations

Hematopoietic growth factor (CSF) prophylaxis
Primary prophylaxis may be indicated
See Chapter 43 for more information

Antimicrobial prophylaxis
Risk of fever and neutropenia is **LOW**
  Antimicrobial primary prophylaxis to be considered:
  • Antibacterial—not indicated
  • Antifungal—not indicated
  • Antiviral—not indicated unless patient previously had an episode of HSV

Additional supportive care
Dexamethasone 8 mg/dose orally every 12 hours for 6 doses after chemotherapy if G ≥2 arthralgias/myalgias occur
Add a **proton pump inhibitor** during dexamethasone use to prevent gastritis and duodenitis

Note: carboplatin dose is based on Calvert's formula to achieve a target area under the plasma concentration versus time curve (AUC) (AUC units = mg/mL × min)

$$\text{Total carboplatin dose (mg)} = (\text{target AUC}) \times (\text{GFR} + 25)$$

In practice, creatinine clearance (CrCl) is used in place of glomerular filtration rate (GFR). CrCl can be calculated from the equation of Cockcroft and Gault:

$$\text{For males, Clcr} = \frac{(140 - \text{age [years]}) \times \text{body weight (kg)}}{72 \times (\text{Serum creatinine [mg/dL]})}$$

$$\text{For females, Clcr} = \frac{(140 - \text{age [years]}) \times \text{body weight (kg)}}{72 \times (\text{Serum creatinine [mg/dL]})} \times 0.85$$

Calvert AH et al. J Clin Oncol 1989;7:1748–1756
Cockcroft DW, Gault MH. Nephron 1976;16:31–41
Jodrell DI et al. J Clin Oncol 1992;10:520–528
Sorensen BT et al. Cancer Chemother Pharmacol 1991;28:397–401

Treatment Modifications

Adverse Event	Dose Modification
ANC nadir <500/mm³, platelet nadir <50,000/mm³, or febrile neutropenia	Reduce carboplatin dosage to AUC = 5 if previous cycle dose was AUC = 6; or to AUC = 4 if previous cycle dose was AUC = 5
ANC nadir <500/mm³, platelet nadir <50,000/mm³, or febrile neutropenia after 2 carboplatin dose reductions (AUC in previous cycle = 4)	Reduce paclitaxel dosage to 200 mg/m², and decrease carboplatin dosage to AUC = 3
Day 1 ANC <1500/mm³ or platelet <100,000/mm3	Delay chemotherapy until ANC >1500/mm³ and platelet >100,000/mm³, for maximum delay of 2 weeks
Delay of >2 weeks in reaching ANC >1500/mm³ and platelet >100,000/mm3	Discontinue therapy
G2 neurotoxicity	Reduce paclitaxel dosage to 200 mg/m²
G3 neurotoxicity	Reduce paclitaxel dosage to 175 mg/m²
G2 arthralgia/myalgia despite dexamethasone prophylaxis	Reduce paclitaxel dosage to 200 mg/m²
G3 arthralgia/myalgia despite dexamethasone prophylaxis	Reduce paclitaxel dosage to 175 mg/m²
G ≥2 AST or G ≥3 bilirubin	Hold paclitaxel
Moderate hypersensitivity	Patient may be re-treated
Severe hypersensitivity	Discontinue therapy
Chest pain or arrhythmia during chemotherapy	Immediately stop chemotherapy and evaluate the patient
Symptomatic arrhythmias, or ≥2-degree AV block, or an ischemic event	Discontinue therapy

Patient Population Studied

A study of 855 patients with advanced, previously untreated stage IIIB (pleural or pericardial effusion only) NSCLC (non-squamous histologies). A randomized comparison with paclitaxel + carboplatin. ECOG PS 0 (40%) or 1 (60%). INR <1.5 and PTT no greater than upper limit of normal. No history of thrombotic or hemorrhagic disorders. No gross hemoptysis defined as one-half teaspoon or more of bright red blood per day. Brain metastases were not allowed; 43% were age ≥65 years, and 28% had ≥5% weight loss

Toxicity (N = 420)

Hematologic

Toxicity	% G4
Neutropenia	24*
Fever + neutropenia	3.3*
Thrombocytopenia	1.4
Anemia	0

Non-hematologic

	% G ≥3
Hemorrhage	4.5*
Hemoptysis	1.9*
CNS	1*
Gastrointestinal	1.2
Other	1
Hypertension	6*
Venous thrombosis	3.8
Arterial thrombosis	1.9

Treatment-Related Deaths

Hemoptysis	5 (1.2%)
Gastrointestinal bleeding	2 (0.5%)
Fever + neutropenia	1 (0.25%)

*These values were statistically worse than those with paclitaxel + carboplatin alone

Efficacy (N = 357)

Overall response	27.2%
Complete response	1.4%
Partial response	25.8%
6-month progression-free survival	55%
12-month progression-free survival	14.6%
Median survival	12.5 months
1-year survival	51.9%
2-year survival	22.1%

Therapy Monitoring

1. *Every week:* CBC with differential and platelet count
2. *Response evaluation:* every 2–3 cycles

Notes

1. Compared with paclitaxel + carboplatin, overall survival advantage is confined to men; not seen in women (P = 0.8), despite statistically significant advantage for progression-free survival and response rate in women
2. Bevacizumab is associated with a small increase in serious bleeding, including hemoptysis. In a phase 2 trial, apparent risk factors for life-threatening hemorrhages included baseline hemoptysis brain metastases, anticoagulant therapy, and squamous histology (Johnson DH et al. J Clin Oncol 2004;22:2184–2191)
3. This therapy is the ECOG reference standard for first-line treatment of advanced NSCLC and is recommended by NCCN. Confirmatory trials have yet to be performed
4. Only patients with non-squamous histologies were included in this study

ADVANCED NON-SQUAMOUS NSCLC • FIRST-LINE

LUNG CANCER REGIMEN: CISPLATIN + PEMETREXED

Scagliotti GV et al. J Clin Oncol 2008; 26:3543–3551

Ancillary medications:
Folic acid 350–1000 mcg/day; administer orally beginning 1–2 weeks before the first dose of pemetrexed and continuing until 3 weeks after the last dose of pemetrexed
Cyanocobalamin (vitamin B$_{12}$) 1000 mcg; administer intramuscularly every 9 weeks, beginning 1–2 weeks before the first dose of pemetrexed
Dexamethasone 4 mg; administer orally twice daily for 3 consecutive days, starting the day before pemetrexed administration to decrease the risk and severity of severe skin rash associated with pemetrexed

Hydration before cisplatin: ≥1000 mL 0.9% sodium chloride injection (0.9% NS); administer intravenously over a minimum of 2–4 hours
Pemetrexed 500 mg/m^2; administer intravenously in 100 mL 0.9% NS over 10 minutes on day 1 every 21 days for a maximum of 6 cycles (unless there was earlier evidence of disease progression or intolerance of the study treatment) (total dosage/cycle = 500 mg/m^2)
Cisplatin 75 mg/m^2; administer intravenously in 100–250 mL 0.9% NS over 1 hour on day 1, every 21 days for a maximum of 6 cycles (unless there was earlier evidence of disease progression or intolerance of the study treatment) (total dosage/cycle = 75 mg/m^2)

Hydration after cisplatin: ≥1000 mL 0.9% NS; administer intravenously over a minimum of 2–4 hours

Supportive Care
Antiemetic prophylaxis
Emetogenic potential: **HIGH**. *Potential for delayed symptoms*
See Chapter 42 for antiemetic recommendations

Hematopoietic growth factor (CSF) prophylaxis
Primary prophylaxis is **NOT** *indicated*
See Chapter 43 for more information

Antimicrobial prophylaxis
Risk of fever and neutropenia is **LOW**
Antimicrobial primary prophylaxis to be considered:
- Antibacterial—not indicated
- Antifungal—not indicated
- Antiviral—not indicated unless patient previously had an episode of HSV

Treatment Modifications

Adverse Event	Dose Modification
Day1 dose reduction of pemetrexed, or cisplatin required	Reduced dose is administered during subsequent treatment cycles
Patients with 2 dose reductions on day 1 who experience toxicity requiring a third dose reduction	Discontinue therapy
Toxicity G ≥2	Delay start of next cycle up to 42 days

Toxicity* (N = 839)

Toxicity	% G3/4
Neutropenia	15.1%
Anemia	5.6%
Thrombocytopenia	4.1%
Febrile neutropenia	1.3%
Nausea	7.2%
Vomiting	6.1%
Fatigue	6.7%
Alopecia, any grade	11.9%
Dehydration, any grade	3.6%

*NCI CTC, National Cancer Institute (USA) Common Toxicity Criteria, version 2.0. Available at: http://ctep.cancer.gov/protocolDevelopment/electronic_applications/ctc.htm [accessed December 7, 2013]

Patient Population Studied

Noninferiority, phase 3, randomized study comparing the overall survival between treatment arms in 1725 chemotherapy-naïve patients with histologically or cytologically confirmed NSCLC, classified as stage IIIB not amenable to curative treatment or stage IV and an Eastern Cooperative Oncology Group (ECOG) performance status of 0–1. A total of 862 patients were treated with cisplatin + pemetrexed

Efficacy (N = 862)

Objective response rate*	30.6%
Duration of response	4.5 months
Median overall survival	10.3 months
Median progression-free survival	4.8 months
1-year survival	43.5%
2-year survival	18.9%

*RECIST

Therapy Monitoring

Baseline, every other cycle, and then every 6 weeks: history and physical examination; assessment by imaging techniques

ADVANCED NSCLC • FIRST-LINE
LUNG CANCER REGIMEN: PEMBROLIZUMAB

KEYTRUDA (pembrolizumab) injection prescribing information. Whitehouse Station, NJ: Merck & Co., Inc; updated 2019 September

Mok TSK et al. Lancet 2019;393(10183):1819–1830
Supplementary appendix to: Mok TSK et al. Lancet 2019;393(10183):1819–1830
Reck M et al. N Engl J Med 2016;375(19):1823–1833
Protocol for: Reck M et al. N Engl J Med 2016;375(19):1823–1833
Supplementary appendix to: Reck M et al. N Engl J Med 2016;375(19):1823–1833

Pembrolizumab 200 mg; administer intravenously over 30 minutes in a volume of 0.9% sodium chloride injection (0.9% NS) or 5% dextrose injection (D5W) sufficient to produce a pembrolizumab concentration within the range 1–10 mg/mL every 3 weeks for up to 24 months (total dose/3-week cycle = 200 mg)

- Administer pembrolizumab with an administration set that contains a sterile, non-pyrogenic, low-protein-binding in-line or add-on filter with pore size within the range of 0.2–5.0μm

- Pembrolizumab can cause severe or life-threatening infusion-related reactions, including hypersensitivity and anaphylaxis

Alternative pembrolizumab dose and schedule as per the U.S. FDA regimens approved on April 28, 2020:

Pembrolizumab 400 mg; administer intravenously over 30 minutes in a volume of 0.9% NS or D5W sufficient to produce a pembrolizumab concentration within the range 1–10 mg/mL every 6 weeks for up to 24 months (total dose/6-week cycle = 400 mg)

Supportive Care
Antiemetic prophylaxis
Emetogenic potential is **MINIMAL**
See Chapter 42 for antiemetic recommendations

Hematopoietic growth factor (CSF) prophylaxis
Primary prophylaxis is **NOT** *indicated*
See Chapter 43 for more information

Antimicrobial prophylaxis
Risk of fever and neutropenia is **LOW**
   Antimicrobial primary prophylaxis to be considered:
- Antibacterial—not indicated
- Antifungal—not indicated
- Antiviral—not indicated unless patient previously had an episode of HSV

Patient Population Studied

KEYNOTE-042 was a randomized, open-label, phase 3 trial that included 1274 adult patients and compared pembrolizumab to platinum-based chemotherapy as first-line treatment for PD-L1-positive non–small cell lung cancer (NSCLC). Patients were eligible if they had histologically or cytologically confirmed locally advanced or metastatic NSCLC without a sensitizing EGFR mutation or an ALK translocation, if they had at least one measurable lesion according to RECIST v1.1, if they had not previously received treatment for locally advanced or metastatic disease, if they had an Eastern Cooperative Oncology Group (ECOG) performance score of ≤1, if they had a life expectancy of ≥3 months, and if they had a PD-L1 tumor proportion score (TPS) (percentage of viable tumor cells showing partial or complete membrane staining [≥1+] relative to all viable tumor cells present in the sample [positive and negative]) of ≥1%. Patients were excluded if they had known unstable or untreated CNS metastases, if they had a history of non-infectious pneumonitis requiring systemic glucocorticoids, if they had an active autoimmune disease, if they were receiving systemic immunosuppressive therapy, if their NSCLC could be treated with surgical resection or chemoradiation, if they would be expected to require systemic or localized neoplastic therapy during the trial, if they had ever received a checkpoint or T-cell costimulation inhibitor, or if they had active hepatitis B or C infection. The data presented herein include those presented up through the second interim analysis.

Efficacy (N = 1274)

	Pembrolizumab (n = 637)	Chemotherapy (n = 637)	
Median overall survival (TPS ≥50%)	20.0 months (95% CI, 15.4–24.9)	12.2 months (95% CI, 10.4–14.2)	HR 0.69 (95% CI, 0.56–0.85); P = 0.0003
Median overall survival (TPS ≥20%)	17.7 months (95% CI, 15.3–22.1)	13.0 months (95% CI, 11.6–15.3)	HR 0.77 (95% CI, 0.64–0.92); P = 0.0020
Median overall survival (TPS ≥1%)	16.7 months (95% CI, 13.9–19.7)	12.1 months (95% CI, 11.3–13.3)	HR 0.81 (95% CI, 0.71–0.93); P = 0.0018
Overall median survival duration (1% ≤ TPS ≤ 49%)*	13.4 months (95% CI, 10.7–18.2)	12.1 months (95% CI, 11.0–14.0)	HR 0.92 (95% CI, 0.77–1.11)
Estimated overall survival rate (TPS ≥50%) (24 months)	45%	30%	
Estimated overall survival rate (TPS ≥20%) (24 months)	41%	30%	

(continued)

Efficacy (N = 1274) *(continued)*

	Pembrolizumab (n = 637)	Chemotherapy (n = 637)	
Estimated overall survival rate (TPS ≥1%) (24 months)	39%	28%	
Median progression-free survival (TPS ≥50%)	7.1 months (95% CI, 5.9–9.0)	6.4 months (95% CI, 6.1–6.9)	HR 0.81 (95% CI, 0.67–0.99); P = 0.0170 (not significant)
Median progression-free survival (TPS ≥20%)	6.2 months (95% CI, 5.1–7.8)	6.6 months (95% CI, 6.2–7.3)	HR 0.94 (95% CI, 0.80–1.11); significance not tested
Median progression-free survival (TPS ≥1%)	5.4 months (95% CI, 4.3–6.2)	6.5 months (95% CI, 6.3–7.0)	HR 1.07 (95% CI, 0.94–1.21); significance not tested
Objective response rate (TPS ≥50%)	39% (95% CI, 34–45)	32% (95% CI, 27–38)	
Objective response rate (TPS ≥20%)	33% (95% CI, 29–38)	29% (95% CI, 25–34)	
Objective response rate (TPS ≥1%)	27% (95% CI, 24–31)	27% (95% CI, 23–30)	
Objective complete response rate (TPS ≥50%)	<1%	<1%	
Objective complete response rate (TPS ≥20%)	<1%	<1%	
Objective complete response rate (TPS ≥1%)	<1%	<1%	
Objective partial response rate (TPS ≥50%)	39%	32%	
Objective partial response rate (TPS ≥20%)	33%	29%	
Objective partial response rate (TPS ≥1%)	27%	26%	
Median response duration (TPS ≥50%)*	20.2 months (95% CI, 16.6-NR)	10.8 months (95% CI, 6.1–13.4)	
Median response duration (TPS ≥20%)*	20.2 months (95% CI, 16.3-NR)	8.3 months (95% CI, 6.4–13.4)	
Median response duration (TPS ≥1%)*	20.2 months (95% CI, 16.6-NR)	8.3 months (95% CI, 6.5–11.1)	

HR, hazard ratio; CI, confidence interval; NR, not reached; TPS, tumor proportion score for PD-L1
*Considered a protocol-specified exploratory end point
All data presented here are reported in the second interim analysis paper titled "Pembrolizumab versus chemotherapy for previously untreated, PD-L1-expressing, locally advanced or metastatic non–small cell lung cancer (KEYNOTE-042): a randomised, open-label, controlled, phase 3 trial." Overall median follow-up time was 12.8 months (IQR, 6.0–20.0). All analyses were performed on the intention-to-treat populations. Tumor response was graded according to RECIST v1.1 criteria. Response rates in TPS ≥50 and TPS ≥1 were originally considered exploratory end points, but later amended to be secondary end points. Between-group differences in overall and progression-free survival were analyzed with stratified log-rank tests. Hazard ratios and 95% CIs for these end points were analyzed with a stratified Cox regression model with Efron's method of tie handling. The stratified Miettinen and Nurminen method was used to compare between-group differences in response rate

Therapy Monitoring

1. Initially at the time of each dose, and eventually every 6–12 weeks, perform a total-body skin examination with attention to ALL mucous membranes as well as a complete review of systems

2. Monitor patients for signs and symptoms of pneumonitis. Evaluate patients with suspected pneumonitis with chest x-ray, CT, and pulse oximetry. For ≥2 toxicity, may include nasal swab, sputum culture and sensitivity, blood culture and sensitivity, and urine culture and sensitivity

3. Monitor patients for signs and symptoms of colitis. Encourage patients to report diarrhea immediately to any member of the health care team

4. Draw AST, ALT, and bilirubin prior to each infusion and/or weekly if there are Grade 1 liver function test elevations. Note, no treatment is recommended for G1 LFT abnormalities. For ≥2 toxicity, work up for other causes of elevated LFTs including viral hepatitis

5. Use basic metabolic panel (Na, K, CO_2, glucose) and patient history as screening tools for hypophysitis including hypopituitarism and adrenal insufficiency. If in doubt, evaluate AM adrenocorticotropic hormone (ACTH) and cortisol levels. Consider ACTH stimulation test for indeterminate results

6. Assess thyroid function at the start of treatment, periodically during treatment, and as indicated based on clinical evaluation, and for clinical signs and symptoms of thyroid disorders. Test for TSH and free thyroxine (FT4) every 4–6 weeks as part of routine clinical monitoring of therapy or for case detection in symptomatic patients

7. Measure glucose at baseline and with each treatment during the first 12 weeks and every 6 weeks thereafter

8. Obtain a serum creatinine prior to every dose. If creatinine is found to be newly elevated, consider holding therapy while other potential causes are evaluated. Note, routine urinalysis is not necessary other than to rule out urinary tract infections, etc

9. Obtain a complete rheumatologic history and perform an examination of all peripheral joints for tenderness, swelling, and range of motion. Examine the spine. Consider plain x-ray/imaging to exclude metastases and evaluate joint damage (erosions), if appropriate

10. In patients at high risk for infections and in appropriately selected patients based on an infectious disease evaluation, draw screening laboratories (HIV, hepatitis A and B, and blood QuantiFERON for TB) to prepare patients to start infliximab

Treatment Modifications

RECOMMENDED DOSE MODIFICATIONS FOR PEMBROLIZUMAB

Adverse Event	Grade/Severity	Treatment Modification
Infusion reaction	Clinically significant but not severe infusion reaction	Interrupt the infusion in patients with clinically significant infusion reactions and consider resuming at a slower rate following resolution. If decision is made to restart, begin at ≤50% of the rate prior to the reaction and increase in 50% increments every 30 minutes if well tolerated. Infusions may be restarted at the full rate during the next cycle
	G3/4 (severe infusion reaction—pyrexia, chills, flushing, hypotension, dyspnea, wheezing, back pain, abdominal pain, and urticaria). Not rapidly responsive to brief interruption of infusion	Stop infusion and administer appropriate medical therapy (eg, epinephrine, corticosteroids, intravenous antihistamines, bronchodilators, and/or oxygen). Discontinue pembrolizumab
Colitis	G1	Loperamide 4 mg as starting dose then 2 mg before each meal and after each loose stool until without diarrhea for 12 hours, with maximum of 16 mg loperamide per day. If G1 diarrhea or colitis persists >14 days, then add prednisolone 0.5–1 mg/kg (non-enteric-coated) or consider oral budesonide 9 mg daily if no bloody diarrhea
	G2/3 diarrhea or colitis	Withhold pembrolizumab. Loperamide 4 mg as starting dose then 2 mg before each meal and after each loose stool until without diarrhea for 12 hours, with maximum of 16 mg loperamide per day. Administer oral prednisone/prednisolone at a dose of 0.5–2.0 mg/kg/day or its equivalent. When improves to G1, begin a slow corticosteroid taper over at least 4 weeks. Resume pembrolizumab upon symptom control, or when prednisone/prednisolone daily dose <10 mg
	G4 diarrhea or colitis	Permanently discontinue pembrolizumab. Loperamide 4 mg as starting dose then 2 mg before each meal and after each loose stool until without diarrhea for 12 hours, with maximum of 16 mg loperamide per day. Administer 1–2 mg/kg IV (methyl)prednisolone and convert to 0.5–2.0 mg/kg prednisone/prednisolone orally each day or its equivalent only after a response. Taper over at least 4 weeks when symptoms improve. If does not improve over 72 hours or worsens, perform flexible sigmoidoscopy/colonoscopy to document colitis then begin infliximab 5 mg/kg (if no perforation/sepsis/TB/hepatitis/NYHA III/IV CHF). If no response, add MMF 500–1000 mg twice daily. If worse on MMF, consider addition of tacrolimus or ATG

(continued)

Treatment Modifications (*continued*)

Adverse Event	Grade/Severity	Treatment Modification
Pneumonitis	G2	Withhold pembrolizumab. Consider pneumocystis prophylaxis depending on the clinical context and coverage with empiric antibiotics. Administer oral prednisone/prednisolone at a dose of 1–2 mg/kg/day or its equivalent. When improves to G1, begin a slow corticosteroid taper over at least 4 weeks. If does not respond adequately after 48 hours, then administer 2–4 mg/kg IV (methyl)prednisolone and convert to 0.5–2.0 mg/kg prednisone/prednisolone orally each day or its equivalent only after a response, followed by a taper over at least 6 weeks when symptoms improve to G1, titrating to symptoms. Resume pembrolizumab upon symptom control, or when prednisone/prednisolone daily dose <10 mg
	G3/4	Permanently discontinue pembrolizumab. Consider pneumocystis prophylaxis depending on the clinical context; cover with empiric antibiotics. Administer 2–4 mg/kg IV (methyl)prednisolone and convert to 1–2 mg/kg prednisone/prednisolone orally each day or its equivalent only after a response, followed by a taper over at least 8 weeks when symptoms improve to G1, titrating to symptoms. If when initially treated improvement does not occur within 48–72 hours, begin infliximab 5 mg/kg (if no perforation/sepsis/TB/hepatitis/NYHA III/IV CHF). If no response to infliximab, add MMF 500–1000 mg twice daily. Consider MMF especially if has concurrent hepatic toxicity
Hepatitis	G2 (AST or ALT >3–5× ULN or total bilirubin >1.5-3× ULN)	Withhold pembrolizumab. Administer oral prednisone/prednisolone at a dose of 1–2 mg/kg/day or its equivalent. When improves to G1, begin a slow corticosteroid taper over at least 4 weeks. Resume pembrolizumab upon symptom control, or when prednisone/prednisolone daily dose <10 mg
	G3/4 (AST or ALT >5× ULN or total bilirubin >3× ULN)	Permanently discontinue pembrolizumab. Administer 1–2 mg/kg IV (methyl)prednisolone and convert to 0.5–2.0 mg/kg prednisone/prednisolone orally each day or its equivalent only after a response. Taper over at least 6 weeks when symptoms improve. If no response, add MMF 500–1000 mg twice daily. If worse on MMF, consider adding tacrolimus or ATG
Hypophysitis	G2/3 (moderate symptoms, ie, headache but no visual disturbance or fatigue/mood alteration but hemodynamically stable, no electrolyte disturbance)	Administer analgesia as needed for headache. Withhold pembrolizumab. Administer oral prednisone/prednisolone at a dose of 0.5–2.0 mg/kg/day or its equivalent. When improves to G1, begin a slow corticosteroid taper over at least 4 weeks. If no improvement in 48 hours, administer 1–2 mg/kg IV (methyl)prednisolone and convert to 0.5–2.0 mg/kg prednisone/prednisolone orally each day or its equivalent only after a response. Taper over at least 4 weeks when symptoms improve to 5 mg prednisone/prednisolone or equivalent; do not stop steroids. Resume pembrolizumab upon symptom control, or when prednisone/prednisolone daily dose <10 mg
	G4 (severe mass effect symptoms, ie, severe headache, any visual disturbance or severe hypoadrenalism, ie, hypotension, severe electrolyte disturbance)	Permanently discontinue pembrolizumab. Administer analgesia as needed for headache. Administer 1–2 mg/kg IV (methyl)prednisolone and convert to 0.5–2.0 mg/kg prednisone/prednisolone orally each day or its equivalent only after a response. Taper over at least 4 weeks when symptoms improve to 5 mg prednisone/prednisolone or equivalent; do not stop steroids
Adrenal insufficiency	G2	Withhold pembrolizumab. Administer oral prednisone/prednisolone at a dose of 0.5–2.0 mg/kg/day or its equivalent. When improves to G1, begin a slow corticosteroid taper over at least 4 weeks. Serially assess adrenal function and continue steroids at replacement doses (20–40 mg hydrocortisone daily ~2/3 dose in AM upon awakening and ~1/3 at 4:00 PM) until recovery of adrenal function is documented. Resume pembrolizumab upon symptom control, or when prednisone/prednisolone daily dose <10 mg
	G3/4	Permanently discontinue pembrolizumab. Administer oral prednisone/prednisolone at a dose of 0.5–2.0 mg/kg/day or its equivalent. When improves to G1, begin a slow corticosteroid taper over at least 4 weeks. Serially assess adrenal function and continue steroids at replacement doses (20–40 mg hydrocortisone daily ~2/3 dose in AM upon awakening and ~1/3 at 4:00 PM) until recovery of adrenal function is documented
Type 1 diabetes mellitus	G3 hyperglycemia	Withhold pembrolizumab. Admit to hospital to manage hyperglycemia. Role of corticosteroids in preventing complete loss of insulin-producing cells is unknown and not recommended. Resume pembrolizumab upon symptom control, or when prednisone/prednisolone daily dose <10 mg
	G4 hyperglycemia	Permanently discontinue pembrolizumab. Admit to hospital to manage hyperglycemia. Role of corticosteroids in preventing complete loss of insulin-producing cells is unknown and not recommended

(*continued*)

Treatment Modifications (continued)

Adverse Event	Grade/Severity	Treatment Modification
Nephritis and renal dysfunction	G2/3 (serum creatinine 1.5–6× ULN)	Withhold pembrolizumab. Administer oral prednisone/prednisolone at a dose of 0.5–2.0 mg/kg/day or its equivalent. When improves to G1, begin a slow corticosteroid taper over at least 4 weeks. If does not respond adequately, then administer 0.5–1 mg/kg IV (methyl)prednisolone and convert to 0.5–2.0 mg/kg prednisone/prednisolone orally each day or its equivalent only after a response, followed by a taper over at least 4 weeks when improves to G1. Resume pembrolizumab upon symptom control, or when prednisone/prednisolone daily dose <10 mg
	G4 (serum creatinine >6× ULN)	Permanently discontinue pembrolizumab. Administer 0.5–1 mg/kg IV (methyl)prednisolone and convert to 0.5–2.0 mg/kg prednisone/prednisolone orally each day or its equivalent only after a response, followed by a taper over at least 4 weeks when improves to G1
Skin	G1/2	Continue pembrolizumab. Avoid skin irritants, avoid sun exposure, topical emollients recommended. Topical steroid (mild strength for G1, moderate/potent strength for G2) cream once or twice daily ± oral or topical antihistamines for itching
	G3 rash or suspected SJS or TEN	Withhold pembrolizumab. Avoid skin irritants, avoid sun exposure, topical emollients recommended. Administer oral or topical antihistamines for itching. Administer oral prednisone/prednisolone at a dose of 0.5–2.0 mg/kg or its equivalent daily for 3 days followed by a slow corticosteroid taper over at least 4 weeks when the rash improves to G1. If does not respond adequately, then administer 0.5–1 mg/kg IV (methyl)prednisolone and convert to 0.5–2.0 mg/kg prednisone/prednisolone orally each day or its equivalent only after a response, followed by a taper over at least 4 weeks when the rash improves to G1. Resume pembrolizumab upon symptom control, or when prednisone/prednisolone daily dose <10 mg
	G4 rash or confirmed SJS or TEN	Avoid skin irritants, avoid sun exposure, topical emollients recommended. Administer oral or topical antihistamines for itching. Administer 1–2 mg/kg IV (methyl)prednisolone and convert to oral steroids 0.5–2.0 mg/kg prednisone/prednisolone each day or its equivalent only after a response. Taper over at least 4 weeks when the rash improves to G1. Permanently discontinue pembrolizumab
Encephalitis	Confusion or altered behavior, headaches, alteration in Glasgow Coma Scale, motor or sensory deficits, speech abnormality, may or may not be febrile	Initially withhold pembrolizumab, but permanently discontinue pembrolizumab if there is no doubt as to diagnosis. Exclude bacterial and ideally viral infections prior to high-dose steroids. Administer oral prednisone/prednisolone at a dose of 0.5–2.0 mg/kg/day or its equivalent. When symptoms improve, begin a slow corticosteroid taper over at least 4–8 weeks. If symptoms are severe, administer 1–2 mg/kg IV (methyl)prednisolone and convert to 0.5–2.0 mg/kg prednisone/prednisolone orally each day or its equivalent only after a response. Consider concurrent empiric antiviral (IV acyclovir) and antibacterial therapy
Aseptic meningitis	Headache, photophobia, neck stiffness with fever or may be afebrile, vomiting; normal cognition/cerebral function (distinguishes from encephalitis)	
Other syndromes include neurosarcoidosis, posterior reversible leukoencephalopathy syndrome (PRES), Vogt-Koyanagi-Harada syndrome, demyelination, vasculitic encephalopathy, and generalized seizures		
Transverse myelitis	Acute or subacute neurologic signs/symptoms of motor/sensory/autonomic origin; most have sensory level; often bilateral symptoms	Initially withhold pembrolizumab, but permanently discontinue pembrolizumab if there is no doubt as to diagnosis. Administer 2 mg/kg IV (methyl)prednisolone or consider 1 g/day and convert to 0.5–2.0 mg/kg prednisone/prednisolone orally each day or its equivalent only after a response. When symptoms improve, begin a slow corticosteroid taper over at least 4–8 weeks. Plasmapheresis may be required if steroids do not bring about improvement
Myocarditis	G3	Permanently discontinue pembrolizumab. Administer 2 mg/kg IV (methyl)prednisolone or consider 1 g/day and convert to 0.5–2.0 mg/kg prednisone/prednisolone orally each day or its equivalent only after a response. When symptoms improve, begin a slow corticosteroid taper over at least 4–8 weeks. If no response, add MMF 500–1000 mg twice daily. If worse on MMF, consider adding tacrolimus
Peripheral neurologic toxicity	Moderate: some interference with ADL, symptoms concerning to patient	Withhold pembrolizumab. Initial observation reasonable or initiate prednisone/prednisolone 0.5–1 mg/kg (if progressing, eg, from mild) and/or pregabalin or duloxetine for pain. When symptoms improve, begin a slow corticosteroid taper over at least 4 weeks. Resume pembrolizumab upon symptom control, or when prednisone/prednisolone daily dose <10 mg
	Severe: limits self-care and aids warranted, life-threatening, eg, respiratory problems	Permanently discontinue pembrolizumab. Administer 1–2 mg/kg IV (methyl)prednisolone and convert to 0.5–2.0 mg/kg prednisone/prednisolone orally each day or its equivalent only after a response. Taper over at least 4–8 weeks when symptoms improve to G1

(continued)

Treatment Modifications (*continued*)

Adverse Event	Grade/Severity	Treatment Modification
Guillain-Barré syndrome	Progressive symmetrical muscle weakness with absent or reduced tendon reflexes—involves extremities, facial, respiratory, and bulbar and oculomotor muscles; dysregulation of autonomic nerves	Permanently discontinue pembrolizumab. Use of steroids not recommended in idiopathic Guillain-Barré syndrome; however, a trial of (methyl)prednisolone 1–2 mg/kg is reasonable, converting to 0.5–2.0 mg/kg prednisone/prednisolone orally each day or its equivalent only after a response. If no improvement or worsening, plasmapheresis or IVIG indicated
Myasthenia gravis	Fluctuating muscle weakness (proximal limb, trunk, ocular, eg, ptosis/diplopia or bulbar) with fatigability, respiratory muscles may also be involved	Permanently discontinue pembrolizumab. Administer pyridostigmine at an initial dose of 30 mg three times daily. Administer oral prednisone/prednisolone at a dose of 0.5–2.0 mg/kg/day or its equivalent or 1–2 mg/kg IV (methyl)prednisolone depending on the severity of symptoms. If begin with IV, convert to 0.5–2.0 mg/kg prednisone/prednisolone orally each day or its equivalent only after a response. If no improvement or worsening, plasmapheresis or IVIG may be considered. Additional immunosuppressants used in myasthenia gravis include azathioprine, cyclosporine, and mycophenolate. Avoid certain medications, eg, ciprofloxacin, beta-blockers, that may precipitate cholinergic crisis
Other syndromes including motor and sensory peripheral neuropathy, multifocal radicular neuropathy/plexopathy, autonomic neuropathy, phrenic nerve palsy, cranial nerve palsies (eg, facial nerve, optic nerve, hypoglossal nerve)		Permanently discontinue pembrolizumab. Administer oral prednisone/prednisolone at a dose of 0.5–2.0 mg/kg/day or its equivalent or 1–2 mg/kg IV (methyl)prednisolone depending on the severity of symptoms. If begin with IV, convert to 0.5–2.0 mg/kg prednisone/prednisolone orally each day or its equivalent only after a response
Arthralgia	G1 (mild pain with inflammation, erythema or joint swelling)	Continue pembrolizumab. Administer acetaminophen (paracetamol) and ibuprofen
	G2 (moderate pain with inflammation, erythema, or joint swelling that limits ADLs)	Withhold pembrolizumab. Administer higher doses of acetaminophen (paracetamol) and ibuprofen, and use diclofenac or naproxen or etoricoxib. If inadequately controlled, consider intra-articular steroid injections for large joints or administer oral prednisone/prednisolone at a dose of 0.5–2.0 mg/kg/day or its equivalent. When improves to G1, begin a slow corticosteroid taper over at least 4 weeks. If does not respond adequately, then administer 0.5–1 mg/kg IV (methyl)prednisolone and convert to 0.5–2.0 mg/kg prednisone/prednisolone orally each day or its equivalent only after a response, followed by a taper over at least 4 weeks when improves to G1. Resume pembrolizumab upon symptom control, or when prednisone/prednisolone daily dose <10 mg
	G3 (severe pain; irreversible joint damage; disabling; limits self-care ADL)	Withhold pembrolizumab. Administer 0.5–1 mg/kg IV (methyl)prednisolone and convert to 0.5–2.0 mg/kg prednisone/prednisolone orally each day or its equivalent only after a response, followed by a taper over at least 4 weeks when improves to G1. In severe cases, infliximab or another anti–TNF alpha drug may be required for improvement of arthritis. Resume pembrolizumab upon symptom control, or when prednisone/prednisolone daily dose <10 mg
Other	First occurrence of other G3	Withhold pembrolizumab. Administer oral prednisone/prednisolone at a dose of 0.5–2.0 mg/kg/day or its equivalent. When improves to G1, begin a slow corticosteroid taper over at least 4 weeks. Resume pembrolizumab upon symptom control, or when prednisone/prednisolone daily dose <10 mg
	Recurrence of same G3	Permanently discontinue pembrolizumab. Administer 1–2 mg/kg IV (methyl)prednisolone and convert to 0.5–2.0 mg/kg prednisone/prednisolone orally each day or its equivalent only after a response. Taper over at least 4–8 weeks when symptoms improve to G1
	Life-threatening or G4	
	Requirement for ≥10 mg/day prednisone or equivalent for >12 weeks	Permanently discontinue pembrolizumab
	Persistent G2/3 adverse reactions lasting ≥12 weeks	

ADL, activities of daily living; ALT, alanine aminotransferase; AST, aspartate aminotransferase; ATG, anti-thymocyte globulin; SJS, Stevens-Johnson Syndrome; TEN, toxic epidermal necrolysis; ULN, upper limit of normal.

Notes on general supportive care:
• Steroid taper in most cases will proceed over a minimum of 1 month, but if symptoms improve rapidly, a 2-week taper can be considered. If steroids are administered for more than 4 weeks, consider PCP prophylaxis (cotrimoxazole 480 mg twice daily M/W/F or inhaled pentamidine if has cotrimoxazole allergy), regular random blood glucose, vitamin D level and starting calcium/vitamin D supplementation per guidelines

Adverse Events (N = 1251)

Event	Pembrolizumab (n = 636)		Chemotherapy (n = 615)	
Grade (%)	Grade 1 or 2	Grade 3–5	Grade 1 or 2	Grade 3–5
Any event	45	18	49	41
Event leading to discontinuation	1	8	2	7
Event leading to death	0	2	0	2
Hypothyroidism	11	<1	<1	0
Fatigue	7	<1	15	1
Pruritis	7	<1	2	0
Rash	7	<1	4	0
Alanine aminotransferase increased	6	1	8	<1
Pneumonitis	4	3	0	0
Aspartate aminotransferase increased	6	<1	7	<1
Decreased appetite	6	<1	16	1
Hyperthyroidism	6	<1	<1	0
Anemia	5	<1	24	13
Diarrhea	5	<1	7	<1
Nausea	5	0	29	1
Arthralgia	4	0	7	0
Asthenia	4	<1	8	2
Myalgia	3	<1	8	0
Vomiting	2	0	15	<1
Leukopenia	2	0	4	2
Constipation	1	0	11	0
Stomatitis	1	0	5	0
Neutropenia	<1	<1	7	7
Peripheral sensory neuropathy	<1	0	6	1
Thrombocytopenia	<1	<1	7	2
White blood cell count decreased	<1	0	6	5
Alopecia	<1	0	21	1
Neutrophil count decreased	<1	0	5	9
Platelet count decreased	<1	0	7	3
Neuropathy peripheral	<1	0	7	<1

Adverse events were included in the table if they were considered treatment-related and if they were reported by ≥5% of patients in either group (except for events leading to death). All data correspond to the as-treated populations. Adverse events were graded according to the National Cancer Institute Common Terminology Criteria for Adverse Events, v4.0

Adverse events of interest

Event	Pembrolizumab (n = 636)		Chemotherapy (n = 615)	
Grade (%)	Grade 1 or 2	Grade 3–5	Grade 1 or 2	Grade 3–5
Any event	20	8	6	1
Hypothyroidism	12	<1	1	0
Pneumonitis	5	3	<1	<1
Hyperthyroidism	6	<1	<1	0
Severe skin reactions	<1	2	<1	<1
Infusion reactions	1	<1	3	1
Thyroiditis	2	0	0	0
Hepatitis	<1	1	0	0
Colitis	<1	<1	<1	<1
Adrenal insufficiency	<1	<1	<1	0
Hypophysitis	0	<1	0	0
Nephritis	<1	<1	0	0
Myocarditis	0	<1	0	0
Pancreatitis	<1	0	0	0

Adverse events included in this table were adverse events of interest, which are infusion reactions and events with an immune-mediated cause but which are not necessarily attributed to treatment by the investigators. The data included correspond to the as-treated populations. Adverse events were graded according to the National Cancer Institute Common Terminology Criteria for Adverse Events, v4.0

ADVANCED NSCLC • FIRST-LINE
LUNG CANCER REGIMEN: PACLITAXEL + CARBOPLATIN

Kelly K et al. J Clin Oncol 2001;19:3210–3218

Premedication (primary prophylaxis against hypersensitivity reactions from paclitaxel):
Dexamethasone 20 mg/dose for 2 doses; administer orally the evening before and the morning of chemotherapy prior to paclitaxel, *plus:*
Diphenhydramine 50 mg for 1 dose; administer by intravenous injection 30 minutes before paclitaxel, *and:*
Ranitidine 50 mg or **cimetidine** 300 mg for 1 dose; administer intravenously in 25–100 mL 0.9% sodium chloride injection (0.9% NS) or 5% dextrose injection (D5W) over 5–30 minutes, 30 minutes before paclitaxel
Paclitaxel 225 mg/m²; administer intravenously in a volume of 0.9% NS or D5W sufficient to produce a solution with concentration within the range 0.3–1.2 mg/mL over 3 hours on day 1, every 3 weeks (total dosage/cycle = 225 mg/m²)
Carboplatin (calculated dose) AUC = 6 mg/mL × min; administer intravenously in 50–150 mL D5W over 15–30 minutes, on day 1, every 3 weeks (total dosage/cycle calculated to produce an AUC = 6 mg/mL × min) (see equation below)

Supportive Care
Antiemetic prophylaxis
Emetogenic potential: **HIGH**. *Potential for delayed symptoms*
See Chapter 42 for antiemetic recommendations

Hematopoietic growth factor (CSF) prophylaxis
Primary prophylaxis is indicated with one of the following:
Filgrastim (G-CSF) 5mcg/kg per day by subcutaneous injection, *or*
  Pegfilgrastim (pegylated filgrastim) 6mg/0.6mL by subcutaneous injection for 1 dose
  • Begin use from 24–72 hours after myelosuppressive chemotherapy is completed
  • Continue filgrastim until ANC >10,000/mm³ on 2 consecutive daily measurements
See Chapter 43 for more information

Antimicrobial prophylaxis
Risk of fever and neutropenia is **LOW**
  Antimicrobial primary prophylaxis to be considered:
  • Antibacterial—not indicated
  • Antifungal—not indicated
  • Antiviral—not indicated unless patient previously had an episode of HSV

Additional supportive care
Dexamethasone 8 mg/dose orally every 12 hours for 6 doses after chemotherapy if G ≥2 arthralgias/myalgias occur
Add a **proton pump inhibitor** during dexamethasone use to prevent gastritis and duodenitis

Note: carboplatin dose is based on Calvert's formula to achieve a target area under the plasma concentration versus time curve (AUC) [AUC units = mg/mL × min]

$$\text{Total carboplatin dose (mg)} = (\text{Target AUC}) \times (\text{GFR} + 25)$$

In practice, creatinine clearance (CrCl) is used in place of glomerular filtration rate (GFR). CrCl can be calculated from the equation of Cockcroft and Gault:

$$\text{For males, Clcr} = \frac{(140 - \text{age [years]}) \times \text{body weight (kg)}}{72 \times (\text{Serum creatinine [mg/dL]})}$$

$$\text{For females, Clcr} = \frac{(140 - \text{age [years]}) \times \text{body weight (kg)}}{72 \times (\text{Serum creatinine [mg/dL]})} \times 0.85$$

Calvert AH et al. J Clin Oncol 1989;7:1748–1756
Cockcroft DW, Gault MH. Nephron 1976;16:31–41
Jodrell DI et al. J Clin Oncol 1992;10:520–528
Sorensen BT et al. Cancer Chemother Pharmacol 1991;28:397–401

Treatment Modifications

Adverse Event	Dose Modification
ANC nadir <500/mm^3, platelet nadir <50,000/mm^3, or febrile neutropenia	Reduce carboplatin dosage to AUC = 5 if previous cycle dose was AUC = 6; or to AUC = 4 if previous cycle dose was AUC = 5
ANC nadir <500/mm^3, platelet nadir <50,000/mm^3, or febrile neutropenia after 2 carboplatin dose reductions (AUC in previous cycle = 4)	Reduce paclitaxel dosage to 200 mg/m^2, and decrease carboplatin dosage to AUC = 3
Day 1 ANC <1500/mm^3 or platelets <100,000/mm^3	Delay chemotherapy until ANC >1500/mm^3 and platelets >100,000/mm^3, for maximum delay of 2 weeks
Delay of >2 weeks in reaching ANC >1500/mm^3 and platelet nadir >100,000/mm^3	Discontinue therapy
G2 neurotoxicity	Reduce paclitaxel dosage to 200 mg/m^2
G3 neurotoxicity	Reduce paclitaxel dosage to 175 mg/m^2
G2 arthralgia/myalgia despite dexamethasone prophylaxis	Reduce paclitaxel dosage to 200 mg/m^2
G3 arthralgia/myalgia despite dexamethasone prophylaxis	Reduce paclitaxel dosage to 175 mg/m^2
G ≥2 AST or G ≥3 total bilirubin	Hold paclitaxel
Moderate hypersensitivity	Patient may be re-treated
Severe hypersensitivity	Discontinue therapy
Chest pain or arrhythmia during chemotherapy	Immediately stop chemotherapy and evaluate the patient
Symptomatic arrhythmias, or ≥2-degree AV block, or an ischemic event	Discontinue therapy

Patient Population Studied

The study compared paclitaxel + carboplatin, the regimen here to a combination of vinorelbine and cisplatin in 206 patients with advanced, previously untreated NSCLC

Efficacy (N = 203)*

Response rate (CR + PR)	25%
Median progression-free survival	4 months
Median survival	8.6 months
1-year survival	38%
2-year survival	15%

*WHO criteria

Toxicity (N = 203)*

Adverse Event	% G3	% G4
Hematologic		
Leukopenia	26	5
Neutropenia	21	36
Thrombocytopenia	10	0
Anemia	11	2
Non-hematologic		
Nausea	7	0
Sensory neuropathy	13	0
Vomiting	4	0
Dehydration	4	0
Fatigue	8	0
Hyponatremia	3	0
Weakness (motor neuropathy)	8	0
Respiratory infection/neutropenia	1	0

*NCI CTC, National Cancer Institute (USA) Common Toxicity Criteria, version 2.0. Available at: http://ctep.cancer.gov/protocolDevelopment/electronic_applications/ctc.htm [accessed December 7, 2013]

Therapy Monitoring

1. *Before each cycle:* H&P, PS evaluation, CBC with differential, LFTs, BUN, and creatinine
2. *Every week:* CBC with differential and platelet count
3. *Response evaluation:* every 2–3 cycles

ADVANCED NSCLC • FIRST-LINE
LUNG CANCER REGIMEN: GEMCITABINE + CISPLATIN

Sandler AB et al. J Clin Oncol 2000;18:122–130

Gemcitabine 1000 mg/m^2; administer intravenously in 50–250 mL 0.9% sodium chloride injection (0.9% NS) over 30–60 minutes, on days 1, 8, and 15, every 28 days (total dosage/cycle = 3000 mg/m^2). On day 1, administer after or during hydration for cisplatin and follow with cisplatin
Hydration before cisplatin: ≥1000 mL 0.9% NS; administer intravenously over a minimum of 2–4 hours

Cisplatin 100 mg/m^2; administer intravenously in 100–250 mL 0.9% NS over 30–120 minutes, on day 1 every 28 days (total dosage/cycle = 100 mg/m^2)
Hydration after cisplatin: ≥1000 mL 0.9% NS; administer intravenously over a minimum of 2–4 hours. Also encourage patients to increase oral intake of nonalcoholic fluids. Monitor serum electrolytes and replace as needed (potassium, magnesium, sodium)

Supportive Care
Antiemetic prophylaxis
Emetogenic potential on day 1 is **HIGH**. *Potential for delayed symptoms*
Emetogenic potential on days 8 and 15 is **LOW**
See Chapter 42 for antiemetic recommendations

Hematopoietic growth factor (CSF) prophylaxis
Primary prophylaxis is **NOT** *indicated*
See Chapter 43 for more information

Antimicrobial prophylaxis
Risk of fever and neutropenia is **LOW**
   Antimicrobial primary prophylaxis to be considered:
   • Antibacterial—not indicated
   • Antifungal—not indicated
   • Antiviral—not indicated unless patient previously had an episode of HSV

Patient Population Studied

A randomized comparison with single-agent cisplatin in 260 patients with advanced (stage III/IV) previously untreated NSCLC

Efficacy (N = 260)

Complete response	1.2%
Partial response	29.2%
Estimated median progression-free survival	5.6 months
Estimated median survival	9.1 months
Estimated 1-year survival	39%

Toxicity (N = 260)[*]

	% G3	% G4
Hematologic		
Granulocytopenia	21.5	35.3
Thrombocytopenia	25	25.4
Anemia	21.9	3.1
Febrile neutropenia	4.6% of patients	
Platelet transfusions	20.4% of patients	
Erythrocyte transfusions	37.7% of patients	
Non-hematologic		
Nausea	25	2
Vomiting	11	12
Increased creatinine	4.4	0.4
Neurologic (hearing)	5.6	0.4
Neurologic (motor)	11.5	0
Dyspnea	4	3
Increased transaminases	2	1
Increased bilirubin	0.8	0.8

[*]WHO criteria

Treatment Modifications

Adverse Event	Dose Modification
ANC <1500/mm³, or platelets <100,000/mm³	Hold chemotherapy until ANC >1500/mm³ and platelets >100,000/mm³
Febrile granulocytopenia that requires antibiotics	Reduce cisplatin and gemcitabine dosages by 25% in subsequent cycles
Bleeding associated with thrombocytopenia	
Intracycle: G1/2 non-hematologic toxicity or G1–3 nausea or vomiting	100% gemcitabine dosage on days 8 and 15
Intracycle: G3 non-hematologic toxicity, except nausea, vomiting, and alopecia	Reduce gemcitabine dosage by 25% on days 8 and 15, or hold treatment at clinician's discretion
Intracycle: G4 non-hematologic toxicity	Hold gemcitabine
Day 1 serum creatinine 1.6–2.0 mg/dL (141–177 µmol/L)	Reduce cisplatin dosage by 25%
Day 1 serum creatinine >2.0 mg/dL (>177 µmol/L)	Hold cisplatin until serum creatinine ≤2.0 mg/dL (≤177 µmol/L)
G3/4 neurotoxicity	Delay treatment until toxicity resolves to G1
Treatment delay >2 weeks	Discontinue therapy according to clinician's discretion

----

Therapy Monitoring

1. *Each cycle on day 1:* H&P, performance status reevaluation, CBC with differential andplatelet count, serum electrolytes, magnesium, serum creatinine, hepatic transaminases, and bilirubin
2. *Cycle days 8 and 15:* CBC with differential and platelet count
3. *Response evaluation:* every 2–3 cycles

ADVANCED NSCLC • FIRST-LINE
LUNG CANCER REGIMEN: DOCETAXEL + CISPLATIN

Fossella F et al. J Clin Oncol 2003;21:3016–3024

Prophylaxis for fluid retention and hypersensitivity reactions from docetaxel:
Dexamethasone 8 mg/dose; administer orally twice daily for 3 days, starting the day before docetaxel is administered (total dose/cycle = 48 mg)

Hydration before cisplatin: ≥1000 mL 0.9% sodium chloride injection (0.9% NS); administer intravenously over a minimum of 2–4 hours
Docetaxel 75 mg/m²; administer intravenously in a volume of 0.9% NS or 5% dextrose injection (D5W) sufficient to produce a solution with concentration within the range 0.3–0.74 mg/mL over 1 hour on day 1, every 3 weeks (total dosage/cycle = 75 mg/m²), *followed immediately by:*
Cisplatin 75 mg/m²; administer intravenously in 100–250 mL 0.9% NS over 1 hour on day 1, every 3 weeks (total dosage/cycle = 75 mg/m²)

Hydration after cisplatin: ≥1000 mL 0.9% NS; administer intravenously over a minimum of 2–4 hours. Encourage patients to increase oral intake of nonalcoholic fluids. Monitor serum electrolytes and replace as needed (potassium, magnesium, sodium)

Supportive Care
Antiemetic prophylaxis
Emetogenic potential: **HIGH**. *Potential for delayed symptoms*
See Chapter 42 for antiemetic recommendations

Hematopoietic growth factor (CSF) prophylaxis
Primary prophylaxis is indicated with one of the following:
Filgrastim (G-CSF) 5 mcg/kg per day by subcutaneous injection, *or*
Pegfilgrastim (pegylated filgrastim) 6 mg/0.6mL by subcutaneous injection for 1 dose
• Begin use from 24–72 hours after myelosuppressive chemotherapy is completed
• Continue filgrastim until ANC >10,000/mm³ on 2 consecutive daily measurements
See Chapter 43 for more information

Antimicrobial prophylaxis
Risk of fever and neutropenia is **LOW**
Antimicrobial primary prophylaxis to be considered:
• Antibacterial—not indicated
• Antifungal—not indicated
• Antiviral—not indicated unless patient previously had an episode of HSV

Patient Population Studied

A multicenter, international, prospective, open-label, randomized phase 3 comparison with vinorelbine + cisplatin in 408 patients with locally advanced or recurrent (stage IIIB) or metastatic (stage IV) NSCLC

Efficacy (N = 408)

Complete response	2.0%
Partial response	29.7%
Overall median survival	11.3 months
1-year survival	46%
2-year survival	21%

Therapy Monitoring

1. *Each cycle on day 1:* H&P, PS evaluation, CBC with differential, serum electrolytes, magnesium, BUN, creatinine, and LFTs
2. *Every week:* CBC with differential and platelet count
3. *Response evaluation:* every 2–3 cycles

Toxicity (N = 406)*

Toxicity[†]	% G3/4
Hematologic	
Leukopenia	42.8
Neutropenia	74.8
Thrombocytopenia	2.7
Anemia	6.9
Erythrocyte transfusions	10.3% of patients
Non-hematologic	
Infection	8.4
Asthenia	12.3
Nausea	9.9
Pulmonary	9.6
Pain	7.9
Vomiting	7.9
Diarrhea	6.7
Anorexia	5.4

*NCI CTC, National Cancer Institute (USA) Common Toxicity Criteria, version 2.0. Available at: http://ctep.cancer.gov/protocolDevelopment/electronic_applications/ctc.htm [accessed December 7, 2013]
[†]G3/4 adverse event in >5% of patients

Treatment Modifications

Adverse Event	Dose Modification
ANC <1500/mm^3 or platelet count <100,000/mm^3	Hold chemotherapy until ANC >1500/mm^3 and platelets >100,000/mm^3
Febrile granulocytopenia that requires antibiotics	Reduce cisplatin and docetaxel dosages by 25% during subsequent cycles*
Bleeding associated with thrombocytopenia	
Day 1 serum creatinine 1.6–2.0 mg/dL (141–177 μmol/L)	Reduce cisplatin dosage* by 25%
Day 1 serum creatinine >2.0 mg/dL (>177 μmol/L)	Hold cisplatin until serum creatinine ≤2.0 mg/dL (≤177 μmol/L)
G3/4 neurotoxicity	Delay treatment
Treatment delay ≥2 weeks	Discontinue therapy or according to clinician's criteria

*A maximum of 2 docetaxel or cisplatin dosage reductions are permitted

ADVANCED NSCLC • FIRST-LINE

LUNG CANCER REGIMEN: VINORELBINE + CISPLATIN

Wozniak AJ et al. J Clin Oncol 1998;16:2459–2465

Vinorelbine 25 mg/m^2 per dose; administer intravenously in a volume of 0.9% sodium chloride injection (0.9% NS) or 5% dextrose injection (D5W) sufficient to produce a solution with concentration within the range 0.5–3 mg/mL over 6–10 minutes, once weekly on days 1, 8, 15, and 22, every 4 weeks (total dosage/cycle = 100 mg/m^2)
Hydration before cisplatin: ≥1000 mL 0.9% NS; administer intravenously over a minimum of 2–4 hours
Cisplatin 100 mg/m^2; administer intravenously in 100–250 mL 0.9% NS over 1 hour on day 1, every 4 weeks (total dosage/cycle = 100 mg/m^2)
Hydration after cisplatin: ≥1000 mL 0.9% NS; administer intravenously over a minimum of 2–4 hours. Encourage patients to increase oral intake of nonalcoholic fluids. Monitor serum electrolytes and replace as needed (potassium, magnesium, sodium)

Supportive Care
Antiemetic prophylaxis
Emetogenic potential: **HIGH**. *Potential for delayed symptoms*
See Chapter 42 for antiemetic recommendations

Hematopoietic growth factor (CSF) prophylaxis
Primary prophylaxis may be indicated
See Chapter 43 for more information

Antimicrobial prophylaxis
Risk of fever and neutropenia is **LOW**
   Antimicrobial primary prophylaxis to be considered:
   • Antibacterial—not indicated
   • Antifungal—not indicated
   • Antiviral—not indicated unless patient previously had an episode of HSV

Patient Population Studied

A randomized comparison with cisplatin of 206 patients with advanced previously untreated NSCLC

Efficacy

Complete response	2%
Partial response	24%
Median progression-free survival	4 months
Median survival	8 months
1-year survival	36%
2-year survival	12%

Toxicity (N = 204)*

Hematologic

	% G3	% G4
Granulocytopenia	22	59
Thrombocytopenia	4	1
Anemia	21	3

Non-hematologic

	% G3/4
Fever/sepsis with granulocytopenia	10
Nausea/vomiting	20
Malaise/weakness	15
Constipation	3
Diarrhea	3
Electrolyte imbalance	6
Hearing	4
Vision	1
Neurologic (peripheral)	2
Neurologic (central)	2
Renal	5
Phlebitis/thrombosis	3

*SWOG criteria

Treatment Modifications

Treatment day ANC must be ≥1500/mm^3 and platelets ≥100,000/mm^3 to treat on schedule at 100% dosages

Adverse Event	Dose Modification
Treatment day ANC 1000–1499/mm^3 or platelets 75,000–99,999/mm^3	Reduce cisplatin and vinorelbine dosages by 50%
Treatment day ANC <1000 or platelets <75,000/mm^3	Hold cisplatin* and vinorelbine
Treatment delay >2 weeks but <3 weeks	Reduce subsequent cisplatin and vinorelbine dosages by 50%
Fever or sepsis with neutropenia in any cycle	
ANC nadir <500/mm^3 or platelet nadir <50,000/mm^3	Reduce cisplatin dosage by 50% in subsequent cycles
Serum creatinine ≥1.6 mg/dL (≥141 μmol/L), but creatinine clearance ≥50 mL/min (≥0.83 mL/s)	Reduce cisplatin dosage by 50%
Creatinine clearance <50 mL/min (<0.83 mL/s)	Hold cisplatin*
Serum total bilirubin 2.1–3.0 mg/dL (35.9–51.3 μmol/L)	Reduce vinorelbine dosage by 50%
Serum total bilirubin >3.0 mg/dL (>51.3 μmol/L)	Reduce vinorelbine dosage by 75%
Treatment delay >4 weeks	Discontinue therapy

*If cisplatin treatment is held for any period of time, reduce cisplatin dosage 50% when treatment resumes

Therapy Monitoring

1. *Before repeated cycles:* H&P, PS evaluation, serum creatinine and calculated creatinine clearance; serum electrolytes, magnesium, hepatic transaminases, and bilirubin
2. *Weekly:* CBC with differential and platelet count
3. *Response evaluation:* every 2–3 cycles

ADVANCED NSCLC • FIRST-LINE
LUNG CANCER REGIMEN: WEEKLY *NAB*-PACLITAXEL + CARBOPLATIN

Socinski MA et al. J Clin Oncol 2012;30:2055–2062

Paclitaxel protein-bound particles for injectable suspension (nab-paclitaxel) 100 mg/m² per dose; administer intravenously over 30 minutes, once weekly for 3 doses, on days 1, 8, and 15 every 3 weeks (total dosage/cycle = 300 mg/m²)

Carboplatin [calculated dose] AUC = 6 mg/mL × min*; administer intravenously diluted to concentrations as low as 0.5 mg/mL with either 5% dextrose injection or 0.9% sodium chloride injection over 15–30 minutes on day 1, every 3 weeks (total dosage/cycle calculated to produce an AUC = 6 mg/mL × min)

*Carboplatin dose is based on a formula described by Calvert et al. to achieve a target area under the plasma concentration versus time curve (AUC)

Recommendations for Initial nab-Paclitaxel Dosage in Hepatically Impaired Patients

	SGOT (AST) Levels		Total Bilirubin Levels	nab-Paclitaxel Dosage*
Mild	<10 × ULN	*and*	> ULN to ≤1.25 × ULN	100mg/m²
Moderate	<10 × ULN		1.26–2 × ULN	75mg/m²
Severe	<10 × ULN		2.01–5 × ULN	50mg/m²†
	>10 × ULN	*or*	>5 × ULN	Do not administer

*A need for dosage adjustments during repeated treatment cycles should be based on individual tolerance for previous treatment
†Increase dose to 75mg/m² during subsequent courses, as tolerated

$$\text{Total carboplatin dose (mg)} = (\text{Target AUC}) \times (\text{GFR} + 25)$$

In practice, creatinine clearance (CrCl) is used in place of glomerular filtration rate (GFR). CrCl can be estimated from the equation of Cockcroft and Gault, thus:

$$\text{For males, Clcr} = \frac{(140 - \text{age [years]}) \times \text{body weight (kg)}}{72 \times (\text{Serum creatinine } \lceil mg/dL \rceil)}$$

$$\text{For females, Clcr} = \frac{(140 - \text{age [years]}) \times \text{body weight (kg)}}{72 \times (\text{Serum creatinine } \lceil mg/dL \rceil)} \times 0.85$$

Calvert AH et al. J Clin Oncol 1989;7:1748–1756
Cockcroft DW, Gault MH. Nephron 1976;16:31–41
Jodrell DI et al. J Clin Oncol 1992;10:520–528
Sorensen BT et al. Cancer Chemother Pharmacol 1991;28:397–401

Supportive Care
Antiemetic prophylaxis
Emetogenic potential on with nab-*paclitaxel alone is* **LOW**
Emetogenic potential on days with carboplatin *alone is* **MODERATE–HIGH**. *Potential for delayed symptoms*
See Chapter 42 for antiemetic recommendations
Hematopoietic growth factor (CSF) prophylaxis
Primary prophylaxis may be indicated
See Chapter 43 for more information

Antimicrobial prophylaxis
Risk of fever and neutropenia is **LOW**
  Antimicrobial primary prophylaxis to be considered:
  • Antibacterial—not indicated
  • Antifungal—not indicated
  • Antiviral—not indicated unless patient previously had an episode of HSV

Toxicity

Most Common Treatment-Related G $\geq$ 3 Adverse Events According to NCI CTCAE

	nab-PC (%) (N = 514)		Sb-PC (%) (N = 524)		P
	G3	G4	G3	G4	
Hematologic Adverse Events					
Neutropenia	33	14	32	26	<0.001*
Thrombocytopenia	13	5	7	2	<0.00†
Anemia	22	5	6	<1	<0.001†
Febrile neutropenia	<1	<1	1	<1	N/S
Non-hematologic Adverse Events					
Fatigue	4	<1	6	<1	N/S
Sensory neuropathy	3	0	11	<1	<0.001*
Anorexia	2	0	<1	0	N/S
Nausea	<1	0	<1	0	N/S
Myalgia	<1	0	2	0	0.011*
Arthralgia	0	0	2	0	0.008*

N/S, not significant; nab-PC, 130-nm albumin-bound paclitaxel + carboplatin; NCI CTCAE, National Cancer Institute Common Terminology Criteria for Adverse Events; sb-PC, conventional (solvent-based) paclitaxel + carboplatin
*P<0.05 in favor of nab-PC
†P<0.05 in favor of sb-PC

Patient Population Studied

Patients with histologically/cytologically confirmed nonresectable stage IIIB (± pleural effusion) or stage IV NSCLC, Eastern Cooperative Oncology Group performance status of 0–1, who had not previously received treatment for metastatic disease and had no radiotherapy within 4 weeks before enrollment. Prior adjuvant chemotherapy was allowed if it had been completed 12 months prior to enrollment. Patients with CNS metastases and those with neuropathy G≥1 were excluded

Dose Adjustments

Adapted in part from Abraxane for Injectable Suspension (paclitaxel protein-bound particles for injectable suspension) (albumin-bound); October 2012 product label. Celgene Corporation, Summit, NJ

Adverse Event	Treatment Modification
On day 1 of a cycle, ANC <1500/mm^3 or platelet count <100,000/mm^3	Withhold nab-paclitaxel and carboplatin until ANC ≥1500/mm^3 and platelet count ≥100,000/mm^3
On day 8 of a cycle, ANC <500/mm^3 or platelet count <50,000/mm^3	Withhold nab-paclitaxel and carboplatin until ANC ≥500/mm^3 and platelet count ≥50,000/mm^3
On day 15 of a cycle, ANC <500/mm^3 or platelet count <50,000/mm^3	Withhold nab-paclitaxel and carboplatin until ANC ≥500/mm^3 and platelet count ≥50,000/mm^3
Fever and neutropenia (ANC <500/mm^3 with fever >38°C [>100.4°F]), or delay of next cycle >7 days for ANC <1500/mm^3, or ANC <500/mm^3 >7 days at a weekly nab-paclitaxel dose of 100 mg/m^2 and carboplatin dose of AUC = 6 mg/mL × min	Reduce weekly nab-paclitaxel dose to 75 mg/m^2 and carboplatin dose to AUC = 4.5 mg/mL × min every 3 weeks
Fever and neutropenia (ANC <500/mm^3 with fever >38°C [>100.4°F]), or delay of next cycle >7 days for ANC <1500/mm^3, or ANC <500/mm^3 >7 days at a weekly *nab*-paclitaxel dose of 75 mg/m^2 and carboplatin dose of AUC = 4.5 mg/mL × min	Reduce weekly nab-paclitaxel dose to 50 mg/m^2 and carboplatin dose to AUC = 3 mg/mL × min every 3 weeks
Fever and neutropenia (ANC <500/mm^3 with fever >38°C [>100.4°F]), or delay of next cycle >7 days for ANC <1500/mm^3, or ANC <500/mm^3 >7 days at a weekly nab-paclitaxel dose of 50 mg/m^2 and carboplatin dose of AUC = 3 mg/mL × min	Discontinue nab-paclitaxel and carboplatin
Platelet count <50,000/mm^3 at a weekly nab-paclitaxel dose of 100 mg/m^2 and carboplatin dose of AUC >6 mg/mL × min	Reduce weekly nab-paclitaxel dose to 75 mg/m^2 and carboplatin dose to AUC = 4.5 mg/mL × min every 3 weeks
Platelet count <50,000/mm^3 at a weekly nab-paclitaxel dose of 75 mg/m^2 and carboplatin dose of AUC = 4.5 mg/mL × min	Discontinue nab-paclitaxel and carboplatin
G3/4 sensory neuropathy at a weekly nab-paclitaxel dose of 100 mg/m^2 and carboplatin dose of AUC = 6 mg/mL × min	Withhold nab-paclitaxel and carboplatin until toxicity G ≤1, then reduce weekly nab-paclitaxel dose to 75 mg/m^2 and carboplatin dose to AUC = 4.5 mg/mL × min every 3 weeks
G3/4 sensory neuropathy at a weekly nab-paclitaxel dose of 75 mg/m^2 and carboplatin dose of AUC = 4.5 mg/mL × min	Withhold nab-paclitaxel and carboplatin until toxicity G ≤1, then reduce weekly nab-paclitaxel dose to 50 mg/m^2 and carboplatin dose to AUC = 3.0 mg/mL × min every 3 weeks
G3/4 sensory neuropathy at a weekly nab-paclitaxel dose of 50 mg/m^2 and carboplatin dose of AUC = 3 mg/mL × min	Discontinue nab-paclitaxel and carboplatin

Efficacy

Response Rates for the Intent-to-Treat Population and Histologic Subset Based on Independent Radiologic Assessment

	nab-PC		sb-PC				
	%	95% CI	%	95% CI	RR Ratio	95% CI	P
Intent-to-treat	N = 521		N = 531				
Overall response	33%	28.6–36.7%	25%	21.2–28.5%	1.313	1.082–1.593	0.005
Complete response	0		<1%				
Partial response	33%		25%				
Stable disease	20%		24%				
Progressive disease	16%		16%				
Squamous subset	N = 229		N = 221				
Overall response	41	34.7–47.4%	24	18.8–30.1%	1.680	1.271–2.221	<0.001
Non-squamous subset	N = 292		N = 310				
Overall response	26	21.0–31.1	25	20.3–30.0	1.034	0.788–1.358	0.808

Progression-free Survival (PFS) and Overall Survival (OS)

	nab-PC		sb-PC				
	Months	95% CI	Months	95% CI	HR	95% CI	P
Median PFS	6.3	5.6–7.0	5.8	5.6–6.7	0.902	0.767–1.060	0.214
Median OS, ITT	12.1	10.8–12.9	11.2	10.3–12.6	0.922	0.797–1.066	0.271
Median OS, squamous subset	10.7	9.4–12.5	9.5	8.6–11.6	0.890	0.719–1.101	0.284
Median OS, non-squamous subset	13.1		13.0		0.950		
Median OS, <70 years	11.4		11.3		0.999		
Median OS, ≥70 years	19.9		10.4		0.583		0.009

HR, hazard ratio; nab-PC, 130-nm albumin-bound paclitaxel + carboplatin; RR ratio, response rate ratio; sb-PC, conventional (solvent-based) paclitaxel + carboplatin

Treatment Monitoring

1. *Monthly and as clinically indicated:* Complete blood counts (CBC) including differential white blood cell counts and liver function tests
2. *If G3/4 clinical or laboratory abnormalities are observed or if fever or infection occurs:* Frequent monitoring of complete blood counts (CBC) including differential white blood cell counts and liver function tests

ADVANCED NSCLC • FIRST-LINE
LUNG CANCER REGIMEN: VINORELBINE

Gridelli C et al. J Natl Cancer Inst 2003;95:362–372

Vinorelbine 30 mg/m² per dose; administer intravenously in a volume of 0.9% sodium chloride injection or 5% dextrose injection sufficient to produce a solution with concentration within the range 0.5–3 mg/mL over 6–10 minutes for 2 doses, on days 1 and 8 every 3 weeks for a maximum of 6 cycles (total dosage/cycle = 60 mg/m²)

Supportive Care
Antiemetic prophylaxis
Emetogenic potential is MINIMAL
See Chapter 42 for antiemetic recommendations

Hematopoietic growth factor (CSF) prophylaxis
Primary prophylaxis is NOT indicated
See Chapter 43 for more information

Antimicrobial prophylaxis
Risk of fever and neutropenia is LOW
Antimicrobial primary prophylaxis to be considered:
- Antibacterial—not indicated
- Antifungal—not indicated
- Antiviral—not indicated unless patient previously had an episode of HSV

Patient Population Studied

A randomized comparison of gemcitabine + vinorelbine in 233 patients age 70 years and older with advanced (stage IIIB/IV) untreated NSCLC

Efficacy
(Intent-to-Treat, N = 233)

Response rate	18%
Median survival	36 weeks
6-month survival	60%
Estimated 1-year survival	38%

Treatment Modifications

Adverse Event	Dose Modification
Days 1 and 8 ANC ≥1500/mm³, platelet count ≥100,000/mm³, and no organ toxicity (other than alopecia)	Vinorelbine given at 100% dosage
Days 1 and 8 ANC <1500/mm³, platelet count <100,000/mm³, or organ toxicity (other than alopecia)	Delay treatment for up to 2 weeks
Serum total bilirubin 2.1–3.0 mg/dL (35.9–51.3 µmol/L)	Reduce vinorelbine dosage by 50%
Serum total bilirubin >3.0 mg/dL (51.3 µmol/L)	Reduce vinorelbine dosage by 75%

Therapy Monitoring

1. *Days 1* and *8:* CBC with differential and platelet count. Serum electrolytes, BUN, creatinine, and LFTs
2. *Weekly:* CBC with differential and platelet count
3. *Response evaluation:* every 2–3 cycles

Toxicity (N = 229)*

	% G3	% G4
Hematologic		
Anemia	3	<1
Neutropenia	14	11
Thrombocytopenia	<1	—
Infection	3	—
Bleeding	1	—
Non-hematologic		
Nausea/vomiting	<1	—
Mucositis	1	—
Fatigue	7	—
Fever	2	—
Cardiac	1	<1
Pulmonary	1	—
Hepatic	<1	—
Constipation	3	<1
Peripheral neuropathy	1	—
Central neurotoxicity	—	<1

*WHO criteria

ADVANCED NON-SQUAMOUS NSCLC • MAINTENANCE
LUNG CANCER REGIMEN: PEMETREXED

Ciuleanu T et al. Lancet 2009;374:1432–1440

Ancillary medications:

Folic acid 350–1000 mcg per day; administer orally beginning 1–2 weeks before the first dose of pemetrexed and continuing until 3 weeks after the last dose of pemetrexed

Cyanocobalamin (vitamin B$_{12}$) 1000 mcg; administer intramuscularly every 9 weeks, beginning 1–2 weeks before the first dose of pemetrexed

Dexamethasone 4mg; administer orally twice daily for 3 consecutive days (6 doses), starting the day before pemetrexed administration to decrease the risk and severity of severe skin rash associated with pemetrexed (total dose/cycle = 24 mg)

Pemetrexed disodium 500 mg/m²; administer intravenously in 100 mL 0.9% sodium chloride injection over 10 minutes on day 1, every 21 days until disease progression (total dosage/cycle = 500 mg/m²), *plus*

Best Supportive Care
Supportive Care
Antiemetic prophylaxis
Emetogenic potential is **LOW**
See Chapter 42 for antiemetic recommendations

Hematopoietic growth factor (CSF) prophylaxis
Primary prophylaxis is **NOT** indicated
See Chapter 43 for more information

Antimicrobial prophylaxis
Risk of fever and neutropenia is **LOW**
   Antimicrobial primary prophylaxis to be considered:
   • Antibacterial—not indicated
   • Antifungal—not indicated
   • Antiviral—not indicated unless patient previously had an episode of HSV

Treatment Modifications

Adapted in part from Alimta (pemetrexed for injection) Lyophilized Powder, for Solution for Intravenous Use; 05/2013 product label. Lilly USA, LLC, Indianapolis, IN

Nadir ANC <500/mm³ and nadir platelets ≥50,000/mm³	75% of the previous pemetrexed dose
Nadir platelets <50,000/mm³ without bleeding regardless of nadir ANC	75% of the previous pemetrexed dose
Nadir platelets <50,000/mm³ with bleeding*, regardless of nadir ANC	50% of the previous pemetrexed dose
Any G3/4 toxicities except mucositis	Withhold treatment until toxicity resolves to the same or less than pretreatment status. Then, resume treatment with pemetrexed dosage decreased by 75%
Any G3/4 toxicities except mucositis after two dose reductions	Discontinue therapy
Any diarrhea requiring hospitalization (irrespective of grade) or G3/4 diarrhea	Withhold treatment until toxicity resolves to the same or less than pretreatment status. Then, resume treatment with pemetrexed dosage decreased by 75%
Any diarrhea requiring hospitalization (irrespective of grade) or G3/4 diarrhea after 2 dose reductions	Discontinue therapy
G3/4 mucositis	Withhold treatment until toxicity resolves to the same or less than pretreatment status. Then, resume treatment with pemetrexed dosage decreased by 50%
G3/4 mucositis after 2 dose reductions	Discontinue therapy

*These criteria meet the National Cancer Institute Common Toxicity Criteria, version 2.0 (1998) definition of bleeding G≥2. Available at: http://ctep.cancer.gov/protocolDevelopment/electronic_applications/ctc.htm [accessed December 7, 2013]

Patient Population Studied

Patients were enrolled no earlier than 21 days and no later than 42 days after the first day of their last cycle of induction therapy. Inclusion criteria included an Eastern Cooperative Oncology Group performance status of 0 or 1, histologic or cytologic diagnosis of stage IIIB (with pleural effusion, positive supraclavicular lymph nodes, or both) or stage IV non–small cell lung cancer before induction therapy, and adequate organ function. Patients must not have progressed during four 21-day cycles of 1 of the following 6 initial doublet chemotherapy regimens: gemcitabine + carboplatin, gemcitabine + cisplatin, paclitaxel + carboplatin, paclitaxel + cisplatin, docetaxel + carboplatin, or docetaxel + cisplatin. Induction regimens did not include pemetrexed. Previous radiotherapy was completed ≥4 weeks before study enrollment

Patient Characteristics

Sex	
Men	73%
Women	27%
Disease Stage	
IIIB	18%
IV	82%
Smoking status	
Smoker	73%
Never-smoker	26%
ECOG* Performance Status	
0	40%
1	60%
Histologies	
Non-squamous	74%
Adenocarcinoma	50%
Large cell	2%
Other or indeterminate	21%
Squamous	26%
Induction regimen	
Docetaxel-carboplatin	5%
Docetaxel-cisplatin	2%
Paclitaxel-carboplatin	30%
Paclitaxel-cisplatin	6%
Gemcitabine-carboplatin	24%
Gemcitabine-cisplatin	33%

*Eastern Cooperative Oncology Group

Treatment Monitoring

1. *Monthly and as clinically indicated:* Complete blood counts (CBC) including differential white blood cell counts and liver function tests
2. *If G3/4 clinical or laboratory abnormalities are observed or if fever or infection occurs:* Frequent monitoring of complete blood counts (CBC) including differential white blood cell counts and liver function tests

Efficacy

	Median PFS*,† (months, 95% CI)		HR (95% CI) P Value	Median OS (months, 95% CI)		HR (95% CI) P Value	Patients with CR+PR+SD (%)		P Value
	PMTX	Placebo		PMTX	Placebo		PMTX	Placebo	
Overall population	4.3 (4.1–4.7)	2.6 (1.7–2.8)	0.50 (0.42–0.61) <0.0001	13.4 (11.9–15.9)	10.6 (8.7–12.0)	0.79 (0.65–0.95) 0.012	228 (52%)	74 (33%)	<0.0001
Non-squamous (n = 481)‡	4.5 (4.2–5.6)	2.6 (1.6–2.8)	0.44 (0.36–0.55) <0.0001	15.5 (13.2–18.1)	10.3 (8.1–12.0)	0.70 (0.56–0.88) 0.002	188 (58%)	51 (33%)	<0.0001
Adenocarcinoma (n = 328)	4.7 (4.2–6.1)	2.6 (1.6–2.8)	0.45 (0.35–0.59) <0.0001	16.8 (14.0–19.7)	11.5 (9.1–15.3)	0.73 (0.56–0.96) 0.026	136 (61%)	35 (33%)	<0.0001
Large cell (n = 20)	3.5 (1.6–6.9)	2.1 (1.4–2.9)	0.40 (0.13–1.22) 0.109	8.4 (6.4–10.3)	7.9 (4.1–13.2)	0.98 (0.36–2.65) 0.964	5 (46%)	3 (33%)	0.670
Other (n = 133)	4.2 (3.1–5.6)	2.8 (1.5–3.6)	0.43 (0.28–0.68) 0.0002	11.3 (9.5–18.3)	7.7 (6.6–11.0)	0.61 (0.40–0.94) 0.025	47 (51%)	13 (32%)	0.041
Squamous (n = 182)	2.8 (2.4–4.0)	2.6 (1.6–3.2)	0.69 (0.49–0.98) 0.039	9.9 (7.5–11.5)	10.8 (8.5–13.2)	1.07 (0.77–1.50) 0.678	40 (35%)	23 (35%)	>0.999

CR, complete response; HR, hazard ratio; OS, overall survival; PFS, progression-free survival; PMTX, pemetrexed; PR, partial response; SD, stable disease

*Investigator-assessed PFS in intention-to-treat population

†PFS based on independently reviewed population (N = 581: pemetrexed = 387, placebo = 194)

‡Non-squamous histology included patients with adenocarcinoma, large cell carcinoma, and other or unknown histology (ie, all patients without a diagnosis of predominantly squamous cell carcinoma)

Toxicity*

	Pemetrexed		Placebo	
	All Grades	G3/4	All Grades	G3/4
Hematologic Toxicities				
Neutropenia†	26 (6%)	13 (3%)	0	0
Anemia	67 (15%)	12 (3%)	12 (5%)	1 (<1%)
Leukopenia	27 (6%)	7 (2%)	3 (1%)	1 (<1%)
Non-hematologic Toxicities				
ALT	42 (10%)	1 (<1%)	8 (4%)	0
AST	36 (8%)	0	8 (4%)	0
Fatigue†	108 (24%)	22 (5%)	23 (10%)	1 (<1%)
Anorexia	82 (19%)	8 (2%)	11 (5%)	0
Infection	23 (5%)	7 (2%)	4 (2%)	0
Diarrhea	23 (5%)	2 (<1%)	6 (3%)	0
Nausea	83 (19%)	4 (<1%)	12 (5%)	1 (<1%)
Vomiting	38 (9%)	1 (<1%)	3 (1%)	0
Sensory neuropathy	39 (9%)	3 (<1%)	9 (4%)	0
Mucositis/stomatitis	31 (7%)	3 (<1%)	4 (2%)	0
Rash	9 (2%)	1 (<1%)	2 (<1%)	0

ALT, alanine aminotransferase; AST, aspartate aminotransferase

*A cutoff of 5% was used for inclusion of all events for which the investigator considered a possible link with pemetrexed

†P<0.05 for Grade 3 or 4 rates of neutropenia and fatigue between study groups

ADVANCED NSCLC • SUBSEQUENT THERAPY

LUNG CANCER REGIMEN: RAMUCIRUMAB + DOCETAXEL

FDA and EMA prescribing information and miscellaneous sources
Garon EB et al. Lancet. 2014;384:665–673

Prophylaxis for infusion-related reaction from ramucirumab:
Diphenhydramine 25–50 mg; administer intravenously, 30–60 minutes before starting ramucirumab, *plus*
Acetaminophen 650–1000 mg; administer orally, 30–60 minutes before starting ramucirumab (only if history of Grade 1/2 infusion reaction), *plus*
Dexamethasone 8 mg; administer orally or intravenously, 30–60 minutes before starting ramucirumab (only if history of Grade 1/2 infusion reaction; note dexamethasone is also indicated for prophylaxis with docetaxel, as described below)
Ramucirumab 10 mg/kg; administer intravenously in 250 mL of 0.9% sodium chloride injection (0.9% NS) over 1 hour on day 1 before docetaxel, every 3 weeks (total dosage/cycle = 10 mg/kg)

Prophylaxis for fluid retention and hypersensitivity reactions from docetaxel:
Dexamethasone 8 mg/dose; administer orally twice daily for 3 days, starting the day before docetaxel is administered (total dose/cycle = 48 mg)
Docetaxel 75 mg/m²; administer intravenously in a volume of 0.9% sodium chloride injection (0.9% NS) or 5% dextrose injection, USP, sufficient to produce a solution with concentration within the range of 0.3–0.74 mg/mL over 1 hour on day 1, every 3 weeks (total dosage/cycle = 75 mg/m²)

Notes:
• Consider a starting docetaxel dose of 60 mg/m² rather than 75 mg/m² in East Asian patients based on findings of higher rates of neutropenia in this group in the REVEL study
• Some formulations of docetaxel contain alcohol; use caution or consider using a non-alcohol-containing formulation in patients who are sensitive to alcohol

Supportive Care
Antiemetic prophylaxis
Emetogenic potential is **LOW**
See Chapter 42 for antiemetic recommendations

Hematopoietic growth factor (CSF) prophylaxis
Primary prophylaxis **MAY** be indicated
See Chapter 43 for more information

Antimicrobial prophylaxis
Risk of fever and neutropenia is **MODERATE**
Antimicrobial primary prophylaxis to be considered:
• Antibacterial—not indicated
• Antifungal—not indicated
• Antiviral—not indicated unless patient previously had an episode of HSV

Patient Population Studied

A multicenter, double-blind, randomized, phase 3 study of 1253 patients with pathologically confirmed, squamous or non-squamous, stage IV NSCLC who had progressed during or after a first-line platinum-based chemotherapy. Eligible patients were age ≥18 years, with an Eastern Cooperative Oncology Group (ECOG) performance status score ≤1. Patients were not eligible if their only previous therapy for advanced or metastatic disease was EGFR tyrosine kinase inhibitor monotherapy. Patients received docetaxel with (1:1) ramucirumab or placebo.

Efficacy (N = 1253)

Median overall survival	10.5 months with docetaxel + ramucirumab 9.1 months with docetaxel + placebo HR 0.86, 95% CI 0.75–0.98, P = 0.023
Median progression-free survival	4.5 months with docetaxel + ramucirumab 3.0 months with docetaxel + placebo HR 0.76, 95% CI 0.68–0.86, P<0.0001
Objective response rate*	23% with docetaxel + ramucirumab 14% with docetaxel + placebo OR 1.89, 95% CI 1.41–2.54, P<0.0001

*Overall response rate is the percentage of patients who experienced a confirmed partial or complete response to the study drug

Therapy Monitoring

1. Draw serum bilirubin, AST or ALT, and alkaline phosphatase prior to each cycle
2. Obtain CBC with differential at a minimum once per cycle, but initially also at days 10–14
3. Observe closely for hypersensitivity reactions, especially during the first and second ramucirumab infusions
4. Monitor patients with preexisting effusions closely for possible exacerbation of effusions
5. Monitor all patients for fluid retention. Median cumulative dose to onset of moderate/severe fluid retention was 819 mg/m² of docetaxel
6. Check blood pressure every 2 weeks or more frequently as indicated during treatment.
7. Assess proteinuria by urine dipstick and/or urinary protein creatinine ratio at baseline and every 2 cycles. If protein ≥2+, then collect a 24-hour urine for protein measurement
8. Assess thyroid function at outset and every 3 months while on therapy

Treatment Modifications

RAMUCIRUMAB DOSE MODIFICATIONS

Starting dose	10 mg/kg (starting ramucirumab dose for lung cancer)
Dose level −1	8 mg/kg
Dose level −2	6 mg/kg
G1/2 infusion-related	Stop ramucirumab. Administer dexamethasone intravenously at commonly used antiemetic doses of 8–20 mg (or equivalent) and acetaminophen, then resume infusion at 50% of previous rate. Use the 50% infusion rate for all subsequent administrations
Prior G1/2 infusion-related reaction	Premedicate with dexamethasone intravenously at commonly used antiemetic doses of 8–20 mg (or equivalent) and acetaminophen prior to each ramucirumab infusion. Continue diphenhydramine 25–50 mg intravenously
G3/4 infusion-related reaction	Permanently discontinue ramucirumab
G3/4 hypertension	Interrupt ramucirumab until symptoms controlled with medical management; if unable to control with medical management, discontinue ramucirumab
PRES	Permanently discontinue ramucirumab
Urine protein ≥2 g/24 hours	Interrupt ramucirumab. Reinitiate treatment at a reduced dose once the urine protein level returns to <2 g/24 hours
Reoccurrence of urine protein ≥2 g/24 hours	Interrupt ramucirumab and reduce the dose once the urine protein level returns to <2 g/24 hours
Urine protein >3 g/24 hours or nephrotic syndrome	Permanently discontinue ramucirumab
Anticipated wound healing	Stop ramucirumab ≥4 weeks prior to a scheduled surgery and until wound is fully healed; discontinue ramucirumab if patient develops wound healing complications
G3/4 bleeding, arterial thromboembolic event, gastrointestinal perforation	Permanently discontinue ramucirumab
G3/4 fatigue/asthenia	Interrupt ramucirumab. Reinstitute treatment at a reduced dose once toxicity is G1
G3/4 stomatitis/mucosal inflammation	

DOCETAXEL DOSE MODIFICATIONS

Starting docetaxel dose	75 mg/m² (recommended starting dose in East Asian patients = 60 mg/m²)
Dose level −1*	65 mg/m²
Dose level −2*	50 mg/m²
Serum bilirubin > ULN	Do not administer docetaxel
AST and/or ALT >1.5× ULN with concomitant with alkaline phosphatase >2.5× ULN	Do not administer docetaxel
ANC <1500/mm³; platelet count <100,000/mm³	Withhold docetaxel until ANC >1500/mm³ and platelet count <100,000/mm³
ANC nadir <500 cells/mm³ for >1 week	Reduce dose by 1 level in subsequent cycle
Platelet nadir <25,000 cells/mm³	
Febrile neutropenia	
Severe or cumulative cutaneous reactions from docetaxel	Withhold treatment until toxicity improves, then resume with dose reduced by 1 level
G3/4 non-hematologic toxicities	Withhold treatment until toxicity improves to G1, then resume with dose reduced by 1 level

(continued)

Treatment Modifications (*continued*)

DOCETAXEL DOSE MODIFICATIONS

Severe hypersensitivity reaction	Immediately discontinue docetaxel infusion and administer dexamethasone intravenously at commonly used antiemetic doses 8–20 mg
History of severe hypersensitivity to docetaxel or other drugs formulated with polysorbate 80	Do not administer docetaxel
Minor flushing or localized skin reactions	Interruption of therapy is not required
G ≥3 peripheral neuropathy	Discontinue docetaxel
Fluid retention	Treat with salt restriction and oral diuretics; reduce dose by 1 level
Mild peripheral edema	Treat with salt restriction and oral diuretics

ALT, alanine transaminase; ANC, absolute neutrophil count; AST, aspartate transaminase; PRES, posterior reversible leukoencephalopathy syndrome; ULN, upper limit of normal
*The U.S. FDA-approved package insert for docetaxel recommends only 1 dose reduction of docetaxel to 55 mg/m² in patients with NSCLC after platinum failure; the dose levels listed above were included to allow for greater physician discretion

Notes:
- Patients who are pregnant or who become pregnant should be apprised of the potential hazard to the fetus. Females of childbearing potential should be advised to avoid becoming pregnant during therapy
- No dose adjustments for docetaxel or ramucirumab are recommended for patients with renal impairment
- Dose adjustments for hepatic impairment:
  - Ramucirumab: No dose adjustment is recommended for patients with mild (total bilirubin within ULN and AST >ULN, or total bilirubin >1.0–1.5× ULN and any AST) or moderate (total bilirubin >1.5–3.0× ULN and any AST) hepatic impairment
  - Docetaxel: Use is not recommended for patients with total bilirubin > ULN, or AST and/or ALT >1.5× ULN concomitant with alkaline phosphatase >2.5× ULN

Adverse Events (N = 1245)

Grade (%)*	Docetaxel + Ramucirumab		Docetaxel + Placebo	
	Grade 1/2	Grade 3/4	Grade 1/2	Grade 3/4
Non-hematologic Adverse Events				
Fatigue	41	14	39	10
Diarrhea	27	5	25	3
Decreased appetite	27	2	24	1
Nausea	26	1	26	1
Alopecia	26	—	26	—
Stomatitis	19	4	11	2
Neuropathy	20	3	19	2
Dyspnea	18	4	16	8
Cough	21	<1	20	1
Pyrexia	16	<1	13	<1
Peripheral edema	16	0	8	<1
Mucosal inflammation	13	3	6	<1

(*continued*)

Adverse Events (N = 1245) (continued)

Grade (%)*	Docetaxel + Ramucirumab		Docetaxel + Placebo	
	Grade 1/2	Grade 3/4	Grade 1/2	Grade 3/4
Non-hematologic Adverse Events				
Constipation	16	<1	17	1
Vomiting	13	1	12	2
Lacrimation increased	13	<1	4	0
Myalgia	12	1	10	1
Arthralgia	10	1	7	1
Back pain	10	1	8	<1
Abdominal pain	10	1	9	1
Insomnia	10	<1	8	<1
Dysgeusia	11	—	7	—
Headache	10	<1	10	1
Hypertension[†]	5	6	3	2
Infusion-related reaction[†]	3	1	4	1
Proteinuria[†]	3	<1	1	0
Renal failure[†]	2	<1	2	<1
Congestive heart failure[†]	<1	1	<1	<1
Gastrointestinal perforation[†]	<1	1	0	<1
Hematologic Adverse Events				
Neutropenia	6	49	6	39
Febrile neutropenia	0	16	0	10
Bleeding or hemorrhage[†]	26	2	13	2
Leukopenia	8	14	6	12
Anemia	18	3	22	6
Epistaxis[†]	18	<1	6	<1
Thrombocytopenia	11	3	5	1
Pulmonary hemorrhage[†]	7	1	6	1
Hemoptysis[†]	5	1	5	1
Gastrointestinal hemorrhage[†]	2	1	1	<1
Venous thromboembolic[†]	<1	2	3	3
Arterial thromboembolic[†]	<1	1	<1	1

*According to the National Cancer Institute Common Terminology Criteria for Adverse Events, version 4.0
[†]Denotes those events of special interest
Note: toxicities are included in the table if all-grade events occurred in ≥10% of patients or were of special interest. Events are included regardless of whether they were caused by the study treatment

ADVANCED NSCLC • SUBSEQUENT THERAPY

LUNG CANCER REGIMEN: DOCETAXEL

Shepherd FA et al. J Clin Oncol 2000;18:2095–2103

Prophylaxis for fluid retention and hypersensitivity reactions from docetaxel:
Dexamethasone 8 mg/dose; administer orally twice daily for 3 days, starting the day before docetaxel is administered (total dose/cycle = 48 mg)
Docetaxel 75 mg/m^2; administer intravenously in a volume of 0.9% sodium chloride injection or 5% dextrose injection sufficient to produce a solution with concentration within the range 0.3–0.74 mg/mL over 1 hour on day 1, every 3 weeks (total dosage/cycle = 75 mg/m^2)

Supportive Care
Antiemetic prophylaxis
Emetogenic potential: **LOW**
See Chapter 42 for antiemetic recommendations

Hematopoietic growth factor (CSF) prophylaxis
Primary prophylaxis is **NOT** indicated
See Chapter 43 for more information

Antimicrobial prophylaxis
Risk of fever and neutropenia is **LOW**
  Antimicrobial primary prophylaxis to be considered:
  • Antibacterial—not indicated
  • Antifungal—not indicated
  • Antiviral—not indicated unless patient previously had an episode of HSV

Patient Population Studied

A randomized comparison with best supportive care of 55 patients with advanced (stage III/IV) NSCLC previously treated with platinum-containing chemotherapy

Efficacy (N = 55)

Complete response	—
Partial response	7.1%
Median survival	7.5 months
1-year survival	37%

Treatment Modifications

Adverse Event	Dose Modification
G4 neutropenia for >7 days, alone, or accompanied by fever >38°C (>100.4°F)	Reduce docetaxel dosage by 25% in all subsequent treatments
G4 thrombocytopenia	Resume docetaxel after platelet count recovers with docetaxel dosage decreased by 25%
G4 vomiting not controlled by antiemetics	Reduce docetaxel dosage by 25%
G ≥3 diarrhea	
G ≥3 neuropathy	Discontinue therapy

Therapy Monitoring

1. *Before treatment:* H&P, PS evaluation, CBC with differential, and LFTs
2. *Weekly:* CBC with differential and platelet count
3. *Response evaluation:* every 2–3 cycles

Toxicity (N = 55)

	% G3/4
Neutropenia	67.3
Anemia	5.5
Febrile neutropenia	1.8
Thrombocytopenia	0
Pulmonary	20
Asthenia	18.2
Infection	5.5
Nausea	3.6
Vomiting	3.6
Diarrhea	1.8
Neuromotor	1.8
Neurosensory	1.8

ADVANCED NSCLC • SUBSEQUENT THERAPY
LUNG CANCER REGIMEN: NIVOLUMAB

Borghaei H et al. N Engl J Med 2015;373:1627–1639
Brahmer JR et al. J Clin Oncol 2018;36(17):1714–1768
FDA and EMA prescribing information
Garon E et al. J Thorac Oncol 2018;13:S117–S118
Haanen JB et al. Ann Oncol 2017;28(suppl 4):iv119–iv142
Waterhouse D et al. Cancer Chemother Pharmacol 2018;81:679–686
Zhao X et al. Ann Oncol 2017;28:2002–2008
Zhao X et al. Cancer Res 2017;77(suppl 13):abstract CT101

Notes:
- The U.S. FDA-approved regimen for lung cancer includes fixed doses of nivolumab and allows for a shortened infusion duration of 30 minutes, consistent with the regimens approved on March 5, 2018, thus:

Nivolumab 240 mg; administer intravenously over 30–60 minutes in a volume of 0.9% sodium chloride injection (0.9% NS) or 5% dextrose injection, USP, not to exceed 160 mL and sufficient to produce a nivolumab concentration within the range of 1–10 mg/mL, every 2 weeks (total dosage/2-week course = 240 mg)
  - Administer nivolumab through an administration set that contains a sterile, nonpyrogenic, low-protein-binding in-line filter with pore size within the range of 0.2–1.2 μm

OR

Nivolumab 480 mg; administer intravenously over 30–60 minutes in a volume of 0.9% sodium chloride injection (0.9% NS) or 5% dextrose injection, USP, not to exceed 160 mL and sufficient to produce a nivolumab concentration within the range of 1–10 mg/mL, every 4 weeks (total dosage/4-week course = 480 mg)
  - Administer nivolumab through an administration set that contains a sterile, nonpyrogenic, low-protein-binding in-line filter with pore size within the range of 0.2–1.2 μm
- Nivolumab can cause severe infusion-related reactions
  - Interrupt or slow the administration rate in patients with mild or moderate infusion-related reactions
  - Discontinue nivolumab in patients who experience severe or life-threatening infusion-related reactions
- Patients who require systemic corticosteroids must be on a dose of ≤10 mg daily prednisone (or equivalent) before initiating treatment with nivolumab

Supportive Care
Antiemetic prophylaxis
Emetogenic potential is **MINIMAL**
See Chapter 42 for antiemetic recommendations

Hematopoietic growth factor (CSF) prophylaxis
Primary prophylaxis is **NOT** indicated
See Chapter 43 for more information

Antimicrobial prophylaxis
Risk of fever and neutropenia is **LOW**
  Antimicrobial primary prophylaxis to be considered:
  - Antibacterial—not indicated
  - Antifungal—not indicated
  - Antiviral—not indicated unless patient previously had an episode of HSV

Patient Population Studied

A multicenter, open-label, randomized, phase 3 study involved 582 patients with documented stage IIIB or IV or recurrent non-squamous NSCLC after radiation therapy or surgical resection, who had also had disease recurrence or progression during or after a platinum-based doublet chemotherapy regimen. Eligible patients were age ≥18 years, with Eastern Cooperative Oncology Group (ECOG) performance status score ≤1. Patients with autoimmune disease, symptomatic ILD, or systemic immunosuppression were not eligible. Patients who had previously been treated with an immune-stimulatory antitumor agent or docetaxel were also not eligible. Patients received (1:1) nivolumab or docetaxel

Efficacy (N = 582)

Median overall survival*	12.2 months with nivolumab 9.4 months with docetaxel HR for death 0.73, 95% CI 0.59–0.89, P = 0.002
Overall survival at 1 year*	51% with nivolumab 39% with docetaxel
Median progression-free survival	2.3 months with nivolumab 4.2 months with docetaxel HR for disease progression or death 0.92, 95% CI 0.77–1.11, P = 0.39
Progression-free survival at 1 year*	19% with nivolumab 8% with docetaxel
Objective response rate†	19% with nivolumab 12% with docetaxel OR 1.7, 95% CI 1.1–2.6, P = 0.02

*At time of interim analysis (minimum follow-up 13.2 months)
†Overall response rate is the percentage of patients who experienced an investigator-assessed confirmed partial or complete response to the study drug

Therapy Monitoring

1. Initially at the time of each dose, and eventually every 6–12 weeks, perform a total-body skin examination with attention to *all* mucous membranes as well as a complete review of systems

2. Monitor patients for signs and symptoms of pneumonitis. Evaluate patients with suspected pneumonitis, with chest x-ray, CT scan, and pulse oximetry. For ≥2 toxicity, may include nasal swab, sputum culture and sensitivity, blood culture and sensitivity, and urine culture and sensitivity

3. Monitor patients for signs and symptoms of colitis. Encourage patients to report diarrhea immediately to any member of the health care team

4. Draw AST, ALT, and bilirubin prior to each infusion and/or weekly if there are Grade 1 LFT elevations. Note, no treatment is recommended for G1 LFT abnormalities. For ≥2 toxicity, implement work-up for other causes of elevated LFTs, including viral hepatitis

5. Use basic metabolic panel (Na, K, CO_2, glucose) and patient history as screening tools for hypophysitis, including hypopituitarism and adrenal insufficiency. If in doubt, evaluate morning adrenocorticotropic hormone (ACTH) and cortisol levels. Consider ACTH stimulation test for indeterminate results

6. Assess thyroid function at the start of treatment, periodically during treatment, and as indicated based on clinical evaluation, and for clinical signs and symptoms of thyroid disorders. Test for TSH and free thyroxine (FT4) every 4–6 weeks as part of routine clinical monitoring of therapy or for case detection in symptomatic patients

7. Measure glucose at baseline and with each treatment during the first 12 weeks and every 6 weeks thereafter

8. Obtain a serum creatinine level prior to every dose. If creatinine is found to be newly elevated, consider holding therapy while other potential causes are evaluated. Note, routine urinalysis is not necessary other than to rule out urinary tract infections, etc

9. Obtain a complete rheumatologic history and perform an examination of all peripheral joints for tenderness, swelling, and range of motion. Examine the spine. Consider plain x-ray/imaging to exclude metastases and evaluate joint damage (erosions), if appropriate

10. In patients at high risk for infections and in appropriately selected patients based on an infectious disease evaluation, draw screening laboratories (HIV, hepatitis A and B, and blood QuantiFERON for TB) to prepare patients to start infliximab

Treatment Modifications

Adverse Reaction	Grade/Severity	Dose Modification
Colitis	G1	Loperamide 4 mg as starting dose then 2 mg before each meal and after each loose stool until without diarrhea for 12 hours, with maximum of 16 mg loperamide per day. If G1 diarrhea or colitis persists for >14 days, then add prednisolone 0.5–1 mg/kg (non-enteric-coated) or consider oral budesonide 9 mg daily if no bloody diarrhea
	G2/3 diarrhea or colitis	Withhold nivolumab. Loperamide 4 mg as starting dose then 2 mg before each meal and after each loose stool until without diarrhea for 12 hours, with maximum of 16 mg loperamide per day. Administer oral prednisone/prednisolone at a dose of 0.5–2 mg/kg/day or its equivalent. When symptoms improve to G1, begin a slow corticosteroid taper over at least 4 weeks. Resume nivolumab upon symptom control, or when prednisone/prednisolone daily dose <10 mg
	G4 diarrhea or colitis	Permanently discontinue nivolumab. Loperamide 4 mg as starting dose then 2 mg before each meal and after each loose stool until without diarrhea for 12 hours, with maximum of 16 mg loperamide per day. Administer 1–2 mg/kg intravenous (methyl)prednisolone and convert to 0.5–2 mg/kg prednisone/prednisolone orally each day or its equivalent only after a response. Taper over at least 4 weeks when symptoms improve. If symptoms do not improve over 72 hours or worsen, perform flexible sigmoidoscopy/colonoscopy to document colitis then begin infliximab 5 mg/kg (if no perforation, sepsis, TB, hepatitis, NYHA III/IV CHF). If no response, add MMF 500–1000 mg twice daily. If worse on MMF, consider addition of tacrolimus or ATG

(continued)

Treatment Modifications (continued)

Adverse Reaction	Grade/Severity	Dose Modification
Pneumonitis	G2	Withhold nivolumab. Consider pneumocystis prophylaxis depending on the clinical context and cover with empiric antibiotics. Administer oral prednisone/prednisolone at a dose of 1–2 mg/kg/day or its equivalent. When symptoms improve to G1, begin a slow corticosteroid taper over at least 4 weeks. If response is not adequate after 48 hours, then administer 2–4 mg/kg intravenous (methyl) prednisolone and convert to 0.5–2 mg/kg prednisone/prednisolone orally each day or its equivalent only after a response, followed by a taper over at least 6 weeks when symptoms improve to G1, titrating to symptoms. Resume nivolumab upon symptom control, or when prednisone/prednisolone daily dose <10 mg
	G3/4	Permanently discontinue nivolumab. Consider pneumocystis prophylaxis depending on the clinical context; cover with empiric antibiotics. Administer 2–4 mg/kg intravenous (methyl)prednisolone and convert to 1–2 mg/kg prednisone/prednisolone orally each day or its equivalent only after a response, followed by a taper over at least 8 weeks when symptoms improve to G1, titrating to symptoms. If, when initially treated, improvement does not occur within 48–72 hours, begin infliximab 5 mg/kg (if no perforation, sepsis, TB, hepatitis, NYHA III/IV CHF). If no response to infliximab, add MMF 500–1000 mg twice daily. Consider MMF especially if concurrent hepatic toxicity
Hepatitis	G2 (AST or ALT >3–5× ULN or total bilirubin >1.5–3× ULN)	Withhold nivolumab. Administer oral prednisone/prednisolone at a dose of 1–2 mg/kg/day or its equivalent. When symptoms improve to G1, begin a slow corticosteroid taper over at least 4 weeks. Resume nivolumab upon symptom control, or when prednisone/prednisolone daily dose <10 mg
	G3/4 (AST or ALT >5× ULN or total bilirubin >3× ULN)	Permanently discontinue nivolumab. Administer 1–2 mg/kg intravenous (methyl) prednisolone and convert to 0.5–2 mg/kg prednisone/prednisolone orally each day or its equivalent only after a response. Taper over at least 6 weeks when symptoms improve. If no response, add MMF 500–1000 mg twice daily. If worse on MMF, consider adding tacrolimus or ATG
Hypophysitis	G2/3 (moderate symptoms, ie, headache but no visual disturbance or fatigue/mood alteration but hemodynamically stable, no electrolyte disturbance)	Administer analgesia as needed for headache. Withhold nivolumab. Administer oral prednisone/prednisolone at a dose of 0.5–2 mg/kg/day or its equivalent. When symptoms improve to G1, begin a slow corticosteroid taper over at least 4 weeks. If no improvement in 48 hours, administer 1–2 mg/kg intravenous (methyl) prednisolone and convert to 0.5–2 mg/kg prednisone/prednisolone orally each day or its equivalent only after a response. Taper over at least 4 weeks when symptoms improve to 5 mg prednisone/prednisolone or equivalent; do not stop steroids. Resume nivolumab upon symptom control, or when prednisone/prednisolone daily dose <10 mg
	G4 (severe mass effect symptoms, ie, severe headache, any visual disturbance or severe hypoadrenalism, ie, hypotension, severe electrolyte disturbance)	Permanently discontinue nivolumab. Administer analgesia as needed for headache. Administer 1–2 mg/kg intravenous (methyl)prednisolone and convert to 0.5–2 mg/kg prednisone/prednisolone orally each day or its equivalent only after a response. Taper over at least 4 weeks when symptoms improve to 5 mg prednisone/prednisolone or equivalent; do not stop steroids
Adrenal insufficiency	G2	Withhold nivolumab. Administer oral prednisone/prednisolone at a dose of 0.5–2 mg/kg/day or its equivalent. When symptoms improve to G1, begin a slow corticosteroid taper over at least 4 weeks. Serially assess adrenal function and continue steroids at replacement doses (20–40 mg hydrocortisone daily ~2/3 dose in morning upon awakening and ~1/3 at 4:00 PM) until recovery of adrenal function is documented. Resume nivolumab upon symptom control, or when prednisone/prednisolone daily dose <10 mg
	G3/4	Permanently discontinue nivolumab. Administer oral prednisone/prednisolone at a dose of 0.5–2 mg/kg/day or its equivalent. When symptoms improve to G1, begin a slow corticosteroid taper over at least 4 weeks. Serially assess adrenal function and continue steroids at replacement doses (20–40 mg hydrocortisone daily ~2/3 dose in morning upon awakening and ~1/3 at 4:00 PM) until recovery of adrenal function is documented

(continued)

Treatment Modifications (*continued*)

Adverse Reaction	Grade/Severity	Dose Modification
Type 1 diabetes mellitus	G3 hyperglycemia	Withhold nivolumab. Admit to hospital to manage hyperglycemia. Role of corticosteroids in preventing complete loss of insulin-producing cells is unknown and not recommended. Resume nivolumab upon symptom control, or when prednisone/prednisolone daily dose <10 mg
	G4 hyperglycemia	Permanently discontinue nivolumab. Admit to hospital to manage hyperglycemia. Role of corticosteroids in preventing complete loss of insulin-producing cells is unknown and not recommended
Nephritis and renal dysfunction	G2/3 (serum creatinine 1.5–6× ULN)	Withhold nivolumab. Administer oral prednisone/prednisolone at a dose of 0.5–2 mg/kg/day or its equivalent. When symptoms improve to G1, begin a slow corticosteroid taper over at least 4 weeks. If response is not adequate, then administer 0.5–1 mg/kg intravenous (methyl)prednisolone and convert to 0.5–2 mg/kg prednisone/prednisolone orally each day or its equivalent only after a response, followed by a taper over at least 4 weeks when symptoms improve to G1. Resume nivolumab upon symptom control, or when prednisone/prednisolone daily dose <10 mg
	G4 (serum creatinine >6× ULN)	Permanently discontinue nivolumab. Administer 0.5–1 mg/kg intravenous (methyl) prednisolone and convert to 0.5–2 mg/kg prednisone/prednisolone orally each day or its equivalent only after a response, followed by a taper over at least 4 weeks when symptoms improve to G1
Skin	G1/2	Continue nivolumab. Avoid skin irritants, avoid sun exposure; topical emollients recommended. Topical steroid (mild strength for G1, moderate/potent strength for G2) cream once or twice daily ± oral or topical antihistamines for itching
	G3 rash or suspected SJS or TEN	Withhold nivolumab. Avoid skin irritants, avoid sun exposure; topical emollients recommended. Administer oral or topical antihistamines for itching. Administer oral prednisone/prednisolone at a dose of 0.5–2 mg/kg or its equivalent daily for 3 days followed by a slow corticosteroid taper over at least 4 weeks when the rash improves to G1. If rash does not respond adequately, then administer 0.5–1 mg/kg intravenous (methyl)prednisolone and convert to 0.5–2 mg/kg prednisone/prednisolone orally each day or its equivalent only after a response, followed by a taper over at least 4 weeks when the rash improves to G1. Resume nivolumab upon symptom control, or when prednisone/prednisolone daily dose <10 mg
	G4 rash or confirmed SJS or TEN	Avoid skin irritants, avoid sun exposure; topical emollients recommended. Administer oral or topical antihistamines for itching. Administer 1–2 mg/kg intravenous (methyl)prednisolone and convert to oral steroids 0.5–2 mg/kg prednisone/prednisolone each day or its equivalent only after a response. Taper over at least 4 weeks when the rash improves to G1. Permanently discontinue nivolumab
Encephalitis	Confusion or altered behavior, headaches, alteration in Glasgow Coma Scale, motor or sensory deficits, speech abnormality, may or may not be febrile	Initially withhold nivolumab, but permanently discontinue nivolumab if there is no doubt as to diagnosis. Exclude bacterial and ideally viral infections prior to high-dose steroids. Administer oral prednisone/prednisolone at a dose of 0.5–2 mg/kg/day or its equivalent. When symptoms improve, begin a slow corticosteroid taper over at least 4–8 weeks. If symptoms are severe, administer 1–2 mg/kg intravenous (methyl)prednisolone and convert to 0.5–2 mg/kg prednisone/prednisolone orally each day or its equivalent only after a response. Consider concurrent empiric antiviral (intravenous acyclovir) and antibacterial therapy
Aseptic meningitis	Headache, photophobia, neck stiffness with fever or may be afebrile, vomiting; normal cognition/cerebral function (distinguishes from encephalitis)	
Other syndromes include neurosarcoidosis, posterior reversible leukoencephalopathy syndrome (PRES), Vogt-Koyanagi-Harada syndrome, demyelination, vasculitic encephalopathy, and generalized seizures		

(continued)

Treatment Modifications (continued)

Adverse Reaction	Grade/Severity	Dose Modification
Transverse myelitis	Acute or subacute neurologic signs/symptoms of motor, sensory, or autonomic origin; most have sensory level; often bilateral symptoms	Initially withhold nivolumab, but permanently discontinue nivolumab if there is no doubt as to diagnosis. Administer 2 mg/kg intravenous (methyl)prednisolone or consider 1 g/day and convert to 0.5–2 mg/kg prednisone/prednisolone orally each day or its equivalent only after a response. When symptoms improve, begin a slow corticosteroid taper over at least 4–8 weeks. Plasmapheresis may be required if steroids do not bring about improvement
Myocarditis	G3	Permanently discontinue nivolumab. Administer 2 mg/kg intravenous (methyl)prednisolone or consider 1 g/day and convert to 0.5–2 mg/kg prednisone/prednisolone orally each day or its equivalent only after a response. When symptoms improve, begin a slow corticosteroid taper over at least 4–8 weeks. If no response, add MMF 500–1000 mg twice daily. If worse on MMF, consider adding tacrolimus
Peripheral neurologic toxicity	Moderate: some interference with ADLs, symptoms concerning to patient	Withhold nivolumab. Initial observation reasonable or initiate prednisone/prednisolone 0.5–1 mg/kg (if progressing, eg, from mild) and/or pregabalin or duloxetine for pain. When symptoms improve, begin a slow corticosteroid taper over at least 4 weeks. Resume nivolumab upon symptom control, or when prednisone/prednisolone daily dose <10 mg
	Severe: limits self-care and aids warranted, life-threatening, eg, respiratory problems	Permanently discontinue nivolumab. Administer 1–2 mg/kg intravenous (methyl)prednisolone and convert to 0.5–2 mg/kg prednisone/prednisolone orally each day or its equivalent only after a response. Taper over at least 4–8 weeks when symptoms improve to G1
Guillain-Barré syndrome	Progressive symmetrical muscle weakness with absent or reduced tendon reflexes—involves extremities; facial, respiratory, bulbar, and oculomotor muscles; dysregulation of autonomic nerves	Permanently discontinue nivolumab. Use of steroids not recommended in idiopathic Guillain-Barré syndrome; however, a trial of (methyl)prednisolone 1–2 mg/kg is reasonable, converting to 0.5–2 mg/kg prednisone/prednisolone orally each day or its equivalent only after a response. If no improvement or worsening, plasmapheresis or IVIG indicated
Myasthenia gravis	Fluctuating muscle weakness (proximal limb, trunk, ocular, eg, ptosis/diplopia or bulbar) with fatigability; respiratory muscles may also be involved	Permanently discontinue nivolumab. Administer pyridostigmine at an initial dose of 30 mg 3 times daily. Administer oral prednisone/prednisolone at a dose of 0.5–2 mg/kg/day or its equivalent or 1–2 mg/kg intravenous (methyl)prednisolone depending on the severity of symptoms. If treatment begins with intravenous drug, convert to 0.5–2 mg/kg prednisone/prednisolone orally each day or its equivalent only after a response. If no improvement or worsening, plasmapheresis or IVIG may be considered. Additional immunosuppressants used in myasthenia gravis include azathioprine, cyclosporine, and mycophenolate. Avoid certain medications (eg, ciprofloxacin, beta-blockers) that may precipitate cholinergic crisis
Other syndromes including motor and sensory peripheral neuropathy, multifocal radicular neuropathy/plexopathy, autonomic neuropathy, phrenic nerve palsy, cranial nerve palsies (eg, facial nerve, optic nerve, hypoglossal nerve)		Permanently discontinue nivolumab. Administer oral prednisone/prednisolone at a dose of 0.5–2 mg/kg/day or its equivalent or 1–2 mg/kg intravenous (methyl)prednisolone depending on the severity of symptoms. If treatment begins with intravenous drug, convert to 0.5–2 mg/kg prednisone/prednisolone orally each day or its equivalent only after a response

(continued)

Treatment Modifications (*continued*)

Adverse Reaction	Grade/Severity	Dose Modification
Arthralgia	G1 (mild pain with inflammation, erythema, or joint swelling)	Continue nivolumab. Administer acetaminophen (paracetamol) and ibuprofen
	G2 (moderate pain with inflammation, erythema, or joint swelling that limits ADLs)	Withhold nivolumab. Administer higher doses of acetaminophen (paracetamol) and ibuprofen, and use diclofenac or naproxen or etoricoxib. If inadequately controlled, consider intra-articular steroid injections for large joints or administer oral prednisone/prednisolone at a dose of 0.5–2 mg/kg/day or its equivalent. When symptoms improve to G1, begin a slow corticosteroid taper over at least 4 weeks. If response is not adequate, then administer 0.5–1 mg/kg intravenous (methyl)prednisolone and convert to 0.52 mg/kg prednisone/prednisolone orally each day or its equivalent only after a response, followed by a taper over at least 4 weeks when symptoms improve to G1. Resume nivolumab upon symptom control, or when prednisone/prednisolone daily dose <10 mg
	G3 (severe pain; irreversible joint damage; disabling; limits self-care ADLs)	Withhold nivolumab. Administer 0.5–1 mg/kg intravenous (methyl)prednisolone and convert to 0.5–2 mg/kg prednisone/prednisolone orally each day or its equivalent only after a response, followed by a taper over at least 4 weeks when symptoms improve to G1. In severe cases, infliximab or another anti–TNF alpha drug may be required for improvement of arthritis. Resume nivolumab upon symptom control, or when prednisone/prednisolone daily dose <10 mg
Other	First occurrence of other G3	Withhold nivolumab. Administer oral prednisone/prednisolone at a dose of 0.5–2 mg/kg/day or its equivalent. When symptoms improve to G1, begin a slow corticosteroid taper over at least 4 weeks. Resume nivolumab upon symptom control, or when prednisone/prednisolone daily dose <10 mg
	Recurrence of same G3	Permanently discontinue nivolumab. Administer 1–2 mg/kg intravenous (methyl)prednisolone and convert to 0.5–2 mg/kg prednisone/prednisolone orally each day or its equivalent only after a response. Taper over at least 4–8 weeks when symptoms improve to G1
	Life-threatening or G4	
	Requirement for ≥10 mg/day prednisone or equivalent for >12 weeks	Permanently discontinue nivolumab
	Persistent G2/3 adverse reactions lasting ≥12 weeks	

ADL, activities of daily living; ALT, alanine aminotransferase; AST, aspartate aminotransferase; ATG, anti-thymocyte globulin; CHF, congestive heart failure; IVIG, intravenous immunoglobulin; MMF, mycophenolate mofetil; NYHA, New York Heart Association; SJS, Stevens-Johnson syndrome; TB, tuberculosis; TEN, toxic epidermal necrolysis; TNF, tumor necrosis factor; ULN, upper limit of normal

Notes on general supportive care:
• Steroid taper in most cases will proceed over a minimum of 1 month, but if symptoms improve rapidly, a 2-week taper can be considered. If steroids are administered for more than 4 weeks, consider PCP prophylaxis (cotrimoxazole 480 mg twice daily M/W/F or inhaled pentamidine if cotrimoxazole allergy), regular random blood glucose, vitamin D level, and starting calcium/vitamin D supplementation per guidelines

Adverse Events (N = 555)

Grade (%)*	Nivolumab		Docetaxel	
	Grade 1/2	Grade 3/4	Grade 1/2	Grade 3/4
Any event	59	10	34	54
Non-hematologic Adverse Events				
Fatigue	15	1	24	5
Nausea	11	1	25	1
Decreased appetite	10	0	15	1
Asthenia	10	<1	15	2
Diarrhea	7	1	22	1
Peripheral edema	3	0	10	<1
Myalgia	2	<1	11	0
Alopecia	<1	0	25	0
Hematologic Adverse Events				
Anemia	2	<1	17	3
Neutropenia	<1	0	4	27
Febrile neutropenia	0	0	<1	10
Leukopenia	0	0	2	8

*According to the National Cancer Institute Common Terminology Criteria for Adverse Events, version 4.0
Note: toxicities are included in the table if all-grade events occurred in ≥10% of patients and were deemed to be related to the study treatment. Although no treatment-related deaths were reported at the time of the database lock, the death of 1 patient from encephalitis in the nivolumab group was later determined to be caused by the study drug, and 1 patient in the docetaxel group later died from Grade 4 febrile neutropenia reported at the time of the database lock

ADVANCED NSCLC • SUBSEQUENT THERAPY

LUNG CANCER REGIMEN: PEMBROLIZUMAB

Brahmer JR et al. J Clin Oncol 2018;36(17):1714–1768
FDA and EMA prescribing information
Freshwater T et al. J Immunother Cancer 2017;5:43
Haanen JB et al. Ann Oncol 2017;28(suppl 4):iv119–iv142
Herbst RS et al. Lancet 2016;387:1540–1550

Notes:
- The U.S. FDA approved pembrolizumab as a single agent for treatment of metastatic NSCLC patients with progression on or after platinum-based chemotherapy whose tumors express programmed death-ligand 1 (PD-L1) with a proportion score of ≥1% as determined using an FDA-approved test. The FDA approved a *fixed-dose* regimen of pembrolizumab for this indication on October 24, 2016, thus:

  Pembrolizumab 200 mg; administer intravenously over 30 minutes in a volume of 0.9% sodium chloride injection (0.9% NS) or 5% dextrose injection (D5W), USP, sufficient to produce a pembrolizumab concentration within the range of 1–10 mg/mL every 3 weeks for up to 24 months (total dose/3-week cycle = 200 mg)
- Administer pembrolizumab with an administration set that contains a sterile, nonpyrogenic, low-protein-binding in-line or add-on filter with pore size within the range of 0.2–5.0 μm
- Pembrolizumab can cause severe or life-threatening infusion-related reactions, including hypersensitivity and anaphylaxis

Alternative pembrolizumab dose and schedule as per the U.S. FDA regimens approved on April 28, 2020:

Pembrolizumab 400 mg; administer intravenously over 30 minutes in a volume of 0.9% NS or D5W sufficient to produce a pembrolizumab concentration within the range 1–10 mg/mL every 6 weeks, for up to 24 months (total dose/6-week cycle = 400 mg)

Supportive Care
Antiemetic prophylaxis
Emetogenic potential is **MINIMAL**
See Chapter 42 for antiemetic recommendations

Hematopoietic growth factor (CSF) prophylaxis
Primary prophylaxis is **NOT** indicated
See Chapter 43 for more information

Antimicrobial prophylaxis
Risk of fever and neutropenia is **LOW**
  Antimicrobial primary prophylaxis to be considered:
  - Antibacterial—not indicated
  - Antifungal—not indicated
  - Antiviral—not indicated, unless patient previously had an episode of HSV

Efficacy (N = 1034)

Median overall survival	10.4 months with 2 mg/kg pembrolizumab 12.7 months with 10 mg/kg pembrolizumab 8.5 months with 75 mg/m² docetaxel
Median progression-free survival	3.9 months with 2 mg/kg pembrolizumab 4.0 months with 10 mg/kg pembrolizumab 4.0 months with 75 mg/m² docetaxel
Overall response rate*	18% with 2 mg/kg pembrolizumab 18% with 10 mg/kg pembrolizumab 9% with 75 mg/m² docetaxel
Median overall survival in patients with ≥50% tumor cell PD-L1 positivity	14.9 months with 2 mg/kg pembrolizumab 17.3 months with 10 mg/kg pembrolizumab 8.2 months with 75 mg/m² docetaxel
Median progression-free survival in patients with ≥50% tumor cell PD-L1 positivity	5.0 months with 2 mg/kg pembrolizumab 5.2 months with 10 mg/kg pembrolizumab 4.1 months with 75 mg/m² docetaxel
Overall response rate* in patients with ≥50% tumor cell PD-L1 positivity	30% with 2 mg/kg pembrolizumab 29% with 10 mg/kg pembrolizumab 8% with 75 mg/m² docetaxel

*Overall response rate is the percentage of patients who experienced a confirmed partial or complete response to the study drug
Note: median follow-up time was 13.1 months

Patient Population Studied

A multicenter, open-label, randomized, phase 2/3 study involved 1034 patients with previously treated, PD-L1-positive, advanced NSCLC. Eligible patients were age ≥18 years, with Eastern Cooperative Oncology Group (ECOG) performance status score ≤1, with progression after ≥2 cycles of platinum-doublet chemotherapy. Patients who had previously been treated with PD-1 checkpoint inhibitors or docetaxel were not eligible. Patients were assigned (1:1:1) to receive 2 mg/kg pembrolizumab, 10 mg/kg pembrolizumab, or 75 mg/m² docetaxel. Of all patients randomly assigned to treatment, 43% had ≥50% tumor cell PD-L1 positivity

Therapy Monitoring

1. Initially at the time of each dose, and eventually every 6–12 weeks, perform a total-body skin examination with attention to *all* mucous membranes as well as a complete review of systems

2. Monitor patients for signs and symptoms of pneumonitis. Evaluate patients with suspected pneumonitis with chest x-ray, CT scan, and pulse oximetry. For ≥2 toxicity, may include nasal swab, sputum culture and sensitivity, blood culture and sensitivity, and urine culture and sensitivity

3. Monitor patients for signs and symptoms of colitis. Encourage patients to report diarrhea immediately to any member of the health care team

4. Draw AST, ALT, and bilirubin prior to each infusion and/or weekly if there are Grade 1 LFT elevations. Note, no treatment is recommended for G1 LFT abnormalities. For ≥2 toxicity, implement work-up for other causes of elevated LFTs, including viral hepatitis

5. Use basic metabolic panel (Na, K, CO_2, glucose) and patient history as screening tools for hypophysitis including hypopituitarism and adrenal insufficiency. If in doubt, evaluate morning adrenocorticotropic hormone (ACTH) and cortisol levels. Consider ACTH stimulation test for indeterminate results

6. Assess thyroid function at the start of treatment, periodically during treatment, and as indicated based on clinical evaluation, and for clinical signs and symptoms of thyroid disorders. Test for TSH and free thyroxine (FT4) every 4–6 weeks as part of routine clinical monitoring of therapy or for case detection in symptomatic patients

7. Measure glucose at baseline and with each treatment during the first 12 weeks and every 6 weeks thereafter

8. Obtain a serum creatinine level prior to every dose. If creatinine is found to be newly elevated, consider holding therapy while other potential causes are evaluated. Note, routine urinalysis is not necessary other than to rule out urinary tract infections, etc

9. Obtain a complete rheumatologic history and perform an examination of all peripheral joints for tenderness, swelling, and range of motion. Examine the spine. Consider plain x-ray/imaging to exclude metastases and evaluate joint damage (erosions), if appropriate

10. In patients at high risk for infections and in appropriately selected patients based on an infectious disease evaluation, draw screening laboratories (HIV, hepatitis A and B, and blood QuantiFERON for TB) to prepare patients to start infliximab

Treatment Modifications

Adverse Reaction	Grade/Severity	Dose Modification
Colitis	G1	Loperamide 4 mg as starting dose then 2 mg before each meal and after each loose stool until without diarrhea for 12 hours, with maximum of 16 mg loperamide per day. If G1 diarrhea or colitis persists for >14 days, then add prednisolone 0.5–1 mg/kg (non-enteric-coated) or consider oral budesonide 9 mg daily if no bloody diarrhea
	G2/3 diarrhea or colitis	Withhold pembrolizumab. Loperamide 4 mg as starting dose then 2 mg before each meal and after each loose stool until without diarrhea for 12 hours, with maximum of 16 mg loperamide per day. Administer oral prednisone/prednisolone at a dose of 0.5–2 mg/kg/day or its equivalent. When symptoms improve to G1, begin a slow corticosteroid taper over at least 4 weeks. Resume pembrolizumab upon symptom control, or when prednisone/prednisolone daily dose <10 mg
	G4 diarrhea or colitis	Permanently discontinue pembrolizumab. Loperamide 4 mg as starting dose then 2 mg before each meal and after each loose stool until without diarrhea for 12 hours, with maximum of 16 mg loperamide per day. Administer 1–2 mg/kg intravenous (methyl)prednisolone and convert to 0.5–2 mg/kg prednisone/prednisolone orally each day or its equivalent only after a response. Taper over at least 4 weeks when symptoms improve. If symptoms do not improve over 72 hours or worsen, perform flexible sigmoidoscopy/colonoscopy to document colitis then begin infliximab 5 mg/kg (if no perforation, sepsis, TB, hepatitis, NYHA III/IV CHF). If no response, add MMF 500–1000 mg twice daily. If worse on MMF, consider addition of tacrolimus or ATG

(continued)

Treatment Modifications (*continued*)

Adverse Reaction	Grade/Severity	Dose Modification
Pneumonitis	G2	Withhold pembrolizumab. Consider pneumocystis prophylaxis depending on the clinical context and coverage with empiric antibiotics. Administer oral prednisone/prednisolone at a dose of 1–2 mg/kg/day or its equivalent. When symptoms improve to G1, begin a slow corticosteroid taper over at least 4 weeks. If response is not adequate after 48 hours, administer 2–4 mg/kg intravenous (methyl)prednisolone and convert to 0.5–2 mg/kg prednisone/prednisolone orally each day or its equivalent only after a response, followed by a taper over at least 6 weeks when symptoms improve to G1, titrating to symptoms. Resume pembrolizumab upon symptom control, or when prednisone/prednisolone daily dose <10 mg
	G3/4	Permanently discontinue pembrolizumab. Consider pneumocystis prophylaxis depending on the clinical context; cover with empiric antibiotics. Administer 2–4 mg/kg intravenous (methyl)prednisolone and convert to 1–2 mg/kg prednisone/prednisolone orally each day or its equivalent only after a response, followed by a taper over at least 8 weeks when symptoms improve to G1, titrating to symptoms. If, when initially treated, improvement does not occur within 48–72 hours, begin infliximab 5 mg/kg (if no perforation, sepsis, TB, hepatitis, NYHA III/IV CHF). If no response to infliximab, add MMF 500–1000 mg twice daily. Consider MMF especially if concurrent hepatic toxicity
Hepatitis	G2 (AST or ALT >3–5× ULN or total bilirubin >1.5–3× ULN)	Withhold pembrolizumab. Administer oral prednisone/prednisolone at a dose of 1–2 mg/kg/day or its equivalent. When symptoms improve to G1, begin a slow corticosteroid taper over at least 4 weeks. Resume pembrolizumab upon symptom control, or when prednisone/prednisolone daily dose <10 mg
	G3/4 (AST or ALT >5× ULN or total bilirubin >3× ULN)	Permanently discontinue pembrolizumab. Administer 1–2 mg/kg intravenous (methyl) prednisolone and convert to 0.5–2 mg/kg prednisone/prednisolone orally each day or its equivalent only after a response. Taper over at least 6 weeks when symptoms improve. If no response, add MMF 500–1000 mg twice daily. If worse on MMF, consider adding tacrolimus or ATG
Hypophysitis	G2/3 (moderate symptoms, ie, headache but no visual disturbance or fatigue/mood alteration but hemodynamically stable, no electrolyte disturbance)	Administer analgesia as needed for headache. Withhold pembrolizumab. Administer oral prednisone/prednisolone at a dose of 0.5–2 mg/kg/day or its equivalent. When symptoms improve to G1, begin a slow corticosteroid taper over at least 4 weeks. If no improvement in 48 hours, administer 1–2 mg/kg intravenous (methyl)prednisolone and convert to 0.5–2 mg/kg prednisone/prednisolone orally each day or its equivalent only after a response. Taper over at least 4 weeks when symptoms improve to 5 mg prednisone/prednisolone or equivalent; do not stop steroids. Resume pembrolizumab upon symptom control, or when prednisone/prednisolone daily dose <10 mg
	G4 (severe mass effect symptoms, ie, severe headache, any visual disturbance or severe hypoadrenalism, ie, hypotension, severe electrolyte disturbance)	Permanently discontinue pembrolizumab. Administer analgesia as needed for headache. Administer 1–2 mg/kg intravenous (methyl)prednisolone and convert to 0.5–2 mg/kg prednisone/prednisolone orally each day or its equivalent only after a response. Taper over at least 4 weeks when symptoms improve to 5 mg prednisone/prednisolone or equivalent; do not stop steroids
Adrenal insufficiency	G2	Withhold pembrolizumab. Administer oral prednisone/prednisolone at a dose of 0.5–2 mg/kg/day or its equivalent. When symptoms improve to G1, begin a slow corticosteroid taper over at least 4 weeks. Serially assess adrenal function and continue steroids at replacement doses (20–40 mg hydrocortisone daily ~2/3 dose in morning upon awakening and ~1/3 at 4:00 PM) until recovery of adrenal function is documented. Resume pembrolizumab upon symptom control, or when prednisone/prednisolone daily dose <10 mg
	G3/4	Permanently discontinue pembrolizumab. Administer oral prednisone/prednisolone at a dose of 0.5–2 mg/kg/day or its equivalent. When symptoms improve to G1, begin a slow corticosteroid taper over at least 4 weeks. Serially assess adrenal function and continue steroids at replacement doses (20–40 mg hydrocortisone daily ~2/3 dose in morning upon awakening and ~1/3 at 4:00 PM) until recovery of adrenal function is documented

(*continued*)

Treatment Modifications (continued)

Adverse Reaction	Grade/Severity	Dose Modification
Type 1 diabetes mellitus	G3 hyperglycemia	Withhold pembrolizumab. Admit to hospital to manage hyperglycemia. Role of corticosteroids in preventing complete loss of insulin-producing cells is unknown and not recommended. Resume pembrolizumab upon symptom control, or when prednisone/prednisolone daily dose <10 mg
	G4 hyperglycemia	Permanently discontinue pembrolizumab. Admit to hospital to manage hyperglycemia. Role of corticosteroids in preventing complete loss of insulin-producing cells is unknown and not recommended
Nephritis and renal dysfunction	G2/3 (serum creatinine 1.5–6× ULN)	Withhold pembrolizumab. Administer oral prednisone/prednisolone at a dose of 0.5–2 mg/kg/day or its equivalent. When symptoms improve to G1, begin a slow corticosteroid taper over at least 4 weeks. If response is not adequate, administer 0.5–1 mg/kg intravenous (methyl)prednisolone and convert to 0.5–2 mg/kg prednisone/prednisolone orally each day or its equivalent only after a response, followed by a taper over at least 4 weeks when symptoms improve to G1. Resume pembrolizumab upon symptom control, or when prednisone/prednisolone daily dose <10 mg
	G4 (serum creatinine >6× ULN)	Permanently discontinue pembrolizumab. Administer 0.5–1 mg/kg intravenous (methyl)prednisolone and convert to 0.5–2 mg/kg prednisone/prednisolone orally each day or its equivalent only after a response, followed by a taper over at least 4 weeks when improves to G1
Skin	G1/2	Continue pembrolizumab. Avoid skin irritants and sun exposure; topical emollients recommended. Topical steroid (mild strength for G1, moderate/potent strength for G2) cream once or twice daily ± oral or topical antihistamines for itching
	G3 rash or suspected SJS or TEN	Withhold pembrolizumab. Avoid skin irritants and sun exposure; topical emollients recommended. Administer oral or topical antihistamines for itching. Administer oral prednisone/prednisolone at a dose of 0.5–2 mg/kg or its equivalent daily for 3 days followed by a slow corticosteroid taper over at least 4 weeks when the rash improves to G1. If rash does not respond adequately, administer 0.5–1 mg/kg intravenous (methyl)prednisolone and convert to 0.5–2 mg/kg prednisone/prednisolone orally each day or its equivalent only after a response, followed by a taper over at least 4 weeks when the rash improves to G1. Resume pembrolizumab upon symptom control, or when prednisone/prednisolone daily dose <10 mg
	G4 rash or confirmed SJS or TEN	Avoid skin irritants and sun exposure; topical emollients recommended. Administer oral or topical antihistamines for itching. Administer 1–2 mg/kg intravenous (methyl)prednisolone and convert to oral steroids 0.5–2 mg/kg prednisone/prednisolone each day or its equivalent only after a response. Taper over at least 4 weeks when the rash improves to G1. Permanently discontinue pembrolizumab
Encephalitis	Confusion or altered behavior, headaches, alteration in Glasgow Coma Scale, motor or sensory deficits, speech abnormality, may or may not be febrile	Initially withhold pembrolizumab, but permanently discontinue pembrolizumab if there is no doubt as to diagnosis. Exclude bacterial and ideally viral infections prior to high-dose steroids. Administer oral prednisone/prednisolone at a dose of 0.5–2 mg/kg/day or its equivalent. When symptoms improve, begin a slow corticosteroid taper over at least 4–8 weeks. If symptoms are severe, administer 1–2 mg/kg intravenous (methyl)prednisolone and convert to 0.5–2 mg/kg prednisone/prednisolone orally each day or its equivalent only after a response. Consider concurrent empiric antiviral (intravenous acyclovir) and antibacterial therapy
Aseptic meningitis	Headache, photophobia, neck stiffness with fever or may be afebrile, vomiting; normal cognition/cerebral function (distinguishes from encephalitis)	
Other syndromes include neurosarcoidosis, posterior reversible leukoencephalopathy syndrome (PRES), Vogt-Koyanagi-Harada syndrome, demyelination, vasculitic encephalopathy, and generalized seizures		

(continued)

Treatment Modifications (*continued*)

Adverse Reaction	Grade/Severity	Dose Modification
Transverse myelitis	Acute or subacute neurologic signs/symptoms of motor, sensory, or autonomic origin; most have sensory level; often bilateral symptoms	Initially withhold pembrolizumab, but permanently discontinue pembrolizumab if there is no doubt as to diagnosis. Administer 2 mg/kg intravenous (methyl)prednisolone or consider 1 g/day and convert to 0.5–2 mg/kg prednisone/prednisolone orally each day or its equivalent only after a response. When symptoms improve, begin a slow corticosteroid taper over at least 4–8 weeks. Plasmapheresis may be required if steroids do not bring about improvement
Myocarditis	G3	Permanently discontinue pembrolizumab. Administer 2 mg/kg intravenous (methyl) prednisolone or consider 1 g/day and convert to 0.5–2 mg/kg prednisone/prednisolone orally each day or its equivalent only after a response. When symptoms improve, begin a slow corticosteroid taper over at least 4–8 weeks. If no response, add MMF 500–1000 mg twice daily. If worse on MMF, consider adding tacrolimus
Peripheral neurologic toxicity	Moderate: some interference with ADLs, symptoms concerning to patient	Withhold pembrolizumab. Initial observation reasonable or initiate prednisone/ prednisolone 0.5–1 mg/kg (if progressing, eg, from mild) and/or pregabalin or duloxetine for pain. When symptoms improve, begin a slow corticosteroid taper over at least 4 weeks. Resume pembrolizumab upon symptom control, or when prednisone/ prednisolone daily dose <10 mg
	Severe: limits self-care and aids warranted, life-threatening, eg, respiratory problems	Permanently discontinue pembrolizumab. Administer 1–2 mg/kg intravenous (methyl) prednisolone and convert to 0.5–2 mg/kg prednisone/prednisolone orally each day or its equivalent only after a response. Taper over at least 4–8 weeks when symptoms improve to G1
Guillain-Barré syndrome	Progressive symmetrical muscle weakness with absent or reduced tendon reflexes—involves extremities; facial, respiratory, bulbar, and oculomotor muscles; dysregulation of autonomic nerves	Permanently discontinue pembrolizumab. Use of steroids not recommended in idiopathic Guillain-Barré syndrome; however, a trial of (methyl)prednisolone 1–2 mg/ kg is reasonable, converting to 0.5–2 mg/kg prednisone/prednisolone orally each day or its equivalent only after a response. If no improvement or worsening, plasmapheresis or IVIG indicated
Myasthenia gravis	Fluctuating muscle weakness (proximal limb, trunk, ocular, eg, ptosis/diplopia or bulbar) with fatigability; respiratory muscles may also be involved	Permanently discontinue pembrolizumab. Administer pyridostigmine at an initial dose of 30 mg 3 times daily. Administer oral prednisone/prednisolone at a dose of 0.5–2 mg/ kg/day or its equivalent or 1–2 mg/kg intravenous (methyl)prednisolone depending on the severity of symptoms. If treatment begins with intravenous drug, convert to 0.5–2 mg/kg prednisone/prednisolone orally each day or its equivalent only after a response. If no improvement or worsening, plasmapheresis or IVIG may be considered. Additional immunosuppressants used in myasthenia gravis include azathioprine, cyclosporine, and mycophenolate. Avoid certain medications (eg, ciprofloxacin, beta-blockers) that may precipitate cholinergic crisis
Other syndromes, including motor and sensory peripheral neuropathy, multifocal radicular neuropathy/plexopathy, autonomic neuropathy, phrenic nerve palsy, cranial nerve palsies (eg, facial nerve, optic nerve, hypoglossal nerve)		Permanently discontinue pembrolizumab. Administer oral prednisone/prednisolone at a dose of 0.5–2 mg/kg/day or its equivalent or 1–2 mg/kg intravenous (methyl) prednisolone depending on the severity of symptoms. If treatment begins with intravenous drug, convert to 0.5–2 mg/kg prednisone/prednisolone orally each day or its equivalent only after a response

(*continued*)

Treatment Modifications (continued)

Adverse Reaction	Grade/Severity	Dose Modification
Arthralgia	G1 (mild pain with inflammation, erythema, or joint swelling)	Continue pembrolizumab. Administer acetaminophen (paracetamol) and ibuprofen
	G2 (moderate pain with inflammation, erythema, or joint swelling that limits ADLs)	Withhold pembrolizumab. Administer higher doses of acetaminophen (paracetamol) and ibuprofen, and use diclofenac or naproxen or etoricoxib. If inadequately controlled, consider intra-articular steroid injections for large joints or administer oral prednisone/prednisolone at a dose of 0.5–2 mg/kg/day or its equivalent. When symptoms improve to G1, begin a slow corticosteroid taper over at least 4 weeks. If response is not adequate, administer 0.5–1 mg/kg intravenous (methyl)prednisolone and convert to 0.5–2 mg/kg prednisone/prednisolone orally each day or its equivalent only after a response, followed by a taper over at least 4 weeks when improves to G1. Resume pembrolizumab upon symptom control, or when prednisone/prednisolone daily dose <10 mg
	G3 (severe pain; irreversible joint damage; disabling; limits self-care ADLs)	Withhold pembrolizumab. Administer 0.5–1 mg/kg intravenous (methyl)prednisolone and convert to 0.5–2 mg/kg prednisone/prednisolone orally each day or its equivalent only after a response, followed by a taper over at least 4 weeks when improves to G1. In severe cases, infliximab or another anti–TNF alpha drug may be required for improvement of arthritis. Resume pembrolizumab upon symptom control, or when prednisone/prednisolone daily dose <10 mg
Other	First occurrence of other G3	Withhold pembrolizumab. Administer oral prednisone/prednisolone at a dose of 0.5–2 mg/kg/day or its equivalent. When symptoms improve to G1, begin a slow corticosteroid taper over at least 4 weeks. Resume pembrolizumab upon symptom control, or when prednisone/prednisolone daily dose <10 mg
	Recurrence of same G3	Permanently discontinue pembrolizumab. Administer 1–2 mg/kg intravenous (methyl)prednisolone and convert to 0.5–2 mg/kg prednisone/prednisolone orally each day or its equivalent only after a response. Taper over at least 4–8 weeks when symptoms improve to G1
	Life-threatening or G4	
	Requirement for ≥10 mg/day prednisone or equivalent for >12 weeks	Permanently discontinue pembrolizumab
	Persistent G2/3 adverse reactions lasting ≥12 weeks	

ADL, activities of daily living; ALT, alanine aminotransferase; AST, aspartate aminotransferase; ATG, anti-thymocyte globulin; CHF, congestive heart failure; IVIG, intravenous immunoglobulin; MMF, mycophenolate mofetil; NYHA, New York Heart Association; SJS, Stevens-Johnson syndrome; TB, tuberculosis; TEN, toxic epidermal necrolysis; TNF, tumor necrosis factor; ULN, upper limit of normal

Notes on general supportive care:
• Steroid taper in most cases will proceed over a minimum of 1 month, but if symptoms improve rapidly, a 2-week taper can be considered. If steroids are administered for more than 4 weeks, consider PCP prophylaxis (cotrimoxazole 480 mg twice daily M/W/F or inhaled pentamidine if has cotrimoxazole allergy), regular random blood glucose, vitamin D level, and starting calcium/vitamin D supplementation per guidelines

Notes on pregnancy and breastfeeding:
• Pembrolizumab can cause fetal harm. If used during pregnancy, or if the patient becomes pregnant during treatment, apprise the patient of the potential hazard to a fetus. Females of reproductive potential should use highly effective contraception during treatment and for 4 months after the last dose of pembrolizumab
• It is not known whether pembrolizumab is excreted in human milk. Therefore, it is recommended that women discontinue nursing during treatment with and for 4 months after the final dose of pembrolizumab

Adverse Events (N = 991)

Grade (%)*	Pembrolizumab 2 mg/kg		Pembrolizumab 10 mg/kg		Docetaxel 75 mg/m²	
	Grade 1/2	Grade 3–5	Grade 1/2	Grade 3–5	Grade 1/2	Grade 3–5
Any event	51	13	50	16	46	35
Non-hematologic Adverse Events						
Fatigue	12	1	13	2	21	4
Decreased appetite	13	<1	9	<1	15	<1
Nausea	11	<1	8	<1	14	<1
Rash	8	<1	13	<1	5	0
Hypothyroidism[†]	8	0	8	0	<1	0
Diarrhea	6	<1	6	0	16	2
Asthenia	6	<1	5	<1	9	2
Hyperthyroidism[†]	4	0	6	<1	<1	0
Pneumonitis[†]	3	2	2	2	1	<1
Stomatitis	4	0	2	<1	13	<1
Severe skin reactions[†]	<1	<1	<1	2	<1	<1
Colitis[†]	<1	<1	<1	<1	0	0
Alopecia	<1	0	<1	0	32	<1
Adrenal insufficiency[†]	<1	0	<1	<1	0	0
Pancreatitis[†]	<1	<1	0	0	0	0
Myositis[†]	<1	0	<1	0	<1	0
Autoimmune hepatitis[†]	0	<1	<1	0	0	0
Type 1 diabetes[†]	0	<1	<1	<1	0	0
Thyroiditis[†]	<1	0	0	0	0	0
Hypophysitis	0	<1	0	<1	0	0
Hematologic Adverse Events						
Anemia	2	<1	4	<1	11	2
Neutropenia	<1	0	<1	0	2	12

*According to the National Cancer Institute Common Terminology Criteria for Adverse Events, version 4.0
[†]Denotes those events of special interest
Note: toxicities are included in the table if all-grade events occurred in ≥10% of patients in any group and were deemed to be related to the study treatment, or occurred in ≥2 patients in the pembrolizumab groups and were of special interest

ADVANCED NSCLC • SUBSEQUENT THERAPY

LUNG CANCER REGIMEN: ATEZOLIZUMAB

Brahmer JR et al. J Clin Oncol 2018;36(17):1714–1768
FDA and EMA prescribing information
Haanen JB et al. Ann Oncol 2017;28(suppl 4):iv119–iv142
Rittmeyer A et al. Lancet 2017;389:255–265

Atezolizumab 1200 mg; administer intravenously in a volume of 0.9% Sodium Chloride (0.9% NS)sufficient to produce a final concentration within the range 3.2 mg/mL to 16.8 mg/mL over 60 minutes every 3 weeks (total dosage/3-week cycle = 1200 mg)

Alternative atezolizumab dosage regimens as per the U.S. FDA regimens approved on May 6, 2019:

Atezolizumab 840 mg; administer intravenously in a volume of 0.9% NS sufficient to produce a final concentration within the range 3.2 mg/mL to 16.8 mg/mL over 60 minutes every 2 weeks (total dosage/2-week cycle = 840 mg)

Atezolizumab 1680 mg; administer intravenously in a volume of 0.9% NS sufficient to produce a final concentration within the range 3.2 mg/mL to 16.8 mg/mL over 60 minutes every 4 weeks (total dosage/4-week cycle = 1680 mg)

- Atezolizumab may be administered through an administration set either with or without a low-protein binding in-line filter with pore sizes of 0.2–0.22 μm
- If the initial infusion is well tolerated, subsequent administration may be completed over 30 minutes
- Severe infusion reactions have occurred in patients in clinical trials of atezolizumab
  - Interrupt or slow the administration rate in patients with mild or moderate infusion reactions
  - Permanently discontinue atezolizumab in patients who experience infusion reactions G ≥3

Supportive Care

Antiemetic prophylaxis
Emetogenic potential is **LOW**
See Chapter 42 for antiemetic recommendations

Hematopoietic growth factor (CSF) prophylaxis
Primary prophylaxis is **NOT** *indicated*
See Chapter 43 for more information

Antimicrobial prophylaxis
Risk of fever and neutropenia is **LOW**
Antimicrobial primary prophylaxis to be considered:
- Antibacterial—not indicated
- Antifungal—not indicated
- Antiviral—not indicated, unless patient previously had an episode of HSV

Patient Population Studied

A multicenter, open-label, randomized, phase 3 trial involved 1225 patients with squamous or non-squamous NSCLC. Eligible patients were age ≥18 years, with an Eastern Cooperative Oncology Group (ECOG) performance status score ≤1, and had previously received 1–2 cytotoxic chemotherapy regimens (of which at least one regimen involved platinum-based combination therapy) for stage IIIB or IV NSCLC. Patients with a history of autoimmune disease were not eligible. Patients who had previously been treated with docetaxel, CD137 agonists, anti-CTLA4, or therapies targeting the PD-L1 and PD-1 pathways were also not eligible. Patients were assigned (1:1) to receive atezolizumab or docetaxel.

Efficacy (N = 850)

Median overall survival	13.8 months with atezolizumab 9.6 months with docetaxel HR 0.73, 95% CI 0.62–0.87, P = 0.0003
Median progression-free survival	2.8 months with atezolizumab 4.0 months with docetaxel HR 0.95, 95% CI 0.82–1.10, P = 0.49
Overall response rate*	14% with atezolizumab 13% with docetaxel
Median duration of response	16.3 months with atezolizumab 6.2 months with docetaxel HR 0.34, 95% CI 0.21–0.55, P<0.0001
Median overall survival in patients with PD-L1 positivity in ≥1% tumor cells or tumor-infiltrating immune cells	15.7 months with atezolizumab 10.3 months with docetaxel HR 0.74, 95% CI 0.58–0.93, P = 0.0102
Median progression-free survival in patients with PD-L1 positivity in ≥1% tumor cells or tumor-infiltrating immune cells	2.8 months with atezolizumab 4.1 months with docetaxel HR 0.91, 95% CI 0.74–1.12, P = 0.38
Overall response rate* in patients with PD-L1 positivity in ≥1% tumor cells or tumor-infiltrating immune cells	18% with atezolizumab 16% with docetaxel
Median duration of response in patients with PD-L1 positivity in ≥1% tumor cells or tumor-infiltrating immune cells	16.0 months with atezolizumab 6.2 months with docetaxel HR 0.38, 95% CI 0.22–0.65, P = 0.0003

Overall response rate is the percentage of patients who experienced a confirmed partial or complete response to the study drug
Note: median follow-up time was 21 months

Therapy Monitoring

1. Initially at the time of each dose, and eventually every 6–12 weeks, perform a total-body skin examination with attention to *all* mucous membranes as well as a complete review of systems

2. Monitor patients for signs and symptoms of pneumonitis. Evaluate patients with suspected pneumonitis with chest x-ray, CT scan, and pulse oximetry. For ≥2 toxicity, may include nasal swab, sputum culture and sensitivity, blood culture and sensitivity, and urine culture and sensitivity

3. Monitor patients for signs and symptoms of colitis. Encourage patients to report diarrhea immediately to any member of the health care team

4. Draw AST, ALT, and bilirubin prior to each infusion and/or weekly if there are Grade 1 LFT elevations. Note, no treatment is recommended for G1 LFT abnormalities. For ≥2 toxicity, implement work-up for other causes of elevated LFTs, including viral hepatitis

5. Use basic metabolic panel (Na, K, CO_2, glucose) and patient history as screening tools for hypophysitis including hypopituitarism and adrenal insufficiency. If in doubt, evaluate morning adrenocorticotropic hormone (ACTH) and cortisol levels. Consider ACTH stimulation test for indeterminate results

6. Assess thyroid function at the start of treatment, periodically during treatment and as indicated based on clinical evaluation, and for clinical signs and symptoms of thyroid disorders. Test for TSH and free thyroxine (FT4) every 4–6 weeks as part of routine clinical monitoring of therapy or for case detection in symptomatic patients

7. Measure glucose at baseline and with each treatment during the first 12 weeks and every 6 weeks thereafter

8. Obtain a serum creatinine level prior to every dose. If creatinine is found to be newly elevated, consider holding therapy while other potential causes are evaluated. Note, routine urinalysis is not necessary other than to rule out urinary tract infections, etc

9. Obtain a complete rheumatologic history and perform an examination of all peripheral joints for tenderness, swelling, and range of motion. Examine the spine. Consider plain x-ray/imaging to exclude metastases and evaluate joint damage (erosions), if appropriate

10. In patients at high risk for infections and in appropriately selected patients based on an infectious disease evaluation, draw screening laboratories (HIV, hepatitis A and B, and blood QuantiFERON for TB) to prepare patients to start infliximab

Treatment Modifications

Adverse Reaction	Grade/Severity	Dose Modification
Colitis	G1	Loperamide 4 mg as starting dose then 2 mg before each meal and after each loose stool until without diarrhea for 12 hours, with maximum of 16 mg loperamide per day. If G1 diarrhea or colitis persists for >14 days, then add prednisolone 0.5–1 mg/kg (non-enteric-coated) or consider oral budesonide 9 mg daily if no bloody diarrhea
	G2/3 diarrhea or colitis	Withhold atezolizumab. Loperamide 4 mg as starting dose then 2 mg before each meal and after each loose stool until without diarrhea for 12 hours, with maximum of 16 mg loperamide per day. Administer oral prednisone/prednisolone at a dose of 0.5–2 mg/kg/day or its equivalent. When symptoms improve to G1, begin a slow corticosteroid taper over at least 4 weeks. Resume atezolizumab upon symptom control, or when prednisone/prednisolone daily dose <10 mg
	G4 diarrhea or colitis	Permanently discontinue atezolizumab. Loperamide 4 mg as starting dose then 2 mg before each meal and after each loose stool until without diarrhea for 12 hours, with maximum of 16 mg loperamide per day. Administer 1–2 mg/kg intravenous (methyl)prednisolone and convert to 0.5–2 mg/kg prednisone/prednisolone orally each day or its equivalent only after a response. Taper over at least 4 weeks when symptoms improve. If symptoms do not improve over 72 hours or worsen, perform flexible sigmoidoscopy/colonoscopy to document colitis then begin infliximab 5 mg/kg (if no perforation, sepsis, TB, hepatitis, NYHA III/IV CHF). If no response, add MMF 500–1000 mg twice daily. If worse on MMF, consider addition of tacrolimus or ATG

(continued)

Treatment Modifications (*continued*)

Adverse Reaction	Grade/Severity	Dose Modification
Pneumonitis	G2	Withhold atezolizumab. Consider pneumocystis prophylaxis depending on the clinical context and cover with empiric antibiotics. Administer oral prednisone/prednisolone at a dose of 1–2 mg/kg/day or its equivalent. When symptoms improve to G1, begin a slow corticosteroid taper over at least 4 weeks. If response is not adequate after 48 hours, then administer 2–4 mg/kg intravenous (methyl)prednisolone and convert to 0.5–2 mg/kg prednisone/prednisolone orally each day or its equivalent only after a response, followed by a taper over at least 6 weeks when symptoms improve to G1, titrating to symptoms. Resume atezolizumab upon symptom control, or when prednisone/prednisolone daily dose <10 mg
	G3/4	Permanently discontinue atezolizumab. Consider pneumocystis prophylaxis depending on the clinical context; cover with empiric antibiotics. Administer 2–4 mg/kg intravenous (methyl)prednisolone and convert to 1–2 mg/kg prednisone/prednisolone orally each day or its equivalent only after a response, followed by a taper over at least 8 weeks when symptoms improve to G1, titrating to symptoms. If, when initially treated, improvement does not occur within 48–72 hours, begin infliximab 5 mg/kg (if no perforation, sepsis, TB, hepatitis, NYHA III/IV CHF). If no response to infliximab, add MMF 500–1000 mg twice daily. Consider MMF especially if concurrent hepatic toxicity
Hepatitis	G2 (AST or ALT >3–5× ULN or total bilirubin >1.5–3× ULN)	Withhold atezolizumab. Administer oral prednisone/prednisolone at a dose of 1–2 mg/kg/day or its equivalent. When symptoms improve to G1, begin a slow corticosteroid taper over at least 4 weeks. Resume atezolizumab upon symptom control, or when prednisone/prednisolone daily dose <10 mg
	G3/4 (AST or ALT >5× ULN or total bilirubin >3× ULN)	Permanently discontinue atezolizumab. Administer 1–2 mg/kg intravenous (methyl)prednisolone and convert to 0.5–2 mg/kg prednisone/prednisolone orally each day or its equivalent only after a response. Taper over at least 6 weeks when symptoms improve. If no response, add MMF 500–1000 mg twice daily. If worse on MMF, consider adding tacrolimus or ATG
Hypophysitis	G2/3 (moderate symptoms, ie, headache but no visual disturbance or fatigue/mood alteration but hemodynamically stable, no electrolyte disturbance)	Administer analgesia as needed for headache. Withhold atezolizumab. Administer oral prednisone/prednisolone at a dose of 0.5–2 mg/kg/day or its equivalent. When symptoms improve to G1, begin a slow corticosteroid taper over at least 4 weeks. If no improvement in 48 hours, administer 1–2 mg/kg intravenous (methyl)prednisolone and convert to 0.5–2 mg/kg prednisone/prednisolone orally each day or its equivalent only after a response. Taper over at least 4 weeks when symptoms improve to 5 mg prednisone/prednisolone or equivalent; do not stop steroids. Resume atezolizumab upon symptom control, or when prednisone/prednisolone daily dose <10 mg
	G4 (severe mass effect symptoms, ie, severe headache, any visual disturbance or severe hypoadrenalism, ie, hypotension, severe electrolyte disturbance)	Permanently discontinue atezolizumab. Administer analgesia as needed for headache. Administer 1–2 mg/kg intravenous (methyl)prednisolone and convert to 0.5–2 mg/kg prednisone/prednisolone orally each day or its equivalent only after a response. Taper over at least 4 weeks when symptoms improve to 5 mg prednisone/prednisolone or equivalent; do not stop steroids
Adrenal insufficiency	G2	Withhold atezolizumab. Administer oral prednisone/prednisolone at a dose of 0.5–2 mg/kg/day or its equivalent. When symptoms improve to G1, begin a slow corticosteroid taper over at least 4 weeks. Serially assess adrenal function and continue steroids at replacement doses (20–40 mg hydrocortisone daily ~2/3 dose in morning upon awakening and ~1/3 at 4:00 PM) until recovery of adrenal function is documented. Resume atezolizumab upon symptom control, or when prednisone/prednisolone daily dose <10 mg
	G3/4	Permanently discontinue atezolizumab. Administer oral prednisone/prednisolone at a dose of 0.5–2 mg/kg/day or its equivalent. When symptoms improve to G1, begin a slow corticosteroid taper over at least 4 weeks. Serially assess adrenal function and continue steroids at replacement doses (20–40 mg hydrocortisone daily ~2/3 dose in morning upon awakening and ~1/3 at 4:00 PM) until recovery of adrenal function is documented

(*continued*)

Treatment Modifications (*continued*)

Adverse Reaction	Grade/Severity	Dose Modification
Type 1 diabetes mellitus	G3 hyperglycemia	Withhold atezolizumab. Admit to hospital to manage hyperglycemia. Role of corticosteroids in preventing complete loss of insulin-producing cells is unknown and not recommended. Resume atezolizumab upon symptom control, or when prednisone/prednisolone daily dose <10 mg
	G4 hyperglycemia	Permanently discontinue atezolizumab. Admit to hospital to manage hyperglycemia. Role of corticosteroids in preventing complete loss of insulin-producing cells is unknown and not recommended
Nephritis and renal dysfunction	G2/3 (serum creatinine 1.5–6× ULN)	Withhold atezolizumab. Administer oral prednisone/prednisolone at a dose of 0.5–2 mg/kg/day or its equivalent. When symptoms improve to G1, begin a slow corticosteroid taper over at least 4 weeks. If response is not adequate, then administer 0.5–1 mg/kg intravenous (methyl)prednisolone and convert to 0.5–2 mg/kg prednisone/prednisolone orally each day or its equivalent only after a response, followed by a taper over at least 4 weeks when symptoms improve to G1. Resume atezolizumab upon symptom control, or when prednisone/prednisolone daily dose <10 mg
	G4 (serum creatinine >6× ULN)	Permanently discontinue atezolizumab. Administer 0.5–1 mg/kg intravenous (methyl)prednisolone and convert to 0.5–2 mg/kg prednisone/prednisolone orally each day or its equivalent only after a response, followed by a taper over at least 4 weeks when symptoms improve to G1
Skin	G1/2	Continue atezolizumab. Avoid skin irritants, avoid sun exposure; topical emollients recommended. Topical steroid (mild strength for G1, moderate/potent strength for G2) cream once or twice daily ± oral or topical antihistamines for itching
	G3 rash or suspected SJS or TEN	Withhold atezolizumab. Avoid skin irritants, avoid sun exposure; topical emollients recommended. Administer oral or topical antihistamines for itching. Administer oral prednisone/prednisolone at a dose of 0.5–2 mg/kg or its equivalent daily for 3 days followed by a slow corticosteroid taper over at least 4 weeks when the rash improves to G1. If rash does not respond adequately, then administer 0.5–1 mg/kg intravenous (methyl)prednisolone and convert to 0.5–2 mg/kg prednisone/prednisolone orally each day or its equivalent only after a response, followed by a taper over at least 4 weeks when the rash improves to G1. Resume atezolizumab upon symptom control, or when prednisone/prednisolone daily dose <10 mg
	G4 rash or confirmed SJS or TEN	Avoid skin irritants, avoid sun exposure; topical emollients recommended. Administer oral or topical antihistamines for itching. Administer 1–2 mg/kg intravenous (methyl)prednisolone and convert to oral steroids 0.5–2 mg/kg prednisone/prednisolone each day or its equivalent only after a response. Taper over at least 4 weeks when the rash improves to G1. Permanently discontinue atezolizumab
Encephalitis	Confusion or altered behavior, headaches, alteration in Glasgow Coma Scale, motor or sensory deficits, speech abnormality, may or may not be febrile	Initially withhold atezolizumab, but permanently discontinue atezolizumab if there is no doubt as to diagnosis. Exclude bacterial and ideally viral infections prior to high-dose steroids. Administer oral prednisone/prednisolone at a dose of 0.5–2 mg/kg/day or its equivalent. When symptoms improve, begin a slow corticosteroid taper over at least 4–8 weeks. If symptoms are severe, administer 1–2 mg/kg intravenous (methyl)prednisolone and convert to 0.5–2 mg/kg prednisone/prednisolone orally each day or its equivalent only after a response. Consider concurrent empiric antiviral (intravenous acyclovir) and antibacterial therapy
Aseptic meningitis	Headache, photophobia, neck stiffness with fever or may be afebrile, vomiting; normal cognition/cerebral function (distinguishes from encephalitis)	
Other syndromes include neurosarcoidosis, posterior reversible leukoencephalopathy syndrome (PRES), Vogt-Koyanagi-Harada syndrome, demyelination, vasculitic encephalopathy, and generalized seizures		
Transverse myelitis	Acute or subacute neurologic signs/ symptoms of motor, sensory, or autonomic origin; most have sensory level; often bilateral symptoms	Initially withhold atezolizumab, but permanently discontinue atezolizumab if there is no doubt as to diagnosis. Administer 2 mg/kg intravenous (methyl)prednisolone or consider 1 g/day and convert to 0.5–2 mg/kg prednisone/prednisolone orally each day or its equivalent only after a response. When symptoms improve, begin a slow corticosteroid taper over at least 4–8 weeks. Plasmapheresis may be required if steroids do not bring about improvement

(*continued*)

Treatment Modifications (continued)

Adverse Reaction	Grade/Severity	Dose Modification
Myocarditis	G3	Permanently discontinue atezolizumab. Administer 2 mg/kg intravenous (methyl) prednisolone or consider 1 g/day and convert to 0.5–2 mg/kg prednisone/ prednisolone orally each day or its equivalent only after a response. When symptoms improve, begin a slow corticosteroid taper over at least 4–8 weeks. If no response, add MMF 500–1000 mg twice daily. If worse on MMF, consider adding tacrolimus
Peripheral neurologic toxicity	Moderate: some interference with ADLs, symptoms concerning to patient	Withhold atezolizumab. Initial observation reasonable or initiate prednisone/ prednisolone 0.5–1 mg/kg (if progressing, eg, from mild) and/or pregabalin or duloxetine for pain. When symptoms improve, begin a slow corticosteroid taper over at least 4 weeks. Resume atezolizumab upon symptom control, or when prednisone/prednisolone daily dose <10 mg
	Severe: limits self-care and aids warranted, life-threatening, eg, respiratory problems	Permanently discontinue atezolizumab. Administer 1–2 mg/kg intravenous (methyl)prednisolone and convert to 0.5–2 mg/kg prednisone/prednisolone orally each day or its equivalent only after a response. Taper over at least 4–8 weeks when symptoms improve to G1
Guillain-Barré syndrome	Progressive symmetrical muscle weakness with absent or reduced tendon reflexes— involves extremities; facial, respiratory, bulbar, and oculomotor muscles; dysregulation of autonomic nerves	Permanently discontinue atezolizumab. Use of steroids not recommended in idiopathic Guillain-Barré syndrome; however, a trial of (methyl)prednisolone 1–2 mg/kg is reasonable, converting to 0.5–2 mg/kg prednisone/prednisolone orally each day or its equivalent only after a response. If no improvement or worsening, plasmapheresis or IVIG indicated
Myasthenia gravis	Fluctuating muscle weakness (proximal limb, trunk, ocular, eg, ptosis/diplopia or bulbar) with fatigability; respiratory muscles may also be involved	Permanently discontinue atezolizumab. Administer pyridostigmine at an initial dose of 30 mg 3 times daily. Administer oral prednisone/prednisolone at a dose of 0.5–2 mg/kg/day or its equivalent or 1–2 mg/kg intravenous (methyl) prednisolone depending on the severity of symptoms. If treatment begins with intravenous drug, convert to 0.5–2 mg/kg prednisone/prednisolone orally each day or its equivalent only after a response. If no improvement or worsening, plasmapheresis or IVIG may be considered. Additional immunosuppressants used in myasthenia gravis include azathioprine, cyclosporine, and mycophenolate. Avoid certain medications (eg, ciprofloxacin, beta-blockers) that may precipitate cholinergic crisis
Other syndromes, including motor and sensory peripheral neuropathy, multifocal radicular neuropathy/plexopathy, autonomic neuropathy, phrenic nerve palsy, cranial nerve palsies (eg, facial nerve, optic nerve, hypoglossal nerve)		Permanently discontinue atezolizumab. Administer oral prednisone/prednisolone at a dose of 0.5–2 mg/kg/day or its equivalent or 1–2 mg/kg intravenous (methyl) prednisolone depending on the severity of symptoms. If treatment begins with intravenous drug, convert to 0.5–2 mg/kg prednisone/prednisolone orally each day or its equivalent only after a response
Arthralgia	G1 (mild pain with inflammation, erythema, or joint swelling)	Continue atezolizumab. Administer acetaminophen (paracetamol) and ibuprofen
	G2 (moderate pain with inflammation, erythema, or joint swelling that limits ADLs)	Withhold atezolizumab. Administer higher doses of acetaminophen (paracetamol) and ibuprofen, and use diclofenac or naproxen or etoricoxib. If inadequately controlled, consider intra-articular steroid injections for large joints or administer oral prednisone/prednisolone at a dose of 0.5–2 mg/kg/day or its equivalent. When symptoms improve to G1, begin a slow corticosteroid taper over at least 4 weeks. If response is not adequate, then administer 0.5–1 mg/kg intravenous (methyl)prednisolone and convert to 0.5–2 mg/kg prednisone/prednisolone orally each day or its equivalent only after a response, followed by a taper over at least 4 weeks when symptoms improve to G1. Resume atezolizumab upon symptom control, or when prednisone/prednisolone daily dose <10 mg
	G3 (severe pain; irreversible joint damage; disabling; limits self-care ADLs)	Withhold atezolizumab. Administer 0.5–1 mg/kg intravenous (methyl) prednisolone and convert to 0.5–2 mg/kg prednisone/prednisolone orally each day or its equivalent only after a response, followed by a taper over at least 4 weeks when symptoms improve to G1. In severe cases, infliximab or another anti–TNF alpha drug may be required for improvement of arthritis. Resume atezolizumab upon symptom control, or when prednisone/prednisolone daily dose <10 mg

(continued)

Treatment Modifications (continued)

Adverse Reaction	Grade/Severity	Dose Modification
Other	First occurrence of other G3	Withhold atezolizumab. Administer oral prednisone/prednisolone at a dose of 0.5–2 mg/kg/day or its equivalent. When symptoms improve to G1, begin a slow corticosteroid taper over at least 4 weeks. Resume atezolizumab upon symptom control, or when prednisone/prednisolone daily dose <10 mg
	Recurrence of same G3	Permanently discontinue atezolizumab. Administer 1–2 mg/kg intravenous (methyl)prednisolone and convert to 0.5–2 mg/kg prednisone/prednisolone orally each day or its equivalent only after a response. Taper over at least 4–8 weeks when symptoms improve to G1
	Life-threatening or G4	
	Requirement for ≥10 mg/day prednisone or equivalent for >12 weeks	Permanently discontinue atezolizumab
	Persistent G2/3 adverse reactions lasting ≥12 weeks	

ADL, activities of daily living; ALT, alanine aminotransferase; AST, aspartate aminotransferase; ATG, antithymocyte globulin; CHF, congestive heart failure; IVIG, intravenous immunoglobulin; MMF, mycophenolate mofetil; NYHA, New York Heart Association; SJS, Stevens-Johnson syndrome; TB, tuberculosis; TEN, toxic epidermal necrolysis; TNF, tumor necrosis factor; ULN, upper limit of normal

Notes on general supportive care:
• Steroid taper in most cases will proceed over a minimum of 1 month, but if symptoms improve rapidly, a 2-week taper can be considered. If steroids are administered for more than 4 weeks, consider PCP prophylaxis (cotrimoxazole 480 mg twice daily M/W/F or inhaled pentamidine if cotrimoxazole allergy), regular random blood glucose, vitamin D level, and starting calcium/vitamin D supplementation per guidelines

Notes on pregnancy and breastfeeding:
• Atezolizumab can cause fetal harm. If used during pregnancy, or if the patient becomes pregnant during treatment, apprise the patient of the potential hazard to a fetus. Females of reproductive potential should use highly effective contraception during treatment and for 5 months after the last dose of atezolizumab
• It is not known whether atezolizumab is excreted in human milk. Therefore, it is recommended that women discontinue nursing during treatment with and for 5 months after the final dose of atezolizumab

Adverse Events (N = 1187)

Grade (%)*	Atezolizumab			Docetaxel		
	Grade 1/2	Grade 3/4	Grade 5	Grade 1/2	Grade 3/4	Grade 5
Any event	55	37	2	40	54	2
Any treatment-related event	49	15	0	43	43	<1
Fatigue	24	3	0	31	4	0
Decreased appetite	23	<1	0	22	2	0
Cough	23	<1	0	18	<1	0
Dyspnea	17	2	0	17	2	0
Asthenia	18	1	0	17	2	0
Nausea	17	<1	0	22	<1	0
Pyrexia	18	<1	0	13	<1	0
Constipation	17	<1	0	14	<1	0
Diarrhea	15	<1	0	22	2	0
Vomiting	12	<1	0	10	<1	0
Arthralgia	11	<1	0	10	<1	0

(continued)

Adverse Events (N = 1187) *(continued)*

Grade (%)*	Atezolizumab			Docetaxel		
	Grade 1/2	Grade 3/4	Grade 5	Grade 1/2	Grade 3/4	Grade 5
Anemia	9	2	0	18	6	0
Back pain	10	1	0	7	<1	0
Musculoskeletal pain	10	<1	0	4	<1	0
Peripheral edema	9	<1	0	14	<1	0
Myalgia	6	<1	0	15	<1	0
Peripheral neuropathy	4	0	0	10	1	0
Stomatitis	3	<1	0	9	2	0
Dysgeusia	3	0	0	10	0	0
Neutropenia	1	<1	0	3	13	0
Febrile neutropenia	0	<1	0	0	10	0
Alopecia	<1	0	0	35	<1	0

*According to the National Cancer Institute Common Terminology Criteria for Adverse Events, version 4.0
Note: toxicities are included in the table if all-grade events occurred in ≥10% of patients in any group. Events are included regardless of whether they were caused by the study treatment

ADVANCED NON-SQUAMOUS NSCLC • SUBSEQUENT THERAPY

LUNG CANCER REGIMEN: PEMETREXED

Hanna N et al. J Clin Oncol 2004;22:1589–1597

Folic acid 350–1000 mcg per day; administer orally beginning 1–2 weeks before the first dose of pemetrexed and continuing until 3 weeks after the last dose of pemetrexed
Cyanocobalamin (vitamin B$_{12}$) 1000 mcg; administer intramuscularly every 9 weeks, beginning 1–2 weeks before the first dose of pemetrexed
Dexamethasone 4 mg/dose; administer orally twice daily for 3 consecutive days (6 doses), starting the day before pemetrexed administration to decrease the risk and severity of severe skin rash associated with pemetrexed (total dose/cycle = 24 mg)
Pemetrexed 500 mg/m²; administer intravenously in 100 mL 0.9% sodium chloride injection over 10 minutes on day 1, every 21 days (total dosage/cycle = 500 mg/m²)

Supportive Care
Antiemetic prophylaxis
Emetogenic potential: **LOW**
See Chapter 42 for antiemetic recommendations

Hematopoietic growth factor (CSF) prophylaxis
Primary prophylaxis is **NOT** indicated
See Chapter 43 for more information

Antimicrobial prophylaxis
Risk of fever and neutropenia is **LOW**
Antimicrobial primary prophylaxis to be considered:
- Antibacterial—not indicated
- Antifungal—not indicated
- Antiviral—not indicated unless patient previously had an episode of HSV

Patient Population Studied

A study of 283 patients with stage III–IV NSCLC

Therapy Monitoring

1. *Before each 21-day cycle:* CBC with differential, LFTs, BUN, and creatinine
2. *Weekly:* CBC with differential
3. *Response evaluation every 2 cycles:* continue treatment until disease progression or unacceptable toxicity
4. *Every 2–3 months:* consider plasma homocysteine levels. (High homocysteine concentrations are a sensitive indicator of folate deficiency and may predict pemetrexed toxicity)

Efficacy (N = 265)

Overall response rate	9.1%
1-year overall survival	29.7%
Median survival time	8.3 months
Median progression-free survival	2.9 months
Median time to progression	3.4 months
Median duration of response	4.6 months

Toxicity (N = 265)*

	% Any G	% G3/4
Hematologic		
Neutropenia	Not given	5.3
Febrile neutropenia	Not given	1.9
Neutropenia with infection	Not given	0
Anemia	Not given	4.2
Thrombocytopenia	Not given	1.9
Non-hematologic		
Fatigue	34	5.3
Nausea	30.9	2.6
Vomiting	16.2	1.5
Pulmonary	0.8	0
Neurosensory	4.9	0
Stomatitis	14.7	1.1
Alopecia	6.4	0
Diarrhea	12.8	0.4
Rash	14	0.8
Weight loss	1.1	0
Edema	4.5	0

*NCI CTC, National Cancer Institute (USA) Common Toxicity Criteria, version 2.0. Available at: http://ctep.cancer.gov/protocolDevelopment/electronic_applications/ctc.htm [accessed December 7, 2013]

Treatment Modifications

Adverse Event	Dose Modification
G3 hematologic toxicities	Hold therapy until toxicity returns to baseline, then reduce pemetrexed dosage by 25%
G4 hematologic toxicities (thrombocytopenia)	Hold therapy until toxicity returns to baseline, then reduce pemetrexed dosage by 50%
Increased serum creatinine to 1.6–2 mg/dL (141–177 μmol/L)	Reduce pemetrexed dosage by 25%
Serum creatinine increased to ≤2 mg/dL (≤177 μmol/L)	Hold pemetrexed until serum creatinine <1.5 mg/dL (<133 μmol/L), then resume with pemetrexed dosage reduced by 25%
G ≥2 diarrhea	Hold pemetrexed until toxicity resolves to G <2, then resume with pemetrexed dosage reduced by 25%
G3/4 mucositis	Reduce pemetrexed dosage by 50%
Increased liver transaminases	Hold therapy until toxicity resolves, then resume with pemetrexed dosage reduced by 25%
Other G ≥3 non-hematologic toxicities (except nausea, vomiting, elevated transaminases, and alopecia)	Delay treatment until toxicity resolves to baseline, then resume with pemetrexed dosage reduced by 25% from previous dose level

Note: if a patient requires 3 dose reductions, discontinue pemetrexed

Notes

In the study reported by Hanna et al. (J Clin Oncol 2004;22:1589–1597), 288 patients were treated with docetaxel 75 mg/m² by intravenous infusion every 21 days. Treatment with docetaxel resulted in clinically equivalent efficacy outcomes, but had significantly greater side effects compared with pemetrexed.

ADVANCED NSCLC • EGFR MUTATED • FIRST-LINE
LUNG CANCER REGIMEN: OSIMERTINIB

Ramalingam SS et al. N Engl J Med 2020;382(1):41–50
Soria JC et al. N Engl J Med 2018;378:113–125
Protocol for: Soria JC et al. N Engl J Med 2018;378:113–125
Supplementary appendix to: Soria JC et al. N Engl J Med 2018;378:113–125
TAGRISSO (osimertinib) prescribing information. Wilmington, DE: AstraZeneca Pharmaceuticals LP; revised 2018 April

Osimertinib 80 mg/dose; administer orally, once daily, without regard to food, continuously until disease progression (total dose/week = 560 mg)

Notes:

- Patients who delay taking osimertinib at a regularly scheduled time should take the next dose at the next regularly scheduled time
- If patients have difficulty swallowing whole osimertinib tablets:
  - Disperse tablet in 60 mL of non-carbonated water only. Stir until tablet is dispersed into small pieces (note: the tablet will not completely dissolve) and swallow immediately. Do not crush, heat, or ultrasonicate during preparation. Rinse the container with 120–240 mL of water and drink immediately
  - If administration via a nasogastric tube is required, disperse the tablet in 15 mL of non-carbonated water. Stir until tablet is dispersed into small pieces (note: the tablet will not completely dissolve). Use an additional 15 mL of water to transfer any residues to the syringe. The resulting 30 mL liquid should be administered per the nasogastric tube instructions with appropriate water flushes (approximately 30 mL)
- In vitro studies suggest that osimertinib is a substrate for CYP3A4, that osimertinib is a substrate and inhibitor of BCRP and P-glycoprotein (P-gp), and that osimertinib is an inducer of CYP1A2
  - Coadministration of osimertinib with rifampin (a strong CYP3A inducer) reduced the steady-state AUC of osimertinib by 78%. Therefore, if coadministration of a strong CYP3A inducer is unavoidable, then increase the osimertinib dose to 160 mg daily. Resume at 80 mg daily 3 weeks after discontinuation of the strong CYP3A inducer. No dose adjustment is necessary when coadministered with weak/moderate CYP3A inducers
  - Coadministration of osimertinib with itraconazole (a strong CYP3A4 inhibitor) increased the osimertinib AUC by 24% and decreased the osimertinib C_{max} by 20%. Therefore, no adjustment to the osimertinib dose is needed with CYP3A4 inhibitors
  - Coadministration of osimertinib with omeprazole had no effect on the exposure to osimertinib. Therefore, no adjustment to the osimertinib dose and/or schedule is needed with acid-reducing medications
  - Coadministration of osimertinib with rosuvastatin (a BCRP substrate) increased rosuvastatin AUC by 35% and Cmax by 72%. Therefore, if concomitant use of osimertinib with a BCRP substrate is unavoidable, then monitor closely for adverse reactions related to the BCRP substrate
  - Coadministration of osimertinib with fexofenadine (a P-gp substrate) increased fexofenadine AUC and Cmax by 56% and 76% after a single dose and by 27% and 25% at steady state, respectively. Therefore, if concomitant use of osimertinib with a P-gp substrate is unavoidable, then monitor closely for adverse reactions related to the P-gp substrate
  - Coadministration of osimertinib with simvastatin (a CYP3A4 substrate) had no clinically significant effect on the exposure of simvastatin. Therefore, no dose modification of CYP3A4 substrates is needed when coadministered with osimertinib

Supportive Care

Antiemetic prophylaxis
Emetogenic potential is **MINIMAL TO LOW**
See Chapter 42 for antiemetic recommendations

Hematopoietic growth factor (CSF) prophylaxis
Primary prophylaxis is **NOT** *indicated*
See Chapter 43 for more information

Antimicrobial prophylaxis
Risk of fever and neutropenia is **LOW**
  Antimicrobial primary prophylaxis to be considered:
  - Antibacterial—not indicated
  - Antifungal—not indicated
  - Antiviral—not indicated unless patient previously had an episode of HSV

Diarrhea management
Latent or delayed-onset diarrhea:

  Loperamide 4 mg orally initially after the first loose or liquid stool, *then*

  Loperamide 2 mg orally every 2 hours during waking hours, *plus*

  Loperamide 4 mg orally every 4 hours during hours of sleep

- Continue for at least 12 hours after diarrhea resolves
- Recurrent diarrhea after a 12-hour diarrhea-free interval is treated as a new episode

(continued)

(*continued*)

- Rehydrate orally with fluids and electrolytes during a diarrheal episode
- If a patient develops blood or mucus in stool, dehydration, or hemodynamic instability, or if diarrhea persists >48 hours despiteloperamide, stop loperamide and hospitalize the patient for IV hydration

Alternatively, a trial of **diphenoxylate hydrochloride** 2.5 mg with **atropine sulfate** 0.025 mg (eg, Lomotil)
- Initial adult dose is 2 tablets 4 times daily until control has been achieved, after which the dose may be reduced to meet individual requirements. Control may often be maintained with as little as 2 tablets daily
- Clinical improvement of acute diarrhea is usually observed within 48 hours. If improvement of chronic diarrhea after treatment with a maximum daily dose of 8 tablets is not observed within 10 days, control is unlikely with further administration

Persistent diarrhea:
Octreotide 100–150 mcg subcutaneously 3 times daily. Maximum total daily dose is 1500 mcg

Antibiotic therapy during latent or delayed-onset diarrhea:
A fluoroquinolone (eg, ciprofloxacin 500 mg orally every 12 hours) if absolute neutrophil count is <500/mm^3 with or without accompanying fever in association with diarrhea
- Antibiotics should also be administered if patient is hospitalized with prolonged diarrhea and should be continued until diarrhea resolves

Patient Population Studied

This randomized, double-blind, phase 3 trial included 556 patients with epidermal growth factor receptor (EGFR) mutation–positive advanced non–small cell lung cancer (NSCLC). Study participants had not previously received treatment for advanced disease and were eligible to receive first-line treatment with gefitinib or erlotinib. Confirmation of the EGFR exon 19 deletion (Ex19del) or p.Leu858Arg (L858R) mutation, alone or with other EGFR mutations, was required for enrollment. Patients with CNS metastases who were neurologically stable also were eligible. Participants were randomized 1:1 to receive either osimertinib or a standard EGFR tyrosine kinase inhibitor (gefitinib or erlotinib).

Efficacy (N = 556)

End Point	Osimertinib (N=279)	Comparator EGFR-TKI (N=277)	Between-Group Comparison
Median progression-free survival among all patients*	18.9 months (95% CI 15.2–21.4)	10.2 months (95% CI 9.6–11.1)	HR 0.46 (95% CI 0.37–0.57) P<0.001
Median progression-free survival in patients with CNS metastases*	15.2 months (95% CI 12.1–21.4)	9.6 months (95% CI 7.0–12.4)	HR 0.47 (95% CI 0.30–0.74) P<0.001
Median progression-free survival in patients without CNS metastases*	19.1 months (95% CI 15.2–23.5)	10.9 months (95% CI 9.6–12.3)	HR 0.46 (95% CI 0.36–0.59) P<0.001
Median overall survival†	38.6 months (95% CI 34.5–41.8)	31.8 months (95% CI 26.6–36.0)	HR 0.80 (95% CI 0.64–1.0) P=0.046
Objective response rate	80% (95% CI 75–85)	76% (95% CI 70–81)	—
Complete response‡	3%	1%	—
Partial response	77%	74%	—
Stable disease for ³6 weeks	17%	17%	—
Disease control rate§	97% (95% CI 94–99)	92% (95% CI 89–95)	—

HR, hazard ratio, CI, confidence interval
*Results reported from the interim analysis. At the time of data cutoff, the median duration of treatment exposure was 16.2 months in the osimertinib group and 11.5 months in the comparator group
†Updated results reported from the complete analysis. At the time of data cutoff, the median duration of treatment exposure was 20.7 months in the osimertinib group and 11.5 months in the comparator group. All patients had the opportunity for 43 months of follow-up, with a median duration of follow-up of 35.8 months for the osimertinib group and 27.0 months for the comparator
‡Tumor response was assessed according to the Response Evaluation Criteria in Solid Tumors (RECIST) version 1.1. RECIST assessments occurred every 6 weeks for 18 months, then every 12 weeks until disease progression per the protocol
§The disease-control rate represents the proportion of patients who had complete response, partial response, or stable disease lasting at least 6 weeks before any disease-progression event

Therapy Monitoring

1. Advise patients to promptly report new or worsening respiratory symptoms (eg, dyspnea, cough, fever), which could be indicative of interstitial lung disease (ILD)/pneumonitis. ILD/pneumonitis occurred in 3.9% of 1142 osimertinib-treated patients described in the FDA-approved prescribing information

2. Periodically monitor electrocardiograms in patients who are prone to heart rate-corrected QT (QTc) interval prolongation (eg, patients with congenital long QTc syndrome, congestive heart failure, electrolyte abnormalities, or those who are taking concomitant medications known to prolong the QTc interval). QTc interval prolongation to >500 msec occurred in 0.9%, and an increase from baseline by >60 msec occurred in 3.6% of 1142 patients described in the FDA-approved prescribing information. Osimertinib clinical trials excluded patients with a baseline QTc of >470 msec

3. Consider cardiac monitoring, including assessment of left ventricular ejection fraction (LVEF) at baseline and periodically during treatment in patients with cardiac risk factors. Consider assessing LVEF in patients who develop relevant cardiac signs or symptoms during treatment

4. Advise patients to report any signs or symptoms of keratitis (eg, eye inflammation, lacrimation, light sensitivity, blurred vision, eye pain, and/ or red eye). If symptoms of keratitis are present, perform an ophthalmological evaluation

5. Advise patients to report any new or worsening rashes. Perform a skin examination at each visit. Any-grade rash occurred in 58% of patients receiving osimertinib in the FLAURA study; G ≥3 rash occurred in 1.1% of patients

6. Advise patients to report any new or worsening diarrhea. Any-grade diarrhea occurred in 58% of patients receiving osimertinib in the FLAURA study; G ≥3 diarrhea occurred in 2.2% of patients

Treatment Modifications

OSIMERTINIB

Starting dose	80 mg by mouth once daily
Dose level −1	40 mg by mouth once daily

Pulmonary Toxicities

Adverse Event	Treatment Modification
ILD/pneumonitis (any grade)	Permanently discontinue osimertinib

Cardiovascular Adverse Events

QTc interval >500 msec on at least 2 separate ECGs	Withhold osimertinib until QTc interval is <481 msec or recovery to baseline if baseline QTc is ≥481 msec, then resume at 40 mg
QTc interval prolongation with signs/symptoms of a life-threatening arrhythmia	Permanently discontinue osimertinib
Symptomatic congestive heart failure	Permanently discontinue osimertinib

Other Adverse Events

Other G ≥3 adverse event	Withhold osimertinib for up to 3 weeks. If improvement to G ≤2 occurs within 3 weeks, then resume osimertinib at either 80 mg daily or 40 mg daily, at the discretion of the medically responsible health care provider. If no improvement occurs within 3 weeks, then permanently discontinue osimertinib

Drug-Drug Interactions

Concomitant therapy with a strong CYP3A inducer is required	If coadministration of a strong CYP3A inducer is unavoidable, then increase the osimertinib dose to 160 mg daily. Resume at 80 mg daily 3 weeks after discontinuation of the strong CYP3A inducer
Concomitant therapy with a sensitive P-glycoprotein substrate is required	If coadministration of a sensitive P-glycoprotein substrate is unavoidable, then monitor more closely for adverse reactions attributable to the P-glycoprotein substrate
Concomitant therapy with a sensitive BCRP substrate is required	If coadministration of a sensitive BCRP substrate is unavoidable, then monitor more closely for adverse reactions attributable to the BCRP substrate

ILD, interstitial lung disease; QTc, heart rate-corrected QT interval
Grading of adverse events per National Cancer Institute Common Terminology Criteria for Adverse Events. Version 4.0

Adverse Events (N = 556)

Grade (%)	Osimertinib (N = 279)		Standard EGFR-TKI (N = 277)	
	Grade 1–2	Grade 3–4	Grade 1–2	Grade 3–4
Rash or acne*	57	1	71	7
Diarrhea	56	2	55	2
Dry skin*	35	<1	35	1
Paronychia*	35	<1	33	1
Stomatitis	28	1	20	<1
Decreased appetite	18	3	17	2
Pruritus	17	<1	16	0
Cough	16	0	15	<1
Constipation	15	0	13	0
Nausea	14	0	19	0
Fatigue	13	1	11	1
Dyspnea	13	<1	6	1
Anemia	11	1	7	1
Headache	11	<1	7	0
Vomiting	11	0	9	1
Upper respiratory tract infection	10	0	6	0
Pyrexia	11	0	4	<1
Prolonged QT interval	8	3	3	1
AST elevation	8	1	20	4
Alopecia	7	0	12	0
ALT elevation	6	<1	18	9

AST, aspartate aminotransferase; ALT, alanine aminotransferase
Listed adverse events were reported in at least 10% of the patients in any group. The safety analysis included all patients who received at least one dose of trial drug
*Adverse event categories representing a grouped term for the event. For patients experiencing multiple events within a specified grouped term adverse event, the maximum grade across those events was reported

ADVANCED NSCLC • EGFR MUTATED • FIRST-LINE

LUNG CANCER REGIMEN: GEFITINIB

Maemondo M et al. N Engl J Med 2010;362:2380–2388

Gefitinib 250 mg per day; administer orally with or without food, continually (total dose/week = 1750 mg)*

*Gefitinib availability in the United States is limited to participation in the Iressa Access Program. Postmarket Drug Safety Information for Patients and Providers may be acquired online from the U.S. Food and Drug Administration at http://www.fda.gov/Drugs/DrugSafety/PostmarketDrugSafetyInformationforPatientsandProviders/ucm110476.htm (last accessed June 7, 2013) or from AstraZeneca

Supportive Care

Antiemetic prophylaxis
Emetogenic potential is **MINIMAL–LOW**
See Chapter 42 for antiemetic recommendations

Hematopoietic growth factor (CSF) prophylaxis
Primary prophylaxis is **NOT** indicated
See Chapter 43 for more information

Antimicrobial prophylaxis
Risk of fever and neutropenia is **LOW**
   Antimicrobial primary prophylaxis to be considered:
- Antibacterial—not indicated
- Antifungal—not indicated
- Antiviral—not indicated unless patient previously had an episode of HSV

Diarrhea management

Latent or delayed-onset diarrhea:
Loperamide 4 mg orally initially after the first loose or liquid stool, *then*
Loperamide 2 mg orally every 2 hours during waking hours, *plus*
Loperamide 4 mg orally every 4 hours during hours of sleep
- Continue for at least 12 hours after diarrhea resolves
- Recurrent diarrhea after a 12-hour diarrhea-free interval is treated as a new episode
- Rehydrate orally with fluids and electrolytes during a diarrheal episode
- If a patient develops blood or mucus in stool, dehydration, or hemodynamic instability, or if diarrhea persists >48 hours despite loperamide, stop loperamide and hospitalize the patient for IV hydration. Alternatively, a trial of **diphenoxylate hydrochloride** 2.5mg with **atropine sulfate** 0.025 mg (eg, Lomotil)
- Initial adult dose is 2 tablets 4 times daily until control has been achieved, after which the dose may be reduced to meet individual requirements. Control may often be maintained with as little as 2 tablets daily
- Clinical improvement of acute diarrhea is usually observed within 48 hours. If improvement of chronic diarrhea after treatment with a maximum daily dose of 8 tablets is not observed within 10 days, control is unlikely with further administration

Persistent diarrhea:
Octreotide 100–150 mcg subcutaneously 3 times daily. Maximum total daily dose is 1500 mcg

Antibiotic therapy during latent or delayed-onset diarrhea:
- A fluoroquinolone (eg, **ciprofloxacin** 500 mg orally every 12 hours) if absolute neutrophil count <500/mm^3 with or without accompanying fever in association with diarrhea
- Antibiotics should also be administered if patient is hospitalized with prolonged diarrhea and should be continued until diarrhea resolves

*Abigerges D et al. J Natl Cancer Inst 1994;86:446–449
Rothenberg ML et al. J Clin Oncol 2001;19:3801–3807
Wadler S et al. J Clin Oncol 1998;16:3169–3178

Patient Population Studied

Patients with advanced NSCLC (stage IIIB or IV, or postoperative relapse) harboring *sensitive EGFR mutations*, which excludes the resistant EGFR mutation T790M (threonine at amino acid 790 is substituted by methionine), without a previous history of chemotherapy, and ages ≤75 years

Patient Characteristics

Sex	Number (%)
Male	42 (36.8)
Female	72 (63.2)

Age (years)	
Mean	63.9 ± 7.7
Range	43–75

Smoking Status	
Never smoked	75 (65.8)
Previous or current smoker	39 (34.2)

ECOG performance status score	
0	54 (47.4)
1	59 (51.8)
2	1 (0.9)

Histologic diagnosis	
Adenocarcinoma	103 (90.4)
Large cell carcinoma	1 (0.9)
Adenosquamous carcinoma	2 (1.8)
Squamous cell carcinoma	3 (2.6)
Other	5 (4.4)

Clinical stage	
IIIB	15 (13.2)
IV	88 (77.2)
Postoperative relapse	11 (9.6)

Type of EGFR mutation	
Exon 19 deletion	58 (50.9)
L858R	49 (43.0)
Other	7 (6.1)

Dose Adjustments

Summary of product characteristics for IRESSA 250-mg film-coated tablets. Available at: http://www.iressa.com/ [accessed March 21, 2014]

Acute onset of new or progressive pulmonary symptoms, such as dyspnea, cough, or fever	Interrupt treatment with gefitinib pending diagnostic evaluation
Interstitial lung disease (ILD)	Discontinue gefitinib and institute appropriate treatment as necessary
Hepatic failure or gastrointestinal perforation	Discontinue gefitinib
Dehydration, severe bullous, blistering or exfoliative skin conditions, or acute worsening ocular disorders	Interrupt or discontinue gefitinib
G1/2 diarrhea	Interrupt gefitinib temporarily and institute loperamide therapy. Resume gefitinib if symptoms resolve to G≤1
G3/4 diarrhea	Discontinue or interrupt gefitinib temporarily. Institute symptomatic therapy. If the patient is receiving benefit from gefitinib, and treatment is interrupted only temporarily, resume gefitinib only if symptoms resolve to G≤1
G3/4 diarrhea despite loperamide	Discontinue gefitinib
G1/2 skin reaction	Interrupt gefitinib temporarily and institute symptomatic therapy; resume gefitinib if symptoms resolve to G≤1
G3/4 skin reaction	Discontinue or interrupt gefitinib temporarily. Institute symptomatic therapy. If the patient is receiving benefit from gefitinib, and treatment is interrupted only temporarily, resume gefitinib only if symptoms resolve to G≤1
Total bilirubin >3 × ULN and/or transaminases a >5 × ULN in the setting of normal pretreatment values	Interrupt or discontinue gefitinib

Note: gefitinib plasma concentrations may increase by administration concurrently with potent inhibitors of CYP3A4 activity (eg, clarithromycin, itraconazole, ketoconazole, posaconazole, protease inhibitors, telithromycin, voriconazole). The increase may be clinically relevant as adverse reactions are related to dose and exposure. Patients who receive gefitinib concomitantly with potent CYP3A4 inhibitors should be closely monitored for adverse reactions referable to gefitinib
Gefitinib systemic concentrations also may be increased in individuals with CYP2D6 poor metabolizer genotypes

Toxicity*

	Gefitinib (N = 114)					Carboplatin + Paclitaxel (N + 113)					
	Number of Patients				# (%)	Number of Patients				# (%)	
Toxic Effect	G1	G2	G3	G4	G ≥3	G1	G2	G3	G4	G≥3	P for G≥3
Diarrhea	32	6	1	0	1 (0.9)	7	0	0	0	0	<0.001
Appetite loss	7	4	6	0	6 (5.3)	39	18	7	0	7	<0.001
Fatigue	8	1	3	0	3 (2.6)	19	11	1	0	1 (0.9)	0.002
Rash	38	37	6	0	6 (5.3	8	14	3	0	3 (2.7)	<0.001
Neuropathy (sensory)	0	1	0	0	0	28	27	7	0	7 (6.2)	<0.001
Arthralgia	1	2	1	0	1 (0.9)	25	21	8	0	8 (7.1)	<0.001
Pneumonitis	3	0	2	1†	3 (2.6)	0	0	0	0	0	0.02
↑ Aminotransferase	20	13	29	1	30 (26)	31	5	0	1	1 (0.9)	<0.001
Neutropenia	5	1	0	1	1 (0.9)	4	9	37	37	74 (66)	<0.001
Anemia	19	2	0	0	0	35	32	6	0	6 (5.3)	<0.001

(continued)

Toxicity* (continued)

Toxic Effect	Gefitinib (N = 114)					Carboplatin + Paclitaxel (N + 113)					P for G≥3
	Number of Patients				# (%)	Number of Patients				# (%)	
	G1	G2	G3	G4	G ≥3	G1	G2	G3	G4	G≥3	
Thrombocytopenia	8	0	0	0	0	25	3	3	1	4 (3.5)	<0.001
Any	17	44	43	4†	47 (41)	4	25	41	40	81 (72)	<0.001

*Grades are based on the National Cancer Institute Common Terminology Criteria for Adverse Events, version 3.0. Available at: http://ctep.cancer.gov/protocolDevelopment/electronic_applications/ctc.htm [accessed December 7, 2013]
†One patient experienced a Grade 5 toxic effect

Efficacy

Response to Treatment in the Intention-to-Treat Population According to Treatment Group*

	Gefitinib (N = 114)	Carboplatin + Paclitaxel (N = 114)	P
	Number of Patients (%)		
Complete response	5 (4.4)	0	<0.001
Partial response	79 (69.3)	35 (30.7)	<0.001
Complete or partial response	84 (73.7)	35 (30.7)	<0.001
Stable disease	18 (15.8)	56 (49.1)	<0.001
Progressive disease	11 (9.6)	16 (14.0)	<0.001
Response could not be evaluated	1 (0.9)	7 (6.1)	
	Gefitinib (N = 114)	Carboplatin + Paclitaxel (N = 114)	HR [95%CI]; P Value
Median progression-free survival (interim analysis)	10.4 months	5.5 months	0.36 [0.25–0.51]; <0.001
Median progression-free survival (final analysis)	10.8 months	5.4 months	0.30 [0.22–0.41]; <0.001
1-year progression-free survival rate	42.1%	3.2%	
2-year progression-free survival rate	8.4%	0%	
Median overall survival*	30.5 months	23.6 months	
2-year survival rate	61.4%	46.7%	P = 0.31
	Men	Women	HR [95%CI]; P Value
Median progression-free survival	6.5 months	6.0 months	0.68 [0.51–0.92; 0.01
	Exon 19 Deletion	L858R Point Mutation	P Value
Median progression-free survival	11.5 months	10.8 months	0.90
Response rate	82.8%)	67.3%)	

*Neither sex nor clinical stage had a significant effect on overall survival

Treatment Monitoring

1. *Weekly, then monthly, then every 3 months:* history and physical exam, pulse O_2
2. *Weekly, then monthly, then every 3 months:* serum creatinine, LFTs

ADVANCED NSCL • EGFR MUTATED • FIRST-LINE
LUNG CANCER REGIMEN: ERLOTINIB

Rosell R et al. Lancet Oncol 2012;13:239–246

Erlotinib 150 mg per day; administer orally at least 1 hour before or 2 hours after food, continually (total dose/week = 1050 mg)

Supportive Care
Antiemetic prophylaxis
Emetogenic potential is **MINIMAL–LOW**
See Chapter 42 for antiemetic recommendations

Hematopoietic growth factor (CSF) prophylaxis
Primary prophylaxis is **NOT** *indicated*
See Chapter 43 for more information

Antimicrobial prophylaxis
Risk of fever and neutropenia is **LOW**
Antimicrobial primary prophylaxis to be considered:
- Antibacterial—not indicated
- Antifungal—not indicated
- Antiviral—not indicated unless patient previously had an episode of HSV

Diarrhea management
Latent or delayed-onset diarrhea:
Loperamide 4 mg orally initially after the first loose or liquid stool, *then*
Loperamide 2 mg orally every 2 hours during waking hours, *plus*
Loperamide 4 mg orally every 4 hours during hours of sleep
- Continue for at least 12 hours after diarrhea resolves
- Recurrent diarrhea after a 12-hour diarrhea-free interval is treated as a new episode
- Rehydrate orally with fluids and electrolytes during a diarrheal episode
- If a patient develops blood or mucus in stool, dehydration, or hemodynamic instability, or if diarrhea persists >48 hours despite loperamide, stop loperamide and hospitalize the patient for IV hydration. Alternatively, a trial of **diphenoxylate hydrochloride** 2.5mg with **atropine sulfate** 0.025 mg (eg, Lomotil)
- Initial adult dose is 2 tablets 4 times daily until control has been achieved, after which the dose may be reduced to meet individual requirements. Control may often be maintained with as little as 2 tablets daily
- Clinical improvement of acute diarrhea is usually observed within 48 hours. If improvement of chronic diarrhea after treatment with a maximum daily dose of 8 tablets is not observed within 10 days, control is unlikely with further administration

Persistent diarrhea:
Octreotide 100–150 mcg subcutaneously 3 times daily. Maximum total daily dose is 1500 mcg
Antibiotic therapy during latent or delayed-onset diarrhea:
- A fluoroquinolone (eg, **ciprofloxacin** 500 mg orally every 12 hours) if absolute neutrophil count <500/mm^3 with or without accompanying fever in association with diarrhea
- Antibiotics should also be administered if patient is hospitalized with prolonged diarrhea and should be continued until diarrhea resolves

*Abigerges D et al. J Natl Cancer Inst 1994;86:446–449
Rothenberg ML et al. J Clin Oncol 2001;19:3801–3807
Wadler S et al. J Clin Oncol 1998;16:3169–178

Patient Population Studied

Eligibility criteria included histologic diagnosis of stage IIIB (with pleural effusion) or stage IV NSCLC (based on the sixth TNM staging system), presence of activating EGFR mutations (exon 19 deletion or L858R mutation in exon 21), and no history of chemotherapy for metastatic disease (neoadjuvant or adjuvant chemotherapy was allowed if it ended ≥6 months before study entry). Patients with asymptomatic, stable brain metastases were eligible to participate

Baseline Demographic and Clinical Characteristics of the Intention-to-Treat Population Randomized to Erlotinib (n = 86)	
Sex, female	58 (67%)
Age, Years	
Mean (SD)	63.44 (10.95)
Median (range, IQR)	65 (24–82, 56–72)
Smoking Status	
Never smoked	57 (66%)
Previous smoker	22 (26%)
Current smoker	7 (8%)
Eastern Cooperative Oncology Group (ECOG) Performance Status	
0	27 (31%)
1	47 (55%)
2	12 (14%)
Histologic Diagnosis	
Adenocarcinoma	82 (95%)
Bronchoalveolar adenocarcinoma	0
Large cell carcinoma	3 (3%)
Squamous cell carcinoma	1 (1%)
Other*	0
Clinical Stage	
N3 (not candidate for thoracic radiotherapy)	1 (1%)
IIIA	1 (1%)
IIIB (malignant pleural effusion)	6 (7%)
IV	78 (91%)
Bone Metastasis	
Yes	28 (33%)
No	58 (67%)
Brain Metastasis	
Yes	9 (10%)
No	77 (90%)
Type of *EGFR* Mutation	
Deletion of exon 19	57 (66%)
L858R mutation in exon 21	29 (34%)

*Four undifferentiated carcinomas, 1 pleomorphic carcinoma, and 1 adenosquamous carcinoma

Efficacy

	Erlotinib n = 86	Chemotherapy n = 87	HR (95% CI) P Value
Median follow-up (months)	18.9 (10.7–29.0*)	14.4 (7.1–24.8*)	—
Median duration of treatment (months)	8.2 (0.3–32.9)	2.8 (0.7–5.1)	—
Median number of chemotherapy cycles administered	4 (1–6)	4 (2–4)	—
Median PFS (preplanned interim analysis) (months)	9.4 (7.9–12.3)	5.2 (4.4–5.8)	0.42 (0.27–0.64) P<0.0001
Median PFS (final analysis) (months)	9.7 (8.4–12.3)	5.2 (4.5–5.8)	0.37 (0.25–0.54) P<0.0001
1-year PFS (95% CI)	40% (28–52)	10% (4–20)	—
2-year PFS (95% CI)	11% (5–26)	0% (NA†)	—
Median PFS (months)			
ECOG PS 0	23.9 (9.7–NA†)	6 (4.3–8.0)	P = 0.0006
ECOG PS 1	8.8 (7.5–10.8)	5.0 (4.1–5.5)	P<0.0001
ECOG PS 2	8.3 (1.0–16.4)	4.4 (0.3–6.0)	P = 0.191
Never smokers	9.7 (8.3–15.5)	5.1 (4.4–5.6)	0.24 (0.15–0.39) P<0.0001
Current	8.7 (5.7–15.8)	4.2 (1.0–15.4)	—
Previous smokers	10.7 (2.7–13.8)	8.0 (1.2–NA)	—
Exon 19 deletion	11.0 (8.8–16.4)	4.6 (4.1–5.6)	0.30 (0.18–0.50) P<0.0001
L858R mutation	8.4 (5.2–10.8)	6.0 (4.9–6.8)	0.55 (0.29–1.02) P = 0.0539
Intention-to-treat population			
	N = 86	N = 87	—
CR	2 (2%)	—	—
PR	48 (56%)	13 (15%)	—
Per-protocol population			
	N = 77 (90%)	N = 73 (84%)	—
CR	2 (3%)	—	—
PR	47 (61%)	13 (18%)	7.5 (3.6–15.6)† P<0.0001
Median overall survival (months)‡	19.3 (14.7–26.8)	19.5 (16.1–NA)	1.04 (0.65–1.68) P = 0.87

95% CI, 95% confidence interval; CR, complete response; ECOG PS, Eastern Cooperative Oncology Group Performance Status; NA, not assessable; PFS, progression-free survival; PR, partial response
*IQR, interquartile range in parentheses
†Odds ratio
‡Sixty-six (76%) of 87 patients in the standard chemotherapy group crossed over to receive EGFR tyrosine kinase inhibitors, primarily erlotinib

Treatment Monitoring

1. *Weekly, then monthly, then every 3 months:* history and physical exam, pulse O_2
2. *Weekly, then monthly, then every 3 months:* serum creatinine
   - Especially in patient at risk of dehydration
3. *Weekly, then monthly, then every 3 months:* LFTs
   - More frequent monitoring in patients with biliary obstruction or hepatic impairment

Dose Adjustments

Adapted in part from: Tarceva (erlotinib) tablets, for oral use; 05/2013 product label. Genentech USA, Inc., 1 DNA Way, South San Francisco, CA

Acute onset of new or progressive pulmonary symptoms, such as dyspnea, cough, or fever	Interrupt treatment with erlotinib pending diagnostic evaluation
Interstitial lung disease (ILD)	Discontinue erlotinib and institute appropriate treatment as necessary
Hepatic failure or gastrointestinal perforation	Discontinue erlotinib
Dehydration, severe bullous, blistering or exfoliative skin conditions, or acute worsening ocular disorders	Interrupt or discontinue erlotinib
G1/2 diarrhea	Interrupt erlotinib temporarily and institute loperamide therapy. Resume erlotinib at same dose or with a dose reduction in 50-mg increments
G3/4 diarrhea	Interrupt erlotinib temporarily and institute loperamide therapy. Resume erlotinib with a dose reduction in 50-mg increments
G3/4 diarrhea despite loperamide	Discontinue erlotinib
G1/2 skin reaction	Interrupt erlotinib temporarily and institute symptomatic therapy. Resume erlotinib at same dose or with a dose reduction in 50-mg increments
G3/4 skin reaction	Interrupt erlotinib temporarily and institute symptomatic therapy. Resume erlotinib with a dose reduction in 50-mg increments
Total bilirubin >3 × ULN and/or transaminases >5 × ULN in the setting of normal pretreatment values	Interrupt or discontinue erlotinib

Note: in patients who are taking erlotinib with a strong CYP3A4 inhibitor such as, but not limited to, atazanavir, clarithromycin, indinavir, itraconazole, ketoconazole, nefazodone, nelfinavir, ritonavir, saquinavir, telithromycin, troleandomycin (TAO), voriconazole, or grapefruit products, a dose reduction should be considered if severe adverse reactions occur. Similarly, in patients who are taking erlotinib with an inhibitor of both CYP3A4 and CYP1A2 like ciprofloxacin, a dose reduction of erlotinib should be considered if severe adverse reactions occur

Toxicity

Common Adverse Events in the Safety Population*

	Erlotinib (n = 84)			Standard Chemotherapy (n = 82)			P Value for G3/4
	G1/2	G3	G4	G1/2	G3	G4	0.0086
Fatigue	43 (51%)	5 (6%)	0	43 (52%)	16 (20%)	0	—
Rash	56 (67%)	11 (13%)	0	4 (5%)	0	0	0.0007
Diarrhea	44 (52%)	4 (5%)	0	15 (18%)	0	0	0.1206
Appetite loss	26 (31%)	0	0	26 (32%)	2 (2%)	0	0.2425
Alopecia	12 (14%)	0	0	—	2 (2%)	0	0.2425
Neuropathy	7 (8%)	0	1 (1%)	11 (13%)	1 (1%)	0	1.0000
Arthralgia	8 (10%)	0	0	—	1 (1%)	0	1.0000
Aminotransferase rise	3 (4%)	0	0	—	0	0	0.4970
Pneumonitis	0	1 (1%)	0	0	1 (1%)	0	1.0000
Anemia	9 (11%)	0	1 (1%)	—	—	—	0.3644
Neutropenia	0	0	0	15 (18%)	12 (15%)	6 (7%)	<0.0001
Thrombocytopenia	1 (1%)	0	0	1 (1%)	6 (7%)	6 (7%)	0.0003
Febrile neutropenia	0	0	0	1 (1%)	1 (1%)	2 (2%)	0.1183

*Adverse events were assessed according to the National Cancer Institute (USA) Common Terminology Criteria for Adverse Events, version 3.0. Available at: http://ctep.cancer.gov/protocolDevelopment/electronic_applications/ctc.htm [accessed December 7, 2013]

(continued)

Toxicity (continued)

Safety Data

	Erlotinib (n = 84)	Standard Chemotherapy (n = 82)
Any adverse event (all grades)	82 (98%)	81 (99%)
Treatment-related adverse event (all grades)	78 (93%)	78 (95%)
Grade 3 or 4 adverse event	38 (45%)	55 (67%)
Dose reduction because of adverse event	18 (21%)	23 (28%)
Dose reduction because of drug-related adverse event	18 (21%)	21 (26%)
Discontinuation because of an adverse event	11 (13%)	19 (23%)
Discontinuation because of drug-related adverse event	5 (6%)	16 (20%)
Any severe adverse event	27 (32%)	25 (30%)
Treatment-related severe adverse event	5 (6%)	16 (20%)
Treatment-related death[†]	1 (1%)	2 (2%)
Interstitial lung disease-like events	1 (1%)	1 (1%)

*The safety analysis included all patients who were randomly allocated to treatment groups and received at least 1 dose of study drug
[†]One patient in the erlotinib group experienced hepatotoxicity, 2 patients in the chemotherapy group had cerebrovascular accidents (1 after a Grade 5 infection)

ADVANCED NSCLC • EGFR MUTATED • SUBSEQUENT THERAPY
LUNG CANCER REGIMEN: OSIMERTINIB

Mok TS et al. N Engl J Med 2017;376:629–640
Protocol for: Mok TS et al. N Engl J Med 2017;376:629–640
Supplementary appendix to: Mok TS et al. N Engl J Med 2017;376:629–640
TAGRISSO (osimertinib) prescribing information. Wilmington, DE: AstraZeneca Pharmaceuticals LP; revised 2018 April

Osimertinib 80 mg/dose; administer orally, once daily, without regard to food, continuously until disease progression (total dose/week = 560 mg)

Notes:

- Patients who delay taking osimertinib at a regularly scheduled time should take the next dose at the next regularly scheduled time

- If patients have difficulty swallowing whole osimertinib tablets:

  - Disperse tablet in 60 mL of non-carbonated water only. Stir until tablet is dispersed into small pieces (note: the tablet will not completely dissolve) and swallow immediately. Do not crush, heat, or ultrasonicate during preparation. Rinse the container with 120–240 mL of water and drink immediately

  - If administration via a nasogastric tube is required, disperse the tablet in 15 mL of non-carbonated water. Stir until tablet is dispersed into small pieces (note: the tablet will not completely dissolve). Use an additional 15 mL of water to transfer any residues to the syringe. The resulting 30 mL liquid should be administered per the nasogastric tube instructions with appropriate water flushes (approximately 30 mL)

- In vitro studies suggest that osimertinib is a substrate for CYP3A4, that osimertinib is a substrate and inhibitor of BCRP and P-glycoprotein (P-gp), and that osimertinib is an inducer of CYP1A2

  - Coadministration of osimertinib with rifampin (a strong CYP3A inducer) reduced the steady-state AUC of osimertinib by 78%. Therefore, if coadministration of a strong CYP3A inducer is unavoidable, then increase the osimertinib dose to 160 mg daily. Resume at 80 mg daily 3 weeks after discontinuation of the strong CYP3A inducer. No dose adjustment is necessary when coadministered with weak/moderate CYP3A inducers

  - Coadministration of osimertinib with itraconazole (a strong CYP3A4 inhibitor) increased the osimertinib AUC by 24% and decreased the osimertinib C_{max} by 20%. Therefore, no adjustment to the osimertinib dose is needed with CYP3A4 inhibitors

  - Coadministration of osimertinib with omeprazole had no effect on the exposure to osimertinib. Therefore, no adjustment to the osimertinib dose and/or schedule is needed with acid-reducing medications

  - Coadministration of osimertinib with rosuvastatin (a BCRP substrate) increased rosuvastatin AUC by 35% and Cmax by 72%. Therefore, if concomitant use of osimertinib with a BCRP substrate is unavoidable, then monitor closely for adverse reactions related to the BCRP substrate

  - Coadministration of osimertinib with fexofenadine (a P-gp substrate) increased fexofenadine AUC and Cmax by 56% and 76% after a single dose and by 27% and 25% at steady state, respectively. Therefore, if concomitant use of osimertinib with a P-gp substrate is unavoidable, then monitor closely for adverse reactions related to the P-gp substrate

  - Coadministration of osimertinib with simvastatin (a CYP3A4 substrate) had no clinically significant effect on the exposure of simvastatin. Therefore, no dose modification of CYP3A4 substrates is needed when coadministered with osimertinib

Supportive Care
Antiemetic prophylaxis
Emetogenic potential is **MINIMAL TO LOW**
See Chapter 42 for antiemetic recommendations

Hematopoietic growth factor (CSF) prophylaxis
Primary prophylaxis is **NOT** *indicated*
See Chapter 43 for more information

Antimicrobial prophylaxis
Risk of fever and neutropenia is LOW
   Antimicrobial primary prophylaxis to be considered:
- Antibacterial—not indicated

- Antifungal—not indicated

- Antiviral—not indicated unless patient previously had an episode of HSV

Diarrhea management
Latent or delayed-onset diarrhea:

Loperamide 4 mg orally initially after the first loose or liquid stool,*t hen*

Loperamide 2 mg orally every 2 hours during waking hours, *plus*

Loperamide 4 mg orally every 4 hours during hours of sleep

- Continue for at least 12 hours after diarrhea resolves

- Recurrent diarrhea after a 12-hour diarrhea-free interval is treated as a new episode

- Rehydrate orally with fluids and electrolytes during a diarrheal episode

- If a patient develops blood or mucus in stool, dehydration, or hemodynamic instability, or if diarrhea persists >48 hours despiteloperamide, stoploperamideand hospitalize the patient for IV hydration

(continued)

(*continued*)

Alternatively, a trial of **diphenoxylate hydrochloride** 2.5 mg with **atropine sulfate** 0.025 mg (eg, Lomotil)
- Initial adult dose is 2 tablets 4 times daily until control has been achieved, after which the dose may be reduced to meet individual requirements. Control may often be maintained with as little as 2 tablets daily
- Clinical improvement of acute diarrhea is usually observed within 48 hours. If improvement of chronic diarrhea after treatment with a maximum daily dose of 8 tablets is not observed within 10 days, control us unlikely with further administration

Persistent diarrhea:
  Octreotide 100–150 mcg subcutaneously 3 times daily. Maximum total daily dose is 1500 mcg

Antibiotic therapy during latent or delayed-onset diarrhea:
  A fluoroquinolone (eg, **ciprofloxacin** 500 mg orally every 12 hours) if absolute neutrophil count is <500/mm^3 with or without accompanying fever in association with diarrhea
  - Antibiotics should also be administered if patient is hospitalized with prolonged diarrhea and should be continued until diarrhea resolves

Patient Population Studied

This randomized, international, open-label, phase 3 trial involved 419 adult patients with histologically or cytologically confirmed locally advanced or metastatic non–small cell lung cancer. Eligible patients had experienced disease progression after treatment with a first-line epidermal growth factor receptor tyrosine kinase inhibitor (EGFR-TKI). Documentation of an EGFR mutation and confirmation of the T790M variant after first-line EGFR-TKI therapy was required. Patients with stable, asymptomatic CNS metastases were eligible if they had not been treated with glucocorticoids for at least 4 weeks prior to the first dose of the study drug. Participants were stratified by Asian or non-Asian race and randomized 2:1 to receive oral osimertinib or intravenous pemetrexed plus either carboplatin or cisplatin.

Efficacy (N = 419)

End Point	Osimertinib (N=279)	Platinum-Pemetrexed (N=140)	Between-Group Comparison
Median progression-free survival in intent-to-treat population*	10.1 months (95% CI 8.3–12.3)	4.4 months (95% CI 4.2–5.6)	HR 0.30 (95% CI 0.23–0.41) P<0.001
Median progression-free survival in patients with CNS metastases*	8.5 months (95% CI 6.8–12.3)	4.2 months (95% CI 4.1–5.4)	HR 0.32 (95% CI 0.21–0.49)
Median progression-free survival in patients with EGFR T790M-positive status in both tumor and plasma*	8.2 months (95% CI 6.8–9.7)	4.2 months (95% CI 4.1–5.1)	HR 0.42 (95% CI 0.29–0.61)
Objective response rate	71% (95% CI 65–76)	31% (95% CI 24–40)	OR 5.39 (95% CI 3.47–8.48) P<0.001
Complete response†	1%	1%	—
Partial response†	69%	30%	—
Stable disease for ³6 weeks†	23%	43%	—
Disease control rate‡	93% (95% CI 90–96)	74% (95% CI 66–81)	OR 4.76 (95% CI 2.64–8.84) P<0.001
Median time to response§	6.1 weeks (95% CI NC-NC)	6.4 weeks (95% CI 6.3–7.0)	—
Median duration of response‛	9.7 months (95% CI 8.3–11.6)	4.1 months (95% CI 3.0–5.6)	—

HR, hazard ratio, CI, confidence interval; OR, odds ratio; NC, could not be calculated
*The median follow-up at the time of data cutoff was 8.3 months. Progression events occurred in 140 patients (50%) in the osimertinib group and in 110 (79%) of the platinum-pemetrexed group
†Tumor response was assessed according to Response Evaluation Criteria in Solid Tumors (RECIST) version 1.1
‡Disease control rate represents the proportion of patients who had a complete response, partial response, or stable disease for at least 6 weeks before any disease-progression event
§Time to response was calculated from the date of randomization to the date of the first documentation of partial or complete response
‛Duration of response was determined with the use of the Kaplan-Meier method from the time of first documented response until the date of disease progression or the last RECIST assessment for patients who did not have disease progression

Therapy Monitoring

1. Advise patients to promptly report new or worsening respiratory symptoms (eg, dyspnea, cough, fever), which could be indicative of interstitial lung disease (ILD)/pneumonitis. ILD/pneumonitis occurred in 3.9% of 1142 osimertinib-treated patients described in the FDA-approved prescribing information

2. Periodically monitor electrocardiograms in patients who are prone to heart rate-corrected QT (QTc) interval prolongation (eg, patients with congenital long QTc syndrome, congestive heart failure, electrolyte abnormalities, or those who are taking concomitant medications known to prolong the QTc interval). QTc interval prolongation to >500 msec occurred in 0.9% and an increase from baseline by >60 msec occurred in 3.6% out of 1142 patients described in the FDA-approved prescribing information. Osimertinib clinical trials excluded patients with a baseline QTc of >470 msec

3. Consider cardiac monitoring, including assessment of left ventricular ejection fraction (LVEF) at baseline and periodically during treatment in patients with cardiac risk factors. Consider assessing LVEF in patients who develop relevant cardiac signs or symptoms during treatment

4. Advise patients to report any signs or symptoms of keratitis (eg, eye inflammation, lacrimation, light sensitivity, blurred vision, eye pain, and/or red eye). If symptoms of keratitis are present, perform an ophthalmological evaluation

5. Advise patients to report any new or worsening rashes. Perform a skin examination at each visit. Any-grade rash occurred in 34% of patients receiving osimertinib in the AURA3 study; G ≥3 rash occurred in 0.7% of patients

6. Advise patients to report any new or worsening diarrhea. Any-grade diarrhea occurred in 41% of patients receiving osimertinib in the AURA3 study; G ≥3 diarrhea occurred in 1.1% of patients

Treatment Modifications

OSIMERTINIB

Starting dose	80 mg by mouth once daily
Dose level −1	40 mg by mouth once daily

Pulmonary Toxicities

Adverse Event	Treatment Modification
ILD/pneumonitis (any grade)	Permanently discontinue osimertinib

Cardiovascular Adverse Events

QTc interval >500 msec on at least 2 separate ECGs	Withhold osimertinib until QTc interval is <481 msec or recovery to baseline if baseline QTc is ≥481 msec, then resume at 40 mg
QTc interval prolongation with signs/symptoms of a life-threatening arrhythmia	Permanently discontinue osimertinib
Symptomatic congestive heart failure	Permanently discontinue osimertinib

Other Adverse Events

Other G ≥3 adverse event	Withhold osimertinib for up to 3 weeks. If improvement to G ≤2 occurs within 3 weeks, then resume osimertinib at either 80 mg daily or 40 mg daily, at the discretion of the medically responsible health care provider. If no improvement occurs within 3 weeks, then permanently discontinue osimertinib

Drug-Drug Interactions

Concomitant therapy with a strong CYP3A inducer is required	If coadministration of a strong CYP3A inducer is unavoidable, then increase the osimertinib dose to 160 mg daily. Resume at 80 mg daily 3 weeks after discontinuation of the strong CYP3A inducer
Concomitant therapy with a sensitive P-glycoprotein substrate is required	If coadministration of a sensitive P-glycoprotein substrate is unavoidable, then monitor more closely for adverse reactions attributable to the P-glycoprotein substrate
Concomitant therapy with a sensitive BCRP substrate is required	If coadministration of a sensitive BCRP substrate is unavoidable, then monitor more closely for adverse reactions attributable to the BCRP substrate

Grading of adverse events per National Cancer Institute Common Terminology Criteria for Adverse Events. Version 4.0
ILD, interstitial lung disease; QTc, heart rate-corrected QT interval

Adverse Events (N = 415)

Grade (%)	Osimertinib (n = 279)		Platinum-Pemetrexed (n = 136)	
	Grade 1–2	Grade 3–5	Grade 1–2	Grade 3–5
Diarrhea	40	1	10	1
Rash*	33	1	6	0
Dry skin*	23	0	4	0
Paronychia*	22	0	1	0
Decreased appetite	17	1	33	3
Cough	16	0	14	0
Nausea	15	1	45	4
Fatigue	15	1	27	1
Stomatitis	15	0	14	1
Constipation	14	0	35	0
Pruritis	13	0	4	0
Vomiting	11	<1	18	2
Back pain	10	<1	8	1
Thrombocytopenia*	10	<1	13	7
Nasopharyngitis	10	0	5	0
Headache	10	0	11	0
Dyspnea	8	1	13	0
Neutropenia*	7	1	11	12
Leukopenia*	8	0	11	4
Anemia*	7	1	18	12
Asthenia	6	1	11	4
Pyrexia	6	0	10	0
ALT elevation	5	1	10	1
AST elevation	4	1	10	1
Malaise	4	0	10	0

ALT, alanine aminotransferase; AST, aspartate aminotransferase
The table includes adverse events reported in ≥10% of patients in either group. Safety information was collected for all patients who received at least one dose of a trial drug.
Adverse events were included in the safety analysis if the onset date was on or after the date of the first dose, up to and including 28 days after discontinuation of the trial drug
*Adverse event categories representing a grouped term for the event. For patients experiencing multiple events within a specified grouped term adverse event, the maximum grade across those events was reported

ADVANCED NSCLC • ALK-REARRANGED • FIRST-LINE

LUNG CANCER REGIMEN: ALECTINIB

FDA and EMA prescribing information and miscellaneous sources
Ou SH et al. J Clin Oncol 2016;34:661–668

Alectinib 600 mg/dose; administer orally twice daily (approximately every 12 hours) with food, continually (total dose/week = 8400 mg)

Notes:

• Patients who delay taking alectinib at a regularly scheduled time or who vomit after taking a dose of alectinib should take the next dose at the next regularly scheduled time

• Alectinib may cause photosensitivity. Counsel patients to apply sunscreen and avoid prolonged sun exposure during treatment and for a minimum of 7 days following the last dose of alectinib

Supportive Care
Antiemetic prophylaxis
*Emetogenic potential is **LOW***
See Chapter 42 for antiemetic recommendations

Hematopoietic growth factor (CSF) prophylaxis
*Primary prophylaxis is **NOT** indicated*
See Chapter 43 for more information
Antimicrobial prophylaxis
*Risk of fever and neutropenia is **LOW***
    Antimicrobial primary prophylaxis to be considered:
    • Antibacterial—not indicated

    • Antifungal—not indicated

    • Antiviral—not indicated unless patient previously had an episode of HSV

Patient Population Studied

A multicenter, single-arm, phase 2 study involved 138 patients with crizotinib-refractory, locally advanced or metastatic, *ALK*-rearranged non–small cell lung cancer. Eligible patients were age ≥18 years, with an Eastern Cooperative Oncology Group (ECOG) performance status score ≤2. All patients received 600 mg alectinib twice daily

Efficacy (N = 122)

Objective response rate*	50%
Median duration of response	11.2 months
Median progression-free survival	8.9 months

*Overall response rate is the percentage of patients who experienced a confirmed partial or complete response to the study drug

Therapy Monitoring

1. Monitor liver function tests, including ALT, AST, and total bilirubin, every 2 weeks during the first 3 months of treatment, then once a month and as clinically indicated, with more frequent testing in patients who develop transaminase and bilirubin elevations

2. Promptly investigate for ILD/pneumonitis in any patient who presents with worsening of respiratory symptoms indicative of ILD/pneumonitis (eg, dyspnea, cough, and fever)

3. Monitor renal function at least monthly during entire duration of drug administration. The median time to Grade ≥3 renal impairment in clinical trials was 3.7 months (range 0.5–14.7 months)

4. Monitor heart rate and blood pressure regularly

5. Advise patients to report any unexplained muscle pain, tenderness, or weakness. Assess CPK levels every 2 weeks for the first month of treatment and as clinically indicated in patients reporting symptoms

Treatment Modifications

Dose Reduction Schedule	Dose Level
Starting dose	600 mg taken orally twice daily
Dose level −1	450 mg taken orally twice daily
Dose level −2	300 mg taken orally twice daily
Dose level −3	Discontinue alectinib

Adverse Event	Dose Modification
G ≥3 ALT or AST elevation (>5× ULN) + total bilirubin ≤2× ULN	Withhold alectinib until recovery to baseline or ALT and AST ≤3× ULN, then resume alectinib but reduce the dose by 150 mg
G ≥2 ALT or AST elevation (>3× ULN) + total bilirubin >2× ULN	Permanently discontinue alectinib
Total bilirubin elevation of >3× ULN	Temporarily withhold alectinib until recovery to baseline or to ≤1.5× ULN, then resume at 1 lower dose level
Any grade treatment-related ILD/ pneumonitis	Permanently discontinue alectinib
G3 renal impairment	Temporarily withhold alectinib until serum creatinine recovers to ≤1.5× ULN, then resume at 1 lower dose level
G4 renal impairment	Permanently discontinue alectinib
Asymptomatic bradycardia	Dose modification is not required
Symptomatic bradycardia	Withhold alectinib until recovery to asymptomatic bradycardia or to a heart rate ≥60 bpm. If contributing concomitant medication is identified and discontinued, or its dose is adjusted, resume alectinib at previous dose upon recovery to asymptomatic bradycardia or to a heart rate ≥60 bpm. If no contributing concomitant medication is identified, or if contributing concomitant medications are not discontinued or dose modified, resume alectinib at 1 lower dose level upon recovery to asymptomatic bradycardia or to a heart rate ≥60 bpm
Life-threatening bradycardia requiring urgent intervention	Permanently discontinue alectinib if no contributing concomitant medication is identified. If contributing concomitant medication is identified and discontinued, or its dose is adjusted, resume alectinib at 1 lower dose level upon recovery to asymptomatic bradycardia or to a heart rate ≥60 bpm, with frequent monitoring as clinically indicated. Permanently discontinue alectinib in case of recurrence
CPK elevation >5× ULN	Temporarily withhold alectinib until recovery to baseline or to ≤2.5× ULN, then resume at same dose
CPK elevation >10× ULN or second occurrence of CPK elevation of >5× ULN	Temporarily withhold alectinib until recovery to baseline or to ≤2.5× ULN, then resume at 1 lower dose level
G ≥2 constipation, fatigue, edema, myalgia, and anemia	Temporarily withhold alectinib until recovery to baseline or to G ≤1, then resume at same dose

ALT, alanine aminotransferase; AST, aspartate aminotransferase; CPK, creatine phosphokinase; ILD, interstitial lung disease; ULN, upper limit of normal

Notes:
- Advise females of reproductive potential to use effective contraception during treatment with alectinib and for at least 2 weeks following completion of therapy
- No dose adjustment is recommended for patients with mild or moderate renal impairment. The safety of alectinib in patients with creatinine clearance <30 mL/min has not been studied
- No dose adjustment is recommended for patients with mild hepatic impairment. The safety of alectinib in patients with moderate or severe hepatic impairment has not been studied

Adverse Events (N = 138)

Grade (%)*	Grade 1	Grade 2	Grade 3	Grade 4
Myalgia	14	2	1	0
Constipation	12	2	0	0
Fatigue	12	1	1	0
Asthenia	9	1	1	0
Elevated AST level	8	1	1	1
Elevated ALT level	4	4	1	1
Peripheral edema	7	1	1	0
Rash	8	1	0	0
Photosensitivity reaction	9	0	0	0
Elevated bilirubin level	1	5	1	0
Nausea	5	1	0	0
Diarrhea	4	0	1	0
Dry skin	5	0	0	0

*According to the National Cancer Institute Common Terminology Criteria for Adverse Events, version 4.0
Note: toxicities included in the table are those deemed to have been related to treatment and to have occurred in ≥5% of patients. No treatment-related deaths occurred

ADVANCED NSCLC • ALK-REARRANGED • FIRST-LINE
LUNG CANCER REGIMEN: BRIGATINIB

ALUNBRIG (brigatinib) tablet prescribing information. Cambridge, MA: Ariad Pharmaceuticals, Inc.; updated 2018 December
Camidge DR et al. N Engl J Med 2018;379(21):2027–2039.
Protocol for: Camidge DR et al. N Engl J Med 2018;379(21):2027–2039.
Supplementary appendix to: Camidge DR et al. N Engl J Med 2018;379(21):2027–2039.

7-Day Lead-in Phase:
   Brigatinib 90 mg/dose; administer orally, once daily, without regard to food, for 7 consecutive days (total dose/week during lead-in phase = 630 mg)

Continuation phase (if brigatinib was tolerated during the initial 7 day lead-in phase [see Treatment Modifications section]):
   Brigatinib 180 mg/dose; administer orally, once daily, without regard to food, continuously until disease progression (total dose/week during continuation phase = 1260 mg)

Notes:
- Patients who delay taking brigatinib at a regularly scheduled time or who vomit after taking a dose of brigatinib should take the next dose at the next regularly scheduled time
- Brigatinib tablets should be swallowed whole. Do not crush or chew tablets
- If brigatinib is interrupted for ≥14 days for reasons other than adverse reactions, resume treatment at 90 mg once daily for 7 days before increasing to the previously tolerated dose
- In vitro studies suggest that brigatinib is a substrate for CYP2C8 and CYP3A4, that brigatinib may induce CYP3A and CYP2C expression, and that brigatinib is an inhibitor of P-glycoprotein (P-gp), BCRP, OCT1, MATE1, and MATE2K
  - Coadministration of brigatinib with itraconazole (a strong CYP3A inhibitor) increased brigatinib C_{max} by 21% and AUC_{0-inf} by 101%. Moderate CYP3A4 inhibitors are estimated to increase the AUC of brigatinib by about 40%. If coadministration of a strong CYP3A inhibitor is unavoidable, then reduce the brigatinib dose by approximately 50% (ie, from 180 mg to 90 mg, or from 90 mg to 60 mg). If coadministration of a moderate CYP3A inhibitor is unavoidable, then reduce the brigatinib dose by approximately 40% (ie, from 180 mg to 120 mg, from 120 mg to 90 mg, or from 90 mg to 60 mg)
  - Coadministration of brigatinib with gemfibrozil (a strong CYP2C8 inhibitor) decreased brigatinib C_{max} by 41% and AUC_{0-inf} by 12%. No dose modification is necessary when brigatinib is coadministered with a CYP2C8 inhibitor
  - Coadministration of brigatinib with rifampin (a strong CYP3A inducer) decreased brigatinib C_{max} by 60% and AUC_{0-inf} by 80%. Moderate CYP3A inducers are estimated to reduce the AUC of brigatinib by about 50%. Avoid coadministration of brigatinib with strong CYP3A inducers. If coadministration of brigatinib with a moderate CYP3A inducer is unavoidable, then increase the brigatinib dose in 30-mg increments after 7 days of treatment with the current brigatinib dose, as tolerated, to a maximum of twice the brigatinib dose that was tolerated prior to initiation of the moderate CYP3A inducer
  - Based on in vitro data, brigatinib may decrease concentrations of medications metabolized by CYP3A. Monitor for loss of efficacy of sensitive CYP3A substrates when coadministered with brigatinib
- Patients with severe hepatic impairment (Child-Pugh C) had a 37% higher unbound brigatinib systemic exposure (AUC_{0-inf}) compared to patients with normal hepatic function. Thus, in patients with severe hepatic impairment (Child-Pugh C), reduce the brigatinib dose by approximately 40% (ie, from 180 mg to 120 mg, from 120 mg to 90 mg, or from 90 mg to 60 mg)
- Patients with severe renal impairment (CrCl 15–29 mL/min) had a 86% higher unbound brigatinib systemic exposure (AUC_{0-inf}) compared to patients with normal renal function. Therefore, in patients with severe renal impairment (CrCl 15–29 mL/min), reduce the brigatinib dose by approximately 50% (ie, from 180 mg to 90 mg, or from 90 mg to 60 mg)

Supportive Care

Antiemetic prophylaxis
*Emetogenic potential is **MINIMAL TO LOW***
See Chapter 42 for antiemetic recommendations

Hematopoietic growth factor (CSF) prophylaxis
*Primary prophylaxis is **NOT** indicated*
See Chapter 43 for more information

Antimicrobial prophylaxis
Risk of fever and neutropenia is LOW
   Antimicrobial primary prophylaxis to be considered:
   - Antibacterial—not indicated
   - Antifungal—not indicated
   - Antiviral—not indicated unless patient previously had an episode of HSV

Patient Population Studied

The ALTA-1L study was a randomized, open-label, multicenter, international, phase 3 trial that included 275 adult patients with ALK-positive non–small cell lung cancer (NSCLC) who were naïve to ALK inhibitors. Patients were randomized 1:1 to receive brigatinib or crizotinib. Patients were included if they had histologically or cytologically confirmed stage IIIB (and not a candidate for definitive therapy) or stage IV NSCLC with at least one measurable lesion according to RECIST v1.1 criteria, laboratory-confirmed ALK rearrangement, an Eastern Cooperative Oncology Group (ECOG) performance status of ≤2, and adequate organ function. Patients were excluded if they had previously received an investigational antineoplastic drug or tyrosine kinase inhibitor for NSCLC, if they had received more than one systemic anticancer treatment for advanced disease, or if they had received chemotherapy or radiation therapy within 14 days of the first dose of trial drug. Additional exclusion criteria included symptomatic CNS metastases and cardiovascular disease, including uncontrolled hypertension. Patients with untreated asymptomatic brain metastases were not excluded.

Efficacy (N = 275)

	Brigatinib (n = 137)	Crizotinib (n = 138)	
Median progression-free survival (months)*†‡	NR	9.8 (95% CI, 9.0–12.9)	HR 0.49 (95% CI, 0.33–0.74); P<0.001
Estimated progression-free survival, 12 months*	67% (95% CI, 56–75)	43% (95% CI, 32–53)	
Overall survival rate, 12 months*	85% (95% CI, 76–91)	86% (95% CI, 77–91)	HR 0.98 (95% CI, 0.50–1.93)
Median intracranial progression-free survival (months)‡	NR (95% CI, 11-NR)	5.6 (95% CI, 4.1–9.2)	HR 0.27 (95% CI, 0.13–0.54)
Estimated survival rate without intracranial disease progression, 12 months‡	67% (95% CI, 47–80)	21% (95% CI, 6–42)	
Confirmed objective response rate	71% (95% CI, 62–78)	60% (95% CI, 51–68)	OR 1.59 (95% CI, 0.96–2.62)
Confirmed complete response rate	4%	5%	
Confirmed partial response rate	67%	55%	
Confirmed intracranial response‡	78% (95% CI, 52–94)	29% (95% CI, 11–52)	OR 10.42 (95% CI, 1.90–57.05)

HR, hazard ratio; CI, confidence interval; NR, not reached; OR, odds ratio
*In the intention-to-treat population
†Log-rank test with a two-sided alpha of 0.0031
‡Among patients with measurable brain metastases at baseline
All data are from the interim analysis with a median follow-up of 11.0 months in the brigatinib group and 9.3 months in the crizotinib group

Therapy Monitoring

1. Monitor ALT, AST, alkaline phosphatase, bilirubin, serum creatinine, and BUN prior to initiation of therapy with brigatinib, and then periodically or as clinically indicated
2. Monitor for new or worsening respiratory symptoms (eg, dyspnea, cough), especially during the first week of therapy. Interstitial lung disease or pneumonitis occurred in 4% (all-grade) and 3% (G ≥3) of patients treated with brigatinib in the ALTA-1L trial. Early-onset (defined as <14 days after initiating treatment) interstitial lung disease or pneumonitis was observed in 4 of the 5 patients who developed pneumonitis (onset between days 3–8)
3. Control blood pressure prior to initiation of brigatinib treatment. Monitor blood pressure 2 weeks after initiation of brigatinib and then at least monthly thereafter. Use caution with coadministration of antihypertensive agents that can cause bradycardia. All-grade hypertension occurred in 23% of patients treated with brigatinib in the ALTA-1L trial and Grade ≥3 hypertension occurred in 10% of patients
4. Monitor heart rate periodically during treatment with brigatinib; consider more frequent monitoring in patients where other medications known to cause bradycardia are unavoidable. Bradycardia occurred in 5% (all-grade) and 1% (G ≥3) of patients treated with brigatinib in the ALTA-1L study
5. Advise patients to report any visual symptoms during treatment with brigatinib. Withhold brigatinib and obtain an ophthalmologic evaluation in patients with new or worsening G ≥2 visual symptoms. In the ALTA study, visual disturbances observed included blurred vision, diplopia, and reduced visual acuity. Grade 3 macular edema and Grade 3 cataract were each observed in 1 patient
6. Advise patients to report unexplained muscle pain, tenderness, or weakness. Monitor creatine phosphokinase (CPK) levels periodically during brigatinib treatment. In the ALTA-1L study, increased CPK levels occurred in 39% (all-grade) and 16% (G ≥3) of patients receiving brigatinib. Elevated CPK levels were not associated with the frequency or severity of myalgias or musculoskeletal pain
7. Monitor lipase and amylase levels periodically during brigatinib treatment. In the ALTA-1L study, increased amylase levels occurred in 14% (all-grade) and 5% (G ≥3) of patients receiving brigatinib. In the same study, increased lipase levels occurred in 19% (all-grade) and 13% (G ≥3) of patients receiving brigatinib. No cases of clinical pancreatitis were observed in the ALTA-1L study
8. Monitor fasting blood glucose prior to initiation of brigatinib and then periodically thereafter (or more frequently as clinically indicated). In the ALTA study, 43% of patients experienced new or worsening hyperglycemia during brigatinib treatment. Grade 3 hyperglycemia occurred in 3.7% of patients. Ten percent of patients who had baseline diabetes or glucose intolerance required the initiation of insulin while receiving brigatinib treatment

Treatment Modifications

BRIGATINIB

	7-Day Lead-in Phase	Continuation Phase
Starting dose	90 mg by mouth once daily	180 mg by mouth once daily
Dose level −1	60 mg by mouth once daily	120 mg by mouth once daily
Dose level −2	Permanently discontinue	90 mg by mouth once daily
Dose level −3	—	60 mg by mouth once daily
Dose level −4	—	Permanently discontinue

Note: if brigatinib is interrupted for ≥14 days for reasons other than adverse reactions, resume treatment at 90 mg once daily for 7 days before increasing to the previously tolerated dose. Once the dose of brigatinib has been reduced for adverse reactions, do not subsequently increase the dosage

Pulmonary Toxicities

Adverse Event	Treatment Modification
ILD/pneumonitis, Grade 1 (asymptomatic; clinical or diagnostic observations only; intervention not indicated)	If new symptoms occur during the first 7 days of treatment, withhold brigatinib until recovery to baseline, then resume at the same dose and do not escalate to 180 mg if ILD/pneumonitis is suspected If new pulmonary symptoms occur after the first 7 days of treatment, withhold brigatinib until recovery to baseline, then resume at the same dose If ILD/pneumonitis recurs, then permanently discontinue brigatinib

(continued)

Treatment Modifications (continued)

Adverse Event	Treatment Modification
ILD/pneumonitis, Grade 2 (symptomatic; medical intervention indicated; limiting instrumental ADL)	If new symptoms occur during the first 7 days of treatment, withhold brigatinib until recovery to baseline. Resume at the next lower dose level and do not dose escalate if ILD/pneumonitis is suspected If new pulmonary symptoms occur after the first 7 days of treatment, withhold brigatinib until recovery to baseline. If ILD/pneumonitis is suspected, resume at the next lower dose; otherwise, resume at the same dose If ILD/pneumonitis recurs, then permanently discontinue brigatinib
ILD/pneumonitis, Grade 3 (severe symptoms; limiting self-care ADL; oxygen indicated)	Permanently discontinue brigatinib for ILD/pneumonitis
ILD/pneumonitis, Grade 4 (life-threatening respiratory compromise; urgent intervention indicated [eg, tracheotomy or intubation])	
Cardiovascular Adverse Events	
Grade 3 hypertension despite optimal antihypertensive therapy (SBP ≥160 mmHg or DBP ≥100 mmHg, medical intervention indicated, more than one antihypertensive drug, or more intensive therapy than previously used indicated)	Withhold brigatinib until hypertension has recovered to G ≤1 (SBP <140 mmHg and DBP <90 mmHg), then resume brigatinib at next lower dose Recurrence: withhold brigatinib until recovery to G ≤1, and resume at next lower dose or permanently discontinue treatment
Grade 4 hypertension (life-threatening consequences, urgent intervention indicated)	Withhold brigatinib until recovery to G ≤1 (SBP <140 mmHg and DBP <90 mmHg), and resume at next lower dose or permanently discontinue treatment Recurrence: permanently discontinue brigatinib for recurrence of G4 hypertension
Symptomatic bradycardia (heart rate <60 bpm)	Withhold brigatinib until recovery to asymptomatic bradycardia or to a resting heart rate of ≥60 bpm If a concomitant medication known to cause bradycardia is identified and discontinued or dose-adjusted, then resume brigatinib at the same dose upon recovery to asymptomatic bradycardia or to a resting heart rate of ≥60 bpm If no concomitant medication known to cause bradycardia is identified, or if contributing medications are not discontinued or dose-adjusted, then resume brigatinib at the next lower dose upon recovery to asymptomatic bradycardia or to a resting heart rate of ≥60 bpm
Bradycardia (heart rate <60 bpm) with life-threatening consequences, urgent intervention indicated	Permanently discontinue brigatinib if no contributing concomitant medication known to cause bradycardia is identified If a contributing concomitant medication known to cause bradycardia is identified and discontinued or dose-adjusted, then resume brigatinib at the next lower dose upon recovery to asymptomatic bradycardia or to a resting heart rate of ≥60 bpm, with frequent monitoring as clinically indicated Recurrence: permanently discontinue brigatinib
Other Adverse Events	
G2/3 visual disturbance	Withhold brigatinib until recovery to G ≤1 or baseline. Obtain an ophthalmologic evaluation, then resume at the next lower dose level
G4 visual disturbance	Permanently discontinue brigatinib. Obtain an ophthalmologic evaluation
G3 CPK elevation (>5× ULN to ≤10× ULN)	Withhold brigatinib until recovery to G ≤1 (≤2.5× ULN) or to baseline, then resume brigatinib at the same dose Recurrence: withhold brigatinib until recovery to G ≤1 (≤2.5× ULN) or to baseline, then resume brigatinib at the next lower dose
G4 CPK elevation (>10× ULN)	Withhold brigatinib until recovery to G ≤1 (≤2.5× ULN) or to baseline, then resume brigatinib at the next lower dose
G3 lipase or amylase elevation (>2× ULN to ≤5× ULN)	Withhold brigatinib until recovery to G ≤1 (≤1.5× ULN) or to baseline, then resume brigatinib at the same dose Recurrence: withhold brigatinib until recovery to G ≤1 (≤1.5× ULN) or to baseline, then resume brigatinib at the next lower dose

(continued)

Treatment Modifications (*continued*)

Other Adverse Events

G4 lipase or amylase elevation (>5× ULN)	Withhold brigatinib until recovery to G ≤1 (≤1.5× ULN) or to baseline, then resume brigatinib at the next lower dose
G ≥3 hyperglycemia (blood glucose >250 mg/dL) despite optimal medical management	Withhold brigatinib until adequate hyperglycemic control is achieved and consider reduction to the next lower dose, or permanently discontinue brigatinib
Other G3 adverse effects	Withhold brigatinib until recovery to baseline, then resume at the same dose Recurrence: withhold brigatinib until recovery to baseline, then resume at the next lower dose or discontinue brigatinib
Other G4 adverse effects	First occurrence: either withhold brigatinib until recovery to baseline and resume at the next lower dose or permanently discontinue brigatinib Recurrence: permanently discontinue brigatinib

Hepatic Impairment

Severe hepatic impairment (Child-Pugh C)	Reduce the brigatinib dose by approximately 40% (ie, from 180 mg to 120 mg, from 120 mg to 90 mg, or from 90 mg to 60 mg)

Renal Impairment

Severe renal impairment (CrCl 15–29 mL/min)	Reduce the brigatinib dose by approximately 50% (ie, from 180 mg to 90 mg, or from 90 mg to 60 mg)

Drug-Drug Interactions

Concomitant therapy with a strong CYP3A inhibitor is required	If coadministration of a strong CYP3A inhibitor is unavoidable, then reduce the brigatinib dose by approximately 50% (ie, from 180 mg to 90 mg, or from 90 mg to 60 mg)
Concomitant therapy with a moderate CYP3A inhibitor is required	If coadministration of a moderate CYP3A inhibitor is unavoidable, then reduce the brigatinib dose by approximately 40% (ie, from 180 mg to 120 mg, from 120 mg to 90 mg, or from 90 mg to 60 mg)
Concomitant therapy with a strong CYP3A inducer is required	Avoid coadministration of a strong CYP3A inducer with brigatinib
Concomitant therapy with a moderate CYP3A inducer is required	If coadministration of brigatinib with a moderate CYP3A inducer is unavoidable, then increase the brigatinib dose in 30 mg increments after 7 days of treatment with the current brigatinib dose, as tolerated, to a maximum of twice the brigatinib dose that was tolerated prior to initiation of the moderate CYP3A inducer
Concomitant therapy with a sensitive CYP3A substrate is required	Based on in vitro data, brigatinib may decrease concentrations of medications metabolized by CYP3A. Monitor for loss of efficacy of sensitive CYP3A substrates when coadministered with brigatinib

Grading of adverse events per National Cancer Institute Common Terminology Criteria for Adverse Events. Version 4.0
ILD, interstitial lung disease; ADL, activities of daily living; SBP, systolic blood pressure; DBP, diastolic blood pressure; bpm, beats per minute; ULN, upper limit of normal; CrCl, creatinine clearance

Adverse Events (N = 273)

Event	Brigatinib (n = 136)		Crizotinib (n = 137)	
Grade (%)	Grade 1 or 2	Grade 3–5	Grade 1 or 2	Grade 3–5
Any adverse effect	36	61	45	55
Diarrhea	48	1	53	2
Increased blood creatine kinase level*	23	16	7	1

(*continued*)

Adverse Events (N = 273) (continued)

Event	Brigatinib (n = 136)		Crizotinib (n = 137)	
Grade (%)	Grade 1 or 2	Grade 3–5	Grade 1 or 2	Grade 3–5
Nausea	25	1	53	3
Cough	25	0	16	0
Hypertension	13	10	4	3
Increased alanine aminotransferase level	18	1	23	9
Increased lipase level[†]	6	13	7	5
Vomiting	18	<1	37	2
Constipation	15	0	41	<1
Increased amylase level[†]	9	5	6	<1
Pruritis	13	<1	4	<1
Rash	10	0	2	0
Decreased appetite	7	<1	17	3
Dermatitis acneiform	7	0	1	0
Dyspepsia	6	0	13	0
Epistaxis	6	0	0	0
Bradycardia	4	<1	12	0
Peripheral edema	4	<1	38	<1
Dysgeusia	4	0	19	0
Upper abdominal pain	4	<1	12	1
Pain in extremity	4	0	12	<1
Increased blood creatinine level	2	0	13	<1
Neutropenia	1	0	4	4
Pleural effusion	<1	<1	5	1
Photopsia	<1	0	20	<1
Gastroesophageal reflux disease	<1	0	9	0
Visual impairment	0	0	16	0
Deep-vein thrombosis	0	0	6	0

*Myalgia was reported in 6% of patients in the brigatinib group and 4% of patients in the crizotinib group. Musculoskeletal pain was reported in 4% and 6% of patients in these groups, respectively. None of these reported events occurred at Grade 3 or greater in either group

[†]There were no reported cases of pancreatitis in either group

Adverse events were included in the table if the incidence rate differed by at least 5 percent between treatment groups. Interstitial lung disease or pneumonitis (all-grade) occurred in 4% of patients in the brigatinib arm versus 2% of patients in the crizotinib arm. Grade 3–4 interstitial lung disease or pneumonitis occurred in 3% of patients in the brigatinib arm and 0.7% of patients in the crizotinib arm. Fourteen patients (7 [5%] of brigatinib patients and 7 [5%] of crizotinib patients) had adverse events that led to death within 30 days after the last dose of trial drug, but none of these events was considered related to the trial treatment by the investigators. Investigator- or protocol-mandated dose reduction due to adverse event occurred in 29% of patients in the brigatinib group and 21% of the crizotinib group. The most common reasons for dose reductions were increased blood creatine phosphokinase in the brigatinib group (10.3% of all patients or 36% of patients with dose reduction) and increased alanine aminotransferase (5.8% of all patients or 28% of patients with dose reduction) and nausea (4.4% of all patients or 21% of patients with dose reduction) in the crizotinib group. A total of 12% of patients in the brigatinib group and 9% of patients in the crizotinib group discontinued treatment due to adverse events

ADVANCED NSCLC • ALK-REARRANGED • FIRST-LINE
LUNG CANCER REGIMEN: CERITINIB

Cho BC et al. J Thorac Oncol 2017;12(9):1357–1367
FDA and EMA prescribing information and miscellaneous sources
Shaw AT et al. N Engl J Med 2014;370(13):1189–1197

Ceritinib 450 mg/dose; administer orally once daily, *continually,* *with* food (total dose/week = 3150 mg)

Notes:
- On December 21, 2017, the U.S. FDA revised the approved dosage regimen to 450 mg administered orally once daily *with* food based on similar systemic exposure and improved gastrointestinal tolerability compared to the 750-mg dose administered *without* food found in the ASCEND–8 study. The study found similar systemic exposure between the 450 mg (fed state) and 750 mg (fasting state) regimens, but improved gastrointestinal tolerability with the former
- Patients who delay taking ceritinib at a regularly scheduled time may take a missed dose if the interval remaining before the next regularly scheduled dose is ≥12 hours. If vomiting occurs after a dose of ceritinib, take the next dose at the next regularly scheduled time
- In patients with a history of diabetes mellitus, optimize antihyperglycemic medications prior to initiating ceritinib. If ceritinib therapy is interrupted, patients receiving antihyperglycemic medications should be monitored for hypoglycemia
- Ceritinib is metabolized by cytochrome P450 (CYP) CYP3A subfamily enzymes. Avoid using ceritinib with strong CYP3A4 inhibitors (eg, ketoconazole, itraconazole, voriconazole, ritonavir, clarithromycin) when possible. If concurrent use with a strong CYP3A4 inhibitor is required, reduce the ceritinib dose by approximately 33%. Avoid using ceritinib with strong CYP3A4 inducers (eg, carbamazepine, rifampin, phenytoin, phenobarbital, St John's Wort).
- Advise patients to not consume grapefruit and grapefruit juice as they may inhibit CYP3A in the gut wall and increase the bioavailability of ceritinib
- Ceritinib may inhibit CYP3A4 and CYP2C9; use caution and consider dose reduction, when appropriate, of concurrently used CYP3A4 and CYP2C9 substrates, especially if the substrate has a narrow therapeutic index (eg, alfentanil, cyclosporine, dihydroergotamine, ergotamine, fentanyl, pimozide, quinidine, sirolimus, tacrolimus, warfarin, phenytoin)

Supportive Care
Antiemetic prophylaxis
Emetogenic potential is **MODERATE**
See Chapter 42 for antiemetic recommendations

Hematopoietic growth factor (CSF) prophylaxis
Primary prophylaxis is **NOT** indicated
See Chapter 43 for more information

Antimicrobial prophylaxis
Risk of fever and neutropenia is **LOW**
   Antimicrobial primary prophylaxis to be considered:
- Antibacterial—not indicated
- Antifungal—not indicated
- Antiviral—not indicated unless patient previously had an episode of HSV

Diarrhea management
Latent or delayed-onset diarrhea:
- **Loperamide** 4 mg orally initially after the first loose or liquid stool, *then*
- **Loperamide** 2 mg orally every 2 hours during waking hours, *plus*
- **Loperamide** 4 mg orally every 4 hours during hours of sleep
  - Continue for at least 12 hours after diarrhea resolves
  - Recurrent diarrhea after a 12-hour diarrhea-free interval is treated as a new episode
  - Rehydrate orally with fluids and electrolytes during a diarrheal episode
  - If a patient develops blood or mucus in stool, dehydration, or hemodynamic instability, or if diarrhea persists <48 hours despite loperamide, stop loperamide and hospitalize the patient for IV hydration
    Alternatively, a trial of **diphenoxylate hydrochloride** 2.5 mg with **atropine sulfate** 0.025 mg (eg, Lomotil)
  - Initial adult dose is 2 tablets 4 times daily until control has been achieved, after which the dose may be reduced to meet individual requirements. Control may often be maintained with as little as 2 tablets daily
  - Clinical improvement of acute diarrhea is usually observed within 48 hours. If improvement of chronic diarrhea after treatment with a maximum daily dose of 8 tablets is not observed within 10 days, control is unlikely with further administration

(continued)

(continued)

Persistent diarrhea:
Octreotide 100–150 mcg subcutaneously 3 times daily. Maximum total daily dose is 1500 mcg

Antibiotic therapy during latent or delayed-onset diarrhea:

A fluoroquinolone (eg, **ciprofloxacin** 500 mg orally every 12 hours) if absolute neutrophil count <500/mm^3 with or without accompanying fever in association with diarrhea
  • Antibiotics should also be administered if patient is hospitalized with prolonged diarrhea and should be continued until diarrhea resolves

Patient Population Studied

A phase 1 study involved 130 patients with locally advanced or metastatic, *ALK*-rearranged, cancer. The majority of patients (122; 94%) had advanced NSCLC. Eligible patients were age ≥18 years, with an Eastern Cooperative Oncology Group (ECOG) performance status score ≤2. A total of 59 patients underwent a dose-escalation phase. An additional 71 patients were then treated at the maximum tolerated dose (750 mg daily) determined in the dose-escalation phase

Efficacy (N = 122)

Overall response rate*	58%
Overall response rate* for patients who received 750 mg daily	59%

Overall response rate is the percentage of patients who experienced a confirmed partial or complete response to the study drug
Note: results are shown for the patients with advanced NSCLC. Of the 8 patients who had other types of advanced cancer, 2 had a response to the study drug

Therapy Monitoring

1. Monitor and manage patients using standards of care, including antidiarrheals, antiemetics, or fluid replacement, as indicated
2. Monitor with liver laboratory tests including ALT, AST, and total bilirubin once a month and as clinically indicated, with more frequent testing in patients who develop transaminase elevations
3. Monitor patients for pulmonary symptoms indicative of ILD/pneumonitis
4. Obtain an ECG and evaluate electrolytes at baseline. Conduct periodic monitoring with ECGs and electrolytes in patients with congestive heart failure, bradyarrhythmias, electrolyte abnormalities, or those who are taking medications that are known to prolong the QTc interval
5. Monitor fasting serum glucose prior to the start of ceritinib treatment and periodically thereafter as clinically indicated
6. Monitor lipase and amylase prior to the start of ceritinib treatment and periodically thereafter as clinically indicated

Treatment Modifications

Starting dose = 450 mg once daily with food
Dose levels 450 mg/300 mg/150 mg

Adverse Event	Treatment Modification
G ≥3 ALT or AST elevation (>5× ULN) + total bilirubin ≤2× ULN	Withhold ceritinib until recovery to baseline or ALT and AST ≤3× ULN, then resume ceritinib but reduce the dose by 150 mg
G ≥2 ALT or AST elevation (>3× ULN) + total bilirubin >2× ULN	Permanently discontinue ceritinib
Any grade treatment-related ILD/pneumonitis	Permanently discontinue ceritinib
Severe or intolerable nausea, vomiting, or diarrhea despite optimal antiemetic or antidiarrheal therapy	Withhold until improved, then resume ceritinib but reduce the dose by 150 mg
Persistent hyperglycemia >250 mg/dL despite optimal antihyperglycemic therapy	Withhold ceritinib until hyperglycemia is adequately controlled, then resume ceritinib but reduce the dose by 150 mg. If adequate hyperglycemic control cannot be achieved with optimal medical management, discontinue ceritinib
G 3 lipase or amylase elevation (>2× ULN)	Withhold ceritinib and monitor serum lipase and amylase. After recovery to <1.5× ULN, resume ceritinib but reduce the dose by 150 mg
Concomitant use of a strong CYP3A inhibitor is unavoidable	Reduce the ceritinib dose by ~1/3, rounded to the nearest multiple of the 150 mg dosage strength. After discontinuation of a strong CYP3A inhibitor, resume the ceritinib dose taken prior to initiating the strong CYP3A4 inhibitor
Dose adjustments for cardiac adverse events	
QTc interval >500 msec on ≥2 separate ECGs	Withhold ceritinib until QTc interval <481 msec or recovery to baseline if baseline QTc ≥481 msec, then resume ceritinib but reduce the dose by 150 mg
QTc interval prolongation in combination with torsades de pointes or polymorphic ventricular tachycardia or signs/symptoms of serious arrhythmia	Permanently discontinue ceritinib
Symptomatic bradycardia that is not life-threatening	Withhold ceritinib until recovery to asymptomatic bradycardia or to a heart rate ≥60 bpm. Evaluate concomitant medications known to cause bradycardia. Resume ceritinib but reduce the dose by 150 mg
Clinically significant bradycardia requiring intervention or life-threatening bradycardia in patients taking a concomitant medication also known to cause bradycardia or a medication known to cause hypotension	Withhold ceritinib until recovery to asymptomatic bradycardia or to a heart rate ≥60 bpm. If the concomitant medication can be adjusted or discontinued, then resume ceritinib but reduce the dose by 150 mg
Life-threatening bradycardia in patients who are not taking a concomitant medication also known to cause bradycardia or known to cause hypotension	Permanently discontinue ceritinib

ALT, alanine aminotransferase; AST, aspartate aminotransferase; ECG, electrocardiogram; ILD, interstitial lung disease; ULN, upper limit of normal

Notes:
- Advise the use of effective contraception during treatment with ceritinib and for at least 2 weeks following completion of therapy
- Ceritinib is eliminated primarily via the liver and drug exposure may be increased in patients with hepatic impairment. Patients with mild hepatic impairment do not require dose adjustments. A recommended dose for patients with moderate to severe hepatic impairment has not been determined
- No dose adjustment is recommended for patients with mild or moderate renal impairment. The safety of alectinib in patients with creatinine clearance <30 mL/min has not been studied

Adverse Events (N = 130)

	Grade 3/4* (%)
Any event	49
Elevated ALT level	21
Elevated AST level	11
Elevated lipase level	7
Diarrhea	7
Nausea	5
Vomiting	5
Fatigue	5
Hypophosphatemia	3
Elevated amylase level	2
Elevated blood alkaline phosphatase level	2
Hyperglycemia	2

*According to the National Cancer Institute Common Terminology Criteria for Adverse Events, version 4.0
Note: only events reported in ≥2% and suspected to be related to the study drug are included in this table. All events were reversible on discontinuation of ceritinib treatment. Four cases of interstitial lung disease and 1 case of asymptomatic Grade 3 prolongation of the QT interval were thought to possibly be related to ceritinib treatment. Dose reduction was required in 51% of patients, and permanent discontinuation of the study drug owing to an adverse event occurred in 6% of patients. Of the patients receiving the maximum tolerated dose of 750 mg daily, 62% required dose reduction. No treatment-related deaths occurred

ADVANCED NSCLC • ALK-REARRANGED • FIRST-LINE
LUNG CANCER REGIMEN: CRIZOTINIB

Kwak EL et al. N Engl J Med 2010;363:1693–1703
Shaw AT et al. Lancet Oncol 2011;12:1004–1012

Crizotinib 250 mg/dose; administer orally twice daily, continually, with or without food (total dose/week = 3500 mg; total dose/28-day cycle = 14,000 mg)

Supportive Care
Antiemetic prophylaxis
Emetogenic potential is at least **MODERATE**
See Chapter 42 for antiemetic recommendations

Hematopoietic growth factor (CSF) prophylaxis
Primary prophylaxis is **NOT** indicated
See Chapter 43 for more information

Antimicrobial prophylaxis
Risk of fever and neutropenia is **LOW**
   Antimicrobial primary prophylaxis to be considered:
   • Antibacterial—not indicated
   • Antifungal—not indicated
   • Antiviral—not indicated unless patient previously had an episode of HSV

Diarrhea management
Latent or delayed-onset diarrhea:
   Loperamide 4 mg orally initially after the first loose or liquid stool, *then*
   Loperamide 2 mg orally every 2 hours during waking hours, *plus*
   Loperamide 4 mg orally every 4 hours during hours of sleep
   • Continue for at least 12 hours after diarrhea resolves
   • Recurrent diarrhea after a 12-hour diarrhea-free interval is treated as a new episode
   • Rehydrate orally with fluids and electrolytes during a diarrheal episode
   • If a patient develops blood or mucus in stool, dehydration, or hemodynamic instability, or if diarrhea persists <48 hours despite loperamide, stop loperamide and hospitalize the patient for IV hydration
      Alternatively, a trial of **diphenoxylate hydrochloride** 2.5mg with **atropine sulfate** 0.025 mg (eg, Lomotil)
   • Initial adult dose is 2 tablets 4 times daily until control has been achieved, after which the dose may be reduced to meet individual requirements. Control may often be maintained with as little as 2 tablets daily
   • Clinical improvement of acute diarrhea is usually observed within 48 hours. If improvement of chronic diarrhea after treatment with a maximum daily dose of 8 tablets is not observed within 10 days, control is unlikely with further administration

Persistent diarrhea:
   Octreotide 100–150 mcg subcutaneously 3 times daily. Maximum total daily dose is 1500 mcg

Antibiotic therapy during latent or delayed-onset diarrhea:
   A fluoroquinolone (eg, **ciprofloxacin** 500 mg orally every 12 hours) if absolute neutrophil count <500/mm^3 with or without accompanying fever in association with diarrhea
   • Antibiotics should also be administered if patient is hospitalized with prolonged diarrhea and should be continued until diarrhea resolves

*Abigerges D et al. J Natl Cancer Inst 1994;86:446–449
Rothenberg ML et al. J Clin Oncol 2001;19:3801–3807
Wadler S et al. J Clin Oncol 1998;16:3169–3178

Notes:
1. Detection of ALK-positive NSCLC using an FDA-approved test indicated for this use is necessary for selection of patients for treatment with crizotinib
2. Assessment for ALK-positive NSCLC should be performed by laboratories with demonstrated proficiency in the specific technology being utilized. Improper assay performance can lead to unreliable test results

Drugs That May Increase Crizotinib Plasma Concentrations
Coadministration of crizotinib with strong CYP3A inhibitors increases crizotinib plasma concentrations
• Avoid concomitant use of strong CYP3A inhibitors, including but not limited to atazanavir, clarithromycin, indinavir, itraconazole, ketoconazole, nefazodone, nelfinavir, ritonavir, saquinavir, telithromycin, troleandomycin, and voriconazole
• Avoid grapefruit or grapefruit juice, which may increase plasma concentrations of crizotinib
• Exercise caution with concomitant use of moderate CYP3A inhibitors

(continued)

(*continued*)

Drugs That May Decrease Crizotinib Plasma Concentrations
Coadministration of crizotinib with strong CYP3A inducers decreases crizotinib plasma concentrations
• Avoid concurrent use of strong CYP3A inducers, including but not limited to carbamazepine, phenobarbital, phenytoin, rifabutin, rifampin, and St. John's Wort

Dose Adjustments

Adverse Event	Dose Modification
Hematologic Toxicity*	
G3 hematologic toxicity	Withhold until recovery to G ≤2, then resume at the same dose schedule
G4 hematologic toxicity	Withhold until recovery to G ≤2, then resume at 200 mg twice daily
G4 hematologic toxicity at a dose of 200 mg twice daily	Withhold until recovery to G ≤2, then resume at 250 mg once daily
G4 hematologic toxicity at a dose of 250 mg once daily	Permanently discontinue crizotinib
Non-hematologic Toxicity	
G3/4 alanine aminotransferase (ALT) or aspartate aminotransferase (AST) elevation with G ≤1 total bilirubin	Withhold until recovery to G ≤1 or baseline, then resume at 200 mg twice daily
G3/4 ALT or AST elevation with G ≤1 total bilirubin on a dose of 200 mg twice daily	Withhold until recovery to G ≤1 or baseline, then resume 250 mg once daily
G3/4 ALT or AST elevation with G ≤1 total bilirubin on a dose of 250 mg once daily	Permanently discontinue crizotinib
G2/3/4 ALT or AST elevation with concurrent G2/3/4 total bilirubin elevation (in the absence of cholestasis or hemolysis)	Permanently discontinue crizotinib
Any grade pneumonitis[†]	Permanently discontinue crizotinib
G3 QTc prolongation	Withhold until recovery to G ≤1, then resume at 200 mg twice daily
G3 QTc prolongation on a dose of 200 mg twice daily	Withhold until recovery to G ≤1 or baseline, then resume 250 mg once daily
G3 QTc prolongation on a dose of 250 mg once daily	Permanently discontinue crizotinib
Grade 4 QTc prolongation	Permanently discontinue crizotinib

*Except lymphopenia (unless associated with clinical events, eg, opportunistic infections)
[†]Not attributable to NSCLC progression, other pulmonary disease, infection, or radiation effect

Patient Population Studied

Eighty-two patients with advanced ALK-positive NSCLC who had received crizotinib in the phase 1 clinical trial. For all patients, ALK positivity was confirmed by fluorescence in situ hybridization (FISH). ALK FISH was done before trial enrollment, using the initial diagnostic or surgical specimen, or a repeat biopsy specimen obtained for the purposes of genetic testing. These patients were mainly young (median age: 51 years [range: 25–78years]), never smokers with adenocarcinoma histology. Among the 82 patients, 50 (61%) were enrolled at U.S. study sites, 26 (32%) at the Korean site, and the remaining 6 (7%) in Australia. Because the protocol placed no restriction on the number of previous therapies, the number varied widely among patients, ranging from 0 to 7 previous lines (median: 2) of therapy for metastatic disease. Seventy-three (89%) of 82 patients had received at least 1 previous therapy for metastatic disease. An additional 36 patients with advanced, ALK-positive NSCLC who had not received crizotinib were identified through retrospective and prospective screening efforts

Efficacy

	ALK(+) Patients*	ALK(+) Patients†	ALK(+) Controls‡	ALK(+) Patients§	ALK(−) EGFR(+) Patients𝄒	Crizotinib-naïve, ALK(+) Controls**	Wild-type Controls††
Number of patients	82	30	23	56	63	36	253
Median OS [95% CI]‡‡	NR [17mo–NR]§§	NR [14mo–NR]	6 mo [4–17 mo]	NR [17mo–NR]	24 mo [15–34mo]	20 mo [13–26mo]	15 mo [13–17mo]
	—			—		HR 0.77, 95% CI 0.50–1.19; P = 0.244	
1-year OS [95% CI]	74% [63–82%]	70% [50–83%]	44% [23–64%]	71% [58–81%]	74% [61–83]	72% [54–84%]	
2-year OS [95% CI]	54% [40–66%]	55% [33–72%]	12% [2–30%]	57% [40–71%]	52% [38–65%]	36% [19–54%]	
	HR 0.36, 95% CI 0.17–0.75; P = 0.004			P = 0.786		—	

Mo, months; NR, not reached; OS, overall survival

*Patients with advanced, ALK-positive NSCLC who had enrolled on the multicenter phase 1 clinical trial of crizotinib. Median follow-up was 18 months (IQR 16–22)

†ALK-positive patients given crizotinib in the second- or third-line setting

‡ALK+ controls given any second-line therapy

§Fifty-six crizotinib-treated, ALK+ patients; 20 (36%) of the 56 crizotinib-treated patients received 3 to 7 previous lines of therapy. This could overestimate the survival benefit associated with crizotinib

𝄒Sixty-three ALK-negative, EGFR-positive patients given EGFR TKI therapy

**Thirty-six crizotinib-naïve, ALK-positive controls

††Two hundred fifty-three wild-type controls

‡Median OS from date of first crizotinib dose in months

§§OS did not differ based on age (≤50 years vs. >50 years, P = 0.692), sex (P = 0.975), smoking history (never vs. any smoking, P = 0.857), or ethnic origin (Asian vs. non-Asian, P = 0.857)

Toxicity

Adapted from XALKORI (crizotinib) Capsules, oral; 05/2013 product label. Pfizer Labs, Division of Pfizer Inc., New York, NY

Adverse Reactions in ≥10% of Patients with Locally Advanced or Metastatic ALK-Positive NSCLC Enrolled in 2 Studies*

Adverse Event	Treatment Emergent N = 255		Treatment Related N = 255	
	All G, n (%)	G3/4, n (%)	All G, n (%)	G3/4, n (%)
Eye Disorders				
Vision disorder†	163 (64%)	0	159 (62%)	0
Gastrointestinal Disorders				
Nausea	145 (57%)	2 (<1%)	136 (53%)	0
Diarrhea	124 (49%)	1 (<1%)	109 (43%)	0
Vomiting	116 (45%)	3 (1%)	101 (40%)	0
Constipation	98 (38%)	2 (<1%)	69 (27%)	1 (<1%)
Esophageal disorder‡	51 (20%)	3 (1%)	29 (11%)	0
Abdominal pain§	40 (16%)	1 (<1%)	20 (8%)	0
Stomatitis𝄒	27 (11%)	1 (<1%)	15 (6%)	1 (<1%)
General Disorders				
Edema**	97 (38%)	2 (<1%)	72 (28%)	0
Fatigue	80 (31%)	6 (2%)	51 (20%)	4 (2%)
Chest pain/discomfort††	30 (12%)	1 (<1%)	3 (1%)	0
Fever	30 (12%)	1 (<1%)	2 (<1%)	0
Infections and Infestations				
Upper respiratory infection‡	50 (20%)	1 (<1%)	4 (2%)	0

(continued)

Toxicity (continued)

Investigations

↑ Alanine aminotransferase	38 (15%)	17 (7%)	34 (13%)	14 (5%)
↑ Aspartate aminotransferase	29 (11%)	7 (3%)	24 (9%)	5 (2%)

Metabolism and Nutrition

Decreased appetite	69 (27%)	3 (1%)	49 (19%)	0

Musculoskeletal

Arthralgia	29 (11%)	3 (1%)	4 (2%)	0
Back pain	28 (11%)	0	2 (<1%)	0

Nervous System Disorders

Dizziness§§	60 (24%)	0	42 (16%)	0
Neuropathy‶	58 (23%)	1 (<1%)	34 (13%)***	1 (<1%)
Headache	34 (13%)	1 (<1%)	10 (4%)	0
Dysgeusia	33 (13%)	0	30 (12%)	0

Psychiatric Disorders

Insomnia	30 (12%)	0	8 (3%)	0

Respiratory Disorders

Dyspnea	57 (22%)	16 (6%)	5 (2%)	3 (1%)
Cough	54 (21%)	3 (1%)	9 (4%)	0

Skin Disorders

Rash	41 (16%)	0	25 (10%)	0

Cardiovascular

G1/2 bradycardia	12 (5%)

Hematologic Toxicities

G3/4 neutropenia	5.2%
G3/4 thrombocytopenia	0.4%
G3/4 lymphopenia	11.4%

*One study used NCI Common Terminology Criteria for Adverse Events (CTCAE) v4.0; the other used CTCAE v3.0. All CTCAE versions available at: http://ctep.cancer.gov/protocolDevelopment/electronic_applications/ctc.htm [accessed December 7, 2013]
†Includes diplopia, photopsia, photophobia, vision blurred, visual field defect, visual impairment, vitreous floaters, visual brightness, and visual acuity reduced. Consider ophthalmologic evaluation, particularly if patients experience photopsia or experience new or increased vitreous floaters. Severe or worsening vitreous floaters and/or photopsia could also be signs of a retinal hole or pending retinal detachment
‡Includes dyspepsia, dysphagia, epigastric discomfort/pain/burning, esophagitis, esophageal obstruction/pain/spasm/ulcer, gastroesophageal reflux, odynophagia, and reflux esophagitis
§Includes abdominal discomfort, abdominal pain, abdominal pain upper, and abdominal tenderness
‶Includes mouth ulceration, glossodynia, glossitis, cheilitis, mucosal inflammation, oropharyngeal pain/discomfort, oral pain, and stomatitis
**Includes edema, edema localized, and peripheral edema
††Includes chest pain, chest discomfort, and musculoskeletal chest pain
‡‡Includes nasopharyngitis, rhinitis, pharyngitis, and upper respiratory tract infection
§§Includes balance disorder, dizziness, and presyncope
‶Includes burning sensation, dysesthesia, hyperesthesia, hypoesthesia, neuralgia, paresthesia, peripheral neuropathy, peripheral motor neuropathy, and peripheral sensory neuropathy
***Although most events were G1, G2 motor neuropathy and G3 peripheral neuropathy were reported in 1 patient each

Treatment Monitoring

1. *Monthly and as clinically indicated:* complete blood counts (CBC) including differential white blood cell counts and liver function tests
2. *If G3/4 clinical or laboratory abnormalities are observed or if fever or infection occurs:* frequent monitoring of complete blood counts (CBC) including differential white blood cell counts and liver function tests
3. Consider periodic monitoring with electrocardiograms (ECGs) and electrolytes in patients with congestive heart failure, bradyarrhythmias, electrolyte abnormalities, or who are taking medications that are known to prolong the QT interval

ADVANCED NSCLC • ALK-REARRANGED • SUBSEQUENT THERAPY

LUNG CANCER REGIMEN: BRIGATINIB

ALUNBRIG (brigatinib) tablet prescribing information. Cambridge, MA: Ariad Pharmaceuticals, Inc.; updated 2018 December
Camidge DR et al. J Clin Oncol 2018;36(26):2693–2701
Kim DW et al. J Clin Oncol 2017;35(22):2490–2498
Protocol for: Kim DW et al. J Clin Oncol 2017;35(22):2490–2498
Supplementary appendix to: Kim DW et al. J Clin Oncol 2017;35(22):2490–2498

7-Day Lead-in Phase:

Brigatinib 90 mg/dose; administer orally, once daily, without regard to food, for 7 consecutive days (total dose/week during lead-in phase = 630 mg)

Continuation phase (if brigatinib was tolerated during the initial 7 day lead-in phase [see Treatment Modifications section]):

Brigatinib 180 mg/dose; administer orally, once daily, without regard to food, continuously until disease progression (total dose/week during continuation phase = 1260 mg)

Notes:

- Patients who delay taking brigatinib at a regularly scheduled time or who vomit after taking a dose of brigatinib should take the next dose at the next regularly scheduled time

- Brigatinib tablets should be swallowed whole. Do not crush or chew tablets

- If brigatinib is interrupted for ≥14 days for reasons other than adverse reactions, resume treatment at 90 mg once daily for 7 days before increasing to the previously tolerated dose

- In vitro studies suggest that brigatinib is a substrate for CYP2C8 and CYP3A4, that brigatinib may induce CYP3A and CYP2C expression, and that brigatinib is an inhibitor of P-glycoprotein (P-gp), BCRP, OCT1, MATE1, and MATE2K

  - Coadministration of brigatinib with itraconazole (a strong CYP3A inhibitor) increased brigatinib C_{max} by 21% and AUC_{0-inf} by 101%. Moderate CYP3A4 inhibitors are estimated to increase the AUC of brigatinib by about 40%. If coadministration of a strong CYP3A inhibitor is unavoidable, then reduce the brigatinib dose by approximately 50% (ie, from 180 mg to 90 mg, or from 90 mg to 60 mg). If coadministration of a moderate CYP3A inhibitor is unavoidable, then reduce the brigatinib dose by approximately 40% (ie, from 180 mg to 120 mg, from 120 mg to 90 mg, or from 90 mg to 60 mg)

  - Coadministration of brigatinib with gemfibrozil (a strong CYP2C8 inhibitor) decreased brigatinib C_{max} by 41% and AUC_{0-inf} by 12%. No dose modification is necessary when brigatinib is coadministered with a CYP2C8 inhibitor

  - Coadministration of brigatinib with rifampin (a strong CYP3A inducer) decreased brigatinib C_{max} by 60% and AUC_{0-inf} by 80%. Moderate CYP3A inducers are estimated to reduce the AUC of brigatinib by about 50%. Avoid coadministration of brigatinib with strong CYP3A inducers. If coadministration of brigatinib with a moderate CYP3A inducer is unavoidable, then increase the brigatinib dose in 30 mg increments after 7 days of treatment with the current brigatinib dose, as tolerated, to a maximum of twice the brigatinib dose that was tolerated prior to initiation of the moderate CYP3A inducer

  - Based on in vitro data, brigatinib may decrease concentrations of medications metabolized by CYP3A. Monitor for loss of efficacy of sensitive CYP3A substrates when coadministered with brigatinib

- Patients with severe hepatic impairment (Child-Pugh C) had a 37% higher unbound brigatinib systemic exposure (AUC_{0-inf}) compared to patients with normal hepatic function. Thus, in patients with severe hepatic impairment (Child-Pugh C), reduce the brigatinib dose by approximately 40% (ie, from 180 mg to 120 mg, from 120 mg to 90 mg, or from 90 mg to 60 mg)

- Patients with severe renal impairment (CrCl 15–29 mL/min) had a 86% higher unbound brigatinib systemic exposure (AUC_{0-inf}) compared to patients with normal renal function. Therefore, in patients with severe renal impairment (CrCl 15–29 mL/min), reduce the brigatinib dose by approximately 50% (ie, from 180 mg to 90 mg, or from 90 mg to 60 mg)

Supportive Care
Antiemetic prophylaxis
Emetogenic potential is **MINIMAL TO LOW**
See Chapter 42 for antiemetic recommendations

Hematopoietic growth factor (CSF) prophylaxis
Primary prophylaxis is **NOT** *indicated*
See Chapter 43 for more information

Antimicrobial prophylaxis
Risk of fever and neutropenia is LOW
Antimicrobial primary prophylaxis to be considered:

- Antibacterial—not indicated

- Antifungal—not indicated

- Antiviral—not indicated unless patient previously had an episode of HSV

Patient Population Studied

This randomized, open-label, phase 2 trial included 222 adult patients and compared 2 different doses of brigatinib for ALK-positive, crizotinib-refractory non–small cell lung cancer (NSCLC). Patients were eligible if they had histologically or cytologically confirmed, locally advanced or metastatic NSCLC, investigator-determined disease progression while receiving crizotinib, at least one measurable lesion according to RECIST v1.1 criteria, adequate organ and hematologic function, an ECOG performance status of ≤2, and a life expectancy of ≥3 months. Patients were excluded if they had ever received an ALK inhibitor other than crizotinib, if they had received crizotinib within 3 days of the first brigatinib dose; cytotoxic chemotherapy, investigational agents, or radiation therapy (except stereotactic radiosurgery) within 14 days; or monoclonal antibodies within 30 days. They were also ineligible if they had present or past history of active or uncontrolled cardiovascular disease, another primary malignancy (with exceptions), pulmonary interstitial disease or drug-related pneumonitis, or symptomatic, neurologically unstable CNS metastases or those requiring increasing doses of corticosteroids, or active infection. Make it other conventional chemotherapy regimens were acceptable. Data included herein were reported in the primary clinical trial paper and in the subsequent exploratory analysis paper.

Efficacy (N = 222)

	Brigatinib 90 mg (n = 112)	Brigatinib 180 mg (n = 110)	
Overall confirmed objective response rate (investigator-assessed)	45% (97.5% CI, 34–56)	54% (97.5% CI, 43–65)	
Complete response rate (investigator-assessed)	1%	4%	
Partial response rate (investigator-assessed)	44%	50%	
Median time to response (investigator-assessed)	1.8 months (range, 1.7–9.1)	1.9 months (range, 1.0–11.0)	
Median duration of response (investigator-assessed)	13.8 months (95% CI, 5.6–13.8)	11.1 months (95% CI, 9.2–13.8)	
Disease control rate (investigator-assessed)	82% (95% CI, 74–89)	86% (95% CI, 79–92)	
Overall confirmed objective response rate (IRC-assessed)	48% (95% CI, 39–58)	53% (95% CI, 43–62)	
Complete response rate (IRC-assessed)	4%	5%	
Partial response rate (IRC-assessed)	45%	48%	
Median duration of response (IRC-assessed)	13.8 months (95% CI, 7.4–NR)	13.8 months (95% CI, 9.3–NR)	
Disease control rate (IRC-assessed)	78% (95% CI, 69–85)	84% (95% CI, 75–90)	
Median progression-free survival (investigator-assessed)*†‡	9.2 months (95% CI, 7.4–15.6)	12.9 months (95% CI, 11.1–NR)	HR for progression or death (180 mg vs. 90 mg) 0.55 (95% CI, 0.35–0.86)
Median progression-free survival (IRC-assessed)*†‡	9.2 months (95% CI, 7.4–NR)	15.6 months (95% CI, 11.0–NR)	
Estimated progression-free survival (6 months)	63% (95% CI, 53–72)	78% (95% CI, 68–85)	
Estimated overall survival (12 months)	71% (95% CI, 60–79)	80% (95% CI, 67–88)	
Intracranial objective response rate (IRC-assessed)*†	46% (95% CI, 27–67)	67% (95% CI, 41–87)	
Intracranial complete objective response rate (IRC-assessed)*†	8%	0%	

(continued)

Efficacy (N = 222) (continued)

	Brigatinib 90 mg (n = 112)	Brigatinib 180 mg (n = 110)	
Intracranial partial objective response rate (IRC-assessed)*†	38%	67%	
Intracranial disease control rate (IRC-assessed)*†	85% (95% CI, 65–96)	83% (95% CI, 59–96)	
Median intracranial progression-free survival (IRC-assessed)*	15.6 months (95% CI, 9.0–18.3)	18.4 months (95% CI, 12.8–NR)	HR for intracranial progression or death (180 mg vs. 90 mg) 0.64 (95% CI, 0.35–1.18)
Systemic objective response rate (in patients with brain metastases at baseline) (investigator-assessed)*	40% (95% CI, 29–52)	59% (95% CI, 47–70)	
Median systemic progression-free survival (in patients with brain metastases at baseline) (investigator-assessed)*	8.8 months (95% CI, 5.6–11.1)	12.9 months (95% CI, 9.3–NR)	
Overall survival (in patients with brain metastases at baseline) (investigator-assessed) (12 months)*	72% (95% CI, 59–81)	85% (95% CI, 73–92)	

HR, hazard ratio; CI, confidence interval; IRC, independent review committee; NR, not reached

*Data from the update paper titled "Brigatinib in ALK-Positive NSCLC and Brain Metastases" with a median follow-up time of 9.6 months (range, 0.1–19.7) in the 90-mg group and 11.0 months (range, 0.1–22.0) in the 180-mg group

†Intracranial response defined as ≥30% decrease in measurable lesions

All data are from the paper titled "Brigatinib in Crizotinib-Refractory ALK-Positive NSCLC" unless noted. Data in this paper were generated with a median follow-up time of 7.8 months (range, 0.1–16.7) in the 90-mg group and 8.3 months (range, 0.1–20.2) in the 180-mg group. Tumor response was graded according to RECIST v1.1 criteria. All efficacy measures analyzed the intention-to-treat population

Therapy Monitoring

1. Monitor ALT, AST, alkaline phosphatase, bilirubin, serum creatinine, and BUN prior to initiation of therapy with brigatinib, and then periodically or as clinically indicated

2. Monitor for new or worsening respiratory symptoms (eg, dyspnea, cough), especially during the first week of therapy. In the ALTA study, all-grade interstitial lung disease or pneumonitis occurred in 3.7% of patients in the 90-mg once-daily group, and in 9.1% of patients in the group that escalated to 180 mg. Grade 3–4 events occurred in 2.7% of patients. Interstitial lung disease/pneumonitis occurred early (within 9 days) in 6.4% of patients, with a median onset of 2 days

3. Control blood pressure prior to initiation of brigatinib treatment. Monitor blood pressure 2 weeks after initiation of brigatinib and then at least monthly thereafter. Use caution with coadministration of antihypertensive agents that can cause bradycardia. All-grade hypertension occurred in 11% of patients in the 90-mg group and in 21% of patients in the group that escalated to 180 mg. Grade 3 hypertension occurred in 5.9% of patients

4. Monitor heart rate periodically during treatment with brigatinib; consider more frequent monitoring in patients where other medications known to cause bradycardia are unavoidable. All-grade bradycardia occurred in 5.7% of patients in the 90-mg group and in 7.6% of patients in the group that escalated to 180 mg. Grade 2 bradycardia occurred in 1 patient in the 90-mg group

5. Advise patients to report any visual symptoms during treatment with brigatinib. Withhold brigatinib and obtain an ophthalmologic evaluation in patients with new or worsening G ≥2 visual symptoms. In the ALTA study, visual disturbances observed included blurred vision, diplopia, and reduced visual acuity. Grade 3 macular edema and grade 3 cataract were each observed in 1 patient

6. Advise patients to report unexplained muscle pain, tenderness, or weakness. Monitor creatine phosphokinase (CPK) levels periodically during brigatinib treatment. In the ALTA study, increased CPK levels occurred in 27% of patients in the 90-mg group and in 48% of patients in the group that escalated to 180 mg. Grade 3/4 elevations occurred in 2.8% of patients in the 90-mg group and in 12% of patients in the group that escalated to 180 mg

7. Monitor lipase and amylase levels periodically during brigatinib treatment. In the ALTA study, increased amylase levels occurred in 27% of patients in the 90-mg group and in 39% of patients in the group that escalated to 180 mg. Increased lipase levels occurred in 21% of patients in the 90-mg group and in 45% of patients in the group that escalated to 180 mg. Grade 3/4 amylase elevation occurred in 3.7% of patients in the 90-mg group and in 2.7% of patients in the group that escalated to 180 mg. Grade 3/4 lipase elevation occurred in 4.6% of patients in the 90-mg group and in 5.5% of patients in the group that escalated to 180 mg

8. Monitor fasting blood glucose prior to initiation of brigatinib and then periodically thereafter (or more frequently as clinically indicated). In the ALTA study, 43% of patients experienced new or worsening hyperglycemia during brigatinib treatment. Grade 3 hyperglycemia occurred in 3.7% of patients. Ten percent of patients who had baseline diabetes or glucose intolerance required the initiation of insulin while receiving brigatinib treatment

Treatment Modifications

BRIGATINIB		
	7-Day Lead-in Phase	**Continuation Phase**
Starting dose	90 mg by mouth once daily	180 mg by mouth once daily
Dose level −1	60 mg by mouth once daily	120 mg by mouth once daily
Dose level −2	Permanently discontinue	90 mg by mouth once daily
Dose level −3	—	60 mg by mouth once daily
Dose level −4	—	Permanently discontinue

Note: if brigatinib is interrupted for ≥14 days for reasons other than adverse reactions, resume treatment at 90 mg once daily for 7 days before increasing to the previously tolerated dose. Once the dose of brigatinib has been reduced for adverse reactions, do not subsequently increase the dosage

Pulmonary Toxicities

Adverse Event	Treatment Modification
ILD/pneumonitis, Grade 1 (asymptomatic; clinical or diagnostic observations only; intervention not indicated)	If new symptoms occur during the first 7 days of treatment, withhold brigatinib until recovery to baseline, then resume at the same dose and do not escalate to 180 mg if ILD/pneumonitis is suspected If new pulmonary symptoms occur after the first 7 days of treatment, withhold brigatinib until recovery to baseline, then resume at the same dose If ILD/pneumonitis recurs, then permanently discontinue brigatinib
ILD/pneumonitis, Grade 2 (symptomatic; medical intervention indicated; limiting instrumental ADL)	If new symptoms occur during the first 7 days of treatment, withhold brigatinib until recovery to baseline. Resume at the next lower dose level and do not dose escalate if ILD/pneumonitis is suspected If new pulmonary symptoms occur after the first 7 days of treatment, withhold brigatinib until recovery to baseline. If ILD/pneumonitis is suspected, resume at the next lower dose; otherwise, resume at the same dose If ILD/pneumonitis recurs, then permanently discontinue brigatinib
ILD/pneumonitis, Grade 3 (severe symptoms; limiting self care ADL; oxygen indicated) ILD/pneumonitis, Grade 4 (life-threatening respiratory compromise; urgent intervention indicated [eg, tracheotomy or intubation])	Permanently discontinue brigatinib for ILD/pneumonitis

Cardiovascular Adverse Events

Grade 3 hypertension despite optimal antihypertensive therapy (SBP ≥160 mmHg or DBP ≥100 mmHg, medical intervention indicated, more than one antihypertensive drug, or more intensive therapy than previously used indicated)	Withhold brigatinib until hypertension has recovered to G ≤1 (SBP <140 mmHg and DBP <90 mmHg), then resume brigatinib at next lower dose Recurrence: withhold brigatinib until recovery to G ≤1, and resume at next lower dose or permanently discontinue treatment
Grade 4 hypertension (life-threatening consequences, urgent intervention indicated)	Withhold brigatinib until recovery to G ≤1 (SBP <140 mmHg and DBP <90 mmHg), and resume at next lower dose or permanently discontinue treatment. Recurrence: permanently discontinue brigatinib for recurrence of G4 hypertension
Symptomatic bradycardia (heart rate <60 bpm)	Withhold brigatinib until recovery to asymptomatic bradycardia or to a resting heart rate of ≥60 bpm If a concomitant medication known to cause bradycardia is identified and discontinued or dose-adjusted, then resume brigatinib at the same dose upon recovery to asymptomatic bradycardia or to a resting heart rate of ≥60 bpm If no concomitant medication known to cause bradycardia is identified, or if contributing medications are not discontinued or dose-adjusted, then resume brigatinib at the next lower dose upon recovery to asymptomatic bradycardia or to a resting heart rate of ≥60 bpm

(continued)

Treatment Modifications (*continued*)

Cardiovascular Adverse Events

Bradycardia (heart rate <60 bpm) with life-threatening consequences, urgent intervention indicated	Permanently discontinue brigatinib if no contributing concomitant medication known to cause bradycardia is identified If a contributing concomitant medication known to cause bradycardia is identified and discontinued or dose-adjusted, then resume brigatinib at the next lower dose upon recovery to asymptomatic bradycardia or to a resting heart rate of ≥60 bpm, with frequent monitoring as clinically indicated Recurrence: permanently discontinue brigatinib

Other Adverse Events

G2/3 visual disturbance	Withhold brigatinib until recovery to G ≤1 or baseline. Obtain an ophthalmologic evaluation, then resume at the next lower dose level
G4 visual disturbance	Permanently discontinue brigatinib. Obtain an ophthalmologic evaluation
G3 CPK elevation (>5× ULN to ≤10× ULN)	Withhold brigatinib until recovery to G ≤1 (≤2.5× ULN) or to baseline, then resume brigatinib at the same dose Recurrence: withhold brigatinib until recovery to G ≤1 (≤2.5× ULN) or to baseline, then resume brigatinib at the next lower dose
G4 CPK elevation (>10× ULN)	Withhold brigatinib until recovery to G ≤1 (≤2.5× ULN) or to baseline, then resume brigatinib at the next lower dose
G3 lipase or amylase elevation (>2X ULN to ≤5× ULN)	Withhold brigatinib until recovery to G ≤1 (≤1.5× ULN) or to baseline, then resume brigatinib at the same dose Recurrence: withhold brigatinib until recovery to G ≤1 (≤1.5× ULN) or to baseline, then resume brigatinib at the next lower dose
G4 lipase or amylase elevation (>5× ULN)	Withhold brigatinib until recovery to G ≤1 (≤1.5× ULN) or to baseline, then resume brigatinib at the next lower dose
G ≥3 hyperglycemia (blood glucose >250 mg/dL) despite optimal medical management	Withhold brigatinib until adequate hyperglycemic control is achieved and consider reduction to the next lower dose, or permanently discontinue brigatinib
Other G3 adverse effects	Withhold brigatinib until recovery to baseline, then resume at the same dose Recurrence: withhold brigatinib until recovery to baseline, then resume at the next lower dose or discontinue brigatinib
Other G4 adverse effects	First occurrence: either withhold brigatinib until recovery to baseline and resume at the next lower dose or permanently discontinue brigatinib Recurrence: permanently discontinue brigatinib

Hepatic Impairment

Severe hepatic impairment (Child-Pugh C)	Reduce the brigatinib dose by approximately 40% (ie, from 180 mg to 120 mg, from 120 mg to 90 mg, or from 90 mg to 60 mg)

Renal Impairment

Severe renal impairment (CrCl 15–29 mL/min)	Reduce the brigatinib dose by approximately 50% (ie, from 180 mg to 90 mg, or from 90 mg to 60 mg)

Drug-Drug Interactions

Concomitant therapy with a strong CYP3A inhibitor is required	If coadministration of a strong CYP3A inhibitor is unavoidable, then reduce the brigatinib dose by approximately 50% (ie, from 180 mg to 90 mg, or from 90 mg to 60 mg)
Concomitant therapy with a moderate CYP3A inhibitor is required	If coadministration of a moderate CYP3A inhibitor is unavoidable, then reduce the brigatinib dose by approximately 40% (ie, from 180 mg to 120 mg, from 120 mg to 90 mg, or from 90 mg to 60 mg)
Concomitant therapy with a strong CYP3A inducer is required	Avoid coadministration of a strong CYP3A inducer with brigatinib

(*continued*)

Treatment Modifications (continued)

Drug-Drug Interactions

Concomitant therapy with a moderate CYP3A inducer is required	If coadministration of brigatinib with a moderate CYP3A inducer is unavoidable, then increase the brigatinib dose in 30 mg increments after 7 days of treatment with the current brigatinib dose, as tolerated, to a maximum of twice the brigatinib dose that was tolerated prior to initiation of the moderate CYP3A inducer
Concomitant therapy with a sensitive CYP3A substrate is required	Based on in vitro data, brigatinib may decrease concentrations of medications metabolized by CYP3A. Monitor for loss of efficacy of sensitive CYP3A substrates when coadministered with brigatinib

Grading of adverse events per National Cancer Institute Common Terminology Criteria for Adverse Events. Version 4.0
ILD, interstitial lung disease; ADL, activities of daily living; SBP, systolic blood pressure; DBP, diastolic blood pressure; bpm, beats per minute; ULN, upper limit of normal; CrCl, creatinine clearance

Adverse Events (N = 219)

Event	Brigatinib 90 mg (n = 109)		Brigatinib 180 mg (n = 110)	
Grade (%)	Grade 1 or 2	Grade 3–5	Grade 1 or 2	Grade 3–5
Nausea	32	<1	39	<1
Diarrhea	19	0	38	0
Vomiting	22	2	23	0
Constipation	18	<1	15	0
Abdominal pain	17	0	8	0
Headache	28	0	26	<1
Fatigue	19	<1	27	0
Pyrexia	14	0	5	<1
Cough	18	0	34	0
Dyspnea	18	3	19	2
Muscle spasms	12	0	17	0
Arthralgia	13	<1	14	0
Back pain	8	2	14	2
Increased blood creatine phosphokinase	8	3	21	9
Increased amylase	7	<1	14	<1
Increased aspartate aminotransferase	8	0	15	0
Rash	6	<1	14	3
Decreased appetite	21	<1	15	<1
Hypertension	6	6	15	6

Adverse events were included in the table if they were considered treatment-emergent and if they were reported by ≥10% of all patients. Median time on treatment was 7.5 months for the 90-mg group and 7.8 months for the 180-mg group. The most common treatment-emergent adverse effects of Grade ≥3 were hypertension (6% each group), increased blood creatine phosphokinase (3%/9% for 90-mg/180-mg groups), pneumonia (3%/5% for 90-mg/180-mg groups), and increased lipase (4%/3% for 90-mg/180-mg groups). Dose reduction as a result of an adverse event occurred in 7% of patients in the 90-mg brigatinib group and 20% of those in the 180-mg group. Dose interruption of ≥3 days occurred in 18% of patients in the 90-mg brigatinib group and 36% of those in the 180-mg group. Eight patients died within 30 days of the last dose of trial drug (excluding those who died from neoplasm progression, malignant pleural effusion, or meningeal metastases), with 2 deaths from pneumonia and 1 death each from bacterial meningitis, dyspnea, pulmonary embolism, respiratory failure, sudden death, and urosepsis

ADVANCED NSCLC • ALK-REARRANGED • SUBSEQUENT THERAPY
LUNG CANCER REGIMEN: LORLATINIB

LORBRENA (lorlatinib) prescribing information. New York, NY: Pfizer Labs; revised 2018 November
Solomon BJ et al. Lancet Oncol 2018;19(12):1654–1667
Protocol for: Solomon BJ et al. Lancet Oncol 2018;19(12):1654–1667
Supplementary appendix to: Solomon BJ et al. Lancet Oncol 2018;19(12):1654–1667

Lorlatinib 100 mg/dose; administer orally, once daily, without regard to food, continuously until disease progression (total dose/week = 700 mg)

Notes:
- Patients who delay taking lorlatinib at a regularly scheduled time may take the missed dose unless the next dose is due within 4 hours. Advise patients not to take 2 doses at the same time to make up for a missed dose. Patients who vomit after taking a dose of lorlatinib should not take another dose, but rather take the next dose at the next regularly scheduled time
- Lorlatinib tablets should be swallowed whole. Do not chew, crush, or split tablets
- In vitro studies suggest that lorlatinib is a major substrate for CYP3A4 and UGT1A4 and a minor substrate of CYP2C8, CYP2C19, CYP3A5, and UGT1A3. In vitro studies suggest that lorlatinib is a time-dependent inhibitor and an inducer of CYP3A (net inducing effect); an inducer of CYP2B6; and an inhibitor of P-glycoprotein, OCT1, OAT3, MATE1, and BCRP
  - In drug-drug interaction study involving 12 healthy volunteers, coadministration of lorlatinib with rifampin (a strong CYP3A inducer) decreased the mean lorlatinib AUC_{inf} by 85% and C_{max} by 76%. Notably, serious hepatotoxicity was observed in 10 out of the 12 subjects. Grade 4 alanine aminotransferase (ALT) or aspartate aminotransferase (AST) elevations occurred in 50% of subjects, Grade 3 elevations in 33%, and Grade 2 elevations in 8%. Therefore, the use of strong CYP3A4 inducers is contraindicated with lorlatinib. It is unknown what effect concomitant use of moderate CYP3A4 inducers would have on the risk of hepatotoxicity or on the pharmacokinetics of lorlatinib; therefore, avoid concomitant use of moderate CYP3A inducers. If concomitant use of a moderate CYP3A inducer with lorlatinib is unavoidable, then monitor AST, ALT, and bilirubin within 48 hours after initiating lorlatinib and at least 3 times during the first week after initiating lorlatinib
  - Coadministration of lorlatinib with itraconazole (a strong CYP3A inhibitor) increased the lorlatinib AUC_{inf} by 42% and increased C_{max} by 24%. Therefore, when concomitant use of lorlatinib with a strong CYP3A inhibitor is unavoidable, reduce the lorlatinib dose from 100 mg once daily to 75 mg once daily. If the lorlatinib dose had already been reduced to 75 mg daily due to adverse reactions, then reduce the dose further to 50 mg once daily. If the strong CYP3A inhibitor is subsequently discontinued, then increase the lorlatinib dose back to the dose used prior to introduction of the strong CYP3A inhibitor after 3 half-lives of the strong CYP3A inhibitor have elapsed
  - Coadministration of lorlatinib with midazolam (a sensitive CYP3A substrate) decreased midazolam AUC_{inf} by 64% and C_{max} by 50%. Therefore, avoid concomitant use of lorlatinib with CYP3A substrates where minimal concentration changes of the substrate may result in serious therapeutic failure
  - Coadministration of lorlatinib with rabeprazole (a proton pump inhibitor) had no effect on lorlatinib pharmacokinetics

Supportive Care
Antiemetic prophylaxis
Emetogenic potential is **MINIMAL TO LOW**
See Chapter 42 for antiemetic recommendations

Hematopoietic growth factor (CSF) prophylaxis
Primary prophylaxis is **NOT** *indicated*
See Chapter 43 for more information

Antimicrobial prophylaxis
Risk of fever and neutropenia is LOW
Antimicrobial primary prophylaxis to be considered:
- Antibacterial—not indicated
- Antifungal—not indicated
- Antiviral—not indicated unless patient previously had an episode of HSV

Patient Population Studied

This international, multicenter, open-label, single-arm, phase 2 trial included 276 adult patients with histologically or cytologically confirmed, *ALK*-positive or *ROS1*-positive, advanced, non–small cell lung cancer. Eligible patients were with or without CNS metastases and had an Eastern Cooperative Oncology Group (ECOG) performance status of ≤2. Patients were enrolled into six different expansion cohorts on the basis of previous therapy and *ALK* and *ROS1* status. Participants were required to have at least one measurable extracranial lesion according to Response Evaluation Criteria in Solid Tumors (RECIST) version 1.1. Patients were required to have sufficient organ function, including adequate bone marrow (absolute neutrophil count $^3 1.5{\times}10^9$/L, platelets $^3 100{\times}10^9$/L, and hemoglobin $^3 9$ g/dL) to be eligible. Patients with spinal cord compression and active infection were excluded. A total of 275 patients received at least one dose of lorlatinib, with 228 patients having *ALK*-positive disease and 47 patients with *ROS1*-positive disease.

Efficacy (N = 228*)

	Treatment Naïve [EXP1] (n = 30)	Previous Crizotinib ± Chemotherapy [EXP2–3A] (n = 59)	Previous Non-crizotinib ALK TKI ± Chemotherapy [EXP3B] (n = 28)	≥2 Previous ALK TKIs ± Chemotherapy [EXP4–5] (n = 111)	≥1 Previous ALK TKI ± Chemotherapy [Pooled EXP2–5] (n = 198)
Complete response	3%	2%	4%	2%	2%
Partial response	87%	68%	29%	37%	45%
Stable disease	7%	17%	36%	34%	29%
Objective progression	3%	10%	25%	18%	17%
Indeterminate response	0	3%	7%	9%	7%
Patients with confirmed objective response	90% (95% CI 73.5–97.9%)	69.5% (95% CI 56.1–80.8%)	32.1% (95% CI 15.9–52.4%)	38.7% (95% CI 29.6–48.5%)	47% (95% CI 39.9–54.2%)
Median time to first tumor response, months (IQR)	1.4 (1.3–2.7)	1.4 (1.3–2.6)	1.4 (1.4–2.7)	1.4 (1.4–2.9)	1.4 (1.3–2.7)
Median duration of response	NR	NR	NR	NR	NR
Median duration of follow-up for response, months (IQR)	6.9 (5.6–12.5)	6.9 (4.2–7.0)	7.0 (5.6–8.3)	7.2 (5.6–9.8)	6.9 (5.6–8.3)
Number of patients with CNS lesion at baseline†	3	23	9	49	81
Patients with confirmed intracranial objective response	66.7% (95% CI 9.4–99.2%)	87% (95% CI 66.4–97.2%)	55.6% (95% CI 21.2–86.3%)	53.1% (95% CI 38.3–67.5%)	63% (95% CI 51.5–73.4%)
Median time to first intracranial response, months (IQR)	2 (1.2–2.7)	1.4 (1.3–1.4)	1.4 (1.4–2.6)	1.4 (1.3–3.1)	1.4 (1.3–2.7)

ALK, anaplastic lymphoma kinase; EXP, expansion cohort; TKI, tyrosine kinase inhibitor; CI, confidence interval; IQR, interquartile range; NR, not reached
*Efficacy data reported for all cohorts of patients with *ALK*-positive disease (EXP1–5). Antitumor activity for the cohort with *ROS1*-positive disease was reported separately
†Number of patients within each expansion cohort with at least one measurable CNS lesion present at baseline

Therapy Monitoring

1. Monitor ALT, AST, alkaline phosphatase, bilirubin, serum creatinine, and BUN prior to initiation of therapy with lorlatinib, and then periodically or as clinically indicated

2. Review the patient's concomitant medications carefully for the presence of interacting medications
   a. Concomitant use of lorlatinib with strong CYP3A inducers is associated with a high risk of serious hepatotoxicity and is contraindicated
   b. Concomitant use of moderate CYP3A inducers should also be avoided whenever possible. If concomitant use of a moderate CYP3A inducer with lorlatinib is unavoidable, then monitor AST, ALT, and bilirubin within 48 hours of initiation of lorlatinib and then at least 3 times during the first week of therapy
   c. Unavoidable concomitant use of a strong CYP3A inhibitor requires a lorlatinib dose modification (see Treatment Modifications section)
   d. Lorlatinib may reduce the efficacy of sensitive CYP3A substrates. Therefore, avoid concomitant use of lorlatinib with CYP3A substrates where minimal concentration changes of the substrate may result in serious therapeutic failure

3. Monitor for central nervous system (CNS) adverse effects including seizures (3% incidence), hallucinations (7% incidence), and changes in cognitive function (29% incidence), mood (24% incidence), speech (14% incidence), mental status (2.1% incidence), and sleep (10% incidence). The incidence of any CNS adverse effect was 54%, with a median (range) onset of 1.2 months (1 day to 1.7 years)

4. Monitor fasting serum cholesterol and triglycerides before initiation of lorlatinib and repeat 1–2 months later, then periodically. Grade 3–4 elevation in total cholesterol was noted in 17% of patients and Grade 3–4 elevations in triglycerides in 17%, with a median onset of 15 days. In the study, about 7% of patients had to temporarily interrupt lorlatinib therapy and 3% had a lorlatinib dose reduction for elevation in cholesterol or triglycerides; 80% of patients required initiation of a lipid-lowering medication

5. Monitor an electrocardiogram (ECG) prior to initiation of lorlatinib and periodically thereafter. PR interval prolongation and atrioventricular (AV) block has occurred in patients treated with lorlatinib. Among 295 patients in the study who had a baseline ECG, the incidence of AV block was 1% and 0.3% experienced Grade 3 AV block requiring placement of a pacemaker

6. Monitor for new or worsening respiratory symptoms (eg, dyspnea, cough, fever). The incidence of all grade (Grade 3/4) interstitial lung disease (ILD)/pneumonitis was 1.5% (1.2%) in the study

Treatment Modifications

LORLATINIB

Starting dose	100 mg orally once daily
Dose level −1	75 mg orally once daily
Dose level −2	50 mg orally once daily
Dose level −3	Permanently discontinue

Central Nervous System (CNS) Effects

Adverse Event	Treatment Modification
Grade 1 CNS effect	Continue lorlatinib at the same dose, or interrupt dosing until recovery to baseline. Resume lorlatinib at either the same dose or with the dose reduced by 1 dosage level at the discretion of the medically responsible health care provider
Grade 2–3 CNS effect	Interrupt lorlatinib until improvement to G ≤1, then resume lorlatinib with the dosage reduced by 1 dose level
Grade 4 CNS effect	Permanently discontinue lorlatinib

Hyperlipidemia

Grade 1–3 elevation in cholesterol (>ULN–500 mg/dL; >ULN –12.92 mmol/L) OR Grade 1–3 hypertriglyceridemia (150–1000 mg/dL; 1.71–11.4 mmol/L)	Continue lorlatinib at the same dose. Initiate or optimize the dosage of lipid-lowering agents and increase the frequency of monitoring
Grade 4 elevation in cholesterol (>500 mg/dL; >12.92 mmol/L) OR Grade 4 hypertriglyceridemia (>1000 mg/dL; >11.4 mmol/L; life-threatening consequences)	Interrupt lorlatinib until improvement of cholesterol to ≤G2 (≤400 mg/dL; ≤10.34 mmol/L) and/or improvement of hypertriglyceridemia to ≤G2 (≤500 mg/dL; ≤5.7 mmol/L), then resume lorlatinib at the same dose. Initiate or optimize the dosage of lipid-lowering agents and increase the frequency of monitoring
Recurrent Grade 4 elevation in cholesterol (>500 mg/dL; >12.92 mmol/L) OR Recurrent Grade 4 hypertriglyceridemia (>1000 mg/dL; >11.4 mmol/L; life-threatening consequences)	Interrupt lorlatinib until improvement of cholesterol to ≤G2 (≤400 mg/dL; ≤10.34 mmol/L) and/or improvement of hypertriglyceridemia to ≤G2 (≤500 mg/dL; ≤5.7 mmol/L), then resume lorlatinib with the dosage reduced by 1 dose level. Optimize lipid-lowering therapy and increase the frequency of monitoring

Cardiovascular Adverse Effects

Second-degree atrioventricular block	Interrupt lorlatinib until PR interval is <200 msec, then resume lorlatinib with the dosage reduced by 1 dose level

(continued)

Treatment Modifications (continued)

Cardiovascular Adverse Effects

First occurrence of complete atrioventricular block	Withhold lorlatinib until either a pacemaker has been placed or until PR interval is <200 msec. If a pacemaker has been placed, then resume lorlatinib at the same dose. If no pacemaker was placed, then resume lorlatinib with the dosage reduced by 1 dose level
Recurrent complete atrioventricular block	Place a pacemaker and then resume lorlatinib at the full dose of 100 mg orally once daily unless the dose had previously been reduced for reasons other than atrioventricular block. Alternatively, if no pacemaker is placed, then permanently discontinue lorlatinib

Interstitial lung disease/pneumonitis

Any-grade treatment-related interstitial lung disease/pneumonitis	Permanently discontinue lorlatinib

Other Adverse Reactions

Other Grade 1 or 2 reaction	Continue lorlatinib at either the same dose or with the dosage reduced by 1 dose level at the discretion of the medically responsible health care provider
Other Grade 3 or 4 reaction	Interrupt lorlatinib until symptoms improve to ≤G2 or baseline, then resume lorlatinib with the dosage reduced by 1 dose level

Drug-Drug Interactions

Patient is taking a strong CYP3A inducer	The use of strong CYP3A inducers is contraindicated with lorlatinib due to a high rate of serious hepatotoxicity. Discontinue the strong CYP3A inducer for at least 3 plasma half-lives of the inducer before initiation of lorlatinib
Concomitant use of a moderate CYP3A inducer is unavoidable	It is unknown what effect concomitant use of moderate CYP3A4 inducers would have on the risk of hepatotoxicity or on the pharmacokinetics of lorlatinib; therefore, avoid concomitant use of moderate CYP3A inducers and ideally discontinue the moderate CYP3A inducer for at least 3 plasma half-lives of the inducer before initiation of lorlatinib If concomitant use of a moderate CYP3A inducer with lorlatinib is unavoidable, then monitor AST, ALT, and bilirubin within 48 hours after initiating lorlatinib and at least 3 times during the first week after initiating lorlatinib. If persistent G ≥2 hepatotoxicity occurs with concomitant use of the moderate CYP3A inducer and lorlatinib, then either discontinue the moderate CYP3A inducer or discontinue lorlatinib at the discretion of the medically responsible health care provider
Concomitant therapy with a strong CYP3A inhibitor is unavoidable	When concomitant use of lorlatinib with a strong CYP3A inhibitor is unavoidable, reduce the lorlatinib dose from 100 mg once daily to 75 mg once daily. If the lorlatinib dose had already been reduced to 75 mg daily due to adverse reactions, then reduce the dose further to 50 mg once daily. If the strong CYP3A inhibitor is subsequently discontinued, then increase the lorlatinib dose back to the dose used prior to introduction of the strong CYP3A inhibitor after 3 half-lives of the strong CYP3A inhibitor have elapsed
Concomitant therapy with a sensitive CYP3A substrate is required (ie, it is predicted that minimal reductions in the CYP3A substrate plasma concentration/exposure may be associated with a risk of serious therapeutic failure)	Avoid concomitant use of lorlatinib with sensitive CYP3A substrates

Grading of adverse events per National Cancer Institute Common Terminology Criteria for Adverse Events. Version 4.0
CNS, central nervous system; ULN, upper limit of normal

Adverse Events (N = 275)

Grade (%)	Lorlatinib (All Cohorts*)		
	Grade 1–2	Grade 3	Grade 4
Hypercholesterolemia	66	14	1
Hypertriglyceridemia	45	13	3
Edema	41	2	0
Peripheral neuropathy	28	2	0
Weight gain	16	2	0
Cognitive effects	17	1	0
Mood effects	14	1	0
Fatigue	13	<1	0
Diarrhea	10	<1	0
Arthralgia	10	0	0
AST increased	10	<1	0
Dizziness	8	1	0
ALT increased	8	1	0
Speech effects	7	<1	0
Lipase increased	4	3	<1
Anemia	5	1	0
Amylase increased	4	1	0
Rash	5	<1	0
Vomiting	4	<1	0
Dyspnea	3	<1	0
Hypertension	1	1	0
Ejection fraction decreased	2	<1	0
Hyperglycemia	1	1	0
Localized edema	1	1	0
Hallucination, auditory	1	<1	0
Abdominal pain	1	<1	0
Hypophosphatemia	1	1	0
Hypoxia	<1	1	0
Night sweats	1	<1	0
Pulmonary edema	1	<1	0
Acute respiratory failure	0	<1	<1
Hyponatremia	<1	<1	0

(continued)

Adverse Events (N = 275) *(continued)*

Grade (%)	Lorlatinib (All Cohorts*)		
	Grade 1–2	Grade 3	Grade 4
Presyncope	<1	<1	0
Respiratory failure	0	1	0
Ascites	0	<1	0
Rise in serum potassium	0	0	<1
Diabetes mellitus	0	<1	0
Erysipelas	0	<1	0
Gastritis	0	<1	0
Glossitis	0	<1	0
Hydrocephalus	0	<1	0
Hypermagnesemia	0	<1	0
Interstitial lung disease	0	<1	0
Leukocytosis	0	<1	0
Mental status changes	0	<1	0
Mucocutaneous candidiasis	0	<1	0
Pancreatitis	0	<1	0
Pneumonia	0	<1	0
Pneumonitis	0	0	<1
Thrombosis	0	<1	0

AST, aspartate aminotransferase; ALT, alanine aminotransferase
*Adverse event information was collected from the pooled population of all of the patients from each expansion cohort (EXP 1–6), including the patients with *ROS1*-positive disease
No Grade 5 treatment-related adverse events were reported

Small Cell Lung Cancer (SCLC)

Work-up

General work-up

1. History and physical examination
2. Complete blood count, liver and renal function tests, LDH, and serum electrolytes with special attention to serum sodium
3. Chest x-ray
4. CT scan of chest and upper abdomen including adrenals
5. Brain MRI (or CT scan)
6. Bone scan
7. FDG-PET scan (optional)

Individualized work-up

1. Bone marrow biopsy in selected patients
2. Pulmonary function tests and cardiac function assessment if thoracic radiation therapy is going to be performed
3. If a patient presents with pleural effusion, a diagnostic thoracocentesis is recommended. Consider thoracoscopy if thoracocentesis is inconclusive
4. Plain-film x-rays of bone scan abnormalities

Staging

Limited disease	Disease confined to ipsilateral hemithorax within a single radiation port
Extensive disease	Disease beyond ipsilateral hemithorax or obvious metastatic disease

Østerlind K et al. Cancer Treat Rep 1983;67:3–9

Five-Year Survival for Each Stage

Limited Disease	
Median survival	14–20 months
2-year survival	40%

Extensive Disease	
Median survival	8–12 months
2-year survival	5%

More information at http://www.seer.cancer.gov

Expert Opinion

Treatment of limited disease

1. Etoposide + cisplatin combination for 4–6 cycles is the regimen of choice to combine with concurrent chest radiation therapy
2. Chest radiation therapy increases local control and survival. Several studies suggest starting chest radiotherapy early
3. Prophylactic cranial irradiation is indicated in patients with complete remission; it reduces the risk of cerebral metastases and improves survival

Treatment of extensive disease

1. Etoposide + platinum or cyclophosphamide + doxorubicin regimens for 4–6 cycles
2. Prophylactic cranial irradiation should be considered in patients with response after chemotherapy

Second-line chemotherapy for both limited and extensive disease

1. Patients who relapse after a response to first-line chemotherapy should be considered for second-line chemotherapy with topotecan

LIMITED-STAGE SCLC • CHEMORADIOTHERAPY

LUNG CANCER REGIMEN: ETOPOSIDE + CISPLATIN WITH CONCURRENT THORACIC RADIATION THERAPY

Turrisi AT et al. N Engl J Med 1999;340:265–271

Hydration before cisplatin: ≥1000 mL 0.9% sodium chloride injection (0.9% NS); administer intravenously over a minimum of 2–4 hours

Cisplatin 60 mg/m², administer intravenously in 50–150 mL 0.9% NS over 60 minutes, on day 1, every 3 weeks for 4 cycles (total dosage/cycle = 60 mg/m²)

Hydration after cisplatin: ≥1000 mL 0.9% NS; administer intravenously over a minimum of 2–4 hours. Encourage patients to increase oral intake of nonalcoholic fluids. Monitor serum electrolytes and replace as needed (potassium, magnesium, sodium)

Etoposide 120 mg/m² per dose; administer intravenously, diluted in 0.9% NS or 5% dextrose injection to a concentration within the range of 0.2–0.4 mg/mL over 60 minutes, for 3 consecutive days, on days 1, 2, and 3, every 3 weeks for 4 cycles (total dosage/cycle = 360 mg/m²)

Thoracic RT begins concurrently with the first cycle of chemotherapy to a total dose of 45 Gy delivered as:

1. Once daily in 1.8-Gy fractions for 25 treatments over 5 weeks, *or*

2. Twice daily in 1.5-Gy fractions for 30 treatments over 3 weeks

Prophylactic cranial RT is offered to patients who achieve a CR after completing systemic chemotherapy

Supportive Care

Antiemetic prophylaxis

Emetogenic potential on day 1 is **HIGH**. *Potential for delayed symptoms*
Emetogenic potential on days 2 and 3 is **LOW**
See Chapter 42 for antiemetic recommendations

Hematopoietic growth factor (CSF) prophylaxis

Primary prophylaxis is **NOT** *indicated*
See Chapter 43 for more information

Antimicrobial prophylaxis

Risk of fever and neutropenia is **LOW**
  Antimicrobial primary prophylaxis to be considered:
  • Antibacterial—not indicated
  • Antifungal—not indicated
  • Antiviral—not indicated unless patient previously had an episode of HSV

Patient Population Studied

A study of 417 patients with previously untreated limited SCLC. A randomized comparison between twice-daily and once-daily thoracic radiation therapy, both combined with etoposide and cisplatin given at fixed dosages

Therapy Monitoring

1. *Before each cycle:* H&P, CBC with differential, LFTs, BUN, creatinine, and serum electrolytes

2. *Response evaluation:* evaluate therapy at the end of treatment

Efficacy (N = 206/211)

	RT Fractionation	
	Once Daily (N = 206)	**Twice Daily** (N = 211)
Complete response	49%	56%
Partial response	38%	31%
Local failure	52%	36%
Median survival	19 months	23 months
2-year survival	41%	47%
5-year survival	16%	26%

Treatment Modifications

Adverse Event	Dose Modification
G4 toxicities, febrile neutropenia, documented infection, or thrombocytopenia with bleeding during cycles 3 and 4	Reduce etoposide dosage by 25%
Serum creatinine = 1.6–2.5 mg/dL (141–221 µmol/L) during cycles 3 and 4	Reduce cisplatin dosage by 25%
Platelets ≤50,000/mm³	Interrupt radiation therapy
G2 weight loss (≥4.5 kg or ≥10 pounds)	
Hospitalization for febrile neutropenia or sepsis	
Difficulty swallowing	Do not interrupt radiation therapy*
Fever with low ANC	

*In general, interruptions of thoracic radiation therapy are discouraged
Note: DO NOT modify chemotherapy during the first 2 cycles

Toxicity (N = 206/211)

Toxicity	% G3	% G4	% G5
Once-Daily RT (N = 206)			
Overall toxicity	23	63	2
Esophagitis	11	5	0
Granulocytopenia	15	60	0
Thrombocytopenia	16	8	0
Anemia	23	3	0
Infection	6	1	1
Vomiting	8	2	0
Pulmonary effects	3	0.5	0.5
Weight loss	3	0	0
Twice-Daily RT (N = 211)			
Overall toxicity	25	62	3
Esophagitis	27	5	0
Granulocytopenia	21	59	0
Thrombocytopenia	13	8	0
Anemia	23	5	0
Infection	6	2	1
Vomiting	8	1	0
Pulmonary effects	4	1	1
Weight loss	2	0	0

EXTENSIVE-STAGE SCLC • FIRST-LINE
LUNG CANCER REGIMEN: ATEZOLIZUMAB + CARBOPLATIN + ETOPOSIDE

Horn L et al. N Engl J Med 2018;379:2220–2229
Protocol for: Horn L et al. N Engl J Med 2018;379:2220–2229
Supplementary appendix to: Horn L et al. N Engl J Med 2018;379:2220–2229
TECENTRIQ (atezolizumab) prescribing information. South San Francisco, CA: Genentech, Inc; revised 2019 May

Induction phase

Atezolizumab 1200 mg per dose; administer intravenously in 250 mL 0.9% sodium chloride injection, USP (0.9% NS) over 60 minutes on day 1, every 3 weeks, for 4 cycles (total dosage/3-week cycle = 1200 mg)

Notes:
- Atezolizumab may be administered through an administration set either with or without a low-protein-binding in-line filter with pore size within the range of 0.2–0.22μm. Infusion bag may be composed of polyvinyl chloride (PVC), polyethylene (PE), or polyolefin (PO).
- If the initial infusion is well tolerated, subsequent administration may be completed over 30 minutes
- Severe infusion-related reactions have occurred in patients in clinical trials of atezolizumab
  - Interrupt or slow the administration rate in patients with mild or moderate infusion-related reactions
  - Permanently discontinue atezolizumab in patients who experience infusion reactions Grade ≥3

Carboplatin (calculated dose) AUC = 5 mg/mL × min; administer intravenously diluted in 5% dextrose injection (D5W) or 0.9% NS to a concentration as low as 0.5 mg/mL over 30 minutes on day 1, every 3 weeks, for 4 cycles (total dosage/3-week cycle calculated to produce an AUC = 5 mg/mL × min; see equation below)

Etoposide 100 mg/m^2 per dose; administer intravenously, diluted in 0.9% NS or 5% dextrose injection to a concentration within the range of 0.2–0.4 mg/mL over 60 minutes, for 3 consecutive days, on days 1, 2, and 3, every 3 weeks for 4 cycles (total dosage/3-week cycle = 300 mg/m^2)

Supportive Care (Induction Phase)
Antiemetic prophylaxis
Note: premedication with corticosteroids should be minimized to the extent possible due to the potential for attenuation of atezolizumab-mediated anti-tumor immune activity
*Emetogenic potential on days with carboplatin is **HIGH**. Potential for delayed symptoms*
*Emetogenic potential on days with etoposide only is **LOW***
See Chapter 42 for antiemetic recommendations

Hematopoietic growth factor (CSF) prophylaxis
*Primary prophylaxis **MAY** be indicated*
See Chapter 43 for more information

Antimicrobial prophylaxis
*Risk of fever and neutropenia is **LOW***
Antimicrobial primary prophylaxis to be considered:
- Antibacterial—not indicated
- Antifungal—not indicated
- Antiviral—not indicated, unless patient previously had an episode of HSV

Maintenance phase (choose one of the following 3 dosing schedules):

Atezolizumab 840 mg per dose; administer intravenously in 250 mL 0.9% sodium chloride injection, USP (0.9% NS) over 60 minutes on day 1, every 2 weeks, until disease progression (total dosage/2-week cycle = 840 mg), *or:*

Atezolizumab 1200 mg per dose; administer intravenously in 250 mL 0.9% NS over 60 minutes on day 1, every 3 weeks, until disease progression (total dosage/3-week cycle = 1200 mg), *or:*

Atezolizumab 1680 mg per dose; administer intravenously in 250 mL 0.9% NS over 60 minutes on day 1, every 4 weeks, until disease progression (total dosage/4-week cycle = 1680 mg)

Notes:
- Consider prophylactic cranial irradiation during maintenance treatment with atezolizumab
- Atezolizumab may be administered through an administration set either with or without a low-protein-binding in-line filter with pore size within the range of 0.2–0.22μm. Infusion bag may be composed of polyvinyl chloride (PVC), polyethylene (PE), or polyolefin (PO)
- If the initial infusion is well tolerated, subsequent administration may be completed over 30 minutes
- Severe infusion-related reactions have occurred in patients in clinical trials of atezolizumab
  - Interrupt or slow the administration rate in patients with mild or moderate infusion-related reactions
  - Permanently discontinue atezolizumab in patients who experience infusion reactions Grade ≥3

(continued)

(continued)

Supportive Care (Maintenance phase)
Antiemetic prophylaxis
Emetogenic potential on days with atezolizumab only is **MINIMAL**
See Chapter 42 for antiemetic recommendations

Hematopoietic growth factor (CSF) prophylaxis
Primary prophylaxis is **NOT** *indicated*
See Chapter 43 for more information

Antimicrobial prophylaxis
Risk of fever and neutropenia is **LOW**
  Antimicrobial primary prophylaxis to be considered:
  • Antibacterial—not indicated
  • Antifungal—not indicated
  • Antiviral—not indicated, unless patient previously had an episode of HSV

Carboplatin dose
Carboplatin dose is based on a formula described by Calvert et al. to achieve a target area under the plasma concentration versus time curve (AUC)

$$\text{Total carboplatin dose (mg)} = (\text{target AUC})(\text{GFR} + 25)$$

In practice, creatinine clearance (CrCl) is used in place of glomerular filtration rate (GFR). CrCl can be estimated from the equation of Cockcroft and Gault, thus:

$$\text{For males, Clcr} = \frac{(140 - \text{age [years]}) \times (\text{body weight [kg]})}{72 \times (\text{serum creatinine [mg/dL]})}$$

$$\text{For females, Clcr} = \frac{(140 - \text{age [years]}) \times (\text{body weight [kg]})}{72 \times (\text{serum creatinine [mg/dL]})} \times 0.85$$

Calvert AH et al. J Clin Oncol 1989;7:1748–1756
Cockcroft DW, Gault MH. Nephron 1976;16:31–41
Jodrell DI et al. J Clin Oncol 1992;10:520–528
Sorensen BT et al. Cancer Chemother Pharmacol 1991;28:397–401

Patient Population Studied

IMpower133 was a multinational, double-blind, placebo-controlled, phase 3 trial that involved 403 adult patients with previously untreated small cell lung cancer (SCLC). Eligible patients had histologically or cytologically confirmed extensive-stage SCLC according to the Veterans Administration Lung Study Group staging system, measurable disease according to Response Evaluation Criteria in Solid Tumors (RECIST), and an Eastern Cooperative Oncology Group (ECOG) performance status score of 0 or 1. Patients with a history of autoimmune disease and previous treatment with CD137 agonists or immune-checkpoint inhibitors were excluded. Patients were randomized in a 1:1 ratio to receive induction therapy with carboplatin and etoposide plus either atezolizumab or placebo for four 21-day cycles, followed by maintenance therapy with either atezolizumab or placebo.

Efficacy (N = 403)

End Point	Carboplatin + Etoposide + Atezolizumab (n = 201)	Carboplatin + Etoposide + Placebo (n = 202)	Between-Group Comparison
Median overall survival*	12.3 months (95% CI 10.8–15.9)	10.3 months (95% CI 9.3–11.3)	HR 0.70 (95% CI 0.54–0.91) P = 0.007
12-month survival rate	51.7% (95% CI 44.4–59.0)	38.2% (95% CI, 31.2–45.3)	
Median progression-free survival†	5.2 months (95% CI 4.4–5.6)	4.3 months (95% CI 4.2–4.5)	HR 0.77 (95% CI 0.62–0.96) P = 0.02
6-month progression-free survival rate	30.9% (95% CI, 24.3–37.5)	22.4% (95% CI, 16.6–28.2)	
12-month progression-free survival rate	12.6% (95% CI, 7.9–17.4)	5.4% (95% CI, 2.1–8.6)	
Patients with objective confirmed response‡	60.2% (95% CI 53.1–67.0)	64.4% (95% CI 57.3–71.0)	—
Patients with complete response‡	2.5% (95% CI 0.8–5.7)	1.0% (95% CI 0.1–3.5)	—
Patients with partial response‡	57.7% (95% CI 50.6–64.6)	63.4% (95% CI 56.3–70.0)	—
Median (range) duration of response§	4.2 months (1.4–19.5)	3.9 months (2.0–16.1)	—
Patients with stable disease	20.9% (95% CI 15.5–27.2)	21.3% (95% CI 15.9–27.6)	—
Patients with progressive disease	10.9% (95% CI 7.0–16.1)	6.9% (95% CI 3.8–11.4)	—

NR, not reached; HR, hazard ratio, CI, confidence interval; OR, odds ratio

Median follow-up period was 13.9 months

*Overall survival was defined as the time from randomization to death from any cause. At the time of data cutoff, 104 patients in the atezolizumab group (51.7%) and 134 patients in the placebo group (66.3%) had died

†Progression-free survival was defined as the time from randomization to disease progression according to RECIST or death from any cause. A total of 171 patients in the atezolizumab group (85.1%) and 189 patients in the placebo group (93.6%) had disease progression or died

‡The objective confirmed response rate was assessed in patients in the intent-to-treat population who had measurable disease at baseline. Response was classified as complete response or partial response according to RECIST version 1.1

§Duration of response was assessed for patients who had an objective confirmed response and was defined as the time from the first occurrence of documented objective response to the time of disease progression or death from any cause, whichever occurred first

Therapy Monitoring

1. *Prior to each cycle of carboplatin + etoposide + atezolizumab (induction phase):* CBC with differential and platelet count, liver function tests, serum creatinine, BUN, serum electrolytes

2. *Monitoring for atezolizumab (induction and maintenance phases):*

    a. Initially at the time of each atezolizumab dose, and eventually every 6–12 weeks, perform a total-body skin examination with attention to ALL mucous membranes as well as a complete review of systems

    b. Monitor patients for signs and symptoms of pneumonitis. Evaluate patients with suspected pneumonitis with chest x-ray, CT, and pulse oximetry. For ≥2 toxicity, may include nasal swab, sputum culture and sensitivity, blood culture and sensitivity, and urine culture and sensitivity

    c. Monitor patients for signs and symptoms of colitis. Encourage patients to report diarrhea immediately to any member of the health care team

    d. Draw AST, ALT, and bilirubin prior to each atezolizumab infusion and/or weekly if there are Grade 1 liver function test elevations. Note, no intervention is recommended for G1 LFT abnormalities. For ≥2 toxicity, work up for other causes of elevated LFTs including viral hepatitis

    e. Use basic metabolic panel (Na, K, CO_2, glucose) and patient history as screening tools for hypophysitis including hypopituitarism and adrenal insufficiency. If in doubt, evaluate AM adrenocorticotropic hormone (ACTH) and cortisol levels. Consider ACTH stimulation test for indeterminate results

(*continued*)

Therapy Monitoring (*continued*)

f. Assess thyroid function at the start of treatment, periodically during atezolizumab treatment and as indicated based on clinical evaluation, and for clinical signs and symptoms of thyroid disorders. Test for TSH and free thyroxine (FT4) every 4–6 weeks as part of routine clinical monitoring of therapy or for case detection in symptomatic patients

g. Measure glucose at baseline and with each atezolizumab treatment during the first 12 weeks and every 6 weeks thereafter

h. Obtain a serum creatinine prior to every atezolizumab dose. If creatinine is found to be newly elevated, consider holding therapy while other potential causes are evaluated. Note, routine urinalysis is not necessary other than to rule out urinary tract infections, etc

i. Obtain a complete rheumatologic history and perform an examination of all peripheral joints for tenderness, swelling, and range of motion. Examine the spine. Consider plain x-ray/imaging to exclude metastases and evaluate joint damage (erosions), if appropriate

j. In patients at high risk for infections and in appropriately selected patients based on an infectious disease evaluation, draw screening laboratories (HIV, hepatitis A and B, and blood QuantiFERON for TB) to prepare patients to start infliximab

Treatment Modifications

CARBOPLATIN + ETOPOSIDE DOSE MODIFICATIONS

	Carboplatin	Etoposide
Starting dose	AUC = 5 mg/mL × min	100 mg/m^2 per dose
Dose level −1	AUC = 4 mg/mL × min	80 mg/m^2 per dose
Dose level −2	AUC = 3 mg/mL × min	60 mg/m^2 per dose
Dose level −3	Discontinue	Discontinue

Adverse Reaction	Dose Modification
Hematologic Toxicity	
Day 1 ANC <1500/mm^3	Delay the start of the cycle until ANC ≥1500/mm^3
Day 1 platelet count <100,000/mm^3	Delay the start of the cycle until platelet count ≥100,000/mm^3
ANC nadir <500/mm^3 persisting for >7 days	Reduce the carboplatin dosage by 1 dose level. Do not modify the etoposide dosage. Consider use of prophylactic colony-stimulating factor with subsequent cycles
Platelet nadir <25,000/mm^3	Reduce the carboplatin dosage by 1 dose level. Do not modify the etoposide dosage
Platelet nadir <50,000/mm^3 with Grade ≥2 bleeding	Reduce the carboplatin dosage by 2 dose levels. Do not modify the etoposide dosage
ANC nadir <1000/mm^3 plus fever of ≥38.5°C	Reduce the carboplatin dosage by 1 dose level. Do not modify the etoposide dosage. Consider use of prophylactic colony stimulating factor with subsequent cycles
Non-Hematologic Toxicity	
Oral mucositis (any grade) present on day 1 of a treatment cycle	Delay treatment with carboplatin and etoposide until oral mucositis has resolved
G ≥3 mucositis at any time (severe pain; interfering with oral intake; or worse)	Reduce both the carboplatin dosage and etoposide dosage by 1 dose level

(*continued*)

Treatment Modifications (*continued*)

ATEZOLIZUMAB DOSE MODIFICATIONS

Adverse Reaction	Grade/Severity	Dose Modification
Colitis	G1	Loperamide 4 mg as starting dose then 2 mg before each meal and after each loose stool until without diarrhea for 12 hours, with maximum of 16 mg loperamide per day. If G1 diarrhea or colitis persists for >14 days, then add prednisolone 0.5–1 mg/kg (non-enteric-coated) or consider oral budesonide 9 mg daily if no bloody diarrhea
	G2/3 diarrhea or colitis	Withhold atezolizumab. Loperamide 4 mg as starting dose then 2 mg before each meal and after each loose stool until without diarrhea for 12 hours, with maximum of 16 mg loperamide per day. Administer oral prednisone/prednisolone at a dose of 0.5–2 mg/kg/day or its equivalent. When improves to G1, begin a slow corticosteroid taper over at least 4 weeks. Resume atezolizumab upon symptom control, or when prednisone/prednisolone daily dose <10 mg
	G4 diarrhea or colitis	Permanently discontinue atezolizumab. Loperamide 4 mg as starting dose then 2 mg before each meal and after each loose stool until without diarrhea for 12 hours, with maximum of 16 mg loperamide per day. Administer 1–2 mg/kg IV (methyl)prednisolone and convert to 0.5–2.0 mg/kg prednisone/prednisolone orally each day or its equivalent only after a response. Taper over at least 4 weeks when symptoms improve. If does not improve over 72 hours or worsens, perform flexible sigmoidoscopy/colonoscopy to document colitis then begin infliximab 5 mg/kg (if no perforation/sepsis/TB/hepatitis/NYHA III/IV CHF). If no response, add MMF 500–1000 mg twice daily. If worse on MMF, consider addition of tacrolimus or ATG
Pneumonitis	G2	Withhold atezolizumab. Consider pneumocystis prophylaxis depending on the clinical context and cover with empiric antibiotics. Administer oral prednisone/prednisolone at a dose of 1–2 mg/kg/day or its equivalent. When improves to G1, begin a slow corticosteroid taper over at least 4 weeks. If does not respond adequately after 48 hours, then administer 2–4 mg/kg IV (methyl)prednisolone and convert to 0.5–2.0 mg/kg prednisone/prednisolone orally each day or its equivalent only after a response, followed by a taper over at least 6 weeks when symptoms improve to G1, titrating to symptoms. Resume atezolizumab upon symptom control, or when prednisone/prednisolone daily dose <10 mg
	G3/4	Permanently discontinue atezolizumab. Consider pneumocystis prophylaxis depending on the clinical context; cover with empiric antibiotics. Administer 2–4 mg/kg IV (methyl)prednisolone and convert to 1–2 mg/kg prednisone/prednisolone orally each day or its equivalent only after a response, followed by a taper over at least 8 weeks when symptoms improve to G1, titrating to symptoms. If when initially treated improvement does not occur within 48–72 hours, begin infliximab 5 mg/kg (if no perforation/sepsis/TB/hepatitis/NYHA III/IV CHF). If no response to infliximab, add MMF 500–1000 mg twice daily. Consider MMF especially if has concurrent hepatic toxicity

(continued)

Treatment Modifications (continued)

Adverse Reaction	Grade/Severity	Dose Modification
Hepatitis	G2 (AST or ALT >3–5× ULN or total bilirubin >1.5-3× ULN)	Withhold atezolizumab. Administer oral prednisone/prednisolone at a dose of 1–2 mg/kg/day or its equivalent. When improves to G1, begin a slow corticosteroid taper over at least 4 weeks. Resume atezolizumab upon symptom control, or when prednisone/prednisolone daily dose <10 mg
	G3/4 (AST or ALT >5× ULN or total bilirubin >3× ULN)	Permanently discontinue atezolizumab. Administer 1–2 mg/kg IV (methyl)prednisolone and convert to 0.5–2.0 mg/kg prednisone/prednisolone orally each day or its equivalent only after a response. Taper over at least 6 weeks when symptoms improve. If no response, add MMF 500–1000 mg twice daily. If worse on MMF, consider adding tacrolimus or ATG
Hypophysitis	G2/3 (Moderate symptoms, ie, headache but no visual disturbance or fatigue/mood alteration but hemodynamically stable, no electrolyte disturbance)	Administer analgesia as needed for headache. Withhold atezolizumab. Administer oral prednisone/prednisolone at a dose of 0.5–2 mg/kg/day or its equivalent. When improves to G1, begin a slow corticosteroid taper over at least 4 weeks. If no improvement in 48 hours, administer 1–2 mg/kg IV (methyl)prednisolone and convert to 0.5–2.0 mg/kg prednisone/prednisolone orally each day or its equivalent only after a response. Taper over at least 4 weeks when symptoms improve to 5 mg prednisone/prednisolone or equivalent; do not stop steroids. Resume atezolizumab upon symptom control, or when prednisone/prednisolone daily dose <10 mg
	G4 (Severe mass effect symptoms, ie, severe headache, any visual disturbance or severe hypoadrenalism, ie, hypotension, severe electrolyte disturbance)	Permanently discontinue atezolizumab. Administer analgesia as needed for headache. Administer 1–2 mg/kg IV (methyl)prednisolone and convert to 0.5–2 mg/kg prednisone/prednisolone orally each day or its equivalent only after a response. Taper over at least 4 weeks when symptoms improve to 5 mg prednisone/prednisolone or equivalent; do not stop steroids
Adrenal insufficiency	G2	Withhold atezolizumab. Administer oral prednisone/prednisolone at a dose of 0.5–2 mg/kg/day or its equivalent. When improves to G1, begin a slow corticosteroid taper over at least 4 weeks. Serially assess adrenal function and continue steroids at replacement doses (20–40 mg hydrocortisone daily ~2/3 dose in AM upon awakening and ~1/3 at 4:00 PM) until recovery of adrenal function is documented. Resume atezolizumab upon symptom control, or when prednisone/prednisolone daily dose <10 mg
	G3/4	Permanently discontinue atezolizumab. Administer oral prednisone/prednisolone at a dose of 0.5–2 mg/kg/day or its equivalent. When improves to G1, begin a slow corticosteroid taper over at least 4 weeks. Serially assess adrenal function and continue steroids at replacement doses (20–40 mg hydrocortisone daily ~2/3 dose in AM upon awakening and ~1/3 at 4:00 PM) until recovery of adrenal function is documented
Type 1 diabetes mellitus	G3 hyperglycemia	Withhold atezolizumab. Admit to hospital to manage hyperglycemia. Role of corticosteroids in preventing complete loss of insulin-producing cells is unknown and not recommended. Resume atezolizumab upon symptom control, or when prednisone/prednisolone daily dose <10 mg
	G4 hyperglycemia	Permanently discontinue atezolizumab. Admit to hospital to manage hyperglycemia. Role of corticosteroids in preventing complete loss of insulin-producing cells is unknown and not recommended

(continued)

Treatment Modifications (*continued*)

Adverse Reaction	Grade/Severity	Dose Modification
Nephritis and renal dysfunction	G2/3 (serum creatinine 1.5–6× ULN)	Withhold atezolizumab. Administer oral prednisone/prednisolone at a dose of 0.5–2 mg/kg/day or its equivalent. When improves to G1, begin a slow corticosteroid taper over at least 4 weeks. If does not respond adequately, then administer 0.5–1 mg/kg IV (methyl)prednisolone and convert to 0.5–2 mg/kg prednisone/prednisolone orally each day or its equivalent only after a response, followed by a taper over at least 4 weeks when improves to G1. Resume atezolizumab upon symptom control, or when prednisone/prednisolone daily dose <10 mg
	G4 (serum creatinine >6× ULN)	Permanently discontinue atezolizumab. Administer 0.5–1 mg/kg IV (methyl)prednisolone and convert to 0.5–2 mg/kg prednisone/prednisolone orally each day or its equivalent only after a response, followed by a taper over at least 4 weeks when improves to G1
Skin	G1/2	Continue atezolizumab. Avoid skin irritants, avoid sun exposure, topical emollients recommended. Topical steroid (mild strength for G1, moderate/potent strength for G2) cream once or twice daily ± oral or topical antihistamines for itching
	G3 rash or suspected SJS or TEN	Withhold atezolizumab. Avoid skin irritants, avoid sun exposure, topical emollients recommended. Administer oral or topical antihistamines for itching. Administer oral prednisone/prednisolone at a dose of 0.5–2 mg/kg or its equivalent daily for 3 days followed by a slow corticosteroid taper over at least 4 weeks when the rash improves to G1. If does not respond adequately, then administer 0.5–1 mg/kg IV (methyl)prednisolone and convert to 0.5–2 mg/kg prednisone/prednisolone orally each day or its equivalent only after a response, followed by a taper over at least 4 weeks when the rash improves to G1. Resume atezolizumab upon symptom control, or when prednisone/prednisolone daily dose <10 mg
	G4 rash or confirmed SJS or TEN	Avoid skin irritants, avoid sun exposure, topical emollients recommended. Administer oral or topical antihistamines for itching. Administer 1–2 mg/kg IV (methyl)prednisolone and convert to oral steroids 0.5–2 mg/kg prednisone/prednisolone each day or its equivalent only after a response. Taper over at least 4 weeks when the rash improves to G1. Permanently discontinue atezolizumab
Encephalitis	Confusion or altered behavior, headaches, alteration in Glasgow Coma Scale, motor or sensory deficits, speech abnormality, may or may not be febrile	Initially withhold atezolizumab, but permanently discontinue atezolizumab if there is no doubt as to diagnosis. Exclude bacterial and ideally viral infections prior to high-dose steroids. Administer oral prednisone/prednisolone at a dose of 0.5–2 mg/kg/day or its equivalent. When symptoms improve, begin a slow corticosteroid taper over at least 4–8 weeks. If symptoms are severe, administer 1–2 mg/kg IV (methyl)prednisolone and convert to 0.5–2 mg/kg prednisone/prednisolone orally each day or its equivalent only after a response. Consider concurrent empiric antiviral (IV acyclovir) and antibacterial therapy
Aseptic meningitis	Headache, photophobia, neck stiffness with fever or may be afebrile, vomiting; normal cognition/cerebral function (distinguishes from encephalitis)	
Other syndromes include neurosarcoidosis, posterior reversible leukoencephalopathy syndrome (PRES), Vogt-Koyanagi-Harada syndrome, demyelination, vasculitic encephalopathy, and generalized seizures		
Transverse myelitis	Acute or subacute neurologic signs/ symptoms of motor/sensory/ autonomic origin; most have sensory level; often bilateral symptoms	Initially withhold atezolizumab, but permanently discontinue atezolizumab if there is no doubt as to diagnosis. Administer 2 mg/kg IV (methyl)prednisolone or consider 1 g/day and convert to 0.5–2.0 mg/kg prednisone/prednisolone orally each day or its equivalent only after a response. When symptoms improve, begin a slow corticosteroid taper over at least 4–8 weeks. Plasmapheresis may be required if steroids do not bring about improvement

(*continued*)

Treatment Modifications (continued)

Adverse Reaction	Grade/Severity	Dose Modification
Myocarditis	G3	Permanently discontinue atezolizumab. Administer 2 mg/kg IV (methyl)prednisolone or consider 1 g/day and convert to 0.5–2.0 mg/kg prednisone/prednisolone orally each day or its equivalent only after a response. When symptoms improve, begin a slow corticosteroid taper over at least 4–8 weeks. If no response, add MMF 500–1000 mg twice daily. If worse on MMF, consider adding tacrolimus
Peripheral neurologic toxicity	Moderate: some interference with ADL, symptoms concerning to patient	Withhold atezolizumab. Initial observation reasonable or initiate prednisone/prednisolone 0.5–1 mg/kg (if progressing, eg, from mild) and/or pregabalin or duloxetine for pain. When symptoms improve, begin a slow corticosteroid taper over at least 4 weeks. Resume atezolizumab upon symptom control, or when prednisone/prednisolone daily dose <10 mg
	Severe: limits self-care and aids warranted, life-threatening, eg, respiratory problems	Permanently discontinue atezolizumab. Administer 1–2 mg/kg IV (methyl)prednisolone and convert to 0.5–2.0 mg/kg prednisone/prednisolone orally each day or its equivalent only after a response. Taper over at least 4–8 weeks when symptoms improve to G1
Guillain-Barré syndrome	Progressive symmetrical muscle weakness with absent or reduced tendon reflexes—involves extremities, facial, respiratory, and bulbar and oculomotor muscles; dysregulation of autonomic nerves	Permanently discontinue atezolizumab. Use of steroids not recommended in idiopathic Guillain-Barré syndrome; however, a trial of (methyl)prednisolone 1–2 mg/kg is reasonable, converting to 0.5–2.0 mg/kg prednisone/prednisolone orally each day or its equivalent only after a response. If no improvement or worsening, plasmapheresis or IVIG indicated
Myasthenia gravis	Fluctuating muscle weakness (proximal limb, trunk, ocular, eg, ptosis/diplopia or bulbar) with fatigability, respiratory muscles may also be involved	Permanently discontinue atezolizumab. Administer pyridostigmine at an initial dose of 30 mg three times daily. Administer oral prednisone/prednisolone at a dose of 0.5–2.0 mg/kg/day or its equivalent or 1–2 mg/kg IV (methyl)prednisolone depending on the severity of symptoms. If begin with IV, convert to 0.5–2.0 mg/kg prednisone/prednisolone orally each day or its equivalent only after a response. If no improvement or worsening, plasmapheresis or IVIG may be considered. Additional immunosuppressants used in myasthenia gravis include azathioprine, cyclosporine, and mycophenolate. Avoid certain medications, eg, ciprofloxacin, beta-blockers, that may precipitate cholinergic crisis
Other syndromes including motor and sensory peripheral neuropathy, multifocal radicular neuropathy/plexopathy, autonomic neuropathy, phrenic nerve palsy, cranial nerve palsies (eg, facial nerve, optic nerve, hypoglossal nerve)		Permanently discontinue atezolizumab. Administer oral prednisone/prednisolone at a dose of 0.5–2.0 mg/kg/day or its equivalent or 1–2 mg/kg IV (methyl)prednisolone depending on the severity of symptoms. If begin with IV, convert to 0.5–2.0 mg/kg prednisone/prednisolone orally each day or its equivalent only after a response
Arthralgia	G1 (mild pain with inflammation, erythema, or joint swelling)	Continue atezolizumab. Administer acetaminophen (paracetamol) and ibuprofen
	G2 (moderate pain with inflammation, erythema, or joint swelling that limits ADLs)	Withhold atezolizumab. Administer higher doses of acetaminophen (paracetamol) and ibuprofen, and use diclofenac or naproxen or etoricoxib. If inadequately controlled, consider intra-articular steroid injections for large joints or administer oral prednisone/prednisolone at a dose of 0.5–2.0 mg/kg/day or its equivalent. When improves to G1, begin a slow corticosteroid taper over at least 4 weeks. If does not respond adequately, then administer 0.5–1 mg/kg IV (methyl)prednisolone and convert to 0.5–2.0 mg/kg prednisone/prednisolone orally each day or its equivalent only after a response, followed by a taper over at least 4 weeks when improves to G1. Resume atezolizumab upon symptom control, or when prednisone/prednisolone daily dose <10 mg
	G3 (severe pain; irreversible joint damage; disabling; limits self-care ADL)	Withhold atezolizumab. Administer 0.5–1 mg/kg IV (methyl)prednisolone and convert to 0.5–2.0 mg/kg prednisone/prednisolone orally each day or its equivalent only after a response, followed by a taper over at least 4 weeks when improves to G1. In severe cases, infliximab or another anti–TNF alpha drug may be required for improvement of arthritis. Resume atezolizumab upon symptom control, or when prednisone/prednisolone daily dose <10 mg

(continued)

Treatment Modifications (*continued*)

Adverse Reaction	Grade/Severity	Dose Modification
Other	First occurrence of other G3	Withhold atezolizumab. Administer oral prednisone/prednisolone at a dose of 0.5–2.0 mg/kg/day or its equivalent. When improves to G1, begin a slow corticosteroid taper over at least 4 weeks. Resume atezolizumab upon symptom control, or when prednisone/prednisolone daily dose <10 mg
	Recurrence of same G3	Permanently discontinue atezolizumab. Administer 1–2 mg/kg IV (methyl)prednisolone and convert to 0.5–2.0 mg/kg prednisone/prednisolone orally each day or its equivalent only after a response. Taper over at least 4–8 weeks when symptoms improve to G1
	Life-threatening or G4	
	Requirement for ≥10 mg/day prednisone or equivalent for >12 weeks	Permanently discontinue atezolizumab
	Persistent G2/3 adverse reactions lasting ≥12 weeks	

ADL, activities of daily living; ALT, alanine aminotransferase; AST, aspartate aminotransferase; ATG, anti-thymocyte globulin; SJS, Stevens-Johnson Syndrome; TEN, toxic epidermal necrolysis; ULN, upper limit of normal

Notes on general supportive care:
• Steroid taper in most cases will proceed over a minimum of 1 month, but if symptoms improve rapidly, a 2-week taper can be considered. If steroids are administered for more than 4 weeks, consider PCP prophylaxis (cotrimoxazole 480 mg twice daily M/W/F or inhaled pentamidine if has cotrimoxazole allergy), regular random blood glucose, vitamin D level and starting calcium/vitamin D supplementation per guidelines

Adverse Events* (N = 394)

Grade (%)	Carboplatin + Etoposide + Atezolizumab (n = 198)		Carboplatin + Etoposide + Placebo (n = 196)	
	Grade 1–2	Grade 3–5	Grade 1–2	Grade 3–5
Neutropenia	13.1	23.2	10.2	24.5
Anemia	24.7	14.1	20.9	12.2
Alopecia	34.8	0	33.7	0
Nausea	31.3	0.5	29.6	0.5
Fatigue	19.7	1.5	18.9	0.5
Decreased neutrophil count	3.5	14.1	6.1	16.8
Decreased appetite	19.7	1	13.3	0
Thrombocytopenia	6.1	10.1	7.1	7.7
Decreased platelet count	8.6	3.5	10.7	3.6
Vomiting	12.6	1	9.7	1.5
Constipation	9.6	0.5	12.8	0
Leukopenia	7.6	5.1	5.1	4.1
Decreased WBC count	5.1	3	8.2	4.6
Diarrhea	7.6	2	9.2	0.5
Febrile neutropenia	0	3	0	6.1
Infusion-related reaction	3	2	4.6	0.5

WBC, white blood cell
Adverse events related to any component of the trial regimen are included in the table
*Multiple occurrences of the same adverse event in the same patient were counted once at the highest grade
There were 3 deaths related to the trial regimen in the atezolizumab group (1.5%) (death due to neutropenia in 1 patient, pneumonia in 1 patient, and 1 unspecified cause) and 3 patients in the placebo group (1.5%) (death due to pneumonia in 1 patient, septic shock in 1 patient, and cardiopulmonary failure in 1 patient)

EXTENSIVE-STAGE SCLC • SUBSEQUENT THERAPY

LUNG CANCER REGIMEN: TOPOTECAN

von Pawel J et al. J Clin Oncol 1999;17:658–667

Topotecan HCl 1.5 mg/m² per day; administer intravenously in 50–250 mL 0.9% sodium chloride injection or 5% dextrose injection over 30 minutes, for 5 consecutive days, on days 1 through 5, every 21 days (total dosage/cycle = 7.5 mg/m²)

Supportive Care
Antiemetic prophylaxis
Emetogenic potential on days 1–5 is **LOW**
See Chapter 42 for antiemetic recommendations

Hematopoietic growth factor (CSF) prophylaxis
Primary prophylaxis is indicated with one of the following:

Filgrastim (G-CSF) 5 mcg/kg per day by subcutaneous injection, *or*
Pegfilgrastim (pegylated filgrastim) 6 mg/0.6 mL by subcutaneous injection for 1 dose
- Begin use from 24–72 hours after myelosuppressive chemotherapy is completed
- Continue filgrastim until ANC >10,000/mm³ on 2 consecutive daily measurements

See Chapter 43 for more information

Antimicrobial prophylaxis
Risk of fever and neutropenia is **LOW**
Antimicrobial primary prophylaxis to be considered:
- Antibacterial—not indicated
- Antifungal—not indicated
- Antiviral—not indicated unless patient previously had an episode of HSV

Patient Population Studied

A study of 107 patients with SCLC and disease progression at least 60 days after having completed first-line chemotherapy. A randomized comparison with combination chemotherapy, including cyclophosphamide, doxorubicin, and vincristine

Efficacy (N = 107)

Intention-to-treat response rate	24.3%*
Median survival	25 weeks
6-month survival	46.7%
1-year survival	14.2%

*Partial responses

Toxicity (N = 107)*

	% G3/4
Neutropenia	88
Thrombocytopenia	58
Anemia	42
Nausea	3.7
Fatigue	4.7
Vomiting	1.9
Stomatitis	1.9
Fever†	1.9
Diarrhea	0.9
Worsening LVEF: 2 of 26 patients (7.7%)	

*NCI CTC, National Cancer Institute (USA) Common Toxicity Criteria, version 2.0. Available at: http://ctep.cancer.gov/protocolDevelopment/electronic_applications/ctc.htm [accessed December 7, 2013]
†Excludes patients with febrile neutropenia

Treatment Modifications

Adverse Event	Dose Modification
Day 1 ANC <1000/mm³, platelets <100,000/mm³	Delay treatment until ANC >1000/mm³, platelets >100,000/mm³
Toxicity G <2 during the previous cycle	Increase topotecan dosage to a maximum daily dose of 2 mg/m² during repeated cycles (ie, first cycle escalated to 1.75 mg/m² per d for 5 days; second cycle escalated to 2 mg/m² per d for 5 days)
G4 neutropenia with fever or infection, or of duration ≥7 days	Decrease daily topotecan dosage from the previous cycle by 0.25 mg/m²*
G3 neutropenia during the preceding cycle persisting after day 21	
G4 thrombocytopenia	
G3/4 non-hematologic toxicity, excluding Grade 3 nausea	Decrease daily topotecan dosage from the previous cycle by 0.25 mg/m² or discontinue treatment*
Treatment delay >2 weeks	Discontinue treatment

*The minimum permissible daily topotecan dosage is 1 mg/m² per day for 5 days

Notes

Patients with objective responses continue treatment until disease progression or unacceptable toxicity, or for 6 additional cycles after maximal response

Therapy Monitoring

1. *Before day 1 chemotherapy:* CBC with differential, LFTs, serum BUN, and creatinine and electrolytes
2. *Weekly:* CBC with differential
3. *Day 15:* LFTs, serum BUN, and creatinine
4. *Before starting and after completing treatment:* ECG and multiple-gated acquisition or echocardiogram assessment of left ventricular ejection fraction (LVEF)
5. *Response evaluation:* every 2–3 cycles

EXTENSIVE-STAGE SCLC • SUBSEQUENT THERAPY

LUNG CANCER REGIMEN: PEMBROLIZUMAB

Chung HC et al. J Clin Oncol 2018;36(15 suppl):8506
KEYTRUDA (pembrolizumab) prescribing information. Whitehouse Station, NJ: Merck & Co.; revised 2019 September

Pembrolizumab 200 mg; administer intravenously over 30 minutes in a volume of 0.9% sodium chloride injection (0.9% NS) or 5% dextrose injection (D5W) sufficient to produce a pembrolizumab concentration within the range 1–10 mg/mL every 3 weeks for up to 24 months (total dose/3-week cycle = 200 mg)

Alternative pembrolizumab dose and schedule as per the U.S. FDA regimens approved on April 28, 2020:

Pembrolizumab 400 mg; administer intravenously over 30 minutes in a volume of 0.9% NS or D5W sufficient to produce a pembrolizumab concentration within the range 1–10 mg/mL every 6 weeks, for up to 24 months (total dose/6-week cycle = 400 mg)

- Administer pembrolizumab with an administration set that contains a sterile, non-pyrogenic, low-protein-binding in-line or add-on filter with pore size within the range of 0.2–5.0μm
- Pembrolizumab can cause severe or life-threatening infusion-related reactions, including hypersensitivity and anaphylaxis

Supportive Care
Antiemetic prophylaxis
Emetogenic potential is **MINIMAL**
See Chapter 42 for antiemetic recommendations

Hematopoietic growth factor (CSF) prophylaxis
Primary prophylaxis is **NOT** indicated
See Chapter 43 for more information

Antimicrobial prophylaxis
Risk of fever and neutropenia is **LOW**
Antimicrobial primary prophylaxis to be considered:
- Antibacterial—not indicated
- Antifungal—not indicated
- Antiviral—not indicated unless patient previously had an episode of HSV

Patient Population Studied

KEYNOTE-158 was a phase 2 multicenter, single-arm basket study involving patients with 11 different cancer types, including 107 adult patients with advanced incurable small cell lung cancer (cohort G). Eligible patients had an Eastern Cooperative Oncology Group performance status of ≤1 and had failed, progressed on, or were intolerant to standard therapy. Patients must have had a tumor sample evaluable for PD-L1. All patients were treated with pembrolizumab.

Efficacy (N = 107)

End Point	Pembrolizumab All Patients N = 107	Pembrolizumab PD-L1 Combined Positive Score ≥1 N = 42	Pembrolizumab PD-L1 Combined Positive Score <1 N = 50
Overall response rate	18.7% (95% CI, 11.8–27.4)	35.7% (95% CI, 21.6–52.0)	6.0% (95% CI, 1.3–16.5)
Median progression-free survival	2.0 months (95% CI, 1.9–2.1)	2.1 months (95% CI, 2.0–9.9)	1.9 months (95% CI, 1.6–2.0)
Median overall survival	9.1 months (95% CI, 5.7–14.6)	14.6 months (95% CI, 5.6-not estimable)	7.7 months (95% CI, 3.9–10.4)

CI, confidence interval
Data presented are with a median follow-up of 10.1 months (range, 0.5–17.5) and with a data cutoff date of August 23, 2017
Overall, median duration of response had not been reached (range, 2.1+ to 13.2+ months). Twelve patients had a duration of response of 9 months or longer

Therapy Monitoring

1. Initially at the time of each dose, and eventually every 6–12 weeks, perform a total-body skin examination with attention to ALL mucous membranes as well as a complete review of systems
2. Monitor patients for signs and symptoms of pneumonitis. Evaluate patients with suspected pneumonitis with chest x-ray, CT, and pulse oximetry. For ≥2 toxicity, may include nasal swab, sputum culture and sensitivity, blood culture and sensitivity, and urine culture and sensitivity
3. Monitor patients for signs and symptoms of colitis. Encourage patients to report diarrhea immediately to any member of the health care team
4. Draw AST, ALT, and bilirubin prior to each infusion and/or weekly if there are Grade 1 liver function test elevations. Note, no treatment is recommended for G1 LFT abnormalities. For ≥2 toxicity, work up for other causes of elevated LFTs including viral hepatitis
5. Use basic metabolic panel (Na, K, CO2, glucose) and patient history as screening tools for hypophysitis including hypopituitarism and adrenal insufficiency. If in doubt, evaluate AM adrenocorticotropic hormone (ACTH) and cortisol levels. Consider ACTH stimulation test for indeterminate results
6. Assess thyroid function at the start of treatment, periodically during treatment, and as indicated based on clinical evaluation, and for clinical signs and symptoms of thyroid disorders. Test for TSH and free thyroxine (FT4) every 4–6 weeks as part of routine clinical monitoring of therapy or for case detection in symptomatic patients
7. Measure glucose at baseline and with each treatment during the first 12 weeks and every 6 weeks thereafter
8. Obtain a serum creatinine prior to every dose. If creatinine is found to be newly elevated, consider holding therapy while other potential causes are evaluated. Note, routine urinalysis is not necessary other than to rule out urinary tract infections, etc

(continued)

Therapy Monitoring (*continued*)

9. Obtain a complete rheumatologic history and perform an examination of all peripheral joints for tenderness, swelling, and range of motion. Examine the spine. Consider plain x-ray/imaging to exclude metastases and evaluate joint damage (erosions), if appropriate
10. In patients at high risk for infections and in appropriately selected patients based on an infectious disease evaluation, draw screening laboratories (HIV, hepatitis A and B, and blood QuantiFERON for TB) to prepare patients to start infliximab

Treatment Modifications

RECOMMENDED DOSE MODIFICATIONS FOR PEMBROLIZUMAB

Adverse Event	Grade/Severity	Treatment Modification
Infusion reaction	Clinically significant but not severe infusion reaction	Interrupt the infusion in patients with clinically significant infusion reactions and consider resuming at a slower rate following resolution. If decision is made to restart, begin at ≤50% of the rate prior to the reaction and increase in 50% increments every 30 minutes if well tolerated. Infusions may be restarted at the full rate during the next cycle
	G3/4 (severe infusion reaction—pyrexia, chills, flushing, hypotension, dyspnea, wheezing, back pain, abdominal pain, and urticaria). Not rapidly responsive to brief interruption of infusion	Stop infusion and administer appropriate medical therapy (eg, epinephrine, corticosteroids, intravenous antihistamines, bronchodilators, and/or oxygen). Discontinue pembrolizumab
Colitis	G1	Loperamide 4 mg as starting dose then 2 mg before each meal and after each loose stool until without diarrhea for 12 hours, with maximum of 16 mg loperamide per day. If G1 diarrhea or colitis persists >14 days, then add prednisolone 0.5–1 mg/kg (non-enteric-coated) or consider oral budesonide 9 mg daily if no bloody diarrhea
	G2/3 diarrhea or colitis	Withhold pembrolizumab. Loperamide 4 mg as starting dose then 2 mg before each meal and after each loose stool until without diarrhea for 12 hours, with maximum of 16 mg loperamide per day. Administer oral prednisone/prednisolone at a dose of 0.5–2.0 mg/kg/day or its equivalent. When improves to G1, begin a slow corticosteroid taper over at least 4 weeks. Resume pembrolizumab upon symptom control, or when prednisone/prednisolone daily dose <10 mg
	G4 diarrhea or colitis	Permanently discontinue pembrolizumab. Loperamide 4 mg as starting dose then 2 mg before each meal and after each loose stool until without diarrhea for 12 hours, with maximum of 16 mg loperamide per day. Administer 1–2 mg/kg IV (methyl)prednisolone and convert to 0.5–2.0 mg/kg prednisone/prednisolone orally each day or its equivalent only after a response. Taper over at least 4 weeks when symptoms improve. If does not improve over 72 hours or worsens, perform flexible sigmoidoscopy/colonoscopy to document colitis then begin infliximab 5 mg/kg (if no perforation/sepsis/TB/hepatitis/NYHA III/IV CHF). If no response, add MMF 500–1000 mg twice daily. If worse on MMF, consider addition of tacrolimus or ATG
Pneumonitis	G2	Withhold pembrolizumab. Consider pneumocystis prophylaxis depending on the clinical context and coverage with empiric antibiotics. Administer oral prednisone/prednisolone at a dose of 1–2 mg/kg/day or its equivalent. When improves to G1, begin a slow corticosteroid taper over at least 4 weeks. If does not respond adequately after 48 hours, then administer 2–4 mg/kg IV (methyl)prednisolone and convert to 0.5–2.0 mg/kg prednisone/prednisolone orally each day or its equivalent only after a response, followed by a taper over at least 6 weeks when symptoms improve to G1, titrating to symptoms. Resume pembrolizumab upon symptom control, or when prednisone/prednisolone daily dose <10 mg
	G3/4	Permanently discontinue pembrolizumab. Consider pneumocystis prophylaxis depending on the clinical context; cover with empiric antibiotics. Administer 2–4 mg/kg IV (methyl)prednisolone and convert to 1–2 mg/kg prednisone/prednisolone orally each day or its equivalent only after a response, followed by a taper over at least 8 weeks when symptoms improve to G1, titrating to symptoms. If when initially treated improvement does not occur within 48–72 hours, begin infliximab 5 mg/kg (if no perforation/sepsis/TB/hepatitis/NYHA III/IV CHF). If no response to infliximab, add MMF 500–1000 mg twice daily. Consider MMF especially if has concurrent hepatic toxicity

(*continued*)

Treatment Modifications (continued)

RECOMMENDED DOSE MODIFICATIONS FOR PEMBROLIZUMAB

Adverse Event	Grade/Severity	Treatment Modification
Hepatitis	G2 (AST or ALT >3–5× ULN or total bilirubin >1.5-3× ULN)	Withhold pembrolizumab. Administer oral prednisone/prednisolone at a dose of 1–2 mg/kg/day or its equivalent. When improves to G1, begin a slow corticosteroid taper over at least 4 weeks. Resume pembrolizumab upon symptom control, or when prednisone/prednisolone daily dose <10 mg
	G3/4 (AST or ALT >5× ULN or total bilirubin >3× ULN)	Permanently discontinue pembrolizumab. Administer 1–2 mg/kg IV (methyl)prednisolone and convert to 0.5–2.0 mg/kg prednisone/prednisolone orally each day or its equivalent only after a response. Taper over at least 6 weeks when symptoms improve. If no response, add MMF 500–1000 mg twice daily. If worse on MMF, consider adding tacrolimus or ATG
Hypophysitis	G2/3 (moderate symptoms, ie, headache but no visual disturbance or fatigue/mood alteration but hemodynamically stable, no electrolyte disturbance)	Administer analgesia as needed for headache. Withhold pembrolizumab. Administer oral prednisone/prednisolone at a dose of 0.5–2.0 mg/kg/day or its equivalent. When improves to G1, begin a slow corticosteroid taper over at least 4 weeks. If no improvement in 48 hours, administer 1–2 mg/kg IV (methyl)prednisolone and convert to 0.5–2.0 mg/kg prednisone/prednisolone orally each day or its equivalent only after a response. Taper over at least 4 weeks when symptoms improve to 5 mg prednisone/prednisolone or equivalent; do not stop steroids. Resume pembrolizumab upon symptom control, or when prednisone/prednisolone daily dose <10 mg
	G4 (severe mass effect symptoms, ie, severe headache, any visual disturbance or severe hypoadrenalism, ie, hypotension, severe electrolyte disturbance)	Permanently discontinue pembrolizumab. Administer analgesia as needed for headache. Administer 1–2 mg/kg IV (methyl)prednisolone and convert to 0.5–2.0 mg/kg prednisone/prednisolone orally each day or its equivalent only after a response. Taper over at least 4 weeks when symptoms improve to 5 mg prednisone/prednisolone or equivalent; do not stop steroids
Adrenal insufficiency	G2	Withhold pembrolizumab. Administer oral prednisone/prednisolone at a dose of 0.5–2.0 mg/kg/day or its equivalent. When improves to G1, begin a slow corticosteroid taper over at least 4 weeks. Serially assess adrenal function and continue steroids at replacement doses (20–40 mg hydrocortisone daily ~2/3 dose in AM upon awakening and ~1/3 at 4:00 PM) until recovery of adrenal function is documented. Resume pembrolizumab upon symptom control, or when prednisone/prednisolone daily dose <10 mg
	G3/4	Permanently discontinue pembrolizumab. Administer oral prednisone/prednisolone at a dose of 0.5–2.0 mg/kg/day or its equivalent. When improves to G1, begin a slow corticosteroid taper over at least 4 weeks. Serially assess adrenal function and continue steroids at replacement doses (20–40 mg hydrocortisone daily ~2/3 dose in AM upon awakening and ~1/3 at 4:00 PM) until recovery of adrenal function is documented
Type 1 diabetes mellitus	G3 hyperglycemia	Withhold pembrolizumab. Admit to hospital to manage hyperglycemia. Role of corticosteroids in preventing complete loss of insulin-producing cells is unknown and not recommended. Resume pembrolizumab upon symptom control, or when prednisone/prednisolone daily dose <10 mg
	G4 hyperglycemia	Permanently discontinue pembrolizumab. Admit to hospital to manage hyperglycemia. Role of corticosteroids in preventing complete loss of insulin-producing cells is unknown and not recommended
Nephritis and renal dysfunction	G2/3 (serum creatinine 1.5–6× ULN)	Withhold pembrolizumab. Administer oral prednisone/prednisolone at a dose of 0.5–2.0 mg/kg/day or its equivalent. When improves to G1, begin a slow corticosteroid taper over at least 4 weeks. If does not respond adequately, then administer 0.5–1 mg/kg IV (methyl)prednisolone and convert to 0.5–2.0 mg/kg prednisone/prednisolone orally each day or its equivalent only after a response, followed by a taper over at least 4 weeks when improves to G1. Resume pembrolizumab upon symptom control, or when prednisone/prednisolone daily dose <10 mg
	G4 (serum creatinine >6× ULN)	Permanently discontinue pembrolizumab. Administer 0.5–1 mg/kg IV (methyl)prednisolone and convert to 0.5–2.0 mg/kg prednisone/prednisolone orally each day or its equivalent only after a response, followed by a taper over at least 4 weeks when improves to G1

(continued)

Treatment Modifications (continued)

RECOMMENDED DOSE MODIFICATIONS FOR PEMBROLIZUMAB

Adverse Event	Grade/Severity	Treatment Modification
Skin	G1/2	Continue pembrolizumab. Avoid skin irritants, avoid sun exposure, topical emollients recommended. Topical steroid (mild strength for G1, moderate/potent strength for G2) cream once or twice daily ± oral or topical antihistamines for itching
	G3 rash or suspected SJS or TEN	Withhold pembrolizumab. Avoid skin irritants, avoid sun exposure, topical emollients recommended. Administer oral or topical antihistamines for itching. Administer oral prednisone/prednisolone at a dose of 0.5–2.0 mg/kg or its equivalent daily for 3 days followed by a slow corticosteroid taper over at least 4 weeks when the rash improves to G1. If does not respond adequately, then administer 0.5–1 mg/kg IV (methyl)prednisolone and convert to 0.5–2.0 mg/kg prednisone/prednisolone orally each day or its equivalent only after a response, followed by a taper over at least 4 weeks when the rash improves to G1. Resume pembrolizumab upon symptom control, or when prednisone/prednisolone daily dose <10 mg
	G4 rash or confirmed SJS or TEN	Avoid skin irritants, avoid sun exposure, topical emollients recommended. Administer oral or topical antihistamines for itching. Administer 1–2 mg/kg IV (methyl)prednisolone and convert to oral steroids 0.5–2.0 mg/kg prednisone/prednisolone each day or its equivalent only after a response. Taper over at least 4 weeks when the rash improves to G1. Permanently discontinue pembrolizumab
Encephalitis	Confusion or altered behavior, headaches, alteration in Glasgow Coma Scale, motor or sensory deficits, speech abnormality, may or may not be febrile	Initially withhold pembrolizumab, but permanently discontinue pembrolizumab if there is no doubt as to diagnosis. Exclude bacterial and ideally viral infections prior to high-dose steroids. Administer oral prednisone/prednisolone at a dose of 0.5–2.0 mg/kg/day or its equivalent. When symptoms improve, begin a slow corticosteroid taper over at least 4–8 weeks. If symptoms are severe, administer 1–2 mg/kg IV (methyl)prednisolone and convert to 0.5–2.0 mg/kg prednisone/prednisolone orally each day or its equivalent only after a response. Consider concurrent empiric antiviral (IV acyclovir) and antibacterial therapy
Aseptic meningitis	Headache, photophobia, neck stiffness with fever or may be afebrile, vomiting; normal cognition/cerebral function (distinguishes from encephalitis)	
Other syndromes include neurosarcoidosis, posterior reversible leukoencephalopathy syndrome (PRES), Vogt-Koyanagi-Harada syndrome, demyelination, vasculitic encephalopathy, and generalized seizures		
Transverse myelitis	Acute or subacute neurologic signs/symptoms of motor/sensory/autonomic origin; most have sensory level; often bilateral symptoms	Initially withhold pembrolizumab, but permanently discontinue pembrolizumab if there is no doubt as to diagnosis. Administer 2 mg/kg IV (methyl)prednisolone or consider 1 g/day and convert to 0.5–2.0 mg/kg prednisone/prednisolone orally each day or its equivalent only after a response. When symptoms improve, begin a slow corticosteroid taper over at least 4–8 weeks. Plasmapheresis may be required if steroids do not bring about improvement
Myocarditis	G3	Permanently discontinue pembrolizumab. Administer 2 mg/kg IV (methyl)prednisolone or consider 1 g/day and convert to 0.5–2.0 mg/kg prednisone/prednisolone orally each day or its equivalent only after a response. When symptoms improve, begin a slow corticosteroid taper over at least 4–8 weeks. If no response, add MMF 500–1000 mg twice daily. If worse on MMF, consider adding tacrolimus
Peripheral neurologic toxicity	Moderate: some interference with ADL, symptoms concerning to patient	Withhold pembrolizumab. Initial observation reasonable or initiate prednisone/prednisolone 0.5–1 mg/kg (if progressing, eg, from mild) and/or pregabalin or duloxetine for pain. When symptoms improve, begin a slow corticosteroid taper over at least 4 weeks. Resume pembrolizumab upon symptom control, or when prednisone/prednisolone daily dose <10 mg
	Severe: limits self-care and aids warranted, life-threatening, eg, respiratory problems	Permanently discontinue pembrolizumab. Administer 1–2 mg/kg IV (methyl)prednisolone and convert to 0.5–2.0 mg/kg prednisone/prednisolone orally each day or its equivalent only after a response. Taper over at least 4–8 weeks when symptoms improve to G1
Guillain-Barré syndrome	Progressive symmetrical muscle weakness with absent or reduced tendon reflexes—involves extremities, facial, respiratory, and bulbar and oculomotor muscles; dysregulation of autonomic nerves	Permanently discontinue pembrolizumab. Use of steroids not recommended in idiopathic Guillain-Barré syndrome; however, a trial of (methyl)prednisolone 1–2 mg/kg is reasonable, converting to 0.5–2.0 mg/kg prednisone/prednisolone orally each day or its equivalent only after a response. If no improvement or worsening, plasmapheresis or IVIG indicated

(*continued*)

Treatment Modifications (*continued*)

RECOMMENDED DOSE MODIFICATIONS FOR PEMBROLIZUMAB

Adverse Event	Grade/Severity	Treatment Modification
Myasthenia gravis	Fluctuating muscle weakness (proximal limb, trunk, ocular, eg, ptosis/diplopia or bulbar) with fatigability, respiratory muscles may also be involved	Permanently discontinue pembrolizumab. Administer pyridostigmine at an initial dose of 30 mg three times daily. Administer oral prednisone/prednisolone at a dose of 0.5–2.0 mg/kg/day or its equivalent or 1–2 mg/kg IV (methyl)prednisolone depending on the severity of symptoms. If begin with IV, convert to 0.5–2.0 mg/kg prednisone/prednisolone orally each day or its equivalent only after a response. If no improvement or worsening, plasmapheresis or IVIG may be considered. Additional immunosuppressants used in myasthenia gravis include azathioprine, cyclosporine, and mycophenolate. Avoid certain medications, eg, ciprofloxacin, beta-blockers, that may precipitate cholinergic crisis
Other syndromes including motor and sensory peripheral neuropathy, multifocal radicular neuropathy/plexopathy, autonomic neuropathy, phrenic nerve palsy, cranial nerve palsies (eg, facial nerve, optic nerve, hypoglossal nerve)		Permanently discontinue pembrolizumab. Administer oral prednisone/prednisolone at a dose of 0.5–2.0 mg/kg/day or its equivalent or 1–2 mg/kg IV (methyl)prednisolone depending on the severity of symptoms. If begin with IV, convert to 0.5–2.0 mg/kg prednisone/prednisolone orally each day or its equivalent only after a response
Arthralgia	G1 (mild pain with inflammation, erythema, or joint swelling)	Continue pembrolizumab. Administer acetaminophen (paracetamol) and ibuprofen
	G2 (moderate pain with inflammation, erythema, or joint swelling that limits ADLs)	Withhold pembrolizumab. Administer higher doses of acetaminophen (paracetamol) and ibuprofen, and use diclofenac or naproxen or etoricoxib. If inadequately controlled, consider intra-articular steroid injections for large joints or administer oral prednisone/prednisolone at a dose of 0.5–2.0 mg/kg/day or its equivalent. When improves to G1, begin a slow corticosteroid taper over at least 4 weeks. If does not respond adequately, then administer 0.5–1 mg/kg IV (methyl)prednisolone and convert to 0.5–2.0 mg/kg prednisone/prednisolone orally each day or its equivalent only after a response, followed by a taper over at least 4 weeks when improves to G1. Resume pembrolizumab upon symptom control, or when prednisone/prednisolone daily dose <10 mg
	G3 (severe pain; irreversible joint damage; disabling; limits self-care ADL)	Withhold pembrolizumab. Administer 0.5–1 mg/kg IV (methyl)prednisolone and convert to 0.5–2.0 mg/kg prednisone/prednisolone orally each day or its equivalent only after a response, followed by a taper over at least 4 weeks when improves to G1. In severe cases, infliximab or another anti–TNF alpha drug may be required for improvement of arthritis. Resume pembrolizumab upon symptom control, or when prednisone/prednisolone daily dose <10 mg
Other	First occurrence of other G3	Withhold pembrolizumab. Administer oral prednisone/prednisolone at a dose of 0.5–2.0 mg/kg/day or its equivalent. When improves to G1, begin a slow corticosteroid taper over at least 4 weeks. Resume pembrolizumab upon symptom control, or when prednisone/prednisolone daily dose <10 mg
	Recurrence of same G3	Permanently discontinue pembrolizumab. Administer 1–2 mg/kg IV (methyl)prednisolone and convert to 0.5–2.0 mg/kg prednisone/prednisolone orally each day or its equivalent only after a response. Taper over at least 4–8 weeks when symptoms improve to G1
	Life-threatening or G4	
	Requirement for ≥10 mg/day prednisone or equivalent for >12 weeks	Permanently discontinue pembrolizumab
	Persistent G2/3 adverse reactions lasting ≥12 weeks	

ADL, activities of daily living; ALT, alanine aminotransferase; AST, aspartate aminotransferase; ATG, anti-thymocyte globulin; SJS, Stevens-Johnson Syndrome; TEN, toxic epidermal necrolysis; ULN, upper limit of normal.

Notes on general supportive care:
• Steroid taper in most cases will proceed over a minimum of 1 month, but if symptoms improve rapidly, a 2-week taper can be considered. If steroids are administered for more than 4 weeks, consider PCP prophylaxis (cotrimoxazole 480 mg twice daily M/W/F or inhaled pentamidine if has cotrimoxazole allergy), regular random blood glucose, vitamin D level and starting calcium/vitamin D supplementation per guidelines

Adverse Events (N = 107)

Treatment-related adverse events occurred in 63 patients (59%). Four patients discontinued protocol therapy due to adverse events, and one patient had a Grade 5 event (pneumonia).

24. Melanoma

Ahmad A. Tarhini, MD, PhD and John M. Kirkwood, MD

Epidemiology

Incidence: 100,350 (male: 60,190; female: 40,160. Estimated new cases for 2020 in the United States)

22.2 per 100,000 male and female per year (28.8 per 100,000 male 17.5 per 100,000 female)

Deaths: Estimated 6850 in 2020 (male: 4610; female: 2240)

Median age: 65 years

Male to female ratio: 1.6:1

Stage at Presentation	
Localized	81.0%
Regional	8.6%
Distant	4.2%
Unstaged	6.1%

Koh HK. N Engl J Med 1991;325:171–182

Siegel R et al. CA Cancer J Clin 2020;70:7–30

Surveillance, Epidemiology and End Results (SEER) Program, available from http://seer.cancer.gov [accessed in 2020]

Work-up

Stage IB Stage II	Chest x-ray (optional), LDH Further imaging as clinically indicated for Stage IIB, IIC patients (CT scan ± PET/MRI brain)
Stage IIIA	Chest x-ray, LDH. Further imaging as clinically indicated (CT scan ± PET, and/or MRI brain) BRAF mutation testing
Stage IIIB Stage IIIC Stage IIID	FNA of clinically palpable lymph node preferred, if feasible, otherwise lymph node or other accessible metastatic disease biopsy Chest x-ray, LDH. Further imaging as clinically indicated (CT scan ± PET, and/or MRI brain) BRAF mutation testing
Stage IV	FNA preferred, if feasible, otherwise lymph node or other accessible metastatic disease biopsy LDH; CT scan ± PET, and/or MRI brain Further imaging as clinically indicated BRAF mutation testing

Note:

1. Consider sentinel lymph node biopsy (SLNB) for Stage IA with adverse features (positive deep margins, lympho-vascular invasion, mitotic rate ≥1 mm²)
2. Encourage SLNB for Stage IB and II
3. Discuss the impact of SLNB as an important staging tool and that the impact on survival is still unclear

Pathology

Melanoma Types	
1. Superficial spreading melanoma	60–70%
2. Nodular melanoma	15–30%
3. Lentigo malignant melanoma	5%
4. Acral lentiginous melanoma	2–8%

Lotze MT et al. Cutaneous melanoma. In: DeVita VT et al (editors). Cancer: Principles & Practice of Oncology, 6th ed. Philadelphia: Lippincott Williams & Wilkins; 2001

Survival

	5-Year Melanoma-specific Survival	10-Year Melanoma-specific Survival
Stage IA	99%	98%
Stage IB	97%	94%
Stage IIA	94%	88%
Stage IIB	87%	82%
Stage IIC	82%	75%
Stage IIIA	93%	88%
Stage IIIB	83%	77%
Stage IIIC	69%	60%
Stage IIID	32%	24%

Gershenwald JE et al. CA Cancer J Clin 2017;67:472–492

Staging

Primary Tumor (T)		
Classification	Thickness (mm)	Ulceration Status/ Mitoses
TX: primary tumor thickness cannot be assessed (eg, diagnosis by curettage)	NA	NA
T0: no evidence of primary tumor (eg, unknown primary or completely regressed melanoma)	NA	NA
Tis (melanoma in situ)	NA	NA
T1	≤1.0	Unknown or unspecified
T1a	<0.8 mm	Without ulceration
T1b	<0.8 mm	With ulceration
	0.8–1.0 mm	With or without ulceration
T2	>1.0–2.0 mm	Unknown or unspecified
T2a	>1.0–2.0 mm	Without ulceration
T2b	>1.0–2.0 mm	With ulceration
T3	>2.0–4.0 mm	Unknown or unspecified
T3a	>2.0–4.0 mm	Without ulceration
T3b	>2.0–4.0 mm	With ulceration
T4	>4.0 mm	Unknown or unspecified
T4a	>4.0 mm	Without ulceration
T4b	>4.0 mm	With ulceration

NA, Not applicable

Regional Lymph Nodes (N)		
N	Number of Tumor-involved Regional Lymph Nodes	Presence of In-transit, Satellite, and/ or Microsatellite Metastases
NX	Regional nodes not assessed (eg, SLN biopsy not performed, regional nodes previously removed for another reason)	No
	Exception: pathological N category is not required for T1 melanomas, use cN	
N0	No regional metastases detected	No
N1	One tumor-involved node or in-transit, satellite, and/or microsatellite metastases with no tumor-involved nodes	—
N1a	One clinically occult (ie, detected by SLN biopsy)	No
N1b	One clinically detected	No
N1c	No regional lymph node disease	Yes
N2	Two or three tumor-involved nodes or in-transit, satellite, and/or microsatellite metastases with one tumor-involved node	—
N2a	Two or three clinically occult (ie, detected by SLN biopsy)	No
N2b	Two or three, at least one of which was clinically detected	No
N2c	One clinically occult or clinically detected	Yes
N3	Four or more tumor-involved nodes or in-transit, satellite, and/or microsatellite metastases with two or more tumor-involved nodes, or any number of matted nodes without or with in-transit, satellite, and/or microsatellite metastases	—
N3a	Four or more clinically occult (ie, detected by SLN biopsy)	No
N3b	Four or more, at least one of which was clinically detected, or presence of any number of matted nodes	No
N3c	Two or more clinically occult or clinically detected and/or presence of any number of matted nodes	Yes

Amin MB et al (editors). AJCC Cancer Staging Manual, 8th ed. New York: Springer; 2017

Expert Opinion

Tumor Thickness	Recommended Margins*
In situ	0.5 cm
≤1.0 mm	1.0 cm
1.01–2.0 mm	1–2 cm
2.01–4.0 mm	2.0 cm
>4.0 mm	2.0 cm

*The recommended surgical margin in the treatment of melanoma depends on the tumor thickness and is affected by anatomic constraints and optimal functional outcome

- **Prognosis according to stage:**
  - *Stage I:* Excellent prognosis with surgical treatment alone and a 95% 10-year survival rate
  - *Stages IIA, IIB, and IIC:* There is increased risk of melanoma relapse with increasing stage. Enrollment in adjuvant clinical trials testing immune checkpoint inhibitors or BRAF-MEK inhibitors can be offered
  - *Stage III:* Patients with regional lymph node involvement have a 5-year relapse rate of 37–89%. Adjuvant therapy with pembrolizumab, nivolumab, and the combination of dabrafenib and trametinib (for BRAF-mutated) significantly reduces the risk of relapse
  - *Stage IV:* Prognosis has significantly improved with the introduction of immune checkpoint inhibitors and BRAF-MEK inhibitors (for BRAF-mutated). The 5-year survival rate is currently estimated to approach 50%
- Diagnosis and initial surgical management:
  - For patients with a suspicious pigmented lesion, an **excisional biopsy** is preferred
  - When an excisional biopsy is thought inappropriate because of location (eg, face, ear, palm, sole, digit, subungual), a full-thickness **incisional biopsy** or a punch biopsy rather than a shave is acceptable
  - Patients with initial presentation of melanoma T1–4 should be treated by wide excision of the primary. Definitive surgery should include **wide excision of the primary and lymphadenectomy**. For subungual melanoma, a distal interphalangeal amputation with histologically negative margins constitutes an adequate **wide excision**
  - Consider **sentinel lymph node biopsy (SLNB)** for Stage IA with adverse features (positive deep margins, lymphovascular invasion, mitotic rate ≥1/mm²). Encourage SLNB for Stage IB and II. SLNB is an important staging tool, but its effect on survival is still unclear
- **Adjuvant therapy**
  - For the adjuvant treatment of malignant melanoma, the current U.S. Food and Drug Administration (FDA)-approved regimens are high-dose interferon alfa-2b (HDI), which was approved in 1995, pegylated interferon alfa-2b, which was approved in 2011 for the treatment of Stage III disease based on the EORTC 18991 study, ipilimumab, which was approved in 2015 based on the EORTC 18071 study, nivolumab, which was approved in 2017 based on the CHECKMATE–238 study, pembrolizumab, which was approved in 2019 based on the KEYNOTE–054 study, and the combination of dabrafenib and trametinib, which was approved in 2018 based on the COMBI-AD study
  - HDI is the only form of adjuvant therapy that has ever shown a consistent, significant, and durable relapse-free survival benefit in multicenter randomized controlled trials from U.S. Cooperative Groups. Estimated relapse frequency reductions of 24–38% and mortality reductions of 22–32% based on the hazard ratios for patients treated with interferon alfa versus observation or the GMK vaccine have been demonstrated
  - Based on the EORTC 18991 study, pegylated interferon alfa-2b has recurrence-free survival benefits that seem to be confined to the subpopulation of patients with microscopic nodal disease, and therefore, it can be offered to patients who cannot undertake high-dose interferon alfa-2b treatment
  - As tested in EORTC 18071 and North American Intergroup E1609, ipilimumab improves relapse-free survival compared with placebo and improves overall survival compared with placebo and HDI, albeit with a high toxicity and discontinuation rate. In cases where adjuvant therapy with ipilimumab represents an option, ipilimumab at 3 mg/kg has an advantage over the approved dosage of ipilimumab 10 mg/kg
  - Nivolumab, pembrolizumab, and the combination of dabrafenib and trametinib (for BRAF-mutated melanoma) represent the current first-line standard of care adjuvant therapy as tested in Checkmate-238, KeyNote-054, and COMBI-AD trials, respectively. Nivolumab and pembrolizumab prolong relapse-free survival compared with ipilimumab or placebo, respectively. In BRAF-mutated melanoma, dabrafenib and trametinib prolong relapse-free survival compared with placebo
- **Metastatic melanoma**
  - For metastatic melanoma, survival is currently estimated to approach 50% at 5 or more years. Major improvements in patient survival have been demonstrated with recently approved immune checkpoint inhibitors and BRAF-MEK inhibitors. First-line systemic therapy consisting of pembrolizumab, nivolumab, and the combination of nivolumab and ipilimumab has been shown to significantly improve survival. BRAF-MEK inhibitors (vemurafenib-cobimetinib, dabrafenib-trametinib, and encorafenib-binimetinib) for patients with documented melanoma BRAF mutation also have been shown to significantly improve survival

Dummer R et al. Lancet Oncol 2018;19:603–615
Hodi et al. Lancet Oncol 2018;19:1480–1492
Long GV et al. Lancet 2015;386:444–451

Robert C et al. N Engl J Med 2015;372:30–39
Robert C et al. N Engl J Med 2015;372:2521–2532
Wolchok et al. N Engl J Med 2017;377:1345–1356

(continued)

Expert Opinion (continued)

- Ipilimumab as monotherapy is the current preferred second-line systemic therapy option in patients failing prior anti-PD1 monotherapy. In 2011, the FDA approved ipilimumab for late-stage (metastatic) melanoma. Ipilimumab (Yervoy; Bristol-Myers Squibb Company, Princeton, NJ) is a monoclonal antibody to cytotoxic T-lymphocyte antigen 4 (CTLA4), which is also known as CD152 (cluster of differentiation 152). CTLA4, a member of the immunoglobulin superfamily, is expressed on the surface of T cells and transmits an inhibitory signal. CTLA4 is similar to CD28, a costimulatory protein that is also present on the surface of T cells. Both CTLA4 and CD28 bind to CD80 (B7-1) and CD86 (B7-2) on antigen-presenting cells (APCs). Response to an antigen begins when an APC loads a peptide on its major histocompatibility complex (MHC) antigen and presents this to a resting T cell through its T-cell receptor (TCR). The outcome depends in part on the interaction of CD80 and CD86 on the APC with CTLA4 and CD28 on the T-cell surface. An interaction with CTLA4 transmits an inhibitory signal to T cells, whereas CD28 transmits a stimulatory signal. By targeting CTLA4, ipilimumab reduces inhibitory signals and may augment the immune response. Ipilimumab's safety and effectiveness were established in a single international study of 676 patients. All patients in the study had stopped responding to other FDA-approved or commonly used treatments for melanoma. Because of the unusual and severe side effects associated with ipilimumab, it was approved with a Risk Evaluation and Mitigation Strategy to inform health care professionals about these serious risks. A medication guide is also provided to patients to inform them about potential side effects

Hodi FS et al. N Engl J Med 2010;363:711–723

- Single-agent **dacarbazine** is the only *cytotoxic* chemotherapy agent approved by the FDA for metastatic melanoma. Response rates range from 20% in early trials to 6.7% in one of the largest recent phase 3 trials. Median response durations range from 4–6 months. Higher response rates have been achieved with strategies involving combination chemotherapy and autologous bone marrow transplant, but with higher toxicities and no benefit in terms of relapse or survival

Bedikian AY et al. J Clin Oncol 2006;24:4738–4745
Chapman PB et al. J Clin Oncol 1999;17:2745–2751
Kirkwood JM. [General Principles of Oncology]. In: DeVita VT et al (editors). Cancer: Principles & Practice of Oncology, 4th ed. Philadelphia: J.B. Lippincott; 1993:1–16

- Temozolomide (TMZ) is transformed in vivo to monomethyltriazenoimidazole carboxamide (MTIC), the same active metabolite derived from hepatic metabolism of dacarbazine. Temozolomide crosses the blood-brain barrier and does not require metabolic activation; it undergoes spontaneous chemical degradation to MTIC at physiologic pH. A large randomized trial compared temozolomide with dacarbazine in patients with melanoma after the first presentation of metastatic disease. The median overall survival was 7.7 months with temozolomide and 6.4 months with dacarbazine (HR = 1.18; P = 0.2). The 6-month overall survival rate for temozolomide compared to dacarbazine was 61% versus 51%, respectively (HR = 1.36; P = 0.063). The difference between the treatment groups for overall survival did not reach statistical significance (P = 0.20), and the 95% confidence interval for the HR (0.92–1.52) indicated temozolomide was at least equivalent to dacarbazine. Continuous prolonged daily administration of temozolomide has been found to more effectively deplete the activity of the DNA repair enzyme O_6-methylguanine-DNA-methyltransferase (MGMT) (73% after 21 days, with low levels persisting up to day 28). In phase 1 studies of daily temozolomide use, including a trial in which the drug was administered for 21 days during a 28-day cycle, temozolomide 75 mg/m² per day resulted in a 2.1-fold greater exposure to drug per 28-day period than a 5-day schedule. A recent phase 3 trial described temozolomide use on an extended schedule (150 mg/m² per day orally on days 1–7, repeated every 14 days). There was no significant difference in overall survival (HR = 0.99, median 9.13 months [temozolomide] vs 9.36 months [dacarbazine]), progression-free survival (HR = 0.92, median 2.30 months [temozolomide] vs 2.17 months [dacarbazine]), or overall response rates (CR/PR) (14% temozolomide vs 10 % dacarbazine)

Brock CS et al. Cancer Res 1998;58:4363–4367
Middleton MR et al. J Clin Oncol 2000;18:158–166
Patel PM et al. In: Proceedings of the 33rd ESMO Congress; 2008 Sept 12–16; Stockholm, Sweden. (EORTC 18032). Available from: Eur J Cancer. 2011; 47:1476–83.

- **High-dose aldesleukin** (high-dose IL-2, HD IL-2) is approved by the U.S. Food and Drug Administration for metastatic melanoma based on a retrospective analysis of 8 phase 2 trials that demonstrated an objective response rate of 16% with durable responses in approximately 4% of patients. However, the major toxicities associated with this regimen, including a capillary leak syndrome leading to hypotension, renal insufficiency, and hypoxia, have precluded its widespread application. The use of high-dose aldesleukin is currently limited to specialized programs with experienced personnel, and it is generally offered to patients with good performance and excellent organ function

Atkins MB et al. J Clin Oncol 1999;17:2105–2116

- Promising results from a single-arm study of **paclitaxel and carboplatin plus sorafenib (PC + SOR)** in advanced melanoma has led to further investigation in a randomized phase 3 trial as second-line treatment. The addition of SOR to PC did not improve PFS or ORR, but overall, PC showed an improvement in the disease control rate (DCR) compared with historical data (DCR 62%; ORR 11%; SD 51%)

Agarwala SS et al. J Clin Oncol 2007;25(June 20 Suppl):abstract 8510

ADJUVANT

MELANOMA REGIMEN: NIVOLUMAB

Weber J et al. N Engl J Med 2017;377(19):1824–1835

The U.S. Food and Drug Administration (FDA)-approved regimens for melanoma include fixed doses of nivolumab and allow for a shortened infusion duration of 30 minutes, consistent with the regimens approved on March 5, 2018, thus:

Nivolumab 240 mg; administer intravenously over 30 minutes in a volume of 0.9% sodium chloride injection (0.9% NS) or 5% dextrose injection (D5W), not to exceed 160 mL and sufficient to produce a nivolumab concentration within the range 1–10 mg/mL, every 2 weeks for 1 year (total dosage/2-week course = 240 mg)

- Administer nivolumab through an administration set that contains a sterile, non-pyrogenic, low-protein-binding in-line filter with pore size within the range of 0.2–1.2 μm
- Nivolumab can cause severe infusion-related reactions

OR

Nivolumab 480 mg; administer intravenously over 30 minutes in a volume of 0.9% NS or D5W not to exceed 160 mL and sufficient to produce a nivolumab concentration within the range 1–10 mg/mL, every 4 weeks for 1 year (total dosage/4-week course = 480 mg)

- Administer nivolumab through an administration set that contains a sterile, non-pyrogenic, low-protein-binding in-line filter with pore size within the range of 0.2–1.2 μm
- Nivolumab can cause severe infusion-related reactions

Supportive Care

Antiemetic prophylaxis
Emetogenic potential with nivolumab is **MINIMAL**
See Chapter 42 for antiemetic recommendations

Hematopoietic growth factor (CSF) prophylaxis
Primary prophylaxis is **NOT** *indicated*
See Chapter 43 for more information

Antimicrobial prophylaxis
Risk of fever and neutropenia is **LOW**
Antimicrobial primary prophylaxis to be considered:
- Antibacterial—not indicated
- Antifungal—not indicated
- Antiviral—not indicated unless patient previously had an episode of HSV

Patient Population Studied

An international, multicenter, randomized, double-blind, phase 3 study (CheckMate 238) involving 906 patients with histologically confirmed Stage IIIB, IIIC, or IV melanoma with metastases to regional lymph nodes or distant metastases that had been surgically resected. Eligible patients were aged ≥15 years, had an Eastern Cooperative Oncology Group (ECOG) performance status score of ≤1, and had undergone complete regional lymphadenectomy or resection within 12 weeks before randomization. Patients who had previously received a systemic therapy for melanoma were not eligible for inclusion in the study. Participants were randomly assigned in a 1:1 ratio to receive nivolumab or ipilimumab for up to 1 year

Efficacy (N = 906)

	Nivolumab (N = 453)	Ipilimumab (N = 453)	HR (97.56% CI); P Value
Recurrence-free survival at 18 months	66.4%	52.7%	0.65 (0.51–0.83); P<0.001

Note: Minimum follow-up was 18 months. Median duration of follow-up was 19.5 months. By clinical data cut-off, the median recurrence-free survival had not been reached in either group

Therapy Monitoring

1. Initially at the time of each dose, and eventually every 6–12 weeks, perform a total body skin examination with attention to ALL mucous membranes as well as a complete review of systems
2. Monitor patients for signs and symptoms of pneumonitis. Evaluate patients with suspected pneumonitis with chest x-ray, CT, and pulse oximetry. For ≥2 toxicity, may include nasal swab, sputum culture and sensitivity, blood culture and sensitivity, and urine culture and sensitivity
3. Monitor patients for signs and symptoms of colitis. Encourage patients to report diarrhea immediately to any member of the health care team
4. Draw AST, ALT, and bilirubin prior to each infusion and/or weekly if there are Grade 1 liver function test elevations. Note, no treatment is recommended for G1 LFT abnormalities. For ≥2 toxicity, work up for other causes of elevated LFTs including viral hepatitis
5. Use basic metabolic panel (Na, K, CO_2, glucose) and patient history as screening tools for hypophysitis including hypopituitarism and adrenal insufficiency. If in doubt, evaluate AM adrenocorticotropic hormone (ACTH) and cortisol levels. Consider ACTH stimulation test for indeterminate results
6. Assess thyroid function at the start of treatment, periodically during treatment, and as indicated based on clinical evaluation and for clinical signs and symptoms of thyroid disorders. Test for TSH and free thyroxine (FT4) every 4–6 weeks as part of routine clinical monitoring of therapy or for case detection in symptomatic patients
7. Measure glucose at baseline and with each treatment during the first 12 weeks and every 6 weeks thereafter
8. Obtain a serum creatinine prior to every dose. If creatinine is found to be newly elevated, consider holding therapy while other potential causes are evaluated. Note, routine urinalysis is not necessary other than to rule out urinary tract infections, etc
9. Obtain a complete rheumatologic history and perform an examination of all peripheral joints for tenderness, swelling, and range of motion. Examine the spine. Consider plain x-ray/imaging to exclude metastases and evaluate joint damage (erosions), if appropriate
10. In patients at high risk for infections and in appropriately selected patients based on an infectious disease evaluation, draw screening laboratories (HIV, hepatitis A and B, and blood QuantiFERON for TB) to prepare patients to start infliximab

Treatment Modifications

RECOMMENDED DOSE MODIFICATIONS FOR NIVOLUMAB

Adverse Event	Grade/Severity	Treatment Modification
Infusion reaction	Clinically significant but not severe infusion reaction	Interrupt the infusion in patients with clinically significant infusion reactions and consider resuming at a slower rate following resolution. If decision is made to restart, begin at ≤50% of the rate prior to the reaction and increase in 50% increments every 30 minutes if well tolerated. Infusions may be restarted at the full rate during the next cycle
	G3/4 (severe infusion reaction—pyrexia, chills, flushing, hypotension, dyspnea, wheezing, back pain, abdominal pain, and urticaria). Not rapidly responsive to brief interruption of infusion	Stop infusion and administer appropriate medical therapy (eg, epinephrine, corticosteroids, intravenous antihistamines, bronchodilators, and/or oxygen). Discontinue nivolumab
Colitis	G1	Loperamide 4 mg as starting dose then 2 mg before each meal and after each loose stool until without diarrhea for 12 hours, with maximum of 16 mg loperamide per day. If G1 diarrhea or colitis persists >14 days, then add prednisolone 0.5–1 mg/kg (non-enteric-coated) or consider oral budesonide 9 mg daily if no bloody diarrhea
	G2/3 diarrhea or colitis	Withhold nivolumab. Loperamide 4 mg as starting dose then 2 mg before each meal and after each loose stool until without diarrhea for 12 hours, with maximum of 16 mg loperamide per day. Administer oral prednisone/prednisolone at a dose of 0.5–2 mg/kg/day or its equivalent. When improves to G1, begin a slow corticosteroid taper over at least 4 weeks. Resume nivolumab upon symptom control, or when prednisone/prednisolone daily dose <10 mg
	G4 diarrhea or colitis	Permanently discontinue nivolumab. Loperamide 4 mg as starting dose then 2 mg before each meal and after each loose stool until without diarrhea for 12 hours, with maximum of 16 mg loperamide per day. Administer 1–2 mg/kg intravenously (methyl)prednisolone and convert to 0.5–2 mg/kg prednisone/prednisolone orally each day or its equivalent only after a response. Taper over at least 4 weeks when symptoms improve. If does not improve over 72 hours or worsens, perform flexible sigmoidoscopy/colonoscopy to document colitis then begin infliximab 5 mg/kg (if no perforation/sepsis/TB/hepatitis/NYHA III/IV CHF). If no response, add MMF 500–1000 mg twice daily. If worse on MMF, consider addition of tacrolimus or ATG
Pneumonitis	G2	Withhold nivolumab. Consider *Pneumocystis* prophylaxis depending on the clinical context and coverage with empiric antibiotics. Administer oral prednisone/prednisolone at a dose of 1–2 mg/kg/day or its equivalent. When improves to G1, begin a slow corticosteroid taper over at least 4 weeks. If does not respond adequately after 48 hours, then administer 2–4 mg/kg intravenously (methyl)prednisolone and convert to 0.5–2 mg/kg prednisone/prednisolone orally each day or its equivalent only after a response, followed by a taper over at least 6 weeks when symptoms improve to G1, titrating to symptoms. Resume nivolumab upon symptom control, or when prednisone/prednisolone daily dose <10 mg
	G3/4	Permanently discontinue nivolumab. Consider *Pneumocystis* prophylaxis depending on the clinical context; cover with empiric antibiotics. Administer 2–4 mg/kg intravenously (methyl)prednisolone and convert to 1–2 mg/kg prednisone/prednisolone orally each day or its equivalent only after a response, followed by a taper over at least 8 weeks when symptoms improve to G1, titrating to symptoms. If when initially treated improvement does not occur within 48–72 hours, begin infliximab 5 mg/kg (if no perforation/sepsis/TB/hepatitis/NYHA III/IV CHF). If no response to infliximab, add MMF 500–1000 mg twice daily. Consider MMF especially if has concurrent hepatic toxicity
Hepatitis	G2 (AST or ALT >3–5× ULN or total bilirubin >1.5–3× ULN)	Withhold nivolumab. Administer oral prednisone/prednisolone at a dose of 1–2 mg/kg/day or its equivalent. When improves to G1, begin a slow corticosteroid taper over at least 4 weeks. Resume nivolumab upon symptom control, or when prednisone/prednisolone daily dose <10 mg
	G3/4 (AST or ALT >5× ULN or total bilirubin >3× ULN)	Permanently discontinue nivolumab. Administer 1–2 mg/kg intravenously (methyl)prednisolone and convert to 0.5–2 mg/kg prednisone/prednisolone orally each day or its equivalent only after a response. Taper over at least 6 weeks when symptoms improve. If no response, add MMF 500–1000 mg twice daily. If worse on MMF, consider adding tacrolimus or ATG

(continued)

Treatment Modifications (*continued*)

RECOMMENDED DOSE MODIFICATIONS FOR NIVOLUMAB

Adverse Event	Grade/Severity	Treatment Modification
Hypophysitis	G2/3 (moderate symptoms, ie, headache but no visual disturbance or fatigue/mood alteration but hemodynamically stable, no electrolyte disturbance)	Administer analgesia as needed for headache. Withhold nivolumab. Administer oral prednisone/prednisolone at a dose of 0.5–2 mg/kg/day or its equivalent. When improves to G1, begin a slow corticosteroid taper over at least 4 weeks. If no improvement in 48 hours, administer 1–2 mg/kg intravenously (methyl)prednisolone and convert to 0.5–2 mg/kg prednisone/prednisolone orally each day or its equivalent only after a response. Taper over at least 4 weeks when symptoms improve to 5 mg prednisone/prednisolone or equivalent; do not stop steroids. Resume nivolumab upon symptom control, or when prednisone/prednisolone daily dose <10 mg
	G4 (severe mass effect symptoms, ie, severe headache, any visual disturbance or severe hypoadrenalism, ie, hypotension, severe electrolyte disturbance)	Permanently discontinue nivolumab. Administer analgesia as needed for headache. Administer 1–2 mg/kg intravenously (methyl)prednisolone and convert to 0.5–2 mg/kg prednisone/prednisolone orally each day or its equivalent only after a response. Taper over at least 4 weeks when symptoms improve to 5 mg prednisone/prednisolone or equivalent; do not stop steroids
Adrenal insufficiency	G2	Withhold nivolumab. Administer oral prednisone/prednisolone at a dose of 0.5–2 mg/kg/day or its equivalent. When improves to G1, begin a slow corticosteroid taper over at least 4 weeks. Serially assess adrenal function and continue steroids at replacement doses (20–40 mg hydrocortisone daily ~2/3 dose in AM upon awakening and ~1/3 at 4 PM) until recovery of adrenal function is documented. Resume nivolumab upon symptom control, or when prednisone/prednisolone daily dose <10 mg
	G3/4	Permanently discontinue nivolumab. Administer oral prednisone/prednisolone at a dose of 0.5–2 mg/kg/day or its equivalent. When improves to G1, begin a slow corticosteroid taper over at least 4 weeks. Serially assess adrenal function and continue steroids at replacement doses (20–40 mg hydrocortisone daily ~2/3 dose in AM upon awakening and ~1/3 at 4 PM) until recovery of adrenal function is documented
Type 1 diabetes mellitus	G3 hyperglycemia	Withhold nivolumab. Admit to hospital to manage hyperglycemia. Role of corticosteroids in preventing complete loss of insulin-producing cells is unknown and not recommended. Resume nivolumab upon symptom control, or when prednisone/prednisolone daily dose <10 mg
	G4 hyperglycemia	Permanently discontinue nivolumab. Admit to hospital to manage hyperglycemia. Role of corticosteroids in preventing complete loss of insulin-producing cells is unknown and not recommended
Nephritis and renal dysfunction	G2/3 (serum creatinine 1.5–6× ULN)	Withhold nivolumab. Administer oral prednisone/prednisolone at a dose of 0.5–2 mg/kg/day or its equivalent. When improves to G1, begin a slow corticosteroid taper over at least 4 weeks. If does not respond adequately, then administer 0.5–1 mg/kg intravenously (methyl)prednisolone and convert to 0.5–2 mg/kg prednisone/prednisolone orally each day or its equivalent only after a response, followed by a taper over at least 4 weeks when improves to G1. Resume nivolumab upon symptom control, or when prednisone/prednisolone daily dose <10 mg
	G4 (serum creatinine >6× ULN)	Permanently discontinue nivolumab. Administer 0.5–1 mg/kg intravenously (methyl)prednisolone and convert to 0.5–2 mg/kg prednisone/prednisolone orally each day or its equivalent only after a response, followed by a taper over at least 4 weeks when improves to G1

(*continued*)

Treatment Modifications (*continued*)

RECOMMENDED DOSE MODIFICATIONS FOR NIVOLUMAB

Adverse Event	Grade/Severity	Treatment Modification
Skin	G1/2	Continue nivolumab. Avoid skin irritants, avoid sun exposure, topical emollients recommended. Topical steroid (mild strength for G1, moderate/potent strength for G2) cream once or twice daily ± oral or topical antihistamines for itching
	G3 rash or suspected SJS or TEN	Withhold nivolumab. Avoid skin irritants, avoid sun exposure, topical emollients recommended. Administer oral or topical antihistamines for itching. Administer oral prednisone/prednisolone at a dose of 0.5–2 mg/kg or its equivalent daily for 3 days followed by a slow corticosteroid taper over at least 4 weeks when the rash improves to G1. If does not respond adequately, then administer 0.5–1 mg/kg intravenously (methyl)prednisolone and convert to 0.5–2 mg/kg prednisone/prednisolone orally each day or its equivalent only after a response, followed by a taper over at least 4 weeks when the rash improves to G1. Resume nivolumab upon symptom control, or when prednisone/prednisolone daily dose <10 mg
	G4 rash or confirmed SJS or TEN	Avoid skin irritants, avoid sun exposure, topical emollients recommended. Administer oral or topical antihistamines for itching. Administer 1–2 mg/kg intravenously (methyl)prednisolone and convert to oral steroids 0.5–2 mg/kg prednisone/prednisolone each day or its equivalent only after a response. Taper over at least 4 weeks when the rash improves to G1. Permanently discontinue nivolumab
Encephalitis	Confusion or altered behavior, headaches, alteration in Glasgow Coma Scale, motor or sensory deficits, speech abnormality, may or may not be febrile	Initially withhold nivolumab, but permanently discontinue nivolumab if there is no doubt as to diagnosis. Exclude bacterial and ideally viral infections prior to high-dose steroids. Administer oral prednisone/prednisolone at a dose of 0.5–2 mg/kg/day or its equivalent. When symptoms improve, begin a slow corticosteroid taper over at least 4–8 weeks. If symptoms are severe, administer 1–2 mg/kg intravenously (methyl)prednisolone and convert to 0.5–2 mg/kg prednisone/prednisolone orally each day or its equivalent only after a response. Consider concurrent empiric antiviral (intravenous acyclovir) and antibacterial therapy
Aseptic meningitis	Headache, photophobia, neck stiffness with fever or may be afebrile, vomiting; normal cognition/cerebral function (distinguishes from encephalitis)	
Other syndromes include neurosarcoidosis, posterior reversible leukoencephalopathy syndrome (PRES), Vogt-Koyanagi-Harada syndrome, demyelination, vasculitic encephalopathy, and generalized seizures		
Transverse myelitis	Acute or subacute neurologic signs/symptoms of motor/sensory/autonomic origin; most have sensory level; often bilateral symptoms	Initially withhold nivolumab, but permanently discontinue nivolumab if there is no doubt as to diagnosis. Administer 2 mg/kg intravenously (methyl)prednisolone or consider 1 g/day and convert to 0.5–2 mg/kg prednisone/prednisolone orally each day or its equivalent only after a response. When symptoms improve, begin a slow corticosteroid taper over at least 4–8 weeks. Plasmapheresis may be required if steroids do not bring about improvement
Myocarditis	G3	Permanently discontinue nivolumab. Administer 2 mg/kg intravenously (methyl)prednisolone or consider 1 g/day and convert to 0.5–2 mg/kg prednisone/prednisolone orally each day or its equivalent only after a response. When symptoms improve, begin a slow corticosteroid taper over at least 4–8 weeks. If no response, add MMF 500–1000 mg twice daily. If worse on MMF, consider adding tacrolimus
Peripheral neurologic toxicity	Moderate: some interference with ADL, symptoms concerning to patient	Withhold nivolumab. Initial observation reasonable or initiate prednisone/prednisolone 0.5–1 mg/kg (if progressing, eg, from mild) and/or pregabalin or duloxetine for pain. When symptoms improve, begin a slow corticosteroid taper over at least 4 weeks. Resume nivolumab upon symptom control, or when prednisone/prednisolone daily dose <10 mg
	Severe: limits self-care and aids warranted, life-threatening, eg, respiratory problems	Permanently discontinue nivolumab. Administer 1–2 mg/kg intravenously (methyl)prednisolone and convert to 0.5–2 mg/kg prednisone/prednisolone orally each day or its equivalent only after a response. Taper over at least 4–8 weeks when symptoms improve to G1

(*continued*)

Treatment Modifications (*continued*)

RECOMMENDED DOSE MODIFICATIONS FOR NIVOLUMAB

Adverse Event	Grade/Severity	Treatment Modification
Guillain-Barré syndrome	Progressive symmetrical muscle weakness with absent or reduced tendon reflexes—involves extremities, facial, respiratory, and bulbar and oculomotor muscles; dysregulation of autonomic nerves	Permanently discontinue nivolumab. Use of steroids not recommended in idiopathic Guillain-Barré syndrome; however, a trial of (methyl)prednisolone 1–2 mg/kg is reasonable, converting to 0.5–2 mg/kg prednisone/prednisolone orally each day or its equivalent only after a response. If no improvement or worsening, plasmapheresis or IVIG indicated
Myasthenia gravis	Fluctuating muscle weakness (proximal limb, trunk, ocular, eg, ptosis/diplopia or bulbar) with fatigability, respiratory muscles may also be involved	Permanently discontinue nivolumab. Administer pyridostigmine at an initial dose of 30 mg three times daily. Administer oral prednisone/prednisolone at a dose of 0.5–2 mg/kg/day or its equivalent or 1–2 mg/kg intravenously (methyl)prednisolone depending on the severity of symptoms. If begin with IV, convert to 0.5–2 mg/kg prednisone/prednisolone orally each day or its equivalent only after a response. If no improvement or worsening, plasmapheresis or IVIG may be considered. Additional immunosuppressants used in myasthenia gravis include azathioprine, cyclosporine, and mycophenolate. Avoid certain medications, eg, ciprofloxacin, beta-blockers, that may precipitate cholinergic crisis
Other syndromes including motor and sensory peripheral neuropathy, multifocal radicular neuropathy/plexopathy, autonomic neuropathy, phrenic nerve palsy, cranial nerve palsies (eg, facial nerve, optic nerve, hypoglossal nerve)		Permanently discontinue nivolumab. Administer oral prednisone/prednisolone at a dose of 0.5–2 mg/kg/day or its equivalent or 1–2 mg/kg intravenously (methyl)prednisolone depending on the severity of symptoms. If begin with IV, convert to 0.5–2 mg/kg prednisone/prednisolone orally each day or its equivalent only after a response
Arthralgia	G1 (mild pain with inflammation, erythema, or joint swelling)	Continue nivolumab. Administer acetaminophen (paracetamol) and ibuprofen
	G2 (moderate pain with inflammation, erythema, or joint swelling that limits ADLs)	Withhold nivolumab. Administer higher doses of acetaminophen (paracetamol) and ibuprofen and use diclofenac or naproxen or etoricoxib. If inadequately controlled, consider intra-articular steroid injections for large joints or administer oral prednisone/prednisolone at a dose of 0.5–2 mg/kg/day or its equivalent. When improves to G1, begin a slow corticosteroid taper over at least 4 weeks. If does not respond adequately, then administer 0.5–1 mg/kg intravenously (methyl)prednisolone and convert to 0.5–2 mg/kg prednisone/prednisolone orally each day or its equivalent only after a response, followed by a taper over at least 4 weeks when improves to G1. Resume nivolumab upon symptom control, or when prednisone/prednisolone daily dose <10 mg
	G3 (severe pain; irreversible joint damage; disabling; limits self-care ADL)	Withhold nivolumab. Administer 0.5–1 mg/kg intravenously (methyl)prednisolone and convert to 0.5–2 mg/kg prednisone/prednisolone orally each day or its equivalent only after a response, followed by a taper over at least 4 weeks when improves to G1. In severe cases, infliximab or another anti–TNF-alpha drug may be required for improvement of arthritis. Resume nivolumab upon symptom control, or when prednisone/prednisolone daily dose <10 mg
Other	First occurrence of other G3	Withhold nivolumab. Administer oral prednisone/prednisolone at a dose of 0.5–2 mg/kg/day or its equivalent. When improves to G1, begin a slow corticosteroid taper over at least 4 weeks. Resume nivolumab upon symptom control, or when prednisone/prednisolone daily dose <10 mg
	Recurrence of same G3	Permanently discontinue nivolumab. Administer 1–2 mg/kg intravenously (methyl)prednisolone and convert to 0.5–2 mg/kg prednisone/prednisolone orally each day or its equivalent only after a response. Taper over at least 4–8 weeks when symptoms improve to G1
	Life-threatening or G4	
	Requirement for ≥10 mg/day prednisone or equivalent for >12 weeks	Permanently discontinue nivolumab
	Persistent G2/3 adverse reactions lasting ≥12 weeks	

ADL, activities of daily living; ALT, alanine aminotransferase; AST, aspartate aminotransferase; ATG, anti-thymocyte globulin; SJS, Stevens-Johnson Syndrome; TEN, toxic epidermal necrolysis; ULN, upper limit of normal.

Notes on general supportive care:
- Steroid taper in most cases will proceed over a minimum of 1 month but if symptoms improve rapidly, a 2-week taper can be considered. If steroids are administered for more than 4 weeks, consider PCP prophylaxis (cotrimoxazole 480 mg twice daily M/W/F or inhaled pentamidine if has cotrimoxazole allergy), regular random blood glucose, VitD level, and starting calcium/VitD supplementation per guidelines

Adverse Events (N = 905)

Grade (%)*	Nivolumab (n = 452)		Ipilimumab (n = 453)	
	Grade 1–2	Grade 3–4	Grade 1–2	Grade 3–4
Any adverse event	71	14	50	46
Fatigue	34	<1	32	<1
Diarrhea	23	2	36	9
Pruritus	23	0	32	1
Rash	19	1	26	3
Nausea	15	<1	20	0
Asthenia	12	<1	11	<1
Arthralgia	12	<1	10	<1
Hypothyroidism	11	<1	6	<1
Headache	10	<1	16	2
Abdominal pain	6	0	10	<1
Increased alanine aminotransferase level	5	1	9	6
Increased aspartate aminotransferase level	5	<1	9	4
Maculopapular rash	5	0	9	2
Hypophysitis	1	<1	8	2
Pyrexia	2	0	11	<1

*According to the National Cancer Institute Common Terminology Criteria for Adverse Events, version 4.0
Note: Treatment-related adverse events that occurred in ≥10% of patients in either treatment group are included in the table. Treatment-related adverse events leading to discontinuation occurred in 7.7% of the nivolumab group and 41.7% of the ipilimumab group. Two patients in the ipilimumab group died as a result of toxic effects (marrow aplasia and colitis, both >100 days after the last dose)

ADJUVANT

MELANOMA REGIMEN: PEMBROLIZUMAB

Eggermont AMM et al. N Engl J Med. 2018;378(19):1789–1801

Pembrolizumab 200 mg; administer intravenously over 30 minutes in a volume of 0.9% sodium chloride injection (0.9% NS) or 5% dextrose injection (D5W) sufficient to produce a pembrolizumab concentration within the range 1–10 mg/mL every 3 weeks for 18 cycles, not to exceed 1 year of therapy (total dose/3-week cycle = 200 mg)

Alternative pembrolizumab dose and schedule as per the U.S. FDA regimens approved on April 28, 2020:

Pembrolizumab 400 mg; administer intravenously over 30 minutes in a volume of 0.9% NS or D5W sufficient to produce a pembrolizumab concentration within the range 1–10 mg/mL every 6 weeks for up to 12 months (total dose/6-week cycle = 400 mg)

- Administer pembrolizumab with an administration set that contains a sterile, non-pyrogenic, low-protein-binding in-line or add-on filter with pore size within the range of 0.2–5 μm
- Pembrolizumab can cause severe or life-threatening infusion-related reactions, including hypersensitivity and anaphylaxis

Supportive Care
Antiemetic prophylaxis
Emetogenic potential is **MINIMAL**
See Chapter 42 for antiemetic recommendations

Hematopoietic growth factor (CSF) prophylaxis
Primary prophylaxis is **NOT** indicated
See Chapter 43 for more information

Antimicrobial prophylaxis
Risk of fever and neutropenia is **LOW**
Antimicrobial primary prophylaxis to be considered:
- Antibacterial—not indicated
- Antifungal—not indicated
- Antiviral—not indicated unless patient previously had an episode of HSV

Patient Population Studied

An international, multicenter, randomized, double-blind, placebo-controlled, phase 3 study (EORTC 1325) involving 1019 patients with resected, histologically confirmed, high-risk, Stage III melanoma with metastasis to regional lymph nodes. Eligible patients were aged ≥18 years, had an Eastern Cooperative Oncology Group (ECOG) performance status score of ≤1, and had undergone complete regional lymphadenectomy within 13 weeks before start of treatment. Patients who had previously received a systemic therapy for melanoma were not eligible for inclusion in the study. Participants were randomly assigned in a 1:1 ratio to receive pembrolizumab or placebo for 1 year

Efficacy (N = 1019)

	Pembrolizumab (N = 514)	Control (N = 505)	HR (95% CI); P Value
Relapse-free survival at 12 months	75.4%	61.0%	0.57 (0.43–0.74); P<0.001

Note: Median duration of follow-up was 14.7 months in the pembrolizumab group and 15.4 months in the placebo group

Therapy Monitoring

1. Initially at the time of each dose, and eventually every 6–12 weeks, perform a total body skin examination with attention to ALL mucous membranes as well as a complete review of systems

2. Monitor patients for signs and symptoms of pneumonitis. Evaluate patients with suspected pneumonitis with chest x-ray, CT, and pulse oximetry. For ≥2 toxicity, may include nasal swab, sputum culture and sensitivity, blood culture and sensitivity, and urine culture and sensitivity

3. Monitor patients for signs and symptoms of colitis. Encourage patients to report diarrhea immediately to any member of the health care team

4. Draw AST, ALT, and bilirubin prior to each infusion and/or weekly if there are Grade 1 liver function test elevations. Note, no treatment is recommended for G1 LFT abnormalities. For ≥2 toxicity, work up for other causes of elevated LFTs including viral hepatitis

5. Use basic metabolic panel (Na, K, CO_2, glucose) and patient history as screening tools for hypophysitis including hypopituitarism and adrenal insufficiency. If in doubt, evaluate AM adrenocorticotropic hormone (ACTH) and cortisol levels. Consider ACTH stimulation test for indeterminate results

6. Assess thyroid function at the start of treatment, periodically during treatment, and as indicated based on clinical evaluation and for clinical signs and symptoms of thyroid disorders. Test for TSH and free thyroxine (FT4) every 4–6 weeks as part of routine clinical monitoring of therapy or for case detection in symptomatic patients

7. Measure glucose at baseline and with each treatment during the first 12 weeks and every 6 weeks thereafter

8. Obtain a serum creatinine prior to every dose. If creatinine is found to be newly elevated, consider holding therapy while other potential causes are evaluated. Note, routine urinalysis is not necessary other than to rule out urinary tract infections, etc

9. Obtain a complete rheumatologic history and perform an examination of all peripheral joints for tenderness, swelling, and range of motion. Examine the spine. Consider plain x-ray/imaging to exclude metastases and evaluate joint damage (erosions), if appropriate

10. In patients at high risk for infections and in appropriately selected patients based on an infectious disease evaluation, draw screening laboratories (HIV, hepatitis A and B, and blood QuantiFERON for TB) to prepare patients to start infliximab

Treatment Modifications

RECOMMENDED DOSE MODIFICATIONS FOR PEMBROLIZUMAB

Adverse Event	Grade/Severity	Treatment Modification
Infusion reaction	Clinically significant but not severe infusion reaction	Interrupt the infusion in patients with clinically significant infusion reactions and consider resuming at a slower rate following resolution. If decision is made to restart, begin at ≤50% of the rate prior to the reaction and increase in 50% increments every 30 minutes if well tolerated. Infusions may be restarted at the full rate during the next cycle
	G3/4 (severe infusion reaction—pyrexia, chills, flushing, hypotension, dyspnea, wheezing, back pain, abdominal pain, and urticaria). Not rapidly responsive to brief interruption of infusion	Stop infusion and administer appropriate medical therapy (eg, epinephrine, corticosteroids, intravenous antihistamines, bronchodilators, and/or oxygen). Discontinue pembrolizumab
Colitis	G1	Loperamide 4 mg as starting dose then 2 mg before each meal and after each loose stool until without diarrhea for 12 hours, with maximum of 16 mg loperamide per day. If G1 diarrhea or colitis persists >14 days, then add prednisolone 0.5–1 mg/kg (non-enteric-coated) or consider oral budesonide 9 mg daily if no bloody diarrhea
	G2/3 diarrhea or colitis	Withhold pembrolizumab. Loperamide 4 mg as starting dose then 2 mg before each meal and after each loose stool until without diarrhea for 12 hours, with maximum of 16 mg loperamide per day. Administer oral prednisone/prednisolone at a dose of 0.5–2 mg/kg/day or its equivalent. When improves to G1, begin a slow corticosteroid taper over at least 4 weeks. Resume pembrolizumab upon symptom control, or when prednisone/prednisolone daily dose <10 mg
	G4 diarrhea or colitis	Permanently discontinue pembrolizumab. Loperamide 4 mg as starting dose then 2 mg before each meal and after each loose stool until without diarrhea for 12 hours, with maximum of 16 mg loperamide per day. Administer 1–2 mg/kg intravenously (methyl)prednisolone and convert to 0.5–2 mg/kg prednisone/prednisolone orally each day or its equivalent only after a response. Taper over at least 4 weeks when symptoms improve. If does not improve over 72 hours or worsens, perform flexible sigmoidoscopy/colonoscopy to document colitis then begin infliximab 5 mg/kg (if no perforation/sepsis/TB/hepatitis/NYHA III/IV CHF). If no response, add MMF 500–1000 mg twice daily. If worse on MMF, consider addition of tacrolimus or ATG
Pneumonitis	G2	Withhold pembrolizumab. Consider *Pneumocystis* prophylaxis depending on the clinical context and coverage with empiric antibiotics. Administer oral prednisone/prednisolone at a dose of 1–2 mg/kg/day or its equivalent. When improves to G1, begin a slow corticosteroid taper over at least 4 weeks. If does not respond adequately after 48 hours, then administer 2–4 mg/kg intravenously (methyl)prednisolone and convert to 0.5–2 mg/kg prednisone/prednisolone orally each day or its equivalent only after a response, followed by a taper over at least 6 weeks when symptoms improve to G1, titrating to symptoms. Resume pembrolizumab upon symptom control, or when prednisone/prednisolone daily dose <10 mg
	G3/4	Permanently discontinue pembrolizumab. Consider *Pneumocystis* prophylaxis depending on the clinical context; cover with empiric antibiotics. Administer 2–4 mg/kg intravenously (methyl)prednisolone and convert to 1–2 mg/kg prednisone/prednisolone orally each day or its equivalent only after a response, followed by a taper over at least 8 weeks when symptoms improve to G1, titrating to symptoms. If when initially treated improvement does not occur within 48–72 hours, begin infliximab 5 mg/kg (if no perforation/sepsis/TB/hepatitis/NYHA III/IV CHF). If no response to infliximab, add MMF 500–1000 mg twice daily. Consider MMF especially if has concurrent hepatic toxicity

(continued)

Treatment Modifications (*continued*)

RECOMMENDED DOSE MODIFICATIONS FOR PEMBROLIZUMAB

Adverse Event	Grade/Severity	Treatment Modification
Hepatitis	G2 (AST or ALT >3–5× ULN or total bilirubin >1.5–3× ULN)	Withhold pembrolizumab. Administer oral prednisone/prednisolone at a dose of 1–2 mg/kg/day or its equivalent. When improves to G1, begin a slow corticosteroid taper over at least 4 weeks. Resume pembrolizumab upon symptom control, or when prednisone/prednisolone daily dose <10 mg
	G3/4 (AST or ALT >5× ULN or total bilirubin >3× ULN)	Permanently discontinue pembrolizumab. Administer 1–2 mg/kg intravenously (methyl)prednisolone and convert to 0.5–2 mg/kg prednisone/prednisolone orally each day or its equivalent only after a response. Taper over at least 6 weeks when symptoms improve. If no response, add MMF 500–1000 mg twice daily. If worse on MMF, consider adding tacrolimus or ATG
Hypophysitis	G2/3 (moderate symptoms, ie, headache but no visual disturbance or fatigue/mood alteration but hemodynamically stable, no electrolyte disturbance)	Administer analgesia as needed for headache. Withhold pembrolizumab. Administer oral prednisone/prednisolone at a dose of 0.5–2 mg/kg/day or its equivalent. When improves to G1, begin a slow corticosteroid taper over at least 4 weeks. If no improvement in 48 hours, administer 1–2 mg/kg intravenously (methyl)prednisolone and convert to 0.5–2 mg/kg prednisone/prednisolone orally each day or its equivalent only after a response. Taper over at least 4 weeks when symptoms improve to 5 mg prednisone/prednisolone or equivalent; do not stop steroids. Resume pembrolizumab upon symptom control, or when prednisone/prednisolone daily dose <10 mg
	G4 (severe mass effect symptoms, ie, severe headache, any visual disturbance or severe hypoadrenalism, ie, hypotension, severe electrolyte disturbance)	Permanently discontinue pembrolizumab. Administer analgesia as needed for headache. Administer 1–2 mg/kg intravenously (methyl)prednisolone and convert to 0.5–2 mg/kg prednisone/prednisolone orally each day or its equivalent only after a response. Taper over at least 4 weeks when symptoms improve to 5 mg prednisone/prednisolone or equivalent; do not stop steroids
Adrenal insufficiency	G2	Withhold pembrolizumab. Administer oral prednisone/prednisolone at a dose of 0.5–2 mg/kg/day or its equivalent. When improves to G1, begin a slow corticosteroid taper over at least 4 weeks. Serially assess adrenal function and continue steroids at replacement doses (20–40 mg hydrocortisone daily ~2/3 dose in AM upon awakening and ~1/3 at 4 PM) until recovery of adrenal function is documented. Resume pembrolizumab upon symptom control, or when prednisone/prednisolone daily dose <10 mg
	G3/4	Permanently discontinue pembrolizumab. Administer oral prednisone/prednisolone at a dose of 0.5–2 mg/kg/day or its equivalent. When improves to G1, begin a slow corticosteroid taper over at least 4 weeks. Serially assess adrenal function and continue steroids at replacement doses (20–40 mg hydrocortisone daily ~2/3 dose in AM upon awakening and ~1/3 at 4 PM) until recovery of adrenal function is documented
Type 1 diabetes mellitus	G3 hyperglycemia	Withhold pembrolizumab. Admit to hospital to manage hyperglycemia. Role of corticosteroids in preventing complete loss of insulin-producing cells is unknown and not recommended. Resume pembrolizumab upon symptom control, or when prednisone/prednisolone daily dose <10 mg
	G4 hyperglycemia	Permanently discontinue pembrolizumab. Admit to hospital to manage hyperglycemia. Role of corticosteroids in preventing complete loss of insulin-producing cells is unknown and not recommended
Nephritis and renal dysfunction	G2/3 (serum creatinine 1.5–6× ULN)	Withhold pembrolizumab. Administer oral prednisone/prednisolone at a dose of 0.5–2 mg/kg/day or its equivalent. When improves to G1, begin a slow corticosteroid taper over at least 4 weeks. If does not respond adequately, then administer 0.5–1 mg/kg intravenously (methyl)prednisolone and convert to 0.5–2 mg/kg prednisone/prednisolone orally each day or its equivalent only after a response, followed by a taper over at least 4 weeks when improves to G1. Resume pembrolizumab upon symptom control, or when prednisone/prednisolone daily dose <10 mg
	G4 (serum creatinine >6× ULN)	Permanently discontinue pembrolizumab. Administer 0.5–1 mg/kg intravenously (methyl)prednisolone and convert to 0.5–2 mg/kg prednisone/prednisolone orally each day or its equivalent only after a response, followed by a taper over at least 4 weeks when improves to G1

(*continued*)

Treatment Modifications (*continued*)

RECOMMENDED DOSE MODIFICATIONS FOR PEMBROLIZUMAB

Adverse Event	Grade/Severity	Treatment Modification
Skin	G1/2	Continue pembrolizumab. Avoid skin irritants, avoid sun exposure, topical emollients recommended. Topical steroid (mild strength for G1, moderate/potent strength for G2) cream once or twice daily ± oral or topical antihistamines for itching
	G3 rash or suspected SJS or TEN	Withhold pembrolizumab. Avoid skin irritants, avoid sun exposure, topical emollients recommended. Administer oral or topical antihistamines for itching. Administer oral prednisone/prednisolone at a dose of 0.5–2 mg/kg or its equivalent daily for 3 days followed by a slow corticosteroid taper over at least 4 weeks when the rash improves to G1. If does not respond adequately, then administer 0.5–1 mg/kg intravenously (methyl) prednisolone and convert to 0.5–2 mg/kg prednisone/prednisolone orally each day or its equivalent only after a response, followed by a taper over at least 4 weeks when the rash improves to G1. Resume pembrolizumab upon symptom control, or when prednisone/prednisolone daily dose <10 mg
	G4 rash or confirmed SJS or TEN	Avoid skin irritants, avoid sun exposure, topical emollients recommended. Administer oral or topical antihistamines for itching. Administer 1–2 mg/kg intravenously (methyl) prednisolone and convert to oral steroids 0.5–2 mg/kg prednisone/prednisolone each day or its equivalent only after a response. Taper over at least 4 weeks when the rash improves to G1. Permanently discontinue pembrolizumab
Encephalitis	Confusion or altered behavior, headaches, alteration in Glasgow Coma Scale, motor or sensory deficits, speech abnormality, may or may not be febrile	Initially withhold pembrolizumab, but permanently discontinue pembrolizumab if there is no doubt as to diagnosis. Exclude bacterial and ideally viral infections prior to high-dose steroids. Administer oral prednisone/prednisolone at a dose of 0.5–2 mg/kg/day or its equivalent. When symptoms improve, begin a slow corticosteroid taper over at least 4–8 weeks. If symptoms are severe, administer 1–2 mg/kg intravenously (methyl) prednisolone and convert to 0.5–2 mg/kg prednisone/prednisolone orally each day or its equivalent only after a response. Consider concurrent empiric antiviral (intravenous acyclovir) and antibacterial therapy
Aseptic meningitis	Headache, photophobia, neck stiffness with fever or may be afebrile, vomiting; normal cognition/cerebral function (distinguishes from encephalitis)	
Other syndromes include neurosarcoidosis, posterior reversible leukoencephalopathy syndrome (PRES), Vogt-Koyanagi-Harada syndrome, demyelination, vasculitic encephalopathy, and generalized seizures		
Transverse myelitis	Acute or subacute neurologic signs/symptoms of motor/sensory/autonomic origin; most have sensory level; often bilateral symptoms	Initially withhold pembrolizumab, but permanently discontinue pembrolizumab if there is no doubt as to diagnosis. Administer 2 mg/kg intravenously (methyl)prednisolone or consider 1 g/day and convert to 0.5–2 mg/kg prednisone/prednisolone orally each day or its equivalent only after a response. When symptoms improve, begin a slow corticosteroid taper over at least 4–8 weeks. Plasmapheresis may be required if steroids do not bring about improvement
Myocarditis	G3	Permanently discontinue pembrolizumab. Administer 2 mg/kg intravenously (methyl) prednisolone or consider 1 g/day and convert to 0.5–2 mg/kg prednisone/prednisolone orally each day or its equivalent only after a response. When symptoms improve, begin a slow corticosteroid taper over at least 4–8 weeks. If no response, add MMF 500–1000 mg twice daily. If worse on MMF, consider adding tacrolimus
Peripheral neurologic toxicity	Moderate: some interference with ADL, symptoms concerning to patient	Withhold pembrolizumab. Initial observation reasonable or initiate prednisone/prednisolone 0.5–1 mg/kg (if progressing, eg, from mild) and/or pregabalin or duloxetine for pain. When symptoms improve, begin a slow corticosteroid taper over at least 4 weeks. Resume pembrolizumab upon symptom control, or when prednisone/prednisolone daily dose <10 mg
	Severe: limits self-care and aids warranted, life-threatening, eg, respiratory problems	Permanently discontinue pembrolizumab. Administer 1–2 mg/kg intravenously (methyl) prednisolone and convert to 0.5–2 mg/kg prednisone/prednisolone orally each day or its equivalent only after a response. Taper over at least 4–8 weeks when symptoms improve to G1

(*continued*)

Treatment Modifications (*continued*)

RECOMMENDED DOSE MODIFICATIONS FOR PEMBROLIZUMAB

Adverse Event	Grade/Severity	Treatment Modification
Guillain-Barré syndrome	Progressive symmetrical muscle weakness with absent or reduced tendon reflexes—involves extremities, facial, respiratory, and bulbar and oculomotor muscles; dysregulation of autonomic nerves	Permanently discontinue pembrolizumab. Use of steroids not recommended in idiopathic Guillain-Barré syndrome; however, a trial of (methyl)prednisolone 1–2 mg/kg is reasonable, converting to 0.5–2 mg/kg prednisone/prednisolone orally each day or its equivalent only after a response. If no improvement or worsening, plasmapheresis or IVIG indicated
Myasthenia gravis	Fluctuating muscle weakness (proximal limb, trunk, ocular, eg, ptosis/diplopia or bulbar) with fatigability, respiratory muscles may also be involved	Permanently discontinue pembrolizumab. Administer pyridostigmine at an initial dose of 30 mg three times daily. Administer oral prednisone/prednisolone at a dose of 0.5–2 mg/kg/day or its equivalent or 1–2 mg/kg intravenously (methyl)prednisolone depending on the severity of symptoms. If begin with intravenous, convert to 0.5–2 mg/kg prednisone/prednisolone orally each day or its equivalent only after a response. If no improvement or worsening, plasmapheresis or IVIG may be considered. Additional immunosuppressants used in myasthenia gravis include azathioprine, cyclosporine, and mycophenolate. Avoid certain medications, eg, ciprofloxacin, beta-blockers, that may precipitate cholinergic crisis
Other syndromes including motor and sensory peripheral neuropathy, multifocal radicular neuropathy/plexopathy, autonomic neuropathy, phrenic nerve palsy, cranial nerve palsies (eg, facial nerve, optic nerve, hypoglossal nerve)		Permanently discontinue pembrolizumab. Administer oral prednisone/prednisolone at a dose of 0.5–2 mg/kg/day or its equivalent or 1–2 mg/kg intravenously (methyl)prednisolone depending on the severity of symptoms. If begin with intravenous, convert to 0.5–2 mg/kg prednisone/prednisolone orally each day or its equivalent only after a response
Arthralgia	G1 (mild pain with inflammation, erythema, or joint swelling)	Continue pembrolizumab. Administer acetaminophen (paracetamol) and ibuprofen
	G2 (moderate pain with inflammation, erythema, or joint swelling that limits ADLs)	Withhold pembrolizumab. Administer higher doses of acetaminophen (paracetamol) and ibuprofen and use diclofenac or naproxen or etoricoxib. If inadequately controlled, consider intra-articular steroid injections for large joints or administer oral prednisone/prednisolone at a dose of 0.5–2 mg/kg/day or its equivalent. When improves to G1, begin a slow corticosteroid taper over at least 4 weeks. If does not respond adequately, then administer 0.5–1 mg/kg intravenously (methyl)prednisolone and convert to 0.5–2 mg/kg prednisone/prednisolone orally each day or its equivalent only after a response, followed by a taper over at least 4 weeks when improves to G1. Resume pembrolizumab upon symptom control, or when prednisone/prednisolone daily dose <10 mg
	G3 (severe pain; irreversible joint damage; disabling; limits self-care ADL)	Withhold pembrolizumab. Administer 0.5–1 mg/kg intravenously (methyl)prednisolone and convert to 0.5–2 mg/kg prednisone/prednisolone orally each day or its equivalent only after a response, followed by a taper over at least 4 weeks when improves to G1. In severe cases, infliximab or another anti–TNF-alpha drug may be required for improvement of arthritis. Resume pembrolizumab upon symptom control, or when prednisone/prednisolone daily dose <10 mg
Other	First occurrence of other G3	Withhold pembrolizumab. Administer oral prednisone/prednisolone at a dose of 0.5–2 mg/kg/day or its equivalent. When improves to G1, begin a slow corticosteroid taper over at least 4 weeks. Resume pembrolizumab upon symptom control, or when prednisone/prednisolone daily dose <10 mg
	Recurrence of same G3	Permanently discontinue pembrolizumab. Administer 1–2 mg/kg intravenously (methyl)prednisolone and convert to 0.5–2 mg/kg prednisone/prednisolone orally each day or its equivalent only after a response. Taper over at least 4–8 weeks when symptoms improve to G1
	Life-threatening or G4	
	Requirement for ≥10 mg/day prednisone or equivalent for >12 weeks	Permanently discontinue pembrolizumab
	Persistent G2/3 adverse reactions lasting ≥12 weeks	

ADL, activities of daily living; ALT, alanine aminotransferase; AST, aspartate aminotransferase; ATG, anti-thymocyte globulin; SJS, Stevens-Johnson Syndrome; TEN, toxic epidermal necrolysis; ULN, upper limit of normal

Notes on general supportive care:
• Steroid taper in most cases will proceed over a minimum of 1 month but if symptoms improve rapidly, a 2-week taper can be considered. If steroids are administered for more than 4 weeks, consider PCP prophylaxis (cotrimoxazole 480 mg twice daily M/W/F or inhaled pentamidine if has cotrimoxazole allergy), regular random blood glucose, VitD level, and starting calcium/VitD supplementation per guidelines

Adverse Events (N = 1011)

Grade (%)*	Pembrolizumab (N = 509)		Control (N = 502)	
	Grade 1–2	Grade ≥3	Grade 1–2	Grade ≥3
Any adverse event	63	15	63	3
Fatigue or asthenia	36	<1	33	<1
Skin reactions	28	<1	18	0
Diarrhea	18	<1	16	<1
Pruritus	18	0	10	0
Rash	16	<1	11	0
Arthralgia	11	<1	11	0
Nausea	11	0	9	0
Dyspnea	6	<1	3	0

*According to the National Cancer Institute Common Terminology Criteria for Adverse Events, version 4.0
Note: Treatment-related adverse events that occurred in ≥10% of patients or that were considered medically relevant are included in the table. Treatment-related adverse events resulting in study discontinuation occurred in 13% of the pembrolizumab group and 2% of the controls. One patient in the pembrolizumab group died owing to treatment-related myositis

ADJUVANT

MELANOMA REGIMEN: DABRAFENIB + TRAMETINIB

Long GV et al. N Engl J Med 2017;377(19):1813–1823
Protocol for: Long GV et al. N Engl J Med 2017;377(19):1813–1823
Supplementary appendix to: Long GV et al. N Engl J Med 2017;377(19):1813–1823

Dabrafenib 150 mg per dose; administer orally twice daily, at least 1 hour before or 2 hours after meals, continuously for 1 year (total dose/week = 2100 mg), *plus:*

Treatment notes:
- Advise patients NOT to open, crush, or break dabrafenib capsules
- Missed doses may be taken up to 6 hours before a subsequently scheduled dose
- Dabrafenib is a substrate for metabolism catalyzed by CYP2C8 and CYP3A4. Avoid concomitant use of dabrafenib with strong CYP3A4 or strong CYP2C8 inhibitors (eg, ketoconazole, nefazodone, clarithromycin, gemfibrozil), when possible. If concomitant use of a strong CYP3A4 or CYP2C8 inhibitor is unavoidable, monitor closely for toxicities. If concomitant use of a strong CYP3A4 or strong CYP2C8 inducer (eg, rifampin, phenytoin, carbamazepine, phenobarbital, St John's wort) is unavoidable, monitor closely for loss of efficacy
- Dabrafenib has been shown in experimental studies in vitro to induce CYP3A4 and CYP2C9. As a result, dabrafenib decreases systemic exposure to *S*-warfarin and *R*-warfarin. Monitor international normalized ratio (INR) levels closely in patients receiving warfarin during the initiation or discontinuation of dabrafenib

Trametinib 2 mg per dose; administer orally once daily, at least 1 hour before or 2 hours after a meal at approximately the same time each day, continuously for 1 year (total dose/week = 14 mg)

Treatment note:
- Missed doses may be taken up to 12 hours before a subsequently scheduled dose

Supportive Care
Antiemetic prophylaxis
Emetogenic potential is **LOW**
See Chapter 42 for antiemetic recommendations

Hematopoietic growth factor (CSF) prophylaxis
Primary prophylaxis is **NOT** indicated
See Chapter 43 for more information

Antimicrobial prophylaxis
Risk of fever and neutropenia is **LOW**
Antimicrobial primary prophylaxis to be considered:
- Antibacterial—not indicated
- Antifungal—not indicated
- Antiviral—not indicated unless patient previously had an episode of HSV

Patient Population Studied

An international, multicenter, randomized, double-blind, placebo-controlled, phase 3 study (COMBI-AD) involving 870 patients with histologically confirmed Stage III BRAF^{V600}-mutant melanoma that had been completely surgically resected. Eligible patients were aged ≥18 years, had an Eastern Cooperative Oncology Group (ECOG) performance status score of ≤1, and had undergone complete regional lymphadenectomy within 12 weeks before randomization. Patients who had previously received a systemic anticancer therapy or radiotherapy for melanoma were not eligible for inclusion in the study. Participants were randomly assigned to receive oral dabrafenib + trametinib or matching placebo tablets for 12 months

Therapy Monitoring

1. *Prior to the start of therapy in women of childbearing potential:* pregnancy test
2. *Prior to the start of therapy and repeated every 2 months during therapy and for 6 months after cessation of therapy:* dermatologic evaluation
3. *Prior to the start of therapy, 1 month after the start of therapy, and then every 2–3 months while on therapy:* assess left ventricular ejection fraction
4. *Periodically:*
   a. Monitor for signs and symptoms of uveitis (eg, changes in vision, photophobia, ocular pain) and perform an ophthalmologic examination in patients with new visual symptoms
   b. Monitor for febrile reactions and advise patients to promptly report fevers
   c. Monitor blood glucose at baseline and then as clinically necessary, especially in patients with pre-existing diabetes mellitus or hyperglycemia
   d. Monitor for signs and symptoms of colitis and/or gastrointestinal perforation
   e. Monitor for signs and symptoms of venous thromboembolism
   f. Monitor for signs and symptoms of hemorrhage
   g. In patients with known glucose-6-phosphate dehydrogenase deficiency, monitor for signs of hemolytic anemia
   h. Monitor for signs and symptoms of interstitial lung disease

Efficacy (N = 870)

	Dabrafenib + Trametinib (n = 438)	Control (n = 432)	HR (95% CI); P Value
Relapse-free survival rate	62%	43%	0.47 (0.39–0.58); P<0.001
Overall survival rate	86%	78%	0.57 (0.42–0.79); P = 0.0006
Distant-metastasis-free survival	75%	65%	0.51 (0.40–0.65); P<0.001

Note: Minimum follow-up was 2.5 years. Median duration of follow-up was 2.8 years. By clinical data cut-off, the median relapse-free survival had not been reached in the combination group and was 16.6 months in the placebo group

Treatment Modifications

DABRAFENIB + TRAMETINIB

Dabrafenib

Starting dose	150 mg by mouth twice a day
Dose Level −1	100 mg by mouth twice a day
Dose Level −2	75 mg by mouth twice a day
Dose Level −3	50 mg by mouth twice a day
Dose Level −4	Permanently discontinue dabrafenib

Trametinib

Starting dose	2 mg by mouth once daily
Dose Level −1	1.5 mg by mouth once daily
Dose Level −2	1 mg by mouth once daily
Dose Level −3	Permanently discontinue trametinib

Adverse Event	Dose Modification
New Primary Malignancy Adverse Events	
New primary non-cutaneous RAS mutation–positive malignancy	Permanently discontinue dabrafenib. Continue trametinib without modification, if appropriate
New primary non-melanoma cutaneous malignancy	Continue dabrafenib and trametinib at the same dose. Refer patient to dermatologist for management of non-melanoma cutaneous malignancy
Cardiac Adverse Events	
Asymptomatic, absolute decrease in LVEF of ≥10% but <20% from baseline that is below LLN	Interrupt trametinib for up to 4 weeks. If LVEF improves to ≥LLN, then resume trametinib at one lower dose level. If LVEF does not improve to ≥ LLN, then permanently discontinue trametinib. Continue dabrafenib without modification
Symptomatic CHF Absolute decrease in LVEF by ≥20% from baseline that is below LLN	Permanently discontinue trametinib. Interrupt dabrafenib. If LVEF improves to ≥LLN and an absolute decrease ≤10% compared to baseline, then resume dabrafenib at the same dose
Ocular Adverse Events	
Patient reports loss of vision or other visual disturbances.	Interrupt dabrafenib and trametinib until ophthalmologic status is clarified. Urgently (within 24 hours) perform ophthalmologic evaluation
Uveitis, including iritis and iridocyclitis	If mild or moderate uveitis does not respond to ocular therapy, or for severe uveitis, interrupt dabrafenib for up to 6 weeks. If improved to G0/1, then resume at the same dose or at a lower dose level. If G ≥2 uveitis persists for >6 weeks, then permanently discontinue dabrafenib. Continue trametinib without modification
Retinal pigment epithelial detachments	Interrupt trametinib for up to 3 weeks. If improved, resume trametinib at the same or lower dose level. If not improved, then resume trametinib at one lower dose level, or permanently discontinue trametinib. Continue dabrafenib without modification
Retinal vein occlusion	Permanently discontinue trametinib. Continue dabrafenib without modification
Pulmonary Adverse Events	
Dyspnea, cough, fever, and radiologic abnormalities—pneumonitis is suspected	Interrupt trametinib until pulmonary status is clarified. Continue dabrafenib without modification
Interstitial lung disease/pneumonitis is confirmed	Permanently discontinue trametinib. Continue dabrafenib without modification

(*continued*)

Treatment Modifications (continued)

Febrile Adverse Events

Fever of 38.5°C to 40°C	Interrupt dabrafenib and trametinib until fever resolves. Increase fluid intake and administer antipyretics (eg, acetaminophen) as needed. Consider monitoring renal function as clinically indicated. Upon resolution of fever, resume dabrafenib at the same or a lower dose level and resume trametinib at the same dose
Fever of >40°C	Interrupt dabrafenib and trametinib until fever resolves. Increase fluid intake, administer antipyretics (eg, acetaminophen) as needed, and monitor renal function closely. Upon resolution of fever, resume dabrafenib at a lower dose level along with prophylactic antipyretics, or permanently discontinue dabrafenib. Upon resolution of fever, resume trametinib at the same or a lower dose level
Fever ≥38.5°C complicated by rigors, hypotension, dehydration, or renal failure	Interrupt dabrafenib and trametinib until fever resolves. Increase fluid intake, administer antipyretics (eg, acetaminophen) as needed, and monitor renal function closely. Administer corticosteroids (eg, prednisone 10 mg daily) for ≥5 days if there is no evidence of active infection. Upon resolution of fever, resume dabrafenib at a lower dose level along with prophylactic antipyretics, or permanently discontinue dabrafenib. Upon resolution of fever, resume trametinib at the same or a lower dose level
Recurrent fever ≥38.5°C	Interrupt dabrafenib and trametinib until fever resolves. Increase fluid intake and administer antipyretics (eg, acetaminophen) as needed. In the absence of evidence of active infection, administer corticosteroids (eg, prednisone 10 mg daily) for ≥5 days if fever persists for >3 days or if fever is associated with complications such as dehydration, hypotension, renal failure, or severe chills/rigors. Upon resolution of fever, resume dabrafenib at a lower dose level along with prophylactic antipyretics, or permanently discontinue dabrafenib. Upon resolution of fever, resume trametinib at the same dose level, or optionally at a lower dose level if temperature was ≥40°C or associated with complications

Dermatologic Adverse Events

Intolerable G2 dermatologic toxicity G3/4 dermatologic toxicity	Interrupt dabrafenib and trametinib for up to 3 weeks. If improved, resume dabrafenib at one lower dose level and resume trametinib at one lower dose level. If not improved, permanently discontinue both dabrafenib and trametinib

Hemorrhagic Adverse Events

G3 hemorrhage	Interrupt dabrafenib and trametinib. If bleeding is improved to G0/1, resume dabrafenib at the next lower dose level and resume trametinib at the next lower dose level
G4 hemorrhage	Permanently discontinue dabrafenib and trametinib

Venous Thromboembolism Events

Uncomplicated DVT or PE	Interrupt trametinib for up to 3 weeks. If improved to G0/1 within 3 weeks, resume trametinib at one lower dose level. Continue dabrafenib without modification
Life-threatening PE	Permanently discontinue trametinib. Interrupt dabrafenib until toxicity resolves to G0/1, then resume at a lower dose level, or permanently discontinue dabrafenib

Other Adverse Events

Other intolerable G2 toxicities*† Other G3 toxicities*†	Interrupt dabrafenib and trametinib. If improved to G0/1, resume dabrafenib at one lower dose level and resume trametinib at one lower dose level. If not improved, permanently discontinue dabrafenib and trametinib
First occurrence of any other G4 toxicity*†	Interrupt dabrafenib and trametinib until toxicity improves to G0/1. If toxicity improves to G0/1, then resume at dabrafenib at one lower dose level or permanently discontinue dabrafenib. If toxicity improves to G0/1, then resume trametinib at one lower dose level or permanently discontinue trametinib
Recurrent other G4 toxicity*†	Permanently discontinue dabrafenib and trametinib
Known G6PD deficiency	Monitor closely for hemolytic anemia with dabrafenib

Note: Advise patients of potential risk to a fetus with dabrafenib and trametinib and to use effective contraception. Advise female patients of reproductive potential to use an effective *nonhormonal* method of contraception during dabrafenib treatment and for 2 weeks after the last dabrafenib dose, since dabrafenib can render hormonal contraceptives ineffective. Advise female patients to use effective contraception during treatment with trametinib and for 4 months after the last trametinib dose

(continued)

Treatment Modifications (*continued*)

*Dose modifications are not recommended for dabrafenib when administered with trametinib for the following adverse reactions attributable to trametinib: retinal vein occlusion, retinal pigment epithelial detachment, interstitial lung disease/pneumonitis, and uncomplicated venous thromboembolism. Dose modification of dabrafenib is not required for new primary cutaneous malignancies

†Dose modifications are not recommended for trametinib when administered with dabrafenib for the following adverse reactions attributable to dabrafenib: noncutaneous malignancies and uveitis. Dose modification of trametinib is not required for new primary cutaneous malignancies

LVEF, left ventricular ejection fraction; LLN, lower limit of normal; CHF, congestive heart failure; G6PD, glucose-6-phosphate dehydrogenase; DVT, deep vein thrombosis; PE, pulmonary embolism

Tafinlar (dabrafenib) prescribing information. East Hanover, NJ: Novartis Pharmaceuticals Corporation; revised 2018 May
Mekinist (trametinib) prescribing information. East Hanover, NJ: Novartis Pharmaceuticals Corporation; revised 2018 May

Adverse Events (N = 867)

Grade (%)*	Dabrafenib + Trametinib N = 435)		Control (N = 432)	
	Grade 1–2	Grade 3–4	Grade 1–2	Grade 3–4
Any adverse event	56	41	74	14
Pyrexia	57	5	10	<1
Fatigue	43	4	28	<1
Nausea	39	<1	20	0
Headache	38	1	24	0
Chills	36	1	4	0
Diarrhea	32	<1	15	<1
Vomiting	27	<1	10	0
Arthralgia	27	<1	14	0
Rash	24	0	11	<1
Cough	17	0	8	0
Myalgia	16	<1	9	0
Increased alanine aminotransferase level	12	4	1	<1
Influenza-like illness	15	<1	7	0
Increased aspartate aminotransferase level	11	4	1	<1
Pain in limb	13	<1	9	0
Asthenia	13	<1	9	<1
Peripheral edema	13	<1	4	0
Dry skin	13	0	7	0
Dermatitis acneiform	12	<1	2	0
Constipation	12	0	6	0
Hypertension	6	6	6	2
Decreased appetite	11	<1	6	0
Erythema	11	0	3	0

*According to the National Cancer Institute Common Terminology Criteria for Adverse Events, version 4.0
Note: Adverse events that were reported for >10% of patients in the combination therapy group are included in the table. One fatal adverse event (pneumonia) was reported in the combination therapy group. Adverse events leading to permanent discontinuation of the trial drug occurred in 26% of the combination therapy group and 3% of the placebo group

ADJUVANT

MELANOMA REGIMEN: INTERFERON ALFA–2B

Kirkwood JM et al. J Clin Oncol 1996;14:7–17 [Trial E1684]

Interferon alfa–2b 20 million units/m^2 per dose; administer intravenously over 20 minutes in 0.9% sodium chloride injection (0.9% NS), sufficient to produce a solution with an interferon concentration ≥10 million units/100 mL, 5 consecutive days/week for 4 weeks (total dosage/week = 100 million units/m^2), *then:*

Interferon alfa–2b 10 million units/m^2 per dose; administer subcutaneously 3 days/week for 48 weeks (total dosage/week = 30 million units/m^2)

Supportive Care
Antiemetic prophylaxis
Emetogenic potential is **MINIMAL**
See Chapter 42 for antiemetic recommendations

Hematopoietic growth factor (CSF) prophylaxis
Primary prophylaxis is **NOT** *indicated*
See Chapter 43 for more information

Antimicrobial prophylaxis
Risk of fever and neutropenia is **LOW**
  Antimicrobial primary prophylaxis to be considered:
  • Antibacterial—not indicated
  • Antifungal—not indicated
  • Antiviral—not indicated unless patient previously had an episode of HSV

Treatment Modifications

Adverse Event	Dose Modification
First occurrence of a DLT*	Hold dose until resolution, then reduce interferon alfa dosage by 33%
Second occurrence of a DLT*	Hold dose until resolution, then decrease interferon alfa dosage by 66%
Third occurrence of a DLT*	Discontinue interferon alfa therapy

*Definitions of dose-limiting toxicities (DLTs): hematologic DLT, granulocyte count <500/mm^3; hepatic DLT, SGPT (ALT) or SGOT (AST) >5× ULN (upper limit of normal)

Notes:
1. Dose reductions or delays are usually required at least once for 50% of patients during the IV treatment phase and for 48% during the subcutaneous treatment phase
2. Of patients with appropriate dose reductions, 74–90% continue treatment on protocol for 1 year or until relapse
3. Dose delays and reductions as a result of adverse events occur in 28–44% of patients during the induction phase and in 36–52% of patients during the maintenance phase
4. A response to other adverse events is determined largely by the patient and treating physician. Side effects are rarely life-threatening and should not lead to discontinuation if appropriate and proactive supportive care is provided

Kirkwood JM et al. J Clin Oncol 2002;20:3703–3718

Patient Population Studied

ECOG 1684 was a study of 143 patients with deep primary (T4) or regionally metastatic (N1) cutaneous melanoma who had no evidence of distant metastatic disease or significant medical or psychiatric comorbidity and who had not previously received systemic adjuvant therapy

Efficacy (N = 143)

Median relapse-free survival	1.72 years
Overall median survival	3.8 years
5-year relapse-free survival rate	37%

Three U.S. national cooperative group studies have evaluated the benefit of HDI as an adjuvant for high-risk melanoma. All demonstrate significant and durable reduction in the frequency of relapse, while the first and third trials demonstrated significant improvement in the fraction of patients surviving compared to observation (E1684) or to GMK that was a promising vaccine in 1994. E1684 showed a median relapse-free survival (RFS) of 1.72 years for HDI versus 0.98 year with observation (P1 = 0.0023), and a median OS of 3.82 versus 2.78 years (P1 = 0.0237), respectively. E1694 was closed early, based on analysis demonstrating significantly increased mortality and relapse risk for patients who did not receive HDI. E1690 was inconsistent in that mortality benefit did not track with RFS benefit as it did in the E1684 and E1694 trials, but was unique in that it began before FDA approval of HDI but was completed after FDA approval of HDI for treatment of high-risk melanoma. Not surprisingly, patients who were assigned observation in this trial, where no nodal staging by either elective or sentinel lymph node surgery was required, were associated with systematic crossover from observation to posttrial treatment at nodal relapse with HDI. This may explain why this trial showed RFS, but not OS differences that were observed in the prior and subsequent U.S. Cooperative Group trials. The analysis of each of the foregoing studies has been updated to April 2001, representing a median follow-up of 12.6 years for E1684, where significant clinical benefit of HDI versus observation is evident with respect to RFS (HR = 1.38; P2 = 0.02). Improvement of OS with HDI over observation remains, with diminished magnitude, at this most recent update (HR = 1.22; P2 = 0.18). The changes observed with late reanalysis of this study do not detract from the meaning of the mature observation published at a median follow-up of 6.9 years—considerably longer than many other trial reports. It raises interesting questions regarding competing causes of mortality, because the differences in RFS for the HDI group remain stable out to more than 15 years—and may be a result of deaths from vascular or other events, among the treatment cohort now well into the eighth decade of life (median age now >70 years). In E1694, at a median follow-up of 2.1 years, HDI continued to demonstrate superiority to the GMK in terms of both RFS (HR = 1.33; P2 = 0.006) and OS (HR = 1.32; P2 = 0.04).

Toxicity (N = 143)

	% G1/2	% G3/4
Constitutional*	50	48
Myelosuppression	66	24
Neutropenia		26
Neurologic	55	28
Depression		10
Hepatotoxicity	48	14

*Fever, chills, fatigue, malaise, diaphoresis

Notes:
1. Other adverse effects of IFN alfa-2b: anorexia, weight loss, alopecia, transient mild rash-like erythema, exacerbation of psoriasis, erythema or induration at the site of injection, impaired cognitive function, alternating episodes of manic depression
2. Rare adverse effects of IFN alfa-2b: rhabdomyolysis, delirium, cutaneous necrosis at the site of injection
3. Thyroid dysfunction (hypothyroidism or hyperthyroidism) occurs in 8–20% of patients

Kirkwood JM et al. J Clin Oncol 1996;14:7–17
Kirkwood JM et al. J Clin Oncol 2002;20:3703–3718

Therapy Monitoring

1. *WBC, LFTs, electrolytes, and mineral panel:* Weekly during induction, monthly during maintenance therapy for at least 3 months, then no less frequently than every 3 months in patients who are stable with no new complaints
2. *Other standard tests (eg, serum electrolytes, thyroid-stimulating hormone [TSH] creatine kinase [CK] levels):* Recommended at baseline and at least every 3 months during treatment

Note

Developed as an adjuvant regimen

ADJUVANT

MELANOMA REGIMEN: PEGYLATED INTERFERON ALFA–2B

Eggermont AMM et al. J Clin Oncol 2012;30:3810–3818
Eggermont AMM et al. Lancet 2008;372:117–126

Premedication:
Acetaminophen 650–1000 mg; administer orally 30 minutes before the first dose and as needed prior to subsequent doses of peginterferon alfa-2b
Peginterferon alfa–2b 6 mcg/kg per dose; administer subcutaneously, once weekly for 8 consecutive weeks (induction phase; total dosage/week = 6 mcg/kg), *and then:*
Peginterferon alfa–2b 3 mcg/kg per dose; administer subcutaneously, once weekly for 5 years (maintenance phase; total dosage/week = 3 mcg/kg)

Supportive Care
Antiemetic prophylaxis
Emetogenic potential is **LOW**
See Chapter 42 for antiemetic recommendations

Hematopoietic growth factor (CSF) prophylaxis
Primary prophylaxis is **NOT** indicated
See Chapter 43 for more information

Antimicrobial prophylaxis
Risk of fever and neutropenia is **LOW**
   Antimicrobial primary prophylaxis to be considered:
   • Antibacterial—not indicated
   • Antifungal—not indicated
   • Antiviral—not indicated unless patient previously had an episode of HSV

Treatment Modifications

Adverse Event	Dose Modification
Absolute neutrophil count (ANC) <500/mm³, platelet count <50,000/mm³, ECOG PS ≥2, or nonhematologic toxicity G ≥3	Hold dose until ANC ≥500/mm³, platelet count ≥50,000/mm³, ECOG PS 0–1, and nonhematologic toxicity G ≤1. Then, resume at a reduced dose (see below)
Persistent or worsening severe neuropsychiatric disorders, G4 nonhematologic toxicity, inability to tolerate a dose of 1 mcg/kg per week, or new or worsening retinopathy	Permanently discontinue treatment

ECOG PS, Eastern Cooperative Oncology Group Performance Status

Starting Dose	Dose Modification
6 mcg/kg per week	**For doses 1 to 8** First modification: 3 mcg/kg per week Second modification: 2 mcg/kg per week Third modification: 1 mcg/kg per week Permanently discontinue peginterferon if patient is unable to tolerate 1 mcg/kg per week
3 mcg/kg per week	**For doses 9 to 260** First modification: 2 mcg/kg per week Second modification: 1 mcg/kg per week Permanently discontinue peginterferon if patient is unable to tolerate 1 mcg/kg per week

Toxicity (N = 608)

	% All Grades	% G3	% G4
Any	99	40	5
Fatigue	94	15	1
Liver abnormalities	79	10	<1
Pyrexia	75	4	<1
Headache	70	4	0
Myalgia	67	4	<1
Depression	59	6	<1

Patient Population Studied

Included in the study were 627 patients with histologically confirmed Stage III melanoma (Tx N1–2 M0) whose primary cutaneous melanoma was completely excised with adequate surgical margins and complete regional lymphadenectomy. Patients with ocular or mucous membrane melanoma, evidence of distant metastasis or in-transit metastasis, prior malignancy within the past 5 years, autoimmune disease, uncontrolled infections, cardiovascular disease, liver or renal disease, use of systemic corticosteroids, and previous use of systemic therapy for melanoma were excluded

Efficacy

	Recurrence-Free Survival		Distant Metastasis-Free Survival		Overall Survival	
	3.8 Years	7.6 Years	3.8 Years	7.6 Years	3.8 Years	7.6 Years
Number of events	328	384	304	370	262	332
Rate of recurrence-free survival	45.6%	39.1%	48.2%	41.7%	56.8%	47.8%
Median time to event	months	years	months	years	NR	years
Hazard ratio	0.82	0.87	0.88	0.93	0.98	0.96
P Value	0.01	0.055	0.11	0.33	0.78	0.57

NR, Not reported

Therapy Monitoring

Every 3 months for 3 years and then every 6 months for 2 years: CBC with differential, LFTs, basic metabolic panel, LDH, physical examination, chest x-ray, and CT scans

METASTATIC • IMMUNE THERAPY

MELANOMA REGIMEN: IPILIMUMAB

Hodi FS et al. N Engl J Med 2010;363:711–723

Ipilimumab 3 mg/kg; administer intravenously, diluted in 0.9% sodium chloride injection or 5% dextrose injection to a concentration between 1 and 2 mg/mL, over 90 minutes, once every 3 weeks, for a total of 4 doses (total dosage/3-week cycle = 3 mg/kg)

Note: Adverse events associated with the administration of ipilimumab consist primarily of reactions that are immune in nature. Almost all immune-related adverse events can be managed with supportive care or corticosteroids. Corticosteroids do not appear to adversely affect patients who had an immune-related adverse event or alter objective antitumor responses. Glucocorticoids do not appear to alter the activity of activated CD8+ cells, and, therefore, may explain this unique characteristic of CTLA4 inhibition. Rash and colitis are reported most often during early use, whereas hypophysitis is reported with later doses. Ipilimumab immune-related adverse events are dose-dependent in incidence and occurred more frequently after 10-mg/kg doses than with lower dosages

Patient Population Studied

Patients with a diagnosis of unresectable Stage III or IV melanoma who had previously received therapy, including one or more of the following: dacarbazine, temozolomide, fotemustine, carboplatin, or aldesleukin. Other inclusion criteria were Eastern Cooperative Oncology Group performance status of 0 or 1, and positive status for HLA-A*0201. Exclusion criteria included long-term use of systemic corticosteroids

Therapy Monitoring

1. Monitor patients for signs and symptoms of infusion-related reactions including pyrexia, chills, flushing, hypotension, dyspnea, wheezing, back pain, abdominal pain, and urticaria
2. Initially at the time of each dose, and eventually every 6–12 weeks, perform a total-body skin examination with attention to ALL mucous membranes as well as a complete review of systems
3. Monitor patients for signs and symptoms of pneumonitis. Evaluate patients with suspected pneumonitis with chest x-ray, CT, and pulse oximetry. For ≥2 toxicity, may include nasal swab, sputum culture and sensitivity, blood culture and sensitivity, and urine culture and sensitivity
4. Monitor patients for signs and symptoms of colitis. Encourage patients to report diarrhea immediately to any member of the health care team
5. Draw AST, ALT, and bilirubin prior to each infusion and/or weekly if there are Grade 1 liver function test elevations. Note, no treatment is recommended for G1 LFT abnormalities. For ≥2 toxicity, work up for other causes of elevated LFTs including viral hepatitis
6. Use basic metabolic panel (Na, K, CO_2, glucose) and patient history as screening tools for hypophysitis including hypopituitarism and adrenal insufficiency. If in doubt, evaluate am adrenocorticotropic hormone (ACTH) and cortisol levels. Consider ACTH stimulation test for indeterminate results
7. Assess thyroid function at the start of treatment, periodically during treatment, and as indicated based on clinical evaluation and for clinical signs and symptoms of thyroid disorders. Test for TSH and free thyroxine (FT4) every 4–6 weeks as part of routine clinical monitoring of therapy or for case detection in symptomatic patients
8. Measure glucose at baseline and with each treatment during the first 12 weeks and every 6 weeks thereafter
9. Obtain a serum creatinine prior to every dose. If creatinine is found to be newly elevated, consider holding therapy while other potential causes are evaluated. Note, routine urinalysis is not necessary other than to rule out urinary tract infections, etc
10. Obtain a complete rheumatologic history and perform an examination of all peripheral joints for tenderness, swelling, and range of motion. Examine the spine. Consider plain x-ray/imaging to exclude metastases and evaluate joint damage (erosions), if appropriate
11. In patients at high risk for infections and in appropriately selected patients based on an infectious disease evaluation, draw screening laboratories (HIV, hepatitis A and B, and blood QuantiFERON for TB) to prepare patients to start infliximab

Treatment Modifications

RECOMMENDED DOSE MODIFICATIONS FOR IPILIMUMAB

Adverse Event	Grade/Severity	Treatment Modification
Infusion reaction	Clinically significant but not severe infusion reaction	Interrupt the infusion in patients with clinically significant infusion reactions and consider resuming at a slower rate following resolution. If decision is made to restart, begin at ≤50% of the rate prior to the reaction and increase in 50% increments every 30 minutes if well tolerated. Infusions may be restarted at the full rate during the next cycle
	G3/4 (severe infusion reaction—pyrexia, chills, flushing, hypotension, dyspnea, wheezing, back pain, abdominal pain, and urticaria). Not rapidly responsive to brief interruption of infusion	Stop infusion and administer appropriate medical therapy (eg, epinephrine, corticosteroids, intravenous antihistamines, bronchodilators, and/or oxygen). Discontinue ipilimumab
COLITIS	G1	Loperamide 4 mg as starting dose then 2 mg before each meal and after each loose stool until without diarrhea for 12 hours, with maximum of 16 mg loperamide per day. If G1 diarrhea or colitis persists >14 days, then add prednisolone 0.5–1 mg/kg (non-enteric-coated) or consider oral budesonide 9 mg daily if no bloody diarrhea
	G2/3 diarrhea or colitis	Withhold ipilimumab. Loperamide 4 mg as starting dose then 2 mg before each meal and after each loose stool until without diarrhea for 12 hours, with maximum of 16 mg loperamide per day. Administer oral prednisone/prednisolone at a dose of 0.5–2 mg/kg/day or its equivalent. When improves to G1, begin a slow corticosteroid taper over at least 4 weeks. Resume ipilimumab upon symptom control, or when prednisone/prednisolone daily dose <10 mg
	G4 diarrhea or colitis	Permanently discontinue ipilimumab. Loperamide 4 mg as starting dose then 2 mg before each meal and after each loose stool until without diarrhea for 12 hours, with maximum of 16 mg loperamide per day. Administer 1–2 mg/kg intravenously (methyl)prednisolone and convert to 0.5–2 mg/kg prednisone/prednisolone orally each day or its equivalent only after a response. Taper over at least 4 weeks when symptoms improve. If does not improve over 72 hours or worsens, perform flexible sigmoidoscopy/colonoscopy to document colitis then begin infliximab 5 mg/kg (if no perforation/sepsis/TB/hepatitis/NYHA III/IV CHF). If no response, add MMF 500–1000 mg twice daily. If worse on MMF, consider addition of tacrolimus or ATG
Pneumonitis	G2	Withhold ipilimumab. Consider *Pneumocystis* prophylaxis depending on the clinical context and coverage with empiric antibiotics. Administer oral prednisone/prednisolone at a dose of 1–2 mg/kg/day or its equivalent. When improves to G1, begin a slow corticosteroid taper over at least 4 weeks. If does not respond adequately after 48 hours, then administer 2–4 mg/kg intravenously (methyl)prednisolone and convert to 0.5–2 mg/kg prednisone/prednisolone orally each day or its equivalent only after a response, followed by a taper over at least 6 weeks when symptoms improve to G1, titrating to symptoms. Resume ipilimumab upon symptom control, or when prednisone/prednisolone daily dose <10 mg
	G3/4	Permanently discontinue ipilimumab. Consider *Pneumocystis* prophylaxis depending on the clinical context; cover with empiric antibiotics. Administer 2–4 mg/kg intravenously (methyl)prednisolone and convert to 1–2 mg/kg prednisone/prednisolone orally each day or its equivalent only after a response, followed by a taper over at least 8 weeks when symptoms improve to G1, titrating to symptoms. If when initially treated improvement does not occur within 48–72 hours, begin infliximab 5 mg/kg (if no perforation/sepsis/TB/hepatitis/NYHA III/IV CHF). If no response to infliximab, add MMF 500–1000 mg twice daily. Consider MMF especially if has concurrent hepatic toxicity

(continued)

Treatment Modifications (*continued*)

RECOMMENDED DOSE MODIFICATIONS FOR IPILIMUMAB

Adverse Event	Grade/Severity	Treatment Modification
HEPATITIS	G2 (AST or ALT >3–5× ULN or total bilirubin >1.5–3× ULN)	Withhold ipilimumab. Administer oral prednisone/prednisolone at a dose of 1–2 mg/kg/day or its equivalent. When improves to G1, begin a slow corticosteroid taper over at least 4 weeks. Resume ipilimumab upon symptom control, or when prednisone/prednisolone daily dose <10 mg
	G3/4 (AST or ALT >5× ULN or total bilirubin >3× ULN)	Permanently discontinue ipilimumab. Administer 1–2 mg/kg intravenously (methyl)prednisolone and convert to 0.5–2 mg/kg prednisone/prednisolone orally each day or its equivalent only after a response. Taper over at least 6 weeks when symptoms improve. If no response, add MMF 500–1000 mg twice daily. If worse on MMF, consider adding tacrolimus or ATG
Hypophysitis	G2/3 (moderate symptoms, ie, headache but no visual disturbance or fatigue/mood alteration but hemodynamically stable, no electrolyte disturbance)	Administer analgesia as needed for headache. Withhold ipilimumab. Administer oral prednisone/prednisolone at a dose of 0.5–2 mg/kg/day or its equivalent. When improves to G1, begin a slow corticosteroid taper over at least 4 weeks. If no improvement in 48 hours, administer 1–2 mg/kg intravenously (methyl)prednisolone and convert to 0.5–2 mg/kg prednisone/prednisolone orally each day or its equivalent only after a response. Taper over at least 4 weeks when symptoms improve to 5 mg prednisone/prednisolone or equivalent; do not stop steroids. Resume ipilimumab upon symptom control, or when prednisone/prednisolone daily dose <10 mg
	G4 (severe mass effect symptoms, ie, severe headache, any visual disturbance or severe hypoadrenalism, ie, hypotension, severe electrolyte disturbance)	Permanently discontinue ipilimumab. Administer analgesia as needed for headache. Administer 1–2 mg/kg intravenously (methyl)prednisolone and convert to 0.5–2 mg/kg prednisone/prednisolone orally each day or its equivalent only after a response. Taper over at least 4 weeks when symptoms improve to 5 mg prednisone/prednisolone or equivalent; do not stop steroids
Adrenal insufficiency	G2	Withhold ipilimumab. Administer oral prednisone/prednisolone at a dose of 0.5–2 mg/kg/day or its equivalent. When improves to G1, begin a slow corticosteroid taper over at least 4 weeks. Serially assess adrenal function and continue steroids at replacement doses (20–40 mg hydrocortisone daily ~2/3 dose in AM upon awakening and ~1/3 at 4 PM) until recovery of adrenal function is documented. Resume ipilimumab upon symptom control, or when prednisone/prednisolone daily dose <10 mg
	G3/4	Permanently discontinue ipilimumab. Administer oral prednisone/prednisolone at a dose of 0.5–2 mg/kg/day or its equivalent. When improves to G1, begin a slow corticosteroid taper over at least 4 weeks. Serially assess adrenal function and continue steroids at replacement doses (20–40 mg hydrocortisone daily ~2/3 dose in AM upon awakening and ~1/3 at 4 PM) until recovery of adrenal function is documented
Type 1 diabetes mellitus	G3 hyperglycemia	Withhold ipilimumab. Admit to hospital to manage hyperglycemia. Role of corticosteroids in preventing complete loss of insulin-producing cells is unknown and not recommended. Resume ipilimumab upon symptom control, or when prednisone/prednisolone daily dose <10 mg
	G4 hyperglycemia	Permanently discontinue ipilimumab. Admit to hospital to manage hyperglycemia. Role of corticosteroids in preventing complete loss of insulin-producing cells is unknown and not recommended
Nephritis and renal dysfunction	G2/3 (serum creatinine 1.5–6× ULN)	Withhold ipilimumab. Administer oral prednisone/prednisolone at a dose of 0.5–2 mg/kg/day or its equivalent. When improves to G1, begin a slow corticosteroid taper over at least 4 weeks. If does not respond adequately, then administer 0.5–1 mg/kg intravenously (methyl)prednisolone and convert to 0.5–2 mg/kg prednisone/prednisolone orally each day or its equivalent only after a response, followed by a taper over at least 4 weeks when improves to G1. Resume ipilimumab upon symptom control, or when prednisone/prednisolone daily dose <10 mg
	G4 (serum creatinine >6× ULN)	Permanently discontinue ipilimumab. Administer 0.5–1 mg/kg intravenously (methyl)prednisolone and convert to 0.5–2 mg/kg prednisone/prednisolone orally each day or its equivalent only after a response, followed by a taper over at least 4 weeks when improves to G1

(*continued*)

Treatment Modifications (*continued*)

RECOMMENDED DOSE MODIFICATIONS FOR IPILIMUMAB

Adverse Event	Grade/Severity	Treatment Modification
Skin	G1/2	Continue ipilimumab. Avoid skin irritants, avoid sun exposure, topical emollients recommended. Topical steroid (mild strength for G1, moderate/potent strength for G2) cream once or twice daily ± oral or topical antihistamines for itching
	G3 rash or suspected SJS or TEN	Withhold ipilimumab. Avoid skin irritants, avoid sun exposure, topical emollients recommended. Administer oral or topical antihistamines for itching. Administer oral prednisone/prednisolone at a dose of 0.5–2 mg/kg or its equivalent daily for 3 days followed by a slow corticosteroid taper over at least 4 weeks when the rash improves to G1. If does not respond adequately, then administer 0.5–1 mg/kg intravenously (methyl) prednisolone and convert to 0.5–2 mg/kg prednisone/prednisolone orally each day or its equivalent only after a response, followed by a taper over at least 4 weeks when the rash improves to G1. Resume ipilimumab upon symptom control, or when prednisone/prednisolone daily dose <10 mg
	G4 rash or confirmed SJS or TEN	Avoid skin irritants, avoid sun exposure, topical emollients recommended. Administer oral or topical antihistamines for itching. Administer 1–2 mg/kg intravenously (methyl)prednisolone and convert to oral steroids 0.5–2 mg/kg prednisone/prednisolone each day or its equivalent only after a response. Taper over at least 4 weeks when the rash improves to G1. Permanently discontinue ipilimumab
Encephalitis	Confusion or altered behavior, headaches, alteration in Glasgow Coma Scale, motor or sensory deficits, speech abnormality, may or may not be febrile	Initially withhold ipilimumab, but permanently discontinue ipilimumab if there is no doubt as to diagnosis. Exclude bacterial and ideally viral infections prior to high-dose steroids. Administer oral prednisone/prednisolone at a dose of 0.5–2 mg/kg/day or its equivalent. When symptoms improve, begin a slow corticosteroid taper over at least 4–8 weeks. If symptoms are severe, administer 1–2 mg/kg intravenously (methyl)prednisolone and convert to 0.5–2 mg/kg prednisone/prednisolone orally each day or its equivalent only after a response. Consider concurrent empiric antiviral (intravenous acyclovir) and antibacterial therapy
Aseptic meningitis	Headache, photophobia, neck stiffness with fever or may be afebrile, vomiting; normal cognition/cerebral function (distinguishes from encephalitis)	
Other syndromes include neurosarcoidosis, posterior reversible leukoencephalopathy syndrome (PRES), Vogt-Koyanagi-Harada syndrome, demyelination, vasculitic encephalopathy, and generalized seizures		
Transverse myelitis	Acute or subacute neurologic signs/symptoms of motor/sensory/autonomic origin; most have sensory level; often bilateral symptoms	Initially withhold ipilimumab, but permanently discontinue ipilimumab if there is no doubt as to diagnosis. Administer 2 mg/kg intravenously (methyl)prednisolone or consider 1 g/day and convert to 0.5–2 mg/kg prednisone/prednisolone orally each day or its equivalent only after a response. When symptoms improve, begin a slow corticosteroid taper over at least 4–8 weeks. Plasmapheresis may be required if steroids do not bring about improvement
Myocarditis	G3	Permanently discontinue ipilimumab. Administer 2 mg/kg intravenously (methyl)prednisolone or consider 1 g/day and convert to 0.5–2 mg/kg prednisone/prednisolone orally each day or its equivalent only after a response. When symptoms improve, begin a slow corticosteroid taper over at least 4–8 weeks. If no response, add MMF 500–1000 mg twice daily. If worse on MMF, consider adding tacrolimus
Peripheral neurologic toxicity	Moderate: some interference with ADL, symptoms concerning to patient	Withhold ipilimumab. Initial observation reasonable or initiate prednisone/prednisolone 0.5–1 mg/kg (if progressing, eg, from mild) and/or pregabalin or duloxetine for pain. When symptoms improve, begin a slow corticosteroid taper over at least 4 weeks. Resume ipilimumab upon symptom control, or when prednisone/prednisolone daily dose <10 mg
	Severe: limits self-care and aids warranted, life-threatening, eg, respiratory problems	Permanently discontinue ipilimumab. Administer 1–2 mg/kg intravenously (methyl)prednisolone and convert to 0.5–2 mg/kg prednisone/prednisolone orally each day or its equivalent only after a response. Taper over at least 4–8 weeks when symptoms improve to G1

(*continued*)

Treatment Modifications (*continued*)

RECOMMENDED DOSE MODIFICATIONS FOR IPILIMUMAB

Adverse Event	Grade/Severity	Treatment Modification
Guillain-Barré syndrome	Progressive symmetrical muscle weakness with absent or reduced tendon reflexes—involves extremities, facial, respiratory, and bulbar and oculomotor muscles; dysregulation of autonomic nerves	Permanently discontinue ipilimumab. Use of steroids not recommended in idiopathic Guillain-Barré syndrome; however, a trial of (methyl)prednisolone 1–2 mg/kg is reasonable, converting to 0.5–2 mg/kg prednisone/prednisolone orally each day or its equivalent only after a response. If no improvement or worsening, plasmapheresis or IVIG indicated
Myasthenia gravis	Fluctuating muscle weakness (proximal limb, trunk, ocular, eg, ptosis/diplopia or bulbar) with fatigability, respiratory muscles also may be involved	Permanently discontinue ipilimumab. Administer pyridostigmine at an initial dose of 30 mg three times daily. Administer oral prednisone/prednisolone at a dose of 0.5–2 mg/kg/day or its equivalent or 1–2 mg/kg intravenously (methyl)prednisolone depending on the severity of symptoms. If begin with intravenous, convert to 0.5–2 mg/kg prednisone/prednisolone orally each day or its equivalent only after a response. If no improvement or worsening, plasmapheresis or IVIG may be considered. Additional immunosuppressants used in myasthenia gravis include azathioprine, cyclosporine, and mycophenolate. Avoid certain medications, eg, ciprofloxacin, beta-blockers, that may precipitate cholinergic crisis
Other syndromes including motor and sensory peripheral neuropathy, multifocal radicular neuropathy/plexopathy, autonomic neuropathy, phrenic nerve palsy, cranial nerve palsies (eg, facial nerve, optic nerve, hypoglossal nerve)		Permanently discontinue ipilimumab. Administer oral prednisone/prednisolone at a dose of 0.5–2 mg/kg/day or its equivalent or 1–2 mg/kg intravenously (methyl)prednisolone depending on the severity of symptoms. If begin with intravenous, convert to 0.5–2 mg/kg prednisone/prednisolone orally each day or its equivalent only after a response
Arthralgia	G1 (mild pain with inflammation, erythema, or joint swelling)	Continue ipilimumab. Administer acetaminophen (paracetamol) and ibuprofen
	G2 (moderate pain with inflammation, erythema, or joint swelling that limits ADLs)	Withhold ipilimumab. Administer higher doses of acetaminophen (paracetamol) and ibuprofen and use diclofenac or naproxen or etoricoxib. If inadequately controlled, consider intra-articular steroid injections for large joints or administer oral prednisone/prednisolone at a dose of 0.5–2 mg/kg/day or its equivalent. When improves to G1, begin a slow corticosteroid taper over at least 4 weeks. If does not respond adequately, then administer 0.5–1 mg/kg intravenously (methyl)prednisolone and convert to 0.5–2 mg/kg prednisone/prednisolone orally each day or its equivalent only after a response, followed by a taper over at least 4 weeks when improves to G1. Resume ipilimumab upon symptom control, or when prednisone/prednisolone daily dose <10 mg
	G3 (severe pain; irreversible joint damage; disabling; limits self-care ADL)	Withhold ipilimumab. Administer 0.5–1 mg/kg intravenously (methyl)prednisolone and convert to 0.5–2 mg/kg prednisone/prednisolone orally each day or its equivalent only after a response, followed by a taper over at least 4 weeks when improves to G1. In severe cases, infliximab or another anti–TNF-alpha drug may be required for improvement of arthritis. Resume ipilimumab upon symptom control, or when prednisone/prednisolone daily dose <10 mg
Other	First occurrence of other G3	Withhold ipilimumab. Administer oral prednisone/prednisolone at a dose of 0.5–2 mg/kg/day or its equivalent. When improves to G1, begin a slow corticosteroid taper over at least 4 weeks. Resume ipilimumab upon symptom control, or when prednisone/prednisolone daily dose <10 mg
	Recurrence of same G3	Permanently discontinue ipilimumab. Administer 1–2 mg/kg intravenously (methyl)prednisolone and convert to 0.5–2 mg/kg prednisone/prednisolone orally each day or its equivalent only after a response. Taper over at least 4–8 weeks when symptoms improve to G1
	Life-threatening or G4	
	Requirement for ≥10 mg/day prednisone or equivalent for >12 weeks	Permanently discontinue ipilimumab
	Persistent G2/3 adverse reactions lasting ≥12 weeks	

ADL, activities of daily living; ALT, alanine aminotransferase; AST, aspartate aminotransferase; ATG, anti-thymocyte globulin; SJS, Stevens-Johnson Syndrome; TEN, toxic epidermal necrolysis; ULN, upper limit of normal

Notes on general supportive care:
- Steroid taper in most cases will proceed over a minimum of 1 month but if symptoms improve rapidly, a 2-week taper can be considered. If steroids are administered for more than 4 weeks, consider PCP prophylaxis (cotrimoxazole 480 mg twice daily M/W/F or inhaled pentamidine if has cotrimoxazole allergy), regular random blood glucose, VitD level, and starting calcium/VitD supplementation per guidelines

Efficacy (N = 137)

Median overall survival	10.1 months (95% CI, 8.0–13.8)
Rate of overall survival at 12 months	45.6%
Rate of overall survival at 18 months	33.2%
Rate of overall survival at 24 months	23.5%
Objective response*,†	10.9%
Complete response†	1.5%
Partial response†	9.5%
Stable disease†	17.5%

Reinduction (n = 8)

Complete response	12.5% (1/8)
Partial response	25% (2/8)
Stable disease	37.5% (3/8)

*Responses to ipilimumab continued to improve beyond week 24: 2 patients with SD improved to a PR, and 3 patients with a PR improved to a CR. Among 31 patients given reinduction therapy with ipilimumab, 21 patients achieved a CR, PR, or SD

†Duration of response: 60.0% maintained an objective response for at least 2 years (26.5–44 months, ongoing)

Toxicity (N = 131)

Adverse Event	Total % (All Grades)	% G3	% G4
Any event	96.9	37.4	8.4
Any drug-related event	80.2	19.1	3.8
Gastrointestinal disorders			
Diarrhea	32.8	5.3	0
Nausea	35.1	2.3	0
Constipation	20.6	2.3	0
Vomiting	23.7	2.3	0
Abdominal pain	15.3	1.5	0
Other			
Fatigue	42.0	6.9	0
Decrease appetite	26.7	1.5	0
Pyrexia	12.2	0	0
Headache	14.5	2.3	0
Cough	16.0	0	0
Dyspnea	14.5	3.1	0.8
Anemia	11.5	3.1	0
Any immune-related event			
Any immune-related event	61.1	12.2	2.3
Dermatologic	43.5	1.5	0
Pruritus	24.4	0	0
Rash	19.1	0.8	0
Vitiligo	2.3	0	0
Gastrointestinal	29.0	7.6	0
Diarrhea	27.5	4.6	0
Colitis	7.6	5.3	0
Endocrine	7.6	2.3	1.5
Hypothyroidism	1.5	0	0
Hypopituitarism	2.3	0.8	0.8
Hypophysitis	1.5	1.5	0
Adrenal insufficiency	1.5	0	0
Long-term adverse effects in survivors for >2 years (N = 94)			
Injection-site reactions	17%		
Vitiligo	12.8%		
Proctocolitis with rectal pain	4.3%		
Endocrine immune-related adverse event*	8.5%		

*Required hormone-replacement therapy

(continued)

Toxicity (N = 131) *(continued)*

Toxicity—General Notes:

1. All immune-related events occurred during the induction and reinduction periods
2. Median time to the resolution of immune-related adverse events of G2–4 was 4.9 weeks (95% CI, 3.1–6.4)
3. After administration of corticosteroids, median time to resolution of diarrhea G ≥2 was 2.3 weeks for 14 of 15 patients
4. In addition to corticosteroids, 4 patients received infliximab (antitumor necrosis factor-α antibody) for diarrhea G ≥3 or colitis
5. Ongoing events in 94 persons who survived ≥2 years included rash, pruritus, diarrhea, anorexia, and fatigue, generally G1/2 (5–15% of patients) and G3 leukocytosis (1 patient)
6. There were 14 deaths related to the study drugs (2.1%), of which 7 were associated with immune-related adverse events

Toxicity—Specific Notes:

Skin:

1. Rash is the most common immune-related toxicity associated with ipilimumab (incidence ~20%)
2. Median time to onset of moderate, severe, or life-threatening immune-mediated dermatitis was 3.1 weeks (range: days to 17.3 weeks after initiation)

Gastrointestinal:

1. Most common serious adverse event affects the lower gastrointestinal tract and manifests as diarrhea and/or intestinal bleeding
2. Serious lower intestinal toxicity was reported in ~13% of patients treated at 10 mg ipilimumab/kg of body weight
3. *Onset of diarrhea occurred within first 12 weeks after starting treatment and was generally reversible*

Hepatic:

1. Immune-related hepatotoxicity consists of elevated LFTs and immune hepatitis
2. Patients with right upper quadrant pain, nausea, or vomiting should have LFTs evaluated immediately, although hepatotoxicity can occur in the absence of symptoms
3. In patients with hepatotoxicity, rule out infectious or malignant causes and increase frequency of LFT monitoring until resolution

Endocrine:

1. Most patients with hypophysitis/hypopituitarism present with headache; however, visual disturbances, fatigue, confusion, and impotency are common symptoms
2. Median time to onset of moderate to severe immune-mediated endocrinopathy was 11 weeks (range: days to 19.3 weeks after initiation)
3. Of 21 patients with moderate to life-threatening endocrinopathy, 17 required long-term hormone replacement therapy, most commonly adrenal (n = 10) and thyroid (n = 13) replacement

Neurologic:

1. Myasthenia gravis and cases of Guillain-Barré syndrome have been reported in association with ipilimumab use
2. Monitor for symptoms of motor and sensory neuropathy

METASTATIC • IMMUNE THERAPY

MELANOMA REGIMEN: PEMBROLIZUMAB

Brahmer JR et al. J Clin Oncol 2018;36(17):1714–1768
Robert C et al. N Engl J Med 2015;372:2521–2532.
Comment in: Nat Rev Clin Oncol 2015;12:371
Freshwater T et al. J Immunother Cancer 2017;5:43
Haanen JB et al. Ann Oncol 2017;28(suppl_4):iv119–iv142
FDA and EMA prescribing information

The U.S. Food and Drug Administration (FDA)-approved regimen for melanoma includes a fixed dose of pembrolizumab, consistent with the regimen approved on May 10, 2017, thus:

Pembrolizumab 200 mg; administer intravenously over 30 minutes in a volume of 0.9% sodium chloride injection (0.9% NS) or 5% dextrose injection (D5W) sufficient to produce a pembrolizumab concentration within the range 1–10 mg/mL every 3 weeks for up to 24 months (total dose/3-week cycle = 200 mg)

Alternative pembrolizumab dose and schedule as per the U.S. FDA regimens approved on April 28, 2020:

Pembrolizumab 400 mg; administer intravenously over 30 minutes in a volume of 0.9% NS or D5W sufficient to produce a pembrolizumab concentration within the range 1–10 mg/mL every 6 weeks for up to 24 months (total dose/6-week cycle = 400 mg)

- Administer pembrolizumab with an administration set that contains a sterile, non-pyrogenic, low-protein-binding in-line or add-on filter with pore size within the range of 0.2–5 μm
- Patients who achieved a confirmed complete response after receiving at least 6 months of pembrolizumab could discontinue treatment after receiving two doses beyond the determination of complete response
- Pembrolizumab can cause severe or life-threatening infusion-related reactions, including hypersensitivity and anaphylaxis

Supportive Care

Antiemetic prophylaxis
*Emetogenic potential is **MINIMAL***
See Chapter 42 for antiemetic recommendations

Hematopoietic growth factor (CSF) prophylaxis
*Primary prophylaxis is **NOT** indicated*
See Chapter 43 for more information

Antimicrobial prophylaxis
*Risk of fever and neutropenia is **LOW***
Antimicrobial primary prophylaxis to be considered:
- Antibacterial—not indicated
- Antifungal—not indicated
- Antiviral—not indicated unless patient previously had an episode of HSV

Patient Population Studied

An international, multicenter, randomized, controlled, phase 3 study involving 834 patients with histologically confirmed Stage III or IV melanoma not amenable to resection. Patients who had previously received more than one systemic therapy for advanced disease, patients who had previously received therapy with CTLA-4, PD-1, or PD-L1 inhibitors, and patients who had ocular melanoma, active brain metastases, or a history of serious autoimmune disease were not eligible for inclusion in the study. Participants were randomly assigned in a 1:1:1 ratio to receive pembrolizumab every 2 weeks, pembrolizumab every 3 weeks, or ipilimumab every 3 weeks

Efficacy (N = 834)

Median progression-free survival (primary end point)*	5.5 months for pembrolizumab every 2 weeks 4.1 months for pembrolizumab every 3 weeks 2.8 months for ipilimumab every 3 weeks	Compared with ipilimumab, HR for disease progression (95% CI) was 0.58 (0.46–0.72) for pembrolizumab every 2 weeks (P<0.001) and 0.58 (0.47–0.72) for pembrolizumab every 3 weeks (P<0.001)
1-year survival (primary end point)†	74.1% for pembrolizumab every 2 weeks 68.4% for pembrolizumab every 3 weeks 58.2% for ipilimumab every 3 weeks	Compared with ipilimumab, HR for death (95% CI) was 0.63 (0.47–0.83) for pembrolizumab every 2 weeks (P<0.0005) and 0.69 (0.52–0.90) for pembrolizumab every 3 weeks (P = 0.0036)
Objective response rate (secondary end point)‡	33.7% for pembrolizumab every 2 weeks 32.9% for pembrolizumab every 3 weeks 11.9% for ipilimumab every 3 weeks	P<0.001 for pembrolizumab every 2 weeks vs ipilimumab and for pembrolizumab every 3 weeks vs ipilimumab
Median duration of response (secondary end point)§	Not reached in any group	

*Progression-free survival was defined as the time from randomization to documented disease progression according to RECIST or death from any cause, in the intention-to-treat population. These results are from the first interim analysis, which was conducted after at least 260 patients had disease progression or died in all study groups and all patients had been followed for at least 6 months

†Overall survival was defined as the time from randomization to death from any cause, in the intention-to-treat population. These results are from the second interim analysis, which was conducted after all patients had been followed for at least 12 months

‡Objective response rate was defined as the percentage of patients with complete or partial response according to RECIST, in the intention-to-treat population. These results are from the first interim analysis, which was conducted after at least 260 patients had disease progression or died in all study groups and all patients had been followed for at least 6 months

§Duration of response was defined as the time from the first documented response to radiologic progression according to RECIST, in the intention-to-treat population. These results are from the first interim analysis, which was conducted after at least 260 patients had disease progression or died in all study groups and all patients had been followed for at least 6 months

Therapy Monitoring

1. Initially at the time of each dose, and eventually every 6–12 weeks, perform a total body skin examination with attention to ALL mucous membranes as well as a complete review of systems

2. Monitor patients for signs and symptoms of pneumonitis. Evaluate patients with suspected pneumonitis with chest x-ray, CT, and pulse oximetry. For ≥2 toxicity, may include nasal swab, sputum culture and sensitivity, blood culture and sensitivity, and urine culture and sensitivity

3. Monitor patients for signs and symptoms of colitis. Encourage patients to report diarrhea immediately to any member of the health care team

4. Draw AST, ALT, and bilirubin prior to each infusion and/or weekly if there are Grade 1 liver function test elevations. Note, no treatment is recommended for G1 LFT abnormalities. For ≥2 toxicity, work up for other causes of elevated LFTs including viral hepatitis

5. Use basic metabolic panel (Na, K, CO_2, glucose) and patient history as screening tools for hypophysitis including hypopituitarism and adrenal insufficiency. If in doubt, evaluate am adrenocorticotropic hormone (ACTH) and cortisol levels. Consider ACTH stimulation test for indeterminate results

6. Assess thyroid function at the start of treatment, periodically during treatment, and as indicated based on clinical evaluation and for clinical signs and symptoms of thyroid disorders. Test for TSH and free thyroxine (FT4) every 4–6 weeks as part of routine clinical monitoring of therapy or for case detection in symptomatic patients

7. Measure glucose at baseline and with each treatment during the first 12 weeks and every 6 weeks thereafter

8. Obtain a serum creatinine prior to every dose. If creatinine is found to be newly elevated, consider holding therapy while other potential causes are evaluated. Note, routine urinalysis is not necessary other than to rule out urinary tract infections, etc

9. Obtain a complete rheumatologic history and perform an examination of all peripheral joints for tenderness, swelling, and range of motion. Examine the spine. Consider plain x-ray/imaging to exclude metastases and evaluate joint damage (erosions), if appropriate

10. In patients at high risk for infections and in appropriately selected patients based on an infectious disease evaluation, draw screening laboratories (HIV, hepatitis A and B, and blood QuantiFERON for TB) to prepare patients to start infliximab

11. Response evaluation: Every 2–4 months

Treatment Modifications

RECOMMENDED DOSE MODIFICATIONS FOR PEMBROLIZUMAB

Adverse Event	Grade/Severity	Treatment Modification
Infusion reaction	Clinically significant but not severe infusion reaction	Interrupt the infusion in patients with clinically significant infusion reactions and consider resuming at a slower rate following resolution. If decision is made to restart, begin at ≤50% of the rate prior to the reaction and increase in 50% increments every 30 minutes if well tolerated. Infusions may be restarted at the full rate during the next cycle
	G3/4 (severe infusion reaction—pyrexia, chills, flushing, hypotension, dyspnea, wheezing, back pain, abdominal pain, and urticaria). Not rapidly responsive to brief interruption of infusion	Stop infusion and administer appropriate medical therapy (eg, epinephrine, corticosteroids, intravenous antihistamines, bronchodilators, and/or oxygen). Discontinue pembrolizumab
Colitis	G1	Loperamide 4 mg as starting dose then 2 mg before each meal and after each loose stool until without diarrhea for 12 hours, with maximum of 16 mg loperamide per day. If G1 diarrhea or colitis persists >14 days, then add prednisolone 0.5–1 mg/kg (non-enteric-coated) or consider oral budesonide 9 mg daily if no bloody diarrhea
	G2/3 diarrhea or colitis	Withhold pembrolizumab. Loperamide 4 mg as starting dose then 2 mg before each meal and after each loose stool until without diarrhea for 12 hours, with maximum of 16 mg loperamide per day. Administer oral prednisone/prednisolone at a dose of 0.5–2 mg/kg/day or its equivalent. When improves to G1, begin a slow corticosteroid taper over at least 4 weeks. Resume pembrolizumab upon symptom control, or when prednisone/prednisolone daily dose <10 mg
	G4 diarrhea or colitis	Permanently discontinue pembrolizumab. Loperamide 4 mg as starting dose then 2 mg before each meal and after each loose stool until without diarrhea for 12 hours, with maximum of 16 mg loperamide per day. Administer 1–2 mg/kg intravenously (methyl)prednisolone and convert to 0.5–2 mg/kg prednisone/prednisolone orally each day or its equivalent only after a response. Taper over at least 4 weeks when symptoms improve. If does not improve over 72 hours or worsens, perform flexible sigmoidoscopy/colonoscopy to document colitis then begin infliximab 5 mg/kg (if no perforation/sepsis/TB/hepatitis/NYHA III/IV CHF). If no response, add MMF 500–1000 mg twice daily. If worse on MMF, consider addition of tacrolimus or ATG

(continued)

Treatment Modifications (*continued*)

RECOMMENDED DOSE MODIFICATIONS FOR PEMBROLIZUMAB

Adverse Event	Grade/Severity	Treatment Modification
Pneumonitis	G2	Withhold pembrolizumab. Consider *Pneumocystis* prophylaxis depending on the clinical context and coverage with empiric antibiotics. Administer oral prednisone/prednisolone at a dose of 1–2 mg/kg/day or its equivalent. When improves to G1, begin a slow corticosteroid taper over at least 4 weeks. If does not respond adequately after 48 hours, then administer 2–4 mg/kg intravenously (methyl)prednisolone and convert to 0.5–2 mg/kg prednisone/prednisolone orally each day or its equivalent only after a response, followed by a taper over at least 6 weeks when symptoms improve to G1, titrating to symptoms. Resume pembrolizumab upon symptom control, or when prednisone/prednisolone daily dose <10 mg
	G3/4	Permanently discontinue pembrolizumab. Consider *Pneumocystis* prophylaxis depending on the clinical context; cover with empiric antibiotics. Administer 2–4 mg/kg intravenously (methyl)prednisolone and convert to 1–2 mg/kg prednisone/prednisolone orally each day or its equivalent only after a response, followed by a taper over at least 8 weeks when symptoms improve to G1, titrating to symptoms. If when initially treated improvement does not occur within 48–72 hours, begin infliximab 5 mg/kg (if no perforation/sepsis/TB/hepatitis/NYHA III/IV CHF). If no response to infliximab, add MMF 500–1000 mg twice daily. Consider MMF especially if has concurrent hepatic toxicity
Hepatitis	G2 (AST or ALT >3–5× ULN or total bilirubin >1.5–3× ULN)	Withhold pembrolizumab. Administer oral prednisone/prednisolone at a dose of 1–2 mg/kg/day or its equivalent. When improves to G1, begin a slow corticosteroid taper over at least 4 weeks. Resume pembrolizumab upon symptom control, or when prednisone/prednisolone daily dose <10 mg
	G3/4 (AST or ALT >5× ULN or total bilirubin >3× ULN)	Permanently discontinue pembrolizumab. Administer 1–2 mg/kg intravenously (methyl)prednisolone and convert to 0.5–2 mg/kg prednisone/prednisolone orally each day or its equivalent only after a response. Taper over at least 6 weeks when symptoms improve. If no response, add MMF 500–1000 mg twice daily. If worse on MMF, consider adding tacrolimus or ATG
Hypophysitis	G2/3 (moderate symptoms, ie, headache but no visual disturbance or fatigue/mood alteration but hemodynamically stable, no electrolyte disturbance)	Administer analgesia as needed for headache. Withhold pembrolizumab. Administer oral prednisone/prednisolone at a dose of 0.5–2 mg/kg/day or its equivalent. When improves to G1, begin a slow corticosteroid taper over at least 4 weeks. If no improvement in 48 hours, administer 1–2 mg/kg intravenously (methyl)prednisolone and convert to 0.5–2 mg/kg prednisone/prednisolone orally each day or its equivalent only after a response. Taper over at least 4 weeks when symptoms improve to 5 mg prednisone/prednisolone or equivalent; do not stop steroids. Resume pembrolizumab upon symptom control, or when prednisone/prednisolone daily dose <10 mg
	G4 (severe mass effect symptoms, ie, severe headache, any visual disturbance or severe hypoadrenalism, ie, hypotension, severe electrolyte disturbance)	Permanently discontinue pembrolizumab. Administer analgesia as needed for headache. Administer 1–2 mg/kg intravenously (methyl)prednisolone and convert to 0.5–2 mg/kg prednisone/prednisolone orally each day or its equivalent only after a response. Taper over at least 4 weeks when symptoms improve to 5 mg prednisone/prednisolone or equivalent; do not stop steroids
Adrenal insufficiency	G2	Withhold pembrolizumab. Administer oral prednisone/prednisolone at a dose of 0.5–2 mg/kg/day or its equivalent. When improves to G1, begin a slow corticosteroid taper over at least 4 weeks. Serially assess adrenal function and continue steroids at replacement doses (20–40 mg hydrocortisone daily ~2/3 dose in AM upon awakening and ~1/3 at 4 PM) until recovery of adrenal function is documented. Resume pembrolizumab upon symptom control, or when prednisone/prednisolone daily dose <10 mg
	G3/4	Permanently discontinue pembrolizumab. Administer oral prednisone/prednisolone at a dose of 0.5–2 mg/kg/day or its equivalent. When improves to G1, begin a slow corticosteroid taper over at least 4 weeks. Serially assess adrenal function and continue steroids at replacement doses (20–40 mg hydrocortisone daily ~2/3 dose in AM upon awakening and ~1/3 at 4 PM) until recovery of adrenal function is documented

(*continued*)

Treatment Modifications (continued)

RECOMMENDED DOSE MODIFICATIONS FOR PEMBROLIZUMAB

Adverse Event	Grade/Severity	Treatment Modification
Type 1 diabetes mellitus	G3 hyperglycemia	Withhold pembrolizumab. Admit to hospital to manage hyperglycemia. Role of corticosteroids in preventing complete loss of insulin-producing cells is unknown and not recommended. Resume pembrolizumab upon symptom control, or when prednisone/prednisolone daily dose <10 mg
	G4 hyperglycemia	Permanently discontinue pembrolizumab. Admit to hospital to manage hyperglycemia. Role of corticosteroids in preventing complete loss of insulin-producing cells is unknown and not recommended
Nephritis and renal dysfunction	G2/3 (serum creatinine 1.5–6× ULN)	Withhold pembrolizumab. Administer oral prednisone/prednisolone at a dose of 0.5–2 mg/kg/day or its equivalent. When improves to G1, begin a slow corticosteroid taper over at least 4 weeks. If does not respond adequately, then administer 0.5–1 mg/kg intravenously (methyl)prednisolone and convert to 0.5–2 mg/kg prednisone/prednisolone orally each day or its equivalent only after a response, followed by a taper over at least 4 weeks when improves to G1. Resume pembrolizumab upon symptom control, or when prednisone/prednisolone daily dose <10 mg
	G4 (serum creatinine >6× ULN)	Permanently discontinue pembrolizumab. Administer 0.5–1 mg/kg intravenously (methyl) prednisolone and convert to 0.5–2 mg/kg prednisone/prednisolone orally each day or its equivalent only after a response, followed by a taper over at least 4 weeks when improves to G1
Skin	G1/2	Continue pembrolizumab. Avoid skin irritants, avoid sun exposure, topical emollients recommended. Topical steroid (mild strength for G1, moderate/potent strength for G2) cream once or twice daily ± oral or topical antihistamines for itching
	G3 rash or suspected SJS or TEN	Withhold pembrolizumab. Avoid skin irritants, avoid sun exposure, topical emollients recommended. Administer oral or topical antihistamines for itching. Administer oral prednisone/prednisolone at a dose of 0.5–2 mg/kg or its equivalent daily for 3 days followed by a slow corticosteroid taper over at least 4 weeks when the rash improves to G1. If does not respond adequately, then administer 0.5–1 mg/kg intravenously (methyl)prednisolone and convert to 0.5 intravenously 2 mg/kg prednisone/prednisolone orally each day or its equivalent only after a response, followed by a taper over at least 4 weeks when the rash improves to G1. Resume pembrolizumab upon symptom control, or when prednisone/prednisolone daily dose <10 mg
	G4 rash or confirmed SJS or TEN	Avoid skin irritants, avoid sun exposure, topical emollients recommended. Administer oral or topical antihistamines for itching. Administer 1–2 mg/kg intravenously (methyl)prednisolone and convert to oral steroids 0.5–2 mg/kg prednisone/prednisolone each day or its equivalent only after a response. Taper over at least 4 weeks when the rash improves to G1. Permanently discontinue pembrolizumab
Encephalitis	Confusion or altered behavior, headaches, alteration in Glasgow Coma Scale, motor or sensory deficits, speech abnormality, may or may not be febrile	Initially withhold pembrolizumab, but permanently discontinue pembrolizumab if there is no doubt as to diagnosis. Exclude bacterial and ideally viral infections prior to high-dose steroids. Administer oral prednisone/prednisolone at a dose of 0.5–2 mg/kg/day or its equivalent. When symptoms improve, begin a slow corticosteroid taper over at least 4–8 weeks. If symptoms are severe, administer 1–2 mg/kg intravenously (methyl)prednisolone and convert to 0.5–2 mg/kg prednisone/prednisolone orally each day or its equivalent only after a response. Consider concurrent empiric antiviral (intravenous acyclovir) and antibacterial therapy
Aseptic meningitis	Headache, photophobia, neck stiffness with fever or may be afebrile, vomiting; normal cognition/cerebral function (distinguishes from encephalitis)	
	Other syndromes include neurosarcoidosis, posterior reversible leukoencephalopathy syndrome (PRES), Vogt-Koyanagi-Harada syndrome, demyelination, vasculitic encephalopathy, and generalized seizures	
Transverse myelitis	Acute or subacute neurologic signs/symptoms of motor/ sensory/autonomic origin; most have sensory level; often bilateral symptoms	Initially withhold pembrolizumab, but permanently discontinue pembrolizumab if there is no doubt as to diagnosis. Administer 2 mg/kg intravenously (methyl)prednisolone or consider 1 g/day and convert to 0.5–2 mg/kg prednisone/prednisolone orally each day or its equivalent only after a response. When symptoms improve, begin a slow corticosteroid taper over at least 4–8 weeks. Plasmapheresis may be required if steroids do not bring about improvement

(continued)

Treatment Modifications (continued)

RECOMMENDED DOSE MODIFICATIONS FOR PEMBROLIZUMAB

Adverse Event	Grade/Severity	Treatment Modification
Myocarditis	G3	Permanently discontinue pembrolizumab. Administer 2 mg/kg intravenously (methyl) prednisolone or consider 1 g/day and convert to 0.5–2 mg/kg prednisone/prednisolone orally each day or its equivalent only after a response. When symptoms improve, begin a slow corticosteroid taper over at least 4–8 weeks. If no response, add MMF 500–1000 mg twice daily. If worse on MMF, consider adding tacrolimus
Peripheral neurologic toxicity	Moderate: some interference with ADL, symptoms concerning to patient	Withhold pembrolizumab. Initial observation reasonable or initiate prednisone/prednisolone 0.5–1 mg/kg (if progressing, eg, from mild) and/or pregabalin or duloxetine for pain. When symptoms improve begin a slow corticosteroid taper over at least 4 weeks. Resume pembrolizumab upon symptom control, or when prednisone/prednisolone daily dose <10 mg
	Severe: limits self-care and aids warranted, life-threatening, eg, respiratory problems	Permanently discontinue pembrolizumab. Administer 1–2 mg/kg intravenously (methyl) prednisolone and convert to 0.5–2 mg/kg prednisone/prednisolone orally each day or its equivalent only after a response. Taper over at least 4–8 weeks when symptoms improve to G1
Guillain-Barré syndrome	Progressive symmetrical muscle weakness with absent or reduced tendon reflexes—involves extremities, facial, respiratory, and bulbar and oculomotor muscles; dysregulation of autonomic nerves	Permanently discontinue pembrolizumab. Use of steroids not recommended in idiopathic Guillain-Barré syndrome; however, a trial of (methyl)prednisolone 1–2 mg/kg is reasonable, converting to 0.5–2 mg/kg prednisone/prednisolone orally each day or its equivalent only after a response. If no improvement or worsening, plasmapheresis or IVIG indicated
Myasthenia gravis	Fluctuating muscle weakness (proximal limb, trunk, ocular, eg, ptosis/diplopia or bulbar) with fatigability, respiratory muscles also may be involved	Permanently discontinue pembrolizumab. Administer pyridostigmine at an initial dose of 30 mg 3 times daily. Administer oral prednisone/prednisolone at a dose of 0.5–2 mg/kg/day or its equivalent or 1–2 mg/kg intravenously (methyl)prednisolone depending on the severity of symptoms. If begin with intravenously, convert to 0.5–2 mg/kg prednisone/prednisolone orally each day or its equivalent only after a response. If no improvement or worsening, plasmapheresis or IVIG may be considered. Additional immunosuppressants used in myasthenia gravis include azathioprine, cyclosporine, and mycophenolate. Avoid certain medications, eg, ciprofloxacin, beta-blockers, that may precipitate cholinergic crisis
Other syndromes including motor and sensory peripheral neuropathy, multifocal radicular neuropathy/plexopathy, autonomic neuropathy, phrenic nerve palsy, cranial nerve palsies (eg, facial nerve, optic nerve, hypoglossal nerve)		Permanently discontinue pembrolizumab. Administer oral prednisone/prednisolone at a dose of 0.5–2 mg/kg/day or its equivalent or 1–2 mg/kg intravenously (methyl)prednisolone depending on the severity of symptoms. If begin with IV, convert to 0.5–2 mg/kg prednisone/prednisolone orally each day or its equivalent only after a response
Arthralgia	G1 (mild pain with inflammation, erythema, or joint swelling)	Continue pembrolizumab. Administer acetaminophen (paracetamol) and ibuprofen
	G2 (moderate pain with inflammation, erythema, or joint swelling that limits ADLs)	Withhold pembrolizumab. Administer higher doses of acetaminophen (paracetamol) and ibuprofen and use diclofenac or naproxen or etoricoxib. If inadequately controlled, consider intra-articular steroid injections for large joints or administer oral prednisone/prednisolone at a dose of 0.5–2 mg/kg/day or its equivalent. When improves to G1, begin a slow corticosteroid taper over at least 4 weeks. If does not respond adequately, then administer 0.5–1 mg/kg intravenously (methyl)prednisolone and convert to 0.5–2 mg/kg prednisone/prednisolone orally each day or its equivalent only after a response, followed by a taper over at least 4 weeks when improves to G1. Resume pembrolizumab upon symptom control, or when prednisone/prednisolone daily dose <10 mg
	G3 (severe pain; irreversible joint damage; disabling; limits self-care ADL)	Withhold pembrolizumab. Administer 0.5–1 mg/kg intravenously (methyl)prednisolone and convert to 0.5–2 mg/kg prednisone/prednisolone orally each day or its equivalent only after a response, followed by a taper over at least 4 weeks when improves to G1. In severe cases, infliximab or another anti–TNF-alpha drug may be required for improvement of arthritis. Resume pembrolizumab upon symptom control, or when prednisone/prednisolone daily dose <10 mg

(continued)

Treatment Modifications (*continued*)

RECOMMENDED DOSE MODIFICATIONS FOR PEMBROLIZUMAB

Adverse Event	Grade/Severity	Treatment Modification
Other	First occurrence of other G3	Withhold pembrolizumab. Administer oral prednisone/prednisolone at a dose of 0.5–2 mg/kg/day or its equivalent. When improves to G1, begin a slow corticosteroid taper over at least 4 weeks. Resume pembrolizumab upon symptom control, or when prednisone/prednisolone daily dose <10 mg
	Recurrence of same G3	Permanently discontinue pembrolizumab. Administer 1–2 mg/kg intravenously (methyl)prednisolone and convert to 0.5–2 mg/kg prednisone/prednisolone orally each day or its equivalent only after a response. Taper over at least 4–8 weeks when symptoms improve to G1
	Life-threatening or G4	
	Requirement for ≥10 mg/day prednisone or equivalent for >12 weeks	Permanently discontinue pembrolizumab
	Persistent G2/3 adverse reactions lasting ≥12 weeks	

ADL, activities of daily living; ALT, alanine aminotransferase; AST, aspartate aminotransferase; ATG, anti-thymocyte globulin; SJS, Stevens-Johnson Syndrome; TEN, toxic epidermal necrolysis; ULN, upper limit of normal

Notes on general supportive care:
• Steroid taper in most cases will proceed over a minimum of 1 month but if symptoms improve rapidly, a 2-week taper can be considered. If steroids are administered for more than 4 weeks, consider PCP prophylaxis (cotrimoxazole 480 mg twice daily M/W/F or inhaled pentamidine if has cotrimoxazole allergy), regular random blood glucose, VitD level, and starting calcium/VitD supplementation per guidelines

Adverse Events (N = 811)

Grade* (%)	Pembrolizumab Every 2 Weeks (n = 278)		Pembrolizumab Every 3 Weeks (n = 277)		Ipilimumab Every 3 Weeks (n = 256)	
	Any Grade	Grade 3–5	Any Grade	Grade 3–5	Any Grade	Grade 3–5
Any adverse event[†]	79.5	13.3	72.9	10.1	73.0	19.9
Occurring in at least 10% of patients in any one study group[†]						
Fatigue	20.9	0	19.1	0.4	15.2	1.2
Diarrhea	16.9	2.5	14.4	1.1	22.7	3.1
Rash	14.7	0	13.4	0	14.5	0.8
Pruritis	14.4	0	14.1	0	25.4	0.4
Asthenia	11.5	0.4	11.2	0	6.8	0.8
Nausea	10.1	0	11.2	0.4	8.6	0.4
Arthralgia	9.4	0	11.6	0.4	5.1	0.8
Vitiligo	9.0	0	11.2	0	1.6	0
Other selected adverse events[‡]						
Hypothyroidism	10.1	0.4	8.7	0	2.0	0
Hyperthyroidism	6.5	0	3.2	0	2.3	0.4
Colitis	1.8	1.4	3.6	2.5	8.2	7.0
Hepatitis	1.1	1.1	1.8	1.8	1.2	0.4
Pneumonitis	0.4	0	1.8	0.4	0.4	0.4
Hypophysitis	0.4	0.4	0.7	0.4	2.3	1.6
Uveitis	0.4	0	1.1	0	0	0
Type 1 diabetes mellitus	0.4	0.4	0.4	0.4	0	0
Myositis	0	0	0.7	0	0.4	0
Nephritis	0	0	0.4	0	0.4	0.4

*According to the National Cancer Institute Common Terminology Criteria for Adverse Events (NCI-CTCAE), version 4.0. At: https://ctep.cancer.gov/protocolDevelopment/electronic_applications/ctc.htm [accessed January 19, 2017]
[†]Attributed to the study drug by the investigator
[‡]Not necessarily related to treatment
Note: Safety was analyzed according to the study treatment received. Deaths attributed to adverse events: 1 in the ipilimumab group. Rate of adverse events leading to the permanent withdrawal from treatment: 4.0% in the pembrolizumab every 2 weeks group, 6.9% in the pembrolizumab every 3 weeks group, and 9.4% in the ipilimumab group

METASTATIC DISEASE • IMMUNE THERAPY

MELANOMA REGIMEN: NIVOLUMAB

Larkin J et al. N Engl J Med 2015;373:23–34. Comment in: Nat Rev Clin Oncol 2015;12:435, N Engl J Med 2015;373:1270–1271

The U.S. Food and Drug Administration (FDA)-approved regimens for melanoma include fixed doses of nivolumab and allow for a shortened infusion duration of 30 minutes, consistent with the regimens approved on March 5, 2018, thus:

Nivolumab 240 mg; administer intravenously over 30 minutes in a volume of 0.9% sodium chloride injection (0.9% NS) or 5% dextrose injection (D5W), not to exceed 160 mL and sufficient to produce a nivolumab concentration within the range 1–10 mg/mL, every 2 weeks until disease progression (total dosage/2-week course = 240 mg)

- Administer nivolumab through an administration set that contains a sterile, non-pyrogenic, low-protein-binding in-line filter with pore size within the range of 0.2–1.2 μm
- Nivolumab can cause severe infusion-related reactions

OR

Nivolumab 480 mg; administer intravenously over 30 minutes in a volume of 0.9% NS or D5W not to exceed 160 mL and sufficient to produce a nivolumab concentration within the range 1–10 mg/mL, every 4 weeks until disease progression (total dosage/4-week course = 480 mg)

- Administer nivolumab through an administration set that contains a sterile, non-pyrogenic, low-protein-binding in-line filter with pore size within the range of 0.2–1.2 μm
- Nivolumab can cause severe infusion-related reactions

Supportive Care

Antiemetic prophylaxis
Emetogenic potential with nivolumab is **MINIMAL**
See Chapter 42 for antiemetic recommendations

Hematopoietic growth factor (CSF) prophylaxis
Primary prophylaxis is **NOT** indicated
See Chapter 43 for more information

Antimicrobial prophylaxis
Risk of fever and neutropenia is **LOW**
Antimicrobial primary prophylaxis to be considered:

- Antibacterial—not indicated
- Antifungal—not indicated
- Antiviral—not indicated unless patient previously had an episode of HSV

Patient Population Studied

An international, multicenter, randomized, controlled, double-blind, phase 3 study involving 945 patients with histologically confirmed Stage III or IV melanoma not amenable to resection. Patients who had previously received a systemic therapy for advanced disease, patients with an Eastern Cooperative Oncology Group (ECOG) performance status score of ≥2, and patients who had ocular melanoma, active brain metastases, or autoimmune disease were not eligible for inclusion in the study. Participants were randomly assigned in a 1:1:1 ratio to receive nivolumab (+ ipilimumab-matched placebo), nivolumab + ipilimumab, or ipilimumab (+ nivolumab-matched placebo). The data presented below relate only to the nivolumab (+ ipilimumab-matched placebo) and the ipilimumab (+ nivolumab-matched placebo) groups

Efficacy (N = 631)

Median progression-free survival (primary end point)*	6.9 months in the nivolumab group 2.9 months in the ipilimumab group	Compared with ipilimumab, HR for death or disease progression (95% CI) with nivolumab was 0.57 (0.43–0.76); P<0.001
Objective response rate (secondary end point)†	43.7% in the nivolumab group 19.0% in the ipilimumab group	Compared with ipilimumab, the estimated OR (95% CI) with nivolumab was 3.40 (2.02–5.72); P<0.001

*Progression-free survival was defined as the time from randomization to documented disease progression or death, whichever came first, in the intention-to-treat population
†Objective response rate was defined as the percentage of patients with complete or partial response, in the intention-to-treat population

Therapy Monitoring

1. Initially at the time of each dose, and eventually every 6–12 weeks, perform a total body skin examination with attention to ALL mucous membranes as well as a complete review of systems
2. Monitor patients for signs and symptoms of pneumonitis. Evaluate patients with suspected pneumonitis with chest x-ray, CT, and pulse oximetry. For ≥2 toxicity, may include nasal swab, sputum culture and sensitivity, blood culture and sensitivity, and urine culture and sensitivity
3. Monitor patients for signs and symptoms of colitis. Encourage patients to report diarrhea immediately to any member of the health care team
4. Draw AST, ALT, and bilirubin prior to each infusion and/or weekly if there are Grade 1 liver function test elevations. Note, no treatment is recommended for G1 LFT abnormalities. For ≥2 toxicity, work up for other causes of elevated LFTs including viral hepatitis
5. Use basic metabolic panel (Na, K, CO_2, glucose) and patient history as screening tools for hypophysitis including hypopituitarism and adrenal insufficiency. If in doubt, evaluate AM adrenocorticotropic hormone (ACTH) and cortisol levels. Consider ACTH stimulation test for indeterminate results
6. Assess thyroid function at the start of treatment, periodically during treatment, and as indicated based on clinical evaluation and for clinical signs and symptoms of thyroid disorders. Test for TSH and free thyroxine (FT4) every 4–6 weeks as part of routine clinical monitoring of therapy or for case detection in symptomatic patients
7. Measure glucose at baseline and with each treatment during the first 12 weeks and every 6 weeks thereafter
8. Obtain a serum creatinine prior to every dose. If creatinine is found to be newly elevated, consider holding therapy while other potential causes are evaluated. Note, routine urinalysis is not necessary other than to rule out urinary tract infections, etc
9. Obtain a complete rheumatologic history and perform an examination of all peripheral joints for tenderness, swelling, and range of motion. Examine the spine. Consider plain x-ray/imaging to exclude metastases and evaluate joint damage (erosions), if appropriate

(continued)

Therapy Monitoring (*continued*)

10. In patients at high risk for infections and in appropriately selected patients based on an infectious disease evaluation, draw screening laboratories (HIV, hepatitis A and B, and blood QuantiFERON for TB) to prepare patients to start infliximab
11. Response evaluation: Every 2–4 months

Treatment Modifications

RECOMMENDED DOSE MODIFICATIONS FOR NIVOLUMAB

Adverse Event	Grade/Severity	Treatment Modification
Infusion reaction	Clinically significant but not severe infusion reaction	Interrupt the infusion in patients with clinically significant infusion reactions and consider resuming at a slower rate following resolution. If decision is made to restart, begin at ≤50% of the rate prior to the reaction and increase in 50% increments every 30 minutes if well tolerated. Infusions may be restarted at the full rate during the next cycle
	G3/4 (severe infusion reaction—pyrexia, chills, flushing, hypotension, dyspnea, wheezing, back pain, abdominal pain, and urticaria). Not rapidly responsive to brief interruption of infusion	Stop infusion and administer appropriate medical therapy (eg, epinephrine, corticosteroids, intravenous antihistamines, bronchodilators, and/or oxygen). Discontinue nivolumab
Colitis	G1	Loperamide 4 mg as starting dose then 2 mg before each meal and after each loose stool until without diarrhea for 12 hours, with maximum of 16 mg loperamide per day. If G1 diarrhea or colitis persists >14 days, then add prednisolone 0.5–1 mg/kg (non-enteric-coated) or consider oral budesonide 9 mg daily if no bloody diarrhea
	G2/3 diarrhea or colitis	Withhold nivolumab. Loperamide 4 mg as starting dose then 2 mg before each meal and after each loose stool until without diarrhea for 12 hours, with maximum of 16 mg loperamide per day. Administer oral prednisone/prednisolone at a dose of 0.5–2 mg/kg/day or its equivalent. When improves to G1, begin a slow corticosteroid taper over at least 4 weeks. Resume nivolumab upon symptom control, or when prednisone/prednisolone daily dose <10 mg
	G4 diarrhea or colitis	Permanently discontinue nivolumab. Loperamide 4 mg as starting dose then 2 mg before each meal and after each loose stool until without diarrhea for 12 hours, with maximum of 16 mg loperamide per day. Administer 1–2 mg/kg intravenously (methyl)prednisolone and convert to 0.5–2 mg/kg prednisone/prednisolone orally each day or its equivalent only after a response. Taper over at least 4 weeks when symptoms improve. If does not improve over 72 hours or worsens, perform flexible sigmoidoscopy/colonoscopy to document colitis then begin infliximab 5 mg/kg (if no perforation/sepsis/TB/hepatitis/NYHA III/IV CHF). If no response, add MMF 500–1000 mg twice daily. If worse on MMF, consider addition of tacrolimus or ATG
Pneumonitis	G2	Withhold nivolumab. Consider *Pneumocystis* prophylaxis depending on the clinical context and coverage with empiric antibiotics. Administer oral prednisone/prednisolone at a dose of 1–2 mg/kg/day or its equivalent. When improves to G1, begin a slow corticosteroid taper over at least 4 weeks. If does not respond adequately after 48 hours, then administer 2–4 mg/kg intravenously (methyl)prednisolone and convert to 0.5–2 mg/kg prednisone/prednisolone orally each day or its equivalent only after a response, followed by a taper over at least 6 weeks when symptoms improve to G1, titrating to symptoms. Resume nivolumab upon symptom control, or when prednisone/prednisolone daily dose <10 mg
	G3/4	Permanently discontinue nivolumab. Consider *Pneumocystis* prophylaxis depending on the clinical context; cover with empiric antibiotics. Administer 2–4 mg/kg intravenously (methyl)prednisolone and convert to 1–2 mg/kg prednisone/prednisolone orally each day or its equivalent only after a response, followed by a taper over at least 8 weeks when symptoms improve to G1, titrating to symptoms. If when initially treated improvement does not occur within 48–72 hours, begin infliximab 5 mg/kg (if no perforation/sepsis/TB/hepatitis/NYHA III/IV CHF). If no response to infliximab, add MMF 500–1000 mg twice daily. Consider MMF especially if has concurrent hepatic toxicity

(*continued*)

Treatment Modifications (*continued*)

RECOMMENDED DOSE MODIFICATIONS FOR NIVOLUMAB

Adverse Event	Grade/Severity	Treatment Modification
Hepatitis	G2 (AST or ALT >3–5× ULN or total bilirubin >1.5–3× ULN)	Withhold nivolumab. Administer oral prednisone/prednisolone at a dose of 1–2 mg/kg/day or its equivalent. When improves to G1, begin a slow corticosteroid taper over at least 4 weeks. Resume nivolumab upon symptom control, or when prednisone/prednisolone daily dose <10 mg
	G3/4 (AST or ALT >5× ULN or total bilirubin >3× ULN)	Permanently discontinue nivolumab. Administer 1–2 mg/kg intravenously (methyl)prednisolone and convert to 0.5–2 mg/kg prednisone/prednisolone orally each day or its equivalent only after a response. Taper over at least 6 weeks when symptoms improve. If no response, add MMF 500–1000 mg twice daily. If worse on MMF, consider adding tacrolimus or ATG
Hypophysitis	G2/3 (moderate symptoms, ie, headache but no visual disturbance or fatigue/mood alteration but hemodynamically stable, no electrolyte disturbance)	Administer analgesia as needed for headache. Withhold nivolumab. Administer oral prednisone/prednisolone at a dose of 0.5–2 mg/kg/day or its equivalent. When improves to G1, begin a slow corticosteroid taper over at least 4 weeks. If no improvement in 48 hours, administer 1–2 mg/kg intravenously (methyl)prednisolone and convert to 0.5–2 mg/kg prednisone/prednisolone orally each day or its equivalent only after a response. Taper over at least 4 weeks when symptoms improve to 5 mg prednisone/prednisolone or equivalent; do not stop steroids. Resume nivolumab upon symptom control, or when prednisone/prednisolone daily dose <10 mg
	G4 (severe mass effect symptoms, ie, severe headache, any visual disturbance or severe hypoadrenalism, ie, hypotension, severe electrolyte disturbance)	Permanently discontinue nivolumab. Administer analgesia as needed for headache. Administer 1–2 mg/kg intravenously (methyl)prednisolone and convert to 0.5–2 mg/kg prednisone/prednisolone orally each day or its equivalent only after a response. Taper over at least 4 weeks when symptoms improve to 5 mg prednisone/prednisolone or equivalent; do not stop steroids
Adrenal insufficiency	G2	Withhold nivolumab. Administer oral prednisone/prednisolone at a dose of 0.5–2 mg/kg/day or its equivalent. When improves to G1, begin a slow corticosteroid taper over at least 4 weeks. Serially assess adrenal function and continue steroids at replacement doses (20–40 mg hydrocortisone daily ~2/3 dose in AM upon awakening and ~1/3 at 4 PM) until recovery of adrenal function is documented. Resume nivolumab upon symptom control, or when prednisone/prednisolone daily dose <10 mg
	G3/4	Permanently discontinue nivolumab. Administer oral prednisone/prednisolone at a dose of 0.5–2 mg/kg/day or its equivalent. When improves to G1, begin a slow corticosteroid taper over at least 4 weeks. Serially assess adrenal function and continue steroids at replacement doses (20–40 mg hydrocortisone daily ~2/3 dose in AM upon awakening and ~1/3 at 4 PM) until recovery of adrenal function is documented
Type 1 diabetes mellitus	G3 hyperglycemia	Withhold nivolumab. Admit to hospital to manage hyperglycemia. Role of corticosteroids in preventing complete loss of insulin-producing cells is unknown and not recommended. Resume nivolumab upon symptom control, or when prednisone/prednisolone daily dose <10 mg
	G4 hyperglycemia	Permanently discontinue nivolumab. Admit to hospital to manage hyperglycemia. Role of corticosteroids in preventing complete loss of insulin-producing cells is unknown and not recommended
Nephritis and renal dysfunction	G2/3 (serum creatinine 1.5–6× ULN)	Withhold nivolumab. Administer oral prednisone/prednisolone at a dose of 0.5–2 mg/kg/day or its equivalent. When improves to G1, begin a slow corticosteroid taper over at least 4 weeks. If does not respond adequately, then administer 0.5–1 mg/kg intravenously (methyl)prednisolone and convert to 0.5–2 mg/kg prednisone/prednisolone orally each day or its equivalent only after a response, followed by a taper over at least 4 weeks when improves to G1. Resume nivolumab upon symptom control, or when prednisone/prednisolone daily dose <10 mg
	G4 (serum creatinine >6× ULN)	Permanently discontinue nivolumab. Administer 0.5–1 mg/kg intravenously (methyl)prednisolone and convert to 0.5–2 mg/kg prednisone/prednisolone orally each day or its equivalent only after a response, followed by a taper over at least 4 weeks when improves to G1

(*continued*)

Treatment Modifications (*continued*)

RECOMMENDED DOSE MODIFICATIONS FOR NIVOLUMAB

Adverse Event	Grade/Severity	Treatment Modification
Skin	G1/2	Continue nivolumab. Avoid skin irritants, avoid sun exposure, topical emollients recommended. Topical steroid (mild strength for G1, moderate/potent strength for G2) cream once or twice daily ± oral or topical antihistamines for itching
	G3 rash or suspected SJS or TEN	Withhold nivolumab. Avoid skin irritants, avoid sun exposure, topical emollients recommended. Administer oral or topical antihistamines for itching. Administer oral prednisone/prednisolone at a dose of 0.5–2 mg/kg or its equivalent daily for 3 days followed by a slow corticosteroid taper over at least 4 weeks when the rash improves to G1. If does not respond adequately, then administer 0.5–1 mg/kg intravenously (methyl)prednisolone and convert to 0.5–2 mg/kg prednisone/prednisolone orally each day or its equivalent only after a response, followed by a taper over at least 4 weeks when the rash improves to G1. Resume nivolumab upon symptom control, or when prednisone/prednisolone daily dose <10 mg
	G4 rash or confirmed SJS or TEN	Avoid skin irritants, avoid sun exposure, topical emollients recommended. Administer oral or topical antihistamines for itching. Administer 1–2 mg/kg intravenously (methyl)prednisolone and convert to oral steroids 0.5–2 mg/kg prednisone/prednisolone each day or its equivalent only after a response. Taper over at least 4 weeks when the rash improves to G1. Permanently discontinue nivolumab
Encephalitis	Confusion or altered behavior, headaches, alteration in Glasgow Coma Scale, motor or sensory deficits, speech abnormality, may or may not be febrile	Initially withhold nivolumab, but permanently discontinue nivolumab if there is no doubt as to diagnosis. Exclude bacterial and ideally viral infections prior to high-dose steroids. Administer oral prednisone/prednisolone at a dose of 0.5–2 mg/kg/day or its equivalent. When symptoms improve, begin a slow corticosteroid taper over at least 4–8 weeks. If symptoms are severe, administer 1–2 mg/kg intravenously (methyl)prednisolone and convert to 0.5–2 mg/kg prednisone/prednisolone orally each day or its equivalent only after a response. Consider concurrent empiric antiviral (intravenous acyclovir) and antibacterial therapy
Aseptic meningitis	Headache, photophobia, neck stiffness with fever or may be afebrile, vomiting; normal cognition/cerebral function (distinguishes from encephalitis)	
Other syndromes include neurosarcoidosis, posterior reversible leukoencephalopathy syndrome (PRES), Vogt-Koyanagi-Harada syndrome, demyelination, vasculitic encephalopathy, and generalized seizures		
Transverse myelitis	Acute or subacute neurologic signs/symptoms of motor/sensory/autonomic origin; most have sensory level; often bilateral symptoms	Initially withhold nivolumab, but permanently discontinue nivolumab if there is no doubt as to diagnosis. Administer 2 mg/kg intravenously (methyl)prednisolone or consider 1 g/day and convert to 0.5–2 mg/kg prednisone/prednisolone orally each day or its equivalent only after a response. When symptoms improve, begin a slow corticosteroid taper over at least 4–8 weeks. Plasmapheresis may be required if steroids do not bring about improvement
Myocarditis	G3	Permanently discontinue nivolumab. Administer 2 mg/kg intravenously (methyl)prednisolone or consider 1 g/day and convert to 0.5–2 mg/kg prednisone/prednisolone orally each day or its equivalent only after a response. When symptoms improve, begin a slow corticosteroid taper over at least 4–8 weeks. If no response, add MMF 500–1000 mg twice daily. If worse on MMF, consider adding tacrolimus
Peripheral neurologic toxicity	Moderate: some interference with ADL, symptoms concerning to patient	Withhold nivolumab. Initial observation reasonable or initiate prednisone/prednisolone 0.5–1 mg/kg (if progressing, eg, from mild) and/or pregabalin or duloxetine for pain. When symptoms improve, begin a slow corticosteroid taper over at least 4 weeks. Resume nivolumab upon symptom control, or when prednisone/prednisolone daily dose <10 mg
	Severe: limits self-care and aids warranted, life-threatening, eg, respiratory problems	Permanently discontinue nivolumab. Administer 1–2 mg/kg intravenously (methyl)prednisolone and convert to 0.5–2 mg/kg prednisone/prednisolone orally each day or its equivalent only after a response. Taper over at least 4–8 weeks when symptoms improve to G1
Guillain-Barré syndrome	Progressive symmetrical muscle weakness with absent or reduced tendon reflexes—involves extremities, facial, respiratory, and bulbar and oculomotor muscles; dysregulation of autonomic nerves	Permanently discontinue nivolumab. Use of steroids not recommended in idiopathic Guillain-Barré syndrome; however, a trial of (methyl)prednisolone 1–2 mg/kg is reasonable, converting to 0.5–2 mg/kg prednisone/prednisolone orally each day or its equivalent only after a response. If no improvement or worsening, plasmapheresis or IVIG indicated

(*continued*)

Treatment Modifications (*continued*)

RECOMMENDED DOSE MODIFICATIONS FOR NIVOLUMAB

Adverse Event	Grade/Severity	Treatment Modification
Myasthenia gravis	Fluctuating muscle weakness (proximal limb, trunk, ocular, eg, ptosis/diplopia or bulbar) with fatigability, respiratory muscles also may be involved	Permanently discontinue nivolumab. Administer pyridostigmine at an initial dose of 30 mg three times daily. Administer oral prednisone/prednisolone at a dose of 0.5–2 mg/kg/day or its equivalent or 1–2 mg/kg intravenously (methyl)prednisolone depending on the severity of symptoms. If begin with intravenously, convert to 0.5–2 mg/kg prednisone/prednisolone orally each day or its equivalent only after a response. If no improvement or worsening, plasmapheresis or IVIG may be considered. Additional immunosuppressants used in myasthenia gravis include azathioprine, cyclosporine, and mycophenolate. Avoid certain medications, eg, ciprofloxacin, beta-blockers, that may precipitate cholinergic crisis
Other syndromes including motor and sensory peripheral neuropathy, multifocal radicular neuropathy/plexopathy, autonomic neuropathy, phrenic nerve palsy, cranial nerve palsies (eg, facial nerve, optic nerve, hypoglossal nerve)		Permanently discontinue nivolumab. Administer oral prednisone/prednisolone at a dose of 0.5–2 mg/kg/day or its equivalent or 1–2 mg/kg intravenously (methyl)prednisolone depending on the severity of symptoms. If begin with intravenously convert to 0.5–2 mg/kg prednisone/prednisolone orally each day or its equivalent only after a response
Arthralgia	G1 (mild pain with inflammation, erythema, or joint swelling)	Continue nivolumab. Administer acetaminophen (paracetamol) and ibuprofen
	G2 (moderate pain with inflammation, erythema, or joint swelling that limits ADLs)	Withhold nivolumab. Administer higher doses of acetaminophen (paracetamol) and ibuprofen and use diclofenac or naproxen or etoricoxib. If inadequately controlled, consider intra-articular steroid injections for large joints or administer oral prednisone/prednisolone at a dose of 0.5–2 mg/kg/day or its equivalent. When improves to G1, begin a slow corticosteroid taper over at least 4 weeks. If does not respond adequately, then administer 0.5–1 mg/kg intravenously (methyl)prednisolone and convert to 0.5–2 mg/kg prednisone/prednisolone orally each day or its equivalent only after a response, followed by a taper over at least 4 weeks when improves to G1. Resume nivolumab upon symptom control, or when prednisone/prednisolone daily dose <10 mg
	G3 (severe pain; irreversible joint damage; disabling; limits self-care ADL)	Withhold nivolumab. Administer 0.5–1 mg/kg intravenously (methyl)prednisolone and convert to 0.5–2 mg/kg prednisone/prednisolone orally each day or its equivalent only after a response, followed by a taper over at least 4 weeks when improves to G1. In severe cases, infliximab or another anti–TNF-alpha drug may be required for improvement of arthritis. Resume nivolumab upon symptom control, or when prednisone/prednisolone daily dose <10 mg
Other	First occurrence of other G3	Withhold nivolumab. Administer oral prednisone/prednisolone at a dose of 0.5–2 mg/kg/day or its equivalent. When improves to G1, begin a slow corticosteroid taper over at least 4 weeks. Resume nivolumab upon symptom control, or when prednisone/prednisolone daily dose <10 mg
	Recurrence of same G3	Permanently discontinue nivolumab. Administer 1–2 mg/kg intravenously (methyl)prednisolone and convert to 0.5–2 mg/kg prednisone/prednisolone orally each day or its equivalent only after a response. Taper over at least 4–8 weeks when symptoms improve to G1
	Life-threatening or G4	
	Requirement for ≥10 mg/day prednisone or equivalent for >12 weeks	Permanently discontinue nivolumab
	Persistent G2/3 adverse reactions lasting ≥12 weeks	

ADL, activities of daily living; ALT, alanine aminotransferase; AST, aspartate aminotransferase; ATG, anti-thymocyte globulin; SJS, Stevens-Johnson Syndrome; TEN, toxic epidermal necrolysis; ULN, upper limit of normal

Notes on general supportive care:
• Steroid taper in most cases will proceed over a minimum of 1 month but if symptoms improve rapidly, a 2-week taper can be considered. If steroids are administered for more than 4 weeks, consider PCP prophylaxis (cotrimoxazole 480 mg twice daily M/W/F or inhaled pentamidine if has cotrimoxazole allergy), regular random blood glucose, VitD level, and starting calcium/VitD supplementation per guidelines

Adverse Events (N = 624)

Grade* (%)	Nivolumab (n = 313)		Ipilimumab (n = 311)	
	Any Grade	Grade 3–4	Any Grade	Grade 3–4
Any adverse event	99.4	43.5	99.0	55.6
Any treatment-related adverse event	82.1	16.3	86.2	27.3
Occurring in at least 10% of patients in any one study group[†]				
Fatigue	34.2	1.3	28.0	1.0
Rash	25.9	0.6	32.8	1.9
Diarrhea	19.2	2.2	33.1	6.1
Pruritus	18.8	0	35.4	0.3
Nausea	13.1	0	16.1	0.6
Decreased appetite	10.9	0	12.5	0.3
Colitis	1.3	0.6	11.6	8.7

*According to the National Cancer Institute Common Terminology Criteria for Adverse Events (NCI-CTCAE), version 4.0. At: https://ctep.cancer.gov/protocolDevelopment/electronic_applications/ctc.htm [accessed January 19, 2017]

[†]Attributed to the study drug by the investigator

Note: Safety was analyzed according to the study treatment received. Deaths attributed to adverse events: 1 in the nivolumab group and 1 in the ipilimumab group. Rate of adverse events leading to the permanent withdrawal from treatment: 7.7% in the nivolumab group and 14.8% in the ipilimumab group

METASTATIC • IMMUNE THERAPY
MELANOMA REGIMEN: NIVOLUMAB + IPILIMUMAB

Larkin J et al. N Engl J Med 2015;373:23–34. Comment in: Nat Rev Clin Oncol 2015;12:435, N Engl J Med 2015;373:1270–1271
Wolchok JD et al. N Engl J Med 2017;377:1345–1356

Concurrent treatment with Nivolumab and Ipilimumab:
Nivolumab 1 mg/kg; administer intravenously over 30 minutes in a volume of 0.9% sodium chloride injection (0.9% NS) or 5% dextrose injection (D5W) not to exceed 160 mL and sufficient to produce a nivolumab concentration within the range 1–10 mg/mL on day 1, every 3 weeks for a maximum of 4 doses (total dosage/3-wk cycle = 1 mg/kg)
- Administer nivolumab through an administration set that contains a sterile, non-pyrogenic, low-protein-binding in-line filter with pore size within the range of 0.2–1.2 μm
- Nivolumab can cause severe infusion-related reactions

Followed on the same day by:
Ipilimumab 3 mg/kg; administer intravenously over 90 minutes in a volume of 0.9% NS or D5W sufficient to produce an ipilimumab concentration within the range 1–2 mg/mL on day 1, every 3 weeks for a maximum of 4 doses (total dose/3-week cycle = 3 mg/kg)
- Administer ipilimumab through an administration set containing a sterile, non-pyrogenic, low-protein-binding in-line filter

After completing treatment with Ipilimumab (up to 4 doses):
The U.S. Food and Drug Administration (FDA)-approved regimens for melanoma include fixed doses of nivolumab and allows for a shortened infusion duration of 30 minutes, consistent with the regimens approved on March 5, 2018. Note that fixed dosing of nivolumab may only be used *after completion* of concurrent treatment with nivolumab and ipilimumab, thus:

Nivolumab 240 mg; administer intravenously over 30 minutes in a volume of 0.9% sodium chloride injection (0.9% NS) or 5% dextrose injection (D5W), not to exceed 160 mL and sufficient to produce a nivolumab concentration within the range 1–10 mg/mL, every 2 weeks until disease progression (total dosage/2-week course = 240 mg)
- Administer nivolumab through an administration set that contains a sterile, non-pyrogenic, low-protein-binding in-line filter with pore size within the range of 0.2–1.2 μm
- Nivolumab can cause severe infusion-related reactions

OR
Nivolumab 480 mg; administer intravenously over 30 minutes in a volume of 0.9% NS or D5W not to exceed 160 mL and sufficient to produce a nivolumab concentration within the range 1–10 mg/mL, every 4 weeks until disease progression (total dosage/4-week course = 480 mg)
- Administer nivolumab through an administration set that contains a sterile, non-pyrogenic, low-protein-binding in-line filter with pore size within the range of 0.2–1.2 μm
- Nivolumab can cause severe infusion-related reactions

Supportive Care
Antiemetic prophylaxis
Emetogenic potential with nivolumab ± ipilimumab is **MINIMAL**
See Chapter 42 for antiemetic recommendations

Hematopoietic growth factor (CSF) prophylaxis
Primary prophylaxis is **NOT** *indicated*
See Chapter 43 for more information

Antimicrobial prophylaxis
Risk of fever and neutropenia is **LOW**
   Antimicrobial primary prophylaxis to be considered:
- Antibacterial—not indicated
- Antifungal—not indicated
- Antiviral—not indicated unless patient previously had an episode of HSV

Patient Population Studied

An international, multicenter, randomized, controlled, double-blind, phase 3 study involving 945 patients with histologically confirmed Stage III or IV melanoma not amenable to resection. Patients who had previously received a systemic therapy for advanced disease, patients with an Eastern Cooperative Oncology Group (ECOG) performance status score of ≥2, and patients who had ocular melanoma, active brain metastases, or autoimmune disease were not eligible for inclusion in the study. Participants were randomly assigned in a 1:1:1 ratio to receive nivolumab (+ ipilimumab-matched placebo), nivolumab + ipilimumab, or ipilimumab (+ nivolumab-matched placebo). The data presented below relate only to the nivolumab + ipilimumab and the ipilimumab (+ nivolumab-matched placebo) groups

Efficacy (N = 629)

Median progression-free survival (primary end point)*	11.5 months in the nivolumab + ipilimumab group 2.9 months in the ipilimumab group	Compared with ipilimumab, HR for death or disease progression (95% CI) with nivolumab + ipilimumab was 0.42 (0.31–0.57); P<0.001
Overall survival at 3 years (primary end point)	58% in the nivolumab + ipilimumab group 34% in the ipilimumab group	Compared with ipilimumab, HR for death (95% CI) with nivolumab + ipilimumab was 0.55 (0.45–0.69); P<0.001
Objective response rate (secondary end point)†	57.6% in the nivolumab + ipilimumab group 19.0% in the ipilimumab group	Compared with ipilimumab, the estimated OR (95% CI) with nivolumab + ipilimumab was 6.11 (3.59–10.38); P<0.001

*Progression-free survival was defined as the time from randomization to documented disease progression or death, whichever came first, in the intention-to-treat population
†Objective response rate was defined as the percentage of patients with complete or partial response, in the intention-to-treat population
Note: Progression-free survival and objective response rate data was reported in the 2015 publication of the Checkmate 067 trial. The overall survival data were reported in the 2017 publication. At the minimum follow-up or 36 months, the median overall survival had not yet been reached in the nivolumab + ipilimumab group

Therapy Monitoring

1. Monitor patients for signs and symptoms of infusion-related reactions including pyrexia, chills, flushing, hypotension, dyspnea, wheezing, back pain, abdominal pain, and urticaria

2. Initially at the time of each dose, and eventually every 6–12 weeks, perform a total body skin examination with attention to ALL mucous membranes as well as a complete review of systems

3. Monitor patients for signs and symptoms of pneumonitis. Evaluate patients with suspected pneumonitis with chest x-ray, CT, and pulse oximetry. For ≥2 toxicity, may include nasal swab, sputum culture and sensitivity, blood culture and sensitivity, and urine culture and sensitivity

4. Monitor patients for signs and symptoms of colitis. Encourage patients to report diarrhea immediately to any member of the health care team

5. Draw AST, ALT, and bilirubin prior to each infusion and/or weekly if there are Grade 1 liver function test elevations. Note, no treatment is recommended for G1 LFT abnormalities. For ≥2 toxicity, work up for other causes of elevated LFTs including viral hepatitis

6. Use basic metabolic panel (Na, K, CO_2, glucose) and patient history as screening tools for hypophysitis including hypopituitarism and adrenal insufficiency. If in doubt, evaluate AM adrenocorticotropic hormone (ACTH) and cortisol levels. Consider ACTH stimulation test for indeterminate results

7. Assess thyroid function at the start of treatment, periodically during treatment, and as indicated based on clinical evaluation and for clinical signs and symptoms of thyroid disorders. Test for TSH and free thyroxine (FT4) every 4–6 weeks as part of routine clinical monitoring of therapy or for case detection in symptomatic patients

8. Measure glucose at baseline and with each treatment during the first 12 weeks and every 6 weeks thereafter

9. Obtain a serum creatinine prior to every dose. If creatinine is found to be newly elevated, consider holding therapy while other potential causes are evaluated. Note, routine urinalysis is not necessary other than to rule out urinary tract infections, etc

10. Obtain a complete rheumatologic history and perform an examination of all peripheral joints for tenderness, swelling, and range of motion. Examine the spine. Consider plain x-ray/imaging to exclude metastases and evaluate joint damage (erosions), if appropriate

11. In patients at high risk for infections and in appropriately selected patients based on an infectious disease evaluation, draw screening laboratories (HIV, hepatitis A and B, and blood QuantiFERON for TB) to prepare patients to start infliximab

12. Response evaluation: Every 2–4 months

Treatment Modifications

RECOMMENDED DOSE MODIFICATIONS FOR NIVOLUMAB AND IPILIMUMAB

Note: Immune modulatory agents, including topical agents, were used to manage AEs in 47% of patients receiving nivolumab alone in the randomized study and 83.4% of those in the nivolumab + ipilimumab group, with secondary immunosuppressive agents (eg, infliximab) used in 0.6% and 6.1% of the patients, respectively. Resolution rates for select G3/4 AEs were 85–100% in the nivolumab + ipilimumab group for most organs. Most endocrine events did not resolve

Adverse Event	Grade/Severity	Treatment Modification
Infusion reaction	Clinically significant but not severe infusion reaction	Interrupt the infusion in patients with clinically significant infusion reactions and consider resuming at a slower rate following resolution. If decision is made to restart, begin at ≤50% of the rate prior to the reaction and increase in 50% increments every 30 minutes if well tolerated. Infusions may be restarted at the full rate during the next cycle
	G3/4 (severe infusion reaction—pyrexia, chills, flushing, hypotension, dyspnea, wheezing, back pain, abdominal pain, and urticaria). Not rapidly responsive to brief interruption of infusion	Stop infusion and administer appropriate medical therapy (eg, epinephrine, corticosteroids, intravenous antihistamines, bronchodilators, and/or oxygen). Discontinue nivolumab and ipilimumab
COLITIS	G1	Loperamide 4 mg as starting dose then 2 mg before each meal and after each loose stool until without diarrhea for 12 hours, with maximum of 16 mg loperamide per day. If G1 diarrhea or colitis persists >14 days, then add prednisolone 0.5–1 mg/kg (non-enteric-coated) or consider oral budesonide 9 mg daily if no bloody diarrhea
	G2/3 diarrhea or colitis	Withhold nivolumab and ipilimumab. Loperamide 4 mg as starting dose then 2 mg before each meal and after each loose stool until without diarrhea for 12 hours, with maximum of 16 mg loperamide per day. Administer oral prednisone/prednisolone at a dose of 0.5–2 mg/kg/day or its equivalent. When improves to G1, begin a slow corticosteroid taper over at least 4 weeks. Resume nivolumab and ipilimumab upon symptom control, or when prednisone/prednisolone daily dose <10 mg
	G4 diarrhea or colitis	Permanently discontinue nivolumab and ipilimumab. Loperamide 4 mg as starting dose then 2 mg before each meal and after each loose stool until without diarrhea for 12 hours, with maximum of 16 mg loperamide per day. Administer 1–2 mg/kg intravenously (methyl)prednisolone and convert to 0.5–2 mg/kg prednisone/prednisolone orally each day or its equivalent only after a response. Taper over at least 4 weeks when symptoms improve. If does not improve over 72 hours or worsens, perform flexible sigmoidoscopy/colonoscopy to document colitis then begin infliximab 5 mg/kg (if no perforation/sepsis/TB/hepatitis/NYHA III/IV CHF). If no response, add MMF 500–1000 mg twice daily. If worse on MMF, consider addition of tacrolimus or ATG
Pneumonitis	G2	Withhold nivolumab and ipilimumab. Consider *Pneumocystis* prophylaxis depending on the clinical context and coverage with empiric antibiotics. Administer oral prednisone/prednisolone at a dose of 1–2 mg/kg/day or its equivalent. When improves to G1, begin a slow corticosteroid taper over at least 4 weeks. If does not respond adequately after 48 hours, then administer 2–4 mg/kg intravenously (methyl)prednisolone and convert to 0.5–2 mg/kg prednisone/prednisolone orally each day or its equivalent only after a response, followed by a taper over at least 6 weeks when symptoms improve to G1, titrating to symptoms. Resume nivolumab and ipilimumab upon symptom control, or when prednisone/prednisolone daily dose <10 mg
	G3/4	Permanently discontinue nivolumab and ipilimumab. Consider *Pneumocystis* prophylaxis depending on the clinical context; cover with empiric antibiotics. Administer 2–4 mg/kg intravenously (methyl)prednisolone and convert to 1–2 mg/kg prednisone/prednisolone orally each day or its equivalent only after a response, followed by a taper over at least 8 weeks when symptoms improve to G1, titrating to symptoms. If when initially treated improvement does not occur within 48–72 hours, begin infliximab 5 mg/kg (if no perforation/sepsis/TB/hepatitis/NYHA III/IV CHF). If no response to infliximab, add MMF 500–1000 mg twice daily. Consider MMF especially if has concurrent hepatic toxicity

(continued)

Treatment Modifications (*continued*)

Adverse Event	Grade/Severity	Treatment Modification
HEPATITIS	G2 (AST or ALT >3–5× ULN or total bilirubin >1.5–3× ULN)	Withhold nivolumab and ipilimumab. Administer oral prednisone/prednisolone at a dose of 1–2 mg/kg/day or its equivalent. When improves to G1, begin a slow corticosteroid taper over at least 4 weeks. Resume nivolumab and ipilimumab upon symptom control, or when prednisone/prednisolone daily dose <10 mg
	G3/4 (AST or ALT >5× ULN or total bilirubin >3× ULN)	Permanently discontinue nivolumab and ipilimumab. Administer 1–2 mg/kg intravenously (methyl)prednisolone and convert to 0.5–2 mg/kg prednisone/prednisolone orally each day or its equivalent only after a response. Taper over at least 6 weeks when symptoms improve. If no response, add MMF 500–1000 mg twice daily. If worse on MMF, consider adding tacrolimus or ATG
Hypophysitis	G2/3 (moderate symptoms, ie, headache but no visual disturbance or fatigue/mood alteration but hemodynamically stable, no electrolyte disturbance)	Administer analgesia as needed for headache. Withhold nivolumab and ipilimumab. Administer oral prednisone/prednisolone at a dose of 0.5–2 mg/kg/day or its equivalent. When improves to G1, begin a slow corticosteroid taper over at least 4 weeks. If no improvement in 48 hours, administer 1–2 mg/kg intravenously (methyl)prednisolone and convert to 0.5–2 mg/kg prednisone/prednisolone orally each day or its equivalent only after a response. Taper over at least 4 weeks when symptoms improve to 5 mg prednisone/prednisolone or equivalent; do not stop steroids. Resume nivolumab and ipilimumab upon symptom control, or when prednisone/prednisolone daily dose <10 mg
	G4 (severe mass effect symptoms, ie, severe headache, any visual disturbance or severe hypoadrenalism, ie, hypotension, severe electrolyte disturbance)	Permanently discontinue nivolumab and ipilimumab. Administer analgesia as needed for headache. Administer 1–2 mg/kg intravenously (methyl)prednisolone and convert to 0.5–2 mg/kg prednisone/prednisolone orally each day or its equivalent only after a response. Taper over at least 4 weeks when symptoms improve to 5 mg prednisone/prednisolone or equivalent; do not stop steroids
Adrenal insufficiency	G2	Withhold nivolumab and ipilimumab. Administer oral prednisone/prednisolone at a dose of 0.5–2 mg/kg/day or its equivalent. When improves to G1, begin a slow corticosteroid taper over at least 4 weeks. Serially assess adrenal function and continue steroids at replacement doses (20–40 mg hydrocortisone daily ~2/3 dose in AM upon awakening and ~1/3 at 4 PM) until recovery of adrenal function is documented. Resume nivolumab and ipilimumab upon symptom control, or when prednisone/prednisolone daily dose <10 mg
	G3/4	Permanently discontinue nivolumab and ipilimumab. Administer oral prednisone/prednisolone at a dose of 0.5–2 mg/kg/day or its equivalent. When improves to G1, begin a slow corticosteroid taper over at least 4 weeks. Serially assess adrenal function and continue steroids at replacement doses (20–40 mg hydrocortisone daily ~2/3 dose in AM upon awakening and ~1/3 at 4 PM) until recovery of adrenal function is documented
Type 1 diabetes mellitus	G3 hyperglycemia	Withhold nivolumab and ipilimumab. Admit to hospital to manage hyperglycemia. Role of corticosteroids in preventing complete loss of insulin-producing cells is unknown and not recommended. Resume nivolumab and ipilimumab upon symptom control, or when prednisone/prednisolone daily dose <10 mg
	G4 hyperglycemia	Permanently discontinue nivolumab and ipilimumab. Admit to hospital to manage hyperglycemia. Role of corticosteroids in preventing complete loss of insulin-producing cells is unknown and not recommended
Nephritis and renal dysfunction	G2/3 (serum creatinine 1.5–6× ULN)	Withhold nivolumab and ipilimumab. Administer oral prednisone/prednisolone at a dose of 0.5–2 mg/kg/day or its equivalent. When improves to G1, begin a slow corticosteroid taper over at least 4 weeks. If does not respond adequately, then administer 0.5–1 mg/kg intravenously (methyl)prednisolone and convert to 0.5–2 mg/kg prednisone/prednisolone orally each day or its equivalent only after a response, followed by a taper over at least 4 weeks when improves to G1. Resume nivolumab and ipilimumab upon symptom control, or when prednisone/prednisolone daily dose <10 mg
	G4 (serum creatinine >6× ULN)	Permanently discontinue nivolumab and ipilimumab. Administer 0.5–1 mg/kg intravenously (methyl)prednisolone and convert to 0.5–2 mg/kg prednisone/prednisolone orally each day or its equivalent only after a response, followed by a taper over at least 4 weeks when improves to G1

(*continue*

Treatment Modifications (*continued*)

Adverse Event	Grade/Severity	Treatment Modification
Skin	G1/2	Continue nivolumab and ipilimumab. Avoid skin irritants, avoid sun exposure, topical emollients recommended. Topical steroid (mild strength for G1, moderate/potent strength for G2) cream once or twice daily ± oral or topical antihistamines for itching
	G3 rash or suspected SJS or TEN	Withhold nivolumab and ipilimumab. Avoid skin irritants, avoid sun exposure, topical emollients recommended. Administer oral or topical antihistamines for itching. Administer oral prednisone/prednisolone at a dose of 0.5–2 mg/kg or its equivalent daily for 3 days followed by a slow corticosteroid taper over at least 4 weeks when the rash improves to G1. If does not respond adequately then administer 0.5–1 mg/kg intravenously (methyl) prednisolone and convert to 0.5–2 mg/kg prednisone/prednisolone orally each day or its equivalent only after a response, followed by a taper over at least 4 weeks when the rash improves to G1. Resume nivolumab and ipilimumab upon symptom control, or when prednisone/prednisolone daily dose <10 mg
	G4 rash or confirmed SJS or TEN	Avoid skin irritants, avoid sun exposure, topical emollients recommended. Administer oral or topical antihistamines for itching. Administer 1–2 mg/kg intravenously (methyl)prednisolone and convert to oral steroids 0.5–2 mg/kg prednisone/prednisolone each day or its equivalent only after a response. Taper over at least 4 weeks when the rash improves to G1. Permanently discontinue nivolumab and ipilimumab
Encephalitis	Confusion or altered behavior, headaches, alteration in Glasgow Coma Scale, motor or sensory deficits, speech abnormality, may or may not be febrile	Initially withhold nivolumab and ipilimumab, but permanently discontinue nivolumab and ipilimumab if there is no doubt as to diagnosis. Exclude bacterial and ideally viral infections prior to high-dose steroids. Administer oral prednisone/prednisolone at a dose of 0.5–2 mg/kg/day or its equivalent. When symptoms improve, begin a slow corticosteroid taper over at least 4–8 weeks. If symptoms are severe, administer 1–2 mg/kg intravenously (methyl)prednisolone and convert to 0.5–2 mg/kg prednisone/prednisolone orally each day or its equivalent only after a response. Consider concurrent empiric antiviral (intravenous acyclovir) and antibacterial therapy
Aseptic meningitis	Headache, photophobia, neck stiffness with fever or may be afebrile, vomiting; normal cognition/cerebral function (distinguishes from encephalitis)	
Other syndromes include neurosarcoidosis, posterior reversible leukoencephalopathy syndrome (PRES), Vogt-Koyanagi-Harada syndrome, demyelination, vasculitic encephalopathy, and generalized seizures		
Transverse myelitis	Acute or subacute neurologic signs/symptoms of motor/sensory/autonomic origin; most have sensory level; often bilateral symptoms	Initially withhold nivolumab and ipilimumab, but permanently discontinue nivolumab and ipilimumab if there is no doubt as to diagnosis. Administer 2 mg/kg intravenously (methyl) prednisolone or consider 1 g/day and convert to 0.5–2 mg/kg prednisone/prednisolone orally each day or its equivalent only after a response. When symptoms improve, begin a slow corticosteroid taper over at least 4–8 weeks. Plasmapheresis may be required if steroids do not bring about improvement
Myocarditis	G3	Permanently discontinue nivolumab and ipilimumab. Administer 2 mg/kg intravenously (methyl)prednisolone or consider 1 g/day and convert to 0.5–2 mg/kg prednisone/prednisolone orally each day or its equivalent only after a response. When symptoms improve, begin a slow corticosteroid taper over at least 4–8 weeks. If no response, add MMF 500–1000 mg twice daily. If worse on MMF, consider adding tacrolimus
Peripheral neurologic toxicity	Moderate: some interference with ADL, symptoms concerning to patient	Withhold nivolumab and ipilimumab. Initial observation reasonable or initiate prednisone/prednisolone 0.5–1 mg/kg (if progressing, eg, from mild) and/or pregabalin or duloxetine for pain. When symptoms improve, begin a slow corticosteroid taper over at least 4 weeks. Resume nivolumab and ipilimumab upon symptom control, or when prednisone/prednisolone daily dose <10 mg
	Severe: limits self-care and aids warranted, life-threatening, eg, respiratory problems	Permanently discontinue nivolumab and ipilimumab. Administer 1–2 mg/kg intravenously (methyl)prednisolone and convert to 0.5–2 mg/kg prednisone/prednisolone orally each day or its equivalent only after a response. Taper over at least 4–8 weeks when symptoms improve to G1

(continued)

Treatment Modifications (continued)

Adverse Event	Grade/Severity	Treatment Modification
Guillain-Barré syndrome	Progressive symmetrical muscle weakness with absent or reduced tendon reflexes—involves extremities, facial, respiratory, and bulbar and oculomotor muscles; dysregulation of autonomic nerves	Permanently discontinue nivolumab and ipilimumab. Use of steroids not recommended in idiopathic Guillain-Barré syndrome; however, a trial of (methyl)prednisolone 1–2 mg/kg is reasonable, converting to 0.5–2 mg/kg prednisone/prednisolone orally each day or its equivalent only after a response. If no improvement or worsening, plasmapheresis or IVIG indicated
Myasthenia gravis	Fluctuating muscle weakness (proximal limb, trunk, ocular, eg, ptosis/diplopia or bulbar) with fatigability, respiratory muscles may also be involved	Permanently discontinue nivolumab and ipilimumab. Administer pyridostigmine at an initial dose of 30 mg three times daily. Administer oral prednisone/prednisolone at a dose of 0.5–2 mg/kg/day or its equivalent or 1–2 mg/kg intravenously (methyl)prednisolone depending on the severity of symptoms. If begin with intravenous, convert to 0.5–2 mg/kg prednisone/prednisolone orally each day or its equivalent only after a response. If no improvement or worsening, plasmapheresis or IVIG may be considered. Additional immunosuppressants used in myasthenia gravis include azathioprine, cyclosporine, and mycophenolate. Avoid certain medications, eg, ciprofloxacin, beta-blockers, that may precipitate cholinergic crisis
Other syndromes including motor and sensory peripheral neuropathy, multifocal radicular neuropathy/plexopathy, autonomic neuropathy, phrenic nerve palsy, cranial nerve palsies (eg, facial nerve, optic nerve, hypoglossal nerve)		Permanently discontinue nivolumab and ipilimumab. Administer oral prednisone/prednisolone at a dose of 0.5–2 mg/kg/day or its equivalent or 1–2 mg/kg intravenously (methyl)prednisolone depending on the severity of symptoms. If begin with intravenous, convert to 0.5–2 mg/kg prednisone/prednisolone orally each day or its equivalent only after a response
Arthralgia	G1 (mild pain with inflammation, erythema, or joint swelling)	Continue nivolumab and ipilimumab. Administer acetaminophen (paracetamol) and ibuprofen
	G2 (moderate pain with inflammation, erythema, or joint swelling that limits ADLs)	Withhold nivolumab and ipilimumab. Administer higher doses of acetaminophen (paracetamol) and ibuprofen and use diclofenac or naproxen or etoricoxib. If inadequately controlled, consider intra-articular steroid injections for large joints or administer oral prednisone/prednisolone at a dose of 0.5–2 mg/kg/day or its equivalent. When improves to G1, begin a slow corticosteroid taper over at least 4 weeks. If does not respond adequately, then administer 0.5–1 mg/kg intravenously (methyl)prednisolone and convert to 0.5–2 mg/kg prednisone/prednisolone orally each day or its equivalent only after a response, followed by a taper over at least 4 weeks when improves to G1. Resume nivolumab and ipilimumab upon symptom control, or when prednisone/prednisolone daily dose <10 mg
	G3 (severe pain; irreversible joint damage; disabling; limits self-care ADL)	Withhold nivolumab and ipilimumab. Administer 0.5–1 mg/kg intravenously (methyl)prednisolone and convert to 0.5–2 mg/kg prednisone/prednisolone orally each day or its equivalent only after a response, followed by a taper over at least 4 weeks when improves to G1. In severe cases, infliximab or another anti–TNF-alpha drug may be required for improvement of arthritis. Resume nivolumab and ipilimumab upon symptom control, or when prednisone/prednisolone daily dose <10 mg
Other	First occurrence of other G3	Withhold nivolumab and ipilimumab. Administer oral prednisone/prednisolone at a dose of 0.5–2 mg/kg/day or its equivalent. When improves to G1, begin a slow corticosteroid taper over at least 4 weeks. Resume nivolumab and ipilimumab upon symptom control, or when prednisone/prednisolone daily dose <10 mg
	Recurrence of same G3	Permanently discontinue nivolumab and ipilimumab. Administer 1–2 mg/kg intravenously (methyl)prednisolone and convert to 0.5–2 mg/kg prednisone/prednisolone orally each day or its equivalent only after a response. Taper over at least 4–8 weeks when symptoms improve to G1
	Life-threatening or G4	
	Requirement for ≥10 mg/day prednisone or equivalent for >12 weeks	Permanently discontinue nivolumab and ipilimumab
	Persistent G2/3 adverse reactions lasting ≥12 weeks	

ADL, activities of daily living; ALT, alanine aminotransferase; AST, aspartate aminotransferase; ATG, anti-thymocyte globulin; SJS, Stevens-Johnson Syndrome; TEN, toxic epidermal necrolysis; ULN, upper limit of normal

Notes on general supportive care:
• Steroid taper in most cases will proceed over a minimum of 1 month but if symptoms improve rapidly, a 2-week taper can be considered. If steroids are administered for more than 4 weeks, consider PCP prophylaxis (cotrimoxazole 480 mg twice daily M/W/F or inhaled pentamidine if has cotrimoxazole allergy), regular random blood glucose, VitD level, and starting calcium/VitD supplementation per guidelines

Adverse Events (N = 624)

Grade* (%)	Nivolumab + Ipilimumab (N = 313)		Ipilimumab (N = 311)	
	Any Grade	Grade 3–4	Any Grade	Grade 3–4
Any adverse event	99.7	68.7	99.0	55.6
Any treatment-related adverse event	95.5	55.0	86.2	27.3
Occurring in at least 10% of patients in any one study group[†]				
Diarrhea	44.1	9.3	33.1	6.1
Rash	40.3	4.8	32.8	1.9
Fatigue	35.1	4.2	28.0	1.0
Pruritis	33.2	1.9	35.4	0.3
Nausea	25.9	2.2	16.1	0.6
Pyrexia	18.5	0.6	6.8	0.3
Decreased appetite	17.9	1.3	12.5	0.3
Elevated alanine aminotransferase level	17.6	8.3	3.9	1.6
Elevated aspartate aminotransferase level	15.3	6.1	3.5	0.6
Vomiting	15.3	2.6	7.4	0.3
Hypothyroidism	15.0	0.3	4.2	0
Colitis	11.8	7.7	11.6	8.7
Arthralgia	10.5	0.3	6.1	0
Headache	10.2	0.3	7.7	0.3
Dyspnea	10.2	0.6	4.2	0

*According to the National Cancer Institute Common Terminology Criteria for Adverse Events (NCI-CTCAE), version 4.0. At: https://ctep.cancer.gov/protocolDevelopment/electronic_applications/ctc.htm [accessed January 19, 2017]

[†]Attributed to the study drug by the investigator

Note: Safety data reported in the 2015 publication of the Checkmate 067 trial are shown. In the 2017 publication, the authors indicated that the safety profile was unchanged from the initial report. Rate of adverse events leading to the permanent withdrawal from treatment: 36.4% in the nivolumab + ipilimumab group and 14.8% in the ipilimumab group. Deaths attributed to adverse events: 1 in the ipilimumab group

METASTATIC • BRAF V600E TARGETED THERAPY

MELANOMA REGIMEN: VEMURAFENIB

Chapman PB et al. N Engl J Med 2011;364:2507–2516

Vemurafenib 960 mg/dose; administer orally, twice daily without regard to food, continually (total dose/week = 13,440 mg)

Supportive Care

Antiemetic prophylaxis
Emetogenic potential is **MINIMAL–LOW**
See Chapter 42 for antiemetic recommendations

Hematopoietic growth factor (CSF) prophylaxis
Primary prophylaxis is **NOT** indicated
See Chapter 43 for more information

Antimicrobial prophylaxis
Risk of fever and neutropenia is **LOW**
Antimicrobial primary prophylaxis to be considered:
- Antibacterial—not indicated
- Antifungal—not indicated
- Antiviral—not indicated unless patient previously had an episode of HSV

Toxicity

Adverse Event	Dose Modification
G1 or G2 (tolerable)	None; maintain dose at 960 mg twice daily
G2 (intolerable) or G3	Hold dose until G ≤1, then resume vemurafenib at 720 mg twice daily. If the adverse event recurs, hold dose until G ≤1, then further reduce the vemurafenib dose to 480 mg twice daily. If the adverse event occurs a third time, permanently discontinue vemurafenib
G4	Discontinue permanently or hold dose until G ≤1 and then resume vemurafenib at 480 mg twice daily. If the adverse event recurs, discontinue permanently
Cutaneous squamous cell carcinoma	None; maintain dose at 960 mg twice daily; resect lesion

Patient Population Studied

The study evaluated 337 patients with unresectable, previously untreated Stage IIIC or Stage IV melanoma that tested positive for the BRAF V600E mutation. Patients were excluded if they had a history of cancer within the past 5 years (except basal or squamous cell carcinoma of the skin or carcinoma of the cervix), metastases to the central nervous system (unless such metastases were definitively treated more than 3 months previously with no progression and no requirement for continued glucocorticoid therapy), or if they were on any other concomitant anticancer therapy

Therapy Monitoring

1. *At baseline:* Contrast CT or MRI of the brain, chest, abdomen, pelvis, and other anatomic regions as clinically indicated; physical and dermatologic examination; electrocardiography; CBC with differential; LFTs; basic metabolic panel; and LDH
2. *Every 3 weeks:* Physical examination, CBC with differential, LFTs, basic metabolic panel, and LDH
3. *Every 6 weeks:* Electrocardiography
4. Tumor assessments are performed at baseline, at weeks 6 and 12, and every 9 weeks thereafter

Therapy Modifications

Dose Levels	Vemurafenib Dose
Initial dose	960 mg twice daily
First dose reduction	720 mg twice daily
Second dose reduction	480 mg twice daily

Efficacy

Overall Survival (N = 336)

Hazard ratio	0.37
P Value	<0.001
6-month OS	84%

Progression-Free Survival (N = 275)

Hazard ratio	0.26
P Value	<0.001
Median PFS	5.3 months

Tumor Response (N = 219)

Complete response	2 (1%)
Partial response	104 (47%)
Median time to response	1.45 months

Toxicity (N = 336)

	% G2	% G3	% G4
Arthralgia	18	3	
Rash	10	8	
Fatigue	11	2	
Cutaneous squamous cell carcinoma		12	
Keratoacanthoma	2	6	
Nausea	7	1	
Alopecia	8		
Pruritus	6	1	
Hyperkeratosis	5	1	
Diarrhea	5	<1	
Headache	4	<1	
Vomiting	3	1	
Neutropenia	<1	0	<1

METASTATIC • BRAF V600E TARGETED THERAPY

MELANOMA REGIMEN: VEMURAFENIB + COBIMETINIB

Larkin J et al. N Engl J Med 2014;371:1867–1876
Comment in: Nat Rev Clin Oncol 2014;11:683, N Engl J Med 2014;371:1929–1930
Protocol for: Larkin J et al. N Engl J Med 2014;371:1867–1876

Vemurafenib 960 mg per dose; administer orally twice daily, continuously, without regard to food, every 28 days (total dose/28-day cycle = 53,760 mg)

• Advise patients NOT to crush or chew vemurafenib tablets

• Missed doses may be taken up to four hours before a subsequently scheduled dose

• Patients should not take an additional dose if vomiting occurs after administration, but should continue use with the next scheduled dose

• Vemurafenib is a substrate for metabolism catalyzed by CYP3A4 and has been shown in experimental studies in vitro to inhibit CYP1A2, CYP2A6, CYP2B6, CYP2C8/9, CYP2C19, CYP2D6, and CYP3A4/5. Avoid concomitant use of vemurafenib with strong CYP3A4 inhibitors and, when possible, with strong CY P3A4 inducers. If concomitant use of a strong CYP3A4 inducer is unavoidable, increase each dose of vemurafenib by 240 mg if tolerated. If the strong CYP3A4 inducer is subsequently discontinued, 2 weeks later reduce the vemurafenib dose back to the dose taken before initiation of the strong CYP3A4 inducer

• Vemurafenib has been shown in experimental studies in vitro to be a substrate and inhibitor of P-glycoprotein (P-gp, MDR1, ABCB1) and BRCP (MXR1, ABCG2) efflux transport proteins

plus

Cobimetinib fumarate 60 mg/dose, administer orally, once daily, without regard to food, for 21 consecutive days on days 1–21, followed by 7 days without treatment, every 28 days (total dose/28-day cycle = 1260 mg)

• If a patient misses a dose, or vomits following administration of a dose, advise the patient to take the next dose at the next regularly scheduled time

• Cobimetinib is a substrate for metabolism catalyzed by CYP3A subfamily enzymes. Avoid concomitant use with moderate or strong CYP3A4 inhibitors. If short-term use (<2 weeks) of a moderate CYP3A4 inhibitor is unavoidable, then reduce the cobimetinib dose from 60 mg to 20 mg during concomitant therapy, and then increase the dose back to 60 mg following discontinuation of the moderate CYP3A4 inhibitor

• Experimental studies in vitro indicate cobimetinib may inhibit CYP2D6 and CYP3A subfamily enzymes

• Cobimetinib is a substrate for efflux transport by P-glycoprotein

Supportive Care

Antiemetic prophylaxis
Emetogenic potential with vemurafenib ± cobimetinib is **MINIMAL–LOW**
See Chapter 42 for antiemetic recommendations

Hematopoietic growth factor (CSF) prophylaxis
Primary prophylaxis is **NOT** indicated
See Chapter 43 for more information

Antimicrobial prophylaxis
Risk of fever and neutropenia is **LOW**
   Antimicrobial primary prophylaxis to be considered:
    • Antibacterial—not indicated
    • Antifungal—not indicated
    • Antiviral—not indicated unless patient previously had an episode of HSV

Patient Population Studied

An international, multicenter, randomized, phase 3 study involving 495 patients with previously untreated, but histologically confirmed, locally advanced Stage IIIC or Stage IV BRAF V600 mutation–positive melanoma that was not amenable to resection. Only patients with adequate hematologic, hepatic, renal, and cardiac function were eligible for inclusion in the study. Patients were randomly assigned to receive vemurafenib and cobimetinib (the combination group) or vemurafenib and placebo (control group)

Efficacy (N = 495)

Median progression-free survival as assessed by the investigator (primary end point)*	9.9 months vs 6.2 months in the control group; HR for death or disease progression (95% CI): 0.51 (0.39–0.68); P<0.001
Overall survival (secondary end point)†	Median survival not reached in either group; HR for death (95% CI): 0.65 (0.42–1.00); P = 0.046
Rate of confirmed objective response according to RECIST criteria, version 1.1 (secondary end point)	68% vs 45% in the control group; P<0.001
Duration of response (secondary end point)	Not reached vs 7.3 months in the control group
Progression-free survival as assessed by an independent review facility (secondary end point)	11.3 months vs 6.0 months in the control group; HR for death or disease progression (95% CI): 0.60 (0.45–0.79); P<0.001

*Progression-free survival was defined as the time between the date of randomization and the date of the first documented event of disease progression or death, whichever occurred first, in the intention-to-treat population
†These results are from the first interim analysis, which was performed at the time of the final analysis of progression-free survival. A second interim analysis of overall survival will be reported after 256 deaths have occurred. The final analysis of overall survival will be reported after 385 deaths have occurred

Therapy Monitoring

1. Perform dermatologic evaluations prior to initiation of therapy and every two months while on therapy. Monitor for cutaneous squamous cell carcinomas (cuSCC) and malignant melanomas. Excise any suspicious skin lesions, send for dermatopathologic evaluation, and treat per standard of care. Continue monitoring for 6 months following discontinuation of vemurafenib

2. QT interval prolongation has been reported with vemurafenib. Monitor ECG and electrolytes including potassium, magnesium, and calcium before treatment and after every dose modification. Monitor ECGs at day 15, monthly during the first 3 months of treatment, every 3 months thereafter, or more often as clinically indicated

3. Evaluate LVEF before treatment, after 1 month of treatment, then every 3 months thereafter during treatment with cobimetinib

4. Liver laboratory abnormalities may occur. Monitor liver enzymes and bilirubin before initiation of treatment and monthly during treatment, or as clinically indicated

5. Photosensitivity has been reported with vemurafenib. Advise patients to avoid sun exposure while taking vemurafenib and to wear protective clothing and use a broad-spectrum UVA/UVB sunscreen and lip balm (SPF ≥30)

6. Serious ophthalmologic reactions, including uveitis, iritis, and retinal vein occlusion, have been reported with both vemurafenib and cobimetinib. Monitor patients routinely for ophthalmologic reactions. Perform an ophthalmologic evaluation at regular intervals and for any visual disturbances

7. Major hemorrhagic events can occur with cobimetinib. Monitor for signs and symptoms of bleeding

8. Rhabdomyolysis has been reported with cobimetinib. Monitor creatine phosphokinase periodically and as clinically indicated for signs and symptoms of rhabdomyolysis

9. Response assessment: Imaging every 2–3 months

Treatment Modifications

VEMURAFENIB + COBIMETINIB	
VEMURAFENIB	
Starting dose	960 mg twice daily continuously
Dose Level −1	720 mg twice daily continuously
Dose Level −2	480 mg twice daily continuously
Dose Level −3	Discontinue vemurafenib
New primary malignant melanomas	Manage with excision, and continue treatment without dose modification
Cutaneous squamous cell carcinomas (cuSCC)	
Serious hypersensitivity reactions	Permanently discontinue vemurafenib. Do not attempt to re-treat
Stevens-Johnson syndrome or toxic epidermal necrolysis (TEN)	Permanently discontinue vemurafenib
Patient with uncorrectable electrolyte abnormalities, QTc >500 ms, or who are taking medicinal products known to prolong the QT interval.	Do not administer vemurafenib
QTc >500 ms occurring during vemurafenib treatment	Withhold vemurafenib, correct electrolyte abnormalities, and control for cardiac risk factors for QT prolongation. If QT improves to <500 ms, resume vemurafenib at a lower dose level
QTc both >500 ms and >60 ms longer than pre-treatment values while receiving vemurafenib despite correction of electrolyte abnormalities, and control for cardiac risk factors	Permanently discontinue vemurafenib
Other Nonhematologic Toxicities Due to Vemurafenib	
G1 or G2 (tolerable)	Continue administration; do not alter dose
First occurrence of G2 (intolerable) or G3	Interrupt treatment until toxicity G ≤1. Resume dosing at one lower dose level unless current dose is 480 mg twice a day in which case discontinue vemurafenib
Second occurrence of G2 (intolerable) or G3	Interrupt treatment until toxicity G ≤1. Resume dosing at one lower dose level unless current dose is 480 mg twice a day in which case discontinue vemurafenib
Third occurrence of G2 (intolerable) or G3	Discontinue vemurafenib
First occurrence of G4	Discontinue vemurafenib or interrupt treatment until toxicity G ≤1 then resume dosing at 480 mg twice a day
Second occurrence of G4	Discontinue vemurafenib

(continued)

Treatment Modifications (*continued*)

COBIMETINIB	
Starting dose	60 mg once daily on days 1–21 of each 28-day cycle
Dose Level −1	40 mg once daily on days 1–21 of each 28-day cycle
Dose Level −2	20 mg once daily on days 1–21 of each 28-day cycle
Dose Level −3	Discontinue cobimetinib
New primary malignancy	Manage with excision, and continue treatment without dose modification
G2 (intolerable), G3/4 dermatologic toxicity	Withhold cobimetinib. When symptoms improve to G ≤1 resume with dose one lower level
G3 hemorrhage	Withhold cobimetinib up to 4 weeks. If improved to G ≤1, resume at the next lower dose level. If not improved within 4 weeks, permanently discontinue
G4 hemorrhage	Permanently discontinue cobimetinib
Serous retinopathy	Withhold cobimetinib for up to 4 weeks. If signs and symptoms improve, resume at the next lower dose level. If not improved within 4 weeks, permanently discontinue
Recurrence of serous retinopathy at a reduced dose within four weeks	Permanently discontinue cobimetinib
Retinal vein occlusion	Discontinue cobimetinib
Asymptomatic, absolute decrease in LVEF from baseline of >10% and less than institutional LLN	Withhold cobimetinib for 2 weeks and repeat LVEF. Resume at next lower dose if (a) LVEF is ≥LLN *and* (b) absolute decrease from baseline LVEF is ≤10%. Permanently discontinue if (a) LVEF is < LLN *or* (b) absolute decrease from baseline LVEF is >10%
Symptomatic LVEF decrease from baseline	Withhold cobimetinib for up to 4 weeks and repeat LVEF. Resume at next lower dose if (a) symptoms resolve *and* (b) LVEF is ≥LLN *and* (c) absolute decrease from baseline LVEF is ≤10%. Permanently discontinue if (a) symptoms persist, *or* (b) LVEF is < LLN, *or* (c) absolute decrease from baseline LVEF is >10%
First occurrence of G4 hepatotoxicity	Withhold cobimetinib for up to 4 weeks. If improved to G ≤1, resume at the next lower dose level. If not improved to G ≤1 within 4 weeks, permanently discontinue cobimetinib
Recurrence of G4 hepatotoxicity	Permanently discontinue cobimetinib
G4 CPK elevation or any CPK elevation and myalgia	Withhold cobimetinib for up to 4 weeks. If improved to G ≤3, resume at the next lower dose level. If not improved to G ≤3 within 4 weeks, permanently discontinue cobimetinib
G2 (intolerable), or G3/4 photosensitivity	Withhold cobimetinib for up to 4 weeks. If improved to G ≤1, resume at next lower dose level. If not improved to G ≤1 within 4 weeks, permanently discontinue cobimetinib
Drug that is a strong CYP3A inhibitor is needed	Discontinue cobimetinib
Concurrent short-term (14 days or less) use of moderate CYP3A inhibitors is unavoidable	Adjust the vemurafenib dose. In patients taking vemurafenib 60 mg, reduce the dose to 20 mg. After discontinuation of a moderate CYP3A inhibitor, resume previous 60 mg dose of cobimetinib
...d for a moderate CYP3A inhibitor in patient taking 20 or 40 mg ...netinib	Use an alternative to a strong or moderate CYP3A inhibitor or if not possible discontinue cobimetinib
Other Nonhematologic Toxicities Due to Cobimetinib	
...tolerable) or G3 adverse event	Withhold cobimetinib for up to 4 weeks. If improves to G ≤1, resume at the next lower dose level. If not improved to G ≤1 within 4 weeks, permanently discontinue cobimetinib
...currence of any G4 adverse event	Withhold cobimetinib until improves to G ≤1. Then resume at the next lower dose level *or* permanently discontinue.
...t G4 adverse event	Permanently discontinue cobimetinib

May cause fetal harm. Advise women of potential risk to the fetus

Adverse Events (N = 493)

Grade* (%)	Vemurafenib + Cobimetinib (n = 254)				Vemurafenib + Placebo (Control; n = 239)			
	Grade 1	Grade 2	Grade 3	Grade 4	Grade 1	Grade 2	Grade 3	Grade 4
Any adverse event	7	26	49	13	9	29	49	9
Occurring in at least 20% of patients in any one study group								
Diarrhea	39	11	6	0	21	7	0	0
Nausea	30	9	1	0	18	5	1	0
Rash	22	11	5	1	19	11	5	0
Arthralgia	21	9	2	0	22	13	5	0
Fatigue	19	9	4	0	18	10	3	0
Pyrexia	19	5	2	0	18	4	0	0
Photosensitivity reaction	19	7	2	0	10	5	0	0
Vomiting	16	4	1	0	9	3	1	0
Alopecia	13	<1	<1	0	23	6	<1	0
Hyperkeratosis	9	1	0	0	21	6	2	0
Elevated creatine kinase level	9	11	7	4	3	<1	0	0
Elevated aspartate aminotransferase level	7	7	8	0	6	4	2	<1
Elevated alanine aminotransferase level	6	6	11	<1	7	5	6	<1
Other selected adverse events								
Chorioretinopathy	7	5	<1	0	<1	0	0	0
Retinal detachment	4	2	2	<1	0	0	0	0
QT-interval prolongation	2	1	<1	0	3	1	1	0
Decreased ejection fraction	1	6	1	0	0	2	1	0
Cutaneous squamous cell carcinoma	0	<1	2	0	0	0	11	0
Keratoacanthoma	0	0	1	0	<1	<1	8	0

*According to the National Cancer Institute Common Terminology Criteria for Adverse Events (NCI-CTCAE), version 4.0. At: https://ctep.cancer.gov/protocolDevelopment/electronic_applications/ctc.htm [accessed January 19, 2017]

Note: Safety was analyzed according to the study treatment received. For patients in whom multiple occurrences of a specific adverse event occurred, only the highest grade event was recorded. Deaths attributed to adverse events: 6 in the combination group vs 3 in the control group. Incidence of toxic events leading to the withdrawal from treatment: 13% in the combination group vs 12% in the control group

METASTATIC • BRAF V600E TARGETED THERAPY
MELANOMA REGIMEN: DABRAFENIB + TRAMETINIB

Flaherty KT et al. N Engl J Med 2012;367:1694–1703

Dabrafenib 150 mg per dose; administer orally twice daily, at least 1 hour before or 2 hours after meals, continuously, until disease progression (total dose/week = 2100 mg), *plus:*

Treatment notes:

- Advise patients NOT to open, crush, or break dabrafenib capsules
- Missed doses may be taken up to 6 hours before a subsequently scheduled dose
- Dabrafenib is a substrate for metabolism catalyzed by CYP2C8 and CYP3A4. Avoid concomitant use of dabrafenib with strong CYP3A4 or strong CYP2C8 inhibitors (eg, ketoconazole, nefazodone, clarithromycin, gemfibrozil), when possible. If concomitant use of a strong CYP3A4 or CYP2C8 inhibitor is unavoidable, monitor closely for toxicities. If concomitant use of a strong CYP3A4 or strong CYP2C8 inducer (eg, rifampin, phenytoin, carbamazepine, phenobarbital, St John's wort) is unavoidable, monitor closely for loss of efficacy
- Dabrafenib has been shown in experimental studies in vitro to induce CYP3A4 and CYP2C9. As a result, dabrafenib decreases systemic exposure to *S*-warfarin and *R*-warfarin. Monitor international normalized ratio (INR) levels closely in patients receiving warfarin during the initiation or discontinuation of dabrafenib

Trametinib 2 mg per dose; administer orally once daily, at least 1 hour before or 2 hours after a meal at approximately the same time each day, continuously, until disease progression (total dose/week = 14 mg)

Treatment note:

- Missed doses may be taken up to 12 hours before a subsequently scheduled dose

Supportive Care

Antiemetic prophylaxis
Emetogenic potential is **LOW**
See Chapter 42 for antiemetic recommendations

Hematopoietic growth factor (CSF) prophylaxis
Primary prophylaxis is **NOT** indicated
See Chapter 43 for more information

Antimicrobial prophylaxis
Risk of fever and neutropenia is **LOW**
  Antimicrobial primary prophylaxis to be considered:
- Antibacterial—not indicated
- Antifungal—not indicated
- Antiviral—not indicated unless patient previously had an episode of HSV

Patient Population Studied

Patients with histologically confirmed metastatic melanoma with either BRAF V600E or BRAF V600K mutations were eligible for inclusion. Eligible patients had measurable disease, an ECOG PS of 0 or 1. Patients with treated brain metastases and at least a 3-month history of stable disease were allowed to enroll. Patients were randomly assigned to receive 150 mg of dabrafenib twice daily plus once-daily trametinib at a dose of either 1 mg (combination 150/1) or 2 mg (combination 150/2) or 150 mg of dabrafenib monotherapy twice daily. There were no significant differences among groups except that patients in the combination 150/2 group were older than those in the monotherapy group (P = 0.04)

Treatment Modifications

DABRAFENIB + TRAMETINIB

Dabrafenib

Starting dose	150 mg by mouth twice a day
Dose Level −1	100 mg by mouth twice a day
Dose Level −2	75 mg by mouth twice a day
Dose Level −3	50 mg by mouth twice a day
Dose Level −4	Permanently discontinue dabrafenib

Trametinib

Starting dose	2 mg by mouth once daily
Dose Level −1	1.5 mg by mouth once daily
Dose Level −2	1 mg by mouth once daily
Dose Level −3	Permanently discontinue trametinib

Adverse Event	Dose Modification
New Primary Malignancy Adverse Events	
New primary non-cutaneous RAS mutation–positive malignancy	Permanently discontinue dabrafenib. Continue trametinib without modification, if appropriate
New primary non-melanoma cutaneous malignancy	Continue dabrafenib and trametinib at the same dose. Refer patient to dermatologist for management of non-melanoma cutaneous malignancy
Cardiac Adverse Events	
Asymptomatic, absolute decrease in LVEF of ≥10% but <20% from baseline that is below LLN	Interrupt trametinib for up to 4 weeks. If LVEF improves to ≥LLN, then resume trametinib at one lower dose level. If LVEF does not improve to ≥LLN, then permanently discontinue trametinib. Continue dabrafenib without modification
Symptomatic CHF Absolute decrease in LVEF by ≥20% from baseline that is below LLN	Permanently discontinue trametinib. Interrupt dabrafenib. If LVEF improves to ≥LLN and an absolute decrease ≤10% compared to baseline, then resume dabrafenib at the same dose
Ocular Adverse Events	
Patient reports loss of vision or other visual disturbances.	Interrupt dabrafenib and trametinib until ophthalmologic status is clarified. Urgently (within 24 hours) perform ophthalmologic evaluation
Uveitis, including iritis and iridocyclitis	If mild or moderate uveitis does not respond to ocular therapy, or for severe uveitis, interrupt dabrafenib for up to 6 weeks. If improved to G0/1, then resume at the same dose or at a lower dose level. If G ≥2 uveitis persists for >6 weeks, then permanently discontinue dabrafenib. Continue trametinib without modification
Retinal pigment epithelial detachments	Interrupt trametinib for up to 3 weeks. If improved, resume trametinib at the same or lower dose level. If not improved, then resume trametinib at one lower dose level, or permanently discontinue trametinib. Continue dabrafenib without modification
Retinal vein occlusion	Permanently discontinue trametinib. Continue dabrafenib without modification
Pulmonary Adverse Events	
Dyspnea, cough, fever, and radiologic abnormalities—pneumonitis is suspected	Interrupt trametinib until pulmonary status is clarified. Continue dabrafenib without modification
Interstitial lung disease/pneumonitis is confirmed	Permanently discontinue trametinib. Continue dabrafenib without modification

(continued)

Treatment Modifications (continued)

Febrile Adverse Events

Fever of 38.5°C to 40°C	Interrupt dabrafenib and trametinib until fever resolves. Increase fluid intake and administer antipyretics (eg, acetaminophen) as needed. Consider monitoring renal function as clinically indicated. Upon resolution of fever, resume dabrafenib at the same or a lower dose level and resume trametinib at the same dose
Fever of >40°C	Interrupt dabrafenib and trametinib until fever resolves. Increase fluid intake, administer antipyretics (eg, acetaminophen) as needed, and monitor renal function closely. Upon resolution of fever, resume dabrafenib at a lower dose level along with prophylactic antipyretics, or permanently discontinue dabrafenib. Upon resolution of fever, resume trametinib at the same or a lower dose level
Fever ≥38.5°C complicated by rigors, hypotension, dehydration, or renal failure	Interrupt dabrafenib and trametinib until fever resolves. Increase fluid intake, administer antipyretics (eg, acetaminophen) as needed, and monitor renal function closely. Administer corticosteroids (eg, prednisone 10 mg daily) for ≥5 days if there is no evidence of active infection. Upon resolution of fever, resume dabrafenib at a lower dose level along with prophylactic antipyretics, or permanently discontinue dabrafenib. Upon resolution of fever, resume trametinib at the same or a lower dose level
Recurrent fever ≥38.5°C	Interrupt dabrafenib and trametinib until fever resolves. Increase fluid intake and administer antipyretics (eg, acetaminophen) as needed. In the absence of evidence of active infection, administer corticosteroids (eg, prednisone 10 mg daily) for ≥5 days if fever persists for >3 days or if fever is associated with complications such as dehydration, hypotension, renal failure, or severe chills/rigors. Upon resolution of fever, resume dabrafenib at a lower dose level along with prophylactic antipyretics, or permanently discontinue dabrafenib. Upon resolution of fever, resume trametinib at the same dose level, or optionally at a lower dose level if temperature was ≥40°C or associated with complications

Dermatologic Adverse Events

Intolerable G2 dermatologic toxicity G3/4 dermatologic toxicity	Interrupt dabrafenib and trametinib for up to 3 weeks. If improved, resume dabrafenib at one lower dose level and resume trametinib at one lower dose level. If not improved, permanently discontinue both dabrafenib and trametinib

Hemorrhagic Adverse Events

G3 hemorrhage	Interrupt dabrafenib and trametinib. If bleeding is improved to G0/1, resume dabrafenib at the next lower dose level and resume trametinib at the next lower dose level
G4 hemorrhage	Permanently discontinue dabrafenib and trametinib

Venous Thromboembolism Events

Uncomplicated DVT or PE	Interrupt trametinib for up to 3 weeks. If improved to G0/1 within 3 weeks, resume trametinib at one lower dose level. Continue dabrafenib without modification
Life-threatening PE	Permanently discontinue trametinib. Interrupt dabrafenib until toxicity resolves to G0/1, then resume at a lower dose level, or permanently discontinue dabrafenib

Other Adverse Events

Other intolerable G2 toxicities*† Other G3 toxicities*†	Interrupt dabrafenib and trametinib. If improved to G0/1, resume dabrafenib at one lower dose level and resume trametinib at one lower dose level. If not improved, permanently discontinue dabrafenib and trametinib
First occurrence of any other G4 toxicity*†	Interrupt dabrafenib and trametinib until toxicity improves to G0/1. If toxicity improves to G0/1, then resume at dabrafenib at one lower dose level or permanently discontinue dabrafenib. If toxicity improves to G0/1, then resume trametinib at one lower dose level or permanently discontinue trametinib
Recurrent other G4 toxicity*†	Permanently discontinue dabrafenib and trametinib
Known G6PD deficiency	Monitor closely for hemolytic anemia with dabrafenib

(continued)

Treatment Modifications (*continued*)

Note: Advise patients of potential risk to a fetus with dabrafenib and trametinib and to use effective contraception. Advise female patients of reproductive potential to use an effective *nonhormonal* method of contraception during dabrafenib treatment and for 2 weeks after the last dabrafenib dose, since dabrafenib can render hormonal contraceptives ineffective. Advise female patients to use effective contraception during treatment with trametinib and for 4 months after the last trametinib dose

*Dose modifications are not recommended for dabrafenib when administered with trametinib for the following adverse reactions attributable to trametinib: retinal vein occlusion, retinal pigment epithelial detachment, interstitial lung disease/pneumonitis, and uncomplicated venous thromboembolism. Dose modification of dabrafenib is not required for new primary cutaneous malignancies

†Dose modifications are not recommended for trametinib when administered with dabrafenib for the following adverse reactions attributable to dabrafenib: noncutaneous malignancies and uveitis. Dose modification of trametinib is not required for new primary cutaneous malignancies

LVEF, left ventricular ejection fraction; LLN, lower limit of normal; CHF, congestive heart failure; G6PD, glucose–6-phosphate dehydrogenase; DVT, deep vein thrombosis; PE, pulmonary embolism

Tafinlar (dabrafenib) prescribing information. East Hanover, NJ: Novartis Pharmaceuticals Corporation; revised 2018 May

Mekinist (trametinib) prescribing information. East Hanover, NJ: Novartis Pharmaceuticals Corporation; revised 2018 May

Efficacy End Points as Assessed by the Site Investigators (Intention-to-Treat Population)*

End Point	Dabrafenib Monotherapy (N = 54)	Dabrafenib 150 mg + Trametinib 1 mg (N = 54)	Dabrafenib 150 mg + Trametinib 2 mg (N = 54)
Progression-free survival, months			
Median (95% CI)	5.8 (4.6–7.4)	9.2 (6.4–11.0)	9.4 (8.6–16.7)
HR for death or progression (95% CI)	Reference	0.56 (0.37–0.87)	0.39 (0.25–0.62)
P value	Reference	0.006	<0.001
PFS at 12 months, % (95% CI)	9 (3–20)	26 (15–39)	41 (27–54)
Best response—no. (%)			
Complete response	2 (4)	3 (6)	5 (9)
Partial response	27 (50)	24 (44)	36 (67)
Stable disease	22 (41)	24 (44)	13 (24)
Progressive disease	3 (6)	2 (4)	0
Could not be evaluated	0	1 (2)	0
Complete or partial response			
Number of patients	29	27	41
Percentage of patients (95% CI)	54 (40–67)	50 (36–64)	76 (62–86)
P value	Reference	0.77	0.03
Duration of response, months			
Median (95% CI)	5.6 (4.5–7.4)	9.5 (7.4–NA)	10.5 (7.4–14.9)

HR, hazard ratio; PFS, progression-free survival; NA, not achieved
*Hazard ratios and P values are for the comparison between each combination-therapy group and the monotherapy group

Adverse Events*

Adverse Event	Dabrafenib Monotherapy (n = 53)[†]		Dabrafenib 150 mg + Trametinib 1 mg (n = 54)		Dabrafenib 150 mg + Trametinib 2 mg (n = 55)[†]	
	G3/4	All Grades	G3/4	All Grades	G3/4	All Grades
	Number of Patients (Percentage)					
Any event	23 (43)	53 (100)	26 (48)	53 (98)	32 (58)	55 (100)
Pyrexia	0	14 (26)	5 (9)	37 (69)	3 (5)	39 (71)
Chills	0	9 (17)	1 (2)	27 (50)	1 (2)	32 (58)
Fatigue	3 (6)	21 (40)	1 (2)	31 (57)	2 (4)	29 (53)
Nausea	0	11 (21)	3 (6)	25 (46)	1 (2)	24 (44)
Vomiting	0	8 (15)	2 (4)	23 (43)	1 (2)	22 (40)
Diarrhea	0	15 (28)	0	14 (26)	1 (2)	20 (36)
Headache	0	15 (28)	1 (2)	20 (37)	0	16 (29)
Peripheral edema	0	9 (17)	0	13 (24	0	16 (29)
Cough	0	11 (21)	0	6 (11)	0	16 (29)
Arthralgia	0	18 (34)	0	24 (44)	0	15 (27)
Rash	0	19 (36)	0	11 (20)	0	15 (27)
Night sweats	0	3 (6)	0	8 (15)	0	13 (24)
↓ Appetite	0	10 (19)	0	16 (30)	0	12 (22)
Myalgia	1 (2)	12 (23)	0	13 (24)	1 (2)	12 (22)
Constipation	0	6 (11)	1 (2)	9 (17)	0	12 (22)
↑ Alkaline phosphatase	0	1 (2)	3 (6)	12 (22)	0	5 (9)
Hyperkeratosis	0	16 (30)	0	3 (6)	0	5 (9)
Alopecia	0	18 (34)	0	5 (9)	0	3 (5)
	G3[‡]	All Grades	G3[‡]	All Grades	G3[‡]	All Grades
Cutaneous squamous cell carcinoma[§]	9 (17)	10 (19)	1 (2)	1 (2)	3 (5)	4 (7)
Skin papilloma	0	8 (15)	0	4 (7)	0	2 (4)
Hyperkeratosis	0	16 (30)	0	3 (6)	0	5 (9)
↑ Ejection fraction	0	0	1 (2)	2 (4)	0	5 (9)
Cardiac failure	0	0	1 (2)	1 (2)	0	0
Hypertension	0	2 (4)	0	2 (4)	1 (2)	5 (9)
Chorioretinopathy	0	0	0	0	1 (2)	1 (2)

*Adverse events reported in ≥20% of patients in any group, regardless of whether a causal relationship was likely. In addition to these events, there was one death from sepsis in 150/1 combination group and three deaths in the 150/2 combination group (two from brain hemorrhage and one from pulmonary embolism). None were considered related to study drug. Neutropenia (G3/4) occurred in 11% of patients in the 150/2 combination group, with one case of febrile neutropenia. Acneiform dermatitis occurred in 11% of patients in the 150/1 combination group, 16% in the combination group, and 4% in the 150/2 monotherapy group, with no G3/4 events reported

[†]One patient who was assigned to the monotherapy group received combination 150/2 and so was included in the combination 150/2 safety analyses

[‡]For these categories, no G4 events were reported

[§]Keratoacanthoma was classified as cutaneous squamous cell carcinoma

Treatment Monitoring

1. *Prior to the start of therapy in women of childbearing potential:* pregnancy test
2. *Prior to the start of therapy and repeated every 2 months during therapy and for 6 months after cessation of therapy:* dermatologic evaluation
3. *Prior to the start of therapy, 1 month after the start of therapy, and then every 2–3 months while on therapy:* assess left ventricular ejection fraction
4. *Periodically:*
   a. Monitor for signs and symptoms of uveitis (eg, changes in vision, photophobia, ocular pain) and perform an ophthalmologic examination in patients with new visual symptoms
   b. Monitor for febrile reactions and advise patients to promptly report fevers
   c. Monitor blood glucose at baseline and then as clinically necessary, especially in patients with pre-existing diabetes mellitus or hyperglycemia
   d. Monitor for signs and symptoms of colitis and/or gastrointestinal perforation
   e. Monitor for signs and symptoms of venous thromboembolism
   f. Monitor for signs and symptoms of hemorrhage
   g. In patients with known glucose-6-phosphate dehydrogenase deficiency, monitor for signs of hemolytic anemia
   h. Monitor for signs and symptoms of interstitial lung disease
5. *Tumor assessments:* performed at baseline, at weeks 6 and 12, and every 9 weeks thereafter

METASTATIC • BRAF V600E TARGETED THERAPY
MELANOMA REGIMEN: ENCORAFENIB + BINIMETINIB

Dummer R et al. Lancet Oncol 2018;19:603–615

Encorafenib 450 mg per dose; administer orally once daily, without regard to food, continuously until disease progression (total dosage/week = 3150 mg)
- Missed doses may be taken up to 12 hours before a subsequently scheduled dose
- Patients should not take an additional dose if vomiting occurs after administration, but should continue use with the next regularly scheduled dose
- Encorafenib is a substrate for metabolism catalyzed by CYP3A4. Avoid concomitant use of encorafenib with moderate or strong CYP3A4 inhibitors when possible. If concomitant use of a moderate or strong CYP3A4 inhibitor is unavoidable, decrease the encorafenib dose as described in the Treatment Modifications section. If the moderate or strong CYP3A4 inhibitor is subsequently discontinued, resume the encorafenib dose that was taken prior to initiation of the CYP3A4 inhibitor after approximately 3–5 inhibitor half-lives have elapsed. Avoid concomitant use of encorafenib with moderate or strong CYP3A4 inducers
- Advise patients to not consume grapefruit or grapefruit juice, as they may inhibit CYP3A in the gut wall and increase the bioavailability of encorafenib
- Encorafenib is a reversible inhibitor of UGT1A1, CYP1A2, CYP2B6, CYP2C8/9, CYP2D6, and CYP3A, and a time-dependent inhibitor of CYP3A4. Encorafenib induced CYP2B6, CYP2C9, and CYP3A4 at clinically relevant plasma concentrations
- Encorafenib may decrease the effectiveness of oral contraceptives (CYP3A4 substrates) which may lead to loss of oral contraceptive efficacy

plus:

Binimetinib 45 mg/dose, administer orally, twice daily (approximately 12 hours apart), without regard to food, continuously until disease progression (total dosage/week = 630 mg)
- Missed doses may be taken up to 6 hours before a subsequently scheduled dose
- Patients should not take an additional dose if vomiting occurs after administration, but should continue use with the next regularly scheduled dose
- Reduce the binimetinib starting dose to 30 mg per dose, orally twice daily for moderate (total bilirubin >1.5× ULN and ≤3× ULN and any AST) or severe (total bilirubin >3× ULN and any AST) hepatic impairment

Supportive Care
Antiemetic prophylaxis
Emetogenic potential with encorafenib + binimetinib is **MODERATE–HIGH**
See Chapter 42 for antiemetic recommendations

Hematopoietic growth factor (CSF) prophylaxis
Primary prophylaxis is **NOT** *indicated*
See Chapter 43 for more information

Antimicrobial prophylaxis
Risk of fever and neutropenia is **LOW**
 Antimicrobial primary prophylaxis to be considered:
  - Antibacterial—not indicated
  - Antifungal—not indicated
  - Antiviral—not indicated unless patient previously had an episode of HSV

Diarrhea management
Latent or delayed-onset diarrhea*:
 Loperamide 4 mg orally initially after the first loose or liquid stool, *then*
 Loperamide 2 mg orally every 2 hours during waking hours, *plus*
 Loperamide 4 mg orally every 4 hours during hours of sleep
  - Continue for at least 12 hours after diarrhea resolves
  - Recurrent diarrhea after a 12-hour diarrhea-free interval is treated as a new episode
  - Rehydrate orally with fluids and electrolytes during a diarrheal episode
  - If diarrhea persists >48 hours despite loperamide, stop loperamide and hospitalize the patient for IV hydration

Patient Population Studied

An international, multicenter, randomized, open-label, phase 3 study (COLUMBUS) involving 577 patients with histologically confirmed, locally advanced (Stage IIIB, IIIC, or IV), unresectable or metastatic cutaneous melanoma (or unknown primary melanoma) with a BRAF^{V600} mutation. Eligible patients were aged ≥18 years and had an Eastern Cooperative Oncology Group (ECOG) performance status score of ≤1. Patients who had previously received a systemic chemotherapy, extensive radiotherapy, or used an investigational agent other than previous immunotherapy for locally advanced, unresectable, or metastatic melanoma were not eligible for inclusion in the study. Participants were randomly assigned in a 1:1:1 ratio to receive encorafenib + binimetinib, encorafenib alone, or vemurafenib alone

Efficacy (N = 577)

	Encorafenib + Binimetinib (n = 192)	Encorafenib Alone (n = 194)	Vemurafenib Alone (n = 191)	HR (95% CI); P Value
Median progression-free survival	14.9 months	9.6 months	7.3 months	0.54 (0.41–0.71); P<0.0001 for combined therapy vs vemurafenib 0.75 (0.56–1.00); P = 0.051 for combined therapy vs encorafenib
Overall response rate*	63%	51%	40%	

*Overall response rate includes patients with either a complete or partial response to treatment
Note: Median duration of follow-up was 16.7 months for the encorafenib + binimetinib group, 16.6 months for the encorafenib group, and 14.4 months for the vemurafenib group

Therapy Monitoring

1. *Laboratory testing:*
   a. *Prior to initiation of encorafenib:* serum potassium, serum magnesium, pregnancy test (women of child-bearing potential). Correct hypokalemia and hypomagnesemia prior to initiation of encorafenib
      i. *Periodically during therapy with encorafenib in patients with baseline hypomagnesemia, baseline hypokalemia, or at risk for QTc interval prolongation:* consider interval measurements of serum potassium and serum magnesium and maintain values within the normal range
   b. *Prior to initiation of binimetinib:* liver function tests, creatine phosphokinase, serum creatinine, pregnancy test
      i. *At least monthly during binimetinib therapy:* liver function tests
      ii. *Periodically during binimetinib therapy, or as clinically indicated for signs/symptoms of rhabdomyolysis:* creatine phosphokinase, serum creatinine
2. *Cardiovascular testing:*
   a. *Patients receiving encorafenib who are at increased risk for developing QTcF interval prolongation (eg, long QT syndrome, bradyarrhythmias, heart failure, concomitant use of medications known to prolong the QTcF interval, hypokalemia and/or hypomagnesemia):* electrocardiogram for QTcF interval measurement prior to initiation of encorafenib and then periodically during treatment with encorafenib
   b. *Prior to initiation of binimetinib, 1 month after initiation of binimetinib, and every 2–3 months during treatment with binimetinib:* echocardiogram or MUGA to determine left ventricular ejection fraction (LVEF). The safety of binimetinib has not been established in patients with a baseline LVEF <50% or below the institutional lower limit of normal
3. *Dermatologic evaluations:*
   a. *Prior to initiation of encorafenib and repeated every 2 months during therapy and for 6 months after cessation of therapy:* dermatologic evaluation for detection of new primary cutaneous malignancies
4. *Ophthalmologic evaluations:*
   a. Binimetinib in combination with encorafenib has been associated with serous retinopathy with an incidence of 20% (median time to onset 1.2 months [range, 0–17.5 months]). Encorafenib, in combination with binimetinib, has been associated with uveitis with an incidence of 4%. Binimetinib, in combination with encorafenib, has been associated with retinal vein occlusion with an incidence of 0.1%.
      i. *At every visit:* assess for visual symptoms.
      ii. *At regular intervals and within 24 hours of patient-reported acute vision loss or other visual disturbance:* perform an ophthalmologic evaluation
5. *Periodically:*
   a. Monitor for signs and symptoms of hemorrhage associated with encorafenib
   b. Monitor for signs and symptoms of venous thromboembolism associated with binimetinib
   c. Monitor for signs and symptoms of interstitial lung disease associated with binimetinib

Treatment Modifications

ENCORAFENIB + BINIMETINIB

Encorafenib

	Without concomitant use of a moderate CYP3A4 inhibitor or strong CYP3A4 inhibitor	Concomitant use of a moderate CYP3A4 inhibitor	Concomitant use of a strong CYP3A4 inhibitor
Starting dose	450 mg by mouth once daily	225 mg by mouth once daily	150 mg by mouth once daily
Dose Level −1	300 mg by mouth once daily	150 mg by mouth once daily	75 mg by mouth once daily
Dose Level −2	225 mg by mouth once daily	75 mg by mouth once daily	75 mg by mouth once daily
Dose Level −3	Discontinue encorafenib	Discontinue encorafenib	Discontinue encorafenib

Note: If binimetinib is withheld, reduce the encorafenib dose to a maximum dose of 300 mg once daily until binimetinib is resumed

Binimetinib

Starting dose	45 mg by mouth twice per day
Dose Level −1	30 mg by mouth twice per day
Dose Level −2	Discontinue binimetinib

Note: If encorafenib is permanently discontinued, binimetinib should also be permanently discontinued

Adverse Event	Dose Modification
New Primary Malignancy Adverse Events	
New primary non-cutaneous RAS mutation–positive malignancy	Permanently discontinue encorafenib and binimetinib
New primary cutaneous malignancy	Continue encorafenib and binimetinib at the same dose. Refer patient to dermatologist for management of new primary cutaneous malignancy
Cardiac Adverse Events	
Asymptomatic, absolute decrease in LVEF of ≥10% but ≤20% from baseline that is below LLN	Interrupt binimetinib for up to 4 weeks and evaluate LVEF every 2 weeks. If within 4 weeks the LVEF improves to ≥LLN to a value within 10% of the patient's baseline and the patient is asymptomatic, then resume binimetinib with the dosage reduced by 1 dose level. If the patient does not recover to the above conditions within 4 weeks, then permanently discontinue binimetinib. Continue encorafenib; during periods when binimetinib is withheld or permanently discontinued, the encorafenib dose should not exceed 300 mg daily
Symptomatic CHF or Absolute decrease in LVEF by >20% from baseline that is below LLN	Permanently discontinue binimetinib. Continue encorafenib at a dose not exceeding 300 mg daily
QTcF >500 ms and ≤60 ms increase from baseline, first occurrence	Withhold encorafenib until QTcF is ≤500 ms, then resume encorafenib at 1 lower dose level. Continue binimetinib at the same dosage
QTcF >500 ms and ≤60 ms increase from baseline, second occurrence	Withhold encorafenib until QTcF is ≤500 ms, then resume encorafenib at 1 lower dose level. Continue binimetinib at the same dosage
QTcF >500 ms and ≤60 ms increase from baseline, third occurrence	Permanently discontinue encorafenib and binimetinib
QTcF >500 ms and >60 ms increase from baseline	Permanently discontinue encorafenib and binimetinib

Treatment Modifications (*continued*)

Ocular Adverse Events

Patient reports loss of vision or other visual disturbances	Interrupt encorafenib and binimetinib until ophthalmologic status is clarified. Urgently (within 24 hours) perform ophthalmologic evaluation
G1/G2 uveitis not responding to specific ocular therapy, or G3 uveitis	Withhold binimetinib for up to 6 weeks. If improved, resume binimetinib at the same dose or at 1 lower dosage level. If not improved, permanently discontinue binimetinib. Continue encorafenib; during periods when binimetinib is withheld or permanently discontinued, the encorafenib dose should not exceed 300 mg daily
G4 uveitis (blindness [20/200 or worse] in the affected eye)	Permanently discontinue binimetinib. Continue encorafenib at a dose not exceeding 300 mg daily
Serous retinopathy/retinal pigment epithelial detachments	Withhold binimetinib for up to 10 days. If improved and asymptomatic, resume binimetinib at the same dose. If not improved, then resume binimetinib at one lower dose level, or permanently discontinue binimetinib. Continue encorafenib; during periods when binimetinib is withheld or permanently discontinued, the encorafenib dose should not exceed 300 mg daily
Retinal vein occlusion	Permanently discontinue binimetinib. Continue encorafenib at a dose not exceeding 300 mg daily

Pulmonary Adverse Events

Dyspnea, cough, fever, and radiologic abnormalities—pneumonitis is suspected	Interrupt binimetinib until pulmonary status is clarified. Continue encorafenib; during periods when binimetinib is withheld or permanently discontinued, the encorafenib dose should not exceed 300 mg daily
G2 interstitial lung disease (symptomatic; medical intervention indicated; limiting instrumental ADL) is confirmed	Withhold binimetinib for up to 4 weeks. If improved to G ≤1 (asymptomatic; clinical or diagnostic observations only; intervention not indicated), then resume binimetinib at 1 lower dose level. If not improved to G ≤1 within 4 weeks, then permanently discontinue binimetinib. Continue encorafenib; during periods when binimetinib is withheld or permanently discontinued, the encorafenib dose should not exceed 300 mg daily
G ≥3 interstitial lung disease (severe symptoms; limiting self-care ADL; oxygen indicated; or worse) is confirmed	Permanently discontinue binimetinib. Continue encorafenib at a dose not exceeding 300 mg daily

Dermatologic Adverse Events

G2 dermatologic toxicity, first occurrence	If no improvement within 2 weeks, withhold encorafenib and binimetinib until improvement to G ≤1, then resume encorafenib and binimetinib at the same dosages
G2 dermatologic toxicity, recurrent	If no improvement within 2 weeks, withhold encorafenib and binimetinib until improvement to G ≤1, then resume encorafenib at the same dose and resume binimetinib at 1 lower dose level
G3 dermatologic toxicity, first occurrence	Withhold encorafenib and binimetinib until improvement to G ≤1, then resume encorafenib and binimetinib at the same dosages
G3 dermatologic toxicity, recurrent	Withhold encorafenib and binimetinib until improvement to G ≤1, then resume encorafenib at 1 lower dose level and resume binimetinib at 1 lower dose level
G4 dermatologic toxicity	Permanently discontinue encorafenib and binimetinib.

Hemorrhagic Adverse Events

Recurrent G2 hemorrhage or first occurrence of G3 hemorrhage	Interrupt encorafenib and binimetinib for up to 4 weeks. If improves to G ≤1, then resume encorafenib at 1 lower dose level and resume binimetinib at 1 lower dose level. If no improvement, then permanently discontinue encorafenib and binimetinib
Recurrent G3 hemorrhage	Consider permanently discontinuing binimetinib. Consider permanently discontinuing encorafenib. Note that if encorafenib is permanently discontinued, then binimetinib should also be permanently discontinued. Note that if binimetinib is discontinued and the decision is made to continue encorafenib monotherapy, then the encorafenib dose should not exceed 300 mg daily

(*continued*)

Treatment Modifications (continued)

Hemorrhagic Adverse Events	
G4 hemorrhage, first occurrence	*Binimetinib:* at the medically responsible health care provider's discretion, either: • Permanently discontinue binimetinib *or* • Withhold binimetinib for up to 4 weeks If improves to G ≤1, then resume binimetinib at 1 lower dose level. Note that if encorafenib is permanently discontinued, then binimetinib should also be permanently discontinued. *Encorafenib:* at the medically responsible health care provider's discretion, either: • Permanently discontinue encorafenib *or* • Withhold encorafenib for up to 4 weeks If improves to G ≤1, then resume encorafenib at 1 lower dose level. Note that during periods when binimetinib is withheld or permanently discontinued (if applicable), the encorafenib dose should not exceed 300 mg daily
Recurrent G4 hemorrhage	Permanently discontinue encorafenib and binimetinib

Venous Thromboembolism Events	
Uncomplicated DVT or PE	Withhold binimetinib. If improves to G ≤1, then resume binimetinib at 1 lower dose level. If no improvement, then permanently discontinue binimetinib. Continue encorafenib; during periods when binimetinib is withheld or permanently discontinued, the encorafenib dose should not exceed 300 mg daily
Life-threatening PE	Permanently discontinue binimetinib. Continue encorafenib at a dose not exceeding 300 mg daily

Hepatotoxicity and Hepatic Impairment	
Moderate (total bilirubin >1.5× ULN and ≤3× ULN and any AST) or severe (total bilirubin >3× ULN and any AST) hepatic impairment	Reduce the binimetinib starting dose to 30 mg per dose, orally twice daily. The recommended dose of encorafenib has not been determined in patients with moderate or severe hepatic impairment
G2 AST or ALT increased (>3–5× ULN)	Continue binimetinib at the same dosage and increase the frequency of liver function test monitoring to at least once per week. If no improvement within 2 weeks, then withhold binimetinib until improved to G ≤1 or to pretreatment/baseline values and then resume at the same dose. Continue encorafenib at the same dosage and increase the frequency of liver function test monitoring to at least once per week. If no improvement within 4 weeks, then withhold encorafenib until improved to G ≤1 or to pretreatment/baseline values and then resume at the same dose. Note that during periods when binimetinib is withheld and encorafenib is continued, the encorafenib dose should not exceed 300 mg daily
First occurrence of G3 AST or ALT increased (>5–20× ULN)	Interrupt encorafenib and binimetinib for up to 4 weeks. If improves to G ≤1, then resume encorafenib at 1 lower dose level and resume binimetinib at 1 lower dose level. If no improvement, then permanently discontinue encorafenib and binimetinib
Recurrent G3 AST or ALT increased (>5 – 20× ULN)	Consider permanently discontinuing binimetinib. Consider permanently discontinuing encorafenib. Note that if encorafenib is permanently discontinued, then binimetinib should also be permanently discontinued. Note that if binimetinib is discontinued and the decision is made to continue encorafenib monotherapy, then the encorafenib dose should not exceed 300 mg daily
G4 AST or ALT increased (>20× ULN), first occurrence	*Binimetinib:* at the medically responsible health care provider's discretion, either: • Permanently discontinue binimetinib *or* • Withhold binimetinib for up to 4 weeks If improves to G ≤1, then resume binimetinib at 1 lower dose level. Note that if encorafenib is permanently discontinued, then binimetinib should also be permanently discontinued. *Encorafenib:* at the medically responsible health care provider's discretion, either: • Permanently discontinue encorafenib *or* • Withhold encorafenib for up to 4 weeks If improves to G ≤1, then resume encorafenib at 1 lower dose level. Note that during periods when binimetinib is withheld or permanently discontinued (if applicable), the encorafenib dose should not exceed 300 mg daily
Recurrent G4 AST or ALT increased (>20× ULN)	Permanently discontinue encorafenib and binimetinib

(continued)

Treatment Modifications (continued)

Rhabdomyolysis or Creatine Phosphokinase Elevation

G4 asymptomatic CPK elevation (>10× ULN) or Any grade CPK elevation (> ULN) with symptoms or with renal impairment	Withhold binimetinib for up to 4 weeks. If improved to G ≤1, asymptomatic, and renal function returned to baseline, then resume binimetinib at the same dose. If not resolved within 4 weeks, then permanently discontinue binimetinib. Continue encorafenib; during periods when binimetinib is withheld or permanently discontinued, the encorafenib dose should not exceed 300 mg daily

Drug Interactions

Concomitant administration of a moderate CYP3A4 inhibitor or strong CYP3A4 inhibitor is unavoidable	See above for encorafenib dose reduction recommendations. Do not modify the dose of binimetinib
Concomitant administration of a moderate CYP3A4 inducer or strong CYP3A4 inducer is unavoidable	Avoid moderate CYP3A4 inducers and strong CYP3A4 inducers with encorafenib. Do not modify the binimetinib dose
Patient is taking a hormonal contraceptive concomitantly with encorafenib	Advise women of child-bearing potential that encorafenib may render hormonal contraceptives ineffective and to use an effective nonhormonal method of contraception
Concomitant use of a medication known to prolong the QTcF interval is unavoidable	Consider periodic electrocardiogram monitoring for measurement of the QTcF interval while the patient is taking encorafenib concomitantly with a medication known to prolong the QTcF interval. Maintain serum potassium and magnesium within the higher end of the normal range
Concomitant use of a sensitive CYP3A4 substrate is unavoidable	Encorafenib may result in increased toxicity or decreased efficacy of sensitive CYP3A4 substrates. Consider increased monitoring

Other Adverse Reactions[*][†]

Recurrent G2 adverse reaction[*][†] or first occurrence of G3 adverse reaction[*][†]	Interrupt encorafenib and binimetinib for up to 4 weeks. If improves to G ≤1, then resume encorafenib at 1 lower dose level and resume binimetinib at 1 lower dose level. If no improvement, then permanently discontinue encorafenib and binimetinib
Recurrent G3 adverse reaction[*][†]	Consider permanently discontinuing binimetinib. Consider permanently discontinuing encorafenib. Note that if encorafenib is permanently discontinued, then binimetinib should also be permanently discontinued. Note that if binimetinib is discontinued and the decision is made to continue encorafenib monotherapy, then the encorafenib dose should not exceed 300 mg daily
G4 adverse reaction, first occurrence[*][†]	*Binimetinib:* at the medically responsible health care provider's discretion, either: • Permanently discontinue binimetinib *or* • Withhold binimetinib for up to 4 weeks If improves to G ≤1, then resume binimetinib at 1 lower dose level. Note that if encorafenib is permanently discontinued, then binimetinib should also be permanently discontinued. *Encorafenib:* at the medically responsible health care provider's discretion, either: • Permanently discontinue encorafenib *or* • Withhold encorafenib for up to 4 weeks If improves to G ≤1, then resume encorafenib at 1 lower dose level. Note that during periods when binimetinib is withheld or permanently discontinued (if applicable), the encorafenib dose should not exceed 300 mg daily
Recurrent G4 adverse reaction[*][†]	Permanently discontinue encorafenib and binimetinib

Note: Advise patients of potential risk to a fetus with encorafenib and binimetinib and to use effective contraception. Advise female patients of reproductive potential to use an effective nonhormonal method of contraception during encorafenib treatment and for 2 weeks after the last encorafenib dose, since encorafenib can render hormonal contraceptives ineffective. Advise female patients to use effective contraception during treatment with binimetinib and for at least 30 days after the last binimetinib dose

[*]Dose modifications are not recommended for encorafenib when administered with binimetinib for the following adverse reactions: new primary cutaneous malignancies; ocular events other than uveitis, iritis, and iridocyclitis; interstitial lung disease/pneumonitis; cardiac dysfunction; creatine phosphokinase elevation; rhabdomyolysis; and venous thromboembolism

[†]Dose modifications are not recommended for binimetinib when administered with encorafenib for the following adverse reactions: palmar-plantar erythrodysesthesia syndrome, non-cutaneous RAS mutation–positive malignancies, and QTc prolongation

LVEF, left ventricular ejection fraction; LLN, lower limit of normal; CHF, congestive heart failure; QTcF, QT interval corrected by the Fridericia formula; ADL, activity of daily living; DVT, deep vein thrombosis; PE, pulmonary embolism; ULN, upper limit of normal; AST, aspartate aminotransferase; ALT, alanine aminotransferase; CPK, creatine phosphokinase

BRAFTOVI (encorafenib) prescribing information. Boulder, CO: Array BioPharma Inc; revised 2019 May

MEKTOVI (binimetinib) prescribing information. Boulder, CO: Array BioPharma Inc; revised 2019 January

Adverse Events

Grade (%)*	Encorafenib + Binimetinib (n = 192)		Encorafenib Alone (n = 192)		Vemurafenib Alone (n = 186)	
	Grade 1–2	Grade 3–4	Grade 1–2	Grade 3–4	Grade 1–2	Grade 3–4
Nausea	40	2	34	4	32	2
Diarrhea	34	3	12	2	32	2
Vomiting	28	2	22	5	14	1
Fatigue	27	2	24	<1	28	2
Arthralgia	25	<1	34	9	39	6
Increased blood creatine phosphokinase level	16	7	1	0	2	0
Headache	20	2	24	3	18	<1
Constipation	22	0	14	0	6	<1
Asthenia	17	2	17	3	14	4
Pyrexia	15	4	14	1	28	0
Abdominal pain	14	3	5	2	6	<1
Vision blurred	16	0	2	0	2	0
Increased gamma-glutamyltransferase level	6	9	6	5	8	3
Anemia	11	4	3	3	5	2
Rash	13	1	19	2	26	3
Hyperkeratosis	14	<1	34	4	29	0
Dry skin	14	0	30	0	23	0
Alopecia	14	0	56	0	37	0
Myalgia	14	0	18	10	18	<1
Dizziness	11	2	5	0	3	0
Hypertension	5	6	3	3	8	3
Increased alanine aminotransferase level	6	5	4	1	6	2
Pruritus	10	<1	21	<1	11	0
Back pain	9	<1	13	3	4	2
Insomnia	9	0	16	3	8	0
Palmoplantar keratoderma	9	0	24	2	15	1
Decreased appetite	8	0	20	<1	18	1
Erythema	7	0	12	<1	16	<1
Palmoplantar erythrodysesthesia	7	0	38	14	13	1
Skin papilloma	6	0	9	0	17	0
Musculoskeletal pain	6	0	14	3	5	1
Keratosis pilaris	5	0	17	0	23	0
Photosensitivity reaction	4	<1	4	0	23	1
Keratoacanthoma	2	0	6	0	8	3
Rash maculopapular	2	0	9	<1	10	4

*According to the National Cancer Institute Common Terminology Criteria for Adverse Events, version 4.03
Note: Grade 1–2 adverse events that occurred in ≥10% and Grade 3–4 adverse events that occurred in ≥2% of patients in any of the treatment groups are included in the table, irrespective of causality. Adverse events were monitored during the study and for at least 30 days after the last dose of study drug. Adverse events leading to discontinuation and suspected to be related to study treatment occurred in 6% of the combined therapy group, 10% of the encorafenib group, and 14% of the vemurafenib group. No deaths were considered likely related to study treatment, but one death in the combined therapy group was considered possibly related to the study treatment by the investigator; the patient stopped treatment on study day 9 and committed suicide on day 24

METASTATIC
• CYTOTOXIC THERAPY

MELANOMA REGIMEN: DACARBAZINE (DTIC)

Middleton MR et al. J Clin Oncol 2000;18:158–166

Dacarbazine 250 mg/m² (initial dosage) per day; administer intravenously in 50–250 mL of either 5% dextrose injection (D5W) or 0.9% sodium chloride injection (0.9% NS) over 30 minutes for 5 consecutive days on days 1–5, every 21 days (total dosage/cycle = 1250 mg/m²)

Alternative regimen:
Eggermont AMM, Kirkwood JM. Eur J Cancer 2004;40:1825–1836

Dacarbazine 1000 mg/m²; administer intravenously in 50–250 mL D5W or 0.9% NS over 30 minutes on day 1, every 28 days, for 2 cycles (total dosage/cycle = 1000 mg/m²)

Supportive Care
Antiemetic prophylaxis
Emetogenic potential on days of chemotherapy is **HIGH**
Potential for delayed symptoms
See Chapter 42 for antiemetic recommendations

Hematopoietic growth factor (CSF) prophylaxis
Primary prophylaxis is **NOT** indicated
See Chapter 43 for more information

Antimicrobial prophylaxis
Risk of fever and neutropenia is **LOW**
  Antimicrobial primary prophylaxis to be considered:
  • Antibacterial—not indicated
  • Antifungal—not indicated
  • Antiviral—not indicated unless patient previously had an episode of HSV

Patient Population Studied

A study of 136 patients with histologically confirmed incurable or unresectable advanced metastatic melanoma. Patients with nonmeasurable disease, ocular melanoma, or CNS metastases were excluded

Efficacy (N = 136)

Complete response	2.9%
Partial response	10.3%
Stable disease	17.7%
Progressive disease	69.1%
Median overall survival	6.4 months

Toxicity (N = 136)

	% All Grades	% G3	% G4
Hematologic			
Anemia	11	0	1
Neutropenia	3	1	1
Thrombocytopenia	9	4	4
Nonhematologic			
Asthenia	14	1	0
Fatigue	18	2	0
Fever	18	2	0
Headache	12	1	0
Pain	39	13	0
Anorexia	20	2	0
Constipation	29	3	0
Nausea	38	4	0
Vomiting	24	4	0
Somnolence	13	1	0

Treatment Modifications

Retreatment allowed if ANC ≥1500/mm³ and platelet count ≥100,000/mm³

Adverse Event	Dose Modification
Retreatment delayed by ≥2 weeks	Reduce dacarbazine dosage by 25%
G3/4 nonhematologic toxicity	Reduce dacarbazine dosage by 50%
>2 Dosage reductions	Discontinue therapy

Therapy Monitoring

1. *Before each cycle:* CBC with differential, LFTs, mineral panel, and electrolytes
2. *Response evaluation every 2 cycles:* PE, chest x-ray, and CT scans

METASTATIC • CYTOTOXIC THERAPY

MELANOMA REGIMEN: TEMOZOLOMIDE

Middleton MR et al. J Clin Oncol 2000;18:158–166

Temozolomide 200 mg/m² per day; administer orally for 5 consecutive days on days 1–5, every 28 days (total dosage/cycle = 1000 mg/m²)

Alternative regimens:

Brock CS et al. Cancer Res 1998;58:4363–4367

Temozolomide 75 mg/m² per day; administer orally for 21 consecutive days, every 28 days, for 2 cycles, followed by reevaluation of index measurable disease (total dosage/week = 525 mg/m²; total dosage/28-day cycle = 1575 mg/m²)

Patel PM et al. EORTC 18032 (poster). In: 33rd Annual ESMO Congress. Stockholm, Sweden; 2008

Temozolomide 150 mg/m² per day; administer orally for 7 consecutive days, on days 1–7, every 14 days ("7 days on/ 7 days off"; total dosage/14-day cycle = 1050 mg/m²)

Supportive Care
Antiemetic prophylaxis
*Emetogenic potential is **MODERATE***
See Chapter 42 for antiemetic recommendations

Hematopoietic growth factor (CSF) prophylaxis
*Primary prophylaxis is **NOT** indicated*
See Chapter 43 for more information

Antimicrobial prophylaxis
*Risk of fever and neutropenia is **LOW***
  Antimicrobial primary prophylaxis to be considered:
  • Antibacterial—not indicated
  • Antifungal—not indicated
  • Antiviral—not indicated unless patient previously had an episode of HSV

Patient Population Studied

A study of 144 patients with histologically confirmed incurable or unresectable advanced metastatic melanoma. Patients with nonmeasurable disease, ocular melanoma, or CNS metastases were excluded

Efficacy (N = 144)

Complete response	2.8%
Partial response	11.8%
Stable disease	19.4%
Progressive disease	66%
Median overall survival	7.7 months

Toxicity (N = 144)

	% All Grades	% G3	% G4
Asthenia	12	3	0
Fatigue	20	3	0
Fever	11	1	1
Headache	22	5	1
Pain	34	7	0
Anorexia	15	0	0
Constipation	30	3	0
Nausea	52	4	0
Vomiting	34	4	1
Somnolence	12	0	0
Anemia	8	1	1
Neutropenia	5	1	2
Thrombocytopenia	9	2	5

Treatment Modifications

Retreatment allowed if ANC ≥1500/mm³ and platelet count ≥100,000/mm³

Adverse Event	Dose Modification
Retreatment delayed by ≥2 weeks	Reduce temozolomide dosage by 25%
G3/4 hematologic toxicity	Reduce temozolomide dosage by 25%
G3/4 nonhematologic toxicity	Reduce temozolomide dosage by 50%
>2 Dosage reductions	Discontinue therapy

Therapy Monitoring

1. *Before each cycle:* CBC with differential, LFTs, mineral panel, and electrolytes
2. *Response evaluation every 2 cycles:* PE, chest x-ray, and CT scans

METASTATIC • CYTOTOXIC THERAPY

MELANOMA REGIMEN: CARBOPLATIN + PACLITAXEL

Hauschild A et al. J Clin Oncol 2009;27:2823–2830

Premedications:
Dexamethasone 20 mg per dose; administered orally or intravenously for 2 doses: the first dose between 12 and 14 hours before starting paclitaxel, and a second dose 6–7 hours before starting paclitaxel
Diphenhydramine 50 mg; administer intravenously per push 30 minutes before starting paclitaxel
Ranitidine 50 mg; administer intravenously in 25–100 mL of 0.9% sodium chloride injection (0.9% NS) or 5% dextrose injection (D5W) over 15–30 minutes, 30–60 minutes before starting paclitaxel

Cycles 1 through 4
Paclitaxel 225 mg/m^2; administer intravenously, diluted in 0.9% sodium chloride injection (0.9% NS) or 5% dextrose injection (D5W) to a concentration between 0.3 and 1.2 mg/mL, over 3 hours before carboplatin on day 1, every 21 days cycle (total dosage/cycle = 225 mg/m^2)
Carboplatin AUC = 6 mg/mL × min*; administer intravenously, diluted in 0.9% NS or D5W to a concentration >0.5 mg/mL, over 30 minutes on day 1 every 21 days (total dose/cycle calculated to produce an AUC = 6 mg/mL × min*)

Cycles 5 through 10
Paclitaxel 175 mg/m^2; administer intravenously, diluted in 0.9% NS or D5W to a concentration between 0.3 and 1.2 mg/mL, over 3 hours on day 1, every 21 days (total dosage/cycle = 175 mg/m^2)
Carboplatin AUC = 5 mg/mL × min*; administer intravenously, diluted in 0.9% NS or D5W to a concentration >0.5 mg/mL, over 30 minutes on day 1, every 21 days (total dose/cycle calculated to produce an AUC = 5 mg/mL × min*)

*Carboplatin dose is based on a formula described by Calvert et al. to achieve a target area under the plasma concentration versus time curve (AUC)

$$\text{Total Carboplatin Dose (mg)} = (\text{target AUC}) \times (\text{GFR} + 25)$$

In practice, creatinine clearance (CrCl) is used in place of glomerular filtration rate (GFR). CrCl can be estimated from the equation of Cockcroft and Gault, thus:

$$\text{For males, CrCl} = \frac{(140 - \text{age [years]}) \times (\text{body weight [kg]})}{72 \times (\text{serum creatinine [mg/dL]})}$$

$$\text{For females, CrCl} = \frac{(140 - \text{age [years]} \times (\text{body weight [kg]})}{72 \times (\text{serum creatinine [mg/dL]})} \times 0.85$$

Note: A carboplatin dose calculated with an IDMS-measured serum creatinine result using the Calvert formula could exceed an expected exposure (AUC) and result in increased drug-related toxicity. The FDA recommends capping an estimated GFR at 125 mL/min for any targeted AUC value. No greater estimated GFR values should be used (online) May 23, 2013. Available from: http://www.fda.gov/AboutFDA/CentersOffices/OfficeofMedicalProductsandTobacco/CDER/ucm228974.htm (accessed February 26, 2014)

Notes:
1. If paclitaxel is discontinued because of hypersensitivity, carboplatin may be continued
2. If carboplatin is discontinued because of hypersensitivity, tinnitus, or hearing loss, paclitaxel may be continued
3. After 4 cycles of chemotherapy, the dose of both chemotherapy agents will be reduced to carboplatin AUC of = 5 mg/mL × min and paclitaxel 175 mg/m^2. Patients who had a dose reduction during the first 4 chemotherapy cycles will continue at reduced doses. There is no additional dose reduction at cycle 5; a second dose reduction would be triggered by an occurrence of toxicity
4. In the absence of unacceptable toxicity, patients may continue to receive chemotherapy until disease progression. After completing 10 cycles of chemotherapy, carboplatin and paclitaxel may be discontinued at the discretion of a treating physician

Supportive Care
Antiemetic prophylaxis
Emetogenic potential is **HIGH** *with potential for delayed symptoms*
See Chapter 42 for antiemetic recommendations

Hematopoietic growth factor (CSF) prophylaxis
Primary prophylaxis is indicated with one of the following:
Filgrastim (G-CSF) 5 mcg/kg per day by subcutaneous injection, *or*
Pegfilgrastim (pegylated filgrastim) 6 mg/0.6 mL by subcutaneous injection for 1 dose
• Begin use from 24–72 hours after myelosuppressive chemotherapy is completed
See Chapter 43 for more information

Antimicrobial prophylaxis
Risk of fever and neutropenia is **LOW**

Dose Modifications

Adverse Event	Dose Modification
If carboplatin target dose is an AUC = 6 mg/mL × min and paclitaxel dose is 225 mg/m² and one of the following occurs: • G4 neutropenia (ANC <500/mm³) lasting >7 days • G4 neutropenia (ANC <500/mm³) with fever (≥38°C [≥100.5°F]) • G4 thrombocytopenia (<25,000/mm³) • Lack of ANC or platelet count recovery to pretreatment levels by day 28 of each cycle • Any G3/4 nonhematologic toxicity (including neuropathy) attributed to carboplatin or paclitaxel, with the exception of G4 hypersensitivity reactions	Reduce carboplatin dose to AUC = 5 mg/mL × min and paclitaxel dose to 175 mg/m² on the same administration schedule *Note:* This dose reduction is permanent. Do not increase doses during subsequent cycles
If carboplatin target dose is an AUC = 5 mg/mL × min and paclitaxel dose is 175 mg/m² and one of the following occurs: • G4 neutropenia (ANC <500/mm³) lasting >7 days • G4 neutropenia (ANC <500/mm³) with fever (≥38°C [≥100.5°F]) • G4 thrombocytopenia (<25,000/mm³) • Lack of ANC or platelet count recovery to pretreatment levels by day 28 of each cycle • Any G3/4 nonhematologic toxicity (including neuropathy) attributed to carboplatin or paclitaxel, with the exception of G4 hypersensitivity reaction	Reduce carboplatin dose to AUC = 4 mg/mL × min and paclitaxel dose to 125 mg/m² on the same administration schedule *Note:* This dose reduction is permanent. Do not increase doses during subsequent cycles *Note:* If any of the criteria for dose reduction are met after this second dose reduction, discontinue carboplatin and paclitaxel
G4 hypersensitivity reactions to either paclitaxel or carboplatin	Discontinue the agent responsible for the hypersensitivity reaction *Note:* Continue the remaining chemotherapy agent at the same dose and administration schedule, in the absence of the discontinued agent

Toxicity (N = 134)

Adverse Event	% G3	% G4
Any event	31%	39%
Hematologic events	25%	34%
Neutrophils	13%	32%
Platelets	9%	3%
Hemoglobin	12%	2%
Infection	11%	4%
Febrile neutropenia	5%	2%
Constitutional symptoms	11%	2%
Fatigue	8%	2%
Gastrointestinal	12%	2%
Diarrhea	3%	0
Metabolic/laboratory	6%	5%
Lipase	1%	2%
Neurology	19%	2%
Neuropathy, sensory	13%	1%
Pain	16%	2%

Patient Population Studied

A study of 270 patients with unresectable Stages III/IV melanoma with disease progression on a dacarbazine- or temozolomide-containing regimen. Prior adjuvant immunotherapy was allowed. Patients with active brain metastases were excluded

Efficacy (N = 135)

Response	N (%)
CR	0
PR	15 (11%)
SD	69 (51%)
PD	48 (36%)
Not evaluated	3 (2%)
Median PFS	17.9 weeks
Median OS	42.0 weeks

Therapy Monitoring

1. *Before each cycle:* CBC with differential, serum sodium, potassium, BUN, creatinine, glucose, SGOT (AST), SGPT (ALT), total bilirubin, alkaline phosphatase, LDH, albumin, amylase, lipase
2. *Response evaluation:* Every 2 cycles

25. Mesothelioma

Mohamed M. Azab, MD, Tamarah A. Al-Dawoodi, MD, and Nicholas J. Vogelzang, MD

Pleural Mesothelioma

Epidemiology

Incidence:	Approximately 3000 new cases per year in the U.S. Incidence of 0.8 per 100,000 in the U.S. in 2016; decreased from 1.1 per 100,000 in 2000
Median age:	72 years
Male to female incidence rate ratio:	3.5:1

Surveillance, Epidemiology and End Results (SEER) Program, available from http://seer.cancer.gov [accessed January 20, 2020]
Key Statistics About Malignant Mesothelioma. American Cancer Society. Available from https://www.cancer.org/cancer/malignant-mesothelioma/about/key-statistics.html [accessed January 20, 2020]
Peto J et al. Lancet 1995;345:535–539
Vogelzang NJ et al. Cancer 1984;53:377–383

Staging

	TNM Descriptors for Diffuse Malignant Pleural Mesothelioma
TX	Primary tumor cannot be assessed
T0	No evidence of primary tumor
T1	Limited to the ipsilateral parietal, ± visceral, ± mediastinal, ± diaphragmatic pleura
T2	Involves each of the ipsilateral pleural surfaces (parietal, mediastinal, diaphragmatic, and visceral pleura) with either involvement of diaphragmatic muscle, or extension of tumor from visceral pleura into the underlying pulmonary parenchyma, or both
T3	Locally advanced but potentially resectable, involving all of the ipsilateral pleural surfaces (parietal, mediastinal, diaphragmatic, and visceral pleura) with involvement of the endothoracic fascia, extension into the mediastinal fat, with solitary focus of completely resectable tumor extending into the soft tissues of the chest wall and/or nontransmural involvement of the pericardium
T4	Locally advanced and technically unresectable, involving all of the ipsilateral pleural surfaces (parietal, mediastinal, diaphragmatic, and visceral) with diffuse extension or multifocal masses of tumor in the chest wall with or without rib destruction, direct transdiaphragmatic extension of tumor to the peritoneum, direct extension to the contralateral pleura, direct extension to mediastinal organs, direct extension to the spine, or extension through the internal surface of the pericardium with or without a pericardial effusion, and/or myocardium involvement
NX	Regional lymph nodes cannot be assessed
N0	No regional lymph node metastases
N1	Metastases in the ipsilateral bronchopulmonary, hilar, or mediastinal (including the internal mammary, peridiaphragmatic, pericardial fat pad, or intercostal) lymph nodes

(continued)

Pathology

H & E staining

1. Epithelioid: 60% of cases = tubulopapillary, granular, solid (~5% 5-year survival)
2. Sarcomatoid/mixed: 40% of cases (0% 5-year survival)

Immunohistochemical staining: Keratin positive, CEA negative, Leu M negative, calretinin positive

Cytogenetics: Deletion of short arm of chromosome 1 and 3 and long arm of chromosome 22

Chaihinan AP et al. In: Holland JC, Frei E, eds. Cancer Medicine. 5th ed. Hamilton, ON: BC Decker; 2000:1293–1312
Corson JM. Semin Thorac Cardiovasc Surg 1997;9:347–355

Staging (continued)

TNM Descriptors for Diffuse Malignant Pleural Mesothelioma

N2	Metastases in the contralateral mediastinal, ipsilateral, or contralateral supraclavicular lymph nodes
M0	No distant metastasis
M1	Distant metastasis present

AJCC Prognostic Stage Groups for Diffuse Malignant Pleural Mesothelioma

	T (Primary)	N	M
Stage IA	T1	N0	M0
Stage IB	T2	N0	M0
	T3	N0	M0
Stage II	T1	N1	M0
	T2	N1	M0
Stage IIIA	T3	N1	M0
Stage IIIB	T1	N2	M0
	T2	N2	M0
	T3	N2	M0
	T4	Any N	M0
Stage IV	Any T	Any N	M1

Amin MB et al. (editors). AJCC Cancer Staging Manual, 8th ed. New York: Springer; 2017

Survival

AJCC 8th Edition Stage	2-year Overall Survival	5-year Overall Survival
Stage IA	46%	16%
Stage IB	41%	13%
Stage II	38%	10%
Stage IIIA	30%	8%
Stage IIIB	26%	5%
Stage IV	17%	0%

Amin MB et al. (editors). AJCC Cancer Staging Manual, 8th ed. New York: Springer; 2017

Work-up

1. *Chest x-ray:* Initial tool for diagnosing pleural plaques and effusion
2. *CT scan or MRI:* CT scan or MRI can be used to assess the extent of disease. Calcifications are not generally visible on CT scan. Furthermore, the CT scan is less sensitive than the MRI in depicting diaphragmatic, pericardial, and chest wall involvement
3. *PET scan:* Has shown benefit in assessing lymph node involvement but is useful in only 50–70% of cases
4. *Thoracentesis:* Used when there is a pleural effusion (30% diagnostic yield)
5. *CT-guided biopsy:* Depends on CT findings. If tumor is thick and easily biopsied, do a CT-directed biopsy
6. *Video-assisted thoracoscopic (VAT) surgery:* Do if on CT scan disease is thin or minimal or in a difficult location and thoracentesis is negative (90% diagnostic yield)
7. *Endobronchial ultrasound (EBUS) guided biopsy:* Use to biopsy mediastinal lesions for staging
8. *Mediastinoscopy:* Data suggest extra-pleural nodal metastases confer a poor survival. Because pathologic nodal involvement cannot be predicted from nodal dimensions and especially if mediastinal nodes are suspicious or equivocal on PET/CT, all patients being considered for radical resection should undergo preoperative cervical mediastinoscopy irrespective of radiologic findings

Ghigna MR et al. Cytopathology 2016;27:284–288
Patz EF Jr et al. AJR Am J Roentgenol 1992;159:961–966
Pilling JE et al. Eur J Cardiothoracr Surg 2004;25:497–501
Schneider DB et al. J Thorac Cardiovasc Surg 2000;120:128–133
Steele JPC. Semin Oncol 2002;29:36–40

Expert Opinion

Surgical management
Data regarding the choice of surgical procedure are derived mostly from observational studies involving selected patient populations treated with a variety of surgical techniques and adjuvant chemotherapies

- Pleurectomy and decortication (lung-sparing surgery): Indicated for minimal bulky disease associated with massive or recurrent pleural effusions
- Extrapleural pneumonectomy (en bloc resection of ipsilateral lung, pleura [parietal and visceral], pericardium, and hemidiaphragm): Indicated for highly selected patients with early-stage epithelioid type disease with extensive involvement of the diaphragm and visceral pleural surfaces, no nodal metastases, good performance status, and no comorbidities
- In a large observational cohort study of 20,561 patients with malignant pleural mesothelioma, 2655 patients underwent surgical treatment. Surgery was alone, with chemotherapy, or with chemotherapy and radiotherapy. The surgical cohort showed 15.5% mortality at 90 days postoperative and a small survival benefit. Overall median survival in patients who underwent surgical treatment was 13.9 months versus 10.5 months in patients who did not. The greatest survival benefit was observed in the subgroup of patients who underwent surgical treatment in addition to chemotherapy and radiotherapy

Nelson DB et al. J Clin Oncol 2017;35:3354–3362

Radiation therapy
- Because of the large volume of lung in the radiation field, delivery of tumoricidal doses of radiation is difficult without causing serious toxicities. Hence, radiation is not usually recommended as single-modality treatment. It is, however, recommended for palliating pain and to prevent or treat chest wall masses that are the result of seeding from sites of invasive procedures, such as prior thoracocentesis or thoracoscopic surgery. It is also used as part of a combined modality approach in patients with surgically resectable disease
- In a large observational cohort study of 20,561 patients with malignant pleural mesothelioma, patients who underwent radiation therapy alone had no overall survival benefit over supportive treatment alone. The greatest survival benefit was achieved with combination of surgery, chemotherapy, and radiation therapy

Nelson DB et al. J Clin Oncol 2017;35:3354–3362

Chemotherapy
- Chemotherapy or immunotherapy is indicated in virtually all mesothelioma patients with performance status 0-2. Systemic treatment can be administered before or after surgery. It is best to administer it before radiation therapy if radiation is planned. Chemotherapy alone was shown to improve overall survival versus no therapy. Best overall survival benefit was observed in patients who underwent combined therapy with chemotherapy, surgery, and radiation therapy
- Pemetrexed in combination with cisplatin is the standard first-line chemotherapy, with vitamin B_{12} and folic acid given prophylactically to mitigate leukopenia and gastrointestinal adverse effects associated with pemetrexed. Although the phase 3 MAPS trial showed slightly improved overall survival with the addition of bevacizumab to pemetrexed and cisplatin, no regulatory agency has yet approved bevacizumab for treatment of mesothelioma. New trials of immunotherapies as second-/third-line treatment show promising results At the August 2020 World Conference on Lung Cancer's virtual presidential symposium, Bristol Myers unveiled phase 3 data showing the nivolumab/ipilimumab combination decreased the risk of death among previously untreated mesothelioma patients by 26%, or a median four months longer than those treated with pemetrexed/cisplatin. When peer-reviewed and published, these data will likely make immunotherapy with nivolumab/ipilimumab the standard first line therapy

Boutin C et al. Chest 1995;108:754–758
Flores RM. Semin Thorac Cardiovasc Surg 2009;2:149–153
Flores RM et al. J Thorac Cardiovasc Surg 2008;135:620–626
Maasilta P et al. Int J Radiat Oncol Biol Phys 1991;20:433–438
Nelson DB et al. J Clin Oncol 2017;35:3354–3362
Rice D. Ann Diagn Pathol 2009;13:65–72
Vogelzang NJ et al. J Clin Oncol 2003;21:2636–2644
Yanagawa J, Rusch V. Thorac Surg Clin 2013;23:73–78
Zalcman G et al. Lancet 2016;387:1405–1414

OTHER INVESTIGATIONAL THERAPIES
Thalidomide has shown antiangiogenic activity and was used as second-line treatment in a randomized control trial of 222 patients assigned to thalidomide or supportive care. Results showed no benefit in median time to progression in the thalidomide group compared with the supportive care group

Buikhuisen WA et al. Thalidomide versus active supportive care for maintenance in patients with malignant mesothelioma after first-line chemotherapy (NVALT 5): an open-label, multicentre, randomised phase 3 study Lancet Oncol 2013;14:543–51

Vorinostat is a histone deacetylase inhibitor. It is FDA approved for treatment of cutaneous T-cell lymphoma. It was used as a second-/third-line treatment in a randomized controlled trial of 661 patients assigned to vorinostat or placebo. Results showed no overall survival benefit. Other studies showed vorinostat to enhance the expression of immune relevant antigens and have synergistic effects to other immunotherapies

Krug LM et al. Lancet Oncol 2015;16:447–456
Kroesen M et al. Oncoimmunology 2016;5;e1164919

PERITONEAL MESOTHELIOMA

Epidemiology

Incidence:	10% of all mesothelioma (200–400 new cases per year)
Median age:	53 years
Male to female ratio:	1:1

Survival

Overall survival rates: 1-, 3- and 5-year survival of 84%, 59%, and 42%, respectively

Expert Opinion

1. No standard treatment
2. Resectable disease
   a. *In women:* Treatment is the same as for ovarian cancer because these tumors behave and respond similarly to cytoreduction followed by cisplatin-based chemotherapy. Intraperitoneal (IP) chemotherapy has shown superiority over intravenous chemotherapy for advanced ovarian cancer. Cytoreduction surgery and hyperthermic intraperitoneal chemotherapy have seen improved outcomes
   b. *In men:* Treatment is the same as for pleural mesothelioma, or if disease is not related to asbestos exposure, it can be treated with IP chemotherapy or cytoreduction surgery and hyperthermic intraperitoneal chemotherapy
3. Locally advanced or recurrent disease: Give systemic chemotherapy as for pleural mesothelioma

Alberts DS et al. (Editorial). J Clin Oncol 2002;20:3944–3949
Eltabbakh GH et al. J Surg Oncol 1999;70:6–12
Helm JH et al. Ann Surg Oncol 2015;22:1686–1693
Markman M et al. J Clin Oncol 2001;19:1001–1007
Markman M, Kelsen D. J Cancer Res Clin Oncol 1992;118:547–550

Passot G et al. J Surg Oncol 2016;113:796–803

ADVANCED DISEASE • FIRST-LINE

MESOTHELIOMA REGIMEN: PEMETREXED + CISPLATIN

Vogelzang NJ et al. J Clin Oncol 2003;21:2636–2644

Pemetrexed 500 mg/m²; administer intravenously in 100 mL 0.9% NS over 10 minutes, given before cisplatin on day 1, every 21 days (total dosage/cycle = 500 mg/m²)
Cisplatin 75 mg/m²; administer intravenously in 1000 mL 0.9% NS over 2 hours on day 1, beginning 30 minutes after pemetrexed has been administered, every 21 days (total dosage/cycle = 75 mg/m²)
Folic acid 350–1000 mcg daily; administer orally, beginning 1–3 weeks before chemotherapy and continuing throughout treatment with pemetrexed + cisplatin, *and*
Cyanocobalamin (vitamin B$_{12}$) 1000 mcg; administer intramuscularly every 9 weeks, beginning 1–3 weeks before chemotherapy and continuing throughout treatment with pemetrexed + cisplatin
Dexamethasone 4 mg; administer intravenously or orally twice daily for 3 consecutive days, starting the day before pemetrexed administration to decrease the risk of severe skin rash associated with pemetrexed (total dose/cycle = 24 mg)
Hydration: 0.9% sodium chloride injection (0.9% NS), ≥1000 mL before and after cisplatin; administer intravenously over a minimum of 2–4 hours. Encourage patients to increase oral nonalcoholic fluid intake. Monitor and replace magnesium/electrolytes as needed

Supportive Care
Antiemetic prophylaxis
Emetogenic potential is HIGH. Potential for delayed symptoms
See Chapter 42 for antiemetic recommendations

Hematopoietic growth factor (CSF) prophylaxis
Primary prophylaxis is NOT indicated
See Chapter 43 for more information

Antimicrobial prophylaxis
Risk of fever and neutropenia is LOW
Antimicrobial primary prophylaxis to be considered:
- Antibacterial—not indicated
- Antifungal—not indicated
- Antiviral—not indicated unless patient previously had an episode of HSV

Additional supportive care
Add a **proton pump inhibitor** during dexamethasone use to prevent gastritis and duodenitis

Treatment Modifications

Delay cycle until ANC is >1500/mm³ and platelet >100,000/mm³

Adverse Event	Dose Modification
G3 hematologic toxicities	Hold therapy until returns to baseline. Then decrease both drug dosages by 25%
G4 hematologic toxicities (thrombocytopenia)	Hold therapy until returns to baseline. Then decrease both drug dosages by 50%
Serum creatinine 1.6–2 mg/dL (141–177 μmol/L)	Decrease cisplatin dosage by 25%
Serum creatinine ≥2 mg/dL (≥177 μmol/L)	Hold therapy until serum creatinine <2 mg/dL (<177 μmol/L), then decrease cisplatin dosage by 25%
G ≥2 diarrhea	Hold chemotherapy until toxicity resolves to Grade <2, then decrease both drug dosages by 25%
G3/4 mucositis	Decrease pemetrexed dosage 50%
Increased liver transaminases	Hold therapy until toxicity resolves, then decrease pemetrexed dosage by 25%
Other G ≥3 nonhematologic toxicities (except N/V, elevated transaminases and alopecia)	Delay treatment until toxicity resolves to baseline, then decrease both drug dosages by 25% from previous dose levels

Delays of ≤42 days are permitted for recovery from pemetrexed- and cisplatin-related toxicities. Patients requiring 3 dose reductions: discontinue therapy

Patient Population Studied

A study of 456 patients with advanced measurable pleural mesothelioma

Efficacy

Response rate	40–45%
Median time to progression	5–6 months
1-year survival	50%
Median survival	12–13 months

Toxicity (N = 168 Fully Supplemented with Vitamins)

	% CTC Grade 3/4
Hematologic	
Hemoglobin	4.2
Leukocytes	14.9
Neutrophils	23.2
Platelets	5.4
Febrile neutropenia	0.6
Nonhematologic	
Nausea	11.9
Fatigue	10.1
Vomiting	10.7
Diarrhea	3.6
Dehydration	4.2
Stomatitis	3
Anorexia	1.2
Rash	0.6

Three deaths thought possibly related to pemetrexed + cisplatin occurred before folic acid and vitamin B12 supplementation was added; none occurred thereafter

Therapy Monitoring

1. *Before initial and repeated treatments:* H&P, CBC with differential, calculated creatinine clearance, serum electrolytes, glucose, calcium, LFTs, and vitamin metabolites
2. *Treatment evaluation:* Every 2 cycles

Notes

1. G2 neutropenia and anemia secondary to pemetrexed are brief and not cumulative
2. Anemia is cumulative with cisplatin. Consider using erythropoietin therapy if anemia G <1 occurs
3. Folate deficiency is best measured with homocysteine levels
4. Vitamin B$_{12}$ deficiency can be tested most readily with methylmalonic acid (MMA) levels

ADVANCED DISEASE • FIRST-LINE
MESOTHELIOMA REGIMEN: PEMETREXED + CARBOPLATIN

Ceresoli GL et al. J Clin Oncol 2006;24:1443–1448

Pemetrexed 500 mg/m^2; administer intravenously in 100 mL 0.9% sodium chloride injection over 10 minutes on day 1, every 21 days (total dosage/cycle = 500 mg/m^2), *followed 30 minutes later by:*

Carboplatin AUC 5 mg/mL per min; administer intravenously in 50–250 mL D5W over 30 minutes on day 1, every 21 days (total dosage/cycle calculated to produce an AUC = 5 mg/mL per min)

Folic acid 350–1000 mcg/day orally beginning at least 1 week before the first dose of pemetrexed and continued throughout the duration of treatment

Cyanocobalamin (vitamin B$_{12}$) 1000 mcg intramuscularly at least 1 week before the first dose of pemetrexed and repeated every 9 weeks (every 3 cycles) throughout treatment

Dexamethasone 4 mg/dose orally twice daily for 3 consecutive days (6 doses), starting the day before pemetrexed administration to decrease the risk of severe skin rash associated with pemetrexed (total dose/cycle = 24 mg)

Notes:

• Salicylates and nonsteroidal anti-inflammatory agents (NSAIDs) were not allowed during the 2 days before (5 days for NSAIDs with a long half-life), the day of, and for 2 days after chemotherapy

• Carboplatin dose calculation is based on formulas developed to achieve consistent drug exposure within and among patients. In the method that follows, area under the plasma concentration versus time curve (AUC) is the targeted pharmacokinetic end point used to obtain consistent exposure

• Current product labeling for carboplatin approved by the U.S. Food and Drug Administration describes dose calculation based on a formula described by Calvert et al.[*,†,‡]:

$$\text{Total Carboplatin Dose (mg)} = (\text{target AUC}) \times (\text{GFR} + 25)$$

• In practice, creatinine clearance (Clcr) is used in place of glomerular filtration rate (GFR). Clcr can be measured from a 24-hour urine collection or estimated from 1 among several equations, such as the method of Cockcroft and Gault[§]:

$$\text{For males, Clcr} = \frac{(140 - \text{age [years]}) \times \text{body weight (kg)}}{72 \times (\text{Serum creatinine [mg/dL]})}$$

$$\text{For females, Clcr} = \frac{(140 - \text{age [years]}) \times \text{body weight (kg)}}{72 \times (\text{Serum creatinine [mg/dL]})} \times 0.85$$

• *Note:* On October 8, 2010, the U.S. Food and Drug Administration (FDA) identified a potential safety issue with carboplatin dosing based on recent changes in the measurement of serum creatinine. Since the end of 2010, all clinical laboratories in the United States use the standardized Isotope Dilution Mass Spectrometry (IDMS) method to measure serum creatinine, which could result in an overestimation of the GFR in some patients with normal renal function. A carboplatin dose calculated with an IDMS-measured serum creatinine result using the Calvert formula could exceed an expected exposure (AUC) and result in increased drug-related toxicity

• Provided actual GFR measurements are made to assess renal function, carboplatin can be safely dosed according to the Calvert formula described in product labeling

• If GFR (or creatinine clearance) is estimated based on serum creatinine measurements by the IDMS method, the FDA recommends capping an estimated GFR at 125 mL/min for any targeted AUC value for patients with normal renal function. No greater estimated GFR values should be used

U.S. FDA. Carboplatin dosing. (online) October 8, 2010. Available from: http://www.fda.gov/aboutfda/centersoffices/officeofmedicalproductsandtobacco/cder/ucm228974.htm (last accessed September 4, 2013)

[*]Calvert AH et al. J Clin Oncol 1989;7:1748–1756
[†]Sørensen BT et al. Cancer Chemother Pharmacol 1991;28:397–401
[‡]Jodrell DI et al. J Clin Oncol 1992;10:520–528
[§]Cockcroft DW, Gault MH. Prediction of creatinine clearance from serum creatinine. Nephron 1976;16:31–41

Supportive Care
Antiemetic prophylaxis
Emetogenic potential is at least **MODERATE**. *Potential for delayed emetic symptoms*
See Chapter 42 for antiemetic recommendations

Hematopoietic growth factor (CSF) prophylaxis
Primary prophylaxis may be indicated
See Chapter 43 for more information

(continued)

(*continued*)

Antimicrobial prophylaxis
Risk of fever and neutropenia is **LOW**
  Antimicrobial primary prophylaxis to be considered:
  • Antibacterial—not indicated
  • Antifungal—not indicated
  • Antiviral—not indicated unless patient previously had an episode of HSV

Oral care
Prophylaxis and treatment for mucositis/stomatitis
  General advice:
  • Encourage patients to maintain intake of nonalcoholic fluids
  • Evaluate patients for oral pain and provide analgesic medications
  • Consider histamine (H_2-subtype) receptor antagonists (eg, ranitidine, famotidine), or a proton pump inhibitor for epigastric pain
  • *Lactobacillus* sp.—containing probiotics may be beneficial in preventing diarrhea
  Patients with intact oral mucosa:
  • Clean the mouth, tongue, and gums by brushing after every meal and at bedtime with an ultrasoft toothbrush with fluoride toothpaste
  • Floss teeth gently every day unless contraindicated. If gums bleed and hurt, avoid bleeding or sore areas, but floss other teeth
  • Patients may use saline or commercial brand, nonalcoholic rinses
    ▪ Do not use mouthwashes that contain alcohols
  If mucositis or stomatitis is present:
  • Keep the mouth moist utilizing water, ice chips, sugarless gum, sugar-free hard candies, or a saliva substitute
  • Rinse mouth several times a day to remove debris
    ▪ Use a solution of ¼ teaspoon (1.25 g) each of baking soda and table salt (sodium chloride) in 1 quart (~950 mL) of warm water. Follow with a plain water rinse
    ▪ Do not use mouthwashes that contain alcohols
  • Foam-tipped swabs (eg, Toothettes) are useful in moisturizing oral mucosa, but ineffective for cleansing teeth and removing plaque
  • Advise patients who develop mucositis to:
    ▪ Choose foods that are easy to chew and swallow
    ▪ Take small bites of food, chew slowly, and sip liquids with meals
    ▪ Encourage soft, moist foods such as cooked cereals, mashed potatoes, and scrambled eggs
    ▪ For trouble swallowing, soften food with gravies, sauces, broths, yogurt, or other bland liquids
    ▪ Avoid sharp, crunchy foods; hot, spicy, or highly acidic foods (eg, citrus fruits and juices); sugary foods; toothpicks; tobacco products; alcoholic drinks

Treatment Modifications

Adverse Event	Dose Modification
ANC <1500/mm³ or platelet count <100,000/mm³	Delay start of cycle up to 42 days until ANC ≥1500/mm³ and platelet count ≥100,000/mm³
ANC nadir <500/mm³ *and* platelets ≥50,000/mm³	Administer 75% of the previous pemetrexed dose, *or* carboplatin AUC = 4 mg/mL per min
Platelet nadir count <50,000/mm³ *and* any ANC	Administer 50% of the previous pemetrexed dose, *or* carboplatin AUC = 3 mg/mL per min
Recurrence of G3/4 thrombocytopenia or neutropenia after 2 dose reductions	Discontinue therapy
G3/4 nonhematologic toxicities	Delay treatment until there is resolution to G ≤1 then proceed with pemetrexed reduced to 75% of the previous dose and carboplatin at AUC = 4 mg/mL per min
Creatinine clearance* <45 mL/min (<0.75 mL/s)	Delay the next cycle until creatinine clearance ≥45 mL/min (≥0.75 mL/s)

*Calculated by the Cockcroft and Gault formula before each dose

Patient Population Studied

Patients with histologically proven malignant pleural mesothelioma who were not candidates for curative surgery. Eligibility criteria included ages >18 years, Eastern Cooperative Oncology Group (ECOG) performance status (PS) ≤2, and an estimated life expectancy of ≥12 weeks. Creatinine clearance ≥45 mL/min. Patients were excluded if they were unable to discontinue administration of aspirin and/or other nonsteroidal anti-inflammatory agents for 2 days before (5 days for long-acting agents), the day of, and 2 days after the dose of pemetrexed

Patient Characteristics

Characteristic	Number of Patients (N = 102)	Percentage
Sex		
Male	76	74.5
Female	26	25.5
Age, years		
Median	65	
Range	38–79	
ECOG performance status		
0	33	32
1	61	60
2	8	8
Histologic subtype		
Mixed cell	8	8
Unspecified	7	7
Epithelial	80	78
Sarcomatoid	7	7
EORTC prognostic score		
Good	25	24.5
Poor	77	75.5
IMIG stage		
II	11	11
III	34	33
IV	49	48
Relapse after EPP	8	8

Efficacy (N = 102)

Response Rate[*],[†]

Objective response rate	18.6% (95% CI, 11.6–27.5%)
Complete response	1.96% (2 patients) (10+ and 11 months)
Partial response	16.66% (17 patients)
Stable disease	47% (95% CI, 37.1–57.2%) (48 patients)
Progressive disease	34.3% (35 patients)

Response According to Histology

Epithelial MPM	15/80 (18.8%)
Mixed histotype MPM	4/8 (50%)
Sarcomatoid MPM	0/7

Effect on ECOG Performance Status[‡]

Patients with OR/baseline PS (N = 19)	0 (3)/1 (16)
Patients with OR/posttreatment PS	0 (10)/1 (9)
Patients with SD/baseline PS (N = 48)	0 (21)/1 (25)/2 (2)
Patients with SD/posttreatment PS	0 (23)/1 (22)/2 (3)

Median Follow-Up Time of 14.2 Months (95% CI, 12.2–15 Months) 26 without any Evidence of Disease Progression

Median TTP[§]	6.5 months
Median OS[ϵ]	12.7 months
6-month survival estimates	70.0% (95% CI, 60.0–78.0%)
1-year survival estimates	51.6% (95% CI, 40.7–61.5%)

*Best tumor response was assessed according to an intent-to-treat analysis
†Response to treatment showed a trend that correlated with OS in univariate analysis (P = 0.069) and reached statistical significance in the multivariate model (P = 0.024). When SD patients were grouped with responders, the correlation with OS was much more significant (P<0.001)
‡Sixty-nine patients (68%) were symptomatic at the time of study enrollment. ECOG PS improved or was stable in the majority of patients who achieved response or SD
§TTP was significantly related to good PS (P = 0.047) and epithelial histology (P = 0.02) in both univariate and multivariate analyses
ϵPatients' PS was the only factor significantly related to OS in univariate and multivariate analyses (P = 0.04)

Toxicity

Hematologic Toxicity by Cycle (N = 482)

Toxicity	Toxicity Grade (Number of Patients)				G3/4
	G1	G2	G3	G4	
Neutropenia	60	59	36	11	9.7
Thrombocytopenia	51	12	7*	3*	2
Anemia	166	79	16†	1†	3.5

Toxicity (continued)

Toxicity	Toxicity Grade (Number of Patients) %				G3/4
	G1	G2	G3	G4	
Hematologic Toxicity by Patient (N = 102)					
Neutropenia	17	25	9	11‡	19.6
Thrombocytopenia	17	3	6	2	7.8
Anemia	33	30	11	1	11.7
Nonhematologic Toxicity by Patient (N = 102)§					
Nausea/vomiting	47	17	1	0	1
Fatigue	31	13	1	0	1
Stomatitis	3	7	0	0	0
Conjunctivitis	20	3	0	0	0
Diarrhea	2	0	3	0	3
Constipation	5	1	0	0	0

*G3/4 thrombocytopenia occurred after the second cycle in 7 of 10 patients (70%)
†G3/4 anemia occurred after the second cycle in 15 of 17 patients (88%)
‡Febrile neutropenia was reported in 2 patients
§Other toxicities reported as rare events included G4 rhabdomyolysis (1 patient), G2 hepatotoxicity (1 patient), G2 arthralgia-myalgia (2 patients), G2 genitourinary mucositis (2 patients), and G1 skin rash (2 patients)

Therapy Monitoring

1. *Before initial and repeated treatments:* H&P, CBC with differential, calculated or measured creatinine clearance, serum electrolytes, glucose, calcium, LFTs, and vitamin metabolites
2. *Treatment evaluation:* every 2 cycles

ADVANCED DISEASE • FIRST-LINE

MESOTHELIOMA REGIMEN: GEMCITABINE + CISPLATIN

Byrne MJ et al. J Clin Oncol 1999;17:25–30
Castagneto B et al. Am J Clin Oncol 2005;28:223–226
van Haarst JW et al. Br J Cancer 2002;86(3):342–345

Cisplatin 80 mg/m^2; administer intravenously in 100–250 mL 0.9% NS over 60 minutes, given before gemcitabine on day 1, every 21 days for 6 cycles (total dosage/cycle = 80 mg/m^2), *plus*:

Gemcitabine 1250 mg/m^2 per dose; administer intravenously in 50–250 mL 0.9% NS over 30 minutes, given on days 1 and 8, every 21 days for 6 cycles (total dosage/cycle = 2500 mg/m^2)

Hydration: 0.9% sodium chloride injection (0.9% NS) ≥1000 mL before and after cisplatin; administer intravenously over a minimum of 2–4 hours. Monitor and replace magnesium/electrolytes as needed

Supportive Care

Antiemetic prophylaxis
Emetogenic potential on day 1 is **HIGH**. *Potential for delayed symptoms*
Emetogenic potential with gemcitabine alone is **LOW**
See Chapter 42 for antiemetic recommendations

Hematopoietic growth factor (CSF) prophylaxis
Primary prophylaxis is **NOT** *indicated*
See Chapter 43 for more information

Antimicrobial prophylaxis
Risk of fever and neutropenia is **LOW**
   Antimicrobial primary prophylaxis to be considered:
   • Antibacterial—not indicated
   • Antifungal—not indicated
   • Antiviral—not indicated unless patient previously had an episode of HSV

Treatment Modifications

Serum creatinine >1.4 mg/dL (>124 µmol/L), but <1.7 mg/dL (<150 µmol/L)	Decrease cisplatin by 50% and gemcitabine by 25%
Serum creatinine >1.7 mg/dL (>150 µmol/L)	Withhold cisplatin and gemcitabine until serum creatinine <1.7 mg/dL (<150 µmol/L), then administer 50% of the previous cisplatin dosage and 75% of the previous gemcitabine dosage
WBC <3000/mm^3 or platelet <100,000/mm^3 on days 1 and 8 or days 1, 8, and 15 when gemcitabine treatment is planned	Decrease gemcitabine by 25%
WBC <2000/mm^3 or platelet <75,000/mm^3 when gemcitabine treatment is planned for day 8 or days 8 and 15	Omit gemcitabine

Byrne MJ et al. J Clin Oncol 1999;17:25–30

Patient Population Studied

A study of 21 patients with advanced measurable pleural mesothelioma (Byrne MJ et al.)
A study of 25 patients with advanced measurable pleural mesothelioma (van Haarst JW et al.)
A study of 35 patients with advanced measurable pleural mesothelioma (Castagneto B et al.)

Castagneto B et al. Am J Clin Oncol 2005;28:223–226
Byrne MJ et al. J Clin Oncol 1999;17:25–30
van Haarst JW et al. Br J Cancer 2002;86(3):342–345

Therapy Monitoring

1. *Before chemotherapy on cycle days 1 and 8:* CBC with differential, serum electrolytes, creatinine, bilirubin, ALT, and alkaline phosphatase
2. *Treatment evaluation:* every 2 cycles

Efficacy (N = 46)

Response rate	18–47%
Duration of response	5–7 months
Estimated median survival	9.5–12 months
Estimated 1-year survival	41%

Of 10 responding patients, 9 achieved substantial or complete symptomatic improvement. Symptoms decreased significantly in 3 additional patients who achieved disease stabilization
From Byrne MJ et al. J Clin Oncol 1999;17:25–30 and van Haarst JW et al. Br J Cancer 2002;86(3):342–345

Toxicity (N = 21)

	Worst Toxicity Grade (%)				
	0	1	2	3	4
Hematologic					
Leukopenia	29	10	24	38	0
Thrombocytopenia*	24	14	29	14	19
Anemia	14	29	57	0	0
Nonhematologic					
Nausea/vomiting[†]	0	14	52	33	0
Stomatitis	62	38	0	0	0
Alopecia	71	24	5	0	0
Hearing loss	57	33	5	5	0
Neurologic	90	10	0	0	0

*Thrombocytopenia on days 8 and 15 was the major cause of dose modification
[†]One-third of patients had ≥1 episodes of severe nausea and vomiting, and symptoms were worse >24 hours after treatment
From Byrne MJ et al. J Clin Oncol 1999;17:25–30

ADVANCED DISEASE • FIRST-LINE
MESOTHELIOMA REGIMEN: BEVACIZUMAB + GEMCITABINE + CISPLATIN

Kindler HL et al. J Clin Oncol 2012;30:2509–2515

Gemcitabine 1250 mg/m^2 per dose; administer intravenously in 50–250 mL 0.9% sodium chloride injection (0.9% NS) over 30 minutes, on days 1 and 8, every 3 weeks for up to 6 cycles (total dosage/3-week cycle = 2500 mg/m^2), *followed by:*

Hydration before cisplatin: ≥1000 mL 0.9% NS; administer intravenously over a minimum of 1 hour before commencing cisplatin administration

Cisplatin 75 mg/m^2; administer intravenously in 1000 mL 0.9% NS over 1 hour, following gemcitabine administration and prior to bevacizumab administration, on day 1 every 3 weeks for up to 6 cycles (total dosage/3-week cycle = 75 mg/m^2), *followed by:*

Hydration after cisplatin: Administer by intravenous infusion ≥1000 mL 0.9% NS over a minimum of 2 hours. Encourage patients to increase oral intake of nonalcoholic fluids and provide electrolyte replacement as needed (potassium, magnesium, sodium)

Bevacizumab 15 mg/kg; administer intravenously in 100 mL 0.9% NS on day 1, following cisplatin administration, every 3 weeks for up to 6 cycles (total dosage/3-week cycle = 15 mg/kg)

Notes:
- Duration of administration for the initial dose of bevacizumab is 90 minutes. If administration is well tolerated, the administration duration may be decreased stepwise during subsequent administrations to 60 minutes and, finally, to a minimum duration of 30 minutes
- In the absence of disease progression following completion of 6 cycles of bevacizumab + gemcitabine + cisplatin, maintenance therapy with bevacizumab monotherapy is allowed, *thus:*
  - **Bevacizumab** 15 mg/kg; administer intravenously in 100 mL 0.9% NS on day 1, every 3 weeks as maintenance therapy (total dosage/3-week cycle = 15 mg/kg)

Supportive Care
Antiemetic prophylaxis
Emetogenic potential on day 1 (of cycles 1–6) is **HIGH**. *Potential for delayed symptoms*
Emetogenic potential on day 8 (of cycles 1–6) is **LOW**
Emetogenic potential on day 1 (during bevacizumab maintenance therapy) is **MINIMAL**
See Chapter 42 for antiemetic recommendations

Hematopoietic growth factor (CSF) prophylaxis
Primary prophylaxis is **NOT** *indicated*
See Chapter 43 for more information

Antimicrobial prophylaxis
Risk of fever and neutropenia is **LOW**
Antimicrobial primary prophylaxis to be considered:
- Antibacterial—not indicated
- Antifungal—not indicated
- Antiviral—not indicated unless patient previously had an episode of HSV

Treatment Modifications

BEVACIZUMAB DOSAGE MODIFICATIONS

Adverse Event	Treatment Modification
Gastrointestinal perforations (gastrointestinal perforations, fistula formation in the gastrointestinal tract, intra-abdominal abscess), fistula formation involving an internal organ	Discontinue bevacizumab permanently
Serious bleeding	
Wound dehiscence requiring medical intervention	
Nephrotic syndrome	
Hypertensive crisis or hypertensive encephalopathy or reversible posterior leukoencephalopathy syndrome (RPLS)	

(continued)

Treatment Modifications (*continued*)

Adverse Event	Treatment Modification
Congestive heart failure	
Necrotizing fasciitis	
Severe arterial or venous thromboembolic events	Discontinue bevacizumab permanently; the safety of reinitiating bevacizumab after a thromboembolic event is resolved is not known
Moderate to severe proteinuria	Patients with a urine dipstick reading ≥2+ should undergo further assessment, eg, 24-hour urine collection. Suspend bevacizumab administration for ≥2 g of proteinuria/24 h and resume when proteinuria is <2 g/24 h
Severe hypertension not controlled with medical management	Hold bevacizumab pending further evaluation and treatment of hypertension
Mild, clinically insignificant infusion reaction	Decrease the rate of infusion
Clinically significant but not severe infusion reaction	Interrupt the infusion in patients with clinically significant infusion reactions and consider resuming at a slower rate following resolution. If decision is made to restart, the infusion may be continued at ≤50% of the rate prior to the reaction and increased in 50% increments every 30 minutes if well tolerated. Infusions may be restarted at the full rate during the next cycle
Severe infusion reaction—hypertension, hypertensive crises associated with neurologic signs and symptoms, wheezing, oxygen desaturation, G3 hypersensitivity, chest pain, headaches, rigors, and diaphoresis)	Stop infusion and administer appropriate medical therapy (eg, epinephrine, corticosteroids, intravenous antihistamines, bronchodilators, and/or oxygen). Discontinue bevacizumab
Planned elective surgery	Suspend bevacizumab at least 28 days before elective surgery and do not resume for at least 28 days after surgery or until surgical incision is fully healed
Recent hemoptysis	Do not administer bevacizumab
Evidence of rectosigmoid involvement by pelvic examination or bowel involvement on CT scan or clinical symptoms of bowel obstruction	

CISPLATIN + GEMCITABINE

Dose Levels

	Gemcitabine	Cisplatin
Starting dose	1250 mg/m² per dose on days 1 and 8	75 mg/m² on day 1
Dose level −1	1000 mg/m² per dose on days 1 and 8	60 mg/m² on day 1
Dose level −2	800 mg/m² per dose on days 1 and 8	50 mg/m² on day 1
Dose level −3	600 mg/m² per dose on days 1 and 8	40 mg/m² on day 1

Delay cycle until ANC is >1500/mm³ and platelet count is >100,000/mm³

Adverse Event	Treatment Modification
G3 hematologic toxicities (ANC <1000/mm³; platelet count <50,000/mm³)	Hold therapy until ANC and platelets return to baseline. Then decrease both drug dosages by 1 dose level
G4 hematologic toxicities (ANC <500/mm³; platelet count <25,000/mm³)	Hold therapy until ANC and platelets return to baseline. Then decrease both drug dosages by 2 dose levels. Consider use of hematopoietic growth factor (CSF) prophylaxis in subsequent cycles for dose-limiting neutropenia

(*continued*)

Treatment Modifications (*continued*)

Adverse Event	Treatment Modification
Day 8 ANC ≥1500/mm^3 and/or platelet count >100,000/mm^3	Administer full dose of gemcitabine
Day 8 ANC 1000–1499/mm^3 and/or platelet count 75,000–99,999/mm^3	Administer 50% of day 1 gemcitabine dose
Day 8 ANC <1000/mm^3 and or platelet count <100,000/mm^3	Withhold day 8 gemcitabine dose. Consider use of hematopoietic growth factor (CSF) prophylaxis in subsequent cycles for dose-limiting neutropenia
Serum creatinine ≥1.5 mg/dL (≥130 μmol/L) and/or BUN ≥25 mg/dL (≥8.92 mmol/L).	Withhold cisplatin until serum creatinine <1.5 mg/dL (<130 μmol/L) and BUN <25 mg/dL (<8.92 mmol/L). Then decrease cisplatin dosage by 1 dose level; if already reduced, then reduce again
G ≥2 diarrhea	Hold chemotherapy until toxicity resolves to G <2, then decrease gemcitabine 1 dose level
G3/4 mucositis	Decrease gemcitabine dosage by 2 dose levels
ALT and AST >1.5× ULN in a patient without liver metastasis	Withhold gemcitabine until ALT and AST ≤1.5× ULN
ALT and AST >2.5× ULN in a patient with liver metastasis with alkaline phosphatase >2.5× ULN	Withhold gemcitabine until ALT and AST ≤2.5× ULN and alkaline phosphatase ≤2.5× ULN
Peripheral neuropathy G ≥3	G4 discontinue cisplatin permanently; G3 may reinstitute if toxicity resolves within 2–3 weeks to G ≤1
Cisplatin-induced hearing loss G ≥3	
Severe hypersensitivity reaction to gemcitabine or cisplatin is noted	Permanently discontinue gemcitabine or cisplatin
Other G ≥3 nonhematologic toxicities (except nausea, vomiting, elevated transaminases, and alopecia)	Delay treatment until toxicity resolves to baseline, then decrease both drug dosages by 1 dose level from previous levels
Unexplained new or worsening dyspnea or evidence of severe pulmonary toxicity	Discontinue gemcitabine immediately and assess for gemcitabine pulmonary toxicity
HUS	Discontinue gemcitabine for HUS or severe renal impairment
Capillary leak syndrome	Discontinue gemcitabine
PRES	Discontinue gemcitabine

Notes:
- Patients who are pregnant or become pregnant should be apprised of the potential hazard to the fetus; women of childbearing potential should be advised to avoid becoming pregnant during therapy
- Gemcitabine may cause severe and life-threatening toxicity when administered during or within 7 days of radiation therapy

Patient Population Studied

This multicenter, double-blind, placebo-controlled, randomized, phase 2 trial included 108 patients with histologically or cytologically confirmed malignant mesothelioma not amenable to curative surgery. Eligible patients were aged >18 years, with an Eastern Cooperative Oncology Group (ECOG) performance status score ≤1, and life expectancy >3 months. Patients who had previous systemic cytotoxic chemotherapy, and patients on anticoagulation, were not eligible. On day 1 of a 21-day cycle, all patients received intravenous gemcitabine (1250 mg/m^2) and then cisplatin (75 mg/m^2), and then either bevacizumab (15 mg/kg) or placebo. All patients also received intravenous gemcitabine (1250 mg/m^2) on day 8. Combination therapy was administered for 6 cycles. Bevacizumab or placebo was continued every 21 days after the 6 cycles until disease progression, unacceptable adverse effects, or withdrawal of consent

Efficacy (N = 108)

	Bevacizumab + Gemcitabine + Cisplatin (n = 53)	Placebo + Gemcitabine + Cisplatin (n = 55)	
Estimated median progression-free survival	6.9 months	6.0 months	HR 0.90, 95% CI 0.61–1.34; P = 0.62
Estimated median survival	15.6 months	14.7 months	HR 1.04, 95% CI 0.68–1.59; P = 0.87
Objective response rate*	24.5%	21.8%	P = 0.74

Objective response rate is the percentage of patients who experienced a confirmed partial or complete response to the study drug. In this study, no patients experienced a complete response

Adverse Events (N = 108)

	Bevacizumab + Gemcitabine + Cisplatin (n = 53)	Placebo + Gemcitabine + Cisplatin (n = 55)
Neutropenia	42	40
Thrombocytopenia	38	25
Hypertension	23	9
Venous thrombosis	17	9
Epistaxis	8	2
Infection without neutropenia	6	2
Proteinuria	6	2
Anemia	4	15
Febrile neutropenia	4	2
Cerebrovascular accident	2	0

*According to the National Cancer Institute Common Terminology Criteria for Adverse Events, version 3.0
Note: G3/4 toxicities are included in the table. No significant differences in G ≥3 events were observed

Therapy Monitoring

1. *Before therapy:* history and physical examination. CBC with differential, renal and liver function tests, serum electrolytes
2. Assess proteinuria by urine dipstick and/or urinary protein-to-creatinine ratio. Patients with a urine dipstick reading ≥2+ should undergo further assessment with 24-hour urine collection
3. Blood pressure every 2 weeks or more frequently as indicated during treatment
4. Monitor hepatic function prior to initiation and during therapy with gemcitabine
5. Pulmonary toxicity and respiratory failure: discontinue gemcitabine immediately for unexplained new or worsening dyspnea or evidence of severe pulmonary toxicity
6. Monitor renal function and electrolytes prior to initiation and during therapy with cisplatin and gemcitabine, including hemolytic uremic syndrome (HUS) secondary to gemcitabine
7. Increased toxicity with infusion time >30 minutes or dosing more frequently than once weekly may occur with gemcitabine; monitor carefully
8. *Response evaluation:* CT scan every 8 weeks for 6 months (modified RECIST 1.1 for mesothelioma), then every 12 weeks

ADVANCED DISEASE • FIRST-LINE

MESOTHELIOMA REGIMEN: BEVACIZUMAB + PEMETREXED + CISPLATIN

Zalcman G et al. Lancet 2016;387:1405–1414

Premedications for Pemetrexed

Folic acid 350–1000 mcg daily; administer orally, beginning 1–3 weeks before chemotherapy and continuing throughout treatment with pemetrexed and for 21 days after the last pemetrexed dose, *and*

Cyanocobalamin (vitamin B$_{12}$) 1000 mcg; administer intramuscularly every 9 weeks, beginning 1–3 weeks before chemotherapy and continuing throughout treatment with pemetrexed, *and*

Dexamethasone 4 mg; administer intravenously or orally twice daily for 3 consecutive days, starting the day before pemetrexed administration to decrease the risk of severe skin rash associated with pemetrexed (total dose/cycle = 24 mg)

Bevacizumab 15 mg/kg; administer intravenously in 100 mL 0.9% sodium chloride injection (0.9% NS) on day 1, every 3 weeks for up to 6 cycles (total dosage/3-week cycle = 15 mg/kg)

Notes:

• Duration of administration for the initial dose of bevacizumab is 90 minutes. If administration is well tolerated, the administration duration may be decreased stepwise during subsequent administrations to 60 minutes and, finally, to a minimum duration of 30 minutes

• In the absence of disease progression following completion of 6 cycles of bevacizumab + pemetrexed + cisplatin, maintenance therapy with bevacizumab monotherapy is allowed, *thus:*

  ▪ **Bevacizumab** 15 mg/kg; administer intravenously in 100 mL 0.9% NS on day 1, every 3 weeks as maintenance therapy (total dosage/3-week cycle = 15 mg/kg)

Pemetrexed 500 mg/m^2; administer intravenously in 100 mL 0.9% NS over 10 minutes, given before cisplatin, on day 1, every 21 days for up to 6 cycles (total dosage/3-week cycle = 500 mg/m^2)

Hydration before cisplatin: ≥1000 mL 0.9% NS; administer intravenously over a minimum of 1 hour before commencing cisplatin administration

Cisplatin 75 mg/m^2; administer intravenously in 1000 mL 0.9% NS over 2 hours, beginning 30 minutes after pemetrexed has been administered, on day 1 every 21 days for up to 6 cycles (total dosage/3-week cycle = 75 mg/m^2)

Note: In case of Grade ≥2 renal toxicity with cisplatin, substitution with carboplatin (AUC = 5) was allowed (Zalcman et al.)

Hydration after cisplatin: Administer by intravenous infusion ≥1000 mL 0.9% NS over a minimum of 2 hours. Encourage patients to increase oral intake of nonalcoholic fluids and provide electrolyte replacement as needed (potassium, magnesium, sodium)

Supportive Care

Antiemetic prophylaxis

Emetogenic potential on day 1 (of cycles 1–6) is **HIGH**. *Potential for delayed symptoms*

Emetogenic potential on day 1 (during bevacizumab maintenance therapy) is **MINIMAL**

See Chapter 42 for antiemetic recommendations

Hematopoietic growth factor (CSF) prophylaxis

Primary prophylaxis is **NOT** indicated

See Chapter 43 for more information

Antimicrobial prophylaxis

Risk of fever and neutropenia is **LOW**

  Antimicrobial primary prophylaxis to be considered:

• Antibacterial—not indicated

• Antifungal—not indicated

• Antiviral—not indicated unless patient previously had an episode of HSV

Additional supportive care

Add a **proton pump inhibitor** during dexamethasone use to prevent gastritis and duodenitis

Patient Population Studied

This multicenter, randomized, open-label, phase 3 trial (MAPS) included 448 patients with histologically confirmed malignant pleural mesothelioma who had not previously received chemotherapy. Eligible patients were aged 18–75 years, with an Eastern Cooperative Oncology Group (ECOG) performance status score ≤2 and life expectancy >12 weeks. Patients who had central nervous system metastases were not eligible. On day 1 of a 21-day cycle, all patients received intravenous pemetrexed (500 mg/m^2) and cisplatin (75 mg/m^2), and those randomly assigned to receive triple therapy also received bevacizumab (15 mg/kg). Combination therapy was administered for a maximum of 6 cycles. Patients in the triple-therapy group were allowed to receive maintenance bevacizumab after the 6 cycles until disease progression or toxic effects

Treatment Modifications

BEVACIZUMAB + PEMETREXED + CISPLATIN

BEVACIZUMAB DOSAGE MODIFICATIONS

Adverse Event	Treatment Modification
Gastrointestinal perforations (gastrointestinal perforations, fistula formation in the gastrointestinal tract, intra-abdominal abscess), fistula formation involving an internal organ	Discontinue bevacizumab permanently
Serious bleeding	
Wound dehiscence requiring medical intervention	
Nephrotic syndrome	
Hypertensive crisis or hypertensive encephalopathy or reversible posterior leukoencephalopathy syndrome (RPLS)	
Congestive heart failure	
Necrotizing fasciitis	
Severe arterial or venous thromboembolic events	Discontinue bevacizumab permanently; the safety of reinitiating bevacizumab after a thromboembolic event is resolved is not known
Moderate to severe proteinuria	Patients with a urine dipstick reading ≥2+ should undergo further assessment, eg, 24-hour urine collection. Suspend bevacizumab administration for ≥2 g of proteinuria/24 h and resume when proteinuria is <2 g/24 h
Severe hypertension not controlled with medical management	Hold bevacizumab pending further evaluation and treatment of hypertension
Mild, clinically insignificant infusion reaction	Decrease the rate of infusion
Clinically significant but not severe infusion reaction	Interrupt the infusion in patients with clinically significant infusion reactions and consider resuming at a slower rate following resolution. If decision is made to restart, the infusion may be continued at ≤50% of the rate prior to the reaction and increased in 50% increments every 30 minutes if well tolerated. Infusions may be restarted at the full rate during the next cycle
Severe infusion reaction—hypertension, hypertensive crises associated with neurologic signs and symptoms, wheezing, oxygen desaturation, G3 hypersensitivity, chest pain, headaches, rigors, and diaphoresis)	Stop infusion and administer appropriate medical therapy (eg, epinephrine, corticosteroids, intravenous antihistamines, bronchodilators, and/or oxygen). Discontinue bevacizumab
Planned elective surgery	Suspend bevacizumab at least 28 days before elective surgery and do not resume for at least 28 days after surgery or until surgical incision is fully healed
Recent hemoptysis	Do not administer bevacizumab
Evidence of rectosigmoid involvement by pelvic examination or bowel involvement on CT scan or clinical symptoms of bowel obstruction	

CISPLATIN + PEMETREXED

Delay cycle until ANC is >1500/mm³ and platelet count is >100,000/mm³

G3 hematologic toxicities	Hold therapy until values return to baseline. Then decrease both drug dosages by 25%
G4 hematologic toxicities	Hold therapy until values return to baseline. Then decrease both drug dosages by 50%

(continued)

Treatment Modifications (*continued*)

Adverse Event	Treatment Modification
Serum creatinine ≥1.5 mg/dL (≥130 μmol/L) and/or BUN ≥25 mg/dL (≥8.92 mmol/L)	Withhold cisplatin until serum creatinine <1.5 mg/dL (<130 μmol/L) and BUN <25 mg/dL (<8.92 mmol/L). Then consider a decrease in cisplatin dosage by 25%
G ≥2 renal toxicity due to cisplatin	Consider substituting carboplatin (AUC = 5) for cisplatin in subsequent cycles
G ≥2 diarrhea	Hold chemotherapy until toxicity resolves to <G2, then decrease both drug dosages by 25%
G3/4 mucositis	Decrease pemetrexed dosage by 50%
ALT and AST >1.5× ULN in a patient without liver metastasis	Withhold cisplatin and pemetrexed until ALT and AST ≤1.5× ULN
ALT and AST >2.5× ULN in a patient with liver metastasis with alkaline phosphatase >2.5× ULN	Withhold cisplatin and pemetrexed until ALT and AST ≤2.5× ULN and alkaline phosphatase ≤2.5× ULN
Peripheral neuropathy of G ≥3	Permanently discontinue cisplatin + pemetrexed
Cisplatin-induced hearing loss G ≥3	
Severe hypersensitivity reaction to pemetrexed or cisplatin is noted	
Occurrence of an adverse event requiring a third dose reduction	
Other G ≥3 nonhematologic toxicities (except nausea, vomiting, and alopecia)	Delay treatment until toxicity resolves to baseline, then decrease both drug dosages by 25% from previous levels

Delays of ≤42 days are permitted for recovery from pemetrexed- and cisplatin-related toxicities
Patients requiring 3 dose reductions: Discontinue therapy

Efficacy (N = 448)

	Bevacizumab + Pemetrexed + Cisplatin (n = 223)	Pemetrexed + Cisplatin (n = 225)	
Median survival	18.8 months	16.1 months	HR 0.77, 95% CI 0.62–0.95; P = 0.0167
Median progression-free survival	9.2 months	7.3 months	HR 0.61, 95% CI 0.50–0.75; *P* < 0.0001

Note: The median duration of follow-up was 39.4 months

Adverse Events (N = 446)

	Bevacizumab + Pemetrexed + Cisplatin (n = 222)		Pemetrexed + Cisplatin (n = 224)	
Grade (%)*	Grade 1/2	Grade 3–5	Grade 1/2	Grade 3–5
Nausea or vomiting	70	8	69	8
Neutropenia	34	44	34	45
Anemia	66	7	70	13

(*continued*)

Adverse Events (N = 446) *(continued)*

Grade (%)*	Bevacizumab + Pemetrexed + Cisplatin (n = 222)		Pemetrexed + Cisplatin (n = 224)	
	Grade 1/2	Grade 3–5	Grade 1/2	Grade 3–5
Asthenia or fatigue	56	14	55	13
Cardiovascular adverse events	33	29	2	<1
Thrombocytopenia	49	10	44	9
Hypertension	33	23	1	0
Hemorrhage	40	<1	7	0
Elevated creatinine level	35	4	26	2
Anorexia	32	2	29	4
Constipation	21	<1	19	<1
Oral mucositis	16	<1	14	<1
Diarrhea	16	<1	11	<1
Weight loss	10	0	10	0
Arterial and venous thromboembolic events	<1	6	<1	<1
Hepatic enzymes	2	0	<1	<1
Febrile neutropenia	0	2	0	3
Sepsis	0	1	0	1

*According to the National Cancer Institute Common Terminology Criteria for Adverse Events, version 3.0

Therapy Monitoring

1. *Once per week:* CBC with differential and platelet count
2. *Before the start of a cycle:* CBC with differential, serum electrolytes, serum bilirubin, AST or ALT, and alkaline phosphatase, BUN, and creatinine
3. Observe closely for hypersensitivity reactions, especially during the first and second bevacizumab infusions
4. Blood pressure every 2 weeks or more frequently as indicated during treatment
5. Assess proteinuria by urine dipstick and/or urinary protein-to-creatinine ratio. Patients with a urine dipstick reading ≥2+ should undergo further assessment with 24-hour urine collection
6. *Response evaluation:* CT scan every 8 weeks for 6 months (modified RECIST 1.1 for mesothelioma), then every 12 weeks

ADVANCED DISEASE · SUBSEQUENT THERAPY
MESOTHELIOMA REGIMEN: PEMBROLIZUMAB

Alley EW et al. Lancet Oncol 2017;18:623–630
Kindler H et al. Thorac Oncol 2017;12:S293
ClinicalTrials.gov. Study of Pembrolizumab (MK–3475) in Participants With Advanced Solid Tumors (MK–3475–158/KEYNOTE–158). Available from: https://clinicaltrials.gov/ct2/show/record/NCT02628067

Pembrolizumab 10 mg/kg; administer intravenously over 30 minutes in a volume of 0.9% sodium chloride injection (0.9% NS) or 5% dextrose injection (D5W), USP, sufficient to produce a pembrolizumab concentration within the range of 1–10 mg/mL every 2 weeks for up to 24 months (total dosage/2-week cycle = 10 mg/kg)
- Administer pembrolizumab with an administration set that contains a sterile, nonpyrogenic, low-protein-binding in-line or add-on filter with pore size within the range of 0.2–5 μm

Notes:
- Eligibility required PD-L1 expression in ≥1% of tumor cells (Alley et al.)
- A 200-mg fixed-dose regimen of pembrolizumab is currently under study for malignant mesothelioma (eg, Kindler et al. NCT02628067), *thus consider:*
  - **Pembrolizumab** 200 mg; administer intravenously over 30 minutes in a volume of 0.9% NS or D5W sufficient to produce a pembrolizumab concentration within the range of 1–10 mg/mL every 3 weeks for up to 24 months (total dosage/3-week cycle = 200 mg)
    - Administer pembrolizumab with an administration set that contains a sterile, nonpyrogenic, low-protein-binding in-line or add-on filter with pore size within the range of 0.2–5 μm

Supportive Care
Antiemetic prophylaxis
Emetogenic potential is **MINIMAL**
See Chapter 42 for antiemetic recommendations

Hematopoietic growth factor (CSF) prophylaxis
Primary prophylaxis is **NOT** *indicated*
See Chapter 43 for more information

Antimicrobial prophylaxis
Risk of fever and neutropenia is **LOW**
Antimicrobial primary prophylaxis to be considered:
- Antibacterial—not indicated
- Antifungal—not indicated
- Antiviral—not indicated, unless patient previously had an episode of HSV

Treatment Modifications

RECOMMENDED DOSAGE MODIFICATIONS FOR PEMBROLIZUMAB

Adverse Event	Grade/Severity	Treatment Modification
Infusion reaction	Clinically significant but not severe infusion reaction	Interrupt the infusion in patients with clinically significant infusion reactions and consider resuming at a slower rate following resolution. If decision is made to restart, begin at ≤50% of the rate prior to the reaction and increase in 50% increments every 30 minutes if well tolerated. Infusions may be restarted at the full rate during the next cycle
	G3/4 (severe infusion reaction—pyrexia, chills, flushing, hypotension, dyspnea, wheezing, back pain, abdominal pain, and urticaria). Not rapidly responsive to brief interruption of infusion	Stop infusion and administer appropriate medical therapy (eg, epinephrine, corticosteroids, intravenous antihistamines, bronchodilators, and/or oxygen). Discontinue pembrolizumab

(continued)

Treatment Modifications (continued)

Adverse Event	Grade/Severity	Treatment Modification
Colitis	G1	Loperamide 4 mg as starting dose, then 2 mg before each meal and after each loose stool until without diarrhea for 12 hours, with maximum of 16 mg loperamide per day. If G1 diarrhea or colitis persists >14 days, add prednisolone 0.5–1 mg/kg (non-enteric-coated) or consider oral budesonide 9 mg daily if no bloody diarrhea
	G2/3 diarrhea or colitis	Withhold pembrolizumab. Loperamide 4 mg as starting dose, then 2 mg before each meal and after each loose stool until without diarrhea for 12 hours, with maximum of 16 mg loperamide per day. Administer oral prednisone/prednisolone at a dosage of 0.5–2 mg/kg per day or its equivalent. When symptoms improve to G1, begin a slow corticosteroid taper over at least 4 weeks. Resume pembrolizumab upon symptom control, or when prednisone/prednisolone daily dosage <10 mg
	G4 diarrhea or colitis	Permanently discontinue pembrolizumab. Loperamide 4 mg as starting dose, then 2 mg before each meal and after each loose stool until without diarrhea for 12 hours, with maximum of 16 mg loperamide per day. Administer 1–2 mg/kg intravenous (methyl)prednisolone and convert to 0.5–2 mg/kg prednisone/prednisolone orally each day or its equivalent only after a response. Taper over at least 4 weeks when symptoms improve. If symptoms do not improve over 72 hours or worsen, perform flexible sigmoidoscopy/colonoscopy to document colitis, then begin infliximab 5 mg/kg (if no perforation, sepsis, TB, hepatitis, NYHA III/IV CHF). If no response, add MMF 500–1000 mg twice daily. If worse on MMF, consider addition of tacrolimus or ATG
Pneumonitis	G2	Withhold pembrolizumab. Consider pneumocystis prophylaxis depending on the clinical context and coverage with empiric antibiotics. Administer oral prednisone/prednisolone at a dosage of 1–2 mg/kg per day or its equivalent. When symptoms improve to G1, begin a slow corticosteroid taper over at least 4 weeks. If response is not adequate after 48 hours, administer 2–4 mg/kg intravenous (methyl)prednisolone and convert to 0.5–2 mg/kg prednisone/prednisolone orally each day or its equivalent only after a response, followed by a taper over at least 6 weeks when symptoms improve to G1, titrating to symptoms. Resume pembrolizumab upon symptom control, or when prednisone/prednisolone daily dosage <10 mg
	G3/4	Permanently discontinue pembrolizumab. Consider pneumocystis prophylaxis depending on the clinical context; cover with empiric antibiotics. Administer 2–4 mg/kg intravenous (methyl)prednisolone and convert to 1–2 mg/kg prednisone/prednisolone orally each day or its equivalent only after a response, followed by a taper over at least 8 weeks when symptoms improve to G1, titrating to symptoms. If, when initially treated, improvement does not occur within 48–72 hours, begin infliximab 5 mg/kg (if no perforation, sepsis, TB, hepatitis, NYHA III/IV CHF). If no response to infliximab, add MMF 500–1000 mg twice daily. Consider MMF especially if concurrent hepatic toxicity
Hepatitis	G2 (AST or ALT >3–5× ULN or total bilirubin >1.5–3× ULN)	Withhold pembrolizumab. Administer oral prednisone/prednisolone at a dosage of 1–2 mg/kg per day or its equivalent. When symptoms improve to G1, begin a slow corticosteroid taper over at least 4 weeks. Resume pembrolizumab upon symptom control, or when prednisone/prednisolone daily dosage <10 mg
	G3/4 (AST or ALT >5× ULN or total bilirubin >3× ULN)	Permanently discontinue pembrolizumab. Administer 1–2 mg/kg intravenous (methyl)prednisolone and convert to 0.5–2 mg/kg prednisone/prednisolone orally each day or its equivalent only after a response. Taper over at least 6 weeks when symptoms improve. If no response, add MMF 500–1000 mg twice daily. If worse on MMF, consider adding tacrolimus or ATG
Hypophysitis	G2/3 (moderate symptoms, ie, headache but no visual disturbance or fatigue/mood alteration but hemodynamically stable, no electrolyte disturbance)	Administer analgesia as needed for headache. Withhold pembrolizumab. Administer oral prednisone/prednisolone at a dosage of 0.5–2 mg/kg per day or its equivalent. When improves to G1, begin a slow corticosteroid taper over at least 4 weeks. If no improvement in 48 hours, administer 1–2 mg/kg intravenous (methyl)prednisolone and convert to 0.5–2 mg/kg prednisone/prednisolone orally each day or its equivalent only after a response. Taper over at least 4 weeks when symptoms improve to 5 mg prednisone/prednisolone or equivalent; do not stop steroids. Resume pembrolizumab upon symptom control, or when prednisone/prednisolone daily dosage <10 mg
	G4 (severe mass effect symptoms, ie, severe headache, any visual disturbance or severe hypoadrenalism, ie, hypotension, severe electrolyte disturbance)	Permanently discontinue pembrolizumab. Administer analgesia as needed for headache. Administer 1–2 mg/kg intravenous (methyl)prednisolone and convert to 0.5–2 mg/kg prednisone/prednisolone orally each day or its equivalent only after a response. Taper over at least 4 weeks when symptoms improve to 5 mg prednisone prednisolone or equivalent; do not stop steroids

(continued)

Treatment Modifications (continued)

Adverse Event	Grade/Severity	Treatment Modification
Adrenal insufficiency	G2	Withhold pembrolizumab. Administer oral prednisone/prednisolone at a dosage of 0.5–2 mg/kg per day or its equivalent. When symptoms improve to G1, begin a slow corticosteroid taper over at least 4 weeks. Serially assess adrenal function and continue steroids at replacement doses (20–40 mg hydrocortisone daily ~2/3 dose in morning upon awakening and ~1/3 at 4 PM) until recovery of adrenal function is documented. Resume pembrolizumab upon symptom control, or when prednisone/prednisolone daily dosage <10 mg
	G3/4	Permanently discontinue pembrolizumab. Administer oral prednisone/prednisolone at a dosage of 0.5–2 mg/kg per day or its equivalent. When symptoms improve to G1, begin a slow corticosteroid taper over at least 4 weeks. Serially assess adrenal function and continue steroids at replacement doses (20–40 mg hydrocortisone daily ~2/3 dose in morning upon awakening and ~1/3 at 4 PM) until recovery of adrenal function is documented
Type 1 diabetes mellitus	G3 hyperglycemia	Withhold pembrolizumab. Admit to hospital to manage hyperglycemia. Role of corticosteroids in preventing complete loss of insulin-producing cells is unknown, and use is not recommended. Resume pembrolizumab upon symptom control, or when prednisone/prednisolone daily dosage <10 mg
	G4 hyperglycemia	Permanently discontinue pembrolizumab. Admit to hospital to manage hyperglycemia. Role of corticosteroids in preventing complete loss of insulin-producing cells is unknown, and use is not recommended
Nephritis and renal dysfunction	G2/3 (serum creatinine 1.5–6× ULN)	Withhold pembrolizumab. Administer oral prednisone/prednisolone at a dosage of 0.5–2 mg/kg per day or its equivalent. When symptoms improve to G1, begin a slow corticosteroid taper over at least 4 weeks. If response is not adequate, administer 0.5–1 mg/kg intravenous (methyl)prednisolone and convert to 0.5–2 mg/kg prednisone/prednisolone orally each day or its equivalent only after a response, followed by a taper over at least 4 weeks when symptoms improve to G1. Resume pembrolizumab upon symptom control, or when prednisone/prednisolone daily dosage <10 mg
	G4 (serum creatinine >6× ULN)	Permanently discontinue pembrolizumab. Administer 0.5–1 mg/kg intravenous (methyl)prednisolone and convert to 0.5–2 mg/kg prednisone/prednisolone orally each day or its equivalent only after a response, followed by a taper over at least 4 weeks when symptoms improve to G1
Skin	G1/2	Continue pembrolizumab. Avoid skin irritants, avoid sun exposure; topical emollients recommended. Topical steroid (mild strength for G1, moderate/potent strength for G2) cream once or twice daily ± oral or topical antihistamines for itching
	G3 rash or suspected SJS or TEN	Withhold pembrolizumab. Avoid skin irritants, avoid sun exposure; topical emollients recommended. Administer oral or topical antihistamines for itching. Administer oral prednisone/prednisolone at a dosage of 0.5–2 mg/kg or its equivalent daily for 3 days followed by a slow corticosteroid taper over at least 4 weeks when the rash improves to G1. If rash does not respond adequately, administer 0.5–1 mg/kg intravenous (methyl)prednisolone and convert to 0.5–2 mg/kg prednisone/prednisolone orally each day or its equivalent only after a response, followed by a taper over at least 4 weeks when the rash improves to G1. Resume pembrolizumab upon symptom control, or when prednisone/prednisolone daily dosage <10 mg
	G4 rash or confirmed SJS or TEN	Avoid skin irritants, avoid sun exposure; topical emollients recommended. Administer oral or topical antihistamines for itching. Administer 1–2 mg/kg intravenous (methyl)prednisolone and convert to oral steroids 0.5–2 mg/kg prednisone/prednisolone each day or its equivalent only after a response. Taper over at least 4 weeks when the rash improves to G1. Permanently discontinue pembrolizumab
Encephalitis	Confusion or altered behavior, headaches, alteration in Glasgow Coma Scale, motor or sensory deficits, speech abnormality; may or may not be febrile	Initially withhold pembrolizumab, but permanently discontinue pembrolizumab if there is no doubt as to diagnosis. Exclude bacterial and ideally viral infections prior to high-dose steroids. Administer oral prednisone/prednisolone at a dosage of 0.5–2 mg/kg per day or its equivalent. When symptoms improve, begin a slow corticosteroid taper over at least 4–8 weeks. If symptoms are severe, administer 1–2 mg/kg intravenous (methyl)prednisolone and convert to 0.5–2 mg/kg prednisone/prednisolone orally each day or its equivalent only after a response. Consider concurrent empiric antiviral (intravenous acyclovir) and antibacterial therapy

(continued)

Treatment Modifications (continued)

Adverse Event	Grade/Severity	Treatment Modification
Aseptic meningitis	Headache, photophobia, neck stiffness with fever, or may be afebrile, vomiting; normal cognition/cerebral function (distinguishes from encephalitis)	
Other syndromes include neurosarcoidosis, posterior reversible leukoencephalopathy syndrome (PRES), Vogt-Koyanagi-Harada syndrome, demyelination, vasculitic encephalopathy, and generalized seizures		
Transverse myelitis	Acute or subacute neurologic signs/symptoms of motor, sensory, autonomic origin; most have sensory level; often bilateral symptoms	Initially withhold pembrolizumab, but permanently discontinue pembrolizumab if there is no doubt as to diagnosis. Administer 2 mg/kg intravenous (methyl)prednisolone or consider 1 g/day and convert to 0.5–2 mg/kg prednisone/prednisolone orally each day or its equivalent only after a response. When symptoms improve, begin a slow corticosteroid taper over at least 4–8 weeks. Plasmapheresis may be required if steroids do not bring about improvement
Myocarditis	G3	Permanently discontinue pembrolizumab. Administer 2 mg/kg intravenous (methyl)prednisolone or consider 1 g/day and convert to 0.5–2 mg/kg prednisone/prednisolone orally each day or its equivalent only after a response. When symptoms improve, begin a slow corticosteroid taper over at least 4–8 weeks. If no response, add MMF 500–1000 mg twice daily. If worse on MMF, consider adding tacrolimus
Peripheral neurologic toxicity	Moderate: some interference with ADL, symptoms concerning to patient	Withhold pembrolizumab. Initial observation reasonable or initiate prednisone/prednisolone 0.5–1 mg/kg (if progressing, eg, from mild) and/or pregabalin or duloxetine for pain. When symptoms improve, begin a slow corticosteroid taper over at least 4 weeks. Resume pembrolizumab upon symptom control, or when prednisone/prednisolone daily dosage <10 mg
	Severe: limits self-care and aids warranted, life-threatening, eg, respiratory problems	Permanently discontinue pembrolizumab. Administer 1–2 mg/kg intravenous (methyl)prednisolone and convert to 0.5–2 mg/kg prednisone/prednisolone orally each day or its equivalent only after a response. Taper over at least 4–8 weeks when symptoms improve to G1
Guillain-Barré syndrome	Progressive symmetrical muscle weakness with absent or reduced tendon reflexes—involves extremities; facial, respiratory, and bulbar and oculomotor muscles; dysregulation of autonomic nerves	Permanently discontinue pembrolizumab. Use of steroids not recommended in idiopathic Guillain-Barré syndrome; however, a trial of (methyl)prednisolone 1–2 mg/kg is reasonable, converting to 0.5–2 mg/kg prednisone/prednisolone orally each day or its equivalent only after a response. If no improvement or worsening, plasmapheresis or IVIG is indicated
Myasthenia gravis	Fluctuating muscle weakness (proximal limb, trunk, ocular, eg, ptosis/diplopia or bulbar) with fatigability; respiratory muscles may also be involved	Permanently discontinue pembrolizumab. Administer pyridostigmine at an initial dosage of 30 mg 3 times daily. Administer oral prednisone/prednisolone at a dosage of 0.5–2 mg/kg per day or its equivalent or 1–2 mg/kg intravenous (methyl)prednisolone, depending on the severity of symptoms. If treatment begins with intravenous drug, convert to 0.5–2 mg/kg prednisone/prednisolone orally each day or its equivalent only after a response. If no improvement or worsening, plasmapheresis or IVIG may be considered. Additional immunosuppressants used in myasthenia gravis include azathioprine, cyclosporine, and mycophenolate. Avoid certain medications, eg, ciprofloxacin and beta-blockers, that may precipitate cholinergic crisis
Other syndromes, including motor and sensory peripheral neuropathy, multifocal radicular neuropathy/plexopathy, autonomic neuropathy, phrenic nerve palsy, cranial nerve palsies (eg, facial nerve, optic nerve, hypoglossal nerve)		Permanently discontinue pembrolizumab. Administer oral prednisone/prednisolone at a dosage of 0.5–2 mg/kg per day or its equivalent or 1–2 mg/kg intravenous (methyl)prednisolone, depending on the severity of symptoms. If treatment begins with intravenous drug, convert to 0.5–2 mg/kg prednisone/prednisolone orally each day or its equivalent only after a response

(continued)

Treatment Modifications (*continued*)

Adverse Event	Grade/Severity	Treatment Modification
Arthralgia	G1 (mild pain with inflammation, erythema, or joint swelling)	Continue pembrolizumab. Administer acetaminophen (paracetamol) and ibuprofen
	G2 (moderate pain with inflammation, erythema, or joint swelling that limits ADLs)	Withhold pembrolizumab. Administer higher doses of acetaminophen (paracetamol) and ibuprofen and use diclofenac or naproxen or etoricoxib. If inadequately controlled, consider intra-articular steroid injections for large joints or administer oral prednisone/prednisolone at a dosage of 0.5–2 mg/kg per day or its equivalent. When symptoms improve to G1, begin a slow corticosteroid taper over at least 4 weeks. If response is not adequate, administer 0.5–1 mg/kg intravenous (methyl) prednisolone and convert to 0.5–2 mg/kg prednisone/prednisolone orally each day or its equivalent only after a response, followed by a taper over at least 4 weeks when symptoms improve to G1. Resume pembrolizumab upon symptom control, or when prednisone/prednisolone daily dosage <10 mg
	G3 (severe pain; irreversible joint damage; disabling; limits self-care ADLs)	Withhold pembrolizumab. Administer 0.5–1 mg/kg intravenous (methyl)prednisolone and convert to 0.5–2 mg/kg prednisone/prednisolone orally each day or its equivalent only after a response, followed by a taper over at least 4 weeks when symptoms improve to G1. In severe cases, infliximab or another anti-TNF-alpha drug may be required for improvement of arthritis. Resume pembrolizumab upon symptom control, or when prednisone/prednisolone daily dosage <10 mg
Other	First occurrence of other G3	Withhold pembrolizumab. Administer oral prednisone/prednisolone at a dosage of 0.5–2 mg/kg per day or its equivalent. When symptoms improve to G1, begin a slow corticosteroid taper over at least 4 weeks. Resume pembrolizumab upon symptom control, or when prednisone/prednisolone daily dosage <10 mg
	Recurrence of same G3	Permanently discontinue pembrolizumab. Administer 1–2 mg/kg intravenous (methyl)prednisolone and convert to 0.5–2 mg/kg prednisone/prednisolone orally each day or its equivalent only after a response. Taper over at least 4–8 weeks when symptoms improve to G1
	Life-threatening or G4	
	Requirement for ³10 mg/day prednisone or equivalent for >12 weeks	Permanently discontinue pembrolizumab
	Persistent G2/3 adverse reactions lasting ³12 weeks	

ADL, activities of daily living; ALT, alanine aminotransferase; AST, aspartate aminotransferase; ATG, anti-thymocyte globulin; CHF, congestive heart failure; IVIG, intravenous immunoglobulin; MMF, mycophenolate mofetil; NYHA, New York Heart Association; PRES, posterior reversible leukoencephalopathy syndrome; SJS, Stevens-Johnson syndrome; TB, tuberculosis; TEN, toxic epidermal necrolysis; TNF, tumor necrosis factor; ULN, upper limit of normal

Notes on general supportive care:
• Steroid taper in most cases will proceed over a minimum of 1 month, but if symptoms improve rapidly, a 2-week taper can be considered. If steroids are administered for >4 weeks, consider PCP prophylaxis (cotrimoxazole 480 mg twice daily M/W/F or inhaled pentamidine if cotrimoxazole allergy), regular random blood glucose, vitamin D level, and starting calcium/vitamin D supplementation per guidelines

Patient Population Studied

This ongoing, multicenter, nonrandomized, open-label, multicohort, phase 1b trial (KEYNOTE–028) included 25 patients with incurable, histologically confirmed, locally advanced, or metastatic malignant pleural mesothelioma that was PD-L1-positive. Eligible patients were aged ≥18 years, with an Eastern Cooperative Oncology Group (ECOG) performance status score ≤1, and had failed or were unable to receive standard therapy. Patients who had previously received treatment with PD-1 and PD-L1 checkpoint inhibitors were not eligible. All patients received intravenous pembrolizumab (10 mg/kg) every 2 weeks.

Efficacy (N = 25)

Objective response rate*	20%
Median progression-free survival	5.4 months (95% CI 3.4–7.5)
Median survival	18 months (95% CI 9.4–not reached)
Median duration of response	12 months (95% CI 3.7–not reached)

*Objective response rate is the percentage of patients who experienced a confirmed partial or complete response to the study drug
Note: The median duration of follow-up was 18.7 months, and the median duration of therapy was 5.1 months

Adverse Events (N = 25)

Grade (%)*	Grade 1	Grade 2	Grade 3
Nausea	20	4	0
Fatigue	12	12	0
Arthralgia	8	12	0
Pruritus	8	8	0
Decreased appetite	4	4	4
Dry mouth	12	0	0
Dyspnea	0	4	4
Pyrexia	4	0	4
Asthenia	0	8	0
Diarrhea	4	4	0
Headache	4	4	0
Constipation	8	0	0
Dry skin	8	0	0
Mucosal inflammation	8	0	0
Rash maculopapular	8	0	0
Decreased neutrophil count	0	0	4
Elevated ALT level	0	0	4
Iridocyclitis	0	0	4
Thrombocytopenia	0	0	4
Cancer pain	0	4	0
Decreased white blood cell count	0	4	0
Dysgeusia	0	4	0
Elevated AST level	0	4	0
Elevated γ-glutamyltransferase level	0	4	0
Infusion-related reaction	0	4	0

(continued)

Therapy Monitoring

1. Monitor patients for signs and symptoms of infusion-related reactions, including pyrexia, chills, flushing, hypotension, dyspnea, wheezing, back pain, abdominal pain, and urticaria

2. Initially at the time of each dose, and eventually every 6–12 weeks, perform a total body skin examination with attention to *all* mucous membranes as well as a complete review of systems

3. Monitor patients for signs and symptoms of pneumonitis. Evaluate patients with suspected pneumonitis with chest x-ray, CT scan, and pulse oximetry. For toxicity ≥2, may include nasal swab, sputum culture and sensitivity, blood culture and sensitivity, and urine culture and sensitivity

4. Monitor patients for signs and symptoms of colitis. Encourage patients to report diarrhea immediately to any member of the health care team

5. Draw AST, ALT, and bilirubin prior to each infusion and/or weekly if there are G1 LFT elevations. Note, no treatment is recommended for G1 LFT abnormalities. For toxicity ≥2, work up for other causes of elevated LFTs, including viral hepatitis

6. Use basic metabolic panel (Na, K, CO_2, glucose) and patient history as screening tools for hypophysitis, including hypopituitarism and adrenal insufficiency. If in doubt, evaluate morning adrenocorticotropic hormone (ACTH) and cortisol levels. Consider ACTH stimulation test for indeterminate results

7. Assess thyroid function at the start of treatment, periodically during treatment, and, as indicated, based on clinical evaluation and for clinical signs and symptoms of thyroid disorders. Test for TSH and free thyroxine (FT4) every 4–6 weeks as part of routine clinical monitoring on therapy or for case detection in symptomatic patients

8. Measure glucose at baseline and with each treatment during the first 12 weeks and every 6 weeks thereafter

9. Obtain a serum creatinine level prior to every dose. If creatinine is found to be newly elevated, consider holding therapy while other potential causes are evaluated. *Note:* Routine urinalysis is not necessary other than to rule out urinary tract infections, etc

(continued)

Adverse Events (N = 25) (continued)

Grade (%)*	Grade 1	Grade 2	Grade 3
Pleuritic pain	0	4	0
Rash pruritic	0	4	0
Thrombosis	0	4	0
Balance disorder	4	0	0
Burning sensation	4	0	0
Chest pain	4	0	0
Cough	4	0	0
Decreased hemoglobin level	4	0	0
Decreased platelet count	4	0	0
Elevated blood alkaline phosphatase	4	0	0
Hypocalcemia	4	0	0
Irritability	4	0	0
Joint stiffness	4	0	0
Musculoskeletal stiffness	4	0	0
Myalgia	4	0	0
Paresthesia	4	0	0
Rash	4	0	0
Rash generalized	4	0	0
Vitreous floaters	4	0	0

*According to the National Cancer Institute Common Terminology Criteria for Adverse Events, version 4.0
Note: Toxicities are included in the table if the events were deemed to be related to the study treatment. No G4 or G5 treatment-related adverse events occurred. In total, 64% of patients reported treatment-related adverse events. No one discontinued treatment as a result of a treatment-related adverse event

Therapy Monitoring
(continued)

10. Obtain a complete rheumatologic history and perform an examination of all peripheral joints for tenderness, swelling, and range of motion. Examine the spine. Consider plain x-ray/imaging to exclude metastases and evaluate joint damage (erosions), if appropriate

11. In patients at high risk for infections and in appropriately selected patients based on an infectious disease evaluation, draw screening laboratories (HIV, hepatitis A and B, and blood QuantiFERON for TB) to prepare patients to start infliximab

12. *Response evaluation:* CT scan every 8 weeks for 6 months (modified RECIST 1.1 for mesothelioma), then every 12 weeks

ADVANCED DISEASE • SUBSEQUENT THERAPY
MESOTHELIOMA REGIMEN: NIVOLUMAB

Scherpereel A et al. Lancet 2019;20:239:253
Supplement to: Scherpereel A et al. Lancet 2019;20:239–253
OPDIVO (nivolumab) prescribing information. Princeton, NJ: Bristol-Myers Squibb Company; revised September 2019

Nivolumab 3 mg/kg; administer intravenously over 60 minutes in a volume of 0.9% sodium chloride (0.9% NS) or 5% dextrose injection (D5W), not to exceed 160 mL and sufficient to produce a nivolumab concentration within the range 1–10 mg/mL, every 2 weeks until disease progression or for a maximum duration of 2 years (total dosage/2-week cycle = 240 mg)

- Note that the U.S. Food and Drug Administration (FDA)-approved regimens for other indications include fixed doses of nivolumab and allow for a shortened infusion duration of 30 minutes, consistent with the regimens approved on March 5, 2018, thus consider:

  - **Nivolumab** 240 mg; administer intravenously over 30 minutes in a volume of 0.9% NS or D5W, not to exceed 160 mL and sufficient to produce a nivolumab concentration within the range 1–10 mg/mL, every 2 weeks until disease progression or for a maximum duration of 2 years (total dosage/2-week cycle = 240 mg)
    - Administer nivolumab through an administration set that contains a sterile, non-pyrogenic, low-protein-binding in-line filter with pore size within the range of 0.2–1.2 μm
    - Nivolumab can cause severe infusion-related reactions

  OR

  - **Nivolumab** 480 mg; administer intravenously over 30 minutes in a volume of 0.9% NS or D5W, not to exceed 160 mL and sufficient to produce a nivolumab concentration within the range 1–10 mg/mL, every 4 weeks until disease progression or for a maximum duration of 2 years (total dosage/4-week cycle = 480 mg)
    - Administer nivolumab through an administration set that contains a sterile, non-pyrogenic, low-protein-binding in-line filter with pore size within the range of 0.2–1.2 μm
    - Nivolumab can cause severe infusion-related reactions

Supportive Care
Antiemetic prophylaxis
Emetogenic potential with nivolumab is **MINIMAL**
See Chapter 42 for antiemetic recommendations

Hematopoietic growth factor (CSF) prophylaxis
Primary prophylaxis is **NOT** *indicated*
See Chapter 43 for more information

Antimicrobial prophylaxis
Risk of fever and neutropenia is **LOW**
Antimicrobial primary prophylaxis to be considered:
- Antibacterial—not indicated
- Antifungal—not indicated
- Antiviral—not indicated unless patient previously had an episode of HSV

Treatment Modifications

RECOMMENDED DOSE MODIFICATIONS FOR NIVOLUMAB

Adverse Event	Grade/Severity	Treatment Modification
Infusion reaction	Clinically significant but not severe infusion reaction	Interrupt the infusion in patients with clinically significant infusion reactions and consider resuming at a slower rate following resolution. If decision is made to restart, begin at ≤50% of the rate prior to the reaction and increase in 50% increments every 30 minutes if well tolerated. Infusions may be restarted at the full rate during the next cycle
	G3/4 (severe infusion reaction—pyrexia, chills, flushing, hypotension, dyspnea, wheezing, back pain, abdominal pain, and urticaria). Not rapidly responsive to brief interruption of infusion	Stop infusion and administer appropriate medical therapy (eg, epinephrine, corticosteroids, intravenous antihistamines, bronchodilators, and/or oxygen). Discontinue nivolumab

(continued)

Treatment Modifications (continued)

Adverse Event	Grade/Severity	Treatment Modification
Colitis	G1	Loperamide 4 mg as starting dose then 2 mg before each meal and after each loose stool until without diarrhea for 12 hours, with maximum of 16 mg loperamide per day. If G1 diarrhea or colitis persists >14 days, then add prednisolone 0.5–1 mg/kg (non-enteric-coated) or consider oral budesonide 9 mg daily if no bloody diarrhea
	G2/3 diarrhea or colitis	Withhold nivolumab. Loperamide 4 mg as starting dose then 2 mg before each meal and after each loose stool until without diarrhea for 12 hours, with maximum of 16 mg loperamide per day. Administer oral prednisone/prednisolone at a dose of 0.5–2 mg/kg/day or its equivalent. When improves to G1, begin a slow corticosteroid taper over at least 4 weeks. Resume nivolumab upon symptom control, or when prednisone/prednisolone daily dose <10 mg
	G4 diarrhea or colitis	Permanently discontinue nivolumab. Loperamide 4 mg as starting dose then 2 mg before each meal and after each loose stool until without diarrhea for 12 hours, with maximum of 16 mg loperamide per day. Administer 1–2 mg/kg IV (methyl)prednisolone and convert to 0.5–2 mg/kg prednisone/prednisolone orally each day or its equivalent only after a response. Taper over at least 4 weeks when symptoms improve. If does not improve over 72 hours or worsens, perform flexible sigmoidoscopy/colonoscopy to document colitis then begin infliximab 5 mg/kg (if no perforation/sepsis/TB/hepatitis/NYHA III/IV CHF). If no response, add MMF 500–1000 mg twice daily. If worse on MMF, consider addition of tacrolimus or ATG
Pneumonitis	G2	Withhold nivolumab. Consider pneumocystis prophylaxis depending on the clinical context and coverage with empiric antibiotics. Administer oral prednisone/prednisolone at a dose of 1–2 mg/kg/day or its equivalent. When improves to G1, begin a slow corticosteroid taper over at least 4 weeks. If does not respond adequately after 48 hours, then administer 2–4 mg/kg IV (methyl)prednisolone and convert to 0.5–2 mg/kg prednisone/prednisolone orally each day or its equivalent only after a response, followed by a taper over at least 6 weeks when symptoms improve to G1, titrating to symptoms. Resume nivolumab upon symptom control, or when prednisone/prednisolone daily dose <10 mg
	G3/4	Permanently discontinue nivolumab. Consider pneumocystis prophylaxis depending on the clinical context; cover with empiric antibiotics. Administer 2–4 mg/kg IV (methyl)prednisolone and convert to 1–2 mg/kg prednisone/prednisolone orally each day or its equivalent only after a response, followed by a taper over at least 8 weeks when symptoms improve to G1, titrating to symptoms. If when initially treated improvement does not occur within 48–72 hours, begin infliximab 5 mg/kg (if no perforation/sepsis/TB/hepatitis/NYHA III/IV CHF). If no response to infliximab, add MMF 500–1000 mg twice daily. Consider MMF especially if has concurrent hepatic toxicity
Hepatitis	G2 (AST or ALT >3–5× ULN or total bilirubin >1.5–3× ULN)	Withhold nivolumab. Administer oral prednisone/prednisolone at a dose of 1–2 mg/kg/day or its equivalent. When improves to G1, begin a slow corticosteroid taper over at least 4 weeks. Resume nivolumab upon symptom control, or when prednisone/prednisolone daily dose <10 mg
	G3/4 (AST or ALT >5× ULN or total bilirubin >3× ULN)	Permanently discontinue nivolumab. Administer 1–2 mg/kg IV (methyl)prednisolone and convert to 0.5–2 mg/kg prednisone/prednisolone orally each day or its equivalent only after a response. Taper over at least 6 weeks when symptoms improve. If no response, add MMF 500–1000 mg twice daily. If worse on MMF, consider adding tacrolimus or ATG
Hypophysitis	G2/3 (moderate symptoms, ie, headache but no visual disturbance or fatigue/mood alteration but hemodynamically stable, no electrolyte disturbance)	Administer analgesia as needed for headache. Withhold nivolumab. Administer oral prednisone/prednisolone at a dose of 0.5–2 mg/kg/day or its equivalent. When improves to G1, begin a slow corticosteroid taper over at least 4 weeks. If no improvement in 48 hours, administer 1–2 mg/kg IV (methyl)prednisolone and convert to 0.5–2 mg/kg prednisone/prednisolone orally each day or its equivalent only after a response. Taper over at least 4 weeks when symptoms improve to 5 mg prednisone/prednisolone or equivalent; do not stop steroids. Resume nivolumab upon symptom control, or when prednisone/prednisolone daily dose <10 mg

(continued)

Treatment Modifications (continued)

Adverse Event	Grade/Severity	Treatment Modification
	G4 (severe mass effect symptoms, ie, severe headache, any visual disturbance or severe hypoadrenalism, ie, hypotension, severe electrolyte disturbance)	Permanently discontinue nivolumab. Administer analgesia as needed for headache. Administer 1–2 mg/kg IV (methyl)prednisolone and convert to 0.5–2 mg/kg prednisone/prednisolone orally each day or its equivalent only after a response. Taper over at least 4 weeks when symptoms improve to 5 mg prednisone/prednisolone or equivalent; do not stop steroids
Adrenal Insufficiency	G2	Withhold nivolumab. Administer oral prednisone/prednisolone at a dose of 0.5–2 mg/kg/day or its equivalent. When improves to G1, begin a slow corticosteroid taper over at least 4 weeks. Serially assess adrenal function and continue steroids at replacement doses (20–40 mg hydrocortisone daily ~2/3 dose in AM upon awakening and ~1/3 at 4 PM) until recovery of adrenal function is documented. Resume nivolumab upon symptom control, or when prednisone/prednisolone daily dose <10 mg
	G3/4	Permanently discontinue nivolumab. Administer oral prednisone/prednisolone at a dose of 0.5–2 mg/kg/day or its equivalent. When improves to G1, begin a slow corticosteroid taper over at least 4 weeks. Serially assess adrenal function and continue steroids at replacement doses (20–40 mg hydrocortisone daily ~2/3 dose in AM upon awakening and ~1/3 at 4 PM) until recovery of adrenal function is documented
Type 1 diabetes mellitus	G3 hyperglycemia	Withhold nivolumab. Admit to hospital to manage hyperglycemia. Role of corticosteroids in preventing complete loss of insulin-producing cells is unknown and not recommended. Resume nivolumab upon symptom control, or when prednisone/prednisolone daily dose <10 mg
	G4 hyperglycemia	Permanently discontinue nivolumab. Admit to hospital to manage hyperglycemia. Role of corticosteroids in preventing complete loss of insulin-producing cells is unknown and not recommended
Nephritis and renal dysfunction	G2/3 (serum creatinine 1.5–6× ULN)	Withhold nivolumab. Administer oral prednisone/prednisolone at a dose of 0.5–2 mg/kg/day or its equivalent. When improves to G1, begin a slow corticosteroid taper over at least 4 weeks. If does not respond adequately, then administer 0.5–1 mg/kg IV (methyl)prednisolone and convert to 0.5–2 mg/kg prednisone/prednisolone orally each day or its equivalent only after a response, followed by a taper over at least 4 weeks when improves to G1. Resume nivolumab upon symptom control, or when prednisone/prednisolone daily dose <10 mg
	G4 (serum creatinine >6× ULN)	Permanently discontinue nivolumab. Administer 0.5–1 mg/kg IV (methyl)prednisolone and convert to 0.5–2 mg/kg prednisone/prednisolone orally each day or its equivalent only after a response, followed by a taper over at least 4 weeks when improves to G1
Skin	G1/2	Continue nivolumab. Avoid skin irritants, avoid sun exposure, topical emollients recommended. Topical steroid (mild strength for G1, moderate/potent strength for G2) cream once or twice daily ± oral or topical antihistamines for itching
	G3 rash or suspected SJS or TEN	Withhold nivolumab. Avoid skin irritants, avoid sun exposure, topical emollients recommended. Administer oral or topical antihistamines for itching. Administer oral prednisone/prednisolone at a dose of 0.5–2 mg/kg or its equivalent daily for 3 days followed by a slow corticosteroid taper over at least 4 weeks when the rash improves to G1. If does not respond adequately, then administer 0.5–1 mg/kg IV (methyl)prednisolone and convert to 0.5–2 mg/kg prednisone/prednisolone orally each day or its equivalent only after a response, followed by a taper over at least 4 weeks when the rash improves to G1. Resume nivolumab upon symptom control, or when prednisone/prednisolone daily dose <10 mg
	G4 rash or confirmed SJS or TEN	Avoid skin irritants, avoid sun exposure, topical emollients recommended. Administer oral or topical antihistamines for itching. Administer 1–2 mg/kg IV (methyl)prednisolone and convert to oral steroids 0.5–2 mg/kg prednisone/prednisolone each day or its equivalent only after a response. Taper over at least 4 weeks when the rash improves to G1. Permanently discontinue nivolumab

(continued)

Treatment Modifications (*continued*)

Adverse Event	Grade/Severity	Treatment Modification
Encephalitis	Confusion or altered behavior, headaches, alteration in Glasgow Coma Scale, motor or sensory deficits, speech abnormality, may or may not be febrile	Initially withhold nivolumab, but permanently discontinue nivolumab if there is no doubt as to diagnosis. Exclude bacterial and ideally viral infections prior to high-dose steroids. Administer oral prednisone/prednisolone at a dose of 0.5–2 mg/kg/day or its equivalent. When symptoms improve, begin a slow corticosteroid taper over at least 4–8 weeks. If symptoms are severe, administer 1–2 mg/kg IV (methyl)prednisolone and convert to 0.5–2 mg/kg prednisone/prednisolone orally each day or its equivalent only after a response. Consider concurrent empiric antiviral (IV acyclovir) and antibacterial therapy
Aseptic meningitis	Headache, photophobia, neck stiffness with fever or may be afebrile, vomiting; normal cognition/cerebral function (distinguishes from encephalitis)	
Other syndromes include neurosarcoidosis, posterior reversible leukoencephalopathy syndrome (PRES), Vogt-Koyanagi-Harada syndrome, demyelination, vasculitic encephalopathy, and generalized seizures		
Transverse myelitis	Acute or subacute neurologic signs/symptoms of motor/sensory/autonomic origin; most have sensory level; often bilateral symptoms	Initially withhold nivolumab, but permanently discontinue nivolumab if there is no doubt as to diagnosis. Administer 2 mg/kg IV (methyl)prednisolone or consider 1 g/day and convert to 0.5–2 mg/kg prednisone/prednisolone orally each day or its equivalent only after a response. When symptoms improve, begin a slow corticosteroid taper over at least 4–8 weeks. Plasmapheresis may be required if steroids do not bring about improvement
Myocarditis	G3	Permanently discontinue nivolumab. Administer 2 mg/kg IV (methyl)prednisolone or consider 1 g/day and convert to 0.5–2 mg/kg prednisone/prednisolone orally each day or its equivalent only after a response. When symptoms improve, begin a slow corticosteroid taper over at least 4–8 weeks. If no response, add MMF 500–1000 mg twice daily. If worse on MMF, consider adding tacrolimus
Peripheral neurologic toxicity	Moderate: some interference with ADL, symptoms concerning to patient	Withhold nivolumab. Initial observation reasonable or initiate prednisone/prednisolone 0.5–1 mg/kg (if progressing, eg, from mild) and/or pregabalin or duloxetine for pain. When symptoms improve, begin a slow corticosteroid taper over at least 4 weeks. Resume nivolumab upon symptom control, or when prednisone/prednisolone daily dose <10 mg
	Severe: limits self-care and aids warranted, life-threatening, eg, respiratory problems	Permanently discontinue nivolumab. Administer 1–2 mg/kg IV (methyl)prednisolone and convert to 0.5–2 mg/kg prednisone/prednisolone orally each day or its equivalent only after a response. Taper over at least 4–8 weeks when symptoms improve to G1
Guillain-Barré syndrome	Progressive symmetrical muscle weakness with absent or reduced tendon reflexes—involves extremities, facial, respiratory, and bulbar and oculomotor muscles; dysregulation of autonomic nerves	Permanently discontinue nivolumab. Use of steroids not recommended in idiopathic Guillain-Barré syndrome; however, a trial of (methyl)prednisolone 1–2 mg/kg is reasonable, converting to 0.5–2 mg/kg prednisone/prednisolone orally each day or its equivalent only after a response. If no improvement or worsening, plasmapheresis or IVIG indicated
Myasthenia gravis	Fluctuating muscle weakness (proximal limb, trunk, ocular, eg, ptosis/diplopia or bulbar) with fatigability, respiratory muscles may also be involved	Permanently discontinue nivolumab. Administer pyridostigmine at an initial dose of 30 mg three times daily. Administer oral prednisone/prednisolone at a dose of 0.5–2 mg/kg/day or its equivalent or 1–2 mg/kg IV (methyl)prednisolone depending on the severity of symptoms. If begin with IV, convert to 0.5–2 mg/kg prednisone/prednisolone orally each day or its equivalent only after a response. If no improvement or worsening, plasmapheresis or IVIG may be considered. Additional immunosuppressants used in myasthenia gravis include azathioprine, cyclosporine, and mycophenolate. Avoid certain medications, eg, ciprofloxacin, beta-blockers, that may precipitate cholinergic crisis
Other syndromes including motor and sensory peripheral neuropathy, multifocal radicular neuropathy/plexopathy, autonomic neuropathy, phrenic nerve palsy, cranial nerve palsies (eg, facial nerve, optic nerve, hypoglossal nerve)		Permanently discontinue nivolumab. Administer oral prednisone/prednisolone at a dose of 0.5–2 mg/kg/day or its equivalent or 1–2 mg/kg IV (methyl)prednisolone depending on the severity of symptoms. If begin with IV, convert to 0.5–2 mg/kg prednisone/prednisolone orally each day or its equivalent only after a response

(*continued*)

Treatment Modifications (*continued*)

Adverse Event	Grade/Severity	Treatment Modification
Arthralgia	G1 (mild pain with inflammation, erythema, or joint swelling)	Continue nivolumab. Administer acetaminophen (paracetamol) and ibuprofen
	G2 (moderate pain with inflammation, erythema, or joint swelling that limits ADLs)	Withhold nivolumab. Administer higher doses of acetaminophen (paracetamol) and ibuprofen and use diclofenac or naproxen or etoricoxib. If inadequately controlled, consider intra-articular steroid injections for large joints or administer oral prednisone/prednisolone at a dose of 0.5–2 mg/kg/day or its equivalent. When improves to G1, begin a slow corticosteroid taper over at least 4 weeks. If does not respond adequately, then administer 0.5–1 mg/kg IV (methyl)prednisolone and convert to 0.5–2 mg/kg prednisone/prednisolone orally each day or its equivalent only after a response, followed by a taper over at least 4 weeks when improves to G1. Resume nivolumab upon symptom control, or when prednisone/prednisolone daily dose <10 mg
	G3 (severe pain; irreversible joint damage; disabling; limits self-care ADL)	Withhold nivolumab. Administer 0.5–1 mg/kg IV (methyl)prednisolone and convert to 0.5–2 mg/kg prednisone/prednisolone orally each day or its equivalent only after a response, followed by a taper over at least 4 weeks when improves to G1. In severe cases, infliximab or another anti-TNF-alpha drug may be required for improvement of arthritis. Resume nivolumab upon symptom control, or when prednisone/prednisolone daily dose <10 mg
Other	First occurrence of other G3	Withhold nivolumab. Administer oral prednisone/prednisolone at a dose of 0.5–2 mg/kg/day or its equivalent. When improves to G1, begin a slow corticosteroid taper over at least 4 weeks. Resume nivolumab upon symptom control, or when prednisone/prednisolone daily dose <10 mg
	Recurrence of same G3	Permanently discontinue nivolumab. Administer 1–2 mg/kg IV (methyl)prednisolone and convert to 0.5–2 mg/kg prednisone/prednisolone orally each day or its equivalent only after a response. Taper over at least 4–8 weeks when symptoms improve to G1
	Life-threatening or G4	
	Requirement for ≥10 mg/day prednisone or equivalent for >12 weeks	Permanently discontinue nivolumab
	Persistent G2/3 adverse reactions lasting ≥12 weeks	

ADL, activities of daily living; ALT, alanine aminotransferase; AST, aspartate aminotransferase; ATG, anti-thymocyte globulin; SJS, Stevens-Johnson Syndrome; TEN, toxic epidermal necrolysis; ULN, upper limit of normal

Notes on general supportive care:
- Steroid taper in most cases will proceed over a minimum of 1 month but if symptoms improve rapidly, a 2-week taper can be considered. If steroids are administered for more than 4 weeks, consider PCP prophylaxis (cotrimoxazole 480 mg twice daily M/W/F or inhaled pentamidine if has cotrimoxazole allergy), regular random blood glucose, VitD level, and starting calcium/VitD supplementation per guidelines

Patient Population Studied

Eligible patients had an ECOG performance status of 0–1, histologically proven malignant pleural mesothelioma progressing after first-line or second-line pemetrexed and platinum-based treatments, measurable disease by CT, and life expectancy greater than 12 weeks. Central randomization was stratified by histology (epithelioid vs non-epithelioid), treatment line (second line vs third line), and chemosensitivity to previous treatment (progression ≥3 months vs <3 months after pemetrexed treatment) and used a minimization method with a 0·8 random factor

	Nivolumab Group (n = 63)	Nivolumab Plus Ipilimumab Group (n = 62)
Sex		
Female	16 (25%)	9 (15%)
Male	47 (75%)	53 (85%)

(*continued*)

Patient Population Studied (*continued*)

	Nivolumab Group (n = 63)	Nivolumab Plus Ipilimumab Group (n = 62)
Age, years		
Mean (SD)	71.2 (9.5)	70.4 (9.0)
Median (IQR)	72.3 (32.5–87.2)	71.2 (48.1–88.1)
Histologic subtype		
Epithelioid	52 (83%)	53 (85%)
Sarcomatoid or biphasic	11 (17%)	9 (15%)
ECOG performance status*		
0	19 (30%)	25 (40%)
1	42 (67%)	36 (58%)
2	0	1 (2%)
Pemetrexed chemosensitivity		
Progression before 3 months	26 (41%)	21 (34%)
Progression after 3 months	37 (59%)	41 (66%)
Smoking status		
Smoker	34 (54%)	36 (58%)
Never smoker	29 (46%)	26 (42%)
Number of previous lines of treatment		
One (second-line patients)	44 (70%)	42 (68%)
Two (third-line patients)	17 (27%)	19 (31%)
More than two	2 (3%)	1 (2%)
Tumor-node-metastasis classification		
Stages I–II	7 (11%)	11 (18%)
Stages III–IV	56 (89%)	51 (82%)
Leukocytes		
$<8.3 \times 10^9$ per L	43 (68%)	41 (66%)
$\geq 8.3 \times 10^9$ per L	20 (32%)	21 (34%)
Hemoglobin		
≤ 12 g/L	30 (48%)	25 (40%)
>12 g/L	33 (52%)	37 (60%)
Platelets		
$<350 \times 10^9$ per L	46 (73%)	43 (69%)
$\geq 350 \times 10^9$ per L	17 (27%)	19 (31%)

(*continued*)

Patient Population Studied (*continued*)

	Nivolumab Group (n = 63)	Nivolumab Plus Ipilimumab Group (n = 62)
PD-L1 status available (28–8 monoclonal antibody, Dako PharmDx)		
Negative	31 (49%)	27 (44%)
≥1%	19 (30%)	22 (35%)
≥25%	2 (3%)	5 (8%)
≥50%	0	3 (5%)
Data not available	13 (21%)	13 (21%)

Data are n (%) unless otherwise stated. ECOG, Eastern Cooperative Oncology Group; PD-L1, programmed cell death ligand 1
*Performance status was not available for two patients in the nivolumab group
Scherpereel A et al. Lancet 2019;20:239–253

Efficacy

Efficacy (Assessable population = 108; ITT population = 125)
Scherpereel A et al. Lancet 2019;20:239–253

	Nivolumab	Nivolumab Plus Ipilimumab
DCR 12 weeks > randomization centrally assessed by independent radiology in assessable population	24/54 (44%; 95% CI 31–58)	27/54 (50%; 95% CI 37–63)
DCR 12 weeks > randomization centrally assessed by independent radiology in ITT population	25/63 (40%; 95% CI 28–52)	32/62 (52%; 95% CI 39–64)
Objective responses	10/54 (19%; 95% CI 8–29)	15/54 (28%; 95% CI 16–40)
>80% increase in size of target lesions, suggesting hyperprogression, at week 12 first tumor response evaluation	6/59 (10%)	2/55 (4%)
ORR at data cutoff (Dec 28, 2017)	11%	19%
Median DOR	7.4 months (95% CI 4.1–11.9) 4 still responding at 15 months	8.3 months (95% CI 3.0–14.0) 7 still responding at 15 months
Median PFS (median follow-up 20.1 months; IQR 19.6–20.3)	4.0 months (95% CI 2.8–5.7)	5.6 months (95% CI, 3.1–8.3)
Disease progression or death by study cutoff	58/63 (92%)	53/62 (85%)
Death by data cutoff	41/63 (65%)	32/62 (52%)
1-year PFS estimates	15.9% (95% CI 6.8–24.9)	22.6% (95% CI, 12.2–33.0)
Median OS	11.9 months (95% CI 6.7–17.7)	15.9 months (95% CI, 10.7–not reached
1-year survival estimates	49.2% (36.9–61.6)	58.1% (45.8–70.3)

DCR, disease control rate; DOR, duration of response; ITT, intention to treat; ORR, objective response rate; OS, overall survival; PFS, progression-free survival

Adverse Events

Adverse event Scherpereel et al. 2019	Nivolumab Group (n = 63)			Nivolumab + Ipilimumab Group (n = 61)		
	G1/2	G3	G4	G1/2	G3	G4
Any adverse event	47 (75%)	8 (13%)	1 (2%)	38 (62%)	14 (23%)	2 (3%)
Serious adverse event	1 (2%)	2 (3%)	0	7 (11%)	6 (10%)	1 (2%)
Led to discontinuation	2 (3%)	1 (2%)	0	4 (7%)	7 (11%)	2 (3%)
Led to death	0	0	0	0	0	0
Immune-related adverse events						
Stomatitis	4 (6%)	1 (2%)	0	4 (7%)	0	0
Arthritis	3 (5%)	0	0	7 (11%)	0	0
Aspartate aminotransferase increase	2 (3%)	0	0	3 (5%)	4 (7%)	0
Alanine aminotransferase increase	1 (2%)	0	0	4 (7%)	4 (7%)	0
Lipase increase	1 (2%)	2 (3%)	1 (2%)	2 (3%)	1 (2%)	1 (2%)
Edema peripheral	4 (6%)	0	0	3 (5%)	1 (2%)	0
γ-Glutamyltransferase increased	1 (2%)	0	0	3 (5%)	3 (5%)	0
Amylase increased	1 (2%)	1 (2%)	0	3 (5%)	0	0
General physical health deterioration	3 (5%)	0	0	0	2 (3%)	0
Acute kidney failure	0	0	0	0	0	1 (2%)
Blood alkaline phosphatase increased	0	0	0	2 (3%)	2 (3%)	0
Colitis	1 (2%)	0	0	1 (2%)	1 (2%)	0
Pneumonitis	1 (2%)	0	0	1 (2%)	1 (2%)	0
Polyneuropathy	0	0	0	0	1 (2%)	0
Acute respiratory distress syndrome	0	0	0	0	1 (2%)	0
Cardiac failure	0	0	0	0	1 (2%)	0
Dermatitis bullous	0	0	0	0	1 (2%)	0
Encephalitis	0	0	0	0	0	0
Hepatitis	0	0	0	0	2 (3%)	0
Hyperbilirubinemia	0	0	0	0	1 (2%)	0
Hyponatremia	0	0	0	0	1 (2%)	0
Hypophysitis	0	0	0	0	1 (2%)	0
Interstitial lung disease	0	0	0	0	1 (2%)	0
Pericardial effusion	0	1 (2%)	0	0	0	0
Pleural effusion	0	1 (2%)	0	0	0	0

All Grade 3 and 4 events are shown as well as Grade 1 and 2 occurrences of these events. For other Grade 1–2 events, only events occurring in more than ten people are included
Three serious Grade 5 events (deaths) occurred in the nivolumab plus ipilimumab group: one acute kidney failure, one fulminant hepatitis, and one encephalitis

Therapy Monitoring

1. Initially at the time of each dose, and eventually every 6–12 weeks, perform a total body skin examination with attention to ALL mucous membranes as well as a complete review of systems

2. Monitor patients for signs and symptoms of pneumonitis. Evaluate patients with suspected pneumonitis with chest x-ray, CT, and pulse oximetry. For ≥2 toxicity, may include nasal swab, sputum culture and sensitivity, blood culture and sensitivity, and urine culture and sensitivity

3. Monitor patients for signs and symptoms of colitis. Encourage patients to report diarrhea immediately to any member of the health care team

4. Draw AST, ALT, and bilirubin prior to each infusion and/or weekly if there are Grade 1 liver function test elevations. Note, no treatment is recommended for G1 LFT abnormalities. For ≥2 toxicity, work up for other causes of elevated LFTs including viral hepatitis

5. Use basic metabolic panel (Na, K, CO_2, glucose) and patient history as screening tools for hypophysitis including hypopituitarism and adrenal insufficiency. If in doubt, evaluate AM adrenocorticotropic hormone (ACTH) and cortisol levels. Consider ACTH stimulation test for indeterminate results

6. Assess thyroid function at the start of treatment, periodically during treatment, and, as indicated, based on clinical evaluation and for clinical signs and symptoms of thyroid disorders. Test for TSH and free thyroxine (FT4) every 4–6 weeks as part of routine clinical monitoring on therapy or for case detection in symptomatic patients

7. Measure glucose at baseline and with each treatment during the first 12 weeks and every 6 weeks thereafter

8. Obtain a serum creatinine prior to every dose. If creatinine is found to be newly elevated, consider holding therapy while other potential causes are evaluated. Note, routine urinalysis is not necessary other than to rule out urinary tract infections, etc

9. Obtain a complete rheumatologic history and perform an examination of all peripheral joints for tenderness, swelling, and range of motion. Examine the spine. Consider plain x-ray/imaging to exclude metastases and evaluate joint damage (erosions), if appropriate

10. In patients at high risk for infections and in appropriately selected patients based on an infectious disease evaluation, draw screening laboratories (HIV, hepatitis A and B, and blood QuantiFERON for TB) to prepare patients to start infliximab

ADVANCED DISEASE • SUBSEQUENT THERAPY

MESOTHELIOMA REGIMEN: NIVOLUMAB + IPILIMUMAB

Disselhorst MJ et al. Lancet Respir Med 2019;7:260–270
Supplement to: Disselhorst MJ et al. Lancet Respir Med 2019;7:260–70
Scherpereel A et al. Lancet 2019;20:239–253
Supplement to: Scherpereel A et al. Lancet 2019;20:239–253
OPDIVO (nivolumab) prescribing information. Princeton, NJ: Bristol-Myers Squibb Company; revised September 2019
YERVOY (ipilimumab) prescribing information. Princeton, NJ: Bristol-Myers Squibb Company; revised September 2019

Induction phase (four cycles of concurrent treatment with nivolumab and ipilimumab):
Nivolumab 240 mg per dose; administer intravenously over 30 minutes in a volume of 0.9% sodium chloride injection (0.9% NS) or 5% dextrose injection (D5W) not to exceed 160 mL and sufficient to produce a nivolumab concentration within the range 1–10 mg/mL for 3 doses on days 1, 15, and 29, every 6 weeks, for four induction cycles (total dosage/6-week induction cycle = 720 mg)
- Administer nivolumab through an administration set that contains a sterile, non-pyrogenic, low-protein-binding in-line filter with pore size within the range of 0.2–1.2 μm
- Nivolumab can cause severe infusion-related reactions

Ipilimumab 1 mg/kg; administer intravenously over 30 minutes in a volume of 0.9% NS or D5W sufficient to produce an ipilimumab concentration within the range 1–2 mg/mL on day 1, every 6 weeks, for four induction cycles (total dose/6-week induction cycle = 1 mg/kg)
- Administer ipilimumab after nivolumab through an administration set containing a sterile, non-pyrogenic, low-protein-binding in-line filter

Maintenance phase (single agent nivolumab):
Nivolumab 240 mg; administer intravenously over 30 minutes in a volume of 0.9% NS or D5W, not to exceed 160 mL and sufficient to produce a nivolumab concentration within the range 1–10 mg/mL, every 2 weeks until disease progression and for a maximum total duration of 2 years (total dosage/2-week maintenance cycle = 240 mg)
- Administer nivolumab through an administration set that contains a sterile, non-pyrogenic, low-protein-binding in-line filter with pore size within the range of 0.2–1.2 μm
- Nivolumab can cause severe infusion-related reactions
- Note that U.S. Food and Drug Administration (FDA)-approved regimens for other indications include an option for nivolumab to be administered at a fixed dose of 480 mg every 4 weeks, consistent with the regimens approved on March 5, 2018, thus consider:
  - **Nivolumab** 480 mg; administer intravenously over 30 minutes in a volume of 0.9% NS or D5W not to exceed 160 mL and sufficient to produce a nivolumab concentration within the range 1–10 mg/mL, every 4 weeks until disease progression (total dosage/4-week cycle = 480 mg)
    ○ Administer nivolumab through an administration set that contains a sterile, non-pyrogenic, low-protein-binding in-line filter with pore size within the range of 0.2–1.2 μm
    ○ Nivolumab can cause severe infusion-related reactions

Supportive Care
Antiemetic prophylaxis
Emetogenic potential with nivolumab ± ipilimumab is **MINIMAL**
See Chapter 42 for antiemetic recommendations
Hematopoietic growth factor (CSF) prophylaxis
Primary prophylaxis is **NOT** indicated
See Chapter 43 for more information

Antimicrobial prophylaxis
Risk of fever and neutropenia is **LOW**
  Antimicrobial primary prophylaxis to be considered:
- Antibacterial—not indicated
- Antifungal—not indicated
- Antiviral—not indicated unless patient previously had an episode of HSV

Efficacy

Clinical Activity	
Radiologic response at 12 weeks	
Complete response	0
Partial response	10 (29%)
Stable disease	13 (38%)
Progressive disease	11 (32%)
Disease control	23 (68%; 50–83)*
Objective response at 6 months	13 (38%; 22–56)
Ongoing response†	11 (32%; 17–51)
Median follow-up time, months	14.3 (12.7–15.7)
Median duration of response, months‡	14.3 (6.4–NR)
Median progression-free survival, months	6.2 (4.1–NR)
Progression-free survival at 6 months	50% (36–70)
Median overall survival, months	NR (12.7–NR)
Overall survival at 1 year	64% (50–83)ϵ

Data are n (%), n (%; 95% CI), median (95% CI), or % (95% CI)
NR, not reached
*CI calculated accounting for the planned interim analysis after 12 patients
†Patients with partial response or stable disease for more than 6 months, on study drugs or at end of treatment
‡Time from start of response to progression
ϵEstimated from Kaplan-Meier analysis
Disselhorst MJ et al. Lancet Respir Med 2019;7:260–270

Treatment Modifications

RECOMMENDED DOSE MODIFICATIONS FOR NIVOLUMAB AND IPILIMUMAB

Adverse Event	Grade/Severity	Treatment Modification
Infusion reaction	Clinically significant but not severe infusion reaction	Interrupt the infusion in patients with clinically significant infusion reactions and consider resuming at a slower rate following resolution. If decision is made to restart, begin at ≤50% of the rate prior to the reaction and increase in 50% increments every 30 minutes if well tolerated. Infusions may be restarted at the full rate during the next cycle
	G3/4 (severe infusion reaction—pyrexia, chills, flushing, hypotension, dyspnea, wheezing, back pain, abdominal pain, and urticaria). Not rapidly responsive to brief interruption of infusion	Stop infusion and administer appropriate medical therapy (eg, epinephrine, corticosteroids, intravenous antihistamines, bronchodilators, and/or oxygen). Discontinue nivolumab and ipilimumab
Colitis	G1	Loperamide 4 mg as starting dose then 2 mg before each meal and after each loose stool until without diarrhea for 12 hours, with maximum of 16 mg loperamide per day. If G1 diarrhea or colitis persists >14 days, then add prednisolone 0.5–1 mg/kg (non-enteric-coated) or consider oral budesonide 9 mg daily if no bloody diarrhea
	G2/3 diarrhea or colitis	Withhold nivolumab and ipilimumab. Loperamide 4 mg as starting dose then 2 mg before each meal and after each loose stool until without diarrhea for 12 hours, with maximum of 16 mg loperamide per day. Administer oral prednisone/prednisolone at a dose of 0.5–2 mg/kg/day or its equivalent. When improves to G1, begin a slow corticosteroid taper over at least 4 weeks. Resume nivolumab and ipilimumab upon symptom control, or when prednisone/prednisolone daily dose <10 mg
	G4 diarrhea or colitis	Permanently discontinue nivolumab and ipilimumab. Loperamide 4 mg as starting dose then 2 mg before each meal and after each loose stool until without diarrhea for 12 hours, with maximum of 16 mg loperamide per day. Administer 1–2 mg/kg intravenously (methyl)prednisolone and convert to 0.5–2 mg/kg prednisone/prednisolone orally each day or its equivalent only after a response. Taper over at least 4 weeks when symptoms improve. If does not improve over 72 hours or worsens, perform flexible sigmoidoscopy/colonoscopy to document colitis then begin infliximab 5 mg/kg (if no perforation/sepsis/TB/hepatitis/NYHA III/IV CHF). If no response, add MMF 500–1000 mg twice daily. If worse on MMF, consider addition of tacrolimus or ATG
Pneumonitis	G2	Withhold nivolumab and ipilimumab. Consider pneumocystis prophylaxis depending on the clinical context and coverage with empiric antibiotics. Administer oral prednisone/prednisolone at a dose of 1–2 mg/kg/day or its equivalent. When improves to G1, begin a slow corticosteroid taper over at least 4 weeks. If does not respond adequately after 48 hours, then administer 2–4 mg/kg intravenously (methyl)prednisolone and convert to 0.5–2 mg/kg prednisone/prednisolone orally each day or its equivalent only after a response, followed by a taper over at least 6 weeks when symptoms improve to G1, titrating to symptoms. Resume nivolumab and ipilimumab upon symptom control, or when prednisone/prednisolone daily dose <10 mg
	G3/4	Permanently discontinue nivolumab and ipilimumab. Consider pneumocystis prophylaxis depending on the clinical context; cover with empiric antibiotics. Administer 2–4 mg/kg intravenously (methyl)prednisolone and convert to 1–2 mg/kg prednisone/prednisolone orally each day or its equivalent only after a response, followed by a taper over at least 8 weeks when symptoms improve to G1, titrating to symptoms. If when initially treated improvement does not occur within 48–72 hours, begin infliximab 5 mg/kg (if no perforation/sepsis/TB/hepatitis/NYHA III/IV CHF). If no response to infliximab, add MMF 500–1000 mg twice daily. Consider MMF especially if has concurrent hepatic toxicity
Hepatitis	G2 (AST or ALT >3–5× ULN or total bilirubin >1.5–3× ULN)	Withhold nivolumab and ipilimumab. Administer oral prednisone/prednisolone at a dose of 1–2 mg/kg/day or its equivalent. When improves to G1, begin a slow corticosteroid taper over at least 4 weeks. Resume nivolumab and ipilimumab upon symptom control, or when prednisone/prednisolone daily dose <10 mg

(continued)

Treatment Modifications (continued)

Adverse Event	Grade/Severity	Treatment Modification
	G3/4 (AST or ALT >5× ULN or total bilirubin >3× ULN)	Permanently discontinue nivolumab and ipilimumab. Administer 1–2 mg/kg intravenously (methyl)prednisolone and convert to 0.5–2 mg/kg prednisone/prednisolone orally each day or its equivalent only after a response. Taper over at least 6 weeks when symptoms improve. If no response, add MMF 500–1000 mg twice daily. If worse on MMF, consider adding tacrolimus or ATG
Hypophysitis	G2/3 (moderate symptoms, ie, headache but no visual disturbance or fatigue/mood alteration but hemodynamically stable, no electrolyte disturbance)	Administer analgesia as needed for headache. Withhold nivolumab and ipilimumab. Administer oral prednisone/prednisolone at a dose of 0.5–2 mg/kg/day or its equivalent. When improves to G1, begin a slow corticosteroid taper over at least 4 weeks. If no improvement in 48 hours, administer 1–2 mg/kg intravenously (methyl)prednisolone and convert to 0.5–2 mg/kg prednisone/prednisolone orally each day or its equivalent only after a response. Taper over at least 4 weeks when symptoms improve to 5 mg prednisone/prednisolone or equivalent; do not stop steroids. Resume nivolumab and ipilimumab upon symptom control, or when prednisone/prednisolone daily dose <10 mg
	G4 (severe mass effect symptoms, ie, severe headache, any visual disturbance or severe hypoadrenalism, ie, hypotension, severe electrolyte disturbance)	Permanently discontinue nivolumab and ipilimumab. Administer analgesia as needed for headache. Administer 1–2 mg/kg intravenously (methyl)prednisolone and convert to 0.5–2 mg/kg prednisone/prednisolone orally each day or its equivalent only after a response. Taper over at least 4 weeks when symptoms improve to 5 mg prednisone/prednisolone or equivalent; do not stop steroids
Adrenal Insufficiency	G2	Withhold nivolumab and ipilimumab. Administer oral prednisone/prednisolone at a dose of 0.5–2 mg/kg/day or its equivalent. When improves to G1, begin a slow corticosteroid taper over at least 4 weeks. Serially assess adrenal function and continue steroids at replacement doses (20–40 mg hydrocortisone daily ~2/3 dose in AM upon awakening and ~1/3 at 4 PM) until recovery of adrenal function is documented. Resume nivolumab and ipilimumab upon symptom control, or when prednisone/prednisolone daily dose <10 mg
	G3/4	Permanently discontinue nivolumab and ipilimumab. Administer oral prednisone/prednisolone at a dose of 0.5–2 mg/kg/day or its equivalent. When improves to G1, begin a slow corticosteroid taper over at least 4 weeks. Serially assess adrenal function and continue steroids at replacement doses (20–40 mg hydrocortisone daily ~2/3 dose in AM upon awakening and ~1/3 at 4 PM) until recovery of adrenal function is documented
Type 1 diabetes mellitus	G3 hyperglycemia	Withhold nivolumab and ipilimumab. Admit to hospital to manage hyperglycemia. Role of corticosteroids in preventing complete loss of insulin-producing cells is unknown and not recommended. Resume nivolumab and ipilimumab upon symptom control, or when prednisone/prednisolone daily dose <10 mg
	G4 hyperglycemia	Permanently discontinue nivolumab and ipilimumab. Admit to hospital to manage hyperglycemia. Role of corticosteroids in preventing complete loss of insulin-producing cells is unknown and not recommended
Nephritis and renal dysfunction	G2/3 (serum creatinine 1.5–6× ULN)	Withhold nivolumab and ipilimumab. Administer oral prednisone/prednisolone at a dose of 0.5–2 mg/kg/day or its equivalent. When improves to G1, begin a slow corticosteroid taper over at least 4 weeks. If does not respond adequately, then administer 0.5–1 mg/kg intravenously (methyl)prednisolone and convert to 0.5–2 mg/kg prednisone/prednisolone orally each day or its equivalent only after a response, followed by a taper over at least 4 weeks when improves to G1. Resume nivolumab and ipilimumab upon symptom control, or when prednisone/prednisolone daily dose <10 mg
	G4 (serum creatinine >6× ULN)	Permanently discontinue nivolumab and ipilimumab. Administer 0.5–1 mg/kg intravenously (methyl)prednisolone and convert to 0.5–2 mg/kg prednisone/prednisolone orally each day or its equivalent only after a response, followed by a taper over at least 4 weeks when improves to G1
Skin	G1/2	Continue nivolumab and ipilimumab. Avoid skin irritants, avoid sun exposure, topical emollients recommended. Topical steroid (mild strength for G1, moderate/potent strength for G2) cream once or twice daily ± oral or topical antihistamines for itching.

(continued)

Treatment Modifications (*continued*)

Adverse Event	Grade/Severity	Treatment Modification
	G3 rash or suspected SJS or TEN	Withhold nivolumab and ipilimumab. Avoid skin irritants, avoid sun exposure, topical emollients recommended. Administer oral or topical antihistamines for itching. Administer oral prednisone/prednisolone at a dose of 0.5–2 mg/kg or its equivalent daily for 3 days followed by a slow corticosteroid taper over at least 4 weeks when the rash improves to G1. If does not respond adequately, then administer 0.5–1 mg/kg intravenously (methyl) prednisolone and convert to 0.5–2 mg/kg prednisone/prednisolone orally each day or its equivalent only after a response, followed by a taper over at least 4 weeks when the rash improves to G1. Resume nivolumab and ipilimumab upon symptom control, or when prednisone/prednisolone daily dose <10 mg
	G4 rash or confirmed SJS or TEN	Avoid skin irritants, avoid sun exposure, topical emollients recommended. Administer oral or topical antihistamines for itching. Administer 1–2 mg/kg intravenously (methyl) prednisolone and convert to oral steroids 0.5–2 mg/kg prednisone/prednisolone each day or its equivalent only after a response. Taper over at least 4 weeks when the rash improves to G1. Permanently discontinue nivolumab and ipilimumab
Encephalitis	Confusion or altered behavior, headaches, alteration in Glasgow Coma Scale, motor or sensory deficits, speech abnormality, may or may not be febrile	Initially withhold nivolumab and ipilimumab, but permanently discontinue nivolumab and ipilimumab if there is no doubt as to diagnosis. Exclude bacterial and ideally viral infections prior to high-dose steroids. Administer oral prednisone/prednisolone at a dose of 0.5–2 mg/kg/day or its equivalent. When symptoms improve, begin a slow corticosteroid taper over at least 4–8 weeks. If symptoms are severe, administer 1–2 mg/kg intravenously (methyl)prednisolone and convert to 0.5–2 mg/kg prednisone/prednisolone orally each day or its equivalent only after a response. Consider concurrent empiric antiviral (intravenous acyclovir) and antibacterial therapy
Aseptic meningitis	Headache, photophobia, neck stiffness with fever or may be afebrile, vomiting; normal cognition/cerebral function (distinguishes from encephalitis)	
Other syndromes include neurosarcoidosis, posterior reversible leukoencephalopathy syndrome (PRES), Vogt-Koyanagi-Harada syndrome, demyelination, vasculitic encephalopathy, and generalized seizures		
Transverse myelitis	Acute or subacute neurologic signs/ symptoms of motor/sensory/ autonomic origin; most have sensory level; often bilateral symptoms	Initially withhold nivolumab and ipilimumab, but permanently discontinue nivolumab and ipilimumab if there is no doubt as to diagnosis. Administer 2 mg/kg intravenously (methyl)prednisolone or consider 1 g/day and convert to 0.5–2 mg/kg prednisone/ prednisolone orally each day or its equivalent only after a response. When symptoms improve, begin a slow corticosteroid taper over at least 4–8 weeks. Plasmapheresis may be required if steroids do not bring about improvement
Myocarditis	G3	Permanently discontinue nivolumab and ipilimumab. Administer 2 mg/kg intravenously (methyl)prednisolone or consider 1 g/day and convert to 0.5–2 mg/kg prednisone/ prednisolone orally each day or its equivalent only after a response. When symptoms improve, begin a slow corticosteroid taper over at least 4–8 weeks. If no response, add MMF 500–1000 mg twice daily. If worse on MMF, consider adding tacrolimus
Peripheral neurologic toxicity	Moderate: some interference with ADL, symptoms concerning to patient	Withhold nivolumab and ipilimumab. Initial observation reasonable or initiate prednisone/ prednisolone 0.5–1 mg/kg (if progressing, eg, from mild) and/or pregabalin or duloxetine for pain. When symptoms improve, begin a slow corticosteroid taper over at least 4 weeks. Resume nivolumab and ipilimumab upon symptom control, or when prednisone/ prednisolone daily dose <10 mg
	Severe: limits self-care and aids warranted, life-threatening, eg, respiratory problems	Permanently discontinue nivolumab and ipilimumab. Administer 1–2 mg/kg intravenously (methyl)prednisolone and convert to 0.5–2 mg/kg prednisone/prednisolone orally each day or its equivalent only after a response. Taper over at least 4–8 weeks when symptoms improve to G1
Guillain-Barré syndrome	Progressive symmetrical muscle weakness with absent or reduced tendon reflexes—involves extremities, facial, respiratory, and bulbar and oculomotor muscles; dysregulation of autonomic nerves	Permanently discontinue nivolumab and ipilimumab. Use of steroids not recommended in idiopathic Guillain-Barré syndrome; however, a trial of (methyl)prednisolone 1–2 mg/kg is reasonable, converting to 0.5–2 mg/kg prednisone/prednisolone orally each day or its equivalent only after a response. If no improvement or worsening, plasmapheresis or IVIG indicated

(*continued*)

Treatment Modifications (*continued*)

Adverse Event	Grade/Severity	Treatment Modification
Myasthenia gravis	Fluctuating muscle weakness (proximal limb, trunk, ocular, eg, ptosis/diplopia or bulbar) with fatigability, respiratory muscles also may be involved	Permanently discontinue nivolumab and ipilimumab. Administer pyridostigmine at an initial dose of 30 mg three times daily. Administer oral prednisone/prednisolone at a dose of 0.5–2 mg/kg/day or its equivalent or 1–2 mg/kg intravenously (methyl)prednisolone depending on the severity of symptoms. If begin with intravenous, convert to 0.5–2 mg/kg prednisone/prednisolone orally each day or its equivalent only after a response. If no improvement or worsening, plasmapheresis or IVIG may be considered. Additional immunosuppressants used in myasthenia gravis include azathioprine, cyclosporine, and mycophenolate. Avoid certain medications, eg, ciprofloxacin, beta-blockers, that may precipitate cholinergic crisis
Other syndromes including motor and sensory peripheral neuropathy, multifocal radicular neuropathy/plexopathy, autonomic neuropathy, phrenic nerve palsy, cranial nerve palsies (eg, facial nerve, optic nerve, hypoglossal nerve)		Permanently discontinue nivolumab and ipilimumab. Administer oral prednisone/prednisolone at a dose of 0.5–2 mg/kg/day or its equivalent or 1–2 mg/kg intravenously (methyl)prednisolone depending on the severity of symptoms. If begin with intravenous, convert to 0.5–2 mg/kg prednisone/prednisolone orally each day or its equivalent only after a response
Arthralgia	G1 (mild pain with inflammation, erythema, or joint swelling)	Continue nivolumab and ipilimumab. Administer acetaminophen (paracetamol) and ibuprofen
	G2 (moderate pain with inflammation, erythema, or joint swelling that limits ADLs)	Withhold nivolumab and ipilimumab. Administer higher doses of acetaminophen (paracetamol) and ibuprofen and use diclofenac or naproxen or etoricoxib. If inadequately controlled, consider intra-articular steroid injections for large joints or administer oral prednisone/prednisolone at a dose of 0.5–2 mg/kg/day or its equivalent. When improves to G1, begin a slow corticosteroid taper over at least 4 weeks. If does not respond adequately, then administer 0.5–1 mg/kg intravenously (methyl)prednisolone and convert to 0.5–2 mg/kg prednisone/prednisolone orally each day or its equivalent only after a response, followed by a taper over at least 4 weeks when improves to G1. Resume nivolumab and ipilimumab upon symptom control, or when prednisone/prednisolone daily dose <10 mg
	G3 (severe pain; irreversible joint damage; disabling; limits self-care ADL)	Withhold nivolumab and ipilimumab. Administer 0.5–1 mg/kg intravenously (methyl)prednisolone and convert to 0.5–2 mg/kg prednisone/prednisolone orally each day or its equivalent only after a response, followed by a taper over at least 4 weeks when improves to G1. In severe cases, infliximab or another anti-TNF-alpha drug may be required for improvement of arthritis. Resume nivolumab and ipilimumab upon symptom control, or when prednisone/prednisolone daily dose <10 mg
Other	First occurrence of other G3	Withhold nivolumab and ipilimumab. Administer oral prednisone/prednisolone at a dose of 0.5–2 mg/kg/day or its equivalent. When improves to G1, begin a slow corticosteroid taper over at least 4 weeks. Resume nivolumab and ipilimumab upon symptom control, or when prednisone/prednisolone daily dose <10 mg
	Recurrence of same G3	Permanently discontinue nivolumab and ipilimumab. Administer 1–2 mg/kg intravenously (methyl)prednisolone and convert to 0.5–2 mg/kg prednisone/prednisolone orally each day or its equivalent only after a response. Taper over at least 4–8 weeks when symptoms improve to G1
	Life-threatening or G4	
	Requirement for ≥10 mg/day prednisone or equivalent for >12 weeks	Permanently discontinue nivolumab and ipilimumab
	Persistent G2/3 adverse reactions lasting ≥12 weeks	

ADL, activities of daily living; ALT, alanine aminotransferase; AST, aspartate aminotransferase; ATG, anti-thymocyte globulin; SJS, Stevens-Johnson Syndrome; TEN, toxic epidermal necrolysis; ULN, upper limit of normal

Notes on general supportive care:
• Steroid taper in most cases will proceed over a minimum of 1 month but if symptoms improve rapidly, a 2-week taper can be considered. If steroids are administered for more than 4 weeks, consider PCP prophylaxis (cotrimoxazole 480 mg twice daily M/W/F or inhaled pentamidine if has cotrimoxazole allergy), regular random blood glucose, VitD level, and starting calcium/VitD supplementation per guidelines

Patient Population Studied

Patients with previously treated and relapsed malignant pleural mesothelioma.

Characteristic	
Age, years	
Median (IQR)	65 (62–71)
Range	37–79
Sex	
Men	27 (77%)
Women	8 (23%)
Histology	
Epithelioid	30 (86%)
Sarcomatoid	3 (9%)
Mixed	2 (6%)
Eastern Cooperative Oncology Group performance status	
0	10 (29%)
1	25 (71%)
Ethnicity	
White	34 (97%)
Black	1 (3%)
Previous lines of therapy	
1	29 (83%)
2	4 (11%)
3	1 (3%)
4	1 (3%)
Disease stage	
I–III	21 (60%)
IV	14 (40%)
Smoking status	
Never	12 (34%)
Former	17 (49%)
Current	6 (17%)
PD-L1 expression on tumor cells	
Negative (<1%)	19 (54%)
Positive (≥1%)	15 (43%)
Not scored	1 (3%)

Data are n (%) unless otherwise stated
PD-L1, programmed cell death ligand 1
Disselhorst MJ et al. Lancet Respir Med 2019;7:260–270

Therapy Monitoring

1. Monitor patients for signs and symptoms of infusion-related reactions including pyrexia, chills, flushing, hypotension, dyspnea, wheezing, back pain, abdominal pain, and urticaria

2. Initially at the time of each dose, and eventually every 6–12 weeks, perform a total body skin examination with attention to ALL mucous membranes as well as a complete review of systems

3. Monitor patients for signs and symptoms of pneumonitis. Evaluate patients with suspected pneumonitis with chest x-ray, CT, and pulse oximetry. For ≥2 toxicity, may include nasal swab, sputum culture and sensitivity, blood culture and sensitivity, and urine culture and sensitivity

4. Monitor patients for signs and symptoms of colitis. Encourage patients to report diarrhea immediately to any member of the health care team

5. Draw AST, ALT, and bilirubin prior to each infusion and/or weekly if there are Grade 1 liver function test elevations. Note, no treatment is recommended for G1 LFT abnormalities. For ≥2 toxicity, work up for other causes of elevated LFTs including viral hepatitis

6. Use basic metabolic panel (Na, K, CO_2, glucose) and patient history as screening tools for hypophysitis including hypopituitarism and adrenal insufficiency. If in doubt evaluate AM adrenocorticotropic hormone (ACTH) and cortisol levels. Consider ACTH stimulation test for indeterminate results

7. Assess thyroid function at the start of treatment, periodically during treatment, and, as indicated, based on clinical evaluation and for clinical signs and symptoms of thyroid disorders. Test for TSH and free thyroxine (FT4) every 4–6 weeks as part of routine clinical monitoring on therapy or for case detection in symptomatic patients

8. Measure glucose at baseline and with each treatment during the first 12 weeks and every 6 weeks thereafter

9. Obtain a serum creatinine prior to every dose. If creatinine is found to be newly elevated, consider holding therapy while other potential causes are evaluated. Note, routine urinalysis is not necessary other than to rule out urinary tract infections, etc

(continued)

Adverse Events

Adverse event	All Grades	Grade 1	Grade 2	Grade 3	Grade 4
Any	33 (94%)	30 (88%)	26 (77%)	12 (35%)	1 (3%)
Adrenal insufficiency	3 (9%)	0	2 (6%)	1 (3%)	0
Alanine aminotransferase increased	3 (9%)	1 (3%)	0	2 (6%)	0
Anorexia	7 (20%)	4 (11%)	1 (3%)	2 (6%)	0
Arthralgia	4 (11%)	1 (3%)	3 (9%)	0	0
Aspartate transaminase increased	5 (14%)	2 (6%)	1 (3%)	2 (6%)	0
Cardiac asthma	1 (3%)	0	0	1 (3%)	0
Diarrhea	7 (20%)	3 (9%)	1 (3%)	3 (9%)	0
Dyspnea	4 (11%)	2 (6%)	1 (3%)	1 (3%)	0
Fatigue	9 (26%)	5 (14%)	4 (11%)	0	0
γ-Glutamyltransferase increased	1 (3%)	0	0	0	1 (3%)
Infusion-related reaction	17 (49%)	2 (6%)	15 (43%)	0	0
Malaise*	3 (9%)	0	3 (9%)	0	0
Mucositis oral	1 (3%)	0	0	1 (3%)	0
Myalgia	4 (11%)	2 (6%)	2 (6%)	0	0
Nausea	6 (17%)	0	6 (17%)	0	0
Pleural effusion	2 (6%)	2 (6%)	0	2 (6%)	0
Pleural infection	1 (3%)	0	0	1 (3%)	0
Skin disorders	17 (49%)	10 (29%)	6 (17%)	1 (3%)	0
Pruritus	11 (31%)	10 (29%)	1 (3%)	0	0
Dry skin	8 (23%)	5 (14%)	3 (9%)	0	0
Rash	10 (29%)	5 (14%)	4 (11%)	1 (3%)	0

Data are n (%). For Grade 1–2 events, only those that occurred in 10% or more patients are reported. All Grade 3 and 4 events are reported. No Grade 5 events occurred
*Resulted in treatment discontinuation for one patient
Disselhorst MJ et al. Lancet Respir Med 2019;7:260–270

Therapy Monitoring
(continued)

10. Obtain a complete rheumatologic history and perform an examination of all peripheral joints for tenderness, swelling, and range of motion. Examine the spine. Consider plain x-ray/imaging to exclude metastases and evaluate joint damage (erosions), if appropriate

11. In patients at high risk for infections and in appropriately selected patients based on an infectious disease evaluation, draw screening laboratories (HIV, hepatitis A and B, and blood QuantiFERON for TB) to prepare patients to start infliximab

RESECTABLE DISEASE

MESOTHELIOMA (PERITONEAL) REGIMEN: INTRAPERITONEAL (IP) CISPLATIN + PACLITAXEL

Rothenberg ML et al. J Clin Oncol 2003; 21:1313–1319

Paclitaxel 135 mg/m²; administer intravenously in a volume of 0.9% NS or D5W sufficient to produce a solution with concentration within the range 0.3–1.2 mg/mL over 24 hours on day 1, every 21 days for 6 cycles (total paclitaxel dosage/cycle given intravenously = 135 mg/m²)

Cisplatin 100 mg/m²; administer intraperitoneally in 2000 mL 0.9% NS warmed to body temperature on day 2, every 21 days for 6 cycles (total dosage/cycle = 100 mg/m²)

Paclitaxel 60 mg/m²; administer intraperitoneally in 2000 mL 0.9% NS, warmed to body temperature on day 8, every 21 days for 6 cycles (total paclitaxel dosage/cycle from IP route = 60 mg/m²)

Dexamethasone 20 mg/dose; administer orally for 2 doses, 12 hours and 6 hours before paclitaxel on days 1 and 8, *plus*

Diphenhydramine 50 mg; administer by intravenous injection 30–60 minutes before paclitaxel on days 1 and 8, *plus*

Ranitidine 50 mg or **cimetidine** 300 mg; administer intravenously in 25–100 mL of a compatible solution; for example, 0.9% sodium chloride injection (0.9% NS) or 5% dextrose injection (D5W) over 5–30 minutes beginning 30–60 minutes before paclitaxel on days 1 and 8

Additional information: Drug distribution is facilitated by sequentially placing patients R side down, L side down, in Trendelenburg and in reverse Trendelenburg position for 15 minutes each after drugs are instilled IP. Cisplatin- and paclitaxel-containing fluids are not drained after instillation

Supportive Care
Antiemetic prophylaxis
Emetogenic potential on days *1 and 8 is* **LOW**
Emetogenic potential on day *2 is* **HIGH**. *Potential for delayed symptoms*
See Chapter 42 for antiemetic recommendations

Hematopoietic growth factor (CSF) prophylaxis
Primary prophylaxis may be indicated
See Chapter 43 for more information

Antimicrobial prophylaxis
Risk of fever and neutropenia is **LOW**
   Antimicrobial primary prophylaxis to be considered:
   • Antibacterial—not indicated
   • Antifungal—not indicated
   • Antiviral—not indicated unless patient previously had an episode of HSV

Treatment Modifications

ANC ≥3000/mm³ and platelet ≥100,000/mm³ required to start cycle. Delay therapy up to 2 weeks to allow hematologic recovery

Adverse Event	Dose Modification
Hematologic toxicity	No dose modifications. Day 8 paclitaxel given without regard for CBC
G >2 peripheral neuropathy	Delay therapy until toxicity G ≤2, then decrease all drug dosages by 20%
G2 abdominal pain	Decrease IP drug dosages by 20%
G3/4 abdominal pain	Decrease IP drug dosages by 40%
CrCl <50 mL/min	Hold cisplatin until CrCl >50 mL/min (>0.83 mL/s), then decrease cisplatin dosage to 75 mg/m² during all subsequent cycles
Peritoneal catheter dysfunction or inability to administer therapy IP	Modify regimen schedule and route of administration for all remaining cycles: Paclitaxel 135 mg/m² intravenously over 24 hours on day 1, every 21 days; cisplatin 100 mg/m² intravenously over 60 minutes on day 2, every 21 days

Patient Population Studied

A study of 68 patients with FIGO stage III epithelial ovarian cancer (tumor extending outside the pelvis and/or positive retroperitoneal or inguinal lymph nodes) with residual peritoneal disease ≤1 cm in largest dimension after surgical staging by GOG standards

Efficacy (N = 68)

Median disease-free survival	33 months
Median survival	51 months
2-year survival rate	91%

Toxicity (N = 68)

	% G3	% G4
Hematologic		
Neutropenia	21	59
Anemia	15	4
Thrombocytopenia	9	0
Infection with neutropenia	12	0
Nonhematologic		
Nausea	50	0
Vomiting	29	4
Abdominal pain	12	1
Diarrhea	4	1
Fatigue/malaise/lethargy	24	0
Sensory neuropathy	3	0
Catheter-related infection	10	0
	% G1	**% G2**
Alopecia	10	66

96% of patients experienced ≥1 G3/4 toxicity

Therapy Monitoring

1. *Before each treatment cycle:* PE, CBC with differential, serum creatinine, and serum bilirubin
2. *Weekly:* CBC, serum electrolytes, serum creatinine, calcium, magnesium, and LFTs

26. Multiple Myeloma

Giada Bianchi, MD, Aldo Roccaro, MD, PhD, Irene M. Ghobrial, MD, and Kenneth C. Anderson, MD

Epidemiology

Incidence: 32,270 (male: 17,530; female: 14,740) estimated new cases for 2020 in the United States

Gender Differences 8.7 per 100,000 males, 5.6 per 100,000 females

Ethnic Differences 1:1.7:3.3 for Asian/Pacific Islander vs White vs Black males
1:1.6:4 for Asian/Pacific Islander vs White vs Black females

Deaths: Estimated 12,830 in 2020
4.2 per 100,000 males, 2.7 per 100,000 females

Median age: 69 years

Durie-Salmon stage at presentation	
Stage I	6%
Stage II	21%
Stage III	73%

Durie BGM, Salmon SE. Cancer 1975;36:842–854
Siegel R et al. CA Cancer J Clin 2020;70:7–30
Surveillance, Epidemiology and End Results (SEER) Program, available from http://seer.cancer.gov (accessed in 2020)

Pathology

Monoclonal gammopathy of uncertain significance (MGUS), all criteria must be met
- Serum M-protein level <3 g/dL and bone marrow clonal plasma cells <10%
- Urine monoclonal protein <500 mg/24 hours
- Abnormal sFLC ratio (<0.26 but >0.01 or >1.65 but <100) in light chain MGUS with absolute increase in affected light chain
- No myeloma-defining events (MDE)
- No evidence of other B-lymphoproliferative disorders/AL amyloidosis
- Progression to multiple myeloma (MM) in ~1% per year (0.3%/year in light chain MGUS)

Smoldering (asymptomatic) myeloma
- M-protein in serum ≥3 g/dL and/or
- Urine monoclonal protein ≥500 mg/24 hour and/or
- Abnormal sFLC ratio (<0.26 but >0.01 or >1.65 but <100) and/or
- Bone marrow clonal plasma cells 10–60% and
- No MDE or AL amyloidosis
Progression to MM in 10%/year in first 5 years (5%/year for light chain SMM)

Active (symptomatic) myeloma[†]
Requires one or more of the following MDE:
- Evidence of end organ damage (CRAB criteria)
  - Calcium elevation (>11.5 mg/dL [>2.88 mmol/L])
  - Renal insufficiency (creatinine >2 mg/dL [>177 μmol/L])
  - Anemia (hemoglobin <10 g/dL or 2 g less than normal)
  - Bone disease (one or more lytic lesions on x-ray, CT/PET-CT scan, or MRI)
- Presence of biomarker of active disease
  - Clonal BM plasmacytosis ≥60%
  - Affected:unaffected sFLC ratio ≥100 with absolute value of affected sFLC≥100 mg/L
  - >1 focal lesions on MRI imaging

Work-up

All patients
1. H&P
2. CBC with differential; serum electrolytes, BUN, creatinine, calcium and albumin, LDH
3. Quantitative immunoglobulins, serum protein electrophoresis, and immunofixation
4. Twenty-four-hour urine protein electrophoresis, immunofixation, and Bence Jones quantitation
5. Serum free light-chain assay
6. Skeletal survey
7. Unilateral bone marrow aspirate and biopsy with flow and immunohistochemistry
8. Bone marrow cytogenetics and interphase FISH
9. Albumin and β_2-microglobulin (see staging system)

Selected patients
1. MRI of the spine (evaluate for solitary plasmacytoma of bone or suspected cord compression)
2. FDG-PET/CT scan in selected patients to evaluate for radiographically occult bone lesions and/or extramedullary disease

(continued)

(continued)

Pathology (continued)

Solitary Plasmacytoma
- Biopsy proven tumor of clonal plasma cells affecting soft tissue (extramedullary) or bone (medullary)
- Normal bone marrow aspirate/biopsy with no evidence of clonal plasma cells
- Normal skeletal survey + MRI/CT spine and pelvis, excluding the plasmacytoma
- Absence of MDE

It represents 3–5% of cases of plasma cell dyscrasia
Progression to MM in ~10% patients within 3 years
Local treatment (radiation therapy and/or surgical excision) is treatment of choice

Solitary plasmacytoma with minimal bone marrow involvement
- Biopsy proven tumor of clonal plasma cells affecting soft tissue (extraosseous) or bone (osseous)
- Clonal BM plasmacytosis <10%*
- Normal skeletal survey + MRI/CT spine and pelvis, excluding the plasmacytoma
- Absence of MDE

Progression to MM in ~60% (osseous) and 20% (extraosseous) of patients within 3 years
*If more than 10% clonal plasmacytosis, then it is defined as active MM

Rajkumar et al. Lancet Oncol 2014;15:e538–e548

Plasma cell leukemia—defined as primary in the setting of de novo presentation (60% cases), secondary as terminal stage of advanced MM
- Peripheral blood absolute plasma cell count $\geq 2 \times 10^9/L$
- Peripheral blood plasma cell count ≥20% white blood cell differential count

Five percent of newly presenting MM patients

AL amyloidosis (all criteria must be met)
- Amyloid-related syndrome (ie, nephrotic syndrome, diastolic heart failure, etc)
- Biopsy-proven, positive Congo red stain (in any tissue)
- Presence of a plasma cell disorder based on abnormal sFLC, SPEP/UPEP, and/or BM biopsy
- Mass spectrometry confirmation of light chain identity in amyloid fibrils

Incidence: 1/100,000 individuals/year, likely underestimation based on missed diagnosis

Staging

Durie-Salmon Staging System

	Stage I	Stage II*	Stage III†
Myeloma cell mass	Low	Intermediate	High
Hemoglobin	>10 g/dL	8.5–10 g/dL	<8.5 g/dL
Serum calcium	≤12 mg/dL (≤3 mmol/L)	Fitting neither stage I nor stage II	>12 mg/dL (>3 mmol/L)
Skeletal survey	Normal‡		Advanced lytic bone lesions
Serum M-protein levels: IgG	<5 g/dL	5–7 g/dL	>7 g/dL
Serum M-protein levels: IgA	<3 g/dL	3–5 g/dL	>5 g/dL
24-hour urinary light chain excretion	<4 g/24 hours	4–12 g/24 hours	>12 g/24 hours

*Not meeting criteria for either stage I or stage III
†Need to meet 1 or more of the criteria listed
‡Or solitary plasmacytoma
Note: subclassification: For each stage, A denotes serum creatinine <2 mg/dL (<177 μmol/L) and B denotes serum creatinine ≥2 mg/dL (≥177 μmol/L)

Work-up (continued)

3. Tissue biopsy (evaluate for solitary plasmacytoma)
4. Serum viscosity (if M-protein level is markedly elevated or symptoms of hyperviscosity are present)
5. Fat pad aspirate or biopsy (to rule out AL amyloidosis)
6. *Additional tests (prognostic markers):* plasma cell labeling index, C-reactive protein, and LDH

Response Criteria

International Myeloma Working Group Uniform Response Criteria CR and Other Response Categories

Minimal Residual Disease (MRD) Negative Disease

sCR as described below, PLUS:
- Negative MRD assessment with a sensitivity of at least 10^{-5} via next-generation sequencing (nGS) or flow cytometry

CR = Complete Response

- Negative immunofixation on the serum and urine
- Disappearance of any soft tissue plasmacytomas
- ≤5% plasma cells in bone marrow

VGPR = Very Good Partial Response

- Serum and urine M-protein detectable by immunofluorescence but not on electrophoresis *or*

≥90% reduction in serum M-protein + urine M-protein level <100 mg/24 hours

PR = Partial Response

- ≥50% reduction of serum M-protein + reduction in 24-hour urinary M-protein by ≥90% or to <200 mg/24 hours. If the serum and urine M-protein are unmeasurable:

A ≥50% decrease in the difference between involved and uninvolved FLC levels is required in place of the M-protein criteria
If serum and urine M-protein are unmeasurable, and serum FLC assay also is unmeasurable:
- ≥50% reduction in plasma cells is required in place of M-protein, provided baseline bone marrow plasma cell percentage was ≥30%

Note: in addition to the above listed criteria, if present at baseline, a ≥50% reduction in the size of soft-tissue plasmacytomas is also required

(continued)

Staging (continued)

International Staging System

	Stage I	Stage II		Stage III
Serum β_2-microglobulin	<3.5 mg/L	<3.5 mg/L	3.5 to <5.5 mg/mL	≥5.5 mg/L
Serum albumin	≥3.5 g/dL (≥35 g/L)	<3.5 g/dL	—	—

Durie BGM, Salmon SE. Cancer 1975;36:842–854
Greipp PR et al. J Clin Oncol 2005;23:3412–3420

Revised ISS (R-ISS)

	Stage I	Stage II	Stage III
ISS	I	Not fulfilling criteria for Stage I or III	III
Chromosomal abnormalities by iFISH*	Standard risk		High risk†
LDH	Normal		High†

*High-risk chromosomal abnormalities: del(17p) and/or translocation t(4;14) and/or translocation t(14;16)
†Either high-risk CA or high LDH is sufficient for stage III classification
Palumbo A et al. J Clin Oncol 2015;33:2863–2869

Response Criteria (continued)

SD = Stable Disease*

- Not meeting criteria for CR, VGPR, PR, or progressive disease

*Not recommended for use as an indicator of response; stability of disease is best described by providing the time-to-progression estimates

Median Survival

Treatments for myeloma have expanded in the last two decades. A recent study[1] examined the changes in survival across 1038 patients diagnosed between the year 2001 and 2010 at the Mayo Clinic. For the purpose of the analysis, patients were divided into 2 groups: patients diagnosed between 2001 and 2005 and patients diagnosed between 2006 and 2010. Results showed that:
- Median overall survival (OS) improved from 4.6 years to 6.1 years in the 2006–2010 cohort compared with the 2001–2005 cohort (P = 0.002)
- Patients older than 65 enjoyed the most significant improvement in OS, with 6-year OS improving from 31% to 56% (P <0.001)
- Early mortality was significantly decreased in the 2006–2010 cohort (10%) versus the 2001–2005 cohort (16%), P <0.01, suggestive of improved outcome for patients with high-risk disease
- Of patients in the 2006–2010 cohort, 89% received at least one novel agent (thalidomide, lenalidomide, bortezomib) as part of initial induction therapy compared to 29% of the earlier cohort (P <0.001). Median OS of patients receiving at least novel agent was not reached versus 3.8 years (P <0.001) with a median follow-up of 5.9 years

A second study[2,3] estimated trends in age-specific 5- and 10-year relative survival of patients with multiple myeloma (MM) in the United States from 1990–1992 to 2002–2004 from the 1973–2004 database of the Surveillance, Epidemiology, and End Results (SEER) Program. Techniques of period analysis were used to show most recent developments:

Five- and 10-Year Estimates of Relative Survival of Patients with MM by Age Group and Calendar Period

	1990–1992		2002–2004		Increase†	P‡
	PE*	SE*	PE	SE		
5-Year Relative Survival						
All ages	28.8	0.9	34.7	0.9	5.9	<0.001
Younger than 50 years	44.8	3.5	56.7	3.0	11.9	0.001
50–59 years	38.8	2.5	48.2	2.1	9.4	0.001
60–69 years	30.6	1.8	36.3	1.8	5.7	0.09
70–79 years	27.1	1.7	28.7	1.6	1.6	0.21
80 years and older	13.8	2.0	15.2	1.9	1.4	0.96

(continued)

Median Survival (continued)

	1990–1992		2002–2004		Increase[†]	P[‡]
	PE*	SE*	PE	SE		
10-Year Relative Survival						
All ages	11.1	0.8	17.4	0.8	6.3	<0.001
Younger than 50 years	24.5	3.4	41.3	3.2	16.8	<0.001
50–59 years	17.2	2.1	28.6	2.2	11.4	<0.001
60–69 years	10.8	1.3	15.4	1.5	4.6	0.03
70–79 years	7.4	1.4	10.4	1.4	3.0	0.09
80 years and older	7.1	2.3	5.7	1.7	−1.4	0.94

*PE indicates point estimate; SE, standard error
[†]Increase from 1990–1992 to 2002–2004 in percentage points
[‡]P for trend from 1990–1992 to the last period 2002–2004

1. Kumar SK et al. Leukemia 2014;28:1122–1128
2. Brenner H et al. Blood 2008;111:2521–2526
3. Ghobrial IM, Anderson KC. Blood 2008;111:2503

A number of recent studies report ethnical disparities in survival benefit in patients with MM, with racial/ethnic minority patients deriving less survival benefit when compared to non-Hispanic whites. This outcome appears mostly related to under-allocation/under-use of standard therapies, such as autologous stem cell transplant and novel agents, as the OS of minority patients enrolled in clinical trials with novel agents was similar to non-Hispanic whites

Five- and 10-Year Relative Survival by Ethnic/Racial Group for All Age Groups

	Unadjusted Relative Survival (SE)			Adjusted Relative Survival (SE)*		
Period	1998–2001	2002–2005	2006–2009	1998–2001	2002–2005	2006–2009
5-Year Survival						
All	34.8 (0.6)	39.7 (0.4)	44.6 (0.6)	35.6 (0.6)	39.8 (0.4)	44 (0.6)
δ/P value[†]	+9.8/<0.0001			+8.4/<0.0001		
NHW	34.2 (0.7)	39.6 (0.5)	44.9 (0.8)	36.4 (0.7)	40.9 (0.5)	45.3 (0.7)
δ/P value[†]	+10.7/<0.0001			+8.9/<0.0001		
All nonwhite	35.4 (1)	39.5 (0.7)	43.5 (1)	33.8 (1)	37.6 (0.7)	41.4 (1)
δ/P value[†]	+8.1/<0.0001			+7.6/<0.0001		
AA	35.1 (1.5)	39.7 (1)	44.3 (1.4)	33.4 (1.4)	37.4 (0.9)	41.5 (1.4)
δ/P value[†]	+9.2/<0.0001			+8.1/<0.0001		
Hispanic	35.3 (1.9)	38.9 (1.2)	42.5 (1.8)	32.6 (1.8)	36.2 (1.2)	39.8 (1.8)
δ/P value[†]	+7.2/0.01			+7.2/0.007		
API	37.3 (2.5)	39.8 (1.6)	42.4 (2.3)	37.5 (2.3)	40.4 (1.5)	43.3 (2.2)
δ/P value[†]	+5.1/0.16			+5.8/0.09		

(continued)

Median Survival (continued)

Period	Unadjusted Relative Survival (SE)			Adjusted Relative Survival (SE)*		
	1998–2001	2002–2005	2006–2009	1998–2001	2002–2005	2006–2009
10-Year Survival						
All	16.1 (0.5)	20.4 (0.4)	25 (0.6)	16.6 (0.5)	20.2 (0.4)	24.1 (0.5)
δ/P value†	+8.9/<0.0001			+7.7/<0.0001		
NHW	15.3 (0.6)	19.7 (0.5)	24.5 (0.7)	17 (0.6)	20.5 (0.5)	24.6 (0.7)
δ/P value†	+9.2/<0.0001			+7.8/<0.0001		
All nonwhite	17.4 (1)	21.3 (0.8)	25.6 (1.2)	16.1 (0.8)	19.4 (0.6)	23 (0.9)
δ/P value†	+8.2/<0.0001			+7.3/<0.0001		
AA	16.1 (1.2)	20.1 (1)	24.5 (1.4)	14.8 (1.1)	18.2 (0.9)	21.6 (1.2)
δ/P value†	+8.4/<0.0001			+7.0/<0.0001		
Hispanic	17.4 (1.7)	21.1 (1.3)	25.2 (1.8)	15.3 (1.5)	18.6 (1.2)	22 (1.6)
δ/P value†	+7.8/0.001			+6.9/0.0006		
API	22 (2.3)	24.9 (1.7)	27.8 (2.3)	21.4 (2.1)	24.4 (1.6)	28.1 (2.2)
δ/P value†	+5.8/0.07			+7.0/0.03		

*Age adjusted to International Cancer Survival Standard
†δ = Delta or difference between 1998–2001 and 2006–2009 periods and P value for trend
AA, African American; API, Asian and Pacific Islander; NHW, non-Hispanic white
Adapted from Pulte D et al. Leuk Lymphoma 2014;55:1083–1089

Five- and 10-year Relative Survival by Ethnic and Age Groups

Period	15–49		50–69		70 and Older	
	5-Year Relative Survival (SE)		5-Year Relative Survival (SE)		5-Year Relative Survival (SE)	
	1998–2001	2006–2009	1998–2001	2006–2009	1998–2001	2006–2009
5-Year Survival						
All	52.9 (1.9)	66.1 (1.7)	39.9 (0.9)	52.2 (0.9)	26 (0.8)	30.8 (0.9)
δ/P value*	+13.2/<0.0001		+12.5/<0.0001		+4.8/<0.0001	
NHW	54.4 (2.6)	71.2 (2.2)	40.8 (1.2)	53.7 (1.1)	25.6 (1)	31 (1.1)
δ/P value*	+16.8/<0.0001		+13.3/<0.0001		+5.4/<0.0001	
All nonwhite	50.7 (2.9)	60.1 (2.6)	38.1 (1.5)	49 (1.4)	26.7 (1.9)	29.9 (1.8)
δ/P value*	+9.4/0.03		+11.7/<0.0001		+3.2/0.23	
AA	46.1 (4)	60.5 (3.6)	39 (2.1)	48.9 (2)	25.9 (2.3)	30 (2.3)
δ/P value*	+14.4/0.01		+10.3/0.0007		+4.1/0.21	
Hispanic	52.4 (5)	58.2 (4.5)	36.6 (2.7)	47.4 (2.6)	25.2 (3.1)	29.3 (2.9)
δ/P value*	+5.8/0.42		+9.2/0.02		+4.1/0.34	
API	60.3 (7.3)	63.4 (8)	39 (3.8)	51.3 (3.4)	30.1 (3.5)	30.5 (3.2)
δ/P value*	+3.1/0.79		+14.2/0.01		+0.4/0.93	

(continued)

Median Survival (continued)

Period	15–49 5-Year Relative Survival (SE)		50–69 5-Year Relative Survival (SE)		70 and Older 5-Year Relative Survival (SE)	
	1998–2001	2006–2009	1998–2001	2006–2009	1998–2001	2006–2009
10-Year Survival						
All	34.6 (1.9)	47.3 (1.9)	17.6 (0.8)	30 (0.9)	9.8 (0.6)	13 (0.7)
δ/P value*	+12.7/<0.0001		+12.4/<0.0001		+3.2/<0.0001	
NHW	36.6 (2.7)	53.7 (2.6)	17.7 (1)	30.1 (1.1)	9 (0.7)	12.4 (0.9)
δ/P value*	+17.1/<0.0001		+12.4/<0.0001		+3.4/<0.0001	
All nonwhite	30 (3.3)	39.4 (3.4)	17.4 (1.5)	29.6 (1.7)	12.5 (1.6)	14.7 (1.7)
δ/P value*	+9.4/0.06		+12.2/<0.0001		+2.2/0.25	
AA	27 (3.6)	38.9 (3.9)	16.6 (1.7)	27.5 (2)	10.5 (1.8)	12.7 (2)
δ/P value*	+11.9/0.03		+10.9/<0.0001		+2.2/0.31	
Hispanic	36.6 (5.5)	41.3 (4.7)	16.4 (2.3)	28.2 (2.6)	8.5 (2.4)	11.8 (2.6)
δ/P value*	+4.7/0.54		+1.8/<0.0001		+3.3/0.24	
API	37.8 (7.3)	39.3 (7.8)	21.6 (3.5)	35 (3.6)	18 (3.4)	19.2 (3.1)
δ/P value*	+1.5/0.89		+13.4/0.008		+1.2/0.78	

*δ = Delta or difference between 1998–2001 and 2006–2009 periods and P value for trend
AA, African American; API, Asian and Pacific Islander; NHW , non-Hispanic white
Adapted from Pulte D et al. Leuk Lymphoma 2014;55:1083–1089
Pulte D et al. Blood Adv 2018;2:116–119

International Myeloma Working Group Uniform Response Criteria

Disease Progression and Relapse

Progressive Disease*

Any one or more of the following:
- Increase of ≥25% from baseline in serum M-component (absolute increase must be 0.5 g/dL)
- Increase of ≥25% from baseline in urine M-component (absolute increase must be 200 mg/24 hours)
- Increase of ≥25% from baseline in the difference between involved and uninvolved FLC levels—only in patients without measurable serum and urine M-protein levels (absolute increase must be ≥10 mg/dL)
- Increase of ≥25% from baseline in bone marrow plasma cell percentage (absolute percentage must be ≥10%)
- Definite development of new bone lesions or soft-tissue plasmacytomas or definite increase in the size of existing bone lesions or soft-tissue plasmacytomas

Development of hypercalcemia (corrected serum calcium >11.5 mg/dL or >2.88 mmol/L) that can be attributed solely to the plasma cell proliferative disorder

Clinical Relapse

One or more of the following:
- Development of new soft-tissue plasmacytomas or bone lesions
- Definite increase in the size of existing plasmacytomas or bone lesions. A definite increase is defined as a 50% (and at least 1 cm) increase as measured serially by the sum of the products of the cross-diameters of the measurable lesion
- Hypercalcemia >11.5 mg/dL (>2.88 mmol/L)
- Decrease in hemoglobin of ≥2 g/dL
- Rise in serum creatinine by ≥2 mg/dL (≥177 μmol/L)

(continued)

International Myeloma Working Group Uniform Response Criteria (continued)

Relapse from CR[†]

One or more of the following:
- Reappearance of serum or urine M-protein by immunofixation or electrophoresis
- Development of ≥5% plasma cells in the bone marrow

Appearance of any other sign of progression (ie, new plasmacytoma, lytic bone lesion, or hypercalcemia)

*Used for calculation of time to progression and progression-free survival outcomes for all patients, including those in CR (includes primary progressive and disease progression on or off therapy)
[†]Used only if the outcome studied is disease-free survival (DFS)
Kumar S et al. Lancet Oncol 2016;17:e328–e346

Expert Opinion

1. *Treatment by stage:*

   Asymptomatic MGUS and smoldering MM. These patients do not need primary therapy and should be *monitored without therapy* unless they have evidence of disease progression. Alternatively, patients can be offered the opportunity to enroll in clinical trials evaluating the effect of early treatment on PFS and OS of precursor condition patients. Follow-up every 3–6 months is recommended. Bisphosphonate treatment every 3 months may be considered in patients with SMM. Progression of disease is defined as follows:
   - 25% increase in the monoclonal component (serum or urine)
   - >25% increase in plasma cells bone marrow infiltration
   - Increased size of bone lesions or development of new lytic lesions
   - Hypercalcemia
   - Increased plasmacytoma tumor volume

   Mateos MV et al. N Engl J Med 2013;369(5):438–447

   Symptomatic patients (Active MM)
   These patients are identified as discussed in the diagnostic criteria, by the presence of myeloma-defining events (MDE), either CRAB criteria or biomarker of disease.
   These patients should be *treated with combination therapy followed by consideration for stem cell transplantation* if eligible. Determine whether a patient is a candidate for high-dose therapy with autologous peripheral blood stem cell (PBSC) transplantation before initiating chemotherapy. Avoid alkylating agents in such patients before autologous PBSCs are collected, because exposure to alkylating agents may prevent the collection of an adequate number of PBSCs for autologous transplantation

Regimens

Newly Diagnosed Multiple Myeloma—Transplantation Candidates

Bortezomib + lenalidomide + dexamethasone	Richardson PG et al. Blood 2010;116:679–686
Carfilzomib + lenalidomide + dexamethasone	Jakubowlak AJ et al. Blood 2012;120:1801–1809
Carfilzomib + thalidomide + dexamethasone	Sonneveld P et al. Blood 2015;125:449–456
Cyclophosphamide + bortezomib + dexamethasone	Reeder CB et al. Leukemia 2009;23:1337–1341
Bortezomib + thalidomide + dexamethasone	Cavo M et al. Lancet 2010;376:2075–2085
Bortezomib + doxorubicin + dexamethasone	Sonneveld P et al. J Clin Oncol 2012;30:2946–2955
Lenalidomide + low-dose dexamethasone	Rajkumar SV et al. Lancet Oncol 2010;11:29–37
Bortezomib + dexamethasone	Harousseau J-L et al. J Clin Oncol 2010;28:4621–4629
Bortezomib + thalidomide + dexamethasone + cisplatin + doxorubicin + cyclophosphamide + etoposide (VTD-PACE)	Barlogie B et al. Br J Haematol 2007;138:176–185
Ixazomib + lenalidomide + dexamethasone	Kumar SK et al. Lancet Oncol 2014;15:1503–1512

(continued)

Expert Opinion (*continued*)

Newly Diagnosed Multiple Myeloma—Those Not Transplantation Candidates	
Lenalidomide + dexamethasone	Benboubker L et al. N Engl J Med 2014;371:906–917
Modified lenalidomide + bortezomib + dexamethasone (RVD-lite)	O'Donnell EK et al. Br J Haematol 2018;182:222–230
Daratumumab + lenalidomide + dexamethasone	Facon T et al. N Engl J Med 2019;380:2104–2115
Melphalan + prednisone + lenalidomide	Palumbo A et al. J Clin Oncol 2007;25:4459–4465
Bortezomib + melphalan + prednisone	San Miguel JF et al. N Engl J Med 2008;359:906–917
Daratumumab + melphalan + bortezomib + dexamethasone	Mateos MV et al. N Engl J Med 2018; 378:518–528
Melphalan + prednisone + thalidomide	Palumbo A et al. Lancet 2006;367:825–831
Carfilzomib + cyclophosphamide + dexamethasone	Bringhen S et al. Blood 2014;124:63–69
Relapsed/Refractory Multiple Myeloma	
Daratumumab	Lokhorst HM et al. N Engl J Med 2015;373:1207–1219
Daratumumab + lenalidomide + low-dose dexamethasone	Dimopoulos MA et al. N Engl J Med 2016;375:1319–1331
Daratumumab + bortezomib + dexamethasone	Palumbo A et al. N Engl J Med 2016;375:754–766
Isatuximab + pomalidomide + dexamethasone	Attal M et al. Lancet 2019;394:2096–2107
Elotuzumab + lenalidomide + dexamethasone	Lonial S et al. N Engl J Med 2015;373:621–631
Elotuzumab + pomalidomide + dexamethasone	Dimopoulos MA et al. N Engl J Med 2018;379:1811–1822
Carfilzomib	Vij R et al. Blood 2012;119:5661–5670
Carfilzomib + dexamethasone	Dimopoulos MA et al. Lancet Oncol 2016;17:27–38
Carfilzomib + lenalidomide + dexamethasone	Stewart AK et al. N Engl J Med 2015;372:142–152
Ixazomib + lenalidomide + dexamethasone	Moreau P et al. N Engl J Med 2016;374:1621–1634
Pomalidomide + dexamethasone	Leleu X et al. Blood 2013;121:1968–1975
Pomalidomide + cyclophosphamide + prednisone	Larocca A et al. Blood 2013;122:2799–2806
Bendamustine + lenalidomide + dexamethasone	Lentzsch S et al. Blood 2012;119:4608–4613
Bendamustine + pomalidomide + dexamethasone	Sivaraj D et al. Blood Cancer J 2018;8:71
Selinexor + dexamethasone	Chari A et al. N Engl J Med 2019;381:727–738
Lenalidomide + dexamethasone	Weber DM et al. N Engl J Med 2007;357:2133–2142
Bortezomib ± dexamethasone	Richardson PG et al. N Engl J Med 2003;348:2609–2617
Dexamethasone + cyclophosphamide + etoposide + cisplatin (DCEP)	Lazzarino M et al. Bone Marrow Transplant 2001;28:835–839
Liposomal doxorubicin + bortezomib	Orlowski RZ et al. J Clin Oncol 2007;25:3892–3901
High-Dose Conditioning for Stem Cell Transplantation in Relapsed/Refractory Multiple Myeloma	
High-dose melphalan	Moreau P et al. Blood 2002;99:731–735
Maintenance Therapy Multiple Myeloma	
Bortezomib	Sonneveld P et al. J Clin Oncol 2012;30:2946–2955
Lenalidomide	Attal M et al. N Engl J Med 2012;366:1782–1791 Dimopoulos MA et al. Haematologica 2013;98:784–788 McCarthy PL et al. N Engl J Med 2012;366:1770–1781 Palumbo A et al. N Engl J Med 2012;366:1759–1769
Thalidomide	Morgan GJ et al. Blood 2012;119:7–15

(*continued*)

Expert Opinion (*continued*)

2. *Solitary plasmacytoma:*
- Primary radiation therapy (≥45 Gy) to the involved fields represents the initial treatment for patients diagnosed with osseous plasmacytoma
- Same approach and/or surgery represent the initial treatment for patients with extraosseous plasmacytomas
- Follow-up for either solitary or extraosseous plasmacytomas includes blood and urine tests every 4 weeks to monitor response to radiation treatment
- If a complete disappearance of the monoclonal component is demonstrated, blood and urine tests will be performed every 3–6 months
- If the monoclonal component persists, follow-up should continue every 4 weeks
- If a progression in the disease is documented, a reevaluation for recurrent extraosseous plasmacytomas and/or myeloma should be considered

Dimopoulos MA et al. J Clin Oncol 1992;10:587–590
Hu K, Yahalom J. Oncology (Williston Park) 2000;14:101–108, 111; discussion 111–112, 115

3. Treatment with monthly bisphosphonate is recommended to reduce skeletal events for all myeloma patients. Denosumab is a monoclonal antibody targeting RANKL. Based on the results of a noninferiority trial comparing denosumab to zoledronic acid in preventing skeletal related events, denosumab was FDA approved for use in MM in January 2018 and represents a safe alternative to bisphosphonates in patients with advanced renal impairment. Patients with SMM may be offered bisphosphonate every 3 months as a protective strategy against bone events. Alternatives that have demonstrated efficacy in this setting include

- Pamidronate, *or*
- Zoledronic acid, *or*
- Clodronate
- Denosumab

Notes:
- Because renal toxicity can result from bisphosphonate therapy, renal function should be monitored closely. Bisphosphonate doses may need to be modified or discontinued in renally impaired individuals. Denosumab is safe in renal failure and can be used as an alternative in MM patients with advanced eGFR impairment
- Current recommendations are to administer standard doses of bisphosphonates every 4 weeks. The duration for which repeated doses should be administered is unclear. Currently, there are no data from randomized studies to guide bisphosphonate use for more than 2 years. The risks and benefits of continuing bisphosphonate treatment after 2 years must be considered in each patient. To prevent osteonecrosis of the jaw, patients treated with bisphosphonates should maintain good dental hygiene and should stop bisphosphonate treatment for 90 days before and after invasive dental procedures. Caregivers must ensure that myeloma patients get enough vitamin D and calcium. This is a concern because 60% of myeloma patients are vitamin D and calcium deficient. U.S. Food and Drug Administration product labeling for both zoledronic acid and pamidronate disodium recommend vitamin D and calcium supplementation in conjunction with bisphosphonate treatment, but calcium supplementation should be used cautiously for patients with kidney problems

4. Anemia is present in most patients with multiple myeloma. Reversible causes of anemia should be evaluated and treated
5. Waldenström macroglobulinemia presents with lymphoplasmacytic bone marrow infiltration and IgM paraproteinemia. Therapeutic regimens include rituximab alone or in combination with alkylating agents such as cyclophosphamide, bortezomib, or nucleoside analogs such as fludarabine. Bruton tyrosine kinase inhibitor ibrutinib is FDA approved for treatment of WM. Other management considerations focus on complications caused by macroglobulinemia, such as hyperviscosity, cryoglobulinemia, and hemolytic anemia
6. Primary amyloidosis is characterized by organ dysfunction resulting from monoclonal light-chain production and tissue deposition. Carefully selected patients may benefit from high-dose melphalan with autologous PBSC support, which can result in sustained hematologic remission followed by organ response. Therapeutic options in frontline and relapsed/refractory settings include bortezomib alone or in combination with cyclophosphamide and dexamethasone (CyBorD) or lenalidomide and dexamethasone (RVd), pomalidomide plus dexamethasone, daratumumab, and most recently ixazomib. If t(11;14) is present, patients may be amenable to therapy with the BCL2 inhibitor venetoclax
7. Patients receiving combinatory treatment including an IMiD must receive venous thromboembolic event (VTE) prophylaxis. The optimal prophylaxis strategy for thromboembolic complications of IMiD therapy (thalidomide and lenalidomide) is not clear, and a careful assessment of risk factors must be carried out for each individual patient. Therapy with low-molecular-weight heparin, full-dose warfarin anticoagulation, and possibly direct oral anticoagulants should be considered in patients with a prior history of VTE, inherited procoagulable diathesis, and/or limited mobility. Aspirin alone at a dose between 81 mg and 325 mg daily is considered standard VTE prophylaxis in patients with no other VTE risk factors beyond MM diagnosis and IMiD-containing regimen

Anderson KC et al. J Clin Oncol 2018;36:812–818
Palumbo A et al. J Thromb Haemost 2006;4:1842–1845
Palumbo A et al. Leukemia 2008;22:414–423

TRANSPLANT-ELIGIBLE • FIRST-LINE INDUCTION

MULTIPLE MYELOMA REGIMEN: BORTEZOMIB + LENALIDOMIDE + DEXAMETHASONE INDUCTION PRIOR TO AUTOLOGOUS STEM CELL TRANSPLANTATION (ASCT)

Richardson PG et al. Blood 2010;116:679–686
Durie BGM et al. Lancet. 2017;289:519–527

All Cycles:
Bortezomib 1.3 mg/m^2 per dose; administer by intravenous injection over 3–5 seconds for 4 doses on days 1, 4, 8, and 11, every 3 weeks for 8 cycles (total dosage/cycle = 5.2 mg/m^2)
Lenalidomide 25 mg per day; administer orally for 14 consecutive days on days 1–14, every 3 weeks for 8 cycles (total dose/cycle = 350 mg)
Dexamethasone 20 mg per dose; administer orally for 8 doses on days 1, 2, 4, 5, 8, 9, 11, and 12, every 3 weeks for 8 cycles (total dose/cycle = 160 mg)

Supportive Care
Antiemetic prophylaxis
Emetogenic potential is **MINIMAL**
See Chapter 42 for antiemetic recommendations

Hematopoietic growth factor (CSF) prophylaxis
Primary prophylaxis is **NOT** *indicated*
See Chapter 43 for more information

Antimicrobial prophylaxis
Risk of fever and neutropenia is **HIGH**
   Antimicrobial primary prophylaxis is recommended:
   • Antibacterial—consider fluoroquinolone prophylaxis; *P. jirovecii* prophylaxis is recommended (eg, cotrimoxazole)
   • Antifungal—recommended
   • Antiviral—antiherpes antivirals (eg, acyclovir, famciclovir, valacyclovir)

Decreased bowel motility prophylaxis
Give a bowel regimen to prevent constipation based initially on **stool softeners**

Bisphosphonates
All patients receiving primary therapy for symptomatic multiple myeloma should receive a bisphosphonate adjunctively.

(continued)

Treatment Modifications

Adverse Event	Treatment Modification
Platelet count <30,000/mm^3	Interrupt lenalidomide treatment, follow CBC weekly. Resume lenalidomide at 15 mg/day after platelet count is ≥30,000/mm^3
For each subsequent platelet count <30,000/mm^3	Interrupt lenalidomide treatment, follow CBC weekly. After platelet count recovers to ≥30,000/mm^3, resume lenalidomide at a dose decreased from the previous dose by 5 mg/day, but the daily dose should not be less than 5 mg/day
ANC <1000/mm^3	Interrupt lenalidomide treatment, follow CBC weekly. Resume lenalidomide at 15 mg/day after ANC ≥1000/mm^3
For each subsequent ANC <1000/mm^3	Interrupt lenalidomide treatment, follow CBC weekly. After ANC recovers to ≥1000/mm^3, resume lenalidomide at a dose decreased from the previous dose by 5 mg/day, but the daily dose should not be less than 5 mg/day
Febrile neutropenia	Interrupt lenalidomide treatment, follow closely, and resume lenalidomide at 15 mg/day after fever abates
G3/4 nonhematologic toxicity	Interrupt lenalidomide treatment and follow clinically. After toxicity abates to G ≤2, resume lenalidomide at a dose decreased from the previous dose by 5 mg/day, but the daily dose should not be less than 5 mg/day
Toxicities ascribed to dexamethasone such as severe manifestations of hypercorticism, including hyperglycemia, irritability, insomnia, and oral candidiasis	Reduce dexamethasone dose to 20 mg per day

(continued)

(*continued*)

Thromboprophylaxis

Risk assessment and recommendations for VTE prophylaxis in patients with multiple myeloma with individual or myeloma-related risk factors, or risk factors related to treatment

Individual risk factors	

• Obesity (BMI ≥30 kg/m²)
 • H/O VTE
 • CVC or pacemaker
 • Comorbid pathologies
   ■ Cardiac disease
   ■ Chronic renal disease
   ■ Diabetes
   ■ Acute infection
   ■ Immobilization
 • Surgery
   ■ General surgery
   ■ Any anesthesia
   ■ Trauma
 • Medications
   ■ Erythropoietin (epoetin alfa, darbepoetin)
   ■ Estrogenic compounds
   ■ Bevacizumab
 • Clotting disorders
   ■ Thrombophilia
 Myeloma-related risk factors
 • Diagnosis of multiple myeloma
 • Hyperviscosity
	≤1 Individual or myeloma-related risk factor present:
	 • **Aspirin** 81–325 mg daily
	
	 ≥2 Individual or myeloma-related risk factors present:
	 • **LMWH,** * equivalent to enoxaparin sodium 40 mg/day or **dalteparin sodium** 5000 IU/day; administer subcutaneously, *or*
	 • **Warfarin,** targeting an INR = 2–3

Concomitant treatment-related risk factors Thalidomide or lenalidomide in combination with: • High-dose dexamethasone (≥480 mg/month) • Doxorubicin • Multiagent chemotherapy	• **LMWH,** * equivalent to enoxaparin sodium 40 mg/day or **dalteparin sodium** 5000 IU/day; administer subcutaneously, *or* • **Warfarin,** targeting an INR = 2–3

*LMWHs should be used with caution in individuals with impaired renal function (creatinine clearance <30 mL/min). Refer to product labeling for information about doses and administration schedules in renally impaired patients, and guidance for monitoring anti-Factor Xa concentrations

Abbreviations: CVC, central venous catheter; INR, international normalized ratio; LMWH, low-molecular-weight heparin; VTE, venous thromboembolic disease

References: Geerts WH et al. Chest 2008;133(6 Suppl):381S–453S

National Comprehensive Cancer Network. Multiple Myeloma, V.1.2014. (Accessed October 8, 2013, at http://www.nccn.org)

National Comprehensive Cancer Network. Venous Thromboembolic Disease, V.2.2013. (Accessed October 8, 2013, at http://www.nccn.org)

Palumbo A et al. Leukemia 2008;22:414–423

Patient Population Studied

A phase 1/2 study of 66 patients with newly diagnosed symptomatic multiple myeloma who had not previously received systemic antimyeloma therapy, and had a Karnofsky Performance Status ≥60%. Patients were excluded if they had G ≥2 peripheral neuropathy, serum creatinine >2.5 mg/dL (>221 μmol/L), platelets <50,000/mm³, ANC <1000/mm³, hemoglobin <8 g/dL, or transaminases ≥2× the upper limit of normal range

Treatment Modifications
(*continued*)

Treatment Modification for Bortezomib-Induced Peripheral Neuropathy*

Severity of Peripheral Neuropathy	Modifications of Dose and Schedule
G1 (paresthesias or loss of reflexes) without pain or loss of function	No action
G1 with pain or G2 (interferes with function but not with activities of daily living)	Reduce bortezomib dosage to 1 mg/m² per dose
G2 with pain or G3 (interferes with activities of daily living)	Withhold bortezomib treatment until toxicity resolves, then reinitiate at a dosage of 0.7 mg/m² per dose once weekly
G4 (permanent sensory loss that interferes with function)	Discontinue treatment

Lenalidomide Starting Dose Adjustment for Renal Impairment in Multiple Myeloma (Days 1–21 of Each 28-Day Cycle)

Moderate renal impairment CrCl 30–60 mL/min (0.5–1 mL/s)	10 mg lenalidomide every 24 hours
Severe renal impairment CrCl <30 mL/min (<0.5 mL/s), not requiring dialysis	15 mg lenalidomide every 48 hours
End-stage renal disease CrCl <30 mL/min (<0.5 mL/s), requiring dialysis	Lenalidomide 5 mg/day. On dialysis days, administer a daily dose following dialysis

CrCl, Creatinine clearance
*Richardson PG et al. J Clin Oncol 2006;24:3113–3120

Efficacy

Best Response to Treatment for Treated and Phase 2 Populations

Response	All Patients (n = 66)		Phase 2 Population (n = 35)	
	Percentage	90% CI	Percentage	90% CI
CR	29	20–39	37	24–52
nCR	11	5–19	20	10–34
VGPR	27	18–38	17	8–31
PR	33	24–44	26	14–41
CR + nCR	39	29–50	57	42–71
CR + nCR + VGPR	67	56–76	74	59–86
At least PR	100	96–100	100	92–100
Estimated 18-month duration of response	68% (95% CI, 55–79%)			

Percentages of Patients Achieving a Best Response of VGPR or Better, and Estimated 18-Month PFS Rates

Characteristic/Value	n	Response ≥VGPR n (%)	Estimated 18-Month PFS, % (95% CI)
Baseline Characteristic			
All patients	66	100 (96–100)	75 (63–84)
ISS disease stage I	29	21 (72)	89 (70–96)
ISS disease stage II/III	37	23 (62)	65 (47–78)
Durie-Salmon disease stage I	22	12 (55)	82 (59–93)
Durie-Salmon disease stage II/III	44	32 (73)	72 (56–83)
β_2-Microglobulin <3.5 mg/L	44	32 (73)	77 (61–87)
β_2-Microglobulin ≥3.5 mg/L	22	12 (55)	73 (49–87)
Albumin <3.5 g/dL	24	17 (71)	63 (40–78)
Albumin ≥3.5 g/dL	42	27 (64)	83 (67–91)
Cytogenetics Present			
Abnormal metaphase cytogenetics = Yes	6	5 (83)	(27–97)
Abnormal metaphase cytogenetics = No	60	39 (65)	75 (62–84)
Del 13/13q by FISH = Yes	24	79 (57–91)	18 (75)
Del 13/13q by FISH = No	27	16 (59)	65 (43–80)
Del 17p by FISH = Yes	5	3 (60)	100
Del 17p by FISH = No	45	30 (67)	68 (52–80)
t(4;14) by FISH = Yes	2	2 (100)	100
t(4;14) by FISH = No	39	24 (62)	63 (46–77)

(continued)

Toxicity

Adverse Events in ≥ 15% of Patients and All G3/4 (n = 66)

Event	% Total	% G3	% G4
Neuropathy, sensory*	80	2	0
Fatigue	64	3	0
Constipation	61	0	0
Edema limb	45	0	0
Muscle pain	44	2	0
Rash/desquamation	36	2	0
Diarrhea	35	0	0
Nausea	32	0	0
Neuropathic pain	32	3	0
Extremity, limb pain	30	3	0
Insomnia	30	2	0
Hyperglycemia	27	2	0
Dizziness	26	3	0
Constitutional	18	0	0
Dyspnea	18	0	0
Neuropathy, motor	18	2	0
Platelets	18	2	5
Pruritus/itching	18	0	0
Neutrophils	15	8	2
Anxiety	14	2	0
Dry skin	14	2	0
Lymphopenia	14	11	3
Vision, blurred	12	2	0
Alanine transaminase	12	3	0
Hypokalemia	11	5	0
Mental status	11	2	0
Hyperkalemia	9	2	0
Hyponatremia	9	2	0
Hypophosphatemia	9	5	0
Pulmonary/upper respiratory, other	9	3	0
Agitation	6	2	0

(continued)

Treatment Modifications (*continued*)

Characteristic/Value	n	Response ≥VGPR n (%)	Estimated 18-Month PFS, % (95% CI)
Cytogenetics Present			
t(11;14) by FISH = Yes	11	7 (64)	73 (37–90)
t(11;14) by FISH = No	40	28 (70)	72 (55–83)
Del 17p and/or t(4;14) by FISH = Yes	6	4 (67)	100
Del 17p and/or t(4;14) by = No	44	29 (66)	68 (51–79)
Estimated 18-month OS (with/without ASCT)		97% (95% CI, 88–99%)	

Note: per European Group for Blood and Marrow Transplant criteria, all response categories required 2 confirmatory assessments at least 6 weeks apart

CI, confidence interval; CR, complete response; FISH, fluorescence in situ hybridization; ISS, International Staging System; nCR, near-complete response; OS, overall survival; PFS, progression-free survival; PR, partial response; VGPR, very good partial response

Toxicity (*continued*)

Event	% Total	% G3	% G4
Hearing	6	2	0
Hemoglobin	6	2	0
QTc interval	6	3	0
Thrombosis/ thrombus/embolism	6	3	2
Creatinine	3	2	0
Leukocytes	3	3	0
Atrial fibrillation	2	2	0
Infection, other	2	2	0
Stomach hemorrhage	2	2	0

*Including 34 (52%) = G1 and 18 (27%) = G2

Therapy Monitoring

1. *Before each cycle:* CBC with differential and blood chemistries (including BUN, creatinine, and calcium)
2. *Every 6 weeks to 3 months:* Measure serum and urine M-protein

TRANSPLANT-ELIGIBLE • FIRST-LINE INDUCTION

MULTIPLE MYELOMA REGIMEN: CARFILZOMIB + LENALIDOMIDE + DEXAMETHASONE (CRd) INDUCTION PRIOR TO AUTOLOGOUS STEM CELL TRANSPLANTATION (ASCT)

Jakubowlak AJ et al. Blood 2012;120:1801–1809

Hydration with carfilzomib: During cycle 1, days 1 and 2, administer intravenously 250–500 mL 0.9% NS before each carfilzomib dose, *and* an additional 250–500 mL of fluid after carfilzomib. During repeated treatments, continue intravenous hydration as needed. Encourage oral hydration

Carfilzomib (see dose below); intravenously in 50-mL 5% dextrose injection
Cycle 1, days 1 and 2: 20 mg/m^2 per dose, for 2 doses, infused over 5–10 minutes, on days 1 and 2 of cycle 1 only, then:
  Cycle 1, days 8, 9, 15 and 16: 36 mg/m^2 per dose; infused over 30 minutes, for 4 doses on days 8, 9, 15, and 16 of cycle 1 only (total dosage in cycle 1 = 184 mg/m^2; cycle length = 28 days)
  Cycles 2–8: 36 mg/m^2 per dose; infused over 30 minutes, for 6 doses, on days 1, 2, 8, 9, 15, and 16, every 28 days (total dosage/cycle = 216 mg/m^2)
  Cycle 9 and subsequent cycles: 36 mg/m^2 per dose; for 4 doses, on days 1, 2, 15, and 16, every 28 days (total dosage/ cycle = 144 mg/m^2)

Lenalidomide 25 mg/day orally, continually for 21 consecutive days on days 1–21, every 28 days (total dose/cycle = 525 mg)

Dexamethasone administer orally or intravenously for 4 doses on days 1, 8, 15, and 22, every 28 days
• *Cycles 1–4*: 40 mg/dose (total dose/cycle = 160 mg)
• *Cycle 5 and subsequent cycles*: 20 mg/dose (total dose/cycle = 80 mg)

Notes:
• After cycle 4, transplantation-eligible candidates underwent stem cell collection (SCC) then continued CRd with the option of transplantation
• Thirty-five patients underwent SCC, 7 proceeded to transplantation, and the remainder resumed CRd
• After 8 cycles, patients received maintenance CRd. Per initial design, CRd maintenance was planned for an indefinite period of time, but because progression events were limited and no maintenance treatments were discontinued because of toxicity, the study was amended to 24 total cycles of CRd. After completion of 24 cycles, single-agent lenalidomide off protocol was recommended

Lenalidomide Starting Dose Adjustment for Renal Impairment in Multiple Myeloma

CrCl 30–60 mL/min	Lenalidomide 10 mg q24h days 1–21 very 28 days
CrCl <30 mL/min not requiring dialysis	Lenalidomide 15 mg q48h days 1–21 very 28 days
End-stage renal disease: requiring dialysis	Lenalidomide 5 mg/day. On dialysis days, administer the daily dose following dialysis

CrCl, creatinine clearance
*Richardson PG et al. J Clin Oncol 2006;24:3113–3120

Carfilzomib Dose Adjustments

BSA >2.2 m^2	Use BSA of 2.2 m^2 to calculate carfilzomib
• Bilirubin 1–1.5× ULN and any AST, *or* • Bilirubin 1.5–3× ULN and any AST, *or* • Bilirubin ≤ULN and AST >ULN	Reduce initial carfilzomib dose by 25%
Bilirubin >3× ULN	No dose recommendation available
Creatinine clearance <15 mL/minute	Full dose carfilzomib at discretion of physician
End-stage renal disease on hemodialysis	No dose adjustment necessary; administer carfilzomib after hemodialysis

(continued)

Treatment Modifications

Carfilzomib Dose Levels

Starting dose	36 mg/m^2 per dose
Level −1	27 mg/m^2 per dose
Level −2	20 mg/m^2 per dose
Level −3	15 mg/m^2 per dose
Level −4	11 mg/m^2 per dose
Level −5	Discontinue

Adverse Event	Treatment Modification
Hematologic Toxicity	
G3/4 neutropenia Febrile neutropenia (ANC <1000/mm^3 with fever ≥38°C) G4 thrombocytopenia G3/4 thrombocytopenia associated with bleeding	Hold carfilzomib dosing for up to 21 days to resolve toxicity and then restart at the same dosage, or reduce the carfilzomib dosage by 1 dose level. If counts recover to G2 neutropenia or G3 thrombocytopenia, reduce carfilzomib dosage by 1 dose level. If tolerated, the reduced dose may be escalated to the previous dose level
Nonhematologic Toxicity	
G3/4 cardiac toxicity New onset or worsening: • Congestive heart failure • Decreased left ventricular function • Myocardial ischemia Pulmonary hypertension G3/4 pulmonary complications G3/4 elevation of transaminases, bilirubin, or other liver abnormalities	Hold carfilzomib dosing for up to 21 days to resolve toxicity and then restart at the same dosage or reduce the carfilzomib dosage by 1 dose level. If tolerated, the reduced dosage may be escalated to the previous dose level

(continued)

(continued)

Supportive Care

Antiemetic prophylaxis
Emetogenic potential on days with lenalidomide ± carfilzomib is **LOW**
See Chapter 42 for antiemetic recommendations

Hematopoietic growth factor (CSF) prophylaxis
Primary prophylaxis may be indicated
See Chapter 43 for more information

Antimicrobial prophylaxis
Risk of fever and neutropenia is INTERMEDIATE
Antimicrobial primary prophylaxis to be considered:
- Antibacterial—consider a fluoroquinolone or no prophylaxis; *P. jirovecii* prophylaxis is recommended (eg, cotrimoxazole)
- Antifungal—recommended; consider use during periods of neutropenia
- Antiviral—antiherpes antivirals (eg, acyclovir, famciclovir, valacyclovir)

Bisphosphonates
All patients receiving primary therapy for symptomatic multiple myeloma should receive a bisphosphonate adjunctively.

Steroid-associated gastritis
Add a **proton pump inhibitor** during steroid use to prevent gastritis and duodenitis

Diarrhea management
Loperamide or **diphenoxylate hydrochloride** 2.5 mg with **atropine sulfate** 0.025 mg (eg, Lomotil)

Thromboprophylaxis
Risk assessment and recommendations for VTE prophylaxis in patients with multiple myeloma with individual or myeloma-related risk factors, or risk factors related to treatment

Individual risk factors	
• Obesity (BMI ≥30 kg/m²)	
• H/O VTE	
• CVC or pacemaker	
• Comorbid pathologies	
▪ Cardiac disease	
▪ Chronic renal disease	≤1 Individual or myeloma-related risk factor present:
▪ Diabetes	• **Aspirin** 81–325 mg daily
▪ Acute infection	
▪ Immobilization	
• Surgery	
▪ General surgery	≥2 Individual or myeloma-related risk factors present:
▪ Any anesthesia	• **LMWH,*** equivalent to enoxaparin sodium 40 mg/day *or* **dalteparin sodium** 5000 IU/day; administer subcutaneously, *or*
▪ Trauma	
• Medications	• **Warfarin**, targeting an INR = 2–3
▪ Erythropoietin (epoetin alfa, darbepoetin)	
▪ Estrogenic compounds	
▪ Bevacizumab	
• Clotting disorders	
▪ Thrombophilia	
Myeloma-related risk factors	
• Diagnosis of multiple myeloma	
• Hyperviscosity	

(continued)

Treatment Modifications
(continued)

Nonhematologic Toxicity

Serum creatinine ≥2× baseline	If attributable to carfilzomib, hold carfilzomib doses for up to 21 days to resolve toxicity to G1 or to baseline and then restart at the same dosage, or reduce the carfilzomib dosage by 1 dose level. If tolerated, the reduced dosage may be escalated to the previous dose level
G2 neuropathy with pain G3/4 peripheral neuropathy	Hold carfilzomib dosing for up to 21 days to resolve toxicity and then restart at the same dose, or reduce the carfilzomib dosage by 1 dose level. If tolerated, the reduced dosage may be escalated to the previous dose level
Other G3/4 nonhematologic toxicities	If attributable to carfilzomib, hold carfilzomib doses for up to 21 days to resolve toxicity to G1 or to baseline and then restart at the same dosage or reduce the carfilzomib dosage by 1 dose level. If tolerated, the reduced dosage may be escalated to the previous dose level

Lenalidomide Dose Levels

Starting dose	25 mg/day
Level −1	20 mg/day
Level −2	15 mg/day
Level −3	10 mg/day
Level −4	5 mg/day
Level −5	Discontinue

Adverse Event	Treatment Modification
G3/4 neutropenia Febrile neutropenia (ANC <1000/mm³ with fever ≥38°C)	Hold lenalidomide dosing for up to 21 days to resolve toxicity and then restart at the same dosage or reduce the lenalidomide dosage by 1 dose level
G3/4 nonhematologic toxicity	Hold lenalidomide dosing for up to 21 days to resolve toxicity to G ≤2 and then restart at the same dosage or reduce the lenalidomide dosage by 1 dose level

(continued)

(*continued*)

Concomitant treatment-related risk factors	
Thalidomide or lenalidomide in combination with: • High-dose dexamethasone (≥480 mg/month) • Doxorubicin • Multiagent chemotherapy	• **LMWH,** * equivalent to enoxaparin sodium 40 mg/day *or* **dalteparin sodium** 5000 IU/day; administer subcutaneously, *or* • **Warfarin**, targeting an INR = 2–3

*LMWHs should be used with caution in individuals with impaired renal function (creatinine clearance <30 mL/min). Refer to product labeling for information about doses and administration schedules in renally impaired patients, and guidance for monitoring anti-Factor Xa concentrations

Abbreviations: CVC, central venous catheter; INR, international normalized ratio; LMWH, low-molecular-weight heparin; VTE, venous thromboembolic disease

References: Geerts WH et al. Chest 2008;133(6 Suppl):381S–453S

National Comprehensive Cancer Network. Multiple Myeloma, V.1.2014. (Accessed October 8, 2013, at http://www.nccn.org)

National Comprehensive Cancer Network. Venous Thromboembolic Disease, V.2.2013. (Accessed October 8, 2013, at http://www.nccn.org)

Palumbo A et al. Leukemia 2008;22:414–423

Efficacy

Best Response to Treatment in Evaluable Patients

	Responses, n (%)			
	≥PR	≥VGPR	≥nCR	sCR
All patients (n = 53)	52 (98)	43 (81)	33 (62)	22 (42)
Treatment duration				
>4 cycles (n = 49)	49 (100)	43 (88)	33 (67)	22 (45)
>8 cycles (n = 36)	36 (100)	33 (92)	28 (78)	22 (61)
>12 cycles (n = 29)	29 (100)	25 (86)	21 (72)	18 (62)

nCR, near-complete response; PR, partial response; sCR, stringent complete response; VGPR, very good partial response

Best response to treatment by carfilzomib dose, ISS stage, and cytogenetics (n = 53)*

Responses, n (%)

	≥PR	≥VGPR	≥nCR	sCR
Carfilzomib dose, mg/m²				
20 (n = 4)	4 (100)	4 (100)	3 (75)	1 (25)
27 (n = 13)	13 (100)	13 (100)	10 (77)	7 (54)
36 (n = 36)	35 (97)	26 (72)	20 (55)	14 (39)
ISS stage				
I (n = 21)	21 (100)	16 (76)	12 (57)	7 (33)
II (n = 18)	18 (100)	15 (75)	10 (55)	8 (44)
III (n = 14)	13 (93)	12 (86)	11 (79)	7 (50)
Cytogenetics				
Normal/favorable (n = 34)†	34 (100)	26 (76)	20 (59)	13 (38)
Unfavorable (n = 17)†	16 (94)	13 (76)	11 (65)	9 (53)

*Assessed by Modified International Myeloma Working Group (IMWG) Uniform Criteria with the addition of nCR
†Any of del 13 by metaphase or hypodiploidy or t(4;14) or t(14;16) or del 17p considered as unfavorable; all others considered normal/favorable
ISS, International Staging System; nCR, near-complete response; PR, partial response; sCR, stringent complete response; VGPR, very good partial response

Treatment Modifications
(*continued*)

Adverse Event	Treatment Modification
• Any adverse event G ≥3 (excluding nausea, vomiting, diarrhea, lenalidomide-induced maculopapular rash or dexamethasone-induced hyperglycemia) • G ≥3 nausea, vomiting, or diarrhea despite maximal therapy • G4 fatigue lasting >7 days	Hold carfilzomib and lenalidomide dosing for up to 21 days to resolve toxicity to G ≤2 and then, depending on presumed attribution of toxicity, restart at the same dosage or reduce the carfilzomib dosage and/or lenalidomide daily dose by 1 dose level
Toxicities ascribed to dexamethasone such as severe manifestations of hypercorticism, including hyperglycemia, irritability, insomnia, or oral candidiasis	Hold dexamethasone dosing for up to 21 days to resolve toxicity and then restart at the same dose, or reduce dexamethasone doses by 50%

Patient Population Studied

Enrolled both transplantation-eligible and -ineligible patients with newly diagnosed, symptomatic MM. Patients were required to have an Eastern Cooperative Oncology Group performance status of 0–2. Patients were ineligible if they had G3/4 neuropathy, and an estimated creatinine clearance <50 mL/min (<0.83 mL/s) or serum creatinine ≥2 g/dL (>177 μmol/L)

Baseline Characteristics

Characteristics	N = 53
Age	
Median, years (range)	59 (35–81)
≥65 years, n (%)	23 (43)
Sex	
Male, n (%)	39 (74)
Female	14 (26)

(*continued*)

Toxicity

Treatment-Emergent Adverse Events During Induction (Cycles 1–8; n = 53)

	Any Grade, n (%)	G3/4, n (%)
Nonhematologic		
Hyperglycemia	38 (72)	12 (23)
Edema	25 (47)	2 (4)
Hypophosphatemia	24 (45)	13 (25)
Fatigue	20 (38)	1 (2)
Muscle cramping	17 (32)	0
Rash	15 (28)	4 (8)
Elevated liver function test	15 (28)	4 (8)
Diarrhea	14 (26)	0
Infection*	12 (23)	2 (4)
Phlebitis	12 (23)	0
Peripheral neuropathy	12 (23)[†]	0
Dyspnea	8 (15)	2 (4)
Deep-vein thrombosis	6 (11)	2 (4)
Pulmonary embolism	3 (6)	3 (6)
Nausea	7 (13)	0
Renal	5 (9)	1 (2)
Constipation	5 (9)	0
Mood alterations	5 (9)	1 (2)
Hematologic		
Thrombocytopenia	36 (68)	9 (17)
Anemia	32 (60)	11 (21)
Neutropenia	16 (30)	9 (17)

*Grade 3/4 events were pneumonia, and Grade 1/2 events were upper respiratory infections
[†]Three (6%) Grade 2, remaining Grade 1

Therapy Monitoring

1. Blood counts and physical examinations on day 1 of each cycle
2. Serum and urinary protein electrophoresis studies on day 1 of each cycle as indicated and at the end of treatment

Patient Population Studied
(continued)

ISS stage, n (%)	
I	21 (40)
II	18 (34)
III	14 (26)
Durie-Salmon stage, n (%)	
I	7 (13)
II	12 (24)
III	34 (63)
Unfavorable cytogenetics, n (%)*	17/51 (33)
del 13[†]/hypodiploidy	10/50 (20)
t(4;14)	5/49 (10)
t(14;16)	0/48
del 17p	7/48 (15)

*One or more of the abnormalities listed
[†]del 13 by metaphase only
ISS, International Staging System

TRANSPLANT-ELIGIBLE • FIRST-LINE INDUCTION

MULTIPLE MYELOMA REGIMEN: CYCLOPHOSPHAMIDE + BORTEZOMIB + DEXAMETHASONE (CYBORD) INDUCTION PRIOR TO AUTOLOGOUS STEM CELL TRANSPLANTATION (ASCT)

Reeder CB et al. Leukemia 2009;23:1337–1341

Bortezomib 1.3 mg/m² per dose intravenously over 3–5 seconds for 4 doses on days 1, 4, 8, and 11, every 28 days, for 4 cycles (total dosage/cycle = 5.2 mg/m²)

Cyclophosphamide 300 mg/m² per dose orally for 4 doses on days 1, 8, 15, and 22, every 28 days, for 4 cycles (total dosage/cycle = 1200 mg/m²)

Dexamethasone 40 mg/dose orally for 12 doses on days 1–4, days 9–12, and days 17–20 for 3 cycles (total dose/cycle = 480 mg)

Notes:
• Dose escalation was not allowed
• At the end of 4 cycles, patients proceeded to stem cell mobilization and harvest

Supportive Care
Antiemetic prophylaxis
Emetogenic potential on days with cyclophosphamide is **MODERATE–HIGH**
Emetogenic potential on days with bortezomib ± dexamethasone is **MINIMAL**
See Chapter 42 for antiemetic recommendations

Hematopoietic growth factor (CSF) prophylaxis
Primary prophylaxis may be indicated
See Chapter 43 for more information

Antimicrobial prophylaxis
Risk of fever and neutropenia is **INTERMEDIATE**
  Antimicrobial primary prophylaxis to be considered:
  • Antibacterial—consider a fluoroquinolone or no prophylaxis; *P. jirovecii* prophylaxis is recommended (eg, cotrimoxazole)
  • Antifungal—recommended; consider use during periods of neutropenia
  • Antiviral—antiherpes antivirals (eg, acyclovir, famciclovir, valacyclovir) throughout bortezomib induction

Steroid-associated gastritis
  Add a **proton pump inhibitor** during steroid use to prevent gastritis and duodenitis
Bisphosphonates
  All patients receiving primary therapy for symptomatic multiple myeloma should receive a bisphosphonate adjunctively.

Thromboprophylaxis
Risk assessment and recommendations for VTE prophylaxis in patients with multiple myeloma with individual or myeloma-related risk factors, or risk factors related to treatment

(continued)

Treatment Modifications

Note: dose reduction was allowed after the first cycle, but cyclophosphamide and bortezomib can be held during cycle 1 for neutropenia or thrombocytopenia G ≥3

Cyclophosphamide Dose Levels	
Starting dose	300 mg/m² per dose on days 1, 8, 15, and 22
Level −1	300 mg/m² per dose on days 1, 8, and 15
Level −2	300 mg/m² per dose on days 1 and 8
Level −3	300 mg/m² on day 1

Adverse Event	Treatment Modification
G3 hematologic toxicity	Reduce cyclophosphamide 1 dose level
G1/2 cystitis	Reduce cyclophosphamide 1 dose level
G3/4 cystitis	Discontinue cyclophosphamide

Bortezomib Dose Levels	
Starting dose	1.3 mg/m² per dose on days 1, 4, 8, and 11
Level −1	1 mg/m² per dose on days 1, 4, 8, and 11
Level −2	0.7 mg/m² per dose on days 1, 4, 8, and 11
Level −3	1.3 mg/m² per dose on days 1 and 8

Adverse Event	Treatment Modification
G3 thrombocytopenia (platelet count <50,000/mm³)	Reduce bortezomib dosage by 1 dose level

(continued)

(*continued*)

Individual risk factors
- Obesity (BMI ≥30 kg/m²)
- H/O VTE
- CVC or pacemaker
- Comorbid pathologies
  - Cardiac disease
  - Chronic renal disease
  - Diabetes
  - Acute infection
  - Immobilization
- Surgery
  - General surgery
  - Any anesthesia
  - Trauma
- Medications
  - Erythropoietin (epoetin alfa, darbepoetin)
  - Estrogenic compounds
  - Bevacizumab
- Clotting disorders
  - Thrombophilia

Myeloma-related risk factors
- Diagnosis of multiple myeloma
- Hyperviscosity

≤1 Individual or myeloma-related risk factor present:
- **Aspirin** 81–325 mg daily

≥2 Individual or myeloma-related risk factors present:
- **LMWH,*** equivalent to enoxaparin sodium 40 mg/day *or* **dalteparin sodium** 5000 IU/day; administer subcutaneously, *or*
- **Warfarin**, targeting an INR = 2–3

Concomitant treatment-related risk factors
Thalidomide or lenalidomide in combination with:
- High-dose dexamethasone (≥480 mg/month)
- Doxorubicin
- Multiagent chemotherapy

- **LMWH,*** equivalent to enoxaparin sodium 40 mg/day *or* **dalteparin sodium** 5000 IU/day; administer subcutaneously, *or*
- **Warfarin**, targeting an INR = 2–3

*LMWHs should be used with caution in individuals with impaired renal function (creatinine clearance <30 mL/min). Refer to product labeling for information about doses and administration schedules in renally impaired patients, and guidance for monitoring anti-Factor Xa concentrations

Abbreviations: CVC, central venous catheter; INR, international normalized ratio; LMWH, low-molecular-weight heparin; VTE, venous thromboembolic disease

References: Geerts WH et al. Chest 2008;133(6 Suppl):381S–453S
National Comprehensive Cancer Network. Multiple Myeloma, V.1.2014. (Accessed October 8, 2013, at http://www.nccn.org)
National Comprehensive Cancer Network. Venous Thromboembolic Disease, V.2.2013. (Accessed October 8, 2013, at http://www.nccn.org)
Palumbo A et al. Leukemia 2008;22:414–423

Patient Population Studied

Newly diagnosed, symptomatic MM of Durie-Salmon stage II or III, Eastern Cooperative Oncology Group performance status ≤2, creatinine ≤3.5 mg/dL (≤309 μmol/L), absolute neutrophil count ≥1000/mm³, platelets ≥100,000/mm³

Patient Characteristics

Mean age	60 (38–75) years
Gender: M/F	52%/48%
International Staging System, stages I/II/III	33/36/30%
Durie-Salmon stage II or III; symptomatic disease	100%
del13 in 16/32	16/32 (50%)
del17*	4/31 (13%)
t(4;14)*	6/33 (18%)
Favorable hyperdiploid karyotype	7/33 (21%)

*Genetic high-risk categories

Treatment Modifications
(*continued*)

Treatment Modification for Bortezomib-Induced Peripheral Neuropathy*

Severity of Peripheral Neuropathy	Modification of Dose and Schedule
G1 (paresthesias or loss of reflexes) without pain or loss of function	No action
G1 with pain or G2 (interferes with function but not with activities of daily living)	Reduce bortezomib dosage 1 dose level
G2 with pain or G3 (interferes with activities of daily living)	Withhold bortezomib treatment until toxicity resolves, then reinitiate reducing bortezomib dosage 1 dose level
G4 (permanent sensory loss that interferes with function)	Discontinue treatment

Dexamethasone Dose Levels

Starting dose	40 mg per dose on days 1–4, 9–12, and 17–20
Level −1	20 mg per dose on days 1–4, 9–12, and 17–20
Level −2	20 mg per dose on days 1–4
Level −3	10 mg per dose on days 1–4

Adverse Event	Treatment Modification
G2 muscle weakness, G3 gastrointestinal tract, hyperglycemia, confusion or mood alteration	Reduce dexamethasone dose by 1 dose level

*Richardson PG et al. J Clin Oncol 2006;24:3113–3120

Efficacy

Responses	By ITT (n = 33)	By ITT if Completed 4 Cycles (n = 28)	After SCT (n = 23)
ORR (≥PR)	29 (88%)	27 (96%)	23 (100%)
≥VGPR	20 (61%)*	20 (71%)	17 (74%)
PR	9 (27%)	7 (25%)	6 (26%)

ITT, intention to treat; ORR, overall response (partial response or better); PR, partial response; SCT, stem cell transplantation; ≥VGPR, very good partial response or better
*One in CR, 12 in nCR, and 7 in VGPR

Risk Category as Assessed by Bone Marrow Plasma Cell FISH Analysis and ISS Stage, and Corresponding Response After 4 Cycles

Risk Category	Frequency	ORR	≥VGPR
Deletion 13	50% (16/32)	94% (15/16)	63% (10/16)
Deletion 17	13% (4/31)	75% (3/4)	50% (2/4)
t(4;14)	18% (6/33)	83% (5/6)	50% (3/6)
Hyperdiploid	21% (7/33)	100% (7/7)	71% (5/7)
ISS stage 3	30% (10/33)	80% (8/10)	60% (6/10)

FISH, fluorescent in situ hybridization; ISS, international staging system; ORR, overall response; VGPR, very good partial response

Toxicity

Adverse Events	G3/4*
Anemia	12%
Neutropenia	13%
Thrombocytopenia	25%
Hyperglycemia	13%
Diarrhea	6%
Hypokalemia	9%
Neuropathy	7%
Thrombosis	7%

*National Cancer Institute Common Terminology Criteria for Adverse Events (version 3.0) severity grades

Therapy Monitoring

1. Blood counts and physical examinations on day 1 of each cycle
2. Serum and urinary protein electrophoresis studies on day 1 of each cycle as indicated and at the end of treatment

TRANSPLANT-ELIGIBLE • FIRST LINE INDUCTION

MULTIPLE MYELOMA REGIMEN: BORTEZOMIB + THALIDOMIDE + DEXAMETHASONE INDUCTION PRIOR TO AUTOLOGOUS STEM CELL TRANSPLANTATION (ASCT)

Cavo M et al. Lancet 2010;376:2075–2085

Bortezomib 1.3 mg/m^2 per dose; administer by intravenous injection over 3–5 seconds for 4 doses on days 1, 4, 8, and 11, every 21 days for 3 cycles (total dosage/cycle = 5.2 mg/m^2)
Thalidomide 200 mg/day; administer orally, continually, for 21 consecutive days on days 1–21, every 21 days for 3 cycles (total dose/cycle = 4200 mg)
Dexamethasone 40 mg per dose; administer orally for 8 doses on days 1, 2, 4, 5, 8, 9, 11, and 12, every 21 days for 3 cycles (total dose/cycle = 320 mg)

Supportive Care
Antiemetic prophylaxis
Emetogenic potential is **MINIMAL**
See Chapter 42 for antiemetic recommendations

Hematopoietic growth factor (CSF) prophylaxis
Primary prophylaxis is **NOT** indicated
See Chapter 43 for more information

Antimicrobial prophylaxis
Risk of fever and neutropenia is **HIGH**
  Antimicrobial primary prophylaxis is recommended:
  • Antibacterial—consider fluoroquinolone prophylaxis; *P. jirovecii* prophylaxis is recommended (eg, cotrimoxazole)
  • Antifungal—recommended
  • Antiviral—antiherpes antivirals (eg, acyclovir, famciclovir, valacyclovir)

Bisphosphonates
All patients receiving primary therapy for symptomatic multiple myeloma should receive a bisphosphonate adjunctively.

Thromboprophylaxis
Risk assessment and recommendations for VTE prophylaxis in patients with multiple myeloma with individual or myeloma-related risk factors, or risk factors related to treatment

(continued)

Treatment Modifications

Bortezomib Dosage Levels	
Dose Level 1	1.3 mg/m^2
Dose Level −1	1 mg/m^2
Dose Level −2	0.7 mg/m^2

Thalidomide Dose Levels	
Dose Level 1	200 mg daily
Dose Level −1	100 mg daily
Dose Level −2	50 mg daily

Adverse Event	Treatment Modification
Febrile neutropenia	Withhold therapy until fever abates then resume therapy
G4 hematologic toxicity	Withhold therapy until ANC >750/mm^3 and platelets >50,000/mm^3, then resume therapy at a dose decreased by 1 dose level
G3/4 nonhematologic toxicity	Interrupt therapy, follow clinically. After toxicity abates to G ≤2, resume therapy at a dose decreased by 1 dose level
G ≥3 thalidomide neuropathy	Interrupt therapy and follow clinically. After toxicity abates to G ≤2, resume therapy at a dose decreased by 1 dose level
Toxicities ascribed to dexamethasone such as severe manifestations of hypercorticism, including hyperglycemia, irritability, insomnia, and oral candidiasis	Reduce dexamethasone dose to 20 mg per dose

(continued)

(*continued*)

Individual risk factors
• Obesity (BMI ≥30 kg/m²)
• H/O VTE
• CVC or pacemaker
• Comorbid pathologies
  ▪ Cardiac disease
  ▪ Chronic renal disease
  ▪ Diabetes
  ▪ Acute infection
  ▪ Immobilization
• Surgery
  ▪ General surgery
  ▪ Any anesthesia
  ▪ Trauma
• Medications
  ▪ Erythropoietin (epoetin alfa, darbepoetin)
  ▪ Estrogenic compounds
  ▪ Bevacizumab
• Clotting disorders
  ▪ Thrombophilia
Myeloma-related risk factors
• Diagnosis of multiple myeloma
• Hyperviscosity
	≤1 Individual or myeloma-related risk factor present:
	• **Aspirin** 81–325 mg daily
	
	≥2 Individual or myeloma-related risk factors present:
	• **LMWH,** * equivalent to enoxaparin sodium 40 mg/day *or* **dalteparin sodium** 5000 IU/day; administer subcutaneously, *or*
	• **Warfarin**, targeting an INR = 2–3

Concomitant treatment-related risk factors Thalidomide or lenalidomide in combination with: • High-dose dexamethasone (≥480 mg/month) • Doxorubicin • Multiagent chemotherapy	• **LMWH,** * equivalent to enoxaparin sodium 40 mg/day *or* **dalteparin sodium** 5000 IU/day; administer subcutaneously, *or* • **Warfarin**, targeting an INR = 2–3

*LMWHs should be used with caution in individuals with impaired renal function (creatinine clearance <30 mL/min). Refer to product labeling for information about doses and administration schedules in renally impaired patients, and guidance for monitoring anti-Factor Xa concentrations

Abbreviations: CVC, central venous catheter; INR, international normalized ratio; LMWH, low-molecular-weight heparin; VTE, venous thromboembolic disease

References: Geerts WH et al. Chest 2008;133(6 Suppl):381S–453S

National Comprehensive Cancer Network. Multiple Myeloma, V.1.2014. (Accessed October 8, 2013, at http://www.nccn.org)

National Comprehensive Cancer Network. Venous Thromboembolic Disease, V.2.2013. (Accessed October 8, 2013, at http://www.nccn.org)

Palumbo A et al. Leukemia 2008;22:414–423

Treatment Modifications
(*continued*)

Treatment Modification for Bortezomib-Induced Peripheral Neuropathy*

Severity of Peripheral Neuropathy	Modification of Dose and Schedule
G1 (paresthesias or loss of reflexes) without pain or loss of function	No action
G1 with pain or G2 (interferes with function, but not with activities of daily living)	Reduce bortezomib dosage to 1 mg/m² per dose
G2 with pain or G3 (interferes with activities of daily living)	Withhold bortezomib treatment until toxicity resolves, then reinitiate at a dosage of 0.7 mg/m² per dose once weekly
G4 (permanent sensory loss that interferes with function)	Discontinue treatment

*Richardson PG et al. J Clin Oncol 2006;24:3113–3120

Patient Population Studied

A phase 3 study of 480 patients, aged 18–65 years, with previously untreated, symptomatic, newly diagnosed multiple myeloma who were eligible for stem cell transplantation. Eligible subjects demonstrated a Karnofsky performance status ≥60%. Patients with peripheral neuropathy G ≥2, a history of venous thromboembolism, or a previous diagnosis of thrombophilic alterations were ineligible

Efficacy

Response to Different Treatment Phases and Best Response

N = 236	% (95% CI)
After induction therapy	
Complete response	19% (13.7–23.6)
Complete or near complete response	31% (25–36.8)
Very good partial response or better	62% (55.7–68.1)
Partial response or better	93% (90–96.4)
Minimal response or stable disease	7% (3.6–10)
Progressive disease	5% (2.3–7.8)
After first autologous stem cell transplantation	
Complete response	38% (31.5–43.9)
Complete or near complete response	52% (45.7–58.5)
Very good partial response or better	79% (73.6–84)
Partial response or better	93% (90–96.4)
Minimal response or stable disease	6% (3.2–9.5)
Progressive disease	<1% (0–1.3)
After second autologous stem cell transplantation	
Complete response	42% (35.2–47.8)
Complete or near complete response	55% (48.7–61.4)
Very good partial response or better	82% (76.9–86.7)
Partial response or better	93% (90–96.4)
Minimal response or stable disease	6% (2.9–8.9)
Progressive disease	8% (4.9–11.9)
After consolidation therapy	
Complete response	49% (42.8–55.5)
Complete or near complete response	62% (56.1–68.5)
Very good partial response or better	85% (80.6–89.7)
Partial response or better	92% (89–95.8)
Minimal response or stable disease	5% (2.3–7.9)
Progressive disease	9% (5.2–12.4)
Best response to overall treatment protocol	
Complete response	58% (51.3–63.9)
Complete or near complete response	71% (65.4–77)
Very good partial response or better	89% (85–93)
Partial response or better	96% (93.7–98.6)
Minimal response, stable disease, or progressive disease	4% (1.4–6.3)

Toxicity

Serious and G3/4 adverse events reported in ≥2% of patients during induction therapy

Any serious adverse event	13%
Any Grade 3 or 4 adverse event	56%
Any Grade 3 or 4 nonhematologic adverse event	51%
Skin rash	10%
Peripheral neuropathy	10%
Deep-vein thrombosis	3%
Constipation	4%
Infections excluding herpes zoster	3%
Gastrointestinal events (excluding constipation)	2%
Cardiac toxicity	2%
Liver toxicity	2%
Discontinuation during or after induction therapy	6%
Toxic effects	4%
Disease progression	0
Other reasons	1%
Early death	<1%

Nonhematologic adverse events of any grade reported in at least 10% of patients during induction therapy (n = 236)

	% G1–4	% G3/4
Constipation	42	4
Neuropathy	34	10
Skin rash	28	10
Fever	12	1
Infections	10	3
Edema	11	1
Gastrointestinal events (excluding constipation)	19	2

Therapy Monitoring

1. *Before each cycle:* CBC with differential and blood chemistries (including BUN, creatinine, and calcium)
2. *Every 6 weeks to 3 months:* Measure serum and urine M-protein

TRANSPLANT-ELIGIBLE • FIRST-LINE INDUCTION

MULTIPLE MYELOMA REGIMEN: BORTEZOMIB + DOXORUBICIN + DEXAMETHASONE INDUCTION PRIOR TO AUTOLOGOUS STEM CELL TRANSPLANTATION (ASCT)

Sonneveld P et al. J Clin Oncol 2012;30:2946–2955

Induction:
Bortezomib 1.3 mg/m^2 per dose intravenously over 3–5 seconds for 4 doses on days 1, 4, 8, and 11, every 28 days for 3 cycles (total dosage/cycle = 5.2 mg/m^2)
Doxorubicin 9 mg/m^2 per day by slow intravenous injection over 3–5 minutes for 4 consecutive days on days 1–4, every 28 days for 3 cycles (total dosage/cycle = 36 mg/m^2)
Dexamethasone 40 mg/dose orally for 12 doses on days 1–4, days 9–12, and days 17–20 for 3 cycles, every 28 days, (total dose/cycle = 480 mg)
Notes:
- Stem cell collection was performed 4–6 weeks after induction
- High-dose melphalan (HDM) 200 mg/m^2, and autologous stem cell transplantation (ASCT) were administered
- Starting 4 weeks after HDM, patients received maintenance with bortezomib 1.3 mg/m^2 intravenously every 2 weeks for 2 years
- Patients with an HLA-identical sibling could proceed to nonmyeloablative allogeneic stem cell transplantation (alloSCT) after HDM
- Maintenance therapy was not given after alloSCT

Supportive Care
Antiemetic prophylaxis
Emetogenic potential on days with doxorubicin is **LOW**
Emetogenic potential on days with bortezomib ± dexamethasone is **MINIMAL**
See Chapter 42 for antiemetic recommendations

Hematopoietic growth factor (CSF) prophylaxis
Primary prophylaxis is **NOT** indicated
See Chapter 43 for more information

Antimicrobial prophylaxis
Risk of fever and neutropenia is **INTERMEDIATE**
  Antimicrobial primary prophylaxis to be considered:
  - Antibacterial—consider a fluoroquinolone or no prophylaxis; *P. jirovecii* prophylaxis is recommended (eg, cotrimoxazole)
  - Antifungal—recommended; consider use during periods of neutropenia
  - Antiviral—antiherpes antivirals (eg, acyclovir, famciclovir, valacyclovir) throughout bortezomib induction

Steroid-associated gastritis
  Add a **proton pump inhibitor** during steroid use to prevent gastritis and duodenitis
Bisphosphonates
  All patients receiving primary therapy for symptomatic multiple myeloma should receive a bisphosphonate adjunctively.

Thromboprophylaxis
Risk assessment and recommendations for VTE prophylaxis in patients with multiple myeloma with individual or myeloma-related risk factors, or risk factors related to treatment

(continued)

Treatment Modifications

Adverse Event	Treatment Modification
G3 nonhematologic toxicity or G4 hematologic toxicity	Hold treatment until toxicity resolves to G ≤1, then resume with bortezomib 1 mg/m^2 per dose and/or 25% reduction in doxorubicin dosage
G3 nonhematologic toxicity or G4 hematologic toxicity in a patient receiving bortezomib 1 mg/m^2	Hold treatment until toxicity resolves to G ≤1, then resume with bortezomib 0.7 mg/m^2 per dose and/or 25% reduction in doxorubicin dosage
Severe manifestations of hypercorticism, including severe hyperglycemia, irritability, insomnia, or oral candidiasis	Reduce daily dexamethasone dose by 20% for G3 toxicity, and by 40% for G4 or recurrent G3 toxicity

Treatment Modification for Bortezomib-Induced Peripheral Neuropathy*

Severity of Peripheral Neuropathy	Modification of Dose and Schedule
G1 (paresthesias or loss of reflexes) without pain or loss of function	No action
G1 with pain or G2 (interferes with function but not with activities of daily living)	Reduce bortezomib dosage to 1 mg/m^2 per dose
G2 with pain or G3 (interferes with activities of daily living)	Withhold bortezomib treatment until toxicity resolves, then reinitiate with bortezomib 0.7 mg/m^2 per dose once weekly
G4 (permanent sensory loss that interferes with function)	Discontinue treatment

*Richardson PG et al. J Clin Oncol 2006;24:3113–3120

(continued)

Individual risk factors
• Obesity (BMI ≥30 kg/m²)
• H/O VTE
• CVC or pacemaker
• Comorbid pathologies
  ▪ Cardiac disease
  ▪ Chronic renal disease
  ▪ Diabetes
  ▪ Acute infection
  ▪ Immobilization
• Surgery
  ▪ General surgery
  ▪ Any anesthesia
  ▪ Trauma
• Medications
  ▪ Erythropoietin (epoetin alfa, darbepoetin)
  ▪ Estrogenic compounds
  ▪ Bevacizumab
• Clotting disorders
  ▪ Thrombophilia
Myeloma-related risk factors
• Diagnosis of multiple myeloma
• Hyperviscosity
	≤1 Individual or myeloma-related risk factor present:
	• **Aspirin** 81–325 mg daily
	
	≥2 Individual or myeloma-related risk factors present:
	• **LMWH,*** equivalent to enoxaparin sodium 40 mg/day *or* **dalteparin sodium** 5000 IU/day; administer subcutaneously, *or*
	• **Warfarin,** targeting an INR = 2–3

Concomitant treatment-related risk factors Thalidomide or lenalidomide in combination with: • High-dose dexamethasone (≥480 mg/month) • Doxorubicin • Multiagent chemotherapy	• **LMWH,*** equivalent to enoxaparin sodium 40 mg/day *or* **dalteparin sodium** 5000 IU/day; administer subcutaneously, *or* • **Warfarin,** targeting an INR = 2–3

*LMWHs should be used with caution in individuals with impaired renal function (creatinine clearance <30 mL/min). Refer to product labeling for information about doses and administration schedules in renally impaired patients, and guidance for monitoring anti-Factor Xa concentrations

Abbreviations: CVC, central venous catheter; INR, international normalized ratio; LMWH, low-molecular-weight heparin; VTE, venous thromboembolic disease

References: Geerts WH et al. Chest 2008;133(6 Suppl):381S–453S

National Comprehensive Cancer Network. Multiple Myeloma, V.1.2014. (Accessed October 8, 2013, at http://www.nccn.org)

National Comprehensive Cancer Network. Venous Thromboembolic Disease, V.2.2013. (Accessed October 8, 2013, at http://www.nccn.org)

Palumbo A et al. Leukemia 2008;22:414–423

Patient Population Studied

Patients 18–65 years of age with newly diagnosed MM (Durie-Salmon stage II to III) WHO performance status 0 to 2, or WHO 3 when caused by MM. Exclusion criteria were systemic amyloid light-chain amyloidosis, nonsecretory MM, neuropathy G ≥2. Prior corticosteroids were allowed for a maximum of 5 days. Patients with renal impairment were not excluded. Local radiotherapy for painful MM lesions was allowed

Patient Characteristic (n = 413)	No. (%)
ISIS stage	
I	144 (35)
II	150 (36)
III	81 (20)
IV	38 (9)

(continued)

Efficacy (n = 413)

Response	No. (%)
Response after induction	
CR	29 (7)
≥nCR	46 (11)
≥VGPR	174 (42)
≥PR	322 (78)
Response after high-dose melphalan (HDM)	
CR	85 (21)
≥nCR	127 (31)
≥VGPR	254 (62)
≥PR	363 (88)
Response overall	
CR	147 (36)
≥nCR	201 (49)
≥VGPR	312 (76)
≥PR	373 (90)
Response upgrade during maintenance	
Any response upgrade*	93 (23)
<CR → CR	48 (12)
<nCR → nCR	23 (6)
<VGPR → VGPR	20 (5)
<PR → PR	2*
ISS stage I (n = 144)	
CR	59 (41)
≥nCR	78 (54)
≥VGPR	115 (80)
≥PR	132 (92)
ISS stage II (n = 150)	
CR	51 (34)
≥nCR	70 (47)
≥VGPR	109 (73)
≥PR	134 (89)
ISS stage III (n = 81)	
CR	26 (32)
≥nCR	35 (43)
≥VGPR	56 (69)
≥PR	70 (86)

(continued)

Patient Population Studied (continued)

M-protein isotype	
IgA	92 (22)
IgG	251 (61)
IgD	5 (1)
LCD	63 (15)
Other	2
M-protein light chain (unknown = 1 [0%])	
Kappa	277 (67)
Lambda	135 (33)
Creatinine, mg/dL (unknown = 1 [0%])	
≤2	376 (91)
>2	36 (9)
Number of skeletal lesions (unknown = 12 [3%])	
0	102 (25)
1–2	44 (11)
≥3	255 (62)
Serum LDH (unknown = 12 [3%])	
≤ULN	329 (80)
>ULN	72 (17)
Genetic abnormalities	
del(13q) done in 361 (88%)	148/361 (41)
t(4;14) done in 250 (615)	35/250 (14)
del(17p13) done in 289 (70%)	25/289 (9)
Hematologic abnormalities	
Median β_2-microglobulin, mg/L	3.40
Median hemoglobin, mmol/L	6.6
Median calcium, mmol/L	2.34
Median number of bone marrow plasma cells	40

Efficacy (n = 413) *continued*

ISS stage unknown (n = 38)

CR	11 (29)
≥nCR	18 (47)
≥VGPR	32 (84)
≥PR	37 (97)

β₂-microglobulin >3 mg/L (n = 223)

CR	77 (35)
≥nCR	103 (46)
≥VGPR	163 (73)
≥PR	189 (79)

Creatinine >2 mg/dL (n = 36)

CR	13 (36)
≥nCR	19 (53)
≥VGPR	28 (78)
≥PR	31 (86)

Genetic abnormalities

del(13/13q14) (n = 148)

≥nCR	76 (51)
≥VGPR	124 (84)

t(4;14) (n = 35)

≥nCR	20 (57)
≥VGPR	30 (86)

del(17p13) (δ = 25)

≥nCR	13 (52)
≥VGPR	18 (72)

CR, complete response; ISS, International Staging System; nCR, near complete response; PR, partial response; VGPR, very good partial response
*Median time to any response upgrade after start of maintenance was 7 months (range, 1–57 months)

Median PFS	35 months
Median PFSA (ie, without censoring of alloSCT)	34 months
Median OS	Not reached at 66 months
5-year OS	61%
PFS calculated from the time of last HDM	31 months

Toxicity

Variable	Induction (n = 410)		Bortezomib Maintenance (n = 229)	
	No.	%	No.	%
Any AE	400	98	222	97
AE G3/4	258	63	110	48
AE classified as SAE	187	46	77	34
AE leading to discontinuation, dose reduction, or delay of bortezomib	112	27	81	35
Death from AE	7	2	0	0

	All Grades	G3/4	All Grades	G3/4
Hematologic Toxicities (%)				
Anemia	28	8	27	1
Neutropenia	4	3	2	0
Thrombocytopenia	39	10	37	4
Infections	56	26	75	24
Herpes zoster	2	0	2	0
Nonhematologic Toxicities (%)				
Wasting, fatigue	27	4	20	1
GI symptoms	67	11	48	5
Cardiac disorders	27	8	19	3
Thrombosis	6	4	1	1
Peripheral neuropathy	37	24	33	5

AE, adverse event (including infection); SAE, serious adverse event

Therapy Monitoring

1. Blood counts and physical examinations on day 1 of each cycle
2. Serum and urinary protein electrophoresis studies on day 1 of each cycle as indicated and at the end of treatment

TRANSPLANT-ELIGIBLE • FIRST-LINE INDUCTION

MULTIPLE MYELOMA REGIMEN: LENALIDOMIDE + LOW-DOSE DEXAMETHASONE INDUCTION PRIOR TO AUTOLOGOUS STEM CELL TRANSPLANTATION (ASCT)

Rajkumar SV et al. Lancet Oncol 2010;11:29–37

Lenalidomide 25 mg/day; administer orally, continually, for 21 consecutive days on days 1–21, every 28 days (total dose/cycle = 525 mg)

Dexamethasone 40 mg/dose; administer orally for 4 doses on days 1, 8, 15, and 22, every 28 days (total dose/cycle = 160 mg)

Supportive Care

Antiemetic prophylaxis
Emetogenic potential is **MINIMAL–LOW**
See Chapter 42 for antiemetic recommendations

Hematopoietic growth factor (CSF) prophylaxis
Primary prophylaxis may be indicated
See Chapter 43 for more information

Antimicrobial prophylaxis
Risk of fever and neutropenia is **INTERMEDIATE**
  Antimicrobial primary prophylaxis to be considered:
  • Antibacterial—consider a fluoroquinolone or no prophylaxis; *P. jirovecii* prophylaxis is recommended (eg, cotrimoxazole)
  • Antifungal—recommended; consider use during periods of neutropenia
  • Antiviral—antiherpes antivirals (eg, acyclovir, famciclovir, valacyclovir) throughout bortezomib induction

Bisphosphonates

All patients receiving primary therapy for symptomatic multiple myeloma should receive a bisphosphonate adjunctively.

Thromboprophylaxis

Risk assessment and recommendations for VTE prophylaxis in patients with multiple myeloma with individual or myeloma-related risk factors, or risk factors related to treatment

Individual risk factors
• Obesity (BMI ≥30 kg/m²)
• H/O VTE
• CVC or pacemaker
• Comorbid pathologies
  ▪ Cardiac disease
  ▪ Chronic renal disease
  ▪ Diabetes
  ▪ Acute infection
  ▪ Immobilization
• Surgery
  ▪ General surgery
  ▪ Any anesthesia
  ▪ Trauma
• Medications
  ▪ Erythropoietin (epoetin alfa, darbepoetin)
  ▪ Estrogenic compounds
  ▪ Bevacizumab
• Clotting disorders
  ▪ Thrombophilia

Myeloma-related risk factors
• Diagnosis of multiple myeloma
• Hyperviscosity

≤1 Individual or myeloma-related risk factor present:
• **Aspirin** 81–325 mg daily

≥2 Individual or myeloma-related risk factors present:
• **LMWH,** * **equivalent to enoxaparin sodium** 40 mg/day *or* **dalteparin sodium** 5000 IU/day; administer subcutaneously, *or*
• **Warfarin**, targeting an INR = 2–3

Treatment Modifications

Adverse Event	Treatment Modification
Platelet count <30,000/mm³	Interrupt lenalidomide treatment, follow CBC weekly. Resume lenalidomide at 15 mg/day after platelet count is ≥30,000/mm³
For each subsequent platelet count <30,000/mm³	Interrupt lenalidomide treatment, follow CBC weekly. After platelet count recovers to ≥30,000/mm³, resume lenalidomide at a dose decreased from the previous dose by 5 mg/day, but the daily dose should not be less than 5 mg/day
ANC <1000/mm³	Interrupt lenalidomide treatment, follow CBC weekly. Resume lenalidomide at 15 mg/day after ANC ≥1000/mm³
For each subsequent ANC <1000/mm³	Interrupt lenalidomide treatment, follow CBC weekly. After ANC recovers to ≥1000/mm³, resume lenalidomide at a dose decreased from the previous dose by 5 mg/day, but the daily dose should not be less than 5 mg/day
Febrile neutropenia	Interrupt lenalidomide treatment, follow closely, and resume lenalidomide at 15 mg/day after fever abates
G3/4 nonhematologic toxicity	Interrupt lenalidomide treatment, follow clinically. After toxicity abates to G ≤2, resume lenalidomide at a dose decreased from the previous dose by 5 mg/day, but the daily dose should not be less than 5 mg/day

(continued)

(continued)

(*continued*)

Concomitant treatment-related risk factors Thalidomide or lenalidomide in combination with: • High-dose dexamethasone (≥480 mg/month) • Doxorubicin • Multiagent chemotherapy	• **LMWH,*** equivalent to enoxaparin **sodium** 40 mg/day *or* **dalteparin sodium** 5000 IU/day; administer subcutaneously, *or* • **Warfarin**, targeting an INR = 2–3

*LMWHs should be used with caution in individuals with impaired renal function (creatinine clearance <30 mL/min). Refer to product labeling for information about doses and administration schedules in renally impaired patients, and guidance for monitoring anti-Factor Xa concentrations
Abbreviations: CVC, central venous catheter; INR, international normalized ratio; LMWH, low-molecular-weight heparin; VTE, venous thromboembolic disease
References: Geerts WH et al. Chest 2008;133(6 Suppl):381S–453S
National Comprehensive Cancer Network. Multiple Myeloma, V.1.2014. (Accessed October 8, 2013, at http://www.nccn.org)
National Comprehensive Cancer Network. Venous Thromboembolic Disease, V.2.2013. (Accessed October 8, 2013, at http://www.nccn.org)
Palumbo A et al. Leukemia 2008;22:414–423

Efficacy (n = 208)

Best overall Response to Therapy	Percentage of Patients
Overall response rate (partial response or better)	70%
Complete plus very good partial response	40%
Complete response	4%
Immunofixation-negative complete response	10%
Very good partial response	26%
Partial response	30%
Minimal response	13%
No response/stable disease	8%
Progressive disease	2%
Unevaluable	7%

1-year overall survival*	96% (95% CI, 94–99)
2-year overall survival*	87% (95% CI, 81–93)
1-year overall survival, ages <65 years old	98% (95% CI, 92–99)
1-year overall survival, ages ≥65 years old	94% (95% CI, 89–99)
Median time to partial response or better	1 month[†]
Median response duration	24.1 months (95% CI, 21.5–28.1)
Median progression-free survival	25.3 months (22.3–not reached)

*Overall survival was not a protocol-specified end point in this study. However, the study was stopped on recommendations of the independent data monitoring committee at a median follow-up of 12.5 months (95% CI, 11.5–14.6), because overall survival was significantly higher with low-dose dexamethasone than with high-dose dexamethasone (P = 0.0002). All patients in the high-dose group were instructed to cross over to receive low-dose dexamethasone
[†]Among patients who responded

Treatment Modifications
(*continued*)

Toxicities ascribed to dexamethasone such as severe manifestations of hypercorticism, including hyperglycemia, irritability, insomnia, and oral candidiasis	Reduce dexamethasone dose to 20 mg per day

Lenalidomide starting dose adjustment for renal impairment in multiple myeloma (days 1–21 of each 28-day cycle)

Moderate renal impairment CrCl 30–60 mL/min (0.5–1 mL/s)	10 mg lenalidomide every 24 hours
Severe renal impairment CrCl <30 mL/min (<0.5 mL/s), not requiring dialysis	15 mg lenalidomide every 48 hours
End-stage renal disease CrCl <30 mL/min (<0.5 mL/s), requiring dialysis	5 mg/day. On dialysis days, administer a daily dose following dialysis

CrCl, Creatinine clearance

Patient Population Studied

Randomized phase 3 trial of 445 patients with newly diagnosed multiple myeloma. Patients were eligible if they had previously untreated symptomatic multiple myeloma, bone marrow plasmacytosis (≥10% plasma cells or sheets of plasma cells), or a biopsy-proven plasmacytoma, and measurable disease defined as serum monoclonal protein >10 g/L or urine monoclonal protein ≥0.2 g/day or more. Patients were excluded if they had G ≥2 peripheral neuropathy, active infection, current or prior deep-vein thrombosis, or Eastern Cooperative Oncology Group performance status 3/4

Toxicity

G ≥3 Toxicities (n = 220)

Toxicity	Percentage of Patients
Hematologic	
Hemoglobin	7%
Platelets	5%
Neutrophils	20%
Nonhematologic	
Deep-vein thrombosis or pulmonary embolism	12%
Infection or pneumonia	9%
Hyperglycemia	6%
Cardiac ischemia	<1%
Atrial fibrillation or flutter	<1%
Fatigue	9%
Neuropathy	2%
Nonneuropathic weakness	4%
Summary	
Any G ≥3 toxicity in first 4 months	35%
Any G ≥3 nonhematologic toxicity at any time during therapy	48%
Any G ≥4 nonhematologic toxicity at any time during therapy	14%
Early mortality (first 4 months)	<1%
Reason for discontinuation (n = 222)	
Treatment completed per protocol	25%
Disease progression	17%
Adverse events or complications	23%
Death on study	3%
Patient withdrawal or refusal	5%
Alternative therapy	17%
Other complicating disease	1%
Other	8%

Therapy Monitoring

1. *Before each cycle:* CBC with differential and blood chemistries (including BUN, creatinine, and calcium)
2. *Every 6 weeks to 3 months:* Measure serum and urine M-protein

TRANSPLANT-ELIGIBLE • FIRST-LINE INDUCTION

MULTIPLE MYELOMA REGIMEN: BORTEZOMIB + DEXAMETHASONE INDUCTION PRIOR TO AUTOLOGOUS STEM CELL TRANSPLANTATION (ASCT)

Harousseau J-L et al. J Clin Oncol 2010;28:4621–4629

Bortezomib 1.3 mg/m^2 per dose; administer by intravenous injection over 3–5 seconds for 4 doses on days 1, 4, 8, and 11, every 3 weeks for 4 cycles (total dosage/cycle = 5.2 mg/m^2)

Dexamethasone 40 mg/dose; administer orally, as follows:

• *Cycles 1 and 2:* For 4 consecutive days on days 1–4, and for 4 consecutive days on days 9–12, every 3 weeks for 2 cycles (total dose/cycle = 320 mg)

• *Cycles 3 and 4:* For 4 consecutive days on days 1–4, every 3 weeks for 2 cycles (total dose/cycle = 160 mg)

Supportive Care

Antiemetic prophylaxis
Emetogenic potential is **MINIMAL**
See Chapter 42 for antiemetic recommendations

Hematopoietic growth factor (CSF) prophylaxis
Primary prophylaxis is **NOT** indicated
See Chapter 43 for more information

Antimicrobial prophylaxis
Risk of fever and neutropenia is **HIGH**
  Antimicrobial primary prophylaxis is recommended:
• Antibacterial—consider fluoroquinolone prophylaxis; *P. jirovecii* prophylaxis is recommended (eg, cotrimoxazole)
• Antifungal—recommended
• Antiviral—antiherpes antivirals (eg, acyclovir, famciclovir, valacyclovir)

Bisphosphonates
All patients receiving primary therapy for symptomatic multiple myeloma should receive a bisphosphonate adjunctively.

Thromboprophylaxis
Risk assessment and recommendations for VTE prophylaxis in patients with multiple myeloma with individual or myeloma-related risk factors, or risk factors related to treatment

(continued)

Treatment Modifications

Adverse Event	Treatment Modification
Febrile neutropenia	Withhold therapy until fever abates, then resume therapy at the same dosages and schedules
G4 hematologic toxicity	Withhold therapy until counts recover to ANC >750/mm^3 and platelets >50,000/mm^3, then resume therapy
G3/4 nonhematologic toxicity	Interrupt therapy, follow clinically, and resume therapy when toxicity G ≤2
Toxicities ascribed to dexamethasone such as severe manifestations of hypercorticism, including hyperglycemia, irritability and insomnia, oral candidiasis	Reduce dexamethasone dose to 20 mg per dose

Treatment Modification for Bortezomib-Induced Peripheral Neuropathy*

Severity of Peripheral Neuropathy	Modification of Dose and Schedule
G1 (paresthesias or loss of reflexes) without pain or loss of function	No action
G1 with pain or G2 (interferes with function, but not with activities of daily living)	Reduce bortezomib dosage to 1 mg/m^2 per dose
G2 with pain or G3 (interferes with activities of daily living)	Withhold bortezomib treatment until toxicity resolves, then reinitiate at a dosage of 0.7 mg/m^2 per dose once weekly
G4 (permanent sensory loss that interferes with function)	Discontinue treatment

*Richardson PG et al. J Clin Oncol 2006;24:3113–3120

(continued)

Individual risk factors	
• Obesity (BMI ≥30 kg/m²)	
• H/O VTE	
• CVC or pacemaker	
• Comorbid pathologies	
▪ Cardiac disease	
▪ Chronic renal disease	**≤1 Individual or myeloma-related risk**
▪ Diabetes	**factor present:**
▪ Acute infection	• **Aspirin** 81–325 mg daily
▪ Immobilization	
• Surgery	
▪ General surgery	**≥2 Individual or myeloma-related risk**
▪ Any anesthesia	**factors present:**
▪ Trauma	• **LMWH,** * equivalent to enoxaparin
• Medications	sodium 40 mg/day *or* **dalteparin**
▪ Erythropoietin (epoetin alfa, darbepoetin)	sodium 5000 IU/day; administer
▪ Estrogenic compounds	subcutaneously, *or*
▪ Bevacizumab	• **Warfarin,** targeting an INR = 2–3
• Clotting disorders	
▪ Thrombophilia	
Myeloma-related risk factors	
• Diagnosis of multiple myeloma	
• Hyperviscosity	
Concomitant treatment-related risk factors	• **LMWH,** * equivalent to enoxaparin
Thalidomide or lenalidomide in combination with:	sodium 40 mg/day *or* **dalteparin**
• High-dose dexamethasone (≥480 mg/month)	sodium 5000 IU/day; administer
• Doxorubicin	subcutaneously, *or*
• Multiagent chemotherapy	• **Warfarin,** targeting an INR = 2–3

*LMWHs should be used with caution in individuals with impaired renal function (creatinine clearance <30 mL/min). Refer to product labeling for information about doses and administration schedules in renally impaired patients, and guidance for monitoring anti-Factor Xa concentrations

Abbreviations: CVC, central venous catheter; INR, international normalized ratio; LMWH, low-molecular-weight heparin; VTE, venous thromboembolic disease

References: Geerts WH et al. Chest 2008;133(6 Suppl):381S–453S

National Comprehensive Cancer Network. Multiple Myeloma, V.1.2014. (Accessed October 8, 2013, at http://www.nccn.org)

National Comprehensive Cancer Network. Venous Thromboembolic Disease, V.2.2013. (Accessed October 8, 2013, at http://www.nccn.org)

Palumbo A et al. Leukemia 2008;22:414–423

Patient Population Studied

Phase 3 study of 482 patients with multiple myeloma who were ≤65 years of age and eligible for autologous stem cell transplantation. All patients had untreated symptomatic MM with measurable paraprotein in serum (>10 g/L) or urine (>0.2 g/24 hours). Patients with confirmed diagnosis of amyloidosis and G ≥2 peripheral neuropathy were excluded

Efficacy

Response to Induction Therapy Overall and According to Baseline Disease Stage and Prognostic Factors

Evaluable Population (n = 223)	
ORR (at least PR)	78.5%
At least VGPR	37.7%
CR/nCR	14.8%
CR	5.8%
MR + SD	12.6%
PD	4.5%
Death	0.5%
Not assessable	4%

ORR and at Least VGPR and CR/nCR Response Rates by Disease Stage

ISS 1	
ORR	81.4%
At least VGPR	37.3%
CR/nCR	15.7%
ISS 2	
ORR	71.6%
At least VGPR	35.8%
CR/nCR	14.8%
ISS 3	
ORR	76.9%
At least VGPR	40.4%
CR/nCR	13.5%

(continued)

Toxicity (n = 239)

Toxicity	Percentage of Patients
Any AE	96.7%
Any G ≥3 AE	46.9%
Any grade ≥4 AE	11.3%
Any serious AE	27.2%
Toxicity leading to study drug discontinuation or delay	18.4%
Toxicity leading to bortezomib dose reduction	6.9% (64/931 cycles)
Death related to toxicity	0

Hematologic Toxicity	G1–4	G3/4
Anemia	15.9%	4.2%
Neutropenia	8%	5%
Thrombocytopenia	10.9%	2.9%
Infections	48.1%	8.8%
Herpes zoster*	9.2%	—
Thrombosis	4.6%	1.7%

Nonhematologic Toxicities	G1–4
Fatigue	28.5%
Rash	11.7%
GI symptoms	26.8%
Cardiac disorders	5.9%
Pneumopathy	3.4%
G1 Peripheral neuropathy†	21.3%
G2 Peripheral neuropathy†	15.5%
G3 Peripheral neuropathy†	7.1%

*No antiviral prophylaxis for *Herpes zoster* was specified in the protocol
†Medical Dictionary for Regulatory Activities (MedDRA) Preferred Terms used by investigators that were considered related to neurologic toxicity included accommodation disorder, anosmia, areflexia, difficulty in walking, dysesthesia, fall, formication, hypoesthesia, hyperreflexia, muscle spasms, pain in limb, paraparesis, paresthesia, peripheral motor neuropathy, peripheral neuropathy, sensory loss, vertigo, and vision blurred

Efficacy (continued)

Response to First Transplantation and Overall at Least VGPR and CR/nCR Rates, Including Second Transplantation, Among All Evaluable Patients

Response to First Transplantation	
ORR (at least PR)	80.3%
At least VGPR	54.3%
CR/nCR	35%
CR	16.1%
MR + SD + PD	2.7%
Death	0.5%
No transplantation	11.7%

Overall, Including Second Transplantation	
At least VGPR	67.7%
CR/nCR	39.5%

CR, complete response; CR/nCR, complete response/near complete response; ISS, International Staging System; MR, minimal response; ORR, overall response rate; PD, progressive disease; PR, partial response; SD, stable disease; VGPR, very good partial response

Therapy Monitoring

1. *Before each cycle:* CBC with differential and blood chemistries (including BUN, creatinine, and calcium)
2. *Every 6 weeks to 3 months:* Measure serum and urine M-protein

TRANSPLANT-ELIGIBLE • FIRST-LINE INDUCTION

MULTIPLE MYELOMA REGIMEN: BORTEZOMIB + THALIDOMIDE + DEXAMETHASONE + CISPLATIN + DOXORUBICIN + CYCLOPHOSPHAMIDE + ETOPOSIDE (VTD-PACE)

Barlogie B et al. Br J Haematol 2007;138:176–185
Lee CK et al. J Clin Oncol 2003;21:2732–2739

INDUCTION VTD-PACE (2 cycles, administered ≤8 weeks apart)
Hydration:
0.9% Sodium chloride injection (0.9% NS) 500–1000 mL; administer intravenously over 1–2 hours prior to starting cisplatin infusion on day 1, every 28–56 days, for 2 cycles, *then:*
0.9% NS; following completion of the bolus dose, administer intravenously by continuous infusion initially at a rate of 100–150 mL/hour for 4 consecutive days throughout chemotherapy administration on days 1–4, every 28–56 days, for 2 cycles

Notes:
- May increase rate of 0.9% NS infusion if needed to maintain a goal urine output of ≥100 mL/hour throughout chemotherapy administration
- Monitor and replace magnesium/electrolytes as needed

Bortezomib 1 mg/m^2 per dose; administer subcutaneously in a volume of 0.9% NS sufficient to produce a final bortezomib concentration of 2.5 mg/mL on days 1, 4, 8, and 11, every 28–56 days, for 2 cycles (total dosage/ cycle = 4 mg/m^2)
Note: in the regimen described by Barlogie et al, a test dose of single-agent bortezomib was administered on day 1 of induction cycle 1, and TD-PACE was delayed until day 4 to allow for correlative research sample collection. In routine clinical practice, treatment with bortezomib is started together with TD-PACE on day 1 of cycle 1
Thalidomide 200 mg/day; administer orally, once daily at bedtime, at least 1 hour after the evening meal, for 4 consecutive days on days 1–4, every 28–56 days, for 2 cycles (total dose/cycle = 800 mg)
Dexamethasone 40 mg; administer orally once daily for 4 consecutive days on days 1–4, every 28–56 days, for 2 cycles (total dosage/cycle = 160 mg)
Cisplatin 10 mg/m^2 per day; administer by continuous intravenous infusion in 1000 mL 0.9% NS over 24 hours for 4 consecutive days on days 1–4, every 28–56 days, for 2 cycles (total dosage/cycle = 40 mg/m^2)
Note for patients with renal dysfunction: the cisplatin dose is reduced to 5 mg/m^2 per day if the SCr is between 132.6–176.8 μmol/L (1.5–2 mg/dL), and is omitted if the SCr is >176.8 μmol/L (>2 mg/dL).
Doxorubicin 10 mg/m^2 per day; administer by continuous intravenous infusion in 50–1000 mL 5% dextrose injection, USP (D5W) over 24 hours, for 4 consecutive days, on days 1–4, every 28–56 days, for 2 cycles (total dosage/cycle = 40 mg/m^2)
Cyclophosphamide 400 mg/m^2 per day; administer by continuous intravenous infusion in 1000 mL 0.9% NS over 24 hours for 4 consecutive days on days 1–4, every 28–56 days, for 2 cycles (total dosage/cycle = 1600 mg/m^2)
Etoposide 40 mg/m^2 per day; administer by continuous intravenous infusion in 1000 mL 0.9% NS over 24 hours for 4 consecutive days on days 1–4, every 28–56 days, for 2 cycles (total dosage/cycle = 160 mg/m^2)
Notes for VTD-PACE Induction Treatment:
- Consider beginning cycle 2 of induction VTD-PACE between 4–8 weeks after the start of cycle 1 upon recovery of ANC to >1000/mm^3, platelet count to >100,000/mm^3 and resolution of all nonhematologic toxicities to Grade ≤2
- See comment below regarding a 3-in-1 admixture of cisplatin, etoposide, and cyclophosphamide
- Upon post-nadir platelet recovery to >50,000/mm^3 following VTD-PACE induction cycle 1, thalidomide and dexamethasone "bridging" therapy is administered until the start of VTD-PACE induction cycle 2. Similarly, upon post-nadir platelet recovery to >50,000/mm^3 following VTD-PACE induction cycle 2, thalidomide and dexamethasone "bridging" therapy is administered until the start of conditioning chemotherapy with high-dose melphalan prior to the first of two planned tandem autologous stem cell transplants. *Thus:*

Thalidomide 50 mg/day; administer orally, once daily at bedtime, at least 1 hour after the evening meal, continually, on days 1–21, every 21 days, until the next treatment phase (either VTD-PACE or autologous stem cell transplantation) is initiated (total dose/cycle = 1050 mg), *plus:*
Dexamethasone 20 mg; administer orally once daily for 4 consecutive days on days 1–4, every 21 days, until the next treatment phase (either VTD-PACE or autologous stem cell transplantation) is initiated (total dosage/cycle = 80 mg)

CONSOLIDATION VTD-PACE (start after recovery from tandem autologous stem cell transplantation, 2 cycles, administered ≤8 weeks apart)
Hydration:
0.9% NS 500–1000 mL; administer intravenously over 1–2 hours prior to starting cisplatin infusion on day 1, every 28–56 days, for 2 cycles, *then:*
0.9% NS; following completion of the bolus dose, administer intravenously by continuous infusion initially at a rate of 100–150 mL/hour for 4 consecutive days throughout chemotherapy administration on days 1–4, every 28–56 days, for 2 cycles

Notes:
- May increase rate of 0.9% NS infusion if needed to maintain a goal urinary output of ≥100 mL/hour throughout chemotherapy administration
- Monitor and replace magnesium/electrolytes as needed

Bortezomib 1 mg/m^2 per dose; administer subcutaneously in a volume of 0.9% NS sufficient to produce a final bortezomib concentration of 2.5 mg/mL on days 1, 4, 8, and 11, every 28–56 days, for 2 cycles (total dosage/cycle = 4 mg/m^2)

(continued)

(*continued*)

Thalidomide 200 mg/day; administer orally, once daily at bedtime, at least 1 hour after the evening meal, for 4 consecutive days on days 1–4, every 28–56 days, for 2 cycles (total dose/cycle = 800 mg)
Dexamethasone 40 mg; administer orally once daily for 4 consecutive days on days 1–4, every 28–56 days, for 2 cycles (total dosage/cycle = 160 mg)
Cisplatin 7.5 mg/m² per day; administer by continuous intravenous infusion in 1000 mL 0.9% NS over 24 hours for 4 consecutive days on days 1–4, every 28–56 days, for 2 cycles (total dosage/cycle = 30 mg/m²)
Note for patients with renal dysfunction: the cisplatin dose is reduced to 5 mg/m² per day if the SCr is between 132.6–176.8 μmol/L (1.5–2 mg/dL), and is omitted if the SCr is >176.8 μmol/L (>2 mg/dL)
Doxorubicin 7.5 mg/m² per day; administer by continuous intravenous infusion in 50–1000 mL D5W over 24 hours, for 4 consecutive days, on days 1–4, every 28–56 days, for 2 cycles (total dosage/cycle = 30 mg/m²)
Cyclophosphamide 300 mg/m² per day; administer by continuous intravenous infusion in 1000 mL 0.9% NS over 24 hours for 4 consecutive days on days 1–4, every 28–56 days, for 2 cycles (total dosage/cycle = 1200 mg/m²)
Etoposide 30 mg/m² per day; administer by continuous intravenous infusion in 1000 mL 0.9% NS over 24 hours for 4 consecutive days on days 1–4, every 28–56 days, for 2 cycles (total dosage/cycle = 120 mg/m²)

Notes for VTD-PACE Consolidation Treatment:
• Consider beginning cycle 2 of consolidation VTD-PACE between 4 and 8 weeks after the start of cycle 1 upon recovery of ANC to >1000/mm³, recovery of platelet count to >100,000/mm³, and resolution of all nonhematologic toxicities to Grade ≤2
• See comment below regarding a 3-in-1 admixture of cisplatin, etoposide, and cyclophosphamide
• Upon post-nadir platelet recovery to >50,000/mm³ following VTD-PACE consolidation cycle 1, thalidomide and dexamethasone "bridging" therapy is administered until the start of VTD-PACE consolidation cycle 2. Similarly, upon post-nadir platelet recovery to >50,000/mm³ following VTD-PACE induction cycle 2, thalidomide and dexamethasone "bridging" therapy is administered until the start of the next phase of treatment. *Thus:*

Thalidomide 50 mg/day; administer orally, once daily at bedtime, at least 1 hour after the evening meal, continually, on days 1–21, every 21 days, until the next phase of treatment is initiated (total dose/cycle = 1050 mg), *plus:*
Dexamethasone 20 mg; administer orally once daily for 4 consecutive days on days 1–4, every 21 days, until the next phase of treatment is initiated (total dosage/cycle = 80 mg)

Supportive Care
Antiemetic prophylaxis
Emetogenic potential on days 1–4 of VTD-PACE cycles is **HIGH**. *Potential for delayed symptoms*
Emetogenic potential during thalidomide + dexamethasone bridging therapy is **LOW**
See Chapter 42 for antiemetic recommendations

Hematopoietic growth factor (CSF) prophylaxis
Primary prophylaxis is indicated with one of the following after each cycle of VTD-PACE:
Filgrastim (G-CSF) 5 μg/kg per day, by subcutaneous injection, or
Pegfilgrastim (pegylated filgrastim) 6 mg/0.6 mL, by subcutaneous injection for one dose
• Begin use from 24–72 h after myelosuppressive chemotherapy is completed
• Continue daily filgrastim use until ANC ≥5000/mm³ after the leukocyte nadir
• Discontinue daily filgrastim use at least 24 hours before administering myelosuppressive treatment. Do not administer pegfilgrastim within 14 days before administering myelosuppressive treatment
See Chapter 43 for more information

Antimicrobial prophylaxis
Risk of fever and neutropenia is **HIGH**
Antimicrobial primary prophylaxis to be considered:
• Antibacterial—consider a fluoroquinolone during periods of neutropenia, or no prophylaxis; *P. jirovecii* prophylaxis is recommended (eg, cotrimoxazole)
• Antifungal—consider concomitant use of fluconazole during periods of neutropenia
• Antiviral—anti-herpes antivirals (eg, acyclovir, famciclovir, valacyclovir)

Steroid-associated gastritis
Add a proton pump inhibitor or H₂-receptor antagonist during dexamethasone use to prevent gastritis and duodenitis

Bisphosphonates
All patients receiving primary therapy for symptomatic multiple myeloma should receive a bisphosphonate adjunctively.

Thromboprophylaxis
Risk assessment and recommendations for VTE prophylaxis in patients with multiple myeloma with individual or myeloma-related risk factors, or risk factors related to treatment

(*continued*)

(continued)

| **Individual risk factors**
• Obesity (BMI ≥30 kg/m²)
• H/O VTE
• CVC or pacemaker
• Comorbid pathologies
  ▪ Cardiac disease
  ▪ Chronic renal disease
  ▪ Diabetes
  ▪ Acute infection
  ▪ Immobilization
• Surgery
  ▪ General surgery
  ▪ Any anesthesia
  ▪ Trauma
• Medications
  ▪ Erythropoietin (epoetin alfa, darbepoetin)
  ▪ Estrogenic compounds
  ▪ Bevacizumab
• Clotting disorders
  ▪ Thrombophilia
Myeloma-related risk factors
• Diagnosis of multiple myeloma
• Hyperviscosity | ≤1 Individual or myeloma-related risk factor present:
• **Aspirin** 81–325 mg daily

≥2 Individual or myeloma-related risk factors present:
• **LMWH,*** equivalent to enoxaparin sodium 40 mg/day *or* **dalteparin sodium** 5000 IU/day; administer subcutaneously, *or*
• **Warfarin,** targeting an INR = 2–3 |
| **Concomitant treatment-related risk factors**
Thalidomide or lenalidomide in combination with:
• High-dose dexamethasone (≥480 mg/month)
• Doxorubicin
• Multiagent chemotherapy | • **LMWH,*** equivalent to enoxaparin sodium 40 mg/day *or* **dalteparin sodium** 5000 IU/day; administer subcutaneously, *or*
• **Warfarin,** targeting an INR = 2–3 |

*LMWHs should be used with caution in individuals with impaired renal function (creatinine clearance <30 mL/min). Refer to product labeling for information about doses and administration schedules in renally impaired patients, and guidance for monitoring anti-Factor Xa concentrations
Abbreviations: CVC, central venous catheter; INR, international normalized ratio; LMWH, low-molecular-weight heparin; VTE, venous thromboembolic disease
References: Geerts WH et al. Chest 2008;133(6 Suppl):381S–453S
National Comprehensive Cancer Network. Multiple Myeloma, V.1.2014. (Accessed October 8, 2013, at http://www.nccn.org)
National Comprehensive Cancer Network. Venous Thromboembolic Disease, V.2.2013. (Accessed October 8, 2013, at http://www.nccn.org)
Palumbo A et al. Leukemia 2008;22:414–423

Cisplatin + Etoposide + Cyclophosphamide 3-in–1 Admixture

• Cisplatin, etoposide, and cyclophosphamide may be mixed together in the same 1000 mL 0.9% NS admixture. Etoposide 0.2 mg/mL, cisplatin 0.2 mg/mL, and cyclophosphamide 2 mg/mL, diluted in 0.9% NS, is stable for 7 days at 20°–25°C (68°–77°F) when protected from exposure to light.

Williams DA et al. Cancer Chemother Pharmacol 1992;31:171–181

• A 3-in-1 admixture does not prevent microbial growth after exposure to bacterial and fungal contamination. With respect to product sterility, expiration dating should be determined by the aseptic techniques used in preparation and local and national guidelines

Treatment Modifications

BORTEZOMIB

Starting dose	1 mg/m^2/dose
Dose level −1	0.7 mg/m^2/dose

Adverse Event	Treatment Modification
G1 (paresthesias, weakness, and/or loss of reflexes) without pain or loss of function	No action
G1 with pain or G2 (interferes with function but not with activities of daily living)	Reduce bortezomib dosage one dose level
G2 with pain or G3 (interferes with activities of daily living)	Withhold bortezomib treatment until toxicity resolves to G1 or baseline, then reinitiate reducing bortezomib dosage one dose level
G4 (sensory neuropathy that is disabling or motor neuropathy that is life-threatening or leads to paralysis)	Discontinue treatment*
Hepatotoxicity	Monitor liver function. Stop bortezomib and evaluate if hepatotoxicity is suspected
Bilirubin level greater than 1.5× ULN and any AST level	Reduce bortezomib to 0.7 mg/m^2 in the first cycle; consider dose escalation to 1 mg/m^2 based on tolerability
If several bortezomib doses in consecutive cycles are withheld due to toxicity	Reduce bortezomib by 1 dosage level
G ≥2 nonhematologic toxicity on day 1 of a cycle	Hold bortezomib until toxicity has resolved to G1 or baseline
G ≥3 nonhematologic toxicities	Hold bortezomib until toxicity has resolved to G1 or baseline; then, may be reinitiated with 1 dosage level reduction

THALIDOMIDE

	Dosing with VTD-PACE cycles	Bridging Dose
Starting dose	200 mg/day	50 mg/day
Dose Level −1	150 mg/day	
Dose Level −2	100 mg/day	Discontinue thalidomide
Dose Level −3	50 mg/day	
Dose Level −4	Discontinue thalidomide	

Adverse Event	Treatment Modification
Platelet count <50,000/mm^3 during "bridging" phase of treatment	Hold thalidomide and dexamethasone bridging treatment until platelet count recovers to ≥50,000/mm^3
Bradycardia and possible syncope	Dose reduction or discontinuation may be required*
Any thromboembolic events	Discontinue treatment and start standard anticoagulation therapy. Once stabilized on the anticoagulation treatment and complications of the thromboembolic event have been managed, thalidomide treatment may be restarted at the original dose dependent upon a benefit-risk assessment, continuing anticoagulation therapy during thalidomide treatment
Mild to moderate skin rash	Withhold thalidomide until toxicity resolves to baseline G ≤1, and then restart treatment with a reduction of thalidomide dose by one dose level
Stevens-Johnson syndrome and toxic epidermal necrolysis (TEN)	Permanently discontinue thalidomide*
Symptoms of dizziness and orthostatic hypotension	Counsel patient to sit upright for a few minutes prior to standing up from a recumbent position

(continued)

Treatment Modifications (continued)

Adverse Event	Treatment Modification
G1 (paresthesia, weakness, and/or loss of reflexes) with no loss of function	Continue to monitor the patient with clinical examination. Consider reducing dose if symptoms worsen. However, dose reduction is not necessarily followed by improvement of symptoms
G2 (interfering with function but not with activities of daily living)	Reduce dose or interrupt treatment and continue to monitor the patient with clinical and neurologic examination. If no improvement or continued worsening of the neuropathy, discontinue treatment. If the neuropathy resolves to G ≤1, treatment may be restarted if the benefit/risk is favorable
G3 (interfering with activities of daily living)	Discontinue treatment
G4 (neuropathy which is disabling)	
Somnolence	Instruct patients to take total daily dose at bedtime. Advise against use of concurrent medications that may cause drowsiness. If obtundation, stupor, or coma occurs, withhold thalidomide until toxicity resolves to baseline, then restart with a reduction of thalidomide dose by one dose level
Constipation	Prescribe prophylactic measures. In cases of obstipation, obstruction, and toxic megacolon, withhold thalidomide until condition resolves, then resume thalidomide with prophylactic laxatives and/or a reduction of thalidomide dose by one dose level

DEXAMETHASONE

	Dosing with VTD-PACE cycles	Bridging Dose
Starting dose	40 mg/dose/day	20 mg/dose/day
Dose level −1	20 mg/dose/day	12 mg/dose/day
Dose level −2	12 mg/dose/day	8 mg/dose/day
Dose level −3	Discontinue dexamethasone	Discontinue dexamethasone

Adverse Event	Treatment Modification
Platelet count <50,000/mm³ during "bridging" phase of treatment	Hold thalidomide and dexamethasone bridging treatment until platelet count recovers to ≥50,000/mm³
G1/2 dyspepsia (moderate symptoms; medical intervention indicated; limiting instrumental ADL), gastric or duodenal ulcer, or gastritis	Continue dexamethasone at the same dose. Treat with therapeutic doses of an H₂-receptor antagonist or proton pump inhibitor. If symptoms persist, then reduce the dexamethasone dose by one level
G ≥3 dyspepsia, gastric or duodenal ulcer, or gastritis (surgery or hospitalization indicated)	Withhold dexamethasone until symptoms return to baseline. Resume dexamethasone reduced by one dose level along with concurrent treatment with therapeutic doses of an H₂-receptor antagonist or proton pump inhibitor. If symptoms recur, then permanently discontinue dexamethasone[†]
Acute pancreatitis	Permanently discontinue dexamethasone[†]
G ≥3 edema	Withhold dexamethasone until symptoms return to baseline. Consider treatment with diuretics. Resume dexamethasone reduced by one dose level. If edema persists, reduce by another dose level. Discontinue dexamethasone permanently if symptoms persist despite two prior dose reductions[†]
G ≥2 mood alteration (moderate mood alteration) or confusion (moderate disorientation; limiting instrumental ADL)	Withhold dexamethasone until symptoms return to baseline. Resume dexamethasone reduced by one dose level. If symptoms persist, reduce by another dose level
G ≥2 muscle weakness (symptomatic; evident on physical exam; limiting instrumental ADL)	Withhold dexamethasone until symptoms return to baseline. Resume dexamethasone reduced by one dose level. If weakness persists, reduce by another dose level. If weakness still persists, then permanently discontinue dexamethasone[†]

(continued)

Treatment Modifications (*continued*)

Adverse Event	Treatment Modification
G ≥3 hyperglycemia (insulin therapy initiated; hospitalization indicated)	Withhold dexamethasone until glucose is ≤250 mg/dL. Treat with insulin or other hypoglycemic agents as clinically appropriate and then resume dexamethasone at the same dose. If hyperglycemia is uncontrolled despite above measures, decrease dexamethasone by one dose level
Other G ≥2 nonhematologic toxicity attributable to dexamethasone including severe irritability, insomnia, or oral candidiasis	Withhold dexamethasone until toxicity resolves to G ≤1, then resume at a lower dose. Consider reduction by one dose level for G2/G3 toxicity, and by two dose levels for G4 or recurrent G3 toxicity
CISPLATIN + DOXORUBICIN + CYCLOPHOSPHAMIDE + ETOPOSIDE	
Day 1 ANC <1000/mm³, or platelets <100,000/mm³, or unresolved G ≥3 nonhematologic toxicity	Delay initiation of cycle (bortezomib, thalidomide, dexamethasone, cisplatin, doxorubicin, cyclophosphamide, and etoposide) by 1 week or until ANC >1000/mm³, platelets >100,000/mm³, and nonhematologic toxicity G ≤2
G4 neutropenia (ANC <500/mm³) at nadir	Continue to administer filgrastim or pegfilgrastim during subsequent cycles as described in the therapy administration section. Consider decreasing cyclophosphamide, etoposide, doxorubicin, and/or cisplatin dosages by 25%
G4 thrombocytopenia (platelet count <25,000/mm³) at nadir	Consider decreasing cyclophosphamide, etoposide, doxorubicin, and/or cisplatin dosages by 25%
Hypersensitivity reaction	Immediately interrupt etoposide and/or cisplatin infusion—whichever is deemed responsible—and institute supportive management as appropriate. In patients who experience a severe hypersensitivity reaction, permanently discontinue etoposide or cisplatin—whichever is deemed responsible
Hypoalbuminemia	Albumin <3.2 g/dL consider reducing etoposide dosage by 50%. Albumin <2.5 g/dL consider discontinuing etoposide until albumin >2.5 g/dL
Severe hemorrhagic cystitis	Discontinue cyclophosphamide therapy
Serum bilirubin ≥1.2 mg/dL and ≤3 mg/dL	Administer 50% of the doxorubicin dose
Serum bilirubin >3 mg/dL and ≤5 mg/dL	Administer 25% of the doxorubicin dose
Serum bilirubin >5 mg/dL, or Child-Pugh class C hepatic impairment	Omit doxorubicin
Serum creatinine ≥1.5 mg/dL (132.6 μmol/L) and ≤2 mg/dL (176.8 μmol/L)	Reduce the cisplatin dose to 5 mg/m²/day
Serum creatinine ≥2 mg/dL (176.8 μmol/L)	Omit cisplatin
Peripheral neuropathy G ≥3	G4 discontinue cisplatin permanently; G3 may reinstitute if toxicity resolves within 2–3 weeks to G ≤1
Cisplatin induced hearing loss G ≥3	
Other G ≥3 nonhematologic toxicities (except nausea, vomiting, elevated transaminases, and alopecia)	Delay treatment until toxicity resolves to baseline, then decrease cyclophosphamide, etoposide, doxorubicin, and/or cisplatin dosages by 25–50% from previous dose levels
On serial multi-gated radionuclide angiography (MUGA) or echocardiography (ECHO), a 10% decline in LVEF to below the lower limit of normal or an absolute LVEF of 45%, or a 20% decline in LVEF at any level	Considered indicative of deterioration in cardiac function. Benefit of continued therapy with doxorubicin should be carefully evaluated against the risk of producing irreversible cardiac damage
Evidence of mucositis (stomatitis, esophagitis, or colitis)	Reduce dose of doxorubicin in subsequent cycles by 25–50%. Alternately, reduce the duration of administration by one day. Monitor carefully

Patient Population Studied

A phase 2 study of 303 patients with newly diagnosed progressive or symptomatic multiple myeloma. Eligible patients were aged ≤75 years, and had ≤1 cycle of prior therapy, Southwest Oncology Group (SWOG) performance status <3 (unless based solely on pain), adequate cardio-pulmonary functions and serum creatinine levels ≤265.2 μmol/L (3 mg/dL)

Efficacy (n = 303)

Event-free survival at 2 years	84%
Overall survival at 2 years	86%
Treatment-related mortality	5%
Near-complete response at 2 years	83%
Complete response at 2 years	56%

Note: median follow-up was 20 months

Adverse Events (n = 303)

Treatment-related mortality was 5%. Grade >2 thromboembolic events and peripheral neuropathy, respectively, occurred in 11% and 14% of patients at the end of induction therapy, 12% and 11% of patients after tandem transplantation, 6% and 11% of patients at the end of consolidation therapy, and 2% and 13% of patients after maintenance therapy

Therapy Monitoring

1. *Prior to the start of treatment:*
   a. Cardiac function (left ventricular ejection fraction, LVEF) assessment measured by multi-gated radionuclide angiography (MUGA) or echocardiography (ECHO). Repeat interval measurement(s) while receiving treatment if administered for prolonged duration
   b. Pregnancy test (in women of child-bearing potential)
2. *Prior to each cycle of VTD-PACE:* CBC with differential, liver function tests, serum chemistries, serum electrolytes, and serum glucose
3. *Once or twice weekly (ie, between cycles of VTD-PACE):* CBC with differential, serum chemistries, serum electrolytes
4. *In patients at high risk for tumor lysis syndrome (eg, high tumor burden, renal dysfunction, rapidly progressing disease, markedly elevated LDH, baseline abnormalities in laboratory indices of tumor lysis syndrome [potassium, phosphate, uric acid, calcium, serum creatinine]):* consider frequent monitoring of laboratory indices of tumor lysis syndrome, intravenous hydration, and prophylaxis with a xanthine oxidase inhibitor (eg, allopurinol) during the first cycle
5. Ensure adequate hydration of patients to reduce the risk of cisplatin-induced renal toxicity and of tumor lysis syndrome
6. With abdominal pain, check serum amylase/lipase
7. Monitor for bortezomib toxicities including neuropathy and hypotension
   a. *Note:* patients with pre-existing severe neuropathy should be treated with bortezomib only after careful risk-benefit assessment
8. Monitor for thalidomide toxicities including:
   a. Cardiac complications (bradycardia and syncope), severe skin reactions, peripheral neuropathy, seizures (in patients with history of seizures or other risk factors for the development of seizures), and signs/symptoms of venous thromboembolism
   b. **Pregnancy must be excluded before start of treatment. Prevent pregnancy thereafter by the use of two reliable methods of contraception**

Note on thalidomide:
THALOMID (thalidomide) is only available through a restricted distribution program, the THALOMID REMS program

TRANSPLANT-ELIGIBLE OR TRANSPLANT-INELIGIBLE • FIRST-LINE INDUCTION

MULTIPLE MYELOMA REGIMEN: IXAZOMIB + LENALIDOMIDE + DEXAMETHASONE

Kumar SK et al. Lancet Oncol 2014;15:1503–1512
Supplement to: Kumar SK et al. Lancet Oncol 2014;15:1503–1512

The regimen consists of up to twelve 28-day cycles of induction therapy with ixazomib, lenalidomide, and dexamethasone. Patients could temporarily interrupt therapy any time after 3 cycles to undergo stem cell collection. Patients could discontinue ixazomib, lenalidomide, and dexamethasone therapy after 6 cycles to undergo autologous stem cell transplantation. Patients who did not undergo autologous stem cell transplantation completed up to twelve cycles of induction therapy and were then allowed to undergo maintenance therapy with single-agent ixazomib

Induction therapy with ixazomib + lenalidomide + dexamethasone (up to 12 cycles):
Ixazomib 4 mg/dose; administer orally for 3 doses, at least 1 hour prior to food or at least 2 hours after food, with water, on day 1, 8, and 15, every 28 days, for up to 12 cycles (total dosage/4-week cycle = 12 mg)
• Patients who delay taking an ixazomib dose at a regularly scheduled time may take the missed dose if the time to the next regularly scheduled dose is >72 hours away
• If a patient vomits after taking a dose of ixazomib, the patient should take the next dose at the next regularly scheduled time
• Avoid concomitant administration with strong CYP3A4 inducers (eg, rifampin, carbamazepine, phenytoin, phenobarbital, and St. John's Wort)
• Reduce the starting dose to 3 mg on days 1, 8, and 15 for moderate (total bilirubin >1.5–3× ULN) or severe (total bilirubin >3× ULN) hepatic impairment
• Reduce the starting dose to 3 mg on days 1, 8, and 15 for patients with severe renal impairment (creatinine clearance <30 mL/minute) or end-stage renal disease requiring hemodialysis. In patients undergoing hemodialysis, ixazomib can be administered without regard to dialysis timing

Lenalidomide 25 mg/dose; administer orally, without regard to meals, once daily for 21 consecutive days on days 1–21, followed by 7 days with no treatment, every 28 days, for up to 12 cycles (total dosage/4-week cycle = 525 mg)
• Patients who delay taking a lenalidomide dose at a regularly scheduled time may take the missed dose if the time to the next regularly scheduled dose is >12 hours away
• Consider doses in Treatment Modifications table for dose adjustments for renal function

Dexamethasone 40 mg/dose; administer orally once daily for 4 doses on days 1, 8, 15, and 22, every 28 days, for 12 cycles (total dosage/4-week cycle = 160 mg)

Maintenance therapy with ixazomib monotherapy:
Ixazomib 4 mg/dose; administer orally for 3 doses, at least 1 hour prior to food or at least 2 hours after food, with water, on day 1, 8, and 15, every 28 days, as maintenance therapy until disease progression (total dosage/4-week cycle = 12 mg). See guidelines above
• Patients who underwent ixazomib dose reduction during induction therapy should continue with the last tolerated dose of ixazomib during maintenance therapy
• Patients who delay taking an ixazomib dose at a regularly scheduled time may take the missed dose if the time to the next regularly scheduled dose is >72 hours away
• If a patient vomits after taking a dose of ixazomib, the patient should take the next dose at the next regularly scheduled time
• Avoid concomitant administration with strong CYP3A4 inducers (eg, rifampin, carbamazepine, phenytoin, phenobarbital, and St. John's Wort)
• Reduce the starting dose to 3 mg on days 1, 8, and 15 for total bilirubin >1.5
• Reduce the starting dose to 3 mg on days 1, 8, and 15 for patients with severe renal impairment (creatinine clearance <30 mL/minute) or end-stage renal disease requiring hemodialysis. In patients undergoing hemodialysis, ixazomib can be administered without regard to dialysis timing

Supportive Care
Antiemetic prophylaxis
Emetogenic potential on days with lenalidomide and/or ixazomib is **LOW**
See Chapter 42 for antiemetic recommendations

Hematopoietic growth factor (CSF) prophylaxis
Primary prophylaxis is **NOT** *indicated*
See Chapter 43 for more information

Antimicrobial prophylaxis
Risk of fever and neutropenia is **INTERMEDIATE**
  Antimicrobial primary prophylaxis to be considered:
  • Antibacterial—consider a fluoroquinolone during periods of neutropenia, or no prophylaxis; *P. jirovecii* prophylaxis is recommended (eg, cotrimoxazole)
  • Antifungal—consider fluconazole during periods of neutropenia
  • Antiviral—antiherpes antivirals (eg, acyclovir, famciclovir, valacyclovir)

(continued)

(continued)

Diarrhea management
Loperamide or **diphenoxylate hydrochloride** 2.5 mg with **atropine sulfate** 0.025 mg (eg, Lomotil)

Bisphosphonates
All patients receiving primary therapy for symptomatic multiple myeloma should receive a bisphosphonate adjunctively.

Thromboprophylaxis
Risk assessment and recommendations for VTE prophylaxis in patients with multiple myeloma with individual or myeloma-related risk factors, or risk factors related to treatment

Individual risk factors
• Obesity (BMI ≥30 kg/m^2)
• H/O VTE
• CVC or pacemaker
• Comorbid pathologies
  ▪ Cardiac disease
  ▪ Chronic renal disease
  ▪ Diabetes
  ▪ Acute infection
  ▪ Immobilization
• Surgery
  ▪ General surgery
  ▪ Any anesthesia
  ▪ Trauma
• Medications
  ▪ Erythropoietin (epoetin alfa, darbepoetin)
  ▪ Estrogenic compounds
  ▪ Bevacizumab
• Clotting disorders
  ▪ Thrombophilia
Myeloma-related risk factors
• Diagnosis of multiple myeloma
• Hyperviscosity
	≤1 Individual or myeloma-related risk factor present:
	• **Aspirin** 81–325 mg daily
	
	≥2 Individual or myeloma-related risk factors present:
	• **LMWH,*** equivalent to **enoxaparin sodium** 40 mg/day *or* **dalteparin sodium** 5000 IU/day; administer subcutaneously, *or*
	• **Warfarin,** targeting an INR = 2–3

Concomitant treatment-related risk factors Thalidomide or lenalidomide in combination with: • High-dose dexamethasone (≥480 mg/month) • Doxorubicin • Multiagent chemotherapy	• **LMWH,*** equivalent to **enoxaparin sodium** 40 mg/day *or* **dalteparin sodium** 5000 IU/day; administer subcutaneously, *or* • **Warfarin,** targeting an INR = 2–3

*LMWHs should be used with caution in individuals with impaired renal function (creatinine clearance <30 mL/min). Refer to product labeling for information about doses and administration schedules in renally impaired patients, and guidance for monitoring anti-Factor Xa concentrations

Abbreviations: CVC, central venous catheter; INR, international normalized ratio; LMWH, low-molecular-weight heparin; VTE, venous thromboembolic disease

References: Geerts WH et al. Chest 2008;133(6 Suppl):381S–453S
National Comprehensive Cancer Network. Multiple Myeloma, V.1.2014. (Accessed October 8, 2013, at http://www.nccn.org)
National Comprehensive Cancer Network. Venous Thromboembolic Disease, V.2.2013. (Accessed October 8, 2013, at http://www.nccn.org)
Palumbo A et al. Leukemia 2008;22:414–423

Treatment Modifications

IXAZOMIB

Ixazomib dose levels (Days 1, 8, and 15 of every 28-day cycle)

	CrCl ≥30 mL/min, normal hepatic function	CrCl <30 mL/min, end-stage renal disease requiring dialysis, moderate hepatic impairment (total bilirubin >1.5–3× ULN), or severe hepatic impairment (total bilirubin >3× ULN)
Starting dose	4 mg/dose	3 mg/dose (irrespective of hemodialysis timing, if applicable)
Dose Level −1	3 mg/dose	2.3 mg/dose (irrespective of hemodialysis timing, if applicable)
Dose Level −2	2.3 mg/dose	Discontinue ixazomib
Dose Level −3	Discontinue ixazomib	

Adverse Event	Treatment Modification
Day 1 ANC <1000/mm^3 and/or platelet count <75,000/mm^3 and/or nonhematologic toxicities G ≥2	Delay administration of ixazomib and lenalidomide until ANC ≥1000/mm^3 and platelet count ≥75,000/mm^3. Consider treatment with filgrastim and/or platelet transfusion according to local guidelines. If the start of a new cycle is delayed >14 days, then reduce the lenalidomide by one dose level and also consider reducing the ixazomib dose by one dose level
ANC <500/mm^3 and/or platelet count <30,000/mm^3	Withhold ixazomib and lenalidomide until platelet count ≥30,000/mm^3 and/or ANC >500/mm^3. Consider adding G-CSF per clinical guidelines. Following recovery, resume lenalidomide at the next lower dose, and resume ixazomib at its most recent dose
Recurrence of ANC <500/mm^3 and/or platelet count <30,000/mm^3 despite a reduction in lenalidomide dose	Withhold ixazomib and lenalidomide until platelet count ≥30,000/mm^3 and/or ANC >500/mm^3. Consider adding G-CSF per clinical guidelines. Following recovery, resume ixazomib at the next lower dose and resume lenalidomide at its most recent dose For additional occurrences, alternate dose modification of lenalidomide and ixazomib
G2/3 rash	Withhold lenalidomide until rash recovers to G ≤1. Following recovery, resume lenalidomide at one lower dose level
Recurrence of G2/3 rash despite a reduction in lenalidomide dose	Withhold ixazomib and lenalidomide until rash recovers to G ≤1. Following recovery, resume ixazomib at the next lower dose and resume lenalidomide at its most recent dose For additional occurrences, alternate dose modification of lenalidomide and ixazomib
G1 peripheral neuropathy with pain or G2 peripheral neuropathy	Withhold ixazomib until peripheral neuropathy recovers to G ≤1 without pain or patient's baseline. Following recovery, resume ixazomib at its most recent dose
G2 peripheral neuropathy with pain or G3 peripheral neuropathy	Withhold ixazomib until peripheral neuropathy recovers to G ≤1 without pain or patient's baseline. Following recovery, resume ixazomib at the next lower dose level
G4 peripheral neuropathy	Discontinue ixazomib
Other G3/4 nonhematologic toxicities	Withhold ixazomib. Toxicities should recover to G ≤1 prior to resuming ixazomib. If attributable to ixazomib resume with ixazomib dose at one lower level

LENALIDOMIDE

Lenalidomide dose levels (Days 1–21 of each 28 day cycle)

	CrCl ≥60 mL/min	CrCl ≥30 mL/min and <60 mL/min	CrCl <30 mL/min (not on hemodialysis)	ESRD on hemodialysis
Starting dose	25 mg each day	10 mg each day	15 mg every other day	5 mg each day (after dialysis on dialysis days)
Dose level −1	15 mg each day	5 mg each day	10 mg every other day	2.5 mg each day (after dialysis on dialysis days)
Dose level −2	10 mg each day	2.5 mg each day	5 mg every other day	Discontinue[†]
Dose level −3	5 mg each day	Discontinue[†]	Discontinue[†]	
Dose level −4	Discontinue[†]			

(continued)

Treatment Modifications (*continued*)

Adverse Event	Treatment Modification
Hematologic Toxicity	
Day 1 ANC <1000/mm^3 and/or platelet count <75,000/mm^3 and/or nonhematologic toxicities G ≥2	Delay administration of ixazomib and lenalidomide until ANC ≥1000/mm^3 and platelet count ≥75,000/mm^3. Consider treatment with filgrastim and/or platelet transfusion according to local guidelines. If the start of a new cycle is delayed >14 days, then reduce the lenalidomide by one dose level and also consider reducing the ixazomib dose by one dose level
ANC <500/mm^3 and/or platelet count <30,000/mm^3	Withhold ixazomib and lenalidomide until platelet count ≥30,000/mm^3 and/or ANC >500/mm^3. Following recovery, resume lenalidomide at the next lower dose, but not lower than 2.5 mg/day, and resume ixazomib at its most recent dose
ANC <500/mm^3 and/or platelet count <30,000/mm^3 despite a reduction in lenalidomide dose	Withhold ixazomib and lenalidomide until platelet count ≥30,000/mm^3 and/or ANC >500/mm^3. Following recovery, resume ixazomib at the next lower dose and resume lenalidomide at its most recent dose For additional occurrences, alternate dose modification of lenalidomide and ixazomib
Nonhematologic Toxicity	
G3/4 hepatotoxicity (ALT/AST >5× ULN and/or bilirubin >3× ULN)	Withhold lenalidomide and ixazomib until hepatotoxicity resolves to G ≤1 (ALT/AST ≤3× ULN and/or bilirubin ≤1.5× ULN), then resume lenalidomide at one lower dose level and ixazomib at one lower dose level
G2/3 rash	Withhold lenalidomide until rash recovers to G ≤1. Following recovery, resume lenalidomide at one lower dose level
Recurrence of G2/3 rash despite a reduction in lenalidomide dose	Withhold ixazomib and lenalidomide until rash recovers to G ≤1. Following recovery, resume ixazomib at the next lower dose and resume lenalidomide at its most recent dose For additional occurrences, alternate dose modification of lenalidomide and ixazomib
Allergic reactions, including hypersensitivity, angioedema, Stevens-Johnson syndrome, toxic epidermal necrolysis (TEN), and drug reaction with eosinophilia and systemic symptoms (DRESS)	Discontinue lenalidomide if reactions are suspected. Do not resume lenalidomide if these reactions are confirmed
Tumor lysis syndrome (TLS)	Monitor patients at risk of TLS (ie, those with high tumor burden) and take appropriate precautions including aggressive hydration and allopurinol
G3/4 venous thromboembolism (VTE) during aspirin monotherapy or inadequate anticoagulation	Continue lenalidomide at the current dose and initiate adequate anticoagulation
G3/4 venous thromboembolism (VTE) during adequate anticoagulation (eg, prophylactic or therapeutic doses of LMWH, UFH, or warfarin)	Discontinue lenalidomide
G ≥2 hypothyroidism or G ≥2 hyperthyroidism	Continue lenalidomide at current dose and initiate appropriate medical treatment
Other G ≥3 lenalidomide-related toxicities	Withhold lenalidomide for the remainder of the cycle. Delay initiation of the next cycle until toxicity resolves to G ≤2, then resume lenalidomide at one lower dose level
DEXAMETHASONE	
Dexamethasone dose levels (Days 1, 8, 15, and 22 of each 28-day cycle)	
Starting dose	40 mg/dose
Dose Level −1	20 mg/dose
Dose Level −2	8 mg/dose
Dose Level −3	Discontinue dexamethasone

(*continued*)

Treatment Modifications (*continued*)

Adverse Event	Treatment Modification
G1/2 dyspepsia (moderate symptoms; medical intervention indicated; limiting instrumental ADL), gastric or duodenal ulcer, or gastritis	Continue dexamethasone at the same dose. Treat with therapeutic doses of an H_2-receptor antagonist or proton pump inhibitor. If symptoms persist, then reduce the dexamethasone dose by one level
G ≥3 dyspepsia, gastric or duodenal ulcer, or gastritis (surgery or hospitalization indicated)	Withhold dexamethasone until symptoms return to baseline. Resume dexamethasone reduced by one dose level along with concurrent treatment with therapeutic doses of an H_2-receptor antagonist or proton pump inhibitor. If symptoms recur, then permanently discontinue dexamethasone
Acute pancreatitis	Permanently discontinue dexamethasone
G ≥3 edema	Withhold dexamethasone until symptoms return to baseline. Consider treatment with diuretics. Resume dexamethasone reduced by one dose level. If edema persists, reduce by another dose level. Discontinue dexamethasone permanently if symptoms persist despite two prior dose reductions
G ≥2 mood alteration (moderate mood alteration) or confusion (moderate disorientation; limiting instrumental ADL)	Withhold dexamethasone until symptoms return to baseline. Resume dexamethasone reduced by one dose level. If symptoms persist, reduce by another dose level
G ≥2 muscle weakness (symptomatic; evident on physical exam; limiting instrumental ADL)	Withhold dexamethasone until symptoms return to baseline. Resume dexamethasone reduced by one dose level. If weakness persists, reduce by another dose level. If weakness still persists, then permanently discontinue dexamethasone
G ≥3 hyperglycemia (insulin therapy initiated; hospitalization indicated)	Withhold dexamethasone until glucose is ≤250 mg/dL. Treat with insulin or other hypoglycemic agents as clinically appropriate and then resume dexamethasone at the same dose. If hyperglycemia is uncontrolled despite above measures, decrease dexamethasone by one dose level
Other G ≥2 nonhematologic toxicity attributable to dexamethasone including severe irritability, insomnia, or oral candidiasis	Withhold dexamethasone until toxicity resolves to G ≤1, then resume at a lower dose. Consider reduction by one dose level for G2/G3 toxicity, and by two dose levels for G4 or recurrent G3 toxicity

If the dose of one drug in the regimen (ie, lenalidomide, dexamethasone, or ixazomib) is delayed, interrupted, or discontinued, the treatment with the other drugs may continue as scheduled.

Patient Population Studied

The multicenter, non-randomized, open-label, dose-escalation, phase 1/2 trial involved 65 patients with newly diagnosed multiple myeloma. Eligible patients were aged ≥18 years and had Eastern Cooperative Oncology Group (ECOG) performance score ≤2. Patients who had Grade ≥2 peripheral neuropathy, previous deep-vein thrombosis, prolonged QT interval, or known HIV or hepatitis infection were ineligible

Efficacy (n = 65)

Complete or very good partial response*	58%
Complete response	27%

*The primary end point
Note: the median duration of follow-up was 14.3 months

Adverse Events

Grade (%)*	Phase 1/2 (n = 65)		Patients Receiving Maintenance (n = 25)	
	Grade 1–2	Grade 3–4	Grade 1–2	Grade 3–4
Skin and subcutaneous tissue disorders	38	17	8	0
Diarrhea	45	6	28	0
Nausea	45	5	12	0
Fatigue	38	9	0	0
Peripheral neuropathy not elsewhere classified	32	6	0	0
Vomiting	29	6	0	0
Insomnia	25	2	4	0
Thrombocytopenia	18	8	4	4
Constipation	25	0	0	0
Dizziness	20	2	0	0

(*continued*)

Therapy Monitoring

1. *Prior to each cycle:* CBC with differential, liver function tests, serum creatinine, and serum glucose. Consider more frequent CBC monitoring during the first 3 cycles
2. With abdominal pain, check serum amylase/lipase
3. Ensure adequate hydration of patients
4. Monitor thyroid function
5. Monitor for signs/symptoms of thromboembolism, peripheral neuropathy, gastrointestinal toxicities (eg, diarrhea, constipation, nausea, and vomiting), edema, and cutaneous reactions

Lenalidomide notes:
• Higher incidences of second primary malignancies were observed in controlled trials of patients with MM receiving lenalidomide. While no routine monitoring is indicated, awareness of this potential complication is necessary

• A decrease in the number of CD34+ cells collected after treatment has been reported in patients who have received >4 cycles of lenalidomide. In patients who may undergo transplant, consider early referral to transplant center

• Because of the embryo-fetal risk, lenalidomide is available only through a restricted program under a Risk Evaluation and Mitigation Strategy (REMS), the REVLIMID REMS program

Adverse Events (continued)

Grade (%)*	Phase 1/2 (n = 65)		Patients Receiving Maintenance (n = 25)	
	Grade 1–2	Grade 3–4	Grade 1–2	Grade 3–4
Neutropenia	9	12	0	0
Peripheral edema	18	2	4	0
Dysgeusia	20	0	0	0
Anemia	14	3	4	0
Muscle spasms	17	0	0	0
Hypokalemia	6	6	4	0
Decreased appetite	11	2	0	0
Dyspnea	12	0	0	0
Leukopenia	6	5	0	0
Abdominal distention	9	2	0	0
Gastro-esophageal reflux disease	9	2	0	0
Lymphopenia	3	9	0	0
Increased alanine aminotransferase level	8	2	0	0
Hypophosphatemia	3	5	4	0
Increased aspartate aminotransferase level	5	2	0	0
Hypertension	0	5	0	4
Increased blood creatinine level	3	2	4	0
Hyperglycemia	3	2	0	0
Dehydration	0	3	0	0
Syncope	0	3	0	0
Agitation	2	2	0	0
Non-cardiac chest pain	2	2	0	0
Orthostatic hypotension	2	2	0	0
Decreased platelet count	2	2	0	0
Atrial fibrillation	0	2	0	0
Hyponatremia	0	2	0	4
Hypovolemia	0	2	0	0
Mood swings	0	2	0	0
Bone abscess	0	2	0	0
Embolism	0	2	0	0
Intestinal perforation	0	2	0	0
Decreased neutrophil count	0	2	0	0
Pneumonia	0	2	0	0
Rash pustules	0	2	0	0
Decreased white blood cell count	0	2	0	0

*According to the National Cancer Institute Common Terminology Criteria for Adverse Events, version 4.02
Note: drug-related adverse events that occurred in >10% of the total population and all G ≥3 adverse events are included. Treatment was discontinued owing to adverse events in eight (12%) patients. One patient died as a result of drug-related respiratory syncytial viral pneumonia

TRANSPLANT-INELIGIBLE • FIRST-LINE INDUCTION
MULTIPLE MYELOMA REGIMEN: LENALIDOMIDE + DEXAMETHASONE (Rd)

Benboubker L et al. N Engl J Med 2014;371:906–917
Supplement to: Benboubker L et al. N Engl J Med 2014;371:906–917
Protocol for: Benboubker L et al. N Engl J Med 2014;371:906–917

Lenalidomide 25 mg/dose; administer orally, without regard to meals, once daily for 21 consecutive days on days 1–21, followed by 7 days without treatment, every 28 days until disease progression (total dosage/28-day cycle = 525 mg)

Treatment notes:
- Patients who delay taking a lenalidomide dose at a regularly scheduled time may take the missed dose if the time to the next regularly scheduled dose is >12 hours away
- Lenalidomide initial dosing in renal impairment—see Dose Modification table

Dexamethasone 40 mg/dose; administer orally or intravenously for 4 doses on days 1, 8, 15, and 22, every 28 days until disease progression (total dosage/28-day cycle = 160 mg)

Treatment notes:
- For patients ≥75 years of age: reduce the initial dexamethasone dose to 20 mg/dose; administered orally or intravenously for 4 doses on days 1, 8, 15, and 22, every 28 days (total dosage/28-day cycle = 80 mg)

Supportive Care
Antiemetic prophylaxis
Emetogenic potential on days 1–21 is **LOW**
See Chapter 42 for antiemetic recommendations

Hematopoietic growth factor (CSF) prophylaxis
Primary prophylaxis is **NOT** *indicated*
See Chapter 43 for more information

Antimicrobial prophylaxis
Risk of fever and neutropenia is **INTERMEDIATE**
Antimicrobial primary prophylaxis to be considered:
- Antibacterial—consider a fluoroquinolone during periods of neutropenia or no prophylaxis; *P. jirovecii* prophylaxis is recommended (eg, cotrimoxazole)
- Antifungal—consider fluconazole during periods of neutropenia
- Antiviral—antiherpes antivirals (eg, acyclovir, famciclovir, valacyclovir)

Bisphosphonates
All patients receiving primary therapy for symptomatic multiple myeloma should receive a bisphosphonate adjunctively.

Thromboprophylaxis
In the study by Benboubker et al, patients were required to take low-dose aspirin (70–100 mg per day) throughout the study. Patients with a history of deep-vein thrombosis or pulmonary embolism within the past 5 years were required to be treated with low-molecular-weight heparin, heparin, or warfarin during the first 4 months of the study instead of aspirin. After 4 months, these patients could optionally be switched to low-dose aspirin (70–100 mg per day)

Risk assessment and recommendations for VTE prophylaxis in patients with multiple myeloma with individual or myeloma-related risk factors, or risk factors related to treatment

(continued)

(continued)

Individual risk factors
• Obesity (BMI ≥30 kg/m²)
• H/O VTE
• CVC or pacemaker
• Comorbid pathologies
  ▪ Cardiac disease
  ▪ Chronic renal disease
  ▪ Diabetes
  ▪ Acute infection
  ▪ Immobilization
• Surgery
  ▪ General surgery
  ▪ Any anesthesia
  ▪ Trauma
• Medications
  ▪ Erythropoietin (epoetin alfa, darbepoetin)
  ▪ Estrogenic compounds
  ▪ Bevacizumab
• Clotting disorders
  ▪ Thrombophilia
Myeloma-related risk factors
• Diagnosis of multiple myeloma
• Hyperviscosity
	≤1 Individual or myeloma-related risk factor present:
	• **Aspirin** 81–325 mg daily
	
	≥2 Individual or myeloma-related risk factors present:
	• **LMWH,*** equivalent to enoxaparin sodium 40 mg/day *or* **dalteparin sodium** 5000 IU/day; administer subcutaneously, *or*
	• **Warfarin,** targeting an INR = 2–3

Concomitant treatment-related risk factors Thalidomide or lenalidomide in combination with: • High-dose dexamethasone (≥480 mg/month) • Doxorubicin • Multiagent chemotherapy	• **LMWH,*** equivalent to enoxaparin sodium 40 mg/day *or* **dalteparin sodium** 5000 IU/day; administer subcutaneously, *or* • **Warfarin,** targeting an INR = 2–3

*LMWHs should be used with caution in individuals with impaired renal function (creatinine clearance <30 mL/min). Refer to product labeling for information about doses and administration schedules in renally impaired patients, and guidance for monitoring anti-Factor Xa concentrations
Abbreviations: CVC, central venous catheter; INR, international normalized ratio; LMWH, low-molecular-weight heparin; VTE, venous thromboembolic disease

References: Geerts WH et al. Chest 2008;133(6 Suppl):381S–453S
National Comprehensive Cancer Network. Multiple Myeloma, V.1.2014. (Accessed October 8, 2013, at http://www.nccn.org)
National Comprehensive Cancer Network. Venous Thromboembolic Disease, V.2.2013. (Accessed October 8, 2013, at http://www.nccn.org)
Palumbo A et al. Leukemia 2008;22:414–423

Treatment Modifications

LENALIDOMIDE + DEXAMETHASONE

LENALIDOMIDE

Lenalidomide dose levels (Days 1–21 of each 28-day cycle)

	CrCl ≥50 mL/min	CrCl ≥30 mL/min and <50 mL/min	CrCl <30 mL/min (not on hemodialysis)	ESRD on hemodialysis
Starting dose	25 mg each day	10 mg each day (advance to 15 mg if 10 tolerated)	15 mg every other day	5 mg each day (after dialysis on dialysis days)
Dose level −1	20 mg each day	5 mg each day	10 mg every other day	2.5 mg each day (after dialysis on dialysis days)
Dose level −2	15 mg each day	2.5 mg each day	5 mg every other day	Discontinue†
Dose level −3	10 mg each day	Discontinue†	2.5 mg every other day	
Dose level −4	5 mg each day		Discontinue†	
Dose level −5	2.5 mg each day			
Dose level −6	Discontinue†			

(continued)

Treatment Modifications (*continued*)

Adverse Event	Treatment Modification
Hematologic Toxicity	
Day 1 ANC <1000/mm³ or platelet count <50,000/mm³	Delay the next cycle until ANC ≥1000/mm³ and platelet count ≥50,000/mm³. Consider treatment with filgrastim and/or platelet transfusion according to local guidelines. If the start of a new cycle is delayed >14 days for lenalidomide-related toxicity, then reduce the lenalidomide dosage by one dose level
Either of the following: G4 neutropenia (ANC <500/mm³) Neutropenic fever (ANC <1000/mm³ + a single temperature >38.5°C)	Withhold lenalidomide for the remainder of the cycle* and delay initiation of the next cycle until ANC ≥1000/mm³ and platelet count ≥50,000/mm³, if necessary. Consider treatment with filgrastim according to local guidelines. If neutropenia was the only dose-limiting toxicity AND if filgrastim is continued AND if the next cycle was delayed by ≤14 days, then resume lenalidomide at the same dose. Otherwise, reduce the lenalidomide dose by one dose level at the start of the next cycle
G3 neutropenia (ANC ≥500/mm³ and less than 1000/mm³) during a cycle	Interrupt lenalidomide treatment and follow weekly CBC. When ANC ≥1000/mm³ and there are no other toxicities, resume lenalidomide treatment at same dose. If other toxicities are still present, then resume lenalidomide with dose reduced one dose level
Recurrent G3 neutropenia (ANC ≥500/mm³ and less than 1000/mm³) during a cycle	Interrupt lenalidomide treatment and follow weekly CBC. When ANC ≥1000/mm³, resume with dose reduced one dosage level
G4 thrombocytopenia (platelet count <25,000/mm³)	Interrupt lenalidomide treatment and follow weekly CBC. When platelet count ≥25,000/mm³, resume lenalidomide with dose reduced one dosage level
Recurrent G4 thrombocytopenia (platelet count <25,000/mm³)	
Nonhematologic Toxicity	
G3/4 hepatotoxicity (ALT/AST >5× ULN and/or bilirubin >3× ULN)	Withhold lenalidomide for the remainder of the cycle.* Delay initiation of the next cycle until hepatotoxicity resolves to G ≤2 (ALT/AST ≤5× ULN and/or bilirubin ≤3× ULN), then resume lenalidomide at one lower dose level
G3 rash	Hold dose for remainder of cycle.* Decrease by one dosage level when dosing resumed at next cycle (rash must resolve to G ≤1)
Allergic reactions, including hypersensitivity, angioedema, Stevens-Johnson syndrome, toxic epidermal necrolysis (TEN), and drug reaction with eosinophilia and systemic symptoms (DRESS)	Discontinue lenalidomide if reactions are suspected. Do not resume lenalidomide if these reactions are confirmed
Tumor lysis syndrome (TLS)	Monitor patients at risk of TLS (ie, those with high tumor burden) and take appropriate precautions including aggressive hydration and allopurinol
G3 peripheral neuropathy	Withhold lenalidomide for the remainder of the cycle.* Delay initiation of the next cycle until neuropathy resolves to G ≤1, then resume lenalidomide at one lower dose level
G4 peripheral neuropathy	Discontinue lenalidomide[†]
G3/4 venous thromboembolism (VTE) during aspirin monotherapy or inadequate anticoagulation	Continue lenalidomide at the current dose and initiate adequate anticoagulation
G3/4 venous thromboembolism (VTE) during adequate anticoagulation (eg, prophylactic or therapeutic doses of LMWH, UFH, or warfarin)	Discontinue lenalidomide[†]
G ≥2 hypothyroidism or G ≥2 hyperthyroidism	Continue lenalidomide at current dose and initiate appropriate medical treatment
Other G ≥3 lenalidomide-related toxicities	Withhold lenalidomide for the remainder of the cycle.* Delay initiation of the next cycle until toxicity resolves to G ≤2, then resume lenalidomide at one lower dosage level

(*continued*)

Treatment Modifications (continued)

DEXAMETHASONE

	Age ≤75 years	Age >75 years
Starting dose	40 mg/dose/day	20 mg/dose/day
Dose Level −1	20 mg/dose/day	12 mg/dose/day
Dose Level −2	12 mg/dose/day	8 mg/dose/day
Dose Level −3	8 mg/dose/day	4 mg/dose/day
Dose Level −4	4 mg/dose/day	Discontinue dexamethasone
Dose Level −5	Discontinue dexamethasone	

Adverse Event	Treatment Modification
G1/2 dyspepsia (moderate symptoms; medical intervention indicated; limiting instrumental ADL), gastric or duodenal ulcer, or gastritis	Continue dexamethasone at the same dose. Treat with therapeutic doses of an H_2-receptor antagonist or proton pump inhibitor. If symptoms persist, then reduce the dexamethasone dosage by one level
G ≥3 dyspepsia, gastric or duodenal ulcer, or gastritis (surgery or hospitalization indicated)	Withhold dexamethasone until symptoms return to baseline. Resume dexamethasone reduced by one dosage level along with concurrent treatment with therapeutic doses of an H_2-receptor antagonist or proton pump inhibitor. If symptoms recur, then permanently discontinue dexamethasone[‡]
Acute pancreatitis	Permanently discontinue dexamethasone[‡]
G ≥3 edema	Withhold dexamethasone until symptoms return to baseline. Consider treatment with diuretics. Resume dexamethasone reduced by one dose level. If edema persists, reduce by another dose level. Discontinue dexamethasone permanently if symptoms persist despite two prior dose reductions[‡]
G ≥2 mood alteration (moderate mood alteration) or confusion (moderate disorientation; limiting instrumental ADL)	Withhold dexamethasone until symptoms return to baseline. Resume dexamethasone reduced by one dose level. If symptoms persist, reduce by another dose level
G ≥2 muscle weakness (symptomatic; evident on physical exam; limiting instrumental ADL)	Withhold dexamethasone until symptoms return to baseline. Resume dexamethasone reduced by one dose level. If weakness persists, reduce by another dose level. If weakness still persists, then permanently discontinue dexamethasone[‡]
G ≥3 hyperglycemia (insulin therapy initiated; hospitalization indicated)	Withhold dexamethasone until glucose is ≤250 mg/dL. Treat with insulin or other hypoglycemic agents as clinically appropriate and then resume dexamethasone at the same dose. If hyperglycemia is uncontrolled despite above measures, decrease dexamethasone by one dose level
Other G ≥2 nonhematologic toxicity attributable to dexamethasone including severe irritability, insomnia, or oral candidiasis	Withhold dexamethasone until toxicity resolves to G ≤1, then resume at a lower dose. Consider reduction by one dose level for G2/G3 toxicity, and by two dose levels for G4 or recurrent G3 toxicity

*If a dose-limiting toxicity occurs on day ≤15 of a cycle, the new cycle may begin as soon as 7 days after lenalidomide was stopped if the dose-limiting toxicity resolves. If the dose-limiting toxicity occurs on day >15 of a cycle, lenalidomide dosing should be interrupted for at least the remainder of that cycle
[†]If lenalidomide is permanently discontinued, then also consider discontinuation of dexamethasone
[‡]If dexamethasone is permanently discontinued, continued administration of lenalidomide may be considered at the discretion of the treating physician

Patient Population Studied

The international, multicenter, open-label, phase 3 trial (FIRST) involved 1623 patients with previously untreated, symptomatic, and measurable multiple myeloma. Eligible patients were either ≥65 years or <65 years and ineligible for stem-cell transplantation, and had Eastern Cooperative Oncology Group (ECOG) performance score ≤2. Patients who had undergone prior antimyeloma treatment (except for radiotherapy and treatment with bisphosphonates or a single course of glucocorticoids), or had renal failure requiring dialysis, or Grade ≥2 peripheral neuropathy were ineligible. Patients were randomly assigned (1:1:1) to receive 28-day cycles of lenalidomide (25 mg on days 1 to 21) plus dexamethasone (40 mg on days 1, 8, 15, and 22) until disease progression, the same regimen for 72 weeks (18 cycles), or 42-day cycles of standard therapy of melphalan (0.25 mg/kg on days 1 to 4) plus prednisone (2 mg/kg on days 1 to 4) plus thalidomide (200 mg/day) for 72 weeks (12 cycles). All patients received protocol-specified antithrombotic prophylaxis

Efficacy (n = 1623)

	Lenalidomide + Dexamethasone Until Disease Progression (n = 535)	Lenalidomide + Dexamethasone for 18 Cycles (n = 541)	Melphalan + Prednisone + Thalidomide for 12 Cycles (n = 547)
Median progression-free survival*	25.5 months	20.7 months	21.2 months
Overall survival at 3 years	70%	66%	62%
Overall survival at 4 years	59%	56%	51%
Overall response rate†	75%	73%	62%

*The comparison between the lenalidomide + dexamethasone until disease progression and melphalan + prednisone + thalidomide for 12 cycles groups was the primary end point; the hazard ratio (HR) for this comparison was 0.72 (95% CI 0.61–0.85); P <0.001. For comparison between the lenalidomide + dexamethasone until disease progression and lenalidomide + dexamethasone for 18 cycles groups: HR 0.70 (95% CI 0.60–0.82); P <0.001. For comparison between the lenalidomide + dexamethasone for 18 cycles and melphalan + prednisone + thalidomide for 12 cycles groups: HR 1.03 (95% CI 0.89–1.20); P = 0.70
†Overall response rate was the proportion of patients who experienced a partial or complete response according to the International Uniform Response Criteria for Multiple Myeloma
Note: the median duration of treatment was 18.4 months, 16.6 months, and 15.4 months, respectively, for the lenalidomide + dexamethasone until disease progression, lenalidomide + dexamethasone for 18 cycles, and melphalan + prednisone + thalidomide for 12 cycles groups. Among surviving patients at data cut-off, the median duration of follow-up was 37.0 months

Adverse Events (n = 1613)

Grade 3–4 adverse event*	Lenalidomide + Dexamethasone Until Disease Progression (n = 532)	Lenalidomide + Dexamethasone for 18 Cycles (n = 540)	Melphalan + Prednisone + Thalidomide for 12 Cycles (n = 541)
Any Grade 3–4 event	85	80	89
Infection	29	22	17
Neutropenia	28	26	45
Anemia	18	16	19
Cardiac disorder	12	7	9
Thrombocytopenia	8	8	11
Pneumonia	8	8	6
Deep-vein thrombosis, pulmonary embolism, or both	8	6	5
Asthenia	8	6	6
Fatigue	7	9	6
Back pain	7	6	5
Hypokalemia	7	4	2
Rash	6	5	5
Dyspnea	6	4	3
Lymphopenia	6	3	7
Cataracts	6	3	<1
Leukopenia	5	6	10
Hyperglycemia	5	4	2
Constipation	2	2	5
Peripheral sensory neuropathy	1	<1	9

*According to the National Cancer Institute Common Terminology Criteria for Adverse Events, version 3.0
Note: adverse events reported for 5% of any study group are included

Therapy Monitoring

1. CBC with differential, liver function tests, serum creatinine, and serum glucose prior to each cycle
2. With abdominal pain, check serum amylase/lipase
3. Ensure adequate hydration of patients to reduce the risk of renal toxicity and of tumor lysis syndrome

Lenalidomide notes:
- Higher incidences of second primary malignancies were observed in controlled trials of patients with MM receiving lenalidomide. While no routine monitoring is indicated, awareness of this potential complication is necessary
- A decrease in the number of CD34+ cells collected after treatment has been reported in patients who have received >4 cycles of lenalidomide. In patients who may undergo autologous stem cell transplantation, consider early referral to transplant center
- Because of the embryo-fetal risk lenalidomide is available only through a restricted program under a Risk Evaluation and Mitigation Strategy (REMS), the REVLIMID REMS program

TRANSPLANT-INELIGIBLE • FIRST-LINE INDUCTION
MULTIPLE MYELOMA REGIMEN: MODIFIED LENALIDOMIDE + BORTEZOMIB + DEXAMETHASONE (RVD-LITE)

O'Donnell EK et al. Br J Haematol 2018;182:222–230

Induction therapy (RVD-lite, nine 35-day cycles)

Bortezomib 1.3 mg/m^2 per dose; administer subcutaneously in a volume of 0.9% sodium chloride injection (0.9% NS) sufficient to produce a final bortezomib concentration of 2.5 mg/mL, for 4 doses on days 1, 8, 15, and 22, every 35 days for 9 cycles of induction therapy (total dosage/35-day induction cycle = 5.2 mg/m^2)

Lenalidomide 15 mg/dose; administer orally, without regard to meals, once daily for 21 consecutive days on days 1–21, followed by 14 days without treatment, every 35 days for 9 cycles of induction therapy (total dosage/35-day induction cycle = 315 mg)

- Patients who delay taking a lenalidomide dose at a regularly scheduled time may take the missed dose if the time to the next regularly scheduled dose is >12 hours away

- Lenalidomide dosing in renal impairment was prespecified in the trial (O'Donnell et al) but the specific dose adjustment guidelines followed were not published in the manuscript. Consider doses in Treatment Modifications table

Dexamethasone 20 mg/dose; administer orally or intravenously for 8 doses on days 1, 2, 8, 9, 15, 16, 22, and 23, every 35 days for 9 cycles of induction therapy (total dosage/35-day induction cycle for patients <75 years of age = 160 mg)

Note: patients ≥75 years of age received a reduced dose of dexamethasone, thus:

- **Dexamethasone** 20 mg/dose; administer orally or intravenously for 4 doses on days 1, 8, 15, and 22, every 35 days for 9 cycles of induction therapy (total dosage/35-day induction cycle for patients ≥75 years of age = 80 mg)

Consolidation therapy (lenalidomide + bortezomib, six 28-day cycles)

Lenalidomide 15 mg/dose; administer orally, without regard to meals, once daily for 21 consecutive days on days 1–21, followed by 7 days without treatment, every 28 days for 6 cycles of consolidation therapy (total dosage/28-day consolidation cycle = 315 mg)

- Patients who underwent a lenalidomide dose reduction during induction therapy should continue receiving the same reduced dose of lenalidomide during consolidation therapy (according to the consolidation schedule)

- Patients who delay taking a lenalidomide dose at a regularly scheduled time may take the missed dose if the time to the next regularly scheduled dose is >12 hours away

- Lenalidomide dosing in renal impairment was pre-specified in the trial (O'Donnell et al), but the specific dose adjustment guidelines followed were not published in the manuscript. Consider doses in Treatment Modifications table

Bortezomib 1.3 mg/m^2 per dose; administer subcutaneously in a volume of 0.9% NS sufficient to produce a final bortezomib concentration of 2.5 mg/mL, for 2 doses on days 1 and 15, every 28 days for 6 cycles of consolidation therapy (total dosage/28-day consolidation cycle = 2.6 mg/m^2)

Note: patients who underwent a bortezomib dose reduction during induction therapy should continue receiving the same reduced dose of bortezomib during consolidation

Optional maintenance therapy (lenalidomide, 28-day cycles until disease progression)

Lenalidomide 15 mg/dose; administer orally, without regard to meals, once daily for 21 consecutive days on days 1–21, followed by 7 days without treatment, every 28 days as maintenance therapy until disease progression (total dosage/28-day maintenance cycle = 315 mg)

- Maintenance therapy with lenalidomide was optional in the trial by O'Donnell et al

- Patients who underwent a lenalidomide dose reduction during consolidation therapy should continue receiving the same reduced dose of lenalidomide during maintenance therapy

- Patients who delay taking a lenalidomide dose at a regularly scheduled time may take the missed dose if the time to the next regularly scheduled dose is >12 hours away

- Lenalidomide dosing in renal impairment was pre-specified in the trial (O'Donnell et al) but the specific dose adjustment guidelines followed were not published in the manuscript. Consider doses in Treatment Modifications table

Supportive Care

Antiemetic prophylaxis

Emetogenic potential on days with lenalidomide and/or bortezomib is **LOW**

See Chapter 42 for antiemetic recommendations

Hematopoietic growth factor (CSF) prophylaxis

Primary prophylaxis is NOT indicated

See Chapter 43 for more information

(continued)

(*continued*)

Antimicrobial prophylaxis
Risk of fever and neutropenia is **INTERMEDIATE**
Antimicrobial primary prophylaxis to be considered:
- Antibacterial—consider a fluoroquinolone during periods of neutropenia or no prophylaxis; *P. jirovecii* prophylaxis is recommended (eg, cotrimoxazole)
- Antifungal—consider fluconazole during periods of neutropenia
- Antiviral—antiherpes antivirals (eg, acyclovir, famciclovir, valacyclovir) is recommended during therapy with bortezomib

Bisphosphonates
All patients receiving primary therapy for symptomatic multiple myeloma should receive a bisphosphonate adjunctively.

Thromboprophylaxis
Risk assessment and recommendations for VTE prophylaxis in patients with multiple myeloma with individual or myeloma-related risk factors, or risk factors related to treatment

Individual risk factors	
• Obesity (BMI ≥30 kg/m²)	
• H/O VTE	
• CVC or pacemaker	
• Comorbid pathologies	
▪ Cardiac disease	
▪ Chronic renal disease	
▪ Diabetes	≤1 Individual or myeloma-related risk factor present:
▪ Acute infection	• **Aspirin** 81–325 mg daily
▪ Immobilization	
• Surgery	
▪ General surgery	≥2 Individual or myeloma-related risk factors present:
▪ Any anesthesia	• **LMWH,*** equivalent to enoxaparin sodium 40 mg/day *or* **dalteparin sodium** 5000 IU/day; administer subcutaneously, *or*
▪ Trauma	• **Warfarin**, targeting an INR = 2–3
• Medications	
▪ Erythropoietin (epoetin alfa, darbepoetin)	
▪ Estrogenic compounds	
▪ Bevacizumab	
• Clotting disorders	
▪ Thrombophilia	
Myeloma-related risk factors	
• Diagnosis of multiple myeloma	
• Hyperviscosity	
Concomitant treatment-related risk factors	
Thalidomide or lenalidomide in combination with:	• **LMWH,*** equivalent to enoxaparin sodium 40 mg/day *or* **dalteparin sodium** 5000 IU/day; administer subcutaneously, *or*
• High-dose dexamethasone (≥480 mg/month)	• **Warfarin**, targeting an INR = 2–3
• Doxorubicin	
• Multiagent chemotherapy	

*LMWHs should be used with caution in individuals with impaired renal function (creatinine clearance <30 mL/min). Refer to product labeling for information about doses and administration schedules in renally impaired patients, and guidance for monitoring anti-Factor Xa concentrations

Abbreviations: CVC, central venous catheter; INR, international normalized ratio; LMWH, low-molecular-weight heparin; VTE, venous thromboembolic disease

References: Geerts WH et al. Chest 2008;133(6 Suppl):381S–453S
National Comprehensive Cancer Network. Multiple Myeloma, V.1.2014. (Accessed October 8, 2013, at http://www.nccn.org)
National Comprehensive Cancer Network. Venous Thromboembolic Disease, V.2.2013. (Accessed October 8, 2013, at http://www.nccn.org)
Palumbo A et al. Leukemia 2008;22:414–423

Treatment Modifications

LENALIDOMIDE

Lenalidomide dose levels (Days 1–21 of each cycle only)

	CrCl ≥60 mL/min	CrCl ≥30 mL/min and <60 mL/min	CrCl <30 mL/min (not on hemodialysis)	ESRD on hemodialysis
Starting dose	15 mg each day	7.5 mg each day	7.5 mg every other day	2.5 mg each day (after dialysis on dialysis days)
Dose level −1	10 mg each day	5 mg each day	5 mg every other day	Discontinue†
Dose level −2	5 mg each day	2.5 mg each day	2.5 mg every other day	
Dose level −3	2.5 mg each day	Discontinue†	Discontinue†	
Dose level −4	Discontinue†			

Adverse Event	Treatment Modification
Hematologic Toxicity	
Day 1 ANC <1000/mm³ or platelet count <70,000/mm³	Delay the next cycle until ANC ≥1000/mm³ and platelet count ≥70,000/mm³. Consider treatment with filgrastim and/or platelet transfusion according to local guidelines. If the start of a new cycle is delayed >14 days for lenalidomide-related toxicity, then reduce the lenalidomide dosage by one dose level
Either of the following: • G4 neutropenia (ANC <500/mm³) • Neutropenic fever (ANC <1000/mm³ + a single temperature >38.5°C)	Withhold lenalidomide for the remainder of the cycle and delay initiation of the next cycle until ANC ≥1000/mm³ and platelet count ≥50,000/mm³, if necessary. Consider treatment with filgrastim according to local guidelines. If neutropenia was the only dose-limiting toxicity AND if filgrastim is continued AND if the next cycle was delayed by ≤14 days, then resume lenalidomide at the same dose. Otherwise, reduce the lenalidomide dose by one dose level at the start of the next cycle
G3 neutropenia (ANC ≥500/mm³ and <1000/mm³) during a cycle	Interrupt lenalidomide treatment and follow weekly CBC. When ANC ≥1000/mm³, and there are no other toxicities, resume lenalidomide treatment at same dose. If other toxicities are still present then resume lenalidomide with dose reduced one dose level
Recurrent G3 neutropenia (ANC ≥500/mm³ and <1000/mm³) during a cycle	Interrupt lenalidomide treatment and follow weekly CBC. When ANC ≥1000/mm³, resume with dose reduced one dose level
G4 thrombocytopenia (platelet count <25,000/mm³)	Interrupt lenalidomide treatment and follow weekly CBC. When platelet count ≥25,000/mm³ resume lenalidomide with dose reduced one dose level
Recurrent G4 thrombocytopenia (platelet count <25,000/mm³)	
Nonhematologic Toxicity	
G3/4 hepatotoxicity (ALT/AST >5× ULN and/or bilirubin >3× ULN)	Withhold lenalidomide for remainder of the cycle. Delay initiation of next cycle until hepatotoxicity resolves to G ≤2 (ALT/AST ≤5× ULN and/or bilirubin ≤3× ULN), then resume lenalidomide at one lower dose level
G3 rash	Hold dose for remainder of cycle. Decrease by one dose level when dosing resumed at next cycle (rash must resolve to G ≤1)
Allergic reactions, including hypersensitivity, angioedema, Stevens-Johnson syndrome, toxic epidermal necrolysis (TEN), and drug reaction with eosinophilia and systemic symptoms (DRESS)	Discontinue lenalidomide if reactions are suspected. Do not resume lenalidomide if these reactions are confirmed
Tumor lysis syndrome (TLS)	Monitor patients at risk of TLS (ie, those with high tumor burden) and take appropriate precautions including aggressive hydration and allopurinol
G3 peripheral neuropathy	If neuropathy is considered to be attributable to lenalidomide, then withhold lenalidomide for the remainder of the cycle. Delay initiation of the next cycle until neuropathy resolves to G ≤1, then resume lenalidomide at one lower dose level
G4 peripheral neuropathy	If neuropathy is considered to be attributable to lenalidomide, then discontinue lenalidomide
G3/4 venous thromboembolism (VTE) during aspirin monotherapy or inadequate anticoagulation	Continue lenalidomide at the current dose and initiate adequate anticoagulation
G3/4 venous thromboembolism (VTE) during adequate anticoagulation (eg, prophylactic or therapeutic doses of LMWH, UFH, or warfarin)	Discontinue lenalidomide

(continued)

Treatment Modifications (continued)

Nonhematologic Toxicity

G ≥2 hypothyroidism or G ≥2 hyperthyroidism	Continue lenalidomide at current dose and initiate appropriate medical treatment
Other G ≥3 lenalidomide-related toxicities	Withhold lenalidomide for the remainder of the cycle. Delay initiation of the next cycle until toxicity resolves to G ≤2, then resume lenalidomide at one lower dose level

BORTEZOMIB

Starting dose	1.3 mg/m^2/dose
Dose level −1	1 mg/m^2/dose
Dose level −2	0.7 mg/m^2/dose

Adverse Event	Treatment Modification
Platelet count <70,000/mm^3 or ANC <1000/mm^3 on day 1 of a cycle	Hold therapy until platelet count ≥70,000/mm^3 and ANC ≥1000/mm^3
G3 thrombocytopenia (platelet count <50,000/mm^3)	Reduce bortezomib dosage by one dose level
G1 neuropathy (paresthesias, weakness, and/or loss of reflexes) without pain or loss of function	No action
G1 neuropathy with pain or G2 neuropathy (interferes with function but not with activities of daily living)	Reduce bortezomib dosage one dose level
G2 neuropathy with pain or G3 neuropathy (interferes with activities of daily living)	Withhold bortezomib treatment until toxicity resolves to G1 or baseline, then reinitiate reducing bortezomib dosage one dose level
G4 neuropathy (sensory neuropathy that is disabling or motor neuropathy that is life-threatening or leads to paralysis)	Discontinue treatment
Hepatotoxicity	Monitor liver function. Stop bortezomib and evaluate if hepatotoxicity is suspected
Bilirubin level greater than 1.5× ULN and any AST level	Reduce bortezomib to 0.7 mg/m^2 in the first cycle; consider dose escalation to 1 mg/m^2 based on tolerability
If several bortezomib doses in consecutive cycles are withheld due to toxicity	Reduce bortezomib by 1 dosage level
G ≥2 nonhematologic toxicity on day 1 of a cycle	Hold bortezomib until toxicity has resolved to G1 or baseline
G ≥3 nonhematologic toxicities	Hold bortezomib until toxicity has resolved to G1 or baseline; then, may be reinitiated with 1 dosage level reduction

DEXAMETHASONE

Starting dose	20 mg/dose/day
Dose Level −1	12 mg/dose/day
Dose Level −2	8 mg/dose/day
Dose Level −3	4 mg/dose/day
Dose Level −4	Discontinue dexamethasone

Adverse Event	Treatment Modification
G1/2 dyspepsia (moderate symptoms; medical intervention indicated; limiting instrumental ADL), gastric or duodenal ulcer, or gastritis	Continue dexamethasone at the same dose. Treat with therapeutic doses of an H$_2$-receptor antagonist or proton pump inhibitor. If symptoms persist, then reduce the dexamethasone dose by one level
G ≥3 dyspepsia, gastric or duodenal ulcer, or gastritis (surgery or hospitalization indicated)	Withhold dexamethasone until symptoms return to baseline. Resume dexamethasone reduced by one dose level along with concurrent treatment with therapeutic doses of an H$_2$-receptor antagonist or proton pump inhibitor. If symptoms recur, then permanently discontinue dexamethasone
Acute pancreatitis	Permanently discontinue dexamethasone
G ≥3 edema	Withhold dexamethasone until symptoms return to baseline. Consider treatment with diuretics. Resume dexamethasone reduced by one dose level. If edema persists, reduce by another dose level. Discontinue dexamethasone permanently if symptoms persist despite two prior dose reductions

(continued)

Treatment Modifications (continued)

Adverse Event	Treatment Modification
G ≥2 mood alteration (moderate mood alteration) or confusion (moderate disorientation; limiting instrumental ADL)	Withhold dexamethasone until symptoms return to baseline. Resume dexamethasone reduced by one dose level. If symptoms persist, reduce by another dose level
G ≥2 muscle weakness (symptomatic; evident on physical exam; limiting instrumental ADL)	Withhold dexamethasone until symptoms return to baseline. Resume dexamethasone reduced by one dose level. If weakness persists, reduce by another dose level. If weakness still persists, then permanently discontinue dexamethasone
G ≥3 hyperglycemia (insulin therapy initiated; hospitalization indicated)	Withhold dexamethasone until glucose is ≤250 mg/dL. Treat with insulin or other hypoglycemic agents as clinically appropriate and then resume dexamethasone at the same dose. If hyperglycemia is uncontrolled despite above measures, decrease dexamethasone by one dose level
Other G ≥2 nonhematologic toxicity attributable to dexamethasone including severe irritability, insomnia, or oral candidiasis	Withhold dexamethasone until toxicity resolves to G ≤1, then resume at a lower dose. Consider reduction by one dose level for G2/G3 toxicity, and by two dose levels for G4 or recurrent G3 toxicity

If the dose of one drug in the regimen (ie, lenalidomide, dexamethasone, or bortezomib) is delayed, interrupted, or discontinued, the treatment with the other drugs may continue as scheduled.

Patient Population Studied

The multicenter, single-arm, phase 2 trial involved 50 transplant-ineligible patients with newly diagnosed multiple myeloma. Eligible patients were either ≥65 years or <65 years and ineligible for autologous stem-cell transplantation, and had Eastern Cooperative Oncology Group (ECOG) performance score ≤2. Patients who had received prior systemic therapy for multiple myeloma, or Grade ≥2 peripheral neuropathy were ineligible

Efficacy (n = 50)

Overall response rate*	86%
Median progression-free survival	35.1 months

*Overall response rate was the proportion of patients who experienced a partial or complete response according to the International Myeloma Working Group Uniform Response Criteria after four cycles of RVD-lite; this was the primary end point
Note: median duration of follow-up was 30 months

Adverse Events (n = 50)

Grade (%)*	Grade 1–2	G ≥3
Fatigue	58	16
Peripheral neuropathy	58	2
Hypophosphatemia	12	34
Neutropenia	30	14
Diarrhea	38	0
Peripheral edema	34	2
Rash	24	10
Insomnia	32	2
Anemia	26	2
Hyperglycemia	20	4
Thrombocytopenia	22	2
Constipation	24	0
Dysgeusia	24	0
Nausea	18	0
Psychiatric disorder, other	12	4
Generalized muscle weakness	12	4
Depression	16	0

*According to the National Cancer Institute Common Terminology Criteria for Adverse Events, version 4.0
Note: treatment-related adverse events that occurred in >15% of patient are included. Two (4%) patients discontinued treatment owing to toxicity

Therapy Monitoring

1. CBC with differential, liver function tests, serum creatinine, and serum glucose prior to the start of each cycle and prior to each bortezomib dose
2. With abdominal pain, check serum amylase/lipase
3. Ensure adequate hydration of patients to reduce the risk of renal toxicity
4. Monitor for bortezomib toxicities including neuropathy and hypotension
5. In a patient who is a potential candidate for future auto-HSCT, consider mobilization and collection of autologous stem cells within the first 4 cycles of lenalidomide
6. Monitor thyroid function

Lenalidomide notes:

• Higher incidences of second primary malignancies were observed in controlled trials of patients with MM receiving lenalidomide. While no routine monitoring is indicated, awareness of this potential complication is necessary

• A decrease in the number of CD34+ cells collected after treatment has been reported in patients who have received >4 cycles of lenalidomide. In patients who may undergo transplant, consider early referral to transplant center

• Because of the embryo-fetal risk lenalidomide is available only through a restricted program under a Risk Evaluation and Mitigation Strategy (REMS), the REVLIMID REMS program

Bortezomib note:

• Patients with pre-existing severe neuropathy should be treated with bortezomib only after careful risk-benefit assessment

TRANSPLANT-INELIGIBLE • FIRST-LINE INDUCTION
MULTIPLE MYELOMA REGIMEN: DARATUMUMAB + LENALIDOMIDE + DEXAMETHASONE

Chari A et al. Blood 2016;128:2142
Facon T et al. N Engl J Med 2019;380:2104–2115
Protocol for: Facon T et al. N Engl J Med 2019;380:2104–2115
Supplementary appendix to: Facon T et al. N Engl J Med 2019;380:2104–2115
DARZALEX (daratumumab) prescribing information. Horsham, PA: Janssen Biotech, Inc; revised September 2019
DARZALEX FASPRO (daratumumab and hyaluronidase-fihj) prescribing information. Horsham, PA: Janssen Biotech, Inc; revised May 2020

All cycles (28-day cycles):
Lenalidomide 25 mg per dose; administer orally, without regard to meals, once daily for 21 consecutive days on days 1–21, followed by 7 days without treatment, every 28 days, until disease progression (total dosage/28-day cycle = 525 mg)
- Patients who delay taking a lenalidomide dose at a regularly scheduled time may take the missed dose if the time to the next regularly scheduled dose is >12 hours away
- Consider doses in Treatment Modifications table for dose adjustments for renal function

Dexamethasone (age ≤75 years and body mass index (BMI) ≥18.5 kg/m^2, 40 mg per dose; age >75 years or BMI <18.5 kg/m^2, 20 mg per dose); administer orally or intravenously for 4 doses on days 1, 8, 15, and 22, every 28 days, until disease progression (total dosage/28-day cycle = 160 mg [age ≤75 years and BMI ≥18.5 kg/m^2] or 80 mg [age >75 years or BMI <18.5 kg/m^2])
- During weeks when daratumumab is administered, dexamethasone serves a dual purpose as (1) a component of the anti-myeloma therapy backbone and (2) a component of the daratumumab premedication regimen. Therefore, during weeks when daratumumab is administered, dexamethasone should be administered between 1–3 hours prior to daratumumab

Cycles 1–2 (28-day cycles):
May choose to administer either DARZALEX (daratumumab) intravenously, or DARZALEX FASPRO (daratumumab and hyaluronidase-fihj) subcutaneously:

DARZALEX (daratumumab) 16 mg/kg per dose; administer intravenously for 4 doses on days 1, 8, 15, and 22, every 28 days, for 2 cycles (cycles 1–2) (total dosage/28-day cycle during cycles 1–2 = 64 mg/kg), or:
Notes:
- The first daratumumab dose may optionally be split over two consecutive days (ie, in cycle 1 administer 8 mg/kg on day 1 and 8 mg/kg on day 2) to facilitate administration
- Refer to the table titled "Administration Instructions" for instructions regarding daratumumab premedication, infusion rate, dilution, and post-infusion medication

DARZALEX FASPRO *(daratumumab and hyaluronidase-fihj)* 1800 mg/30,000 units in 15 mL of ready-to-use solution per dose; administer by a health care provider subcutaneously into the abdomen over approximately 3–5 minutes for 4 doses on days 1, 8, 15, and 22, every 28 days, for 2 cycles (cycles 1–2) (total dosage/28-day cycle during cycles 1–2 = 7200 mg/120,000 units)
Note: refer to the table titled "Administration Instructions" for instructions regarding premedications, post-administration medications, and administration

Cycles 3–6 (28-day cycles):
May choose to administer either DARZALEX (daratumumab) intravenously, or DARZALEX FASPRO (daratumumab and hyaluronidase-fihj) subcutaneously:

DARZALEX (daratumumab) 16 mg/kg per dose; administer intravenously for 2 doses on days 1 and 15, every 28 days, for 4 cycles (cycles 3–6) (total dosage/28-day cycle during cycles 3–6 = 32 mg/kg), or:
Note: refer to the table titled "Administration Instructions" for instructions regarding daratumumab premedication, infusion rate, dilution, and post-infusion medication

DARZALEX FASPRO *(daratumumab and hyaluronidase-fihj)* 1800 mg/30,000 units in 15 mL of ready-to-use solution per dose; administer by a health care provider subcutaneously into the abdomen over approximately 3–5 minutes for 2 doses on days 1 and 15, every 28 days, for 4 cycles (cycles 3–6) (total dosage/28-day cycle during cycles 3–6 = 3,600 mg/60,000 units)
Note: refer to the table titled "Administration Instructions" for instructions regarding premedications, post-administration medications, and administration

Cycle 7 and beyond (28-day cycles):
May choose to administer either DARZALEX (daratumumab) intravenously, or DARZALEX FASPRO (daratumumab and hyaluronidase-fihj) subcutaneously:

Daratumumab 16 mg/kg per dose; administer intravenously for 1 dose on day 1, every 28 days, until disease progression (cycle 7 and beyond) (total dosage/28-day cycle during cycle 7 and beyond = 16 mg/kg), or:
Note: refer to the table titled "Daratumumab Administration" for instructions regarding daratumumab premedication, infusion rate, dilution, and post-infusion medication

DARZALEX FASPRO *(daratumumab and hyaluronidase-fihj)* 1800 mg/30,000 units in 15 mL of ready-to-use solution per dose; administer by a health care provider subcutaneously into the abdomen over approximately 3–5 minutes for 4 doses on days 1, 8, 15, and 22, every 28 days, for 2 cycles (cycles 1–2) (total dosage/28-day cycle during cycles 1–2 = 7200 mg/120,000 units)
Note: Refer to the table titled "Administration Instructions" for instructions regarding premedications, post-administration medications, and administration

(continued)

(continued)

ADMINISTRATION INSTRUCTIONS

Premedications
(applies to DARZALEX (daratumumab) and DARZALEX FASPRO (daratumumab and hyaluronidase-fihj))

Antipyretic	**Acetaminophen** 650–1000 mg; administer orally 1–3 hours before each DARZALEX (daratumumab) or DARZALEX FASPRO (daratumumab and hyaluronidase-fihj) dose
H$_1$-subtype antihistamine	**Diphenhydramine** 25–50 mg; administer orally or intravenously 1–3 hours before each DARZALEX (daratumumab) or DARZALEX FASPRO (daratumumab and hyaluronidase-fihj) dose
Corticosteroid	**Dexamethasone** (age ≤75 years and BMI ≥18.5 kg/m^2, 40 mg; age >75 years or BMI <18.5 kg/m^2, 20 mg); administer intravenously or orally 1–3 hours before each DARZALEX (daratumumab) or DARZALEX FASPRO (daratumumab and hyaluronidase-fihj) dose • May administer dexamethasone orally beginning with the second dose
Leukotriene receptor antagonist *(optional)**	**Montelukast** 10 mg; administer orally 1–3 hours before each DARZALEX (daratumumab) or DARZALEX FASPRO (daratumumab and hyaluronidase-fihj) dose

Dilution volume and infusion rate
(applies to DARZALEX [daratumumab] only)

DARZALEX (daratumumab) must be administered through an administration set with a flow regulator and with an in-line, sterile, nonpyrogenic, low-protein-binding polyethersulfone filter with a pore size of 0.2 or 0.22 μm

First infusion	Dilute in 1000 mL 0.9% NS. Infuse initially at 50 mL/hour. If hypersensitivity or infusion reactions do not occur during the first hour, increase the rate by 50 mL/hour every hour as tolerated to a maximum rate of 200 mL/hour *Note:* if splitting the first daratumumab over two consecutive days (ie, 8 mg/kg on day 1 and 8 mg/kg on day 2), then dilute each 8 mg/kg dose in 500 mL 0.9% NS. Infuse initially at 50 mL/hour. If hypersensitivity or infusion reactions do not occur during the first hour, increase the rate by 50 mL/hour every hour as tolerated to a maximum rate of 200 mL/hour
Second infusion†	Dilute in 500 mL 0.9% NS. Infuse initially at 50 mL/hour. If hypersensitivity or infusion reactions do not occur during the first hour, increase the rate by 50 mL/hour every hour as tolerated to a maximum rate of 200 mL/hour
Subsequent infusions‡	Dilute in 500 mL 0.9% NS. Infuse initially at 100 mL/hour. If hypersensitivity or infusion reactions do not occur during the first hour, increase the rate by 50 mL/hour every hour as tolerated to a maximum rate of 200 mL/hour

Subcutaneous Injection
(applies to DARZALEX FASPRO [daratumumab and hyaluronidase-fihj] only)

• Attach the hypodermic injection needle or subcutaneous infusion set to the syringe immediately prior to injection in order to reduce the chances of needle clogging

• Choose a site for administration approximately 3 inches (7.5 cm) to the right or left of the navel; rotate administration sites. Do not inject into areas where the skin is red, bruised, tender, hard, or scarred, or into areas used for administration of other subcutaneous medications

• A health care provider should administer the 15 mL dose subcutaneously into the abdomen over approximately 3–5 minutes

• If the injection causes pain, temporarily interrupt or reduce the rate of injection. If this does not relieve the pain, then choose another injection site on the opposite side of the abdomen in which to deliver the remainder of the dose

• Among low-body-weight (<50 kg) patients, the mean maximum trough concentration after the 8th dose was 81% higher in patients who received the fixed subcutaneous doses of DARZALEX FASPRO (daratumumab and hyaluronidase-fihj) compared to those who received 16 mg/kg per dose of intravenously administered DARZALEX (daratumumab). Higher rates of G3/4 neutropenia were observed in low-body-weight patients who received the formulation for subcutaneous injection

Post-administration medications
(applies to DARZALEX [daratumumab] and DARZALEX FASPRO [daratumumab and hyaluronidase-fihj])

Corticosteroid *(optional)*	**Methylprednisolone** 20 mg; administer orally once on the day after each DARZALEX (daratumumab) or DARZALEX FASPRO (daratumumab and hyaluronidase-fihj) dose is administered
Short-acting β–2 agonist§	**Albuterol** inhalation aerosol, metered, 90 μg/actuation, administer 2 inhalations every 4 hours as needed for bronchospasm for 3 days, starting on the day of each of the first 4 DARZALEX (daratumumab) or DARZALEX FASPRO (daratumumab and hyaluronidase-fihj) doses
Long-acting β–2 agonist§	**Salmeterol xinafoate** aerosol powder, metered, 50 μg/actuation, administer 1 inhalation twice a day for 3 days, starting the day of each of the first 4 DARZALEX (daratumumab) or DARZALEX FASPRO (daratumumab and hyaluronidase-fihj) doses
Inhaled corticosteroid§	**Fluticasone propionate** inhalation aerosol, metered, 220 μg/actuation, administer 2 inhalations twice a day for 3 days, starting on the day of each of the first 4 DARZALEX (daratumumab) or DARZALEX FASPRO (daratumumab and hyaluronidase-fihj) doses

(continued)

(continued)

*Some institutions consider adding an optional leukotriene receptor antagonist based on data by Chari et al, 2016

†Use a dilution volume of 500 mL only if there were no infusion reactions during the first 3 hours of the first infusion. Otherwise, continue to use a dilution volume of 1000 mL and instructions for the first infusion

‡Use an initial rate of 100 mL/hour for subsequent infusions only if there were no infusion reactions during a final infusion rate of ≥100 mL/hour in the first two infusions. Otherwise, start infusion at 50 mL/hour per instructions for second infusion

§For patients with a history of chronic obstructive pulmonary disease, consider prescribing additional post-infusion inhaled medications for approximately 48 hours following the first 4 daratumumab infusions. Note that availability of inhalational medication formulations may vary by country; representative examples are included in the table

Note: DARZALEX (daratumumab) and DARZALEX FASPRO (daratumumab and hyaluronidase-fihj) can cause severe administration-related reactions. Symptoms of an administration-related reaction may include respiratory symptoms, chills, nausea/vomiting, fever, chest discomfort, hypotension, or pruritus. Only administer the products under medical supervision in a facility with immediate access to medical support and emergency equipment. Closely monitor patients throughout each administration. Most reactions occur during the first dose, when the all-grade systemic administration-related reaction incidence approaches 50% for the intravenous formulation and 10% for the subcutaneous formulation. Reactions may also occur during or following subsequent administrations. Delayed reactions may occur up to 48 hours following each dose; incidence of delayed reactions is reduced when post-infusion corticosteroids are administered. See Treatment Modifications section for management recommendations

Supportive Care

Antiemetic prophylaxis

Emetogenic potential of lenalidomide is **MINIMAL TO LOW**

Emetogenic potential of daratumumab is **MINIMAL**

See Chapter 42 for antiemetic recommendations

Hematopoietic growth factor (CSF) prophylaxis

Primary prophylaxis is NOT indicated

See Chapter 43 for more information

Antimicrobial prophylaxis

Risk of fever and neutropenia is **INTERMEDIATE**

Antimicrobial primary prophylaxis to be considered:

- Antibacterial—consider a fluoroquinolone during periods of neutropenia or no prophylaxis; *P. jirovecii* prophylaxis is recommended (eg, cotrimoxazole)
- Antifungal—recommended; consider use during periods of neutropenia
- Antiviral—antiherpes antivirals (eg, acyclovir, famciclovir, valacyclovir) should be initiated within 1 week of starting daratumumab or daratumumab and hyaluronidase-fihj, and continued for at least 3 months after completion of the last dose

Bisphosphonates

All patients receiving primary therapy for symptomatic multiple myeloma should receive a bisphosphonate adjunctively.

Thromboprophylaxis

Risk assessment and recommendations for VTE prophylaxis in patients with multiple myeloma with individual or myeloma-related risk factors, or risk factors related to treatment

Individual risk factors
• Obesity (BMI ≥30 kg/m²)
• H/O VTE
• CVC or pacemaker
• Comorbid pathologies
  ▪ Cardiac disease
  ▪ Chronic renal disease
  ▪ Diabetes
  ▪ Acute infection
  ▪ Immobilization
• Surgery
  ▪ General surgery
  ▪ Any anesthesia
  ▪ Trauma
• Medications
  ▪ Erythropoietin (epoetin alfa, darbepoetin)
  ▪ Estrogenic compounds
  ▪ Bevacizumab
• Clotting disorders
  ▪ Thrombophilia
Myeloma-related risk factors
• Diagnosis of multiple myeloma
• Hyperviscosity
	≤1 Individual or myeloma-related risk factor present:
	• **Aspirin** 81–325 mg daily
	
	≥2 Individual or myeloma-related risk factors present:
	• **LMWH,*** equivalent to enoxaparin sodium 40 mg/day *or* **dalteparin sodium** 5000 IU/day; administer subcutaneously, *or*
	• **Warfarin**, targeting an INR = 2–3

(continued)

(*continued*)

Concomitant treatment-related risk factors	
Thalidomide or lenalidomide in combination with: • High-dose dexamethasone (≥480 mg/month) • Doxorubicin • Multiagent chemotherapy	• **LMWH,** * equivalent to enoxaparin sodium 40 mg/day *or* **dalteparin sodium** 5000 IU/day; administer subcutaneously, *or* • **Warfarin**, targeting an INR = 2–3

*LMWHs should be used with caution in individuals with impaired renal function (creatinine clearance <30 mL/min). Refer to product labeling for information about doses and administration schedules in renally impaired patients, and guidance for monitoring anti-Factor Xa concentrations

Abbreviations: CVC, central venous catheter; INR, international normalized ratio; LMWH, low-molecular-weight heparin; VTE, venous thromboembolic disease

References: Geerts WH et al. Chest 2008;133(6 Suppl):381S–453S
National Comprehensive Cancer Network. Multiple Myeloma, V.1.2014. (Accessed October 8, 2013, at http://www.nccn.org)
National Comprehensive Cancer Network. Venous Thromboembolic Disease, V.2.2013. (Accessed October 8, 2013, at http://www.nccn.org)
Palumbo A et al. Leukemia 2008;22:414–423

Treatment Modifications

DARATUMUMAB OR DARATUMUMAB AND HYALURONIDASE-FIHJ

Adverse Event	Dose Modification
Infusion-Related Reaction and Anaphylactic Reaction Adverse Events	
• G1/2 infusion-related reaction to intravenous daratumumab. (G1/2 IRR) • First occurrence of G3 infusion-related reaction (G3 IRR) to intravenous daratumumab • Second occurrence of G3 infusion-related reaction to intravenous daratumumab G1 IRR = Mild transient reaction; infusion interruption not indicated; intervention not indicated G2 IRR = Therapy or infusion interruption indicated but responds promptly to symptomatic treatment (eg, antihistamines, NSAIDS, narcotics, IV fluids); prophylactic medications indicated for ≤24 hours G3 IRR = Prolonged (eg, not rapidly responsive to symptomatic medication and/or brief interruption of infusion); recurrence of symptoms following initial improvement; hospitalization indicated for clinical sequelae	Immediately interrupt the daratumumab infusion for infusion-related reactions of *any* severity and manage symptoms as clinically appropriate with additional intravenous corticosteroid (50–150 mg hydrocortisone IVP), an H$_1$-receptor antagonist (diphenhydramine 50 mg IVP), inhaled short-acting ß–2 agonist (albuterol 2 puffs, may repeat in 4 hours) plus epinephrine 0.5 mg IM for hypotension or airway obstructive symptoms. Upon resolution of symptoms, resume the daratumumab infusion at no more than 50% of the rate at which the reaction occurred. If tolerated, escalate the infusion by 50 mL/hour every hour up to a maximum rate of 200 mL/hour
• Third occurrence of G3 infusion-related reaction (IRR) to intravenous daratumumab • G4 infusion-related reaction (G4 IRR) to intravenous daratumumab or subcutaneous daratumumab and hyaluronidase-fihj • Anaphylactic reaction (AR) to intravenous daratumumab or subcutaneous daratumumab and hyaluronidase-fihj G3 IRR = Prolonged (eg, not rapidly responsive to symptomatic medication and/or brief interruption of infusion); recurrence of symptoms following initial improvement; hospitalization indicated for clinical sequelae G4 IRR = Life-threatening consequences; urgent intervention indicated G3 AR = Symptomatic bronchospasm, with or without urticaria; parenteral intervention indicated; allergy-related edema/angioedema; hypotension G4 AR = Life-threatening consequences; urgent intervention indicated	Immediately interrupt administration for infusion-related reactions of *any* severity and manage symptoms as clinically appropriate with additional intravenous corticosteroid (50–150 mg hydrocortisone IVP), an H$_1$-receptor antagonist (diphenhydramine 50 mg IVP), inhaled short-acting ß-2 agonist (albuterol 2 puffs, may repeat in 4 hours) plus epinephrine 0.5 mg IM for hypotension or airway obstructive symptoms Permanently discontinue*
Hematologic Adverse Events	
G3/4 neutropenia G3/4 thrombocytopenia	Consider delaying the dose until recovery to G ≤2 or baseline; or, continue without interruption as clinically appropriate. In the case of neutropenia, consider administration of granulocyte-colony stimulating factor (G-CSF)
Blood transfusion within 6 months following a daratumumab infusion	Notify blood bank the patient has received daratumumab or daratumumab and hyaluronidase-fihj within the past 6 months since either product may result in a positive indirect antiglobulin test (indirect Coombs test) that can persist for up to 6 months and may mask detection of antibodies to minor antigens in the patient's serum. Determination of ABO and Rh blood type is not affected

Note: dose reductions are not recommended for daratumumab or daratumumab and hyaluronidase-fihj

(*continued*)

Treatment Modifications (*continued*)

LENALIDOMIDE TREATMENT MODIFICATIONS

Lenalidomide dose levels (Days 1–21 of each 28-day cycle)

	CrCl ≥50 mL/min	CrCl ≥30 mL/min and <50 mL/min	CrCl <30 mL/min (not on hemodialysis)	ESRD on hemodialysis
Starting dose	25 mg each day	10 mg each day	15 mg every other day	5 mg each day (after dialysis on dialysis days)
Dose level −1	15 mg each day	5 mg each day	10 mg every other day	2.5 mg each day (after dialysis on dialysis days)
Dose level −2	10 mg each day	2.5 mg each day	5 mg every other day	Discontinue*
Dose level −3	5 mg each day	Discontinue*	Discontinue*	
Dose level −4	Discontinue*			

Adverse Event	Treatment Modification
Hematologic Toxicity	
Day 1 ANC <1000/mm³ or platelet count <50,000/mm³	Delay the next cycle until ANC ≥1000/mm³ and platelet count ≥50,000/mm³. Consider treatment with filgrastim and/or platelet transfusion according to local guidelines. If the start of a new cycle is delayed >14 days for lenalidomide-related toxicity, then reduce the lenalidomide by one dose level
G ≥3 neutropenia (ANC <1000/mm³) during a cycle	Interrupt lenalidomide treatment and follow weekly CBC. When ANC ≥1000/mm³ and there are no other toxicities, resume lenalidomide treatment at same dose. If other toxicities are still present, then resume lenalidomide with dose reduced one dose level
Recurrent G ≥3 neutropenia (ANC <1000/mm³) during a cycle	Interrupt lenalidomide treatment and follow weekly CBC. When ANC ≥1000/mm³, resume with dose reduced one dose level
Febrile neutropenia (ANC <1000/mm³ with fever ≥38.3°C)	Hold lenalidomide dosing for up to 21 days to resolve toxicity and then restart at the same dose or reduce the lenalidomide dose by one dose level
Platelet count <30,000/mm³	Interrupt lenalidomide treatment and follow weekly CBC. When platelet count ≥30,000/mm³, resume lenalidomide with dose reduced one dose level
Recurrent platelet count <30,000/mm³	
Nonhematologic Toxicity	
G3/4 hepatotoxicity (ALT/AST >5× ULN and/or bilirubin >3× ULN)	Withhold lenalidomide for remainder of the cycle. Delay initiation of next cycle until hepatotoxicity resolves to G ≤2 (ALT/AST ≤5× ULN and/or bilirubin ≤3× ULN), then resume lenalidomide at one lower dose level
G3 rash	Hold dose for remainder of cycle. Decrease by one dose level when dosing resumed at next cycle (rash must resolve to G ≤1)
Allergic reactions, including hypersensitivity, angioedema, Stevens-Johnson syndrome, toxic epidermal necrolysis (TEN), and drug reaction with eosinophilia and systemic symptoms (DRESS)	Discontinue lenalidomide if reactions are suspected. Do not resume lenalidomide if these reactions are confirmed
Tumor lysis syndrome (TLS)	Monitor patients at risk of TLS (eg, those with high tumor burden) and take appropriate precautions including aggressive hydration and allopurinol
G3 peripheral neuropathy	If neuropathy is considered to be attributable to lenalidomide, then withhold lenalidomide for the remainder of the cycle. Delay initiation of the next cycle until neuropathy resolves to G ≤1, then resume lenalidomide at one lower dose level
G4 peripheral neuropathy	If neuropathy is considered to be attributable to lenalidomide, then discontinue lenalidomide*
G3/4 venous thromboembolism (VTE) during aspirin monotherapy or inadequate anticoagulation	Continue lenalidomide at the current dose and initiate adequate anticoagulation
G3/4 venous thromboembolism (VTE) during adequate anticoagulation (eg, prophylactic or therapeutic doses of LMWH, UFH, or warfarin)	Discontinue lenalidomide*
G ≥2 hypothyroidism or G ≥2 hyperthyroidism	Continue lenalidomide at current dose and initiate appropriate medical treatment
Other G ≥3 lenalidomide-related toxicities	Withhold lenalidomide for the remainder of the cycle. Delay initiation of the next cycle until toxicity resolves to G ≤2, then resume lenalidomide at one lower dose level

(*continued*)

Treatment Modifications (continued)

DEXAMETHASONE TREATMENT MODIFICATIONS

Dexamethasone Dose Levels

	Age ≤75 Years and Body Mass Index ≥18.5 kg/m²	Age >75 Years or Body Mass Index <18.5 kg/m²
Starting dose	40 mg/dose/day days 1, 8, 15, and 22 every 28 days	20 mg/dose/day days 1, 8, 15, and 22 every 28 days
Dose Level −1	20 mg/dose/day days 1, 8, 15, and 22 every 28 days	10 mg/dose/day days 1, 8, 15, and 22 every 28 days
Dose Level −2	10 mg/dose/day days 1, 8, 15, and 22 every 28 days	-

Adverse Event	Treatment Modification
G1/2 dyspepsia (moderate symptoms; medical intervention indicated; limiting instrumental ADL), gastric or duodenal ulcer, or gastritis	Continue dexamethasone at the same dose. Treat with therapeutic doses of an H₂-receptor antagonist or proton pump inhibitor. If symptoms persist, then reduce the dexamethasone dose by one level
G ≥3 dyspepsia, gastric or duodenal ulcer, or gastritis (surgery or hospitalization indicated)	Withhold dexamethasone until symptoms return to baseline. Resume dexamethasone reduced by one dose level along with concurrent treatment with therapeutic doses of an H₂-receptor antagonist or proton pump inhibitor. If symptoms recur, then reduce dexamethasone to dose level −2
Acute pancreatitis	Reduce dexamethasone to dose level −2
G ≥3 edema	Withhold dexamethasone until symptoms return to baseline. Consider treatment with diuretics. Resume dexamethasone reduced by one dose level. If edema persists, reduce to dose level −2
G ≥2 mood alteration (moderate mood alteration) or confusion (moderate disorientation; limiting instrumental ADL)	Withhold dexamethasone until symptoms return to baseline. Resume dexamethasone reduced by one dose level. If symptoms persist, reduce by another dose level
G ≥2 muscle weakness (symptomatic; evident on physical exam; limiting instrumental ADL)	Withhold dexamethasone until symptoms return to baseline. Resume dexamethasone reduced by one dose level. If weakness persists, reduce by another dose level
G ≥3 hyperglycemia (insulin therapy initiated; hospitalization indicated)	Withhold dexamethasone until blood glucose is ≤250 mg/dL. Treat with insulin or other hypoglycemic agents as clinically appropriate and then resume dexamethasone at the same dose. If hyperglycemia is uncontrolled despite above measures, decrease dexamethasone by one dose level
Other G ≥2 nonhematologic toxicity attributable to dexamethasone including severe irritability, insomnia, or oral candidiasis	Withhold dexamethasone until toxicity resolves to G ≤1, then resume at a lower dose. Consider reduction by one dose level for G2/G3 toxicity, and two dose levels for G4 or recurrent G3 toxicity

*If daratumumab and lenalidomide are permanently discontinued, then also consider discontinuing dexamethasone
IRR, infusion-related reactions; AR, anaphylactic reactions

Patient Population Studied

The MAIA trial was a randomized, open-label, international, phase 3 study involving 737 patients with newly diagnosed multiple myeloma who were ineligible for transplant. The study randomized patients 1:1 to receive lenalidomide and dexamethasone either with or without daratumumab. Patients were required to have an Eastern Cooperative Oncology Group performance status (ECOG PS) of ≤2, and to be ineligible for transplant (ie, ≥65 years of age, or younger patients with comorbidities precluding transplant). Patients were required to have a creatinine clearance of ≥30 mL/minute. Among the 368 patients randomized to the daratumumab-containing arm, the median age was 73 years (range, 50–90 years); the ECOG PS was 0 in 34.5%, 1 in 48.4%, and 2 in 17.1%; 15% of patients had high-risk cytogenetics; and the International Staging System disease stage was I in 26.6%, II in 44.3%, and III in 29.1%. Baseline characteristics were well balanced in both arms

Efficacy (n = 737)

Efficacy Variable	Dara + Rd (n = 368)	Rd (n = 369)	Between-group Comparison
PFS (n = 368 in dara + Rd arm, n = 369 in Rd arm)			
Median PFS—months (95% CI)	NR	31.9 (28.9-NR)	HR 0.56 (95% CI, 0.43–0.73); P <0.001
PFS rate at 30 months—% (95% CI)	70.6 (65.0–75.4)	55.6 (49.5–61.3)	—
Response*			
Overall response—n/N (%) (95% CI)	342/368 (92.9) (89.8–95.3)	300/369 (81.3) (76.9–85.1)	P <0.001[†]
CR or better—n/N (%)	175/368 (47.6)	92/369 (24.9)	P <0.001[†]
Stringent CR[‡]—n/N (%)	112/368 (30.4)	46/369 (12.5)	—
CR—n/N (%)	63/368 (17.1)	46/369 (12.5)	—
VGPR or better—n/N (%)	292/368 (79.3)	196/369 (53.1)	P <0.001[†]
VGPR—n/N (%)	117/368 (31.8)	104/369 (28.2)	—
Partial response—n/N (%)	50/368 (13.6)	104/369 (28.2)	—
Stable disease—n/N (%)	11/368 (3.0)	56/369 (15.2)	—
Progressive disease—n/N (%)	1/368 (0.3)	0	—
Response not evaluable—n/N (%)	14/368 (3.8)	13/369 (3.5)	—
Negative for MRD[§]—n/N (%)	89/368 (24.2)	27/369 (7.3)	P <0.001[|]

*Responses were defined according to the International Myeloma Working Group. Response rates were secondary end points and were tested sequentially, each with an overall two-sided alpha level of 0.05, with a hierarchical approach: CR or better, then VGPR or better, then negative status for MRD, and then finally overall response
[†]Cochran-Mantel-Haenszel chi-square test
[‡]Criteria for a stringent CR included criteria for CR plus a normal free light-chain ratio and absence of clonal plasma cells as assessed by immunofluorescence or immunohisto-chemical analysis or by two- to four-color flow cytometry
[§]MRD based on a threshold of 1 cell per 10^5 white cells using a validated next-generation sequencing assay (clonoSEQ Assay v2.0) performed on bone marrow samples
[|]Fisher's exact test
Note: efficacy end points were assessed in the intention-to-treat population. At the primary analysis data cutoff date of 24 September 2018, the median follow-up time was 28.0 months (range, 0–41.4). At data cutoff, disease progression or death had occurred in 240 patients overall (26.4% in the daratumumab-containing arm and 38.8% of the control arm), and death had occurred in 138 patients overall (16.8% in the daratumumab group and 20.6% in the control group); median overall survival was not reached in either group, and long-term follow-up for survival was ongoing at the time of publication. Prespecified subgroup analyses demonstrated the superiority of Dara + Rd over Rd for PFS in all subgroups with the exception of those who had hepatic impairment at baseline (n = 60 patients total)
Dara, daratumumab; Rd, lenalidomide + dexamethasone; PFS, progression-free survival; CI, confidence interval; NR, not reached; HR, hazard ratio; CR, complete response; VGPR, very good partial response; MRD, minimal residual disease

Adverse Events (n = 729)

Grade* (%)	Daratumumab + Lenalidomide + Dexamethasone (n = 364)		Lenalidomide + Dexamethasone (n = 365)	
	Any Grade	Grade 3–4	Any Grade	Grade 3–4
Neutropenia	56.9	50.0	42.2	35.3
Anemia	34.6	11.8	37.8	19.7
Leukopenia	18.7	11.0	9.3	4.9
Lymphopenia	18.1	15.1	12.3	10.7
Infections	86.3	32.1	73.4	23.3
Pneumonia	22.5	13.7	12.6	7.9

(*continued*)

Adverse Events (n = 729) *(continued)*

Grade* (%)	Daratumumab + Lenalidomide + Dexamethasone (n = 364)		Lenalidomide + Dexamethasone (n = 365)	
	Any Grade	Grade 3–4	Any Grade	Grade 3–4
Diarrhea	56.9	6.6	46.0	4.1
Constipation	40.9	1.6	35.6	0.3
Fatigue	40.4	8.0	28.5	3.8
Peripheral edema	38.5	1.9	29.3	0.5
Back pain	33.8	3.0	26.3	3.0
Asthenia	32.1	4.4	24.7	3.6
Nausea	31.6	1.4	23.0	0.5
Second primary cancer†	8.8	NA	7.1	NA
Invasive second primary cancer	3.3	NA	3.6	NA
Any infusion-related reaction	40.9	2.7	NA	NA

*Adverse events were graded according to the National Cancer Institute Common Terminology Criteria for Adverse Events (NCI CTCAE) v4
†Prespecified as an adverse event of clinical interest
Note: adverse events were reported in the safety population, which included all patients who received at least 1 dose of study treatment. The table includes all-grade adverse events that were reported in >30% of patients in either group, Grade 3/4 adverse events that were reported in >10% of patients in either group, and second primary cancers which was prespecified as an adverse event of clinical interest

Therapy Monitoring

1. Type and screen prior to first dose of daratumumab or daratumumab and hyaluronidase-fihj
2. CBC with differential, liver function tests, serum creatinine, and serum glucose prior to each cycle
3. CBC with differential, liver function tests and serum glucose prior to each daratumumab dose
4. Monitor for infusion related daratumumab reaction symptoms frequently during infusion; check vital signs frequently during infusion and at least prior to each scheduled rate increase, ensure medications are available for post-infusion prophylaxis as applicable

Daratumumab note: daratumumab, a human IgG1 kappa monoclonal antibody, may be detected by serum protein electrophoresis and immunofixation assays routinely used to monitor endogenous M-protein. Thus, daratumumab may interfere with disease monitoring in patients with plasma cell neoplasms that produce an IgG kappa M-protein

Lenalidomide notes:
• Higher incidences of second primary malignancies were observed in controlled trials of patients with multiple myeloma receiving lenalidomide. While no routine monitoring is indicated, awareness of this potential complication is necessary
• A decrease in the number of CD34+ cells collected after treatment has been reported in patients who have received >4 cycles of lenalidomide. In patients who may undergo transplant, consider early referral to transplant center
• Because of the embryo-fetal risk, lenalidomide is available only through a restricted program under a Risk Evaluation and Mitigation Strategy (REMS), the REVLIMID REMS program

TRANSPLANT-INELIGIBLE • FIRST-LINE INDUCTION

MULTIPLE MYELOMA REGIMEN: MELPHALAN + PREDNISONE + LENALIDOMIDE

Palumbo A et al. J Clin Oncol 2007;25:4459–4465

Induction:

Melphalan 0.18 mg/kg per day; administer orally for 4 consecutive days on days 1–4, every 4 weeks, for 9 cycles (total dosage/cycle = 0.72 mg/kg)

Prednisone 2 mg/kg per day; administer orally for 4 consecutive days on days 1–4, every 4 weeks, for 9 cycles (total dosage/cycle = 8 mg/kg)

Lenalidomide 10 mg per day; administer orally for 21 consecutive days on days 1–21, every 4 weeks, for 9 cycles (total dose/cycle = 210 mg)

Maintenance:

Lenalidomide 10 mg/day; administer orally for 21 consecutive days on days 1–21, every 4 weeks until signs of relapse or disease progression (total dose/cycle = 210 mg)

Supportive Care

Antiemetic prophylaxis

Emetogenic potential is **MINIMAL–LOW**

See Chapter 42 for antiemetic recommendations

Hematopoietic growth factor (CSF) prophylaxis

Primary prophylaxis is **NOT** indicated

See Chapter 43 for more information

Antimicrobial prophylaxis

Risk of fever and neutropenia is **INTERMEDIATE**

   Antimicrobial primary prophylaxis to be considered:

- Antibacterial—consider a fluoroquinolone or no prophylaxis; *P. jirovecii* prophylaxis is recommended (eg, cotrimoxazole)
- Antifungal—consider concomitant use of clotrimazole during periods of neutropenia
- Antiviral—antiherpes antivirals (eg, acyclovir, famciclovir, valacyclovir)

Decreased bowel motility prophylaxis

Give a bowel regimen to prevent constipation based initially on **stool softeners**

Bisphosphonates

All patients receiving primary therapy for symptomatic multiple myeloma should receive a bisphosphonate adjunctively.

Thromboprophylaxis

Risk assessment and recommendations for VTE prophylaxis in patients with multiple myeloma with individual or myeloma-related risk factors, or risk factors related to treatment

(continued)

Treatment Modifications

Lenalidomide Dose Levels	
Dose Level 1	10 mg/day
Dose Level −1	5 mg/day
Melphalan Dose Levels	
Dosage Level 1	0.18 mg/kg
Dosage Level −1	0.135 mg/kg

Adverse Event	Treatment Modification
Febrile neutropenia	Withhold therapy until fever abates, then resume therapy
G4 neutropenia for ≥7 days despite filgrastim administration, any other G4 hematologic toxicities, or any G ≥3 nonhematologic toxicities	Withhold therapy until toxicities resolve to G ≤2, then resume therapy with a subsequent dose/dosage reduction in lenalidomide and melphalan at the start of the following cycle
G ≥3 neuropathy	Interrupt therapy and follow clinically. After toxicity abates to G ≤2, resume lenalidomide with a dose decreased by 1 dose level
G3/4 nonhematologic toxicity	Interrupt lenalidomide treatment and follow clinically. Resume lenalidomide at 5 mg/day after toxicity abates to G ≤2
ANC <1000/mm³, platelet count <50,000/mm³, or nonhematologic adverse events G ≥2	Withhold therapy as long as 2 weeks until ANC ≥1000/mm³, platelet count is ≥50,000/mm³, and nonhematologic toxicities are G ≤1, then resume therapy. A delay of 2 weeks is allowed without any dose modification. A new cycle delay beyond a maximum of 2 weeks requires a dose/dosage reduction in lenalidomide and melphalan by 1 dose level

(continued)

(continued)

Individual risk factors
• Obesity (BMI ≥30 kg/m²)
• H/O VTE
• CVC or pacemaker
• Comorbid pathologies
  ▪ Cardiac disease
  ▪ Chronic renal disease
  ▪ Diabetes
  ▪ Acute infection
  ▪ Immobilization
• Surgery
  ▪ General surgery
  ▪ Any anesthesia
  ▪ Trauma
• Medications
  ▪ Erythropoietin (epoetin alfa, darbepoetin)
  ▪ Estrogenic compounds
  ▪ Bevacizumab
• Clotting disorders
  ▪ Thrombophilia
Myeloma-related risk factors
• Diagnosis of multiple myeloma
• Hyperviscosity
	≤1 Individual or myeloma-related risk factor present:
	• **Aspirin** 81–325 mg daily
	
	≥2 Individual or myeloma-related risk factors present:
	• **LMWH,*** equivalent to **enoxaparin sodium** 40 mg/day *or* **dalteparin sodium** 5000 IU/day; administer subcutaneously, *or*
	• **Warfarin,** targeting an INR = 2–3

Concomitant treatment-related risk factors Thalidomide or lenalidomide in combination with: • High-dose dexamethasone (≥480 mg/month) • Doxorubicin • Multiagent chemotherapy	• **LMWH,*** equivalent to **enoxaparin sodium** 40 mg/day *or* **dalteparin sodium** 5000 IU/day; administer subcutaneously, *or* • **Warfarin,** targeting an INR = 2–3

*LMWHs should be used with caution in individuals with impaired renal function (creatinine clearance <30 mL/min). Refer to product labeling for information about doses and administration schedules in renally impaired patients, and guidance for monitoring anti-Factor Xa concentrations

Abbreviations: CVC, central venous catheter; INR, international normalized ratio; LMWH, low-molecular-weight heparin; VTE, venous thromboembolic disease

References: Geerts WH et al. Chest 2008;133(6 Suppl):381S–453S

National Comprehensive Cancer Network. Multiple Myeloma, V.1.2014. (Accessed October 8, 2013, at http://www.nccn.org)

National Comprehensive Cancer Network. Venous Thromboembolic Disease, V.2.2013. (Accessed October 8, 2013, at http://www.nccn.org)

Palumbo A et al. Leukemia 2008;22:414–423

Treatment Modifications
(continued)

Adverse Event	Treatment Modification
Toxicities ascribed to prednisone such as severe manifestations of hypercorticism, including: hyperglycemia, irritability, insomnia, or oral candidiasis	Reduce prednisone dose to 20 mg/day

Lenalidomide Starting Dose Adjustment for Renal Impairment in Multiple Myeloma (Days 1–21 of Each 28-Day Cycle)*

Moderate renal impairment CrCl 30–60 mL/min (0.5–1 mL/s)	10 mg lenalidomide every 24 hours
Severe renal impairment CrCl <30 mL/min, not requiring dialysis	15 mg lenalidomide every 48 hours
End-stage renal disease CrCl <30 mL/min, requiring dialysis	Lenalidomide 5 mg/day. On dialysis days, administer a daily dose following dialysis

CrCl, Creatinine clearance

*Richardson PG et al. J Clin Oncol 2006;24:3113–3120

Patient Population Studied

Phase 1/2 trial of 54 patients aged ≥65 years or younger if ineligible for high-dose therapy for newly diagnosed multiple myeloma. Karnofsky performance status ≥60%; platelet count ≥75,000/mm³; absolute neutrophil count ≥1500/mm³; corrected serum calcium ≤3.5 mmol/L (≤14 mg/dL)

Efficacy

	Dose Levels Evaluated			
	1	2	3 (MTD)	4
Lenalidomide (mg)	5	5	10	10
Melphalan (mg/kg)	0.18	0.25	0.18	0.25
Number of patients	6	6	21	20
Complete or partial response	66.7	83.3	81	85
CR, immunofixation negative	—	—	23.8	10
VGPR	—	33.3	23.8	30
Partial response	66.7	50	33.3	45
Minimal response	33.3	16.7	19	15
No response	—	—	—	—
Progressive Disease	—	—	—	—

Median Time to Best Response	4 Months
PR > first cycle	52.9%
PR > third cycle	66%
PR > sixth cycle	79.2%
1-year event-free survival	92.3% (95% CI, 85.1–99.5)
1-year event-free survival at MTD	95.2% (95% CI, 93.2–97.3)
1-year overall survival in all patients	100% (95% CI, 91.8–100)

CR, complete response; MTD, maximum tolerated doses; PR, partial response; VGPR, very good partial response

Therapy Monitoring

1. *Before each cycle:* CBC with differential and blood chemistries (including BUN, creatinine, and calcium)
2. *Every 6 weeks to 3 months:* Measure serum and urine M-protein

Toxicity

	Total G3/4 Events	Total G1/2 Events
Hematologic Events		
Neutropenia	67.9%	ND
Thrombocytopenia	32.1%	ND
Anemia	17%	ND
Nonhematologic Events		
Infective		
Febrile neutropenia	9.4%	—
Pneumonia	1.9%	5.7%
Upper respiratory	—	13.2%
Dermatologic events		
Rash	3.8%	35.8%
Vasculitis	3.8%	1.9%
Thromboembolism		
Deep venous thrombosis	3.8%	—
Pulmonary embolism	1.9%	—
Constitutional events		
Fatigue	3.8%	43.4%
Fever	—	18.9%
Gastrointestinal events		
Constipation	—	24.5%
Diarrhea	1.9%	22.6%
Nausea	—	18.9%
Anorexia	—	17%
Neurologic events		
Mood alterations	1.9%	9.4%
Dizziness	—	3.8%

ND, Not determined
Note: G1/2 adverse events reported by ≥10% of patients or G3/4 adverse events reported by ≥3% of patients

TRANSPLANT-INELIGIBLE • FIRST-LINE INDUCTION

MULTIPLE MYELOMA REGIMEN: BORTEZOMIB + MELPHALAN + PREDNISONE

San Miguel JF et al. N Engl J Med 2008;359:906–917

All Cycles:
Melphalan 9 mg/m^2 per day; administer orally for 4 consecutive days on days 1–4, every 6 weeks, for 9 cycles (total dosage/cycle = 36 mg/m^2)
Prednisone 60 mg/m^2 per day; administer orally for 4 consecutive days on days 1–4, every 6 weeks, for 9 cycles (total dosage/cycle = 240 mg/m^2), *plus*
Cycles 1–4:
Bortezomib 1.3 mg/m^2 per dose; administer by intravenous injection over 3–5 seconds for 8 doses, on days 1, 4, 8, 11, 22, 25, 29, and 32, every 6 weeks, for 4 cycles (total dosage/cycle = 10.4 mg/m^2)
Cycles 5–9:
Bortezomib 1.3 mg/m^2 per dose; administer by intravenous injection over 3–5 seconds for 4 doses on days 1, 8, 22, and 29, every 6 weeks, for 5 cycles (total dosage/cycle = 5.2 mg/m^2)

Supportive Care
Antiemetic prophylaxis
Emetogenic potential is **MINIMAL–LOW**
See Chapter 42 for antiemetic recommendations

Hematopoietic growth factor (CSF) prophylaxis
Primary prophylaxis is **NOT** indicated
See Chapter 43 for more information

Antimicrobial prophylaxis
Risk of fever and neutropenia is **HIGH**
  Antimicrobial primary prophylaxis is recommended:
  • Antibacterial—consider fluoroquinolone prophylaxis; *P. jirovecii* prophylaxis is recommended (eg, cotrimoxazole)
  • Antifungal—recommended
  • Antiviral—antiherpes antivirals (eg, acyclovir, famciclovir, valacyclovir)

Decreased bowel motility prophylaxis
Give a bowel regimen to prevent constipation based initially on **stool softeners**

Bisphosphonates
All patients receiving primary therapy for symptomatic multiple myeloma should receive a bisphosphonate adjunctively.

Thromboprophylaxis
Risk assessment and recommendations for VTE prophylaxis in patients with multiple myeloma with individual or myeloma-related risk factors, or risk factors related to treatment

(continued)

Treatment Modifications

Bortezomib Dosage Levels (per Dose)	
Dosage Level 1	1.3 mg/m^2
Dosage Level −1	1 mg/m^2
Dosage Level −2	0.7 mg/m^2

Melphalan Dose Levels (per Day)	
Dosage Level 1	9 mg/m^2
Dosage Level −1	6.75 mg/m^2
Dosage Level −2	4.5 mg/m^2

Adverse Event	Treatment Modification
Febrile neutropenia	Withhold therapy until fever abates then resume therapy
G4 hematologic toxicity	Withhold therapy until ANC >750/mm^3 and platelets >50,000/mm^3, then resume therapy with bortezomib and melphalan dosages decreased by 1 dose level
G3/4 nonhematologic toxicity	Withhold therapy. After toxicity abates to G ≤2, resume therapy with bortezomib and melphalan dosages decreased by 1 dose level
G≥3 thalidomide neuropathy	Continue treatment, but reduce thalidomide dose by 1 dose level
If ANC nadir is ≤1000/mm^3 or platelets nadir is ≤50,000/mm^3	Continue treatment, but reduce bortezomib and melphalan dosages by 1 level
G3 toxicities ascribed to prednisone such as severe manifestations of hypercorticism, including hyperglycemia, irritability, insomnia, or oral candidiasis	Reduce daily prednisone dosage by 20%

(continued)

(continued)

Individual risk factors
- Obesity (BMI ≥30 kg/m²)
- H/O VTE
- CVC or pacemaker
- Comorbid pathologies
  - Cardiac disease
  - Chronic renal disease
  - Diabetes
  - Acute infection
  - Immobilization
- Surgery
  - General surgery
  - Any anesthesia
  - Trauma
- Medications
  - Erythropoietin (epoetin alfa, darbepoetin)
  - Estrogenic compounds
  - Bevacizumab
- Clotting disorders
  - Thrombophilia

Myeloma-related risk factors
- Diagnosis of multiple myeloma
- Hyperviscosity

≤1 Individual or myeloma-related risk factor present:
- **Aspirin** 81–325 mg daily

≥2 Individual or myeloma-related risk factors present:
- **LMWH,*** equivalent to enoxaparin sodium 40 mg/day *or* **dalteparin sodium** 5000 IU/day; administer subcutaneously, *or*
- **Warfarin,** targeting an INR = 2–3

Concomitant treatment-related risk factors
Thalidomide or lenalidomide in combination with:
- High-dose dexamethasone (≥480 mg/month)
- Doxorubicin
- Multiagent chemotherapy

- **LMWH,*** equivalent to enoxaparin sodium 40 mg/day *or* **dalteparin sodium** 5000 IU/day; administer subcutaneously, *or*
- **Warfarin,** targeting an INR = 2–3

*LMWHs should be used with caution in individuals with impaired renal function (creatinine clearance <30 mL/min). Refer to product labeling for information about doses and administration schedules in renally impaired patients, and guidance for monitoring anti-Factor Xa concentrations

Abbreviations: CVC, central venous catheter; INR, international normalized ratio; LMWH, low-molecular-weight heparin; VTE, venous thromboembolic disease

References: Geerts WH et al. Chest 2008;133(6 Suppl):381S–453S

National Comprehensive Cancer Network. Multiple Myeloma, V.1.2014. (Accessed October 8, 2013, at http://www.nccn.org)

National Comprehensive Cancer Network. Venous Thromboembolic Disease, V.2.2013. (Accessed October 8, 2013, at http://www.nccn.org)

Palumbo A et al. Leukemia 2008;22:414–423

Treatment Modifications
(continued)

Adverse Event	Treatment Modification
G4 or recurrent G3 toxicities ascribed to prednisone such as severe manifestations of hypercorticism, including hyperglycemia, irritability, insomnia, or oral candidiasis	Reduce daily prednisone dosage by 40%

Treatment Modification for Bortezomib-Induced Peripheral Neuropathy*

Severity of Peripheral Neuropathy	Modification of Dose and Schedule
G1 (paresthesias or loss of reflexes) without pain or loss of function	No action
G1 with pain, or G2 (interferes with function but not with activities of daily living)	Reduce bortezomib dosage to 1 mg/m² per dose
G2 with pain, or G3 (interferes with activities of daily living)	Withhold bortezomib treatment until toxicity resolves, then reinitiate at a dosage of 0.7 mg/m² per dose once weekly
G4 (permanent sensory loss that interferes with function)	Discontinue treatment

*Richardson PG et al. J Clin Oncol 2006;24:3113–3120

Patient Population Studied

A randomized, open-label, phase 3 trial of 682 patients with newly diagnosed, untreated, symptomatic, measurable myeloma who, because of age (≥65 years), were not candidates for high-dose therapy plus stem cell transplantation

Efficacy (n = 337)*

European Group for Blood and Marrow Transplantation (EBMT) Criteria

Complete or partial response	71%
Complete response	30%
Partial response	40%
Minimal response	9%
Stable disease	18%
Progressive disease	1%

Time to Event

Median time to response†	
First response (months)	1.4
Complete response	4.2
Median duration of response†	
Complete or partial response	19.9
Complete response	24
Time to subsequent myeloma therapy‡	Not reached
Treatment-free interval‡	Not reached

International Uniform Response Criteria§

Complete, very good partial, or partial response	74%
Complete response	33%
Very good partial response	8%
Partial response	33%
Stable disease	23%
Progressive disease	1%

*Seven patients could not be evaluated for a response. Among patients evaluated, responses were not determined for 4. Percentages may not total 100 because of rounding
†Data determined by computer algorithm, applying EBMT criteria
‡Data based on 344 patients
§Of 79 patients considered to have stable disease on the basis of International Uniform Response Criteria who could be evaluated, 4 patients (1%) had negative results on immunofixation (complete response) and 19 (6%) had a reduction of at least 50% in M-protein (partial response). These patients were not recorded as having a complete or partial response because confirmatory results were missing. If these patients are included, the response rate is 81% and the complete-response rate is 34%. Patients could not be assessed for the category of stringent complete response because immunohistochemical, immunofluorescence, and free light-chain assays were not performed. International Uniform Response Criteria do not require changes in M-protein be confirmed a minimum of 6 weeks after the initial assessment

Toxicity (n = 340)*

	G1/2	G3	G4
Any Event	18	53	28
Hematologic Events†			
Thrombocytopenia	15	20	17
Neutropenia	9	30	10
Anemia	24	16	3
Leukopenia	10	20	3
Lymphopenia	5	14	5
Gastrointestinal Events			
Nausea	44	4	0
Diarrhea	38	7	1
Constipation	36	1	0
Vomiting	29	4	0
Infections			
Pneumonia	9	5	2
Herpes zoster	10	3	0
Nervous System Disorders			
Peripheral sensory neuropathy	31	13	<1
Neuralgia	27	8	1
Dizziness	14	2	0
Other Conditions			
Pyrexia	26	2	1
Fatigue	21	7	1
Asthenia	20	3	<1
Cough	21	0	0
Insomnia	20	<1	0
Peripheral edema	19	1	0
Rash	18	1	0
Back pain	14	3	<1
Dyspnea	11	3	1
Hypokalemia	6	6	1
Arthralgia	10	1	0
Deep venous thrombosis	1	1	0

*Listed adverse events were reported in ≥15% of patients, and G3 or G4 events were reported in ≥5% of patients. Patients may have more than 1 adverse event. Included are all patients who received at least 1 dose of a study drug
†Rates of red cell transfusions were 26%; erythropoiesis-stimulating agents for treatment-related anemia were used in 30% of patients

Therapy Monitoring

1. *Before each cycle:* CBC with differential and blood chemistries (including BUN, creatinine, and calcium)
2. *Every 6 weeks to 3 months:* Measure serum and urine M-protein

TRANSPLANT-INELIGIBLE • FIRST-LINE INDUCTION

MULTIPLE MYELOMA REGIMEN: DARATUMUMAB + BORTEZOMIB + MELPHALAN + PREDNISONE

Chari A et al. Blood 2016;128:2142
Mateos MV et al. Lancet 2020;395:132–141
Supplement to: Mateos MV et al. Lancet 2020;395:132–141
Mateos MV et al. N Engl J Med 2018;378:518–528
Supplement to: Mateos MV et al. N Engl J Med 2018;378:518–528
Protocol for: Mateos MV et al. N Engl J Med 2018;378:518–528
DARZALEX (daratumumab) prescribing information. Horsham, PA: Janssen Biotech, Inc; revised September 2019
DARZALEX FASPRO (daratumumab and hyaluronidase-fihj) prescribing information. Horsham, PA: Janssen Biotech, Inc; revised May 2020

Induction therapy (9 cycles)

All induction cycles (cycles 1–9; cycle length = 6 weeks):

Melphalan 9 mg/m^2 per day; administer orally for 4 consecutive days on days 1–4, every 42 days, for 9 cycles (total dosage/cycle during cycles 1–9 = 36 mg/m^2), *plus:*

Note: round dose to the nearest 2 mg tablet

Prednisone 60 mg/m^2 per day; administer orally for 4 consecutive days on days 1–4, every 42 days, for 9 cycles (total dosage/42-day cycle during cycles 1–9 = 240 mg/m^2)

Note: on days when daratumumab and prednisone are both scheduled for administration, omit the prednisone dose in lieu of dexamethasone premedication

Induction cycle 1 only (cycle length = 6 weeks):

Bortezomib 1.3 mg/m^2 per dose; administer subcutaneously in a volume of 0.9% sodium chloride injection (0.9% NS) sufficient to produce a final bortezomib concentration of 2.5 mg/mL for 8 doses on days 1, 4, 8, 11, 22, 25, 29, and 32 during cycle 1 (total dosage/42-day cycle during cycle 1 = 10.4 mg/m^2)

May choose to administer either DARZALEX (daratumumab) intravenously, or DARZALEX FASPRO (daratumumab and hyaluronidase-fihj) subcutaneously:

DARZALEX (daratumumab) 16 mg/kg per dose; administer intravenously for 6 doses on days 1, 8, 15, 22, 29, and 36 during cycle 1 (total dosage/42-day cycle during cycle 1 = 96 mg/kg), or:

Notes:
- The first daratumumab dose may optionally be split over two consecutive days (ie, in cycle 1 administer 8 mg/kg on day 1 and 8 mg/kg on day 2) to facilitate administration
- Refer to the table titled "Administration Instructions" for instructions regarding daratumumab premedication, infusion rate, dilution, and post-infusion medication

DARZALEX FASPRO (daratumumab and hyaluronidase-fihj) 1800 mg/30,000 units in 15 mL of ready-to-use solution per dose; administer by a health care provider subcutaneously into the abdomen over approximately 3–5 minutes for 6 doses on days 1, 8, 15, 22, 29, and 36 during cycle 1 (total dosage/42-day cycle during cycle 1 = 1800 mg/30,000 units)

Notes:
- Refer to the table titled "Administration Instructions" for instructions regarding premedications, post-administration medications, and administration

Induction cycles 2–9 only (cycle length = 6 weeks):

Bortezomib 1.3 mg/m^2 per dose; administer subcutaneously in a volume of 0.9% NS sufficient to produce a final bortezomib concentration of 2.5 mg/mL for 4 doses on days 1, 8, 22 and 29, every 42 days, for 8 cycles during cycles 2–9 (total dosage/42-day cycle during cycles 2–9 = 5.2 mg/m^2

May choose to administer either DARZALEX (daratumumab) intravenously, or DARZALEX FASPRO (daratumumab and hyaluronidase-fihj) subcutaneously:

DARZALEX (daratumumab) 16 mg/kg per dose; administer intravenously for 2 doses on days 1 and 22, every 42 days, for 8 cycles during cycles 2–9 (total dosage/42-day cycle during cycles 2–9 = 32 mg/kg), or:

Note: refer to the table below titled "Administration Instructions" for instructions regarding daratumumab premedication, infusion rate, dilution, and post-infusion medication

DARZALEX FASPRO (daratumumab and hyaluronidase-fihj) 1800 mg/30,000 units in 15 mL of ready-to-use solution per dose; administer by a health care provider subcutaneously into the abdomen over approximately 3–5 minutes for 2 doses on days 1 and 22, every 42 days, for 8 cycles during cycles 2–9 (total dosage/42-day cycle during cycles 2–9 = 3,600 mg/60,000 units)

Note: refer to the table titled "Administration Instructions" for instructions regarding premedications, post-administration medications, and administration

Maintenance therapy (begin after completion of 9 induction cycles)

All maintenance cycles (cycle length = 4 weeks):

May choose to administer either DARZALEX (daratumumab) intravenously, or DARZALEX FASPRO (daratumumab and hyaluronidase-fihj) subcutaneously:

(continued)

(continued)

DARZALEX (daratumumab) 16 mg/kg per dose; administer intravenously on day 1, every 28 days, until disease progression (total dosage/28-day cycle during maintenance = 16 mg/kg), or:

Note: refer to the table titled "Administration Instructions: for instructions regarding daratumumab premedication, infusion rate, dilution, and post-infusion medication

DARZALEX FASPRO (daratumumab and hyaluronidase-fihj) 1800 mg/30,000 units in 15 mL of ready-to-use solution per dose; administer by a health care provider subcutaneously into the abdomen over approximately 3–5 minutes for 4 doses on day 1, every 28 days, until disease progression (total dosage/28-day cycle during maintenance = 1800 mg/30,000 units)

Note: refer to the table titled "Administration Instructions" for instructions regarding premedications, post-administration medications, and administration

ADMINISTRATION INSTRUCTIONS

Premedications
(applies to DARZALEX (daratumumab) and DARZALEX FASPRO (daratumumab and hyaluronidase-fihj)

Antipyretic	**Acetaminophen** 650–1000 mg; administer orally 1–3 hours before each DARZALEX (daratumumab) or DARZALEX FASPRO (daratumumab and hyaluronidase-fihj) dose
H$_1$-subtype antihistamine	**Diphenhydramine** 25–50 mg; administer orally or intravenously 1–3 hours before each DARZALEX (daratumumab) or DARZALEX FASPRO (daratumumab and hyaluronidase-fihj) dose
Corticosteroid	**Dexamethasone** 20 mg; administer intravenously 1–3 hours before each DARZALEX (daratumumab) or DARZALEX FASPRO (daratumumab and hyaluronidase-fihj) dose • May administer dexamethasone orally beginning with the second dose
Leukotriene receptor antagonist *(optional)**	**Montelukast** 10 mg; administer orally 1–3 hours before each DARZALEX (daratumumab) or DARZALEX FASPRO (daratumumab and hyaluronidase-fihj) dose

Dilution volume and infusion rate
(applies to DARZALEX [daratumumab] only)

Daratumumab must be administered through an administration set with a flow regulator and with an in-line, sterile, nonpyrogenic, low-protein-binding, polyethersulfone filter with a pore size of 0.2 or 0.22 μm

First infusion	Dilute in 1000 mL 0.9% NS. Infuse initially at 50 mL/hour. If hypersensitivity or infusion reactions do not occur during the first hour, increase the rate by 50 mL/hour every hour as tolerated to a maximum rate of 200 mL/hour *Note:* if splitting the first daratumumab over two consecutive days (ie, 8 mg/kg on day 1 and 8 mg/kg on day 2), then dilute each 8 mg/kg dose in 500 mL 0.9% NS. Infuse initially at 50 mL/hour. If hypersensitivity or infusion reactions do not occur during the first hour, increase the rate by 50 mL/hour every hour as tolerated to a maximum rate of 200 mL/hour
Second infusion†	Dilute in 500 mL 0.9% NS. Infuse initially at 50 mL/hour. If hypersensitivity or infusion reactions do not occur during the first hour, increase the rate by 50 mL/hour every hour as tolerated to a maximum rate of 200 mL/hour
Subsequent infusions‡	Dilute in 500 mL 0.9% NS. Infuse initially at 100 mL/hour. If hypersensitivity or infusion reactions do not occur during the first hour, increase the rate by 50 mL/hour every hour as tolerated to a maximum rate of 200 mL/hour

Subcutaneous injection
(applies to DARZALEX FASPRO [daratumumab and hyaluronidase-fihj] only)

• Attach the hypodermic injection needle or subcutaneous infusion set to the syringe immediately prior to injection in order to reduce the chances of needle clogging

• Choose a site for administration approximately 3 inches (7.5 cm) to the right or left of the navel; rotate administration sites. Do not inject into areas where the skin is red, bruised, tender, hard, or scarred, or into areas used for administration of other subcutaneous medications

• A health care provider should administer the 15 mL dose subcutaneously into the abdomen over approximately 3–5 minutes

• If the injection causes pain, temporarily interrupt or reduce the rate of injection. If this does not relieve the pain, then choose another injection site on the opposite side of the abdomen in which to deliver the remainder of the dose

• Among low-body-weight (<50 kg) patients, the mean maximum trough concentration after the 8th dose was 81% higher in patients who received the fixed subcutaneous doses of DARZALEX FASPRO (daratumumab and hyaluronidase-fihj) compared to those who received 16 mg/kg per dose of intravenously administered DARZALEX (daratumumab). Higher rates of G3/4 neutropenia were observed in low-body-weight patients who received the formulation for subcutaneous injection

(continued)

(*continued*)

	Post-administration medications (*applies to DARZALEX [daratumumab] and DARZALEX FASPRO [daratumumab and hyaluronidase-fihj]*)
Corticosteroid	Methylprednisolone 20 mg; administer orally once on the day after each DARZALEX (daratumumab) or DARZALEX FASPRO (daratumumab and hyaluronidase-fihj) dose is administered • *Note:* on days when a regimen-specified prednisone dose is administered on the following day, then the post-administration methylprednisolone dose should be omitted
Short-acting β–2 agonist[§]	**Albuterol inhalation aerosol, metered**, 90 μg/actuation, administer 2 inhalations every 4 hours as needed for bronchospasm for 3 days, starting on the day of each of the first 4 DARZALEX (daratumumab) or DARZALEX FASPRO (daratumumab and hyaluronidase-fihj) doses
Long-acting β–2 agonist[§]	**Salmeterol xinafoate aerosol powder, metered**, 50 μg/actuation, administer 1 inhalation twice a day for 3 days, starting the day of each of the first 4 DARZALEX (daratumumab) or DARZALEX FASPRO (daratumumab and hyaluronidase-fihj) doses
Inhaled corticosteroid[§]	**Fluticasone propionate inhalation aerosol, metered**, 220 μg/actuation, administer 2 inhalations twice a day for 3 days, starting on the day of each of the first 4 DARZALEX (daratumumab) or DARZALEX FASPRO (daratumumab and hyaluronidase-fihj) doses

*Some institutions consider adding an optional leukotriene receptor antagonist based on data by Chari et al, 2016

[†]Use a dilution volume of 500 mL only if there were no infusion reactions during the first 3 hours of the first infusion. Otherwise, continue to use a dilution volume of 1000 mL and instructions for the first infusion

[‡]Use an initial rate of 100 mL/hour for subsequent infusions only if there were no infusion reactions during a final infusion rate of ≥100 mL/hour in the first two infusions. Otherwise, start infusion at 50 mL/hour per instructions for second infusion

[§]For patients with a history of chronic obstructive pulmonary disease, consider prescribing additional post-infusion inhaled medications for approximately 48 hours following the first 4 daratumumab infusions. Note that availability of inhalational medication formulations may vary by country; representative examples are included in the table

Note: DARZALEX (daratumumab) and DARZALEX FASPRO (daratumumab and hyaluronidase-fihj) can cause severe administration-related reactions. Symptoms of an administration-related reaction may include respiratory symptoms, chills, nausea/vomiting, fever, chest discomfort, hypotension, or pruritus. Only administer the products under medical supervision in a facility with immediate access to medical support and emergency equipment. Closely monitor patients throughout each administration. Most reactions occur during the first dose, when the all-grade systemic administration-related reaction incidence approaches 50% for the intravenous formulation and 10% for the subcutaneous formulation. Reactions may also occur during or following subsequent administrations. Delayed reactions may occur up to 48 hours following each dose; incidence of delayed reactions is reduced when post-infusion corticosteroids are administered. See Treatment Modifications section for management recommendations

Supportive Care
Antiemetic prophylaxis
Emetogenic potential of bortezomib and daratumumab is **MINIMAL**
Emetogenic potential of oral melphalan is **MINIMAL–LOW**
See Chapter 42 for antiemetic recommendations

Hematopoietic growth factor (CSF) prophylaxis
Primary prophylaxis is **NOT** *indicated*
See Chapter 43 for more information

Antimicrobial prophylaxis
Risk of fever and neutropenia is **INTERMEDIATE**
Antimicrobial primary prophylaxis to be considered:
- Antibacterial—consider a fluoroquinolone during periods of neutropenia or no prophylaxis; *P. jirovecii* prophylaxis is recommended (eg, cotrimoxazole)
- Antifungal—recommended; consider use during periods of neutropenia
- Antiviral—antiherpes antivirals (eg, acyclovir, famciclovir, valacyclovir) should be initiated within 1 week of starting daratumumab or daratumumab and hyaluronidase-fihj, and continued for at least 3 months after completion of the last dose

Bisphosphonates
All patients receiving primary therapy for symptomatic multiple myeloma should receive a bisphosphonate adjunctively.

Treatment Modifications

BORTEZOMIB, MELPHALAN, AND PREDNISONE DOSE MODIFICATIONS

Bortezomib, melphalan, and prednisone dose levels

	Bortezomib	Melphalan	Prednisone
Starting dose	1.3 mg/m² per dose	9 mg/m²	60 mg/m² orally on days 1–4
Dose level −1	1 mg/m² per dose	6.75 mg/m²	45 mg/m² orally on days 1–4
Dose level −2	0.7 mg/m² per dose	4.5 mg/m²	30 mg/m² orally on days 1–4
Dose level −3	Discontinue bortezomib	Discontinue melphalan	Discontinue prednisone

Allergic Reactions

Adverse Event	Treatment Modification		
	Bortezomib	Melphalan	Prednisone
Allergic reaction or hypersensitivity, G2/3	Hold all treatment. If the toxicity resolves to G ≤1, then resume VMP incorporating clinically appropriate prophylaxis for hypersensitivity. Consider reducing the dosage of the suspected medication(s) by 1 dosage level. For an anaphylactic-type reaction, do not resume VMP		
Allergic reaction or hypersensitivity, G4	Discontinue VMP		

Constitutional Toxicities

Adverse Event	Treatment Modification		
	Bortezomib	Melphalan	Prednisone
Edema that limits function and that is unresponsive to therapy	No change	No change	Treat with diuretics as indicated. Decrease the prednisone dosage by 1 dose level
Anasarca			
Fatigue G ≥3, therapy-related (severe, interfering with ADLs)	Reduce the dosage by 1 dose level	No change	No change

Cutaneous Toxicities

Adverse Event	Treatment Modification		
	Bortezomib	Melphalan	Prednisone
Non-blistering G2 rash	Withhold bortezomib. Consider treatment with antihistamines and/or low-dose steroids. Upon improvement to G ≤1, resume with the dosage reduced by 1 dose level	No change	No change
Non-blistering G3/4 rash, first occurrence	Withhold bortezomib. Consider treatment with antihistamines and/or low-dose corticosteroids. Upon improvement to G ≤1, resume with the dosage reduced by 1 dose level and consider continuing antihistamine and low-dose steroids prophylactically	No change	No change
Non-blistering G3/4 rash, second occurrence	Permanently discontinue bortezomib	No change	No change
Desquamating (blistering) rash (any grade), or G3/4 erythema multiforme	Withhold all treatment. Discontinue bortezomib permanently. Treat with antihistamines and/or low-dose corticosteroids as clinically appropriate. Upon improvement to G ≤1, then resume daratumumab, prednisone, and melphalan		

(continued)

Treatment Modifications (continued)

Gastrointestinal Toxicities

Adverse Event	Bortezomib	Melphalan	Prednisone
Constipation G3/4	Withhold bortezomib until recovery to G ≤1, then resume with the dosage reduced by 1 dose level	No change	No change
Diarrhea G3/4	Withhold bortezomib until recovery to G ≤1, then resume with the dosage reduced by 1 dose level. Optimize supportive care (eg, with loperamide)	No change	No change
G1/2 dyspepsia, gastric or duodenal ulcer, or gastritis (requiring medical management)	No change	No change	Optimize supportive care (eg, with H2-antagonist, sucralfate, and/or proton pump inhibitor therapy). If symptoms persist despite above measures, then reduce the dosage by 1 dose level
G3/4 dyspepsia, gastric or duodenal ulcer, or gastritis (requiring hospitalization or surgery)	No change	No change	Withhold prednisone and optimize supportive care (eg, with H2-antagonist, sucralfate, and/or proton pump inhibitor therapy). Upon adequate control of symptoms, resume prednisone with the dosage reduced by 1 dose level. If symptoms persist, discontinue prednisone

Hematologic Toxicities

	Treatment Modification		
Adverse Event	**Bortezomib**	**Melphalan**	**Prednisone**
G3 neutropenia (ANC ≥500/mm³ and <1000/mm³) without complications	No change. Consider adding filgrastim	No change. Consider adding filgrastim	No change
First occurrence of either: G3 neutropenia (ANC ≥500/mm³ and <1000/mm³) with fever (≥38.5°C), *or:* G4 neutropenia (ANC <500/mm³)	Consider use of filgrastim. Withhold treatment until improvement to G ≤2 or baseline, then continue at full dose	Consider use of filgrastim. Withhold treatment until improvement to G ≤2 or baseline, then continue with the dosage reduced by 1 dose level	Consider use of filgrastim. Withhold treatment until improvement to G ≤2 or baseline, then continue at full dose
Recurrence of either: G3 neutropenia (ANC ≥500/mm³ and <1000/mm³) with fever (≥38.5°C), *or:* G4 neutropenia (ANC <500/mm³)	Consider use of filgrastim. Withhold until improvement to G ≤2 or baseline, then reduce the dosage by 1 dose level	Consider use of filgrastim. Withhold until improvement to G ≤2 or baseline, then reduce the dosage by 1 dose level	Consider use of filgrastim. Withhold until improvement to G ≤2 or baseline, continue at the same dose
G3 thrombocytopenia (platelet count ≥25,000/mm³ and <50,000/mm³) without bleeding	No change	Reduce dosage by 1 dose level for the remainder of the cycle	No change
G3 thrombocytopenia (platelet count ≥25,000/mm³ and <50,000/mm³) with bleeding	Withhold until improvement to G ≤2 or baseline, then reduce the dosage by 1 dose level	Withhold until improvement to G ≤2 or baseline, then reduce the dosage by 1 dose level	Withhold until improvement to G ≤2 or baseline, then continue at the same dose
G4 thrombocytopenia (platelet count <25,000/mm³)			

(continued)

Treatment Modifications (continued)

Peripheral Neuropathy

Adverse Event	Treatment Modification		
	Bortezomib	Melphalan	Prednisone
G1 (paresthesias and/or loss of reflexes without pain or loss of function)	No change	No change	No change
G1 with pain G2 (interfering with function but not with ADLs)	Reduce dosage by 1 dose level	No change	No change
G2 with pain G3 (interfering with ADLs)	Withhold until toxicity improves to G ≤1, then resume with the dosage reduced by 1 dose level. If the patient is receiving bortezomib on a twice per week schedule, then also change to once per week	No change	No change
G4 (permanent sensory loss that interferes with function)	Permanently discontinue	No change	No change

Other Toxicities

Adverse Event	Treatment Modification		
	Bortezomib	Melphalan	Prednisone
Herpes zoster infection	Withhold all therapies until lesions are crusted over. Begin antiviral treatment. Upon resolution, resume therapies at the same dosages and with continued prophylaxis		
Muscle weakness G3/4 (symptomatic and interfering with function ± ADLs)	No change	No change	Reduce the dosage by 1 dose level. If persistent, decrease by another dose level. If still persistent, then discontinue until resolution of symptoms
Hyperglycemia G ≥3 (blood glucose >250–500 mg/dL; hospitalization indicated)	No change	No change	Optimize antihyperglycemic therapy. If hyperglycemia persists, then reduce the dosage by 1 dose level
Confusion or mood alteration G3/4 (interfering with function ± ADLs)	No change	No change	Withhold until resolution of symptoms, then resume with the dosage reduced by 1 dose level. If symptoms recur, then permanently discontinue prednisone
Venous and/or pulmonary thromboembolism G ≥3 (DVT or cardiac thrombosis with intervention indicated such as anticoagulation, thrombolysis, filter placement, or invasive procedure)	No change	No change	Withhold until acute effects of toxicity have resolved and patient is stable on anticoagulation therapy, then resume prednisone at the same dose
SCr value is >2 mg/dL, but is ≤3X baseline and ≤3X ULN	No change	Reduce the melphalan dosage to 4.5 mg/m²	No change
Bilirubin >1 mg/dL	If bilirubin is >1.5× ULN, then reduce the bortezomib dosage to 0.7 mg/m² in the first cycle and, if tolerated, consider escalation to a maximum dose of 1 mg/m²	Reduce the melphalan dosage to 4.5 mg/m²	No change
ALT, AST, and alkaline phosphatase >2× ULN	No change	Reduce the melphalan dosage to 4.5 mg/m²	No change
Other toxicities G ≥3	Withhold the attributable medication(s) until resolution to G ≤1, then resume treatment with the dosage of the attributable medication(s) reduced by 1 dose level, if clinically appropriate		

(continued)

Treatment Modifications (continued)

DARATUMUMAB OR DARATUMUMAB AND HYALURONIDASE-FIHJ

Adverse Event	Dose Modification
Infusion-Related Reaction and Anaphylactic Reaction Adverse Events	
• G1/2 infusion-related reaction to intravenous daratumumab. (G1/2 IRR) • First occurrence of G3 infusion-related reaction (G3 IRR) to intravenous daratumumab • Second occurrence of G3 infusion-related reaction to intravenous daratumumab	Immediately interrupt the daratumumab infusion for infusion-related reactions of *any* severity and manage symptoms as clinically appropriate with additional intravenous corticosteroid (50–150 mg hydrocortisone IVP), an H_1-receptor antagonist (diphenhydramine 50 mg IVP), inhaled short-acting ß–2 agonist (albuterol 2 puffs, may repeat in 4 hours) plus epinephrine 0.5 mg IM for hypotension or airway obstructive symptoms
G1 IRR = mild transient reaction; infusion interruption not indicated; intervention not indicated G2 IRR = therapy or infusion interruption indicated but responds promptly to symptomatic treatment (eg, antihistamines, NSAIDs, narcotics, IV fluids); prophylactic medications indicated for ≤24 hours G3 IRR = prolonged (eg, not rapidly responsive to symptomatic medication and/or brief interruption of infusion); recurrence of symptoms following initial improvement; hospitalization indicated for clinical sequelae	Upon resolution of symptoms, resume the daratumumab infusion at no more than 50% of the rate at which the reaction occurred. If tolerated, escalate the infusion by 50 mL/hour every hour up to a maximum rate of 200 mL/hour *Note:* dose reductions are not recommended for daratumumab
• Third occurrence of G3 infusion-related reaction (IRR) to intravenous daratumumab • G4 infusion-related reaction (G4 IRR) to intravenous daratumumab or subcutaneous daratumumab and hyaluronidase-fihj • Anaphylactic reaction (AR) to intravenous daratumumab or subcutaneous daratumumab and hyaluronidase-fihj	Immediately interrupt the administration for infusion-related reactions of *any* severity and manage symptoms as clinically appropriate with additional intravenous corticosteroid (50–150 mg hydrocortisone IVP), an H_1-receptor antagonist (diphenhydramine 50 mg IVP), inhaled short-acting ß–2 agonist (albuterol 2 puffs, may repeat in 4 hours) plus epinephrine 0.5 mg IM for hypotension or airway obstructive symptoms
G3 IRR = prolonged (eg, not rapidly responsive to symptomatic medication and/or brief interruption of infusion); recurrence of symptoms following initial improvement; hospitalization indicated for clinical sequelae G4 IRR = life-threatening consequences; urgent intervention indicated G3 AR = symptomatic bronchospasm, with or without urticaria; parenteral intervention indicated; allergy-related edema/angioedema; hypotension G4 AR = life-threatening consequences; urgent intervention indicated	Permanently discontinue
Hematologic Adverse Events	
G3/4 neutropenia G3/4 thrombocytopenia	Consider delaying the dose until recovery to G ≤2 or baseline; or, continue without interruption as clinically appropriate. In the case of neutropenia, consider administration of granulocyte-colony stimulating factor (G-CSF)
Blood transfusion within 6 months following a daratumumab infusion	Notify blood bank the patient has received daratumumab or daratumumab and hyaluronidase-fihj within the past 6 months since either product may result in a positive indirect antiglobulin test (indirect Coombs test) that can persist for up to 6 months and may mask detection of antibodies to minor antigens in the patient's serum. Determination of ABO and Rh blood type is not affected

Note: dose reductions are not recommended for daratumumab or daratumumab and hyaluronidase-fihj. Withhold all therapy (including daratumumab and daratumumab and hyaluronidase-fihj) for G3 neutropenia with fever, G4 neutropenia, G4 thrombocytopenia, active herpes zoster infection, desquamating rash (any grade) or erythema multiforme G3/4, and allergic reaction/hypersensitivity

VMP, bortezomib + melphalan + prednisone; ADL, activities of daily living; ANC, absolute neutrophil count; DVT, deep-vein thrombosis; SCr, serum creatinine; ULN, upper limit of normal; ALT, alanine aminotransferase; AST, aspartate aminotransferase; IRR, infusion-related reactions; IVP, intravenous push; NSAID, non-steroidal anti-inflammatory drug; IM, intramuscular; AR, anaphylactic reaction

Patient Population Studied

The ALCYONE trial was a randomized, open-label, active-controlled, phase 3 trial that included 706 adult patients with newly diagnosed multiple myeloma and compared treatment between bortezomib plus melphalan plus prednisone either alone (VMP) or with daratumumab (D-VMP). Patients were eligible if they had newly diagnosed multiple myeloma satisfying the CRAB criteria, if they were ineligible for high-dose chemotherapy with stem cell transplant due to age or presence of comorbid conditions, if they had an ECOG performance status of 0–2, and if they had adequate organ function. Subjects were excluded if they had primary amyloidosis, monoclonal gammopathy of undetermined significance, smoldering multiple myeloma, Waldenström macroglobulinemia, previous systemic therapy or stem cell transplantation, cancer within 3 years before randomization (except squamous- and basal-cell carcinomas of the skin, carcinoma in situ of the cervix, or other cured cancers with minimal risk of recurrence within 3 years), peripheral neuropathy, or Grade 2 or higher neuropathic pain (according to NCI CTCAE v4.0 criteria)

Efficacy (n = 706)

Efficacy Variable	D-VMP (n = 350)	VMP (n = 356)	Between-group Comparison
PFS			
Median PFS—months (95% CI)	36.4 (32.1–45.9)	19.3 (18.0–20.4)	HR 0.42 (95% CI, 0.34–0.51); P <0.0001
Estimated PFS rate at 36 months—% (95% CI)	50.7 (45.1–55.9)	18.5 (14.4–23.1)	
PFS2*			
Median PFS2—months (95% CI)	NR	42.3 (35.8-NR)	HR 0.55 (95% CI, 0.43–0.71); p < 0.0001
Estimated PFS2 rate at 36 months—% (95% CI)	73.2 (68.1–77.7)	55.2 (49.4–60.6)	
OS†			
Median OS—months (95% CI)	NR	NR	HR 0.60 (95% CI, 0.46–0.80); P = 0.0003†
Estimated OS rate at 36 months—% (95% CI)	78.0 (73.2–82.0)	67.9 (62.6–72.6)	
Response‡			
ORR—n/N (%) (95% CI)	318/350 (90.9) (87.3–93.7)	263/356 (73.9) (69.0–78.4)	OR 3.55 (95% CI, 2.30–5.49); p < 0.0001
CR or better rate—n/N (%)	160/350 (46)	90/356 (25)	OR 2.50 (95% CI, 1.82–3.45); p < 0.0001
Stringent CR rate—n/N (%)	81/350 (23)	28/356 (8)	
CR rate—n/N (%)	79/350 (23)	62/356 (17)	
VGPR or better rate—n/N (%)	255/350 (73)	177/356 (50)	OR 2.71 (95% CI, 1.98–3.71); p < 0.0001
VGPR rate—n/N (%)	95/350 (27)	87/356 (24)	
PR rate—n/N (%)	63/350 (18)	86/356 (24)	
Stable disease rate—n/N (%)	20/350 (6)	76/356 (21)	
Progressive disease rate—n/N (%)	0/350 (0)	2/356 (<1)	
Response could not be measured—n/N (%)	12/350 (3)	15/356 (4)	
Negative status for MRD—n/N (%)	99/350 (28)	25/356 (7)	OR 5.23 (95% CI, 3.27–8.36); p < 0.0001
Sustained negative status for MRD for ≥ 6 months—n/N (%)	55/350 (16)	16/356 (5)	OR 3.96 (95% CI, 2.22–7.06); p < 0.0001
Sustained negative status for MRD for ≥ 12 months—n/N (%)▫	49/350 (14)	10/356 (3)	OR 5.63 (95% CI, 2.80–11.31); p < 0.0001

*PFS2 is the PFS on a subsequent line of therapy and corresponds to the time from randomization to death or progression

†A sensitivity analysis in the per-protocol population, including all patients who were randomized and met all eligibility criteria (344 patients in the D-VMP group and 351 in the VMP group) generated similar results: HR 0.61 (95% CI, 0.46–0.80); P = 0.0004

(continued)

Therapy Monitoring

1. Type and screen prior to first dose of daratumumab or daratumumab and hyaluronidase-fihj
2. CBC with differential, liver function tests, serum creatinine, and serum glucose prior to each dose of daratumumab and bortezomib
3. Monitor for infusion related daratumumab reaction symptoms frequently during infusion; check vital signs frequently during infusion and at least prior to each scheduled rate increase, ensure medications are available for post-infusion prophylaxis as applicable
4. Monitor for bortezomib toxicities including neuropathy and hypotension

Daratumumab note: daratumumab, a human IgG1 kappa monoclonal antibody, may be detected by serum protein electrophoresis and immunofixation assays routinely used to monitor endogenous M-protein. Thus, daratumumab may interfere with disease monitoring in patients with plasma cell neoplasms that produce an IgG kappa M-protein.

Bortezomib note: patients with pre-existing severe neuropathy should be treated with bortezomib only after careful risk-benefit assessment

Efficacy (n = 706) *(continued)*

[‡]Response was assessed according to the International Myeloma Working Group criteria. Stringent CR includes the criteria for CR plus a normal free light chain ratio and absence of clonal plasma cells. Negative status for MRD was defined as <1 tumor cell per 100,000 white blood cells in a bone marrow sample. P Values for MRD negativity were calculated with Fisher's exact test and P Values for response rates were calculated using the Cochran-Mantel-Haenszel X^2 test

[□]Sustained MRD for ≥12 months was associated with a significantly increased PFS and OS

Note: all efficacy outcome assessments were performed in the intention-to-treat population, which included all patients who were randomized to treatment, regardless of drug reception. PFS and OS rates were estimated using Kaplan-Meier methods. A Cox regression model was used to estimate treatment effect, presented as Hours and 95% CIs. The primary outcome was PFS. A prespecified subgroup analysis of response rates and OS by age (<75 or ≥75 years), cytogenetic risk (standard vs high), and other factors was also performed and the results consistently showed a significant benefit of D-VMP over VMP across all subgroups. Effects across age and cytogenetic risk subgroups were similar to the whole intention-to-treat population but there was slightly lower benefit of D-VMP over VMP in the age ≥75 subgroup for OS and response and in the high cytogenetic risk groups for OS. All data included in the table were published in Mateos et al, 2020 and its supplementary appendix. Data were collected with a median follow-up time of 40.1 months (IQR, 37.4–43.1)

D-VMP, daratumumab + bortezomib + melphalan + prednisone; VMP, bortezomib + melphalan + prednisone; CI, confidence interval; HR, hazard ratio; NR, not reached; PFS, progression-free survival; OS, overall survival; OR, odds ratio; ORR, objective response rate; CR, complete response; VGPR, very good partial response; PR, partial response; MRD, minimum residual disease

Adverse Events (n = 700)

Event	D-VMP (n = 346)		VMP (n = 354)	
Grade (%)	Any Grade	Grade 3 or 4	Any Grade	Grade 3 or 4
Neutropenia	50	40	53	39
Thrombocytopenia	49	34	53	38
Anemia	28	16	38	20
Peripheral sensory neuropathy	28	1	34	4
Diarrhea	24	3	25	3
Pyrexia	23	<1	21	<1
Nausea	21	<1	21	1
Any infection	67	23	48	15
Upper respiratory tract infection	26	2	14	1
Pneumonia	15	11	5	4
Second primary cancer*	2	N/A	3	N/A
Any infusion-related reaction	28	5	N/A	N/A

*The presence of a second primary cancer was a prespecified adverse event of clinical interest

Adverse events of any grade were included in the table if they were reported in ≥20% of patients in either treatment group, and Grade 3 or 4 adverse events were included if they were reported in ≥10% of patients in either group except for second primary cancer. Adverse events were graded according to the National Cancer Institute Common Terminology Criteria for Adverse Events (NCI CTCAE) v4 in all patients who received at least one dose of study drug treatment. Most infections, including pneumonia, resolved (87.9% of D-VMP patients and 86.5% of VMP patients), and the rates of discontinuation of trial treatment due to infection were similar (0.9% and 1.4%, respectively). One patient in each group (0.3% each) discontinued trial treatment due to pneumonia. Death due to infection occurred in 5 patients (1.4%) in the D-VMP group (2 from pneumonia, 1 each from peritonitis, septic shock, and upper respiratory tract infection) and in 4 patients (1.1%) in the VMP group (1 each from septic shock, candida sepsis, bacterial pneumonia, and sepsis). Serious adverse events occurred in 41.6% of patients in the D-VMP group and 32.5% of patients in the VMP group. Discontinuation of trial treatment due to adverse events occurred in 4.9% of D-VMP patients and 9.0% of VMP patients. Adverse events that occurred within 30 days after the last trial treatment and led to death occurred in 4.0% of patients in the D-VMP group and 4.5% of patients in the VMP group. The majority of daratumumab-related infusion reactions occurred during the first infusion. Tumor lysis syndrome was reported in 0.6% of patients in each group. All safety data included in this table were reported in Mateos et al, 2018

TRANSPLANT-INELIGIBLE • FIRST-LINE INDUCTION

MULTIPLE MYELOMA REGIMEN: MELPHALAN + PREDNISONE + THALIDOMIDE (MPT)

Palumbo A et al. Lancet 2006;367:825–831
Palumbo A et al. Blood 2008;112:3107–3114

Induction:

Melphalan 4 mg/m² per day; administer orally for 7 consecutive days on days 1–7, every 4 weeks, for 6 cycles (total dosage/cycle = 28 mg/m²)

Prednisone 40 mg/m² per day; administer orally for 7 consecutive days on days 1–7, every 4 weeks, for 6 cycles (total dosage/cycle = 280 mg/m²)

Thalidomide 100 mg/day; administer orally for 28 consecutive day on days 1–28, every 4 weeks for 6 cycles (total dose/cycle = 2800 mg)

Maintenance:

Thalidomide 100 mg/day; administer orally, continually, until confirmation of relapsed or refractory disease (total dose/week = 700 mg)

Supportive Care

Antiemetic prophylaxis
Emetogenic potential is **MINIMAL–LOW**
See Chapter 42 for antiemetic recommendations

Hematopoietic growth factor (CSF) prophylaxis
Primary prophylaxis is **NOT** *indicated*
See Chapter 43 for more information

Antimicrobial prophylaxis
Risk of fever and neutropenia is **INTERMEDIATE**
  Antimicrobial primary prophylaxis to be considered:
  • Antibacterial—consider a fluoroquinolone or no prophylaxis; *P. jirovecii* prophylaxis is recommended (eg, cotrimoxazole)
  • Antifungal—consider concomitant use of clotrimazole during periods of neutropenia
  • Antiviral—antiherpes antivirals (eg, acyclovir, famciclovir, valacyclovir)

Bisphosphonates

All patients receiving primary therapy for symptomatic multiple myeloma should receive a bisphosphonate adjunctively.

Thromboprophylaxis

Risk assessment and recommendations for VTE prophylaxis in patients with multiple myeloma with individual or myeloma-related risk factors, or risk factors related to treatment

(continued)

Treatment Modifications

Melphalan Dosage Levels	
Dosage Level 1	4 mg/m²
Dosage Level −1	3 mg/m²
Dosage Level −2	2 mg/m²

Adverse Event	Treatment Modification
Febrile neutropenia	Withhold therapy until fever abates, then resume therapy
G4 hematologic toxicity	Withhold therapy until ANC >750/mm³ and platelets >50,000/mm³, then resume therapy with the melphalan dose decreased by 1 dose level
G3/4 nonhematologic toxicity	Interrupt therapy and follow clinically. After toxicity abates to G ≤2, resume therapy with thalidomide dose decreased by 1 dose level
G ≥3 thalidomide neuropathy	
If ANC nadir is ≤1000/mm³ or platelets nadir is ≤50,000/mm³	Continue treatment, but reduce melphalan dosage by 1 level
G2 nonhematologic toxicity	Reduce thalidomide dose by 50% to 50 mg/day
G ≥3 nonhematologic toxicity	Discontinue thalidomide
G3 toxicities ascribed to prednisone such as severe manifestations of hypercorticism, including hyperglycemia, irritability, insomnia, and oral candidiasis	Reduce daily prednisone dosage by 20%
G4 or recurrent G3 toxicities ascribed to prednisone such as severe manifestations of hypercorticism, including hyperglycemia, irritability, insomnia, and oral candidiasis	Reduce daily prednisone dosage by 40%

(*continued*)

Individual risk factors
• Obesity (BMI ≥30 kg/m²)
• H/O VTE
• CVC or pacemaker
• Comorbid pathologies
  ▪ Cardiac disease
  ▪ Chronic renal disease
  ▪ Diabetes
  ▪ Acute infection
  ▪ Immobilization
• Surgery
  ▪ General surgery
  ▪ Any anesthesia
  ▪ Trauma
• Medications
  ▪ Erythropoietin (epoetin alfa, darbepoetin)
  ▪ Estrogenic compounds
  ▪ Bevacizumab
• Clotting disorders
  ▪ Thrombophilia
Myeloma-related risk factors
• Diagnosis of multiple myeloma
• Hyperviscosity
	≤1 Individual or myeloma-related risk factor present:
	• **Aspirin** 81–325 mg daily
	
	≥2 Individual or myeloma-related risk factors present:
	• **LMWH,*** equivalent to enoxaparin sodium 40 mg/day *or* **dalteparin sodium** 5000 IU/day; administer subcutaneously, *or*
	• **Warfarin**, targeting an INR = 2–3

Concomitant treatment-related risk factors Thalidomide or lenalidomide in combination with: • High-dose dexamethasone (≥480 mg/month) • Doxorubicin • Multiagent chemotherapy	• **LMWH,*** equivalent to enoxaparin sodium 40 mg/day *or* **dalteparin sodium** 5000 IU/day; administer subcutaneously, *or* • **Warfarin**, targeting an INR = 2–3

*LMWHs should be used with caution in individuals with impaired renal function (creatinine clearance <30 mL/min). Refer to product labeling for information about doses and administration schedules in renally impaired patients, and guidance for monitoring anti-Factor Xa concentrations

Abbreviations: CVC, central venous catheter; INR, international normalized ratio; LMWH, low-molecular-weight heparin; VTE, venous thromboembolic disease

References: Geerts WH et al. Chest 2008;133(6 Suppl):381S–453S
National Comprehensive Cancer Network. Multiple Myeloma, V.1.2014. (Accessed October 8, 2013, at http://www.nccn.org)
National Comprehensive Cancer Network. Venous Thromboembolic Disease, V.2.2013. (Accessed October 8, 2013, at http://www.nccn.org)
Palumbo A et al. Leukemia 2008;22:414–423

Patient Population Studied

A multicenter randomized trial of 331 previously untreated patients with Durie-Salmon stage II or III multiple myeloma who were older than 65 years (or younger but unable to undergo transplantation), and had measurable disease. Exclusion criteria included any G2 peripheral neuropathy. Abnormal cardiac function, chronic respiratory disease, and abnormal liver or renal function were not criteria for exclusion

Efficacy (n = 129)

Complete or partial response	76%
Complete response	15.5%
Partial response	60.4%
Near-complete response	12.4%
90% to 99% myeloma protein reduction	8.5%
50% to 89% myeloma protein reduction	39.5%
Minimal response	5.4%
No response	5.4%
Progressive disease	7.8%
Responses not available	5.4%
Progression free survival*	21.8 months
Median overall survival†	45 months

*After a median follow-up of 38.1 months. The magnitude of PFS benefit was consistent irrespective of age, serum concentrations of β_2-microglobulin, or high International Staging System
†The median OS of 45 months for melphalan + prednisone (MP) + thalidomide (T) compared to a median OS of 47.6 months for MP was not statistically significant (P = 0.79). New agents in the management of relapsed disease could explain this finding

Toxicity (n = 129)

Adverse Event	G3/4 Adverse Events Percentage of Patients
≥1 Event	48%
Hematologic	22%
Neutropenia	16%
Anemia	3%
Thrombocytopenia	3%
Thrombosis/embolism	12%
Deep venous thrombosis	9%
Pulmonary embolism	2%
Neurologic	10%
Peripheral neuropathy	8%
Somnolence or fatigue	3%
Infection	10%
Pneumonia	5%
Fever of unknown origin	2%
Herpes zoster	1%
Upper respiratory	2%
Cardiac	7%
Arrhythmia	2%
Myocardial infarction/angina	2%
Cardiac failure	3%
Hypertension	1%
Gastrointestinal	6%
Constipation	6%
Mucositis	0
Dermatologic	3%
Rash	2%
Toxic epidermal necrolysis	1%
Renal	1%
Creatinine increase	1%
Edema	1%
Bleeding	0%

Therapy Monitoring

1. *Before each cycle:* CBC with differential and blood chemistries (including BUN, creatinine, and calcium)
2. *Every 6 weeks to 3 months:* Measure serum and urine M-protein

TRANSPLANT-INELIGIBLE • FIRST-LINE INDUCTION

MULTIPLE MYELOMA REGIMEN: CARFILZOMIB + CYCLOPHOSPHAMIDE + DEXAMETHASONE (CCyd)

Bringhen S et al. Blood 2014;124(1):63–69

The regimen consists of carfilzomib, cyclophosphamide, and dexamethasone (CCyd) given for 9 cycles as induction therapy, followed by a maintenance schedule of single-agent carfilzomib administered until disease progression

Induction:
Hydration with carfilzomib during induction: During cycle 1 of induction, on days 1, 2, 8, 9, 15, and 16, administer intravenously 250–500 mL 0.9% sodium chloride injection (0.9% NS) before each carfilzomib dose, *and* an additional 250–500 mL of 0.9% NS intravenously after carfilzomib. During repeated treatments, continue intravenous hydration as needed. Encourage oral hydration
Premedication for carfilzomib during induction: During cycle 1 of induction, on days 1, 8, and 15, administer dexamethasone 40 mg (as specified in the regimen) orally or intravenously between 0.5 and 4 hours before the carfilzomib dose. Additionally, during cycle 1 of induction on days 2, 9, and 16, administer dexamethasone 8 mg orally or intravenously between 0.5 and 4 hours before the carfilzomib dose. Reinstate dexamethasone premedication in subsequent cycles if infusion-related reaction symptoms occur

Carfilzomib; intravenously in 50–100 mL 5% dextrose injection (D5W) for 6 doses, on days 1, 2, 8, 9, 15, and 16, every 28 days, for 9 cycles of induction therapy, *as follows:*

Induction cycle 1 days 1 and 2	20 mg/m² per dose intravenously over 30 minutes	Total dosage in induction cycle 1= 184 mg/m²)
Induction cycle 1 days 8, 9, 15, and 16	36 mg/m² per dose intravenously over 30 minutes	
Induction cycles 2–9 days 1, 2, 8, 9, 15, and 16	36 mg/m² per dose intravenously over 30 minutes	Total dosage per cycle (induction cycles 2–9) = 216 mg/m²

Carfilzomib Dose Adjustments

BSA >2.2 m²	Use BSA of 2.2 m² to calculate carfilzomib
• Bilirubin 1–1.5× ULN and any AST, *or* • Bilirubin 1.5–3× ULN and any AST, *or* • Bilirubin ≤ ULN and AST > ULN	Reduce initial carfilzomib dose by 25%
Bilirubin >3× ULN	No dose recommendation available
Creatinine clearance <15 mL/minute	Full dose carfilzomib at discretion of physician
End-stage renal disease on hemodialysis	No dose adjustment necessary; administer carfilzomib after hemodialysis

Cyclophosphamide 300 mg/m² per dose; administer orally, preferably in the morning, for 3 doses on days 1, 8, and 15, every 28 days, for 9 cycles of induction therapy (total dosage/cycle = 900 mg/m²)
Dexamethasone 40 mg/dose; administer orally once daily for 4 doses on days 1, 8, 15, and 22, every 28 days, for 9 cycles of induction therapy (total dose/induction cycle = 160 mg)

After completion of 9 cycles of induction, patients proceeded to receiving single-agent carfilzomib maintenance. Note that the schedule for maintenance carfilzomib differs from the schedule used during induction therapy

Maintenance:
Hydration with carfilzomib during maintenance: Intravenous hydration as needed. Encourage oral hydration.
Premedication for carfilzomib during maintenance: Reinstate premedication with dexamethasone 8 mg, administered orally 0.5–4 hours prior to each carfilzomib dose, in subsequent cycles only if infusion-related reaction symptoms occur

Carfilzomib 36 mg/m² per dose; administer intravenously in 50–100 mL D5W over 30 minutes for 4 doses on days 1, 2, 15, and 16, every 28 days, as maintenance therapy until progression of disease (total dosage/maintenance cycle = 144 mg/m²)

BSA >2.2 m²	Use BSA of 2.2 m² to calculate carfilzomib
• Bilirubin 1–1.5× ULN and any AST, or • Bilirubin 1.5–3× ULN and any AST, *or* • Bilirubin ≤ ULN and AST > ULN	Reduce initial carfilzomib dose by 25%
Bilirubin >3× ULN	No dose recommendation available

(continued)

(continued)

Creatinine clearance <15 mL/minute	Full dose carfilzomib at discretion of physician
End-stage renal disease on hemodialysis	No dose adjustment necessary; administer carfilzomib after hemodialysis

Supportive Care

Antiemetic prophylaxis
*Emetogenic potential on days with cyclophosphamide is **MODERATE-HIGH***
*Emetogenic potential on days with carfilzomib ± dexamethasone is **LOW***
See Chapter 42 for antiemetic recommendations

Hematopoietic growth factor (CSF) prophylaxis
*Primary prophylaxis is **NOT** indicated*
See Chapter 43 for more information

Antimicrobial prophylaxis
*Risk of fever and neutropenia is **INTERMEDIATE***
Antimicrobial primary prophylaxis to be considered:
- Antibacterial—consider a fluoroquinolone during periods of neutropenia, or no prophylaxis; *P. jirovecii* prophylaxis is recommended (eg, cotrimoxazole)
- Antifungal—consider fluconazole during periods of neutropenia
- Antiviral—antiherpes antivirals (eg, acyclovir, famciclovir, valacyclovir)

Steroid-associated gastritis
Add a proton pump inhibitor or H_2-receptor antagonist during dexamethasone use to prevent gastritis and duodenitis

Diarrhea management
Loperamide or **diphenoxylate hydrochloride** 2.5 mg **with atropine sulfate** 0.025 mg (eg, Lomotil)

Bisphosphonates
All patients receiving primary therapy for symptomatic multiple myeloma should receive a bisphosphonate adjunctively.

Thromboprophylaxis
Risk assessment and recommendations for VTE prophylaxis in patients with multiple myeloma with individual or myeloma-related risk factors, or risk factors related to treatment

Individual risk factors
• Obesity (BMI ≥30 kg/m²)
• H/O VTE
• CVC or pacemaker
• Comorbid pathologies
  ▪ Cardiac disease
  ▪ Chronic renal disease
  ▪ Diabetes
  ▪ Acute infection
  ▪ Immobilization
• Surgery
  ▪ General surgery
  ▪ Any anesthesia
  ▪ Trauma
• Medications
  ▪ Erythropoietin (epoetin alfa, darbepoetin)
  ▪ Estrogenic compounds
  ▪ Bevacizumab
• Clotting disorders
  ▪ Thrombophilia
Myeloma-related risk factors
• Diagnosis of multiple myeloma
• Hyperviscosity
	≤1 Individual or myeloma-related risk factor present:
	• **Aspirin** 81–325 mg daily
	
	≥2 Individual or myeloma-related risk factors present:
	• **LMWH,*** equivalent to enoxaparin sodium 40 mg/day or **dalteparin sodium** 5000 IU/day; administer subcutaneously, *or*
	• **Warfarin**, targeting an INR = 2–3

(continued)

(*continued*)

Concomitant treatment-related risk factors	
Thalidomide or lenalidomide in combination with: • High-dose dexamethasone (≥480 mg/month) • Doxorubicin • Multiagent chemotherapy	• **LMWH,*** equivalent to **enoxaparin sodium** 40 mg/day *or* **dalteparin sodium** 5000 IU/day; administer subcutaneously, *or* • **Warfarin,** targeting an INR = 2–3

*LMWHs should be used with caution in individuals with impaired renal function (creatinine clearance <30 mL/min). Refer to product labeling for information about doses and administration schedules in renally impaired patients, and guidance for monitoring anti-Factor Xa concentrations

Abbreviations: CVC, central venous catheter; INR, international normalized ratio; LMWH, low-molecular-weight heparin; VTE, venous thromboembolic disease

References: Geerts WH et al. Chest 2008;133(6 Suppl):381S–453S

National Comprehensive Cancer Network. Multiple Myeloma, V.1.2014. (Accessed October 8, 2013, at http://www.nccn.org)

National Comprehensive Cancer Network. Venous Thromboembolic Disease, V.2.2013. (Accessed October 8, 2013, at http://www.nccn.org)

Palumbo A et al. Leukemia 2008;22:414–423

Treatment Modifications

CARFILZOMIB

Starting dose	36 mg/m² per dose
Level −1	27 mg/m² per dose
Level −2	20 mg/m² per dose
Level −3	15 mg/m² per dose
Level −4	Discontinue

Hematologic Toxicity

G3/4 neutropenia (<1000/mm³) Febrile neutropenia (ANC <1000/mm³ with a single temperature of >38.3°C [101°F] or a sustained temperature of ≥38°C [100.4°F] for >1 hour) G4 thrombocytopenia (<25,000/mm³) G3/4 thrombocytopenia (<50,000/mm³) associated with bleeding	• Hold carfilzomib dosing for up to 21 days to resolve toxicity and then restart at the same dosage, or reduce the carfilzomib dosage by 1 dose level • If recover to G2 neutropenia or G3 thrombocytopenia, reduce carfilzomib dosage by 1 dose level • If tolerated, the reduced dose may be escalated to the previous dose level
Confirmed TTP or HUS	Permanently discontinue carfilzomib. (The safety of reinitiating carfilzomib in patients previously experiencing TTP or HUS is unknown)*

Nonhematologic Toxicity

G3/4 cardiac toxicity New onset or worsening: • Congestive heart failure • Decreased left ventricular function • Myocardial ischemia Pulmonary hypertension G3/4 pulmonary complications G3/4 elevation of transaminases, bilirubin, or other liver abnormalities (ALT/AST >5× ULN or bilirubin >3× ULN)	Hold carfilzomib dosing for up to 21 days to resolve toxicity to G1 or to baseline and then, at the discretion of the medically responsible health care provider, consider either permanently discontinuing carfilzomib or restarting carfilzomib at 1 lower dose level. If tolerated, the reduced dosage may be escalated to the previous dose level

(*continued*)

Patient Population Studied

The multicenter, nonrandomized, open-label, phase 2 study involved 58 patients with symptomatic newly diagnosed multiple myeloma who were aged ≥65 years or ineligible for autologous stem cell transplantation. Eligible patients had measurable disease, a Karnofsky performance status ≥60%, creatinine clearance ≥15 mL/min, platelet count ≥50 × 10⁹/L (or ≥30 × 10⁹/L if myeloma involvement in the bone marrow was >50%), and an absolute neutrophil count ≥1 × 10⁹/L without growth factor use. Patients who had nonsecretory multiple myeloma (unless serum-free light chains were present and the ratio was abnormal), peripheral neuropathy of Grade >2, active viral infection, or various clinically significant heart diseases, were not eligible

Efficacy (n = 55)

Proportion who experienced at least a partial response*	95%
Proportion who experienced at least a very good partial response*	71%
Proportion who experienced a complete response or near complete response*	49%
Proportion who experienced a stringent complete response*	20%
Median duration of response*	14.0 months
Progression-free survival at 2 years	76%
Overall survival at 2 survival at 2 years	87%

*Response was assessed according to the International Myeloma Working Group criteria

Note: for the survival analysis (progression-free survival and overall survival), median follow-up was 18 months

Treatment Modifications (continued)

Serum creatinine ≥2× baseline or CrCl decreased to ≤50% of baseline	If attributable to carfilzomib, hold carfilzomib doses for up to 21 days to resolve toxicity to G1 or to baseline and then restart at the same dosage, or reduce the carfilzomib dosage by 1 dose level. If tolerated, the reduced dosage may be escalated to the previous dose level
G2 neuropathy with pain G3/4 peripheral neuropathy	Hold carfilzomib dosing for up to 21 days to resolve toxicity to G1 or to baseline and then restart at the same dose, or reduce the carfilzomib dosage by 1 dose level. If tolerated, the reduced dosage may be escalated to the previous dose level
Confirmed PRES (posterior reversible encephalopathy syndrome) eg, seizure, headache, lethargy, confusion, blindness, altered consciousness, visual and neurologic disturbances, hypertension	Permanently discontinue carfilzomib. The safety of reinitiating carfilzomib in patients previously experiencing PRES is unknown*
Tumor lysis syndrome (TLS)	Withhold carfilzomib until resolution of TLS, then resume carfilzomib at the same dose
Other G3/4 nonhematologic toxicities	If attributable to carfilzomib, hold carfilzomib doses for up to 21 days to resolve toxicity to G1 or to baseline and then restart at the same dosage or reduce the carfilzomib dosage by 1 dose level. If tolerated, the reduced dosage may be escalated to the previous dose level

CYCLOPHOSPHAMIDE

ANC ≤1500/mm^3 and/or platelets <50,000/mm^3	Withhold cyclophosphamide
Patients who have or who develop a serious infection	Withhold cyclophosphamide; consider reducing dose in subsequent cycles. Consider using filgrastim
Severe hemorrhagic cystitis	Discontinue cyclophosphamide therapy
Urotoxicity (bladder ulceration, necrosis, fibrosis, contracture, and secondary cancer)	May require interruption of cyclophosphamide treatment or cystectomy
Hyponatremia and a syndrome resembling SIADH (syndrome of inappropriate antidiuretic hormone)	Hold cyclophosphamide and treat hyponatremia

DEXAMETHASONE

Starting dose	40 mg/dose/day
Dose Level −1	20 mg/dose/day
Dose Level −2	12 mg/dose/day
Dose Level −3	8 mg/dose/day
Dose Level −4	4 mg/dose/day
Dose Level −5	Discontinue dexamethasone

Adverse Event	**Treatment Modification**
G1/2 dyspepsia (moderate symptoms; medical intervention indicated; limiting instrumental ADL), gastric or duodenal ulcer, or gastritis	Continue dexamethasone at the same dose. Treat with therapeutic doses of an H$_2$-receptor antagonist or proton pump inhibitor. If symptoms persist, then reduce the dexamethasone dose by one level

(continued)

Adverse Events (n = 56)

Grade (%)*	Grade 1–2	Grade 3–5
Anemia	59	11
Thrombocytopenia	34	4
Neutropenia	16	20
Fever	23	2
Fatigue	18	2
Nausea/vomiting	20	0
Diarrhea	14	0
Other neurologic events (not listed elsewhere in this table)	14	0
Hyperglycemia	11	2
Edema	13	0
Upper respiratory tract infection	9	2
Other events (not listed elsewhere in this table)	11	0
Lymphopenia	2	7
Hypertension	7	2
Dermatologic events	9	0
Increased levels of alanine or aspartate aminotransferase	7	0
Sensitive peripheral neuropathy	7	0
Dyspnea	7	0
Renal events	2	4
Constipation	5	0
Other respiratory events (not listed elsewhere in table)	5	0
Pneumonia	0	4
Arrhythmia	2	2
Other gastrointestinal events (not listed elsewhere in table)	4	0
Other metabolic events (not listed elsewhere in table)	4	0
Phlebitis	4	0

(continued)

Treatment Modifications (continued)

Adverse Event	Treatment Modification
G ≥3 dyspepsia, gastric or duodenal ulcer, or gastritis (surgery or hospitalization indicated)	Withhold dexamethasone until symptoms return to baseline. Resume dexamethasone reduced by one dose level along with concurrent treatment with therapeutic doses of an H₂-receptor antagonist or proton pump inhibitor. If symptoms recur, then permanently discontinue dexamethasone[†]
Acute pancreatitis	Permanently discontinue dexamethasone[†]
G ≥3 edema	Withhold dexamethasone until symptoms return to baseline. Consider treatment with diuretics. Resume dexamethasone reduced by one dose level. If edema persists, reduce by another dose level. Discontinue dexamethasone permanently if symptoms persist despite two prior dose reductions[†]
G ≥2 mood alteration (moderate mood alteration) or confusion (moderate disorientation; limiting instrumental ADL)	Withhold dexamethasone until symptoms return to baseline. Resume dexamethasone reduced by one dose level. If symptoms persist, reduce by another dose level
G ≥2 muscle weakness (symptomatic; evident on physical exam; limiting instrumental ADL)	Withhold dexamethasone until symptoms return to baseline. Resume dexamethasone reduced by one dose level. If weakness persists, reduce by another dose level. If weakness still persists, then permanently discontinue dexamethasone[†]
G ≥3 hyperglycemia (insulin therapy initiated; hospitalization indicated)	Withhold dexamethasone until blood glucose is ≤250 mg/dL. Treat with insulin or other hypoglycemic agents as clinically appropriate and then resume dexamethasone at the same dose. If hyperglycemia is uncontrolled despite above measures, decrease dexamethasone by one dose level
Other G ≥2 nonhematologic toxicity attributable to dexamethasone including severe irritability, insomnia, or oral candidiasis	Withhold dexamethasone until toxicity resolves to G ≤1, then resume at a lower dose. Consider reduction by one dose level for G2/G3 toxicity, and by two dose levels for G4 or recurrent G3 toxicity

*If carfilzomib is permanently discontinued, then also consider discontinuing dexamethasone and cyclophosphamide
[†]If dexamethasone is permanently discontinued, continued administration of carfilzomib and cyclophosphamide may be considered at the discretion of the treating physician

Adverse Events (n = 56) (continued)

Grade (%)*	Grade 1–2	Grade 3–5
Myocardial infarction	0	2
Heart failure	0	2
Pulmonary thromboembolism	0	2
Stroke	0	2
Febrile neutropenia	0	2
Intestinal perforation	0	2
Acute pulmonary edema	0	2
Mood alteration	0	2
Respiratory failure	2	0
Genitourinary tract infection	2	0
Motor peripheral neuropathy	2	0
Hypoglycemia	2	0

*According to the National Cancer Institute Common Terminology Criteria for Adverse Events, version 4.0
Note: treatment-related adverse events that occurred while on the triple therapy are included in the table. Seven deaths occurred during the trial: two due to disease progression, two owing to conditions thought to be related to carfilzomib (one intestinal perforation and one heart failure), two due to conditions not thought to be related to carfilzomib (one atrial fibrillation and one pneumonia) and one owing to an unknown cause

Therapy Monitoring

1. CBC with differential, liver function tests, serum electrolytes, and serum glucose prior to each dose
2. Monitor for cardiac complications
3. Monitor for and manage dyspnea immediately
4. With abdominal pain, check serum amylase/lipase
5. Ensure adequate hydration of patients to reduce the risk of renal toxicity and of tumor lysis syndrome
6. Check urinary sediment regularly for the presence of erythrocytes and other signs of urotoxicity
7. Treat all urinary tract infections aggressively

MAINTENANCE THERAPY

MULTIPLE MYELOMA REGIMEN: LENALIDOMIDE + BORTEZOMIB + DEXAMETHASONE (RVD)

Nooka AK et al. Leukemia 2014;28:690–693

Bortezomib 1.3 mg/m² per dose; administer subcutaneously in a volume of 0.9% sodium chloride injection (0.9% NS) sufficient to produce a final bortezomib concentration of 2.5 mg/mL, for 4 doses on days 1, 8, 15, and 22, every 28 days for up to 3 years (total dosage/28-day cycle = 5.2 mg/m²)

Note: the protocol allowed for bortezomib to be administer either subcutaneously or intravenously, although the subcutaneous route is preferred since it is associated with a lower rate of peripheral neuropathy (Moreau P et al. Lancet Oncol 2011;12:431–440). If the intravenous route is chosen, bortezomib 1.3 mg/m² per dose is instead diluted in a volume of 0.9% NS sufficient to produce a final bortezomib concentration of *1 mg/mL* and administered intravenously as a 3- to 5-second bolus injection on days 1, 8, 15, and 22, every 28 days for up to 3 years (total dosage/28-day cycle = 5.2 mg/m²)

Lenalidomide 10 mg/dose; administer orally, without regard to meals, once daily for 21 consecutive days on days 1–21, every 28 days until disease progression (total dosage/28-day cycle = 210 mg)
- Patients who delay taking a lenalidomide dose at a regularly scheduled time may take the missed dose if the time to the next regularly scheduled dose is >12 hours away
- Consider doses in Treatment Modifications table for dose adjustments for renal function

Dexamethasone 40 mg/dose; administer orally or intravenously for 4 doses on days 1, 8, 15, and 22, every 28 days for up to 3 years (total dosage/cycle = 160 mg)

Note: lenalidomide, bortezomib, and dexamethasone cycles were repeated every 28 days for up to 3 years, followed by single agent lenalidomide maintenance, administered as described above, until disease progression

Supportive Care
Antiemetic prophylaxis
Emetogenic potential on days 1–21 is **LOW**
See Chapter 42 for antiemetic recommendations

Hematopoietic growth factor (CSF) prophylaxis
Primary prophylaxis is **NOT** *indicated*
See Chapter 43 for more information

Antimicrobial prophylaxis
Risk of fever and neutropenia is **INTERMEDIATE**
  Antimicrobial primary prophylaxis to be considered:
- Antibacterial—consider a fluoroquinolone during periods of neutropenia or no prophylaxis; *P. jirovecii* prophylaxis is recommended (eg, cotrimoxazole)
- Antifungal—consider fluconazole during periods of neutropenia
- Antiviral—antiherpes antivirals (eg, acyclovir, famciclovir, valacyclovir)

Bisphosphonates
All patients receiving primary therapy for symptomatic multiple myeloma should receive a bisphosphonate adjunctively.

Thromboprophylaxis
Risk assessment and recommendations for VTE prophylaxis in patients with multiple myeloma with individual or myeloma-related risk factors, or risk factors related to treatment

(*continued*)

(continued)

Individual risk factors
• Obesity (BMI ≥30 kg/m²)
• H/O VTE
• CVC or pacemaker
• Comorbid pathologies
  ▪ Cardiac disease
  ▪ Chronic renal disease
  ▪ Diabetes
  ▪ Acute infection
  ▪ Immobilization
• Surgery
  ▪ General surgery
  ▪ Any anesthesia
  ▪ Trauma
• Medications
  ▪ Erythropoietin (epoetin alfa, darbepoetin)
  ▪ Estrogenic compounds
  ▪ Bevacizumab
• Clotting disorders
  ▪ Thrombophilia
Myeloma-related risk factors
• Diagnosis of multiple myeloma
• Hyperviscosity
	≤1 Individual or myeloma-related risk factor present:
	• **Aspirin** 81–325 mg daily
	
	≥2 Individual or myeloma-related risk factors present:
	• **LMWH,** * equivalent to enoxaparin sodium 40 mg/day *or* **dalteparin sodium** 5000 IU/day; administer subcutaneously, *or*
	• **Warfarin,** targeting an INR = 2–3

Concomitant treatment-related risk factors Thalidomide or lenalidomide in combination with: • High-dose dexamethasone (≥480 mg/month) • Doxorubicin • Multiagent chemotherapy	• **LMWH,** * equivalent to enoxaparin sodium 40 mg/day *or* **dalteparin sodium** 5000 IU/day; administer subcutaneously, *or* • **Warfarin,** targeting an INR = 2–3

*LMWHs should be used with caution in individuals with impaired renal function (creatinine clearance <30 mL/min). Refer to product labeling for information about doses and administration schedules in renally impaired patients, and guidance for monitoring anti-Factor Xa concentrations

Abbreviations: CVC, central venous catheter; INR, international normalized ratio; LMWH, low-molecular-weight heparin; VTE, venous thromboembolic disease

References: Geerts WH et al. Chest 2008;133(6 Suppl):381S–453S
National Comprehensive Cancer Network. Multiple Myeloma, V.1.2014. (Accessed October 8, 2013, at http://www.nccn.org)
National Comprehensive Cancer Network. Venous Thromboembolic Disease, V.2.2013. (Accessed October 8, 2013, at http://www.nccn.org)
Palumbo A et al. Leukemia 2008;22:414–423

Treatment Modifications

LENALIDOMIDE + BORTEZIMB + DEXAMETHASONE

LENALIDOMIDE

Lenalidomide dose levels (Days 1–21 of each 28-day cycle)

	CrCl ≥60 mL/min	CrCl ≥30 mL/min and <60 mL/min	CrCl <30 mL/minor end-stage renal disease on hemodialysis
Starting dose	10 mg each day	5 mg each day	2.5 mg each day (administered after dialysis on dialysis days, if applicable)
Dose level −1	7.5 mg each day	2.5 mg each day	2.5 mg every other day (administered after dialysis on dialysis days, if applicable)
Dose level −2	5 mg each day	Discontinue†	Discontinue†
Dose level −3	Discontinue†		

(continued)

Treatment Modifications (continued)

Adverse Event	Treatment Modification
Hematologic Toxicity	
Day 1 ANC <1000/mm³ or platelet count <70,000/mm³	Delay the next cycle until ANC ≥1000/mm³ and platelet count ≥70,000/mm³. Consider treatment with filgrastim and/or platelet transfusion according to local guidelines. If the start of a new cycle is delayed >14 days for lenalidomide-related toxicity, then reduce the lenalidomide dosage by one dose level
Either of the following: • G4 neutropenia (ANC <500/mm³) • Neutropenic fever (ANC <1000/mm³ + a single temperature >38.5°C)	Withhold lenalidomide for the remainder of the cycle and delay initiation of the next cycle until ANC ≥1000/mm³ and platelet count ≥50,000/mm³, if necessary. Consider treatment with filgrastim according to local guidelines. If neutropenia was the only dose-limiting toxicity AND if filgrastim is continued AND if the next cycle was delayed by ≤14 days, then resume lenalidomide at the same dose. Otherwise, reduce the lenalidomide dose by one dose level at the start of the next cycle
G3 neutropenia (ANC ≥500/mm³ and less than 1000/mm³) during a cycle	Interrupt lenalidomide treatment and follow weekly CBC. When ANC ≥1000/mm³ and there are no other toxicities, resume lenalidomide treatment at same dose. If other toxicities are still present, then resume lenalidomide with dose reduced one dose level
Recurrent G3 neutropenia (ANC ≥500/mm³ and less than 1000/mm³) during a cycle	Interrupt lenalidomide treatment and follow weekly CBC. When ANC ≥1000/mm³, resume with dose reduced one dose level
G4 thrombocytopenia (platelet count <25,000/mm³)	Interrupt lenalidomide treatment and follow weekly CBC. When platelet count ≥25,000/mm³, resume lenalidomide with dose reduced one dose level
Recurrent G4 thrombocytopenia (platelet count <25,000/mm³)	
Nonhematologic Toxicity	
G3/4 hepatotoxicity (ALT/AST >5× ULN and/or bilirubin >3× ULN)	Withhold lenalidomide for the remainder of the cycle. Delay initiation of the next cycle until hepatotoxicity resolves to G ≤2 (ALT/AST ≤5× ULN and/or bilirubin ≤3× ULN), then resume lenalidomide at one lower dose level
G3 rash	Hold dose for remainder of cycle. Decrease by one dose level when dosing resumed at next cycle (rash must resolve to G ≤1)
Allergic reactions, including hypersensitivity, angioedema, Stevens-Johnson syndrome, toxic epidermal necrolysis (TEN), and drug reaction with eosinophilia and systemic symptoms (DRESS)	Discontinue lenalidomide if reactions are suspected. Do not resume lenalidomide if these reactions are confirmed
Tumor lysis syndrome (TLS)	Monitor patients at risk of TLS (ie, those with high tumor burden) and take appropriate precautions including aggressive hydration and allopurinol
G3 peripheral neuropathy	If neuropathy is considered to be attributable to lenalidomide, then withhold lenalidomide for the remainder of the cycle. Delay initiation of the next cycle until neuropathy resolves to G ≤1, then resume lenalidomide at one lower dose level
G4 peripheral neuropathy	If neuropathy is considered to be attributable to lenalidomide, then discontinue lenalidomide[†]
G3/4 venous thromboembolism (VTE) during aspirin monotherapy or inadequate anticoagulation	Continue lenalidomide at the current dose and initiate adequate anticoagulation
G3/4 venous thromboembolism (VTE) during adequate anticoagulation (eg, prophylactic or therapeutic doses of LMWH, UFH, or warfarin)	Discontinue lenalidomide[†]
G ≥2 hypothyroidism or G ≥2 hyperthyroidism	Continue lenalidomide at current dose and initiate appropriate medical treatment
Other G ≥3 lenalidomide-related toxicities	Withhold lenalidomide for the remainder of the cycle. Delay initiation of the next cycle until toxicity resolves to G ≤2, then resume lenalidomide at one lower dose level

(continued)

Treatment Modifications (*continued*)

BORTEZOMIB

Starting dose	1.3 mg/m²/dose
Dose level −1	1 mg/m²/dose
Dose level −2	0.7 mg/m²/dose

Adverse Event	**Treatment Modification**
Platelet count <70,000/mm³ or ANC <1000/mm³ on day 1 of a cycle	Hold therapy until platelet count ≥70,000/mm³ and ANC ≥1,000/mm³
G3 thrombocytopenia (platelet count <50,000/mm³)	Reduce bortezomib dosage by one dose level
G1 neuropathy (paresthesias, weakness, and/or loss of reflexes) without pain or loss of function	No action
G1 neuropathy with pain or G2 neuropathy (interferes with function but not with activities of daily living)	Reduce bortezomib dosage one dose level
G2 neuropathy with pain or G3 (interferes with activities of daily living)	Withhold bortezomib treatment until toxicity resolves to G1 or baseline, then reinitiate reducing bortezomib dosage one dose level
G4 neuropathy (sensory neuropathy that is disabling or motor neuropathy that is life-threatening or leads to paralysis)	Discontinue treatment
Hepatotoxicity	Monitor liver function. Stop bortezomib and evaluate if hepatotoxicity is suspected
Bilirubin level greater than 1.5× ULN and any AST level	Reduce bortezomib to 0.7 mg/m² in the first cycle; consider dose escalation to 1 mg/m² based on tolerability
If several bortezomib doses in consecutive cycles are withheld due to toxicity	Reduce bortezomib by 1 dosage level
G ≥2 nonhematologic toxicity on day 1 of a cycle	Hold bortezomib until toxicity has resolved to G1 or baseline
G ≥3 nonhematologic toxicities	Hold bortezomib until toxicity has resolved to G1 or baseline; then, may be reinitiated with 1 dosage level reduction

DEXAMETHASONE

Starting dose	40 mg/dose/day
Dose Level −1	20 mg/dose/day
Dose Level −2	12 mg/dose/day
Dose Level −3	8 mg/dose/day
Dose Level −4	4 mg/dose/day
Dose Level −5	Discontinue dexamethasone

Adverse Event	**Treatment Modification**
G1/2 dyspepsia (moderate symptoms; medical intervention indicated; limiting instrumental ADL), gastric or duodenal ulcer, or gastritis	Continue dexamethasone at the same dose. Treat with therapeutic doses of an H₂-receptor antagonist or proton pump inhibitor. If symptoms persist, then reduce the dexamethasone dose by one level
G ≥3 dyspepsia, gastric or duodenal ulcer, or gastritis (surgery or hospitalization indicated)	Withhold dexamethasone until symptoms return to baseline. Resume dexamethasone reduced by one dose level along with concurrent treatment with therapeutic doses of an H₂-receptor antagonist or proton pump inhibitor. If symptoms recur, then permanently discontinue dexamethasone‡
Acute pancreatitis	Permanently discontinue dexamethasone‡

(*continued*)

Treatment Modifications (continued)

Adverse Event	Treatment Modification
G ≥3 edema	Withhold dexamethasone until symptoms return to baseline. Consider treatment with diuretics. Resume dexamethasone reduced by one dose level. If edema persists, reduce by another dose level. Discontinue dexamethasone permanently if symptoms persist despite two prior dose reductions[‡]
G ≥2 mood alteration (moderate mood alteration) or confusion (moderate disorientation; limiting instrumental ADL)	Withhold dexamethasone until symptoms return to baseline. Resume dexamethasone reduced by one dose level. If symptoms persist, reduce by another dose level
G ≥2 muscle weakness (symptomatic; evident on physical exam; limiting instrumental ADL)	Withhold dexamethasone until symptoms return to baseline. Resume dexamethasone reduced by one dose level. If weakness persists, reduce by another dose level. If weakness still persists, then permanently discontinue dexamethasone[‡]
G ≥3 hyperglycemia (insulin therapy initiated; hospitalization indicated)	Withhold dexamethasone until blood glucose is ≤250 mg/dL. Treat with insulin or other hypoglycemic agents as clinically appropriate and then resume dexamethasone at the same dose. If hyperglycemia is uncontrolled despite above measures, decrease dexamethasone by one dose level
Other G ≥2 nonhematologic toxicity attributable to dexamethasone including severe irritability, insomnia, or oral candidiasis	Withhold dexamethasone until toxicity resolves to G ≤1, then resume at a lower dose. Consider reduction by one dose level for G2/G3 toxicity, and by two dose levels for G4 or recurrent G3 toxicity

[†]If lenalidomide and bortezomib are permanently discontinued, then also consider discontinuation of dexamethasone
[‡]If dexamethasone is permanently discontinued, continued administration of lenalidomide and/or bortezomib may be considered at the discretion of the treating physician

Patient Population Studied

A study of 45 high-risk patients with multiple myeloma. Eligible patients had deletion of *p53* (locus *17p13*), deletion of 1p, immunoglobulin heavy chain translocations (t[4;14] or t[14;16]) by fluorescence in situ hybridization or by metaphase cytogenetics, or presentation as plasma cell leukemia (≥20% circulating plasma cells in peripheral blood).

Efficacy (n = 45)

Best response of stringent complete response*	51%
Best response of at least very good partial response*	96%
Overall response rate[†]	100%
Median progression-free survival	32 months
Overall survival at 3 years	93%

*Response was determined according to the International Myeloma Working Group Uniform Response Criteria
[†]Overall response rate was the proportion of patients who experienced at least a partial response
Note: median follow-up time was 26 months

Adverse Events (n = 45)

No Grade 3 or 4 neuropathy was observed. Dose modifications were needed in 40% of patients. No patients discontinued therapy owing to adverse events.

Therapy Monitoring

1. CBC with differential, liver function tests, serum creatinine, and serum glucose prior to each dose of bortezomib
2. With abdominal pain, check serum amylase/lipase
3. Ensure adequate hydration of patients to reduce the risk of renal toxicity
4. Monitor for bortezomib toxicities including neuropathy and hypotension

Lenalidomide notes:
- Higher incidences of second primary malignancies were observed in controlled trials of patients with MM receiving lenalidomide. While no routine monitoring is indicated, awareness of this potential complication is necessary
- A decrease in the number of CD34+ cells collected after treatment has been reported in patients who have received >4 cycles of lenalidomide. In patients who may undergo transplant, consider early referral to transplant center
- Because of the embryo-fetal risk, lenalidomide is available only through a restricted program under a Risk Evaluation and Mitigation Strategy (REMS), the REVLIMID REMS program

Bortezomib note:
- Patients with pre-existing severe neuropathy should be treated with bortezomib only after careful risk-benefit assessment

MAINTENANCE THERAPY
MULTIPLE MYELOMA REGIMEN: BORTEZOMIB

Sonneveld P et al. J Clin Oncol 2012;30:2946–2955

Note: the post-transplant maintenance regimen outlined below was evaluated within the context of a broader protocol involving induction therapy with bortezomib + doxorubicin + dexamethasone followed by 1–2 cycles of high-dose melphalan and autologous stem cell transplant

Maintenance therapy (starting 4 weeks after high-dose melphalan):
Bortezomib 1.3 mg/m^2 per dose by intravenous injection over 3–5 seconds, continually, every 2 weeks for 2 years (total dosage/2-week course = 1.3 mg/m^2)

Supportive Care
Antiemetic prophylaxis
*Emetogenic potential with bortezomib is **MINIMAL***
See Chapter 42 for antiemetic recommendations

Hematopoietic growth factor (CSF) prophylaxis
*Primary prophylaxis is **NOT** indicated*
See Chapter 43 for more information

Antimicrobial prophylaxis
*Risk of fever and neutropenia is **LOW***
   Antimicrobial primary prophylaxis to be considered:
   • Antibacterial—not indicated
   • Antifungal—not indicated
   • Antiviral—antiherpes antivirals (eg, acyclovir, famciclovir, valacyclovir) throughout bortezomib therapy

Bisphosphonates
All patients receiving primary therapy for symptomatic multiple myeloma should receive a bisphosphonate adjunctively.

Thromboprophylaxis
Risk assessment and recommendations for VTE prophylaxis in patients with multiple myeloma with individual or myeloma-related risk factors, or risk factors related to treatment

Individual risk factors
 • Obesity (BMI ≥30 kg/m^2)
 • H/O VTE
 • CVC or pacemaker
 • Comorbid pathologies
   ■ Cardiac disease
   ■ Chronic renal disease
   ■ Diabetes
   ■ Acute infection
   ■ Immobilization
 • Surgery
   ■ General surgery
   ■ Any anesthesia
   ■ Trauma
 • Medications
   ■ Erythropoietin (epoetin alfa, darbepoetin)
   ■ Estrogenic compounds
   ■ Bevacizumab
 • Clotting disorders
   ■ Thrombophilia
 Myeloma-related risk factors
 • Diagnosis of multiple myeloma
 • Hyperviscosity
	≤1 Individual or myeloma-related risk factor present:
	 • **Aspirin** 81–325 mg daily
	
	 ≥2 Individual or myeloma-related risk factors present:
	 • **LMWH,*** **equivalent to enoxaparin sodium** 40 mg/day *or* **dalteparin sodium** 5000 IU/day; administer subcutaneously, *or*
	 • **Warfarin**, targeting an INR = 2–3

Treatment Modifications

Bortezomib Dose Level	
Starting dose	1.3 mg/m^2 per dose every 2 weeks
Level −1	1 mg/m^2 per dose every 2 weeks
Level −2	0.7 mg/m^2 per dose every 2 weeks

Adverse Event	Treatment Modification
G3 thrombocytopenia (<50,000/mm^3)	Reduce bortezomib dosage by 1 dose level

Treatment Modification for Bortezomib-Induced Peripheral Neuropathy*

Severity of Peripheral Neuropathy	Modification of Dose and Schedule
G1 (paresthesias or loss of reflexes) without pain or loss of function	No action
G1 with pain or G2 (interferes with function but not with activities of daily living)	Reduce bortezomib dosage by 1 dose level
G2 with pain or G3 (interferes with activities of daily living)	Withhold bortezomib treatment until toxicity resolves, then reinitiate reducing bortezomib dosage by 1 dose level
G4 (permanent sensory loss that interferes with function)	Discontinue treatment

*Richardson PG et al. J Clin Oncol 2006;24:3113–3120

(continued)

(continued)

Concomitant treatment-related risk factors	
Thalidomide or lenalidomide in combination with: • High-dose dexamethasone (≥480 mg/month) • Doxorubicin • Multiagent chemotherapy	• **LMWH,*** equivalent to enoxaparin sodium 40 mg/day *or* **dalteparin sodium** 5000 IU/day; administer subcutaneously, *or* • **Warfarin**, targeting an INR = 2–3

*LMWHs should be used with caution in individuals with impaired renal function (creatinine clearance <30 mL/min). Refer to product labeling for information about doses and administration schedules in renally impaired patients, and guidance for monitoring anti-Factor Xa concentrations

Abbreviations: CVC, central venous catheter; INR, international normalized ratio; LMWH, low-molecular-weight heparin; VTE, venous thromboembolic disease

References: Geerts WH et al. Chest 2008;133(6 Suppl):381S–453S

National Comprehensive Cancer Network. Multiple Myeloma, V.1.2014. (Accessed October 8, 2013, at http://www.nccn.org)

National Comprehensive Cancer Network. Venous Thromboembolic Disease, V.2.2013. (Accessed October 8, 2013, at http://www.nccn.org)

Palumbo A et al. Leukemia 2008;22:414–423

Toxicity

- Bortezomib-emergent peripheral neuropathy (BiPN) was the prevalent toxicity during induction, preventing a substantial number of patients from starting maintenance therapy
- In those who started maintenance, 5% experienced G3/4 BiPN
- Prolonged administration of bortezomib on the once-every-2-weeks schedule was deemed feasible; therefore, it is important to prevent BiPN during induction, which enables patients to continue into maintenance
- The tolerability of bortezomib given every 2 weeks is similar to the weekly schedule
- Subcutaneous bortezomib administration may further improve tolerability

Bortezomib Maintenance After Bortezomib + Doxorubicin 1 Dexamethasone Induction (n = 229)

Still on treatment after 6 months	90%
Still on treatment after 12 months	76%
Still on treatment after 18 months	64%
Still on treatment after 24 months	47%

Safety Profile and Toxicities

Variable	Bortezomib + Doxorubicin + Dexamethasone Induction (n = 410)		Bortezomib Maintenance (n = 229)	
	No.	%	No.	%
Any AE	400	98	222	97
AE Grades 3 to 4	258	63	110	48
AE classified as SAE	187	46	77	34
AE leading to discontinuation, dose reduction, or delay of bortezomib	112	27	81	35
Death from AE	7	2	0	0

(continued)

Patient Population Studied

Patients were newly diagnosed with MM Durie-Salmon stages II–III, WHO PS 0–2, or WHO 3 when caused by MM. Exclusion criteria included systemic amyloid light-chain amyloidosis, nonsecretory MM, and neuropathy G ≥2. Local RT was allowed for painful MM lesions

Baseline Patient and Disease Characteristics (n = 413)

	No.	%
Age, years: median (range)	57 (31–65)	
Male sex	253	61
WHO performance stage		
0	193	47
1	170	41
2	31	8
3	15	4
ISS stage		
I	144	35
II	150	36
III	81	20
M-protein isotype		
IgA	92	22
IgG	251	61
IgD	5	1
LCD	63	15
M-protein light chain		
Kappa	277	67
Lambda	135	33
Number of skeletal lesions		
0	102	25
1–2	44	11
≥3	255	62
Genetic abnormalities (positive/# assessed, %)		
del(13q)	148/361	41%
t(4;14)	35/250	14%
del(17p13)	25/289	9%

(continued)

Toxicity (*continued*)

	All G	G3/4	All G	G3/4
Hematologic Toxicities				
Anemia	28	8	27	1
Neutropenia	4	3	2	0
Thrombocytopenia	39	10	37	4
Infections	56	26	75	24
Herpes zoster	2	0	2	0
Nonhematologic Toxicities				
Wasting, fatigue	27	4	20	1
GI symptoms	67	11	48	5
Cardiac disorders	27	8	19	3
Thrombosis	6	4	1	1
Peripheral neuropathy	37	24	33	5

AE, adverse event (including infection); N/A, not applicable; SAE, serious adverse event

Therapy Monitoring

1. Blood counts and physical examinations at regular intervals (1–3 months)
2. Serum and urinary protein electrophoresis studies as indicated at regular intervals (1–3 months)

Patient Population Studied (*continued*)

Creatinine >2 mg/dL	36	9
Median β$_2$-microglobulin, mg/L	3.40	
Median hemoglobin, mmol/L (g/dL)	6.6 (10.6)	
Median calcium, mmol/L (mg/dL)	2.34 (9.4)	
Median number of bone marrow plasma cells	40	

Ig, immunoglobulin; ISS, International Staging System
*WHO performance stage, 4 = 1% unknown; ISS stage, 38 = 9% unknown; M-protein isotype, 2 = 0% other; M-protein light chain, 1 = 0% unknown; number of skeletal lesions, 12 = 3% unknown

Efficacy

An analysis of PFS calculated in 645 patients from the time of last high-dose melphalan (HDM) indicated that posttransplantation bortezomib contributed to improvement of PFS

MAINTENANCE THERAPY
MULTIPLE MYELOMA REGIMEN : LENALIDOMIDE

Attal M et al. N Engl J Med 2012;366:1782–1791
Dimopoulos MA et al. Haematologica 2013;98:784–788
McCarthy PL et al. N Engl J Med 2012;366:1770–1781
Palumbo A et al. N Engl J Med 2012;366:1759–1769

Lenalidomide 10 mg/day orally, continually, for 21 consecutive days, on days 1–21, every 28 days (total dose/cycle = 210 mg)

or

Lenalidomide 15 mg/day orally, continually, for 21 consecutive days, on days 1–21, every 28 days (total dose/cycle = 315 mg)
Notes:
- Maintenance treatment may begin with lenalidomide 10 mg/day for 21 consecutive days every 28 days, and if tolerated, escalated to lenalidomide 15 mg/day for 21 consecutive days every 28 days
- Maintenance therapy is continued until disease progression or the development of unacceptable rates of adverse effects

Supportive Care
Antiemetic prophylaxis
Emetogenic potential is **MINIMAL–LOW**
See Chapter 42 for antiemetic recommendations

Hematopoietic growth factor (CSF) prophylaxis
Primary prophylaxis is **NOT** indicated
See Chapter 43 for more information

Antimicrobial prophylaxis
Risk of fever and neutropenia is **INTERMEDIATE**
  Antimicrobial primary prophylaxis to be considered:
  - Antibacterial—consider a fluoroquinolone or no prophylaxis; *P. jirovecii* prophylaxis is recommended (eg, cotrimoxazole)
  - Antifungal—recommended; consider use during periods of neutropenia
  - Antiviral—antiherpes antivirals (eg, acyclovir, famciclovir, valacyclovir)

Diarrhea management
Loperamide or **diphenoxylate hydrochloride** 2.5 mg with **atropine sulfate** 0.025 mg (eg, Lomotil)

Bisphosphonates
All patients receiving primary therapy for symptomatic multiple myeloma should receive a bisphosphonate adjunctively.

Thromboprophylaxis
Risk assessment and recommendations for VTE prophylaxis in patients with multiple myeloma with individual or myeloma-related risk factors, or risk factors related to treatment

(continued)

Treatment Modifications

Lenalidomide Dose Levels	
Starting dose	25 mg/dose
Level –1	20 mg/dose
Level –2	15 mg/dose
Level –3	10 mg/dose
Level –4	5 mg/dose
Level –5	Discontinue

Adverse Event	Treatment Modification
G3/4 neutropenia; Febrile neutropenia (ANC <1000/mm³ + fever ≥38°C)	Hold lenalidomide dosing for up to 21 days to resolve toxicity and then restart at the same dose or reduce the lenalidomide dose by 1 dose level
G3/4 nonhematologic toxicity	Hold lenalidomide dosing for up to 21 days to resolve toxicity to G ≤2 and then restart at the same dose or reduce the lenalidomide dose by 1 dose level

Patient Population Studied

Patients with symptomatic, measurable, newly diagnosed MM who were not candidates for transplantation (≥65 years of age) were eligible for this trial. Exclusion criteria were an ANC <1500/mm³, platelet count <75,000/mm³, a hemoglobin level <8.0 g/dL, a serum creatinine level of >2.5 mg/dL (>221 μmol/L), and peripheral neuropathy of G ≥2. A total of 459 patients were randomly assigned to receive nine 4-week cycles of melphalan-prednisone-lenalidomide induction (MPR) followed by lenalidomide maintenance therapy until a relapse or disease progression occurred (152 patients) or to receive MPR (153 patients) or melphalan-prednisone (MP) (154 patients) without maintenance therapy. Maintenance consisted of lenalidomide 10 mg daily for the first 21 days of 28-day cycles until disease progression or the development of unacceptable toxicity. The primary end point was progression-free survival

Palumbo A et al. N Engl J Med 2012;366:1759–1769

(continued)

(*continued*)

Individual risk factors	
• Obesity (BMI ≥30 kg/m²)	
• H/O VTE	
• CVC or pacemaker	
• Comorbid pathologies	≤1 Individual or myeloma-related risk factor present:
▪ Cardiac disease	• **Aspirin** 81–325 mg daily
▪ Chronic renal disease	
▪ Diabetes	
▪ Acute infection	
▪ Immobilization	
• Surgery	≥2 Individual or myeloma-related risk factors present:
▪ General surgery	• **LMWH,*** equivalent to enoxaparin sodium 40 mg/day *or* **dalteparin sodium** 5000 IU/day; administer subcutaneously, *or*
▪ Any anesthesia	
▪ Trauma	• **Warfarin,** targeting an INR = 2–3
• Medications	
▪ Erythropoietin (epoetin alfa, darbepoetin)	
▪ Estrogenic compounds	
▪ Bevacizumab	
• Clotting disorders	
▪ Thrombophilia	
Myeloma-related risk factors	
• Diagnosis of multiple myeloma	
• Hyperviscosity	
Concomitant treatment-related risk factors Thalidomide or lenalidomide in combination with:	• **LMWH,*** equivalent to enoxaparin sodium 40 mg/day *or* **dalteparin sodium** 5000 IU/day; administer subcutaneously, *or*
• High-dose dexamethasone (≥480 mg/month)	
• Doxorubicin	• **Warfarin,** targeting an INR = 2–3
• Multiagent chemotherapy	

*LMWHs should be used with caution in individuals with impaired renal function (creatinine clearance <30 mL/min). Refer to product labeling for information about doses and administration schedules in renally impaired patients, and guidance for monitoring anti-Factor Xa concentrations
Abbreviations: CVC, central venous catheter; INR, international normalized ratio; LMWH, low-molecular-weight heparin; VTE, venous thromboembolic disease
References: Geerts WH et al. Chest 2008;133(6 Suppl):381S–453S
National Comprehensive Cancer Network. Multiple Myeloma, V.1.2014. (Accessed October 8, 2013, at http://www.nccn.org)
National Comprehensive Cancer Network. Venous Thromboembolic Disease, V.2.2013. (Accessed October 8, 2013, at http://www.nccn.org)
Palumbo A et al. Leukemia 2008;22:414–423

Efficacy

Variable	MPR-R (n = 152)	MPR (n = 153)	MP (n = 154)
Best Response			
Complete or partial response—no. (%)	117 (77.0) *	104 (68.0) †	77 (50.0)
Complete response	15 (9.9)	5 (3.3)	5 (3.2)
Partial response‡	102 (67.1)	99 (64.7)	72 (46.8)
Very good partial response§	35 (23.0)	45 (29.4)	14 (9.1)
Stable disease—no. (%)	28 (18.4)	40 (26.1)	70 (45.5)
Progressive disease—no. (%)	0	2 (1.3)	0
Response could not be evaluated—no. (%)	7 (4.6)	7 (4.6)	7 (4.5)

Patient Population Studied (*continued*)

Patients with MM between 18 and 70 years of age, an Eastern Cooperative Oncology Group performance status of 0 or 1, symptomatic disease requiring treatment (Durie-Salmon stage ≥1), and any induction regimen of 2 to 12 months' duration, who had received ≤2 induction regimens (excluding dexamethasone alone). Patients with stable disease or a marginal, partial, or complete response during the first 100 days after stem cell transplantation were eligible. After disease restaging, patients were randomly assigned in a blinded manner to lenalidomide or placebo between days 100 and 110 after transplantation. A total of 460 patients <71 years of age with stable disease or a marginal, partial, or complete response 100 days after undergoing stem cell transplantation were randomly assigned to lenalidomide or placebo, which was administered until disease progression. The starting dose of lenalidomide was 10 mg/day (range, 5–15 mg/day). The time to disease progression was the primary end point

McCarthy PL et al. N Engl J Med 2012;366:1770–1781

Study patients were <65 years of age with MM that had not progressed during the interval between first-line autologous stem cell transplantation (1 or 2 procedures) within the previous 6 months, serum creatinine <1.8 mg/dL (<160 μmol/L), an ANC ≥1000/mm³, and platelet count >75,000/mm³. After undergoing transplantation, patients received consolidation treatment with 2 cycles of lenalidomide 25 mg daily for the first 21 days of 28-day cycles, and then, based on prior random assignment, received maintenance therapy with either placebo or lenalidomide 10 mg daily for the first 3 months, which, if tolerated, could be increased to 15 mg daily on the same administration schedule. Treatment was continued until the patient withdrew consent, disease progressed, or toxicity was unacceptable. Randomization was stratified according to baseline levels of serum β_2-microglobulin (≤3 mg/L or >3 mg/L), the presence or absence of a 13q deletion by FISH, and treatment response after transplantation (a complete or very good partial response vs a partial response or stable disease). The primary end point was progression-free survival

Attal M et al. N Engl J Med 2012;366:1782–1791

Efficacy (continued)

Variable	MPR-R (n = 152)	MPR (n = 153)	MP (n = 154)
Time to Event			
Median time to first evidence of response: months (range)	2* (1–9)	2* (1–6)	3 (1–15)
Duration of response—months			
Median complete or partial response (95% CI)	29$^\epsilon$ (22–NR)	13 (12–15)	13 (10–18)
Median complete response (95% CI)	NR$^\epsilon$ (36–NR)	31 (23–33)	22 (10–24)
Median partial response‡ (95% CI)	19 (11–NR)	11 (9–13)	10 (9–15)
Median very good partial response§ (95% CI)	28* (22–NR)	15 (13–22)	18 (10–22)

*P <0.001 for the comparison with the MP group
†P = 0.002 for the comparison with the MP group
‡Partial response defined as 50–99% reduction in serum/urinary levels of myeloma protein
§Very good partial response defined as 90–99% reduction in serum/urinary levels of myeloma protein
$^\epsilon$P <0.001 for the comparison with the MPR group and the comparison with the MP group
MP, melphalan–prednisone induction without lenalidomide maintenance; MPR, melphalan–prednisone–lenalidomide induction without lenalidomide maintenance; MPR-R, melphalan–prednisone–lenalidomide induction followed by lenalidomide maintenance; NR, not reached
Palumbo A et al. N Engl J Med 2012;366:1759–1769

	Lenalidomide	Placebo	HR	P Value
At a Median of 18 Months				
Progression/death	47/231 (20%)	101/229 (44%)	0.37; 95% CI, 0.26–0.53	P <0.001
Median time to progression	39 months	21 months		P <0.001
Deaths	13/231	24/229	0.52; 95% CI, 0.26–1.02	P = 0.05
Median overall survival	NR	NR	—	—
At a Median of 34 Months				
Progression/death	86/231 (37%)	132/229 (58%)	0.48; 95% CI, 0.36–0.63	—
Median time to progression	46 months	27 months	—	P <0.001
Deaths	35 (15%)	53 (23%)	—	P = 0.03
3-year rate freedom from progression/death	66%; 95% CI, 59–73	39%; 95% CI, 33–48	—	—
Overall survival at 3 years	88%; 95% CI, 84–93	80%; 95% CI, 74–86	0.62; 95% CI, 0.40–0.95	P = 0.03

McCarthy PL et al. N Engl J Med 2012;366:1770–1781

(continued)

Efficacy (continued)

Response to Treatment as Assessed by the Independent Review Committee*

Variable	Lenalidomide (n = 307)	Placebo (n = 307)	P Value
Response at randomization			
Evaluable for response—# (%) of patients	266 (87)	274 (89)	0.18
Percent complete response	5	8	
Percent VGPR[†]	56	51	
Percent partial response	38	39	
Percent stable disease	1	2	
Percent complete response or VGPR	61	59	0.55
Best response during maintenance			
Evaluable for response—# (%) of patients	300 (98)	293 (95)	0.07
Percent complete response	29	27	
Percent VGPR[‡]	55	49	
Percent partial response	15	23	
Percent stable disease	1	1	
Percent complete response or VGPR	84	76	0.009

VGPR, very good partial response
*Responses assessed according to International Uniform Response Criteria for MM
[†]Includes 4 patients (2%) in lenalidomide group and 5 (2%) in placebo group with disappearance of M protein on immunofixation but no BM marrow evaluation
[‡]Includes 6 patients (2%) in lenalidomide group and 9 (3%) in placebo group with disappearance of M protein on immunofixation but no BM marrow evaluation
Attal M et al. N Engl J Med 2012;366:1782–1791

Survival End Points

	Lenalidomide (n = 307)	Placebo (n = 307)	HR, P Value
Progressive disease	104	160	HR 1.25, P = 0.29
Median progression-free survival	41 months	23 months	P <0.001
Overall survival 3 years after randomization	80%	84%	

Rate of Progression-Free Survival 3 Years After Randomization*

Probability 3-year progression-free survival	59%	35%	
With VGPR at randomization	64%	49%	P = 0.006
Without VGPR at randomization	51%	18%	P <0.001
Baseline serum β_2-microglobulin ≤3 mg/L	71%	41%,	P <0.001
Baseline serum β_2-microglobulin >3 mg/L	50%	29%	P <0.001
With 13q deletion	53%	24%	P <0.001
Without 13q deletion	67%	44%	P <0.001

VGPR, very good partial response. Median follow-up = 30 months
*Age, sex, isotype of the monoclonal component, International Staging System stage, induction regimen, or number of transplantations did not modify the progression-free survival benefit with lenalidomide
Attal M et al. N Engl J Med 2012;366:1782–1791

Toxicity

Maintenance Therapy

	G3	G4
Hematologic Adverse Events—Number/Total (%)		
Neutropenia	4/88 (5)	2/88 (2)
Thrombocytopenia	0/88	5/88 (6)
Anemia	2/88 (2)	2/88 (2)
Nonhematologic Adverse Events—Number/Total (%)		
Infection*	3/88 (3)	2/88 (2)
Fatigue	2/88 (2)	1/88 (1)
Deep-vein thrombosis	2/88 (2)	0/88
Diarrhea	3/88 (3)	1/88 (1)
Bone pain	4/88 (5)	0/88
Diabetes mellitus	2/88 (2)	0/88

*Infection was described in the following terms: pneumonia, lower respiratory tract infection, upper respiratory tract infection, bronchitis, sepsis, urinary tract infection, diverticulitis, herpes zoster, infective arthritis, bacteriuria, cellulitis, gastrointestinal tract infection, oral infection, tooth infection, septic shock, appendicitis, sinusitis, postprocedural infection, streptococcal bacteremia, *Escherichia coli* infection, and meningitis
Palumbo A et al. N Engl J Med 2012;366:1759–1769

Hematologic Adverse Events Following Randomization to Placebo or Maintenance Lenalidomide

Event	Lenalidomide (n = 231)		Placebo (n = 229)		P Value
	G3	G4	G3	G4	
	Number of Patients (%)				
Neutropenia	74 (32)	30 (13)	27 (12)	7 (3)	<0.001
Thrombocytopenia	21 (9)	11 (5)	3 (1)	8 (3)	0.001
Lymphopenia	15 (6)	1 (<1)	3 (1)	1 (<1)	0.01
Anemia	9 (4)	2 (1)	1 (<1)	0	0.006
Leukopenia	24 (10)	3 (1)	7 (3)	1 (<1)	0.001
Any event	74 (32)	36 (16)	27 (12)	12 (5)	<0.001

McCarthy PL et al. N Engl J Med 2012;366:1770–1781

Adverse Events After Randomization in the Treated Population

Event	Lenalidomide Group (n = 306)		Placebo Group (n = 302)	
	All Events	G3/4	All Events	G3/4
	Number of Patients (%)			
Any event	305 (>99)	225 (74)	297 (98)	130 (43)
Hematologic Events				
Hematologic events	210 (69)	179 (58)	107 (35)	68 (22)
Neutropenia	180 (59)	157 (51)	78 (26)	53 (18)
Febrile neutropenia	6 (2)	4 (1)	1 (<1)	1 (<1)
Anemia	31 (10)	10 (3)	28 (9)	7 (2)
Thrombocytopenia	74 (24)	44 (14)	45 (15)	20 (7)

(continued)

Toxicity (continued)

Nonhematologic Events

Nausea and vomiting	48 (16)	1 (<1)	54 (18)	0
Constipation	61 (20)	2 (1)	58 (19)	0
Diarrhea	123 (40)	5 (2)	61 (20)	1 (<1)
Fatigue	145 (47)	15 (5)	122 (40)	6 (2)
Pyrexia	62 (20)	1 (<1)	33 (11)	0
Peripheral edema	20 (7)	0	19 (6)	0
Upper respiratory infection	215 (70)	7 (2)	194 (64)	2 (1)
Pneumonia	35 (11)	11 (4)	14 (5)	5 (2)
Herpes zoster	51 (17)	7 (2)	53 (18)	4 (1)

Nonhematologic Events

Deep-vein thrombosis	14 (5)	7 (2)	6 (2)	3 (1)
Pulmonary embolism	5 (2)	4 (1)	0	0
Ischemic stroke	2 (1)	2 (1)	0	0
Peripheral neuropathy	71 (23)	4 (1)	49 (16)	3 (1)
Rash	61 (20)	10 (3)	51 (17)	6 (2)
Decreased appetite	18 (6)	0	12 (4)	1 (<1)
Dyspnea	20 (6)	1 (<1)	13 (4)	0
Muscle spasms	119 (39)	2 (1)	70 (23)	1 (<1)

Attal M et al. N Engl J Med 2012;366:1782–1791

Reasons for Discontinuing Treatment

Number in Lenalidomide Group Who Discontinued	Event (Disorder)	Number in Placebo Group Who Discontinued
10	Blood disorders	7
13	Gastrointestinal disorders	3
13	General disorders	3
8	Neoplasms	2
11	Nervous system disorders	6
12	Skin/subcutaneous tissue	8
6	Vascular disorders	3
4	Infections	4
17	Other events	17
83 (27.1%)	**All events**	**44 (14.6%)**

(continued)

Toxicity (continued)

	Second Primary Cancers			
	McCarthy et al		Attal et al*	
	Lenalidomide (n = 231)	Placebo (n = 229)	Lenalidomide (n = 306)	Placebo (n = 302)
Second Cancer	Number of Patients		Number of Patients (Percentage)	
Hematologic Cancers[†]				
Acute lymphoblastic leukemia	1	0	3	0
Acute myeloid leukemia	5	0	5[†]	4[‡]
Hodgkin lymphoma	1	0	4	0
Myelodysplastic syndrome	1	0	1	1
Non-Hodgkin lymphoma	0	1	—	—
Total	8	1	13 (4)	5 (2)
Solid Tumor Cancers				
Breast cancer	3	0	2	0
Carcinoid tumor	0	1	—	—
Central nervous system cancer	1	0	—	—
Colorectal cancer	—	—	3	0
Esophageal cancer	—	—	1	0
Gastrointestinal cancer	2	1	—	—
Gynecologic cancer	1	1	—	—
Lung cancer	—	—	0	1
Malignant melanoma	1	2	0	1
Prostate cancer	1	0	2	1
Renal cell carcinoma	—	—	1	1
Sinus cancer	—	—	1	0
Thyroid cancer	1	0	—	—
Total	10	5	10 (3)	4 (1)
Nonmelanoma Skin Cancers				
Basal-cell carcinoma	2	1	5 (2)	3 (1)
Squamous-cell carcinoma	2	2		

*Thirty-two second primary cancers in 26 patients were reported in the lenalidomide group versus 12 second primary cancers in 11 patients in the placebo group. The incidence of second primary cancers was 3.1 per 100 patient-years in the lenalidomide group versus 1.2 per 100 patient-years in the placebo group (P = 0.002). In the multivariate analysis, the incidence of second primary cancers was significantly related to study-group assignment, age, sex, and International Staging System stage
[†]Median time to diagnosis of a hematologic cancer after randomization was 28 months (range, 12–46 months) in patients in the lenalidomide group, and 30 months in the 1 hematologic cancer in the placebo group. The median time to the diagnosis of a solid tumor cancer after randomization was 15 months (range, 3–51 months) in the lenalidomide group and 21 months (range, 6–34 months) in the placebo group
[‡]AML or MDS

Therapy Monitoring

1. Blood counts and physical examinations at regular intervals (1–3 months)
2. Serum and urinary protein electrophoresis studies as indicated at regular intervals (1–3 months)

SUBSEQUENT THERAPY
MULTIPLE MYELOMA REGIMEN: DARATUMUMAB

Chari A et al. Blood 2016;128(22):2142
Lokhorst HM et al. N Engl J Med 2015;373:1207–1219
Protocol for: Lokhorst HM et al. N Engl J Med 2015;373:1207–1219
Supplemental appendix to: Lokhorst HM et al. N Engl J Med 2015;373:1207–1219
DARZALEX (daratumumab) prescribing information. Horsham, PA: Janssen Biotech, Inc; revised February 2019
DARZALEX FASPRO (daratumumab and hyaluronidase-fihj) prescribing information. Horsham, PA: Janssen Biotech, Inc; revised May 2020

May choose to administer either DARZALEX (daratumumab) intravenously, or DARZALEX FASPRO (daratumumab and hyaluronidase-fihj) subcutaneously:

DARZALEX (daratumumab) 16 mg/kg per dose; administer intravenously in 0.9% sodium chloride injection (0.9% NS), or:
Notes:
- The first daratumumab dose may optionally be split over two consecutive days (ie, in cycle 1 administer 8 mg/kg on day 1 and 8 mg/kg on day 2) to facilitate administration
- Refer to the table titled "Dosing Schedule" for schedule information
- Refer to the table titled "Administration Instructions" for instructions regarding daratumumab premedication, infusion rate, dilution, and post-infusion medication

DARZALEX FASPRO (daratumumab and hyaluronidase-fihj) 1800 mg/30,000 units in 15 mL of ready-to-use solution per dose; administer by a health care provider subcutaneously into the abdomen over approximately 3–5 minutes
Notes:
- Refer to the table titled "Dosing Schedule" for schedule information
- Refer to the table titled "Administration Instructions" for instructions regarding premedications, post-administration medications, and administration

DOSING SCHEDULE

Week of Treatment	Frequency	
	DARZALEX (daratumumab)	**DARZALEX FASPRO (daratumumab and hyaluronidase-fihj)**
Weeks 1, 2, 3, 4, 5, 6, 7, 8	16 mg/kg every 7 days for 8 doses (total dosage/week = 16 mg/kg; total dosage/8-week course = 128 mg/kg) *Note:* the first daratumumab dose (ie, week 1 dose) may optionally be split over two consecutive days (ie, 8 mg/kg on day 1 and 8 mg/kg on day 2) to facilitate administration	1800 mg/30,000 units every 7 days for 8 doses (total dosage/week = 1800 mg/30,000 units); total dosage/8-week course = 14,400 mg/240,000 units)
Weeks* 9, 11, 13, 15, 17, 19, 21, 23	16 mg/kg every 14 days for 8 doses (total dose/2-week cycle = 16 mg/kg; total dose/15-week course = 128 mg/kg)	1800 mg/30,000 units every 14 days for 8 doses (total dosage/2-week cycle = 1800 mg/30,000 units); total dosage/15-week course = 14,400 mg/240,000 units)
Week 25† onward	16 mg/kg every 28 days until disease progression (total dose/28-day cycle = 16 mg/kg)	1800 mg/30,000 units every 28 days until disease progression (total dose/28-day cycle = 1800 mg/30,000 units)

*Every-14-day dosing starts on week 9
†Every-28-day dosing starts on week 25

ADMINISTRATION INSTRUCTIONS

Premedications
(applies to DARZALEX [daratumumab] and DARZALEX FASPRO [daratumumab and hyaluronidase-fihj])

Antipyretic	**Acetaminophen** 650–1000 mg; administer orally 1–3 hours before each DARZALEX (daratumumab) or DARZALEX FASPRO (daratumumab and hyaluronidase-fihj) dose
H$_1$-subtype antihistamine	**Diphenhydramine** 25–50 mg; administer orally or intravenously 1–3 hours before each DARZALEX (daratumumab) or DARZALEX FASPRO (daratumumab and hyaluronidase-fihj) dose
Corticosteroid	**Methylprednisolone** 100 mg; administer intravenously 1–3 hours before each DARZALEX (daratumumab) or DARZALEX FASPRO (daratumumab and hyaluronidase-fihj) dose • May reduce methylprednisolone dose to 60 mg; administered orally or intravenously 1–3 hours before each dose, beginning with the third dose • May substitute another intermediate- or long-acting equivalent dose corticosteroid for methylprednisolone

(continued)

(*continued*)

Leukotriene receptor antagonist (*optional*)*	**Montelukast** 10 mg; administer orally 1–3 hours before each DARZALEX (daratumumab) or DARZALEX FASPRO (daratumumab and hyaluronidase-fihj) dose

Dilution volume and infusion rate
(*applies to DARZALEX [daratumumab] only*)

DARZALEX (daratumumab) must be administered through an administration set with a flow regulator and with an in-line, sterile, nonpyrogenic, low-protein-binding, polyethersulfone filter with a pore size of 0.2 or 0.22 μm

First infusion	Dilute in 1000 mL 0.9% NS. Infuse initially at 50 mL/hour. If hypersensitivity or infusion reactions do not occur during the first hour, increase the rate by 50 mL/hour every hour as tolerated to a maximum rate of 200 mL/hour *Note:* if splitting the first daratumumab over two consecutive days (ie, 8 mg/kg on day 1 and 8 mg/kg on day 2), then dilute each 8 mg/kg dose in 500 mL 0.9% NS. Infuse initially at 50 mL/hour. If hypersensitivity or infusion reactions do not occur during the first hour, increase the rate by 50 mL/hour every hour as tolerated to a maximum rate of 200 mL/hour
Second infusion†	Dilute in 500 mL 0.9% NS. Infuse initially at 50 mL/hour. If hypersensitivity or infusion reactions do not occur during the first hour, increase the rate by 50 mL/hour every hour as tolerated to a maximum rate of 200 mL/hour
Subsequent infusions‡	Dilute in 500 mL 0.9% NS. Infuse initially at 100 mL/hour. If hypersensitivity or infusion reactions do not occur during the first hour, increase the rate by 50 mL/hour every hour as tolerated to a maximum rate of 200 mL/hour

Subcutaneous Injection
(*applies to DARZALEX FASPRO [daratumumab and hyaluronidase-fihj] only*)

- Attach the hypodermic injection needle or subcutaneous infusion set to the syringe immediately prior to injection in order to reduce the chances of needle clogging
- Choose a site for administration approximately 3 inches (7.5 cm) to the right or left of the navel; rotate administration sites. Do not inject into areas where the skin is red, bruised, tender, hard, or scarred, or into areas used for administration of other subcutaneous medications
- A health care provider should administer the 15-mL dose subcutaneously into the abdomen over approximately 3–5 minutes
- If the injection causes pain, temporarily interrupt or reduce the rate of injection. If this does not relieve the pain, then choose another injection site on the opposite side of the abdomen in which to deliver the remainder of the dose
- Among low-body-weight (<50 kg) patients, the mean maximum trough concentration after the 8th dose was 81% higher in patients who received the fixed subcutaneous doses of DARZALEX FASPRO (daratumumab and hyaluronidase-fihj) compared with those who received 16 mg/kg per dose of intravenously administered DARZALEX (daratumumab). Higher rates of G3/4 neutropenia were observed in low-body-weight patients who received the formulation for subcutaneous injection

Post-administration medications
(*applies to DARZALEX [daratumumab] and DARZALEX FASPRO [daratumumab and hyaluronidase-fihj]*)

Corticosteroid	**Methylprednisolone 20 mg**; administer orally once daily for 2 days starting on the day after each DARZALEX (daratumumab) or DARZALEX FASPRO (daratumumab and hyaluronidase-fihj) dose is administered • For patients receiving DARZALEX FASPRO (daratumumab and hyaluronidase-fihj), post-administration methylprednisolone may optionally be omitted after the first 3 doses in the absence of a prior major systemic administration-related reaction
Short-acting β–2 agonist§	**Albuterol inhalation aerosol, metered**, 90 μg/actuation, administer 2 inhalations every 4 hours as needed for bronchospasm for 3 days, starting on the day of each of the first 4 DARZALEX (daratumumab) or DARZALEX FASPRO (daratumumab and hyaluronidase-fihj) doses
Long-acting β–2 agonist§	**Salmeterol xinafoate aerosol powder, metered**, 50 μg/actuation, administer 1 inhalation twice a day for 3 days, starting the day of each of the first 4 DARZALEX (daratumumab) or DARZALEX FASPRO (daratumumab and hyaluronidase-fihj) doses
Inhaled corticosteroid§	**Fluticasone propionate inhalation aerosol, metered**, 220 μg/actuation, administer 2 inhalations twice a day for 3 days, starting on the day of each of the first 4 DARZALEX (daratumumab) or DARZALEX FASPRO (daratumumab and hyaluronidase-fihj) doses

*Some institutions consider adding an optional leukotriene receptor antagonist based on data by Chari et al, 2016
†Use a dilution volume of 500 mL only if there were no infusion reactions during the first 3 hours of the first infusion. Otherwise, continue to use a dilution volume of 1000 mL and instructions for the first infusion
‡Use an initial rate of 100 mL/hour for subsequent infusions only if there were no infusion reactions during a final infusion rate of ≥100 mL/hour in the first two infusions. Otherwise, start infusion at 50 mL/hour per instructions for second infusion
§For patients with a history of chronic obstructive pulmonary disease, consider prescribing additional post-infusion inhaled medications for approximately 48 hours following the first 4 daratumumab infusions. Note that availability of inhalational medication formulations may vary by country; representative examples are included in the table
Note: DARZALEX (daratumumab) and DARZALEX FASPRO (daratumumab and hyaluronidase-fihj) can cause severe administration-related reactions. Symptoms of an administration-related reaction may include respiratory symptoms, chills, nausea/vomiting, fever, chest discomfort, hypotension, or pruritus. Only administer the products under medical supervision in a facility with immediate access to medical support and emergency equipment. Closely monitor patients throughout each administration. Most reactions occur during the first dose, when the all-grade systemic administration-related reaction incidence approaches 50% for the intravenous formulation and 10% for the subcutaneous formulation. Reactions may also occur during or following subsequent administrations. Delayed reactions may occur up to 48 hours following each dose; incidence of delayed reactions is reduced when post-infusion corticosteroids are administered. See Treatment Modifications section for management recommendations

(*continued*)

(*continued*)

Supportive Care
Antiemetic prophylaxis
Emetogenic potential is **MINIMAL**
See Chapter 42 for antiemetic recommendations

Hematopoietic growth factor (CSF) prophylaxis
Primary prophylaxis is **NOT** *indicated*
See Chapter 43 for more information

Antimicrobial prophylaxis
Risk of fever and neutropenia is **INTERMEDIATE**
  Antimicrobial primary prophylaxis to be considered:
  • Antibacterial—consider a fluoroquinolone during periods of neutropenia or no prophylaxis; *P. jirovecii* prophylaxis is recommended (eg, cotrimoxazole)
  • Antifungal—recommended; consider use during periods of neutropenia
  • Antiviral—antiherpes antivirals (eg, acyclovir, famciclovir, valacyclovir) should be initiated within 1 week of starting daratumumab or daratumumab and hyaluronidase-fihj, and continued for at least 3 months after completion of the last dose

Bisphosphonates
All patients receiving primary therapy for symptomatic multiple myeloma should receive a bisphosphonate adjunctively.

Treatment Modifications

DARATUMUMAB OR DARATUMUMAB AND HYALURONIDASE-FIHJ

Adverse Event	Dose Modification
Infusion-Related Reaction and Anaphylactic Reaction Adverse Events	
• G1/2 infusion-related reaction to intravenous daratumumab (G1/2 IRR) • First occurrence of G3 infusion-related reaction (G3 IRR) to intravenous daratumumab • Second occurrence of G3 infusion-related reaction to intravenous daratumumab G1 IRR = mild transient reaction; infusion interruption not indicated; intervention not indicated G2 IRR = therapy or infusion interruption indicated but responds promptly to symptomatic treatment (eg, antihistamines, NSAIDS, narcotics, IV fluids); prophylactic medications indicated for ≤24 hours G3 IRR = prolonged (eg, not rapidly responsive to symptomatic medication and/or brief interruption of infusion); recurrence of symptoms following initial improvement; hospitalization indicated for clinical sequelae	Immediately interrupt the daratumumab infusion for infusion-related reactions of *any* severity and manage symptoms as clinically appropriate with additional intravenous corticosteroid (50–150 mg hydrocortisone IVP), an H_1-receptor antagonist (diphenhydramine 50 mg IVP), inhaled short-acting ß–2 agonist (albuterol 2 puffs, may repeat in 4 hours), plus epinephrine 0.5 mg IM for hypotension or airway obstructive symptoms. Upon resolution of symptoms, resume the daratumumab infusion at no more than 50% of the rate at which the reaction occurred. If tolerated, escalate the infusion by 50 mL/hour every hour up to a maximum rate of 200 mL/hour. *Note:* dose reductions are not recommended for daratumumab
• Third occurrence of G3 infusion-related reaction (IRR) to intravenous daratumumab • G4 infusion-related reaction (G4 IRR) to intravenous daratumumab or subcutaneous daratumumab and hyaluronidase-fihj • Anaphylactic reaction (AR) to intravenous daratumumab or subcutaneous daratumumab and hyaluronidase-fihj G3 IRR = prolonged (eg, not rapidly responsive to symptomatic medication and/or brief interruption of infusion); recurrence of symptoms following initial improvement; hospitalization indicated for clinical sequelae G4 IRR = life-threatening consequences; urgent intervention indicated G3 AR = symptomatic bronchospasm, with or without urticaria; parenteral intervention indicated; allergy-related edema/angioedema; hypotension G4 AR = Life-threatening consequences; urgent intervention indicated	Immediately interrupt the administration for infusion-related reactions of *any* severity and manage symptoms as clinically appropriate with additional intravenous corticosteroid (50–150 mg hydrocortisone IVP), an H_1-receptor antagonist (diphenhydramine 50 mg IVP), inhaled short-acting ß–2 agonist (albuterol 2 puffs, may repeat in 4 hours), plus epinephrine 0.5 mg IM for hypotension or airway obstructive symptoms Permanently discontinue

(*continued*)

Treatment Modifications (*continued*)

Hematologic Adverse Events

G3/4 neutropenia G3/4 thrombocytopenia	Consider delaying the dose until recovery to G ≤2 or baseline; or, continue without interruption as clinically appropriate. In the case of neutropenia, consider administration of granulocyte-colony stimulating factor (G-CSF)
Blood transfusion within 6 months following a daratumumab infusion	Notify blood bank the patient has received daratumumab or daratumumab and hyaluronidase-fihj within the past 6 months since either product may result in a positive indirect antiglobulin test (indirect Coombs test) that can persist for up to 6 months and may mask detection of antibodies to minor antigens in the patient's serum. Determination of ABO and Rh blood type is not affected

Note: dose reductions are not recommended for daratumumab or daratumumab and hyaluronidase-fihj
IRR, infusion-related reactions; AR, anaphylactic reactions

Patient Population Studied

The multicenter, open-label, dose-escalation/dose-expansion, phase 1/2 study involved 104 patients with relapsed or refractory myeloma requiring systemic therapy (32 patients enrolled in the phase 1 part of the study and 72 patients enrolled in the phase 2 part of the study). In the phase 1 part of the study, 32 patients were divided into 10 cohorts and received daratumumab at doses of 0.0005 to 24 mg/kg body weight. In the phase 2 part of the study, 30 patients received daratumumab 8 mg/kg in eight once-weekly infusions followed by twice-monthly infusions for 16 weeks and then monthly infusions until disease progression or unmanageable toxic events. An additional 42 patients received an infusion of daratumumab 16 mg/kg followed by a 3-week washout period and then seven once-weekly infusions followed by twice-monthly infusions for 14 weeks and then monthly infusions until disease progression or unmanageable toxic events

Efficacy (n = 72)

	Daratumumab 8 mg/kg (n = 30)	Daratumumab 16 mg/kg (n = 42)
Objective response rate*	10%	36%
Proportion who experienced ≥50% reduction in level of M protein or free light chains	15%	46%
Median progression-free survival	2.4 months	5.6 months
Overall survival at 12 months	77%	77%

*Objective response rate was the proportion of patients who experienced a partial or complete response according to the International Myeloma Working Group Uniform Response Criteria
Note: median follow-up time was 16.9 months in the patients that received daratumumab 8mg/kg and 10.2 months in the cohort that received daratumumab 16 mg/kg. All 30 patients who received daratumumab 8 mg/kg discontinued treatment owing to disease progression. Of the 42 patients who received daratumumab 16 mg/kg, 28 discontinued treatment during the study; 23 owing to disease progression, 4 due to physician decision and 1 because of an adverse event (Grade 5 pneumonia not considered to be related to study treatment)

Adverse Events (n = 72)

Grade (%)*	Daratumumab 8 mg/kg (n = 30)		Daratumumab 16 mg/kg (n = 42)	
	Grade 1–2	Grade 3–4	Grade 1–2	Grade 3–4
Fatigue	40	3	40	0
Allergic rhinitis	40	0	24	0
Pyrexia	43	0	14	2
Diarrhea	30	0	14	0
Upper respiratory tract infection	27	0	17	0
Dyspnea	27	0	14	0

*According to the National Cancer Institute Common Terminology Criteria for Adverse Events, version 4.03
Note: adverse events that occurred in ≥25% of patients in either cohort are included in the table. Grade 3 or 4 adverse events occurred in 53% of patients in the daratumumab 8 mg/kg cohort and 26% of patients in the daratumumab 16 mg/kg cohort (the most frequent Grade 3 or 4 adverse events were pneumonia and thrombocytopenia). Serious adverse events occurred in 40% of patients in the daratumumab 8 mg/kg cohort and 33% of patients in the daratumumab 16 mg/kg cohort (the most frequent serious adverse events were related to infection). No treatment-related deaths occurred

Therapy Monitoring

1. Type and screen prior to first dose
2. CBC with differential prior to each dose
3. Monitor for infusion-related reaction symptoms frequently during infusion; check vital signs frequently during infusion and at least prior to each scheduled rate increase, and ensure medications are available for post-infusion prophylaxis as applicable

Note: daratumumab, a human IgG1 kappa monoclonal antibody, may be detected by serum protein electrophoresis and immunofixation assays routinely used to monitor endogenous M-protein. Thus, daratumumab may interfere with disease monitoring in patients with plasma cell neoplasms that produce an IgG kappa M-protein

SUBSEQUENT THERAPY

MULTIPLE MYELOMA REGIMEN: DARATUMUMAB + LENALIDOMIDE + LOW-DOSE DEXAMETHASONE

Chari A et al. Blood 2016;128(22):2142
Dimopoulos MA et al. N Engl J Med 2016;375:1319–1331
DARZALEX (daratumumab) prescribing information. Horsham, PA: Janssen Biotech, Inc; revised September 2019
DARZALEX FASPRO (daratumumab and hyaluronidase-fihj) prescribing information. Horsham, PA: Janssen Biotech, Inc; revised May 2020

All cycles (28-day cycles):

   Lenalidomide 25 mg/dose; administer orally, without regard to meals, once daily for 21 consecutive days on days 1–21, followed by 7 days without treatment, every 28 days, until disease progression (total dosage/28-day cycle = 525 mg)
   • Patients who delay taking a lenalidomide dose at a regularly scheduled time may take the missed dose if the time to the next regularly scheduled dose is >12 hours away
   • Consider doses in Treatment Modifications table for dose adjustments for renal function

   Dexamethasone 40 mg/dose; administer orally or intravenously for 4 doses on days 1, 8, 15, and 22, every 28 days, until disease progression (total dosage/28-day cycle = 160 mg)
   • During weeks when daratumumab is administered, the dexamethasone dose should instead be split into two equally divided doses (ie, 20 mg/dose), with the first 20-mg dose administered either orally or intravenously 1–3 hours prior to daratumumab on the day of daratumumab infusion (pre-infusion medication) and the second 20-mg dose given on the day after the daratumumab infusion (post-infusion medication)
   • The dose of dexamethasone may be reduced to 20 mg/dose for patients who were older than 75 years of age or whose body mass index was less than 18.5 kg/m² at the discretion of the medically responsible health care provider. In this case, during weeks when daratumumab is administered, the entire 20-mg dose of dexamethasone should be administered either orally or intravenously 1–3 hours prior to daratumumab on the day of daratumumab infusion (pre-infusion medication) and the patient should be prescribed low-dose oral methylprednisolone 20 mg (or equivalent) to be taken as a post-infusion medication on the day following the daratumumab infusion (post-infusion medication)

Cycles 1–2 (28-day cycles):
May choose to administer either DARZALEX (daratumumab) intravenously, or DARZALEX FASPRO (daratumumab and hyaluronidase-fihj) subcutaneously:

DARZALEX (daratumumab) 16 mg/kg per dose; administer intravenously for 4 doses on days 1, 8, 15, and 22, every 28 days, for 2 cycles (cycles 1–2) (total dosage/28-day cycle during cycles 1–2 = 64 mg/kg), or:

Notes:
• The first daratumumab dose may optionally be split over two consecutive days (ie, in cycle 1 administer 8 mg/kg on day 1 and 8 mg/kg on day 2) to facilitate administration
• Refer to the table titled "Administration Instructions" for instructions regarding daratumumab premedication, infusion rate, dilution, and post-infusion medication

DARZALEX FASPRO *(daratumumab and hyaluronidase-fihj)* 1800 mg/30,000 units in 15 mL of ready-to-use solution per dose; administer by a health care provider subcutaneously into the abdomen over approximately 3–5 minutes for 4 doses on days 1, 8, 15, and 22, every 28 days, for 2 cycles (cycles 1–2) (total dosage/28-day cycle during cycles 1–2 = 7200 mg/120,000 units)
Note: refer to the table titled "Administration Instructions" for instructions regarding premedications, post-administration medications, and administration

Cycles 3–6 (28-day cycles):
May choose to administer either DARZALEX (daratumumab) intravenously, or DARZALEX FASPRO (daratumumab and hyaluronidase-fihj) subcutaneously:

DARZALEX (daratumumab) 16 mg/kg per dose; administer intravenously for 2 doses on days 1 and 15, every 28 days, for 4 cycles (cycles 3–6) (total dosage/28-day cycle during cycles 3–6 = 32 mg/kg), or:
Note: refer to the table titled "Administration Instructions" for instructions regarding daratumumab premedication, infusion rate, dilution, and post-infusion medication

DARZALEX FASPRO *(daratumumab and hyaluronidase-fihj)* 1800 mg/30,000 units in 15 mL of ready-to-use solution per dose; administer by a health care provider subcutaneously into the abdomen over approximately 3–5 minutes for 2 doses on days 1 and 15, every 28 days, for 4 cycles (cycles 3–6) (total dosage/28-day cycle during cycles 3–6 = 3600 mg/60,000 units)
Note: refer to the table titled "Administration Instructions" for instructions regarding premedications, post-administration medications, and administration

Cycle 7 and beyond (28-day cycles):
May choose to administer either DARZALEX (daratumumab) intravenously, or DARZALEX FASPRO (daratumumab and hyaluronidase-fihj) subcutaneously:

DARZALEX (daratumumab) 16 mg/kg per dose; administer intravenously for 1 dose on day 1, every 28 days, until disease progression (cycle 7 and beyond) (total dosage/28-day cycle during cycle 7 and beyond = 16 mg/kg), or:
Note: refer to the table titled "Administration Instructions" for instructions regarding daratumumab premedication, infusion rate, dilution, and post-infusion medication

(continued)

(continued)

DARZALEX FASPRO *(daratumumab and hyaluronidase-fihj)* 1800 mg/30,000 units in 15 mL of ready-to-use solution per dose; administer by a health care provider subcutaneously into the abdomen over approximately 3–5 minutes for 1 dose on day 1, every 28 days, until disease progression (cycle 7 and beyond) (total dosage/28-day cycle during cycle 7 and beyond = 1800 mg/30,000 units)

Note: refer to the table titled "Administration Instructions" for instructions regarding premedications, post-administration medications, and administration

ADMINISTRATION INSTRUCTIONS

Premedications
(applies to DARZALEX (daratumumab) and DARZALEX FASPRO (daratumumab and hyaluronidase-fihj))

Antipyretic	**Acetaminophen** 650–1000 mg; administer orally 1–3 hours before each DARZALEX (daratumumab) or DARZALEX FASPRO (daratumumab and hyaluronidase-fihj) dose
H$_1$-subtype antihistamine	**Diphenhydramine** 25–50 mg; administer orally or intravenously 1–3 hours before each DARZALEX (daratumumab) or DARZALEX FASPRO (daratumumab and hyaluronidase-fihj) dose
Corticosteroid	**Dexamethasone** (age ≤75 years and BMI ≥18.5 kg/m², 40 mg; age >75 years or BMI <18.5 kg/m², 20 mg); administer intravenously or orally 1–3 hours before each DARZALEX (daratumumab) or DARZALEX FASPRO (daratumumab and hyaluronidase-fihj) dose • May administer dexamethasone orally beginning with the second dose
Leukotriene receptor antagonist *(optional)**	**Montelukast** 10 mg; administer orally 1–3 hours before each DARZALEX (daratumumab) or DARZALEX FASPRO (daratumumab and hyaluronidase-fihj) dose

Dilution volume and infusion rate
(applies to DARZALEX [daratumumab] only)

DARZALEX (daratumumab) must be administered through an administration set with a flow regulator and with an in-line, sterile, nonpyrogenic, low-protein-binding, polyethersulfone filter with a pore size of 0.2 or 0.22 μm

First infusion	Dilute in 1000 mL 0.9% NS. Infuse initially at 50 mL/hour. If hypersensitivity or infusion reactions do not occur during the first hour, increase the rate by 50 mL/hour every hour as tolerated to a maximum rate of 200 mL/hour *Note:* if splitting the first daratumumab over 2 consecutive days (ie, 8 mg/kg on day 1 and 8 mg/kg on day 2), then dilute each 8 mg/kg dose in 500 mL 0.9% NS. Infuse initially at 50 mL/hour. If hypersensitivity or infusion reactions do not occur during the first hour, increase the rate by 50 mL/hour every hour as tolerated to a maximum rate of 200 mL/hour
Second infusion†	Dilute in 500 mL 0.9% NS. Infuse initially at 50 mL/hour. If hypersensitivity or infusion reactions do not occur during the first hour, increase the rate by 50 mL/hour every hour as tolerated to a maximum rate of 200 mL/hour
Subsequent infusions‡	Dilute in 500 mL 0.9% NS. Infuse initially at 100 mL/hour. If hypersensitivity or infusion reactions do not occur during the first hour, increase the rate by 50 mL/hour every hour as tolerated to a maximum rate of 200 mL/hour

Subcutaneous Injection
(applies to DARZALEX FASPRO [daratumumab and hyaluronidase-fihj] only)

• Attach the hypodermic injection needle or subcutaneous infusion set to the syringe immediately prior to injection in order to reduce the chances of needle clogging
• Choose a site for administration approximately 3 inches (7.5 cm) to the right or left of the navel; rotate administration sites. Do not inject into areas where the skin is red, bruised, tender, hard, or scarred, or into areas used for administration of other subcutaneous medications
• A health care provider should administer the 15-mL dose subcutaneously into the abdomen over approximately 3–5 minutes
• If the injection causes pain, temporarily interrupt or reduce the rate of injection. If this does not relieve the pain, then choose another injection site on the opposite side of the abdomen in which to deliver the remainder of the dose
• Among low-body-weight (<50 kg) patients, the mean maximum trough concentration after the 8th dose was 81% higher in patients who received the fixed subcutaneous doses of DARZALEX FASPRO (daratumumab and hyaluronidase-fihj) compared with those who received 16 mg/kg per dose of intravenously administered DARZALEX (daratumumab). Higher rates of G3/4 neutropenia were observed in low-body-weight patients who received the formulation for subcutaneous injection

Post-administration medications
(applies to DARZALEX [daratumumab] and DARZALEX FASPRO [daratumumab and hyaluronidase-fihj])

Corticosteroid *(optional)*	**Dexamethasone** 20 mg; administer orally once on the day after each DARZALEX (daratumumab) or DARZALEX FASPRO (daratumumab and hyaluronidase-fihj) dose is administered • As described above, for patients receiving a reduced dose of dexamethasone, methylprednisolone 20 mg (or equivalent) may instead be administered orally for 1 dose on the day following each dose

(continued)

(*continued*)

Short-acting β-2 agonist§	**Albuterol inhalation aerosol, metered**, 90 μg/actuation, administer 2 inhalations every 4 hours as needed for bronchospasm for 3 days, starting on the day of each of the first 4 DARZALEX (daratumumab) or DARZALEX FASPRO (daratumumab and hyaluronidase-fihj) doses
Long-acting β-2 agonist§	**Salmeterol xinafoate aerosol powder, metered**, 50 μg/actuation, administer 1 inhalation twice a day for 3 days, starting the day of each of the first 4 DARZALEX (daratumumab) or DARZALEX FASPRO (daratumumab and hyaluronidase-fihj) doses
Inhaled corticosteroid§	**Fluticasone propionate inhalation aerosol, metered**, 220 μg/actuation, administer 2 inhalations twice a day for 3 days, starting on the day of each of the first 4 DARZALEX (daratumumab) or DARZALEX FASPRO (daratumumab and hyaluronidase-fihj) doses

*Some institutions consider adding an optional leukotriene receptor antagonist based on data by Chari et al, 2016
†Use a dilution volume of 500 mL only if there were no infusion reactions during the first 3 hours of the first infusion. Otherwise, continue to use a dilution volume of 1000 mL and instructions for the first infusion
‡Use an initial rate of 100 mL/hour for subsequent infusions only if there were no infusion reactions during a final infusion rate of ≥100 mL/hour in the first two infusions. Otherwise, start infusion at 50 mL/hour per instructions for second infusion
§For patients with a history of chronic obstructive pulmonary disease, consider prescribing additional post-infusion inhaled medications for approximately 48 hours following the first 4 daratumumab infusions. Note that availability of inhalational medication formulations may vary by country; representative examples are included in the table
Note: DARZALEX (daratumumab) and DARZALEX FASPRO (daratumumab and hyaluronidase-fihj) can cause severe administration-related reactions. Symptoms of an administration-related reaction may include respiratory symptoms, chills, nausea/vomiting, fever, chest discomfort, hypotension, or pruritus. Only administer the products under medical supervision in a facility with immediate access to medical support and emergency equipment. Closely monitor patients throughout each administration. Most reactions occur during the first dose, when the all-grade systemic administration-related reaction incidence approaches 50% for the intravenous formulation and 10% for the subcutaneous formulation. Reactions may also occur during or following subsequent administrations. Delayed reactions may occur up to 48 hours following each dose; incidence of delayed reactions is reduced when post-infusion corticosteroids are administered. See Treatment Modifications section for management recommendations

Supportive Care

Antiemetic prophylaxis
Emetogenic potential on days with lenalidomide is **LOW**
Emetogenic potential on days when daratumumab is administered without lenalidomide is **MINIMAL**
See Chapter 42 for antiemetic recommendations

Hematopoietic growth factor (CSF) prophylaxis
Primary prophylaxis is **NOT** indicated
See Chapter 43 for more information

Antimicrobial prophylaxis
Risk of fever and neutropenia is **INTERMEDIATE**
Antimicrobial primary prophylaxis to be considered:
- Antibacterial—consider a fluoroquinolone during periods of neutropenia or no prophylaxis; *P. jirovecii* prophylaxis is recommended (eg, cotrimoxazole)
- Antifungal—recommended; consider use during periods of neutropenia
- Antiviral—antiherpes antivirals (eg, acyclovir, famciclovir, valacyclovir) should be initiated within 1 week of starting DARZALEX (daratumumab) or DARZALEX FASPRO (daratumumab and hyaluronidase-fihj), and continued for at least 3 months after completion of the last dose

Bisphosphonates
All patients receiving primary therapy for symptomatic multiple myeloma should receive a bisphosphonate adjunctively.

Thromboprophylaxis
Risk assessment and recommendations for VTE prophylaxis in patients with multiple myeloma with individual or myeloma-related risk factors, or risk factors related to treatment

(*continued*)

(*continued*)

Individual risk factors • Obesity (BMI ≥30 kg/m²) • H/O VTE • CVC or pacemaker • Comorbid pathologies 　▪ Cardiac disease 　▪ Chronic renal disease 　▪ Diabetes 　▪ Acute infection 　▪ Immobilization • Surgery 　▪ General surgery 　▪ Any anesthesia 　▪ Trauma • Medications 　▪ Erythropoietin (epoetin alfa, darbepoetin) 　▪ Estrogenic compounds 　▪ Bevacizumab • Clotting disorders 　▪ Thrombophilia **Myeloma-related risk factors** • Diagnosis of multiple myeloma • Hyperviscosity	≤1 Individual or myeloma-related risk factor present: • **Aspirin** 81–325 mg daily ≥2 Individual or myeloma-related risk factors present: • **LMWH,*** equivalent to enoxaparin sodium 40 mg/day *or* **dalteparin sodium** 5000 IU/day; administer subcutaneously, *or* • **Warfarin**, targeting an INR = 2–3
Concomitant treatment-related risk factors Thalidomide or lenalidomide in combination with: • High-dose dexamethasone (≥480 mg/month) • Doxorubicin • Multiagent chemotherapy	• **LMWH,*** equivalent to enoxaparin sodium 40 mg/day *or* **dalteparin sodium** 5000 IU/day; administer subcutaneously, *or* • **Warfarin**, targeting an INR = 2–3

*LMWHs should be used with caution in individuals with impaired renal function (creatinine clearance <30 mL/min). Refer to product labeling for information about doses and administration schedules in renally impaired patients, and guidance for monitoring anti-Factor Xa concentrations

Abbreviations: CVC, central venous catheter; INR, international normalized ratio; LMWH, low-molecular-weight heparin; VTE, venous thromboembolic disease

References: Geerts WH et al. Chest 2008;133(6 Suppl):381S–453S
National Comprehensive Cancer Network. Multiple Myeloma, V.1.2014. (Accessed October 8, 2013, at http://www.nccn.org)
National Comprehensive Cancer Network. Venous Thromboembolic Disease, V.2.2013. (Accessed October 8, 2013, at http://www.nccn.org)
Palumbo A et al. Leukemia 2008;22:414–423

Treatment Modifications

DARATUMUMAB OR DARATUMUMAB AND HYALURONIDASE-FIHJ

Adverse Event	Dose Modification
Infusion-Related Reaction and Anaphylactic Reaction Adverse Events	
• G1/2 infusion-related reaction to intravenous daratumumab (G1/2 IRR) • First occurrence of G3 infusion-related reaction (G3 IRR) to intravenous daratumumab • Second occurrence of G3 infusion-related reaction to intravenous daratumumab	Immediately interrupt the daratumumab infusion for infusion-related reactions of *any* severity and manage symptoms as clinically appropriate with additional intravenous corticosteroid (50–150 mg hydrocortisone IVP), an H₁-receptor antagonist (diphenhydramine 50 mg IVP), inhaled short-acting ß-2 agonist (albuterol 2 puffs, may repeat in 4 hours) plus epinephrine 0.5 mg IM for hypotension or airway obstructive symptoms
G1 IRR = mild transient reaction; infusion interruption not indicated; intervention not indicated G2 IRR = therapy or infusion interruption indicated but responds promptly to symptomatic treatment (eg, antihistamines, NSAIDS, narcotics, IV fluids); prophylactic medications indicated for ≤24 hours G3 IRR = prolonged (eg, not rapidly responsive to symptomatic medication and/or brief interruption of infusion); recurrence of symptoms following initial improvement; hospitalization indicated for clinical sequelae	Upon resolution of symptoms, resume the daratumumab infusion at no more than 50% of the rate at which the reaction occurred. If tolerated, escalate the infusion by 50 mL/hour every hour up to a maximum rate of 200 mL/hour

(*continued*)

Treatment Modifications (continued)

Adverse Event	Dose Modification
Infusion-Related Reaction and Anaphylactic Reaction Adverse Events	
• Third occurrence of G3 infusion-related reaction (IRR) to intravenous daratumumab • G4 infusion-related reaction (G4 IRR) to intravenous daratumumab or subcutaneous daratumumab and hyaluronidase-fihj • Anaphylactic reaction (AR) to intravenous daratumumab or subcutaneous daratumumab and hyaluronidase-fihj	Immediately interrupt administration for infusion-related reactions of *any* severity and manage symptoms as clinically appropriate with additional intravenous corticosteroid (50–150 mg hydrocortisone IVP), an H_1-receptor antagonist (diphenhydramine 50 mg IVP), inhaled short-acting ß-2 agonist (albuterol 2 puffs, may repeat in 4 hours) plus epinephrine 0.5 mg IM for hypotension or airway obstructive symptoms
G3 IRR = prolonged (eg, not rapidly responsive to symptomatic medication and/or brief interruption of infusion); recurrence of symptoms following initial improvement; hospitalization indicated for clinical sequelae G4 IRR = life-threatening consequences; urgent intervention indicated G3 AR = symptomatic bronchospasm, with or without urticaria; parenteral intervention indicated; allergy-related edema/angioedema; hypotension G4 AR = life-threatening consequences; urgent intervention indicated	Permanently discontinue[†]
Hematologic Adverse Events	
G3/4 neutropenia G3/4 thrombocytopenia	Consider delaying the dose until recovery to G ≤2 or baseline; or, continue without interruption as clinically appropriate. In the case of neutropenia, consider administration of granulocyte-colony stimulating factor (G-CSF)
Blood transfusion within 6 months following a daratumumab infusion	Notify blood bank the patient has received daratumumab or daratumumab and hyaluronidase-fihj within the past 6 months since either product may result in a positive indirect antiglobulin test (indirect Coombs test) that can persist for up to 6 months and may mask detection of antibodies to minor antigens in the patient's serum. Determination of ABO and Rh blood type is not affected

Note: dose reductions are not recommended for daratumumab or daratumumab and hyaluronidase-fihj

---

LENALIDOMIDE

Lenalidomide dose levels (Days 1–21 of each 28-day cycle)

	CrCl ≥60 mL/min	CrCl ≥30 mL/min and <60 mL/min	CrCl <30 mL/min (not on hemodialysis)	ESRD on hemodialysis
Starting dose	25 mg each day	10 mg each day	15 mg every other day	5 mg each day (after dialysis on dialysis days)
Dose level −1	15 mg each day	5 mg each day	10 mg every other day	2.5 mg each day (after dialysis on dialysis days)
Dose level −2	10 mg each day	2.5 mg each day	5 mg every other day	Discontinue[†]
Dose level −3	5 mg each day	Discontinue[†]	Discontinue[†]	
Dose level −4	Discontinue[†]			

Adverse Event	Treatment Modification
Hematologic Toxicity	
Day 1 ANC <1000/mm³ or platelet count <50,000/mm³	Delay the next cycle until ANC ≥1000/mm³ and platelet count ≥50,000/mm³. Consider treatment with filgrastim and/or platelet transfusion according to local guidelines. If the start of a new cycle is delayed >14 days for lenalidomide-related toxicity, then reduce the lenalidomide by one dose level
G ≥3 neutropenia (ANC <1000/mm³) during a cycle	Interrupt lenalidomide treatment and follow weekly CBC. When ANC ≥1000/mm³ and there are no other toxicities, resume lenalidomide treatment at same dose. If other toxicities are still present, then resume lenalidomide with dose reduced one dose level

(continued)

Treatment Modifications (*continued*)

Adverse Event	Treatment Modification
Hematologic Toxicity	
Recurrent G ≥3 neutropenia (ANC <1000/mm³) during a cycle	Interrupt lenalidomide treatment and follow weekly CBC. When ANC ≥1000/mm³, resume with dose reduced one dose level
Febrile neutropenia (ANC <1000/mm³ with fever ≥38.3°C)	Hold lenalidomide dosing for up to 21 days to resolve toxicity and then restart at the same dose or reduce the lenalidomide dose by one dose level
Platelet count <30,000/mm³	Interrupt lenalidomide treatment and follow weekly CBC. When platelet count ≥30,000/mm³, resume lenalidomide with dose reduced one dose level
Recurrent platelet count <30,000/mm³	
Nonhematologic Toxicity	
G3/4 hepatotoxicity (ALT/AST >5× ULN and/or bilirubin >3× ULN)	Withhold lenalidomide for remainder of the cycle. Delay initiation of next cycle until hepatotoxicity resolves to G ≤2 (ALT/AST ≤5× ULN and/or bilirubin ≤3× ULN), then resume lenalidomide at one lower dose level
G3 rash	Hold dose for remainder of cycle. Decrease by one dose level when dosing resumed at next cycle (rash must resolve to G≤1)
Allergic reactions, including hypersensitivity, angioedema, Stevens-Johnson syndrome, toxic epidermal necrolysis (TEN), and drug reaction with eosinophilia and systemic symptoms (DRESS)	Discontinue lenalidomide if reactions are suspected. Do not resume lenalidomide if these reactions are confirmed
Tumor lysis syndrome (TLS)	Monitor patients at risk of TLS (ie, those with high tumor burden) and take appropriate precautions including aggressive hydration and allopurinol
G3 peripheral neuropathy	If neuropathy is considered to be attributable to lenalidomide, then withhold lenalidomide for the remainder of the cycle. Delay initiation of the next cycle until neuropathy resolves to G ≤1, then resume lenalidomide at one lower dose level
G4 peripheral neuropathy	If neuropathy is considered to be attributable to lenalidomide, then discontinue lenalidomide[†]
G3/4 venous thromboembolism (VTE) during aspirin monotherapy or inadequate anticoagulation	Continue lenalidomide at the current dose and initiate adequate anticoagulation
G3/4 venous thromboembolism (VTE) during adequate anticoagulation (eg, prophylactic or therapeutic doses of LMWH, UFH, or warfarin)	Discontinue lenalidomide[†]
G ≥2 hypothyroidism or G ≥2 hyperthyroidism	Continue lenalidomide at current dose and initiate appropriate medical treatment
Other G ≥3 lenalidomide-related toxicities	Withhold lenalidomide for the remainder of the cycle. Delay initiation of the next cycle until toxicity resolves to G ≤2, then resume lenalidomide at one lower dose level

	DEXAMETHASONE	
	Age ≤75 years, body mass index ≥18.5 kg/m², and no prior steroid intolerance	Age >75 years of age, body mass index <18.5 kg/m², or with prior steroid intolerance
Starting dose	40 mg/dose/day on days 1, 8, 15, and 22 every 28 days	20 mg/dose/day on days 1, 8, 15, and 22 every 28 days*
Dose Level −1	20 mg/dose/day on days 1, 8, 15, and 22 every 28 days*	10 mg/dose/day on days 1, 8, 15, and 22 every 28 days*
Dose Level −2	Discontinue dexamethasone doses on days when daratumumab is not administered*	Discontinue dexamethasone doses on days when daratumumab is not administered*

*Note: the 20-mg dose of dexamethasone given 1–3 hours before the infusion on the day of daratumumab infusions must not be reduced or omitted. For patients on a reduced dexamethasone dose, the entire 20-mg dose may be given as a daratumumab pre-infusion medication

(*continued*)

Treatment Modifications (continued)

Adverse Event	Treatment Modification
G1/2 dyspepsia (moderate symptoms; medical intervention indicated; limiting instrumental ADL), gastric or duodenal ulcer, or gastritis	Continue dexamethasone at the same dose. Treat with therapeutic doses of an H_2-receptor antagonist or proton pump inhibitor. If symptoms persist, then reduce the dexamethasone dose by one level
G ≥3 dyspepsia, gastric or duodenal ulcer, or gastritis (surgery or hospitalization indicated)	Withhold dexamethasone until symptoms return to baseline. Resume dexamethasone reduced by one dose level along with concurrent treatment with therapeutic doses of an H_2-receptor antagonist or proton pump inhibitor. If symptoms recur, then reduce dexamethasone to dose level −2
Acute pancreatitis	Reduce dexamethasone to dose level −2
G ≥3 edema	Withhold dexamethasone until symptoms return to baseline. Consider treatment with diuretics. Resume dexamethasone reduced by one dose level. If edema persists, reduce to dose level −2
G ≥2 mood alteration (moderate mood alteration) or confusion (moderate disorientation; limiting instrumental ADL)	Withhold dexamethasone until symptoms return to baseline. Resume dexamethasone reduced by one dose level. If symptoms persist, reduce by another dose level
G ≥2 muscle weakness (symptomatic; evident on physical exam; limiting instrumental ADL)	Withhold dexamethasone until symptoms return to baseline. Resume dexamethasone reduced by one dose level. If weakness persists, reduce by another dose level
G ≥3 hyperglycemia (insulin therapy initiated; hospitalization indicated)	Withhold dexamethasone until blood glucose is ≤250 mg/dL. Treat with insulin or other hypoglycemic agents as clinically appropriate and then resume dexamethasone at the same dose. If hyperglycemia is uncontrolled despite above measures, decrease dexamethasone by one dose level
Other G ≥2 nonhematologic toxicity attributable to dexamethasone including severe irritability, insomnia, or oral candidiasis	Withhold dexamethasone until toxicity resolves to G ≤1, then resume at a lower dose. Consider reduction by one dose level for G2/G3 toxicity, and two dose levels for G4 or recurrent G3 toxicity

[†]If daratumumab and lenalidomide are permanently discontinued, then also consider discontinuing dexamethasone
IRR, infusion-related reactions; AR, anaphylactic reactions

Patient Population Studied

The multicenter, randomized, open-label, phase 3 study involved 569 patients with relapsed or refractory symptomatic multiple myeloma. Patients with lenalidomide-refractory disease or had discontinued lenalidomide previously owing to adverse events were not eligible. All patients received oral lenalidomide on days 1 to 21 of a 28-day cycle and dexamethasone 40 mg weekly (although this dose could be reduced to 20 mg weekly at the physician's discretion for patients aged >75 years or who had a body mass index of <18.5). Patients randomly assigned to daratumumab also received intravenous daratumumab 16 mg/kg on days 1, 8, 15, and 22 of the first two cycles, days 1 and 15 of the next four cycles, and then once every 4 weeks thereafter, and their dexamethasone was divided into a 20-mg dose before daratumumab infusion (as prophylaxis for infusion-related reactions) and a 20-mg dose the following day. Cycles were continued until disease progression, unacceptable toxic events, withdrawal of consent, or death

Efficacy (n = 569)

	Daratumumab Group (n = 286)	Control Group (n = 283)	
Kaplan-Meier progression-free survival at 12 months*	83.2%	60.1%	
Disease progression or death	18.5%	41.0%	HR 0.37 (95% CI 0.27–0.52; P <0.001)
Overall response rate[†]	92.9%	76.4%	P <0.001
Proportion who experienced at least a very good partial response	75.8%	44.2%	P <0.001
Proportion who experienced at least a complete response	43.1%	19.2%	P <0.001
Proportion who had below the threshold[‡] for minimal residual disease	22.4%	4.6%	P <0.001
Overall survival at 12 months	92.1%	86.8%	

*Progression and response were determined according to the International Myeloma Working Group criteria
[†]Overall response rate was the proportion of patients who experienced at least a partial response
[‡]At a threshold of 1 tumor cell per 10^5 white cells
Note: median follow-up time was 13.5 months

Adverse Events (n = 564)

	Daratumumab Group (n = 283)		Control Group (n = 281)	
	Grade 1–2 (%)	Grade 3–4 (%)	Grade 1–2 (%)	Grade 3–4 (%)
Neutropenia	7	52	6	37
Diarrhea	37	5	21	3
Fatigue	29	6	25	2
Upper respiratory tract infection	31	1	20	1
Anemia	19	12	15	20
Constipation	28	1	25	<1
Cough	29	0	12	0
Thrombocytopenia	14	13	14	14
Muscle spasms	25	<1	17	2
Nasopharyngitis	24	0	15	0
Nausea	23	1	14	0
Pyrexia	18	2	10	1
Insomnia	19	<1	19	<1
Dyspnea	15	3	11	<1
Back pain	16	1	16	1
Vomiting	16	1	5	<1
Asthenia	13	3	10	2
Peripheral edema	14	<1	12	1
Pneumonia	6	8	4	8
Febrile neutropenia	0	6	0	2
Lymphopenia	<1	5	2	4

Note: adverse events that occurred in >15% of patients in either cohort are included in the table. Grade 3–4 adverse events that occurred in >5% of patients in either cohort are additionally listed. In total, 6.7% of patients in the daratumumab group and 7.8% of controls discontinued treatment owing to adverse events, and 3.9% of patients in the daratumumab group and 5.3% of controls died owing to adverse events (the most common causes were acute kidney disease, septic shock, and pneumonia)

Therapy Monitoring

1. Type and screen prior to first dose of daratumumab or daratumumab and hyaluronidase-fihj
2. CBC with differential, liver function tests, serum creatinine, and serum glucose prior to each cycle
3. CBC with differential, liver function tests, and serum glucose prior to each daratumumab infusion
4. Monitor for infusion-related daratumumab reaction symptoms frequently during infusion; check vital signs frequently during infusion and at least prior to each schedule rate increase, ensure medications are available for post-infusion prophylaxis as applicable

Daratumumab note: daratumumab, a human IgG1 kappa monoclonal antibody, may be detected by serum protein electrophoresis and immunofixation assays routinely used to monitor endogenous M-protein. Thus, daratumumab may interfere with disease monitoring in patients with plasma cell neoplasms that produce an IgG kappa M-protein.

Lenalidomide notes:
- Higher incidences of second primary malignancies were observed in controlled trials of patients with multiple myeloma receiving lenalidomide. While no routine monitoring is indicated, awareness of this potential complication is necessary
- A decrease in the number of CD34+ cells collected after treatment has been reported in patients who have received >4 cycles of lenalidomide. In patients who may undergo transplant, consider early referral to transplant center
- Because of the embryo-fetal risk, lenalidomide is available only through a restricted program under a Risk Evaluation and Mitigation Strategy (REMS), the REVLIMID REMS program

SUBSEQUENT THERAPY

MULTIPLE MYELOMA REGIMEN: DARATUMUMAB + BORTEZOMIB + DEXAMETHASONE

Chari A et al. Blood 2016;128(22):2142
Palumbo A et al. N Engl J Med 2016;375:754–766
Supplement to: Palumbo A et al. N Engl J Med 2016;375:754–766
Protocol for: Palumbo A et al. N Engl J Med 2016;375:754–766
Darzalex (daratumumab) prescribing information. Horsham, PA: Janssen Biotech, Inc; revised June 2018

Bortezomib 1.3 mg/m^2 per dose; administer subcutaneously in a volume of 0.9% sodium chloride injection (0.9% NS) sufficient to produce a final bortezomib concentration of 2.5 mg/mL on days 1, 4, 8, and 11, every 21 days for up to 8 cycles (total dosage/21-day cycle = 5.2 mg/m^2)

Dexamethasone 20 mg per dose; administer orally or intravenously once daily for 8 doses on days 1, 2, 4, 5, 8, 9, 11, and 12, every 21 days for up to 8 cycles (total dosage/21-day cycle = 160 mg)
Note: patients >75 years of age, with body mass index <18.5 kg/m^2, or with prior steroid intolerance may receive a reduced initial dose of dexamethasone, *as follows:*
• **Dexamethasone** 20 mg per dose; administer orally or intravenously for 3 doses on days 1, 8, and 15, every 21 days for up to 8 cycles (total dosage/21-day cycle = 60 mg)

May choose to administer either DARZALEX (daratumumab) intravenously, or DARZALEX FASPRO (daratumumab and hyaluronidase-fihj) subcutaneously:

DARZALEX (daratumumab) 16 mg/kg per dose; administer intravenously in 0.9% sodium chloride injection (0.9% NS), or:
Notes:
• The first daratumumab dose may optionally be split over two consecutive days (ie, in cycle 1 administer 8 mg/kg on day 1 and 8 mg/kg on day 2) to facilitate administration
• Refer to the table titled "Dosing Schedule" for schedule information
• Refer to the table titled "Administration Instructions" for instructions regarding daratumumab premedication, infusion rate, dilution, and post-infusion medication

DARZALEX FASPRO *(daratumumab and hyaluronidase-fihj)* 1800 mg/30,000 units in 15 mL of ready-to-use solution per dose; administer by a health care provider subcutaneously into the abdomen over approximately 3–5 minutes
Notes:
• Refer to the table titled "Dosing Schedule" for schedule information
• Refer to the table titled "Administration Instructions" for instructions regarding premedications, post-administration medications, and administration

DOSING SCHEDULE

Week of Treatment	Frequency	
	DARZALEX (daratumumab)	**DARZALEX FASPRO (daratumumab and hyaluronidase-fihj)**
Weeks 1, 2, 3, 4, 5, 6, 7, 8, 9	16 mg/kg every 7 days for 9 doses (total dosage/week = 16 mg/kg; total dosage/9-week course = 144 mg/kg) *Note:* the first daratumumab dose (ie, week 1 dose) may optionally be split over two consecutive days (ie, 8 mg/kg on day 1 and 8 mg/kg on day 2) to facilitate administration	1800 mg/30,000 units every 7 days for 9 doses (total dosage/week = 1800 mg/30,000 units); total dosage/9-week course = 16,200 mg/270,000 units)
Weeks* 10, 13, 16, 19, 22	16 mg/kg every 21 days for 5 doses (total dose/3-week cycle = 16 mg/kg; total dose/13-week course = 80 mg/kg)	1800 mg/30,000 units every 21 days for 5 doses (total dosage/3-week cycle = 1800 mg/30,000 units); total dosage/13-week course = 9000 mg/150,000 units)
Week 25† onward	16 mg/kg every 28 days until disease progression (total dose/28-day cycle = 16 mg/kg)	1800 mg/30,000 units every 28 days until disease progression (total dose/28-day cycle = 1800 mg/30,000 units)

*Every-21-day dosing starts on week 10
†Every-28-day dosing starts on week 25

(continued)

(*continued*)

ADMINISTRATION INSTRUCTIONS

Premedications
(*applies to DARZALEX [daratumumab] and DARZALEX FASPRO [daratumumab and hyaluronidase-fihj]*)

Antipyretic	**Acetaminophen** 650–1000 mg; administer orally 1–3 hours before each DARZALEX (daratumumab) or DARZALEX FASPRO (daratumumab and hyaluronidase-fihj) dose
H$_1$-subtype antihistamine	**Diphenhydramine** 25–50 mg; administer orally or intravenously 1–3 hours before each DARZALEX (daratumumab) or DARZALEX FASPRO (daratumumab and hyaluronidase-fihj) dose
Corticosteroid	**Dexamethasone** 20 mg; administer intravenously or orally 1–3 hours before each DARZALEX (daratumumab) or DARZALEX FASPRO (daratumumab and hyaluronidase-fihj) dose • May administer dexamethasone orally beginning with the second dose
Leukotriene receptor antagonist (*optional*)*	**Montelukast** 10 mg; administer orally 1–3 hours before each DARZALEX (daratumumab) or DARZALEX FASPRO (daratumumab and hyaluronidase-fihj) dose

Dilution volume and infusion rate
(*applies to DARZALEX [daratumumab] only*)

DARZALEX (daratumumab) must be administered through an administration set with a flow regulator and with an in-line, sterile, nonpyrogenic, low-protein-binding, polyethersulfone filter with a pore size of 0.2 or 0.22 μm

First infusion	Dilute in 1000 mL 0.9% NS. Infuse initially at 50 mL/hour. If hypersensitivity or infusion reactions do not occur during the first hour, increase the rate by 50 mL/hour every hour as tolerated to a maximum rate of 200 mL/hour *Note:* if splitting the first daratumumab over two consecutive days (ie, 8 mg/kg on day 1 and 8 mg/kg on day 2), then dilute each 8 mg/kg dose in 500 mL 0.9% NS. Infuse initially at 50 mL/hour. If hypersensitivity or infusion reactions do not occur during the first hour, increase the rate by 50 mL/hour every hour as tolerated to a maximum rate of 200 mL/hour
Second infusion†	Dilute in 500 mL 0.9% NS. Infuse initially at 50 mL/hour. If hypersensitivity or infusion reactions do not occur during the first hour, increase the rate by 50 mL/hour every hour as tolerated to a maximum rate of 200 mL/hour
Subsequent infusions‡	Dilute in 500 mL 0.9% NS. Infuse initially at 100 mL/hour. If hypersensitivity or infusion reactions do not occur during the first hour, increase the rate by 50 mL/hour every hour as tolerated to a maximum rate of 200 mL/hour

Subcutaneous Injection
(*applies to DARZALEX FASPRO [daratumumab and hyaluronidase-fihj] only*)

• Attach the hypodermic injection needle or subcutaneous infusion set to the syringe immediately prior to injection in order to reduce the chances of needle clogging
• Choose a site for administration approximately 3 inches (7.5 cm) to the right or left of the navel; rotate administration sites. Do not inject into areas where the skin is red, bruised, tender, hard, or scarred, or into areas used for administration of other subcutaneous medications
• A health care provider should administer the 15-mL dose subcutaneously into the abdomen over approximately 3–5 minutes
• If the injection causes pain, temporarily interrupt or reduce the rate of injection. If this does not relieve the pain, then choose another injection site on the opposite side of the abdomen in which to deliver the remainder of the dose
• Among low-body-weight (<50 kg) patients, the mean maximum trough concentration after the 8th dose was 81% higher in patients who received the fixed subcutaneous doses of DARZALEX FASPRO (daratumumab and hyaluronidase-fihj) compared to those who received 16 mg/kg per dose of intravenously administered DARZALEX (daratumumab). Higher rates of G3/4 neutropenia were observed in low-body-weight patients who received the formulation for subcutaneous injection

Post-administration medications
(*applies to DARZALEX [daratumumab] and DARZALEX FASPRO [daratumumab and hyaluronidase-fihj]*)

Corticosteroid (*optional*)	**Methylprednisolone 20 mg**; administer orally once on the day after each DARZALEX (daratumumab) or DARZALEX FASPRO (daratumumab and hyaluronidase-fihj) dose is administered *Note:* on days when a regimen-specified dexamethasone dose is administered the day after the daratumumab infusion, then the post-infusion methylprednisolone dose should be omitted
Short-acting β-2 agonist§	**Albuterol inhalation aerosol, metered**, 90 μg/actuation, administer 2 inhalations every 4 hours as needed for bronchospasm for 3 days, starting on the day of each of the first 4 DARZALEX (daratumumab) or DARZALEX FASPRO (daratumumab and hyaluronidase-fihj) doses
Long-acting β-2 agonist§	**Salmeterol xinafoate aerosol powder, metered**, 50 μg/actuation, administer 1 inhalation twice a day for 3 days, starting the day of each of the first 4 DARZALEX (daratumumab) or DARZALEX FASPRO (daratumumab and hyaluronidase-fihj) doses

(*continued*)

(continued)

Inhaled corticosteroid§	Fluticasone propionate inhalation aerosol, metered, 220 µg/actuation, administer 2 inhalations twice a day for 3 days, starting on the day of each of the first 4 DARZALEX (daratumumab) or DARZALEX FASPRO (daratumumab and hyaluronidase-fihj) doses

*Some institutions consider adding an optional leukotriene receptor antagonist based on data by Chari et al, 2016
†Use a dilution volume of 500 mL only if there were no infusion reactions during the first 3 hours of the first infusion. Otherwise, continue to use a dilution volume of 1000 mL and instructions for the first infusion
‡Use an initial rate of 100 mL/hour for subsequent infusions only if there were no infusion reactions during a final infusion rate of ≥100 mL/hour in the first two infusions. Otherwise, start infusion at 50 mL/hour per instructions for second infusion
§For patients with a history of chronic obstructive pulmonary disease, consider prescribing additional post-infusion inhaled medications for approximately 48 hours following the first 4 daratumumab infusions. Note that availability of inhalational medication formulations may vary by country; representative examples are included in the table
Note: DARZALEX (daratumumab) and DARZALEX FASPRO (daratumumab and hyaluronidase-fihj) can cause severe administration-related reactions. Symptoms of an administration-related reaction may include respiratory symptoms, chills, nausea/vomiting, fever, chest discomfort, hypotension, or pruritus. Only administer the products under medical supervision in a facility with immediate access to medical support and emergency equipment. Closely monitor patients throughout each administration. Most reactions occur during the first dose, when the all-grade systemic administration-related reaction incidence approaches 50% for the intravenous formulation and 10% for the subcutaneous formulation. Reactions may also occur during or following subsequent administrations. Delayed reactions may occur up to 48 hours following each dose; incidence of delayed reactions is reduced when post-infusion corticosteroids are administered. See Treatment Modifications section for management recommendations

Supportive Care
Antiemetic prophylaxis
Emetogenic potential on days with bortezomib is **LOW**
Emetogenic potential on days when daratumumab is administered without bortezomib is **MINIMAL**
See Chapter 42 for antiemetic recommendations

Hematopoietic growth factor (CSF) prophylaxis
Primary prophylaxis is **NOT** *indicated*
See Chapter 43 for more information

Antimicrobial prophylaxis
Risk of fever and neutropenia is **INTERMEDIATE**
  Antimicrobial primary prophylaxis to be considered:
  • Antibacterial—consider a fluoroquinolone during periods of neutropenia or no prophylaxis; *P. jirovecii* prophylaxis is recommended (eg, cotrimoxazole)
  • Antifungal—recommended; consider use during periods of neutropenia
  • Antiviral—antiherpes antivirals (eg, acyclovir, famciclovir, valacyclovir) should be initiated within 1 week of starting daratumumab or daratumumab and hyaluronidase-fihj, and continued for at least 3 months after completion of the last dose and for the duration of bortezomib use, whichever is longer

Bisphosphonates
All patients receiving primary therapy for symptomatic multiple myeloma should receive a bisphosphonate adjunctively.

Treatment Modifications

DARATUMUMAB OR DARATUMUMAB AND HYALURONIDASE-FIHJ

Adverse Event	Dose Modification
Infusion-Related Reaction and Anaphylactic Reaction Adverse Events	
• G1/2 infusion-related reaction to intravenous daratumumab. (G1/2 IRR) • First occurrence of G3 infusion-related reaction (G3 IRR) to intravenous daratumumab • Second occurrence of G3 infusion-related reaction	Immediately interrupt the daratumumab infusion for infusion-related reactions of *any* severity and manage symptoms as clinically appropriate with additional intravenous corticosteroid (50–150 mg hydrocortisone IVP), an H$_1$-receptor antagonist (diphenhydramine 50 mg IVP), inhaled short-acting ß-2 agonist (albuterol 2 puffs, may repeat in 4 hours) plus epinephrine 0.5 mg IM for hypotension or airway obstructive symptoms
G1 IRR = mild transient reaction; infusion interruption not indicated; intervention not indicated G2 IRR = therapy or infusion interruption indicated but responds promptly to symptomatic treatment (eg, antihistamines, NSAIDS, narcotics, IV fluids); prophylactic medications indicated for ≤24 hours G3 IRR = prolonged (eg, not rapidly responsive to symptomatic medication and/or brief interruption of infusion); recurrence of symptoms following initial improvement; hospitalization indicated for clinical sequelae	Upon resolution of symptoms, resume the daratumumab infusion at no more than 50% of the rate at which the reaction occurred. If tolerated, escalate the infusion by 50 mL/hour every hour up to a maximum rate of 200 mL/hour

(continued)

Treatment Modifications (continued)

Adverse Event	Dose Modification
Infusion-Related Reaction and Anaphylactic Reaction Adverse Events	
• Third occurrence of G3 infusion-related reaction (IRR) to intravenous daratumumab • G4 infusion-related reaction (G4 IRR) to intravenous daratumumab or subcutaneous daratumumab and hyaluronidase-fihj • Anaphylactic reaction (AR) to intravenous daratumumab or subcutaneous daratumumab and hyaluronidase-fihj	Immediately interrupt the administration for infusion-related reactions of *any* severity and manage symptoms as clinically appropriate with additional intravenous corticosteroid (50–150 mg hydrocortisone IVP), an H$_1$-receptor antagonist (diphenhydramine 50 mg IVP), inhaled short-acting ß–2 agonist (albuterol 2 puffs, may repeat in 4 hours) plus epinephrine 0.5 mg IM for hypotension or airway obstructive symptoms
G3 IRR = prolonged (eg, not rapidly responsive to symptomatic medication and/or brief interruption of infusion); recurrence of symptoms following initial improvement; hospitalization indicated for clinical sequelae G4 IRR = life-threatening consequences; urgent intervention indicated G3 AR = symptomatic bronchospasm, with or without urticaria; parenteral intervention indicated; allergy-related edema/angioedema; hypotension G4 AR = life-threatening consequences; urgent intervention indicated	Permanently discontinue
Hematologic Adverse Events	
G3/4 neutropenia G3/4 thrombocytopenia	Consider delaying the dose until recovery to G ≤2 or baseline; or, continue without interruption as clinically appropriate. In the case of neutropenia, consider administration of granulocyte-colony stimulating factor (G-CSF)
Blood transfusion within 6 months following a daratumumab infusion	Notify blood bank the patient has received daratumumab or daratumumab and hyaluronidase-fihj within the past 6 months since either product may result in a positive indirect antiglobulin test (indirect Coombs test) that can persist for up to 6 months and may mask detection of antibodies to minor antigens in the patient's serum. Determination of ABO and Rh blood type is not affected

IRR, infusion-related reactions; AR, anaphylactic reactions
Note: dose reductions are not recommended for daratumumab or daratumumab and hyaluronidase

BORTEZOMIB

Starting dose	1.3 mg/m^2 per dose on days 1, 4, 8, and 11
Dose level −1	1 mg/m^2 per dose on days 1, 4, 8, and 11
Dose level −2	0.7 mg/m^2 per dose on days 1, 4, 8, and 11
Dose level −3	1.3 mg/m^2 per dose on days 1 and 8

Adverse Event	Treatment Modification
Platelet count <70,000/mm^3 or ANC <1000/mm^3 on day 1 of a cycle	Hold therapy until platelet count ≥70,000/mm^3 and ANC ≥1000/mm^3
G3 thrombocytopenia (platelet count <50,000/mm^3)	Reduce bortezomib dosage by one dose level
G1 neuropathy (paresthesias, weakness, and/or loss of reflexes) without pain or loss of function	No action
G1 neuropathy with pain or G2 neuropathy (interferes with function but not with activities of daily living)	Reduce bortezomib dosage one dose level
G2 neuropathy with pain or G3 neuropathy (interferes with activities of daily living)	Withhold bortezomib treatment until toxicity resolves to G1 or baseline, then reinitiate reducing bortezomib dosage one dose level
G4 neuropathy (sensory neuropathy that is disabling or motor neuropathy that is life-threatening or leads to paralysis)	Discontinue treatment
Hepatotoxicity	Monitor liver function. Stop bortezomib and evaluate if hepatotoxicity is suspected

(continued)

Treatment Modifications (*continued*)

Adverse Event	Treatment Modification
Bilirubin level greater than 1.5× ULN and any AST level	Reduce bortezomib to 0.7 mg/m² in the first cycle; consider dose escalation to 1 mg/m² based on tolerability
If several bortezomib doses in consecutive cycles are withheld due to toxicity	Reduce bortezomib by 1 dosage level
G ≥2 nonhematologic toxicity on day 1 of a cycle	Hold bortezomib until toxicity has resolved to G1 or baseline
G ≥3 nonhematologic toxicities	Hold bortezomib until toxicity has resolved to G1 or baseline; then, may be reinitiated with 1 dosage level reduction

DEXAMETHASONE

	Age ≤75 years of age, body mass index ≥18.5 kg/m², and no prior steroid intolerance	Age >75 years of age, body mass index <18.5 kg/m², or with prior steroid intolerance
Starting dose	20 mg/dose/day on days 1, 2, 4, 5, 8, 9, 11, and 12 every 21 days	20 mg/dose/day on days 1, 8, and 15 every 21 days
Dose Level −1	10 mg/dose/day on days 1, 2, 4, 5, 8, 9, 11, and 12 every 21 days*	10 mg/dose/day on days 1, 8, and 15 every 21 days*
Dose Level −2	Discontinue dexamethasone doses on days when daratumumab is not administered*	Discontinue dexamethasone doses on days when daratumumab is not administered*

*Note: the 20-mg dose of dexamethasone given 1–3 hours before the infusion on the day of daratumumab infusions must not be reduced or omitted. For patients on a reduced dexamethasone dose, the entire 20-mg dose may be given as a daratumumab pre-infusion medication

Adverse Event	Adverse Event
G1/2 dyspepsia (moderate symptoms; medical intervention indicated; limiting instrumental ADL), gastric or duodenal ulcer, or gastritis	Continue dexamethasone at the same dose. Treat with therapeutic doses of an H₂-receptor antagonist or proton pump inhibitor. If symptoms persist, then reduce the dexamethasone dose by one level
G ≥3 dyspepsia, gastric or duodenal ulcer, or gastritis (surgery or hospitalization indicated)	Withhold dexamethasone until symptoms return to baseline. Resume dexamethasone reduced by one dose level along with concurrent treatment with therapeutic doses of an H₂-receptor antagonist or proton pump inhibitor. If symptoms recur, then reduce dexamethasone to dose level −2
Acute pancreatitis	Reduce dexamethasone to dose level −2
G ≥3 edema	Withhold dexamethasone until symptoms return to baseline. Consider treatment with diuretics. Resume dexamethasone reduced by one dose level. If edema persists, reduce to dose level −2
G ≥2 mood alteration (moderate mood alteration) or confusion (moderate disorientation; limiting instrumental ADL)	Withhold dexamethasone until symptoms return to baseline. Resume dexamethasone reduced by one dose level. If symptoms persist, reduce by another dose level
G ≥2 muscle weakness (symptomatic; evident on physical exam; limiting instrumental ADL)	Withhold dexamethasone until symptoms return to baseline. Resume dexamethasone reduced by one dose level. If weakness persists, reduce by another dose level
G ≥3 hyperglycemia (insulin therapy initiated; hospitalization indicated)	Withhold dexamethasone until blood glucose is ≤250 mg/dL. Treat with insulin or other hypoglycemic agents as clinically appropriate and then resume dexamethasone at the same dose. If hyperglycemia is uncontrolled despite above measures, decrease dexamethasone by one dose level
Other G ≥2 nonhematologic toxicity attributable to dexamethasone including severe irritability, insomnia, or oral candidiasis	Withhold dexamethasone until toxicity resolves to G ≤1, then resume at a lower dose. Consider reduction by one dose level for G2/G3 toxicity, and by two dose levels for G4 or recurrent G3 toxicity

Patient Population Studied

The multicenter, randomized, open-label, active-controlled, phase 3 study involved 498 patients with relapsed or refractory symptomatic multiple myeloma. Patients who had disease refractory to bortezomib or another proteasome inhibitor, had previously experienced unacceptable toxic events owing to bortezomib, or had neuropathic pain or peripheral neuropathy of Grade ≥2, were not eligible. All patients received up to eight 21-day cycles of subcutaneous bortezomib 1.3 mg/m² on days 1, 4, 8, and 11 and oral or intravenous dexamethasone 20 mg on days 1, 2, 4, 5, 8, 9, 11, and 12 (for a total dose of 160 mg per 21-day cycle; this dose could be reduced to 20 mg weekly for patients aged >75 years, who had a body mass index of <18.5, or who had previously experienced unacceptable adverse events from glucocorticoid therapy). Patients randomly assigned to daratumumab also received intravenous daratumumab 16 mg/kg on days 1, 8, and 15 of the first three cycles, day 1 of the next five cycles, and then once every 4 weeks thereafter until disease progression, unacceptable toxic events, or withdrawal of consent

Therapy Monitoring

1. Type and screen prior to first dose of daratumumab or daratumumab and hyaluronidase-fihj
2. CBC with differential, liver function tests, and serum glucose prior to each dose of bortezomib and daratumumab or daratumumab and hyaluronidase-fihj
3. Monitor for infusion-related daratumumab reaction symptoms frequently during infusion; check vital signs frequently during infusion and at least prior to each scheduled rate increase, ensure medications are available for post-infusion prophylaxis as applicable
4. Monitor for bortezomib toxicities including neuropathy and hypotension

Daratumumab note: daratumumab, a human IgG1 kappa monoclonal antibody, may be detected by serum protein electrophoresis and immunofixation assays routinely used to monitor endogenous M-protein. Thus, daratumumab may interfere with disease monitoring in patients with plasma cell neoplasms that produce an IgG kappa M-protein

Bortezomib note: patients with pre-existing severe neuropathy should be treated with bortezomib only after careful risk-benefit assessment

Efficacy (n = 498)

	Daratumumab Group (n = 251)	Control Group (n = 247)	
Kaplan-Meier progression-free survival at 12 months*	60.7%	26.9%	
Disease progression or death			HR 0.39 (95% CI 0.28–0.53; P <0.001)
Overall response rate†	82.9%	63.2%	P <0.001
Proportion who experienced at least a very good partial response	59.2%	29.1%	P <0.001
Proportion who experienced at least a complete response	19.2%	9.0%	P = 0.001

*Progression and response were determined according to the International Myeloma Working Group criteria
†Overall response rate was the proportion of patients who experienced at least a partial response
Note: median follow-up time was 7.4 months

Adverse Events (n = 480)

	Daratumumab Group (n = 243)		Control Group (n = 237)	
	Grade 1–2 (%)*	Grade 3–4 (%)*	Grade 1–2 (%)*	Grade 3–4 (%)*
Thrombocytopenia	14	45	11	33
Peripheral sensory neuropathy	43	5	31	7
Diarrhea	28	4	21	1
Anemia	12	14	15	16
Upper respiratory tract infection	23	2	17	<1
Fatigue	17	5	21	3
Cough	24	0	13	0
Constipation	20	0	15	<1
Dyspnea	15	4	8	<1
Neutropenia	5	13	5	4
Insomnia	17	0	14	1
Peripheral edema	16	<1	8	0
Pyrexia	14	1	10	1
Lymphopenia	4	9	1	3
Pneumonia	3	8	2	10
Hypertension	2	7	3	<1
Asthenia	8	<1	14	2
Secondary primary cancer	2	NA	<1	NA

*According to the National Cancer Institute Common Terminology Criteria for Adverse Events, version 4.03
Note: adverse events that occurred in ≥15% of patients in either cohort are included in the table. Grade 3–4 adverse events that occurred in ≥5% of patients in either cohort are additionally listed. In total, 7.4% of patients in the daratumumab group and 9.3% of controls discontinued treatment owing to adverse events (the most common causes were peripheral sensitive neuropathy and pneumonia), and 5.3% of patients in the daratumumab group and 5.9% of controls died owing to adverse events (mainly a result of general deterioration of patient physical health, but the next most common causes were pneumonia, ischemic stroke, and respiratory failure)

SUBSEQUENT THERAPY

MULTIPLE MYELOMA REGIMEN: ISATUXIMAB + POMALIDOMIDE + DEXAMETHASONE

Attal M et al. Lancet 2019;394:2096–2107 (also, for supplementary appendix)
SARCLISA (elotuzumab) prescribing information. Bridgewater, NJ: Sanofi-Aventis U.S. LLC; March 2020
POMALYST (pomalidomide) prescribing information. Summit, NJ: Celgene Corporation; October 2019

All cycles (28-day cycles):

Pomalidomide 4 mg per dose; administer orally, once daily, without regard to food, for 21 consecutive days on days 1–21, followed by 7 days without treatment, every 28 days, until disease progression (total dose/4-week cycle (all cycles) = 84 mg)

Notes:

- Patients who delay taking pomalidomide at a regularly scheduled time may take a missed dose if the interval remaining before the next regularly scheduled dose is ≥12 hours

- Do not break, chew, or open pomalidomide capsules

- Women of childbearing potential must not become pregnant while taking pomalidomide, and for at least 4 weeks following the last dose, due to the risk of severe birth defects. Either abstinence from heterosexual contact must be practiced, or at least 2 forms of reliable birth control must be utilized

- Men taking pomalidomide must wear a synthetic or latex condom during sexual contact with a woman of childbearing potential, and must avoid sperm donation during pomalidomide therapy and for at least 4 weeks after discontinuation

- Pomalidomide exposure is reduced in smokers; encourage patients to quit smoking during pomalidomide treatment

- If possible, avoid concomitant use of strong CYP1A2 inhibitors (eg, fluvoxamine, ciprofloxacin). If patients must receive a strong CYP1A2 inhibitor concomitantly, reduce the pomalidomide dose by approximately 50%. If coadministration of the strong inhibitor is discontinued, the pomalidomide dose should be returned to the dose used prior to initiation of a strong CYP1A2 inhibitor

Cycle 1 (28-day cycle):

Premedications for Isatuximab:

Acetaminophen 650–1000 mg; administer orally 15–60 minutes prior to each isatuximab dose for 4 doses on days 1, 8, 15, and 22 for 1 cycle (cycle 1)

Diphenhydramine 25–50 mg; administer intravenously 15–60 minutes prior to each isatuximab dose for 4 doses on days 1, 8, 15, and 22 for 1 cycle (cycle 1)

Note: the intravenous route is preferred prior to the first 4 isatuximab infusions

Ranitidine 50 mg (or an equivalent histamine receptor [H_2]-subtype antagonist); administer intravenously (or an equivalent dosage, ie, ranitidine 150 mg, administered orally) 15–60 minutes prior to each isatuximab dose for 4 doses on days 1, 8, 15, and 22 for 1 cycle (cycle 1)

Dexamethasone (age <75 years, 40 mg per dose; age ≥75 years, 20 mg per dose); administer orally or intravenously 15–60 minutes prior to each isatuximab dose for 4 doses on days 1, 8, 15, and 22 for 1 cycle (cycle 1) (total dosage/4-week cycle during cycle 1 = 160 mg [age <75 years] or 80 mg [age ≥75 years])

Isatuximab 10 mg/kg per dose; administer intravenously in 250 mL of 0.9% sodium chloride injection (0.9% NS) or 5% dextrose injection (D5W) for 4 doses on days 1, 8, 15, and 22 for 1 cycle (cycle 1) (total dosage/4-week cycle during cycle 1 = 40 mg/kg)
- Refer to table titled "Isatuximab Infusion Instructions"

Cycle 2 and beyond (28-day cycles):

Premedications for Isatuximab:

Acetaminophen 650–1000 mg; administer orally 15–60 minutes prior to each isatuximab dose for 2 doses on days 1 and 15, every 28 days, until disease progression (cycle 2 and beyond)

Diphenhydramine 25–50 mg; administer intravenously or orally 15–60 minutes prior to each isatuximab dose for 2 doses on days 1 and 15, every 28 days, until disease progression (cycle 2 and beyond)

Note: the intravenous route is preferred prior to the first isatuximab 4 infusions

Ranitidine 50 mg (or an equivalent histamine receptor [H_2]-subtype antagonist); administer intravenously (or an equivalent dosage, ie, ranitidine 150 mg, administered orally) 15–60 minutes prior to each isatuximab dose for 2 doses on days 1 and 15, every 28 days, until disease progression (cycle 2 and beyond)

Dexamethasone (age <75 years, 40 mg per dose; age ≥75 years, 20 mg per dose); administer orally or intravenously 15–60 minutes prior to each isatuximab dose for 2 doses on days 1 and 15, every 28 days, until disease progression (cycle 2 and beyond)

Isatuximab 10 mg/kg per dose; administer intravenously in 250 mL of 0.9% NS or D5W for 2 doses on days 1 and 15, every 28 days, until disease progression (cycle 2 and beyond) (total dosage/4-week cycle during cycle 2 and beyond = 20 mg/kg)
- Refer to table titled "Isatuximab Infusion Instructions"

(continued)

(continued)

Dexamethasone (age >75 years, 20 mg per dose; age ≤75 years, 40 mg per dose); administer orally for 2 doses on days 8 and 22, every 28 days, until disease progression (cycle 2 and beyond) (total dexamethasone dosage including isatuximab premedication/4-week cycle during cycle 2 and beyond = 80 mg [age >75 years] or 160 mg [age ≤75 years])

Isatuximab Infusion Instructions

First infusion (ie, cycle 1, day 1)	Infuse initially at 25 mL/hour for the first 60 minutes. If tolerated, increase the rate by 25 mL/hour, every 30 minutes, to a maximum rate of 150 mL/hour
Second infusion (ie, cycle 1, day 8)	Infuse initially at 50 mL/hour for the first 30 minutes. If tolerated, increase the rate by 50 mL/hour for 30 minutes. If tolerated, increase the rate by 100 mL/hour, every 30 minutes, to a maximum rate of 200 mL/hour
Subsequent infusions (ie, cycle 1, day 15 and beyond)	Infuse at 200 mL/hour for the entire infusion

Notes:
- If a planned dose of isatuximab is missed, administer the dose as soon as possible and adjust the treatment schedule accordingly, maintaining the treatment interval
- Isatuximab can cause severe infusion-related reactions. Symptoms may include dyspnea, cough, chills, nausea, and/or hypertension. Refer to the Treatment Modifications section for management of infusion-related reactions

Supportive Care
Antiemetic prophylaxis
Emetogenic potential is **MINIMAL**
See Chapter 42 for antiemetic recommendations

Hematopoietic growth factor (CSF) prophylaxis
Primary prophylaxis **MAY** *be indicated*
See Chapter 43 for more information

Antimicrobial prophylaxis
Risk of fever and neutropenia is **INTERMEDIATE**
   Antimicrobial primary prophylaxis to be considered:
- Antibacterial—consider a fluoroquinolone during periods of prolonged neutropenia (ANC <500/mm³ for ≥7 days) or no prophylaxis; *P. jirovecii* prophylaxis is recommended (eg, cotrimoxazole)
- Antifungal—consider fluconazole during periods of prolonged neutropenia (ANC <500/mm³ for ≥7 days) or no prophylaxis
- Antiviral—antiherpes antivirals (eg, acyclovir, famciclovir, valacyclovir)

Bisphosphonates
All patients receiving primary therapy for symptomatic multiple myeloma should receive a bisphosphonate adjunctively.
Steroid-associated gastritis
Add a proton pump inhibitor or H$_2$-receptor antagonist during dexamethasone use to prevent gastritis and duodenitis

Thromboprophylaxis
Risk assessment and recommendations for VTE prophylaxis in patients with multiple myeloma with individual or myeloma-related risk factors, or risk factors related to treatment

(continued)

(*continued*)

Individual risk factors
• Obesity (BMI ≥30 kg/m²)
• H/O VTE
• CVC or pacemaker
• Comorbid pathologies
  ■ Cardiac disease
  ■ Chronic renal disease
  ■ Diabetes
  ■ Acute infection
  ■ Immobilization
• Surgery
  ■ General surgery
  ■ Any anesthesia
  ■ Trauma
• Medications
  ■ Erythropoietin (epoetin alfa, darbepoetin)
  ■ Estrogenic compounds
  ■ Bevacizumab
• Clotting disorders
  ■ Thrombophilia
Myeloma-related risk factors
  ■ Diagnosis of multiple myeloma
  ■ Hyperviscosity
	≤1 Individual or myeloma-related risk factor present:
	• **Aspirin** 81–325 mg daily
	
	≥2 Individual or myeloma-related risk factors present:
	• **LMWH,*** equivalent to **enoxaparin sodium** 40 mg/day *or* **dalteparin sodium** 5000 IU/day; administer subcutaneously, *or*
	• **Warfarin**, targeting an INR = 2–3

Concomitant treatment-related risk factors Thalidomide or lenalidomide in combination with: • High-dose dexamethasone (≥480 mg/month) • Doxorubicin • Multiagent chemotherapy	• **LMWH,*** equivalent to **enoxaparin sodium** 40 mg/day *or* **dalteparin sodium** 5000 IU/day; administer subcutaneously, *or* • **Warfarin**, targeting an INR = 2–3

*LMWHs should be used with caution in individuals with impaired renal function (creatinine clearance <30 mL/min). Refer to product labeling for information about doses and administration schedules in renally impaired patients, and guidance for monitoring anti-Factor Xa concentrations

Abbreviations: CVC, central venous catheter; INR, international normalized ratio; LMWH, low-molecular-weight heparin; VTE, venous thromboembolic disease

References: Geerts WH et al. Chest 2008;133(6 Suppl):381S–453S
National Comprehensive Cancer Network. Multiple Myeloma, V.1.2014. (Accessed October 8, 2013, at http://www.nccn.org)
National Comprehensive Cancer Network. Venous Thromboembolic Disease, V.2.2013. (Accessed October 8, 2013, at http://www.nccn.org)
Palumbo A et al. Leukemia 2008;22:414–423

Treatment Modifications

ISATUXIMAB TREATMENT MODIFICATIONS

Isatuximab Dose Levels	
Isatuximab starting dose	10 mg/kg per dose (No dose reduction is allowed)
Adverse Event	**Treatment Modification**
G1 IRR (mild transient reaction; infusion interruption not indicated; intervention not indicated) or G2 IRR (therapy or infusion interruption indicated but responds promptly to symptomatic treatment [eg, antihistamines, NSAIDS, narcotics, IV fluids]; prophylactic medications indicated for ≤24 hours)	Interrupt the isatuximab infusion and provide appropriate supportive care. When symptoms improve, resume the isatuximab infusion with the infusion rate reduced to 50% of the initial infusion rate and monitor carefully for recurrent symptoms. If tolerated for 30 minutes, increase the infusion rate to the initial rate, and then increase incrementally as described in the above table titled "Isatuximab Infusion Instructions" as tolerated. If symptoms do not improve or recur, then permanently discontinue isatuximab

(*continued*)

Treatment Modifications (*continued*)

Adverse Event	Treatment Modification
G3 IRR (prolonged [eg, not rapidly responsive to symptomatic medication and/or brief interruption of infusion]; recurrence of symptoms following initial improvement; hospitalization indicated for clinical sequelae) or G4 IRR (life-threatening consequences; urgent intervention indicated)	Permanently discontinue isatuximab and provide appropriate supportive care
G4 neutropenia (ANC <500/mm^3)	Delay isatuximab until ANC recovers to ≥1000/mm^3. Consider prescribing prophylactic antibiotics and granulocyte-colony stimulating factor
Patient receiving isatuximab requires a blood transfusion	Notify blood bank the patient has received isatuximab since isatuximab may result in a positive indirect antiglobulin test (indirect Coombs test) that may mask detection of antibodies to minor antigens in the patient's serum. Determination of ABO and Rh blood type is not affected. Interference with blood compatibility testing can be resolved using dithiothreitol-treated red blood cells. If an emergency transfusion is required, non-cross-matched ABO/RhD-compatible RBCs may be given per local blood bank practices

POMALIDOMIDE TREATMENT MODIFICATIONS

Note: because of the embryo-fetal risk, pomalidomide is available only through a restricted program under a Risk Evaluation and Mitigation Strategy (REMS) called "POMALYST REMS"

Pomalidomide Dose Levels

Dose level 1 (starting dose)	4 mg
Dose level −1	3 mg
Dose level −2	2 mg
Dose level −3	1 mg

Adverse Event	Treatment Modification
First occurrence of ANC <500/mm^3 and/or platelet count between 25,000/mm^3 and 50,000/mm^3 at start of a new cycle	Withhold start of pomalidomide cycle until ANC ≥500/mm^3 and platelet count ≥50,000/mm^3, then resume pomalidomide at the same dose
Recurrence of ANC <500/mm^3 or platelet count between 25,000/mm^3 and 50,000/mm^3 at start of a subsequent cycle	Withhold start of pomalidomide cycle until ANC ≥500/mm^3 and platelet count ≥50,000/mm^3, and then resume pomalidomide reduced by 1 mg/dose
Febrile neutropenia (fever ≥38.5°C and ANC <500/mm^3) or severe infection during a cycle	Withhold pomalidomide. When ANC ≥500/mm^3 and infection adequately controlled, resume pomalidomide reduced by 2 mg/dose
Platelet count <25,000/mm^3 at start of a new cycle	Withhold start of pomalidomide cycle until ANC ≥500/mm^3 and platelet count ≥50,000/mm^3, then resume pomalidomide reduced by 1 mg/dose
Any recurrence of platelet count <25,000/mm^3 at start of a subsequent cycle	Withhold start of pomalidomide cycle until ANC ≥500/mm^3 and platelet count ≥50,000/mm^3, then resume pomalidomide reduced by 1 mg/dose
ANC <500/mm^3 or platelet count <25,000/mm^3 occurring *within* a pomalidomide cycle	Hold pomalidomide until ANC >500/mm^3 and platelet count >50,000/mm^3, then resume pomalidomide reduced by 1 mg/dose
ANC <500/mm^3 or platelet count <25,000/mm^3 at any time while on a pomalidomide dose of 1 mg daily	Discontinue pomalidomide
Any other G3/4 adverse event at start of a new cycle or at any time during a cycle	Withhold pomalidomide and restart treatment reduced by 1 mg/dose less than the previous dose when toxicity has resolved to ≤G2 at the physician's discretion
Patient considered to be at higher risk of DVT or PE	Consider anticoagulation prophylaxis after an assessment of each patient's underlying risk factors

Note: pomalidomide is a thalidomide analogue and is contraindicated in pregnancy. Thalidomide is a known human teratogen that causes severe life-threatening birth defects. For females of reproductive potential, exclude pregnancy before start of treatment and prevent pregnancy during treatment by the use of two reliable methods of contraception

(*continued*)

Treatment Modifications (continued)

DEXAMETHASONE TREATMENT MODIFICATIONS

Dexamethasone Dose Levels

	Age <75 years	Age ≥75 years
Starting dose	40 mg	20 mg
Dose level −1	20 mg	12 mg
Dose level −2	12 mg	8 mg

Note: if the dexamethasone dose is delayed, discontinued, or reduced during a week in which isatuximab is administered, then base the decision on whether to administer isatuximab on clinical judgement (ie, risk of hypersensitivity)

Adverse Event	Treatment Modification
G1/2 dyspepsia (moderate symptoms; medical intervention indicated; limiting instrumental ADL), gastric or duodenal ulcer, or gastritis	Continue dexamethasone at the same dose. Treat with therapeutic doses of an H_2-receptor antagonist or proton pump inhibitor. If symptoms persist, then reduce the dexamethasone dose by one level
G ≥3 dyspepsia, gastric or duodenal ulcer, or gastritis (surgery or hospitalization indicated)	Withhold dexamethasone until symptoms return to baseline. Resume dexamethasone reduced by one dose level along with concurrent treatment with therapeutic doses of an H_2-receptor antagonist or proton pump inhibitor. If symptoms recur, then permanently discontinue dexamethasone
Acute pancreatitis	Permanently discontinue dexamethasone
G ≥3 edema	Withhold dexamethasone until symptoms return to baseline. Consider treatment with diuretics. Resume dexamethasone reduced by one dose level. If edema persists, reduce by another dose level. Discontinue dexamethasone permanently if symptoms persist despite two prior dose reductions
G ≥2 mood alteration (moderate mood alteration) or confusion (moderate disorientation; limiting instrumental ADL)	Withhold dexamethasone until symptoms return to baseline. Resume dexamethasone reduced by one dose level. If symptoms persist, reduce by another dose level
G ≥2 muscle weakness (symptomatic; evident on physical exam; limiting instrumental ADL)	Withhold dexamethasone until symptoms return to baseline. Resume dexamethasone reduced by one dose level. If weakness persists, reduce by another dose level. If weakness still persists, then permanently discontinue dexamethasone
G ≥3 hyperglycemia (insulin therapy initiated; hospitalization indicated)	Withhold dexamethasone until blood glucose is ≤250 mg/dL. Treat with insulin or other hypoglycemic agents as clinically appropriate and then resume dexamethasone at the same dose. If hyperglycemia is uncontrolled despite above measures, decrease dexamethasone by one dose level
Other G ≥2 nonhematologic toxicity attributable to dexamethasone including severe irritability, insomnia, or oral candidiasis	Withhold dexamethasone until toxicity resolves to G ≤1, then resume at a lower dose. Consider reduction by one dose level for G2/G3 toxicity, and by two dose levels for G4 or recurrent G3 toxicity

If the dose of one drug in the regimen (ie, pomalidomide, dexamethasone, or isatuximab) is delayed, interrupted, or discontinued, the treatment with the other drugs may continue as scheduled

IRR, infusion-related reaction; NSAIDs, non-steroidal anti-inflammatory drugs; ANC, absolute neutrophil count; RBCs, red blood cells; DVT, deep-vein thrombosis; PE, pulmonary embolism; ADL, activities of daily living

Patient Population Studied

This international, multicenter, open-label, randomized phase 3 trial included 307 adult patients with multiple myeloma. Eligible patients had relapsed and refractory multiple myeloma and had received at least two previous lines of therapy which included lenalidomide and a proteasome inhibitor (given alone or in combination). Non-response to therapy was classified as progression on or within 60 days of therapy, intolerance to either drug, or disease progression within 6 months after achieving at least a partial response. Patients were excluded if they were refractory to previous therapy with an anti-CD38 monoclonal antibody, had experienced prior therapy with pomalidomide, or had an ongoing toxic effect greater than Grade 1 from a previous antimyeloma therapy. Participants with active primary amyloid light-chain amyloidosis or concomitant plasma cell leukemia were ineligible

Efficacy (n = 307)

Efficacy Variable	Isatuximab + Pomalidomide + Dexamethasone (n = 154)	Pomalidomide + Dexamethasone (n = 153)	Between-group Comparison
Survival Outcomes			
Median progression-free survival	11.53 months	6.47 months	HR 0.596 (95% CI 0.436–0.814) P=0.001
Overall survival rate at 12 months*	72%	63%	HR 0.687 (95% CI 0.461–1.023) P=0.0631
Overall Response Rate			
Responders†	60% (95% CI 52.2–68.2)	35% (95% CI 27.8–43.4)	OR 2.795 (95% CI 1.75–4.56) P <0.0001
Very good partial response or better	32% (95% CI 24.6–39.8)	9% (95% CI 4.6–14.1)	OR 5.026 (95% CI 2.514–10.586) P <0.0001
Best Overall Response			
Complete response	5%	1%	—
Stringent complete response	0	<1%	—
Very good partial response	27%	7%	—
Partial response	29%	27%	—
Minimal response	7%	11%	—
Stable disease	21%	29%	—
Non-progressive disease	4%	9%	—
Unconfirmed progressive disease	<1%	3%	—
Not evaluable or not assessed	5%	11%	—

*Median overall survival was not reached in either treatment group based on data with a cutoff date of October 11, 2018
†Responders included patients experiencing stringent complete response, complete response, very good partial response, or partial response
HR, hazard ratio; CI, confidence interval; OR, odds ratio

Adverse Events (n = 301)

	Isatuximab + Pomalidomide + Dexamethasone (n = 152)		Pomalidomide + Dexamethasone (n = 149)	
Most common adverse effects (in ≥15% of patients with isatuximab, worst grade)				
	Grade 1–2 (%)	Grade 3–4 (%)	Grade 1–2 (%)	Grade 3–4 (%)
Infusion reaction*	36%	2%	0%	0%
Upper respiratory tract infection	25%	3%	16%	<1%
Diarrhea	24%	2%	19%	<1%
Bronchitis	21%	3%	8%	<1%
Pneumonia	4%	16%	3%	14%
Fatigue	13%	4%	22%	0%
Back pain	14%	2%	14%	1%
Constipation	16%	0%	17%	0%
Asthenia	12%	3%	15%	3%
Dyspnea	11%	4%	9%	1%
Nausea	15%	0%	9%	0%

(*continued*)

Adverse Events (n = 301) (continued)

Hematologic laboratory abnormalities (worst grade in evaluable patients)				
	Grade 1–2 (%)	Grade 3–4 (%)	Grade 1–2 (%)	Grade 3–4 (%)
Neutropenia	11%	85%	23%	70%
Thrombocytopenia	53%	31%	55%	25%
Anemia	67%	32%	71%	28%

Other adverse event of interest		
	All Grades	All Grades
Secondary primary malignancy[†]	6 patients (4%)	1 patient (<1%)

* Infusion reactions were reported by the investigator and included infusion-related reactions, cytokine release syndrome, and drug hypersensitivity
[†]In the isatuximab + pomalidomide + dexamethasone group, there was one patient with myelodysplastic syndrome, one patient with post-radiation angiosarcoma, and four patients with squamous cell carcinoma of the skin. In the pomalidomide + dexamethasone group, there was one patient with squamous cell carcinoma of the skin

Therapy Monitoring

1. Type and screen prior to first dose of isatuximab; consider phenotyping prior to the start of isatuximab. Inform blood banks that a patient has received isatuximab

2. *Periodically and as clinically indicated:* CBC with differential, liver function tests, BUN, serum creatinine, and serum glucose

3. Monitor for infusion-related reaction symptoms frequently during each isatuximab infusion; check vital signs frequently during each infusion and at least prior to each scheduled rate increase, when applicable

4. Monitor patients for the development of second primary malignancies per International Myeloma Working Group guidelines (Musto P et al. Ann Oncol 2017;28:228–245)

Isatuximab note: isatuximab, a human IgG1 kappa monoclonal antibody, may be detected by serum protein electrophoresis and immunofixation assays routinely used to monitor endogenous M-protein. Thus, isatuximab may interfere with disease monitoring in patients with plasma cell neoplasms that produce an IgG kappa M-protein

Pomalidomide note:

• Because of the embryo-fetal risk, pomalidomide is available only through a restricted program under a Risk Evaluation and Mitigation Strategy (REMS), the POMALYST REMS program

SUBSEQUENT THERAPY

MULTIPLE MYELOMA REGIMEN: ELOTUZUMAB + LENALIDOMIDE + DEXAMETHASONE

Lonial S et al. N Engl J Med 2015;373:621–631
Protocol for: Lonial S et al. N Engl J Med 2015;373:621–631
EMPLICITI (elotuzumab) prescribing information. Princeton, NJ: Bristol-Myers Squibb Company; November 2018

Premedications for Elotuzumab:

Acetaminophen 650–1000 mg; administer orally 45–90 minutes prior to each elotuzumab dose for 4 doses on days 1, 8, 15, and 22, every 28 days for 2 cycles (cycles 1–2 only), and then 45–90 minutes prior to each elotuzumab dose for 2 doses on days 1 and 15, every 28 days until disease progression, beginning with cycle 3

Diphenhydramine 25–50 mg; administer orally or intravenously 45–90 minutes prior to each elotuzumab dose for 4 doses on days 1, 8, 15, and 22, every 28 days for 2 cycles (cycles 1–2 only), and then 45–90 minutes prior to each elotuzumab dose for 2 doses on days 1 and 15, every 28 days until disease progression, beginning with cycle 3

Ranitidine 50 mg (or an equivalent histamine receptor [H_2]–subtype antagonist); administer intravenously (or an equivalent dosage, ie, ranitidine 150 mg, administered orally) 45–90 minutes prior to each elotuzumab dose for 4 doses on days 1, 8, 15, and 22, every 28 days for 2 cycles (cycles 1–2 only), and then 45–90 minutes prior to each elotuzumab dose for 2 doses on days 1 and 15, every 28 days until disease progression, beginning with cycle 3

Dexamethasone 8 mg; administer intravenously 45–90 minutes prior to each elotuzumab dose for 4 doses on days 1, 8, 15, and 22, every 28 days for 2 cycles (cycles 1–2 only), and then 45–90 minutes prior to each elotuzumab dose for 2 doses on days 1 and 15, every 28 days until disease progression, beginning with cycle 3

Elotuzumab 10 mg/kg per dose; administer intravenously in a volume of 0.9% sodium chloride injection (0.9% NS) or 5% dextrose injection (D5W) not to exceed 5 mL/kg body weight and also sufficient to produce a final concentration between 1 mg/mL and 6 mg/mL, for 4 doses on days 1, 8, 15, and 22, every 28 days for 2 cycles (cycles 1–2 only), and then for 2 doses on days 1 and 15, every 28 days until disease progression, beginning with cycle 3 (total dosage/cycle in cycles 1–2 = 40 mg/kg; total dosage/cycle in cycle 3 and thereafter = 20 mg/kg). *Infuse as follows:*

Elotuzumab Infusion Instructions	
Cycle 1, day 1	Infuse initially at 0.5 mL/min (30 mL/hour) for the first 30 minutes. If tolerated, increase to 1 mL/min (60 mL/hour) for 30 minutes. If tolerated, increase to 2 mL/min (120 mL/hour) for the remainder of the infusion
Cycle 1, day 8	Infuse initially at 3 mL/min (180 mL/hour) for the first 30 minutes. If tolerated, increase to 4 mL/min (240 mL/hour) for the remainder of the infusion
Cycle 1, day 15 and 22, and all subsequent doses	Infuse at 5 mL/min (300 mL/hour) for the entire infusion

- **Elotuzumab can cause severe infusion-related reactions**

  Symptoms of an infusion-related reaction may include fever, chills, hypertension or hypotension, and bradycardia. The incidence of all-grade infusion-related reactions was 10%. The incidence of Grade 3 infusion-related reactions was 1% and no patients experienced a Grade 4 or 5 infusion-related reaction. Most reactions (70%) occur during the first elotuzumab infusion.

  See Treatment Modifications table for guidance

Lenalidomide 25 mg/dose; administer orally, without regard to meals, once daily for 21 consecutive days on days 1–21, followed by 7 days without treatment, every 28 days, until disease progression (total dosage/28-day cycle = 525 mg)
- Patients who delay taking a lenalidomide dose at a regularly scheduled time may take the missed dose if the time to the next regularly scheduled dose is >12 hours away
- Consider doses in Treatment Modifications table for dose adjustments for renal function

Dexamethasone, *as follows:*
- During weeks when elotuzumab is administered:

  Dexamethasone 28 mg; administer orally between 3 and 24 hours prior to each elotuzumab dose for 4 doses on days 1, 8, 15, and 22 (ie, during weeks when elotuzumab is administered), every 28 days for 2 cycles (cycles 1–2 only), and then between 3 and 24 hours prior to each elotuzumab dose for 2 doses on days 1 and 15 (ie, during weeks when elotuzumab is administered), every 28 days until disease progression, beginning with cycle 3
  - *Note:* patients must also receive dexamethasone 8 mg intravenously 45–90 minutes prior to each elotuzumab infusion as described in the premedication section
- During weeks when elotuzumab is *not* administered:

  Dexamethasone 40 mg/dose; administer orally for 2 doses on days 8 and 22 (ie, during weeks when elotuzumab is not administered), every 28 days, until disease progression, beginning with cycle 3
  - Total dexamethasone dosage/28-day cycle, during cycles 1–2 = 112 mg administered orally and 32 mg administered intravenously (total of 144 mg/28-day cycle including both routes of administration)
  - Total dexamethasone dosage/28-day cycle, during cycles 3 and thereafter = 136 mg administered orally and 16 mg administered intravenously (total of 152 mg/28-day cycle including both routes of administration)

(continued)

(continued)

Supportive Care

Antiemetic prophylaxis
Emetogenic potential is **MINIMAL**
See Chapter 42 for antiemetic recommendations

Hematopoietic growth factor (CSF) prophylaxis
Primary prophylaxis is **NOT** *indicated*
See Chapter 43 for more information

Antimicrobial prophylaxis
Risk of fever and neutropenia is **INTERMEDIATE**
Antimicrobial primary prophylaxis to be considered:
- Antibacterial—consider a fluoroquinolone or no prophylaxis; *P. jirovecii* prophylaxis is recommended (eg, cotrimoxazole)
- Antifungal—consider fluconazole during periods of neutropenia
- Antiviral—antiherpes antivirals (eg, acyclovir, famciclovir, valacyclovir)

Bisphosphonates
All patients receiving primary therapy for symptomatic multiple myeloma should receive a bisphosphonate adjunctively.

Steroid-associated gastritis
Add a proton pump inhibitor or H_2-receptor antagonist during dexamethasone use to prevent gastritis and duodenitis

Thromboprophylaxis
Risk assessment and recommendations for VTE prophylaxis in patients with multiple myeloma with individual or myeloma-related risk factors, or risk factors related to treatment

Individual risk factors	
• Obesity (BMI ≥30 kg/m²)	
• H/O VTE	
• CVC or pacemaker	
• Comorbid pathologies	
▪ Cardiac disease	
▪ Chronic renal disease	
▪ Diabetes	
▪ Acute infection	≤1 Individual or myeloma-related risk factor present:
▪ Immobilization	• **Aspirin** 81–325 mg daily
• Surgery	
▪ General surgery	
▪ Any anesthesia	≥2 Individual or myeloma-related risk factors present:
▪ Trauma	• **LMWH,*** equivalent to enoxaparin sodium 40 mg/day *or* **dalteparin sodium** 5000 IU/day; administer subcutaneously, *or*
• Medications	• **Warfarin**, targeting an INR = 2–3
▪ Erythropoietin (epoetin alfa, darbepoetin)	
▪ Estrogenic compounds	
▪ Bevacizumab	
• Clotting disorders	
▪ Thrombophilia	
Myeloma-related risk factors	
• Diagnosis of multiple myeloma	
• Hyperviscosity	
Concomitant treatment-related risk factors Thalidomide or lenalidomide in combination with:	
• High-dose dexamethasone (≥480 mg/month)	• **LMWH,*** equivalent to enoxaparin sodium 40 mg/day *or* **dalteparin sodium** 5000 IU/day; administer subcutaneously, *or*
• Doxorubicin	• **Warfarin**, targeting an INR = 2–3
• Multiagent chemotherapy	

*LMWHs should be used with caution in individuals with impaired renal function (creatinine clearance <30 mL/min). Refer to product labeling for information about doses and administration schedules in renally impaired patients, and guidance for monitoring anti-Factor Xa concentrations

Abbreviations: CVC, central venous catheter; INR, international normalized ratio; LMWH, low-molecular-weight heparin; VTE, venous thromboembolic disease

References: Geerts WH et al. Chest 2008;133(6 Suppl):381S–453S
National Comprehensive Cancer Network. Multiple Myeloma, V.1.2014. (Accessed October 8, 2013, at http://www.nccn.org)
National Comprehensive Cancer Network. Venous Thromboembolic Disease, V.2.2013. (Accessed October 8, 2013, at http://www.nccn.org)
Palumbo A et al. Leukemia 2008;22:414–423

Treatment Modifications

ELOTUZUMAB

Starting dose	10 mg/kg (no dose reduction is allowed)
G1 infusion-related reaction	Continue elotuzumab infusion and provide supportive care. Monitor vital signs every 30 minutes during the infusion and for 2 hours after infusion completion
G2–4 infusion-related reactions	Interrupt elotuzumab infusion and provide supportive care. Consider permanent discontinuation of elotuzumab and emergency care for severe reactions. Monitor vital signs every 30 minutes during the infusion and for 2 hours after infusion completion. Upon resolution G ≤1, resume elotuzumab infusion at 0.5 mL/min (30 mL/hour) and gradually increase the infusion rate every 30 minutes, as tolerated, in increments of 0.5 mL/min (30 mL/hour) until the rate at which the infusion-related reaction occurred is reached. In the absence of a recurrent infusion-related reaction, continue the standard dose escalation regimen as described in the therapy section. If the infusion-related reaction recurs, discontinue the remainder of the elotuzumab infusion for that day
Discontinuation of dexamethasone	Base decision to continue elotuzumab on clinical judgment (ie, risk of hypersensitivity)
G ≥3 elevation of liver enzymes	Stop elotuzumab. After return to baseline values, continuation of treatment may be considered

LENALIDOMIDE

Lenalidomide dose levels (Days 1–21 of each 28-day cycle)

	CrCl ≥60 mL/min	CrCl ≥30 mL/min and <60 mL/min	CrCl <30 mL/min (not on hemodialysis)	ESRD on hemodialysis
Starting dose	25 mg each day	10 mg each day	15 mg every other day	5 mg each day (after dialysis on dialysis days)
Dose level −1	15 mg each day	5 mg each day	10 mg every other day	2.5 mg each day (after dialysis on dialysis days)
Dose level −2	10 mg each day	2.5 mg each day	5 mg every other day	Discontinue†
Dose level −3	5 mg each day	Discontinue†	Discontinue†	
Dose level −4	Discontinue†			

Adverse Event	Treatment Modification
Hematologic Toxicity	
Day 1 ANC <1000/mm³ or platelet count <50,000/mm³	Delay the next cycle until ANC ≥1000/mm³ and platelet count ≥50,000/mm³. Consider treatment with filgrastim and/or platelet transfusion according to local guidelines. If the start of a new cycle is delayed >14 days for lenalidomide-related toxicity, then reduce the lenalidomide by one dose level
G ≥3 neutropenia (ANC <1000/mm³) during a cycle	Interrupt lenalidomide treatment and follow weekly CBC. When ANC ≥1000/mm³ and there are no other toxicities, resume lenalidomide treatment at same dose. If other toxicities are still present, then resume lenalidomide with dose reduced one dose level
Recurrent G ≥3 neutropenia (ANC <1000/mm³) during a cycle	Interrupt lenalidomide treatment and follow weekly CBC. When ANC ≥1000/mm³ resume with dose reduced one dose level
Febrile neutropenia (ANC <1000/mm³ with fever ≥38.3°C)	Hold lenalidomide dosing for up to 21 days to resolve toxicity and then restart at the same dose or reduce the lenalidomide dose by one dose level
Platelet count <30,000/mm³	Interrupt lenalidomide treatment and follow weekly CBC. When platelet count ≥30,000/mm³, resume lenalidomide with dose reduced one dose level
Recurrent platelet count <30,000/mm³	
Nonhematologic Toxicity	
G3/4 hepatotoxicity (ALT/AST >5× ULN and/or bilirubin >3× ULN)	Withhold lenalidomide for remainder of the cycle. Delay initiation of next cycle until hepatotoxicity resolves to G ≤2 (ALT/AST ≤5× ULN and/or bilirubin ≤3× ULN), then resume lenalidomide at one lower dose level

(continued)

Treatment Modifications (continued)

Nonhematologic Toxicity

G3 rash	Hold dose for remainder of cycle. Decrease by one dose level when dosing resumed at next cycle (rash must resolve to G ≤1)
Allergic reactions, including hypersensitivity, angioedema, Stevens-Johnson syndrome, toxic epidermal necrolysis (TEN), and drug reaction with eosinophilia and systemic symptoms (DRESS)	Discontinue lenalidomide if reactions are suspected. Do not resume lenalidomide if these reactions are confirmed
Tumor lysis syndrome (TLS)	Monitor patients at risk of TLS (ie, those with high tumor burden) and take appropriate precautions including aggressive hydration and allopurinol
G3 peripheral neuropathy	If neuropathy is considered to be attributable to lenalidomide, then withhold lenalidomide for the remainder of the cycle. Delay initiation of the next cycle until neuropathy resolves to G ≤1, then resume lenalidomide at one lower dose level
G4 peripheral neuropathy	If neuropathy is considered to be attributable to lenalidomide, then discontinue lenalidomide
G3/4 venous thromboembolism (VTE) during aspirin monotherapy or inadequate anticoagulation	Continue lenalidomide at the current dose and initiate adequate anticoagulation
G3/4 venous thromboembolism (VTE) during adequate anticoagulation (eg, prophylactic or therapeutic doses of LMWH, UFH, or warfarin)	Discontinue lenalidomide
G ≥2 hypothyroidism or G ≥2 hyperthyroidism	Continue lenalidomide at current dose and initiate appropriate medical treatment
Other G ≥3 lenalidomide-related toxicities	Withhold lenalidomide for the remainder of the cycle. Delay initiation of the next cycle until toxicity resolves to G ≤2, then resume lenalidomide at one lower dose level

DEXAMETHASONE

Dose Level	Dexamethasone Doses During Weeks with Elotuzumab		Dexamethasone Doses During Weeks Without Elotuzumab	
	Oral dose	Intravenous Dose	Oral dose	Intravenous Dose
Starting dose	28 mg	8 mg	40 mg	0 mg
Dose level −1	12 mg	8 mg	20 mg	0 mg
Dose level −2	0 mg	8 mg	12 mg	0 mg
Dose level −3	0 mg	0 mg	0 mg	0 mg

Note: if the dexamethasone dose is delayed or discontinued during a week in which elotuzumab is administered, then base the decision on whether to administer elotuzumab on clinical judgement (ie, risk of hypersensitivity)

Adverse Event	Treatment Modification
G1/2 dyspepsia (moderate symptoms; medical intervention indicated; limiting instrumental ADL), gastric or duodenal ulcer, or gastritis	Continue dexamethasone at the same dose. Treat with therapeutic doses of an H$_2$-receptor antagonist or proton pump inhibitor. If symptoms persist, then reduce the dexamethasone dose by one level
G ≥3 dyspepsia, gastric or duodenal ulcer, or gastritis (surgery or hospitalization indicated)	Withhold dexamethasone until symptoms return to baseline. Resume dexamethasone reduced by one dose level along with concurrent treatment with therapeutic doses of an H$_2$-receptor antagonist or proton pump inhibitor. If symptoms recur, then permanently discontinue dexamethasone
Acute pancreatitis	Permanently discontinue dexamethasone
G ≥3 edema	Withhold dexamethasone until symptoms return to baseline. Consider treatment with diuretics. Resume dexamethasone reduced by one dose level. If edema persists, reduce by another dose level. Discontinue dexamethasone permanently if symptoms persist despite two prior dose reductions
G ≥2 mood alteration (moderate mood alteration) or confusion (moderate disorientation; limiting instrumental ADL)	Withhold dexamethasone until symptoms return to baseline. Resume dexamethasone reduced by one dose level. If symptoms persist, reduce by another dose level

(continued)

Treatment Modifications (*continued*)

Adverse Event	Treatment Modification
G ≥2 muscle weakness (symptomatic; evident on physical exam; limiting instrumental ADL)	Withhold dexamethasone until symptoms return to baseline. Resume dexamethasone reduced by one dose level. If weakness persists, reduce by another dose level. If weakness still persists, then permanently discontinue dexamethasone
G ≥3 hyperglycemia (insulin therapy initiated; hospitalization indicated)	Withhold dexamethasone until blood glucose is ≤250 mg/dL. Treat with insulin or other hypoglycemic agents as clinically appropriate and then resume dexamethasone at the same dose. If hyperglycemia is uncontrolled despite above measures, decrease dexamethasone by one dose level
Other G ≥2 nonhematologic toxicity attributable to dexamethasone including severe irritability, insomnia, or oral candidiasis	Withhold dexamethasone until toxicity resolves to G ≤1, then resume at a lower dose. Consider reduction by one dose level for G2/G3 toxicity, and by two dose levels for G4 or recurrent G3 toxicity

If the dose of one drug in the regimen (ie, lenalidomide, dexamethasone, or elotuzumab) is delayed, interrupted, or discontinued, the treatment with the other drugs may continue as scheduled

Patient Population Studied

The multicenter, randomized, open-label, phase 3 study involved 646 patients with relapsed or refractory symptomatic multiple myeloma. Patients randomly assigned to elotuzumab received intravenous elotuzumab 10 mg/kg on days 1, 8, 15, and 22 of the first two 28-day cycles and on days 1 and 15 of the subsequent cycles, oral lenalidomide 25 mg on days 1 to 21 of each cycle, and dexamethasone (40 mg administered orally on days not also administered elotuzumab and 28 mg orally plus 8 mg intravenously on days that elotuzumab was administered) on days 1, 8, 15, and 22 of each cycle. Controls received oral lenalidomide 25 mg on days 1 to 21 of each 28-day cycle, and dexamethasone 40 mg on days 1, 8, 15, and 22 of each cycle. Cycles were continued until disease progression, unacceptable toxic events, or withdrawal of consent

Efficacy (n = 646)

	Elotuzumab Group (n = 321)	Control Group (n = 325)	
Progression-free survival at 1 year*	68%	57%	
Progression-free survival at 2 year*	41%	27%	
Median progression-free survival*	19.4 months	14.9 months	HR 0.70 (95% CI 0.57–0.85; P <0.001)
Overall response rate†	79%	66%	OR 1.9 (95% CI 1.4–2.8; P <0.001)

*Progression and response were determined through blinded review of tumor assessments by an independent review committee
†Overall response rate was the proportion of patients who experienced at least a partial response according to the International Myeloma Working Group Uniform Response Criteria
Note: median follow-up time was 24.5 months

Adverse Events (n = 635)

	Elotuzumab Group (n = 318)		Control Group (n = 317)	
	Grade 1–2 (%)*	Grade 3–4 (%)*	Grade 1–2 (%)*	Grade 3–4 (%)*
Lymphocytopenia	23	77	50	49
Anemia	77	19	74	21
Thrombocytopenia	64	19	57	20
Neutropenia	48	34	45	44
Fatigue	38	8	31	8
Diarrhea	42	5	32	4
Pyrexia	35	3	22	3
Constipation	34	1	27	<1
Cough	31	<1	18	0
Muscle spasms	30	<1	26	<1
Back pain	23	5	24	4
Peripheral edema	25	1	22	<1
Nasopharyngitis	25	0	19	0
Insomnia	21	2	23	3

*According to the National Cancer Institute Common Terminology Criteria for Adverse Events, version 3.0
Note: adverse events that occurred in ≥25% of patients in either cohort are included in the table. In each study group, 2% of patients died owing to adverse events (the most common cause was infection)

Therapy Monitoring

1. CBC with differential, liver function tests, serum creatinine, and serum glucose prior to the start of each cycle, weekly during cycles 1–2, and every 2 weeks during cycles 3 and beyond
2. With abdominal pain, check serum amylase/lipase
3. Ensure adequate hydration of patients to reduce the risk of renal toxicity
4. Monitor patients for development of infections and treat promptly
5. In a patient who is a potential candidate for future auto-HSCT, consider mobilization and collection of autologous stem cells within the first 4 cycles of lenalidomide
6. Monitor thyroid function
7. Monitor for infusion-related reaction symptoms frequently during the elotuzumab infusion; check vital signs frequently during infusion and at least prior to each scheduled rate increase

Note: elotuzumab, a humanized IgG1 kappa monoclonal antibody, may be detected by serum protein electrophoresis and immunofixation assays routinely used to monitor endogenous M-protein. Thus, elotuzumab may interfere with disease monitoring in patients with plasma cell neoplasms that produce an IgG kappa M-protein

Lenalidomide notes:
• Higher incidences of second primary malignancies were observed in controlled trials of patients with multiple myeloma receiving lenalidomide. While no routine monitoring is indicated, awareness of this potential complication is necessary
• A decrease in the number of CD34+ cells collected after treatment has been reported in patients who have received >4 cycles of lenalidomide. In patients who may undergo transplant, consider early referral to transplant center
• Because of the embryo-fetal risk, lenalidomide is available only through a restricted program under a Risk Evaluation and Mitigation Strategy (REMS), the REVLIMID REMS program

SUBSEQUENT THERAPY

MULTIPLE MYELOMA REGIMEN: ELOTUZUMAB + POMALIDOMIDE + DEXAMETHASONE

Dimopoulos MA et al. N Engl J Med 2018;379:1811–1822
Protocol for: Dimopoulos MA et al. N Engl J Med 2018;379:1811–1822
Supplementary appendix to: Dimopoulos MA et al. N Engl J Med 2018;379:1811–1822
EMPLICITI (elotuzumab) prescribing information. Princeton, NJ: Bristol-Myers Squibb Company; October 2019

All cycles:
Pomalidomide 4 mg per dose; administer orally, once daily, without regard to food, for 21 consecutive days on days 1–21, followed by 7 days without treatment, every 28 days until disease progression (total dose/4-week cycle = 84 mg)
Notes:
- Patients who delay taking pomalidomide at a regularly scheduled time may take a missed dose if the interval remaining before the next regularly scheduled dose is ≥12 hours
- Do not break, chew, or open pomalidomide capsules
- Women of childbearing potential must not become pregnant while taking pomalidomide, and for at least 4 weeks following the last dose, due to the risk of severe birth defects. Either abstinence from heterosexual contact must be practiced or at least 2 forms of reliable birth control must be utilized
- Men taking pomalidomide must wear a synthetic or latex condom during sexual contact with a woman of childbearing potential, and must avoid sperm donation during pomalidomide therapy and for at least 4 weeks after discontinuation
- Pomalidomide exposure is reduced in smokers; encourage patients to quit smoking during pomalidomide treatment
- If possible, avoid concomitant use of strong CYP1A2 inhibitors (eg, fluvoxamine, ciprofloxacin). If patients must receive a strong CYP1A2 inhibitor concomitantly, reduce the pomalidomide dose by approximately 50%. If coadministration of the strong inhibitor is discontinued, the pomalidomide dose should be returned to the dose used prior to initiation of a strong CYP1A2 inhibitor

Cycles 1–2:
Premedications for Elotuzumab:
Acetaminophen 650–1000 mg; administer orally 45–90 minutes prior to each elotuzumab dose for 4 doses on days 1, 8, 15, and 22, every 28 days for 2 cycles (cycles 1–2)
Diphenhydramine 25–50 mg; administer orally or intravenously 45–90 minutes prior to each elotuzumab dose for 4 doses on days 1, 8, 15, and 22, every 28 days for 2 cycles (cycles 1–2)
Ranitidine 50 mg (or an equivalent histamine receptor [H$_2$]–subtype antagonist); administer intravenously (or an equivalent dosage, ie, ranitidine 150 mg, administered orally) 45–90 minutes prior to each elotuzumab dose for 4 doses on days 1, 8, 15, and 22, every 28 days for 2 cycles (cycles 1–2)
Dexamethasone 8 mg; administer intravenously 45–90 minutes prior to each elotuzumab dose for 4 doses on days 1, 8, 15, and 22, every 28 days for 2 cycles (cycles 1–2)
Dexamethasone (age >75 years, 8 mg per dose; age ≤75 years, 24 mg per dose); administer orally between 3 and 24 hours prior to each elotuzumab dose for 4 doses on days 1, 8, 15, and 22, every 28 days for 2 cycles (cycles 1–2) (total dosage including oral and intravenous formulations/4-week cycle during cycles 1–2 = 128 mg [age ≤75 years] or 64 mg [age >75 years])

Elotuzumab 10 mg/kg per dose; administer intravenously in a volume of 0.9% sodium chloride injection (0.9% NS) or 5% dextrose injection (D5W) not to exceed 5 mL/kg body weight and also sufficient to produce a final concentration between 1 mg/mL and 6 mg/mL, for 4 doses on days 1, 8, 15, and 22, every 28 days for 2 cycles (cycles 1–2) (total dosage/4-week cycle during cycles 1–2 = 40 mg/kg)
- Refer to table titled "Elotuzumab Infusion Instructions"

Cycles 3 and beyond:
Premedications for Elotuzumab:
Acetaminophen 650–1000 mg; administer orally 45–90 minutes prior to each elotuzumab dose for 1 dose on day 1, every 28 days, until disease progression (cycle 3 and beyond)
Diphenhydramine 25–50 mg; administer orally or intravenously 45–90 minutes prior to each elotuzumab dose for 1 dose on day 1, every 28 days, until disease progression (cycle 3 and beyond)
Ranitidine 50 mg (or an equivalent histamine receptor [H$_2$]–subtype antagonist); administer intravenously (or an equivalent dosage, ie, ranitidine 150 mg, administered orally) 45–90 minutes prior to each elotuzumab dose for 1 dose on day 1, every 28 days, until disease progression (cycle 3 and beyond)
Dexamethasone 8 mg; administer intravenously 45–90 minutes prior to each elotuzumab dose for 1 dose on day 1, every 28 days, until disease progression (cycle 3 and beyond)
Dexamethasone (age >75 years, 8 mg per dose; age ≤75 years, 24 mg per dose); administer orally between 3 and 24 hours prior to each elotuzumab dose for 1 dose on day 1, every 28 days, until disease progression (cycle 3 and beyond)

Elotuzumab 20 mg/kg per dose; administer intravenously in a volume of 0.9% NS or D5W not to exceed 5 mL/kg body weight and also sufficient to produce a final concentration between 1 mg/mL and 6 mg/mL, for 1 dose on day 1, every 28 days, until disease progression (cycle 3 and beyond) (total dosage/4-week cycle during cycle 3 and beyond = 20 mg/kg)
- Refer to table titled "Elotuzumab Infusion Instructions"

(continued)

(continued)

Dexamethasone (age >75 years, 20 mg per dose; age ≤75 years, 40 mg per dose); administer orally for 3 doses on days 8, 15, and 22 every 28 days, until disease progression (cycle 3 and beyond) (total dexamethasone dosage including day 1 elotuzumab premedication/4-week cycle during cycle 3 and beyond = 152 mg [age ≤75 years] or 76 mg [age >75 years])

Elotuzumab Infusion Instructions

Elotuzumab 10 mg/kg	Cycle 1, day 1 only	Infuse initially at 0.5 mL/min (30 mL/hour) for the first 30 minutes. If tolerated, increase to 1 mL/min (60 mL/hour) for 30 minutes. If tolerated, increase to 2 mL/min (120 mL/hour) for the remainder of the infusion
	Cycle 1, day 8 only	Infuse initially at 3 mL/min (180 mL/hour) for the first 30 minutes. If tolerated, increase to 4 mL/min (240 mL/hour) for the remainder of the infusion
	Cycle 1, days 15 and 22 *and* cycle 2, days 1, 8, 15, and 22	Infuse at 5 mL/min (300 mL/hour) for the entire infusion
Elotuzumab 20 mg/kg	Cycle 3, day 1 only	Infuse at 3 mL/min (180 mL/hour) for the first 30 minutes. If tolerated, increase to 4 mL/min (240 mL/hour) for the remainder of the infusion
	Cycle 4 and beyond, day 1	Infuse at 5 mL/min (300 mL/hour) for the entire infusion

Notes:
- Elotuzumab must be prepared in an infusion bag composed of either polyvinyl chloride or polyolefin
- Administer elotuzumab through an administration set that contains a sterile, nonpyrogenic, low-protein-binding, in-line filter with pore size within the range of 0.2–1.2 μm
- **Elotuzumab can cause severe infusion-related reactions**
  - Symptoms may include fever, chills, hypertension or hypotension, and bradycardia. The incidence of all-grade infusion-related reactions in the ELOQUENT-3 study was 5%; all reactions were Grade 1 or 2, and all occurred during the first cycle. Refer to the Treatment Modifications section for management of infusion-related reactions

Supportive Care
Antiemetic prophylaxis
Emetogenic potential is **MINIMAL**
See Chapter 42 for antiemetic recommendations

Hematopoietic growth factor (CSF) prophylaxis
Primary prophylaxis is **NOT** *indicated*
See Chapter 43 for more information

Antimicrobial prophylaxis
Risk of fever and neutropenia is **INTERMEDIATE**
Antimicrobial primary prophylaxis to be considered:
- Antibacterial—consider a fluoroquinolone during periods of prolonged neutropenia (ANC <500/mm³ for ≥7 days) or no prophylaxis; *P. jirovecii* prophylaxis is recommended (eg, cotrimoxazole)
- Antifungal—consider fluconazole during periods of prolonged neutropenia (ANC <500/mm³ for ≥7 days) or no prophylaxis
- Antiviral—antiherpes antivirals (eg, acyclovir, famciclovir, valacyclovir)

Bisphosphonates
All patients receiving primary therapy for symptomatic multiple myeloma should receive a bisphosphonate adjunctively.
Steroid-associated gastritis
Add a proton pump inhibitor or H₂-receptor antagonist during dexamethasone use to prevent gastritis and duodenitis

Thromboprophylaxis
Risk assessment and recommendations for VTE prophylaxis in patients with multiple myeloma with individual or myeloma-related risk factors, or risk factors related to treatment

(continued)

(*continued*)

Individual risk factors • Obesity (BMI ≥30 kg/m²) • H/O VTE • CVC or pacemaker • Comorbid pathologies 　▪ Cardiac disease 　▪ Chronic renal disease 　▪ Diabetes 　▪ Acute infection 　▪ Immobilization • Surgery 　▪ General surgery 　▪ Any anesthesia 　▪ Trauma • Medications 　▪ Erythropoietin (epoetin alfa, darbepoetin) 　▪ Estrogenic compounds 　▪ Bevacizumab • Clotting disorders 　▪ Thrombophilia **Myeloma-related risk factors** • Diagnosis of multiple myeloma • Hyperviscosity	≤1 Individual or myeloma-related risk factor present: • **Aspirin** 81–325 mg daily ≥2 Individual or myeloma-related risk factors present: • **LMWH,** * equivalent to enoxaparin sodium 40 mg/day *or* **dalteparin sodium** 5000 IU/day; administer subcutaneously, *or* • **Warfarin**, targeting an INR = 2–3
Concomitant treatment-related risk factors Thalidomide or lenalidomide in combination with: • High-dose dexamethasone (≥480 mg/month) • Doxorubicin • Multiagent chemotherapy	• **LMWH,** * equivalent to enoxaparin sodium 40 mg/day *or* **dalteparin sodium** 5000 IU/day; administer subcutaneously, *or* • **Warfarin**, targeting an INR = 2–3

*LMWHs should be used with caution in individuals with impaired renal function (creatinine clearance <30 mL/min). Refer to product labeling for information about doses and administration schedules in renally impaired patients, and guidance for monitoring anti-Factor Xa concentrations

Abbreviations: CVC, central venous catheter; INR, international normalized ratio; LMWH, low-molecular-weight heparin; VTE, venous thromboembolic disease

References: Geerts WH et al. Chest 2008;133(6 Suppl):381S–453S
National Comprehensive Cancer Network. Multiple Myeloma, V.1.2014. (Accessed October 8, 2013, at http://www.nccn.org)
National Comprehensive Cancer Network. Venous Thromboembolic Disease, V.2.2013. (Accessed October 8, 2013, at http://www.nccn.org)
Palumbo A et al. Leukemia 2008;22:414–423

Treatment Modifications

ELOTUZUMAB TREATMENT MODIFICATIONS

Elotuzumab Dose Levels	
Starting dose	10 mg/kg (cycles 1–2) or 20 mg/kg (cycles 3 and beyond) (No dose reduction is allowed)
Adverse event	**Treatment Modification**
G1 infusion-related reaction	Continue elotuzumab infusion and provide supportive care. Monitor vital signs every 30 minutes during the infusion and for 2 hours after infusion completion

(*continued*)

Treatment Modifications (continued)

G2–4 infusion-related reactions	Interrupt elotuzumab infusion and provide supportive care. Consider permanent discontinuation of elotuzumab and emergency care for severe reactions. Monitor vital signs every 30 minutes during the infusion and for 2 hours after infusion completion. Upon resolution to G ≤1, resume elotuzumab infusion at 0.5 mL/min (30 mL/hour) and gradually increase the infusion rate every 30 minutes, as tolerated, in increments of 0.5 mL/min (30 mL/hour) until the rate at which the infusion-related reaction occurred is reached. In the absence of a recurrent infusion-related reaction, continue the standard dose escalation regimen as described in the therapy section. If the infusion-related reaction recurs, discontinue the remainder of the elotuzumab infusion for that day
Discontinuation of dexamethasone	Base decision to continue elotuzumab on clinical judgment (ie, risk of hypersensitivity)
G ≥3 elevation of liver enzymes	Stop elotuzumab. After return to baseline values, continuation of treatment may be considered

POMALIDOMIDE TREATMENT MODIFICATIONS

Note: because of the embryo-fetal risk, pomalidomide is available only through a restricted program under a Risk Evaluation and Mitigation Strategy (REMS) called POMALYST REMS

Pomalidomide Dose Levels

Dose level 1 (starting dose)	4 mg
Dose level −1	3 mg
Dose level −2	2 mg
Dose level −3	1 mg

Adverse Event	Treatment Modification
First occurrence of ANC <500/mm³ and/or platelet count between 25,000/mm³ and 50,000/mm³ at start of a new cycle	Withhold start of cycle until ANC ≥500/mm³ and platelet count ≥50,000/mm³, then resume pomalidomide at the same dose
Recurrence of ANC <500/mm³ or platelet count between 25,000/mm³ and 50,000/mm³ at start of a subsequent cycle	Withhold start of cycle until ANC ≥500/mm³ and platelet count ≥50,000/mm³, and then resume pomalidomide reduced by 1 mg/dose
Febrile neutropenia (fever ≥38.5°C and ANC <500/mm³) or severe infection during a cycle	Withhold pomalidomide. When ANC ≥500/mm³ and infection adequately controlled, resume pomalidomide reduced by 2 mg/dose
Platelet count <25,000/mm³ at start of a new cycle	Withhold start of cycle until ANC ≥500/mm³ and platelet count ≥50,000/mm³, then resume pomalidomide reduced by 1 mg/dose
Any recurrence of platelet count <25,000/mm³ at start of a subsequent cycle	Withhold start of cycle until ANC ≥500/mm³ and platelet count ≥50,000/mm³, then resume pomalidomide reduced by 1 mg/dose
ANC <500/mm³ or platelet count <25,000/mm³ occurring *within* a pomalidomide cycle	Hold pomalidomide until ANC >500/mm³ and platelet count >50,000/mm³, then resume pomalidomide reduced by 1 mg/dose
ANC <500/mm³ or platelet count <25,000/mm³ at any time while on a pomalidomide dose of 1 mg daily	Discontinue pomalidomide
Any other G3/4 adverse event at start of a new cycle or at any time during a cycle	Withhold pomalidomide and restart treatment reduced by 1 mg/dose less than the previous dose when toxicity has resolved to G ≤2 at the physician's discretion
Patient considered to be at higher risk of deep venous thrombosis (DVT) or pulmonary embolism (PE)	Consider anticoagulation prophylaxis after an assessment of each patient's underlying risk factors

Note: pomalidomide is a thalidomide analogue and is contraindicated in pregnancy. Thalidomide is a known human teratogen that causes severe life-threatening birth defects. For females of reproductive potential, exclude pregnancy before start of treatment and prevent pregnancy during treatment by the use of two reliable methods of contraception

(continued)

Treatment Modifications (*continued*)

DEXAMETHASONE TREATMENT MODIFICATIONS

Dose Level	Dexamethasone Doses During Weeks With Elotuzumab			Dexamethasone Doses During Weeks Without Elotuzumab		
	Oral Dose		Intravenous Dose	Oral Dose		Intravenous Dose
	Age ≤75 Years	Age >75 Years		Age ≤75 Years	Age >75 Years	
Starting dose	28 mg	8 mg	8 mg	40 mg	20 mg	Not applicable
Dose level −1	12 mg	2 mg	8 mg	20 mg	12 mg	
Dose level −2	0 mg	0 mg	8 mg	12 mg	8 mg	

Note: if the dexamethasone dose is delayed or discontinued during a week in which elotuzumab is administered, then base the decision on whether to administer elotuzumab on clinical judgement (ie, risk of hypersensitivity)

Adverse Event	Treatment Modification
G1/2 dyspepsia (moderate symptoms; medical intervention indicated; limiting instrumental ADL), gastric or duodenal ulcer, or gastritis	Continue dexamethasone at the same dose. Treat with therapeutic doses of an H_2-receptor antagonist or proton pump inhibitor. If symptoms persist, then reduce the dexamethasone dose by one level
G ≥3 dyspepsia, gastric or duodenal ulcer, or gastritis (surgery or hospitalization indicated)	Withhold dexamethasone until symptoms return to baseline. Resume dexamethasone reduced by one dose level along with concurrent treatment with therapeutic doses of an H_2-receptor antagonist or proton pump inhibitor. If symptoms recur, then permanently discontinue dexamethasone
Acute pancreatitis	Permanently discontinue dexamethasone
G ≥3 edema	Withhold dexamethasone until symptoms return to baseline. Consider treatment with diuretics. Resume dexamethasone reduced by one dose level. If edema persists, reduce by another dose level. Discontinue dexamethasone permanently if symptoms persist despite two prior dose reductions
G ≥2 mood alteration (moderate mood alteration) or confusion (moderate disorientation; limiting instrumental ADL)	Withhold dexamethasone until symptoms return to baseline. Resume dexamethasone reduced by one dose level. If symptoms persist, reduce by another dose level
G ≥2 muscle weakness (symptomatic; evident on physical exam; limiting instrumental ADL)	Withhold dexamethasone until symptoms return to baseline. Resume dexamethasone reduced by one dose level. If weakness persists, reduce by another dose level. If weakness still persists, then permanently discontinue dexamethasone
G ≥3 hyperglycemia (insulin therapy initiated; hospitalization indicated)	Withhold dexamethasone until blood glucose is ≤250 mg/dL. Treat with insulin or other hypoglycemic agents as clinically appropriate and then resume dexamethasone at the same dose. If hyperglycemia is uncontrolled despite above measures, decrease dexamethasone by one dose level
Other G ≥2 nonhematologic toxicity attributable to dexamethasone including severe irritability, insomnia, or oral candidiasis	Withhold dexamethasone until toxicity resolves to G ≤1, then resume at a lower dose. Consider reduction by one dose level for G2/G3 toxicity, and by two dose levels for G4 or recurrent G3 toxicity

If the dose of one drug in the regimen (ie, pomalidomide, dexamethasone, or elotuzumab) is delayed, interrupted, or discontinued, the treatment with the other drugs may continue as scheduled

Patient Population Studied

ELOQUENT-3 was a randomized, open-label, phase 2 trial that included 117 adult patients with refractory or relapsed and refractory multiple myeloma and evaluated treatment with elotuzumab plus pomalidomide plus dexamethasone. Patients were eligible for the trial if they had received at least 2 prior lines of therapy for multiple myeloma, which must have included at least 2 consecutive cycles of lenalidomide and a proteasome inhibitor alone or in combination, if they had documented refractory or relapsed and refractory disease, if they were refractory to their last treatment (defined as progression during or within 60 days of treatment), if they had measurable disease, and if they had an ECOG performance status of ≤2. Patients were excluded if their only evidence of plasma cell dyscrasia was solitary bone or extramedullary plasmacytoma, if they had monoclonal gammopathy of undetermined significance, smoldering multiple myeloma, amyloidosis, Waldenström macroglobulinemia, POEMS syndrome, or active plasma cell leukemia, if they had any uncontrolled or severe cardiovascular or pulmonary disease, or active infection requiring parenteral anti-infective treatment, if they couldn't tolerate antithrombotic prophylaxis while in the trial, if they had Grade ≥ 2 peripheral neuropathy, active hepatitis A, B, or C, HIV, malabsorptive GI disease, prior concurrent malignancy, prior treatment with pomalidomide, or treatment with melphalan or monoclonal antibodies within 6 weeks of the first dose of trial drug, or if they had inadequate organ function

Efficacy (n = 117)

Efficacy Variable	Elotuzumab + Pomalidomide + Dexamethasone (n = 60)	Pomalidomide + Dexamethasone (n = 57)	Between-group Comparison
Investigator-assessed PFS*			
Median PFS—months (95% CI)	10.3 (5.6-NR)	4.7 (2.8–7.2)	HR 0.54 (95% CI, 0.34–0.86); P = 0.008*
IRC-assessed PFS			
Median PFS—months (95% CI)	10.3 (6.5-NR)	4.7 (2.8–7.6)	HR 0.51 (95% CI, 0.32–0.82)
OS†			
Median OS—months (95% CI)	Not reported†	Not reported†	HR 0.62 (95% CI, 0.30–1.28)
TTR and DOR			
Median TTR—months (95% CI)	2.0	1.9	
Median DOR—months (95% CI)	NR (8.3–NR)	8.3 (4.6–NR)	
Investigator-assessed Response‡			
ORR—n/N (%) (95% CI)	32/60 (53) (40–66)	15/57 (26) (16–40)	OR 3.25 (95% CI, 1.49–7.11)
Stringent CR rate—n/N (%)	2/60 (3)	0/57 (0)	
CR rate—n/N (%)	3/60 (5)	1/57 (2)	
VGPR rate—n/N (%)	7/60 (12)	4/57 (7)	
VGPR or better rate—n/N (%)	12/60 (20)	5/57 (9)	
PR rate—n/N (%)	20/60 (33)	10/57 (18)	
Minor response rate—n/N (%)‡	4/60 (7)	8/57 (14)	
Stable disease rate—n/N (%)	13/60 (22)	16/57 (28)	
Progressive disease—n/N (%)	7/60 (12)	9/57 (16)	
Response could not be measured or was not reported—n/N (%)	4/60 (7)	9/57 (16)	
IRC-assessed Response			
ORR—n/N (%) (95% CI)	35/60 (58) (45–71)	14/57 (25) (14–38)	OR 4.62 (95% CI, 2.05–10.43)

A subgroup analysis showed that there was benefit of elotuzumab treatment across all groups evaluated

*P value was calculated using a two-sided stratified log-rank test

†Median OS was not reached in either group. At time of analysis, the data on OS were immature. There were 13 deaths in the elotuzumab group and 18 in the control group; 78 deaths were required for final analysis of OS. Disease progression was the main cause of death in both groups (13% of treated patients in the elotuzumab group and 25% of treated patients in the control group)

‡Response was assessed according to a modified version of the International Myeloma Working Group criteria, except for minor (minimal) response, which was derived from the European Society for Blood and Marrow Transplantation criteria. Complete descriptions of the characterizations were reported in the supplementary appendix. Estimated ORs and P values for between-group comparisons of ORR were performed between groups using the Cochran-Mantel-Haenszel X^2 test

Note: all analyses were performed in the intention-to-treat population, which included all patients randomized, regardless of drug reception. OS, PFS, TTR, and DOR were estimated using Kaplan-Meier methods. Hours for PFS and OS were estimated using a stratified Cox proportional-hazards model, with treatment as the single covariate. TTR and DOR were exploratory end points. All data included in the table were published in Dimopoulos et al, 2018, and its supplementary appendix. Data in this paper were collected with a minimum follow-up time of 9.1 months

CI, confidence interval; HR, hazard ratio; IRC, independent review committee; NR, not reached; PFS, progression-free survival; OS, overall survival; OR, odds ratio; ORR, objective response rate; CR, complete response; VGPR, very good partial response; PR, partial response; TTR, time to response; DOR, duration of response

Adverse Events (n = 115)

Event	Elotuzumab + Pomalidomide + Dexamethasone (n = 60)		Pomalidomide + Dexamethasone (n = 55)	
	Any Grade (%)	Grade 3 or 4 (%)	Any Grade (%)	Grade 3 or 4 (%)
Any adverse event	97	57	95	60
Constipation	22	2	11	0
Hyperglycemia	20	8	15	7
Diarrhea	18	0	9	0
Fatigue	15	0	16	4
Bone pain	15	3	9	0
Dyspnea	15	3	7	2
Pyrexia	13	0	25	0
Insomnia	13	2	11	0
Peripheral edema	13	0	7	0
Muscle spasms	13	0	5	0
Asthenia	12	2	9	4
Rash	10	0	11	2
Hypokalemia	7	0	13	5
Increased blood creatinine	5	0	11	4
Malignant neoplasm progression	2	2	11	4
Any hematologic adverse event	52	38	55	42
Anemia	25	10	36	20
Neutropenia	23	13	31	27
Thrombocytopenia	15	8	18	5
Lymphopenia	10	8	2	2

Adverse events of any cause were included in the table if they were reported in ≥ 10% of patients in either treatment group from the time of the first dose until 60 days after the last dose. Adverse events were graded according to the National Cancer Institute Common Terminology Criteria for Adverse Events (NCI CTCAE) v3.0 in all patients who received at least one dose of study drug treatment. Pomalidomide dose reduction occurred in 20% of patients in each group, and elotuzumab dose delays occurred in 33% of patients in the elotuzumab group. Serious adverse events occurred in 53% of patients in the elotuzumab group and 55% of patients in the control group. The most common treatment-related adverse events were neutropenia (18% in the elotuzumab group, 20% in the control group), hyperglycemia (18% vs 11%), and anemia (10% vs 15%). The complete list of treatment-related adverse events was reported in the supplementary appendix. Adverse events that led to discontinuation were reported in 18% and 24% of patients, respectively. Adverse events that led to death were reported in 8% of patients in the elotuzumab group (3 from infection, and 1 each from cardiac failure and general physical health deterioration) and 15% of patients in the control group (1 from infection, 1 from multiorgan failure and infection, 1 from myocardial infarction, one from plasma-cell myeloma, and 4 from malignant neoplasm progression). No deaths were considered to be caused by trial medication by the investigators. Infusion reactions occurred very infrequently, all were Grade 1 or 2, and all resolved

(*continued*)

Adverse Events (n = 115) (continued)

	Adverse Events of Special Interest (n = 115)			
Event	Elotuzumab + Pomalidomide + Dexamethasone (n = 60)		Pomalidomide + Dexamethasone (n = 55)	
	Any Grade (%)	Grade 3 or 4 (%)	Any Grade (%)	Grade 3 or 4 (%)
Any infection	65	13	65	22
Nasopharyngitis	17	0	15	0
Respiratory tract infection	17	0	9	2
Upper respiratory tract infection	12	0	15	2
Bronchitis	10	2	9	2
Pneumonia	7	5	11	9
Herpes zoster infection	5	0	2	0
Vascular disorders	13	3	9	0
Cardiac disorders	12	7	11	4
Neoplasms*	2	2	22	11

*Includes malignant, benign, and unspecified neoplasms. Grade 5 neoplasms were reported in 9% of patients in the control group and no patients in the elotuzumab group

Therapy Monitoring

1. CBC with differential, liver function tests, BUN, serum creatinine, and serum glucose prior to the start of each cycle
2. With abdominal pain, check serum amylase/lipase
3. Ensure adequate hydration of patients to reduce the risk of renal toxicity
4. Monitor patients for development of infections and treat promptly
5. Monitor for infusion-related reaction symptoms frequently during the elotuzumab infusion; check vital signs frequently during infusion and at least prior to each scheduled rate increase

Note:
• elotuzumab, a humanized IgG1 kappa monoclonal antibody, may be detected by serum protein electrophoresis and immunofixation assays routinely used to monitor endogenous M-protein. Thus, elotuzumab may interfere with disease monitoring in patients with plasma cell neoplasms that produce an IgG kappa M-protein

Pomalidomide note:
• Because of the embryo-fetal risk, pomalidomide is available only through a restricted program under a Risk Evaluation and Mitigation Strategy (REMS), the POMALYST REMS program

SUBSEQUENT THERAPY

MULTIPLE MYELOMA REGIMEN: CARFILZOMIB + DEXAMETHASONE

Dimopoulos MA et al. Lancet Oncol 2016;17:27–38
Supplementary appendix to: Dimopoulos MA et al. Lancet Oncol 2016;17:27–38

Hydration with carfilzomib: During cycle 1, days 1, 2, 8, 9, 15, and 16, administer intravenously 250–500 mL 0.9% sodium chloride injection (0.9% NS) before each carfilzomib dose, *and* an additional 250–500 mL of 0.9% NS intravenously after carfilzomib. During repeated treatments, continue intravenous hydration as needed. Encourage oral hydration

Premedication for carfilzomib: During cycle 1, days 1, 2, 8, 9, 15, and 16, administer dexamethasone 20 mg (as specified in the regimen) orally or intravenously between 0.5 and 4 hours before each carfilzomib dose. If an infusion reaction occurs in subsequent cycles, reinstitute dexamethasone premedication

Carfilzomib; intravenously in 50–100 mL 5% dextrose injection (D5W) over 30 minutes for 6 doses, on days 1, 2, 8, 9, 15, and 16, every 28 days, until disease progression, *as follows:*

Cycle 1 days 1 and 2	20 mg/m² per dose	Total dosage in cycle 1= 264 mg/m²
Cycle 1 days 8, 9, 15, and 16	56 mg/m² per dose	
Cycle 2 and thereafter, days 1, 2, 8, 9, 15, and 16	56 mg/m² per dose	Total dosage per cycle (cycle 2 and thereafter) = 336 mg/m²

Carfilzomib Dose Adjustments

BSA >2.2 m²	Use BSA of 2.2 m² to calculate carfilzomib
• Bilirubin 1–1.5× ULN and any AST, *or* • Bilirubin 1.5–3× *ULN and any AST, or* • Bilirubin ≤ ULN and AST > ULN	Reduce initial carfilzomib dose by 25%
Bilirubin >3× ULN	No dose recommendation available
Creatinine clearance <15 mL/minute	Full dose carfilzomib at discretion of physician
End-stage renal disease on hemodialysis	No dose adjustment necessary; administer carfilzomib after hemodialysis

Dexamethasone 20 mg/dose; administer orally or intravenously once daily for 8 doses on days 1, 2, 8, 9, 15, 16, 22, and 23, every 28 days, until disease progression (total dose/cycle = 160 mg)
Note: during cycle 1, administer dexamethasone between 0.5 and 4 hours before each carfilzomib dose as described in the premedication section above

Supportive Care
Antiemetic prophylaxis
Emetogenic potential is **LOW**
See Chapter 42 for antiemetic recommendations

Hematopoietic growth factor (CSF) prophylaxis
Primary prophylaxis is **NOT** indicated
See Chapter 43 for more information

Antimicrobial prophylaxis
Risk of fever and neutropenia is **INTERMEDIATE**
   Antimicrobial primary prophylaxis to be considered:
   • Antibacterial—consider a fluoroquinolone during periods of neutropenia, or no prophylaxis; *P. jirovecii* prophylaxis is recommended (eg, cotrimoxazole)
   • Antifungal—consider fluconazole during periods of neutropenia
   • Antiviral—antiherpes antivirals (eg, acyclovir, famciclovir, valacyclovir)

(continued)

Treatment Modifications

CARFILZOMIB

Carfilzomib Dose Levels

Starting dose	56 mg/m²/dose
Dose level −1	45 mg/m²/dose
Dose level −2	36 mg/m²/dose
Dose level −3	27 mg/m²/dose
Dose level −4	Discontinue carfilzomib*

Hematologic Toxicity

G3/4 neutropenia (<1000/mm³) Febrile neutropenia (ANC <1000/mm³ with a single temperature of >38.3°C [101°F] or a sustained temperature of ≥38°C [100.4°F] for >1 hour) G4 thrombocytopenia (<25,000/mm³) G3/4 thrombocytopenia (<50,000/mm³) associated with bleeding	• Hold carfilzomib dosing for up to 21 days to resolve toxicity and then restart at the same dosage, or reduce the carfilzomib dosage by 1 dose level • If recover to G2 neutropenia or G3 thrombocytopenia, reduce carfilzomib dosage by 1 dose level • If tolerated, the reduced dose may be escalated to the previous dose level
Confirmed TTP or HUS	Permanently discontinue carfilzomib. (The safety of reinitiating carfilzomib in patients previously experiencing TTP or HUS is unknown)*

Nonhematologic Toxicity

G3/4 cardiac toxicity New onset or worsening: • Congestive heart failure • Decreased left ventricular function • Myocardial ischemia Pulmonary hypertension G3/4 pulmonary complications	Hold carfilzomib dosing for up to 21 days to resolve toxicity to G1 or to baseline and then, at the discretion of the medically responsible health care provider, consider either permanently discontinuing carfilzomib or restarting carfilzomib at 1 lower dose level. If tolerated, the reduced dosage may be escalated to the previous dose level

(continued)

(continued)

Steroid-associated gastritis
Add a proton pump inhibitor or H$_2$-receptor antagonist during dexamethasone use to prevent gastritis and duodenitis

Diarrhea management
Loperamide or **diphenoxylate hydrochloride** 2.5 mg with **atropine sulfate** 0.025 mg (eg, Lomotil)

Bisphosphonates
All patients receiving primary therapy for symptomatic multiple myeloma should receive a bisphosphonate adjunctively.

Thromboprophylaxis
Risk assessment and recommendations for VTE prophylaxis in patients with multiple myeloma with individual or myeloma-related risk factors, or risk factors related to treatment

Individual risk factors	

• Obesity (BMI ≥30 kg/m²)
• H/O VTE
• CVC or pacemaker
• Comorbid pathologies
  ▪ Cardiac disease
  ▪ Chronic renal disease
  ▪ Diabetes
  ▪ Acute infection
  ▪ Immobilization
• Surgery
  ▪ General surgery
  ▪ Any anesthesia
  ▪ Trauma
• Medications
  ▪ Erythropoietin (epoetin alfa, darbepoetin)
  ▪ Estrogenic compounds
  ▪ Bevacizumab
• Clotting disorders
  ▪ Thrombophilia
Myeloma-related risk factors
• Diagnosis of multiple myeloma
• Hyperviscosity
	≤1 Individual or myeloma-related risk factor present:
	• **Aspirin** 81–325 mg daily
	
	≥2 Individual or myeloma-related risk factors present:
	• **LMWH,*** equivalent to enoxaparin sodium 40 mg/day *or* **dalteparin sodium** 5000 IU/day; administer subcutaneously, *or*
	• **Warfarin,** targeting an INR = 2–3

Concomitant treatment-related risk factors Thalidomide or lenalidomide in combination with: • High-dose dexamethasone (≥480 mg/month) • Doxorubicin • Multiagent chemotherapy	• **LMWH,*** equivalent to enoxaparin sodium 40 mg/day *or* **dalteparin sodium** 5000 IU/day; administer subcutaneously, *or* • **Warfarin,** targeting an INR = 2–3

*LMWHs should be used with caution in individuals with impaired renal function (creatinine clearance <30 mL/min). Refer to product labeling for information about doses and administration schedules in renally impaired patients, and guidance for monitoring anti-Factor Xa concentrations

Abbreviations: CVC, central venous catheter; INR, international normalized ratio; LMWH, low-molecular-weight heparin; VTE, venous thromboembolic disease

References: Geerts WH et al. Chest 2008;133(6 Suppl):381S–453S
National Comprehensive Cancer Network. Multiple Myeloma, V.1.2014. (Accessed October 8, 2013, at http://www.nccn.org)
National Comprehensive Cancer Network. Venous Thromboembolic Disease, V.2.2013. (Accessed October 8, 2013, at http://www.nccn.org)
Palumbo A et al. Leukemia 2008;22:414–423

Treatment Modifications
(continued)

Nonhematologic Toxicity

G3/4 elevation of transaminases, bilirubin, or other liver abnormalities (ALT/AST >5× ULN or bilirubin >3× ULN)	
Serum creatinine ≥2× baseline or CrCl decreased to ≤50% of baseline	If attributable to carfilzomib, hold carfilzomib doses for up to 21 days to resolve toxicity to G1 or to baseline and then restart at the same dosage, or reduce the carfilzomib dosage by 1 dose level. If tolerated, the reduced dosage may be escalated to the previous dose level
G2 neuropathy with pain G3/4 peripheral neuropathy	Hold carfilzomib dosing for up to 21 days to resolve toxicity to G1 or to baseline and then restart at the same dose, or reduce the carfilzomib dosage by 1 dose level. If tolerated, the reduced dosage may be escalated to the previous dose level
Confirmed PRES (posterior reversible encephalopathy syndrome) eg, seizure, headache, lethargy, confusion, blindness, altered consciousness, visual and neurologic disturbances, hypertension	Permanently discontinue carfilzomib. The safety of reinitiating carfilzomib in patients previously experiencing PRES is unknown*
Tumor lysis syndrome (TLS)	Withhold carfilzomib until resolution of TLS, then resume carfilzomib at the same dose.
Other G3/4 nonhematologic toxicities	If attributable to carfilzomib, hold carfilzomib doses for up to 21 days to resolve toxicity to G1 or to baseline and then restart at the same dosage or reduce the carfilzomib dosage by 1 dose level. If tolerated, the reduced dosage may be escalated to the previous dose level

(continued)

Patient Population Studied

The multicenter, randomized, open-label, phase 3 study involved 929 patients with relapsed or refractory multiple myeloma. Eligible patients were aged ≥18 years, with an Eastern Cooperative Oncology Group (ECOG) performance status score ≤2, one to three previous treatments, at least partial response to at least one previous treatment, an absolute neutrophil count $≥1 × 10^9$/L, platelet count $≥50 × 10^9$/L ($≥30 × 10^9$/L if myeloma involvement in the bone marrow was >50%), and creatinine clearance ≥15 mL/min. Patients who had peripheral neuropathy of Grade 2 (with pain) to Grade 4 within the past 14 days, myocardial infarction within the past 4 months, or heart failure (New York Heart Association class III/IV) were not eligible. Half of the patients received carfilzomib intravenously on days 1, 2, 8, 9, 15, and 16 of a 28-day cycle (20 mg/m^2 on days 1 and 2 of the first cycle and then 56 mg/m^2 thereafter), and oral or intravenous dexamethasone 20 mg on days 1, 2, 8, 9, 15, 16, 22 and 23. The other patients received an intravenous bolus or subcutaneous injection of bortezomib 1.3 mg/m^2 on days 1, 4, 8, and 11 of a 21-day cycle, and oral or intravenous dexamethasone 20 mg on days 1, 2, 4, 5, 8, 9, 11, and 12. Cycles were repeated until disease progression, withdrawal of consent, or unacceptable toxic effects

Efficacy (n = 929)

	Carfilzomib + Dexamethasone (n = 464)	Bortezomib + Dexamethasone (n = 465)	
Median progression-free survival	18.7 months	9.4 months	HR 0.53 (95% CI 0.44–0.65; P <0.0001)
Objective response rate*	77%	63%	OR 2.03 (95% CI 1.52–2.72; P <0.0001)
Median duration of response†	21.3 months	10.4 months	
Median time to response†	1.1 months	1.1 months	
Median duration of treatment	39.9 weeks	26.8 weeks	

*Objective response rate was the proportion of patients who experienced a partial or complete response according to the International Myeloma Working Group Uniform Response Criteria
†Determined for those patients who experienced at least a partial response
Note: median follow-up time for the primary analysis (progression-free survival) was 11.9 months in the carfilzomib group and 11.1 months in the bortezomib group

Adverse Events (n = 919)

	Carfilzomib + Dexamethasone (n = 463)		Bortezomib + Dexamethasone (n = 456)	
	Grade 1–2 (%)*	Grade 3–5 (%)*	Grade 1–2 (%)*	Grade 3–5 (%)*
Anemia	25	14	17	10
Diarrhea	27	3	31	7
Fatigue	24	5	21	7
Dyspnea	23	5	11	2
Pyrexia	26	2	13	<1
Insomnia	24	2	24	2
Cough	25	0	14	<1
Hypertension	16	9	6	3

(continued)

Treatment Modifications
(continued)

DEXAMETHASONE

Dexamethasone Dose Levels

Starting dose	20 mg/dose/day
Dose level −1	12 mg/dose/day
Dose level −2	8 mg/dose/day
Dose level −3	4 mg/dose/day
Dose level −4	Discontinue dexamethasone

Adverse Event	Treatment Modification
G1/2 dyspepsia (moderate symptoms; medical intervention indicated; limiting instrumental ADL), gastric or duodenal ulcer, or gastritis	Continue dexamethasone at the same dose. Treat with therapeutic doses of an H_2-receptor antagonist or proton pump inhibitor. If symptoms persist, then reduce the dexamethasone dose by one level
G ≥3 dyspepsia, gastric or duodenal ulcer, or gastritis (surgery or hospitalization indicated)	Withhold dexamethasone until symptoms return to baseline. Resume dexamethasone reduced by one dose level along with concurrent treatment with therapeutic doses of an H_2-receptor antagonist or proton pump inhibitor. If symptoms recur, then permanently discontinue dexamethasone†
Acute pancreatitis	Permanently discontinue dexamethasone†
G ≥3 edema	Withhold dexamethasone until symptoms return to baseline. Consider treatment with diuretics. Resume dexamethasone reduced by one dose level. If edema persists, reduce by another dose level. Discontinue dexamethasone permanently if symptoms persist despite two prior dose reductions†

(continued)

Adverse Events (n = 919) (continued)

	Carfilzomib + Dexamethasone (n = 463)		Bortezomib + Dexamethasone (n = 456)	
	Grade 1–2 (%)*	Grade 3–5 (%)*	Grade 1–2 (%)*	Grade 3–5 (%)*
Peripheral edema	21	<1	16	<1
Thrombocytopenia	12	8	8	9
Asthenia	17	3	13	3
Upper respiratory tract infection	18	2	14	<1
Nausea	18	1	17	<1
Back pain	17	2	13	3
Muscle spasms	18	<1	5	<1
Headache	16	<1	9	<1
Bronchitis	14	2	8	<1
Constipation	14	<1	25	2
Nasopharyngitis	14	0	11	<1
Vomiting	13	1	7	1
Pain in extremity	10	<1	10	<1
Peripheral neuropathy	8	1	21	5
Decreased appetite	8	<1	11	1
Dizziness	8	<1	14	<1
Paresthesia	8	<1	16	<1
Peripheral sensory neuropathy	6	<1	13	1
Neuralgia	1	<1	14	2
Pneumonia	2	7	3	8
Cardiac failure	3	5	1	3
Acute renal failure	4	4	2	3
Ischemic heart disease	<1	2	<1	2
Pulmonary hypertension	<1	<1	0	<1

*According to the National Cancer Institute Common Terminology Criteria for Adverse Events, version 4.03
Note: all adverse Grade 1–2 events that occurred in ≥10% of patients, as well as some additional adverse events of interest, are included in the table. On-study deaths due to adverse events occurred in 4% of the carfilzomib group and 3% of the bortezomib group

Therapy Monitoring

1. CBC with differential, liver function tests, serum electrolytes, and serum glucose prior to each carfilzomib dose
2. Monitor for cardiac complications
3. Monitor for and manage dyspnea immediately
4. With abdominal pain, check serum amylase/lipase
5. Ensure adequate hydration of patients to reduce the risk of renal toxicity and of tumor lysis syndrome
6. Check urinary sediment regularly for the presence of erythrocytes and other signs of urotoxicity
7. Treat all urinary tract infections aggressively

Treatment Modifications
(continued)

Adverse Event	Treatment Modification
G ≥2 mood alteration (moderate mood alteration) or confusion (moderate disorientation; limiting instrumental ADL)	Withhold dexamethasone until symptoms return to baseline. Resume dexamethasone reduced by one dose level. If symptoms persist, reduce by another dose level
G ≥2 muscle weakness (symptomatic; evident on physical exam; limiting instrumental ADL)	Withhold dexamethasone until symptoms return to baseline. Resume dexamethasone reduced by one dose level. If weakness persists, reduce by another dose level. If weakness still persists, then permanently discontinue dexamethasone†
G ≥3 hyperglycemia (insulin therapy initiated; hospitalization indicated)	Withhold dexamethasone until blood glucose is ≤250 mg/dL. Treat with insulin or other hypoglycemic agents as clinically appropriate and then resume dexamethasone at the same dose. If hyperglycemia is uncontrolled despite above measures, decrease dexamethasone by one dose level
Other G ≥2 nonhematologic toxicity attributable to dexamethasone including severe irritability, insomnia, or oral candidiasis	Withhold dexamethasone until toxicity resolves to G ≤1, then resume at a lower dose. Consider reduction by one dose level for G2/G3 toxicity, and by two dose levels for G4 or recurrent G3 toxicity

*If carfilzomib is permanently discontinued, then also consider discontinuing dexamethasone.
†If dexamethasone is permanently discontinued, continued administration of carfilzomib may be considered at the discretion of the treating physician

SUBSEQUENT THERAPY

MULTIPLE MYELOMA REGIMEN: CARFILZOMIB + LENALIDOMIDE + DEXAMETHASONE

Stewart AK et al. N Engl J Med 2015;372:142–152
Supplement to: Stewart AK et al. N Engl J Med 2015;372:142–152
Protocol for: Stewart AK et al. N Engl J Med 2015;372:142–152

Hydration with carfilzomib: During cycle 1, on days 1, 2, 8, 9, 15, and 16, administer intravenously 250–500 mL 0.9% sodium chloride injection (0.9% NS) before each carfilzomib dose, *and* an additional 250–500 mL of 0.9% NS intravenously after carfilzomib. During repeated treatments, continue intravenous hydration as needed. Encourage oral hydration

Premedication for carfilzomib: During cycle 1, on days 1, 8, and 15, administer dexamethasone 40 mg (as specified in the regimen) orally or intravenously between 0.5 and 4 hours before each carfilzomib dose. If an infusion reaction occurs in subsequent cycles, reinstitute dexamethasone premedication

Carfilzomib; intravenously in 50–100 mL 5% dextrose injection (D5W) over 10 minutes, *according to the following schedule:*

Carfilzomib Dose and Schedule According to Cycle (28-Day Cycles)

Cycle 1 (days 1 and 2)	20 mg/m²/dose*	Total dosage/28-days (cycle 1)=148 mg/m²
Cycle 1 (days 8, 9, 15, 16)	27 mg/m²/dose*	
Cycles 2–12 (days 1, 2, 8, 9, 15, 16)	27 mg/m²/dose*	Total dosage/28-days (cycles 2–12)=162 mg/m²
Cycles 13–18 (days 1, 2, 15, 16)†	27 mg/m²/dose*	Total dosage/28-days (cycle 13–18)=108 mg/m²

*According to the U.S. Food and Drug Administration–approved labeling, for patients with a body surface area (BSA) >2.2 m², use a BSA of 2.2 m² for calculating the dose of carfilzomib
†Carfilzomib is discontinued after cycle 18. Lenalidomide and dexamethasone may be continued beyond cycle 18 until disease progression

Carfilzomib Dose Adjustments

BSA >2.2 m²	Use BSA of 2.2 m² to calculate carfilzomib
• Bilirubin 1–1.5× ULN and any AST, *or* • Bilirubin 1.5–3× *ULN and any AST, or* • Bilirubin ≤ ULN and AST > ULN	Reduce initial carfilzomib dose by 25%
Bilirubin >3× ULN	No dose recommendation available
Creatinine clearance <15 mL/minute	Full dose carfilzomib at discretion of physician
End-stage renal disease on hemodialysis	No dose adjustment necessary; administer carfilzomib after hemodialysis

Lenalidomide 25 mg/dose; administer orally, without regard to meals, once daily for 21 consecutive days on days 1–21, followed by 7 days without treatment, every 28 days until disease progression (total dosage/28-day cycle = 525 mg)
• Patients who delay taking a lenalidomide dose at a regularly scheduled time may take the missed dose if the time to the next regularly scheduled dose is >12 hours away
• Consider doses in Treatment Modifications table for dose adjustments for renal function

Dexamethasone 40 mg/dose; administer orally or intravenously once daily for 4 doses on days 1, 8, 15, and 22, every 28 days, until disease progression (total dosage/28-day cycle = 160 mg)
Note: during cycle 1 on day 1, 8 and 15, administer dexamethasone between 0.5 and 4 hours before the carfilzomib dose as described in the premedication section above

Supportive Care
Antiemetic prophylaxis
Emetogenic potential on days with carfilzomib and/or lenalidomide is **LOW**
See Chapter 42 for antiemetic recommendations

Hematopoietic growth factor (CSF) prophylaxis
Primary prophylaxis is **NOT** *indicated*
See Chapter 43 for more information

(continued)

(continued)

Antimicrobial prophylaxis
Risk of fever and neutropenia is **INTERMEDIATE**
   Antimicrobial primary prophylaxis to be considered:
- Antibacterial—consider a fluoroquinolone during periods of neutropenia, or no prophylaxis; *P. jirovecii* prophylaxis is recommended (eg, cotrimoxazole)
- Antifungal—consider fluconazole during periods of neutropenia
- Antiviral—antiherpes antivirals (eg, acyclovir, famciclovir, valacyclovir) is recommended throughout treatment with carfilzomib

Steroid-associated gastritis
Add a proton pump inhibitor or H_2-receptor antagonist during dexamethasone use to prevent gastritis and duodenitis
Diarrhea management
Loperamide or **diphenoxylate hydrochloride** 2.5 mg with **atropine sulfate** 0.025 mg (eg, Lomotil)
Bisphosphonates
All patients receiving primary therapy for symptomatic multiple myeloma should receive a bisphosphonate adjunctively.

Thromboprophylaxis
Risk assessment and recommendations for VTE prophylaxis in patients with multiple myeloma with individual or myeloma-related risk factors, or risk factors related to treatment

Individual risk factors
 • Obesity (BMI ≥30 kg/m²)
 • H/O VTE
 • CVC or pacemaker
 • Comorbid pathologies
   ▪ Cardiac disease
   ▪ Chronic renal disease
   ▪ Diabetes
   ▪ Acute infection
   ▪ Immobilization
 • Surgery
   ▪ General surgery
   ▪ Any anesthesia
   ▪ Trauma
 • Medications
   ▪ Erythropoietin (epoetin alfa, darbepoetin)
   ▪ Estrogenic compounds
   ▪ Bevacizumab
 • Clotting disorders
   ▪ Thrombophilia
 Myeloma-related risk factors
 • Diagnosis of multiple myeloma
 • Hyperviscosity
	≤1 Individual or myeloma-related risk factor present:
	 • **Aspirin** 81–325 mg daily
	
	 ≥2 Individual or myeloma-related risk factors present:
	 • **LMWH,*** equivalent to enoxaparin sodium 40 mg/day *or* **dalteparin sodium** 5000 IU/day; administer subcutaneously, *or*
	 • **Warfarin**, targeting an INR = 2–3

Concomitant treatment-related risk factors Thalidomide or lenalidomide in combination with: • High-dose dexamethasone (≥480 mg/month) • Doxorubicin • Multiagent chemotherapy	• **LMWH,*** equivalent to enoxaparin sodium 40 mg/day *or* **dalteparin sodium** 5000 IU/day; administer subcutaneously, *or* • **Warfarin**, targeting an INR = 2–3

*LMWHs should be used with caution in individuals with impaired renal function (creatinine clearance <30 mL/min). Refer to product labeling for information about doses and administration schedules in renally impaired patients, and guidance for monitoring anti-Factor Xa concentrations
Abbreviations: CVC, central venous catheter; INR, international normalized ratio; LMWH, low-molecular-weight heparin; VTE, venous thromboembolic disease
References: Geerts WH et al. Chest 2008;133(6 Suppl):381S–453S
National Comprehensive Cancer Network. Multiple Myeloma, V.1.2014. (Accessed October 8, 2013, at http://www.nccn.org)
National Comprehensive Cancer Network. Venous Thromboembolic Disease, V.2.2013. (Accessed October 8, 2013, at http://www.nccn.org)
Palumbo A et al. Leukemia 2008;22:414–423

Treatment Modifications

CARFILZOMIB

Starting dose	27 mg/m²/dose
Level −1	20 mg/m²/dose
Level −2	15 mg/m²/dose
Level −3	Discontinue

Hematologic Toxicity

G3/4 neutropenia (<1000/mm³)	• Hold carfilzomib dosing for up to 21 days to resolve toxicity and then restart at the same dosage, or reduce the carfilzomib dosage by 1 dose level
Febrile neutropenia (ANC <1000/mm³ with a single temperature of >38.3°C [101°F] or a sustained temperature of ≥38°C [100.4°F] for >1 hour)	• If recover to G2 neutropenia or G3 thrombocytopenia, reduce carfilzomib dosage by 1 dose level
G4 thrombocytopenia (<25,000/mm³)	• If tolerated, the reduced dose may be escalated to the previous dose level
G3/4 thrombocytopenia (<50,000/mm³) associated with bleeding	
Confirmed TTP or HUS	Permanently discontinue carfilzomib. (The safety of reinitiating carfilzomib in patients previously experiencing TTP or HUS is unknown)†

Nonhematologic Toxicity

G3/4 cardiac toxicity New onset or worsening: • Congestive heart failure • Decreased left ventricular function • Myocardial ischemia	Hold carfilzomib dosing for up to 21 days to resolve toxicity to G1 or to baseline and then, at the discretion of the medically responsible health care provider, consider either permanently discontinuing carfilzomib or restarting carfilzomib at 1 lower dose level. If tolerated, the reduced dosage may be escalated to the previous dose level
Pulmonary hypertension	
G3/4 pulmonary complications	
G3/4 elevation of transaminases, bilirubin, or other liver abnormalities (ALT/AST >5× ULN or bilirubin >3× ULN)	
Serum creatinine ≥2× baseline or CrCl decreased to ≤50% of baseline	If attributable to carfilzomib, hold carfilzomib doses for up to 21 days to resolve toxicity to G1 or to baseline and then restart at the same dosage, or reduce the carfilzomib dosage by 1 dose level. If tolerated, the reduced dosage may be escalated to the previous dose level
G2 peripheral neuropathy with pain	Hold carfilzomib dosing for up to 21 days to resolve toxicity to G1 or to baseline and then restart at the same dose, or reduce the carfilzomib dosage by 1 dose level. If tolerated, the reduced dosage may be escalated to the previous dose level
G3/4 peripheral neuropathy	
Confirmed PRES (posterior reversible encephalopathy syndrome) eg, seizure, headache, lethargy, confusion, blindness, altered consciousness, visual and neurologic disturbances, hypertension	Permanently discontinue carfilzomib. The safety of reinitiating carfilzomib in patients previously experiencing PRES is unknown†
Tumor lysis syndrome (TLS)	Withhold carfilzomib until resolution of TLS, then resume carfilzomib at the same dose
Other G3/4 nonhematologic toxicities	If attributable to carfilzomib, hold carfilzomib doses for up to 21 days to resolve toxicity to G1 or to baseline and then restart at the same dosage or reduce the carfilzomib dosage by 1 dose level. If tolerated, the reduced dosage may be escalated to the previous dose level

(continued)

Treatment Modifications (continued)

LENALIDOMIDE

Lenalidomide dose levels (Days 1–21 of each 28-day cycle)

	CrCl ≥60 mL/min	CrCl ≥30 mL/min and <60 mL/min	CrCl <30 mL/min (not on hemodialysis)	ESRD on hemodialysis
Starting dose	25 mg each day	10 mg each day	15 mg every other day	5 mg each day (after dialysis on dialysis days)
Dose level −1	20 mg each day	5 mg each day	10 mg every other day	2.5 mg each day (after dialysis on dialysis days)
Dose level −2	15 mg each day	2.5 mg each day	5 mg every other day	Discontinue†
Dose level −3	10 mg each day	Discontinue†	2.5 mg every other day	
Dose level −4	5 mg each day		Discontinue†	
Dose level −5	2.5 mg each day			
Dose level −6	Discontinue†			

Adverse Event	Treatment Modification
Hematologic Toxicity	
Day 1 ANC <1000/mm³ or platelet count <50,000/mm³	Delay the next cycle until ANC ≥1000/mm³ and platelet count ≥50,000/mm³. Consider treatment with filgrastim and/or platelet transfusion according to local guidelines. If the start of a new cycle is delayed >14 days for lenalidomide-related toxicity, then reduce the lenalidomide dosage by one dose level
Either of the following: • G4 neutropenia (ANC <500/mm³) • Neutropenic fever (ANC <1000/mm³ + a single temperature >38.5°C)	Withhold lenalidomide for the remainder of the cycle and delay initiation of the next cycle until ANC ≥1000/mm³ and platelet count ≥50,000/mm³, if necessary. Consider treatment with filgrastim according to local guidelines. If neutropenia was the only dose-limiting toxicity *and* if filgrastim is continued *and* if the next cycle was delayed by ≤14 days, then resume lenalidomide at the same dose. Otherwise, reduce the lenalidomide dose by one dose level at the start of the next cycle
G3 neutropenia (ANC ≥500 and <1000/mm³) during a cycle	Interrupt lenalidomide treatment and follow weekly CBC. When ANC ≥1000/mm³ and there are no other toxicities, resume lenalidomide treatment at same dose. If other toxicities are still present, then resume lenalidomide with dose reduced one dose level
Recurrent G3 neutropenia (ANC ≥500 and <1000/mm³) during a cycle	Interrupt lenalidomide treatment and follow weekly CBC. When ANC ≥1000/mm³, resume with dose reduced one dose level
G4 thrombocytopenia (platelet count <25,000/mm³)	Interrupt lenalidomide treatment and follow weekly CBC. When platelet count ≥25,000/mm³, resume lenalidomide with dose reduced one dose level
Recurrent G4 thrombocytopenia (platelet count <25,000/mm³)	
Nonhematologic Toxicity	
G3/4 hepatotoxicity (ALT/AST >5× ULN and/or bilirubin >3× ULN)	Withhold lenalidomide for remainder of the cycle. Delay initiation of next cycle until hepatotoxicity resolves to G ≤2 (ALT/AST ≤5× ULN and/or bilirubin ≤3× ULN), then resume lenalidomide at one lower dose level
G3 rash	Hold dose for remainder of cycle. Decrease by one dose level when dosing resumed at next cycle (rash must resolve to G ≤1)
Allergic reactions, including hypersensitivity, angioedema, Stevens-Johnson syndrome, toxic epidermal necrolysis (TEN), and drug reaction with eosinophilia and systemic symptoms (DRESS)	Discontinue lenalidomide if reactions are suspected. Do not resume lenalidomide if these reactions are confirmed
Tumor lysis syndrome (TLS)	Monitor patients at risk of TLS (ie, those with high tumor burden) and take appropriate precautions including aggressive hydration and allopurinol

(continued)

Treatment Modifications (continued)

Nonhematologic Toxicity

G3 peripheral neuropathy	Withhold lenalidomide for the remainder of the cycle. Delay initiation of the next cycle until neuropathy resolves to G ≤1, then resume lenalidomide at one lower dose level
G4 peripheral neuropathy	Discontinue lenalidomide[†]
G3/4 venous thromboembolism (VTE) during aspirin monotherapy or inadequate anticoagulation	Continue lenalidomide at the current dose and initiate adequate anticoagulation
G3/4 venous thromboembolism (VTE) during adequate anticoagulation (eg, prophylactic or therapeutic doses of LMWH, UFH, or warfarin)	Discontinue lenalidomide[†]
G ≥2 hypothyroidism or G ≥2 hyperthyroidism	Continue lenalidomide at current dose and initiate appropriate medical treatment
Other G ≥3 lenalidomide-related toxicities	Withhold lenalidomide for the remainder of the cycle. Delay initiation of the next cycle until toxicity resolves to G ≤2, then resume lenalidomide at one lower dose level

DEXAMETHASONE

Starting dose	40 mg/dose/day
Dose Level −1	20 mg/dose/day
Dose Level −2	12 mg/dose/day
Dose Level −3	8 mg/dose/day
Dose Level −4	4 mg/dose/day
Dose Level −5	Discontinue dexamethasone

Adverse Event	Treatment Modification
G1/2 dyspepsia (moderate symptoms; medical intervention indicated; limiting instrumental ADL), gastric or duodenal ulcer, or gastritis	Continue dexamethasone at the same dose. Treat with therapeutic doses of an H_2-receptor antagonist or proton pump inhibitor. If symptoms persist, then reduce the dexamethasone dosage by one level
G ≥3 dyspepsia, gastric or duodenal ulcer, or gastritis (surgery or hospitalization indicated)	Withhold dexamethasone until symptoms return to baseline. Resume dexamethasone reduced by one dose level along with concurrent treatment with therapeutic doses of an H_2-receptor antagonist or proton pump inhibitor. If symptoms recur, then permanently discontinue dexamethasone[ϵ]
Acute pancreatitis	Permanently discontinue dexamethasone[ϵ]
G ≥3 edema	Withhold dexamethasone until symptoms return to baseline. Consider treatment with diuretics. Resume dexamethasone reduced by one dose level. If edema persists, reduce by another dose level. Discontinue dexamethasone permanently if symptoms persist despite two prior dose reductions[ϵ]
G ≥2 mood alteration (moderate mood alteration) or confusion (moderate disorientation; limiting instrumental ADL)	Withhold dexamethasone until symptoms return to baseline. Resume dexamethasone reduced by one dose level. If symptoms persist, reduce by another dose level
G ≥2 muscle weakness (symptomatic; evident on physical exam; limiting instrumental ADL)	Withhold dexamethasone until symptoms return to baseline. Resume dexamethasone reduced by one dose level. If weakness persists, reduce by another dose level. If weakness still persists, then permanently discontinue dexamethasone[ϵ]
G ≥3 hyperglycemia (insulin therapy initiated; hospitalization indicated)	Withhold dexamethasone until blood glucose is ≤250 mg/dL. Treat with insulin or other hypoglycemic agents as clinically appropriate and then resume dexamethasone at the same dose. If hyperglycemia is uncontrolled despite above measures, decrease dexamethasone by one dose level
Other G ≥2 nonhematologic toxicity attributable to dexamethasone including severe irritability, insomnia, or oral candidiasis	Withhold dexamethasone until toxicity resolves to G ≤1, then resume at a lower dose. Consider reduction by one dose level for G2/G3 toxicity, and by two dose levels for G4 or recurrent G3 toxicity

[†]If carfilzomib and lenalidomide are permanently discontinued, then also consider discontinuing dexamethasone
[ϵ]If dexamethasone is permanently discontinued, continued administration of carfilzomib and/or lenalidomide may be considered at the discretion of the treating physician

Patient Population Studied

The international, multicenter, open-label, phase 3 trial (ASPIRE) involved 792 patients with relapsed and measurable multiple myeloma. Eligible patients had received 1–3 prior treatments and had adequate hepatic, hematologic, and renal function. Patients with Grade 3–4 peripheral neuropathy, or Grade 2 with pain, within 14 days before randomization and those with New York Heart Association class III–IV heart failure were ineligible. Patients were randomly assigned (1:1) to receive 28-day cycles of lenalidomide (25 mg on days 1 to 21) plus dexamethasone (40 mg on days 1, 8, 15, and 22) with or without carfilzomib until disease progression, unacceptable toxicity, or withdrawal of consent. During cycles 1–12, carfilzomib was administered in 10-minute infusion on days 1, 2, 8, 9, 15, and 16 (starting dose 20 mg/m² on days 1 and 2 of cycle 1; target dose 27 mg/m² thereafter). During cycles 13–18, carfilzomib was administered in 10-minute infusion on days 1, 2, 15, and 16. No carfilzomib was administered after cycle 18. All patients received antiviral and antithrombotic prophylaxis. Pretreatment and post-treatment intravenous hydration was required on cycle 1

Efficacy (n = 792)

	Carfilzomib + Lenalidomide + Dexamethasone (n = 396)	Lenalidomide + Dexamethasone (n = 396)	
Median progression-free survival	26.3 months	17.6 months	HR 0.69 (95% CI 0.57–0.83); P = 0.0001
Overall response rates*	87.1%	66.7%	P <0.001

*Overall response rate was the proportion of patients who experienced a partial or complete response according to the International Myeloma Working Group Uniform Response Criteria

Adverse Events (n = 781)

	Carfilzomib + Lenalidomide + Dexamethasone (n = 392)		Lenalidomide + Dexamethasone (n = 389)	
	Grade 1–2 (%)*	G ≥3 (%)*	Grade 1–2 (%)*	G ≥3 (%)*
Diarrhea	39	4	30	4
Fatigue	25	8	24	6
Cough	29	<1	17	0
Pyrexia	27	2	20	<1
Upper respiratory tract infection	27	2	18	1
Hypokalemia	18	9	8	5
Muscle spasms	26	1	20	<1
Dyspnea	17	3	13	2
Hypertension	10	4	5	2
Acute renal failure	5	3	4	3
Cardiac failure	3	4	2	2
Ischemic heart disease	3	3	3	2

*According to the National Cancer Institute Common Terminology Criteria for Adverse Events, version 4.0
Note: adverse events that occurred in ≥25% of either treatment group or that were of particular clinical relevance are included. Treatment was discontinued owing to adverse events in 15.3% and 17.7% of the carfilzomib and control groups, respectively. Treatment-related deaths occurred in six of the carfilzomib and eight of the control group

Therapy Monitoring

1. CBC with differential, liver function tests, and serum glucose prior to each carfilzomib dose
2. Monitor for cardiac complications
3. Monitor for and manage dyspnea immediately
4. With abdominal pain, check serum amylase/lipase
5. Ensure adequate hydration of patients to reduce the risk of renal toxicity and of tumor lysis syndrome

Lenalidomide notes:
• Higher incidences of second primary malignancies were observed in controlled trials of patients with MM receiving lenalidomide. While no routine monitoring is indicated, awareness of this potential complication is necessary
• A decrease in the number of CD34+ cells collected after treatment has been reported in patients who have received >4 cycles of lenalidomide. In patients who may undergo transplant, consider early referral to transplant center
• Because of the embryo-fetal risk lenalidomide is available only through a restricted program under a Risk Evaluation and Mitigation Strategy (REMS), the REVLIMID REMS program

SUBSEQUENT THERAPY

MULTIPLE MYELOMA REGIMEN: IXAZOMIB + LENALIDOMIDE + DEXAMETHASONE

Moreau P et al. N Engl J Med 2016;374:1621–1634
Protocol for: Moreau P et al. N Engl J Med 2016;374:1621–1634

Ixazomib 4 mg/dose; administer orally for 3 doses, at least 1 hour prior to food or at least 2 hours after food, with water, on day 1, 8, and 15, every 28 days, until disease progression (total dosage/cycle = 12 mg)
- Patients who delay taking an ixazomib dose at a regularly scheduled time may take the missed dose if the time to the next regularly scheduled dose is >72 hours away
- If a patient vomits after taking a dose of ixazomib, the patient should take the next dose at the next regularly scheduled time
- Avoid concomitant administration with strong CYP3A4 inducers (eg, rifampin, carbamazepine, phenytoin, phenobarbital, and St. John's Wort)
- Reduce the starting dose to 3 mg on days 1, 8, and 15 for moderate (total bilirubin >1.5–3× ULN) or severe (total bilirubin >3× ULN) hepatic impairment
- Reduce the starting dose to 3 mg on days 1, 8, and 15 for patients with severe renal impairment (creatinine clearance <30 mL/minute) or end-stage renal disease requiring hemodialysis. In patients undergoing hemodialysis, ixazomib can be administered without regard to dialysis timing

Lenalidomide 25 mg/dose; administer orally, without regard to meals, once daily for 21 consecutive days on days 1–21, followed by 7 days with no treatment, every 28 days, until disease progression (total dosage/cycle = 525 mg)
- Patients who delay taking a lenalidomide dose at a regularly scheduled time may take the missed dose if the time to the next regularly scheduled dose is >12 hours away
- Consider doses in Treatment Modifications table for dose adjustments for renal function

Dexamethasone 40 mg/dose; administer orally once daily for 4 doses on days 1, 8, 15, and 22, every 28 days, until disease progression (total dosage/ cycle = 160 mg)

Supportive Care
Antiemetic prophylaxis
Emetogenic potential is **LOW**
See Chapter 42 for antiemetic recommendations

Hematopoietic growth factor (CSF) prophylaxis
Primary prophylaxis is **NOT** *indicated*
See Chapter 43 for more information

Antimicrobial prophylaxis
Risk of fever and neutropenia is **INTERMEDIATE**
Antimicrobial primary prophylaxis to be considered:
- Antibacterial—consider a fluoroquinolone during periods of neutropenia, or no prophylaxis; *Pneumocystis jirovecii* prophylaxis is recommended (eg, cotrimoxazole)
- Antifungal—consider fluconazole during periods of neutropenia
- Antiviral—antiherpes antivirals (eg, acyclovir, famciclovir, valacyclovir)

Diarrhea management
Loperamide or **diphenoxylate hydrochloride** 2.5 mg with **atropine sulfate** 0.025 mg (eg, Lomotil)
Bisphosphonates
All patients receiving primary therapy for symptomatic multiple myeloma should receive a bisphosphonate adjunctively.

(continued)

(*continued*)

Thromboprophylaxis

Risk assessment and recommendations for VTE prophylaxis in patients with multiple myeloma with individual or myeloma-related risk factors, or risk factors related to treatment

Individual risk factors
• Obesity (BMI ≥30 kg/m²)
• H/O VTE
• CVC or pacemaker
• Comorbid pathologies
  ▪ Cardiac disease
  ▪ Chronic renal disease
  ▪ Diabetes
  ▪ Acute infection
  ▪ Immobilization
• Surgery
  ▪ General surgery
  ▪ Any anesthesia
  ▪ Trauma
• Medications
  ▪ Erythropoietin (epoetin alfa, darbepoetin)
  ▪ Estrogenic compounds
  ▪ Bevacizumab
• Clotting disorders
  ▪ Thrombophilia
Myeloma-related risk factors
• Diagnosis of multiple myeloma
• Hyperviscosity
	≤1 Individual or myeloma-related risk factor present:
	• **Aspirin** 81–325 mg daily
	
	≥2 Individual or myeloma-related risk factors present:
	• **LMWH,*** equivalent to enoxaparin sodium 40 mg/day *or* **dalteparin sodium** 5000 IU/day; administer subcutaneously, *or*
	• **Warfarin,** targeting an INR = 2–3

Concomitant treatment-related risk factors Thalidomide or lenalidomide in combination with: • High-dose dexamethasone (≥480 mg/month) • Doxorubicin • Multiagent chemotherapy	• **LMWH,*** equivalent to enoxaparin sodium 40 mg/day *or* **dalteparin sodium** 5000 IU/day; administer subcutaneously, *or* • **Warfarin,** targeting an INR = 2–3

*LMWHs should be used with caution in individuals with impaired renal function (creatinine clearance <30 mL/min). Refer to product labeling for information about doses and administration schedules in renally impaired patients, and guidance for monitoring anti-Factor Xa concentrations
Abbreviations: CVC, central venous catheter; INR, international normalized ratio; LMWH, low-molecular-weight heparin; VTE, venous thromboembolic disease
References: Geerts WH et al. Chest 2008;133(6 Suppl):381S–453S
National Comprehensive Cancer Network. Multiple Myeloma, V.1.2014. (Accessed October 8, 2013, at http://www.nccn.org)
National Comprehensive Cancer Network. Venous Thromboembolic Disease, V.2.2013. (Accessed October 8, 2013, at http://www.nccn.org)
Palumbo A et al. Leukemia 2008;22:414–423

Treatment Modifications

IXAZOMIB

Ixazomib Dose Levels (Days 1, 8, and 15 of Every 28-Day Cycle)

	CrCl ≥30 mL/min, normal hepatic function	CrCl <30 mL/min, end-stage renal disease requiring dialysis, moderate hepatic impairment (**total bilirubin >1.5–3× ULN**), or severe hepatic impairment (**total bilirubin >3× ULN**)
Starting dose	4 mg/dose	3 mg/dose (irrespective of hemodialysis timing, if applicable)
Dose Level −1	3 mg/dose	2.3 mg/dose (irrespective of hemodialysis timing, if applicable)
Dose Level −2	2.3 mg/dose	Discontinue ixazomib
Dose Level −3	Discontinue ixazomib	

(*continued*)

Treatment Modifications (*continued*)

Adverse Event	Treatment Modification
Day 1 ANC <1000/mm^3 and/or platelet count <75,000/mm^3 and/or nonhematologic toxicities G ≥2	Delay administration of ixazomib and lenalidomide until ANC ≥1000/mm^3 and platelet count ≥75,000/mm^3. Consider treatment with filgrastim and/or platelet transfusion according to local guidelines. If the start of a new cycle is delayed >14 days, then reduce the lenalidomide by one dose level and also consider reducing the ixazomib dose by one dose level
ANC <500/mm^3 and/or platelet count <30,000/mm^3	Withhold ixazomib and lenalidomide until platelet count ≥30,000/mm^3 and/or ANC >500/mm^3. Consider adding G-CSF per clinical guidelines. Following recovery, resume lenalidomide at the next lower dose, and resume ixazomib at its most recent dose
Recurrence of ANC <500/mm^3 and/or platelet count <30,000/mm^3 despite a reduction in lenalidomide dose	Withhold ixazomib and lenalidomide until platelet count ≥30,000/mm^3 and/or ANC >500/mm^3. Consider adding G-CSF per clinical guidelines. Following recovery, resume ixazomib at the next lower dose and resume lenalidomide at its most recent dose. For additional occurrences, alternate dose modification of lenalidomide and ixazomib
G2/3 rash	Withhold lenalidomide until rash recovers to G ≤1. Following recovery, resume lenalidomide at one lower dose level
Recurrence of G2/3 rash despite a reduction in lenalidomide dose	Withhold ixazomib and lenalidomide until rash recovers to G ≤1. Following recovery, resume ixazomib at the next lower dose and resume lenalidomide at its most recent dose For additional occurrences, alternate dose modification of lenalidomide and ixazomib
G1 peripheral neuropathy with pain or G2 peripheral neuropathy	Withhold ixazomib until peripheral neuropathy recovers to G ≤1 without pain or patient's baseline. Following recovery, resume ixazomib at its most recent dose
G2 peripheral neuropathy with pain or G3 peripheral neuropathy	Withhold ixazomib until peripheral neuropathy recovers to G ≤1 without pain or patient's baseline. Following recovery, resume ixazomib at the next lower dose level
G4 peripheral neuropathy	Discontinue ixazomib
Other G3/4 nonhematologic toxicities	Withhold ixazomib. Toxicities should recover to G ≤1 prior to resuming ixazomib. If attributable to ixazomib, resume with ixazomib dose at one lower level

LENALIDOMIDE

Lenalidomide Dose Levels (Days 1–21 of Each 28-day Cycle)

	CrCl ≥60 mL/min	CrCl ≥30 mL/min and <60 mL/min	CrCl <30 mL/min (not on hemodialysis)	ESRD on hemodialysis
Starting dose	25 mg each day	10 mg each day	15 mg every other day	5 mg each day (after dialysis on dialysis days)
Dose level −1	15 mg each day	5 mg each day	10 mg every other day	2.5 mg each day (after dialysis on dialysis days)
Dose level −2	10 mg each day	2.5 mg each day	5 mg every other day	Discontinue†
Dose level −3	5 mg each day	Discontinue†	Discontinue†	
Dose level −4	Discontinue†			

Adverse Event	Treatment Modification
Hematologic Toxicity	
Day 1 ANC <1000/mm^3 and/or platelet count <75,000/mm^3 and/or nonhematologic toxicities G ≥2	Delay administration of ixazomib and lenalidomide until ANC ≥1000/mm^3 and platelet count ≥75,000/mm^3. Consider treatment with filgrastim and/or platelet transfusion according to local guidelines. If the start of a new cycle is delayed >14 days, then reduce the lenalidomide by one dose level and also consider reducing the ixazomib dose by one dose level
ANC <500/mm^3 and/or platelet count <30,000/mm^3	Withhold ixazomib and lenalidomide until platelet count ≥30,000/mm^3 and/or ANC >500/mm^3. Following recovery, resume lenalidomide at the next lower dose, but not lower than 2.5 mg/day, and resume ixazomib at its most recent dose
ANC <500/mm^3 and/or platelet count <30,000/mm^3 despite a reduction in lenalidomide dose	Withhold ixazomib and lenalidomide until platelet count ≥30,000/mm^3 and/or ANC >500/mm^3. Following recovery, resume ixazomib at the next lower dose and resume lenalidomide at its most recent dose For additional occurrences, alternate dose modification of lenalidomide and ixazomib

(*continued*)

Treatment Modifications (continued)

Nonhematologic Toxicity	
G3/4 hepatotoxicity (ALT/AST >5× ULN and/or bilirubin >3× ULN)	Withhold lenalidomide and ixazomib until hepatotoxicity resolves to G ≤1 (ALT/AST ≤3× ULN and/or bilirubin ≤1.5× ULN), then resume lenalidomide at one lower dose level and ixazomib at one lower dose level
G2/3 rash	Withhold lenalidomide until rash recovers to G ≤1. Following recovery, resume lenalidomide at one lower dose level
Recurrence of G2/3 rash despite a reduction in lenalidomide dose	Withhold ixazomib and lenalidomide until rash recovers to G ≤1. Following recovery, resume ixazomib at the next lower dose and resume lenalidomide at its most recent dose For additional occurrences, alternate dose modification of lenalidomide and ixazomib
Allergic reactions, including hypersensitivity, angioedema, Stevens-Johnson syndrome, toxic epidermal necrolysis (TEN), and drug reaction with eosinophilia and systemic symptoms (DRESS)	Discontinue lenalidomide if reactions are suspected. Do not resume lenalidomide if these reactions are confirmed
Tumor lysis syndrome (TLS)	Monitor patients at risk of TLS (ie, those with high tumor burden) and take appropriate precautions including aggressive hydration and allopurinol
G3/4 venous thromboembolism (VTE) during aspirin monotherapy or inadequate anticoagulation	Continue lenalidomide at the current dose and initiate adequate anticoagulation
G3/4 venous thromboembolism (VTE) during adequate anticoagulation (eg, prophylactic or therapeutic doses of LMWH, UFH, or warfarin)	Discontinue lenalidomide
G ≥2 hypothyroidism or G ≥2 hyperthyroidism	Continue lenalidomide at current dose and initiate appropriate medical treatment
Other G ≥3 lenalidomide-related toxicities	Withhold lenalidomide for the remainder of the cycle. Delay initiation of the next cycle until toxicity resolves to G ≤2, then resume lenalidomide at one lower dose level

DEXAMETHASONE

Dexamethasone Dose Levels (Days 1, 8, 15, and 22 of Each 28-Day Cycle)

Starting dose	40 mg/dose
Dose Level −1	20 mg/dose
Dose Level −2	8 mg/dose
Dose Level −3	Discontinue dexamethasone

Adverse Event	Treatment Modification
G1/2 dyspepsia (moderate symptoms; medical intervention indicated; limiting instrumental ADL), gastric or duodenal ulcer, or gastritis	Continue dexamethasone at the same dose. Treat with therapeutic doses of an H_2-receptor antagonist or proton pump inhibitor. If symptoms persist, then reduce the dexamethasone dose by one level
G ≥3 dyspepsia, gastric or duodenal ulcer, or gastritis (surgery or hospitalization indicated)	Withhold dexamethasone until symptoms return to baseline. Resume dexamethasone reduced by one dose level along with concurrent treatment with therapeutic doses of an H_2-receptor antagonist or proton pump inhibitor. If symptoms recur, then permanently discontinue dexamethasone
Acute pancreatitis	Permanently discontinue dexamethasone
G ≥3 edema	Withhold dexamethasone until symptoms return to baseline. Consider treatment with diuretics. Resume dexamethasone reduced by one dose level. If edema persists, reduce by another dose level. Discontinue dexamethasone permanently if symptoms persist despite two prior dose reductions
G ≥2 mood alteration (moderate mood alteration) or confusion (moderate disorientation; limiting instrumental ADL)	Withhold dexamethasone until symptoms return to baseline. Resume dexamethasone reduced by one dose level. If symptoms persist, reduce by another dose level
G ≥2 muscle weakness (symptomatic; evident on physical exam; limiting instrumental ADL)	Withhold dexamethasone until symptoms return to baseline. Resume dexamethasone reduced by one dose level. If weakness persists, reduce by another dose level. If weakness still persists, then permanently discontinue dexamethasone

(continued)

Treatment Modifications (*continued*)

Adverse Event	Treatment Modification
G ≥3 hyperglycemia (insulin therapy initiated; hospitalization indicated)	Withhold dexamethasone until glucose is ≤250 mg/dL. Treat with insulin or other hypoglycemic agents as clinically appropriate and then resume dexamethasone at the same dose. If hyperglycemia is uncontrolled despite above measures, decrease dexamethasone by one dose level
Other G ≥2 nonhematologic toxicity attributable to dexamethasone including severe irritability, insomnia, or oral candidiasis	Withhold dexamethasone until toxicity resolves to G ≤1, then resume at a lower dose. Consider reduction by one dose level for G2/G3 toxicity, and by two dose levels for G4 or recurrent G3 toxicity

If the dose of one drug in the regimen (ie, lenalidomide, dexamethasone, or ixazomib) is delayed, interrupted, or discontinued, the treatment with the other drugs may continue as scheduled

Patient Population Studied

The multicenter, double-blind, placebo-controlled, randomized, phase 3 study involved 722 patients with relapsed and/or refractory multiple myeloma. Eligible patients had an Eastern Cooperative Oncology Group (ECOG) performance status score ≤2 and had received one to three prior treatments. Patients who had Grade 1 with pain or Grade 2 or higher peripheral neuropathy, or had disease refractory to lenalidomide or proteasome inhibitor–based therapy, were not eligible. All patients were required to have thromboprophylaxis. Treatment continued until disease progression or unacceptable toxic events

Efficacy (n = 722)

	Ixazomib + Lenalidomide + Dexamethasone (n = 360)	Placebo + Lenalidomide + Dexamethasone (n = 362)	
Median progression-free survival	20.6 months	14.7 months	HR 0.74 (95% CI 0.59–0.94; P = 0.01)
Objective response rate*	78.3%	71.5%	P = 0.04
Median duration of response	20.5 months	15.0	
Median time to response†	1.1 months	1.9 months	P = 0.009
Median time to disease progression	21.4 months	15.7 months	HR 0.71 (95% CI 0.56–0.91; P = 0.007)

*Objective response rate was the proportion of patients who experienced a partial or complete response according to the International Myeloma Working Group 2011 Criteria
Note: median follow-up time for the first analysis was 14.8 months in the ixazomib group and 14.6 months in the control group

Adverse Events (n = 720)

	Ixazomib + Lenalidomide + Dexamethasone (n = 361)			Placebo + Lenalidomide + Dexamethasone (n = 359)		
	Grade 1–2 (%)*	Grade 3 (%)*	Grade 4 (%)*	Grade 1–2 (%)*	Grade 3 (%)*	Grade 4 (%)*
Diarrhea	39	6	0	36	3	0
Rash (standardized MedDRA query)	31	5	0	21	2	0
Constipation	35	<1	0	26	<1	0
Neutropenia	10	18	5	7	18	6
Thrombocytopenia	12	12	7	7	5	4
Fatigue	26	4	0	26	3	0

(*continued*)

Adverse Events (n = 720) (continued)

Nausea	27	2	0	22	0	0
Anemia	19	9	0	14	13	0
Peripheral edema	26	2	0	19	1	0
Peripheral neuropathy	24	2	0	20	2	0
Back pain	23	<1	0	15	3	0
Vomiting	22	1	0	11	<1	0
Upper respiratory tract infection	22	<1	0	19	<1	0
Nasopharyngitis	22	0	0	20	0	0
Insomnia	18	2	0	24	3	0
Rash (high-level term)	17	2	0	11	2	0
Muscle spasms	18	0	0	26	<1	0
Arrhythmias	10	5	<1	12	3	<1
Acute renal failure	6	2	<1	7	3	1
Thromboembolism	5	2	<1	7	3	<1
Liver impairment	5	2	0	5	1	0
Hypertension	3	3	0	4	1	0
Hypotension	5	1	0	6	<1	0
New primary malignant tumor	5	NA	NA	4	NA	NA
Heart failure	2	2	<1	2	1	<1
Myocardial infarction	<1	0	<1	1	<1	<1
Encephalopathy	0	<1	0	1	0	0
Interstitial lung disease	<1	<1	<1	1	<1	0
Hypertensive crisis	<1	0	0	0	0	0

*According to the National Cancer Institute Common Terminology Criteria for Adverse Events, version 4.03
Note: adverse events that occurred in ≥20% patients in either group, as well as some additional adverse events of clinical interest, are included in the table. Median follow-up was 23.3 months for the ixazomib group and 22.9 months for the control group. Adverse events resulting in discontinuation of any agent occurred in 25% of the ixazomib group and 20% of the control group. In total, 4% of the ixazomib group and 6% of the control group died during the treatment period

Therapy Monitoring

1. *Prior to each cycle:* CBC with differential, liver function tests, serum creatinine, and serum glucose. Consider more frequent CBC monitoring during the first 3 cycles
2. With abdominal pain, check serum amylase/lipase
3. Ensure adequate hydration of patients
4. Monitor thyroid function
5. Monitor for signs/symptoms of thromboembolism, peripheral neuropathy, gastrointestinal toxicities (eg, diarrhea, constipation, nausea, and vomiting), edema, and cutaneous reactions

Lenalidomide notes:
• Higher incidences of second primary malignancies were observed in controlled trials of patients with MM receiving lenalidomide. While no routine monitoring is indicated, awareness of this potential complication is necessary
• A decrease in the number of CD34+ cells collected after treatment has been reported in patients who have received >4 cycles of lenalidomide. In patients who may undergo transplant, consider early referral to transplant center
• Because of the embryo-fetal risk, lenalidomide is available only through a restricted program under a Risk Evaluation and Mitigation Strategy (REMS), the REVLIMID REMS program

SUBSEQUENT THERAPY

MULTIPLE MYELOMA REGIMEN: POMALIDOMIDE + DEXAMETHASONE

Leleu X et al. Blood 2013;121:1968–1975
Lacy MQ et al. Leukemia 2010;24:1934–1939

Pomalidomide 4 mg/day orally, continually, for 21 consecutive days, on days 1–21, every 28 days (total dose/cycle = 84 mg)
Dexamethasone 40 mg/dose; orally for 4 doses on days 1, 8, 15, and 22, every 28 days (total dose/cycle = 160 mg)
or
Pomalidomide 2 mg/day; orally, continually, for 28 consecutive days, on days 1–28, every 28 days (total dose/cycle = 56 mg)
Dexamethasone 40 mg daily orally on days 1, 8, 15, and 22, every 28 days (total dose/cycle = 160 mg)

Supportive Care
Antiemetic prophylaxis
Emetogenic potential is **MINIMAL–LOW**
See Chapter 42 for antiemetic recommendations

Hematopoietic growth factor (CSF) prophylaxis
Primary prophylaxis may be indicated
See Chapter 43 for more information

Antimicrobial prophylaxis
Risk of fever and neutropenia is **INTERMEDIATE**
   Antimicrobial primary prophylaxis to be considered:
   • Antibacterial—consider a fluoroquinolone or no prophylaxis; *P. jirovecii* prophylaxis is recommended (eg, cotrimoxazole)
   • Antifungal—recommended; consider use during periods of neutropenia
   • Antiviral—antiherpes antivirals (eg, acyclovir, famciclovir, valacyclovir)

Bisphosphonates
All patients receiving primary therapy for symptomatic multiple myeloma should receive a bisphosphonate adjunctively.

Thromboprophylaxis
Risk assessment and recommendations for VTE prophylaxis in patients with multiple myeloma with individual or myeloma-related risk factors, or risk factors related to treatment

Individual risk factors
• Obesity (BMI ≥30 kg/m^2)
• H/O VTE
• CVC or pacemaker
• Comorbid pathologies
  ▪ Cardiac disease
  ▪ Chronic renal disease
  ▪ Diabetes
  ▪ Acute infection
  ▪ Immobilization
• Surgery
  ▪ General surgery
  ▪ Any anesthesia
  ▪ Trauma
• Medications
  ▪ Erythropoietin (epoetin alfa, darbepoetin)
  ▪ Estrogenic compounds
  ▪ Bevacizumab
• Clotting disorders
  ▪ Thrombophilia
Myeloma-related risk factors
• Diagnosis of multiple myeloma
• Hyperviscosity
	≤1 Individual or myeloma-related risk factor present:
	• **Aspirin** 81–325 mg daily
	
	≥2 Individual or myeloma-related risk factors present:
	• **LMWH,*** equivalent to enoxaparin sodium 40 mg/day *or* **dalteparin sodium** 5000 IU/day; administer subcutaneously, *or*
	• **Warfarin**, targeting an INR = 2–3

(continued)

(*continued*)

| Concomitant treatment-related risk factors
Thalidomide or lenalidomide in combination with:
• High-dose dexamethasone (≥480 mg/month)
• Doxorubicin
• Multiagent chemotherapy | • **LMWH,** equivalent to enoxaparin sodium 40 mg/day *or* **dalteparin sodium** 5000 IU/day; administer subcutaneously, *or*
• **Warfarin**, targeting an INR = 2–3 |

*LMWHs should be used with caution in individuals with impaired renal function (creatinine clearance <30 mL/min). Refer to product labeling for information about doses and administration schedules in renally impaired patients, and guidance for monitoring anti-Factor Xa concentrations

Abbreviations: CVC, central venous catheter; INR, international normalized ratio; LMWH, low-molecular-weight heparin; VTE, venous thromboembolic disease

References: Geerts WH et al. Chest 2008;133(6 Suppl):381S–453S
National Comprehensive Cancer Network. Multiple Myeloma, V.1.2014. (Accessed October 8, 2013, at http://www.nccn.org)
National Comprehensive Cancer Network. Venous Thromboembolic Disease, V.2.2013. (Accessed October 8, 2013, at http://www.nccn.org)
Palumbo A et al. Leukemia 2008;22:414–423

Treatment Modifications

Pomalidomide Dose Levels

Starting dose	4 mg/day
Level −1	3 mg/day
Level −2	2 mg/day
Level −3	1 mg/day
Level −4	Discontinue

Dexamethasone Dose Levels

Starting dose	40 mg/dose
Level −1	20 mg/dose
Level −2	12 mg/dose
Level −3	8 mg/dose
Level −4	4 mg/dose
Level −5	Discontinue

Adverse Event	Treatment Modification
ANC <500/mm^3 Febrile neutropenia (fever ≥38.5°C + ANC <1000/mm^3) Platelets <25,000/mm^3	Interrupt pomalidomide treatment, and follow CBC weekly. When ANC ≥500/mm^3 and platelet count 50,000/mm^3, resume pomalidomide 1 dose level lower
Nonhematologic G3/4 toxicity	Interrupt pomalidomide treatment, and follow weekly or more frequently. Restart treatment 1 dose level lower than the previous dose when toxicity has resolved G ≤2
G4 rash, neuropathy, hypersensitivity, or G ≥3 bradycardia or cardiac arrhythmia	Permanently discontinue pomalidomide
G3/4 adverse events occurring on or after day 15 during a single cycle	Withhold pomalidomide for the remainder of the cycle and reduce by 1 dose level beginning with the next cycle
Toxicities ascribed to dexamethasone such as severe manifestations of hypercorticism, including hyperglycemia, irritability, insomnia, or oral candidiasis	Hold dexamethasone dosing for up to 21 days to resolve toxicity and then restart at the same dose or reduce the dexamethasone dose by 50%

Patient Population Studied

Patients were eligible if they had relapsed MM after at least 1 prior regimen. Patients were considered to be "nonresponders" to the last line of lenalidomide or bortezomib after having received ≥2 cycles of either drug if they did not achieve a response defined by International Myeloma Working Group (IMWG) criteria (stable disease [stable disease and minor response]) within 2 cycles of treatment

Characteristic	21/28 (n = 43)*	28/28 (n = 41)*
Median time from diagnosis to randomization, years (range)	5.1 (0.9–8.7)	6.5 (0.8–23.1)
≤3 years, n (%)	13 (30)	4 (10)
Median age, years (range)	60 (45–81)	60 (42–83)
Age ≥65 years, n (%)	11 (26)	15 (37)
ISS stage II/III (%)[†]	32/24	42/17
Myeloma type, n (%)		
Intact Ig	36 (84)	34 (83)
Light chain	4 (9)	5 (12)
Freelite measurable only[‡]	3 (7)	2 (5)
Lytic bone lesions, n (%)	37 (86)	37 (90)
Number of lytic lesions: (3–6)	9 (25)	8 (22)
Number of lytic lesions: >6	11 (31)	17 (46)
Osseous fracture	10 (29)	11 (32)
Medullary compression	0	3 (9)
Plasmacytoma	9 (21)	5 (12)
Median β_2-microglobulin, mg/L (range)	3.9 (1.0–13.2)	3.7 (1.6–12.0)
(3.5–5.5) mg/L, n (%)	19 (44)	11 (27.5)
>5.5 mg/L, n (%)	10 (23)	11 (27.5)
Median serum creatinine, (µmol/L) (range)	80.0 (0.9 mg/dL) (44.0–193.0)	87.0 (0.98 mg/dL) (42.0–196)
>115 µmol/L (1.3 mg/dL), n (%)	6 (14)	4 (10)
Median hemoglobin, g/dL (range)	10.5 (7.2–14.1)	10.5 (6.4–14.1)
<10 g/dL, n (%)	18 (42)	15 (37.5)
Median neutrophils, × 10^9/L (range)	2.6 (0.04–10.4)	2.3 (0.9–8.3)
Median platelets, × 10^9/L (range)	161 (51–366)	147 (33–269)
<100 × 10^9/L, n (%)	8 (19)	10 (25)
Median number of lines (min-max)	5 (1–13)	5 (2–10)

*Pomalidomide was given orally either daily on days 1 to 21 of each 28-day cycle (arm 21/28 days) or continuously of each 28-day cycle (arm 28/28 days)
[†]ISS classification at diagnosis
[‡]Patients whose disease was considered "not measurable" based on intact serum immunoglobulin and urine light-chain excretion but had serum immunoglobulin free light chain >100 mg/L and an abnormal free light-chain ratio
Leleu X et al. Blood 2013;121:1968–1975

Incidence Rate (Number and Percentage) of Patients with Various Adverse Prognostic Factors by Arm (n = 84)

Prognostic Factor	21/28 (n = 43)	28/28 (n = 41)	Total (n = 84)
Patients >6 lines of therapy, n (%)	12 (28)	7 (17)	19 (23)
Refractory* to, n (%)			
Lenalidomide	36 (84)	39 (95)	75 (89)
Lenalidomide last prior therapy	15 (35)	11 (27)	26 (31)
Bortezomib	34 (79)	34 (83)	68 (81)
Both lenalidomide and bortezomib	32 (74)	32 (78)	64 (76)
Last prior therapy	36 (70)	35 (68)	71 (84.5)

(continued)

Patient Population Studied (continued)

FISH cytogenetics, n (%)[†]	N = 33	N = 32	
Deletion 17p	6 (21)	9 (33)	—
Translocation (4;14)	2 (7)	4 (17)	—

*Refractory by International Myeloma Working Group (IMWG) criteria
[†]High-risk cytogenetics by FISH consisted of deletion 17p or t(4;14) at diagnosis and/or at entry in the trial
Leleu X et al. Blood 2013;121:1968–1975

Efficacy

Response to Treatment and Survival End Points by Arm Based on Independent Review Committee Assessment			
	21/28	28/28	Total
ITT (n = 84)			
	N = 43	N = 41	N = 84
ORR (≥PR), n (%)	15 (35)	14 (34)	29 (34.5)
CR*, n (%)	1 (2)	2 (5)	3 (4)
VGPR, n (%)	1 (2)	1 (2)	2 (2)
PR, n (%)	13 (30)	11 (27)	24 (27)
Stable disease, n (%)	19 (44)	21 (51)	40 (48)
Progressive disease, n (%)	5 (12)	3 (7)	8 (9.5)
Not evaluable, n (%)	4 (9)	3 (7)	7 (8)
Median time to first response (95% CI), months	2.7 (0.8, 9.5)	1.1 (0.6, 8)	1.8 (0.6, 9.5)
Median duration of response (95% CI), months	6.4 (4,—)	8.3 (6.5, 16)	7.3 (5, 15)
1 year free of relapse	42%	47%	44%
Efficacy-Evaluable Population (n = 66)			
	N = 34	N = 32	N = 66
ORR (CR + PR), n (%)	15 (44)	12 (37.5)	27 (41)
≥VGPR, n (%)	2 (6)	3 (9)	5 (7.5)
Median survival (95% CI), months	21/28 (n = 43)	28/28 (n = 41)	Total
Time to progression	5.8 (3, 10)	4.8 (3, 7)	5.4 (4, 8)
At 1 year, %	31	25	28
Progression-free survival	5.4 (3, 9)	3.7 (2, 7)	4.6 (4, 7)
At 1 year, %	29	22	25.5
Overall survival	14.9 (9,—)	14.8 (9, 20)	14.9 (11, 20)
At 12 months, %	58	56	57
At 18 months, %	49	39	44

Abbreviations: CR, complete response; ORR, overall response rate; PR, partial response; VGPR, very good partial response
*CR confirmed by bone marrow assessment
Leleu X et al. Blood 2013;121:1968–1975

(continued)

Efficacy (continued)

Patient Outcomes	
Confirmed response rate*,†	32% (95% CI 19–53)
*Confirmed response rate**	32% (95% CI 17–51)
Number of responders*	11
VGPR	2
PR	9
MR	4
Best response	
VGPR	3 (9%)
PR	8 (23%)
MR	5 (15%)
SD	12 (35%)
PD	6 (18%)
Median time to response*	2.0 months (range, 0.7–3.9)
Duration of response*,‡	9.1 months (95% CI 6.5–NA)
Overall survival‡	13.9 months (95% CI NA)
Progression free survival‡	4.8 months (95% CI 2.7–10.1)

Abbreviations: CI, confidence interval; MR, best response; NA, not attained; PD, progressive disease; PR, partial response; SD, stable disease; VGPR, very good partial response
*Does not include MR per study design
†Study design uses the first 32 patients
‡Kaplan-Meier method
Lacy MQ et al. Leukemia 2010;24:1934–1939

Toxicity

Summary of G3/4 (nCI-CTC*) Adverse Events That Occurred in > 5% of Cases

Adverse Events, n (%)	21/28 (n = 43)	28/28 (n = 41)	Total (n = 84)
SAEs	32 (74)	33 (80)	65 (77)
Study drug–related SAEs	14 (33)	18 (44)	32 (38)
Any G3 or G4 AE	40 (93)	35 (85)	75 (89)
Hematologic			
Blood and lymphatic system	32 (74)	30 (73)	62 (74)
Anemia	16 (37)	14 (34)	30 (36)
Neutropenia	28 (65)	24 (58.5)	52 (62)
Thrombocytopenia	12 (28)	11 (27)	23 (27)
Nonhematologic			
General disorders	10 (23)	10 (24)	20 (24)
Asthenia	6 (14)	2 (5)	8 (9.5)

(continued)

Toxicity (continued)

Nonhematologic			
Infections and infestations	8 (19)	11 (27)	19 (23)
Pneumonia	3 (7)	8 (19.5)	11 (13)
Musculoskeletal/connective tissue	9 (21)	8 (19.5)	17 (20)
Bone pain	6 (14)	3 (7)	9 (11)
Renal and urinary disorders	7 (16)	2 (5)	9 (11)
Renal failure	7 (16)	2 (5)	9 (11)
Respiratory disorders	8 (19)	2 (5)	10 (12)
Dyspnea	5 (12)	0	5 (6)

*National Cancer Institute Common Terminology Criteria for Adverse Events, version 3.0
Leleu X et al. Blood 2013;121:1968–1975

Maximum Severity of Toxicities* (n = 34)

Toxicity[†]	G1	G2	G3	G4	All Grades
Hematologic					
Anemia	15	9	4	0	28
Lymphocyte count decreased	0	3	0	0	3
Neutrophil count decreased	5	7	6	4	22
Platelet count decreased	8	4	3	0	15
Leukopenia	9	5	7	1	22
Nonhematologic					
Edema limbs	0	2	0	0	2
Musculoskeletal	0	1	0	0	1
Muscle weakness lower limb	0	1	0	0	1
Agitation	0	2	0	0	2
Anxiety	0	1	0	0	1
Confusion	0	1	0	0	1
Peripheral sensory neuropathy	6	3	0	0	9
Tremor	0	1	0	0	1
Myalgia	0	1	0	0	1
Dyspnea	0	1	0	0	1
Pneumonitis	0	0	1	0	1
Edema	0	0	1	0	1
Fatigue	8	9	3	0	20
Dermatology	0	0	1	0	1
Anorexia	5	1	0	0	6
Constipation	0	1	0	0	1
Diarrhea	4	0	0	0	4
Gastritis	0	1	0	0	1
Nausea	2	2	0	0	4

(continued)

Toxicity (*continued*)

Metabolic/Laboratory					
Hyperglycemia	0	3	0	1	4
Infection/Febrile Neutropenia					
Infection—no ANC	0	1	0	0	1
Upper airway infection	0	1	0	0	1
Bladder infection	0	1	0	0	1
Pneumonia G0 to G2 ANC	0	0	1	0	1
Respiratory tract infection	0	2	0	0	2
Skin infection	0	1	0	0	1

*Possibly, probably, or definitely related
†National Cancer Institute Common Terminology Criteria for Adverse Events, version 3.0
Lacy MQ et al. Leukemia 2010;24:1934–1939

Therapy Monitoring

1. Blood counts and physical examinations on day 1 of each cycle
2. Serum and urinary protein electrophoresis studies on day 1 of each cycle as indicated and at the end of treatment

SUBSEQUENT THERAPY

MULTIPLE MYELOMA REGIMEN: POMALIDOMIDE + CYCLOPHOSPHAMIDE + PREDNISONE

Larocca A et al. Blood 2013;122:2799–2806

Induction:

Cyclophosphamide 50 mg/dose orally, every other day (eg, days 1, 3, 5…, etc. *or* days 2, 4, 6…, etc.) continually, for 14 doses every 28 days (total dose/cycle = 700 mg)

Prednisone 50 mg/dose orally, every other day (eg, days 1, 3, 5…, etc. *or* days 2, 4, 6…, etc.) continually, for 14 doses every 28 days (total dose/cycle = 700 mg)

plus

Pomalidomide 2–3 mg/day orally, continually, for 28 consecutive days, on days 1–28, every 28 days (total dose/cycle = 56–84 mg), *or*

Pomalidomide 4 mg/day orally, continually, for 21 consecutive days, on days 1–21, every 28 days (total dose/cycle = 84 mg)

Maintenance:

Pomalidomide 1 mg/day orally, continually, until disease relapse or progression (total dose/week = 7 mg)

Prednisone 25 mg/dose orally, every other day (eg, days 1, 3, 5…, etc. *or* days 2, 4, 6…, etc.) continually, until disease relapse or progression

Supportive Care

Antiemetic prophylaxis

Emetogenic potential is **MINIMAL–LOW**

See Chapter 42 for antiemetic recommendations

Hematopoietic growth factor (CSF) prophylaxis

Primary prophylaxis may be indicated

See Chapter 43 for more information

Antimicrobial prophylaxis

Risk of fever and neutropenia is INTERMEDIATE

Antimicrobial primary prophylaxis to be considered:

- Antibacterial—consider a fluoroquinolone or no prophylaxis; *P. jirovecii* prophylaxis is recommended (eg, cotrimoxazole)
- Antifungal—recommended; consider use during periods of neutropenia, and in anticipation of mucositis
- Antiviral—antiherpes antivirals (eg, acyclovir, famciclovir, valacyclovir)

Bisphosphonates

All patients receiving primary therapy for symptomatic multiple myeloma should receive a bisphosphonate adjunctively.

Thromboprophylaxis

Risk assessment and recommendations for VTE prophylaxis in patients with multiple myeloma with individual or myeloma-related risk factors, or risk factors related to treatment

(continued)

Treatment Modifications

Pomalidomide Dose Levels	
Starting dose	2.5 mg/day
Level −1	2 mg/day
Level −2	1.5 mg/day
Level −3	1 mg/day
Level −4	0.5 mg/day
Level −5	Discontinue

Prednisone Dose Levels	
Starting dose	50 mg/dose
Level −1	25 mg/dose
Level −2	20 mg/dose
Level −3	10 mg/dose
Level −4	5 mg/dose
Level −5	Discontinue

Adverse Event	Treatment Modification
ANC <500/mm^3 Febrile neutropenia (fever ≥38.5°C + ANC <1000/mm^3) Platelets <25,000/mm^3	Interrupt pomalidomide and cyclophosphamide treatment, and follow CBC weekly. When ANC ≥500/mm^3 and platelet count ≥50,000/mm^3, resume pomalidomide 1 dose level lower and cyclophosphamide at a dose of 25 mg every other day
Nonhematologic G3/4 toxicity	Interrupt pomalidomide treatment, and follow weekly or more frequently. Restart treatment 1 dose level lower than the previous dose when toxicity has resolved G ≤2
ANC <1000/mm^3, platelet count <50,000/mm^3, hemoglobin <8 g/dL, and/or nonhematologic adverse events G ≥3	Delay the start of a new cycle. If delayed by ≥2 weeks, reduce the dose of pomalidomide by 1 dose level
G4 rash, neuropathy, or hypersensitivity, or G ≥3 bradycardia or cardiac arrhythmia	Permanently discontinue pomalidomide

(continued)

(*continued*)

Individual risk factors
• Obesity (BMI ≥30 kg/m²)
• H/O VTE
• CVC or pacemaker
• Comorbid pathologies
  ▪ Cardiac disease
  ▪ Chronic renal disease
  ▪ Diabetes
  ▪ Acute infection
  ▪ Immobilization
• Surgery
  ▪ General surgery
  ▪ Any anesthesia
  ▪ Trauma
• Medications
  ▪ Erythropoietin (epoetin alfa, darbepoetin)
  ▪ Estrogenic compounds
  ▪ Bevacizumab
• Clotting disorders
  ▪ Thrombophilia
Myeloma-related risk factors
• Diagnosis of multiple myeloma
• Hyperviscosity
	≤1 Individual or myeloma-related risk factor present:
	• **Aspirin** 81–325 mg daily
	
	≥2 Individual or myeloma-related risk factors present:
	• **LMWH,* equivalent to enoxaparin sodium** 40 mg/day *or* **dalteparin sodium** 5000 IU/day; administer subcutaneously, *or*
	• **Warfarin**, targeting an INR = 2–3

Concomitant treatment-related risk factors Thalidomide or lenalidomide in combination with: • High-dose dexamethasone (≥480 mg/month) • Doxorubicin • Multiagent chemotherapy	• **LMWH,* equivalent to enoxaparin sodium** 40 mg/day *or* **dalteparin sodium** 5000 IU/day; administer subcutaneously, *or* • **Warfarin**, targeting an INR = 2–3

*LMWHs should be used with caution in individuals with impaired renal function (creatinine clearance <30 mL/min). Refer to product labeling for information about doses and administration schedules in renally impaired patients, and guidance for monitoring anti-Factor Xa concentrations
Abbreviations: CVC, central venous catheter; INR, international normalized ratio; LMWH, low-molecular-weight heparin; VTE, venous thromboembolic disease
References: Geerts WH et al. Chest 2008;133(6 Suppl):381S–453S
National Comprehensive Cancer Network. Multiple Myeloma, V.1.2014. (Accessed October 8, 2013, at http://www.nccn.org)
National Comprehensive Cancer Network. Venous Thromboembolic Disease, V.2.2013. (Accessed October 8, 2013, at http://www.nccn.org)
Palumbo A et al. Leukemia 2008;22:414–423

Treatment Modifications
(*continued*)

G3/4 adverse events occurring on or after day 15 during a single cycle	Withhold pomalidomide for the remainder of the cycle, and reduce pomalidomide dose by 1 dose level beginning with the next cycle
Toxicities ascribed to prednisone such as severe manifestations of hypercorticism, including: hyperglycemia, irritability, insomnia, or oral candidiasis	Hold prednisone doses for up to 21 days to resolve toxicity and then restart at the same dose level or reduce the prednisone dose by 50%

Patient Population Studied

Patients with MM who had received 1–3 prior lines of therapy and whose disease had relapsed after lenalidomide or was refractory. Relapse was defined as reoccurrence of disease requiring the initiation of a salvage therapy. Refractory disease was defined as relapse while on salvage therapy or progression within 60 days after the most recent therapy. Patients were required to have Karnofsky performance status ≥60%

Baseline Patients Characteristics (n = 66)

Median age, years (range)	69 (41–84)
Gender (F/M)	33 (48%)/36 (52%)
International Staging System stage I/II/III	34 (49%)/27 (39%)/8 (12%)
Myeloma protein class	
IgG	42 (61%)
IgA 4	16 (23%)
Bence-Jones protein	10 (15%)
Non-secretory	1 (1%)
Karnofsky performance status 60–70/80/90–100	10 (14%)/13 (19%)/46 (67%)
Serum β_2-microglobulin level: median (mg/L)	3 (1.6–12)

(*continued*)

Efficacy

Best Responses to Pomalidomide + Cyclophosphamide + Prednisone

POL Dose	1 mg (n = 4)	1.5 mg (n = 4)	2 mg (n = 4)	Relapsed >LEN		Refractory to LEN	Refractory to LEN/BOR
				mg (n = 55)	mg (n = 18)	mg (n = 37)	mg (n = 16)
Response							
CR/PR	1 (25%)	2 (50%)	2 (50%)	28 (51%)	11 (61%)	17 (46%)	8 (50%)
CR	—	—	—	3	1	2	2
VGPR	—	—	—	10	6	4	1
PR	1	2	2	15	4	11	5
MR	1	-	1	11	2	9	5
SD	1	1	1	15	5	10	3
PD	1	1	—	1	0	1	—

BOR, bortezomib; CR, complete response; LEN, lenalidomide; MR, minimal response; PD, progressive disease; POL, pomalidomide; PR, partial response; SD, stable disease; VGPR, very good partial response

Time to Event Analysis

	N	Median Follow-Up	Median PFS	Median OS	12-Month OS
		Months (Range)	Months (95% CI)		
All patients	67	15.0 (3.7–26.4)	8.6 (7.5–13.9)	NR	65% (51–76%)
LEN 1–2 mg	12	24.1 (3.7–26.4)	4.6 (3.3–8.0)	9 (5.2–NR)	44% (15–70%)
LEN 2.5 mg	55	14.8 (6.1–21.4)	10.4 (7.8–15.8)	NR	69% (54–81%)
Relapsed > LEN	18	12.7 (7.2–21.4)	15.7 (12.8–20.7)	NR	88% (60–97%)
Refractory to LEN	37	15.3 (6.1–21.4)	8.6 (7.5–13.9)	NR	60% (41–75%)
Refractory to LEN/BOR	16	15.8 (6.6–21.4)	8.6 (4.8–NR)	NR	67% (37–85%)

BOR, bortezomib; LEN, lenalidomide; NR, not reached; OS, overall survival; PFS, progression-free survival

Treatment Modifications
(continued)

Baseline Patients Characteristics (n = 66)

Months from diagnosis to on study: median (range)	53 (11–203)
Prior lines of therapy: median (range)	3 (1–3)
Prior therapies	
Lenalidomide	69 (100%)
Bortezomib	58 (84%)
Thalidomide	14 (20%)
Autologous transplant	23 (33%)
Allogeneic transplant	10 (15%)
Previous lenalidomide	
Relapsed	23 (33%)
Refractory	46 (67%)
Previous bortezomib (data not available for 14 [20%])	
Relapsed	17 (25%)
Refractory	27 (39%)
FISH*	
High risk	18 (26%)
Standard risk	35 (51%)
Not available	16 (23%)
Chromosome abnormalities	
Del 13	24 (35%)
(4;14)	8 (12%)
t(11;14)	12 (17%)
t(14;16)	3 (4%)
Del17	8 (12%)

*High-risk FISH = presence of at least 1 of the following: t(4;14), t(14;16), or del17

Toxicity

Treatment—Related Adverse Events During Salvage Therapy Phase 2 (n = 55)

Event	G1	G2	G3	G4	G5	All Grades
Hematologic						
Neutropenia	6	10	14	9	—	33
Thrombocytopenia	15	5	3	3	—	26
Anemia	10	22	5	—	—	37
Nonhematologic						
Ischemia	—	—	—	1	—	1
Arrhythmia	—	3	—	—	—	3
Sensory neuropathy	6	2	—	—	—	8
Neuralgia	2	1	1	—	—	4
Motor neuropathy	—	—	1	—	—	1
Tremor	—	1	—	—	—	1
Confusion	—	1	—	1	—	2
Mood depression	—	1	—	—	—	1
Other neurologic	3	—	1	—	—	4
Upper respiratory	2	5	—	—	—	7
Pneumonia	2	5	3	—	1	11
Sepsis	—	—	—	—	1	1
Other infective	1	4	—	—	—	5
Diarrhea	1	—	—	—	—	1
Constipation	—	5	—	—	—	5
Nausea/vomiting	1	—	—	—	—	1
Other gastrointestinal	1	2	1	—	—	4
Increased transaminase	2	1	—	—	—	3
Liver failure	—	—	1	—	—	1
Pancreatitis	—	1	—	—	—	1
Deep-vein thrombosis	—	1	—	1	—	2
Phlebitis	1	—	—	—	—	1
Nonhematologic						
Fatigue	5	7	2	—	—	14
Fever	2	—	—	—	—	2
Drowsiness	1	—	—	—	—	1
Weight gain	—	1	—	—	—	1
Rash	—	2	4	—	—	6
Other dermatologic	—	1	—	—	—	1
Other	7	6	3	—	—	16

Therapy Monitoring

1. Blood counts and physical examinations on day 1 of each cycle
2. Serum and urinary protein electrophoresis studies on day 1 of each cycle as indicated and at the end of treatment

SUBSEQUENT THERAPY
MULTIPLE MYELOMA REGIMEN: SELINEXOR + DEXAMETHASONE

Chari A et al. N Engl J Med 2019;381:727–738
Supplementary appendix to: Chari A et al. N Engl J Med 2019;381:727–738
Protocol for: Chari A et al. N Engl J Med 2019;381:727–738
XPOVIO (selinexor) prescribing information. Newton, MA: Karyopharm Therapeutics Inc; revised July 2019

Selinexor 80 mg per dose; administer orally twice per week on days 1 and 3, every 7 days, until disease progression (total dosage/week = 160 mg)
- Patients should swallow selinexor tablets whole. Do not break, chew, crush, or divide tablets
- If a patient misses or delays a dose of selinexor, instruct the patient to take the next dose on the next regularly scheduled day. The dose should not be made up
- If a patient vomits after taking selinexor, instruct the patient to take the next dose on the next regularly scheduled day. The dose should not be repeated
- In vitro studies indicate that selinexor is a substrate for CYP3A4, multiple UDP-glucuronosyltransferases (UGTs), and glutathione S-transferases (GSTs), and that selinexor inhibits OATP1B3. Clinical drug interaction studies have not been performed

Dexamethasone 20 mg per dose; administer orally twice per week on days 1 and 3, every 7 days, until disease progression (total dosage/week = 40 mg)

Supportive Care
Antiemetic prophylaxis
*Emetogenic potential is **MODERATE TO HIGH**.* The U.S. FDA-approved prescribing information for selinexor recommends that patients receive prophylactic treatment with a 5-HT3 antagonist and/or other anti-nausea agents prior to and during treatment with selinexor
See Chapter 42 for antiemetic recommendation

Hematopoietic growth factor (CSF) prophylaxis
*Primary prophylaxis is **NOT** indicated*
See Chapter 43 for more information

Antimicrobial prophylaxis
*Risk of fever and neutropenia is **INTERMEDIATE***
   Antimicrobial primary prophylaxis to be considered:
   - Antibacterial—consider a fluoroquinolone during periods of prolonged neutropenia (ANC <500/mm³ for ≥7 days) or no prophylaxis; *P. jirovecii* prophylaxis is recommended (eg, cotrimoxazole)
   - Antifungal—consider fluconazole during periods of prolonged neutropenia (ANC <500/mm³ for ≥7 days) or no prophylaxis
   - Antiviral—antiherpes antivirals (eg, acyclovir, famciclovir, valacyclovir)

Diarrhea management
Loperamide or **diphenoxylate hydrochloride** 2.5 mg **with atropine sulfate** 0.025 mg (eg, Lomotil)
Hydration and nutrition
Instruct patients to maintain adequate intake of oral fluids and calories during treatment with selinexor. Consider administration of intravenous fluids for patients at higher risk for dehydration

Bisphosphonates
All patients receiving primary therapy for symptomatic multiple myeloma should receive a bisphosphonate adjunctively.
Steroid-associated gastritis
Add a proton pump inhibitor or H₂-receptor antagonist during dexamethasone use to prevent gastritis and duodenitis

Treatment Modifications

SELINEXOR TREATMENT MODIFICATIONS

Selinexor Dose Levels	
Dose level 1 (starting dose)	80 mg twice per week
Dose level −1	100 mg once per week
Dose level −2	80 mg once per week
Dose level −3	60 mg once per week
Dose level −4	Discontinue selinexor

(continued)

Treatment Modifications (*continued*)

Adverse Event	Treatment Modification
Thrombocytopenia	
Platelet count ≥25,000/mm³ to <75,000/mm³ *without* bleeding	Reduce the selinexor dosage by 1 dose level
Platelet count ≥25,000/mm³ to <75,000/mm³ *with* bleeding	Withhold selinexor until resolution of bleeding, then resume selinexor with the dosage reduced by 1 dose level
Platelet count <25,000/mm³	Withhold selinexor until recovery of platelet count to ≥50,000/mm³, then resume selinexor with the dosage reduced by 1 dose level
Neutropenia	
ANC ≥500/mm³ to <1000/mm³ *without* fever	Reduce the selinexor dosage by 1 dose level
ANC ≥500/mm³ to <1000/mm³ *with* fever *or* Febrile neutropenia	Monitor CBC with differential frequently. Withhold selinexor until ANC improves to ≥1000/mm³, then resume selinexor with the dosage reduced by 1 dose level
Anemia	
Hemoglobin <8 g/dL	Reduce the selinexor dosage by 1 dose level. Alternately, transfuse and maintain dosage unchanged
Anemia with life-threatening consequences (urgent intervention indicated)	Monitor CBC frequently. Transfuse and/or administer other treatments as indicated. Withhold selinexor until hemoglobin improves to ≥8 g/dL, then resume selinexor with the dosage reduced by 1 dose level
Gastrointestinal toxicities	
G1/2 nausea (oral intake decreased without significant weight loss, dehydration, or malnutrition) *or* G1/2 vomiting (≤5 episodes per day)	Continue selinexor at the same dose and optimize prophylactic and rescue anti-nausea medication regimen
G3 nausea (inadequate oral caloric or fluid intake) *or* G3/4 vomiting (6 or more episodes per day)	Withhold selinexor. Optimize prophylactic and rescue anti-nausea medication regimen. Resume selinexor when nausea and/or vomiting has resolved to G ≤2 or baseline with the dosage reduced by 1 dose level
G2 diarrhea (increase of 4–6 stools per day above baseline), first occurrence	Continue selinexor at the same dose and optimize supportive care, including antidiarrheal medications
G2 diarrhea (increase of 4–6 stools per day above baseline), second and subsequent occurrence	Reduce the selinexor dosage by 1 dose level and optimize supportive care, including antidiarrheal medications
G3/4 diarrhea (increase of ≥7 stools per day over baseline; hospitalization indicated)	Withhold selinexor. Optimize supportive care, including antidiarrheal medications. Resume selinexor when diarrhea has resolved to G ≤2 with the dosage reduced by 1 dose level
Other Toxicities	
Hyponatremia (sodium ≤130 mmol/L)	Provide appropriate supportive care. Correct sodium level for hyperglycemia and high serum paraprotein levels, if applicable. Monitor sodium levels frequently as clinically indicated. Withhold selinexor until sodium improves to ≥130 mmol/L, then resume selinexor with the dosage reduced by 1 dose level
G2 fatigue* (not relieved by rest; limits instrumental ADL) lasting >7 days *or* G3 fatigue* (not relieved by rest, limits self-care ADL) of any duration	Withhold selinexor until fatigue resolves to G ≤1 (fatigue relieved by rest) or baseline, then resume selinexor with the dosage reduced by 1 dose level
Weight loss of ≥10% to <20% *or* Anorexia associated with significant weight loss or malnutrition	Withhold selinexor and provide supportive care. Monitor until weight returns to >90% of baseline weight, then resume selinexor with the dosage reduced by 1 dose level
Other G3/4 life-threatening nonhematologic toxicities	Withhold selinexor until toxicity improves to G ≤2, then resume selinexor with the dosage reduced by 1 dose level, if clinically appropriate

(*continued*)

Treatment Modifications (continued)

DEXAMETHASONE TREATMENT MODIFICATIONS

Dexamethasone Dose Levels

Starting dose	20 mg twice per week
Dose Level −1	10 mg twice per week
Dose Level −2	6 mg twice per week
Dose Level −3	4 mg twice per week
Dose Level −4	Discontinue dexamethasone

Adverse Event	Treatment Modification
G1/2 dyspepsia (moderate symptoms; medical intervention indicated; limiting instrumental ADL), gastric or duodenal ulcer, or gastritis	Continue dexamethasone at the same dose. Treat with therapeutic doses of an H_2-receptor antagonist or proton pump inhibitor. If symptoms persist, then reduce the dexamethasone dose by one level
G ≥3 dyspepsia, gastric or duodenal ulcer, or gastritis (surgery or hospitalization indicated)	Withhold dexamethasone until symptoms return to baseline. Resume dexamethasone reduced by one dose level along with concurrent treatment with therapeutic doses of an H_2-receptor antagonist or proton pump inhibitor. If symptoms recur, then permanently discontinue dexamethasone
Acute pancreatitis	Permanently discontinue dexamethasone
G ≥3 edema	Withhold dexamethasone until symptoms return to baseline. Consider treatment with diuretics. Resume dexamethasone reduced by one dose level. If edema persists, reduce by another dose level. Discontinue dexamethasone permanently if symptoms persist despite two prior dose reductions
G ≥2 mood alteration (moderate mood alteration) or confusion (moderate disorientation; limiting instrumental ADL)	Withhold dexamethasone until symptoms return to baseline. Resume dexamethasone reduced by one dose level. If symptoms persist, reduce by another dose level
G ≥2 muscle weakness (symptomatic; evident on physical exam; limiting instrumental ADL)	Withhold dexamethasone until symptoms return to baseline. Resume dexamethasone reduced by one dose level. If weakness persists, reduce by another dose level. If weakness still persists, then permanently discontinue dexamethasone
G ≥3 hyperglycemia (insulin therapy initiated; hospitalization indicated)	Withhold dexamethasone until blood glucose is ≤250 mg/dL. Treat with insulin or other hypoglycemic agents as clinically appropriate and then resume dexamethasone at the same dose. If hyperglycemia is uncontrolled despite above measures, decrease dexamethasone by one dose level
Other G ≥2 nonhematologic toxicity attributable to dexamethasone including severe irritability, insomnia, or oral candidiasis	Withhold dexamethasone until toxicity resolves to G ≤1, then resume at a lower dose. Consider reduction by one dose level for G2/G3 toxicity, and by two dose levels for G4 or recurrent G3 toxicity

Note: if the dose of one drug in the regimen is delayed, interrupted, or discontinued, treatment with the other drug may continue as scheduled
*According to the National Cancer Institute Common Terminology Criteria for Adverse Events (NCI CTCAE) v4.0
ANC, absolute neutrophil count; CBC, complete blood count; ADL, activities of daily living

Patient Population Studied

The STORM trial was an open-label, phase 2b study that included 122 adult patients with previously treated multiple myeloma (MM) and evaluated treatment with selinexor plus dexamethasone. Patients were eligible for the trial if they had measurable, progressive, symptomatic MM (according to International Myeloma Working Group Uniform Response Criteria); if they had received ≥ 3 prior regimens including (alone or in combination) an alkylating agent, bortezomib, carfilzomib, lenalidomide, pomalidomide, and a glucocorticoid; if their disease was "triple-class refractory" (ie, refractory to ≥1 immunomodulatory drug, refractory to ≥1 proteasome inhibitor, refractory to daratumumab, and refractory to glucocorticoids, and also refractory to the most recent anti-myeloma regimen); if they had an ECOG performance status of ≤2; and if they had adequate organ function

Efficacy (n = 122)

Efficacy Variable	Selinexor + Dexamethasone (n = 122)
PFS	
Median PFS—months (95% CI)	3.7 (3.0–5.3)
Median OS in various groups (as denoted below)—months (95% CI)	
Modified ITT population (n = 122)	8.6 (6.2–11.3)
Patients with PR or better (n = 32)	15.6 (15.6–NE)
Patients with MR or better (n = 48)	15.6 (12.9–NE)
Patients with a best response of SD (n = 48)	5.9 (4.3–10.4)
Patients with a best response of PD or NE (n = 32)	1.7 (1.2–NE)
DOR and TTR in patients with a PR or better (n = 32)	
Median DOR—months (95% CI)	4.4 (3.7–10.8)
Median TTR—weeks (range)	4.1 (1–14)
Response in modified ITT population (n = 122)*	
Stringent CR rate—n/N (%)	2/122 (2)
VGPR rate—n/N (%)	6/122 (5)
PR or better rate—n/N (%) (95% CI)[†]	32/122 (26) (19–35)[†]
PR rate—n/N (%)	24/122 (20)
MR or better rate—n/N (%) (95% CI)	48/122 (39) (31–49)
MR rate—n/N (%)	16/122 (13)
SD rate—n/N (%)	48/122 (39)
PD or NE rate—n/N (%)	32/122 (26)
Response in patients with R-ISS disease stage I (n = 20)	
PR or better rate—n/N (%)	7/20 (35)
MR or better rate—n/N (%)	10/20 (50)
Response in patients with R-ISS disease stage II (n = 78)	
PR or better rate—n/N (%)	21/78 (27)
MR or better rate—n/N (%)	32/78 (41)
Response in patients with R-ISS disease stage III (n = 23)	
PR or better rate—n/N (%)	4/23 (17)
MR or better rate—n/N (%)	6/23 (26)
Response in patients with measurable free light chains (n = 35)	
PR or better rate—n/N (%)	15/35 (43)
MR or better rate—n/N (%)	19/35 (54)

(continued)

Adverse Events (n = 123)

Event	Selinexor + Dexamethasone (n = 123)	
	Grade 1 or 2 (%)	Grade 3 or 4 (%)
Thrombocytopenia	15	59
Anemia	24	44
Neutropenia	19	21
Leukopenia	20	14
Lymphopenia	5	11
Fatigue	48	25
Nausea	62	10
Decreased appetite	51	5
Decreased weight	50	1
Diarrhea	38	7
Vomiting	35	3
Hyponatremia	15	22
Upper respiratory tract infection	21	2
Constipation	20	2
Dyspnea	18	4
Cough	17	0
Hypokalemia	11	7
Insomnia	15	2
Mental status changes	11	6
Pneumonia	7	9
Dizziness	15	0
Pyrexia	15	0
Epistaxis	11	1

(continued)

Efficacy (n = 122) *(continued)*

Response in patients without measurable free light chains (n = 87)	
PR or better rate—n/N (%)	17/87 (20)
MR or better rate—n/N (%)	29/87 (33)
Response in patients with a high-risk cytogenetic abnormality (n = 65)‡	
PR or better rate—n/N (%)	12/65 (18)
MR or better rate—n/N (%)	24/65 (37)

*Response was assessed according to International Myeloma Working Group Uniform Response Criteria and adjudicated by an independent review committee. Overall response was defined as a confirmed PR (≥50% reduction in the serum level of myeloma protein) or better; clinical benefit was defined as a confirmed MR (≥25% to <50% reduction in the serum level of myeloma protein) or better

†This was the primary outcome and was analyzed for statistical significance by calculating a two-sided, exact 95% CI; if the lower boundary of the CI was >10%, then the result was considered significant

‡This category included any of: del(17p)/p53, t(14;16), t(4;14), or 1q21 (1q gain >2)

CI, confidence interval; HR, hazard ratio; IRC, independent review committee; NR, not reached; PFS, progression-free survival; OS, overall survival; ITT, intention-to-treat; CR, complete response; VGPR, very good partial response; PR, partial response; MR, minimal response; SD, stable disease; PD, progressive disease; NE, not able to be evaluated; TTR, time to response; DOR, duration of response; R-ISS, Revised International Staging System

Note: all efficacy analyses were performed in the modified ITT population (122 patients), which included all patients who met all enrollment criteria or received a waiver to enroll from the sponsor (12 patients) and who received at least one dose of selinexor plus dexamethasone. Kaplan-Meier methods were used to analyze PFS, OS, DOR, and TTR. All data included in the table were published in Chari, 2019, and its supplementary appendix

Therapy Monitoring

1. *At baseline and periodically (more frequent during initial 2 months):* CBC with differential and platelet count, serum chemistries (especially sodium), and body weight
2. *Monitor periodically for, and advise patients to report symptoms of:*
   a. Dehydration, malnutrition, gastrointestinal adverse effects (eg, nausea/vomiting, diarrhea, anorexia), and infection
   b. Neurologic adverse reactions (eg, dizziness, confusion) may occur with selinexor. Avoid concomitant use with other medications that may cause dizziness or confusion and avoid situations where dizziness or a confused state may be problematic. Maintenance of optimal hydration status, correction of anemia, and minimization of polypharmacy may reduce the incidence and severity of neurologic adverse reactions

Adverse Events (n = 123) *(continued)*

Event	Selinexor + Dexamethasone (n = 123)	
	Grade 1 or 2 (%)	Grade 3 or 4 (%)
Fall	11	2
Hyperglycemia	4	7
Peripheral edema	9	2
Blurred vision	9	2

Adverse events that emerged during treatment were included in the table if they were reported in ≥10% of all patients. Adverse events were graded according to the National Cancer Institute Common Terminology Criteria for Adverse Events (NCI CTCAE) v4.03 in all patients who received at least one dose of study drug treatment. Adverse events of any grade were reported in 100% of patients in the trial. Study treatment was discontinued in 18% of patients because of an adverse event considered by the investigator to be related to selinexor or dexamethasone (full list of adverse events considered by the investigator to be possibly, probably, or definitely related to study drug treatment was reported in the supplementary appendix). Adverse events leading to dose modification or interruption were reported in 80% of patients, with the majority being reported in the first two cycles. The most common adverse events leading to dose reduction or interruption were thrombocytopenia (43%), fatigue (16%), and neutropenia (11%). Thrombocytopenia was reported more frequently in patients who had thrombocytopenia at baseline than in those who did not and 6 patients with Grade ≥3 thrombocytopenia had a concurrent bleeding event of Grade ≥3. Adverse events were reversible and lacked cumulative toxic effects except for 1 report of irreversible acute kidney injury. Serious adverse events occurred in 63% of patients, with pneumonia (11%) and sepsis (9%) being the most common. A total of 28 patients died during the study, 16 from disease progression and 12 from adverse events; only 2 adverse events that led to death were considered by the investigator to be related to treatment (pneumonia with concurrent disease progression and sepsis)

SUBSEQUENT THERAPY

MULTIPLE MYELOMA REGIMEN: LENALIDOMIDE + DEXAMETHASONE

Dimopoulos M et al. N Engl J Med 2007;357:2123–2132
Weber DM et al. N Engl J Med 2007;357:2133–2142

Lenalidomide 25 mg per day; administer orally for 21 consecutive days on days 1–21, every 28 days (total dose/cycle = 525 mg)

Cycles 1–4:

Dexamethasone 40 mg per dose; administer orally for 12 doses on days 1–4, 9–12, and 17–20, every 28 days for 4 cycles (total dose/cycle = 480 mg)

Cycle 5 and subsequently:

Dexamethasone 40 mg per dose; administer orally for 4 doses on days 1–4, every 28 days, until the occurrence of disease progression or unacceptable toxic effects (total dose/cycle = 160 mg)

Supportive Care

Antiemetic prophylaxis

Emetogenic potential is **MINIMAL–LOW**

See Chapter 42 for antiemetic recommendations

Hematopoietic growth factor (CSF) prophylaxis

Primary prophylaxis is **NOT** indicated

See Chapter 43 for more information

Antimicrobial prophylaxis

Risk of fever and neutropenia is **INTERMEDIATE**

Antimicrobial primary prophylaxis to be considered:

- Antibacterial—consider a fluoroquinolone or no prophylaxis; *P. jirovecii* prophylaxis is recommended (eg, cotrimoxazole)
- Antifungal—consider concomitant use of clotrimazole during periods of neutropenia
- Antiviral—antiherpes antivirals (eg, acyclovir, famciclovir, valacyclovir)

Bisphosphonates

All patients receiving primary therapy for symptomatic multiple myeloma should receive a bisphosphonate adjunctively.

Thromboprophylaxis

Risk assessment and recommendations for VTE prophylaxis in patients with multiple myeloma with individual or myeloma-related risk factors, or risk factors related to treatment

(continued)

Treatment Modifications

Lenalidomide Dose Levels	
Dose Level 1	25 mg
Dose Level −1	15 mg
Dose Level −2	10 mg
Dose Level −3	5 mg

Dexamethasone Dose Levels	
Dose Level 1	40 mg/dose for 12 doses on days 1 to 4, 9 to 12, and 17 to 20
Dose Level −1	40 mg daily for 4 days every 2 weeks (days 1–4 and 15–18)
Dose Level −2	40 mg daily for 4 days every 4 weeks (days 1–4)
Dose Level −3	20 mg daily for 4 days every 4 weeks (days 1–4)

Adverse Event	Treatment Modification
G3/4 neutropenia	Interrupt lenalidomide treatment and follow clinically. After ANC recovers to ≥1000/mm³, resume lenalidomide at a dose decreased from the previous dose by 5 mg/day, but the daily dose should not be less than 5 mg/day
Febrile neutropenia	Interrupt lenalidomide treatment and follow closely. After fever abates, resume lenalidomide at a dose decreased from the previous dose by 5 mg/day, but the daily dose should not be less than 5 mg/day
G3/4 nonhematologic toxicity	Interrupt lenalidomide treatment and follow clinically. After toxicity abates to G ≤2, resume lenalidomide at a dose decreased from the previous dose by 5 mg/day, but the daily dose should not be less than 5 mg/day

(continued)

(continued)

Individual risk factors
- Obesity (BMI ≥30 kg/m²)
- H/O VTE
- CVC or pacemaker
- Comorbid pathologies
  - Cardiac disease
  - Chronic renal disease
  - Diabetes
  - Acute infection
  - Immobilization
- Surgery
  - General surgery
  - Any anesthesia
  - Trauma
- Medications
  - Erythropoietin (epoetin alfa, darbepoetin)
  - Estrogenic compounds
  - Bevacizumab
- Clotting disorders
  - Thrombophilia

Myeloma-related risk factors
- Diagnosis of multiple myeloma
- Hyperviscosity

≤1 Individual or myeloma-related risk factor present:
- **Aspirin** 81–325 mg daily

≥2 Individual or myeloma-related risk factors present:
- **LMWH,** * equivalent to enoxaparin sodium 40 mg/day *or* **dalteparin sodium** 5000 IU/day; administer subcutaneously, *or*
- **Warfarin**, targeting an INR = 2–3

Concomitant treatment-related risk factors
Thalidomide or lenalidomide in combination with:
- High-dose dexamethasone (≥480 mg/month)
- Doxorubicin
- Multiagent chemotherapy

- **LMWH,** * equivalent to enoxaparin sodium 40 mg/day *or* **dalteparin sodium** 5000 IU/day; administer subcutaneously, *or*
- **Warfarin**, targeting an INR = 2–3

*LMWHs should be used with caution in individuals with impaired renal function (creatinine clearance <30 mL/min). Refer to product labeling for information about doses and administration schedules in renally impaired patients, and guidance for monitoring anti-Factor Xa concentrations

Abbreviations: CVC, central venous catheter; INR, international normalized ratio; LMWH, low-molecular-weight heparin; VTE, venous thromboembolic disease

References: Geerts WH et al. Chest 2008;133(6 Suppl):381S–453S

National Comprehensive Cancer Network. Multiple Myeloma, V.1.2014. (Accessed October 8, 2013, at http://www.nccn.org)

National Comprehensive Cancer Network. Venous Thromboembolic Disease, V.2.2013. (Accessed October 8, 2013, at http://www.nccn.org)

Palumbo A et al. Leukemia 2008;22:414–423

Treatment Modifications
(continued)

Adverse Event	Treatment Modification
Toxicities ascribed to dexamethasone such as severe manifestations of hypercorticism, including hyperglycemia, irritability, insomnia, or oral candidiasis	Reduce dexamethasone dose to the next lowest dose level

Lenalidomide Starting Dose Adjustment for Renal Impairment in Multiple Myeloma (Days 1–21 of Each 28-Day Cycle)*

CrCl 30–60 mL/min	10 mg lenalidomide every 24 hours
CrCl <30 mL/min, not requiring dialysis	15 mg lenalidomide every 48 hours
CrCl <30 mL/min, requiring dialysis	Lenalidomide 5 mg/day. On dialysis days, administer daily dose following dialysis

CrCl, Creatinine clearance
*Richardson PG et al. J Clin Oncol 2006;24:3113–3120

Patient Population Studied

Two multicenter, randomized, phase 3 studies that enrolled patients with progressive multiple myeloma not resistant to dexamethasone who had received at least 1 previous treatment. Patients were considered to have disease that was resistant to dexamethasone if they had had progression during previous therapy containing high-dose dexamethasone (total monthly dose >200 mg). Measurable disease was defined as a serum monoclonal protein (M-protein) level of ≥0.5 g/dL or a urinary Bence Jones protein level ≥0.2 g/day. Additional eligibility criteria included an Eastern Cooperative Oncology Group performance status ≤2

European Study
(Dimopoulos M et al. N Engl J Med 2007;357:2123–2132)
(351 patients: n = 176 lenalidomide group; n = 175 placebo group)

North America Study
(Weber DM et al. N Engl J Med 2007;357:2133–2142)
(353 patients: n = 177 lenalidomide group; n = 176 placebo group)

Efficacy

	North American Study (Weber et al)		European Study (Dimopoulos et al)	
	Lenalidomide n = 177	Placebo n = 176	Lenalidomide n = 176	Placebo n = 175
Overall response	61	19.9	60.2	24
Complete response	14.1	0.6	15.9	3.4
Near-complete response	10.2	1.1	8.5	1.7
Partial response	36.7	18.2	35.8	18.9
Stable disease	30.5	58	30.1	55.4
Progressive disease	2.8	14.2	1.7	14.3
Response not evaluable	5.6	8	8	6.3
Previous Thalidomide, Response Rate, and Time to Progression (TTP)				
Yes	56.8	12.5	49.1	16.4
Median TTP (months)	8.5	4.1	8.4	4.6
No	64.1	26	65	28.7
Median TTP (months)	—	—	13.5	4.7
β_2-Microglobulin Level, Response Rate				
<2.5 mg/L	75	27.5	70.6	37.5
≥2.5 mg/L	55.2	16.8	56	18.9
Previous Therapies (Number), Response Rate, and Time to Progression (TTP)				
1	64.7	22.4	66.1	29.8
Median TTP (months)	NR	5.1	—	—
≥2	58.7	18.3	57.5	21.2
Median TTP (months)	10.2	4.6	—	—
Previous Stem Cell Transplant, Response Rate				
Yes	66.1	19.4	61.9	28.4
No	52.9	20.6	58.2	18.8
Previous Use of Bortezomib, Response Rate, and Time to Progression (TTP)				
Yes	68.4	10	—	—
No	60.1	21.2	—	—
Median TTP (months)	10.3	3.3	—	—
Median TTP, All Patients (Months)	11.1	4.7	11.3	4.7
Median Overall Survival (Months)	26.2	12.9	NR	20.6

NR, not reached; TTP, Time to progression

Toxicity

	North America Study (Weber et al) G3/4 (n = 177)	European Study (Dimopoulos et al) G3/4 (n = 176)
Hematologic Events		
Neutropenia	41.2	29.5
Anemia	13	8.6
Thrombocytopenia	14.7	11.4
Febrile neutropenia	3.4	3.4
Gastrointestinal Events		
Constipation	2.8	1.7
Diarrhea	3.4	2.8
Nausea	2.8	1.1
General Disorders		
Asthenia	3.4	6.2
Fatigue	6.2	6.8
Pyrexia	2.3	0.6
Peripheral edema	2.3	1.1
Infections		
Upper respiratory	1.1	1.7
Any infection	21.4	9.6
Pneumonia	12.4	Not reported
Neurologic Disorders		
Headache	Not reported	0.6
Tremor	Not reported	1.1
Dizziness	Not reported	0.6
Paresthesia	Not reported	0.6
Insomnia	Not reported	1.1
Musculoskeletal or Connective Tissue Disorder		
Muscle cramp	Not reported	0.6
Back pain	Not reported	2.3
Bone pain	Not reported	2.8
Muscle weakness	Not reported	7.4
Arthralgia	Not reported	0.6
Vascular Disorders		
Deep-vein thrombosis	Not reported	4
Pulmonary embolism	Not reported	4.5
Venous thromboembolism	Not reported	11.4

Therapy Monitoring

1. Blood counts and physical examinations
   - Cycle 1: days 1, 8, and 15
   - Cycles 2 and 3: days 1 and 15
   - Cycle 4, and subsequently: day 1
2. Serum and urinary protein electrophoresis studies on day 1 of each cycle and at the end of treatment
3. Serum electrolytes and creatinine before beginning each treatment cycle

SUBSEQUENT THERAPY

MULTIPLE MYELOMA REGIMEN: DEXAMETHASONE + CYCLOPHOSPHAMIDE + ETOPOSIDE + CISPLATIN (DCEP)

Lazzarino M et al. Bone Marrow Transplant 2001;28:835–839
Park S et al. Ann Hematol 2014;93:99–110

Hydration:
0.9% sodium chloride injection (0.9% NS) 500–1000 mL; administer intravenously over 1–2 hours prior to starting cisplatin infusion on day 1, every 21 days, *then:*
0.9% NS; following completion of the bolus dose, administer intravenously by continuous infusion initially at a rate of 100–150 mL/hour for 4 consecutive days throughout chemotherapy administration on days 1–4, every 21 days
Notes:
• May increase rate of 0.9% NS infusion if needed to maintain a goal urine output of ≥100 mL/hour throughout chemotherapy administration
• Monitor and replace magnesium/electrolytes as needed

Dexamethasone 40 mg; administer orally once daily for 4 consecutive days on days 1–4, every 21 days (total dosage/21-day cycle = 160 mg)
Cyclophosphamide 400 mg/m^2 per day; administer by continuous intravenous infusion in 1000 mL 0.9% NS over 24 hours for 4 consecutive days on days 1–4, every 21 days (total dosage/cycle = 1600 mg/m^2)
Etoposide 40 mg/m^2 per day; administer by continuous intravenous infusion in 1000 mL 0.9% NS over 24 hours for 4 consecutive days on days 1–4, every 21 days (total dosage/cycle = 160 mg/m^2)
Cisplatin 10 mg/m^2 per day; administer by continuous intravenous infusion in 1000 mL 0.9% NS over 24 hours for 4 consecutive days on days 1–4, every 21 days (total dosage/cycle = 40 mg/m^2)
Notes:
• Cisplatin, etoposide, and cyclophosphamide may be mixed together in the same 1000 mL 0.9% NS admixture. Etoposide 0.2 mg/mL, cisplatin 0.2 mg/mL, and cyclophosphamide 2 mg/mL, diluted in 0.9% NS, is stable for 7 days at 20°–25°C (68°–77°F) when protected from exposure to light. Williams DA et al. Cancer Chemother Pharmacol 1992;31:171–181
• A 3-in-1 admixture does not prevent microbial growth after exposure to bacterial and fungal contamination. With respect to product sterility, expiration dating should be determined by the aseptic techniques used in preparation and local and national guidelines

Supportive Care
Antiemetic prophylaxis
Emetogenic potential on Days 1–4 is **HIGH**. *Potential for delayed symptoms*
See Chapter 42 for antiemetic recommendations

Hematopoietic growth factor (CSF) prophylaxis
  Primary prophylaxis is indicated with one of the following:
  Filgrastim (G-CSF) 5 μg/kg per day, by subcutaneous injection, or
  Pegfilgrastim (pegylated filgrastim) 6 mg/0.6 mL, by subcutaneous injection for one dose
  • Begin use from 24–72 h after myelosuppressive chemotherapy is completed
  • Continue daily filgrastim use until ANC ≥5000/mm^3 after the leukocyte nadir
  • Discontinue daily filgrastim use at least 24 hours before administering myelosuppressive treatment. Do not administer pegfilgrastim within 14 days before administering myelosuppressive treatment
  See Chapter 43 for more information

Antimicrobial prophylaxis
Risk of fever and neutropenia is **HIGH**
  Antimicrobial primary prophylaxis to be considered:
  • Antibacterial—consider a fluoroquinolone during periods of neutropenia, or no prophylaxis; *P. jirovecii* prophylaxis is recommended (eg, cotrimoxazole)
  • Antifungal—consider concomitant use of fluconazole during periods of neutropenia
  • Antiviral—anti-herpes antivirals (eg, acyclovir, famciclovir, valacyclovir)

Steroid-associated gastritis
Add a proton pump inhibitor or H$_2$-receptor antagonist during dexamethasone use to prevent gastritis and duodenitis
Bisphosphonates
All patients receiving primary therapy for symptomatic multiple myeloma should receive a bisphosphonate adjunctively.

Treatment Modifications

DEXAMETHASONE

Starting dose	40 mg/dose/day
Dose Level −1	20 mg/dose/day
Dose Level −2	12 mg/dose/day
Dose Level −3	Discontinue dexamethasone

Adverse Event	Treatment Modification
G1/2 dyspepsia (moderate symptoms; medical intervention indicated; limiting instrumental ADL), gastric or duodenal ulcer, or gastritis	Continue dexamethasone at the same dose. Treat with therapeutic doses of an H_2-receptor antagonist or proton pump inhibitor. If symptoms persist, then reduce the dexamethasone dose by one level
G ≥3 dyspepsia, gastric or duodenal ulcer, or gastritis (surgery or hospitalization indicated)	Withhold dexamethasone until symptoms return to baseline. Resume dexamethasone reduced by one dose level along with concurrent treatment with therapeutic doses of an H_2-receptor antagonist or proton pump inhibitor. If symptoms recur, then permanently discontinue dexamethasone[†]
Acute pancreatitis	Permanently discontinue dexamethasone[†]
G ≥3 edema	Withhold dexamethasone until symptoms return to baseline. Consider treatment with diuretics. Resume dexamethasone reduced by one dose level. If edema persists, reduce by another dose level. Discontinue dexamethasone permanently if symptoms persist despite two prior dose reductions[†]
G ≥2 mood alteration (moderate mood alteration) or confusion (moderate disorientation; limiting instrumental ADL)	Withhold dexamethasone until symptoms return to baseline. Resume dexamethasone reduced by one dose level. If symptoms persist, reduce by another dose level
G ≥2 muscle weakness (symptomatic; evident on physical exam; limiting instrumental ADL)	Withhold dexamethasone until symptoms return to baseline. Resume dexamethasone reduced by one dose level. If weakness persists, reduce by another dose level. If weakness still persists, then permanently discontinue dexamethasone[†]
G ≥3 hyperglycemia (insulin therapy initiated; hospitalization indicated)	Withhold dexamethasone until glucose is ≤250 mg/dL. Treat with insulin or other hypoglycemic agents as clinically appropriate and then resume dexamethasone at the same dose. If hyperglycemia is uncontrolled despite above measures, decrease dexamethasone by one dose level
Other G ≥2 nonhematologic toxicity attributable to dexamethasone including severe irritability, insomnia, or oral candidiasis	Withhold dexamethasone until toxicity resolves to G ≤1, then resume at a lower dose. Consider reduction by one dose level for G2/G3 toxicity, and by two dose levels for G4 or recurrent G3 toxicity

CYCLOPHOSPHAMIDE + ETOPOSIDE + CISPLATIN

Day 1 ANC <1500/mm³ or platelets <100,000/mm³	Delay dexamethasone, cyclophosphamide, etoposide, and cisplatin treatment 1 week or until ANC >1500/mm³ and platelets >100,000/mm³, then administer full doses

(continued)

Patient Population Studied

Study of 55 patients with multiple myeloma. Of the enrolled patients, 40 had previously received the VAD regimen only and 15 had received alkylating agents. At the start of the study, 36 patients were classified as stage I according to the Durie-Salmon criteria, 6 were classified as stage II, and 13 were classified as stage III

Efficacy (n = 55)

Successful mobilization*	87%
≥4 × 10⁶ CD34+ cells per kg collected	75%
Median number of CD34+ cells per kg collected	5.82 × 10⁶

*Mobilization was considered successful if ≥2 × 10⁶ CD34+ cells per kg were collected

Adverse Events (n = 55)

Toxicities were mild and tolerable. No patient experienced a drop in granulocyte count to <1.0 × 10⁹/L or hemoglobin level to <10 g/dL as a result of treatment. No patient had thrombocytopenia <50,000 × 10⁹/L or needed hospitalization for septic complications. The most frequent nonhematologic adverse event was nausea related to cisplatin, but this was mild or moderate and easily controlled with antiemetic therapy. No treatment-related deaths occurred

Treatment Modifications (*continued*)

CYCLOPHOSPHAMIDE + ETOPOSIDE + CISPLATIN

G4 neutropenia (ANC <500/mm^3) at nadir	Continue to administer filgrastim or pegfilgrastim during subsequent cycles as described in the therapy administration section. Consider decreasing cyclophosphamide, etoposide, and/or cisplatin dosages by 25%
G4 thrombocytopenia (platelet count <25,000/mm^3) at nadir	Consider decreasing cyclophosphamide, etoposide, and/or cisplatin dosages by 25%
Hypersensitivity reaction	Immediately interrupt etoposide and/or cisplatin infusion—whichever is deemed responsible—and institute supportive management as appropriate. In patients who experience a severe hypersensitivity reaction, permanently discontinue etoposide or cisplatin—whichever is deemed responsible
Hypoalbuminemia	Albumin <3.2 g/dL consider reducing etoposide dosage by 50%. Albumin <2.5 g/dL consider discontinuing etoposide until albumin >2.5 g/dL
Severe hemorrhagic cystitis	Discontinue cyclophosphamide therapy
Serum creatinine ≥1.5 mg/dL (≥130 μmol/L) and/or BUN ≥25 mg/dL (≥8.92 mmol/L).	Withhold cisplatin until serum creatinine <1.5 mg/dL (<130 μmol/L) and BUN <25 mg/dL (<8.92 mmol/L). Then decrease cisplatin dosage by 25%; if already reduced, then reduce again
Peripheral neuropathy G ≥3	G4 discontinue cisplatin permanently; G3 may reinstitute if toxicity resolves within 2–3 weeks to G ≤1
Cisplatin-induced hearing loss G ≥3	
Other G ≥3 nonhematologic toxicities (except nausea, vomiting, elevated transaminases, and alopecia)	Delay treatment until toxicity resolves to baseline, then decrease cyclophosphamide, etoposide, and/or cisplatin dosages by 25% from previous dose levels

Therapy Monitoring

1. CBC with differential, liver function tests, serum electrolytes, serum chemistries, and serum glucose prior to each cycle

2. *In patients at high risk for tumor lysis syndrome (eg, high tumor burden, renal dysfunction, rapidly progressing disease, markedly elevated LDH, baseline abnormalities in laboratory indices of tumor lysis syndrome [potassium, phosphate, uric acid, calcium, serum creatinine]): consider frequent monitoring of laboratory indices of tumor lysis syndrome, intravenous hydration, and prophylaxis with a xanthine oxidase inhibitor (eg, allopurinol) during the first cycle*

3. With abdominal pain, check serum amylase/lipase

4. Ensure adequate hydration of patients to reduce the risk of cisplatin-induced renal toxicity and of tumor lysis syndrome

5. Check urinary sediment regularly for the presence of erythrocytes and other signs of urotoxicity

6. Treat all urinary tract infections aggressively

SUBSEQUENT THERAPY

MULTIPLE MYELOMA REGIMEN: LIPOSOMAL DOXORUBICIN + BORTEZOMIB

Orlowski RZ et al. J Clin Oncol 2007;25:3892–3901

Bortezomib 1.3 mg/m² per dose; administer by intravenous injection over 3–5 seconds for 4 doses on days 1, 4, 8, and 11, every 3 weeks (total dosage/cycle = 5.2 mg/m²)

Doxorubicin HCl Liposome Injection ([pegylated] liposomal doxorubicin) 30 mg/m²; administer intravenously in 250 mL (doses ≤90 mg) or 500 mL (doses ≤90 mg) 5% dextrose injection over 60 minutes after bortezomib on day 4, every 3 weeks (total dosage/cycle = 30 mg/m²)

Notes:

1. Liposomal doxorubicin doses >60 mg are administered at an initial rate of 1 mg/min to minimize the risk of infusion reactions. If no infusion-related adverse reactions are observed within 15 minutes after starting administration, the infusion rate may be increased to complete administration over 1 hour

2. Treatment on study continued until disease progression, unacceptable treatment-related toxicities, or for 8 cycles. Patients still responding after 8 cycles were permitted to continue, provided treatment was well tolerated

Supportive Care

Antiemetic prophylaxis

Emetogenic potential on days with bortezomib alone is **MINIMAL–LOW**

Emetogenic potential on days with liposomal doxorubicin is **LOW**

See Chapter 42 for antiemetic recommendations

Hematopoietic growth factor (CSF) prophylaxis

Primary prophylaxis may be indicated

See Chapter 43 for more information

Antimicrobial prophylaxis

Risk of fever and neutropenia is **HIGH**

    Antimicrobial primary prophylaxis is recommended:

- Antibacterial—consider fluoroquinolone prophylaxis; *P. jirovecii* prophylaxis is recommended (eg, cotrimoxazole)

- Antifungal—recommended

- Antiviral—antiherpes antivirals (eg, acyclovir, famciclovir, valacyclovir)

Hand-foot reaction (palmar-plantar erythrodysesthesia)

For patients who develop a hand-foot reaction, use topical emollients (eg, Aquaphor), topical or orally administered steroids, antihistamine agents (H_1-receptor antagonists), or pyridoxine

Pyridoxine may provide relief for discomfort/pain associated with PPE, although the mechanism through which this occurs remains unclear
• The suggested pyridoxine starting dose is 50 mg/day, which may be increased to a maximum of 200 mg/day

Patients who have developed G1/2 PPE while receiving doxorubicin HCl liposome injection may receive a fixed daily dose of pyridoxine 200 mg. This may allow for treatment to be completed without dosage reduction, treatment delay, or recurrence of PPE

Diarrhea management

Latent or delayed-onset diarrhea*:

Loperamide or **diphenoxylate hydrochloride** 2.5 mg with **atropine sulfate** 0.025 mg (eg, Lomotil)

Oral care

Prophylaxis and treatment for mucositis/stomatitis

Bisphosphonates

All patients receiving primary therapy for symptomatic multiple myeloma should receive a bisphosphonate adjunctively.

Thromboprophylaxis

Risk assessment and recommendations for VTE prophylaxis in patients with multiple myeloma with individual or myeloma-related risk factors, or risk factors related to treatment

(continued)

(*continued*)

Individual risk factors
• Obesity (BMI ≥30 kg/m²)
• H/O VTE
• CVC or pacemaker
• Comorbid pathologies
  ■ Cardiac disease
  ■ Chronic renal disease
  ■ Diabetes
  ■ Acute infection
  ■ Immobilization
• Surgery
  ■ General surgery
  ■ Any anesthesia
  ■ Trauma
• Medications
  ■ Erythropoietin (epoetin alfa, darbepoetin)
  ■ Estrogenic compounds
  ■ Bevacizumab
• Clotting disorders
  ■ Thrombophilia
Myeloma-related risk factors
• Diagnosis of multiple myeloma
• Hyperviscosity
	≤1 Individual or myeloma-related risk factor present:
	• **Aspirin** 81–325 mg daily
	
	≥2 Individual or myeloma-related risk factors present:
	• **LMWH,*** equivalent to enoxaparin sodium 40 mg/day *or* **dalteparin sodium** 5000 IU/day; administer subcutaneously, *or*
	• **Warfarin**, targeting an INR = 2–3

Concomitant treatment-related risk factors Thalidomide or lenalidomide in combination with: • High-dose dexamethasone (≥480 mg/month) • Doxorubicin • Multiagent chemotherapy	• **LMWH,*** equivalent to enoxaparin sodium 40 mg/day *or* **dalteparin sodium** 5000 IU/day; administer subcutaneously, *or* • **Warfarin**, targeting an INR = 2–3

*LMWHs should be used with caution in individuals with impaired renal function (creatinine clearance <30 mL/min). Refer to product labeling for information about doses and administration schedules in renally impaired patients, and guidance for monitoring anti-Factor Xa concentrations

Abbreviations: CVC, central venous catheter; INR, international normalized ratio; LMWH, low-molecular-weight heparin; VTE, venous thromboembolic disease

References: Geerts WH et al. Chest 2008;133(6 Suppl):381S–453S

National Comprehensive Cancer Network. Multiple Myeloma, V.1.2014. (Accessed October 8, 2013, at http://www.nccn.org)

National Comprehensive Cancer Network. Venous Thromboembolic Disease, V.2.2013. (Accessed October 8, 2013, at http://www.nccn.org)

Palumbo A et al. Leukemia 2008;22:414–423

Treatment Modifications

Bortezomib Dosage Levels

Dosage Level 1	1.3 mg/m²
Dosage Level −1	1 mg/m²
Dosage Level −2	0.7 mg/m²

Modification Guidelines for Hematologic Toxicity on Day 1 of Planned Therapy

Toxicity	Treatment Modification
ANC 1000–1500/mm³ or platelets 75,000–100,000/mm³	Resume treatment with no dosage reduction
ANC 500–999/mm³ or platelets 50,000–75,000/mm³	Hold treatment until toxicity resolves to G ≤1 or 75% of the counts measured at the start of the previous cycle, then resume without dosage reduction

(*continued*)

Treatment Modifications (*continued*)

Toxicity	Treatment Modification
ANC <500/mm³ or platelets <25,000/mm³	First episode: Hold treatment until toxicity resolves to G ≤1, then resume with a 25% dosage reduction of both liposomal doxorubicin and bortezomib or continue full dose with hematopoietic growth factor support (filgrastim, sargramostim) Reduce dose by 25% if neutropenia occurs despite growth factor use
Febrile neutropenia	Withhold therapy until fever abates then resume therapy

Treatment Modification for Bortezomib-Induced Peripheral Neuropathy*

Severity of Peripheral Neuropathy	Modification of Dose and Schedule
G1 (paresthesias or loss of reflexes) without pain or loss of function	No action
G1 with pain or G2 (interferes with function but not with activities of daily living)	Reduce bortezomib dosage to 1 mg/m² per dose
G2 with pain or G3 (interferes with activities of daily living)	Withhold bortezomib treatment until toxicity resolves, then reinitiate at a dosage of 0.7 mg/m² per dose once weekly
G4 (permanent sensory loss that interferes with function)	Discontinue treatment

*Richardson PG et al. J Clin Oncol 2006;24:3113–3120

Liposomal Doxorubicin: Treatment Modification Guidelines for Cardiac Toxicity

Toxicity	Treatment Modification
LVEF decreases by ≥15% from baseline, or to <45%	Discontinue liposomal doxorubicin

LVEF, left ventricular ejection fraction

Treatment Modification Guidelines for Palmar-Plantar Erythrodysesthesia (PPE, Hand-Foot Syndrome)

Grade of Toxicity	Liposomal Doxorubicin Dosing Interval		
	4 Weeks	5 Weeks	6 Weeks
G1: Mild erythema, swelling, or desquamation not interfering with daily activities	Resume unless patient has previous G3/4 skin toxicity. If so, delay an additional week	Resume unless patient has previous G3/4 skin toxicity. If so, delay an additional week	Resume liposomal doxorubicin at a 25% dose reduction; return to a 4-week dosing interval or discontinue therapy
G2: Erythema, desquamation, or swelling interfering with, but not precluding, normal physical activities; small blisters or ulcerations <2 cm in diameter	Delay treatment 1 week	Delay treatment 1 week	Resume liposomal doxorubicin at a 25% dose reduction; return to 4-week dosing interval or discontinue therapy
G3: Blistering, ulceration, or swelling interfering with walking or normal daily activities; cannot wear regular clothing	Delay treatment 1 week	Delay treatment 1 week	Discontinue therapy
G4: Diffuse or local process causing infectious complications, or a bedridden state, or hospitalization	Delay treatment 1 week	Delay treatment 1 week	Discontinue therapy

Patient Population Studied

A randomized phase 3 study of 646 patients with relapsed refractory multiple myeloma. Eligible subjects had an Eastern Cooperative Oncology Group performance status ≤1, had experienced disease progression after a response to 1 or more lines of therapy or were refractory to initial treatment, but were bortezomib naïve. Subjects were excluded if their disease progressed while receiving anthracycline-containing therapy, if they had already received >240 mg/m² doxorubicin, or if they had clinically significant cardiac disease, a left ventricular ejection fraction less than institutional normal limits, or peripheral neuropathy G ≥2

Efficacy (n = 324)

Total response (CR + PR)	44%
CR	4%
PR	40%
nCR	9%
CR + VGPR	27%

Median time to first response	43 days
Median number of cycles administered	5 cycles
Median treatment duration	105 days
Median duration of response	10.2 months
Median time to progression	9.3 months
Median progression-free survival	9 months
Median duration of overall survival	311 days
15-month survival rate	76%

CR, complete response; nCR, near-complete response; PR, partial response; VGPR, very good partial response

Therapy Monitoring

1. Blood counts with differential leukocyte count and physical examinations on day 1 of each cycle
2. Serum and urinary protein electrophoresis studies on day 1 of each cycle and at the end of treatment

Toxicity (n = 318)

Overview of Treatment-Emergent Adverse Events	Percentage of Patients
Any adverse event	98
Drug-related adverse events	94
Serious adverse events	36
Drug-related serious adverse events	22
G3/4 adverse events	80
Drug-related G3/4 adverse events	68
Adverse event leading to bortezomib discontinuation	30
Adverse event leading to liposomal doxorubicin discontinuation	36
Adverse event with fatal outcome	4
Drug-related adverse event with fatal outcome	2

Adverse Events During Treatment Reported by at Least 15% of Patients

	% Total	% G3/4
Hematologic Events		
Thrombocytopenia	30	23
Anemia	23	9
Neutropenia	35	29
Febrile neutropenia	3	3
Gastrointestinal Events		
Nausea	46	2
Diarrhea	43	7
Constipation	28	1
Vomiting	31	4
Constitutional Symptoms		
Fatigue	31	6
Pyrexia	29	1
Asthenia	19	6
Anorexia	18	2
Other		
Thromboembolic event	1	1
Bleeding/hemorrhage	14	4
Cough	16	0
Stomatitis	18	2
Hand-foot syndrome	16	5
Cardiac events	10	2
Neuralgia	14	3
Headache	18	1
Peripheral neuropathy	35	4
Alopecia	2	N/A

27. Myelodysplastic Syndromes

Michael M. Boyiadzis, MD, MHSc, and Neal S. Young, MD

Epidemiology

Incidence: Increases with Age

Mean age: 71 years	Male-to-female ratio: 1.5:1
Overall:	4.1 per 100,000
Ages 50–59 years	0.3 per 100,000
Ages 60–69 years	15 per 100,000
Ages 70–79 years	49 per 100,000
Ages >80 years	89 per 100,000

Dunbar CE, Saunthararajah Y. Myelodysplastic syndromes. In: Young NS (editor). Bone Marrow Failure Syndromes. Philadelphia, PA: WB Saunders; 2000:69–98

Greenberg P et al. Blood 2012;120:2454–2465

Work-up

CBC with differential, reticulocyte count

Serum liver function tests, electrolytes, serum creatinine, lactate dehydrogenase

Bone marrow biopsy and aspiration with iron stains, flow cytometry, cytogenetics, molecular studies

HLA typing for patients who are candidates for allogeneic cell transplantation

RBC folate, serum B_{12}, serum iron/TIBC/ferritin, serum erythropoietin level (prior to RBC transfusion)

HIV testing if clinically indicated

Thyroid function tests to rule out hypothyroidism

Evaluation of patients with chronic myelomonocytic leukemia (CMML) for PDGFRβ gene rearrangements at 5q32

Frequent Chromosomal Aberrations in MDS

Numerical		Translocations		Deletions	
Cytogenetics	(%)	Cytogenetics	(%)	Cytogenetics	(%)
+8	19	inv 3	7	del 5q	27
−7	15	t(1;7)	2	del 11q	7
+21	7	t(1;3)	1	del 12q	5
−5	7	t(3;3)	1	del 20q	5
		t(6;9)	<1	del 7q	4
		t(5;12)	<1	del 13q	2

−, Loss of chromosome; +, additional chromosome; inv, inversion; t, translocation; del, deletion
- Clonal cytogenetic abnormalities: 30–79%
- Deletions are more frequent than translocations

Commonly mutated genes in MDS

Mutated Gene	Frequency (%)
TET2	20–30
SF3B1	20–30
ASXL1	15–25
SRSF2	10–15
DNMT3A	10–15
RUNX1	10–15
TP53	5–10
EZH2	5–10
IDH1/IDH2	<5

(continued)

Work-up (continued)

Peripheral and bone marrow findings and cytogenetics of MDS

Name	Dysplastic Lineages	Cytopenias*	Ring Sideroblasts as % of Marrow Erythroid Elements	BM and PB Blasts	Cytogenetics by Conventional Karyotype Analysis
MDS with single-lineage dysplasia (MDS-SLD)	1	1 or 2	<15%/<5[†]	BM <5%, PB <1%, no Auer rods	Any, unless fulfills all criteria for MDS with isolated del(5q)
MDS with multilineage dysplasia (MDS-MLD)	2 or 3	1–3	<15%/<5[†]	BM <5%, PB <1%, no Auer rods	Any, unless fulfills all criteria for MDS with isolated del(5q)
MDS with ring sideroblasts (MDS-RS)					
MDS-RS with single lineage dysplasia (MDS-RS-SLD)	1	1 or 2	≥15%/≥5[†]	BM <5%, PB <1%, no Auer rods	Any, unless fulfills all criteria for MDS with isolated del(5q)
MDS-RS with multilineage dysplasia (MDS-RS-MLD)	2 or 3	1–3	≥15%/≥5[†]	BM <5%, PB <1%, no Auer rods	Any, unless fulfills all criteria for MDS with isolated del(5q)
MDS with isolated del(5q)	1–3	1–2	None or any	BM <5%, PB <1%, no Auer rods	del(5q) alone or with 1 additional abnormality except −7 or del(7q)
MDS with excess blasts (MDS-EB)					
MDS-EB-1	0–3	1–3	None or any	BM 5%–9% or PB 2%–4%, no Auer rods	Any
MDS-EB-2	0–3	1–3	None or any	BM 10%–19% or PB 5%–19% or Auer rods	Any
MDS, unclassifiable (MDS-U)					
With 1% blood blasts	1–3	1–3	None or any	BM <5%, PB = 1%,[‡] no Auer rods	Any
With single-lineage dysplasia and pancytopenia	1	3	None or any	BM <5%, PB <1%, no Auer rods	Any
Based on defining cytogenetic abnormality	0	1–3	<15%[§]	BM <5%, PB <1%, no Auer rods	MDS-defining abnormality
Refractory cytopenia of childhood	1–3	1–3	None	BM <5%, PB <2%	Any

*Cytopenias defined as: hemoglobin, <10 g/dL; platelet count, <100 × 10^9/L; and absolute neutrophil count, <1.8 × 10^9/L. Rarely, MDS may present with mild anemia or thrombocytopenia above these levels. PB monocytes must be <1 × 10^9/L

[†]If *SF3B1* mutation is present

[‡]One percent PB blasts must be recorded on at least 2 separate occasions

[§]Cases with ≥15% ring sideroblasts by definition have significant erythroid dysplasia, and are classified as MDS-RS-SLD

Arber A. Blood 2016;127:2391–2405

Classification Systems for De Novo MDS

International Prognostic Scoring System (IPSS)

Survival and AML Evolution

Prognostic Variable	Score Value				
	0	0.5	1.0	1.5	2.0
Marrow blasts (%)	<5	5–10	—	11–20	21–30
Karyotype*	Good	Intermediate	Poor		
Cytopenia†	0/1	2/3			

Risk Category (% IPSS Pop.)	Overall Score	Median Survival (Years) in the Absence of Therapy	25% AML Progression (Years) in the Absence of Therapy
LOW (33)	0	5.7	9.4
INT-1 (38)	0.5–1.0	3.5	3.3
INT-2 (22)	1.5–2.0	1.1	1.1
HIGH (7)	≥2.5	0.4	0.2

*Cytogenetics: Good = normal, −Y alone, del (5q) alone, del (20q) alone; Poor = complex (≥3 abnormalities) or chromosome 7 anomalies; Intermediate = other abnormalities
†Cytopenias: neutrophil count <1800/μL, platelets <100,000/μL, Hb<10 g/dL
Note: categorization excludes karyotypes t(8;21), inv 16, and t(15;17), which are considered to be AML not MDS

Greenberg P et al. Blood 1997;89:2079–2088. Erratum in: Blood 1998;91:1100. Comment in: Blood 1997;90:2843–2846, Blood 2001;98:1985

IPSS-R, Revised International Prognostic Scoring System

Prognostic Variable	0	0.5	1	1.5	2	3	4
Cytogenetics*	Very good	—	Good	—	Intermediate	Poor	Very poor
BM blast, %	≤2%	—	>2% to <5%	—	5–10%	>10%	—
Hemoglobin	≥10	—	8 to <10	<8	—	—	—
Platelets	≥100	50 to <100	<50	—	—	—	—
ANC	≥0.8	<0.8	—	—	—	—	—

*Cytogenetics: Very good = −Y, del(11q); Good = normal, del(5q), del(12p), del(20q), double including del(5q); Intermediate = del(7q), +8, +19, i(17q), any other single or double independent clones; Poor = −7, inv(3)/t(3q)/del(3q), double including −7/del(7q), complex: 3 abnormalities; Very poor = complex >3 abnormalities

Risk Category	Risk Score
Very low	≤1.5
Low	>1.5–3
Intermediate	>3–4.5
High	>4.5–6
Very high	>6

(continued)

Classification Systems for De Novo MDS (continued)

	Very Low	Low	Intermediate	High	Very High
Median survival, years	8.8	5.3	3.0	1.6	0.8
	(7.8–9.9)	(5.1–5.7)	(2.7–3.3)	(1.5–1.7)	(0.7–0.8)
25% AML progression, years	NR	10.8	3.2	1.4	0.73
	(14.5–NR)	(9.2–NR)	(2.8–4.4)	(1.1–1.7)	(0.7–0.9)

NR, not reached

Greenberg PL et al. Blood 2012;120:245–2465

WHO-based Prognostic Scoring System (WPSS)

Variable	Variable Scores			
	0	1	2	3
WHO category	RCUD, RARS, MDS, with isolated deletion (5q)	RCMD	RAEB–1	RAEB–2
Karyotype*	Good	Intermediate	Poor	—
Severe anemia (Hb <9 g/dL in males or <8 g/dL in females)	Absent	Present	—	—

WPSS Risk	Sum of Individual Variable Scores
Very low	0
Low	1
Intermediate	2
High	3–4
Very high	5–6

*Cytogenetics: Good = normal, −Y alone, del (5q) alone, del (20q) alone; Poor = complex (≥3 abnormalities) or chromosome 7 anomalies; Intermediate = other abnormalities

Malcovati L et al. Hematologica 2011;95:1433–1440

Differential Diagnosis of Hypo-Productive Cytopenias

Hematologic Conditions	Nonhematologic Conditions
1. Congenital hereditary sideroblastic anemia, congenital dyserythropoietic anemia Fanconi anemia, Diamond-Blackfan syndrome, Shwachman syndrome, Kostmann syndrome 2. Nutritional vitamin B_{12} deficiency, folate deficiency, iron deficiency 3. Aplastic anemia 4. Paroxysmal nocturnal hemoglobinuria 5. Systemic mastocytosis 6. Hairy cell leukemia 7. Large granular lymphocyte disease 8. Myeloproliferative neoplasms, idiopathic myelofibrosis. polycythemia vera chronic myeloid leukemia, essential thrombocytosis	1. Toxins, alcohol, post-chemotherapy or radiation, medications 2. Chronic diseases, renal failure collagen-vascular diseases, chronic infections 3. Viral infections, parvovirus B19, cytomegalovirus, human immunodeficiency virus 4. Malignancy, marrow infiltration paraneoplastic syndrome

Expert Opinion

Lower-risk patients

Patients with symptomatic anemia and del(5q) chromosomal abnormalities with or without other cytogenetic abnormalities (except those involving chromosome 7) should receive lenalidomide. Response should be assessed 2–4 months after therapy is started. Patients with del(5q) may also be treated with erythropoiesis-stimulating agent (ESA) if the serum erythropoietin (sEPO) levels are ≤500 mU/mL. Other patients with symptomatic anemia can be treated based on their levels of sEPO. Patients with levels of ≤500 mU/mL may be treated with recombinant human epoetin alfa or darbepoetin alfa either with or without colony-stimulating factor. Iron depletion needs to be verified before instituting epoetin alfa or darbepoetin alfa therapy. G-CSF and, to a lesser extent, granulocyte-macrophage colony-stimulating factor (GM-CSF) show synergistic erythropoietic activity when used in combination with ESAs and markedly enhanced erythroid responses. Erythroid responses occur after 6–8 weeks of treatment

Luspatercept has been approved for anemia failing an ESA requiring 2 or more RBC units over 8 weeks in adult patients with very low- to intermediate-risk myelodysplastic syndromes with ring sideroblasts (MDS-RS) or with myelodysplastic/myeloproliferative neoplasm with ring sideroblasts and thrombocytosis (MDS/MPN-RS-T). Decitabine/cedazuridine is a combination of decitabine and cedazuridine, a cytidine deaminase inhibitor, indicated for treatment of adult patients with MDS including previously treated and untreated, de novo and secondary MDS with the following French-American-British subtypes (refractory anemia, refractory anemia with ringed sideroblasts, refractory anemia with excess blasts, and chronic myelomonocytic leukemia [CMML]) and intermediate-1, intermediate-2, and high-risk International Prognostic Scoring System groups.

Patients not responding after 4–6 months of therapy should be considered for immunosuppressive therapy with thymocyte immune globulin and cyclosporine. Response rates to immunosuppressive therapy are higher among patients who have ≤5% marrow blasts, a hypocellular marrow, a PNH-positive clone, STAT3 mutant cytotoxic T-cell clone, or who are ≤60 years old. Patients who have a low probability for responding to immunosuppressive therapy should be considered for treatment with lenalidomide, decitabine, or azacytidine

Patients without symptomatic anemia but with other serious cytopenias (eg, thrombocytopenia) should be considered for treatment with decitabine or azacytidine, or immunosuppressive therapy with ATG and cyclosporine. TPO agonists also may be used in these patients. For patients who do not respond to these therapies, allogeneic hematopoietic cell transplantation (allo-HCT) may be considered

Anemic patients with sEPO levels >500 mU/mL should be considered for immunosuppressive therapy if they have a high likelihood for response. Patients not responding to immunosuppressive therapy should be treated with decitabine or azacytidine. Patients not responding to these agents should be considered for allo-HCT

For patients with chronic RBC transfusion needs, serum ferritin levels and associated organ dysfunction should be monitored. Iron chelation therapy should also be considered in patients with MDS

High-risk patients

Allogeneic HCT is the only treatment that can induce long-term remission in patients with MDS. Such therapy, however, is not applicable for many patients because the median age at diagnosis exceeds 65 years with associated comorbidities. Allo-HCT for MDS is associated with a high rate of treatment-related death and suboptimal disease-free survival. The decision to offer HCT as therapy for MDS remains an individual "personalized" decision. Age and presence of comorbid disease are among the most relevant clinical variables to be considered when judging a patient's eligibility for allo-HCT. For patients who are eligible for intensive therapy but lack a stem cell donor, or those whose marrow blast count requires reduction, intensive chemotherapy should be considered. Patients who are not candidates for allo-HCT should receive hypomethylating agents and supportive care therapies similar to those used in low-risk patients

Fenaux P et al. Lancet Oncol 2009;10:223–232
Fenaux P et al. N Engl J Med 2020;382:140–151
Greenberg P et al. Blood 2012;120: 2454–2465
Malcovati L et al. Hematologica 2011;95:1433–1440
Ogawa S. Blood 2019;133:1049–1059
Platzbecker U et al. Blood 2019;133:1096–1107
Savona MR et al. Lancet Haematol 2019;6:e194–e203
Silverman LR et al. J Clin Oncol 2002;20:2429–2440
Silverman LR et al. J Clin Oncol 2006;24:3895–3903
Sloand EM et al. J Clin Oncol 2008;26:2505–2511
Steensma DP et al. J Clin Oncol 2009;27:3842–3848

MYELODYSPLASTIC SYNDROME REGIMEN: DECITABINE

Kantarjian H et al. Blood 2007;109:52–57
Kantarjian H et al. Cancer 2006;106:1794–1803
Steensma DP et al. J Clin Oncol 2009;27:3842–3848

Decitabine 20 mg/m² per day; administer intravenously in a volume of cold* 0.9% sodium chloride injection (0.9% NS), 5% dextrose injection (D5W), or lactated Ringer's injection (LRI) sufficient to result in a solution concentration within the range of 0.1–1 mg/mL, over 60 minutes for 5 consecutive days, on days 1–5, every 4 weeks (total dosage per 5-day course = 100 mg/m²)

or

Decitabine 15 mg/m² per dose; administer intravenously in a volume of cold* 0.9% NS, D5W, or LRI sufficient to result in a solution concentration within the range of 0.1–1 mg/mL, over 3 hours, every 8 hours for 3 consecutive days (total dosage/day = 45 mg/m²; total dosage/3-day course = 135 mg/m²)

- Patients should receive either regimen for a minimum of 4 cycles; however, it may take longer than 4 cycles to achieve a complete or partial response

*Cold vehicle solutions must be used if a decitabine product will not be used within 15 minutes after preparation is completed. See Chapter 45 for more information

Supportive Care

Antiemetic prophylaxis
Emetogenic potential is **MINIMAL**
See Chapter 42 for antiemetic recommendations

Hematopoietic growth factor (CSF) prophylaxis
Primary prophylaxis may be indicated for patients with refractory symptomatic cytopenias
See Chapter 43 for more information

Antimicrobial prophylaxis
Risk of fever and neutropenia is **HIGH**
  Antimicrobial primary prophylaxis is recommended:
- Antibacterial—consider fluoroquinolone prophylaxis; *P. jirovecii* prophylaxis is recommended (eg, cotrimoxazole)
- Antifungal—recommended
- Antiviral—anti-herpes antivirals (eg, acyclovir, famciclovir, valacyclovir)

Patient Population Studied

Ninety-nine patients with MDS (median age: 72 years; range: 34–87 years) including IPPS risk groups: high (24%), intermediate-2 (32%), intermediate-1 (28%), and low (4%). FAB classifications: RA plus RARS (37%), RAEB plus RAEB-T (52%), CMML (11%). At baseline, 67% of patients were RBC transfusion dependent and 15% were platelet transfusion dependent

Efficacy

Response by 2006 IWG Criteria	ITT (N = 99) %
Overall complete response rate, CR + mCR	32
Overall response rate, CR + mCR + PR	32
Overall improvement rate, CR + mCR + PR + HI	51
Rate of stable disease or better, CR + mCR + PR + HI + SD	75
CR	17
mCR	15
PR	0
HI	18
SD	24
PD	10
Not assessable	15

IWG, International Working Group; ITT, intention to treat; CR, complete response; mCR, marrow CR; PR, partial response; HI, hematologic improvement; SD, stable disease; PD, progressive disease

Activity was demonstrated across investigator-assessed IPSS risk groups, with an overall improvement rate of 50% for intermediate-1 patients, 61% for intermediate-2 patients, and 43% for high-risk patients

The 1-year survival rate for patients treated with decitabine was 66%. Median survival was 19.4 months. Patients who were classified as having CMML (n = 11) had a 73% improvement rate. Among 66 patients who were RBC transfusion dependent at baseline, 22 patients (33%) became RBC transfusion independent during the study. Of the 15 patients who were platelet transfusion dependent at baseline, 6 patients (40%) became transfusion independent during the course of the study

Adverse Effects

Event	% of Patients	
	Grades 1–2	Grades ≥3
Hematologic		
Neutropenia	1	31
Thrombocytopenia	2	18
Febrile neutropenia	3	14
Anemia	5	12

(continued)

Adverse Effects (continued)

Nonhematologic		
Fatigue	26	5
Nausea	26	1
Pyrexia	17	0
Diarrhea	12	0
Anorexia	12	0
Constipation	11	0
Pneumonia	1	11
Vomiting	10	1
Chills	10	0

Of the 619 cycles administered, 198 (32%) were delayed, primarily because of myelosuppression, with a median delay of 8 days, and there were 119 hospitalizations (19% of cycles were associated with a hospitalization)
Eleven patients (11%) died within 30 days after receiving decitabine

Treatment Modifications

REGIMEN 1: Decitabine 20 mg/m² per day; administer intravenously over 60 minutes, once daily for 5 consecutive, days 1–5, every 4 weeks (100 mg/m² per 5-day course)

Hematologic Adverse Effects

Cycles ≥2 (4-week cycles):

Day 1 ANC ≥1000/μL and platelets ≥50,000/μL	Begin a new treatment cycle at the same decitabine dosage and schedule previously given
Day 1 ANC <1000/μL or platelets <50,000/μL	Delay treatment and continually monitor ANC and platelet counts until recovery to ANC ≥1000/μL and platelets ≥50,000/μL, then: Begin a new treatment cycle at the same decitabine dosage and schedule previously given

Nonhematologic Adverse Effects

Cycles ≥2, for:	
• Serum creatinine ≥2 mg/dL (≥177 μmol/L) • Serum ALT (SGPT) or total bilirubin ≥2 times ULN • Active or uncontrolled infection	Withhold decitabine treatment until the toxicity is resolved, *then* Begin a new treatment cycle at the same decitabine dosage and schedule previously given

REGIMEN 2: Decitabine 15 mg/m² per dose; administer intravenously over 3 hours, every 8 hours for 3 consecutive days, days 1–3 (45 mg/m² per day; 135 mg/m² per 3-day course)

Hematologic Adverse Effects

Cycles ≥2, 4 weeks after a previous cycle:

If ANC ≥1000/μL and platelets ≥50,000/μL	Begin a new treatment cycle at the same decitabine dosage and schedule previously given
If ANC <1000/μL or platelets <50,000/μL	Delay treatment for up to 6 weeks after the last cycle began, and continually monitor ANC and platelet counts

(continued)

Treatment Modifications (*continued*)

Hematologic Adverse Effects

Cycles ≥2, 6–8 weeks after a previous cycle:

Recovery to ANC ≥1000/μL and platelets ≥50,000/μL requiring >6 weeks, but <8 weeks	Delay treatment for up to 8 weeks after the last cycle began until ANC ≥1000/μL and platelets ≥50,000/μL, *then* Begin a new treatment cycle with decitabine dosage decreased to 11 mg/m² per dose every 8 hours for 3 consecutive days (33 mg/m² per day; 99 mg/m² per 3-day course)
If ANC <1000/μL or platelets <50,000/μL	Delay treatment for up to 10 weeks after the last cycle began, and continually monitor ANC and platelet counts

Cycles ≥2, 8–10 weeks after a previous cycle:

Recovery to ANC ≥1000/μL and platelets ≥50,000/μL requiring >8 weeks, but <10 weeks	1. Delay treatment for up to 8 weeks after the last cycle began until ANC ≥1000/μL and platelets ≥50,000/μL 2. Evaluate bone marrow (BM) aspirate for evidence of disease progression (PD). If BM aspirate is negative for PD, *then:* 3. Begin a new treatment cycle with decitabine dosage decreased to 11 mg/m² per dose every 8 hours for 3 consecutive days (33 mg/m² per day; 99 mg/m² per 3-day course) 4. Maintain or increase decitabine dosage during subsequent cycles as clinically indicated

Nonhematologic Adverse Effects

Cycles ≥2, for: • Serum creatinine ≥2 mg/dL (≥177 μmol/L) • Serum ALT (SGPT) or total bilirubin ≥2 times ULN • Active or uncontrolled infection	Withhold decitabine treatment until the toxicity is resolved, *then* Begin a new treatment cycle at the same decitabine dosage and schedule previously given

Therapy Monitoring

1. Complete blood counts, leukocyte differential, and platelet counts should be performed as needed to monitor response and toxicity; that is, at least once weekly
2. Consider bone marrow biopsy every 2 cycles until CR is confirmed
3. Liver chemistries and serum creatinine should be obtained prior to initiation of treatment

MYELODYSPLASTIC SYNDROME REGIMEN: DECITABINE + CEDAZURIDINE TABLETS

Garcia-Manero G et al. Blood 2019;134(1_suppl):846
Garcia-Manero G et al. Blood 2020;136:674–683
Savona MR et al. Lancet Haematol 2019;6:e194–e203
INQOVI (decitabine and cedazuridine) package insert. Princeton, NJ: Taiho Oncology, Inc.; July 2020

Decitabine/cedazuridine tablet (INQOVI) 35 mg/100 mg per dose; administer orally once per day, on an empty stomach, for 5 consecutive days on days 1–5, every 28 days, until disease progression (total dose of decitabine per 28 day cycle = 175 mg; total dose of cedazuridine per 28 day cycle = 500 mg)

Notes:
- Consider prescribing a prophylactic antiemetic medication to be administered prior to each dose of decitabine/cedazuridine

- A minimum of 4 cycles is recommended; a partial or complete response may require >4 cycles

- Advise patients not to eat for 2 hours before and for 2 hours following each dose of decitabine/cedazuridine

- Advise patients to take decitabine/cedazuridine doses at approximately the same time each day

- Swallow decitabine/cedazuridine tablets whole. Do not cut, crush, or chew tablets

- Patients who delay taking decitabine/cedazuridine at a regularly scheduled time may take a missed dose if the interval remaining before the next regularly scheduled dose is ≥12 hours and then resume the normal daily dosing schedule. If the time to the next regularly scheduled dose is <12 hours, then the patient should delay taking the dose until the next regularly scheduled time but should extend the dosing period by 1 day for every missed dose so that 5 daily doses are administered for each cycle

- Patients who vomit following a dose of decitabine/cedazuridine should not take an additional dose

- Within a cycle, do not substitute decitabine/cedazuridine (INQOVI) for intravenous decitabine (DACOGEN)

- Decitabine/cedazuridine is a hazardous drug. Follow applicable special handling and disposal procedures

- Avoid coadministration of decitabine/cedazuridine with drugs that are metabolized by cytidine deaminase

Supportive Care
Antiemetic prophylaxis
Emetogenic potential is **MINIMAL–LOW**
Note: the U.S. FDA-approved prescribing information for decitabine/cedazuridine recommends to consider administering an antiemetic medication prior to each dose to minimize nausea and vomiting
See Chapter 42 for antiemetic recommendations

Hematopoietic growth factor (CSF) prophylaxis
Primary prophylaxis may be indicated for patients with refractory symptomatic cytopenias
See Chapter 43 for more information

Antimicrobial prophylaxis
Risk of fever and neutropenia is **HIGH**
  Antimicrobial primary prophylaxis is recommended:
  - Antibacterial—consider fluoroquinolone prophylaxis

  - Antifungal—recommended

  - Antiviral—anti-herpes antivirals (eg, acyclovir, famciclovir, valacyclovir)

Patient Population Studied

Trials ASTX727-01 and ASTX727-02 were multicenter, open-label, randomized, crossover studies designed to draw comparisons about the pharmacokinetics, pharmacodynamics, efficacy, and safety of oral cedazuridine/decitabine compared to intravenous decitabine in adults with myelodysplastic syndrome (MDS). Eligible participants were ≥18 years of age with intermediate-1, intermediate-2, or high-risk MDS based on the International Prognostic Scoring System, or with chronic myelomonocytic leukemia. Additionally, patients had to have an ECOG performance status of 0–2 with adequate hepatic and renal function. Patients were permitted to have received one prior cycle of either decitabine or azacitidine. Patients who had received allogenic hematopoietic cell transplants were able to enroll if they were free of graft-vs-host disease and off immunosuppressive therapy. Patients were randomized 1:1 to receive oral decitabine/cedazuridine in cycle 1 followed by IV decitabine in cycle 2 (sequence A) or to receive the reverse sequence (sequence B). Starting with cycle 3, all patients received oral decitabine/cedazuridine

Efficacy

Results from Phase 2 PK/PD Study (NCT02103748), n = 80

Parameter	C-DEC	IV-DEC	Between-group Comparison
Exposure			
Primary paired population			
Decitabine 5-day AUC$_{last}$ (geometric least squares mean), h*ng/mL			
DC cohort (n = 40)	750.82	802.81	LSM ratio oral/IV 93.52 (80% CI 82.1–106.5)
FDC cohort (n = 24)	727.29	745.26	LSM ratio oral/IV 97.59 (80% CI 80.48–118.3)
Secondary unpaired population			
Decitabine 5-day AUC$_{last}$ (geometric least squares mean), h*ng/mL			
DC cohort	735.62 (n = 48)	795.41 (n = 42)	LSM ratio oral/IV 92.48 (80% CI 81.37–105.1)
FDC cohort	760.43 (n = 28)	742.26 (n = 26)	LSM ratio oral/IV 102.45 (80% CI 85.35–123)
Decitabine 5-day AUC$_{0-24}$ (geometric least squares mean), h*ng/mL			
DC cohort	753.68 (n = 45)	794.73 (n = 40)	LSM ratio oral/IV 94.83 (80% CI 83.97–107.1)
FDC cohort	846.82 (n = 26)	696.90 (n = 20)	LSM ratio oral/IV 121.51 (80% CI 97.15–152)
Decitabine 5-day AUC$_{\infty}$ (geometric least squares mean), h*ng/mL			
DC cohort	733.26 (n = 42)	794.73 (n = 40)	LSM ratio oral/IV 92.27 (80% CI 81.27–104.7)
FDC cohort	845.57 (n = 26)	687.08 (n = 40)	LSM ratio oral/IV 121.30 (80% CI 97–151.7)

Hypomethylating Activity

Cycle	Difference (oral-IV) in mean maximum %LINE-1 demethylation (95% CI)
Phase 2 cycle 1 (n = 78)	−1.079 (−3.320 to 1.163)
Phase 2 cycle 2 (n = 64)	−0.017 (−2.736 to 2.701)

Best Response (Overall Population, n = 80)	Number of Patients (%)
Complete response (CR)	17 (21)
Partial response (PR)	0
Marrow complete response (mCR) mCR + hematologic improvement (HI)	18 (22) 6 (7)

Hematologic improvement (HI)
    HI-erythroid response
    HI-neutrophil response
    HI-platelet response
	13 (16)
	8 (10)
	2 (2)
	11 (14)

Overall response (CR + PR + mCR + HI)	48 (60)

(continued)

Treatment Modifications (continued)

Updated Results from Phase 3 PK Equivalence/Efficacy Study (ASCERTAIN study), n = 133

Parameter	C-DEC	IV-DEC	Between-group Comparison
Exposure			
Decitabine 5-day AUC_{0-24} (geometric mean estimate), h*ng/mL	856	865	Oral/IV AUC ratio 98.9% 90% CI (92.7–105.6)

Hypomethylating Activity

Comparison of hypomethylating activity by *LINE–1* demethylation showed difference between oral C-DEC and IV-DEC demethylation of <1% and 95% CI of difference included 0

Best Response (n = 101 Evaluable Patients)	Number of Patients (%)
Complete response (CR)	12 (11.9)
Marrow complete response (mCR) mCR + hematologic improvement (HI)	46 (45.5) 14 (13.9)
Hematologic improvement (HI)	7 (6.9)
Objective response rate (CR + mCR + HI)	65 (64)

C-DEC, oral cedazuridine/decitabine; IV-DEC, intravenous decitabine; AUC_{last}, area under the curve from time 0 to last measurable concentration; AUC_{0-24}, area under the curve from time 0 to 24 hours; AUC_{∞}, area under the curve from time 0 to ∞; DC, dose confirmation cohort (2 separate capsules of cedazuridine and decitabine); FDC, fixed-dose combination cohort; LSM, least squares mean; CI, confidence interval

Therapy Monitoring

1. Complete blood counts, leukocyte differential, and platelet counts prior to each cycle and as needed to monitor response and toxicity—that is, at least once weekly
2. Liver chemistries and serum creatinine should be obtained prior to each cycle
3. Consider bone marrow biopsy every 2 cycles until CR is confirmed

Notes

Decitabine/cedazuridine is indicated for treatment of adult patients with myelodysplastic syndromes (MDS), including previously treated and untreated, de novo and secondary MDS with the following French-American-British subtypes (refractory anemia, refractory anemia with ringed sideroblasts, refractory anemia with excess blasts, and chronic myelomonocytic leukemia [CMML]) and intermediate-1, intermediate-2, and high-risk International Prognostic Scoring System groups

Treatment Modifications

RECOMMENDED DOSE MODIFICATIONS FOR DECITABINE/CEDAZURIDINE

Starting dose	1 tablet orally once daily on days 1–5
Dose level −1	1 tablet orally once daily on days 1–4
Dose level −2	1 tablet orally once daily on days 1–3
Dose level −3	1 tablet orally once daily on days 1, 3, and 5

(continued)

Treatment Modifications (*continued*)

Adverse Event	Treatment Modification
Day 1 ANC <1000/mm³ or platelets <50,000/mm³ in a patient without active disease	Delay the next cycle until ANC ≥1000/mm³ and platelets ≥50,000/mm³. For patients with persistent severe neutropenia (ANC <500/mm³) and/or neutropenic fever, provide appropriate supportive care with growth factors and antimicrobial prophylaxis/treatment as clinically indicated. If hematologic recovery occurs within 2 weeks of achieving remission, then continue the same dose. If hematologic recovery does not occur within 2 weeks of achieving remission, then delay the next cycle for up to an additional 2 weeks and then resume decitabine/cedazuridine with the dosage reduced by 1 dose level*
Day 1 SCr ≥2 mg/dL	Delay the next cycle until serum creatinine is <2 mg/dL, serum bilirubin is <2× ULN, and AST and ALT are <2× ULN, then proceed with decitabine/cedazuridine at the same dosage or at a reduced dosage per the discretion of the medically responsible health care provider
Day 1 serum bilirubin >2× ULN	
Day 1 AST or ALT >2× ULN	
Active or uncontrolled infection	Withhold decitabine/cedazuridine until infection has resolved or is determined to be responding to antimicrobial therapy

*Maintain or increase the dose in subsequent cycles as clinically indicated
ANC, absolute neutrophil count; SCr, serum creatinine; ULN, upper limit of normal; AST, aspartate aminotransferase; ALT, alanine aminotransferase

Adverse Events—Pooled Safety Population

Grade (%)	INQOVI (Oral Decitabine-Cedazuridine) Cycle 1 N = 107		Intravenous Decitabine Cycle 1 N = 106		INQOVI (Oral Decitabine-Cedazuridine) All Cycles N = 208*	
	All Grades	Grades 3–4	All Grades	Grads 3–4	All Grades	Grades 3–4
General disorders and administration site conditions						
Fatigue	29	2	25	0	55	5
Hemorrhage	24	2	17	0	43	3
Edema	10	0	11	0	30	0.5
Pyrexia	7	0	7	0	19	1
Gastrointestinal disorders						
Constipation	20	0	23	0	44	0
Mucositis	18	1	24	2	41	4
Nausea	25	0	16	0	40	0.5
Diarrhea	16	0	11	0	37	1
Transaminase increased	12	1	3	0	21	3
Abdominal pain	9	0	7	0	19	1
Vomiting	5	0	5	0	15	0
Musculoskeletal and connective tissue disorders						
Myalgia	9	2	16	1	42	3
Arthralgia	9	1	13	1	40	3

(*continued*)

Adverse Events—Pooled Safety Population (continued)

Respiratory, thoracic, and mediastinal disorders						
Dyspnea	17	3	9	3	38	6
Cough	7	0	8	0	28	0
Blood and lymphatic system disorders						
Febrile neutropenia	10	10	13	13	33	32
Skin and subcutaneous tissue disorders						
Rash	12	1	11	1	33	0.5
Nervous system disorders						
Dizziness	16	1	11	0	33	2
Headache	22	0	13	0	13	0
Neuropathy	4	0	8	0	13	0
Metabolism and nutritional disorders						
Decreased appetite	10	1	6	0	24	2
Infections and infestations						
Upper respiratory tract infection	6	0	3	0	23	1
Pneumonia	7	7	7	5	21	15
Sepsis	6	6	2	1	14	11
Cellulitis	4	1	3	2	12	5
Investigations						
Renal impairment	9	0	8	1	18	0
Weight decreased	5	0	3	0	10	1
Injury, poisoning, and procedural complications						
Fall	4	0	1	0	12	1
Psychiatric disorders						
Insomnia	6	0	2	0	12	0.5
Vascular disorders						
Hypotension	4	0	6	1	11	2
Cardiac disorders						
Arrhythmia	3	0	2	0	11	1
Hematology lab abnormalities						
Leukocytes decreased	79	65	77	59	87	81
Platelet count decreased	79	65	77	67	82	76
Neutrophil count decreased	70	65	62	59	73	71
Hemoglobin decreased	58	41	59	36	71	55

(continued)

Adverse Events—Pooled Safety Population (*continued*)

Chemistry lab abnormalities

Glucose increased	19	0	11	0	54	7
Albumin decreased	22	1	20	0	45	2
Alkaline phosphatase increased	22	1	12	0	42	0.5
Glucose decreased	14	0	17	0	40	1
ALT increased	13	1	7	0	37	2
Sodium decreased	9	2	8	0	30	4
Calcium decreased	16	0	12	0	30	2
AST increased	6	1	2	0	30	2
Creatinine increased	7	0	8	0	29	0.5

*Includes adverse reactions that occurred during all cycles, including during treatment with 1 cycle of intravenous decitabine therapy
Note: table denotes adverse reactions in ≥10 of patients who received INQOVI (decitabine/cedazuridine) in the pooled safety population
INQOVI (decitabine and cedazuridine) package insert. Princeton, NJ: Taiho Oncology, Inc.; July 2020

MYELODYSPLASTIC SYNDROME REGIMEN: AZACITIDINE

Fenaux P et al. Lancet Oncol 2009;10:223–232
VIDAZA (azacitidine) prescribing information. Summit, NJ: Celgene Corporation; March 2020

Azacitidine 75 mg/m^2 per dose; administer either intravenously or subcutaneously once daily for 7 consecutive days on days 1–7, every 28 days, for a minimum of 6 cycles and until disease progression (total dosage/28-day cycle = 525 mg/m^2)

Administration by subcutaneous injection
- Azacitidine is reconstituted with sterile water for injection (SWFI) to obtain a solution with concentration equal to 25 mg/mL that is suitable for subcutaneous injection
- Doses >100 mg (>4 mL) should be equally divided into 2 (or more) syringes and injected into 2 (or more) separate sites
- Rotate sites for each injection (thigh, abdomen, or upper arm) and administer new injections ≥2.5 cm from an old site and never into areas where the site is tender, bruised, red, or hard
- If azacitidine was stored in refrigerated conditions (2–8°C), then allow the suspension to equilibrate to room temperature for up to 30 minutes following removal from the refrigerator
- Immediately prior to injection, roll the syringe between the palms until a uniform, cloudy suspension is achieved
- Stability varies based on temperature of diluent used for reconstitution and storage conditions. Refer to Chapter 44 for details

Intravenous administration
- Azacitidine is reconstituted with 10 mL SWFI to obtain a solution with concentration equal to 10 mg/mL that is then further diluted in 50–100 mL 0.9% sodium chloride injection or lactated Ringer's injection
- Administer a dose over 10–40 minutes. Dose administration must be completed within 60 minutes after product preparation

Supportive Care
Antiemetic prophylaxis
Emetogenic potential is **MODERATE**
See Chapter 42 for antiemetic recommendations

Hematopoietic growth factor (CSF) prophylaxis
Primary prophylaxis may be indicated for patients with refractory symptomatic cytopenias
Antimicrobial prophylaxis
Risk of fever and neutropenia is **HIGH**
Antimicrobial primary prophylaxis is recommended:
- Antibacterial—recommended during periods of prolonged (>7 days) neutropenia
- Antifungal—recommended during periods of prolonged (>7 days) neutropenia
- Antiviral—anti-herpes antivirals (eg, acyclovir, famciclovir, valacyclovir)

Patient Population Studied

In a phase 3, multicenter, controlled, parallel-group, open-label trial, patients with higher-risk myelodysplastic syndromes were randomly assigned 1:1 to receive azacitidine or conventional care (best supportive care, low-dose cytarabine, or intensive chemotherapy as selected by investigators before randomization). Patients were stratified by French-American-British and international prognostic scoring system classifications

Efficacy (N = 358)

Efficacy Variable	Azacitidine (n = 179)	Conventional Care* (n = 179)	P Value
Overall survival[†]	24.5 months (9.9–not reached)	15 months (5.6–24.1)	0.0001
Time to transformation to AML	17.8 months	11.5 months	0.0001
Any remission	51 (29%)	21 (12%)	0.0001
Complete remission	30 (17%)	14 (8%)	0.015
Partial remission	21 (12%)	7 (4%)	0.0094
Stable disease	75 (42%)	65 (36%)	0.33

(continued)

Efficacy (N = 358) *(continued)*

Efficacy Variable	Azacitidine (n = 179)	Conventional Care* (n = 179)	P Value
Hematologic improvement	87/177 (49%)	51/178 (29%)	<0.0001
Major erythroid improvement	62/157 (40%)	17/160 (11%)	<0.0001
Major platelet improvement	46/141 (33%)	18/129 (14%)	0.0003
Major neutrophil improvement	25/131 (19%)	20/111 (18%)	0.87

*Conventional care: best supportive care, low-dose cytarabine, or intensive chemotherapy
†Overall survival was better for azacitidine than conventional care in all the cytogenetic subgroups on the international prognosis scoring system

Therapy Monitoring

1. Serum liver chemistries and creatinine should be obtained prior to initiation of treatment
2. Complete blood counts, leukocyte differential, and platelet count should be performed as needed to monitor response and toxicity; that is, at least once weekly
3. Consider bone marrow biopsy after 2–4 cycles of therapy. Patients should receive treatment for a minimum of 4–6 cycles; however, it may take longer than 4 cycles to achieve a complete or partial response

Treatment Modifications

For patients with baseline (start of treatment) WBC ≥3000/μL, ANC ≥1500/μL, and platelets ≥75,000/μL, adjust the dose as follows, based on nadir counts for any given cycle:

Nadir Counts		% Dose During the Next Course
ANC (/μL)	Platelets (/μL)	
<500	<25,000	50%
500–1500	25,000–50,000	67%
>1500	>50,000	100%

For patients whose baseline counts are WBC <3000/μL, ANC <1500/μL, or platelets <75,000/μL, dose adjustments should be based on nadir counts and bone marrow biopsy cellularity at the time of the nadir as noted below, unless there is clear improvement in differentiation (percentage of mature granulocytes is higher and ANC is higher than at the onset of that course) at the time of the next cycle, in which case the dose of the current treatment should be continued:

WBC or Platelet Nadir % Decrease in Counts from Baseline	Bone Marrow Biopsy Cellularity at Time of Nadir (%)		
	30–60	15–30	<15
	% Dosage During the Next Course		
50–75	100	50	33
>75	75	50	33

Notes:
- If a nadir has occurred as defined in the above table, the next course of treatment should be given 28 days after the start of the preceding course, provided that both the WBC and platelet counts are >25% above the nadir and rising
- If a >25% increase above the nadir is not seen by day 28, counts should be reassessed every 7 days
- If a 25% increase is not seen by day 42, then the patient should be treated with 50% of the scheduled dose

(continued)

Treatment Modifications (*continued*)

Renal Toxicity

Adverse Effect	Dose Modification
Unexplained reduction in serum bicarbonate levels to <20 mEq/L in a patient receiving azacitidine	Reduce the azacitidine dosage by 50% in the subsequent course. If the toxicity does not recur, consider administering full-dose azacitidine thereafter
Unexplained elevations of BUN or serum creatinine in a patient receiving azacitidine	Withhold the next cycle of azacitidine until serum creatinine and BUN values return to normal or baseline, then reduce the azacitidine dosage by 50% for the next cycle. If the toxicity does not recur, consider administering full dose azacitidine thereafter

Dermatologic Toxicity

Intolerable injection site adverse reaction (erythema, pain, bruising, reaction) in a patient receiving subcutaneous azacitidine	Consider switching the route of azacitidine administration from subcutaneous to intravenous

Adverse Events

	Azacitidine (n = 179)	Conventional Care (n = 179)
Deaths	82 (46%)	113 (63%)
Deaths during first 3 months of treatment	20 (11%)	16 (9%)
Safety population	n = 175	n = 165
Discontinuation before study completion due to hematologic adverse events	8 (5%)	4 (2%)
Grade 3 or 4 toxicity		
Neutropenia	159 (91%)	126 (76%)
Thrombocytopenia	149 (85%)	132 (80%)
Anemia	100 (57%)	112 (68%)
Baseline Grade 0–2 progressed to Grade 3 or 4 during treatment		
Neutropenia	67/80 (84%)	46/76 (61%)
Thrombocytopenia	72/97 (74%)	68/94 (72%)
Anemia	84/156 (54%)	83/130 (64%)

MYELODYSPLASTIC SYNDROME REGIMEN: LENALIDOMIDE

List A et al. N Engl J Med 2006;355:1456–1465

Lenalidomide 10 mg per day; administer orally, continually (total dose/week = 70 mg)

Supportive Care
Antiemetic prophylaxis
Emetogenic potential is **MINIMAL–LOW**
See Chapter 42 for antiemetic recommendations

Hematopoietic growth factor (CSF) prophylaxis
Primary prophylaxis may be indicated for patients with refractory symptomatic cytopenias
See Chapter 43 for more information

Antimicrobial prophylaxis
Risk of fever and neutropenia is **HIGH**
Antimicrobial primary prophylaxis is recommended:
- Antibacterial—*P. jirovecii* prophylaxis is recommended (eg, cotrimoxazole)
- Antifungal—recommended
- Antiviral—anti-herpes antivirals (eg, acyclovir, famciclovir, valacyclovir)

Patient Population Studied

A study of 148 patients with MDS who were treated with lenalidomide, of whom 46 were treated on the 21-day schedule and 102 received continuous daily dosing. Of the patients, 64% had either refractory anemia or refractory anemia with ringed sideroblasts, and 81% were at low or intermediate-1 risk according to the IPSS scores

Treatment Modifications

Dose Adjustments for Hematologic Toxicities During MDS Treatment

Platelet Counts

If thrombocytopenia develops WITHIN 4 weeks of starting treatment at 10 mg daily in MDS

If baseline ≥100,000/μL

When Platelets	Recommended Course
Fall to <50,000/μL	Interrupt **lenalidomide** treatment
Return to ≥50,000/μL	Resume **lenalidomide** at 5 mg daily

If baseline <100,000/μL

When Platelets	Recommended Course
Fall to 50% of the baseline value	Interrupt **lenalidomide** treatment
If baseline ≥60,000/μL and returns to ≥50,000/μL	Resume **lenalidomide** at 5 mg daily
If baseline <60,000/μL and returns ≥30,000/μL	Resume **lenalidomide** at 5 mg daily

If thrombocytopenia develops *after* 4 weeks of starting treatment at 10 mg daily in MDS

When Platelets	Recommended Course
<30,000/μL or <50,000/μL with platelet transfusions	Interrupt **lenalidomide** treatment
Return to ≥30,000/μL (without hemostatic failure)	Resume **lenalidomide** at 5 mg daily

Patients who experience thrombocytopenia at 5 mg daily should have their dosage adjusted as follows:

If thrombocytopenia develops during treatment at 5 mg daily in MDS

When Platelets	Recommended Course
<30,000/μL or <50,000/μL with platelet transfusions	Interrupt **lenalidomide** treatment
Return to ≥30,000/μL (without hemostatic failure)	Resume **lenalidomide** at 2.5 mg daily

(*continued*)

Treatment Modifications (*continued*)

Patients who are dosed initially at 10 mg and experience neutropenia should have their dosage adjusted as follows:

Absolute neutrophil counts (ANC)
If neutropenia develops WITHIN 4 weeks of starting treatment at 10 mg daily in MDS

If baseline ANC ≥1000/μL

When Neutrophils	Recommended Course
Fall to <750/μL	Interrupt **lenalidomide** treatment
Return to ≥1000/μL	Resume **lenalidomide** at 5 mg daily

If baseline ANC <1000/μL

When Neutrophils	Recommended Course
Fall to <500/μL	Interrupt **lenalidomide** treatment
Return to ≥500/μL	Resume **lenalidomide** at 5 mg daily

If neutropenia develops 4 weeks AFTER starting treatment at 10 mg daily in MDS

When Neutrophils	Recommended Course
<500/μL for ≥7 days or <500/μL associated with fever (≥38.5°C)	Interrupt **lenalidomide** treatment
Return to ≥500/μL	Resume **lenalidomide** at 5 mg daily

Patients who experience neutropenia at 5 mg daily should have their dosage adjusted as follows:

If neutropenia develops during treatment at 5 mg daily in MDS

When Neutrophils	Recommended Course
<500/μL for ≥7 days or < 500/μL associated with fever (≥38.5°C)	Interrupt lenalidomide
Return to ≥500/μL	Resume lenalidomide at 2.5 mg daily

Other Grade 3/4 Toxicities in MDS
For other Grade 3/4 toxicities judged to be related to **lenalidomide**, hold treatment and restart at next lower dose level when toxicity has resolved to Grade ≤ 2

Starting Dose Adjustment for Renal Impairment in Myelodysplastic Syndromes (Days 1–28 of Each 28-Day Cycle)

Category	Renal Function (Cockcroft-Gault)	Dose
Moderate renal impairment	Clcr 30–60 mL/min (0.5–1 mL/s)	5 mg every 24 hours
Severe renal impairment	Clcr <30 mL/min (not requiring dialysis)	2.5 mg every 24 hours
End-stage renal disease	Clcr <30 mL/min (requiring dialysis)	2.5 mg once daily. On dialysis days, administer the dose following dialysis

Therapy Monitoring

1. Serum liver chemistries and creatinine should be obtained prior to initiation of treatment
2. Complete blood counts, leukocyte differential, and platelet count should be performed as needed to monitor response and toxicity—that is, at least once weekly
3. Consider bone marrow biopsy every 2 cycles until CR is confirmed

Efficacy

Frequency of Cytogenetic Response According to Karyotype Complexity

Complexity	Patients Who Could be Evaluated*	Cytogenetic Response	Complete Cytogenetic Remission
Isolated 5q deletion—no. (%)	64	49 (77)	29 (45)
5q deletion + 1 additional abnormality—no. (%)	15	10 (67)	6 (40)
Complex (≥3 abnormalities) —no. (%)	6	3 (50)	3 (50)
P value		0.27	0.93

*Patients who could be evaluated were those with at least 20 analyzable cells in metaphase at baseline and at least 1 follow-up assessment. P values are for the association between karyotypic complexity and cytogenic response or complete cytogenetic remission

Among 148 patients, 99 (67%) no longer needed transfusions by week 24; the remaining 13 patients had a reduction of 50% or greater in the number of transfusions required. The median time to transfusion independence was 4.6 weeks (range: 1–49)

The rate of transfusion independence was significantly lower among patients with baseline thrombocytopenia than among patients with platelet counts >100,000/μL at baseline (39% vs 73%, P = 0.001)

Toxicity

Grade 3 and 4 Treatment-Related Adverse Events

	Grade 3		Grade 4		Grades 3 and 4
	Continuous Daily Dosing*	21-Day Dosing*	Continuous Daily Dosing*	21-Day Dosing*	Both Schedules
	(N = 102)	(N = 46)	(N = 102)	(N = 46)	(N = 148)
Adverse Event	Number of Patients (%)				
Neutropenia	20 (20)	8 (17)	45 (44)	8 (17)	81 (55)
Thrombocytopenia	37 (36)	14 (30)	7 (7)	7 (15)	65 (44)
Anemia (not otherwise specified)	4 (4)	2 (4)	4 (4)	0	10 (7)
Leukopenia (not otherwise specified)	3 (3)	2 (4)	4 (4)	0	9 (6)
Rash	5 (5)	4 (9)	0	0	9 (6)
Febrile neutropenia	2 (2)	1 (2)	2 (2)	1 (2)	1 (1)
Pruritus	2 (2)	2 (4)	0	0	4 (3)
Fatigue	2 (2)	2 (4)	0	0	4 (3)
Muscle cramp	3 (3)	0	0	0	3 (2)
Pneumonia	1 (1)	2 (4)	1 (1)	0	4 (3)
Nausea	3 (3)	1 (2)	0	0	4 (3)
Diarrhea	4 (4)	0	0	0	4 (3)
Deep-vein thrombosis	3 (3)	1 (2)	0	0	4 (3)
Hemorrhage	1 (1)	2 (4)	1 (1)	1 (2)	4 (3)
Hypokalemia	1 (1)	1 (2)	0	0	2 (1)
Pyrexia	1 (1)	0	0	0	1 (1)

*Lenalidomide 10 mg/day

Notes

A phase 3, randomized, double-blind study assessed the efficacy and safety of lenalidomide in 205 red blood cell (RBC) transfusion–dependent patients with International Prognostic Scoring System low-/intermediate-1–risk del5q31 MDS. Patients received lenalidomide 10 mg/day on days 1–21 (n = 69) or 5 mg/day on days 1–28 (n = 69) of 28-day cycles; or placebo (n = 67). Crossover to lenalidomide or higher dose was allowed after 16 weeks. More patients in the lenalidomide 10- and 5-mg groups achieved RBC-transfusion independence (TI) for ≥26 weeks (primary end point) versus placebo (56.1% and 42.6% vs 5.9%; both P <0.001)

The median duration of RBC-TI was not reached (median follow-up: 1.55 years), with 60–67% of responses ongoing in patients without progression to acute myeloid leukemia (AML). Cytogenetic response rates were 50% (10 mg) vs 25% (5 mg; P = 0.066)

For the lenalidomide groups combined, 3-year overall survival and AML risk were 56.5% and 25.1%, respectively

RBC-TI for ≥8 weeks was associated with 47% and 42% reductions in the relative risks of death and AML progression or death, respectively (P = 0.021 and 0.048)

Fenaux P et al. Blood 2011;118:3765–3776

MYELODYSPLASTIC SYNDROME REGIMEN: LYMPHOCYTE IMMUNE GLOBULIN, ANTI-THYMOCYTE GLOBULIN (EQUINE) (ATG)

Atgam (lymphocyte immune globulin, anti-thymocyte globulin, [equine] sterile solution) product labeling. New York, NY: Pharmacia & Upjohn Co., Division of Pfizer Inc.; November 2005
Molldrem JJ et al. Ann Intern Med 2002;137:156–163
Molldrem JJ et al. Br J Haematol 1997;99:699–705
Sloand EM et al. J Clin Oncol 2008;26:2505–2511
Saunthararajah Y et al. Blood 2003;102:3025–3027
U.S. National Heart, Lung, and Blood Institute. Clinical trial 09-H–0183. Available from clinicalstudies.info.nih.gov/ProtocolDetails.aspx?id=2009-H–0183

Premedication:

Acetaminophen 650 mg; administer orally 60 minutes before each antithymocyte globulin treatment, *plus*

Diphenhydramine 25–50 mg; administer orally 60 minutes before each antithymocyte globulin treatment

Prednisone 1 mg/kg per day or 40 mg/day (whichever dose is greater); administer orally starting prior to the first dose of ATG

- The daily prednisone dose is gradually decreased (tapered) starting on day 10 or when signs of serum sickness have resolved, whichever occurs later
- Prednisone dose is tapered with a dose decrement every 2 days over the following 8 days, and then is discontinued
- Patients with serum sickness may require greater prednisone doses to achieve clinical resolution and dose tapering over a longer duration

Lymphocyte immune globulin, anti-thymocyte globulin (equine) (see Note 1 below) 40 mg/kg per day administered through a high-flow (central) vein, vascular shunt, or arteriovenous fistula in a volume of 0.9% sodium chloride injection (0.9% NS), 5% dextrose and 0.2% sodium chloride injection (D5W/0.2% NS), or 5% dextrose and 0.45% sodium chloride injection (D5W/0.45% NS) sufficient to produce a solution with antithymocyte globulin concentration ≤4 mg/mL, over at least 4 hours for 4 consecutive days, on days 1–4 (total dosage/course = 160 mg/kg)

Notes:

1. Lymphocyte immune globulin, anti-thymocyte globulin [equine] (ATG) product labeling recommends intradermal skin testing prior to administration. Patients with a reactive skin test may still receive antithymocyte globulin after desensitization
2. Always administer anti-thymocyte globulin through an inline filter with 0.2- to 1.0-μm pore size
3. After dilution, ATG should be allowed to come to room temperature before administration begins
4. The initial infusion rate should be 10% of the total volume per hour. For example, for a total volume of 500 mL, start at a rate of 50 mL/hour for the first 30 minutes. If there are no signs of an adverse reaction, the infusion rate can be advanced to complete the infusion over no less than 4 hours

Cyclosporine orally every 12 hours, continually, starting on day 14

Patients ≥12 years of age: **cyclosporine** 3 mg/kg per dose; administer orally every 12 hours (total daily dose = 6 mg/kg)

- Dosing is based on actual body weight (ABW) except in obese patients (defined as a body mass index >35 kg/m² in patients >20 years of age and >95th percentile for ages 12–20 years)
- For obese patients, cyclosporine dosage is based on an *adjusted body weight* that is calculated as the midpoint between the ideal body weight (IBW) and ABW, thus:

$$\text{Adjusted Body Weight} = \text{IBW} + (\text{ABW} - \text{IBW})/2$$

- Cyclosporine is continued for 6 months, after which:
  - In responding patients, the dose is gradually decreased by 5% per week, and then is discontinued
  - In nonresponding patients, cyclosporine is discontinued
- Cyclosporine doses are adjusted for increases in serum creatinine and to maintain serum cyclosporine concentrations within the range of 200–400 μg/L (166–333 nmol/L) by radioimmunoassay
- *Notes:*
  - Avoid other nephrotoxic drugs concurrent with cyclosporine treatment
  - Granulocyte colony-stimulating factors (G-CSF) should be administered as clinically indicated, usually for evidence of infection such as fever or localized inflammation in the setting of severe inflammation. Emergence of monosomy 7 has been linked to use of exogenous G-CSF

Allergy skin testing prior to ATG administration:

1. Anti-thymocyte globulin [equine] is freshly diluted (1:1000) with 0.9% sodium chloride injection (0.9% NS), to a concentration of 5 μg/0.1 mL, and administered intradermally
2. Administer 0.1 mL 0.9% NS, intradermally in a contralateral extremity as a control
3. Observe every 15–20 minutes during the first hour after intradermal injection
   a. A local reaction ≥10 mm with a wheal, erythema, or both, ± pseudopod formation and itching or a marked local swelling is considered a positive test. For patients who exhibit a positive test result, consider desensitization prior to therapy
   Notes:
   - Advise patients to avoid using H_1-receptor antagonists for 72 hours before skin testing

(continued)

(*continued*)

- The predictive value of skin testing has not been proved clinically; that is, allergic reactions including anaphylaxis have occurred in patients whose skin test result is negative
- If anti-thymocyte globulin is administered after a locally positive skin test, administration should only be attempted in a setting where intensive life-support facilities are immediately available and with the attendance of a physician familiar with the treatment of potentially life-threatening allergic reactions
- Systemic reactions preclude antithymocyte globulin administration—for example, generalized rash, tachycardia, dyspnea, hypotension, or anaphylaxis

Guidelines for administering antithymocyte globulin (ATG):
- Severity and frequency of toxicities (rigors, fevers, oxygen desaturation, hypotension, nausea, vomiting, anaphylaxis) are greatest during the first day of infusion and diminish with each subsequent day. Toxicities generally subside after completing treatment
- Adverse effects generally can be managed while continuing antithymocyte globulin infusion
- Most patients receiving ATG will develop fever. Most fevers are not infectious in origin

Monitoring during ATG administration:
- Patients should remain under continual surveillance
- Assess peripheral vascular access sites for thrombophlebitis every 8 hours
- Monitor vital signs and assess for adverse reactions (flushing, hives, itching, SOB, difficulty breathing, chest tightness) before starting administration, *then:*
  - *During initial dose:* continually during the first 15 minutes, then every 30 minutes × 2, then at least every hour until administration is completed
  - *During subsequent doses:* 30 minutes after initiating ATG infusion

Supportive Care
Antimicrobial prophylaxis
Risk of fever and neutropenia is **HIGH**
  Antimicrobial primary prophylaxis is recommended:
  - Antibacterial—*P. jirovecii* prophylaxis is recommended (eg, cotrimoxazole or aerosolized pentamidine)
    - Begin during the first month of therapy, and continue throughout the duration of cyclosporine use
  - Antifungal—recommended
  - Antiviral—anti-herpes antivirals (eg, acyclovir, famciclovir, valacyclovir)

Toxicity

Twelve patients required temporary admission to an intensive care unit during ATG treatment. Six patients did not complete 4 planned days of ATG treatment: 3 developed shaking chills, 2 experienced hypotension associated with shaking chills, and 1 died from alveolar hemorrhage associated with leukemic pulmonary infiltrates. One patient died shortly after receiving ATG from alveolar hemorrhage

Infusional toxicities of antithymocyte globulin:
- Severity and frequency of toxicities are greatest during the first day of ATG administration and diminish with each subsequent day. Toxicities generally subside after completing treatment

Adverse Events	Interventions
Rigors	Antihistamines (eg, diphenhydramine 25–50 mg, intravenously or orally every 6 hours as needed) Meperidine 12.5–50 mg, intravenously may be repeated every 10 minutes
Nausea, vomiting	Antiemetic rescue. Then give antiemetic prophylaxis during subsequent antithymocyte globulin treatments (secondary prophylaxis)
Anaphylaxis*	Immediately STOP administration; administer steroids; assist respiration; and provide other resuscitative measures. DO NOT resume treatment

Patient Population Studied

Sixteen patients had low IPSS risk, 94 patients intermediate-1 (int-1) IPSS, 13 patients int-2 IPSS, and 6 patients high IPSS risk. Seventy-four patients received equine ATG, 42 patients received a combination of ATG and cyclosporine (maintaining cyclosporine levels >100 µg/L [>83 nmol/L] for up to 6 months), and 13 patients received cyclosporine alone on the same schedule

(*continued*)

Toxicity (*continued*)

Adverse Events	Interventions
Thrombocytopenia, anemia	Blood product transfusions as needed[†]
Fever and neutropenia[‡]	Broad-spectrum antibiotics empirically, if ANC <500/mm³. May give acetaminophen 650 mg orally every 4 hours
Hypotension	Fluid resuscitation
Refractory hypotension	May indicate anaphylaxis. Stop antithymocyte globulin administration and stabilize blood pressure. Intensive care unit support
Oxygen desaturation	Oxygen therapy
Refractory oxygen desaturation	Discontinue antithymocyte globulin. Intensive care unit support
Respiratory distress	Discontinue antithymocyte globulin. If distress persists, administer an antihistamine, epinephrine, steroids
Rash, pruritus, urticaria	Administer antihistamines and/or topical steroids for prophylaxis and treatment
Serum sickness-like symptoms[§]	Administer prophylactic glucocorticoids
Hepatotoxicity[ϵ]	Monitor LFTs

*Anaphylaxis (<3% of patients) more frequently occurs within the first hour after starting antithymocyte globulin infusion. After the first hour, adverse effects occur as result of a delayed immune response and generally can be managed while continuing the antithymocyte globulin infusion

[†]Concurrent administration of blood products should be avoided with antithymocyte globulin infusions to avoid confusing transfusion reactions with reactions to antithymocyte globulin

[‡]Most patients who receive antithymocyte globulin will develop fever as a result of the drug. Most fevers are not infectious in origin

[§]Type II hypersensitivity reactions/serum sickness consisting of fever, rash, and arthralgia develops in approximately 85% of patients between 7 and 14 days after ATG treatment. These symptoms can be managed with steroids

[ϵ]An isolated increase in serum alanine aminotransferase (ALT) frequently has no clinical significance. Generally, liver function abnormalities are transient and return to normal within 1 month

Bevans MF, Shalabi RA. Clin J Oncol Nurs 2004;8:377–382

Efficacy

Eighteen (24%) of 74 patients (95% CI, 14–34) responded to ATG, 20 (45%) of 42 patients (95% CI, 32–63) responded to ATG plus cyclosporine (P = 0.01), and 1 (8%) of 13 patients responded to cyclosporine. Thirty-one percent (12 of 39 patients; 95% CI, 16–46) of the responses were complete, resulting in near-normal blood counts and transfusion independence; 32 (82%) of 39 (95% CI, 70–94) of the responders achieved either bi-lineage or tri-lineage responses. Of the partial responders, all but 1 became transfusion independent. In multivariate analysis, young age was the most significant factor favoring response to therapy. Other favorable factors affecting response were HLA-DR15 positivity and combination ATG plus cyclosporine treatment (P = 0.001 and P = 0.048, respectively). Patients were seen at yearly follow-up from the start of IST. Seventy patients survive with a median follow-up of 3 years. Patients treated with ATG plus cyclosporine had superior response rates compared with patients treated with ATG alone, although there were no survival differences between these groups

Therapy Monitoring

1. *During antithymocyte globulin infusion:* CBC with differential, LFTs, electrolytes
2. *After antithymocyte globulin therapy:* CBC monitoring is dependent on blood counts. If WBC, ANC, and platelet counts are stable, a CBC with differential may be as infrequent as once every 2–3 weeks. Patients who require platelets may need more frequent CBCs, but not more than twice weekly and usually only once weekly
3. *Six months after the start of therapy:* bone marrow biopsy and aspiration. If patients are stable based on blood counts, bone marrow biopsy may not need to be repeated

Therapeutic drug monitoring for cyclosporine:
- When initiating cyclosporine treatment and after any dose adjustments, monitor cyclosporine trough concentrations (sampled at the end of a dosing interval) every 4–7 days until stable concentrations are achieved
- For patients on a stable cyclosporine regimen, monitor trough levels every 2 weeks
- More frequent cyclosporine monitoring is recommended whenever cyclosporine dosage adjustments are made, serum creatinine increases, and when a patient's concomitantly administered medication regimen is changed (be wary of drugs that potentially perturb cytochrome P450 CYP3A subfamily enzymes expression, availability, or activity)
- Cyclosporine doses are adjusted to maintain blood concentrations with the range of 200–400 µg/L (166–333 nmol/L) by radioimmunoassay

MYELODYSPLASTIC SYNDROME REGIMEN: LUSPATERCEPT

Fenaux P et al. N Engl J Med 2020;382:140–151
Supplementary appendix to: Fenaux P et al. N Engl J Med 2020;382:140–151
Protocol for: Fenaux P et al. N Engl J Med 2020;382:140–151
REBLOZYL (luspatercept-aamt) prescribing information. Summit, NJ: Celgene Corporation; April 2020

Luspatercept-aamt 1 mg/kg; administer in a volume of sterile water for injection, USP sufficient to produce a final concentration of 50 mg/mL, as a subcutaneous injection into the upper arm, thigh, and/or abdomen, by a health care professional, on day 1, every 21 days (total dosage/21-day cycle = 1 mg/kg)

Notes:

- Doses >60 mg (1.2 mL) should be divided equally into two separate syringes and injected into separate sites

- The U.S. Food and Drug Administration-approved indication for luspatercept is for the treatment of anemia failing an erythropoiesis stimulating agent and requiring ≥2 red blood cell (RBC) units over 8 weeks in adults with very low- to intermediate-risk myelodysplastic syndrome with ring sideroblasts (MDS-RS) or with myelodysplastic/myeloproliferative neoplasms with ring sideroblasts and thrombocytosis (MDS/MPN-RS-T). Luspatercept should not be used as a substitute for transfusion in patients who require immediate treatment of anemia

- Doses should be adjusted for insufficient hemoglobin response, for overcorrection of anemia, and for toxicity as described in the "Treatment Modifications" section

Supportive Care

Antiemetic prophylaxis
Emetogenic potential is **MINIMAL**
See Chapter 42 for antiemetic recommendations

Hematopoietic growth factor (CSF) prophylaxis
Prophylaxis is **NOT** *indicated*
See Chapter 43 for more information

Antimicrobial prophylaxis
Risk of fever and neutropenia is **LOW**
  Antimicrobial primary prophylaxis to be considered:
  - Antibacterial—not indicated
  - Antifungal—not indicated
  - Antiviral—not indicated unless patient previously had an episode of HSV

Patient Population Studied

The MEDALIST trial was a double blind, placebo-controlled, international, phase 3 study involving 229 adult patients with myelodysplastic syndrome (MDS) who were randomized (2:1) to receive either luspatercept (n = 153) or placebo (n = 76). Patients were required to have MDS with ring sideroblasts according to World Health Organization criteria (ie, with either ≥15% ring sideroblasts or ≥5% ring sideroblasts if an *SF3B1* mutation was present, and with <5% bone marrow blasts); to have disease classified as very low-, low-, or intermediate-risk per the International Prognostic Scoring System (IPSS); to have been receiving regular red blood cell transfusions (≥2 units per 8 weeks during the 16 weeks prior to randomization); and to have disease that was refractory to erythropoiesis-stimulating agents (ESAs), to have disease that was unlikely to respond to ESAs (based on a serum erythropoietin level of >200 U/L), or to have been intolerant of prior ESA therapy

Efficacy (N = 229)

Efficacy Variable	Luspatercept (n = 153)	Placebo (n = 76)	Between-group Comparison
Response (n = 153 luspatercept arm, n = 76 placebo arm)			
RBC transfusion independence for ≥8 weeks in weeks 1–24*—n/N (%) [95% CI]	58/153 (38) [30–46]	10/76 (13) [6–23]	OR 5.07 (95% CI, 2.28–11.26); P <0.001[†]
RBC transfusion independence for ≥12 weeks in weeks 1–24‡—n/N (%) [95% CI]	43/153 (28) [21–36]	6/76 (8) [3–16]	OR 5.07 (95% CI, 2.00–12.84); P <0.001[†]
RBC transfusion independence for ≥12 weeks in weeks 1–48‡—n/N (%) [95% CI]	51/153 (33) [26–41]	9/76 (12) [6–21]	OR 4.05 (95% CI, 1.83–8.96); P <0.001[†]
RBC transfusion independence for ≥16 weeks in weeks 1–24—n/N (%) [95% CI]	29/153 (19) [13–26]	3/76 (4) [1–11]	—
RBC transfusion independence for ≥16 weeks in weeks 1–48—n/N (%) [95% CI]	43/153 (28) [21–36]	5/76 (7) [2–15]	—

*Primary end point
[†]Cochran-Mantel-Haenszel test with stratification for average baseline RBC transfusion burden (≥6 units per 8 weeks vs <6 units per 8 weeks) and baseline R-IPSS category (very low or low risk vs intermediate risk)
‡Key secondary end point
RBC, red blood cell; CI, confidence interval; OR, odds ratio; R-IPSS, Revised International Prognostic Scoring System
Note: transfusion independence was defined as the absence of an RBC transfusion. The efficacy end points were assessed in the intention-to-treat population. The data cutoff date was 8 May 2018

Therapy Monitoring

1. *Prior to initiation of therapy in females of reproductive potential:* pregnancy test
2. *Prior to each dose:* hemoglobin, blood pressure
3. *Periodically:* monitor for signs and symptoms of thromboembolic events, hypersensitivity reactions, and injection-site reactions

Treatment Modifications

Luspatercept Dose Modifications	
Dose level	Luspatercept
Dose level +2	1.75 mg/kg every 3 weeks
Dose level +1	1.33 mg/kg every 3 weeks
Starting dose	1 mg/kg every 3 weeks
Dose level −1	0.8 mg/kg every 3 weeks
Dose level −2	0.6 mg/kg every 3 weeks
Dose level −3	Discontinue treatment
Insufficient Response at Initiation of Treatment	
Not RBC transfusion-free after ≥2 consecutive doses (6 weeks) at the 1 mg/kg starting dose	Increase the dose to 1.33 mg/kg every 3 weeks*
Not RBC transfusion-free after ≥2 consecutive doses (6 weeks) at 1.33 mg/kg	Increase the dose to 1.75 mg/kg every 3 weeks*
No reduction in RBC transfusion burden after ≥3 consecutive doses (9 weeks) at 1.75 mg/kg	Discontinue treatment
Over-correction of Hemoglobin	
Predose Hgb is ≥11.5 g/dL in the absence of transfusions	Withhold treatment until hemoglobin is ≤11 g/dL
Increase in Hgb >2 g/dL within 3 weeks in the absence of transfusions	Reduce the dose by 1 dosage level
Toxicities	
G ≥3 hypersensitivity reaction	Discontinue treatment
Other G ≥3 adverse reactions	Withhold treatment until resolution to G ≤1, then resume treatment with the dosage reduced by 1 dose level

*Do not increase the dose if the patient is experiencing a Grade ≥3 toxicity
RBC, red blood cell; Hgb, hemoglobin

Adverse Events (N = 229)

Event*	Luspatercept (n = 153)		Placebo (n = 76)	
	Any Grade (%)	Grade 3 (%)	Any Grade (%)	Grade 3 (%)
Fatigue	27	5	13	3
Asthenia	20	3	12	0
Peripheral edema	16	0	17	1
Diarrhea	22	0	9	0
Nausea*	20	1	8	0
Constipation	11	0	9	0
Dizziness	20	0	5	0
Headache	16	1	7	0
Back pain*	19	2	7	0

Event*	Luspatercept (n = 153)		Placebo (n = 76)	
	Any Grade (%)	Grade 3 (%)	Any Grade (%)	Grade 3 (%)
Arthralgia	5	1	12	3
Dyspnea*	15	1	7	0
Cough	18	0	13	0
Bronchitis*	11	1	1	0
Urinary tract infection*	11	1	5	4
Fall	10	5	12	3

*At least 1 serious AE occurred: nausea (in 1 patient receiving luspatercept), back pain (in 3 receiving luspatercept), dyspnea (in 1 receiving luspatercept), bronchitis (in 1 receiving luspatercept), and urinary tract infection (in 1 receiving luspatercept)
Note: the table includes adverse events (AEs) reported in ≥10% of patients. AEs were not adjusted for treatment exposure

28. Myeloproliferative Neoplasms

Naseema Gangat, MD, and Ayalew Tefferi, MD

Myeloproliferative neoplasms (MPN) are clonal disorders of hematopoietic stem cells that manifest clinically as overproduction of cells that contribute to the myeloid lineage

Classification WHO Myeloproliferative Neoplasm (MPN) Categories

1. Classic MPN
   - Chronic myeloid leukemia (CML), *BCRI-ABL1*+; see Chapter 12
   - **Polycythemia vera (PV)***
   - **Essential thrombocythemia (ET)***
   - **Primary myelofibrosis (PMF)***
     - PMF, prefibrotic/early stage
     - PMF, overt fibrotic stage
2. "Nonclassic" MPNs
   - Chronic neutrophilic leukemia (CNL)
   - Chronic eosinophilic leukemia not otherwise specified (CEL-NOS)
   - "MPN unclassifiable"

*BCR-ABL—negative classic MPN (PV, ET, and PMF)
Arber DA et al. Blood 2016;127:2391

Epidemiology

BCR-ABL—negative classic MPN
Polycythemia vera (PV), essential thrombocythemia (ET), and primary myelofibrosis (PMF)

Polycythemia vera (PV)

1. Incidence: 0.8–2.6/100,000
2. Median age at diagnosis: ~60 years
3. Median survival: >15 years
4. 10-year risk of myelofibrosis: <4%
5. 10-year risk of AML: <2%

Note: longer disease duration and evolution into myelofibrosis significantly increase the risk of leukemic transformation

Essential thrombocythemia (ET)

1. Incidence: 0.2–2.5/100,000
2. Median age at diagnosis: ~60 years
3. Median survival: >15 years
4. 10-year risk of myelofibrosis: ~10%
5. 10-year risk of AML: ~6%

Note: longer disease duration and evolution into myelofibrosis significantly increase the risk of leukemic transformation

Ania BJ et al. Am J Hematol 1994;47:89–93
Gangat N et al. Br J Haematol 2007;138:354–358
Gangat N et al. Leukemia 2007;21:270–276
Mesa RA et al. Am J Hematol 1999;61:10–15
Tefferi A et al. Leukemia 2013;27:1874–1881
Tefferi A et al. Blood 2014;124:2507–2513

Primary myelofibrosis (PMF)

1. Incidence: 0.4–1.5/100,000
2. Median age at diagnosis: ~60 years
3. Median survival: <3 years to >10 years
4. 10-year risk of myelofibrosis: N/A
5. 10-year risk of AML: ~20% based on the presence or absence of well-defined prognostic determinants
6. Indicators of adverse prognosis as in Dynamic International Prognostic Scoring System (DIPSS-Plus):
   - Age >65 years
   - Hemoglobin <10 g/dL
   - Leukocyte count >25,000/mm^3
   - Circulating blasts ≥1%
   - Constitutional symptoms
   - Unfavorable karyotype included complex karyotype or single or two abnormalities including +8, −7/7q-, i(17q), −5/5q-, 12p-, inv(3), or 11q23 rearrangement
   - Thrombocytopenia <100,000/mm^3

(continued)

Epidemiology (*continued*)

7. Revised cytogenetic risk stratification: very high-risk (VHR) karyotype includes single/ multiple abnormalities of −7, inv(3)/3q21, i(17q), 12p−/12p11.2 or 11q−/11q23, single/multiple autosomal trisomies other than +9 and +8, unfavorable karyotype comprises of any abnormal karyotype other than normal karyotype or sole abnormalities of 20q−, 13q−, +9, chromosome 1 translocation/duplication, −Y, or sex chromosome abnormality other than −Y

8. High-molecular-risk (HMR) genetic abnormalities encompass *ASXL1*, *EZH2*, *SRSF2*, *IDH1/2*, and *U2AF1Q157* mutations and absence of type 1 *CALR* mutation

Cervantes F et al. Br J Haematol 1997;97:635–640
Dupriez B et al. Blood 1996;88:1013–1018
Gangat N et al. J Clin Oncol 2011;29:392–397
Passamonti F et al. Blood 2010;115:1703–1708
Tefferi A et al. Cancer 2007;109:2083–2088
Tefferi A et al. J Clin Oncol 2018;36:1769–1770
Tefferi A et al. Leukemia 2018;32:1189–1199
Tefferi A et al. Leukemia 2018;32:1631–1642

Mutations in MPN

Chronology:

- *1951:* CML, PV, ET, and PMF recognized to have significant overlap in both clinical and biological features and felt to be related diseases
- *1960:* CML recognized as distinct entity after discovery of Philadelphia chromosome
- *Early 1980s:* analysis of X chromosome inactivation patterns in women with CML, PV, ET, or PMF carrying a polymorphic variant of the glucose-6-phosphate dehydrogenase gene establishes all 4 diseases as clonal stem-cell disorders
- *2005:* somatic mutation involving Janus kinase 2 (*JAK2*) identified in patients with PV, ET, and PMF. Mutation at codon 617, (*JAK2*V617F) is a G→T transversion at nucleotide 1849 in exon 14 of *JAK2* gene, with substitution of valine by phenylalanine at codon 617
- *2006–2007:* additional *JAK2* and *MPL* (thrombopoietin receptor) mutations described in these diseases; some induce PV-like (*JAK2*) or PMF-like (*MPL*) phenotype in mice

2013: CALR (*calreticulin*) mutations encoding an endoplasmic reticulum chaperone discovered in the majority of *JAK2* or *MPL* wild type ET and PMF patients (frequency 23%). *CALR* mutations constitute 1 of 2 variants: type 1, a 52-bp deletion (p.L367fs*46), or type 2, a 5-bp TTGTC insertion (p.K385fs*47), generating a one-base-pair frameshift whereby the canonical highly acidic C-terminal with calcium-binding sites and the KDEL retrieval sequence is replaced by a novel basic protein sequence sans KDEL and calcium-binding sites

Adamson JW et al. N Engl J Med 1976;295:913–916
Baxter E et al. Lancet 2005;365:1054–1061
Dameshek W. Blood 1951;6:372–375
Fialkow PJ et al. Blood 1981;58:916–919
James C et al. Nature 2005;434:1144–1148
Klampfl T et al. N Engl J Med 2013;369:2379–2390
Kralovics R et al. N Engl J Med 2005;352:1779–1790
Levine R et al. Cancer Cell 2005;7:387–397
Nangalia J et al. N Engl J Med 2013;369:2391–2405
Pikmam Y et al. PLoS Med 2006;3:e270

Mutations

1. *JAK2*V617F **mutations:** 20–95% (most frequent mutation in *BCR-ABL*-negative chronic myeloid malignancies)
   - 95% in PV
   - 50% in ET
   - 50% in PMF
   - 20% in RARS-T
   - 20% in other "MPN or MDS/MPN, unclassifiable"
   - <5% in AML
   - <5% in MDS
2. *JAK2* **exon 12 mutations (eg, N542-E543del):** 3%
   - 3% of all PV cases (relatively specific to PV); occur in virtually all *JAK2*V617F-negative PV cases

(*continued*)

Mutations in MPN (continued)

3. *MPL* (thrombopoietin receptor) mutations (eg, *MPL*W515L/K): 1–10%
   - 5–10% in PMF
   - 1–5% in ET
4. *CALR* (calreticulin) mutations type 1, 52-bp deletion (p.L367fs*46), or type 2, 5-bp TTGTC insertion (p.K385fs*47):
   - 22% in ET
   - 23% in PMF

Baxter EJ et al. Lancet 2005;365:1054–1061. Erratum in: Lancet 2005;366:122
James C et al. Nature 2005;434:1144–1148
Kralovics R et al. N Engl J Med 2005;352:1779–1790
Klampfl T et al. N Engl J Med 2013;369:2379–2390
Levine RL et al. Cancer Cell 2005;7:387–397
Nangalia J et al N Engl J Med 2013;369:2391–2405
Pardanani AD et al. Blood 2006;108:3472–3476
Pikman Y et al. PLoS Med 2006;3:e270
Scott LM et al. N Engl J Med 2007;356:459–468

Thrombosis in MPN

Thrombosis in ET and PV
- Incidence of major thrombosis, mostly arterial: 11–25% at diagnosis and 11–22% during follow-up
- As regards the pathogenesis of thrombosis, an increased presence of neutrophil-platelet aggregates has been demonstrated in ET patients. Moreover, it has been shown that neutrophils are activated and endothelial dysfunction occurs, which is indicated by increased neutrophil activation parameters such as CD11b and leukocyte alkaline phosphatase, as well as markers of endothelial damage
- These observations have been confirmed in recent clinical studies, suggesting that leukocytosis is associated with an increased risk of thrombosis in both PV and ET

Barbui T et al. Blood 2012;120:5128–5133
Carobbio A et al. Blood 2007;109:2310–2313
Falanga A et al. Blood 2000;96:4261–4266
Landolfi R et al. Blood 2007;109:2446–2452

Thrombohemorrhagic events in ET
- Incidence of major hemorrhage: 2–5% at diagnosis and 6–12% during follow-up
- Pathogenesis of thrombohemorrhagic events in ET remains unclear
- A frequently accepted mechanism for hemorrhage in ET patients has been the association of extreme thrombocytosis (platelet count >1,000,000/mm^3) with acquired von Willebrand disease characterized by loss of the large von Willebrand factor multimers

Note: an elevated platelet count >1,000,000/mm^3 has been loosely associated with an increased risk of hemorrhage but has not been shown to correlate with thrombotic complications

Elliott MA et al. Br J Haematol 2005;128:275–290
Finazzi G et al. Leukemia 2012;26:716–719
Tefferi A et al. Blood 2006;108:2493–2494
van Genderen PJJ et al. Br J Haematol 1997;99:832–836

Table 28–1. 2016 World Health Organization Diagnostic Criteria

Polycythemia Vera (PV)	Essential Thrombocythemia (ET)	Pre-Primary Myelofibrosis (prePMF)	Overt PMF
Diagnosis of PV requires meeting all 3 major criteria *or* The first 2 major criteria and the minor criterion*	Diagnosis of ET requires meeting all 4 major criteria *or* The first 3 major criteria and the minor criterion	Diagnosis of prePMF requires meeting all 3 major criteria, and at least 1 minor criterion. The minor criterion must be confirmed in 2 consecutive determinations	Diagnosis of overt PMF requires meeting all 3 major criteria, and at least 1 minor criterion. The minor criterion must be confirmed in 2 consecutive determinations
Major Criteria			
1. Hgb >16.5 g/dL (men) Hgb >16.0 g/dL (women) *or* Hematocrit >49% (men) Hematocrit >48% (women) *or* Red cell mass >25% above mean normal predicted 2. Bone marrow biopsy hypercellular for age with trilineage growth including prominent erythroid, granulocytic, and megakaryocytic proliferation with pleomorphic, mature megakaryocytes 3. Presence of *JAK2*V617F or *JAK2* exon 12 mutation	1. Platelet count ≥450,000/mm³ 2. Bone marrow biopsy showing proliferation mainly of the megakaryocyte lineage with increased numbers of enlarged, mature megakaryocytes with hyperlobulated nuclei. No significant increase or left shift in neutrophil granulopoiesis or erythropoiesis and very rarely minor (Grade 1) increase in reticulin fibers. 3. Not meeting WHO criteria for *BCR-ABL1*⁺ CML, PV, PMF, MDS, or other myeloid neoplasm 4. Demonstration of *JAK2*, *CALR*, or *MPL* mutation	1. Megakaryocyte proliferation and atypia, without reticulin fibrosis Grade >1, accompanied by increased age-adjusted bone marrow cellularity, granulocytic proliferation, and often decreased erythropoiesis 2. Not meeting WHO criteria for *BCR-ABL1*⁺ CML, PV, ET, MDS, or other myeloid neoplasm 3. Presence of *JAK2*, *CALR*, or *MPL* mutation or in the absence of these mutations, presence of another clonal marker,[†] or absence of minor reactive bone marrow reticulin fibrosis[‡]	1. Presence of megakaryocytic proliferation and atypia, accompanied by either reticulin and/or collagen fibrosis Grades 2 or 3 2. Not meeting WHO criteria for *BCR-ABL1*⁺ CML, PV, ET, MDS, or other myeloid neoplasm 3. Presence of *JAK2*, *CALR*, or *MPL* mutation or in the absence of these mutations, presence of another clonal marker,[†] or absence of reactive myelofibrosis[§]
Minor Criteria			
1. Subnormal serum Epo level	1. Presence of a clonal marker or absence of evidence for reactive thrombocytosis	1. Anemia not attributed to a comorbid condition 2. Leukocytosis ≥11,000/mm³ 3. Palpable splenomegaly 4. LDH increased to >ULN of institutional reference range	1. Anemia not attributed to a comorbid condition 2. Leukocytosis ≥11,000/mm³ 3. Palpable splenomegaly 4. LDH increased to >ULN of institutional reference range 5. Leukoerythroblastosis

Hgb, hemoglobin; Hct, hematocrit; Epo, erythropoietin; EEC, endogenous erythroid colony; WHO, World Health Organization; CML, chronic myelogenous leukemia; MDS, myelodysplastic syndrome; LDH, lactate dehydrogenase; ULN, upper limit of normal

*Criterion number 2 (bone marrow biopsy) may not be required in cases with sustained absolute erythrocytosis: hemoglobin levels >18.5 g/dL in men (hematocrit, 55.5%) or >16.5 g/dL in women (hematocrit, 49.5%) if major criterion 3 and the minor criterion are present. However, initial myelofibrosis (present in up to 20% of patients) can only be detected by performing a bone marrow biopsy; this finding may predict a more rapid progression to overt myelofibrosis (post-PV MF)

[†]In the absence of any of the 3 major clonal mutations, the search for the most frequent accompanying mutations (eg, *ASXL1, EZH2, TET2, IDH1/IDH2, SRSF2, SF3B1*) are of help in determining the clonal nature of the disease

[‡]Minor (Grade 1) reticulin fibrosis secondary to infection, autoimmune disorder or other chronic inflammatory conditions, hairy cell leukemia or other lymphoid neoplasm, metastatic malignancy, or toxic (chronic) myelopathies

[§]Bone marrow fibrosis secondary to infection, autoimmune disorder or other chronic inflammatory conditions, hairy cell leukemia or other lymphoid neoplasm, metastatic malignancy, or toxic (chronic) myelopathies

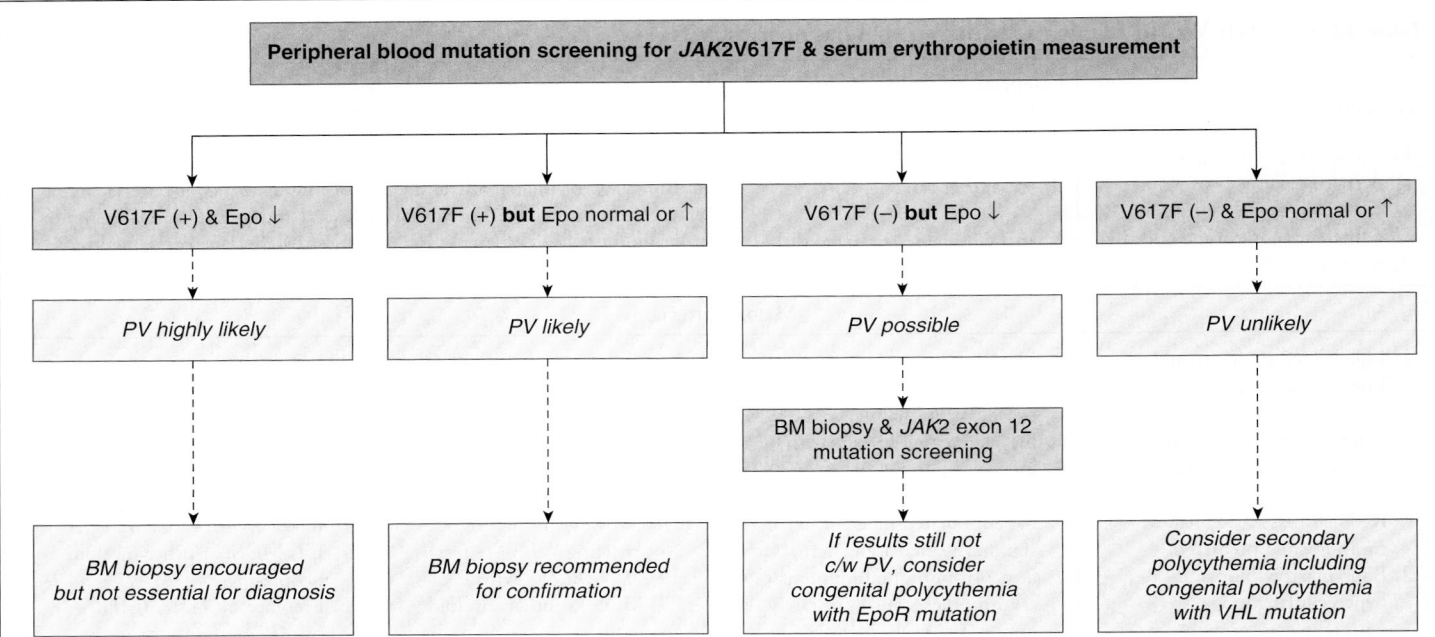

Figure 28-1. Diagnostic algorithm for suspected polycythemia vera.
PV, polycythemia vera; SP, secondary polycythemia; CP, congenital polycythemia; BM, bone marrow; V617F, JAK2V617F; Epo, erythropoietin; EpoR, erythropoietin receptor; VHL, von Hippel-Lindau; c/w, consistent with

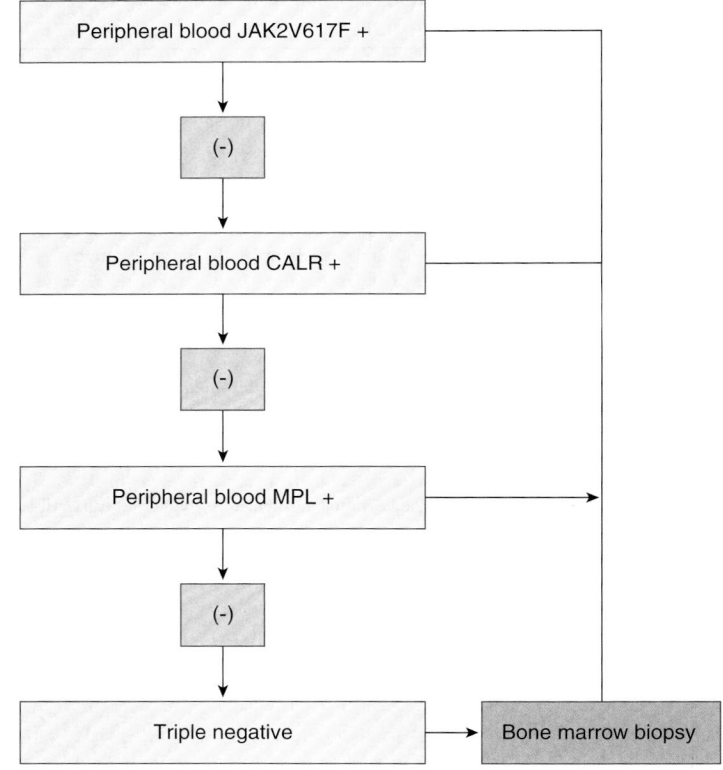

Figure 28-2. Diagnostic algorithm for suspected essential thrombocythemia.
PV, polycythemia vera; ET, essential thrombocythemia; PMF, primary myelofibrosis; CML, chronic myeloid leukemia; MDS, myelodysplastic syndrome; MPN, myeloproliferative neoplasm; WHO, World Health Organization; RT, reactive thrombocytosis; FISH, fluorescent in situ hybridization; Ph, Philadelphia; BM, bone marrow; V617F, JAK2V617F

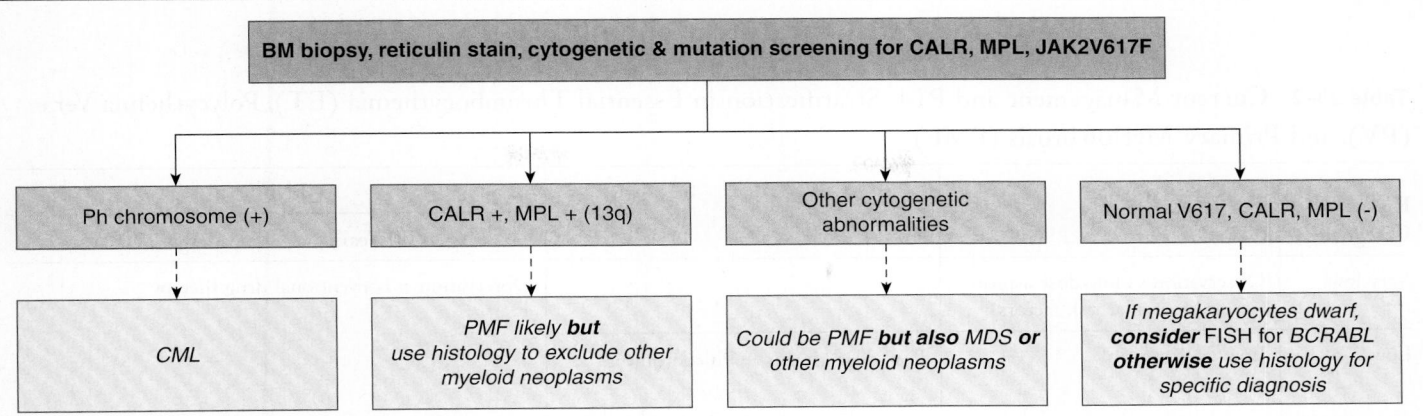

Figure 28-3. Diagnostic algorithm for suspected primary myelofibrosis.
PMF, primary myelofibrosis; CML, chronic myeloid leukemia; MDS, myelodysplastic syndrome; FISH, fluorescent in situ hybridization; Ph, Philadelphia; BM, bone marrow; V617F, JAK2V617F

Mutational Analysis and Bone Marrow Examination

Polycythemia vera (PV)

- Almost all patients with PV carry a *JAK2* mutation (either *JAK2*V617F or *JAK2* exon 12 mutations). Therefore, *JAK2* mutation screening in PV has a high negative predictive value, and, in general, the presence of either a *JAK2* or *MPL*, or *CALR* mutation reliably excludes the possibility of nonclonal myeloproliferation, such as secondary polycythemia or reactive thrombocytosis
- Peripheral blood *JAK2*V617F screening is currently the preferred initial test for evaluating a patient with suspected PV (see Figure 28-1)
- The concomitant determination of serum erythropoietin (Epo) level is encouraged to minimize the consequences of false-positive or false-negative molecular test results, and also address the infrequent but possible occurrence of *JAK2*V617F-negative PV
- Mutation screening for an exon 12 *JAK2* mutation and bone marrow examination should be considered in a *JAK2*V617F-negative patient who displays a subnormal serum Epo level (see Figure 28-1)

Essential thrombocythemia (ET)

- Because *JAK2*V617F also occurs in approximately 60% of patients with ET, *CALR* in 22%, *MPL* in 3%, triple negative in 15%, it is reasonable to include mutation screening in the diagnostic work-up of both thrombocytosis (see Figure 28-2) and bone marrow fibrosis (see Figure 28-3); the presence of the mutation excludes reactive myeloproliferation whereas its absence does not exclude an underlying MPN
- Bone marrow morphologic examination is often required for making the diagnosis of ET (see Figures 28-2 and 29-3)
- ET is the only MPN currently diagnosed by exclusion. ET may be diagnosed in patients with persistent thrombocytosis only in the absence of a known cause of reactive or clonal thrombocytosis

Primary myelofibrosis (PMF)

- Because *JAK2*V617F also occurs in approximately 60% of patients with PMF, *CALR* in 23%, *MPL* in 7%, triple negative in 10%, it is reasonable to include mutation screening in the diagnostic work-up of bone marrow fibrosis (see Figure 28-3); the presence of the mutation excludes reactive myeloproliferation whereas its absence does not exclude an underlying MPN
- Bone marrow morphologic examination is often required for making the diagnosis of PMF (see Figures 28-2 and 29-3)
- Bone marrow examination is critical in distinguishing between the causes of both myelophthisis and bone marrow fibrosis. In PMF, peripheral blood myelophthisis is associated with:
  - Bone marrow megakaryocytic hyperplasia
  - Collagen fibers
  - Osteosclerosis
  - Intramedullary sinusoidal hematopoiesis

Risk stratification in MPN

Table 28–2. Current Management and Risk Stratification in Essential Thrombocythemia (ET), Polycythemia Vera (PV), and Primary Myelofibrosis (PMF)

Risk Categories	ET	PV	PMF*	
			Age <70 Years	Age ≥70 Years
Very low	Observation vs low-dose aspirin (if cardiovascular risk factors)		Observation *or* conventional drug therapy	
Low	Low-dose aspirin†	Low-dose aspirin† + Phlebotomy		
Intermediate	Low-dose aspirin Hydroxyurea (optional)		Experimental drug therapy *or* Conventional drug therapy	Experimental drug therapy *or* Conventional drug therapy
High	Low-dose aspirin + Hydroxyurea Anticoagulation (if venous thrombosis)	Low-dose aspirin + Phlebotomy + Hydroxyurea Anticoagulation (if venous thrombosis)	Allogeneic transplant *or* Experimental drug therapy	Experimental drug therapy
Very high			Allogeneic transplant *or* Experimental drug therapy	Experimental drug therapy

Risk stratification for ET:
High risk: Age ≥60 years *or* previous thrombosis, *JAK2/MPL* mutated
Intermediate risk: No thrombosis history, age >60 years, *JAK2/MPL* unmutated
Low-risk: No thrombosis history, age ≤60 years, JAK2/MPL mutated
Very low risk: No thrombosis history, age ≤60 years, *JAK2/MPL* unmutated

Risk stratification for PV
High risk: History of thrombosis *or* age >60 years
Low risk: No history of thrombosis, age ≤60 years

Tefferi A et al. Blood Cancer J 2018;8:2

Risk Stratification of Primary Myelofibrosis According to the Dynamic International Prognostic Scoring System Plus (DIPSS-plus):
Age >65 years, hemoglobin <10 g/dL, leukocytes >25,000/mm³, circulating blasts ≥1%, constitutional symptoms, unfavorable karyotype, platelet count <100,000/mm³, transfusion status
Low risk: 0 adverse points (median survival, 180 months)
Intermediate–1 risk: 1 adverse point (median survival, 80 months)
Intermediate–2 risk: 2–3 adverse points (median survival, 35 months)
High risk: 4–6 adverse points (median survival, 16 months)

Mutation enhanced prognostic scoring system 2.0 (MIPSS70+ version 2.0):
Sex adjusted categories for severe anemia (hemoglobin <8 g/dL in women and <9 g/dL in men) *(2 points)*
Moderate anemia (hemoglobin 8–9.9 g/dL in women and 9–10.9 g/dL in men) *(1 point)*
Circulating blasts ≥2% *(1 point)*
Constitutional symptoms *(2 points)*
VHR (very high-risk) karyotype (4 points)
Unfavorable karyotype (3 points)
≥2 HMR (high-molecular-risk) mutations (3 points)
One HMR mutation (2 points)
Type 1/like CALR absent (2 points)

Very low risk (median survival)	Zero points (not reached)
Low risk (median survival)	1–2 points (16.4 years)
Intermediate risk (median survival)	3–4 points (7.7 years)
High risk (median survival)	5–8 points (4.1 years)
Very high risk (median survival)	≥9 points (1.8 years)

(continued)

Risk stratification in MPN (*continued*)

Genetically inspired prognostic scoring system (GIPSS)

VHR karyotype (2 points)
Unfavorable karyotype (1 point)

Type 1/like CALR absent (1 point)

ASXL1 mutation (1 point)
SRSF2 mutation (1 point)
*U2AF1*Q157 mutation (1 point

Low risk (median survival)	Zero points (26.4 years)
Intermediate 1 risk (median survival)	One point (8 years)
Intermediate 2 risk (median survival)	Two points (4.2 years)
High risk (median survival)	≥3 points (2 years)

*PMF risk stratification by MIPSS–70 Plus Version 2.0
†Clinically significant acquired von Willebrand syndrome (ristocetin cofactor activity <30%) should be excluded before using aspirin in patients with a platelet count ≥1,000,000/mm³

Risk Stratification

Polycythemia Vera, Essential Thrombocythemia, and Primary Myelofibrosis
Risk factors for thrombotic complications in ET and PV patients

- Advanced age (age >60 years)
- Prior history of thrombosis
- Well-established cardiovascular risk; there is conflicting evidence

Cortelazzo S et al. J Clin Oncol 1990;8:556–562

*JAK2*V617F Mutational Analysis—Prognostic Significance

Notes:

- Although data suggest *JAK2*V617F mutational status may have prognostic significance in PV, ET, and PMF, additional studies of large cohorts are needed for confirmation
- *JAK2* (*calreticulin [CALR], and myeloproliferative leukemia virus oncogene [MPL] mutations*) are neither disease-specific nor contemporaneous with the ancestral clone of myeloproliferative neoplasms. Instead, they *appear to constitute phenotype-modifying subclones that do not necessarily contribute to leukemic transformation*

ET and *JAK2*V617F

- Prognostic significance of the *JAK2*V617F mutation has not been precisely delineated. Although *JAK2*V617F mutant and wild-type patients differ in regard to laboratory parameters and clinical features, there were no differences in overall survival or myelofibrotic and leukemic transformations
- *JAK2*V617F is associated with:
  - Advanced age
  - Higher hemoglobin level
  - Higher leukocyte counts
  - Lower platelet counts
- In patients with *JAK2*V617F mutation, *allele burden* is directly correlated with:
  - Leukocyte count
  - Platelet count
  - Presence of palpable splenomegaly

Kittur J et al. Cancer 2007;109:2279–2284

(*continued*)

Risk Stratification (*continued*)

ET and *CALR*

80% of *CALR* mutations constitute 1 of 2 variants: type 1, a 52-bp deletion (p.L367fs*46), or type 2, a 5-bp TTGTC insertion (p.K385fs*47)
CALR mutation associated with higher platelet (type 2 as opposed to type 1), lower hemoglobin and leukocyte counts compared with mutant *JAK2*
Male sex associated with type 1 and younger age with type 2 variants

Tefferi A et al. Am J Hematol 2014;89:E121–E124

PV and *JAK2*V617F

- *JAK2*V617F homozygous patients have:
  - Higher hemoglobin level
  - Higher leukocyte count
  - Lower platelet count
  - Increased incidence of pruritus
  - NO increased risk of thrombosis
- In patients with *JAK2*V617F mutation, *allele burden* is directly correlated with:
  - Higher hemoglobin level
  - Higher leukocyte count
  - Lower platelet count
  - Increased incidence of pruritus
  - NO increased risk of thrombosis

Vannucchi AM et al. Blood 2007;110:840–846

PMF and *JAK2*V617F

- *JAK2*V617F mutation is associated with:
  - Poorer overall survival
  - Older age at diagnosis
  - Higher leukocyte count
  - Presence of pruritus
- *JAK2*V617F "homozygous" PMF patients have:
  - Even higher leukocyte count
  - Larger spleen size

PMF and *CALR*

CALR mutation is associated with:
  - Younger age
  - Higher platelet count
  - Lower leukocyte count
  - Higher hemoglobin level
  - Longer survival with type 1/like CALR, compared to *JAK2*, type 2/like *CALR*, *MPL* and triple-negative
  - Survival similar between the non–type 1/like *CALR* mutational states

Tefferi A et al. Am J Hematol 2018;93:348–355
Tefferi A et al. Leukemia 2008;22:756–761
Tefferi A et al. Leukemia 2014;28:1472–1477

Treatment Options

Treatment of Essential Thrombocythemia (ET)

Treatment recommendations:

1. Low-dose aspirin for all patients
2. Add hydroxyurea in high-risk patients

Barbui T et al. N Engl J Med 2005;353:85–86

Treatment options:

1. Antiplatelet therapy (eg, low-dose aspirin)
2. Cytoreductive therapy—hydroxyurea
3. Cytoreductive therapy—anagrelide
4. Cytoreductive therapy—interferon alfa (interferon α, IFN-α)
5. Cytoreductive therapy—pipobroman
6. Cytoreductive therapy—busulfan

Note: there is no hard evidence to implicate any one of these agents, including hydroxyurea, as being leukemogenic in the treatment of ET

1. *Antiplatelet therapy (eg, low-dose aspirin)*
   - Has not been shown to influence survival or lower risk of disease transformation
   - Used to either alleviate microvascular symptoms or to prevent thrombohemorrhagic complications
2. *Cytoreductive therapy—hydroxyurea*
   - Treatment of choice in high-risk ET patients because of superior efficacy and less toxicity (see Table 28-1)
   - Has not been shown to influence survival or lower risk of disease transformation
   - Used to either alleviate microvascular symptoms or prevent thrombohemorrhagic complications
   - Two randomized controlled trials have evaluated hydroxyurea efficacy—*Hydroxyurea vs No Cytoreductive Therapy*—the first study to demonstrate the benefit of cytoreductive therapy in ET patients:
     - N = 114
     - High-risk ET patients (age >60 years, or prior thrombosis)
     - Randomized to hydroxyurea (n = 56) or no cytoreductive therapy (n = 58)
     - Median follow-up = 27 months:
       - Two thromboses in hydroxyurea group (1.6% per patient-year)
       - Fourteen thromboses in control group (10.7% per patient-year; P = 0.003)
3. *Cytoreductive therapy—anagrelide*
   - Anagrelide is inferior to hydroxyurea in every respect. The evidence does not support its role as first-line therapy. Can be considered for use as a third-line agent in patients who have failed or are intolerant to hydroxyurea or interferon-α therapy—*Hydroxyurea + Aspirin vs Anagrelide + Aspirin (MRC PT-I trial)*
   - Superiority of hydroxyurea over anagrelide as first therapy for high-risk ET patients
     - N = >800 patients
     - High-risk ET patients (age >60 years, prior thrombosis or platelets >1,000,000/mm^3)
     - Randomized to hydroxyurea + aspirin or anagrelide + aspirin
     - Anagrelide plus aspirin
       - Decreased rate of venous thrombosis

- Increased rate of arterial thrombosis
- Increased rate of major hemorrhage
- Increased rate of transformation to MF
- Increased rate of withdrawal from treatment

4. *Cytoreductive therapy—interferon alfa (IFN-α)*
   - Single-agent activity
   - Sometimes associated with modest reductions in *JAK2V617F* allele burden
5. *Cytoreductive therapy—pipobroman*
   - Several single-arm studies have confirmed the efficacy of pipobroman in ET
6. *Cytoreductive therapy—busulfan*
   - Several single-arm studies have confirmed the efficacy of busulfan in ET

Cortelazzo S et al. N Engl J Med 1995;332:1132–1136
Harrison CN et al. N Engl J Med 2005;353:33–45
Kiladjian J-J et al. Blood 2006;108:2037–2040

Treatment of Polycythemia Vera (PV)

Treatment options:

1. Phlebotomy
2. Antiplatelet therapy (eg, low-dose aspirin)
3. Cytoreductive therapy—hydroxyurea
4. Cytoreductive therapy—interferon alfa (interferon α, IFN-α)
5. Cytoreductive therapy—pipobroman
6. Cytoreductive therapy—busulfan
7. Cytoreductive therapy—ruxolitinib

Note: there is no hard evidence to implicate any one of these agents, including hydroxyurea, as being leukemogenic in the treatment of PV

Treatment recommendations:

1. Phlebotomy for all patients
2. Low-dose aspirin for all patients
3. Add hydroxyurea in high-risk patients

Barbui N Engl J Med 2013; 368:22–33.
Barbui T et al. N Engl J Med 2005;353:85–86

1. *Phlebotomy*
   - Generally recommended to keep hematocrit levels at <45% in men and <42% in women
   - There is compelling evidence to support the use of phlebotomy in all patients
2. *Antiplatelet therapy (eg, low-dose aspirin)*
   - Has not been shown to influence survival or lower risk of disease transformation
   - Used to either alleviate microvascular symptoms or to prevent thrombohemorrhagic complications
3. *Cytoreductive therapy—hydroxyurea*
   - Treatment of choice in high-risk PV patients because of superior efficacy and less toxicity (see Table 28-1)
   - Has not been shown to influence survival or lower risk of disease transformation
   - Used to either alleviate microvascular symptoms or to prevent thrombohemorrhagic complications

(continued)

Treatment Options (continued)

- Studies have evaluated hydroxyurea efficacy of hydroxyurea vs pipobroman:
  - Similar survival
  - Similar thrombosis risk
  - Similar leukemic transformation rate
  - Pipobroman associated with a lesser incidence of transformation into post-PV MF
  - Pipobroman is leukemogenic and is unsuitable for first-line therapy
4. *Interferon alfa (IFN-α)*
  - Single-agent activity
  - Sometimes associated with modest reductions in *JAK2*V617F allele burden
5. *Pipobroman*
  - Several studies have confirmed the efficacy of pipobroman in PV
  - Pipobroman is leukemogenic and is unsuitable for first-line therapy
6. *Busulfan*
  - Several single-arm studies have confirmed the efficacy of busulfan in PV
7. *Ruxolitinib (JAK1/2 inhibitor)*
  - Approved for PV patients who had an inadequate response to or had unacceptable side effects from hydroxyurea
  - Ruxolitinib superior to standard therapy in controlling hematocrit, reducing splenomegaly, and improving symptoms

Finazzi G et al. Blood 2007;109:5104–5111
Kiladjian J-J et al. Blood 2006;108:2037–2040
Najean Y et al. Blood 1997;90:3370–3377
Vannucchi A et al. N Engl J Med 2015;372:426–435

Treatment of (Primary) Myelofibrosis

- At present, only allogeneic hematopoietic stem cell transplantation (HSCT) is potentially curative in primary myelofibrosis (PMF). **However, the majority of patients are of advanced age, and, therefore, not good candidates for allogeneic HSCT, and such patients rely on palliative therapy to improve quality of life,** although it may not prolong life
- Therapeutic options:
  - Allogeneic HSCT
  - Drug therapy
  - Splenectomy
  - Radiation therapy

Hematopoietic stem-cell transplantation

- In a retrospective, multicenter study of 66 consecutive patients, age was the major determinant of transplant outcome; 5-year survival was 62% in patients younger than 45 years of age and 14% in those who were older
- Other investigators have reported better survival in patients older than 44 years, and data suggest that transplant-related morbidity (TRM) in older patients may be positively influenced by the use of reduced-intensity conditioning regimens
- In the most recent communication of reduced-intensity, conditioning transplantation in myelofibrosis (n = 104; median age: 55 years [range, 32–68 years]; unrelated donors in 71 patients), 1-year mortality was 19% (27% if one excludes low-risk patients), and 32% of patients experienced chronic graft-versus-host disease. The 3-year

overall survival, event-free survival, and relapse rate were 70%, 55%, and 29%, respectively

Conclusions: At present, it is reasonable to consider allogeneic HSCT (related or unrelated donor) *in high-risk patients who are younger than age 70 years*

Drug treatment

- Conventional drug therapy for anemia includes a combination of:
  - An **androgen** preparation (eg, fluoxymesterone 10 mg; administer orally twice daily, continually)
  - **Prednisone** 0.5 mg/kg per day; administer orally, continually
  - **Epoetin alfa** 40,000 units/week; administer subcutaneously in the presence of an endogenous blood erythropoietin concentration <100 mU/mL (<100 IU/L)
  - **Danazol** 200–800 mg/day; administer orally, continually
- **Low-dose thalidomide in combination with prednisone** has been identified as an effective combination for myelofibrosis-associated anemia, thrombocytopenia, and splenomegaly, with an approximate 50% overall response rate
- **Lenalidomide**, a thalidomide analog, also has been evaluated in myelofibrosis with 20–30% response rates in both anemia and splenomegaly. Lenalidomide response rates were increased in patients with myelofibrosis with the del(5q) abnormality. Therapy for symptomatic anemia in myelofibrosis should include lenalidomide in the presence of del(5q), and, in its absence, low-dose thalidomide and prednisone
- **Ruxolitinib**, a JAK1/JAK2 inhibitor, is approved for the treatment of patients with intermediate or high-risk myelofibrosis, including primary myelofibrosis, post–polycythemia vera myelofibrosis, and post–essential thrombocythemia myelofibrosis. Two randomized studies (COMFORT–1 and 2) confirmed the palliative value of ruxolitinib in terms of a partial response in splenomegaly and alleviation of constitutional symptoms. However, they did not show histopathologic, cytogenetic, or molecular remissions, and the drug was more likely to cause anemia and thrombocytopenia than to correct them. Notwithstanding the above, JAK–STAT remains an important drug target by virtue of its role in the production and activity of proinflammatory cytokines, which are overexpressed in myelofibrosis and probably contribute to disease symptoms. Ruxolitinib induces a rapid and marked suppression of these cytokines, in conjunction with its salutary effect on constitutional symptoms. Therefore, cytokine modulation might constitute its primary mode of action, although nonspecific myelosuppression probably contributes to the drug's effect on splenomegaly and blood counts. In line with this assumption, cytokine rebound after drug withdrawal might explain the immediate and florid relapse of symptoms when ruxolitinib is discontinued; this relapse is sometimes accompanied by hemodynamic decompensation. Approximately 30% of patients with myelofibrosis present with ruxolitinib-sensitive symptoms, and the drug can be considered in these patients if they are not candidates for stem cell transplantation
- **Fedratinib**, a JAK2/FLT3 inhibitor is approved for intermediate-2 or high-risk primary or secondary (post–polycythemia vera or post–essential thrombocythemia) myelofibrosis (MF) based on the JAKARTA2 study, which confirmed a palliative value of fedratinib in terms of splenomegaly and alleviation of symptoms. The most common adverse events were diarrhea, nausea, anemia, and vomiting. The risk of serious and fatal encephalopathy, including Wernicke

(continued)

Treatment Options (*continued*)

encephalopathy, is to be considered by prescribing physicians and it is advised to assess thiamine levels in all patients prior to starting fedratinib, periodically during treatment, and as clinically indicated. If encephalopathy is suspected, fedratinib should be immediately discontinued and parenteral thiamine initiated. In a recent analysis conducted on the JAKARTA2 study patients by Harrison et al, one-third of patients achieved a spleen response with fedratinib regardless of whether they were relapsed, refractory, or intolerant to ruxolitinib. Hydroxyurea can also be used to control splenomegaly, leukocytosis, or thrombocytosis. Other drugs that have been used in a similar setting include pegylated interferon alfa, busulfan, and cladribine

Surgical treatment

- Splenectomy in myelofibrosis is indicated in the presence of drug-refractory mechanical discomfort, portal hypertension, severe hypercatabolic symptoms, and heavy red blood cell transfusion requirements
- Operative mortality is approximately 9%, and 25% of patients may experience postsplenectomy thrombocytosis and progressive hepatomegaly

Radiation treatment

- Splenic irradiation (a total dose of 100–500 cGy in 5–10 fractions) may be considered an alternative treatment to splenectomy in poor surgical candidates
- Symptomatic pulmonary hypertension not secondary to a thromboembolic process has been associated with PMF and is believed to arise from diffuse pulmonary extramedullary hematopoiesis. Diagnosis is confirmed by a technetium–99m sulfur colloid scintigraphy, which shows diffuse pulmonary uptake, and treatment with single-fraction (100 cGy) whole-lung irradiation has been shown to be effective

Björkholm M et al. J Clin Oncol 2011;29:2410–2415
Cervantes F et al. Br J Haematol 2006;134:184–186
Cervantes F et al. Haematologica 2000;85:595–599
Deeg HJ et al. Blood 2003;102:3912–3918
Guardiola P et al. Blood 1999;93:2831–2838
Kroeger N et al. Proc Am Soc Hematol 2007;110:683 (abstract)
Mesa RA et al. Blood 2003;101:2534–2541
Silver RT. Semin Hematol 1997;34:40–50
Tefferi A et al. Blood 2006;108:1158–1164

PRIMARY THERAPY

POLYCYTHEMIA VERA (PV) REGIMEN: PHLEBOTOMY

Marchioli R et al. N Engl J Med 2013;368:22–33
Streiff MB et al. Blood 2002;99:1144–1149
Barbui N Engl J Med 2013; 368:22–33.

Indications:	• Prevent thrombosis by reducing the RBC mass. Indicated for all patients to normalize hematocrit • Treatment of choice for patients ages <50 years and all women during childbearing years
Goal:	• Achieve and maintain a hematocrit of 40–45% (Hct <45% in men and <42% in women)
Initial therapy:	• *Most patients:* 250–500 mL every other day to achieve a hematocrit of 40–45% • *Elderly and those with hemodynamic compromise:* 250–300 mL twice per week
Maintenance therapy:	• CBC every 4–8 weeks • Phlebotomy if hematocrit >45% in men; >42% in women
Limitations:	• Phlebotomy unable to control leukocytosis, hyperuricemia, hypermetabolism, pruritus, and complications of splenomegaly seen in PV patients • Patients treated with phlebotomy alone have a higher incidence of serious thrombotic complications during the first 3 years of therapy when compared to patients treated with myelosuppression. True especially in those >60 years old • Elderly should be treated with cytoreduction in addition to phlebotomy

ANTIPLATELET THERAPY

POLYCYTHEMIA VERA (PV) AND ESSENTIAL THROMBOCYTHEMIA (ET) REGIMEN: ASPIRIN

Landolfi R et al. N Engl J Med 2004;350:114–124

Aspirin 50–100 mg/day; administer orally, continually

Notes:

- Dose used in clinical trial was 100 mg per day
- Although clinical trial enrolled patients with PV, the data is thought to support its use in ET as well

Patient Population Studied

Conducted by a network of 94 hematologic centers in 12 countries. Of the 1638 patients included in the ECLAP project, 1120 were entered into a prospective, observational cohort study, and the other 518 (32%) were enrolled in a double-blind, placebo-controlled, randomized trial to assess the efficacy and safety of low-dose aspirin (100 mg daily in an enteric-coated formulation [Bayer]). The main reasons for excluding patients in the ECLAP project from this aspirin trial were an indication for antithrombotic therapy (742 patients [66%]), a contraindication to aspirin therapy (271 patients [24%]), and a patient's unwillingness to participate (197 patients [18%]). Polycythemia vera was diagnosed on the basis of standard clinical and laboratory findings and criteria. Patients were eligible if they had no clear indication for aspirin treatment and no clear contraindication to it. There were no age limits. A total of 253 patients were randomly assigned to receive aspirin (100 mg daily), and 265 were randomly assigned to receive placebo. All patients received other recommended treatments: phlebotomy, cytoreductive drugs, and standard cardiovascular drugs as required. Data collection was recorded at follow-up visits at 12, 24, 36, 48, and 60 months. Compliance was monitored with the use of counts of aspirin or placebo pills and through attendance at follow-up visits

Efficacy

Rates and Relative Risks of Major Study End Points in the Two Groups*

End Point	Aspirin (N = 253) Number (%)	Placebo (N = 265) Number (%)	Relative Risk (95% CI)	P Value
Primary End Points				
Nonfatal myocardial infarction, nonfatal stroke, or death from cardiovascular causes	5 (2.0)	13 (4.9)	0.41 (0.15–1.15)	0.09
Nonfatal myocardial infarction, nonfatal stroke, pulmonary embolism, major venous thrombosis, or death from cardiovascular causes	8 (3.2)	21 (7.9)	0.40 (0.18–0.91)	0.03
Secondary End Points				
Nonfatal myocardial infarction, nonfatal stroke, or death from any cause	11 (4.3)	22 (8.3)	0.54 (0.26–1.11)	0.09
Nonfatal myocardial infarction, nonfatal stroke, pulmonary embolism, deep venous thrombosis, or death from any cause	13 (5.1)	29 (10.9)	0.47 (0.25–0.91)	0.02
Death from any cause	9 (3.6)	18 (6.8)	0.54 (0.24–1.20)	0.13
Death from cardiovascular causes	3 (1.2)	8 (3.0)	0.41 (0.11–1.53)	0.18
Cardiac	2 (0.8)	2 (0.8)	1.07 (0.15–7.58)	0.95
Acute myocardial infarction	1 (0.4)	1 (0.4)		
Other cardiac causes	1 (0.4)	1 (0.4)		
Vascular	1 (0.4)	6 (2.3)	0.18 (0.02–1.50)	0.11
Nonhemorrhagic stroke	0	4 (1.5)		
Intracranial hemorrhage	0	1 (0.4)		
Pulmonary embolism	0	1 (0.4)		
Other vascular causes	1 (0.4)	0		
Death from noncardiovascular causes	6 (2.4)	10 (3.8)	0.65 (0.24–1.79)	0.40
Major cerebrovascular events	3 (1.2)	10 (3.8)	0.32 (0.09–1.16)	0.08
Myocardial infarction	1 (0.4)	2 (0.8)	0.54 (0.09–23.57)	0.81
Major venous thrombosis	4 (1.6)	10 (3.8)	0.49 (0.13–1.78)	0.28
Deep venous thrombosis	2 (0.8)	6 (2.3)		
Pulmonary embolism	2 (0.8)	5 (1.9)		
Major or minor thrombosis	17 (6.7)	41 (15.5)	0.42 (0.24–0.74)	0.003
Minor thrombotic complications	10 (4.0)	22 (8.3)	0.47 (0.22–0.99)	0.049
Transient ischemic attack	4 (1.6)	9 (3.4)		
Peripheral arterial thrombosis	0	3 (1.1)		
Superficial venous thrombosis	2 (0.8)	6 (2.3)		
Erythromelalgia	4 (1.6)	5 (1.9)		

CI, Confidence interval

*Major cerebrovascular events include fatal and nonfatal stroke plus episodes of intracranial bleeding; minor thrombotic complications include transient ischemic attacks, superficial thrombophlebitis, peripheral arterial thrombosis, and erythromelalgia. Totals for categories may not equal the sum of the values for subcategories because some patients had more than 1 type of event

Toxicity

Rates and Relative Risks of Bleeding Episodes in the Two Groups*

Type of Bleeding Episode	Aspirin (N = 253)	Placebo (N = 265)	Relative Risk (95% CI)	P Value
	Number (%)			
Any bleeding	23 (9.1)	14 (5.3)	1.82 (0.94–3.53)	0.08
Major bleeding	3 (1.2)	2 (0.8)	1.62 (0.27–9.71)	0.60
Gastrointestinal	2 (0.8)	0		
Intracranial	1 (0.4)	2 (0.8)		
Minor bleeding	20 (7.9)	12 (4.5)	1.83 (0.90–3.75)	0.10
Hematoma	2 (0.8)	2 (0.8)		
Gastrointestinal	7 (2.8)	3 (1.1)		
Hematuria	1 (0.4)	3 (1.1)		
Epistaxis	9 (3.6)	1 (0.4)		
Other	2 (0.8)	4 (1.5)		

CI, confidence interval

*Major bleeding was defined as any bleeding episode that was fatal or necessitated transfusions or hospitalization. Totals for categories may not equal the sum of the values for subcategories because some patients had more than one type of bleeding episode

Study Conclusion

The authors noted the moderate increase in the risk of bleeding episodes associated with the long-term use of aspirin in polycythemia vera. The relative risk of major bleeding complications of 1.62 was felt to be consistent with estimates from 5 primary prevention trials involving subjects who did not have polycythemia, although the occurrence of a limited number of events precluded the precise estimation of the risk of bleeding. The authors concluded they believed that the risk of aspirin-induced bleeding in patients with PV has been overemphasized and recommended the use of aspirin to prevent thrombotic complications in patients with polycythemia vera who have no contraindication to this treatment

Notes:

- **Low-dose aspirin** 50–100 mg/day orally, continually, is beneficial in reducing arterial thrombosis in patients with PV and ET
- Microcirculatory disturbances, particularly erythromelalgia, are alleviated by aspirin. However, the use of aspirin in PV and ET requires the absence of clinically relevant acquired von Willebrand syndrome (AvWS), which might occur in patients with extreme thrombocytosis (platelet count >1,000,000/mm^3). Use a ristocetin cofactor activity cutoff level of 30% to decide on aspirin therapy
- Aspirin significantly lowered the combined risk of cardiovascular death, nonfatal myocardial infarction, nonfatal stroke, pulmonary embolism, or major venous thrombosis (relative risk 0.40; 95% CI, 0.18–0.91)
- The study was insufficiently powered to detect significant differences between aspirin and placebo in the rates of any bleeding

CYTOREDUCTIVE THERAPY

POLYCYTHEMIA VERA (PV) AND ESSENTIAL THROMBOCYTHEMIA (ET) REGIMEN: HYDROXYUREA

Cortelazzo S et al. N Engl J Med 1995;332:1132–1136 (ET)
(Editorial) Haematologica 1999;84:673–674 (PV)
Fruchtman SM et al. Semin Hematol 1997;34:17–23 (PV)

Note: mechanism of action is believed to be inhibition of ribonucleotide reductase that is required for DNA repair by scavenging tyrosyl free radicals as they are involved in the reduction of nucleotide diphosphates

Initial dose:
Hydroxyurea 15–20 mg/kg; administer orally, every day after meals, as a single dose or divided into 2 doses (total dosage per week = 105–140 mg/kg)

Chronic therapy—optimal dose:
- Determined **empirically.** Adjust without causing leukopenia
- *Frequent monitoring of CBC:* Every 1–2 weeks for the first 2 months, every month thereafter, and after reaching a steady state, every 3 months
- Increase total daily dose by 25% to 50%, and assess effect after 7 days before further escalation. A dose of hydroxyurea 500–1000 mg/day is sufficient for the majority of patients; however, the total daily dose is extremely variable

Therapeutic goals:
Polycythemia Vera

1. Control the hematocrit without causing leukopenia (<3500/mm^3) or thrombocytopenia (<100,000/mm^3). This may require significantly higher or lower doses than the initial dose
2. Patients requiring frequent phlebotomies or those with platelet counts >600,000/mm^3, increase the hydroxyurea dosage by 5 mg/kg per day at monthly intervals, with frequent monitoring until control is achieved
3. Supplemental phlebotomy is preferable to increased myelosuppression in controlling the hematocrit

Emergency situations in polycythemia vera patients: **Decreased cerebral perfusion in setting of an elevated hematocrit or marked thrombocytosis:**
- *Phlebotomy:* Daily to a hematocrit of 45% in men and 42% in women
- *Initial (loading) dose:* **Hydroxyurea** 30 mg/kg per day; administer orally every day, after meals, as single dose or divided into 2 doses for 7 days (total dosage/week = 210 mg/kg), *followed by:*
- *Maintenance dose:* **Hydroxyurea** 15 mg/kg per day; administer orally every day, after meals, as single dose or divided into 2 doses with close monitoring of CBC (total dosage/week = 105 mg/kg)

Note: treatment of choice in high-risk PV and ET patients because of its superior efficacy and decreased toxicity

Essential Thrombocythemia

1. Achieve a target platelet count <600,000/mm^3 (greater protection from thrombosis if platelet count <450,000/mm^3) with care to avoid the development of significant leukopenia

Note: very high doses carry a risk of prolonged aplasia

Supportive Care
Antiemetic prophylaxis
Emetogenic potential is **MINIMAL–LOW**
See Chapter 42 for antiemetic recommendations

Hematopoietic growth factor (CSF) prophylaxis
Primary prophylaxis is **NOT** indicated
See Chapter 43 for more information

Antimicrobial prophylaxis
Risk of fever and neutropenia is **LOW**
 Antimicrobial primary prophylaxis to be considered:
 - Antibacterial—*P. jirovecii* prophylaxis is recommended (eg, cotrimoxazole)
 - Antifungal—not indicated
 - Antiviral—not indicated unless patient previously had an episode of HSV

Treatment Modifications

Adverse Event	Treatment Modification
Hematologic Toxicity	
WBC <3500/mm^3 or platelet <100,000/mm^3	Hold hydroxyurea until WBC >3500/mm^3 and platelet >100,000/mm^3, then restart hydroxyurea at 50% of prior dose
Nonhematologic Toxicity	
G1	No dose modifications
G2/3	Hold hydroxyurea until toxicity G ≤1; restart at prior dose
Recurrent G2/3	Hold hydroxyurea until toxicity G ≤1; restart at 75% of prior dose
G4	Hold hydroxyurea until toxicity G ≤1; restart at 50% of prior dose
Recurrent G4	Discontinue hydroxyurea

Patient Population Studied

Polycythemia Vera (Fruchtman SM et al. Semin Hematol 1997;34:17–23)
Patients with Philadelphia chromosome (Ph)-positive and Ph-negative myeloproliferative disorders

Essential Thrombocythemia (Cortelazzo S et al. N Engl J Med 1995;332:1132–1136)
Fifty-six patients with essential thrombocythemia with median platelet count of 788,000/mm^3

Toxicity

Hematologic side effects

1. Neutropenia is common
2. Thrombocytopenia is rare
3. Cytopenias often are rapidly reversible within 3–4 days but may take 7–21 days to recover after hydroxyurea is discontinued
4. High doses and/or failure to interrupt treatment despite cytopenia may result in prolonged aplasia

Nonhematologic Side Effects

Relatively Common	Rare

1. Gastrointestinal symptoms:
  • Stomatitis/mucositis
  • Anorexia
  • Mild nausea/vomiting
  • Diarrhea
  • Constipation
2. Acute skin reactions
  • Rash
  • Painful lower extremity ulcerations
  • Dermatomyositis-like changes
  • Erythema
  • Nail ridging or discoloration
	1. Chronic skin reactions
	  • Hyperpigmentation
	  • Atrophy of skin and nails
	2. Skin cancer
	3. Alopecia
	4. Headache
	5. Drowsiness
	6. Convulsions
	7. Constitutional symptoms:
	  • Fever
	  • Chills
	  • Asthenia
	8. Renal impairment
	9. Hepatic impairment

Boxed Warning (FDA approved product label):
Hydroxyurea is mutagenic and clastogenic, and causes cellular transformation to a tumorigenic phenotype. Hydroxyurea is thus unequivocally genotoxic and a presumed trans-species carcinogen that implies a carcinogenic risk to humans. Secondary leukemias have been reported in patients who received long-term hydroxyurea for myeloproliferative disorders, such as polycythemia vera and thrombocythemia. It is unknown whether this leukemogenic effect is secondary to hydroxyurea or is associated with a patients' underlying disease. Physicians and their patients must very carefully consider the potential benefits of hydroxyurea relative to the undefined risk of developing secondary malignancies

Efficacy

Polycythemia Vera (Fruchtman SM et al. Semin Hematol 1997;34:17–23)

• Eighty percent of patients achieved control of blood counts with hydroxyurea and phlebotomy

• The other 20% of patients had refractory disease, could not tolerate therapy, or may develop leukopenia preventing further dose escalation

Essential Thrombocythemia (Cortelazzo S et al. N Engl J Med 1995;332:1132–1136)

• Patients treated with hydroxyurea had a lower incidence of thrombotic events compared to patients who received placebo

• Hydroxyurea is not universally successful in controlling thrombocytosis

• Resistance to hydroxyurea has been reported in 11–17% of cases

Therapy Monitoring

Frequent monitoring of CBC is necessary to prevent excessive marrow suppression. Obtain a CBC every 1–2 weeks for the first 2 months, every month thereafter, and, after reaching a steady state, every 3 months

CYTOREDUCTIVE THERAPY

POLYCYTHEMIA VERA (PV) AND ESSENTIAL THROMBOCYTHEMIA (ET) REGIMEN: ANAGRELIDE HCL

Anagrelide Study Group. Am J Med 1992;92:69–76 (ET)
Fruchtman SM et al. Annual Meeting of the American Society of Hematology, Philadelphia, PA, 2002; Abstract #256 (PV)
Storen EC, Tefferi A. Blood 2001;97:863–866 (PV, ET)
Tomer A. Blood 2002;99:1602–1609 (ET)

Note:
• Oral imidazoquinazoline compound for treatment of thrombocytosis associated with MPN

Initial dose:
Anagrelide HCl 0.5 mg/dose; administer orally every 12 hours for 7 consecutive days
Usual maintenance dose:
After 1 week at a dose of 0.5 mg orally every 12 hours, the dose should be increased by 0.5 mg/day at weekly intervals until response is achieved. The optimal dose is determined **empirically**, with frequent monitoring of platelet counts

Anagrelide HCl 0.5–1 mg/dose; administer orally, 2–4 doses/day to provide a total daily dose = 2–2.5 mg/day (doses need not be equal)

Note: individual anagrelide doses should not exceed 2.5 mg; daily doses should not exceed 10 mg

Efficacy

Polycythemia Vera
More than 75% of patients will achieve good platelet control. The remaining 25% will be either intolerant or have disease that is refractory to anagrelide

Essential Thrombocythemia
• Anagrelide Study Group
• Purpose:
  ▪ Evaluate the safety and efficacy of anagrelide when used to reduce platelet counts in patients with thrombocytosis and a diagnosis of a chronic myeloproliferative disease
  ▪ **Anagrelide** 0.5–1 mg given orally 4 times per day

Patients and methods:
• 577 patients (504/577 previously but unsuccessfully treated with other modalities)
  ▪ Essential thrombocythemia = 355
  ▪ Chronic granulocytic leukemia = 114
  ▪ Polycythemia vera = 68
  ▪ Undifferentiated myeloproliferative diseases = 60

Results:
• 424/577 evaluable for response
• 396/424 (93%): Platelet count reduced by 50%, or to <600,000/mm3, for ≥28 days
• Acquired resistance was not observed
• Major side effects: neurologic, gastrointestinal, and cardiac
• In >5 years, 16% of patients discontinued treatment because of side effects
• The MRC PT–1 trial (Medical Research Council clinical trial in patients with Primary Thrombocythemia) showed anagrelide is inferior to hydroxyurea in every respect, and does not support its role as first-line therapy; instead, *use as a third-line agent in patients who have failed or are intolerant to hydroxyurea or interferon* α *therapy*

Notes:
• Initial studies suggested a specific effect on megakaryopoiesis and thrombocytosis. Anagrelide works by inhibiting the maturation of platelets from megakaryocytes. The exact mechanism of action is unclear, although it is known to be a potent inhibitor of phosphodiesterase-III (IC_{50} = 36 nmol/L)

Patient Population Studied

PV (Storen EC, Tefferi A. Blood 2001;97:863–866)
More than 2000 patients with both Philadelphia chromosome-positive and -negative MPDs have been studied

ET (Anagrelide Study Group. Am J Med 1992;92:69–76)
The Anagrelide Study Group included 335 patients with essential thrombocythemia

Treatment Modifications

Adverse Event	Treatment Modification
Hematologic Toxicity	
Platelet count <100,000/mm³	Hold anagrelide until platelet count >100,000/mm³; then restart at 50% of prior dose
Nonhematologic Toxicity > Initial 2 Weeks	
G1	No dose modifications
G2/3	Hold anagrelide until toxicity G ≤1; then restart at prior dose
Recurrent G2/3	Hold anagrelide until toxicity G ≤1; then restart at 75% of prior dose
G4	Hold anagrelide until toxicity G ≤1; then restart at 50% of prior dose
Recurrent G4	Discontinue anagrelide

Toxicity*

Toxicity	Percentage	Notes
Hematologic Toxicities		
↓ Hemoglobin[†]	36	
↓ WBC	—	
Leukemogenic	(2.6)[‡]	
Nonhematologic Toxicities		
Palpitations[§]	26	Administer carefully to elderly; avoid in patients with cardiac disease
Fluid retention[§]	20	
Headaches	43	Usually within 2 weeks after starting therapy; often diminishes in severity or resolves in 2 weeks with continued therapy
Diarrhea[ϵ]	25	
Nausea	17	
Abdominal pain	16	
Dizziness	15	

Less Common Nonhematologic Toxicities

Atrial fibrillation	Gastric/duodenal ulceration	Pulmonary hypertension
Cardiomegaly	Hair loss	Pulmonary infiltrates
Cardiomyopathy	Myocardial infarction	Renal impairment/failure
Cerebrovascular accident	Pancreatitis	Seizure
Complete heart block	Pericarditis	Weakness/fatigue
Congestive heart failure	Pulmonary fibrosis	

*Not to be used during pregnancy
[†]With long-term therapy, ↓ hemoglobin level up to 3 g/dL in 24% of patients
[‡]All patients who developed acute leukemia were previously exposed to other cytoreductive agents. There were no patients who transformed who were exposed only to anagrelide
[§]Related to drug's vasodilatory and inotropic properties. Minimize by starting with a low dose (0.5 mg twice daily), and gradually increase the dose until control of the platelet count is achieved
[ϵ]Occurs in patients with lactose intolerance because of the presence of lactose in commercially available products

Therapy Monitoring

Frequent platelet count monitoring is necessary to prevent excessive marrow suppression

1. *During period of initial dose adjustment:* Platelet count every 5–7 days
2. *When the peripheral blood count is maintained within acceptable range on a stable dose of anagrelide:* Lengthen interval to 2 weeks and then to 4 weeks

CYTOREDUCTIVE THERAPY

POLYCYTHEMIA VERA (PV) AND ESSENTIAL THROMBOCYTHEMIA (ET) REGIMEN: INTERFERON ALFA—2B

Elliott MA, Tefferi A. Semin Thromb Hemost 1997;23:463–472
Sacchi S et al. Ann Hematol 1991;63:206–209
Sacchi S. Leuk Lymphoma 1995;19:13–20
Silver RT. Cancer 2006;107:451–458
Silver RT. Semin Hematol 1997;34:40–50
Gisslinger: Lancet Haematol 2020 Mar;7(3):e196–e208.

Antipyretic primary prophylaxis:
Acetaminophen 650–1000 mg; administer orally, 1 hour before interferon administration, and then every 4 hours for a total of 3 doses, *or*
Ibuprofen 400–600 mg; administer orally, 1 hour before interferon administration, and then every 4 hours for a total of 3 doses

Secondary antiemetic prophylaxis:
If needed, use as primary prophylaxis with subsequent doses
Note: have patients take interferon at bedtime, so they sleep through the period when symptoms are likely to be most severe

pegylated interferon alfa 2a- 45 mcg subcutaneous weekly, may uptitrate to 90 mcg weekly followed by 180 mcg weekly.

Pegylated interferon alpha may be administered subcutaneously every 2 weeks (dose 45 mcg, 90 or 180 mcg) depending on response.
Note: interferon alfa is the agent of choice for PV and ET in high-risk women of childbearing age. It has been safely used in pregnant women because it does not cross the placenta

Supportive Care
Antiemetic prophylaxis
Emetogenic potential is **MINIMAL**
See Chapter 42 for antiemetic recommendations

Hematopoietic growth factor (CSF) prophylaxis
Primary prophylaxis is **NOT** indicated
See Chapter 43 for more information

Antimicrobial prophylaxis
Risk of fever and neutropenia is **LOW**
   Antimicrobial primary prophylaxis to be considered:
   • Antibacterial—not indicated
   • Antifungal—not indicated
   • Antiviral—not indicated unless patient previously had an episode of HSV

Treatment Modifications

Adverse Event	Treatment Modification
Hematologic Toxicity	
ANC 1000–1500/mm^3	Reduce interferon dose by 50%; consider dose reescalation if ANC then increases to >1500/mm^3
ANC <500/mm^3 or platelet counts <25000/mm^3	Discontinue interferon therapy
Nonhematologic Toxicity > Initial 2 Weeks	
ALT/AST >5–10× upper limit of normal	Withhold therapy until ALT and AST return to pretreatment values, then resume interferon at 50% of the dose previously administered
G1	No dose modifications
G2/3	Withhold therapy until toxicity G ≤1, then resume interferon at 50% of the dose previously administered
Recurrent G2/3 at reduced interferon dosage	Discontinue therapy
G4	Withhold therapy until toxicity G ≤1, then resume interferon at 50% of the dose previously administered
Recurrent G4 at reduced interferon dosage	Discontinue therapy

Efficacy

Studied extensively in PV and ET with satisfactory responses in >80% of patients

Polycythemia Vera

- Interferon alfa (IFN-α) has myelosuppressive activity and antagonizes the action of platelet-derived growth factor (PDGF), a product of megakaryopoiesis that initiates fibroblast proliferation

- In general, control of erythrocytosis occurs in approximately 76% of patients receiving subcutaneous IFN-α in doses ranging from 4.5 to 27 million units per week (usual dose: 3 million units subcutaneously 3 times per week)

- A similar degree of benefit was achieved in terms of reduction in spleen size and relief from intractable pruritus in other series

(Silver RT. Cancer 2006;107:451–458)

- Report of long-term use (median: 13 years) of IFN-α in 55 patients previously treated with phlebotomy alone or with phlebotomy + hydroxyurea

- Patients achieved partial response of their disease by 6 months, and complete response by 1–2 years (phlebotomy-free, Hct ≤45%, platelets ≤600,000/mm³); spleen size was reduced in 27 of 30 patients with prior splenomegaly

- Prefered treatment: Pegylated-interferon alfa-2a induces complete hematologic and molecular response rates of 76–95 and 18%, respectively

Kiladjian, et al. *Blood.* 2008;112;3065-3072
Quintas-Cardama, et al. *Blood.* 2013;122;893;

- Initial dose: pegylated interferon alfa 2a- 45 mcg subcutaneous weekly, may uptitrate to 90 mcg weekly followed by 180 mcg weekly.

- Maintenance dose: Pegylated interferon alpha may be administered subcutaneously every 2 weeks (dose 45 mcg, 90 or 180 mcg) depending on response.

Essential Thrombocythemia

- Single-agent activity associated with modest reductions in JAK2*V617F* allele burden has been demonstrated in ET

- Results of several series indicate platelet counts can be reduced to <600,000/mm³ after approximately 3 months of therapy

(Sacchi S et al. Leuk Lymphoma 1995;19:13–20)

- In a total of 212 patients treated in 11 different clinical trials, a response rate of approximately 90% has been reported. At a dose of 3 million IU per dose, administered subcutaneously, 5 days/week, the median time to complete response with this dose is 3 months

Toxicity

General Comments

Drawback: IFN-α use is associated with many side effects and is not tolerated by a significant proportion of patients

Most frequent adverse effects are flu-like symptoms: increased body temperature, feeling ill, fatigue, headache, muscle pain, convulsion, dizziness, hair thinning, and depression. Erythema, pain, and injection site induration are also frequently observed. Interferon therapy also causes immunosuppression and can result in infections manifesting in unusual ways. All known adverse effects are usually reversible and disappear a few days after the therapy has been discontinued

General Recommendations Causes and Management of Acute Symptoms During Induction Therapy

Fever	Frequently controlled with acetaminophen
Bone and muscle pain	
Fatigue	
Lethargy	
Depression	

Symptoms Following Long-Term Administration

Mild weight loss	
Alopecia	
Thyroiditis and hypothyroidism	Autoimmune disorders
Hemolytic anemia	

Summary of Toxicities*

Application Site Disorders

Injection site inflammation	3% (1–5%)
All others	<5%

Blood Disorders

Anemia, leukopenia, neutropenia, thrombocytopenia	All ≤5%

Body as a Whole

Facial edema	<1% (<1–10%)
Weight decrease	3% (<1–13%)
All others	≤5%

Cardiovascular System Disorders

Angina, arrhythmia, cardiac failure, hypertension, hypotension	All <5%

Endocrine System Disorders

All toxicities	<5%

Flu-like Symptoms

Arthralgia	8% (3–19%)	Asthenia	11% (5–63%)	Back pain	6% (1–19%)
Chest pain	3% (1–28%)	Chills	46% (45–54%)	Dizziness	10% (7–24%)
Dry mouth	6% (1–28%)	Fatigue	65% (8–96%)	Fever	60% (34–94%)
Headache	52% (21–62%)	Influenza-like symptoms		65 (3–18%)	
Malaise	6% (3–14%)	Myalgia	40% (16–75%)	Rigors	23% (2–42%)
↑ Sweating	4% (1–21%)	Pain, unspecified	22% (<1–79%)	All others	<5%

(continued)

Therapy Monitoring

1. *Prior to initiation of therapy:* CBC and platelet counts, thyroid function tests including TSH
2. *Weeks 1 and 2 following initiation of therapy, and monthly thereafter:* CBC and platelet counts
3. LFTs at approximately 3-month intervals
4. Thyroid function tests at 3 and 6 months

Toxicity (continued)

Gastrointestinal System Disorders

Abdominal Pain	5% (1–21%)	Anorexia	40% (1–69%)	Constipation	3% (<1–14%)
Diarrhea	19% (2–45%)	Dyspepsia	4% (2–8%)	Gingivitis	5% (1–14%)
Loose stools	2% (<1–10%)	Nausea	23% (17–66%)	Taste altered	6% (<1–24%)
Vomiting	10% (2–32%)	All others	<5%		

Liver and Biliary Systems Disorders

Abnormal liver function tests	All <5%

Musculoskeletal Systems Disorders

Musculoskeletal pain	9% (1–21%)	All others	<5%

Nervous System and Psychiatric Disorders

Amnesia	<5% (1–14%)	Anxiety	3% (<1–9%)	Confusion	<5% (2–10%)
Decreased libido	1% (1–5%)			Depression	9% (3–40%)
Hypoesthesia	<5% (1–10%)	Impaired concentration		3% (<1–14%)	
Insomnia	5% (<1–12%)	Irritability	12% (1–13%)	Nervousness	2% (1–3%)
Paresthesia	6% (1–21%)	Somnolence	<5% (1–33%)	All others	<5%

Reproduction System

All toxicities	<5%

Resistance Mechanisms Disorders

Moniliasis	1% (<1–17%)	Herpes simplex	1% (1–5%)

Respiratory System Disorders

Coughing	5% (<1–31%)	Dyspnea	5% (<1–34%)	Nasal congestion	3% (1–10%)
Nonproductive cough	2% (0–14%)			Pharyngitis	<5% (1–31%)
Sinusitis	3% (1–21%)	All other		<5%	

Skin and Appendages Disorders

Alopecia	26% (8–31%)	Dermatitis	2% (1–8%)	Dry skin	4% (<1–10%)
Pruritus	7% (1–11%)	Rash	9% (1–25%)	All others	<5%

Urinary Systems Disorders

↑ BUN	<5%	All other		<5%

Vision Disorders

All toxicities	<5%

*Excerpts from INTRON A, interferon alfa–2b, recombinant for injection; Aug. 2012 product labeling. Schering Corporation, a subsidiary of Merck & Co., Inc., Whitehouse Station, NJ. Percent toxicities are presented as median percent (range) reported for 3 to as many as 10 evaluations in a diverse group of disease states including malignant melanoma, follicular lymphoma, hairy cell leukemia, condylomata acuminata, AIDS-related Kaposi sarcoma, chronic hepatitis C, and chronic hepatitis B. The doses of interferon alfa–2b used ranged from 1 million IU/lesion to 30 million IU/m^2

CYTOREDUCTIVE THERAPY

ESSENTIAL THROMBOCYTHEMIA (ET) REGIMEN: BUSULFAN

Shvidel L et al. Leukemia 2007;21:2071–2072
Van de Pette JEW et al. Br J Haematol 1986;62:229–237

Notes:

- Busulfan is an alkylating agent with a specific action on megakaryocytic proliferation
- Because of concerns about leukemogenic potential busulfan use should be limited to older patients (>60 years of age) or patients intolerant of hydroxyurea

Busulfan 2–4 mg per day; administer orally, continually, until platelet count decreases to <400,000/mm³ (total dose/week = 14–28 mg)

Note: once platelet count normalizes, long-term control of platelet count can be achieved with intermittent courses of busulfan given as follows:
Busulfan 2–4 mg per day; administer orally, continually, for 2 weeks after the platelet count increases to >400,000/mm³ (total dose/2-week cycle = 28–56 mg)

Supportive Care

Antiemetic prophylaxis
Emetogenic potential is **MINIMAL–LOW**
See Chapter 42 for antiemetic recommendations

Hematopoietic growth factor (CSF) prophylaxis
Primary prophylaxis is **NOT** indicated
See Chapter 43 for more information

Antimicrobial prophylaxis
Risk of fever and neutropenia is **LOW**
   Antimicrobial primary prophylaxis to be considered:
- Antibacterial—*P. jirovecii* prophylaxis is recommended (eg, cotrimoxazole)
- Antifungal—not indicated
- Antiviral—not indicated unless patient previously had an episode of HSV

Patient Population Studied

Shvidel L et al. Leukemia 2007;21:2071–2072

Long-term outcome of 36 elderly patients with ET treated with busulfan and evaluated for thrombotic complications and blastic transformation. Thirteen men and 23 women; median age at treatment = 73 years (range: 60–91 years). Diagnosis of ET established according to Polycythemia Vera (PV) Study Group Criteria. Major risk factors for thrombosis: (a) old age (100%); (b) platelet count >1,500,000/mm³ or history of thrombosis (16/36, 44%); (c) at least 1 thrombotic event (12/36, 33%); (d) disturbances such as dizziness, headache, syncope, angina pectoris, erythromelalgia, or leg ulcers before busulfan therapy (21/36, 58%). The median platelet count at start of busulfan was 994,000/mm³ (range: 783,000–1,768,000/mm³)

Van de Pette JEW et al. Br J Haematol 1986;62:229–237

Thirty-seven patients with essential thrombocythemia treated with busulfan and followed for periods up to 25 years

Treatment Modifications

Adverse Events	Treatment Modifications
WBC* <4000/mm³ but >3500/mm³	Reduce busulfan dose by 50%
WBC* <3500/mm³	Discontinue busulfan
LFTs 2–3 × UNL	Reduce busulfan dose by 50%
LFTs >3 × UNL	Hold busulfan until LFTs have returned to baseline values

*Regarding WBC monitoring and treatment modification. The product label for Myleran, a film-coated busulfan tablet (January 2004. GlaxoSmithKline, Research Triangle Park, NC), states: "A decrease in the leukocyte count is not usually seen during the first 10–15 days of treatment; the leukocyte count may actually increase during this period and it should not be interpreted as resistance to the drug, nor should the dose be increased. Since the leukocyte count may continue to fall for more than 1 month after discontinuing the drug, it is important that busulfan be discontinued prior to the total leukocyte count falling into the normal range. When the total leukocyte count has declined to approximately 15,000/μL, the drug should be withheld. With a constant dose of busulfan, the total leukocyte count declines exponentially . . . .
A decision to increase, decrease, continue, or discontinue a given dose of busulfan must be based not only on the absolute hematologic values, but also on the rapidity with which changes are occurring (in response to treatment)." Plotting weekly WBC counts on a semilogarithmic graph (WBC counts on the log axis; time on the linear axis) may aid in planning when to discontinue therapy

Efficacy (N = 36)

Shvidel et al. Leukemia 2007;21:2071–2072*

Median follow-up time after therapy	72 months (range: 30–300 months)
Hematologic response (platelet count <400,000/mm³)	100%
Disappearance of thrombocytosis-related symptoms	100%
Cycles of busulfan administered	47[†]
Median duration of response in all the cycles given	38 months (range: 8+ to 207+ months)
Response duration following the first cycle	36 months[‡]
Response duration following subsequent cycles	38 months[‡]
Percent relapsed	47% (17/36)
Percent requiring additional treatment	33% (12/36)
Median time for next treatment	56 months (range: 22–116 months)
Actual survival at 7 years	78%
Percentage dead during follow-up	36% (13/36)[§]
Leukemic transformation/other malignancies during follow-up	0

*To avoid the combination of multiple cytotoxic drugs, only 1 patient received hydroxyurea following busulfan. Two other patients in relapse were subsequently treated with anagrelide
[†]Twenty-six patients received 1 cycle, 9 patients received 2 cycles, and 1 patient received 3 cycles
[‡]No difference between response duration following the first and subsequent cycles
[§]One patient who was sequentially treated with busulfan and hydroxyurea died of myelofibrosis with splenomegaly, thrombocytopenia, and bleeding 7 years after busulfan therapy. Among the other 12 patients, 9 >80 years of age died of cardiovascular disorders; all had normal platelet count at the time of death and causes of their death were thought to be related to old age/underlying diseases

Toxicity

Toxicity	Percent/Comment
Myelosuppression, all cell lines are equally affected*	Platelets can drop precipitously*
G1/2 nausea	>80%
G1/2 vomiting	>80%
G1/2 diarrhea	>80%
Skin hyperpigmentation	5–10%
Insomnia	Rare
Anxiety	Rare
Dizziness	Rare
Depression	Rare
Elevated LFTs	Rare
Pulmonary symptoms, cough, dyspnea, and fever	With long-term use in <5% of patients
Increased risk of secondary malignancy, especially AML	

*Failure to stop busulfan treatment may result in bone marrow failure with severe prolonged pancytopenia. Pancytopenia is potentially reversible, but recovery may take 1 month to 2 years

Efficacy (N = 37)

Van de Pette JEW et al. Br J Haematol 1986;62:229–237

Cox regression analysis indicated only 2 prognostically important presenting features:

• Age → Strong inverse correlation with survival
• Vascular occlusive symptoms → Correlated with a better survival

Platelet count to <400,000/mm³	100%
Resolution of vascular occlusive symptoms	100%*
Median duration of survival on treatment	9.8 years
Deaths from thrombosis and malignant diseases, including leukemia	Not significantly different from the number expected
Progression of PT into myelofibrosis	24%
Development of polycythemia	9%

*Hemorrhagic symptoms often remained unaltered

Therapy Monitoring

1. *Weekly:* CBC with differential and platelet count, and LFTs during period of busulfan therapy. (*Note:* because sudden, unexpected marrow suppression may occur, frequent CBC monitoring is mandatory)
2. *CXR as indicated:* For insidious onset of cough, dyspnea, and low-grade fever after months to years of therapy, consider busulfan-related lung toxicity in differential diagnosis

HYDROXYUREA-INTOLERANT OR -RESISTANT

POLYCYTHEMIA VERA (PV) REGIMEN: RUXOLITINIB

Vannucchi A et al. N Engl J Med 2015;372:426–443
Protocol for: Vannucchi A et al. N Engl J Med 2015;372:426–443
Supplementary appendix to: Vannucchi A et al. N Engl J Med 2015;372:426–443
JAKAFI (ruxolitinib) prescribing information. Wilmington, DE: Incyte Corporation; revised January 2020

Ruxolitinib 10 mg per dose; administer orally, twice daily, without regard to food, continuously (total dosage/week = 140 mg)
Notes:
- Patients who miss a dose of ruxolitinib should be advised not to take an additional dose, but instead to take the next usual prescribed dose at the next regularly scheduled time
- Ruxolitinib may be administered through a nasogastric tube (≥8 French):
  - Suspend 1 tablet in 40 mL of water and stir for 10 minutes
  - Within 6 hours after the tablet has dispersed, administer through tube using an appropriate syringe
  - Rinse the tube with 75 mL of water
- If discontinuing ruxolitinib for reasons other than thrombocytopenia, consider gradual tapering by 5 mg twice daily each week to minimize the risk of myeloproliferative neoplasm symptom exacerbation. Advise patients not to interrupt or discontinue ruxolitinib treatment without consulting their treating health care provider
- See Treatment Modifications section for recommended dose modifications for adverse events, insufficient response, drug interactions, renal impairment, and hepatic impairment

Supportive Care
Antiemetic prophylaxis
Emetogenic potential is **MINIMAL–LOW**
See Chapter 42 for antiemetic recommendations

Hematopoietic growth factor (CSF) prophylaxis
Primary prophylaxis is **NOT** indicated
See Chapter 43 for more information

Antimicrobial prophylaxis
Risk of fever and neutropenia is **LOW**
   Antimicrobial primary prophylaxis to be considered:
- Antibacterial—not indicated
- Antifungal—not indicated
- Antiviral—not indicated unless patient previously had an episode of HSV

Treatment Modifications

Ruxolitinib Dose Reductions for Adverse Events

Adverse Event	Treatment Modification
Bleeding requiring intervention, irrespective of platelet count	Withhold ruxolitinib therapy. Upon resolution of bleeding, consider resuming treatment at the prior dose if the underlying cause of bleeding has been controlled. If the underlying cause persists, consider resuming treatment at a lower dose
Withdrawal syndrome: patient with symptom exacerbation following interruption, discontinuation. or tapering of ruxolitinib treatment (fever, respiratory distress, hypotension, DIC, MOF)	Evaluate for and treat any intercurrent illness and consider restarting or increasing the dose of ruxolitinib
Hb ≥12 g/dL AND platelet count ≥100,000/mm^3	No change required
Hb 10 to <12 g/dL AND platelet count 75,000 to <100,000/mm^3	Consider dose reduction with the goal of avoiding dose interruptions for anemia and thrombocytopenia
Hb 8 to <10 g/dL OR platelet count 50,000 to <75,000/mm^3	Reduce dose by 5 mg twice daily. For patients on 5 mg twice daily, decrease dose to 5 mg once daily

(continued)

Treatment Modifications (*continued*)

Adverse Event	Treatment Modification
Hb <8 g/dL OR platelet count <50,000/mm^3 OR ANC <1000/mm^3	Withhold ruxolitinib dosing until recovery of hematologic parameters to acceptable levels (Hb ≥8 g/dL, platelet count ≥50,000/mm^3, and ANC ≥1000/mm^3), then resume at a dose based on the most severe category of a patient's recovery Hb, platelet count, or ANC as follows: <ul><li>If recovery Hb is 8 to <10 g/dL, OR platelet count 50,000 to <75,000/mm^3, OR ANC 1000 to <1500/mm^3, then resume ruxolitinib at 5 mg orally twice daily* or no more than 5 mg twice daily less than the dose which resulted in dose interruption</li><li>If recovery Hb is 10 to <12 g/dL, OR platelet count 75,000 to <100,000/mm^3, OR ANC 1,500 to <2,000/mm^3, then resume ruxolitinib at 10 mb twice daily* or no more than 5 mg twice daily less than the dose which resulted in dose interruption</li><li>If recovery Hb is ≥12 g/dL, OR platelet count ≥100,000/mm^3, OR ANC ≥2,000/mm^3, then resume ruxolitinib at 15 mb twice daily* or no more than 5 mg twice daily less than the dose which resulted in dose interruption</li></ul> Patients who had required dose interruption while receiving a dose of 5 mg twice daily may restart at a dose of 5 mg twice daily or 5 mg once daily, but not higher, once Hb is ≥10 g/dL, platelet count is ≥75,000/mm^3, and ANC is ≥1500/mm^3 *Continue treatment for ≥2 weeks; if stable, may increase dose by 5 mg twice daily After resuming, doses may be titrated, but the maximum total daily dose should not exceed 5 mg less than the dose that resulted in the dose interruption. An exception to this is dose interruption following phlebotomy-associated anemia, in which case the maximal total daily dose allowed after restarting would not be limited

Ruxolitinib Dose Increases for Insufficient Response

Parameter	Treatment Modification

Efficacy considered insufficient in a patient who meets all of the following conditions:
1. Inadequate efficacy as demonstrated by ≥1 of the following:
  a. Continued need for phlebotomy
  b. WBC >ULN
  c. Platelet count >ULN
  d. Palpable spleen reduced by <25% from baseline
2. Platelet count ≥140,000/mm^3
3. Hb ≥12 g/dL
4. ANC ≥1500/mm^3
	Consider a dose increase in 5 mg twice daily increments to a maximum of 25 mg twice daily. Doses should not be increased during the first 4 weeks of therapy and doses should not be increased more frequently than every 2 weeks

Ruxolitinib Dose Modifications for Drug Interactions, Renal Impairment, or Hepatic Impairment

Parameter	Treatment Modification
Ruxolitinib is to be newly initiated in a patient where use of a strong CYP3A4 inhibitor or fluconazole dose ≤200 mg* is unavoidable	Reduce the starting dose of ruxolitinib to 5 mg twice daily
A strong CYP3A4 inhibitor or fluconazole dose ≤200 mg* is to be initiated in a patient on a stable dose of ruxolitinib ≥10 mg twice daily	Decrease ruxolitinib dose by 50% (round up to the closest available tablet strength)
A strong CYP3A4 inhibitor or fluconazole dose ≤200 mg* is to be initiated in a patient on a stable dose of ruxolitinib 5 mg twice daily	Decrease ruxolitinib dose to 5 mg once daily
A strong CYP3A4 inhibitor or fluconazole dose ≤200 mg is to be initiated in a patient on a stable dose of ruxolitinib 5 mg once daily	Avoid strong CYP3A4 inhibitor or fluconazole treatment or interrupt ruxolitinib treatment for the duration of strong CYP3A4 inhibitor or fluconazole use
Moderate (CrCl = 30–59 mL/min; 0.5–0.98 mL/s) or severe (CrCl = 15–29 mL/min; 0.25–0.48 mL/s) renal impairment	Reduce the starting dose to 5 mg orally twice daily

(*continued*)

Treatment Modifications (*continued*)

Adverse Event	Treatment Modification
ESRD (CrCl <15 mL/min; <0.25 mL/s) on hemodialysis	Reduce the starting dose to 10 mg orally once after each dialysis session
ESRD (CrCl <15 mL/min; <0.25 mL/s) not requiring dialysis	Avoid ruxolitinib use
Hepatic impairment of any severity (ie, mild [Child-Pugh class A], moderate [Child-Pugh class B], or severe [Child-Pugh class C])	Reduce the starting dose to 5 mg orally, twice daily

*Avoid use of fluconazole at doses >200 mg
DIC, disseminated intravascular coagulation; MOF, multiorgan failure; Hb, hemoglobin; ANC, absolute neutrophil count; WBC, white blood cell; ULN, upper limit of normal; CrCl, creatinine clearance; ESRD, end-stage renal disease

Patient Population Studied

The RESPONSE study was a phase 3, open-label, international, multicenter, randomized controlled trial that evaluated ruxolitinib (n = 110) vs standard therapy (n = 112) in adult patients with phlebotomy-dependent polycythemia vera who had either resistance or intolerance to prior hydroxyurea treatment. Patients were required to be phlebotomy-dependent (≥2 phlebotomies within 24 weeks and ≥1 phlebotomy within 16 weeks before screening), have a spleen volume of ≥450 cm^3 assessed by MRI or CT, no prior JAK inhibitor treatment, and resistance or intolerance to prior hydroxyurea. Single-agent standard therapy was determined by the treating physician and could include hydroxyurea (58.9%), interferon or pegylated interferon (11.6%), pipobroman (1.8%), anagrelide (7.1%), lenalidomide or thalidomide (4.5%), or no medication (15.2%). Notably, phosphorus-32, busulfan, and chlorambucil were prohibited. All patients were to receive low-dose aspirin when not contraindicated. Standard therapy could be changed if needed (n = 6) based on tolerance or lack of efficacy, and patients randomized to the standard therapy arm could cross over to ruxolitinib (85.7%) at week 32 if the primary end point was not met, or at a later timepoint if disease progressed

Efficacy (N = 222)

Efficacy Variable	Ruxolitinib (N = 110)	Standard Therapy (N = 112)	Between-group Comparison
Response			
Composite primary endpoint of both HCT control* and ≥35% reduction in spleen volume at week 32—n/N (%)	23/110 (20.9)	1/112 (0.9)	OR 28.6 (95% CI, 4.5–1206); *P*<0.001
HCT control* at week 32—n/N (%)	66/110 (60.0)	22/112 (19.6)	—
≥35% reduction in spleen volume at week 32—n/N (%)	42/110 (38.2)	1/112 (0.9)	—
Patients with a primary HCT and spleen response at week 32 also maintained at week 48—n/N (%)	21/110 (19.1)	1/112 (0.9)	*P*<0.001
≥1 phlebotomy procedure(s) between weeks 8–32—n/N (%)	21/106 (19.8)	68/109 (62.4)	—
≥3 phlebotomy procedures between weeks 8–32—n/N (%)	3/106 (2.8)	22/109 (20.2)	—
≥50% reduction in MPN-SAF† symptom score at week 32	36/74 (49)	4/81 (5)	—

*Hematocrit control was defined as protocol-specified ineligibility for phlebotomy from week 8–32 and ≤1 instance of phlebotomy eligibility between randomization and week 8. Phlebotomy eligibility was defined as a hematocrit >45% that was ≥3 percentage points higher than baseline or a hematocrit >48%, whichever was lower
†MPN-SAF assesses 14 disease-related symptoms each on a scale of 0 (absent) to 10 (worst possible)
HCT, hematocrit; OR, odds ratio; MPN-SAF, Myeloproliferative Neoplasm Symptom Assessment Form

Adverse Events (N = 221)

Nonhematologic Adverse Events Occurring in ≥10% of Patients in Either Treatment Group

Event*	Ruxolitinib (N = 110)		Standard Therapy (N = 111)	
Grade (%)	All Grades	Grade 3–4	All Grades	Grade 3–4
Headache	16.4	0.9	18.9	0.9
Diarrhea	14.5	0	7.2	0.9
Fatigue	14.5	0	15.3	2.7
Pruritus	13.6	0.9	22.5	3.6
Dizziness	11.8	0	9.9	0
Muscle spasms	11.8	0.9	4.5	0
Dyspnea	10.0	2.7	1.8	0
Abdominal pain	9.1	0.9	11.7	0
Asthenia	7.3	1.8	10.8	0

Hematologic Adverse Events, New or Worsening Laboratory Abnormalities

Event*	Ruxolitinib (N = 110)			Standard Therapy (N = 111)		
Grade (%)	All Grades	Grade 3	Grade 4	All Grades	Grade 3	Grade 4
Anemia	43.6	0.9	0.9	30.6	0	0
Thrombocytopenia	24.5	4.5	0.9	18.9	2.7	0.9
Lymphopenia	43.6	15.5	0.9	50.5	16.2	1.8
Leukopenia	9.1	0.9	0	12.6	1.8	0
Neutropenia	1.8	0	0.9	8.1	0.9	0

Therapy Monitoring

1. A complete blood count (CBC) with leukocyte differential and platelet count must be performed before initiating therapy, every 2–4 weeks until doses are stabilized, and then as clinically indicated

2. Renal and liver function tests before starting treatment with ruxolitinib (baseline), with serial reassessment as clinically indicated

3. Assess for the presence of tuberculosis risk factors (eg, prior residence in or travel to countries with a high prevalence of tuberculosis, close contact with a person with active tuberculosis, and a history of active or latent tuberculosis where an adequate course of treatment cannot be confirmed). If a risk factor is present, screen for latent tuberculosis prior to initiation of ruxolitinib. For patients with evidence of active or latent tuberculosis, consult a physician with expertise in the treatment of tuberculosis before starting ruxolitinib. The decision to continue ruxolitinib during treatment of active tuberculosis should be based on the overall risk-benefit determination

4. Between 8–12 weeks after initiation of ruxolitinib, obtain a fasting lipid panel

5. When doses are interrupted, discontinued, or reduced, monitor for exacerbation of symptoms associated with the underlying myeloproliferative neoplasm such as fever, respiratory distress, hypotension, diffuse intravascular coagulation, and multiorgan failure

6. Advise patients to report and periodically assess for signs and symptoms of:
   a. Infection
   b. Progressive multifocal leukoencephalopathy
   c. Non-melanoma skin cancers

PRIMARY MYELOFIBROSIS (PMF) REGIMEN: LOW-DOSE THALIDOMIDE IN COMBINATION WITH PREDNISONE (THAL-PRED)

Mesa RA et al. Blood 2003;101:2534–2541

Thalidomide 50 mg; administer orally, daily, by rigorously adhering to the Celgene *S.T.E.P.S.* **program** for thalidomide safety
Prednisone 0.5 mg/kg per day; administer orally for 1 month, *followed by:*
Prednisone 0.25 mg/kg per day; administer orally for 1 month, *followed by:*
Prednisone 0.125 mg/kg per day; administer orally for 1 month

Note: patients showing any evidence of response after 3 months of combination therapy are treated for an additional 3 months with only 50 mg thalidomide daily
The System for Thalidomide Education and Prescribing Safety (*S.T.E.P.S.*) program is a Risk Evaluation and Mitigation Strategy program against the toxicity associated with fetal exposure to thalidomide, and designed to minimize the chance of fetal exposure to thalidomide

- To avoid fetal exposure, thalidomide is available only under a special restricted distribution program called *S.T.E.P.S. S.T.E.P.S.* requirements include, but are not limited to, the following:
  - Thalidomide must not be prescribed for female patients who are pregnant
  - Female patients taking thalidomide must not become pregnant, breastfeed a baby, or donate blood
  - Female patients able to become pregnant must use 2 methods of contraception 4 weeks before starting to use thalidomide and undergo pregnancy testing before receiving thalidomide and at prescribed intervals and during treatment
  - Male patients taking thalidomide must not impregnate a female, must not have unprotected sexual contact with a woman who is pregnant, and must use a latex condom every time they have sexual contact with women during thalidomide treatment and for 4 weeks after completing treatment
  - Only prescribers registered with *S.T.E.P.S.* can prescribe thalidomide
  - To receive thalidomide, patients must enroll in *S.T.E.P.S.* and agree to comply with the requirements of the *S.T.E.P.S.* program
- Information about thalidomide (THALOMID) and the *S.T.E.P.S.* program can be obtained by calling the Celgene Customer Care Center toll-free at (888) 423-5436, or online from the U.S. Food and Drug Administration website for Postmarket Drug Safety Information for Patients and Providers, Approved Risk Evaluation and Mitigation Strategies (REMS) at: www.fda.gov/Drugs/DrugSafety/PostmarketDrugSafetyInformationforPatientsandProviders/ [accessed April 12, 2021]

Supportive Care
Antiemetic prophylaxis
Emetogenic potential is **MINIMAL–LOW**
See Chapter 42 for antiemetic recommendations

Hematopoietic growth factor (CSF) prophylaxis
Primary prophylaxis is **NOT** indicated
See Chapter 43 for more information

Antimicrobial prophylaxis
Risk of fever and neutropenia is **LOW**
  Antimicrobial primary prophylaxis to be considered:
  - Antibacterial—not indicated
  - Antifungal—not indicated
  - Antiviral—not indicated unless patient previously had an episode of HSV

Thromboprophylaxis
Primary prophylaxis is not indicated

- Instruct patients to seek medical care if they develop shortness of breath, chest pain, or arm or leg swelling
- Consider thromboprophylaxis based on an assessment of an individual patient's underlying risk factors

Treatment Modifications

Adverse Event	Treatment Modification
Febrile neutropenia	Withhold therapy until fever abates, then resume therapy
G4 hematologic toxicity	Withhold therapy until ANC >750/mm³ and platelets >500,00/mm³, then resume therapy at a dose of thalidomide 25 mg/day
G3/4 nonhematologic toxicity	Interrupt therapy, follow clinically until toxicity remits to G ≤2, then resume therapy at a dose of thalidomide 25 mg/day
G ≥3 thalidomide neuropathy	Interrupt therapy, follow clinically until toxicity remits to G ≤2, then resume therapy at a dose of thalidomide 25 mg/day
If ANC nadir ≤1000/mm³ or platelets nadir ≤50,000/mm³	Continue treatment, but reduce thalidomide doses to 25 mg/day
G2 nonhematologic toxicity	Reduce thalidomide dose to 25 mg/day
G ≥3 nonhematologic toxicity	Discontinue thalidomide

Patient Population Studied

Patients met standard diagnostic criteria for myelofibrosis with myeloid metaplasia (MMM). All subtypes of MMM were eligible (agnogenic myeloid metaplasia [AMM], postpolycythemic myeloid metaplasia [PPMM], and postthrombocythemic myeloid metaplasia [PTMM]). All patients underwent bone marrow examination with cytogenetic and fluorescent in situ hybridization (FISH) studies to exclude occult chronic myeloid leukemia

Efficacy (N = 21)

Objective and sustained clinical response in anemia	13 (62%; 95% CI, 38%–82%)*
Median increase in hemoglobin value	1.8 g/dL (range: 0.1–5.1 g/dL)
Response in RBC transfusion-dependent patients (n = 10)	7/10 (70%)†
Response in RBC transfusion-independent patients (n = 11; 7 patients (64%) with hemoglobin level <10 g/dL)	Hemoglobin increased by 2.1 g/dL (range: 0.1–5.1 g/dL)
Response in patients with clinically relevant thrombocytopenia (n = 8; platelet count <100,000/mm^3)	8/8 (100%)‡,§,¶
>50% decrease in palpable splenomegaly	4 (19%)¶

*Improvements in anemia correlated with lower pretherapy CD34 cell counts in the peripheral blood (median: 81.2 CD34 cells/mm^3 in responders vs 554 CD34 cells/mm^3 in nonresponders; P = 0.03) as well as lower numbers of circulating blasts (median: 0.8% in responders vs 4.7% in nonresponders; P = 0.03)
†Four patients (40%) became transfusion independent and 3 (30%) had ≥50% decrease in transfusion requirements
‡Six patients (75%) had a >50% increase in their platelet count
§Improvements in clinically significant thrombocytopenia were associated with older ages (median: 71.4 years vs 61.7 years; P = 0.04), smaller pretreatment spleens (median: 6.5 cm vs 16.1 cm below the left costal margin; P <0.01), and hypocellular marrows (median cellularity: 18% vs 58% for nonresponders; P <0.01)
¶Responses in either splenomegaly or thrombocytopenia were strongly correlated with a concurrent response in anemia (P <0.01)

Therapy Monitoring

1. Monitor white blood cell count and differential on an ongoing basis, especially in patients who may be predisposed to develop neutropenia
2. Pregnancy testing
   - Females of childbearing potential
     - Within 24 hours before commencing thalidomide treatment and at intervals explicitly prescribed by the *S.T.E.P.S.* program
3. Neurologic testing before starting thalidomide treatment (baseline), then every 3 months while receiving treatment

Toxicity

Toxicity	Number of Patients Affected (Percentage Affected)		
	Thalidomide + Prednisone	G2/G3 or Higher	Thalidomide 100–400 mg*
Leukocytosis†	8 (38)	6/2 (29/10)	2 (13)
Thrombocytosis‡	4 (19)	3/2 (14/10)	3 (20)
Constipation	8 (38)	3 (14)	9 (60)
Edema	5 (24)	2 (10)	3 (20)
Visual disturbance	4 (19)	2 (10)	2 (13)
Fatigue	2 (10)	2 (10)	10 (67)
Thrombosis	1 (5)	1/1 (5/5)	0
Paresthesias	6 (29)	1 (5)	4 (27)
Sedation	6 (29)	1 (5)	3 (20)
Neutropenia <1500/mm^3	5 (24)	1 (5)	6 (40)
Neutropenia <1000/mm^3	4 (19)	4 (19)	4 (27)
Anxiety	4 (19)	0	3 (20)
Rash	3 (14)	0	4 (27)
Orthostatic symptoms	0	0	5 (33)
Tremor	0	0	3 (20)
Myeloproliferative reaction	0	0	3 (20)
Dry mouth	0	0	2 (13)
Sinus bradycardia	0	0	2 (13)
Abdominal pain	0	0	2 (13)
Decreased hearing	0	0	2 (13)
Anorexia	0	0	1 (7)
Confusion	0	0	1 (7)
Dry eyes	0	0	1 (7)
Depression	0	0	1 (7)

*Elliott MA et al. Br J Haematol 2002;117:288–296
†One patient developed acute myeloid leukemia
‡A clinical consequence was observed in only 1 patient (deep venous thrombosis)

PRIMARY MYELOFIBROSIS (PMF) REGIMEN: LENALIDOMIDE

Tefferi A et al. Blood 2006;108:1158–1164

Lenalidomide 10 mg/day; administer orally for 28 days, continually for 3–4 months (total dose/week = 70 mg)
• If initial platelet count is <100,000/mm³, give **lenalidomide** 5 mg/day; administer orally for 28 days, continually for 3–4 months (total dose/week = 35 mg)

Note: continue treatment for 6–24 months if response is observed

Supportive Care
Antiemetic prophylaxis
Emetogenic potential is **MINIMAL–LOW**
See Chapter 42 for antiemetic recommendations

Hematopoietic growth factor (CSF) prophylaxis
Primary prophylaxis is **NOT** indicated
See Chapter 43 for more information

Antimicrobial prophylaxis
Risk of fever and neutropenia is **LOW**
  Antimicrobial primary prophylaxis to be considered:
  • Antibacterial—not indicated
  • Antifungal—not indicated
  • Antiviral—not indicated unless patient previously had an episode of HSV

Thromboprophylaxis
Primary prophylaxis is not indicated
• Instruct patients to seek medical care if they develop shortness of breath, chest pain, or arm or leg swelling
• Consider thromboprophylaxis based on an assessment of an individual patient's underlying risk factors

Dose Modifications

Adverse Event	Dose Modification
Platelet count <30,000/mm³ on a lenalidomide dose of 10 mg/day	Interrupt lenalidomide treatment, follow CBC weekly, and when platelet count ≥30,000/mm³, resume lenalidomide at 5 mg/day
Platelet count <30,000/mm³ on a lenalidomide dose of 5 mg/day	Discontinue lenalidomide treatment
ANC <1000/mm³ on a lenalidomide dose of 10 mg/day	Interrupt lenalidomide treatment, follow CBC weekly and resume lenalidomide when ANC ≥1000/mm³ at 5 mg/day
ANC <1000/mm³ on a lenalidomide dose of 5 mg/day	Discontinue lenalidomide treatment
Febrile neutropenia on a lenalidomide dose of 10 mg/day	Interrupt lenalidomide treatment, follow closely, and when fever is abated, resume lenalidomide at 5 mg/day
Febrile neutropenia on a lenalidomide dose of 5 mg/day	Discontinue lenalidomide treatment
G3/4 nonhematologic toxicity on a lenalidomide dose of 10 mg/day	Interrupt lenalidomide treatment, follow clinically, and when toxicity G ≤2, resume lenalidomide at 5 mg/day
G3/4 nonhematologic toxicity on a lenalidomide dose of 5 mg/day	Discontinue lenalidomide treatment

Starting Dose Adjustment for Renal Impairment in Multiple Myeloma (Days 1–21 of Each 28-Day Cycle)

Moderate renal impairment (30–60 mL/min [0.5–1 mL/s])	Lenalidomide 10 mg every 24 hours
Severe renal impairment (not requiring dialysis) (<30 mL/min [<0.5 mL/s])	Lenalidomide 15 mg every 48 hours
End-stage renal disease (requiring dialysis) (<30 mL/min [<0.5 mL/s])	Lenalidomide 5 mg/day. On dialysis days, administer a dose following dialysis

Patient Population Studied

Two separate phase 2 studies involving single-agent lenalidomide therapy in patients with myelofibrosis with myeloid metaplasia (MMM). Conventional criteria were used for the diagnosis of MMM including all subtypes of myeloid metaplasia: agnogenic (AMM), postpolycythemic (PPMM), and postthrombocythemic (PTMM). Patients with acute myelofibrosis or myelodysplastic syndrome with myelofibrosis were not eligible for participation

Efficacy

	Combined (n = 68)	Mayo Clinic* (n = 27)	MDACC† (n = 41)
	Number of Patients (% with Each Finding)		
Response‡ in anemia (patients with baseline hemoglobin <10 g/dL)	10/46 (22)	6/27 (22)	4/19 (21)
Major‡	8 (17)	4 (15)	4 (21)
Minor‡	2 (4)	2 (7)	0
Response‡ in palpable splenomegaly	14/42 (33)	6/22 (27)	8/20 (40)
Major‡	1 (2)	1 (5)	1 (5)
Minor‡	13 (31)	5 (23)	7 (35)
Response‡ in thrombocytopenia (patients with baseline platelet count <100,000/mm³)	6/12 (50)	Not available	6/12 (50)
Response‡ in hypercatabolic symptoms	4/10 (40)	4/10 (40)	Not available
More than 25% decrease in serum LDH	39/59 (66)	16/27 (67)	21/32 (66)
LDH normalized	20 (34)	8 (30)	12 (38)

*Treated at Mayo Clinic (lenalidomide dose = 10 mg/day)
†Treated at M.D. Anderson Cancer Center (MDACC lenalidomide dose = 10 mg or 5 mg/day)
‡Response criteria
- *Anemia*: Patients who entered the study as transfusion-dependent needed to maintain response for at least 3 months. Transfusion-independent patients needed to maintain response for at least 1 month to be considered responses. Major response indicates normalization of hemoglobin; minor response means either becoming transfusion-independent or having an increase in hemoglobin ≥2 g/dL
- *Spleen*: Patients needed to maintain response for ≥1 month to be considered responses. Major response indicates either becoming nonpalpable if baseline is palpable at >5 cm in maximum distance below left costal margin (LCM) or >50% decrease if baseline is ≥10 cm palpable below LCM. Minor response means either >50% decrease if baseline is <10 cm from LCM or >30% decrease if baseline is ≥10 cm from LCM
- *Thrombocytopenia*: Response indicates >50% increase from baseline and an absolute platelet count of 50,000/mm³
- *Hypercatabolic symptoms*: Patients needed to maintain response for ≥1 month to be considered responses. Response indicates complete resolution in patients with baseline fever, weight loss, or drenching night sweats

Therapy Monitoring

Monitor white blood cell count and differential on an ongoing basis, especially in patients who may be more prone to develop neutropenia

Toxicity*,†

	G1	G2	G3	G4	All Grades
Neutropenia					
Mayo Clinic‡	1 (4)	6 (22)	7 (23)	1 (4)	15 (56)
MDACC§	0	0	4 (10)	9 (22)	13 (32)
Fatigue					
Mayo Clinic	2 (7)	8 (30)	2 (7)	2 (7)	14 (52)
MDACC	0	0	3 (7)	0	3 (7)
Thrombocytopenia					
Mayo Clinic	5 (19)	3 (11)	2 (7)	0	10 (37)
MDACC	0	0	4 (10)	7 (17)	11 (27)
Pruritus					
Mayo Clinic	8 (30)	2 (7)	0	0	190 (37)
MDACC	8 (20)	0	1 (2)	0	9 (22)
Anemia					
Mayo Clinic	0	4 (15)	2 (7)	1 (4)	7 (26)
MDACC	0	0	0	0	0
Dyspnea/Hypoxia					
Mayo Clinic	0	1 (4)	4 (15)	0	5 (19)
MDACC	0	0	0	0	0
Rash					
Mayo Clinic	0	1 (4)	1 (4)	1 (4)	3 (11)
MDACC	8 (20)	6 (15)	2 (5)	0	16 (39)

*Adverse event episodes that occurred in more than 1 patient and were attributed as being possibly, probably, or definitely related to drug in patients with MMM
†Toxicity grades are according to the U.S. National Cancer Institute Common Terminology Criteria for Adverse Events, version 3.0
‡Treated at Mayo Clinic (lenalidomide 10 mg/day; n = 27)
§Treated at M.D. Anderson Cancer Center (MDACC; n = 41; lenalidomide 10 mg or 5 mg/day)

PRIMARY MYELOFIBROSIS (PMF) REGIMEN: HYDROXYUREA

Löfvenberg E, Wahlin A. Eur J Haematol 1988;41:375–381
Martínez-Trillos A et al. Ann Hematol 2010;89:1233–1237

Hydroxyurea 500 mg/day; administer orally, continually (initial total dose/week = 3500 mg)
Notes:
- Modify dosage according to the efficacy and tolerability in each patient
- In the study by Martínez-Trillos et al, median maintenance daily hydroxyurea dose in responding patients was 700 mg (range: 500–2000 mg)
- Clinical end points for titrating the hydroxyurea dosage:
  - Disappearance of symptoms that motivated starting hydroxyurea
  - Improvement or normalization of clinical and hematologic parameters that led to using hydroxyurea (spleen size in case of symptomatic splenomegaly, and leukocyte and platelet counts in case of leukocytosis or thrombocytosis)

Cervantes F et al. Haematologica 2000;85:595–599

Supportive Care
Antiemetic prophylaxis
Emetogenic potential is **MINIMAL–LOW**
See Chapter 42 for antiemetic recommendations

Hematopoietic growth factor (CSF) prophylaxis
Primary prophylaxis is **NOT** *indicated*
See Chapter 43 for more information

Antimicrobial prophylaxis
Risk of fever and neutropenia is **LOW**
  Antimicrobial primary prophylaxis to be considered:
  - Antibacterial—not indicated
  - Antifungal—not indicated
  - Antiviral—not indicated unless patient previously had an episode of HSV

Treatment Modifications

Adverse Event	Treatment Modification
Hematologic Toxicity	
WBC count <3500/mm³ or platelet count <100,000/mm³	Hold hydroxyurea until WBC >3500/mm³ and platelet >100,000/mm³, then restart hydroxyurea at 50% of prior dose
Nonhematologic Toxicity	
G1	No dose modifications
G2/3	Hold hydroxyurea until toxicity G ≤1, then restart at prior dose
Recurrent G2/3	Hold hydroxyurea until toxicity G ≤1, then restart at 75% of prior dose
G4	Hold hydroxyurea until toxicity G ≤1, then restart at 50% of prior dose
Recurrent G4	Discontinue hydroxyurea

Patient Population Studied

Martínez-Trillos A et al. Ann Hematol 2010;89:1233–1237

Forty from among 157 subjects consecutively diagnosed with primary myelofibrosis (n = 127), or post-ET (n = 20), or post-PV (n = 10) myelofibrosis. Patients received hydroxyurea as treatment for hyperproliferative manifestations of myelofibrosis, including constitutional symptoms (weight loss, night sweats, low-grade fevers), symptomatic splenomegaly, pruritus, bone pain, leukocytosis, and thrombocytosis. The diagnosis of myelofibrosis was made according to the criteria accepted at the time patients were diagnosed, but in all cases, current WHO criteria were fulfilled

Efficacy

Martínez-Trillos A et al. Ann Hematol 2010;89:1233–1237

	Number of Patients	Response Rate (%)*
Overall Clinical and Hematologic Responses According to EUMNET Criteria*		
Complete plus major response		30%
Moderate plus minor response		32%
Failure		38%†
Overall Clinical and Hematologic Responses According IWG-MRT Criteria*		
Clinical improvement	16/40	40%
Disappearance of palpable splenomegaly	4/40	10%
Reduction in spleen size ≥50%	12/40	30%
Hemoglobin value increase >2 g/dL	5/40	12.5%
Median duration of the response	13.2 months (range: 3–126.2 months)	
Alive‡	14 (35%)	
Dead§	26 (65%)	
Response by Specific Features in 40 Patients with Myelofibrosis Treated with Hydroxyurea*		
Constitutional symptoms	18	82
Symptomatic splenomegaly	8	45
Pruritus	2	50
Bone pain	2	100
Leukocytosis	9	81
Thrombocytosis	11	71

*The response was evaluated using the criteria of the European Myelofibrosis Network (EUMNET) and those of the International Working Group for Myelofibrosis Research and Treatment (IWG-MRT). The minimum time to assess the response was 3 months. Responses include complete plus partial responses according to EUMNET criteria
†Among patients whose disease did not respond, 5 eventually developed acute transformation at a median of 18.8 months (range: 11.9–25.3 months) after the start of hydroxyurea, 2 received allo-HSCT and died from complications related to the procedure, and 2 required splenectomy or splenic radiation as salvage therapy for symptomatic splenomegaly
‡Thirteen patients were still receiving hydroxyurea maintenance
§Causes of death included disease progression (n = 8, including acute transformation in 5 patients), infection (n = 5), bleeding (n = 3), thrombosis (n = 3), complications of allo-HSCT (n = 2), liver failure and cardiac insufficiency (n = 1 each), and unknown causes (n = 3)

Toxicity

Hematologic Toxicity	18/40 (45%)
Appearance or worsening of a preexisting anemia*	14/40 (35%)
Required concomitant treatment for anemia*,†	26/40 (65%)
Concomitant epoetin alfa or darbepoetin alfa†	17/40 (42.5)
Concomitant danazol†	9/40 (22.5%)
Pancytopenia	4/40 (10%)
Nonhematologic Toxicity	6/40 (15%)
Oral or leg ulcers‡	5/40 (12.5%)
Gastrointestinal symptoms	1/40 (2.5%)

Toxicities Included in Product Labeling§

Hematologic Side Effects
1. Neutropenia common
2. Thrombocytopenia and anemia are less common than neutropenia, and seldom occur without preceding leukopenia
   a. Hydroxyurea causes macrocytosis which may mask incidental folic acid deficiency
      (1) Folic acid supplementation is recommended during treatment with hydroxyurea
3. Cytopenias often are rapidly reversible within 3–4 days but may take 7–21 days to recover after drug discontinued
4. High doses and/or failure to interrupt treatment despite cytopenia may result in prolonged aplasia

Nonhematologic Side Effects

Relatively common
1. Gastrointestinal symptoms:
   - Stomatitis/mucositis
   - Anorexia
   - Mild nausea/vomiting
   - Diarrhea
   - Constipation
2. Acute skin reactions
   - Rash
   - Painful lower extremity ulcerations
   - Dermatomyositis-like changes
   - Erythema
   - Nail ridging or discoloration

Rare
1. Chronic skin reactions
   - Hyperpigmentation
   - Atrophy of skin and nails
2. Skin cancer
3. Alopecia
4. Headache
5. Drowsiness
6. Convulsions
7. Constitutional symptoms:
   - Fever
   - Chills
   - Asthenia
8. Renal impairment
9. Hepatic impairment

*Median hydroxyurea dose received by patients who developed hydroxyurea-induced anemia was 643 mg/day (range: 143–1500 mg) versus 1000 mg/day (range: 143–1500 mg) for patients who did not require a specific treatment for anemia. The difference between groups was not significant (Mann-Whitney U test)
†Twelve patients responded to epoetin alfa or darbepoetin alfa, 7 patients responded to danazol, but in all cases, responses were short-lived
‡Median daily hydroxyurea dose in patients developing ulcers was 1340 mg (range: 500–2000 mg)
§Droxia—hydroxyurea capsule; product labeling, January 2012. Bristol-Myers Squibb Company, Princeton, NJ

Boxed warning (FDA-approved product label):
Hydroxyurea is mutagenic and clastogenic, and causes cellular transformation to a tumorigenic phenotype. Hydroxyurea is thus unequivocally genotoxic and a presumed trans-species carcinogen that implies a carcinogenic risk to humans. Secondary leukemias have been reported in patients receiving hydroxyurea for long periods for myeloproliferative disorders, such as polycythemia vera and thrombocythemia. It is not known whether the leukemogenic effect is secondary to hydroxyurea or is associated with the underlying disease. Physicians and patients must very carefully consider the potential benefits of hydroxyurea relative to the undefined risk of developing secondary malignancies

Therapy Monitoring

Frequent monitoring of CBC is necessary to prevent excessive marrow suppression. Obtain CBC with leukocyte differential every 1–2 weeks for the first 2 months, every month thereafter, and every 3 months after reaching a steady state

PRIMARY MYELOFIBROSIS (PMF) REGIMEN: RUXOLITINIB

Harrison C et al. N Engl J Med 2012;366:787–798
Verstovsek S et al. N Engl J Med 2012;366:799–807

Ruxolitinib (see dose in table below); administer orally, twice daily, without regard to food, continuously

Notes:

- The recommended starting dose of **ruxolitinib** is based on platelet count (see table below). A complete blood count (CBC) and platelet count must be performed before initiating therapy

Platelet Count	Ruxolitinib Starting Dose
>200,000/mm^3	20 mg; administer orally twice daily (total dosage/week = 280 mg)
100,000–200,000/mm^3	15 mg; administer orally twice daily (total dosage/week = 210 mg)
50,000 to <100,000/mm^3	5 mg; administer orally twice daily (total dosage/week = 70 mg)

- Patients who miss a dose of ruxolitinib should be advised not to take an additional dose, but instead to take the next usual prescribed dose at the next regularly scheduled time

- Ruxolitinib may be administered through a nasogastric tube (≥8 French):
  - Suspend 1 tablet in 40 mL of water and stir for 10 minutes
  - Within 6 hours after the tablet has dispersed, administer through tube using an appropriate syringe
  - Rinse the tube with 75 mL of water

- If discontinuing ruxolitinib for reasons other than thrombocytopenia, consider gradual tapering by 5 mg twice daily each week to minimize the risk of myeloproliferative neoplasm symptom exacerbation. Advise patients not to interrupt or discontinue ruxolitinib treatment without consulting their treating health care provider

- See Treatment Modifications section for recommended dose modifications for adverse events, insufficient response, drug interactions, renal impairment, and hepatic impairment

Supportive Care

Antiemetic prophylaxis
Emetogenic potential is **MINIMAL–LOW**
See Chapter 42 for antiemetic recommendations

Hematopoietic growth factor (CSF) prophylaxis
Primary prophylaxis is **NOT** indicated
See Chapter 43 for more information

Antimicrobial prophylaxis
Risk of fever and neutropenia is **LOW**
  Antimicrobial primary prophylaxis to be considered:
  - Antibacterial—not indicated
  - Antifungal—not indicated
  - Antiviral—not indicated unless patient previously had an episode of HSV

Treatment Modifications

Ruxolitinib Dose Reductions for Adverse Events

Adverse Event	Treatment Modification	
Bleeding		
Bleeding requiring intervention, irrespective of platelet count	Withhold ruxolitinib therapy. Upon resolution of bleeding, consider resuming treatment at the prior dose if the underlying cause of bleeding has been controlled. If the underlying cause persists, consider resuming treatment at a lower dose	
Withdrawal Syndrome		
Patient with symptom exacerbation following interruption, discontinuation. or tapering of ruxolitinib treatment (fever, respiratory distress, hypotension, DIC, MOF)	Evaluate for and treat any intercurrent illness and consider restarting or increasing the dose of ruxolitinib. DIC, disseminated intravascular coagulation; MOF, multiorgan failure	
Hematologic Toxicity in Patients with a Pre-treatment Platelet Count of $\geq100,000/mm^3$		
Platelet count 100,000 to <125,000/mm^3	*Current dose 25 mg twice daily*	Reduce dose to 20 mg twice daily
	Current dose 20 mg twice daily	Reduce dose to 15 mg twice daily
	Current dose between 5 mg twice daily and 15 mg twice daily	No change
Platelet count 75,000 to <100,000/mm^3	*Current dose between 15 mg twice daily and 25 mg twice daily*	Reduce dose to 10 mg twice daily
	Current dose between 5 mg twice daily and 10 mg twice daily	No change
Platelet count 50,000 to <75,000/mm^3	*Current dose between 10 mg twice daily and 25 mg twice daily*	Reduce dose to 5 mg twice daily
	Current dose is 5 mg twice daily	No change
Platelet count <50,000/mm^3	Withhold ruxolitinib dosing until recovery of platelet count to >50,000/mm^3, then resume at a dose based on the current recovery platelet count as follows: • *Platelet count $\geq125,000/mm^3$*: resume at 20 mg twice daily • *Platelet count 100,000 to <125,000/mm^3*: resume at 15 mg twice daily • *Platelet count 75,000 to <100,000/mm^3*: resume at 10 mg twice daily for ≥2 weeks; if stable, may increase to 15 mg twice daily • *Platelet count 50,000 to <75,000/mm^3*: resume at 5 mg twice daily for ≥2 weeks; if stable, may increase to 10 mg twice daily • *Platelet count <50,000/mm^3*: continue holding	
ANC <500/mm^3	Withhold ruxolitinib dosing until recovery of ANC to >750/mm^3, then resume dosing at the higher of 5 mg once daily or 5 mg twice daily below the largest dose in the week prior to the treatment interruption	
Hematologic Toxicity in Patients with a Pre-treatment Platelet Count Between 50,000 and <100,000/mm^3		
Platelet count 25,000 to <35,000/mm^3 AND the platelet count decline is $\geq20\%$ during the prior 4 weeks	Decrease the dose by 5 mg twice daily. For patients on 5 mg twice daily, decrease the dose to 5 mg once daily. For patients on 5 mg once daily, maintain the dose at 5 mg once daily	
Platelet count 25,000 to <35,000/mm^3 AND the platelet count decline is <20% during the prior 4 weeks	Decrease the dose by 5 mg once daily. For patients on 5 mg once daily, maintain the dose at 5 mg once daily	
Platelet count <25,000/mm^3	Withhold ruxolitinib dosing until recovery of platelet count to >35,000/mm^3, then resume dosing at the higher of 5 mg once daily or 5 mg twice daily below the largest dose in the week prior to the decrease in platelet count to <25,000/mm^3 that led to dose interruption	
ANC <500/mm^3	Withhold ruxolitinib dosing until recovery of ANC to >750/mm^3, then resume dosing at the higher of 5 mg once daily or 5 mg twice daily below the largest dose in the week prior to the decrease in ANC below <500/mm^3 that led to dose interruption	

(continued)

Treatment Modifications (continued)

Ruxolitinib Dose Increases for Insufficient Response

Parameter	Treatment Modification
Efficacy considered insufficient in a patient with a pre-treatment platelet count ≥100,000/mm³ who meets all of the following conditions: 1. Failure to achieve either a reduction of 50% in palpable spleen length or a 35% reduction in spleen volume as measured by CT or MRI in comparison with pretreatment baseline 2. Platelet count >125,000/mm³ at 4 weeks and platelet count never <100,000/mm³ 3. ANC >750/mm³	Consider a dose increase in 5-mg twice-daily increments to a maximum of 25 mg twice daily. Doses should not be increased during the first 4 weeks of therapy and doses should not be increased more frequently than every 2 weeks
Efficacy considered insufficient in a patient with a pre-treatment platelet count between 50,000 and <100,000/mm³ who meets all of the following conditions: 1. Failure to achieve either a reduction of 50% in palpable spleen length or a 35% reduction in spleen volume as measured by CT or MRI in comparison with pretreatment baseline 2. Platelet count has remained >40,000/mm³ 3. Platelet count has not fallen by >20% in the prior 4 weeks 4. ANC >1000/mm³ 5. Dose has not been reduced or interrupted for an adverse event or hematologic toxicity in the prior 4 weeks	Consider a dose increase in 5-mg daily increments to a maximum of 10 mg twice daily. Doses should not be increased during the first 4 weeks of therapy and doses should not be increased more frequently than every 2 weeks

Ruxolitinib Dose Modifications for Drug Interactions, Renal Impairment, or Hepatic Impairment

Parameter	Treatment Modification	
Ruxolitinib is to be newly initiated in a patient where use of a strong CYP3A4 inhibitor or fluconazole dose ≤200 mg* is unavoidable	*Baseline platelet count is ≥100,000/mm³*	Reduce the starting dose of ruxolitinib to 10 mg twice daily
	Baseline platelet count is between 50,000 and <100,000/mm³	Reduce the starting dose of ruxolitinib to 5 mg once daily
A strong CYP3A4 inhibitor or fluconazole dose ≤200 mg* is to be initiated in a patient on a stable dose of ruxolitinib	*Ruxolitinib dose before starting the CYP3A4 inhibitor is ≥10 mg twice daily*	Decrease ruxolitinib dose by 50% (round up to the closest available tablet strength)
	Ruxolitinib dose before starting the CYP3A4 inhibitor is 5 mg twice daily	Decrease ruxolitinib dose to 5 mg once daily
	Ruxolitinib dose before starting the CYP3A4 inhibitor is 5 mg once daily	Avoid strong CYP3A4 inhibitor or fluconazole treatment or interrupt ruxolitinib treatment for the duration of strong CYP3A4 inhibitor or fluconazole use

(continued)

Treatment Modifications (*continued*)

Parameter	Treatment Modification	
Moderate (CrCl = 30–59 mL/min; 0.5–0.98 mL/s) or severe (CrCl = 15–29 mL/min; 0.25–0.48 mL/s) renal impairment	*Baseline platelet count >150,000/mm³*	No treatment modification needed
	Baseline platelet count between 100,000 and ≤150,000/ mm³	Reduce starting dose to 10 mg twice daily
	Baseline platelet count between 50,000 and <100,000/mm³	Reduce starting dose to 5 mg once daily
	Baseline platelet count <50,000/mm³	Avoid use
ESRD (CrCl <15 mL/min; <0.25 mL/s) on hemodialysis	*Baseline platelet count between 100,000 and ≤200,000/ mm³*	Reduce starting dosage to 15 mg once after each dialysis session
	Baseline platelet count >200,000/mm³	Reduce starting dosage to 20 mg once after each dialysis session
ESRD (CrCl <15 mL/min; <0.25 mL/s) not requiring dialysis	Avoid ruxolitinib use	
Hepatic impairment of any severity (ie, mild [Child-Pugh class A], moderate [Child-Pugh class B], or severe [Child-Pugh class C])	*Baseline platelet count >150,000/mm³*	No treatment modification needed
	Baseline platelet count between 100,000 and ≤150,000/mm³	Reduce starting dose to 10 mg twice daily
	Baseline platelet count between 50,000 and <100,000/mm³	Reduce starting dose to 5 mg once daily
	Baseline platelet count <50,000/mm³	Avoid use

*Avoid use of fluconazole at doses >200 mg

DIC, disseminated intravascular coagulation; MOF, multiorgan failure; ANC, absolute neutrophil count; CT, computed tomography; MRI, magnetic resonance imaging; CrCl, creatinine clearance; ESRD, end-stage renal disease

Patient Population Studied

International Prognostic Scoring System—prognostic factors:

1. Age >65 years
2. Hemoglobin level <10 g/dL
3. Leukocyte count of >25,000/mm³
4. ≥1% circulating myeloblasts
5. Presence of constitutional symptoms

Verstovsek S et al. N Engl J Med 2012;366:799–807

Patients with primary myelofibrosis, post–polycythemia vera myelofibrosis, or post–essential thrombocythemia myelofibrosis according to 2008 World Health Organization criteria, with a life expectancy of ≥6 months, an International Prognostic Scoring System (IPSS) score of 2 (intermediate–2 risk) or 3 or more (high risk), an Eastern Cooperative Oncology Group (ECOG) performance status ≤3 (on a scale from 0 to 5, with higher scores indicating greater disability), <10% peripheral blood blasts, an absolute peripheral blood CD34+ cell count >20/mm³, a platelet count >100,000/mm³, and palpable splenomegaly (≥5 cm below the left costal margin). Patients had disease that was refractory to available therapies, had side effects requiring their discontinuation, or were not candidates for available therapies and had disease-requiring treatment

Harrison C et al. N Engl J Med 2012;366:787–798

Patients who had primary myelofibrosis, post–polycythemia vera myelofibrosis, or post–essential thrombocythemia myelofibrosis and a palpable spleen ≥5 cm below the costal margin, irrespective of their JAK2 V617F mutation status. Eligible patients had 2 prognostic factors (intermediate–2 risk) or ≥3 prognostic factors (high risk) according to the International Prognostic Scoring System, a peripheral blood blast count <10%, a platelet count ≥100,000/mm³, an ECOG performance status ≤3, and no prior treatment with a JAK inhibitor. In addition, eligible patients were not considered to be suitable candidates for allogeneic stem cell transplantation at the time of enrollment

Efficacy

Verstovsek S et al. N Engl J Med 2012;366:799–807

	Ruxolitinib N = 129–139	Placebo N = 103–106	
Proportion of patients with ≥35% reduction in spleen volume at week 24	41.9%	0.7%	OR 134.4 P<0.001
Mean percentage change in spleen volume	−31.6%	+8.1%	
Median percentage change in spleen volume	−33.0%	+8.5%	
35% reduction in spleen volume maintained ≥48 weeks	67.0%		
Proportion of patients with ≥50% reduction in total symptom score from baseline to week 24	45.9%	5.3%	OR 15.3 P<0.001
Mean change symptom score from baseline to week 24	−46.1%*	+41.8%*	
Median change symptom score from baseline to week 24	−56.2%*	+14.6%*	P<0.001
Subgroups[†]			
≥50% improvement in spleen-related symptoms[‡] with a reduction in spleen volume of ≥35%	62.7%		
≥50% improvement in spleen-related symptoms[‡] with a reduction in spleen volume of <35%	46.9%		
≥50% improvement in non-abdominal symptoms[§] with a reduction in spleen volume of ≥35%	58.6%		
≥50% improvement in non-abdominal symptoms[§] with a reduction in spleen volume of <35%	54.1%		
Mean percentage change in spleen volume, patients with JAK2 V617F mutation	−34.6%	+8.1%	P = 0.07 For interaction
Mean percentage change in spleen volume, patients without JAK2 V617F mutation	−23.8%	+8.4%	
Mean change symptom score from baseline to week 24, patients with JAK2 V617F	−52.6%*	+42.8%*	P = 0.11 For interaction
Mean change symptom score from baseline to week 24, patients without JAK2 V617F	−28.1%*	+37.2%*	
Biomarkers[¶]			
Mean change in JAK2 V617F allele burden at week 24	−10.9%	+3.5%	
Mean change in JAK2 V617F allele burden at week 48	−21.5%	+6.3%	

*− means improvement in symptoms; + means worsening of symptoms
[†]Across myelofibrosis subtypes (primary myelofibrosis, post–polycythemia vera myelofibrosis, and post–essential thrombocythemia myelofibrosis), patients who received ruxolitinib had a decrease in spleen volume and improvement in the total symptom score; patients receiving placebo had increases in spleen volume (P = 0.52 for interaction) and worsening of the total symptom score (P = 0.46 for interaction)
[‡]As indicated by the sum of Myelofibrosis Symptom Assessment Form (version 2.0) scores for abdominal discomfort, pain under the ribs on the left side, and a feeling of fullness (early satiety)
[§]Night sweats, bone or muscle pain, and pruritus
[¶]Patients receiving ruxolitinib also had reductions in plasma levels of C-reactive protein and the proinflammatory cytokines, tumor necrosis factor α, and interleukin 6, and increases in levels of plasma leptin and erythropoietin

Harrison C et al. N Engl J Med 2012;366:787–798

(continued)

Efficacy (continued)

	Ruxolitinib N = 149	Best Available N = 73
Proportion of patients with ≥35% reduction in spleen volume at week 24	32%*	0*
Proportion of patients with ≥35% reduction in spleen volume at week 48	28%*	0*
Mean percentage change in spleen volume*,†	−29.2%*	+2.7%*
Mean percentage change in spleen volume*,†	−30.1%*	+7.3%*
Median time to first observation on MRI or CT of a reduction ≥35% reduction in spleen volume from baseline	12 weeks	
The median duration of response	>12 months (80% at 12 months)	
Progression at 48 weeks	30%	26%
Mean Change from Baseline at 48 Weeks—EORTC QLQ-C30 Core Model Scores‡,§		
Global health status and quality of life§	+9.1	+3.4
Role functioning§	+3.4	−5.4
Mean Change from Baseline at 48 Weeks—EORTC QLQ-C30 Symptom Scores∊		
Fatigue∊	−12.8	+0.4
Pain∊	−1.9	+3.0
Dyspnea∊	−6.3	+4.8
Insomnia∊	−12.3	+6.0
Appetite loss∊	−8.2	+9.5
Mean Change from Baseline at 48 Weeks—FACT-Lym Scores§		
FACT-Lym Total Scores§ (6.5–11.2)**	+11.3	−0.9
FACT-TOI†† Score§ (5.5–11)**	+9.1	−0.9
FACT-G Total Scores§ (3–7)**	+8.9	+0.1
LymS Score§,‡‡ (2.9–5.4)**	+6.0	+0.7
Subgroups		
≥35% reduction in spleen volume at week 24 in patients with JAK2 V617F mutation	33%	0
≥35% reduction in spleen volume at week 24 in patients without JAK2 V617F mutation	14%	0

EORTC, European Organization for Research and Treatment of Cancer; FACT, Functional Assessment of Cancer Therapy; FACT-Lym, FACT–Lymphoma; FACT-TOI, FACT–Trial Outcome Index

*P<0.001
†Note: + means reduction in size; − means increase of size
‡For EORTC QLQ-C30 functioning and symptom subscales that are not shown, there were minimal between-group differences (ie, a difference of <10 points in the mean change in scores between the ruxolitinib group and the best-available-therapy (BAT) group at weeks 24 and 48)
§Note: + means improvement in symptoms; − means worsening of symptoms
∊Note: − means improvement in symptoms; + means worsening of symptoms
**The ranges in parentheses represent values for minimal clinically important differences
††FACT-TOI Scores: A summary of physical, functional, and disease-specific outcomes
‡‡FACT-LymS: Disease-specific subscale
Note: levels of several proinflammatory cytokines, including interleukin 6, tumor necrosis factor α, and C-reactive protein were reduced, whereas erythropoietin and leptin levels were increased

Toxicity*

Verstovsek S et al. N Engl J Med 2012;366:799–807

	Ruxolitinib (N = 155)		Placebo (N = 151)	
	% All Grades	% G3/4	% All Grades	% G3/4
Nonhematologic fatigue	25.2	5.2	33.8	6.6
Diarrhea	23.2	1.9	21.2	0
Peripheral edema	18.7	0	22.5	1.3
Bruising[†]	23.2	0.6	14.6	0
Dyspnea	17.4	1.3	17.2	4.0
Dizziness[‡]	18.1	0.6	7.3	0
Nausea	14.8	0	19.2	0.7
Headache	14.8	0	5.3	0
Constipation	12.9	0	11.9	0
Vomiting	12.3	0.6	9.9	0.7
Pain in extremity	12.3	1.3	9.9	0
Insomnia	11.6	0	9.9	0
Arthralgia	11.0	1.9	8.6	0.7
Pyrexia	11.0	0.6	7.3	0.7
Abdominal pain	10.3	2.6	41.1	11.3
Weight gain	7.1	0.6	1.3	0.7
Flatulence	5.2	0	0.7	0
Hematologic Abnormalities				
Anemia[§]	96.1	45.2	86.8	19.2
Thrombocytopenia[§]	69.7	12.9	30.5	1.3
Neutropenia[§]	18.7	7.1	4.0	2.0
↑Alanine transaminase (ALT)	25.2	1.3	7.3	—
↑Aspartate transaminase (AST)	17.4	0	6	—
↑Cholesterol	16.8	0	0.7	—

*National Cancer Institute Common Terminology Criteria for Adverse Events (CTCAE), version 3.0
[†]Includes contusion, ecchymosis, hematoma, injection site hematoma, periorbital hematoma, vessel puncture site hematoma, increased tendency to bruise, petechiae, purpura
[‡]Includes dizziness, postural dizziness, vertigo, balance disorder, Meniere disease, labyrinthitis
[§]Presented as worst-grade values regardless of baseline
Data from Verstovsek et al., and from JAKAFI (ruxolitinib) tablets, for oral use; product label, November 2011. Incyte Corporation, Wilmington, DE

Harrison C et al. N Engl J Med 2012;366:787–798

(continued)

Toxicity* (continued)

Adverse Event	Ruxolitinib (N = 146)		Best Available Therapy (N = 73)	
	All Grades	G3/4	All Grades	G3/4
	Number of Patients (Percentage)			
Nonhematologic				
Diarrhea	34 (23)	2 (1)	9 (12)	0
Peripheral edema	32 (22)	0	19 (26)	0
Asthenia	26 (18)	2 (1)	7 (10)	1 (1)
Dyspnea	23 (16)	1 (1)	13 (18)	3 (4)
Nasopharyngitis	23 (16)	0	10 (14)	0
Pyrexia	20 (14)	3 (2)	7 (10)	0
Cough	20 (14)	0	11 (15)	1 (1)
Nausea	19 (13)	1 (1)	5 (7)	0
Arthralgia	18 (12)	1 (1)	5 (7)	0
Fatigue	18 (12)	1 (1)	6 (8)	0
Pain in extremity	17 (12)	1 (1)	3 (4)	0
Abdominal pain	16 (11)	5 (3)	10 (14)	2 (3)
Headache	15 (10)	2 (1)	3 (4)	0
Back pain	14 (10)	3 (2)	8 (11)	0
Pruritus	7 (5)	0	9 (12)	0

Hematologic

	G1	G2	G3	G4	G1	G2	G3	G4
Anemia	24 (16)	55 (38)	50 (34)	12 (8)	16 (23)	28 (40)	15 (21)	7 (10)
Thrombocytopenia	46 (32)	42 (28)	9 (6)	3 (2)	11 (16)	4 (6)	3 (4)	2 (3)

Serious

Adverse Event	Ruxolitinib	Best Available Therapy
Abdominal pain	3 (2)	1 (1)
Pyrexia	3 (2)	1 (1)
Esophageal varices	3 (2)	0
Dyspnea	2 (1)	3 (4)
Pneumonia	1 (1)	4 (5)
Actinic keratosis	0	2 (3)
Ascites	0	2 (3)
Peritoneal hemorrhage	0	2 (3)
Respiratory failure	0	2 (3)

Therapy Monitoring

1. A complete blood count (CBC) with leukocyte differential and platelet count must be performed before initiating therapy, every 2–4 weeks until doses are stabilized, and then as clinically indicated

2. Renal and liver function tests before starting treatment with ruxolitinib (baseline), with serial reassessment as clinically indicated

3. Assess for the presence of tuberculosis risk factors (eg, prior residence in or travel to countries with a high prevalence of tuberculosis, close contact with a person with active tuberculosis, and a history of active or latent tuberculosis where an adequate course of treatment cannot be confirmed). If a risk factor is present, screen for latent tuberculosis prior to initiation of ruxolitinib. For patients with evidence of active or latent tuberculosis, consult a physician with expertise in the treatment of tuberculosis before starting ruxolitinib. The decision to continue ruxolitinib during treatment of active tuberculosis should be based on the overall risk-benefit determination

4. Between 8–12 weeks after initiation of ruxolitinib, obtain a fasting lipid panel

5. When doses are interrupted, discontinued, or reduced, monitor for exacerbation of symptoms associated with the underlying myeloproliferative neoplasm such as fever, respiratory distress, hypotension, diffuse intravascular coagulation, and multiorgan failure

6. Advise patients to report and periodically assess for signs and symptoms of:
   a. Infection
   b. Progressive multifocal leukoencephalopathy
   c. Non-melanoma skin cancers

PRIMARY MYELOFIBROSIS (PMF) REGIMEN: FEDRATINIB

Pardanani A et al. JAMA Oncol 2015;1:643–651
Trial protocol for: Pardanani A et al. JAMA Oncol 2015;1:643–651
Supplementary online content to: Pardanani A et al. JAMA Oncol 2015;1:643–651
INREBIC (fedratinib) capsules. Summit, NJ: Celgene Corporation; revised August 2019

Fedratinib 400 mg; administer orally once daily, continually (total dosage/week = 2800 mg)
Notes:

• Advise patients that administration with a high-fat meal may reduce the incidence or severity of nausea or vomiting

• Patients who delay taking fedratinib at a regularly scheduled time should take the next dose at the next regularly scheduled time

• Patients who are being transitioned from ruxolitinib to fedratinib should taper and discontinue ruxolitinib prior to initiation of fedratinib. Refer to the U.S. Food and Drug Administration approved prescribing information for ruxolitinib

• Avoid concomitant use of moderate or strong CYP3A4 inducers with fedratinib

• Avoid concomitant use of dual CYP3A4 and CYP2C19 inhibitors with fedratinib

• If concomitant use of a strong CYP3A4 inhibitor with fedratinib is unavoidable, then reduce the initial dose of fedratinib to 200 mg once daily. If the strong CYP3A4 inhibitor is subsequently discontinued, then increase the fedratinib dosage to 300 mg once daily for 2 weeks, and then to 400 mg once daily thereafter, if tolerated

• In patients with severe renal impairment (creatinine clearance 15–29 mL/min per the Cockcroft-Gault equation), reduce the initial dose of fedratinib to 200 mg once daily

Antiemetic prophylaxis
Emetogenic potential is **MODERATE–HIGH**

• The U.S. Food and Drug Administration-approved prescribing information states to consider providing appropriate anti-emetic therapy (eg, 5-HT3 receptor antagonists) during fedratinib treatment
See Chapter 42 for antiemetic recommendations

Hematopoietic growth factor (CSF) prophylaxis
Primary prophylaxis is **NOT** indicated
See Chapter 43 for more information

Antimicrobial prophylaxis
Risk of fever and neutropenia is **LOW**
Antimicrobial primary prophylaxis to be considered:

• Antibacterial—not indicated

• Antifungal—not indicated

• Antiviral—not indicated unless patient previously had an episode of HSV

Diarrhea management
Latent or delayed-onset diarrhea:
Loperamide 4 mg orally initially after the first loose or liquid stool, *then*
Loperamide 2 mg orally every 2 hours during waking hours, *plus*
Loperamide 4 mg orally every 4 hours during hours of sleep

• Continue for at least 12 hours after diarrhea resolves

• Recurrent diarrhea after a 12-hour diarrhea-free interval is treated as a new episode

• Rehydrate orally with fluids and electrolytes during a diarrheal episode

• If a patient develops blood or mucus in stool, dehydration, or hemodynamic instability, or if diarrhea persists >48 hours despite loperamide, stop loperamide and hospitalize the patient for intravenous hydration

Treatment Modifications

RECOMMENDED DOSE MODIFICATIONS FOR FEDRATINIB

Starting dose (level 1)	400 mg orally once daily
Dose level −1	300 mg orally once daily
Dose level −2	200 mg orally once daily
Dose level −3	Discontinue fedratinib

Grade/Severity	Treatment Modification
Hematologic toxicity	
Baseline platelet count <50,000/mm³	Avoid use of fedratinib
G4 thrombocytopenia (platelet count <25,000/mm³) during therapy	Withhold fedratinib until toxicity has improved to G ≤2 or baseline, then resume fedratinib with the dosage reduced by 1 dose level
G3 thrombocytopenia (platelet count ≥25,000/mm³ and <50,000/mm³) during therapy with active bleeding	
G4 neutropenia (ANC <500/mm³) during therapy	
Patient with new or worsening anemia during therapy and becomes transfusion-dependent	Consider reducing the fedratinib dosage by 1 dose level
Hepatic toxicity	
G ≥3 increase in ALT, AST, or bilirubin, first occurrence	Withhold fedratinib until toxicity has improved to G ≤1 or baseline, then resume fedratinib with the dosage reduced by 1 dose level. Increase the frequency of ALT, AST, direct bilirubin, and total bilirubin monitoring
G ≥3 increase in ALT, AST, or bilirubin, second occurrence	Permanently discontinue fedratinib
CNS toxicity	
Whole blood thiamine level is < LLN in a patient without CNS symptoms concerning for Wernicke encephalopathy	Continue fedratinib. Administer oral thiamine supplementation. Increase the frequency of fasting whole blood thiamine levels until normalization
Wernicke encephalopathy is suspected	Permanently discontinue fedratinib, perform a full neurologic examination, assess a whole blood thiamine level, perform a brain MRI and administer empiric parenteral thiamine. Monitor closely until resolution of symptoms and improvement of thiamine levels to > LLN
Gastrointestinal toxicity	
G ≥3 nausea, vomiting, or diarrhea unresponsive to supportive measures within 48 hours	Withhold fedratinib until toxicity has improved to G ≤1 or baseline, then resume fedratinib with the dosage reduced by 1 dose level. Maximize supportive antiemetic and antidiarrheal therapies. Monitor a whole blood thiamine level in patients with poor nutritional status and replete if needed
Pancreatic toxicity	
G ≥3 elevation of amylase and/or lipase	Withhold fedratinib until toxicity has improved to G ≤1 or baseline, then resume fedratinib with the dosage reduced by 1 dose level
Other nonhematologic toxicities	
G ≥3 other nonhematologic toxicity	Withhold fedratinib until toxicity has improved to G ≤1 or baseline, then resume fedratinib with the dosage reduced by 1 dose level, if clinically appropriate
Hepatic impairment	
Severe hepatic impairment (total bilirubin <3× ULN and any AST)	Avoid fedratinib use

(continued)

Treatment Modifications (continued)

Renal impairment

Moderate renal impairment (CrCl 15–29 mL/min by Cockcroft-Gault equation)	Administer the full dose of fedratinib but monitor more closely for toxicity
Severe renal impairment (CrCl 15–29 mL/min by Cockcroft-Gault equation)	Reduce the initial fedratinib dose to 200 mg orally once daily

Drug interactions

Patient is being transitioned from ruxolitinib to fedratinib	Taper and discontinue ruxolitinib according to its package labeling prior to initiation of fedratinib
Concomitant use of a strong CYP3A4 inhibitor is unavoidable	Reduce the fedratinib starting dose to 200 mg orally once daily
A concurrently administered strong CYP3A4 inhibitor is discontinued in a patient taking fedratinib 200 mg orally once daily	Increase the fedratinib dose to 300 mg orally once daily for the initial 2 weeks following discontinuation of the strong CYP3A4 inhibitor. If tolerated, then increase the dose to 400 mg orally once daily
Patient must take a moderate or strong CYP3A4 inducer	Avoid use of fedratinib
Patient must take a dual inhibitor of CYP3A4 and CYP2C19	

ALT, alanine aminotransferase; AST, aspartate aminotransferase; CNS, central nervous system; LLN, lower limit of normal; MRI, magnetic resonance imaging; ULN, upper limit of normal; CrCl, creatinine clearance

Efficacy (N = 289)

Efficacy Variable by Group	Fedratinib 400 mg (N = 96)		Fedratinib 500 mg (N = 97)		Placebo (N = 96)	
	Week 24	Confirmed Week 24*	Week 24	Confirmed Week 24*	Week 24	Confirmed Week 24*
Splenic response—n/N (%) (95% CI)						
All patients	45/96 (47) (37–57)†	35/96 (36) (27–46)†	48/97 (49) (40–59)†	39/97 (40) (30–50)†	1/96 (1) (0–3)	1/96 (1) (0–3)
Splenic response by baseline platelet count—n/ subgroup N (%)						
≥ 100 × 10³/μL	40/82 (49)	32/82 (39)	42/82 (51)	34/82 (42)	1/77 (<1)	1/77 (<1)
> 100 × 10³/μL	5/14 (36)	3/14 (21)	6/15 (40)	5/15 (33)	0/18 (0)	0/18 (0)
Splenic response by baseline disease subtype—n/ subgroup N (%)						
Primary MF	29/62 (47)	21/62 (34)	32/63 (51)	25/63 (40)	1/58 (2)	1/58 (2)
Post-ET MF	6/10 (60)	5/10 (50)	4/9 (44)	4/9 (44)	0/11 (0)	0/11 (0)
Post-PV MF	10/24 (42)	9/24 (38)	12/25 (48)	10/25 (40)	0/27 (0)	0/27 (0)
Splenic response by baseline risk status‡—n/ subgroup N (%)						
Intermediate-2 risk‡	30/57 (53)	23/57 (40)	26/47 (55)	21/47 (45)	1/46 (2)	1/46 (2)
High risk‡	15/39 (38)	12/39 (31)	22/50 (44)	18/50 (36)	0/50 (0)	0/50 (0)
Splenic response by JAK2 mutational status—n/ subgroup N (%)						
Wild type	10/30 (33)	9/30 (30)	8/20 (40)	7/20 (35)	1/32 (3)	1/32 (3)
Mutant	34/62 (55)	25/62 (40)	37/72 (51)	31/72 (43)	0/59 (0)	0/59 (0)

(continued)

Efficacy (N = 289) *(continued)*

Symptom response (n = 267 total evaluable patients)—n/N (%) (95% CI)§

Group	Fedratinib 400 mg (N = 91 evaluable patients)§	Fedratinib 500 mg (N = 91 evaluable patients)§	Placebo (N = 85 evaluable patients)§
TSS reduction ≥ 50% from baseline to week 24§	33/91 (36) (26–46)ᶜ	31/91 (34) (24–44)ᶜ	6/85 (7) (2–12)

JAK2 V617F allele burden—median % (range)**

Group	Fedratinib 400 mg (N = 62 with baseline positive allele burden)	Fedratinib 500 mg (N = 72 with baseline positive allele burden)	Placebo (N = 59 with baseline positive allele burden)
Change from baseline to 24 weeks	+0.4 (−99 to +196)	+0.8 (−77 to +115)	+2 (−74 to +96)

*Indicates the splenic response in patients who had their splenic response confirmed at week 28, 4 weeks after the initial measurement at week 24 via MRI or CT. A lack of confirmation was due to either the reduction in spleen volume at week 28 being less than 35% despite being ≥ 35% on first measurement or because a confirmatory measurement at week 28 was not available

†Significant difference vs placebo: P<0.001 using a X^2 test with a 2-sided alpha of 0.025

‡Risk status was characterized according to 2008 World Health Organization and modified International Working Group for Myelofibrosis Research and Treatment (IWG-MRT) criteria

§Only patients with baseline TSS were evaluable here, accounting for the lower n per treatment group than the full-group n. TSS was graded using the modified Myelofibrosis Symptom Assessment Form e-diary

ᶜReported as both clinically and statistically significant. Using a step-down procedure for controlling multiplicity of statistical comparisons, P<0.001 using a X^2 test with a 2-sided alpha of 0.025 for each comparison

**Exploratory end point. Burden was determined by collection of whole blood followed by granulocyte isolation and nucleic acid analysis for presence of the JAK2 V617F mutation, a common gain-of-function mutation in MF patients that causes constitutive activation of JAK2. Fedratinib has shown activity against this mutant JAK2 isoform in preclinical work. Allele burden only measured in patients positive for the JAK2 V617F mutation at baseline

CI, confidence interval; MF, myelofibrosis; post-ET, post-essential thrombocythemia; post-PV, post-polycythemia vera; TSS, total symptom score

Note: all patients randomized were included in analyses (intention-to-treat approach). All patients received their assigned treatment except for 1 placebo group patient who died before treatment initiation. Splenic response was defined as a ≥ 35% reduction in spleen volume as measured by MRI or CT from baseline to 24 weeks (end of cycle 6). Patients whose spleen volume was not measured at week 24 or who experienced disease progression before week 24 were considered non-responders for splenic response analyses. The authors indicate that splenic response was greater across all subgroups for both fedratinib groups vs placebo. The protocol notes that progression-free survival and overall survival analyses were planned, but the discussion mentions that the study was terminated early, leaving insufficient follow-up time to analyze these outcomes

Adverse Events (N = 288)

Event	Fedratinib 400 mg (N = 96) All Grades (%)	G3/4 (%)	Fedratinib 500 mg (N = 97) All Grades (%)	G3/4 (%)	Placebo (N = 95) All Grades (%)	G3/4 (%)
Any adverse event	100	54	98	70	94	32
Adverse event leading to treatment discontinuation by week 24	14	13	25	16	8	4
Serious adverse event	27	18	31	24	23	15
Diarrhea	66	5	56	5	16	0
Vomiting	42	3	55	9	5	0
Nausea	64	0	51	6	15	0
Constipation	10	2	18	0	7	0
Asthenia	9	2	16	4	6	1

(continued)

Adverse Events (N = 288) *(continued)*

Event	Fedratinib 400 mg (N = 96)		Fedratinib 500 mg (N = 97)		Placebo (N = 95)	
	All Grades (%)	G3/4 (%)	All Grades (%)	G3/4 (%)	All Grades (%)	G3/4 (%)
Abdominal pain	15	0	12	1	16	1
Fatigue	16	6	10	5	10	0
Dyspnea	8	0	10	1	6	2
Weight decrease	4	0	10	0	5	0
Anemia	99	43	98	60	91	25
Thrombocytopenia	63	17	57	27	51	9
Lymphopenia	57	21	66	27	54	21
Leukopenia	47	6	53	16	19	3
Neutropenia	28	8	44	18	15	4
Infections and infestations*	42	2	39	12	27	4
Increased alanine transaminase	53	3	46	3	17	0
Increased aspartate transaminase	60	2	48	2	29	1
Hyperbilirubinemia	31	2	28	1	40	2
Increased serum creatinine	54	3	63	0	30	1
Increased amylase	26	2	23	3	7	0
Increased lipase	45	13	36	9	6	2

*System organ class
- The most common adverse events leading to discontinuation of study treatment were:
  - Thrombocytopenia (7 patients total) — fedratinib discontinuation due to thrombocytopenia was more frequent among patients with baseline platelet levels < 100 × 10³/μL
  - Cardiac failure (4 patients)
  - Vomiting (4 patients)
  - Diarrhea (4 patients)
- Fedratinib treatment was associated with a decrease in hemoglobin levels, with a nadir reached after 12–16 weeks; there was a partial recovery in the 400-mg fedratinib group but not in the 500-mg fedratinib group
- Alanine aminotransferase and aspartate aminotransferase elevations were generally mild to moderate, asymptomatic, and reversible with fedratinib dose reduction or interruption
- Transition to acute myeloid leukemia occurred in 1 patient in each fedratinib group and 2 patients in the placebo group
- Death attributed to adverse events of study treatment occurred in 1% of patients in the fedratinib 400-mg group and 4% of patients in each of the fedratinib 500-mg and placebo groups
- Wernicke encephalopathy (WE) and encephalopathy of unknown origin each occurred in 1 patient before the data cutoff point and 2 additional cases of WE were identified after database lock; all 4 cases occurred in women who received 500 mg fedratinib. Intravenous thiamine was administered to all patients and each showed some response to treatment, but some cognitive deficits remained in each patient

Therapy Monitoring

1. *Prior to initiation of fedratinib:* CBC with differential and platelet count, whole blood fasting thiamine level, BUN, serum creatinine, liver function tests, amylase, and lipase. Assess baseline nutritional status
   a. Patients with baseline thiamine deficiency should have thiamine repleted prior to initiation of fedratinib
   b. Patients were required to have a baseline platelet count >50,000/mm³ to be eligible for the clinical study
2. *Periodically:*
   a. *Encephalopathy:* serious encephalopathy events (including Wernicke encephalopathy) occurred in 8/608 patients (1.3%) treated with fedratinib in clinical trials. Monitor for ataxia, mental status changes, nystagmus, diplopia, altered mental status, confusion, and memory impairment. In patients with suspected encephalopathy, immediately and permanently discontinue fedratinib, perform a full neurologic examination, assess a whole blood thiamine level, perform a brain MRI, and administer empiric parenteral thiamine
   b. *Myelosuppression:* monitor CBC with differential and platelet count periodically and as clinically indicated
   c. *Gastrointestinal toxicities:* monitor for nausea, vomiting, and diarrhea
   d. *Hepatic and renal toxicity:* monitor liver function tests, BUN, and serum creatinine periodically and as clinically indicated
   e. *Pancreatic toxicity:* monitor amylase and lipase periodically and as clinically indicated

29. Neuroendocrine Tumors

Sara Ekeblad, MD, PhD, and Britt Skogseid, MD, PhD

Epidemiology

Incidence: 1/100,000

~85% sporadic

~15% hereditary, for example, multiple endocrine neoplasia (MEN1), von Hippel-Lindau disease

Median age: 53–57 years

Male to female ratio: 0.8–1.3:1

Ekeblad SB et al. Clin Cancer Res 2008;14:7798–7803
Fischer L et al. Br J Surg 2008;95:627–635
Hochwald SN et al. J Clin Oncol 2002;20:2633–2642
Öberg K, Eriksson B. Best Pract Res Clin Gastroenterol 2005;19:753–781
Tomassetti PD et al. Ann Oncol 2005;16:1806–1810

Pathology

2017 WHO Classification: Gastroenteropancreatic Neuroendocrine Neoplasms (GEP-NEN)

Morphology	Grade	Ki–67 Index (%)	Mitotic Count (2 mm²)
Well-differentiated *neuroendocrine tumor*	Grade 1	<3% of cells Ki67+	Mitotic index <2
Well-differentiated *neuroendocrine tumor*	Grade 2	2–20% of cells Ki67+	Mitotic index 2–20
Well-differentiated *neuroendocrine tumor*	Grade 3	>20% of cells Ki67+	Mitotic index >20
Poorly differentiated *neuroendocrine carcinoma*			
Small cell type	Grade 3	>20% of cells Ki67+	Mitotic index >20
Large cell type	Grade 3	>20% of cells Ki67+	Mitotic index >20
Mixed neuroendocrine-non-neuroendocrine neoplasm			
Tumor-like lesions			

Note: Final grading is assigned based on whichever index (Ki67 or mitotic) places the tumor in the higher grade category
Lloyd RV et al (editors). WHO Classification of Tumors of Endocrine Organs, 4th ed, Volume 10. Lyon: IARC Press; 2017:211

Functional status:
Intestinal NETs
- Presenting with carcinoid syndrome: 20%
- Presenting without carcinoid syndrome: 80%

Notes: Carcinoid syndrome—symptoms and (secreted products):
- Flushing (prostaglandin, kinins, substance P)
- Diarrhea (serotonin)
- Wheezing (histamine, kinins)
- Endocardial fibrosis (serotonin)

Work-up

Radiology
1. Body CT or MRI
2. Positron emission tomography (PET) scan—as part of the staging and preoperative imaging and in selected cases at restaging
   - ^{68}Ga/^{64}Cu-labeled somatostatin analog PET/CT
   - (^{11}C)5-hydroxy-l-tryptophan (5-HTP) PET/CT for well-differentiated tumors
   - Fluorodeoxyglucose (FDG) PET/CT for poorly differentiated tumors
3. If the above not available, then use somatostatin receptor scintigraphy (SRS): Uses *radioactive octreotide*, a drug similar to somatostatin that attaches to tumor cells that have somatostatin receptors. It is less sensitive
4. Serum chromogranin levels may be helpful in following patient
5. Endoscopic ultrasound
6. Intraoperative ultrasound
   - To localize small tumors not visualized by other modalities but suspected because of biochemical findings
   - To localize multiple tumors in MEN1 patients

Biochemistry
1. In all patients with suspected pancreatic endocrine tumor obtain fasting levels of:
   - Insulin, proinsulin, blood glucose
   - Gastrin
   - Glucagon
   - Pancreatic polypeptide
   - Vasoactive intestinal peptide (VIP)
   - Chromogranin A
2. If insulinoma is suspected (high fasting insulin or symptoms of hypoglycemia):
   - 72-hour fast with measurements of insulin, C-peptide, proinsulin, and plasma glucose
   - Consider differential diagnoses, for example, measurement of sulfonylurea in blood to exclude abuse of oral hypoglycemic drugs

(continued)

(continued)

Pathology (continued)

Pancreatic NETs
Nonfunctioning: 59–76%
Functioning: 24–41%
Insulinoma: 8–17%
Gastrinoma: 10–14%
Glucagonoma: 1–6%
VIPoma: 2–5%

Notes: Functioning tumors—symptoms and (secreted products):
- Zollinger-Ellison syndrome (gastrin)
- Hypoglycemia (insulin)
- Necrolytic erythema (glucagon)
- Hyperglycemia
- WDHA (watery diarrhea, hypokalemia, and achlorhydria) syndrome (vasoactive intestinal polypeptide [VIP])
- Diabetes, gallstones, diarrhea (somatostatin)
- Cushing syndrome (corticotropin-releasing hormone [CRH], adrenocorticotropic hormone [ACTH])
- Acromegaly (growth hormone releasing hormone [GHRH], growth hormone [GH])
- Hypercalcemia (parathyroid hormone related protein [PTHrP])
- Flushing (calcitonin)
- Diarrhea (serotonin)

Ekeblad SB et al. Clin Cancer Res 2008;14:7798–7803
Fischer L et al. Br J Surg 2008;95:627–635
Pape U-F et al. Cancer 2008;113:256–265
Rindi G, Klöppel G. Neuroendocrinology 2004;80(Suppl 1):12–15

Work-up (continued)

3. If gastrinoma is suspected (high fasting gastrin in the absence of treatment with proton pump inhibitors, multiple ulcers, and/or steatorrhea):
   - Measure gastrin after *secretin stimulation test* (after withdrawal of proton pump inhibitors, ideally for 1 week)
   - Measure gastric pH together with fasting gastrin
4. If ectopic Cushing syndrome is suspected to be caused by a pancreatic tumor:
   - Measure 24-hour urine free cortisol excretion, *or* free cortisol to creatinine ratio. A ratio of cortisol >95 μg per gram of creatinine helps confirm hypercortisolism
   - Measure adrenocorticotropic hormone (ACTH) and corticotropin-releasing factor (CRF)

Biopsies
1. If possible, radiologically verified tumors should be biopsied under ultrasound guidance
2. Ideally, biopsy specimens should be evaluated by pathologists knowledgeable in endocrine pathology and stained for:
   - *General markers for pancreatic endocrine tumors:* chromogranin A, synaptophysin
   - *Specific hormones:* Insulin, gastrin, glucagon, VIP, pancreatic polypeptide
   - *Markers of proliferation:* Ki67

MEN1 investigation
1. If MEN1 is suspected (family history, hyperparathyroidism)
   - Measure serum calcium, PTH, prolactin
   - Perform genetic testing

Staging

Stage	Location/Size/Extension	Percentage of Cases
I	Limited to pancreas, <2 cm	5–31
IIa	Limited to pancreas, 2–4 cm	8–9
IIb	Limited to pancreas, >4 cm, *or* Invading duodenum or bile duct	5–7
IIIa	Invading adjacent organs (stomach, spleen, colon, adrenal gland), *or* Invading the wall of large vessels (celiac axis or superior mesenteric artery)	3–8
IIIb	Regional lymph node metastasis	14–15
IV	Distant metastasis	29–60

Ekeblad SB et al. Clin Cancer Res 2008;14:7798–7803
Fischer L et al. Br J Surg 2008;95:627–635
Pape U-F et al. Cancer 2008;113:256–265
Rindi G, Klöppel G. Virchows Arch 2006;449:395–401

Survival

5-Year: 55–64%
10-Year: 44%
Median survival: 90–99 months

Stage	Mean Survival
I	231 months (~19 years)
IIa	222 months (~18.5 years)
IIb	153 months (~13 years)
IIIa	94 months (~8 years)
IIIb	133 months (~11 years)
IV	76 months (~6 years)

Expert Opinion

Pancreatic endocrine tumors are rare, and there is a lack of solid evidence on treatment and outcomes. The following is our view of their management, based on available evidence and many years of clinical experience. Similar general principles apply to intestinal NETs

Diagnosis and work-up

1. Always measure hormone levels if symptoms of a functioning tumor occur or a pancreatic mass is demonstrated
2. Obtain an MRI or CT scan if hormone levels are elevated
   - Obtain somatostatin receptor scintigraphy (radioactive octreotide scan), ^{68}Ga/^{64}Cu-labeled somatostatin analog PET/CT or 5-HTP PET/CT if unclear
3. Patient history: Always probe for family history, history of kidney stones, and history of hyperparathyroidism (MEN1)
4. If MEN1 is suspected, discuss performing genetic testing
   - For known MEN1 carriers, perform annual biochemical screening beginning in adolescence. MRI or CT and/or ^{68}Ga-labeled somatostatin analog PET/CT if hormone levels are elevated
5. Radiologically visualized tumor: Biopsy if radical surgery seems impossible

Surgery

1. Preferably performed by experienced endocrine surgeon at a high-volume center
2. Radical surgery of tumors that can be demonstrated by imaging
3. For tumors that can only be detected biochemically, if fully confident of the analyses, perform a surgical exploration. If a tumor is identified, proceed to resection if possible
4. Aim for pancreas-preserving surgery. If MEN1, distal pancreatectomy in combination with enucleation of lesions in the head of the pancreas is preferable. In addition, consider duodenotomy in case of MEN1 gastrinoma
5. Use intraoperative ultrasound to localize possible additional tumors or very small functioning tumors (especially important for MEN1 tumors)
6. If there is evidence of disease dissemination, consider:
   - Radiofrequency ablation of liver metastases
     - Useful for limited numbers of liver metastases
     - One study showed 45% of patients rendered tumor-free with relatively few complications (Eriksson J et al. World J Surg 2008;32:930–938)
     - Metastases usually recur, but radiofrequency ablation can be performed repeatedly
     - Can alleviate hormonal symptoms
   - Liver embolization
     - Useful if there are a larger number of liver metastases than can be treated with radiofrequency ablation
     - Lessens tumor burden in many patients
     - Can alleviate hormonal symptoms

Systemic treatment

Treat inoperable tumors at once; do not wait for tumor progression to initiate treatment
1. Streptozocin + fluorouracil or streptozocin + doxorubicin have long been considered the first choice for patients with *well-differentiated tumors*
2. Carboplatin + etoposide (or cisplatin plus etoposide) is effective, and, generally, the first choice in patients with *poorly differentiated carcinomas*
3. Temozolomide used as second-line treatment after the combinations mentioned above, or for patients who cannot tolerate more intensive chemotherapy. Temozolomide may be combined with capecitabine (CAP-TEM)
   - Easy to use for the patient as it is taken orally; thus, it can easily be taken in an outpatient setting
   - Test tumor material for O_6-methylguanine-methyltranferase, low levels of which might predict a favorable response to temozolomide
4. Two additional options that may prolong progression-free survival for patients with well and moderately differentiated tumors include sunitinib malate and everolimus. There is no consensus on whether these agents should be used before or after cytotoxic chemotherapy regimens such as streptozocin + fluorouracil
5. Somatostatin analogs should be used to alleviate hormonal symptoms, and might possibly also have antitumor effects, by means of prolonged progression-free survival. Somatostatin analogs can be used in combination with chemotherapy
6. Radionuclide-tagged somatostatin analogs (^{177}Lu-DOTA^0, Tyr^3) are increasingly used
   - A recent study showed a 42% response rate with an acceptable safety profile

(continued)

Expert Opinion (continued)

Supportive care:

Regardless of the therapy used, attention should be given to symptom management as many patients present with debilitating symptoms for which amelioration can significantly improve the quality of their lives:

- *Gastric hyperacidity (patients with a diagnosis of gastrinoma):* **Omeprazole** 40–60 mg per day orally, or an equivalent **proton pump inhibitor** or **histamine (H2)-receptor antagonist** may be used
- *Steatorrhea:* Consider supplementation with **pancreatic enzymes** whenever steatorrhea or changes in bowel habits suggest malabsorption
- *Diarrhea*:*

  Loperamide 4 mg; administer orally initially after the first loose or liquid stool, *then*
  Loperamide 2 mg; administer orally every 2 hours during waking hours, *plus*
  Loperamide 4 mg; administer orally every 4 hours during hours of sleep

  - Continue for at least 12 hours after diarrhea resolves
  - Recurrent diarrhea after a 12-hour diarrhea-free interval is treated as a new episode
  - Rehydrate orally with fluids and electrolytes during a diarrheal episode
  - If a patient develops blood or mucus in stool, dehydration, or hemodynamic instability, or if diarrhea persists >48 hours despite loperamide, stop loperamide and hospitalize the patient for IV hydration

- *Persistent diarrhea:*

  Tincture of opium: Doses are individually titrated. Begin with 2–4 drops mixed in water; administer orally 2–3 times per day, and titrate by decreasing or increasing the number of drops per dose as needed
  Octreotide 50–500 μg; administer subcutaneously 3 times daily. Maximum total daily dose is 1500 μg. Long-acting somatostatin analogs are frequently used

- *Diarrhea in patients who have undergone ileocecal resection:*

  Cholestyramine 4 g/dose; administer orally for 2–6 doses per day (up to 24 g/day)

*Abigerges D et al. J Natl Cancer Inst 1994;86:446–449
Arnold R et al. Gut 1996;38:430–438
Caplin ME et al. N Engl J Med 2014;371:224–233
de Keizer B et al. Eur J Nucl Med Mol Imaging 2008;35:749–755
Ekeblad S et al. Clin Cancer Res 2007;13:2986–2991
Ekeblad SB et al. Clin Cancer Res 2008;14:7798–7803
Eriksson B et al. Cancer 1990;65:1883–1890
Eriksson J et al. World J Surg 2008;32:930–938
Fischer L et al. Br J Surg 2008;95:627–635
Fjällskog M–LH et al. Cancer 2001;92:1101–1107
Hochwald SN et al. J Clin Oncol 2002;20:2633–2642
Kulke MH et al. J Clin Oncol 2008;26:3403–3410
Kwekkeboom DJ et al. J Clin Oncol 2008;26:2124–2130
Moertel CG et al. Cancer 1991;68:227–232
Moertel CG et al. N Engl J Med 1980;303:1189–1194
Moertel CG et al. N Engl J Med 1992;326:519–523
Öberg K, Eriksson B. Best Pract Res Clin Gastroenterol 2005;19:753–781
Pape U-F et al. Cancer 2008;113:256–265
Rindi G, Klöppel G. Neuroendocrinology 2004;80(Suppl 1):12–15
Rindi G, Klöppel G. Virchows Arch 2006;449:395–401
Rothenberg ML et al. J Clin Oncol 2001;19:3801–3807
Strosberg JR et al. Cancer 2011;117:268–275
Tomassetti PD et al. Ann Oncol 2005;16:1806–1810
Wadler S et al. J Clin Oncol 1998;16:3169–3178
Yao JC et al. N Engl J Med 2011; 364:514–523

METASTATIC • LOCALLY ADVANCED

NEUROENDOCRINE TUMORS REGIMEN: SHORT-ACTING OCTREOTIDE ACETATE

Arnold R et al. Gut 1996;38:430–438

Starting dose:	**Octreotide acetate** 50 µg; administer by subcutaneous injection 3 times daily for 3 days
Followed by:	**Octreotide acetate** 100 µg; administer by subcutaneous injection 3 times daily for 3 days
Followed by:	**Octreotide acetate** 200 µg; administer by subcutaneous injection 3 times daily continually, starting on day 7

Duration of treatment: Treatment is continued indefinitely

Supportive Care

Supplemental therapy for all somatostatin analogs:
Pancreatic enzymes to avoid steatorrhea. Individualize dosage by giving the number of tablets or capsules that optimally minimize steatorrhea

Antiemetic prophylaxis
Emetogenic potential is **MINIMAL**
See Chapter 42 for antiemetic recommendations

Hematopoietic growth factor (CSF) prophylaxis
Primary prophylaxis is **NOT** indicated
See Chapter 43 for more information

Antimicrobial prophylaxis
Risk of fever and neutropenia is **LOW**
  Antimicrobial primary prophylaxis to be considered:
  • Antibacterial—not indicated
  • Antifungal—not indicated
  • Antiviral—not indicated unless patient previously had an episode of HSV

Treatment Modifications

Adverse Event	Treatment Modification
Steatorrhea	Increase dose of pancreatic enzyme supplement to 3 capsules with every meal

Patient Population Studied

- One-hundred three patients with gastroenteropancreatic neuroendocrine tumors given somatostatin analogs in a multicenter phase 2 trial
- Patients with functional or nonfunctional, poorly differentiated, intermediate, or small cell carcinoma with high-grade malignant behavior were not included

Efficacy (N = 52)

- No objective tumor regression was seen
- Of patients with progressive pancreatic endocrine tumor, 28% had stabilization of tumor growth for ≥3 months

Tumor Growth in 52 Patients with Confirmed Progression Before Treatment

Responses at Month 3	Responses Reassessed During Months 6–12			
	Death	Progression	Stable Disease	Regression
Death (8)	8			
Progression (30)	11	14	5	0
Stable disease (14)	3	4	7	0
Regression (0)	0	0	0	0
Total (52)	22	18	12	0

Response to octreotide occurred in 19 patients according to the study protocol. WHO criteria used. However, tumors growing slowly but continuously with progression of ≤25% within 3 months also were judged as "progression" if progression ≥25% occurred within 12 months. Response = stable disease or decrease in tumor growth after confirmed progression before treatment, or decrease in tumor growth after stable disease within the pretreatment period, if lasting for at least 3 months

Effect of Octreotide on Flushing, Diarrhea, and Hormone Secretion in Patients with Functional Endocrine GEP Tumors

Symptoms	Normalization	Improvement >50%	No Change	Worse
Diarrhea*				
Month 3 (n = 28)	32.1%	32.1%	21.5%	14.3%
Month 12 (n = 20)	45%	40%	5%	10%
Flushing*				
Month 3 (n = 40)	35%	40%	22.5%	2.5%
Month 12 (n = 27)	44.4%	40.8%	11.1%	3.7%
Hormone secretion				
Month 3 (n = 61)	11.5%	29.5%	34.4%	24.6%
Month 12 (n = 39)	5.1%	28.2%	38.5%	28.2%

GEP tumors, gastroenteropancreatic neuroendocrine tumors
*Patients with carcinoid syndrome, patients with functional tumors

Toxicity

Symptom	All Grades
Diarrhea	34%
Flatulence	27%
Pain at injection site	27%
Vomiting	11%
Steatorrhea	8%
Hyperglycemia	3%
Gall stones	2%
Septicemia	1%

Therapy Monitoring

1. *Every 3 months:* Complete history and physical examination
2. *Every 3–6 months:* Conventional imaging (CT, MRI, or ultrasound), serum electrolytes, and serum glucose
3. *Every year:* Somatostatin receptor scintigraphy (OctreoScan Kit for the Preparation of Indium In–111 Pentetreotide; Mallinckrodt Inc., St. Louis, MO) is controversial
4. *New symptoms:* Somatostatin receptor scintigraphy (OctreoScan)

METASTATIC • LOCALLY ADVANCED

NEUROENDOCRINE TUMORS REGIMEN: LONG-ACTING OCTREOTIDE

Caplin ME et al. N Engl J Med 2014;371:224–233
Kvols LK et al. N Engl J Med 1986;315:663–666
Öberg K et al. Ann Oncol 2004;15:966–973

Octreotide acetate for injectable suspension 10–30 mg per dose intragluteally every 4 weeks (avoid intramuscular injection into the deltoids)

Supportive Care
Supplemental therapy for all somatostatin analogs:
Pancreatic enzymes to avoid steatorrhea. Individualize dosage by giving the number of tablets or capsules that optimally minimize steatorrhea

Antiemetic prophylaxis
Emetogenic potential is **MINIMAL**
See Chapter 42 for antiemetic recommendations

Hematopoietic growth factor (CSF) prophylaxis
Primary prophylaxis is **NOT** *indicated*
See Chapter 43 for more information

Antimicrobial prophylaxis
Risk of fever and neutropenia is **LOW**
  Antimicrobial primary prophylaxis to be considered:
  • Antibacterial—not indicated
  • Antifungal—not indicated
  • Antiviral—not indicated unless patient previously had an episode of HSV

Treatment Modifications

Patients Receiving Octreotide Acetate for Injectable Suspension

Escape from antisecretory response	Administer octreotide acetate injection 100–500 μg per dose subcutaneously 2 or 3 times daily. Increase dose or reduce interval between doses of the long-acting preparation as needed
Steatorrhea	Increase dose of pancreatic enzyme supplement to 3 capsules with every meal

Patient Population Studied

Primary symptomatic treatment in 25 patients with hormonally active tumors

Efficacy (N = 25)

Octreotide 150 μg/Dose 3 Times Daily—18-month Follow-up

Biochemical response*	72%
Biochemical stable disease	28%
Tumor size stable (n = 13)	100%
Symptomatic relief†	76%

*>50% decrease in 24-hour urinary 5-HIAA
†>50% decrease in flushing and diarrhea
Kvols LK et al. N Engl J Med 1986;315:663–666

Toxicity (N = 25)

Steatorrhea*,†	Frequent (~66%)
Loose stools†	Common
Nausea†	Common
Abdominal cramps†	Common
Flatulence†	Common
Hyperglycemia‡/hypoglycemia	<10%
Gallbladder stone/sludge	50%
Bradycardia	<2%
Pain/erythema at injection site	Occasional
Gastric atony	Very rare

*Occurs frequently unless pancreatic enzyme supplements are administered. Etiology is presumed to be transient inhibition of pancreatic exocrine function and malabsorption of fat
†Starts within hours of the first subcutaneous injection and usually subsides spontaneously within the first few weeks of treatment
‡From transient inhibition of insulin secretion
Kvols LK et al. N Engl J Med 1986;315:663–666
Öberg K et al. Ann Oncol 2004;15:966–973

Therapy Monitoring

1. *Every 3 months:* Complete history and physical examination
2. *Every 3–6 months:* Conventional imaging (CT, MRI, or ultrasound), serum electrolytes, and serum glucose
3. *Every year:* Somatostatin receptor scintigraphy (OctreoScan Kit for the Preparation of Indium In–111 Pentetreotide; Mallinckrodt Inc., St. Louis, MO) is controversial
4. *New symptoms:* Somatostatin receptor scintigraphy (OctreoScan)

Notes

1. Performing a ^{68}Ga/^{64}Cu-labeled somatostatin analog PET/CT provides information about the somatostatin receptor status of the patient's tumor and should be performed before treatment with a somatostatin analog is initiated. Patients with receptor-positive tumors more frequently respond to such treatment than those with receptor-negative tumors

2. Because of adverse events, administration of the immediate-release octreotide formulation is recommended before administration of the depot formulation

3. Patients should begin therapy with octreotide acetate injection subcutaneously for 3–7 days to test for tolerability before receiving a long-acting formulation (octreotide acetate for injectable suspension) intramuscularly

4. Increase the dosage of the short-acting octreotide acetate injection until control of symptoms is achieved by doubling the dosage at 3- to 4-day intervals

5. Patients who are considered to be "responders" to the drug and who tolerate the short-acting formulation can then receive octreotide acetate for injectable suspension or lanreotide acetate

6. The short-acting octreotide acetate subcutaneous injections should be continued for at least 14 days after the start of the long-acting formulation to allow time for therapeutic levels to be achieved

7. Conversion to the long-acting formulation provides greater patient convenience. If the dose of the short-acting formulation was 200–600 μg per day, begin with a 20-mg dose of the long-acting octreotide formulation, or 60 mg of lanreotide. If the dose of the short-acting formulation was 750–1500 μg per day, begin with a 30-mg dose of the long-acting octreotide formulation or 120 mg of the long-acting lanreotide formulation

8. Supplementary ("rescue") administration of the short-acting octreotide acetate injection should be given to patients "escaping" the antisecretory effects of the long-acting octreotide acetate for injectable suspension. If the rescue therapy is required during the week before the next dose of the long-acting formulation, a reduction in the dosing interval by 1 week is recommended. If the rescue medication is administered sporadically throughout the month, then increasing the dose of octreotide acetate for injectable suspension stepwise in increments of 10 mg per month, up to 60 mg per month, is recommended

9. *Supplemental therapy for all somatostatin analogs:*
   - Pancreatic enzymes to avoid steatorrhea
   - Individualize dosage by giving the number of tablets or capsules that optimally minimize steatorrhea
   - Select pancrelipase products with a high lipase content to avoid steatorrhea. In some patients, enteric-coated enzyme tablets may not dissociate as intended and may pass through the bowel intact
   - Administer pancrelipase with meals or snacks
   - Adjust doses slowly; monitor symptoms and response
   - Do not crush or chew enteric-coated products or the enteric-coated contents of opened capsules
   - Capsules may be opened and shaken onto a small quantity of soft food that is not hot and does not require chewing
   - Pancrelipase should be immediately swallowed without chewing to prevent mucosal irritation
   - Ingested doses should be followed with a glass of juice or water to ensure complete ingestion
   - Avoid mixing pancrelipase with foods that have a pH >5.5, which can dissolve enteric coatings

METASTATIC • LOCALLY ADVANCED

NEUROENDOCRINE TUMORS REGIMEN: LANREOTIDE

Caplin M et al. N Engl J Med 2014;371:224–233
Protocol for: Caplin M et al. N Engl J Med 2014;371:224–233
Supplementary appendix to: Caplin M et al. N Engl J Med 2014;371:224–233
SOMATULINE DEPOT (lanreotide) prescribing information. Basking Ridge, NJ: Ipsen Biopharmaceuticals, Inc;
Revised June 2019

Lanreotide 120 mg, administer by deep subcutaneous injection into the upper outer area of the right or left buttock (alternating from one injection to the next), every 4 weeks (total dosage/4-week cycle = 120 mg)

Follow the administration steps outlined below

1. Remove box from refrigerator
2. Let pouch sit for 30 *minutes* to reach room temperature. *Do not open* pouch until ready to inject.
   Note: Injection of cold medication may be painful
3. Find a clean, comfortable area for the patient to relax during procedure. It's important that the patient remain as still as possible during the injection.
4. *Hold pre-filled syringe by the syringe body* and *pull off* the needle cap to remove it.
5. *Flatten* injection area using the thumb and index finger of your other hand to stretch the skin. *Do not* pinch skin.
6. Insert needle *perpendicular* to the skin (90 degree angle). Use a strong, straight, dart-like motion to quickly *insert the needle all the way into the skin*. It is very important to insert the needle *completely*.
7. When needle is completely inserted, release injection site that has been flattened by hand.
8. Push plunger with *steady, very firm pressure*. The medication is thick and hard to push. While depressing plunger, slowly count to 20 and *continue steady pressure* on the plunger.
   Note: Pushing the plunger too fast may cause discomfort to the patient
9. *Give plunger a final push* to make sure you cannot depress the plunger further. Continue steady pressure with your thumb
10. While continuing to hold down the plunger, remove the needle from the injection site, then allow the needle to retract by removing thumb from the plunger
11. If needed, gently apply a gauze pad to injection area

<u>Important:</u> *Never rub or massage* the injection site

Supportive Care
Antiemetic prophylaxis
Emetogenic potential is **MINIMAL**
See Chapter 42 for antiemetic recommendations

Hematopoietic growth factor (CSF) prophylaxis
Primary prophylaxis is **NOT** *indicated*
See Chapter 43 for more information

Antimicrobial prophylaxis
Risk of fever and neutropenia is **LOW**
   Antimicrobial primary prophylaxis to be considered:
   • Antibacterial—not indicated
   • Antifungal—not indicated
   • Antiviral—not indicated, unless patient previously had an episode of HSV

Treatment Modification

LANREOTIDE TREATMENT MODIFICATION

Adverse Event	Dose Modification
Abdominal pain, diarrhea, and steatorrhea	• In many cases, symptoms are self-limited and may even disappear with time, thus symptomatic management is indicated • If symptoms persist, treat symptomatically including the addition of diphenoxylate hydrochloride 2.5 mg/atropine sulfate 0.025 mg (eg, Lomotil) or loperamide • If severe, assess with serum lipase and amylase
Pancreatitis	• Discontinue lanreotide
Injection-site reactions	• Ensure personnel administering the lanreotide have been properly trained and that the administration is being done properly
Symptoms of hypoglycemia	• Monitor blood glucose levels and treat symptomatically; if severe, discontinue lanreotide
Bradycardia	• Concomitant administration of bradycardia-inducing drugs (eg, beta-blockers) may have an additive effect on the reduction of heart rate associated with lanreotide. Dose adjustments of concomitant medication may be necessary
Severe renal impairment	• Reduce dose of lanreotide to 60 mg every 4 weeks or 120 mg every 6 or 8 weeks
Moderate or severe hepatic impairment	• Reduce dose of lanreotide to 60 mg every 4 weeks

Patient Population Studied

This randomized, multinational, multicenter, double-blind, parallel-group, placebo-controlled, phase 3 trial involved 204 adult patients with advanced, unresectable, moderately or well-differentiated, nonfunctioning, somatostatin receptor–positive neuroendocrine tumors. Patients were randomly assigned to receive lanreotide or placebo. Eligible patients had primary tumors in the pancreas, midgut, or hindgut, with a Ki67 proliferation index of <10% (Grade 1 or 2). Additionally, patients had target lesions classified by somatostatin-receptor scintigraphy as Grade ≥2 within the last 6 months, and a score of ≤2 on the World Health Organization (WHO) performance scale. Exclusion criteria included receipt of chemotherapy or interferon within the previous 6 months, or treatment with a radionucleotide or other somatostatin analog at any time (unless the analog was given >6 months prior to the study and for <15 days). Patients who completed 96 weeks of lanreotide with stable disease or who had received placebo were eligible for a lanreotide extension study.

Efficacy (N = 204)

End point	Lanreotide 120 mg (N = 101)	Placebo (N = 103)	Between-Group Comparison
Median progression-free survival*	NR	18.0 months (95% CI, 12.1–24.0)	HR 0.47 (95% CI 0.30–0.73); P <0.001
Patients alive without disease progression at week 48†	66%	49%	OR 2.11 (95% CI 1.19–3.76); P <0.05
Patients alive without disease progression at week 96†	52%	25%	OR 3.27 (95% CI 1.81–5.93); P <0.001

NR, not reached; HR, hazard ratio, CI, confidence interval; OR, odds ratio
*Progression-free survival defined as the time to disease progression or death within 96 weeks after the first injection of study drug. Disease progression was assessed centrally according to the Response Evaluation Criteria in Solid Tumors, version 1.0 (RECIST)
†Patients who withdrew from the study before the visit were recorded as having disease progression or having died for this outcome

Adverse Events (N = 204)

Grade (%)	Lanreotide 120 mg (N = 101)		Placebo (N = 103)	
	Not Severe	Severe*	Not Severe	Severe*
Abdominal pain	28	6	20	4
Musculoskeletal pain	17	2	11	2
Vomiting	17	2	7	2
Headache	16	0	10	1
Injection site reaction	15	0	7	0
Hyperglycemia	14	0	5	0
Hypertension	13	1	5	0
Cholelithiasis	13	1	7	0
Dizziness	9	0	2	0
Depression	7	0	1	0
Dyspnea	6	0	1	0

*Severe is defined as hazardous to well-being, significant impairment of function, or incapacitation
• Adverse events were defined according to the Medical Dictionary for Regulatory Activities, version 16.0
• Adverse events included. In the table are those with a reported incidence of ≥5% in the lanreotide arm and reported more commonly than in the placebo group

Therapy Monitoring

1. Interval history and physical exam including pulse and blood pressure 1 month after first dose and then at intervals of 3–6 months usually coinciding with planned re-evaluations
2. CBC with differential, serum glucose, LFTs, BUN, creatinine once per month. Thyroid function tests if clinically indicated
3. Efficacy/continued efficacy: CT or MRI at intervals of 3–4 months initially and yearly thereafter
4. In patients treated with lanreotide long-term, check for emerging cholelithiasis. This can usually be accomplished by assessing gallbladder on the imaging studies obtained as part of follow-up at intervals of 1–2 years. Otherwise consider ultrasound or CT at intervals of 1–2 years

METASTATIC
• LOCALLY
ADVANCED

NEUROENDOCRINE TUMORS REGIMEN: STREPTOZOCIN + FLUOROURACIL

Eriksson B et al. Cancer 1990;65:1883–1890
Moertel CG et al. N Engl J Med 1980;303:1189–1194
Moertel CG et al. N Engl J Med 1992;326:519–523

Premedications and hydration:
≥1000 mL 0.9% sodium chloride injection (0.9% NS); administer intravenously, starting 1.5 hours before administration of chemotherapy, continuing during administration, and for approximately 1.5 hours afterward

Induction course:
Streptozocin 500 mg/m^2/day; administer intravenously in 100–1000 mL 0.9% NS or 5% dextrose injection (D5W) over 30–120 minutes for 5 consecutive days, on days 1–5 (total dose/cycle = 2500 mg/m^2)
Fluorouracil 400 mg/m^2 per day; administer by intravenous injection over 1–2 minutes for 5 consecutive days, days 1–5 (total dosage/cycle = 2000 mg/m^2)

Subsequent courses: (beginning 3 weeks after the induction cycle)
Streptozocin 1000 mg/m^2 intravenously in 100–1000 mL 0.9% NS or D5W over 30–120 minutes on day 1, every 3 weeks (total dose/cycle = 1000 mg/m^2)
Fluorouracil 400 mg/m^2 by intravenous injection over 1–2 minutes on day 1, every 3 weeks (total dosage/cycle = 400 mg/m^2)

Supportive Care
Antiemetic prophylaxis
Emetogenic potential on days with streptozocin is **HIGH**
See Chapter 42 for antiemetic recommendations

Hematopoietic growth factor (CSF) prophylaxis
Primary prophylaxis is **NOT** *indicated*
See Chapter 43 for more information

Antimicrobial prophylaxis
Risk of fever and neutropenia is **LOW**
   Antimicrobial primary prophylaxis to be considered:
   • Antibacterial—not indicated
   • Antifungal—not indicated
   • Antiviral—not indicated unless patient previously had an episode of HSV

Treatment Modifications

Adverse Event	Treatment Modification
Creatinine clearance on day 1 of a second and subsequent cycles = 60–75 mL/min (1–1.25 mL/s)	Give streptozocin 500 mg/m^2/day for 2 consecutive days, on days 1 and 2 (total dose/cycle = 1000 mg/m^2)
Creatinine clearance on day 1 of a second and subsequent cycles = 50–60 mL/min (0.83–1 mL/s)	Give streptozocin 500 mg/m^2 on day 1 only (total dose/cycle = 500 mg/m^2)
Creatinine clearance on day 1 of a second and subsequent cycles <50 mL/min (<0.83 mL/s)	Discontinue streptozocin. Resume treatment after creatinine clearance >50 mL/min
Altered LFTs	No streptozocin adjustments recommended since hepatic metabolism does not appear to be important. Hold fluorouracil if total bilirubin >5 mg/dL (>85.5 μmol/L). In individual patients, titrate fluorouracil dosage to keep hematologic toxicities no greater than mild to moderate
Hematologic toxicities	Streptozocin and fluorouracil doses are titrated to produce no greater than mild to moderate hematologic toxicities

Patient Populations Studied

• One-hundred eighteen patients with metastatic carcinoid tumor were randomly assigned to receive treatment with streptozocin combined with cyclophosphamide or with fluorouracil (Moertel CG et al. N Engl J Med 1980;303:1189–1194)
• Of 84 patients with advanced pancreatic endocrine tumor, 19 received streptozocin + fluorouracil in a prospective, nonrandomized trial (Eriksson B et al. Cancer 1990;65:1883–1890)
• A multicenter randomized trial in which responses to streptozocin + fluorouracil, streptozocin + doxorubicin, or chlorozotocin monotherapy were compared in 105 patients with advanced pancreatic endocrine tumors (Moertel CG et al. N Engl J Med 1992;326:519–523)

Efficacy

Study	Objective Response Rate	Median Duration of Response
Moertel et al, 1980	63% (CR 33%)	17 months
Eriksson et al, 1990*	45%	27.5 months
Moertel et al, 1992	45%	6.9 months

*Combined results of streptozocin in combination with fluorouracil or doxorubicin as first-line treatment

Toxicity

	All Grades	Grades 1/2	Grades 3/4
Nausea	54–85%	—	22–41% (severe)
Anemia	9%	N/A	N/A
Leukopenia	2–56%	—	25% G3; 4% G4
Thrombocytopenia	15–25%	4%	6–11%
Elevated creatinine	30–36%	N/A	N/A
Renal failure	—	—	7% (G4)
Diarrhea	—	33% (mild)	2% (severe)
Stomatitis	—	5–19% (mild)	5% (severe)
Urinary albumin >30 mg/day	65%	—	—
>1.25× increase in LFTs	34%	—	—

Therapy Monitoring

Before each cycle of treatment: WBC with differential and platelet count, liver function tests, renal function tests

METASTATIC • LOCALLY ADVANCED

NEUROENDOCRINE TUMORS REGIMEN: STREPTOZOCIN + DOXORUBICIN

Eriksson B et al. Cancer 1990;65:1883–1890
Moertel CG et al. N Engl J Med 1992;326:519–523

Premedications and hydration:
1000 mL 0.9% sodium chloride injection (0.9% NS); administer intravenously, starting 1.5 hours before administration of chemotherapy, continuing during administration and for approximately 1.5 hours afterward

Induction course:
Streptozocin 500 mg/m^2/day; administer intravenously in 100–1000 mL 0.9% NS or 5% dextrose injection (D5W) over 30–120 minutes for 5 consecutive days, on days 1–5 (total dose/cycle = 2500 mg/m^2)
Doxorubicin 40 mg/m^2; administer by intravenous injection over 3–5 minutes on day 3 (total dosage/cycle = 40 mg/m^2)

Subsequent courses: (beginning 3 weeks after the induction cycle)
Streptozocin 1000 mg/m^2; administer intravenously in 100–1000 mL 0.9% NS or D5W over 30–120 minutes on day 1, every 3 weeks (total dose/cycle = 1000 mg/m^2)
Doxorubicin 40 mg/m^2; administer by intravenous injection over 3–5 minutes on day 1 (total dosage/cycle = 40 mg/m^2)

Supportive Care
Antiemetic prophylaxis
Emetogenic potential on days with streptozocin is **HIGH**
See Chapter 42 for antiemetic recommendations

Hematopoietic growth factor (CSF) prophylaxis
Primary prophylaxis is **NOT** indicated
See Chapter 43 for more information

Antimicrobial prophylaxis
Risk of fever and neutropenia is **LOW**
Antimicrobial primary prophylaxis to be considered:
- Antibacterial—not indicated
- Antifungal—not indicated
- Antiviral—not indicated unless patient previously had an episode of HSV

Treatment Modifications

Adverse Event	Treatment Modification
Creatinine clearance on day 1 of a second and subsequent cycles = 60–75 mL/min (1–1.25 mL/s)	Give streptozocin 500 mg/m^2/day for 2 consecutive days, on days 1 and 2 (total dose/cycle = 1000 mg/m^2)
Creatinine clearance on day 1 of a second and subsequent cycles = 50–60 mL/min (0.83–1 mL/s)	Give streptozocin 500 mg/m^2 on day 1 only (total dose/cycle = 500 mg/m^2)
Creatinine clearance on day 1 of a second and subsequent cycles <50 mL/min (<0.83 mL/s)	Discontinue streptozocin. Resume treatment after creatinine clearance >50 mL/min
Cumulative dose of doxorubicin ≥550 mg/m^2 (450 mg/m^2 in patients >70 years of age)	Monitor cardiac ejection fraction at baseline and reevaluate before repeating a treatment cycle or every other cycle
Altered LFTs	No streptozocin adjustments recommended since hepatic metabolism does not appear to be important Hold doxorubicin if total bilirubin >5 mg/dL (>85.5 μmol/L)
Hematologic toxicities	Streptozocin and doxorubicin doses are titrated to produce no greater than mild to moderate hematologic toxicities

Patient Populations Studied

- A prospective study of 84 patients with neuroendocrine pancreatic tumors. Fifty-nine (70%) had malignant tumors and received 1 or more types of medical treatment (Eriksson B et al. Cancer 1990;65:1883–1890)
- A multicenter randomized trial comparing streptozocin + fluorouracil, streptozocin + doxorubicin, and chlorozotocin alone. One-hundred five patients with advanced islet-cell carcinoma (Moertel CG et al. N Engl J Med 1992;326:519–523)

Efficacy

Study	Objective Response Rate	Median Duration of Response
Eriksson et al, 1990*	45%	27.5 months
Moertel et al, 1992	69%	20 months

*Combined results of streptozocin in combination with fluorouracil or doxorubicin as first-line treatment

Toxicity

	All Grades	Grades 1/2	Grades 3/4
Nausea	80%	—	20% (severe)
Anemia	9%	N/A	N/A
Leukopenia	57%	—	5%
Elevated creatinine	46%	N/A	N/A
Renal failure	—	—	4% (G4)
Diarrhea	—	5% (mild)	
Stomatitis	—	5% (mild)	—

Therapy Monitoring

1. *Before each cycle of treatment:* WBC with differential and platelet count, liver function tests, renal function tests
2. *Before initiation of treatment with doxorubicin, and before every third cycle:* Myocardial scintigraphy to assess cardiac function

METASTATIC • LOCALLY ADVANCED
NEUROENDOCRINE TUMORS REGIMEN: SUNITINIB MALATE

Raymond E et al. N Engl J Med 2011;364:501–513

Sunitinib malate 37.5 mg per day orally, continually (total dose/week = 262.5 mg)
Notes:
In patients without an objective tumor response who had Grade ≤1 nonhematologic or Grade ≤2 hematologic treatment-related adverse events during the first 8 weeks, the dose may be increased to 50 mg per day
Patients can receive somatostatin analogs as needed

Supportive Care
Antiemetic prophylaxis
Emetogenic potential is **MINIMAL–LOW**
See Chapter 42 for antiemetic recommendations

Hematopoietic growth factor (CSF) prophylaxis
Primary prophylaxis is **NOT** indicated
See Chapter 43 for more information

Antimicrobial prophylaxis
Risk of fever and neutropenia is **LOW**
  Antimicrobial primary prophylaxis to be considered:
  • Antibacterial—not indicated
  • Antifungal—not indicated
  • Antiviral—not indicated unless patient previously had an episode of HSV

Diarrhea management
Latent or delayed-onset diarrhea*:
Loperamide 4 mg orally initially after the first loose or liquid stool, *then* 2–4 mg orally every 2–4 hours or **diphenoxylate hydrochloride** 2.5 mg with **atropine sulfate** 0.025 mg (eg, Lomotil)

*Abigerges D et al. J Natl Cancer Inst 1994; 86:446–449
Rothenberg ML et al. J Clin Oncol 2001; 19:3801–3807
Wadler S et al. J Clin Oncol 1998; 16:3169–3178

Oral care
Standard prophylaxis and treatment for mucositis/stomatitis

Hand-foot reaction (palmar-plantar erythrodysesthesia, PPE)
For patients who develop a hand-foot reaction, use topical emollients (eg, Aquaphor), topical or orally administered steroids, antihistamine agents (H_1-receptor antagonists), or pyridoxine
Pyridoxine may provide relief for discomfort/pain associated with PPE, although the mechanism through which this occurs remains unclear
• The suggested pyridoxine starting dose is 50 mg/day, which may be increased to a maximum of 200 mg/day

Treatment Modifications

Adverse Event	Treatment Modification
Sunitinib Dose Levels	
Starting dose: Level 1	37.5 mg once daily
Level −1	25 mg once daily
Level +1	50 mg once daily
Cutaneous Toxicities	
Rash G ≥2	Hold sunitinib and provide immediate symptomatic treatment
If treatment is withheld for more than 3 weeks because of cutaneous toxicity	Discontinue therapy

(continued)

Treatment Modifications (*continued*)

Cutaneous Toxicities

When cutaneous toxicity resolves to G ≤1	Restart sunitinib at 1 dose level lower than the dose level administered at the time toxicity developed. Treatment for symptoms may continue indefinitely as a preventive measure
If cutaneous toxicity G3/4 recurs at reduced sunitinib doses	Again, hold sunitinib until the toxicity resolves to G ≤1, at which time sunitinib should be restarted at 1 dose level lower than the dose level administered at the time toxicity developed. Treatment for symptoms may continue indefinitely as a preventive measure
If cutaneous toxicity G3/4 recurs at dose level −1	Discontinue therapy
If cutaneous toxicity does not recur at reduced sunitinib doses with or without continued treatment for symptoms	The dose of sunitinib may be increased 1 dose level to the dose level administered at the time the cutaneous toxicity developed. Interrupt treatment by withholding sunitinib if toxicity recurs following the increase. When toxicity again resolves to G ≤1, resume sunitinib at the reduced dose previously tolerated

Diarrhea

G1/2 diarrhea	Focus on treatment for symptoms designed to resolve the diarrhea. No dose modifications will be made for G1/2 diarrhea unless G2 diarrhea persists for >2 weeks
If G2 diarrhea persists for more than 2 weeks	Follow the guidelines below for G3/4 diarrhea
If the diarrhea cannot be controlled with the preventive measures outlined, and is G3/4 or worsens by 1 grade level (G3 to G4) while on sunitinib and is not alleviated within 48 hours by antidiarrheal treatment	Hold sunitinib. Also withhold sunitinib if persistent G2 diarrhea (lasting >2 weeks) is not alleviated by antidiarrheal treatment while sunitinib use continues
If sunitinib is held for more than 3 weeks and the diarrhea does not resolve to G ≤1	Discontinue therapy
If within 3 weeks of holding sunitinib, diarrhea resolves to G ≤1	Restart sunitinib at 1 dose level less than the dose level administered at the time toxicity developed
If G3/4 diarrhea or persistent G2 diarrhea recurs at reduced sunitinib doses and the dose level at which persistent G2 diarrhea occurs is greater than dose level −1 (persistent is defined as lasting for >2 weeks)	Again, withhold sunitinib until the toxicity resolves to G ≤1, at which time sunitinib should be restarted at 1 dose level less than the dose level administered at the time toxicity developed. Treatment for symptoms may continue indefinitely as a preventive measure
If G3/4 diarrhea or persistent G2 diarrhea recurs at dose level −1 (persistent defined as lasting for more >2 weeks)	Discontinue therapy
If diarrhea does not recur at the reduced sunitinib doses with or without continued treatment for symptoms	The dose of sunitinib may be increased 1 dose level to the dose level administered at the time diarrhea developed. Interrupt treatment by withholding sunitinib if toxicity recurs following the increase. When toxicity again resolves to G ≤1, resume sunitinib at the reduced dose previously tolerated

Hypertension

Note: Patients should have their blood pressure checked once weekly during their first 24 weeks of therapy and for an 8-week period after an adjustment in their sunitinib dose

G1 hypertension	Continue sunitinib at same dose and schedule
G2 asymptomatic	Treat with antihypertensive medications and continue sunitinib at same dose and schedule
G2 symptomatic, or persistent G2 despite antihypertensive medications, or diastolic BP >110 mm Hg, or G3 hypertension	Treat with antihypertensive medications. Hold sunitinib (maximum 3 weeks until symptoms resolve and diastolic BP <100 mm Hg); then continue sunitinib at 1 dose level lower. *Note:* Discontinue therapy if sunitinib is withheld >3 weeks
G4 hypertension	Discontinue therapy

Treatment Modifications (continued)

Other Adverse Events

Signs and/or symptoms suggestive of thyroid dysfunction	Perform laboratory monitoring of thyroid function and treat as per standard medical practice.
Any other adverse event	Interrupt treatment. Resume at 25 mg/day when toxicity resolves to G ≤1. If symptoms do not recur, try increasing dose to the starting dose level, 37.5 mg daily
Recurrence of adverse event once dose increased to 37.5 mg/day	Interrupt treatment. Resume at 25 mg/day when toxicity resolves to G ≤1 but do not increase dose to the starting dose level, 37.5 mg daily
Coadministration of potent CYP3A4 inhibitors (eg, atazanavir, clarithromycin, itraconazole, ketoconazole, ritonavir, telithromycin, voriconazole)	Reduce sunitinib dose
Coadministration of potent CYP3A4 inducers (eg, carbamazepine, dexamethasone, phenytoin, phenobarbital, rifampin, St. John's Wort)	Increase sunitinib dose (to a maximum of 87.5 mg daily)

Patient Population Studied

A multinational, double-blind, placebo-controlled, phase 3 trial that randomly assigned patients in a 1:1 ratio to receive orally once-daily placebo or sunitinib 37.5 mg. Patient characteristics are shown below

Demographic and Baseline Characteristics of the Patients	Sunitinib (N = 86)	Placebo (N = 85)
Variable		
Age		
Median—years	56	57
Range—years	25–84	26–78
≥65 y—no. (%)	22 (26)	23 (27)
Sex—no. (%)		
Male	42 (49)	40 (47)
Female	44 (51)	45 (53)
ECOG performance status—no. (%)		
0	53 (62)	41 (48)
1	33 (38)	43 (51)
2	0	1 (1)
Inherited genetic conditions—no. (%)		
Multiple endocrine neoplasia type 1	0	2 (2)
von Hippel–Lindau disease	2 (2)	0
Time since diagnosis—years		
Median	2.4	3.2
Range	0.1–25.6	0.1–21.3
Tumor functionality—no. (%)*		
Nonfunctioning	42 (49)	44 (52)
Functioning	25 (29)	21 (24)
Not specified	19 (22)	20 (24)

(continued)

Efficacy

Summary of Efficacy Measures in the Intention-to-Treat Population*

Outcome	Sunitinib (N = 86)	Placebo (N = 85)	P Value
Progression-Free Survival*			
Patients with events—no. (%)	30 (35)	51 (60)	
Progression	27 (31)	48 (56)	
Death without progression	3 (3)	3 (4)	
Patients with data censored—no. (%)	56 (65)	34 (40)	
Probability event-free at 6 months—% (95% CI)	71.3 (60.0–82.5)	43.2 (30.3–56.1)	
Estimated median progression-free survival, months	11.4 (7.4–19.8)	5.5 (3.6–7.4)	
Hazard ratio for progression or death (95% CI)	0.42 (0.26–0.66)		<0.001
Overall Survival			
Deaths—no. (%)	9 (10)	21 (25)	
Patients with data censored—no. (%)	77 (90)	64 (75)	
Survival probability at 6 months—% (95% CI)	92.6 (86.3–98.9)	85.2 (77.1–93.3)	
Estimated median overall survival	Not reached	Not reached	
Hazard ratio for death (95% CI)	0.41 (0.19–0.89)		0.02
Objective Tumor Response			
Best observed RECIST response—no. (%)			
Complete response	2 (2)	0	
Partial response	6 (7)	0	
Stable disease	54 (63)	51 (60)	
Progressive disease	12 (14)	23 (27)	
Could not be evaluated	12 (14)	11 (13)	
Objective response rate—%	9.3	0	0.007

CI, confidence interval; RECIST, Response Evaluation Criteria in Solid Tumors (Therasse P et al. J Natl Cancer Inst 2000;92:205–216)

*Data for a total of 3 patients (1 in the sunitinib group and 2 in the placebo group) were censored at day 1 in the analysis of PFS because of inadequate baseline tumor assessment

Patient Population Studied
(*continued*)

Demographic and Baseline Characteristics of the Patients	Sunitinib (N = 86)	Placebo (N = 85)
Ki67 index		
Number of patients with data that could be evaluated	36	36
Index—no. (%)		
≤2%	7 (19)	6 (17)
>2%–5%	16 (44)	14 (39)
>5%–10%	5 (14)	10 (28)
>10%	8 (22)	6 (17)
No. of sites of disease—no. (%)°		
1	30 (35)	23 (27)
2	31 (36)	26 (31)
≥3	24 (28)	35 (41)
Not reported	1 (1)	1 (1)
Presence of distant metastases—no. (%)		
Any, including hepatic	82 (95)	80 (94)
Extrahepatic	21 (24)	34 (40)
Previous treatment—no. (%)		
Surgery	76 (88)	77 (91)
Radiation therapy	9 (10)	12 (14)
Chemoembolization	7 (8)	14 (16)
Radiofrequency ablation	3 (3)	6 (7)
Percutaneous ethanol injection	1 (1)	2 (2)
Somatostatin analogs[†]	30 (35)	32 (38)
Previous systemic chemotherapy—no. (%)		
Any	57 (66)	61 (72)
Streptozocin	24 (28)	28 (33)
Anthracyclines	27 (31)	35 (41)
Fluoropyrimidines	20 (23)	25 (29)

*Tumor functionality was reported by investigators. On the basis of the investigators' assessment, patients included in the "unknown" category had clinical symptoms but no identified corresponding neuropeptide secretion

[†]This category includes patients who received somatostatin analogs (predominantly octreotide acetate and lanreotide acetate) before the first dose of study drug, regardless of whether they continued receiving somatostatin analogs concomitantly with the study drug

Toxicity

Common Adverse Events in the Safety Population*

Event	Sunitinib (N = 83)			Placebo (N = 82)		
	All Grades	G1/2	G3/4	All Grades	G1/2	G3/4
Number of Patients (%)						
Diarrhea	49 (59)	45 (54)	4 (5)	32 (39)	30 (37)	2 (2)
Nausea	37 (45)	36 (43)	1 (1)	24 (29)	23 (28)	1 (1)
Asthenia	28 (34)	24 (29)	4 (5)	22 (27)	19 (23)	3 (4)
Vomiting	28 (34)	28 (34)	0	25 (30)	23 (28)	2 (2)
Fatigue	27 (32)	23 (28)	4 (5)	22 (27)	15 (18)	7 (8)
Hair-color changes	24 (29)	23 (28)	1 (1)	1 (1)	1 (1)	0
Neutropenia	24 (29)	14 (17)	10 (12)	3 (4)	3 (4)	0
Abdominal pain	23 (28)	19 (23)	4 (5)	26 (32)	18 (22)	8 (10)
Hypertension	22 (26)	14 (17)	8 (10)	4 (5)	3 (4)	1 (1)
Palmar–plantar erythrodysesthesia	19 (23)	14 (17)	5 (6)	2 (2)	2 (2)	0
Anorexia	18 (22)	16 (19)	2 (2)	17 (21)	16 (20)	1 (1)
Stomatitis	18 (22)	15 (18)	3 (4)	2 (2)	2 (2)	0
Dysgeusia	17 (20)	17 (20)	0	4 (5)	4 (5)	0
Epistaxis	17 (20)	16 (19)	1 (1)	4 (5)	4 (5)	0
Headache	15 (18)	15 (18)	0	11 (13)	10 (12)	1 (1)
Insomnia	15 (18)	15 (18)	0	10 (12)	10 (12)	0
Rash	15 (18)	15 (18)	0	4 (5)	4 (5)	0
Thrombocytopenia	14 (17)	11 (13)	3 (4)	4 (5)	4 (5)	0
Mucosal inflammation	13 (16)	12 (14)	1 (1)	6 (7)	6 (7)	0
Weight loss	13 (16)	12 (14)	1 (1)	9 (11)	9 (11)	0
Constipation	12 (14)	12 (14)	0	16 (20)	15 (18)	1 (1)
Back pain	10 (12)	10 (12)	0	14 (17)	10 (12)	4 (5)

*Adverse events were defined on the basis of the National Cancer Institute, Common Terminology Criteria for Adverse Events, version 3.0. Events listed are those of any grade that occurred in more than 15% of patients in either group

Therapy Monitoring

1. *Every 6 weeks to 3 months:* Physical examination and routine laboratory tests including thyroid function tests
2. *Response assessment:* Every 2–3 cycles. A cycle is defined as a 6-week period

METASTATIC • LOCALLY ADVANCED

NEUROENDOCRINE TUMORS REGIMEN: EVEROLIMUS

Yao JC et al. N Engl J Med 2011;364:514–523

Everolimus 10 mg/day orally, continually (total dose/week = 70 mg)

Notes:
- Everolimus tablets should be swallowed whole (without breaking, crushing, or chewing) with water
- Everolimus tablets and tablets for oral suspension may be taken with or without food, but should be taken consistently either with or without food
- Commercially available formulations, (1) tablets and (2) tablets for oral suspension, should not be used in combination to administer a dose

Supportive Care

Antiemetic prophylaxis
Emetogenic potential is **MINIMAL–LOW**
See Chapter 42 for antiemetic recommendations

Hematopoietic growth factor (CSF) prophylaxis
Primary prophylaxis is **NOT** indicated
See Chapter 43 for more information

Antimicrobial prophylaxis
Risk of fever and neutropenia is **LOW**
  Antimicrobial primary prophylaxis to be considered:
  - Antibacterial—not indicated
  - Antifungal—not indicated
  - Antiviral—not indicated unless patient previously had an episode of HSV

Diarrhea management

Latent or delayed-onset diarrhea*:
Loperamide 4 mg orally initially after the first loose or liquid stool, *then* 2–4 mg orally every 2–4 hours or **diphenoxylate hydrochloride** 2.5 mg with **atropine sulfate** 0.025 mg (eg, Lomotil)

*Abigerges D et al. J Natl Cancer Inst 1994;86:446–449
Rothenberg ML et al. J Clin Oncol 2001;19:3801–3807
Wadler S et al. J Clin Oncol 1998;16:3169–3178

Oral care
Standard prophylaxis and treatment for mucositis/stomatitis

Treatment Modifications

Adverse Event	Treatment Modification
Invasive systemic fungal infection	Discontinue everolimus and treat with appropriate antifungal therapy
Noninfectious pneumonitis without symptoms with only radiologic changes	Observe carefully. Specific therapies or drug interruption may not be necessary
Noninfectious pneumonitis with mild to moderate symptoms	Withhold therapy. Glucocorticoids may be initiated. Resume everolimus at a reduced dose depending on the individual clinical circumstances
Noninfectious pneumonitis with severe symptoms (including a decrease in DL_{CO} on pulmonary function tests)	Discontinue therapy and consider administering high doses of glucocorticoids
ANC <1000/mm^3 or platelet count <75,000/mm^3	Withhold therapy. Resume everolimus when symptoms improve to G ≤2 with everolimus dose reduced to 5 mg/day or 5 mg every other day but not <15 mg/week
Any nonhematologic G3/4 toxicity	Withhold therapy. Restart everolimus when symptoms improve to G ≤2 with everolimus dose reduced to 5 mg/day or 5 mg every other day but not <15 mg/week
G1/2 oral ulcerations	Topical treatments are recommended, but alcohol- or peroxide-containing mouthwashes should be avoided. Focus on pain control, oral hygiene, and IV fluid replacement or parenteral nutrition if severe
Hyperglycemia	Monitor blood sugar levels and institute oral hypoglycemic agent or insulin as needed
Hypertriglyceridemia	Monitor triglycerides, instituting dietary interventions for minor elevations and lipid-lowering agents for levels >500 mg/dL (>5.65 mmol/L)

Patient Population Studied

International, multicenter, double-blind, phase 3 study. Patients were randomly assigned to treatment with oral everolimus 10 mg or matching placebo, both administered once daily in conjunction with best supportive care. Patients initially assigned to placebo who met criteria for disease progression could switch to open-label everolimus. Of the 203 patients initially assigned to receive placebo, 148 (73%) crossed over to open-label everolimus

Demographic and Baseline Clinical Characteristics of the Patients

Characteristic	Everolimus (N = 207)	Placebo (N = 203)
Age—years		
Median	58	57
Range	23–87	20–82
Sex—no. (%)		
Male	110 (53)	117 (58)
Female	97 (47)	86 (42)
WHO performance status—no. (%)		
0	139 (67)	133 (66)
1	62 (30)	64 (32)
2	6 (3)	6 (3)
Histologic status of tumor—no. (%)		
Well differentiated	170 (82)	171 (84)
Moderately differentiated	35 (17)	30 (15)
Unknown	2 (1)	2 (1)
Time from initial diagnosis—no. (%)		
≤6 months	24 (12)	33 (16)
>6 months to ≤2 years	65 (31)	43 (21)
>2 years to ≤5 years	54 (26)	81 (40)
>5 years	64 (31)	46 (23)

(continued)

Efficacy

Variable	Everolimus (N = 207)	Placebo (N = 203)
Progression-Free Survival (PFS)		
Assessment by local investigator		
Progression-free survival events—no. (%)	109 (53)	165 (81)
Censored data—no. (%)	98 (47)	38 (19)
Median progression-free survival—months	11.0	4.6
Hazard ratio for PFS with everolimus (95% CI); P Value	0.35 (0.27–0.45); <0.001	
Review by central adjudication committee		
Progression-free survival events—no. (%)	95 (46)	142 (70)
Censored data—no. (%)	112 (54)	61 (30)
Median progression-free survival—months	11.4	5.4
Hazard ratio for PFS with everolimus (95% CI); P Value	0.34 (0.26–0.44); <0.001	
Estimated proportion of patients alive and progression-free at 18 months—% (95% CI)	34% (26–43)	9% (4–16)
Response According to RECIST Criteria		
Partial response—no. (%)	10 (5)	4 (2)
Percent with stable disease	73%	51%
Percent with some tumor shrinkage	64%	21%
Overall Survival*		
Hazard ratio for death with everolimus	1.05; 95% CI, 0.71–1.55; P = 0.59	

*Median overall survival not reached. Of the 203 patients initially assigned to receive placebo, 148 (73%) crossed over to receive open-label everolimus

Toxicity*,†

	Everolimus (N = 204)		Placebo (N = 203)	
Median treatment duration, months (range)	8.79 (0.25–27.47)		3.74 (0.01–37.79)	
Treatment a minimum of 12 months	31%		11%	
Mean relative dose intensity‡	0.86		0.97	
Percentage requiring dose adjustments§	59%		28%	
	All Grades	G3/4	All G	G3/4
Adverse Event	**Number of Patients (%)**			
Stomatitis℮	131 (64)	14 (7)	34 (17)	0

(continued)

(continued)

Patient Population Studied
(continued)

Demographic and Baseline Clinical Characteristics of the Patients

Characteristic	Everolimus (N = 207)	Placebo (N = 203)
Time from disease progression to randomization—no. (%)		
≤1 months	73 (35)	61 (30)
>1 months to ≤2 months	43 (21)	53 (26)
>2 months to ≤3 months	30 (14)	29 (14)
>3 months to ≤12 months	58 (28)	54 (27)
>12 months	3 (1)	1 (<1)
No. of disease sites—no. of patients (%)		
1	51 (25)	62 (31)
2	85 (41)	64 (32)
≥3	70 (34)	77 (38)
Organ involved—no. (%)		
Liver	190 (92)	187 (92)
Pancreas	92 (44)	84 (41)
Lymph nodes	68 (33)	73 (36)
Lung	28 (14)	30 (15)
Bone	13 (6)	29 (14)

Toxicity*,† (continued)

	Everolimus (N = 204)		Placebo (N = 203)	
Rash	99 (49)	1 (<1)	21 (10)	0
Diarrhea	69 (34)	7 (3)	20 (10)	0
Fatigue	64 (31)	5 (2)	29 (14)	1 (<1)
Infections**	46 (23)	5 (2)	12 (6)	1 (<1)
Nausea	41 (20)	5 (2)	37 (18)	0
Peripheral edema	41 (20)	1 (<1)	7 (3)	0
Decreased appetite	40 (20)	0	14 (7)	2 (1)
Headache	39 (19)	0	13 (6)	0
Dysgeusia	35 (17)	0	8 (4)	0
Anemia	35 (17)	12 (6)	6 (3)	0
Epistaxis	35 (17)	0	0	0
Pneumonitis††	35 (17)	5 (2)	0	0
Weight loss	32 (16)	0	9 (4)	0
Vomiting	31 (15)	0	13 (6)	0
Pruritus	30 (15)	0	18 (9)	0
Hyperglycemia	27 (13)	11 (5)	9 (4)	4 (2)
Thrombocytopenia	27 (13)	8 (4)	1 (<1)	0
Asthenia	26 (13)	2 (1)	17 (8)	2 (1)
Nail disorder	24 (12)	1 (<1)	2 (1)	0
Cough	22 (11)	0	4 (2)	0
Pyrexia	22 (11)	0	0	0
Dry skin	21 (10)	0	9 (4)	0

*Drug-related adverse events occurring in ≥10% of patients
†Median follow-up period of 17 months
‡Ratio of administered doses to planned doses
§Reductions or temporary interruptions
¶Includes stomatitis, aphthous stomatitis, mouth ulceration, and tongue ulceration
**Includes all types of infections
††Includes pneumonitis, interstitial lung disease, lung infiltration, and pulmonary fibrosis

Therapy Monitoring

1. *Prior to starting treatment and periodically thereafter:* renal function, CBC with differential, blood glucose, and serum lipid profiles
2. *ECG:* a 12-lead ECG should be performed before the start of treatment, weekly for at least the first 2 weeks. Additional ECGs may be performed depending on the QTc. If the dose is increased, then at least 1 additional ECG should be obtained
3. *Safety assessment:* every 2–4 weeks for the first 3 cycles; every 4–8 weeks, thereafter
4. *Response assessment:* every 8–12 weeks

METASTATIC • LOCALLY ADVANCED

NEUROENDOCRINE TUMORS REGIMEN: CISPLATIN + ETOPOSIDE

Fjällskog M-LH et al. Cancer 2001;92:1101–1107
Moertel CG et al. Cancer 1991;68:227–232

Hydration days 2 and 3:
≥1000 mL 0.9% sodium chloride injection (0.9% NS); administer intravenously at a rate that produces a diuresis ≥100 mL/h, starting at least 2 hours before chemotherapy administration. Continue hydration during chemotherapy administration and for at least 2 hours afterward. Mannitol or furosemide may be given as needed to enhance diuresis and prevent excessive fluid retention. Encourage increased oral intake of nonalcoholic fluids. Monitor and replace electrolytes as needed (potassium, magnesium, sodium)
Etoposide 100 mg/m² per day; administer intravenously, diluted in a volume of 0.9% NS to a concentration within the range of 0.2–0.4 mg/mL, over 60 minutes on 3 consecutive days, on days 1–3, every 4 weeks (total dosage/cycle = 300 mg/m²)
Cisplatin 45 mg/m² per day; administer intravenously in 100–250 mL 0.9% NS over 1 hour on 2 consecutive days, on days 2 and 3, every 4 weeks (total dosage/cycle = 90 mg/m²)

Supportive Care
Antiemetic prophylaxis
Emetogenic potential on day 1 is **LOW**
Emetogenic potential on days 2 and 3 is **HIGH**, *with a potential for delayed symptoms*
See Chapter 42 for antiemetic recommendations

Hematopoietic growth factor (CSF) prophylaxis
Primary prophylaxis may be indicated
See Chapter 43 for more information

Antimicrobial prophylaxis
Risk of fever and neutropenia is LOW
  Antimicrobial primary prophylaxis to be considered:
  • Antibacterial—not indicated
  • Antifungal—not indicated
  • Antiviral—not indicated unless patient previously had an episode of HSV

Treatment Modifications

Adverse Event	Treatment Modification
Day 1 ANC <1500/mm³ or platelets <100,000/mm³	Delay treatment 1 week or until ANC >1500/mm³ and platelets >100,000/mm³, then administer full doses
ANC at nadir <500/mm³	Administer filgrastim during subsequent cycles: • Administer filgrastim on days 4–11, *or* • Administer pegfilgrastim at least 24 hours after completing chemotherapy, *and/or* • Decrease etoposide dosage by 25%
Albumin <3.2 g/dL (<32 g/L)	Reduce etoposide dosage by 50%
Albumin <2.5 g/dL (<25 g/L)	Discontinue etoposide until albumin ≥2.5 g/dL (≥25 g/L)

Patient Populations Studied

• Nonrandomized study of 15 patients with malignant pancreatic endocrine tumors (4 were poorly differentiated endocrine carcinomas) treated with cisplatin + etoposide as second- or third-line treatment (Fjällskog M-LH et al. Cancer 2001;92:1101–1107)
• Prospective, nonrandomized study of 45 patients with neuroendocrine tumors among whom 14 had well-differentiated pancreatic endocrine tumors (Moertel CG et al. Cancer 1991;68:227–232)

Efficacy

Study	Objective Response Rate	Median Duration of Response
Moertel et al, 1991*	67%	8 months
Fjällskog et al, 2001[†]	53%	9 months

*Tumor response was unrelated to primary site, endocrine hyperfunction, or prior therapy experience. The median survival of all patients with anaplastic tumors was 19 months
[†]Includes foregut carcinoids and endocrine pancreatic tumors. No difference in response between patients with well-differentiated or poorly differentiated endocrine pancreatic carcinoma

Toxicity

	All Grades	Grades 1/2	Grades 3/4
Nephrotoxicity	53–66%	—	2% (severe)
Anemia	89%	Decreased Hb: 1–3 g/dL (38%); 3–4 g/dL (29%); >4 g/dL (22%)	
Leukopenia	100%	35%	65%
Thrombocytopenia	—	49%	35%
Peripheral neuropathy	—	17%	75%
Ototoxicity	—	2–8%	—
Diarrhea	16%	—	—
Stomatitis	13%	11%	2%
Nausea	96%	83%	13%
Alopecia	100%	—	—
Dermatitis	—	4%,	—
Fever	—	—	2%

Therapy Monitoring

1. *Before and during each cycle of treatment:* Body weight to detect excessive fluid retention
2. *Days 7, 10, and 14 of each cycle:* WBC with differential count
3. *Every cycle:* Liver and renal function tests

METASTATIC • LOCALLY ADVANCED
NEUROENDOCRINE TUMORS REGIMEN: CAPTEM (CAPECITABINE + TEMOZOLOMIDE)

Strosberg JR et al. Cancer 2011;117:268–275

Capecitabine 750 mg/m^2 per dose; administer orally twice daily (approximately every 12 hours), within 30 minutes after the end of a meal, for 14 consecutive days (28 doses) on days 1–14, every 28 days (total dosage/28-day cycle = 21,000 mg/m^2)
Temozolomide 200 mg/m^2 per dose, administer orally once daily at bedtime for 5 consecutive days (5 doses) on days 10–14, every 28 days (total dosage/28-day cycle = 1000 mg/m^2)
Notes:
- Temozolomide doses are rounded to use combinations of 5-mg, 20-mg, 100-mg, 140-mg, 180-mg, and 250-mg capsules that most closely approximate calculated values
- Capecitabine doses are rounded to use combinations of 500-mg and 150-mg tablets that most closely approximate calculated values
- Patients who miss a dose of capecitabine should be instructed to continue with the usual dosing schedule without making up the missed dose and to contact their physician for further instructions.
- Patients who take too much (ie, overdose) capecitabine should contact their doctor immediately and present to the emergency department for further care and consideration for timely treatment with the antidote uridine triacetate.
- Although food decreases the rate and extent of drug absorption and the time to peak plasma concentration and systemic exposure (AUC) for capecitabine and fluorouracil, product labeling recommends giving capecitabine within 30 minutes after the end of a meal because established safety and efficacy data are based on administration with food
- Initial capecitabine dosage should be decreased by 25% in patients with moderate renal impairment (baseline creatinine clearance = 30–50 mL/min [0.5–0.83 mL/s]); ie, a dosage reduction from 750 mg/m^2 per dose, to 550 mg/m^2 per dose, twice daily. Capecitabine use is contraindicated in persons with severe renal impairment (creatinine clearance <30 mL/min (<0.5 mL/s))

Supportive Care
Antiemetic prophylaxis
Emetogenic potential on days 1–9 (capecitabine alone) is **MINIMAL–LOW**
Emetogenic potential on days 10–14 (temozolomide + capecitabine) is **MODERATE–HIGH**
See Chapter 42 for antiemetic recommendations

Hematopoietic growth factor (CSF) prophylaxis
Primary prophylaxis is **NOT** *indicated*
See Chapter 43 for more information

Antimicrobial Primary Prophylaxis
Risk of Fever and Neutropenia is **LOW**
  Antimicrobial primary prophylaxis to be considered:
  - Antibacterial—not indicated
  - Antifungal—not indicated
  - Antiviral—not indicated, unless patient previously had an episode of HSV infection and for VZV post-exposure prophylaxis

Hand-foot reaction (palmar-plantar erythrodysesthesia, PPE)
For patients who develop a hand-foot reaction, use topical emollients (eg, Aquaphor), topical or orally administered steroids, antihistamine agents (H$_1$-receptor antagonists), or pyridoxine
Pyridoxine may provide relief for discomfort/pain associated with PPE, although the mechanism through which this occurs remains unclear
- The suggested pyridoxine starting dose is 50 mg/day, which may be increased to a maximum of 200 mg/day

Treatment Modifications

CAPTEM (CAPECITABINE + TEMOZOLOMIDE)

Starting doses: capecitabine 600 to 750 mg/m^2 twice daily (d1-14). Consider a maximum of 1000 mg; temozolomide 200 mg/m^2 once daily or divided into two daily doses Add or divided into two daily doses after the once daily
Note: Doses omitted for toxicity are not replaced or restored; instead patient resumes planned treatment cycles

Adverse Event	Treatment Modification
Baseline ANC <1500/mm^3 or baseline platelets <100,000/mm^3	Delay start of treatment until ANC ≥1500/mm^3 and platelets ≥100,000/mm^3

(continued)

Treatment Modifications (continued)

Adverse Event	Treatment Modification
ANC <1000/mm³ or platelets <50,000/mm³ during cycle	Withhold administration of therapy until resolves to ANC ≥1500/mm³ or baseline platelets ≥75,000/mm³. Administer 66–75% of doses taken at the time toxicity occurred in subsequent cycle(s)
ANC <500/mm³ or platelets <25,000/mm³ during cycle (G4 toxicity)	Discontinue permanently *or* If physician deems it to be in the patient's best interest to continue, interrupt until resolved to G ≤1, then resume therapy with doses ≤50% that at the time G4 toxicity occurred
Drug-related increase in serum bilirubin to >3× ULN (G3)	Stop administration of capecitabine and temozolomide; provide supportive care. Do not resume capecitabine or temozolomide until serum bilirubin <3× ULN. When treatment is resumed, administer 50–66% of the doses taken at the time toxicity occurred. If serum bilirubin >10× ULN, discontinue therapy. Note that once the dose has been reduced, it should not be increased at a later time

Capecitabine-specific dose modifications

Patients receiving phenytoin and coumarin-derivative anticoagulants	Monitor carefully as the dose of phenytoin and coumarin-derivative anticoagulants may need to be reduced when either drug is administered concomitantly with capecitabine
G2/3/4 diarrhea	Stop administration of capecitabine; provide supportive care including fluids and loperamide; if severe, send stool for culture. Do not resume capecitabine until diarrhea resolved to G ≤1. In subsequent cycle(s), administer a fraction of the capecitabine dose taken at the time toxicity occurred or discontinue as follows: G2 = 66–80%; G3 = 50–66%; G4 = discontinue. Note that once the dose has been reduced, it should not be increased at a later time
G2/3/4 mucositis	Stop administration of capecitabine; provide supportive care. Do not resume capecitabine until toxicity resolved to G ≤1. In subsequent cycle(s), administer a fraction of the capecitabine dose taken at the time toxicity occurred or discontinue as follows: G2 = 66–80%; G3 = 50–66%; G4 = discontinue. Note that once the dose has been reduced, it should not be increased at a later time
G2/3/4 dehydration	
Hand-and-foot syndrome (HFS) or palmar-plantar erythrodysesthesia (PPE) or chemotherapy-induced acral erythema*	Stop administration of capecitabine; provide supportive care. Do not resume capecitabine until toxicity resolved to G ≤1. In subsequent cycle(s), administer a fraction of the capecitabine dose taken at the time toxicity occurred or discontinue as follows: G2 = 66–80%; G3 = 50–66%; G4 = discontinue. Note that once the dose has been reduced, it should not be increased at a later time
Stevens-Johnson syndrome and toxic epidermal necrolysis (TEN) (severe mucocutaneous reactions, some with fatal outcome)	Discontinue treatment permanently
Patients with moderate renal impairment (creatinine clearance = 30–50 mL/min)	Administer 75% of the starting capecitabine dose
Toxicity in the setting of DPD deficiency (early-onset severe mucositis, diarrhea, neutropenia, and neurotoxicity)	Occurs in individuals with homozygous or certain compound heterozygous mutations in the DPD gene that result in complete or near complete absence of DPD activity (eg, mucositis, diarrhea, neutropenia, and neurotoxicity). Discontinue capecitabine permanently. There are insufficient data to recommend a specific dose in patients with partial DPD activity as measured by any specific test

Adjustments for other nonhematologic toxicities due to capecitabine, temozolomide, or both

G1	Continue treatment and maintain dose in subsequent cycle
G2 (first occurrence)	Interrupt until resolved to G ≤1; administer 100% of dose in subsequent cycle
G2 (second occurrence)	Interrupt until resolved to G ≤1; administer 75–80% of dose in subsequent cycle. Note that once the dose has been reduced, it should not be increased at a later time
G2 (third occurrence)	Interrupt until resolved to G ≤1; administer 50% of dose in subsequent cycle. Note that once the dose has been reduced, it should not be increased at a later time
G2 (fourth occurrence)	Discontinue treatment permanently
G3 (first occurrence)	Interrupt until resolved to G ≤1; administer 75–80% of dose in subsequent cycle. Note that once the dose has been reduced, it should not be increased at a later time

(continued)

Treatment Modifications (*continued*)

G3 (second occurrence)	Interrupt until resolved to G ≤1; administer 50% of dose in subsequent cycle. Note that once the dose has been reduced, it should not be increased at a later time
G3 (third occurrence)	Discontinue treatment permanently
G4 (first occurrence)	Discontinue permanently *or* If physician deems it to be in the patient's best interest to continue, interrupt until resolved to G ≤1, then resume therapy with doses ≤50% that at the time G4 toxicity occurred. Note that once the dose has been reduced, it should not be increased at a later time

*Median time to onset, 79 days (range, 11–360)
- G1: Numbness, dysesthesia/paresthesia, tingling, painless swelling or erythema of the hands and/or feet, and/or discomfort that does not disrupt normal activities
- G2: Painful erythema and swelling of the hands and/or feet and/or discomfort affecting the patient's activities of daily living
- G3: Moist desquamation, ulceration, blistering or severe pain of the hands and/or feet, and/or severe discomfort that causes the patient to be unable to work or perform activities of daily living

Patient Population Studied

The study involved 30 patients with metastatic, moderately to well-differentiated pancreatic endocrine carcinoma. Patients who had previously received octreotide, interferon-α, or locoregional therapy with hepatic artery embolization were eligible. Patients who had received prior systemic chemotherapy in the metastatic setting were not eligible. Patients received oral capecitabine 750 mg/m^2 twice daily on days 1–14 of a 28-day cycle. Patients also received oral temozolomide 200 mg/m^2 once daily (at bedtime) on days 10–14, with ondansetron 8 mg before each dose of temozolomide

Efficacy (N = 30)

Objective response rate	70% (95% CI 54–86%)
Median progression-free survival	18 months (95% CI 9–31 months)
Overall survival at 2 years	92% (95% CI 72–98%)
Duration of response*	20 months (95% CI 14–26 months)

*Among responding patients.

Adverse Events[†] (N = 30)

Grade (%)	Grade 1	Grade 2	Grade 3	Grade 4
Thrombocytopenia	17	7	0	3
Hand-foot skin reaction	17	7	0	0
Nausea	10	7	0	0
Fatigue	13	0	3	0
Anemia	3	7	0	3
Neutropenia	0	7	0	0
Herpes zoster	7	0	0	0
Vomiting	7	0	0	0
Elevated aspartate aminotransferase level	0	0	3	0
Elevated alanine aminotransferase level	0	3	0	0
Leukopenia	0	3	0	0
Vaginal bleeding	0	3	0	0
Diarrhea	3	0	0	0
Herpes labialis	3	0	0	0

[†]U.S. National Cancer Institute Common Terminology Criteria for Adverse Events, version 3.0. At: https://ctep.cancer.gov/protocolDevelopment/electronic_applications/ctc.htm (accessed 12 December 2017)

Therapy Monitoring

1. During first cycle and in any cycle after a dose adjustment, weekly CBC with differential and platelet count to assess dose
2. *Before each cycle:* physical examination, WBC with differential and platelet count, liver function tests, renal function tests. Serum chromogranin or other serum/urine hormones/peptides if these are being followed
3. *Response assessment:* Every 2–3 cycles. A cycle is defined as a 4-week period
4. Patients receiving concomitant capecitabine and oral coumarin-derivative anticoagulant therapy should have their anticoagulant response (INR or prothrombin time) monitored frequently in order to adjust the anticoagulant dose accordingly

METASTATIC • LOCALLY ADVANCED
NEUROENDOCRINE TUMORS REGIMEN: LUTETIUM LU 177 DOTATATE

Strosberg J et al. N Engl J Med 2017;372:125–135
Protocol for: Strosberg J et al. N Engl J Med 2017;372:125–135
Supplementary appendix to: Strosberg J et al. N Engl J Med 2017;372:125–135
Strosberg JR et al. J Clin Oncol 2018;36(suppl):Abstract 4099
LUTATHERA (lutetium Lu 177 dotatate) injection prescribing information. Millburn, NJ: Advanced Accelerator Applications USA, Inc.; revised July 2018

Premedication:

Granisetron 1–3 mg *or* **ondansetron** 8 mg acetate solution intravenously 30 minutes prior to initiation of the amino acid infusion

Lutetium Lu–177-dotatate 7.4 GBq (200 mCi) per dose, administered intravenously (as outlined below), every 8 weeks, for a total of 4 doses (total dosage/8-week cycle = 7.4 GBq [200 mCi]; total dosage/entire 24-week treatment course = 29.6 GBq [800 mCi])

<u>Notes:</u>
- Use aseptic technique and radiation shielding when administering the lutetium Lu-177-dotatate solution. Use tongs when handling the vial to minimize radiation exposure
- Do not inject lutetium Lu-177-dotatate directly into any other intravenous solution
- Confirm the amount of radioactivity of lutetium Lu-177-dotatate in the vial with a dose calibrator prior to and after administration
- Inspect the product visually for particulate matter and discoloration prior to administration under a shielded screen. Discard vial if particulates or discoloration are present

<u>Administration Instructions</u>
- Insert a 2.5-cm, 20-gauge needle (short needle) into the lutetium Lu-177-dotatate vial and connect via a catheter to 500 mL 0.9% sterile sodium chloride solution (used to transport lutetium Lu-177-dotatate during the infusion). Do not allow the short needle to touch the lutetium Lu-177-dotatate solution in the vial and do not connect this short needle directly to the patient. Do not allow sodium chloride solution to flow into the lutetium Lu-177-dotatate vial prior to the initiation of the lutetium Lu-177-dotatate infusion and do not inject lutetium Lu-177-dotatate directly into the sodium chloride solution
- Insert a second needle that is 9 cm, 18 gauge (long needle) into the lutetium Lu-177-dotatate vial ensuring that this long needle touches and is secured to the bottom of the lutetium Lu-177-dotatate vial during the entire infusion. Connect the long needle to the patient by an intravenous catheter that is prefilled with 0.9% sterile sodium chloride and that is used exclusively for the lutetium Lu-177-dotatate infusion into the patient
- Use a clamp or pump to regulate the flow of the sodium chloride solution via the short needle into the lutetium Lu-177-dotatate vial at a rate of 50 mL/hour to 100 mL/hour for 5–10 minutes and then 200 mL/hour to 300 mL/hour for an additional 25–30 minutes. (The sodium chloride solution entering the vial through the short needle will carry the lutetium Lu-177-dotatate from the vial to the patient via the catheter connected to the long needle over a total duration of 30–40 minutes)
- Do not administer lutetium Lu-177-dotatate as an intravenous bolus
- During the infusion, ensure that the level of solution in the lutetium Lu-177-dotatate vial remains constant
- Disconnect the vial from the long needle line and clamp the saline line once the level of radioactivity is stable for at least 5 minutes
- Follow the infusion with an intravenous flush of 25 mL of 0.9% sterile sodium chloride
- Dispose of any unused medicinal product or waste material in accordance with local and federal laws

<u>Somatostatin Analogs</u>
<u>Prior to the administration of lutetium Lu-177-dotatate:</u>
- Discontinue long-acting somatostatin analogs for at least 4 weeks prior to initiating lutetium Lu-177-dotatate
- In the 4-week period between the administration of a long-acting somatostatin analog and the initiation of lutetium Lu-177-dotatate, administer short-acting octreotide as needed for symptomatic treatment but do not administer short-acting octreotide in the 24 hours prior to initiating lutetium Lu-177-dotatate

<u>After lutetium Lu-177-dotatate treatment:</u>
- Administer long-acting somatostatin analog between 4 and 24 hours after each lutetium Lu–177-dotatate dose
- But do not administer long-acting octreotide within 4 weeks of each subsequent lutetium Lu-177-dotatate dose

<u>After lutetium Lu-177-dotatate treatment is completed:</u>
- Continue long-acting somatostatin analog intramuscularly every 4 weeks until disease progression for a minimum of 18 months following treatment initiation

<u>Amino Acid Solution:</u>
- Administer an amino acid solution containing L-lysine and L-arginine intravenously starting 30 minutes before administering lutetium Lu-177-dotatate
- If using the same access as that used for the administration of lutetium Lu-177-dotatate, then use a three-way valve or administer amino acids through a separate venous access in other arm

(continued)

(*continued*)

- Infuse amino acids during, and for at least 3 hours after, lutetium Lu-177-dotatate infusion
- Do not decrease the dose of the amino acid solution if the dose of lutetium Lu-177-dotatate is reduced

Amino Acid Solution	
Item	**Specification**
Lysine HCl content	Between 18 g and 24 g
Arginine HCl content	Between 18 g and 24 g
Volume	1.5 L to 2.2 L
Osmolarity	<1050 mOsmol

Supportive Care

Antiemetic prophylaxis
Emetogenic potential of the amino acid solution is **LOW**
Emetogenic potential of lutetium Lu-177-dotatate is **MINIMAL**
See Chapter 42 for antiemetic recommendations

Hematopoietic growth factor (CSF) prophylaxis
Primary prophylaxis is **NOT** *indicated*
See Chapter 43 for more information

Antimicrobial prophylaxis
Risk of fever and neutropenia is **LOW**
  Antimicrobial primary prophylaxis to be considered:
  - Antibacterial—not indicated
  - Antifungal—not indicated
  - Antiviral—not indicated unless patient previously had an episode of HSV

Treatment Modification

Adverse Reaction	Dose Modification
Grade 2/3/4 thrombocytopenia	• Withhold dose until complete or partial resolution (Grade 0/1). Resume LUTATHERA at 3.7 GBq (100 mCi) in patients with complete or partial resolution. If reduced dose does not result in Grade 2/3/4 thrombocytopenia, administer LUTATHERA at 7.4 GBq (200 mCi) for next dose • Permanently discontinue LUTATHERA for G ≥2 thrombocytopenia requiring a treatment delay ≥16 weeks
Recurrent Grade 2/3/4 thrombocytopenia	Permanently discontinue LUTATHERA
Grade 3/4 anemia and neutropenia	• Withhold dose until complete or partial resolution (Grade 0/1/2) • Resume LUTATHERA at 3.7 GBq (100 mCi) in patients with complete or partial resolution. If reduced dose does not result in Grade 3/4 anemia or neutropenia, administer LUTATHERA at 7.4 GBq (200 mCi) for next dose • Permanently discontinue LUTATHERA for G ≥3 anemia or neutropenia requiring a treatment delay ≥16 weeks
Recurrent Grade 3/4 anemia and neutropenia	Permanently discontinue LUTATHERA
• Creatinine clearance <40 mL/min; calculate using Cockcroft Gault with actual body weight, or • 40% increase in baseline serum creatinine, or • 40% decrease in baseline creatinine clearance calculated using Cockcroft Gault with actual body weight	• Withhold dose until complete resolution • Resume LUTATHERA at 3.7 GBq (100 mCi) in patients with complete resolution. If reduced dose does not result in renal toxicity, administer LUTATHERA at 7.4 GBq (200 mCi) for next dose • Permanently discontinue LUTATHERA for renal toxicity requiring a treatment delay ≥16 weeks

(*continued*)

Treatment Modification (*continued*)

Adverse Reaction	Dose Modification
Recurrent renal toxicity as above	Permanently discontinue LUTATHERA
• Bilirubinemia >3× ULN (Grade 3/4) or • Hypoalbuminemia <30 g/L with a decreased prothrombin ratio <70%	• Withhold dose until complete resolution • Resume LUTATHERA at 3.7 GBq (100 mCi) in patients with complete resolution. If reduced LUTATHERA dose does not result in hepatotoxicity, administer LUTATHERA at 7.4 GBq (200 mCi) for next dose • Permanently discontinue LUTATHERA for hepatotoxicity requiring a treatment delay ≥16 weeks
Recurrent hepatotoxicity as above	Permanently discontinue LUTATHERA
Other Grade 3/4 nonhematologic toxicity	• Withhold dose until complete or partial resolution (Grade 0 to 2) • Resume LUTATHERA at 3.7 GBq (100 mCi) in patients with complete or partial resolution. If reduced dose does not result in Grade 3/4 toxicity, administer LUTATHERA at 7.4 GBq (200 mCi) for next dose • Permanently discontinue LUTATHERA for Grade 3 or higher toxicity requiring treatment delay ≥16 weeks
Recurrent Grade 3/4 nonhematologic toxicity	Permanently discontinue LUTATHERA
Neuroendocrine hormonal crisis (diarrhea, hypotension, bronchoconstriction, or other signs and symptoms)	Administer somatostatin analogs (octreotide acetate 50–200 μg administered by subcutaneous or intravenous injection), fluids, corticosteroids (50–100 mg hydrocortisone intravenously), and electrolytes as indicated

Patient Population Studied

This open-label, multicenter, randomized, parallel-group, comparator-controlled, phase 3 study included 229 adult patients with neuroendocrine tumors who were randomized to receive either Lu-177 Dotatate plus best supportive care (including continuation of 30 mg octreotide LAR intramuscular [IM] injections) or high-dose (60 mg) octreotide LAR IM injections alone. Patients were eligible if they had inoperable, somatostatin receptor–positive, well-differentiated, histologically proven neuroendocrine tumors of the small bowel (midgut carcinoid tumors) and if they had shown progressive disease over a maximum of 3 years while taking octreotide LAR 20–30 mg every 3–4 weeks for at least 12 weeks before enrollment. Patients were required to have a Karnofsky Performance Score of ≥60 and tumors had to have a Ki67 index of ≤20% (low–intermediate grade) with confirmed presence of somatostatin receptors on all tumor lesions. Exclusion criteria included inadequate organ function and treatment with >30 mg octreotide LAR within 12 weeks before randomization

Efficacy (N = 229)

	Lu–177 Dotatate + Supportive Therapy (N = 116)	Octreotide LAR High-Dose Therapy (N = 113)	
Median progression-free survival*	28.4 months (95% CI, 28.4–NE)	8.5 months (95% CI, 5.8–11.0)	HR 0.21 (95% CI, 0.14–0.33); P <0.0001
20-month progression-free survival†	65.2% (95% CI, 50.0–76.8)	10.8% (95% CI, 3.5–23.0)	
Objective tumor response‡‡	18% (95% CI, 10–25)	3% (95% CI, 0–6)	P <0.001
Median overall survival*	NR (95% CI, NE–NE)	27.4 months (95% CI, 23.1–NE)	HR 0.536

HR, hazard ratio; CI, confidence interval; NR, not reached; NE, not estimable
*Based on an updated analysis with a data cutoff date of 30 June 2016
†Based on an interim analysis with data cutoff date of 24 July 2015
‡Based on RECIST criteria, version 1.1. Data include only patients evaluable for response (n = 101 in the Lu-177 dotatate plus supportive therapy and n = 100 in the octreotide LAR high-dose therapy group).

Adverse Events (N = 221)

Event	Lu-177 Dotatate Plus Supportive Therapy (N = 111)		Octreotide LAR High-Dose Therapy (N = 110)	
Grade (%)	Grade 1/2	Grade 3/4	Grade 1/2	Grade 3/4
Any adverse event	53	41	51	33
Nausea	55	4	10	2
Vomiting	40	7	9	1
Abdominal pain	23	3	21	5
Diarrhea	26	3	17	2
Distension	13	0	14	0
Fatigue or asthenia	38	2	24	2
Peripheral edema	14	0	7	0
Thrombocytopenia	23	2	1	0
Anemia	14	0	5	0
Lymphopenia	9	9	2	0
Leukopenia	9	1	1	0
Neutropenia	5	1	1	0
Musculoskeletal pain	27	2	19	1
Decreased appetite	18	0	5	3
Headache	16	0	5	0
Dizziness	11	0	5	0
Flushing	12	1	9	0
Alopecia	11	0	2	0
Cough	11	0	5	0

- Adverse events are included in the table if they were reported in at least 10% of the patients in the Lu-177 dotatate group, except for leukopenia, which was reported in less than 10% of that group
- Data include all patients randomized and who received treatment. 5% of patients randomized to the investigational therapy withdrew from the trial due to adverse events considered related to treatment, whereas no patients from the control group did
- Nausea and vomiting were attributed to amino acid infusions
- No renal toxic effects were noted in the Lu-177 dotatate group, potentially due to amino acid treatment
- Myelodysplastic syndrome occurred in 0.9% of patients in the Lu-177 dotatate group

Therapy Monitoring

1. CBC with differential every 2 weeks, or weekly if a trend is detected indicating neutropenia, anemia, or thrombocytopenia may occur. BUN, creatinine, and LFTs every 2 weeks
2. Imaging to assess response to therapy before every dose of LUTATHERA. Although not much shrinkage may occur, at least initially, the purpose of monitoring is to exclude progression of disease at a rate that would support discontinuation of treatment
3. Interval history and physical exam before every dose

30. Non-Hodgkin Lymphoma

Jennifer E. Amengual, MD and Philippe Armand, MD, PhD

Pathology (WHO 2016)

Mature B-cell neoplasms
- Chronic Lymphocytic Leukemia/Small Lymphocytic Lymphoma
- Monoclonal B-cell lymphocytosis°
- B-cell prolymphocytic leukemia
- Splenic marginal zone lymphoma
- Hairy cell leukemia
- Splenic B-cell lymphoma/leukemia, unclassifiable†
  - Splenic diffuse red pulp small B-cell lymphoma†
  - Hairy cell leukemia-variant†
- Lymphoplasmacytic lymphoma
  - Waldenström macroglobulinemia
- Monoclonal gammopathy of undetermined significance (MGUS), IgM°
- μ heavy-chain disease
- γ heavy-chain disease
- α heavy-chain disease
- Monoclonal gammopathy of undetermined significance (MGUS), IgG/A°
- Plasma cell myeloma
- Solitary plasmacytoma of bone
- Extraosseous plasmacytoma
- Monoclonal immunoglobulin deposition diseases°
- Extranodal marginal zone lymphoma of mucosa-associated lymphoid tissue (MALT lymphoma)
- Nodal marginal zone lymphoma
  - Pediatric nodal marginal zone lymphoma†
- Follicular lymphoma
  - In situ follicular neoplasia°
  - Duodenal-type follicular lymphoma°
- Pediatric-type follicular lymphoma°
- Large B-cell lymphoma with IRF4 rearrangement°†
- Primary cutaneous follicle center lymphoma
- Mantle cell lymphoma
  - In situ mantle cell neoplasia°
- Diffuse large B-cell lymphoma (DLBCL), NOS
  - Germinal center B-cell type°
  - Activated B-cell type°
- T-cell/histiocyte-rich large B-cell lymphoma
- Primary DLBCL of the central nervous system (CNS)
- Primary cutaneous DLBCL, leg type
- EBV+ DLBCL, NOS°
- EBV+ mucocutaneous ulcer°†
- DLBCL associated with chronic inflammation
- Lymphomatoid granulomatosis
- Primary mediastinal (thymic) large B-cell lymphoma
- Intravascular large B-cell lymphoma
- ALK+ large B-cell lymphoma
- Plasmablastic lymphoma
- Primary effusion lymphoma
- HHV8+ DLBCL, NOS°†
- Burkitt lymphoma

Epidemiology

Incidence:	74,200 (male: 41,090; female: 33,110) Estimated new cases for 2019 in the United States 23.9 per 100,000 male; 16.2 per 100,000 female
Deaths:	Estimated 19,970 in 2019 (male: 11,510; female: 8460)
Median age:	67 years
Male to female ratio:	1.5 for all lymphoid neoplasms

Siegel R et al. CA Cancer J Clin 2019;69:7–34
Surveillance, Epidemiology and End Results (SEER) Program. Available from: http://seer.cancer.gov [accessed 3 October 2019]

Work-up

1. Immunophenotyping
   - DLBCL (Diffuse large B-cell lymphoma)
     - FISH for *MYC*, *BCL2*, *BCL6* to rule out / identify double/triple hit (DH/TH) lymphomas ± Immunohistochemistry for *MYC* and *BCL2* to identify double expressor, although this is not a separate WHO category

     Note: The World Health Organization (WHO) classification defines double-hit lymphoma (DHL) as a high-grade B-cell lymphoma harboring a *MYC* rearrangement occurring with *either* a B-cell CLL/lymphoma 2 (*BCL2*) *and/or* B-cell CLL/lymphoma (*BCL6*) rearrangement. In a triple-hit lymphoma (THL) all three gene rearrangements are present. Double expressor lymphoma (DEL) is DLBCL that exhibits co-expression of the respective proteins in the absence of gene rearrangement
     - IHC to assign cell of origin (COO) category—although there exists some controversy about value of COO

Work-up (continued)

- MCL (mantle cell lymphoma)
  - Immunohistochemistry for p53 or sequencing for TP53 mutation
- CLL (chronic lymphocytic lymphoma)
  - FISH, IGHV mutational status imperative as prognostic marker (mutant *IGHV* correlates with marked improvement in both progression-free survival [PFS] and overall survival [OS])
  - Other prognostic markers less important
- LPL (lymphoplasmacytic lymphoma)
  - MYD88 (myeloid differentiation primary response 88) and CXCR4 (chemokine receptor 4) mutation analysis—for diagnosis and risk stratification
- MZL (marginal zone lymphoma)
  - FISH, ideally MYD88 mutation testing to exclude LPL
- T-cell lymphomas
  - HTLV testing at least based on geographic background to exclude ATLL (adult T-cell leukemia/lymphoma)
- ALCL (anaplastic large cell lymphoma)
  - ALK (anaplastic lymphoma kinase) testing
  - for ALK(−) ALCL, consider DUSP22 and TP63 rearrangement testing
2. Cytogenetics for CLL/SLL and Burkitt lymphoma
3. PET scan in the majority of histologies— value less certain in MCL (mantle cell lymphoma), MZL (marginal zone lymphoma), and SLL (small lymphocytic lymphoma/chronic lymphocytic leukemia)
   - PET scan recommended before and after treatment, mid cycle only appropriate in clinical trial setting
   - Also indicated for relapsed indolent disease when suspect aggressive transformation

Seam P et al. Blood 2007;110:3507–3516

CNS Lymphomas (Non-HIV-Related; Additional Staging Work-up Recommended or To Be Considered)

1. Slit-lamp exam by ophthalmologist
2. HIV testing
3. Lumbar puncture
4. Brain and spine MRI
5. Testicular exam/ultrasound in men
6. Bone marrow biopsy in some cases— depends on the histology; generally has limited therapeutic implication

Other tests that can be considered for staging in specific histologies:

- Lumbar puncture for Burkitt lymphoma (always)
- EGD (esophagogastroduodenoscopy) for marginal zone lymphoma (often)
- Colonoscopy for mantle cell lymphoma (sometimes)

Pathology (WHO 2016) (continued)

- Burkitt-like lymphoma with 11q aberration[*†]
- High-grade B-cell lymphoma, with MYC and BCL2 and/or BCL6 rearrangements[*]
- High-grade B-cell lymphoma, NOS[*]
- B-cell lymphoma, unclassifiable, with features intermediate between DLBCL and classic Hodgkin lymphoma

Mature T And NK Neoplasms

- T-cell prolymphocytic leukemia
- T-cell large granular lymphocytic leukemia
- Chronic lymphoproliferative disorder of NK cells[†]
- Aggressive NK-cell leukemia
- Systemic EBV+ T-cell lymphoma of childhood[*]
- Hydroa vacciniforme–like lymphoproliferative disorder[*]
- Adult T-cell leukemia/lymphoma
- Extranodal NK-/T-cell lymphoma, nasal type
- Enteropathy-associated T-cell lymphoma
- Monomorphic epitheliotropic intestinal T-cell lymphoma[*]
- Indolent T-cell lymphoproliferative disorder of the GI tract[†]
- Hepatosplenic T-cell lymphoma
- Subcutaneous panniculitis-like T-cell lymphoma
- Mycosis fungoides
- Sézary syndrome
- Primary cutaneous CD30+ T-cell lymphoproliferative disorders
  - Lymphomatoid papulosis
  - Primary cutaneous anaplastic large cell lymphoma
- Primary cutaneous γδ T-cell lymphoma
- Primary cutaneous CD8+ aggressive epidermotropic cytotoxic T-cell lymphoma[†]
- Primary cutaneous acral CD8+ T-cell lymphoma[*†]
- Primary cutaneous CD4+ small/medium T-cell lymphoproliferative disorder[*†]
- Peripheral T-cell lymphoma, NOS
- Angioimmunoblastic T-cell lymphoma
- Follicular T-cell lymphoma[*†]
- Nodal peripheral T-cell lymphoma with TFH phenotype[*†]
- Anaplastic large-cell lymphoma, ALK+
- Anaplastic large-cell lymphoma, ALK-[*]
- Breast implant–associated anaplastic large-cell lymphoma[*†]

Posttransplant Lymphoproliferative Disorders (PTLD)

- Plasmacytic hyperplasia PTLD
- Infectious mononucleosis PTLD
- Florid follicular hyperplasia PTLD[*]
- Polymorphic PTLD
- Monomorphic PTLD (B- and T-/NK-cell types)
- Classic Hodgkin lymphoma PTLD

Histiocytic and Dendritic Cell Neoplasms

- Histiocytic sarcoma
- Langerhans cell histiocytosis
- Langerhans cell sarcoma
- Indeterminate dendritic cell tumor
- Interdigitating dendritic cell sarcoma
- Follicular dendritic cell sarcoma
- Fibroblastic reticular cell tumor
- Disseminated juvenile xanthogranuloma
- Erdheim-Chester disease[*]

[*]Changes from the WHO 2008 classification
[†]Provisional entity
Swerdlow SH et al, eds. World Health Organization Classification of Tumours of Haematopoietic and Lymphoid Tissues, Revised 4th Edition. Lyon, France: IARC Press, 2017

Staging

Ann Arbor Staging Classification for Hodgkin and Non-Hodgkin Lymphomas

Stage	Description
I	Involvement of a single lymph node region (I) or involvement of a single extralymphatic organ or site (IE)
II	Involvement of ≥2 lymph node regions or lymphatic structures on the same side of the diaphragm alone (II) or with involvement of limited, contiguous extralymphatic organ or tissue (IIE)
III	Involvement of lymph node regions on both sides of the diaphragm (III), which may include the spleen (IIIS) or limited, contiguous extralymphatic organ or site (IIIE) or both (IIIES)
IV	Diffuse or disseminated foci of involvement of one or more extralymphatic organs or tissues, with or without associated lymphatic involvement

Abbreviations

A	Asymptomatic
B	Unexplained persistent or recurrent fever with temperature higher than 38°C (100.4°F), or recurrent drenching night sweats within 1 month, or unexplained loss of >10% body weight within 6 months
E	Limited direct extension into extralymphatic organ from adjacent lymph node
X	Bulky disease (mediastinal tumor width > one-third of the transthoracic diameter at T5/6, or a tumor diameter >10 cm)

Moormeier JA et al. Semin Oncol 1990;17:43–50

5-Year Survival Rate

NHL Subtype	5-Year Survival Rates
Diffuse large B-cell lymphoma	Varies according to IPI and treatment
Follicular lymphoma	Varies according to FLIPI
Mantle cell lymphoma	Varies according to MIPI

Prognostic Indices
International Prognostic Index (IPI)

A predictive model for aggressive non-Hodgkin's lymphoma
The International Non-Hodgkin's Lymphoma Prognostic Factors Project
Shipp et al. N Engl J Med 1993;329:987–994

The **International Prognostic Index (IPI)** is a clinical tool to aid in predicting the prognosis of patients with aggressive non-Hodgkin lymphoma. First developed in 1993, it replaced the Ann Arbor stage as a prognosis tool. The original report was a retrospective analysis performed on 2031 patients with aggressive non-Hodgkin lymphoma treated between 1982 and 1987. Patients of all ages were included; all had been treated with doxorubicin-based regimens, most commonly CHOP (Shipp et al, 1993). Five patient characteristics emerged as significant. Although the IPI has been shown to be a useful clinical tool, it should be kept in mind that the studies on which it was based did not include rituximab. This has been addressed with other similar scores such as the NCCN-IPI and the R-IPI

Risk Factors	Zero (0) Points	One (1) Point
Age	≤60 years	>60 years
Ann Arbor Stage of Disease III/IV	No	Yes
Serum LDH >ULN	No	Yes
ECOG/Zubrod performance status ≥2	No	Yes
More than one extranodal site	No	Yes

Staging (continued)

Points	Risk Category	5-Year Survival
0–1 points	Low risk	73%
2 points	Low-intermediate risk	51%
3 points	High-intermediate risk	43%
4–5 points	High risk	26%

NCCN IPI

Zhou et al. Blood 2014;123:837–842

The original International Prognostic Index (IPI) was developed was developed by Shipp et al and validated prior to the addition of rituximab to curative chemotherapy. Using a database of 1935 patients in the National Comprehensive Cancer Network (NCCN) database treated with doxorubicin-based regimens in the rituximab era. This enhanced IPI score is able to discriminate individuals based on 5 clinical predictors and an 8-point scoring system. The enhanced NCCN-IPI offers improved discrimination for the overall survival of low- and high-risk patients in the rituximab era

Risk Factors	Zero (0) Points	One (1) Point	Two (2) Points	Three (3) Points
Age	≤40	41–60	61–75	>75
Ann Arbor Stage of	I/II	III/IV	—	—
Serum LDH >ULN	Normal	>1 to ≤3	>3	—
ECOG/Zubrod performance status	0/1	2/3/4	—	—
Extranodal disease in bone marrow, CNS, liver/GI tract or lungs	No	Yes	—	—

Points	Risk Category	5-Year Survival
0–1 points	Low risk	96%
2–3 points	Low-intermediate risk	82%
4–5 points	High-intermediate risk	64%
≥6 points	High risk	33%

R-IPI

Sehn et al. Blood 2007;109:1857–1861

The original International Prognostic Index (IPI) was developed and validated prior to the addition of rituximab to curative anthracycline-based chemotherapy. Clinical trials have confirmed that rituximab improves the survival of individuals with diffuse large B-cell lymphoma. The revised International Prognostic Index (R-IPI) was developed to predict the outcome of individuals receiving rituximab with chemotherapy. The score is able to differentiate patients into three groups (very good, good, poor), all of who have survival >50% in the new era. The enhanced NCCN-IPI offers improved discrimination for the overall survival of low- and high-risk patients in the rituximab era

Risk Factors	Zero (0) Points	One (1) Point
Age	≤60 years	>60 years
Ann Arbor Stage of Disease III/IV	No	Yes
Serum LDH >ULN	No	Yes
ECOG/Zubrod performance status 3/4	No	Yes
More than one extranodal site	No	Yes

Staging (*continued*)

Points	Prognostic Category	4-Year Survival
0	Very good	94%
1–2 points	Good	79%
4–5 points	High risk	55%

Comparison of Alternate DLBCL IPI Models
Diffuse Large B-cell Lymphoma (DLBCL)
One point is assigned for each of the above risk factors
Stratified models for OS[*]

Model	Hazard Ratio (95% CI)	AIC[†]	C-index[‡] (95% CI)
IPI risk group		5455	0.626 (0.557–0.694)
Low (0–1)	Reference		
Low-intermediate (2)	1.99 (1.46–2.72)		
High-intermediate (3)	2.73 (1.99–3.74)		
High (4–5)	4.51 (3.29–6.16)		
R-IPI risk group		5492	0.590 (0.528–0.652)
Very good (0)	Reference		
Good (1–2)	1.68 (0.81–3.48)		
Poor (3–5)	3.67 (1.75–7.67)		
NCCN-IPI risk group		5428	0.632 (0.565–0.700)
Low (0–1)	Reference		
Low-intermediate (2–3)	1.49 (0.83–2.67)		
High-intermediate (4–5)	3.95 (2.17–7.19)		
High (6–8)	6.40 (3.45–11.89)		

[*]Adapted from Ruppert et al. Blood 2020;135:2041–2048. Models were stratified by study and type of induction therapy
[†]The AIC provided a relative measure of model quality; smaller values correspond with a better fitting model. Differences in AIC <2 between models indicate no improvement in fit, differences >2 but <10 indicate increasing improvement in fit, and differences ≥10 indicate substantial improvement in the fit of the model
[‡]The C-index provided a measure of predictive ability of the model, defined as the probability of concordance between predicted and observed survival. The C-index corresponds to the area under the receiver operating characteristics curve for censored data. C-index values of 0.5, 0.7, and 1.0 indicate that the model has completely random, acceptable, or perfect discrimination, respectively, between short and long survival times
Author conclusions:
- The NCCN-IPI had the greatest absolute difference in OS estimates between the highest- and lowest-risk groups and best discriminated OS (concordance index = 0.632 vs 0.626 [IPI] vs 0.590 [R-IPI])
- For each given IPI risk category, NCCN-IPI risk categories were significantly associated with OS ($P \leq 0.01$); the reverse was not true, and the IPI did not provide additional significant prognostic information within all NCCN-IPI risk categories
- Collectively, the NCCN-IPI outperformed the IPI and R-IPI. Patients with low-risk NCCN-IPI had favorable survival outcomes with little room for further improvement
- In the rituximab era, none of the clinical risk scores identified a patient subgroup with long-term survival clearly <50%. Integrating molecular features of the tumor and microenvironment into the NCCN-IPI or IPI might better characterize a high-risk group for which novel treatment approaches are most needed

Age-Adjusted IPI

Hamlin et al. Blood 2003;102:1989–1996

A simplified index can be used when comparing patients within an age group (ie, 60 or younger, or over 60) and includes only 3 of the above risk factors

Risk Factors	Zero (0) Points	One (1) Point
Ann Arbor Stage of Disease III/IV	No	Yes
Serum LDH >ULN	No	Yes
ECOG/Zubrod performance status ≥2	No	Yes

(*continued*)

Staging (*continued*)

Points	Risk Category	5-Year Survival
0 point	Low risk	83%
1 point	Low-intermediate risk	69%
2 points	High-intermediate risk	46%
3 points	High risk	32%

Stage-Adjusted IPI (St-IPI)

Norasetthada et al. Blood 2015;126:5030

A simplified index. Developed in an attempt to better predict PFS for limited stage DLBCL treated with R-CHOP. The model aspires to predict lower risk disease more discriminately than the IPI to tailor therapy and avoid unnecessary treatment related toxicities. Moreover, the St-IPI also attempts to better predict outcomes in patients with high risk of relapses in whom more aggressive treatment is warranted to improve the cure rate of the patients

Risk Factors	Zero (0) Points	One (1) Point
Age	≤60 years	>60 years
Serum LDH >ULN	No	Yes
ECOG/Zubrod performance status ≥2	No	Yes

Points	Risk Category	5-Year Survival
0 point	Low risk	84%
1–2 point	Intermediate risk	73%
3 points	High risk	49%

Follicular Lymphoma International Prognostic Index (FLIPI)

Solal-Céligny et al. Blood 2004;104:1258–1265

Risk Factors	Zero (0) Points	One (1) Point
Age	<60	≥60
Stage of Disease	I, II	III, IV
Lymph node groups involved	≤3	>4
Elevated serum LDH	Within normal range	Elevated
Hemoglobin	≥12 g/dL	<12 g/dL

Risk Category and Prognosis

FLIPI Score	FLIPI Risk Category	5-year PFS	10-year PFS
0–1 points	Low risk	91%	71%
2 points	Intermediate risk	78%	51%
3–5 points	High risk	53%	36%

Staging (continued)

FLIPI–2

Federico et al. J Clin Oncol 2009;27:4555–4562

Risk Factors	Zero (0) Points	One (1) Point
Age	<60	≥60
Serum β₂-microglobulin	Normal	Raised
Bone marrow involvement	Absent	Present
Longest diameter of largest involved node	<6 cm	≥6 cm
Hemoglobin	≥12 g/dL	< 12 g/dL

Risk Category and Prognosis

FLIPI-2 Score	FLIPI-2 Risk Category	5-year PFS
0	Low risk	80%
1—2	Intermediate risk	51%
3—5	High risk	19%

PRIMA-PI

Bachy et al. Blood 2018;132:49–58

Risk Category and Prognosis

PRIMA-PI Risk Category	Parameters	% 5-year PFS°
Low risk	β2m ≤3 mg/L without bone marrow involvement	65 (77)
Intermediate risk	β2m ≤3 mg/L with bone marrow involvement	55 (57)
High risk	β2m > 3 mg/L	37 (44)

°Results of validation cohort in parentheses

m7FLIPI

Pastore et al. Lancet Oncol 2015;16:1111–1122

Improves risk stratification by integrating

— The mutation status of seven genes (*EZH2, ARID1A, MEF2B, EP300, FOXO1, CREBBP,* and *CARD11*)
— The FL International Prognostic Index (FLIPI)
— The ECOG performance status

Note, that this score was established and validated only in patients with

• Follicular lymphoma grade 1, 2, or 3A, advanced stage or bulky disease considered ineligible for curative irradiation
• Symptomatic disease requiring systemic treatment according to published criteria (Hiddemann et al, Blood 2004)
• A lymphoma biopsy obtained less than 12 months prior to therapy initiation
• A history of having received a combination of rituximab and chemotherapy (either CVP or CHOP) as first-line treatment
• FLIPI
  — Low-risk group
  — Intermediate-risk group
  — High-risk group
• ECOG PS
  — 0—Fully active
  — 1—Capable of light work
  — 2—Capable of selfcare

- – 3—Mostly confined to bed or chair
- – 4—Completely disabled
- Mutation status
  - – EZH2: not mutated or mutated
  - – ARID1A: not mutated or mutated
  - – EP300: not mutated or mutated
  - – FOXO1: not mutated or mutated
  - – MEF2B: not mutated or mutated
  - – CREBBP: not mutated or mutated
  - – CARD11: not mutated or mutated

Mantle Cell Lymphoma International Prognostic Index (MIPI and MIPI-c)

Hoster et al. Blood 2008;11:558–565
Hoster et al. J Clin Oncol 2016;34:1386–1394

Mantle Cell Lymphoma International Prognostic Index (MIPI)

	0 Points	1 Point	2 Points	3 Points
Age in years	<50	50–59	60–69	≥70
ECOG performance status	0–1	—	2–4	—
LDH	<0.67 × ULN	0.67–0.99 × ULN	1–1.49 × ULN	≥1.5 × ULN
WBC/mcl	<6700	6700 to 9999	10,000–14,999	≥15,000

Points	Risk Category	Median Survival
0–3 points	Low risk	Not yet reached
4–5 points	Intermediate risk	51 months
6–11 points	High risk	29 months

MIPI-c combined Mantle Cell International Prognostic Index[*]

The modified combination of Ki–67 index and MIPI integrates the most important clinical and biologic markers currently available in clinical routine and provides for additional risk stratification beyond MIPI

Original MIPI	Ki-67 Index, %	MIPI-c Score	Percentage[†]	Median PFS (Years)[†]	Median OS (Years)[†]
Low risk	<30	Low risk	32	7.4	Not reached
	>30	Low-intermediate risk	34	4.4	Not reached
Intermediate risk	<30				
	>30	High-intermediate risk	23	2.0	4.3
High risk	<30				
	>30	High risk	11	1	1.5

[*]Adapted from Hoster et al with additional data provided by Dr. Hoster
[†]Percentage of patients, PFS, and OS, according to MIPI-c from the European MCL Network Younger and Elderly Trials

Expert Opinion

The choice of therapy requires consideration of many factors, including age, comorbid pathologies, and future therapies (eg, stem cell transplantation). Therefore, treatment selection should be individualized

Diffuse Large B-Cell Lymphoma
First-line therapy
- Rituximab-CHOP (rituximab + cyclophosphamide + doxorubicin + vincristine + prednisone)

   Coiffier B et al. N Engl J Med 2002;346:235–242

For older patients:
- R-miniCHOP (cyclophosphamide + doxorubicin + vincristine + prednisone)

   Peyrade F et al. Lancet Oncol 2011;12:460–468
- R-CEOP (MINI-CEOP) (cyclophosphamide + etoposide + vincristine + prednisone)

   Merli et al. Leuk Lymphoma 2007;48:367–373
- RCDOP (rituximab + cyclophosphamide + pegylated liposomal doxorubicin + vincristine + prednisone)

   Martino R et al. Haematologica 2002;87:822–882; Zaja F et al. Leuk Lymphoma 2006;47:2174–2180
- RGCVP (rituximab + gemcitabine + cyclophosphamide + vincristine + prednisolone)

   Fields PA et al. J Clin Oncol 2014;32:282–287
- RCEPP (rituximab + cyclophosphamide + etoposide + procarbazine + prednisone)

   Chao NJ et al. Blood 1990;76:1293–1298
- R-Benda (bendamustine + rituximab)

   Park S et al. Br J Haematol 2016;175:281–289
- R-GemOx (rituximab + gemcitabine + oxaliplatin)

   Shen QD et al. Lancet Haematol 2018;5:e261–e269

Primary mediastinal DLBCL and also in other circumstances (ie, double hit lymphoma [DHL] and triple hit lymphoma [THL])
- Dose-adjusted EPOCH-R (etoposide + prednisone + vincristine + cyclophosphamide + doxorubicin + rituximab) for primary mediastinal DLBCL

   Primary Mediastinal DLBCL: Dunleavy et al. N Engl J Med 2013;368:1408–1416
   DLBCL: Wilson et al. J Clin Oncol 2008;26:2717–2724; Purroy et al. Br J Haematol 2015;169:118–198; Petrich et al. Blood 2014;124:2354–2361

First-line consolidation (option)
- Lenalidomide maintenance for patients 60–80 years old

   Thieblemont et al. J Clin Oncol 2017;35:2473–2481

Second-line therapy
- R-GemOx (rituximab + gemcitabine + oxaliplatin)

   Shen et al. Lancet Haematol 2018;5:e261–e69 (as above); López A et al. Eur J Haematol 2008;80:127–132; Corazzelli G et al. Cancer Chemother Pharmacol 2009;64:907–916

- RICE (rituximab + ifosfamide + carboplatin + etoposide)

   Kewalramani et al. Blood 2004;103:3684–3688
- R-ESHAP (etoposide + methylprednisolone + cytarabine + cisplatin)

   ESHAP: Velasquez et al. J Clin Oncol 1994;12:1169–1176; R-ESHAP: Martín et al. Haematologica 2008;93:1829–1836
- R-DHAP (dexamethasone + high dose cytarabine + cisplatin)

   Gisselbrecht et al. J Clin Oncol 2010;28:4184–4190
- GDP-R (gemcitabine + dexamethasone + cisplatin + rituximab)

   Crump et al. Cancer 2004;101:1835–1842; Crump et al. Clin Lymphoma 2005;6:56–60; Ghio et al. J Cancer Metastasis Treat 2016;2:59–63
- Clinical trials, if available

Second-line refractory disease not eligible for consolidative autologous stem cell transplant
- R-GemOx (rituximab + gemcitabine + oxaliplatin)

   Shen et al. Lancet Haematol 2018;5:e261–e69 (as above)
- R2: (rituximab + lenalidomide)

   Witzig et al. Ann Oncol 2011;22:1622–1627; Wiemik et al. J Clin Oncol 2008;26:4952–4957; Wang et al. Leukemia 2013;27:1902–1909
- R-bendamustine (rituximab + bendamustine)

   Weidmann E et al. Ann Oncol 2002;13:1285–1289; Ohmachi et al. J Clin Oncol 2013;31:2103–2109; Vacirca et al. Ann Hematol 2013;93:403–409
- Tafasitamab + lenalidomide (tafasitamab + lenalidomide)

   Salles et al. Lancet Oncol 2020:21:978–988
- Clinical trials, if available

Salvage beyond second-line refractory disease not eligible for consolidative autologous stem cell transplant
- Regimens in section above that have not been used
- Pola-B-R (polatuzumab vedotin + bendamustine + rituximab)

   Sehn et al. J Clin Oncol 2019;38:155–165
- Selinexor (Selinexor)

   Kalakonda et al. Lancet Hematol 2020;7:e511–e522
- CAR-T (axicabtagene ciloleucel)

   Locke et al. Lancet Oncol 2019;20:31–42; Neelapu et al. N Engl J Med 2017;377:2531–2544
- CAR-T (tisagenlecleucel)

   Schuster et al. N Engl J Med 2019;380:45–56

Follicular Lymphoma
First-line therapy
- CVP ± R (cyclophosphamide + vincristine + prednisone ± rituximab)

   Bagley et al. Ann Intern Med 1972;76:227–234; Flinn et al. Ann Oncol 2000;11:691–695; Marcus R et al. Blood 2005;105:1417–1423
- CVP + obinutuzumab (cyclophosphamide + vincristine + prednisone + obinutuzumab)

   Marcus et al. N Engl J Med 2017;377:1331–1344

- Rituximab-CHOP (rituximab + cyclophosphamide + doxorubicin + vincristine + prednisone)

   Coiffier et al. N Engl J Med 2002;346:235–242 (as above)
- Bendamustine + rituximab

   Rummel et al. Lancet 2013;381:1203–1221
- Bendamustine + obinutuzumab

   Marcus et al. N Engl J Med 2017;377:1331–1334
- Lenalidomide + rituximab

   Morschhauser et al. N Engl J Med 2018;379:934–947; Martin et al. Ann Oncol 2017;28:2806–2812; Fowler et al. Lancet Oncol 2014;15:1311–1318
- Rituximab (selected circumstances)

   Davis et al. J Clin Oncol 1999;17:1851–1857
- Extended-schedule rituximab

   Ghielmini M et al. Blood 2004;103:4416–4442
- Maintenance/extended schedule rituximab after rituximab-containing regimen

   Salles et al. Lancet 2011;377:42–51
- Obinutuzumab maintenance after obinutuzumab-containing regimen

Subsequent therapy
- Treatments listed under *First-line therapy*
- Rituximab (selected circumstances)

   Davis et al. J Clin Oncol 1999;17:1851–1857
- Extended-schedule rituximab

   Ghielmini M et al. Blood 2004;103:4416–4442
- Idelalisib

   Gopal et al. N Engl J Med 2014;370:1008–1018
- Copanlisib

   Dreyling et al. J Clin Oncol 2017;35:3898–3905
- Duvelisib

   Flinn et al. J Clin Oncol 2019;37:912–922
- Tazemetostat

   Morschhauser et al. Lancet Oncol 2020;21:1433–1442
- Obi-Len (obinutuzumab + lenalidomide)

   Morschhauser et al. Lancet Haematol 2019;6:e429–e437
- Bortezomib

   Zinzani et al. Hematol Oncol 2013;31:179–182
- R-GemOx (rituximab + gemcitabine + oxaliplatin)

   Shen et al. Lancet Haematol 2018;5:e261–e69 (as above)
- RICE (rituximab + ifosfamide + carboplatin + etoposide)

   Kewalramani et al. Blood 2004;103:3684–3688 (as above)
- R-ESHAP (etoposide + methylprednisolone + cytarabine + cisplatin)

   ESHAP: Velasquez et al. J Clin Oncol 1994;12:1169–1176; R-ESHAP: Martín et al. Haematologica 2008;93:1829–1836 (as above)
- R-DHAP (dexamethasone + high dose cytarabine + cisplatin)

   Gisselbrecht et al. J Clin Oncol 2010;28:4184–4190 (as above)
- Autologous stem cell transplant (ASCT) or allogeneic hematopoietic progenitor cell transplantation for patients with chemotherapy-sensitive disease
- Clinical trials, if available

Expert Opinion (continued)

Mantle Cell Lymphoma
First-line therapy—aggressive Therapy
- Nordic Regimen
  Geisler et al. Br J Haematol 2012;158:355–362; Geisler et al. Blood 2008;112:2687–2693
- Hyper-CVAD alternating with R-MC (Hyper-CVAD, cyclophosphamide + vincristine + doxorubicin + dexamethasone) (R-MC, high-dose methotrexate + cytarabine + rituximab)
  Romaguera et al. J Clin Oncol 2005;23:7013–7023; Wang et al. Cancer 2008;113:2734–2741
- Alternating R-CHOP + DHAP. (R-CHOP, rituximab + cyclophosphamide + doxorubicin + vincristine + prednisone) (R-DHAP, rituximab + dexamethasone + cytarabine [high-dose Ara-C] + cisplatin)
  Delarue et al. Blood 2013;121:48–53; Pott C et al. Blood 2010;115:3215–3223
- R-Benda (bendamustine plus rituximab)
  Rummel et al. Lancet 2013;381:1203–1210
- R-Benda/R-Cytarabine (rituximab/bendamustine and rituximab/cytarabine)
  Merryman et al. Blood 2020;4:858–867
- Consolidative ASCT

First-line therapy—less-aggressive therapy
- VR-CAP (bortezomib + rituximab + cyclophosphamide + doxorubicin + prednisone)
  Robak et al. N Engl J Med 2015;372:944–953
- R2 (Revlimid [lenalidomide] + rituximab)
  Ruan J et al. N Engl J Med 2015;373:1835–1844; Ruan et al. Blood 2018;132:2016–2025
- RBAC (rituximab + bendamustine + cytarabine)
  Visco et al. J Clin Oncol 2013;31:1442–1449; Ohmachi K et al. J Clin Oncol 2013;31:2103–2109; Vacirca et al. Ann Hematol 2013; 93:403–409

Subsequent therapy
- Treatments listed under *First-line therapy*
- Bortezomib
  Fisher et al. J Clin Oncol 2006;24:4867–4874; Goy A et al. Ann Oncol 2009;20:520–525
- Lenalidomide (with or without rituximab)
  Goy et al. J Clin Oncol 2013;31:3688–3695
- Ibrutinib
  Wang et al. N Engl J Med 2013;369:507–516
- Acalabrutinib
  Wang et al. Lancet 2018;391:659–667

- Zanubrutinib
  Song et al. Clin Can Res 2020;26:4216–4224
- Venetoclax + ibrutinib
  Tam et al. N Engl J Med 2018;378:1211–1123
- Temsirolimus with or without rituximab
  Hess et al. J Clin Oncol 2009;23:3822–3829
- Brexucabtagene
  Wang et al. N Engl J Med 2020;382:13314–13342
- Allogeneic stem cell transplant for patients with chemosensitive tumors

Older patients
- R-Benda (bendamustine plus rituximab)
  Rummel et al. Lancet 2013;381:1203–1210 (as above)

Peripheral T-Cell Lymphomas
Note: There are different and specific treatments for certain subtypes, like ATLL and ENKTL

First-line therapy
- Clinical Trial
- Rituximab-CHOP (rituximab + cyclophosphamide + doxorubicin + vincristine + prednisone)
  Coiffier et al. N Engl J Med 2002;346:235–242 (as above)
- A-CHP (brentuximab vedotin [Adcetris] + cyclophosphamide + doxorubicin + prednisone)
  Horwitz et al. Lancet 2019;393:229–224 (Only for CD30+ disease including ALCL)
- CHOEP (cyclophosphamide, doxorubicin, etoposide, vincristine, prednisone)
  Pfreundschuh et al. Ann Oncol 2008;19:545–552; Schmitz et al. Blood 2010;116:3418–3425
- Consider consolidation with autologous stem cell transplant (ASCT)

Second-line therapy
- Clinical Trial
- Romidepsin
  Coiffier B et al. J Clin Oncol 2012;30:631–663
- Pralatrexate
  O'Connor et al. J Clin Oncol 2011;29:1182–118
- Belinostat
  O'Connor et al. J Clin Oncol 2015;33:2492
- Brentuximab for CD30+ T-cell lymphoma
  Horwitz et al. Blood 2014;123:3095; Pro et al. J Clin Oncol 2012;30:2190–2196
- Bendamustine
  Damaj et al. J Clin Oncol 2013;31:104–110

- Gemcitabine + oxaliplatin
  Lopez et al. Eur J Haematol 2008;80:127–132
- GDP (gemcitabine + dexamethasone + cisplatin)
  Crump et al. Cancer 2004;101:1835–1842; Dong et al. Med Oncol 2013;30:351; Moccia et al. Leuk Lymphoma 2017;58:324–332
- GiFOX (gemcitabine + ifosfamide + oxaliplatin)
  Corazzelli et al. Blood 2010;116:2829; Cozarelli et al. Ann Oncol 2006;17(Suppl 4):iv18–24
- GND (gemcitabine + navelbine + doxorubicin)
  Qian et al. Biomed Res Int 2015;2015:60675
- Lenalidomide
  Morschhauser et al. Eur J Cancer 2013;49:2869–2876; Toumishey et al. Cancer 2015;121:716–723
- Gemcitabine
  Zinzani et al. J Clin Oncol 2000;18:2603–2606; Zinzani et al. Ann Oncol 1998;9:1351–1353
- Bortezomib
  Zinzani et al. J Clin Oncol 2007;25:4293–4297
- Azacitidine (AITL)
  Delarue et al. Blood 2016;128:4164
- Duvelisib
  Pro et al. ASH 2020. Abstract 44. Presented December 5, 2020. NCT03372057

Burkitt's Lymphoma
- DA-EPOCH-R (Dose-adjusted etoposide + prednisone + vincristine + cyclophosphamide + doxorubicin + rituximab)
  Dunleavy K et al. N Engl J Med 2013;369:1915–1925
- CODOX-M + I-VAC—(CODOX-M, cyclophosphamide + vincristine + doxorubicin + methotrexate) + (IVAC, Ifosfamide + etoposide + cytarabine [ARA-C])
  Magrath et al. J Clin Oncol 1996;14:925–934
- R-HYPER-CVAD (rituximab + hyperfractionated cyclophosphamide + vincristine + doxorubicin [Adriamycin] + dexamethasone)
  Thomas et al. J Clin Oncol 1999;17:2461–2470; Thomas et al. Cancer 2006;106:1569–1580
- NHL-BFM 86 (BERLIN-FRANKFURT-MÜNSTER 86)
  Reiter A et al. J Clin Oncol 1995;13:359–372

DIFFUSE LARGE B-CELL LYMPHOMA • FIRST LINE
NON-HODGKIN LYMPHOMA REGIMEN: CYCLOPHOSPHAMIDE, DOXORUBICIN (HYDROXYLDAUNORUBICIN), VINCRISTINE (ONCOVIN), PREDNISONE + RITUXIMAB (CHOP + RITUXIMAB)

Coiffier B et al. N Engl J Med 2002;346:235–242

Rituximab
Premedication for rituximab:
Acetaminophen 650–1000 mg; administer orally, *plus*
Diphenhydramine 25–50 mg; administer orally or intravenously, 30–60 minutes before starting rituximab
Rituximab 375 mg/m^2; administer intravenously in 0.9% sodium chloride injection (0.9% NS) or 5% dextrose injection (D5W), diluted to a concentration of 1–4 mg/mL, on day 1, every 21 days (total dosage/cycle = 375 mg/m^2)
Notes on rituximab administration:
- Infuse initially at 50 mg/hour. If hypersensitivity or infusion reactions do not occur during the first 30 minutes, increase the rate by 50 mg/hour every 30 minutes, as tolerated, to a maximum rate of 400 mg/hour. Subsequently, if previous administration was well tolerated, start at 100 mg/hour and increase by 100 mg/hour every 30 minutes, as tolerated, to a maximum rate of 400 mg/hour

INFUSION REACTIONS ASSOCIATED WITH RITUXIMAB
Note: Medications for the treatment of hypersensitivity reactions should be available for immediate use in the event of a reaction during administration (eg, intravenous fluids, epinephrine, antihistamines, glucocorticoids, and O$_2$)
Fevers, chills, and rigors
1. Interrupt rituximab administration for severe symptoms, and give:
   - **Acetaminophen** 650 mg orally for fever. For persistent or recurrent symptoms, repeat administration every 4–6 hours as needed during rituximab administration
   - **Diphenhydramine** 25–50 mg orally or by intravenous injection for pruritus, hypotension, or angioedema. For persistent or recurrent symptoms, repeat administration every 4–6 hours as needed during rituximab administration
   - **Meperidine** 12.5–25 mg by intravenous injection every 10–20 minutes as needed for shaking chills (generally, cumulative doses >100 mg are not needed; use repeated doses with caution in persons with moderate or more severely impaired renal function)
2. If rituximab administration was interrupted, resume infusion at a slower rate than the maximum rate previously attempted. Rate escalation may be reattempted at smaller incremental steps with close monitoring. Do not exceed the maximum recommended rate of 400 mg/h

Dyspnea or wheezing without allergic findings (urticaria, or tongue or laryngeal edema)
1. Interrupt rituximab administration immediately
2. Give **hydrocortisone** 100 mg by intravenous injection (or an alternative steroid with equivalent glucocorticoid potency)
3. Give a **histamine (H$_2$) receptor antagonist** (ranitidine 50 mg, cimetidine 300 mg, or famotidine 20 mg) intravenously over 15–30 minutes
4. After symptoms resolve, resume rituximab administration at 25 mg/h with close monitoring. Do not increase the administration rate
Note: Medications and equipment for the treatment of hypersensitivity reactions should be available for immediate use in the event of a reaction during administration (eg, intravenous fluids, epinephrine, antihistamines, glucocorticoids, and oxygen)
Rituxan (rituximab) prescribing information. South San Francisco, CA: Genentech, Inc; 2018 October

Intravenous hydration before and after cyclophosphamide administration:
500–1000 mL 0.9% NS
Chemotherapy
Cyclophosphamide 750 mg/m^2; administer intravenously in 25–250 mL 0.9% NS or D5W over 10–30 minutes, given on day 1, every 3 weeks (total dosage/cycle = 750 mg/m^2)
Doxorubicin 50 mg/m^2; administer by intravenous injection over 3–5 minutes, given on day 1, every 3 weeks (total dosage/cycle = 50 mg/m^2)
Vincristine 1.4 mg/m^2 (maximum dose = 2 mg); administer by intravenous infusion over 15 minutes in 50 mL 0.9% NS, given on day 1, every 3 weeks (total dosage/cycle = 1.4 mg/m^2; maximum dose/cycle = 2 mg)
Prednisone 40 mg/m^2 per day; administer orally for 5 consecutive days, days 1–5 every 3 weeks (total dosage/cycle = 200 mg/m^2)

Supportive Care
Antiemetic prophylaxis
Emetogenic potential on day 1 is **MODERATELY HIGH**
See Chapter 42 for antiemetic recommendations

Hematopoietic growth factor (CSF) prophylaxis
Primary prophylaxis is indicated with 1 of the following:
Filgrastim (G-CSF) 5 μg/kg per day; administer by subcutaneous injection, *or*
Pegfilgrastim (pegylated filgrastim) 6 mg/0.6 mL; administer by subcutaneous injection for 1 dose
- Begin use from 24–72 hours after myelosuppressive chemotherapy is completed
See Chapter 43 for more information

(*continued*)

Antimicrobial prophylaxis

Risk of fever and neutropenia is INTERMEDIATE

Antimicrobial primary prophylaxis to be considered:

- Antibacterial—consider a fluoroquinolone or no prophylaxis; *Pneumocystis jirovecii* prophylaxis is recommended (eg, cotrimoxazole)
- Antifungal—consider use during neutropenia and for anticipated mucositis
- Antiviral—antiherpes antivirals (eg, acyclovir)

Steroid-associated gastritis

Add a **proton pump inhibitor** during prednisone use to prevent gastritis and duodenitis

Treatment Modifications

Adverse Event	Dose Modification
G4 ANC or febrile neutropenia after any cycle of chemotherapy	Filgrastim prophylaxis after chemotherapy during subsequent cycles[*]
G4 ANC during a cycle in which filgrastim was administered	Reduce cyclophosphamide and doxorubicin dosages 50% during subsequent cycles
G3/4 thrombocytopenia	
ANC <1500/mm^3 or platelet count <100,000/mm^3 on first day of a repeated cycle	Delay cycle for up to 2 weeks. Stop treatment if recovery has not occurred after a 2-week delay

[*]Filgrastim 5 µg/kg per day; administer subcutaneously, starting on day 2 and continuing beyond ANC nadir until ANC exceeds 5000/mm^3 on 1 reading

Efficacy

	CHOP	RCHOP	
CR and Cru	63%	75%	P = 0.005
PR and SD	6%	8%	
PD during treatment	22%	9.5%	
Death during treatment	6%	6%	
Median OS	3.1 years	Not reached	
5-Year PFS	30%	54%	
5-Year PFS in low aaIPI[*] risk	34%	69%	P = 0.00013
5-Year PFS in high aaIPI[*] risk	29%	47%	P = 0.00078
5-Year DFS	45%	66%	
5-Year OS	45%	58%	
5-Year OS in low aaIPI[*] risk	62%	80%	P = 0.023
5-Year OS in high aaIPI[*] risk	39%	48%	P = 0.062

[*]Age-adjusted International Prognostic Index
Feugier P et al. J Clin Oncol 2005;23:4117–4126

Patient Population Studied

Previously untreated patients with diffuse large B-cell lymphoma 60–80 years of age were randomly assigned to receive 8 cycles of CHOP every 3 weeks (197 patients) or 8 cycles of CHOP plus rituximab given on the first day of each cycle (202 patients). Patients who were serologically positive for HIV and patients with active hepatitis B infection were excluded

Toxicity[*,†] (N = 202)

	% Any Grade	% G3/4
Fever	64	2
Infection	65	12
Mucositis	27	3
Liver toxicity	46	3
Cardiac toxicity	47	8
Neurologic toxicity	51	5
Renal toxicity	11	1
Lung toxicity	33	8
Nausea or vomiting	42	2
Constipation	38	2
Alopecia	97	39
Other toxicities	84	20

[*]NCI CTC
[†]Percentage of patients with event during at least 1 cycle
Coiffier B et al. N Engl J Med 2002;346:235–242

Therapy Monitoring

1. *Prior to treatment initiation*: CBC with differential, serum chemistries, serum bilirubin, ALT or AST, hepatitis B core antibody (IgG or total) and hepatitis B surface antigen, left ventricular ejection fraction (LVEF), and urine pregnancy test (women of child-bearing potential only)

   a. In addition to baseline monitoring, evaluate LVEF during doxorubicin treatment if clinical symptoms of heart failure are present

   b. *In patients at high risk for tumor lysis syndrome (eg, high tumor burden, renal dysfunction, rapidly progressing disease, markedly elevated LDH, baseline abnormalities in laboratory indices of tumor lysis syndrome [potassium, phosphate, uric acid, calcium, serum creatinine])*: consider frequent monitoring of laboratory indices of tumor lysis syndrome, intravenous hydration, and prophylaxis with a xanthine oxidase inhibitor (eg, allopurinol) during the first cycle

2. *Prior to each cycle*: CBC with differential, serum chemistries, serum bilirubin, ALT or AST

3. *Weekly*: CBC with differential

4. *During each rituximab infusion and for at least 1 hour after infusion completion*: Signs and symptoms of infusion-related reaction, vital signs every 30 minutes

5. *Monitor periodically for*: Signs and symptoms of infection (including progressive multifocal leukoencephalopathy), dermatologic toxicity, peripheral neuropathy (vincristine), constipation (vincristine)

6. *Response assessment (after 2–4 cycles and then after cycle 6)*: Physical examination, CBC with differential, CT scan or PET scan, bone marrow evaluation (if clinically indicated)

DIFFUSE LARGE B-CELL LYMPHOMA, OLDER PATIENTS • FIRST LINE

NON-HODGKIN LYMPHOMA REGIMEN: RITUXIMAB + CYCLOPHOSPHAMIDE + DOXORUBICIN (HYDROXYLDAUNORUBICIN) + VINCRISTINE (ONCOVIN) + PREDNISONE (R-MINICHOP)

Peyrade F et al. Lancet Oncol 2011;12:460–468

Rituximab
Premedication for rituximab:
Acetaminophen 650–1000 mg; administer orally, *plus*
Diphenhydramine 25–50 mg; administer orally or intravenously, 30–60 minutes before each dose of rituximab
Rituximab 375 mg/m^2; administer intravenously in 0.9% sodium chloride injection (0.9% NS) or 5% dextrose injection (D5W) diluted to a concentration of 1–4 mg/mL on day 1 every 3 weeks for a total of 6 cycles (total dosage/cycle = 375 mg/m^2)
Notes on rituximab administration:
• Infuse initially at 50 mg/h. If hypersensitivity or infusion reactions do not occur during the first 30 minutes, increase the rate by 50 mg/h every 30 minutes as tolerated to a maximum rate of 400 mg/h. Subsequently, if previous administration was well tolerated, start at 100 mg/h and increase by 100 mg/h every 30 minutes as tolerated to a maximum rate of 400 mg/h

INFUSION REACTIONS ASSOCIATED WITH RITUXIMAB

Note: Medications for the treatment of hypersensitivity reactions should be available for immediate use in the event of a reaction during administration (eg, intravenous fluids, epinephrine, antihistamines, glucocorticoids, and O$_2$)
Fevers, chills, and rigors
3. Interrupt rituximab administration for severe symptoms, and give:
   • **Acetaminophen** 650 mg orally for fever. For persistent or recurrent symptoms, repeat administration every 4–6 hours as needed during rituximab administration
   • **Diphenhydramine** 25–50 mg orally or by intravenous injection for pruritus, hypotension, or angioedema. For persistent or recurrent symptoms, repeat administration every 4–6 hours as needed during rituximab administration
   • **Meperidine** 12.5–25 mg by intravenous injection every 10–20 minutes as needed for shaking chills (generally, cumulative doses >100 mg are not needed; use repeated doses with caution in persons with moderate or more severely impaired renal function)
4. If rituximab administration was interrupted, resume infusion at a slower rate than the maximum rate previously attempted. Rate escalation may be reattempted at smaller incremental steps with close monitoring. Do not exceed the maximum recommended rate of 400 mg/h

Dyspnea or wheezing without allergic findings (urticaria, or tongue or laryngeal edema)
5. Interrupt rituximab administration immediately
6. Give **hydrocortisone** 100 mg by intravenous injection (or an alternative steroid with equivalent glucocorticoid potency)
7. Give a **histamine (H$_2$) receptor antagonist** (ranitidine 50 mg, cimetidine 300 mg, or famotidine 20 mg) intravenously over 15–30 minutes
8. After symptoms resolve, resume rituximab administration at 25 mg/h with close monitoring. Do not increase the administration rate
Note: Medications and equipment for the treatment of hypersensitivity reactions should be available for immediate use in the event of a reaction during administration (eg, intravenous fluids, epinephrine, antihistamines, glucocorticoids, and oxygen)
Rituxan (rituximab) prescribing information. South San Francisco, CA: Genentech, Inc; 2018 October

Hydration: 500–1000 mL 0.9% sodium chloride injection (0.9% NS); administer intravenously before and after cyclophosphamide administration
• May be administered concurrently with rituximab or after completing administration

Chemotherapy
Cyclophosphamide 400 mg/m^2; administer intravenously in 25–250 mL 0.9% NS or D5W over 10–30 minutes on day 1 every 3 weeks for a total of 6 cycles (total dosage/cycle = 400 mg/m^2)
Doxorubicin 25 mg/m^2; administer by intravenous injection over 3–5 minutes on day 1 every 3 weeks for a total of 6 cycles (total dosage/cycle = 25 mg/m^2)
Vincristine 1 mg; administer by intravenous infusion over 15 minutes in 50 mL 0.9% NS on day 1 every 3 weeks for a total of 6 cycles (total dose/cycle = 1 mg)
Prednisone 40 mg/m^2 per dose; administer orally for 5 consecutive days on days 1–5 every 3 weeks for a total of 6 cycles (total dosage/cycle = 200 mg/m^2)

Supportive Care
Antiemetic prophylaxis
Emetogenic potential on day 1 is **HIGH**. *Potential for delayed emetic symptoms*
See Chapter 42 for antiemetic recommendations

Hematopoietic growth factor (CSF) prophylaxis
Primary prophylaxis may be indicated
See Chapter 43 for more information

Antimicrobial prophylaxis

Risk of fever and neutropenia is *INTERMEDIATE*

Antimicrobial primary prophylaxis to be considered:

- Antibacterial—consider a fluoroquinolone or no prophylaxis; *Pneumocystis jirovecii* prophylaxis is recommended (eg, cotrimoxazole)
- Antifungal—consider use during neutropenia and for anticipated mucositis
- Antiviral—antiherpes antivirals (eg, acyclovir)

Steroid-associated gastritis

Add a **proton pump inhibitor** during prednisone use to prevent gastritis and duodenitis

Decreased bowel motility prophylaxis

Give **stool softeners** in a scheduled regimen, and **saline, osmotic, and lubricant laxatives**, as needed to prevent constipation associated with vincristine use. If needed, circumspectly add **stimulant (irritant) laxatives** in the least amounts and for the briefest durations needed cause defecation

Patient Population Studied

Patient Characteristics (N = 149)

	Number of Patients (%)
Age, median (range)	83 years (80–95 years)
Men	51 (34%)
Performance status: 0/1/2	27 (18%)/72 (48%)/50 (34%)
Ann Arbor stage	
I	13 (9%)
II	24 (16%)
III	35 (23%)
IV	77 (52%)
Tumor mass ≥10 cm	30 (20%)
>1 extranodal sites	55 (37%)
LDH concentration >618 U/L	102 (68%)
B symptoms*	49 (33%)
β_2-Microglobulin ≥3 mg/L	82/112 (73%)
Serum albumin <35 g/L	69/137 (50%)
IPI	
0–1	13 (9%)
2	31 (21%)
3	46 (31%)
4–5	59 (40%)
Age-adjusted IPI	
0	15 (10%)
1	36 (24%)
2	66 (44%)
3	32 (21%)

Treatment Modifications

Adverse Event	Treatment Modifications
Severe neutropenia (G3 lasting ≥7 days or G4) or fever + neutropenia	Do not adjust dosages. Administer filgrastim during subsequent cycles from days 6–13 (8 doses) or until ANC is ≥1000/mm³
Any hematologic toxicity	Do not adjust dosages
On day 1 of a cycle, ANC <1000/mm³ or platelet count <100,000/mm³	Delay start of cycle until ANC ≥1000/mm³ and platelet count ≥100,000/mm³ with a maximum of 28 days between two consecutive cycles
ANC <1000/mm³ or platelet count <100,000/mm³ 1 week (day 28) after day 1 of a cycle despite withholding chemotherapy	Discontinue therapy
G2 neurologic vincristine-related toxicity including sensory or motor polyneuritis, constipation, or visual or auditory changes	Discontinue vincristine

(continued)

Patient Population Studied (*continued*)

IADL scale[†]	
Without limitation (score 4)	63 (47%)
With limitation (score <4)	72 (53%)

IADL, instrumental activities of daily living; IPI, International Prognostic Index; LDH, lactate dehydrogenase
*Fever, night sweats, and weight loss
[†]Completed by 135 patients
Note: Percentages do not add up to 100% in some cases because of rounding

Efficacy

Response at End of Treatment (N = 149)

	Number of Patients (%)
Complete response	59 (40%)
Unconfirmed complete response	34 (23%)
Partial response	16 (11%)
Stable disease	2 (1%)
Progression during treatment	8 (5%)
Death	27 (18%)
Not assessed	3 (2%)

Prognostic Factors for Overall Survival: Univariate Analyses

	2-Year Overall Survival	Hazard Ratio (95% CI)	Log-Rank P Value
Performance status ≥2	40.4% vs 68.4%	2.9 (1.8–4.9)	<0.0001
Ann Arbor stages III–IV	55.9% vs 68.5%	1.6 (0.8–2.9)	0.17
LDH concentration >618 U/L	54.4% vs 67.6%	1.6 (0.9–2.9)	0.12
Age-adjusted IPI 2–3	50.4% vs 74.7%	2.6 (1.4–4.9)	0.0024
Number of extranodal sites >1	45.1% vs 67%	2.1 (1.3–3.6)	0.0033
Serum albumin ≤3.5 g/Dl	40.5% vs 80.4%	3.6 (1.9–6.6)	<0.0001
β_2-Microglobulin ≥3 mg/L	59.6% vs 58%	1.1 (0.6–2.2)	0.69
Tumor mass >10 cm	30.3% vs 65.1%	2.2 (1.2–3.8)	0.0071
IADL score <4	52.7% vs 65.6%	1.8 (1.0–3.1)	0.0394

CI, confidence interval; IADL, instrumental activities of daily living; IPI, International Prognostic Index; LDH, lactate dehydrogenase
Note: IADL consisted of a simple questionnaire that included the following items: ability to use a telephone, shopping, medication use, and ability to handle finance. The sum score of all 4 items was calculated and patients were classified as being without limitation in the event of a full sum score (4) and with limitation in the event of a sum score less than 4

Efficacy (continued)

Prognostic Factors for Overall Survival: Multivariate Analyses

	Hazard Ratio (95% CI)	P
Age-adjusted IPI 2–3	1.4 (0.6–3.5)	0.46
Number of extranodal sites >1	1.2 (0.6–2.4)	0.59
Serum albumin ≤3.5 g/dL	3.2 (1.4–7.1)	0.0053
β_2-Microglobulin ≥3 mg/L	0.9 (0.4–1.9)	0.75
Tumor mass >10 cm	1.4 (0.6–2.9)	0.43
IADL score <4	1.9 (1.0–3.9)	0.064

CI, confidence interval; IADL, instrumental activities of daily living; IPI, International Prognostic Index
Note: IADL consisted of a simple questionnaire that included the following items: ability to use a telephone, shopping, medication use, and ability to handle finance. The sum score of all 4 items was calculated and patients were classified as being without limitation in the event of a full sum score (4) and with limitation in the event of a sum score less than 4

Toxicity

Incidence of Nonhematologic Toxicity by Grade (N = 149)

	Number of Patients (%)				
	No Toxicity	G1/2	G3	G4	G5
Infection without neutropenia	113 (76%)	22 (15%)	12 (8%)	0 (0%)	2 (1%)
Febrile neutropenia	138 (93%)	1 (1%)	7 (5%)	0 (0%)	3 (2%)
Constitutional symptoms	69 (46%)	68 (46%)	7 (5%)	2 (1%)	3 (2%)
Neurologic toxicity	109 (73%)	30 (20%)	7 (5%)	3 (2%)	0 (0%)
Pulmonary toxicity	118 (79%)	25 (17%)	4 (3%)	1 (0%)	1 (1%)
Renal toxicity	137 (92%)	8 (5%)	2 (1%)	1 (0%)	1 (1%)
Cardiac arrhythmia	134 (90%)	11 (7%)	2 (1%)	2 (1%)	0 (0%)
Cardiac (other)	133 (89%)	13 (9%)	2 (1%)	0 (0%)	1 (1%)
Vascular toxicity	137 (92%)	8 (5%)	3 (2%)	1 (1%)	0 (0%)
Mucositis	138 (93%)	11 (7%)	0 (0%)	0 (0%)	0 (0%)
Creatinine	117 (79%)	31 (21%)	0 (0%)	1 (1%)	0 (0%)
Transaminases	128 (86%)	20 (13%)	0 (0%)	1 (1%)	0 (0%)

Note: Percentages do not add up to 100% in some cases because of rounding

Serious Adverse Events (N = 70)

	Number of Patients (%)
Infections and infestations	19 (27%)
General disorders	12 (17%)
Respiratory and mediastinal disorders	10 (14%)

(continued)

Toxicity (continued)

Gastrointestinal disorders	7 (10%)
Nervous system disorders	7 (10%)
Renal and urinary disorders	4 (6%)
Cardiac and vascular disorders	4 (6%)
Injury and procedural complications	3 (4%)
Hepatobiliary disorders	2 (3%)
Skin disorders	1 (1%)
Musculoskeletal tissue disorders	1 (1%)

Treatment Monitoring

1. *Within 1 month before the first treatment cycle:* full history, physical examination, instrumental activities of daily living (IADL) scale, thoracic and abdominal computerized scans, electrocardiogram, and assessment of resting left ventricular ejection fraction by echocardiography or an isotopic method, hepatitis B core antibody (IgG or total) and hepatitis B surface antigen
2. *Laboratory assessments within 1 week before first chemotherapy:* lactate dehydrogenase, β_2-microglobulin, serum creatinine, serum transaminases, bilirubin, alkaline phosphatase
3. *Tumor response assessment:* after 3 cycles and at the end of treatment
4. *Follow-up:* every 3 months for the first 2 years after treatment and every 6 months thereafter

DIFFUSE LARGE B-CELL LYMPHOMA, OLDER PATIENTS • FIRST LINE

NON-HODGKIN LYMPHOMA REGIMEN: RITUXIMAB + CYCLOPHOSPHAMIDE + EPIRUBICIN + VINBLASTINE + PREDNISONE (R-MINI-CEOP)

Merli et al. Leuk Lymphoma 2007;48:367–373

Rituximab
Premedication for rituximab:
Acetaminophen 650–1000 mg; administer orally, *plus*
Diphenhydramine 25–50 mg; administer orally or intravenously, 30–60 minutes before each dose of rituximab
Rituximab 375 mg/m²; administer intravenously in 0.9% sodium chloride injection (0.9% NS) or 5% dextrose injection (D5W) diluted to a concentration of 1–4 mg/mL on day 1, every 3 or 4 weeks, according to hematologic toxicity (total dosage/cycle = 375 mg/m²)
Notes on rituximab administration:
- Infuse initially at 50 mg/h. If hypersensitivity or infusion reactions do not occur during the first 30 minutes, increase the rate by 50 mg/h every 30 minutes as tolerated to a maximum rate of 400 mg/h. Subsequently, if previous administration was well tolerated, start at 100 mg/h and increase by 100 mg/h every 30 minutes as tolerated to a maximum rate of 400 mg/h

INFUSION REACTIONS ASSOCIATED WITH RITUXIMAB
Note: Medications for the treatment of hypersensitivity reactions should be available for immediate use in the event of a reaction during administration (eg, intravenous fluids, epinephrine, antihistamines, glucocorticoids, and O₂)
Fevers, chills, and rigors
5. Interrupt rituximab administration for severe symptoms, and give:
- **Acetaminophen** 650 mg orally for fever. For persistent or recurrent symptoms, repeat administration every 4–6 hours as needed during rituximab administration
- **Diphenhydramine** 25–50 mg orally or by intravenous injection for pruritus, hypotension, or angioedema. For persistent or recurrent symptoms, repeat administration every 4–6 hours as needed during rituximab administration
- **Meperidine** 12.5–25 mg by intravenous injection every 10–20 minutes as needed for shaking chills (generally, cumulative doses >100 mg are not needed; use repeated doses with caution in persons with moderate or more severely impaired renal function)
6. If rituximab administration was interrupted, resume infusion at a slower rate than the maximum rate previously attempted. Rate escalation may be reattempted at smaller incremental steps with close monitoring. Do not exceed the maximum recommended rate of 400 mg/h

Dyspnea or wheezing without allergic findings (urticaria, or tongue or laryngeal edema)
9. Interrupt rituximab administration immediately
10. Give **hydrocortisone** 100 mg by intravenous injection (or an alternative steroid with equivalent glucocorticoid potency)
11. Give a **histamine (H₂) receptor antagonist** (ranitidine 50 mg, cimetidine 300 mg, or famotidine 20 mg) intravenously over 15–30 minutes
12. After symptoms resolve, resume rituximab administration at 25 mg/h with close monitoring. Do not increase the administration rate

Note: Medications and equipment for the treatment of hypersensitivity reactions should be available for immediate use in the event of a reaction during administration (eg, intravenous fluids, epinephrine, antihistamines, glucocorticoids, and oxygen)
Rituxan (rituximab) prescribing information. South San Francisco, CA: Genentech, Inc; 2018 October

Hydration: 500–1000 mL 0.9% sodium chloride injection (0.9% NS); administer intravenously before and after cyclophosphamide administration

Chemotherapy
Cyclophosphamide 750 mg/m²; administer intravenously in 25–250 mL 0.9% NS or 5% dextrose injection over 10–30 minutes on day 1 every 3 or 4 weeks, according to hematologic toxicity (total dosage/cycle = 750 mg/m²)

Treatment Modifications

Adverse Event	Treatment Modifications
ANC ≥1000/mm³	Administer full doses of epirubicin and cyclophosphamide
ANC 500–999/mm³	Administer 2/3 doses of epirubicin and cyclophosphamide
Anemia or thrombocytopenia	No reduction in treatment intensity
On day 1 of a cycle, ANC <500/mm³	Delay start of cycle until ANC ≥1000/mm³ with a maximum of 28 days between two consecutive cycles
ANC <500/mm³ 1 week (day 35) after day 1 of a cycle despite withholding chemotherapy	Discontinue therapy
G2 neurologic vinblastine-related toxicity including sensory or motor polyneuritis, constipation, or visual or auditory changes	Discontinue vinblastine

Patient Population Studied

Patient Characteristics R-mini-CEOP (N = 125)

	Number of Patients (%)
Median age (range)	73 years (66–87 years)
Male gender	47 (38)
Performance status 2–4	33 (27)
Ann Arbor stage III–IV	94 (75)
Bulky disease	29 (23)
Extranodal involvement ≥2 sites	38 (31)
Bone marrow involvement	29 (24)
Elevated LDH	66 (55)
Age-adjusted IPI	
Low	17 (15)
Low-intermediate	39 (33)
Intermediate-high	38 (32)
High	23 (20)
NA	8

IPI, International Prognostic Index; LDH, lactate dehydrogenase; NA, not assessed

Epirubicin 50 mg/m²; administer by intravenous injection over 3–5 minutes on day 1 every 3 or 4 weeks, according to hematologic toxicity (total dosage/cycle = 50 mg/m²)
Vinblastine 5 mg/m²; administer by intravenous injection over 1–2 minutes on day 1 every 3 or 4 weeks, according to hematologic toxicity (total dosage/cycle = 5 mg/m²)
Prednisone 50 mg/m² per dose; administer orally for 5 consecutive days on days 1–5 every 3 or 4 weeks, according to hematologic toxicity (total dosage/cycle = 250 mg/m²)

Supportive Care
Antiemetic prophylaxis
Emetogenic potential on day 1 is **HIGH**. Potential for delayed emetic symptoms
See Chapter 42 for antiemetic recommendations

Hematopoietic growth factor (CSF) prophylaxis
Primary prophylaxis is indicated with 1 of the following:
Filgrastim (G-CSF) 5 µg/kg per day; administer by subcutaneous injection, or
Pegfilgrastim (pegylated filgrastim) 6 mg/0.6 mL; administer by subcutaneous injection for 1 dose
- Begin use from 24–72 hours after myelosuppressive chemotherapy is completed
- Continue daily filgrastim use until ANC ≥10,000/mm³ on 2 measurements separated temporally by ≥12 hours
- Discontinue daily filgrastim use at least 24 hours before administering myelosuppressive treatment. Do not administer pegfilgrastim within 14 days before administering myelosuppressive treatment
See Chapter 43 for more information

Antimicrobial prophylaxis
Risk of fever and neutropenia is *INTERMEDIATE*
Antimicrobial primary prophylaxis to be considered:
- Antibacterial—consider a fluoroquinolone or no prophylaxis; *Pneumocystis jirovecii* prophylaxis is recommended (eg, cotrimoxazole)
- Antifungal—recommended; consider use during periods of neutropenia
- Antiviral—antiherpes antivirals (eg, acyclovir, famciclovir, valacyclovir)

Steroid-associated gastritis
Add a **proton pump inhibitor** during steroid use to prevent gastritis and duodenitis

Efficacy

Response to Treatment (N = 104)

	Number of Patients (%)
Complete remission	69 (66)
Partial remission	12 (12)
Overall response	81 (78)
Stable disease/progressive disease	23 (22)

	Number of Patients and/or Percentage
5-Year relapse-free survival*	48%
5-Year failure-free survival†	21%
Number of deaths	93 (89.4%)
Death from lymphoma	73%
Treatment-related deaths	10 (8.8%)
5-Year overall survival	32%
Median overall survival	18 months

(continued)

Efficacy (continued)

Variable	P
Univariate analysis of survival—correlations for entire group	
Age as a continuous variable and ↓ overall survival	<0.001
Bone marrow involvement and ↓ overall survival	0.04
Elevated lactate dehydrogenase (LDH) and ↓ overall survival	<0.001
Age Adjusted International Prognostic Index and ↓ overall survival	0.004
Bone marrow involvement and ↓ relapse-free survival	<0.001
Cox multivariate analysis—correlations for entire group	
Age as a continuous variable and ↓ overall survival	<0.001
Elevated lactate dehydrogenase (LDH) and ↓ overall survival	<0.001
Bone marrow involvement and ↓ relapse-free survival	<0.001
Quality of Life (QoL) Improvements—All Patients	
Pain	0.003
Appetite	0.006
Sleep	0.015
Global health	0.027
Quality of Life (QoL) Improvements—Patients with A Complete Response	
Emotional state	0.10
Role	0.05
Constipation	0.04
Global QoL	0.05

*After a median follow-up for living patients of 72 months (range: 9–104 months)
†Among eligible patients

Toxicity

Adverse Event	Percentage of Patients (Number)
Treatment program stopped for toxicity	2% (2)
Toxic deaths	7% (9)
Grades 3/4 neutropenia	27%
Cardiac events	6%
Nausea and vomiting	5%
Severe infections	10%
Neurologic problems	4%

Treatment Monitoring

1. *Within 1 month before the first treatment cycle:* full history, physical examination, instrumental activities of daily living (IADL) scale, thoracic and abdominal computerized scans, electrocardiogram, and assessment of resting left ventricular ejection fraction by echocardiography or an isotopic method, hepatitis B core antibody (IgG or total) and hepatitis B surface antigen

2. *Laboratory assessments within 1 week before first chemotherapy:* lactate dehydrogenase, β_2-microglobulin, serum creatinine, serum transaminases, bilirubin, alkaline phosphatase

3. *Tumor response assessment:* after 3 cycles and at the end of treatment

4. *Follow-up:* every 3 months for the first 2 years after treatment and every 6 months thereafter

DIFFUSE LARGE B-CELL LYMPHOMA, OLDER PATIENTS • FIRST LINE

NONHODGKIN LYMPHOMA REGIMEN: RITUXIMAB, GEMCITABINE, CYCLOPHOSPHAMIDE, VINCRISTINE, AND PREDNISOLONE (R-GCVP)

Fields PA et al. J Clin Oncol 2014;32:282–287

Rituximab
Premedication for rituximab:
Acetaminophen 650–1000 mg; administer orally 30–60 minutes before starting rituximab, *plus*
Diphenhydramine 25–50 mg; administer orally or intravenously 30–60 minutes before starting rituximab
Rituximab 375 mg/m^2 per dose; administer intravenously in 0.9% sodium chloride injection (0.9% NS) or 5% dextrose injection (D5W), diluted to a concentration within the range 1–4 mg/mL, on day 1, every 21 days, for 6 cycles (total dosage/21-day cycle = 375 mg/m^2)
Notes on rituximab administration:
• Infuse initially at 50 mg/h. If hypersensitivity or infusion reactions do not occur during the first 30 minutes, increase the rate by 50 mg/h every 30 minutes as tolerated to a maximum rate of 400 mg/h. During subsequent treatments if previous rituximab administration was well tolerated, start at 100 mg/h and increase by 100 mg/h every 30 minutes as tolerated to a maximum rate of 400 mg/h

INFUSION REACTIONS ASSOCIATED WITH RITUXIMAB

Note: Medications for the treatment of hypersensitivity reactions should be available for immediate use in the event of a reaction during administration (eg, intravenous fluids, epinephrine, antihistamines, glucocorticoids, and O$_2$)
Fevers, chills, and rigors
1. Interrupt rituximab administration for severe symptoms, and give:
   • **Acetaminophen** 650 mg orally for fever. For persistent or recurrent symptoms, repeat administration every 4–6 hours as needed during rituximab administration
   • **Diphenhydramine** 25–50 mg orally or by intravenous injection for pruritus, hypotension, or angioedema. For persistent or recurrent symptoms, repeat administration every 4–6 hours as needed during rituximab administration
   • **Meperidine** 12.5–25 mg by intravenous injection every 10–20 minutes as needed for shaking chills (generally, cumulative doses >100 mg are not needed; use repeated doses with caution in persons with moderate or more severely impaired renal function)
2. If rituximab administration was interrupted, resume infusion at a slower rate than the maximum rate previously attempted. Rate escalation may be reattempted at smaller incremental steps with close monitoring. Do not exceed the maximum recommended rate of 400 mg/h
Dyspnea or wheezing without allergic findings (urticaria, or tongue or laryngeal edema)
1. Interrupt rituximab administration immediately
2. Give **hydrocortisone** 100 mg by intravenous injection (or an alternative steroid with equivalent glucocorticoid potency)
3. Give a **histamine (H$_2$) receptor antagonist** (ranitidine 50 mg, cimetidine 300 mg, or famotidine 20 mg) intravenously over 15–30 minutes
4. After symptoms resolve, resume rituximab administration at 25 mg/h with close monitoring. Do not increase the administration rate
Note: Medications and equipment for the treatment of hypersensitivity reactions should be available for immediate use in the event of a reaction during administration (eg, intravenous fluids, epinephrine, antihistamines, glucocorticoids, and oxygen)
Rituxan (rituximab) prescribing information. South San Francisco, CA: Genentech, Inc; 2018 October

Chemotherapy

Gemcitabine (dose as per table below); administer intravenously in 0.9% NS diluted to a concentration ≥0.1 mg/mL over 30 minutes on days 1 and 8, every 21 days, for 6 cycles

Cycle	Gemcitabine Dose
1	750 mg/m^2 per dose on days 1 and 8 (total dosage/21-day cycle = 1500 mg/m^2)
2*	875 mg/m^2 per dose on days 1 and 8 (total dosage/21-day cycle = 1750 mg/m^2)
3–6*	1000 mg/m^2 per dose on days 1 and 8 (total dosage/21-day cycle = 2000 mg/m^2) (if 875 mg/m^2 dose was tolerated without G ≥3 neutropenia or G ≥2 thrombocytopenia)

*The gemcitabine dosage was escalated if no G ≥3 neutropenia (ANC <1000/mm^3) or G ≥2 thrombocytopenia (platelet count <75,000/mm^3) occurred in the prior cycle

(continued)

(continued)

Intravenous hydration before and after cyclophosphamide administration:
500–1000 mL 0.9% NS
Cyclophosphamide 750 mg/m²; administer intravenously in 25–250 mL 0.9% NS or D5W over 10–30 minutes, given on day 1, every 21 days, for 6 cycles (total dosage/21-day cycle = 750 mg/m²)
Vincristine 1.4 mg/m² (maximum dose = 2 mg); administer by intravenous infusion over 15 minutes in 50 mL 0.9% NS, given on day 1, every 21 days, for 6 cycles (total dosage/21-day cycle = 1.4 mg/m²; maximum dosage/21-day cycle = 2 mg)
Prednisolone 100 mg per day; administer orally for 5 consecutive days, days 1–5, every 21 days, for 6 cycles (total dosage/21-day cycle = 500 mg)

Supportive Care
Antiemetic prophylaxis
Emetogenic potential on day 1 is **MODERATE**
Emetogenic potential on day 8 is **LOW**
See Chapter 42 for antiemetic recommendations

Hematopoietic growth factor (CSF) prophylaxis
Primary prophylaxis is indicated with one of the following:
Filgrastim (G-CSF) 5 µg/kg per day, by subcutaneous injection, *or*
Pegfilgrastim (pegylated filgrastim) 6 mg/0.6 mL, by subcutaneous injection for 1 dose
• Begin use 24 hours after day 8 gemcitabine is completed
• Continue daily filgrastim use until ANC ≥5000/mm³ after the leukocyte nadir
• Discontinue daily filgrastim use at least 24 hours before administering myelosuppressive treatment. Do not administer pegfilgrastim within 14 days before administering myelosuppressive treatment
See Chapter 43 for more information

Antimicrobial prophylaxis
Risk of fever and neutropenia is *INTERMEDIATE*
Antimicrobial primary prophylaxis to be considered:
• Antibacterial—not indicated
• Antifungal—not indicated
• Antiviral—antiherpes antivirals (eg, acyclovir, famciclovir, valacyclovir)

Treatment Modifications

Gemcitabine + Cyclophosphamide + Vincristine + Prednisolone (GCVP) Dose Modifications

Dose Levels	Gemcitabine	Cyclophosphamide	Vincristine	Prednisolone
Second gemcitabine dose escalation	1000 mg/m²	—	—	—
First gemcitabine dose escalation	875 mg/m²	—	—	—
Starting dose	750 mg/m²	750 mg/m²	1.4 mg/m² (max dose of 2 mg)	100 mg
Dose level 1	500 mg/m²	500 mg/m²	1.05 mg/m² (max dose of 1.5 mg)	80 mg
Dose level 2	375 mg/m²	375 mg/m²	0.7 mg/m² (max dose of 1 mg)	60 mg
Dose level 3	Discontinue R-GCVP			

Note: There are no dose reductions for rituximab

Adverse Event	Treatment Modifications
Hematologic Toxicity	
G3 neutropenia (ANC ≥500 and <1000/mm³) on day 1	Do not delay treatment, but reduce the dosages of gemcitabine and cyclophosphamide by 1 dose level
G2 thrombocytopenia (platelet count ≥50,000 and <75,000/mm³) on day 1	Do not reduce the vincristine dose
	Do not escalate the gemcitabine dose in future cycles

Treatment Modifications (continued)

G3 neutropenia (ANC ≥500 and <1000/mm³) on day 8	Do not delay treatment, but reduce the gemcitabine dosage by 1 dose level
G2 thrombocytopenia (platelet count ≥50,000 and <75,000/mm³) on day 8	Do not escalate the gemcitabine dose in future cycles
G4 neutropenia (ANC <500/mm³) on day 1	Delay start of cycle by 1 week and until ANC ≥1000/mm³ and platelet count ≥75,000/mm³
G ≥3 thrombocytopenia (platelet count <50,000/mm³) on day 1	Do not escalate the gemcitabine dose in future cycles
G4 neutropenia (ANC <500/mm³) on day 8	Omit the gemcitabine dose on day 8. In subsequent cycles, consider reducing the cyclophosphamide or gemcitabine dosage by 1 dose level
G ≥3 thrombocytopenia (platelet count <50,000/mm³) on day 8	Do not escalate the gemcitabine dose in future cycles
ANC nadir ≥1000/mm³ and platelet count nadir ≥75,000/mm³ during cycle 1 administered with a gemcitabine dose of 750 mg/m²	Increase the gemcitabine dosage to 875 mg/m² for subsequent cycles
ANC nadir ≥1000/mm³ and platelet count nadir ≥75,000/mm³ during cycle 2 administered with a gemcitabine dose of 875 mg/m²	Increase the gemcitabine dosage to 1000 mg/m² for subsequent cycles
Infectious Complications	
G2 infection	Interrupt R-GCVP until resolution of infection, then resume R-GCVP at the same dose
G ≥3 infection	Interrupt R-GCVP until resolution of infection, then resume rituximab, vincristine, and prednisolone at the same doses, and resume cyclophosphamide and gemcitabine at either the same dose or with the doses reduced by 1 dose level
New or changes in preexisting neurologic symptoms (eg, confusion, dizziness, loss of balance, vision problems, aphasia, ambulation issues); PML suspected	Interrupt R-GCVP until central nervous system status is clarified. Work-up may include (but is not limited to) consultation with a neurologist, brain MRI, and LP
PML is confirmed	Discontinue R-GCVP
HBV reactivation	Discontinue R-GCVP. Institute appropriate treatment for HBV. Upon resolution of HBV reactivation, resumption of R-GCVP should be discussed with a physician with expertise in management of HBV. Insufficient data exist to determine the safety of resumption of R-GCVP in this setting
Gastrointestinal Toxicities	
G ≥3 ileus (severely altered GI function; TPN indicated; tube placement indicated)	Withhold all chemotherapy until resolution of ileus and constipation, then reduce the next dose of vincristine by 1 dose level with an optimal prophylactic bowel regimen. Do not change the gemcitabine, cyclophosphamide, or prednisolone doses
G ≥3 constipation (obstipation with manual evacuation indicated; limiting self-care ADL)	If symptoms do not recur at the reduced vincristine dose, then the vincristine dose may be re-escalated on subsequent cycles with an appropriate prophylactic bowel regimen
Neurologic Toxicities	
G3 peripheral sensory neuropathy (severe symptoms; limiting self-care ADL)	Proceed with treatment and reduce the dose of vincristine by 1 dose level. Do not change the gemcitabine, cyclophosphamide, or prednisolone doses
G2 peripheral motor neuropathy (moderate symptoms; limiting instrumental ADL)	If symptoms improve, then the vincristine dose may be re-escalated on subsequent cycles
G3 peripheral motor neuropathy (severe symptoms; limiting self-care ADL)	Proceed with treatment and reduce the dose of vincristine by 2 dose levels. Do not change the gemcitabine, cyclophosphamide, or prednisolone doses
	If symptoms improve, then the vincristine dose may be re-escalated on subsequent cycles

(continued)

Treatment Modifications (*continued*)

G4 peripheral sensory neuropathy (life-threatening symptoms; urgent intervention indicated)	Discontinue vincristine
G4 peripheral motor neuropathy (life-threatening consequences; urgent intervention indicated)	Do not change the gemcitabine, cyclophosphamide, or prednisolone doses
G ≥2 mood alteration (moderate mood alteration) or confusion (moderate disorientation; limiting instrumental ADL)	Withhold prednisolone until symptoms return to baseline Resume prednisolone reduced by 1 dose level. If symptoms persist, reduce by another dose level. Do not change the gemcitabine, cyclophosphamide, or vincristine doses

Hepatic Impairment

Serum bilirubin 1.5–3 mg/dL	Decrease the vincristine dose by 50%
Serum bilirubin >3 mg/Dl	Withhold vincristine

Drug Interactions

Patient requires concomitant therapy with antihypertensive medication(s)	On days of rituximab treatment, and especially with the initial dose, weigh the risk versus benefit of delaying administration of the antihypertensive medication(s) until after completion of the rituximab infusion due to the potential risk of rituximab infusion-related hypotension
Patient requires concomitant therapy with a strong CYP3A4 inhibitor	Patient may have earlier onset of neuromuscular side effects of vincristine. If concomitant use of the strong CYP3A4 inhibitor cannot be avoided, consider dose reduction of vincristine and increased monitoring for toxicity
Live attenuated vaccine is indicated during or after rituximab administration	Avoid administration of a live attenuated vaccine during rituximab therapy and following therapy until adequate B-cell recovery has occurred

Other Toxicities

G ≥3 hyperglycemia (insulin therapy initiated; hospitalization indicated)	Withhold prednisolone until blood glucose is ≤250 mg/dL. Treat with insulin or other hypoglycemic agents as clinically appropriate, and then resume prednisolone at the same dose. If hyperglycemia is uncontrolled despite aforementioned measures, decrease prednisolone by 1 dose level
Unexplained new or worsening dyspnea or evidence of severe pulmonary toxicity	Discontinue R-GCVP immediately, and assess for gemcitabine-related pulmonary toxicity
Hemolytic uremic syndrome	Discontinue gemcitabine for hemolytic uremic syndrome or severe renal impairment[*]
Capillary leak syndrome	Discontinue gemcitabine[*]
Posterior reversible encephalopathy syndrome	Discontinue gemcitabine[*]

ADL, activities of daily living; ANC, absolute neutrophil count; GI, gastrointestinal; HBV, hepatitis B virus; LP, lumbar puncture; MRI, magnetic resonance imaging; PML, progressive multifocal leukoencephalopathy; TPN, total parenteral nutrition

[*]If gemcitabine is discontinued, may consider further administration of rituximab, cyclophosphamide, vincristine, and prednisolone

Efficacy (N = 62)

Overall response rate[*]	61.3%
2-year progression-free survival	49.8%
2-year overall survival	55.8%

[*]*Overall response rate includes patients with either a complete or partial response to treatment*
Note: Median follow-up was 24.9 months

Patient Population Studied

This multicenter, two-stage, single-arm, non-randomized, phase 2 trial involved 62 patients with previously untreated, CD20-positive, diffuse large B-cell lymphoma who were considered unsuitable for anthracycline-containing chemoimmunotherapy owing to cardiac comorbidity. Eligible patients had an Eastern Cooperative Oncology Group (ECOG) performance status score ≤3. All patients were scheduled to receive six 21-day cycles of intravenous rituximab (375 mg/m² on day 1), gemcitabine (over 30 minutes on days 1 and 8 at a dose of 750 mg/m² in cycle 1, 875 mg/m² in cycle 2, and 1000 mg/m² in cycles 3–6, if tolerated), cyclophosphamide (750 mg/m² on day 1), and vincristine (1.4 mg/m² on day 1; maximum dose 2 mg), and oral prednisolone (100 mg on days 1–5)

Toxicity

(N = 61)

	Grade 3–5* (%)
Any nonhematologic event	64
Any hematologic event	56
Neutropenia	48
Thrombocytopenia	31
Infection	28
Fatigue	23
Cardiac	16
Anemia	11
Neurologic	8
Bone pain	7
Diarrhea	7
Fever	7

*According to the National Cancer Institute Common Terminology Criteria for Adverse Events, version 3.0
Note: Grade 3–5 toxicities are included if they occurred in >5% of patients. Three patients (with known ischemic heart disease) died, one as a result of pulmonary edema and two owing to myocardial infarctions

Therapy Monitoring

1. *Prior to treatment initiation:* CBC with differential, serum chemistries, serum bilirubin, ALT or AST, hepatitis B core antibody (IgG or total) and hepatitis B surface antigen, and urine pregnancy test (women of child-bearing potential only)
   a. *In patients at high risk for tumor lysis syndrome (eg, high tumor burden, renal dysfunction, rapidly progressing disease, markedly elevated LDH, baseline abnormalities in laboratory indices of tumor lysis syndrome [potassium, phosphate, uric acid, calcium, serum creatinine]):* consider frequent monitoring of laboratory indices of tumor lysis syndrome, intravenous hydration, and prophylaxis with a xanthine oxidase inhibitor (eg, allopurinol) during the first cycle
2. *Prior to each cycle:* CBC with differential, serum chemistries, serum bilirubin, ALT or AST
3. *Weekly during therapy:* CBC with differential
4. *During each rituximab infusion and for at least 1 hour after infusion completion:* Signs and symptoms of infusion-related reaction, vital signs every 30 minutes
5. *Monitor periodically for:* Signs and symptoms of infection (including progressive multifocal leukoencephalopathy), dermatologic toxicity, peripheral neuropathy (vincristine), and constipation (vincristine)
6. *Response assessment (after 2–4 cycles and then after cycle 6):* physical examination, CBC with differential, CT scan or PET scan, bone marrow evaluation (if clinically indicated)

DLBCL (OLDER PATIENTS)—FIRST LINE
RITUXIMAB + BENDAMUSTINE (R-BENDA)

Park SI et al. Br J Haematol 2016;175:281–289

Bendamustine
Premedication for bendamustine HCl: Premedication is not necessary for primary prophylaxis of infusion-related reactions. In the event of a non-severe infusion-related reaction, consider adding a histamine receptor (H_1)-subtype antagonist (eg, diphenhydramine 25–50 mg intravenously or orally), an antipyretic (eg, acetaminophen 650–1000 mg orally), and a corticosteroid (eg, methylprednisolone 100 mg intravenously) administered 30 minutes prior to bendamustine HCl administration in subsequent cycles

Bendamustine HCl 120 mg/m^2 per dose; administer intravenously in a volume of 0.9% sodium chloride injection (0.9% NS) sufficient to produce a concentration with the range 0.2–0.6 mg/mL over 60 minutes, on 2 consecutive days, days 1 and 2, every 21 days for up to 8 cycles (total dosage/21-day cycle = 240 mg/m^2)
Note:

• Patients with ECOG PS of 3 at baseline were allowed to receive bendamustine at a dose of 90 mg/m^2 daily, with a dose increase to 120 mg/m^2 daily if their ECOG PS improved to ≤2 after 3 cycles of BR

• Pre-phase steroid therapy with prednisone 100 mg/d for 5 days was permitted prior to the initiation of R-Benda in patients with poor functional status at the initial presentation (Pfreundschuh et al, 2004)

• Bendamustine HCl can cause severe infusion-related reactions

  – For grade 1–2 infusion-related reactions, consider rechallenge with the addition of antihistamine, antipyretic, and corticosteroid premedications (as described in the Premedication section)

  – For grade 3 infusion-related reactions, consider permanent discontinuation versus rechallenge with the addition of antihistamine, antipyretic, and corticosteroid premedications (as described in the Premedication section) after weighing risks and benefits

  – For grade 4 infusion-related reactions, permanently discontinue bendamustine HCl

• Coadministration of strong CYP1A2 inhibitors (eg, ciprofloxacin, fluvoxamine) may increase exposure to bendamustine HCl and decrease exposure to its active metabolites. Concomitant CYP1A2 inducers (eg, omeprazole, cigarette smoking) may decrease exposure to bendamustine HCl and increase exposure to its active metabolites. Use caution, or select an alternative therapy, when coadministration of bendamustine HCl with strong CYP1A2 inhibitors or inducers is unavoidable

• Bendamustine HCl formulations may vary by country; consult local regulatory-approved labeling for guidance. For example, in the United States, the Food and Drug Administration approved Bendeka under Section 505(b)(2) of the Federal Food, Drug, and Cosmetic Act on 7 December 2015. The Bendeka product labeling contains specific dilution and administration instructions, *thus*:

  – **Bendamustine HCl (Bendeka, where available)** 120 mg/m^2 per dose; administer intravenously in a volume of 0.9% NS or 5% dextrose injection (D5W) sufficient to produce a concentration with the range 1.85–5.6 mg/mL, over 10 minutes, on 2 consecutive days, days 1 and 2, every 21 days for up to 8 cycles (total dosage/21-day cycle = 240 mg/m^2)

Rituximab
Premedication for rituximab:
Acetaminophen 650–1000 mg; administer orally 30–60 minutes before starting rituximab, *plus*
Diphenhydramine 25–50 mg; administer orally or intravenously 30–60 minutes before starting rituximab
Rituximab 375 mg/m^2 per dose; administer intravenously in 0.9% NS or 5% dextrose injection, diluted to a concentration within the range 1–4 mg/mL, on day 1, after bendamustine administration, every 21 days, for up to 8 cycles (total dosage/21-day cycle = 375 mg/m^2)
Notes on rituximab administration:

• Infuse initially at 50 mg/h. If hypersensitivity or infusion reactions do not occur during the first 30 minutes, increase the rate by 50 mg/h every 30 minutes as tolerated to a maximum rate of 400 mg/h. During subsequent treatments, if previous rituximab administration was well tolerated, start at 100 mg/h and increase by 100 mg/h every 30 minutes as tolerated to a maximum rate of 400 mg/h

INFUSION REACTIONS ASSOCIATED WITH RITUXIMAB
Note: Medications for the treatment of hypersensitivity reactions should be available for immediate use in the event of a reaction during administration (eg, intravenous fluids, epinephrine, antihistamines, glucocorticoids, and O_2)
Fevers, chills, and rigors
1. Interrupt rituximab administration for severe symptoms, and give:

  • **Acetaminophen** 650 mg orally for fever. For persistent or recurrent symptoms, repeat administration every 4–6 hours as needed during rituximab administration

  • **Diphenhydramine** 25–50 mg orally or by intravenous injection for pruritus, hypotension, or angioedema. For persistent or recurrent symptoms, repeat administration every 4–6 hours as needed during rituximab administration

  • **Meperidine** 12.5–25 mg by intravenous injection every 10–20 minutes as needed for shaking chills (generally, cumulative doses >100 mg are not needed; use repeated doses with caution in persons with moderate or more severely impaired renal function)

2. If rituximab administration was interrupted, resume infusion at a slower rate than the maximum rate previously attempted. Rate escalation may be reattempted at smaller incremental steps with close monitoring. Do not exceed the maximum recommended rate of 400 mg/h

Dyspnea or wheezing without allergic findings (urticaria, or tongue or laryngeal edema)
1. Interrupt rituximab administration immediately
2. Give **hydrocortisone** 100 mg by intravenous injection (or an alternative steroid with equivalent glucocorticoid potency)
3. Give a **histamine (H₂) receptor antagonist** (ranitidine 50 mg, cimetidine 300 mg, or famotidine 20 mg) intravenously over 15–30 minutes
4. After symptoms resolve, resume rituximab administration at 25 mg/h with close monitoring. Do not increase the administration rate

Note: Medications and equipment for the treatment of hypersensitivity reactions should be available for immediate use in the event of a reaction during administration (eg, intravenous fluids, epinephrine, antihistamines, glucocorticoids, and oxygen)

Rituxan (rituximab) prescribing information. South San Francisco, CA: Genentech, Inc; 2018 October

Supportive Care
Antiemetic prophylaxis
Emetogenic potential on days with bendamustine is **MODERATE**
See Chapter 42 for antiemetic recommendations

Hematopoietic growth factor (CSF) prophylaxis
Primary prophylaxis with granulocyte colony-stimulating factor (pegfilgrastim or filgrastim) was administered as part of the protocol
See Chapter 43 for more information

Antimicrobial prophylaxis
Risk of fever and neutropenia is INTERMEDIATE
Antimicrobial primary prophylaxis to be considered:
- Antibacterial—consider a fluoroquinolone during periods of prolonged neutropenia, or no prophylaxis
- Antifungal—consider use during periods of prolonged neutropenia, or no prophylaxis
- Antiviral—antiherpes antivirals (eg, acyclovir, famciclovir, valacyclovir)

Treatment Modifications

Bendamustine Dose Modifications

Starting dose	120 mg/m² per dose on days 1 and 2
Dose level 1	90 mg/m² per dose on days 1 and 2
Dose level 2	60 mg/m² per dose on days 1 and 2
Dose level 3	Discontinue bendamustine

There are no dose reductions for rituximab

Adverse Event	Treatment Modification
Hematologic Toxicity	
Day 1 platelet count <75,000/mm³ or day 1 ANC <1000/mm³	Delay start of cycle until platelet count ≥75,000/mm³ and ANC ≥1000/ mm³ or until recovery to near baseline values, then reduce the bendamustine dosage by 1 dose level for subsequent cycles. Consider G-CSF use in subsequent cycles for dose-limiting neutropenia
G4 hematologic toxicity occurring in the previous cycle	Delay start of cycle until platelet count ≥75,000/mm³ and ANC ≥1000/mm³ or until recovery to near baseline values, then reduce the bendamustine dosage by 1 dose level for subsequent cycles. Consider G-CSF use in subsequent cycles for dose-limiting neutropenia or severe neutropenic complications
Infectious Complications	
Active infection	Interrupt bendamustine and rituximab until resolution of infection, then resume treatment at either the same dosages, or with the bendamustine dosage reduced by 1 dose level, depending on the severity of infection
New or changes in preexisting neurologic symptoms (eg, confusion, dizziness, loss of balance, vision problems, aphasia, ambulation issues); PML suspected	Interrupt bendamustine and rituximab until central nervous system status is clarified. Work-up may include (but is not limited to) consultation with a neurologist, brain MRI, and LP
PML is confirmed	Discontinue bendamustine and rituximab
HBV reactivation	Discontinue bendamustine and rituximab. Institute appropriate treatment for HBV. Upon resolution of HBV reactivation, resumption of bendamustine and rituximab should be discussed with a physician with expertise in management of HBV

(continued)

Treatment Modifications (*continued*)

Drug Interactions

Patient requires concomitant therapy with antihypertensive medication(s)	On days of rituximab treatment, and especially with the initial dose, weigh the risk versus benefit of delaying administration of the antihypertensive medication(s) until after completion of the rituximab infusion due to the potential risk of rituximab infusion-related hypotension
Live attenuated vaccine is indicated during or after rituximab administration	Avoid administration of a live attenuated vaccine during rituximab therapy and following therapy until adequate B-cell recovery has occurred
Patient requires concomitant therapy with a CYP1A2 inhibitor (eg, fluvoxamine, ciprofloxacin)	Consider alternative treatment instead of the CYP1A2 inhibitor. If the CYP1A2 inhibitor cannot be avoided, use caution and monitor carefully for bendamustine adverse effects. Do not modify the rituximab dose
Patient requires concomitant therapy with a CYP1A2 inducer (eg, omeprazole) or patient is a smoker	Consider alternative treatment instead of the CYP1A2 inducer. Recommend cessation of smoking, if applicable. If the CYP1A2 inducer cannot be avoided, use caution and monitor carefully for reduced bendamustine efficacy. Do not modify the rituximab dose

Other Toxicities

Clinically significant G2 nonhematologic toxicity during the prior cycle	Delay start of cycle until the nonhematologic toxicity resolves to G ≤1 or baseline, then resume treatment at the same dosages
Clinically significant G ≥3 nonhematologic toxicity during the prior cycle	Delay start of cycle until the nonhematologic toxicity resolves to G ≤1 or baseline, then resume treatment with the bendamustine dosage reduced by 1 dose level

ANC, absolute neutrophil count; G-CSF, granulocyte-colony stimulating factor; PML, progressive multifocal leukoencephalopathy; MRI, magnetic resonance imaging; LP, lumbar puncture; HBV, hepatitis B virus
Bendeka (bendamustine hydrochloride injection) prescribing information. North Wales, PA: Teva Pharmaceuticals USA, Inc; 2018 July

Patient Population Studied

Patients aged 65 years or older with ECOG PS 0–3 and previously untreated histologically confirmed CD20+ DLBCL were eligible for the study. Patients were required to be deemed a poor candidate for R-CHOP due to ejection fraction ≤45%, ECOG PS ≥2, or based on the treating physician's discretion. Patients with a history of hepatitis or with central nervous system involvement by lymphoma were excluded from the study

Characteristic	*N* (%)
Age, years (median, range)	80 (65–89)
Gender: male / female	12 (52%) / 11 (48%)
Race: white / other	21 (91%) / 2 (9%)
Stage: II / III / IV	4 (17%) / 7 (30%) / 12 (52%)
ECOG PS: 0 / 1 / 2 / 3	2 (9%) / 9 (39%) / 6 (26%) / 6 (26%)
IPI: 2 / 3 / 4 / 5	5 (22%) / 5 (22%) / 8 (35%) / 5 (22%)
LDH: normal / elevated	8 (35%) / 15 (65%)
Pathology subtype	
Non-germinal center	12 (52%)
Germinal center	7 (30%)
Not classified	4 (17%)

ECOG,-PS, Eastern Cooperative Oncology Group Performance Status; IPI, International Prognostic Index; LDH, lactate dehydrogenase

Efficacy

(N = 23)

Overall response rate (ORR = CR + PR)	18 (78%)
Complete response (CR)	12 (52%, 95% CI: 30.6–73.2%)
Partial response (PR)	6 (26%, 95% CI: 10.2–48.4%).
Stable disease (SD)	1 (4.3%)
Not evaluable for progression due to early death	3 (13%)
Median follow-up	29 months
Median OS	10.2 months (95% CI: 3.8–13.3 months)
Median PFS	5.4 months (95% CI: 3.8–10.2 months
Median OS, ECOG score ≥2	3.7 months	P = 0.17
Median OS, ECOG score 0–1,	10.4 months	
Median OS ≥80 years	6.4 months	P = 0.43
Median OS <80 years	10.2 months	

ECOG, Eastern Cooperative Oncology Group; OS, overall survival; PFS, progression-free survival

Toxicity

Toxicity	Number of Patients with G3	Number of Patients with G ≥4	Patients with G ≥3
Hematologic toxicities			
Lymphopenia	8	8	70%
Anemia	6	0	26%
Neutropenia	1	3	17%
Thrombocytopenia	1	3	17%
Lymphocytosis	1	0	4%
Nonhematologic toxicities			
Fatigue	3	0	13%
Anorexia	0	2	9%
Hyperglycemia	2	0	9%
Urinary tract infection	2	0	9%
Arthralgia	1	0	4%
Atrial fibrillation	1	0	4%
Cognitive disturbance	1	0	4%
Generalized muscle weakness	1	0	4%
Heart failure	0	1	4%
Hypoalbuminemia	1	0	4%
Hyponatremia	1	0	4%
Infusion related reaction	1	0	4%
Myalgia	1	0	4%
Nausea	1	0	4%
Pleural effusion	1	0	4%
Maculopapular rash	1	0	4%
Sepsis	0	1	4%
Skin infection	1	0	4%

Therapy Monitoring

1. *Prior to treatment initiation*: CBC with differential, serum chemistries, serum bilirubin, ALT or AST, hepatitis B core antibody (IgG or total) and hepatitis B core antigen, urine pregnancy test (women of child-bearing potential only)

2. *Prior to each cycle*: CBC with differential, serum chemistries, serum bilirubin, ALT or AST

3. *Weekly during treatment*: CBC with differential

4. *During each rituximab infusion and for at least 1 hour after infusion completion*: Signs and symptoms of infusion-related reaction, vital signs every 30 minutes

5. *In patients at high risk for tumor lysis syndrome (eg, high tumor burden, renal dysfunction, rapidly progressing disease, markedly elevated LDH, baseline abnormalities in laboratory indices of tumor lysis syndrome [potassium, phosphate, uric acid, calcium, serum creatinine])*: Consider frequent monitoring of laboratory indices of tumor lysis syndrome, intravenous hydration, and prophylaxis with a xanthine oxidase inhibitor (eg, allopurinol) during the first cycle

6. *Monitor periodically for*: signs and symptoms of infection (including progressive multifocal leukoencephalopathy) and dermatologic toxicity

7. *Response assessment every 2–3 cycles*: physical examination, CT scan, or PET scan

DIFFUSE LARGE B-CELL LYMPHOMA, OLDER PATIENTS • FIRST LINE

NON-HODGKIN LYMPHOMA REGIMEN: RITUXIMAB, GEMCITABINE, AND OXALIPLATIN (R-GEM-OX)

Shen QD et al. Lancet Haematol 2018;5:e261–e269

Rituximab
Premedication for rituximab:
Acetaminophen 650–1000 mg; administer orally 30–60 minutes before starting rituximab, *plus*
Diphenhydramine 25–50 mg; administer orally or intravenously 30–60 minutes before starting rituximab
Rituximab 375 mg/m² per dose; administer intravenously in 0.9% sodium chloride injection (0.9% NS) or 5% dextrose injection (D5W), diluted to a concentration within the range 1–4 mg/mL, on day 1, every 14 days, for up to 6 cycles (total dosage/14-day cycle = 375 mg/m²)
Notes on rituximab administration:
• Infuse initially at 50 mg/h. If hypersensitivity or infusion reactions do not occur during the first 30 minutes, increase the rate by 50 mg/h every 30 minutes as tolerated to a maximum rate of 400 mg/h. During subsequent treatments, if previous rituximab administration was well tolerated, start at 100 mg/h and increase by 100 mg/h every 30 minutes as tolerated to a maximum rate of 400 mg/h

INFUSION REACTIONS ASSOCIATED WITH RITUXIMAB
Note: Medications for the treatment of hypersensitivity reactions should be available for immediate use in the event of a reaction during administration (eg, intravenous fluids, epinephrine, antihistamines, glucocorticoids, and O₂)
Fevers, chills, and rigors
1. Interrupt rituximab administration for severe symptoms, and give:
   • **Acetaminophen** 650 mg orally for fever. For persistent or recurrent symptoms, repeat administration every 4–6 hours as needed during rituximab administration
   • **Diphenhydramine** 25–50 mg orally or by intravenous injection for pruritus, hypotension, or angioedema. For persistent or recurrent symptoms, repeat administration every 4–6 hours as needed during rituximab administration
   • **Meperidine** 12.5–25 mg by intravenous injection every 10–20 minutes as needed for shaking chills (generally, cumulative doses >100 mg are not needed; use repeated doses with caution in persons with moderate or more severely impaired renal function)
2. If rituximab administration was interrupted, resume infusion at a slower rate than the maximum rate previously attempted. Rate escalation may be reattempted at smaller incremental steps with close monitoring. Do not exceed the maximum recommended rate of 400 mg/h
Dyspnea or wheezing without allergic findings (urticaria, or tongue or laryngeal edema)
1. Interrupt rituximab administration immediately
2. Give **hydrocortisone** 100 mg by intravenous injection (or an alternative steroid with equivalent glucocorticoid potency)
3. Give a **histamine (H₂) receptor antagonist** (ranitidine 50 mg, cimetidine 300 mg, or famotidine 20 mg) intravenously over 15–30 minutes
4. After symptoms resolve, resume rituximab administration at 25 mg/h with close monitoring. Do not increase the administration rate
Note: Medications and equipment for the treatment of hypersensitivity reactions should be available for immediate use in the event of a reaction during administration (eg, intravenous fluids, epinephrine, antihistamines, glucocorticoids, and oxygen)

Rituxan (rituximab) prescribing information. South San Francisco, CA: Genentech, Inc; 2018 October

Chemotherapy
Gemcitabine 1000 mg/m²; administer intravenously in 0.9% NS diluted to a concentration ≥0.1 mg/mL over 30 minutes on day 2, every 14 days, for up to 6 cycles (total dosage/14-day cycle = 1000 mg/m²)
Oxaliplatin 100 mg/m²; administer intravenously over 2 hours in 500 mL D5W on day 2, every 14 days, for up to 6 cycles (total dosage/14-day cycle = 100 mg/m²)
• *Note:* Oxaliplatin must not be mixed with 0.9% sodium chloride injection. Therefore, flush infusion line with D5W prior to and following administration of oxaliplatin

Supportive Care
Antiemetic prophylaxis
Emetogenic potential is **MODERATE**
See Chapter 42 for antiemetic recommendations

Hematopoietic growth factor (CSF) prophylaxis
Primary prophylaxis **MAY** be indicated
See Chapter 43 for more information

Antimicrobial prophylaxis
Risk of fever and neutropenia is *INTERMEDIATE*
Antimicrobial primary prophylaxis to be considered:
• Antibacterial—not indicated
• Antifungal—not indicated
• Antiviral—antiherpes antivirals (eg, acyclovir, famciclovir, valacyclovir)

Treatment Modifications

Gemcitabine + Oxaliplatin

Dose Levels	Gemcitabine	Oxaliplatin
Starting dose	1000 mg/m^2	100 mg/m^2
Dose level 1	750 mg/m^2	75 mg/m^2
Dose level 2	500 mg/m^2	50 mg/m^2

Adverse Event	Treatment Modification
Hematologic Toxicity	
Day 1 ANC <1500/mm^3	Delay start of cycle by 1 week and until ANC >1500/mm^3 *and* platelet count >100,000/mm^3. If delay occurred following a cycle with a cycle length of 14 days, consider prolonging subsequent cycle lengths to 21 days
Day 1 platelet count <100,000/mm^3	
G4 neutropenia (ANC <500/mm^3) at nadir	If toxicity occurred during cycle 1 and patient is known to have lymphoma involving the bone marrow, consider treating at the same dose in the subsequent cycle. Otherwise, reduce the doses of either gemcitabine or oxaliplatin by 1 dose level in subsequent cycles
G4 thrombocytopenia (platelet count <25,000/mm^3) at nadir	
Neurologic Toxicity	
G2 paresthesia (persistent paresthesia or dysesthesia, moderate in nature without functional impairment other than limiting instrumental ADL)	Reduce oxaliplatin dosage by 1 dose level
Persistent G2 paresthesia/dysesthesia	Discontinue oxaliplatin[*]
Persistent painful paresthesia or G3 neuropathy (persistent paresthesia or dysesthesia with persistent functional impairment limiting self-care and ADL)	Discontinue oxaliplatin[*]
Hepatic Impairment and Hepatic Toxicity	
Serum bilirubin >1.6 mg/dL	Consider using an initial gemcitabine dose of 800 mg/m^2. If tolerated, may escalate to full dose in subsequent cycles
Renal Impairment and Renal Toxicity	
Creatinine clearance <30 mL/min	Consider reducing the oxaliplatin dose by 25%
Hypersensitivity Reactions	
Significant hypersensitivity reaction to oxaliplatin (hypotension, dyspnea, and angioedema requiring therapy) *Note:* Allergic reaction to oxaliplatin including anaphylaxis risk is increased in patients previously exposed to platinum therapy	May occur within minutes of administration. Interrupt the oxaliplatin infusion in patients with clinically significant infusion reactions. Discontinue therapy or can consider desensitization and a rechallenge[*]
Other Toxicities	
Unexplained new or worsening dyspnea or evidence of severe pulmonary toxicity	Discontinue gemcitabine and oxaliplatin immediately, and assess for gemcitabine-related pulmonary toxicity
Hemolytic uremic syndrome	Discontinue gemcitabine for hemolytic uremic syndrome or severe renal impairment[*]
Capillary leak syndrome	Discontinue gemcitabine[*]
Posterior reversible encephalopathy syndrome	Discontinue gemcitabine[*]

ANC, absolute neutrophil count; ADL, activities of daily living
[*]If oxaliplatin or gemcitabine is discontinued, consider discontinuing the entire regimen and switching to an alternate regimen, if appropriate

Patient Population Studied

Single-arm, open-label, phase 2 clinical trial, that enrolled patients with previously untreated, histologically confirmed, CD20-positive diffuse large B-cell lymphoma, aged 70 years or older, or aged 60–69 years with an Eastern Cooperative Oncology Group (ECOG) performance status ≥2

Therapy Monitoring

1. *Prior to treatment initiation*: CBC with differential, serum chemistries, serum bilirubin, ALT or AST, hepatitis B core antibody (IgG or total), and hepatitis B surface antigen
2. *Weekly during therapy*: CBC with differential
3. *Before each cycle*: CBC with differential, serum chemistries, serum bilirubin, ALT or AST, signs and symptoms of infection (including progressive multifocal leukoencephalopathy), signs and symptoms of peripheral neuropathy
4. *During each rituximab infusion and for at least 1 hour after infusion completion*: signs and symptoms of infusion-related reaction, vital signs every 30 minutes
5. *Response assessment (every 2–3 cycles)*: physical examination, CT scan, or PET scan

Efficacy

		Complete Response	Partial Response	Stable Disease	Progressive Disease	Overall Response	P
All patients		28 (47%)	17 (28%)	10 (17%)	5 (8%)	45 (75%)	
Sex	Men	18 (47%)	11 (29%)	6 (16%)	3 (8%)	29 (76%)	0.76
	Women	10 (46%)	6 (27%)	4 (18%)	2 (9%)	16 (73%)	
Age	60–69 years	7 (50%)	4 (29%)	2 (14%)	1 (7%)	11 (79%)	0.66
	70–79 years	12 (40%)	9 (30%)	6 (20%)	3 (10%)	21 (70%)	
	≥80 years	9 (56%)	4 (25%)	2 (13%)	1 (6%)	13 (81%)	
IPI score	0–2	20 (57%)	10 (29%)	4 (11%)	1 (3%)	30 (86%)	0.023
	3–5	8 (32%)	7 (28%)	6 (24%)	4 (16%)	15 (60%)	
NCCN-IPI score	2–3	18 (64%)	6 (21%)	4 (14%)	0 (0%)	24 (86%)	0.089
	4–5	7 (37%)	7 (37%)	3 (16%)	2 (11%)	14 (74%)	
	≥6	3 (23%)	4 (31%)	3 (23%)	3 (23%)	7 (54%)	
Subtype							
Germinal center B-like		11 (58%)	5 (26%)	2 (11%)	1 (5%)	16 (84%)	0.63
Non-germinal center B-like		17 (41%)	12 (29%)	8 (20%)	4 (10%)	29 (71%)	

Data are n (%) or %. X² test was used to compare overall response among different groups
IPI, International Prognostic Index; NCCN, National Comprehensive Cancer Network; R-GemOx, rituximab + gemcitabine + oxaliplatin

Toxicity*

(N = 60)

	G1–2	G3	G4
Neutropenia	11 (18%)	7 (12%)	2 (3%)
Thrombocytopenia	13 (22%)	3 (5%)	2 (3%)
Anemia	18 (30%)	4 (7%)	0
Febrile neutropenia	2 (3%)	2 (3%)	1 (2%)
Nausea	8 (13%)	5 (8%)	0
Vomiting	9 (15%)	3 (5%)	0
Diarrhea	2 (3%)	1 (2%)	0
Mucositis	2 (3%)	0	0
Neurologic toxicity	1 (2%)	1 (2%)	0
Aminotransferases elevation	5 (8%)	0	0

Data are n (%). No grade 5 events were observed. Patients could have the same type of adverse events more than once

DIFFUSE LARGE B-CELL LYMPHOMA, PRIMARY MEDIASTINAL*

NON-HODGKIN LYMPHOMA REGIMEN: DOSE-ADJUSTED ETOPOSIDE, PREDNISONE, VINCRISTINE (ONCOVIN), CYCLOPHOSPHAMIDE, AND DOXORUBICIN (HYDROXYLDAUNORUBICIN) WITH RITUXIMAB (DA-EPOCH WITH RITUXIMAB)

Dunleavy K et al. N Engl J Med 2013;368:14089
Bartlett NL et al. J Clin Oncol 2019;37:1790–1799

*Can also be used in other circumstances, such as double hit lymphoma (DHL) and triple hit lymphoma (THL)

Rituximab
Premedications for Rituximab
Acetaminophen 650–1000 mg; administer orally 30–60 minutes before starting rituximab on day 1, every 21 days, for up to 6 cycles, *plus*
Diphenhydramine 25–50 mg; administer orally or intravenously 30–60 minutes before starting rituximab on day 1, every 21 days, for up to 6 cycles

Rituximab 375 mg/m^2; administer intravenously in 0.9% sodium chloride injection (0.9% NS) or 5% dextrose injection (D5W), diluted to a concentration within the range 1–4 mg/mL, on day 1, every 21 days, for up to 6 cycles (total dosage/3-week cycle = 375 mg/m^2)
Rituximab administration:
- Infuse initially at 50 mg/hour. If hypersensitivity or infusion reactions do not occur during the first 30 minutes, increase the rate by 50 mg/hour every 30 minutes as tolerated to a maximum rate of 400 mg/hour. During subsequent treatments if previous rituximab administration was well tolerated, start at 100 mg/hour and increase by 100 mg/hour every 30 minutes as tolerated to a maximum rate of 400 mg/hour

INFUSION REACTIONS ASSOCIATED WITH RITUXIMAB
Note: Medications for the treatment of hypersensitivity reactions should be available for immediate use in the event of a reaction during administration (eg, intravenous fluids, epinephrine, antihistamines, glucocorticoids, and O$_2$)
Fevers, chills, and rigors
1. Interrupt rituximab administration for severe symptoms, and give:
   - **Acetaminophen** 650 mg orally for fever. For persistent or recurrent symptoms, repeat administration every 4–6 hours as needed during rituximab administration
   - **Diphenhydramine** 25–50 mg orally or by intravenous injection for pruritus, hypotension, or angioedema. For persistent or recurrent symptoms, repeat administration every 4–6 hours as needed during rituximab administration
   - **Meperidine** 12.5–25 mg by intravenous injection every 10–20 minutes as needed for shaking chills (generally, cumulative doses >100 mg are not needed; use repeated doses with caution in persons with moderate or more severely impaired renal function)
2. If rituximab administration was interrupted, resume infusion at a slower rate than the maximum rate previously attempted. Rate escalation may be reattempted at smaller incremental steps with close monitoring. Do not exceed the maximum recommended rate of 400 mg/h

Dyspnea or wheezing without allergic findings (urticaria, or tongue or laryngeal edema)
1. Interrupt rituximab administration immediately
2. Give **hydrocortisone** 100 mg by intravenous injection (or an alternative steroid with equivalent glucocorticoid potency)
3. Give a **histamine (H$_2$) receptor antagonist** (ranitidine 50 mg, cimetidine 300 mg, or famotidine 20 mg) intravenously over 15–30 minutes
4. After symptoms resolve, resume rituximab administration at 25 mg/h with close monitoring. Do not increase the administration rate

Note: Medications and equipment for the treatment of hypersensitivity reactions should be available for immediate use in the event of a reaction during administration (eg, intravenous fluids, epinephrine, antihistamines, glucocorticoids, and oxygen)

Rituxan (rituximab) prescribing information. South San Francisco, CA: Genentech, Inc; 2018 October

Chemotherapy
Etoposide 50 mg/m^2 per day; administer by continuous intravenous infusion over 24 hours, for 4 consecutive days, on days 1–4, every 21 days, for up to 6 cycles (total dosage/cycle = 200 mg/m^2) (see Therapy Modifications section for dosage specifications)
Doxorubicin 10 mg/m^2 per day; administer by continuous intravenous infusion over 24 hours, for 4 consecutive days, on days 1–4, every 21 days, for up to 6 cycles (total dosage/cycle = 40 mg/m^2) (see Therapy Modifications section for dosage specifications)
Vincristine 0.4 mg/m^2 per day; administer by continuous intravenous infusion over 24 hours, for 4 consecutive days, on days 1–4, every 21 days, for up to 6 cycles (total dosage/cycle = 1.6 mg/m^2)
Note: See Special Instructions below for preparing a 3-in-1 admixture with etoposide, doxorubicin, and vincristine
Prednisone 60 mg/m^2 per dose; administer orally, twice daily for 5 consecutive days, on days 1–5 (10 doses), every 21 days, for up to 6 cycles (total dosage/cycle = 600 mg/m^2)
- The first prednisone dose should be given at least 1 hour before rituximab administration begins
- Patients who were unable to ingest oral medications may receive a parenterally administered steroid at a glucocorticoid equivalent dosage for the same number of doses on the same administration schedule (eg, methylprednisolone 48 mg/m^2 per dose)

Cyclophosphamide 750 mg/m^2; administer intravenously in 100 mL 0.9% NS or D5W over 30 minutes on day 5 (after completing infusional etoposide + doxorubicin + vincristine) every 21 days, for up to 6 cycles (total dosage/cycle = 750 mg/m^2) (see therapy modifications section for dosage specifications)

(continued)

(continued)

Supportive Care

Antiemetic prophylaxis

Emetogenic potential on Days 1–5 is **MODERATE**

See Chapter 42 for antiemetic recommendations

Hematopoietic growth factor (CSF) prophylaxis

Primary prophylaxis is indicated with one of the following:

Filgrastim (G-CSF) 5 µg/kg per day, by subcutaneous injection, *or:*

Pegfilgrastim (pegylated filgrastim) 6 mg/0.6 mL, by subcutaneous injection for one dose

- Begin use from 24–72 h after myelosuppressive chemotherapy is completed
- Continue daily filgrastim use until ANC ≥5000/mm^3 after the leukocyte nadir
- Discontinue daily filgrastim use at least 24 hours before administering myelosuppressive treatment. Do not administer pegfilgrastim within 14 days before administering myelosuppressive treatment

See Chapter 43 for more information

Antimicrobial prophylaxis

Risk of fever and neutropenia is *INTERMEDIATE*

Antimicrobial primary prophylaxis to be considered:

- Antibacterial—consider a fluoroquinolone during periods of neutropenia; *P. jirovecii* prophylaxis is recommended (eg, cotrimoxazole)
- Antifungal—consider concomitant use of fluconazole during periods of neutropenia, and in anticipation of mucositis
- Antiviral—anti-herpes antivirals (eg, acyclovir, famciclovir, valacyclovir)

Risk of reactivation of viral hepatitis with rituximab administration

- All patients should be tested for active or previous exposure to hepatitis B and C prior to receiving rituximab
- Providers should ensure patients with active previous exposure to hepatitis B are receiving appropriate prophylaxis or treatment prior to initiation of rituximab

Additional prophylaxis

Add a **proton pump inhibitor** during prednisone use to prevent gastritis and duodenitis

Give **stool softeners and/or laxatives** during and after vincristine administration

Suggested CNS prophylaxis for patients who have either ≥2 extranodal sites AND elevated LDH, or bone marrow involvement:

Methotrexate 12 mg per dose; administer intrathecally in a volume of **preservative-free** 0.9% NS equivalent to the amount of cerebrospinal fluid removed via lumbar puncture on day 2, every 21 days, during cycles 3, 4, 5, and 6 only (total dosage/3-week cycle in cycles 3–6 = 12 mg)

General instructions:

To prepare a 3-in-1 admixture with etoposide + doxorubicin + vincristine, dilute all 3 drug products in 0.9% NS as follows:

Total Dose of Etoposide	Volume of 0.9% NS
≤130 mg	500 mL
>130 mg	1000 mL

Etoposide (base) + doxorubicin + vincristine 3-in–1 admixtures:

Etoposide 50 mg/m², doxorubicin hydrochloride 10 mg/m², and vincristine sulfate 0.4 mg/m² admixtures diluted in 0.9% NS to produce a final etoposide concentration <250 µg/mL, in polyolefin-lined infusion bags are stable and compatible for 72 hours at 23°–25°C (73.4°–77°F), and at 31°–33°C (87.8°–91.4°F) when protected from exposure to light

Wolfe JL et al. Am J Health Syst Pharm 1999;56:985–989

Etoposide Phosphate + doxorubicin + vincristine 3-in-1 admixtures:

Etoposide phosphate, doxorubicin hydrochloride, and vincristine sulfate admixtures diluted in 0.9% NS, to produce a final etoposide concentration <250 µg/mL in polyolefin-lined infusion bags are stable and compatible for up to 124 hours at 2°–6°C (35.6°–42.8°F) and 35°–40°C (95°–104°F) in the dark and under fluorescent light. In admixtures stored at 35°–40°C (95°–104°F) and exposed to light, the initial drug concentrations decreased slightly, but remain within acceptable concentrations

Yuan P et al. Am J Health Syst Pharm 2001;58:594–598

A 3-in-1 admixture does not prevent microbial growth after exposure to bacterial and fungal contamination. With respect to product sterility, expiration dating should be determined by the aseptic techniques used in preparation and local and national guidelines

Treatment Modifications

Dose-adjusted EPOCH-R (DA-EPOCH-R)

Drug	Dose Level								
	−3	−2	−1	1 (Starting Dose)	2	3	4	5	6
Prednisone (mg/m²/dose)	60	60	60	60	60	60	60	60	60
Vincristine (mg/m²/day)	0.4	0.4	0.4	0.4	0.4	0.4	0.4	0.4	0.4
Doxorubicin (mg/m²/day)	10	10	10	10	12	14.4	17.3	20.7	24.8
Etoposide (mg/m²/day)	50	50	50	50	60	72	86.4	103.7	124.4
Cyclophosphamide (mg/m²)	384	480	600	750	900	1080	1296	1555	1866
Rituximab (mg/m²)	375	375	375	375	375	375	375	375	375

Dose Modification of Doxorubicin, Etoposide, and Cyclophosphamide Based on Twice-Weekly ANC and Platelet Measurements
Note: ANC and platelets should be measured twice per week (3–4 days apart, ie every Monday and Thursday) beginning 3–4 days after completion of chemotherapy. Dose adjustments for hematologic toxicity only apply to etoposide, doxorubicin, and cyclophosphamide. Only cyclophosphamide is reduced in dose levels −1 through −3

ANC <1000/mm³ or platelets <100,000/mm³ on day 1	Delay the cycle until recovery of ANC >1000/mm³ or platelets >100,00/mm³
Previous cycle ANC >500/mm³ on all measurements AND platelet nadir ≥25,000/ mm³*	Increase etoposide, doxorubicin, and cyclophosphamide dosages by 1 dose level
Previous cycle ANC <500/mm³ on 1 or 2 measurements (3–4 days apart) AND platelet nadir ≥25,000/ mm³*	Maintain the same dose level of etoposide, doxorubicin, and cyclophosphamide
Previous cycle ANC <500/mm³ on ≥3 measurements (3–4 days apart) *or* platelet nadir <25,000/ mm³*	Decrease etoposide, doxorubicin, and cyclophosphamide dosages by 1 dose level

Neuropathy

G2 motor neuropathy	Decrease vincristine dose 25%[†]
G3 sensory neuropathy	Decrease vincristine dose 25%[†]
G3 motor neuropathy	Decrease vincristine 50%[†]
G4 neuropathy (any)	Discontinue vincristine, continue other agents[†]
Ileus or constipation requiring hospitalization	Optimize the prophylactic bowel regimen. Consider reducing the dose of vincristine in the next cycle by 25%. If the ileus or constipation do not recur, then re-escalate the vincristine dose to the full dose in subsequent cycles

Hyperbilirubinemia Secondary to Lymphoma

Total bilirubin >1.5 mg/dL, but <3 mg/dL	Decrease the vincristine dosage by 25%[‡] Do not reduce the doxorubicin dosage
Total bilirubin ≥3.0 mg/dL, but ≤7 mg/dL	Reduce the vincristine dosage by 50%[‡] Do not reduce the doxorubicin dosage
Total bilirubin >7 mg/dL	Reduce vincristine dosage by 50%[‡] Omit doxorubicin until bilirubin improves to ≤7 mg/dL

*ANC and platelet nadir measurements are based on twice-weekly CBC with differential only
[†]Vincristine dosage is increased to 100% if neuropathy resolves to G1
[‡]The vincristine dose may be re-escalated as hyperbilirubinemia improves
Protocol for: Bartlett NL et al. J Clin Oncol 2019;37:1790–1799

Patient Population Studied

Dunleavy K et al. N Engl J Med 2013;368:14089–1416

Baseline Characteristics of the Study Patients

Characteristic	Prospective NCI Cohort (N = 51)	Retrospective Stanford Cohort (N = 16)	P Value Between Study Cohorts
Female sex—no. (%)	30 (59)	9 (56)	1.00
Age (years)—median (range)	30 (19–52)	33 (23–68)	0.04
Bulky tumor, ≥10 cm			0.57
Patients—no. (%)	33 (65)	9 (56)	
Maximal diameter range—cm	5–18	7–18	
Stage IV disease—no. (%)	15 (29)	7 (44)	0.36
Elevated lactate dehydrogenase level—no. (%)	40 (78)	11 (69)	0.51
Extranodal site—no. (%)	27 (53)	3 (19)	0.02
Pleural effusion—no. (%)	24 (47)	10 (62)	0.39
CD20+ malignant cells—no. (%)	51 (100)	16 (100)	1.00
BCL6+ malignant cells—no. (%)	33/37 (89)	ND	ND

*BCL6 denotes the B-cell lymphoma 6 protein, NCI National Cancer Institute, and ND not done

Efficacy

Dunleavy K et al. N Engl J Med 2013;368:14089

Median follow-up of 63 months (range 3 to 156) in the prospective NCI study	
Event-free survival rate	93% (95% CI, 81–98)[†]
Overall survival rate	97% (95% CI, 81 to 99)[†]
Evidence of disease after DA-EPOCH-R treatment	3/51*
Median follow-up of 37 months (range, 5 to 53) in the retrospective Stanford cohort	
Event-free survival rate	100% (95% CI, 79 to 100)
Overall survival rate	100% (95% CI, 79 to 100)
Median follow-up of 16 years, in phase 2 NCI study of DA-EPOCH	
Event-free survival rate	67% (95% CI, 44 to 84)[†]
Overall survival rate	78% (95% CI, 55 to 91)[†]
Long-term complications	No cardiac failure or second tumors observed

*Two with persistent focal disease on FDG-PET-CT, and with disease progression. Two underwent mediastinal radiotherapy, and one excisional biopsy. All three patients became disease-free. One later died from acute myeloid leukemia, while still in remission

[†]The event-free (P = 0.007) and overall survival (P = 0.01) rates were higher with addition of rituximab in the NCI prospective cohort than in the cohort of 18 patients who received DA-EPOCH alone

Selected Treatment-related Toxicities
Comparison of R-CHOP and DA-EPOCH-R

CTCAE Toxicity Grade	Treatment		P
	R-CHOP (N = 243)*	DA-EPOCH-R (N = 237)*	
G3/4/5 AE			<0.001
No	53 (21.8)	4 (1.7)	
Yes	190 (78.2)	233 (98.3)	
G3/4 Hematologic			<0.001
No	64 (26.3)	6 (2.5)	
Yes	179 (73.7)	231 (97.5)	
G3/4 Nonhematologic			<0.001
No	138 (56.8)	66 (27.8)	
Yes	105 (43.2)	171 (72.2)	
G3/4 Infection			0.0494
No	217 (89.3)	197 (83.1)	
Yes	26 (10.7)	40 (16.9)	
G3/4 Febrile neutropenia			<0.001
No	200 (82.3)	154 (65.0)	
Yes	43 (17.7)	83 (35.0)	
G3/4 Mucositis			0.0017
No	238 (97.9)	217 (91.6)	
Yes	5 (2.1)	20 (8.4)	
G1/2 Neuropathy			<0.001
No	128 (52.7)	82 (34.6)	
Yes	115 (47.3)	155 (65.4)	
G3/4 Neuropathy			<0.001
No	235 (96.7)	193 (81.4)	
Yes	8 (3.3)	44 (18.6)	

Note: Data reported as No. (%) unless otherwise indicated
AE, adverse event; CTCAE, National Cancer Institute Common Terminology Criteria for Adverse Events, version 4.0; DA-EPOCH-R, dose-adjusted etoposide, prednisone, vincristine, cyclophosphamide, doxorubicin, and rituximab; R-CHOP, rituximab, cyclophosphamide, doxorubicin, vincristine, and prednisone
*Excludes 10 patients who did not initiate treatment and one patient in the R-CHOP arm without toxicity data submitted
†X² P value

Toxicity

Dunleavy K et al. N Engl J Med 2013;368:14089
In the NCI study, 90% of patients received six cycles, and 10% received eight cycles, of DA-EPOCH-R. More than half the 51 patients had an escalation to at least dose level 4, representing a 73% increase compared to dose level 1; 6% of patients did not have a dose escalation
More than half the patients received 69 mg of doxorubicin per square meter of body-surface area for at least one cycle and cumulative doses of 345 to 507 mg per square meter
Ejection fractions were normal up to 10 years in 10 patients in whom they were measured. There was no significant relationship between the ejection fraction and the length of time since treatment (P = 0.30) or between the ejection fraction and the cumulative doxorubicin dose (P = 0.20), and no significant interaction between the dose and time interval (P = 0.40)

Bartlett NL et al. J Clin Oncol 2019;37:1790–1799

Therapy Monitoring

1. *Before therapy:* CBC with differential, LFTs, BUN, serum creatinine, hepatitis B and C serologies, tumor lysis labs (ie, potassium, phosphate, uric acid, LDH, calcium), and left ventricular ejection fraction (LVEF)
2. Evaluate LVEF during doxorubicin treatment if clinical symptoms of heart failure are present
3. *Day 1 each cycle:* CBC with differential count, LFTs, BUN, and serum creatinine
4. *Twice-weekly during chemotherapy (at least 3 days apart):* CBC with differential

DIFFUSE LARGE B-CELL LYMPHOMA • SUBSEQUENT THERAPY

NON-HODGKIN LYMPHOMA REGIMEN: RITUXIMAB, IFOSFAMIDE, CARBOPLATIN, AND ETOPOSIDE (RICE)

Kewalramani T et al. Blood 2004;103:3684–3688

Rituximab

Premedication for rituximab:

Acetaminophen 650–1000 mg; administer orally 30–60 minutes before starting rituximab, *plus*

Diphenhydramine 25–50 mg; administer orally or intravenously 30–60 minutes before starting rituximab

Rituximab 375 mg/m²; administer intravenously in 0.9% sodium chloride injection (0.9% NS) or 5% dextrose injection (D5W), diluted to a concentration of 1–4 mg/mL, 48 hours before initiation of the first cycle, then every 2 weeks on day 1 of each cycle (total dosage/3 cycles = 1500 mg/m²)

Notes on rituximab administration:

- An initiating dose was given 48 hours before the first cycle of RICE. Subsequently, rituximab was given on the first day of each cycle of RICE

- Infuse initially at 50 mg/hour. If hypersensitivity or infusion reactions do not occur during the first 30 minutes, increase the rate by 50 mg/hour every 30 minutes, as tolerated, to a maximum rate of 400 mg/hour. Subsequently, if previous administration was well tolerated, start at 100 mg/hour and increase by 100 mg/hour every 30 minutes, as tolerated, to a maximum rate of 400 mg/hour

INFUSION REACTIONS ASSOCIATED WITH RITUXIMAB

Note: Medications for the treatment of hypersensitivity reactions should be available for immediate use in the event of a reaction during administration (eg, intravenous fluids, epinephrine, antihistamines, glucocorticoids, and O_2)

Fevers, chills, and rigors

1. Interrupt rituximab administration for severe symptoms, and give:

   - **Acetaminophen** 650 mg orally for fever. For persistent or recurrent symptoms, repeat administration every 4–6 hours as needed during rituximab administration

   - **Diphenhydramine** 25–50 mg orally or by intravenous injection for pruritus, hypotension, or angioedema. For persistent or recurrent symptoms, repeat administration every 4–6 hours as needed during rituximab administration

   - **Meperidine** 12.5–25 mg by intravenous injection every 10–20 minutes as needed for shaking chills (generally, cumulative doses >100 mg are not needed; use repeated doses with caution in persons with moderate or more severely impaired renal function)

2. If rituximab administration was interrupted, resume infusion at a slower rate than the maximum rate previously attempted. Rate escalation may be reattempted at smaller incremental steps with close monitoring. Do not exceed the maximum recommended rate of 400 mg/h

Dyspnea or wheezing without allergic findings (urticaria, or tongue or laryngeal edema)

1. Interrupt rituximab administration immediately

2. Give **hydrocortisone** 100 mg by intravenous injection (or an alternative steroid with equivalent glucocorticoid potency)

3. Give a **histamine (H_2) receptor antagonist** (ranitidine 50 mg, cimetidine 300 mg, or famotidine 20 mg) intravenously over 15–30 minutes

4. After symptoms resolve, resume rituximab administration at 25 mg/h with close monitoring. Do not increase the administration rate

Note: Medications and equipment for the treatment of hypersensitivity reactions should be available for immediate use in the event of a reaction during administration (eg, intravenous fluids, epinephrine, antihistamines, glucocorticoids, and oxygen)

Rituxan (rituximab) prescribing information. South San Francisco, CA: Genentech, Inc; 2018 October

Note: ICE chemotherapy is administered on an inpatient basis beginning on day 3 of each cycle. Cycles are administered at 2-week intervals such that the second and third cycles of RICE would begin on day 15 of the previous cycle

Induction phase:

Etoposide 100 mg/m² per day; administer intravenously diluted in 0.9% NS to a concentration within the range of 0.2–0.4 mg/mL, over 1 hour for 3 consecutive days, days 3–5, every 2 weeks (total dosage/cycle = 300 mg/m²)

Carboplatin (calculated dose) AUC = 5 mg/mL . min* (maximum absolute dose/cycle = 800 mg); administer intravenously in 100–500 mL D5W or 0.9% NS over 15–30 minutes on day 4, every 2 weeks (total dosage/cycle calculated to produce an AUC = 5 mg/mL . min; maximum absolute dose/cycle = 800 mg)

Ifosfamide 5000 mg/m² with **mesna** 5000 mg/m²; administer by continuous intravenous infusion diluted in 0.9% NS or D5W to an ifosfamide concentration within the range of 0.6–20 mg/mL over 24 hours on day 4, every 2 weeks (total ifosfamide and mesna dosages/cycle = 5000 mg/m²)
- Ifosfamide and mesna may be combined in a single container, or may be administered separately

*Carboplatin dose is based on a formula developed by Calvert et al. to achieve a target area under the plasma concentration versus time curve (AUC; AUC units = mg/mL . min)

$$\text{Total Carboplatin Dose (mg)} = (\text{Target AUC}) \times (\text{GFR} + 25)$$

In practice, creatinine clearance (ClCr) is used in place of glomerular filtration rate (GFR). ClCr can be calculated from the equation of Cockcroft and Gault:

$$\text{For males, Clcr} = \frac{(140 \pm \text{age [years]}) \times \text{body weight [kg]}}{72 \times (\text{serum creatinine [mg/dL]})}$$

$$\text{For females, Clcr} = \frac{(140 - \text{age [years]}) \times \text{body weight [kg]}}{72 \times (\text{serum creatinine [mg/dL]})} \times 0.85$$

Calvert AH et al. J Clin Oncol 1989;7:1748–1756
Cockcroft DW , Gault MH. Nephron 1976;16:31–41
Jodrell DI et al. J Clin Oncol 1992;10:520–528
Sorensen BT et al. Cancer Chemother Pharmacol 1991;28:397–401

Supportive Care
Antiemetic prophylaxis
Emetogenic potential on days 1, 3, and 5 is **LOW**
Emetogenic potential on day 4 is **MODERATE–HIGH**. *Potential for delayed symptoms*
See Chapter 42 for antiemetic recommendations

Hematopoietic growth factor (CSF) prophylaxis
Primary prophylaxis is indicated with:
Filgrastim (G-CSF) 5 μg/kg per day; administer by subcutaneous injection for 8 consecutive days, on days 5–12
See Chapter 43 for more information

Antimicrobial prophylaxis
Risk of fever and neutropenia is *LOW*
Antimicrobial primary prophylaxis to be considered:
- Antibacterial—*Pneumocystis jirovecii* prophylaxis is recommended (eg, cotrimoxazole)
- Antifungal—not indicated
- Antiviral—not indicated unless patient previously had an episode of HSV

Treatment Modifications

Adverse Event	Dose Modification
ANC <1000/mm³ and platelet count <50,000/mm³	Delay start of treatment until ANC is >1000/mm³ and platelet count is >50,000/mm³

Patient Population Studied

A study comparing 37 patients 18–72 years of age who had diffuse large B-cell lymphoma (DLBCL), according to the World Health Organization classification, that relapsed after, or was refractory to, a single standard anthracycline-based regimen, to historical control treated with ICE alone

Therapy Monitoring

1. Prior to treatment: hepatitis B core antibody (IgG or total) and hepatitis B surface antigen
2. Before each cycle: CBC with differential, serum BUN, and creatinine

Note:
1. Used for cytoreduction and stem cell mobilization in transplant-eligible patients. There were no dose reductions. Of 381 cycles, 66 were delayed because of hematologic toxicity
2. Four patients developed confusion that resolved without intervention. These patients were not retreated

Efficacy

Response Rates to RICE Compared with ICE Historic Controls						
Patient Subgroup	Overall Response Rate (%)			Complete Response Rate (%)		
	R-ICE	ICE*	P	R-ICE	ICE*	P
All patients	78	71	0.53	53	27	0.01
Relapsed	96	79	0.07	65	34	0.01
Refractory	46	63	0.36	31	19	0.46
sAAIPI L/LI	79	86	0.47	53	39	0.42
sAAIPI H/HI	76	61	0.28	53	19	0.01

sAAIP, Second-line age-adjusted international prognostic index; L, low risk; LI, low–intermediate risk; HI, high–intermediate risk; H, high risk
*ICE historic control

DIFFUSE LARGE B-CELL LYMPHOMA • SUBSEQUENT THERAPY
NON-HODGKIN LYMPHOMA REGIMEN: RITUXIMAB + DEXAMETHASONE, CYTARABINE (HIGH-DOSE ARA-C), AND CISPLATIN (R-DHAP)

Gisselbrecht C et al. J Clin Oncol 2010;28:4184–4190

Rituximab
Premedication for rituximab:
Acetaminophen 650–1000 mg; administer orally 30–60 minutes before starting rituximab, *plus*
Diphenhydramine 25–50 mg; administer orally or intravenously 30–60 minutes before starting rituximab
Rituximab 375 mg/m² per dose; administer intravenously in 0.9% sodium chloride injection (0.9% NS) or 5% dextrose injection (D5W), diluted to a concentration within the range 1–4 mg/mL, on day 0, every 14 days (total dosage/14-day cycle = 375 mg/m²)
Notes on rituximab administration:
• Infuse initially at 50 mg/h. If hypersensitivity or infusion reactions do not occur during the first 30 minutes, increase the rate by 50 mg/h every 30 minutes as tolerated to a maximum rate of 400 mg/h. During subsequent treatments, if previous rituximab administration was well tolerated, start at 100 mg/h and increase by 100 mg/h every 30 minutes as tolerated to a maximum rate of 400 mg/h

INFUSION REACTIONS ASSOCIATED WITH RITUXIMAB
Note: Medications for the treatment of hypersensitivity reactions should be available for immediate use in the event of a reaction during administration (eg, intravenous fluids, epinephrine, antihistamines, glucocorticoids, and O_2)
Fevers, chills, and rigors
Interrupt rituximab administration for severe symptoms, and give:
• **Acetaminophen** 650 mg orally for fever. For persistent or recurrent symptoms, repeat administration every 4–6 hours as needed during rituximab administration
• **Diphenhydramine** 25–50 mg orally or by intravenous injection for pruritus, hypotension, or angioedema. For persistent or recurrent symptoms, repeat administration every 4–6 hours as needed during rituximab administration
• **Meperidine** 12.5–25 mg by intravenous injection every 10–20 minutes as needed for shaking chills (generally, cumulative doses >100 mg are not needed; use repeated doses with caution in persons with moderate or more severely impaired renal function)
If rituximab administration was interrupted, resume infusion at a slower rate than the maximum rate previously attempted. Rate escalation may be reattempted at smaller incremental steps with close monitoring. Do not exceed the maximum recommended rate of 400 mg/h
Dyspnea or wheezing without allergic findings (urticaria, or tongue or laryngeal edema)
1. Interrupt rituximab administration immediately
2. Give **hydrocortisone** 100 mg by intravenous injection (or an alternative steroid with equivalent glucocorticoid potency)
3. Give a **histamine (H_2) receptor antagonist** (ranitidine 50 mg, cimetidine 300 mg, or famotidine 20 mg) intravenously over 15–30 minutes
4. After symptoms resolve, resume rituximab administration at 25 mg/h with close monitoring. Do not increase the administration rate
Note: Medications and equipment for the treatment of hypersensitivity reactions should be available for immediate use in the event of a reaction during administration (eg, intravenous fluids, epinephrine, antihistamines, glucocorticoids, and oxygen)
Rituxan (rituximab) prescribing information. South San Francisco, CA: Genentech, Inc; 2018 October

Hydration: 0.9% sodium chloride injection (0.9% NS) + at a rate of 250 mL/hour for 36 hours; administer intravenously beginning at least 6 hours before starting cisplatin administration, every 3–4 weeks, for 6–10 cycles. Monitor and replace magnesium/electrolytes as needed
Cisplatin 100 mg/m²; administer by continuous intravenous infusion over 24 hours in a volume equivalent to the dose, or diluted in 100 mL to ≥1000 mL 0.9% NS. Begin administration on day 1 after completing 6 hours of hydration, every 3–4 weeks, for 6–10 cycles (total dosage/cycle = 100 mg/m²)
Cytarabine
Patients ≤70 years: **Cytarabine** 2000 mg/m² per dose; administer intravenously over 3 hours in 50–500 mL 0.9% NS or 5% dextrose injection (D5W) every 12 hours for 2 doses, starting after the completion of cisplatin administration on day 2, every 3–4 weeks, for 6–10 cycles (total dosage/cycle = 4000 mg/m²)
Patients >70 years: **Cytarabine** 1000 mg/m² per dose; administer intravenously over 3 hours in 50–500 mL 0.9% NS or D5W every 12 hours for 2 doses, starting after the completion of cisplatin administration on day 2, every 3–4 weeks, for 6–10 cycles (total dosage/cycle = 2000 mg/m²)

Keratitis prophylaxis
• Steroid ophthalmic drops (prednisolone 1% or dexamethasone 0.1%); administer 2 drops by intraocular instillation into each eye every 6 hours starting prior to the first cytarabine dose and continuing until 48 hours after high-dose cytarabine is completed

Dexamethasone 40 mg/day; administer orally or intravenously in 10–100 mL 0.9% NS or D5W over 10–30 minutes for 4 consecutive days on days 1–4, every 3–4 weeks, for 6–10 cycles (total dosage/cycle = 160 mg)

Supportive Care
Antiemetic prophylaxis
Emetogenic potential on day 1 is **HIGH**. *Potential for delayed symptoms*
Emetogenic potential on day 2 is **MODERATE–HIGH**
See Chapter 42 for antiemetic recommendations

(continued)

(continued)

Hematopoietic growth factor (CSF) prophylaxis
Primary prophylaxis is indicated with 1 of the following:
Filgrastim (G-CSF) 5 µg/kg per day; administer by subcutaneous injection, *or*
Pegfilgrastim (pegylated filgrastim) 6 mg/0.6 mL; administer by subcutaneous injection for 1 dose
• Begin use from 24–72 hours after myelosuppressive chemotherapy is completed
See Chapter 43 for more information

Antimicrobial prophylaxis
Risk of fever and neutropenia is *INTERMEDIATE*
Antimicrobial primary prophylaxis to be considered:
• Antibacterial—consider a fluoroquinolone or no prophylaxis; *Pneumocystis jirovecii* prophylaxis is recommended (eg, cotrimoxazole)
• Antifungal—consider use during neutropenia and for anticipated mucositis
• Antiviral—antiherpes antivirals (eg, acyclovir)

Steroid-associated gastritis
Add a **proton pump inhibitor** during dexamethasone use to prevent gastritis and duodenitis

Dexamethasone + High-Dose Cytarabine + Cisplatin Dose Modifications

	Dexamethasone	Cytarabine	Cisplatin
Starting dose	40 mg	2000 mg/m^2	100 mg/m^2
Dose level 1	30 mg	1500 mg/m^2	75 mg/m^2
Dose level 2	20 mg	1000 mg/m^2	50 mg/m^2

Hematologic Toxicity

Day 1 platelet count <100,000/mm^3 or ANC <1500/mm^3	Delay start of cycle until platelet count ≥100,000/mm^3 and ANC ≥1500/mm^3, or until recovery to near baseline value, then continue at the same doses
G4 neutropenia (ANC <500/mm^3) during the prior cycle given without G-CSF (filgrastim, pegfilgrastim) prophylaxis	Administer filgrastim or pegfilgrastim during all subsequent cycles, and continue the same doses
Febrile neutropenia (ANC <1000/mm^3 with temperature >38°C or >100.4°F) during the prior cycle given without G-CSF (filgrastim, pegfilgrastim) prophylaxis	
Febrile neutropenia (ANC <1000/mm^3 with temperature >38°C or >100.4°F) during the prior cycle given with growth factor (filgrastim, pegfilgrastim) prophylaxis	Consider reducing the dose of cytarabine by 1 dose level for subsequent cycles. Do not change the dexamethasone or cisplatin dose
G4 thrombocytopenia (platelets <25,000/mm^3) during the prior cycle	

Neurologic Toxicities

Peripheral sensory neuropathy G ≥3 (severe symptoms; limiting self-care ADL)	Discontinue cisplatin. May continue to administer dexamethasone and cytarabine at the discretion of the medically responsible healthcare provider
Neurologic (cerebellar) toxicity	Discontinue cytarabine. Patients who develop CNS symptoms should not receive subsequent high-dose cytarabine. May continue to administer dexamethasone and cisplatin at the discretion of the medically responsible healthcare provider
G ≥2 mood alteration (moderate mood alteration) or confusion (moderate disorientation; limiting instrumental ADL)	Withhold dexamethasone until symptoms return to baseline. Resume dexamethasone reduced by 1 dose level. If symptoms persist, reduce by another dose level. Do not change the cytarabine or cisplatin doses

Other Toxicities

Serum creatinine ≥1.5 mg/dL (≥130 µmol/L) and/or BUN ≥25 mg/dL (≥8.92 mmol/L)	Withhold dexamethasone, cytarabine, and cisplatin until serum creatinine <1.5 mg/dL (<130 µmol/L) and BUN <25 mg/dL (<8.92 mmol/L). Then, reduce the cisplatin dose by 1 dose level, and continue dexamethasone and cytarabine at the same doses
Cisplatin induced hearing loss G ≥3 (hearing loss with hearing aid or intervention indicated; limiting self-care ADL)	Discontinue cisplatin. May continue to administer dexamethasone and cytarabine at the discretion of the medically responsible healthcare provider

Significant hypersensitivity reaction to cisplatin (hypotension, dyspnea, and angioedema requiring therapy) *Note:* Allergic reaction to cisplatin including anaphylaxis risk is increased in patients previously exposed to platinum therapy	May occur within minutes of cisplatin administration. Interrupt the cisplatin infusion in patients with clinically significant infusion reactions. Discontinue cisplatin or can consider desensitization and a rechallenge. May continue to administer dexamethasone and cytarabine at the discretion of the medically responsible healthcare provider
Fever, myalgia, bone pain, occasionally chest pain, maculopapular rash, conjunctivitis and malaise 6–12 hours following drug administration (cytarabine or Ara-C syndrome)	Corticosteroids are beneficial in treating or preventing this syndrome. If the symptoms deemed treatable, continue therapy with cytarabine and pretreat with corticosteroids If the syndrome occurs in a patient already receiving corticosteroid pretreatment, consider reducing the cytarabine dose by 1 dose level
G ≥3 hyperglycemia (insulin therapy initiated; hospitalization indicated)	Withhold dexamethasone until blood glucose is ≤250 mg/dL. Treat with insulin or other hypoglycemic agents as clinically appropriate, and then resume dexamethasone at the same dose. If hyperglycemia is uncontrolled despite above measures, decrease dexamethasone by 1 dose level

ANC, absolute neutrophil count; G-CSF, granulocyte-colony stimulating factor
Note: Medications and equipment for the treatment of hypersensitivity reactions should be available for immediate use in the event of a reaction during rituximab administration (eg, intravenous fluids, epinephrine, antihistamines, glucocorticoids, oxygen)

Efficacy

Response After Induction Treatment (Including Death) for All Patients (N = 191)

Response	No. of Patients	%
Complete response	53	28
Unconfirmed complete response	22	12
Partial response	45	24
Stable disease	22	12
Progressive disease	35	18
Death	10	5
Premature withdrawal, not evaluated	4	2
Autologous transplantation		
Median CD34+ cells collected, million/kg	4.9	
Collection failure <2,000,000 CD34+ cells	15	8
Mobilization-adjusted response	104	54.5
Consolidation with BEAM performed per protocol	105	55

After a median follow-up time of 27 months

3-year EFS rate	35%
3-year PFS rate	42%
3-year OS rate	51%

For the combined RICE and R-DHAP cohorts in the Gisselbrecht C et al study

Three-year EFS, PFS, and OS	Affected by prior rituximab treatment, early relapse, and saaIP
Three-year EFS, PFS, and OS in the COX model	Prior rituximab treatment, early relapse, and saaIP remained significant ($P<0.001$); the treatment arm RICE or R-DHAP was not significant
Three-year PFS	Early relapse (≤12 months and prior rituximab treatment had lower 3-year PFS; no difference if relapse >12 months)
Three-year EFS, and OS	No difference if relapse >12 months

EFS, event-free survival; OS, overall survival; PFS, progression-free survival; saaIP, second-line age adjusted international prognostic index

Patient Population Studied

Patients with CD20+ DLBCL in first relapse or who were refractory after first-line therapy were randomly assigned to either rituximab, ifosfamide, etoposide, and carboplatin (R-ICE) or rituximab, dexamethasone, high-dose cytarabine, and cisplatin (R-DHAP). Responding patients received high-dose chemotherapy and ASCT

Demographic or Clinical Characteristic	(N = 194)
Age, years (median / range)	55 / 19–65
Sex (male / female)	1189 / 76
Ann Arbor stage (I–II / III–IV)	66 / 121
Extranodal site > 1	64
Bone marrow involvement	19
Elevated LDH	94
saaIPI at relapse (0–1 / 2–3)	107 / 74
< 12 / ≥ 12 months to relapse > diagnosis	87 / 103
Prior rituximab treatment	
Prior first-line CHOP-like chemotherapy	167
Intensified CHOP	23

Therapy Monitoring

1. *Prior to treatment*: hepatitis B core antibody (IgG or total) and hepatitis B surface antigen
2. *Before each cycle*: PE, CBC with differential, serum electrolytes, BUN, creatinine, LFTs
3. *Daily on days of drug administration*: Serum electrolytes. Cardiac, pulmonary, and renal status are carefully monitored during administration of fluids
4. *Prior to each administration of high-dose cytarabine*: Monitor for signs of cerebellar toxicity (nystagmus, dysmetria, and ataxia)
5. *Weekly*: CBC with differential

Toxicity

N = 191

- The median time between salvage cycles was 22 days
- 120 serious events occurred in 68 patients

Hemoglobin, g/dL	
Day 10 (median / range)	11.1 / 7–16
Day 14 (median / range)	10.1 / 7–15

WBC, cells/μL	
Day 10 (median / range)	6 / 0–86
Day 14 (median / range)	6 / 0–68

Platelets, platelets/μL	
Day 10 (median / range)	101 / 2–2,940
Day 14 (median / range)	47 / 1–2,360

	No. of Patients	%
Transfusion	109	57
Patients who received 3 cycles	161	84
Infection with grade 3/4 neutropenia	31	16
Infection without grade 3/4 neutropenia	15	8
G3/4 renal toxicity	11	6
Toxic death	3	1.5

DIFFUSE LARGE B-CELL LYMPHOMA • SUBSEQUENT THERAPY • NOT ELIGIBLE FOR ASCT • RELAPSED/REFRACTORY

NON-HODGKIN LYMPHOMA REGIMEN: RITUXIMAB AND ORAL LENALIDOMIDE (R²)

Wang M et al. Leukemia 2013;27:1902–1909

Rituximab
Premedication for rituximab:
Acetaminophen 650–1000 mg; administer orally 30–60 minutes before each rituximab dose, *plus*
Diphenhydramine 25–50 mg; administer orally or intravenously 30–60 minutes before each rituximab dose
Rituximab 375 mg/m² per dose; administer intravenously in 0.9% NS or D5W, diluted to a concentration within the range 1–4 mg/mL, for 4 doses on days 1, 8, 15, and 22 for 1 cycle, cycle 1, only (total dosage/28-day cycle = 1500 mg/m²)
Notes on rituximab administration:
- Infuse initially at 50 mg/h. If hypersensitivity or infusion reactions do not occur during the first 30 minutes, increase the rate by 50 mg/h every 30 minutes as tolerated to a maximum rate of 400 mg/h. During subsequent treatments if previous rituximab administration was well tolerated, start at 100 mg/h, and increase by 100 mg/h every 30 minutes as tolerated to a maximum rate of 400 mg/h

INFUSION REACTIONS ASSOCIATED WITH RITUXIMAB
Note: Medications for the treatment of hypersensitivity reactions should be available for immediate use in the event of a reaction during administration (eg, intravenous fluids, epinephrine, antihistamines, glucocorticoids, and O₂)
Fevers, chills, and rigors
1. Interrupt rituximab administration for severe symptoms, and give:
   - **Acetaminophen** 650 mg orally for fever. For persistent or recurrent symptoms, repeat administration every 4–6 hours as needed during rituximab administration
   - **Diphenhydramine** 25–50 mg orally or by intravenous injection for pruritus, hypotension, or angioedema. For persistent or recurrent symptoms, repeat administration every 4–6 hours as needed during rituximab administration
   - **Meperidine** 12.5–25 mg by intravenous injection every 10–20 minutes as needed for shaking chills (generally, cumulative doses >100 mg are not needed; use repeated doses with caution in persons with moderate or more severely impaired renal function)
2. If rituximab administration was interrupted, resume infusion at a slower rate than the maximum rate previously attempted. Rate escalation may be reattempted at smaller incremental steps with close monitoring. Do not exceed the maximum recommended rate of 400 mg/h
Dyspnea or wheezing without allergic findings (urticaria, or tongue or laryngeal edema)
1. Interrupt rituximab administration immediately
2. Give **hydrocortisone** 100 mg by intravenous injection (or an alternative steroid with equivalent glucocorticoid potency)
3. Give a **histamine (H₂) receptor antagonist** (ranitidine 50 mg, cimetidine 300 mg, or famotidine 20 mg) intravenously over 15–30 minutes
4. After symptoms resolve, resume rituximab administration at 25 mg/h with close monitoring. Do not increase the administration rate
Note: Medications and equipment for the treatment of hypersensitivity reactions should be available for immediate use in the event of a reaction during administration (eg, intravenous fluids, epinephrine, antihistamines, glucocorticoids, and oxygen)
Rituxan (rituximab) prescribing information. South San Francisco, CA: Genentech, Inc; 2018 October

Lenalidomide
Lenalidomide 20 mg/dose; administer orally, without regard to meals, once daily for 21 consecutive days on days 1–21, followed by 7 days without treatment, starting in cycle 1, every 28 days, until disease progression (total dosage/28-day cycle = 420 mg)
- Patients who delay taking a lenalidomide dose at a regularly scheduled time may take the missed dose if the time to the next regularly scheduled dose is >12 hours away

Supportive Care
Antiemetic prophylaxis
Emetogenic potential is **MINIMAL**
See Chapter 42 for antiemetic recommendations

Hematopoietic growth factor (CSF) prophylaxis
Primary prophylaxis is **NOT** *indicated*
See Chapter 43 for more information

Antimicrobial prophylaxis
Risk of fever and neutropenia is *INTERMEDIATE*
Antimicrobial primary prophylaxis to be considered:
- Antibacterial—not indicated
- Antifungal—not indicated
- Antiviral—antiherpes antivirals (eg, acyclovir, famciclovir, valacyclovir)

Treatment Modifications

Lenalidomide Dose Modifications

	CrCl ≥60 mL/min	CrCl ≥30 and <60 mL/min
Starting dose	20 mg per day	10 mg per day*
Level 1	15 mg per day	5 mg per day
Level 2	10 mg per day	2.5 mg per day
Level 3	5 mg per day	Discontinue†
Level 4	2.5 mg per day	—
Level 5	Discontinue†	—

*If after completion of cycle 2 the patient remains free of G ≥3 toxicity, the lenalidomide dose may be increased to a maximum of 15 mg per day starting on day 1 of cycle 3

Adverse Event	Treatment Modification
Hematologic Toxicity	
Day 1 ANC <1000/mm³ or platelet count <50,000/mm³	Delay the next cycle until ANC ≥1000/mm³ and platelet count ≥50,000/mm³. Consider treatment with filgrastim and/or platelet transfusion according to local guidelines. If the start of a new cycle is delayed >14 days for lenalidomide-related toxicity, reduce the lenalidomide by 1 dose level
G3 neutropenia (ANC ≥500 to <1000/mm³) sustained for ≥7 days G4 neutropenia (ANC <500/mm³) at any time Febrile neutropenia (ANC <1000/mm³ with fever ≥38.3°C)	If neutropenia occurred on or after day 15, withhold lenalidomide for the rest of the cycle, and follow weekly CBC If neutropenia occurred before day 15 and resolves to G ≤2 (ANC ≥1000/mm³), resume lenalidomide at the same dose for the rest of the cycle Consider use of filgrastim according to local guidelines In subsequent cycles, reduce the lenalidomide dosage by 1 dose level
G ≥3 thrombocytopenia (platelet count <50,000/mm³) at any time	If thrombocytopenia occurred on or after day 15, withhold lenalidomide for the rest of the cycle, and follow weekly CBC If thrombocytopenia occurred before day 15 and resolved to G ≤2 (platelet count ≥50,000/mm³), resume lenalidomide at the same dose for the rest of the cycle In subsequent cycles, reduce the lenalidomide dosage by 1 dose level
Nonhematologic Toxicities	
G2/3 non-desquamating rash	Hold lenalidomide. Consider administering antihistamines and/or a short course of steroids. Resume at the same dose when resolved to G ≤1
G ≥3 desquamating (blistering) rash G4 non-desquamating rash Allergic reactions, including hypersensitivity, angioedema, Stevens-Johnson syndrome, toxic epidermal necrolysis (TEN), and drug reaction with eosinophilia and systemic symptoms (DRESS)	Permanently discontinue lenalidomide†
Tumor lysis syndrome (TLS)	Monitor patients at risk of TLS (ie, those with high tumor burden), and take appropriate precautions including aggressive hydration and allopurinol
G ≥3 peripheral neuropathy	If neuropathy is attributable to lenalidomide and occurred on or after day 15, withhold lenalidomide for the remainder of the cycle and reassess weekly If neuropathy is attributable to lenalidomide and occurred before day 15 and resolved to G ≤1, restart lenalidomide at the same dose level for the remainder of the cycle In either case, resume lenalidomide with the dosage reduced by 1 dose level in subsequent cycles provided that the toxicity resolves to G ≤1

Treatment Modifications (*continued*)

G3/4 venous thromboembolism (VTE) during aspirin monotherapy or inadequate anticoagulation	Continue lenalidomide at the current dose, and initiate adequate anticoagulation
G3/4 venous thromboembolism (VTE) during adequate anticoagulation (eg, prophylactic or therapeutic doses of LMWH, UFH, or warfarin)	Discontinue lenalidomide[†]
G ≥2 hypothyroidism or G ≥2 hyperthyroidism	Continue lenalidomide at current dose, and initiate appropriate medical treatment
AST or ALT >3× ULN Total bilirubin ≥3× ULN	If the toxicity occurred on or after day 15, withhold lenalidomide for the rest of the cycle. Reevaluate liver function tests weekly until AST/ALT improve to ≤2.5× ULN and bilirubin improves to ≤1.5× ULN If the toxicity occurred before day 15 and ALT/AST resolve to ≤2.5× ULN and bilirubin improves to ≤1.5× ULN, restart lenalidomide at the same dose level for the rest of the cycle In either case, resume lenalidomide with the dosage reduced by 1 dose level in subsequent cycles if ALT/AST improves to ≤2.5× ULN and bilirubin improves to ≤1.5× ULN
Other G ≥3 lenalidomide-related toxicities	If the toxicity occurred on or after day 15, withhold lenalidomide for the remainder of the cycle, and reassess toxicity at least every 7 day If the toxicity occurred before day 15 and resolved to G ≤2, restart lenalidomide at the same dose for the remainder of the cycle In either case, resume lenalidomide with the dosage reduced by 1 dose level in subsequent cycles provided that the toxicity resolves to G ≤2

Renal Impairment

Moderate renal impairment (CrCl 30–60 mL/min)	Reduce the lenalidomide induction starting dose to 10 mg per dose. If after completion of cycle 2 the patient remains free of G ≥3 toxicity, the lenalidomide dose may be increased to a maximum of 15 mg per day starting on day 2 of cycle 3 Reduce the lenalidomide maintenance starting dose to 5 mg per dose
Severe renal impairment (CrCl <30 mL/min, or requiring hemodialysis)	Patients with creatinine clearance <30 mL/min were excluded from the study. No recommendations available

[*]In general, if a dose-limiting toxicity occurs on or after day 15 of the cycle, treatment will be withheld until the end of the cycle, and the dose will then be reduced (if applicable) beginning in the subsequent cycle. If the toxicity occurs before day 15 of the cycle, treatment will be held until recovery and restarted without dose reduction for the rest of the cycle (ie, continue until day 21; missed doses will not be made up), and then the next cycle will resume at a reduced dose

[†]If lenalidomide or rituximab are discontinued, the medically responsible healthcare provider may decide to either continue the other agent as monotherapy, or switch to an alternative regimen

CrCl, creatinine clearance; ANC, absolute neutrophil count; CBC, complete blood count; LMWH, low molecular weight heparin; UFH, unfractionated heparin; AST, aspartate aminotransferase; ALT, alanine aminotransferase; ULN, upper limit of normal

Efficacy (N = 45)

Overall response rate[*]	33%
Median overall survival	10.7 months
Median progression-free survival	3.7 months

[*]*Overall response rate* includes patients with either a complete or partial response to treatment
Note: Median follow-up was 29.1 months

Patient Population Studied

This second arm of a phase 2 study involved 45 patients with diffuse large B-cell lymphoma (N = 32), grade 3 follicular lymphoma (N = 4), or transformed large cell lymphoma (N = 9). Eligible patients had an Eastern Cooperative Oncology Group (ECOG) performance status score ≤2 and had previously received 1–4 lines of therapy. All patients received intravenous rituximab (375 mg/m² once per week for 4 weeks only during cycle 1) and oral lenalidomide (20 mg on days 1–21 of each 28-day cycle)

Therapy Monitoring

1. *Prior to treatment initiation*: CBC with differential, serum chemistries, serum bilirubin, ALT or AST, hepatitis B core antibody (IgG or total) and hepatitis B surface antigen, and urine pregnancy test (women of child-bearing potential only)

   a. *In patients at high risk for tumor lysis syndrome (eg, high tumor burden, renal dysfunction, rapidly progressing disease, markedly elevated LDH, baseline abnormalities in laboratory indices of tumor lysis syndrome [potassium, phosphate, uric acid, calcium, serum creatinine])*: Consider frequent monitoring of laboratory indices of tumor lysis syndrome, intravenous hydration, and prophylaxis with a xanthine oxidase inhibitor (eg, allopurinol) during the first cycle

2. *Prior to each dose of rituximab, and then every 2 weeks thereafter*: CBC with differential, serum chemistries, serum bilirubin, ALT or AST

3. *During each rituximab infusion and for at least 1 hour after infusion completion*: signs and symptoms of infusion-related reaction, vital signs every 30 minutes

4. *Monitor periodically for*: signs and symptoms of infection (including progressive multifocal leukoencephalopathy) and dermatologic toxicity

5. *Response assessment (every 2–3 cycles)*: physical examination, CBC with differential, CT scan or PET scan

Lenalidomide Notes:
- A decrease in the number of CD34+ cells collected after treatment has been reported in patients who have received >4 cycles of lenalidomide. In patients who may undergo transplant, consider early referral to transplant center
- Because of the embryo-fetal risk, lenalidomide is available only through a restricted program under a Risk Evaluation and Mitigation Strategy (REMS), the REVLIMID REMS program. Required components of the REVLIMID REMS program include the following:
- Patients must sign a patient-physician agreement form and comply with the REMS requirements. In particular, female patients of reproductive potential who are not pregnant must comply with the pregnancy testing and contraception requirements, and males must comply with contraception requirements

Toxicity

(N = 45)

Grade (%)[*]	Grade 1	Grade 2	Grade 3	Grade 4
Neutropenia	24	33	31	22
Lymphopenia	27	33	29	11
Thrombocytopenia	33	27	18	16
Leukopenia	31	33	16	11
Anemia	40	31	13	4
Fatigue	56	20	7	0
Neuropathy	40	16	2	0
Elevated lactate dehydrogenase	31	11	9	2
Dizziness	40	9	2	0
Diarrhea	40	11	0	0
Myalgia	40	9	0	0
Hyperglycemia	36	9	2	0
Nausea	36	7	0	0
Non-neutropenic fever	22	18	2	0
Hypoalbuminemia	22	18	0	0
Constipation	31	7	0	0
Hypophosphatemia	9	18	9	0
Elevated liver function test	24	7	2	0
Blurred vision	31	0	0	0
Hypocalcemia	13	13	4	0
Dyspnea	22	7	0	0
Elevated creatinine	18	7	2	0
Red eyes	22	2	0	0
Hypokalemia	18	0	2	2
Rash	11	7	4	0
Vomiting	18	2	2	0
Elevated alkaline phosphatase	18	4	0	0
Hyponatremia	16	0	4	0
Febrile neutropenia	2	4	7	4
Edema limb	2	7	4	0
Hypercalcemia	4	2	2	4
Thrombosis/embolism	0	0	4	4
Arrhythmia	2	2	2	0
Myelodysplasia	0	0	0	2
Hypermagnesemia	0	0	2	0
Pneumothorax	0	0	2	0
Syncope	0	0	2	0

[*]According to the National Cancer Institute Common Terminology Criteria for Adverse Events, version 3.0
Note: All grade 3–4 toxicities and any grade 1–2 toxicities that occurred in >20% patients are included

DIFFUSE LARGE B-CELL LYMPHOMA • SUBSEQUENT THERAPY • NOT ELIGIBLE FOR ASCT • RELAPSED/REFRACTORY

NON-HODGKIN LYMPHOMA REGIMEN : BENDAMUSTINE + RITUXIMAB (BR)

Ohmachi K et al. J Clin Oncol 2013;31:2103–2109
Vacirca JL et al. Ann Hematol 2013;93:403–409
Weidmann E et al. Ann Oncol 2002;13:1285–1289

Prophylaxis for tumor lysis syndrome
Recommended for high-risk patients (eg, high tumor burden, bulky lymphadenopathy, or renal impairment):
- Hydration; encourage oral hydration (eg, ≥3 L/day) starting 1–2 days prior to the first rituximab dose. Consider administering additional *intravenous* hydration prior to the infusion if needed. Continue hydration prior to subsequent cycles if needed
- **Allopurinol** 300 mg per dose; administer orally twice per day starting 12–24 hours prior to the first rituximab infusion for 7 days. Continue prophylaxis prior to subsequent cycles if needed
  - Reduce allopurinol dose to 300 mg by mouth once daily for 7 days for patients with renal impairment

Rituximab
Premedication for rituximab:
Acetaminophen 650–1000 mg; administer orally 30–60 minutes before each rituximab dose, *plus*
Diphenhydramine 25–50 mg; administer orally or intravenously 30–60 minutes before each rituximab dose
Rituximab 375 mg/m² per dose; administer intravenously in 0.9% sodium chloride injection (0.9% NS) or 5% dextrose injection (D5W), diluted to a concentration within the range 1–4 mg/mL, on day 1, every 21 days, for 6 cycles (total dosage/21-day cycle = 375 mg/m²)
Notes on rituximab administration:
- Infuse initially at 50 mg/h. If hypersensitivity or infusion reactions do not occur during the first 30 minutes, increase the rate by 50 mg/h every 30 minutes as tolerated to a maximum rate of 400 mg/h. During subsequent treatments if previous rituximab administration was well tolerated, start at 100 mg/h, and increase by 100 mg/h every 30 minutes as tolerated to a maximum rate of 400 mg/h

INFUSION REACTIONS ASSOCIATED WITH RITUXIMAB

Note: Medications for the treatment of hypersensitivity reactions should be available for immediate use in the event of a reaction during administration (eg, intravenous fluids, epinephrine, antihistamines, glucocorticoids, and O_2)
Fevers, chills, and rigors
1. Interrupt rituximab administration for severe symptoms, and give:
   - **Acetaminophen** 650 mg orally for fever. For persistent or recurrent symptoms, repeat administration every 4–6 hours as needed during rituximab administration
   - **Diphenhydramine** 25–50 mg orally or by intravenous injection for pruritus, hypotension, or angioedema. For persistent or recurrent symptoms, repeat administration every 4–6 hours as needed during rituximab administration
   - **Meperidine** 12.5–25 mg by intravenous injection every 10–20 minutes as needed for shaking chills (generally, cumulative doses >100 mg are not needed; use repeated doses with caution in persons with moderate or more severely impaired renal function)
2. If rituximab administration was interrupted, resume infusion at a slower rate than the maximum rate previously attempted. Rate escalation may be reattempted at smaller incremental steps with close monitoring. Do not exceed the maximum recommended rate of 400 mg/h
Dyspnea or wheezing without allergic findings (urticaria, or tongue or laryngeal edema)
1. Interrupt rituximab administration immediately
2. Give **hydrocortisone** 100 mg by intravenous injection (or an alternative steroid with equivalent glucocorticoid potency)
3. Give a **histamine (H₂) receptor antagonist** (ranitidine 50 mg, cimetidine 300 mg, or famotidine 20 mg) intravenously over 15–30 minutes
4. After symptoms resolve, resume rituximab administration at 25 mg/h with close monitoring. Do not increase the administration rate
Note: Medications and equipment for the treatment of hypersensitivity reactions should be available for immediate use in the event of a reaction during administration (eg, intravenous fluids, epinephrine, antihistamines, glucocorticoids, and oxygen)
Rituxan (rituximab) prescribing information. South San Francisco, CA: Genentech, Inc; 2018 October

Bendamustine
Premedication for bendamustine HCl: Premedication is not necessary for primary prophylaxis of infusion-related reactions. In the event of a non-severe infusion-related reaction, consider adding a histamine receptor (H_1)-subtype antagonist (eg, diphenhydramine 25–50 mg intravenously or orally), an antipyretic (eg, acetaminophen 650–1000 mg orally), and a corticosteroid (eg, methylprednisolone 100 mg intravenously) administered 30 minutes prior to bendamustine HCl administration in subsequent cycles

Bendamustine HCl 120 mg/m² per dose; administer intravenously in a volume of 0.9% sodium chloride injection (0.9% NS) sufficient to produce a concentration with the range 0.2–0.6 mg/mL over 30–60 minutes, on 2 consecutive days, days 1 and 2, every 21 days for 6 cycles (total dosage/21-day cycle = 240 mg/m²)

(continued)

(continued)

Note:

- Bendamustine HCl can cause severe infusion-related reactions
  - For grade 1–2 infusion-related reactions, consider rechallenge with the addition of antihistamine, antipyretic, and corticosteroid premedications (as described in the Premedication section)
  - For grade 3 infusion-related reactions, consider permanent discontinuation versus rechallenge with the addition of antihistamine, antipyretic, and corticosteroid premedications (as described in the Premedication section) after weighing risks and benefits
  - For grade 4 infusion-related reactions, permanently discontinue bendamustine HCl

Note:

- Coadministration of strong CYP1A2 inhibitors (eg, ciprofloxacin, fluvoxamine) may increase exposure to bendamustine HCl and decrease exposure to its active metabolites. Concomitant CYP1A2 inducers (eg, omeprazole, cigarette smoking) may decrease exposure to bendamustine HCl and increase exposure to its active metabolites. Use caution, or select an alternative therapy, when coadministration of bendamustine HCl with strong CYP1A2 inhibitors or inducers is unavoidable
- Bendamustine HCl formulations may vary by country; consult local regulatory-approved labeling for guidance. For example, in the United States, the Food and Drug Administration approved Bendeka under Section 505(b)(2) of the Federal Food, Drug, and Cosmetic Act on 7 December 2015. The Bendeka product labeling contains specific dilution and administration instructions, *thus*:
  - **Bendamustine HCl (Bendeka, where available)** 120 mg/m^2 per dose; administer intravenously in a volume of 0.9% NS or 5% dextrose injection (D5W) sufficient to produce a concentration with the range 1.85–5.6 mg/mL, over 10 minutes, on 2 consecutive days, days 1 and 2, every 21 days for 6 cycles (total dosage/21-day cycle = 240 mg/m^2)

Supportive Care

Antiemetic prophylaxis

Emetogenic potential on days with bendamustine is **MODERATE**

See Chapter 42 for antiemetic recommendations

Hematopoietic growth factor (CSF) prophylaxis

Primary prophylaxis **MAY** *be indicated*

See Chapter 43 for more information

Antimicrobial prophylaxis

Risk of fever and neutropenia is *INTERMEDIATE*

Antimicrobial primary prophylaxis to be considered:

- Antibacterial—consider a fluoroquinolone during periods of prolonged neutropenia, or no prophylaxis
- Antifungal—consider use during periods of prolonged neutropenia, or no prophylaxis
- Antiviral—antiherpes antivirals (eg, acyclovir, famciclovir, valacyclovir)

Treatment Modifications

Bendamustine Dose Modifications	
Starting dose	120 mg/m^2 per dose on days 1 and 2
Dose level −1	90 mg/m^2 per dose on days 1 and 2
Dose level −2	60 mg/m^2 per dose on days 1 and 2
Dose level −3	Discontinue bendamustine
There are no dose reductions for rituximab	

Adverse Event	Treatment Modification
Hematologic Toxicity	
Day 1 platelet count <75,000/mm^3 or day 1 ANC <1000/mm^3	Delay start of cycle until platelet count ≥75,000/mm^3 and ANC ≥1000/ mm^3 or until recovery to near baseline values, then reduce the bendamustine dosage by 1 dose level for subsequent cycles. Consider G-CSF use in subsequent cycles for dose-limiting neutropenia
G4 hematologic toxicity occurring in the previous cycle	Delay start of cycle until platelet count ≥75,000/mm^3 and ANC ≥1000/mm^3 or until recovery to near baseline values, then reduce the bendamustine dosage by 1 dose level for subsequent cycles. Consider G-CSF use in subsequent cycles for dose-limiting neutropenia or severe neutropenic complications

(continued)

Treatment Modifications (continued)

Infectious Complications

Active infection	Interrupt bendamustine and rituximab until resolution of infection, then resume treatment at either the same dosages, or with the bendamustine dosage reduced by 1 dose level, depending on the severity of infection
New or changes in preexisting neurologic symptoms (eg, confusion, dizziness, loss of balance, vision problems, aphasia, ambulation issues); PML suspected	Interrupt bendamustine and rituximab until central nervous system status is clarified. Work-up may include (but is not limited to) consultation with a neurologist, brain MRI, and LP
PML is confirmed	Discontinue bendamustine and rituximab
HBV reactivation	Discontinue bendamustine and rituximab. Institute appropriate treatment for HBV. Upon resolution of HBV reactivation, resumption of bendamustine and rituximab should be discussed with a physician with expertise in management of HBV

Drug Interactions

Patient requires concomitant therapy with antihypertensive medication(s)	On days of rituximab treatment, and especially with the initial dose, weigh the risk versus benefit of delaying administration of the antihypertensive medication(s) until after completion of the rituximab infusion due to the potential risk of rituximab infusion-related hypotension
Live attenuated vaccine is indicated during or after rituximab administration	Avoid administration of a live attenuated vaccine during rituximab therapy and following therapy until adequate B-cell recovery has occurred
Patient requires concomitant therapy with a CYP1A2 inhibitor (eg, fluvoxamine, ciprofloxacin)	Consider alternative treatment instead of the CYP1A2 inhibitor. If the CYP1A2 inhibitor cannot be avoided, use caution and monitor carefully for bendamustine adverse effects. Do not modify the rituximab dose
Patient requires concomitant therapy with a CYP1A2 inducer (eg, omeprazole) or patient is a smoker	Consider alternative treatment instead of the CYP1A2 inducer. Recommend cessation of smoking, if applicable. If the CYP1A2 inducer cannot be avoided, use caution and monitor carefully for reduced bendamustine efficacy. Do not modify the rituximab dose

Other Toxicities

Clinically significant G2 nonhematologic toxicity during the prior cycle	Delay start of cycle until the nonhematologic toxicity resolves to G ≤1 or baseline, then resume treatment at the same dosages
Clinically significant G ≥3 nonhematologic toxicity during the prior cycle	Delay start of cycle until the nonhematologic toxicity resolves to G ≤1 or baseline, then resume treatment with the bendamustine dosage reduced by 1 dose level

ANC, absolute neutrophil count; G-CSF, granulocyte-colony stimulating factor; PML, progressive multifocal leukoencephalopathy; MRI, magnetic resonance imaging; LP, lumbar puncture; HBV, hepatitis B virus

Bendeka (bendamustine hydrochloride injection) prescribing information. North Wales, PA: Teva Pharmaceuticals USA, Inc; 2018 July

Rituxan (rituximab) prescribing information. South San Francisco, CA: Genentech, Inc; 2018 October

Ohmachi K et al. J Clin Oncol 2013;3:2103–2109

- -

Patient Population Studied

Ohmachi K et al. J Clin Oncol 2013;31:2103–2109

This multicenter, open-label, phase 2 study involved 59 patients with relapsed or refractory, CD20-positive, diffuse large B-cell lymphoma who were not eligible for autologous stem cell transplantation. Eligible patients were aged 20–75 years, had an Eastern Cooperative Oncology Group (ECOG) performance status score ≤1, and had previously received 1–3 chemotherapy regimens. Patients who had not experienced a complete, complete unconfirmed, or partial response with any prior treatment regimen, or who had previously undergone allogeneic stem cell transplantation or radioimmunotherapy were ineligible. Patients received up to six 21-day cycles of intravenous rituximab (375 mg/m² on day 1) and bendamustine (120 mg/m² over 60 minutes on days 2 and 3)

Vacirca JL et al. Ann Hematol 2013; 93:403–409

This multicenter, phase 2 study involved 59 patients with relapsed or refractory, CD20-positive, diffuse large B-cell lymphoma who were not eligible for intensive salvage therapies. Eligible patients had ECOG performance status score ≤2, and had previously received at least one therapeutic regimen. Patients who were candidates for autologous stem cell transplantation or high-dose therapy were ineligible

Efficacy

Ohmachi K et al. J Clin Oncol 2013;31:2103–2109 (N = 59)	
Overall response rate[*]	62.7%
Complete response rate	37.3%
Median progression-free survival	6.7 months

[*]Overall response rate includes patients with either a complete or partial response
Note: Median follow-up was 4.7 months

Vacirca JL et al. Ann Hematol 2013; 93:403–409 (N = 59)	
Overall response rate[*]	45.8%
Median duration of response[†]	17.3 months
Median progression-free survival	3.6 months

[*]Overall response rate includes patients with either a complete or partial response
[†]Among all patients with an objective response

Toxicity

Ohmachi K et al. J Clin Oncol 2013;31:2103–2109 (N = 59)

Grade[*]	Grade 1–2 (%)	Grade 3 (%)	Grade 4 (%)
Neutropenia	12	31	46
Leukopenia	10	63	10
Lymphopenia	0	7	71
Thrombocytopenia	47	15	7
CD4 lymphopenia	3	22	44
Anemia	37	15	2
Constipation	47	3	0
Infection	34	12	0
Anorexia	27	7	0
Nausea	34	0	0
Fatigue	32	0	0
Maculopapular rash	20	5	0
Fever	24	2	0
Insomnia	24	0	0
Malaise	24	0	0
Injection site reaction	22	0	0
Stomatitis	20	0	0
Febrile neutropenia	0	7	0

[*]According to the National Cancer Institute Common Terminology Criteria for Adverse Events, version 4.0
Note: Nonhematologic toxicities that occurred in ≥20% of patients, and common hematologic toxicities are included. Five patients (8.5%) discontinued treatment owing to adverse events. Three deaths occurred during the treatment period: one was due to disease progression, one was a result of respiratory failure owing to tumor-related airway compression, and one was due to hypotensive shock of unknown cause

Treatment Modifications (*continued*)

Vacirca JL et al. Ann Hematol 2013;93:403–409 (N = 59)

Grade*	Grade 1–2 (%)	Grade 3 (%)	Grade 4 (%)
Neutropenia	8	29	7
Thrombocytopenia	22	17	5
Anemia	32	12	0
Nausea	37	2	2
Fatigue	32	3	0
Leukopenia	10	22	2
Diarrhea	27	3	0
Fever	25	2	2
Anorexia	19	5	0
Constipation	22	0	0
Cough	17	2	0
Weight loss	17	2	0
Vomiting	14	2	2
Dizziness	12	3	0
Abdominal pain	8	5	0
Limb edema	12	2	0
Pain	14	0	0
Back pain	10	2	0
Hypotension	8	0	2
Dyspnea	5	5	0
Dehydration	7	3	0
Headache	8	2	0
Chills	10	0	0

*According to the National Cancer Institute Common Terminology Criteria for Adverse Events, version 3.0

Note: Toxicities that occurred in ≥10% of patients are included. Four deaths occurred during the study; two were due to disease-related complications, one was a result of disseminated herpes zoster, and one was due to unknown cause

Therapy Monitoring

1 *Prior to treatment initiation*: CBC with differential, serum chemistries, serum bilirubin, ALT or AST, hepatitis B core antibody (IgG or total) and hepatitis B core antigen, urine pregnancy test (women of child-bearing potential only)

2 *Prior to each cycle*: CBC with differential, serum chemistries, serum bilirubin, ALT or AST

3 *Weekly during treatment*: CBC with differential

4 *During each rituximab infusion and for at least 1 hour after infusion completion*: Signs and symptoms of infusion-related reaction, vital signs every 30 minutes

5 *In patients at high risk for tumor lysis syndrome (eg, high tumor burden, renal dysfunction, rapidly progressing disease, markedly elevated LDH, baseline abnormalities in laboratory indices of tumor lysis syndrome [potassium, phosphate, uric acid, calcium, serum creatinine])*: Consider frequent monitoring of laboratory indices of tumor lysis syndrome, intravenous hydration, and prophylaxis with a xanthine oxidase inhibitor (eg, allopurinol) during the first cycle

6 *Monitor periodically for*: Signs and symptoms of infection (including progressive multifocal leukoencephalopathy) and dermatologic toxicity

7 *Response assessment every 2–3 cycles*: Physical examination, CT scan or PET scan, bone marrow evaluation (if clinically indicated)

DIFFUSE LARGE B-CELL LYMPHOMA • SUBSEQUENT THERAPY • NOT ELIGIBLE FOR ASCT • RELAPSED/REFRACTORY

NON-HODGKIN LYMPHOMA REGIMEN: TAFASITAMAB + LENALIDOMIDE

Salles G et al. Lancet Oncol 2020;21:978–988

Lenalidomide 25 mg/dose; administer orally, without regard to meals, once daily for 21 consecutive days on days 1–21, followed by 7 days without treatment, starting in cycle 1, every 28 days, for up to 12 cycles (total dosage/28-day cycle = 525 mg)

- Patients who delay taking a lenalidomide dose at a regularly scheduled time may take the missed dose if the time to the next regularly scheduled dose is >12 hours away

Tafasitamab

Premedication for tafasitamab:

Acetaminophen 1000 mg; administer orally or intravenously 30 minutes to 2 hours before tafasitamab

Diphenhydramine 25–50 mg; administer orally or intravenously 30 minutes to 2 hours before tafasitamab

Cimetidine 300 mg (or **ranitidine** 150 mg, **famotidine** 20–40 mg, or an equivalent histamine receptor [H$_2$]-subtype antagonist); administer orally 30 minutes to 2 hours before tafasitamab, *or* **cimetidine** 300 mg (or **ranitidine** 50 mg, **famotidine** 20 mg); administer intravenously over 15–30 minutes, 30 minutes to 2 hours before tafasitamab

Methylprednisolone 80–120 mg; administer intravenously 30 minutes to 2 hours before tafasitamab

Note: if no infusion-related reactions occur during infusions 1–3, then may omit premedications for subsequent infusions

Tafasitamab 12 mg/kg per dose; administer intravenously in 250 mL 0.9% sodium chloride, according to the schedule in the below table, until disease progression

Notes on tafasitamab administration:

- The first infusion should be initiated at a rate of 70 mL/h for 30 minutes. If tolerated, the rate may be increased to within the range 107.5–215 mL/h (ie, at a rate calculated so that the infusion is completed within a total of 1.5–2 hours)
- All subsequent infusions should be infused at a fixed rate within the range of 100–166.7 mL/h (ie, at a rate calculated so that the infusion is completed within 1.5–2 hours)
- Calculate the tafasitamab dose based upon the patient's actual body weight
- Do not co-administer other drugs through the same infusion line as tafasitamab
- Lenalidomide is administered for a maximum of 12 cycles; tafasitamab is continued until disease progression

Tafasitamab Dosing Schedule (Cycle Length = 28 Days)

Cycle	Tafasitamab Dosing Schedule	Total Tafasitamab Dosage Per 28-Day Cycle
Cycle 1	Days 1, 4, 8, 15, and 22	(Total dosage in cycle 1 = 60 mg/kg)
Cycles 2 and 3	Days 1, 8, 15, and 22	(Total dosage/cycle during cycles 2 and 3 = 48 mg/kg)
Cycle 4 and beyond (until disease progression)	Days 1 and 15	(Total dosage/cycle during cycle 4 and beyond = 24 mg/kg)

Supportive Care

Antiemetic prophylaxis

Emetogenic potential is **MINIMAL TO LOW**

See Chapter 42 for antiemetic recommendations

Hematopoietic growth factor (CSF) prophylaxis

Primary prophylaxis is **NOT** indicated

See Chapter 43 for more information

Antimicrobial prophylaxis

Risk of fever and neutropenia is *INTERMEDIATE*

Antimicrobial primary prophylaxis to be considered:

- Antibacterial—consider a fluoroquinolone or no prophylaxis during periods of neutropenia
- Antifungal—recommended; consider use during periods of neutropenia
- Antiviral—antiherpes antivirals (eg, acyclovir, famciclovir, valacyclovir)

Treatment Modifications

Lenalidomide Dose Modifications

	CrCl ≥60 mL/min	CrCl ≥30 and <60 mL/min
Starting dose	25 mg/day on days 1–21	10 mg/day on days 1–21
Level −1	20 mg/day on days 1–21	5 mg/day on days 1–21
Level −2	15 mg/day on days 1–21	2.5 mg/day on days 1–21
Level −3	10 mg/day on days 1–21	Discontinue†
Level −4	5 mg/day on days 1–21	—
Level −5	Discontinue†	—

Adverse Event	Treatment Modification

Hematologic Toxicity

Day 1 ANC <1000/mm³ or platelet count <50,000/mm³	Delay the next cycle until ANC ≥1000/mm³ and platelet count ≥50,000/mm³. Consider treatment with filgrastim and/or platelet transfusion according to local guidelines. If the start of a new cycle is delayed >14 days for lenalidomide-related toxicity, reduce the lenalidomide by 1 dose level
G3 neutropenia (ANC ≥500 to <1000/mm³) sustained for ≥7 days	If neutropenia occurred on or after day 15, withhold lenalidomide for the rest of the cycle, and follow weekly CBC
G4 neutropenia (ANC <500/mm³) at any time	If neutropenia occurred before day 15 and resolves to G ≤2 (ANC ≥1000/mm³), resume lenalidomide at the same dose for the rest of the cycle
Febrile neutropenia (ANC <1000/mm³ with fever ≥38.3°C)	Consider use of filgrastim according to local guidelines. In subsequent cycles, reduce the lenalidomide dosage by 1 dose level
G ≥3 thrombocytopenia (platelet count <50,000/mm³) at any time	If thrombocytopenia occurred on or after day 15, withhold lenalidomide for the rest of the cycle, and follow weekly CBC. If thrombocytopenia occurred before day 15 and resolved to G ≤2 (platelet count ≥50,000/mm³), resume lenalidomide at the same dose for the rest of the cycle. In subsequent cycles, reduce the lenalidomide dosage by 1 dose level

Nonhematologic Toxicities

G2/3 non-desquamating rash	Hold lenalidomide. Consider administering antihistamines and/or a short course of steroids. Resume at the same dose when resolved to G ≤1
G ≥3 desquamating (blistering) rash	Permanently discontinue lenalidomide†
G4 non-desquamating rash	
Allergic reactions, including hypersensitivity, angioedema, Stevens-Johnson syndrome, toxic epidermal necrolysis (TEN) and drug reaction with eosinophilia and systemic symptoms (DRESS)	
Tumor lysis syndrome (TLS)	Monitor patients at risk of TLS (ie, those with high tumor burden), and take appropriate precautions including aggressive hydration and allopurinol
G ≥3 peripheral neuropathy	If neuropathy is attributable to lenalidomide and occurred on or after day 15, withhold lenalidomide for the remainder of the cycle and reassess weekly. If neuropathy is attributable to lenalidomide and occurred before day 15 and resolved to G ≤1, restart lenalidomide at the same dose level for the remainder of the cycle. In either case, resume lenalidomide with the dosage reduced by 1 dose level in subsequent cycles provided that the toxicity resolves to G ≤1

(continued)

Treatment Modifications (*continued*)

G3/4 venous thromboembolism (VTE) during aspirin monotherapy or inadequate anticoagulation	Continue lenalidomide at the current dose, and initiate adequate anticoagulation
G3/4 venous thromboembolism (VTE) during adequate anticoagulation (eg, prophylactic or therapeutic doses of LMWH, UFH, or warfarin)	Discontinue lenalidomide†
G ≥2 hypothyroidism or G ≥2 hyperthyroidism	Continue lenalidomide at current dose, and initiate appropriate medical treatment
AST or ALT >3× ULN Total bilirubin ≥3× ULN	If the toxicity occurred on or after day 15, withhold lenalidomide for the rest of the cycle. Re-evaluate liver function tests weekly until AST/ALT improve to ≤2.5× ULN and bilirubin improves to ≤1.5× ULN If the toxicity occurred before day 15 and ALT/AST resolve to ≤2.5× ULN and bilirubin improves to ≤1.5× ULN, restart lenalidomide at the same dose level for the rest of the cycle In either case, resume lenalidomide with the dosage reduced by 1 dose level in subsequent cycles if ALT/AST improves to ≤2.5× ULN and bilirubin improves to ≤1.5× ULN.
Other G ≥3 lenalidomide-related toxicities	If the toxicity occurred on or after day 15, withhold lenalidomide for the remainder of the cycle, and reassess toxicity at least every 7 day If the toxicity occurred before day 15 and resolved to G ≤2, restart lenalidomide at the same dose for the remainder of the cycle In either case, resume lenalidomide with the dosage reduced by 1 dose level in subsequent cycles provided that the toxicity resolves to G ≤2

Renal Impairment

Moderate renal impairment (CrCl 30–60 mL/min)	Reduce the lenalidomide induction starting dose to 10 mg per dose. If after completion of cycle 2 the patient remains free of G ≥3 toxicity, the lenalidomide dose may be increased to a maximum of 15 mg per day starting on day 2 of cycle 3

*In general, if a dose-limiting toxicity occurs on or after day 15 of the cycle, treatment will be withheld until the end of the cycle, and the dose will then be reduced (if applicable) beginning in the subsequent cycle. If the toxicity occurs before day 15 of the cycle, treatment will be held until recovery and restarted without dose reduction for the rest of the cycle (ie, continue until day 21; missed doses will not be made up), and then the next cycle will resume at a reduced dose

†If lenalidomide or tafasitamab are discontinued, the medically responsible healthcare provider may decide to either continue the other agent as monotherapy, or switch to an alternative regimen

CrCl, creatinine clearance; ANC, absolute neutrophil count; CBC, complete blood count; LMWH, low molecular weight heparin; UFH, unfractionated heparin; AST, aspartate aminotransferase; ALT, alanine aminotransferase; ULN, upper limit of normal

Tafasitamab Dosage Modifications for Toxicity

Adverse Reaction	Severity	Dosage Modification
Infusion-related reactions	Grade 2 (moderate)	• Interrupt infusion immediately and manage signs and symptoms • Once signs and symptoms G ≤1, resume infusion at no more than 50% of rate at which reaction occurred. If patient does not experience further reaction within 1 hour and vital signs are stable, the infusion rate may be increased every 30 minutes as tolerated to the rate at which the reaction occurred
	Grade 3 (severe)	Interrupt infusion immediately and manage signs and symptoms • Once signs and symptoms G ≤1, resume infusion at no more than 25% of the rate at which the reaction occurred. If patient does not experience further reaction within 1 hour and vital signs stable, the infusion rate may be increased every 30 minutes as tolerated to a maximum of 50% of the rate at which the reaction occurred If after re-challenge the reaction returns, stop the infusion immediately
	Grade 4 (life-threatening)	• Stop the infusion immediately and permanently discontinue tafasitamab

(*continued*)

Treatment Modifications (*continued*)

Myelosuppression	Platelet count ≤50,000/mcL	• Withhold tafasitamab and lenalidomide and monitor CBC weekly until platelet count ≥50,000/mcL • Resume tafasitamab at the same dose and lenalidomide at a reduced dose. Refer to lenalidomide dose modifications for dosages
	ANC ≤1000/mm³ for ≥7 days *or* ANC ≤1000/mm³ with ≥100.4°F (38°C) or higher *or* ANC <500/mm³	• Withhold tafasitamab and lenalidomide and monitor CBC weekly until ANC ≥1000/μL • Resume tafasitamab at the same dose and lenalidomide at a reduced dose. Refer to lenalidomide dose modifications for dosages

Patient Population Studied

Patient >18 years, with histologically confirmed diffuse large B-cell lymphoma (including transformed indolent lymphoma with a subsequent diffuse large B-cell lymphoma relapse); had disease that relapsed after or was refractory to at least one, but not more than three systemic regimens (with at least one anti-CD20 therapy); and were not candidates for high-dose chemotherapy and subsequent autologous stem-cell transplantation. Relapsed disease defined as appearance of any new lesions or an increase in size of ≥50% of previously involved sites from nadir after the most recent systemic therapy according to the 2007 International Working Group (IWG) response criteria. Refractory disease was defined as disease progression as per IWG response criteria, showing less than a partial response or disease recurrence or progression within <6 months from the completion of 1st line therapy, or showing less than a partial response to the most recently administered systemic therapy. Additional inclusion criteria were ECOG PS 0–2

Exclusion criteria included a history of double-hit or triple-hit diffuse large B-cell lymphoma if already known; previous treatment with anti-CD19 therapy or immunomodulatory drugs such as thalidomide or lenalidomide; and primary refractory diffuse large B-cell lymphoma, defined as no response to, or progression during or within 6 months of frontline therapy. Until a protocol amendment (introduced June 27, 2016), only patients whose disease relapsed within 3 months of a previous anti-CD20-containing regimen were defined as primary refractory and excluded. Thus, patients with disease that relapsed or progressed between 3 and 6 months of frontline therapy were recruited before the protocol amendment, and considered as primary-refractory patients as per B-cell lymphoma National Comprehensive Cancer Network guidelines

Baseline Characteristics of the Safety Population (N = 81)	
Median age, years	72 (62–76)
Sex (male / female)	44 (54%) / 37 (46%)
Race (Asian / White / other / NA)	2 (2%) / 72 (89%) / 1 (1%) / 6 (7%)
Median time since first DLBCL diagnosis, months	26.9 (17–51)
Previous lines of systemic therapy—median (range)	2 (1–4)
Previous lines of systemic therapy (1 / 2 / 3 / 4)	40 (50%) / 35 (43%) / 5 (6%) / 1 (1%)
Previous anti-CD20 therapy (Yes / No)	81 (100%) / 0 (0%)
Previous anthracycline therapy (Yes / No)	81 (100%) / 0 (0%)
Primary refractory (Yes / No)	15 (19%) / 66 (81%)
Rituximab refractory (Yes / No / NA)	34 (42%) / 46 (57%) / 1 (1%)
Refractory to most recent previous therapy (Yes / No)	36 (44%) / 45 (56%)
Previous ASCT (Yes / No)	9 (11%) / 72 (89%)
Ann Arbor stage at screening (I or II / III or IV)	20 (25%) / 61 (75%)
ECOG performance status (0 / 1 / 2)	29 (36%) / 45 (56%) / 7 (9%)
IPI score at screening (0–2 / 3–5)	40 (49%) / 41 (51%)
Bulky disease° (present / absent / NA)	15 (19%) / 65 (80%) / 1 (1%)
LDH at screening (elevated / WNL)	45 (56%) / 36 (44%)

(*continued*)

Cell of origin by immunohistochemistry	
Germinal center B cell	38 (47%)
Non-germinal center B cell	21 (26%)
Unknown	22 (27%)
Cell of origin by gene-expression profiling	
Germinal center B cell	7 (9%)
Non-germinal center B cell	19 (24%)
Unclassified / Unknown	6 (7%) / 49 (60%)
DLBCL arising from a previous indolent lymphoma	7 (9%)
Reasons for ASCT ineligibility	
Age >70 years	37 (46%)
Chemorefractory[†]	19 (23%)
Refusal / comorbidities[‡] / other[§]	13 (16%) / 11 (14%) / 1 (1%)

Data are median (IQR) or n (%) unless otherwise stated
ASCT, autologous stem-cell transplantation; DLBCL, diffuse large B-cell lymphoma; ECOG, Eastern Cooperative Oncology Group; IPI, International Prognostic Index; LDH, lactate dehydrogenase; R-CHOP, rituximab, cyclophosphamide, doxorubicin, vincristine, and prednisone or prednisolone

Efficacy

(N = 80)

Patients Treated with Tafasitamab Plus Lenalidomide (N = 80)[*]	
Objective response[‡]	48 (60%; 48–71)
Complete response	34 (43%; 32–54)
Partial response	14 (18%; 10–28)
Stable disease	11 (14%; 7–23)
Progressive disease	13 (16%; 9–26)
Not evaluable[†]	8 (10%; 4–19)
PET-confirmed complete response	30/34 (88%; 73–97)
Disease control[§]	59 (74%; 63–83)

Median duration of response (N = 48)	21.7 months (95% CI 21.7–NR)
Progression > initial response	13/48 (27%)
Response lasting 12 months	72% (95% CI 55–83%)
Progression-free survival event	39/80 (49%)

Median follow-up of 17.3 months (IQR 11.5–21.2)	
Median progression-free survival	12.1 months (95% CI 5.7–NR)
12-month progression-free survival	50% (95% CI, 38–61)
18-month progression-free survival	46% (95% CI, 33–57)

Post-hoc analysis	
Median progression-free survival > lenalidomide discontinued	12.7 months (95% CI 2.3–NR)
Median time to progression	16.2 months (95% CI 7.4–NR)
Disease progression events	35/80 (44%)
Median time to next treatment	15.4 months (95% CI 7.6–NR)
Received subsequent treatment	43/80 (54%)

Median follow-up of 19.6 months (IQR 15.3–21.9)	
Died	29 (36%)
Median overall survival	NR (95% CI 18.3–NR)
Alive at 12 months	74% (62–82)
Alive at 18 months	64% (51–74)
In remission at data cutoff	30 (38%)

Data are n (%; 95% CI) or n/N (%)
* One patient received tafasitamab only
†Patients had no valid postbaseline response assessments
‡Complete response plus partial response
§Complete response plus partial response plus stable disease
CI, confidence interval; NR, not reached

Toxicity

(N = 80)

	G 1–2	G3	G4	G5
Hematologic events				
Neutropenia	1 (1%)	22 (27%)	17 (21%)	0
Anemia	22 (27%)	6 (7%)	0	0
Thrombocytopenia	11 (14%)	10 (12%)	4 (5%)	0
Leukopenia	5 (6%)	6 (7%)	1 (1%)	0
Febrile neutropenia	0	8 (10%)	2 (2%)	0
Lymphopenia	2 (2%)	2 (2%)	1 (1%)	0
Agranulocytosis	0	0	1 (1%)	0
Nonhematologic events				
All rash*	22 (27%)	7 (9%)	0	0
Diarrhea	26 (32%)	1 (1%)	0	0
Asthenia	17 (21%)	2 (2%)	0	0
Cough	17 (21%)	1 (1%)	0	0
Peripheral oedema	18 (22%)	0	0	0
Pyrexia	16 (20%)	1 (1%)	0	0

(continued)

Therapy Monitoring

1. Prior to treatment initiation: CBC with differential, serum chemistries, serum bilirubin, ALT or AST, hepatitis B core antibody (IgG or total) and hepatitis B core antigen, urine pregnancy test (women of child-bearing potential only)
2. Prior to each cycle: CBC with differential, serum chemistries, serum bilirubin, ALT or AST
3. Weekly during treatment: CBC with differential
4. Response assessment every 2–3 cycles: Physical examination, CT scan or PET scan

Treatment Modifications (*continued*)

Decreased appetite	16 (20%)	0	0	0
Hypokalemia	10 (12%)	4 (5%)	1 (1%)	0
Back pain†	11 (14%)	2 (2%)	0	0
Fatigue	12 (15%)	2 (2%)	0	0
All urinary tract infection*	9 (11%)	3 (4%)	1 (1%)	0
Constipation	13 (16%)	0	0	0
Muscle spasms	12 (15%)	0	0	0
Nausea	12 (15%)	0	0	0
Bronchitis	10 (12%)	0	1 (1%)	0
Vomiting	11 (14%)	0	0	0
Dyspnea	9 (11%)	1 (1%)	0	0
Abdominal pain	7 (9%)	1 (1%)	0	0
Upper respiratory tract infection	6 (7%)	2 (2%)	0	0
Hypertension	4 (5%)	3 (4%)	0	0
Increased blood creatinine†	5 (6%)	1 (1%)	0	0
Mucosal inflammation	5 (6%)	1 (1%)	0	0
Pneumonia	1 (1%)	5 (6%)	0	0
Hypocalcemia	4 (5%)	1 (1%)	0	0
Hypogammaglobulinemia	4 (5%)	1 (1%)	0	0
Increased γ-glutamyltransferase	4 (5%)	1 (1%)	0	0
Sinusitis	3 (4%)	1 (1%)	0	0
Progressive multifocal leukoencephalopathy	0	0	0	1 (1%)
Cerebrovascular accident	0	0	0	1 (1%)
Respiratory failure	0	0	0	1 (1%)
Sudden death	0	0	0	1 (1%)

Lower respiratory tract infection, bronchopulmonary aspergillosis, cytomegalovirus infection, febrile infection, lung infection, neutropenic sepsis, respiratory syncytial virus infection, sepsis, soft tissue infection, streptococcal sepsis, varicella zoster virus infection	G1–4 toxicity all <2% and no G5 toxicity
Hyperbilirubinemia, increased blood bilirubin, increased transaminases, hyperkalemia, hyponatremia	
Atrial fibrillation, deep vein thrombosis, syncope, congestive heart failure, atrial flutter, cardiac failure, myocardial ischemia, pulmonary embolism	
Renal failure, tumor flare, muscle weakness, arthritis, biliary colic, cervicobrachial syndrome, device-related thrombosis, hematuria, hypersensitivity, myositis, osteonecrosis, peripheral sensorimotor neuropathy	

Data are n (%). The table shows treatment-emergent adverse events of grade 1 or 2 occurring in at least 10% of patients and all grade 3, 4, and 5 events
*Defined by customized Medical Dictionary for Regulatory Activities query
†One report of back pain and one report of increased blood creatinine had no toxicity grading

DIFFUSE LARGE B-CELL LYMPHOMA • SALVAGE BEYOND SECOND-LINE REFRACTORY DISEASE • NOT ELIGIBLE FOR CONSOLIDATIVE ASCT

NON-HODGKIN LYMPHOMA REGIMEN: POLATUZUMAB VEDOTIN + BENDAMUSTINE + RITUXIMAB (POLA-BR)

Sehn LH et al. J Clin Oncol 2020;38:155–165
POLIVY (polatuzumab vedotin-piiq) prescribing information. South San Francisco, CA: Genentech, Inc.; Revised 2020 September

Prophylaxis for tumor lysis syndrome
Recommended for high-risk patients (eg, high tumor burden, bulky lymphadenopathy, or renal impairment):

- **Hydration**: Encourage oral hydration (eg, ≥3 L/day) starting 1–2 days prior to the first rituximab dose. Consider administering additional *intravenous* hydration prior to the infusion if needed. Continue hydration prior to subsequent cycles if needed

- **Allopurinol** 300 mg per dose; administer orally twice per day starting 12–24 hours prior to the first rituximab infusion for 7 days. Continue prophylaxis prior to subsequent cycles if needed.
  - Reduce allopurinol dose to 300 mg by mouth once daily for 7 days for patients with renal impairment

Bendamustine HCl
Premedications for bendamustine HCl: Premedications are not necessary for primary prophylaxis of infusion-related reactions. In the event of a non-severe infusion-related reaction, consider adding a histamine receptor (H_1)-subtype antagonist (eg, diphenhydramine 25–50 mg intravenously or orally), an antipyretic (eg, acetaminophen 650–1000 mg orally), and a corticosteroid (eg, methylprednisolone 100 mg intravenously) administered 30 minutes prior to bendamustine HCl administration in subsequent cycles

Bendamustine HCl 90 mg/m^2 per dose; administer intravenously in a volume of 0.9% sodium chloride injection (0.9% NS) sufficient to produce a concentration with the range 0.2–0.7 mg/mL over 30–60 minutes, on 2 consecutive days, days 1 and 2, every 3 weeks for up to 6 cycles (total dosage/21-day cycle = 180 mg/m^2)
Note:
- Bendamustine HCl can cause severe infusion-related reactions
  - For grade 1–2 infusion-related reactions, consider rechallenge with the addition of antihistamine, antipyretic, and corticosteroid premedications (as described in the above premedication section)
  - For grade 3 infusion-related reactions, consider permanent discontinuation versus rechallenge with the addition of antihistamine, antipyretic, and corticosteroid premedications (as described in the above premedication section) after weighing risks and benefits
  - For grade 4 infusion-related reactions, permanently discontinue bendamustine HCl
- Coadministration of strong CYP1A2 inhibitors (eg, ciprofloxacin, fluvoxamine) may increase exposure to bendamustine HCl and decrease exposure to its active metabolites. Concomitant CYP1A2 inducers (eg, omeprazole, cigarette smoking) may decrease exposure to bendamustine HCl and increase exposure to its active metabolites. Use caution, or select an alternative therapy, when coadministration of bendamustine HCl with strong CYP1A2 inhibitors or inducers is unavoidable
- Bendamustine HCl formulations may vary by country; consult local regulatory-approved labeling for guidance. For example, in the U.S., the Food and Drug Administration approved Bendeka under Section 505(b)(2) of the Federal Food, Drug, and Cosmetic Act on 7 December 2015. The Bendeka product labeling contains specific dilution and administration instructions, *thus*:

  Bendamustine HCl (Bendeka, where available) 90 mg/m^2 per dose; administer intravenously in a volume of 0.9% NS or D5W sufficient to produce a concentration with the range 1.85–5.6 mg/mL, over 10 minutes, on 2 consecutive days, days 1 and 2, every 3 weeks for up to 6 cycles (total dosage/21-day cycle = 180 mg/m^2)

Rituximab
Premedication for rituximab (Note: if premedications were given for polatuzumab vedotin-piiq within 4 hours then there is no need to repeat premedications prior to rituximab):
Acetaminophen 650–1000 mg; administer orally *plus* **diphenhydramine** 25–50 mg; administer orally or intravenously 30–60 minutes before each dose of rituximab

Rituximab 375 mg/m^2; administer intravenously in 0.9% NS or 5% dextrose injection diluted to a concentration of 1–4 mg/mL on day 1, every 3 weeks, for up to 6 cycles (total dosage/cycle = 375 mg/m^2)
Notes on rituximab administration:
- Infuse initially at 50 mg/h. If hypersensitivity or infusion reactions do not occur during the first 30 minutes, increase the rate by 50 mg/h every 30 minutes as tolerated to a maximum rate of 400 mg/h. Subsequently, if previous administration was well tolerated, start at 100 mg/h and increase by 100 mg/h every 30 minutes as tolerated to a maximum rate of 400 mg/h
- Interrupt rituximab administration for fever chills, edema, congestion of the head and neck mucosa, hypertension, and other serious adverse events. Resume rituximab administration after adverse events abate

INFUSION REACTIONS ASSOCIATED WITH RITUXIMAB
Note: Medications for the treatment of hypersensitivity reactions should be available for immediate use in the event of a reaction during administration (eg, intravenous fluids, epinephrine, antihistamines, glucocorticoids, and O$_2$)

(continued)

(continued)

Fevers, chills, and rigors
1. Interrupt rituximab administration for severe symptoms, and give:
   - **Acetaminophen** 650 mg orally for fever. For persistent or recurrent symptoms, repeat administration every 4–6 hours as needed during rituximab administration
   - **Diphenhydramine** 25–50 mg orally or by intravenous injection for pruritus, hypotension, or angioedema. For persistent or recurrent symptoms, repeat administration every 4–6 hours as needed during rituximab administration
   - **Meperidine** 12.5–25 mg by intravenous injection every 10–20 minutes as needed for shaking chills (generally, cumulative doses >100 mg are not needed; use repeated doses with caution in persons with moderate or more severely impaired renal function)
2. If rituximab administration was interrupted, resume infusion at a slower rate than the maximum rate previously attempted. Rate escalation may be reattempted at smaller incremental steps with close monitoring. Do not exceed the maximum recommended rate of 400 mg/h

Dyspnea or wheezing without allergic findings (urticaria, or tongue or laryngeal edema)
1. Interrupt rituximab administration immediately
1. Give **hydrocortisone** 100 mg by intravenous injection (or an alternative steroid with equivalent glucocorticoid potency)
2. Give a **histamine (H$_2$) receptor antagonist** (ranitidine 50 mg, cimetidine 300 mg, or famotidine 20 mg) intravenously over 15–30 minutes
3. After symptoms resolve, resume rituximab administration at 25 mg/h with close monitoring. Do not increase the administration rate
Note: Medications and equipment for the treatment of hypersensitivity reactions should be available for immediate use in the event of a reaction during administration (eg, intravenous fluids, epinephrine, antihistamines, glucocorticoids, and oxygen)
Rituxan (rituximab) prescribing information. South San Francisco, CA: Genentech, Inc; 2018 October

Polatuzumab vedotin-piiq
Premedication for polatuzumab vedotin-piiq (Note: if premedications were given for rituximab within 4 hours then there is no need to repeat premedications prior to polatuzumab vedotin-piiq):
Acetaminophen 650–1000 mg; administer orally *plus* **diphenhydramine** 25–50 mg; administer orally or intravenously 30–60 minutes before each dose of polatuzumab vedotin-piiq
Polatuzumab vedotin-piiq 1.8 mg/kg; administer intravenously in a volume of 0.9% NS, 5% dextrose injection, or 0.45% sodium chloride not less than 50 mL and sufficient to produce a final concentration within the range 0.72–2.7 mg/mL, on day 1, every 3 weeks, for up to 6 cycles (total dosage/cycle = 1.8 mg/kg)
Notes on polatuzumab vedotin-piiq administration:
- Infuse the first dose of 90 minutes.
- If the prior infusion was well tolerated, subsequent doses may be administered over 30 minutes
- Polatuzumab vedotin-piiq must be administered using a dedicated infusion line equipped with a sterile, non-pyrogenic, low-protein-binding in-line or add-on filter (0.2- or 0.22-micron pore size) and a catheter
- Do not mix polatuzumab vedotin-piiq with or administer as an Infusion with other drugs

Polatuzumab vedotin-piiq Infusion-Related Reaction
G1–3 Infusion-Related Reaction:
- Interrupt polatuzumab vedotin-piiq infusion and give supportive treatment
- For the first instance of G3 wheezing, bronchospasm, or generalized urticaria, permanently discontinue polatuzumab vedotin-piiq
- For recurrent G2 wheezing or urticaria, or for recurrence of any G3 symptoms, permanently discontinue polatuzumab vedotin-piiq
- Otherwise, upon complete resolution of symptoms, infusion may be resumed at 50% of the rate achieved prior to interruption. In the absence of infusion related symptoms, the rate of infusion may be escalated in increments of 50 mg/hour every 30 minutes
- For the next cycle, infuse polatuzumab vedotin-piiq over 90 minutes. If no infusion-related reaction occurs, subsequent infusions may be administered over 30 minutes. Administer premedication for all cycles
G4 Infusion-Related Reaction
Stop polatuzumab vedotin-piiq infusion immediately. Give supportive treatment. Permanently discontinue polatuzumab vedotin-piiq
Regimen note: On day 1, bendamustine, rituximab, and polatuzumab vedotin-piiq may be given in any order

Supportive Care
Antiemetic prophylaxis
Emetogenic potential is **MODERATE**
See Chapter 42 for antiemetic recommendations

Hematopoietic growth factor (CSF) prophylaxis
Primary prophylaxis **MAY** *be indicated*
See Chapter 43 for more information

Antimicrobial prophylaxis
Risk of fever and neutropenia is INTERMEDIATE
   Antimicrobial primary prophylaxis to be considered:
- Antibacterial—consider a fluoroquinolone or no prophylaxis; *Pneumocystis jirovecii* prophylaxis (eg, cotrimoxazole) is specifically recommended in the polatuzumab vedotin-piiq prescribing information
- Antifungal—antiherpes antivirals (eg, acyclovir, famciclovir, valacyclovir) are specifically recommended in the polatuzumab vedotin-piiq prescribing information

Treatment Modifications

Bendamustine, Polatuzumab Vedotin-piiq, and Rituximab Treatment Modifications

Bendamustine Dose Levels

Starting dose	90 mg/m^2 per dose on days 1 and 2
Dose level −1	70 mg/m^2 per dose on days 1 and 2
Dose level −2	Discontinue bendamustine

Polatuzumab Vedotin-piiq Dose Levels

Starting dose	1.8 mg/kg on day 1
Dose level −1	1.4 mg/kg on day 1
Dose level −2	Discontinue polatuzumab vedotin-piiq

Rituximab Dose Levels

There are no dose reductions for rituximab

Hematologic Toxicity

ANC <1000/mm^3 on day 1 (unrelated to lymphoma)	• Withhold all treatment until ANC improves to ≥1000/mm^3
	• If ANC recovers to ≥1000/mm^3 on or before day 7, resume all treatment without any additional dose reductions. Consider G-CSF prophylaxis for subsequent cycles, if not previously given
	• If ANC recovers to ≥1000/mm^3 after day 7:
	  − Restart all treatment. Consider G-CSF prophylaxis for subsequent cycles, if not previously given. If prophylaxis was given, then consider a dose reduction of bendamustine
	  − If dose reduction of bendamustine has already occurred, consider dose reduction of polatuzumab vedotin-piiq to 1.4 mg/kg

Platelet count <50,000/mm^3 on day 1 (unrelated to lymphoma)	• Withhold all treatment until platelets improves to ≥75,000/mm^3
	• If platelets recover to ≥75,000/mm^3 on or before day 7, resume all treatment without any additional dose reductions
	• If platelets recover to ≥75,000/mm^3 after day 7:
	  − Restart all treatments, with dose reduction of bendamustine
	  − If dose reduction of bendamustine has already occurred, consider dose reduction of polatuzumab vedotin-piiq to 1.4 mg/kg

Peripheral Neuropathy

G2/3 peripheral neuropathy	• Hold polatuzumab vedotin-piiq dosing until improvement to G ≤1 • If recovered to G ≤1 on or before day 14, restart polatuzumab vedotin-piiq with the next cycle at a permanently reduced dose of 1.4 mg/kg • If a prior dose reduction to 1.4 mg/kg has occurred, discontinue polatuzumab vedotin-piiq • If not recovered to G ≤1 on or before day 14, discontinue polatuzumab vedotin-piiq
G4 peripheral neuropathy	Discontinue polatuzumab vedotin-piiq

Infectious Complications

Active infection	Interrupt all therapy until resolution of infection, then resume treatment at either the same doses, or with the bendamustine dose reduced by one dose level, depending on severity of infection
New or changes in pre-existing neurologic symptoms (eg, confusion, dizziness, loss of balance, vision problems, aphasia, ambulation issues)- PML suspected	Interrupt all therapy until central nervous system status clarified. Work-up may include (but is not limited to) consultation with a neurologist, brain MRI, and LP
PML is confirmed	Discontinue all therapy
HBV reactivation	Discontinue all therapy. Institute appropriate treatment for HBV. Upon resolution of HBV reactivation, resumption of polatuzumab vedotin-piiq, bendamustine, and rituximab should be discussed with a physician with expertise in management of HBV

Treatment Modifications (*continued*)

Drug Interactions

Patient requires concomitant therapy with antihypertensive medication(s)	On days of rituximab treatment, and especially with the initial dose, weigh the risk versus benefit of delaying administration of the antihypertensive medication(s) until after completion of the rituximab infusion due to the potential risk of rituximab infusion-related hypotension
Live attenuated vaccine is indicated during or after rituximab administration	Avoid administration of a live attenuated vaccine during rituximab therapy and following therapy until adequate B-cell recovery has occurred
Patient requires concomitant therapy with a CYP1A2 inhibitor (eg, fluvoxamine, ciprofloxacin)	Consider alternative treatment instead of the CYP1A2 inhibitor. If the CYP1A2 inhibitor cannot be avoided, use caution and monitor carefully for bendamustine adverse effects. Do not modify the rituximab dose
Patient requires concomitant therapy with a CYP1A2 inducer (eg, omeprazole), or patient is a smoker	Consider alternative treatment instead of the CYP1A2 inducer. Recommend cessation of smoking, if applicable. If the CYP1A2 inducer cannot be avoided, use caution and monitor carefully for reduced bendamustine efficacy. Do not modify the rituximab dose

Other Toxicities

Clinically significant G2 nonhematologic toxicity during the prior cycle	Delay start of cycle until the nonhematologic toxicity resolves to G ≤1 or baseline, then resume treatment at the same dosages
Clinically significant G ≥3 nonhematologic toxicity during the prior cycle	Delay start of cycle until the nonhematologic toxicity resolves to G ≤1 or baseline, then resume treatment with the bendamustine dosage reduced by one dosage level

Patient Population Studied

International, multicenter, open-label, phase 1b/2 trial involving adult patients with relapsed/refractory diffuse large B-cell lymphoma (DLBCL) after ≥1 prior line of therapy who were deemed to be ineligible for autologous hematopoietic stem cell transplant (auto-HSCT) or who had already undergone prior auto-HSCT. Selected characteristics of patients in the BR + polatuzumab vedotin-piiq arm include: median age of 67 years, 70% male, 77.5% ECOG performance status of 0–1, 47.5% activated B-cell–like phenotype, 37.5% germinal center B-cell–like phenotype, 25% prior auto-HSCT, median of 2 lines of prior therapy, with 97.% having received prior anti-CD20 therapy

Efficacy

Outcome	Pola-BR (n = 40)	BR (n = 40)
ORR* by IRC, n/N (%)	18/40 (45)	7/40 (17.5)
CR* by IRC, n/N (%)	16/40 (40)	7/40 (17.5)
PR* by IRC, n/N (%)	2/40 (5)	0/40 (0)
SD* by IRC, n/N (%)	6/40 (15)	1/40 (2.5)
PD* by IRC, n/N (%)	8/40 (20)	10/40 (25)
Median DOR by IRC, months (95% CI)	12.6 (7.2–NE)	7.7 (4.0–18.9)
Median PFS by IRC, months (95% CI)†	9.5 (6.2–13.9)	3.7 (2.1–4.5)
Median OS, months (95% CI)‡	12.4 (9.0–NE)	4.7 (3.7–8.3)

*Denotes end-of-treatment response rates
†HR, 0.36 (95% CI, 0.21–0.60); log-rank P<0.001
‡HR 0.42 (95% CI, 0.24–0.75); log-rank P = 0.002
BR, bendamustine + rituximab; CI, confidence interval; CR, complete response; DOR, duration of response; IRC, independent review committee; NE, not estimable; ORR, overall response rate; OS, overall survival; PD, progressive disease; PFS, progression-free survival; Pola-BR, polatuzumab vedotin-piiq + bendamustine + rituximab; PR, partial response; SD, stable disease

Toxicity

Adverse Event (%)	Pola-BR		BR	
	All Grades	Grades 3–4	All Grades	Grades 3–4
Blood and lymphatic system disorders				
Anemia	53.8	28.2	25.6	17.9
Neutropenia	53.8	46.2	38.5	33.3
Thrombocytopenia	48.7	41.0	28.2	23.1
Lymphopenia	12.8	12.8	0	0
Febrile neutropenia	10.3	10.3	12.8	12.8
GI disorders				
Diarrhea	38.5	2.6	28.2	2.6
Nausea	30.8	0	41.0	0
Constipation	17.9	0	20.5	2.6
General disorders and administration site conditions				
Fatigue	35.9	2.6	35.9	2.6
Pyrexia	33.3	2.6	23.1	0
Metabolism and nutrition disorders				
Decreased appetite	25.6	2.6	20.5	0
Peripheral neuropathy				
Peripheral neuropathy	43.6	0	7.7	0

Pola-BR, polatuzumab vedotin-piiq + bendamustine + rituximab; BR, bendamustine + rituximab

Therapy Monitoring

1. *Prior to treatment initiation*: CBC with differential, serum chemistries, serum bilirubin, ALT or AST, hepatitis B core antibody (IgG or total) and hepatitis B core antigen, urine pregnancy test (women of child-bearing potential only)

2. *Prior to each cycle*: CBC with differential, serum chemistries, serum bilirubin, ALT or AST, neurologic examination

3. *Weekly during treatment*: CBC with differential

4. *In patients at high risk for tumor lysis syndrome* consider frequent monitoring of laboratory indices of tumor lysis syndrome, intravenous hydration, and prophylaxis with a xanthine oxidase inhibitor (eg, allopurinol) during the first cycle

5. *Response assessment every 2–3 cycles*: Physical examination, CT scan or PET scan, bone marrow evaluation (if clinically indicated)

DIFFUSE LARGE B-CELL LYMPHOMA • SALVAGE BEYOND SECOND-LINE REFRACTORY DISEASE • NOT ELIGIBLE FOR CONSOLIDATIVE ASCT

NON-HODGKIN LYMPHOMA REGIMEN: SELINEXOR

Kalakonda N et al. Lancet Hematol 2020;7:e511–e522
Supplementary appendix to: Kalakonda N et al. Lancet Hematol 2020;7:e511–e522
XPOVIO (selinexor) prescribing information. Newton, MA: Karyopharm Therapeutics Inc; Revised 2020 December

Selinexor 60 mg per dose; administer orally twice per week on days 1 and 3, every 7 days, until disease progression (total dosage/week = 120 mg)
• Patients should swallow selinexor tablets whole. Do not break, chew, crush, or divide tablets

• If a patient misses or delays a dose of selinexor, instruct the patient to take the next dose on the next regularly scheduled day. The dose should not be made up

• If a patient vomits after taking selinexor, instruct the patient to take the next dose on the next regularly scheduled day. The dose should not be repeated

• In vitro studies indicate that selinexor is a substrate for CYP3A4, multiple UDP-glucuronosyltransferases (UGTs), and glutathione S-transferases (GSTs), and that selinexor inhibits OATP1B3. Coadministration of selinexor with acetaminophen (up to 1000 mg/day) had no effect on selinexor pharmacokinetics

Supportive Care
Antiemetic prophylaxis
Emetogenic potential is **MODERATE TO HIGH**. The U.S. FDA-approved prescribing information for selinexor recommends that patients receive prophylactic treatment with a 5-HT3 antagonist and/or other anti-nausea agents prior to and during treatment with selinexor
See Chapter 42 for antiemetic recommendations

Hematopoietic growth factor (CSF) prophylaxis
Primary prophylaxis is **NOT** *indicated*
See Chapter 43 for more information

Antimicrobial prophylaxis
Risk of fever and neutropenia is *INTERMEDIATE*
Antimicrobial primary prophylaxis to be considered:
• Antibacterial—consider a fluoroquinolone during periods of prolonged neutropenia (ANC <500/mm^3 for ≥7 days) or no prophylaxis; *P jirovecii* prophylaxis is recommended (eg, cotrimoxazole)
• Antifungal—consider fluconazole during periods of prolonged neutropenia (ANC <500/mm^3 for ≥7 days) or no prophylaxis
• Antiviral—antiherpes antivirals (eg, acyclovir, famciclovir, valacyclovir)

Diarrhea management
    Loperamide 4 mg orally initially after the first loose or liquid stool, *then*
    Loperamide 2 mg orally every 2 hours during waking hours, *plus*
    Loperamide 4 mg orally every 4 hours during hours of sleep
• Continue for at least 12 hours after diarrhea resolves
• Recurrent diarrhea after a 12-hour diarrhea-free interval is treated as a new episode
• Rehydrate orally with fluids and electrolytes during a diarrheal episode
• If a patient develops blood or mucus in stool, dehydration, or hemodynamic instability, or if diarrhea persists >48 hours despite loperamide, stop loperamide and evaluate urgently in clinic or hospitalize the patient for IV hydration
    Alternatively, a trial of **diphenoxylate hydrochloride** 2.5 mg **with atropine sulfate** 0.025 mg (eg, Lomotil)
• Initial adult dose is 2 tablets 4 times daily until control has been achieved, after which the dose may be reduced to meet individual requirements. Control may often be maintained with as little as 2 tablets daily
• Clinical improvement of acute diarrhea is usually observed within 48 hours. If improvement of chronic diarrhea after treatment with a maximum daily dose of 8 tablets is not observed within 10 days, control is unlikely with further administration

Hydration and Nutrition
Instruct patients to maintain adequate intake of oral fluids and calories during treatment with selinexor. Consider administration of intravenous fluids for patients at higher risk for dehydration

Treatment Modifications

Selinexor Treatment Modifications

Selinexor dose levels

Dose level 1 (starting dose)	60 mg twice per week
Dose level −1	40 mg twice per week
Dose level −2	60 mg once per week
Dose level −3	40 mg once per week
Dose level −4	Discontinue selinexor

Adverse Event	Treatment Modification
Thrombocytopenia	
Platelet count ≥50,000/mm^3 to <75,000/mm^3	Omit one dose of selinexor, then resume at the same dose level
Platelet count ≥25,000/mm^3 to <50,000/mm^3 *without* bleeding	Withhold selinexor until platelets improve to ≥50,000/mm^3, then resume at one lower dose level
Platelet count ≥25,000/mm^3 to <50,000/mm^3 *with* concurrent bleeding	Withhold selinexor until platelets improve to ≥50,000/mm^3, then resume at one lower dose level, after resolution of bleeding. Transfuse platelets as per clinical guidelines
Platelet count <25,000/mm^3	Withhold selinexor until recovery of platelet count to ≥50,000/mm^3, then resume selinexor with the dosage reduced by 1 dose level. Transfuse platelets as per clinical guidelines
Neutropenia	
ANC ≥500/mm^3 to <1000/mm^3 *without* fever, first occurrence	Withhold selinexor until ANC ≥1000/mm^3, then resume selinexor at the same dose level
ANC ≥500/mm^3 to <1000/mm^3 *without* fever, recurrence	Withhold selinexor until ANC ≥1000/mm^3, then resume selinexor at one lower dose level. Administer growth factors as per clinical guidelines
ANC <500/mm^3 or febrile neutropenia	Monitor CBC with differential frequently. Withhold selinexor until ANC improves to ≥1000/mm^3, then resume selinexor at one lower dose level. Administer growth factors as per clinical guidelines
Anemia	
Hemoglobin <8 g/dL	Reduce the selinexor dosage by 1 dose level. Transfuse and/or administer other treatments as indicated
Anemia with life-threatening consequences (urgent intervention indicated)	Monitor CBC frequently. Transfuse and/or administer other treatments as indicated. Withhold selinexor until hemoglobin improves to ≥8 g/dL, then resume selinexor at one lower dose level
Gastrointestinal toxicities	
G1/2 nausea (oral intake decreased without significant weight loss, dehydration or malnutrition) or G1/2 vomiting (≤5 episodes per day)	Continue selinexor at the same dose and optimize prophylactic and rescue anti-nausea medication regimen
G3 nausea (inadequate oral caloric or fluid intake) or G3/4 vomiting (6 or more episodes per day)	Withhold selinexor. Optimize prophylactic and rescue anti-nausea medication regimen. Resume selinexor when nausea and/or vomiting has resolved to G ≤2 or baseline with the dosage reduced by 1 dose level
G2 diarrhea (increase of 4–6 stools per day above baseline), first occurrence	Continue selinexor at the same dose and optimize supportive care, including antidiarrheal medications
G2 diarrhea (increase of 4–6 stools per day above baseline), second and subsequent occurrence	Reduce the selinexor dosage by 1 dose level and optimize supportive care, including antidiarrheal medications
G3/4 diarrhea (increase of ≥7 stools per day over baseline; hospitalization indicated)	Withhold selinexor. Optimize supportive care, including antidiarrheal medications. Resume selinexor when diarrhea has resolved to G ≤2 with the dosage reduced by 1 dose level

(continued)

Treatment Modifications (*continued*)

Other toxicities	
Hyponatremia (sodium ≤130 mmol/L)	Provide appropriate supportive care. Correct sodium level for hyperglycemia and high serum paraprotein levels, if applicable. Monitor sodium levels frequently as clinically indicated. Withhold selinexor until sodium improves to ≥130 mmol/L, then resume selinexor with the dosage reduced by 1 dose level
G2 fatigue* (not relieved by rest; limits instrumental ADL) lasting >7 days or G3 fatigue* (not relieved by rest, limits self care ADL) of any duration	Withhold selinexor until fatigue resolves to G ≤1 (fatigue relieved by rest) or baseline, then resume selinexor with the dosage reduced by 1 dose level
Weight loss of ≥10% to <20% or Anorexia associated with significant weight loss or malnutrition	Withhold selinexor and provide supportive care. Monitor until weight returns to >90% of baseline weight, then resume selinexor with the dosage reduced by 1 dose level
G2 ocular toxicity, excluding cataract	Perform ophthalmologic evaluation. Withhold selinexor and provide supportive care. Monitor until ocular symptoms improve to G ≤1 or baseline, then resume selinexor at one lower dose level
G ≥3 ocular toxicity, excluding cataract	Perform ophthalmologic examination. Permanently discontinue selinexor
Other G3/4 life-threatening nonhematologic toxicities	Withhold selinexor until toxicity improves to G ≤2, then resume selinexor with the dosage reduced by 1 dose level, if clinically appropriate

Patient Population Studied

The SADAL study was a phase 2b, open-label, international, multicenter study that involved adult patients with diffuse large B-cell lymphoma (DLBCL) or DLBCL transformed from a prior indolent lymphoma who had received 2–5 prior lines of treatment and who had either progressed following or were considered ineligible for autologous hematopoietic stem cell transplant (auto-HSCT). A total of 175 patients were assigned to receive selinexor at a dose of 60 mg, of which 127 were included in the analysis. Selected baseline characteristics of the patients include: median age 67 years, 59% male, 89% ECOG PS of 0–1, 74% de novo DLBCL, 24% transformed DLBCL, 47% germinal center B-cell like phenotype, 50% non-germinal center B-cell like phenotype, 4% known double- or triple-hit DLBCL, median of 2 prior lines of therapy, 30% prior auto-HSCT, and 72% refractory to most recent line of therapy

Efficacy (N = 127)

Outcome	Selinexor (n = 127)
ORR, n/N (%) [95% CI]	36/127 (28) [20.7–37.0]
CR, n/N (%) [95% CI]	15/127 (12) [6.8–18.7]
PR, n/N (%) [95% CI]	21/127 (17) [10.5–24.2]
SD, n/N (%) [95% CI]	11/127 (9) [4.4–15.0]
PD or no response recorded, n/N (%) [95% CI]	80/127 (63) [54.0–71.4]
Median DOR among patients with PR or CR (n = 36), months (95% CI)	9.3 (4.8–23.0)
Median DOR among patients with CR only (n = 15), months (95% CI)	23 (10.4–23.0)
Median PFS, months (95% CI)	2.6 (1.9–4.0)
Median OS, months (95% CI)	9.1 (6.6–15.1)

CI, confidence interval; CR, complete response; DOR, duration of response; ORR, overall response rate; OS, overall survival; PD, progressive disease; PFS, progression-free survival; PR, partial response; SD, stable disease

Adverse Events (N = 127)

Adverse Event	Selinexor 60 mg (n = 127)		
	Grade 1–2 (%)	Grade 3 (%)	Grade 4 (%)
Thrombocytopenia	16	31	15
Nausea	52	6	0
Fatigue	36	11	0
Anemia	21	21	1
Decreased appetite	33	4	0
Diarrhea	32	3	0
Neutropenia	6	16	9
Weight loss	30	0	0
Vomiting	28	2	0
Pyrexia	18	4	0
Asthenia	17	5	0
Cough	18	0	0
Upper respiratory tract infection	14	1	0
Dizziness	14	0	0
Hypotension	10	3	0
Peripheral edema	11	1	0
Dyspnea	10	1	1
Hyponatremia	3	8	0

Note: The table includes treatment-emergent adverse events occurring in 10% or more patients. No grade 5 toxicities occurred in >10% of patients

Therapy Monitoring

1. *At baseline and periodically (more frequent during initial 3 months)*: CBC with differential and platelet count, serum chemistries (especially sodium), body weight
2. *Monitor periodically for, and advise patients to report symptoms of:*
   a. Dehydration, malnutrition, gastrointestinal adverse effects (eg, nausea/vomiting, diarrhea, anorexia), and infection
   b. Neurologic adverse reactions (eg, dizziness, confusion) may occur with selinexor. Avoid concomitant use with other medications that may cause dizziness or confusion and avoid situations where dizziness or a confused state may be problematic. Maintenance of optimal hydration status, correction of anemia, and minimization of polypharmacy may reduce the incidence and severity of neurologic adverse reactions

FOLLICULAR LYMPHOMA • FIRST LINE

NON-HODGKIN LYMPHOMA REGIMEN: RITUXIMAB + CYCLOPHOSPHAMIDE, VINCRISTINE, AND PREDNISONE (R-CVP)

Marcus R et al. Blood 2005;105:1417–1423

Rituximab
Premedication for rituximab:
Acetaminophen 650–1000 mg; administer orally, *plus*
Diphenhydramine 25–50 mg; administer orally or intravenously 30–60 minutes before starting rituximab

Rituximab 375 mg/m^2; administer intravenously in 0.9% sodium chloride injection (0.9% NS) or 5% dextrose injection (D5W), diluted to a concentration of 1–4 mg/mL, on day 1, every 3 weeks, for a maximum of 8 cycles (total dosage/cycle = 375 mg/m^2)
Notes on rituximab administration:
• Infuse initially at 50 mg/hour. If hypersensitivity or infusion reactions do not occur during the first 30 minutes, increase the rate by 50 mg/hour every 30 minutes, as tolerated, to a maximum rate of 400 mg/hour. Subsequently, if previous administration was well tolerated, start at 100 mg/hour and increase by 100 mg/hour every 30 minutes, as tolerated, to a maximum rate of 400 mg/hour

INFUSION REACTIONS ASSOCIATED WITH RITUXIMAB
Note: Medications for the treatment of hypersensitivity reactions should be available for immediate use in the event of a reaction during administration (eg, intravenous fluids, epinephrine, antihistamines, glucocorticoids, and O$_2$)
Fevers, chills, and rigors
1. Interrupt rituximab administration for severe symptoms, and give:
   • **Acetaminophen** 650 mg orally for fever. For persistent or recurrent symptoms, repeat administration every 4–6 hours as needed during rituximab administration
   • **Diphenhydramine** 25–50 mg orally or by intravenous injection for pruritus, hypotension, or angioedema. For persistent or recurrent symptoms, repeat administration every 4–6 hours as needed during rituximab administration
   • **Meperidine** 12.5–25 mg by intravenous injection every 10–20 minutes as needed for shaking chills (generally, cumulative doses >100 mg are not needed; use repeated doses with caution in persons with moderate or more severely impaired renal function)
2. If rituximab administration was interrupted, resume infusion at a slower rate than the maximum rate previously attempted. Rate escalation may be reattempted at smaller incremental steps with close monitoring. Do not exceed the maximum recommended rate of 400 mg/h

Dyspnea or wheezing without allergic findings (urticaria, or tongue or laryngeal edema)
1. Interrupt rituximab administration immediately
2. Give **hydrocortisone** 100 mg by intravenous injection (or an alternative steroid with equivalent glucocorticoid potency)
3. Give a **histamine (H$_2$) receptor antagonist** (ranitidine 50 mg, cimetidine 300 mg, or famotidine 20 mg) intravenously over 15–30 minutes
4. After symptoms resolve, resume rituximab administration at 25 mg/h with close monitoring. Do not increase the administration rate
Note: Medications and equipment for the treatment of hypersensitivity reactions should be available for immediate use in the event of a reaction during administration (eg, intravenous fluids, epinephrine, antihistamines, glucocorticoids, and oxygen)
Rituxan (rituximab) prescribing information. South San Francisco, CA: Genentech, Inc; 2018 October

Chemotherapy
Cyclophosphamide 750 mg/m^2; administer intravenously in 25–250 mL 0.9% NS or D5W, over 10–30 minutes on day 1, every 3 weeks, for a maximum of 8 cycles (total dosage/cycle = 750 mg/m^2)
Vincristine 1.4 mg/m^2 (maximum single dose = 2 mg); administer by intravenous infusion over 15 minutes in 50 mL 0.9% NS, on day 1, every 3 weeks, for a maximum of 8 cycles (total dosage/cycle = 1.4 mg/m^2, maximum dose/cycle = 2 mg)
Prednisone 40 mg/m^2 per day; administer orally for 5 consecutive days, days 1–5, every 3 weeks, for a maximum of 8 cycles (total dosage/cycle = 200 mg/m^2)

Supportive Care
Antiemetic prophylaxis
Emetogenic potential on day 1 is **MODERATE**
See Chapter 42 for antiemetic recommendations

Hematopoietic growth factor (CSF) prophylaxis
Primary prophylaxis is indicated with 1 of the following:
   Filgrastim (G-CSF) 5 μg/kg per day, by subcutaneous injection, *or*
   Pegfilgrastim (pegylated filgrastim) 6 mg/0.6 mL, by subcutaneous injection for 1 dose
• Begin use from 24–72 hours after myelosuppressive chemotherapy is completed
See Chapter 43 for more information

Antimicrobial prophylaxis
Risk of fever and neutropenia is *LOW*
Antimicrobial primary prophylaxis to be considered:
• Antibacterial—*Pneumocystis jirovecii* prophylaxis is recommended (eg, cotrimoxazole)
• Antifungal—not indicated
• Antiviral—not indicated unless patient previously had an episode of HSV

Patient Population Studied

A study of 321 patients age 18 years or older with advanced stage untreated CD20+ follicular lymphoma who were randomized to RCVP or CVP for 8 cycles. All patients had stage III or IV disease, an Eastern Clinical Oncology Group (ECOG) performance status of 0–2, and a need for therapy in the opinion of the participating clinician. Median age was 52–53 years. Majority were grade 1 or 2 follicular lymphoma

Toxicity

Adverse Event	CVP	R-CVP
At least 1 adverse event	95%	97%
Life-threatening events	—	3.1%
Adverse event within 24 hours after an infusion	51%	71%
G 3/4, rituximab infusion-related reaction	N/A	9%
G 3/4 neutropenia	14%	24%
Overall infection rate or incidence of neutropenia and sepsis	No difference	

Therapy Monitoring

1. *Prior to treatment*: hepatitis B core antibody (IgG or total) and hepatitis B surface antigen
2. *Prior to each cycle*: PE, CBC with differential, LFTs, serum BUN, and creatinine
3. *Weekly:* CBC with differential and LFTs

Treatment Modification

ANC	Adverse Event — Platelet Count	Dose Modification — Percent of Planned Dosages — Cyclophosphamide	Vincristine	Prednisone
>4000/mm^3	≥100,000/mm^3	100%	100%	100%
3000–4000/mm^3	50,000–100,000/mm^3	75%	100%	100%
2000–3000/mm^3	50,000–100,000/mm^3	50%	100%	100%
1000–2000/mm^3	<50,000/mm^3	25%	50%	100%
0–1000/mm^3	<50,000/mm^3	0	0	0

G2 neurotoxicity	Reduce vincristine dosage 50%
G3/4 neurotoxicity	Discontinue vincristine
Rituximab-induced infusion reaction	Interrupt therapy; resume rituximab and CVP once symptoms resolve

Note: Repeated cycles may be delayed for up to 1 week for incomplete hematologic recovery (ie, day 1 ANC must be >1000/mm^3 from prior treatment)

Efficacy

(Median Follow-up: 30 Months)

	CVP (N = 159)	R-CVP (N = 162)
Tumor Response[*]		
Complete response	8%	30%
Complete response, unconfirmed	3%	11%
Partial response	47%	40%
CR + CRu + PR	57%	81%
Stable disease	21%	7%
Progressive disease	20%	11%
Could not be assessed	3%	1%
Median time to progression[*]	15 months	32 months
Median time to treatment failure[*]	7 months	27 months
Median duration of response[*]	14 months	35 months
Median disease-free survival[†]	21 months	Not reached
Median time to new antilymphoma treatment or death	14 months	Not reached
KM estimates for overall survival at 30 months[‡]	85%	89%

CVP, Cyclophosphamide, vincristine, and prednisone; CR, complete response; CRu, complete response, unconfirmed; PR, partial response; R-CVP, Rituximab + CVP

[*]P<0.001
[†]P = 0.0009
[‡]Not significant

FOLLICULAR LYMPHOMA • FIRST LINE

NON-HODGKIN LYMPHOMA REGIMEN: CYCLOPHOSPHAMIDE, VINCRISTINE, AND PREDNISONE (CVP) + OBINUTUZUMAB

Marcus R et al. N Engl J Med 2017;377:1331–1344
Supplementary Appendix to: Marcus R et al. N Engl J Med 2017;377:1331–1344
Protocol for: Marcus R et al. N Engl J Med 2017;377:1331–1344
Gazyva (obinutuzumab) prescribing information. South San Francisco, CA: Genentech, Inc; 2017 November

Prophylaxis for tumor lysis syndrome is recommended for high-risk patients (eg, high tumor burden, bulky lymphadenopathy, or renal impairment):

• Hydration; encourage *oral* hydration (eg, ≥3 L/day) starting 1–2 days prior to the first obinutuzumab dose. Consider administering additional *intravenous* hydration prior to the infusion if needed. Continue hydration prior to subsequent obinutuzumab infusions if needed

• **Allopurinol** 300 mg per dose; administer orally twice per day starting 12–24 hours prior to the first obinutuzumab infusion for 7 days. Continue prophylaxis prior to subsequent obinutuzumab infusions if needed

  ▪ Reduce allopurinol dose to 300 mg by mouth once daily for 7 days for patients with renal impairment

The regimen consists of eight 21-day cycles of cyclophosphamide + vincristine + prednisone + obinutuzumab. Patients who achieve complete response or partial response to the initial 8 cycles of combination therapy should then continue obinutuzumab monotherapy maintenance every 8 weeks for up to 2 years

Premedication for obinutuzumab:

• **Acetaminophen** 650–1000 mg; administer orally at least 30 minutes prior to each dose of obinutuzumab

• **Diphenhydramine** 50 mg; administer orally or intravenously at least 30 minutes prior to obinutuzumab

  – Required for the cycle 1, day 1 infusion

  – Required for subsequent infusions only if the previous infusion was complicated by a grade 1–3 infusion-related reaction

• **Corticosteroid** premedication is required for the cycle 1, day 1 infusion. For subsequent infusions, administer corticosteroid premedication only if the absolute lymphocyte count is >25 × 10^9/L *or* if the previous dose was complicated by a grade 3 infusion-related reaction. Choose only *one* of the following options, when indicated:

  – **Dexamethasone** 20 mg; administer intravenously at least 1 hour prior to obinutuzumab, *or*

  – **Methylprednisolone** 80 mg; administer intravenously at least 1 hour prior to obinutuzumab, *or*

  – *Note:* if a glucocorticoid-containing chemotherapy regimen is administered on the same day as obinutuzumab, the glucocorticoid can be administered orally if given at least 1 hour prior to obinutuzumab, in which case additional intravenous glucocorticoid premedication is not required. Thus, on days when prednisone is scheduled as part of cyclophosphamide + vincristine + prednisone (CVP) chemotherapy (ie, day 1 of cycles 1–8), may instead administer:

    ▪ **Prednisone** 100 mg; administer orally at least 1 hour prior to obinutuzumab

Obinutuzumab; administer intravenously diluted in 0.9% sodium chloride (0.9% NS) injection to a final concentration ranging from 0.4–4 mg/mL (see table below for dose, dilution, infusion rate, and schedule information)

Note:

• Administer prior to cyclophosphamide + vincristine on days where both obinutuzumab and cyclophosphamide + vincristine are administered

• Hepatitis B virus (HBV) reactivation, in some cases resulting in fulminant hepatitis, hepatic failure, and death, can occur in patients receiving CD20-directed cytolytic antibodies, including obinutuzumab. Screen all patients for HBV infection before treatment initiation. Monitor HBV-positive patients during and after treatment with obinutuzumab, and consider antiviral prophylaxis. Discontinue obinutuzumab and concomitant medications in the event of HBV reactivation

• Obinutuzumab can cause severe and life-threatening infusion reactions. Symptoms may include hypotension, tachycardia, dyspnea, and respiratory symptoms (eg, bronchospasm, larynx and throat irritation, wheezing, laryngeal edema). Other common symptoms include nausea, vomiting, diarrhea, hypertension, flushing, headache, pyrexia, and chills

  ▪ Sixty percent of previously untreated non-Hodgkin lymphoma patients experienced a reaction to the first infusion of obinutuzumab. Infusion reactions can also occur with subsequent infusions

• Hypotension may occur as an infusion reaction. Consider withholding antihypertensive treatments for 12 hours prior to and during each obinutuzumab infusion, and for the first hour after administration until blood pressure is stable

(continued)

(continued)

Obinutuzumab Dosage and Schedule During Combination Therapy with CVP (Eight 21-day cycles)

Cycle and Day[*]	Obinutuzumab Dose	Volume of 0.9% NS for Dilution	Obinutuzumab Administration	Total Dose per Cycle[*]
Cycle 1 Day 1	1000 mg	250 mL	Begin infusion at 50 mg/h, and increase by 50 mg/h every 30 minutes to a maximum rate of 400 mg/h	Cycle 1 = 3000 mg
Cycle 1 Day 8	1000 mg	250 mL	If no infusion reaction occurred during previous dose and the final infusion rate was ≥100 mg/h, start at 100 mg/h, and increase by 100 mg/h every 30 minutes to a maximum rate of 400 mg/h. If an infusion reaction occurred during previous dose, begin infusion at 50 mg/h, and increase by 50 mg/h every 30 minutes to a maximum rate of 400 mg/h	
Cycle 1 Day 15	1000 mg	250 mL		
Cycles 2-8 Day 1 only	1000 mg	250 mL	If no infusion reaction occurred during previous dose and the final infusion rate was ≥100 mg/h, start at 100 mg/h, and increase by 100 mg/h every 30 minutes to a maximum rate of 400 mg/h. If an infusion reaction occurred during previous dose, begin infusion at 50 mg/h, and increase by 50 mg/h every 30 minutes to a maximum rate of 400 mg/h	Cycles 2–8 = 1000 mg

[*]Cycle length = 21 days

Obinutuzumab Dosage and Schedule During Monotherapy Maintenance
Every 8 weeks for up to 2 years, for patients who achieve a complete response or partial response to the initial 8 cycles of combination therapy

Schedule[†]	Obinutuzumab Dose	Volume of 0.9% NS for Dilution	Obinutuzumab Administration	Total Dose per Cycle[†]
Maintenance cycles (every 8 weeks for up to 2 years)	1000 mg	250 mL	If no infusion reaction occurred during previous dose and the final infusion rate was ≥100 mg/h, start at 100 mg/h, and increase by 100 mg/h every 30 minutes to a maximum rate of 400 mg/h. If an infusion reaction occurred during previous dose, begin infusion at 50 mg/h, and increase by 50 mg/h every 30 minutes to a maximum rate of 400 mg/h	Maintenance therapy = 1000 mg

[†]Obinutuzumab maintenance cycle length = 8 weeks (56 days) for up to 2 years

Obinutuzumab Infusion-Related Toxicities

Note: Medications and equipment for the treatment of hypersensitivity reactions should be available for immediate use in the event of a reaction during obinutuzumab administration (eg, intravenous fluids, epinephrine, antihistamines, glucocorticoids, oxygen)

- **G ≤2 obinutuzumab infusion-related reaction**
- **G3 obinutuzumab infusion-related reaction, first occurrence**
  1. Interrupt obinutuzumab infusion
  2. For fever, chills: Give additional dose of acetaminophen 650 mg orally and diphenhydramine 25–50 mg by intravenous push
  3. For dyspnea/wheezing: Give additional dose of diphenhydramine 25–50 mg by intravenous push. Give a histamine H$_2$-antagonist (ranitidine 50 mg or famotidine 20 mg) by intravenous push. Give hydrocortisone 100 mg (or glucocorticoid equivalent) by intravenous push
  4. For rigors: Give meperidine 12.5–25 mg by intravenous push ± promethazine 12.5–25 mg by intravenous infusion in at least 10 mL 0.9% NS or D5W over 5–15 minutes. If after 15–20 minutes the response to a single dose is considered inadequate, the dose may be repeated
  5. After symptoms resolve, resume obinutuzumab infusion at a minimum of 50% reduction in the rate at which the event occurred. If no further infusion-related events, increase the infusion rate at the increments and intervals as appropriate for the treatment cycle dose. If G3 infusion-related reaction recurs during rechallenge, then permanently discontinue obinutuzumab

Refer to the "premedications for obinutuzumab" section within the regimen description to determine appropriate premedications for the subsequent cycle

- **G3 obinutuzumab infusion-related reaction, recurrent (following rechallenge on the same day of treatment)**
- **G4 obinutuzumab infusion-related reaction**
- **Serum sickness or hypersensitivity reaction**
  1. Permanently discontinue obinutuzumab and provide supportive care

Intravenous hydration before and after cyclophosphamide administration:
500–1000 mL 0.9% NS
Chemotherapy
Cyclophosphamide 750 mg/m²; administer intravenously in 25–250 mL 0.9% NS or 5% dextrose injection (D5W) over 10–30 minutes, given on day 1, every 21 days, for 8 cycles (total dosage/21-day cycle = 750 mg/m²)
Vincristine 1.4 mg/m² (maximum dose = 2 mg); administer by intravenous infusion over 15 minutes in 50 mL 0.9% NS, given on day 1, every 21 days, for 8 cycles (total dosage/21-day cycle = 1.4 mg/m²; maximum dosage/21-day cycle = 2 mg)
Prednisone 100 mg per day; administer orally for 5 consecutive days, days 1–5, every 21 days, for 8 cycles (total dosage/21-day cycle = 500 mg)

Supportive Care
Antiemetic prophylaxis
Emetogenic potential on day 1 of cycle 1–8 is **MODERATE**
Emetogenic potential of obinutuzumab monotherapy maintenance is **MINIMAL**
See Chapter 42 for antiemetic recommendations

Hematopoietic growth factor (CSF) prophylaxis
Primary prophylaxis **MAY** *be indicated*
See Chapter 43 for more information

Antimicrobial prophylaxis
Risk of fever and neutropenia is **INTERMEDIATE**
Antimicrobial primary prophylaxis to be considered:
• Antibacterial—consider a fluoroquinolone during periods of prolonged neutropenia, or no prophylaxis
• Antifungal—consider use during periods of prolonged neutropenia, or no prophylaxis
• Antiviral—antiherpes antivirals (eg, acyclovir, famciclovir, valacyclovir)

Treatment Modifications

Obinutuzumab + Cyclophosphamide + Vincristine + Prednisone (G-CVP)

Dose Levels	Cyclophosphamide	Vincristine	Prednisone
Starting dose	750 mg/m²	1.4 mg/m² (max dose of 2 mg)	100 mg
Dose level −1	500 mg/m²	1.05 mg/m² (max dose of 1.5 mg)	80 mg
Dose level −2	375 mg/m²	0.7 mg/m² (max dose of 1 mg)	60 mg
Dose level −3	Discontinue CVPª		

There are no dose reductions for obinutuzumab
ªIf CVP chemotherapy is discontinued due to toxicity, may continue with obinutuzumab induction/maintenance at discretion of healthcare provider

Adverse Event	Dose Modification
Hematologic Toxicity During G-CVP Combination Therapy	
G3 neutropenia (ANC <1000–500/mm³)	Delay doses of G-CVP for a maximum of 3 weeks. Consider administering filgrastim or pegfilgrastim during all subsequent cycles for neutropenia. If improvement to G ≤2 (ANC ≥1000/mm³ and platelet count ≥50,000/mm³), then administer previous dose of G-CVP
G3 thrombocytopenia (platelet count <50,000–25,000/mm³)	
G4 neutropenia (ANC <500/mm³)	Delay doses of G-CVP for a maximum of 3 weeks. Consider administering filgrastim or pegfilgrastim during all subsequent cycles for neutropenia. If improvement to G ≤2 (ANC ≥1000/mm³ and platelet count ≥50,000/mm³), then administer G-CVP with the cyclophosphamide dose reduced by 1 dose level for subsequent cycles
G4 thrombocytopenia (platelet count <25,000/mm³)	
Hematologic Toxicity During Obinutuzumab Monotherapy Maintenance	
G ≥3 hematologic toxicity during obinutuzumab monotherapy maintenance	Delay obinutuzumab for up to 42 days until improvement to G ≤2 or baseline. Consider increasing the frequency of CBC with differential monitoring
	Consider treatment with filgrastim, as indicated. If toxicity improves to G ≤2 or baseline, then administer the same dosage of obinutuzumab

(continued)

Treatment Modifications (continued)

Infectious Complications

G2 infection	Interrupt G-CVP until resolution of infection, then resume G-CVP at the same dose
G ≥3 infection	Interrupt G-CVP until resolution of infection, then resume obinutuzumab, vincristine, and prednisone at the same doses and resume cyclophosphamide at either the same dose, or with the dose reduced by 1 dose level
New or changes in preexisting neurologic symptoms (eg, confusion, dizziness, loss of balance, vision problems, aphasia, ambulation issues); PML suspected	Interrupt G-CVP until central nervous system status clarified. Workup may include (but is not limited to) consultation with a neurologist, brain MRI, and LP
PML is confirmed	Discontinue G-CVP
HBV reactivation	Discontinue G-CVP. Institute appropriate treatment for HBV. Upon resolution of HBV reactivation, resumption of G-CVP should be discussed with a physician with expertise in management of HBV. Insufficient data exist to determine the safety of resumption of G-CVP in this setting

Gastrointestinal Toxicities

G ≥3 ileus (severely altered GI function; TPN indicated; tube placement indicated)	Withhold all chemotherapy until resolution of ileus and constipation, then reduce the next dose of vincristine by 1 dose level with an optimal prophylactic bowel regimen. Do not change the cyclophosphamide or prednisone doses. If symptoms do not recur at the reduced vincristine dose, then the vincristine dose may be re-escalated on subsequent cycles with an appropriate prophylactic bowel regimen
G ≥3 constipation (obstipation with manual evacuation indicated; limiting self-care ADL)	

Neurologic Toxicities

G3 peripheral sensory neuropathy (severe symptoms; limiting self-care ADL)	Proceed with treatment, and reduce the dose of vincristine by 1 dose level. Do not change the cyclophosphamide or prednisone doses. If symptoms improve, then the vincristine dose may be re-escalated on subsequent cycles
G2 peripheral motor neuropathy (moderate symptoms; limiting instrumental ADL)	
G3 peripheral motor neuropathy (severe symptoms; limiting self-care ADL)	Proceed with treatment, and reduce the dose of vincristine by 2 dose levels. Do not change the cyclophosphamide or prednisone doses. If symptoms improve, then the vincristine dose may be re-escalated on subsequent cycles
G4 peripheral sensory neuropathy (life-threatening symptoms; urgent intervention indicated)	Discontinue vincristine. Do not change the cyclophosphamide or prednisone doses
G4 peripheral motor neuropathy (life-threatening consequences; urgent intervention indicated)	
G ≥2 mood alteration (moderate mood alteration) or confusion (moderate disorientation; limiting instrumental ADL)	Withhold prednisone until symptoms return to baseline. Resume prednisone reduced by 1 dose level. If symptoms persist, reduce by another dose level. Do not change the cyclophosphamide or vincristine doses

Hepatic Impairment

Serum bilirubin 1.5–3 mg/dL	Decrease the vincristine dose by 50%
Serum bilirubin >3 mg/dL	Withhold vincristine

Drug Interactions

Patient requires concomitant therapy with antihypertensive medication(s)	On days of obinutuzumab treatment, and especially with the initial dose, weigh the risk versus benefit of delaying administration of the antihypertensive medication(s) until after completion of the obinutuzumab infusion due to the potential risk of obinutuzumab infusion-related hypotension
Patient requires concomitant therapy with a strong CYP3A4 inhibitor	Patient may have earlier onset of neuromuscular side effects of vincristine. If concomitant use of the strong CYP3A4 inhibitor cannot be avoided, consider dose reduction of vincristine and increased monitoring for toxicity
Live attenuated vaccine is indicated during or after obinutuzumab administration	Avoid administration of a live attenuated vaccine during obinutuzumab therapy and following therapy until adequate B-cell recovery has occurred

(continued)

Treatment Modifications (*continued*)

Other Toxicities	
G ≥3 hyperglycemia (insulin therapy initiated; hospitalization indicated)	Withhold prednisone until blood glucose is ≤250 mg/dL. Treat with insulin or other hypoglycemic agents as clinically appropriate, and then resume prednisone at the same dose. If hyperglycemia is uncontrolled despite the aforementioned measures, decrease prednisone by 1 dose level

G-CVP, obinutuzumab + cyclophosphamide + vincristine + prednisone; ANC, absolute neutrophil count; CBC, complete blood count; PML, progressive multifocal leukoencephalopathy; MRI, magnetic resonance imaging; LP, lumbar puncture; HBV, hepatitis B virus; GI, gastrointestinal; TPN, total parenteral nutrition; ADL, activities of daily living

Gazyva (obinutuzumab) prescribing information. South San Francisco, CA: Genentech, Inc; 2017 November
Marcus R et al. N Engl J Med 2017;277:1331–1344
Supplementary Appendix to: Marcus R et al. N Engl J Med 2017;277:1331–1344
Protocol for: Marcus R et al. N Engl J Med 2017;277:1331–1344

Patient Population Studied

This was a post hoc analysis of a multicenter, randomized, open-label, phase 3 trial (GALLIUM) involving 1202 patients with previously untreated, advanced, CD20-positive follicular lymphoma. Eligible patients had an Eastern Cooperative Oncology Group (ECOG) performance status score ≤2. Patients were randomly assigned 1:1 to receive intravenous obinutuzumab (1000 mg on days 1, 8, and 15 of cycle 1 and on day 1 only of subsequent cycles) or rituximab (375 mg/m^2 on day 1) in addition to standard chemotherapy regimens of: intravenous cyclophosphamide (750 mg/m^2 on day 1), doxorubicin (50 mg/m^2 on day 1), and vincristine (1.4 mg/m^2 [maximum dose 2 mg] on day 1), and oral prednisone (100 mg per day on days 1–5) (CHOP) for six 21-day cycles; intravenous cyclophosphamide (750 mg/m^2 on day 1) and vincristine (1.4 mg/m^2 [maximum dose 2 mg] on day 1), and oral prednisone (100 mg per day on days 1–5) (CVP) for eight 21-day cycles; or intravenous bendamustine (90 mg/m^2 on days 1 and 2) for six 28-day cycles. When combined with CHOP or CVP, obinutuzumab and rituximab were administered for eight 21-day cycles; when combined with bendamustine, obinutuzumab and rituximab were administered for six 28-day cycles. At the end of the induction therapy, patients who had a complete or partial response received maintenance treatment of the same study drug (intravenous obinutuzumab 1000 mg or rituximab 375 mg/m^2) every 2 months for 2 years or until disease progression or withdrawal from trial. Of the 1202 patients involved in the trial, 61 were assigned to CVP + obinutuzumab, and 57 were assigned to CVP + rituximab

Efficacy

(N = 118)

	Obinutuzumab + CVP (N = 61)	Rituximab + CVP (N = 57)	
Median progression-free survival	95%	78.9%	HR 0.63, 95% CI 0.32–1.21

Note: The median follow-up among all trial participants was 34.5 months

Toxicity

Grade 3–5 Event (%)[*]	Induction Phase		Maintenance and Observation Phases		Follow-up	
	CVP + Obinutuzumab (N = 61)	CVP + Rituximab (N = 56)	CVP + Obinutuzumab (N = 57)	CVP + Rituximab (N = 43)	CVP + Obinutuzumab (N = 44)	CVP + Rituximab (N = 45)
Neutropenia	39.3	23.2	8.8	4.7	0	0
Infection	4.9	7.1	8.8	2.3	2.3	4.4
Second neoplasm	0	0	0	2.3	0	0

[*]According to the NCI Common Terminology Criteria for Adverse Events, version 4.0

Toxicity (continued)

Induction Phase for Obinutuzumab + Standard Chemotherapy Regimens

Grade 3–5 Event (%)[*]	Bendamustine (N = 338)	CHOP (N = 193)	CVP (N = 61)
Neutropenia	21.6	64.2	39.3
Infection	8.0	7.3	4.9
Second neoplasm	0	0	0

[*]According to the NCI Common Terminology Criteria for Adverse Events, version 4.0

Maintenance and Observation Phases for Obinutuzumab + Standard Chemotherapy Regimens

Grade 3–5 Event (%)[*]	Bendamustine (N = 312)	CHOP (N = 179)	CVP (N = 57)
Neutropenia	15.7	20.1	8.8
Infection	16.7	3.9	8.8
Second neoplasm	6.7	4.5	0

[*]According to the NCI Common Terminology Criteria for Adverse Events, version 4.0

Follow-up for Obinutuzumab + Standard Chemotherapy Regimens

Grade 3–5 Event (%)[*]	Bendamustine (N = 270)	CHOP (N = 128)	CVP (N = 44)
Neutropenia	2.2	1.6	0
Infection	9.3	1.6	2.3
Second neoplasm	5.2	0.8	0

[*]According to the NCI Common Terminology Criteria for Adverse Events, version 4.0

Note: Among all patients in the trial (including those on CHOP, CVP, or bendamustine), 4% of the obinutuzumab group and 3.4% of the rituximab group died as a result of adverse events; non-relapse-related fatal adverse events were less common among the patients who received CVP (1.6% and 1.8%, respectively) or CHOP (1.6% and 2.0%, respectively) than among the patients who received bendamustine (5.6% and 4.4%, respectively)

Therapy Monitoring

1. *Prior to treatment initiation*: CBC with differential, serum chemistries (potassium, uric acid, phosphorus, calcium, serum creatinine, LDH), serum bilirubin, ALT or AST, hepatitis B core antibody (IgG or total) and hepatitis B surface antigen, and urine pregnancy test (women of child-bearing potential only)

   – Hepatitis B virus (HBV) reactivation, in some cases resulting in fulminant hepatitis, hepatic failure, and death, can occur in patients receiving CD20-directed cytolytic antibodies, including obinutuzumab. Monitor HBV-positive patients during and after treatment with obinutuzumab, and consider antiviral prophylaxis. Discontinue obinutuzumab and lenalidomide in the event of HBV reactivation

2. *In patients at high risk for tumor lysis syndrome* consider frequent monitoring of laboratory indices of tumor lysis syndrome, intravenous hydration, and prophylaxis with a xanthine oxidase inhibitor (eg, allopurinol) following the initial dose of obinutuzumab

3. *Prior to each cycle of combination therapy*: CBC with differential and platelet count, serum chemistries, serum bilirubin, ALT or AST

4. *Weekly during combination (cyclophosphamide + vincristine + prednisone + obinutuzumab) treatment*: CBC with differential and platelet count

5. *Prior to each cycle of obinutuzumab monotherapy maintenance*: CBC with differential and platelet count

6. *Response assessment after cycle 4 and 8 of combination therapy, and then every 2–4 months during maintenance therapy*: CT scans or PET scans, physical exam, bone marrow evaluation (as clinically indicated)

FOLLICULAR LYMPHOMA • FIRST LINE
NON-HODGKIN LYMPHOMA REGIMEN: BENDAMUSTINE + RITUXIMAB

Rummel MJ et al. Lancet 2013;381:1203–1210

Note: this regimen was evaluated in follicular lymphoma, mantle cell lymphoma, and small lymphocytic lymphoma

Prophylaxis for tumor lysis syndrome is recommended for high-risk patients (eg, high tumor burden, bulky lymphadenopathy, or renal impairment):

- **Hydration**; encourage oral hydration (eg, ≥3 L/day) starting 1–2 days prior to the first rituximab dose. Consider administering additional *intravenous* hydration prior to the infusion if needed. Continue hydration prior to subsequent cycles if needed.

- **Allopurinol** 300 mg per dose; administer orally twice per day starting 12–24 hours prior to the first rituximab infusion for 7 days. Continue prophylaxis prior to subsequent cycles if needed.
  - Reduce allopurinol dose to 300 mg by mouth once daily for 7 days for patients with renal impairment

Bendamustine
Premedications for Bendamustine HCl: premedications are not necessary for primary prophylaxis of infusion-related reactions. In the event of a non-severe infusion-related reaction, consider adding a histamine receptor (H_1)-subtype antagonist (eg, diphenhydramine 25–50 mg intravenously or orally), an antipyretic (eg, acetaminophen 650–1000 mg orally), and a corticosteroid (eg, methylprednisolone 100 mg intravenously) administered 30 minutes prior to bendamustine HCl administration in subsequent cycles

Bendamustine HCl 90 mg/m^2 per dose; administer intravenously in a volume of 0.9% sodium chloride injection (0.9% NS) sufficient to produce a concentration with the range 0.2–0.7 mg/mL over 30–60 minutes, on 2 consecutive days, days 1 and 2, every 4 weeks for up to 6 cycles (total dosage/28-day cycle = 180 mg/m^2)
Note:
- Bendamustine HCl can cause severe infusion-related reactions
  - For grade 1–2 infusion-related reactions, consider rechallenge with the addition of antihistamine, antipyretic, and corticosteroid premedications (as described in the above premedication section)
  - For grade 3 infusion-related reactions, consider permanent discontinuation versus rechallenge with the addition of antihistamine, antipyretic, and corticosteroid premedications (as described in the above premedication section) after weighing risks and benefits
  - For grade 4 infusion-related reactions, permanently discontinue bendamustine HCl
- Coadministration of strong CYP1A2 inhibitors (eg, ciprofloxacin, fluvoxamine) may increase exposure to bendamustine HCl and decrease exposure to its active metabolites. Concomitant CYP1A2 inducers (eg, omeprazole, cigarette smoking) may decrease exposure to bendamustine HCl and increase exposure to its active metabolites. Use caution, or select an alternative therapy, when coadministration of bendamustine HCl with strong CYP1A2 inhibitors or inducers is unavoidable
- Bendamustine HCl formulations may vary by country; consult local regulatory-approved labeling for guidance. For example, in the U.S., the Food and Drug Administration approved Bendeka under Section 505(b)(2) of the Federal Food, Drug, and Cosmetic Act on 7 December 2015. The Bendeka product labeling contains specific dilution and administration instructions, *thus*:

  Bendamustine HCl (Bendeka, where available) 90 mg/m^2 per dose; administer intravenously in a volume of 0.9% NS or D5W sufficient to produce a concentration with the range 1.85–5.6 mg/mL, over 10 minutes, on 2 consecutive days, days 1 and 2, every 4 weeks for up to 6 cycles (total dosage/28-day cycle = 180 mg/m^2)

Premedication for rituximab:
Acetaminophen 650–1000 mg; administer orally *plus* **diphenhydramine** 25–50 mg; administer orally or intravenously 30–60 minutes before each dose of rituximab

Rituximab 375 mg/m^2; administer intravenously in 0.9% NS or 5% dextrose injection diluted to a concentration of 1–4 mg/mL on day 1, every 4 weeks for up to 6 cycles (total dosage/cycle = 375 mg/m^2)
Notes on rituximab administration:
- Infuse initially at 50 mg/h. If hypersensitivity or infusion reactions do not occur during the first 30 minutes, increase the rate by 50 mg/h every 30 minutes as tolerated to a maximum rate of 400 mg/h. Subsequently, if previous administration was well tolerated, start at 100 mg/h and increase by 100 mg/h every 30 minutes as tolerated to a maximum rate of 400 mg/h
- The regimen did not include maintenance or consolidation treatment with rituximab

INFUSION REACTIONS ASSOCIATED WITH RITUXIMAB
Note: Medications for the treatment of hypersensitivity reactions should be available for immediate use in the event of a reaction during administration (eg, intravenous fluids, epinephrine, antihistamines, glucocorticoids, and O_2)
Fevers, chills, and rigors
1. Interrupt rituximab administration for severe symptoms, and give:
   - **Acetaminophen** 650 mg orally for fever. For persistent or recurrent symptoms, repeat administration every 4–6 hours as needed during rituximab administration
   - **Diphenhydramine** 25–50 mg orally or by intravenous injection for pruritus, hypotension, or angioedema. For persistent or recurrent symptoms, repeat administration every 4–6 hours as needed during rituximab administration

(continued)

(continued)

- **Meperidine** 12.5–25 mg by intravenous injection every 10–20 minutes as needed for shaking chills (generally, cumulative doses >100 mg are not needed; use repeated doses with caution in persons with moderate or more severely impaired renal function)

2. If rituximab administration was interrupted, resume infusion at a slower rate than the maximum rate previously attempted. Rate escalation may be reattempted at smaller incremental steps with close monitoring. Do not exceed the maximum recommended rate of 400 mg/h

Dyspnea or wheezing without allergic findings (urticaria, or tongue or laryngeal edema)

1. Interrupt rituximab administration immediately
2. Give **hydrocortisone** 100 mg by intravenous injection (or an alternative steroid with equivalent glucocorticoid potency)
3. Give a **histamine (H₂) receptor antagonist** (ranitidine 50 mg, cimetidine 300 mg, or famotidine 20 mg) intravenously over 15–30 minutes
4. After symptoms resolve, resume rituximab administration at 25 mg/h with close monitoring. Do not increase the administration rate

Note: Medications and equipment for the treatment of hypersensitivity reactions should be available for immediate use in the event of a reaction during administration (eg, intravenous fluids, epinephrine, antihistamines, glucocorticoids, and oxygen)

Rituxan (rituximab) prescribing information. South San Francisco, CA: Genentech, Inc; 2018 October

Supportive Care

Antiemetic prophylaxis
Emetogenic potential is **MODERATE**
See Chapter 42 for antiemetic recommendations

Hematopoietic growth factor (CSF) prophylaxis
Primary prophylaxis **MAY** be indicated
See Chapter 43 for more information

Antimicrobial prophylaxis
Risk of fever and neutropenia is *INTERMEDIATE*
  Antimicrobial primary prophylaxis to be considered:
- Antibacterial—consider a fluoroquinolone or no prophylaxis; *Pneumocystis jirovecii* prophylaxis is recommended (eg, cotrimoxazole)
- Antifungal—recommended; consider use during periods of neutropenia, and in anticipation of mucositis
- Antiviral—antiherpes antivirals (eg, acyclovir, famciclovir, valacyclovir)

Treatment Modifications

Bendamustine Dose Modifications	
Starting dose	90 mg/m² per dose on days 1 and 2
Dose level –1	70 mg/m² per dose on days 1 and 2
Dose level –2	Discontinue bendamustine
There are no dose reductions for rituximab	

Hematologic Toxicity	
Day 1 platelet count <75,000/mm³ or day 1 ANC <1000/mm³	Delay start of cycle until platelet count ≥75,000/ mm³ and ANC ≥1000/ mm³ or until recovery to near baseline values, then reduce the bendamustine dosage by 1 dose level for subsequent cycles. Consider G-CSF use in subsequent cycles for dose-limiting neutropenia
G4 hematologic toxicity occurring in the previous cycle	Delay start of cycle until platelet count ≥75,000/ mm³ and ANC ≥1000/ mm³ or until recovery to near baseline values, then reduce the bendamustine dose by 1 dose level for subsequent cycles. Consider G-CSF use in subsequent cycles for dose-limiting neutropenia or severe neutropenic complications

Infectious Complications	
Active infection	Interrupt bendamustine and rituximab until resolution of infection, then resume treatment at either the same doses, or with the bendamustine dose reduced by one dose level, depending on the severity of infection
New or changes in pre-existing neurologic symptoms (eg, confusion, dizziness, loss of balance, vision problems, aphasia, ambulation issues)- PML suspected	Interrupt bendamustine and rituximab until central nervous system status clarified. Work-up may include (but is not limited to) consultation with a neurologist, brain MRI, and LP
PML is confirmed	Discontinue bendamustine and rituximab

(continued)

Treatment Modifications (*continued*)

HBV reactivation	Discontinue bendamustine and rituximab. Institute appropriate treatment for HBV. Upon resolution of HBV reactivation, resumption of bendamustine and rituximab should be discussed with a physician with expertise in management of HBV

Drug Interactions

Patient requires concomitant therapy with antihypertensive medication(s)	On days of rituximab treatment, and especially with the initial dose, weigh the risk versus benefit of delaying administration of the antihypertensive medication(s) until after completion of the rituximab infusion due to the potential risk of rituximab infusion-related hypotension
Live attenuated vaccine is indicated during or after rituximab administration	Avoid administration of a live attenuated vaccine during rituximab therapy and following therapy until adequate B-cell recovery has occurred
Patient requires concomitant therapy with a CYP1A2 inhibitor (eg, fluvoxamine, ciprofloxacin)	Consider alternative treatment instead of the CYP1A2 inhibitor. If the CYP1A2 inhibitor cannot be avoided, use caution and monitor carefully for bendamustine adverse effects. Do not modify the rituximab dose
Patient requires concomitant therapy with a CYP1A2 inducer (eg, omeprazole), or patient is a smoker	Consider alternative treatment instead of the CYP1A2 inducer. Recommend cessation of smoking, if applicable. If the CYP1A2 inducer cannot be avoided, use caution and monitor carefully for reduced bendamustine efficacy. Do not modify the rituximab dose

Other Toxicities

Clinically significant G2 nonhematologic toxicity during the prior cycle	Delay start of cycle until the nonhematologic toxicity resolves to G ≤1 or baseline, then resume treatment at the same dosages
Clinically significant G ≥3 nonhematologic toxicity during the prior cycle	Delay start of cycle until the nonhematologic toxicity resolves to G ≤1 or baseline, then resume treatment with the bendamustine dosage reduced by one dosage level

ANC, absolute neutrophil count; G-CSF, granulocyte-colony stimulating factor; PML, progressive multifocal leukoencephalopathy; MRI, magnetic resonance imaging; LP, lumbar puncture; HBV, hepatitis B virus.

Bendeka (bendamustine hydrochloride injection) prescribing information. North Wales, PA: Teva Pharmaceuticals USA, Inc; 2018 July

Patient Characteristics (N = 261 + 253 = 514)

Open-label, Multicenter, Randomized, Phase 3, Noninferiority Trial Comparing Bendamustine Plus Rituximab (B-R) versus Chop Plus Rituximab (Chop-R) as First-line Treatment for Patients with Indolent and Mantle Cell Lymphomas

	B-R (N = 261)	CHOP-R (N = 253)
Age (years)	64 (34–83)	63 (31–82)
<60	94 (36%)	90 (36%)
61–70	107 (41%)	105 (42%)
>70	60 (23%)	58 (23%)
Stage		
II	9 (3%)	9 (4%)
III	50 (19%)	47 (19%)
IV	202 (77%)	197 (78%)
Histology		
Follicular	139 (53%)	140 (55%)
Mantle cell	46 (18%)	48 (19%)
Marginal zone	37 (14%)	30 (12%)
Lymphoplasmacytic[a]	22 (8%)	19 (8%)
Small lymphocytic	10 (4%)	11 (4%)

(*continued*)

Patient Population Studied

Patients with a histologically confirmed mantle cell or indolent non-Hodgkin lymphoma, including CD20-positive subtypes: grades 1/2 follicular, lymphoplasmacytic (Waldenström's macroglobulinemia), small lymphocytic, and marginal-zone lymphoma. All had previously untreated stages III/IV disease, and patients with indolent lymphoma subtypes had at least 1 of the following criteria: impaired hemopoiesis (Hgb <10 g/dL, ANC <1500/mm³, or platelet count <100,000/mm³); presence of B symptoms; large tumor burden (3 areas >5 cm or 1 area >7.5 cm); bulky disease with impingement on internal organs; progressive disease, defined as a more than 50% increase of tumor mass within 6 months; or a hyperviscosity syndrome. Patients younger than 65 years with mantle cell lymphoma were referred to clinical trials incorporating autologous stem cell transplantation

Low grade, unclassifiable	7 (3%)	5 (2%)
B symptoms	100 (38%)	74 (29%)
Bone marrow involved	177 (68%)	170 (67%)
Extranodal involved sites ≥1	212 (81%)	193 (76%)
Lactate dehydrogenase >240 U/L	100 (38%)	84 (33%)
Median β_2-microglobulin (mg/L)	2.6 (0.7–17.8)	2.4 (1.1–23.2)
Prognostic groups for all patients (IPI)		
>2 risk factors	96 (37%)	89 (35%)
Prognostic groups according to FLIPI		
Low risk (0–1 risk factor)	16/139 (12%)	26/140 (19%)
Intermediate risk (2 risk factors)	57/139 (41%)	44/140 (31%)
Poor risk (3–5 risk factors)	63/136 (46%)	64/134 (48%)

FLIPI, Follicular Lymphoma International Prognostic Index

Efficacy

(N = 514)

Open-label, Multicenter, Randomized, Phase 3, Noninferiority Trial Comparing Bendamustine Plus Rituximab versus CHOP Plus Rituximab as First-line Treatment for Patients with Indolent and Mantle Cell Lymphomas

	Bendamustine + R (N = 261)	CHOP + R (N = 253)	HR (95% CI) P Value
Median PFS[*†]	69.5 months (26.1–NR)	31.2 months (15.2–65.7)	0.58 (0.44–0.74) <0.0001
Overall response rate	242 (93%)	231 (91%)	
Complete response	104 (40%)	76 (30)	0.021

Exploratory Subgroup Analysis to Assess the Progression-free Survival Benefit of Bendamustine Plus Rituximab versus CHOP Plus Rituximab

	HR (95% CI)	P Value
Age (years)		
≤60 (N = 199)	0.52 (0.33–0.79)	0.002
>60 (N = 315)	0.62 (0.45–0.84)	0.002
LDH concentration		
Normal (N = 319)	0.48 (0.34–0.67)	<0.0001
Elevated (N = 184)	0.74 (0.50–1.08)	0.118
FLIPI subgroup		
Favorable (0–2 risk factors; N = 143)	0.56 (0.31–0.98)	0.043
Unfavorable (3–5 risk factors; N = 127)	0.63 (0.38–1.04)	0.068

FLIPI, Follicular Lymphoma International Prognostic Index; HR, hazard ratio; LDH, lactate dehydrogenase; NR, not reached; PFS, progression-free survival; R, rituximab

[*]Progression-free survival at median follow-up of 45 months (IQR 25–57)

[†]A significant benefit for PFS was shown with bendamustine + R versus CHOP + R for all histologic subtypes, except for marginal-zone lymphoma

Toxicity

Hematologic Toxic Events in Patients Receiving ≥1 Dose of Study Treatment

Toxicity	G1		G2		G3		G4		G3/4	
	R-C	B-R	R-C	B-R	R-C	B-R	R-C	B-R	R-C	B-R
Leukocytopenia	13 (5%)	52 (19%)	39 (15%)	80 (30%)	110 (44%)	85 (32%)	71 (28%)	13 (5%)	181 (72%)*	98 (37%)*
Neutropenia	6 (2%)	30 (11%)	19 (8%)	61 (23%)	70 (28%)	53 (20%)	103 (41%)	24 (9%)	173 (69%)*	77 (29%)*
Lymphocytopenia	12 (5%)	14 (5%)	72 (29%)	38 (14%)	87 (35%)	122 (46%)	19 (8%)	74 (28%)	106 (43%)	196 (74%)
Anemia	115 (46%)	102 (38%)	84 (33%)	44 (16%)	10 (4%)	6 (2%)	2 (<1%)	2 (<1%)	12 (5%)	8 (3%)
Thrombocytopenia	89 (35%)	104 (39%)	20 (8%)	19 (7%)	11 (4%)	15 (6%)	5 (2%)	2 (<1%)	16 (6%)	13 (5%)

B-R, bendamustine + rituximab; R-C, rituximab + cyclophosphamide + doxorubicin + vincristine + prednisone (R-CHOP)
*P<0.0001 between groups

All Grades of Nonhematologic Toxic Events in Patients Receiving ≥1 Dose of Study Treatment

	Bendamustine + R (N = 261)	CHOP + R (N = 253)	P
Alopecia	0	245 (100%)*	<0.0001
Paresthesia	18 (7%)	73 (29%)	<0.0001
Stomatitis	16 (6%)	47 (19%)	<0.0001
Skin (erythema)	42 (16%)	23 (9%)	0.024
Skin (allergic reaction)	40 (15%)	15 (6%)	0.0006
Infectious episodes	96 (37%)	127 (50%)	0.0025
Sepsis	1 (<1%)	8 (3%)	0.019

CHOP + R, cyclophosphamide + doxorubicin + vincristine + prednisone + rituximab (R-CHOP); R, rituximab
*Includes only patients who received 3 or more cycles

Treatment Monitoring

1. *Before treatment:* physical examination; CBC with differential; assessment of serum chemistry; serum immunoelectrophoresis; measurement of immunoglobulin concentrations; hepatitis B core antibody (IgG or total) and hepatitis B surface antigen; urine pregnancy test in women of child-bearing potential; CT or PET scan of the chest, abdomen, and pelvis; sonography of the abdomen; and bone marrow aspiration and biopsy as indicated. If clinically relevant, endoscopy of the gastrointestinal tract is performed

2. *Prior to each cycle:* CBC with differential, serum chemistries, serum bilirubin, ALT or AST

3. *During each rituximab infusion and for at least 1 hour after infusion completion:* Signs and symptoms of infusion-related reaction, vital signs every 30 minutes

4. *Weekly:* CBC with differential

5. *Monitor periodically for:* Signs and symptoms of infection (including progressive multifocal leukoencephalopathy) and dermatologic toxicity

6. *Assessment of efficacy:* Physical examination, CBC with differential, CT scans or PET scan, bone marrow evaluation (if clinically indicated), endoscopy (if clinically indicated) after cycles 3 and 6, or at the end of treatment

FOLLICULAR LYMPHOMA • FIRST LINE

NON-HODGKIN LYMPHOMA REGIMEN: BENDAMUSTINE + OBINUTUZUMAB

Marcus R et al. N Engl J Med 2017;377:133–1344
Supplementary Appendix to: Marcus R et al. N Engl J Med 2017;377:1331–1344
Protocol for: Marcus R et al. N Engl J Med 2017;377:1331–1344
Gazvya (obinutuzumab) prescribing information. South San Francisco, CA: Genentech, Inc; 2017 November

The regimen consists of six 28-day cycles of bendamustine plus obinutuzumab. Patients who achieve a complete response or partial response to the initial 6 cycles of combination therapy should then continue obinutuzumab monotherapy maintenance every 8 weeks for up to 2 years

Prophylaxis for tumor lysis syndrome is recommended for high-risk patients (eg, high tumor burden, bulky lymphadenopathy, or renal impairment):

• Hydration; encourage oral hydration (eg, ≥3 L/day) starting 1–2 days prior to the first obinutuzumab dose. Consider administering additional *intravenous* hydration prior to the infusion if needed. Continue hydration prior to subsequent obinutuzumab infusions if needed

• **Allopurinol** 300 mg per dose; administer orally twice per day starting 12–24 hours prior to the first obinutuzumab infusion for 7 days. Continue prophylaxis prior to subsequent obinutuzumab infusions if needed

   – Reduce allopurinol dose to 300 mg by mouth once daily for 7 days for patients with renal impairment

Bendamustine

Premedication for bendamustine HCl: Premedication is not necessary for primary prophylaxis of bendamustine infusion-related reactions. In the event of a non-severe infusion-related reaction, consider adding a histamine receptor (H_1)-subtype antagonist (eg, diphenhydramine 25–50 mg intravenously or orally), an antipyretic (eg, acetaminophen 650–1000 mg orally), and a corticosteroid (eg, methylprednisolone 100 mg intravenously) administered 30 minutes prior to bendamustine HCl administration in subsequent cycles

Bendamustine HCl 90 mg/m^2 per dose; administer intravenously in a volume of 0.9% sodium chloride injection (0.9% NS) sufficient to produce a concentration with the range 0.2–0.6 mg/mL over 60 minutes, on 2 consecutive days, days 1 and 2, every 28 days for 6 cycles (total dosage/28-day cycle = 180 mg/m^2)

Note:

• Administer after obinutuzumab on days when both bendamustine and obinutuzumab are administered

• Bendamustine HCl can cause severe infusion-related reactions

   – For grade 1–2 infusion-related reactions, consider rechallenge with the addition of antihistamine, antipyretic, and corticosteroid premedications (as described previously)

   – For grade 3 infusion-related reactions, consider permanent discontinuation versus rechallenge with the addition of antihistamine, antipyretic, and corticosteroid premedications (as described previously) after weighing risks and benefits

   – For grade 4 infusion-related reactions, permanently discontinue bendamustine HCl

Note:

• Coadministration of strong CYP1A2 inhibitors (eg, ciprofloxacin, fluvoxamine) may increase exposure to bendamustine HCl and decrease exposure to its active metabolites. Concomitant CYP1A2 inducers (eg, omeprazole, cigarette smoking) may decrease exposure to bendamustine HCl and increase exposure to its active metabolites. Use caution, or select an alternative therapy, when coadministration of bendamustine HCl with strong CYP1A2 inhibitors or inducers is unavoidable

• Bendamustine HCl formulations may vary by country; consult local regulatory-approved labeling for guidance. For example, in the United States, the Food and Drug Administration approved Bendeka under Section 505(b)(2) of the Federal Food, Drug, and Cosmetic Act on December 7, 2015. The Bendeka product labeling contains specific dilution and administration instructions, *thus*:

   – **Bendamustine HCl (Bendeka, where available)** 90 mg/m^2 per dose; administer intravenously in a volume of 0.9% NS or 5% dextrose injection (D5W) sufficient to produce a concentration with the range 1.85–5.6 mg/mL, over 10 minutes, on 2 consecutive days, days 1 and 2, every 28 days for 6 cycles (total dosage/28-day cycle = 180 mg/m^2)

Premedication for obinutuzumab:

• **Acetaminophen** 650–1000 mg; administer orally at least 30 minutes prior to each dose of obinutuzumab

• **Diphenhydramine** 50 mg; administer orally or intravenously at least 30 minutes prior to obinutuzumab

   – Required for the cycle 1, day 1 infusion

   – Required for subsequent infusions only if the previous infusion was complicated by a grade 1–3 infusion-related reaction

• Corticosteroid premedication is required for the cycle 1, day 1 infusion. For subsequent infusions, administer corticosteroid premedication only if the absolute lymphocyte count is >25 × 10^9/L *or* if the previous dose was complicated by a grade 3 infusion-related reaction. Choose only *one* of the following options, when indicated:

   – **Dexamethasone** 20 mg; administer intravenously at least 1 hour prior to obinutuzumab, *or*

   – **Methylprednisolone** 80 mg; administer intravenously at least 1 hour prior to obinutuzumab

Obinutuzumab; administer intravenously diluted in 0.9% sodium chloride (0.9% NS) injection to a final concentration ranging from 0.4–4 mg/mL (see table for dose, dilution, infusion rate, and schedule information)

Note:

- Administer prior to bendamustine on days where both obinutuzumab and bendamustine are administered
- Hepatitis B virus (HBV) reactivation, in some cases resulting in fulminant hepatitis, hepatic failure, and death, can occur in patients receiving CD20-directed cytolytic antibodies, including obinutuzumab. Screen all patients for HBV infection before treatment initiation. Monitor HBV-positive patients during and after treatment with obinutuzumab, and consider antiviral prophylaxis. Discontinue obinutuzumab and concomitant medications in the event of HBV reactivation
- Obinutuzumab can cause severe and life-threatening infusion reactions. Symptoms may include hypotension, tachycardia, dyspnea, and respiratory symptoms (eg, bronchospasm, larynx and throat irritation, wheezing, laryngeal edema). Other common symptoms include nausea, vomiting, diarrhea, hypertension, flushing, headache, pyrexia, and chills
  - Sixty percent of previously untreated non-Hodgkin lymphoma patients experienced a reaction to the first infusion of obinutuzumab. Infusion reactions can also occur with subsequent infusions
- Hypotension may occur as an infusion reaction. Consider withholding antihypertensive treatments for 12 hours prior to and during each obinutuzumab infusion, and for the first hour after administration until blood pressure is stable

Obinutuzumab Dosage and Schedule During Combination Therapy with Bendamustine (Six 28-day cycles)

Cycle and Day*	Obinutuzumab Dose	Volume of 0.9% NS for Dilution	Obinutuzumab Administration	Total Dose per Cycle*
Cycle 1 Day 1	1000 mg	250 mL	Begin infusion at 50 mg/h, and increase by 50 mg/h every 30 minutes to a maximum rate of 400 mg/h	Cycle 1 = 3000 mg
Cycle 1 Day 8	1000 mg	250 mL	If no infusion reaction occurred during previous dose and the final infusion rate was ≥100 mg/h, start at 100 mg/h, and increase by 100 mg/h every 30 minutes to a maximum rate of 400 mg/h. If an infusion reaction occurred during previous dose, begin infusion at 50 mg/h, and increase by 50 mg/h every 30 minutes to a maximum rate of 400 mg/h	
Cycle 1 Day 15	1000 mg	250 mL		
Cycles 2–6 Day 1 only	1000 mg	250 mL	If no infusion reaction occurred during previous dose and the final infusion rate was ≥100 mg/h, start at 100 mg/h, and increase by 100 mg/h every 30 minutes to a maximum rate of 400 mg/h. If an infusion reaction occurred during previous dose, begin infusion at 50 mg/h, and increase by 50 mg/h every 30 minutes to a maximum rate of 400 mg/h	Cycles 2–6 = 1000 mg

*Cycle length = 28 days

Obinutuzumab Dosage and Schedule During Monotherapy Maintenance—every 8 weeks for up to 2 years, for patients who achieve a complete response or partial response to the initial 6 cycles of combination therapy

Schedule†	Obinutuzumab Dose	Volume of 0.9% NS for Dilution	Obinutuzumab Administration	Total Dose per Cycle†
Maintenance cycles (every 8 weeks for up to 2 years)	1000 mg	250 mL	If no infusion reaction occurred during previous dose and the final infusion rate was ≥100 mg/h, start at 100 mg/h, and increase by 100 mg/h every 30 minutes to a maximum rate of 400 mg/h. If an infusion reaction occurred during the previous dose, begin infusion at 50 mg/h, and increase by 50 mg/h every 30 minutes to a maximum rate of 400 mg/h	Maintenance therapy = 1000 mg

†Obinutuzumab maintenance cycle length = 8 weeks (56 days) for up to 2 years

Obinutuzumab Infusion-Related Toxicities

Note: Medications and equipment for the treatment of hypersensitivity reactions should be available for immediate use in the event of a reaction during obinutuzumab administration (eg, intravenous fluids, epinephrine, antihistamines, glucocorticoids, and oxygen)

- G ≤2 obinutuzumab infusion-related reaction
- G3 obinutuzumab infusion-related reaction, first occurrence
1. Interrupt obinutuzumab infusion
2. For fever, chills: Give additional dose of acetaminophen 650 mg orally and diphenhydramine 25–50 mg by intravenous push

(continued)

(*continued*)

3. For dyspnea/wheezing: Give additional dose of diphenhydramine 25–50 mg by intravenous push. Give a histamine H_2-antagonist (ranitidine 50 mg or famotidine 20 mg) by intravenous push. Give hydrocortisone 100 mg (or glucocorticoid equivalent) by intravenous push

4. For rigors: Give meperidine 12.5–25 mg by intravenous push ± promethazine 12.5–25 mg by intravenous infusion in at least 10 mL 0.9% NS or D5W over 5–15 minutes. If after 15–20 minutes the response to a single dose is considered inadequate, the dose may be repeated

5. After symptoms resolve, resume obinutuzumab infusion at a minimum of 50% reduction in the rate at which the event occurred. If no further infusion-related events, increase the infusion rate at the increments and intervals as appropriate for the treatment cycle dose. If G3 infusion-related reaction recurs during rechallenge, then permanently discontinue obinutuzumab

Refer to the "Premedications for obinutuzumab" section within the regimen description to determine appropriate premedications for the subsequent cycle

– **G3 obinutuzumab infusion-related reaction, recurrent (following rechallenge on the same day of treatment)**
– **G4 obinutuzumab infusion-related reaction**
– **Serum sickness or hypersensitivity reaction**

1. Permanently discontinue obinutuzumab and provide supportive care

Supportive Care
Antiemetic prophylaxis
Emetogenic potential of bendamustine hydrochloride is **MODERATE**
Emetogenic potential of obinutuzumab is **MINIMAL**
See Chapter 42 for antiemetic recommendations

Hematopoietic growth factor (CSF) prophylaxis
Primary prophylaxis **MAY** *be indicated*
See Chapter 43 for more information

Antimicrobial prophylaxis
Risk of fever and neutropenia is *INTERMEDIATE*
Antimicrobial primary prophylaxis to be considered:
• Antibacterial—consider a fluoroquinolone during periods of prolonged neutropenia, or no prophylaxis
• Antifungal—consider use during periods of prolonged neutropenia
• Antiviral—antiherpes antivirals (eg, acyclovir, famciclovir, valacyclovir)

Treatment Modifications

Bendamustine + Obinutuzumab	
Bendamustine starting dose	90 mg/m² per day on days 1 and 2, every 28 days
There are no dose reductions for obinutuzumab	

Adverse Event	Dose Modification
Infectious Complications	
G2 infection	Interrupt both bendamustine and obinutuzumab until resolution of infection, then resume obinutuzumab and bendamustine at the same dose
G ≥3 infection	Interrupt both bendamustine and obinutuzumab until resolution of infection, then resume obinutuzumab at the same dose, and resume bendamustine at a dosage of 60 mg/m² per dose
New or changes in preexisting neurologic symptoms (eg, confusion, dizziness, loss of balance, vision problems, aphasia, ambulation issues); PML suspected	Interrupt both bendamustine and obinutuzumab until central nervous system status is clarified. Work-up may include (but is not limited to) consultation with a neurologist, brain MRI, and LP
PML is confirmed	Discontinue obinutuzumab and bendamustine
HBV reactivation	Discontinue obinutuzumab and bendamustine. Institute appropriate treatment for HBV. Upon resolution of HBV reactivation, resumption of obinutuzumab and bendamustine should be discussed with a physician with expertise in management of HBV. Insufficient data exist to determine the safety of resumption of obinutuzumab and bendamustine in this setting

(*continued*)

Treatment Modifications (*continued*)

Hematologic Toxicity During Combination Therapy	
First episode of any of the following during combination therapy: G3 neutropenia (ANC ≥500/mm³ to <1000/mm³) or G4 neutropenia (ANC <500/mm³) or G3 thrombocytopenia (platelet count ≥25,000/mm³ to <50,000/mm³) or G4 thrombocytopenia (platelet count <25,000/mm³)	Delay bendamustine and obinutuzumab administration until improvement to G ≤2 or baseline. Consider increasing frequency of CBC with differential monitoring. Consider transfusion of platelets or red blood cells, or treatment with G-CSF, as indicated. For G ≥3 neutropenia persisting for >1 week, consider prophylaxis with antibiotic (strongly recommended) (eg, ciprofloxacin), antiviral (eg, acyclovir), and antifungal (eg, fluconazole) until improvement of neutropenia to G ≤2. For G ≥3 thrombocytopenia, consider holding concomitant antiplatelet and anticoagulation medications, if applicable. If toxicity improves to G ≤2 or baseline, decrease the bendamustine dosage to 70 mg/m² per dose for subsequent cycles. Do not reduce the dosage of obinutuzumab
Second episode of any of the following during combination therapy: G3 neutropenia (ANC ≥500/mm³ to <1000/mm³) or G4 neutropenia (ANC <500/mm³) or G3 thrombocytopenia (platelet count ≥25,000/mm³ to <50,000/mm³) or G4 thrombocytopenia (platelet count <25,000/mm³)	Delay bendamustine and obinutuzumab administration until improvement to G ≤2 or baseline. Consider increasing the frequency of CBC with differential monitoring Consider transfusion of platelets or red blood cells, or treatment with G-CSF, as indicated. For G ≥3 neutropenia persisting for >1 week, consider prophylaxis with antibiotic (strongly recommended) (eg, ciprofloxacin), antiviral (eg, acyclovir), and antifungal (eg, fluconazole) until improvement of neutropenia to G ≤2. For G ≥3 thrombocytopenia, consider holding concomitant antiplatelet and anticoagulation medications, if applicable If toxicity improves to G ≤2 or baseline, decrease the bendamustine dosage to 60 mg/m² per dose for subsequent cycles. Do not reduce the dosage of obinutuzumab
Third episode of any of the following during combination therapy: G3 neutropenia (ANC ≥500/mm³ to <1000/mm³) or G4 neutropenia (ANC <500/mm³) or G3 thrombocytopenia (platelet count ≥25,000/mm³ to <50,000/mm³) or G4 thrombocytopenia (platelet count <25,000/mm³)	Delay bendamustine and obinutuzumab administration until improvement to G ≤2 or baseline. Consider increasing the frequency of CBC with differential monitoring Consider transfusion of platelets or red blood cells, or treatment with G-CSF, as indicated. For G ≥3 neutropenia persisting for >1 week, consider prophylaxis with antibiotic (strongly recommended) (eg, ciprofloxacin), antiviral (eg, acyclovir), and antifungal (eg, fluconazole) until improvement of neutropenia to G ≤2. For G ≥3 thrombocytopenia, consider holding concomitant antiplatelet and anticoagulation medications, if applicable If toxicity improves to G ≤2 or baseline, decrease the bendamustine dosage to 50 mg/m² per dose for subsequent cycles. Do not reduce the dosage of obinutuzumab
Fourth episode of any of the following during combination therapy: G3 neutropenia (ANC ≥500/mm³ to <1000/mm³) or G4 neutropenia (ANC <500/mm³) or G3 thrombocytopenia (platelet count ≥25,000/mm³ to <50,000/mm³) or G4 thrombocytopenia (platelet count <25,000/mm³)	Discontinue bendamustine. Delay obinutuzumab administration until improvement to G ≤2 or baseline. Consider increasing the frequency of CBC with differential monitoring Consider transfusion of platelets or red blood cells, or treatment with G-CSF, as indicated. For G ≥3 neutropenia persisting for >1 week, consider prophylaxis with antibiotic (strongly recommended) (eg, ciprofloxacin), antiviral (eg, acyclovir), and antifungal (eg, fluconazole) until improvement of neutropenia to G ≤2. For G ≥3 thrombocytopenia, consider holding concomitant antiplatelet and anticoagulation medications, if applicable If toxicity improves to G ≤2 or baseline, continue full dose of obinutuzumab
Fifth episode of any of the following during combination therapy: G3 neutropenia (ANC ≥500/mm³ to <1000/mm³) or G4 neutropenia (ANC <500/mm³) or G3 thrombocytopenia (platelet count ≥25,000/mm³ to <50,000/mm³) or G4 thrombocytopenia (platelet count <25,000/mm³)	Discontinue all treatment

(*continued*)

Treatment Modifications (continued)

Hematologic Toxicity During Obinutuzumab Monotherapy Maintenance

G ≥3 hematologic toxicity during obinutuzumab monotherapy maintenance	Delay obinutuzumab for up to 42 days until improvement to G ≤2 or baseline. Consider increasing the frequency of CBC with differential monitoring
	Consider transfusion of platelets or red blood cells, or treatment with G-CSF, as indicated. For G ≥3 neutropenia persisting for >1 week, consider prophylaxis with antibiotic (strongly recommended) (eg, ciprofloxacin), antiviral (eg, acyclovir), and antifungal (eg, fluconazole) until improvement of neutropenia to G ≤2. For G ≥3 thrombocytopenia, consider holding concomitant antiplatelet and anticoagulation medications, if applicable
	If toxicity improves to G ≤2 or baseline, administer the same dosage of obinutuzumab

Drug Interactions

Patient requires concomitant therapy with a CYP1A2 inhibitor (eg, fluvoxamine, ciprofloxacin)	Consider alternative treatment instead of the CYP1A2 inhibitor. If the CYP1A2 inhibitor cannot be avoided, use caution, and monitor carefully for bendamustine adverse effects. Do not modify the obinutuzumab dosage
Patient requires concomitant therapy with a CYP1A2 inducer (eg, omeprazole), or patient is a smoker	Consider alternative treatment instead of the CYP1A2 inducer. Recommend cessation of smoking, if applicable. If the CYP1A2 inducer cannot be avoided, use caution, and monitor carefully for reduced bendamustine efficacy. Do not modify the obinutuzumab dosage
Patient requires concomitant therapy with antihypertensive medication(s)	On days of obinutuzumab treatment, and especially with the initial dose, weigh the risk versus benefit of delaying administration of the antihypertensive medication(s) until after completion of the obinutuzumab infusion due to the potential risk of obinutuzumab infusion-related hypotension
Live attenuated vaccine is indicated during or after obinutuzumab and bendamustine administration	Avoid administration of a live attenuated vaccine during obinutuzumab therapy and following therapy until adequate B-cell recovery has occurred

Other Toxicities During Combination Therapy

G2 nonhematologic toxicity during combination therapy	Consider interruption of bendamustine and obinutuzumab. Upon resolution of toxicity to G ≤1 or baseline, resume bendamustine and obinutuzumab at the same dosages
First episode of G ≥3 nonhematologic toxicity during combination therapy	Delay bendamustine and obinutuzumab administration until improvement to G ≤1 or baseline, then decrease the bendamustine dosage to 60 mg/m² per dose for subsequent cycles. Do not reduce the obinutuzumab dosage
Second episode of G ≥3 nonhematologic toxicity during combination therapy	Discontinue bendamustine. Delay obinutuzumab administration until improvement to G ≤1 or baseline, then continue obinutuzumab at the same dosage
Third episode of G ≥3 nonhematologic toxicity during combination therapy	Discontinue all treatment

Other Toxicities During Obinutuzumab Monotherapy Maintenance

G ≥2 nonhematologic toxicity during obinutuzumab monotherapy maintenance	Delay obinutuzumab for up to 42 days. If improvement to G ≤1 or baseline, then administer the same dosage of obinutuzumab

PML, progressive multifocal leukoencephalopathy; MRI, magnetic resonance imaging; LP, lumbar puncture; HBV, hepatitis B virus; ANC, absolute neutrophil count; CBC, complete blood count; G-CSF, granulocyte-colony stimulating factor

Note:

1. Medications and equipment for the treatment of hypersensitivity reactions should be available for immediate use in the event of a reaction during obinutuzumab administration (eg, intravenous fluids, epinephrine, antihistamines, glucocorticoids, and oxygen)
2. Embryo-fetal risk: Obinutuzumab is likely to cause fetal B-cell depletion in pregnant women based on animal studies and its known mechanism of action. There are no data with obinutuzumab use in pregnant women. Advise females of reproductive potential of the potential risk to a fetus with obinutuzumab. Bendamustine hydrochloride may cause fetal harm. Advise females of reproductive potential of the potential risk to a fetus and to use effective contraception during therapy

Gazyva (obinutuzumab) prescribing information. South San Francisco, CA: Genentech, Inc; 2017 November
Bendeka (bendamustine hydrochloride injection) prescribing information. North Wales, PA: Teva Pharmaceuticals USA, Inc; 2018 July
Marcus R et al. N Engl J Med 2017;277:1331–1344
Supplementary Appendix to: Marcus R et al. N Engl J Med 2017;277:1331–1344
Protocol for: Marcus R et al. N Engl J Med 2017;277:1331–1344

Patient Population Studied

This was a post hoc analysis of a multicenter, randomized, open-label, phase 3 trial (GALLIUM) involving 1202 patients with previously untreated, advanced, CD20-positive follicular lymphoma. Eligible patients were aged ≥18 years and had an Eastern Cooperative Oncology Group (ECOG) performance status score ≤2. Patients were randomly assigned 1:1 to receive intravenous obinutuzumab (1000 mg on days 1, 8, and 15 of cycle 1 and on day 1 only of subsequent cycles) or rituximab (375 mg/m² on day 1) in addition to standard chemotherapy regimens of: intravenous cyclophosphamide (750 mg/m² on day 1), doxorubicin (50 mg/m² on day 1), and vincristine (1.4 mg/m² [maximum dose 2 mg] on day 1), and oral prednisone (100 mg per day on days 1–5) (CHOP) for six 21-day cycles; intravenous cyclophosphamide (750 mg/m² on day 1) and vincristine (1.4 mg/m² [maximum dose 2 mg] on day 1), and oral prednisone (100 mg per day on days 1–5) (CVP) for eight 21-day cycles; or intravenous bendamustine (90 mg/m² on days 1 and 2) for six 28-day cycles. When combined with CHOP or CVP, obinutuzumab and rituximab were administered for eight 21-day cycles; when combined with bendamustine, obinutuzumab and rituximab were administered for six 28-day cycles. At the end of the induction therapy, patients who had a complete or partial response received maintenance treatment of the same study drug (intravenous obinutuzumab 1000 mg or rituximab 375 mg/m²) every 2 months for 2 years or until disease progression or withdrawal from trial. Of the 1202 patients involved in the trial, 345 were assigned to bendamustine + obinutuzumab, and 341 were assigned to bendamustine + rituximab

Efficacy

(N = 686)

	Obinutuzumab + Bendamustine (N = 345)	Rituximab + Bendamustine (N = 341)	
1-year progression-free survival	93.9%	89%	HR 0.61 95% CI 0.43–0.86

Note: The median follow-up among all trial participants was 34.5 months

Toxicity

	Induction Phase		Maintenance and Observation Phases		Follow-up	
Grade 3–5 Event (%)[*]	Bendamustine + Obinutuzumab (N = 338)	Bendamustine + Rituximab (N = 338)	Bendamustine + Obinutuzumab (N = 312)	Bendamustine + Rituximab (N = 305)	Bendamustine + Obinutuzumab (N = 270)	Bendamustine + Rituximab (N = 263)
Neutropenia	21.6	25.7	15.7	9.5	2.2	0.4
Infection	8.0	7.7	16.7	12.8	9.3	2.3
Second neoplasm	0	0	6.7	5.9	5.2	0.8

[*]According to the National Cancer Institute Common Terminology Criteria for Adverse Events, version 4.0

Induction Phase for Obinutuzumab + Standard Chemotherapy Regimens

Grade 3–5 Event (%)[*]	Bendamustine (N = 338)	CHOP (N = 193)	CVP (N = 61)
Neutropenia	21.6	64.2	39.3
Infection	8.0	7.3	4.9
Second neoplasm	0	0	0

[*]According to the National Cancer Institute Common Terminology Criteria for Adverse Events, version 4.0

Maintenance and Observation Phases for Obinutuzumab + Standard Chemotherapy Regimens

Grade 3–5 Event (%)[*]	Bendamustine (N = 312)	CHOP (N = 179)	CVP (N = 57)
Neutropenia	15.7	20.1	8.8
Infection	16.7	3.9	8.8
Second neoplasm	6.7	4.5	0

[*]According to the National Cancer Institute Common Terminology Criteria for Adverse Events, version 4.0

(continued)

Toxicity (continued)

Follow-up for Obinutuzumab + Standard Chemotherapy Regimens

Grade 3–5 Event (%)*	Bendamustine (N = 270)	CHOP (N = 128)	CVP (N = 44)
Neutropenia	2.2	1.6	0
Infection	9.3	1.6	2.3
Second neoplasm	5.2	0.8	0

*According to the National Cancer Institute Common Terminology Criteria for Adverse Events, version 4.0

Note: Among the various chemotherapy regimens used, patients treated with bendamustine had higher rates of grade 3–5 infection and second neoplasm during the maintenance and follow-up phases than those treated with CHOP or CVP. Among all patients in the trial (including those on CHOP, CVP, or bendamustine), 4.0% of the obinutuzumab group and 3.4% of the rituximab group died as a result of adverse events; non-relapse-related fatal adverse events were more common among the patients who received bendamustine (5.6% and 4.4%, respectively) than among the patients who received CHOP (1.6% and 2.0%, respectively) or CVP (1.6% and 1.8%, respectively)

Therapy Monitoring

1. *Prior to treatment initiation:* CBC with differential and platelet count, serum chemistries (potassium, uric acid, phosphorus, calcium, serum creatinine, LDH), serum bilirubin, ALT or AST, hepatitis B core antibody (IgG or total) and hepatitis B core antigen, urine pregnancy test (women of child-bearing potential only)
   - Hepatitis B virus (HBV) reactivation, in some cases resulting in fulminant hepatitis, hepatic failure, and death, can occur in patients receiving CD20-directed cytolytic antibodies, including obinutuzumab. Monitor HBV-positive patients during and after treatment with obinutuzumab, and consider antiviral prophylaxis. Discontinue obinutuzumab and lenalidomide in the event of HBV reactivation
2. *During each obinutuzumab infusion and for at least 1 hour after infusion completion:* Signs and symptoms of infusion-related reaction, vital signs every 30 minutes
3. *In patients at high risk for tumor lysis* consider frequent monitoring of laboratory indices of tumor lysis syndrome, intravenous hydration, and prophylaxis with a xanthine oxidase inhibitor (eg, allopurinol) following the initial dose of obinutuzumab
4. *Prior to each cycle of combination therapy:* CBC with differential and platelet count, serum chemistries, serum bilirubin, ALT or AST
5. *Weekly during combination (bendamustine and obinutuzumab) treatment:* CBC with differential and platelet count
6. *Monitor periodically for:* Signs and symptoms of infection (including progressive multifocal leukoencephalopathy) and dermatologic toxicity
7. *Prior to each cycle of obinutuzumab monotherapy maintenance:* CBC with differential and platelet count
8. *Response assessment after cycle 3 and 6 of combination therapy, and then every 2–4 months during maintenance therapy:* CT scan or PET scan, physical exam, bone marrow evaluation (as clinically indicated)

FOLLICULAR LYMPHOMA • FIRST LINE
NON-HODGKIN LYMPHOMA REGIMEN: LENALIDOMIDE + RITUXIMAB

Morschhauser F et al. N Engl J Med 2018;379:934–947
Supplementary appendix to: Morschhauser F et al. N Engl J Med 2018;379:934–947
Protocol for: Morschhauser F et al. N Engl J Med 2018;379:934–947
Martin P et al. Ann Oncol 2017;28:2806–2812
Fowler NH et al. Lancet Oncol 2014;15:1311–1318

RITUXIMAB
Rituximab (cycle 1 [loading cycle]: rituximab weekly × 4 doses)
Premedication for rituximab:
Acetaminophen 650–1000 mg; administer orally 30–60 minutes before each rituximab dose, *plus*
Diphenhydramine 25–50 mg; administer orally or intravenously 30–60 minutes before each rituximab dose
Rituximab 375 mg/m^2 per dose; administer intravenously in 0.9% sodium chloride (0.9% NS) or 5% dextrose injection (D5W), diluted to a concentration within the range 1–4 mg/mL, for 4 doses on days 1, 8, 15, and 22 for 1 loading dose cycle, cycle 1, only (total dosage/28-day cycle during cycle 1 = 1500 mg/m^2), *followed by*

Rituximab (cycles 2–6 [induction cycles]; rituximab every 4 weeks × 5 cycles)
Premedication for rituximab:
Acetaminophen 650–1000 mg; administer orally 30–60 minutes before each rituximab dose, *plus*
Diphenhydramine 25–50 mg; administer orally or intravenously 30–60 minutes before each rituximab dose
Rituximab 375 mg/m^2 per dose; administer intravenously in 0.9% NS or D5W, diluted to a concentration within the range 1–4 mg/mL, on day 1, every 28 days, for 5 induction cycles, cycles 2, 3, 4, 5, and 6 (total dosage/28-day cycle during cycles 2–6 = 375 mg/m^2)

Rituximab (maintenance cycles [starting 8 weeks after cycle 6 induction rituximab dose]): rituximab every 8 weeks × 12 cycles
Premedication for rituximab:
Acetaminophen 650–1000 mg; administer orally 30–60 minutes before each rituximab dose, *plus*
Diphenhydramine 25–50 mg; administer orally or intravenously 30–60 minutes before each rituximab dose
Rituximab 375 mg/m^2 per dose; administer intravenously in 0.9% NS or D5W, diluted to a concentration within the range 1–4 mg/mL, on day 1, every 56 days, for 12 maintenance cycles (total dosage/56-day cycle = 375 mg/m^2)
Notes on rituximab administration:
• Infuse initially at 50 mg/h. If hypersensitivity or infusion reactions do not occur during the first 30 minutes, increase the rate by 50 mg/h every 30 minutes as tolerated to a maximum rate of 400 mg/h. During subsequent treatments if previous rituximab administration was well tolerated, start at 100 mg/h, and increase by 100 mg/h every 30 minutes as tolerated to a maximum rate of 400 mg/h

INFUSION REACTIONS ASSOCIATED WITH RITUXIMAB
Fevers, chills, and rigors
1. Interrupt rituximab administration for severe symptoms, and give:
   • **Acetaminophen** 650 mg orally for fever. For persistent or recurrent symptoms, repeat administration every 4–6 hours as needed during rituximab administration
   • **Diphenhydramine** 25–50 mg orally or by intravenous injection for pruritus, hypotension, or angioedema. For persistent or recurrent symptoms, repeat administration every 4–6 hours as needed during rituximab administration
   • **Meperidine** 12.5–25 mg by intravenous injection every 10–20 minutes as needed for shaking chills (generally, cumulative doses >100 mg are not needed; use repeated doses with caution in persons with moderate or more severely impaired renal function)
2. If rituximab administration was interrupted, resume infusion at a slower rate than the maximum rate previously attempted. Rate escalation may be reattempted at smaller incremental steps with close monitoring. Do not exceed the maximum recommended rate of 400 mg/h

Dyspnea or wheezing without allergic findings (urticaria, or tongue or laryngeal edema)
1. Interrupt rituximab administration immediately
2. Give **hydrocortisone** 100 mg by intravenous injection (or an alternative steroid with equivalent glucocorticoid potency)
3. Give a **histamine (H$_2$) receptor antagonist** (ranitidine 50 mg, cimetidine 300 mg, or famotidine 20 mg) intravenously over 15–30 minutes
4. After symptoms resolve, resume rituximab administration at 25 mg/h with close monitoring. Do not increase the administration rate
Note: Medications and equipment for the treatment of hypersensitivity reactions should be available for immediate use in the event of a reaction during administration (eg, intravenous fluids, epinephrine, antihistamines, glucocorticoids, and oxygen)
Rituxan (rituximab) prescribing information. South San Francisco, CA: Genentech, Inc; 2018 October

LENALIDOMIDE
Lenalidomide Induction Dosing (ie, lenalidomide 20 mg/dose)
Lenalidomide 20 mg/dose; administer orally, without regard to meals, once daily for 21 consecutive days on days 1–21, starting in cycle 1, every 28 days, for 6–12 cycles (total dosage/28-day cycle = 420 mg)
• Patients who delay taking a lenalidomide dose at a regularly scheduled time may take the missed dose if the time to the next regularly scheduled dose is >12 hours away
• If a complete response (CR) is documented after cycle 6, then proceed directly to maintenance lenalidomide to complete a total of eighteen 28-day lenalidomide cycles (ie, 6 induction [20 mg/dose] cycles + 12 maintenance [10 mg/dose] cycles)

(continued)

(*continued*)

- If a partial response (PR) is documented after cycle 6, administer an additional 3 cycles of lenalidomide at induction dosing (ie, proceed with cycles 7–9 at lenalidomide 20 mg/dose), and then reassess response
  - If a CR is documented after cycle 9, proceed to maintenance lenalidomide to complete a total of eighteen 28-day lenalidomide cycles (ie, 9 induction [20 mg/dose] cycles + 9 maintenance [10 mg/dose] cycles)
  - If a PR is documented after cycle 9, administer a final additional 3 cycles of lenalidomide at induction dosing (ie, proceed with cycles 10–12 at lenalidomide 20 mg/dose), followed by a transition to maintenance lenalidomide to complete a total of eighteen 28-day lenalidomide cycles (ie, 12 induction [20 mg/dose] cycles + 6 maintenance [10 mg/dose] cycles)

Lenalidomide Maintenance Dosing (ie, lenalidomide 10 mg/dose)
Lenalidomide 10 mg/dose; administer orally, without regard to meals, once daily for 21 consecutive days on days 1–21, starting after completion of induction lenalidomide cycles as described above, every 28 days, for 6–12 cycles as necessary to complete a total of 18 cycles of lenalidomide (induction + maintenance) therapy (total dosage/28-day cycle = 210 mg)
  - Patients who delay taking a lenalidomide dose at a regularly scheduled time may take the missed dose if the time to the next regularly scheduled dose is >12 hours away

Supportive Care
Antiemetic prophylaxis
Emetogenic potential is **MINIMAL**
See Chapter 42 for antiemetic recommendations

Hematopoietic growth factor (CSF) prophylaxis
Primary prophylaxis is **NOT** *indicated*
See Chapter 43 for more information

Antimicrobial prophylaxis
Risk of fever and neutropenia is INTERMEDIATE
Antimicrobial primary prophylaxis to be considered:
- Antibacterial—not indicated
- Antifungal—not indicated
- Antiviral—antiherpes antivirals (eg, acyclovir, famciclovir, valacyclovir)

Treatment Modifications

Lenalidomide Dose Modifications

	Induction Lenalidomide Dosing		Maintenance Lenalidomide Dosing	
	CrCl ≥60 mL/min	CrCl ≥30 and <60 mL/min	CrCl ≥60 mL/min	CrCl ≥30 and <60 mL/min
Starting dose	20 mg per day	10 mg per day[*]	10 mg per day	5 mg per day
Level −1	15 mg per day	5 mg per day	5 mg per day	2.5 mg per day
Level −2	10 mg per day	2.5 mg per day	2.5 mg per day	Discontinue[†]
Level −3	5 mg per day	Discontinue[†]	Discontinue[†]	—
Level −4	2.5 mg per day	—	—	—
Level −5	Discontinue[†]	—	—	—

[*]If after completion of cycle 2 the patient remains free of G ≥3 toxicity, the lenalidomide dose may be increased to a maximum of 15 mg per day starting on day 2 of cycle 3

Adverse Event	Dose Modification
Hematologic Toxicity	
Day 1 ANC <1000/mm³ or platelet count <50,000/mm³	Delay the next cycle until ANC ≥1000/mm³ and platelet count ≥50,000/mm³. Consider treatment with filgrastim or platelet transfusion according to local guidelines. If the start of a new cycle is delayed >14 days for lenalidomide-related toxicity, reduce the lenalidomide by 1 dose level
G3 neutropenia (ANC ≥500 to <1000/mm³) sustained for ≥7 days	If neutropenia occurred on or after day 15, withhold lenalidomide for the rest of the cycle, and follow weekly CBC.
G4 neutropenia (ANC <500/mm³) at any time	If neutropenia occurred before day 15 and resolves to G ≤2 (ANC ≥1000/mm³), resume lenalidomide at the same dose for the rest of the cycle
Febrile neutropenia (ANC <1000/mm³ with fever ≥38.3°C)	Consider use of filgrastim according to local guidelines. In subsequent cycles, reduce the lenalidomide dosage by 1 dose level

(*continued*)

Treatment Modifications (*continued*)

G ≥3 thrombocytopenia (platelet count <50,000/mm³) at any time	If thrombocytopenia occurred on or after day 15, withhold lenalidomide for the rest of the cycle, and follow weekly CBC. If thrombocytopenia occurred before day 15 and resolved to G ≤2 (platelet count ≥50,000/mm³), resume lenalidomide at the same dose for the rest of the cycle In subsequent cycles, reduce the lenalidomide dosage by 1 dose level
Nonhematologic Toxicities	
G2/3 non-desquamating rash	Hold lenalidomide. Consider administering antihistamines or a short course of steroids. Resume at the same dose when resolved to G ≤1
G ≥3 desquamating (blistering) rash	Permanently discontinue lenalidomide†
G4 non-desquamating rash	
Allergic reactions, including hypersensitivity, angioedema, Stevens-Johnson syndrome, toxic epidermal necrolysis (TEN) and drug reaction with eosinophilia and systemic symptoms (DRESS)	
Tumor lysis syndrome (TLS)	Monitor patients at risk of TLS (ie, those with high tumor burden), and take appropriate precautions including aggressive hydration and allopurinol
G ≥3 peripheral neuropathy	If neuropathy is attributable to lenalidomide and occurred on or after day 15, withhold lenalidomide for the remainder of the cycle, and reassess weekly If neuropathy is attributable to lenalidomide and occurred before day 15 and resolved to G ≤1, restart lenalidomide at the same dose level for the remainder of the cycle In either case, resume lenalidomide with the dosage reduced by 1 dose level in subsequent cycles provided that the toxicity has resolved to G ≤1
G3/4 venous thromboembolism (VTE) during aspirin monotherapy or inadequate anticoagulation	Continue lenalidomide at the current dose and initiate adequate anticoagulation
G3/4 venous thromboembolism (VTE) during adequate anticoagulation (eg, prophylactic or therapeutic doses of LMWH, UFH, or warfarin)	Discontinue lenalidomide†
G ≥2 hypothyroidism or G ≥2 hyperthyroidism	Continue lenalidomide at current dose and initiate appropriate medical treatment
AST or ALT >3× ULN	If the toxicity occurred on or after day 15, withhold lenalidomide for the rest of the cycle. Reevaluate liver function tests weekly until AST/ALT improve to ≤2.5× ULN and bilirubin improves to ≤1.5× ULN If the toxicity occurred before day 15 and ALT/AST resolve to ≤2.5× ULN and bilirubin improves to ≤1.5× ULN, restart lenalidomide at the same dose level for the rest of the cycle. In either case, resume lenalidomide with the dosage reduced by 1 dose level in subsequent cycles if ALT/AST improve to ≤2.5× ULN and bilirubin improves to ≤1.5× ULN
Total bilirubin ≥3× ULN	
Other G ≥3 lenalidomide-related toxicities	If the toxicity occurred on or after day 15, withhold lenalidomide for the remainder of the cycle, and reassess toxicity at least every 7 days If the toxicity occurred before day 15 and resolved to G ≤2, restart lenalidomide at the same dose for the remainder of the cycle In either case, resume lenalidomide with the dosage reduced by 1 dose level in subsequent cycles provided that the toxicity resolves to G ≤2

Renal Impairment	
Moderate renal impairment (CrCl 30–60 mL/min)	Reduce the lenalidomide induction starting dose to 10 mg per dose. If after completion of cycle 2 the patient remains free of G ≥3 toxicity, the lenalidomide dose may be increased to a maximum of 15 mg per day starting on day 2 of cycle 3. Reduce the lenalidomide maintenance starting dose to 5 mg per dose
Severe renal impairment (CrCl <30 mL/min, or requiring hemodialysis)	Patients with creatinine clearance <30 mL/min were excluded from the study. No recommendations available

*In general, if a dose-limiting toxicity occurs on or after day 15 of the cycle, treatment will be withheld until the end of the cycle, and the dose will then be reduced (if applicable) beginning in the subsequent cycle. If the toxicity occurs before day 15 of the cycle, treatment will be held until recovery and restarted without dose reduction for the rest of the cycle (ie, continue until day 21; missed doses will not be made up), and then the next cycle will resume at a reduced dose

CrCl, creatinine clearance; ANC, absolute neutrophil count; CBC, complete blood count; LMWH, low molecular weight heparin; UFH, unfractionated heparin; AST, aspartate aminotransferase; ALT, alanine aminotransferase; ULN, upper limit of normal

†If lenalidomide or rituximab are discontinued, the medically responsible healthcare provider may decide to either continue the other agent as monotherapy, or switch to an alternative regimen

Note: Medications and equipment for the treatment of hypersensitivity reactions should be available for immediate use in the event of a reaction during rituximab administration (eg, intravenous fluids, epinephrine, antihistamines, glucocorticoids, oxygen)

Patient Population Studied

This international, multicenter, randomized, open-label, phase 3 trial (RELEVANCE) involved 1030 patients with previously untreated, CD20-positive follicular lymphoma. Patients were randomly assigned 1:1 to receive lenalidomide plus rituximab, or rituximab plus chemotherapy. Patients randomized to receive lenalidomide plus rituximab received six 28-day induction cycles of rituximab (375 mg/m² on days 1, 8, 15, and 22 of cycle 1 and on day 1 only in cycles 2–6), and then, if they had a response, an additional twelve 56-day maintenance cycles of rituximab (375 mg/m² on day 1 only), plus 18 total 28-day cycles of lenalidomide (6–12 induction cycles [20 mg on days 2–22] followed by 6–12 maintenance cycles [10 mg on days 2–22]). Patients who did not experience a complete response after 6 cycles of induction (20 mg) lenalidomide could receive an additional 3–6 cycles of 20 mg dosing before transitioning to maintenance (10 mg) dosing to complete a total of 18 (induction plus maintenance) cycles. Patients randomized to the rituximab plus chemotherapy arm received the investigator's choice of R-CHOP, R-B, or R-CVP for six 28-day induction cycles, followed by rituximab on day 1 only in twelve 56-day maintenance cycles, followed by rituximab maintenance therapy at standard doses for 2 years. Treatment was administered for a total of 120 weeks in both arms

Efficacy

(N = 1030)

	Rituximab + Lenalidomide (N = 513)	Rituximab + Chemotherapy (N = 517)	
Complete response at 120 weeks	48%	53%	P = 0.13
Overall response rate* at 120 weeks	61%	65%	
3-year progression-free survival	77%	78%	P = 0.48
3-year overall survival	94%	94%	

*Overall response rate includes patients with either a complete or partial response

Note: The median follow-up was 37.9 months

Toxicity

(N = 1010)

	Rituximab + Lenalidomide N = 507)		Rituximab + Chemotherapy (N = 503)	
Grade*	Grade 1–2 (%)	Grade ≥3 (%)	Grade 1–2 (%)	Grade ≥3 (%)
Neutropenia	44	32	27	50
Anemia	66	0	89	0
Thrombocytopenia	51	2	51	2
Cutaneous reactions	36	7	23	<1
Diarrhea	35	2	18	1
Constipation	35	<1	32	<1
Rash	25	4	8	<1
Fatigue	22	<1	28	<1
Nausea	20	0	40	2

Toxicity (continued)

Abdominal pain	15	<1	8	<1
Myalgia	14	0	6	<1
Arthralgia	13	<1	14	<1
Peripheral edema	14	0	9	<1
Muscle spasms	13	0	4	0
Infusion-related reaction	12	1	11	<1
Upper respiratory tract infection	9	0	11	0
Vomiting	6	<1	17	1
Peripheral neuropathy	7	<1	15	<1
Tumor flare reaction	5	1	<1	0
Leukopenia	3	2	4	6
Febrile neutropenia	0	2	<1	7
Tumor lysis syndrome	<1	1	<1	<1
Alopecia	<1	0	8	<1

*According to the NCI Common Terminology Criteria for Adverse Events, version 4.03
Note: Adverse events that occurred during treatment are included. Fatal adverse events that occurred during treatment were reported for 1% of each treatment group. The death of one patient in each group was classified as being related to trial treatment

Therapy Monitoring

1. *Prior to treatment initiation:* CBC with differential, serum chemistries, serum bilirubin, ALT or AST, hepatitis B core antibody (IgG or total) and hepatitis B surface antigen, and urine pregnancy test (women of child-bearing potential only)
   - *In patients at high risk for tumor lysis syndrome* consider frequent monitoring of laboratory indices of tumor lysis syndrome, intravenous hydration, and prophylaxis with a xanthine oxidase inhibitor (eg, allopurinol) during the first cycle
2. *Prior to each dose of rituximab, and then every 2 weeks thereafter:* CBC with differential, serum chemistries, serum bilirubin, ALT or AST
3. *Monitor periodically for:* Signs and symptoms of infection (including progressive multifocal leukoencephalopathy), dermatologic toxicity
4. *Response assessment (every 2–3 cycles):* Physical examination, CBC with differential, CT scan or PET scan

   Lenalidomide Notes:
- A decrease in the number of CD34+ cells collected after treatment has been reported in patients who have received >4 cycles of lenalidomide. In patients who may undergo transplant, consider early referral to transplant center
- Because of the embryo-fetal risk, lenalidomide is available only through a restricted program under a Risk Evaluation and Mitigation Strategy (REMS), the REVLIMID REMS program. Required components of the REVLIMID REMS program include the following:
- Patients must sign a patient-physician agreement form and comply with the REMS requirements. In particular, female patients of reproductive potential who are not pregnant must comply with the pregnancy testing and contraception requirements, and males must comply with contraception requirements

Treatment Modifications

Treatment prerequisites: Within 2 weeks before starting rituximab, study patients were required to have a hemoglobin ≥8.0 g/dL, ANC ≥1500/mm^3, platelet count ≥75,000/mm^3, serum creatinine concentration ≤2 mg/dL (≤177 μmol/L), total bilirubin level ≤2 mg/dL (≤34.2 μmol/L), and alkaline phosphatase and AST ≤2 times the upper limit of normal

Patient Population Studied

A study of 31 patients who had either low-grade or follicular B-cell NHL with either relapsed disease or primary therapy failure and progressive disease that required further treatment. Additional requirements included a demonstrable monoclonal CD20-positive B-cell population in a pathologic lymph node or bone marrow specimen and a WHO PS of 0, 1, or 2. Concurrent steroid use was not permitted

Efficacy

(N = 28)

Complete response	4%
++Partial response	39%
Overall response rate	43%

Toxicity*

	% of Patients
Transient fever	61
Leukopenia	23
Nausea	19
Dizziness	19
Throat irritation	19
G1/2 chills	36
G3/4 chills	3
G3/4 pulmonary disorders	6
G3/4 infusion-related hypotension	3

*NCI Adult Toxicity Criteria (February 1988 guidelines)

Therapy Monitoring

1. *Prior to treatment:* hepatitis B core antibody (IgG or total) and hepatitis B surface antigen
2. *Weekly:* CBC with differential, LFTs, serum BUN, and creatinine
3. *Response assessment (every 2–3 cycles):* Physical examination, CBC with differential, CT scan or PET scan

FOLLICULAR LYMPHOMA • FIRST LINE • SUBSEQUENT THERAPY
NON-HODGKIN LYMPHOMA REGIMEN: RITUXIMAB

Davis TA et al. J Clin Oncol 1999;17:1851–1857
Premedication for rituximab:
Acetaminophen 650–1000 mg; administer orally, *plus*
Diphenhydramine 25–50 mg; administer orally or intravenously 30–60 minutes before starting rituximab
Rituximab 375 mg/m^2; administer intravenously diluted to a concentration of 1–4 mg/mL in 0.9% sodium chloride injection or 5% dextrose injection, weekly, for 4 consecutive weeks (days 1, 8, 15, and 22) (total dosage/course = 1500 mg/m^2)

Notes on rituximab administration:
- Infuse initially at 50 mg/hour. If hypersensitivity or infusion reactions do not occur during the first 30 minutes, increase the rate by 50 mg/hour every 30 minutes, as tolerated, to a maximum rate of 400 mg/hour. Subsequently, if previous administration was well tolerated, start at 100 mg/hour, and increase by 100 mg/hour every 30 minutes, as tolerated, to a maximum rate of 400 mg/hour

INFUSION REACTIONS ASSOCIATED WITH RITUXIMAB
Fevers, chills, and rigors
1. Interrupt rituximab administration for severe symptoms, and give:
   - **Acetaminophen** 650 mg orally for fever. For persistent or recurrent symptoms, repeat administration every 4–6 hours as needed during rituximab administration
   - **Diphenhydramine** 25–50 mg orally or by intravenous injection for pruritus, hypotension, or angioedema. For persistent or recurrent symptoms, repeat administration every 4–6 hours as needed during rituximab administration
   - **Meperidine** 12.5–25 mg by intravenous injection every 10–20 minutes as needed for shaking chills (generally, cumulative doses >100 mg are not needed; use repeated doses with caution in persons with moderate or more severely impaired renal function)
2. If rituximab administration was interrupted, resume infusion at a slower rate than the maximum rate previously attempted. Rate escalation may be reattempted at smaller incremental steps with close monitoring. Do not exceed the maximum recommended rate of 400 mg/h

Dyspnea or wheezing without allergic findings (urticaria, or tongue or laryngeal edema)
1. Interrupt rituximab administration immediately
2. Give **hydrocortisone** 100 mg by intravenous injection (or an alternative steroid with equivalent glucocorticoid potency)
3. Give a **histamine (H$_2$) receptor antagonist** (ranitidine 50 mg, cimetidine 300 mg, or famotidine 20 mg) intravenously over 15–30 minutes
4. After symptoms resolve, resume rituximab administration at 25 mg/h with close monitoring. Do not increase the administration rate

Note: Medications and equipment for the treatment of hypersensitivity reactions should be available for immediate use in the event of a reaction during administration (eg, intravenous fluids, epinephrine, antihistamines, glucocorticoids, and oxygen)
Rituxan (rituximab) prescribing information. South San Francisco, CA: Genentech, Inc; 2018 October

Supportive Care
Antiemetic prophylaxis
Emetogenic potential is **MINIMAL**
See Chapter 42 for antiemetic recommendations

Hematopoietic growth factor (CSF) prophylaxis
Primary prophylaxis is **NOT** indicated
See Chapter 43 for more information

Antimicrobial prophylaxis
Risk of fever and neutropenia is *LOW*
Antimicrobial primary prophylaxis to be considered:
- Antibacterial—*Pneumocystis jirovecii* prophylaxis is recommended (eg, cotrimoxazole)
- Antifungal—not indicated
- Antiviral—not indicated unless patient previously had an episode of HSV

FOLLICULAR LYMPHOMA • FIRST LINE • SUBSEQUENT THERAPY
NON-HODGKIN LYMPHOMA REGIMEN: EXTENDED-SCHEDULE RITUXIMAB

Ghielmini M et al. Blood 2004;103:4416–4423

Premedication for rituximab:
Acetaminophen 650–1000 mg; administer orally, *plus*
Diphenhydramine 25–50 mg; administer orally or intravenously, 30–60 minutes before starting rituximab

Induction phase:
Rituximab 375 mg/m²; administer intravenously in 0.9% sodium chloride injection (0.9% NS) or 5% dextrose injection (D5W), diluted to a concentration of 1–4 mg/mL, once per week for 4 consecutive weeks (total dosage: 1500 mg/m²), *followed by:*

Extended schedule phase:
Rituximab 375 mg/m²; administer intravenously in 0.9% NS or D5W, diluted to a concentration of 1–4 mg/mL, at week 12 (8 weeks after the last *induction phase* dose), and again at months 5, 7, and 9, for a total of 4 doses (total dosage during maintenance phase = 1500 mg/m²; total dosage during induction phase plus extended schedule phase = 3000 mg/m²)
Notes on rituximab administration:
- Infuse initially at 50 mg/hour. If hypersensitivity or infusion reactions do not occur during the first 30 minutes, increase the rate by 50 mg/hour every 30 minutes, as tolerated, to a maximum rate of 400 mg/hour. Subsequently, if previous administration was well tolerated, start at 100 mg/hour and increase by 100 mg/hour every 30 minutes, as tolerated, to a maximum rate of 400 mg/hour

INFUSION REACTIONS ASSOCIATED WITH RITUXIMAB
Fevers, chills, and rigors
1. Interrupt rituximab administration for severe symptoms, and give:
   - **Acetaminophen** 650 mg orally for fever. For persistent or recurrent symptoms, repeat administration every 4–6 hours as needed during rituximab administration
   - **Diphenhydramine** 25–50 mg orally or by intravenous injection for pruritus, hypotension, or angioedema. For persistent or recurrent symptoms, repeat administration every 4–6 hours as needed during rituximab administration
   - **Meperidine** 12.5–25 mg by intravenous injection every 10–20 minutes as needed for shaking chills (generally, cumulative doses >100 mg are not needed; use repeated doses with caution in persons with moderate or more severely impaired renal function)
2. If rituximab administration was interrupted, resume infusion at a slower rate than the maximum rate previously attempted. Rate escalation may be reattempted at smaller incremental steps with close monitoring. Do not exceed the maximum recommended rate of 400 mg/h

Dyspnea or wheezing without allergic findings (urticaria, or tongue or laryngeal edema)
1. Interrupt rituximab administration immediately
2. Give **hydrocortisone** 100 mg by intravenous injection (or an alternative steroid with equivalent glucocorticoid potency)
3. Give a **histamine (H2) receptor antagonist** (ranitidine 50 mg, cimetidine 300 mg, or famotidine 20 mg) intravenously over 15–30 minutes
4. After symptoms resolve, resume rituximab administration at 25 mg/h with close monitoring. Do not increase the administration rate

Note: Medications and equipment for the treatment of hypersensitivity reactions should be available for immediate use in the event of a reaction during administration (eg, intravenous fluids, epinephrine, antihistamines, glucocorticoids, and oxygen)
Rituxan (rituximab) prescribing information. South San Francisco, CA: Genentech, Inc; 2018 October

Supportive Care
Antiemetic prophylaxis
Emetogenic potential is **MINIMAL**
See Chapter 42 for antiemetic recommendations

Hematopoietic growth factor (CSF) prophylaxis
Primary prophylaxis is **NOT** *indicated*
See Chapter 43 for more information

Antimicrobial prophylaxis
Risk of fever and neutropenia is *LOW*
Antimicrobial primary prophylaxis to be considered:
- Antibacterial—*Pneumocystis jirovecii* prophylaxis is recommended (eg, cotrimoxazole)
- Antifungal—not indicated
- Antiviral—not indicated unless patient previously had an episode of HSV

Patient Population Studied

A study of 202 newly diagnosed (32%) or relapsed/refractory follicular lymphoma patients. Biopsy-proven CD20+ follicular lymphoma, grade I (34%), II (45%), or III (12%) according to the REAL classification. ECOG performance status 0 (73%), 1 (21%), or 2 (6%), and a cardiac ejection fraction (EF) of at least 50% as determined by echocardiography. Median age was 57 years

Toxicity

Toxicity After Randomized Phase

	No Maintenance	Maintenance
G3/4 nonhematologic	3%	10%
G3/4 hematologic	17%	18%

Toxicity During Induction Phase

Nonhematologic

Overall	9.5%
Hypotension	2.5%
Asthenia	4%
Other	6.4%

Hematologic

Anemia	2%
Leukocytopenia	3%
Neutropenia	9.4%
Thrombocytopenia	4%

Therapy Monitoring

1. *Prior to treatment*: hepatitis B core antibody (IgG or total) and hepatitis B surface antigen
2. *Before each rituximab administration:* CBC before each rituximab and at months 2 and 12
3. *Response assessment (every 2–3 cycles)*: Physical examination, CBC with differential, CT scan or PET scan

Efficacy

(N = 185; Median follow-up time in 126 living patients = 36 months)
Randomization:
- Rituximab 375 mg/m^2 weekly for 4 weeks then no further treatment *versus*
- Rituximab 375 mg/m^2 weekly for 4 weeks followed by extended schedule with a single infusion of rituximab 375 mg/m^2 at week 12 (3 months) and again at months 5, 7, and 9

	All Evaluable (N = 185)	Chemotherapy-Naïve (N = 57)	Previously Treated (N = 128)
Month 3 RR	52%	67% with 9% CR	46% with 8% CR
	OR = 2.34; P = 0.0097		
	No Maintenance	Maintenance	P
Median EFS (151 randomized patients)	11.8 months	23.2 months	HR = 0.61; P = 0.024
Median EFS (chemotherapy-naïve patients)	19 months	36 months	P = 0.009

EFS by Response to Induction Phase

Response at first restaging	16 months	36 months	P = 0.004
SD at first restaging	8 months	11 months	P = 0.35
Overall best response	77% (31% CR)	75% (38% CR)	NS
Overall best response (chemotherapy-naïve)	81% (31% CR)	92% (52% CR)	NS
Median remission duration among week 12 responders	16 months	36 months	P = 0.0039 (Marginally significant for chemotherapy-naïve vs pretreated patients)

RR Over Time

Month 3	67%	62%	Between-arm differences in RR not significant at months 3 or 7, but become significant after 1 year (P = 0.046)
Month 12	44%	60%	
Month 24	28%	45%	

% in CR Over Time

Month 3	8%	12%	NS at any time point
Month 24	19%	29%	

CR, complete response; EFS, event-free survival; OR, overall response; RR, Response rate; SD, stable disease

FOLLICULAR LYMPHOMA • MAINTENANCE THERAPY
NON-HODGKIN LYMPHOMA REGIMEN: MAINTENANCE RITUXIMAB

Hainsworth JD et al. J Clin Oncol 2005;23:1088–1095 [Minnie Pearl Cancer Research Network]
Salles G et al. Lancet 2011;377:42–51

Rituximab
Premedication for rituximab:

Acetaminophen 650–1000 mg; administer orally, *plus*

Diphenhydramine 25–50 mg; administer orally or intravenously, 30–60 minutes before starting rituximab

Induction phase:

Rituximab 375 mg/m^2; administer intravenously in 0.9% sodium chloride injection (0.9% NS) or 5% dextrose injection (D5W), diluted to a concentration of 1–4 mg/mL, once per week, for 4 weeks (total dosage/4-week course = 1500 mg/m^2), *followed by:*

Maintenance phase:

Rituximab 375 mg/m^2; administer intravenously in 0.9% NS or D5W, diluted to a concentration of 1–4 mg/mL, once per week for 4 weeks, administered at 6-month intervals times 3 cycles (total dosage = 1500 mg/m^2 every 6 months; potential total dosage during maintenance phase (3 cycles) = 4500 mg/m^2

Notes on rituximab administration:
- Infuse initially at 50 mg/hour. If hypersensitivity or infusion reactions do not occur during the first 30 minutes, increase the rate by 50 mg/hour every 30 minutes, as tolerated, to a maximum rate of 400 mg/hour. Subsequently, if previous administration was well tolerated, start at 100 mg/hour and increase by 100 mg/hour every 30 minutes, as tolerated, to a maximum rate of 400 mg/hour

INFUSION REACTIONS ASSOCIATED WITH RITUXIMAB
Fevers, chills, and rigors

1. Interrupt rituximab administration for severe symptoms, and give:
   - **Acetaminophen** 650 mg orally for fever. For persistent or recurrent symptoms, repeat administration every 4–6 hours as needed during rituximab administration
   - **Diphenhydramine** 25–50 mg orally or by intravenous injection for pruritus, hypotension, or angioedema. For persistent or recurrent symptoms, repeat administration every 4–6 hours as needed during rituximab administration
   - **Meperidine** 12.5–25 mg by intravenous injection every 10–20 minutes as needed for shaking chills (generally, cumulative doses >100 mg are not needed; use repeated doses with caution in persons with moderate or more severely impaired renal function)
2. If rituximab administration was interrupted, resume infusion at a slower rate than the maximum rate previously attempted. Rate escalation may be reattempted at smaller incremental steps with close monitoring. Do not exceed the maximum recommended rate of 400 mg/h

Dyspnea or wheezing without allergic findings (urticaria, or tongue or laryngeal edema)

1. Interrupt rituximab administration immediately
2. Give **hydrocortisone** 100 mg by intravenous injection (or an alternative steroid with equivalent glucocorticoid potency)
3. Give a **histamine (H$_2$) receptor antagonist** (ranitidine 50 mg, cimetidine 300 mg, or famotidine 20 mg) intravenously over 15–30 minutes
4. After symptoms resolve, resume rituximab administration at 25 mg/h with close monitoring. Do not increase the administration rate

Note: Medications and equipment for the treatment of hypersensitivity reactions should be available for immediate use in the event of a reaction during administration (eg, intravenous fluids, epinephrine, antihistamines, glucocorticoids, and oxygen)

Rituxan (rituximab) prescribing information. South San Francisco, CA: Genentech, Inc; 2018 October

Supportive Care
Antiemetic prophylaxis

Emetogenic potential is **MINIMAL**

See Chapter 42 for antiemetic recommendations

Hematopoietic growth factor (CSF) prophylaxis

Primary prophylaxis is **NOT** *indicated*

See Chapter 43 for more information

Antimicrobial prophylaxis

Risk of fever and neutropenia is *LOW*

Antimicrobial primary prophylaxis to be considered:
- Antibacterial—*Pneumocystis jirovecii* prophylaxis is recommended (eg, cotrimoxazole)
- Antifungal—not indicated
- Antiviral—not indicated unless patient previously had an episode of HSV

Therapy Monitoring

1. *Prior to treatment*: hepatitis B core antibody (IgG or total) and hepatitis B surface antigen
2. *Every 3 months:* CBC with differential and serum chemistries
3. *Response assessment (every 2–3 cycles)*: Physical examination, CBC with differential, CT scan or PET scan

Patient Population Studied

A study of 114 patients who had received previous chemotherapy (previous rituximab not allowed) for indolent non-Hodgkin lymphoma (follicular and small lymphocytic), who were treated with a standard 4-week course of rituximab. Patients with objective response or stable disease were randomly assigned to receive either maintenance rituximab therapy (standard 4-week courses administered at 6-month intervals) or rituximab retreatment at the time of lymphoma progression. The duration of rituximab benefit was measured from the date of first rituximab treatment until the date other treatment was required

Efficacy

	Retreatment Group (No Maintenance)	Maintenance Group	P
Response to initial rituximab			
CR	0	9	
ORR	15	39	
Response to subsequent treatment			
CR	4	27	0.007
ORR	35	52	—
Median PFS	7.4 months	31.3 months	0.007
Median duration rituximab benefit	27.4 months	31.3 months	0.94
3-year survival	68%	72%	NS

Toxicities

	Retreatment Group (No Maintenance; N = 46)	Maintenance Group (N = 44)
G3 infusion reactions	0%	4.5%
G3 hematologic toxicity	2.2%	2.3%
G3 nonhematologic toxicity	2.2%	2.3%

FOLLICULAR LYMPHOMA • SUBSEQUENT THERAPY

NON-HODGKIN LYMPHOMA REGIMEN: IDELALISIB

Gopal AK et al. N Engl J Med 2014;370:1008–1018
Supplementary appendix to: Gopal AK et al. N Engl J Med 2014;370:1008–1018
Protocol for: Gopal AK et al. N Engl J Med 2014;370:1008–1018
Zydelig (idelalisib) prescribing information. Foster City, CA: Gilead Sciences, Inc; 2018 October
Coutré SE et al. Leuk Lymphoma 2015;56:2779–2786

Idelalisib 150 mg per dose; administer orally twice per day, without regard to food, continually until disease progression (total dosage/week = 2100 mg)

Notes on idelalisib administration:

- Idelalisib tablets should be swallowed whole
- Patients who delay taking an idelalisib dose at a regularly scheduled time may administer the missed dose if within 6 hours of the usual dosing time. If >6 hours, skip the missed dose, and resume treatment at the next regularly scheduled time
- Idelalisib is metabolized by aldehyde oxidase and CYP3A (major routes) and by UGT1A4 (minor route). If concomitant use with a strong CY3A inhibitor is unavoidable, monitor closely for idelalisib side effects. Avoid concomitant use with strong CYP3A inducers
- Idelalisib was shown in vitro to inhibit CYP2C8, CYP2C19, UGT1A1 and to induce CYP2B6. Idelalisib increased the mean C_{max} of midazolam (a sensitive CYP3A substrate) by 2.4-fold and the mean area-under-the-curve of midazolam by 5.4-fold. Thus, avoid concomitant use with sensitive CYP3A substrates

Supportive Care

Antiemetic prophylaxis
Emetogenic potential is **MINIMAL-LOW**
See Chapter 42 for antiemetic recommendations

Hematopoietic growth factor (CSF) prophylaxis
Primary prophylaxis is **NOT** indicated
See Chapter 43 for more information

Antimicrobial prophylaxis
Risk of fever and neutropenia is *LOW*
Antimicrobial primary prophylaxis to be considered:

- Antibacterial—not indicated. *Pneumocystis jirovecii* prophylaxis is recommended (eg, cotrimoxazole)
- Antifungal—not indicated
- Antiviral—antiherpes antivirals (eg, acyclovir, famciclovir, valacyclovir). Consider preemptive cytomegalovirus (CMV) management in CMV seropositive patients treated with idelalisib

Patient Population Studied

The international, multicenter, single-arm, open-label, phase 2 trial (known as DELTA or Study 101-09) involved 125 patients with indolent non-Hodgkin lymphoma that had suffered a relapse after, or whose disease was refractory to both rituximab and an alkylating agent. The patient population included 72 patients with follicular lymphoma, 28 patients with small lymphocytic lymphoma, 15 patients with marginal zone lymphoma, and 10 patients with lymphoplasmacytic lymphoma. Eligible patients had received at least two prior systemic therapies for indolent non-Hodgkin lymphoma. Patients received oral idelalisib (150 mg) twice daily

Treatment Modifications

Idelalisib	
Starting dose	150 mg by mouth twice a day
Dose level 1	100 mg by mouth twice a day
Adverse Event	**Dose Modification**
Pulmonary Toxicity	
Dyspnea, cough, fever, hypoxia (decline by ≥5% O_2 saturation) and/or radiologic abnormalities; pneumonitis is suspected	Interrupt idelalisib until pulmonary status clarified. Perform extensive evaluations for infectious etiology, including testing for PJP
Symptomatic pneumonitis or organizing pneumonia (any grade) is confirmed	Discontinue idelalisib, and initiate appropriate treatment with corticosteroids

(continued)

Treatment Modifications (continued)

Infectious Complications	
G ≥3 sepsis or pneumonia	Interrupt idelalisib until resolution of infection, then resume at the same dose
CMV infection (any grade) or CMV viremia	Interrupt idelalisib until viremia or infection has resolved. Upon resolution, idelalisib may be resumed at the same dose; if resumed, then monitor blood CMV PCR or pp65 antigen detection at least monthly during ongoing treatment
PJP infection is suspected	Interrupt idelalisib during workup for suspected PJP infection
PJP infection is confirmed	Permanently discontinue idelalisib

Gastrointestinal Toxicity	
G1 diarrhea (increase of <4 stools per day over baseline) or early-onset (≤8 weeks), G2 diarrhea (increase of 4–6 stools per day over baseline)	Continue idelalisib at the current dose without interruption. Discontinue other medications which may cause diarrhea, if applicable. Rule out infectious causes of diarrhea (eg, *Campylobacter, Salmonella, Escherichia coli, Clostridium difficile*). Consider colonoscopy in atypical cases (eg, bloody diarrhea), or for refractory diarrhea. Early-onset uncomplicated diarrhea (grade 1 and sometimes grade 2) is often self-limiting and may occasionally respond to antimotility agents (eg, loperamide) and dietary modification (avoidance of lactose, alcohol, and high-osmolar supplements; increase in oral clear liquids; consumption of frequent small, bland meals, etc.). Monitor at least weekly until resolution (median time to resolution in trials ranged from 1 week to 1 month), and then resume normal diet. See below for early-onset G2 diarrhea that does not respond to antimotility agents
Late-onset (>8 weeks), G2 diarrhea (increase of 4–6 stools per day over baseline) or early-onset (>8 weeks), G2 diarrhea (increase of 4–6 stools per day over baseline) unresponsive to antimotility agents or G3 diarrhea (increase of ≥7 stools per day over baseline, or requiring hospitalization) or G4 diarrhea (life-threatening consequences; urgent intervention indicated)	Interrupt idelalisib. Determine the need for hospitalization or IV hydration. Discontinue other medications that may cause diarrhea, if applicable. Rule out infectious causes of diarrhea (eg, *Campylobacter, Clostridium difficile, Salmonella, E. coli*). Consider colonoscopy in atypical cases (eg, bloody diarrhea), or for refractory diarrhea. Diarrhea responds poorly to antimotility (eg, loperamide) agents. Implement dietary modification (avoidance of lactose, alcohol, and high-osmolar supplements; increase in oral clear liquids; consumption of frequent small, bland meals, etc.) After ruling out infectious diarrhea, consider treatment with budesonide 9 mg by mouth once daily until resolution to G ≤1, followed by taper. Alternatively, systemic corticosteroids (initial dose = prednisolone 1 mg/kg or equivalent) may be administered until resolution to G ≤1, followed by taper

Monitor at least weekly until resolution (median time to resolution in trials ranged from 1 week to 1 month) and then resume normal diet

In cases of G2 or G3 diarrhea, upon resolution to G ≤1, consider resumption of idelalisib, per clinical judgement, at dose level 1 with or without concomitant budesonide prophylaxis. In cases of G4 diarrhea, permanently discontinue idelalisib |
| Intestinal perforation | Permanently discontinue idelalisib |

Hematologic Toxicity	
G3 neutropenia (ANC ≥500/mm³ to <1000/mm³)	Continue idelalisib at the current dose without interruption. Monitor ANC at least once per week
G4 neutropenia (ANC <500/mm³)	Interrupt idelalisib. Monitor ANC at least once per week until ANC ≥500/mm³, then resume idelalisib at dose level 1
G3 thrombocytopenia (platelet count ≥25,000/mm³ to <50,000/mm³)	Continue idelalisib at the current dose without interruption. Monitor platelet count at least once per week
G4 thrombocytopenia (platelet count <25,000/mm³)	Interrupt idelalisib. Monitor platelet count at least once per week until platelet count ≥25,000/mm³, then resume idelalisib at dose level 1

Hepatic Toxicity	
G2 elevation in ALT or AST (ALT or AST >3 to ≤5× ULN) or G2 elevation in bilirubin (bilirubin >1.5 to ≤3× ULN)	Continue idelalisib at the current dose without interruption

Monitor liver function tests at least weekly until resolution to ≤1× ULN, then resume normal frequency of monitoring |

(continued)

Treatment Modifications (*continued*)

G3 elevation in ALT or AST (ALT or AST >5 to ≤20× ULN) or G3 elevation in bilirubin (bilirubin >3 to ≤10× ULN)	Interrupt idelalisib. Monitor liver function tests at least weekly until resolution to ≤1× ULN, then resume idelalisib at dose level 1
G4 elevation in ALT or AST (ALT or AST >20× ULN) or G4 elevation in bilirubin (bilirubin >10× ULN)	Permanently discontinue idelalisib
Dermatologic and Immunologic Toxicities	
SJS or TEN is suspected	Interrupt idelalisib until dermatologic status is clarified
SJS or TEN is confirmed	Permanently discontinue idelalisib
Other G ≥3 cutaneous reaction	Permanently discontinue idelalisib
Severe allergic reaction or anaphylactic reaction	Permanently discontinue idelalisib
Drug-Drug Interactions	
Concomitant therapy with a strong CYP3A inhibitor is required	Consider alternative medication. If the strong CYP3A inhibitor is unavoidable, then monitor patients more frequently for idelalisib adverse reactions
Concomitant therapy with a strong CYP3A inducer is required	Do not administer a strong CYP3A inducer with idelalisib
Concomitant therapy with a CYP3A substrate with a narrow therapeutic index is required	Do not administer idelalisib with sensitive CYP3A substrates
Concomitant therapy with other hepatotoxic medications or medications which cause diarrhea	Avoid coadministration of idelalisib with other medications that are hepatotoxic or cause diarrhea
Other Toxicities	
Other severe or life-threatening toxicity, first occurrence	Interrupt idelalisib until resolution of toxicity. Upon resolution, consider resuming idelalisib at dose level 1, per the discretion of the medically responsible healthcare provider
Other severe or life-threatening toxicity, second occurrence	Permanently discontinue idelalisib

Idelalisib may cause fetal harm. Advise women of reproductive potential of the potential risk to a fetus and to use effective contraception during treatment and for at least 1 month after the last dose

ALT, alanine aminotransferase; ANC, absolute neutrophil count; AST, aspartate aminotransferase; CMV, cytomegalovirus; PCR, polymerase chain reaction; PJP, *Pneumocystis jirovecii* pneumonia; SJS, Stevens-Johnson syndrome; TEN, toxic epidermal necrolysis; ULN, upper limit of normal

Zydelig (idelalisib) prescribing information. Foster City, CA: Gilead Sciences, Inc; 2018 October
Coutré SE et al. Leuk Lymphoma 2015;56:2779–2786

Toxicity

(N = 125)

Grade[*]	Grade 1–2 (%)	Grade ≥3 (%)
Any adverse event	28	54
Decreased neutrophils	29	27
Increased alanine aminotransferase level	34	13
Diarrhea	30	13
Increased aspartate aminotransferase level	27	8
Fatigue	28	2
Nausea	28	2

(*continued*)

Efficacy

(N = 125)

Overall response rate[*]	57% (54% in those with follicular lymphoma)
Median progression-free survival	11 months
Median overall survival	20.3 months

[*]*Overall response rate* includes patients with either a complete or partial response
Note: Results are shown for all trial participants (that is, individuals with follicular lymphoma, small lymphocytic lymphoma, marginal zone lymphoma, or lymphoplasmacytic lymphoma). The median follow-up among all was 9.7 months

Therapy Monitoring

1. *Prior to initiation of idelalisib:* CBC with differential, chemistries (potassium, uric acid, phosphorus, calcium, serum creatinine, LDH), liver function tests (serum bilirubin, ALT, AST, alkaline phosphatase), urine pregnancy test (women of child-bearing potential only)

2. *During treatment with idelalisib:*

   a. Monitor liver function tests (ALT, AST, and serum bilirubin) in all patients at least every 2 weeks for the first 3 months of treatment, then at least every 4 weeks for the next 3 months, then at least every 1–3 months thereafter. Monitor at least weekly if ALT or AST increases to >5× ULN or if bilirubin increases to >1.5× ULN until resolution to ≤1× ULN

   b. Monitor CBC with differential at least every 2 weeks for the first 6 months of therapy, and at least weekly while absolute neutrophil count is <1000/mm^3 or platelet count is <50,000/mm^3

   c. Monitor periodically for:
   - Signs and symptoms of diarrhea/colitis
   - Signs and symptoms of intestinal perforation
   - Signs and symptoms of dermatologic toxicity or hypersensitivity reactions
   - Signs and symptoms of pneumonitis
   - Signs and symptoms of infection (including sepsis, pneumonia, *Pneumocystis jirovecii* pneumonia, and cytomegalovirus)

3. *Response assessment every 2–3 months:* Physical examination, CBC with differential, CT scan with contrast

Toxicity (continued)

Cough	29	0
Decreased hemoglobin	26	2
Pyrexia	26	2
Decreased platelets	19	6
Increased alkaline phosphatase level	22	0
Dyspnea	14	3
Decreased appetite	17	<1
Abdominal pain	14	2
Vomiting	13	2
Decreased weight	14	0
Upper respiratory tract infection	14	0
Rash	11	2
Pneumonia	4	7
Asthenia	9	2
Night sweats	11	0
Peripheral edema	8	2
Headache	10	<1
Increased bilirubin level	10	0

*According to the National Cancer Institute Common Terminology Criteria for Adverse Events, version 4.0.3
Note: All-grade toxicities that occurred during treatment in ≥10% patients are included. Treatment discontinuation owing to adverse events was reported for 20% patients. A total of 8.8% patients died while receiving study drug or within 30 days after the last dose, 2.4% were a result of progressive disease, and the remainder were due to pneumonia, cardiac arrest, cardiac failure, splenic infarction, septic shock, or pneumonitis

FOLLICULAR LYMPHOMA • SUBSEQUENT THERAPY
NON-HODGKIN LYMPHOMA REGIMEN: COPANLISIB

Dreyling M et al. J Clin Oncol 2017;35:3898–3905
Appendix (online only) to: Dreyling M et al. J Clin Oncol 2017;35:3898–3905
Aliqopa (copanlisib) prescribing information. Whippany, NJ: Bayer HealthCare Pharmaceuticals Inc; 2017 September

Copanlisib 60 mg per dose; administer intravenously in 100 mL 0.9% sodium chloride injection over 1 hour for 3 doses on days 1, 8, and 15, every 28 days, until disease progression (total dosage/28-day cycle = 180 mg)
Notes on copanlisib administration:

- Coadministration of copanlisib with rifampin (a strong CYP3A4 and P-glycoprotein [P-gp] inducer) decreased the mean copanlisib AUC by 63% and C_{max} by 15%. Coadministration of copanlisib with strong CYP3A4 inducers (eg, carbamazepine, enzalutamide, mitotane, phenytoin, rifampin, and St. John's wort) should be avoided

- Coadministration of copanlisib with itraconazole (a strong CYP3A inhibitor and a P-gp and breast cancer resistance protein [BCRP] inhibitor) increased the mean AUC of copanlisib by 53% (ie, 1.53-fold) with no effect on C_{max} (1.03-fold) in cancer patients. If possible, avoid concomitant use of strong CYP3A inhibitors with copanlisib. If patients must receive a strong CYP3A inhibitor, then reduce the starting dose of copanlisib to 45 mg per dose. If coadministration of the strong inhibitor is discontinued, the copanlisib dose should be returned to the dose used prior to initiation of a strong CYP3A inhibitor

- In a population pharmacokinetic analysis, mild hepatic impairment (bilirubin ≤ULN and AST >ULN, or bilirubin <1–1.5× ULN *and* any AST) had no clinically significant effect on the pharmacokinetics of copanlisib. The effects of moderate to severe hepatic impairment are unknown

- In a population pharmacokinetic analysis, mild to moderate renal impairment (estimated creatinine clearance ≥30 mL/min as calculated by the Cockcroft-Gault equation) had no clinically significant effect on the pharmacokinetics of copanlisib. The effects of severe renal impairment or end stage renal disease with or without hemodialysis is unknown

Supportive Care
Antiemetic prophylaxis
Emetogenic potential is **LOW**
See Chapter 42 for antiemetic recommendations

Hematopoietic growth factor (CSF) prophylaxis
Primary prophylaxis is **NOT** *indicated*
See Chapter 43 for more information

Antimicrobial prophylaxis
Risk of fever and neutropenia is LOW
Antimicrobial primary prophylaxis to be considered:

- Antibacterial—not indicated. Consider *Pneumocystis jirovecii* primary prophylaxis in patients with other risk factors

- Antifungal—not indicated

- Antiviral—not indicated unless patient previously had an episode of HSV

Diarrhea management
Latent or delayed-onset diarrhea*:
Loperamide 4 mg orally initially after the first loose or liquid stool, *then* 2–4 mg orally every 2–4 hours or **diphenoxylate hydrochloride** 2.5 mg **with atropine sulfate** 0.025 mg (eg, Lomotil)

*Abigerges D et al. J Natl Cancer Inst 1994;86:446–449
Rothenberg ML et al. J Clin Oncol 2001;19:3801–3807
Wadler S et al. J Clin Oncol 1998;16:3169–3178

Treatment Modifications

Copanlisib	
Starting dose	60 mg intravenously on days 1, 8, and 15, every 28 days*
Dose level −1	45 mg intravenously on days 1, 8, and 15, every 28 days*
Dose level −2	30 mg intravenously on days 1, 8, and 15, every 28 days*
Dose level −3	Discontinue copanlisib

(continued)

Treatment Modifications (*continued*)

Adverse Event	Treatment Modification
Hematologic Toxicity	
First occurrence of G4 neutropenia (ANC <500/mm^3)	Withhold copanlisib. Continue to monitor CBC with differential and platelet count at least weekly. Resume copanlisib at the same dose when ANC ≥500/mm^3
Second occurrence of G4 neutropenia (ANC <500/mm^3)	Withhold copanlisib. Continue to monitor CBC with differential and platelet count at least weekly. Resume copanlisib at dose level −1 (45 mg) when ANC ≥500/mm^3
G4 thrombocytopenia (platelet count <25,000/mm^3)	Withhold copanlisib. Continue to monitor CBC with differential and platelet count at least weekly. If recovery to platelet count ≥75,000/mm^3 occurs within 21 days, then resume copanlisib with the dose reduced by 1 dose level. If platelet count does not recover to ≥75,000/mm^3 occurs within 21 days, discontinue copanlisib
Infections	
G ≥3 infection	Withhold copanlisib until resolution of infection, then resume copanlisib at the same dosage
Suspected PJP infection of any grade	Withhold copanlisib until pulmonary status is clarified. If PJP infection is confirmed, treat infection until resolution, and then resume copanlisib at the same dosage with concomitant PJP prophylaxis
Hypertension	
Pre-dose blood pressure ≥150/90 mm Hg	Withhold copanlisib until blood pressure is <150/90 mm Hg based on two consecutive measurements obtained at least 15 minutes apart
Post-dose blood pressure ≥150/90 mm Hg (non-life-threatening)	If anti-hypertensive treatment is not required, continue copanlisib at the same dose. If anti-hypertensive treatment is required, consider reducing the copanlisib dosage by 1 dose level
Persistent elevation in blood pressure ≥150/90 mm Hg (non-life-threatening) despite optimal anti-hypertensive treatment and despite at least one copanlisib dose reduction	Discontinue copanlisib
Post-dose elevated blood pressure with life-threatening consequences	Discontinue copanlisib
Hyperglycemia	
Pre-dose fasting blood glucose ≥160 to <500 mg/dL or pre-dose random/non-fasting blood glucose ≥200 to <500 mg/dL	Withhold copanlisib until fasting blood glucose is <160 mg/dL or random/non-fasting blood glucose is <200 mg/dL, then administer copanlisib at the same dose. Monitor closely for signs and symptoms of hyperglycemia, and monitor blood glucose for 1–2 days following each copanlisib infusion. Ensure adequate oral hydration during periods of hyperglycemia and especially for 1–2 days following each copanlisib dose Copanlisib-induced hyperglycemia is typically transient, peaking at 5–8 hours following infusion and resolving within 24 hours. Thus, pre-dose hyperglycemia is unlikely to be related to copanlisib and may require initiation or optimization of antihyperglycemic therapy
Occurrence of G4 hyperglycemia (blood glucose [fasting or random] ≥500 mg/dL) occurring at a copanlisib dose of 60 mg or 45 mg	Withhold copanlisib until fasting blood glucose is <160 mg/dL or random/non-fasting blood glucose is <200 mg/dL, then administer copanlisib at 1 lower dose level. Ensure adequate oral hydration during period of hyperglycemia and especially for 1–2 days following each copanlisib dose. Monitor closely for signs and symptoms of hyperglycemia, and monitor blood glucose for 1–2 days following each copanlisib infusion Patients without a baseline diagnosis of diabetes mellitus who experience transient, *asymptomatic* G4 hyperglycemia following administration of copanlisib can often be managed with oral hydration as described above without the need for antihyperglycemic medication. Consider intravenous hydration for patients unable to tolerate adequate oral fluids Patients without a baseline diagnosis of diabetes mellitus experiencing *symptomatic* hyperglycemia or with persistent hyperglycemia >250 mg/dL despite adequate hydration may require acute antihyperglycemic therapy (eg, rapid- or short-acting insulin). If insulin therapy is required, consider administration of an oral antihyperglycemic medication to cover postprandial hyperglycemia on subsequent copanlisib infusion days. Recommended options include: • A biguanide (eg, metformin 500 mg orally taken twice per day, with breakfast and dinner, for 2 doses on copanlisib infusion days only), *or* • A DPP–4 inhibitor (eg, sitagliptin 100 mg orally as a single daily dose with breakfast on copanlisib infusion days only), *or* • An SGLT2 inhibitor (eg, canagliflozin 100 mg orally as a single daily dose with breakfast on copanlisib infusion days only) Patients with a baseline diagnosis of diabetes may require intensification of their baseline antihyperglycemic regimen and more frequent monitoring of blood glucose for 1–2 days following each dose of copanlisib

(*continued*)

Treatment Modifications (continued)

Occurrence of blood glucose (fasting or random) ≥500 mg/dL at a copanlisib dose of 30 mg	Discontinue copanlisib

Pulmonary

Cough, dyspnea, or hypoxia; pneumonitis is suspected	Withhold copanlisib until pulmonary status is clarified
G2 non-infectious pneumonitis is confirmed	Withhold copanlisib and treat pneumonitis (eg, with systemic corticosteroids). If pneumonitis improves to G ≤1, resume copanlisib at 1 lower dose level
G ≥3 non-infectious pneumonitis is confirmed	Discontinue copanlisib. Treat pneumonitis (eg, with systemic corticosteroids)

Dermatologic

G3 severe cutaneous reactions	Withhold copanlisib until toxicity is resolved. Depending on the severity and persistence of the reaction, either resume copanlisib at 1 lower dose level or discontinue copanlisib
Life-threatening cutaneous reaction	Discontinue copanlisib

Drug Interactions

Strong CYP3A inducer is required	Avoid concomitant administration of a strong CYP3A inducer with copanlisib
Strong CYP3A inhibitor is required	If possible, avoid concomitant use of a strong CYP3A inhibitor with copanlisib. If concomitant use cannot be avoided, reduce the copanlisib dose to 45 mg. If the strong CYP3A inhibitor is subsequently discontinued, increase the copanlisib dosage back to the dosage that was used prior to initiation of the strong CYP3A inhibitor

Other Toxicities

Other severe, non-life-threatening, G3 toxicity	Withhold copanlisib until toxicity is resolved, then resume copanlisib at 1 lower dose level
Other G4 toxicity or life-threatening G3 toxicity	Discontinue copanlisib

ANC, absolute neutrophil count; CBC, complete blood count; PJP, *Pneumocystis jirovecii*; DPP-4, dipeptidyl peptidase-4; SGLT2, sodium-glucose cotransporter-2
*A minimum of 7 days should elapse between two consecutive copanlisib infusions
Copanlisib may cause fetal harm. Advise pregnant women of the potential risk to a fetus. Advise females of reproductive potential and males with female partners of reproductive potential to use effective contraception during treatment and for at least 1 month after the last dose

Dreyling M et al. J Clin Oncol 2017;35:3898–3905
Appendix (online only) to: Dreyling M et al. J Clin Oncol 2017;35:3898–3905
Aliqopa (copanlisib) prescribing information. Whippany, NJ: Bayer HealthCare Pharmaceuticals Inc; 2017 September

Patient Population Studied

The international, multicenter, single-arm, phase 2 trial (CHRONOS-1) enrolled 142 patients with relapsed/refractory indolent B-cell lymphoma, including 104 patients with follicular lymphoma, 23 patients with marginal zone lymphoma, 8 patients with small lymphocytic lymphoma, and 6 patients with lymphoplasmacytic lymphoma. Eligible patients had an Eastern Cooperative Oncology Group (ECOG) performance status score ≤2, and had received at least two prior lines of therapy, including rituximab and alkylating agents. Patients who had received prior treatment with a phosphatidylinositol 3-kinase inhibitor or a prior allogeneic bone marrow transplant were ineligible. Patients received 28-day cycles of intravenous copanlisib (60 mg over 1 hour on days 1, 8, and 15)

Efficacy

(N = 142)

Overall response rate*	59% (59% also in only those with follicular lymphoma)
Median progression-free survival	11.2 months

*Overall response rate includes patients with either a complete or partial response
Note: Results are shown for all trial participants (that is, individuals with follicular lymphoma, marginal zone lymphoma, small lymphocytic lymphoma, or lymphoplasmacytic lymphoma, and the one patient with diffuse large B-cell lymphoma)

Toxicity

(N = 142)

Grade[*]	Grade 1–2 (%)	Grade ≥3 (%)
Any treatment-related adverse event	18	71
Hyperglycemia	8	40
Hypertension	6	23
Decreased neutrophil count	6	19
Diarrhea	14	4
Nausea	15	<1
Lung infection	3	11
Decreased platelet count	9	4
Oral mucositis	9	3
Fatigue	11	1

[*]According to the National Cancer Institute Common Terminology Criteria for Adverse Events, version 4.0.3
Note: All-grade treatment-related toxicities that occurred in ≥10% patients are included. Treatment discontinuation owing to adverse events was reported for 25% patients; the adverse events were considered to be treatment-related in 16% of patients. A total of 4% patients died during treatment or within 35 days after permanent treatment discontinuation; half of these deaths were considered to be treatment-related (one death due to lung infection, one due to respiratory failure, and one due to a cerebral thromboembolic event)

Therapy Monitoring

1. *Prior to initiation of copanlisib:* CBC with differential, serum chemistries (including fasting or random blood glucose), liver function tests, vital signs (including blood pressure), advise patients to report signs/symptoms of hyperglycemia and to ensure adequate oral hydration for 1–2 days following each copanlisib infusion, pregnancy test (women of child-bearing potential only)

2. *Prior to each copanlisib infusion:* CBC with differential, serum chemistries (including fasting or random blood glucose), physical exam, vital signs (including blood pressure)

3. *Fifteen minutes following each copanlisib infusion:* Vital signs (including blood pressure)

4. *In patients with a baseline diagnosis of diabetes mellitus or with a past episode of hyperglycemia following a copanlisib infusion:* Consider self-monitoring of blood glucose (eg, 2–4 times per day for at least 1–2 days) following each copanlisib infusion

5. *At least weekly during therapy:* CBC with differential

6. *Periodically:* monitor for signs and symptoms of: Infection (including *Pneumocystis jirovecii* pneumonia), hyperglycemia, hypertension, non-infectious pneumonitis, and severe cutaneous reactions

7. *Response assessment every 2–3 cycles:* Physical examination, CT scan

FOLLICULAR LYMPHOMA • SUBSEQUENT THERAPY

NON-HODGKIN LYMPHOMA REGIMEN: DUVELISIB

Flinn IW et al. J Clin Oncol 2019;37:912–922
Copiktra (duvelisib) prescribing information. Needham, MA: Verastem, Inc.; 2019 July

Duvelisib 25 mg per dose; administer orally twice per day, without regard to food, continually until disease progression (total dosage/week = 350 mg)
Notes on duvelisib administration:
- Duvelisib capsules should be swallowed whole. Do not break, open, or chew capsules
- Patients who delay taking a duvelisib dose at a regularly scheduled time may administer the missed dose if within 6 hours of the usual dosing time. If >6 hours, skip the missed dose, and resume treatment at the next regularly scheduled time
- Duvelisib is metabolized by CYP3A. If concomitant use with a strong CY3A4 inhibitor is unavoidable, reduce the duvelisib dose to 15 mg twice daily. Avoid concomitant use with strong CYP3A inducers
- Duvelisib inhibits CYP3A4 and increased the mean C_{max} of midazolam (a sensitive CYP3A substrate) by 2.2-fold and the mean area-under-the-curve of midazolam by 4.3-fold. Thus, consider reducing the dose of sensitive CYP3A4 substrates and monitor closely for signs of toxicity of the coadministered sensitive CYP3A4 substrate

Supportive Care
Antiemetic prophylaxis
*Emetogenic potential is **MINIMAL-LOW***
See Chapter 42 for antiemetic recommendations

Hematopoietic growth factor (CSF) prophylaxis
*Primary prophylaxis is **NOT** indicated*
See Chapter 43 for more information

Antimicrobial prophylaxis
Risk of fever and neutropenia is *LOW*
Antimicrobial primary prophylaxis to be considered:
- Antibacterial—not indicated. *Pneumocystis jirovecii* prophylaxis (eg, cotrimoxazole) is specifically recommended in the prescribing information during treatment and until the absolute CD4+ T-cell count is >200 cells/mm³
- Antifungal—not indicated
- Antiviral—antiherpes antivirals (eg, acyclovir, famciclovir, valacyclovir). Consider preemptive or prophylactic cytomegalovirus (CMV) management in CMV seropositive patients treated with duvelisib

Treatment Modifications

Duvelisib	
Starting dose	25 mg by mouth twice a day
Dose level −1	15 mg by mouth twice a day
Dose level −2	Discontinue therapy

Adverse Event	Dose Modification
Pulmonary Toxicity	
Moderate (G2), symptomatic, non-infectious pneumonitis	Withhold duvelisib. Treat with systemic corticosteroids. If improvement to G ≤1 occurs, may resume duvelisib at dose level −1

(continued)

Patient Population Studied

The DYNAMO study was a single-arm, phase II, open-label study involving patients with relapsed indolent non-Hodgkin lymphoma (follicular lymphoma [FL], small lymphocytic lymphoma [SLL], or marginal zone lymphoma [MZL]) that was refractory to rituximab (no response or disease progression within 6 months of therapy completion) and refractory to either chemotherapy or radioimmunotherapy. Patients with grade 3B FL or with evidence of transformation to aggressive lymphoma were excluded. Patients were excluded if they had prior treatment with a Bruton's tyrosine kinase inhibitor or other PI3K inhibitor. Enrolled patients (n = 129) had FL (n = 83), SLL (n = 28), or MZL (n = 18). The median age of patients was 65 years, 90% were white, 68% were male, median time since diagnosis was 54 months, 95% of patients had an ECOG PS of 0 or 1, 67% had an elevated baseline LDH, and the median number of prior regimens was 3. Among the FL patients, the FLIPI score was low (0–1) in 13%, intermediate (2) in 21%, high (>2) in 65%, and missing in 1%

Efficacy

(N = 129)

Overall response rate*	47.3% (42.2% in those with follicular lymphoma)
Median progression-free survival	9.5 months (95% CI, 8.1–11.8)
Median overall survival	28.9 months (95% CI, 21.4 to not estimable)

Overall response rate includes patients with either a complete or partial response
Note: Results are shown for all trial participants (that is, individuals with follicular lymphoma, small lymphocytic lymphoma, or marginal zone lymphoma). Response rates and progression-free survival shown are those from the independent review committee. The median follow-up among all was 32.1 months

Toxicity

N = 129

Adverse Event (%)	All Grades	Grade ≥3
Diarrhea	48.8	14.7
Nausea	29.5	1.6
Neutropenia	28.7	24.8
Fatigue	27.9	4.7
Cough	27.1	0
Anemia	26.4	14.7
Pyrexia	24.8	0
Rash	18.6	4.7
Thrombocytopenia	18.6	11.6
Vomiting	18.6	3.9
Decreased appetite	14.7	0.8
Headache	15.5	0
Peripheral edema	17.1	2.3
ALT increased	14.0	5.4
Back pain	13.2	0.8
Arthralgia	14.7	0
Abdominal pain	14.7	1.6
Hypokalemia	13.2	3.1
Constipation	11.6	0
Asthenia	11.6	2.3
AST increased	10.1	3.1
Night sweats	10.1	0
Febrile neutropenia	9.3	9.9
Lipase increased	9.3	7.0
Pneumonia	7.8	5.4
Colitis	7.8	5.4

Note: the table includes all-grade treatment-emergent adverse events (TEAEs) occurring in >10% of patients and G ≥3 TEAEs occurring in >5% of patients

Treatment Modifications (continued)

Moderate (G2), symptomatic, non-infectious pneumonitis not responsive to steroids or recurrent moderate (G2), symptomatic, non-infectious pneumonitis	Discontinue duvelisib
Severe (G3) or life-threatening (G4) non-infectious pneumonitis	Discontinue duvelisib. Treat with systemic corticosteroids

Infectious Complications

G ≥3 infection	Interrupt duvelisib until resolution of infection, then resume at the same or reduced dose
Clinical CMV infection or CMV viremia	Interrupt duvelisib until viremia or infection has resolved. Upon resolution, duvelisib may be resumed at the same dose or at a reduced dose; if resumed, then monitor blood CMV PCR or pp65 antigen detection at least monthly during ongoing treatment
PJP infection is suspected	Interrupt duvelisib during workup for suspected PJP infection
PJP infection is confirmed	Permanently discontinue duvelisib

Gastrointestinal Toxicity

G1/2 non-infectious diarrhea (up to 6 stools per day over baseline) and responsive to antidiarrhea agent or asymptomatic (G1) colitis	No change in duvelisib dose. Initiate supportive therapy with antidiarrheal agents as appropriate. Discontinue other medications which may cause diarrhea, if applicable. Monitor at least weekly until resolution, and then resume normal diet
G1/2 diarrhea (up to 6 stools per day over baseline) and *not* responsive to antidiarrhea agents	Interrupt duvelisib. Initiate supportive therapy with enteric acting steroids (eg, budesonide). Monitor at least weekly until resolution, then resume duvelisib at a reduced dose
Abdominal pain, stool with mucus or blood, change in bowel habits, peritoneal signs or severe diarrhea (G3, >6 stools per day above baseline)	Interrupt duvelisib. Initiate supportive therapy with enteric acting steroids (eg, budesonide) or systemic steroids. Monitor at least weekly until resolved, then resume duvelisib at a reduced dose
Recurrent G3 diarrhea or recurrent colitis of any grade	Permanently discontinue duvelisib
Life-threatening diarrhea or colitis	

Hematologic Toxicity

G3 neutropenia (ANC ≥500/mm³ to <1000/mm³)	Continue duvelisib at the current dose without interruption. Monitor ANC at least once per week
G4 neutropenia (ANC <500/mm³)	Interrupt duvelisib. Monitor ANC at least once per week until ANC ≥500/mm³, then resume duvelisib at the same dose (for first occurrence)
Recurrent G4 neutropenia (ANC <500/mm³)	Interrupt duvelisib. Monitor ANC at least once per week until ANC ≥500/mm³, then resume duvelisib at a reduced dose
G3 thrombocytopenia (platelet count ≥25,000/mm³ to <50,000/mm³) with G ≤1 bleeding	Continue duvelisib at the current dose without interruption. Monitor platelet count at least once per week

(continued)

Treatment Modifications (continued)

G3 thrombocytopenia (platelet count ≥25,000/mm³ to <50,000/mm³) with G2 bleeding or G4 thrombocytopenia (platelet count <25,000/mm³)	Interrupt duvelisib. Monitor platelet count at least once per week until platelet count ≥25,000/mm³, and resolution of bleeding (if applicable), then resume duvelisib at the same dose
Recurrent G3 thrombocytopenia (platelet count ≥25,000/mm³ to <50,000/mm³) with G2 bleeding or G4 thrombocytopenia (platelet count <25,000/mm³)	Interrupt duvelisib. Monitor platelet count at least once per week until platelet count ≥25,000/mm³, and resolution of bleeding (if applicable), then resume duvelisib at a reduced dose

Hepatic Toxicity

G2 elevation in ALT or AST (ALT or AST >3 to ≤5× ULN)	Continue duvelisib at the current dose without interruption. Monitor liver function tests at least weekly until resolution to ≤3× ULN, then resume normal frequency of monitoring
G3 elevation in ALT or AST (ALT or AST >5 to ≤20× ULN)	Interrupt duvelisib. Monitor liver function tests at least weekly until resolution to ≤3× ULN, then resume duvelisib at the same dose
Recurrent G3 elevation in ALT or AST (ALT or AST >5 to ≤20× ULN)	Interrupt duvelisib. Monitor liver function tests at least weekly until resolution to ≤3× ULN, then resume duvelisib at a reduced dose
G4 elevation in ALT or AST (ALT or AST >20× ULN)	Permanently discontinue duvelisib

Dermatologic and Immunologic Toxicities

SJS, TEN, or DRESS is suspected	Interrupt duvelisib until dermatologic status is clarified
SJS, TEN, or DRESS is confirmed	Permanently discontinue duvelisib
Other G1/2 cutaneous reaction	No change in duvelisib dose. Initiate supportive care with emollients, anti-histamines (for pruritus), or topical steroids. Monitor closely
Other G3 cutaneous reaction	Withhold duvelisib until resolution. Initiate supportive care with emollients, anti-histamines (for pruritus), or topical steroids. Monitor at least weekly until resolved, then resume at a reduced dose. If severe cutaneous reaction does not improve, worsens, or recurs, then discontinue duvelisib
Other life-threatening cutaneous reaction	Permanently discontinue duvelisib

Drug-Drug Interactions

Concomitant therapy with a strong CYP3A inhibitor is required	Consider alternative medication. If the strong CYP3A inhibitor is unavoidable, then reduce the duvelisib dosage to 15 mg twice per day
Concomitant therapy with a strong CYP3A inducer is required	Do not administer a strong CYP3A inducer with duvelisib
Concomitant therapy with a CYP3A substrate with a narrow therapeutic index is required	Consider reducing the dose of the concomitantly administered sensitive CYP3A substrate. Monitor closely for toxicity related to the sensitive CYP3A substrate

ALT, alanine aminotransferase; ANC, absolute neutrophil count; AST, aspartate aminotransferase; CMV, cytomegalovirus; DRESS, drug reaction with eosinophilia and systemic systems; PCR, polymerase chain reaction; PJP, *Pneumocystis jirovecii* pneumonia; SJS, Stevens-Johnson syndrome; TEN, toxic epidermal necrolysis; ULN, upper limit of normal
Copiktra (duvelisib) prescribing information. Needham, MA: Verastem, Inc.; 2019 July

Therapy Monitoring

Prior to initiation of duvelisib:
1. CBC with differential, chemistries (potassium, uric acid, phosphorus, calcium, serum creatinine, LDH), liver function tests (serum bilirubin, ALT, AST, alkaline phosphatase), urine pregnancy test (women of child-bearing potential only)

During treatment with duvelisib:
2. Monitor liver function tests (ALT, AST, and serum bilirubin) in all patients. In patients with normal ALT/AST, consider monitoring at least every 2 weeks for the first 3 months of treatment, then at least every 4 weeks for the next 3 months, then at least every 1–3 months thereafter. Monitor at least weekly if ALT or AST increases to >3× ULN until resolution to ≤3× ULN
3. Monitor CBC with differential at least every 2 weeks for the first 2 months of therapy, and at least weekly while absolute neutrophil count is <1000/mm³ or platelet count is <50,000/mm³
4. Monitor periodically for:
   - Signs and symptoms of diarrhea/colitis
   - Signs and symptoms of intestinal perforation
   - Signs and symptoms of dermatologic toxicity or hypersensitivity reactions
   - Signs and symptoms of pneumonitis
   - Signs and symptoms of infection (including sepsis, pneumonia, *Pneumocystis jirovecii* pneumonia, and cytomegalovirus)
5. *Response assessment every 2–3 months:* Physical examination, CBC with differential, CT scan with contrast

Treatment Modifications

Tazemetostat Treatment Modifications

Tazemetostat Dose Levels

Starting dose	800 mg by mouth twice per day
Dose level −1	600 mg by mouth twice per day
Dose level −2	400 mg by mouth twice per day
Dose level −3	Permanently discontinue tazemetostat

Hematologic Toxicity

ANC <1000/mm³; first occurrence	Withhold tazemetostat until ANC ≥1000/mm³ or baseline, then resume at the same dose
ANC <1000/mm³; second occurrence	Withhold tazemetostat until ANC ≥1000/mm³ or baseline, then resume at one lower dose level
ANC <1000/mm³; third occurrence	
ANC <1000/mm³; fourth occurrence	Permanently discontinue tazemetostat
Platelets <50,000/mm³; first occurrence	Withhold tazemetostat until platelets ≥75,000/mm³ or baseline, then resume at one lower dose level
Platelets <50,000/mm³; second occurrence	Withhold tazemetostat until platelets ≥75,000/mm³ or baseline, then resume at one lower dose level
Platelets <50,000/mm³; third occurrence	Permanently discontinue tazemetostat
Hemoglobin <8 g/dL	Withhold tazemetostat until improvement to G ≤1 (Hgb ≥10 g/dL) or baseline, then resume at either the same or reduced dose

Nonhematologic Toxicities

Other G3 adverse reaction; first occurrence	Withhold tazemetostat until improvement to G ≤1 or baseline, then resume at one lower dose level

FOLLICULAR LYMPHOMA • FIRST LINE • SUBSEQUENT THERAPY
NON-HODGKIN LYMPHOMA REGIMEN: TAZEMETOSTAT

Morschhauser F et al. Lancet Oncol 2020;21:1433–1442
TAZVERIK (tazemetostat) prescribing information. Cambridge, MA: Epizyme, Inc., 2020 July

Tazemetostat 800 mg/dose; administer orally, twice per day, with or without food, continually, until disease progression (total dose/week = 11,200 mg)
- Tazemetostat tablets should be swallowed whole; do not cut, crush, or chew tablets
- Patients who delay taking tazemetostat at a regularly scheduled time or who vomit following administration of a dose should not repeat the dose, but instead should continue with the next scheduled dose
- Tazemetostat is metabolized by CYP3A to form the major inactive major M5 (EPZ-6930) and M3 (EPZ006931) metabolites. Refer to treatment modification section for initial dose adjustment recommendations for patients requiring concurrent treatment with moderate CYP3A inhibitors. Avoid concomitant use of tazemetostat with strong CYP3A4 inhibitors, moderate CYP3A4 inducers, and strong CYP3A inducers
- Advise patients to not consume grapefruit products or St. John's Wort as they may inhibit or induce CYP3A in the gut wall, respectively, thus affecting the bioavailability of tazemetostat
- Coadministration of tazemetostat with oral midazolam (a CYP3A probe substrate) reduced the midazolam AUC_{0-12h} by 40% and Cmax by 21%. Thus, use caution when co-administering tazemetostat with sensitive CYP3A4 substrates, including hormonal contraceptives, where reductions in the concentration of the CYP3A4 substrate may have detrimental clinical effects

Supportive Care
Antiemetic prophylaxis
Emetogenic potential is **MINIMAL**
See Chapter 42 for antiemetic recommendations

Hematopoietic growth factor (CSF) prophylaxis
Primary prophylaxis is **NOT** indicated
See Chapter 43 for more information

Antimicrobial prophylaxis
Risk of fever and neutropenia is *LOW*
Antimicrobial primary prophylaxis to be considered:
- Antibacterial—not indicated
- Antifungal—not indicated
- Antiviral—antiherpes antivirals (eg, acyclovir, famciclovir, valacyclovir)

Patient Population Studied

Baseline Patient and Disease Characteristics

	*EZH2*mut (n = 45)	*EZH2*WT (n = 54)
Age, years	62 (57–68)	61 (53–67)
Sex—male / female	19 (42%) / 26 (58%)	34 (63%) / 20 (37%)
ECOG performance status—0/1/2	21 (47%) / 24 (53%) /0	26 (48%) / 23 (43%) / 4 (7%)
Satisfied GELF criteria*—Yes / No	31 (69%) / 14 (31%)	40 (74%) / 14 (26%)
Time from initial diagnosis, years	4.7 (1.7–6.4)	6.3 (3.4–9.0)
Histology		
Grade 1, 2, or 3a	42 (93%)	51 (94%)[†]
Grade 3b or transformed follicular lymphoma	3 (7%)	6 (11%)[†]

(continued)

Treatment Modifications
(continued)

Other G3 adverse reaction; second occurrence	Withhold tazemetostat until improvement to G ≤1 or baseline, then resume at one lower dose level
Other G3 adverse reaction; third occurrence	Permanently discontinue tazemetostat
Other G4 adverse reaction; first occurrence	Withhold tazemetostat until improvement to G ≤1 or baseline, then resume with the dose reduced by one or two dose levels, if clinically appropriate
Other G4 adverse reaction; second occurrence	Permanently discontinue tazemetostat

ANC, absolute neutrophil count
TAZVERIK (tazemetostat) prescribing information.
Cambridge, MA: Epizyme, Inc., 2020 July

Patient Population Studied *(continued)*

Previous lines of anticancer therapy		
One	2 (4%)	1 (2%)
Two	22 (49%)	16 (30%)
Three	10 (22%)	11 (20%)
Four	4 (9%)	10 (19%)
Five or more	7 (16%)	16 (30%)
Median	2 (2–43)	3 (2–5)
Refractory to last regimen⁶	22 (49%)	22 (41%)
Poor risk features		
Refractory to a rituximab-containing regimen‖	22 (49%)	32 (59%)
Double refractory**	9 (20%)	15 (28%)
Previous hematopoietic stem-cell transplant	4 (9%)	21 (39%)
Disease progression within 24 months of disease diagnosis in patients treated with first-line immunochemotherapy (POD24)	19 (42%)	32 (59%)

Data are median (IQR) or n (%)
ECOG, Eastern Cooperative Oncology Group; GELF, *Groupe d'Etude des Lymphomes Folliculaires*
*Defined as a target lesion of more than 7 cm in diameter, three nodal target lesions of more than 3 cm in diameter each, the presence of B symptoms at baseline, a concentration of serum lactate dehydrogenase higher than the upper limit of normal, a serum hemoglobin concentration of 100 g/L or less, a neutrophil count of 1500 cells per µL or less, or a platelet count of 100 000 platelets per mL or less
†Some patients were counted in more than one category
⁶Patients with stable disease or progressive disease to the most recent previous anticancer therapy
‖Refractory to either rituximab monotherapy or rituximab-containing therapy or progressive disease within 6 months of completion of rituximab-containing therapy
**Refractory to rituximab (as a monotherapy or as part of a combination therapy) and a chemotherapy induction regimen containing one or more alkylating agent or purine nucleoside antagonist and have relapsed within 6 months

Efficacy (N = 99)

	*EZH2*mut (n = 45)	*EZH2*WT (n = 54)
	IRC-assessed	IRC-assessed
Objective response rate*	31 (69%; 53–82)	19 (35%; 23–49)
Overall disease control rate†	44 (98%)	37 (69%)
Complete response	6 (13%)	2 (4%)
Partial response	25 (56%)	17 (31%)
Stable disease	13 (29%)	18 (33%)
Progressive disease	1 (2%)	12 (22%)
Not estimable or unknown	0	5 (9%)

Data are n (%; 95% CI) or n (%)
IRC, independent radiology committee
*Objective response rate includes patients with a complete or partial response
†Overall disease control rate includes patients with a complete response, partial response, or stable disease

Adverse Events

	Treatment-emergent Adverse Events			Treatment-related Adverse Events		
	G1–2	G3	G4	G1–2	G3	G4
Nausea	23 (23%)	0	0	19 (19%)	0	0
Diarrhea	18 (18%)	0	0	12 (12%)	0	0
Alopecia	17 (17%)	0	0	14 (14%)	0	0
Cough	16 (16%)	0	0	2 (2%)	0	0
Asthenia	15 (15%)	3 (3%)	0	13 (13%)	1 (1%)	0
Fatigue	15 (15%)	2 (2%)	0	11 (11%)	1 (1%)	0
Upper respiratory tract infection	15 (15%)	0	0	1 (1%)	0	0
Bronchitis	15 (15%)	0	0	3 (3%)	0	0
Abdominal pain	12 (12%)	1 (1%)	0	2 (2%)	0	0
Headache	12 (12%)	0	0	5 (5%)	0	0
Vomiting	11 (11%)	1 (1%)	0	6 (6%)	0	0
Back pain	11 (11%)	0	0	0	0	0
Pyrexia	10 (10%)	0	0	2 (2%)	0	0
Anemia	9 (9%)	4 (4%)	1 (1%)	7 (7%)	2 (2%)	0
Thrombocytopenia	5 (5%)	4 (4%)	1 (1%)	5 (5%)	3 (3%)	0
Neutropenia	3 (3%)	3 (3%)	1 (1%)	3 (3%)	2 (2%)	1 (1%)
Leucopenia	2 (2%)	1 (1%)	0	2 (2%)	1 (1%)	0
Hypophosphatemia	2 (2%)	1 (1%)	0	2 (2%)	1 (1%)	0
Hypertriglyceridemia	1 (1%)	1 (1%)	0	1 (1%)	1 (1%)	0
↑Serum amylase	1 (1%)	1 (1%)	0	1 (1%)	1 (1%)	0
Presyncope	0	1 (1%)	0	0	1 (1%)	0
Pancytopenia	0	0	1 (1%)	0	0	1 (1%)
↑Serum aminotransferase	0	1 (1%)	0	0	1 (1%)	0
Myelodysplastic syndrome	0	1 (1%)	0	0	1 (1%)	0
Dyspnea	5 (5%)	3 (3%)	0	1 (1%)	0	0
Dizziness	6 (6%)	1 (1%)	0	3 (3%)	0	0
Upper abdominal pain	5 (5%)	1 (1%)	0	4 (4%)	0	0
Urinary tract infection	5 (5%)	1 (1%)	0	1 (1%)	0	0
Hypogammaglobulinemia	3 (3%)	1 (1%)	0	1 (1%)	0	0
Hypertension	3 (3%)	1 (1%)	0	0	0	0
Hyperkalemia	2 (2%)	1 (1%)	0	1 (1%)	1 (1%)	0
Lung infection	2 (2%)	1 (1%)	0	1 (1%)	0	0
Pleural effusion	2 (2%)	1 (1%)	0	0	0	0

(continued)

Patient Population Studied (*continued*)

Herpes zoster	1 (1%)	1 (1%)	0	0	0	0
Sepsis	0	0	2 (2%)	0	0	0
General physical health deterioration	0	0	2 (2%)	0	0	0
Non-cardiac chest pain	1 (1%)	1 (1%)	0	1 (1%)	0	0
Hyperuricemia	1 (1%)	0	1 (1%)	1 (1%)	0	0
Prolonged QT on EKG, hypothyroidism	1 (1%)	1 (1%)	0	1 (1%)	0	0
Lymphopenia	1 (1%)	0	1 (1%)	0	0	0
Lower gastrointestinal hemorrhage, hypokalemia, acute myeloid leukemia, malignant melanoma, chronic kidney disease, bile duct obstruction,	0	0	1 (1%)	0	0	0
Ascites, acute pancreatitis, empyema, cerebrovascular accident, osmotic demyelination syndrome, post-herpetic neuralgia, syncope, hypoxia, hypercalcemia, hyperglycemia, hyponatremia, ↑blood pressure, femoral artery occlusion, subclavian vein thrombosis, squamous cell carcinoma, constrictive pericarditis	0	1 (1%)	0	0	0	0

Therapy Monitoring

1 *Prior to initiation of therapy*: CBC with differential, liver function tests, urine pregnancy test (in women of child-bearing potential), review concomitant medications for drug-drug interaction
2 *Every 2–4 weeks, or as clinically indicated*: CBC with differential
3 *Response assessment (every 2–4 months)*: Physical examination, CBC with differential, CT scan or PET scan

MANTLE CELL LYMPHOMA • FIRST LINE
NON-HODGKIN LYMPHOMA REGIMEN (NORDIC): (R)-MAXI-CHOP ALTERNATING WITH (R)-HIDAC

Geisler CH et al. Br J Haematol 2012;158:355–362
Geisler CH et al. Blood 2008;112:2687–2693

Regimen note: Patients receive 3 cycles of cyclophosphamide + doxorubicin + vincristine + prednisone (Maxi-CHOP) alternating every 3 weeks with 3 cycles of high-dose cytarabine (HiDAC) for a total of 6 cycles of induction therapy. The last cycle (HiDAC) also serves as chemomobilization for peripheral blood hematopoietic stem cell collection. Rituximab is also administered on day 1 of cycles 2–5, and on day 1 and 9 of cycle 6. Patients who respond to Maxi-CHOP-R/R-HiDAC undergo intensification with high dose chemotherapy (carmustine + etoposide + cytarabine + melphalan [BEAM]) or (carmustine + etoposide + cytarabine + cyclophosphamide [BEAC]) followed by autologous hematopoietic stem cell transplantation (not included in this regimen description). Following transplant, Geisler et al performed assessment of minimal residual disease (MRD) and, if converted from negative to positive, initiated preemptive therapy with weekly rituximab 375 mg/m^2 per dose for 4 weeks (not included in this regimen description). **As an alternative to MRD-directed preemptive rituximab, most centers administer maintenance rituximab following autologous transplant** (Le Gouill S et al. N Engl J Med 2017;377:1250–1260) (not included in this regimen description)

Maxi-CHOP (cycle 1):
Intravenous hydration before and after cyclophosphamide administration:
500–1000 mL 0.9% sodium chloride (0.9% NS)

Cyclophosphamide 1200 mg/m^2; administer intravenously in 25–250 mL 0.9% NS or 5% dextrose injection (D5W) over 10–30 minutes, given on day 1, for 1 cycle, cycle 1 (total dosage/21-day cycle = 1200 mg/m^2)
Doxorubicin 75 mg/m^2; administer by intravenous injection over 3–5 minutes, given on day 1, for 1 cycle, cycle 1 (total dosage/21-day cycle = 75 mg/m^2)
Vincristine 2 mg; administer by intravenous infusion over 15 minutes in 50 mL 0.9% NS, given on day 1, for 1 cycle, cycle 1 (total dose/21-day cycle = 2 mg)
Prednisone 100 mg per day; administer orally for 5 consecutive days, days 1–5 for 1 cycle, cycle 1 (total dose/21-day cycle = 500 mg)

R-HiDAC (cycles 2 and 4):
Premedication for Rituximab:
Acetaminophen 650–1000 mg; administer orally 30–60 minutes before each rituximab dose, *plus*
Diphenhydramine 25–50 mg; administer orally or intravenously 30–60 minutes before each rituximab dose
Rituximab 375 mg/m^2 per dose; administer intravenously in 0.9% NS or D5W, diluted to a concentration within the range 1–4 mg/mL, on day 1, for 2 cycles, cycles 2 and 4 (total dosage/21-day cycle = 375 mg/m^2)
Rituximab administration:
• Infuse initially at 50 mg/h. If hypersensitivity or infusion reactions do not occur during the first 30 minutes, increase the rate by 50 mg/h every 30 minutes as tolerated to a maximum rate of 400 mg/h. During subsequent treatments if previous rituximab administration was well tolerated, start at 100 mg/h, and increase by 100 mg/h every 30 minutes as tolerated to a maximum rate of 400 mg/h
• Interrupt rituximab administration for fever, chills, edema, congestion of the head and neck mucosa, hypertension, and other serious adverse events. Resume rituximab administration after adverse events abate

Cytarabine
Patients aged <60 years: **Cytarabine** 3000 mg/m^2 per dose; administer intravenously over 3 hours in 50–500 mL 0.9% NS or D5W every 12 hours for 4 doses on days 1 and 2, for 2 cycles, cycles 2 and 4 (total dosage/21-day cycle = 12,000 mg/m^2)
Patients aged ≥60 years: **Cytarabine** 2000 mg/m^2 per dose; administer intravenously over 3 hours in 50–500 mL 0.9% NS or D5W every 12 hours for 4 doses on days 1 and 2, for 2 cycles, cycles 2 and 4 (total dosage/21-day cycle = 8000 mg/m^2)

Keratitis prophylaxis
Steroid ophthalmic drops (**prednisolone 1% or dexamethasone 0.1%**); administer 2 drops by intraocular instillation into each eye every 6 hours starting prior to the first cytarabine dose and continuing until 48 hours after high-dose cytarabine is completed

Maxi-CHOP-R (cycles 3 and 5):
Premedication for rituximab:
Acetaminophen 650–1000 mg; administer orally 30–60 minutes before each rituximab dose, *plus*
Diphenhydramine 25–50 mg; administer orally or intravenously 30–60 minutes before each rituximab dose
Rituximab 375 mg/m^2 per dose; administer intravenously in 0.9% NS or D5W, diluted to a concentration within the range 1–4 mg/mL, on day 1, for 2 cycles, cycles 3 and 5 (total dosage/21-day cycle = 375 mg/m^2)
Notes on rituximab administration:
• Infuse initially at 50 mg/h. If hypersensitivity or infusion reactions do not occur during the first 30 minutes, increase the rate by 50 mg/h every 30 minutes as tolerated to a maximum rate of 400 mg/h. During subsequent treatments if previous rituximab administration was well tolerated, start at 100 mg/h, and increase by 100 mg/h every 30 minutes as tolerated to a maximum rate of 400 mg/h

INFUSION REACTIONS ASSOCIATED WITH RITUXIMAB

Fevers, chills, and rigors

1. Interrupt rituximab administration for severe symptoms, and give:
   - **Acetaminophen** 650 mg orally for fever. For persistent or recurrent symptoms, repeat administration every 4–6 hours as needed during rituximab administration
   - **Diphenhydramine** 25–50 mg orally or by intravenous injection for pruritus, hypotension, or angioedema. For persistent or recurrent symptoms, repeat administration every 4–6 hours as needed during rituximab administration
   - **Meperidine** 12.5–25 mg by intravenous injection every 10–20 minutes as needed for shaking chills (generally, cumulative doses >100 mg are not needed; use repeated doses with caution in persons with moderate or more severely impaired renal function)
2. If rituximab administration was interrupted, resume infusion at a slower rate than the maximum rate previously attempted. Rate escalation may be reattempted at smaller incremental steps with close monitoring. Do not exceed the maximum recommended rate of 400 mg/h

Dyspnea or wheezing without allergic findings (urticaria, or tongue or laryngeal edema)

1. Interrupt rituximab administration immediately
1. Give **hydrocortisone** 100 mg by intravenous injection (or an alternative steroid with equivalent glucocorticoid potency)
2. Give a **histamine (H$_2$) receptor antagonist** (ranitidine 50 mg, cimetidine 300 mg, or famotidine 20 mg) intravenously over 15–30 minutes
3. After symptoms resolve, resume rituximab administration at 25 mg/h with close monitoring. Do not increase the administration rate

Note: Medications and equipment for the treatment of hypersensitivity reactions should be available for immediate use in the event of a reaction during administration (eg, intravenous fluids, epinephrine, antihistamines, glucocorticoids, and oxygen)

Rituxan (rituximab) prescribing information. South San Francisco, CA: Genentech, Inc; 2018 October

Intravenous hydration before and after cyclophosphamide administration:

500–1000 mL 0.9% NS

Cyclophosphamide 1200 mg/m^2; administer intravenously in 25–250 mL 0.9% NS or D5W over 10–30 minutes, given on day 1, for 2 cycles, cycles 3 and 5 (total dosage/21-day cycle = 1200 mg/m^2)

Doxorubicin 75 mg/m^2; administer by intravenous injection over 3–5 minutes, given on day 1, for 2 cycles, cycles 3 and 5 (total dosage/21-day cycle = 75 mg/m^2)

Vincristine 2 mg; administer by intravenous infusion over 15 minutes in 50 mL 0.9% NS, given on day 1, for 2 cycles, cycles 3 and 5 (total dosage/21-day cycle = 2 mg)

Prednisone 100 mg per day; administer orally for 5 consecutive days, days 1–5 for 2 cycles, cycles 3 and 5 (total dosage/21-day cycle = 500 mg)

R-HiDAC (cycle 6, peripheral blood stem cell chemo-mobilization):

Note during cycle 6: Coordinate growth factor administration and peripheral blood hematopoietic stem cell collection with a stem cell transplant center

Premedication for rituximab:

Acetaminophen 650–1000 mg; administer orally 30–60 minutes before each rituximab dose, *plus*

Diphenhydramine 25–50 mg; administer orally or intravenously 30–60 minutes before each rituximab dose

Rituximab 375 mg/m^2 per dose; administer intravenously in 0.9% NS or D5W, diluted to a concentration within the range 1–4 mg/mL, for 2 doses on days 1 and 9, for 1 cycle, cycle 6 (total dosage/21-day cycle = 750 mg/m^2)

Notes on rituximab administration:
- Infuse initially at 50 mg/h. If hypersensitivity or infusion reactions do not occur during the first 30 minutes, increase the rate by 50 mg/h every 30 minutes as tolerated to a maximum rate of 400 mg/h. During subsequent treatments if previous rituximab administration was well tolerated, start at 100 mg/h, and increase by 100 mg/h every 30 minutes as tolerated to a maximum rate of 400 mg/h

INFUSION REACTIONS ASSOCIATED WITH RITUXIMAB

Fevers, chills, and rigors

1. Interrupt rituximab administration for severe symptoms, and give:
   - **Acetaminophen** 650 mg orally for fever. For persistent or recurrent symptoms, repeat administration every 4–6 hours as needed during rituximab administration
   - **Diphenhydramine** 25–50 mg orally or by intravenous injection for pruritus, hypotension, or angioedema. For persistent or recurrent symptoms, repeat administration every 4–6 hours as needed during rituximab administration
   - **Meperidine** 12.5–25 mg by intravenous injection every 10–20 minutes as needed for shaking chills (generally, cumulative doses >100 mg are not needed; use repeated doses with caution in persons with moderate or more severely impaired renal function)
2. If rituximab administration was interrupted, resume infusion at a slower rate than the maximum rate previously attempted. Rate escalation may be reattempted at smaller incremental steps with close monitoring. Do not exceed the maximum recommended rate of 400 mg/h

Dyspnea or wheezing without allergic findings (urticaria, or tongue or laryngeal edema)

1. Interrupt rituximab administration immediately
2. Give **hydrocortisone** 100 mg by intravenous injection (or an alternative steroid with equivalent glucocorticoid potency)
3. Give a **histamine (H$_2$) receptor antagonist** (ranitidine 50 mg, cimetidine 300 mg, or famotidine 20 mg) intravenously over 15–30 minutes
4. After symptoms resolve, resume rituximab administration at 25 mg/h with close monitoring. Do not increase the administration rate

Note: Medications and equipment for the treatment of hypersensitivity reactions should be available for immediate use in the event of a reaction during administration (eg, intravenous fluids, epinephrine, antihistamines, glucocorticoids, and oxygen)

Rituxan (rituximab) prescribing information. South San Francisco, CA: Genentech, Inc; 2018 October

(continued)

(continued)

Cytarabine

Patients aged <60 years: **Cytarabine** 3000 mg/m² per dose; administer intravenously over 3 hours in 50–500 mL 0.9% NS or D5W every 12 hours for 4 doses on days 1 and 2, for 1 cycle, cycle 6 (total dosage/21-day cycle = 12,000 mg/m²)

Patients aged ≥60 years: **Cytarabine** 2000 mg/m² per dose; administer intravenously over 3 hours in 50–500 mL 0.9% NS or D5W every 12 hours for 4 doses on days 1 and 2, for 1 cycle, cycle 6 (total dosage/21-day cycle = 8000 mg/m²)

Keratitis prophylaxis

Steroid ophthalmic drops **(prednisolone 1% or dexamethasone 0.1%)**; administer 2 drops by intraocular instillation into each eye every 6 hours starting prior to the first cytarabine dose and continuing until 48 hours after high-dose cytarabine is completed

Supportive Care

Antiemetic prophylaxis

Emetogenic potential on day 1 of Maxi-CHOP-(R) cycles: **HIGH, POTENTIAL FOR DELAYED SYMPTOMS**

Emetogenic potential on days 1 and 2 of R-HiDAC cycles: **MODERATE**

Emetogenic potential on days with just rituximab: **MINIMAL**

See Chapter 42 for antiemetic recommendations

Hematopoietic growth factor (CSF) prophylaxis

Primary prophylaxis is indicated prior to cycles 1–5 with one of the following:

Filgrastim (G-CSF) 5 µg/kg per day by subcutaneous injection, *or*

Pegfilgrastim (pegylated filgrastim) 6 mg/0.6 mL by subcutaneous injection for 1 dose

• Begin use 24–72 hours after myelosuppressive chemotherapy is completed

• Continue daily filgrastim use until ANC ≥5000/mm³ after the leukocyte nadir

• Discontinue daily filgrastim use at least 24 hours before administering myelosuppressive treatment. Do not administer pegfilgrastim within 14 days before administering myelosuppressive treatment

Filgrastim is also required during cycle 6 but must be coordinated with a stem cell transplant center for purposes of peripheral blood hematopoietic stem cell collection (follow institutional protocols)

See Chapter 43 for more information

Antimicrobial prophylaxis

Risk of fever and neutropenia is *INTERMEDIATE*

Antimicrobial primary prophylaxis to be considered:

• Antibacterial—consider a fluoroquinolone during periods of prolonged neutropenia, or no prophylaxis

• Antifungal—consider use during periods of prolonged neutropenia, or no prophylaxis

• Antiviral—antiherpes antivirals (eg, acyclovir, famciclovir, valacyclovir)

Treatment Modifications

Cyclophosphamide + Doxorubicin +Vincristine + Prednisone (MAXI-CHOP) Dose Modifications				
Dose Level	Cyclophosphamide	Doxorubicin	Vincristine	Prednisone
Starting	1200 mg/m²	75 mg/m²	2 mg	100 mg
Level −1	1000 mg/m²	60 mg/m²	1.5 mg	80 mg
Level −2	800 mg/m²	45 mg/m²	1 mg	60 mg

Adverse Event	Treatment Modification
Hematologic Toxicity	
Day 1 platelet count <100,000/mm³ or ANC <1500/mm³	Delay start of cycle until platelet count ≥100,000/mm³ and ANC ≥1500/mm³, or until recovery to near baseline value, then continue at the same doses
G4 neutropenia (ANC <500/mm³) during the prior cycle given without growth factor (filgrastim, pegfilgrastim) prophylaxis	Administer filgrastim or pegfilgrastim during all subsequent cycles, and continue the same doses
Febrile neutropenia (ANC <1000/mm³ with temperature >38°C or >100.4°F) during the prior cycle given without growth factor (filgrastim, pegfilgrastim) prophylaxis	

(continued)

Treatment Modifications (*continued*)

Febrile neutropenia (ANC <1000/mm³ with temperature >38°C or >100.4°F) during the prior cycle given with growth factor (filgrastim, pegfilgrastim) prophylaxis	Reduce the dose of cyclophosphamide and doxorubicin by 1 dose level for subsequent cycles. Do not change the prednisone or vincristine dose
G ≥3 thrombocytopenia (platelets <50,000/mm³) during the prior cycle	

Gastrointestinal Toxicities

G ≥3 ileus (severely altered GI function; TPN indicated; tube placement indicated)	Withhold all chemotherapy until resolution of ileus and constipation, then reduce the next dose of vincristine by 1 dose level with an optimal prophylactic bowel regimen. Do not change the cyclophosphamide, doxorubicin, or prednisone doses
G ≥3 constipation (obstipation with manual evacuation indicated; limiting self-care ADL)	If symptoms do not recur at the reduced vincristine dose, then the vincristine dose may be re-escalated on subsequent cycles with an appropriate prophylactic bowel regimen

Neurologic Toxicities

G3 peripheral sensory neuropathy (severe symptoms; limiting self-care ADL)	Proceed with treatment and reduce the dose of vincristine by 1 dose level. Do not change the cyclophosphamide, doxorubicin, or prednisone doses
G2 peripheral motor neuropathy (moderate symptoms; limiting instrumental ADL)	If symptoms improve, the vincristine dose may be re-escalated on subsequent cycles
G3 peripheral motor neuropathy (severe symptoms; limiting self-care ADL)	Proceed with treatment, and reduce the dose of vincristine by 2 dose levels. Do not change the cyclophosphamide, doxorubicin, or prednisone doses
	If symptoms improve, the vincristine dose may be re-escalated on subsequent cycles
G4 peripheral sensory neuropathy (life-threatening symptoms; urgent intervention indicated)	Discontinue vincristine
G4 peripheral motor neuropathy (life-threatening consequences; urgent intervention indicated)	Do not change the cyclophosphamide, doxorubicin, or prednisone doses
G ≥2 mood alteration (moderate mood alteration) or confusion (moderate disorientation; limiting instrumental ADL)	Withhold prednisone until symptoms return to baseline. Resume prednisone reduced by 1 dose level. If symptoms persist, reduce by another dose level. Do not change the cyclophosphamide, doxorubicin, or vincristine doses

Hepatic Impairment

Serum bilirubin 1.2–3 mg/dL	Decrease the doxorubicin dose by 50%
	Additionally, if the bilirubin is 1.5–3 mg/dL, decrease the vincristine dose by 50%
Serum bilirubin 3.1–5 mg/dL	Decrease the doxorubicin by 75%
	Do not administer vincristine
Serum bilirubin >5 mg/dL	Do not administer doxorubicin or vincristine

Drug Interactions

Patient requires concomitant therapy with antihypertensive medication(s)	On days of rituximab treatment, and especially with the initial dose, weigh the risk versus benefit of delaying administration of the antihypertensive medication(s) until after completion of the rituximab infusion due to the potential risk of rituximab infusion-related hypotension
Patient requires concomitant therapy with a strong CYP3A4 inhibitor	Patient may have earlier onset of neuromuscular side effects of vincristine. If concomitant use of the strong CYP3A4 inhibitor cannot be avoided, consider dose reduction of vincristine and increased monitoring for toxicity

(*continued*)

Treatment Modifications (continued)

Other Toxicities

G ≥3 hyperglycemia (insulin therapy initiated; hospitalization indicated)	Withhold prednisone until blood glucose is ≤250 mg/dL. Treat with insulin or other hypoglycemic agents as clinically appropriate, and then resume prednisone at the same dose. If hyperglycemia is uncontrolled despite above measures, decrease prednisone by 1 dose level
LVEF is 40%, or is 40% to 45% with a 10% or greater absolute decrease below the pretreatment	Withhold doxorubicin, and repeat LVEF assessment within approximately 4 weeks. Discontinue doxorubicin if the LVEF has not improved or has declined further, unless the benefits for the individual patient outweigh the risks

High-dose Cytarabine (HIDAC) Dose Modifications

	Patients Aged <60 Years	Patients Aged ≥60 Years
Starting dose	3000 mg/m^2 per dose	2000 mg/m^2 per dose
Dose level 1	2250 mg/m^2 per dose	1500 mg/m^2 per dose
Dose level 2	1500 mg/m^2 per dose	1000 mg/m^2 per dose

Hematologic Toxicity

Day 1 platelet count <100,000/mm^3 or ANC <1500/mm^3	Delay start of cycle until platelet count ≥100,000/mm^3 and ANC ≥1500/mm^3, or until recovery to near baseline value, then continue at the same doses
G4 neutropenia (ANC <500/mm^3) during the prior cycle given without growth factor (filgrastim, pegfilgrastim) prophylaxis	Administer filgrastim or pegfilgrastim during all subsequent cycles, and continue the same doses
Febrile neutropenia (ANC <1000/mm^3 with temperature >38°C or >100.4°F) during the prior cycle given without growth factor (filgrastim, pegfilgrastim) prophylaxis	
Febrile neutropenia (ANC <1000/mm^3 with temperature >38°C or >100.4°F) during the prior cycle given with growth factor (filgrastim, pegfilgrastim) prophylaxis	Reduce the dose of cytarabine by 1 dose level for subsequent cycles
G ≥3 thrombocytopenia (platelets <50,000/mm^3) during the prior cycle	

Neurologic Toxicities

Neurologic (cerebellar) toxicity	Discontinue cytarabine. Patients who develop CNS symptoms should not receive subsequent high-dose cytarabine

Other Toxicities

Fever, myalgia, bone pain, occasionally chest pain, maculopapular rash, conjunctivitis and malaise 6–12 hours following drug administration (cytarabine or Ara-C syndrome)	Corticosteroids are beneficial in treating or preventing this syndrome. If the symptoms deemed treatable, continue therapy with cytarabine and pretreat with corticosteroids. If the syndrome occurs in a patient already receiving corticosteroid pretreatment, consider reducing the cytarabine dose by 1 dose level

ANC, absolute neutrophil count; GI, gastrointestinal; TPN, total parenteral nutrition; ADL, activities of daily living; LVEF, left ventricular ejection fraction
Note: Medications and equipment for the treatment of hypersensitivity reactions should be available for immediate use in the event of a reaction during rituximab administration (eg, intravenous fluids, epinephrine, antihistamines, glucocorticoids, and oxygen)

Patient Population Studied

The international, multicenter, nonrandomized, phase 2 trial (Nordic MCL2) involved 160 patients with newly diagnosed, stage II–IV, cyclin D1–positive mantle cell lymphoma. Eligible patients had received no prior treatment or had just initiated first-line treatment. Patients underwent six 21-day cycles of induction treatment, comprising cycles of intravenous cyclophosphamide (1200 mg/m² on day 1), doxorubicin (75 mg/m² on day 1), and vincristine (2 mg on day 1), and oral prednisone (100 mg/day on days 1–5) (maxi-CHOP) alternating with cycles of high-dose intravenous cytarabine (3 g/m² over 3 hours every 12 hours for a total of 4 doses; patients aged >60 years received a dose of 2 g/m²) (for a total of 3 cycles of each regimen). During the induction treatment, intravenous rituximab (375 mg/m²) was also administered on day 1 of cycles 2–5 and on days 1 and 9 of cycle 6. Subsequently, 1–2 weeks after a sufficient stem cell harvest (≥2 million CD34+ cells/kg), patients underwent high-dose chemotherapy with intravenous carmustine (300 mg/m² on day 1), etoposide (100 mg/m² twice daily on days 2–5), cytarabine (400 mg/m² on days 2–5), and either melphalan (140 mg/m² on day 6) or cyclophosphamide (1.5 g/m² on days 2–5) (BEAM or BEAC), and then stem cell infusion

Efficacy

(N = 160)

Median event-free survival	7.4 years
Projected 10-year event-free survival	43%
Projected 10-year overall survival	58%

Note: Median follow-up was 6.5 years

Toxicity

(N = 160)

- Hospitalization for grade 3–4 adverse events occurred in 17% of the maxi-CHOP cycles and 12% of the high-dose cytarabine cycles; 80% of these hospitalizations were due to neutropenic fever
- A total of five patients (3%) did not proceed to high-dose chemotherapy because of toxicity (an additional 10 patients did not proceed for other reasons)
- After high-dose chemotherapy, 5 cases of late neutropenia were reported, but all resolved after G-CSF treatment, and 2 patients developed hypogammaglobulinemia and recurrent respiratory tract infections, but responded to repeated series of intravenous immunoglobulin infusions
- A total of 7 treatment-related deaths (4.4%) were noted: 4 during autologous stem cell transplantation (one owing to graft failure and three owing to infection) and 3 due to heart failure (8, 20, and 28 months after autologous stem cell transplantation)

Therapy Monitoring

1. *Prior to treatment initiation*: CBC with differential, serum chemistries, serum bilirubin, ALT or AST, hepatitis B core antibody (IgG or total) and hepatitis B surface antigen, left ventricular ejection fraction (LVEF), and urine pregnancy test (women of child-bearing potential only)

   a. In addition to baseline monitoring, evaluate LVEF during doxorubicin treatment if clinical symptoms of heart failure are present. If baseline LVEF is ≥50%, repeat LVEF evaluation after a cumulative lifetime doxorubicin dose between 250 and 300 mg/m² has been reached, after a cumulative lifetime doxorubicin dose of 450 mg/m² has been reached, and then before each cycle beyond a cumulative lifetime doxorubicin dose of 450 mg/m². If the baseline LVEF is <50%, consider repeating LVEF evaluation before each dose of doxorubicin

   b. *In patients at high risk for tumor lysis syndrome* consider frequent monitoring of laboratory indices of tumor lysis syndrome, intravenous hydration, and prophylaxis with a xanthine oxidase inhibitor (eg, allopurinol) during the first cycle

2. *Prior to each cycle and weekly*: CBC with differential, serum chemistries, serum bilirubin, ALT or AST

   a. Patients who receive high-dose cytarabine need to be closely monitored for changes in renal function. Renal dysfunction is highly correlated with an increased risk of cerebellar toxicity

3. *Prior to each dose of cytarabine:* Monitor for signs of cerebellar toxicity (nystagmus, dysmetria, and ataxia)

4. *Monitor periodically for*: Signs and symptoms of infection (including progressive multifocal leukoencephalopathy), dermatologic toxicity, cytarabine syndrome (rash, conjunctivitis, chest pain, malaise, myalgia, arthralgia, fever), peripheral neuropathy (vincristine), and constipation (vincristine)

5. *Response assessment (after cycle 5 and after autologous stem cell transplant)*: Physical examination, CBC with differential, CT scans or PET scan, bone marrow evaluation (if clinically indicated), endoscopy (if clinically indicated)

MANTLE CELL LYMPHOMA • FIRST LINE

NON-HODGKIN LYMPHOMA REGIMEN: RITUXIMAB WITH HYPERFRACTIONATED CYCLOPHOSPHAMIDE + VINCRISTINE + DOXORUBICIN + DEXAMETHASONE (R-HYPER-CVAD) ALTERNATING WITH RITUXIMAB WITH METHOTREXATE + CYTARABINE (R-MC)

Romaguera JE et al. J Clin Oncol 2005;23:7013–7023
Wang M et al. Cancer 2008;113:2734–2741

If indicated: Prophylaxis against tumor lysis syndrome during the first cycle:
Hydration with 2500–3000 mL/day, as tolerated; administer intravenously at 100–125 mL/hour
Note:
- Furosemide 20–40 mg; administer intravenously every 12–24 hours to maintain fluid balance
- Diuresis is maintained for at least the first 72 hours after starting chemotherapy in the absence of metabolic aberrations, or after metabolic complications normalize
- **Allopurinol** 300 mg/day; administer orally for 7 consecutive days on days 1–7 (longer treatment may be needed)
  - Persons who express a variant human leukocyte antigen allele, HLA-B*58:01, are at increased risk for severe cutaneous adverse reactions from allopurinol (Hershfield MS et al. Clin Pharmacol Ther 2013;93:153–158; Zineh I et al. Pharmacogenomics 2011;12:1741–1749)

R-Hyper-CVAD (odd-numbered cycles, ie, 1, 3, 5, ±7)
Premedication for rituximab:
Acetaminophen 650–1000 mg; administer orally, *plus*
Diphenhydramine 25–50 mg; administer orally or intravenously 30–60 minutes before starting rituximab
Rituximab 375 mg/m² per dose; administer intravenously in 0.9% sodium chloride injection (0.9% NS) or 5% dextrose injection (D5W), diluted to a concentration within the range of 1–4 mg/mL on day 1, for 3–4 cycles, cycles 1, 3, 5 (±7). Cycle duration is 21 days (total dosage/cycle = 375 mg/m²)
Notes on rituximab administration:
- Infuse initially at 50 mg/h. If hypersensitivity or infusion reactions do not occur during the first 30 minutes, increase the rate by 50 mg/h every 30 minutes, as tolerated, to a maximum rate of 400 mg/h. Subsequently, if previous administration was well tolerated, start at 100 mg/h and increase by 100 mg/h every 30 minutes, as tolerated, to a maximum rate of 400 mg/h
- *Patients with evidence of peripheral blood involvement (as determined by flow cytometric analysis at the time of initial presentation) may have their first dose of rituximab delayed or omitted when they are believed to be at risk for tumor lysis syndrome or cytokine-release syndrome*

INFUSION REACTIONS ASSOCIATED WITH RITUXIMAB
Fevers, chills, and rigors
1. Interrupt rituximab administration for severe symptoms, and give:
   - **Acetaminophen** 650 mg orally for fever. For persistent or recurrent symptoms, repeat administration every 4–6 hours as needed during rituximab administration
   - **Diphenhydramine** 25–50 mg orally or by intravenous injection for pruritus, hypotension, or angioedema. For persistent or recurrent symptoms, repeat administration every 4–6 hours as needed during rituximab administration
   - **Meperidine** 12.5–25 mg by intravenous injection every 10–20 minutes as needed for shaking chills (generally, cumulative doses >100 mg are not needed; use repeated doses with caution in persons with moderate or more severely impaired renal function)
2. If rituximab administration was interrupted, resume infusion at a slower rate than the maximum rate previously attempted. Rate escalation may be reattempted at smaller incremental steps with close monitoring. Do not exceed the maximum recommended rate of 400 mg/h

Dyspnea or wheezing without allergic findings (urticaria, or tongue or laryngeal edema)
1. Interrupt rituximab administration immediately
2. Give **hydrocortisone** 100 mg by intravenous injection (or an alternative steroid with equivalent glucocorticoid potency)
3. Give a **histamine (H₂) receptor antagonist** (ranitidine 50 mg, cimetidine 300 mg, or famotidine 20 mg) intravenously over 15–30 minutes
4. After symptoms resolve, resume rituximab administration at 25 mg/h with close monitoring. Do not increase the administration rate

Note: Medications and equipment for the treatment of hypersensitivity reactions should be available for immediate use in the event of a reaction during administration (eg, intravenous fluids, epinephrine, antihistamines, glucocorticoids, and oxygen)
Rituxan (rituximab) prescribing information. South San Francisco, CA: Genentech, Inc; 2018 October

Cyclophosphamide 300 mg/m² per dose; administer intravenously in 500 mL 0.9% NS over 3 hours, every 12 hours for 6 doses, on days 2, 3, and 4, for 3–4 cycles, cycles 1, 3, 5 (±7). Cycle duration is 21 days (total dosage/cycle = 1800 mg/m²)
Mesna 600 mg/m² per day; administer by continuous intravenous infusion over 24 hours in 1000–2000 mL 0.9% NS on days 2, 3, and 4, starting 1 hour before cyclophosphamide and continuing until 12 hours after the last dose of cyclophosphamide, for 3–4 cycles, cycles 1, 3, 5 (±7). Cycle duration is 21 days (total duration of mesna administration per cycle is approximately 76 hours; total dosage/cycle is approximately 1900 mg/m²)
Vincristine 1.4 mg/m² per dose (maximum single dose = 2 mg); administer by intravenous infusion over 15 minutes in 50 mL 0.9% NS for 2 doses, 12 hours after the last dose of cyclophosphamide on day 5 and on day 12, for 3–4 cycles, cycles 1, 3, 5 (±7). Cycle duration is 21 days (total dosage/cycle = 2.8 mg/m²; maximum total dose/cycle = 4 mg)

Doxorubicin 16.6 mg/m² per day; administer by continuous intravenous infusion over 24 hours in 25–250 mL 0.9% NS or D5W for 3 consecutive days starting 12 hours after the last dose of cyclophosphamide, on days 5, 6, and 7, for 3–4 cycles, cycles 1, 3, 5 (±7). Cycle duration is 21 days (total dosage/cycle ~50 mg/m²)

Dexamethasone 40 mg/day; administer orally or intravenously in 25–150 mL 0.9% NS or D5W over 15–30 minutes for 8 doses, on days 2–5 and days 12–15 for 3–4 cycles, cycles 1, 3, 5 (±7). Cycle duration is 21 days (total dosage/cycle = 320 mg)

R-MC (even-numbered cycles; ie, 2, 4, 6, ±8)
Premedication for rituximab:

Acetaminophen 650–1000 mg; administer orally, *plus*

Diphenhydramine 25–50 mg; administer orally or intravenously, 30–60 minutes before starting rituximab

Rituximab 375 mg/m² per dose; administer intravenously in 0.9% NS or D5W diluted to a concentration within the range of 1–4 mg/mL on day 1 for 3–4 cycles, cycles 2, 4, 6 (±8). Cycle duration is 21 days (total dosage/cycle = 375 mg/m²)

Notes on rituximab administration:

- Infuse initially at 100 mg/h. If hypersensitivity or infusion reactions do not occur during the first 30 minutes, increase the rate by 100 mg/h every 30 minutes, as tolerated, to a maximum rate of 400 mg/h. Subsequently, if previous administration was well tolerated, start at 100 mg/h and increase by 100 mg/h every 30 minutes, as tolerated, to a maximum rate of 400 mg/h

INFUSION REACTIONS ASSOCIATED WITH RITUXIMAB

Fevers, chills, and rigors

1. Interrupt rituximab administration for severe symptoms, and give:

- **Acetaminophen** 650 mg orally for fever. For persistent or recurrent symptoms, repeat administration every 4–6 hours as needed during rituximab administration
- **Diphenhydramine** 25–50 mg orally or by intravenous injection for pruritus, hypotension, or angioedema. For persistent or recurrent symptoms, repeat administration every 4–6 hours as needed during rituximab administration
- **Meperidine** 12.5–25 mg by intravenous injection every 10–20 minutes as needed for shaking chills (generally, cumulative doses >100 mg are not needed; use repeated doses with caution in persons with moderate or more severely impaired renal function)

2. If rituximab administration was interrupted, resume infusion at a slower rate than the maximum rate previously attempted. Rate escalation may be reattempted at smaller incremental steps with close monitoring. Do not exceed the maximum recommended rate of 400 mg/h

Dyspnea or wheezing without allergic findings (urticaria, or tongue or laryngeal edema)

1. Interrupt rituximab administration immediately

2. Give **hydrocortisone** 100 mg by intravenous injection (or an alternative steroid with equivalent glucocorticoid potency)

3. Give a **histamine (H₂) receptor antagonist** (ranitidine 50 mg, cimetidine 300 mg, or famotidine 20 mg) intravenously over 15–30 minutes

4. After symptoms resolve, resume rituximab administration at 25 mg/h with close monitoring. Do not increase the administration rate

Note: Medications and equipment for the treatment of hypersensitivity reactions should be available for immediate use in the event of a reaction during administration (eg, intravenous fluids, epinephrine, antihistamines, glucocorticoids, and oxygen)

Rituxan (rituximab) prescribing information. South San Francisco, CA: Genentech, Inc; 2018 October

Hydration: 2500–3000 mL/day, as tolerated, with a solution containing a total amount of sodium not >0.9% NS (ie, ≤154 mEq sodium/1000 mL) by intravenous infusion during methotrexate administration and for at least 24 hours afterward

- Commence fluid administration 2–12 hours before starting methotrexate, depending on patient's fluid status
- Urine output should be at least 100 mL/hour before starting methotrexate infusion
- Maintain hydration at a rate that maintains urine output ≥100 mL/hour until the serum methotrexate concentration is <0.1 μmol/L
- Urine pH should be increased within the range ≥7.0 to ≤8.0 to enhance methotrexate solubility and ensure elimination
- Adverse effects attributable to methotrexate are related to systemic methotrexate concentrations *and* the duration for which concentrations are maintained

Sodium Bicarbonate 50–150 mEq/1000 mL is Added to Parenteral Hydration Solutions to Maintain Urine pH ≥7.0 to ≤8.0		
Base Solution Sodium Content	**Sodium Bicarbonate Additive**	**Total Sodium Content**
0.45% Sodium Chloride Injection (0.45% NS)		
77 mEq/L	50–75 mEq	127–152 mEq/L
0.2% Sodium Chloride Injection (0.2% NS)		
34 mEq/L	100–125 mEq	134–159 mEq/L
5% Dextrose Injection (D5W)		
0	125–150 mEq	125–150 mEq/L
D5W/0.45% NS		
77 mEq/L	50–75 mEq	127–152 mEq/L
D5W/0.2% NS		
34 mEq/L	100–125 mEq	134–159 mEq/L

(continued)

(continued)

Methotrexate 200 mg/m²; administer intravenously in 250 mL to >1000 mL 0.9% NS or D5W (or saline and dextrose combinations) over 2 hours, *followed by:*

Methotrexate 800 mg/m²; administer intravenously in 250 mL to >1000 mL 0.9% NS or D5W (or saline and dextrose combinations) over 22 hours, on day 2, for 3–4 cycles, cycles 2, 4, 6 (±8). Cycle duration is 21 days (total dosage/cycle [not including intrathecal methotrexate] = 1000 mg/m²)

Notes on methotrexate administration:
- Patients with an initial serum creatinine level >1.5 mg/dL (>133 μmol/L), reduce the dose of methotrexate by 50%
- Patients with evidence of third spacing of fluids, remove the fluid as completely as possible or, if this is not possible, repeat rituximab plus hyper-CVAD until third spacing of fluid is resolved

Cytarabine 3000 mg/m² per dose; administer intravenously in 50–500 mL 0.9% NS or D5W over 2 hours, every 12 hours, for 4 doses, on days 3 and 4, for 3–4 cycles, cycles 2, 4, 6 (±8). Cycle duration is 21 days (total dosage/cycle [not including intrathecal cytarabine] = 12,000 mg/m²)

Notes on cytarabine administration:
- Reduce the cytarabine dose to 1000 mg/m² in patients whose age is ≥60 years and in those with a serum creatinine level >1.5 mg/dL (>133 μmol/L)

Keratitis prophylaxis
Steroid ophthalmic drops (**prednisolone 1% or dexamethasone 0.1%**); administer 2 drops by intraocular instillation into each eye every 6 hours starting prior to the first cytarabine dose and continuing until 48 hours after high-dose cytarabine is completed

Leucovorin calcium 50 mg; administer intravenously in 10–100 mL 0.9% NS or D5W over 10–20 minutes, on day 3, 36 hours after methotrexate administration began (12 hours after completing methotrexate), followed 6 hours later by:

Leucovorin calcium 15 mg; administer orally *or* intravenously in 10–100 mL 0.9% NS or D5W over 10–20 minutes, every 6 hours, for 8 doses or until blood methotrexate concentrations is <0.1 μmol/L

If methotrexate elimination is delayed or attenuated, both the dose and administration schedule for leucovorin calcium are escalated, thus:
leucovorin calcium 100 mg/dose intravenously every 3 hours, if serum methotrexate concentrations are:

Time After Methotrexate Administration Began	Serum Methotrexate Concentration
24 hours	>20 μmol/L (>20 × 10²⁶ mol/L)
48 hours	>1 μmol/L (>1 × 10²⁶ mol/L)
72 hours	>0.1 μmol/L (>1 × 10²⁷ mol/L)

If methotrexate elimination is delayed, measure serum methotrexate concentrations at daily intervals and continue leucovorin administration until serum methotrexate concentration is ≤0.05 μmol/L (≤5 × 10²⁸ mol/L) or undetectable

Treatment Duration:
- Patients who achieved a CR after the first 2 cycles (1 cycle with rituximab plus hyper-CVAD and 1 cycle with rituximab plus methotrexate and cytarabine) received 4 more cycles, for a total of 6 cycles
- Patients who achieved a partial response (PR) after 2 cycles and a complete remission after 6 cycles received 2 more cycles, for a total of 8 cycles
- Patients with evidence of disease after 6 cycles did not receive further therapy
- Patients whose disease was responding could be referred at any time during treatment for consolidation with stem cell transplantation

Supportive Care
Antiemetic prophylaxis for R-Hyper-CVAD (cycles 1, 3, 5, ±7)
Emetogenic potential on day 1 is **MINIMAL**
Emetogenic potential on days 2, 3, and 4 is **MODERATE**
Emetogenic potential on days 5, 6, and 7 is **LOW–MODERATE**
Emetogenic potential on day 12 is **MINIMAL**
See Chapter 42 for antiemetic recommendations

Antiemetic prophylaxis for R-MC (cycles 2, 4, 6, ±8)
Emetogenic potential on day 1 is **MINIMAL**
Emetogenic potential on day 2 is **MODERATE**
Emetogenic potential on days 3 and 4 is **MODERATE**
See Chapter 42 for antiemetic recommendations

Hematopoietic growth factor (CSF) prophylaxis (all cycles)
Primary prophylaxis is indicated with:
Filgrastim (G-CSF) 5 µg/kg per day; administer by subcutaneous injection for 10 days
• Begin use from 24–36 hours after myelosuppressive chemotherapy is completed
• Discontinue daily filgrastim use at least 24 hours before restarting myelosuppressive treatment
See Chapter 43 for more information

Antimicrobial prophylaxis
Risk of fever and neutropenia is *HIGH*
Antimicrobial primary prophylaxis is recommended:

R-Hyper-CVAD (Cycles 1, 3, 5, ±7)

Antibacterial prophylaxis	**Ciprofloxacin** 500 mg orally, twice daily (or an alternative fluoroquinolone at an equivalent dose and schedule)	Days 8–17 (10 days)
	Cotrimoxazole (160 mg trimethoprim + 800 mg sulfamethoxazole), orally	One dose, 3 days per week, continually throughout all cycles (withhold for 72 hours prior to and during R-MC cycles due to interaction with methotrexate until methotrexate concentration <0.05 micromolar)
Antifungal prophylaxis	**Fluconazole** 100 mg/day, orally	Days 8–17 (10 days)
Antiviral prophylaxis	**Valacyclovir** 500 mg/day, orally (or acyclovir or famciclovir at an equivalent dose and schedule)	Days 8–17 (10 days)

R-MC (Cycles 2, 4, 6, ±8)

Antibacterial prophylaxis	**Ciprofloxacin** 500 mg, orally, twice daily (or an alternative fluoroquinolone at an equivalent dose and schedule)	Days 5–14 (10 days)
	Cotrimoxazole (160 mg trimethoprim + 800 mg sulfamethoxazole), orally	One dose, 3 days per week, continually throughout all cycles (withhold for 72 hours prior to and during R-MC cycles due to interaction with methotrexate until methotrexate concentration <0.05 micromolar)
Antifungal prophylaxis	**Fluconazole** 100 mg/day, orally	Days 5–14 (10 days)
Antiviral prophylaxis	**Valacyclovir** 500 mg/day, orally (or acyclovir or famciclovir at an equivalent dose and schedule)	Days 5–14 (10 days)

Steroid-associated gastritis
Add a **proton pump inhibitor** during steroid use to prevent gastritis and duodenitis

Decreased bowel motility prophylaxis
Give **stool softeners** in a scheduled regimen, and **saline, osmotic, and lubricant laxatives**, as needed to prevent constipation for as long as vincristine use continues. If needed, circumspectly add **stimulant (irritant) laxatives** in the least amounts and for the briefest durations needed to produce defecation

Treatment Modifications

Adverse Event	Treatment Modifications
Platelet count 75,000–100,000/mm³, or an ANC 750–1000/mm³ on day 21 of a treatment cycle	Delay start of next cycle until platelets >100,000/mm³ and ANC >1000/mm³, reevaluating hematologic values every 3 days. Then resume therapy without a decrease in drug dosages
Platelet count was <75,000/mm³ or ANC was <750/mm³ on day 21 of a treatment cycle	Delay start of next cycle until platelet count >100,000/mm³ and ANC >1000/mm³ reevaluating hematologic values every 3 days. Then resume therapy with a decrease in the dose of cyclophosphamide and doxorubicin (cycles 1, 3, 5, ±7) or methotrexate and cytarabine (cycles 2, 4, 6, ± 8) by 25–50%
Patient age ≥60 years	Reduce cytarabine dosage to 1000 mg/m² per dose

(continued)

Treatment Modifications (continued)

Blood methotrexate concentration >20 μmol/L at the start of cytarabine treatment	Reduce cytarabine dosage to 2000 mg/m² per dose and reduce methotrexate dosage by 50% in subsequent cycles
Serum creatinine >2 mg/dL (>177 μmol/L)	
Serum creatinine >3 mg/dL (>265 μmol/L)	Reduce methotrexate dosage by 75%
Delayed methotrexate excretion or nephrotoxicity attributable to previous methotrexate treatment	Reduce methotrexate dosage by 50–75% (commensurate with the severity of nephrotoxicity)
Total bilirubin >2 g/dL (>34.2 μmol/L)	Reduce vincristine dose to 1 mg/dose
Total bilirubin 2–3 g/dL (34.2–51.3 μmol/L)	Reduce doxorubicin dosage by 25%
Total bilirubin 3–4 g/dL (51.3–68.4 μmol/L)	Reduce doxorubicin dosage by 50%
Total bilirubin >4 g/dL (>68.4 μmol/L)	Reduce doxorubicin dosage by 75%
Disease involving the stomach or small bowel	Eliminate doxorubicin during the first hyper-CVAD cycle
If cytarabine is eliminated because of adverse effects	Omit the high-dose methotrexate + cytarabine regimen, replacing it with repeated cycles of hyper-CVAD
Peripheral neuropathy	Discontinue vincristine
Proximal myopathy	Discontinue dexamethasone
Cerebellar neurotoxicity	Reduce cytarabine dosage or omit cytarabine during subsequent treatments
G3 mucositis	Reduce methotrexate dosage

Cycles with Dose Reductions According to Age

Romaguera JE et al. J Clin Oncol 2005;23:7013–7023

Age/Regimen	Number of Patients	Number of Cycles	Reduced Cycles		P
			Number	%	
All ages	97	602	142	24	
≤65 years	65	410	70	17	0.00001
>65 years	32	192	72	38	

Cycles with Dose Reductions According to Regimens

R-hyper-CVAD		302	51	17	0.0002
R-MC		300	91	30	

R-hyper-CVAD, rituximab with fractionated cyclophosphamide, vincristine, doxorubicin, and dexamethasone; R-MC, rituximab with methotrexate and cytarabine

Patient Population Studied

Prior Therapies and Responses to Prior Therapies
in 29 Patients with Relapsed or Refractory Mantle Cell Lymphoma
Wang M et al. Cancer 2008;113:2734–2741
Prior Therapies

Therapy	Number of Patients
Median prior no. of regimens (range)	1 (1–5)
Doxorubicin-containing regimens	21

(continued)

Patient Population Studied (*continued*)

Fludarabine-containing regimens	5
Rituximab-containing regimens	18
Radiotherapy (excluding TBI)	9
Zevalin or Bexxar	2
Rituximab plus hyper-CVAD alternating with rituximab plus methotrexate-cytarabine	4
Autologous stem cell transplantation or TBI	5

Responses to Prior Therapies

	Number of Patients (%)
CR	10 (35)
PR	7 (24)
Less than PR	12 (41)

Bexxar, tositumomab and iodine (^{131}I) tositumomab; TBI indicates total body irradiation; Zevalin, ibritumomab tiuxetan

Patient Characteristics (N = 97)
Romaguera JE et al. J Clin Oncol 2005;23:7013–7023

Characteristic	Number of Patients		
	All Ages	≤65 Years	>65 Years
Number of patients	97	65	32
Age, median (range)	61 years (41–80 years)	—	—
Male-to-female ratio	3:1	3:1	3:1
Ann Arbor stage IV	99	98	100
Bone marrow involvement	91	89	94
GI involvement	88	85	94
Performance status, 0–1 (Zubrod)	98	98	97
Diffuse histologic pattern, N = 83[*]	89	88	88
Blastoid cytologic variant	14	14	16
Serum lactate dehydrogenase > normal	24	20	31
Serum/β_2-microglobulin ≥3 mg/L	55	46	72
Peripheral blood involvement	49	35	41
Large spleen	40	40	41
International Prognostic Index >2	57	34	91

[*]Fourteen patients had no lymph node to biopsy

Efficacy

Response Rates Among 29 Patients with Relapsed or Refractory Mantle Cell Lymphoma
Wang M et al. Cancer 2008;113:2734–2741

Response	Number (%)
Complete response/unconfirmed complete response	13 (45)
Partial response	14 (48)
Complete response/unconfirmed complete response + partial response	27 (93)
No benefit	2 (7)
Failure-free and Overall Survival	
Median failure-free survival (FFS)*	11 months
Median overall survival (OS)	19 months

*Note: No pretreatment variable (number of prior chemotherapy regimens, response to the previous regimen, pretreatment serum levels of β_2-microglobulin or LDH, and age) was associated with better FFS
Romaguera JE et al. J Clin Oncol 2005;23:7013–7023

CR/CRu Rates After 6 Courses
Romaguera JE et al. J Clin Oncol 2005;23:7013–7023

Variable	CR/CRu Response Rate (%) [95% CI (%)]			$X^2 P$
Overall	87 [79 to 93]			
High serum β_2M: No vs Yes	98 [88 to 100]	vs	79 [66 to 89]	0.01
High serum LDH: No vs Yes	91 [81 to 96]	vs	78 [56 to 93]	0.15
GI: Negative vs Positive	91 [59 to 100]	vs	89 [79 to 95]	0.16
IPI score: ≤2 vs >2	93 [81 to 99]	vs	84 [71 to 92]	0.10
BM involvement: No vs Yes	78 [40 to 97]	vs	89 [80 to 94]	0.31
Blastoid cytology: No vs Yes	89 [80 to 95]	vs	79 [49 to 95]	0.37
Age: ≤65 years vs >65 years	89 [79 to 96]	vs	84 [67 to 95]	0.52
Enlarged spleen: No vs Yes	90 [75 to 95]	vs	85 [69 to 94]	0.54
Age: <60 years vs 61–65 years	90 [77 to 97]	vs	88 [64 to 99]	—
Peripheral blood: No vs Yes	89 [75 to 95]	vs	86 [75 to 95]	0.76
IPI score: ≤1 vs >1	89 [52 to 100]	vs	88 [79 to 94]	0.99

3-Year FFS and OS Estimates

Overall	No Patients	% 3-Year FFS			P Value	% 3-Year OS			P Value
		65%				82%			
Serum β_2M ≥3 mg/L: No vs Yes	44/53	79	vs	51	.001	87	vs	78	0.1
Serum LDH normal: No vs Yes	74/23	74	vs	39	.002	84	vs	77	0.87
BM involvement: No vs Yes	9/88	78	vs	62	0.25	83	vs	82	0.86
Blastoid cytology: No vs Yes	83/14	66	vs	50	0.33	86	vs	61	0.06
Age: ≤65 years vs >65 years	65/32	75	vs	50	0.01	85	vs	75	0.05
Enlarged spleen: No vs Yes	58/39	68	vs	66	0.36	81	vs	83	0.52

(*continued*)

Efficacy (continued)

Peripheral blood: No vs Yes	61/36	69	vs	58	0.22	86	vs	76	0.51
IPI score: ≤2 vs >2	42/55	78	vs	54	0.03	87	vs	78	0.41

β_2M, β_2-microglobulin; BM, bone marrow; CR, complete response; CRu, complete response unconfirmed; FFS, failure-free survival; LDH, lactate dehydrogenase; IPI, International Prognostic Index; OS, overall survival

Toxicity

Toxicity Rates in 104 Cycles of Rituximab Plus Hyper-CVAD Alternating with Rituximab Plus Methotrexate + Cytarabine Therapy
Wang M et al. Cancer 2008;113:2734–2741

Toxicity Grade	% G1	% G2	% G3	% G4
Fever and neutropenia	0	3	11	0
Fever without neutropenia	11	0	0	0
Neutropenia	6	6	14	60
Thrombocytopenia	21	15	9	54
Fatigue	36	6	0	0
Sensory loss	18	2	1	0
Nausea	17	21	0	0
Pruritus	15	3	2	0
Edema	13	18	0	0
Diarrhea	10	6	0	0
Muscle weakness	10	0	0	0
Stomatitis	5	6	0	0
Constipation	4	11	0	0
Vomiting	4	10	0	0

Hematologic Toxic Effects After 602 Courses
Romaguera JE et al. J Clin Oncol 2005;23:7013–7023

Course Number	Neutropenia (%)		Thrombocytopenia (%)	
	G3	G4	G3	G4
1	10	51	12.5	2
2	7	64	9	28
3	7	28	23	14
4	5	64	9	42
5	7	31	17	12
6	3	68	5	46
7	14	37	15	17
8	4	55	7	50

(continued)

Therapy Monitoring

1. *Pretreatment evaluation:* determination of LVEF by echocardiogram, hepatitis B core antibody (IgG or total) and hepatitis B surface antigen

2. CMP and CBC with differential and platelet count prior to each cycle

3. Monitor serum methotrexate levels 24, 48, and 72 hours after the start of each methotrexate infusion. In patients with delayed clearance, monitor daily methotrexate levels thereafter until the methotrexate concentration declines to <0.1 micromolar. Monitor serum creatinine daily during each admission for methotrexate. Monitor urine output closely (goal ≥100 mL/hour). Monitor urine pH (goal ≥7.0 to ≤8.0) every 8 hours prior to and during each methotrexate course until the methotrexate concentration declines to <0.1 micromolar

4. Patients who receive high-dose cytarabine need to be closely monitored for changes in renal function. Renal dysfunction is highly correlated with increased risk of cerebellar toxicity associated with cytarabine. Patients need to be monitored for nystagmus, dysmetria, and ataxia before each cytarabine dose

5. *Response assessment every 2 cycles:* CT of the chest, abdomen, and pelvis; gallium scan or PET, and bilateral bone marrow biopsy with unilateral aspiration
   Note: To confirm CR, esophagogastroduodenoscopy and colonoscopy were performed, with biopsies performed randomly

6. *Response assessment upon completion of therapy:* CT of the chest, abdomen, and pelvis every 3 months during the first year, every 4 months during the second year, every 6 months during the third and fourth years, and yearly thereafter

Toxicity (*continued*)

Nonhematologic Toxic Effects After 602 Cycles
Romaguera JE et al. J Clin Oncol 2005;23:7013–7023

G3/4 Toxic Effect	Number of Events (%)
Neutropenic fever[*]	80 (13)
R-hyper-CVAD	20[†]
R-MC	60[†]
Infection[*]	35 (6)
Bacteremia	20 (3)
Pneumonia	6 (1)
Other	9 (1.5)
Fatigue	18 (3)
Stomatitis	6 (1)
Bleeding	3 (0.5)
Pancreatitis	1 (0.1)
Kidney failure	1 (0.1)
CNS	1 (0.1)

R-hyper-CVAD, rituximab plus fractionated cyclophosphamide, vincristine, doxorubicin, and dexamethasone; R-MC, rituximab plus methotrexate and cytarabine
[*]No difference for patients ≤65 years vs patients >65 years
[†]P = 0.00001
Note: Lethal acute toxicity occurred in five patients: sepsis in 3 patients (*Staphylococcus aureus, Escherichia coli, Proteus mirabilis*); pulmonary hemorrhage in 1 patient; unknown cause in 1 patient

MANTLE CELL LYMPHOMA • FIRST LINE
NON-HODGKIN LYMPHOMA REGIMEN: (R)-CHOP + R-DHAP
RITUXIMAB + CYCLOPHOSPHAMIDE, DOXORUBICIN (HYDROXYLDAUNORUBICIN), VINCRISTINE (ONCOVIN), PREDNISONE (R-CHOP) AND RITUXIMAB + DEXAMETHASONE, CYTARABINE (HIGH-DOSE ARA-C), AND CISPLATIN [R-DHAP)

Delarue R et al. Blood 2013;121:48–53

Regimen notes:
- Patients received 2 cycles of cyclophosphamide + doxorubicin + vincristine + prednisone (CHOP); followed by 1 cycle of rituximab + CHOP (R-CHOP); followed by 3 cycles of rituximab + dexamethasone + high dose cytarabine + cisplatin (R-DHAP), the third of which also served as chemo-mobilization for the collection of peripheral blood stem cells
- Patients who experienced disease progression during (R)-CHOP proceeded directly to R-DHAP
- Prophylactic intrathecal chemotherapy was allowed but not mandated by the protocol (not included in this regimen description)
- Patients who responded to R-CHOP/R-DHAP underwent intensification with high-dose radio-chemotherapy followed by autologous hematopoietic stem cell transplantation (not included in this regimen description)

Cycles 1–2 (CHOP):
Intravenous hydration before and after cyclophosphamide administration:
500–1000 mL 0.9% sodium chloride (0.9% NS)
Cyclophosphamide 750 mg/m^2; administer intravenously in 25–250 mL 0.9% NS or 5% dextrose injection (D5W) over 10–30 minutes, given on day 1, every 3 weeks, for 2 cycles (total dosage/21-day cycle = 750 mg/m^2)
Doxorubicin 50 mg/m^2; administer by intravenous injection over 3–5 minutes, given on day 1, every 3 weeks, for 2 cycles (total dosage/21-day cycle = 50 mg/m^2)
Vincristine 1.4 mg/m^2 (maximum dose = 2 mg); administer by intravenous infusion over 15 minutes in 50 mL 0.9% NS, given on day 1, every 3 weeks, for 2 cycles (total dosage/21-day cycle = 1.4 mg/m^2; maximum dose/cycle = 2 mg)
Prednisone 40 mg/m^2 per day; administer orally for 5 consecutive days, days 1–5 every 3 weeks, for 2 cycles (total dosage/21-day cycle = 200 mg/m^2)

Cycle 3 (R-CHOP):
Premedication for rituximab:
Acetaminophen 650–1000 mg; administer orally 30–60 minutes before each rituximab dose, *plus*
Diphenhydramine 25–50 mg; administer orally or intravenously 30–60 minutes before each rituximab dose
Rituximab 375 mg/m^2 per dose; administer intravenously in 0.9% NS or D5W, diluted to a concentration within the range 1–4 mg/mL, on day 1 for 1 cycle (total dosage/21-day cycle = 375 mg/m^2)
Rituximab administration:
- Infuse initially at 50 mg/h. If hypersensitivity or infusion reactions do not occur during the first 30 minutes, increase the rate by 50 mg/h every 30 minutes as tolerated to a maximum rate of 400 mg/h. During subsequent treatments if previous rituximab administration was well tolerated, start at 100 mg/h and increase by 100 mg/h every 30 minutes as tolerated to a maximum rate of 400 mg/h

INFUSION REACTIONS ASSOCIATED WITH RITUXIMAB
Fevers, chills, and rigors
1. Interrupt rituximab administration for severe symptoms, and give:
   - **Acetaminophen** 650 mg orally for fever. For persistent or recurrent symptoms, repeat administration every 4–6 hours as needed during rituximab administration
   - **Diphenhydramine** 25–50 mg orally or by intravenous injection for pruritus, hypotension, or angioedema. For persistent or recurrent symptoms, repeat administration every 4–6 hours as needed during rituximab administration
   - **Meperidine** 12.5–25 mg by intravenous injection every 10–20 minutes as needed for shaking chills (generally, cumulative doses >100 mg are not needed; use repeated doses with caution in persons with moderate or more severely impaired renal function)
2. If rituximab administration was interrupted, resume infusion at a slower rate than the maximum rate previously attempted. Rate escalation may be reattempted at smaller incremental steps with close monitoring. Do not exceed the maximum recommended rate of 400 mg/h

Dyspnea or wheezing without allergic findings (urticaria, or tongue or laryngeal edema)
1. Interrupt rituximab administration immediately
2. Give **hydrocortisone** 100 mg by intravenous injection (or an alternative steroid with equivalent glucocorticoid potency)
3. Give a **histamine (H$_2$) receptor antagonist** (ranitidine 50 mg, cimetidine 300 mg, or famotidine 20 mg) intravenously over 15–30 minutes
4. After symptoms resolve, resume rituximab administration at 25 mg/h with close monitoring. Do not increase the administration rate
Note: Medications and equipment for the treatment of hypersensitivity reactions should be available for immediate use in the event of a reaction during administration (eg, intravenous fluids, epinephrine, antihistamines, glucocorticoids, and oxygen)
Rituxan (rituximab) prescribing information. South San Francisco, CA: Genentech, Inc; 2018 October

(continued)

(continued)

Intravenous hydration before and after cyclophosphamide administration:
500–1000 mL 0.9% sodium chloride (0.9% NS)
Cyclophosphamide 750 mg/m²; administer intravenously in 25–250 mL 0.9% NS or D5W over 10–30 minutes, given on day 1 for 1 cycle (total dosage/21-day cycle = 750 mg/m²)
Doxorubicin 50 mg/m²; administer by intravenous injection over 3–5 minutes, given on day 1 for 1 cycle (total dosage/21-day cycle = 50 mg/m²)
Vincristine 1.4 mg/m² (maximum dose = 2 mg); administer by intravenous infusion over 15 minutes in 50 mL 0.9% NS, given on day 1 for 1 cycle (total dosage/21-day cycle = 1.4 mg/m²; maximum dose/cycle = 2 mg)
Prednisone 40 mg/m² per day; administer orally for 5 consecutive days, days 1–5, for 1 cycle (total dosage/21-day cycle = 200 mg/m²)

Cycles 4–6 (R-DHAP):
Premedication for rituximab:
Acetaminophen 650–1000 mg; administer orally 30–60 minutes before each rituximab dose, *plus*
Diphenhydramine 25–50 mg; administer orally or intravenously 30–60 minutes before each rituximab dose
Rituximab 375 mg/m² per dose; administer intravenously in 0.9% NS or D5W, diluted to a concentration within the range 1–4 mg/mL, on day 1, every 21 days, for 3 cycles (total dosage/21-day cycle = 375 mg/m²)
Notes on rituximab administration:
• Infuse initially at 50 mg/h. If hypersensitivity or infusion reactions do not occur during the first 30 minutes, increase the rate by 50 mg/h every 30 minutes as tolerated to a maximum rate of 400 mg/h. During subsequent treatments if previous rituximab administration was well tolerated, start at 100 mg/h and increase by 100 mg/h every 30 minutes as tolerated to a maximum rate of 400 mg/h
• Interrupt rituximab administration for fever, chills, edema, congestion of the head and neck mucosa, hypertension, and other serious adverse events. Resume rituximab administration after adverse events abate

Hydration:
0.9% NS at a rate of 250 mL/h for 36 hours; administer intravenously beginning at least 6 hours before starting cisplatin administration, every 21 days, for 3 cycles. Monitor and replace magnesium/electrolytes as needed

Cisplatin 100 mg/m²; administer by continuous intravenous infusion over 24 hours in a volume equivalent to the dose, or diluted in 100 mL to ≥1000 mL 0.9% NS. Begin administration on day 1 after completing 6 hours of hydration, every 21 days, for 3 cycles (total dosage/21-day cycle = 100 mg/m²)
Cytarabine 2000 mg/m² per dose; administer intravenously over 3 hours in 50–500 mL 0.9% NS or D5W every 12 hours for 2 doses, starting after the completion of cisplatin administration on day 2, every 21 days, for 3 cycles (total dosage/21-day cycle = 4000 mg/m²)
Dexamethasone 40 mg/day; administer orally or intravenously in 10–100 mL 0.9% NS or D5W over 10–30 minutes for 4 consecutive days on days 1–4, every 21 days, for 3 cycles (total dosage/21-day cycle = 160 mg)

Keratitis prophylaxis
Steroid ophthalmic drops (**prednisolone 1% or dexamethasone 0.1%**); administer 2 drops by intraocular instillation into each eye every 6 hours starting prior to the first cytarabine dose and continuing until 48 hours after high-dose cytarabine is completed

Supportive Care
Antiemetic prophylaxis
Emetogenic potential on day 1 of all cycles (cycles 1–6): **HIGH, POTENTIAL FOR DELAYED SYMPTOMS**
See Chapter 42 for antiemetic recommendations

Hematopoietic growth factor (CSF) prophylaxis
Primary prophylaxis is indicated prior to all cycles with one of the following:
Filgrastim (G-CSF) 5 μg/kg per day, by subcutaneous injection, *or*
Pegfilgrastim (pegylated filgrastim) 6 mg/0.6 mL, by subcutaneous injection for 1 dose
• Begin use from 24–72 hours after myelosuppressive chemotherapy is completed
• Continue daily filgrastim use until ANC ≥5000/mm³ after the leukocyte nadir
• Discontinue daily filgrastim use at least 24 hours before administering myelosuppressive treatment. Do not administer pegfilgrastim within 14 days before administering myelosuppressive treatment
See Chapter 43 for more information

Antimicrobial prophylaxis
Risk of fever and neutropenia is *INTERMEDIATE*
Antimicrobial primary prophylaxis to be considered:
• Antibacterial—consider a fluoroquinolone during periods of prolonged neutropenia, or no prophylaxis
• Antifungal—consider use during periods of prolonged neutropenia, or no prophylaxis
• Antiviral—antiherpes antivirals (eg, acyclovir, famciclovir, valacyclovir)

Treatment Modifications

Cyclophosphamide + Doxorubicin + Vincristine + Prednisone Dose Modifications

Dose Levels	Cyclophosphamide	Doxorubicin	Vincristine	Prednisone
Starting	750 mg/m²	50 mg/m²	1.4 mg/m² (max 2 mg)	40 mg/m²
Level −1	562.5 mg/m²	37.5 mg/m²	1.05 mg/m² (max 1.5 mg)	30 mg/m²
Level −2	375 mg/m²	25 mg/m²	0.7 mg/m² (max 1 mg)	20 mg/m²

Adverse Event	Treatment Modification
Hematologic Toxicity	
Day 1 platelet count <100,000/mm³ or ANC <1500/mm³	Delay start of cycle until platelet count ≥100,000/mm³ and ANC ≥1500/mm³, or until recovery to near baseline value, then continue at the same doses
G4 neutropenia (ANC <500/mm³) during the prior cycle given without growth factor (filgrastim, pegfilgrastim) prophylaxis	Administer filgrastim or pegfilgrastim during all subsequent cycles, and continue the same doses
Febrile neutropenia (ANC <1000/mm³ with temperature >38°C or >100.4°F) during the prior cycle given without growth factor (filgrastim, pegfilgrastim) prophylaxis	
Febrile neutropenia (ANC <1000/mm³ with temperature >38°C or >100.4°F) during the prior cycle given with growth factor (filgrastim, pegfilgrastim) prophylaxis	Reduce the dose of cyclophosphamide and doxorubicin by 1 dose level for subsequent cycles. Do not change the prednisone or vincristine dose
G ≥3 thrombocytopenia (platelets <50,000/mm³) during the prior cycle	
Gastrointestinal Toxicities	
G ≥3 ileus (severely altered GI function; TPN indicated; tube placement indicated)	Withhold all chemotherapy until resolution of ileus and constipation, then reduce vincristine by 1 dose level with an optimal prophylactic bowel regimen. Do not change the cyclophosphamide, doxorubicin, or prednisone doses. If symptoms do not recur at the reduced vincristine dose, then the vincristine dose may be re-escalated on subsequent cycles with an appropriate prophylactic bowel regimen
G ≥3 constipation (obstipation with manual evacuation indicated; limiting self-care ADL)	
Neurologic Toxicities	
G3 peripheral sensory neuropathy (severe symptoms; limiting self-care ADL)	Proceed with treatment, and reduce vincristine by 1 dose level. Do not change cyclophosphamide, doxorubicin, or prednisone doses. If symptoms improve, the vincristine dose may be re-escalated on subsequent cycles
G2 peripheral motor neuropathy (moderate symptoms; limiting instrumental ADL)	
G3 peripheral motor neuropathy (severe symptoms; limiting self-care ADL)	Proceed with treatment, and reduce the dose of vincristine by 2 dose levels. Do not change the cyclophosphamide, doxorubicin, or prednisone doses. If symptoms improve, the vincristine dose may be re-escalated on subsequent cycles
G4 peripheral sensory neuropathy (life-threatening symptoms; urgent intervention indicated)	Discontinue vincristine. Do not change the cyclophosphamide, doxorubicin, or prednisone doses
G4 peripheral motor neuropathy (life-threatening consequences; urgent intervention indicated)	
G ≥2 mood alteration (moderate mood alteration) or confusion (moderate disorientation; limiting instrumental ADL)	Withhold prednisone until symptoms return to baseline. Resume prednisone reduced by 1 dose level. If symptoms persist, reduce by another dose level. Do not change the cyclophosphamide, doxorubicin, or vincristine doses

(continued)

Treatment Modifications (continued)

Hepatic Impairment

Serum bilirubin 1.2–3 mg/dL	Decrease doxorubicin dose by 50%. Additionally, if the bilirubin is 1.5–3 mg/dL, decrease the vincristine dose by 50%
Serum bilirubin 3.1–5 mg/dL	Decrease the doxorubicin by 75%. Do not administer vincristine
Serum bilirubin >5 mg/dL	Do not administer doxorubicin or vincristine

Drug Interactions

Patient requires concomitant therapy with antihypertensive medication(s)	On days of rituximab treatment, and especially with the initial dose, weigh the risk versus benefit of delaying administration of the antihypertensive medication(s) until after completion of the rituximab infusion due to the potential risk of rituximab infusion-related hypotension
Patient requires concomitant therapy with a strong CYP3A4 inhibitor	Patient may have earlier onset of neuromuscular side effects of vincristine. If concomitant use of the strong CYP3A4 inhibitor cannot be avoided, consider dose reduction of vincristine and increased monitoring for toxicity

Other Toxicities

G ≥3 hyperglycemia (insulin therapy initiated; hospitalization indicated)	Withhold prednisone until blood glucose is ≤250 mg/dL. Treat with insulin or other hypoglycemic agents as clinically appropriate, and then resume prednisone at the same dose. If hyperglycemia is uncontrolled despite above measures, decrease prednisone by 1 dose level
LVEF is 40%, or is 40% to 45% with a 10% or greater absolute decrease below the pretreatment	Withhold doxorubicin, and repeat LVEF assessment within approximately 4 weeks. Discontinue doxorubicin if LVEF has not improved or declines further, unless the benefits for the individual patient outweigh the risks

Dexamethasone + High-Dose Cytarabine + Cisplatin Dose Modifications

	Dexamethasone	Cytarabine	Cisplatin
Starting dose	40 mg	2000 mg/m^2	100 mg/m^2
Dose level −1	30 mg	1500 mg/m^2	75 mg/m^2
Dose level −2	20 mg	1000 mg/m^2	50 mg/m^2

Hematologic Toxicity

Day 1 platelet count <100,000/mm^3 or ANC <1500/mm^3	Delay start of cycle until platelet count ≥100,000/mm^3 and ANC ≥1500/mm^3, or until recovery to near baseline value, then continue at the same doses
G4 neutropenia (ANC <500/mm^3) during the prior cycle given without growth factor (filgrastim, pegfilgrastim) prophylaxis	Administer filgrastim or pegfilgrastim during all subsequent cycles, and continue the same doses
Febrile neutropenia (ANC <1000/mm^3 with temperature >38°C or >100.4°F) during the prior cycle given without growth factor (filgrastim, pegfilgrastim) prophylaxis	
Febrile neutropenia (ANC <1000/mm^3 with temperature >38°C or >100.4°F) during the prior cycle given with growth factor (filgrastim, pegfilgrastim) prophylaxis	Reduce the dose of cisplatin and cytarabine by 1 dose level for subsequent cycles. Do not change the dexamethasone dose
G ≥3 thrombocytopenia (platelets <50,000/mm^3) during the prior cycle	

Neurologic Toxicities

Peripheral sensory neuropathy G ≥3 (severe symptoms; limiting self-care ADL)	Discontinue cisplatin. May continue to administer dexamethasone and cytarabine at the discretion of the medically responsible healthcare provider

(continued)

Treatment Modifications (*continued*)

Neurologic (cerebellar) toxicity	Discontinue cytarabine. Patients who develop CNS symptoms should not receive subsequent high-dose cytarabine. May continue to administer dexamethasone and cisplatin at the discretion of the medically responsible healthcare provider
G ≥2 mood alteration (moderate mood alteration) or confusion (moderate disorientation; limiting instrumental ADL)	Withhold dexamethasone until symptoms return to baseline. Resume dexamethasone reduced by 1 dose level. If symptoms persist, reduce by another dose level. Do not change the cytarabine or cisplatin doses

Other Toxicities

Serum creatinine ≥1.5 mg/dL (≥130 μmol/L) and/or BUN ≥25 mg/dL (≥8.92 mmol/L)	Withhold dexamethasone, cytarabine, and cisplatin until serum creatinine <1.5 mg/dL (<130 μmol/L) and BUN <25 mg/dL (<8.92 mmol/L). Then, reduce the cisplatin dose by 1 dose level, and continue dexamethasone and cytarabine at the same doses
Cisplatin induced hearing loss G ≥3 (hearing loss with hearing aid or intervention indicated; limiting self-care ADL)	Discontinue cisplatin. May continue to administer dexamethasone and cytarabine at discretion of the medically responsible healthcare provider
Significant hypersensitivity reaction to cisplatin (hypotension, dyspnea, and angioedema requiring therapy) *Note:* Allergic reaction to cisplatin including anaphylaxis risk is increased in patients previously exposed to platinum therapy	May occur within minutes of cisplatin administration. Interrupt the cisplatin infusion in patients with clinically significant infusion reactions. Discontinue cisplatin or can consider desensitization and a rechallenge. May continue to administer dexamethasone and cytarabine at the discretion of the medically responsible healthcare provider
Fever, myalgia, bone pain, occasionally chest pain, maculopapular rash, conjunctivitis and malaise 6–12 hours following drug administration (cytarabine or Ara-C syndrome)	Corticosteroids are beneficial in treating or preventing this syndrome. If the symptoms deemed treatable, continue therapy with cytarabine and pretreat with corticosteroids If the syndrome occurs in a patient already receiving corticosteroid pretreatment, consider reducing the cytarabine dose by 1 dose level
G ≥3 hyperglycemia (insulin therapy initiated; hospitalization indicated)	Withhold dexamethasone until blood glucose is ≤250 mg/dL. Treat with insulin or other hypoglycemic agents as clinically appropriate, and then resume dexamethasone at the same dose. If hyperglycemia is uncontrolled despite above measures, decrease dexamethasone by 1 dose level

ANC, absolute neutrophil count; G-CSF, granulocyte-colony stimulating factor; HBV, hepatitis B virus; LP, lumbar puncture; MRI, magnetic resonance imaging; PML, progressive multifocal leukoencephalopathy

Note: Medications and equipment for the treatment of hypersensitivity reactions should be available for immediate use in the event of a reaction during rituximab administration (eg, intravenous fluids, epinephrine, antihistamines, glucocorticoids, oxygen)

Efficacy

(N = 60)

Median event-free survival	83.9 months
Median disease-free survival	78 months
Median progression-free survival	84 months
5-year overall survival	75%

Note: Median follow-up was 67 months

Patient Population Studied

The prospective, multicenter, phase 2 trial involved 60 patients with newly diagnosed, Ann Arbor stage 3–4, mantle cell lymphoma. Eligible patients had an Eastern Cooperative Oncology Group (ECOG) performance status score ≤2. Patients with blastoid variants were ineligible. Peripheral blood stem cell harvest was subsequently performed, followed by radiochemotherapy with total body irradiation (10 Gy over 3 days and twice-daily fractions), high-dose cytarabine (1500 mg/m², four infusions every 12 hours), and high-dose melphalan (140 mg/m²), and then reinfusion of peripheral stem cells

Toxicity

(N = 60)

- The main complication during the induction phase was renal toxicity secondary to cisplatin (5 patients [8%] experienced renal insufficiency)
- One patient experienced grade 4 neurologic toxicity, one case of *Pneumocystis jirovecii* infection was reported, and three patients developed idiopathic interstitial pneumonia but recovered without sequelae
- One patient died suddenly 10 days after the first infusion of CHOP; no patients died during the autologous stem cell transplantation phase
- During follow-up, 11 patients experienced 12 second malignancies; no patients were diagnosed with myelodysplasia or secondary acute leukemia

Therapy Monitoring

1. *Prior to treatment initiation*: CBC with differential, serum chemistries, serum bilirubin, ALT or AST, hepatitis B core antibody (IgG or total) and hepatitis B surface antigen, left ventricular ejection fraction (LVEF), and urine pregnancy test (women of child-bearing potential only)

   a. In addition to baseline monitoring, evaluate LVEF during doxorubicin treatment if clinical symptoms of heart failure are present. If baseline LVEF is ≥50%, repeat LVEF evaluation after a cumulative lifetime doxorubicin dose between 250 and 300 mg/m² has been reached, after a cumulative lifetime doxorubicin dose of 450 mg/m² has been reached, and then before each cycle beyond a cumulative lifetime doxorubicin dose of 450 mg/m². If the baseline LVEF is <50%, consider repeating LVEF evaluation before each dose of doxorubicin

   b. *In patients at high risk for tumor lysis syndrome (eg, high tumor burden, renal dysfunction, rapidly progressing disease, markedly elevated LDH, baseline abnormalities in laboratory indices of tumor lysis syndrome [potassium, phosphate, uric acid, calcium, serum creatinine])*: Consider frequent monitoring of laboratory indices of tumor lysis syndrome, intravenous hydration, and prophylaxis with a xanthine oxidase inhibitor (eg, allopurinol) during the first cycle

2. *Prior to each cycle and weekly*: CBC with differential, serum chemistries, serum bilirubin, ALT or AST

3. *During each rituximab infusion and for at least 1 hour after infusion completion*: Signs and symptoms of infusion-related reaction, vital signs every 30 minutes

4. *Monitor periodically for*: Signs and symptoms of infection (including progressive multifocal leukoencephalopathy), dermatologic toxicity, cytarabine syndrome (rash, conjunctivitis, chest pain, malaise, myalgia, arthralgia, fever), cerebellar toxicity (nystagmus, dysmetria, and ataxia) (cytarabine), peripheral neuropathy (vincristine, cisplatin), constipation (vincristine), anaphylaxis (cisplatin), hearing loss/tinnitus (cisplatin)

5. *Response assessment (after cycles 3 and 6)*: Physical examination, CBC with differential, CT scan or PET scan, bone marrow evaluation (if clinically indicated), endoscopy (if clinically indicated)

MANTLE CELL LYMPHOMA • FIRST LINE
NON-HODGKIN LYMPHOMA REGIMEN: BENDAMUSTINE + RITUXIMAB FOLLOWED BY CYTARABINE + RITUXIMAB (BR → R-CYTARABINE)

Merryman RW et al. Blood Adv 2020;4:858–867

Prophylaxis for tumor lysis syndrome is recommended for high-risk patients (eg, high tumor burden, bulky lymphadenopathy, or renal impairment):
- **Hydration**; encourage oral hydration (eg, ≥3 L/day) starting 1–2 days prior to the first rituximab dose. Consider administering additional *intravenous* hydration prior to the infusion if needed. Continue hydration prior to subsequent cycles if needed
- **Allopurinol** 300 mg per dose; administer orally twice per day starting 12–24 hours prior to the first rituximab infusion for 7 days. Continue prophylaxis prior to subsequent cycles if needed.
  - Reduce allopurinol dose to 300 mg by mouth once daily for 7 days for patients with renal impairment

Cycles 1–3: Bendamustine + rituximab (BR) (28-day cycles)

Premedications for Rituximab:
- **Acetaminophen** 650–1000 mg; administer orally 30–60 minutes before each rituximab dose, *plus*
- **Diphenhydramine** 25–50 mg; administer orally or intravenously 30–60 minutes before each rituximab dose

Rituximab 375 mg/m^2; administer intravenously in 0.9% sodium chloride injection (0.9% NS) or 5% dextrose Injection (D5W), diluted to a concentration within the range 1–4 mg/mL, on day 1, every 28 days, for 3 cycles during cycles 1–3 (total dosage/28-day cycle during cycles 1–3 = 375 mg/m^2)
Rituximab administration:
- Infuse initially at 50 mg/hour. If hypersensitivity or infusion reactions do not occur during the first 30 minutes, increase the rate by 50 mg/hour every 30 minutes as tolerated to a maximum rate of 400 mg/hour. During subsequent treatments if previous rituximab administration was well tolerated, start at 100 mg/hour and increase by 100 mg/hour every 30 minutes as tolerated to a maximum rate of 400 mg/hour

INFUSION REACTIONS ASSOCIATED WITH RITUXIMAB
Fevers, chills, and rigors
1. Interrupt rituximab administration for severe symptoms, and give:
   - **Acetaminophen** 650 mg orally for fever. For persistent or recurrent symptoms, repeat administration every 4–6 hours as needed during rituximab administration
   - **Diphenhydramine** 25–50 mg orally or by intravenous injection for pruritus, hypotension, or angioedema. For persistent or recurrent symptoms, repeat administration every 4–6 hours as needed during rituximab administration
   - **Meperidine** 12.5–25 mg by intravenous injection every 10–20 minutes as needed for shaking chills (generally, cumulative doses >100 mg are not needed; use repeated doses with caution in persons with moderate or more severely impaired renal function)
2. If rituximab administration was interrupted, resume infusion at a slower rate than the maximum rate previously attempted. Rate escalation may be reattempted at smaller incremental steps with close monitoring. Do not exceed the maximum recommended rate of 400 mg/h

Dyspnea or wheezing without allergic findings (urticaria, or tongue or laryngeal edema)
1. Interrupt rituximab administration immediately
2. Give **hydrocortisone** 100 mg by intravenous injection (or an alternative steroid with equivalent glucocorticoid potency)
3. Give a **histamine (H$_2$) receptor antagonist** (ranitidine 50 mg, cimetidine 300 mg, or famotidine 20 mg) intravenously over 15–30 minutes
4. After symptoms resolve, resume rituximab administration at 25 mg/h with close monitoring. Do not increase the administration rate
Note: Medications and equipment for the treatment of hypersensitivity reactions should be available for immediate use in the event of a reaction during administration (eg, intravenous fluids, epinephrine, antihistamines, glucocorticoids, and oxygen)
Rituxan (rituximab) prescribing information. South San Francisco, CA: Genentech, Inc; 2018 October

Premedications for Bendamustine HCl: premedications are not necessary for primary prophylaxis of infusion-related reactions. In the event of a non-severe infusion-related reaction, consider adding a histamine receptor (H$_1$)-subtype antagonist (eg, diphenhydramine 25–50 mg intravenously or orally), an antipyretic (eg, acetaminophen 650–1000 mg orally), and a corticosteroid (eg, methylprednisolone 100 mg intravenously) administered 30 minutes prior to Bendamustine HCl administration in subsequent cycles

Bendamustine HCl 90 mg/m^2 per dose; administer intravenously in a volume of 0.9% NS sufficient to produce a concentration with the range 0.2–0.6 mg/mL over 30–60 minutes, on 2 consecutive days, days 1 and 2, every 28 days for 3 cycles during cycles 1–3 (total dosage/28-day cycle during cycles 1–3 = 180 mg/m^2)
Note:
- Bendamustine HCl can cause severe infusion-related reactions
  - For grade 1–2 infusion-related reactions, consider rechallenge with the addition of antihistamine, antipyretic, and corticosteroid premedications (as described in the above premedication section)
  - For grade 3 infusion-related reactions, consider permanent discontinuation versus rechallenge with the addition of antihistamine, antipyretic, and corticosteroid premedications (as described in the above premedication section) after weighing risks and benefits.
  - For grade 4 infusion-related reactions, permanently discontinue bendamustine HCl

(continued)

(continued)

- Coadministration of strong CYP1A2 inhibitors (eg, ciprofloxacin, fluvoxamine) may increase exposure to bendamustine HCl and decrease exposure to its active metabolites. Concomitant CYP1A2 inducers (eg, omeprazole, cigarette smoking) may decrease exposure to bendamustine HCl and increase exposure to its active metabolites. Use caution, or select an alternative therapy, when coadministration of bendamustine HCl with strong CYP1A2 inhibitors or inducers is unavoidable

- Bendamustine HCl formulations may vary by country; consult local regulatory-approved labeling for guidance. For example, in the U.S., the Food and Drug Administration approved Bendeka under Section 505(b)(2) of the Federal Food, Drug, and Cosmetic Act on 7 December 2015. The Bendeka product labeling contains specific dilution and administration instructions, *thus:*

    Bendamustine HCl (Bendeka, where available) 90 mg/m² per dose; administer intravenously in a volume of 0.9% NS or D5W sufficient to produce a concentration with the range 1.85–5.6 mg/mL, over 10 minutes, on 2 consecutive days, days 1 and 2, every 28 days for 3 cycles during cycles 1–3 (total dosage/28-day cycle during cycles 1–3 = 180 mg/m²)

Cycles 4–6: Cytarabine + rituximab (21-day cycles)

Premedications for Rituximab:
- **Acetaminophen** 650–1000 mg; administer orally 30–60 minutes before each rituximab dose, *plus*
- **Diphenhydramine** 25–50 mg; administer orally or intravenously 30–60 minutes before each rituximab dose

Rituximab 375 mg/m²; administer intravenously in 0.9% sodium chloride injection (0.9% NS) or 5% dextrose injection (D5W), diluted to a concentration within the range 1–4 mg/mL, on day 1, every 21 days, for 3 cycles during cycles 4–6 (total dosage/21-day cycle during cycles 4–6 = 375 mg/m²)

Rituximab administration:
- Infuse initially at 50 mg/hour. If hypersensitivity or infusion reactions do not occur during the first 30 minutes, increase the rate by 50 mg/hour every 30 minutes as tolerated to a maximum rate of 400 mg/hour. During subsequent treatments if previous rituximab administration was well tolerated, start at 100 mg/hour and increase by 100 mg/hour every 30 minutes as tolerated to a maximum rate of 400 mg/hour

INFUSION REACTIONS ASSOCIATED WITH RITUXIMAB

Fevers, chills, and rigors
1. Interrupt rituximab administration for severe symptoms, and give:
    - **Acetaminophen** 650 mg orally for fever. For persistent or recurrent symptoms, repeat administration every 4–6 hours as needed during rituximab administration
    - **Diphenhydramine** 25–50 mg orally or by intravenous injection for pruritus, hypotension, or angioedema. For persistent or recurrent symptoms, repeat administration every 4–6 hours as needed during rituximab administration
    - **Meperidine** 12.5–25 mg by intravenous injection every 10–20 minutes as needed for shaking chills (generally, cumulative doses >100 mg are not needed; use repeated doses with caution in persons with moderate or more severely impaired renal function)
2. If rituximab administration was interrupted, resume infusion at a slower rate than the maximum rate previously attempted. Rate escalation may be reattempted at smaller incremental steps with close monitoring. Do not exceed the maximum recommended rate of 400 mg/h

Dyspnea or wheezing without allergic findings (urticaria, or tongue or laryngeal edema)
1. Interrupt rituximab administration immediately
2. Give **hydrocortisone** 100 mg by intravenous injection (or an alternative steroid with equivalent glucocorticoid potency)
3. Give a **histamine (H₂) receptor antagonist** (ranitidine 50 mg, cimetidine 300 mg, or famotidine 20 mg) intravenously over 15–30 minutes
4. After symptoms resolve, resume rituximab administration at 25 mg/h with close monitoring. Do not increase the administration rate

Note: Medications and equipment for the treatment of hypersensitivity reactions should be available for immediate use in the event of a reaction during administration (eg, intravenous fluids, epinephrine, antihistamines, glucocorticoids, and oxygen)
Rituxan (rituximab) prescribing information. South San Francisco, CA: Genentech, Inc; 2018 October

Cytarabine

Patient Group	Recommended Initial Cytarabine Dosage
<60 Years of age	**Cytarabine** 2000 mg/m² per dose; administer intravenously over 3 hours in 50–500 mL 0.9% NS or D5W every 12 hours for 4 doses on days 1 and 2, every 21 days, for 3 cycles during cycles 4–6 (total dosage/21-day cycle during cycles 4–6 = 8000 mg/m²)
≥60 Years of age, serum creatinine <1.3 mg/dL, *and* no preexisting neurotoxicity	
≥60 Years of age with either serum creatinine 1.3–2.0 mg/dL *or* preexisting neurotoxicity	**Cytarabine** 1500 mg/m² per dose; administer intravenously over 3 hours in 50–500 mL 0.9% NS or D5W every 12 hours for 4 doses on days 1 and 2, every 21 days, for 3 cycles during cycles 4–6 (total dosage/21-day cycle during cycles 4–6 = 6000 mg/m²)
≥60 Years of age with *both* serum creatinine ≥1.3–2.0 mg/dL *and* preexisting neurotoxicity	**Cytarabine** 1000 mg/m² per dose; administer intravenously over 3 hours in 50–500 mL 0.9% NS or D5W every 12 hours for 4 doses on days 1 and 2, every 21 days, for 3 cycles during cycles 4–6 (total dosage/21-day cycle during cycles 4–6 = 4000 mg/m²)

(continued)

Keratitis prophylaxis

Steroid ophthalmic drops (**prednisolone 1% or dexamethasone 0.1%**); administer 2 drops by intraocular instillation into each eye every 6 hours starting prior to the first cytarabine dose and continuing until 48 hours after high-dose cytarabine is completed

Supportive Care

Antiemetic prophylaxis

Emetogenic potential on days when bendamustine and/or cytarabine are administered is MODERATE

See Chapter 42 for antiemetic recommendations

Hematopoietic growth factor (CSF) prophylaxis

During cycles 1–3 (bendamustine + rituximab), primary prophylaxis MAY be indicated

During cycles 4–6 (cytarabine + rituximab), primary prophylaxis is indicated with one of the following:

Filgrastim (G-CSF) 5 µg/kg per day, by subcutaneous injection, *or:*

Pegfilgrastim (pegylated filgrastim) 6 mg/0.6 mL, by subcutaneous injection for one dose

• Begin use from 24–72 h after myelosuppressive chemotherapy is completed

• Continue daily filgrastim use until ANC ≥5000/mm³ after the leukocyte nadir

• Discontinue daily filgrastim use at least 24 hours before administering myelosuppressive treatment. Do not administer pegfilgrastim within 14 days before administering myelosuppressive treatment

See Chapter 43 for more information

Antimicrobial prophylaxis

Risk of fever and neutropenia is INTERMEDIATE

Antimicrobial primary prophylaxis to be considered:

• Antibacterial—consider a fluoroquinolone during periods of prolonged neutropenia, or no prophylaxis

• Antifungal—consider use during periods of prolonged neutropenia, or no prophylaxis

• Antiviral—antiherpes antivirals (eg, acyclovir, famciclovir, valacyclovir)

Treatment Modifications

Bendamustine Treatment Modifications	
Starting dose	90 mg/m² per dose on days 1 and 2
Dose level −1	70 mg/m² per dose on days 1 and 2
Dose level −2	Discontinue bendamustine

Hematologic Toxicity	
Day 1 platelet count <75,000/mm³ or day 1 ANC <1000/mm³	Delay start of cycle until platelet count ≥75,000/mm³ and ANC ≥1000/mm³ or until recovery to near baseline values, then reduce bendamustine dosage by 1 dose level for subsequent cycles. Consider G-CSF use in subsequent cycles for dose-limiting neutropenia
G4 hematologic toxicity occurring in the previous cycle	Delay start of cycle until platelet count ≥75,000/mm³ and ANC ≥1000/mm³ or until recovery to near baseline values, then reduce the bendamustine dosage by 1 dose level for subsequent cycles. Consider G-CSF use in subsequent cycles for dose-limiting neutropenia or severe neutropenic complications

Infectious Complications	
Active infection	Interrupt bendamustine and rituximab until resolution of infection, then resume treatment at either the same dosages, or with the bendamustine dosage reduced by 1 dose level, depending on the severity of infection
New or changes in preexisting neurologic symptoms (eg, confusion, dizziness, loss of balance, vision problems, aphasia, ambulation issues); PML suspected	Interrupt all therapy until central nervous system status is clarified. Work-up may include (but is not limited to) consultation with a neurologist, brain MRI, and LP
PML is confirmed	Discontinue all therapy
HBV reactivation	Withhold all therapy. Institute appropriate treatment for HBV. Upon resolution of HBV reactivation, resumption of therapy should be discussed with a physician with expertise in management of HBV

(continued)

Treatment Modifications (continued)

Drug Interactions

Patient requires concomitant therapy with a CYP1A2 inhibitor (eg, fluvoxamine, ciprofloxacin)	Consider alternative treatment instead of the CYP1A2 inhibitor. If the CYP1A2 inhibitor cannot be avoided, use caution and monitor carefully for bendamustine adverse effects. Do not modify the rituximab dose
Patient requires concomitant therapy with a CYP1A2 inducer (eg, omeprazole) or patient is a smoker	Consider alternative treatment instead of the CYP1A2 inducer. Recommend cessation of smoking, if applicable. If the CYP1A2 inducer cannot be avoided, monitor carefully for reduced bendamustine efficacy. Do not modify the rituximab dose

Other Toxicities

Clinically significant G2 nonhematologic toxicity during the prior cycle	Delay start of cycle until the nonhematologic toxicity resolves to G ≤1 or baseline, then resume treatment at the same dose
Clinically significant G ≥3 nonhematologic toxicity during the prior cycle	Delay start of cycle until the nonhematologic toxicity resolves to G ≤1 or baseline, then resume treatment with the bendamustine dosage reduced by 1 dose level

Bendeka (bendamustine hydrochloride injection) prescribing information. North Wales, PA: Teva Pharmaceuticals USA, Inc; 2018 July
Rituxan (rituximab) prescribing information. South San Francisco, CA: Genentech, Inc; 2018 October

High-dose Cytarabine (HiDAC) Treatment Modifications

Dose Level	Age <60 Years, or Age ≥60 Years with Both Serum Creatinine <1.3 mg/dL *and* No Pre-existing Neurotoxicity	Age ≥60 Years with *Either* Serum Creatinine 1.3–2.0 mg/dL *or* Pre-existing Neurotoxicity	Age ≥60 years with *Both* Serum Creatinine ≥1.3–2.0 mg/dL *and* Preexisting Neurotoxicity
Starting	2000 mg/m^2 per dose	1500 mg/m^2 per dose	1000 mg/m^2 per dose
Level −1	1500 mg/m^2 per dose	1000 mg/m^2 per dose	800 mg/m^2 per dose
Level −2	1000 mg/m^2 per dose	800 mg/m^2 per dose	Discontinue therapy

Hematologic Toxicity

Day 1 platelet count <100,000/mm^3 or ANC <1500/mm^3	Delay start of cycle until platelet count ≥100,000/mm^3 and ANC ≥1500/mm^3, or until recovery to near baseline value, then continue at the same dose
G4 neutropenia (ANC <500/mm^3) during the prior cycle given without growth factor (filgrastim, pegfilgrastim) prophylaxis	Administer filgrastim or pegfilgrastim during all subsequent cycles, and continue the same dose
Febrile neutropenia (ANC <1000/mm^3 with temperature >38°C or >100.4°F) during the prior cycle given without growth factor (filgrastim, pegfilgrastim) prophylaxis	
Febrile neutropenia (ANC <1000/mm^3 with temperature >38°C or >100.4°F) during the prior cycle given with growth factor (filgrastim, pegfilgrastim) prophylaxis	Reduce the dose of cytarabine by 1 dose level for subsequent cycles
G ≥3 thrombocytopenia (platelets <50,000/mm^3) during the prior cycle	

Neurologic Toxicities

Neurologic (cerebellar) toxicity	Discontinue cytarabine. Patients who develop CNS symptoms should not receive subsequent high-dose cytarabine

Other Toxicities

Fever, myalgia, bone pain, occasionally chest pain, maculopapular rash, conjunctivitis and malaise 6–12 hours following drug administration (cytarabine or Ara-C syndrome)	Corticosteroids are beneficial in treating or preventing this syndrome. If the symptoms deemed treatable, continue therapy with cytarabine and pretreat with corticosteroids. If the syndrome occurs in a patient already receiving corticosteroid pretreatment, consider reducing the cytarabine dose by 1 dose level

Patient Population Studied

The DFCI trial enrolled 23 patients from August 2012 to March 2014. The WUSTL trial enrolled 18 patients from August 2016 to September 2018. Forty-seven patients initiated RB/RC therapy outside of a clinical trial between July 2014 and August 2018 and were included in the off-trial cohort

Baseline Characteristics					
		Patient Cohort, n (%)			
	Total	DFCI Off-trial	DFCI trial	WUSTL Trial	P
N (% of all)	88 [100%]	47 [53%]	23 [26%]	18 [20%]	
Age, years—median (range)	58 (30–72)	58 (30–72)	57 (42–69)	60 (38–65)	0.97*
Age >60 years–No (%)	36 (41)	20 (43)	8 (35)	8 (44)	0.84†
Male sex	64 (73)	32 (68)	15 (65)	17 (94)	0.056†
Stage at diagnosis					
1	1 (1)	0 (0)	0 (0)	1 (6)	0.80‡
2	1 (1))	1 (2)	0 (0)	0 (0)	
3	11 (12)	7 (15)	3 (13)	1 (6)	
4	75 (85)	39 (83)	20 (87)	16 (89)	
ECOG PS					
0–1	84 (95)	47 (100)	22 (96)	15 (83)	**0.013†**
2	4 (5)	0 (0)	1 (4)	3 (17)	
Days from diagnosis to treatment—median (range)	32 (0–1539)	31 (3–1388)	40 (12–245)	21 (0–1539)	**0.031***
MIPI score					
Low	47 (53)	22 (47)	16 (70)	9 (50)	0.13‡
Intermediate	16 (18)	11 (23)	5 (22)	0 (0)	
High	17 (19)	6 (13)	2 (9)	9 (50)	
Missing	8 (9)	8 (17)	0 (0)	0 (0)	
LDH > ULN					
No	54 (61)	27 (57)	18 (78)	9 (50)	0.16†
Yes	27 (31)	13 (28)	5 (22)	9 (50)	
Missing	7 (8)	7 (15)	0 (0)	0 (0)	
Ki67					
≤30%	49 (56)	27 (57)	12 (52)	10 (56)	>0.99†
>30%	21 (24)	12 (26)	5 (22)	4 (22)	
Missing	18 (20)	8 (17)	6 (26)	4 (22)	
MCL subtype					
Other	76 (86)	40 (85)	23 (100)	13 (72)	**0.037†**
Blastoid/pleomorphic	11 (12)	7 (15)	0 (0)	4 (22)	
Missing	1 (1)	0 (0)	0 (0)	1 (6)	

(continued)

Patient Population Studied (continued)

Treating center					
Community	8 (9)	8 (17)	0 (0)	0 (0)	**0.025**[†]
Academic	80 (91)	39 (83)	23 (100)	18 (100)	

Significant P values (ie, P<0.05) are bolded
LDH, lactate dehydrogenase; MIPI, MCL International Prognostic Index; PS, performance status
[*]Kruskal-Wallis rank-sum test
[†]Fisher's exact test
[‡]Kruskal-Wallis trend test (Monte Carlo simulation with 10 000 replicates)

Efficacy (N = 87)

EOI Response Rates among Response-evaluable Patients

	ORR, n/N (%) [95% CI]	CR, n/N (%) [95% CI]	PR, n/N (%) [95% CI]
Overall	84/87 (97) [90–99]	78/87 (90) [81–95]	6/87 (7) [3–14]
Cohort			
DFCI off trial	47/47 (100) [92–100]	44/47 (94) [82–99]	3/47 (6) [1–18]
DFCI trial[*]	22/23 (96) [78–100]	22/23 (96) [78–100]	0/23 (0) [0–15]
WUSTL trial	15/17 (88) [64–99]	12/17 (71) [44–90]	3/17 (18) [4–43]
MIPI			
Low	47/47 (100) [92–100]	43/47 (91) [80–98]	4/47 (9) [2–20]
Intermediate	15/16 (94) [70–100]	15/16 (94) [70–100]	0/16 (0) [0–21]
High	14/16 (88) [62–98]	12/16 (75) [48–93]	2/16 (12) [2–38]
Ki67			
≤30%	48/49 (98) [89–100]	45/49 (92) [80–98]	3/49 (6) [1–17]
>30%	19/20 (95) [75–100]	17/20 (85) [62–97]	2/20 (10) [1–32]
Histologic subtype			
Other	73/75 (97) [91–100]	69/75 (92) [83–97]	4/75 (5) [1–13]
Blastoid/pleomorphic	10/11 (91) [59–100]	9/11 (82) [4–98]	1/11 (9) [0–41]
Starting cytarabine dose			
3 g/m2	28/28 (100) [88–100]	25/28 (89) [72–98]	3/28 (11) [2–28]
<3 g/m2	53/56 (95) [85–99]	50/56 (89) [78–96]	3/56 (5) [1–15]
Cumulative cytarabine dose[†]			
≤24 g/m2	52/53 (98) [90–100]	51/53 (96) [87–100]	1/53 (2) [0–10]
>24 g/m2 28/28 (100)	28/28 (100) [88–100]	25/28 (89) [72–98]	3/28 (11) [2–28]

[*]Response assessment in the DFCI trial was based on CT using the International Working Group Criteria. Responses in other cohorts were based on PET using the Lugano classification
[†]Among the 81 patients who completed 3 cycles of RC

Adverse Events (N = 87)

Completed 6 cycles of RB/RC	81/87 (93%)
Discontinued therapy	7/87 (8%) Persistent cytopenias during RC cycles (N = 2), Progressive disease (N = 2) Physician preference (N = 1) G3 rash attributed to bendamustine (N = 1) G3 type III hypersensitivity reaction to rituximab (N = 1)

Treatment discontinuation those receiving alternating cycles of RB/RC	17%	P = 0.15
Treatment discontinuation those receiving sequential cycles of RB/RC	6%	

Serious AEs for Trial (DFCI/WUSTL) Patients

Grade toxicity No of patients [% of total]	DFCI			WUSTL			Combined		
	G3/4 23 [56%]	G3	G4	G3/4 18 [44%]	G3	G4	G3/4 41 [100%]	G3	G4
Lymphopenia	21 (91)	—	21 (91)	15 (83)	1 (6)	14 (78)	36 (88)	1 (2)	35 (85)
Thrombocytopenia	19 (83)	—	19 (83)	16 (89)	2 (11)	14 (78)	35 (85)	2 (5)	33 (80)
Neutropenia	20 (87)	2 (9)	18 (78)	14 (78)	4 (22)	10 (56)	34 (83)	6 (15)	28 (68)
Leukopenia	18 (78)	—	18 (78)	13 (72)	1 (6)	12 (67)	31 (76)	1 (2)	30 (73)
Anemia	11 (48)	11 (48)	—	7 (39)	6 (33)	1 (6)	18 (44)	17 (41)	1 (2)
Febrile neutropenia	4 (17)	3 (13)	1 (4)	2 (11)	1 (6)	1 (6)	6 (15)	4 (10)	2 (5)
Fever	2 (9)	2 (9)	—	—	—	—	2 (5)	2 (5)	—
Enterocolitis	—	—	—	1 (6)	1 (6)	—	1 (2)	1 (2)	—
Pneumonia	1 (4)	1 (4)	—	—	—	—	1 (2)	1 (2)	—
Sepsis	1 (4)	1 (4)	—	—	—	—	1 (2)	1 (2)	—
Hyperglycemia	—	—	—	1 (6)	1 (6)	—	1 (2)	1 (2)	—
Hyperuricemia	—	—	—	1 (6)	—	1 (6)	1 (2)	—	1 (2)
IRR	—	—	—	1 (6)	1 (6)	—	1 (2)	1 (2)	—
TTP	1 (4)	—	1 (4)	—	—	—	1 (2)	—	1 (2)

Data are presented as n (%) of patients
Abbreviations: IRR, infusion related reaction; TTP, thrombotic thrombocytopenic purpura

Therapy Monitoring

1. *Prior to treatment initiation*: CBC with differential, serum chemistries, serum bilirubin, ALT or AST, hepatitis B core antibody (IgG or total) and hepatitis B surface antigen, and urine pregnancy test (women of child-bearing potential only)
   - *In patients at high risk for tumor lysis syndrome* consider frequent monitoring of laboratory indices of tumor lysis syndrome, intravenous hydration, and prophylaxis with a xanthine oxidase inhibitor (eg, allopurinol) during the first cycle
2. *Prior to each cycle and at least weekly*: CBC with differential, serum chemistries, serum bilirubin, ALT or AST
   - Patients who receive high-dose cytarabine need to be closely monitored for changes in renal function. Renal dysfunction is highly correlated with an increased risk of cerebellar toxicity
3. *Prior to each dose of cytarabine:* Monitor for signs of cerebellar toxicity (nystagmus, dysmetria, and ataxia)
4. *Monitor periodically for:* Signs and symptoms of infection (including progressive multifocal leukoencephalopathy), dermatologic toxicity, and cytarabine syndrome (rash, conjunctivitis, chest pain, malaise, myalgia, arthralgia, fever)
5. *Response assessment (after cycle 6)*: Physical examination, CBC with differential, CT scans or PET scan, bone marrow evaluation (if clinically indicated), endoscopy (if clinically indicated)

MANTLE CELL LYMPHOMA • FIRST LINE, LESS AGRESSIVE

NON-HODGKIN LYMPHOMA REGIMEN: BORTEZOMIB (VELCADE) + RITUXIMAB + CYCLOPHOSPHAMIDE + DOXORUBICIN (ADRIAMYCIN) + PREDNISONE (VR-CAP)

Robak T et al. N Engl J Med 2015;372:944–953
Supplementary appendix to: Robak T et al. N Engl J Med 2015;372:944–953
Protocol for: Robak T et al. N Engl J Med 2015;372:944–953

Bortezomib 1.3 mg/m^2 per dose; administer intravenously as a 3–5 second bolus injection in a volume of 0.9% sodium chloride (0.9% NS) sufficient to produce a final bortezomib concentration of 1 mg/mL for 4 doses on days 1, 4, 8, and 11, every 21 days, for 6–8 cycles (total dosage/21-day cycle = 5.2 mg/m^2)

Premedication for rituximab:
Acetaminophen 650–1000 mg; administer orally 30–60 minutes before each rituximab dose, *plus*
Diphenhydramine 25–50 mg; administer orally or intravenously 30–60 minutes before each rituximab dose
Rituximab 375 mg/m^2 per dose; administer intravenously in 0.9% NS or 5% dextrose injection (D5W), diluted to a concentration within the range 1–4 mg/mL, on day 1 after the bortezomib infusion, every 21 days, for 6–8 cycles (total dosage/21-day cycle = 375 mg/m^2)
Notes on rituximab administration:
• Infuse initially at 50 mg/h. If hypersensitivity or infusion reactions do not occur during the first 30 minutes, increase the rate by 50 mg/h every 30 minutes as tolerated to a maximum rate of 400 mg/h. During subsequent treatments if previous rituximab administration was well tolerated, start at 100 mg/h, and increase by 100 mg/h every 30 minutes as tolerated to a maximum rate of 400 mg/h

INFUSION REACTIONS ASSOCIATED WITH RITUXIMAB
Fevers, chills, and rigors
1. Interrupt rituximab administration for severe symptoms, and give:
   • **Acetaminophen** 650 mg orally for fever. For persistent or recurrent symptoms, repeat administration every 4–6 hours as needed during rituximab administration
   • **Diphenhydramine** 25–50 mg orally or by intravenous injection for pruritus, hypotension, or angioedema. For persistent or recurrent symptoms, repeat administration every 4–6 hours as needed during rituximab administration
   • **Meperidine** 12.5–25 mg by intravenous injection every 10–20 minutes as needed for shaking chills (generally, cumulative doses >100 mg are not needed; use repeated doses with caution in persons with moderate or more severely impaired renal function)
2. If rituximab administration was interrupted, resume infusion at a slower rate than the maximum rate previously attempted. Rate escalation may be reattempted at smaller incremental steps with close monitoring. Do not exceed the maximum recommended rate of 400 mg/h

Dyspnea or wheezing without allergic findings (urticaria, or tongue or laryngeal edema)
1. Interrupt rituximab administration immediately
2. Give **hydrocortisone** 100 mg by intravenous injection (or an alternative steroid with equivalent glucocorticoid potency)
3. Give a **histamine (H$_2$) receptor antagonist** (ranitidine 50 mg, cimetidine 300 mg, or famotidine 20 mg) intravenously over 15–30 minutes
4. After symptoms resolve, resume rituximab administration at 25 mg/h with close monitoring. Do not increase the administration rate
Note: Medications and equipment for the treatment of hypersensitivity reactions should be available for immediate use in the event of a reaction during administration (eg, intravenous fluids, epinephrine, antihistamines, glucocorticoids, and oxygen)
Rituxan (rituximab) prescribing information. South San Francisco, CA: Genentech, Inc; 2018 October

Intravenous hydration before and after cyclophosphamide administration:
500–1000 mL 0.9% NS
Cyclophosphamide 750 mg/m^2; administer intravenously in 25–250 mL 0.9% NS or D5W over 10–30 minutes on day 1, every 21 days, for 6–8 cycles (total dosage/21-day cycle = 750 mg/m^2)
Doxorubicin 50 mg/m^2; administer by intravenous injection over 3–5 minutes on day 1, every 21 days, for 6–8 cycles (total dosage/21-day cycle = 50 mg/m^2)
Prednisone 100 mg/m^2 per day; administer orally once daily for 5 consecutive days, days 1–5 every 21 days, for 6–8 cycles (total dosage/21-day cycle = 500 mg/m^2)

Supportive Care
Antiemetic prophylaxis
Emetogenic potential on day 1: **HIGH, POTENTIAL FOR DELAYED SYMPTOMS**
See Chapter 42 for antiemetic recommendations

Hematopoietic growth factor (CSF) prophylaxis
Primary prophylaxis **MAY** *be indicated*
See Chapter 43 for more information

Antimicrobial prophylaxis
Risk of fever and neutropenia is INTERMEDIATE
Antimicrobial primary prophylaxis to be considered:
- Antibacterial—consider a fluoroquinolone during periods of prolonged neutropenia, or no prophylaxis
- Antifungal—consider use during periods of prolonged neutropenia, or no prophylaxis
- Antiviral—antiherpes antivirals (eg, acyclovir, famciclovir, valacyclovir)

Treatment Modifications

Cyclophosphamide + Doxorubicin + Prednisone Dose Modifications

Dose Level	Cyclophosphamide	Doxorubicin	Prednisone
Starting	750 mg/m^2	50 mg/m^2	100 mg/m^2 per dose
Level −1	562.5 mg/m^2	37.5 mg/m^2	100 mg/dose (fixed dose)
Level −2	375 mg/m^2	25 mg/m^2	80 mg/dose (fixed dose)

Adverse Event	Treatment Modification
Hematologic Toxicity	
Day 1 platelet count <100,000/mm^3 or ANC <1500/mm^3	Delay start of cycle until platelet count ≥100,000/mm^3 and ANC ≥1500/mm^3, or until recovery to near baseline value, then continue at the same doses of cyclophosphamide, doxorubicin, and prednisone
G4 neutropenia (ANC <500/mm^3) during the prior cycle given without growth factor (filgrastim, pegfilgrastim) prophylaxis	Administer filgrastim or pegfilgrastim during all subsequent cycles, and continue the same doses of cyclophosphamide, doxorubicin, and prednisone
Febrile neutropenia (ANC <1000/mm^3 with temperature >38°C or >100.4°F) during the prior cycle given without growth factor (filgrastim, pegfilgrastim) prophylaxis	
Febrile neutropenia (ANC <1000/mm^3 with temperature >38°C or >100.4°F) during the prior cycle given with growth factor (filgrastim, pegfilgrastim) prophylaxis	Reduce the dose of cyclophosphamide and doxorubicin by 1 dose level for subsequent cycles. Do not change the prednisone dose
G ≥3 thrombocytopenia (platelets <50,000/mm^3) during the prior cycle	
Hepatic Impairment	
Serum bilirubin 1.2–3 mg/dL	Decrease the doxorubicin dose by 50%
Serum bilirubin 3.1–5 mg/dL	Decrease the doxorubicin dose by 75%
Serum bilirubin >5 mg/dL	Do not administer doxorubicin
Other Toxicities	
LVEF is 40%, or is 40% to 45% with a 10% or greater absolute decrease below the pretreatment	Withhold doxorubicin, and repeat LVEF assessment within approximately 4 weeks. Discontinue doxorubicin if the LVEF has not improved or has declined further, unless the benefits for the individual patient outweigh the risks
G ≥3 hyperglycemia (insulin therapy initiated; hospitalization indicated)	Withhold prednisone until blood glucose is ≤250 mg/dL. Treat with insulin or other hypoglycemic agents as clinically appropriate, and then resume prednisone at the same dose. If hyperglycemia is uncontrolled despite above measures, decrease prednisone by 1 dose level
G ≥2 mood alteration (moderate mood alteration) or confusion (moderate disorientation; limiting instrumental ADL)	Withhold prednisone until symptoms return to baseline. Resume prednisone reduced by 1 dose level. If symptoms persist, reduce by another dose level. Do not change the cyclophosphamide or doxorubicin doses

Bortezomib Dose Modifications

Starting dose	1.3 mg/m^2 per dose
Dose level −1	1 mg/m^2 per dose
Dose level −2	0.7 mg/m^2 per dose

(continued)

Treatment Modifications (continued)

Adverse Event	Treatment Modification
Day 1 platelet count <100,000/mm³or ANC <1500/mm³	Delay start of cycle until platelet count ≥100,000/mm³ and ANC ≥1500/mm³, or until recovery to near baseline value
G ≥3 neutropenia (ANC <1000/mm³) G4 thrombocytopenia (platelet count <25,000/mm³)	Withhold bortezomib for up to 2 weeks until ANC ≥750/mm³and platelet count is ≥25,000/mm³ If, after bortezomib has been withheld, the toxicity does not resolve, discontinue bortezomib If ANC recovers to ≥750/mm³ and platelet count recovers to ≥25,000/mm³, reduce the bortezomib dose by 1 dose level
G1 neuropathy (paresthesia, weakness or loss of reflexes) without pain or loss of function	No action
G1 neuropathy with pain or G2 neuropathy (moderate symptoms; limiting instrumental activities of daily living)	Reduce bortezomib dosage by 1 dose level
G2 neuropathy with pain or G3 neuropathy (severe symptoms, limiting self-care activities of daily living)	Withhold bortezomib treatment until toxicity resolves to G1 or baseline, then reinitiate reducing bortezomib dose to 0.7 mg/m² once per week (on days 1 and 8 only of each 21-day cycle)
G4 neuropathy (sensory neuropathy that is disabling or motor neuropathy that is life threatening or leads to paralysis)	Discontinue treatment
Hepatotoxicity	Monitor liver function. Stop bortezomib and evaluate if hepatotoxicity is suspected
Bilirubin level >1.5 × ULN and any AST level	Reduce bortezomib to 0.7 mg/m² in the first cycle; consider dose escalation to 1 mg/m² or dose reduction to 0.5 mg/m² in subsequent cycles based on patient tolerability
If several bortezomib doses in consecutive cycles are withheld due to toxicity	Reduce bortezomib by 1 dose level
G ≥2 nonhematologic toxicity on day 1 of a cycle	Hold bortezomib until toxicity resolved to G1 or baseline
Grade ≥3 nonhematologic toxicities	Hold bortezomib until toxicity resolved to G ≤2 or baseline; then, may be reinitiated with 1 dose level reduction

ANC, absolute neutrophil count; G-CSF, granulocyte-colony stimulating factor; PML, progressive multifocal leukoencephalopathy; MRI, magnetic resonance imaging; LP, lumbar puncture; HBV, hepatitis B virus
Note: Medications and equipment for the treatment of hypersensitivity reactions should be available for immediate use in the event of a reaction during rituximab administration (eg, intravenous fluids, epinephrine, antihistamines, glucocorticoids, oxygen)

Therapy Monitoring

1. *Prior to treatment initiation*: CBC with differential, serum chemistries, serum bilirubin, ALT or AST, hepatitis B core antibody (IgG or total) and hepatitis B surface antigen, left ventricular ejection fraction (LVEF), and urine pregnancy test (women of child-bearing potential only)
   — In addition to baseline monitoring, evaluate LVEF during doxorubicin treatment if clinical symptoms of heart failure are present. If baseline LVEF is ≥50%, repeat LVEF evaluation after a cumulative lifetime doxorubicin dose between 250 and 300 mg/m² has been reached, after a cumulative lifetime doxorubicin dose of 450 mg/m² has been reached, and then before each cycle beyond a cumulative lifetime doxorubicin dose of 450 mg/m². If the baseline LVEF is <50%, consider repeating LVEF evaluation before each dose of doxorubicin
   — *In patients at high risk for tumor lysis syndrome* consider frequent monitoring of laboratory indices of tumor lysis syndrome, intravenous hydration, and prophylaxis with a xanthine oxidase inhibitor (eg, allopurinol) during the first cycle
2. *Prior to each cycle and prior to each dose of bortezomib (ie, on days 1, 4, 8 and 11)*: CBC with differential, serum chemistries, serum bilirubin, ALT or AST
3. *Monitor periodically for*: Signs and symptoms of infection (including progressive multifocal leukoencephalopathy), dermatologic toxicity, peripheral neuropathy (bortezomib)
4. *Response assessment (every 2–3 cycles)*: Physical examination, CBC with differential, CT scans or PET scan, bone marrow evaluation (if clinically indicated), endoscopy (if clinically indicated)

Efficacy

(N = 487)

	R-CHOP (N = 244)	VR-CAP (N = 243)	
Progression-free survival	14.4 months	24.7 months	HR 0.63; P<0.001
Overall response rate*	89%	92%	HR 1.03; 95% CI 0.97–1.09
Complete response rate	42%	53%	HR 1.29; 95% CI 1.07–1.57
Median time to progression	16.1 months	30.5 months	HR 0.58; 95% CI 0.45–0.74
Median overall survival	56.3 months	Not reached	HR 0.80; 95% CI 0.59–1.10

Overall response rate includes patients with either a complete or partial response
Note: Median follow-up was 40 months

Toxicity

(N = 482)

Grade (%)*	R-CHOP (N = 242)		VR-CAP (N = 240)	
	G1–2	G≥3	G1–2	G≥3
Any adverse event	13	85	6	93
Neutropenia	7	67	3	85
Thrombocytopenia	13	6	15	57
Any infection	33	14	38	21
Anemia	24	14	35	15
Leukopenia	9	29	6	44
Lymphocytopenia	5	9	3	28
Peripheral neuropathy not elsewhere classified	24	4	23	8
Diarrhea	7	2	25	5
Pyrexia	13	2	26	3
Constipation	15	<1	25	<1
Nausea	14	0	24	<1
Fatigue	17	2	17	6
Peripheral sensory neuropathy	17	2	18	5
Cough	8	0	19	1
Decreased appetite	9	<1	18	<1
Febrile neutropenia	<1	14	2	15
Asthenia	10	<1	13	3
Peripheral edema	10	<1	15	<1
Pneumonia	2	5	5	7

*According to the National Cancer Institute Common Terminology Criteria for Adverse Events, version 3.0
Note: All-grade toxicities that occurred in ≥15% patients and grade ≥3 toxicities that occurred in ≥5% patients in either study group during treatment are included. Rates of all-grade drug-related adverse events (93% for R-CHOP and 96% for VR-CAP) and treatment discontinuation owing to drug-related adverse events (6% for R-CHOP and 8% for VR-CAP) were similar for the two treatment groups; the rate of grade ≥3 drug-related adverse events was lower in the R-CHOP group than in the VR-CAP group (80% vs 91%). Deaths due to drug-related adverse events occurred in 3% of the R-CHOP group and 2% of the VR-CAP group

Patient Population Studied

The international, multicenter, randomized, phase 3 trial involved 487 patients with newly diagnosed, stage II–IV, mantle cell lymphoma who were ineligible or not considered for stem-cell transplantation. Patients were randomly assigned (1:1) to receive six to eight 21-day cycles of: intravenous rituximab (375 mg/m² on day 1), cyclophosphamide (750 mg/m² on day 1), doxorubicin (50 mg/m² on day 1), and vincristine (1.4 mg/m² [maximum 2 mg] on day 1), and oral prednisone (100 mg/m² on days 1–5) (R-CHOP); or intravenous bortezomib (1.3 mg/m² on days 1, 4, 8, and 11; administered first on day 1), rituximab (375 mg/m² on day 1; administered second), cyclophosphamide (750 mg/m² on day 1), and doxorubicin (50 mg/m² on day 1), and oral prednisone (100 mg/m² on days 1–5) (VR-CAP)

MANTLE CELL LYMPHOMA • FIRST LINE, LESS AGGRESSIVE
NON-HODGKIN LYMPHOMA REGIMEN: REVLIMID (LENALIDOMIDE) + RITUXIMAB (R²)

Ruan J et al. N Engl J Med 2015;373:1835–1844
Ruan J et al. Blood 2018;132:2016–2025

Premedication for rituximab:
Acetaminophen 650–1000 mg; administer orally 30–60 minutes before each rituximab dose, *plus*
Diphenhydramine 25–50 mg; administer orally or intravenously 30–60 minutes before each rituximab dose

Cycle 1:
    Rituximab 375 mg/m² per dose; administer intravenously in 0.9% NS or D5W, diluted to a concentration within the range 1–4 mg/mL, for 4 doses, on days 1, 8, 15, and 22, for 1 cycle, cycle 1, only (total dosage during cycle 1 only = 1500 mg/m²)
Every 8 weeks beginning in cycle 4 on day 1:
    Rituximab 375 mg/m² per dose; administer intravenously in 0.9% NS or D5W, diluted to a concentration within the range 1–4 mg/mL, on day 1, every 8 weeks, starting in cycle 4, until disease progression (total dosage every 8 weeks = 375 mg/m²)

Notes on rituximab administration:
- Infuse initially at 50 mg/h. If hypersensitivity or infusion reactions do not occur during the first 30 minutes, increase the rate by 50 mg/h every 30 minutes as tolerated to a maximum rate of 400 mg/h. During subsequent treatments if previous rituximab administration was well tolerated, start at 100 mg/h, and increase by 100 mg/h every 30 minutes as tolerated to a maximum rate of 400 mg/h
- Interrupt rituximab administration for fever, chills, edema, congestion of the head and neck mucosa, hypertension, and other serious adverse events. Resume rituximab administration after adverse events abate

Induction lenalidomide (cycles 1–12):
    Lenalidomide 20 mg/dose; administer orally, without regard to meals, once daily for 21 consecutive days on days 1–21, followed by 7 days without treatment, starting in cycle 1, every 28 days, for 12 induction cycles (total dosage/28-day cycle during induction cycles 1–12 = 420 mg)
- Patients who tolerate cycle 1 at a dosage of 20 mg/day may escalate the dosage to 25 mg/day on days 1–21 of each 28 day cycle beginning with cycle 2
- Patients with a CrCl between 30–60 mL/minute should initiate lenalidomide at a reduced dosage of 10 mg/day on days 1–21 of each 28 day cycle. If the first cycle is tolerated, subsequent induction cycles may be administered at a dosage of 15 mg/day
- Patients who delay taking a lenalidomide dose at a regularly scheduled time may take the missed dose if the time to the next regularly scheduled dose is >12 hours away

Maintenance lenalidomide (cycles 13+, continued until disease progression):
    Lenalidomide 15 mg/dose; administer orally, without regard to meals, once daily for 21 consecutive days on days 1–21, followed by 7 days without treatment, starting in cycle 13, every 28 days, until disease progression (total dosage/28-day cycle during maintenance cycles 13+ = 315 mg)
- Patients with a CrCl between 30–60 mL/minute should initiate lenalidomide at a reduced dosage of 5 mg/day on days 1–21 of each 28-day maintenance cycle
- Patients who delay taking a lenalidomide dose at a regularly scheduled time may take the missed dose if the time to the next regularly scheduled dose is >12 hours away

Supportive Care
Antiemetic prophylaxis
Emetogenic potential is **MINIMAL**
See Chapter 42 for antiemetic recommendations

Hematopoietic growth factor (CSF) prophylaxis
Primary prophylaxis is **NOT** *indicated*
See Chapter 43 for more information

Antimicrobial prophylaxis
Risk of fever and neutropenia is INTERMEDIATE
Antimicrobial primary prophylaxis to be considered:
- Antibacterial—not indicated
- Antifungal—not indicated
- Antiviral—antiherpes antivirals (eg, acyclovir, famciclovir, valacyclovir)

Thromboprophylaxis (administered to all patients unless already receiving anticoagulation for known thrombosis)
Choose one of the following:
- **Aspirin** 81 mg or 325 mg/dose; administer orally once daily, *or:*
- **Enoxaparin** 40 mg/dose; administer subcutaneously once per day

INFUSION REACTIONS ASSOCIATED WITH RITUXIMAB

Note: Medications for the treatment of hypersensitivity reactions should be available for immediate use in the event of a reaction during administration (eg, intravenous fluids, epinephrine, antihistamines, glucocorticoids, and O_2)

Fevers, chills, and rigors

1. Interrupt rituximab administration for severe symptoms, and give:

   • **Acetaminophen** 650 mg orally for fever. For persistent or recurrent symptoms, repeat administration every 4–6 hours as needed during rituximab administration

   • **Diphenhydramine** 25–50 mg orally or by intravenous injection for pruritus, hypotension, or angioedema. For persistent or recurrent symptoms, repeat administration every 4–6 hours as needed during rituximab administration

   • **Meperidine** 12.5–25 mg by intravenous injection every 10–20 minutes as needed for shaking chills (generally, cumulative doses >100 mg are not needed; use repeated doses with caution in persons with moderate or more severely impaired renal function)

2. If rituximab administration was interrupted, resume infusion at a slower rate than the maximum rate previously attempted. Rate escalation may be reattempted at smaller incremental steps with close monitoring. Do not exceed the maximum recommended rate of 400 mg/h

Dyspnea or wheezing without allergic findings (urticaria, or tongue or laryngeal edema)

1. Interrupt rituximab administration immediately
2. Give **hydrocortisone** 100 mg by intravenous injection (or an alternative steroid with equivalent glucocorticoid potency)
3. Give a **histamine (H₂) receptor antagonist** (ranitidine 50 mg, cimetidine 300 mg, or famotidine 20 mg) intravenously over 15–30 minutes
4. After symptoms resolve, resume rituximab administration at 25 mg/h with close monitoring. Do not increase the administration rate

20 mg per day	10 mg per day*
15 mg per day	5 mg per day
10 mg per day	2.5 mg per day
5 mg per day	Discontinue†
2.5 mg per day	—
Discontinue†	—

Treatment Modifications

Lenalidomide Dose Modifications

	CrCl ≥60 mL/min		CrCl ≥30 and <60 mL/min	
	Induction	Maintenance	Induction	Maintenance
Dose level +1*	25 mg†	N/A	15 mg†	N/A
Starting dose	20 mg†	15 mg†	10 mg†	5 mg†
Level −1	15 mg†	10 mg†	5 mg†	2.5 mg†
Level −2	10 mg†	5 mg†	2.5 mg†	Discontinue
Level −3	5 mg†	2.5 mg†	Discontinue	—
Level −4	2.5 mg†	Discontinue	—	—
Level −5	Discontinue	—	—	—

*If after completion of cycle 1 the patient remains free of G ≥3 toxicity, the lenalidomide dose may be increased to dose level +1
†Represents the once daily dosage administered on days 1–21 of each 28 day cycle

Adverse Event	Treatment Modification
Hematologic Toxicity	
Day 1 ANC <1000/mm³ or platelet count <50,000/mm³	Delay the next cycle until ANC ≥1000/mm³ and platelet count ≥50,000/mm³. Consider treatment with filgrastim and/or platelet transfusion according to local guidelines. If the start of a new cycle is delayed >14 days for lenalidomide-related toxicity, reduce the lenalidomide by 1 dose level

(continued)

Treatment Modifications (continued)

G3 neutropenia (ANC ≥500 to <1000/mm³) sustained for ≥7 days	If neutropenia occurred on or after day 15, withhold lenalidomide for the rest of the cycle, and follow weekly CBC.
G4 neutropenia (ANC <500/mm³) at any time	If neutropenia occurred before day 15 and resolves to G ≤2 (ANC ≥1000/mm³), resume lenalidomide at the same dose for the rest of the cycle
Febrile neutropenia (ANC <1000/mm³ with fever ≥38.3°C)	Consider use of filgrastim according to local guidelines. In subsequent cycles, reduce the lenalidomide dosage by 1 dose level
G ≥3 thrombocytopenia (platelet count <50,000/mm³) at any time	If thrombocytopenia occurred on or after day 15, withhold lenalidomide for the rest of the cycle, and follow weekly CBC. If thrombocytopenia occurred before day 15 and resolved to G ≤2 (platelet count ≥50,000/mm³), resume lenalidomide at the same dose for the rest of the cycle In subsequent cycles, reduce the lenalidomide dosage by 1 dose level
Nonhematologic Toxicities	
G2/3 non-desquamating rash	Hold lenalidomide. Consider administering antihistamines and/or a short course of steroids. Resume at the same dose when resolved to G ≤1
G ≥3 desquamating (blistering) rash	Permanently discontinue lenalidomide‡
G4 non-desquamating rash	
Allergic reactions, including hypersensitivity, angioedema, Stevens-Johnson syndrome, toxic epidermal necrolysis (TEN) and drug reaction with eosinophilia and systemic symptoms (DRESS)	
Tumor lysis syndrome (TLS)	Monitor patients at risk of TLS (ie, those with high tumor burden), and take appropriate precautions including aggressive hydration and allopurinol
G ≥3 peripheral neuropathy	If neuropathy is attributable to lenalidomide and occurred on or after day 15, withhold lenalidomide for the remainder of the cycle and reassess weekly If neuropathy is attributable to lenalidomide and occurred before day 15 and resolved to G ≤1, restart lenalidomide at the same dose level for the remainder of the cycle In either case, resume lenalidomide with the dosage reduced by 1 dose level in subsequent cycles provided that the toxicity resolves to G ≤1
G3/4 venous thromboembolism (VTE) during aspirin monotherapy or inadequate anticoagulation	Continue lenalidomide at the current dose, and initiate adequate anticoagulation
G3/4 venous thromboembolism (VTE) during adequate anticoagulation (eg, prophylactic or therapeutic doses of LMWH, UFH, or warfarin)	Discontinue lenalidomide‡
G ≥2 hypothyroidism or G ≥2 hyperthyroidism	Continue lenalidomide at current dose, and initiate appropriate medical treatment
AST or ALT >3× ULN	If the toxicity occurred on or after day 15, withhold lenalidomide for the rest of the cycle. Reevaluate liver function tests weekly until AST/ALT improve to ≤2.5× ULN and bilirubin improves to ≤1.5× ULN
Total bilirubin ≥3× ULN	If the toxicity occurred before day 15 and ALT/AST resolve to ≤2.5× ULN and bilirubin improves to ≤1.5× ULN, restart lenalidomide at the same dose level for the rest of the cycle In either case, resume lenalidomide with the dosage reduced by 1 dose level in subsequent cycles if ALT/AST improves to ≤2.5× ULN and bilirubin improves to ≤1.5× ULN
Other G ≥3 lenalidomide-related toxicities	If the toxicity occurred on or after day 15, withhold lenalidomide for the remainder of the cycle, and reassess toxicity at least every 7 day If the toxicity occurred before day 15 and resolved to G ≤2, restart lenalidomide at the same dose for the remainder of the cycle In either case, resume lenalidomide with the dosage reduced by 1 dose level in subsequent cycles provided that the toxicity resolves to G ≤2

(continued)

Treatment Modifications (*continued*)

Renal Impairment	
Moderate renal impairment (CrCl 30–60 mL/min)	Reduce the lenalidomide induction starting dose to 10 mg per dose. If after completion of cycle 1 the patient remains free of G ≥3 toxicity, the lenalidomide dose may be increased to a maximum of 15 mg per day starting in cycle 2
	Reduce the lenalidomide maintenance starting dose to 5 mg per dose
Severe renal impairment (CrCl <30 mL/min, or requiring hemodialysis)	Patients with creatinine clearance <30 mL/min were excluded from the study. No recommendations available

Note: In general, if a dose-limiting toxicity occurs on or after day 15 of the cycle, treatment will be withheld until the end of the cycle, and the dose will then be reduced (if applicable) beginning in the subsequent cycle. If the toxicity occurs before day 15 of the cycle, treatment will be held until recovery and restarted without dose reduction for the rest of the cycle (ie, continue until day 21; missed doses will not be made up), and then the next cycle will resume at a reduced dose

CrCl, creatinine clearance; ANC, absolute neutrophil count; CBC, complete blood count; LMWH, low molecular weight heparin; UFH, unfractionated heparin; AST, aspartate aminotransferase; ALT, alanine aminotransferase; ULN, upper limit of normal
‡If lenalidomide or rituximab are discontinued, the medically responsible healthcare provider may decide to either continue the other agent as monotherapy, or switch to an alternative regimen

Patient Population Studied

Sex—no. (%) [M / F]	27 (71) / 11 (29)
Age (years)—median (range)	65 (42–86)
ECOG performance status—no. (%)*—0–1 / >1	37 (97) / 1 (3)
Ann Arbor stage III or IV—no. (%)	38 (100)
Lactate dehydrogenase level—no. (%)–normal / elevated	23 (61) / 15 (39)
Bone marrow involvement—no. (%)—Yes / No	34 (89) / 4 (11)
MIPI score—no. (%)†—<5.7 / 5.7 to <6.2 / ≥6.2	13 (34) / 13 (34) / 12 (32)
IPI score—no. (%)‡—0–1 / 2 / 3 / 4–5	6 (16) / 18 (47) / 10 (26) / 4 (11)
Ki–67 index—no. (%)—<30% / ≥30% / unavailable	26 (68) / 8 (21) / 4 (11)
Indication for treatment—no. (%)	
Symptomatic lymphadenopathy	20 (53)
Cytopenia	7 (18)
Bulky disease (>5 cm)	5 (13)
Gastrointestinal symptom	3 (8)
Patient preference	2 (5)
Rapidly rising white-cell count (>100,000/μL)	1 (3)

*An Eastern Cooperative Oncology Group (ECOG) performance-status score of 0 indicates no symptoms, and a score of 1 indicates mild symptoms; higher scores indicate greater disability
†A Mantle Cell Lymphoma International Prognostic Index (MIPI) score lower than 5.7 indicates low-risk disease, a score of 5.7 to less than 6.2 indicates intermediate-risk disease, and a score of 6.2 or higher indicates high-risk disease
‡A International Prognostic Index (IPI) score of 0 or 1 indicates low-risk disease, a score of 2 indicates low-intermediate–risk disease, a score of 3 indicates high-intermediate-risk disease, and a score of 4 or 5 indicates high-risk disease

Efficacy (N = 36)

Complete response	23/36 (64%)
Partial response	10/36 (28%)
Median PFS	Not reached at a median follow-up of 64 months
Median DOR	**Not reached at a median follow-up of 64 months**
Ongoing responses	21/33 (64%)*
Estimated 3-year PFS	80.3% (95% CI, 63.0–90.1)
Estimated 5-year PFS	63.9% (95% CI, 44.8–77.9)
Estimated 3-year OS	89.5% (95% CI, 74.3–95.9)
Estimated 5-year OS	77.4% (95% CI, 59.4–88.1)
Correlations	
MIPI scores	Not associated with response or PFS
High-risk MIPI	Correlated with unfavorable OS (P = 0.04)
Ki67 proliferation index cutoff of 30%	No difference in PFS (P = 0.72) or OS (P = 0.54)

(*continued*)

Efficacy (N = 36) *continued)*

MDR assessment

MDR assessment at a median of 46 months (range, 42–62)	Among 10 patients[†], 8/9 CR patients, including the 2 patients off therapy, had MRD levels below the detection threshold of 10^{-6}, whereas the remaining 2 patients had detectable MRD levels of 1.2×10^{-5} and 3×10^{-6}

[*]Including 21 patients >3 years, 19 patients >4 years, 16 patients >5 years, and 6 patients >6 years
[†]At time of sampling, 3/10 patients remain on lanreotide/rituximab maintenance, 5/10 remain on maintenance rituximab alone, and 2/10 were off all treatment at 3 and 10 months
DOR, duration of response; MDR, minimal residual disease; OS, overall survival; PFS, progression-free survival

Toxicity

Toxicities[*]	Induction, n (%)		Maintenance (n, %)	
	Any Grade	Grade ≥3	Any Grade	Grade ≥3
Hematologic				
Neutropenia	26 (68)	16 (42)	25 (66)	16 (42)
Anemia	18 (47)	3 (8)	12 (32)	1 (3)
Thrombocytopenia	11 (29)	4 (11)	14 (37)	2 (5)
Febrile neutropenia	1 (3)	1 (3)	2 (5)	2 (5)
Infectious				
URI	9 (24)	0 (0)	17 (45)	0 (0)
UTI	4 (11)	0 (0)	8 (21)	2 (5)
Sinusitis	2 (5)	0 (0)	5 (13)	0 (0)
Cellulitis	2 (5)	0 (0)	4 (11)	1 (3)
Pneumonia	1 (3)	1 (3)	3 (8)	3 (8)
Zoster reactivation	0 (0)	0 (0)	3 (8)	0 (0)
Other				
Fatigue	29 (76)	4 (11)	15 (39)	1 (3)
Rash	26 (68)	11 (29)	6 (16)	0 (0)
Fever	22 (58)	0 (0)	4 (11)	0 (0)
Cough	20 (53)	0 (0)	9 (24)	0 (0)
Diarrhea	20 (53)	0 (0)	21 (55)	0 (0)
Hyperglycemia	13 (34)	2 (5)	16 (42)	0 (0)
Constipation	17 (45)	0 (0)	7 (18)	0 (0)
Edema	15 (39)	0 (0)	5 (13)	0 (0)
Tumor flare	14 (37)	4 (11)	0 (0)	0 (0)
Infusion reaction	13 (34)	1 (3)	0 (0)	0 (0)
Nausea	12 (32)	0 (0)	2 (5)	0 (0)
Anorexia	10 (26)	0 (0)	3 (8)	0 (0)
Dyspnea	10 (26)	1 (3)	2 (5)	0 (0)
Hyponatremia	9 (24)	0 (0)	7 (18)	0 (0)
Elevated ALT	9 (24)	1 (3)	6 (16)	1 (3)
Elevated AST	8 (21)	1 (3)	5 (13)	1 (3)
Arthralgia	8 (21)	1 (3)	5 (13)	0 (0)
Elevated alkaline phosphatase	8 (21)	1 (3)	6 (16)	0 (0)
Headache	7 (18)	0 (0)	5 (13)	0 (0)
Dizziness	7 (18)	0 (0)	3 (8)	0 (0)

Toxicity *(continued)*

Hypothyroidism	6 (16)	0 (0)	1 (3)	0 (0)
Myalgia	6 (16)	1 (3)	4 (11)	0 (0)
Neuropathy	3 (8)	0 (0)	8 (21)	0 (0)
HGG	1 (3)	0 (0)	3 (8)	0 (0)

*Nonhematologic AEs occurring in >10% of 38 patients
ALT, alanine aminotransferase; AST, aspartate aminotransferase; HGG, hypogammaglobulinemia; URI, upper respiratory infection

Severe AE	G3 or 4, n (%)	Phase
Pneumonia	4 (11)	Induction and maintenance
Neutropenic fever	3 (8)	Induction and maintenance
Tumor flare	4 (11)	Induction
Abdominal pain	2 (5)	Induction
Serum sickness	2 (5)	Induction
Syncope	2 (5)	Maintenance
Cholecystitis	2 (5)	Maintenance
UTI	2 (5)	Maintenance
Atrial fibrillation	1 (3)	Induction
Cholangitis	1 (3)	Induction
Dyspnea	1 (3)	Induction
Vertigo	1 (3)	Induction
Ventricular fibrillation	1 (3)	Induction
Rash	1 (3)	Induction
Infusion reaction	1 (3)	Induction
Escherichia coli urosepsis	1 (3)	Maintenance
Hand cellulitis	1 (3)	Maintenance
West Nile viral encephalitis	1 (3)	Maintenance
Car accident	1 (3)	Maintenance
Left femoral neck fracture	1 (3)	Maintenance
Secondary primary malignancies		
Nonmelanoma skin cancers	3 (8)	Induction and maintenance
Melanoma in situ	2 (5)	Induction and maintenance
Merkel cell carcinoma	1 (3)	Maintenance
Pancreatic cancer	1 (3)	Maintenance

Severe AEs are listed, regardless of attribution
Secondary primary malignancies were reported in 6 subjects, including 2 patients with invasive SPMs. One subject had both Merkel cell carcinoma and melanoma in situ

Therapy Monitoring

1. *Prior to treatment initiation:* CBC with differential, serum chemistries, serum bilirubin, ALT or AST, hepatitis B core antibody (IgG or total) and hepatitis B surface antigen, and urine pregnancy test (women of child-bearing potential only)
   a. *In patients at high risk for tumor lysis* consider frequent monitoring of laboratory indices of tumor lysis syndrome, intravenous hydration, and prophylaxis with a xanthine oxidase inhibitor (eg, allopurinol) during the first cycle
2. *Prior to each dose of rituximab, and then every 2 weeks thereafter:* CBC with differential, serum chemistries, serum bilirubin, ALT or AST
3. *Monitor periodically for* signs and symptoms of infection (including progressive multifocal leukoencephalopathy) and dermatologic toxicity

Lenalidomide Notes:
- A decrease in the number of CD34+ cells collected after treatment has been reported in patients who have received >4 cycles of lenalidomide. In patients who may undergo transplant, consider early referral to transplant center
- Because of the embryo-fetal risk, lenalidomide is available only through a restricted program under a Risk Evaluation and Mitigation Strategy (REMS), the REVLIMID REMS program. Required components of the REVLIMID REMS program include the following:
- Patients must sign a patient-physician agreement form and comply with the REMS requirements. In particular, female patients of reproductive potential who are not pregnant must comply with the pregnancy testing and contraception requirements, and males must comply with contraception requirements

MANTLE CELL LYMPHOMA • FIRST LINE, LESS AGGRESSIVE

NON-HODGKIN LYMPHOMA REGIMEN: RITUXIMAB + BENDAMUSTINE + CYTARABINE (R-BAC)

Visco C et al. J Clin Oncol 2013;31:1442–1449
Ohmachi K et al. J Clin Oncol 2013;31:2103–2109
Vacirca JL et al. Ann Hematol 2013;93:403–409

Prophylaxis for tumor lysis syndrome is recommended for high-risk patients (eg, high tumor burden, bulky lymphadenopathy, or renal impairment):

- Hydration; encourage oral hydration (eg, ≥3 L/day) starting 1–2 days prior to the first rituximab dose. Consider administering additional *intravenous* hydration prior to the infusion if needed. Continue hydration prior to subsequent cycles if needed

- **Allopurinol** 300 mg per dose; administer orally twice per day starting 12–24 hours prior to the first rituximab infusion for 7 days. Continue prophylaxis prior to subsequent cycles if needed

  - Reduce allopurinol dose to 300 mg by mouth once daily for 7 days for patients with renal impairment

Rituximab

Premedication for rituximab:

- **Acetaminophen** 650–1000 mg; administer orally 30–60 minutes before each rituximab dose, *plus*

Diphenhydramine 25–50 mg; administer orally or intravenously 30–60 minutes before each rituximab dose

Rituximab Dose

Cycle 1	Rituximab 375 mg/m^2; administer intravenously in 0.9% sodium chloride injection (0.9% NS) or 5% dextrose injection (D5W), diluted to a concentration within the range 1–4 mg/mL, on day 1 of cycle 1 only (total dosage/28-day cycle = 375 mg/m^2)
Cycles 2–6	Rituximab 375 mg/m^2; administer intravenously in 0.9% NS or D5W, diluted to a concentration within the range 1–4 mg/mL, on day 2, every 28 days (total dosage/28-day cycle = 375 mg/m^2)

Notes on rituximab administration:

- Infuse initially at 50 mg/h. If hypersensitivity or infusion reactions do not occur during the first 30 minutes, increase the rate by 50 mg/h every 30 minutes as tolerated to a maximum rate of 400 mg/h. During subsequent treatments if previous rituximab administration was well tolerated, start at 100 mg/h and increase by 100 mg/h every 30 minutes as tolerated to a maximum rate of 400 mg/h

INFUSION REACTIONS ASSOCIATED WITH RITUXIMAB

Fevers, chills, and rigors

1. Interrupt rituximab administration for severe symptoms, and give:

   - **Acetaminophen** 650 mg orally for fever. For persistent or recurrent symptoms, repeat administration every 4–6 hours as needed during rituximab administration

   - **Diphenhydramine** 25–50 mg orally or by intravenous injection for pruritus, hypotension, or angioedema. For persistent or recurrent symptoms, repeat administration every 4–6 hours as needed during rituximab administration

   - **Meperidine** 12.5–25 mg by intravenous injection every 10–20 minutes as needed for shaking chills (generally, cumulative doses >100 mg are not needed; use repeated doses with caution in persons with moderate or more severely impaired renal function)

2. If rituximab administration was interrupted, resume infusion at a slower rate than the maximum rate previously attempted. Rate escalation may be reattempted at smaller incremental steps with close monitoring. Do not exceed the maximum recommended rate of 400 mg/h

Dyspnea or wheezing without allergic findings (urticaria, or tongue or laryngeal edema)

1. Interrupt rituximab administration immediately

2. Give **hydrocortisone** 100 mg by intravenous injection (or an alternative steroid with equivalent glucocorticoid potency)

3. Give a **histamine (H$_2$) receptor antagonist** (ranitidine 50 mg, cimetidine 300 mg, or famotidine 20 mg) intravenously over 15–30 minutes

4. After symptoms resolve, resume rituximab administration at 25 mg/h with close monitoring. Do not increase the administration rate

Note: Medications and equipment for the treatment of hypersensitivity reactions should be available for immediate use in the event of a reaction during administration (eg, intravenous fluids, epinephrine, antihistamines, glucocorticoids, and oxygen)

Rituxan (rituximab) prescribing information. South San Francisco, CA: Genentech, Inc; 2018 October

Bendamustine

Premedication for bendamustine HCl: Premedications are not necessary for primary prophylaxis of infusion-related reactions. In the event of a non-severe infusion-related reaction, consider adding a histamine receptor (H$_1$)-subtype antagonist (eg, diphenhydramine 25–50 mg intravenously or orally), an antipyretic (eg, acetaminophen 650–1000 mg orally), and a corticosteroid (eg, methylprednisolone 100 mg intravenously) administered 30 minutes prior to bendamustine HCl administration in subsequent cycles

Bendamustine HCl 70 mg/m² per dose; administer intravenously in a volume of 0.9% NS sufficient to produce a concentration with the range 0.2–0.6 mg/mL over 30–60 minutes, on 2 consecutive days, days 2 and 3, 2 hours prior to cytarabine administration, every 28 days for up to 6 cycles (total dosage/28-day cycle = 140 mg/m²)
Note:
- On days when both bendamustine and cytarabine are administered (ie, days 2 and 3), bendamustine is administered 2 hours prior to cytarabine administration
- Bendamustine HCl can cause severe infusion-related reactions
  - For grade 1–2 infusion-related reactions, consider rechallenge with the addition of antihistamine, antipyretic, and corticosteroid premedications (as described in the above premedication section)
  - For grade 3 infusion-related reactions, consider permanent discontinuation versus rechallenge with the addition of antihistamine, antipyretic, and corticosteroid premedications (as described in the above premedication section) after weighing risks and benefits
  - For grade 4 infusion-related reactions, permanently discontinue bendamustine HCl
- Coadministration of strong CYP1A2 inhibitors (eg, ciprofloxacin, fluvoxamine) may increase exposure to bendamustine HCl and decrease exposure to its active metabolites. Concomitant CYP1A2 inducers (eg, omeprazole, cigarette smoking) may decrease exposure to bendamustine HCl and increase exposure to its active metabolites. Use caution, or select an alternative therapy, when coadministration of bendamustine HCl with strong CYP1A2 inhibitors or inducers is unavoidable
- Bendamustine HCl formulations may vary by country; consult local regulatory-approved labeling for guidance. For example, in the United States, the Food and Drug Administration–approved Bendeka under Section 505(b)(2) of the Federal Food, Drug, and Cosmetic Act on 7 December 2015. The Bendeka product labeling contains specific dilution and administration instructions, *thus*:
  - **Bendamustine HCl (Bendeka, where available)** 70 mg/m² per dose; administer intravenously in a volume of 0.9% NS or D5W sufficient to produce a concentration with the range 1.85–5.6 mg/mL, over 10 minutes, on 2 consecutive days, days 2 and 3, 2 hours prior to cytarabine administration, every 28 days for up to 6 cycles (total dosage/28-day cycle = 140 mg/m²)

Cytarabine
Cytarabine 800 mg/m² per dose; administer intravenously in 100–1000 mL 0.9% NS over 2 hours, for 3 consecutive days on days 2, 3, and 4, every 28 days for up to 6 cycles (total dosage/28-day cycle = 2400 mg/m²)
Note:
- On days when both cytarabine and bendamustine are administered (ie, days 2 and 3), cytarabine is administered 2 hours after bendamustine administration
- Keratitis prophylaxis (ie, with steroid ophthalmic drops) is not recommended for cytarabine doses <1000 mg/m²

Regimen note: all patients were planned to receive at least 4 cycles of rituximab + bendamustine + cytarabine. Select patients (previously untreated, <80 years of age, responding to therapy, and tolerating treatment well) were eligible to receive up to 6 cycles

Supportive Care
Antiemetic prophylaxis
Emetogenic potential on cycle 1 day 1 (ie, when only rituximab is administered) is **MINIMAL**
Emetogenic potential on days when bendamustine and/or cytarabine are administered is **MODERATE**
See Chapter 42 for antiemetic recommendations

Hematopoietic growth factor (CSF) prophylaxis
Primary prophylaxis is indicated with one of the following:
Filgrastim (G-CSF) 5 μg/kg per day, by subcutaneous injection, *or*
Pegfilgrastim (pegylated filgrastim) 6 mg/0.6 mL, by subcutaneous injection for 1 dose
- Begin use from 24–72 hours after myelosuppressive chemotherapy is completed
- Continue daily filgrastim use until ANC ≥5000/mm³ after the leukocyte nadir
- Discontinue daily filgrastim use at least 24 hours before administering myelosuppressive treatment. Do not administer pegfilgrastim within 14 days before administering myelosuppressive treatment
See Chapter 43 for more information

Antimicrobial prophylaxis
Risk of fever and neutropenia is *INTERMEDIATE*
Antimicrobial primary prophylaxis to be considered:
- Antibacterial—consider a fluoroquinolone during periods of prolonged neutropenia, or no prophylaxis
- Antifungal—consider use during periods of prolonged neutropenia, or no prophylaxis
- Antiviral—antiherpes antivirals (eg, acyclovir, famciclovir, valacyclovir)

Treatment Modifications

Bendamustine + Cytarabine Dose Modifications

	Bendamustine	Cytarabine
Starting dose	70 mg/m^2 per dose on days 2 and 3	800 mg/m^2 per dose on days 2, 3, and 4
Level 1	50 mg/m^2 per dose on days 2 and 3	600 mg/m^2 per dose on days 2, 3, and 4
Level 2	Discontinue bendamustine and cytarabine	

There are no dose reductions for rituximab

Adverse Event	Treatment Modification
Hematologic Toxicity	
Day 1 platelet count <75,000/mm^3 or Day 1 ANC <1000/mm^3	Delay start of cycle until platelet count ≥75,000/ mm^3 and ANC ≥1000/ mm^3 or until recovery to near baseline values, then reduce both the bendamustine dosage and cytarabine dosage by 1 dose level for subsequent cycles
G4 hematologic toxicity occurring in the previous cycle	Delay start of cycle until platelet count ≥75,000/ mm^3 and ANC ≥1000/ mm^3 or until recovery to near baseline values, then reduce both the bendamustine dosage and cytarabine dosage by 1 dose level for subsequent cycles
Infectious Complications	
Active infection	Interrupt bendamustine, cytarabine, and rituximab until resolution of infection, then resume treatment at either the same dosages, or with the bendamustine dosage and/or the cytarabine dosage reduced by 1 dose level, depending on the severity of infection
New or changes in preexisting neurologic symptoms (eg, confusion, dizziness, loss of balance, vision problems, aphasia, ambulation issues); PML suspected	Interrupt bendamustine, cytarabine, and rituximab until central nervous system status clarified. Work-up may include (but is not limited to) consultation with a neurologist, brain MRI, and LP
PML is confirmed	Discontinue bendamustine, cytarabine, and rituximab
HBV reactivation	Discontinue bendamustine, cytarabine, and rituximab. Institute appropriate treatment for HBV. Upon resolution of HBV reactivation, resumption of bendamustine, cytarabine, and rituximab should be discussed with a physician with expertise in management of HBV
Drug Interactions	
Patient requires concomitant therapy with antihypertensive medication(s)	On days of rituximab treatment, and especially with the initial dose, weigh the risk versus benefit of delaying administration of the antihypertensive medication(s) until after completion of the rituximab infusion due to the potential risk of rituximab infusion-related hypotension
Live attenuated vaccine is indicated during or after rituximab administration	Avoid administration of a live attenuated vaccine during rituximab therapy and following therapy until adequate B-cell recovery has occurred
Patient requires concomitant therapy with a CYP1A2 inhibitor (eg, fluvoxamine, ciprofloxacin)	Consider alternative treatment instead of the CYP1A2 inhibitor. If the CYP1A2 inhibitor cannot be avoided, use caution and monitor carefully for bendamustine adverse effects. Do not modify the rituximab dosage or cytarabine dosage
Patient requires concomitant therapy with a CYP1A2 inducer (eg, omeprazole), or patient is a smoker	Consider alternative treatment instead of the CYP1A2 inducer. Recommend cessation of smoking, if applicable. If the CYP1A2 inducer cannot be avoided, use caution and monitor carefully for reduced bendamustine efficacy. Do not modify the rituximab dosage or cytarabine dosage
Other Toxicities	
Fever, myalgia, bone pain, occasionally chest pain, maculopapular rash, conjunctivitis and malaise 6–12 hours following cytarabine administration (cytarabine syndrome)	Corticosteroids beneficial in treating or preventing this syndrome. If the symptoms deemed treatable, continue therapy with cytarabine and pretreat with corticosteroids
Clinically significant G ≥3 nonhematologic toxicity during the prior cycle	Delay start of cycle until the nonhematologic toxicity resolves to G ≤2 or baseline, then resume treatment with the bendamustine dosage and cytarabine dosage reduced by 1 dose level

ANC, absolute neutrophil count; G-CSF, granulocyte-colony stimulating factor; PML, progressive multifocal leukoencephalopathy; MRI, magnetic resonance imaging; LP, lumbar puncture; HBV, hepatitis B virus

Bendeka (bendamustine hydrochloride injection) prescribing information. North Wales, PA: Teva Pharmaceuticals USA, Inc; 2018 July
Rituxan (rituximab) prescribing information. South San Francisco, CA: Genentech, Inc; 2018 October
Ohmachi K et al. J Clin Oncol 2013;31:2103–2109

Patient Population Studied

Stage 2 of the open-label, single-arm, phase 2 trial assessed safety and efficacy in 40 patients with either previously untreated mantle cell lymphoma (age ≥65 years) or relapsed/refractory mantle cell lymphoma after one previous immunochemotherapy treatment (with or without autologous marrow transplantation). Eligible patients had WHO performance status 0–2. Patients received four to six 28-day cycles of intravenous rituximab (375 mg/m² on day 1 of cycle 1 and on day 2 of subsequent cycles), bendamustine (70 mg/m² over 30–60 minutes on days 2 and 3), and cytarabine (800 mg/m² over 2 hours on days 2–4, 2 hours after bendamustine administration) (R-BAC)

Efficacy

(N = 40)

	Previously Untreated Patients (N = 20)	Relapsed/Refractory Patients (N = 20)
Overall response rate*	100%	80%
2-year duration of response	100%	87%
2-year progression-free survival	95%	70%

*Overall response rate includes patients with either a complete or partial response
Note: Median follow-up was 26 months

Toxicity

(N = 40)

Adverse Event	Grade 3/4 (%)*
Thrombocytopenia	87
Leukopenia	57
Anemia	45
Neutropenia	40
Elevated gamma-glutamyl transferase level	23
Infection	13
Febrile neutropenia	13
Cardiac	5
Fatigue	5
Elevated SGOT / SGPT	2

*A total of eight deaths were recorded during the study, with seven being attributed to progressive disease and one being attributed to cerebral stroke
SGOT, serum glutamic-oxaloacetic transaminase; SGPT, serum glutamic-pyruvic transaminase level

Therapy Monitoring

1. *Prior to treatment initiation*: CBC with differential, serum chemistries, serum bilirubin, ALT or AST, hepatitis B core antibody (IgG or total) and hepatitis B core antigen, urine pregnancy test (women of child-bearing potential only)
2. *Prior to each cycle*: CBC with differential, serum chemistries, serum bilirubin, ALT or AST
3. *Weekly during treatment*: CBC with differential
4. *In patients at high risk for tumor lysis syndrome* consider frequent monitoring of laboratory indices of tumor lysis syndrome, intravenous hydration, and prophylaxis with a xanthine oxidase inhibitor (eg, allopurinol) during the first cycle
5. *Monitor periodically for*: signs and symptoms of infection (including progressive multifocal leukoencephalopathy), dermatologic toxicity, and cytarabine syndrome (rash, conjunctivitis, chest pain, malaise, myalgia, arthralgia, fever)
6. *Response assessment every 2–3 cycles*: physical examination, CT scan or PET scan, bone marrow evaluation (if clinically indicated)

MANTLE CELL LYMPHOMA • SUBSEQUENT THERAPY

NON-HODGKIN LYMPHOMA REGIMEN: LENALIDOMIDE

Goy A et al. J Clin Oncol 2013;31:3688–3695

Lenalidomide; administer orally for 21 consecutive days on days 1–21, every 28 days

Note: The investigators based lenalidomide dose on a patient's renal function, thus:

Creatinine Clearance	Lenalidomide Doses	
	Daily Dose	Total Weekly Dose
≥60 mL/min (≥1 mL/s)	25 mg/day	175 mg
≥30 to <60 mL/min (≥0.5 to <1 mL/s)	10 mg/day	70 mg

Supportive Care

Antiemetic prophylaxis

Emetogenic potential is **MINIMAL–LOW**

See Chapter 42 for antiemetic recommendations

Hematopoietic growth factor (CSF) prophylaxis

Primary prophylaxis may be indicated

See Chapter 43 for more information

Antimicrobial prophylaxis

Risk of fever and neutropenia is *LOW*

Antimicrobial primary prophylaxis to be considered:

- Antibacterial—not indicated
- Antifungal—not indicated
- Antiviral—not indicated unless patient previously had an episode of HSV

Lenalidomide Dose Levels

Starting dose	25 mg/day
Level −1	20 mg/day
Level −2	15 mg/day
Level −3	10 mg/day
Level −4	5 mg/day
Level −5	Discontinue

(*continued*)

Patient Population Studied

Characteristic	Number of Patients	Percentage
Age—median (range)	67 years (43–83 years)	
≥65 years	85	63
Male	108	81
Stage III to IV	124	93
ECOG PS		
0–1	116	87
2	18	13
Moderate-severe renal insufficiency*	29	22
Time from original MCL diagnosis to enrollment, years		
<3 years/≥3 years	52/82	39/61
MIPI score group at enrollment		
Intermediate/High	51/39	38/29
Positive bone marrow involvement[†]	55	41
High tumor burden[‡]	77	57
Bulky disease[§]	44	33
Number of prior treatment regimens—median (range)	4 (2–10)	
Number of prior systemic therapies: 2/3/≥4	29/34/71	22/25/53
Prior bortezomib: received/refractory	134/81	100/60
Refractory to last therapy	74	55
Prior high-dose or dose-intensive therapy[ℰ]	44	33
Prior ABMT or ASCT	39	29
Time from prior systemic therapy—median (range)	3.1 months (0.3–37.7 months)	
<6 months/≥6 months	96/38	72/28

ABMT, autologous bone marrow transplantation; ASCT, autologous stem cell transplantation; ECOG PS, Eastern Cooperative Oncology Group performance status; MCL, mantle cell lymphoma; MIPI, MCL International Prognostic Index

*Moderate renal insufficiency was defined as creatinine clearance (CrCl) ≥30 to <60 mL/min; severe renal insufficiency defined as CrCl <30 mL/min

[†]Bone marrow involvement was not required per protocol; prior data for bone marrow biopsy and aspirate were collected in 115 evaluable patients

[‡]Defined as at least 1 lesion ≥5 cm in diameter, or ≥3 lesions that were ≥3 cm in diameter by central radiology review

[§]Defined as at least 1 lesion ≥7 cm in diameter by central radiology review

[ℰ]Includes stem cell transplantation, hyper-CVAD (hyperfractionated cyclophosphamide, vincristine, doxorubicin, dexamethasone), or R-hyper-CVAD (rituximab plus hyper-CVAD)

(*continued*)

Adverse Event (AE)	Treatment Modifications
G ≥2 allergic reaction or hypersensitivity	Hold lenalidomide dosing for up to 21 days to allow toxicity to resolve, then restart at the same dose or reduce the lenalidomide dosage by 1 dose level
>3× upper limit of normal AST, ALT, or bilirubin	
G ≥1 tumor lysis syndrome	
G ≥3 neutropenia for ≥7 days or associated with fever (≥38.5°C [≥101.3°F])	
Platelets <50,000/mm³	
Constipation	
Venous thrombosis/ embolism	
New peripheral neuropathy	
Lenalidomide-related nonhematologic AE	
Tumor flare reaction	
G3/4 neutropenia	Hold lenalidomide dosing for up to 21 days to allow toxicity to resolve to G ≤2, then restart at the same dose or reduce the lenalidomide daily dose by 1 dose level
Febrile neutropenia (ANC <1000/mm³ with fever ≥38°C [≥101.3°F])	
Desquamating (blistering) rash (or G4 non-desquamating rash	
Any AE G ≥3 excluding nausea, vomiting, diarrhea, or lenalidomide-induced maculopapular rash	
G ≥3 nausea, vomiting, or diarrhea despite maximal therapy	
G4 fatigue lasting >7 days	

Efficacy

(N = 134)

Efficacy Parameter	Central Review		Investigator Review	
	Number	Percent	Number	Percent
ORR	37	28	43	32
CR/CRu	10	7.5	22	16
PR	27	20	21	16
SD	39	29	36	27
PD	35	26	43	32
Missing response assessment*	23	17	12	9

Efficacy Parameter	Median	Range	Median	Range
TTR, months	2.2	1.7–13.1	2.0	1.7–15.9
TTCR/CRu, months	3.7	1.9–29.5	5.6	1.8–24.2
	Median	95% CI	Median	95% CI
DOR, months	16.6	7.7–26.7	18.5	12.8–26.7
Duration of CR/CRu, months	16.6	16.6–N/R	26.7	26.7–N/R
Duration of PR, months	9.2	5.7–20.5	7.7	3.7–21.4
PFS, months	4.0	3.6–5.6	3.8	3.5–6.8
TTP, months	5.4	3.7–7.5	4.0	3.6–7.5
TTF months	3.8	2.3–4.5	3.8	2.3–4.5
OS, months	19.0	12.5–23.9	19.0	12.5–23.9

CR, complete response; CRu, unconfirmed complete response; DOR, duration of response; MCL, mantle cell lymphoma; N/R, not reached; ORR, overall response rate; OS, overall survival; PD, progressive disease; PFS, progression-free survival; PR, partial response; SD, stable disease; TTCR/Cru, time to CR/Cru; TTF, time to treatment failure; TTP, time to progression; TTR, time to response
*Includes patients without or with incomplete postbaseline response assessment. For these 23 patients, the investigator's assessment for best ORR included 12 with progressive disease, 10 not assessable, and 1 CR (no identifiable target lesions by the central radiology reviewer who reported this patient as not evaluable, although a single GI [colon] lesion was reported by investigator readings). All 23 patients were included in the centrally reviewed response assessments as nonresponders.

Summary of Subgroup Analyses of ORR and DOR by Baseline Demographics and Patient Characteristics with Lenalidomide in Evaluable Patients with Relapsed/Refractory MCL (Central Review)

Characteristic	Total Patients	ORR			DOR		
		No.	%	95% CI	No.	Median	95% CI
Median age							
<65 years	49	15	31	18–45	15	20.5	5.6–N/A
≥65 years	85	22	26	17–37	22	9.2	5.8–16.7
Sex							
Male	108	28	26	18–35	28	16.7	9.2–N/A

Efficacy (continued)

Female	26	9	35	17–56	9	7.7	2.1–20.5
ECOG PS							
0–1	116	31	27	19–36	31	16.7	14.8–N/A
2–4	18	6	33	13–59	6	7.7	1.7–9.2
Renal function							
Normal	99	28	28	20–38	28	20.5	5.7–N/A
Moderate insufficiency	28	7	25	11–45	7	9.2	7.7–16.6
Time from MCL diagnosis to first dose							
<3 years	52	12	23	13–37	12	16.6	5.1–N/A
≥3 years	82	25	31	21–42	25	14.8	5.8–20.5
MCL (Ann Arbor) stage							
I or II	10	1	10	0.3–45	1	7.7	N/A
III or IV	124	36	29	21–38	36	16.6	9.2–26.7
MIPI score at enrollment							
Low	39	14	36	21–53	14	20.5	5.6–N/A
Intermediate	51	12	23	13–38	12	16.7	5.7–26.7
High	39	10	26	13–42	10	7.7	3.6–N/A
LDH*							
Normal	84	32	38	28–49	32	16.7	14.8–N/A
High	47	5	11	4–23	5	5.8	1.7–7.7
WBC count							
<6.7 × 10^9/L	67	22	33	22–45	22	14.8	5.6–20.5
6.7 to <10 × 10^9/L	41	7	17	7–32	7	26.7	7.7–N/A
10 to <15 × 10^9/L	9	6	67	30–93	6	N/A	3.6–N/A
≥15 × 10^9/L	12	1	8	0.2–39	1	N/A	N/A–N/A
Tumor burden							
High[†]	77	22	29	19–40	22	14.8	5.8–26.7
Low	54	15	28	17–42	15	16.6	5.6–16.6
Bulky disease							
Yes[‡]	44	13	30	17–45	13	14.8	5.7–N/A
No	87	24	28	19–38	24	16.6	5.8–N/A
Prior bone marrow involvement[§]							
Positive	55	13	24	13–37	13	9.2	3.6–N/A
Negative	52	13	25	14–39	13	16.7	5.1–N/A
Indeterminate	8	4	50	16–84	4	14.8	N/A–N/A

Toxicity

All Treatment-Emergent Adverse Events After Lenalidomide (Regardless of Attribution) in ≥10% of Patients with Relapsed/Refractory MCL (N = 134)

Adverse Event (AE)	Any Grade Number (%)	G3 Number (%)	G4 Number (%)
Patients with ≥1 AEs	132 (99)	47 (35)	41 (31)
Hematologic			
Neutropenia	65 (49)	26 (19)	32 (24)
Thrombocytopenia	48 (36)	23 (17)	14 (10)
Anemia	41 (31)	11 (8)	4 (3)
Leukopenia	20 (15)	7 (5)	2 (1)
Nonhematologic			
Fatigue	45 (34)	9 (7)	0
Diarrhea	42 (31)	8 (6)	0
Nausea	40 (30)	0	1 (<1)
Cough	38 (28)	1 (<1)	0
Pyrexia*	31 (23)	1 (<1)	1 (<1)
Rash	30 (22)	2 (1)	0
Dyspnea*	24 (18)	6 (5)	1 (<1)
Pruritus	23 (17)	1 (<1)	0
Constipation	21 (16)	1 (<1)	0
Peripheral edema	21 (16)	0	0
Pneumonia†	19 (14)	10 ()	0
Asthenia*	19 (14)	2 (1)	1 (<1)
Decreased appetite	19 (14)	1 (<1)	0
Back pain	18 (13)	2 (1)	0
Hypokalemia	17 (13)	2 (1)	1 (<1)
Muscle spasms	17 (13)	1 (<1)	0
Upper respiratory tract infection	17 (13)	0	0
Decreased weight	17 (13)	0	0
Vomiting	16 (12)	0	1 (<1)

*One G5 event per AE
† Two G5 events

Treatment Monitoring

1. CBC with differential day 1
2. CT scans every 2 cycles
3. Confirmatory bone marrow aspirate and unilateral biopsy for patients achieving CR (by CT)
4. Risk of peripheral neuropathy: Examine patients at monthly intervals for the first 3 months of lenalidomide therapy and periodically thereafter during treatment
5. Consider thromboprophylaxis based on assessment of individual patients' underlying risk factors for thromboembolism

Efficacy (continued)

Number of prior systemic antilymphoma therapies							
<3	29	9	31	15–51	9	16.6	7.7–N/A
≥3	105	28	27	19–36	28	16.7	5.7–26.7

Received prior stem cell transplantation							
Yes	39	12	31	17–48	12	16.7	3.6–16.7
No	95	25	26	18–36	25	14.8	5.8–26.7

Received prior high-intensity therapy							
Yes	44	12	27	15–43	12	16.7	3.6–16.7
No	90	25	28	19–38	25	14.8	5.8–26.7

Time from last prior systemic anti-lymphoma therapy							
<6 months	96	23	24	16–34	23	7.7	3.6–26.7
≥6 months	38	14	37	22–54	14	16.7	14.8–N/A

Relapsed/refractory to prior bortezomib							
Refractory	81	22	27	18–38	22	20.5	7.7–N/A
Relapsed/progressed	51	15	29	18–44	15	16.6	5.0–16.7

Relapsed/refractory to last prior therapy							
Refractory	74	20	27	17–39	20	26.7	5.6–N/A
Relapsed/progressed	53	16	30	18–44	16	14.8	5.7–20.5

Starting dose of lenalidomide							
10 mg	29	6	21	8–40	6	9.2	7.7–14.8
25 mg	104	31	30	21–40	31	16.7	5.7–N/A

DOR, duration of response; ECOG PS, Eastern Cooperative Oncology Group performance status; LDH, lactate dehydrogenase; MCL, mantle-cell lymphoma; MIPI, MCL International Prognostic Index; N/A, not applicable; ORR, overall response rate

*The only factor that was significant in both the univariate and multivariate models was high lactate dehydrogenase at baseline

†Defined as at least 1 lesion ≥5 cm in diameter or ≥3 lesions that were ≥3 cm in diameter by central radiology review

‡Defined as at least 1 lesion ≥7 cm in diameter by central radiology review

§Bone marrow involvement was assessable in 115 evaluable patients

MANTLE CELL LYMPHOMA • SUBSEQUENT THERAPY
NON-HODGKIN LYMPHOMA REGIMEN: IBRUTINIB

Wang ML et al. N Engl J Med 2013;369:507–516
Protocol for: Wang ML et al. N Engl J Med 2013;369:507–516
Supplementary appendix to: Wang ML et al. N Engl J Med 2013;369:507–516
Wang ML et al. Blood 2015;126:739–745
Supplemental data to: Wang ML et al. Blood 2015;126:739–745
Imbruvica (ibrutinib) prescribing information. Sunnyvale, CA: Pharmacyclics LLC; Revised 2018 August

Ibrutinib 560 mg/dose; administer orally, once daily with a glass of water, without regard to food, continually until disease progression (total dose/week = 3920 mg)

Notes on ibrutinib administration:
- Administration with food increases ibrutinib exposure approximately 2-fold compared with administration after overnight fasting. Clinical studies instructed that ibrutinib be taken at least 30 minutes before eating or at least 2 hours after a meal at approximately the same time each day (Protocol for: Byrd JC et al. N Engl J Med 2014;371:213–223). However, the U.S. Food and Drug Administration–approved prescribing information does not make specific recommendations regarding administration of ibrutinib with regard to food (Imbruvica [ibrutinib] prescribing information. Sunnyvale, CA: Pharmacyclics LLC; Revised 2018 August). **Others have also concluded that no food restrictions are needed given the relative safety profile of ibrutinib and because repeated drug intake in fasted conditions is unlikely** (de Jong J et al. Cancer Chemother Pharmacol. 2015;75:907–916)
- Ibrutinib capsules should be swallowed whole; do not break, open, or chew capsules. Ibrutinib tablets should be swallowed whole; do not cut, crush, or chew tablets
- Patients who delay taking ibrutinib at a regularly scheduled time may administer the missed dose as soon as possible on the same day and then resume the normal schedule the following day. Do not administer an extra dose of ibrutinib to make up for a missed dose
- Ibrutinib is metabolized predominantly by CYP3A. Refer to treatment modification section for initial dose adjustment recommendations for patients requiring concurrent treatment with moderate or strong CYP3A inhibitors. Avoid concomitant use of ibrutinib with strong CYP3A inducers
- Advise patients to not consume grapefruit products or Seville oranges as they may inhibit CYP3A in the gut wall and increase the bioavailability of ibrutinib
- Serious bleeding events, some fatal, have been reported in patients treated with ibrutinib. Ibrutinib may exacerbate the risk of bleeding when administered concurrently with anticoagulant and/or antiplatelet drugs; use caution and monitor closely for bleeding with concomitant use. Consider the risks and benefits of interrupting ibrutinib treatment at least 3–7 days prior to and following elective surgery depending on the risk of bleeding and type of surgery
- After initiation of ibrutinib, lymphocytosis occurs commonly and should not be considered as an indicator of disease progression. An absolute lymphocyte count (ALC) above 5000/µL together with a ≥50% increase from baseline occurred in 34% of patients in the mantle cell lymphoma study (Wang et al, 2013). The peak ALC occurred at a median of 4 weeks after initiation of treatment and lymphocytosis resolved within 16–20 weeks from initiation
- Reduce the ibrutinib starting dose to 140 mg, administered orally once daily for mild (Child-Pugh class A) hepatic impairment. Reduce the ibrutinib starting dose to 70 mg, administered orally once daily for moderate (Child-Pugh class B) hepatic impairment. Avoid ibrutinib in patients with severe (Child-Pugh class C) hepatic impairment
- Tumor lysis syndrome may rarely occur with ibrutinib therapy. Consider appropriate monitoring and precautions (eg, anti-hyperuricemic therapy, hydration) in patients with high baseline risk (eg, high tumor burden, renal impairment)

Supportive Care
Antiemetic prophylaxis
Emetogenic potential is **LOW**
See Chapter 42 for antiemetic recommendations

Hematopoietic growth factor (CSF) prophylaxis
Primary prophylaxis is **NOT** indicated
See Chapter 43 for more information

Antimicrobial prophylaxis
Risk of fever and neutropenia is *LOW*
Antimicrobial primary prophylaxis to be considered:
- Antibacterial—not indicated. Consider prophylaxis for *Pneumocystis jirovecii* (eg, cotrimoxazole)
- Antifungal—not indicated
- Antiviral— not indicated unless patient previously had an episode of HSV

Diarrhea management
Latent or delayed-onset diarrhea*:
- **Loperamide** 4 mg; administer orally initially after the first loose or liquid stool, *then*
- **Loperamide** 2 mg every 2 hours while awake; every 4 hours during sleep
- Alternatively, a trial of **diphenoxylate hydrochloride** 2.5 mg **with atropine sulfate** 0.025 mg (eg, Lomotil) 2 tablets 4 times daily until control has been achieved

(continued)

(*continued*)

Persistent diarrhea:
Octreotide acetate (solution) 100–150 μg; administer subcutaneously 3 times daily

Antibiotic therapy during latent or delayed-onset diarrhea:
A fluoroquinolone (eg, ciprofloxacin 500 mg orally every 12 hours) if absolute neutrophil count <500/mm³

Oral care
Encourage patients to maintain intake of nonalcoholic fluids
If mucositis or stomatitis is present:
• Rinse mouth several times a day with 1/4 teaspoon (1.25 g) each of baking soda and table salt in one quart of warm water. Follow with a plain water rinse
• Do not use mouthwashes that contain alcohols

Patient Population Studied

This international, multicenter, open-label, phase 2 trial involved 111 patients with relapsed/refractory, pathologically confirmed mantle cell lymphoma. Eligible patients had an Eastern Cooperative Oncology Group (ECOG) performance status score ≤2, and 1–5 prior treatment regimens for mantle cell lymphoma. Patients received oral ibrutinib (560 mg/day) until disease progression or unacceptable toxicity

Efficacy

(N = 111)

Overall response rate*	67%
Median duration of response	17.5 months
Median progression-free survival	13 months
Median overall survival	22.5 months

Overall response rate includes patients with either a complete or partial response *Note:* Median follow-up was 26.7 months. Median treatment duration was 8.3 months

Treatment Modifications

Ibrutinib	
Starting dose	560 mg by mouth once a day
Adverse Event	**Treatment Modification**
Drug Interactions	
Treatment with a moderate CYP3A inhibitor is required	Reduce ibrutinib starting dose to 280 mg by mouth once daily during concomitant therapy
Treatment with voriconazole 200 mg by mouth twice a day is required, *or* Treatment with posaconazole suspension 100 mg by mouth once daily is required, *or* Treatment with posaconazole suspension 100–200 mg by mouth twice a day is required	Reduce ibrutinib starting dose to 140 mg by mouth once daily during concomitant therapy
Treatment with posaconazole suspension 200 mg by mouth three times a day is required, *or* Treatment with posaconazole suspension 400 mg by mouth twice a day is required, *or* Treatment with posaconazole 300 mg intravenously once a day is required, *or* Treatment with posaconazole delayed-release tablets 300 mg by mouth once a day is required	Reduce ibrutinib starting dose to 70 mg by mouth once daily during concomitant therapy
Treatment with other strong CYP3A inhibitors besides those listed above is required	Avoid concomitant use of ibrutinib with other strong CYP3A inhibitors. If a strong CYP3A inhibitor is to be used short-term (eg, ≤7 days), interrupt ibrutinib therapy during use of the strong CYP3A inhibitor
Treatment with a strong CYP3A inducer is required	Avoid concomitant use of ibrutinib with strong CYP3A inducers
Treatment with antiplatelet or anticoagulant medications is required	Bleeding risk may be increased. Monitor closely for signs and symptoms of bleeding
Hypertension	
Hypertension	Adjust existing anti-hypertensive medications or initiate anti-hypertensive treatment as appropriate
Hepatic Impairment	
Child-Pugh class A hepatic impairment	Reduce ibrutinib starting dose to 140 mg by mouth once a day
Child-Pugh class B hepatic impairment	Reduce ibrutinib starting dose to 70 mg by mouth once a day
Child-Pugh class C hepatic impairment	Avoid ibrutinib use

(*continued*)

Treatment Modifications (*continued*)

Other Toxicities

Surgical procedure is required during treatment with ibrutinib	Consider benefit-risk of withholding ibrutinib for at least 3–7 days prior to and following surgery depending on the type of surgery and the risk of bleeding
First occurrence of G ≥3 nonhematologic toxicity, G ≥3 neutropenia with infection or fever, or G4 hematologic toxicity	Interrupt ibrutinib until resolution to G1 or baseline, then resume ibrutinib at the same dose (eg, 560 mg by mouth once a day). Consider use of G-CSF for G4 neutropenia lasting >7 days or for life-threatening neutropenic complications
Second occurrence of G ≥3 nonhematologic toxicity, G ≥3 neutropenia with infection or fever, or G4 hematologic toxicity	Interrupt ibrutinib until resolution to G1 or baseline, then resume ibrutinib at 420 mg by mouth once a day. Consider use of G-CSF for G4 neutropenia lasting >7 days or for life-threatening neutropenic complications
Third occurrence of G ≥3 nonhematologic toxicity, G ≥3 neutropenia with infection or fever, or G4 hematologic toxicity	Interrupt ibrutinib until resolution to G1 or baseline, then resume ibrutinib at 280 mg by mouth once a day. Consider use of G-CSF for G4 neutropenia lasting >7 days or for life-threatening neutropenic complications
Fourth occurrence of G ≥3 nonhematologic toxicity, G ≥3 neutropenia with infection or fever, or G4 hematologic toxicity	Discontinue ibrutinib

Ibrutinib can cause fetal harm. Advise females of reproductive potential of the potential risk to a fetus and to use effective contraception and avoid becoming pregnant while taking ibrutinib and for 1 month after cessation of treatment

G-CSF, granulocyte colony-stimulating factor
Imbruvica (ibrutinib) prescribing information. Sunnyvale, CA: Pharmacyclics LLC; Revised 2018 August

Toxicity

(N = 111)

Grade (%)*	Grade 1–2	Grade ≥3
Pneumonia	0	7
Atrial fibrillation	<1	5
Urinary tract infection	<1	3
Acute renal failure	0	3
Abdominal pain	0	3
Febrile neutropenia	0	3
Subdural hematoma	<1	2
Confusional state	2	<1
Pyrexia	2	<1

*According to the National Cancer Institute Common Terminology Criteria for Adverse Events, version 4.0
Note: Serious adverse events that occurred in ≥2% patients, regardless of attribution, are included. The most common all-grade adverse events, regardless of attribution, were diarrhea (54%), fatigue (50%), nausea (33%), and dyspnea (32%). The most common grade ≥3 hematologic adverse events were neutropenia (17%), thrombocytopenia (13%), and anemia (11%). Treatment discontinuation owing to adverse events was recorded for 11% patients. A total of 18 patients (16%) died within 30 days after the last dose of ibrutinib; 8 of these deaths were reported as due to mantle cell lymphoma, 6 were considered associated with disease progression, and the remaining 4 (4%) were due to pneumonia, sepsis, hypovolemic shock, and cardiac arrest in a patient with a history of type 2 diabetes mellitus, hypertension, and heart failure

Therapy Monitoring

1. *Prior to initiation of ibrutinib:* CBC with differential, serum bilirubin, ALT or AST, alkaline phosphatase, potassium, calcium, phosphorus, LDH, uric acid, and serum creatinine
2. *At least monthly:* CBC with differential
3. *Periodically:* Monitor for signs and symptoms of cardiac arrhythmias (eg, atrial fibrillation and atrial flutter) and check electrocardiogram if present, signs and symptoms of bleeding (especially if concomitant antiplatelet or anticoagulant medications are used), signs and symptoms of infection (including progressive multifocal leukoencephalopathy), blood pressure, presence of second primary malignancies, and diarrhea
4. *During initiation of therapy in patients with high tumor burden or renal dysfunction:* Monitor for tumor lysis syndrome (potassium, calcium, phosphorus, LDH, uric acid, and serum creatinine)
5. *Response assessment every 2–3 months:* Physical examination, CBC with differential, CT scan with contrast or PET scan, bone marrow evaluation (as clinically indicated), endoscopy (as clinically indicated)
   a. Note that lymphocytosis occurs commonly in mantle cell lymphoma patients following initiation of ibrutinib and should not be considered as an indicator of disease progression

MANTLE CELL LYMPHOMA • SUBSEQUENT THERAPY
NON-HODGKIN LYMPHOMA REGIMEN: ACALABRUTINIB

Wang M et al. Lancet 2018;391:659–667
Supplementary appendix to: Wang M et al. Lancet 2018;391:659–667

Acalabrutinib 100 mg per dose; administer orally with water twice per day (approximately every 12 hours), without regard to food, continuously until disease progression (total dosage/week = 1400 mg)
Notes on acalabrutinib administration:
- Acalabrutinib capsules should be swallowed whole. Do not break, open, or chew capsules
- Patients who delay taking acalabrutinib at a regularly scheduled time may administer the missed dose if within 3 hours of the usual dosing time. If >3 hours, skip the missed dose, and resume treatment at the next regularly scheduled time
- Acalabrutinib is metabolized predominantly by CYP3A. Avoid concomitant use with strong CYP3A inhibitors. If a strong CYP3A inhibitor must be used short-term (eg, ≤7 days), interrupt acalabrutinib treatment during treatment with the inhibitor. If concomitant use of a moderate CYP3A inhibitor is unavoidable, then reduce the acalabrutinib dose to 100 mg by mouth once daily. If concomitant use of a strong CYP3A inducer is unavoidable, increase the acalabrutinib dose to 200 mg by mouth twice a day
- Among patients with hematologic malignancies treated with acalabrutinib, skin cancer was diagnosed as a secondary primary malignancy in 7% of patients. Thus, counsel patients to apply sunscreen and avoid prolonged sun exposure during treatment with acalabrutinib
- The solubility of acalabrutinib is increased at acidic pH. Thus, gastric acid-reducing medications may interfere with absorption of acalabrutinib and should be avoided when possible
  - A 5-day course of omeprazole reduced acalabrutinib area-under-the-curve (AUC) by 43%. Since proton pump inhibitors (PPIs) have long-lasting effects on gastric pH, avoid concomitant use of PPIs with acalabrutinib
  - A 1000-mg dose of calcium carbonate coadministered with acalabrutinib reduced acalabrutinib AUC by 53%. Thus, if antacid medications are required, separate acalabrutinib administration from antacid administration by ≥2 hours
  - If a histamine receptor (H_2)-subtype antagonist must be used, administer acalabrutinib at least 10 hours following a dose of histamine receptor (H_2)-subtype antagonist and at least 2 hours before the next dose of histamine receptor (H_2)-subtype antagonist
- Serious bleeding events, some fatal, have been reported in patients with hematologic malignancies treated with acalabrutinib. Acalabrutinib may exacerbate the risk of bleeding when administered concurrently with anticoagulant and/or antiplatelet drugs; use caution and monitor closely for bleeding with concomitant use. Consider the risks and benefits of interrupting acalabrutinib treatment 3–7 days prior to and following elective surgery depending on the risk of bleeding and type of surgery
- Hepatitis B virus (HBV) reactivation has been reported in patients treated with acalabrutinib. Monitor HBV positive patients during and after treatment with acalabrutinib and consider antiviral prophylaxis

Supportive Care
Antiemetic prophylaxis
Emetogenic potential is **MINIMAL-LOW**
See Chapter 42 for antiemetic recommendations

Hematopoietic growth factor (CSF) prophylaxis
Primary prophylaxis is **NOT** *indicated*
See Chapter 43 for more information

Antimicrobial prophylaxis
Risk of fever and neutropenia is *LOW*
Antimicrobial primary prophylaxis to be considered:
- Antibacterial—not indicated
- Antifungal—not indicated
- Antiviral— not indicated unless patient previously had an episode of HSV

Diarrhea Management
Latent or delayed-onset diarrhea:
- **Loperamide** 4 mg orally initially after the first loose or liquid stool, *then*
- **Loperamide** 2 mg orally every 2 hours during waking hours, *plus*
- **Loperamide** 4 mg orally every 4 hours during hours of sleep
- Continue for at least 12 hours after diarrhea resolves
- Recurrent diarrhea after a 12-hour diarrhea-free interval is treated as a new episode
- Rehydrate orally with fluids and electrolytes during a diarrheal episode
- If a patient develops blood or mucus in stool, dehydration, or hemodynamic instability, or if diarrhea persists >48 hours despite loperamide, stop loperamide and hospitalize the patient for IV hydration

Alternatively, a trial of **diphenoxylate hydrochloride** 2.5 mg **with atropine sulfate** 0.025 mg (eg, Lomotil)

- Initial adult dose is 2 tablets 4 times daily until control has been achieved, after which the dose may be reduced to meet individual requirements. Control may often be maintained with as little as 2 tablets daily
- Clinical improvement of acute diarrhea is usually observed within 48 hours. If improvement of chronic diarrhea after treatment with a maximum daily dose of 8 tablets is not observed within 10 days, control is unlikely with further administration

Persistent diarrhea:
Octreotide 100–150 µg subcutaneously 3 times daily. Maximum total daily dose is 1500 µg
Antibiotic therapy during latent or delayed onset diarrhea:
A fluoroquinolone (eg, **ciprofloxacin** 500 mg orally every 12 hours) if absolute neutrophil count <500/mm³ with or without accompanying fever in association with diarrhea
- Antibiotics should also be administered if patient is hospitalized with prolonged diarrhea and should be continued until diarrhea resolves

Treatment Modifications

Acalabrutinib

Starting dose	100 mg by mouth twice a day
Dose level 1	100 mg by mouth once daily

Adverse Event	Treatment Modification	
Hematologic Toxicities		
Occurrence of *any* of the following: • G3 thrombocytopenia (platelet count ≥25,000/mm³ and <50,000/mm³) with bleeding *or* • G4 thrombocytopenia (platelet count <25,000/mm³) *or* • G4 neutropenia (ANC <500/mm³) lasting >7 days *or* • G ≥3 nonhematologic toxicity	First occurrence	Interrupt acalabrutinib. Once toxicity resolves to G ≤1 or baseline, then resume acalabrutinib without dose reduction
	Second occurrence	Interrupt acalabrutinib. Once toxicity resolves to G ≤1 or baseline, then resume acalabrutinib without dose reduction
	Third occurrence	Interrupt acalabrutinib. Once toxicity resolves to G ≤1 or baseline, then resume acalabrutinib at a reduced dose of 100 mg by mouth once daily
	Fourth occurrence	Discontinue acalabrutinib
Drug-Drug Interactions		
Concomitant therapy with a strong CYP3A inhibitor is required	Avoid coadministration of a strong CYP3A inhibitor with acalabrutinib. If the strong CYP3A inhibitor is to be used short-term, interrupt acalabrutinib therapy	
Concomitant therapy with a moderate CYP3A inhibitor is required	Reduce the acalabrutinib dose to 100 mg by mouth once daily. If the moderate CYP3A inhibitor is subsequently discontinued, increase the acalabrutinib dose back to the dose that was used prior to initiation of the inhibitor	
Concomitant therapy with a strong CYP3A inducer is required	Consider use of an alternative medication. If concurrent use of a strong CYP3A inducer with acalabrutinib is unavoidable, increase the acalabrutinib dose to 200 mg by mouth twice daily. If the strong CYP3A inducer is subsequently discontinued, reduce the acalabrutinib dose back to the dose that was used prior to initiation of the inducer	
Concomitant therapy with a proton pump inhibitor is required	Avoid coadministration of a proton pump inhibitor with acalabrutinib	
Concomitant therapy with an H₂-receptor antagonist is required	Administer acalabrutinib 2 hours before administration of a H₂-receptor antagonist	
Concomitant therapy with an antacid is required	Separate administration of acalabrutinib from administration of antacid medication by at least 2 hours	
Concomitant therapy with antiplatelet medication(s) or anticoagulants is required	The risk of bleeding with acalabrutinib may be further increased. Monitoring closely for signs of bleeding	
Other		
Planned elective surgery	Consider the benefit-risk of withholding acalabrutinib for 3–7 days before and after surgery depending upon the type of surgery, risk of bleeding, and status of MCL	

(continued)

Treatment Modifications (*continued*)

Severe liver dysfunction (total bilirubin between 3–10× ULN and any AST) or Child-Pugh class C liver dysfunction	Acalabrutinib pharmacokinetics have not been evaluated in patients with severe liver dysfunction, therefore no dose recommendation can be made

Acalabrutinib may cause fetal harm. Advise females of reproductive potential of the potential risk to a fetus

ANC, absolute neutrophil count; ULN, upper limit of normal; AST, aspartate aminotransferase; MCL, mantle cell lymphoma

Wang M et al. Lancet 2018;391:659–667
Supplementary appendix to: Wang M et al. Lancet 2018;391:659–667
Calquence (acalabrutinib) prescribing information. Wilmington, DE: AstraZeneca Pharmaceuticals LP; 2017 November

Patient Population Studied

The international, multicenter, single-arm, open-label, phase 2 trial (ACE-LY–004) involved 124 patients with relapsed/refractory mantle cell lymphoma. Eligible patients were aged ≥18 years, had an Eastern Cooperative Oncology Group (ECOG) performance status score ≤2, and had received 1–5 prior treatment regimens for mantle cell lymphoma. Patients on concomitant treatment with warfarin or equivalent vitamin K antagonists. Patients received 28-day cycles of oral acalabrutinib (100 mg twice daily) until progressive disease or unacceptable toxicity

Efficacy

(N = 124)

Overall response rate*	81%
12-month duration of response	72%
12-month progression-free survival	67%
12-month overall survival	87%

Overall response rate includes patients with either a complete or partial response
Note: Median follow-up was 15.2 months

Adverse Events

(N = 124)

Grade (%)*	Grade 1	Grade 2	Grade 3	Grade 4
Headache	24	12	2	0
Diarrhea	17	10	3	0
Fatigue	19	6	<1	0
Myalgia	15	5	<1	0
Cough	17	2	0	0
Nausea	10	7	<1	0
Pyrexia	11	4	0	0
Anemia	<1	2	8	<1
Neutropenia	0	0	5	6
Pneumonia	0	<1	5	0

*According to the National Cancer Institute Common Terminology Criteria for Adverse Events, version 4.0.3
Note: All-grade adverse events that occurred in ≥15% patients and grade ≥3 adverse events that occurred in ≥5% patients are included. Treatment discontinuation owing to adverse events was reported for seven (6%) patients. One death due to an adverse event (aortic stenosis) was recorded, but was not considered related to treatment

Therapy Monitoring

1. *Prior to initiation of acalabrutinib*: Hepatitis B core antibody (IgG or total), hepatitis B surface antigen
2. *Monthly*: CBC with differential
3. *Periodically*: Monitor for atrial fibrillation and atrial flutter, signs and symptoms of bleeding (especially if concomitant antiplatelet or anticoagulant medications are used), signs and symptoms of infection, presence of second primary malignancies (including skin cancer and other carcinomas)
4. *Response assessment every 1–3 months*: Physical examination, CBC with differential, CT scan with contrast and/or PET scan, bone marrow evaluation (as indicated), endoscopy (as indicated)

MANTLE CELL LYMPHOMA • SUBSEQUENT THERAPY
NON-HODGKIN LYMPHOMA REGIMEN: ZANUBRUTINIB

Song Y et al. Clin Can Res 2020;26:4216–4224
BRUKINSA™ (zanubrutinib) prescribing information. San Mateo, CA: BeiGene USA, Inc; Revised 2019 November

Select one of the following initial dosage regimens:

Once-daily dosing option:
Zanubrutinib 320 mg per dose; administer orally, once per day with water, without regard to food, continually (total dose/week = 2,240 mg), *or:*

Twice-daily dosing option:
Zanubrutinib 160 mg per dose; administer orally, twice per day with water, without regard to food, continually (total dose/week = 2,240 mg)

Zanubrutinib notes:
- Zanubrutinib capsules should be swallowed whole; do not break, open, or chew capsules
- Patients who delay taking zanubrutinib at a regularly scheduled time may administer the missed dose as soon as possible on the same day, and then resume the normal schedule the following day
- Zanubrutinib is metabolized predominantly by CYP3A. Refer to treatment modification section for initial dose adjustment recommendations for patients requiring concurrent treatment with moderate or strong CYP3A inhibitors. Avoid concomitant use of zanubrutinib with moderate or strong CYP3A inducers
- Reduce the zanubrutinib starting dose to 80 mg orally twice per day in patients with severe (Child-Pugh class C) hepatic impairment

Antiemetic prophylaxis
Emetogenic potential is **MINIMAL-LOW**
See Chapter 42 for antiemetic recommendations

Hematopoietic growth factor (CSF) prophylaxis
Primary prophylaxis is **NOT** indicated
See Chapter 43 for more information

Antimicrobial prophylaxis
Risk of fever and neutropenia is *LOW*
Antimicrobial primary prophylaxis to be considered:
- Antibacterial—consider prophylaxis with a fluoroquinolone during periods of prolonged neutropenia only (eg, <500/mm^3 for ≥7 days) until ANC recovery
- Antifungal—not indicated
- Antiviral—antiherpes antivirals (eg, acyclovir, famciclovir, valacyclovir)

Treatment Modifications

ZANUBRUTINIB TREATMENT MODIFICATIONS

Zanubrutinib Dose Levels

Starting dose	160 mg twice per day or 320 mg once per day
Dose level −1	80 mg twice per day or 160 mg once per day
Dose level −2	80 mg once per day
Dose level −3	Discontinue zanubrutinib

Adverse Event		Treatment Modification
• G ≥3 nonhematologic toxicity • G3 febrile neutropenia • G3 thrombocytopenia with significant bleeding • G4 neutropenia lasting >10 consecutive days • G4 thrombocytopenia lasting >10 consecutive days	First occurrence	Withhold zanubrutinib until recovery to G ≤1 or baseline, then resume at the same dosage
	Second occurrence	Withhold zanubrutinib until recovery to G ≤1 or baseline, then resume at dose level −1
	Third occurrence	Withhold zanubrutinib until recovery to G ≤1 or baseline, then resume at dose level −2
	Fourth occurrence	Discontinue zanubrutinib

Note: For dose-limiting neutropenia or neutropenic complications, consider use of granulocyte colony-stimulating factor as clinically appropriate

(continued)

Treatment Modifications (*continued*)

Drug Interactions	
Treatment with a moderate CYP3A inhibitor is required	Reduce zanubrutinib starting dose to 80 mg twice per day. Interrupt and reduce dosing as recommended above for adverse reactions
Treatment with a strong CYP3A inhibitor is required	Reduce zanubrutinib starting dose to 80 mg once per day. Interrupt dosing as recommended above for adverse reactions
Treatment with a moderate or strong CYP3A inducer is required	Avoid concomitant use
Treatment with antiplatelet and/or anticoagulant medications is required	Bleeding risk may be increased. Monitor closely for signs and symptoms of bleeding

Hepatic Impairment	
Severe (Child-Pugh class C) hepatic impairment	Reduce the zanubrutinib starting dose to 80 mg orally twice per day

Other Toxicities	
Surgical procedure is required during treatment with zanubrutinib	Consider benefit-risk of withholding zanubrutinib for at least 3–7 days prior to and following surgery depending on the type of surgery and the risk of bleeding

G-CSF, granulocyte colony stimulating factor
BRUKINSA™ (zanubrutinib) prescribing information. San Mateo, CA: BeiGene USA, Inc; Revised 2019 November

Efficacy (N = 86)

Independent Review Committee–assessed Efficacy Outcomes

Efficacy variable	N = 86
Objective response, n (%)	
Complete	59 (68.6)
Partial	13 (15.1)
No response[*]	14 (16.3)
Overall	72 (84)
95% CI for overall response	(74, 91)
Time to response (months)—median (range)	2.7 (2.5–16.6)
Response duration (months)—median (range)	19.5 (0.9–19.5) / 95% CI (16.6, NE)
Event-free rates at 12 months (%) / 95% CI	78.3% (67, 86)
PFS (months)—median (range) / 95% CI	22.1 (0.0, 22.3) / (17.4, NE)
Event-free rates at 12 months (%) / 95% CI	75.5 / (65, 83)

NE, not estimable; FDG-PET, [18F]-fluorodeoxyglucose positron emission tomography
[*]No response was defined as a best response of stable disease (N = 1) or progressive disease (N = 6). Six patients with no on-treatment response assessments and one with no evidence of disease at baseline are also included in the no response category

Patient Population Studied

Characteristic (N = 86)	
Sex, n (%)—male / female	67 (77.9) / 19 (22.1)
Race, n (%)—Chinese	86 (100)
Age, years—median (range)	60.5 (34–75)
≥65 years, n (%)	22 (25.6)
ECOG performance status, n (%)–0/1 / 2	82 (95.3) / 4 (4.7)
Patients with prior systemic therapies, n (%)	86 (100.0)
Median (range) number of prior therapies	2.0 (1–4)
≥3 prior therapies, n (%)	29 (33.7)
Prior regimens, n (%)	
≥ 1 rituximab-containing regimen	64 (74.4)
R-CHOP, R-CHOP–like	46 (53.5)
CHOP, CHOP-like	31 (36.0)
High-dose cytarabine-containing regimen[*]	33 (38.4)
(R) hyper-CVAD (A)/EPOCH	23 (26.7)
Lenalidomide	12 (14.0)
Bortezomib	7 (8.1)
Stem cell transplant	3 (3.5)
Blastoid histology	12 (14)

(*continued*)

Patient Population Studied (continued)

Bulky disease	
>5 cm tumor mass, n (%)	37 (43)
Extranodal disease, n (%)	61 (70.9)
Bone marrow involvement	39 (45.3)
Gastrointestinal involvement	15 (17.4)
MIPI-b, n (%)[†]	
Low risk	12 (14.0)
Intermediate risk	39 (45.3)
High risk	33 (38.4)
Missing	2 (2.3)
Refractory disease[‡]	45 (52.3)
TP53-mutated (N = 54)	15 (27.8)

Note: Percentages may not add up to 100% because of rounding

CHOP, cyclophosphamide, doxorubicin, vincristine, and prednisone; ECOG, Eastern Cooperative Oncology Group; EPOCH, etoposide, prednisone, vincristine, cyclophosphamide, and doxorubicin; hyper-CVAD, cyclophosphamide, vincristine, doxorubicin, and dexamethasone

[*]High-dose cytarabine-containing regimens included dexamethasone, cytarabine, and cisplatin (DHAP); etoposide, methylprednisolone, cytarabine, and cisplatin (ESHAP); methotrexate and cytarabine (hyper-CVAD B); cyclophosphamide, etoposide, cytarabine, methylprednisolone, vincristine, and nedaplatin (CDEADP)

[†]MIPI-b score was derived with the use of four baseline clinical prognostic factors (age, ECOG performance status, lactate dehydrogenase level, and white blood cell count) plus percent Ki-67 expression in tumor cells, and its range depends on the range of these characteristics. The index classifies patients as having low-, intermediate-, or high-risk disease, as defined by scores of <5.7, ≥5.7 to <6.5, and ≥6.5, respectively

[‡]Refractory disease defined as the lack of at least a partial response to the last therapy before study entry, as assessed by the investigator

Adverse Events (N = 86)

Event[*]	All Grades, n (%)	Grade ≥3, n (%)
Patients with at least one adverse event	83 (96.5)	34 (41.9)
Hematologic events		
Neutropenia	42 (48.8)	17 (19.8)
Leukopenia	30 (34.9)	6 (7.0)
Thrombocytopenia	8 (32.6)	4 (4.7)
Anemia	13 (15.1)	5 (5.8)
Nonhematologic events		
Upper respiratory tract infection	30 (34.9)	0
Rash	29 (33.7)	0
Hypokalemia	14 (16.3)	1 (1.2)
Diarrhea	13 (15.1)	0
Hypertension	13 (15.1)	3 (3.5)
Alanine aminotransferase increased	12 (14.0)	1 (1.2)
Lung infection	11 (12.8)	8 (9.3)

[*]Data are for adverse events reported from first dose date to 30 days following study drug discontinuation or initiation of new anticancer therapy in the 86 patients included in the study. Any-grade events occurred in at least 10% of patients and grade ≥3 events occurred in at least 3% of patients on or before the data cut-off date of February 15, 2019

Therapy Monitoring

1. *Prior to initiation*: CBC with differential, serum bilirubin, ALT or AST, alkaline phosphatase, potassium, calcium, phosphorus, LDH, uric acid, and serum creatinine

2. *At least monthly*: CBC with differential

3. *Periodically*: monitor for signs and symptoms of cardiac arrhythmias (eg, atrial fibrillation and atrial flutter) and check electrocardiogram if present, signs and symptoms of bleeding (especially if concomitant antiplatelet or anticoagulant medication[s] are used), signs and symptoms of infection, presence of second primary malignancies, and diarrhea

   - Serious bleeding events, some fatal, have been reported in patients treated with zanubrutinib. Zanubrutinib may exacerbate the risk of bleeding when administered concurrently with anticoagulant and/or antiplatelet drugs

   - Consider the risks and benefits of interrupting zanubrutinib treatment at least 3–7 days prior to and following elective surgery depending on the risk of bleeding and type of surgery

4. *During initiation of therapy in patients with high tumor burden or renal dysfunction*: monitor for tumor lysis syndrome (potassium, calcium, phosphorus, LDH, uric acid, and serum creatinine)

5. *Response assessment every 2–3 months*: physical examination, CBC with differential, CT scan with contrast and/or PET scan, bone marrow evaluation (as clinically indicated)

Note: After initiation of zanubrutinib, lymphocytosis occurs commonly and should not be considered as an indicator of disease progression

MANTLE CELL LYMPHOMA • SUBSEQUENT THERAPY
NON-HODGKIN LYMPHOMA REGIMEN: VENETOCLAX + IBRUTINIB

Tam CS et al. N Engl J Med 2018;378:1211–1223
Protocol for: Tam CS et al. N Engl J Med 2018;378:1211–1223
Supplementary appendix to: Tam CS et al. N Engl J Med 2018;378:1211–1223

Ibrutinib 560 mg/dose; administer orally, once daily with a glass of water, without regard to food, continually, starting in week 1, until disease progression (total dose/week = 3920 mg)

Ibrutinib notes:

- Administration with food increases ibrutinib exposure approximately 2-fold compared with administration after overnight fasting. Clinical studies instructed that ibrutinib be taken at least 30 minutes before eating or at least 2 hours after a meal at approximately the same time each day (Protocol for: Byrd JC et al. N Engl J Med. 2014;371[3]:213–223). However, the U.S. Food and Drug Administration–approved prescribing information does not make specific recommendations regarding administration of ibrutinib with regard to food. (Imbruvica [ibrutinib] prescribing information. Sunnyvale, CA: Pharmacyclics LLC; Revised 2018 August). Others have also concluded that no food restrictions are needed given the relative safety profile of ibrutinib and because repeated drug intake in fasted conditions is unlikely (de Jong J et al. Cancer Chemother Pharmacol. 2015;75[5]:907–16)
- Ibrutinib capsules should be swallowed whole; do not break, open, or chew capsules. Ibrutinib tablets should be swallowed whole; do not cut, crush, or chew tablets
- Patients who delay taking ibrutinib at a regularly scheduled time may administer the missed dose as soon as possible on the same day, and then resume the normal schedule the following day. Do not administer an extra dose of ibrutinib to make up for a missed dose
- Ibrutinib is metabolized predominantly by CYP3A. Refer to treatment modification section for initial dose adjustment recommendations for patients requiring concurrent treatment with moderate or strong CYP3A inhibitors. Avoid concomitant use of ibrutinib with strong CYP3A inducers
- Advise patients to not consume grapefruit products or Seville oranges as they may inhibit CYP3A in the gut wall and increase the bioavailability of ibrutinib
- Serious bleeding events, some fatal, have been reported in patients treated with ibrutinib. Ibrutinib may exacerbate the risk of bleeding when administered concurrently with anticoagulant and/or antiplatelet drugs; use caution and monitor closely for bleeding with concomitant use. Consider the risks and benefits of interrupting ibrutinib treatment at least 3–7 days prior to and following elective surgery depending on the risk of bleeding and type of surgery
- After initiation of ibrutinib, lymphocytosis occurs commonly and should not be considered as an indicator of disease progression
- Reduce the ibrutinib starting dose to 140 mg dose, administered orally once daily for mild (Child-Pugh class A) hepatic impairment. Reduce the ibrutinib starting dose to 70 mg dose, administered orally once daily for moderate (Child-Pugh class B) hepatic impairment. Avoid ibrutinib in patients with severe (Child-Pugh class C) hepatic impairment
- Tumor lysis syndrome may rarely occur with ibrutinib therapy. Consider appropriate monitoring and precautions (eg, anti-hyperuricemic therapy, hydration) in patients with high baseline risk (eg, high tumor burden, renal impairment)

Venetoclax; administer orally once daily with 240 mL water within 30 minutes of completion of a meal (preferably breakfast), starting during week 5, continuously until disease progression (ibrutinib monotherapy given during weeks 1–4; see table below for venetoclax dosing schedule)

4-Week Venetoclax Dose Escalation Schedule

Week of Treatment	Venetoclax Dose per Day	Total Venetoclax Dosage per Week
Week 5	50 mg	350 mg
Week 6	100 mg	700 mg
Week 7	200 mg	1400 mg
Weeks 8 and beyond*	400 mg	2800 mg

*May increase to 800 mg per day after week 16 if a complete response is not achieved

Venetoclax notes:

- Venetoclax tablets should be swallowed whole. Do not chew, crush, or break venetoclax tablets
- Patients who delay taking venetoclax at a regularly scheduled time may administer the missed dose within 30 minutes of completion of a meal if within 8 hours of the usual dosing time. If >8 hours, skip the missed dose and resume treatment at the next regularly scheduled time. Patients who vomit after a dose of venetoclax should not repeat the dose but rather take the next dose at the next regularly scheduled time
- Venetoclax is a substrate of cytochrome P450 (CYP) CYP3A subfamily enzymes, P-glycoprotein (P-gp), and BCRP. Venetoclax is a weak inhibitor of CYP2C8, CYP2C9, and UGT1A1 in vitro but due to high protein binding is predicted to cause clinically insignificant inhibition of these enzymes in vivo. Venetoclax is a P-gp and BCRP inhibitor and weak OATP1B1 inhibitor in vitro
  - Avoid concurrent use with strong or moderate CYP3A inducers at all times
  - Avoid concurrent use with strong CYP3A4 inhibitors throughout the venetoclax dose escalation period

- For patients who have completed venetoclax dose-escalation and are maintained on a steady dose of venetoclax, reduce the venetoclax dose by approximately 75% (ie, from 400 mg/dose to 100 mg/dose) if concomitant use of a strong CYP3A inhibitor is unavoidable and monitor closely for side effects. If the strong CYP3A inhibitor is subsequently discontinued, resume the venetoclax dose that was administered prior to introduction of the inhibitor 2–3 days after discontinuation of the inhibitor

- For patients who have completed venetoclax dose-escalation and are maintained on a steady dose of venetoclax, reduce the venetoclax dose by approximately 80% (ie, from 400 mg/dose to 70 mg/dose) if concomitant use of posaconazole is unavoidable and monitor closely for side effects. If posaconazole is subsequently discontinued, resume the venetoclax dose that was administered prior to introduction of posaconazole 2–3 days after discontinuation of posaconazole

- Reduce the venetoclax dose by ≥50% if concomitant use of a moderate CYP3A4 inhibitor or P-gp inhibitor is unavoidable and monitor closely for side effects. If the moderate CYP3A4 inhibitor is subsequently discontinued, resume the venetoclax dose that was administered prior to introduction of the inhibitor 2–3 days after discontinuation of the inhibitor

- Advise patients to not consume grapefruit products, Seville oranges, or starfruit as they may inhibit CYP3A in the gut wall and increase the bioavailability of venetoclax

- Coadministration of venetoclax with warfarin caused increased exposure to R-warfarin and S-warfarin. Monitor the international normalized ratio closely in patients coadministered warfarin

- Venetoclax inhibits P-gp. Concomitant use of narrow therapeutic index P-gp substrates (eg, digoxin, everolimus, sirolimus) should be avoided when possible. If use of a P-gp substrate is unavoidable, then administer the P-gp substrate ≥6 hours before venetoclax

Venetoclax can cause rapid death of lymphoma cells leading to rapid onset of tumor lysis syndrome (TLS) during the dose escalation period in some patients. In clinical trials of venetoclax, fatal cases of tumor lysis syndrome have occurred which led to the development of a step-wise dose escalation approach to initiation of venetoclax. Assess tumor burden and TLS laboratory measurements and correct any abnormalities prior to initiation of venetoclax. Based on the tumor burden and baseline renal function assessments, determine the risk of TLS in order to guide decisions regarding optimal setting of therapy initiation (inpatient vs outpatient), hydration requirements, and frequency of TLS laboratory monitoring according to the table below

TLS Risk Assessment and Supportive Care				
		Prophylaxis°		Blood Chemistry† Monitoring
Tumor Burden		Hydration	Hyperuricemia Therapy	Setting and Frequency of Assessment
Low	All LN <5 cm AND ALC <25 × 10⁹/L	Oral (1.5–2 L/day)	Allopurinol	Outpatient: • For the first dose of 50 mg; pre-dose, 6–8 h, 24 h • For subsequent ramp-up doses; pre-dose‡
Medium	Any LN 5–10 cm *or* ALC ≥25 × 10⁹/L	Oral (1.5–2 L/day) and consider additional intravenous	Allopurinol	Outpatient: • For the first dose of 50 mg; pre-dose, 6–8 h, 24 h (for patients with CrCl <80 mL/min consider hospitalization with frequent laboratory monitoring as described below for high-risk patients) • For subsequent ramp-up doses; pre-dose‡
High	Any LN ≥10 cm *or* ALC ≥25 × 10⁹/L *and* Any LN ≥5 cm	Oral (1.5–2 L/day) and IV (150–200 mL/h as tolerated)	Allopurinol. Consider rasburicase if baseline uric acid is elevated	In hospital: • For the first dose of 50 mg; pre-dose, 4, 8, 12, and 24 h Outpatient: • For subsequent ramp-up doses; pre-dose, 6–8 h, 24 h

ALC, absolute lymphocyte count; CrCl, creatinine clearance; LN, lymph node; TLS, tumor lysis syndrome
°Initiate a xanthine oxidase inhibitor (eg, allopurinol) 2–3 days prior to initiation of venetoclax. Continue the xanthine oxidase inhibitor for up to 4 weeks depending upon ongoing risk of TLS. Encourage oral hydration (1.5–2L/day) starting 2 days before and on the day of the first venetoclax dose and each dose escalation
†Blood chemistries = potassium, uric acid, phosphorus, calcium, serum creatinine (evaluate in real-time)
‡For patients at continued risk of TLS, monitor chemistries at 6 to 8 hours and at 24 hours at each subsequent outpatient ramp-up dose
Venclexta (venetoclax tablets) prescribing information. North Chicago, IL: AbbVie Inc; 2018 November
Protocol for: Tam CS et al. N Engl J Med 2018;378:1211–1223

Supportive Care
Antiemetic prophylaxis
Emetogenic potential is **MINIMAL–LOW**
See Chapter 42 for antiemetic recommendations

(*continued*)

Hematopoietic growth factor (CSF) prophylaxis
Primary prophylaxis may be indicated
See Chapter 43 for more information

Antimicrobial prophylaxis
Risk of fever and neutropenia is *LOW*
Antimicrobial primary prophylaxis to be considered:
- Antibacterial—consider prophylaxis with a fluoroquinolone during periods of prolonged neutropenia only (eg, <500/mm³ for ≥7 days) until ANC recovery
- Antifungal—not indicated
- Antiviral—antiherpes antivirals (eg, acyclovir, famciclovir, valacyclovir)

Treatment Modifications

Ibrutinib Treatment Modifications

Starting dose	560 mg by mouth once a day
Adverse Event	**Treatment Modification**

Drug Interactions	
Treatment with a moderate CYP3A inhibitor is required	Reduce ibrutinib starting dose to 280 mg by mouth once daily during concomitant therapy
Treatment with voriconazole 200 mg by mouth twice a day is required, *or:* Treatment with posaconazole suspension 100 mg by mouth once daily is required, *or:* Treatment with posaconazole suspension 100–200 mg by mouth twice a day is required	Reduce ibrutinib starting dose to 140 mg by mouth once daily during concomitant therapy
Treatment with posaconazole suspension 200 mg by mouth three times a day is required, *or:* Treatment with posaconazole suspension 400 mg by mouth twice a day is required, *or:* Treatment with posaconazole 300 mg intravenously once a day is required, *or:* Treatment with posaconazole delayed-release tablets 300 mg by mouth once a day is required	Reduce ibrutinib starting dose to 70 mg by mouth once daily during concomitant therapy
Treatment with strong CYP3A inhibitors is required	Avoid concomitant use of ibrutinib with strong CYP3A inhibitors. If a strong CYP3A inhibitor is to be used short-term (eg, ≤7 days) then interrupt ibrutinib therapy during use of the strong CYP3A inhibitor
Treatment with a strong CYP3A inducer is required	Avoid concomitant use of ibrutinib with strong CYP3A inducers
Treatment with antiplatelet and/or anticoagulant medications is required	Bleeding risk may be increased. Monitor closely for signs and symptoms of bleeding
Hypertension	
Hypertension	Adjust existing anti-hypertensive medications and/or initiate anti-hypertensive treatment as appropriate
Hepatic Impairment	
Child-Pugh class A hepatic impairment	Reduce ibrutinib starting dose to 140 mg by mouth once a day
Child-Pugh class B hepatic impairment	Reduce ibrutinib starting dose to 70 mg by mouth once a day
Child-Pugh class C hepatic impairment	Avoid ibrutinib use
Other Toxicities	
Surgical procedure is required during treatment with ibrutinib	Consider benefit-risk of withholding ibrutinib for at least 3–7 days prior to and following surgery depending on the type of surgery and the risk of bleeding

(*continued*)

Treatment Modifications (*continued*)

First occurrence of G ≥3 nonhematological toxicity, G ≥3 neutropenia with infection or fever, or G4 hematologic toxicity	Interrupt ibrutinib until resolution to G1 or baseline, then resume ibrutinib at the same dose (eg, 560 mg by mouth once a day). Consider use of G-CSF for G4 neutropenia lasting >7 days or for life-threatening neutropenic complications
Second occurrence of G ≥3 nonhematologic toxicity, G ≥3 neutropenia with infection or fever, or G4 hematologic toxicity	Interrupt ibrutinib until resolution to G1 or baseline, then resume ibrutinib at 420 mg by mouth once a day. Consider use of G-CSF for G4 neutropenia lasting >7 days or for life-threatening neutropenic complications
Third occurrence of G ≥3 nonhematologic toxicity, G ≥3 neutropenia with infection or fever, or G4 hematologic toxicity	Interrupt ibrutinib until resolution to G1 or baseline, then resume ibrutinib at 280 mg by mouth once a day. Consider use of G-CSF for G4 neutropenia lasting >7 days or for life-threatening neutropenic complications
Fourth occurrence of G ≥3 nonhematologic toxicity, G ≥3 neutropenia with infection or fever, or G4 hematologic toxicity	Discontinue ibrutinib

G-CSF, granulocyte colony-stimulating factor
Imbruvica (ibrutinib) prescribing information. Sunnyvale, CA: Pharmacyclics LLC; Revised 2018 August

Venetoclax Treatment Modifications

Dose at Interruption	Restart Dose[*†]
400 mg	300 mg
300 mg	200 mg
200 mg	100 mg
100 mg	50 mg[‡]
50 mg	20 mg[‡]
20 mg	10 mg[‡]

[*]If patients interrupt venetoclax for >1 week during the 4-week ramp-up period or interrupt venetoclax for >2 weeks during maintenance therapy, reassess the risk of TLS to determine if reinitiation with a reduced dose of venetoclax is necessary
[†]During the venetoclax ramp-up phase, continue the reduced venetoclax dose for 1 week before further dose escalation
[‡]Consider discontinuing venetoclax for patients who require dose reductions to <100 mg for >2 weeks

Tumor Lysis Syndrome

Adverse Event	Treatment Modification
• Prior to initiation of venetoclax: • Potassium, phosphorus, or uric acid >ULN • Corrected calcium < LLN • Serum creatinine ≥25% above baseline value	Correct pre-existing tumor lysis syndrome abnormalities prior to initiation of venetoclax
Laboratory TLS: Blood chemistry (potassium, phosphorus, uric acid, calcium, serum creatinine) suggestive of TLS *without clinical sequelae*	Withhold venetoclax until resolution. Correct laboratory abnormalities and increase frequency of monitoring. If abnormalities resolve within 48 hours, resume venetoclax at the same dose. If resolution requires >48 hours, then resume venetoclax at a reduced dose
Clinical TLS: Blood chemistry (potassium, phosphorus, uric acid, calcium, serum creatinine) suggestive of TLS *with clinical sequelae* (eg, serum creatinine ≥1.5× ULN, cardiac arrhythmia, seizure, sudden cardiac death)	Correct laboratory abnormalities and increase frequency of monitoring. Withhold venetoclax until resolution and then resume venetoclax at a reduced dose
Potassium > ULN in the setting of TLS	Withhold venetoclax until resolution. Increase frequency of monitoring. If resolution occurs within 24–48 hours of the last dose, resume venetoclax at the same dose. If resolution requires >48 hours, then resume at a reduced dose. Perform STAT ECG and begin telemetry. Consider the following interventions: • Sodium polystyrene sulfonate 15 grams by mouth once • Furosemide 20 mg IV push once • Insulin 10 units IV push once plus 25 grams of 50% dextrose IV push once (may omit glucose if serum glucose is ≥250 mg/dL) • If there is ECG evidence of life-threatening arrhythmia, then administer calcium gluconate 1000 mg in 100 mL D5W IV over 30 minutes once • Consult nephrology for consideration of dialysis for severe, or refractory, or rapidly worsening hyperkalemia, especially in the setting of concomitant AKI

(*continued*)

Treatment Modifications (*continued*)

Uric acid ≥8.0 mg/dL in the setting of TLS	Withhold venetoclax until resolution. Increase frequency of monitoring. If resolution occurs within 24–48 hours of the last dose, resume venetoclax at the same dose. If resolution requires >48 hours, then resume at a reduced dose. Consider a **single dose** of rasburicase 3–6 mg (fixed dose) IV over 30 minutes. Optimize the dose of xanthine oxidase inhibitor (eg, allopurinol) and the rate of IV hydration, as tolerated
Phosphorus ≥5.0 mg/dL in the setting of TLS	Withhold venetoclax until resolution. Increase frequency of monitoring. If resolution occurs within 24–48 hours of the last dose, resume venetoclax at the same dose. If resolution requires >48 hours, then resume at a reduced dose. Administer a phosphate binder (eg, aluminum hydroxide, calcium carbonate, sevelamer carbonate, or lanthanum carbonate) with meals. Place patient on a low phosphate diet. Optimize the rate of IV hydration, as tolerated. Consult nephrology for consideration of hemodialysis, especially if phosphorus ≥10 mg/dL or with concomitant AKI
Serum creatinine increases ≥25% from baseline in the setting of TLS	Withhold venetoclax until resolution. Increase frequency of monitoring. If resolution occurs within 24–48 hours of the last dose, resume venetoclax at the same dose. If resolution requires >48 hours, then resume at a reduced dose. Start or increase rate of IV hydration. For severe AKI, consider nephrology consultation
Corrected calcium ≤7.0 mg/dL and patient is symptomatic (eg, muscle cramps, hypotension, tetany, cardiac arrhythmias) in the setting of TLS	Withhold venetoclax until resolution. Increase frequency of monitoring. If resolution occurs within 24–48 hours of the last dose, resume venetoclax at the same dose. If resolution requires >48 hours, then resume at a reduced dose. Perform STAT ECG and begin telemetry. Administer calcium gluconate 1000 mg in 100 mL D5W IV over 30 minutes once

Hematologic Toxicities

G3 neutropenia (ANC ≥500/mm³ and <1000/mm³) with infection or fever; or G4 neutropenia (ANC <500/mm³); or G4 thrombocytopenia (platelet count <25,000/mm³), first occurrence	Withhold venetoclax until resolution to G ≤1 or baseline, then resume venetoclax at the same dose. G-CSF may be administered with venetoclax if indicated to reduce the risk of infection associated with neutropenia
G3 neutropenia (ANC ≥500/mm³ and <1000/mm³) with infection or fever; or G4 neutropenia (ANC <500/mm³); or G4 thrombocytopenia (platelet count <25,000/mm³), second and subsequent occurrences	Withhold venetoclax until resolution to G ≤1 or baseline, then resume venetoclax at a reduced dose. At the discretion of the medically responsible healthcare provider, a larger dose reduction than that described above may be considered depending on the severity of the toxicity. G-CSF may be administered with venetoclax if indicated to reduce the risk of infection associated with neutropenia

Drug-Drug Interactions

Concomitant therapy with a strong or moderate CYP3A inducer is required	Do not administer a strong or moderate CYP3A inducer with venetoclax
Concomitant therapy with a strong CYP3A4 inhibitor is required during the venetoclax 4-week ramp-up period	Do not administer a strong CYP3A4 inhibitor during the venetoclax ramp-up period
Concomitant therapy with a strong CYP3A4 inhibitor is required in a patient taking a steady daily dosage of venetoclax (after ramp-up phase)	Consider alternative medications. If the strong CYP3A4 inhibitor is unavoidable, then reduce the venetoclax dose by approximately 75% (ie, from 400 mg/dose to 100 mg/dose)
Concomitant therapy with posaconazole is required in a patient taking a steady daily dosage of venetoclax (after ramp-up phase)	Consider alternative medications. If posaconazole is unavoidable, then reduce the venetoclax dose by approximately 80% (ie, from 400 mg/dose to 70 mg/dose)
Concomitant therapy with a moderate CYP3A4 inhibitor or P-gp inhibitor is required (any phase of treatment)	Consider alternative medications. If the moderate CYP3A4 inhibitor or P-gp inhibitor is unavoidable, then reduce the venetoclax dose by at least 50%
Concomitant strong or moderate CYP3A4 inhibitor, posaconazole, or P-gp inhibitor is subsequently discontinued	Resume the venetoclax dosage that was used prior to concomitant use of a strong or moderate CYP3A4 inhibitor, posaconazole, or P-gp inhibitor 2 to 3 days after discontinuation of the inhibitor
Concomitant therapy with warfarin is required	Monitor international normalized ratio frequently

(*continued*)

Treatment Modifications (*continued*)

Concomitant therapy with a P-gp substrate is required	Consider alternative medications. If concomitant use is unavoidable, administer the P-gp substrate at least 6 hours before the administration of venetoclax

Other Toxicities

Other G3/4 nonhematologic toxicity, first occurrence	Withhold venetoclax until resolution to G ≤1 or baseline, then resume venetoclax at the same dose
Other G3/4 nonhematologic toxicity, second and subsequent occurrences	Withhold venetoclax until resolution to G ≤1 or baseline, then resume venetoclax at a lower dose. At the discretion of the medically responsible healthcare provider, a larger dose reduction than that described above may be considered depending on the severity of the toxicity
Immunization with a live attenuated vaccine is indicated prior to, during, or after therapy with venetoclax	Do not administer live attenuated vaccines prior to, during, or after treatment with venetoclax until B-cell recovery occurs

Venetoclax may cause fetal harm. Advise females of reproductive potential of the potential risk to a fetus and to use effective contraception during treatment

TLS, tumor lysis syndrome; ULN, upper limit of normal; LLN, lower limit of normal; ECG, electrocardiogram; IV, intravenous; AKI, acute kidney injury; ANC, absolute neutrophil count; G-CSF, granulocyte-colony stimulating factor; P-gp, P-glycoprotein

Patient Population Studied

Investigator-initiated, open-label, single-group, phase 2 study. Adult patients eligible if they had relapsed or refractory mantle-cell lymphoma or, if they had previously untreated mantle-cell lymphoma, were not suitable candidates for cytotoxic chemotherapy. Patients also had to have an Eastern Cooperative Group Performance Status Score of 0, 1 or 2

Characteristic	Value
Median age (range)—years	68 (47–81)
Sex—no. (%)—female / male	3 (12) / 21 (88)
Previous treatment for mantle-cell lymphoma—no. (%)—Yes / No	23 (96) / 1 (4)
No. previous therapies among patients who received therapy—median (range)‡	2 (1–6)
Disease refractory to most recent therapy—no./total no. (%)	11/23 (48)
Previous therapy—no./total no. (%)	
Autologous transplantation	7/23 (30)
Rituximab	23/23 (100)
Anthracycline	21/23 (91)
High-dose cytarabine	11/23 (48)
Bendamustine	4/23 (17)
ECOG performance-status score—no. (%)—0 / 1 / 2	9 (38) / 10 (42) / 5 (21)
Bone marrow involvement by mantle-cell lymphoma—no. (%)	
Bone marrow involved at study entry	13 (54)
Negative at study entry but positive at week 4	7 (29)
No bone marrow involvement	4 (17)

(*continued*)

Adverse Events (N = 24)

Grade (%)[*]	Any Grade	G ≥3
Any adverse event	100	71
Diarrhea	83	12[†]
Fatigue	75	0
Nausea or vomiting	71	0
Bleeding, bruising, or postoperative hemorrhage	54	4
Musculoskeletal or connective-tissue pain	50	4
Cough or dyspnea	46	4
Soft-tissue infection	42	8[‡]
Upper respiratory tract infection	42	0
Gastroesophageal reflux	38	0
Neutropenia	33	33
Lower respiratory tract infection	33	8
Anemia	29	12
Rash	29	0
Oral mucositis	21	0
Cramps	21	0
Sensory peripheral neuropathy	21	0
Thrombocytopenia	21	17
Tumor lysis syndrome	8	8
Atrial fibrillation	8	8
Any serious adverse event[‡]	58	—
Diarrhea	12	—
Tumor lysis syndrome	8	—
Atrial fibrillation	8	—
Pyrexia	8	—
Pleural effusion	8	—
Cardiac failure	4	—
Soft-tissue infection	4	—

[*]The table includes adverse events reported in ≥15% of patients as well as events of special interest (atrial fibrillation and tumor lysis syndrome)

[†]The 3 cases of grade 3 diarrhea lasted 4 days, 1 week, and 2 weeks

[‡]The table includes serious adverse events reported in ≥2 patients and all fatal events

Patient Population Studied (*continued*)

Bulky adenopathy—no. (%)	
≥5 cm to <10 cm	4 (17)
≥10 cm	2 (8)
Mantle Cell Lymphoma International Prognostic Index score category—no. (%)	
Low risk	1 (4)
Intermediate risk	5 (21)
High risk	18 (75)
Blastic or pleomorphic mantle-cell lymphoma—no./total no. (%)	1/21 (5)
Ki–67 ≥30%—no./total no. (%)	9/21 (43)
TP53 status—no. (%)	
Mutated with deletion	4 (17)
Mutated without deletion	7 (29)
Deletion without mutation	1 (4)
NF-κB pathway mutations in CARD11, BIRC3, or TRAF2—no. (%)	6 (25)
Tumor lysis risk category—no. (%)—Low / Intermediate / High	11 (46) / 6 (25) / 7 (29)

Efficacy

Survival Data		
Estimated 12-month PFS	75% (95% CI, 60–94)	
Estimated 18-month PFS	57% (95% CI, 40–82)	
Estimated 12-month OS	79% (95% CI, 64–97)	
Estimated 18-month OS	74% (95% CI, 57–95)	
Response Data	Without PET (N = 24)	With PET (N = 24)
Overall		
Response at week 4		
CR	0	—
Unconfirmed CR	1 (4%)	—
PR	10 (42%)	—
SD	10 (42)	—
PD	2 (8%)	—
Unevaluable	1 (4%)	—
Response at week 16		
CR	10 (42%)	15 (62%)
Unconfirmed CR	4 (17%)	—

(*continued*)

Efficacy (continued)

PR	4 (17%)	—
SD	2 (8%)	1 (4%)
PD	3 (12%)	4 (17%)
Unevaluable	1 (4%)	2 (8%)
Best response		
CR	16 (67%)	17 (71%)
Unconfirmed CR	1 (4%)	—
PR	1 (4%)	0
SD	4 (17%)	2 (8%)
PD	2 (8%)	3 (12%)
Unevaluable	0	2 (8%)
	With Flow Cytometry	**With ASO-PCR°**
According to MRD clearance		
Tissue tested	*Bone Marrow*	*Blood*
Never MRD positive	4/24	0/16
Could be potentially evaluated for MRD response	19	16
Response at week 4		
MRD negative	0	0
MRD positive	19/19 (100%)	13/13 (100%)
Response at week 16		
MRD negative	12/18 (67%)	2/13 (15%)
MRD positive	6/18 (33%)	11/13 (85%)
Best response		
Among patients who could be evaluated for MRD response		
MRD negative	16/19 (84%)	9/16 (56%)
MRD positive	3/19 (16%)	7/16 (44%)
In the total population		
MRD negative	16 (67%)	9 (38%)
MRD not negative	8 (33%)	15 (62%)

Therapy Monitoring

Ibrutinib monitoring:
1. *Prior to initiation of ibrutinib*: CBC with differential, serum bilirubin, ALT or AST, alkaline phosphatase, potassium, calcium, phosphorus, LDH, uric acid, and serum creatinine
2. *At least monthly*: CBC with differential
3. *Periodically*: monitor for signs and symptoms of cardiac arrhythmias (eg, atrial fibrillation and atrial flutter) and check electrocardiogram if present, signs and symptoms of bleeding (especially if concomitant antiplatelet or anticoagulant medication[s] are used), signs and symptoms of infection (including progressive multifocal leukoencephalopathy)
4. *During initiation of therapy in patients with high tumor burden or renal dysfunction*: monitor for tumor lysis syndrome

Venetoclax monitoring:
1. Prior to initiation of venetoclax: Assess tumor burden (CBC with differential, CT scan) and baseline chemistries (potassium, uric acid, phosphorus, calcium, serum creatinine, LDH) to determine the risk for tumor lysis syndrome (TLS). Decisions regarding treatment setting (inpatient vs outpatient) and frequency of laboratory monitoring depend upon TLS risk assessment (see above table)
2. Tumor lysis syndrome monitoring during venetoclax ramp-up
3. Periodically throughout treatment: CBC with differential

Response assessment:
1. *Response assessment every 2–3 months*: physical examination, CBC with differential, CT scan with contrast and/or PET scan, bone marrow evaluation (as clinically indicated)

Note: Lymphocytosis occurs commonly in mantle cell lymphoma patients following initiation of ibrutinib and should not be considered as an indicator of disease progression

PERIPHERAL T-CELL LYMPHOMA • FIRST LINE

NON-HODGKIN LYMPHOMA REGIMEN: BRENTUXIMAB VEDOTIN (ADCETRIS) + CYCLOPHOSPHAMIDE + DOXORUBICIN (HYDROXYDAUNORUBICIN) + PREDNISONE (A+CHP)

Horwitz S et al. Lancet 2019;393:229–240
Supplementary appendix to: Horwitz S et al. Lancet 2019;393:229–240
Adcetris (brentuximab vedotin) prescribing information. Bothell, WA: Seattle Genetics, Inc; Revised 2018 November

Intravenous hydration before and after cyclophosphamide administration: 500–1000 mL 0.9% sodium chloride (0.9% NS)

Cyclophosphamide 750 mg/m^2; administer intravenously in 25–250 mL 0.9% NS or 5% dextrose injection (D5W) over 10–30 minutes on day 1, every 3 weeks, for 6–8 cycles (total dosage/21-day cycle = 750 mg/m^2)
Doxorubicin 50 mg/m^2; administer by intravenous injection over 3–5 minutes on day 1, every 3 weeks, for 6–8 cycles (total dosage/21-day cycle = 50 mg/m^2)
Prednisone 100 mg per dose; administer orally for 5 consecutive days, days 1–5, every 3 weeks, for 6–8 cycles (total dosage/21-day cycle = 500 mg)
Brentuximab vedotin 1.8 mg/kg (maximum dose = 180 mg); administer intravenously in a volume of 0.9% NS or D5W sufficient to produce a concentration with the range 0.4–1.8 mg/mL (minimum volume, 100 mL) over 30 minutes on day 1, after administration of cyclophosphamide, doxorubicin, and prednisone, every 3 weeks, for 6–8 cycles (total dosage/21-day cycle = 1.8 mg/kg; maximum dose/21-day cycle = 180 mg)

Note:
• The dose for patients whose body weight is >100 kg should be calculated based on a weight of 100 kg (maximum single dose = 180 mg)
• No dose reduction is necessary in patients with mild-moderate renal impairment (creatinine clearance ≥30 mL/min and ≤80 mL/min). Avoid use in patients with severe renal impairment (creatinine clearance <30 mL/min)
• The recommended starting dose in patients with mild hepatic impairment (Child-Pugh A) is 1.2 mg/kg (maximum single dose = 120 mg) intravenously over 30 minutes every 3 weeks. Avoid use in patients with Child-Pugh B or Child-Pugh C hepatic impairment
• Brentuximab vedotin can cause severe or life-threatening infusion-related reactions, including hypersensitivity and anaphylaxis
  – Monitor patients for signs and symptoms of infusion-related reactions including rigors, chills, wheezing, pruritus, flushing, rash, hypotension, hypoxemia, and fever
  – If anaphylaxis occurs, stop administration, and permanently discontinue brentuximab vedotin
  – If an infusion-related reaction occurs, stop the infusion and provide appropriate medical treatment. Consider premedication with acetaminophen, antihistamine, and a corticosteroid with subsequent cycles
• Monomethyl auristatin E (MMAE), the cytotoxic component of brentuximab vedotin, is a substrate of CYP3A4/5 and P-glycoprotein (P-gp). Use caution and monitor closely for brentuximab vedotin side effects when co-administering brentuximab vedotin with strong CYP3A4 inhibitors or P-gp inhibitors

Supportive Care
Antiemetic prophylaxis
Emetogenic potential on day 1 is **HIGH**. *Potential for delayed symptoms*
See Chapter 42 for antiemetic recommendations

Hematopoietic growth factor (CSF) prophylaxis
Primary prophylaxis is indicated with one of the following:
Filgrastim (G-CSF) 5 µg/kg per day, by subcutaneous injection, *or*
Pegfilgrastim (pegylated filgrastim) 6 mg/0.6 mL, by subcutaneous injection for 1 dose
• Begin use from 24–72 hours after myelosuppressive chemotherapy is completed
• Continue daily filgrastim use until ANC ≥5000/mm^3 after the leukocyte nadir
• Discontinue daily filgrastim use at least 24 hours before administering myelosuppressive treatment
• Do not administer pegfilgrastim within 14 days before administering myelosuppressive treatment
See Chapter 43 for more information

Antimicrobial prophylaxis
Risk of fever and neutropenia is *INTERMEDIATE*
Antimicrobial primary prophylaxis to be considered:
• Antibacterial—consider a fluoroquinolone during periods of prolonged neutropenia, or no prophylaxis
• Antifungal—consider use during periods of prolonged neutropenia, or no prophylaxis
• Antiviral—antiherpes antivirals (eg, acyclovir, famciclovir, valacyclovir)

Diarrhea Management
• **Loperamide** 4 mg orally initially after the first loose or liquid stool, *then*
• **Loperamide** 2 mg orally every 2 hours during waking hours, *plus*
• **Loperamide** 4 mg orally every 4 hours during hours of sleep
• Continue for at least 12 hours after diarrhea resolves

(continued)

(continued)

- Recurrent diarrhea after a 12-hour diarrhea-free interval is treated as a new episode
- Rehydrate orally with fluids and electrolytes during a diarrheal episode
- If a patient develops blood or mucus in stool, dehydration, or hemodynamic instability, or if diarrhea persists >48 hours despite loperamide, stop loperamide, and hospitalize the patient for IV hydration

Alternatively, a trial of **diphenoxylate hydrochloride** 2.5 mg **with atropine sulfate** 0.025 mg (eg, Lomotil)

- Initial adult dose is 2 tablets 4 times daily until control has been achieved, after which the dose may be reduced to meet individual requirements. Control may often be maintained with as little as 2 tablets daily
- Clinical improvement of acute diarrhea is usually observed within 48 hours. If improvement of chronic diarrhea after treatment with a maximum daily dose of 8 tablets is not observed within 10 days, control is unlikely with further administration

Treatment Modifications

Cyclophosphamide + Doxorubicin + Prednisone + Brentuximab Vedotin Dose Modifications				
Dose	Cyclophosphamide	Doxorubicin	Brentuximab Vedotin	Prednisone
Starting	750 mg/m^2	50 mg/m^2	1.8 mg/kg	100 mg
Level 1	562.5 mg/m^2	37.5 mg/m^2	1.2 mg/kg	80 mg
Level 2	375 mg/m^2	25 mg/m^2	Discontinue brentuximab vedotin	60 mg

Adverse Event	Dose Modification
General Dose Modification	
Patient weight >100 kg	Use a maximum weight of 100 kg for calculation of the brentuximab vedotin dose. Follow institutional standards and clinical practice guidelines for calculation of cyclophosphamide and doxorubicin doses
Hematologic Toxicity	
Day 1 platelet count <100,000/mm^3 or ANC <1500/mm^3	Delay start of cycle until platelet count ≥100,000/mm^3 and ANC ≥1500/mm^3, or until recovery to near baseline value, then continue all therapy at the same doses If the delay was necessary due to neutropenia and the patient did not receive growth factor (filgrastim, pegfilgrastim) with the prior cycle, administer filgrastim or pegfilgrastim during all subsequent cycles
G4 neutropenia (ANC <500/mm^3) during the prior cycle given *without* growth factor (filgrastim, pegfilgrastim) prophylaxis Febrile neutropenia (ANC <1000/mm^3 with temperature >38°C or >100.4°F) during the prior cycle given *without* growth factor (filgrastim, pegfilgrastim) prophylaxis	Administer filgrastim or pegfilgrastim during all subsequent cycles, and continue the same doses
Febrile neutropenia (ANC <1000/mm^3 with temperature >38°C or >100.4°F) during the prior cycle given *with* growth factor (filgrastim, pegfilgrastim) prophylaxis G ≥3 thrombocytopenia (platelets <50,000/mm^3) during the prior cycle	At the discretion of the medically responsible healthcare provider, consider reducing the dose of cyclophosphamide, and/or doxorubicin, and/or brentuximab vedotin by 1 dose level for subsequent cycles
Neurologic Toxicities	
G2 motor neuropathy G3 sensory neuropathy	Reduce the brentuximab vedotin dosage to dose level 1. Continue cyclophosphamide, doxorubicin, and prednisone at the same dose
G3 motor neuropathy G4 peripheral neuropathy (any)	Permanently discontinue brentuximab vedotin. Continue cyclophosphamide, doxorubicin, and prednisone at the same dose
G ≥2 mood alteration (moderate mood alteration) or confusion (moderate disorientation; limiting instrumental ADL)	Withhold prednisone until symptoms return to baseline. Resume prednisone reduced by 1 dose level. If symptoms persist, reduce by another dose level. Do not change the cyclophosphamide, doxorubicin, or brentuximab vedotin doses

Treatment Modifications (*continued*)

Hepatic Impairment

Patient with mild hepatic impairment (Child-Pugh class A)	Reduce the brentuximab vedotin dose to 1.2 mg/kg (maximum dose = 120 mg). See bilirubin criteria to determine if doxorubicin dose modification is necessary
Patient with moderate-severe hepatic impairment (Child-Pugh class B or C)	Do not administer brentuximab vedotin. See bilirubin criteria to determine if doxorubicin dose modification is necessary
Serum bilirubin 1.2–3 mg/dL	Decrease the doxorubicin dose by 50%. Calculate Child-Pugh score to determine if brentuximab vedotin dose modification is necessary
Serum bilirubin 3.1–5 mg/dL	Decrease the doxorubicin by 75%. Do not administer brentuximab vedotin. Do not adjust the cyclophosphamide or prednisone doses
Serum bilirubin >5 mg/dL	Do not administer doxorubicin or brentuximab vedotin. At the discretion of the medically responsible healthcare provider, may continue cyclophosphamide and prednisone at the same doses

Opportunistic Infection Adverse Events

PML suspected (eg, new neurologic deficit)	Delay all therapy during evaluation
PML confirmed	Permanently discontinue brentuximab vedotin. The safety of resuming chemotherapy (cyclophosphamide, doxorubicin, and prednisone) in patients following recovery from PML has not been determined

Infusion-Related Reaction and Anaphylactic Reaction Adverse Events

Infusion-related reaction during brentuximab vedotin administration	Interrupt the brentuximab vedotin infusion, and initiate appropriate medical management. For subsequent cycles, premedicate with acetaminophen, antihistamine, and corticosteroids
Anaphylactic reaction during brentuximab vedotin administration	Permanently discontinue brentuximab vedotin. Continue cyclophosphamide, doxorubicin, and prednisone at the same dose

Other Toxicities

New or worsening pulmonary symptoms	Delay brentuximab vedotin and all therapy during evaluation and until symptomatic improvement. Upon improvement, depending on the severity of symptoms and results of diagnostic evaluation, consider permanently discontinuing brentuximab vedotin, reducing the brentuximab vedotin dosage to dose level 1, or continuing the same brentuximab vedotin dosage
SJS or TEN	Permanently discontinue brentuximab vedotin
G ≥3 hyperglycemia (insulin therapy initiated; hospitalization indicated)	Withhold prednisone until blood glucose is ≤250 mg/dL. Treat with insulin or other hypoglycemic agents as clinically appropriate, and then resume prednisone at the same dose. If hyperglycemia is uncontrolled despite above measures, decrease prednisone by 1 dose level
LVEF is 40%, or is 40% to 45% with a 10% or greater absolute decrease below the pretreatment	Withhold doxorubicin, and repeat LVEF assessment within approximately 4 weeks. Discontinue doxorubicin if the LVEF has not improved or has declined further, unless the benefits for the individual patient outweigh the risks

Patient Population Studied

This international, multicenter, randomized, phase 3, double-blind, double-dummy trial involved 452 adult patients with treatment-naive CD30-positive (defined as ≥10% of cells) peripheral T-cell lymphoma (eligible histologies were limited to: ALK-positive systemic anaplastic large cell lymphoma with an IPI score ≥2, ALK-negative systemic anaplastic large cell lymphoma, peripheral T-cell lymphoma not otherwise specified, angioimmunoblastic T-cell lymphoma, adult T-cell leukemia or lymphoma, and enteropathy associated T-cell lymphoma). Patients were randomly assigned (1:1) to receive six to eight 21-day cycles of: cyclophosphamide (750 mg/m² on day 1), doxorubicin (50 mg/m² on day 1), oral prednisone (100 mg on days 1–5), and vincristine, plus a placebo form of brentuximab vedotin (CHOP); or cyclophosphamide (750 mg/m² on day 1), doxorubicin (50 mg/m² on day 1), oral prednisone (100 mg on days 1–5), and brentuximab vedotin (1.8 mg/kg [maximum 180 mg] administered last on day 1), plus a placebo form of vincristine (A-CHP)

Therapy Monitoring

1. *Prior to initiation of therapy:* CBC with differential and platelet count, serum electrolytes, liver function tests, serum creatinine, BUN, left ventricular ejection fraction (LVEF), urine pregnancy test (women of child-bearing potential only)

   a. In addition to baseline monitoring, evaluate LVEF during doxorubicin treatment if clinical symptoms of heart failure are present. If baseline LVEF is ≥50%, repeat LVEF evaluation after a cumulative lifetime doxorubicin dose between 250 and 300 mg/m² has been reached, after a cumulative lifetime doxorubicin dose of 450 mg/m² has been reached, and then before each cycle beyond a cumulative lifetime doxorubicin dose of 450 mg/m². If the baseline LVEF is <50%, consider repeating LVEF evaluation before each dose of doxorubicin

   b. *In patients at high risk for tumor lysis syndrome* consider frequent monitoring of laboratory indices of tumor lysis syndrome, intravenous hydration, and prophylaxis with a xanthine oxidase inhibitor (eg, allopurinol)

2. *Weekly during therapy:* CBC with differential and platelet count

3. *Prior to each cycle:* CBC with differential and platelet count, serum electrolytes, liver function tests, serum creatinine, BUN

4. *Periodically assess for:* Peripheral neuropathy, pulmonary toxicity, severe dermatologic toxicity, gastrointestinal toxicity, infection, and progressive multifocal leukoencephalopathy

5. *Response assessment (after cycle 4 and then at end of treatment):* Physical exam, CBC with differential, CT scan or PET scan, bone marrow evaluation (if clinically indicated)

Efficacy

(N = 452)

	CHOP (N = 226)	A-CHP (N = 226)	
Median progression-free survival*	20.8 months	48.2 months	HR 0.71; P = 0.0110
Estimated progression-free survival rate at 36 months	44.4%	57.1%	—
Median overall survival†	Not reached	Not reached	HR 0.66; P = 0.0244
Estimated overall survival rate at 36 months	69.1%	76.8%	—
Objective response rate‡	72%	83%	P = 0.0032
Complete response rate	56%	68%	P = 0.0066

*Analysis performed after 219 progression-free survival events occurred; median follow-up, 36.2 months
†Analysis performed after 124 deaths occurred; median follow-up, 42.1 months
‡Objective response rate includes patients with either a complete or partial response

Toxicity

(N = 449)

Grade*	CHOP (N = 226)		A-CHP (N = 223)	
	Grade 1–2 (%)	Grade ≥3 (%)	Grade 1–2 (%)	Grade ≥3 (%)
Nausea	36	2	44	2
Peripheral sensory neuropathy	38	3	41	4
Neutropenia	4	34	3	35
Diarrhea	19	1	32	6
Constipation	29	1	28	1
Alopecia	24	1	26	0
Pyrexia	19	0	24	2
Vomiting	15	2	25	1
Fatigue	18	2	23	1
Anemia	6	10	8	13

*According to the Medical Dictionary for Regulatory Activities, version 21.0, and the NCI Common Terminology Criteria for Adverse Events, version 4.03
Note: All-grade toxicities that occurred in ≥20% patients in either group during treatment are included. Rates of all-grade adverse events (98% for CHOP and 99% for A+CHP), treatment discontinuation owing to adverse events (7% for CHOP and 6% for A+CHP), grade ≥3 adverse events (65% for CHOP 66% for A+CHOP) and death due to adverse events (4% for CHOP and 3% for A+CHP) were similar in the two treatment groups

PERIPHERAL T-CELL LYMPHOMA • FIRST LINE

NON-HODGKIN LYMPHOMA REGIMEN: CYCLOPHOSPHAMIDE + DOXORUBICIN + VINCRISTINE + ETOPOSIDE + PREDNISOLONE (CHOEP)

Pfreundschuh M et al. Ann Oncol 2008;19:545–552
Schmitz et al. Blood 2010;116:3418–3425

Hydration with 500–1000 mL 0.9% sodium chloride injection (0.9% NS); administer intravenously before starting cyclophosphamide administration and 500–1000 mL 0.9% NS after completing cyclophosphamide

Cyclophosphamide 750 mg/m^2; administer intravenously in 25–250 mL 0.9% NS or 5% dextrose injection (D5W) over 30 minutes on day 1, every 21 days (total dosage/cycle = 750 mg/m^2)

Doxorubicin 50 mg/m^2; administer by intravenous injection over 3–5 minutes on day 1, every 21 days (total dosage/cycle = 50 mg/m^2)

Vincristine 2 mg; administer by intravenous infusion over 15 minutes in 50 mL 0.9% NS on day 1, every 21 days (total dose/cycle = 2 mg)

Etoposide 100 mg/m^2 per day; administer intravenously in a volume of 0.9% NS or D5W sufficient to produce a concentration within the range 0.2–0.4 mg/mL over 60 minutes for 3 consecutive days, on days 1–3, every 21 days (total dosage/cycle = 300 mg/m^2)

Prednisolone *or* **prednisone** 100 mg/day; administer orally for 5 consecutive days, on days 1–5, every 21 days (total dose/cycle = 500 mg)

Note:
- Prednisolone and prednisone may be used interchangeably at the same dose and administration schedule
- In the study reported by Pfreundschuh et al, patients were to receive radiotherapy (36 Gy) to sites of primary bulky and extranodal disease, and 85% of patients received radiotherapy according to protocol

Supportive Care

Antiemetic prophylaxis
Emetogenic potential on day 1 is **HIGH**. *Potential for delayed symptoms*
Emetogenic potential on days 2 and 3 is **LOW**
See Chapter 42 for antiemetic recommendations

Hematopoietic growth factor (CSF) prophylaxis
Primary prophylaxis may be indicated
See Chapter 43 for more information

Antimicrobial prophylaxis
Risk of fever and neutropenia is *LOW*
Antimicrobial primary prophylaxis to be considered:
- Antibacterial—*Pneumocystis jirovecii* prophylaxis is recommended (eg, cotrimoxazole)
- Antifungal—not indicated
- Antiviral—not indicated, unless patient previously had an episode of HSV

Steroid-associated gastritis
Add a **proton pump inhibitor** during steroid use to prevent gastritis and duodenitis

Treatment Modification

Adverse Event	Treatment Modifications
G4 ANC or febrile neutropenia after any cycle	Administer filgrastim during subsequent cycles
G4 neutropenia during a cycle in which filgrastim was administered	Cyclophosphamide, doxorubicin, and etoposide dosages are reduced by 25–50% during subsequent cycles
G3/4 thrombocytopenia	Cyclophosphamide, doxorubicin, and etoposide dosages are reduced by 25–50% during subsequent cycles
ANC <1500/mm^3 or platelets <100,000/mm^3 on day 1 of a scheduled cycle	The cycle is delayed for up to 2 weeks. Treatment is stopped if recovery has not occurred after a 2-week delay

Patient Population Studied

343 patients with mature nodal or extranodal T-cell or NK-cell lymphoma who were enrolled on several protocols of the German High-Grade Non-Hodgkin Lymphoma Study Group between October 1993 and May 2007. Of 343 patients, 320 could be assigned to 1 of the following subtypes:

Anaplastic large cell lymphoma kinase-positive, ALK-positive (ALCL, ALK-positive)	78 (24.4%)
Anaplastic large cell lymphoma kinase-positive, ALK-negative (ALCL, ALK-negative)	113 (35.3%)
Peripheral T-cell lymphoma unspecified (PTCLU)	70 (21.9%)
Angioimmunoblastic T-cell lymphoma (AITL)	28 (8.8%)
NK/T-cell lymphoma	19 (5.9%)
Lymphoblastic lymphoma	7 (2.2%)
Enteropathy-type T-cell lymphoma	2 (0.6%)
Hepatosplenic gamma/delta (γ/δ) T-cell lymphoma	2 (0.6%)
Subcutaneous panniculitis-like T-cell lymphoma	1 (0.3%)

- All patients were treated on either phase 2 or phase 3 trials. The phase 2 studies were dose-finding studies using escalating doses of cyclophosphamide, doxorubicin, and etoposide compared with standard CHOP plus etoposide protocols. The phase 3 trials compared the standard CHOP regimen to 6 or 8 courses of CHOP given every 2 weeks (CHOP–14) or to CHOP plus etoposide (CHOEP-14 or -21), or compared CHOEP to a dose-escalated (Hi-CHOEP), or a mega-dose (Mega CHOEP) variant, the latter regimen necessitated repeated transplantation of hematopoietic stem cells
- Radiotherapy to sites of bulky disease (>7.5 cm) and to extranodal disease was part of all protocols except for the Mega CHOEP phase 2 trial where radiotherapy was optional
- Extranodal disease was common in all subtypes (41–56%)
- Highly significant (P<0.001) differences were seen for involvement of soft tissues (21% in ALK-positive ALCL, 8% in ALK-negative ALCL, 0–1% in other subtypes) and bone marrow (none in ALK-positive ALCL, 4% in ALK-negative ALCL, 11% in PTCLU, 27% in AITL, and 13% in other subtypes) when the 4 major subgroups were compared

Efficacy

N = 289; Median Follow-up of 43.8 Months for the Whole Group					
	ALK-positive ALCL (N = 78)	ALK-negative ALCL (N = 113)	PTCLU (N = 70)	AITL (N = 28)	NK/T (N = 19)
3-Year EFS % (95% CI)	75.8% (65.8–85.8)	45.7% (36.3–55.1)	41.1% (29.5–52.7)	50.0% (31.6–68.4)	36.1% (14.1–58.1)
3-Year OS % (95% CI)	89.8% (82.5–97.1)	62.1% (52.9–71.3)	53.9% (41.7–66.1)	67.5% (50.1–84.9)	46.3% (23.4–69.2)

Younger Patients (<60 years) with Normal LDH NHLB1 Trial[*]			
	CHOP (N = 41)	CHOEP (N = 42)	
3-Year EFS % (95% CI)	75.4% (62.1–88.7)	51.0% (35.7–66.3)	P = 0.003
3-Year OS % (95% CI)	—	—	P = 0.176

Younger Patients (<60 years) with Normal LDH NHLB1 Trial + Hi-CHOEP Phase II/II Trials[*]			
	CHOP (N = 41)	CHOEP (N = 103)	
3-Year EFS % (95% CI)	51.0% (35.7–66.3)	70.5% (61.3–79.7)	P = 0.004
3-Year OS % (95% CI)	75.2% (61.9–88.5)	81.3% (73.5–89.1)	P = 0.285

ALK-positive ALCL			
	CHOP (N = 12)	CHOEP (N = 34)	
3-Year EFS	57.1% (28.5–85.7)	91.2% (81.6–100.0)	P = 0.012

AITL, angioimmunoblastic T-cell lymphoma; ALK-negative ALCL, anaplastic large cell lymphoma kinase ALK-negative; ALK-positive, ALCL, anaplastic large cell lymphoma kinase ALK-positive; CI, confidence interval; EFS, event-free survival; NK/T, NK-/T-cell lymphoma; PTCLU, peripheral T-cell lymphoma, unspecified; OS, overall survival

[*]In patients >60 years of age, 6 courses of CHOP administered every 3 weeks remains the standard therapy

Treatment Monitoring

1. *Prior to treatment initiation*: CBC with differential, serum chemistries, serum bilirubin, ALT or AST, left ventricular ejection fraction (LVEF), and urine pregnancy test (women of child-bearing potential only)
   a. In addition to baseline monitoring, evaluate LVEF during doxorubicin treatment if clinical symptoms of heart failure are present
   b. *In patients at high risk for tumor lysis syndrome (eg, high tumor burden, renal dysfunction, rapidly progressing disease, markedly elevated LDH, baseline abnormalities in laboratory indices of tumor lysis syndrome [potassium, phosphate, uric acid, calcium, serum creatinine])*: consider frequent monitoring of laboratory indices of tumor lysis syndrome, intravenous hydration, and prophylaxis with a xanthine oxidase inhibitor (eg, allopurinol) during the first cycle
2. *Prior to each cycle*: CBC with differential, serum chemistries, serum bilirubin, ALT or AST
3. *Weekly*: CBC with differential
4. *Assessment of efficacy*: Radiographic examination at 2- or 3-cycle intervals and at the end of treatment

Toxicity

N = 194

Pfreundschuh M et al. Ann Oncol 2008;19:545–552

Leukocytopenia	87.2%
Thrombocytopenia	9.6%
Anemia	11.8%
Infection	10.8%
Polyneuropathy	3.3%
Mucositis	2.7%
Cardiac toxicity	0.5%
Renal toxicity	0
Lung toxicity	0
Nausea or vomiting	4.8%
Alopecia	69.8%

Therapeutic Interventions

Red blood cell transfusions (per patient/per cycle)	11.2/4.1
Platelet transfusion (per patient/per cycle)	2.1/0.4
Intravenous antibiotics (per patient/per cycle)	32.6/8.7

PERIPHERAL T-CELL LYMPHOMA • SUBSEQUENT THERAPY

NON-HODGKIN LYMPHOMA REGIMEN: ROMIDEPSIN

Coiffier B et al. J Clin Oncol 2012;30:631–636

Romidepsin 14 mg/m² per dose; administer intravenously in 500 mL 0.9% sodium chloride injection over 4 hours for 3 doses, on days 1, 8, and 15, every 28 days for up to 6 cycles (total dosage/cycle = 43.2 mg/m²)

Note:

- Check serum magnesium and serum potassium before each dose to ensure serum magnesium ≥1.5 mg/dL and serum potassium ≥4 mEq/L. Supplement potassium and magnesium in all patients *before* administering romidepsin if laboratory results do not meet these criteria
- In the study, patients with stable disease (SD), partial response (PR), or CR/CRu could continue to receive romidepsin until they demonstrated disease progression (PD) or met another criterion for withdrawal

Supportive Care

Antiemetic prophylaxis
Emetogenic potential is **LOW–MODERATE**
See Chapter 42 for antiemetic recommendations

Hematopoietic growth factor (CSF) prophylaxis
Primary prophylaxis is **NOT** indicated
See Chapter 43 for more information

Antimicrobial prophylaxis
Risk of fever and neutropenia is *LOW*
Antimicrobial primary prophylaxis to be considered:

- Antibacterial—*Pneumocystis jirovecii* prophylaxis is recommended (eg, cotrimoxazole)
- Antifungal—not indicated
- Antiviral—not indicated unless patient previously had an episode of HSV

Decreased bowel motility prophylaxis

Give a bowel regimen to prevent constipation based initially on **stool softeners**, and **saline, osmotic, and lubricant laxatives**, as needed to prevent constipation for as long as romidepsin use continues. If needed, circumspectly add **stimulant (irritant) laxatives** in the least amounts and for the briefest durations needed to produce defecation

Treatment Modifications

Adverse Event	Treatment Modifications
G2/3 nonhematologic toxicities except alopecia	Withhold treatment with romidepsin until toxicity returns to G ≤1 or baseline. Resume romidepsin therapy at 14 mg/m² per dose
Recurrent G3 nonhematologic toxicities	Withhold treatment with romidepsin until toxicity returns to G ≤1 or baseline. Resume romidepsin therapy at 10 mg/m² per dose. Do not attempt to escalate the dose
G4 nonhematologic toxicity	Withhold treatment with romidepsin until toxicity returns to G ≤1 or baseline. Resume romidepsin therapy at 10 mg/m² per dose. Do not attempt to escalate the dose
Recurrent G3/4 nonhematologic toxicities after romidepsin 10 mg/m²	Discontinue romidepsin
G3/4 neutropenia or thrombocytopenia	Withhold treatment with romidepsin until the specific cytopenia recovers to ANC ≥1500/mm³ and/or platelet count ≥75,000/mm³ or baseline. Resume romidepsin therapy at 14 mg/m per dose²

(continued)

Patient Population Studied

A prospective, single-arm, phase 2 trial that enrolled patients with PTCL. Patients had relapsed or had disease refractory to one or more systemic therapies. Concomitant use of any other anticancer therapy, drugs that could significantly prolong the QTc interval, moderate to significant inhibitors of CYP3A4, or therapeutic warfarin were prohibited. Patients were excluded if they had nontransformed mycosis fungoides or Sézary syndrome, or any known significant cardiac abnormalities (eg, congenital long QT syndrome, QTc interval >480 ms, myocardial infarction within previous 6 months, other significant ECG abnormalities, symptomatic coronary artery disease, congestive heart failure, hypertrophic cardiomyopathy or restrictive cardiomyopathy, uncontrolled hypertension, cardiac arrhythmia requiring antiarrhythmic medications, known history of sustained ventricular tachycardia, ventricular fibrillation, torsades de pointes, or cardiac arrest)

Demographic Characteristics at Study Baseline (Histologically Confirmed Population, N = 130)

	Number (%)
Age, years—median (range)	61 (20–83)
Sex—male-to-female ratio	88 (68%)/42 (32%)
White race/ethnicity	116 (89%)
ECOG performance status*	
0	46 (35)
1	66 (51)
2	17 (13)
International Prognostic Index <2/≥2	31 (24%)/99 (76%)
Time since diagnosis, years—median (range)	1.3 (0.2–17.0)
PTCL subtype based on central diagnosis†	
PTCL NOS	69 (53%)
Angioimmunoblastic T-cell lymphoma	27 (21%)
ALK-1–negative ALCL	21 (16%)
Enteropathy-type T-cell lymphoma	6 (5%)
Subcutaneous panniculitis-like T-cell lymphoma	3 (2%)

(continued)

Patient Population Studied
(continued)

ALK-1–positive ALCL[‡]	1 (1%)
Cutaneous gamma/delta T-cell lymphoma	1 (1%)
Extranodal NK/T-cell lymphoma, nasal type	1 (1%)
Transformed mycosis fungoides	1 (1%)
Type of prior systemic therapy	
Chemotherapy	129 (99%)
Monoclonal antibody therapy	20 (15%)
Other type of immunotherapy	14 (11%)
Number of prior systemic therapies—median (range)	2 (1–8)
1	38 (29%)
2	44 (34%)
3	19 (15%)
4	15 (12%)
>4	14 (11%)
Received prior autologous stem cell transplantation	21 (16%)
Refractory to most recent therapy	49 (38%)

ALCL, anaplastic large-cell lymphoma; ALK–1, anaplastic lymphoma kinase–1; NK, natural killer; NOS, not otherwise specified; PTCL, peripheral T-cell lymphoma
*One patient had missing ECOG performance status at baseline
[†]Also eligible but not enrolled: hepatosplenic TCL
[‡]Eligible because disease progressed after prior autologous bone marrow transplant

Treatment Modifications (continued)

Grade 4 febrile (≥38.5°C [101.3°F]) neutropenia	Withhold treatment with romidepsin until the specific cytopenia recovers to G ≤1 or baseline. Resume romidepsin therapy at 10 mg/m² per dose. Do not attempt to escalate the dose
Thrombocytopenia requiring platelet transfusion	

Note: In patients with congenital long QT syndrome, patients with a history of significant cardiovascular disease, and patients taking antiarrhythmic medicines or medicinal products that lead to significant QT prolongation, appropriate cardiovascular monitoring precautions should be considered, such as the monitoring of electrolytes and ECGs at baseline and periodically during treatment

Efficacy

(N = 130)

Response Rates[*]

Best Response Category

Objective disease response	
(CR/CRu + PR)	38 (29%)
CR/Cru	21 (16%)
CR	19 (15%)
Cru	2 (2%)
PR	17 (13%)
SD	22 (17%)
PD or N/E[†]	70 (54%)
Time to response, months	
All responders (CR/CRu + PR)—median (range)	1.8 (1.0–4.3)
CR/Cru—median (range)	2.4 (1.6–9.6)
Duration of response in months	
All responders (CR/CRu + PR)—median (range)	11.6 (0.5[‡]–34.0)[‡]
CR/Cru—median (range)	N/E (1.2–34.0)[‡]

CR, complete response; CRu, unconfirmed complete response; N/E, not evaluable; PD, progressive disease; PR, partial response; SD, stable disease
*Based on Investigator Assessment. Comparable to Independent Review Committee
[†]Insufficient efficacy data to determine response because of early termination (ie, includes patients determined to have PD by investigators prior to first postbaseline assessment and therefore assessed as N/E according to the IRC)
[‡]Denotes a censored value

CR/CRu Rate and ORR Based on Overall IRC Assessment in Patient Subgroups (Histopathologically Confirmed Population; N = 130)

Subgroup	Total Number of Patients	CR/CRu Rate	P	ORR	P
Sex					
Male	88	12 (14%)	0.79	22 (25%)	1.00
Female	42	7 (17%)		11 (26%)	

(continued)

Efficacy (continued)

Age, years					
>65	81	12 (15%)	1.00	20 (25%)	0.84
≤65	49	7 (14%)		13 (27%)	
PTCL subtype					
PTCL NOS	69	10 (14%)	0.83*	20 (29%)	0.92*
AITL	27	5 (19%)		8 (30%)	
ALK-1–negative ALCL	21	4 (19%)		5 (24%)	
Other subgroups	13	0		0	
International Prognostic Index, baseline					
<2	31	3 (10%)	0.56	7 (23%)	0.81
≥2	99	16 (16%)		26 (26%)	
No. of prior systemic therapies					
≤2	82	11 (13%)	0.62	18 (22%)	0.30
>2	48	8 (17%)		15 (31%)	
Prior stem cell transplantation					
Yes	21	2 (10%)	0.74	5 (24%)	1.00
No	109	17 (16%)		28 (26%)	
Prior monoclonal antibody therapy[†]					
Yes	20	4 (20%)	1.00	5 (25%)	0.49
No	110	15 (14%)		28 (25%)	
Other immunotherapy[‡]					
Yes	14	2 (14%)	1.00	2 (14%)	0.52
No	116	17 (15%)		31 (27%)	
Refractory to last prior therapy					
Yes	49	9 (18%)	0.44	14 (29%)	0.54
No	81	10 (12%)		19 (23%)	

AITL, angioimmunoblastic T-cell lymphoma; ALCL, anaplastic large-cell lymphoma; ALK-1, anaplastic lymphoma kinase-1; CR, complete response; CRu, complete response, unconfirmed; IRC, Independent Review Committee; NOS, not otherwise specified; ORR, objective response rate; PTCL, peripheral T-cell lymphoma
*Based on PTCL NOS, AITL, and ALK-1-negative ALCL
[†]Including alemtuzumab and siplizumab
[‡]Including denileukin diftitox and interferon (type NOS)

Treatment Monitoring

1. *Before treatment:* physical examination; CBC with differential; assessment of serum chemistries; CT scan of the chest, abdomen, and pelvis and bone marrow aspiration and biopsy as indicated
2. *Before each romidepsin dose:* CBC with differential and platelet count; serum electrolytes, including potassium and magnesium
   - Consider cardiovascular monitoring (ie, electrocardiogram at baseline and periodically during treatment) in patients with congenital long QT syndrome, a history of significant cardiovascular disease, and patients taking medicinal products that lead to significant QT prolongation. Ensure that potassium and magnesium are within the normal range before administration of romidepsin
3. *Assessment of efficacy:* radiographic examination at 2- or 3-cycle intervals and at the end of treatment

Toxicity

Adverse Events Reported in at Least 10% of Patients:
All Events and Drug-related Events (as Treated Population, N = 131)

Event	All Events		Drug-related Events	
	All Grades	G ≥3	All Grades	G ≥3
Nausea	77 (59%)	3 (2%)	71 (54%)	2 (2%)
Infections SOC*	72 (55%)	25 (19%)	24 (18%)	8 (6%)
Asthenia/fatigue	72 (55%)	11 (8%)	68 (52%)	7 (5%)
Thrombocytopenia	53 (41%)	32 (24%)	52 (40%)	30 (23%)
Vomiting	51 (39%)	6 (5%)	44 (34%)	5 (4%)
Diarrhea	47 (36%)	3 (2%)	30 (23%)	2 (2%)
Pyrexia	46 (35%)	7 (5%)	22 (17%)	5 (4%)
Neutropenia	39 (30%)	26 (20%)	38 (29%)	24 (18%)
Constipation	39 (30%)	1 (1%)	19 (15%)	0
Anorexia	37 (28%)	2 (2%)	34 (26%)	2 (2%)
Anemia	32 (24%)	14 (11%)	27 (21%)	7 (5%)
Dysgeusia	27 (21%)	0	27 (21%)	0
Cough	23 (18%)	0	2 (2%)	0
Headache	19 (15%)	0	14 (11%)	0
Abdominal pain	18 (14%)	3 (2%)	8 (6%)	0
Dyspnea	17 (13%)	3 (2%)	7 (5%)	1 (1%)
Leukopenia	16 (12%)	8 (6%)	16 (12%)	8 (6%)
Chills	14 (11%))	1 (1%)	6 (5%)	0
Hypokalemia	14 (11%)	3 (2%)	7 (5%)	2 (2%)
Peripheral edema	13 (10%)	1 (1%)	3 (2%)	0
Decreased weight	13 (10%)	0	10 (8%)	0
Stomatitis	13 (10%)	0	9 (7%)	0
Tachycardia	13 (10%)	0	6 (5%)	0

SOC, system organ class (according to Medical Dictionary for Regulatory Activities)
*None of the individual preferred term events in the infections SOC was reported with an incidence ≥10%

PERIPHERAL T-CELL LYMPHOMA • SUBSEQUENT THERAPY

NON-HODGKIN LYMPHOMA REGIMEN: PRALATREXATE

O'Connor OA et al. J Clin Oncol 2011;29:1182–1189

Vitamin supplementation to ameliorate mucositis associated with pralatrexate use:

Cyanocobalamin (vitamin B_{12}) 1 mg; administer by intramuscular injection within 2 weeks before the first dose of pralatrexate repeated every 8–10 weeks after previously administered doses

Folic acid 1–1.25 mg/day; administer orally, continually, starting at least 10 days before the first dose of pralatrexate, and continuing for 30 days after the last dose of pralatrexate

Note:

• Increased methylmalonic acid (>200 nmol/L [>0.2 μmol/L]) or homocysteine (>10 μmol/L) at screening required initiating vitamin supplementation ≥10 days before the first dose of pralatrexate

• Vitamin B_{12} injections may be given on the same day as pralatrexate administration

Pralatrexate 30 mg/m² per dose; administer by intravenous injection over 3–5 minutes once weekly for 6 consecutive weeks followed by 1 week without treatment, every 7 weeks (total dosage/7-week cycle = 180 mg/m²)

Note: Continue treatment until progressive disease (PD) or unacceptable toxicity occurs or at patient/physician discretion

Supportive Care

Antiemetic prophylaxis

Emetogenic potential is **LOW**

See Chapter 42 for antiemetic recommendations

Hematopoietic growth factor (CSF) prophylaxis

Primary prophylaxis may be indicated

See Chapter 43 for more information

Antimicrobial prophylaxis

Risk of fever and neutropenia is *LOW*

Antimicrobial primary prophylaxis to be considered:

• Antibacterial—*Pneumocystis jirovecii* prophylaxis is recommended (eg, cotrimoxazole)

• Antifungal—not indicated

• Antiviral—not indicated unless patient previously had an episode of HSV

Oral care

Standard prophylaxis and treatment for mucositis/stomatitis

Dose Modification

Adverse Event	Treatment Modifications
G2 mucositis	Withhold pralatrexate therapy or omit dose. When toxicity recovers to G ≤1, resume pralatrexate therapy at previous dose
Recurrent G2 mucositis G3 mucositis	Withhold pralatrexate therapy or omit dose. When toxicity recovers to G ≤1, resume pralatrexate therapy at 20 mg/m² per week. Do not attempt to escalate dose
G4 mucositis	Discontinue pralatrexate therapy
G3 nonhematologic toxicity	Withhold pralatrexate therapy or omit dose. When toxicity recovers to G ≤1, resume pralatrexate therapy at 20 mg/m² per week. Do not attempt to escalate dose
G4 nonhematologic toxicity	Discontinue pralatrexate therapy

(continued)

Patient Population Studied

Patients with PTCL according to the Revised European American Lymphoma WHO disease classification were eligible for study (Harris NL et al. Ann Oncol 2000;11[Suppl 1]:S3–S10). Patients were required to have documented disease progression after ≥1 prior treatment. Additional exclusion criteria included prior allogeneic stem cell transplant (SCT), and relapse <75 days after ASCT

Baseline Characteristics of Patients (N = 111)	
Sex, male-to-female ratio	76 (68%)/35 (32%)
Ethnicity	
White	80 (72%)
African American	14 (13%)
Asian	6 (5%)
Hispanic	9 (8%)
Other/unknown	1 (1%)/1 (1%)
Age, years—mean (range)	55.7 (21–85)
≥65 years	40 (36%)
Number of prior therapies for PTCL—median (range)	3 (1–13)
Number of prior systemic therapies for PTCL—median (range)	3 (1–12)
Type of prior therapy for PTCL	
Local therapy	
Radiation therapy	25 (23%)
Photopheresis	10 (9%)
Topical nitrogen mustard	4 (4%)
Systemic therapy	
CHOP	78 (70%)
Platinum-containing multiagent chemotherapy	45 (41%)
Non-platinum-containing multiagent chemotherapy	43 (39%)
Single-agent chemotherapy	36 (32%)
Autologous stem cell transplant	18 (16%)

(continued)

Patient Population Studied
(continued)

Bexarotene	15 (14%)
Other	13 (12%)
Corticosteroids alone	8 (7%)
Hyper-CVAD	8 (7%)
Denileukin diftitox	7 (6%)
Systemic investigational agents	7 (6%)

Histopathology per central review

PTCL unspecified	59 (53%)
Anaplastic large cell lymphoma, primary systemic type[*]	17 (15%)
Angioimmunoblastic T-cell lymphoma	13 (12%)
Transformed mycosis fungoides	12 (11%)
Blastic NK lymphoma (skin, lymph node, or visceral involved)	4 (4%)
Other	2 (2%)
T/NK-cell lymphoma nasal	2 (2%)
Extranodal peripheral T/NK-cell lymphoma unspecified	1 (<1%)
Adult T-cell leukemia/lymphoma (HTLV-1+)	1 (<1%)

CHOP, cyclophosphamide, doxorubicin, vincristine, and prednisone; HTLV, human T-lymphotropic virus; ALK, anaplastic lymphoma kinase; Hyper-CVAD, hyperfractionated cyclophosphamide with vincristine, doxorubicin, and corticosteroids; NK, natural killer; PTCL, peripheral T-cell lymphoma
[*]Eleven ALK-negative, 4 ALK-positive, 2 did not have ALK status determined
Note: Patients treated with corticosteroids alone received other systemic therapies

Dose Modification (continued)

Platelet count <50,000/mm³ for 1 week	Withhold pralatrexate therapy or omit dose. When platelet count >50,000/mm³, resume pralatrexate therapy at previous dose
Platelet count <50,000/mm³ for 2 weeks	Withhold pralatrexate therapy or omit dose. When platelet count >50,000/mm³, resume pralatrexate therapy at 20 mg/m² per week. Do not attempt to escalate dose
Platelet count <50,000/mm³ for ≥3 weeks	Discontinue pralatrexate therapy
ANC 500–1000/mm³ without fever for 1 week	Withhold pralatrexate therapy or omit dose. When ANC >1000/mm³, resume pralatrexate therapy at previous dose
ANC 500–1000/mm³ with fever or ANC <500/mm³ for 1 week	Withhold pralatrexate therapy or omit dose. Administer growth factor support. When ANC >1000/mm³, resume pralatrexate therapy at previous dose with growth factor support
ANC 500–1000/mm³ with fever or ANC <500/mm³ for 2 weeks; Recurrent ANC 500–1000/mm³ with fever or ANC <500/mm³ that lasts 1 week	Withhold pralatrexate therapy or omit dose. Administer growth factor support. When ANC >1000/mm³, resume pralatrexate therapy at 20 mg/m² per week with growth factor support. Do not attempt to escalate dose
ANC 500–1000/mm³ with fever or ANC <500/mm³ that lasts 3 weeks; Second recurrence of ANC 500–1000/mm³ with fever or ANC <500/mm³ that lasts 1 week	Discontinue pralatrexate therapy

Efficacy

Best Response to Treatment and Time-to-event Data (Total N = 109)

	Central Review		Local Investigator
Response and Time to Event	IWC	IWC + PET	
Best response			
CR + CRu + PR	32 (29%)	28 (26%)	43 (39%)
CR	11 (10%)	15 (14%)	17 (16%)
CRu	1 (1%)	0	3 (3%)
PR	20 (18%)	13 (12%)	23 (21%)
SD	21 (19%)	18 (17%)	21 (19%)
PD	40 (37%)	31 (28%)	40 (37%)
UE	2 (2%)	18 (17%)	0
Missing, off treatment in cycle 1	14 (13%)	14 (13%)	5 (5%)
Time to event (number)	32	28	43
Median time to response, days			
First response (range)	46 (37–349)	48 (37–248)	50 (38–358)
Best response (range)	141 (37–726)	136 (37–542)	51 (38–542)

(continued)

Efficacy (*continued*)

Median duration of response, months	10.1	12.7	8.1

CR, complete response; CRu, complete response unconfirmed; IWC, International Workshop Criteria; PD, progressive disease; PET, positron emission tomography; PR, partial response; SD, stable disease; UE, unevaluable

Response Rate by Key Subsets

Parameter	Number (%)	IWC Response Rate Number (%) [95% CI]
Age, years		
<65	70 (64%)	19 (27%) [17 to 39]
≥65	39 (36%)	13 (33%) [19 to 50]
Prior systemic therapy		
1 regimen	23 (21%)	8 (35%) [16 to 57]
2 regimens	29 (27%)	7 (24%) [10 to 44]
>2 regimens	57 (52%)	17 (30%) [18 to 43]
Prior transplant		
Yes	18 (17%)	6 (33%) [13 to 59]
No	91 (83%)	26 (29%) [20 to 39]
Prior methotrexate		
Yes	21 (19%)	5 (24%) [8 to 47]
No	88 (81%)	27 (31%) [21 to 41]
Histology		
PTCL NOS	59 (54%)	19 (32%) [21 to 46]
Angioimmunoblastic	13 (12%)	1 (8%) [0 to 36]
Anaplastic LC	17 (16%)	6 (35%) [14 to 62]
Transformed MF	12 (11%)	3 (25%) [5 to 57]
Other	8 (7%)	3 (38%) [9 to 76]

CI, confidence interval; IWC, International Workshop Criteria; LC, large cell; MF, mycosis fungoides; NOS, not otherwise specified; PTCL, peripheral T-cell lymphoma

Toxicity

Adverse Events in ≥10% of Patients (Safety Population, ≥1 Dose of Study Drug)

Event	Total	G3	G4
Any event[a]	111 (100%)	47 (42%)	35 (32%)
General events and administration site conditions			
Mucositis[†]	79 (71%)	20 (18%)	4 (4%)
Fatigue	40 (36%)	6 (5%)	2 (2%)
Pyrexia	38 (34%)	1 (1%)	1 (1%)
Edema[†]	34 (31%)	1 (1%)	0

(*continued*)

Treatment Monitoring

1. *Before treatment:* physical examination; CBC with differential; assessment of serum chemistries, as well as methylmalonic acid and homocysteine levels; CT scan of the chest, abdomen, and pelvis and bone marrow aspiration and biopsy as indicated
2. *Before each pralatrexate dose:* CBC with differential and platelet count
3. *Assessment of efficacy:* radiographic examination at 2- or 3-cycle intervals and at the end of treatment

Toxicity (*continued*)

Hematologic events			
Thrombocytopenia††	45 (41%)	15 (14%)	21 (19%)
Anemia†	38 (34%)	18 (16%)	2 (2%)
Neutropenia†	28 (25%)	15 (14%)	9 (8%)
Leukopenia†	12 (11%)	4 (4%)	4 (4%)
GI event			
Nausea	46 (41%)	4 (4%)	0
Constipation	38 (34%)	0	0
Vomiting	28 (25%)	2 (2%)	0
Diarrhea	25 (23%)	2 (2%)	0
Dyspepsia†	11 (10%)	0	0
Respiratory, thoracic, and mediastinal events			
Cough	32 (29%)	1 (1%)	0
Epistaxis	29 (26%)	0	0
Dyspnea	21 (19%)	8 (7%)	0
Skin and subcutaneous tissue events			
Rash	17 (15%)	0	0
Pruritus†	16 (14%)	2 (2%)	0
Night sweats	12 (11%)	0	0
Infections			
Upper respiratory tract infection	12 (11%)	1 (1%)	0
Sinusitis	11 (10%)	1 (1%)	0
Other conditions			
Hypokalemia†	18 (16%)	4 (4%)	1 (1%)
Anorexia†	18 (16%)	3 (3%)	0
Pharyngolaryngeal pain	15 (14%)	1 (1%)	0
Liver function test abnormal†	14 (13%)	6 (5%)	0
Back pain	14 (13%)	3 (3%)	0
Abdominal pain	13 (12%)	4 (4%)	0
Headache	13 (12%)	0	0
Pain in extremity	13 (12%)	0	0
Asthenia	12 (11%)	2 (2%)	0
Tachycardia	11 (10%)	0	0

*Twenty-three percent (N = 26) withdrew from treatment because of AEs, most frequently for mucositis (6%) or thrombocytopenia (5%)
†Included a grouping of similar preferred terms
‡Platelet count <10,000/mm³ was seen in 5 patients
Note: Patients could have >1 adverse event

PERIPHERAL T-CELL LYMPHOMA • SUBSEQUENT THERAPY

NON-HODGKIN LYMPHOMA REGIMEN: BELINOSTAT

O'Connor OA et al. J Clin Oncol 2015;33:2492–2499
Beleodaq (belinostat) prescribing information. Irvine, CA: Spectrum Pharmaceuticals, Inc; 2017 April

Belinostat 1000 mg/m² per dose; administer intravenously in 250 mL 0.9% sodium chloride injection over 30 minutes once daily for 5 consecutive days on days 1–5, every 21 days, until disease progression (total dosage/21-day course = 5000 mg/m²)

Supportive Care
Antiemetic prophylaxis
Emetogenic potential is **LOW**
See Chapter 42 for antiemetic recommendations

Hematopoietic growth factor (CSF) prophylaxis
Primary prophylaxis is **NOT** indicated
See Chapter 43 for more information

Antimicrobial prophylaxis
Risk of fever and neutropenia is *LOW*
Antimicrobial primary prophylaxis to be considered:
- Antibacterial—not indicated
- Antifungal—not indicated
- Antiviral—not indicated unless patient previously had an episode of HSV

Diarrhea Management
Latent or delayed onset diarrhea:
- **Loperamide** 4 mg orally initially after the first loose or liquid stool, *then*
- **Loperamide** 2 mg orally every 2 hours during waking hours, *plus*
- **Loperamide** 4 mg orally every 4 hours during hours of sleep
- Continue for at least 12 hours after diarrhea resolves
- Recurrent diarrhea after a 12-hour diarrhea-free interval is treated as a new episode
- Rehydrate orally with fluids and electrolytes during a diarrheal episode
- If a patient develops blood or mucus in stool, dehydration, or hemodynamic instability, or if diarrhea persists >48 hours despite loperamide, stop loperamide and hospitalize the patient for IV hydration

Alternatively, a trial of **diphenoxylate hydrochloride** 2.5 mg **with atropine sulfate** 0.025 mg (eg, Lomotil)
- Initial adult dose is 2 tablets 4 times daily until control has been achieved, after which the dose may be reduced to meet individual requirements. Control may often be maintained with as little as 2 tablets daily
- Clinical improvement of acute diarrhea is usually observed within 48 hours. If improvement of chronic diarrhea after treatment with a maximum daily dose of 8 tablets is not observed within 10 days, control is unlikely with further administration

Treatment Modifications

Belinostat	
Starting dose	1000 mg/m² per dose on days 1–5
Dose level −1	750 mg/m² per dose on days 1–5
Dose level −2	500 mg/m² per dose on days 1–5
Dose level −3	Discontinue belinostat

(continued)

Patient Population Studied

The international, multicenter, nonrandomized, open-label, phase 2 trial (BELIEF) involved 129 patients with relapsed/refractory peripheral T-cell lymphoma. Eligible patients had received at least 1 prior treatment, and were >100 days from hematopoietic stem-cell transplantation. Patients with precursor or adult T-cell lymphoma or leukemia, prolymphocytic leukemia, T-cell large granular lymphocytic leukemia, primary cutaneous anaplastic large-cell lymphoma, mycosis fungoides, or Sézary syndrome were ineligible

Efficacy

(N = 120)

Overall response rate*	25.8%
Median duration of response	13.6 months
Median progression-free survival	1.6 months
Median overall survival	7.9 months

*Overall response rate includes patients with either a complete or partial response

Toxicity

(N = 129)

Grade (%)*	Grade 1–2	Grade 3–4	Grade 5
Pneumonia	<1	5	<1
Pyrexia	5	0	0
Infection	0	3	0
Multiorgan failure	0	0	2
Anemia	0	2	0
Thrombocytopenia	0	2	0
Elevated blood creatinine level	2	0	0

*According to the National Cancer Institute Common Terminology Criteria for Adverse Events, version 3.0
Note: Treatment-emergent serious adverse events that occurred in >2 patients are included. Treatment discontinuation for treatment-emergent adverse events was reported for 19.4% patients, with 10.9% being considered related to treatment. A total of 10 deaths (7.8%) were attributed to treatment-emergent adverse events within 30 days of the last belinostat dose, but all except 1 of these deaths were considered unrelated to belinostat

Therapy Monitoring

1. *Prior to each cycle:* CBC with differential and platelet count, serum chemistries, liver function tests
2. *Weekly during therapy:* CBC with differential and platelet count
3. *Response assessment every 2–4 cycles:* CT scan with contrast and/or PET scan, physical examination

Treatment Modifications (*continued*)

Adverse Event	Treatment Modification
Hematologic Toxicity	
Day 1 ANC <1000/mm^3 or platelet count <50,000/mm^3	Delay initiation of a belinostat cycle until ANC >1000/mm^3 and platelet count >50,000/mm^3
G4 thrombocytopenia (any platelet count <25,000/mm^3) or G4 neutropenia (any ANC <500/mm^3)	Delay belinostat treatment until ANC >1000/mm^3 and platelet count >50,000/mm^3, then decrease the belinostat dosage by 1 dose level
Gastrointestinal Toxicity	
G ≥3 nausea, or G ≥3 vomiting, or G ≥3 diarrhea persisting for >7 days despite maximum supportive management	Delay belinostat treatment until toxicity resolves to G ≤2, then decrease the belinostat dosage by 1 dose level
Hepatic Impairment and Hepatic Toxicity	
G ≥3 increase in AST or ALT (ALT or AST >5× ULN) or G ≥3 increase in bilirubin (bilirubin >3× ULN)	Interrupt therapy until toxicity resolves to G ≤2. Depending on the severity of hepatic toxicity and at the discretion of the medically responsible healthcare provider, may either decrease the belinostat dosage by 1 lower dose level or permanently discontinue belinostat
Patients with moderate or severe baseline hepatic impairment	Patients with total bilirubin >1.5× ULN were excluded from clinical trials. Due to insufficient data, no recommendation for belinostat dosage is available in patients with moderate-severe hepatic impairment
Drug Interactions	
Patient requires concomitant therapy with a strong UGT1A1 inhibitor	Belinostat is primarily metabolized by UGT1A1. Therefore, avoid concomitant administration of belinostat with strong UGT1A1 inhibitors
Pharmacogenomics	
Patient is known to be homozygous for the UGT1A1*28 allele	Belinostat is primarily metabolized by UGT1A1. Therefore, reduce the starting dose of belinostat to 750 mg/m^2 per dose on days 1–5 to minimize toxicity
Other Toxicities	
Other G ≥3 nonhematologic toxicity	Delay treatment until toxicity resolves to G ≤2, then decrease the belinostat dosage by 1 dose level

Belinostat may cause fetal harm. Advise females of reproductive potential of the potential risk to a fetus and to use effective contraception during belinostat therapy

ANC, absolute neutrophil count; AST, aspartate aminotransferase; ALT, alanine aminotransferase; ULN, upper limit of normal

O'Connor OA et al. J Clin Oncol 2015;33:2492–2499

Beleodaq (belinostat) prescribing information. Irvine, CA: Spectrum Pharmaceuticals, Inc; 2017 April

PERIPHERAL T-CELL LYMPHOMA • SUBSEQUENT THERAPY
NON-HODGKIN LYMPHOMA REGIMEN: BRENTUXIMAB VEDOTIN

Horwitz SM et al. Blood 2014;123:3095–3100
Pro B et al. J Clin Oncol 2012;30:2190–2196
Adcetris (brentuximab vedotin) prescribing information. Bothell, WA: Seattle Genetics, Inc; Revised 2018 March

Brentuximab vedotin 1.8 mg/kg (maximum dose = 180 mg); administer intravenously in a volume of 0.9% sodium chloride injection or 5% dextrose injection sufficient to produce a concentration with the range 0.4–1.8 mg/mL (minimum volume, 100 mL) over 30 minutes on day 1, every 3 weeks until disease progression (total dosage/cycle = 1.8 mg/kg; maximum dose/cycle = 180 mg)

Notes on brentuximab vedotin administration:
- The dose for patients whose body weight is >100 kg should be calculated based on a weight of 100 kg (maximum single dose = 180 mg)
- No dose reduction is necessary in patients with mild-moderate renal impairment (creatinine clearance ≥30 mL/min and ≤80 mL/min). Avoid use in patients with severe renal impairment (creatinine clearance <30 mL/min)
- The recommended starting dose in patients with mild hepatic impairment (Child-Pugh A) is 1.2 mg/kg (maximum single dose = 120 mg) intravenously over 30 minutes every 3 weeks. Avoid use in patients with Child-Pugh B or Child-Pugh C hepatic impairment
- Brentuximab vedotin can cause severe or life-threatening infusion-related reactions, including hypersensitivity and anaphylaxis
  - Monitor patients for signs and symptoms of infusion-related reactions including rigors, chills, wheezing, pruritus, flushing, rash, hypotension, hypoxemia, and fever
  - If anaphylaxis occurs, stop administration and permanently discontinue brentuximab vedotin
  - If an infusion related reaction occurs, stop the infusion and provide appropriate medical treatment. Consider premedication with acetaminophen, antihistamine, and a corticosteroid with subsequent cycles
- Monomethyl auristatin E (MMAE), the cytotoxic component of brentuximab vedotin, is a substrate of CYP3A4/5 and P-glycoprotein (P-gp). Use caution, and monitor closely for brentuximab vedotin side effects when co-administering brentuximab vedotin with strong CYP3A4 inhibitors or P-gp inhibitors

Supportive Care
Antiemetic prophylaxis
Emetogenic potential is **LOW**
See Chapter 42 for antiemetic recommendations

Hematopoietic growth factor (CSF) prophylaxis
Primary prophylaxis is **NOT** indicated
See Chapter 43 for more information

Antimicrobial prophylaxis
Risk of fever and neutropenia is *LOW*
Antimicrobial primary prophylaxis to be considered:
- Antibacterial—not indicated
- Antifungal—not indicated
- Antiviral— not indicated unless patient previously had an episode of HSV

Diarrhea management
- **Loperamide** 4 mg orally initially after the first loose or liquid stool, *then*
- **Loperamide** 2 mg orally every 2 hours during waking hours, *plus*
- **Loperamide** 4 mg orally every 4 hours during hours of sleep
- Continue for at least 12 hours after diarrhea resolves
- Recurrent diarrhea after a 12-hour diarrhea-free interval is treated as a new episode
- Rehydrate orally with fluids and electrolytes during a diarrheal episode
- If a patient develops blood or mucus in stool, dehydration, or hemodynamic instability, or if diarrhea persists >48 hours despite loperamide, stop loperamide and hospitalize the patient for IV hydration

Alternatively, a trial of **diphenoxylate hydrochloride** 2.5 mg **with atropine sulfate** 0.025 mg (eg, Lomotil)
- Initial adult dose is 2 tablets 4 times daily until control has been achieved, after which the dose may be reduced to meet individual requirements. Control may often be maintained with as little as 2 tablets daily
- Clinical improvement of acute diarrhea is usually observed within 48 hours. If improvement of chronic diarrhea after treatment with a maximum daily dose of 8 tablets is not observed within 10 days, control is unlikely with further administration

Patient Population Studied

The multicenter, open-label, phase 2 trial involved 35 patients with relapsed/refractory T-cell lymphomas with detectable CD30 expression. Eligible patients were aged ≥12 years, and had an Eastern Cooperative Oncology Group (ECOG) performance status score ≤2, measurable disease, and received at least 1 prior systemic therapy. Patients with Sézary syndrome, mycosis fungoides, or anaplastic large cell lymphoma were ineligible, as were patients who had previously been treated with brentuximab vedotin. Patients received 21-day cycles of intravenous brentuximab vedotin (1.8 mg/kg on day 1) until disease progression, unacceptable toxicity, or study closure

Efficacy

(N = 34)

Objective response rate*	41%
Median duration of response	7.6 months
Median progression-free survival	2.6 months

Overall response rate includes patients with either a complete or partial response
Note: Median follow-up was 2.7 months

Treatment Modifications

Brentuximab Vedotin	
Starting dose	1.8 mg/kg (maximum dose = 180 mg) every 3 weeks
Dose level 1	1.2 mg/kg (maximum dose = 120 mg) every 3 weeks
Adverse Event	**Dose Modification**

General Dose Modification	
Patient weight >100 kg	Use a maximum weight of 100 kg for calculation of the brentuximab vedotin dose

Hepatic Impairment	
Patient with mild hepatic impairment (Child-Pugh class A)	Reduce dose to 1.2 mg/kg (maximum dose = 120 mg) every 3 weeks

Infusion-Related Reaction and Anaphylactic Reaction Adverse Events	
Infusion-related reaction	Interrupt infusion and initiate appropriate medical management. For subsequent cycles, premedicate with acetaminophen, antihistamine, and corticosteroids
Anaphylactic reaction	Permanently discontinue brentuximab vedotin

Neuropathy Adverse Events	
New or worsening G2/3 neuropathy	Delay brentuximab vedotin until improvement to G ≤1 or baseline, then resume at dose level 1
G4 neuropathy	Permanently discontinue brentuximab vedotin

Hematologic Adverse Events	
G3/4 neutropenia	Delay brentuximab vedotin until improvement to G ≤2. Consider G-CSF prophylaxis during subsequent cycles
Recurrent G4 neutropenia despite use of prophylactic G-CSF	Delay brentuximab vedotin until improvement to G ≤2. Continue G-CSF prophylaxis during subsequent cycles, and either reduce brentuximab vedotin to dose level 1 or permanently discontinue brentuximab vedotin
G3 thrombocytopenia First occurrence of G4 thrombocytopenia	Delay brentuximab vedotin until improvement to G ≤2, then resume treatment at the same dose
Second occurrence of G4 thrombocytopenia	Delay brentuximab vedotin until improvement to G ≤2, then resume treatment at dose level 1

Pulmonary Adverse Events	
New or worsening pulmonary symptoms	Delay brentuximab vedotin during evaluation and until symptomatic improvement. Upon improvement, depending on the severity of symptoms and results of diagnostic evaluation, consider permanently discontinuing brentuximab vedotin, reducing to dose level 1, or continuing the same dose

Severe Dermatologic Adverse Events	
SJS or TEN	Permanently discontinue brentuximab vedotin

Opportunistic Infection Adverse Events	
PML suspected (eg, new neurologic deficit)	Delay brentuximab vedotin during evaluation
PML confirmed	Permanently discontinue brentuximab vedotin

(continued)

Treatment Modifications (*continued*)

Other Nonhematologic Adverse Events

Other nonhematologic G3 Adverse Event (excluding electrolyte abnormalities)	Delay brentuximab vedotin until adverse event resolves to G ≤1 or baseline, then resume treatment at the same dose
Other nonhematologic G4 Adverse Event (excluding electrolyte abnormalities)	Delay brentuximab vedotin until adverse event resolves to G ≤1 or baseline, then resume treatment at dose level 1

G-CSF, granulocyte-colony stimulating factor; SJS, Stevens-Johnson Syndrome; TEN, toxic epidermal necrolysis; PML, progressive multifocal leukoencephalopathy

Horwitz SM et al. Blood 2014;123:3095–3100

Adcetris (brentuximab vedotin) prescribing information. Bothell, WA: Seattle Genetics, Inc; Revised 2018 March

Toxicity

(N = 35)

Grade[*]	Grade 3 (%)	Grade 4 (%)	Grade 5 (%)
Neutropenia	14	0	0
Hyperkalemia	6	3	0
Peripheral sensory neuropathy	9	0	0
Disease progression	3	0	3
Pneumonia	3	3	0
Acute renal failure	6	0	0
Anemia	6	0	0
Dehydration	6	0	0
Thrombocytopenia	6	0	0
Tumor lysis syndrome	6	0	0
Urinary tract infection	6	0	0

[*]According to the NCI Common Terminology Criteria for Adverse Events, version 4.0.3

Note: Grade ≥3 adverse events that occurred in at least 2 patients are included. Treatment discontinuation owing to adverse events was reported for 20% patients. One death within 30 days of the last dose was attributed, in part, to study treatment

Therapy Monitoring

1. *Prior to initiation of therapy:* CBC with differential and platelet count, serum electrolytes, liver function tests, serum creatinine, BUN, urine pregnancy test (women of child-bearing potential only)

2. *In patients at high risk for tumor lysis syndrome (eg, high tumor burden, renal dysfunction, rapidly progressing disease, markedly elevated LDH, baseline abnormalities in laboratory indices of tumor lysis syndrome [potassium, phosphate, uric acid, calcium, serum creatinine]):* Consider frequent monitoring of laboratory indices of tumor lysis syndrome, intravenous hydration, and prophylaxis with a xanthine oxidase inhibitor (eg, allopurinol)

3. *During each brentuximab vedotin infusion:* Signs and symptoms of infusion-related reaction, vital signs every 30 minutes

4. *Prior to each cycle:* CBC with differential and platelet count, serum electrolytes, liver function tests, serum creatinine, BUN

5. *Periodically assess for:* Peripheral neuropathy, pulmonary toxicity, severe dermatologic toxicity, gastrointestinal toxicity, infection, and progressive multifocal leukoencephalopathy

6. *Response evaluation:* Physical exam prior to each cycle, CT scan with contrast, and/or PET scan every 2–3 cycles

PERIPHERAL T-CELL LYMPHOMA • SUBSEQUENT THERAPY

NON-HODGKIN LYMPHOMA REGIMEN: BENDAMUSTINE

Damaj G et al. J Clin Oncol 2012;31:104–110

Premedication for bendamustine HCl: Premedications are not necessary for primary prophylaxis of infusion-related reactions. In the event of a non-severe infusion-related reaction, consider adding a histamine receptor (H_1)-subtype antagonist (eg, diphenhydramine 25–50 mg intravenously or orally), an antipyretic (eg, acetaminophen 650–1000 mg orally), and a corticosteroid (eg, methylprednisolone 100 mg intravenously) administered 30 minutes prior to bendamustine HCl administration in subsequent cycles

Bendamustine HCl 120 mg/m² per dose; administer intravenously in a volume of 0.9% sodium chloride injection (0.9% NS) sufficient to produce a concentration with the range 0.2–0.6 mg/mL over 30–60 minutes, on 2 consecutive days, days 1 and 2, every 21 days for 6 cycles (total dosage/21-day cycle = 240 mg/m²)

Notes on bendamustine HCl:

- Bendamustine HCl can cause severe infusion-related reactions
  - For grade 1–2 infusion-related reactions, consider rechallenge with the addition of antihistamine, antipyretic, and corticosteroid premedications (as described in the above premedication section)
  - For grade 3 infusion-related reactions, consider permanent discontinuation versus rechallenge with the addition of antihistamine, antipyretic, and corticosteroid premedications (as described in the above premedication section) after weighing risks and benefits
  - For grade 4 infusion-related reactions, permanently discontinue bendamustine HCl

- Coadministration of strong CYP1A2 inhibitors (eg, ciprofloxacin, fluvoxamine) may increase exposure to bendamustine HCl and decrease exposure to its active metabolites. Concomitant CYP1A2 inducers (eg, omeprazole, cigarette smoking) may decrease exposure to bendamustine HCl and increase exposure to its active metabolites. Use caution, or select an alternative therapy, when coadministration of bendamustine HCl with strong CYP1A2 inhibitors or inducers is unavoidable

- Bendamustine HCl formulations may vary by country; consult local regulatory-approved labeling for guidance. For example, in the United States, the Food and Drug Administration–approved Bendeka under Section 505(b)(2) of the Federal Food, Drug, and Cosmetic Act on 7 December 2015. The Bendeka product labeling contains specific dilution and administration instructions, *thus*:

  Bendamustine HCl (Bendeka, where available) 120 mg/m² per dose; administer intravenously in a volume of 0.9% NS or 5% dextrose injection (D5W) sufficient to produce a concentration with the range 1.85–5.6 mg/mL, over 10 minutes, on 2 consecutive days, days 1 and 2, every 21 days for 6 cycles (total dosage/21-day cycle = 240 mg/m²)

Supportive Care

Antiemetic prophylaxis

Emetogenic potential is **MODERATE**

See Chapter 42 for antiemetic recommendations

Hematopoietic growth factor (CSF) prophylaxis

Primary prophylaxis **MAY** be indicated

See Chapter 43 for more information

Antimicrobial prophylaxis

Risk of fever and neutropenia is *INTERMEDIATE*

Antimicrobial primary prophylaxis to be considered:

- Antibacterial—consider a fluoroquinolone during periods of prolonged neutropenia, or no prophylaxis
- Antifungal—consider use during periods of prolonged neutropenia
- Antiviral—antiherpes antivirals (eg, acyclovir, famciclovir, valacyclovir)

Treatment Modifications

Bendamustine Dose Modifications

Starting dose	120 mg/m² per dose on days 1 and 2
Dose level −1	90 mg/m² per dose on days 1 and 2
Dose level −2	60 mg/m² per dose on days 1 and 2
Dose level −3	Discontinue bendamustine
Adverse Event	**Dose Modification**

Hematologic Toxicity

Day 1 platelet count <75,000/mm³ or Day 1 ANC <1000/mm³	Delay start of cycle until platelet count ≥ 75,000/mm³ and ANC ≥1000/mm³ or until recovery to near baseline values, then reduce by 1 dose level for subsequent cycles. Consider G-CSF use in subsequent cycles for dose-limiting neutropenia
G4 neutropenia (ANC <500/mm³) or G4 thrombocytopenia (platelet count <25,000/mm³)	Delay start of cycle until platelet count ≥75,000/mm³ and ANC ≥1000/mm³ or until recovery to near baseline values, then reduce the bendamustine dosage by 1 dose level for subsequent cycles. Consider G-CSF use in subsequent cycles for dose-limiting neutropenia or severe neutropenic complications

Infectious Complications

Active infection	Interrupt bendamustine until resolution of infection, then resume bendamustine at either the same dose, or reduced by 1 dose level, depending on the severity of infection

Drug Interactions

Patient requires concomitant therapy with a CYP1A2 inhibitor (eg, fluvoxamine, ciprofloxacin)	Consider alternative treatment instead of the CYP1A2 inhibitor. If the CYP1A2 inhibitor cannot be avoided, use caution, and monitor carefully for bendamustine adverse effects
Patient requires concomitant therapy with a CYP1A2 inducer (eg, omeprazole), or patient is a smoker	Consider alternative treatment instead of the CYP1A2 inducer. Recommend cessation of smoking, if applicable. If the CYP1A2 inducer cannot be avoided, use caution and monitor carefully for reduced bendamustine efficacy

Other Toxicities

G ≥3 nonhematologic toxicity during the prior cycle	Delay start of cycle until nonhematologic toxicity resolves to G ≤1 or baseline, then reduce the bendamustine dosage by 1 dose level for subsequent cycles

ANC, absolute neutrophil count; G-CSF, granulocyte colony-stimulating factor

Bendeka (bendamustine hydrochloride injection) prescribing information. North Wales, PA: Teva Pharmaceuticals USA, Inc; 2018 July

Damaj G et al. J Clin Oncol 2012;31:104–110

Patient Population Studied

The prospective, open-label, single-agent, phase 2 trial involved 60 patients with relapsed/refractory, histologically confirmed, stage IIB or higher, peripheral T-cell lymphoma or cutaneous T-cell lymphoma. Eligible patients were aged ≥18 years, and had an Eastern Cooperative Oncology Group (ECOG) performance status score ≤3, measurable disease, and received 1–3 prior lines of chemotherapy. Patients with Sézary syndrome, T-cell leukemia-lymphoma associated with human T-lymphotropic virus, or prior history of malignancies other than T-cell lymphoma within the preceding 3 years were ineligible

Efficacy

(N = 60)

Overall response rate after three cycles*	50%
Median duration of response	3.50 months
Median progression-free survival	3.63 months
Median overall survival	6.27 months

*Overall response rate includes patients with either a complete or partial response

Toxicity

(N = 60)

- Most frequent G3/4 adverse events were neutropenia (which occurred in 57% patients) and thrombocytopenia (occurring in 38% patients)
- The other most frequent G3/4 toxicities included infections, skin reactions, mucositis, and arrhythmia
- Serious adverse events not related to disease progression occurred in 31 (52%) patients. Deaths secondary to infections occurred in four (7%) patients

Therapy Monitoring

1. *Prior to treatment initiation*: CBC with differential, chemistries (potassium, uric acid, phosphorus, calcium, serum creatinine, LDH), serum bilirubin, ALT or AST, urine pregnancy test (women of child-bearing potential only)

2. *Prior to each cycle*: CBC with differential, serum chemistries, serum bilirubin, ALT or AST

3. *Weekly during treatment*: CBC with differential

4. *In patients at high risk for tumor lysis syndrome (eg, high tumor burden, renal dysfunction, rapidly progressing disease, markedly elevated LDH, baseline abnormalities in laboratory indices of tumor lysis syndrome [potassium, phosphate, uric acid, calcium, serum creatinine])*: Consider frequent monitoring of laboratory indices of tumor lysis syndrome, intravenous hydration, and prophylaxis with a xanthine oxidase inhibitor (eg, allopurinol)

5. *Monitor periodically for*: Signs and symptoms of infection and dermatologic toxicity

6. *Response assessment every 2–3 cycles*: Physical examination, CT scans

BURKITT LYMPHOMA—FIRST LINE

DOSE-ADJUSTED ETOPOSIDE + PREDNISONE + VINCRISTINE + CYCLOPHOSPHAMIDE + DOXORUBICIN + RITUXIMAB (DA-EPOCH-R)

Dunleavy K et al. N Engl J Med 2013;369:1915–1925

Prophylaxis against hyperuricemia during cycle 1: **Allopurinol** 600 mg; administer orally for 1 dose 24 hours before administering antineoplastic treatment, *and then:*

Allopurinol 300 mg/day; administer orally for 6 consecutive days, on days 2–7

Note:

• Monitor chemistries (uric acid, potassium, phosphorus, calcium) for tumor lysis

• The initial 600-mg dose may be replaced by a 300-mg dose in patients who are already receiving allopurinol

• Additional measures, such as hospitalization with aggressive intravenous hydration, were used at investigators' discretion

• Persons who express a variant human leukocyte antigen allele, HLA-B*58:01, are at increased risk for severe cutaneous adverse reactions from allopurinol (Hershfield MS et al. Clin Pharmacol Ther 2013;93:153–158; Zineh I et al. Pharmacogenomics 2011;12:1741–1749)

• Consider alternative prophylaxis (rasburicase) in patients at high risk for hyperuricemia, and for treatment

Prednisone 60 mg/m²; administer orally, twice daily for 5 consecutive days, on days 1–5 (10 doses), every 21 days, for 6–8 cycles (total dosage/cycle = 600 mg/m²)

• The first prednisone dose should be given at least 1 hour before rituximab administration begins

• Patients who were unable to ingest oral medications may receive a parenterally administered steroid at a glucocorticoid equivalent dosage for the same number of doses on the same administration schedule (eg, methylprednisolone 48 mg/m² per dose)

Rituximab

Premedication for rituximab:

Acetaminophen 650–1000 mg; administer orally *plus* **diphenhydramine** 25–50 mg; administer orally or intravenously 30–60 minutes before each dose of rituximab

Rituximab 375 mg/m²; administer intravenously in 0.9% sodium chloride injection (0.9% NS) or 5% dextrose injection (D5W) diluted to a concentration within the range of 1–4 mg/mL, on day 1, every 21 days, for 6–8 cycles (total dosage/cycle = 375 mg/m²)

Notes on rituximab administration:

• Infuse initially at 50 mg/h. If hypersensitivity or infusion reactions do not occur during the first 30 minutes, increase the rate by 50 mg/h every 30 minutes as tolerated to a maximum rate of 400 mg/h. Subsequently, if previous administration was well tolerated, start at 100 mg/h and increase by 100 mg/h every 30 minutes as tolerated to a maximum rate of 400 mg/h

INFUSION REACTIONS ASSOCIATED WITH RITUXIMAB

Fevers, chills, and rigors

1. Interrupt rituximab administration for severe symptoms, and give:

   • **Acetaminophen** 650 mg orally for fever. For persistent or recurrent symptoms, repeat administration every 4–6 hours as needed during rituximab administration

   • **Diphenhydramine** 25–50 mg orally or by intravenous injection for pruritus, hypotension, or angioedema. For persistent or recurrent symptoms, repeat administration every 4–6 hours as needed during rituximab administration

   • **Meperidine** 12.5–25 mg by intravenous injection every 10–20 minutes as needed for shaking chills (generally, cumulative doses >100 mg are not needed; use repeated doses with caution in persons with moderate or more severely impaired renal function)

2. If rituximab administration was interrupted, resume infusion at a slower rate than the maximum rate previously attempted. Rate escalation may be reattempted at smaller incremental steps with close monitoring. Do not exceed the maximum recommended rate of 400 mg/h

Dyspnea or wheezing without allergic findings (urticaria, or tongue or laryngeal edema)

1. Interrupt rituximab administration immediately

2. Give **hydrocortisone** 100 mg by intravenous injection (or an alternative steroid with equivalent glucocorticoid potency)

3. Give a **histamine (H₂) receptor antagonist** (ranitidine 50 mg, cimetidine 300 mg, or famotidine 20 mg) intravenously over 15–30 minutes

4. After symptoms resolve, resume rituximab administration at 25 mg/h with close monitoring. Do not increase the administration rate

Note: Medications and equipment for the treatment of hypersensitivity reactions should be available for immediate use in the event of a reaction during administration (eg, intravenous fluids, epinephrine, antihistamines, glucocorticoids, and oxygen)

Rituxan (rituximab) prescribing information. South San Francisco, CA: Genentech, Inc; 2018 October

Etoposide + doxorubicin + vincristine "3-in-1" admixture (preparation instructions appear below*)

Etoposide: administer by continuous intravenous infusion over 24 hours for 4 consecutive days, on days 1–4, every 21 days, for 6–8 cycles (see the table below for daily dosage and total dosage/cycle†)

Doxorubicin: administer by continuous intravenous infusion over 24 hours for 4 consecutive days, on days 1–4, every 21 days, for 6–8 cycles (see the table below for daily dosage and total dosage/cycle†)

Vincristine: administer by continuous intravenous infusion over 24 hours for 4 consecutive days, on days 1–4, every 21 days, for 6–8 cycles (total dosage/cycle = 1.6 mg/m²)

Hydration before and after cyclophosphamide administration: Give 0.9% NS (volumes specified below) at 300–500 mL/h

EPOCH Dose Level	Total Volume of Hydration Fluid[‡]
1 and 2	1000 mL
3, 4, and 5	2000 mL
≥6	2500 mL

Cyclophosphamide 750 mg/m^2; administer intravenously in 100–150 mL 0.9% NS or D5W over 30 minutes on day 5 (after completing infusional etoposide + doxorubicin + vincristine), every 21 days for 6–8 cycles (see the table below for dosage specifications[†])
Filgrastim 480 µg/day; administer by subcutaneous injection, daily for 10 consecutive days, on days 6–15, *or* until postnadir ANC is >5000/mm^3

*Etoposide + doxorubicin + vincristine "3-in-1" admixtures—preparation, storage, and stability
• To prepare a "3-in-1" admixture with etoposide + doxorubicin + vincristine, dilute all 3 drug products in 0.9% sodium chloride injection (0.9% NS) as follows:

Total Dose of Etoposide	0.9% NS Volume to Use
≤130 mg	500 mL
>130 mg	1000 mL

Admixture with etoposide (base):
• Etoposide 50 mg/m^2, doxorubicin hydrochloride 10 mg/m^2, and vincristine sulfate 0.4 mg/m^2 admixtures diluted in 0.9% NS to produce an etoposide concentration <250 µg/mL, in polyolefin-lined infusion bags are stable and compatible for 72 hours at 23°–25°C (73.4°–77°F), and at 31°–33°C (87.8°–91.4°F) when protected from exposure to light (Wolfe JL et al. Am J Health Syst Pharm 1999;56:985–989)

Admixture with etoposide PHOSphate:
• Etoposide PHOSphate, doxorubicin hydrochloride, and vincristine sulfate admixtures diluted in 0.9% NS to produce an etoposide concentration <250 µg/mL, in polyolefin-lined infusion bags are stable and compatible for up to 124 hours at 2°–6°C (35.6°–42.8°F) and 35°–40°C (95°–104°F) in the dark and in regular fluorescent light. In admixtures stored at 35°–40°C (95°–104°F) and exposed to light, the initial drug concentrations decreased slightly, but remained within acceptable concentrations (Yuan P et al. Am J Health Syst Pharm 2001;58:594–598)

The "3-in-1" admixtures described above will not prevent microbial growth after exposure to bacterial and fungal contamination. With respect to product sterility, expiration dating should be determined by the aseptic techniques used in preparation and local and national guidelines

[†]**EPOCH Dosage Levels:**
• At dosage levels 1 through 6, adjustments apply *only* to etoposide, doxorubicin, and cyclophosphamide
• At dosage levels −1 or −2, adjustments apply *only* to cyclophosphamide (20% dosage reductions for each dosage decrement)

	Dosage Levels							
	−2	−1	1	2	3	4	5	6
Drugs	Daily Dosages (mg/m^2 × day)							
Doxorubicin	10	10	10	12	14.4	17.3	20.7	24.8
Etoposide	50	50	50	60	72	86.4	103.7	124.4
Cyclophosphamide	480	600	750	900	1080	1296	1555	1866

	Total Dosage per Cycle (mg/m^2 × 96 hours)							
Doxorubicin	40	40	40	48	57.6	69.2	82.8	99.2
Etoposide	200	200	200	240	288	345.6	414.8	497.6
Cyclophosphamide	480	600	750	900	1080	1296	1555	1866

[‡]Give half the total volume of fluid is before starting cyclophosphamide administration and give half the total volume after completing cyclophosphamide
Note:
• Patients received 2 cycles after complete remission was established, for a total of 6–8 cycles
• HIV-positive patients did not receive antiretroviral therapy during chemotherapy

(continued)

(*continued*)

- DA-EPOCH-R was pharmacodynamically dose-adjusted on the basis of the ANC nadir
- Patients without evidence of cerebrospinal fluid (CSF) involvement received prophylactic intrathecal methotrexate 12 mg via lumbar puncture. Intrathecal treatment was administered on days 1 and 5, every 3 weeks (8 doses), during cycles 3, 4, 5, and 6 (total dose/cycle = 24 mg)
- Patients with evidence of CSF involvement received intrathecal treatment with methotrexate 12 mg via lumbar puncture *or* methotrexate 6 mg via an Ommaya reservoir, twice weekly until 2 weeks after CSF samples are cytologically negative for lymphoma *or* for a minimum duration of 4 weeks, then once weekly for 6 weeks, and then once monthly for 6 months

Antiemetic prophylaxis
Emetogenic potential on Days 1–4 is **LOW**
Emetogenic potential on Day 5 is **MODERATE**
See Chapter 42 for antiemetic recommendations

Hematopoietic growth factor (CSF) prophylaxis
Primary prophylaxis is indicated with:
Filgrastim (G-CSF) use is integral within the R-EPOCH regimen described above

Antimicrobial prophylaxis
Risk of fever and neutropenia is INTERMEDIATE
Antimicrobial primary prophylaxis to be considered:
- Antibacterial—consider a fluoroquinolone or no prophylaxis; *Pneumocystis jirovecii* prophylaxis is recommended (eg, cotrimoxazole)
- Antifungal—recommended; consider use during periods of neutropenia, and in anticipation of mucositis
- Antiviral—antiherpes antivirals (eg, acyclovir, famciclovir, valacyclovir)

Steroid-associated gastritis
Add a **proton pump inhibitor** during steroid use to prevent gastritis and duodenitis

Decreased bowel motility prophylaxis
Give **stool softeners** in a scheduled regimen, and **saline, osmotic, and lubricant laxatives,** as needed to prevent constipation for as long as vincristine use continues. If needed, circumspectly add **stimulant (irritant) laxatives** in the least amounts and for the briefest durations needed to produce defecation

Oral care
Standard prophylaxis and treatment for mucositis/stomatitis

Treatment Modifications

Adverse Events[*]	Treatment Modifications[†]
Creatinine clearance <50 mL/min (<0.83 mL/s)	At any dosage level, decrease etoposide dosage by 50%. If creatinine clearance recovers to >50 mL/min (>0.83 mL/s), etoposide should be given at 100% of planned dosage level
Previous cycle ANC nadir count ≥500/mm³	Increase etoposide, doxorubicin, and cyclophosphamide dosages by 20% greater than the dosages given during the previous cycle (increase by 1 dosage level)
Previous cycle ANC nadir count <500/mm³ on 1 or 2 measurements	Give the same dosages as last cycle
Previous cycle ANC nadir count <500/mm³ on at least 3 measurements	Reduce etoposide, doxorubicin, and cyclophosphamide dosages by 20% less than the dosages given during the previous cycle (decrease by 1 dosage level)
Previous cycle platelet nadir count <25,000/mm³ on 1 measurement	Continue treatment, but withhold vincristine[‡]
Total bilirubin >4.0 mg/dL (>68.4 μmol/L)	Reduce vincristine dosage by 75%[‡]
Total bilirubin >1.5 mg/dL but <3 mg/dL (>25.7 μmol/L but <51.3 μmol/L)	Reduce vincristine dosage by 50%[‡]
G2 neuropathy	Reduce vincristine dosage by 25%[‡]
G3 neuropathy	Reduce vincristine dosage by 50%[‡]

[*]ANC and platelet values based on twice weekly CBC with differential
[†]Dosage adjustment *greater than the starting dose levels* applies only to etoposide, doxorubicin, and cyclophosphamide. Dosage adjustment *less than the starting dose levels* applies only to cyclophosphamide
[‡]Vincristine dosage is increased to 100% if neuropathy resolves to G ≤1 or serum total bilirubin is <1.5 mg/dL (<25.7 μmol/L)

Patient Population Studied

Characteristics of the Patients

Characteristic	All Patients (N = 30)	DA-EPOCH-R (N = 19)	SC-EPOCH-RR (N = 11)
Age in years—median (range)	33 (15–88)[§]	25 (15–88)[§]	44 (24–60)[§]
Age ≥40 years—number (%)	12 (40)	5 (26)	7 (64)
Male sex—number (%)	22 (73)	13 (68)	9 (82)
Ann Arbor stage III or IV—number (%)	20 (67)	11 (58)	9 (82)
ECOG-PS score ≥2—number (%)	9 (30)[ϵ]	3 (16)[ϵ]	6 (55)[ϵ]
Serum LDH >ULN—number (%)	16 (53)[**]	7 (37)[**]	9 (82)[**]
Extranodal site—number (%)[*]	19 (63)	10 (53)	9 (82)
Bowel	15 (50)	9 (47)	6 (55)
Bone marrow or blood	4 (13)	3 (16)	1 (9)
Central nervous system		1 (5)	0
LMB risk group—number (%)[†]			
A	5 (17)	5 (26)	0
B	22 (73)	12 (63)	10 (91)
C	3 (10)	2 (10)	1(9)
Burkitt lymphoma variant—number (%)[**]			
Sporadic	17 (57)	17 (89)	0
Immunodeficiency associated[‡]	13 (43)	2 (11)	11 (100)
Secondary	11 (37)	0	11 (100)
Primary	2 (7)	2 (11)	0
Molecular marker—number/total number (%)			
MYC rearrangement	22/22 (100)	14/14 (100)	8/8 (100)
BCL6 protein expression	24/24 (100)	15/15 (100)	9/9 (100)
BCL2 protein expression	0/26	0/16	0/10
EBER in situ hybridization	6/21 (29)	4/14 (29)	2/7 (29)

DA-EPOCH-R, dose-adjusted infusional therapy with etoposide, doxorubicin, vincristine, with cyclophosphamide, prednisone, and rituximab; ECOG-PS, Eastern Cooperative Oncology Group performance status; EBER, Epstein-Barr virus-encoded RNA; SC-EPOCH-RR short-course infusional therapy with etoposide, doxorubicin, and vincristine, with cyclophosphamide, prednisone, and 2 doses of rituximab; ULN upper limit of the normal range

[*]Patients may have had more than 1 extranodal site

[†]Lymphomes malins B (LMB) risk groups are defined as follows:
- Group A includes patients with low-risk disease (resected stage I or abdominal stage II cancer)
- Group B includes those with intermediate-risk disease (patients not in group A or C)
- Group C includes those with high-risk disease (central nervous system involvement, at least 25% blasts in bone marrow, or both characteristics)

(Société Française d'Oncologie Pédiatrique lymphomes malins B (LMB) prognostic categories [Patte C et al. Blood 2007;109:2773–2780])

[‡]Patients with the immunodeficiency-associated variant may have had HIV infection, the autoimmune lymphoproliferative syndrome, or a deficiency of dedicator of cytokinesis 8

[§]P value = 0.03

[ϵ]P value = 0.04; P value = 0.03

[**]P value <0.001; all other P values >0.06

Efficacy

Clinical Outcome	Immunodeficiency-associated Burkitt Lymphoma	DA-EPOCH-R (N = 19)	SC-EPOCH-RR (N = 11)
Median duration of follow-up	—	86 months	73 months
Rate of freedom from progression	92%	100% (95% CI, 72–100)	95% (95% CI, 75–99)
Overall survival	92%	90% (95% CI, 60–98)	100% (95% CI, 82–100)

CI, confidence interval; DA-EPOCH-R, dose-adjusted infusional therapy with etoposide, doxorubicin, vincristine, with cyclophosphamide, prednisone, and rituximab; SC-EPOCH-RR short-course infusional therapy with etoposide, doxorubicin, and vincristine with cyclophosphamide, prednisone, and 2 doses of rituximab

None of the patients in either group had a recurrence of disease or died from Burkitt lymphoma. However, 1 patient with primary immunodeficiency-associated Burkitt lymphoma did not have a pathologic complete response and received localized radiotherapy. Acute myeloid leukemia developed in 1 HIV-positive patient 2.5 years after the completion of SC-EPOCH-RR, and the patient died 4 months later

Treatment Monitoring

1. *Prior to treatment initiation*: CBC with differential, serum chemistries, serum bilirubin, ALT or AST, hepatitis B core antibody (IgG or total) and hepatitis B surface antigen, left ventricular ejection fraction (LVEF), and urine pregnancy test (women of child-bearing potential only)
   - In addition to baseline monitoring, evaluate LVEF during doxorubicin treatment if clinical symptoms of heart failure are present
   - *In patients at high risk for tumor lysis syndrome* consider frequent monitoring of laboratory indices of tumor lysis syndrome, intravenous hydration, and prophylaxis with a xanthine oxidase inhibitor (eg, allopurinol) during the first cycle
2. *Prior to each cycle*: CBC with differential, serum chemistries, serum bilirubin, ALT or AST
3. *Twice per week (at least 3–4 days apart)*: CBC with differential
4. *Monitor periodically for* signs and symptoms of infection (including progressive multifocal leukoencephalopathy), dermatologic toxicity, peripheral neuropathy (vincristine), constipation (vincristine)

Toxicity

Event	All Cycles (N = 155)	DA-EPOCH-R Cycles (N = 116)	SC-EPOCH-RR Cycles (N = 39)
TLS—no. of cycles (%)	1 (1)	0	1 (3)
Absolute neutropenia—number of cycles (%)			
ANC nadir <500/mm³	72 (46)	60 (52)	12 (31)
ANC nadir <100/mm³	26 (17)	20 (17)	6 (15)
Thrombocytopenia—number of cycles (%)			
Platelets nadir <50,000/mm³	12 (8)	7 (6)	5 (13)
Platelets nadir <25,000/mm³	3 (2)	2 (2)	1 (3)
Fever and neutropenia necessitating hospital admission			
Any patient—number of cycles (%)	30 (19)	26 (22)	4 (10)
Patients ≥40 years of age—number of cycles/total number (%)	4/54 (7)	2/30 (7)	2/24 (8)
Gastrointestinal event—number of cycles (%)*			
Mucositis	8 (5)	7 (6)	1 (9)
Constipation	2 (1)	0	2 (5)
Ileus	2 (1)	2 (2)	0
Neurologic event—number of patients/total number (%)†			
Sensory impairment	5/30 (17)	4/19 (21)	1/11 (9)
Motor impairment	2/30 (7)	2/19 (11)	0/11

NA, not applicable; TLS, Tumor lysis syndrome
*All the gastrointestinal events were G3
†All the sensory-impairment events were G3, and all the motor-impairment events were G2

BURKITT LYMPHOMA • FIRST LINE

NON-HODGKIN LYMPHOMA REGIMEN: CYCLOPHOSPHAMIDE, VINCRISTINE (ONCOVIN), DOXORUBICIN, METHOTREXATE (CODOX-M) + IFOSFAMIDE, ETOPOSIDE (VP–16), AND CYTARABINE (ARA-C) (I-VAC)—(CODOX-M + IVAC)

Magrath I et al. J Clin Oncol 1996;14:925–934

Patients are stratified into high-risk and low-risk groups according to extent of disease and LDH at presentation

Findings at Presentation	Treatment Regimen
Low Risk	
A single extraabdominal mass or completely resected abdominal disease, *and* serum LDH <350 units/L or a concentration within institutional normal range	3 Cycles: A → A → A
High Risk	
All other patients	4 Cycles: A → B → A → B

High- and Low-Risk Patients

Preparation for definitive therapy:

Allopurinol; administer orally or intravenously
- *Initial dosage:* **Allopurinol** 3.3 mg/kg per dose, 3 times daily (daily dosage = 10 mg/kg)
- *Three days after induction treatment commences:* Allopurinol dosage may be decreased to 1.7 mg/kg per dose, 3 times daily (daily dosage = 5 mg/kg)
- *Two weeks after beginning induction treatment:* Allopurinol may be discontinued

Hydration with allopurinol:
3000–4500 mL/m^2 per day, as tolerated; administer intravenously with a solution containing at least 75 mEq sodium/1000 mL
- **Sodium bicarbonate** is added to parenteral hydration solutions in the presence of plasma uric acid ≥9 mg/dL to maintain urine pH ≥7.0

Note:
- Discontinue urinary alkalinization after serum uric acid decreases to <8 mg/dL and before starting chemotherapy
- **Potassium** is not added to parenteral hydration solutions during the first few days of induction therapy unless serum potassium decreases to <3.0 mEq/dL
- **Furosemide** 20–40 mg; administer orally or intravenously, is used to ensure that fluid output is consistent with intake
- Diuresis is maintained for at least the first 72 hours after starting chemotherapy in the absence of metabolic aberrations or after metabolic complications have normalized

High-Risk Patients

4 Cycles A → B → A → B

Regimen A: CODOX-M
Cyclophosphamide 800 mg/m^2; administer intravenously in 50–100 mL 0.9% sodium chloride (0.9% NS) or 5% dextrose injection (D5W) over 30 minutes, given on day 1, *followed by*:
Cyclophosphamide 200 mg/m^2 per day; administer intravenously in 50–100 mL 0.9% NS D5W over 15 minutes for 4 consecutive days, on days 2–5 (total dosage/cycle = 1600 mg/m^2)
Doxorubicin 40 mg/m^2; administer by intravenous injection over 3–5 minutes, given on day 1 (total dosage/cycle = 40 mg/m^2)
Vincristine 1.5 mg/m^2 per dose (maximum single dose is 2.5 mg); administer by intravenous infusion over 15 minutes in 50 mL 0.9% NS, as follows:
- During cycle 1, for 2 doses, on days 1 and 8 (total dosage/cycle = 3 mg/m^2; maximum dose/cycle = 5 mg)
- During cycle 3, for 3 doses, on days 1, 8, and 15 (total dosage/cycle = 4.5 mg/m^2; maximum dose/cycle = 7.5 mg)

Hydration with methotrexate:
3000 mL/m^2 per day with a solution containing at least 75 mEq sodium/1000 mL; administer intravenously during methotrexate administration (day 10) and for at least 24 hours afterward. **Sodium bicarbonate** 50–100 mEq/1000 mL is added to the parenteral solution to maintain urine pH ≥7.0
Methotrexate 1200 mg/m^2; administer intravenously in 25–250 mL dextrose or saline fluids ± 50–100 mEq sodium bicarbonate over 1 hour on day 10, *followed immediately by*:
Methotrexate 240 mg/m^2 per hour; administer by continuous intravenous infusion in 250–6000 mL dextrose or saline fluids ± sodium bicarbonate 50–100 mEq/1000 mL over 23 hours on day 10 (total dosage/cycle [not including intrathecal methotrexate] = 6720 mg/m^2)

(continued)

(continued)

Note:
- For logistical practicality and efficiency, parenteral admixtures containing methotrexate may include a portion or all of the fluid and sodium bicarbonate needed to meet hydration and urinary alkalinization requirements during methotrexate administration
- Methotrexate administration is discontinued after a total duration of 24 hours without regard for any portion not administered

Calcium leucovorin 192 mg/m^2; administer intravenously in 25–250 mL 0.9% NS or D5W over 1 hour at 36 hours after methotrexate administration began, *followed 6 hours later by:*
Calcium leucovorin 12 mg/m^2 per dose; administer intravenously in 25–250 mL 0.9% NS or D5W over 15 minutes every 6 hours until serum methotrexate concentration is <0.05 μmol/L

Note:
- Calcium leucovorin may be administered orally after completing 1 day of parenteral administration if patients are compliant, not vomiting, and without other potentially mitigating complications

Regimen B: IVAC
Ifosfamide 1500 mg/m^2 + **mesna** 360 mg/m^2 per day; administer intravenously in 100–250 mL 0.9% NS or D5W over 1 hour, for 5 consecutive days, on days 1–5 (total ifosfamide dosage/cycle = 7500 mg/m^2)
Mesna 360 mg/m^2 per dose; administer intravenously in 25–150 mL 0.9% NS or D5W over 15 minutes every 3 hours, for 6 doses, starting 3 hours after each ifosfamide + mesna administration is completed (total mesna dosage/day [7 doses/24 hours] = 2520 mg/m^2; total mesna dosage/cycle = 12,600 mg/m^2)
Etoposide 60 mg/m^2 per day; administer intravenously in 150 mL 0.9% NS or D5W over 1 hour for 5 consecutive days, on days 1–5 (total dosage/cycle = 300 mg/m^2)
Cytarabine 2000 mg/m^2 per dose; administer intravenously in 150 mL D5W over 3 hours every 12 hours, for 4 doses, on days 1 and 2 (total dosage/cycle = 8000 mg/m^2)

Keratitis prophylaxis
- Steroid ophthalmic drops (prednisolone 1% or dexamethasone 0.1%); administer 2 drops by intraocular instillation into each eye every 6 hours starting prior to the first cytarabine dose and continuing until 48 hours after high-dose cytarabine is completed

Supportive Care
Antiemetic prophylaxis for Regimen A, CODOX-M
Emetogenic potential on days 1 and 10 is **HIGH**
Emetogenic potential on days 2–5 is **MODERATE**
Emetogenic potential on days 8 and 15 is **MINIMAL**
See Chapter 42 for antiemetic recommendations

Antiemetic prophylaxis for Regimen B, IVAC
Emetogenic potential on days 1–5 is **HIGH**
See Chapter 42 for antiemetic recommendations

Hematopoietic growth factor (CSF) prophylaxis after CODOX-M and IVAC
Primary prophylaxis is indicated with 1 of the following:
   Filgrastim (G-CSF) 5 μg/kg per day; administer by subcutaneous injection, starting on day 13 and continuing until the next treatment cycle (ie, when ANC recovers to ≥1000/mm^3)
See Chapter 43 for more information

Antimicrobial prophylaxis after CODOX-M and IVAC
Risk of fever and neutropenia is *HIGH*
   Antimicrobial primary prophylaxis is recommended:
- Antibacterial—consider fluoroquinolone prophylaxis; *Pneumocystis jirovecii* prophylaxis is recommended (eg, cotrimoxazole). Withhold cotrimoxazole for 72 hours before methotrexate administration and until the methotrexate concentration is <0.1 micromolar
- Antifungal—recommended
- Antiviral—antiherpes antivirals (eg, acyclovir)

Additional prophylaxis
Give **stool softeners** and/or laxatives during and after vincristine administration

Intrathecal Medications for Prophylaxis of High-Risk Patients and Treatment of Patients with CNS Disease						
Dose in Milligrams Adjusted to Patient's Age in Years (y)			**Days of Administration**			
			Prophylaxis		Treatment	
≥3 y	2 y	1 y	A	B	A	B

(continued)

(continued)

			Cytarabine by Lumbar Puncture			
70	50	35	1, 3	—	1, 3, 5	7, 9
			Cytarabine by Intraventricular Route			
15	12	9	1, 3	—	1, 3, 5	7, 9
			Methotrexate by Lumbar Puncture°			
12	10	8	15	5	15, 17	5
			Methotrexate by Intraventricular Route°			
2	1.5	1	15	5	15, 17	5

A, CODOX-M Cycles 1 and 3; B, IVAC cycles 2 and 4

°**Calcium leucovorin** 12 mg/m² orally for 1 dose at 24 hours after each intrathecal dose of methotrexate
Low-Risk Patients

3 Cycles: A → A → A

Modified regimen A: (modified) CODOX-M
Cyclophosphamide 800 mg/m²; administer intravenously in 50–100 mL 0.9% NS or D5W over 30 minutes, given on day 1, *followed by:*
Cyclophosphamide 200 mg/m² per day; administer intravenously in 50–100 mL 0.9% NS D5W over 15 minutes, for 4 consecutive days, on days 2–5 (total dosage/cycle = 1600 mg/m²)
Doxorubicin 40 mg/m²; administer by intravenous injection over 3–5 minutes, given on day 1 (total dosage/cycle = 40 mg/m²)
Vincristine 1.5 mg/m² per dose (maximum single dose is 2.5 mg); administer by intravenous infusion over 15 minutes in 50 mL 0.9% NS, for 2 doses, on days 1 and 8 (total dosage/cycle = 3 mg/m²; maximum dose/cycle = 5 mg)

Hydration with methotrexate:
3000 mL/m² per day with a solution containing at least 75 mEq sodium/1000 mL; administer intravenously during methotrexate administration (day 10) and for at least 24 hours afterward. **Sodium bicarbonate** 50–100 mEq/1000 mL is added to the parenteral solution to maintain urine pH ≥7.0
Methotrexate 1200 mg/m²; administer intravenously in 25–250 mL dextrose or saline fluids ± 50–100 mEq sodium bicarbonate over 1 hour on day 10, *followed immediately by:*
Methotrexate 240 mg/m² per hour; administer by continuous intravenous infusion in 250–6000 mL dextrose or saline fluids ± sodium bicarbonate 50–100 mEq/1000 mL, over 23 hours on day 10 (total dosage/cycle [not including intrathecal methotrexate] = 6720 mg/m²)
Note:
• For logistical practicality and efficiency, parenteral admixtures containing methotrexate may include a portion or all of the fluid and sodium bicarbonate needed to meet hydration and urinary alkalinization requirements during methotrexate administration
• Methotrexate administration is discontinued after a total duration of 24 hours without regard for any portion not administered
Calcium leucovorin 192 mg/m²; administer intravenously in 25–250 mL 0.9% NS or D5W over 1 hour at 36 hours after methotrexate administration began, *followed 6 hours later by:*
Calcium leucovorin 12 mg/m² per dose; administer intravenously in 25–250 mL 0.9% NS or D5W over 15 minutes every 6 hours until serum methotrexate concentration is <0.05 μmol/L
Note:
• Calcium leucovorin may be administered orally after completing 1 day of parenteral administration if patients are compliant, are not vomiting, and have no other potentially mitigating complications

Supportive Care
Antiemetic prophylaxis
Emetogenic potential on days 1 and 10 is **HIGH**
Emetogenic potential on days 2–5 is **MODERATE**
Emetogenic potential on days 8 and 15 is **MINIMAL**
See Chapter 42 for antiemetic recommendations

Hematopoietic growth factor (CSF) prophylaxis
Primary prophylaxis is indicated with
Filgrastim (G-CSF) 5 μg/kg per day; administer by subcutaneous injection, starting on day 13 and continuing until the next treatment cycle (ie, when ANC recovers to ≥1000/mm³)
See Chapter 43 for more information

(continued)

(*continued*)

Antimicrobial prophylaxis
Risk of fever and neutropenia is *HIGH*
Antimicrobial primary prophylaxis is recommended:
• Antibacterial—consider fluoroquinolone prophylaxis; *Pneumocystis jirovecii* prophylaxis is recommended (eg, cotrimoxazole). Withhold cotrimoxazole for 72 hours before methotrexate administration and until the methotrexate concentration is <0.1 micromolar
• Antifungal—recommended
• Antiviral—antiherpes antivirals (eg, acyclovir)

Additional prophylaxis
Give **stool softeners** and/or laxatives during and after vincristine administration

CNS Prophylaxis*		
Cytarabine on Day 1 / Methotrexate on Day 3		
Patient's Age	Cytarabine	Methotrexate
1 year	35 mg	8 mg
2 years	50 mg	10 mg
≥3 years	70 mg	12 mg

Administer intrathecally by lumbar puncture

Patient Population Studied

A study of 41 previously untreated patients with small noncleaved (Burkitt or Burkitt-like) lymphoma. Thirty-four patients (15 adults + 19 children) were considered to be at high risk by the criteria stated above. Seven patients (5 adults + 2 children) were considered low risk

Efficacy

Complete response	95%
Partial response	5%
Event-free survival	92% at 2 years

Treatment Modifications

Treatment prerequisites:
• Cycles 2, 3, and 4 are started, when possible, on the day that the ANC recovers to ≥1000/mm³ after prior treatment
• A platelet count ≥50,000/mm³ without platelet transfusion support is required before starting repeated cycles. If a patient's ANC recovers to ≥1000/mm³, but the platelet count has not recovered to ≥50,000/mm³ without platelet transfusion, the patient should continue to receive daily filgrastim until the platelet count recovers to ≥50,000/mm³
• For CODOX-M, methotrexate is given without regard for blood counts
• Intravenously administered methotrexate is given only if creatinine clearance is >50 mL/min (>0.83 mL/s)

Adverse Event	Dose Modification
Motor weakness or unremitting obstipation	Continue treatment, but hold vincristine. When symptoms resolve, reintroduce vincristine at 50% dosage during subsequent treatments
Severe sensory symptoms	Reduce vincristine dosage by 50% during subsequent treatment
Serum sodium <130 mmol/L	Hold cyclophosphamide. Resume cyclophosphamide after serum sodium recovers to ≥130 mmol/L and change hydration fluid and diluent fluids to 0.9% NS
Hemorrhagic cystitis	Hold cyclophosphamide
Total bilirubin >2.5 mg/dL (42.8 µmol/L)	Reduce doxorubicin dosage by 50%
Total bilirubin >3.0 mg/dL (51.3 µmol/L)	Hold doxorubicin
Cerebellar toxicity	Hold cytarabine
Acute renal failure	Hold ifosfamide

NCI CTC, National Cancer Institute (USA) Common Toxicity Criteria, version 2.0

Toxicity

(N = 41)

A, CODOX-M; B, IVAC
Magrath I et al. J Clin Oncol 1996; 14:925–934
Weintraub M et al. J Clin Oncol 1996; 14:935–940

	Regimen	Patient's Age (Years)	% of Cycles	
			G3	G4
Neutropenia	A	<18	0	97.6
		≥18	2.2	97.8
	B	<18	0	100
		≥18	0	100
Leukopenia	A	<18	0	97.6
		≥18	4.4	95.6
	B	<18	0	100
		≥18	0	100
Thrombocytopenia	A	<18	17.1	53.7
		≥18	9.3	39.5
	B	<18	14.3	82.9
		≥18	3.7	96.3
Liver function abnormalities	A	<18	24.4	2.4
		≥18	24.4	2.4
	B	<18	5.9	0
		≥18	0	0
Stomatitis	A	<18	26.8	41.5
		≥18	28.9	20
	B	<18	5.7	2.9
		≥18	3.4	0
Documented infection	A	All ages	46.6	
	B		54.5	
Fever of unknown origin	A + B	<18	46.3	
		≥18	32.4	
Septicemia	A + B	<18	22.5	
		≥18	21.6	

Neurologic Adverse Events (N = 41 Patients)

Toxicity	% of Patients
Painful disabling neuropathy	26.8
Marked motor/severe sensory neuropathy	19.5
Severe motor weakness	7.3
Mild-moderate neuropathy	29.3

Therapy Monitoring

1. *Prior to treatment initiation:* left ventricular ejection fraction (LVEF)
   - In addition to baseline monitoring, evaluate LVEF during doxorubicin treatment if clinical symptoms of heart failure are present
2. *Before each cycle:* PE, CBC with differential, LFTs, serum BUN, creatinine, creatinine clearance, urinalysis
3. *During the first 3–5 days of induction therapy:*
   - *Every 4–6 hours:* Serum creatinine and electrolytes, calcium, and phosphorus
   - *Daily until normal levels are achieved:* LDH
   - *On days of chemotherapy:* CBC with differential, serum creatinine, electrolytes, calcium, and phosphorus
4. *Weekly during the intervals between treatments:* CBC with differential, serum creatinine and electrolytes, calcium, and phosphorus
5. *After high-dose systemic methotrexate administration:* Daily methotrexate levels, daily BUN and serum creatinine, urine output (goal ≥100 mL/hour), and urine pH every 8 hours (goal ≥7.0 to ≤8.0)

BURKITT LYMPHOMA • FIRST LINE

NON-HODGKIN LYMPHOMA REGIMEN: RITUXIMAB + HYPERFRACTIONATED CYCLOPHOSPHAMIDE, VINCRISTINE, DOXORUBICIN (ADRIAMYCIN), AND DEXAMETHASONE (R-HYPER-CVAD)

Thomas DA et al. J Clin Oncol 1999;17:2461–2470
Thomas DA et al. Cancer 2006; 106:1569–1580

Prophylaxis against tumor lysis syndrome during the first cycle:
Hydration with 2500–3000 mL/day, as tolerated; administer intravenously at 100–125 mL/hour (2500–3000 mL/day)
Note:
Furosemide 20–40 mg; administer intravenously every 12–24 hours to maintain fluid balance
Note: Diuresis is maintained for at least the first 72 hours after starting chemotherapy in the absence of metabolic aberrations, or after metabolic complications normalize
Allopurinol 300 mg/day; administer orally for 7 consecutive days, on days 1–7 (longer treatment may be needed)

Hyper-CVAD (cycles 1 and 3)
Rituximab
Premedication for rituximab:
Acetaminophen 650–1000 mg; administer orally *plus* **diphenhydramine** 25–50 mg; administer orally or intravenously 30–60 minutes before each dose of rituximab
Rituximab 375 mg/m^2 per dose; administer intravenously in 0.9% sodium chloride injection (0.9% NS) or 5% dextrose injection (D5W), diluted to a concentration of 1–4 mg/mL, for 2 doses during cycles 1 and 3, on days 1 and 11 of hyper-CVAD (total dosage/cycle = 750 mg/m^2)
Notes on rituximab administration:
• Infuse initially at 50 mg/hour. If hypersensitivity or infusion reactions do not occur during the first 30 minutes, increase the rate by 50 mg/hour every 30 minutes, as tolerated, to a maximum rate of 400 mg/hour. Subsequently, if previous administration was well tolerated, start at 100 mg/hour and increase by 100 mg/hour every 30 minutes, as tolerated, to a maximum rate of 400 mg/hour

INFUSION REACTIONS ASSOCIATED WITH RITUXIMAB
Fevers, chills, and rigors
1. Interrupt rituximab administration for severe symptoms, and give:
   • **Acetaminophen** 650 mg orally for fever. For persistent or recurrent symptoms, repeat administration every 4–6 hours as needed during rituximab administration
   • **Diphenhydramine** 25–50 mg orally or by intravenous injection for pruritus, hypotension, or angioedema. For persistent or recurrent symptoms, repeat administration every 4–6 hours as needed during rituximab administration
   • **Meperidine** 12.5–25 mg by intravenous injection every 10–20 minutes as needed for shaking chills (generally, cumulative doses >100 mg are not needed; use repeated doses with caution in persons with moderate or more severely impaired renal function)
2. If rituximab administration was interrupted, resume infusion at a slower rate than the maximum rate previously attempted. Rate escalation may be reattempted at smaller incremental steps with close monitoring. Do not exceed the maximum recommended rate of 400 mg/h

Dyspnea or wheezing without allergic findings (urticaria, or tongue or laryngeal edema)
1. Interrupt rituximab administration immediately
2. Give **hydrocortisone** 100 mg by intravenous injection (or an alternative steroid with equivalent glucocorticoid potency)
3. Give a **histamine (H$_2$) receptor antagonist** (ranitidine 50 mg, cimetidine 300 mg, or famotidine 20 mg) intravenously over 15–30 minutes
4. After symptoms resolve, resume rituximab administration at 25 mg/h with close monitoring. Do not increase the administration rate
Note: Medications and equipment for the treatment of hypersensitivity reactions should be available for immediate use in the event of a reaction during administration (eg, intravenous fluids, epinephrine, antihistamines, glucocorticoids, and oxygen)
Rituxan (rituximab) prescribing information. South San Francisco, CA: Genentech, Inc; 2018 October

Hyper-CVAD (cycles 1, 3, 5, and 7)
Cyclophosphamide 300 mg/m^2 per dose; administer intravenously over 2 hours in 500 mL 0.9% sodium chloride injection (0.9% NS) every 12 hours for 6 doses (days 1, 2, and 3), for 4 cycles, cycles 1, 3, 5, and 7 (total dosage/cycle = 1800 mg/m^2)
Mesna 600 mg/m^2 per day; administer by continuous intravenous infusion over 24 hours in 1000–2000 mL 0.9% NS, starting 1 hour before cyclophosphamide and continuing until 12 hours after the last dose of cyclophosphamide (total duration approximately 76 hours/cycle), for 4 cycles, cycles 1, 3, 5, and 7 (total dosage/cycle = 1900 mg/m^2)
Vincristine 2 mg/dose; administer by intravenous infusion over 15 minutes in 50 mL 0.9% NS for 2 doses, on days 4 and 11 (total dose/cycle = 4 mg)
Doxorubicin 50 mg/m^2; administer intravenously via central venous access in 25–250 mL 0.9% NS or 5% dextrose injection (D5W) over 2 hours on day 4 (total dosage/cycle = 50 mg/m^2)
Dexamethasone 40 mg/day; administer orally or by intravenous infusion in 25–150 mL 0.9% NS or D5W over 15–30 minutes for 8 doses, on days 1–4 and days 11–14 (total dosage/cycle = 320 mg)

(continued)

(continued)

High-dose methotrexate and cytarabine (cycles 2 and 4)
Rituximab
Acetaminophen 650–1000 mg; administer orally *plus* **diphenhydramine** 25–50 mg; administer orally or intravenously 30–60 minutes before each dose of rituximab

Rituximab 375 mg/m² per dose; administer intravenously in 0.9% NS or D5W , diluted to a concentration of 1–4 mg/mL, for 2 doses during cycles 2 and 4, on days 2 and 8 of high-dose methotrexate and cytarabine (total dosage/cycle = 750 mg/m²)

Notes on rituximab administration:
• Infuse initially at 100 mg/hour. If hypersensitivity or infusion reactions do not occur during the first 30 minutes, increase the rate by 100 mg/hour every 30 minutes, as tolerated, to a maximum rate of 400 mg/hour. Subsequently if previous administration was well tolerated, start at 100 mg/hour and increase by 100 mg/hour every 30 minutes, as tolerated, to a maximum rate of 400 mg/hour

INFUSION REACTIONS ASSOCIATED WITH RITUXIMAB

Fevers, chills, and rigors

1. Interrupt rituximab administration for severe symptoms, and give:
   • **Acetaminophen** 650 mg orally for fever. For persistent or recurrent symptoms, repeat administration every 4–6 hours as needed during rituximab administration
   • **Diphenhydramine** 25–50 mg orally or by intravenous injection for pruritus, hypotension, or angioedema. For persistent or recurrent symptoms, repeat administration every 4–6 hours as needed during rituximab administration
   • **Meperidine** 12.5–25 mg by intravenous injection every 10–20 minutes as needed for shaking chills (generally, cumulative doses >100 mg are not needed; use repeated doses with caution in persons with moderate or more severely impaired renal function)

2. If rituximab administration was interrupted, resume infusion at a slower rate than the maximum rate previously attempted. Rate escalation may be reattempted at smaller incremental steps with close monitoring. Do not exceed the maximum recommended rate of 400 mg/h

Dyspnea or wheezing without allergic findings (urticaria, or tongue or laryngeal edema)

1. Interrupt rituximab administration immediately

2. Give **hydrocortisone** 100 mg by intravenous injection (or an alternative steroid with equivalent glucocorticoid potency)

3. Give a **histamine (H₂) receptor antagonist** (ranitidine 50 mg, cimetidine 300 mg, or famotidine 20 mg) intravenously over 15–30 minutes

4. After symptoms resolve, resume rituximab administration at 25 mg/h with close monitoring. Do not increase the administration rate

Note: Medications and equipment for the treatment of hypersensitivity reactions should be available for immediate use in the event of a reaction during administration (eg, intravenous fluids, epinephrine, antihistamines, glucocorticoids, and oxygen)

Rituxan (rituximab) prescribing information. South San Francisco, CA: Genentech, Inc; 2018 October

High-dose methotrexate and cytarabine (cycles 2, 4, 6, and 8)

Hydration: 2500–3000 mL/day, as tolerated, with a solution containing a total amount of sodium not >0.9% NS (ie, ≤154 mEq sodium/1000 mL) by intravenous infusion during methotrexate administration and for at least 24 hours afterward

• Commence fluid administration 2–12 hours before starting methotrexate, depending on patient's fluid status

• Urine output should be at least 100 mL/hour before starting methotrexate infusion

• Maintain hydration at a rate that maintains urine output ≥100 mL/hour until the serum methotrexate concentration is <0.1 μmol/L

• Urine pH should be increased within the range ≥7.0 to ≤8.0 to enhance methotrexate solubility and ensure elimination

• Adverse effects attributable to methotrexate are related to systemic methotrexate concentrations *and* the duration for which concentrations are maintained

Sodium Bicarbonate 50–150 mEq/1000 mL Is Added to Parenteral Hydration Solutions to Maintain Urine pH ≥7.0 to ≤8.0		
Base Solution Sodium Content	**Sodium Bicarbonate Additive**	**Total Sodium Content**
0.45% Sodium Chloride Injection (0.45% NS)		
77 mEq/L	50–75 mEq	127–152 mEq/L
0.2% Sodium Chloride Injection (0.2% NS)		
34 mEq/L	100–125 mEq	134–159 mEq/L
5% Dextrose injection (D5W)		
0	125–150 mEq	125–150 mEq/L
D5W/0.45% NS		
77 mEq/L	50–75 mEq	127–152 mEq/L
D5W/0.2% NS		
34 mEq/L	100–125 mEq	134–159 mEq/L

(continued)

(continued)

Methotrexate 1000 mg/m²; administer by continuous intravenous infusion in 250 mL to ≥1000 mL 0.9% NS or D5W (or saline and dextrose combinations) over 24 hours on day 1 (total dosage/cycle [not including intrathecal methotrexate] = 1000 mg/m²)

Cytarabine 3000 mg/m² per dose; administer intravenously in 50–500 mL 0.9% NS or D5W over 2 hours, every 12 hours, for 4 doses, on days 2 and 3 (total dosage/cycle [not including intrathecal cytarabine] = 12,000 mg/m²)

Calcium leucovorin 50 mg; administer intravenously in 10–100 mL 0.9% NS or D5W over 10–20 minutes for 1 dose, 12 hours after methotrexate administration is completed (36 hours after starting methotrexate), *followed 6 hours later by:*

Calcium leucovorin 15 mg; administer intravenously in 10–100 mL 0.9% NS or D5W over 10–20 minutes, every 6 hours, for 8 doses or until blood methotrexate concentrations is <0.1 μmol/L

• Calcium leucovorin doses are escalated to 50–100/dose intravenously every 4–6 hours if serum methotrexate concentrations are:

  ▪ >20 μmol/L at the end of methotrexate administration (hour 24)

  ▪ >1 μmol/L at 24 hours after the end of methotrexate administration (hour 48), *or*

  ▪ >0.1 μmol/L at 48 hours after the end of methotrexate administration (hour 72)

CNS prophylaxis (all patients)

Methotrexate; administer intrathecally on day 2 for 8 cycles (8 doses): 12 mg/dose via lumbar puncture or 6 mg/dose via intraventricular route (eg, Ommaya reservoir; total dose throughout 8 cycles [not including systemic methotrexate] = 96 mg via lumbar puncture or 48 mg intraventricularly)

Cytarabine 100 mg; administer intrathecally via lumbar puncture or intraventricular routes, on day 7 for 8 cycles (total of dose 8 doses throughout 8 cycles [not including systemic cytarabine] = 800 mg)

CNS treatment

Methotrexate 12 mg/dose; administer intrathecally via lumbar puncture or 6 mg/dose via intraventricular route twice weekly until CSF cell count normalizes and cytology becomes negative for malignant disease, then administer intrathecally during subsequent cycles on day 2 per the regimen for CNS prophylaxis

Cytarabine 100 mg; administer intrathecally via lumbar puncture or intraventricular route, twice weekly until CSF cell count normalizes and cytology becomes negative for malignant disease, then administer intrathecally during subsequent cycles on day 7 per the regimen for CNS prophylaxis

Supportive Care

Antiemetic prophylaxis with Hyper-CVAD (cycles 1, 3, 5, and 7)

Emetogenic potential on days 1–4 is **MODERATE**

Antiemetic prophylaxis with high-dose methotrexate and cytarabine (cycles 2, 4, 6, and 8)

Emetogenic potential on days 1, 2, and 3 is **MODERATE**

See Chapter 42 for antiemetic recommendations

Hematopoietic growth factor (CSF) prophylaxis

Primary prophylaxis is indicated with hyper-CVAD (cycles 1, 3, 5, and 7) and with high-dose methotrexate and cytarabine (cycles 2, 4, 6, and 8):

Filgrastim (G-CSF) 10 μg/kg per day; administer by subcutaneous injection starting 24 hours after the last dose of chemotherapy; and continuing until postnadir WBC count ≥3000/mm³

See Chapter 43 for more information

Antimicrobial prophylaxis

Risk of fever and neutropenia is *HIGH*

Antimicrobial primary prophylaxis is recommended:

• Antibacterial—consider fluoroquinolone prophylaxis; *Pneumocystis jirovecii* prophylaxis is recommended (eg, cotrimoxazole). Withhold cotrimoxazole for 3 days prior to each methotrexate dose and during each methotrexate cycle until the methotrexate concentration declines to <0.1 micromolar

• Antifungal—recommended

• Antiviral—antiherpes antivirals (eg, acyclovir)

Additional prophylaxis

Add a **proton pump inhibitor** during dexamethasone use to prevent gastritis and duodenitis

Give **stool softeners** and/or laxatives during and after vincristine administration

Treatment Modifications

Treatment prerequisites
- Second and subsequent cycles are implemented when WBC count ≥3000/mm³ and platelet count ≥60,000/mm³ at least 24 hours after a filgrastim dose was administered
- Subsequent cycles may be repeated at intervals less than every 21 days, but not more frequently than 14 days after the previous cycle

Adverse Event	Dose Modification
On day 21 of a treatment cycle, if WBC count ≥3000/mm³, but platelet count <60,000/mm³	Reevaluate hematologic laboratories every 3 days until platelet count ≥60,000/mm³
On day 21 of a treatment cycle, if WBC count ≥30,000/mm³, but platelet count <60,000/mm³	Hold filgrastim and reevaluate hematologic laboratories every 3 days until platelet count ≥60,000/mm³
Patient age ≥60 years	Reduce cytarabine dosage to 1000 mg/m² per dose
Blood methotrexate concentration >20 μmol/L at the start of treatment	Reduce cytarabine dosage to 2000 mg/m² per dose and reduce methotrexate dosage by 50%
Serum creatinine >2 mg/dL (>177 μmol/L)	
Serum creatinine >3 mg/dL (>265 μmol/L)	Reduce methotrexate dosage by 75%
Delayed methotrexate excretion or nephrotoxicity attributable to previous methotrexate treatment	Reduce methotrexate dosage by 50–75% (commensurate with the severity of nephrotoxicity)
Total bilirubin >2 g/dL (34.2 μmol/L)	Reduce vincristine dose to 1 mg
Total bilirubin 2–3g/dL (34.2–51.3 μmol/L)	Reduce doxorubicin dosage by 25%
Total bilirubin 3–4g/dL (51.3–68.4 μmol/L)	Reduce doxorubicin dosage by 50%
Total bilirubin >4g/dL (68.4 μmol/L)	Reduce doxorubicin dosage by 75%
Disease involving the stomach or small bowel	Eliminate doxorubicin during the first hyper-CVAD cycle
If high-dose cytarabine is eliminated because of adverse effects	Omit the high-dose methotrexate + cytarabine regimen, replacing it with repeated cycles of hyper-CVAD
Peripheral neuropathy	Discontinue vincristine
Proximal myopathy	Discontinue dexamethasone
Cerebellar neurotoxicity	Reduce cytarabine dosage or omit cytarabine during subsequent treatments
Tumor lysis syndrome during induction with renal failure requiring hemodialysis	Reduce methotrexate dosage
G3 mucositis	

Efficacy

Sequential Comparison of Hyper-CVAD Plus Rituximab Versus Hyper-CVAD Alone

Parameter	Hyper-CVAD Plus Rituximab (N = 31)	Hyper-CVAD Alone (N = 48)	P
Percent CR	86%	85%	
Median follow-up	22 months	74 months	
Induction deaths	0%	13%	0.04
Percent relapse	7%	30%	0.008
Percent 3-year survival	89%	53%	<0.01
Percent 3-year EFS	80%	52%	0.02
Percent 3-year DFS	88%	60%	0.03
Percent 3-year CRD	91%	66%	0.024

CRD, complete response duration; DFS, disease-free survival; EFS, Event-free survival

Patient Population Studied

A study of 26 consecutive adult patients with newly diagnosed, untreated Burkitt-type acute lymphoblastic leukemia (23 patients with FAB L3 subtype; 3 patients classified L1 or L2)

1. *Pretreatment evaluation*: determination of LVEF by echocardiogram, hepatitis B core antibody (IgG or total) and hepatitis B surface antigen
2. CMP and CBC with differential and platelet count prior to each cycle
3. Monitor serum methotrexate levels 24, 48, and 72 hours after the start of each methotrexate infusion. In patients with delayed clearance, monitor daily methotrexate levels thereafter until the methotrexate concentration declines to <0.1 micromolar. Monitor serum creatinine daily during each admission for methotrexate. Monitor urine output closely (goal ≥100 mL/hour). Monitor urine pH (goal ≥7.0 to ≤8.0) every 8 hours prior to and during each methotrexate course until the methotrexate concentration declines to <0.1 micromolar
4. Patients who receive high-dose cytarabine need to be closely monitored for changes in renal function. Renal dysfunction is highly correlated with increased risk of cerebellar toxicity associated with cytarabine. Patients need to be monitored for nystagmus, dysmetria, and ataxia before each cytarabine dose

Toxicity*

Toxicities in Patients with CR (N = 21)

	Age <60 Years (N = 13)	Age ≥60 Years (N = 8)
G3/4 neurotoxicity	15%	29%
Tumor lysis in first cycle	8%	25%
Creatinine increased more than 2-fold after methotrexate	23%	12%
Infection with cycle 2	54%	38%

Infectious Complications During First Cycle (N = 37)

Febrile neutropenia	86%
Fever of unknown origin	38%
Pneumonia	32%
Sepsis	11%
Bacterial meningitis	3%
Herpes simplex virus infections	3%

Infectious Complications in Cycles After First (N = 152)

Febrile neutropenia during high-dose methotrexate/cytarabine	47–55%
Febrile neutropenia during hyper-CVAD	30–39%
Herpes simplex virus infections	8%

Events Concurrent with Thrombocytopenia (N = 152)

Hemorrhage with thrombocytopenia (all)	12%
Severe epistaxis	4%
Retinal	2%
Gastrointestinal	2%
CNS	2%
Pulmonary	1%
Antecubital hematoma	1%

Other Toxicities

Deaths during induction	19%
Cerebellar neurotoxicity	3.8%

*NCI CTC

31. Ovarian Cancer

Kunle Odunsi, MD, PhD, and J. Brian Szender MD, MPH

Epidemiology

Incidence: 21,750 (Estimated new cases in 2020 in the United States)
Deaths: Estimated 13,940 in 2020
Median age: 63 years

Stage at presentation	
Limited (stage I–II):	31%
Advanced (stage III–IV):	60%
Unstaged/unknown	8%

American Cancer Society. Cancer Facts & Figures 2020. Atlanta, GA: American Cancer Society; 2020
Surveillance, Epidemiology and End Results (SEER) Program, available from http://seer.cancer.gov [accessed 3 October 2019]

Pathology

WHO classification of malignant ovarian tumors
The World Health Organization histologic classification for ovarian tumors separates ovarian neoplasms according to the most probable tissue of origin
1. Surface epithelial (65%, 90% of malignant tumors)

   Further classified by:
   - Cell type (serous, mucinous, endometrioid, etc)
   - Atypia (benign, borderline [atypical proliferation, low malignant potential] or malignant)
   - Malignant may be invasive or non-invasive
2. Germ cell (15%)
3. Sex cord–stromal (10%)
4. Metastases (5%); miscellaneous (5%)

Tumor Grade
- Grade 1—Well differentiated
- Grade 2—Moderately differentiated
- Grade 3—Poorly differentiated

Ozols RF et al (editors). Cancer: Principles & Practice of Oncology, 6th ed. Philadelphia, PA: Lippincott Williams & Wilkins; 2001:1596–1632

1. **Surface epithelial–stromal tumors**
   - **Serous tumors:**
     - Benign (cystadenoma)
     - Borderline tumors (serous borderline tumor)
     - Malignant (serous adenocarcinoma)
   - **Mucinous tumors, endocervical-like and intestinal type:**
     - Benign (cystadenoma)
     - Borderline tumors (mucinous borderline tumor)
     - Malignant (mucinous adenocarcinoma)
   - **Endometrioid tumors:**
     - Benign (cystadenoma)
     - Borderline tumors (endometrioid borderline tumor)
     - Malignant (endometrioid adenocarcinoma)

Percentage of Cases by Stage

Localized (confined to primary site)	16%
Regional (spread to regional lymph nodes)	21%
Distant (cancer has metastasized)	58%
Unknown	5%

Surveillance, Epidemiology and End Results (SEER) Program, available from http://seer.cancer.gov [accessed in 2020]

(continued)

Pathology (*continued*)

- Clear cell tumors:
  - Benign
  - Borderline tumors
  - Malignant (clear cell adenocarcinoma)
- Transitional cell tumors:
  - Brenner tumor
  - Brenner tumor of borderline malignancy
  - Malignant Brenner tumor
  - Transitional cell carcinoma (non-Brenner type)
- Epithelial-stromal:
  - Adenosarcoma
  - Carcinosarcoma (formerly mixed Müllerian tumors)

2. Germ cell tumors
  - Teratoma:
    - Immature
    - Mature
    - Solid
    - Cystic (dermoid cyst)
  - Monodermal (eg, struma ovarii, carcinoid)
  - Dysgerminoma
  - Yolk sac tumor (endodermal sinus tumor)
  - Mixed germ cell tumors

3. Sex cord–stromal tumors
  - Granulosa tumors:
    - Fibromas
    - Fibrothecomas
    - Thecomas
  - Sertoli cell tumors:
    - Leydig cell tumors
  - Sex cord tumor with annular tubules
  - Gynandroblastoma
  - Steroid (lipid) cell tumors

4. Malignant, not otherwise specified
  - Metastatic cancer from nonovarian primary:
    - Colonic, appendiceal
    - Gastric
    - Breast

5-year Relative Survival by Stage at Diagnosis

Stage at Diagnosis	5-year Relative Survival (%)
Localized (confined to primary site)	92.6
Regional (spread to regional lymph nodes)	74.8
Distant (cancer has metastasized)	30.2
Unknown	25.5

Note: treatment and survival by stage cannot be summarized simply for ovarian cancer. Each stage is strongly influenced by whether the disease is amenable to surgery, by the histologic type and grade, by the bulk of residual disease after the completion of surgery, and by other factors. Differences in survival among patients with the same stage of disease may indicate incomplete staging. When comprehensive staging is performed, a substantial number of patients initially believed to have disease confined to the pelvis will be staged upward Surveillance, Epidemiology and End Results (SEER) Program, available from http://seer.cancer.gov [accessed in 2020]

Work-up

1. Personal and family history, physical examination
2. Liver function tests, BUN, creatinine, LDH
3. CBC with platelets, PT, PTT, INR
4. Tumor markers (CA-125, α-fetoprotein [AFP], HCG)
5. CT scan of abdomen and pelvis, and chest x-ray. CT of chest if chest x-ray is abnormal
6. *Radiographic tests of unclear utility:* MRI of abdomen and pelvis, PET scan

Staging

Primary Tumor (T)

TNM Category	FIGO Stage	
TX		Primary tumor cannot be assessed
T0		No evidence of primary tumor
T1	I	Tumor limited to ovaries (one or both) or fallopian tube(s)
T1a	IA	Tumor limited to one ovary (capsule intact) or fallopian tube, no tumor on ovarian or fallopian tube surface. No malignant cells in ascites or peritoneal washings
T1b	IB	Tumor limited to both ovaries (capsules intact) or fallopian tubes; no tumor on ovarian or fallopian tube surface. No malignant cells in ascites or peritoneal washings
T1c1	IC1	Tumor limited to one or both ovaries or fallopian tubes with surgical spill
T1c2	IC2	Tumor limited to one or both ovaries or fallopian tubes with capsule ruptured before surgery or tumor on ovarian or fallopian tube surface
T1c3	IC3	Tumor limited to one or both ovaries or fallopian tubes with malignant cells in ascites or peritoneal washings
T2	II	Tumor involves 1 or both ovaries or fallopian tubes with pelvic extension below pelvic brim or primary peritoneal cancer
T2a	IIA	Extension and/or implants on uterus and/or fallopian tube(s) and/or ovaries
T2b	IIB	Extension to and/or implants on other pelvic tissues
T3	III	Tumor involves one or both ovaries or fallopian tubes, or primary peritoneal cancer, with microscopically confirmed peritoneal metastasis outside the pelvis and/or metastasis to the retroperitoneal (pelvic and/or para-aortic) lymph nodes
T3a	IIIA2	Microscopic extrapelvic (above the pelvic brim) peritoneal involvement with or without positive retroperitoneal lymph nodes
T3b	IIIB	Macroscopic peritoneal metastasis beyond pelvis 2 cm or less in greatest dimension with or without metastasis to the retroperitoneal lymph nodes
T3c	IIIC	Macroscopic peritoneal metastasis beyond pelvis more than 2 cm in greatest dimension with or without metastasis to the retroperitoneal lymph nodes (includes extension of tumor to capsule of liver and spleen without parenchymal involvement of either organ)

Regional Lymph Nodes (N)

TNM Category	FIGO Stage	
NX		Regional lymph nodes cannot be assessed
N0		No regional lymph node metastasis
N0 (i+)		Isolated tumor cells in regional lymph node(s) no greater than 0.2 mm
N1	IIIA1	Positive retroperitoneal lymph nodes only (histologically confirmed)
N1a	IIIA1i	Metastasis up to and including 10 mm in greatest dimension
N1b	IIIA1ii	Metastasis more than 10 mm in greatest dimension

Distant Metastasis (M)

TNM Category	FIGO Stage	
M0		No distant metastasis
M1	IV	Distant metastasis; including pleural effusion with positive cytology; liver or splenic parenchymal metastasis; metastasis to extra-abdominal organs (including inguinal lymph nodes and lymph nodes outside the abdominal cavity); and transmural involvement of intestine
M1a	IVA	Pleural effusion with positive cytology
M1b	IVB	Liver or splenic parenchymal metastases; metastases to extra-abdominal organs (including inguinal lymph nodes and lymph nodes outside the abdominal cavity); transmural involvement of intestine

Staging

Group	T	N	M
I	T1	N0	M0
IA	T1a	N0	M0
IB	T1b	N0	M0
IC	T1c	N0	M0
II	T2	N0	M0
IIA	T2a	N0	M0
IIB	T2b	N0	M0
IIIA1	T1/T2	N1	M0
IIIA2	T3a	NX/N0/N1	M0
IIIB	T3b	NX/N0/N1	M0
IIIC	T3c	NX/N0/N1	M0
IV	Any T	Any N	M1
IVA	Any T	Any N	M1a
IVB	Any T	Any N	M1b

Amin MB et al (editors). AJCC Cancer Staging Manual. 8th ed. New York: Springer; 2017

Expert Opinion: Chemotherapy

Early-stage Disease

1. In good-prognosis, early-stage disease, surgery alone is adequate therapy: there is a 95% 10-year survival rate (Ia or Ib)
2. In early-stage patients who have an increased risk for recurrence (poorly differentiated histologies):
   - IV chemotherapy with paclitaxel and carboplatin
   - 5-FU/leucovorin/oxaliplatin and capecitabine/oxaliplatin may be of use in patients with mucinous ovarian cancer
   - Hormone therapy such as aromatase inhibitors, leuprolide acetate, and tamoxifen may be of benefit in patients with low-grade serous histologies

Bell J et al. Gynecol Oncol 2006;102:432–439
Fishman A et al. J Reprod Med 1996;41:393–396
Lederman JA et al. Int J Gynecol Cancer 2014;24:S14–S19

Advanced-stage Disease (≥II)

1. Standard of care for advanced-stage disease: depends in part on the amount of residual disease
   - Patients with stage II–III disease that is optimally debulked with no residual mass greater than 1 cm in diameter after surgery may be treated, if possible, with intraperitoneal cisplatin and paclitaxel
   - Six cycles of paclitaxel + carboplatin is used if debulking surgery was not optimal, in stage IV disease, or in patients who may not tolerate IP chemotherapy
   - Poor performance status, age >65, multiple comorbidities portend lack of tolerance of IP regimens
2. Neoadjuvant chemotherapy is recommended in selected patient populations:
   - Patients at risk of significant post-operative morbidity/mortality
   - Patients with disease not amenable to optimal cytoreduction
3. Generally, dose-intense approaches requiring stem cell support are ill advised
4. Benefit of "consolidation" therapy after an initial 6 cycles of systemic treatment is uncertain
   - Consolidation regimens: several additional cycles of paclitaxel or bevacizumab, or transition to a PARP inhibitor such as olaparib, rucaparib, or niraparib

Kohn EC et al. Gynecol Oncol 1996;62:181–191
McGuire WP et al. N Engl J Med 1996;334:1–6
Ozols RF et al. J Clin Oncol 2003;21:3194–200
Sarosy GA, Reed E. Ann Intern Med 2000;133:555–556
Wright AA et al. J Clin Oncol 2016;34:3460–3473

Recurrent Disease

1. Treatment of recurrent disease is complex. Decisions should be based on:
   - Likelihood of sensitivity/resistance to agents given in the past: platinum-sensitive or platinum-resistant disease
   - Residual toxicity from prior treatments
   - Prior treatment with targeted therapies
   - Potential response to immunotherapy
   - Comorbid illnesses, including renal, hepatic, and cardiac function
   - Availability of clinical trials
   - Desires of the patient
2. *Platinum-sensitive disease*
   - Epithelial ovarian cancer that recurs ≥1–2 years after platinum-based chemotherapy
   - Response rate to retreatment with another platinum agent-based regimen tends to be high (>70%)
   - Addition of bevacizumab, especially in patients who have not previously received the drug
3. *Platinum-resistant disease*
   - Disease progression in the face of appropriate initial platinum-based treatment
   - Disease recurrence within the first 6 months after an initial response to platinum-based therapy
   - Poor prognosis, especially if disease progresses during initial 6 cycles of therapy with platinum agents
   - Survival improved in chemotherapy + bevacizumab
   - Use of non-cross-resistant agents in the second-line and third-line setting is critically important
   - Best supportive care and clinical trials should also be offered in this setting

Aghajanian C et al. J Clin Oncol 2012;30:2039–2045
Leitao MM Jr et al. Gynecol Oncol 2003;91:123–129
Markman M et al. Gynecol Oncol 2004;93:699–701
Markman M et al. J Cancer Res Clin Oncol 2004;130:25–28
Pujade-Lauraine E et al. J Clin Oncol 2014;32:1302–1308
Reed E et al. Gynecol Oncol 1992;46:326–329

(continued)

(*continued*)

Platinum Hypersensitivity

1. Platinum hypersensitivity can develop in patients who have received ≥6 cycles of cisplatin or carboplatin
2. A desensitization regimen should be used
3. Rarely, desensitization is unsuccessful. In this situation, oxaliplatin is an acceptable alternative without documented cross-reactivity

Kolomeyevskaya NV et al. Int J Gynecol Cancer 2015;25:42–48
Lee CW et al. Gynecol Oncol 2004;95:370–376

Immunotherapy

1. Importance of the immune system in progression and treatment of cancer has emerged in the last 20 years
2. The tumor microenvironment is an important factor in the response to therapy and development of resistance to treatment
3. Immunotherapy includes immune-modulating therapies (immune checkpoint inhibitors), therapies impacting the tumor microenvironment (amino acid enzyme inhibitors), and antigen-directed therapy (vaccine therapy)
4. Immune checkpoint inhibitors such as pembrolizumab are available outside of clinical trial for patients; however, most immunotherapy is available only in clinical trial setting

PARP Inhibitors

1. The role of genetics in ovarian cancer is another important finding, with poly-ADP ribose polymerase (PARP) inhibitors representing an emerging class of oral therapeutics for ovarian cancer available in multiple settings
   - Patients with tumors harboring BRCA mutations with 3 or more prior lines of chemotherapy
   - Patients with documented homologous recombination deficiency (HRD) on molecular tumor testing
   - Patients with response to salvage therapy in the platinum-sensitive setting
2. Current recommendations are to offer PARP inhibitor maintenance for all patients meeting the above-noted criteria

Gelmon KA et al. Lancet Oncol 2011;12:852–861
Kristeleit R et al. Clin Cancer Res 2017;23:4095–4106
Mirza MR et al. N Engl J Med 2016;375:2154–2164

Surgery

1. Ideally, a gynecologic oncologist should perform all surgical procedures for ovarian cancer, including:
   - Laparoscopic assessment of disease
   - Initial staging and debulking surgery
   - Second-look procedure (if done)
   - Any interval surgical debulking procedure
2. Goals of initial surgical procedure:
   - Define extent of disease and evaluate for resection potential
   - Remove all visible disease from the abdominopelvic cavity; or, if surgeon cannot remove all visible disease, remove all disease possible (debulking surgery)
3. Debulking important because subsequent survival and response to chemotherapy are linked to:
   - Dimension of the largest remaining tumor lesion after completion of surgery
   - Possibly, the overall volume of residual disease
4. Surgery alone is preferred approach to patients with good-prognosis, early-stage epithelial ovarian cancer:
   - Stage: Ia or Ib
   - Any epithelial histology other than clear cell
   - Well-differentiated or moderately well-differentiated histologic grade (low grade). (Any early-stage patient other than the latter should have postsurgery chemotherapy)
5. Neoadjuvant chemotherapy
   - Three to 4 cycles of chemotherapy before an initial staging and debulking procedure
   - Data suggest a less-morbid operation with reduced blood loss and a shorter operative procedure

Aletti GD et al. Obstet Gynecol 2006;107:77–85
Bristow RE et al. J Clin Oncol 2002;20:1248–1259
Brockbank ED et al. Eur J Surg Oncol 2013;39:912–917
Eisenhauer EL et al. Gynecol Oncol 2006;103:1083–1090
Fagotti A et al. Gynecol Oncol 2013;131:341–346
Hoskins WJ et al. Am J Obstet Gynecol 1994;170:974–979; discussion 979–980
Schwartz PE et al. Gynecol Oncol 1999;72:93–99
Schwartz PE, Zheng W. Gynecol Oncol 2003;90:644–650

Germ Cell Tumors

The recommended laboratory evaluation for germ cell tumors should include:
1. A comprehensive metabolic panel, CBC with platelets, magnesium level, LDH, AFP, and HCG levels
2. Pulmonary function studies may be obtained
3. Complete surgical staging is recommended as initial surgery, with fertility-sparing surgery considered in those desiring future fertility

(*continued*)

Toxicities: Ovarian Cancer Chemotherapy

1. **Myelosuppression** Associated with all the agents listed in this chapter except tamoxifen. All 3 lineages are affected. Persistent thrombocytopenia is associated with the platinum compounds

2. **Nausea and vomiting** Preventive treatment is very important. Delayed nausea and vomiting is very common. Steroids, serotonin (HT_3)-receptor antagonists, and neurokinin (NK_1)-receptor antagonists are recommended for routine use with platinum-containing regimens

3. **Renal dysfunction** Seen with cisplatin and with carboplatin, but usually more clinically significant with cisplatin. Serum creatinine may be normal in the face of a markedly reduced creatinine clearance. This is important because other drugs that are eliminated by the kidney may be needed (eg, antibiotics). Platinum-related renal insufficiency is nonoliguric: be vigilant

4. **Neurotoxicity** Clinically occurs before detectable changes on EMG/NCTs. Bilateral paresthesias in stocking-and-glove distribution usually are progressive with repeated platinum doses and can become severe. Cisplatin is more likely than carboplatin to cause this problem

5. **Fatigue/weakness** May be related to anemia, but is a common side effect of several newer agents, including gemcitabine and topotecan

6. **Altered sexual function** A common side effect, but is seldom discussed spontaneously by a patient. It can be an underlying contributing factor to family disruption and clinical reactive depression; usually is a combined function of surgery and effect of neuroactive anticancer agent (platinum agents)

7. **Clinical depression** A common side effect. Many patients request medication for this. Sometimes may be a severe problem

8. **Alopecia** A common side effect, especially with taxane therapy, that can cause significant psychosocial distress. Scalp cooling caps are beneficial in reducing the incidence of this toxicity and may be offered

9. **Rare toxicities** Acute hypersensitivity to paclitaxel. Acute hypersensitivity to cisplatin/carboplatin (usually occurs after 6–8 cycles of therapy). Desensitization is occasionally appropriate and can be successful. On most occasions, switch to another agent right away

Germ Cell Tumors (continued)

Stage I dysgerminoma or stage I grade 1 immature teratoma

1. Patients who have had complete surgical staging and no evidence of disease is found outside the ovary should be observed

2. Patients who have had incomplete surgical staging, for whom observation without chemotherapy is being considered, should undergo a complete staging procedure. If no evidence of disease is found outside the ovary, these patients may be observed. If, at the time of a complete surgical staging, tumor is found outside the ovary, patients should receive bleomycin + etoposide + cisplatin (BEP) in the postoperative period

Stage II–IV dysgerminoma or stage I, grade 2–3 immature teratoma or embryonal tumors or endodermal sinus tumors

1. These patients should receive chemotherapy for 3–4 cycles with bleomycin + etoposide + cisplatin (BEP)

2. Patients achieving a complete clinical response should be observed clinically every 2–4 months with AFP and HCG levels (if initially elevated) for 2 years

3. Patients with radiographic evidence of residual tumor but with normal AFP and HCG levels should be considered for surgical resection of the tumor; observation can be considered

4. Patients with persistently elevated AFP and/or HCG after chemotherapy, or with clinically or radiographically evident disease, should receive chemotherapy or radiation or supportive care. Acceptable regimens for recurrent disease include:
   - Cisplatin + etoposide
   - VIP (etoposide + ifosfamide + cisplatin)
   - VeIP (vinblastine + ifosfamide + cisplatin)
   - VAC (vincristine + dactinomycin + cyclophosphamide)

Radiation

1. External beam radiation therapy:
   - Useful in the management of tumor masses that might cause extreme pain, bleeding, or other medical problems and in cases in which surgery is not a good option
   - Not routinely used in epithelial ovarian cancer due to ubiquitous p53 mutation and poor response rates

2. Intraperitoneal colloidal ^{32}P:
   - May be useful in the treatment of early-stage disease of less common histologies
   - Has fallen out of favor in the United States

3. Gamma-knife, intensity-modulated radiation therapy (IMRT), and standard whole-brain radiation:
   - Metastases to the brain occur uncommonly but are no longer considered rare
   - Several approaches are effective in controlling CNS disease
   - Use of these approaches depends on the clinical setting and the technology available
   - Most useful in patients who cannot receive bevacizumab

Ovarian Stromal Tumors

1. Patients with stages IA–C ovarian stromal tumors desiring fertility may be treated with fertility-sparing surgery. Otherwise, complete staging is recommended to all other patients

2. Those with surgical findings of stage I tumor should be observed

3. Patients having high-risk stage I (tumor rupture, poorly differentiated tumor, tumor size >10–15 cm) or stage II–IV tumors can be observed, or they can receive radiation therapy or undergo cisplatin-based chemotherapy with germ cell regimens preferred

4. Patients subsequently having a clinical relapse may consider secondary cytoreductive surgery, enter a clinical trial, or be offered supportive care

Expert Opinion: Epithelial Ovarian Cancer (EOC), Primary Peritoneal Cancer (PPC), Fallopian Tube Cancer—Chemotherapy

Early-stage disease [IA, IB, IC]

1. IA, grades 1/2 and IB, grades 1/2 (good prognosis, early-stage disease):
   - Surgery alone is adequate therapy with a 95% 10-year survival rate
2. IA, grade 3, IB, grade 3, IC, grades 1/2/3, and some IA/IB grade 2 (early-stage patients who are at increased risk for recurrence):
   - Three to 6 cycles for non-high-grade serous histologies
   - Six cycles recommended for high-grade serous histology

Advanced stage disease (stage II, III, or IV)

1. Standard of care for advanced-stage disease:
   - Six to 8 cycles of paclitaxel 175 mg/m2 + carboplatin AUC 5-6, after debulking surgery
2. Additional standard option in <1 cm, optimally debulked, stage II/III patients:
   - **Intraperitoneal (IP) chemotherapy** every 3 weeks for 6 cycles
     - (Day 1) paclitaxel 135 mg/m^2 by continuous intravenous infusion over 24 hours
     - (Day 2) cisplatin 75–100 mg/m^2 intraperitoneally
     - (Day 8) paclitaxel 60 mg/m^2 intraperitoneally
3. Three-drug combinations in this setting provide no added benefit
   - GOG 182/ICON5: five-arm randomized trial, to determine if adding either topotecan, gemcitabine, or pegylated liposomal doxorubicin in the frontline setting would extend PFS or OS. Control arm = paclitaxel and carboplatin IV every 3 weeks × 8 cycles. Accrual >1200 patients/year; 4312 women enrolled. None of the 3-drug regimens demonstrated an improvement in either PFS or OS. Survival analyses of groups defined by size of residual disease (optimal or suboptimal cytoreduction) also failed to show experimental benefit in any subgroup (Bookman et al, 2009)
4. **Dose-dense weekly paclitaxel**
   - A randomized phase 3 trial comparing a dose-dense regimen of weekly paclitaxel (days 1, 8, and 15) in combination with carboplatin every 3 weeks versus both agents administered once every 3 weeks showed statistically significant improvement with the dose-dense paclitaxel regimen in: (a) PFS (28.0 vs 17.2) and (b) OS at 3 years (72.1% vs 65.1% [HR 0.75; CI 0.57–0.98]). However, patient dropout was higher in the dose-dense group, primarily related to hematologic toxicity (Katsumata et al, 2009)
   - Subsequent studies, especially with bevacizumab added, did not reproduce these findings
5. Generally, **dose-intense approaches requiring stem cell support** are ill advised
6. Maintenance therapy with paclitaxel is a consideration with mixed results and potential increase in toxicity. Pazopanib, bevacizumab, and PARP inhibitors (eg, olaparib, rucaparib, niraparib) are emerging as effective maintenance therapies administered alone or in combination
7. The benefit of adding **bevacizumab** to a standard frontline IV paclitaxel/carboplatin regimen administered every 3 weeks is under debate. Evidence suggests that in standard-risk patients, it does not confer any benefit. It remains to be determined whether it may be beneficial in high-risk patients. The GOG-218 and ICON7 trials suggest a role for maintenance bevacizumab in ovarian cancer; however, the absolute benefit in PFS is very modest, and neither trial showed an OS benefit. There is no level I evidence for (a) *the use of bevacizumab in patients receiving intraperitoneal (IP) chemotherapy*, or (b) *the use of bevacizumab as neoadjuvant chemotherapy prior to surgical cytoreduction.* In addition to resolving whether this therapy is indicated, future trials will need to address (a) an optimal bevacizumab dosage (7.5 mg/kg or 15 mg/kg every 3 weeks); (b) the optimal duration of bevacizumab maintenance (1 year, until progression, or beyond progression); and (c) any biologic predictors given bevacizumab's modest activity and substantial toxicity and cost
   - GOG 218 (3 arms): (a) cyclophosphamide + paclitaxel (CP); (b) CP + concomitant bevacizumab only, and (c) CP + concomitant and maintenance bevacizumab. After a median follow-up of 17.4 months, PFS was significantly prolonged with CP + concomitant and maintenance bevacizumab compared with CP alone (14.1 vs 10.3 months; HR 0.717; P <0.0001). Importantly there was no PFS advantage for CP + *concomitant bevacizumab only* over the CP-alone control arm (11.2 vs 10.3 months; HR 0.908; P = 0.080)
   - ICON7: median PFS 19.8 months for women receiving concurrent and maintenance bevacizumab compared with 17.4 months for those in the control arm (P = 0.039). Overall survival, among all participants was not improved (HR for death of 0.85; 95% CI 0.69–1.04). But in the high-risk subgroup—stage III with ≥1 cm residual tumor after surgery and all stage IV patients—the HR was 0.64; 95% CI 0.48–0.85; P = 0.002

Bookman MA et al. J Clin Oncol 2009;27:1419–1425. Erratum in: J Clin Oncol 2009;27:2305
Burger RA et al. Proc Am Soc Clin Oncol 2010;28(15S, Part I of II):5s [abstract LBA1]
du Bois A et al. Ann Oncol 2005;16(Suppl 8):viii7–viii12
Katsumata N et al. Lancet 2009;374:1331–1338
Kristensen G. Proc Am Soc Clin Oncol 2011;29(18S, Part II of II):781s [abstract LBA5006]
McGuire WP et al. N Engl J Med 1996;334:1–6
Ozols RF et al. J Clin Oncol 2003;21:3194–3200
Papadimitriou C et al. Bone Marrow Transplant 2008;41:547–554
Ray-Coquard I et al. N Engl J Med 2019;381:2416–2428

(continued)

Expert Opinion: Epithelial Ovarian Cancer (EOC), Primary Peritoneal Cancer (PPC), Fallopian Tube Cancer—Chemotherapy (*continued*)

Recurrent disease

1. Treatment of recurrent disease is complex. Decisions should be based on:
   - Likelihood of sensitivity/resistance to agents given in the past: platinum-sensitive or -resistant disease
   - Residual toxicity from prior treatments
   - Prior exposure to immunotherapy and targeted therapies
   - Availability of clinical trials
   - Comorbid illnesses including renal, hepatic, and cardiac function
   - Desires of the patient

Definitions:

Platinum-refractory disease
   - Disease that grows through initial platinum-containing therapy

Platinum-sensitive disease
   - Epithelial ovarian cancer that recurs, $\geq 1–2$ years after platinum-based chemotherapy
   - Response rate to retreatment with another platinum agent-based regimen tends to be high (>70%)

Platinum-resistant disease
   - *Definition:* Disease progression in the face of appropriate initial platinum-based treatment or disease recurrence within the first 6 months after an initial response to platinum-based therapy
   - *Prognosis:* Poor, especially if disease progresses during the initial 6 cycles of therapy with platinum agents
   - *Chemotherapy recommendations:* Use of non-cross-resistant agents in the second-line and third-line settings is critically important

2. Patients with disease progression without evidence of benefit after the initial 2 therapies should either be enrolled on a clinical trial or enroll in hospice

3. Patients who have not received chemotherapy should be approached as discussed above under **Advanced-stage disease (stage II, III, or IV)**

4. Patients with "platinum-sensitive disease" can receive platinum doublets including:
   - **Carboplatin + paclitaxel**
   - **Cisplatin + paclitaxel**
   - **Cisplatin + cyclophosphamide**
   - **Carboplatin + weekly paclitaxel**
   - **Carboplatin + docetaxel**
   - **Carboplatin + gemcitabine**
   - **Carboplatin + liposomal doxorubicin**
   - **Cisplatin + gemcitabine**
   - **Single-agent cisplatin**
   - **Single-agent carboplatin**
   - **Bevacizumab**

5. Agents with activity in both platinum-sensitive and platinum-refractory disease include:
   - **Docetaxel**
   - **Pemetrexed**
   - **Oral etoposide**
   - **Gemcitabine**
   - **Liposomal doxorubicin**
   - **Weekly paclitaxel**
   - **Topotecan**
   - **Fluorouracil**
   - **Altretamine (hexamethylmelamine)**
   - **Olaparib**
   - **Niraparib**
   - **Rucaparib**
   - **Pazopanib**
   - **Pembrolizumab**

(*continued*)

Expert Opinion: Epithelial Ovarian Cancer (EOC), Primary Peritoneal Cancer (PPC), Fallopian Tube Cancer—Chemotherapy (continued)

6. **Bevacizumab** seems to be well tolerated and active in second-line and third-line treatments of patients with EOC/PPC
   - OCEANS: a phase 3 trial comparing carboplatin and gemcitabine ± bevacizumab in women with platinum-sensitive recurrent ovarian cancer. A 3.7-month PFS advantage for women using bevacizumab, with an interim analysis of OS demonstrating a 5.6-month advantage for the bevacizumab arm

Burger RA et al. J Clin Oncol 2007;25:5165–5171
Cannistra SA et al. J Clin Oncol 2007;25:5180–5186
Leitao MM, Jr et al. Gynecol Oncol 2003;91:123–129
Markman M et al. Gynecol Oncol 2004;93:699–701
Markman M et al. J Cancer Res Clin Oncol 2004;130:25–28
Reed E et al. Gynecol Oncol 1992;46:326–329

Expert Opinion: Epithelial Ovarian Cancer (EOC), Primary Peritoneal Cancer (PPC), Fallopian Tube Cancer—Surgery

1. Ideally, a gynecologic oncologist should perform all surgical procedures for ovarian cancer, including:
   - Laparoscopy to evaluate extent of disease and potential for surgical resection
   - Initial staging and debulking surgery
   - "Second look" procedures (if done)
   - Any interval surgical debulking procedure
2. Goals of initial surgical procedure:
   - Stage the disease
   - Remove all visible disease from the abdominopelvic cavity, or
   - If surgeon cannot remove all visible disease, remove all disease possible (debulking surgery)
3. Debulking is important because subsequent survival and response to chemotherapy are linked to:
   - Dimension of the largest remaining tumor lesions after the completion of surgery
   - Possibly the overall volume of residual disease
4. Surgery alone is the preferred approach to patients with good-prognosis early-stage epithelial ovarian cancer:
   - *Stages:* IA or IB
   - *Histology:* any epithelial histology other than clear cell
   - *Histologic grade:* well-differentiated or moderately well-differentiated (any early-stage patient other than these should have chemotherapy after surgery)
5. Neoadjuvant chemotherapy:
   - Three to 4 cycles of chemotherapy before an initial staging and debulking procedure
   - Data suggest a less-morbid operation, with reduced blood loss and a shorter operative procedure
   - Has received widespread acceptance and is regionally offered as standard of care

Bristow RE et al. J Clin Oncol 2002;20:1248–1259
Brockbank ED et al. Eur J Surg Oncol 2013;39:912–917
Eisenhauer EL et al. Gynecol Oncol 2006;103:1083–1090
Fagotti A et al. Gynecol Oncol 2013;131:341–346
Hoskins WJ et al. Am J Obstet Gynecol 1994;170:974–979; discussion 979–980
Schwartz PE et al. Gynecol Oncol 1999;72:93–99
Schwartz PE, Zheng W. Gynecol Oncol 2003;90:644–650

FIRST-LINE

OVARIAN CANCER REGIMEN: INTRAPERITONEAL CISPLATIN AND PACLITAXEL

Armstrong DK et al. N Engl J Med 2006;354:34–43
Walker JL et al. Gynecol Oncol 2006;100:27–32
GOG Protocol #0172

Note: regimen for stage III epithelial ovarian or peritoneal carcinoma optimally debulked with no residual mass greater than 1 cm in diameter after surgery. Suboptimally debulked disease should not be treated with this regimen

Premedication for paclitaxel:
Dexamethasone 10 mg/dose; administer orally for 2 doses 12 hours and 6 hours before paclitaxel, *or*
Dexamethasone 20 mg/dose; administer intravenously over 10–15 minutes, 30–60 minutes before paclitaxel (total dose/cycle = 20 mg)
Diphenhydramine 50 mg; administer by intravenous injection 30 minutes before paclitaxel
Cimetidine 300 mg (or **ranitidine** 50 mg, **famotidine** 20 mg, or an equivalent histamine receptor [H_2]-subtype antagonist); administer intravenously over 15–30 minutes, 30–60 minutes before paclitaxel

Paclitaxel 135 mg/m²; administer intravenously in a volume of 0.9% sodium chloride injection (0.9% NS) or 5% dextrose injection (D5W) sufficient to produce a concentration within the range 0.3–1.2 mg/mL, over 24 hours on day 1, every 21 days, for 6 cycles (total dosage of paclitaxel intravenously/cycle = 135 mg/m²)

Intraperitoneal cisplatin
Hydration before cisplatin: ≥1000 mL 0.9% NS; administer by intravenous infusion over a minimum of 2–4 hours
Note: if a large amount of ascites is present, it should be drained prior to the instillation of cisplatin
Cisplatin 100 mg/m²; administer intraperitoneally as rapidly as possible in warmed (37°C [98.6°F]) 0.9% NS 2000 mL through an implanted peritoneal catheter on day 2, every 21 days, for 6 cycles (total dosage/21-day cycle = 100 mg/m²). Following the infusion, patients alternate position from prone, supine, and left and right lateral decubitus every 15 minutes over 2 hours to maximize drug distribution throughout the peritoneal cavity
Note: do not attempt to retrieve the infusate
Hydration after cisplatin: ≥1000 mL 0.9% NS; administer by intravenous infusion over a minimum of 3–4 hours. Also encourage high oral fluid intake. Goal is to achieve a urine output of ≥100 mL/hour

Intraperitoneal paclitaxel
Note: if a large amount of ascites is present, it should be drained prior to the instillation of paclitaxel
Paclitaxel 60 mg/m²; administer intraperitoneally as rapidly as possible in warmed (37°C [98.6°F]) 0.9% NS or D5W 1000 mL through an implanted peritoneal catheter, followed by an additional 1000 mL of 0.9% NS or D5W on day 8, every 21 days, for 6 cycles (total dosage of paclitaxel administered intraperitoneally/21-day cycle = 60 mg/m²)
Note: do not attempt to retrieve the infusate

Systemic cisplatin
If intraperitoneal therapy is discontinued, substitute:
Cisplatin 75 mg/m²; administer intravenously in 250 mL 0.9% NS over 30–60 minutes on day 2, every 21 days, for 3 cycles (total dosage/cycle = 75 mg/m²)

Supportive Care
Antiemetic prophylaxis
Emetogenic potential on days 1 and 8 is **LOW**
Emetogenic potential on day 2 is **HIGH**. *Potential for delayed symptoms*
See Chapter 42 for antiemetic recommendations

Hematopoietic growth factor (CSF) prophylaxis
Primary prophylaxis is **NOT** *indicated*
See Chapter 43 for more information

Antimicrobial prophylaxis
Risk of fever and neutropenia is **LOW**
  Antimicrobial primary prophylaxis to be considered:
  • Antibacterial—not indicated
  • Antifungal—not indicated
  • Antiviral—not indicated unless patient previously had an episode of HSV

Arthralgia and myalgia G ≤2 associated with chemotherapy
Dexamethasone 4–8 mg/dose orally twice daily for 6 doses after chemotherapy

Treatment Modifications

Dose Modification Levels for Treatment

	IV Paclitaxel	IP Cisplatin	IP Paclitaxel
Starting dose	135 mg/m^2	100 mg/m^2	60 mg/m^2
Level −1	110 mg/m^2	75 mg/m^2	45 mg/m^2

Note: no dose escalations performed

Dose Escalations for Hematologic Toxicity

Adverse Event	Treatment Modification
ANC <1500/mm^3 or platelet count <100,000/mm^3 on day 1 of a cycle	Delay start of next cycle until ANC ≥1500/mm^3 and platelet count ≥100,000/mm^3. Do not adjust dosages or add filgrastim if the delay is less than 2 weeks
>2 weeks, but ≤3 weeks delay to start next cycle because ANC <1500/mm^3 or platelet count <100,000/mm^3 on day 1	Reduce intravenous paclitaxel dosage 1 level
>2 weeks delay in start of a cycle because ANC <1500/mm^3 or platelet count <100,000/mm^3 on day 1 despite 1 dose reduction	Add filgrastim 5 μg/kg per day beginning 24 hours after completion of intravenous chemotherapy and continue use for 14 days
>3 weeks delay to start next cycle because ANC <1500/mm^3 or platelet count <100,000/mm^3 on day 1 regardless of whether filgrastim was or was not used	Discontinue therapy
ANC <1500/mm^3 or platelet count <100,000/mm^3 on day 8 of a cycle	Do not delay nor adjust intraperitoneal paclitaxel dosage
Uncomplicated WBC or ANC nadirs	Do not modify dosages
ANC <500/mm^3 on day 8	Add filgrastim 5 μg/kg per day until ANC >5000–10,000/mm^3
Nadir platelet count <25,000/mm^3	Reduce intravenous paclitaxel dosage 1 dose level
First episode of febrile neutropenia or sepsis requiring intravenous antibiotics	Reduce intravenous paclitaxel dosage 1 dose level. Do not add filgrastim
Febrile neutropenia or sepsis requiring intravenous antibiotics despite reduction of paclitaxel 1 dosage level	Add filgrastim beginning 24 hours after completion of IV chemotherapy and continuing for 14 days without additional dosage modification

Abdominal Pain Score

G0	No pain
G1	Mild pain. Opioid analgesia not required; pain causes minimal interference with daily activities and lasts for less than 72 hours
G2	Moderate pain. Opioid analgesia required; pain causes moderate interference with daily activities and lasts longer than 72 hours
G3	Severe pain. Opioid analgesia required; pain confines patient to bed and causes severe interference with daily activities
G2 abdominal pain	Reduce intraperitoneal cisplatin or paclitaxel, whichever is causing symptoms, by 1 dose level

(continued)

Patient Population Studied

A study of 205 women with stage III epithelial ovarian or peritoneal carcinoma optimally debulked with no residual mass greater than 1 cm in diameter after surgery. All patients had a Gynecologic Oncology Group (GOG) performance status of 0–2

Efficacy (N = 205)

Variable	Months
Median progression-free survival (PFS)	23.8
PFS in patients with gross residual disease	18.3
PFS in patients without visible residual disease	37.6
Median overall survival	65.6

Toxicity (N = 201)

Toxicity	% G3/4
Hematologic Toxicities	
WBC <1000/mm^3	76
Platelet count <25,000/mm^3	12
Other hematologic event	94
Nonhematologic Toxicities	
Gastrointestinal event	46
Metabolic event	27
Neurologic event	19
Fatigue	18
Infection	16
Pain	11
Cardiovascular event	9
Fever	9
Renal or genitourinary event	7
Pulmonary event	3
Hepatic event	3
Other	3
Cutaneous change	1
Event involving lymphatic system	1

(continued)

Treatment Modifications (continued)

Abdominal Pain Score

Recurrent G2 abdominal pain after a dose reduction or G3 abdominal pain or complications involving the intraperitoneal catheter prohibiting further intraperitoneal therapy	Discontinue intraperitoneal therapy and administer intravenous cisplatin instead
Any grade gastrointestinal toxicity	Hospitalize patient if necessary but do not adjust chemotherapy dosages
G2 peripheral neuropathy	Reduce cisplatin dosage by 1 dose level
G3/4 peripheral neuropathy	Hold therapy until peripheral neuropathy G ≤1 then restart therapy with cisplatin dosage reduced by 1 dose level. Consider discontinuing therapy if not recovered to baseline by 2–3 weeks
Increase in serum creatinine >0.7–1.0 mg/dL (>62–88 μmol/L) above baseline	Hold therapy until serum creatinine returns to baseline and reduce intraperitoneal cisplatin 1 dosage level. Consider discontinuing therapy if not recovered to baseline by 2–3 weeks

Notes

1. Among all randomized phase 3 trials conducted by the GOG among patients with advanced ovarian cancer, this therapy yielded the longest median survival (65.6 months)
2. Only 42% of patients received all 6 cycles of intraperitoneal therapy
3. The primary reason for discontinuation of intraperitoneal therapy was catheter-related complications
4. Among 205 patients randomly allocated to the intraperitoneal arm, 58% (119) did not complete all 6 cycles of intraperitoneal therapy. Of these 119 patients, 34% (40/119 = 34%) discontinued intraperitoneal therapy primarily as a result of catheter complications, whereas 29% (34/119 = 29%) discontinued for unrelated reasons. Additionally, 37% (45/119 = 37%) discontinued for reasons that were possibly related to the intraperitoneal treatment (see table under toxicities)
5. Hysterectomy, appendectomy, small bowel resection, and ileocecal resection were not associated with failure to complete 6 cycles
6. There appears to be an association between rectosigmoid colon resection and the ability to initiate intraperitoneal therapy. Intraperitoneal therapy was not initiated in 16% of patients who had a left colon or rectosigmoid colon resection versus 5% of those who did not have such a resection (P = 0.015)
7. Intraperitoneal therapy should begin as soon as possible after surgery. A delay of intraperitoneal therapy allows opportunity for adhesions to develop and may limit intraperitoneal distribution of the IP fluid
8. The 2 L of intraperitoneal fluid administered with the intraperitoneal therapy does not replace the need for intravascular hydration administration and adequate urine output. Administration of at least 1 L of 0.9% sodium chloride injection both prior to and after cisplatin is essential

Armstrong DK et al. N Engl J Med 2006;354:34–43
Walker JL et al. Gynecol Oncol 2006;100:27–32

Toxicity (N = 201) (continued)

Complications of IP Access Devices

Port complications	19.5%
Inflow obstruction	8.8%
Infection	10.2%
Bowel Injury	2%

Armstrong DK et al. N Engl J Med 2006;354:34–43
Walker JL et al. Gynecol Oncol 2006;100:27–32

Discontinuation of IP Therapy (N = 119)

Reason	Primary	Contributing
Catheter related	**40**	**10**
IP catheter infection	21	4
IP catheter blocked	10	0
IP catheter leak	3	2
Access problem	5	3
Fluid leak from vagina	1	1
Not IP catheter related	**34**	**28**
Nausea/vomiting/dehydration	16	16
Renal/metabolic	15	12
Disease progression	3	0
Possibly IP treatment related	**45**	**42**
Other infection (not catheter)	7	5
Abdominal pain	4	16
Patient refusal	19	8
Bowel complication	4	4
Other	11	9

Walker JL et al. Gynecol Oncol 2006;100:27–32

Therapy Monitoring

Before repeated cycles: PE, CBC with differential, and serum electrolytes, magnesium, calcium, BUN, and creatinine

RECURRENT • PLATINUM-SENSITIVE • FIRST-LINE
OVARIAN CANCER REGIMEN: CARBOPLATIN + PACLITAXEL

Ozols RF et al. J Clin Oncol 2003;21:3194–3200

Note: regimen for optimally debulked ovarian cancer and suboptimally debulked disease as well

Premedication for paclitaxel:
Dexamethasone 10 mg/dose; administer orally for 2 doses 12 hours and 6 hours before paclitaxel, *or*
Dexamethasone 20 mg/dose; administer intravenously over 10–15 minutes, 30–60 minutes before paclitaxel (total dose/cycle = 20 mg)
Diphenhydramine 50 mg; administer by intravenous injection 30 minutes before paclitaxel
Cimetidine 300 mg (or **ranitidine** 50 mg, **famotidine** 20 mg, or an equivalent histamine receptor [H_2]-subtype antagonist); administer intravenously over 15–30 minutes, 30–60 minutes before paclitaxel

Paclitaxel 175 mg/m^2; administer intravenously in a volume of 0.9% sodium chloride injection (0.9% NS) or 5% dextrose injection (D5W) sufficient to produce a concentration within the range 0.3–1.2 mg/mL, over 3 hours, on day 1, every 3 weeks (total dosage/cycle = 175 mg/m^2)
Carboplatin (calculated dose) AUC = 7.5*; administer intravenously in 0.9% NS or D5W 100–500 mL over 60 minutes, on day 1 after completing paclitaxel, every 3 weeks for 6 cycles (total dosage/cycle calculated to produce a target AUC = 7.5 mg/mL × min)

*Carboplatin dose is based on a formula described by Calvert et al. to achieve a target area under the plasma concentration versus time curve (AUC)

$$\text{Total carboplatin dose } (\text{mg}) = (\text{target AUC}) \times (\text{GFR} + 25)$$

In practice, creatinine clearance (Clcr) is used in place of glomerular filtration rate (GFR). Clcr can be calculated from the equation of Cockcroft and Gault:

$$\text{For males, Clcr} = \frac{(140 - \text{age [years]}) \times (\text{body weight [kg]})}{72 \times (\text{serum creatinine [mg/dL]})}$$

$$\text{For females, Clcr} = \frac{(140 - \text{age [years]}) \times (\text{body weight [kg]})}{72 \times (\text{serum creatinine [mg/dL]})} \times 0.85$$

Calvert AH et al. J Clin Oncol 1989;7:1748–1756
Cockcroft DW, Gault MH. Nephron 1976;16:31–41
Jodrell DI et al. J Clin Oncol 1992;10:520–528
Sorensen BT et al. Cancer Chemother Pharmacol 1991;28:397–401

- Provided actual GFR measurements are made to assess renal function, carboplatin can be safely dosed according to the Calvert formula described in product labeling
- If GFR (or creatinine clearance) is estimated based on serum creatinine measurements by the IDMS method, the FDA recommends capping an estimated GFR at 125 mL/min for any targeted AUC value for patients with normal renal function. No greater estimated GFR values should be used

Supportive Care
Antiemetic prophylaxis
*Emetogenic potential is **HIGH**. Potential for delayed symptoms*
See Chapter 42 for antiemetic recommendations

Hematopoietic growth factor (CSF) prophylaxis
*Primary prophylaxis is **NOT** indicated*
See Chapter 43 for more information

Antimicrobial prophylaxis
*Risk of fever and neutropenia is **LOW***
  Antimicrobial primary prophylaxis to be considered:
  - Antibacterial—not indicated
  - Antifungal—not indicated
  - Antiviral—not indicated unless patient previously had an episode of HSV

Treatment Modifications

Adverse Event	Dose Modification
At start of a cycle, ANC ≤1000/mm^3 or platelets ≤100,000/mm^3	Delay start of cycle up to 2 weeks until ANC >1000/mm^3 and platelets >100,000/mm^3
ANC ≤1000/mm^3 or platelets ≤100,000/mm^3 for more than 2 but less than 3 weeks after scheduled start of next cycle	Reduce paclitaxel and carboplatin dosages by 20% (140 mg/m^2 and AUC = 6, respectively)
At start of a cycle, ANC ≤1000/mm^3 and platelets ≤100,000/mm^3 despite dose reduction	Delay start of cycle until ANC >1000/mm^3 and platelets >1000/mm^3; then administer filgrastim 5 μg/kg per day subcutaneously for 14 days with same chemotherapy dosages
Serum creatinine >2 mg/dL (>177 μmol/L) or G ≥3 peripheral neuropathy	Delay start of cycle up to 2 weeks; if serum creatinine is not ≤2 mg/dL (≤177 μmol/L) or G <3 peripheral neuropathy, discontinue therapy

Patient Population Studied

A randomized study of 792 women with pathologically verified stage III epithelial ovarian cancer who were left with no residual disease >1 cm in diameter; 400 cisplatin arm and 392 carboplatin arm. McGuire et al (N Engl J Med 1996;334:1–6) had shown that cisplatin plus paclitaxel was superior to cisplatin plus cyclophosphamide in advanced-stage epithelial ovarian cancer. This study was a **noninferiority trial** of cisplatin and paclitaxel versus carboplatin and paclitaxel to show equivalence of the 2 regimens

Efficacy
(Carboplatin: N = 392)

Median progression-free survival	20.7 months
Median overall survival	57.4 months

Toxicity*
(Carboplatin: N = 392)

	% G3	% G4
Hematologic		
Leukopenia	53	6
Granulocytopenia	17	72
Thrombocytopenia	19	20
Nonhematologic		
Gastrointestinal	5	5
Neurologic†	7	0
Alopecia	0	0
Metabolic	2	1
Genitourinary	1	0
Pain	1	0

*GOG toxicity criteria
†Primarily peripheral neuropathy

Therapy Monitoring

Before repeated cycles: PE, CBC with differential, and serum electrolytes, magnesium, calcium, BUN, and creatinine

RECURRENT • PLATINUM-SENSITIVE • FIRST-LINE

OVARIAN CANCER REGIMEN: CISPLATIN + PACLITAXEL

Ozols RF et al. J Clin Oncol 2003;21:3194–3200

Premedication with **dexamethasone** 10 mg/dose; administer orally for 2 doses 12 hours and 6 hours before paclitaxel, *or*
Dexamethasone 20 mg; administer intravenously over 10–15 minutes, 30–60 minutes before paclitaxel (total dose/cycle = 20 mg)
Diphenhydramine 50 mg; administer by intravenous injection 30–60 minutes before paclitaxel
Cimetidine 300 mg (or **ranitidine** 50 mg, **famotidine** 20 mg, or an equivalent histamine receptor $[H_2]$-subtype antagonist); administer intravenously over 15–30 minutes, 30–60 minutes before paclitaxel
Paclitaxel 135 mg/m²; administer intravenously in a volume of 0.9% sodium chloride injection (0.9% NS) or 5% dextrose injection sufficient to produce a concentration within the range 0.3–1.2 mg/mL, over 24 hours on day 1, every 3 weeks, for 6 cycles (total dosage/cycle = 135 mg/m²)
Hydration before cisplatin: ≥1000 mL 0.9% NS; administer by intravenous infusion over a minimum of 2–4 hours
Cisplatin 75 mg/m²; administer intravenously in 0.9% NS 100–250 mL over 1 hour, on day 2 after completing paclitaxel, every 3 weeks, for 6 cycles (total dosage/cycle = 75 mg/m²)
Note: Hydration after cisplatin: ≥1000 mL 0.9% NS; administer by intravenous infusion over a minimum of 3–4 hours. Also encourage high oral fluid intake.

Supportive Care
Antiemetic prophylaxis
Emetogenic potential during paclitaxel administration is **LOW**
Emetogenic potential during and after cisplatin administration is **HIGH**. *Potential for delayed symptoms*
See Chapter 42 for antiemetic recommendations

Hematopoietic growth factor (CSF) prophylaxis
Primary prophylaxis is **NOT** *indicated*
See Chapter 43 for more information

Antimicrobial prophylaxis
Risk of fever and neutropenia is **LOW**
   Antimicrobial primary prophylaxis to be considered:
   • Antibacterial—not indicated
   • Antifungal—not indicated
   • Antiviral—not indicated unless patient previously had an episode of HSV

Treatment Modifications

Adverse Event	Dose Modification
Delay in achieving ANC ≥1000/mm³ and platelets ≥100,000/mm³ <2 weeks	No dose adjustment; no filgrastim
Delay in achieving ANC ≥1000/mm³ and platelets ≥100,000/mm³ ≥2 weeks but ≤3 weeks	Reduce cisplatin dosage by 20%
Recurrent delays in achieving ANC ≥1000/mm³ and platelets ≥100,000/mm³ ≥2 weeks but ≤3 weeks	Add filgrastim 5 µg/kg per day subcutaneously. Start 24 hours after completing chemotherapy, and continue for 14 days without further dosage modification
Episode of febrile neutropenia after earlier delay in achieving ANC and platelets led to a reduction in cisplatin dosage	Add filgrastim 5 µg/kg per day subcutaneously. Start 24 hours after completing chemotherapy, and continue for 14 days without further dosage modification
G3/4 neurologic toxicity that has not resolved even after a 3-week delay	Discontinue therapy
Creatinine clearance* <30 mL/min (<0.5 mL/s)	Discontinue therapy

*Creatinine clearance used as a measure of glomerular filtration rate (GFR)

Patient Population Studied

Patients with advanced ovarian cancer and no residual mass greater than 1.0 cm after surgery were randomly assigned to receive cisplatin 75 mg/m² plus a 24-hour infusion of paclitaxel 135 mg/m² (arm I), or carboplatin area under the curve 7.5 intravenously plus paclitaxel 175 mg/m² over 3 hours (arm II)

Efficacy (Comparison of Regimens)

	Cisplatin (N = 400)	Carboplatin (N = 392)
Median progression-free survival (months)	19.4	20.7
Median overall survival (months)	48.7	57.4

Toxicity

	Cisplatin (N = 400)		Carboplatin (N = 392)	
	% G3	% G4	% G3	% G4
Hematologic				
Leukopenia*	51	12	53	6
Granulocytopenia	15	78	17	72
Thrombocytopenia*	3	2	19	20
Nonhematologic				
Gastrointestinal*	14	9	5	5
Neurologic	8	0	7	0
Alopecia	0	0	0	0
Metabolic*	6	2	2	1
Genitourinary*	3	0	1	0
Pain	1	0	1	0
	% G1/2		% G1/2	
Pain	15		26	

*Statistically significant difference at the 0.05 level

Therapy Monitoring

Before repeated cycles: PE, CBC with differential, and serum electrolytes, magnesium, calcium, BUN, and creatinine

Notes

There were no differences in efficacy between the cisplatin + paclitaxel and the carboplatin + paclitaxel treatment regimens. However, there were differences with respect to toxicities. The authors interpreted the data as showing that the carboplatin + paclitaxel regimen was equally efficacious and significantly less toxic than the cisplatin + paclitaxel regimen

RECURRENT • PLATINUM-SENSITIVE • FIRST-LINE
OVARIAN CANCER REGIMEN: CARBOPLATIN + WEEKLY (DOSE-DENSE) PACLITAXEL

Katsumata N et al. Lancet 2009;374:1331–1338

Note: regimen for optimally debulked ovarian cancer. Suboptimally debulked disease can be treated with this regimen as well

Premedication:
Dexamethasone 10 mg/dose; administer orally for 2 doses 12 hours and 6 hours before paclitaxel, *or*
Dexamethasone 20 mg/dose; administer intravenously over 10–15 minutes, 30–60 minutes before paclitaxel on days 1, 8, and 15 (total dose/cycle = 60 mg)
Diphenhydramine 50 mg; administer by intravenous injection 30–60 minutes before paclitaxel
Cimetidine 300 mg (or **ranitidine** 50 mg, **famotidine** 20 mg, or an equivalent histamine receptor [H_2]-subtype antagonist); administer intravenously over 15–30 minutes, 30–60 minutes before paclitaxel

Paclitaxel 80 mg/m^2 per dose; administer intravenously in a volume of 0.9% sodium chloride injection (0.9% NS) or 5% dextrose injection (D5W) sufficient to produce a concentration within the range 0.3–1.2 mg/mL, over 60 minutes for 3 doses, on days 1, 8, and 15, every 3 weeks (total dosage/cycle = 240 mg/m^2)
Carboplatin (calculated dose) AUC = 6*; administer intravenously in 0.9% NS or D5W 100–500 mL over 60 minutes, on day 1 after completing paclitaxel, every 3 weeks (total dosage/cycle calculated to produce a target AUC = 6 mg/mL × min)

*Carboplatin dose is based on a formula described by Calvert et al. to achieve a target area under the plasma concentration versus time curve (AUC)

$$\text{Total carboplatin dose (mg)} = (\text{target AUC}) \times (\text{GFR} + 25)$$

In practice, creatinine clearance (Clcr) is used in place of glomerular filtration rate (GFR). Clcr can be estimated from the equation of Cockcroft and Gault, thus:

$$\text{For males, Clcr} = \frac{(140 - \text{age [years]}) \times (\text{body weight [kg]})}{72 \times (\text{serum creatinine [mg/dL]})}$$

$$\text{For females, Clcr} = \frac{(140 - \text{age [years]}) \times (\text{body weight [kg]})}{72 \times (\text{serum creatinine [mg/dL]})} \times 0.85$$

Calvert AH et al. J Clin Oncol 1989;7:1748–1756
Cockcroft DW, Gault MH. Nephron 1976;16:31–41
Jodrell DI et al. J Clin Oncol 1992;10:520–528
Sorensen BT et al. Cancer Chemother Pharmacol 1991;28:397–401

Notes:
- Provided actual GFR measurements are made to assess renal function, carboplatin can be safely dosed according to the Calvert formula described in product labeling
- If GFR (or creatinine clearance) is estimated based on serum creatinine measurements by the IDMS method, the FDA recommends capping an estimated GFR at 125 mL/min for any targeted AUC value for patients with normal renal function. No greater estimated GFR values should be used

Supportive Care
Antiemetic prophylaxis
*Emetogenic potential on days with carboplatin is **HIGH**. Potential for delayed symptoms*
*Emetogenic potential on days with paclitaxel alone is **LOW***
See Chapter 42 for antiemetic recommendations

Hematopoietic growth factor (CSF) prophylaxis
*Primary prophylaxis is **NOT** indicated*
See Chapter 43 for more information

Antimicrobial prophylaxis
*Risk of fever and neutropenia is **LOW***
  Antimicrobial primary prophylaxis to be considered:
  - Antibacterial—not indicated
  - Antifungal—not indicated
  - Antiviral—not indicated unless patient previously had an episode of HSV

Dose Modifications

Adverse Event	Dose Modifications
ANC <1000/mm^3 or platelet count <75,000/mm^3	Hold day 1 chemotherapy until ANC ≥1000/mm^3 and platelet count ≥75,000/mm^3
ANC <1000/mm^3 or platelet count <75,000/mm^3 ≥3 weeks	Discontinue therapy
If on days 8 or 15, ANC <500/mm^3 or platelet count <50,000/mm^3	Hold chemotherapy until ANC ≥500/mm^3 and platelet count ≥50,000/mm^3
G3/4 nonhematologic toxicity	Reduce paclitaxel dosage to 70 mg/m^2
G3/4 nonhematologic toxicity with paclitaxel 70 mg/m^2	Reduce paclitaxel dosage to 60 mg/m^2
With carboplatin target AUC = 6 mg/mL × min: Febrile neutropenia, *or* ANC <500/mm^3 for ≥7 days, *or* platelet count <10,000/mm^3, *or* platelet count 10,000–50,000/mm^3 with bleeding, *or* treatment delay for hematologic toxicity <1 week	Reduce carboplatin dosage to target an AUC = 5 mg/mL × min
With carboplatin target AUC = 5 mg/mL × min: Febrile neutropenia, *or* ANC <500/mm^3 for ≥7 days, *or* platelet count <10,000/mm^3, *or* platelet count 10,000–50,000/mm^3 with bleeding, *or* treatment delay for hematologic toxicity <1 week	Reduce carboplatin dosage to target an AUC = 4 mg/mL × min
G ≥2 peripheral neuropathy	Reduce paclitaxel dosage to 70 mg/m^2
G ≥2 peripheral neuropathy with paclitaxel 70 mg/m^2	Reduce paclitaxel dosage to 60 mg/m^2
Significant hypersensitivity reaction to carboplatin (hypotension, dyspnea, and angioedema requiring therapy)*	Discontinue therapy

*Patients who experience G1/2 carboplatin hypersensitivity reactions may continue treatment if there is evidence of tumor response and appropriate preventive measures are instituted

Patient Population Studied

Patients with stage II–IV epithelial ovarian cancer, fallopian tube cancer, or primary peritoneal cancer. Previous chemotherapy was not allowed

Efficacy*

	Dose-Dense Paclitaxel[†] (N = 147)	Conventional Paclitaxel[‡] (N = 135)	P Value
Complete response[§]	20%	16%	0.44
Partial response[§]	36%	38%	0.81
Stable disease[§]	29%	31%	0.8
Progressive disease[§]	3%	7%	0.16
Not evaluable[§]	12%	9%	0.44
Median progression-free survival	28 months	17.2 months	0.0015
Overall survival at 2 years	83.6%	77.7%	0.049
Overall survival at 3 years	72.1%	65.1%	0.03

*Katsumata N et al. Lancet 2009;374:1331–1338
[†]Carboplatin AUC = 6 mg/mL × min + paclitaxel 80 mg/m2 per dose, on days 1, 8, and 15, every 21 days
[‡]Carboplatin AUC = 6 mg/mL × min + paclitaxel 180 mg/m2 on day 1, every 21 days
[§]Clinical response in patients with measurable lesions

Toxicity[*],[†]

	Dose-Dense Paclitaxel[‡] (N = 312)	Conventional Paclitaxel[§] (N = 314)	P Value
Hematologic Toxicity			
Neutropenia	92%	88%	0.15
Thrombocytopenia	44%	38%	0.19
Anemia	69%	44%	<0.0001
Febrile neutropenia	9%	9%	1
Nonhematologic Toxicity			
Nausea	10%	11%	0.7
Vomiting	3%	4%	0.82
Diarrhea	3%	3%	0.64
Fatigue	5%	3%	0.14
Arthralgia	1%	2%	0.72
Myalgia	1%	1%	0.69
Motor neuropathy	5%	4%	0.56
Sensory neuropathy	7%	6%	0.87

[*]Katsumata N et al. Lancet 2009;374:1331–1338
[†]According to NCI Common Toxicity Criteria, version 2.0
[‡]Carboplatin AUC = 6 mg/mL × min + paclitaxel 80 mg/m2 per dose, on days 1, 8, and 15, every 21 days
[§]Carboplatin AUC = 6 mg/mL × min + paclitaxel 180 mg/m2 on day 1, every 21 days

Therapy Monitoring

1. *Baseline:* LFTs, serum chemistry, CBC with differential and platelet count, and CA-125. Complete history and physical examination, including a gynecologic examination
2. *Follow-up:* CBC with differential and platelet count at least weekly through leukocyte and platelet count nadirs, and before beginning *repeated* cycles

Before beginning repeated cycles: Before repeated cycles: PE, CBC with differential, and serum electrolytes, magnesium, calcium, BUN, and creatinine, LFTs

RECURRENT • PLATINUM-SENSITIVE

OVARIAN CANCER REGIMEN: PLATINUM RETREATMENT (CISPLATIN OR CARBOPLATIN)

Leitao M et al. Gynecol Oncol 2003;91:123–129

Hydration before cisplatin: ≥1000 mL 0.9% sodium chloride injection (0.9% NS); administer intravenously over a minimum of 3–4 hours. Monitor and replace magnesium/electrolytes as needed

Cisplatin 80–100 mg/m²; administer intravenously in 100–500 mL 0.9% NS over 30–60 minutes on day 1, every 3 weeks, for a maximum of 8 cycles (total dosage/3-week cycle = 80–100 mg/m²)
Hydration after cisplatin: ≥1000 mL 0.9% NS; administer intravenously over a minimum of 3–4 hours. Also encourage high oral fluid intake. Goal is to achieve a urine output of ≥100 mL/hour
or
Carboplatin (calculated dose) AUC = 6; administer by intravenous infusion in 50–150 mL D5W over 15–30 minutes on day 1, every 3 weeks (total dosage/cycle calculated to produce an AUC = 6 mg/mL × min)

*Carboplatin dose is based on a formula described by Calvert et al. to achieve a target area under the plasma concentration versus time curve (AUC)

$$\text{Total carboplatin dose (mg)} = (\text{target AUC}) \times (\text{GFR} + 25)$$

In practice, creatinine clearance (Clcr) is used in place of glomerular filtration rate (GFR). Clcr can be estimated from the equation of Cockcroft and Gault, thus:

$$\text{For males, Clcr} = \frac{(140 - \text{age [years]}) \times (\text{body weight [kg]})}{72 \times (\text{serum creatinine [mg/dL]})}$$

$$\text{For females, Clcr} = \frac{(140 - \text{age [years]}) \times (\text{body weight [kg]})}{72 \times (\text{serum creatinine [mg/dL]})} \times 0.85$$

Calvert AH et al. J Clin Oncol 1989;7:1748–1756
Cockcroft DW , Gault MH. Nephron 1976;16:31–41
Jodrell DI et al. J Clin Oncol 1992;10:520–528
Sorensen BT et al. Cancer Chemother Pharmacol 1991;28:397–401

Notes:
• Provided actual GFR measurements are made to assess renal function, carboplatin can be safely dosed according to the Calvert formula described in product labeling
• If GFR (or creatinine clearance) is estimated based on serum creatinine measurements by the IDMS method, the FDA recommends capping an estimated GFR at 125 mL/min for any targeted AUC value for patients with normal renal function. No greater estimated GFR values should be used

Supportive Care
Antiemetic prophylaxis
Emetogenic potential is **MODERATE–HIGH** *(carboplatin) or* **HIGH** *(cisplatin). Potential for delayed symptoms with either carboplatin or cisplatin*
See Chapter 42 for antiemetic recommendations

Hematopoietic growth factor (CSF) prophylaxis
   Primary prophylaxis is indicated with 1 of the following:
   Filgrastim (G-CSF) 5 μg/kg per day by subcutaneous injection, *or*
   Pegfilgrastim (pegylated filgrastim) 6 mg/0.6 mL, by subcutaneous injection for 1 dose
   • Begin use from 24–72 hours after myelosuppressive chemotherapy is completed
   • Continue daily filgrastim use until ANC ≥10,000/mm³ on 2 measurements separated temporally by ≥12 hours
   • Discontinue daily filgrastim use at least 24 hours before repeating myelosuppressive treatment. Do not administer pegfilgrastim within 14 days before administering myelosuppressive treatment
See Chapter 43 for more information

Antimicrobial prophylaxis
Risk of fever and neutropenia is **LOW–INTERMEDIATE**
   Antimicrobial primary prophylaxis to be considered:
   • Antibacterial—consider a fluoroquinolone or no prophylaxis
   • Antifungal—not indicated
   • Antiviral—not indicated unless patient previously had an episode of HSV

Arthralgia and myalgia G ≥2 associated with chemotherapy
Dexamethasone 4–8 mg/dose orally twice daily for 6 doses after chemotherapy

Treatment Modifications

Adverse Event	Dose Modification
Cisplatin	
Creatinine clearance 40–60 mL/min (0.66–1 mL/s)	Reduce cisplatin so that dose in milligrams equals the creatinine clearance* value in mL/min[†]
Creatinine clearance <40 mL/min (<0.66 mL/s)	Hold cisplatin
On treatment day 1, serum creatinine 1.6–2 mg/dL (141–177 μmol/L)	Reduce cisplatin dosage by 25%
On treatment day 1, serum creatinine >2 mg/dL (>177 μmol/L)	Hold cisplatin until serum creatinine ≤2.0 mg/dL (≤177 μmol/L)
Day 1 WBC <2000/mm^3 or platelet count <100,000/mm^3	Delay cisplatin for 1 week or until myelosuppression resolves, whichever occurs later
Second treatment delay because of myelosuppression	Delay cisplatin for 1 week, or until myelosuppression resolves, then decrease cisplatin dosage to 60–80 mg/m^2 during subsequent treatments
Sepsis during an episode of neutropenia	
Bleeding associated with thrombocytopenia	Reduce cisplatin dosage to 60–80 mg/m^2
Carboplatin	
ANC nadir <500/mm^3, platelet nadir <50,000/mm^3 or febrile neutropenia	Reduce carboplatin dosage to AUC = 5 mg/mL × min if previous cycle dose was AUC = 6; or to AUC = 4 if previous cycle dose was AUC = 5
ANC nadir <500/mm^3, platelet nadir <50,000/mm^3, or febrile neutropenia after 2 carboplatin dose reductions (AUC in previous cycle = 4 mg/mL × min)	Decrease carboplatin dosage to AUC = 3 mg/mL × min
Day 1 ANC <1500/mm^3 or platelets <100,000/mm^3	Delay chemotherapy until ANC >1500/mm^3 and platelets >100,000/mm^3, for maximum delay of 2 weeks
Delay of >2 weeks in reaching ANC >1500/mm^3 or platelets >100,000/mm^3	Discontinue therapy
Bleeding associated with thrombocytopenia	Reduce carboplatin dosages to AUC 4–5 mg/mL × min

*Creatinine clearance used as a measure of glomerular filtration rate
[†]This also applies to patients with creatinine clearance (GFR) of 40–60 mL/min (0.66–1 mL/s) at the outset of treatment

Efficacy (N = 30)

Variable	No. of Patients	% PR
Best Response to Last Platinum Regimen		
Complete or partial response	14	43
Stable or progressive disease	16	6
Platinum-Free Interval		
≤6 months	2	0
6–12 months	8	63
>12 months	20	10
Number of Intervening Nonplatinum Agents		
≤3	20	35
>3	10	0
Time to Progression After Last Platinum Regimen		
≤6 months	23	17
>4;6 months	6	50
Number of Prior Platinum Regimens		
1 prior regimen	9	33
2 or 3 prior regimens	21	19

Patient Population Studied

A study of 30 patients with platinum-resistant ovarian cancer, who received nonplatinum chemotherapy for recurrent epithelial ovarian cancer before additional platinum therapy. Platinum resistance was defined as less than a partial response to platinum therapy or progression within 6 months of the last platinum therapy

Toxicity

Cisplatin: (PLATINOL-AQ [cisplatin injection] product label, November 2002. Bristol-Myers Squibb)

Individual and cumulative dose-related renal toxicity: increased serum creatinine, uric acid, and BUN *Renal tubular damage with electrolyte wasting:* hypomagnesemia, hypocalcemia, hyponatremia, hypokalemia, and hypophosphatemia	28–36%*
Dose-related, cumulative peripheral neuropathies: bilateral paresthesias, areflexia, loss of proprioception and vibratory sensation, motor neuropathies	30–100% depending on cumulative doses
Optic neuritis, papilledema, and cerebral blindness	Rare
Cumulative ototoxicity: with tinnitus or high frequency hearing loss. Vestibular toxicity	31%*
Nausea and vomiting at any dose: severe and delayed emesis at dosages $\geq$50 mg/m^2	Varies (moderate to severe in virtually all patients without effective antiemetic prophylaxis)
Transiently increased liver transaminases	Rare
Hypersensitivity reactions: anaphylactoid reactions, facial edema, wheezing, tachycardia, and hypotension	1–20%
Coombs-positive hemolytic anemia	Rare
Dose-related leukopenia, thrombocytopenia, anemia	25–30%*

Carboplatin: (PARAPLATIN [carboplatin aqueous solution] Injection product label, January 2004. Bristol-Myers Squibb)

Nausea and vomiting	92%†
Diarrhea, constipation, other GI side effects	21%
Thrombocytopenia <100,000/mm^3 *Thrombocytopenia* <50,000/mm^3	62% 35%
Neutropenia: <1000/mm^3	21%
Anemia <11 g/dL Anemia <8 g/dL	90% 21%
Nephrotoxicity: increased serum creatinine Increased BUN	10% 22%
Hyponatremia, hypomagnesemia, hypocalcemia, hypokalemia	47%, 43%, 31%, 28%
Peripheral neuropathies: paresthesia, ataxia, distal motor deficits; decreased vibratory sense, light touch, pinprick, and joint position; areflexia	
Cumulative ototoxicity: tinnitus, high-frequencies hearing loss, audiogram deficits	1.1%
Increased alkaline phosphatase, AST, total bilirubin	37%
Alopecia	19%
Hypersensitivity reactions: facial flushing, generalized urticaria, hypotension, rash, pruritus, bronchospasm, shortness of breath	5%

*Incidence after a single treatment with cisplatin 50 mg/m^2
†All data are based on the experience of 553 patients with previously treated ovarian carcinoma who received single-agent carboplatin, without regard for their baseline status

Therapy Monitoring

1. *Before repeated cycles:* PE, CBC with differential, serum electrolytes, magnesium, calcium, BUN, and creatinine
2. *Every month:* serum CA-125 level
3. *Every 2–3 months:* restaging radiographic studies

RECURRENT • PLATINUM-SENSITIVE

OVARIAN CANCER REGIMEN: GEMCITABINE + CARBOPLATIN

Pfisterer J et al. J Clin Oncol 2006;24:4699–4707

Gemcitabine 1000 mg/m² per dose; administer intravenously in 50–250 mL 0.9% sodium chloride injection (0.9% NS) over 30–60 minutes for 2 doses, on days 1 and 8, every 21 days (total dosage/cycle = 2000 mg/m²)
Note: on day 1, administer after hydration for carboplatin, then follow with carboplatin
Carboplatin (calculated dose) AUC = 4 mg/mL × min*; administer intravenously in 0.9% NS or 5% dextrose injection 100–500 mL over 1 hour, on day 1 after completing gemcitabine, every 3 weeks (total dosage/cycle calculated to produce a target AUC = 4 mg/mL × min)

*Carboplatin dose is based on a formula described by Calvert et al. to achieve a target area under the plasma concentration versus time curve (AUC)

$$\text{Total carboplatin dose (mg)} = (\text{target AUC}) \times (\text{GFR} + 25)$$

In practice, creatinine clearance (Clcr) is used in place of glomerular filtration rate (GFR). Clcr can be estimated from the equation of Cockcroft and Gault, thus:

$$\text{For males, Clcr} = \frac{(140 - \text{age [years]}) \times (\text{body weight [kg]})}{72 \times (\text{serum creatinine [mg/dL]})}$$

$$\text{For females, Clcr} = \frac{(140 - \text{age [years]}) \times (\text{body weight [kg]})}{72 \times (\text{serum creatinine [mg/dL]})} \times 0.85$$

Calvert AH et al. J Clin Oncol 1989;7:1748–1756
Cockcroft DW , Gault MH. Nephron 1976;16:31–41
Jodrell DI et al. J Clin Oncol 1992;10:520–528
Sorensen BT et al. Cancer Chemother Pharmacol 1991;28:397–401

Notes:
- Provided actual GFR measurements are made to assess renal function, carboplatin can be safely dosed according to the Calvert formula described in product labeling
- If GFR (or creatinine clearance) is estimated based on serum creatinine measurements by the IDMS method, the FDA recommends capping an estimated GFR at 125 mL/min for any targeted AUC value for patients with normal renal function. No greater estimated GFR values should be used

Supportive Care
Antiemetic prophylaxis
Emetogenic potential on days with gemcitabine alone is **LOW**
Emetogenic potential on days with carboplatin is **MODERATE**. *Potential for delayed symptoms*
See Chapter 42 for antiemetic recommendations

Hematopoietic growth factor (CSF) prophylaxis
Primary prophylaxis is **NOT** *indicated*
See Chapter 43 for more information

Antimicrobial prophylaxis
Risk of fever and neutropenia is **LOW**
  Antimicrobial primary prophylaxis to be considered:
- Antibacterial—not indicated
- Antifungal—not indicated
- Antiviral—not indicated unless patient previously had an episode of HSV

Dose Modifications

Adverse Event	Dose Modifications
ANC <1500/mm³ or platelet count <100,000/mm³	Hold day 1 chemotherapy until ANC ≥1500/mm³ and platelet count ≥100,000/mm³
ANC <1500/mm³ or platelet count <100,000/mm³ ≥2 weeks	Discontinue therapy
Intracycle: G1/2 nonhematologic toxicity or G1–3 nausea or vomiting	100% gemcitabine dosage on day 8
Intracycle: G3 nonhematologic toxicity, except nausea, vomiting, and alopecia	Reduce gemcitabine dosage by 50% on day 8, or hold treatment at clinician's discretion
Intracycle: G4 nonhematologic toxicity	Hold gemcitabine
Day 8 ANC ≥1000–1400/mm³ and/or platelet count ≥75,000–99,000/mm³	Reduce gemcitabine dosage by 50%
Day 8 ANC <1000/mm³ and platelet count <75,000/mm³	Hold gemcitabine
Febrile neutropenia, or ANC <500/mm³ for >5 days, or ANC <100/mm³ for >3 days, or platelet count <25,000/mm³, or platelet count <50,000/mm³ with bleeding, or G3/4 nonhematologic toxicity (except nausea/vomiting), or treatment delay for toxicity ≥1 week	Reduce gemcitabine dosage to 800 mg/m² per dose *Note:* if gemcitabine dosage is 800 mg/m² then discontinue gemcitabine
Significant hypersensitivity reaction to carboplatin (hypotension, dyspnea, and angioedema requiring therapy)*	Discontinue therapy

*Patients who experience G1/2 carboplatin hypersensitivity reactions may continue treatment if there is evidence of tumor response and appropriate preventive measures are instituted

Patient Population Studied

Patients with platinum-sensitive recurrent ovarian cancer were randomly assigned to receive either gemcitabine plus carboplatin or carboplatin alone. The primary objective was to compare progression-free survival (PFS)

Efficacy

Efficacy (N = 178)	
Not assessable/not done	6.7
Progressive disease	7.9
Stable disease	38.2
Partial response (PR)	32.6
Complete response (CR)	14.6
Overall response rate: CR + PR (95% CI)	47.2 (39.9–54.5)

Toxicity

Selected Toxicities* and Associated Supportive Care

	% G1	% G2	% G3	% G4
Hematologic				
Anemia	18.3	41.7	22.3	5.1
Neutropenia	5.1	15.4	41.7	28.6
Thrombocytopenia	23.4	20.6	30.3	4.6
Nonhematologic				
Allergic reaction/hypersensitivity	0.6	2.3	1.7	0.6
Alopecia	34.9	14.3	NA[†]	NA[†]
Diarrhea	9.1	4	1.7	0
Dyspnea	0.6	6.9	1.1	0
Fatigue	16.6	20	1.7	0.6
Febrile neutropenia	0	0	1.1	0
Infection without neutropenia	0.6	0.6	0	0.6
Infection with neutropenia	0.6	0	0	0
Neuropathy, motor	5.1	0.6	0.6	0
Neuropathy, sensory	24.6	4	1.1	0
Vomiting	23.4	16	2.9	0
Treatment				
Parenteral Antibiotics	8.4%			
G-CSF or GM-CSF[‡]	23.6%			
RBCs	27%			
EPO[§]	7.3%			

*NCI-CTC, National Cancer Institute Common Toxicity Criteria
[†]NA, not applicable. Grade 3/4 alopecia not recognized by NCI-CTC (version 2.0 and later)
[‡]G-CSF, granulocyte colony-stimulating factor; GM-CSF, granulocyte macrophage colony-stimulating factor
[§]Erythropoietin or epoetin alfa

Therapy Monitoring

1. *Baseline:* LFTs, serum chemistry, CBC with differential and platelet count, and CA-125. Complete history and physical examination including a gynecologic examination
2. *Follow-up:* CBC with differential and platelet count on days 1, 8, and 15 of each cycle

RECURRENT • PLATINUM-SENSITIVE
OVARIAN CANCER REGIMEN: GEMCITABINE + CARBOPLATIN + BEVACIZUMAB

Aghajanian C et al. J Clin Oncol 2012;30:2039–2045
Protocol for: Aghajanian C et al. J Clin Oncol 2012;30:2039–2045
Comment in: Nat Rev Clin Oncol 2012;9:305, J Clin Oncol 2013;31:166–167

Bevacizumab 15 mg/kg; administer intravenously in 100 mL 0.9% sodium chloride injection (0.9% NS) on day 1 before gemcitabine and carboplatin, every 21 days (total dosage/cycle = 15 mg/kg)
Note: the initial bevacizumab dose is administered over 90 minutes. If administration is well tolerated, the administration duration may be decreased stepwise during subsequent administrations to 60 minutes and, finally, to a minimum duration of 30 minutes
Gemcitabine 1000 mg/m² per dose; administer intravenously over 30 minutes in 50–250 mL 0.9% NS for 2 doses on days 1 and 8, every 21 days (total dosage/cycle = 2000 mg/m²)
Carboplatin target AUC = 4 mg/mL min; administer intravenously over 30–60 minutes in a volume of 5% dextrose injection, USP or 0.9% NS sufficient to produce a solution with carboplatin concentration ≥0.5 mg/mL on day 1, every 21 days (total dose/cycle calculated to achieve a target AUC = 4 mg/mL × min)
Notes:

• Planned treatment included six repeated cycles, but patients were permitted to receive up to 10 cycles if continued response was documented

• Hypertension is associated with bevacizumab use. Treat with antihypertensive medications as needed to control blood pressures consistent with general medical practice

Supportive Care
Antiemetic prophylaxis
Emetogenic potential on day 1 is **MODERATE–HIGH**. *Potential for delayed emetic symptoms*
Emetogenic potential on day 8 is **LOW**
See Chapter 42 for antiemetic recommendations

Hematopoietic growth factor (CSF) prophylaxis
Primary prophylaxis may be indicated
See Chapter 43 for more information

Antimicrobial prophylaxis
Risk of fever and neutropenia is **LOW**
  Antimicrobial primary prophylaxis to be considered:
  • Antibacterial—not indicated

  • Antifungal—not indicated

  • Antiviral—not indicated, unless patient previously had an episode of HSV

Treatment plan notes
Carboplatin dose
Carboplatin dose is based on a formula described by Calvert et al to achieve a target area under the plasma concentration versus time curve (AUC):

$$\text{Total Carboplatin Dose (mg)} = (\text{target AUC}) \times (\text{GFR} + 25)$$

In practice, creatinine clearance (Clcr) is used in place of glomerular filtration rate (GFR). Clcr can be estimated from the equation of Cockcroft and Gault, thus:

$$\text{For males, Clcr} = \frac{(140 - \text{age [y]}) \times (\text{body weight [kg]})}{72 \times (\text{serum creatinine [mg/dL]})}$$

$$\text{For females, Clcr} = \frac{(140 - \text{age [y]}) \times (\text{body weight [kg]})}{72 \times (\text{serum creatinine [mg/dL]})} \times 0.85$$

Calvert AH et al. J Clin Oncol 1989;7:1748–1756
Cockcroft DW, Gault MH. Nephron 1976;16:31–41
Jodrell DI et al. J Clin Oncol 1992;10:520–528
Sørensen BT et al. Cancer Chemother Pharmacol 1991;28:397–401

Notes:

• Provided actual GFR measurements are made to assess renal function, carboplatin can be safely dosed according to the Calvert formula described in product labeling

• If GFR (or creatinine clearance) is estimated based on serum creatinine measurements by the IDMS method, the FDA recommends capping an estimated GFR at 125 mL/min for any targeted AUC value for patients with normal renal function. No greater estimated GFR values should be used

Dose Modification

GEMCITABINE + CARBOPLATIN + BEVACIZUMAB
DOSE MODIFICATIONS

Note the protocol document stated the following: No reductions in study drug (bevacizumab) dose are allowed in this study. Criteria for treatment modification and guidelines for the management of toxicities are summarized in Table 1. If adverse events occur that necessitate holding study drug, the dose will remain unchanged once treatment resumes

Bevacizumab	
Adverse Event	**Treatment Modification**
Gastrointestinal perforations (gastrointestinal perforations, fistula formation in the gastrointestinal tract, intra-abdominal abscess), fistula formation involving an internal organ	Discontinue bevacizumab permanently
Serious bleeding	
Wound dehiscence requiring medical intervention	
Nephrotic syndrome	
Hypertensive crisis or hypertensive encephalopathy or reversible posterior leukoencephalopathy syndrome (RPLS)	
Congestive heart failure	
Necrotizing fasciitis	
Severe arterial or venous thromboembolic events	Discontinue bevacizumab permanently; the safety of reinitiating bevacizumab after a thromboembolic event is resolved is not known
Moderate to severe proteinuria	Patients with a ≥2+ urine dipstick reading should undergo further assessment, eg, a 24-hour urine collection. Suspend bevacizumab administration for ≥2 g of proteinuria/24 h and resume when proteinuria is <2 g/24 h
G1/2 hypertension	No dose modification required
G3 hypertension	If not controlled to 150/100 mm Hg with medication, discontinue treatment with bevacizumab
Severe hypertension not controlled with medical management	Hold bevacizumab pending further evaluation and treatment of hypertension
G4 hypertension	Discontinue treatment
Mild, clinically insignificant infusion reaction	Decrease the rate of infusion
Clinically significant but not severe infusion reaction	Interrupt the infusion in patients with clinically significant infusion reactions and consider resuming at a slower rate following resolution. If decision is made to restart, the infusion may be continued at ≤50% of the rate prior to the reaction and increased in 50% increments every 30 minutes if well tolerated. Infusions may be restarted at the full rate during the next cycle
Severe infusion reaction—hypertension, hypertensive crises associated with neurologic signs and symptoms, wheezing, oxygen desaturation, G3 hypersensitivity, chest pain, headaches, rigors, and diaphoresis	Stop infusion and administer appropriate medical therapy (eg, epinephrine, corticosteroids, intravenous antihistamines, bronchodilators, and/or oxygen). Discontinue bevacizumab
Planned elective surgery	Suspend bevacizumab at least 28 days before elective surgery and do not resume for at least 28 days after surgery or until surgical incision is fully healed
Recent hemoptysis	Do not administer bevacizumab
Evidence of rectosigmoid involvement by pelvic examination or bowel involvement on CT scan or clinical symptoms of bowel obstruction	

(continued)

Dose Modification (*continued*)

Gemcitabine + Carboplatin

Starting doses	Gemcitabine 1000 mg/m² days 1 and 8 Carboplatin target AUC = 4 mg/mL × min day 1 only

Adverse Event	**Treatment Modification**
ANC <1500/mm³, hemoglobin <8.5 g/dL, or platelets <100,000/mm³ within 24 hours of scheduled start of a cycle	Delay start of cycle. Consider use of hematopoietic growth factor (CSF) prophylaxis in subsequent cycles for dose-limiting neutropenia. Resume treatment when ANC ≥1500/mm³, hemoglobin ≥8.5 g/dL, or platelets ≥100,000/mm³. If after 3 weeks ANC <1500/mm³, hemoglobin <8.5 g/dL, or platelets <100,000/mm³, discontinue treatment
ANC ≥1500/mm³ and platelets ≥100,000/mm³ within 24 hours of day 8 of a cycle	Administer 100% of day 1 gemcitabine dose
ANC ≥1000–1499/mm³ and platelets ≥75,000–99,999/mm³ within 24 hours of day 8 of a cycle	Administer 50% of day 1 gemcitabine dose
ANC <1000/mm³ or platelets <75,000/mm³ within 24 hours of day 8 of a cycle	Omit day 8 gemcitabine dose. Consider use of hematopoietic growth factor (CSF) prophylaxis in subsequent cycles for dose-limiting neutropenia
Absolute granulocyte count <500/mm³ >5 days, or absolute granulocyte count <100/mm³ >3 days, or febrile neutropenia or platelets <25,000/mm³ >5 days or cycle delay for >1 week during a given cycle	Permanently reduce the dose of gemcitabine to 800 mg/m² on days 1 and 8. Consider use of hematopoietic growth factor (CSF) prophylaxis in subsequent cycles for dose-limiting neutropenia
Absolute granulocyte count <500/mm³ >5 days, or absolute granulocyte count <100/mm³ >3 days, or febrile neutropenia or platelets <25,000/mm³ >5 days or cycle delay for >1 week during a given cycle on a dose of gemcitabine of 800 mg/m² days 1 and 8 of each cycle	Administer 800 mg/m² gemcitabine only on day 1. Omit day 8 gemcitabine dose. Consider use of hematopoietic growth factor (CSF) prophylaxis in subsequent cycles for dose-limiting neutropenia
Severe (G3/4) nonhematologic toxicities, except nausea/vomiting	Hold gemcitabine or decrease by 50%, depending on clinical judgment
Significant hypersensitivity reaction to carboplatin, including anaphylaxis (hypotension, dyspnea, and angioedema requiring therapy)*	Discontinue carboplatin. May also consider desensitization
Unexplained new or worsening dyspnea or evidence of severe pulmonary toxicity	Discontinue gemcitabine
Hemolytic-uremic syndrome (HUS) or severe renal impairment	
Severe hepatic toxicity	
Capillary leak syndrome	
Posterior reversible encephalopathy syndrome (PRES)	

*Allergic reaction to carboplatin, including anaphylaxis, may occur within minutes of administration. Risk is increased in patients previously exposed to platinum therapy
Note: can cause fetal harm. Advise women of potential risk to the fetus

Patient Population Studied

The multicenter, randomized, blinded, placebo-controlled, phase 3 OCEANS study involved 484 patients with histologically confirmed recurrent ovarian, primary peritoneal, or fallopian tube cancer and disease progression ≥6 months after completion of frontline platinum-based chemotherapy. Eligible patients were aged ≥18 years, with an Eastern Cooperative Oncology Group (ECOG) performance status score ≤1 and life expectancy of ≥12 weeks. Patients who had received prior chemotherapy in the recurrent setting, or had received prior treatment with bevacizumab, or other therapies targeting the VEGF pathway, were not eligible. Patients were scheduled to receive 6 cycles of gemcitabine and carboplatin but could receive up to 10 cycles if continued response was documented. Bevacizumab or placebo was administered with each cycle before gemcitabine and carboplatin, and was continued after gemcitabine and carboplatin treatment was discontinued until disease progression or unacceptable toxicity

Efficacy (N = 484)

	Gemcitabine + Carboplatin + Bevacizumab (n = 242)	Gemcitabine + Carboplatin + Placebo (n = 242)	
Median progression-free survival*	12.4 months	8.4 months	HR 0.484 (95% CI 0.388–0.605; P < 0.0001)
Objective response rate†	78.5%	57.4%	P <0.0001
Duration of response for responders	10.4 months	7.4 months	HR 0.534 (95% CI 0.408–0.698)

*Progression was determined on the basis of radiologic evaluation according to RECIST version 1.0
†Objective response rate is the percentage of patients who experienced a partial or complete response. The majority of responses were partial responses
Note: median follow-up time for the primary outcome measure (progression-free survival) was 24 months

Adverse Events (N = 480)

	Gemcitabine + Carboplatin + Bevacizumab (n = 247)		Gemcitabine + Carboplatin + Placebo (n = 233)	
Grade (%)*	Any Grade	Grade 3–5	Any Grade	Grade 3–5
Any adverse event	100	89	100	82
Serious adverse event	35	29	25	20
Neutropenia (Grade ≥4)	0	21	0	22
Hypertension	0	17	0	<1
Proteinuria	0	9	0	<1
Non–central nervous system bleeding	0	6	0	<1
Venous thromboembolic event		4	0	3
Arterial thromboembolic event	3	0	<1	0
Febrile neutropenia	2	0	2	0
Fistula/abscess	2	0	<1	
Left ventricular systolic dysfunction/congestive heart failure	0	1	0	<1
Reverse posterior leukoencephalopathy syndrome	1	0	0	0
Central nervous system bleeding	<1	0	<1	0
Wound-healing complication	0	<1	0	0
Gastrointestinal perforation	0	0	0	0

*According to the National Cancer Institute Common Terminology Criteria for Adverse Events, version 3.0
Note: selected treatment-emergent toxicities (within 30 days of last dose of trial treatment) are included in the table. One death resulting from an adverse event occurred in each group: 1 patient died as a result of intracranial hemorrhage in the context of newly diagnosed brain metastases in the bevacizumab group and 1 patient died from an acute myocardial infarction in the placebo group

Therapy Monitoring

1. *Once per week:* CBC with differential and platelet count
2. *Before the start of a cycle:* CBC with differential, serum electrolytes, serum creatinine
3. Monitor renal function for HUS prior to initiation and during therapy with gemcitabine
4. Monitor hepatic function prior to initiation and during therapy with gemcitabine
5. Observe closely for hypersensitivity reactions, especially during the first and second infusions and especially if prior history of platinum therapy
6. Monitor blood pressure every 2 weeks or more frequently as indicated during treatment
7. Assess proteinuria by urine dipstick and/or urinary protein creatinine ratio. Patients with a urine dipstick reading ≥2+ should undergo further assessment with a 24-hour urine collection
8. *Every 2–3 months:* imaging to assess response. Serum markers can be considered/obtained at each visit if they have been shown to be of value in following the patient's disease status

RECURRENT • PLATINUM-SENSITIVE
OVARIAN CANCER REGIMEN: LIPOSOMAL DOXORUBICIN + CARBOPLATIN

Pujade-Lauraine E et al. J Clin Oncol 2010;28:3323–3329

Doxorubicin HCl liposome injection (liposomal doxorubicin) 30 mg/m²; administer intravenously in 250 mL (doses ≤90 mg) 5% dextrose injection over 60 minutes, on day 1 before carboplatin, every 4 weeks (total dosage/cycle = 30 mg/m²)
Note: doxorubicin HCl liposome injection should be administered at an initial rate of 1 mg/min to minimize the risk of infusion reactions. If no infusion-related adverse events are observed, the rate of infusion can be increased to complete administration of the drug over 1 hour
Note: experience with doxorubicin HCl liposome injection at high cumulative doses is too limited to have established its effects on the myocardium. Therefore, it should be assumed that it will have myocardial toxicity similar to conventional formulations of doxorubicin HCl. Irreversible myocardial toxicity leading to congestive heart failure often unresponsive to cardiac supportive therapy may be encountered as the total cumulative lifetime dosage of doxorubicin HCl approaches **450–550 mg/m²**. Prior anthracyclines or anthracenediones will reduce the total dose of doxorubicin HCl that can be given without associated cardiac toxicity. Cardiac toxicity also may occur at lower cumulative doses in patients receiving concurrent cyclophosphamide therapy
Carboplatin (calculated dose) AUC = 5*; administer intravenously in 0.9% sodium chloride injection or D5W 100–500 mL over 60 minutes, on day 1 after completing liposomal doxorubicin administration, every 4 weeks (total dosage/cycle calculated to produce a target AUC = 5 mg/mL × min)

*Carboplatin dose is based on a formula described by Calvert et al. to achieve a target area under the plasma concentration versus time curve (AUC)

$$\text{Total carboplatin dose (mg)} = (\text{target AUC}) \times (\text{GFR} + 25)$$

In practice, creatinine clearance (Clcr) is used in place of glomerular filtration rate (GFR). Clcr can be estimated from the equation of Cockcroft and Gault, thus:

$$\text{For males, Clcr} = \frac{(140 - \text{age [years]}) \times (\text{body weight [kg]})}{72 \times (\text{serum creatinine [mg/dL]})}$$

$$\text{For females, Clcr} = \frac{(140 - \text{age [years]}) \times (\text{body weight [kg]})}{72 \times (\text{serum creatinine [mg/dL]})} \times 0.85$$

Calvert AH et al. J Clin Oncol 1989;7:1748–1756
Cockcroft DW, Gault MH. Nephron 1976;16:31–41
Jodrell DI et al. J Clin Oncol 1992;10:520–528
Sorensen BT et al. Cancer Chemother Pharmacol 1991;28:397–401

Notes:
• Provided actual GFR measurements are made to assess renal function, carboplatin can be safely dosed according to the Calvert formula described in product labeling
• If GFR (or creatinine clearance) is estimated based on serum creatinine measurements by the IDMS method, the FDA recommends capping an estimated GFR at 125 mL/min for any targeted AUC value for patients with normal renal function. No greater estimated GFR values should be used

Supportive Care
Antiemetic prophylaxis
Emetogenic potential is **MODERATE**. *Potential for delayed symptoms*
See Chapter 42 for antiemetic recommendations

Hematopoietic growth factor (CSF) prophylaxis
Primary prophylaxis is **NOT** *indicated*
See Chapter 43 for more information

Antimicrobial prophylaxis
Risk of fever and neutropenia is **LOW**
    Antimicrobial primary prophylaxis to be considered:
• Antibacterial—not indicated
• Antifungal—not indicated
• Antiviral—not indicated unless patient previously had an episode of HSV

Hand-foot reaction (palmar-plantar erythrodysesthesia, PPE)
For patients who develop a hand-foot reaction, use topical emollients (eg, Aquaphor), topical or orally administered steroids, antihistamine agents (H₁-receptor antagonists), or pyridoxine
• The suggested pyridoxine starting dose is 50 mg/day, which may be increased to a maximum of 200 mg/day
Note: patients who have developed G1/2 PPE while receiving doxorubicin HCl liposome injection may receive a fixed daily dose of pyridoxine 200 mg. This may allow for treatment to be completed without dosage reduction, treatment delay, or recurrence of PPE

Patient Population Studied

Patients with histologically proven ovarian cancer with recurrence ≥6 months after first- or second-line platinum and taxane-based therapies. Randomization against paclitaxel + carboplatin. Primary end point was progression-free survival (PFS); secondary end points were toxicity, quality of life, and overall survival

Efficacy

Efficacy (> Median Follow-up of 22 Months)*

PFS (intent-to-treat population)	11.3 months
Progression according to RECIST	79%
Progression according to CA-125 GCIG criteria	21%

*In the absence of unacceptable toxicity or disease progression, patients were treated for a total of 6 courses of therapy. In the event disease stabilization or partial response was achieved after 6 courses of therapy, patients were allowed to remain on therapy until progression

Therapy Monitoring

1. *Baseline:* LFTs, serum chemistry, CBC with differential and platelet count, and CA-125. Complete history and physical examination including a gynecologic examination
2. Baseline ECG and left ventricular ejection fraction measurement by echocardiogram or multigated angiography. A left ventricular ejection fraction measurement before each course of therapy if cumulative anthracycline dose exceeds 450 mg/m^2
3. *Follow-up:* CBC with differential and platelet count on days 1, 8, and 15 of each cycle, and LFTs prior to commencing repeated cycles

Toxicity

Toxicity (N = 466)*

Adverse Event	% Any Grade	%G ≥2	%G 3–4
Hematologic Toxicity			
Neutropenia	79.6		35.2
Febrile neutropenia			2.6
Infection	20.4		2.6
Thrombocytopenia	38.4		15.9
Anemia	66.3		7.9
Bleeding			0.6
Nonhematologic Toxicity			
Alopecia	34.7		
Nausea	78.3	35.2‡	
Vomiting	48.9	22.5‡	
Constipation	55.4	21.5	
Diarrhea	23.2	5.4‡	
Fatigue	77.9	36.9‡	
Mucositis	39.1	13.9‡	
Neuropathy, Sensory	39.9	4.9‡	
Neuropathy, Motor	7.3	1.5	
Cardiovascular	10.5	2.1‡	
Allergic reaction	15.5	5.6‡	
Hand-foot syndrome	38.6	12‡	
Arthralgia/myalgia	22.3	4‡	

*NCI Common Terminology Criteria for Adverse Events, version 3.0
†Graded as 1, partial hair loss, or 2, complete hair loss
‡Grades 2 and 3 only (no reported Grade 4 toxicities)
Note: because of rounding, percentages may not total 100

RECURRENT • PLATINUM-SENSITIVE
OVARIAN CANCER REGIMEN: CARBOPLATIN + DOCETAXEL

Strauss HG et al. Gynecol Oncol 2007;104:612–616

Premedication with **dexamethasone** 8 mg/dose; administer orally twice daily for 3 days (6 doses), starting on the day before docetaxel administration (total dose/cycle = 48 mg)

Docetaxel 75 mg/m²; administer intravenously in a volume of 0.9% sodium chloride injection (0.9% NS) or 5% dextrose injection (D5W) sufficient to produce a docetaxel concentration within the range 0.3–0.74 mg/mL over 30 minutes on day 1 before carboplatin, every 3 weeks for 6 cycles (total dosage/cycle = 75 mg/m²), *followed by:*

Carboplatin (calculated dose) AUC = 5*; administer intravenously in 0.9% NS or D5W 100–500 mL over 60 minutes, on day 1 after completing docetaxel, every 3 weeks for 6 cycles (total dosage/cycle calculated to produce a target AUC = 5 mg/mL × min)

*Carboplatin dose is based on a formula described by Calvert et al. to achieve a target Area Under the plasma concentration versus time Curve (AUC)

$$\text{Total carboplatin dose (mg)} = (\text{target AUC}) \times (\text{GFR} + 25)$$

In practice, creatinine clearance (Clcr) is used in place of glomerular filtration rate (GFR). Clcr can be estimated from the equation of Cockcroft and Gault, thus:

$$\text{For males, Clcr} = \frac{(140 - \text{age [years]}) \times (\text{body weight [kg]})}{72 \times (\text{serum creatinine [mg/dL]})}$$

$$\text{For females, Clcr} = \frac{(140 - \text{age [years]}) \times (\text{body weight [kg]})}{72 \times (\text{serum creatinine [mg/dL]})} \times 0.85$$

Calvert AH et al. J Clin Oncol 1989;7:1748–1756
Cockcroft DW, Gault MH. Nephron 1976;16:31–41
Jodrell DI et al. J Clin Oncol 1992;10:520–528
Sorensen BT et al. Cancer Chemother Pharmacol 1991;28:397–401

Notes:
- Provided actual GFR measurements are made to assess renal function, carboplatin can be safely dosed according to the Calvert formula described in product labeling
- If GFR (or creatinine clearance) is estimated based on serum creatinine measurements by the IDMS method, the FDA recommends capping an estimated GFR at 125 mL/min for any targeted AUC value for patients with normal renal function. No greater estimated GFR values should be used

Supportive Care
Antiemetic prophylaxis
Emetogenic potential is **MODERATE**. *Potential for delayed symptoms*
See Chapter 42 for antiemetic recommendations

Hematopoietic growth factor (CSF) prophylaxis
Primary prophylaxis is **NOT** *indicated*
See Chapter 43 for more information

Antimicrobial prophylaxis
Risk of fever and neutropenia is **LOW**
Antimicrobial primary prophylaxis to be considered:
- Antibacterial—not indicated
- Antifungal—not indicated
- Antiviral—not indicated unless patient previously had an episode of HSV

Patient Population Studied

Eligible patients had recurrent ovarian, peritoneal, or tubal cancer (platinum-free interval >6 months), performance status 0–2. Patients who had undergone surgical debulking for recurrent disease were excluded from the study. First-line chemotherapy in 25 patients included carboplatin/paclitaxel (21), carboplatin/docetaxel (1), carboplatin/cyclophosphamide (1), and carboplatin alone (2). Patients with preexisting peripheral neuropathy G ≥2 (NCI Common Toxicity Criteria, version 2.0; 1998) were excluded

Efficacy

Efficacy (N = 25)*	
Strauss HG et al. Gynecol Oncol 2007;104:612–616	
Intent-to-Treat Population (N = 25)	
Overall response rate*,†	72% (95% CI 60%–84%)
Median progression-free survival	19 months (95% CI 4–40 months)
Overall survival‡	26 months (95% CI 11–44 months)
Efficacy-Evaluable Patients (N = 23)	
Overall response rate*,†	78.3% (95% CI 64–86%)
Complete response*	69.6% (16/23)
Partial response†	8.7 % (2/23)
Remission duration	50% (8/16 CR) at a median follow-up of 40.4 months

*Complete response: disappearance of all measurable disease assessed by imaging, disappearance of clinical signs and symptoms and normalization of CA-125 serum values without clinical evidence of progression for ≥4 weeks

†Partial response: reduction of ≥50% in the sum of the greatest perpendicular diameters of all measurable lesions without appearance of new lesions for ≥4 weeks, no enlargement of any existing lesion, and decrease of elevated CA-125 values ≥50% from the pretherapeutic level

‡In an unplanned retrospective analysis, patients with a platinum-free interval ≥12 months showed significantly better OS than those with a platinum-free interval <12 months (P = 0.003; HR 8.6 [95% CI, 5.4–10.8])

Dose Modifications

Adverse Event	Dose Modifications
ANC <1000/mm^3 or platelet count <75,000/mm^3	Hold day 1 chemotherapy until ANC ≥1000/mm^3 and platelet count ≥75,000/mm^3
ANC <1000/mm^3 or platelet count <75,000/mm^3 ≥3 weeks	Discontinue therapy
G3/4 nonhematologic toxicity	Reduce carboplatin dosage to AUC 4 mg/mL × min. If toxicity occurred at carboplatin dosage of AUC = 4 mg/mL × min, consider discontinuing therapy. Reduce docetaxel dosage to 60 mg/m^2
ANC <1500/mm^3 or platelet count <100,000/mm^3 on day 1 of a cycle, *or* febrile neutropenia, *or* ANC <500/mm^3 despite filgrastim prophylaxis, *or* ANC <500/mm^3 for ≥7 days, *or* platelet count <25,000/mm^3	Reduce carboplatin dosage to AUC = 4 mg/mL × min. Reduce docetaxel dosage to 60 mg/m^2
Second episode of febrile neutropenia	Continue docetaxel 60 mg/m^2, carboplatin AUC = 4 mg/mL × min, and give filgrastim* during subsequent cycles
ANC <1500/mm^3 or platelet count <100,000/mm^3 on despite 2-week delay, *or* febrile neutropenic despite filgrastim support, *or* febrile neutropenia at docetaxel dosage of 60 mg/m^2 and carboplatin AUC 4 mg/mL × min, *or* nonhematologic toxicity G >2 except mucositis, nausea, or alopecia, *or* significant hypersensitivity reaction to docetaxel or carboplatin (hypotension, dyspnea, and angioedema requiring therapy)†	Discontinue therapy
G ≥3 peripheral neuropathy	Hold therapy for a maximum of 2 weeks, until toxicity G ≤2. Reinstitute therapy reducing docetaxel dosage to 30 mg/m^2. If toxicity recurs at docetaxel dosage = 30 mg/m^2, reduce carboplatin dosage to AUC = 4 mg/mL × min
Second episode of febrile neutropenia	Continue docetaxel 60 mg/m^2, carboplatin AUC = 4 mg/mL × min, and give filgrastim* during subsequent cycles
Significant hypersensitivity reaction to carboplatin (hypotension, dyspnea and angioedema requiring therapy)‡	Discontinue therapy

*For patients with a history of asthma or allergic reactions to drugs, consider parenteral pre-medication with 100 mg hydrocortisone with or without 25–50 mg diphenhydramine

†Preventive measures for PPE include wearing loose-fitting clothes, avoiding activities that can lead to trauma to the vasculature of palms or soles, and use of ice packs to promote vasoconstriction and reduce inflammation. Patients should be advised to avoid hot baths and showers (Jacuzzis and steam baths included) for 24 hours before and 72 hours after liposomal doxorubicin. Cool baths are recommended. Topical steroid creams provide no benefit. Topical antihistamine and anesthetic preparations may aggravate skin toxicity. Emollients and petroleum-based balms may provide some relief

‡Patients who experience G1/2 carboplatin hypersensitivity reactions may continue treatment if there is evidence of tumor response and appropriate preventive measures are instituted

Toxicity

Acute Toxicity (N = 25)*

Strauss HG et al. Gynecol Oncol 2007;104:612–616

Toxicity	% G1	% G2	% G3	% G4
Neutropenia	12	16	28	32
Thrombocytopenia	4	12	20	4
Anemia	28	44	4	0
Infection	16	8	4	0
Nausea	48	32	4	4
Vomiting	32	16	4	0
Diarrhea	12	32	12	0
Stomatitis	16	20	0	0
Sensory neuropathy	20	20	0	0
Mood alteration (depression)	0	8	4	0
Alopecia	12	88	—	—
Epiphora	0	8	0	0
Skin	12	12	0	0
Peripheral edema	0	12	0	0
Joint pain	8	4	0	0

*NCI Clinical Trials Group Common Toxicity Criteria, version 2.0 (1998)

Therapy Monitoring

1. *Baseline:* LFTs, serum chemistry, CBC with differential and platelet count, and CA-125. Complete history and physical examination, including a gynecologic examination

2. *Follow-up:* CBC with differential and platelet count at least weekly through leukocyte and platelet count nadirs, and prior to beginning repeated cycles, and LFTs before commencing repeated cycles

RECURRENT • PLATINUM-SENSITIVE
OVARIAN CANCER REGIMEN: WEEKLY CARBOPLATIN + DOCETAXEL

Kushner DM et al. Gynecol Oncol 2007;105:358–364

Premedication:

Dexamethasone 4 mg/dose; administer orally for 3 doses during the evening before, morning of, and evening after docetaxel administration (total dose/cycle = 12 mg)

Docetaxel 35 mg/m^2 per dose (maximum single dose limited to 70 mg)*; administer intravenously in a volume of 0.9% sodium chloride injection (0.9% NS) or 5% dextrose injection (D5W) sufficient to produce a final docetaxel concentration within the range 0.3–0.74 mg/mL, over 60 minutes for 3 doses, before carboplatin on days 1, 8, and 15, every 28 days (total dosage/cycle = 105 mg/m^2; maximum dose/cycle = 210 mg), *followed by:*

Carboplatin (calculated dose) AUC = 2†; administer intravenously in 0.9% NS or D5W 100–500 mL over 30 minutes for 3 doses, after completing docetaxel on days 1, 8, and 15, every 28 days (total dosage/cycle calculated to produce a cumulative target AUC = 6 mg/mL × min)

Notes: carboplatin hypersensitivity led to 11 subjects coming off trial (31%). Diphenhydramine premedication produced a nonsignificant decrease in reaction rate

In the clinical trial, treatment was continued until evidence of disease progression, intolerable toxicity, patient refusal of further treatment, or physician decision that it was in the best interest of a patient to discontinue therapy. Patients who achieved a complete response (CR) continued therapy for 2 cycles following documentation of CR

*Patients with G2 neurotoxicity were treated at an initial docetaxel dosage of 30 mg/m^2

†Carboplatin dose is based on a formula described by Calvert et al. to achieve a target area under the plasma concentration versus time curve (AUC)

$$\text{Total carboplatin dose (mg)} = (\text{target AUC}) \times (\text{GFR} + 25)$$

In practice, creatinine clearance (Clcr) is used in place of glomerular filtration rate (GFR). Clcr can be estimated from the equation of Cockcroft and Gault, thus:

$$\text{For males, Clcr} = \frac{(140 - \text{age [years]}) \times (\text{body weight [kg]})}{72 \times (\text{serum creatinine [mg/dL]})}$$

$$\text{For females, Clcr} = \frac{(140 - \text{age [years]}) \times (\text{body weight [kg]})}{72 \times (\text{serum creatinine [mg/dL]})} \times 0.85$$

Calvert AH et al. J Clin Oncol 1989;7:1748–1756
Cockcroft DW , Gault MH. Nephron 1976;16:31–41
Jodrell DI et al. J Clin Oncol 1992;10:520–528
Sorensen BT et al. Cancer Chemother Pharmacol 1991;28:397–401

Notes:

• Provided actual GFR measurements are made to assess renal function, carboplatin can be safely dosed according to the Calvert formula described in product labeling

• If GFR (or creatinine clearance) is estimated based on serum creatinine measurements by the IDMS method, the FDA recommends capping an estimated GFR at 125 mL/min for any targeted AUC value for patients with normal renal function. No greater estimated GFR values should be used

Supportive Care
Antiemetic prophylaxis
Emetogenic potential is **MODERATE**
See Chapter 42 for antiemetic recommendations

Hematopoietic growth factor (CSF) prophylaxis
Primary prophylaxis is **NOT** *indicated*
See Chapter 43 for more information

Antimicrobial prophylaxis
Risk of fever and neutropenia is **LOW**
Antimicrobial primary prophylaxis to be considered:
  • Antibacterial—not indicated
  • Antifungal—not indicated
  • Antiviral—not indicated unless patient previously had an episode of HSV

Dose Modifications

Adverse Event	Dose Modifications
ANC <1000/mm³ or platelet count <75,000/mm³*	Hold day 1 chemotherapy until ANC ≥1000/mm³ and platelet count ≥75,000/mm³
ANC <1500/mm³ or platelet count <100,000/mm³ on day 1 of a cycle	Reduce docetaxel dosage to 30 mg/m². If adverse effect occurred with docetaxel 30 mg/m², reduce each carboplatin dosage to AUC = 1 mg/mL × min per dose on the same administration schedule
ANC <1000/mm³ or platelet count <75,000/mm³ ≥3 weeks	Discontinue therapy
ANC <1000/mm³, or platelet count <100,000/mm³, or G ≥3 renal toxicity, or G ≥2 toxicities with an adverse effect on organ function	Omit the scheduled weekly dose
ANC <500/mm³ or platelet count <25,000/mm³ for ≥7 days, or ANC <500/mm³ despite filgrastim prophylaxis, or G4 neutropenia associated with fever, or G ≥3 anemia, or G ≥3 renal toxicity, or G ≥3 hepatic toxicity (bilirubin > ULN or transaminases >5 × ULN), or uncontrolled G ≥3 nausea/vomiting, or G ≥2 stomatitis, or other G ≥2 nonhematologic toxicities with an adverse effect on organ function, or omission of 2 consecutive weekly doses	Reduce docetaxel dosage to 30 mg/m² per dose. If adverse effect occurred with docetaxel 30 mg/m², reduce carboplatin dosage to AUC = 1 mg/mL × min per dose on the same administration schedule
ANC <1500/mm³ or platelet count <100,000/mm³ despite 2-week delay, or febrile neutropenia despite filgrastim support, or febrile neutropenia at docetaxel dosages of 30 mg/m² and carboplatin AUC = 1 mg/mL × min, or significant hypersensitivity reaction to docetaxel or carboplatin (hypotension, dyspnea, and angioedema requiring therapy)*	Discontinue therapy
G ≥3 peripheral neuropathy	Hold therapy for a maximum of 2 weeks until toxicity G ≤2. Reinstitute therapy but reduce docetaxel dosage to 30 mg/m² per dose. If adverse effect occurred with docetaxel 30 mg/m², reduce carboplatin dosage to AUC = 1 mg/mL × min per dose on the same administration schedule

*Patients who experience G1/2 carboplatin hypersensitivity reactions may continue treatment if there is evidence of tumor response and appropriate preventive measures are instituted
ULN, upper limit of normal range

Patient Population Studied

Thirty-six patients were enrolled in a prospective phase 2 study of a weekly docetaxel and carboplatin regimen. Patients eligible for the trial had an initial diagnosis of ovarian or primary peritoneal carcinoma. Initial treatment with a platinum-based regimen was required, with a treatment-free interval of at least 3 months. Patients could have received 1 prior regimen for recurrence. At the time of enrollment, patients were required to have a Gynecologic Oncology Group performance status of <2, neuropathy (sensory and motor) Grade ≤2 (NCI Common Toxicity Criteria), and recovered from effects of recent surgery, radiotherapy, or chemotherapy. Biologically evaluable disease (CA-125) could be followed only if measurable disease was not present. The majority of patients had ovarian cancer (89%) and stage III/IV (97%) disease, with a median initial disease-free interval of 12 months. Most subjects were treated for first recurrence (81%) and had measurable disease (58%)

Efficacy*

Intention to Treat (N = 36)[†]	
Overall response rate (ORR)	50% (18/36)
Complete response	11% (4/36)
Partial response	39% (14/36)

Evaluable for Response (N = 27)[†]	
Overall response rate (ORR)	67% (18/27)
Complete response	15% (4/27)
Partial response	52% (14/27)
ORR biologically evaluable	65% (11/17)
ORR measurable disease	70% (7/10)
ORR platinum-resistant (treatment-free interval <6 months)	60% (3/5)
ORR platinum-sensitive disease (treatment-free interval >6 months)	68% (15/22)

Note: data were not available concerning time to progression or survival

*RECIST (Response Evaluation Criteria in Solid Tumors) criteria were used to define response. If CA-125 was increased at baseline, normalization was required for a complete response (CR). Patients without measurable disease were evaluated by CA-125 values as described by Rustin GJ et al. J Clin Oncol 1996;14:1545–1551. Complete response = normalization of CA-125 lasting ≥4 weeks, documented with at least 3 normal values. Partial response (PR) = 50–75% improvement in the CA-125 level, lasting ≥4 weeks. This could be documented in 1 of 2 ways: (a) 4 CA-125 levels, 2 initial elevated and 1 showing a 50% decrease requiring confirmation by a fourth sample, or (b) 3 CA-125 levels with a serial decrease of at least 75%. Progressive disease = a rise ≥50% documented on 2 separate occasions 1 week apart. Stable disease = any condition not meeting the above parameters
[†]Patients who received 1 or more cycles of drug and lived at least 3 weeks were evaluable for response. Twenty-seven patients were evaluable for response. Nine subjects were removed from study prior to the first response evaluation. Eight of these were removed because of toxicity, and 1 subject withdrew consent for reasons other than toxicity

Toxicity

Hematologic and Nonhematologic Toxicity*

Toxicity	Grade of Worst Event (Per Patient, N = 36)				
	% No Toxicity	% G1	% G2	% G3	% G4
Leukopenia	17	23	29	31	0
Neutropenia	26	9	17	34	14
Anemia	31	46	17	6	0
Thrombocytopenia	69	23	6	3	0
Gastrointestinal	14	43	34	3	6
Neurologic	63	20	17	0	0
Carboplatin reaction[†]	63	11	11	14	0

*There was no detectable difference in quality of life as a consequence of therapy
[†]Carboplatin hypersensitivity reactions led to 11 subjects coming off trial (31%)

Therapy Monitoring

1. *Baseline:* LFTs, serum chemistry, CBC with differential and platelet count, and CA-125. Complete history and physical examination, including a gynecologic examination
2. *Follow-up:* CBC with differential and platelet count on days 1, 8, and 15, and LFTs before commencing repeated cycles

RECURRENT • PLATINUM-SENSITIVE

OVARIAN CANCER REGIMEN: CISPLATIN + GEMCITABINE

Rose PG et al. Gynecol Oncol 2003;88:17–21

Gemcitabine 750 mg/m^2 per dose; administer intravenously in 50–250 mL sodium chloride injection (0.9% NS) over 30–60 minutes for 2 doses, on days 1 and 8, every 21 days (total dosage/cycle = 1500 mg/m^2), followed by:
Hydration before cisplatin with ≥1000 mL 0.9% NS; administer intravenously over a minimum of 3–4 hours
Cisplatin 30 mg/m^2 per dose; administer intravenously in 100–500 mL 0.9% NS over 30–60 minutes for 2 doses, on days 1and 8, every 21 days (total dosage/cycle = 60 mg/m^2)
Hydration after cisplatin with ≥1000 mL 0.9% NS; administer intravenously over a minimum of 3–4 hours
Notes: encourage increased oral intake of nonalcoholic fluids. Goal is to achieve a urine output ≥100 mL/hour. Monitor and replace electrolytes as needed (potassium, magnesium, sodium)

Supportive Care
Antiemetic prophylaxis
Emetogenic potential is MODERATE–HIGH.
Potential for delayed symptoms
See Chapter 42 for antiemetic recommendations

Hematopoietic growth factor (CSF) prophylaxis
Primary prophylaxis is NOT indicated
See Chapter 43 for more information

Antimicrobial prophylaxis
Risk of fever and neutropenia is LOW
   Antimicrobial primary prophylaxis to be considered:
   • Antibacterial—not indicated
   • Antifungal—not indicated
   • Antiviral—not indicated unless patient previously had an episode of HSV

Dose Modifications

Adverse Event	Dose Modifications
ANC <1500/mm^3 or platelet count <100,000/mm^3	Hold day 1 chemotherapy until ANC ≥1500/mm^3 and platelet count ≥100,000/mm^3
ANC <1500/mm^3 or platelet count <100,000/mm^3 ≥2 weeks	Discontinue therapy
Intracycle: G1/2 nonhematologic toxicity or G1–3 nausea or vomiting	100% gemcitabine dosage on day 8
Intracycle: G3 nonhematologic toxicity, except nausea, vomiting, and alopecia	Reduce gemcitabine dosage by 50% on day 8, or hold treatment at clinician's discretion
Intracycle: G4 nonhematologic toxicity	Hold gemcitabine
Intracycle: Day 8 ANC <1000/mm^3 or platelet count <75,000/mm^3	Do not administer day 8 therapy. In subsequent cycles, administer gemcitabine 600 mg/m^2 per dose on days 1 and 8. If adverse event occurred with gemcitabine 600 mg/m^2, administer gemcitabine 400 mg/m^2 per dose on days 1 and 8. If adverse event occurred with gemcitabine 400 mg/m^2, administer gemcitabine 300 mg/m^2 per dose on days 1 and 8
Intracycle: Day 8 ANC 1000–1400/mm^3 and/or platelet count 75,000–100,000/mm^3	Reduce gemcitabine dosage to 600 mg/m^2. If adverse event occurred with gemcitabine 600 mg/m^2, administer gemcitabine 400 mg/m^2 per dose on days 1 and 8. If adverse event occurred with gemcitabine 400 mg/m^2, administer gemcitabine 300 mg/m^2 per dose on days 1 and 8
Neutropenia and sepsis, *or* severe thrombocytopenia (platelets <20,000/mm^3)	Administer gemcitabine 600 mg/m^2. If adverse event occurred with gemcitabine 600 mg/m^2, administer gemcitabine 400 mg/m^2 per dose on days 1 and 8. If adverse event occurred with gemcitabine 400 mg/m^2, administer gemcitabine 300 mg/m^2 per dose on days 1 and 8
G2 peripheral neuropathy	Reduce cisplatin dosage to 25 mg/m^2 per dose on days 1 and 8
G3/4 peripheral neuropathy	Hold therapy until peripheral neuropathy G ≤1, then restart therapy with cisplatin dosage reduced to cisplatin 20–25 mg/m^2 per dose on days 1 and 8. Consider discontinuing therapy if not recovered to baseline by 2–3 weeks
Creatinine clearance 40–60 mL/min (0.66–1 mL/s)	Reduce cisplatin so that dose in milligrams equals the creatinine clearance* value in mL/min†
Creatinine clearance <40 mL/min (<0.66 mL/s)	Hold cisplatin
On treatment day, serum creatinine 1.6–2 mg/dL (141–177 μmol/L)	Reduce cisplatin dosage by 25%
On treatment day 1, serum creatinine >2 mg/dL (>177 μmol/L)	Hold cisplatin until serum creatinine ≤2 mg/dL (≤177 μmol/L)

*Creatinine clearance is used as a measure of glomerular filtration rate
†This also applies to patients with creatinine clearance of 40–60 mL/min (0.66–1 mL/s) at the outset of treatment

Patient Population Studied

Thirty-six patients with ovarian or peritoneal cancers whose disease was platinum- and paclitaxel-refractory, and who had failed to benefit from multiple second-line agents, were treated with a combination of gemcitabine and cisplatin. Tumors were defined as platinum-resistant if disease had progressed on or within 6 months after patients had completed their most recent platinum regimen. Patients had received a median of 2 (range: 1–5) prior platinum- or paclitaxel-based regimens, were heavily pretreated, and had received a median of 3 non-platinum/non-paclitaxel regimens (range: 0–6 regimens). Despite this, the majority of patients had an excellent performance status: ECOG = 0

Efficacy

Intention to Treat (N = 36)	
Overall response rate	41.6% (15/36)
Complete response	11.1% (4/36)
Partial response	30.5% (11/36)

Duration of Benefit (N = 35)	
Progression-free survival	6 months (range: 1–14 months)
Overall survival	12 months
Median response duration, responding patients	11 months (range: 4–14 months)

Intention to Treat/Evaluable Disease (N = 5)*,†	
Overall response rate	40% (2/5)

Intention to Treat/Measurable Disease (N = 31)†	
Overall response rate	42% (13/31)

Response According to Platinum-Free Interval	
<6 months	16.6% (1/6)
6–12 months	37.5% (3/8)
>12 months	50% (11/22)

Progression on Prior Gemcitabine (N = 6)	
Partial response	66% (4/6)

*In patients with "nonmeasurable" disease with only increased CA-125, a partial response was defined as a reduction in CA-125 value by ≥50%
†Neither maximum disease diameter nor a pretreatment CA-125 level correlated with response

Toxicity

Adverse Effects (First Cycle)

Adverse Effect	Grade				
	% G0	% G1	% G2	% G3	% G4
Leukopenia	27.8	11.1	36.1	22.2	2.8
Thrombocytopenia	8.3	22.2	50	16.7	2.8
Neutropenia	25	8.3	30.5	30.5	5.6
Anemia	5.6	38.9	47.2	8.8	—
Nausea/vomiting	86.1	—	5.6	—	8.3
Dermatologic	100	—	—	—	—
Renal	100	—	—	—	—
Peripheral neurotoxicity	100	—	—	—	—
Fever	100	—	—	—	—
Fatigue	100	—	—	—	—
Tinnitus	100	—	—	—	—
Hypomagnesemia	100	—	—	—	—
Pulmonary	100	—	—	—	—

Adverse Effects (All Cycles)

Adverse Effect	% G0	% G1	% G2	% G3	% G4
Leukopenia	25	13.9	16.7	41.7	2.8
Thrombocytopenia	8.8	19.4	38.9	30.6	5.6
Neutropenia	22.2	8.8	16.7	38.9	13.9
Anemia	—	22.2	58.3	19.4	—
Nausea/vomiting	86.1	—	5.6	—	8.8
Dermatologic	100	—	—	—	—
Renal	100	—	—	—	—
Peripheral neurotoxicity*	94.4	2.8	2.8	—	—
Fever	97.2	—	2.8	—	—
Fatigue	—	100	—	—	—
Tinnitus†	97.2	—	—	2.8†	—
Hypomagnesemia	100	—	—	—	—
Pulmonary	100	—	—	—	—

Dose Reductions with Repeated Administrations

Toxicity Responsible for Reduction	Number of Dose Reductions			
	0	1	2	3
Thrombocytopenia and/or neutropenia	47.2	36.1	5.6	11.1

*Grade 1 peripheral neurotoxicity developed in all patients who received more than 8 cycles
†After 6 courses of therapy

Therapy Monitoring

1. *Baseline:* LFTs, serum chemistry (including potassium, magnesium, and sodium), CBC with differential and platelet count, and CA-125. Complete history and physical examination, including a gynecologic examination
2. *Follow-up:* CBC with differential and platelet count at least weekly through leukocyte and platelet count nadirs, and serum potassium, magnesium, and sodium before repeated treatment
3. Repeat LFTs before commencing repeated cycles

RECURRENT • PLATINUM-SENSITIVE • MAINTENANCE

OVARIAN CANCER REGIMEN: NIRAPARIB

Mirza MR et al. N Engl J Med 2016;375:2154–2164
Protocol for: Mirza MR et al. N Engl J Med 2016;375:2154–2164
Supplementary appendix to: Mirza MR et al. N Engl J Med 2016;375:2154–2164
Lord R et al. SGO Annual Meeting on Women's Cancer. March 24–27, 2018. New Orleans, LA. Abstract 20

Start niraparib maintenance therapy within 8 weeks following completion of the last dose of platinum-based chemotherapy Niraparib 300 mg per dose; administer orally once daily at bedtime, without regard to food, continually until disease progression (total dosage/week = 2100 mg)

- Patients with low body weight (<77 kg) or baseline thrombocytopenia (platelet count <150,000/mm³) are at higher risk for early G ≥3 thrombocytopenia requiring dose interruption and reduction. Thus, for patients with either of these baseline characteristics, initiate niraparib at a reduced starting dosage as follows:

  ▪ **Niraparib** 200 mg per dose; administer orally once daily at bedtime, without regard to food, continually until disease progression (total dosage/week = 1400 mg)

- Patients who delay taking a niraparib dose at a regularly scheduled time or who vomit after taking a niraparib dose should take the next dose at the next regularly scheduled time
- Niraparib capsules should be swallowed whole. Do not crush, chew, dissolve, or open capsules
- Starting dosage in hepatic impairment: No dosage adjustment is recommended in patients with mild hepatic impairment (total bilirubin ≤ULN and aspartate aminotransferase [AST] >ULN, or total bilirubin > 1× ULN and <1.5× ULN with any AST). No recommendation for dosing can be made for patients with moderate or severe hepatic impairment due to lack of data in these populations
- Starting dosage in renal impairment: No dosage adjustment is recommended in patients with mild to moderate renal impairment (creatinine clearance ≥30 mL/min and ≤89 mL/min). No recommendation for dosing can be made for patients with severe renal impairment or for those undergoing hemodialysis due to lack of data in these populations

(continued)

Treatment Modifications

NIRAPARIB DOSAGE MODIFICATIONS

Starting dose	300 mg by mouth once daily at bedtime
Dose Level − 1	200 mg by mouth once daily at bedtime
Dose Level − 2	100 mg by mouth once daily at bedtime
Dose Level − 3	Discontinue niraparib

Adverse Event	Treatment Modification
G ≥3 nonhematologic toxicity where prophylaxis is not considered feasible or toxicity persists despite treatment	Interrupt niraparib for up to 28 days or until resolution of toxicity to G ≤1 or baseline. Then reduce niraparib by 1 dose level
First occurrence of platelet count <100,000/mm³	Interrupt niraparib treatment for up to 28 days and monitor CBC with differential and platelet count weekly until platelet count ≥100,000/mm³. Resume niraparib when platelet count recovers to ≥100,000/mm³: If the platelet nadir was ≥75,000/mm³, niraparib may be continued at the same dose or reduced by 1 dose level If the platelet nadir was <75,000/mm³, reduce by 1 dose level If the platelet count does not return to baseline or G ≤1 within 28 days, permanently discontinue niraparib
Second occurrence of platelet count <100,000/mm³	Interrupt niraparib treatment for up to 28 days and monitor CBC with differential and platelet count weekly until platelet count improves to ≥100,000/mm³. Resume niraparib at 1 dose level lower when platelet count recovers to ≥100,000/mm³. If the platelet count does not return to baseline or G ≤1 within 28 days, permanently discontinue niraparib
ANC <1000/mm³ or hemoglobin <8 g/dL	Interrupt niraparib for up to 28 days and monitor CBC with differential and platelet count weekly until neutrophil count returns to ≥1500/mm³ or hemoglobin returns to ≥9 g/dL. Resume niraparib at 1 dose level lower when neutrophil count returns to ≥1500/mm³ or hemoglobin returns to ≥9 g/dL. Permanently discontinue niraparib if ANC and/or hemoglobin have not returned to baseline or G ≤1 within 28 days of the dose interruption period
Hematologic adverse reaction requiring transfusion	For patients with platelet count ≤10,000/mm³, platelet transfusion should be considered. If there are other risk factors such as co-administration of anticoagulation or antiplatelet drugs, consider interrupting these drugs and/or transfusion at a higher platelet count. Resume niraparib at 1 dose level lower
MDS/AML confirmed	Discontinue niraparib

ANC, absolute neutrophil count; CBC, complete blood count; MDS, myelodysplastic syndrome; AML, acute myelogenous leukemia
Zejula (niraparib) prescribing information. Waltham, MA: Tesaro, Inc; revised May 2018

Patient Population Studied

This international, multicenter, randomized, double-blind, placebo-controlled, phase 3 trial (ENGOT-OV16/NOVA) involved 553 patients with platinum-sensitive, histologically diagnosed, high-grade ovarian cancer, fallopian tube cancer, or primary peritoneal cancer. Eligible patients were aged ≥18 years, had an Eastern Cooperative Oncology Group (ECOG) performance status of ≤1, had received at least 2 previous platinum-based chemotherapy regimens, and had taken their last dose of platinum within 8 weeks of the start of the study. Patients were randomly assigned (2:1) to receive niraparib (300 g once daily) or placebo in continuous 28-day cycles until disease progression, unacceptable toxicity, death, withdrawal of consent, or loss to follow-up

(continued)

Supportive care

Antiemetic prophylaxis
Emetogenic potential is **MODERATE-HIGH**
See Chapter 42 for antiemetic recommendations

Hematopoietic growth factor (CSF) prophylaxis
Primary prophylaxis is **NOT** *indicated*
See Chapter 43 for more information

Antimicrobial prophylaxis
Risk of fever and neutropenia is **LOW**
  Antimicrobial primary prophylaxis to be considered:
  • Antibacterial—not indicated
  • Antifungal—not indicated
  • Antiviral—not indicated, unless patient previously had an episode of HSV

Oral care
Standard prophylaxis and treatment for mucositis/stomatitis

Therapy Monitoring

1. CBC weekly for the first month, then monthly for the next 11 months and periodically thereafter for clinically significant changes

2. Myelodysplastic syndrome/acute myeloid leukemia (MDS/AML) has occurred in patients exposed to niraparib, and some cases were fatal. Monitor patients for hematologic toxicity and discontinue if MDS/AML is confirmed

3. Monitor blood pressure and heart rate monthly for the first year and periodically thereafter. Manage elevations in blood pressure with antihypertensive medications as well as adjustment of the niraparib dose, if necessary

4. Apprise pregnant women of the potential risk to a fetus. Advise females of reproductive potential to use effective contraception during treatment and for 6 months after the last dose of niraparib

5. *Every 2–3 months:* obtain imaging to assess response. Serum markers can be considered/obtained at each visit if they have been shown to be of value in following the patient's disease status

Efficacy (N = 553)

	Niraparib	Placebo	
Median progression-free survival in the gBRCA cohort	21.0 months	5.5 months	HR 0.27 (95% CI 0.17–0.41); P <0.001
Median progression-free survival in the homologous recombination deficiency subgroup of the non-gBRCA cohort	12.9 months	3.8 months	HR 0.38 (95% CI 0.24–0.59); P <0.001
Median progression-free survival in the non-gBRCA cohort	9.3 months	3.9 months	HR 0.45 (95% CI 0.34–0.61); P <0.001

Note: the median duration of follow-up was 16.9 months

Adverse Events (N = 546)

Grade (%)*	Niraparib (n = 367)		Placebo (n = 179)	
	Grade 1/2	Grade 3/4	Grade 1/2	Grade 3/4
Nausea	71	3	34	1
Thrombocytopenia	28	34	5	<1
Fatigue	51	8	41	<1
Anemia	25	25	7	0
Constipation	39	<1	20	<1
Vomiting	32	2	16	<1
Neutropenia	11	20	4	2
Headache	26	<1	9	0
Decreased appetite	25	<1	14	<1
Insomnia	24	<1	7	0
Abdominal pain	22	1	28	2
Dyspnea	18	1	7	1
Hypertension	11	8	2	2
Diarrhea	19	<1	20	1
Dizziness	17	0	7	0
Cough	15	0	4	0
Back pain	13	<1	12	0
Arthralgia	11	<1	12	0
Dyspepsia	11	0	9	0
Nasopharyngitis	11	0	7	0
Urinary tract infection	10	<1	5	1
Palpitations	10	0	2	0
Dysgeusia	10	0	4	0
Myalgia	8	<1	10	0
Abdominal distention	8	0	12	<1

*According to the National Cancer Institute Common Terminology Criteria for Adverse Events, version 4.03
Note: treatment-emergent adverse events that occurred in ≥10% of patients in either group are included in the table. During the follow-up period, 1 patient in each group died as a result of treatment-related MDS or AML. Treatment was discontinued owing to adverse events in 14.7% of the niraparib group and 2.2% of the placebo group

RECURRENT • PLATINUM-SENSITIVE • MAINTENANCE

OVARIAN CANCER REGIMEN: OLAPARIB

Ledermann J et al. N Engl J Med 2012;366:1382–1392
Protocol for: Ledermann J et al. N Engl J Med 2012;366:1382–1392
Supplementary appendix to: Ledermann J et al. N Engl J Med 2012;366:1382–1392

Start olaparib maintenance therapy within 8 weeks of completion of the last dose of platinum-based chemotherapy
Olaparib tablets 300 mg per dose; administer orally every 12 hours, without regard to food, continually until disease progression (total dosage/week with the tablet formulation is 4200 mg)
- Patients who delay taking olaparib tablets at a regularly scheduled time or who vomit after taking olaparib tablets should take the next dose at the next regularly scheduled time
- Olaparib tablets should be swallowed whole. Do not crush, chew, dissolve, or divide tablets
- Olaparib is metabolized by cytochrome P450 (CYP) CYP3A subfamily enzymes. Avoid concurrent use with moderate or strong CYP3A4 inhibitors whenever possible. If concurrent use with a *moderate* CYP3A4 inhibitor is required, reduce olaparib tablet dose to 150 mg orally twice daily. If concurrent use with a *strong* CYP3A4 inhibitor is required, reduce olaparib tablet dosage to 100 mg orally twice daily. Avoid concurrent use with moderate or strong CYP3A4 inducers (eg, rifampin, carbamazepine, phenytoin, phenobarbital, St John's Wort)
- Advise patients not to consume grapefruit, grapefruit juice, Seville oranges, or Seville orange juice, as they may inhibit CYP3A in the gut wall and increase the bioavailability of olaparib
- CAUTION: olaparib is currently marketed in the United States in only a tablet formulation. Olaparib was previously marketed as both capsule and tablet formulations. Tablets and capsules cannot be substituted one for the other on a milligram-to-milligram basis. The bioavailability of the tablet formulation is greater than that of the capsule formulation
- "Population pharmacokinetic analyses have shown that the steady state exposure (AUC) following 300-mg **tablet** twice daily was 77% higher compared to that following 400-mg **capsule** twice daily." (LYNPARZA [olaparib] tablets, for oral use; 08/2017 product label. AstraZeneca Pharmaceuticals LP, Wilmington, DE)

Supportive Care
Antiemetic prophylaxis
Emetogenic potential is **MODERATE**
See Chapter 42 for antiemetic recommendations

Hematopoietic growth factor (CSF) prophylaxis
Primary prophylaxis is **NOT** *indicated*
See Chapter 43 for more information

Antimicrobial prophylaxis
Risk of fever and neutropenia is **LOW**
  Antimicrobial primary prophylaxis to be considered:
  - Antibacterial—not indicated
  - Antifungal—not indicated
  - Antiviral—not indicated, unless patient previously had an episode of HSV

Diarrhea management
Latent or delayed-onset diarrhea*:
Loperamide 4 mg orally initially after the first loose or liquid stool, *then* 2–4 mg orally every 2–4 hours or **diphenoxylate hydrochloride** 2.5 mg **with atropine sulfate** 0.025 mg (eg, Lomotil)

*Abigerges D et al. J Natl Cancer Inst 1994;86:446–449
Rothenberg ML et al. J Clin Oncol 2001;19:3801–3807
Wadler S et al. J Clin Oncol 1998;16:3169–3178

Treatment Modifications

OLAPARIB TABLETS DOSAGE MODIFICATIONS

Note: **DO NOT substitute Lynparza (olaparib) tablets (100 mg and 150 mg) with Lynparza (olaparib) capsules (50 mg) on a milligram-to-milligram basis due to differences in the dosing and bioavailability of each formulation**

Starting dose	300 mg twice daily in tablet form
Dose level −1	250 mg twice daily in tablet form
Dose level −2	200 mg twice daily in tablet form

Adverse Event	Treatment Modification
Dyspnea, cough, fever, and radiologic abnormalities—pneumonitis suspected	Interrupt olaparib until pulmonary status clarified
Pneumonitis confirmed	Discontinue olaparib
Creatinine clearance 31–50 mL/min	Reduce olaparib dosage to 200 mg twice daily in tablet form
Administration of a moderate CYP3A inhibitor required	Reduce olaparib dosage to 150 mg twice daily in tablet form
Administration of a strong CYP3A inhibitor required	Reduce olaparib dosage to 100 mg twice daily in tablet form
G ≥2 nonhematologic toxicity	Wait for toxicity to resolve to G1, then reduce olaparib 1 dose level
G ≥2 hematologic toxicity	Wait for toxicity to resolve to G1 then reduce olaparib 1 dose level
MDS/AML confirmed	Discontinue olaparib

Note: olaparib can cause fetal harm. Advise females of reproductive potential of the potential risk to a fetus and to use effective contraception

Patient Population Studied

A randomized, double-blind, placebo-controlled, phase 2 trial involved 265 patients with relapsed, platinum-sensitive, high-grade serous ovarian cancer, fallopian tube cancer, or primary peritoneal cancer. Eligible patients were aged ≥18 years, had received at least 2 previous platinum-based chemotherapy regimens, and had taken their last dose of platinum within 8 weeks of the start of the study. Patients were randomly assigned (1:1) to receive olaparib capsules (400 mg twice daily) or matching placebo until disease progression or unacceptable toxicity

Therapy Monitoring

1. *Once per week initially, then once per month:* CBC with differential and platelet count
2. *Before the start of a cycle:* CBC with differential, serum electrolytes
3. Monitor patients for pneumonitis. Query symptoms of cough, dyspnea, or fever. Obtain radiologic investigations as needed
4. Monitor patients for hematologic toxicity at baseline and monthly thereafter. Discontinue if myelodysplastic syndrome/acute myeloid leukemia (MDS/AML) is confirmed
5. *Every 2–3 months:* imaging to assess response. Serum markers can be considered/obtained at each visit if they have been shown to be of value in following patient's disease status

Efficacy (N = 265)

	Olaparib (N = 136)	Placebo (N = 129)	
Median progression-free survival	8.4 months	4.8 months	HR 0.35 (95% CI 0.25 0.49); P <0.001
Objective response rate*	12%	4%	OR 3.36 (95% CI 0.75–23.72); P = 0.12

*Objective response rate includes patients with either a complete or partial response to treatment; measured for the 40% of the overall study population who had measurable disease and could be assessed according to RECIST guidelines

Adverse Events (N = 264)

Grade (%)*	Olaparib (N = 136)		Placebo (N = 128)	
	Grade 1/2	Grade 3/4	Grade 1/2	Grade 3/4
Nausea	66	2	35	0
Fatigue	42	7	34	3
Vomiting	29	2	13	<1
Diarrhea	21	2	20	2
Headache	18	0	11	<1
Decreased appetite	18	0	13	0
Abdominal pain	16	1	23	3
Anemia	12	5	4	<1
Dyspepsia	15	0	9	0
Dysgeusia	14	0	6	0
Cough	13	0	9	0
Upper abdominal pain	13	0	7	<1
Nasopharyngitis	13	0	11	0
Constipation	13	0	10	0
Dizziness	13	0	7	0
Arthralgia	12	0	13	0
Asthenia	11	<1	9	0
Back pain	10	2	8	0
Hot flush	4	0	12	0
Abdominal distention	10	0	9	0

*According to the National Cancer Institute Common Terminology Criteria for Adverse Events, version 3.0
Note: adverse events that occurred in ≥10% of patients in either group are included in the table. Treatment was permanently discontinued owing to treatment-related adverse events in 2 of the olaparib group and 1 of the placebo group

RECURRENT • PLATINUM-SENSITIVE • MAINTENANCE

OVARIAN CANCER REGIMEN: RUCAPARIB

Coleman RL et al. Lancet 2017;390:1949–1961
Supplementary appendix to: Coleman RL et al. Lancet 2017;390:1949–1961

Start rucaparib maintenance therapy between 2 and 8 weeks following completion of the last dose of platinum-based chemotherapy
Rucaparib 600 mg per dose; administer orally every 12 hours, without regard to food, continually until disease progression (total dosage/week = 8400 mg)

- Patients who delay taking a rucaparib dose at a regularly scheduled time or who vomit after taking a rucaparib dose should take the next dose at the next regularly scheduled time
- Rucaparib may cause photosensitivity. Counsel patients to apply sunscreen and avoid prolonged sun exposure during treatment with rucaparib
- Rucaparib may inhibit cytochrome P450 (CYP) enzymes CYP1A2, CYP3A4, and CYP2C9; use caution and consider dosage reduction, when appropriate, of concurrently used CYP1A2, CYP3A4, and CYP2C9 substrates, especially if the substrate has a narrow therapeutic index. Patients who are concurrently prescribed warfarin (a CYP2C9 substrate) should undergo frequent international normalized ratio (INR) monitoring following initiation or discontinuation of rucaparib
- Starting dosage in hepatic impairment: No dosage adjustment is recommended in patients with mild hepatic impairment (total bilirubin ≤ULN and aspartate aminotransferase [AST] >ULN, or total bilirubin >1× ULN and <1.5× ULN with any AST). No recommendation for dosing can be made for patients with moderate or severe hepatic impairment due to lack of data in these populations
- Starting dosage in renal impairment: No dosage adjustment is recommended in patients with mild to moderate renal impairment (creatinine clearance ≥30 mL/min and ≤89 mL/min). No recommendation for dosing can be made for patients with severe renal impairment or for those undergoing hemodialysis due to lack of data in these populations

Supportive Care
Antiemetic prophylaxis
*Emetogenic potential is **MODERATE–HIGH***
See Chapter 42 for antiemetic recommendations

Hematopoietic growth factor (CSF) prophylaxis
*Primary prophylaxis is **NOT** indicated*
See Chapter 43 for more information

Antimicrobial prophylaxis
*Risk of fever and neutropenia is **LOW***
  Antimicrobial primary prophylaxis to be considered:
- Antibacterial—not indicated
- Antifungal—not indicated
- Antiviral—not indicated, unless patient previously had an episode of HSV

Oral care
Standard prophylaxis and treatment for mucositis/stomatitis

Treatment Modifications

RUCAPARIB DOSAGE MODIFICATIONS	
Starting dose	600 mg by mouth twice a day
Dose level − 1	500 mg by mouth twice a day
Dose level − 2	400 mg by mouth twice a day
Dose level − 3	300 mg by mouth twice a day

Adverse Event	Treatment Modification
G ≥2 nonhematologic toxicity	Withhold rucaparib. Wait for toxicity to resolve to G ≤1, then reduce rucaparib by 1 dose level
G ≥2 hematologic toxicity	Interrupt rucaparib or reduce dosage by 1 level. Monitor CBC with differential at least weekly until recovery. If the toxicity dose not resolve to G ≤1 after 4 weeks or if MDS/AML is suspected, refer the patient to a hematologist for further evaluation including a bone marrow analysis
MDS/AML confirmed	Discontinue rucaparib

CBC, complete blood count; MDS, myelodysplastic syndrome; AML, acute myelogenous leukemia
Rubraca (rucaparib) prescribing information. Boulder, CO: Clovis Oncology, Inc; revised April 2018

Efficacy (N = 564)

	Rucaparib	Placebo	
Median progression-free survival in the *BRCA*-mutant cohort	16.6 months	5.4 months	HR 0.23 (95% CI 0.16–0.34); P <0.0001
Median progression-free survival in the homologous recombination deficiency cohort	13.6 months	5.4 months	HR 0.32 (95% CI 0.24–0.42); P <0.0001
Median progression-free survival in the intention-to-treat population	10.8 months	5.4 months	HR 0.36 (95% CI 0.30–0.45); P <0.0001

Adverse Events (N = 561)

	Rucaparib (n = 372)		Placebo (n = 189)	
Grade (%)*	Grade 1/2	Grade 3/4	Grade 1/2	Grade 3/4
Nausea	72	4	36	<1
Fatigue (asthenia)	63	7	41	3
Dysgeusia	39	0	7	0
Decreased hemoglobin concentration	19	19	5	<1
Vomiting	33	4	14	1
Constipation	35	2	23	1
Increased ALT or AST concentration	23	10	4	0
Diarrhea	31	<1	21	1
Abdominal pain	27	2	25	<1
Thrombocytopenia	23	5	3	0
Decreased appetite	23	<1	14	0
Headache	18	<1	15	<1
Decreased neutrophil count (neutropenia)	11	7	4	1
Photosensitivity reaction	17	<1	<1	0
Arthralgia	15	<1	13	0
Increased blood creatinine concentration	15	<1	2	0
Cough	15	0	13	0
Dizziness	15	0	7	<1
Dyspepsia	14	<1	5	0
Insomnia	14	0	8	0
Upper abdominal pain	13	<1	5	0
Pruritus	13	0	10	0
Dyspnea	13	0	7	0
Rash	12	<1	9	0
Back pain	12	0	15	0
Pyrexia	12	0	4	0

(continued)

Patient Population Studied

This international, multicenter, randomized, double-blind, placebo-controlled, phase 3 trial (ARIEL3) involved 564 patients with platinum-sensitive, high-grade serous or endometrioid ovarian, primary peritoneal, or fallopian tube carcinoma. Eligible patients were aged ≥18 years, had an Eastern Cooperative Oncology Group (ECOG) performance status of ≤1, had received at least 2 previous platinum-based chemotherapy regimens, and had taken their last dose of platinum within 8 weeks of the start of the study. Patients who had received anticancer therapy ≤14 days before the start of the study or had received previous treatment with a poly (ADP-ribose) polymerase inhibitor were ineligible. Patients were randomly assigned (2:1) to receive rucaparib (600 mg twice daily) or matching placebo in continuous 28-day cycles until disease progression, death, or discontinuation for another reason.

Adverse Events (N = 561) (continued)

Grade (%)*	Rucaparib (n = 372)		Placebo (n = 189)	
	Grade 1/2	Grade 3/4	Grade 1/2	Grade 3/4
Abdominal distention	11	0	12	0
Upper respiratory tract infection	11	0	2	1
Peripheral edema	10	<1	7	0
Hypomagnesemia	10	<1	6	0

*According to the National Cancer Institute Common Terminology Criteria for Adverse Events, version 4.03
Note: treatment-emergent adverse events that occurred in ≥10% of patients in either group are included in the table. Deaths resulting from a treatment-emergent adverse event occurred in 6 (2%) patients in the rucaparib group and 2 (1%) patients in the placebo group; 2 of the deaths in the rucaparib group were considered to be treatment related (1 from myelodysplastic syndrome and 1 from acute myeloid leukemia). Treatment was discontinued owing to treatment-emergent adverse events in 13% of the rucaparib group and 2% of the placebo group

Therapy Monitoring

1. Monitor patients for hematologic toxicity at baseline and monthly thereafter
2. *Myelodysplastic syndrome/acute myeloid leukemia (MDS/AML):* MDS/AML has occurred in patients exposed to rucaparib, including 1 fatal event of AML. Discontinue if MDS/AML is confirmed
3. Rucaparib can cause fetal harm. Advise females of reproductive potential of the potential risk to a fetus and to use effective contraception during treatment with rucaparib and for 6 months after the last dose
4. *Every 2–3 months:* imaging to assess response. Serum markers can be considered/obtained at each visit if they have been shown to be of value in following the patient's disease status

RECURRENT PLATINUM-REFRACTORY/ PLATINUM-RESISTANT

OVARIAN CANCER REGIMEN: DOCETAXEL

Kaye SB et al. Eur J Cancer 1995;31A(Suppl 4):S14–S17

Premedication:
Dexamethasone 8 mg/dose; administer orally twice daily for 3 days (6 doses) starting on the day before docetaxel administration (total dose/cycle = 48 mg)
Docetaxel 75–100 mg/m²; administer intravenously in a volume of 0.9% sodium chloride injection or 5% dextrose injection sufficient to produce a docetaxel concentration within the range of 0.3–0.74 mg/mL over 60 minutes on day 1, every 21 days, for 4 cycles (total dosage per cycle = 75–100 mg/m²)

Supportive Care
Antiemetic prophylaxis
*Emetogenic potential is **LOW–MODERATE***
See Chapter 42 for antiemetic recommendations

Hematopoietic growth factor (CSF) prophylaxis
*Primary prophylaxis is **NOT** indicated*
See Chapter 43 for more information

Antimicrobial prophylaxis
*Risk of fever and neutropenia is **LOW***
   Antimicrobial primary prophylaxis to be considered:
• Antibacterial—not indicated
• Antifungal—not indicated
• Antiviral—not indicated unless patient previously had an episode of HSV

Treatment Modifications

Adverse Events	Treatment Modifications
ANC <1500/mm³ on day of planned treatment*	Delay treatment until ANC ≥1500/mm³; administer filgrastim during subsequent cycles[†]
ANC <500/mm³ ≥7 days	Reduce docetaxel dosage by 20% during subsequent cycles (or add filgrastim[†])
First episode of febrile neutropenia	Reduce docetaxel dosage by 20% during subsequent cycles (or add filgrastim[†])
Second episode of febrile neutropenia	Continue docetaxel and give filgrastim[†] during subsequent cycles
Third episode of febrile neutropenia	Add ciprofloxacin[‡]
First episode of G4 documented infection	Reduce docetaxel dosage by 20% during subsequent cycles
Second episode of G4 documented infection	Continue docetaxel and give filgrastim[†] and ciprofloxacin[‡] during subsequent cycles
Third episode of G4 documented infection	Discontinue docetaxel

*Although an ANC of 1500/mm³ is often identified as a minimum acceptable ANC to safely proceed with treatment, recent data show that an ANC ≥1000/mm³ is acceptable if filgrastim is given after chemotherapy
[†]Filgrastim 5 μg/kg per day subcutaneously for 8 consecutive days, days 3–10
[‡]Ciprofloxacin 500 mg orally twice daily for 7 consecutive days starting on day 5

Patient Population Studied

Evaluation of docetaxel administration in 293 patients with advanced ovarian cancer in 3 phase 2 trials. All patients had previously received cisplatin and/or carboplatin as first-line treatment. In all 3 studies, docetaxel 100 mg/m² was administered every 3 weeks, without premedication for hypersensitivity reactions or emesis. At the time of the analysis, 200 patients were evaluable for response

Efficacy*

Results of Phase 2 Trials of 100 mg/m² Docetaxel by Study and Type of Response

Response	Study (Number of Patients)				Percentage of Evaluable Patients E = 200	Percentage of Enrolled Patients N = 293
	ECTG N = 123 E = 85	CSG N = 126 E = 75	MDACC N = 44 E = 40	All Studies N = 293 E = 200		
Complete response	3	6	1	10	5	3.4
Partial response	23	17	13	53	26.5	18.1
Progressive disease	21	22	3	46	23	15.7
Evaluable, ORR	31	31	35	31.5	—	—
Enrolled ORR	21	18	32	21.5	—	—

*Response criteria were those accepted by UICC. Although CA-125 measurements were made with every course of treatment, the results were not used in the response assessment
ECTG, Early Clinical Trials Group of the European Organisation for Research and Treatment of Cancer; CSG, Clinical Screening Group of the EORTC; MDACC, The University of Texas MD Anderson Cancer Center, Houston, Texas, USA; N, number of patients enrolled; E, number of patients evaluable; ORR, overall response rate

Toxicity

Incidence and Severity of Major Adverse Effects of 100 mg/m² Docetaxel

Adverse Effect	Incidence
Neutropenia (Grade 3 or 4)	83/99 patients (84%)
Acute hypersensitivity (Grades 2–4)	13/207 patients (6%)
Skin reactions (Grades 2–4)	98/188 patients (52%)
Fluid retention or effusions	102/181 patients (56%)*
Neuropathy (Grades 2–3)	11/95 patients (12%)

*Incidence was 66% in patients who received 6 courses of docetaxel

Therapy Monitoring

1. *Baseline:* LFTs, serum chemistry, CBC with differential and platelet count, and CA-125. Complete history and physical examination including a gynecologic examination
2. *Follow-up:* CBC with differential and platelet count at least weekly through leukocyte and platelet count nadirs, and prior to beginning *repeated cycles*
3. *Before beginning repeated cycles:* repeat LFTs

RECURRENT • PLATINUM-REFRACTORY/ PLATIUM-RESISTANT

OVARIAN CANCER REGIMEN: FLUOROURACIL + LEUCOVORIN

Reed E et al. Gynecol Oncol 1992;46:326–329

Leucovorin 500 mg/m² per dose; administer intravenously in 25–100 mL 0.9% sodium chloride injection or 5% dextrose injection over 30 minutes, daily for 5 consecutive days, on days 1–5, every 21 days (total dosage/ cycle = 2500 mg/m²), *followed after 1 hour by:* **Fluorouracil** 375 mg/m² per dose; administer by intravenous injection over 3–5 minutes, daily, 1 hour after the completion of leucovorin, for 5 consecutive days, days 1–5, every 21 days (total dosage/cycle = 1875 mg/m²)

Supportive Care
Antiemetic prophylaxis
Emetogenic potential is **LOW**
See Chapter 42 for antiemetic recommendations

Hematopoietic growth factor (CSF) prophylaxis
Primary prophylaxis is **NOT** *indicated*
See Chapter 43 for more information

Antimicrobial prophylaxis
Risk of fever and neutropenia is **LOW**
   Antimicrobial primary prophylaxis to be considered:
   • Antibacterial—not indicated
   • Antifungal—not indicated
   • Antiviral—not indicated unless patient previously had an episode of HSV

Treatment Modifications

Adverse Event	Dose Modification
G2 nonhematologic toxicity	Reduce fluorouracil daily dosage by 25% on the same administration schedule
WBC <3000/mm³ or platelet count <75,000/mm³ on treatment day	Delay cycle 1 week until WBC >3000/mm³ and platelet count >75,000/ mm³

If no toxicity G <1 is documented in a cycle, then increase fluorouracil daily dosage by 25% on the same administration schedule

Patient Population Studied

A study of 29 patients with recurrent advanced-stage ovarian cancer of epithelial histology who had progressive disease while receiving or had suffered relapse after high-dose cisplatin therapy

Efficacy (N = 29)

	Relapsed After Response to Platinum-Based Therapy (n = 8)	Progressive Disease on Platinum-Based Therapy (n = 21)
CR	13%	5%
PR	—	5%
SD*	38%	38%
PD	50%	52%

*SD: 5, 5, 7, 8, 8, 8, 10, 13, 14, 21, and 27 months

Toxicity* (N = 29/204 Cycles)

	Number of Cycles			
	G1	G2	G3	G4
Hematologic				
Neutropenia	1	5	7	4
Thrombocytopenia	7	2	4	4
Anemia	4	6	5	1
Nonhematologic				
Nausea/vomiting	9	3	2	0
Stomatitis	9	5	4	2
Diarrhea	11	3	3	0

*National Cancer Institute Common Toxicity Criteria, version 2

Therapy Monitoring

Before repeated cycles: PE, CBC with differential, and serum electrolytes

Notes

Because this regimen is well tolerated, it represents an option for patients when more attractive options have been exhausted

RECURRENT • PLATINUM-REFRACTORY/ PATINUM-RESISTANT

OVARIAN CANCER REGIMEN: GEMCITABINE

Markman M et al. Gynecol Oncol 2003;90:593–596

Gemcitabine 1000 mg/m^2 per dose; administer intravenously diluted to a concentration $\geq$0.1 mg/mL in 0.9% sodium chloride injection over 30 minutes for 3 doses, on days 1, 8, and 15, every 28 days (total dosage/cycle = 3000 mg/m^2)

Supportive Care
Antiemetic prophylaxis
Emetogenic potential is **LOW**
See Chapter 42 for antiemetic recommendations

Hematopoietic growth factor (CSF) prophylaxis
Primary prophylaxis is **NOT** *indicated*
See Chapter 43 for more information

Antimicrobial prophylaxis
Risk of fever and neutropenia is **LOW**
   Antimicrobial primary prophylaxis to be considered:
   • Antibacterial—not indicated
   • Antifungal—not indicated
   • Antiviral—not indicated unless patient previously had an episode of HSV

Treatment Modifications

Adverse Event	Dose Modification
ANC nadir <1000/mm^3 or platelet count nadir $\leq$100,000/mm^3	Hold treatment until ANC recovers to $\geq$1000/mm^3 and platelets to >100,000/mm^3, then resume with gemcitabine dosage decreased by 200 mg/m^2 per dose
Second occurrence of ANC nadir $\leq$1000/mm^3 or platelet count nadir $\leq$100,000/mm^3	Hold treatment until ANC recovers to >1000/mm^3 and platelets to >100,000/mm^3, then resume with gemcitabine dosage decreased by an additional 200 mg/m^2 per dose
Third occurrence of ANC nadir $\leq$1000/mm^3 or platelet count nadir $\leq$100,000/mm^3	Discontinue gemcitabine therapy
G3 nonhematologic toxicity	Hold treatment until toxicities resolve to G <1, then resume with gemcitabine dosage decreased by 200 mg/m^2 per dose
Second occurrence of G3 nonhematologic toxicity	Hold treatment until toxicities resolve to G $\leq$1, then resume with gemcitabine dosage decreased by an additional 200 mg/m^2 per dose

Patient Population Studied

A study of 51 patients with ovarian (41), fallopian tube (1), and primary peritoneal cancer (9) and prior chemotherapy with a platinum agent (cisplatin or carboplatin) and a taxane (paclitaxel or docetaxel). If a patient had previously responded to such therapy, and the treatment-free interval had been 3 months, the patient had to be re-treated with a platinum agent or a taxane to confirm clinical resistance

Efficacy (N = 51)

Partial response	8%
$\geq$75% decrease in CA-125	8%
Median duration of response	4 months
Survival (all patients)	7 months
Survival (patients with response)	15 months

Toxicity (N = 51)

	% Patients
Hematologic	
G4 neutropenia	24
G3 thrombocytopenia	7
Nonhematologic	
G3 fatigue	10
Fever/chills (no neutropenia)	15
Rash	4
Conjunctivitis	4

Therapy Monitoring

Before repeated cycles: PE, CBC with differential, and serum electrolytes, magnesium, calcium, BUN, creatinine, and LFTs

Notes

Gemcitabine dosages of 1250 mg/m^2 resulted in excessive toxicity

RECURRENT • PLATINUM-REFRACTORY/PLATINUM-RESISTANT

OVARIAN CANCER REGIMEN: LIPOSOMAL DOXORUBICIN

Lorusso D et al. Oncology 2004;67:243–249
Thigpen JT et al. Gynecol Oncol 2005;96:10–18

Doxorubicin HCl liposome injection 40–50 mg/m^2; administer intravenously diluted in 250 mL 5% dextrose injection (D5W) for doses ≤90 mg and in 500 mL D5W for doses >90 mg every 3–4 weeks (total dosage/cycle = 40–50 mg/m^2)
Note: administer at an initial rate of 1 mg/min for 10–15 minutes. If infusion reactions are not observed, the rate may be increased to complete drug administration over 60 minutes

Supportive Care
Antiemetic prophylaxis
Emetogenic potential is **LOW**
See Chapter 42 for antiemetic recommendations

Hematopoietic growth factor (CSF) prophylaxis
Primary prophylaxis is **NOT** indicated
See Chapter 43 for more information

Antimicrobial prophylaxis
Risk of fever and neutropenia is **LOW**
Antimicrobial primary prophylaxis to be considered:
- Antibacterial—not indicated
- Antifungal—not indicated
- Antiviral—not indicated, unless patient previously had an episode of HSV

Hand-foot reaction (palmar-plantar erythrodysesthesia)
For patients who develop a hand-foot reaction, use topical emollients (eg, Aquaphor), topical or orally administered steroids, antihistamine agents (H$_1$-receptor antagonists), or pyridoxine
- The suggested pyridoxine starting dose is 50 mg/day, which may be increased to a maximum of 200 mg/day

Patients who have developed G1/2 PPE while receiving doxorubicin HCl liposome injection may receive a fixed daily dose of pyridoxine, 200 mg. This may allow for treatment to be completed without dosage reduction, treatment delay, or recurrence of PPE

Treatment Modifications

Adverse Event	Dose Modification
Hand-foot syndrome	Reduce dosage to 40 mg/m^2
G3/4 nonhematologic toxicity	
Stomatitis G ≥2	
Persistent (>3 weeks) G1/2 toxicity	Increase dosing interval to 4 weeks
Persistent (>4 weeks) G3/4 toxicity	Discontinue therapy

Patient Population Studied

A study of 37 patients with advanced ovarian cancer in whom first-line therapy had failed to provide benefit

Efficacy

Response rates of 7.7–26% have been reported in several studies with a median progression-free survival of 4–6 months

Therapy Monitoring

Before repeated cycles: PE, CBC with differential, and serum electrolytes, magnesium, calcium, BUN, and creatinine

Notes

The consensus of experts in the management of ovarian carcinoma:
1. Based on survival and toxicity advantages and a once-monthly administration schedule, liposomal doxorubicin is considered by some to be the first-choice nonplatinum agent for relapsed ovarian cancer
2. Tolerability is improved with the use of liposomal doxorubicin 40 mg/m^2 on an every-4-week schedule. Hand-foot syndrome (PPE) is the most commonly reported adverse event associated with liposomal doxorubicin. Avoid this toxicity by using lower dosages of liposomal doxorubicin (40 mg/m^2 every 4 weeks, or 10 mg/m^2 weekly), rather than omitting or decreasing doses as a consequence of adverse events

Thigpen JT et al. Gynecol Oncol 2005;96:10–18

Toxicity (N = 37)

	% G1	% G2	% G3	% G4
Hematologic				
Neutropenia	—	—	—	—
Thrombocytopenia	3	—	—	—
Anemia	24	—	—	—
Febrile neutropenia	—	—	—	—
Nonhematologic				
PPE	11	8	3	—
Stomatitis/mucositis	8	—	—	—
Nausea/vomiting	14	—	—	—
Asthenia	24	—	—	—
Hair loss	16	—	—	—
Anaphylactic reactions	5	—	—	—
Liver toxicity	—	—	—	—
Cardiac toxicity	—	—	—	—

Note: toxicity grades for palmar-plantar erythrodysesthesia (PPE):
- G1: mild erythema, swelling, or desquamation not interfering with daily activities
- G2: erythema, swelling, or desquamation interfering with daily activities; small blisters or ulcerations <2 cm
- G3: blistering, ulcerations, or swelling interfering with daily activities; patient cannot wear regular clothing
- G4: diffuse or local process causing infectious complications, a bedridden state, or hospitalization
Lorusso D et al. Oncology 2004;67:243–249

RECURRENT • PLATINUM-REFRACTORY/ PLATINUM-RESISTANT

OVARIAN CANCER REGIMEN: VINORELBINE

Rothenberg ML et al. Gynecol Oncol 2004;95:506–512

Vinorelbine 30 mg/m^2 per dose; administer by intravenous injection over 1–2 minutes for 2 doses, on days 1 and 8, every 21 days (total dosage/cycle = 60 mg/m^2)

Supportive Care
Antiemetic prophylaxis
*Emetogenic potential is **MINIMAL***
See Chapter 42 for antiemetic recommendations

Hematopoietic growth factor (CSF) prophylaxis
*Primary prophylaxis is **NOT** indicated*
See Chapter 43 for more information

Antimicrobial prophylaxis
*Risk of fever and neutropenia is **LOW***
   Antimicrobial primary prophylaxis to be considered:
   • Antibacterial—not indicated
   • Antifungal—not indicated
   • Antiviral—not indicated unless patient previously had an episode of HSV

Decreased bowel motility
Give a bowel regimen to prevent constipation based initially on stool softeners

Treatment Modifications

Adverse Event	Dose Modification
ANC <1000/mm^3 or platelet count <75,000/mm^3 on the day before or the day of vinorelbine administration	Hold vinorelbine dose on this day
ANC 1000–1499/mm^3 or platelet count 75,000–99,999/mm^3 on the day before or the day of vinorelbine administration	Administer vinorelbine, but reduce vinorelbine dosage by 7.5 mg/m^2
On the day before or the day of repeated vinorelbine administration, ANC 1000–1499/mm^3 or platelet count 75,000–99,999/mm^3 after vinorelbine 15 mg/m^2	Discontinue therapy

Patient Population Studied

A study of 79 patients with recurrent or resistant epithelial ovarian cancer after treatment with platinum and paclitaxel

Efficacy (N = 79)

Partial response (n = 71)	3%
Median time to progression	3 months
6-month survival rate	65%

Median Survival

All patients (N = 79)	10.1 months
Chemotherapy-resistant (n = 52)	8 months
Chemotherapy-sensitive (n = 27)	16 months

Toxicity* (N = 79)

	% G0	% G1	% G2	% G3	% G4
Hematologic					
Anemia	27	23	38	13	0
Granulocytopenia	24	4	16	28	28
Leukopenia	11	19	23	39	8
Thrombocytopenia	78	19	3	0	0
Nonhematologic					
Abdominal pain	72	10	13	5	0
Alopecia	71	16	13	0	0
Anorexia	76	24	0	0	0
Constipation	51	28	15	6	0
Dyspnea	78	0	18	3	1
Fever without infection	79	13	8	0	0
Insomnia	89	11	0	0	0
Malaise/fatigue/lethargy	34	27	28	11	0
Nausea	42	39	11	8	0
Numbness/other symptoms of peripheral neuropathy	75	0	25	0	0
Pain	69	15	11	5	0
Paresthesia	89	5	6	0	0
Vomiting	71	14	13	1	0
Weakness	86	8	3	3	0

*National Cancer Institute Common Toxicity Criteria, version 2

Therapy Monitoring

Before repeated cycles: CBC with differential

Notes

During the initial 10 weeks of treatment, vinorelbine did not appear to be effective in relieving the symptom-related distress or progressive impairment of physical functioning associated with refractory ovarian cancer

RECURRENT • PLATINUM-REFRACTORY/ PLATINUM-RESISTANT

OVARIAN CANCER REGIMEN: PACLITAXEL (24-HOUR PACLITAXEL INFUSION EVERY 3 WEEKS; WEEKLY PACLITAXEL)

Ghamande S et al. Int J Gynecol Cancer 2003;13:142–147
Omura GA et al. J Clin Oncol 2003;21:2843–2848

For both treatment strategies, give premedication for paclitaxel with:
Dexamethasone 10 mg/dose; administer orally for 2 doses 12 hours and 6 hours before paclitaxel, *or*
Dexamethasone 20 mg/dose; administer intravenously over 10–15 minutes, 30–60 minutes before paclitaxel (total dose/cycle = 20 mg)
Diphenhydramine 50 mg; administer by intravenous injection 30 minutes before paclitaxel
Cimetidine 300 mg (or **ranitidine** 50 mg, **famotidine** 20 mg, or an equivalent histamine receptor [H_2]-subtype antagonist); administer intravenously over 15–30 minutes, 30–60 minutes before paclitaxel

24-Hour Paclitaxel
Omura GA et al. J Clin Oncol 2003;21:2843–2848
Paclitaxel 175 mg/m^2; administer intravenously in a volume of 0.9% sodium chloride injection (0.9% NS) or 5% dextrose injection (D5W) sufficient to produce a concentration within the range 0.3–1.2 mg/mL, over 3 hours, on day 1, every 3 weeks (total dosage/cycle = 175 mg/m^2)
or

Weekly Paclitaxel Regimens
Ghamande S et al. Int J Gynecol Cancer 2003;13:142–147
Paclitaxel 70–80 mg/m^2 per dose; administer intravenously in a volume of 0.9% NS or D5W sufficient to produce a concentration within the range 0.3–1.2 mg/mL, over 60 minutes, weekly for a minimum of 6 consecutive weeks (total dosage/6-week cycle = 420–480 mg/m^2), *or*
Paclitaxel 70–80 mg/m^2 per dose; administer intravenously in a volume of 0.9% NS or D5W sufficient to produce a concentration within the range 0.3–1.2 mg/mL, over 60 minutes for 3 doses, on days 1, 8, and 15, every 28 days (total dosage/28-day cycle = 210–240 mg/m^2)

Supportive Care
Antiemetic prophylaxis for 24-hour (every-3-weeks) and weekly paclitaxel regimens
Emetogenic potential is **LOW**
See Chapter 42 for antiemetic recommendations

Hematopoietic growth factor (CSF) prophylaxis for the 24-hour regimen
Primary prophylaxis is indicated with one of the following:
Filgrastim (G-CSF) 5 µg/kg per day, by subcutaneous injection, *or*
Pegfilgrastim (pegylated filgrastim) 6 mg/0.6 mL, by subcutaneous injection for 1 dose
• Begin use from 24–72 hours after myelosuppressive chemotherapy is completed
• Continue daily filgrastim use until ANC ≥10,000/mm^3 on 2 measurements temporally separated by ≥12 hours
• Discontinue daily filgrastim use at least 24 hours before administering another dose of paclitaxel. Do not administer pegfilgrastim within 14 days before a dose of paclitaxel
See Chapter 43 for more information

Hematopoietic growth factor (CSF) prophylaxis for the weekly regimen
Primary prophylaxis is indicated with:
Filgrastim (G-CSF) 5 µg/kg per day by subcutaneous injection
• Begin use approximately 24 hours after myelosuppressive chemotherapy is completed
• Discontinue use at least 24 hours before administering subsequent paclitaxel doses
See Chapter 43 for more information

Antimicrobial prophylaxis
Risk of fever and neutropenia is LOW–INTERMEDIATE
Antimicrobial primary prophylaxis to be considered:
• Antibacterial—consider a fluoroquinolone or no prophylaxis
• Antifungal—not indicated
• Antiviral—not indicated unless patient previously had an episode of HSV

Treatment Modifications

Adverse Event	Dose Modification
24-Hour Paclitaxel Infusion Every 3 Weeks	
G ≥3 Nonhematologic toxicity	Reduce paclitaxel dose to 135 mg/m^2
Delay in achieving ANC ≥1000/mm^3 and platelets ≥100,000/mm^3 <2 weeks	No dose adjustment
Recurrent delays in achieving ANC ≥1000/mm^3 and platelets ≥100,000/mm^3 ≥2 weeks but ≤3 weeks	Add filgrastim 5 µg/kg per day without further dosage modification. If already using filgrastim, reduce paclitaxel dose to 135 mg/m^2
G3/4 neurologic toxicity that has not resolved even after a 3-week delay	Discontinue therapy
Weekly Paclitaxel Regimen	
WBC <2500/mm^3	Hold chemotherapy until WBC <2500/mm^3
ANC <1500/mm^3	Hold chemotherapy until ANC <1500/mm^3
Platelets <75,000/mm^3	Hold chemotherapy until platelets <75,000/mm^3
G3/4 neurologic toxicity that has not resolved even after a 3-week delay	Discontinue therapy

Patient Population Studied

A study of 164 patients with epithelial ovarian cancer who had been treated with not more than 1 platinum-based regimen and no prior taxane

Omura GA et al. J Clin Oncol 2003;21:2843–2848

A study of 23 patients with advanced recurrent ovarian cancer with disease deemed resistant to platinum agents and paclitaxel (defined as either progression of disease while on therapy or progression within 12 months of prior paclitaxel therapy)

Ghamande S et al. Int J Gynecol Cancer 2003;13:142–147

Efficacy

24-Hour Paclitaxel Infusion Every 3 Weeks (N = 164)

Median time to death	13.1 months

Platinum-Resistant Disease

Complete response	5%
Partial response	17%
No response	78%

Platinum-Sensitive Disease

Complete response	15%
Partial response	33%
No response	52%

Omura GA et al. J Clin Oncol 2003;21:2843–2848

Weekly Paclitaxel (N = 23)

	Paclitaxel-Free Interval	
	<12 Months (n = 10)	>12 Months (n = 13)
Partial response*	0	70%
Stable disease	30%	15%
Progressive disease	70%	15%

*Partial response based on Rustin's criteria with more than 50% reduction in CA-125 levels
Ghamande S et al. Int J Gynecol Cancer 2003;13:142–147

Toxicity (N = 164)

24-Hour Paclitaxel Infusion Every 3 Weeks

% G3/4	
Anemia	7
Thrombocytopenia	5
Nausea/vomiting	5
Neuropathy	7
Myalgia/arthralgia	3
G4 neutropenia	22 (first cycle without filgrastim)

Omura GA et al. J Clin Oncol 2003;21:2843–2848

Weekly Paclitaxel (N = 28)

	% Patients
G2 neutropenia	10.7
G3 neutropenia	21.4
G1 thrombocytopenia	3.6
G2 anemia	32.1
G2 neuropathy	7.1
G >2 neuropathy	3.6

Ghamande S et al. Int J Gynecol Cancer 2003;13:142–147

Therapy Monitoring

1. *Before repeated cycles:* CBC with differential
2. *Twice per week:* obtain CBC with differential in patients treated with the weekly regimen

RECURRENT • PLATINUM-REFRACTORY/PLATINUM-RESISTANT

OVARIAN CANCER REGIMEN: TOPOTECAN HCL

Bhoola SM et al. Gynecol Oncol 2004;95:564–569

Topotecan HCl 2.25–4 mg/m² (median: 3.7 mg/m²) per dose; administer intravenously in 50–250 mL 0.9% sodium chloride injection or 5% dextrose injection over 30 minutes, weekly, continually (total dosage/week = 2.25–4 mg/m²)
Or
Topotecan HCl 1.5 mg/m² per dose; administer intravenously in 50–250 mL 0.9% NS or D5W over 30 minutes for 5 consecutive days, on days 1–5, every 21 days (total dosage/cycle = 7.5 mg/m²)

Supportive Care for Both Weekly and Every-3-Weeks Regimens
Antiemetic prophylaxis
Emetogenic potential is **LOW**
See Chapter 42 for antiemetic recommendations

Hematopoietic growth factor (CSF) prophylaxis
Primary prophylaxis may be indicated
See Chapter 43 for more information

Antimicrobial prophylaxis
Risk of fever and neutropenia is **LOW**
   Antimicrobial primary prophylaxis to be considered:
   • Antibacterial—not indicated
   • Antifungal—not indicated
   • Antiviral—not indicated unless patient previously had an episode of HSV

Treatment Modifications

Adverse Event	Dose Modification
G3/4 neutropenia on treatment day 1 (every-21-day regimen)	Hold topotecan until ANC ≥1000/mm³ ± reduce topotecan dose 10–20% ± administer filgrastim in subsequent cycles*
G3/4 neutropenia on treatment day 1 (weekly regimen)	Hold topotecan until ANC ≥1000/mm³ ± reduce topotecan dose 10–20% ± administer filgrastim in subsequent cycles* ± change schedule to 2 weeks on/1 week off
G ≥2 anemia	Administer erythropoietin
G ≥2 fatigue	Administer erythropoietin

*With every-21-day administration schedule, administer filgrastim 5 μg/kg per day subcutaneously beginning 24 hours after the day 5 dose and continuing until ANC <10,000/mm³ on 2 consecutive measurements

Toxicity: Weekly Regimen (N = 50)

	% G2	% G3	% G4
Hematologic			
Anemia	42	24	0
Leukopenia	38	2	2
Neutropenia	24	14	4
Thrombocytopenia	4	10	0

	% G1/2	% G3/4	
Nonhematologic			
Fatigue	14	4	
Neuropathy	6	0	
Nausea	2	0	
Dehydration	2	0	
Diarrhea	2	0	
Alopecia	2	0	

Patient Population Studied

A study of 50 patients with ovarian cancer who had received multiple prior regimens

Efficacy: Weekly Regimen (N = 42*)

Measurable Disease (n = 35)	
Partial response	31%
Stable disease	43%
Progressive disease	26%

↑CA-125†		
	All with↑ CA-125 (n = 41)	↑CA-125† Only (n = 7)
Partial response	27	29
Stable disease	24	29
Progressive disease	49	42

Platinum-Sensitive Disease	
Partial response	39
Stable disease	43
Progressive disease	18

Platinum-Resistant or Platinum-Refractory Disease	
Partial response	21
Stable disease	37
Progressive disease	42

*Includes only patients who received ≥2 cycles
†Partial response defined as a 50% reduction in CA-125 levels maintained for ≥1 month. Progressive disease defined as a 25% increase in CA-125 levels

Therapy Monitoring

Before repeated cycles: CBC with differential

Notes

A retrospective chart review of patients with rapidly progressive disease or clinical deterioration excluded from analysis. Efficacy of both regimens is comparable; toxicity of weekly regimen tolerable

RECURRENT • PLATINUM-REFRACTORY/ PLATINUM RESISTANT

OVARIAN CANCER REGIMEN: LIPOSOMAL DOXORUBICIN + BEVACIZUMAB

Pujade-Lauraine E et al. J Clin Oncol
2014;32:1302–1308
Protocol for: Pujade-Lauraine E et al. J Clin Oncol
2014;32:1302–1308
Erratum in: J Clin Oncol 2014;32:4025
Comment in: Nat Rev Clin Oncol 2014;11:242,
J Clin Oncol 2014;32:1287–1289, J Clin Oncol
2014;32:3580

Bevacizumab 10 mg/kg per dose; administer intravenously in 100 mL 0.9% sodium chloride injection (0.9% NS) for 2 doses, on days 1 and 15 before liposomal doxorubicin, every 4 weeks (total dosage/4-week cycle = 20 mg/kg)
Note: the initial bevacizumab dose is administered over 90 minutes. If administration is well tolerated, the administration duration may be decreased stepwise during subsequent administrations to 60 minutes and, finally, to a minimum duration of 30 minutes
Doxorubicin HCl liposome injection (pegylated liposomal doxorubicin) 40 mg/m^2; administer intravenously over 60 minutes in 250 mL (doses ≤90 mg) or 500 mL (doses >90 mg) 5% dextrose injection on day 1, every 4 weeks (total dosage/4-week cycle = 40 mg/m^2)
Note: liposomal doxorubicin is administered at an initial rate of 1 mg/min to minimize the risk of infusion reactions. If no infusion-related adverse reactions are observed within 15 minutes after starting administration, the infusion rate may be increased to complete administration over 1 hour

Supportive Care
Antiemetic prophylaxis
Emetogenic potential on days of treatment with liposomal doxorubicin is **LOW**
Emetogenic potential on days with bevacizumab alone is **MINIMAL**
See Chapter 42 for antiemetic recommendations

Hematopoietic growth factor (CSF) prophylaxis
Primary prophylaxis is **NOT** *indicated*
See Chapter 43 for more information

(continued)

Treatment Modifications

BEVACIZUMAB AND LIPOSOMAL DOXORUBICIN DOSE MODIFICATIONS

Bevacizumab	
Adverse Event	**Treatment Modification**
Gastrointestinal perforations (gastrointestinal perforations, fistula formation in the gastrointestinal tract, intra-abdominal abscess), fistula formation involving an internal organ	Discontinue bevacizumab permanently
Serious bleeding	
Wound dehiscence requiring medical intervention	
Nephrotic syndrome	
Hypertensive crisis or hypertensive encephalopathy or reversible posterior leukoencephalopathy syndrome (RPLS)	
Congestive heart failure	
Necrotizing fasciitis	
Severe arterial or venous thromboembolic events	Discontinue bevacizumab permanently; the safety of reinitiating bevacizumab after a thromboembolic event is resolved is not known
Moderate to severe proteinuria	Patients with a 2+ or greater urine dipstick reading should undergo further assessment, eg, 24-hour urine collection. Suspend bevacizumab administration for ≥2 g of proteinuria/24 h and resume when proteinuria is <2 g/24 h
Severe hypertension not controlled with medical management	Hold bevacizumab pending further evaluation and treatment of hypertension
Mild, clinically insignificant infusion reaction	Decrease the rate of infusion
Clinically significant but not severe infusion reaction	Interrupt the infusion in patients with clinically significant infusion reactions and consider resuming at a slower rate following resolution. If decision is made to restart, the infusion may be continued at ≤50% of the rate prior to the reaction and increased in 50% increments every 30 minutes if well tolerated. Infusions may be restarted at the full rate during the next cycle
Severe infusion reaction—hypertension, hypertensive crises associated with neurologic signs and symptoms, wheezing, oxygen desaturation, G3 hypersensitivity, chest pain, headaches, rigors, and diaphoresis	Stop infusion and administer appropriate medical therapy (eg, epinephrine, corticosteroids, intravenous antihistamines, bronchodilators, and/or oxygen). Discontinue bevacizumab
Planned elective surgery	Suspend bevacizumab at least 28 days before elective surgery and do not resume for at least 28 days after surgery or until surgical incision is fully healed
Recent hemoptysis	Do not administer bevacizumab
Evidence of rectosigmoid involvement by pelvic examination or bowel involvement on CT scan, or clinical symptoms of bowel obstruction	

(continued)

(continued)

Antimicrobial prophylaxis
Risk of fever and neutropenia is **LOW**
  Antimicrobial primary prophylaxis to be considered:
  • Antibacterial—not indicated
  • Antifungal—not indicated
  • Antiviral—not indicated, unless patient previously had an episode of HSV

Hand-foot syndrome (palmar-plantar erythrodysesthesia, PPE)
For patients who develop a hand-foot syndrome, use topical emollients (eg, Aquaphor), topical or orally administered steroids, antihistamine agents (H$_1$-receptor antagonists), or pyridoxine
Pyridoxine may provide relief for discomfort/pain associated with PPE, although the mechanism through which this occurs remains unclear
• The suggested pyridoxine starting dosage is 50 mg/day, which may be increased to a maximum of 200 mg/day
• Patients who develop G1/2 PPE while receiving doxorubicin HCl liposome injection may receive a fixed daily dose of pyridoxine 200 mg. This may allow for treatment to be completed without dosage reduction, treatment delay, or recurrence of PPE

Liposomal Doxorubicin

Adverse Event	Treatment Modification
Signs or symptoms of extravasation	Liposomal doxorubicin should be considered an irritant, and precautions should be taken to avoid extravasation. Immediately terminate the infusion and restart in another vein. Apply ice over the site of extravasation for approximately 30 minutes
Day of treatment ANC <500/mm^3 or platelets <25,000/mm^3	Do not administer liposomal doxorubicin; wait 1 week and recheck ANC and platelet count; when ANC >1500 and platelet count >100,000, begin next cycle with dosage reduced by 25%
Febrile neutropenia (ANC <1000/mm^3 with temperature >38°C or >100.4°F), or ANC <1000/mm^3 for ≥7 days	Reduce liposomal doxorubicin dosage by 25% and consider adding filgrastim in subsequent cycles, if applicable
Febrile neutropenia (ANC <1000/mm^3 with temperature >38°C or >100.4°F), or ANC <1000/mm^3 for ≥7 days despite 1 dose reduction	Administer filgrastim in subsequent cycles. If already administering filgrastim, reduce liposomal doxorubicin dosage by 25%
Platelet nadir <50,000/mm^3, or platelets <100,000/mm^3 for ≥7 days	Reduce liposomal doxorubicin dosage by 25%
G1 ANC/platelet count (ANC 1500–1900; platelet count 75,000–150,000)	Resume treatment with no dosage reduction
G2 ANC/platelet count (ANC 1000 to <1500 and platelet count 50,000 to <75,000)	Wait until ANC ≥1500 and platelets ≥75,000; redose with no dosage reduction
G3 ANC/platelet count (ANC 500–999 and platelet count 25,000 to <50,000)	Wait until ANC ≥1500 and platelets ≥75,000; redose with no dosage reduction
G4 ANC/platelet count (ANC <500 and platelet count <25,000)	Wait until ANC ≥1500 and platelets ≥75,000; redose at 25% dose reduction or continue full dose with cytokine support
G1 hand-foot syndrome (HFS) (mild erythema, swelling, or desquamation not interfering with daily activities)	Redose unless patient has experienced previous G3/4 HFS. If so, delay up to 2 weeks and decrease dose by 25%. Return to original dose interval
G2 HFS (erythema, desquamation, or swelling interfering with, but not precluding, normal physical activities; small blisters or ulcerations <2 cm in diameter)	Delay dosing up to 2 weeks or until resolved to G0/1. If after 2 weeks there is no resolution, discontinue liposomal doxorubicin. If resolved to G0/1 within 2 weeks and there are no prior G3/4 HFS, continue treatment at previous dose and return to original dose interval. If patient experienced previous G3/4 toxicity, continue treatment with a 25% dose reduction and return to original dose interval
G3 HFS (blistering, ulceration, or swelling interfering with walking or normal daily activities; cannot wear regular clothing)	Delay dosing up to 2 weeks or until resolved to G0/1. Decrease dosage by 25% and return to original dose interval. If after 2 weeks there is no resolution, discontinue liposomal doxorubicin
G4 HFS (diffuse or local process causing infectious complications, or a bedridden state or hospitalization)	Delay dosing up to 2 weeks or until resolved to G0/1. Decrease dose by 25% and return to original dose interval. If after 2 weeks there is no resolution, discontinue liposomal doxorubicin

(continued)

Patient Population Studied

The open-label, randomized, phase 3 AURELIA study involved 361 patients with histologically confirmed epithelial ovarian, primary peritoneal, or fallopian tube cancer that had progressed <6 months after completing ≥4 cycles of platinum-based therapy. Eligible patients were aged ≥18 years, with an Eastern Cooperative Oncology Group (ECOG) performance status score ≤2. Patients who received >2 prior anticancer regimens or had progression during previous platinum-containing therapy were not eligible. Patients received one of the following single-agent chemotherapies (selected by an investigator): pegylated liposomal doxorubicin 40 mg/m^2 intravenously on day 1 every 4 weeks (N = 126); paclitaxel 80 mg/m^2 intravenously on days 1, 8, 15, and 22 every 4 weeks (N = 115); or topotecan 4 mg/m^2 intravenously on days 1, 8, and 15 every 4 weeks or 1.25 mg/m^2 intravenously on days 1 to 5 every 3 weeks (N = 120). Patients were then randomly assigned to receive either chemotherapy alone or with bevacizumab 10 mg/kg every 2 weeks (or 15 mg/kg every 3 weeks in patients receiving topotecan in a 3-week schedule). Trial therapy was continued until disease progression, unacceptable toxicity, or consent withdrawal. Patients receiving chemotherapy + bevacizumab and experiencing toxicity necessitating discontinuation of 1 agent could continue receiving the nonimplicated agent as monotherapy

Treatment Modifications (*continued*)

Liposomal Doxorubicin

Adverse Event	Treatment Modification
G1 stomatitis (painless ulcers, erythema, or mild soreness)	Redose unless patient has experienced previous G3/4 toxicity. If so, delay up to 2 weeks and decrease dosage by 25%. Return to original dose interval
G2 stomatitis (painful erythema, edema, or ulcers, but can eat)	Delay dosing up to 2 weeks or until resolved to G0/1. If after 2 weeks there is no resolution, discontinue liposomal doxorubicin. If resolved to G0/1 within 2 weeks and there was no prior G3/4 stomatitis, continue treatment at previous dose and return to original dose interval. If patient experienced previous G3/4 toxicity, continue treatment with a 25% dosage reduction and return to original dose interval
G3 stomatitis (painful erythema, edema, or ulcers, and cannot eat)	Delay dosing up to 2 weeks or until resolved to G0/1. Decrease dose by 25% and return to original dose interval. If after 2 weeks there is no resolution, discontinue liposomal doxorubicin
G4 stomatitis (requires parenteral or enteral support)	Delay dosing up to 2 weeks or until resolved to G0/1. Decrease dosage by 25% and return to liposomal doxorubicin original dose interval. If after 2 weeks there is no resolution, discontinue liposomal doxorubicin
Serum bilirubin 1.2–3 mg/dL	Administer 30 mg/m^2 liposomal doxorubicin
Serum bilirubin >3 mg/dL	Administer 20 mg/m^2 liposomal doxorubicin
Any other G3/4 nonhematologic drug-related toxicity	Do not dose until recovered to <G2 and reduce dosage by 25% for all subsequent cycles
Any other G3/4 nonhematologic drug-related toxicity despite reduced dose	Do not dose until recovered to <G2 and reduce dosage by an additional 25% for all subsequent cycles

Note:
- The bevacizumab package insert states the following: bevacizumab is not indicated for use with anthracycline-based chemotherapy. The incidence of G>3 left ventricular dysfunction was 1% in patients receiving bevacizumab compared to 0.6% of patients receiving chemotherapy alone. Among patients who received prior anthracycline treatment, the rate of CHF was 4% for patients receiving bevacizumab with chemotherapy as compared to 0.6% for patients receiving chemotherapy alone.
- The liposomal doxorubicin package insert states the following: cardiac function should be carefully monitored in patients treated with liposomal doxorubicin … endomyocardial biopsy … echocardiography or multigated radionuclide scans, have been used to monitor cardiac function and any of these methods should be employed to monitor potential cardiac toxicity in patients treated with liposomal doxorubicin. If these test results indicate possible cardiac injury associated with liposomal doxorubicin therapy, the benefit of continued therapy must be carefully weighed against the risk of myocardial injury

Efficacy (N = 361)

	Single-Agent Chemotherapy + Bevacizumab (n = 179)	Single-Agent Chemotherapy Alone (n = 182)	
Progression-free survival*	6.7 months	3.4 months	HR 0.48 (95% CI 0.38–0.60; P <0.001)
Objective response rate†	30.9%	12.6%	P <0.001
Overall survival	16.6 months	13.3 months	HR 0.85 (95% CI 0.66–1.08; P <0.174)
Median duration of therapy	6 cycles	3 cycles	

*Progression-free survival (the primary end point) was investigator-assessed and determined on the basis of radiologic evaluation according to RECIST version 1.0
†Objective response rate is the percentage of patients who experienced a partial or complete response according to RECIST version 1.0 and/or Gynecologic Cancer Intergroup (GCIG) cancer antigen (CA)-125 criteria
Note: median follow-up time for the primary analysis was 13.0 months in patients receiving chemotherapy + bevacizumab and 13.9 months in patients receiving chemotherapy alone

Adverse Events (N = 360)

	Single-Agent Chemotherapy + Bevacizumab (n = 179)	Single-Agent Chemotherapy Alone (n = 181)
Grade (%)*	Grade 3–5	Grade 3–5
Neutropenia	16	17
Hypertension	7	1
Leukopenia	5	7
Peripheral sensory neuropathy	5	3
HFS	5	2
Fatigue	4	10
Abdominal pain	3	6
Venous thromboembolic event	3	4
Diarrhea	3	3
Dyspnea	2	5
Anemia	2	3
Thrombocytopenia	2	3
Arterial thromboembolic event	2	0
Proteinuria	2	0
Gastrointestinal perforation	2	0
Vomiting	1	5
Bleeding	1	1
Congestive heart failure	1	1
Fistula/abscess	1	0
RPLS	1	0

*According to the National Cancer Institute Common Terminology Criteria for Adverse Events, version 3.0
Note: all reported G3–5 toxicities are included in the table. The single-agent chemotherapy + bevacizumab treatment was associated with more G ≥2 hypertension (20 [zero] vs 7%), gastrointestinal perforation (2% vs 0), and fistula/abscess (2% vs 0) than the single-agent chemotherapy alone. During the trial, 5 deaths thought not to be primarily caused by progressive disease were reported for each treatment group

Therapy Monitoring

1. *Once per week:* CBC with differential and platelet count
2. *Before the start of a cycle:* CBC with differential, serum electrolytes, serum bilirubin, AST or ALT, and alkaline phosphatase, BUN, and creatinine
3. Observe closely for hypersensitivity reactions, especially during the first and second bevacizumab infusions
4. Blood pressure every 2 weeks or more frequently as indicated during treatment
5. Assess proteinuria by urine dipstick and/or urinary protein–creatinine ratio. Patients with a urine dipstick reading ≥2+ should undergo further assessment with a 24-hour urine collection
6. Evaluate LVEF before initiation of liposomal doxorubicin and during treatment if clinical symptoms of heart failure are present. If baseline LVEF is ≥50%, repeat LVEF evaluation after a cumulative lifetime doxorubicin dose between 250 and 300 mg/m² has been reached, after a cumulative lifetime doxorubicin dose of 450 mg/m² has been reached, and then before each cycle beyond a cumulative lifetime doxorubicin dose of 450 mg/m². If the baseline LVEF is <50%, then consider repeating LVEF evaluation before each dose of liposomal doxorubicin
7. *Every 2–3 months:* imaging to assess response. Serum markers can be considered/obtained at each visit if they have been shown to be of value in following the patient's disease status

RECURRENT • PLATINUM-REFRACTORY/ PLATINUM-RESISTANT

OVARIAN CANCER REGIMEN: OLAPARIB

Kaufman B et al. J Clin Oncol 2015;33:244–250
Comment in: J Clin Oncol 2015;33:229–231, J Clin Oncol 2015;33:2581–2584

Olaparib tablets 300 mg per dose; administer orally every 12 hours, without regard to food, continually until disease progression (total dose per week with the tablet formulation is 4200 mg)

- Patients who delay taking olaparib tablets at a regularly scheduled time or who vomit after taking olaparib tablets should take the next dose at the next regularly scheduled time
- Olaparib tablets should be swallowed whole. Do not crush, chew, dissolve, or divide tablets
- Olaparib is metabolized by cytochrome P450 (CYP) CYP3A subfamily enzymes. Avoid concurrent use with moderate or strong CYP3A4 inhibitors whenever possible. If concurrent use with a *moderate* CYP3A4 inhibitor is required, reduce olaparib tablet dose to 150 mg orally twice daily. If concurrent use with a *strong* CYP3A4 inhibitor is required, reduce olaparib tablet dose to 100 mg orally twice daily. Avoid concurrent use with moderate or strong CYP3A4 inducers (eg, rifampin, carbamazepine, phenytoin, phenobarbital, St John's Wort)
- Advise patients not to consume grapefruit, grapefruit juice, Seville oranges, or Seville orange juice, as they may inhibit CYP3A in the gut wall and increase the bioavailability of olaparib
- **CAUTION: Olaparib is currently marketed in the United States in only a tablet formulation. Olaparib was previously marketed as both capsule and tablet formulations. Tablets and capsules cannot be substituted one for the other on a milligram-to-milligram basis. The bioavailability of the tablet formulation is greater than that of the capsule formulation**
  - "Population pharmacokinetic analyses have shown that the steady-state exposure (AUC) following 300 mg **tablet** twice daily was 77% higher compared to that following 400 mg **capsule** twice daily." (LYNPARZA [olaparib] tablets, for oral use; 08/2017 product label. AstraZeneca Pharmaceuticals LP, Wilmington, DE)

Supportive Care
Antiemetic prophylaxis
Emetogenic potential is **MODERATE**
See Chapter 42 for antiemetic recommendations

Hematopoietic growth factor (CSF) prophylaxis
Primary prophylaxis is **NOT** *indicated*
See Chapter 43 for more information

Antimicrobial prophylaxis
Risk of fever and neutropenia is **LOW**
  Antimicrobial primary prophylaxis to be considered:
  - Antibacterial—not indicated
  - Antifungal—not indicated
  - Antiviral—not indicated, unless patient previously had an episode of HSV

Diarrhea management
Latent or delayed-onset diarrhea*:
Loperamide 4 mg orally initially after the first loose or liquid stool, *then* 2-4 mg orally every 2-4 hours or **diphenoxylate hydrochloride** 2.5 mg **with atropine sulfate** 0.025 mg (eg, Lomotil)

*Abigerges D et al. J Natl Cancer Inst 1994;86:446–449
Rothenberg ML et al. J Clin Oncol 2001;19:3801–3807
Wadler S et al. J Clin Oncol 1998;16:3169–3178

Treatment Modifications

Olaparib Tablets

Note: **DO NOT substitute Lynparza (olaparib) tablets (100 mg and 150 mg) with Lynparza (olaparib) capsules (50 mg) on a milligram-to-milligram basis due to differences in the dosing and bioavailability of each formulation**	
Starting dose	300 mg twice daily in tablet form
Dose level −1	250 mg twice daily in tablet form
Dose level −2	200 mg twice daily in tablet form

Adverse Event	Treatment Modification
Dyspnea, cough, fever, and radiologic abnormalities—pneumonitis suspected	Interrupt olaparib until pulmonary status clarified
Pneumonitis confirmed	Discontinue olaparib
Creatinine clearance 31–50 mL/min	Reduce olaparib dosage to 200 mg twice daily in tablet form
Administration of a moderate CYP3A inhibitor required	Reduce olaparib dosage to 150 mg twice daily in tablet form
Administration of a strong CYP3A inhibitor required	Reduce olaparib dosage to 100 mg twice daily in tablet form
G ≥2 nonhematologic toxicity	Wait for toxicity to resolve to G1 then reduce olaparib 1 dose level
G ≥2 hematologic toxicity	Wait for toxicity to resolve to G1 then reduce olaparib 1 dose level
MDS/AML confirmed	Discontinue olaparib

Patient Population Studied

A multicenter, nonrandomized, phase 2 study involved 298 patients with known deleterious germline mutation in *BRCA1/2* and advanced solid tumor. Of the 298 patients enrolled in the trial, 193 had platinum-resistant (relapse within 6 months of platinum therapy) epithelial ovarian (N = 178), primary peritoneal (N = 11), or fallopian tube (N = 4) cancer. Eligible patients were aged ≥18 years, with an Eastern Cooperative Oncology Group (ECOG) performance status score ≤2 and life expectancy ≥16 weeks. All patients received olaparib (oral capsule formulation) until disease progression.

Efficacy

	Patients with Epithelial Ovarian, Primary Peritoneal, or Fallopian Tube Cancer (n = 193)	All Patients (N = 298)
Tumor response rate*	31.1%	26.2%
Median progression-free survival	7.0 months	
Median overall survival	16.6 months	
Median duration of response	225 days	208 days

*Tumor response rate is according to RECIST version 1.1, with confirmation at least 28 days later, and includes partial and complete responses. The majority of responses were partial responses
Note: median total duration of olaparib treatment (for all 298 patients) was 166.5 days

Adverse Events

Grade (%)*	Patients with Epithelial Ovarian, Primary Peritoneal, or Fallopian Tube Cancer (n = 193)		All Patients (N = 298)	
	Grade 1/2	Grade 3–5	Grade 1/2	Grade 3–5
Anemia	13	19	15	17
Abdominal pain	23	7	20	6
Fatigue	54	6	53	6
Vomiting	36	3	35	2
Diarrhea	27	2	26	1
Nausea	61	<1	59	<1
Decreased appetite	18	<1	20	<1
Dysgeusia	20	0	16	0
Dyspepsia	20	0	17	0
Headache	17	0	16	<1

*According to the National Cancer Institute Common Terminology Criteria for Adverse Events, version 3
Note: any-grade adverse events reported in >15% of all 298 patients, or G3–5 adverse events reported in >5% of all 298 patients are included in the table. Of the 298 patients in the trial, 9 died as a result of adverse events; 2 of these events (sepsis and myelodysplastic syndrome) were considered to be causally related to olaparib treatment. Eleven patients experienced adverse events that led to discontinuation of olaparib treatment. Of 298 patients, 120 experienced adverse events that led to olaparib dose modification (dose interruptions or reductions to 200 mg twice daily or 100 mg twice daily were permitted if toxicities occurred)

Therapy Monitoring

1. *Once per week initially then once per month:* CBC with differential and platelet count
2. *Before the start of a cycle:* CBC with differential, serum electrolytes
3. Monitor patients for pneumonitis. Query symptoms of cough, dyspnea, or fever. Obtain radiologic investigations as needed
4. Monitor patients for hematologic toxicity at baseline and monthly thereafter. Discontinue if MDS/AML is confirmed
5. *Every 2–3 months:* imaging to assess response. Serum markers can be considered/obtained at each visit if they have been shown to be of value in following the patient's disease status

RECURRENT • PLATINUM-REFRACTORY/ PLATINUM-RESISTANT

OVARIAN CANCER REGIMEN: TOPOTECAN HCL + BEVACIZUMAB

Pujade-Lauraine E et al. J Clin Oncol 2014;32:1302–1308
Erratum in: J Clin Oncol 2014;32:4025
Comment in: Nat Rev Clin Oncol 2014;11:242, J Clin Oncol 2014;32:1287–1289, J Clin Oncol 2014;32:3580

Four-week cycles
Bevacizumab 10 mg/kg per dose; administer intravenously in 100 mL 0.9% sodium chloride injection (0.9% NS) for 2 doses, on days 1 and 15 before topotecan, every 4 weeks (total dosage/4-week cycle = 20 mg/kg)
Note: the initial bevacizumab dose is administered over 90 minutes. If administration is well tolerated, the administration duration may be decreased stepwise during subsequent administrations to 60 minutes and, finally, to a minimum duration of 30 minutes
Topotecan HCl 4 mg/m^2 per dose; administer intravenously over 30 minutes in 50–250 mL 0.9% NS or 5% dextrose injection (D5W) for 3 doses on days 1, 8, and 15, every 4 weeks (total dosage/4-week cycle = 12 mg/m^2)
or
Three-week cycles
Bevacizumab 15 mg/kg; administer intravenously in 100 mL 0.9% NS on day 1 before topotecan, every 3 weeks (total dosage/3-week cycle = 15 mg/kg)
Note: the initial bevacizumab dose is administered over 90 minutes. If administration is well tolerated, the administration duration may be decreased stepwise during subsequent administrations to 60 minutes and, finally, to a minimum duration of 30 minutes
Topotecan HCl 1.25 mg/m^2 per day; administer intravenously over 30 minutes in 50–250 mL 0.9% NS or D5W for 5 consecutive days, on days 1–5, every 3 weeks (total dosage/3-week cycle = 6.25 mg/m^2)

(continued)

Treatment Modifications

BEVACIZUMAB AND TOPOTECAN DOSE MODIFICATIONS

Adverse Event	Treatment Modification
Gastrointestinal perforations (gastrointestinal perforations, fistula formation in the gastrointestinal tract, intra-abdominal abscess), fistula formation involving an internal organ	Discontinue bevacizumab permanently
Serious bleeding	
Wound dehiscence requiring medical intervention	
Nephrotic syndrome	
Hypertensive crisis or hypertensive encephalopathy or reversible posterior leukoencephalopathy syndrome (RPLS)	
Congestive heart failure	
Necrotizing fasciitis	
Severe arterial or venous thromboembolic events	Discontinue bevacizumab permanently; the safety of reinitiating bevacizumab after a thromboembolic event is resolved is not known
Moderate to severe proteinuria	Patients with a 2+ or greater urine dipstick reading should undergo further assessment, eg, 24-hour urine collection. Suspend bevacizumab administration for ≥2 g of proteinuria/24 h and resume when proteinuria is <2 g/24 h
Severe hypertension not controlled with medical management	Hold bevacizumab pending further evaluation and treatment of hypertension
Mild, clinically insignificant bevacizumab infusion reaction	Decrease the rate of bevacizumab infusion
Clinically significant but not severe bevacizumab infusion reaction	Interrupt the bevacizumab infusion in patients with clinically significant infusion reactions and consider resuming at a slower rate following resolution. If decision is made to restart, the infusion may be continued at ≤50% of the rate prior to the reaction and increased in 50% increments every 30 minutes if well tolerated. Infusions may be restarted at the full rate during the next cycle
Severe bevacizumab infusion reaction— hypertension, hypertensive crises associated with neurologic signs and symptoms, wheezing, oxygen desaturation, G3 hypersensitivity, chest pain, headaches, rigors, and diaphoresis	Stop bevacizumab infusion and administer appropriate medical therapy (eg, epinephrine, corticosteroids, intravenous antihistamines, bronchodilators, and/or oxygen). Discontinue bevacizumab
Planned elective surgery	Suspend bevacizumab at least 28 days before elective surgery and do not resume for at least 28 days after surgery or until surgical incision is fully healed
Recent hemoptysis	Do not administer bevacizumab
Evidence of rectosigmoid involvement by pelvic examination or bowel involvement on CT scan, or clinical symptoms of bowel obstruction	

(continued)

(*continued*)

Supportive Care

Antiemetic prophylaxis
Emetogenic potential on days of treatment with topotecan is **LOW**
Emetogenic potential on days with bevacizumab alone is **MINIMAL**
See Chapter 42 for antiemetic recommendations

Hematopoietic growth factor (CSF) prophylaxis
Primary prophylaxis is **NOT** indicated
See Chapter 43 for more information

Antimicrobial prophylaxis
Risk of fever and neutropenia is **LOW**
Antimicrobial primary prophylaxis to be considered:
- Antibacterial—not indicated
- Antifungal—not indicated
- Antiviral—not indicated, unless patient previously had an episode of HSV

Patient Population Studied

The open-label, randomized, phase 3 AURELIA study involved 361 patients with histologically confirmed epithelial ovarian, primary peritoneal, or fallopian tube cancer that had progressed <6 months after completing ≥4 cycles of platinum-based therapy. Patients whose age was ≥18 years with an Eastern Cooperative Oncology Group (ECOG) performance status score ≤2 were eligible. Patients who received >2 prior anticancer regimens or who developed disease progression during previous platinum-containing therapy were not eligible. Patients received one of the following single-agent chemotherapies (selected by an investigator): topotecan (N = 120), paclitaxel (N = 115), or (pegylated) liposomal doxorubicin (N = 126). Patients were then randomly assigned to receive either chemotherapy alone or with bevacizumab. Trial therapy was continued until disease progression, unacceptable toxicity, or consent withdrawal. Patients who received chemotherapy + bevacizumab and experienced toxicity that necessitated discontinuing 1 agent could continue receiving monotherapy with the drug not implicated in causing toxicity

Treatment Modifications (*continued*)

Topotecan	
Topotecan starting dose	4 mg/m² days 1, 8, and 15, every 4 weeks or 1.25 mg/m² days 1–5, every 3 weeks
Topotecan dose level −1	3 mg/m² days 1, 8, and 15, every 4 weeks or 0.75 mg/m² days 1–5, every 3 weeks
Topotecan dose level −2	2 mg/m² days 1, 8, and 15, every 4 weeks; no dose for days 1–5, every 3 weeks

Adverse Event	Treatment Modifications
Day of treatment in first cycle (day 1, 8, or 15) ANC ≤1500/mm³ or platelets ≤100,000/mm³, or serum creatinine >1.5 mg/Dl	Delay topotecan treatment by 1 week until ANC >1500/mm³ or platelets >100,000/mm³, or serum creatinine ≤1.5 mg/dL
Day of treatment in any cycle after the first cycle (day 1, 8, or 15) ANC ≤1000/mm³ or platelets ≤100,000/mm³, or serum creatinine >1.5 mg/dL	Delay topotecan treatment by 1 week until ANC >1000/mm³ or platelets >100,000/mm³, or serum creatinine ≤1.5 mg/dL
Febrile neutropenia (ANC <1000/mm³ with temperature >38°C or >100.4°F), or ANC <1000/mm³ for ≥7 days	Reduce topotecan dose by 1 level and consider adding filgrastim in subsequent cycles, if applicable
Febrile neutropenia (ANC <1000/mm³ with temperature >38°C or >100.4°F), or ANC <1000/mm³ for ≥7 days despite 1 dose reduction; or ANC <500 at any time	Administer filgrastim in subsequent cycles. If already administering filgrastim, reduce topotecan dosage by 1 level
Platelet nadir <50,000/mm³, or platelets <100,000/mm³ for ≥7 days; or platelet nadir <25,000/mm³ at any time	Reduce topotecan dosage by 1 level
G2/3 mucositis or diarrhea	Reduce topotecan dosage by 1 level
G4 mucositis or diarrhea	Reduce topotecan dosage by 1 level or consider discontinuing topotecan
Recurrent mucositis or diarrhea despite dosage reduction or persistence of mucositis/diarrhea >2 weeks beyond scheduled start of next cycle	Discontinue topotecan
Other G3/4 nonhematologic toxicity	Delay topotecan until resolution to G ≤1, then reduce dosage of topotecan by 1 level

Topotecan dose adjustments for renal impairment:
Creatinine clearance 46–60 mL/min: reduce topotecan dosage by 20%
Creatinine clearance 31–45 mL/min: reduce topotecan dosage by 25%
Creatinine clearance ≤30 mL/min: reduce topotecan dosage by 30%

Efficacy (N = 361)

	Single-Agent Chemotherapy + Bevacizumab (n = 179)	Single-Agent Chemotherapy Alone (n = 182)	
Progression-free survival*	6.7 months	3.4 months	HR 0.48 (95% CI 0.38–0.60; P <0.001)
Objective response rate†	30.9%	12.6%	P <0.001
Overall survival	16.6 months	13.3 months	HR 0.85 (95% CI 0.66–1.08; P <0.174)
Median duration of therapy	6 cycles	3 cycles	

*Progression-free survival (the primary end point) was investigator-assessed and determined on the basis of radiologic evaluation according to RECIST version 1.0
†Objective response rate is the percentage of patients who experienced a partial or complete response according to RECIST version 1.0 and/or Gynecologic Cancer Intergroup (GCIG) cancer antigen (CA)-125 criteria
Note: median follow-up time for the primary analysis was 13.0 months in the patients receiving chemotherapy + bevacizumab and 13.9 months in the patients receiving chemotherapy alone

Adverse Events (N = 360)

	Single-Agent Chemotherapy + Bevacizumab (n = 179)	Single-Agent Chemotherapy Alone (n = 181)
Grade (%)*	Grades 3–5	Grades 3–5
Neutropenia	16	17
Hypertension	7	1
Leukopenia	5	7
Peripheral sensory neuropathy	5	3
Hand-foot syndrome	5	2
Fatigue	4	10
Abdominal pain	3	6
Venous thromboembolic event	3	4
Diarrhea	3	3
Dyspnea	2	5
Anemia	2	3
Thrombocytopenia	2	3
Arterial thromboembolic event	2	0
Proteinuria	2	0
Gastrointestinal perforation	2	0
Vomiting	1	5
Bleeding	1	1
Congestive heart failure	1	1
Fistula/abscess	1	0
Reversible posterior leukoencephalopathy syndrome	1	0

*According to the National Cancer Institute Common Terminology Criteria for Adverse Events, version 3.0
Note: all reported G3–5 toxicities are included in the table. The single-agent chemotherapy + bevacizumab treatment was associated with more G ≥2 hypertension (20% vs 7%), gastrointestinal perforation (2% vs 0), and fistula/abscess (2% vs 0) than the single-agent chemotherapy alone. During the trial, 5 deaths thought not to be primarily caused by progressive disease were reported for each treatment group

Therapy Monitoring

1. *Once per week:* CBC with differential and platelet count
2. *Before the start of a cycle:* CBC with differential, serum electrolytes, serum bilirubin, AST or ALT, and alkaline phosphatase, BUN, and creatinine
3. Observe closely for hypersensitivity reactions, especially during the first and second bevacizumab infusions
4. Blood pressure every 2 weeks or more frequently as indicated during treatment
5. Assess proteinuria by urine dipstick and/or urinary protein creatinine ratio. Patients with a urine dipstick reading ≥2+ should undergo further assessment with a 24-hour urine collection
6. *Every 2–3 months:* imaging to assess response. Serum markers can be considered/obtained at each visit if they have been shown to be of value in following the patient's disease status

RECURRENT • PLATINUM-REFRACTORY/ PLATINUM-RESISTANT

OVARIAN CANCER REGIMEN: WEEKLY PACLITAXEL + BEVACIZUMAB

Pujade-Lauraine E et al. J Clin Oncol
2014;32:1302–1308
Erratum in: J Clin Oncol 2014;32:4025
Comment in: Nat Rev Clin Oncol 2014;11:242,
J Clin Oncol 2014;32:1287–1289, J Clin Oncol
2014;32:3580

Bevacizumab 10 mg/kg per dose; administer intravenously in 100 mL 0.9% sodium chloride injection (0.9% NS) for 2 doses, on days 1 and 15 before paclitaxel, every 4 weeks (total dosage/cycle = 20 mg/kg)
Note: the initial bevacizumab dose is administered over 90 minutes. If administration is well tolerated, the administration duration may be decreased stepwise during subsequent administrations to 60 minutes and, finally, to a minimum duration of 30 minutes
Premedication for Paclitaxel
Dexamethasone 10 mg/dose; administer orally for 2 doses 12 hours and 6 hours before each paclitaxel dose,
or
Dexamethasone 20 mg; administer intravenously over 10–15 minutes, 30–60 minutes before each paclitaxel dose
Note: dexamethasone doses may be gradually decreased in the absence of hypersensitivity reactions during repeated paclitaxel treatments
Diphenhydramine 25–50 mg; administered orally 60 minutes before each paclitaxel dose or by intravenous injection 30–60 minutes before each paclitaxel dose
Cimetidine 300 mg (*or* **ranitidine** 150 mg, *or* **famotidine** 20–40 mg, or an equivalent histamine receptor (H$_2$)-subtype antagonist); administer orally 60 minutes before each paclitaxel dose, *or* cimetidine 300 mg (*or* **ranitidine** 50 mg *or* **famotidine** 20 mg); administer intravenously over 15–30 minutes, 30–60 minutes before each paclitaxel dose
Paclitaxel 80 mg/m² per dose; administer intravenously over 60 minutes in a volume of 0.9% NS or 5% dextrose injection (D5W) sufficient to produce a concentration within the range 0.3–1.2 mg/mL for 4 doses, on days 1, 8, 15, and 22, every 4 weeks (total dosage/cycle = 320 mg/m²)

(continued)

Treatment Modifications

BEVACIZUMAB AND WEEKLY PACLITAXEL DOSE MODIFICATIONS

Adverse Event	Treatment Modification
Gastrointestinal perforations (gastrointestinal perforations, fistula formation in the gastrointestinal tract, intra-abdominal abscess), fistula formation involving an internal organ	Discontinue bevacizumab permanently
Serious bleeding	
Wound dehiscence requiring medical intervention	
Nephrotic syndrome	
Hypertensive crisis or hypertensive encephalopathy or reversible posterior leukoencephalopathy syndrome (RPLS)	
Congestive heart failure	
Necrotizing fasciitis	
Severe arterial or venous thromboembolic events	Discontinue bevacizumab permanently; the safety of reinitiating bevacizumab after a thromboembolic event is resolved is not known
Moderate to severe proteinuria	Patients with a 2+ or greater urine dipstick reading should undergo further assessment, eg, 24-hour urine collection. Suspend bevacizumab administration for ≥2 g of proteinuria/24 h and resume when proteinuria is <2 g/24 h
Severe hypertension not controlled with medical management	Hold bevacizumab pending further evaluation and treatment of hypertension
Mild, clinically insignificant bevacizumab infusion reaction	Decrease the rate of bevacizumab infusion
Clinically significant but not severe bevacizumab infusion reaction	Interrupt the bevacizumab infusion in patients with clinically significant infusion reactions and consider resuming at a slower rate following resolution. If decision is made to restart, the infusion may be continued at ≤50% of the rate prior to the reaction and increased in 50% increments every 30 minutes if well tolerated. Infusions may be restarted at the full rate during the next cycle
Severe bevacizumab infusion reaction— hypertension, hypertensive crises associated with neurologic signs and symptoms, wheezing, oxygen desaturation, G3 hypersensitivity, chest pain, headaches, rigors, and diaphoresis	Stop bevacizumab infusion and administer appropriate medical therapy (eg, epinephrine, corticosteroids, intravenous antihistamines, bronchodilators, and/or oxygen). Discontinue bevacizumab
Planned elective surgery	Suspend bevacizumab at least 28 days before elective surgery and do not resume for at least 28 days after surgery or until surgical incision is fully healed
Recent hemoptysis	Do not administer bevacizumab
Evidence of rectosigmoid involvement by pelvic examination or bowel involvement on CT scan, or clinical symptoms of bowel obstruction	

(continued)

(continued)

Supportive Care
Antiemetic prophylaxis
Emetogenic potential is LOW
See Chapter 42 for antiemetic recommendations

Hematopoietic growth factor (CSF) prophylaxis
Primary prophylaxis is NOT indicated
See Chapter 43 for more information

Antimicrobial prophylaxis
Risk of fever and neutropenia is LOW
  Antimicrobial primary prophylaxis to be considered:
  • Antibacterial—not indicated
  • Antifungal—not indicated
  • Antiviral—not indicated, unless patient previously had an episode of HSV

Patient Population Studied

The open-label, randomized, phase 3 AURELIA study involved 361 patients with histologically confirmed epithelial ovarian, primary peritoneal, or fallopian tube cancer that had progressed <6 months after completing ≥4 cycles of platinum-based therapy. Eligible patients were aged ≥18 years, with an Eastern Cooperative Oncology Group (ECOG) performance status score ≤2. Patients who received >2 prior anticancer regimens or who experienced progression during previous platinum-containing therapy were not eligible. Patients received one of the following single-agent chemotherapies (selected by an investigator): paclitaxel 80 mg/m² intravenously on days 1, 8, 15, and 22 every 4 weeks (n = 115); pegylated liposomal doxorubicin 40 mg/m² intravenously on day 1 every 4 weeks (n = 126); or topotecan 4 mg/m² intravenously on days 1, 8, and 15 every 4 weeks or 1.25 mg/m² intravenously on days 1 to 5 every 3 weeks (n = 120). Patients were then randomly assigned to receive either chemotherapy alone or with bevacizumab 10 mg/kg every 2 weeks (or 15 mg/kg every 3 weeks in patients receiving topotecan in a 3-week schedule). Trial therapy was continued until disease progression, unacceptable toxicity, or consent withdrawal. Patients receiving chemotherapy + bevacizumab and experiencing toxicity necessitating discontinuation of 1 agent could continue receiving the nonimplicated agent as monotherapy

Treatment Modifications (continued)

Weekly Paclitaxel	
Paclitaxel starting dose	80 mg/m² on days 1, 8, 15, and 22
Paclitaxel dose level −1	70 mg/m² on days 1, 8, 15, and 22
Paclitaxel dose level −2	60 mg/m² on days 1, 8, 15, and 22

Adverse Event	Treatment Modifications
Febrile neutropenia (ANC <1000/mm³ with temperature >38°C or >100.4°F), or ANC <1000/mm³ for ≥7 days	Reduce paclitaxel dosage by 10 mg/m² and consider adding filgrastim in subsequent cycles, if applicable
Febrile neutropenia (ANC <1000/mm³ with temperature >38°C or >100.4°F), or ANC <1000/mm³ for ≥7 days despite dosage reduction of 10 mg/m²	Administer filgrastim in subsequent cycles. If already administering filgrastim, reduce paclitaxel dosage an additional 10 mg/m²
Platelet nadir <50,000/mm³, or platelets <100,000/mm³ for ≥7 days	Reduce paclitaxel dose by 1 level
ANC <800/mm³ or platelets <50,000/mm³ at the start of a cycle	Hold treatment until ANC >800/mm³ and platelets >50,000/mm³, then resume with weekly paclitaxel dosage reduced by 10 mg/m²
G2 motor or sensory neuropathies	Reduce weekly paclitaxel dosage by 10 mg/m² without interrupting planned treatment
Other nonhematologic adverse events G2/3	Hold treatment until adverse events resolve to <G1, then resume with weekly paclitaxel dosage reduced by 10 mg/m²
Patients who cannot tolerate paclitaxel at 60 mg/m² per week	Discontinue treatment
Treatment delay >2 weeks	Decrease weekly paclitaxel dosage by 10 mg/m² or consider discontinuing treatment

Efficacy (N = 361)

	Single-Agent Chemotherapy + Bevacizumab (n = 179)	Single-Agent Chemotherapy Alone (n = 182)	
Progression-free survival*	6.7 months	3.4 months	HR 0.48 (95% CI 0.38–0.60; P <0.001)
Objective response rate†	30.9%	12.6%	P <0.001
Overall survival	16.6 months	13.3 months	HR 0.85 (95% CI 0.66–1.08; P <0.174)
Median duration of therapy	6 cycles	3 cycles	

*Progression-free survival (the primary end point) was investigator-assessed and determined on the basis of radiologic evaluation according to RECIST version 1.0
†Objective response rate is the percentage of patients who experienced a partial or complete response according to RECIST version 1.0 and/or Gynecologic Cancer Intergroup (GCIG) cancer antigen (CA)-125 criteria
Note: median follow-up time for the primary analysis was 13.0 months in the patients receiving chemotherapy + bevacizumab and 13.9 months in the patients receiving chemotherapy alone

Adverse Events (N = 360)

Grade (%)*	Single-Agent Chemotherapy + Bevacizumab (n = 179)	Single-Agent Chemotherapy Alone (n = 181)
	Grade 3–5	Grade 3–5
Neutropenia	16	17
Hypertension	7	1
Leukopenia	5	7
Peripheral sensory neuropathy	5	3
Hand-foot syndrome	5	2
Fatigue	4	10
Abdominal pain	3	6
Venous thromboembolic event	3	4
Diarrhea	3	3
Dyspnea	2	5
Anemia	2	3
Thrombocytopenia	2	3
Arterial thromboembolic event	2	0
Proteinuria	2	0
Gastrointestinal perforation	2	0
Vomiting	1	5
Bleeding	1	1
Congestive heart failure	1	1
Fistula/abscess	1	0
Reversible posterior leukoencephalopathy syndrome	1	0

*According to the National Cancer Institute Common Terminology Criteria for Adverse Events, version 3.0
Note: all reported Grade 3–5 toxicities are included in the table. The single-agent chemotherapy + bevacizumab treatment regimen was associated with more Grade ≥2 hypertension (20% vs 7%), gastrointestinal perforation (2% vs 0), and fistula/abscess (2% vs 0) than the single-agent chemotherapy alone. During the trial, 5 deaths thought not to be primarily caused by progressive disease were reported for each treatment group

Therapy Monitoring

1. *Once per week:* CBC with differential and platelet count
2. *Before the start of a cycle:* CBC with differential, serum electrolytes, serum bilirubin, AST or ALT, and alkaline phosphatase, BUN, creatinine, and neurologic exam
3. Observe closely for hypersensitivity reactions, especially during the first and second infusions
4. Blood pressure every 2 weeks or more frequently as indicated during treatment
5. Assess proteinuria by urine dipstick and/or urinary protein creatinine ratio. Patients with a urine dipstick reading ≥2+ should undergo further assessment with a 24-hour urine collection
6. *Every 2–3 months:* imaging to assess response. Serum markers can be considered/obtained at each visit if they have been shown to be of value in following the patient's disease status

32. Pancreatic Cancer

Susan E. Bates, MD and Daniel D. Von Hoff, MD, FACP

Epidemiology

Incidence	• 3.2% of all new cancer cases • Estimated new cases for 2019 in the United States: 56,770 (male: 29,940; female: 26,830) • 12.6 per 100,000 men and women
Deaths	Estimated 57,600 in 2020 (male: 30,400; female: 27,200)
Median age	70 years
Male to female ratio	~1:1

Stage at presentation		
	Stage I:	10%
	Stage II:	22%
	Stage III:	13%
	Stage IV:	55%

Location at Presentation and Surgical Resection

Location	Percent of all presentations	Percent amenable to surgical resection at each disease site
Head of pancreas	67%	27.9%
Pancreas body	16%	10.7%
Tail of pancreas	17%	17%

Surgical resection	Overall 25% of patients undergo surgery
Survival	5-year survival, all patients = 9.3% 5-year survival following resection = 25%

Bilimoria et al. Cancer 2007;110:1227–1234
Huang L et al. Gut 2019;68:130–139
Siegel RL et al. CA Cancer J Clin 2019;69:7–34
Surveillance, Epidemiology, and End Results (SEER) Program, available from http://seer.cancer.gov [accessed in 2019]
Winer LK et al. J Surg Res 2019;239:60–66

Pathology

Malignant tumors of the pancreatic origin*

Histology	Percent
Ductal adenocarcinoma	85–90%
Adenosquamous carcinoma	1–4%
Colloid carcinoma (mucinous noncystic carcinoma)	1–3%
Acinar cell carcinoma	1–2%
Undifferentiated carcinoma without or with osteoclast-like giant cells	<1%
Mixed acinar-ductal carcinoma; mixed acinar-neuroendocrine carcinoma; mixed acinar-neuroendocrine-ductal carcinoma; pancreatoblastoma	<1%
Sarcoma	<1%
Small cell carcinoma	<1%
Squamous cell carcinoma	<1%
Other (hepatoid carcinoma; medullary carcinoma; signet ring cell carcinoma; acinar cell cystadenocarcinoma; intraductal papillary mucinous neoplasm with an associated invasive carcinoma; mucinous cystic neoplasm with an associated invasive carcinoma; serous cystadenocarcinoma; solid-pseudopapillary carcinoma)	<1%

*Adapted from the WHO classification of tumors

Work-up

General and tumor markers

The diagnosis of pancreatic cancer is based on imaging studies and histologic confirmation performed by fine-needle aspiration by endoscopic ultrasonography (EUS), biopsy under CT or US guidance, or during laparotomy. In some clinical situations, relying on fine needle aspiration alone is not recommended.

- History and physical examination
- CBC and differential, serum electrolytes, creatinine, LFTs, PT, PTT, CA19–9
- Measure CA19–9, CEA, and CA125 at baseline. While CA19–9 is often elevated in pancreatic cancer, the other serum tumor markers should be measured at baseline, as 8% of patients carry genetic variants in the Fucosyltransferase 3 gene, which results in a negative test for CA19–9 (the Lewis antigen). In PDAC, CEA or CA125 have a sensitivity of 63.8 and 51.1%, respectively. These markers may be valuable if elevated

Luo G et al. Ann Surg 2017;265:800–805
Vestergaard EM et al. Clin Chem 1999;45:54–61

Imaging

- Spiral CT: spiral or helical CT of the abdomen according to a defined triple-phase pancreas protocol is essential. CT provides localization, size of the primary tumor, and evidence of metastasis and evaluates major vessels adjacent to the pancreas for neoplastic invasion or thrombosis. CT is almost 100% accurate in predicting unresectable disease. However, the positive predictive value of the test is low and approximately 25–50% of patients predicted to have resectable disease on CT have unresectable lesions at laparotomy
- Endoscopic retrograde cholangiopancreatography (ERCP) also can be useful in patients for whom a CT scan is equivocal. Fewer than 3% of patients with pancreatic adenocarcinoma have normal pancreatograms
- EUS is useful for characterizing cystic lesions and assessing vascular invasion by tumor. In addition, an aspirate or core biopsy can be done for histologic diagnosis. *It is important to request additional cores for molecular testing in patients who may never undergo surgical resection*

Agawam B. Am J Gastroenterol 2004;99:844–850
Tamm EP et al. Radiographic imaging. In: Von Hoff DD et al (editors). Pancreatic Cancer, 1st ed. Burlington, MA: Jones & Bartlett; 2005:165–180

Staging

Primary Tumor (T)

TX	Primary tumor cannot be assessed
T0	No evidence of primary tumor
Tis	Carcinoma *in situ*. This includes high-grade intraepithelial neoplasia (PanIn–3), intraductal papillary mucinous neoplasm with high-grade dysplasia, intraductal tubulopapillary neoplasm with high-grade dysplasia, and mucinous cystic neoplasm with high-grade dysplasia
T1a	Tumor 0.5 cm or less in greatest dimension
T1b	Tumor >0.5 cm and <1 cm in greatest dimension
T1c	Tumor 1–2 cm in greatest dimension
T2	Maximum tumor diameter > 2 cm but < 4 cm
T3	Tumor >4 cm in greatest dimension
T4	Tumor involves celiac axis, superior mesenteric artery, and/or common hepatic artery, regardless of size

Regional Lymph Nodes (N)

NX	Regional lymph nodes cannot be assessed
N0	No regional lymph node metastasis
N1	Metastasis in one to three regional lymph nodes
N2	Metastasis in four or more regional lymph nodes

Distant Metastasis (M)

M0	No distant metastasis
M1	Distant metastasis

Stage	T	N	M
0	Tis	N0	M0
IA	T1	N0	M0
IB	T2	N0	M0
IIA	T3	N0	M0
IIB	T1	N1	M0
IIB	T2	N1	M0
IIB	T3	N1	M0
III	T1	N2	M0
III	T2	N2	M0
III	T3	N2	M0
III	T4	Any N	M0
IV	Any T	Any N	M1

Amin MB et al (editors). AJCC Cancer Staging Manual. 8th ed. New York: Springer; 2017

Expert Opinion

General

- Pancreatic cancer at presentation is typically divided into four major groups with the focus on resection of the disease: (1) surgically resectable, (2) borderline resectable, (3) locally advanced, and (4) metastatic disease. Prognosis varies among these four groups, with complete surgical resection offering the only potential chance of cure. Patients should be enrolled to suitable clinical trials for all stages of pancreatic cancer if possible
- Precision oncology is an evolving discipline in which mutational analysis is performed to identify potentially targetable lesions. Best done in the context of a clinical trial, molecular analysis of PDAC finds mutations in DNA repair proteins in approximately 15% of samples. For patients with BRCA1 or 2 mutation, and potentially other mutations in the homologous recombination repair pathway, this offers the PARP inhibitors as an additional therapeutic option. In approximately 1% of cases, patients are found to have mutations in one of the mismatch repair proteins (Lynch syndrome genes), opening the possibility of successful immunotherapy. Investigators are presently searching for other genetic profiles that raise the tumor mutational burden, and for combinations to improve the success of immunotherapy

Surgery

Approximately half of patients who present with localized disease go to surgery.
Neoadjuvant therapy as discussed below aims to convert locally advanced, unresectable disease to resectable

Abbreviated NCCN Guidelines Defining Surgical Resectability

National Comprehensive Cancer Network. Pancreatic Adenocarcinoma (Version 2.2021). https://www.nccn.org/professionals/physician_gls/pdf/pancreatic.pdf. Accessed May 6, 2021.

	Arterial	Venous
Resectable	• No arterial tumor contact (celiac axis, SMA or CHA)	• No tumor contact with SMV or PV or ≤180° contact
Borderline resectable	**Head/uncinate process:** • Solid tumor contact with CHA <180° • Solid tumor contact with SMA of ≤180° **Body/tail:** • Contact with CA of >180° without involvement of aorta or GDA	• Solid tumor contact with SMV or PV of >180° • Solid tumor contact with IVC
Unresectable	**Head/uncinate process:** • Solid tumor contact with SMA >180° • Solid tumor contact with CA >180° **Body/tail:** • Solid tumor contact with SMA or CA >180° • Solid tumor contact with CA or aorta	**Head/uncinate process:** • Unreconstructible SMV/PV due to tumor involvement or occlusion • Contact with most proximal draining jejunal branch into SMV **Body/tail:** • Unreconstructible SMV/PV due to tumor involvement or occlusion

CA, celiac axis; CHA, common hepatic artery; GDA, gastroduodenal artery; IVC, inferior vena cava; PV, portal vein; SMA, superior mesenteric artery; SMV, superior mesenteric vein

Neoadjuvant therapy

- Neoadjuvant therapy is well accepted for patients with locally advanced or borderline resectable disease, as it offers the potential to improve R0 resection rates, downstage tumors, and treat micrometastatic disease (Raufi et al, 2019). One advantage is that as many as 20–25% of patients have postoperative complications that delay the onset of adjuvant chemotherapy, and neoadjuvant therapy provides systemic therapy upfront. Some centers utilize neoadjuvant therapy in all patients prior to resection

Raufi AG et al. Semin Oncol 2019;46:19–27

- Neoadjuvant regimens are typically selected from those used in metastatic disease: FOLFIRINOX or modified FOLFIRINOX for patients with greater likelihood of DNA repair abnormalities (e.g., younger patients), and gemcitabine/nab-paclitaxel for those who may be older or poorer performance status, or where FOLFIRINOX is planned as adjuvant therapy. Several meta-analyses have concluded that neoadjuvant therapy improves outcomes in PDAC, with resection rates at 65–70%, when patients with both borderline resectable and locally advanced disease at diagnosis are included (Raufi et al, 2019). Resection rates are much higher when studies are confined to patients with borderline resectable disease at diagnosis (Versteijne 2018)

Raufi AG et al. Semin Oncol 2019;46:19–27
Versteijne E et al. Br J Surg 2018;105:946–958

- Stereotactic body radiation therapy (SBRT) has been used to improve the rates of R0 resection, along with neoadjuvant chemotherapy. Definitive data are needed to define the population of patients most likely to benefit (Murphy et al, 2018). A randomized Alliance trial of SBRT combined with neoadjuvant chemotherapy with FOLFIRINOX in the setting of borderline resectable PDAC is ongoing

Murphy JE et al. JAMA Oncol 2018;4:963–969

(continued)

Expert Opinion (*continued*)

Adjuvant therapy

- Following surgery, adjuvant therapy should be considered for patients who have recovered from surgery. Approximately 20–25% of patients will have a prolonged convalescence and/or a suboptimal performance status following surgery and will not be candidates for adjuvant therapy. Every effort should be made to get these patients to adjuvant chemotherapy. Both the PRODIGE 24 and the ESPAC–4 trials discussed below allowed patients to enroll up to 12 weeks following surgery

- All patients should be considered for adjuvant chemotherapy. There are three regimens to be considered. The PRODIGE 24 trial demonstrated an overall survival advantage for modified FOLFIRINOX (54.4 months median OS) vs gemcitabine (35.0 months) (stratified hazard ratio for death, 0.64; 95% CI, 0.48 to 0.86; P = 0.003) (Conroy et al 2018). This was a significant improvement over results from ESPAC–4, which randomized gemcitabine with capecitabine vs gemcitabine alone. In that trial, the median overall survival was 28.0 months for patients in the gemcitabine plus capecitabine group compared with 25.5 months for the gemcitabine monotherapy group (HR 0.82, 95% CI 0.68–0.98; P = 0.032) (Neoptolemus 2017)

- The third regimen that can be utilized is gemcitabine plus nab-paclitaxel, based on efficacy data obtained in the metastatic setting. Results from the APACT clinical trial randomizing this combination against gemcitabine alone in the adjuvant setting were presented at the 2019 ASCO annual meeting (NCT01964430). Results were disappointing with a 19.4-month DFS for gemcitabine/nab-paclitaxel by independent review vs 18.8 months for gemcitabine monotherapy (HR, 0.88, 95% CI 0.729–1.063, stratified log-rank P = 0.1824) (Tempero et al, 2019). Interim OS was 40.5 months (nab-P/G) vs 36.2 months (G) (HR, 0.82, 95% CI 0.680–0.996, nominal P = 0.045). However, there was a statistical benefit in the investigator analysis of DFS, so follow-up survival data will be important

- Although mFOLFIRINOX yielded the best data to date, it should be noted that not all patients are candidates for even the modified regimen. It should also be noted that the control arm for both new studies markedly exceeded previous results (eg, 35 months vs 25.5 months in ESPAC–4 and 23.6 months in ESPAC–3) (Conroy et al 2018; Neoptolemos et al, 2017; Neoptolemos et al, 2010), suggesting increasing benefit for salvage therapy after recurrence

Conroy T et al. N Engl J Med 2018;379:2395–2406
Neoptolemos JP et al. JAMA 2010;304:1073–1081
Neoptolemos JP et al. Lancet 2017;389:1011–1024
Tempero M et al. J Clin Oncol 2019;37(15 Suppl):4000

- The choice of adjuvant regimen may be individualized. Modification of the original FOLFIRINOX schedule has led to a more tolerable regimen designated mFOLFIRINOX. Patients were enrolled on adjuvant modified FOLFIRINOX up to age 79. The relative dose intensity was 0.7 in about half of patients randomized to mFOLFIRINOX. For gemcitabine/capecitabine there remains a concern about the toxicity of capecitabine administered for 21 consecutive days, particularly in patients who have undergone the Whipple procedure, with its impact on gastrointestinal functional status and the potential impact of dose reduction limiting efficacy. Most patients have some level of gastrointestinal disturbance following the Whipple procedure (Rashid and Velanovich, 2012)

Rashid L, Velanovich V. HPB (Oxford) 2012;14:9–13

- **Note regarding proton pump inhibitors (PPIs):** if gemcitabine/capecitabine is selected for adjuvant therapy, please note a recent report on reduced efficacy of oral capecitabine in patients with ERBB2/HER2-positive metastatic gastroesophageal cancer receiving **proton pump inhibitors (PPI)** (Chu et al 2017), reducing PFS, 4.2 vs 5.7 months (P<.001) and OS, 9.2 vs 11.3 months (P=0.04) in 545 patients. This is thought to be due to altered absorption of capecitabine due to the higher gastric pH levels

Chu MP et al. JAMA Oncol 2017;3:767–773

Role of radiation therapy in the adjuvant setting

- The European Study Group for Pancreatic Cancer (ESPAC 1, 2, and 3) evaluated the role of fluorouracil, gemcitabine, and RT as adjuvant therapy, establishing the role of chemotherapy alone as adjuvant therapy. The role of RT and the detrimental effect of RT seen in these studies has been controversial as a result of the lack of quality control and central review

Neoptolemos JP et al. Br J Cancer 2009;100:246–250
Neoptolemos JP et al. N Engl J Med 2004;350:1200–1210
Neoptolemos JP et al. Proc Am Soc Clin Oncol 2009;27(Suppl):18s [abstract LBA–4505]

- Following adjuvant chemotherapy, radiation with chemosensitizing fluorouracil or capecitabine may be given as a component of adjuvant therapy for patients at high risk of recurrence. These are patients with a microscopic positive margin (R1 resection), extracapsular lymph node extension, and multiple involved regional nodes (≥4) at resection

- Chemoradiation therapy with concurrent capecitabine: 850 mg/m^2 twice daily for 5 weeks in combination with 1.8 Gy fractions/day × 5 days, for 5 weeks. Significant gastrointestinal toxicity can be observed, with Grade 3 enteritis

Kim HS et al. Anticancer Drugs 2010;21:107–112

Locally advanced disease: Role of radiation therapy

- Surgical resection is the only approach for curative therapy of pancreatic cancer. However, with only 25% of patients able to undergo surgical resection, the question of using radiation therapy to achieve local control in the setting of locally advanced, non-metastatic disease has been

(*continued*)

Expert Opinion (*continued*)

raised. High-dose, definitive radiation therapy, has been attempted in specialized treatment centers with some evidence that durable local control can be obtained in the absence of major toxicity. This needs prospective validation; one early report noted a 22.6-month median overall survival following definitive doses (IMRT to 63–70 Gy in 28 fractions or 67.5 Gy in 15 fractions; BED, 77.2–97.9 Gy) (Crane et al, 2015)

Crane CH. Oncology (Williston Park) 2015;29:561–562
Crane CH et al. J Clin Oncol 2015;33(3 suppl):354–354
Kim SK et al. J Gastrointest Oncol 2016;7:479–486

Metastatic pancreatic cancer

First-Line Regimens:

There are two established first-line regimens for pancreatic cancer. These are based on randomized clinical trials against gemcitabine monotherapy. Both have been shown to have activity in the second-line setting as well

- **nab-PACLITAXEL + GEMCITABINE:** MPACT was a large, international study that enrolled 861 patients and demonstrated that nab-**Paclitaxel + gemcitabine** was superior to gemcitabine monotherapy across all efficacy endpoints, with an acceptable toxicity profile. Median overall survival and progression-free survival were 8.5 months and 4.5 months for nab-paclitaxel + gemcitabine compared with 5.5 months and 3.7 months for gemcitabine monotherapy, respectively. There was no cut-off for age; the oldest patient enrolled was 86 years of age

Von Hoff DD et al. N Engl J Med 2013;369:1691–703

- Many patients with metastatic pancreatic cancer have rapid declines in performance status due to biliary and pancreatic duct obstruction, weight loss, liver dysfunction, and portal hypertension. A study of nab-paclitaxel + gemcitabine in patients with a performance status of 2, a patient population known to have poor outcomes, demonstrated 24–28% response rate and 5.7- to 6.7-month median overall survival

Macarulla T et al. J Clin Oncol 2019;37:230–238

- **FOLFIRINOX:** Compared with gemcitabine, **FOLFIRINOX** (fluorouracil + leucovorin + irinotecan + oxaliplatin) was associated with a survival advantage. Median overall survival and progression-free survival were 11.1 months and 6.4 months for FOLFIRINOX compared with 6.8 months and 3.3 months for gemcitabine monotherapy, respectively. As originally described, FOLFIRINOX is associated with significant toxicity and is thus an option for the treatment of patients with metastatic pancreatic cancer and a good performance status, no cardiac ischemia, and normal or nearly normal bilirubin levels. This trial excluded patients age 76 and above

Conroy T et al. N Engl J Med 2011;364:1817–1825

- **MODIFIED FOLFIRINOX:** Full-dose FOLFIRINOX as administered in Conroy et al, 2011, in the PRODIGE report, was associated with significant toxicity, particularly in older patients or those with GI complications of pancreatic cancer. This was addressed in a number of ways in different trials—reducing the dose of irinotecan, or dropping the 5-FU bolus, or reducing the dose of all drugs (Table 6 in Raufi et al lists these variations), and it has not been clear which of these "modified" regimens offered the greatest efficacy with reduced toxicity. However, the recent publication of a marked benefit of a modified FOLFIRINOX in the adjuvant setting provides some rationale for the choice of the modified regimen used there. In that study, 247 patients with resected pancreatic ductal adenocarcinoma received oxaliplatin (85 mg/m^2), irinotecan (reduced to 150 mg/m^2 after a protocol-specified safety analysis), leucovorin (400 mg/m^2), and fluorouracil (2400 mg/m^2) every 2 weeks, with the bolus 5-FU dose omitted

Conroy T et al. N Engl J Med 2018;379:2395–2406
Raufi AG et al. Semin Oncol. 2019;46:19–27

- **OLAPARIB and PARP INHIBITORS:** A randomized trial conducted in patients with pancreatic cancer who had a germline BRCA1 or BRCA2 mutation and disease that had not progressed on first-line platinum-containing chemotherapy found that olaparib extended the progression-free interval from 3.8 to 7.4 months (Golan et al, 2019). Although no difference in overall survival was noted at interim analysis, follow-up from this trial continues. The discontinuation of first-line therapy at a median 5 months before randomization to placebo or olaparib and subsequent second-line therapy may have impacted this outcome. The activity of PARP inhibitors in the setting of mutations in other genes involved in homologous recombination, such as ATM and PALB2, is currently being explored. Additional PARP inhibitors will need to be tested in this and other trial designs and disease settings before their role in pancreatic cancer is fully known

Golan T et al: N Engl J Med 2019;381:317–327

Therapeutic Strategy of Interest:

- **GEMCITABINE + nab-PACLITAXEL + CISPLATIN:** A phase 1b/2 pilot trial in patients with metastatic pancreatic cancer with no prior systemic therapy combined gemcitabine, nab-paclitaxel, and cisplatin based on the day 1 and 8 gemcitabine/cisplatin regimen. With 25 patients enrolled, the pilot trial demonstrated that the combination could be administered together safely and generated a high overall response rate at 70% and a median overall survival of 16.5 months. In patients with BRCA1/2 or PALB2 mutation, this could be an excellent choice to exploit the impaired DNA damage pathway

Jameson GS et al. JAMA Oncol 2019;6:125–132

(*continued*)

Expert Opinion (*continued*)

Second-Line Regimens:

- Clinical trials should be the first consideration for patients with disease progression following first-line therapy. Although pancreatic cancer is considered a refractory malignancy, there is evidence that 5-FU and gemcitabine-based regimens are not cross-resistant. Second-line choices thus depend upon the first-line regimen used, and performance status at the time of second-line therapy. If patients received a gemcitabine regimen in first line, then consideration should be given to FOLFIRINOX or other 5-FU based regimen in second line. If a patient has been found to have a mutation in BRCA1/2 or PALB2, then consideration should be given to a cisplatin-containing regimen, or perhaps to olaparib as single-agent therapy

- **LIPOSOMAL IRINOTECAN + 5-FLUOROURACIL/LEUCOVORIN:** Most clinical trials in pancreatic cancer are conducted in the first-line setting. Only one regimen has been developed for the second-line setting. The NAPOLI trial randomized patients between liposomal irinotecan (Onivyde) + 5-FU/LV; liposomal irinotecan alone, or 5-FU/LV alone, after progression on gemcitabine-based chemotherapy. Median overall survival in patients treated with liposomal irinotecan plus 5-FU/LV was significantly better at 6.1 months (95% CI 4.8–8.9) compared with 5-FU/LV monotherapy at 4.2 months (3.3–5.3) (HR 0.67, 95% CI 0.49–0.92; P = 0.012) (Wang-Gillam et al 2010). Median overall survival for nanoliposomal irinotecan monotherapy was 4.9 months (4.2–5.6). Liposomal irinotecan is able to induce objective responses with good duration in a subset of patients. However, the drug does come with a black box warning regarding febrile neutropenia and diarrhea in a subset of patients. The FDA-approved labeling notes that patients with known UGT1A1*28 homozygous variant alleles should initiate the drug at a reduced dose of 50 mg/m². Other variants of UGT1A1 are also known to be deleterious and are not tested in the commercial assays and may be associated with increased toxicity. Patients must be prepared for the possiblity of severe diarrhea and instructed in its management.

  Wang-Gillam A et al. Lancet 2016;387:545–557
  Wang-Gillam A et al. Eur J Cancer 2019;108:78–87

- **FOLFIRI and FOLFOX:** FOLFIRI and FOLFOX have been successfully used after gemcitabine-based therapy (Bupati et al, 2016; Neuzillet et al, 2012; Zaanan et al, 2014). FOLFIRI in the setting of prior gemcitabine-containing therapy was associated with a 6.6-month OS (Neuzillet et al, 2012), and a similar OS at 4.3 months was noted with FOLFOX in second line that included some patients treated with FOLFIRI in first line (Zaanan et al, 2014). Finally, the OFF regimen also was shown to have benefit, differing from FOLFOX in the inclusion of weekly 5-FU/LV infusions over 24 hours (Pelzer et al, 2011). Gemcitabine and nab-paclitaxel are active after FOLFIRINOX failure, demonstrating a 17.5% objective response rate and 58% disease control rate (Portal et al, 2015)

  Bupati M et al. Med Oncol 2016;33:37
  Neuzillet C et al. World J Gastroenterol 2012;18:4533–4541
  Pelzer U et al. Eur J Cancer 2011;47:1676–1681
  Portal A et al. Br J Cancer 2015;113:989–995
  Zaanan A et al. BMC Cancer 2014;14:441

- **GEMCITABINE + CISPLATIN** should be considered, particularly in patients with known DNA repair protein mutations in BRCA1/2 and PALB2 to exploit the reduced DNA repair capacity (O'Reilly et al. 2020). A meta-analysis of eight randomized trials exploring gemcitabine-cisplatin regimens in unselected patients with PDAC concluded that gemcitabine-cisplatin regimens improved response rate and 6-month survival rate without improving median OS, which ranged from 5.5 to 22 months among the studies ((Ouyang et al, 2016). This study highlighted that there is no established consensus dose and schedule for gemcitabine-cisplatin regimens in pancreatic cancer, and more recent studies continue that pattern. The Gem/Cis regimen studied in biliary cancer is well-tolerated and can be administered for a long duration, making it a reasonable choice in pancreatic cancer (Valle et al 2010). In this regimen, gemcitabine is administered at 1000 mg/m² with cisplatin at 25 mg/m² on days 1 and 8

  O'Reilly EM et al. J Clin Oncol 2020; 38:1378–1388
  Lundberg J et al. Med Oncol 2016;33:4
  Ouyang G et al. World J Surg Oncol 2016;14:59
  Palmer DH et al. Ann Surg Oncol 2007;14:2088–2096
  Valle J et al. N Engl J Med 2010;362:1273–1281

Other Regimens to Consider:

- There is no established therapy for the third-line setting. However, increasing numbers of patients reach this point with good performance status and it is a space in which clinical trial data are needed.

- Outcome and survival are poor for a patient with an ECOG performance status ≥2 with severe fatigue, rapid weight loss, and/or biliary obstruction. Palliative care with symptom management should be discussed with the patient and family. The use of the gemcitabine/erlotinib regimen has declined with the identification of more effective regimens and agents

- **MITOMYCIN + IRINOTECAN + CISPLATIN (MIC):** While the most recent publication of this regimen included a failed attempt to add olaparib, the basic MIC regimen has been found to be a reasonable salvage regimen in some patients, and it has been of interest as another regimen for those in whom DNA repair mutations are identified. Evidence is anecdotal at present

  Yarchoan M et al. Oncotarget 2017;8:44073–44081

(*continued*)

Expert Opinion *(continued)*

- **OXALIPLATIN + FOLINIC ACID (LEUCOVORIN) + FLUOROURACIL (OFF):** This was a randomized trial against best supportive care in second line after gemcitabine. OFF comprised leucovorin 200 mg/m^2 followed by 5-fluorouracil 2 g/m^2 (24h) weekly × 4 and oxaliplatin 85 mg/m^2 on days 8 and 22 followed by a 3-week rest. Although the trial was terminated due to poor accrual, median survival for patients treated with OFF was 4.82 months vs 2.3 months with BSC

Pelzer U et al. Eur J Cancer 2011;47:1676–1681

- **GEMCITABINE + DOCETAXEL + CAPECITABINE (GTX):** GTX offers the advantage of pulling from both platforms and, for a patient with good performance status without clinical trial options, may be a reasonable salvage therapy. GTX includes capecitabine 750 mg/m^2 PO BID on days 1–14, gemcitabine 750 mg/m^2 over 75 min, and docetaxel 30 mg/m^2 on days 4 and 11 in repeating 21-day cycles. Retrospective information suggested this was an effective regimen (10% CR in primary or metastatic lesions), but it was never studied in a randomized trial

Fine RL. Cancer Chemother Pharmacol 2008;61:167–175. Erratum in: Cancer Chemother Pharmacol 2008;61:177

- **GEMCITABINE MONOTHERAPY:** This was the first trial to demonstrate an effective therapy for pancreatic cancer and the first to describe "clinical benefit" as a response metric in a clinical trial, randomizing patients to gemcitabine 1000 mg/m^2 weekly × 3 vs weekly 5-FU. The study improved median survival by 1.2 months and demonstrated a clinical benefit response in 23.8% of patients treated with gemcitabine monotherapy, bringing in the modern era of treatment for pancreatic cancer

Burris HA et al. J Clin Oncol 1997;15:2403–2413

- **Immunotherapy:** The success of immune checkpoint inhibitors in several tumor types has raised the question of its role in pancreatic cancer. To date, pancreatic cancer responses to immunotherapy have been reported only in the 0.8% of patients whose tumors carry mismatch repair defects (Hu et al, 2018; Le et al, 2017; Cavalieri et al, 2017). These patients can be treated with immune checkpoint inhibitors (regimens found in Chapter 9). Other patients who are candidates for immunotherapy should be enrolled on clinical trials, rather than treated with monotherapy given the low response rate, affirmed in a report of 3.1% response rate for combined PD-L1/CTLA4 inhibition (O'Reilly 2019)

Cavalieri CC et al. J Clin Oncol 2017;35(4_suppl):792–792 [Abstract]
Hu ZI et al. Clin Cancer Res 2018;24:1326–1336
Le DT et al. Science 2017;357:409–413
O'Reilly EM et al. JAMA Oncol 2019;5:1431–1438

ADJUVANT
PANCREATIC CANCER REGIMEN: mFOLFIRINOX (MODIFIED FOLFIRINOX)

Conroy T et al. N Engl J Med 2018;379:2395–2406
Supplementary appendix to: Conroy T et al. N Engl J Med 2018;379:2395–2406
Protocol for: Conroy T et al. N Engl J Med 2018;379:2395–2406

Oxaliplatin 85 mg/m^2; administer intravenously in 250 mL 5% dextrose injection (D5W) over 2 hours on day 1, every 2 weeks, for 12 cycles (total dosage/cycle = 85 mg/m^2), *followed immediately by:*

Either: **(racemic) leucovorin calcium** 400 mg/m^2 *or* **levoleucovorin calcium** 200 mg/m^2; administer intravenously in 25–500 mL D5W over 2 hours, on day 1, every 2 weeks, for 12 cycles (total dosage/2-week cycle for racemic leucovorin = 400 mg/m^2, for levoleucovorin = 200 mg/m^2), *followed by:*

Irinotecan 150 mg/m^2; administer intravenously in 500 mL D5W over 90 minutes on day 1, concurrently during the final 90 minutes of either the leucovorin or levoleucovorin infusion, every 2 weeks, for 12 cycles (total dosage/2-week cycle = 150 mg/m^2), *followed immediately by:*

Fluorouracil 2400 mg/m^2; administer by continuous intravenous infusion over 46 hours in 100–1000 mL 0.9% NS or D5W, starting on day 1 immediately after completion of the irinotecan and either leucovorin or levoleucovorin infusions, every 2 weeks, for 12 cycles (total dosage/2-week cycle = 2400 mg/m^2)

Notes:
- Patients must be instructed in the use of loperamide as treatment for diarrhea, and must have a supply of this drug upon starting modified FOLFIRINOX
- Hematopoietic growth factor (G-CSF) is not generally recommended as primary prophylaxis, but it could be considered for patients with additional risk factors. Secondary prophylaxis should be considered in case of prior febrile neutropenia episode or delay of planned therapy due to neutropenia

Supportive Care
Antiemetic prophylaxis
Emetogenic potential on day 1 is **MODERATE**
Emetogenic potential on day 2 is **LOW**
See Chapter 42 for antiemetic recommendations

Hematopoietic growth factor (CSF) prophylaxis
Primary prophylaxis **MAY** be indicated
See Chapter 43 for more information

Antimicrobial prophylaxis
Risk of fever and neutropenia is **MODERATE**
  Antimicrobial primary prophylaxis to be *CONSIDERED*:
  - Antibacterial—not indicated
  - Antifungal—not indicated
  - Antiviral—not indicated unless patient previously had an episode of HSV

Acute cholinergic syndrome
Atropine sulfate 0.25–1 mg subcutaneously or intravenously if abdominal cramping or diarrhea develop during or within 1 hour after irinotecan administration
  - If symptoms are severe, add as primary prophylaxis at least 30 minutes before irinotecan during subsequent cycles
  - For irinotecan, acute cholinergic syndrome may be characterized by: abdominal cramping, diarrhea, diaphoresis, hypotension, flushing, bradycardia, rhinitis, increased salivation, meiosis, and lacrimation

Diarrhea management
Latent or delayed-onset diarrhea*:
  Loperamide 4 mg orally initially after the first loose or liquid stool, *then*
  Loperamide 2 mg orally every 2 hours during waking hours, *plus*
  Loperamide 4 mg orally every 4 hours during hours of sleep
  - Continue for at least 12 hours after diarrhea resolves
  - Recurrent diarrhea after a 12-hour diarrhea-free interval is treated as a new episode
  - Rehydrate orally with fluids and electrolytes during a diarrheal episode
  - If a patient develops blood or mucus in stool, dehydration, or hemodynamic instability, or if diarrhea persists >48 hours despite loperamide, stop loperamide and hospitalize the patient for IV hydration

(continued)

(*continued*)

Alternatively, a trial of **diphenoxylate hydrochloride** 2.5 mg with **atropine sulfate** 0.025 mg (eg, Lomotil)
- Initial adult dose is 2 tablets 4 times daily until control has been achieved, after which the dose may be reduced to meet individual requirements. Control may often be maintained with as little as 2 tablets daily
- Clinical improvement of acute diarrhea is usually observed within 48 hours. If improvement of chronic diarrhea after treatment with a maximum daily dose of 8 tablets is not observed within 10 days, control is unlikely with further administration

Persistent diarrhea:
Octreotide 100–150 mcg subcutaneously 3 times daily. Maximum total daily dose is 1500 mcg
Antibiotic therapy during latent or delayed-onset diarrhea:
A fluoroquinolone (eg, **ciprofloxacin** 500 mg orally every 12 hours) if absolute neutrophil count <500/mm^3 with or without accompanying fever in association with diarrhea
- Antibiotics should also be administered if patient is hospitalized with prolonged diarrhea and should be continued until diarrhea resolves

Treatment Modifications

Modified FOLFIRINOX DOSE MODIFICATIONS	
Adverse Event	**Treatment Modification**
Hematologic Toxicity	
Day 1 ANC <1500/mm^3, first episode	Withhold the start of the cycle. Consider treatment with filgrastim, and consider prophylactic filgrastim in subsequent cycles. Repeat CBC with differential and platelet count at least weekly. When ANC recovers to >1500/mm^3, proceed with treatment, but reduce the dosage of irinotecan to 120 mg/m^2. Do not reduce the dosages of oxaliplatin, leucovorin, or fluorouracil
Day 1 ANC <1500/mm^3, second episode	Withhold the start of the cycle. Consider treatment with filgrastim, and consider prophylactic G-CSF in subsequent cycles. Repeat CBC with differential and platelet count at least weekly. When ANC recovers to >1500/mm^3, proceed with treatment, maintaining the irinotecan dosage at 120 mg/m^2. Reduce the oxaliplatin dosage to 60 mg/m^2. Do not reduce the dose of leucovorin or fluorouracil
Day 1 ANC <1500/mm^3, third episode	Withhold the start of the cycle. Consider treatment with filgrastim, and consider prophylactic filgrastim in subsequent cycles. Repeat CBC with differential and platelet count at least weekly. Discontinue therapy with irinotecan and oxaliplatin. When ANC recovers to >1500/mm^3, proceed with treatment containing only leucovorin and fluorouracil at full dosages, or consider alternative therapy at the discretion of the medically responsible health care provider
Day 1 platelet count <100,000/mm^3, first episode	Withhold the start of the cycle. Repeat CBC with differential and platelet count at least weekly. When the platelet count recovers to >100,000/mm^3, proceed with treatment, but reduce the dosage of oxaliplatin to 60 mg/m^2. Do not reduce the dosages of irinotecan, leucovorin, or fluorouracil
Day 1 platelet count <100,000/mm^3, second episode	Withhold the start of the cycle. Repeat CBC with differential and platelet count at least weekly. When the platelet count recovers to >100,000/mm^3, proceed with treatment, maintaining the dosage of oxaliplatin at 60 mg/m^2. Reduce the dosage of irinotecan to 120 mg/m^2. Reduce the dosage of fluorouracil to 1800 mg/m^2. Do not reduce the dosage of leucovorin
Day 1 platelet count <100,000/mm^3, third episode	Withhold the start of the cycle. Repeat CBC with differential and platelet count at least weekly. Discontinue therapy with irinotecan and oxaliplatin. When the platelet count recovers to >100,000/mm^3, proceed with treatment containing fluorouracil at 1800 mg/m^2 and leucovorin at full dosage, or consider alternative therapy at the discretion of the medically responsible health care provider

(*continued*)

Treatment Modifications (*continued*)

Modified FOLFIRINOX DOSE MODIFICATIONS

Adverse Event	Treatment Modification
Neutropenic fever (ANC <500/mm³ and temperature >38.5°C) without documented infection occurring in the prior cycle administered without filgrastim prophylaxis	Continue the same dosages of irinotecan, oxaliplatin, leucovorin, and fluorouracil in subsequent cycles and add filgrastim prophylaxis
First episode of any of the following neutropenia complications: • Neutropenic fever (ANC <500/mm³ and temperature >38.5°C) during the prior cycle administered with filgrastim prophylaxis, *or:* • Documented infection during a period of G ≥3 neutropenia (ANC <1000/mm³), *or:* • G4 neutropenia (ANC <500/mm³) lasting >7 days at any time	Reduce the dosage of irinotecan to 120 mg/m² and add or continue prophylactic filgrastim during subsequent cycles. Do not reduce the dosages of oxaliplatin, leucovorin, or fluorouracil
Second episode of any of the following neutropenia complications: • Neutropenic fever (ANC <500/mm³ and temperature >38.5°C) during the prior cycle administered with filgrastim prophylaxis, *or:* • Documented infection during a period of G ≥3 neutropenia (ANC <1000/mm³), *or:* • G4 neutropenia (ANC <500/mm³) lasting >7 days at any time	Maintain the dosage of irinotecan at 120 mg/m². Reduce the dosage of oxaliplatin to 60 mg/m². Do not reduce the dosages of leucovorin or fluorouracil. Continue or institute prophylaxis with filgrastim
Third episode of any of the following neutropenia complications: • Neutropenic fever (ANC <500/mm³ and temperature >38.5°C) during the prior cycle administered with filgrastim prophylaxis, *or:* • Documented infection during a period of G ≥3 neutropenia (ANC <1000/mm³), *or:* • G4 neutropenia (ANC <500/mm³) lasting >7 days at any time	Discontinue irinotecan and oxaliplatin. Continue treatment with full dosages of leucovorin and fluorouracil, and continue or institute prophylaxis with filgrastim

Gastrointestinal Toxicities and Hepatic Impairment

Adverse Event	Treatment Modification
First episode of either of the following: • G ≥3 isolated diarrhea (≥7 stools per day over baseline; incontinence; hospitalization indicated; severe increase in ostomy output compared to baseline; limiting self-care ADL; life-threatening consequences; urgent intervention indicated), *or:* • Any diarrhea with and/or fever (temperature >38.5°C) and/or occurring during an episode of G ≥3 neutropenia (ANC <1000/mm³)	Reduce the irinotecan dosage to 120 mg/m² in subsequent cycles. Do not modify the dosages of oxaliplatin, leucovorin, or fluorouracil
Second episode of either of the following: • G ≥3 isolated diarrhea (≥7 stools per day over baseline; incontinence; hospitalization indicated; severe increase in ostomy output compared to baseline; limiting self-care ADL; life-threatening consequences; urgent intervention indicated), *or:* • Any diarrhea with and/or fever (temperature >38.5°C) and/or occurring during an episode of G ≥3 neutropenia (ANC <1000/mm³)	Maintain the irinotecan dosage at 120 mg/m² in subsequent cycles. Reduce the oxaliplatin dosage to 60 mg/m² and reduce the fluorouracil dosage to 1800 mg/m² in subsequent cycles. Do not modify the dosage of leucovorin in subsequent cycles
Third episode of either of the following: • G ≥3 isolated diarrhea (≥7 stools per day over baseline; incontinence; hospitalization indicated; severe increase in ostomy output compared to baseline; limiting self-care ADL; life-threatening consequences; urgent intervention indicated), *or:* • Any diarrhea with and/or fever (temperature >38.5°C) and/or occurring during an episode of G ≥3 neutropenia (ANC <1000/mm³)	Discontinue irinotecan. Maintain the oxaliplatin dosage at 60 mg/m² and maintain the fluorouracil dosage at 1800 mg/m² in subsequent cycles
G ≥3 mucositis (severe pain interfering with oral intake; or worse)	Withhold all treatment until resolution to G ≤1, then reduce the dosage of fluorouracil by 25% in subsequent cycles. Do not modify the dosages of irinotecan, oxaliplatin, or leucovorin
Total bilirubin >1.5× ULN	Withhold all chemotherapy. Evaluate for possible biliary anastomosis obstruction and/or pancreatic tumor relapse. If elevation in total bilirubin is unrelated to either of these, then withhold irinotecan until total bilirubin is ≤1.5× ULN. May continue full dosages of oxaliplatin, leucovorin, and fluorouracil

(*continued*)

Treatment Modifications (*continued*)

Modified FOLFIRINOX DOSE MODIFICATIONS

Adverse Event	Treatment Modification
Neurotoxicity	
G2 paresthesia (paresthesia or dysesthesia, moderate in nature without functional impairment other than limiting instrumental ADL) that persists ≥14 days (ie, persists between cycles)	Reduce oxaliplatin dosage to 65 mg/m² in subsequent cycles. Do not modify the dosages of irinotecan, fluorouracil, or leucovorin
G2 paresthesia (paresthesia or dysesthesia, moderate in nature without functional impairment other than limiting instrumental ADL) that improves to G ≤1 (asymptomatic) within <14 days (ie, improves before the next cycle is administered)	Proceed with full dosages of oxaliplatin, irinotecan, fluorouracil, and leucovorin
G3 paresthesia (paresthesia or dysesthesia with functional impairment limiting self-care ADL) that persists ≥14 days (ie, persists between cycles)	Discontinue oxaliplatin. Do not modify the dosages of irinotecan, fluorouracil, or leucovorin
G3 paresthesia (paresthesia or dysesthesia with functional impairment limiting self-care ADL) that improves to G ≤1 (asymptomatic) within <14 days (ie, improves before the next cycle is administered)	Reduce oxaliplatin dosage to 65 mg/m² in subsequent cycles. Do not modify the dosages of irinotecan, fluorouracil, or leucovorin
G4 paresthesia (life-threatening consequences; urgent intervention indicated) at any time	Discontinue oxaliplatin. Do not modify the dosages of irinotecan, fluorouracil, or leucovorin
Other Nonhematologic Toxicities	
G3 palmar-plantar erythrodysesthesia syndrome (severe skin changes [eg, peeling, blisters, bleeding, edema, or hyperkeratosis] with pain; limiting self-care ADL)	Withhold all treatment until resolution to G ≤1, then reduce the dosage of fluorouracil by 25% in subsequent cycles. Do not modify the dosages of irinotecan, oxaliplatin, or leucovorin
Coronary vasospasm related to fluorouracil	Immediately and permanently discontinue fluorouracil and leucovorin and perform emergent cardiac workup and appropriate treatment. Upon recovery, continue treatment with irinotecan and oxaliplatin at full dosages, or consider alternative therapy, at the discretion of the medically responsible health care provider
Other significant nonhematologic G ≥2 toxicity	Withhold chemotherapy until improvement to G ≤1 or baseline. At the discretion of the medically responsible health care provider and depending on the type and severity of the toxicity, reduce the dosage(s) of the agent(s) likely responsible for the toxicity by 25% in subsequent cycles, or consider alternative therapy
Recurrence of other G4 nonhematologic toxicity despite prior dosage reduction in the attributable agent(s)	Permanently discontinue the attributable agent(s). Either continue therapy with the remaining agents at full dosages or consider alternative therapy at the discretion of the medically responsible health care provider

ANC, absolute neutrophil count; CBC, complete blood count; ADL, activities of daily living; ULN, upper limit of normal

Note: patients who are pregnant or who become pregnant should be apprised of the potential hazard to the fetus; women of childbearing potential should be advised to avoid becoming pregnant during therapy

Patient Population Studied

This international, multicenter, randomized, open-label, phase 3 trial involved 493 patients with histologically confirmed pancreatic ductal adenocarcinoma who had previously undergone either an R0 (no cancer cells within 1 mm of all margins) or R1 (cancer cells present within 1 mm of ≥1 margin) resection within the past 3–12 weeks and who were without evidence of metastatic disease, malignant ascites, or pleural effusions. Patients had to have been classified as World Health Organization performance status 0–1, had adequate organ function, and had a serum CA 19–9 level not exceeding 180 units/mL within 21 days before randomization.

(*continued*)

Patient Population Studied (continued)

Patients were randomized 1:1 to begin 24 weeks of adjuvant chemotherapy with either modified FOLFIRINOX or adjuvant gemcitabine within 1 week of enrollment

Characteristic	Modified FOLFIRINOX (N = 247)	Gemcitabine (N = 246)
Age		
Median (range)—years	63 (30–79)	64 (30–81)
≥70 years—no. (%)	47 (19.0)	54 (22.0)
Male sex—no. (%)	142 (57.5)	135 (54.9)
WHO performance-status score—no./total no. (%)†		
0	122/245 (49.8)	127/242 (52.5)
1	123/245 (50.2)	115/242 (47.5)
Status of surgical margins—no. (%)‡		
R0	148 (59.9)	134 (54.5)
R1	99 (40.1)	112 (45.5)
Tumor histologic findings—no./total no. (%)		
Ductal adenocarcinoma	244/247 (98.8)	242/245 (98.8)
Nonductal carcinoma	3/247 (1.2)	3/245 (1.2)
Tumor stage—no. (%)§		
I	12 (4.9))	14 (5.7
IIA	43 (17.4)	47 (19.1)
IIB	183 (74.1)	179 (72.8)
III	1 (0.4)	1 (0.4)
IV	8 (3.2)	5 (2.0)
Lymphovascular invasion—no./total no. (%)	154/209 (73.7)	135/214 (63.1)
Perineural invasion—no. (%)	205/221 (92.8)	207/231 (89.6)
Surgery		
Venous resection—no./total no. (%)	53/245 (21.6)	69/245 (28.2)
Portal-vein resection—no. (%)	32 (13.0)	42 (17.1)
Superior-mesenteric-vein resection—no. (%)	19 (7.7)	25 (10.2)
Arterial resection—no./total no. (%)	8/247 (3.2)	7/245 (2.9)

Efficacy (n = 493)

	Modified FOLFIRINOX (N = 247)	Gemcitabine (N = 246)	
Median overall survival	54.4 months (95% CI, 41.8–not reached)	35.0 months (95% CI, 28.7–43.9)	HR 0.64 (95% CI, 0.48–0.86); P = 0.003
Median disease-free survival	21.6 months (95% CI, 17.7–27.6)	12.8 months (95% CI, 11.7–15.2)	HR 0.58 (95% CI, 0.46–0.73); P<0.001

Note: median follow-up in the intention-to-treat population was 33.6 months

Adverse Events (n = 481)

Grade (%)*	Modified FOLFIRINOX (N = 238)		Gemcitabine (N = 243)	
	Grade 1–2	Grade 3–4	Grade 1–2	Grade 3–4
Anemia	81%	3%	86%	3%
Thrombocytopenia	45%	1%	46%	5%
Hyperleukocytosis	42%	5%	48%	7%
Neutropenia	38%	28%	37%	26%
Lymphopenia	35%	1%	45%	3%
Neutropenic fever	0%	3%	0.4%	4%
Nausea	73%	6%	54%	1%
Fatigue	73%	11%	72%	5%
Diarrhea	66%	19%	45%	4%
Peripheral neuropathy, sensory	52%	9%	9%	0%
Paresthesia	45%	13%	5%	0%
Abdominal pain	43%	3%	47%	0.4%
Anorexia	42%	3%	24%	1%
Vomiting	40%	5%	28%	1%
Weight loss	37%	1%	20%	0.4%
Mucositis	31%	3%	15%	0%
Alopecia	27%	0%	19%	0%
Constipation	21%	0%	21%	0%
Fever	16%	0.4%	32%	0.4%
Hand-foot syndrome	5%	0.4%	0.8%	0%
Thrombosis or embolism	3%	3%	7%	0.4%
Alkaline phosphatase level increased	71%	2%	44%	2%
Aspartate aminotransferase level increased	63%	4%	65%	3%
Alanine aminotransferase level increased	59%	4%	68%	5%
Gamma-glutamyltransferase level increased	45%	18%	37%	8%
Hyperglycemia	22%	3%	22%	2%

According to the National Cancer Institute Common Terminology Criteria for Adverse Events, version 4.0
Note: only one Grade 5 toxicity was reported: interstitial pneumonitis occurring in a patient randomized to gemcitabine

Therapy Monitoring

1. *Before each cycle:* history and physical examination with attention to neurologic exam
2. CBC with differential at a minimum once per cycle, but initially also at day 10–14
3. Serum bilirubin, AST, ALT, and alkaline phosphatase prior to each cycle
4. CA 19–9 and/or CEA prior to each cycle if detectable and being used to monitor disease
5. *Every 3–6 months for 2 years, then as clinically indicated:* CT scans and CA 19–9 (if being used to follow disease) to assess for recurrence

ADJUVANT

PANCREATIC CANCER REGIMEN: GEMCITABINE + CAPECITABINE

Neoptolemos JP et al. Lancet 2017;389:1011–1024
Protocol for: Neoptolemos JP et al. Lancet 2017;389:1011–1024

Gemcitabine HCl 1000 mg/m² per dose; administer intravenously in 50–250 mL 0.9% sodium chloride injection for 3 doses on days 1, 8, and 15, every 28 days, for 6 cycles (total dosage/4-week cycle = 3000 mg/m²)

Capecitabine 830 mg/m² per dose; administer orally twice daily within 30 minutes after a meal for 21 consecutive days (42 doses) on days 1–21, followed by 7 days without treatment, repeated every 28 days, for 6 cycles (total dosage/4-week cycle = 34,860 mg/m²)

Notes:
- Doses are rounded to use combinations of 500-mg and 150-mg tablets that most closely approximate calculated values
- Patients who miss a dose of capecitabine should be instructed to continue with the usual dosing schedule without making up the missed dose and to contact their physician for further instructions.
- Patients who take too much (ie, overdose) capecitabine should contact their doctor immediately and present to the emergency department for further care and consideration for timely treatment with the antidote uridine triacetate
- Initial capecitabine dosage should be decreased by 25% in patients with moderate renal impairment (baseline creatinine clearance = 30–50 mL/min [0.5–0.83 mL/s]); ie, a dosage reduction from 830 mg/m² per dose, to 623 mg/m² per dose, twice daily. Capecitabine use is contraindicated in persons with severe renal impairment (creatinine clearance <30 mL/min [<0.5 mL/s])
- Although food decreases the rate and extent of drug absorption and the time to peak plasma concentration and systemic exposure (AUC) for both capecitabine and fluorouracil, product labeling recommends giving capecitabine within 30 minutes after the end of a meal because established safety and efficacy data are based on administration with food

Supportive Care
Antiemetic prophylaxis
Emetogenic potential on days when gemcitabine is administered (ie, days 1, 8, and 15) is **LOW**
Emetogenic potential on days when only capecitabine is administered is **MINIMAL–LOW**
See Chapter 42 for antiemetic recommendations

Hematopoietic growth factor (CSF) prophylaxis
Primary prophylaxis is **NOT** *indicated*
See Chapter 43 for more information

Antimicrobial prophylaxis
Risk of fever and neutropenia is **LOW**
   Antimicrobial primary prophylaxis to be considered:
- Antibacterial—not indicated
- Antifungal—not indicated
- Antiviral—not indicated unless patient previously had an episode of HSV

Diarrhea management
Latent or delayed-onset diarrhea
Loperamide 4 mg orally initially after the first loose or liquid stool, *then*
Loperamide 2 mg orally every 2 hours during waking hours, *plus*
Loperamide 4 mg orally every 4 hours during hours of sleep
- Continue for at least 12 hours after diarrhea resolves
- Recurrent diarrhea after a 12-hour diarrhea-free interval is treated as a new episode
- Rehydrate orally with fluids and electrolytes during a diarrheal episode
- If a patient develops blood or mucus in stool, dehydration, or hemodynamic instability, or if diarrhea persists >48 hours despite loperamide, stop loperamide and hospitalize the patient for IV hydration
- Alternatively, a trial of **diphenoxylate hydrochloride** 2.5 mg with **atropine sulfate** 0.025 mg (eg, Lomotil)
- Initial adult dose is 2 tablets 4 times daily until control has been achieved, after which the dose may be reduced to meet individual requirements. Control may often be maintained with as little as 2 tablets daily
- Clinical improvement of acute diarrhea is usually observed within 48 hours. If improvement of chronic diarrhea after treatment with a maximum daily dose of 8 tablets is not observed within 10 days, control is unlikely with further administration

Persistent diarrhea:
Octreotide 100–150 mcg subcutaneously 3 times daily. Maximum total daily dose is 1500 mcg

(continued)

(*continued*)

Antibiotic therapy during latent or delayed-onset diarrhea:

A fluoroquinolone (eg, **ciprofloxacin** 500 mg orally every 12 hours) if absolute neutrophil count <500/mm^3 with or without accompanying fever in association with diarrhea

• Antibiotics should also be administered if patient is hospitalized with prolonged diarrhea and should be continued until diarrhea resolves

Abigerges D et al. J Natl Cancer Inst 1994;86:446–449
Rothenberg ML et al. J Clin Oncol 2001;19:3801–3807
Wadler S et al. J Clin Oncol 1998;16:3169–3178

Hand-foot syndrome

For patients who develop a hand-foot syndrome, use topical emollients (eg, Aquaphor), topical or orally administered steroids, antihistamine agents (H$_1$-receptor antagonists), or pyridoxine 50–150 mg/day administer orally

Dose Modifications

GEMCITABINE AND CAPECITABINE DOSE MODIFICATIONS

	Gemcitabine Dose	Capecitabine Dose
Starting dose	1,000 mg/m^2	830 mg/m^2/dose twice per day
Dose level −1	750 mg/m^2	622.5 mg/m^2/dose twice per day
Dose level −2	500 mg/m^2	415 mg/m^2/dose twice per day

Adverse Event	Treatment Modification
Hematologic Toxicities	
ANC 500–1,000/mm^3 and/or platelet count 50,000–100,000/mm^3 on day of gemcitabine administration (with immediate prior week ANC and platelet count *not* requiring gemcitabine dose reduction)	Administer gemcitabine at dose level −1 without delay. Administer subsequent gemcitabine dose based on ANC and platelet count measured on that day (ie, consider increasing subsequent dose back to full dose if hematologic parameters allow) If the gemcitabine dose had previously been *permanently* reduced to dose level −1, then administer gemcitabine without delay, but permanently reduce the dose further to dose level −2 for all subsequent doses Do not modify the capecitabine dose
ANC 500–1000/mm^3 and/or platelet count 50,000–100,000/mm^3 on day of gemcitabine administration (for *second consecutive* week)	Administer gemcitabine without delay, but *permanently* reduce the gemcitabine dosage to dose level −1 Do not modify the capecitabine dose
ANC <500/mm^3 and/or platelet count <50,000/mm^3 on day of gemcitabine administration (*first* episode)	Omit gemcitabine and do not make up the dose. Continue capecitabine without interruption. Repeat CBC with differential weekly until ANC ≥500/mm^3 and platelet count >50,000/mm^3 If recovery occurs within 1 week, then *permanently* reduce the gemcitabine dosage to dose level −1. Continue capecitabine at full dose If recovery requires ≥2 weeks, then *permanently* reduce the gemcitabine dosage to dose level −1 and *permanently* reduce the capecitabine dosage to dose level −1
ANC <500/mm^3 and/or platelet count <50,000/mm^3 on day of gemcitabine administration (*recurrent* episode occurring at gemcitabine dose level −1)	Omit gemcitabine and do not make up the dose. Continue capecitabine without interruption. Repeat CBC with differential weekly until ANC ≥500/mm^3 and platelet count >50,000/mm^3, then *permanently* reduce the gemcitabine dosage to dose level −2 and *permanently* reduce the capecitabine dosage by one dose level
Prior episode of neutropenic fever (single temperature ≥38.3°C or a temperature ≥38.0°C sustained for ≥1 hour with an ANC <500/mm^3 or predicted to be <500/mm^3 within 48 hours)	Withhold both gemcitabine and capecitabine until recovery, then *permanently* reduce the dosages of both medications by one dosage level. Consider use of filgrastim to treat neutropenic fever and/or for secondary prophylaxis with subsequent cycles according to local practice

(*continued*)

Dose Modifications (continued)

Adverse Event	Treatment Modification
	Other Toxicities
G2/3/4 diarrhea	Withhold capecitabine; provide supportive care. Do not resume capecitabine until toxicity resolved to G ≤1. If toxicity is G3/4, then also consider omitting gemcitabine until toxicity resolved to G ≤1 as appropriate. If toxicity is G4, then *permanently* discontinue capecitabine. Otherwise, in subsequent cycle(s) *permanently* reduce the capecitabine dosage by 1 dose level
G2/3/4 mucositis	
G2/3/4 dehydration	
G2/3 hand-and-foot syndrome or palmar-plantar erythrodysesthesia or chemotherapy-induced acral erythema*	
Stevens-Johnson syndrome and toxic epidermal necrolysis (severe mucocutaneous reactions, some with fatal outcome)	Permanently discontinue capecitabine
Capecitabine-induced coronary vasospasm/cardiac ischemia	Permanently discontinue capecitabine
Unexplained new or worsening dyspnea or evidence of severe pulmonary toxicity	Withhold gemcitabine and capecitabine and assess for gemcitabine-related pulmonary toxicity. If confirmed, permanently discontinue gemcitabine
Hemolytic-uremic syndrome	Permanently discontinue gemcitabine for hemolytic uremic syndrome or severe renal impairment
Capillary leak syndrome	Permanently discontinue gemcitabine
Posterior reversible encephalopathy syndrome	Permanently discontinue gemcitabine
Creatinine clearance 30–50 mL/minute	Reduce the capecitabine dosage by 1 dose level
Creatinine clearance <30 mL/minute	Withhold capecitabine

ANC, absolute neutrophil count; CBC, complete blood count
*Grading of hand-foot syndrome
- G1: Numbness, dysesthesia/paresthesia, tingling, painless swelling, or erythema of the hands and/or feet and/or discomfort that does not disrupt normal activities
- G2: Painful erythema and swelling of the hands and/or feet and/or discomfort affecting the patient's activities of daily living
- G3: Moist desquamation, ulceration, blistering, or severe pain of the hands and/or feet and/or severe discomfort that causes the patient to be unable to work or perform activities of daily living

Patient Population Studied

The ESPAC–4 study was a phase 3, open label, multicenter, multinational, randomized, active-controlled trial that involved 730 adult patients who had undergone complete macroscopic (R0 or R1 resection) of ductal adenocarcinoma of the pancreas within the prior 12 weeks. Patients were required to have no evidence of metastatic disease or malignant ascites. Patients were required to have fully recovered from surgery, to have a WHO PS of ≤2, to have a creatinine clearance of ≥50 mL/minute, and to have a life expectancy of ≥3 months. Patients were excluded if they had undergone prior neoadjuvant therapy, if they had macroscopic residual disease (R2 resection), or if they had stage IV disease based on the UICC 7th edition TNM criteria. Patients were randomly assigned 1:1 to receive adjuvant treatment with gemcitabine plus capecitabine or gemcitabine alone

Participant Characteristics			
	Gemcitabine (n = 366)	Gemcitabine Plus Capecitabine (n = 364)	Total Participants (n = 730)
Sex			
Male	212 (58%)	202 (55%)	414 (57%)
Female	154 (42%)	162 (45%)	316 (43%)
Age (years)	65 (37–80)	65 (39–81)	65 (37–81)
WHO status			
0	158 (43%)	150 (41%)	308 (42%)
1	199 (54%)	202 (55%)	401 (55%)

(continued)

Patient Population Studied (*continued*)

Participant Characteristics			
	Gemcitabine (n = 366)	Gemcitabine Plus Capecitabine (n = 364)	Total Participants (n = 730)
2	9 (2%)	12 (3%)	21 (3%)
Smoking status			
Never	151 (41%)	146 (40%)	297 (41%)
Past	136 (37%)	148 (41%)	284 (39%)
Present	62 (17%)	61 (17%)	123 (17%)
Unknown	17 (5%)	9 (2%)	26 (4%)
Concurrent conditions			
None	82 (22%)	106 (29%)	188 (26%)
Yes	280 (77%)	257 (71%)	537 (74%)
Unknown	4 (1%)	1 (<1%)	5 (1%)
Diabetes			
No	266 (73%)	272 (75%)	538 (74%)
Non-insulin-dependent	52 (14%)	45 (12%)	97 (13%)
Insulin-dependent	47 (13%)	46 (13%)	93 (13%)
Preoperative carbohydrate antigen 19–9 (KU/L)			
Number of patients with measurements	234	224	458
Median	142·5 (0·9–10 761·0)	154·5 (0·8–76 549·0)	150·5 (0·8–76 549·0)
Postoperative carbohydrate antigen 19–9 (KU/L)			
Number of patients with measurements	341	321	662
Median	20·5 (0·1–2448·3)	17·6 (0·6–8112·0)	18·7 (0·1–8112·0)
Preoperative C-reactive protein (mg/L)			
Number of patients with measurements	275	271	546
Median	8·0 (0·1–343·0)	8·0 (0·3–190·0)	8·0 (0·1– 343·0)
Postoperative C-reactive protein (mg/L)			
Number of patients with measurements	344	348	692
Median	5·0 (0·1–345·0)	5·0 (0·0–296·0)	5·0 (0·0–345·0)
Time from surgery to randomization (days)			
Median	65 (23–111)	64 (21–111)	64 (21–111)
Hospital stay (days)			
Number of patients with measurements	363	357	720
Median	12 (1–89)	12 (3–58)	12 (1–89)
Resection margin status			
Number of patients with negative status	147 (40%)	143 (39%)	290 (40%)

(*continued*)

Patient Population Studied (*continued*)

Participant Characteristics			
	Gemcitabine (n = 366)	Gemcitabine Plus Capecitabine (n = 364)	Total Participants (n = 730)
Number of patients with positive status	219 (60%)	221 (61%)	440 (60%)
Country			
France	12 (3%)	12 (3%)	24 (3%)
Germany	34 (10%)	33 (9%)	67 (9%)
Sweden	40 (11%)	43 (12%)	83 (11%)
England	257 (70%)	254 (70%)	511 (70%)
Scotland	12 (3%)	9 (2%)	21 (3%)
Wales	11 (3%)	13 (4%)	24 (3%)
Tumor grade			
Well differentiated	30 (8%)	32 (9%)	62 (8%)
Moderately differentiated	192 (52%)	175 (48%)	367 (50%)
Poorly differentiated	140 (38%)	147 (40%)	287 (39%)
Undifferentiated	2 (1%)	2 (1%)	4 (1%)
Lymph nodes			
Negative	67 (18%)	76 (21%)	143 (20%)
Positive	299 (82%)	288 (79%)	587 (80%)
Maximum tumor size (mm)			
Number of patients with measurements	361	352	713
Median	30 (0–110)	30 (6–105)	30 (0–110)
Tumor stage			
I	7 (2%)	15 (4%)	22 (3%)
II	29 (8%)	20 (5%)	49 (7%)
III	325 (89%)	326 (90%)	651 (89%)
IV	5 (1%)	3 (1%)	8 (1%)
Surgery			
Whipple resection	188 (51%)	182 (50%)	370 (51%)
Total pancreatectomy	27 (7%)	22 (6%)	49 (7%)
Pylorus-preserving resection	122 (33%)	129 (35%)	251 (34%)
Distal pancreatectomy	29 (8%)	31 (9%)	60 (8%)
Venous resection			
No	298 (81%)	323 (89%)	621 (85%)
Yes	63 (17%)	39 (11%)	102 (14%)
Unknown	5 (1%)	2 (1%)	7 (1%)
Extent of resection			
Standard	289 (79%)	279 (77%)	568 (78%)
Radical	53 (14%)	56 (15%)	109 (15%)

(*continued*)

Patient Population Studied (*continued*)

Participant Characteristics			
	Gemcitabine (n = 366)	Gemcitabine Plus Capecitabine (n = 364)	Total Participants (n = 730)
Extended lymphadenectomy	18 (5%)	28 (8%)	46 (6%)
Unknown	6 (2%)	1 (<1%)	7 (1%)
Cholecystectomy			
No	78 (21%)	90 (25%)	168 (23%)
No, already excised	18 (5%)	16 (4%)	34 (5%)
Yes	270 (74%)	257 (71%)	527 (72%)
Local invasion			
No	189 (52%)	189 (52%)	378 (52%)
Yes	176 (48%)	173 (48%)	349 (48%)
Unknown	1 (0%)	2 (1%)	3 (<1%)
Postoperative complications			
No	271 (74%)	250 (69%)	521 (71%)
Yes	93 (25%)	113 (31%)	206 (28%)
Unknown	2 (1%)	1 (<1%)	3 (<1%)

Efficacy (N = 730)

Efficacy Variable	Gemcitabine + Capecitabine (N = 364)	Gemcitabine (N = 366)	Hazard Ratio (95% CI) and P Value
Overall survival (OS)			
Median OS—months (95% CI)	28.0 (23.5–31.5)	25.5 (22.7–27.9)	0.82 (0.68–0.98); 0.032
Overall survival rate—% (95% CI)			
12 months	84.1 (79.9–87.5)	80.5 (76.0–84.3)	
24 months	53.8 (48.4–58.8)	52.1 (46.7–57.2)	
OS in patients with R1 resection (n = 221 in gemcitabine + capecitabine arm and n = 219 in gemcitabine arm)			
Median OS—months (95% CI)	23.7 (20.7–27.1)	23.0 (21.6–26.2)	
OS in patients with R0 resection (n = 143 in gemcitabine + capecitabine arm and n = 147 in gemcitabine arm)			
Median OS—months (95% CI)	39.5 (32.0–58.0)	27.9 (23.8–34.6)	
Relapse-free survival (RFS)			
Median RFS—months (95% CI)	13.9 (12.1–16.6)	13.1 (11.6–15.3)	0.86 (0.73–1.02); 0.082
Relapse-free survival rate—% (95% CI)			
3-year	23.8 (19.2–28.6)	20.9 (16.5–25.7)	
5-year	18.6 (13.8–24.0)	11.9 (7.8–16.9)	

Adverse Events (N = 725)

Grade (%)*	Gemcitabine Plus Capecitabine (n = 359)			Gemcitabine (n = 366)		
	Grade 1–2	Grade 3–4	Grade 5	Grade 1–2	Grade 3–4	Grade 5
Anemia	56	2	0	58	4	0
Diarrhea	45	5	0	41	2	0
Fatigue	64	6	0	66	5	0
Fever	17	2	0	20	2	0
Infections and infestations, other	10	3	<1	15	7	0
Lymphocyte count decreased	22	3	0	27	3	0
Neutropenia	49	38	0	40	24	0
Hand-foot syndrome	31	7	0	2	0	0
Platelet count decreased	29	2	0	24	2	0
Thromboembolic events	4	2	0	2	2	0
White blood cell count decreased	39	10	0	37	8	0
Acute kidney injury	<1	0	0	1	1	0
Multi-organ failure	0	0	0	0	0	<1
Cardiac disorders	1	0	0	1	<1	<1
Benign, malignant, and unspecified neoplasms (including cysts and polyps), other	0	<1	0	<1	0	1

*According to the National Cancer Institute Common Terminology Criteria for Adverse Events, version 4.03

Therapy Monitoring

1. *Prior to each cycle:* history and physical exam, CBC with differential, BUN, serum creatinine, serum electrolytes, ALT, AST, total bilirubin, and alkaline phosphate
2. *On day 8 and 15:* CBC with differential, BUN, serum creatinine, serum electrolytes, ALT, AST, total bilirubin, and alkaline phosphate
3. Patients receiving concomitant capecitabine and oral coumarin-derivative anticoagulant therapy should have their anticoagulant response (INR or prothrombin time) monitored frequently in order to adjust the anticoagulant dose accordingly
4. Monitor for signs/symptoms of hand-foot syndrome (capecitabine), Stevens-Johnson syndrome and toxic epidermal necrolysis (capecitabine), hydration status (capecitabine), diarrhea (capecitabine), mucositis (capecitabine), coronary vasospasm (capecitabine), pulmonary toxicity (gemcitabine), capillary leak syndrome (gemcitabine), hemolytic uremic syndrome (gemcitabine), posterior reversible encephalopathy syndrome (gemcitabine), and signs of infection

Note: toxicity in the setting of DPD deficiency occurs early and is characterized by severe mucositis, diarrhea, neutropenia, and neurotoxicity. It occurs in individuals with homozygous or certain compound heterozygous mutations in the DPD gene that result in complete or near complete absence of DPD activity. Discontinue capecitabine permanently. There is insufficient data to recommend a specific dose in patients with partial DPD activity as measured by any specific test

METASTATIC • FIRST-LINE

PANCREATIC CANCER REGIMEN: GEMCITABINE + NAB-PACLITAXEL

Von Hoff DD et al. J Clin Oncol 2011;29:4548–4554
Von Hoff DD et al. J Clin Oncol 2013;31(Suppl):Abstract 4005
Von Hoff DD et al. N Engl J Med 2013;369:1691–703

Paclitaxel protein-bound particles for injectable suspension (nab-paclitaxel) 125 mg/m² per dose intravenously once weekly for 3 doses on days 1, 8, and 15, every 28 days (total dosage/4-week cycle = 375 mg/m²), *followed by:*

Gemcitabine HCl 1000 mg/m² per dose intravenously in 50–250 mL 0.9% sodium chloride injection for 3 doses on days 1, 8, and 15, every 28 days (total dosage/4-week cycle = 3000 mg/m²)

Supportive Care *Antiemetic prophylaxis*
Emetogenic potential is **LOW**
See Chapter 42 for antiemetic recommendations

Hematopoietic growth factor (CSF) prophylaxis
Primary prophylaxis may be indicated
See Chapter 43 for more information

Antimicrobial prophylaxis
Risk of fever and neutropenia is **LOW**
  Antimicrobial primary prophylaxis to be considered:
  • Antibacterial—not indicated
  • Antifungal—not indicated
  • Antiviral—not indicated unless patient previously had an episode of HSV

Treatment Modifications

Dose Levels

	nab-Paclitaxel (mg/m²)	Gemcitabine HCl (mg/m²)
Starting dose	125	1000
Dose level −1	100	800
Dose level −2	75	600

Dose Adjustments on Day 1 of Each Treatment Cycle for Hematologic Toxicity

ANC		Platelets	Timing
≥1500/mm³	AND	≥100,000/mm³	Treat on time
<1500/mm³	OR	<100,000/mm³	Delay by 1 week intervals until recovery

Dose Adjustments Within a Treatment Cycle for Hematologic Toxicity

Day 8			Day 15		
Blood Counts	nab-Paclitaxel	Gemcitabine	Blood Counts	nab-Paclitaxel	Gemcitabine
ANC >1000/mm³ *and* platelets ≥75,000/mm³	100%		ANC >1000/mm³ *and* platelets ≥75,000/mm³	100%	
			ANC 500–1000/mm³ *or* platelets 50,000–74,999/mm³	Full dose (treat on time) and administer filgrastim*	
			ANC <500/mm³ *or* platelets <50,000/mm³	Hold and administer filgrastim*	

(continued)

Treatment Modifications (continued)

Dose Adjustments Within a Treatment Cycle for Hematologic Toxicity

	Day 8		Day 15		
Blood Counts	nab-Paclitaxel	Gemcitabine	Blood Counts	nab-Paclitaxel	Gemcitabine
ANC 500–1000/mm³ or platelets 50,000–74,999/mm³	Decrease dose by 1 level (treat on time)		ANC >1000/mm³ *and* platelets ≥75,000/mm³	Return to previous dose level (treat on time) and administer filgrastim*	
			ANC 500–1000/mm³ *or* platelets 50,000–74,999/mm³	Same dose as day 8 (treat on time) and administer filgrastim*	
			ANC <500/mm³ *or* platelets <50,000/mm³	Hold and administer filgrastim*	
ANC <500/mm³ *or* platelets <50,000/mm³	Hold		ANC >1000/mm³ *and* platelets ≥75,000/mm³	Decrease day 8 dose by 1 level (treat on time) and administer filgrastim*	
			ANC 500–1000/mm³ *or* platelets 50,000–74,999/mm³	Decrease day 8 dose by 1 level (treat on time) and administer filgrastim*	
			ANC <500/mm³ *or* platelets <50,000/mm³	Hold and administer filgrastim*	

*Febrile patients (regardless of ANC) should have chemotherapy treatment interrupted. A full sepsis diagnostic work-up should be performed while continuing broad-spectrum antibiotics. If cultures are positive, guide antibiotic therapy by the sensitivity profile of the isolated organism. Patients with persisting fever after 3 weeks, despite uninterrupted antibiotic treatment, should discontinue therapy. Febrile neutropenic patients can also receive filgrastim, in addition to antibiotic treatment, to hasten resolution of their febrile neutropenia

Dose Adjustments on Day 1 of Each Treatment Cycle for Nonhematologic Toxicity and/or Dose Hold with Previous Cycle

Toxicity/Dose Held	nab-Paclitaxel + Gemcitabine Dose This Cycle
G1 peripheral neuropathy	Dose adjustment not needed but follow carefully
G2 peripheral neuropathy	Reduce nab-paclitaxel one dose level but continue gemcitabine administration
G≥3 peripheral neuropathy	Hold nab-paclitaxel treatment but continue gemcitabine administration if indicated. Resume nab-paclitaxel treatment at next lower dose level after the peripheral neuropathy improves to G ≤1
Other G1/2 toxicity†	Same as day 1 previous cycle (except for G2 cutaneous toxicity where doses of gemcitabine and nab-paclitaxel should be reduced to next lower dose level)
Other G3 toxicity†	Decrease nab-paclitaxel and gemcitabine to next lower dose level*
Other G4 toxicity†	Hold therapy†

†The decision as to which drug should be modified depends upon the type of nonhematologic toxicity seen and which course is medically most sound in the judgment of the physician

Dose Adjustments within a Treatment Cycle for Nonhematologic Toxicity

CTC Grade	Percent of Day 1 nab-Paclitaxel + Gemcitabine Dose
G1/2, G3 nausea/vomiting and alopecia	100%*
G3 (except G3 nausea/vomiting and alopecia)	Hold either 1 or both drugs until resolution to G ≤1. Then resume treatment at the next lower dose level
G ≥3 peripheral neuropathy	Hold nab-paclitaxel treatment but continue gemcitabine administration if indicated. Resume *nab*–paclitaxel treatment at next lower dose level after the peripheral neuropathy improves to G ≤1
G4	Hold therapy†

Patient Population Studied

MPACT Trial

A total of 861 patients with metastatic pancreatic ductal adenocarcinoma (PDA) and a Karnofsky performance status (KPS) ≥70 were randomized at 151 community and academic centers 1:1 to receive nab-paclitaxel 125 mg/m² + gemcitabine 1000 mg/m² days 1, 8, and 15 every 4 weeks or gemcitabine alone 1000 mg/m² weekly for 7 weeks followed by 1 week of rest (cycle 1) and then days 1, 8, and 15 every 4 weeks (cycle ≥2). The median age was 63 years (range: 27–88 years). KPS was 100 (16%), 90 (44%), 80 (32%), and 70 (7%). Patients had advanced disease with liver metastases (84%), ≥3 metastatic sites (46%), and CA19–9 ≥59 × upper limit of normal (46%)

Characteristics of the Patients at Baseline*			
Characteristic	nab-Paclitaxel plus Gemcitabine (N = 431)	Gemcitabine Alone (N = 430)	Total (N = 861)
Age			
Median	62 years	63 years	63 years
Range	27–86	32–88	27–88
<65 years	254 (59)	242 (56)	496 (58)
≥65 years	177 (41)	188 (44)	365 (42)
Sex—no. (%)			
Female	186 (43)	173 (40)	359 (42)
Male	245 (57)	257 (60)	502 (58)
Race or ethnic group—no. (%)†			
Asian	8 (2)	9 (2)	17 (2)
Black	16 (4)	16 (4)	32 (4)
White	378 (88)	375 (87)	753 (87)
Hispanic	25 (6)	26 (6)	51 (6)
Other	4 (1)	4 (1)	8 (1)
Karnofsky performance-status score—no./total no. (%)‡			
100	69/429 (16)	69/429 (16)	138/858 (16)
90	179/429 (42)	199/429 (46)	378/858 (44)
80	149/429 (35)	128/429 (30)	277/858 (32)
70	30/429 (7)	33/429 (8)	63/858 (7)
60	2/429 (<1)	0/429	2/858 (<1)
Pancreatic tumor location—no. (%)			
Head	191 (44)	180 (42)	371 (43)
Body	132 (31)	136 (32)	268 (31)
Tail	105 (24)	110 (26)	215 (25)
Unknown	3 (1)	4 (1)	7 (1)
Site of metastatic disease—no. (%)			
Liver	365 (85)	360 (84)	725 (84)
Lung	153 (35)	184 (43)	337 (39)
Peritoneum	19 (4)	10 (2)	29 (3)
No. of metastatic sites—no. (%)			
1	33 (8)	21 (5)	54 (6)
2	202 (47)	206 (48)	408 (47)

(*continued*)

Patient Population Studied (continued)

Characteristics of the Patients at Baseline*

Characteristic	nab-Paclitaxel plus Gemcitabine (N = 431)	Gemcitabine Alone (N = 430)	Total (N = 861)
3	136 (32)	140 (33)	276 (32)
>3	60 (14)	63 (15)	123 (14)
Level of CA19–9—no./total no. (%)			
Normal ᶜ	60/379 (16)	56/371 (15)	116/750 (15)
ULN to <59ᶜ × ULN	122/379 (32)	120/371 (32)	242/750 (32)
≥59 × ULN	197/379 (52)	195/371 (53)	392/750 (52)
CA19–9—U/mL			
Median	2293.7	2759.2	2469.7
Range	1.9–6,159,233.0	0.3–12,207,654.2	0.3–12,207,654.2
Previous therapy—no. (%)			
Radiation therapy	19 (4)	11 (3)	30 (3)
Chemotherapy	23 (5)	12 (3)	35 (4)
Whipple procedure	32 (7)	30 (7)	62 (7)
Biliary stent	80 (19)	68 (16)	148 (17)

nab-paclitaxel, 130-nm albumin-bound paclitaxel; ULN, upper limit of the normal range; CA19–9, carbohydrate antigen 19–9
*No significant between-group differences at baseline
†Race or ethnic group self-reported
‡Karnofsky performance-status scores range from 0–100, with higher scores indicating better performance status. Two patients in the nab-paclitaxel–gemcitabine group had a score 70 at screening but a score of 60 on day 1 of cycle 1
ᶜNormal range = 0–35 U/mL. Approximately 10–15% of patients with pancreatic cancer do not have Lewis antigens and thus do not have the ability to secrete CA19–9. Data missing for 52 patients in the nab-paclitaxel–gemcitabine group and for 59 in the gemcitabine group

Efficacy

Overall Survival, Progression-free Survival, and Response Rates in the Intention-to-Treat Population

Efficacy Variable	nab-Paclitaxel plus Gemcitabine (N = 431)	Gemcitabine Alone (N = 430)	Hazard Ratio or Response-Rate Ratio (95% CI)* and P Value
Overall survival (OS)			
Median OS—months (95% CI)	8.5 (7.9–9.5)	6.7 (6.0–7.2)	0.72 (0.62–0.83); <0.001
Survival rate—% (95% CI)			
6 months	67 (62–71)	55 (50–60)	<0.001
12 months	35 (30–39)	22 (18–27)	<0.001
18 months	16 (12–20)	9 (6–12)	0.008
24 months	9 (6–13)	4 (2–7)	0.02
Progression-free survival (PFS)			
Median PFS—months (95% CI)	5.5 (4.5–5.9)	3.7 (3.6–4.0)	0.69 (0.58–0.82); <0.001

(continued)

Efficacy (continued)

Overall Survival, Progression-free Survival, and Response Rates in the Intention-to-Treat Population

Efficacy Variable	nab-Paclitaxel plus Gemcitabine (N = 431)	Gemcitabine Alone (N = 430)	Hazard Ratio or Response-Rate Ratio (95% CI)* and P Value
Rate of progression-free survival—% (95% CI)			
6 months	44 (39–50)	25 (20–30)	—
12 months	16 (12–21)	9 (5–14)	—
Response			
Rate of objective response			
Independent review—% (95% CI)	23% (19–27)	7% (5–10)	3.19 (2.18–4.66); <0.001
Investigator review—% (95% CI)	29% (25–34)	8% (5–11)	3.81 (2.66–5.46); <0.001
Rate of disease control[†]			
No. patients—% (95% CI)	206—48 (43–53)	141—33 (28–37)	1.46 (1.23–1.72); <0.001
% (95% CI)			
Best response according to independent review—no. (%)			
Complete response	1 (<1)	0	—
Partial response	98 (23)	31 (7)	—
Stable disease	118 (27)	122 (28)	—
Progressive disease	86 (20)	110 (26)	—
Could not be evaluated[‡]	128 (30)	167 (39)	—

Adverse Events

Toxicity—Common Adverse Events of Grade 3 or Higher and Growth-Factor Use*

von Hoff et al. N Engl J Med 2013;369:1691–1703

Event	Gemcitabine 1000 mg/m² + nab-Paclitaxel 125 mg/m² (N = 421)	Gemcitabine Alone (N = 402)
Adverse event leading to death—no. (%)	18 (4)	18 (4)
Grade ≥3 hematologic adverse event—no./total no. (%)[†]		
Neutropenia	153/405 (38)	103/388 (27)
Leukopenia	124/405 (31)	63/388 (16)
Thrombocytopenia	52/405 (13)	36/388 (9)
Anemia	53/405 (13)	48/388 (12)
Receipt of growth factors—no./total no. (%)	110/431 (26)	63/431 (15)
Febrile neutropenia—no. (%)[‡]	14 (3)	6 (1)
Grade ≥3 nonhematologic adverse event occurring in >5% of patients—no. (%)[‡]		

(*continued*)

Adverse Events (*continued*)

Event	Gemcitabine 1000 mg/m² + nab-Paclitaxel 125 mg/m² (N = 421)	Gemcitabine Alone (N = 402)
Fatigue	70 (17)	27 (7)
Peripheral neuropathy[c]	70 (17)	3 (1)
Diarrhea	24 (6)	3 (1)
Grade ≥3 peripheral neuropathy		
Median time to onset—days	140	113
Median time to improvement by one grade—days	21	29
Median time to improvement to Grade ≤1—days	29	NR
Use of nab-paclitaxel resumed—no./total no. (%)	31/70 (44)	NA

*NA denotes not applicable, and NR not reached
[†]Assessment of the event was made on the basis of laboratory values
[‡]Assessment of the event was made on the basis of investigator assessment of treatment-related adverse events
[c]Peripheral neuropathy was reported on the basis of groupings of preferred terms defined by standardized queries in the Medical Dictionary for Regulatory Activities

Treatment Monitoring

1. *Before each cycle:* history and physical examination. CBC with differential, total bilirubin, AST or ALT, alkaline phosphatase, BUN, serum creatinine, and electrolytes. CA 19–9 and/or CEA if detectable and being used to monitor disease. Monitor for hemolytic uremic syndrome (gemcitabine), interstitial lung disease (gemcitabine), and peripheral neuropathy (nab-paclitaxel)

Note: Interstitial Pneumonitis

Monitor patients carefully for signs and symptoms of pneumonitis (ie, episodes of transient or repeated dyspnea with unproductive persistent cough or fever) and, if observed, perform immediate clinical evaluation and timely institution of appropriate management (emphasizing the need for corticosteroids if an infectious process has been ruled out, as well as appropriate ventilation and oxygen support when required)

2. *Days 8 and 15:* CBC with differential
3. *Every 1–3 months:* CT scans to assess response

METASTATIC • FIRST-LINE

PANCREATIC CANCER REGIMEN: FLUOROURACIL + LEUCOVORIN + IRINOTECAN + OXALIPLATIN (FOLFIRINOX)

Conroy T et al. N Engl J Med 2011;364:1817–1825

Oxaliplatin 85 mg/m^2 intravenously in 250 mL 5% dextrose injection (D5W) over 2 hours on day 1, every 2 weeks (total dosage/cycle = 85 mg/m^2)
Note: Oxaliplatin must not be mixed with sodium chloride injection

Either: **(racemic) leucovorin calcium** 400 mg/m^2 *or* **levoleucovorin calcium** 200 mg/m^2 intravenously in 25–500 mL D5W or 0.9% sodium chloride injection over 2 hours on day 1, every 2 weeks (total dosage/cycle for racemic leucovorin = 400 mg/m^2, for levoleucovorin = 200 mg/m^2), *followed 30 minutes after administration begins by:*

Irinotecan 180 mg/m^2 intravenously over 90 minutes in 500 mL D5W on day 1, 30 minutes after leucovorin (or levoleucovorin) administration begins, every 2 weeks (total dosage/cycle = 180 mg/m^2), *followed by:*

(bolus) **Fluorouracil** 400 mg/m^2 by intravenous injection over 1–2 minutes after leucovorin (or levoleucovorin) and irinotecan administration are completed on day 1, every 2 weeks, *followed by:*

Fluorouracil 2400 mg/m^2 by continuous intravenous infusion over 46 hours in 100–1000 mL 0.9% NS or D5W, starting on day 1 every 2 weeks (total dosage/cycle = 2800 mg/m^2)

Important note: this regimen is difficult for patients. Thus, FOLFIRINOX is a first-line option for patients with metastatic pancreatic cancer who are younger than 76 years and who have a good performance status (ECOG 0 or 1), no cardiac ischemia, and normal or nearly normal bilirubin levels

Notes:
• Patients must be instructed in the use of loperamide as treatment for diarrhea, and must have a supply of this drug upon starting FOLFIRINOX
• Filgrastim is not recommended as primary prophylaxis, but it could be considered for high-risk patients
• The dose of leucovorin is not modified for toxicity, but is omitted if fluorouracil is omitted. Once a fluorouracil dose is decreased, it is not re-escalated

Supportive Care
Antiemetic prophylaxis
Emetogenic potential is **MODERATE**
See Chapter 42 for antiemetic recommendations

Hematopoietic growth factor (CSF) prophylaxis
Primary prophylaxis may be indicated
See Chapter 43 for more information

Antimicrobial prophylaxis
Risk of fever and neutropenia is **LOW**
  Antimicrobial primary prophylaxis to be considered:
  • Antibacterial—not indicated
  • Antifungal—not indicated
  • Antiviral—not indicated unless patient previously had an episode of HSV

Acute cholinergic syndrome
Atropine sulfate 0.25–1 mg subcutaneously or intravenously if abdominal cramping or diarrhea develop during or within 1 hour after irinotecan administration

• If symptoms are severe, add as primary prophylaxis at least 30 minutes before irinotecan during subsequent cycles
• For irinotecan, acute cholinergic syndrome may be characterized by: abdominal cramping, diarrhea, diaphoresis, hypotension, flushing, bradycardia, rhinitis, increased salivation, meiosis, and lacrimation

Diarrhea management
Latent or delayed-onset diarrhea:
  Loperamide 4 mg orally initially after the first loose or liquid stool, *then*
  Loperamide 2 mg orally every 2 hours during waking hours, *plus*
  Loperamide 4 mg orally every 4 hours during hours of sleep
  • Continue for at least 12 hours after diarrhea resolves
  • Recurrent diarrhea after a 12-hour diarrhea-free interval is treated as a new episode

(continued)

- Rehydrate orally with fluids and electrolytes during a diarrheal episode
- If a patient develops blood or mucus in stool, dehydration, or hemodynamic instability, or if diarrhea persists >48 hours despite loperamide, stop loperamide and hospitalize the patient for IV hydration

  Alternatively, a trial of **diphenoxylate hydrochloride** 2.5 mg with **atropine sulfate** 0.025 mg (eg, Lomotil)
- Initial adult dose is 2 tablets 4 times daily until control has been achieved, after which the dose may be reduced to meet individual requirements. Control may often be maintained with as little as 2 tablets daily
- Clinical improvement of acute diarrhea is usually observed within 48 hours. If improvement of chronic diarrhea after treatment with a maximum daily dose of 8 tablets is not observed within 10 days, control is unlikely with further administration

Persistent diarrhea:
   Octreotide 100–150 mcg subcutaneously 3 times daily. Maximum total daily dose is 1500 mcg
Antibiotic therapy during latent or delayed-onset diarrhea:
   A fluoroquinolone (eg, **ciprofloxacin** 500 mg orally every 12 hours) if absolute neutrophil count <500/mm³ with or without accompanying fever in association with diarrhea
- Antibiotics should also be administered if patient is hospitalized with prolonged diarrhea and should be continued until diarrhea resolves

*Abigerges D et al. J Natl Cancer Inst 1994;86:446–449
Rothenberg ML et al. J Clin Oncol 2001;19:3801–3807
Wadler S et al. J Clin Oncol 1998;16:3169–3178

Treatment Modifications

Event	Delay of Cycle	Dosage Reductions		
		Irinotecan	Oxaliplatin	Fluorouracil
First occurrence of ANC <1500/mm³ on day 1	Hold treatment up to 2 weeks until granulocytes ≥1500/mm³. In case of nonrecovery >2 weeks delay, stop treatment	Reduce dosage to 150 mg/m²	Do not reduce dosage	Delete bolus fluorouracil
Second occurrence of ANC <1500/mm³ on day 1		Maintain the dosage at 150 mg/m²	Reduce the dosage to 60 mg/m²	Continue without bolus fluorouracil
Third occurrence of ANC <1500/mm³ on day 1	Discontinue treatment			
First occurrence of platelets <75,000/mm³ on day 1	Hold treatment up to 2 weeks until platelets ≥75,000/mm³. In case of nonrecovery >2 weeks delay, stop treatment	Do not reduce dosage	Reduce the dosage to 60 mg/m²	Reduce both bolus and CI by 25% of original dosages
Second occurrence of platelets <75,000/mm³ on day 1		Reduce the dosage to 150 mg/m²	Maintain the dosage at 60 mg/m²	Continue both bolus and CI at 75% of original dosages
Third occurrence of platelets <75,000/mm³ on day 1	Discontinue treatment			
First occurrence febrile neutropenia or G4 neutropenia >7 days or infection with concomitant G3/4 neutropenia		Reduce the dosage to 150 mg/m²	Do not reduce dosage	Delete bolus fluorouracil
Second occurrence febrile neutropenia or G4 neutropenia >7 days or infection with concomitant G3/4 neutropenia		Maintain the dosage at 150 mg/m²	Reduce the dosage to 60 mg/m²	Continue without bolus fluorouracil
		Note: consider the use of filgrastim for recurrent G3/4 neutropenia despite a first dose reduction or after febrile neutropenia		

(continued)

Treatment Modifications (*continued*)

Event	Delay of Cycle	Dosage Reductions		
		Irinotecan	Oxaliplatin	Fluorouracil
Third occurrence febrile neutropenia or G4 neutropenia >7 days or infection with concomitant G3/4 neutropenia	Discontinue treatment			
First occurrence G3/4 thrombocytopenia		Do not reduce dosage	Reduce the dosage to 60 mg/m²	Reduce both bolus and CI fluorouracil by 25% of the original dosages
Second occurrence G3/4 thrombocytopenia		Reduce the dosage to 150 mg/m²	Maintain the dosage at 60 mg/m²	Continue with bolus fluorouracil at 75% of the original dosage and reduce CI by an additional 25–50% of the original dosage
Third occurrence G3/4 thrombocytopenia	Discontinue treatment			
First occurrence G3/4 diarrhea, or diarrhea + fever and/or diarrhea + G3/4 neutropenia		Reduce the dosage to 150 mg/m². Do not re-treat with irinotecan until recovered from diarrhea without loperamide for at least 24 hours	Do not reduce dosage	Delete bolus fluorouracil
Second occurrence G3/4 diarrhea, or diarrhea + fever and/ or diarrhea + G3/4 neutropenia		Maintain the dosage at 150 mg/m². Do not re-treat with irinotecan until recovered from diarrhea without loperamide for at least 24 hours	Reduce the dosage to 60 mg/m²	Continue without bolus fluorouracil and reduce the CI by 25% of the original dosage
Third occurrence G3/4 diarrhea or diarrhea + fever and/or diarrhea + G3/4 neutropenia	Discontinue treatment			
Diarrhea ≥48 hours despite high doses of loperamide	No systematic reduction of the irinotecan, oxaliplatin, or fluorouracil doses after complete recovery, unless G3/4 diarrhea, or diarrhea + fever, and/or concomitant neutropenia G3/4			
G3/4 mucositis or "hand-foot" syndrome		Do not reduce dosage	Do not reduce dosage	Reduce both bolus and CI fluorouracil by 25% of the original dosages
Angina pectoris or myocardial infarction		Do not reduce dosage	Do not reduce dosage	Discontinue fluorouracil
Any toxicity G ≥2, except anemia and alopecia		Consider reducing the dosage to 150 mg/m²	Consider reducing the dosage to 60 mg/m²	Consider reducing both bolus and CI fluorouracil by 25% of the original dosages
Total bilirubin ≥1.5× ULN		Do not administer	Do not reduce dosage	Do not reduce dosage

CI, continuous infusion; ULN, upper limit of normal of laboratory value

Patient Population Studied

Patients with histologically and cytologically confirmed metastatic pancreatic adenocarcinoma not previously treated with chemotherapy. Other inclusion criteria were an Eastern Cooperative Oncology Group (ECOG) performance status score of 0 or 1 and adequate bone marrow, liver function (total bilirubin ≤1.5 times the upper limit of normal range), and renal function. Exclusion criteria included an age ≥76 years and previous radiotherapy for measurable lesions

Patient Characteristics

Age (years)	
Median	61
Range	25–76
Sex—number (%)	
Male	106 (62.0)
Female	65 (38.0)
ECOG performance status score—number (%)	
0	64 (37.4)
1	106 (61.9)
2	(0.6)
Pancreatic tumor location—number (%)	
Head	67 (39.2)
Body	53 (31.0)
Tail	45 (26.3)
Multicentric	6 (3.5)
Biliary stent—number (%)	
Yes	27 (15.8)
No	144 (84.2)
Number of metastatic sites involved	
Median	2
Range	1–6
Number of measurable metastatic sites—number of patients/total number (%)	
Liver	149/170 (87.6)
Pancreas	90/170 (52.9)
Lymph node	49/170 (28.8)
Lung	33/170 (19.4)
Peritoneal	33/170 (19.4)
Other	18/170 (10.6)

Efficacy

Objective Responses in the Intention-to-Treat Population

Variable	FOLFIRINOX* (N = 171)	Gemcitabine (N = 171)	P Value
	Response—Number (%)		
Complete response	1 (0.6)	0	
Partial response	53 (31.0)	16 (9.4)	
Stable disease	66 (38.6)	71 (41.5)	
Progressive disease	26 (15.2)	59 (34.5)	
Could not be evaluated	25 (14.6)	25 (14.6)	
Rate of objective response[†]			<0.001
No. (%)	54 (31.6)	16 (9.4)	
95% CI	24.7–39.1	5.4–14.7	
Rate of disease control[‡]			<0.001
No. (%)	120 (70.2)	87 (50.9)	
95% CI	62.7–76.9	43.1–58.6	
Response duration—months			0.57
Median	5.9	3.9	
95% CI	4.9–7.1	3.1–7.1	

Variable	FOLFIRINOX* (N = 171)	Gemcitabine (N = 171)	HR (95% CI) P Value
Progression-free survival	6.4 months 95% CI, 5.5–7.2	3.3 months 95% CI, 2.2–3.6	0.47 (0.37–0.59) p <0.001
6-month PFS rate	52.8%	17.2%	—
12-month PFS rate	12.1%	3.5%	—
18-month PFS rate	3.3%	0%	—
Overall survival[§]	11.1 months	6.8 months	0.57 (0.45–0.73) p <0.001
6-month OS rate	75.9%	57.6%	—
12-month OS rate	48.4%	20.6%	—
18-month OS rate	18.6%	6.0%	—

95% CI, 95% confidence interval; HR, hazard ratio; OS, overall survival; PFS, progression-free survival
*FOLFIRINOX = oxaliplatin + irinotecan + fluorouracil + leucovorin
[†]Defined as percentage of patients who had a complete response or partial response
[‡]Defined as the percentage of patients who had a complete response, partial response, or stable disease
[§]Synchronous metastases, albumin level <3.5 g/dL (<35 g/L), hepatic metastases, and age >65 years were identified as independent adverse prognostic factors for overall survival

Toxicity

Most Common G3/4 Adverse Events*

Event	FOLFIRINOX (N = 171)	Gemcitabine (N = 171)	P Value
	Number of Patients/Total Number (%)		
Hematologic			
Neutropenia	75/164 (45.7)	35/167 (21.0)	<0.001
Febrile neutropenia	9/166 (5.4)	2/169 (1.2)	0.03
Thrombocytopenia	15/165 (9.1)	6/168 (3.6)	0.04
Anemia	13/166 (7.8)	10/168 (6.0)	NS†
Nonhematologic			
Fatigue	39/165 (23.6)	30/169 (17.8)	NS†
Vomiting	24/166 (14.5)	14/169 (8.3)	NS†
Diarrhea	21/165 (12.7)	3/169 (1.8)	<0.001
Sensory neuropathy	15/166 (9.0)	0/169	<0.001
↑ Alanine aminotransferase	12/165 (7.3)	35/168 (20.8)	<0.001
Thromboembolism	11/166 (6.6)	7/169 (4.1)	NS†

*Events listed are those that occurred in more than 5% of patients in either group
†Not significant
Note: despite the higher incidence of adverse events associated with the FOLFIRINOX regimen, a significant increase in the time to definitive deterioration of the quality of life was observed in the FOLFIRINOX group as compared with the gemcitabine group

Treatment Monitoring

1. *At start of every cycle:* medical history, complete physical examination, CBC with differential and serum electrolytes and LFTs
2. *Weekly:* CBC with differential

METASTATIC • FIRST-LINE

PANCREATIC CANCER REGIMEN: GEMCITABINE MONOTHERAPY

Burris HA et al. J Clin Oncol 1997;15:2403–2413

Gemcitabine 1000 mg/m^2 per dose; administer by intravenous infusion in 50–250 mL 0.9% sodium chloride injection over 30 minutes on days 1, 8, and 15, every 28 days (total dosage/cycle = 3000 mg/m^2)

- In the referenced trial, for the first cycle, patients received gemcitabine 1000 mg/m^2 once weekly for up to 7 weeks. Thereafter, gemcitabine was administered once weekly for 3 consecutive weeks out of every 4 weeks
- Single-agent gemcitabine given at the dose of 1500 mg/m^2 at the rate of 10 mg/min over 150 minutes is an alternative regimen

Tempero M et al. J Clin Oncol 2003;15:3402–3408

Supportive Care
Antiemetic prophylaxis
Emetogenic potential with gemcitabine: **LOW**
See Chapter 42 for antiemetic recommendations

Hematopoietic growth factor (CSF) prophylaxis
Primary prophylaxis is **NOT** *indicated*
See Chapter 43 for more information

Antimicrobial prophylaxis
Risk of fever and neutropenia is **LOW**
  Antimicrobial primary prophylaxis to be considered:
  - Antibacterial—not indicated
  - Antifungal—not indicated
  - Antiviral—not indicated unless patient previously had an episode of HSV

Persistent rash or flulike symptoms after gemcitabine:
Consider dexamethasone 10 mg orally or intravenously before starting gemcitabine

Treatment Modifications

Adverse Events	Treatment Modifications
WBC <1000/mm^3 to 500/mm^3 or platelets <99,000/mm^3 to 50,000/mm^3 on day of treatment	Reduce gemcitabine dosages by 25%
G ≥3 nonhematologic adverse event during the previous treatment cycle	
WBC <500/mm^3 or platelet <50,000/mm^3 on day of treatment	Delay chemotherapy for up to 2 weeks
Treatment delay >2 weeks for recovery from hematologic adverse event	Discontinue treatment

Patient Population Studied

Study of 63 patients with locally advanced or metastatic pancreatic cancer not amenable to curative surgical resection treated with single-agent gemcitabine. Patients who had received previous chemotherapy were not eligible

Efficacy (N = 63)

Median survival	5.65 months
Survival rate at 12 months	18%
Clinical benefit response*	23.8%

*Clinical benefit response (CBR) is a composite measurement of pain, performance status, and weight that was sustained more than 4 weeks in at least 1 parameter without the worsening in any other parameter. The median time to achieve CBR in gemcitabine-treated patients was 7 weeks and duration of benefit was 18 weeks
Note: in this pivotal phase 3 clinical trial, gemcitabine was compared in a randomized fashion with fluorouracil (600 mg/m^2 per week). The median survival in the fluorouracil arm was 4.41 months, survival rate at 12 months was 2%, and clinical benefit response was 4.8%

Adverse Events (N = 63)

WHO Grade (%)	Grade I	Grade II	Grade III	Grade IV
WBC	26	36	10	0
Platelets	16	21	10	0
Hemoglobin	31	24	7	3
Bilirubin	3	10	2	2
Alkaline phosphatase	33	22	16	0
Aspartate transaminase	41	20	10	1.6
BUN	8	0	0	0
Creatinine	2	0	0	0
Diarrhea	18	5	2	0
Constipation	5	2	3	0
Pain	2	6	2	0
Fever	22	8	0	0
Infection	5	3	0	0
Pulmonary	3	3	0	0
Hair	16	2	0	0
Proteinuria	10	0	0	0
Hematuria	12.7	0	0	0
Nausea/ vomiting	29	22	10	3

Therapy Monitoring

1. *Every week:* CBC with differential
2. *Before each cycle:* CBC with differential, serum electrolytes, creatinine, mineral panel, and LFT
3. *Response assessment:* CT scans every 2 months and CA19–9 monthly

METASTATIC • SUBSEQUENT THERAPY

PANCREATIC CANCER REGIMEN: LIPOSOMAL IRINOTECAN + FLUOROURACIL + LEUCOVORIN

Wang-Gillam A et al. Lancet 2016;387:545–557
Supplementary appendix to: Wang-Gillam A et al. Lancet 2016;387:545–557

Premedication for irinotecan liposome injection:

Dexamethasone 8 mg (or equivalent corticosteroid); administer orally or intravenously 30 minutes prior to irinotecan liposome injection on day 1, every 2 weeks, until disease progression

Irinotecan liposome injection 70 mg/m^2; administer intravenously over 90 minutes in 500 mL 0.9% sodium chloride (0.9% NS) or 5% dextrose injection (D5W) on day 1, every 2 weeks, until disease progression (total dosage/2-week cycle = 70 mg/m^2), *followed by:*

Notes:
- In addition to dexamethasone, another antiemetic medication should be given prior to irinotecan liposomal injection (see antiemetic prophylaxis section).
- Allow diluted solution to come to room temperature prior to administration, protect diluted solution from light, and avoid use of an in-line filter for administration
- Liposomal irinotecan is not interchangeable with other drugs containing irinotecan
- **Patients known to be homozygous for UGT1A1*28 should be treated with a starting liposomal irinotecan dosage of 50 mg/m^2.** If the patient tolerates the initial dose without G ≥2 toxicity, then consider escalating the dosage to 70 mg/m^2 in subsequent cycles

Leucovorin calcium 400 mg/m^2; administer intravenously over 30 minutes in 25–500 mL 0.9% NS or D5W on day 1, every 2 weeks, until disease progression (total dosage/2-week cycle = 400 mg/m^2), *followed by:*

Fluorouracil 2400 mg/m^2; administer by continuous intravenous infusion over 46 hours in 100–1000 mL 0.9% NS or D5W, starting on day 1, every 2 weeks, until disease progression (total dosage/2-week cycle = 2400 mg/m^2)

Supportive Care
Antiemetic prophylaxis
Emetogenic potential on day 1 is **MODERATE**
Emetogenic potential on day 2 is **LOW**
See Chapter 42 for antiemetic recommendations

Hematopoietic growth factor (CSF) prophylaxis
Primary prophylaxis is **NOT** indicated
See Chapter 43 for more information

Antimicrobial prophylaxis
Risk of fever and neutropenia is **LOW**
  Antimicrobial primary prophylaxis to be CONSIDERED:
  - *Antibacterial—not indicated*
  - *Antifungal—not indicated*
  - *Antiviral—not indicated unless patient previously had an episode of HSV*

Acute cholinergic syndrome
Atropine sulfate 0.25—1 mg administer subcutaneously or intravenously if abdominal cramping or diarrhea develop during or within 1 hour after irinotecan liposome injection administration
- If symptoms are severe, add as primary prophylaxis at least 30 min before irinotecan liposome injection during subsequent cycles
- For irinotecan liposome injection, acute cholinergic syndrome may be characterized by: abdominal cramping, diarrhea, diaphoresis, hypotension, flushing, bradycardia, rhinitis, increased salivation, meiosis, and lacrimation

Diarrhea management
Latent or delayed-onset diarrhea*:
  Loperamide 4 mg orally initially after the first loose or liquid stool, *then*
  Loperamide 2 mg orally every 2 hours during waking hours, *plus*
  Loperamide 4 mg orally every 4 hours during hours of sleep
  - Continue for at least 12 hours after diarrhea resolves
  - Recurrent diarrhea after a 12-hour diarrhea-free interval is treated as a new episode
  - Rehydrate orally with fluids and electrolytes during a diarrheal episode
  - If diarrhea persists >48 hours despite loperamide, stop loperamide and hospitalize the patient for IV hydration

Persistent diarrhea:
  Octreotide 100–150 mcg subcutaneously 3 times daily. Maximum total daily dose is 1500 mcg

(*continued*)

Antibiotic therapy during latent or delayed-onset diarrhea:

A fluoroquinolone (eg, **ciprofloxacin** 500 mg orally every 12 hours) if absolute neutrophil count is <500/mm³ with or without accompanying fever in association with diarrhea
- Antibiotics should also be administered if patient is hospitalized with prolonged diarrhea and should be continued until diarrhea resolves

Oral care
Prophylaxis and treatment for mucositis/stomatitis

Oral care
Prophylaxis and treatment for mucositis/stomatitis
General advice:
- Encourage patients to maintain intake of nonalcoholic fluids
- Evaluate patients for oral pain and provide analgesic medications
- Consider histamine (H$_2$-subtype) receptor antagonists (eg, ranitidine, famotidine), or a proton pump inhibitor for epigastric pain
- *Lactobacillus* sp.—containing probiotics may be beneficial in preventing diarrhea

Patients with intact oral mucosa:
- Clean the mouth, tongue, and gums by brushing after every meal and at bedtime with an ultra-soft toothbrush with fluoride toothpaste
- Floss teeth gently every day unless contraindicated. If gums bleed and hurt, avoid bleeding or sore areas, but floss other teeth
- Patients may use saline or commercial bland, nonalcoholic rinses
  - Do not use mouthwashes that contain alcohols

If mucositis or stomatitis is present:
- Keep the mouth moist utilizing water, ice chips, sugarless gum, sugar-free hard candies, or a saliva substitute
- Rinse mouth several times a day to remove debris
  - Use a solution of ¼ teaspoon (1.25 g) each of baking soda and table salt (sodium chloride) in 1 quart (~950 mL) of warm water. Follow with a plain water rinse
  - Do not use mouthwashes that contain alcohols
- Foam-tipped swabs (eg, Toothettes) are useful in moisturizing oral mucosa, but ineffective for cleansing teeth and removing plaque
- Advise patients who develop mucositis to:
  - Choose foods that are easy to chew and swallow
  - Take small bites of food, chew slowly, and sip liquids with meals
  - Encourage soft, moist foods such as cooked cereals, mashed potatoes, and scrambled eggs
  - For trouble swallowing, soften food with gravies, sauces, broths, yogurt, or other bland liquids
  - Avoid sharp, crunchy foods; hot, spicy, or highly acidic foods (eg, citrus fruits and juices); sugary foods; toothpicks; tobacco products; alcoholic drinks

Hand-foot reaction (palmar-plantar erythrodysesthesia, PPE)
For patients who develop a hand-foot reaction, use topical emollients (eg, Aquaphor), topical or orally administered steroids, antihistamine agents (H$_1$-receptor antagonists), or pyridoxine

Pyridoxine may provide relief for discomfort/pain associated with PPE although the mechanism through which this occurs remains unclear
- The suggested pyridoxine starting dose is 50 mg/day, which may be increased to a maximum of 200 mg/day

Treatment Modifications

LIPOSOMAL IRINOTECAN + FLUOROURACIL + LEUCOVORIN DOSE MODIFICATIONS

	Dose Level +1	Initial Dose Level	Dose Level −1	Dose Level −2
Liposomal irinotecan (patients not known to be homozygous for UGT1A1*28)	Not applicable	70 mg/m²	50 mg/m²	43 mg/m²
Liposomal irinotecan (patients known to be homozygous for UGT1A1*28)	70 mg/m²	50 mg/m²	43 mg/m²	35 mg/m²
Infusional fluorouracil	2400 mg/m²		1800 mg/m²	1350 mg/m²

(*continued*)

Treatment Modifications (*continued*)

Notes:
- There are no dose reductions for leucovorin with this regimen
- Before beginning a treatment cycle, patients should have baseline bowel function (similar to that before the start of treatment) without antidiarrheal therapy for 24 hours, ANC ≥1500/mm³, and platelet count ≥100,000/mm³
- Treatment should be delayed 1–2 weeks to allow for recovery from treatment-related toxicities. If a patient has not recovered after 2 weeks, consider stopping therapy
- If toxicity occurs despite 2 dose reductions (ie, on Dose Level –2), discontinue therapy
- If fluorouracil is discontinued, then also discontinue leucovorin and liposomal irinotecan
- If liposomal irinotecan is discontinued, then treatment with fluorouracil + leucovorin may be continued at the discretion of the medically responsible health care provider
- Dose modifications are based on the National Cancer Institute Common Terminology Criteria for Adverse Events v4.0. At: http://ctep.cancer.gov/protocolDevelopment/electronic_applications/ctc.htm [accessed May 31, 2019]

Adverse Event	Treatment Modification for Liposomal Irinotecan and Fluorouracil
Neutropenia/Thrombocytopenia	
G ≥3 neutropenia (ANC <1000/mm³) at any time	Reduce the dosage of liposomal irinotecan and fluorouracil by 1 dosage level in subsequent cycles. Consider adding filgrastim prophylaxis in subsequent cycles
Febrile neutropenia (ANC <500/mm³ with single temperature >38.3°C [101°F] or a temperature of ≥38°C [100.4°F] sustained for ≥1 hour)	
Gastrointestinal Toxicities	
Patient with bowel obstruction	Withhold all therapy until complete recovery of bowel function
G2 diarrhea (4–6 stools/day > baseline; moderate increase in ostomy output over baseline)	Withhold all therapy until diarrhea has improved to baseline without the need for antidiarrheal therapy for at least 24 hours. Administer atropine for early-onset (≤24 hours) diarrhea or loperamide for late-onset (>24 hours) diarrhea as described in the therapy administration section. Do not modify the doses of liposomal irinotecan or fluorouracil in subsequent cycles
G ≥3 diarrhea (≥7 stools/day > baseline; incontinence; hospitalization indicated; severe increase in ostomy output over baseline; limiting self-care ADLs; or worse)	Withhold all therapy until diarrhea has improved to baseline without the need for antidiarrheal therapy for at least 24 hours. Administer atropine for early-onset (≤24 hours) diarrhea or loperamide for late-onset (>24 hours) as described in the therapy administration section. Reduce the dosages of liposomal irinotecan and fluorouracil by 1 dose level in subsequent cycles
Pulmonary Toxicity	
Patient with new or worsening cough, dyspnea, and/or fever—interstitial lung disease is suspected	Withhold all therapy until pulmonary status is clarified
Interstitial lung disease possibly related to liposomal irinotecan is confirmed	Permanently discontinue liposomal irinotecan. At the discretion of the medically responsible health care provider, either consider alternative therapy or continue treatment with leucovorin and fluorouracil at the same dosages
Hepatic Impairment	
Serum bilirubin >ULN	No dose recommendations for liposomal irinotecan are available. Do not administer fluorouracil if the total bilirubin is >5 mg/dL
Drug-Drug Interactions	
Patient is receiving a strong CYP3A4 inducer (eg, rifampin, phenytoin, carbamazepine, rifabutin, phenobarbital, St. John's Wort)	If possible, substitute an appropriate non-enzyme-inducing medication for the strong CYP3A4 inducer ≥2 weeks prior to initiation of liposomal irinotecan
Patient is receiving a strong CYP3A4 inhibitor (eg, clarithromycin, indinavir, itraconazole, lopinavir, nefazodone, nelfinavir, ritonavir, saquinavir, telaprevir, voriconazole)	If possible, discontinue the strong CYP3A4 inhibitor at least 1 week prior to initiation of liposomal irinotecan

(*continu*

Treatment Modifications (*continued*)

Adverse Event	Treatment Modification for Liposomal Irinotecan and Fluorouracil
Patient is receiving a strong UGT1A1 inhibitor (eg, atazanavir, gemfibrozil, indinavir)	If possible, discontinue the strong UGT1A1 inhibitor prior to initiation of liposomal irinotecan
Patient is receiving anticoagulation with warfarin	Fluorouracil may increase the international normalized ratio (INR). Warfarin dose requirements may be unpredictable. Consider an alternative anticoagulant, when feasible. Otherwise, consider more frequent monitoring of the INR
Pharmacogenomics	
Patient is homozygous for UGT1A1*28 and completed the initial cycle of liposomal irinotecan at a starting dose of 50 mg/m² without experiencing any G ≥2 toxicity	Increase the dose of liposomal irinotecan by 1 dosage level (ie, to 70 mg/m²) in subsequent cycles
Other Nonhematologic Toxicities	
Patient experiences cardiac toxicity (eg, coronary vasospasm) related to fluorouracil	Discontinue all therapy
Anaphylactic reaction to liposomal irinotecan	Permanently discontinue liposomal irinotecan. At the discretion of the medically responsible health care provider, either consider alternative therapy or continue treatment with leucovorin and fluorouracil at the same dosages
Other nonhematologic G ≥3 toxicity	Withhold all treatment until toxicity resolves to G ≤1, then reduce the dosages of liposomal irinotecan and fluorouracil by 1 dosage level

ANC, absolute neutrophil count; ADL, activities of daily living; ULN, upper limit of normal

Patient Population Studied

This international, multicenter, open-label, phase 3 study involved 417 patients with histologically or cytologically confirmed metastatic pancreatic ductal adenocarcinoma which had progressed following gemcitabine-based therapy. Patients were required to have a Karnofsky performance status ≥70, absolute neutrophil count >1,500/mm³, total bilirubin ≤ upper limit of normal, serum albumin ≥3.0 g/dL, and normal renal function. Patients who had received prior irinotecan and/or fluorouracil were allowed. The first 63 patients were randomized 1:1 to treatment with either single-agent liposomal irinotecan or fluorouracil + leucovorin, administered until disease progression. Following a protocol amendment, a third arm was added containing liposomal irinotecan + fluorouracil + leucovorin. Results will be presented for the liposomal irinotecan + fluorouracil + leucovorin arm and the fluorouracil + leucovorin arm only

Characteristics	Nanoliposomal Irinotecan Plus Fluorouracil and Folinic Acid Combination Therapy (n = 117)	Fluorouracil and Folinic Acid used as Combination Therapy Control (n = 119*)	Nanoliposomal Irinotecan Monotherapy (n = 151)	Fluorouracil and Folinic Acid used as Monotherapy Control (n = 149)
Men	69 (59%)	67 (56%)	87 (58%)	81 (54%)
Women	48 (41%)	52 (44%)	64 (42%)	68 (46%)
Age (years)	63 (57–70)	62 (55–69)	65 (58–70)	63 (55–69)
Ethnic origin				
East Asian	34 (29%)	36 (30%)	52 (34%)	50 (34%)
Black or AA	4 (3%)	3 (3%)	3 (2%)	3 (2%)
White	72 (62%)	76 (64%)	89 (59%)	92 (62%)
Other	7 (6%)	4 (3%)	7 (5%)	4 (3%)
Karnofsky performance status score†				
100	18 (15%)	17 (14%)	22 (15%)	22 (15%)

(*continued*)

Patient Population Studied (continued)

Characteristics	Nanoliposomal Irinotecan Plus Fluorouracil and Folinic Acid Combination Therapy (n = 117)	Fluorouracil and Folinic Acid used as Combination Therapy Control (n = 119*)	Nanoliposomal Irinotecan Monotherapy (n = 151)	Fluorouracil and Folinic Acid used as Monotherapy Control (n = 149)
90	51 (44%)	40 (34%)	64 (42%)	54 (36%)
80	38 (32%)	51 (43%)	50 (33%)	61 (41%)
70	7 (6%)	10 (8%)	15 (10%)	11 (7%)
50–60	3 (3%)	0	0	0
Pancreatic tumor location				
Head	76 (65%)	69 (58%)	99 (66%)	81 (54%)
Other	41 (35%)	50 (42%)	52 (34%)	68 (46%)
Amount of CA19–9¥				
≥40 U/mL	92/114 (81%)	91/114 (80%)	125/146 (86%)	116/144 (81%)
<40 U/mL	22/114 (19%)	23/114 (20%)	21/146 (14%)	28/144 (39%)
Site of metastatic lesions‡				
Liver	75 (64%)	83 (70%)	101 (67%)	108 (72%)
Lung	36 (31%)	36 (30%)	49 (32%)	44 (30%)
Lymph node, distant	32 (27%)	31 (26%)	44 (29%)	40 (27%)
Lymph node, regional	13 (11%)	14 (12%)	19 (13%)	20 (13%)
Pancreas	75 (64%)	72 (61%)	99 (66%)	97 (65%)
Peritoneum	28 (24%)	32 (27%)	48 (32%)	39 (26%)
Other	27 (23%)	39 (33%)	38 (25%)	48 (32%)
Measurable metastatic sites (n)				
1	19 (16%)	22 (18%)	36 (24%)	26 (17%)
2	49 (42%)	58 (49%)	63 (42%)	72 (48%)
3	22 (19%)	15 (13%)	22 (15%)	21 (14%)
≥4	7 (6%)	8 (7%)	7 (5%)	10 (7%)
Previous therapies or procedures				
Radiotherapy	24 (21%)	27 (23%)	40 (26%)	33 (22%)
Whipple procedure	30 (26%)	33 (28%)	47 (31%)	36 (24%)
Biliary stent	15 (13%)	8 (7%)	13 (9%)	9 (6%)
Previous lines of metastatic therapy				
0ϵ	15 (13%)	15 (13%)	17 (11%)	19 (13%)
1	62 (53%)	67 (56%)	86 (57%)	86 (58%)
≥2	40 (34%)	37 (31%)	48 (32%)	44 (30%)

(continued`

Patient Population Studied (continued)

Characteristics	Nanoliposomal Irinotecan Plus Fluorouracil and Folinic Acid Combination Therapy (n = 117)	Fluorouracil and Folinic Acid used as Combination Therapy Control (n = 119*)	Nanoliposomal Irinotecan Monotherapy (n = 151)	Fluorouracil and Folinic Acid used as Monotherapy Control (n = 149)
Previous anticancer therapy‖				
Gemcitabine alone	53 (45%)	55 (46%)	67 (44%)	66 (44%)
Gemcitabine combination	64 (55%)	64 (54%)	84 (56%)	83 (56%)
Fluorouracil based	50 (43%)	52 (44%)	70 (46%)	63 (42%)
Irinotecan based	12 (10%)	17 (14%)	17 (11%)	17 (11%)
Platinum based	38 (32%)	41 (34%)	54 (36%)	45 (30%)

CA19–9, carbohydrate antigen 19–9.
Note: data are number of patients (%) or median (IQR). Some patients had multiple metastatic sites and are listed in more than one group
*Fluorouracil and folinic acid combination control group randomized and accrued as one of the three treatment arms during protocol version 2, when the nanoliposomal irinotecan plus fluorouracil and folinic acid arm (n=117) was accruing.
†Baseline Karnofsky performance status score was missing for one patient in the fluorouracil and folinic acid group (enrolled under protocol 2) who was subsequently stratified as having a score ≥90
‡Data were missing for three patients in the nanoliposomal irinotecan plus fluorouracil and folinic acid group and in five patients each in the nanoliposomal irinotecan monotherapy and fluorouracil and folinic acid groups (enrolled under protocol 2)
¥Investigator-reported with review by the funder's medical team
ᵉPatients received neoadjuvant, adjuvant, or locally advanced treatment, but no previous therapy for metastatic disease
‖Columns add up to greater than 100% because some patients received more than one line of therapy and are listed in more than one group, and regimens might include multiple drug classes, but at least one gemcitabine based

Efficacy (N = 236)

	Liposomal Irinotecan + Fluorouracil + Leucovorin (n = 117)	Fluorouracil + Leucovorin (n = 119)	
Median overall survival*	6.1 months (95% CI, 4.8–8.9)	4.2 months (95% CI, 3.3–5.3)	HR 0.67 (95% CI, 0.49–0.92), P = 0.012
Median progression-free survival*	3.1 months (95% CI, 2.7–4.2)	1.5 months (95% CI, 1.4–1.8)	HR 0.56 (95% CI, 0.41–0.75), P = 0.0001
Objective response rate† (%)	16%	1%	P<0.0001

*Analysis performed after a total of 313 deaths had occurred
†According to RECIST v1.1

Adverse Events (N = 251)

Grade 3 or 4 neutropenic sepsis or neutropenic fever occurred in 3 patients (3%) in the liposomal irinotecan + fluorouracil + leucovorin arm as compared to zero patients in the fluorouracil + leucovorin arm. Twenty patients (17%) in the liposomal irinotecan + fluorouracil + leucovorin arm received treatment with granulocyte colony-stimulating factors compared to 1 patient (1%) in the fluorouracil + leucovorin arm. One treatment-related fatal adverse event occurred in a patient receiving liposomal irinotecan + fluorouracil + leucovorin (septic shock) compared to 0 events in the fluorouracil + leucovorin arm

(continued)

Adverse Events (N = 251) *(continued)*

Grade (%)*	Liposomal Irinotecan + Fluorouracil + Leucovorin		Fluorouracil + Leucovorin	
	Grade 1–2	Grade 3–4	Grade 1–2	Grade 3–4
Diarrhea	46	13	22	4
Vomiting	41	11	23	3
Nausea	44	8	31	3
Decreased appetite	40	4	30	2
Fatigue	26	14	24	4
Neutropenia	12	27	4	1
Anemia	28	9	16	7
Hypokalemia	9	3	7	2

The table includes G3/4 adverse events reported in at least 5% of patients who received liposomal irinotecan with at least a 2% higher incidence compared to patients receiving fluorouracil + leucovorin

Therapy Monitoring

1. *Before each cycle:* history and physical examination
2. Serum bilirubin, AST or ALT, alkaline phosphatase, serum chemistries, electrolytes prior to each cycle
3. CBC with differential and platelet count on day 1 and day 8 of each cycle
4. CA 19–9 and/or CEA prior to each cycle if detectable and being used to monitor disease
5. Where available, consider genotyping for UGT1A1 prior to therapy; patients who are homozygous for the UGT1A1*28 allele may be at higher risk for toxicity related to liposomal irinotecan and should initiate therapy at a lower dosage
6. *Monitor for signs and symptoms of:* diarrhea (liposomal irinotecan), infection (liposomal irinotecan and fluorouracil), nausea/vomiting (liposomal irinotecan), dehydration (liposomal irinotecan and fluorouracil), hypersensitivity reaction (liposomal irinotecan), interstitial lung disease (liposomal irinotecan), coronary vasospasm (fluorouracil), palmar-plantar erythrodysesthesia (fluorouracil), mucositis (liposomal irinotecan and fluorouracil)
7. Population pharmacokinetic data suggest that Asian patients have 56% lower total irinotecan average steady state concentration and 8% higher total SN–38 (active metabolite) average steady state concentration than White patients. Correspondingly, higher rates of G ≥3 neutropenia were observed in Asian patients (18/33, 55%) compared to White patients (13/73, 18%) and higher rates of neutropenia or neutropenic sepsis were observed in Asian patients (6%) compared to White patients (1%)
8. *Every 1–3 months:* CT scans to assess response, CA 19–9 if being used to monitor disease

METASTATIC • SUBSEQUENT THERAPY
PANCREATIC CANCER REGIMEN: FOLFOX

Zaanan et al. BMC Cancer 2014;14:441

Oxaliplatin 85 mg/m^2; administer intravenously over 2 hours in 500 mL 5% dextrose injection (D5W) on day 1, every 2 weeks, concurrently with leucovorin (or levoleucovorin) administration, until disease progression (total dosage/2-week cycle = 85 mg/m^2)
Note: oxaliplatin must not be mixed with sodium chloride injection. Therefore, when leucovorin and oxaliplatin are given concurrently via the same administration set tubing, both drugs must be administered in D5W

Plus either: **(racemic) leucovorin calcium** 400 mg/m^2 *or* **levoleucovorin calcium** 200 mg/m^2; administer intravenously over 2 hours in 25–500 mL D5W on day 1, every 2 weeks, concurrently with oxaliplatin, until disease progression (total dosage/2-week cycle for racemic leucovorin = 400 mg/m^2, for levoleucovorin = 200 mg/m^2), *followed by:*

Fluorouracil 400 mg/m^2; administer by intravenous injection over 1–2 minutes after leucovorin (or levoleucovorin) on day 1, every 2 weeks, until disease progression, *followed by:*
Note: the fluorouracil bolus dose (400 mg/m^2) can be omitted for better hematologic tolerance

Fluorouracil 2400 mg/m^2; administer by continuous intravenous infusion over 46 hours in 100–1000 mL 0.9% sodium chloride injection (0.9% NS) or D5W, starting on day 1 every 2 weeks, until disease progression (total fluorouracil dosage/2-week cycle = 2800 mg/m^2)

Supportive Care
Antiemetic prophylaxis
Emetogenic potential on day 1 is **MODERATE**
Emetogenic potential on day 2 is **LOW**
See Chapter 42 for antiemetic recommendations

Hematopoietic growth factor (G-CSF) prophylaxis
Primary prophylaxis is **NOT** *indicated*
See Chapter 43 for more information

Antimicrobial prophylaxis
Risk of fever and neutropenia is **LOW**
   Antimicrobial primary prophylaxis to be considered:
- *Antibacterial—not indicated*
- *Antifungal—not indicated*
- *Antiviral—not indicated unless patient previously had an episode of HSV*

Diarrhea management
Latent or delayed-onset diarrhea*:
   Loperamide 4 mg orally initially after the first loose or liquid stool, *then*
   Loperamide 2 mg orally every 2 hours during waking hours, *plus*
   Loperamide 4 mg orally every 4 hours during hours of sleep
- Continue for at least 12 hours after diarrhea resolves
- Recurrent diarrhea after a 12-hour diarrhea-free interval is treated as a new episode
- Rehydrate orally with fluids and electrolytes during a diarrheal episode
- If a patient develops blood or mucus in stool, dehydration, or hemodynamic instability, or if diarrhea persists >48 hours despite loperamide, stop loperamide and hospitalize the patient for IV hydration

   Alternatively, a trial of **diphenoxylate hydrochloride** 2.5 mg with **atropine sulfate** 0.025 mg (eg, Lomotil)
- Initial adult dose is 2 tablets 4 times daily until control has been achieved, after which the dose may be reduced to meet individual requirements. Control may often be maintained with as little as 2 tablets daily
- Clinical improvement of acute diarrhea is usually observed within 48 hours. If improvement of chronic diarrhea after treatment with a maximum daily dose of 8 tablets is not observed within 10 days, control is unlikely with further administration

Persistent diarrhea:
   Octreotide 100–150 mcg subcutaneously 3 times daily. Maximum total daily dose is 1500 mcg
Antibiotic therapy during latent or delayed-onset diarrhea:
A fluoroquinolone (eg, **ciprofloxacin** 500 mg orally every 12 hours) if absolute neutrophil count <500/mm^3 with or without accompanying fever in association with diarrhea
- Antibiotics should also be administered if patient is hospitalized with prolonged diarrhea and should be continued until diarrhea resolves

Oral care
Prophylaxis and treatment for mucositis/stomatitis

(continued)

(continued)

General advice:
- Encourage patients to maintain intake of nonalcoholic fluids
- Evaluate patients for oral pain and provide analgesic medications
- Consider histamine (H_2-subtype) receptor antagonists (eg, ranitidine, famotidine), or a proton pump inhibitor for epigastric pain
- *Lactobacillus* sp.–containing probiotics may be beneficial in preventing diarrhea

Patients with intact oral mucosa:
- Clean the mouth, tongue, and gums by brushing after every meal and at bedtime with an ultra-soft toothbrush with fluoride toothpaste
- Floss teeth gently every day unless contraindicated. If gums bleed and hurt, avoid bleeding or sore areas, but floss other teeth
- Patients may use saline or commercial bland, nonalcoholic rinses
  - Do not use mouthwashes that contain alcohols

If mucositis or stomatitis is present:
- Keep the mouth moist utilizing water, ice chips, sugarless gum, sugar-free hard candies, or a saliva substitute
- Rinse mouth several times a day to remove debris
  - Use a solution of ¼ teaspoon (1.25 g) each of baking soda and table salt (sodium chloride) in 1 quart (~950 mL) of warm water. Follow with a plain water rinse
  - Do not use mouthwashes that contain alcohols
- Foam-tipped swabs (eg, Toothettes) are useful in moisturizing oral mucosa, but ineffective for cleansing teeth and removing plaque
- Advise patients who develop mucositis to:
  - Choose foods that are easy to chew and swallow
  - Take small bites of food, chew slowly, and sip liquids with meals
  - Encourage soft, moist foods such as cooked cereals, mashed potatoes, and scrambled eggs
  - For trouble swallowing, soften food with gravies, sauces, broths, yogurt, or other bland liquids
  - Avoid sharp, crunchy foods; hot, spicy, or highly acidic foods (eg, citrus fruits and juices); sugary foods; toothpicks; tobacco products; alcoholic drinks

Treatment Modifications

Treatment Modifications (FOLFOX)	
Adverse Event	**Treatment Modification**

Notes:
- Before beginning a treatment cycle, patients should have baseline bowel function (similar to that before the start of treatment) without antidiarrheal therapy for 24 hours, ANC ≥1500/mm³, and platelet count ≥100,000/mm³
- Treatment should be delayed 1–2 weeks to allow for recovery from treatment-related toxicities. If toxicities have not resolved after 2 weeks, consider stopping therapy
- Dose modifications are based on the National Cancer Institute (USA) Common Toxicity Criteria V5.0. At: http://ctep.cancer.gov/protocolDevelopment/electronic_applications/ctc.htm

Neutropenia/Thrombocytopenia	
G1 ANC (1500–1999/mm³) or G1 thrombocytopenia (<LLN–75,000/mm³)	Maintain dose and schedule
G2 ANC (1000–1499/mm³) or G2 thrombocytopenia (<75,000–50,000/mm³)	Reduce oxaliplatin dosage to 70 mg/m² and fluorouracil by intravenous bolus injection to 300 mg/m²
G3 ANC (500–999/mm³) or G3 thrombocytopenia (<50,000–25,000/mm³)	Hold treatment until toxicity resolves to G ≤2, then reduce oxaliplatin dosage to 70 mg/m² and omit fluorouracil by intravenous bolus injection in subsequent cycles
G4 ANC (<500/mm³) or G4 thrombocytopenia (<25,000/mm³)	Hold treatment until toxicity resolves to G ≤2, then reduce oxaliplatin dosage to 60–70 mg/m², reduce infusional fluorouracil to 2000 mg/m² and omit fluorouracil by intravenous bolus injection in subsequent cycles
Febrile neutropenia (ANC <1000/mm³ with single temperature >38.3°C [101°F] or a sustained temperature of ≥38°C [100.4°F] for more than 1 hour)	Hold treatment until neutropenia resolves, then reduce oxaliplatin dosage to 60–70 mg/m², reduce infusional fluorouracil to 2000 mg/m², and omit fluorouracil by intravenous bolus injection in subsequent cycles

(continued)

Treatment Modifications (*continued*)

Adverse Event	Treatment Modification
Day 1 ANC ≤1500/mm^3 *or* platelet count ≤100,000/mm^3	Delay start of next cycle until ANC >1500/mm^3 *and* platelet count >100,000/mm^3; omit fluorouracil by intravenous bolus injection in subsequent cycles

Diarrhea

Notes: before beginning a treatment cycle, patients should have baseline bowel function (similar to that before the start of treatment) without antidiarrheal therapy for 24 hours

G1 (2–3 stools/day > baseline)	Maintain dose and schedule
G2 (4–6 stools/day > baseline)	Delay until diarrhea resolves to baseline, then reduce oxaliplatin dosage to 70 mg/m^2 and fluorouracil by intravenous bolus injection to 300 mg/m^2
G3 (7–9 stools/day > baseline)	Delay until diarrhea resolves to baseline, then reduce oxaliplatin dosage to 60–70 mg/m^2, infusional fluorouracil to 1600–2000 mg/m^2, and omit fluorouracil by intravenous bolus injection
G4 (≥10 stools/day > baseline; life-threatening; urgent intervention required)	Delay until diarrhea resolves to baseline, then reduce oxaliplatin dosage to 60 mg/m^2, infusional fluorouracil to 1600 mg/m^2, and omit fluorouracil by intravenous bolus injection

Other Nonhematologic Toxicities

Day 1 persistent nonhematologic toxicity G ≥2	Delay start of next cycle until the severity of all toxicities is G ≤1; omit fluorouracil by intravenous bolus injection in subsequent cycles
G ≥3 non-neurologic toxicity	Reduce infusional fluorouracil dosage to 2000 mg/m^2
G2 paresthesia (persistent paresthesia or dysesthesia, moderate in nature without functional impairment other than limiting instrumental ADL)	Reduce oxaliplatin dosage to 60–70 mg/m^2
Persistent G2 paresthesia/dysesthesia	Discontinue oxaliplatin
Persistent painful paresthesia or G3 neuropathy (persistent paresthesia or dysesthesia with persistent functional impairment limiting self-care and ADL)	

Adapted from Tournigand C et al. J Clin Oncol 2004;22:229–237

Patient Population Studied

This was a prospective observational cohort study involving all consecutive patients with metastatic pancreatic cancer enrolled in the FIRGEM trial (Trouilloud I et al. Ann Oncol 2012. Abstract 710P) who subsequently received second-line chemotherapy with FOLFOX (n = 27). During the FIRGEM portion of the study, patients had previously either undergone first-line treatment with FOLFIRI–3 alternating with gemcitabine (n = 7) or gemcitabine monotherapy (n = 20)

Efficacy (N = 27)

Complete response rate*	0%
Partial response rate*	0%
Stable disease rate*	36.4%
Median progression free survival	1.7 months (95% CI, 1.0–2.5)
Median overall survival	4.3 months (95% CI, 2.2–5.9)
6-month overall survival rate	25.9% (95% CI, 11.5–43.1)
12-month overall survival rate	18.5% (95% CI, 6.8–34.8)

*Tumor response rates were only evaluable in 22 patients; patients were excluded due to early death (n = 4) and due to dose-limiting toxicity (n = 1) after 2 cycles. These patients are included in the above overall survival analyses

Adverse Events (N = 27)

	Grade 1–2 Event* (%)	Grade 3 Event*† (%)
Anemia	56%	7%
Thrombocytopenia	48%	11%
Neutropenia	19%	7%
Neutropenic fever	Not applicable	0%
Nausea/vomiting	59%	0%
Sensory neuropathy	44%	7%
Asthenia	67%	15%
Diarrhea	37%	0%
Mucositis	11%	0%

*According to the National Cancer Institute Common Toxicity Criteria for Adverse Events, version 3.0
†No patients experienced Grade 4 toxicity. No patients died from neutropenic fever or sepsis

Therapy Monitoring

1. *Before each cycle:* history and physical examination with attention to neurologic exam
2. CBC with differential at a minimum once per cycle, but initially also at day 10–14
3. Serum bilirubin, AST, ALT, and alkaline phosphatase prior to each cycle
4. CA 19–9 and/or CEA prior to each cycle if detectable and being used to monitor disease
5. *Every 2–3 months:* CT scans to assess response

METASTATIC • SUBSEQUENT THERAPY

PANCREATIC CANCER REGIMEN: GEMCITABINE + CISPLATIN

O'Reilly EM et al. J Clin Oncol 2020;38:1378–1388
Lundberg J et al. Med Oncol 2016;33:4
Ouyang G et al. World J Surg Oncol 2016;14:59
Palmer DH et al. Ann Surg Oncol 2007;14:2088–2096
Valle J et al. N Engl J Med 2010;362:1273–1281

Hydration before cisplatin: ≥1000 mL 0.9% sodium chloride injection (0.9% NS); administer by intravenous infusion over ≥1 hour
Cisplatin 25 mg/m² per dose; administer intravenously in 50–1000 mL 0.9% NS over 1 hour for 2 doses on days 1 and 8, every 3 weeks for 4 cycles (total dosage/3-week cycle = 50 mg/m²), *followed by:*
Hydration after cisplatin: ≥1000 mL 0.9% NS; administer by intravenous infusion over ≥1 hour
Gemcitabine 1000 mg/m² per dose; administer intravenously in 50–250 mL 0.9% NS over 30 minutes for 2 doses on days 1 and 8, every 3 weeks, for 4 cycles (total dosage/3-week cycle = 2000 mg/m²)

• Gemcitabine may be administered concurrently with hydration after cisplatin administration is completed

Note: in the absence of disease progression at 12 weeks, treatment with the same regimen may continue for an additional 12 weeks

Supportive Care
Antiemetic prophylaxis
Emetogenic potential is **HIGH**. Potential for delayed symptoms
See Chapter 42 for antiemetic recommendations

Hematopoietic growth factor (CSF) prophylaxis
Primary prophylaxis is **NOT** *indicated*
See Chapter 43 for more information

Antimicrobial prophylaxis
Risk of fever and neutropenia is **LOW**
  Antimicrobial primary prophylaxis to be considered:
• Antibacterial—not indicated
• Antifungal—not indicated
• Antiviral—not indicated, unless patient previously had an episode of HSV

Treatment Modifications

Adverse Event	Dose Modification
Any G3 adverse event including hematologic toxicity, abnormal renal function, nausea, vomiting, edema, or tinnitus	Decrease cisplatin dosage by 25%
Reduction in creatinine clearance* to 60% of on study value	Delay therapy 1 week. If creatinine clearance does not recover to pretreatment values, then consider reducing cisplatin dose
Creatinine clearance* 40–60 mL/min (0.66–1 mL/s)	Decrease cisplatin dosage by 25%†
Creatinine clearance* <40 mL/min (<0.66 mL/s)	Hold cisplatin
Clinically significant ototoxicity	Discontinue cisplatin
Persistent (>14 days) peripheral neuropathy without functional impairment	Decrease cisplatin dosage by 50%
Clinically significant sensory loss—persistent (>14 days) peripheral neuropathy with functional impairment	Discontinue cisplatin
Day 1 WBC count <2000/mm³ or platelet count <100,000/mm³	Delay cisplatin and gemcitabine for 1 week or until myelosuppression resolves
Recurrent treatment delay because of myelosuppression	Delay cisplatin for 1 week, or until myelosuppression resolves, then decrease cisplatin and gemcitabine dosages by 25% during subsequent treatments
Sepsis during an episode of neutropenia	

*Creatinine clearance is used as a measure of glomerular filtration rate
†This also applies to patients with creatinine clearance (GFR) of 40–60 mL/min at the outset of treatment

Patient Population Studied

The studies included in the meta-analysis by Ouyang et al fulfilled the following inclusion criteria: (1) cytologically or histologically confirmed advanced stage and/or metastatic pancreatic cancer; (2) baseline Karnofsky performance status score ≥50 % (or ECOG performance status <2) and adequate renal, hematologic, hepatic, and cardiac functions; (3) aged over 18 years; and (4) without antitumor therapy within 6 months before study

Ouyang G et al. World J Surg Oncol 2016;14:59

Efficacy

A total of 9 randomized controlled trials involving 1354 patients were included for systematic evaluations. The authors concluded that "despite a higher incidence of G3/4 toxicities, GemCis offered better outcomes of ORR, PFS/TTP, and 6-month survival, which indicates GemCis may be a promising therapy for pancreatic cancer"

Efficacy of Gemcitabine + Cisplatin Compared with Gemcitabine Alone
Meta-analysis Results of Nine Randomized Controlled Trials Involving 1354 Patients*

End Point	Relative Risk (RR)/Hazard Ratio (HR)	P Value
End points with favorable outcomes		
6-month survival rate	RR = 1.303, 95% CI 1.090–1.558	0.004
ORR	RR = 1.482, 95% CI 1.148 1.913	0.003
PFS/TTP	HR = 0.87; 95 % CI 0.78–0.93	0.022
End points without favorable outcomes		
OS	HR = 0.90, 95 % CI 0.80–1.42	1.02
1-year survival rate	RR = 0.956, 95 % CI 0.770–1.187	0.684
CBR†	RR = 0.854, 95 % CI 0.681–1.072	0.175

CBR, clinical benefit rate; ORR, overall response rate; OS, overall survival; PFS, progression-free survival; TTP, time to progression

*Ouyang G et al. World J Surg Oncol 2016;14:59
†Arbitrary and not uniformly defined; usefulness limited

Adverse Events

As compared with gemcitabine alone, gemcitabine + cisplatin significantly increased the incidence of neutropenia, anemia, nausea, and vomiting, but not of leukopenia, thrombocytopenia, and diarrhea

Toxicity of Gemcitabine + Cisplatin Compared with Gemcitabine Alone
Meta-analysis Results of Nine Randomized Controlled Trials Involving 1354 Patients†

Toxicity	GemCis n/N	Gem n/N	RR	95%CI
Overall toxicities	624	537	2.164	1.837–2.549
Leukopenia	29/603	20/518	1.496	0.865–2.586
Neutropenia	124/529	52/442	2.02	**1.493–2.732**
Thrombocytopenia	68/552	28/465	1.871	0.724–4.831
Anemia	72/624	29/537	2.022	**1.336–3.060**
Nausea	80/624	25/537	2.492	**1.629–3.811**
Vomiting	59/552	15/465	3.051	**1.773–5.253**
Diarrhea	32/603	13/518	1.82	0.961–3.446

†Ouyang G et al. World J Surg Oncol 2016;14:59

Treatment Monitoring

1. *Before each cycle:* history and physical examination, electrolytes, BUN, serum creatinine, total bilirubin, ALT or AST, alkaline phosphatase, CA 19–9 and/or CEA if detectable and being used to monitor disease
2. *On day 8:* CBC with differential
3. *Every 2–3 cycles:* CT scans to assess response

METASTATIC • SUBSEQUENT THERAPY
PANCREATIC CANCER REGIMEN: GEMCITABINE + NAB-PACLITAXEL + CISPLATIN

Jameson GS et al. JAMA Oncol 2019;6:125–132

Hydration before each dose of cisplatin: ≥1000 mL 0.9% sodium chloride (0.9% NS); administer by intravenous infusion over ≥1 hour prior to cisplatin on days 1 and 8

Paclitaxel protein-bound particles for injectable suspension (nab-paclitaxel) 125 mg/m² per dose intravenously once weekly for 2 doses on days 1 and 8, every 21 days (total dosage/3-week cycle = 250 mg/m²), *followed by:*

Cisplatin 25 mg/m² per dose; administer intravenously in 50–1000 mL 0.9% NS over 1 hour for 2 doses on days 1 and 8, every 21 days (total dosage/3-week cycle = 50 mg/m²), *followed by:*

Gemcitabine HCl 1000 mg/m² per dose intravenously in 50–250 mL 0.9% sodium chloride injection for 2 doses on days 1 and 8, every 21 days (total dosage/cycle = 2000 mg/m²), *followed by:*

Hydration after cisplatin: ≥1000 mL 0.9% NS; administer by intravenous infusion over ≥1 hour following cisplatin on days 1 and 8

Supportive Care
Antiemetic prophylaxis
Emetogenic potential is **HIGH**. *Potential for delayed symptoms.*
See Chapter 42 for antiemetic recommendations

Hematopoietic growth factor (CSF) prophylaxis
Primary prophylaxis is indicated with:
Pegfilgrastim 6 mg subcutaneously on day 9 of each cycle
See Chapter 43 for more information

Antimicrobial prophylaxis
Risk of fever and neutropenia is **LOW**
  Antimicrobial primary prophylaxis to be considered:
  • Antibacterial—not indicated

  • Antifungal—not indicated

  • Antiviral—not indicated unless patient previously had an episode of HSV

Diarrhea management
Latent or delayed-onset diarrhea*:
  Loperamide 4 mg orally initially after the first loose or liquid stool, *then*
  Loperamide 2 mg orally every 2 hours during waking hours, *plus*
  Loperamide 4 mg orally every 4 hours during hours of sleep
  • Continue for at least 12 hours after diarrhea resolves

  • Recurrent diarrhea after a 12-hour diarrhea-free interval is treated as a new episode

  • Rehydrate orally with fluids and electrolytes during a diarrheal episode

  • If a patient develops blood or mucus in stool, dehydration, or hemodynamic instability, or if diarrhea persists >48 hours despite loperamide, stop loperamide and hospitalize the patient for IV hydration

  Alternatively, a trial of **diphenoxylate hydrochloride** 2.5 mg with **atropine sulfate** 0.025 mg (eg, Lomotil)
  • Initial adult dose is 2 tablets 4 times daily until control has been achieved, after which the dose may be reduced to meet individual requirements. Control may often be maintained with as little as 2 tablets daily

  • Clinical improvement of acute diarrhea is usually observed within 48 hours. If improvement of chronic diarrhea after treatment with a maximum daily dose of 8 tablets is not observed within 10 days, control is unlikely with further administration

Persistent diarrhea:
  Octreotide 100–150 mcg subcutaneously 3 times daily. Maximum total daily dose is 1500 mcg

Antibiotic therapy during latent or delayed-onset diarrhea:
  A fluoroquinolone (eg, **ciprofloxacin** 500 mg orally every 12 hours) if absolute neutrophil count <500/mm³ with or without accompanying fever in association with diarrhea
  • Antibiotics should also be administered if patient is hospitalized with prolonged diarrhea and should be continued until diarrhea resolves

*Abigerges D et al. J Natl Cancer Inst 1994;86:446–449
Rothenberg ML et al. J Clin Oncol 2001;19:3801–3807
Wadler S et al. J Clin Oncol 1998;16:3169–3178

Treatment Modifications

Dose Levels

	nab-Paclitaxel (mg/m²)	Gemcitabine HCl (mg/m²)	Cisplatin (mg/m²)
Starting dose	125	1000	25
Dose level −1	100	800	20
Dose level −2	75	600	15

Dose Adjustments on Day 1 of Each Treatment Cycle for Hematologic Toxicity

ANC		Platelets	Timing
≥1500/mm³	AND	≥100,000/mm³	Treat on time
<1500/mm³	OR	<100,000/mm³	Delay by 1 week intervals until recovery

Dose Adjustments on Day 8 of a Treatment Cycle for Hematologic Toxicity

Blood Counts	nab-Paclitaxel, Gemcitabine, and Cisplatin
ANC >1000/mm³ *and* platelets ≥75,000/mm³	100%
ANC 500–1000/mm³ *or* platelets 50,000–74,999/mm³	Decrease dose by 1 level (treat on time)
ANC <500/mm³ *or* platelets <50,000/mm³	Hold and administer filgrastim*

Note: febrile patients (regardless of ANC) should have chemotherapy treatment interrupted

Dose Adjustments on Day 1 of Each Treatment Cycle for Nonhematologic Toxicity and/or Dose Hold Based on Previous Cycle Toxicity

Toxicity/Dose Held	nab-Paclitaxel + Gemcitabine + Cisplatin Dose This Cycle
G1 peripheral neuropathy	Dose adjustment not needed but follow carefully
G2 peripheral neuropathy	Reduce nab-paclitaxel one dose level and cisplatin by one dose level but continue gemcitabine administration
G≥3 peripheral neuropathy	Hold nab-paclitaxel and cisplatin treatment but continue gemcitabine administration if indicated. Resume nab-paclitaxel and cisplatin treatment at next lower dose level after the peripheral neuropathy improves to G≤1
Serum creatinine >1.7 mg/dL	Do not administer cisplatin
Other G1/2 toxicity†	Same as day 1 previous cycle (except for G2 cutaneous toxicity where doses of gemcitabine and nab-paclitaxel should be reduced to next lower dose level)
Other G3 toxicity†	Decrease nab-paclitaxel and gemcitabine to next lower dose level*
Other G4 toxicity†	Hold therapy†

†The decision as to which drug should be modified depends upon the type of nonhematologic toxicity seen and which course is medically most sound in the judgment of the physician

Dose Adjustments within a Treatment Cycle for Nonhematologic Toxicity

CTC Grade	Percent of Day 1 nab-Paclitaxel + Gemcitabine + Cisplatin Dose
G1/2, G3 nausea/vomiting and alopecia	100%
G3 (except G3 nausea/vomiting and alopecia)	Hold either 1 or more drugs until resolution to G ≤1. Then resume treatment at the next lower dose level
G ≥3 peripheral neuropathy	Hold nab-paclitaxel and cisplatin treatment but continue gemcitabine administration if indicated. Resume nab-paclitaxel and cisplatin treatment at next lower dose level after the peripheral neuropathy improves to G ≤1
G4	Hold therapy†

Patient Population Studied

25 patients with a median (range) age 65.0 (47.0–79.0) years, 14 (56%) were males, and the majority (24) were white (96%). Nine patients were enrolled in the phase 1b dose escalation portion, and 16 in the phase 2 cohort expansion. One patient died of a serious AE prior to post-baseline tumor assessment. Therefore, 24 patients were evaluable for efficacy

Patient Demographic and Disease Characteristics	
Characteristic	No. (%)
No.	25 (100%)
Age, y	
Median (range)	65.0 (47.0–79.0)
>65	13 (52)
Sex	
Female	11 (44)
Male	14 (56)
Race/ethnicity	
White	24 (96)
Asian	1 (4)
KPS score	
100%	10 (40)
90%	12 (48)
80%	3 (12)
Baseline tumor markers	
Elevated CA19–9	19 (76)
Normal CA19–9	6 (24)
Primary tumor location on pancreas	
Head	10 (40)
Body	9 (36)
Tail	6 (24)
Prior surgery	
Whipple	5 (20)
Adjuvant treatment	4 (16)
Gem, fluorouracil/RT, Gem	2
FOLFIRINOX, RT	1
Gem + PBT	1

CA19–9, carbohydrate antigen 19–9; FOLFIRINOX, leucovorin, fluorouracil, irinotecan, and oxaliplatin; Gem, gemcitabine; KPS, Karnofsky Performance Status; PBT, proton beam therapy; RT, radiation

Efficacy N = 24

Response rate

Overall response rate (ORR)	71%
Complete response (CR)	2 (8%)
Partial response (PR)	15 (62%)
Stable disease (SD)	4 (17%)
Progressive disease (PD)	3 (12%)

Median progression-free survival (PFS)

Median PFS	10.1 months (95% CI, 6.0–12.5)

Overall survival (OS)

Median OS	16.4 months (95% CI, 10.2–25.3)
Alive at 1 year	16 (64%)
Alive at 2 years	10 (40%)
Alive at 3 years	4 (16%)
Alive >4 years	2 (8%)

CA19–9 Levels*

Normalization of CA19–9 levels	5/18 (28%)
Decrease 90% CA19–9 levels	8/18 (44%)
Decrease 50% CA19–9 levels	16/18 (89%)

*Nineteen of 25 patients (76%) had elevated CA19–9 levels measured at baseline, and 18 patients were followed up with subsequent CA19–9 measurements. The majority of patients with a baseline elevation in the CA19–9 levels experienced a rapid decrease in the levels of this tumor marker, consistent with radiologic findings of a decrease in tumor size as assessed by RECIST 1.1

Treatment Monitoring

1. *Before each cycle:* history and physical examination. CBC with differential, total bilirubin, AST or ALT, alkaline phosphatase, BUN, serum creatinine, and electrolytes. CA 19–9 and/or CEA if detectable and being used to monitor disease. Monitor for hemolytic uremic syndrome (gemcitabine), interstitial lung disease (gemcitabine), ototoxicity (cisplatin), and peripheral neuropathy (nab-paclitaxel and cisplatin)

   Note: Interstitial Pneumonitis
   Monitor patients carefully for signs and symptoms of pneumonitis (ie, episodes of transient or repeated dyspnea with unproductive persistent cough or fever) and, if observed, perform immediate clinical evaluation and timely institution of appropriate management (emphasizing the need for corticosteroids if an infectious process has been ruled out, as well as appropriate ventilation and oxygen support when required)

2. *Day 8:* CBC with differential

3. *Every 1–3 months:* CT scans to assess response

Toxicity

Treatment-Related Adverse Events Occurring in More Than 5% of Patients*

Jameson GS et al. JAMA Oncol 2019;6:125–132

System Organ Class/Preferred Term	No. (%) of Patients[†]		
	Grade 3 (n = 25)	Grade 4 (n = 25)	Grade 5 (n = 25)
Total patients with adverse events by maximum grade	12 (48)	9 (36)	2 (8)
Platelet count decreased	8 (32)	9 (36)	0
Neutrophil count decreased	5 (20)	1 (4)	0
Anemia	8 (32)	0	0
Diarrhea	2 (8)	0	0
Dehydration	2 (8)	0	0
Acute cryptosporidiosis	0	0	1 (4)
Stroke	0	0	1 (4)

*Worst grade ever as assessed by patient
[†]Percentages are based on the total number of patients in the analysis population. A patient who experienced multiple events within a system organ class or preferred term was counted once for that class and once for the preferred term at the maximum observed grade

METASTATIC • SUBSEQUENT THERAPY

PANCREATIC CANCER REGIMEN: OXALIPLATIN + FOLINIC ACID (LEUCOVORIN) + FLUOROURACIL (OFF)

Pelzer U et al. Eur J Cancer 2011;47:1676–1681

Days 1, 8, 15, and 22 during 6-week cycles:
Leucovorin calcium 200 mg/m^2 per dose intravenously in 25–100 mL 0.9% sodium chloride injection (0.9% NS) or 5% dextrose injection (D5W) over 30 minutes for 4 doses on days 1, 8, 15, and 22, every 6 weeks (total dosage/6-week cycle = 800 mg/m^2), *followed by:*
Fluorouracil 2000 mg/m^2 per dose by continuous intravenous infusion in 100–1000 mL 0.9% NS or D5W over 24 hours for 4 doses on days 1, 8, 15, and 22, every 6 weeks (total dosage/6-week cycle = 8000 mg/m^2)

Days 8 and 22 during 6-week cycles:
Oxaliplatin 85 mg/m^2 per dose administer intravenously in 250 mL D5W over 2–4 hours for 2 doses prior to leucovorin and fluorouracil on days 8 and 22 (total dosage/6-week cycle = 170 mg/m^2)

Note: oxaliplatin must not be mixed with sodium chloride injection. If leucovorin or fluorouracil are diluted in solutions containing sodium chloride injection and administered through the same tubing or vascular access device as oxaliplatin, the fluid pathway should be flushed with D5W before administering oxaliplatin

Best supportive care (BSC) according to current palliative care guidelines includes:
• Adequate pain management

• Therapy of infection

• Biliary stent intervention if needed

• Social support and on-demand psychooncologic intervention

• Nutrition consultation/intervention

Supportive Care
Antiemetic prophylaxis
Emetogenic potential on days with fluorouracil and leucovorin is **LOW**
Emetogenic potential on days with oxaliplatin is **MODERATE**
See Chapter 42 for antiemetic recommendations

Hematopoietic growth factor (CSF) prophylaxis
Primary prophylaxis may be indicated
See Chapter 43 for more information

Antimicrobial prophylaxis
Risk of fever and neutropenia is **LOW**
   Antimicrobial primary prophylaxis to be considered:
   • Antibacterial—not indicated

   • Antifungal—not indicated

   • Antiviral—not indicated unless patient previously had an episode of HSV

Diarrhea management
Latent or delayed-onset diarrhea*:
   Loperamide 4 mg orally initially after the first loose or liquid stool, *then*
   Loperamide 2 mg orally every 2 hours during waking hours, *plus*
   Loperamide 4 mg orally every 4 hours during hours of sleep
   • Continue for at least 12 hours after diarrhea resolves

   • Recurrent diarrhea after a 12-hour diarrhea-free interval is treated as a new episode

   • Rehydrate orally with fluids and electrolytes during a diarrheal episode

   • If a patient develops blood or mucus in stool, dehydration, or hemodynamic instability, or if diarrhea persists >48 hours despite loperamide, stop loperamide and hospitalize the patient for IV hydration
Alternatively, a trial of **diphenoxylate hydrochloride** 2.5 mg with **atropine sulfate** 0.025 mg (eg, Lomotil)
   • Initial adult dose is 2 tablets 4 times daily until control has been achieved, after which the dose may be reduced to meet individual requirements. Control may often be maintained with as little as 2 tablets daily

   • Clinical improvement of acute diarrhea is usually observed within 48 hours. If improvement of chronic diarrhea after treatment with a maximum daily dose of 8 tablets is not observed within 10 days, control is unlikely with further administration

Persistent diarrhea:
   Octreotide 100–150 mcg subcutaneously 3 times daily. Maximum total daily dose is 1500 mcg

(continued)

(*continued*)

Antibiotic therapy during latent or delayed-onset diarrhea:

A fluoroquinolone (eg, **ciprofloxacin** 500 mg orally every 12 hours) if absolute neutrophil count <500/mm^3 with or without accompanying fever in association with diarrhea

• Antibiotics should also be administered if patient is hospitalized with prolonged diarrhea and should be continued until diarrhea resolves

*Abigerges D et al. J Natl Cancer Inst 1994;86:446–449
Rothenberg ML et al. J Clin Oncol 2001;19:3801–3807
Wadler S et al. J Clin Oncol 1998;16:3169–3178

Efficacy

	OFF	Best Supportive Care	Statistics
Median survival with therapy	4.82 months (95% CI, 4.29–5.35)	2.30 months (95% CI, 1.76–2.83)	HR 0.45 (95% CI, 0.24–0.83) P = 0.008
Median survival since diagnosis	9.09 months (95% CI, 6.97–11.21)	7.90 months (95% CI, 4.95–10.84)	HR 0.50 (95% CI, 0.27–0.95) P = 0.031

Patient Population Studied

Patients with histologically confirmed advanced pancreatic cancer whose disease had progressed during first-line gemcitabine therapy. Patients had a Karnofsky performance status (KPS) >60% and good hepatic function, defined as AST (aspartate aminotransferase) and ALT (alanine aminotransferase) <2.5× the upper normal limit (UNL), or, in case of liver metastasis <5× UNL

Total number of patients	23
Sex, male-to-female ratio	14/9
Median age (range)	60 (38–76)
Karnofsky performance status 70–80%	12
Karnofsky performance status 90–100%	11
Gemcitabine first-line therapy	23/23
PFS on gemcitabine <3 months	6
PFS on gemcitabine 3–6 months	10
PFS on gemcitabine >6 months	7
M0/M1 disease	6/17

Toxicity (NCI CTC 2.0)

	G1	G2	G3	G4
	(Number of Patients)			
Hemoglobin	5	1	1	0
Leukopenia	4	0	0	0
Thrombocytopenia	2	2	0	0
Diarrhea	5	1	2	0
Nausea/emesis	6	4	1	0
Paresthesia	10	1	0	0

Mean (range) cumulative doses administered:
Oxaliplatin 281 mg (0–850 mg)
Folinic acid 1591 mg (200–8000 mg)
Fluorouracil 15, 630 mg (2000–20,000 mg)

Treatment Monitoring

1. *At start of every cycle:* medical history, complete physical examination, CBC with differential and serum electrolytes and LFTs
2. *Weekly:* CBC with differential

Dose Modifications

Fluorouracil and Oxaliplatin	
Any G2/3/4 nonhematologic toxicity	Delay start of next cycle until the severity of all toxicities are G ≤1
ANC >1500/mm^3 or platelet count >100,000/mm^3	Delay start of next cycle until ANC >1500/mm^3 and platelet count >100,000/mm^3
G3/4 non-neurologic	Reduce fluorouracil and oxaliplatin dosages by 20%
G3/4 ANC	Reduce oxaliplatin dosage by 20%
Persistent (≥14 days) paresthesias	Reduce oxaliplatin dosage by 20%
Temporary (7–14 days) painful paresthesias	
Temporary (7–14 days) functional impairment	
Persistent (≥14 days) painful paresthesias	Discontinue oxaliplatin
Persistent (≥14 days) functional impairment	

Adapted in part from de Gramont A et al. J Clin Oncol 2000;18:2938–2947

33. Pheochromocytoma

Karel Pacak, MD, PhD, DSc, and Tito Fojo, MD, PhD

Epidemiology

Incidence*:	3–8 cases per one million population
Median age:	42 years
Male to female ratio:	1:1

*The annual incidence of pheochromocytoma in the United States is not precisely known, but the high prevalence (0.05%) of pheochromocytomas found in autopsy series indicates that the tumor is underdiagnosed and that the annual incidence is likely to be higher than indicated

Beard CM et al. Mayo Clin Proc 1983;58:802–804
Eisenhofer G et al. Endocr Relat Cancer 2004;11:423–436
Neumann HPH et al. N Engl J Med 2002;346:1459–1466
Pacak K et al. Nat Clin Pract Endocrinol Metab 2007;3:91–102
Stenstrom et al. Acta Med Scand 1986;220:225–232

Pathology

- Approximately 80–85% of pheochromocytomas are located in the adrenal gland. The remaining 15–20% are located along the paraaortic sympathetic chain, aortic bifurcation, and urinary bladder
- Bilateral tumors occur in ~10% of patients and are much more common in familial pheochromocytomas
- 5–36% of pheochromocytomas are metastatic, but no widely accepted pathologic criteria or biomarkers exist for differentiating between benign and metastatic pheochromocytoma
- A diagnosis of malignancy requires evidence of metastases at nonchromaffin sites (only bones or lymph nodes) distant from that of the primary tumor
- Although most cases of pheochromocytomas are sporadic, a significant proportion occur secondary to several hereditary syndromes. Hereditary contribution is approximately 30%. The propensity of malignancy in hereditary pheochromocytoma syndromes is highly variable

Pheochromocytoma in Common Hereditary Syndromes

Hereditary Syndrome	Gene	Frequency*	Predisposition to Malignancy	Adrenal Disease	Extraadrenal Disease
Von Hippel-Lindau disease (VHL)	VHL	6–20%	3–5%	++	–/+
Multiple endocrine neoplasia types IIA and IIB (MEN IIA, MEN IIB)	RET	30–50%	<3%	++	–
Neurofibromatosis type 1 (NF1)	NF	1–5%	<3%	++	–
Familial paraganglioma and/or pheochromocytoma caused by mutation of succinate dehydrogenase gene family members	SDHB	20–50%	50–80%	+	++
	SDHD	15–43%	5–15%	+	++
	SDHC	<1%	10–20%	–	+ (Head and neck)
	SDHA	<1%	15–20	+	+
	SDHAF2	Extremely rare	Not described	–	+ (Head and neck)
None described	TMEM127	3%	Not described	+	–/+
	MAX	1%	10%	+	+

++, very common; +, common; –, rare (there are various reports and data are presented as the best estimate)
*Frequency in sporadic tumors

Andrews KA et al. J Med Genet 2018; 55:384–394
Burnichon N et al. Hum Mol Genet 2010;19:3011–3020
Crona J et al. Endocr Rev 2017;38:489–515
Eisenhofer G et al. Endocr Relat Cancer 2004;11:423–436
Fishbein L et al. Cancer Cell 2017; 31:181–193
Hao H-X et al. Science 2009;325:1139–1142
Jha A et al. Front Oncol 2019;9:53
Jochmanobva et al. J Cancer Res Clin Oncol 2017;143:1421–1435
John H et al. Urology 1999;53:679–683
Lee H et al. J Med Genet 2020;57:217–225
Mannelli M et al. J Med Genet 2007;44:586–587
O'Riordain DS et al. World J Surg 1996;20:916–921; discussion 922
Pacak K et al. Ann Intern Med 2001;134:315–329
Qin Y et al. Nat Genet 2010;42:229–233

Evaluation

The diagnosis of pheochromocytoma is confirmed by biochemical evidence of elevated catecholamine production (preferably with measurement of plasma metanephrines and methoxytyramine) and by radiologic studies (Figure 33–1)

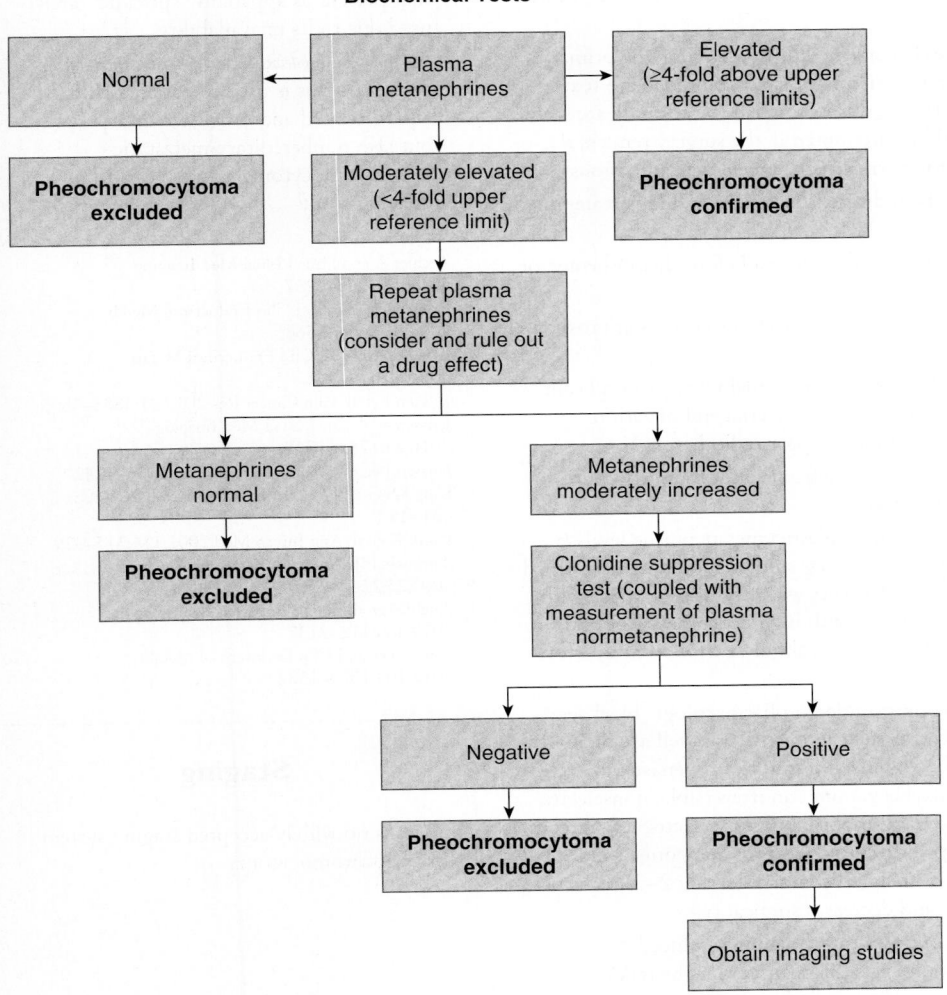

Figure 33–1. Biochemical tests.

Acetaminophen may interfere with measurement of plasma metanephrines if the HPLC method is used. Other drugs, including benzodiazepines, buspirone, diuretics, carbidopa and levodopa, tricyclic antidepressants, SSRIs, MOA inhibitors, sympathomimetics, and α- and β-adrenergic and Ca channel blockers, may cause false-positive elevations of plasma or urine catecholamines or metanephrines. Currently, there is no drug interference using the new liquid chromatography tandem mass spectrometry method

de Jong WHA et al. Clin Chem 2007;53:1684–1693
Eisenhofer G et al. Drugs 2007;30:1031–1062
Eisenhofer G et al. Eur J Cancer 2012;48:1739–1749
Hannah-Shmouni et al. JAMA 2017;318:385–386
Lenders et al. JAMA 2002;20:1427–1434

Survival

For patients with resectable pheochromocytoma, the overall survival is almost equal to that of the age-matched normal population if no long-standing effects of elevated catecholamines on cardiovascular or other systems are present. The 5-year survival of metastatic pheochromocytomas varies between 75% to less than 30%; however, some metastatic pheochromocytomas can be slow-growing, and patients may have minimal morbidity and survive as long as 20 years

Bravo EL, Tagle R. Endocr Rev 2003;24:539–553
Hamidi O et al. Clin Endocrinol 2017;87:440–450
John H et al. Urology 1999;53:679–683
Remine WH et al. Ann Surg 1974;179:740–748
Stolk RF et al. J Clin Endocrinol Metab 2013;98:1100–1106
Turkova H et al. Endocr Pract 2016;22:302–314
van Heerden JA et al. Surgery 1982;91:367–373

Imaging Studies

- *CT or MRI of abdomen (90–100% sensitivity):* because of inadequate specificity, detection of a mass by these tests does not justify a diagnosis. One of the functional imaging modalities [68Ga]-DOTATATE PET/CT, 6-[18F]-Fluorodopa PET/CT, or 123I metaiodobenzylguanidine (MIBG) scintigraphy is needed for confirmation

- *6-[18F]-Fluorodopa PET/CT:* this is now recommended to be used as the first-line imaging modality to confirm diagnosis when CT or MRI detects a tumor mass when no family history is present and in all *MAX*- and *HIF2A*-related pheochromocytoma and as the second-line imaging modality in head and neck paragangliomas

- *[68Ga]-DOTATATE PET/CT:* this is now recommended to be used as the first-line imaging modality in all *SDHx*-related pheochromocytoma and any head and neck paragangliomas. Other DOTA analogues could be used, but no large studies have been published.

- *[123I]-MIBG scintigraphy:* used now only if radiotherapy for metastatic, locally aggressive, or unresectable pheochromocytoma is considered. Drugs that may interfere with MIBG study include labetalol, calcium channel blockers, guanethidine, reserpine, sympathomimetics, and tricyclic antidepressants

(continued)

Treatment Notes

Surgery

- The definitive treatment for pheochromocytoma is surgical excision of the tumor. Surgical removal can cure pheochromocytoma in up to 90% of cases, whereas if left untreated, the tumor can prove fatal. Laparoscopic adrenalectomy is now considered the standard approach for excision of most pheochromocytomas with the exception of very large (≤10 cm) tumors. The survival rates after surgery are 97.7–100%
- Surgery for **metastatic** pheochromocytoma is rarely curative, but resection of the primary mass or metastases can reduce exposure of the cardiovascular system and organs to toxic levels of circulating catecholamines. Consequently, aggressive surgical resection of accessible primary or recurrent disease or metastases should be attempted if the surgery renders the patient free of gross disease with the potential for normal biochemical determinations
- Surgery for **metastatic** pheochromocytoma may be indicated for lesions in life-threatening or debilitating anatomic locations
- The value of surgical debulking for **metastatic** pheochromocytoma before chemotherapy or radiation therapy is not proved
- The median time for recurrence of pheochromocytoma after initial resection is approximately 6 years and may be as long as 20 years
- Alternatives to surgical resection include external beam radiation (including proton beam radiation), cryoablation, radiofrequency ablation, transcatheter arterial embolization, chemotherapy, and radiopharmaceutical therapy (peptide receptor radiotherapy)
- Biochemical testing should always be repeated after recovery from surgical resection of a primary mass to exclude any remaining disease or metastasis
- Postoperative follow-up of patients includes evaluation of plasma metanephrine levels 6 weeks and 6 and 12 months after surgery, then yearly. Imaging studies should be performed on the basis of follow-up test results. Exceptions: (a) Patients with SDHB, (b) those with an extraadrenal tumor or a primary >5 cm, and (c) those with high norepinephrine and/or dopamine levels because they have a higher risk of metastasis, should be followed up more frequently (every 6 months for the first 5 years)
- Before surgery, patients with pheochromocytoma must undergo pharmacologic blockage of catecholamine synthesis and their effects on end-organs and activity as well as volume expansion because they have reduced intravascular volume as a result of a persistent vasoconstricted state. The combination of phenoxybenzamine (an irreversible, nonselective α-adrenergic receptor antagonist) or doxazosin, terazosin, or prazosin (selective α_1-adrenergic receptor antagonists), with atenolol (a selective β_1-adrenergic receptor antagonist) and metyrosine (a tyrosine hydroxylase inhibitor), and liberal salt intake starting 2–3 weeks before surgery leads to better control of blood pressure and decreases surgical risks
- Routine preoperative use of phenoxybenzamine opposes catecholamine-induced vasoconstriction. A β-adrenoceptor blocker (atenolol) is added to prevent the reflex tachycardia associated with α-blockade. The pressor effects of pheochromocytoma must be controlled by α-blockade before β-blockers are initiated *Note:* β-Blockade **alone** can be dangerous in patients with pheochromocytoma and is contraindicated because it does not prevent and can actually augment effects of catecholamines at α-adrenoceptors
- Metyrosine is used to reduce the synthesis of new catecholamines by the tumor

Drug	Mechanism	Oral Dose	Side Effects
Phenoxybenzamine hydrochloride	Long-acting nonselective α-adrenergic antagonist	Initial dose: 10 mg twice daily, gradually increased to 20 and 40 mg 2 or 3 times daily (approximately 1–2 mg/kg per day). Final dose is determined by the patient's blood pressure	Tachycardia, orthostatic hypotension, nausea, abdominal pain, nasal congestion, fatigue, and retrograde or difficulty in ejaculation
Atenolol	Long-acting β_1-selective (cardioselective) β-adrenergic antagonist	Initial dose: 25 mg once a day. This can be increased to 25 mg twice daily and 50 mg twice daily if needed. Dose should be decreased in renal impairment	Hypotension, bradycardia, postural hypotension, cardiac failure, dizziness, tiredness, fatigue, and depression

(continued)

Imaging Studies (continued)

- *6-[^{18}F] Fluorodopamine positron emission tomography:* this is used when biochemical tests are positive but conventional studies cannot locate the tumor, especially those that present as apparently sporadic, rarely used due to its unavailability
- *6-[^{18}F]-Fluorodeoxyglucose positron emission tomography:* this is used in patients with *SDHB*-related and other hereditary but also nonhereditary metastatic pheochromocytoma as the second-line imaging study

Archier A et al. Eur J Nucl Med Imaging 2016;43:1248–1257
Eisenhofer G et al. J Clin Endocrinol Metab 2003;88:2656–2666
Ilias I, Pacak K. J Clin Endocrinol Metab 2004;89:479–491
Janssen I et al. Clin Cancer Res 2015;21:3888–3895
Janssen et al. Eur J Nucl Med Imaging 2016;43:1784–1791
Janssen I et al. J Nucl Med 2017;58:1236–1242
King KS et al. J Clin Endocrinol Metab 2010;95: 481–482
Pacak K et al. Ann Intern Med 2001;134:315–329
Timmers HJLM et al. J Clin Oncol 2007;25:2262–2269
Taieb D et al. Eur J Nucl Med Mol Imaging 2019;46:2112–2137
Taieb D et al. J Clin Endocrinol Metabl 2018;103:1574–1582

Staging

There is no widely accepted staging system for pheochromocytoma

Treatment Notes (*continued*)

Drug	Mechanism	Oral Dose	Side Effects
Metyrosine	Competitively inhibits tyrosine hydroxylase, the rate-limiting enzyme in catecholamine synthesis	Initially, 250 mg 4 times daily. This may be increased by 250–500 mg daily to a maximum dose of 66.7 mg/kg per day or 4000 mg/day (whichever is less); eg, 1000 mg 4 times daily. Doses should be decreased in renal failure and given as divided doses	Extrapyramidal neurologic symptoms, crystalluria, diarrhea, anxiety, depression, headache, fatigue, and xerostomia
Doxazosin mesylate	Short-acting α_1-antagonist	Initial dose: 1–2 mg daily. This can be gradually increased to 10–30 mg/day Recommended maximum daily dose is 16 mg as a single daily dose with either immediate- or extended-release formulations	Postural dizziness and vertigo, postural hypotension, syncope
Terazosin hydrochloride	Short-acting α_1-antagonist	Initial dose: 1–2 mg daily. This can be gradually increased to 5 mg/day Recommended maximum daily dose is 20 mg, either as a single daily dose or 10 mg every 12 hours	
Prazosin hydrochloride	Short-acting α_1-antagonist	Initial dose: 1 mg 2 or 3 times daily. This can be gradually increased to 2–5 mg/dose, 2 or 3 times daily Recommended maximum daily dose is 20 mg given in 2 or 3 divided doses	

Important note:

Several drugs (including some commonly used by oncologists) may lead to a hypertensive crisis in a patient with a diagnosis of pheochromocytoma and should be avoided. These include:

- ACTH
- Amphetamines and other sympathomimetics
- Antibiotics such as linezolid
- Cocaine
- Droperidol*
- Glucagon*
- Glucocorticoids
- Histamine*
- MAO inhibitors
- **Morphine**
- **Metoclopramide***, chlorpromazine, prochlorperazine
- Saralasin
- **Tricyclic and other antidepressants**
- Tyramine
- Weight-loss medications

*Has been used as a provocative test for pheochromocytoma

Ayala-Ramirez M et al. J Clin Endocrinol Metab 2011;96:717–725
2019; 26:539–550
Eigelberger MS, Duh Q-Y. Curr Treat Options Oncol 2001;2:321–329
Eisenhofer G et al. Endocr Relat Cancer 2004;11:423–436
Hamidi O et al. J Clin Endocrinol Metab 2017;102:3296–3305
Hescot S et al. J Clin Endocrinol Metab 2019;104:2367–2374
Pacak K. J Clin Endocrinol Metab 2007;92:4069–4079
Pacak K et al. Ann Intern Med 2001;134:315–329
Turkova H et al. Endocr Pract 2016;22:302–314

Westphal SA. Am J Med Sci 2005;329:18–21

ADVANCED / UNRESECTABLE • METASTATIC

PHEOCHROMOCYTOMA REGIMEN: CYCLOPHOSPHAMIDE + VINCRISTINE + DACARBAZINE (CVD)

[CAN BE USED TO RENDER UNRESECTABLE DISEASE POTENTIALLY RESECTABLE]

Averbuch SD et al. Ann Intern Med 1988;109:267–273
Huang H et al. Cancer 2008;113:2020–2028
Turkova H et al. Endocr Pract 2016;22:302–314

Recommendation: Hospitalization while first cycle is administered given that a rare patient may have worsening of their hypertension or even a hypertensive crisis during administration or shortly thereafter

Cyclophosphamide 750 mg/m²; administer intravenously in 100–250 mL 0.9% sodium chloride injection (0.9% NS) or 5% dextrose injection (D5W) over 15–30 minutes on day 1, every 21 days (total dosage/cycle = 750 mg/m²)

Vincristine 1.4 mg/m²; administer by intravenous injection over 1–2 minutes on day 1, every 21 days (total dosage/cycle = 1.4 mg/m²)

Dacarbazine 600 mg/m² per dose; administer intravenously in 100–250 mL 0.9% NS or D5W over 15–30 minutes for 2 doses on days 1 and 2, every 21 days (total dosage/cycle = 1200 mg/m²)

Supportive Care
Antiemetic prophylaxis
*Emetogenic potential on days 1 and 2 is **HIGH**. Potential for delayed symptoms*
See Chapter 42 for antiemetic recommendations

Hematopoietic growth factor (CSF) prophylaxis
*Primary prophylaxis is **NOT** indicated*
See Chapter 43 for more information

Antimicrobial prophylaxis
*Risk of fever and neutropenia is **LOW***
  Antimicrobial primary prophylaxis to be considered:
  • Antibacterial—not indicated
  • Antifungal—not indicated
  • Antiviral—not indicated unless patient previously had an episode of HSV

Treatment Modifications

Counts on Day 1 of Repeated Cycles

WBC 3000–3999/mm³ or platelets 75,000–100,000/mm³	Vincristine 100%. Reduce cyclophosphamide and dacarbazine dosages by 25%
WBC 2000–2999/mm³ or platelets 50,000–75,000/mm³	Vincristine 100%. Reduce cyclophosphamide and dacarbazine dosages by 50%
WBC 1000–1999/mm³ or platelets 25,000–50,000/mm³	Vincristine 100%. Hold cyclophosphamide and dacarbazine
Total bilirubin 1.5–2 mg/dL (25.7–34.2 µmol/L) or serum AST 75–150 units/L	Reduce vincristine dosage by 50%
Total bilirubin 3–5.9 mg/dL (51.3–100.9 µmol/L) or serum AST 151–300 units/L	Reduce vincristine dosage by 75%
Total bilirubin >6 mg/dL (>102.6 µmol/L) or serum AST >300 units/L	Hold vincristine
G1/2 neuropathy	Decrease vincristine dosage by 50%
G3/4 neuropathy	Hold vincristine

Nadir Counts During the Previous Cycle

WBC 1000–1999/mm³ or platelets 50,000–75,000/mm³	Vincristine 100%. Reduce cyclophosphamide and dacarbazine dosages by 50%
WBC <1000/mm³ or platelets <50,000/mm³	Vincristine 100%. Reduce cyclophosphamide and dacarbazine dosages by 75%

Patient Population
A study of 14 patients with advanced metastatic pheochromocytoma

Efficacy (N = 14)

Averbuch et al, 1988

Tumor Response

Complete response	2 (14%)
Partial response	6 (43%)
Overall response	57%
Median duration	21 months

Biochemical Response

Complete response	3 (21%)
Partial response	8 (57%)
Overall response	78%
Median duration	22 months

Toxicity (N = 14)

Hematologic

WBC nadir <1000/mm³	21% (3/14)
Mean nadir WBC	2100/mm³
Platelet count nadir <50,000/mm³	29% (4/14)
Mean nadir platelet count	144,000/mm³

Nonhematologic

Mild sensory impairment	Mean grade 0.9/4
Paresthesias	Mean grade 0.9/4
Nausea and vomiting	Mean grade 1.6/4
Hypotension	4 episodes

Therapy Monitoring

1. *During initial treatment cycles:* careful hemodynamic monitoring
2. *Before each cycle:* plasma/serum metanephrines and catecholamines, CBC with differential, LFTs, and neurologic exam

Notes

Several drugs (including some commonly used by oncologists) may lead to a hypertensive crisis in a patient with a diagnosis of pheochromocytoma and should be avoided:

1. ACTH
2. Amphetamines and other sympathomimetics
3. Antibiotics such as linezolid
4. Cocaine
5. Droperidol
6. Glucagon*
7. Glucocorticoids
8. Histamine*
9. **Morphine**
10. **MAO inhibitors**
11. **Metoclopramide***, chlorpromazine, prochlorperazine
12. Saralasin
13. **Tricyclic and other antidepressants**
14. Tyramine
15. Weight-loss medications

*Used as a provocative test for pheochromocytoma

34. Prostate Cancer

Fatima Karzai, MD, Wenhui Zhu, MD, PhD, and William L. Dahut, MD

Epidemiology

Incidence: 159,120 cases
Estimated 33,330 deaths (Estimated new cases for 2020 in the United States)
Estimated
Median age: 66 years

Stage at Presentation

Stage	%
Stage I:	50%
Stage II:	20%
Stage III:	17%
Stage IV:	13%

Siegel R et al. CA Cancer J Clin. 2020;70(1):7–30.
Surveillance, Epidemiology and End Results (SEER) Program, available from http://seer.cancer.gov

Pathology

Adenocarcinoma (acinar):	>95%
Ductal adenocarcinoma*:	<1%
Mucinous*:	<1%
Small cell*:	<1%
Transitional cell*:	<1%
Small cell*:	<1%

Gleason Score at Presentation
(Radical prostatectomy specimens)

Score	%
2–4:	6%
5–6:	54%
7:	30%
8–9:	10%

*Poor prognosis

Kantoff PW et al. Prostate Cancer: Principles & Practice. Philadelphia: Lippincott; 2002

Work-up

Bone scan if:
  T1 and PSA >20
  T2 and PSA >10
  Gleason > or = 8
  T3/T4 disease
  Symptomatic
Pelvic CT/MRI if:
  T3/T4
  T1/2 and nomogram indicates probability of LN invasion >10%

Staging

Primary Tumor (T)

Clinical T (*cT*)

T Category	T Criteria
TX	Primary tumor cannot be assessed
T0	No evidence of primary tumor
T1	Clinically inapparent tumor that is not palpable
T1a	Tumor incidental histologic finding in 5% or less of tissue resected
T1b	Tumor incidental histologic finding in more than 5% of tissue resected
T1c	Tumor identified by needle biopsy found in one or both sides, but not palpable
T2	Tumor is palpable and confined within prostate
T2a	Tumor involves one-half of one side or less
T2b	Tumor involves more than one-half of one side but not both sides
T2c	Tumor involves both sides
T3	Extraprostatic tumor that is not fixed or does not invade adjacent structures
T3a	Extraprostatic extension (unilateral or bilateral)
T3b	Tumor invades seminal vesicle(s)
T4	Tumor is fixed or invades adjacent structures other than seminal vesicles such as external sphincter, rectum, bladder, levator muscles, and/or pelvic wall

Pathological T (*pT*)

T Category	T Criteria
T2	Organ confined
T3	Extraprostatic extension
T3a	Extraprostatic extension (unilateral or bilateral) or microscopic invasion of bladder neck
T3b	Tumor invades seminal vesicle(s)
T4	Tumor is fixed or invades adjacent structures other than seminal vesicles such as external sphincter, rectum, bladder, levator muscles, and/or pelvic wall

Note: There is no pathological T1 classification.
Note: Positive surgical margin should be indicated by an R1 descriptor, indicating residual microscopic disease.

Regional Lymph Node (N)

N	Category N Criteria
NX	Regional lymph nodes cannot be assessed
N0	No positive regional nodes
N1	Metastases in regional node(s)

Distant Metastasis (M)

M Category	M Criteria
M0	No distant metastasis
M1	Distant metastasis
M1a	Nonregional lymph node(s)
M1b	Bone(s)
M1c	Other site(s) with or without bone disease

Note: When more than one site of metastasis is present, the most advanced category is used. M1c is most advanced.

Prostate-Specific Antigen (PSA)

PSA values are used to assign this category.

PSA values
< 10
≥ 10 < 20
< 20
≥ 20
Any value

Histologic Grade Group (G)

Recently, the Gleason system has been compressed into so-called Grade Groups.[44]

Grade Group	Gleason Score	Gleason Pattern
1	≤ 6	≤ 3 + 3
2	7	3 + 4
3	7	4 + 3
4	8	4 + 4, 3 + 5, 5 + 3
5	9 or 10	4 + 5, 5 + 4, or 5 + 5

Prognostic Stage Groups

When T is...	And N is...	And M is...	And PSA is...	And Grade Group is...	Then the stage group is...
cT1a-c, cT2a	N0	M0	< 10	1	I
pT2	N0	M0	< 10	1	I
cT1a-c, cT2a, pT2	N0	M0	≥ 10 < 20	1	IIA
cT2b-c	N0	M0	< 20	1	IIA
T1-2	N0	M0	< 20	2	IIB
T1-2	N0	M0	< 20	3	IIC
T1-2	N0	M0	< 20	4	IIC
T1-2	N0	M0	≥ 20	1–4	IIIA
T3-4	N0	M0	Any	1–4	IIIB
Any T	N0	M0	Any	5	IIIC
Any T	N1	M0	Any	Any	IVA
Any T	Any N	M1	Any	Any	IVB

Note: When either PSA or Grade Group is not available, grouping should be determined by T category and/or either PSA or Grade Group as available.

15-Year Relative Survival

Stages I–II	81%
Stage III	57%
Stage IV	6%

Johansson JE et al. JAMA 1997;277:467–471

Predicting 15-year Prostate Cancer Specific Mortality After Radical Prostatectomy

Gleason Score	Mortality (from PrCa)
<6	0.2%–1.2%
3 + 4/4 + 3	4.2%–6.5%/6.6%–11%
8–10	26%–37%

Eggener SE et al. J Urol 2011;185:869–875

Distant Metastasis (M)

M0	No distant metastasis
M1	Distant metastasis
M1a	Nonregional lymph node(s)
M1b	Bone(s)
M1c	Other site(s) with or without bone disease

Note: When more than 1 site of metastasis is present, the most advanced category is used. pM1c is most advanced

Amin MB et al, editors. AJCC Cancer Staging Manual. 8th ed. New York: Springer; 2017

10 Year Disease Free Survival

(After radical prostatectomy for localized disease)

Gleason score 2–4	96%
Gleason score 5–6	82%
Gleason score 7	52%
Gleason score 8–9	35%

Epstein JI et al. Am J Surg Pathol 1996; 20:286–292.

Expert Opinion

Screening for prostate cancer:
The optimal use of PSA in the diagnosis of prostate cancer remains a subject of continued controversy. In 2012 the USPSTF recommended against the use of PSA-based screening for prostate cancer to the general population, regardless of age. The American Urological Association also has revised their guidelines in response, advising against routine PSA-based screening. However, in high-risk men ages 40–54 or all men between 55–69 the AUA advises the test to be a man's decision after a discussion of the full understanding of the risks and benefits of testing. Both groups agree that men above the age of 70 or under the age of 40 do not undergo screening

Moyer VA. Ann Intern Med 2012;157:120–134
http://www.auanet.org/education/guidelines/prostate-cancer-detection.cfm [AUA guidelines]

The traditionally employed PSA threshold of 4 ng/mL has only a 70–80% sensitivity and 60–70% specificity. The positive predictive value of a PSA between 4 and 10 ng/mL is only 25%, and approximately 20% of patients with PSA between 2 and 4 ng/mL will have prostate cancer on biopsy. Free PSA percentage (<10%) has been shown to improve the positive predictive value in patients with total PSA between 4 and 10 ng/mL. In the Prostate Cancer Prevention Trial, 21.1% of prostate cancers were diagnosed in men with a PSA level between 2.6 and 3.9 ng/mL and 15.4% of the prostate cancers had a Gleason score of 7–10 when PSA was ≤2.5 ng/mL

Initial assessment and staging evaluation:
Patients are stratified at diagnosis for an initial treatment plan based on anticipated life expectancy and clinical symptoms
• For asymptomatic patients with life expectancy <10 years, treatment may be delayed until symptoms appear
• Once an abnormal digital rectal exam and/or an elevated PSA suggest prostate cancer is present, an ultrasound-guided prostate core biopsy with 10–12 cores is performed to help establish the diagnosis, and the 2 most common cellular patterns of the tumor are graded pathologically using the Gleason scale
• Pelvic CT or MRI is recommended for patients with T3/T4 tumor or T1/T2 tumor with a predicted probability of lymph node involvement >20%
• Bone scan is recommended for patients with T3/T4 tumor, symptomatic disease, or a T1/T2 tumor with PSA >20 ng/mL or a Gleason score ≥8

Current Guidelines for Germline Testing in Prostate Cancer
• Inquire about known high-risk family history/genes
• Test patients with metastatic disease regardless of family history
• Test patients with high-risk regional disease per NCCN risk categories regardless of family history
• Test patients with very low to unfavorable intermediate-risk disease with a history of a diagnosis of prostate cancer in the family (brother, father, or multiple male relatives diagnosed at <60 years old), known germline repair mutation(s) in the family, or more than 1 relative with family history suggestive of hereditary breast or ovarian cancer (HBOC) or Lynch syndrome
• Test patients with Gleason score ≥7 who have any of the following: one or more relatives with ovarian cancer, pancreatic cancer, metastatic prostate cancer, or breast cancer younger than 50 years of age or two or more relatives with breast or prostate cancer (any grade) at any age, or Ashkenazi Jewish ancestry
• BRCA mutations in tumor profiling

(continued)

Expert Opinion (*continued*)

Localized prostate cancer:
Patients with newly diagnosed clinically localized prostate cancer are divided into 3 risk groups of occult metastasis and relapse after local initial therapy
- *Low risk:* PSA <10 ng/mL, Gleason score ≤6, T1/T2a tumor
- *Intermediate risk:* PSA 10–20 ng/mL, Gleason score 7, T2b/T2c tumor
- *High risk:* PSA >20 ng/mL, Gleason score 8–10, T3/T4 tumor

Treatment options for localized prostate cancer include active surveillance, radical prostatectomy (RP; including open surgery, laparoscopic, and robot-assisted procedures), and radiation therapy (RT; including high-dose external beam radiation therapy with 3D conformal or intensity-modulated radiation therapy, and brachytherapy with or without external beam therapy)
- The treatment decision is based on the probability of organ-confined disease, patient's life expectancy, and risk of relapse and metastasis
- Active surveillance is an option for patients with low-risk prostate cancer. Serial biopsy and close PSA monitoring are used to attempt to identify patients who may benefit from definitive local treatment. Some have suggested intervention if PSA doubling time is less than 3 years or Gleason grade progression to a predominant Gleason 4 pattern
- For patients with organ-confined disease, both RT and RP remain the standard of care, although surgery is not commonly performed in patients ≤70 years of age
- In nonrandomized patient cohort studies, RP and RT appear to provide equivalent PSA-free relapse, but differ in the type and frequency of side effects. At 5 years, the rate of event-free survival was 81% for RP, 81% for high-dose external beam radiation therapy, and 83% for brachytherapy in 2991 patients with clinical stage T1–T2 localized prostate cancer treated between 1990 and 1998
- Patients undergoing RP should have extended pelvic lymph node dissection (PLND), except those with a low predicted probability of nodal metastasis by nomograms
- For T3/T4 disease, RP may be considered for selected patients with well-differentiated tumors. Most high-risk patients will receive XRT plus hormonal ablation
- For RP, nerve-sparing procedures with radical retropubic and robotic-assisted laparoscopic prostatectomy are the most common techniques. The main determinants of outcome are PSA level, Gleason score, and the TNM clinical stage. Adverse effects from surgery include incontinence, erectile dysfunction, bladder neck stricture, and bowel incontinence
- The biochemical control rate after RT depends largely upon the risk features associated with individual tumors. The probability of biochemical control 5 years after RT without hormonal ablation is 84% for low-risk disease, 62% for intermediate-risk disease, and 43% for high-risk disease

Adjuvant therapies after initial definitive therapies
- Adjuvant RT after RP should be considered for patients with positive surgical margins, seminal vesicle involvement, or pathological evidence of T3/T4 disease
- Immediate postoperative RT for patients with pathologic T3 disease improves PSA progression-free survival significantly (74% vs 53% for placebo after 5 years of follow-up), although there is no overall survival benefit
- Due to exclusion of patients with node-positive disease in most clinical trials, it remains unclear whether adjuvant RT after RP should be considered in this subset of patients
- Immediate androgen-deprivation therapy (ADT) provides significant overall survival benefit in patients with microscopically positive lymph nodes treated with RP, compared to hormonal therapy started at the time of symptomatic local recurrence or metastasis
- Neoadjuvant/adjuvant ADT of 2–3 years in combination with RT is the standard for high-risk patients. Neoadjuvant/adjuvant ADT (for 6 months) in combination with RT may improve progression-free disease and prostate cancer-specific and overall survival for patients with PSA ≤10 ng/mL, a Gleason score ≥7, or radiographic evidence of extraprostatic disease. This needs confirmation in a larger study limited only to intermediate-risk patients

Androgen-deprivation therapy
- Optimal ADT includes medical castration with a GnRH antagonist, an LHRH agonist, or surgical castration with bilateral orchiectomy. The addition of an antiandrogen can reduce the initial disease flare that may follow introduction of a LHRH agonist, but does not appear to add significantly to survival
- Side effects of ADT include osteoporosis, hot flashes, loss of libido, erectile dysfunction, fatigue, gynecomastia, cognitive dysfunction, depression, anemia, loss of muscle mass, glucose intolerance, and changes in lipids profile and increased risk of cardiovascular disease
- Hot flashes from hormonal therapy can be treated with clonidine (0.1 mg daily, orally), low-dose estrogens, or antidepressants
- Prophylactic breast XRT can reduce the incidence of painful gynecomastia
- Patients receiving long-term ADT should have a baseline bone density scan and supplemental vitamin D and calcium. Consider bisphosphonates if an evaluation demonstrates evidence of either osteopenia or osteoporosis

PSA Failure
PSA failure after RP:
- Following RP, it is expected that PSA will be undetectable. Biochemical recurrence following RP is defined as either failure to achieve an undetectable PSA level or a PSA rise after surgery on 2 or more laboratory determinations. The American Urological Association Prostate Guideline Update Panel has chosen a PSA level ≥0.2 ng/mL as the threshold

(*continued*)

Expert Opinion (continued)

- Patients with biochemical recurrence because of local failure and without distant metastasis (clinical features include PSA <2 ng/mL, slow PSA doubling time, a long interval to failure after surgery) should be evaluated for salvage RT. Salvage RT provides durable disease-free survival in 60–70% of patients, but no confirmed overall survival benefits. Predictors of progression after salvage RT include a Gleason score of 8–10, pre-RT PSA ≤2 ng/mL, negative surgical margins, and a PSA doubling time <10 months

PSA failure after RT:
- PSA failure after RT is defined as a PSA rise ≥2 ng/mL above the nadir (the Phoenix definition)
- Patients with original clinical stage T1–T2, a life expectancy ≤10 years, and a current PSA <10 ng/mL may be candidates for local therapy such as salvage RP, cryotherapy, or brachytherapy. However, morbidity is high and there are no randomized trials that demonstrate improved survival. Further work-up is indicated to rule out distant metastasis before local therapy

For patients with PSA failure, timing of ADT is affected by PSA velocity, patient preference, and other medical comorbidities. Early implementation of ADT may delay the appearance of metastases; however, there are no data indicating early ADT provides any overall survival benefit

Advanced prostate cancer
- In patients with metastatic prostate cancer, local therapies are used primarily for symptom management. There are no conclusive data that local therapies improve survival
- ADT should begin immediately in the presence of tumor-related symptoms or overt metastasis
- **Combined androgen blockage** (castration combined with an antiandrogen) provides no definite survival improvement over castration alone in patients with metastatic disease
- Initiation of treatment with LHRH agonists is associated with a transient increase in testosterone production with initial use (tumor flare). For patients with overt metastases who are at risk of developing symptoms (such as spinal cord compression, worsening pain, or urinary outlet obstruction), an antiandrogen should be given concurrently with a LHRH agonist for at least 7 days after initiating treatment with the latter to competitively block testosterone at androgen receptors, and prevent potential exacerbation of disease. **Ketoconazole** also may be used in patients who are at high risk for complications associated with tumor flare
- Intermittent ADT can be used to reduce side effects and cost of ADT, but its long-term efficacy remains unproven
- **Abiraterone acetate** has been approved in patients pre-chemotherapy based on improved progression-free survival. The study was stopped before an overall-survival benefit could be seen, but there was a trend toward OS improvement as well (Ryan CJ et al. N Engl J Med 2013;368:138–148). **Enzalutamide** has been approved in patients pre-chemotherapy based on improved OS and radiographic progression-free survival compared with placebo (Beer TM et al. N Engl J Med 2014;371:424–433)
- **Abiraterone acetate** targets cytochrome P450 17A1 (CYP17A1), leading to a decrease in the production of testosterone. It received FDA approval based on a study that demonstrated improved survival in patients who received it after docetaxel chemotherapy. **Abiraterone acetate** is administered daily in combination with prednisone. **Enzalutamide**, a potent anti-androgen, has also been approved for use post-chemotherapy based on an OS benefit. One advantage of enzalutamide over abiraterone acetate is that it does not require concomitant prednisone, which can have side effects in patients with prostate cancer. Selected patients may respond to sequential hormonal manipulations
- **Sipuleucel-T** is a cellular immunotherapy consisting of peripheral blood mononuclear cells obtained by leukapheresis and cultured (activated) with a recombinant human protein consisting of prostatic acid phosphatase linked to granulocyte-macrophage colony-stimulating factor (PAP-GM-CSF). In a randomized trial, this product had no effect on time to progression, but it led to an improvement in overall survival
- Chemotherapy with **docetaxel** every 3 weeks plus prednisone is the preferred first-line chemotherapy for advanced prostate cancer, providing improved survival. **Cabazitaxel** is a semisynthetic derivative of a natural taxoid, which, when combined with prednisone, improved survival in patients who had progressed on docetaxel and prednisone. Alternative regimens include **every-3-week docetaxel and estramustine**, **weekly docetaxel and prednisone**, and **every-3-week mitoxantrone and prednisone**
- **Cabazitaxel** is approved as a second-line chemotherapeutic agent
- *Metastatic small cell carcinoma of the prostate* should be treated with a platinum-containing regimen, but mixed tumors (adenocarcinoma and small cell) may have some initial response to hormonal ablation
- **Zoledronic acid** prevents skeletal-related events in patients with castrate-resistant prostate cancer and bone metastases
- **Radium-223** has been approved by the FDA for prostate cancer and selectively targets bone metastases with alpha particles. It has been shown to improve overall survival but it remains to be seen where exactly it will be used in patients and whether it will be combined with other approved agents

American Cancer Society Guidelines for the Early Detection of Cancer. Prostate Cancer Early Detection. Available from: http://www.cancer.org/Cancer/ProstateCancer/MoreInformation/ProstateCancerEarlyDetection/prostate-cancer-early-detection-toc

Gulley JL, Dahut WL. Prostate cancer. In: Abraham J et al (editors). Bethesda Handbook of Clinical Oncology 2nd ed. Philadelphia, PA: Lippincott Williams & Wilkins; 2005:185–201

Parker et al. N Engl J Med. 2013;369:213–223

Pazdur R et al. Cancer Management: A Multidisciplinary Approach. 13th ed. Manhasset, NY: CMP Healthcare Media, Inc; 2010

The Partin Tables. Available from: https://www.hopkinsmedicine.org/brady-urology-institute/specialties/conditions-and-treatments/prostate-cancer/fighting-prostate-cancer/partin-table.html [accessed July 8, 2011]

U.S. Preventive Services Task Force. Screening for prostate cancer: U.S. Preventive Services Task Force recommendation statement. Ann Intern Med 2008;149:185–191, W–42

LOCALLY ADVANCED • METASTATIC
PROSTATE CANCER REGIMEN: HORMONAL AGENTS

Bolla M et al. Lancet 2002;360:103–108
Delaere KPJ, Van Thillo EL. Semin Oncol 1991;18(5 Suppl 6):13–18
Iversen P et al. J Urol 2000;164:1579–1582
Janknegt RA. Cancer 1993;72(12 Suppl 17):3874–3877
Janknegt RA et al. J Urol 1993;149:77–83
Periti P et al. Clin Pharmacokinet 2002;41:485–504
Tyrrell CJ. Eur Urol 1994;26(Suppl 1):15–19

Treatment options:
1. Surgical castration: Orchiectomy
2. Medical castration: LHRH agonists
3. Nonsteroidal antiandrogens
4. Androgen-deprivation therapy (ADT)
   - GnRH antagonist
   - Orchiectomy + antiandrogen
   - LHRH agonist + antiandrogen

LHRH agonists:
1. **Leuprolide depot** 7.5 mg intramuscularly every month
2. **Leuprolide depot** 22.5 mg intramuscularly every 3 months
3. **Leuprolide depot** 30 mg intramuscularly every 4 months
4. **Leuprolide depot** 45 mg intramuscularly every 6 months
5. **Goserelin implant** 3.6 mg subcutaneously every 4 weeks
6. **Goserelin implant** 10.8 mg subcutaneously every 3 months

Nonsteroidal antiandrogens:
1. **Flutamide** 250 mg/dose orally 3 times per day, continually
2. **Bicalutamide** 50 mg or 150 mg/day if given as monotherapy orally, continually
3. **Nilutamide** 300 mg/day orally for 1 month with castration, followed by nilutamide 150 mg/day orally, continually

GnRH antagonist
Degarelix, starting dose, 240 mg given as two subcutaneous injections of 120 mg in the first month followed by maintenance dose of 80 mg given as one subcutaneous injection monthly thereafter

Supportive Care
Antiemetic prophylaxis
The regimens are not emetogenic. Primary prophylaxis is not indicated
See Chapter 42 for antiemetic recommendations

Hematopoietic growth factor (CSF) prophylaxis
Primary prophylaxis is NOT indicated
See Chapter 43 for more information

Antimicrobial prophylaxis
Risk of fever and neutropenia is LOW
   Antimicrobial primary prophylaxis to be considered:
   - Antibacterial—not indicated
   - Antifungal—not indicated
   - Antiviral—not indicated unless patient previously had an episode of HSV

Efficacy

Metastatic disease
1. LHRH agonists ≤85% response rate
2. No significant differences among LHRH agonists
3. Single-agent antiandrogen therapy may be inferior to medical (LHRH agonist) or surgical castration
4. Use of combined androgen blockade (CAB) as frontline therapy is controversial with limited evidence of clinical benefit

Locally advanced disease
Concurrent radiation and hormonal therapy in locally advanced disease appears to have a survival benefit. LHRH agonist + an antiandrogen are used for up to 3 months before, during, and for 3 years after radiation treatment

Bolla M et al. Lancet 2002;360:103–108
Laverdière J et al. Int J Radiat Oncol Biol Phys 1997;37:247–252
Prostate Cancer Trialists' Collaborative Group. Lancet 2000;355:1491–1498
Seidenfeld J et al. Ann Intern Med 2000;132:566–577. Erratum in: Ann Intern Med 2005;143:764–765; comment in: Ann Intern Med 2000;132:584–585

Patient Population Studied

Patients with metastatic and locally advanced prostate cancer treated with hormonal therapy

Therapy Monitoring

All antiandrogens
1. *Monthly for the first 4 months:* LFTs
2. *Every 2–3 months after the first 4 months:* LFTs

Nilutamide
1. Baseline chest x-ray before therapy
2. *For respiratory symptoms:* Discontinue therapy pending evaluation

Wysowski DK, Fourcroy JL. J Urol 1996;155:209–212

Toxicity

Common Toxicities of Androgen Deprivation

Hot flashes	LHRH Ag > AA
Loss of libido, impotence	LHRH Ag >> AA
Bone and muscle loss	LHRH Ag >> AA
Breast tenderness	AA >> LHRH Ag
Gynecomastia	AA >> LHRH Ag
Skin and hair changes	N/A
Weight gain	N/A
Asthenia	N/A

AA, antiandrogens; LHRH Ag, LHRH agonists

Toxicities of Individual Androgen Therapies

	% Patients
LHRH Agonists	
Tumor flare	Variable
Injection-site reactions	Variable
Flutamide	
Gynecomastia	45–50
Diarrhea	20
Nausea/vomiting	5
Hepatitis	2.5
Vertigo	2.5
Hot flashes	2.5
Bicalutamide	
Gynecomastia	49
Breast tenderness	40
Constipation	14
Aggravation reaction	13
Hot flashes	13
Asthenia	12
Urinary retention	10
Diarrhea	6
Nausea/vomiting	5
Nilutamide	
Hot flashes	28
Visual disturbance*	27–50
Nausea	10 (7–20)
Dyspnea	6
Interstitial pneumonitis	1-2
Gynecomastia	4
Alcohol intolerance	5–19
Increased LFTs†	4–8
Anemia	4

*Includes decreased adaptation to darkness, blurred vision
†Transient in a majority of patients

Notes

1. For patients with metastatic prostate cancer being treated with an LHRH agonist alone, a testosterone level should be checked at 1 month. If it is >20 ng/dL, consider orchiectomy or adding antiandrogen
2. Concurrent antiandrogen therapy can be used with LHRH agonist for the first 2–4 weeks of treatment to avoid tumor flare
3. Antiandrogen withdrawal should be considered the first therapeutic maneuver in men whose disease has progressed after treatment with combined androgen blockade. Approximately 20% of patients have a significant decrease in serum PSA when antiandrogen is withdrawn
4. Degarelix binds to the GnRH receptor in the pituitary gland and blocks LH/FSH release from the pituitary. Patients typically achieve castrate levels of testosterone by day 3 of treatment without a testosterone surge. A phase 3, 1-year, multicenter, randomized, open-label trial compared the efficacy and safety of degarelix with leuprolide. In all, 610 patients with all stages of histologically confirmed prostate cancer for whom androgen deprivation therapy was indicated were enrolled. Patients receiving degarelix showed a significantly lower risk of PSA progression or death compared with leuprolide (P = 0.05). PSA recurrences occurred primarily in patients with advanced disease and exclusively in those with baseline PSA >20 ng/mL. The latter had a significantly longer time to PSA recurrence with degarelix. The results suggest degarelix offers improved PSA control compared with leuprolide. However, further studies are warranted to confirm these findings
5. With acute cord compression or other oncologic emergency caused by a growing prostate tumor, degarelix is the preferred treatment

Kelly WK, Scher HI. J Urol 1993;149:607–609
Pont A. J Urol 1987;137:902–904
Tombal B et al. Eur Urol 2010;57:836–842

NON-METASTATIC • CASTRATION-RESISTANT
PROSTATE CANCER REGIMEN: APALUTAMIDE

Smith MR et al. N Engl J Med 2018;378:1408–1418
Supplementary appendix to: Smith MR et al. N Engl J Med 2018;378:1408–1418
Protocol for: Smith MR et al. N Engl J Med 2018;378:1408–1418
ERLEADA (apalutamide) prescribing information. Horsham, PA: Janssen Products, LP; revised September 2019
Food and Drug Administration Center for Drug Evaluation and Research. NDA/BLA Multi-Disciplinary Review and Evaluation NDA 210951 Erleada (apalutamide) (February 1, 2016) www.accessdata.fda.gov/drugsatfda_docs/nda/2018/210951Orig1s000MultidisciplineR.pdf [accessed 22 Sep 2019]

Apalutamide 240 mg per dose; administer orally once daily at about the same time each day either with or without food, continually, until radiographic or clinical progression of disease (total dose/week = 1680 mg)

Notes:

• Patients receiving apalutamide should have undergone bilateral orchiectomy or should receive concurrent treatment with a gonadotropin-releasing hormone (GnRH) analogue

• Instruct patients who miss a regularly scheduled dose of apalutamide to take the next dose as soon as possible on the same day, and then return to the usual administration schedule on the following day. Patients should be instructed not to take extra tablets to make up missed doses

• Instruct patients to swallow apalutamide tablets whole

• Drug interactions:

  ▪ Apalutamide is a strong inducer of CYP3A4, a strong inducer of CYP2C19, a weak inducer of CYP2C9, a weak inducer of P-glycoprotein (P-gp), a weak inducer of BCRP, and a weak inducer of OATPB1. In vitro experiments suggest that apalutamide may inhibit organic cation transporter 2 (OCT2), organic anion transporter 3 (OAT3), and multidrug and toxin extrusions (MATEs). It is predicted that apalutamide has the potential to induce UDP-glucuronosyltransferase (UGT)

    ○ Coadministration of a CYP3A4 substrate (midazolam) following repeated doses of apalutamide was associated with a 92% reduction in the midazolam AUC. If possible, substitute another medication for a CYP3A4 substrate, or monitor for loss of CYP3A4 substrate efficacy

    ○ Coadministration of a CYP2C19 substrate (omeprazole) following repeated doses of apalutamide was associated with an 85% reduction in the AUC of omeprazole. If possible, substitute another medication for a CYP2C19 substrate, or monitor for loss of CYP2C19 substrate efficacy

    ○ Coadministration of a CYP2C9 substrate (S-warfarin) following repeated doses of apalutamide was associated with a 46% reduction in the AUC of S-warfarin. If possible, substitute another medication for a CYP2C9 substrate, or monitor for loss of CYP2C9 substrate efficacy

    ○ Coadministration of a CYP2C8 substrate (pioglitazone) following repeated doses of apalutamide was associated with an 18% reduction in pioglitazone AUC. It is not necessary to avoid CYP2C8 substrates with apalutamide

    ○ Coadministration of a P-gp substrate (fexofenadine) following repeated doses of apalutamide was associated with a 30% reduction in fexofenadine AUC. If possible, substitute another medication for a P-gp substrate, or monitor for loss of P-gp substrate efficacy

    ○ Coadministration of a BCRP/OATP1B1 substrate (rosuvastatin) following repeated doses of apalutamide was associated with a 41% reduction in rosuvastatin AUC. If possible, substitute another medication for a BCRP or OATP1B1 substrate, or monitor for loss of BCRP/OATP1B1 substrate efficacy

  ▪ Apalutamide is primarily metabolized by CYP2C8 and CYP3A4 to an active metabolite, *N*-desmethyl apalutamide. Because apalutamide is a strong CYP3A4 inducer, it induces its own metabolism. At steady state, it is estimated that the relative contribution of CYP2C8 to apalutamide metabolism is 40% and that of CYP3A4 is 37%

    ○ Coadministration of a strong CYP3A4 inhibitor (itraconazole) with a single dose of apalutamide decreased apalutamide C_{max} by 22%, caused no change in apalutamide AUC, decreased *N*-desmethyl apalutamide C_{max} by 15%, and caused no change in *N*-desmethyl apalutamide AUC. Physiologically based pharmacokinetic simulations predict that ketoconazole (another strong CYP3A4 inhibitor) would increase steady-state apalutamide C_{max} by 38%, increase steady-state apalutamide AUC_{0-24} by 51%, increase active unbound fraction (defined as unbound apalutamide plus one-third of unbound *N*-desmethyl apalutamide) C_{max} by 23%, and increase active unbound fraction AUC_{0-24} by 28%. No initial adjustment in the apalutamide dose is necessary in patients receiving strong CYP3A4 inhibitors

    ○ Coadministration of a single dose of apalutamide with a strong CYP2C8 inhibitor (gemfibrozil 600 mg by mouth twice a day) was associated with a decrease in apalutamide C_{max} of 21%, an increase in apalutamide AUC_{inf} of 68%, a decrease in *N*-desmethyl apalutamide C_{max} of 45%, and a decrease in AUC_{inf} of 15%. Physiologically based pharmacokinetic simulations predict that gemfibrozil will lead to an increase in apalutamide steady-state C_{max} by 32%, an increase in apalutamide steady-state AUC_{0-24} by 44%, an increase in active unbound fraction C_{max} by 19%, and an increase in active unbound fraction AUC_{0-24} by 23%. No initial adjustment in the apalutamide dose is necessary in patients receiving strong CYP2C8 inhibitors

    ○ There have been no clinical studies prospectively evaluating the effects of strong CYP3A4 inducers or strong CYP2C8 inducers on the pharmacokinetics of apalutamide. Physiologically based pharmacokinetic simulations predict that rifampin (a strong CYP3A4 inducer and moderate CYP2C8 inducer) will decrease the apalutamide steady-state C_{max} by 25%, decrease the apalutamide steady-state AUC_{0-24} by 34%, decrease the active unbound fraction C_{max} by 15%, and decrease the active unbound fraction AUC_{0-24} by 19%. No adjustment in the apalutamide dose is necessary in patients receiving strong CYP3A4 inducers or strong CYP2C8 inducers

(continued)

(*continued*)
Supportive Care
Antiemetic prophylaxis
Emetogenic potential is MINIMAL
See Chapter 42 for antiemetic recommendations

Hematopoietic growth factor (CSF) prophylaxis
Primary prophylaxis is NOT indicated
See Chapter 43 for more information

Antimicrobial prophylaxis
Risk of fever and neutropenia is *LOW*
   Antimicrobial primary prophylaxis to be considered:
   • Antibacterial—not indicated
   • Antifungal—not indicated
   • Antiviral—not indicated unless patient previously had an episode of HSV

Patient Population Studied

The multinational, multicenter, randomized, double-blind, placebo-controlled, phase 3 trial involved 1207 men with pathologically confirmed, nonmetastatic, castration-resistant adenocarcinoma of the prostate with a prostate-specific antigen (PSA) doubling time of ≤10 months despite ongoing androgen deprivation therapy (ie, gonadotropin-releasing hormone [GnRH] analogue or prior bilateral orchiectomy). Eligible patients were required to have either no local or regional nodal disease (ie, N0 per the TNM staging system) or malignant pelvic lymph nodes <2 cm in the short axis (ie, N1 per the TNM staging system) located below the aortic bifurcation, an Eastern Cooperative Oncology Group (ECOG) performance status of 0–1, and adequate organ function. Patients with a history of seizure or with a condition that conferred a predisposition to seizures were excluded. All patients continued androgen deprivation therapy throughout the study and were randomized (2:1) to receive apalutamide or placebo after stratification according to PSA doubling time (>6 months vs ≤6 months), use of bone modifying agents, and node staging (N0 vs N1)

Efficacy (N = 1207)

	Apalutamide (n = 806)	Placebo (n = 401)	Statistics
Median metastasis-free survival	40.5 months	16.2 months	HR 0.28 (95% CI, 0.23–0.35); P<0.001
Median time to metastasis	40.5 months	16.6 months	HR 0.27 (95% CI, 0.22–0.34); P<0.001
Median progression-free survival	40.5 months	14.7 months	HR 0.29 (95% CI, 0.24–0.36); P<0.001
Median time to symptomatic progression*	Not reached	Not reached	HR 0.45 (95% CI, 0.32–0.63); P<0.001
Median overall survival†	Not reached	39.0 months	HR 0.70 (95% CI, 0.47–1.04); P=0.07
Median time to the initiation of cytotoxic chemotherapy	Not reached	Not reached	HR 0.44 (95% CI, 0.29–0.66)
Median second-progression—free survival	Not reached	39.0 months	HR 9.49 (95% CI, 0.36–0.66)
Median time to PSA progression‡	Not reached	3.7 months	HR 0.06 (95% CI, 0.05–0.08)
Patients with a PSA response§	89.7%	2.2%	Relative risk 40 (95% CI, 21–77)

Median follow-up of 20.3 months
*Defined as the time from randomization to a skeletal-related event, pain progression, or worsening of disease-related symptoms leading to the initiation of a new systemic anticancer therapy or the time to the development of clinically significant symptoms due to local or regional tumor progression leading to surgery or radiation therapy. The P value for this outcome crossed the O'Brien-Fleming efficacy boundary of 0.00008
†The P value for this outcome did not cross the O'Brien-Fleming efficacy boundary of 0.00008
‡Defined as time from randomization to PSA progression according to the Prostate Cancer Working Group 2 criteria (J Clin Oncol 2008;26:1148–1159)
§Defined as a decline from baseline in the PSA level of ≥50% according to the Prostate Cancer Working Group 2 criteria (J Clin Oncol 2008;26:1148–1159)

Therapy Monitoring

1. Obtain TSH prior to the start of therapy and then every 4 months, or as clinically appropriate. The incidence of hypothyroidism in the apalutamide arm was 8.1% versus 2% in the placebo arm, with a median onset of 16 weeks. All events reported in the trial were grade ≤2

2. Optimize management of cardiovascular risk factors, such as hypertension, diabetes, or dyslipidemia

3. Evaluate patients for fracture and fall risk. The incidence of fracture was 12% in the apalutamide arm and was 7% in the placebo arm which suggests that apalutamide increases risk of fracture beyond that associated with background androgen deprivation therapy. The overall incidence of falls was 16% in the apalutamide arm and 9% in the placebo arm. Among patients who received apalutamide in combined studies, falls occurred in 8% of patients <65 years of age, in 10% of patients between 65–74 years of age, and in 19% of patients ≥75 years of age. Monitor and manage patients at risk for fractures according to established treatment guidelines and consider use of bone-targeted agents. Consider interventions to reduce fall risk in patients at risk for falls, especially in the elderly

4. Advise patients who have a history of seizure of the risk of developing a seizure and of engaging in any activity where sudden loss of consciousness could cause serious harm to themselves or others

5. Obtain serum PSA at every visit; monitor radiographic imaging if PSA is increasing or as clinically indicated

Treatment Modifications

APALUTAMIDE	
Starting Dose	240 mg by mouth once daily
Dose Level −1	180 mg by mouth once daily
Dose Level −2	120 mg by mouth once daily
Dose Level −3	Discontinue therapy

General dose adjustments	
Any grade Seizure	Permanently discontinue apalutamide
G ≤2 ischemic heart disease event	Continue apalutamide at current dose and optimize management of cardiovascular risk factors
G3/4 ischemic heart disease event	Consider permanent discontinuation of apalutamide
G ≤2 rash without intolerable symptoms	Optimize supportive management with oral antihistamines and topical corticosteroids, as clinically appropriate Continue apalutamide at the same dose
G3 rash, or any grade rash with intolerable symptoms	Optimize supportive management with oral antihistamines, topical corticosteroids, and (in select patients) systemic corticosteroids, as clinically appropriateInterrupt apalutamide dosing until rash resolves to G ≤1 or baseline, then resume at the same or a reduced dose (180 mg or 120 mg) if warranted
Hypothyroidism	Initiate or adjust thyroid replacement therapy as clinically indicated Continue apalutamide at the same dose
Other G ≥3 toxicity or intolerable side effect	Interrupt apalutamide dosing until symptoms resolve to G ≤1 or baseline, then resume at the same or a reduced dose (180 mg or 120 mg) if warranted
A sensitive medication which is a substrate of any of the following enzymes or transporters is required: CYP3A4, CYP2C19, CYP2C9, P-glycoprotein, BCRP, or OATP1B1	Consider substituting another medication which is not a substrate for any of these enzymes or transporters. If this is not possible, then monitor closely for loss of activity of the sensitive medication

Note: Advise patients of potential risk to a developing fetus. Advise male patients with female partners of reproductive potential to use effective contraception during treatment and for 3 months after the last dose of apalutamide. Advise male patients to use a condom if having sex with a pregnant woman

ERLEADA (apalutamide) prescribing information. Horsham, PA: Janssen Products, LP; revised September 2019

Adverse Events (N = 1201)

	Apalutamide (n = 803)		Placebo (n = 398)	
	Grade 1–2 (%)	Grade 3–4 (%)	Grade 1–2 (%)	Grade 3–4 (%)
Any AE	51	45	59	34
Fatigue	27	1	21	<1
Hypertension	10	14	8	12
Rash	19	5	5	<1
Diarrhea	19	1	15	1
Nausea	18	0	16	0
Weight loss	15	1	6	<1
Arthralgia	16	0	8	0
Falls	14	2	8	1
Fracture*	9	3	6	1
Dizziness*	9	1	6	0
Hypothyroidism*	8	0	2	0
Metal-impairment disorder*	5	0	3	0
Seizure*	<1	0	0	0

Note: Toxicities were included in the table if they occurred in at least 15% of patients in either group, or if they were deemed to be of special interest

*Denotes adverse event of special interest

There were 10 grade 5 adverse events reported in the apalutamide arm (myocardial infarction, n = 2; cardiopulmonary arrest, n = 1; cerebral hemorrhage, n = 1; multiple organ dysfunction, n = 1; pneumonia, n = 1; prostate cancer, n = 2; and sepsis, n = 2) and 1 grade 5 adverse event reported in the placebo arm (cardiopulmonary arrest, n = 1). Serious adverse events occurred in 25% of patients in the apalutamide arm and in 23% of patients in the placebo arm.

Adverse events that led to discontinuation of trial therapy occurred in 11% of patients in the apalutamide arm and in 7% of patients in the placebo arm

NON-METASTATIC • CASTRATION-RESISTANT

PROSTATE CANCER REGIMEN: ENZALUTAMIDE

Hussain M et al. N Engl J Med 2018;378:2465–2474
Protocol for: Hussain M et al. N Engl J Med 2018;378:2465–2474
Supplementary appendix to: Hussain M et al. N Engl J Med 2018;378:2465–2474
XTANDI (enzalutamide) prescribing information. New York, NY: Astellas Pharma US, Inc; revised July 2018

Enzalutamide 160 mg per dose; administer orally once daily at about the same time each day either with or without food, continually, until radiographic or clinical progression of disease (total dose/week = 1120 mg)

Notes:
- Patients receiving enzalutamide should have undergone bilateral orchiectomy or should also receive concurrent treatment with a gonadotropin-releasing hormone (GnRH) analogue
- If possible, avoid concomitant use of strong CYP2C8 inhibitors. If patients must receive a strong CYP2C8 inhibitor concomitantly, reduce the enzalutamide dose to 80 mg once daily. If coadministration of the strong inhibitor is discontinued, the enzalutamide dose should be returned to the dose used prior to initiation of a strong CYP2C8 inhibitor
- Coadministration of a strong CYP3A4 inhibitor (e.g., itraconazole) increased the composite AUC of enzalutamide plus *N*-desmethyl enzalutamide 1.3-fold in healthy volunteers
- Coadministration of enzalutamide with rifampin (a strong CYP4A4 inducer and moderate CYP2C8 inducer) decrease the composite AUC of enzalutamide pus *N*-desmethyl enzalutamide by 37%. Coadministration of enzalutamide with strong CYP3A4 inducers and St John's wort should be avoided if possible. If coadministration of a strong CYP3A4 inducer with enzalutamide is required, increase the dose of enzalutamide from 160 mg by mouth once daily to 240 mg by mouth once daily
- Enzalutamide is a strong CYP3A4 inducer and a moderate CYP2C9 and CYP2C19 inducer in humans. At steady state, enzalutamide reduced the plasma exposure to midazolam (CYP3A4 substrate), warfarin (CYP2C9 substrate), and omeprazole (CYP2C19 substrate). Concomitant use of enzalutamide with narrow-therapeutic-index drugs that are metabolized by CYP3A4, CYP2C9 (eg, phenytoin, warfarin) and CYP2C19 should be avoided, as enzalutamide may decrease their exposure. If coadministration with warfarin cannot be avoided, conduct additional INR monitoring

Supportive Care
Antiemetic prophylaxis
Emetogenic potential is **MINIMAL**
See Chapter 42 for antiemetic recommendations

Hematopoietic growth factor (CSF) prophylaxis
Primary prophylaxis is NOT indicated
See Chapter 43 for more information

Antimicrobial prophylaxis
Risk of fever and neutropenia is *LOW*
   Antimicrobial primary prophylaxis to be considered:
   - Antibacterial—not indicated
   - Antifungal—not indicated
   - Antiviral—not indicated unless patient previously had an episode of HSV

Patient Population Studied

The international, multicenter, randomized, double-blind, phase 3 trial involved 1401 patients with pathologically confirmed adenocarcinoma of the prostate. Eligible patients had an Eastern Cooperative Oncology Group (ECOG) performance status of ≤1, no evidence of metastatic disease, a rising prostate-specific antigen (PSA) measurement on ≥3 samples collected at least 1 week apart, a baseline PSA value of ≥2 ng/mL, a PSA doubling time of ≤10 months as calculated using the method described by Pound et al (JAMA 1999;281:1591–1597), and castrate levels of testosterone (≤0.5 ng/mL) due to gonadotropin-releasing hormone (GRH) agonist therapy, GRH antagonist therapy, or prior bilateral orchiectomy. Patients who had a history of seizure or a condition that could confer a predisposition to seizure were not eligible. Patients were randomly assigned to receive oral enzalutamide 160 mg or placebo once daily

Efficacy (N = 1401)

	Enzalutamide (n = 933)	Placebo (n = 468)	Statistics
Median metastasis-free survival*	36.6 months	14.7 months	HR 0.29 (95% CI, 0.24–0.35); P<0.001
Metastasis or death	23%	49%	—
Radiographic progression	20%	48%	—
Death without evidence of radiographic progression†	3%	1%	—
PSA progression	22%	69%	—
Median time to PSA progression	37.2 months	3.9 months	HR 0.07 (95% CI, 0.05–0.08); P<0.001
Use of subsequent antineoplastic therapy	15%	48%	—
Median time to use of subsequent antineoplastic therapy	39.6 months	17.7 months	HR 0.21 (95% CI, 0.17–0.26); P<0.001
Median overall survival‡	Not reached	Not reached	HR 0.80 (95% CI, 0.58–1.09); P=0.15
Confirmed PSA response ≥50%	76%	2%	—

Median follow-up of 18.5 months in the enzalutamide arm and 15.1 months in the placebo arm
*Hazard ratio is for metastasis or death
†Death is defined as death occurring between randomization and 112 days after discontinuation of the trial regimen in the absence of radiographic progression
‡Hazard ratio is for death

Therapy Monitoring

1. Obtain CBC with differential prior to start of therapy
2. Optimize management of cardiovascular risk factors, such as hypertension, diabetes, or dyslipidemia
3. Monitor blood pressure at least monthly. Encourage patients to monitor their blood pressure
4. Evaluate patients for fracture and fall risk. Monitor and manage patients at risk for fractures according to established treatment guidelines and consider use of bone-targeted agents
5. Advise patients who have a history of seizure of the risk of developing a seizure and of engaging in any activity where sudden loss of consciousness could cause serious harm to themselves or others
6. Obtain serum PSA at every visit; monitor radiographic imaging if PSA is increasing or as clinically indicated

Treatment Modifications

ENZALUTAMIDE

Starting Dose	160 mg by mouth once daily
Dose Level −1	120 mg by mouth once daily
Dose Level −2	80 mg by mouth once daily
Dose Level −3	Discontinue therapy

General dose adjustments

Seizure	Permanently discontinue enzalutamide
Posterior reversible encephalopathy syndrome (PRES)	Permanently discontinue enzalutamide
Hypersensitivity to enzalutamide	Permanently discontinue enzalutamide
G ≤2 ischemic heart disease event	Continue enzalutamide at current dose and optimize management of cardiovascular risk factors
G3/4 ischemic heart disease event	Permanently discontinue enzalutamide
Other G ≥3 toxicity or intolerable side effect	Interrupt enzalutamide dosing for 1 week or until symptoms resolve to G ≤2, then resume at the same or a reduced dose (120 mg or 80 mg) if warranted
Strong CYP2C8 inhibitor is required	Reduce the enzalutamide dose to 80 mg by mouth once daily

(continued)

Treatment Modifications (*continued*)

General dose adjustments

Strong CYP2C8 inhibitors is discontinued	Resume the enzalutamide dose that was used prior to initiation of the strong CYP2C8 inhibitors
Strong CYP3A4 inducer is required	Increase the enzalutamide dose from 160 mg to 240 mg by mouth once daily
Strong CYP3A4 inducer is discontinued	Resume the enzalutamide dose that was used prior to initiation of the strong CYP3A4 inducer

Note: Advise patients of potential risk to a developing fetus. Advise females who are or may become pregnant not to handle enzalutamide. Advise male patients with female partners of reproductive potential to use effective contraception during treatment and for 3 months after the last dose of enzalutamide. Advise male patients to use a condom if having sex with a pregnant woman

Xtandi (enzalutamide) prescribing information. New York, NY: Astellas Pharma US, Inc; revised July 2018

Adverse Events (N = 1395)

	Enzalutamide (n = 930)		Placebo (n = 465)	
	Grade 1–2 (%)	Grade 3–5 (%)	Grade 1–2 (%)	Grade 3–5 (%)
Any adverse event	55.5	31.4	54	23.4
Fatigue	29.7	2.9	13.1	0.6
Hot flush	12.9	0.1	7.7	0
Nausea	11.1	0.3	8.6	0
Diarrhea	9.5	0.3	9.2	0.4
Fall	10.1	1.3	3.4	0.6
Constipation	8.9	0.2	6.5	0.4
Dizziness	9.4	0.4	4.3	0
Arthralgia	8.3	0.1	6.7	0.2
Asthenia	7.6	1.2	5.8	0.2
Decreased appetite	9.4	0.2	3.7	0.2
Back pain	7.6	0.2	6.9	0.2
Headache	8.9	0.2	4.5	0
Hematuria	4.9	1.7	4.9	2.8
Urinary tract infection	3.3	0.8	5.8	0.6
Weight loss	5.7	0.2	1.5	0
Urinary retention	1.7	0.4	4.9	1.1

	Enzalutamide (n = 930)		Placebo (n = 465)	
	Grade 1–2 (%)	Grade 3–5 (%)	Grade 1–2 (%)	Grade 3–5 (%)
Hypertension*	7.3	4.6	3	2.2
Major adverse cardiovascular event*†	1.5	3.7	1.1	1.7
Mental impairment disorders*	5.1	0.1	1.9	0
Hepatic impairment*	0.6	0.5	1.5	0.4
Neutropenia*	0.4	0.5	0	0.2
Convulsion*	0.1	0.2	0	0
Posterior reversible encephalopathy syndrome	0	0	0	0

Note: Toxicities are included in the table if all-grade events were reported in at least 5% of the patients in either group or if they were denoted as being of special interest. Serious adverse events (ie, those that resulted in death, were life-threatening, resulted in or prolonged hospitalization, resulted in inability to conduct normal life functions, or led to a congenital anomaly or birth defect) occurred in 24% of patients in the enzalutamide group and in 18% of patients in the placebo group. Adverse events leading to discontinuation of the trial regimen occurred in 9% of patients in the enzalutamide group and in 6% of patients in the placebo group. Grade 5 adverse events occurred in 3% of patients in the enzalutamide group and in 1% of patients in the placebo group
*Denotes adverse events of special interest
†Includes acute myocardial infarction, hemorrhagic cerebrovascular conditions, ischemic cerebrovascular conditions, and heart failure

NON-METASTATIC • CASTRATION-RESISTANT

PROSTATE CANCER REGIMEN: DAROLUTAMIDE

Fizazi K et al. N Engl J Med 2019;380:1235–1246
Supplementary appendix to: Fizazi K et al. N Engl J Med 2019;380:1235–1246
Protocol for: Fizazi K et al. N Engl J Med 2019;380:1235–1246
NUBEQA (darolutamide) prescribing information. Whippany, NJ: Bayer HealthCare Pharmaceuticals Inc; revised July 2019

Darolutamide 600 mg per dose; administer orally twice per day with food, continually, until radiographic or clinical progression of disease (total dose/week = 8400 mg)

Notes:
- Patients receiving darolutamide should have undergone bilateral orchiectomy or should receive concurrent treatment with a gonadotropin-releasing hormone (GnRH) analogue
- Instruct patients who miss a regularly scheduled dose of darolutamide to take the next dose as soon as possible prior to the next regularly scheduled dose. Patients should be instructed not to take extra tablets to make up missed doses
- Instruct patients to swallow darolutamide tablets whole and with food. The bioavailability of darolutamide in the fasted state is approximately 30% and is increased 2.0- to 2.5-fold when administered with food
- Non-cancer subjects with severe renal impairment (eGFR 15–29 mL/min/1.73m^2 not on hemodialysis) had 2.5-fold higher exposure to darolutamide. Therefore, reduce the darolutamide dose to 300 mg per dose administered orally twice per day with food in patients with severe renal impairment. There are no data to support a recommended darolutamide dose in patients undergoing hemodialysis
- Non-cancer subjects with moderate hepatic dysfunction (Child-Pugh Class B) had 1.9-fold higher exposure to darolutamide. Therefore, reduce the darolutamide dose to 300 mg per dose administered orally twice per day with food in patients with moderate hepatic dysfunction. There are no data to support a recommended darolutamide dose in patients with severe hepatic impairment (Child-Pugh C)
- Drug interactions:
  - Darolutamide is an inhibitor of BCRP. In vitro experiments also suggest that darolutamide inhibits OATP1B1 and OATP1B3
    - Coadministration of rosuvastatin (a BCRP substrate) with darolutamide was associated with a 5-fold increase in the mean rosuvastatin AUC and C$_{max}$. Therefore, if possible, avoid concomitant use of darolutamide with BCRP substrates. If concomitant use is unavoidable, monitor more closely for side effects of the BCRP substrate medication and consider reducing the dose of the BCRP substrate medication as appropriate
  - Darolutamide is primarily metabolized by CYP3A4 to an active metabolite, keto-darolutamide. UGT1A9 and UGT1A1 also contribute to darolutamide metabolism
    - Coadministration of darolutamide with rifampin (a combined P-glycoprotein and strong CYP3A4 inducer) decreased mean darolutamide AUC$_{0-72}$ by 72% and decreased C$_{max}$ by 52%. A moderate CYP3A4 inducer is predicted to decrease darolutamide exposure by 36–58%. Therefore, avoid concomitant use of darolutamide with combined P-gp and strong or moderate CYP3A4 inducers
    - Coadministration of darolutamide with itraconazole (a combined P-gp inhibitor and strong CYP3A4 inhibitor) increased mean darolutamide AUC$_{0-72}$ 1.7-fold and increased darolutamide C$_{max}$ 1.4-fold. It is not necessary to adjust the initial dose of darolutamide when concomitant use with a combined P-gp and strong CYP3A4 inhibitor is unavoidable; however, monitor more frequently for darolutamide adverse reactions

Supportive Care
Antiemetic prophylaxis
Emetogenic potential is **MINIMAL**
See Chapter 42 for antiemetic recommendations

Hematopoietic growth factor (CSF) prophylaxis
Primary prophylaxis is NOT indicated
See Chapter 43 for more information

(continued)

Patient Population Studied

The multinational, multicenter, randomized, double-blind, placebo-controlled, phase 3 trial involved 1509 men with pathologically confirmed, nonmetastatic, castration-resistant adenocarcinoma of the prostate with a prostate-specific antigen (PSA) of ≥2 ng/mL and a PSA doubling time of ≤10 months despite ongoing androgen deprivation. Eligible patients were required to have either no local or regional nodal disease (ie, N0 per the TNM staging system) or malignant pelvic lymph nodes <2 cm in the short axis (ie, N1 per the TNM staging system) located below the aortic bifurcation, an Eastern Cooperative Oncology Group (ECOG) performance status of 0–1, and adequate organ function. Patients with a history of seizure or with a condition that conferred a predisposition to seizures were permitted to enroll. All patients continued androgen deprivation therapy throughout the study and were randomized (2:1) to receive darolutamide or placebo after stratification according to PSA doubling time (>6 months vs ≤6 months) and the use of bone-modifying agents

(*continued*)

Antimicrobial prophylaxis
Risk of fever and neutropenia is *LOW*
Antimicrobial primary prophylaxis to be considered:
- Antibacterial—not indicated
- Antifungal—not indicated
- Antiviral—not indicated unless patient previously had an episode of HSV

Efficacy (N = 1509)

	Darolutamide (n = 955)	Placebo (n = 554)	Statistics
Median metastasis-free survival*	40.4 months (95% CI, 34.3–not reached)	18.4 months (95% CI, 15.5–22.3)	HR 0.41 (95% CI, 0.34–0.50); P<0.001
Median overall survival	Not reached	Not reached	HR 0.71 (95% CI, 0.50–0.99); P=0.045
Median time to pain progression	40.3 months	25.4 months	HR 0.65 (95% CI, 0.53–0.79); P<0.001
Median time to initiation of cytotoxic chemotherapy	Not reached	38.2 months	HR 0.43 (95% CI, 0.31–0.60); P<0.001
Median time to first symptomatic skeletal event‡	Not reached	Not reached	HR 0.43 (95% CI, 0.22–0.84); P=0.01
Median progression-free survival	36.8 months	14.8 months	HR 0.38 (95% CI, 0.32–0.45); P<0.001
Median time to PSA progression§	33.2 months	7.3 months	HR 0.13 (95% CI, 0.11–0.16); P<0.001
Median time to first prostate cancer-related invasive procedure	Not reached	Not reached	HR 0.39 (95% CI, 0.25–0.61); P<0.001
Median time to initiation of subsequent antineoplastic therapy	Not reached	Not reached	HR 0.33 (95% CI, 0.23–0.47); P<0.001

Median follow-up of 17.9 months
*Defined as the time from randomization to confirmed evidence of distant metastasis on imaging or death
†Defined as either an increase of ≥2 points from baseline in pain score on the Brief Pain Inventory (Short Form) or initiation of opioid treatment for cancer-related pain
‡Defined as external beam radiation therapy for skeletal symptoms, new symptomatic pathologic fracture, spinal cord compression, or tumor-related orthopedic surgical intervention
§Defined according to the Prostate Cancer Working Group 2 criteria (J Clin Oncol 2008;26:1148–1159)

Therapy Monitoring

1. Check liver function tests and serum creatinine prior to initiation of therapy
2. Monitor periodically for rash
3. Obtain serum PSA at every visit; monitor radiographic imaging if PSA is increasing or as clinically indicated

Treatment Modifications

DAROLUTAMIDE	
Starting Dose	600 mg by mouth twice per day
Dose Level −1	300 mg by mouth twice per day
Dose Level −2	Discontinue therapy

General dose adjustments	
G ≥3 toxicity or intolerable side effect	Interrupt darolutamide dosing, or reduce the dose to 300 mg by mouth twice per day until symptoms improve. Then, resume the treatment at the dose of 600 mg by mouth twice per day
A sensitive medication that is a substrate of BCRP is required	Consider substituting another medication that is not a substrate for BCRP. If this is not possible, then monitor closely for side effects related to the BCRP substrate medication and consider reducing the dose of the BCRP substrate medication as clinically appropriate

Treatment Modifications (*continued*)

General dose adjustments	
Patient is taking a combined P-glycoprotein and strong or moderate CYP3A4 inducer	Do not administer darolutamide with a combined P-glycoprotein and strong or moderately CYP3A4 inducer
Severe renal impairment (eGFR 15–29 mL/min/1.73m2 not on hemodialysis)	Reduce the darolutamide dose to 300 mg per dose administered orally twice per day with food
Moderate hepatic impairment (Child-Pugh Class B)	Reduce the darolutamide dose to 300 mg per dose administered orally twice per day with food

Note: Advise patients of potential risk to a developing fetus. Advise male patients with female partners of reproductive potential to use effective contraception during treatment and for 1 week after the last dose of darolutamide
NUBEQA (darolutamide) prescribing information. Whippany, NJ: Bayer HealthCare Pharmaceuticals Inc; revised 2019 July

Adverse Events (N = 1508)

	Darolutamide (n = 954)		Placebo (n = 554)	
	Grade 1–2 (%)	Grade 3–4 (%)	Grade 1–2 (%)	Grade 3–4 (%)
Any	58	25	57	19
Fatigue	12	<1	8	1
Back pain	8	<1	9	<1
Arthralgia	8	<1	9	<1
Diarrhea	7	0	5	<1
Hypertension	3	3	3	2
Constipation	6	0	6	0
Pain in an extremity	6	0	3	<1
Anemia	5	1	4	<1
Hot flush	5	0	4	0
Nausea	5	<1	6	0
Urinary tract infection	4	1	5	1
Urinary retention	2	2	5	2
Fatigue or asthenia*	15	1	10	1
Bone fracture*	3	1	3	1
Falls, including accident*	3	1	4	1

	Darolutamide (n = 954)		Placebo (n = 554)	
	Grade 1–2 (%)	Grade 3–4 (%)	Grade 1–2 (%)	Grade 3–4 (%)
Seizure*	<1	0	<1	0
Rash*	3	<1	1	0
Weight decrease*	4	0	2	0
Dizziness or vertigo*	4	<1	4	<1
Cognitive disorder*	<1	0	<1	0
Memory impairment*	1	0	1	0
Change in metal status*	0	0	<1	0
Hypothyroidism*	0	0	0	0
Cerebral ischemia*	1	1	1	1
Coronary-artery disorder*	2	2	2	<1
Heart failure*	1	1	1	0

Note: Toxicities were included in the table if they occurred in at least 5% of patients in either group, or if they were deemed to be of special interest
*Denotes adverse event of special interest
There were 37 grade 5 adverse events reported in the darolutamide and 18 grade 5 adverse events reported in the placebo arm. Serious adverse events occurred in 25% of patients in the darolutamide arm and in 20% of patients in the placebo arm. Adverse events which led to discontinuation of trial therapy occurred in 9% of patients in the darolutamide arm and in 9% of patients in the placebo arm

METASTATIC • HORMONE-SENSITIVE
PROSTATE CANCER REGIMEN: ABIRATERONE + PREDNISONE

Fizazi K et al. N Engl J Med 2017;377:352–360
Protocol for: Fizazi K et al. N Engl J Med 2017;377:352–360
Supplementary appendix to: Fizazi K et al. N Engl J Med 2017;377:352–360
Fizazi K et al. Lancet Oncol 2019;20:686–700
Supplementary appendix to: Fizazi K et al. Lancet Oncol 2019;20:686–700
ZYTIGA (abiraterone acetate) prescribing information. Horsham, PA: Janssen Biotech, Inc; revised June 2019

Abiraterone acetate 1000 mg orally once daily, continually for 28 consecutive days (total dosage/28-day cycle = 28,000 mg)

Note: No food should be consumed for at least 2 hours before a dose of abiraterone acetate is taken and for at least 1 hour after a dose of abiraterone acetate is taken. Exposure (area under the curve) of abiraterone acetate increases up to 10-fold when abiraterone acetate is taken with meals

Prednisone 5 mg orally once daily, continually for 28 consecutive days (total dosage/28-day cycle = 140 mg)

Notes:
- For patients with baseline moderate hepatic impairment (Child-Pugh Class B), reduce the dose of abiraterone acetate to 250 mg once daily
- Avoid abiraterone acetate in patients with baseline severe hepatic impairment (Child-Pugh Class C), as abiraterone acetate has not been studied in this population, and no dose adjustment can be predicted
- Abiraterone acetate is an inhibitor of the polymorphically expressed cytochrome P450 (CYP) enzyme CYP2D6
  - Avoid coadministration of abiraterone acetate with CYP2D6 substrates that have a low therapeutic index. If an alternative treatment cannot be used, exercise caution and consider a dose reduction of concomitantly used CYP2D6 substrates
- Monitor for symptoms and signs of adrenocortical insufficiency. Increased dosage of corticosteroids may be indicated before, during, and after stressful situations
- Monitor for signs and symptoms of mineralocorticoid excess, including hypokalemia, fluid retention, and hypertension. Prednisone dose may have to be supplemented in some patients or augmented with an aldosterone antagonist such as eplerenone
- Use abiraterone acetate with caution in patients with a history of cardiovascular disease. Control hypertension and correct hypokalemia before initiating treatment
- Abiraterone acetate is a substrate of CYP3A4. Avoid or use with caution strong CYP3A4 inhibitors (eg, atazanavir, clarithromycin, indinavir, itraconazole, ketoconazole, nefazodone, nelfinavir, ritonavir, saquinavir, telithromycin, voriconazole) or inducers (eg, carbamazepine, phenobarbital, phenytoin, rifabutin, rifapentine, rifampin) during abiraterone acetate treatment
- Abiraterone acetate was a strong inhibitor of CYP1A2 and CYP2D6, and a moderate inhibitor of CYP2C9, CYP2C19, and CYP3A4/5 in experimental systems. It is not yet known whether its effects on CYP1A2, CYP2C subfamily, or CYP3A subfamily enzymes in in vitro systems are representative of a potential for clinically important drug interactions
- Use abiraterone acetate with caution in patients with a history of cardiovascular disease. The safety of abiraterone acetate in patients with LVEF <50% or NYHA Class III or IV heart failure is not established. Control hypertension and correct hypokalemia before treatment

Supportive Care
Antiemetic prophylaxis
Emetogenic potential is **MINIMAL**
See Chapter 42 for antiemetic recommendations

Hematopoietic growth factor (CSF) prophylaxis
Primary prophylaxis is **NOT** *indicated*
See Chapter 43 for more information

Antimicrobial prophylaxis
Risk of fever and neutropenia is *LOW*
Antimicrobial primary prophylaxis to be considered:
- Antibacterial—not indicated
- Antifungal—not indicated
- Antiviral—not indicated unless patient previously had an episode of HSV

Patient Population Studied

The international, multicenter, randomized, double-blind, phase 3 trial involved 1199 adult patients with pathologically confirmed, newly diagnosed (≤3 months), high-risk prostate cancer. Eligible patients had at least 2 of the following high risk features: Gleason score of 8 or higher, 3 or more bone lesions, and/or measurable visceral metastases. Patients must have additionally had an ECOG (Eastern Cooperative Oncology Group) performance status of ≤2. Exclusion criteria included prior chemotherapy, radiation therapy, or surgery for metastatic disease (except 1 course of radiation or surgery for palliative treatment of symptoms was allowed); or significant cardiac, adrenal, or hepatic dysfunction. All patients underwent gonadotropin releasing hormone (GRH) analogue therapy or bilateral orchiectomy. Patients were randomly assigned to receive abiraterone 1000 mg orally daily plus prednisone 5 mg orally daily or placebos

Efficacy (N = 1199)

Endpoint	Abiraterone Acetate and Prednisone Plus Androgen-deprivation Therapy (n = 597)		Placebo Plus Androgen-deprivation Therapy (n = 602)		Hazard Ratio (95% CI)
	Events	Median, Months (95% CI)	Events	Median, Months (95% CI)	
Overall survival*	46%	53.3 (48.2–NR)	57%	36.5 months (33.5–40.0)	0.66 (0.56–0.78); P<0.0001
Radiographic progression†	239	33.0	354	14.8	0.47 (0.39–0.55); P<0.001
Pain progression*‡	41%	47.4 months (33.2–NR)	49%	16.6 months (11.1–24.0)	0.72 (0.61–0.86); P=0.00024
Skeletal-related events*§	22%	22%	25%	25%	0.75 (0.60–0.95); P=0.0181
Chemotherapy initiation*	25%	NR (62.6 months–NR)	36%	57.6 months (38.2–NR)	0.51 (0.41–0.63); P<0.0001
Subsequent prostate cancer therapy*|	42%	54.9 months (45.4–NR)	59%	21.2 months (18.6–23.5)	0.45 (0.38–0.53); P<0.0001
PSA progression*€	46%	33.3 months (29.4–46.1)	74%	7.4 months (7.2–9.2)	0.31 (0.27–0.36); P<0.0001

NR, not reached; PSA, prostate-specific antigen
*Data are from the final analysis with median follow-up of 51.8 months (IQR 47.2–57.0). Fizazi K et al. Lancet Oncol 2019;20:686–700
†Based on modified Prostate Cancer Working Group 2 criteria or RECIST, version 1.1. Data are from a planned interim analysis after a median follow-up of 30.4 months
‡Pain progression defined as the time from randomization to first increase of ≥30% from baseline in item 3 of the Brief Pain Inventory—Short Form
§Skeletal-related events defined as time from randomization to any of the following events: clinical or pathologic fracture, spinal cord compression, palliative radiotherapy to bone, or surgery to bone
\|Subsequent prostate cancer therapy includes hormonal therapy, chemotherapy, surgery, or radiotherapy
€PSA progression defined according to Prostate Cancer Working Group 3 criteria

Therapy Monitoring

1. Monitor blood pressure, serum potassium, and symptoms of fluid retention at least monthly
2. Measure serum transaminases (ALT and AST) and bilirubin levels prior to starting treatment with abiraterone acetate, every 2 weeks for the first 3 months of treatment, and monthly thereafter. Modify, interrupt, or discontinue abiraterone acetate dosing as recommended
3. In patients with baseline moderate hepatic impairment receiving a reduced abiraterone acetate dose of 250 mg/day, measure ALT, AST, and bilirubin prior to the start of treatment, every week for the first month, every 2 weeks for the following 2 months of treatment, and monthly thereafter. Promptly measure serum total bilirubin, AST, and ALT if clinical symptoms or signs suggestive of hepatotoxicity develop
4. For patients who resume treatment after LFTs return to G ≤1 from a G2–4 toxicity, monitor serum transaminases and bilirubin at a minimum of every 2 weeks for 3 months and monthly thereafter
5. Monitor for symptoms and signs of adrenocortical insufficiency. Increased dosage of corticosteroids may be indicated before, during, and after stressful situations
6. Obtain serum PSA and perform physical exam every 3–6 months. Monitor radiographic imaging every 6–12 months as clinically indicated

Treatment Modification

Adverse Event	Dose Modification
G3 hepatotoxicity (elevations in ALT and/or AST >5 × upper limit of normal [ULN] or total bilirubin >3 × ULN) in a patient with baseline normal hepatic function	Withhold abiraterone acetate. Treatment may be restarted at a dose of 750 mg once daily following return of liver function tests to a patient's baseline or to AST and ALT G ≤1 (2.5 × ULN) and total bilirubin G ≤1 (≤1.5 × ULN). For patients who resume treatment, monitor serum transaminases and bilirubin every 2 weeks for 3 months and then monthly
G3 hepatotoxicity (elevations in ALT and/or AST >5 × upper limit of normal [ULN] or total bilirubin >3 × ULN) in a patient with baseline normal hepatic impairment on a reduced dose of 750 mg/day because of prior hepatotoxicity at 1000 mg/day	Withhold abiraterone acetate. Treatment may be restarted at a dose of 500 mg once daily following return of liver function tests to a patient's baseline or to AST and ALT G ≤1 (2.5 × ULN) and total bilirubin G ≤1 (≤1.5 × ULN). For patients who resume treatment, monitor serum transaminases and bilirubin every 2 weeks for 3 months and then monthly
G3 hepatotoxicity (elevations in ALT and/or AST >5 × upper limit of normal or total bilirubin >3 × ULN) in a patient with baseline normal hepatic impairment on a reduced dose of 500 mg/day because of prior hepatotoxicity at 750 mg/day	Discontinue abiraterone acetate
G3 hepatotoxicity (elevations in ALT and/or AST >5 × ULN or total bilirubin >3 × ULN) in a patient with baseline moderate hepatic impairment on a reduced dose of 750 mg abiraterone acetate daily	Discontinue abiraterone acetate
G4 hepatotoxicity (elevations in ALT and/or AST >20 × ULN or total bilirubin >10 × ULN) in a patient with baseline moderate hepatic impairment	Discontinue abiraterone acetate
Hypertension, hypokalemia, and fluid retention caused by mineralocorticoid excess	Withhold abiraterone acetate. Ensure corticosteroids are being administered appropriately. Manage hypokalemia and hypertension
Suspicion of adrenocortical insufficiency	Perform appropriate tests to confirm the diagnosis of adrenocortical insufficiency. Consider administering increased corticosteroid doses during and after stressful situations

Adverse Events (N = 1199)

	Abiraterone Acetate and Prednisone Plus Androgen-deprivation Therapy (n = 597)		Placebo Plus Androgen-deprivation Therapy (n = 602)	
	Grade 1–2 (%)	Grade 3–5 (%)	Grade 1–2 (%)	Grade 3–5 (%)
Hypertension	16	20	12	10
Hypokalemia	10	10	2	1
ALT increased	11	6	11	1
Hyperglycemia	8	5	8	3
AST increased	10	4	10	1
Bone pain	9	3	12	3
Any cardiac disorder	7	5	6	2
Atrial fibrillation	1	<1	<1	<1

	Abiraterone Acetate and Prednisone Plus Androgen-deprivation Therapy (n = 597)		Placebo Plus Androgen-deprivation Therapy (n = 602)	
	Grade 1–2 (%)	Grade 3–5 (%)	Grade 1–2 (%)	Grade 3–5 (%)
Anemia	7	3	10	4
Back pain	16	2	17	3
Fatigue	11	2	12	2
Spinal-cord compression	<1	2	<1	2

ALT, alanine aminotransferase; AST, aspartate aminotransferase
Toxicities are included in the table if they were reported in at least 2% of the patients in either group or if they were denoted as being of special interest. Other toxicities of interest included grade 3 peripheral edema, which occurred in 0.3% of patients in the abiraterone group and 0.5% in the placebo group; grade 3–4 fluid retention of congestive heart failure, which did not occur in either group; grade 3 hot flush in 1 patient in the placebo group only; and grade 1 irritability in 3 patients in the abiraterone group only. Grade 5 adverse events occurred in 5% of patients in the abiraterone group and in 4% of patients in the placebo group. Grade 5 cardiac events occurred in 2% of patients in the abiraterone group and in 1% of patients in the placebo group

METASTATIC • HORMONE-SENSITIVE
PROSTATE CANCER REGIMEN: APALUTAMIDE

Chi KN et al. N Engl J Med 2019;381:13–24
Supplementary appendix to: Chi KN et al. N Engl J Med 2019;381:13–24
Protocol for: Chi KN et al. N Engl J Med 2019;381:13–24
ERLEADA (apalutamide) prescribing information. Horsham, PA: Janssen Products, LP; revised September 2019
Food and Drug Administration Center for Drug Evaluation and Research. NDA/BLA Multi-Disciplinary Review and Evaluation
NDA 210951 Erleada (apalutamide) (February 1, 2016) www.accessdata.fda.gov/drugsatfda_docs/nda/2018/210951Orig1s000MultidisciplineR.pdf [accessed 22 Sep 2019]

Apalutamide 240 mg per dose; administer orally once daily at about the same time each day either with or without food, continually, until radiographic or clinical progression of disease (total dose/week = 1680 mg)

Notes:

- Patients receiving apalutamide should have undergone bilateral orchiectomy or should receive concurrent treatment with a gonadotropin-releasing hormone (GnRH) analogue
- Instruct patients who miss a regularly scheduled dose of apalutamide to take the next dose as soon as possible on the same day, and then return to the usual administration schedule on the following day. Patients should be instructed not to take extra tablets to make up missed doses
- Instruct patients to swallow apalutamide tablets whole
- Drug interactions:

  ■ Apalutamide is a strong inducer of CYP3A4, a strong inducer of CYP2C19, a weak inducer of CYP2C9, a weak inducer of P-glycoprotein (P-gp), a weak inducer of BCRP, and a weak inducer of OATPB1. In vitro experiments suggest that apalutamide may inhibit organic cation transporter 2 (OCT2), organic anion transporter 3 (OAT3), and multidrug and toxin extrusions (MATEs). It is predicted that apalutamide has the potential to induce UDP-glucuronosyltransferase (UGT)

  ○ Coadministration of a CYP3A4 substrate (midazolam) following repeated doses of apalutamide was associated with a 92% reduction in the midazolam AUC. If possible, substitute another medication for a CYP3A4 substrate, or monitor for loss of CYP3A4 substrate efficacy

  ○ Coadministration of a CYP2C19 substrate (omeprazole) following repeated doses of apalutamide was associated with an 85% reduction in the AUC of omeprazole. If possible, substitute another medication for a CYP2C19 substrate, or monitor for loss of CYP2C19 substrate efficacy

  ○ Coadministration of a CYP2C9 substrate (S-warfarin) following repeated doses of apalutamide was associated with a 46% reduction in the AUC of S-warfarin. If possible, substitute another medication for a CYP2C9 substrate, or monitor for loss of CYP2C9 substrate efficacy

  ○ Coadministration of a CYP2C8 substrate (pioglitazone) following repeated doses of apalutamide was associated with an 18% reduction in pioglitazone AUC. It is not necessary to avoid CYP2C8 substrates with apalutamide

  ○ Coadministration of a P-gp substrate (fexofenadine) following repeated doses of apalutamide was associated with a 30% reduction in fexofenadine AUC. If possible, substitute another medication for a P-gp substrate, or monitor for loss of P-gp substrate efficacy

  ○ Coadministration of a BCRP/OATP1B1 substrate (rosuvastatin) following repeated doses of apalutamide was associated with a 41% reduction in rosuvastatin AUC. If possible, substitute another medication for a BCRP or OATP1B1 substrate, or monitor for loss of BCRP/OATP1B1 substrate efficacy

  ■ Apalutamide is primarily metabolized by CYP2C8 and CYP3A4 to an active metabolite, N-desmethyl apalutamide. Because apalutamide is a strong CYP3A4 inducer, it induces its own metabolism. At steady state, it is estimated that the relative contribution of CYP2C8 to apalutamide metabolism is 40% and that of CYP3A4 is 37%

  ○ Coadministration of a strong CYP3A4 inhibitor (itraconazole) with a single dose of apalutamide decreased apalutamide C_{max} by 22%, caused no change in apalutamide AUC, decreased N-desmethyl apalutamide C_{max} by 15%, and caused no change in N-desmethyl apalutamide AUC. Physiologically based pharmacokinetic simulations predict that ketoconazole (another strong CYP3A4 inhibitor) would increase steady-state apalutamide C_{max} by 38%, increase steady-state apalutamide AUC_{0-24} by 51%, increase active unbound fraction (defined as unbound apalutamide plus one-third of unbound N-desmethyl apalutamide) C_{max} by 23%, and increase active unbound fraction AUC_{0-24} by 28%. No initial adjustment in the apalutamide dose is necessary in patients receiving strong CYP3A4 inhibitors

  ○ Coadministration of a single dose of apalutamide with a strong CYP2C8 inhibitor (gemfibrozil 600 mg by mouth twice a day) was associated with a decrease in apalutamide C_{max} of 21%, an increase in apalutamide AUCinf of 68%, a decrease in N-desmethyl apalutamide C_{max} of 45%, and a decrease in AUCinf of 15%. Physiologically based pharmacokinetic simulations predict that gemfibrozil will lead to an increase in apalutamide steady-state C_{max} by 32%, an increase in apalutamide steady-state AUC_{0-24} by 44%, an increase in active unbound fraction C_{max} by 19%, and an increase in active unbound fraction AUC_{0-24} by 23%. No initial adjustment in the apalutamide dose is necessary in patients receiving strong CYP2C8 inhibitors

  ○ There have been no clinical studies prospectively evaluating the effects of strong CYP3A4 inducers or strong CYP2C8 inducers on the pharmacokinetics of apalutamide. Physiologically based pharmacokinetic simulations predict that rifampin (a strong CYP3A4 inducer and moderate CYP2C8 inducer) will decrease the apalutamide steady-state C_{max} by 25%, decrease the apalutamide steady-state AUC_{0-24} by 34%, decrease the active unbound fraction C_{max} by 15%, and decrease the active unbound fraction AUC_{0-24} by 19%. No adjustment in the apalutamide dose is necessary in patients receiving strong CYP3A4 inducers or strong CYP2C8 inducers

Supportive Care
Antiemetic prophylaxis
Emetogenic potential is *MINIMAL*
See Chapter 42 for antiemetic recommendations

(continued)

(continued)

Hematopoietic growth factor (CSF) prophylaxis
Primary prophylaxis is NOT indicated
See Chapter 43 for more information

Antimicrobial prophylaxis
Risk of fever and neutropenia is ***LOW***
  Antimicrobial primary prophylaxis to be considered:
  • Antibacterial—not indicated
  • Antifungal—not indicated
  • Antiviral—not indicated unless patient previously had an episode of HSV

Patient Population Studied

The multinational, multicenter, randomized, double-blind, placebo-controlled, phase 3 trial involved 1052 men with metastatic, castration-sensitive adenocarcinoma of the prostate. Prior allowed treatments included ≤6 cycles of docetaxel (with no disease progression during or after treatment), ≤6 months of androgen deprivation therapy (ADT) for metastatic castration-sensitive prostate cancer, ≤3 years of ADT for localized prostate cancer, ≤1 course of radiation or surgery for symptoms related to metastatic prostate cancer, and prior localized treatments for prostate cancer (eg, prostatectomy or radiation). Eligible patients were required to have an Eastern Cooperative Oncology Group (ECOG) performance status of 0–1. Patients were excluded if they had severe angina, myocardial infarction, congestive heart failure, arterial thromboembolic event, venous thromboembolic event, or recent ventricular arrhythmia. All patients received ADT throughout the study and were randomized (1:1) to receive apalutamide or placebo after stratification according to Gleason score at diagnosis (≤7 vs >7), geographic region (North American/European Union vs. other), and prior docetaxel treatment

Efficacy (N = 1052)

	Apalutamide (n = 525)	Placebo (n = 527)	Statistics
Median radiographic progression-free survival	Not estimated	22.1 months (95% CI, 18.5–32.9)	HR 0.48 (95% CI, 0.39–0.60); P<0.001
Patients with radiographic progression-free survival at 24 months	68.2% (95% CI, 62.9–72.9)	47.5% (95% CI, 42.1–52.8)	—
Median overall survival	Not estimated	Not estimated	HR 0.67 (95% CI, 0.51–0.89); P=0.005
Patients alive at 24 months	82.4% (95% CI, 78.4–85.8)	73.5% (95% CI, 68.7–77.8)	—
Median time to cytotoxic chemotherapy	Not estimated	Not estimated	HR 0.39 (95% CI, 0.27–0.56); P<0.001
Median time to pain progression*	Not estimated	Not estimated	HR 0.83 (95% CI, 0.65–1.05); P=0.12
Median time to chronic opioid use	Not estimated	Not estimated	HR 0.77 (95% CI 0.54–1.11)†
Median time to skeletal-related event‡	Not estimated	Not estimated	HR 0.80 (95% CI, 0.56–1.15)†
Median time to symptomatic local progression	Not estimated	Not estimated	HR 1.20 (95% CI, 0.71–2.02)†
Median time to PSA progression§	Not estimated	12.9 months	HR 0.26 (95% CI, 0.21–0.32)†
Median second progression-free survival‖	Not estimated	Not estimated	HR 0.66 (95% CI, 0.50–0.87)†

Median follow-up of 22.7 months
*An increase in ≥2 of worst pain reported on the Brief Pain Inventory (Short Form) item 3
†No P value reported; not formally tested
‡Skeletal-related event is a composite endpoint of symptomatic pathologic fracture, spinal cord compression, radiation to bone, or surgery to bone
§Defined as time from randomization to PSA progression according to the Prostate Cancer Working Group 2 criteria (J Clin Oncol 2008;26:1148–1159)
‖Second progression-free survival was defined as the time from randomization until investigator-determined disease progression (ie, PSA progression, radiographic progression, or clinical progression) or death while on the first subsequent therapy after the trial regimen

Therapy Monitoring

1. Obtain TSH prior to the start of therapy and then every 4 months, or as clinically appropriate. The incidence of hypothyroidism in the apalutamide arm was 6.5% versus 1.1% in the placebo arm. All events reported in the trial were grade ≤2

2. Optimize management of cardiovascular risk factors, such as hypertension, diabetes, or dyslipidemia

3. Evaluate patients for fracture and fall risk. The incidence of fracture was 6.3% in the apalutamide arm and 1.3% in the placebo arm, which suggests that apalutamide increases risk of fracture beyond that associated with background androgen deprivation therapy. The overall incidence of falls was 7.4% in the apalutamide arm and 0.8% in the placebo arm. Among patients who received apalutamide in combined studies, falls occurred in 8% of patients <65 years of age, in 10% of patients between 65–74 years of age, and in 19% of patients ≥75 years of age. Monitor and manage patients at risk for fractures according to established treatment guidelines and consider use of bone-targeted agents. Consider interventions to reduce fall risk in patients at risk for falls, especially in the elderly

4. Advise patients who have a history of seizure of the risk of developing a seizure and of engaging in any activity where sudden loss of consciousness could cause serious harm to themselves or others

5. Obtain serum PSA and perform physical exam every 3–6 months. Monitor radiographic imaging every 6–12 months as clinically indicated

Treatment Modifications

APALUTAMIDE	
Starting dose	240 mg by mouth once daily
Dose Level −1	180 mg by mouth once daily
Dose Level −2	120 mg by mouth once daily
Dose Level −3	Discontinue therapy

General dose adjustments	
Any grade Seizure	Permanently discontinue apalutamide
G ≤2 ischemic heart disease event	Continue apalutamide at current dose and optimize management of cardiovascular risk factors
G3/4 ischemic heart disease event	Consider permanent discontinuation of apalutamide
G ≤2 rash without intolerable symptoms	Optimize supportive management with oral antihistamines and topical corticosteroids, as clinically appropriate Continue apalutamide at the same dose
G3 rash, or any grade rash with intolerable symptoms	Optimize supportive management with oral antihistamines, topical corticosteroids, and (in select patients) systemic corticosteroids, as clinically appropriate Interrupt apalutamide dosing until rash resolves to G ≤1 or baseline, then resume at the same or a reduced dose (180 mg or 120 mg) if warranted
Hypothyroidism	Initiate or adjust thyroid replacement therapy as clinically indicated Continue apalutamide at the same dose
Other G ≥3 toxicity or intolerable side effect	Interrupt apalutamide dosing until symptoms resolve to G ≤1 or baseline, then resume at the same or a reduced dose (180 mg or 120 mg) if warranted
A sensitive medication which is a substrate of any of the following enzymes or transporters is required: CYP3A4, CYP2C19, CYP2C9, P-glycoprotein, BCRP, or OATP1B1	Consider substituting another medication that is not a substrate for any of these enzymes or transporters. If this is not possible, then monitor closely for loss of activity of the sensitive medication

Note: Advise patients of potential risk to a developing fetus. Advise male patients with female partners of reproductive potential to use effective contraception during treatment and for 3 months after the last dose of apalutamide. Advise male patients to use a condom if having sex with a pregnant woman

ERLEADA (apalutamide) prescribing information. Horsham, PA: Janssen Products, LP; revised September 2019

Adverse Events (N = 1051)

	Apalutamide (n = 524)		Placebo (n = 527)	
	Grade 1–2 (%)	Grade 3–5 (%)	Grade 1–2 (%)	Grade 3–5 (%)
Hot flush	23	0	16	0
Fatigue	18	2	16	1
Hypertension	9	8	6	9
Back pain	15	2	17	3
Arthralgia	17	<1	14	1
Pain in an arm or leg	12	1	12	1
Pruritus	10	0	4	<1
Weight increased	9	1	15	2
Anemia	7	2	10	3
Constipation	9	0	11	0
Asthenia	5	2	8	1
Bone pain	5	1	8	2
Rash, generalized	4	3	1	<1
Blood alkaline phosphatase increased	3	<1	3	2
Urinary retention	2	1	2	2
Rash*	21	6	8	1
Fall*	7	1	6	1
Fracture*	5	1	4	1
Hypothyroidism*	6	0	1	0
Seizure*	<1	<1	<1	0

Note: Toxicities were included in the table if they occurred in at least 10% of patients in either group (all grade), if G ≥3 events were reported in ≥10 patients in either group, or if they were deemed to be of special interest. Grading of adverse events was according to the National Cancer Institute Common Terminology Criteria for Adverse Events, version 4.0.3. There were 10 grade 5 adverse events reported in the apalutamide arm and 16 grade 5 adverse events reported in the placebo arm. Serious adverse events occurred in 19.8% of patients in the apalutamide arm and in 20.3% of patients in the placebo arm. Adverse events that led to discontinuation of trial therapy occurred in 8.0% of patients in the apalutamide arm and in 5.3% of patients in the placebo arm. Ischemic heart disease was reported in 4.4% of patients in the apalutamide arm and in 1.5% of patients in the placebo arm

*Denotes adverse event deemed to be of special interest

METASTATIC • HORMONE-SENSITIVE
PROSTATE CANCER REGIMEN: DOCETAXEL

Sweeney CJ et al. N Engl J Med 2015;373:737–746
Supplementary appendix to: Sweeney CJ et al. N Engl J Med 2015;373:737–746
Protocol for: Sweeney CJ et al. Sweeney CJ et al. N Engl J Med 2015;373:737–746
Kyriakopoulos CE et al. J Clin Oncol 2018;36:1080–1087
Supplementary appendix to: Kyriakopoulos CE et al. J Clin Oncol 2018;36:1080–1087
Protocol for: Kyriakopoulos CE et al. J Clin Oncol 2018;36:1080–1087
James ND et al. Lancet 2016;387:1163–1177
Supplementary appendix to: James ND et al. Lancet 2016;387:1163–1177
TAXOTERE (docetaxel) prescribing information. Bridgewater, NJ: Sanofi-Aventis U.S. LLC; revised 2019 June

Dexamethasone 8 mg/dose orally for 3 doses at 12 hours, 3 hours, and 1 hour before docetaxel treatment commences, every 21 days, for 6 cycles (total dose/cycle = 24 mg)

Docetaxel 75 mg/m² intravenously over 1 hour, in a volume of 0.9% sodium chloride injection or 5% dextrose injection sufficient to produce a solution with concentration within the range 0.3–0.74 mg/mL, on day 1, every 21 days, for 6 cycles (total dosage/cycle = 75 mg/m²)

Notes:

- Patients receiving docetaxel in this setting should have undergone bilateral orchiectomy or should also receive concurrent treatment with a gonadotropin-releasing hormone (GnRH) analogue. Use of nonsteroidal antiandrogens (ie, flutamide or bicalutamide) was at the discretion of the treating physician

- Treatment with prednisone along with docetaxel was not required in the study

- Some formulations of docetaxel contain alcohol; use caution or consider using a non-alcohol-containing formulation in patients who are sensitive to alcohol

Supportive Care
Antiemetic prophylaxis
*Emetogenic potential is **LOW***
See Chapter 42 for antiemetic recommendations

Hematopoietic growth factor (CSF) prophylaxis
*Primary prophylaxis is **NOT** indicated*
See Chapter 43 for more information

Antimicrobial prophylaxis
Risk of fever and neutropenia is *LOW*
Antimicrobial primary prophylaxis to be considered:
- Antibacterial—not indicated

- Antifungal—not indicated

- Antiviral—not indicated unless patient previously had an episode of HSV

Patient Population Studied

The multicenter, randomized, open-label, phase 3 cooperative group trial involved 790 patients with metastatic hormone-sensitive prostate cancer. Eligible patients had an Eastern Cooperative Oncology Group (ECOG) performance status of ≤2, total bilirubin ≤ upper limit of normal (ULN), absolute neutrophil count (ANC) ≥1500/mm³, platelet count ≥100,000/mm³, alanine aminotransferase (ALT) ≤2.5 × ULN, and creatinine clearance ≥30 mL/minute. Androgen deprivation therapy was continued throughout the entire course of study treatment and was permitted to have been initiated within 120 days prior to randomization. Prior adjuvant ADT was allowed if the duration was ≤24 months and if progression occurred >12 months after completion. Patients were randomized to either docetaxel plus ADT or ADT alone after stratification for age (<70 vs ≥70 years), ECOG performance status (0 or 1 vs 2), planned use of combined androgen blockade for >30 days (yes or no), planned use of zoledronic acid or denosumab (yes or no), duration of prior adjuvant ADT (<12 vs ≥12 months), and extent of metastases (high volume vs low volume). High-volume disease was defined as the presence of visceral (extranodal) metastases or ≥4 bone lesions with ≥1 bone lesion beyond the vertebral bodies and pelvis

Efficacy (N = 790)

	Docetaxel + ADT (n = 397)	ADT Alone (n = 393)	Statistics
Median overall survival (all patients)	57.6 months	47.2 months	HR 0.72 (95% CI, 0.59–0.89); P=0.0018
Median overall survival (high-volume disease)*	51.2 months	34.4 months	HR 0.63 (95% CI, 0.50–0.79); P<0.001
Median overall survival (low-volume disease)†	63.5 months	Not reached	HR 1.04 (95% CI, 0.70–1.55); P=0.86
PSA level <0.2 ng/mL at 6 months	32%	19.6%	P<0.001
PSA level <0.2 ng/mL at 12 months	27.7%	16.8%	P<0.001
Median time to development of castration-resistant prostate cancer (all patients)‡	19.4 months	11.7 months	HR 0.61 (95% CI, 0.52–0.73); P<0.001

(continued)

Efficacy (N = 790) (continued)

	Docetaxel + ADT (n = 397)	ADT Alone (n = 393)	Statistics
Median time to development of castration-resistant prostate cancer (high-volume disease)[*‡]	14.9 months	8.6 months	HR 0.58 (95% CI, 0.47–0.71); P<0.001
Median time to development of castration-resistant prostate cancer (low-volume disease)[†‡]	31.0 months	22.7 months	HR 0.70 (95% CI, 0.50–0.96); P=0.03
Median time to clinical progression (all patients)[§]	33.0 months	19.8 months	HR 0.62 (95% CI, 0.51–0.75); P<0.001
Median time to clinical progression (high-volume disease)[*§]	27.3 months	13.0 months	HR 0.53 (95% CI, 0.42–0.67); P<0.001
Median time to clinical progression (low-volume disease)[†§]	42.5 months	44.3 months	HR 0.86 (95% CI, 0.60–1.25); P=0.43

Survival and time to event data are based on a final analysis conducted with a data cutoff date for survival of April 23, 2016 with a median follow-up of 53.7 months (Kyriakopoulos CE et al. J Clin Oncol 2018;36:1080–1087)
[*]513 patients were classified as high-volume disease (n = 263 in the ADT + docetaxel arm and n = 250 in the ADT alone arm)
[†]277 patients were classified as low-volume disease (n = 134 in the ADT + docetaxel arm and n = 143 in the ADT alone arm)
[‡]Defined as time until documented clinical or serologic progression with a testosterone level of <50 ng/dL or documentation of medical or surgical castration
[§]Defined as time until increasing symptoms of bone metastases, progression according to RECIST v1.0, or clinical deterioration due to cancer in the opinion of the investigator

Therapy Monitoring

1. Before each cycle: CBC with differential, liver function tests
2. Obtain serum PSA and perform physical exam every 3–6 months. Monitor radiographic imaging every 6–12 months as clinically indicated

Treatment Modifications

DOCETAXEL	
Starting Dose	75 mg/m^2
Dose Level −1	65 mg/m^2
Dose Level −2	55 mg/m^2
Dose Level −3	Discontinue docetaxel

Hematologic Toxicity	
ANC ≥1500/mm^3 and platelet count ≥100,000/mm^3 on day 1 of a cycle	Proceed with docetaxel at the same dose
ANC ≥1000/mm^3 and <1500/mm^3 on day 1 of a cycle	Proceed with docetaxel but reduce the dosage by 1 dose level. Do not re-escalate the docetaxel dose in subsequent cycles
Platelet count ≥75,000/mm3 and <100,000 on day 1 of a cycle	Proceed with docetaxel but reduce the dosage by 1 dose level. Do not re-escalate the docetaxel dose in subsequent cycles
ANC <1000/mm^3 on day 1 of a cycle	Withhold docetaxel and perform weekly CBC until the ANC recovers to ≥1500/mm^3, then reduce the docetaxel dosage by 1 dose level. Do not re-escalate the docetaxel dose in subsequent cycles If recovery does not occur within 3 weeks, then discontinue docetaxel
Platelet count <75,000/mm^3 on day 1 of a cycle	Withhold docetaxel and check weekly CBC until the platelet count recovers to ≥100,000/mm^3, then reduce the docetaxel dosage by 1 dose level. Do not re-escalate the docetaxel dose in subsequent cycles If recovery does not occur within 3 weeks, then discontinue docetaxel

(continued)

Treatment Modifications (*continued*)

Hematologic Toxicity

Neutropenic fever (one episode of temperature >38.5°C or three episodes of temperature >38.0°C in a 24-hour period in conjunction with an ANC <1000/mm³, or occurring in a prior cycle	Withhold docetaxel until ANC ≥1500/mm³, afebrile (temperature <38.0°C), and completion of adequate treatment for infection (if applicable), then reduce the docetaxel dosage by 1 dose level. Consider use of growth factor support in future cycles
Prolonged grade 4 neutropenia (ANC <500/mm³ for ≥7 days) occurring in a prior cycle	

Hepatic Impairment

Total bilirubin >ULN or ALT >5 × ULN on day 1 of a cycle	Withhold docetaxel and check weekly LFTs until total bilirubin improves to ≤ULN and ALT improves to ≤3X ULN, then reduce the docetaxel dosage by 1 dose level. Do not re-escalate the docetaxel dose in subsequent cycles If recovery does not occur within 3 weeks, then discontinue docetaxel
Total bilirubin ≤ULN and ALT >3 × ULN	Proceed with docetaxel but reduce the dosage by 1 dose level. Do not re-escalate the docetaxel dose in subsequent cycles

Gastrointestinal Toxicity

Stomatitis, grade 2 (moderate pain; not interfering with oral intake; modified diet indicated)	Withhold docetaxel until resolution of stomatitis, then proceed with docetaxel at the same doseIf recovery does not occur within 3 weeks, then discontinue docetaxel
Stomatitis grade ≥3 (severe pain; interfering with oral intake; or worse)	Withhold docetaxel until resolution of stomatitis, then proceed with docetaxel with the dosage reduced by 1 dose level. Do not re-escalate the docetaxel dose in subsequent cyclesIf recovery does not occur within 3 weeks, then discontinue docetaxel
Diarrhea grade ≥3 with concurrent G ≥3 neutropenia (ANC <1000/mm³), first episode	Withhold docetaxel until ANC >1000/mm³ and diarrhea improves to G ≤2, then continue docetaxel at the same dose. Consider prophylactic treatment with loperamide or diphenoxylate in subsequent cycles If recovery does not occur within 3 weeks, then discontinue docetaxel
Diarrhea grade ≥3 with concurrent G ≥3 neutropenia (ANC <1000/mm³), second episode (despite prophylaxis with loperamide or diphenoxylate)	Withhold docetaxel until ANC >1000/mm³ and diarrhea improves to G ≤2, then continue docetaxel with the dosage reduced by 1 dose level. Do not re-escalate the docetaxel dose in subsequent cycles Continue prophylactic treatment with loperamide or diphenoxylate in subsequent cyclesIf recovery does not occur within 3 weeks, then discontinue docetaxel
Diarrhea grade ≥3 with concurrent G ≥3 neutropenia (ANC <1000/mm³), third episode (despite prophylaxis with loperamide or diphenoxylate and prior dose reduction of docetaxel)	Discontinue docetaxel

Peripheral Neuropathy

Neuropathy grade 2 (moderate symptoms; limiting instrumental ADL)	Withhold docetaxel until improvement to G ≤1, then reduce the docetaxel dosage by 1 dose level. Do not re-escalate the docetaxel dose in subsequent cyclesIf recovery does not occur within 3 weeks, then discontinue docetaxel
Neuropathy grade ≥3 (severe symptoms; limiting self-care ADL; or worse)	Permanently discontinue docetaxel

Hypersensitivity Reaction

Severe hypersensitivity reaction	Discontinue infusion immediately and administer appropriate support. For hypersensitivity reaction G ≤3, initial management includes temporary discontinuation of infusion for 30 minutes, and administration of additional intravenous antihistamines and glucocorticoids. Upon resolution of symptoms, infusion may be restarted at a slower rate if deemed safe If G4 hypersensitivity is experienced stabilize the cardiorespiratory system and use epinephrine as needed, then permanently discontinue docetaxel

Other Toxicities

Other clinically significant toxicity G ≥3 (except anemia)	Withhold docetaxel until improvement to G ≤1 or baseline, then reduce the docetaxel dosage by 1 dose level. Do not re-escalate the docetaxel dose in subsequent cycles If recovery does not occur within 3 weeks, then discontinue docetaxel

Adverse Events (N = 390)

	Docetaxel + ADT (N = 390)
	Grade 3–5 (%)
Any adverse event	29
Allergic reaction	2
Fatigue	4
Diarrhea	1
Stomatitis	1
Neuropathy, motor	1
Neuropathy, sensory	1
Thromboembolism	1
Sudden death	<1
Anemia	1
Thrombocytopenia	<1
Neutropenia	12
Febrile neutropenia	6
Infection with neutropenia	2

METASTATIC • HORMONE-SENSITIVE
PROSTATE CANCER REGIMEN: ENZALUTAMIDE

Davis ID et al. N Engl J Med 2019;381:121–131
Supplementary appendix to: Davis ID et al. N Engl J Med 2019;381:121–131
Protocol for: Davis ID et al. N Engl J Med 2019;381:121–131
Armstrong AJ et al. J Clin Oncol 2019;37:2974–2986
Data supplement to: Armstrong AJ et al. J Clin Oncol 2019;37:2974–2986
Protocol for: Armstrong AJ et al. Armstrong AJ et al. J Clin Oncol 2019;37:2974–2986
XTANDI (enzalutamide) prescribing information. New York, NY: Astellas Pharma US, Inc; revised July 2018

Enzalutamide 160 mg per dose; administer orally once daily at about the same time each day either with or without food, continually, until radiographic or clinical progression of disease (total dose/week = 1120 mg)

Notes:

- Patients receiving enzalutamide should have undergone bilateral orchiectomy or should also receive concurrent treatment with a gonadotropin-releasing hormone (GnRH) analogue

- If possible, avoid concomitant use of strong CYP2C8 inhibitors. If patients must receive a strong CYP2C8 inhibitor concomitantly, reduce the enzalutamide dose to 80 mg once daily. If coadministration of the strong inhibitor is discontinued, the enzalutamide dose should be returned to the dose used prior to initiation of a strong CYP2C8 inhibitor

- Coadministration of a strong CYP3A4 inhibitor (eg, itraconazole) increased the composite AUC of enzalutamide plus *N*-desmethyl enzalutamide by 1.3-fold in healthy volunteers

- Coadministration of enzalutamide with rifampin (a strong CYP4A4 inducer and moderate CYP2C8 inducer) decrease the composite AUC of enzalutamide pus *N*-desmethyl enzalutamide by 37%. Coadministration of enzalutamide with strong CYP3A4 inducers and St John's wort should be avoided if possible. If coadministration of a strong CYP3A4 inducer with enzalutamide is required, increase the dose of enzalutamide from 160 mg by mouth once daily to 240 mg by mouth once daily

- Enzalutamide is a strong CYP3A4 inducer and a moderate CYP2C9 and CYP2C19 inducer in humans. At steady state, enzalutamide reduced the plasma exposure to midazolam (CYP3A4 substrate), warfarin (CYP2C9 substrate), and omeprazole (CYP2C19 substrate). Concomitant use of enzalutamide with narrow-therapeutic-index drugs that are metabolized by CYP3A4, CYP2C9 (eg, phenytoin, warfarin), and CYP2C19 should be avoided, as enzalutamide may decrease their exposure. If coadministration with warfarin cannot be avoided, conduct additional INR monitoring

Supportive Care
Antiemetic prophylaxis
Emetogenic potential is **MINIMAL**
See Chapter 42 for antiemetic recommendations

Hematopoietic growth factor (CSF) prophylaxis
Primary prophylaxis is NOT indicated
See Chapter 43 for more information

Antimicrobial prophylaxis
Risk of fever and neutropenia is *LOW*
Antimicrobial primary prophylaxis to be considered:
- Antibacterial—not indicated
- Antifungal—not indicated
- Antiviral—not indicated unless patient previously had an episode of HSV

Patient Population Studied

The multinational, multicenter, randomized, open-label, phase 3 trial involved 1125 patients with metastatic adenocarcinoma of the prostate. Eligible patients had initiated testosterone suppression therapy or had undergone bilateral orchiectomy within 12 weeks prior to randomization and had an Eastern Cooperative Oncology Group (ECOG) performance status of ≤2. Androgen deprivation therapy was continued throughout the entire course of study treatment. Patients were excluded if they had suspected brain metastases, active leptomeningeal carcinomatosis, history of seizures, or a condition that might confer a predisposition to seizures. Patients were randomized to either enzalutamide 160 mg by mouth daily or a nonsteroidal antiandrogen control arm consisting of bicalutamide, nilutamide, or flutamide. A protocol revision allowed patients to receive early docetaxel treatment (75 mg/m² without prednisone or prednisolone administered every 3 weeks for up to 6 cycles) in addition to protocol-directed therapy

Efficacy (N = 1125)

	Enzalutamide (n = 563)	Standard Therapy Arm (Bicalutamide, Nilutamide, or Flutamide) (n = 562)	Statistics
3-year overall survival	80%	72%	HR 0.67 (95% CI, 0.52–0.86); P=0.002
3-year PSA progression-free survival*	67%	37%	HR 0.39 (95% CI, 0.33–0.47); P<0.001
3-year clinical progression-free survival†	68%	41%	HR 0.40 (95% CI, 0.33–0.49); P<0.001

Data presented are based on an interim analysis conducted on February 28, 2019 after a median follow-up of 34 months and a total of 245 deaths
*Defined according to the criteria of the Prostate Cancer Working Group 2 (a confirmed relative increase in the prostate-specific antigen (PSA) level from the nadir value by ≥25% and by ≥2 ng/mL)
†Defined as the earliest sign of radiographic progression according to the criteria of the Prostate Cancer Working Group 2 for bone lesions and according to the Response Evaluation Criteria in Solid Tumors, version 1.1, for soft tissue metastasesJ Clin Oncol 2008;26:1148–1159; Eur J Cancer 2009;45:228–247

Therapy Monitoring

1. Obtain CBC with differential prior to start of therapy
2. Optimize management of cardiovascular risk factors, such as hypertension, diabetes, or dyslipidemia
3. Monitor blood pressure at least monthly. Encourage patients to monitor their blood pressure
4. Evaluate patients for fracture and fall risk. Monitor and manage patients at risk for fractures according to established treatment guidelines and consider use of bone-targeted agents
5. Advise patients who have a history of seizure of the risk of developing a seizure and of engaging in any activity where sudden loss of consciousness could cause serious harm to themselves or others
6. Obtain serum PSA and perform physical exam every 3–6 months. Monitor radiographic imaging every 6–12 months as clinically indicated

Treatment Modifications

ENZALUTAMIDE

Starting Dose	160 mg by mouth once daily
Dose Level −1	120 mg by mouth once daily
Dose Level −2	80 mg by mouth once daily
Dose Level −3	Discontinue therapy

General dose adjustments

Seizure	Permanently discontinue enzalutamide
Posterior reversible encephalopathy syndrome (PRES)	Permanently discontinue enzalutamide
Hypersensitivity to enzalutamide	Permanently discontinue enzalutamide
G ≤2 ischemic heart disease event	Continue enzalutamide at current dose and optimize management of cardiovascular risk factors
G3/4 ischemic heart disease event	Permanently discontinue enzalutamide
Other G ≥3 toxicity or intolerable side effect	Interrupt enzalutamide dosing for 1 week or until symptoms resolve to G ≤2, then resume at the same or a reduced dose (120 mg or 80 mg) if warranted
Strong CYP2C8 inhibitor is required	Reduce the enzalutamide dose to 80 mg by mouth once daily
Strong CYP2C8 inhibitor is discontinued	Resume the enzalutamide dose that was used prior to initiation of the strong CYP2C8 inhibitors
Strong CYP3A4 inducer is required	Increase the enzalutamide dose from 160 mg to 240 mg by mouth once daily
Strong CYP3A4 inducer is discontinued	Resume the enzalutamide dose that was used prior to initiation of the strong CYP3A4 inducer

Note: Advise patients of potential risk to a developing fetus. Advise females who are or may become pregnant not to handle enzalutamide. Advise male patients with female partners of reproductive potential to use effective contraception during treatment and for 3 months after the last dose of enzalutamide. Advise male patients to use a condom if having sex with a pregnant woman

Xtandi (enzalutamide) prescribing information. New York, NY: Astellas Pharma US, Inc; revised July 2018

Adverse Events (N = 1121)

	Enzalutamide (n = 563)	Standard Therapy Arm (Bicalutamide, Nilutamide, or Flutamide) (n = 558)
	Grade 3–5 (%)	Grade 3–5 (%)
Febrile neutropenia	7%	6%
Hypertension	8%	4%
Neutrophil count decreased	6%	3%
Fatigue	6%	1%
Syncope	4%	1%
Surgical or medical procedure	2%	2%
Anemia	1%	1%
Fall	1%	<1%
Thromboembolic event	1%	1%
Acute coronary syndrome	1%	1%
Myocardial infarction	1%	<1%
Chest pain from cardiac cause	1%	<1%
Stroke	<1%	<1%
Seizure	<1%	0%
Delirium	0%	<1%

Note: Toxicities are included in the table if they occurred in at least 2% of patients in either group or if they were deemed to be of special interest. There were six grade 5 adverse events reported in the enzalutamide arm and seven grade 5 adverse events reported in the standard arm. Adverse events leading to treatment discontinuation occurred in 6% of patients in the enzalutamide group and in 3% of patients in the standard therapy group

*All-grade seizures occurred in seven patients (1.2%) in the enzalutamide group and in zero patients in the standard therapy group

METASTATIC • CASTRATION-RESISTANT • FIRST-LINE

PROSTATE CANCER REGIMEN: SIPULEUCEL-T

Kantoff PW et al. N Engl J Med 2010;363:411–422

General notes:
- Patients are scheduled for 3 leukapheresis procedures (at weeks 0, 2, and 4), each followed approximately 3 days later by infusion of sipuleucel-T
- Infusions are prepared from PBMCs collected by means of a single standard leukapheresis processing 1.5 to 2 times a patient's estimated blood volume
- Sipuleucel-T is prepared at a designated manufacturing facility by culturing APCs for 36–44 hours at 37°C (98.6°F) with media containing PA2024. The cells are washed before final formulation

Premedication:
Acetaminophen 650 mg orally approximately 30 minutes prior to the administration of sipuleucel-T, *and*
Diphenhydramine 25–50 mg, or an equivalent H$_1$-receptor antihistamine orally approximately 30 minutes prior to the administration of sipuleucel-T
Sipuleucel-T suspension for intravenous infusion containing a minimum of 50 million autologous CD54+ cells activated with PAP-GM-CSF/dose in 250 mL lactated Ringer injection, intravenously over a period of approximately 60 minutes. Administer a total of 3 doses at approximately 2-week intervals (total dose/single treatment is at least 50 million autologous CD54+ cells activated with PAP-GM-CSF)

Notes for acute infusion reactions: Interrupt or slow infusion depending on the severity of the reaction. Administer appropriate medical therapy including:
- **Diphenhydramine** 25–50 mg, or an equivalent H$_1$-receptor antihistamine, intravenously
- **Ranitidine** 50 mg, **cimetidine** 300 mg, **famotidine** 20 mg, or an equivalent histamine receptor [H$_2$]-subtype antagonist, intravenously over 15–30 minutes
- *Note:* In healthy subjects, cimetidine reduces the clearance and volume of distribution of meperidine; thus, use caution when these drugs are used concomitantly
- **Meperidine** 10–25 mg intravenously as needed for chills

Important:
- Sipuleucel-T is for *autologous use only*. Before infusion, confirm that a patient's identity matches patient identifiers on the infusion containers
- Do not initiate infusion of expired sipuleucel-T. If, for any reason, a patient is unable to receive a scheduled infusion of sipuleucel-T, the patient will need to undergo an additional leukapheresis procedure if the course of treatment is to be continued. Patients should be advised of this possibility prior to initiating treatment
- The sipuleucel-T infusion bag must remain within its insulated polyurethane container until the time of administration. Do not remove the insulated polyurethane container from its outer cardboard shipping box
- DO NOT USE a cell filter to administer sipuleucel-T

Supportive Care
Antiemetic prophylaxis
Emetogenic potential is **MINIMAL**
See Chapter 42 for antiemetic recommendations

Hematopoietic growth factor (CSF) prophylaxis
Primary prophylaxis is **NOT** *indicated*
See Chapter 43 for more information

Antimicrobial prophylaxis
Risk of fever and neutropenia is **LOW**
   Antimicrobial primary prophylaxis to be considered:
- Antibacterial—not indicated
- Antifungal—not indicated
- Antiviral—not indicated unless patient previously had an episode of HSV

Treatment Modifications

Adverse Event	Dose Modification
Acute infusion reactions	Interrupt or slow infusion depending on the severity of the reaction and administer appropriate medical therapy including intravenous H$_1$/H$_2$ antagonists ± low-dose meperidine

Patient Population Studied

A study of 512 patients with metastatic castration-resistant prostate cancer and an expected survival ≥6 months (341 randomized to sipuleucel-T and 171 to placebo). Initially, only men without disease-related symptoms and a Gleason score ≤7 were enrolled. Eligibility criteria were later amended to include men with any Gleason score, as well as those with minimal disease-related symptoms. Additional eligibility criteria were a serum PSA ≥5 mcg/L, a serum testosterone level <50 ng/dL (<1.7 nmol/L), and progressive disease on the basis of imaging studies or PSA measurements. Exclusion criteria included an Eastern Cooperative Oncology Group (ECOG) performance status ≥2, visceral metastases, pathologic long-bone fractures, spinal cord compression, and treatment within the previous 28 days with systemic glucocorticoids, external beam radiation, surgery, or systemic therapy for prostate cancer (except medical or surgical castration). Patients were also excluded if they had undergone chemotherapy within the previous 3 months. Continuation of medical castration or bisphosphonate therapy was required at least until the time of disease progression

Efficacy*

Median time to objective disease progression	14.6 weeks[†]
Adjusted HR for death, sipuleucel-T vs placebo	0.78 (95% CI, 0.61–0.98)
Median overall survival	25.8 months[‡]
Estimated probability of survival at 36 months	31.7%[§]
Reductions of PSA ≥50% on two visits ≥4 weeks apart	2.6%[ϵ]
Antibody titers against the immunizing antigen, PA2024 ≤400 at any time after baseline	66.2%[**,‡‡]
Antibody titers against prostatic acid phosphatase >400 at any time after baseline	28.5%[††,‡‡]

*Median follow up time: 34.1 months
[†]Placebo group: 14.4 weeks
[‡]Placebo group: 21.7 months
[§]Placebo group: 23%
[ϵ]Placebo group: 1.3%
[**]Placebo group: 2.9%
[††]Placebo group: 1.4%
[‡‡]In prespecified analyses, patients in the sipuleucel-T group who had an antibody titer >400 against PA2024 or prostatic acid phosphatase at any time after baseline lived longer than those who had an antibody titer ≤400 (P<0.001 and P = 0.08, respectively, by the log-rank test)

Therapy Monitoring

1. *Before each cycle:* CBC with LFTs
2. *Evaluation including PSA:* Every 6 weeks

Toxicity*

Toxicity	Sipuleucel-T (N = 338)		Placebo (N = 168)	
	% All Grades	% G3/4/5	% All Grades	% G3/4/5
Any	98.8	31.7	96.4	35.1
Chills	54.1	1.2	12.5	0
Fatigue	39.1	1.1	38.1	1.8
Back pain	34.3	3.6	36.3	4.8
Pyrexia	29.3	0.3	13.7	1.8
Nausea	28.1	0.6	20.8	0
Arthralgia	20.7	2.1	23.8	3.0
Citrate toxicity[†]	20.1	0	20.2	0
Vomiting	17.8	0	11.9	0
Headache	16.0	0.3	4.8	0
Dizziness	14.5	0	9.5	0
Pain	13.0	1.8	7.1	1.2
Influenza-like illness	9.8	0	3.6	0
Bone pain	9.5	0.9	10.7	1.2
Hypertension	7.4	0.6	3.0	0
Anorexia	7.1	0.3	16.1	1.8
Weight loss	5.9	0.6	10.7	0.6
Hyperhidrosis	5.3	0	0.6	0
Groin pain	5.0	0	2.4	0
Anxiety	3.8	0	8.3	0
Flank pain	2.7	0	6.0	0
Depression	2.4	0.3	6.5	0
	% Mild/moderate (G1/2)		% Severe (G3)[§]	
Acute infusion reactions[‡]	67.7		3.5	

*NCI Common Terminology Criteria for Adverse Events, version 3
[†]Citrate toxicity has been associated with leukapheresis; paresthesia and oral paresthesia are likely symptoms of citrate toxicity
[‡]Acute infusion reactions (*reported within 1 day after infusion*) included chills, fever, fatigue, asthenia, dyspnea, hypoxia, bronchospasm, dizziness, headache, hypertension, tachycardia, muscle ache, nausea, and vomiting. The most common events (≥20%) were chills, fever, and fatigue. Fevers and chills generally resolved within 2 days (71.9% and 89.0%, respectively)
[§]The incidence of severe events was greater following the second sipuleucel-T infusion in comparison with the first infusion (2.1% vs 0.8%, respectively), and decreased to 1.3% following the third infusion. Some (1.2%) patients in the sipuleucel-T group were hospitalized within 1 day after infusion for management of acute infusion reactions. No G4/5 acute infusion reactions were reported with sipuleucel-T

METASTATIC • CASTRATION-RESISTANT • FIRST-LINE

PROSTATE CANCER REGIMEN: ABIRATERONE ACETATE

Ryan CJ et al. N Engl J Med 2013;368:138–148

Abiraterone acetate 1000 mg orally once daily, continually for 28 consecutive days (total dose/28-day cycle = 28,000 mg)
Note: No food should be consumed for at least 2 hours before a dose of abiraterone acetate is taken and for at least 1 hour after a dose of abiraterone acetate is taken. Exposure (area under the curve) of abiraterone acetate increases up to 10-fold when abiraterone acetate is taken with meals
Prednisone 5 mg orally twice daily, continually for 28 consecutive days (total dose/28-day cycle = 280 mg)

Notes:
- For patients with baseline moderate hepatic impairment (Child-Pugh Class B), reduce the dose of abiraterone acetate to 250 mg once daily
- Avoid abiraterone acetate in patients with baseline severe hepatic impairment (Child-Pugh Class C), as abiraterone acetate has not been studied in this population, and no dose adjustment can be predicted
- Abiraterone acetate is an inhibitor of the polymorphically expressed cytochrome P450 (CYP) enzyme, CYP2D6
  - **Avoid coadministration** of abiraterone acetate with CYP2D6 substrates that have a low therapeutic index. If an alternative treatment cannot be used, exercise caution and consider a dose reduction of concomitantly used CYP2D6 substrates
- Monitor for symptoms and signs of adrenocortical insufficiency. Increased dosage of corticosteroids may be indicated before, during, and after stressful situations
- Monitor for signs and symptoms of mineralocorticoid excess, including hypokalemia, fluid retention, and hypertension. Prednisone dose may have to be supplemented in some patients or augmented with an aldosterone antagonist such as eplerenone
- Use abiraterone acetate with caution in patients with a history of cardiovascular disease. Control hypertension and correct hypokalemia before initiating treatment
- Abiraterone acetate is a substrate of CYP3A4. Avoid or use with caution strong CYP3A4 inhibitors (eg, atazanavir, clarithromycin, indinavir, itraconazole, ketoconazole, nefazodone, nelfinavir, ritonavir, saquinavir, telithromycin, voriconazole) or inducers (eg, carbamazepine, phenobarbital, phenytoin, rifabutin, rifapentine, rifampin) during abiraterone acetate treatment
- Abiraterone acetate was a strong inhibitor of CYP1A2 and CYP2D6, and a moderate inhibitor of CYP2C9, CYP2C19, and CYP3A4/5 in experimental systems. It is not yet known whether its effects on CYP1A2, CYP2C subfamily, or CYP3A subfamily enzymes in in vitro systems are representative of a potential for clinically important drug interactions
- Use abiraterone acetate with caution in patients with a history of cardiovascular disease. The safety of abiraterone acetate in patients with LVEF <50% or NYHA Class III or IV heart failure is not established. Control hypertension and correct hypokalemia before treatment

Supportive Care
Antiemetic prophylaxis
Emetogenic potential is **MINIMAL–LOW**
See Chapter 42 for antiemetic recommendations

Hematopoietic growth factor (CSF) prophylaxis
Primary prophylaxis is **NOT** *indicated*
See Chapter 43 for more information

Antimicrobial prophylaxis
Risk of fever and neutropenia is **LOW**
  Antimicrobial primary prophylaxis to be considered:
  - Antibacterial—not indicated
  - Antifungal—not indicated
  - Antiviral—not indicated unless patient previously had an episode of HSV

Treatment Modification

Adverse Event	Dose Modification
G2 hepatotoxicity	Hold abiraterone acetate until toxicity remits to G ≤1, then resume treatment at a dose of 750 mg once daily
G3 hepatotoxicity (elevations in ALT and/or AST >5 × upper limit of normal [ULN] or total bilirubin >3 × ULN) in a patient with baseline normal hepatic function	Withhold abiraterone acetate. Treatment may be restarted at a dose of 750 mg once daily following return of liver function tests to a patient's baseline or to AST and ALT G ≤1 (2.5 × ULN) and total bilirubin G ≤1 (≤1.5 × ULN). For patients who resume treatment, monitor serum transaminases
G3 hepatotoxicity (elevations in ALT and/or AST >5 × upper limit of normal [ULN] or total bilirubin >3 × ULN) in a patient with baseline normal hepatic impairment on a reduced dose of 750 mg/day because of prior hepatotoxicity at 1000 mg/day	Withhold abiraterone acetate. Treatment may be restarted at a dose of 500 mg once daily following return of liver function tests to a patient's baseline or to AST and ALT G ≤1 (2.5 × ULN) and total bilirubin G ≤1 (≤1.5 × ULN). For patients who resume treatment, monitor serum transaminases
G3 hepatotoxicity (elevations in ALT and/or AST >5 × upper limit of normal or total bilirubin >3 × ULN) in a patient with baseline normal hepatic impairment on a reduced dose of 500 mg/day because of prior hepatotoxicity at 750 mg/day	Discontinue abiraterone acetate

(continued)

Efficacy

Prespecified Secondary and Exploratory Efficacy End Points*

	Abiraterone + Prednisone (N = 546)	Prednisone Alone (N = 542)	Value (95% CI)[†]	P Value
End Point				
Secondary End Points				
Median Times in Months to:				
Opioid use for cancer-related pain	Not Reached	23.7	0.69 (0.57–0.83)	<0.001
Starting cytotoxic chemotherapy	25.2	16.8	0.58 (0.49–0.69)	<0.001
Decline in ECOG PS by ≥1 point	12.3	10.9	0.82 (0.71–0.94)	0.005
PSA progression[‡]	11.1	5.6	0.49 (0.42–0.57)	<0.001
Exploratory End Points[§]				
Median Times in Months to:				
Increase in pain[¶]	26.7	18.4	0.82 (0.67–1.00)	0.049
Functional status decline[**]	12.7	8.3	0.78 (0.66–0.92)	0.003
Decline of ≥50% in PSA level (%)[††]	62	24	2.59 (2.19–3.05)[‡‡]	<0.001
Patients with Measurable Disease at Baseline and a RECIST Response (%)				
	N = 220	N = 218		
Defined objective response	36	16	2.27 (1.59–3.25)[‡‡]	<0.001
Stable disease	61	69		
Progressive disease	2	15		

CI, Confidence interval; FACT-P, Functional Assessment of Cancer Therapy–Prostate; HR, hazard ratio; PS, performance score; PSA, prostate-specific antigen; RECIST, Response Evaluation Criteria in Solid Tumors

*Percentages may not sum to 100 because of rounding
[†]Values are hazard ratios unless otherwise specified
[‡]Based on Prostate Cancer Clinical Trials Working Group 2 (PCWG2) criteria
[§]The exploratory analyses are reported with no adjustment for multiplicity
[¶]Increase in pain is defined as an increase in the baseline pain level by 30% or more, as measured by the average of the pain scores on the Brief Pain Inventory–Short Form (range: 0–10, with higher scores indicating worse average pain) at 2 consecutive visits, without a decrease in analgesic use
[**]Defined as months from randomization to the first date a patient has a decrease of 10 points or more on the FACT-P instrument (range: 0–156, with higher scores indicating better overall quality of life)
[††]A decline ≥50% in the PSA level was based on modified PCWG2 criteria
[‡‡]Values are relative risks

Treatment Modification
(continued)

G3 hepatotoxicity (elevations in ALT and/or AST >5 × ULN or total bilirubin >3 × ULN) in a patient with baseline moderate hepatic impairment on a reduced dose of 750 mg abiraterone acetate daily	Discontinue abiraterone acetate
G4 hepatotoxicity (elevations in ALT and/or AST >20 × ULN or total bilirubin >10 × ULN) in a patient with baseline moderate hepatic impairment	Discontinue abiraterone acetate
Hypertension, hypokalemia, and fluid retention caused by mineralocorticoid excess	Withhold abiraterone acetate. Ensure corticosteroids are being administered appropriately. Manage hypokalemia and hypertension
Suspicion of adrenocortical insufficiency	Perform appropriate tests to confirm the diagnosis of adrenocortical insufficiency. Consider administering increased corticosteroid doses during and after stressful situations

Toxicity

Adverse Events

Adverse Event	Abiraterone + Prednisone (N = 542)	Prednisone Alone (N = 540)
	Number of Patients (%)	
Any adverse event	537 (99)	524 (97)
G3/4 adverse event	258 (48)	225 (42)
Any serious adverse event	178 (33)	142 (26)
Adverse event leading to treatment discontinuation	55 (10)	49 (9)
Adverse event leading to death*	20 (4)	12 (2)
G1–4 adverse event ≥15% of patients in either group		
Fatigue	212 (39)	185 (34)
Back pain	173 (32)	173 (32)
Arthralgia	154 (28)	129 (24)
Nausea	120 (22)	118 (22)
Constipation	125 (23)	103 (19)
Hot flush	121 (22)	98 (18)
Diarrhea	117 (22)	96 (18)
Bone pain	106 (20)	103 (19)
Muscle spasm	75 (14)	110 (20)
Pain in extremity	90 (17)	85 (16)
Cough	94 (17)	73 (14)

Adverse Events of Special Interest[†]

Adverse Event	Abiraterone + Prednisone (N = 542)		Prednisone Alone (N = 540)	
	G 1–4	G 3 or 4	G 1–4	G 3 or 4
Fluid retention or edema	150 (28)	4 (<1)	127 (24)	9 (2)
Hypokalemia	91 (17)	13 (2)	68 (13)	10 (2)
Hypertension	118 (22)	21 (4)	71 (13)	16 (3)
Cardiac disorder[‡]	102 (19)	31 (6)	84 (16)	18 (3)
Atrial fibrillation	22 (4)	7 (1)	26 (5)	5 (<1)
ALT increased	63 (12)	29 (5)	27 (5)	4 (<1)
AST increased	58 (11)	16 (3)	26 (5)	5 (<1)

ALT, alanine aminotransferase; AST, aspartate aminotransferase
*Most common adverse events leading to death were general disorders, including disease progression, decline in physical health, and infections including pneumonia and respiratory tract infection
[†]Adverse events of special interest were selected on the basis of the safety profile of phase 2 and phase 3 studies of abiraterone
[‡]Cardiac disorders included ischemic heart disease, myocardial infarction, supraventricular tachyarrhythmia, ventricular tachyarrhythmia, cardiac failure, and possible arrhythmia-related investigations, signs, and symptoms

Patient Population Studied

Inclusion criteria: (a) metastatic, histologically or cytologically confirmed adenocarcinoma of the prostate; (b) PSA progression according to Prostate Cancer Clinical Trials Working Group 2 (PCWG2) criteria or radiographic progression in soft tissue or bone ± PSA progression; (c) ongoing androgen deprivation with a serum testosterone level <50 ng/dL (<1.7 nmol/L); (d) ECOG performance status grade of 0 or 1; (e) no symptoms or mild symptoms, as defined according to the Brief Pain Inventory—Short Form (BPI-SF; scores of 0 to 1 [asymptomatic] or 2 to 3 [mildly symptomatic], respectively). Exclusion criteria: (a) No previous therapy with an antiandrogen; (b) visceral metastases; (c) previous ketoconazole >7 days

Treatment Monitoring

1. CBC every 8 weeks for the first 24 weeks, and then, every 12 weeks
2. *Evaluation including PSA:* Every 8 weeks for the first 24 weeks, and then, every 12 weeks
3. Monitor blood pressure, serum potassium, and symptoms of fluid retention at least every 8 weeks
4. Measure serum transaminases (ALT and AST) and bilirubin levels prior to starting treatment with abiraterone acetate, every 2 weeks for the first 3 months of treatment, and monthly thereafter. Modify, interrupt, or discontinue abiraterone acetate dosing as recommended
5. In patients with baseline moderate hepatic impairment receiving a reduced abiraterone acetate dose of 250 mg/day, measure ALT, AST, and bilirubin prior to the start of treatment, every week for the first month, every 2 weeks for the following 2 months of treatment, and monthly, thereafter. Promptly measure serum total bilirubin, AST, and ALT if clinical symptoms or signs suggestive of hepatotoxicity develop
6. For patients who resume treatment after LFTs return to G ≤1 from a G2/3/4 toxicity, monitor serum transaminases and bilirubin at a minimum of every 2 weeks for 3 months and monthly thereafter
7. Monitor for symptoms and signs of adrenocortical insufficiency. Increased dosage of corticosteroids may be indicated before, during, and after stressful situations

METASTATIC • CASTRATION-RESISTANT • FIRST-LINE

PROSTATE CANCER REGIMEN: ENZALUTAMIDE

Beer TM et al. N Engl J Med 2014;371:424–433
Comments in: Nat Rev Urol. 2014;11:361; N Engl J Med. 2014;371:1755–1756; Eur Urol 2014;66:785–786; Asian J Androl 2014;16:803–804, 807–808; Eur Urol 2015;67:174; Cancer Biol Ther 2015;16:201;203
Protocol for: Beer TM et al. N Engl J Med 2014;371:424–433
Supplementary appendix to: Beer TM et al. N Engl J Med 2014;371:424–433

Enzalutamide 160 mg per dose; administer orally once daily at about the same time each day either with or without food, continually (total dose/week = 1120 mg)

Notes:

- Patients receiving enzalutamide should have undergone bilateral orchiectomy or should also receive concurrent treatment with a gonadotropin-releasing hormone (GnRH) analogue or GnRH antagonist
- Coadministration of a strong CYP2C8 inhibitor (eg, gemfibrozil) increased the composite area under the curve (AUC) of enzalutamide plus *N*-desmethyl enzalutamide by 2.2-fold in healthy volunteers. If possible, avoid concomitant use of strong CYP2C8 inhibitors. If patients must receive a strong CYP2C8 inhibitor concomitantly, reduce the enzalutamide dose to 80 mg once daily. If coadministration of the strong inhibitor is discontinued, the enzalutamide dose should be returned to the dose used prior to initiation of a strong CYP2C8 inhibitor
- Coadministration of a strong CYP3A4 inhibitor (eg, itraconazole) increased the composite AUC of enzalutamide plus *N*-desmethyl enzalutamide by 1.3-fold in healthy volunteers
- Coadministration of enzalutamide with rifampin (a strong CYP3A4 inducer and moderate CYP2C8 inducer) decreased the composite AUC of enzalutamide pus *N*-desmethyl enzalutamide by 37%. Coadministration of enzalutamide with strong CYP3A4 inducers and St John's Wort should be avoided if possible. If coadministration of a strong CYP3A4 inducer with enzalutamide is required, increase the dosage of enzalutamide from 160 mg by mouth once daily to 240 mg by mouth once daily
- Enzalutamide is a strong CYP3A4 inducer and a moderate CYP2C9 and CYP2C19 inducer in humans. At steady state, enzalutamide reduced the plasma exposure to midazolam (CYP3A4 substrate), warfarin (CYP2C9 substrate), and omeprazole (CYP2C19 substrate). Concomitant use of enzalutamide with narrow therapeutic index drugs that are metabolized by CYP3A4, CYP2C9 (eg, phenytoin, warfarin), and CYP2C19 should be avoided, as enzalutamide may decrease their exposure. If coadministration with warfarin cannot be avoided, conduct additional INR monitoring

Supportive Care

Antiemetic prophylaxis
Emetogenic potential is **MINIMAL**
See Chapter 42 for antiemetic recommendations

Hematopoietic growth factor (CSF) prophylaxis
Primary prophylaxis is **NOT** *indicated*
See Chapter 43 for more information

Efficacy (N = 1717)

Median overall survival*	32.4 months with enzalutamide 30.2 months with placebo HR for death 0.71, 95% CI 0.60–0.84, P <0.001
Radiographic progression-free survival at 12 months	65% with enzalutamide 14% with placebo HR for radiographic progression or death 0.19, 95% CI 0.15–0.23, P <0.001

*Estimated at the planned interim analysis, when median duration of follow-up for survival was ~22 months

Therapy Monitoring

1. Obtain CBC with differential prior to start of therapy
2. Optimize management of cardiovascular risk factors, such as hypertension, diabetes, or dyslipidemia
3. Monitor blood pressure at least monthly. Encourage patients to monitor their blood pressure
4. Evaluate patients for fracture and fall risk. Monitor and manage patients at risk for fractures according to established treatment guidelines and consider use of bone-targeted agents
5. Advise patients who have a history of seizure of the risk of developing a seizure and of engaging in any activity where sudden loss of consciousness could cause serious harm to themselves or others
6. Obtain serum PSA at every visit; monitor radiographic imaging every 3 months initially and then every 4 months in patients with radiographically evaluable disease

Patient Population Studied

An international, multicenter, randomized, double-blind, phase 3 trial (PREVAIL) involved 1717 patients with histologically or cytologically confirmed adenocarcinoma of the prostate. Eligible patients had documented metastases, prostate-specific antigen, and/or radiographic progression in bone or soft tissue despite receiving luteinizing hormone-releasing hormone analogue therapy or undergoing orchiectomy; serum testosterone level ≤1.73 nmol/L, Eastern Cooperative Oncology Group (ECOG) performance status ≤1, and Brief Pain Inventory Short Form question 3 score ≤3, and had to be on continued androgen-deprivation therapy. Patients who had received cytotoxic chemotherapy, ketoconazole, or abiraterone acetate, or who had a history of seizure or a condition that could confer a predisposition to seizure, were not eligible. Patients were randomly assigned to receive oral enzalutamide 160 mg or placebo once daily

Treatment Modifications

ENZALUTAMIDE

Starting dose	160 mg by mouth once daily
Dose level −1	120 mg by mouth once daily
Dose level −2	80 mg by mouth once daily
Dose level −3	Discontinue therapy

General Dosage Adjustments

Seizure	Permanently discontinue enzalutamide
Posterior reversible encephalopathy syndrome (PRES)	Permanently discontinue enzalutamide
Hypersensitivity to enzalutamide	Permanently discontinue enzalutamide
G ≤2 ischemic heart disease event	Continue enzalutamide at current dosage and optimize management of cardiovascular risk factors
G3/4 ischemic heart disease event	Permanently discontinue enzalutamide
Other G ≥3 toxicity or intolerable side effect	Interrupt enzalutamide dosing for 1 week or until symptoms resolve to G ≤2, then resume at the same or a reduced dose (120 mg or 80 mg) if warranted
Strong CYP2C8 inhibitor is required	Reduce the enzalutamide dosage to 80 mg by mouth once daily
Strong CYP2C8 inhibitor is discontinued	Resume the enzalutamide dosage that was used prior to initiation of the strong CYP2C8 inhibitor
Strong CYP3A4 inducer is required	Increase the enzalutamide dosage from 160 mg to 240 mg by mouth once daily
Strong CYP3A4 inducer is discontinued	Resume the enzalutamide dosage that was used prior to initiation of the strong CYP3A4 inducer

Note: Advise patients of potential risk to a developing fetus. Advise women who are or may become pregnant not to handle enzalutamide. Advise male patients with female partners of reproductive potential to use effective contraception during treatment and for 3 months after the last dose of enzalutamide. Advise male patients to use a condom if having sex with a pregnant woman

Adverse Events (N = 1057)

Grade (%)*	Enzalutamide (N = 871)		Placebo (N = 844)	
	Grade 1/2	Grade 3–5	Grade 1/2	Grade 3–5
Fatigue	34	2	24	2
Back pain	24	3	19	3
Constipation	22	<1	17	<1
Arthralgia	19	1	15	1
Decreased appetite	18	<1	15	<1
Hot flush	18	<1	8	0
Diarrhea	16	<1	13	<1
Hypertension	7	7	2	2
Asthenia	12	1	7	<1
Fall	10	1	5	<1
Weight loss	11	<1	8	<1
Peripheral edema	10	<1	8	<1
Headache	10	<1	7	<1
Any cardiac adverse event*	7	3	6	2
Acute renal failure*	2	1	3	1
Atrial fibrillation*	1	<1	<1	<1
Ischemic or hemorrhagic cerebrovascular event*	<1	<1	<1	<1
Elevated ALT level*	<1	<1	<1	<1
Acute coronary syndrome*	<1	<1	<1	<1
Seizure*	<1	<1	<1	0

*Denotes those events of special interest
Note: Toxicities are included in the table if all-grade events occurred in ≥10% of patients and were ≥2 percentage points or higher than in the placebo group, or they were of special interest

METASTATIC • CASTRATION-RESISTANT • FIRST-LINE

PROSTATE CANCER REGIMEN: DOCETAXEL + PREDNISONE

Tannock IF et al. N Engl J Med 2004;351:1502–1512

Dexamethasone 8 mg/dose orally for 3 doses at 12 hours, 3 hours, and 1 hour before docetaxel treatment commences (total dose/cycle = 24 mg)

Docetaxel 75 mg/m^2 intravenously over 1 hour, in a volume of 0.9% sodium chloride injection or 5% dextrose injection sufficient to produce a solution with concentration within the range 0.3–0.74 mg/mL, on day 1, every 21 days (total dosage/cycle = 75 mg/m^2)

Prednisone 5 mg/dose orally twice daily, continually, for 21 consecutive days, on days 1–21, every 3 weeks (total dose/cycle = 210 mg)

Supportive Care

Antiemetic prophylaxis
*Emetogenic potential on day 1 is **LOW***
See Chapter 42 for antiemetic recommendations

Hematopoietic growth factor (CSF) prophylaxis
*Primary prophylaxis is **NOT** indicated*
See Chapter 43 for more information

Antimicrobial prophylaxis
*Risk of fever and neutropenia is **LOW***
 Antimicrobial primary prophylaxis to be considered:
- Antibacterial—not indicated
- Antifungal—not indicated
- Antiviral—not indicated unless patient previously had an episode of HSV

Patient Population Studied

A study of 335 patients with castration-refractory metastatic prostate cancer and no prior chemotherapy other than estramustine

Efficacy

	Docetaxel + Prednisone	Mitoxantrone + Prednisone
Median survival	18.9 months (n = 335)	16.5 months (n = 357)
Pain response	35% (n = 153)	22% (n = 157)
50% ↓ PSA	45% (n = 291)	32% (n = 300)

Toxicity (N = 332)

	% All Grades	% G3/4
Hematologic		
Neutropenia	—	32
Anemia	—	5
Thrombocytopenia	—	1
Febrile neutropenia	3	—
Infection	—	6
Nonhematologic		
Fatigue	53	5
Nausea/vomiting	42	—
Diarrhea	32	2
Sensory neuropathy	30	—
Stomatitis	20	—
Dyspnea	15	—
Peripheral edema	15	—
Myalgia	14	—

Treatment Modifications

Adverse Event	Dose Modification
G4 Neutropenia ≥7 days duration, febrile neutropenia, infection, or ANC <1500/mm^3 on day of therapy	Delay therapy until ANC >1500/mm^3 *or* reduce dose of docetaxel by 25%
G3/4 thrombocytopenia	Delay therapy until thrombocytopenia G ≤2, or reduce dosage of docetaxel by 25%
G3/4 toxicities other than those listed above	Wait for toxicity to recover to G ≤1, then reduce docetaxel dosage to 60 mg/m^2
G3/4 neurotoxicity	Stop therapy
G4 nonhematologic toxicity that occurs with 60 mg/m^2 docetaxel	
Aspartate/alanine aminotransferase (AST/ALT) >1.5 × upper limits of normal (ULN) and alkaline phosphatase >2.5 × ULN Bilirubin ≤ ULN	Hold docetaxel until resolved

Therapy Monitoring

Before each cycle: CBC with differential, liver function tests, PSA if indicated

METASTATIC • CASTRATION-RESISTANT • SUBSEQUENT THERAPY

PROSTATE CANCER REGIMEN: ABIRATERONE ACETATE

Fizazi K et al. Lancet Oncol 2012;13:983–992

Abiraterone acetate 1000 mg orally once daily on an empty stomach, continually for 28 consecutive days (total dose/28-day cycle = 28,000 mg)
Note: No food should be consumed for at least 2 hours before a dose of abiraterone acetate is taken and for at least 1 hour after a dose of abiraterone acetate is taken. Exposure (area under the curve) of abiraterone increases up to 10-fold when abiraterone acetate is taken with meals
Prednisone 5 mg orally, twice daily, continually for 28 consecutive days (total dose/28-day cycle = 280 mg)

Notes:
- For patients with baseline moderate hepatic impairment (Child-Pugh Class B), reduce the dose of abiraterone acetate to 250 mg once daily
- Avoid abiraterone acetate in patients with baseline severe hepatic impairment (Child-Pugh Class C), as abiraterone acetate has not been studied in this population, and no dose adjustment can be predicted
- Abiraterone acetate is an inhibitor of the polymorphically expressed cytochrome P450 (CYP) enzyme, CYP2D6
  - **Avoid coadministration** of abiraterone acetate with CYP2D6 substrates that have a low therapeutic index. If an alternative treatment cannot be used, exercise caution and consider a dose reduction of concomitantly used CYP2D6 substrates
- Monitor for symptoms and signs of adrenocortical insufficiency. Increased dosage of corticosteroids may be indicated before, during, and after stressful situations
- Monitor for signs and symptoms of mineralocorticoid excess, including hypokalemia, fluid retention, and hypertension. Prednisone dose may have to be supplemented in some patients or augmented with an aldosterone antagonist such as eplerenone
- Use abiraterone acetate with caution in patients with a history of cardiovascular disease. Control hypertension and correct hypokalemia before initiating treatment
- Abiraterone acetate is a substrate of CYP3A4. Avoid or use with caution strong CYP3A4 inhibitors (eg, atazanavir, clarithromycin, indinavir, itraconazole, ketoconazole, nefazodone, nelfinavir, ritonavir, saquinavir, telithromycin, voriconazole) or inducers (eg, carbamazepine, phenobarbital, phenytoin, rifabutin, rifapentine, rifampin) during abiraterone acetate treatment
- Abiraterone acetate was a strong inhibitor of CYP1A2 and CYP2D6, and a moderate inhibitor of CYP2C9, CYP2C19, and CYP3A4/5 in experimental systems. It is not yet known whether its effects on CYP1A2, CYP2C subfamily, or CYP3A subfamily enzymes in in vitro systems are representative of a potential for clinically important drug interactions
- Use abiraterone acetate with caution in patients with a history of cardiovascular disease. The safety of abiraterone acetate in patients with LVEF <50% or NYHA Class III or IV heart failure is not established. Control hypertension and correct hypokalemia before treatment

Supportive Care
Antiemetic prophylaxis
Emetogenic potential is **MINIMAL–LOW**
See Chapter 42 for antiemetic recommendations

Hematopoietic growth factor (CSF) prophylaxis
Primary prophylaxis is **NOT** indicated
See Chapter 43 for more information

Antimicrobial prophylaxis
Risk of fever and neutropenia is **LOW**
  Antimicrobial primary prophylaxis to be considered:
  - Antibacterial—not indicated
  - Antifungal—not indicated
  - Antiviral—not indicated unless patient previously had an episode of HSV

Treatment Modification

Adverse Event	Dose Modification
G2 hepatotoxicity	Hold abiraterone acetate until toxicity remits to G ≤1, then resume treatment at a dose of 750 mg once daily
G3 hepatotoxicity (elevations in ALT and/or AST >5 × upper limit of normal [ULN] or total bilirubin >3 × ULN) in a patient with baseline normal hepatic function	Withhold abiraterone acetate. Treatment may be restarted at a dose of 750 mg once daily following return of liver function tests to a patient's baseline or to AST and ALT G ≤1 (2.5 × ULN) and total bilirubin G ≤1 (≤1.5 × ULN). For patients who resume treatment, monitor serum transaminases
G3 hepatotoxicity (elevations in ALT and/or AST >5 × upper limit of normal [ULN] or total bilirubin >3 × ULN) in a patient with baseline normal hepatic impairment on a reduced dose of 750 mg/day because of prior hepatotoxicity at 1000 mg/day	Withhold abiraterone acetate. Treatment may be restarted at a dose of 500 mg once daily following return of liver function tests to a patient's baseline or to AST and ALT G ≤1 (2.5 × ULN) and total bilirubin G ≤1 (≤1.5 × ULN). For patients who resume treatment, monitor serum transaminases
G3 hepatotoxicity (elevations in ALT and/or AST >5 × upper limit of normal [ULN] or total bilirubin >3 × ULN) in a patient with baseline normal hepatic impairment on a reduced dose of 500 mg/day because of prior hepatotoxicity at 750 mg/day	Discontinue abiraterone acetate

(continued)

Patient Population Studied

A phase 3, double-blind, randomized, placebo-controlled trial in which men with histologically or cytologically confirmed metastatic castration-resistant prostate cancer were enrolled if they had (a) previous treatment with docetaxel and a maximum of 2 previous chemotherapies; (b) PSA progression according to Prostate Cancer Working Group criteria, or radiographic progression in soft tissue or bone ± PSA progression; (c) ongoing androgen deprivation to maintain serum testosterone concentration lower <50 ng/dL (<2.0 nmol/L by radioimmunoassay); and (d) ECOG performance status ≤2

	Abiraterone Acetate + Prednisone	Placebo + Prednisone
Age (years)		
Median (range)	69 (42–95)	69 (39–90)
≥75 years	220/797 (28%)	111/397 (28%)
Disease location		
Bone	709/797 (89%)	357/397 (90%)
Node	361/797 (45%)	164/397 (41%)
Liver	90/797 (11%)	30/397 (8%)
BPI-SF score for pain*		
Number of patients	792	394
Median score (range)	3.0 (0–10)	3.0 (0–10)
Number of previous cytotoxic chemotherapy regimens		
1	558/797 (70%)	275/398 (69%)
2	239/797 (30%)	123/398 (31%)
ECOG performance status		
0 or 1	715/797 (90%)	353/398 (89%)
2	82/797 (10%)	45/398 (11%)
Prostate-specific antigen		
Number of patients	788	393
Median (range), ng/mL	128.8 (0.4–9253.0)	137.7 (0.6–10114.0)
Gleason score at initial diagnosis		
≤7	341/697 (49%)	161/350 (46%)
≥8	356/697 (51%)	189/350 (54%)
PSA at initial diagnosis (ng/mL)		
Number of patients	619	311
Median (range)	27.0 (0.1–16065.9)	35.5 (1.1–7378.0)
Previous cancer therapy		
Surgery	429/797 (54%)	193/398 (49%)
Radiotherapy	570/797 (72%)	285/398 (72%)
Hormonal	796/797 (100%)	396/398 (100%)
Other†	797/797 (100%)	398/398 (100%)
Extent of disease‡		
Viscera, not otherwise specified	1 (0%)	0 (0%)
Lungs	103 (13%)	45 (11%)
Prostate mass	60 (8%)	23 (6%)
Other viscera	46 (6%)	21 (5%)
Other tissue	40 (5%)	20 (5%)

BPI-SF, Brief Pain Inventory-Short Form
*The BPI-SF rates pain on a scale of 0–10: 0–3 = clinically significant pain is absent; 4–10 = clinically significant pain is present; the scores shown are for the worst pain over the previous 24 hours
†Including chemotherapy
‡Data are for the extent of disease in specific/relevant organs; therefore, numbers ≠ 797 and 398

Treatment Modification
(*continued*)

G3 hepatotoxicity (elevations in ALT and/or AST >5 × ULN or total bilirubin >3 × ULN) in a patient with baseline moderate hepatic impairment on a reduced dose of 750 mg abiraterone acetate daily	Discontinue abiraterone acetate
G4 hepatotoxicity (elevations in ALT and/or AST >20 × ULN or total bilirubin >10 × ULN) in a patient with baseline moderate hepatic impairment	Discontinue abiraterone acetate
Hypertension, hypokalemia, and fluid retention caused by mineralocorticoid excess	Withhold abiraterone acetate. Ensure corticosteroids are being administered appropriately. Manage hypokalemia and hypertension
Suspicion of adrenocortical insufficiency	Perform appropriate tests to confirm the diagnosis of adrenocortical insufficiency. Consider administering increased corticosteroid doses during and after stressful situations

Efficacy

Progression-Free Survival (PFS) and Objective Response (OR)

	Abiraterone Acetate + Prednisone N = 797 (95% CI)	Placebo + Prednisone N = 398 (95% CI)	Hazard Ratio (95% CI)	P Value
Time to PSA progression (months)*	8.5 (8.3–11.1)	6.6 (5.6–8.3)	0.63 (0.52–0.78)	<0.0001
Radiographic PFS (months)*	5.6 (5.6–6.5)	3.6 (2.9–5.5)	0.66 (0.58–0.76)	<0.0001
PSA response (%)†	235 (29.5%)	22 (5.5%)	—	<0.0001
OR by RECIST (%)‡	118 (14.8%)	13 (3.3%)	—	<0.0001

RECIST, Response Evaluation Criteria in Solid Tumors
Data are median (95% CI) or number (%)
*Calculated from date of randomization to date of PSA progression (per Prostate Specific Antigen Working Group criteria) or date of radiographically documented disease progression or death
†Proportion of patients with a PSA decline of 50% or higher according to Prostate Specific Antigen Working Group criteria; unstratified analysis
‡Additional (not secondary) end point

Overall Survival by Subgroup (Univariate Analysis)

	Abiraterone Acetate + Prednisone		Placebo + Prednisone		
	Events (N)	Median OS (Months; 95% CI)	Events (N)	Median OS (Months; 95% CI)	HR (95% CI)
Baseline ECOG status					
0–1	432/715	17.0 (15.6–17.7)	237/353	12.3 (10.8–14.5)	0.74 (0.63–0.87)
2	69/82	7.3 (6.4–8.6)	37/45	7.0 (4.0–8.1)	0.77 (0.50–1.17)
Pain at study entry					
Pain absent (0–3)	244/440	18.4 (17.2–19.9)	137/219	13.9 (11.7–15.9)	0.69 (0.56–0.85)
Pain present (4–10)	257/357	13.3 (11.1–14.7)	137/179	9.3 (7.9–10.7)	0.78 (0.63–0.96)
Previous lines of chemotherapy					
1	329/557	17.1 (15.6–18.2)	185/275	11.7 (10.4–13.9)	0.71 (0.59–0.85)
2	172/240	14.2 (11.8–15.3)	89/123	10.4 (8.8–13.5)	0.80 (0.61–1.02)
Type of progression before study entry					
PSA progression	126/238	18.3 (16.7–20.8)	79/125	13.6 (10.8–16.8)	0.63 (0.47–0.84)
Radiographic progression ± PSA progression	375/559	14.8 (14.0–16.1)	195/273	10.5 (8.9–12.5)	0.78 (0.65–0.93)
Previous docetaxel usage					
From first docetaxel dose	494/787	32.6 (30.7–35.0)	274/397	27.6 (25.9–30.3)	0.75 (0.65–0.88)
From last docetaxel dose	494/787	23.2 (22.4–24.5)	274/397	19.4 (17.5–20.8)	0.74 (0.64–0.86)
Reason for discontinuation of docetaxel					
Progressive disease	241/362	14.2 (12.0–15.8)	129/182	10.5 (9.3–11.8)	0.77 (0.62–0.97)
All other reasons	258/431	17.0 (15.6–18.2)	145/215	12.6 (10.4–14.9)	0.73 (0.59–0.89)
Treatment of abiraterone acetate plus prednisone started					
≤3 months after last docetaxel dose	144/227	15.0 (13.7–17.4)	82/112	10.7 (8.9–13.0)	0.62 (0.47–0.83)
>3 months after last docetaxel dose	346/554	16.1 (14.9–17.3)	190/282	11.8 (10.3–14.6)	0.77 (0.64–0.92)

(continued)

Efficacy (continued)

Docetaxel exposure time					
≤3 Months	98/140	14.6 (11.9–16.7)	51/69	10.8 (8.4–14.9)	0.76 (0.53–1.08)
>3 Months	252/401	16.2 (14.9–17.3)	223/328	11.2 (10.3–13.6)	0.74 (0.63–0.87)

Patients who were not deceased at the time of analysis were censored on the last date the patient was known to be alive or lost to follow-up
Every test was done at a significance level of 0.05
Patient numbers are not consistent across subgroups because of missing data

Toxicity

	Abiraterone Acetate + Prednisone (n = 791)			Placebo + Prednisone (n = 394)		
	All Grades N (%)	G3 N (%)	G4 N (%)	All Grades N (%)	G3 N (%)	G4 N (%)
Hematologic						
Anemia	198 (25%)	53 (7%)	9 (1%)	110 (28%)	26 (7%)	6 (2%)
Thrombocytopenia	30 (4%)	8 (1%)	3 (<1%)	15 (4%)	1 (<1%)	1 (<1%)
Neutropenia	8 (1%)	1 (<1%)	0	2 (<1%)	1 (<1%)	0
Febrile neutropenia	3 (<1%)	0	3 (<1%)	0	0	0
Nonhematologic						
Diarrhea	156 (20%)	8 (1%)	1 (<1%)	58 (15%)	5 (1%)	0
Fatigue	372 (47%)	70 (9%)	2 (<1%)	174 (44%)	38 (10%)	3 (<1%)
Asthenia	122 (15%)	26 (3%)	0	54 (14%)	7 (2%)	1 (<1%)
Back pain	262 (33%)	53 (7%)	3 (<1%)	141 (36%)	39 (10%)	1 (<1%)
Nausea	258 (33%)	16 (2%)	1 (<1%)	130 (33%)	11 (3%)	0
Vomiting	191 (24%)	20 (3%)	1 (<1%)	101 (26%)	12 (3%)	0
Hematuria	73 (9%)	12 (2%)	0	34 (9%)	9 (2%)	0
Abdominal pain	102 (13%)	18 (2%)	0	47 (12%)	8 (2%)	0
Pain in extremity	156 (20%)	23 (3%)	1 (<1%)	82 (21%)	20 (5%)	0
Dyspnea	116 (15%)	12 (2%)	2 (<1%)	49 (12%)	7 (2%)	2 (<1%)
Constipation	223 (28%)	10 (1%)	0	126 (32%)	4 (1%)	0
Pyrexia	80 (10%)	3 (<1%)	0	36 (9%)	5 (1%)	0
Arthralgia	239 (30%)	40 (5%)	0	95 (24%)	17 (4%)	0
Urinary tract infection	105 (13%)	12 (2%)	0	29 (7%)	3 (<1%)	0
Pain	38 (5%)	7 (<1%)	0	21 (5%)	7 (2%)	1 (<1%)
Bone pain	216 (27%)	49 (6%)	2 (<1%)	117 (30%)	27 (7%)	4 (1%)

(continued)

Toxicity (continued)

Adverse Events of Special Interest

Fluid retention or edema	261 (33%)	18 (2%)	2 (<1%)	94 (24%)	4 (1%)	0
Hypokalemia	143 (18%)	31 (4%)	4 (<1%)	36 (9%)	3 (<1%)	0
Cardiac disorders*	126 (16%)	32 (4%)	9 (1%)	46 (12%)	7 (2%)	2 (<1%)
Abnormalities in LFTs	89 (11%)	28 (4%)	2 (<1%)	35 (9%)	11 (3%)	3 (<1%)
Hypertension	88 (11%)	10 (1%)	0	32 (8%)	1 (<1%)	0

LFTs, liver function tests
*Cardiac disorders associated with abiraterone acetate treatment as defined by the standardized *Medical Dictionary for Regulatory Activities Queries* included ischemic heart disease, myocardial infarction, supraventricular tachyarrhythmias, ventricular tachyarrhythmias, cardiac failure, and possible arrhythmia-related investigations, signs, and symptoms

Treatment Monitoring

1. CBC before each cycle
2. *Evaluation including PSA:* Every 6 weeks
3. Monitor blood pressure, serum potassium, and symptoms of fluid retention at least monthly
4. Measure serum transaminases (ALT and AST) and bilirubin levels prior to starting treatment with abiraterone acetate, every 2 weeks for the first 3 months of treatment, and monthly thereafter. Modify, interrupt, or discontinue abiraterone acetate dosing as recommended
5. In patients with baseline moderate hepatic impairment receiving a reduced abiraterone acetate dose of 250 mg/day, measure ALT, AST, and bilirubin prior to the start of treatment, every week for the first month, every 2 weeks for the following 2 months of treatment, and monthly thereafter. Promptly measure serum total bilirubin, AST, and ALT if clinical symptoms or signs suggestive of hepatotoxicity develop
6. For patients who resume treatment after LFTs return to G ≤1 from a G2/3/4 toxicity, monitor serum transaminases and bilirubin at a minimum of every 2 weeks for 3 months and monthly thereafter
7. Monitor for symptoms and signs of adrenocortical insufficiency. Increased dosage of corticosteroids may be indicated before, during, and after stressful situations

METASTATIC • CASTRATION-RESISTANT • SUBSEQUENT THERAPY

PROSTATE CANCER REGIMEN: ENZALUTAMIDE

Scher HI et al. N Engl J Med 2012;367:1187–1197

Enzalutamide 160 mg orally, once daily, continually

Notes:
• Can be taken with or without food
• Swallow capsules whole. Do not chew, dissolve, or open the capsules

Notes:
• If possible, avoid concomitant use of strong CYP2C8 inhibitors. If patients must receive a strong CYP2C8 inhibitor concomitantly, reduce the enzalutamide dose to 80 mg once daily. If coadministration of the strong inhibitor is discontinued, the enzalutamide dose should be returned to the dose used prior to initiation of a strong CYP2C8 inhibitor
• Coadministration of a strong CYP3A4 inhibitor (eg, itraconazole) increased the composite AUC of enzalutamide plus *N*-desmethyl enzalutamide by 1.3-fold in healthy volunteers
• The effects of CYP3A4 inducers on the pharmacokinetics of enzalutamide have not been evaluated in vivo
• Coadministration of enzalutamide with strong CYP3A4 inducers may decrease the plasma exposure of enzalutamide and should be avoided if possible
• Moderate CYP3A4 inducers and St. John's Wort may also reduce the plasma exposure of enzalutamide and should be avoided if possible
• Enzalutamide is a strong CYP3A4 inducer and a moderate CYP2C9 and CYP2C19 inducer in humans. At steady state, enzalutamide reduced the plasma exposure to midazolam (CYP3A4 substrate), warfarin (CYP2C9 substrate), and omeprazole (CYP2C19 substrate). Concomitant use of enzalutamide with narrow therapeutic index drugs that are metabolized by CYP3A4, CYP2C9 (eg, phenytoin, warfarin) and CYP2C19 should be avoided, as enzalutamide may decrease their exposure. If coadministration with warfarin cannot be avoided, conduct additional INR monitoring

Treatment Modification

Adverse Event	Treatment Modification
G ≥3 adverse event or an intolerable side effect	Withhold dosing for 1 week or until symptoms improve to G ≤2, then resume at the same or a reduced dose (120 mg or 80 mg daily), if warranted
Occurrence of a seizure	Discontinue enzalutamide

Patient Population Studied

Patients had (a) a histologically or cytologically confirmed diagnosis of prostate cancer; (b) castrate levels of testosterone (<50 ng/dL; [<1.7 nmol/L]); (c) previous treatment with docetaxel; and (d) progressive disease defined according to Prostate Cancer Working Group 2 criteria (including 3 increasing values for PSA or radiographically confirmed progression with or without a rise in the PSA level)

Efficacy

Multivariate Analysis of Hazard Ratios for Death*

Variable	Measurement Estimates		Hazard Ratio for Death (95% CI)†
	Coefficient	P Value	
Study treatment (enzalutamide vs placebo)	−0.54 ± 0.09	<0.001	0.58 (0.49–0.70)
ECOG performance score (0 or 1 vs 2)	−0.33 ± 0.14	0.02	0.72 (0.55–0.95)
BPI-SF mean pain score (question no. 3) (<4 vs ≥4)‡	−0.23 ± 0.10	0.02	0.79 (0.65–0.97)
Progression at study entry (PSA only vs radiographic)	−0.29 ± 0.09	0.002	0.75 (0.62–0.90)
Visceral disease at screening (no vs yes)	−0.47 ± 0.10	<0.001	0.63 (0.52–0.76)

Secondary End Points Related to Response and Disease Progression§

End Point	Enzalutamide (N = 800)	Placebo (N = 399)	Hazard Ratio (95% CI)	P Value
Confirmed PSA decline§				
≥1 Postbaseline PSA assessment—no. (%)	731 (91)	330 (83)		
PSA response—no./total no. (%)				
Decline ≥50% from baseline	395/731 (54)	5/330 (2)		<0.001
Decline ≥90% from baseline	181/731 (25)	3/330 (1)		<0.001
Soft-tissue objective response				
Patients with measurable disease—no. (%)	446 (56)	208 (52)		
CR or PR—no./total no. (%)	129/446 (29)	8/208 (4)		<0.001
FACT-P quality-of-life response§				
No (%) with ≥1 postbaseline assessment	651 (81)	257 (64)		
Quality-of-life response—no./total no. (%)ᶜ	281/651 (43)	47/257 (18)		<0.001
Progression indicators				
Time to PSA progression			0.25 (0.20–0.30)	<0.001
Median, months	8.3	3.0		
95% CI	5.8–8.3	2.9–3.7		
Radiographic progression-free survival			0.40 (0.35–0.47)	<0.001
Median, months	8.3	2.9		
95% CI	8.2–9.4	2.8–3.4		
Time to first skeletal-related event			0.69 (0.57–0.84)	<0.001
Median, months	16.7	13.3		
95% CI	14.6–19.1	9.9–NYR		

BPI-SF, Brief Pain Inventory–Short Form; CI, confidence interval; CR, complete response; ECOG, Eastern Cooperative Oncology Group; FACT-P, Functional Assessment of Cancer Therapy–Prostate; LDH, lactate dehydrogenase; NYR, not yet reached; PR, partial response

*Patients alive at the time of analysis were censored at the date patient was last known to be alive

†Hazard ratios for death were calculated after adjustment for prognostic factors. These included age (<65 years vs ≥65 years), region (North America vs other), number of previous che-motherapy regimens (1 vs 2), and baseline serum PSA level (per increase of 1 ng/mL). The Gleason score for prostate tumors was excluded owing to a large number of missing values

‡On the Brief Pain Inventory–Short Form (BPI-SF) scores of 0–3 indicate clinically significant pain is absent and scores of 4–10 indicate clinically significant pain is present. Higher scores indicate greater pain

§Only patients with both baseline and postbaseline assessments are included

ᶜDefined as 10-point improvement in the global score on the FACT-P questionnaire, as compared with baseline, on 2 consecutive measurements obtained at least 3 weeks apart

Toxicity

Adverse Events, According to Grade

	Enzalutamide (N = 800)		Placebo (N = 399)	
	Any Grade	G ≥3	Any Grade	G ≥3
Adverse Event	Number of Patients (Percent)			
≥1 Adverse event	785 (98)	362 (45)	390 (98)	212 (53)
Any serious adverse event	268 (34)	227 (28)	154 (39)	134 (34)
Discontinuation owing to adverse event	61 (8)	37 (5)	39 (10)	28 (7)
Adverse event leading to death	23 (3)	23 (3)	14 (4)	14 (4)
Frequent adverse events more common with enzalutamide*				
Fatigue	269 (34)	50 (6)	116 (29)	29 (7)
Diarrhea	171 (21)	9 (1)	70 (18)	1 (<1)
Hot flash	162 (20)	0	41 (10)	0
Musculoskeletal pain	109 (14)	8 (1)	40 (10)	1 (<1)
Headache	93 (12)	6 (<1)	22 (6)	0
Clinically significant adverse events				
Cardiac disorder				
Any	49 (6)	7 (1)	30 (8)	8 (2)
Myocardial infarction	2 (<1)	2 (<1)	2 (<1)	2 (<1)
Abnormality on liver-function testing†	8 (1)	3 (<1)	6 (2)	3 (<1)
Seizure	5 (<1)	5 (<1)	0	0

*Includes adverse events that occurred in >10% of patients in the enzalutamide group and those that occurred in the enzalutamide group at a rate ≥2% higher than in the placebo group
†Includes hyperbilirubinemia and increased levels of aspartate or alanine aminotransferases

Treatment Monitoring

Evaluation including PSA: Every 6 weeks

METASTATIC • CASTRATION-RESISTANT • SUBSEQUENT THERAPY

PROSTATE CANCER REGIMEN: CABAZITAXEL + PREDNISONE

de Bono JS et al. Lancet 2010;376:1147–1154
Eisenberger M et al. J Clin Oncol. 2017;35:3198–3206

Note: Severe hypersensitivity reactions can occur with cabazitaxel administration. These may include generalized rash/erythema, hypotension, and bronchospasm. Severe hypersensitivity reactions require immediate discontinuation of cabazitaxel infusion and administration of appropriate therapy. Patients should receive primary prophylaxis against hypersensitivity reactions as described below. Cabazitaxel must not be given to patients who have a history of severe hypersensitivity reactions to other drugs formulated with polysorbate 80, such as fosaprepitant dimeglumine (the parenteral formulation of aprepitant [Emend]), darbepoetin alfa, docetaxel, etoposide, recombinant human papillomavirus quadrivalent vaccine (Gardasil), and various vaccines. Patients should be observed closely for hypersensitivity reactions, especially during the first and second infusions. Hypersensitivity reactions may occur within a few minutes following the initiation of the cabazitaxel infusion, and thus facilities and equipment for the treatment of hypotension and bronchospasm should be available

Premedication:
At least 30 minutes prior to each cabazitaxel dose, administer the following medications to reduce the risk and/or severity of hypersensitivity:
• **Diphenhydramine** 25 mg, or an equivalent H_1-receptor antihistamine, orally or intravenously
• **Dexamethasone** 8 mg or an equipotent glucocorticoid
• **Ranitidine** 50 mg intravenously or 150 mg orally, or an equivalent histamine (H_2)-receptor antagonist

Cabazitaxel 20 mg/m² intravenously over 60 minutes, diluted in a volume of 0.9% sodium chloride injection or 5% dextrose injection sufficient to produce a solution with concentration within the range 0.1–0.26 mg/mL, on day 1, every 3 weeks (total dosage/cycle = 20 mg/m²)
Prednisone 10 mg/day orally, continually for 21 consecutive days (total dose/21-day cycle = 210 mg)

Note:
• Cabazitaxel is extensively metabolized in the liver (>95%), primarily by cytochrome P450 (CYP) CYP3A4/5 enzymes (80–90%), and, to a lesser extent, by the polymorphically expressed enzyme, CYP2C8. Consequently hepatic impairment is likely to increase cabazitaxel concentrations
• Although no formal drug interaction trials with cabazitaxel have been conducted, clinicians should use caution with respect to the following:
  ▪ *CYP3A4 inhibitors:* Concomitant administration of strong CYP3A subfamily inhibitors (eg, atazanavir, clarithromycin, indinavir, itraconazole, ketoconazole, nefazodone, nelfinavir, ritonavir, saquinavir, telithromycin, voriconazole) is expected to increase concentrations of cabazitaxel. Therefore, coadministration with strong CYP3A inhibitors should be avoided. Caution should be exercised with concomitant use of moderate CYP3A subfamily inhibitors
  ▪ *CYP3A4 inducers:* The concomitant administration of strong CYP3A subfamily inducers (eg, carbamazepine, phenobarbital, phenytoin, rifabutin, rifapentine, rifampin) is expected to decrease cabazitaxel concentrations. Therefore, coadministration with strong CYP3A inducers should be avoided. In addition, patients should also refrain from taking St. John's Wort

Supportive Care
Antiemetic prophylaxis
Emetogenic potential is **LOW**
See Chapter 42 for antiemetic recommendations

Hematopoietic growth factor (CSF) prophylaxis
Primary prophylaxis **MAY BE** *indicated. The FDA-approved prescribing information "Black Box Warning" indicates that primary prophylaxis is recommended in patients with high-risk clinical features, and should be considered in all patients receiving a cabazitaxel dose of 25 mg/m²*
See Chapter 43 for more information

Antimicrobial prophylaxis
Risk of fever and neutropenia is **LOW**
  Antimicrobial primary prophylaxis to be considered:
  • Antibacterial—not indicated
  • Antifungal—not indicated
  • Antiviral—not indicated unless patient previously had an episode of HSV

Treatment Modifications

Adverse Event	Dose Modification
Prolonged grade ≥3 neutropenia (>1 week) despite appropriate medication including filgrastim	Delay treatment until neutrophil count is >1500 cells/mm³, then reduce cabazitaxel dosage to 15 mg/m². Use filgrastim for secondary prophylaxis
Prolonged grade ≥3 neutropenia (>1 week) despite appropriate medication including filgrastim at a cabazitaxel dosage of 20 mg/m²	Discontinue cabazitaxel
Febrile neutropenia	Delay treatment until improvement or resolution, and until neutrophil count is >1500 cells/mm³, then resume treatment with cabazitaxel dosage decreased to 15 mg/m². Use filgrastim for secondary prophylaxis
Febrile neutropenia at a cabazitaxel dosage of 20 mg/m²	Discontinue cabazitaxel
Grade ≥3 diarrhea or diarrhea that persists despite appropriate medication, fluid, and electrolytes replacement	Delay treatment until improvement or resolution, then resume treatment with cabazitaxel dosage decreased to 15 mg/m²
Grade ≥3 diarrhea or diarrhea that persists despite appropriate medication, fluid, and electrolytes replacement at a cabazitaxel dosage of 20 mg/m²	Discontinue cabazitaxel
Total bilirubin ≥ ULN, or AST and/or ALT ≥1.5 times ULN)	Discontinue cabazitaxel

Toxicity* (N = 371)

	% All Grades	% G ≥3
Hematologic		
Neutropenia	94	82
Febrile neutropenia	—	8
Leukopenia	96	68
Anemia	97	11
Thrombocytopenia	47	4
Nonhematologic		
Diarrhea	47	6
Fatigue	37	5
Asthenia	20	5
Back pain	16	4
Nausea	34	2
Vomiting	23	2
Hematuria	17	2
Abdominal pain	12	2
Pain in extremity	8	2
Dyspnea	12	1
Constipation	20	1
Pyrexia	12	1
Arthralgia	11	1
Urinary tract infection	7	1
Pain	5	1
Bone pain	5	1

*NCI Common Terminology Criteria for Adverse Events, version 3

Efficacy

	Mitoxantrone	Cabazitaxel	P Value
Tumor Response Rate*			
Number of evaluable patients	204	201	
Response rate (%)	4.4%	14.4%	0.0005
PSA Response Rate†			
Number of evaluable patients	325	329	
Response rate (%)	17.8%	39.2%	0.0002
Pain Response Rate‡			
Number of evaluable patients	168	174	
Response rate (%)	7.7%	9.2%	0.63
Progression			
Number pts in intention-to-treat analysis	377	378	
Median time to tumor progression (months)	5.4	8.8	<0.0001
Median time to PSA progression (months)	3.1	6.4	0.001
Median time to pain progression (months)§	NR	11.1 (2.9–NR)	0.52

NR, Not reached
*Tumor response was evaluated only for patients with measurable disease according to RECIST
†PSA response was defined as ≥50% reduction in serum PSA concentrations, established only for patients with a serum PSA concentration of 20 mcg/L or more at baseline, confirmed by a repeat PSA measurement after at least 3 weeks
‡Pain response was established only for patients with a median present pain intensity (PPI) score ≥2, a mean analgesic score (AS) ≥10 points at baseline, or both, and was defined as a reduction from baseline median PPI score ≥2 points without an increased AS or a decrease ≥50% in the AS without an increase in the PPI score, maintained for at least 3 weeks
§Data for 265 patients in the cabazitaxel group and 279 patients in the mitoxantrone group were censored as a result of ≥2 PPI or AS assessments or both, being missed during the same week (unless a complete evaluation of ≥5 values showed pain progression)

Patient Population Studied

A study of 755 patients with pathologically proven castration-refractory prostate cancer with documented disease progression during or after completion of docetaxel treatment. Eligible patients had an Eastern Cooperative Oncology Group performance status of 0–2. Patients with measurable disease were required to have documented disease progression by Response Evaluation Criteria in Solid Tumors (RECIST) criteria with at least 1 metastatic visceral or soft-tissue lesion. Patients with nonmeasurable disease were required to have rising serum prostate-specific antigen (PSA) concentrations (at least 2 consecutive increases relative to a reference value measured at least a week apart) or the appearance of at least 1 new demonstrable radiographic lesion. Additional inclusion criteria were: previous and ongoing castration by orchiectomy, LHRH agonists, or both interventions

Therapy Monitoring

1. *Before each cycle:* Physical exam, CBC and LFTs
2. *Evaluation including PSA:* Every 6 weeks to every 3 months

METASTATIC • CASTRATION-RESISTANT • SUBSEQUENT THERAPY

PROSTATE CANCER REGIMEN: RADIUM-223

Parker et al. N Engl J Med 2013;369:213–223
XOFIGO (radium 223) Package Insert. Available from: http://labeling.bayerhealthcare.com/html/products/pi/Xofigo_PI.pdf

Radium (Ra)-223 dichloride 55 kBq (^{223}Ra 1.49 µCi) per kilogram of body weight by slow intravenous injection over 1 minute every 4 weeks for 6 injections

Note:
• Flush the intravenous access line or cannula with 0.9% sodium chloride injection before and after injection of radium-223
• Safety and efficacy beyond 6 injections with radium-223 have not been studied

Calculate volume to be administered to a given patient using the:
• Patient's body weight (kg)
• Dosage level 55 kBq/kg body weight or 1.49 µCi/kg body weight
• Radioactivity concentration of the product (1100 kBq/mL; 30 µCi/mL) at the reference date
• Decay correction factor to correct for physical decay of radium-223

Calculate total volume to be administered as follows:

$$\text{Volume to be administered (mL)} = \frac{\text{Body weight in kg} \times 50 \text{ kBq/kg body weight}}{\text{Decay factor} \times 1000 \text{ kBq/mL}}$$

OR

$$\text{Volume to be administered (mL)} = \frac{\text{Body weight in kg} \times 1.35 \mu \text{ Ci/kg body weight}}{\text{Decay factor} \times 27 \mu \text{ Ci/mL}}$$

Decay Correction Factor Table

Days from Reference Date	Decay Factor	Days from Reference Date	Decay Factor
−14	2.296	0	0.982
−13	2.161	1	0.925
−12	2.034	2	0.870
−11	1.914	3	0.819
−10	1.802	4	0.771
−9	1.696	5	0.725
−8	1.596	6	0.683
−7	1.502	7	0.643
−6	1.414	8	0.605
−5	1.330	9	0.569
−4	1.252	10	0.536
−3	1.178	11	0.504
−2	1.109	12	0.475
−1	1.044	13	0.447
		14	0.420

The Decay Correction Factor Table is corrected to 12 noon Central Standard Time (CST). To determine the decay correction factor, count the number before or after the reference date. The Decay Correction Factor Table includes a correction to account for the 7-hour time difference between 12 noon European Time (CET) at the site of manufacture and 12 noon U.S. CST, which is 7 hours earlier than CET

(continued)

(*continued*)

Note: Immediately before and after administration, the net patient dose of administered radium-223 should be determined by measurement in an appropriate radioisotope dose calibrator that has been calibrated with a National Institute of Standards and Technology (NIST) traceable radium-223 standard and corrected for decay using the date and time of calibration

Safety Information: Radium-223 is primarily an alpha emitter, with 95.3% of energy emitted as alpha particles. Only 3.6% is emitted as beta particles and 1.1% as gamma radiation. Thus the external radiation exposure associated with handling of patient doses is expected to be low, because the typical treatment activity will be <8000 kBq (<216 µCi). Nevertheless, care should be used as follows:

Precautions:
- The administration of radium-223 is associated with potential risks to other persons from radiation or contamination from spills of bodily fluids such as urine, feces, or vomit. Therefore, radiation protection precautions must be taken in accordance with national and local regulations
- Whenever possible, patients should use a toilet (commode) and the toilet should be flushed several times after each use. When handling bodily fluids, simply wearing gloves and hand washing will protect caregivers. Clothing soiled with radium-223 or patient fecal matter or urine should be washed promptly and separately from other clothing

Instructions to Patients:
- Stay well hydrated and monitor oral intake, fluid status, and urine output. Report signs of dehydration
- There are no restrictions regarding contact with other people after receiving radium-223. Follow good hygiene practices for at least 1 week after the last injection so as to minimize radiation exposure from bodily fluids to household members and caregivers
- Flush toilets several times after each use
- Promptly wash clothing soiled with fecal matter or urine separately from other clothing
- Caregivers should use universal precautions when handling body fluids to avoid contamination. When handling bodily fluids, wearing gloves and hand washing will protect caregivers
- Patients who are sexually active should use condoms and their female partners of reproductive potential should use a highly effective method of birth control during treatment and for 6 months following completion of radium-223 treatment

Toxicity

Adverse Events That Occurred in at Least 5% of Patients in Either Study Group in the Safety Population*

Adverse Event	Radium-223 (N = 600)				Placebo (N = 301)			
	% All Grades	% G3	% G4	% G5	% All Grades	% G3	% G4	% G5
Hematologic								
Anemia	31	11	2	0	31	12	1	<1
Thrombocytopenia	12	3	3	<1	6	2	<1	0
Neutropenia	5	2	1	0	1	1	0	0
Nonhematologic								
Constipation	18	1	0	0	15	2	0	0
Diarrhea	25	2	0	0	15	2	0	0
Nausea	36	2	0	0	35	2	0	0
Vomiting	18	2	0	0	14	2	0	0
Asthenia	6	1	0	0	6	1	0	0
Fatigue	26	4	1	0	26	5	1	0
Deterioration general physical health	4	2	<1	1	7	3	1	1
Peripheral edema	13	2	0	0	10	1	<1	0
Pyrexia	6	1	0	0	6	1	0	0
Pneumonia	3	2	0	1	5	2	1	0

(*continued*)

Toxicity (continued)

Nonhematologic								
Urinary tract infection	8	1	0	0	9	1	<1	<1
Weight loss	12	1	0	0	15	2	0	0
Anorexia	17	2	0	0	18	1	0	0
Decreased appetite	6	<1	0	0	4	0	0	0
Bone pain	50	20	1	0	62	25	1	0
Muscular weakness	2	<1	<1	0	6	2	0	0
Pathologic fracture	4	2	0	0	5	3	<1	0
Progression malignant neoplasm	13	2	1	9	15	1	<1	11
Dizziness	7	<1	0	0	9	1	0	0
Spinal cord compression	4	2	1	<1	8	5	<1	0
Insomnia	4	0	0	0	7	<1	0	0
Hematuria	5	1	0	0	5	1	0	0
Urinary retention	4	2	0	0	6	2	0	0
Dyspnea	8	2	<1	<1	9	2	0	1

*Only 1 G5 hematologic adverse event was considered possibly related to study drug: thrombocytopenia in 1 patient in the radium-223 group

Patient Population Studied

Inclusion criteria: (a) histologically confirmed, progressive, castration-resistant prostate cancer; (b) 2 or more bone metastases detected on skeletal scintigraphy and no known visceral metastases; (c) received docetaxel, or were not healthy enough or declined to receive it, or it was not available; (d) symptomatic disease with regular use of analgesic medication or treatment with external beam radiation therapy required for cancer-related bone pain within the previous 12 weeks; (e) a baseline PSA ≥5 ng/mL or with evidence of progressively increasing PSA values (2 consecutive increases over the previous reference value); (f) an ECOG performance-status score of 0–2; and (g) a life expectancy ≥6 months. Exclusion criteria: (a) chemotherapy within the previous 4 weeks; (b) previous hemibody external radiotherapy; (c) systemic radiotherapy with radioisotopes within the previous 24 weeks; (d) a blood transfusion or use of erythropoietin-stimulating agents within the previous 4 weeks; (e) malignant lymphadenopathy ≥3 cm in the short-axis diameter; (f) history of or the presence of visceral metastases; and (g) imminent or established spinal cord compression

Castration-resistant disease was defined as a serum testosterone level ≤50 ng/dL (≤1.7 nmol/L) after bilateral orchiectomy or during maintenance treatment consisting of androgen-ablation therapy with a luteinizing hormone-releasing hormone agonist or polyestradiol phosphate. Patients with castration-resistant disease during maintenance treatment were required to continue that treatment throughout the study

Baseline Characteristics of the Patients*

Characteristic	Radium-223 (N = 614)	Placebo (N = 307)
Age		
Median (range)—years	71 (49–90)	71 (44–94)
>75 years—no. (%)	171 (28)	90 (29)
Total alkaline phosphatase—no. (%)		
<220 U/L	348 (57)	169 (55)
≥220 U/L	266 (43)	138 (45)

(continued)

Patient Population Studied (*continued*)

Current use of bisphosphonates—no. (%)		
Yes	250 (41)	124 (40)
No	364 (59)	183 (60)
Any previous use of docetaxel—no. (%)		
Yes	352 (57)	174 (57)
No	262 (43)	133 (43)
ECOG performance-status score—no. (%)		
0	165 (27)	78 (25)
1	371 (60)	187 (61)
≥2	77 (13)	41 (13)
WHO ladder for cancer pain—no. (%)[†]		
1 (mild pain/no opioid use)	257 (42)	137 (45)
2 (moderate pain/occasional opioid use)	151 (25)	78 (25)
3 (severe pain/regular daily opioid use)	194 (32)	90 (29)
Extent of disease—no. (%)		
<6 metastases	100 (16)	38 (12)
6–20 metastases	262 (43)	147 (48)
>20 metastases	195 (32)	91 (30)
Superscan[‡]	54 (9)	30 (10)
External beam radiation therapy within 12 weeks after screening—no. (%)		
Yes	99 (16)	48 (16)
No	515 (84)	259 (84)
Median biochemical values (range)		
Hemoglobin (normal range = 13.4–17.0 g/dL)	12.2 (8.5–15.7)	12.1 (8.5–16.4)
Albumin (normal range: 36–45 g/L)	40 (24–53)	40 (23–50)
Total alkaline phosphatase >105 U/L	211 (32–6431)	223 (29–4805)
Lactate dehydrogenase >255 U/L	315 (76–2171)	336 (132–3856)
PSA >3.999 ng/mL	146 (3.8–6026)	173 (1.5–14500)

ECOG, Eastern Cooperative Oncology Group
*Percentages may not sum to 100 due to rounding
[†]A total of 12 patients in the radium-223 group (2%) and 2 patients in the placebo group (1%) had no pain or analgesic use at baseline
[‡]Superscan refers to a bone scan showing diffuse, intense skeletal uptake of the tracer without renal and background activity

Treatment Modifications

None

Treatment Monitoring

1. Weekly CBC with differential and platelet count
2. Monitor oral intake, fluid status, and urine output during treatment with radium-223
   • Instruct patients to report signs of dehydration, hypovolemia, urinary retention, or renal failure or insufficiency

Efficacy

Overall Survival and Subgroup Analyses of Hazard Ratios for Death

End Point	Radium-223 (N = 614)	Placebo (N = 307)	Hazard Ratio (95% CI)	P Value
Median overall survival, months	14.9	11.3	0.70 (0.58–0.83)	<0.001
Total AP at baseline				
<220 U/L	—	—	0.82 (0.64–1.07)	—
≥220 U/L	—	—	0.62 (0.49–0.79)	—
Current bisphosphonate use				
Yes	—	—	0.70 (0.52–0.93)	—
No	—	—	0.74 (0.59–0.92)	—
Previous docetaxel use				
Yes	—	—	0.71 (0.56–0.89)	—
No	—	—	0.74 (0.56–0.99)	—
ECOG performance-status score				
0 or 1	—	—	0.68 (0.56–0.82)	—
≥2	—	—	0.82 (0.50–1.35)	—
Extent of disease				
<6 metastases	—	—	0.95 (0.46–1.95)	—
6–20 metastases	—	—	0.71 (0.54–0.92)	—
>20 metastases	—	—	0.64 (0.47–0.88)	—
Superscan*	—	—	0.71 (0.40–1.27)	—
Opioid use				
Yes	—	—	0.68 (0.54–0.86)	—
No	—	—	0.70 (0.52–0.93)	—

Main Secondary Efficacy End Points in the Intention-to-Treat Population

End Point	Radium-223 (N = 614)	Placebo (N = 307)	Hazard Ratio (95% CI)	P Value
Median time to first symptomatic skeletal event	15.6 months	9.8 months	0.66 (0.52–0.83)	<0.001
Median time to increase in total alkaline phosphatase	7.4 months	3.8 months	0.17 (0.13–0.22)	<0.001
Median time to increase in PSA level	3.6 months	3.4 months	0.64 (0.54–0.77)	<0.001
≥30% reduction in total alkaline phosphatase	233/497 (47)	7/211 (3)	—	<0.001
Normalization of total alkaline phosphatase	109/321 (34)	2/140 (1)	—	<0.001

*Superscan refers to a bone scan showing diffuse, intense skeletal uptake of the tracer without renal and background activity

35. Renal Cell Cancer

David H. Aggen, MD, PhD, and Martin H. Voss, MD

Epidemiology

Incidence: Estimated new cases for 2020 in the United States: 73,750 (male: 45,520; female: 28,230) Men: 22.1/100,000 Women: 10.9/100,000

Deaths: Estimated deaths in 2020: 14,830 (Men: 9860; Women: 4970)

Median age: 64 years

Male to female ratio: 1.6:1

Stage at Presentation:

Localized	66.2%
Regional	15.8%
Distant	13.9%
Unstaged	4.1%

Siegel R et al. CA Cancer J Clin 2020;70:7–30

Surveillance, Epidemiology and End Results (SEER) Program, available from http://seer.cancer.gov [accessed in 2020]

Pathology

Clear cell	70–80%
Papillary	10–15%
Chromophobe	5%
Collecting duct	0.4–2.6%

Zambrano NR et al. J Urol 1999;162:1246–1258

Work-up (For Suspicious Renal Mass)

1. H&P
2. CBC, chemistry profile, LDH
3. Urinalysis
4. Chest x-ray
5. Abdominal and pelvic CT with contrast
6. Chest CT if abnormal chest x-ray or advanced lesion
7. MRI if CT suggests caval thrombosis or renal insufficiency
8. Bone scan or brain MRI if clinically indicated

Staging

Primary Tumor (T)

TX	Primary tumor cannot be assessed
T0	No evidence of primary tumor
T1	Tumor 7 cm or less in greatest dimension, limited to the kidney
T1a	Tumor 4 cm or less in greatest dimension, limited to the kidney
T1b	Tumor more than 4 cm but not more than 7 cm in greatest dimension, limited to the kidney
T2	Tumor more than 7 cm in greatest dimension, limited to the kidney
T2a	Tumor more than 7 cm but less than or equal to 10 cm in greatest dimension, limited to the kidney
T2b	Tumor more than 10 cm, limited to the kidney
T3	Tumor extends into major veins or perinephric tissues but not into the ipsilateral adrenal gland and not beyond Gerota's fascia
T3a	Tumor extends into the renal vein or its segmental branches, or invades the pelvicalyceal system, or invades perirenal and/or renal sinus fat but not beyond Gerota's fascia
T3b	Tumor grossly extends into the vena cava below the diaphragm
T3c	Tumor extends into the vena cava above the diaphragm or invades the wall of the vena cava
T4	Tumor invades beyond Gerota's fascia (including contiguous extension into the ipsilateral adrenal gland)

Regional Lymph Nodes (N)

NX	Regional lymph nodes cannot be assessed
N0	No regional lymph node metastasis
N1	Regional lymph node metastasis

Distant Metastasis (M)

M0	No distant metastasis
M1	Distant metastasis

Staging Groups

	T	N	M
I	T1	N0	M0
II	T2	N0	M0
III	T1 or T2	N1	M0
	T3	NX, N0, or N1	M0
IV	T4	Any N	M0
	Any T	Any N	M1

Amin MB et al (editors). AJCC Cancer Staging Manual. 8th ed. New York: Springer; 2017

Relative 5-Year Survival

Localized	93%
Regional	70%
Distant	12%

National Cancer Institute, Surveillance, Epidemiology, and End Results (SEER) Program, 2009–2015

Risk Group Criteria

Memorial Sloan-Kettering Cancer Center (MSKCC) Criteria*

(Motzer RJ et al. J Clin Oncol 2002;20:289–296)

1. <12 Months from initial RCC diagnosis to start of therapy
2. Lactate dehydrogenase $>1.5 \times$ ULN
3. Hemoglobin < lower limit of normal range
4. Corrected serum calcium >10 mg/dL (>2.5 mmol/L)
5. Karnofsky performance score <80
6. ≥2 Metastatic sites

Favorable	0 risk factors
Intermediate	1 or 2 risk factors
Poor	≥3 risk factors

*MSKCC criteria are intended for use in stratifying risk in first line only

International Metastatic Renal Cell Carcinoma Database Consortium Criteria* (IMDC)

(Heng DYC et al. Lancet Oncol 2013;14:141–148)

1. Karnofsky performance status score <80%
2. Time from original diagnosis to initiation of targeted therapy <1 year
3. Hemoglobin less than the lower limit of normal
4. Serum calcium greater than the upper limit of normal
5. Neutrophil count greater than the upper limit of normal
6. Platelet count greater than the upper limit of normal

*This model has been validated for first-, second-, and third-line therapy, for combination immunotherapy and TKI, and in non–clear cell RCC

Risk Category	Number of Risk Factors	Median Overall Survival*
Favorable	0 risk factors	43.2 months (95% CI 31.4–50.1)
Intermediate	1 or 2 risk factors	22.5 months (95% CI 18.7–25.1)
Poor	≥3 risk factors	7.8 months (95% CI 6.5–97)

*in patients receiving first line TKI therapy

Expert Opinion

Primary Treatment:

Surgical candidates: treatment-naïve patients. Important factors include:

1. Histologic subtype
2. Patient-specific factors

Stage 1A:

1. Partial nephrectomy (preferred)
2. Radical nephrectomy (in patients with centrally located tumors, or when other reasons make partial nephrectomy impossible)
3. Thermal ablation or cryoablation (in nonsurgical candidates), although must be prepared to proceed to open resection if needed
4. Active surveillance (AS) in selected patients: although the standard of care for treatment of renal masses has been surgical removal, many elderly patients are at high risk for perioperative morbidity and mortality. AS has emerged as a management option for these patients and for those who choose not to have surgery. Many studies show that most renal masses grow slowly and do not display aggressive behavior. The risk of AS is progression to metastatic disease, but, fortunately, the rate of metastases for renal masses during AS appears to be low

Stage 1B/II:

1. Partial nephrectomy (preferred)
2. Radical nephrectomy (in patients with centrally located tumors, or when other reasons make partial nephrectomy impossible)

Stages III:

1. Radical nephrectomy

Stage IV:

1. Systemic therapy
2. Partial or radical nephrectomy for cytoreduction prior to or after upfront systemic therapy in select cases
3. Partial or radical nephrectomy plus metastasectomy if oligometastases are surgically resectable

Primary Treatment References:
Flanigan RC et al. J Urol 2004;171:1071–1076
Mason RJ et al. Eur Urol 2011;59:863–867
Mejean A et al. N Engl J Med 2018;379:417–427

Systemic Therapy:

High-risk localized disease, adjuvant therapy:

- Sunitinib 50 mg PO daily 4 weeks on 2 weeks off for 1 year*[1]

Metastatic clear cell renal cell carcinoma, first-line therapy:

- Pembrolizumab 200 mg Q3 weeks IV + axitinib 5 mg PO BID‡ [2]

- Nivolumab 3 mg/kg Q3weeks IV + ipilimumab 1 mg/kg Q3 weeks IV§ [3] x 4 cycles, followed by maintenance Nivolumab IV Q2wks at 240mg or Q4 weeks at 480mg

- Avelumab 800mg Q2 weeks IV + axitinib 5 mg PO BID‡ [4]

- Pazopanib 800 mg PO daily [5]

- Sunitinib 50 mg PO daily, 4 weeks on 2 weeks off* [6]

- Cabozantinib 60 mg PO daily [7]

- Temsirolimus 25 mg IV weekly [8]

Metastatic clear cell renal cell carcinoma, subsequent therapy:

- Lenvatinib 18 mg PO daily + everolimus 5 mg PO daily [9]

- Nivolumab IV Q2weeks at 240 mg or Q4 weeks at 480 mg [10]

- Everolimus 10 mg PO daily [11]

- Bevacizumab 10 mg/kg IV Q2weeks [12]

- Axitinib 5 mg PO BID‡ [13]

- Bevacizumab 10 mg/kg IV Q2weeks + interferon 9 million IU subq 3×/week [14]

- Consider any first line regimen which has not yet been utilized

(continued)

Expert Opinion (*continued*)

Systemic Therapy:

Metastatic non–clear cell renal cell carcinoma, first-line therapy:

• Sunitinib 50 mg PO daily, 4 weeks on 2 weeks off* [15]

• Cabozantinib 60 mg PO daily [16]

• Everolimus 10 mg PO daily [17]

• Bevacizumab 10 mg/kg IV Q2 weeks + everolimus 10 mg PO daily [18]

Metastatic non–clear cell renal cell carcinoma, subsequent therapy:

• Lenvatinib 18 mg PO daily + everolimus 5 mg PO daily [19]

• Nivolumab IV Q2weeks at 240 mg or Q4 weeks at 480 mg [20]

• Bevacizumab 10 mg/kg IV Q2weeks [21]

• Pazopanib 800 mg PO daily[22]

• Axitinib 5 mg PO BID‡ [23]

• Temsirolimus 25 mg IV weekly [24]

• Consider any first line regimen which has not yet been utilized

*Alternative dosing strategies for sunitinib, including 50 mg daily PO, 2 weeks on 1 week off, have shown safety and activity in phase 2 trials in the metastatic setting. This dosing has not shown benefit in the adjuvant setting in randomized phase 3 trials[23]
†For IMDC favorable-, intermediate-, or poor-risk patients. Pembrolizumab 400 mg Q6 weeks is a suitable alternative to pembrolizumab Q3 weeks if patients demonstrate tolerability on Q3 week dosing. Pembrolizumab and axitinib is given for a maximum of 2 years
‡Axitinib dosing can be titrated based on side effects. If axitinib is well tolerated without any Grade 2 adverse event, can increase the dose from 5 mg BID to 7 mg BID and then 10 mg BID in combination with pembrolizumab. If any adverse events on axitinib, can also dose decrease to 3 mg or 2 mg BID
§For intermediate- or poor-risk patients. Nivolumab and ipilimumab are given Q3weeks × 4 doses. If continued clinical benefit, nivolumab is continued either at 240 mg Q2weeks or 480 mg Q4weeks. A maximum of 4 doses of ipilimumab should be given

1. Ravaud A et al. N Engl J Med 2016;375:2246–2254
2. Rini BI et al. N Engl J Med 2019;380:1116–1127
3. Motzer RJ et al. N Engl J Med 2018;378:1277–1290
4. Motzer RJ et al. N Engl J Med 2019;380:1103–1115
5. Sternberg CN et al. J Clin Oncol 2010;28:1061–1068
6. Motzer RJ et al. N Engl J Med 2013;369:722–731
7. Choueiri TK et al. J Clin Oncol 2017;35:591–597
8. Hudes G et al. N Engl J Med, 2007;356:2271–2281
9. Motzer RJ et al. Lancet Oncol 2015;16:1473–1482
10. Motzer RJ et al. N Engl J Med 2015;373:1803–1813
11. Motzer RJ et al. Ann Oncol 2016;27:441–448
12. Lee CH et al. Clin Genitourin Cancer 2016;14:56–62
13. Rini BI et al. Clin Genitourin Cancer 2015;13:540–547 e1–7
14. Rini B et al. J Clin Oncol 2008;26:5422–5428
15. Tannir NM et al. Eur Urol 2012;62:1013–1019
16. Martínez Chanzá N et al. Lancet Oncol 2019;20:581–590
17. Escudier B et al. Eur J Cancer 2016;69:226–235
18. Voss M. J Clin Oncol 2016;34:3846–3853
19. Schwartz C et al. Clin Genitourin Cancer 2017;15:e903–e906
20. Koshkin VS et al. J Immunother Cancer 2018;6:9
21. Irshad T et al. J Clin Oncol 2011;29(15_suppl): e15158–e15158
22. Buti S et al. Clin Genitourin Cancer 2017;15:e609–e614
23. Park I et al. Clin Genitourin Cancer 2018;16:e997–e1002
24. Venugopal B et al. BMC Urol 2013;13:26
25. Jonasch E et al. J Clin Oncol 2018;36:1588–1593

US FDA-Approved Indications:
• **Axitinib (Inlyta):** advanced renal cell carcinoma after failure of one prior systemic therapy, or as first line treatment for advanced clear cell RCC in combination with avelumab or pembrolizumab

• **Bevacizumab (Avastin):** metastatic renal cell carcinoma in combination with interferon alfa

• **Everolimus (Afinitor):** advanced renal cell carcinoma after failure of treatment with sunitinib or sorafenib

• **Pazopanib (Votrient):** advanced renal cell carcinoma

• **Sunitinib (Sutent):** (1) advanced renal cell carcinoma and (2) adjuvant treatment of adult patients at high risk of recurrent renal cell carcinoma following nephrectomy

(*continued*)

Expert Opinion (*continued*)

- **Temsirolimus (Torisel):** advanced renal cell carcinoma
- **Avelumab (Bavencio):** advanced renal cell carcinoma as first-line treatment in combination with axitinib
- **Pembrolizumab (Keytruda):** advanced renal cell carcinoma as first-line treatment in combination with axitinib
- **Nivolumab (Opdivo):** (1) intermediate or poor risk, previously untreated advanced renal cell carcinoma, in combination with ipilimumab and (2) advanced renal cell carcinoma who have received prior anti-angiogenic therapy
- **Ipilimumab (Yervoy):** intermediate- or poor-risk, previously untreated advanced renal cell carcinoma, in combination with nivolumab
- **Cabozantinib (Cabometyx):** advanced renal cell carcinoma
- **Lenvatinib (Lenvima):** advanced renal cell carcinoma following one prior antiangiogenic therapy, in combination with everolimus

Considerations in Selecting First- and Second-Line Therapies for Clear Cell and Non–Clear Cell Histologies

1. Co-morbidities that could be exacerbated by agent-specific toxicities such as hypertension with VEGF-targeting agents (sunitinib, sorafenib, pazopanib, axitinib, bevacizumab)
2. Convenience of oral agents
3. Tolerance to prior lines of therapy (which may motivate a change in mechanism of action)
4. Pre-existing autoimmune disease may prohibit use of an immune checkpoint inhibitor. Do not routinely offer immune checkpoint therapy with anti-PD-1 as monotherapy or in combination therapy for patients who are on chronic doses of steroids >10 mg/day or the equivalent in other immunosuppressive therapy
5. In considering immunotherapy-based regimen, particularly combinations, consider the likelihood of requiring high-dose systemic corticosteroids for possible immune-mediated adverse events and how well the patient would tolerate such intervention
6. Do not offer immune checkpoint inhibitor therapy to patients with solid organ transplants

Managing Hypertension Associated with Inhibitors of the VEGF Signaling Pathway Inhibitors (VEGFi)[1,2]

Graded Severity	Antihypertensive Therapy	Blood Pressure Monitoring	VEGFi Dose Modification
CTCAE G1 *Prehypertension* (SBP 120–139 mm Hg or DBP 80–89 mm Hg)	None	At least weekly initially and after changes in dose and administration schedule of the VEGFi. Ideally check blood pressure daily initially. After stable BP is achieved, increase monitoring intervals to weekly, then every 2–3 wks or schedule to coincide with clinical evaluations	No change
CTCAE G2 *Stage 1 HTN* (SBP 140–159 mm Hg or DBP 90–99 mm Hg); recurrent or persistent (≥24 h) HTN; medical intervention indicated; symptomatic increase by >20 mm Hg (diastolic) or to >140/90 mm Hg if previously WNL; monotherapy indicated	*Step 1*: initiate DHP-CCB treatment, and, if needed, after 24–48 h, increase the dose in incremental steps every 24–48 h until BP is controlled or a maximum antihypertensive dose is reached. In diabetic patients, may use an ACE/ARB as first anti-hypertensive *Step 2*: if BP still is not controlled, add another antihypertensive, a BB, ACEI, ARB, or ABB. Increase dose of second drug as described in step 1 (above) *Step 3*: if BP still is not controlled, add third drug from categories listed in step 2; increase dose of third drug as described in step 1 (above) *Step 4*: if BP is still not controlled, consider either decreasing VEGFi dose one dose level or discontinuing VEGFi *Note*: if the dose of the VEGFi is reduced or the VEGFi is stopped, BP is expected to decrease. Monitor patient for hypotension and adjust number and doses of antihypertensive medications accordingly	Monitor BP as recommended by treating clinician	No changes except as described for step 4 (if BP is still not controlled, consider either decreasing VEGFi dose one dose level or discontinuing VEGFi)

(continued)

Managing Hypertension Associated with Inhibitors of the VEGF Signaling Pathway Inhibitors (VEGFi)[1,2] (continued)

Graded Severity	Antihypertensive Therapy	Blood Pressure Monitoring	VEGFi Dose Modification
CTCAE G3 *Stage 2 HTN* (SBP ≥160 mm Hg or DBP ≥100 mm Hg); medical intervention indicated; more than one drug or more intensive therapy than previously used indicated	Withhold VEGFi until systolic BP <159 mm Hg and diastolic BP <99 mm Hg. BP management identical to that for G2 *(stage 1) HTN (see steps 1–4 above)* with two exceptions: 1. If SBP >180 mm Hg or DBP >110 mm Hg *and patient is symptomatic*, optimal management should include management in a monitored setting. Discontinue VEGFi and notify other medically responsible health care providers that stopping VEGFi may result in a decrease in BP 2. If SBP >180 mm Hg or DBP >110 mm Hg *and the patient is asymptomatic*, two new antihypertensives must be given together in step 1, and dose escalated as in step 1 *Note:* if the dose of the VEGFi is reduced or the VEGFi is stopped, BP is expected to decrease. Monitor patient for hypotension and adjust number and doses of antihypertensive medications accordingly	BP should be monitored as recommended by the treating clinician unless the patient is symptomatic with SBP >180 mm Hg or DBP >110 mm Hg, in which case monitoring should be intensive	1. Withhold the VEGFi until SBP <159 mm Hg and DBP <99 mm Hg 2. If BP cannot be controlled after an optimal trial of antihypertensive medications, consider either reducing the dose of the VEGFi or discontinuing its use 3. If a patient requires hospitalization for symptomatic SBP >180 mm Hg or DBP >110 mm Hg, permanently discontinue the VEGFi, or if BP is controlled, resume the VEGFi at a reduced dose
CTCAE G4 Life-threatening consequences (eg, malignant hypertension, transient or permanent neurologic deficit, hypertensive crisis)	1. Optimal management with intensive parenteral support in an ICU setting 2. Discontinue the VEGFi and notify other medically responsible health care providers that stopping a VEGFi may result in a decrease in BP	Intensive	Permanently discontinue the VEGFi, or if BP is controlled, resume the VEGFi at a reduced dose

ABB, α/β-adrenergic blockers; ACEI, angiotensin converting enzyme inhibitors; ARB, angiotensin II receptor blockers; BB, selective β-adrenergic blockers; CTCAE, National Cancer Institute (USA), Common Terminology Criteria for Adverse Events; DBP, diastolic blood pressure; DHP-CCB, dihydropyridine calcium-channel blockers; HTN, hypertension; ICU, intensive (or critical) care unit; SBP, systolic blood pressure; VEGF, vascular endothelial growth factor; VEGFi, VEGF signaling pathway inhibitor

Note:
• Hypertension grading is based on CTCAE, version 4.0 criteria
• When SBP and DBP fall into different categories, the higher category should be selected in classifying blood pressure status
• Discontinue the VEGFi if patients require delaying treatment ≤2 weeks for management of hypertension
• Discontinue the VEGFi if patients require ≤2 VEGFi dose reductions
• Patients may receive up to two drugs for managing hypertension prior to decreasing VEGFi doses
• Allow an interval of at least 24 hours between modifications of antihypertensive therapy
• Treatment with a VEGFi, including aflibercept, axitinib, bevacizumab, cediranib, pazopanib, sunitinib, sorafenib, and vandetanib, has rarely been associated with developing reversible posterior leukoencephalopathy syndrome (RPLS). Presenting symptoms associated with RPLS have included mild to severe hypertension, headache, lethargy, decreased alertness, confusion, altered mental functioning, and visual loss, seizure, and other neurologic disturbances
• Discontinue the VEGFi in patients experiencing signs and symptoms referable to RPLS
• MRI is the most sensitive imaging modality for detecting RPLS, and is recommended in suspected cases to confirm the diagnosis
• RPLS usually is reversible upon removal of precipitating factors and application of measures to alleviate symptoms and control blood pressure; however, some patients have experienced ongoing neurologic effects and death

Commercially Available Orally Administered Antihypertensives

Pharmacologic Categories	Drug Name[†] (Formulation)	Doses and Administration Schedules*			Metabolism
		Initial	Intermediate	Maximum Recommended	
Dihydropyridine calcium-channel blockers (DHP-CCB)	Nifedipine (extended release)	30 mg daily	60 mg daily	90 mg daily	CYP3A4 substrate
	Amlodipine besylate[3]	2.5 mg daily	5 mg daily	10 mg daily	CYP3A4 substrate
	Felodipine (extended release)	2.5 mg daily	5 mg daily	10 mg daily	CYP3A4 substrate and inhibitor[4]
Selective β-adrenergic blockers (BB)	Metoprolol tartrate[3]	25 mg twice daily	50 mg twice daily	100 mg twice daily	CYP2D6 substrate
	Atenolol	25 mg daily	50 mg daily	100 mg daily	Eliminated unchanged in urine and feces
	Acebutolol HCl	100 mg twice daily	200–300 mg twice daily	400 mg twice daily	Yes (CYP450 unknown)
	Bisoprolol fumarate	2.5 mg daily	5–10 mg daily	20 mg daily	Substrate for CYP2D6 and CYP3A4; ~50% renally eliminated as intact bisoprolol
	Nebivolol HCl[5,6]	5 mg daily	—	40 mg daily	Substrate for CYP2D6 and UGT enzymes
		Caution: consider use for BP maintenance rather than titration. Product labeling recommends dose adjustments not more frequently than every 2 weeks			
Angiotensin-converting enzyme inhibitors (ACEIs)	Captopril	12.5 mg three times daily	25 mg three times daily	50 mg three times daily	CYP2D6 substrate
	Enalapril maleate[7]	5 mg daily	10–20 mg daily	40 mg daily	CYP3A4 substrate
	Ramipril	2.5 mg daily	5 mg daily	10 mg daily	Metabolism by liver esterases and phase 2 metabolism; ie, not CYP450
	Lisinopril	5 mg daily	10–20 mg daily	40 mg daily	Minimally, not CYP450
	Fosinopril sodium	10 mg daily	20 mg daily	40 mg daily	Hydrolyzed by intestinal and hepatic esterases; ie, not CYP450
	Perindopril erbumine	4 mg daily	none	8 mg daily	Hydrolysis and phase 2 metabolism; ie, not CYP450
	Quinapril	10 mg daily	20 mg daily	40 mg daily	Hydrolysis to quinaprilat, which is renally eliminated
Angiotensin II receptor blockers (ARBs)	Losartan	25 mg daily	50 mg daily	100 mg daily	CYP3A4 substrate
	Candesartan	4 mg daily	8–16 mg daily	32 mg daily	CYP2C9 substrate
	Irbesartan[7]	75 mg daily	150 mg daily	300 mg daily	CYP2C9 substrate
	Telmisartan	40 mg daily	none	80 mg daily	Phase 2 metabolism; ie, not CYP450
α−/β-Adrenergic blocker	Labetolol HCl	100 mg twice daily	200 mg twice daily	400 mg twice daily	CYP2D6 substrate and inhibitor

ABC, ATP binding cassette proteins; CYP450, cytochrome P450 superfamily microsomal enzymes; FMO, flavin-containing monooxygenase family microsomal enzymes; UGT, uridine diphosphate-glucuronosyltransferase

*Recommendations for use are for adult patients without renal or hepatic impairment. Consult complete prescribing information for use in persons with impaired renal and/or hepatic function and other special populations

[†]Drugs in emboldened characters are suggested as optimal choices to avoid or minimize potential drug interactions with VEGFi through unilateral or mutual effects on CYP3A4

Commercially Available Orally Administered Antihypertensives

Note:

Axitinib
- A substrate for metabolism by CYP3A4/5 (primary catalyst) and, to a lesser extent, CYP1A2, CYP2C19, and UGT1A1 in an in vitro system
- In an in vitro system is an inhibitor of ABCB1 (P-glycoprotein, MDR1); however, it is not expected to inhibit ABCB1-mediated transport at therapeutic plasma concentrations

Pazopanib
- A substrate for metabolism by CYP3A4 (primary catalyst) with minor contributions from CYP1A2 and CYP2C8
- Drug interaction trials conducted in patients with cancer suggest that pazopanib is a weak inhibitor of CYP3A4, CYP2C8, and CYP2D6 in vivo, but had no effect on CYP1A2, CYP2C9, or CYP2C19. Consequently, concomitant use of pazopanib with CYP3A4, CYP2D6, or CYP2C8 substrates that have low therapeutic indices or narrow ranges of therapeutic concentrations is not recommended
- Pazopanib has been shown to inhibit UGT1A1 and OATP1B1 in an in vitro system with IC_{50} of 1.2 μmol/L and 0.79 μmol/L, respectively, ie, systemically achievable concentrations. Thus, drugs eliminated by UGT1A1 and OATP1B1 may be increased during concomitant use with pazopanib

Sorafenib
- A substrate for phase I and II metabolism by CYP3A4 and UGT1A9, respectively
- Sorafenib inhibits UGT1A1[8] and UGT1A9, and ABCB1 (P-glycoprotein, MDR1) in vitro, and may increase the systemic exposure of concomitantly administered drug substrates for metabolism and/or transport by these proteins

Sunitinib and its primary active (N-deethylated) metabolite, SU12662
- Substrates for metabolism by CYP3A4. Consequently, concomitant administration of sunitinib with strong CYP3A4 inhibitors or inducers should be avoided

1. Maitland ML et al. J Natl Cancer Inst 2010;102:596–604
2. de Jesus-Gonzalez N et al. Hypertension 2012;60:607–615
3. Szmit S et al. Acta Oncol 2009;48:921–925
4. Gomo C et al. Invest New Drugs 2011;29:1511–1514
5. Bamias A et al. Eur J Cancer 2011;47:1660–1668
6. Bamias A et al. J Chemother 2009;21:347–350
7. Costero O et al. Nephrol Dial Transplant 2010;25:1001–1003
8. Liu Y et al. Br J Clin Pharmacol 2011;71:917–920

HIGH-RISK • LOCALIZED CLEAR-CELL • ADJUVANT THERAPY
RENAL CELL CARCINOMA REGIMEN: SUNITINIB

Ravaud A et al. N Engl J Med 2016;375:2246–2254
Motzer RJ et al. Eur Urol 2018;73:62–68

Initiate adjuvant sunitinib within 3–12 weeks following nephrectomy:
Sunitinib malate 50 mg; administer orally once daily, continually, without regard for meals, in 6-week cycles consisting of 4 consecutive weeks of daily treatment followed by 2 weeks without treatment, for 1 year (total dose/6-week cycle = 1400 mg)
Notes:
• Patients who delay taking sunitinib malate at a regularly scheduled time may take a missed dose if the interval remaining before the next regularly scheduled dose is ≥12 hours
• If possible, avoid concomitant use of strong CYP3A4 inhibitors and inducers. If a concomitant strong CYP3A4 inhibitor must be used, decrease sunitinib malate to 37.5 mg/dose. If a concomitant strong CYP3A4 inducer must be used, consider increasing sunitinib malate to 87.5 mg/dose while monitoring closely for side effects
• Advise patients to avoid consuming grapefruit juice for as long as they continue to use sunitinib malate

Supportive Care: Hand-Foot Reaction
For patients who develop a hand-foot reaction, use topical emollients (eg, Aquaphor), topical and/or oral steroids, antihistamine agents (H$_1$-receptor antagonists), or pyridoxine 50–150 mg/day orally

Antiemetic prophylaxis
Emetogenic potential is **LOW**
See Chapter 42 for antiemetic recommendations

Hematopoietic growth factor (CSF) prophylaxis
Primary prophylaxis is **NOT** indicated
See Chapter 43 for more information

Antimicrobial prophylaxis
Risk of fever and neutropenia is **LOW**
    Antimicrobial primary prophylaxis to be considered:
    • Antibacterial—not indicated
    • Antifungal—not indicated
    • Antiviral—not indicated unless patient previously had an episode of HSV

Diarrhea management
Latent or delayed-onset diarrhea*:
    Loperamide 4 mg orally initially after the first loose or liquid stool, *then* 2–4 mg orally every 2–4 hours or **diphenoxylate hydrochloride**
    2.5 mg **with atropine sulfate** 0.025 mg (eg, Lomotil)

*Abigerges D et al. J Natl Cancer Inst 1994;86:446–449
Rothenberg ML et al. J Clin Oncol 2001;19:3801–3807
Wadler S et al. J Clin Oncol 1998;16:3169–3178

Treatment Modification

SUNITINIB	
Sunitinib Dose Levels	
Starting dose (Level 1)	50 mg once daily, 4 weeks on/2 weeks off
Dose Level −1	37.5 mg once daily, 4 weeks on/2 weeks off
Dose Level −2	Discontinue sunitinib

Treatment Modification (*continued*)

Adverse Event	Treatment Modification
Cutaneous Toxicities	
Rash G ≥2	Withhold sunitinib and provide immediate symptomatic treatment. When toxicity resolves to G ≤1, restart sunitinib at 1 dose level lower than the dose level administered at the time toxicity developed. Treatment for symptoms may continue indefinitely as a preventive measure *Note: discontinue therapy if sunitinib is withheld >3 weeks*
Recurrence of G3/4 cutaneous toxicity at dose level −1 of sunitinib	Discontinue therapy
Cutaneous toxicity does not recur at reduced sunitinib doses with or without continued treatment for symptoms	Sunitinib dose may be increased 1 dose level to that administered at the time cutaneous toxicity developed. If toxicity recurs following the increase, then again withhold sunitinib and provide immediate symptomatic treatment. When toxicity resolves to G ≤1. restart sunitinib at 1 dose level lower than the dose level administered at the time toxicity developed. Treatment for symptoms may continue indefinitely as a preventive measure
Diarrhea	
G1/2 diarrhea (increase of 4–6 stools/day over baseline; limiting instrumental ADLs)	Focus on treatment for symptoms designed to resolve the diarrhea. No dose modifications are made for G1/2 diarrhea unless G2 diarrhea persists >2 weeks
G2 diarrhea persisting >2 weeks	Follow the guidelines below for G3/4 diarrhea
G2 diarrhea lasting >2 weeks *or* G3/4 diarrhea *or* diarrhea that worsens by 1 grade while on sunitinib	Withhold sunitinib until diarrhea resolves to G ≤1. If resolution occurs within 3 weeks of holding treatment, restart sunitinib at 1 dose level lower than the dose level administered at the time diarrhea developed *Note: discontinue therapy if sunitinib is withheld >3 weeks*
Recurrence of G2 diarrhea lasting >2 weeks or G3/4 diarrhea at dose level −1	Discontinue therapy
Diarrhea does not recur at reduced sunitinib doses with or without continued treatment for symptoms	Sunitinib dose may be increased 1 dose level to the dose level administered at the time the diarrhea developed. If toxicity recurs following the increase, then again withhold sunitinib and provide immediate symptomatic treatment. When toxicity resolves to G ≤1, restart sunitinib at 1 dose level lower than the dose level administered at the time toxicity developed. Treatment for symptoms may continue indefinitely as a preventive measure
Hypertension	
Note: patients should have their blood pressure checked once weekly during their first 24 weeks of therapy and for an 8-week period after an adjustment in their sunitinib dose	
G1 hypertension (SBP 120–139 or DBP 80–89 mm Hg)	Continue sunitinib at same dose and schedule
G2 asymptomatic hypertension (SBP140–159 or DBP 90–99 mm Hg if previously WNL; change in baseline medical intervention indicated; recurrent or persistent [≥24 hours]; symptomatic increase DBP >20 mm Hg or to >140/90 mm Hg; monotherapy indicated initiated)	Treat with antihypertensive medications and continue sunitinib at same dose and schedule
G2 symptomatic, or persistent G2 despite antihypertensive medications, or DBP ≥110 mm Hg, or G3 hypertension (SBP ≥160 or DBP ≥100 mm Hg; medical intervention indicated; >1 drug or more intensive therapy than previously used indicated)	Withhold sunitinib and treat with antihypertensive medications until symptoms resolve and diastolic BP <100 mm Hg. Then continue sunitinib at 1 dose level lower *Note: discontinue therapy if sunitinib is withheld >3 weeks*
G4 hypertension (life-threatening consequences; urgent intervention indicated)	Discontinue therapy

Treatment Modification (continued)

Miscellaneous

G3/4 hepatotoxicity (ALT/AST >5× ULN if baseline was normal; >5× baseline if baseline was abnormal; bilirubin >3× ULN if baseline was normal; >3× baseline if baseline was abnormal)	Withhold sunitinib until LFTs resolve to baseline or G ≤1. If resolution occurs within 3 weeks of holding treatment, restart sunitinib at 1 dose level lower than the dose level administered at the time hepatotoxicity was noted *Note: discontinue therapy if sunitinib is withheld >3 weeks or if worsening occurs during the period of observation off therapy*
Any other G3/4 nonhematologic toxicity (eg, persistent nausea, vomiting, despite maximum supportive treatment)	Withhold treatment until toxicity improves to G ≤1, then resume with dose reduced by 1 level
Wound dehiscence or poor wound healing	Interrupt sunitinib until wound has adequately healed
LVEF decrease by ≥10% to <LLN, clinical heart failure syndrome, necrotizing fasciitis, EM, SJS, TEN, or TMA	Permanently discontinue sunitinib
Proteinuria	If urine dipstick ≥2+, obtain 24-hour urine protein. If 24-hour urine protein ≥3 g, interrupt treatment. Resume treatment when 24-hour urine protein ≤1 g. Resume sunitinib at 1 dose level lower
Repeat episodes of 24-hour urine protein ≥3 g despite dose reductions or nephrotic syndrome	Discontinue sunitinib
Coadministration of potent CYP3A4 inhibitors (eg, ketoconazole, itraconazole, voriconazole, clarithromycin, atazanavir, ritonavir, telithromycin)	Reduce sunitinib dose
Coadministration of potent CYP3A inducers (eg, rifampin, phenytoin, phenobarbital, carbamazepine)	Increase sunitinib dose (to a maximum of 87.5 mg daily)

EM, erythema multiforme; LLN, lower limit of normal; LVEF, left ventricular ejection fraction; SJS, Stevens-Johnson syndrome; TEN, toxic epidermal necrolysis; TMA, thrombotic microangiopathy

Dose adjustment for renal impairment:
- Creatinine clearance ≥30 mL/min: no initial adjustment necessary
- End-stage renal disease (ESRD) on hemodialysis: no initial adjustment necessary. Sunitinib exposure is 47% lower in patients with ESRD on hemodialysis, and doses may need to be increased gradually up to 2-fold based on tolerability

Patient Population Studied

This randomized, double-blind, international, placebo-controlled phase 3 trial included 615 adult patients with locoregional high-risk clear cell RCC and compared 1 year of adjuvant treatment with sunitinib or placebo. Patients with histologically confirmed clear cell RCC were eligible if they had locoregional disease with a tumor stage ≥3 (per modified University of California Los Angeles Integrated Staging System [UISS] criteria), regional lymph node metastasis, or both. Additionally, patients must have had no previous systemic treatment, an Eastern Cooperative Oncology Group (ECOG) score of ≤2 before nephrectomy, and treatment initiation within 3–12 weeks after nephrectomy. Patients were excluded if they had confirmed macroscopic residual or metastatic disease after nephrectomy, renal metastasis or histologically undifferentiated tumors, a diagnosis of a second cancer within 5 years before randomization, a major cardiovascular event or disease within 6 months of enrollment, or uncontrolled hypertension

Efficacy (N = 615)

	Sunitinib (N = 309)	Placebo (N = 306)	—
Median disease-free survival (ICR assessed)	6.8 years (95% CI 5.8–NR)	5.6 years (95% CI 3.8–6.6)	HR 0.76 (95% CI 0.59–0.98); P = 0.03
Disease-free survival at 3 years (ICR assessed)	64.9%	59.5%	—
Disease-free survival at 5 years (ICR assessed)	59.3%	51.3%	—
Median disease-free survival in higher-risk patients (ICR assessed)*	6.2 years (95% CI 4.9–NR)	4.0 years (95% CI 2.6–6.0)	HR 0.74 (95% CI 0.55–0.99); P = 0.04

(continued)

Efficacy (N = 615) *(continued)*

	Sunitinib (N = 309)	Placebo (N = 306)	—
Median disease-free survival (investigator assessed)	6.5 years (95% CI 4.7–7.0)	4.5 years (95% CI 3.8–5.9)	HR 0.81 (95% CI 0.64–1.02); P = 0.08
Median disease-free survival in higher-risk patients (investigator assessed)*	5.9 years (95% CI 4.4–7.0)	3.9 years (95% CI 2.8–5.6)	HR 0.76 (95% CI 0.58–1.01); P = 0.06
Median overall survival†	NR (95% CI NR–NR)	NR (95% CI NR–NR)	HR 0.92 (95% CI 0.66–1.28); P = 0.61

HR, hazard ratio; CI, confidence interval; NR, not reached; ICR, independent central review
*Higher risk defined as patients with a stage 3 tumor, no or undetermined nodal involvement, no metastasis, Fuhrman Grade 2 or higher, and an ECOG score of 1 or higher or a stage 4 tumor, local nodal involvement, or both
†Data are updated results published in Motzer RJ et al. Eur Urol 2018;73:62–68
Note: all efficacy analyses were performed in the intention-to-treat population. All estimates of disease-free survival and overall survival were generated using the Kaplan-Meier method and between-group differences were compared using a two-sided log-rank test. All data included in this table were reported in the paper titled "Adjuvant Sunitinib in High-Risk Renal-Cell Carcinoma after Nephrectomy" except where noted. Data in this paper were generated with a median duration of follow-up of 5.4 years (95% CI 5.2–5.6) in the sunitinib group and 5.4 years (95% CI 5.3–5.6) in the placebo group. In the update paper, median follow-up was 6.6 years for the sunitinib group and 6.7 years for the placebo group (no range or CI reported)

Adverse Events (N = 610)

Event	Sunitinib (N = 306) Grade 1/2 (%)	Grade 3/4 (%)	Placebo (N = 304) Grade 1/2 (%)	Grade 3/4 (%)
Any adverse event	39	60	69	19
Diarrhea	53	4	21	<1
Palmar-plantar erythrodysesthesia	34	16	10	<1
Hypertension	29	8	11	1
Fatigue	32	5	23	1
Nausea	32	2	14	0
Dysgeusia	34	0	6	0
Mucosal inflammation	29	5	8	0
Dyspepsia	25	1	6	0
Stomatitis	24	2	4	0
Neutropenia	15	8	<1	0
Asthenia	19	4	11	<1

Event	Sunitinib (N = 306) Grade 1/2 (%)	Grade 3/4 (%)	Placebo (N = 304) Grade 1/2 (%)	Grade 3/4 (%)
Hair-color change	22	0	2	0
Thrombocytopenia	15	6	1	<1
Decreased appetite	19	<1	5	0
Rash	19	<1	10	0
Vomiting	17	2	7	0
Headache	18	<1	12	0
Hypothyroidism	18	0	1	0
Epistaxis	18	0	3	0

Adverse events were included in the table if they were reported in ≥15% of patients in either group. Adverse events included in the table were considered treatment-emergent, but not necessarily attributed to drug treatment. Adverse events attributed by the investigators to drug treatment were reported by 98.4% of patients in the sunitinib group and 75.7% of patients in the placebo group. Rates of serious adverse events were similar between groups: 21.9% of patients in the sunitinib group and 17.1% of patients in the placebo group. Study drug was discontinued due to adverse events in 28.1% of patients in the sunitinib group and 5.6% of patients in the placebo group. Grade 5 treatment-emergent adverse events were reported in 1.6% of patients in each group. No deaths were attributed by the investigators to toxic effects of a study drug treatment

Therapy Monitoring

1. *Prior to the first cycle of sunitinib:* electrocardiogram (for assessment of QTc interval), echocardiogram, CBC with differential, platelet count, LFTs, serum chemistries, blood glucose, blood pressure, thyroid-stimulating hormone, urine dipstick and/or urinary protein–creatinine ratio, physical examination (including dermatologic examination)

2. *Prior to each cycle of sunitinib:* CBC with differential, platelet count, LFTs, serum chemistries, blood glucose, blood pressure, thyroid-stimulating hormone, urine dipstick and/or urinary protein–creatinine ratio, physical examination (including dermatologic examination)

3. Hepatotoxicity, including liver failure, has been observed. Monitor LFTs before initiation of treatment, during each cycle of treatment, and as clinically indicated

4. Cardiac toxicity including declines in LVEF to below LLN and cardiac failure including death have occurred. Monitor patients for signs and symptoms of congestive heart failure

5. Prolonged QT intervals and torsades de pointes have been observed. Use with caution in patients at higher risk for developing QT interval prolongation. When using sunitinib, monitoring with on-treatment electrocardiograms and electrolytes should be considered monthly at first or when the dose is increased and less frequently thereafter

6. Hypertension may occur. Monitor blood pressure and treat as indicated under Treatment Modifications

7. Thyroid dysfunction may occur. Monitor thyroid function tests every 3 months. Treat hypothyroidism accordingly

8. Temporary interruption of therapy with sunitinib is recommended in patients undergoing major surgical procedures. *Note:* there is limited clinical experience regarding the timing of re-initiation of therapy following major surgical intervention. Therefore, the decision to resume sunitinib therapy following a major surgical intervention should be based on clinical judgment of recovery from surgery

9. Monitor adrenal function in case of stress such as surgery, trauma, or severe infection

METASTATIC • CLEAR-CELL • FIRST-LINE
RENAL CELL CARCINOMA REGIMEN: PEMBROLIZUMAB + AXITINIB

Rini BI et al. N Engl J Med 2019;380:1116–1127
Protocol for: Rini BI et al. N Engl J Med 2019;380:1116–1127
Supplementary appendix to: Rini BI et al. N Engl J Med 2019;380:1116–1127
KEYTRUDA (pembrolizumab) prescribing information. Whitehouse Station, NJ: Merck & Co., Inc; revised June 2020
INLYTA (axitinib) prescribing information. New York, NY: Pfizer Labs; revised January 2020

Pembrolizumab 200 mg; administer intravenously over 30 minutes in a volume of 0.9% sodium chloride injection (0.9% NS) or 5% dextrose injection (D5W) sufficient to produce a pembrolizumab concentration within the range 1–10 mg/mL every 3 weeks, until disease progression and for up to a maximum of 24 months (total dose/3-week cycle = 200 mg)

Alternative pembrolizumab dose and schedule per the U.S. FDA regimens approved on April 28, 2020:
Pembrolizumab 400 mg; administer intravenously over 30 minutes in a volume of 0.9% NS or D5W sufficient to produce a pembrolizumab concentration within the range 1–10 mg/mL every 6 weeks until disease progression and for up to a maximum of 24 months (total dose/6-week cycle = 400 mg)

Notes:
- Administer pembrolizumab with an administration set that contains a sterile, non-pyrogenic, low-protein-binding in-line or add-on filter with pore size within the range of 0.2–5 μm
- Pembrolizumab can cause severe or life-threatening infusion-related reactions, including hypersensitivity and anaphylaxis

Axitinib 5 mg; administer orally twice daily (approximately every 12 hours), continually, until disease progression (total dose/week = 70 mg)

Notes:
- Axitinib should be swallowed whole (no breaking, crushing, or chewing) with water
- Axitinib may be administered without respect to food ingestion
- Advise patients to avoid grapefruit products while taking axitinib
- Instruct patients who vomit or miss a dose of axitinib to avoid taking an additional dose. Take the next prescribed dose at the usual time
- Patients who tolerate axitinib for at least 6 consecutive weeks with no adverse reactions G >2, who remain normotensive (blood pressure ≤150/90 mm Hg), and are not receiving anti-hypertension medications may have their dose increased to 7 mg twice daily, and further to 10 mg twice daily using the same criteria
- Avoid use of concomitant strong CYP3A4/5 inhibitors. If a strong CYP3A4/5 inhibitor must be co-administered, a dose decrease of axitinib by approximately half is recommended. Subsequent doses can be increased or decreased based on individual safety and tolerability. If co-administration of a strong inhibitor is discontinued, the axitinib dose should be returned (after 3–5 elimination half-lives of the inhibitor) to that used prior to initiation of the strong CYP3A4/5 inhibitor
- The axitinib starting dose should be reduced by approximately half in patients with baseline moderate hepatic impairment (Child-Pugh class B)
- If axitinib is interrupted, patients receiving antihypertensive medications should be monitored for hypotension. The plasma half-life of axitinib is 2–4 hours and blood pressure usually decreases within 1–2 days following dose interruption

Regimen note: in the clinical trial, patients who achieved a confirmed complete response after a minimum of 24 weeks of treatment could, at the discretion of the investigator, discontinue treatment with axitinib + pembrolizumab

Antiemetic prophylaxis
Emetogenic potential of axitinib is **MINIMAL TO LOW**
Emetogenic potential of pembrolizumab is **MINIMAL**
See Chapter 42 for antiemetic recommendations

Hematopoietic growth factor (CSF) prophylaxis
Primary prophylaxis is NOT indicated
See Chapter 43 for more information

(continued)

Patient Population Studied (N = 861)

This open-label, multinational, phase 3 trial included 861 adult patients with previously untreated advanced clear cell RCC. Eligible patients had newly diagnosed or recurrent stage IV clear cell RCC and had received no previous systemic therapy for advanced disease. Participants had a Karnofsky performance status score of ≥70, ≥1 measurable lesion according to Response Evaluation Criteria in Solid Tumors (RECIST) version 1.1, and had an available tumor sample for biomarker testing. Patients were excluded if they had symptomatic central nervous system metastases, active autoimmune disease, poorly controlled hypertension (defined as systolic blood pressure ≥150 mmHg or diastolic blood pressure ≥90 mmHg), a history of an ischemic cardiovascular event or heart failure (NYHA class III or IV) within 1 year of screening, or if they were receiving systemic immunosuppressive treatment. Patients were randomized in a 1:1 ratio to receive the combination of pembrolizumab + axitinib or single-agent sunitinib. Randomization was stratified based on International Metastatic Renal Cell Carcinoma Database Consortium (IMDC) risk group and geographic region

(continued)

Antimicrobial prophylaxis

Risk of fever and neutropenia is LOW

Antimicrobial primary prophylaxis to be considered:

- Antibacterial—not indicated
- Antifungal—not indicated
- Antiviral—not indicated unless patient previously had an episode of HSV

Diarrhea management

Latent or delayed-onset diarrhea*:

Loperamide 4 mg orally initially after the first loose or liquid stool, *then* 2–4 mg orally every 2–4 hours or **diphenoxylate hydrochloride** 2.5 mg with **atropine sulfate** 0.025 mg (eg, Lomotil)

*Abigerges D et al. J Natl Cancer Inst 1994;86:446–449
Rothenberg ML et al. J Clin Oncol 2001;19:3801–3807
Wadler S et al. J Clin Oncol 1998;16:3169–3178

Treatment Modifications

RECOMMENDED DOSE MODIFICATIONS FOR AXITINIB

Dose level +2	10 mg orally twice per day
Dose level + 1	7 mg orally twice per day
Starting dose (level 1)	5 mg orally twice per day
Dose level −1	3 mg orally twice per day
Dose level −2	2 mg orally twice per day
Dose level −3	Discontinue axitinib*

Grade/Severity	Treatment Modification
The patient has tolerated axitinib at a dose of 5 mg twice per day for ≥6 weeks without G >2 treatment-related adverse reactions, is normotensive (blood pressure ≤150/90 mm Hg), and is not receiving anti-hypertension medication	Increase the dose of axitinib to dose level +1 (7 mg orally twice per day)
The patient has tolerated axitinib at a dose of 7 mg twice per day for ≥6 weeks without G >2 treatment-related adverse reactions, is normotensive (blood pressure ≤150/90 mm Hg), and is not receiving anti-hypertension medication	Increase the dose of axitinib to dose level +2 (10 mg orally twice per day)
Any hypertension	Treat as needed with standard anti-hypertensive therapy
Persistent hypertension despite use of maximal anti-hypertensive medications	Reduce the dosage of axitinib by 1 dosage level
Evidence of hypertensive crisis	Discontinue axitinib*
Urine dipstick >1+ for protein	Continue axitinib at the same dose pending results of a 24-hour urine protein
Urine protein ≥3 g/24 hours	Withhold axitinib until urine protein is <3 g/24 hours, then resume axitinib at 1 lower dose level*
Grade 3 diarrhea (not immune-related[†])	Optimize antidiarrheal regimen and reduce the dose of axitinib by 1 dose level
Grade 4 diarrhea (not immune-related[†])	Withhold axitinib until recovery to G ≤1, then resume axitinib with the dose reduced by 1 dose level and with optimization of the antidiarrheal regimen

(continued)

Treatment Modifications (*continued*)

Grade/Severity	Treatment Modification
Grade 2 AST, ALT, or bilirubin elevation (not immune-related[†])	Increase the frequency of LFT monitoring. Withhold axitinib until improvement to G ≤1 or baseline, then resume axitinib at the same dosage
Grade ≥3 AST, ALT, or bilirubin elevation (not immune-related[†])	Increase the frequency of LFT monitoring. Withhold axitinib until improvement to G ≤1 or baseline, then resume axitinib with the dosage reduced by 1 dose level
Bleeding occurs that requires medical intervention	Withhold axitinib until resolution of bleeding*
Patient requires elective surgery	Withhold axitinib for ≥2 days prior to elective surgery. Do not resume axitinib for at least 2 weeks following major surgery and until adequate wound healing has occurred*
RPLS is suspected (symptoms of headache, seizure, lethargy, confusion, blindness, and/or other visual and neurologic disturbances along with hypertension of any severity)	Withhold axitinib until clarification of the patient's neurologic status (ie, with an emergent brain MRI) has occurred*
RPLS is confirmed	Discontinue axitinib.* The safety of reinitiating axitinib in a patient who has experienced RPLS is unknown
Patient has moderate hepatic impairment (Child-Pugh class B)	Decrease the starting dose of axitinib by approximately 50% and then increase or decrease the dose based on individual safety and tolerability
Patient requires concomitant use of a strong CYP3A4/5 inhibitor (eg, ketoconazole, itraconazole, posaconazole, clarithromycin, atazanavir, indinavir, nefazodone, nelfinavir, ritonavir, saquinavir, telithromycin, and voriconazole)	If concomitant use of the CYP3A4/5 inhibitor is unavoidable, then decrease the dose of axitinib by approximately 50% and then increase or decrease the dose based on individual safety and tolerability. If the strong CYP3A4/5 inhibitor is subsequently discontinued, then resume the axitinib dose that was used prior to initiation of the CYP3A4/5 inhibitor after 3–5 CYP3A4/5 inhibitor half-lives have transpired
Patient requires concomitant use of a moderate or strong CYP3A4/5 inducer (eg, rifampin, dexamethasone, phenytoin, carbamazepine, rifabutin, rifapentine, phenobarbital, St. John's Wort, bosentan, efavirenz, etravirine, modafinil, nafcillin)	Avoid concomitant use of a moderate or strong CYP3A4/5 inducer with axitinib

*If the patient is receiving antihypertensive medications, monitor closely for development of hypotension if axitinib is withheld or discontinued
[†]Distinguishing immune-mediated toxicity vs TKI toxicity: considering the short half-life of axitinib, a practical strategy in patients with new toxicities that may be due to either drug is to consider withholding axitinib without immediate initiation of empiric corticosteroids; the patient is then monitored closely for improvement (eg, repeat laboratory assessment 48 h later), which would make axitinib the more likely cause of the new toxicity; in the setting of rapid clinical deterioration, however, corticosteroids should be initiated promptly
AST, aspartate aminotransferase; ALT, alanine aminotransferase; LFT, liver function test; RPLS, reversible posterior leukoencephalopathy syndrome; MRI, magnetic resonance imaging

RECOMMENDED DOSE MODIFICATIONS FOR PEMBROLIZUMAB

Adverse Event	Grade/Severity	Treatment Modification
Infusion reaction	Clinically significant but not severe infusion reaction	Interrupt the infusion in patients with clinically significant infusion reactions and consider resuming at a slower rate following resolution. If decision is made to restart, begin at ≤50% of the rate prior to the reaction and increase in 50% increments every 30 minutes if well tolerated. Infusions may be restarted at the full rate during the next cycle
	G3/4 (severe infusion reaction—pyrexia, chills, flushing, hypotension, dyspnea, wheezing, back pain, abdominal pain, and urticaria). Not rapidly responsive to brief interruption of infusion	Stop infusion and administer appropriate medical therapy (eg, epinephrine, corticosteroids, intravenous antihistamines, bronchodilators, and/or oxygen). Discontinue pembrolizumab

(*continued*)

Treatment Modifications (*continued*)

Adverse Event	Grade/Severity	Treatment Modification
Colitis	G1	Loperamide 4 mg as starting dose then 2 mg before each meal and after each loose stool until without diarrhea for 12 hours, with maximum of 16 mg loperamide per day. If G1 diarrhea or colitis persists >14 days, then add prednisolone 0.5–1 mg/kg (non-enteric-coated) or consider oral budesonide 9 mg daily if no bloody diarrhea
	G2/3 diarrhea or colitis	Withhold pembrolizumab. Loperamide 4 mg as starting dose then 2 mg before each meal and after each loose stool until without diarrhea for 12 hours, with maximum of 16 mg loperamide per day. Administer oral prednisone/prednisolone at a dose of 0.5 to 2 mg/kg/day or its equivalent. When improves to G1, begin a slow corticosteroid taper over at least 4 weeks. Resume pembrolizumab upon symptom control, or when prednisone/prednisolone daily dose <10 mg
	G4 diarrhea or colitis	Permanently discontinue pembrolizumab. Loperamide 4 mg as starting dose then 2 mg before each meal and after each loose stool until without diarrhea for 12 hours, with maximum of 16 mg loperamide per day. Administer 1–2 mg/kg IV (methyl)prednisolone and convert to 0.5–2 mg/kg prednisone/prednisolone orally each day or its equivalent only after a response. Taper over at least 4 weeks when symptoms improve. If does not improve over 72 hours or worsens, perform flexible sigmoidoscopy/colonoscopy to document colitis then begin infliximab 5 mg/kg (if no perforation/sepsis/TB/hepatitis/NYHA III/IV CHF). If no response, add MMF 500–1000 mg twice daily. If worse on MMF, consider addition of tacrolimus or ATG
Pneumonitis	G2	Withhold pembrolizumab. Consider *Pneumocystis* prophylaxis depending on the clinical context and coverage with empiric antibiotics. Administer oral prednisone/prednisolone at a dose of 1–2 mg/kg/day or its equivalent. When improves to G1, begin a slow corticosteroid taper over at least 4 weeks. If does not respond adequately after 48 hours, then administer 2–4 mg/kg IV (methyl)prednisolone and convert to 0.5–2 mg/kg prednisone/prednisolone orally each day or its equivalent only after a response, followed by a taper over at least 6 weeks when symptoms improve to G1, titrating to symptoms. Resume pembrolizumab upon symptom control, or when prednisone/prednisolone daily dose <10 mg
	G3/4	Permanently discontinue pembrolizumab. Consider *Pneumocystis* prophylaxis depending on the clinical context; cover with empiric antibiotics. Administer 2–4 mg/kg IV (methyl)prednisolone and convert to 1–2 mg/kg prednisone/prednisolone orally each day or its equivalent only after a response, followed by a taper over at least 8 weeks when symptoms improve to G1, titrating to symptoms. If when initially treated improvement does not occur within 48–72 hours, begin infliximab 5 mg/kg (if no perforation/sepsis/TB/hepatitis/NYHA III/IV CHF). If no response to infliximab, add MMF 500–1000 mg twice daily. Consider MMF especially if has concurrent hepatic toxicity
Hepatitis	G2 (AST or ALT >3–5× ULN or total bilirubin >1.5–3× ULN)	Withhold pembrolizumab. Administer oral prednisone/prednisolone at a dose of 1 to 2 mg/kg/day or its equivalent. When improves to G1, begin a slow corticosteroid taper over at least 4 weeks. Resume pembrolizumab upon symptom control, or when prednisone/prednisolone daily dose <10 mg
	G3/4 (AST or ALT >5× ULN or total bilirubin >3× ULN)	Permanently discontinue pembrolizumab. Administer 1–2 mg/kg IV (methyl)prednisolone and convert to 0.5–2 mg/kg prednisone/prednisolone orally each day or its equivalent only after a response. Taper over at least 6 weeks when symptoms improve. If no response, add MMF 500–1000 mg twice daily. If worse on MMF, consider adding tacrolimus or ATG

(*continued*)

Treatment Modifications (*continued*)

Adverse Event	Grade/Severity	Treatment Modification
Hypophysitis	G2/3 (moderate symptoms, ie, headache but no visual disturbance or fatigue/mood alteration but hemodynamically stable, no electrolyte disturbance)	Administer analgesia as needed for headache. Withhold pembrolizumab. Administer oral prednisone/prednisolone at a dose of 0.5 to 2 mg/kg/day or its equivalent. When improves to G1, begin a slow corticosteroid taper over at least 4 weeks. If no improvement in 48 hours, administer 1–2 mg/kg IV (methyl) prednisolone and convert to 0.5–2 mg/kg prednisone/prednisolone orally each day or its equivalent only after a response. Taper over at least 4 weeks when symptoms improve to 5 mg prednisone/prednisolone or equivalent; do not stop steroids. Resume pembrolizumab upon symptom control, or when prednisone/prednisolone daily dose <10 mg
	G4 (severe mass effect symptoms, ie, severe headache, any visual disturbance or severe hypoadrenalism, ie, hypotension, severe electrolyte disturbance)	Permanently discontinue pembrolizumab. Administer analgesia as needed for headache. Administer 1–2 mg/kg IV (methyl)prednisolone and convert to 0.5–2 mg/kg prednisone/prednisolone orally each day or its equivalent only after a response. Taper over at least 4 weeks when symptoms improve to 5 mg prednisone/prednisolone or equivalent; do not stop steroids
Adrenal insufficiency	G2	Withhold pembrolizumab. Administer oral prednisone/prednisolone at a dose of 0.5 to 2 mg/kg/day or its equivalent. When improves to G1, begin a slow corticosteroid taper over at least 4 weeks. Serially assess adrenal function and continue steroids at replacement doses (20–40 mg hydrocortisone daily ~2/3 dose in AM upon awakening and ~1/3 at 4 PM) until recovery of adrenal function is documented. Resume pembrolizumab upon symptom control, or when prednisone/prednisolone daily dose <10 mg
	G3/4	Permanently discontinue pembrolizumab. Administer oral prednisone/prednisolone at a dose of 0.5 to 2 mg/kg/day or its equivalent. When improves to G1, begin a slow corticosteroid taper over at least 4 weeks. Serially assess adrenal function and continue steroids at replacement doses (20–40 mg hydrocortisone daily ~2/3 dose in AM upon awakening and ~1/3 at 4 PM) until recovery of adrenal function is documented
Type 1 diabetes mellitus	G3 hyperglycemia	Withhold pembrolizumab. Admit to hospital to manage hyperglycemia. Role of corticosteroids in preventing complete loss of insulin-producing cells is unknown and not recommended. Resume pembrolizumab upon symptom control, or when prednisone/prednisolone daily dose <10 mg
	G4 hyperglycemia	Permanently discontinue pembrolizumab. Admit to hospital to manage hyperglycemia. Role of corticosteroids in preventing complete loss of insulin-producing cells is unknown and not recommended
Nephritis and renal dysfunction	G2/3 (serum creatinine 1.5–6× ULN)	Withhold pembrolizumab. Administer oral prednisone/prednisolone at a dose of 0.5 to 2 mg/kg/day or its equivalent. When improves to G1, begin a slow corticosteroid taper over at least 4 weeks. If does not respond adequately, then administer 0.5–1 mg/kg IV (methyl)prednisolone and convert to 0.5–2 mg/kg prednisone/prednisolone orally each day or its equivalent only after a response, followed by a taper over at least 4 weeks when improves to G1. Resume pembrolizumab upon symptom control, or when prednisone/prednisolone daily dose <10 mg
	G4 (serum creatinine >6× ULN)	Permanently discontinue pembrolizumab. Administer 0.5–1 mg/kg IV (methyl)prednisolone and convert to 0.5–2 mg/kg prednisone/prednisolone orally each day or its equivalent only after a response, followed by a taper over at least 4 weeks when improves to G1.
Skin	G1/2	Continue pembrolizumab. Avoid skin irritants, avoid sun exposure, topical emollients recommended. Topical steroid (mild strength for G1, moderate/potent strength for G2) cream once or twice daily ± oral or topical antihistamines for itching.

(*continued*)

Treatment Modifications (*continued*)

Adverse Event	Grade/Severity	Treatment Modification
	G3 rash or suspected SJS or TEN	Withhold pembrolizumab. Avoid skin irritants, avoid sun exposure, topical emollients recommended. Administer oral or topical antihistamines for itching. Administer oral prednisone/prednisolone at a dose of 0.5–2 mg/kg or its equivalent daily for 3 days followed by a slow corticosteroid taper over at least 4 weeks when the rash improves to G1. If does not respond adequately, then administer 0.5–1 mg/kg IV (methyl)prednisolone and convert to 0.5–2 mg/kg prednisone/prednisolone orally each day or its equivalent only after a response, followed by a taper over at least 4 weeks when the rash improves to G1. Resume pembrolizumab upon symptom control, or when prednisone/prednisolone daily dose <10 mg
	G4 rash or confirmed SJS or TEN	Avoid skin irritants, avoid sun exposure, topical emollients recommended. Administer oral or topical antihistamines for itching. Administer 1–2 mg/kg IV (methyl)prednisolone and convert to oral steroids 0.5–2 mg/kg prednisone/prednisolone each day or its equivalent only after a response. Taper over at least 4 weeks when the rash improves to G1. Permanently discontinue pembrolizumab
Encephalitis	Confusion or altered behavior, headaches, alteration in Glasgow Coma Scale, motor or sensory deficits, speech abnormality, may or may not be febrile	Initially withhold pembrolizumab, but permanently discontinue pembrolizumab if there is no doubt as to diagnosis. Exclude bacterial and ideally viral infections prior to high-dose steroids. Administer oral prednisone/prednisolone at a dose of 0.5–2 mg/kg/day or its equivalent. When symptoms improve, begin a slow corticosteroid taper over at least 4–8 weeks. If symptoms are severe, administer 1–2 mg/kg IV (methyl)prednisolone and convert to 0.5–2 mg/kg prednisone/prednisolone orally each day or its equivalent only after a response. Consider concurrent empiric antiviral (IV acyclovir) and antibacterial therapy
Aseptic meningitis	Headache, photophobia, neck stiffness with fever or may be afebrile, vomiting; normal cognition/cerebral function (distinguishes from encephalitis)	
Other syndromes include neurosarcoidosis, posterior reversible leukoencephalopathy syndrome (PRES), Vogt-Koyanagi-Harada syndrome, demyelination, vasculitic encephalopathy, and generalized seizures		
Transverse myelitis	Acute or subacute neurologic signs/symptoms of motor/sensory/autonomic origin; most have sensory level; often bilateral symptoms	Initially withhold pembrolizumab, but permanently discontinue pembrolizumab if there is no doubt as to diagnosis. Administer 2 mg/kg IV (methyl)prednisolone or consider 1 g/day and convert to 0.5–2 mg/kg prednisone/prednisolone orally each day or its equivalent only after a response. When symptoms improve, begin a slow corticosteroid taper over at least 4–8 weeks. Plasmapheresis may be required if steroids do not bring about improvement
Myocarditis	G3	Permanently discontinue pembrolizumab. Administer 2 mg/kg IV (methyl)prednisolone or consider 1 g/day and convert to 0.5–2 mg/kg prednisone/prednisolone orally each day or its equivalent only after a response. When symptoms improve, begin a slow corticosteroid taper over at least 4–8 weeks. If no response, add MMF 500–1000 mg twice daily. If worse on MMF, consider adding tacrolimus
Peripheral neurologic toxicity	Moderate: some interference with ADL, symptoms concerning to patient	Withhold pembrolizumab. Initial observation reasonable or initiate prednisone/prednisolone 0.5–1 mg/kg (if progressing, eg, from mild) and/or pregabalin or duloxetine for pain. When symptoms improve, begin a slow corticosteroid taper over at least 4 weeks. Resume pembrolizumab upon symptom control, or when prednisone/prednisolone daily dose <10 mg
	Severe: limits self-care and aids warranted, life-threatening, eg, respiratory problems	Permanently discontinue pembrolizumab. Administer 1–2 mg/kg IV (methyl)prednisolone and convert to 0.5–2 mg/kg prednisone/prednisolone orally each day or its equivalent only after a response. Taper over at least 4–8 weeks when symptoms improve to G1
Guillain-Barré syndrome	Progressive symmetrical muscle weakness with absent or reduced tendon reflexes—involves extremities, facial, respiratory, and bulbar and oculomotor muscles; dysregulation of autonomic nerves	Permanently discontinue pembrolizumab. Use of steroids not recommended in idiopathic Guillain-Barré syndrome; however, a trial of (methyl)prednisolone 1–2 mg/kg is reasonable, converting to 0.5–2 mg/kg prednisone/prednisolone orally each day or its equivalent only after a response. If no improvement or worsening, plasmapheresis or IVIG indicated

(*continued*)

Treatment Modifications (*continued*)

Adverse Event	Grade/Severity	Treatment Modification
Myasthenia gravis	Fluctuating muscle weakness (proximal limb, trunk, ocular, eg, ptosis/diplopia or bulbar) with fatigability, respiratory muscles may also be involved	Permanently discontinue pembrolizumab. Administer pyridostigmine at an initial dose of 30 mg three times daily. Administer oral prednisone/prednisolone at a dose of 0.5 to 2 mg/kg/day or its equivalent or 1–2 mg/kg IV (methyl) prednisolone depending on the severity of symptoms. If begin with IV, convert to 0.5–2 mg/kg prednisone/prednisolone orally each day or its equivalent only after a response. If no improvement or worsening, plasmapheresis or IVIG may be considered. Additional immunosuppressants used in myasthenia gravis include azathioprine, cyclosporine, and mycophenolate. Avoid certain medications, eg, ciprofloxacin, beta-blockers, that may precipitate cholinergic crisis
	Other syndromes including motor and sensory peripheral neuropathy, multifocal radicular neuropathy/plexopathy, autonomic neuropathy, phrenic nerve palsy, cranial nerve palsies (eg, facial nerve, optic nerve, hypoglossal nerve)	Permanently discontinue pembrolizumab. Administer oral prednisone/prednisolone at a dose of 0.5 to 2 mg/kg/day or its equivalent or 1–2 mg/kg IV (methyl)prednisolone depending on the severity of symptoms. If begin with IV, convert to 0.5–2 mg/kg prednisone/prednisolone orally each day or its equivalent only after a response
Arthralgia	G1 (mild pain with inflammation, erythema, or joint swelling)	Continue pembrolizumab. Administer acetaminophen (paracetamol) and ibuprofen
	G2 (moderate pain with inflammation, erythema, or joint swelling that limits ADLs)	Withhold pembrolizumab. Administer higher doses of acetaminophen (paracetamol) and ibuprofen and use diclofenac or naproxen or etoricoxib. If inadequately controlled, consider intra-articular steroid injections for large joints or administer oral prednisone/prednisolone at a dose of 0.5 to 2 mg/kg/day or its equivalent. When improves to G1, begin a slow corticosteroid taper over at least 4 weeks. If does not respond adequately, then administer 0.5–1 mg/kg IV (methyl)prednisolone and convert to 0.5–2 mg/kg prednisone/prednisolone orally each day or its equivalent only after a response, followed by a taper over at least 4 weeks when improves to G1. Resume pembrolizumab upon symptom control, or when prednisone/prednisolone daily dose <10 mg
	G3 (severe pain; irreversible joint damage; disabling; limits self-care ADL)	Withhold pembrolizumab. Administer 0.5–1 mg/kg IV (methyl)prednisolone and convert to 0.5–2 mg/kg prednisone/prednisolone orally each day or its equivalent only after a response, followed by a taper over at least 4 weeks when improves to G1. In severe cases, infliximab or another anti–TNF alpha drug may be required for improvement of arthritis. Resume pembrolizumab upon symptom control, or when prednisone/prednisolone daily dose <10 mg
Other	First occurrence of other G3	Withhold pembrolizumab. Administer oral prednisone/prednisolone at a dose of 0.5 to 2 mg/kg/day or its equivalent. When improves to G1, begin a slow corticosteroid taper over at least 4 weeks. Resume pembrolizumab upon symptom control, or when prednisone/prednisolone daily dose <10 mg
	Recurrence of same G3	Permanently discontinue pembrolizumab. Administer 1–2 mg/kg IV (methyl) prednisolone and convert to 0.5–2 mg/kg prednisone/prednisolone orally each day or its equivalent only after a response. Taper over at least 4–8 weeks when symptoms improve to G1
	Life-threatening or G4	
	Requirement for ≥10 mg/day prednisone or equivalent for >12 weeks	Permanently discontinue pembrolizumab
	Persistent G2/3 adverse reactions lasting ≥12 weeks	

ADL, activities of daily living; ALT, alanine aminotransferase; AST, aspartate aminotransferase; ATG, anti–thymocyte globulin; SJS, Stevens-Johnson syndrome; TEN, toxic epidermal necrolysis; ULN, upper limit of normal

Notes on general supportive care:
• Steroid taper in most cases will proceed over a minimum of 1 month but if symptoms improve rapidly, a 2-week taper can be considered. If steroids are administered for more than 4 weeks, consider PCP prophylaxis (cotrimoxazole 480 mg twice daily M/W/F or inhaled pentamidine if has cotrimoxazole allergy), regular random blood glucose, Vitamin D level, and starting calcium/Vitamin D supplementation per guidelines

Efficacy (N = 861)

Endpoint	Pembrolizumab + Axitinib (N = 432)	Sunitinib (N = 429)	Between-group Comparison
Overall survival at 12 months	89.9% (95% CI 86.4–92.4)	78.3% (95% CI 73.8–82.1)	HR 0.53 (95% CI 0.38–0.74); P <0.001
Median progression-free survival	15.1 months (95% CI 12.6–17.7)	11.1 months (95% CI 8.7–12.5)	HR 0.69 (95% CI 0.57–0.84); P <0.001
Objective response rate	59.3% (95% CI 54.5–63.9)	35.7% (95% CI 31.1–40.4)	P <0.001
Complete response	5.8%	1.9%	—
Partial response	53.5%	33.8%	—
Stable disease	24.5%	39.4%	—
Median time to response*	2.8 months (range, 1.5 to 16.6)	2.9 months (range, 2.1 to 15.1)	—
Median duration of response†	NR (range, 1.4+ to 18.4+)	15.2 months (range, 1.1+ to 15.4+)	—

HR, hazard ratio; CI, confidence interval; NR, not reached
*The median time to response was only calculated for patients who had a complete or partial response. The numbers in parentheses represent the range
†The median duration response was determined for patients who had a complete or partial response. Plus signs indicate that responses were ongoing at the time of data cutoff

Adverse Events (N = 854)

Event	Pembrolizumab + Axitinib (N = 429)		Sunitinib (N = 425)	
	Grade 1–2 (%)	Grade 3–5* (%)	Grade 1–2 (%)	Grade 3–5† (%)
Diarrhea	45.2	9.1	40.2	4.7
Hypertension	22.4	22.1	26.1	19.3
Fatigue	35.7	2.8	31.3	6.6
Hypothyroidism	35.2	0.2	31.3	0.2
Decreased appetite	26.8	2.8	28.7	0.7
Palmar-plantar erythrodysesthesia	22.9	5.1	36.2	3.8
Nausea	26.8	0.9	30.6	0.9
ALT increased	13.5	13.3	12.0	3.1
AST increased	19.1	7.0	13.8	2.4
Dysphonia	25.2	0.2	3.3	0
Cough	21.0	0.2	13.1	0.5
Constipation	20.7	0	14.4	0.2
Arthralgia	17.3	0.9	5.4	0.7
Weight decreased	14.7	3.0	10.9	0.2
Proteinuria	14.7	2.8	9.7	1.4
Dyspnea	14.5	1.6	9.6	1.2
Headache	15.0	0.9	15.7	0.5
Stomatitis	14.9	0.7	18.8	2.1

(continued)

Adverse Events (N = 854) (continued)

Event	Pembrolizumab + Axitinib (N = 429)		Sunitinib (N = 425)	
	Grade 1–2 (%)	Grade 3–5* (%)	Grade 1–2 (%)	Grade 3–5† (%)
Asthenia	12.6	2.6	11.7	3.1
Pruritis	15.0	0.2	5.9	0
Vomiting	15.0	0.2	17.7	0.9
Rash	14.0	0.2	10.6	0.5
Back pain	12.4	0.9	8.5	1.6
Mucosal inflammation	12.4	0.9	20.0	1.9
Hyperthyroidism	11.6	1.2	3.8	0
Pyrexia	12.8	0	10.1	0
Pain in extremity	11.0	0.9	9.0	0.9
Abdominal pain	10.2	1.2	6.6	0.2
Blood creatinine increased	10.7	0.5	11.3	0.7
Dysgeusia	10.8	0.2	30.8	0
Anemia	7.2	0.7	18.6	4.9
Dyspepsia	5.1	0	14.4	0.2
Gastroesophageal reflux disease	4.2	0	10.6	0.7
Platelet count decreased	3.5	0.2	10.8	7.3
Thrombocytopenia	2.6	0	17.4	5.9
Neutropenia	1.7	0.2	12.7	6.6
Neutrophil count decreased	0.7	0.2	5.0	6.8
White-cell count decreased	0.5	0	7.3	2.8

ALT, alanine aminotransferase; AST, aspartate aminotransferase

Shown are the adverse events that occurred while patients were receiving the assigned treatment, or within 30 days after the end of the treatment period (90 days for serious events). The as-treated population included all patients who underwent randomization and received at least one dose of trial treatment

*There were 11 deaths (2.6%) in the pembrolizumab-axitinib group: 1 patient each from cardiac arrest, myasthenia gravis, myocarditis, necrotizing fasciitis, plasma-cell myeloma, pneumonitis, pulmonary embolism, pulmonary thrombosis, respiratory failure, sudden cardiac death, and death otherwise not specified

†There were 15 deaths (3.5%) in the sunitinib group: 2 patients from pneumonia, 1 patient from both pneumonia and cardiac amyloidosis, and 1 patient each from acute myocardial infarction, cardiac arrest, chronic cardiac failure, fulminant hepatitis, gastric hemorrhage, gastrointestinal hemorrhage, intracranial hemorrhage, malignant neoplasm progression, sepsis, sudden death, urinary tract infection, and death otherwise not specified

Therapy Monitoring

Monitoring for Pembrolizumab:

1. Initially at the time of each dose, and eventually every 6–12 weeks, perform a total body skin examination with attention to *all* mucous membranes as well as a complete review of systems
2. Monitor patients for signs and symptoms of pneumonitis. Evaluate patients with suspected pneumonitis with chest x-ray, CT, and pulse oximetry. For ≥2 toxicity, may include nasal swab, sputum culture and sensitivity, blood culture and sensitivity, and urine culture and sensitivity
3. Monitor patients for signs and symptoms of colitis. Encourage patients to report diarrhea immediately to any member of the health care team

(*continued*)

Therapy Monitoring (*continued*)

4. Draw AST, ALT, and bilirubin prior to each infusion and/or weekly if there are Grade 1 liver function test elevations. Note, no treatment is recommended for G1 LFT abnormalities. For ≥2 toxicity, work up for other causes of elevated LFTs including viral hepatitis

5. Use basic metabolic panel (Na, K, CO_2, glucose) and patient history as screening tools for hypophysitis including hypopituitarism and adrenal insufficiency. If in doubt, evaluate AM adrenocorticotropic hormone (ACTH) and cortisol levels. Consider ACTH stimulation test for indeterminate results

6. Assess thyroid function at the start of treatment, periodically during treatment, and as indicated based on clinical evaluation, and for clinical signs and symptoms of thyroid disorders. Test for TSH and free thyroxine (FT4) every 4–6 weeks as part of routine clinical monitoring of therapy or for case detection in symptomatic patients

7. Measure glucose at baseline and with each treatment during the first 12 weeks and every 6 weeks thereafter

8. Obtain a serum creatinine prior to every dose. If creatinine is found to be newly elevated, consider holding therapy while other potential causes are evaluated. Note, routine urinalysis is not necessary other than to rule out urinary tract infections, etc

9. Obtain a complete rheumatologic history and perform an examination of all peripheral joints for tenderness, swelling, and range of motion. Examine the spine. Consider plain x-ray/imaging to exclude metastases and evaluate joint damage (erosions), if appropriate

10. In patients at high risk for infections and in appropriately selected patients based on an infectious disease evaluation, draw screening laboratories (HIV, hepatitis A and B, and blood QuantiFERON for TB) to prepare patients to start infliximab

Monitoring for Axitinib:

1. *At baseline, week 2, week 4, and every 4 weeks thereafter:* clinical assessments including medical history and physical examination, vital signs, ALT, AST, total bilirubin, and CBC with differential. Control blood pressure prior to initiation of axitinib

2. *At screening, after 6 and 12 weeks of therapy, and every 8 weeks thereafter:* tumor assessments. Thyroid function tests. Spot urine for protein measurement (if spot urine dipstick >1+ for protein, perform a 24-hour urine protein)

METASTATIC • CLEAR-CELL • FIRST-LINE
RENAL CELL CARCINOMA REGIMEN: NIVOLUMAB + IPILIMUMAB

Motzer RJ et al. N Engl J Med 2018;378:1277–1290
Protocol for: Motzer RJ et al. N Engl J Med 2018;378:1277–1290
Supplementary appendix to: Motzer RJ et al. N Engl J Med 2018;378:1277–1290
Motzer RJ et al. Lancet Oncol 2019;20:1370–1385
Supplementary appendix to: Motzer RJ et al. Lancet Oncol 2019;20:1370–1385
Erratum in: Lancet Oncol 2019;20:e559
OPDIVO (nivolumab) prescribing information. Princeton, NJ: Bristol-Myers Squibb Company; revised September 2019
YERVOY (ipilimumab) prescribing information. Princeton, NJ: Bristol-Myers Squibb Company; revised September 2019

Induction phase (concurrent treatment with nivolumab and ipilimumab):

Nivolumab 3 mg/kg; administer intravenously over 30 minutes in a volume of 0.9% sodium chloride injection (0.9% NS) or 5% dextrose injection (D5W) not to exceed 160 mL and sufficient to produce a nivolumab concentration within the range 1–10 mg/mL on day 1, every 3 weeks for a maximum of 4 doses (total dosage/3-week cycle = 3 mg/kg)

- Administer nivolumab through an administration set that contains a sterile, non-pyrogenic, low-protein-binding in-line filter with pore size within the range of 0.2–1.2 μm
- Nivolumab can cause severe infusion-related reactions

followed on the same day by:

Ipilimumab 1 mg/kg; administer intravenously over 30 minutes in a volume of 0.9% NS or D5W sufficient to produce an ipilimumab concentration within the range 1–2 mg/mL on day 1, every 3 weeks for a maximum of 4 doses (total dose/3-week cycle = 1 mg/kg)

- Administer ipilimumab through an administration set containing a sterile, non-pyrogenic, low-protein-binding in-line filter

Maintenance phase (single-agent nivolumab):

Note that the U.S. Food and Drug Administration (FDA)-approved regimens for renal cell carcinoma include fixed doses of nivolumab and allow for a shortened infusion duration of 30 minutes. Note that fixed dosing of nivolumab may only be used *after completion* of concurrent treatment with nivolumab and ipilimumab, thus:

Nivolumab 240 mg; administer intravenously over 30 minutes in a volume of 0.9% NS or D5W, not to exceed 160 mL and sufficient to produce a nivolumab concentration within the range 1–10 mg/mL, every 2 weeks until disease progression (total dosage/2-week cycle = 240 mg)

- Administer nivolumab through an administration set that contains a sterile, non-pyrogenic, low-protein-binding in-line filter with pore size within the range of 0.2–1.2 μm
- Nivolumab can cause severe infusion-related reactions

or

Nivolumab 480 mg; administer intravenously over 30 minutes in a volume of 0.9% NS or D5W not to exceed 160 mL and sufficient to produce a nivolumab concentration within the range 1–10 mg/mL, every 4 weeks until disease progression (total dosage/4-week cycle = 480 mg)

- Administer nivolumab through an administration set that contains a sterile, non-pyrogenic, low-protein-binding in-line filter with pore size within the range of 0.2–1.2 μm
- Nivolumab can cause severe infusion-related reactions

Supportive Care

Antiemetic prophylaxis
Emetogenic potential with nivolumab ± ipilimumab is **MINIMAL**
See Chapter 42 for antiemetic recommendations

Hematopoietic growth factor (CSF) prophylaxis
Primary prophylaxis is **NOT** *indicated*
See Chapter 43 for more information

Antimicrobial prophylaxis
Risk of fever and neutropenia is **LOW**
   Antimicrobial primary prophylaxis to be considered:
   - Antibacterial—not indicated
   - Antifungal—not indicated
   - Antiviral—not indicated unless patient previously had an episode of HSV

Treatment Modifications

RECOMMENDED DOSE MODIFICATIONS FOR NIVOLUMAB AND IPILIMUMAB

Adverse Event	Grade/Severity	Treatment Modification
Infusion reaction	Clinically significant but not severe infusion reaction	Interrupt the infusion in patients with clinically significant infusion reactions and consider resuming at a slower rate following resolution. If decision is made to restart, begin at ≤50% of the rate prior to the reaction and increase in 50% increments every 30 minutes if well tolerated. Infusions may be restarted at the full rate during the next cycle
	G3/4 (severe infusion reaction—pyrexia, chills, flushing, hypotension, dyspnea, wheezing, back pain, abdominal pain, and urticaria). Not rapidly responsive to brief interruption of infusion	Stop infusion and administer appropriate medical therapy (eg, epinephrine, corticosteroids, intravenous antihistamines, bronchodilators, and/or oxygen). Discontinue nivolumab and ipilimumab
Colitis	G1	Loperamide 4 mg as starting dose then 2 mg before each meal and after each loose stool until without diarrhea for 12 hours, with maximum of 16 mg loperamide per day. If G1 diarrhea or colitis persists >14 days, then add prednisolone 0.5–1 mg/kg (non-enteric-coated) or consider oral budesonide 9 mg daily if no bloody diarrhea
	G2/3 diarrhea or colitis	Withhold nivolumab and ipilimumab. Loperamide 4 mg as starting dose then 2 mg before each meal and after each loose stool until without diarrhea for 12 hours, with maximum of 16 mg loperamide per day. Administer oral prednisone/prednisolone at a dose of 0.5–2 mg/kg/day or its equivalent. When improves to G1, begin a slow corticosteroid taper over at least 4 weeks. Resume nivolumab and ipilimumab upon symptom control, or when prednisone/prednisolone daily dose <10 mg
	G4 diarrhea or colitis	Permanently discontinue nivolumab and ipilimumab. Loperamide 4 mg as starting dose then 2 mg before each meal and after each loose stool until without diarrhea for 12 hours, with maximum of 16 mg loperamide per day. Administer 1–2 mg/kg intravenously (methyl)prednisolone and convert to 0.5–2 mg/kg prednisone/prednisolone orally each day or its equivalent only after a response. Taper over at least 4 weeks when symptoms improve. If does not improve over 72 hours or worsens, perform flexible sigmoidoscopy/colonoscopy to document colitis then begin infliximab 5 mg/kg (if no perforation/sepsis/TB/hepatitis/NYHA III/IV CHF). If no response, add MMF 500–1000 mg twice daily. If worse on MMF, consider addition of tacrolimus or ATG
Pneumonitis	G2	Withhold nivolumab and ipilimumab. Consider *Pneumocystis* prophylaxis depending on the clinical context and coverage with empiric antibiotics. Administer oral prednisone/prednisolone at a dose of 1–2 mg/kg/day or its equivalent. When improves to G1, begin a slow corticosteroid taper over at least 4 weeks. If does not respond adequately after 48 hours, then administer 2–4 mg/kg intravenously (methyl)prednisolone and convert to 0.5–2 mg/kg prednisone/prednisolone orally each day or its equivalent only after a response, followed by a taper over at least 6 weeks when symptoms improve to G1, titrating to symptoms. Resume nivolumab and ipilimumab upon symptom control, or when prednisone/prednisolone daily dose <10 mg
	G3/4	Permanently discontinue nivolumab and ipilimumab. Consider *Pneumocystis* prophylaxis depending on the clinical context; cover with empiric antibiotics. Administer 2–4 mg/kg intravenously (methyl)prednisolone and convert to 1–2 mg/kg prednisone/prednisolone orally each day or its equivalent only after a response, followed by a taper over at least 8 weeks when symptoms improve to G1, titrating to symptoms. If when initially treated improvement does not occur within 48–72 hours, begin infliximab 5 mg/kg (if no perforation/sepsis/TB/hepatitis/NYHA III/IV CHF). If no response to infliximab, add MMF 500–1000 mg twice daily. Consider MMF especially if has concurrent hepatic toxicity
Hepatitis	G2 (AST or ALT >3–5× ULN or total bilirubin >1.5–3× ULN)	Withhold nivolumab and ipilimumab. Administer oral prednisone/prednisolone at a dose of 1–2 mg/kg/day or its equivalent. When improves to G1, begin a slow corticosteroid taper over at least 4 weeks. Resume nivolumab and ipilimumab upon symptom control, or when prednisone/prednisolone daily dose <10 mg
	G3/4 (AST or ALT >5× ULN or total bilirubin >3× ULN)	Permanently discontinue nivolumab and ipilimumab. Administer 1–2 mg/kg intravenously (methyl)prednisolone and convert to 0.5–2 mg/kg prednisone/prednisolone orally each day or its equivalent only after a response. Taper over at least 6 weeks when symptoms improve. If no response, add MMF 500–1000 mg twice daily. If worse on MMF, consider adding tacrolimus or ATG

(continued)

Treatment Modifications (continued)

Adverse Event	Grade/Severity	Treatment Modification
Hypophysitis	G2/3 (moderate symptoms, ie, headache but no visual disturbance or fatigue/mood alteration but hemodynamically stable, no electrolyte disturbance)	Administer analgesia as needed for headache. Withhold nivolumab and ipilimumab. Administer oral prednisone/prednisolone at a dose of 0.5–2 mg/kg/day or its equivalent. When improves to G1, begin a slow corticosteroid taper over at least 4 weeks. If no improvement in 48 hours, administer 1–2 mg/kg intravenously (methyl)prednisolone and convert to 0.5–2 mg/kg prednisone/prednisolone orally each day or its equivalent only after a response. Taper over at least 4 weeks when symptoms improve to 5 mg prednisone/prednisolone or equivalent; do not stop steroids. Resume nivolumab and ipilimumab upon symptom control, or when prednisone/prednisolone daily dose <10 mg
	G4 (severe mass effect symptoms, ie, severe headache, any visual disturbance or severe hypoadrenalism, ie, hypotension, severe electrolyte disturbance)	Permanently discontinue nivolumab and ipilimumab. Administer analgesia as needed for headache. Administer 1–2 mg/kg intravenously (methyl)prednisolone and convert to 0.5–2 mg/kg prednisone/prednisolone orally each day or its equivalent only after a response. Taper over at least 4 weeks when symptoms improve to 5 mg prednisone/prednisolone or equivalent; do not stop steroids
Adrenal insufficiency	G2	Withhold nivolumab and ipilimumab. Administer oral prednisone/prednisolone at a dose of 0.5–2 mg/kg/day or its equivalent. When improves to G1, begin a slow corticosteroid taper over at least 4 weeks. Serially assess adrenal function and continue steroids at replacement doses (20–40 mg hydrocortisone daily ~2/3 dose in AM upon awakening and ~1/3 at 4 PM) until recovery of adrenal function is documented. Resume nivolumab and ipilimumab upon symptom control, or when prednisone/prednisolone daily dose <10 mg
	G3/4	Permanently discontinue nivolumab and ipilimumab. Administer oral prednisone/prednisolone at a dose of 0.5–2 mg/kg/day or its equivalent. When improves to G1, begin a slow corticosteroid taper over at least 4 weeks. Serially assess adrenal function and continue steroids at replacement doses (20–40 mg hydrocortisone daily ~2/3 dose in AM upon awakening and ~1/3 at 4 PM) until recovery of adrenal function is documented
Type 1 diabetes mellitus	G3 hyperglycemia	Withhold nivolumab and ipilimumab. Admit to hospital to manage hyperglycemia. Role of corticosteroids in preventing complete loss of insulin-producing cells is unknown and not recommended. Resume nivolumab and ipilimumab upon symptom control, or when prednisone/prednisolone daily dose <10 mg
	G4 hyperglycemia	Permanently discontinue nivolumab and ipilimumab. Admit to hospital to manage hyperglycemia. Role of corticosteroids in preventing complete loss of insulin-producing cells is unknown and not recommended
Nephritis and renal dysfunction	G2/3 (serum creatinine 1.5–6× ULN)	Withhold nivolumab and ipilimumab. Administer oral prednisone/prednisolone at a dose of 0.5–2 mg/kg/day or its equivalent. When improves to G1, begin a slow corticosteroid taper over at least 4 weeks. If does not respond adequately, then administer 0.5–1 mg/kg intravenously (methyl)prednisolone and convert to 0.5–2 mg/kg prednisone/prednisolone orally each day or its equivalent only after a response, followed by a taper over at least 4 weeks when improves to G1. Resume nivolumab and ipilimumab upon symptom control, or when prednisone/prednisolone daily dose <10 mg
	G4 (serum creatinine >6× ULN)	Permanently discontinue nivolumab and ipilimumab. Administer 0.5–1 mg/kg intravenously (methyl)prednisolone and convert to 0.5–2 mg/kg prednisone/prednisolone orally each day or its equivalent only after a response, followed by a taper over at least 4 weeks when improves to G1
Skin	G1/2	Continue nivolumab and ipilimumab. Avoid skin irritants, avoid sun exposure, topical emollients recommended. Topical steroid (mild strength for G1, moderate/potent strength for G2) cream once or twice daily ± oral or topical antihistamines for itching
	G3 rash or suspected SJS or TEN	Withhold nivolumab and ipilimumab. Avoid skin irritants, avoid sun exposure, topical emollients recommended. Administer oral or topical antihistamines for itching. Administer oral prednisone/prednisolone at a dose of 0.5–2 mg/kg or its equivalent daily for 3 days followed by a slow corticosteroid taper over at least 4 weeks when the rash improves to G1. If does not respond adequately, then administer 0.5–1 mg/kg intravenously (methyl)prednisolone and convert to 0.5–2 mg/kg prednisone/prednisolone orally each day or its equivalent only after a response, followed by a taper over at least 4 weeks when the rash improves to G1. Resume nivolumab and ipilimumab upon symptom control, or when prednisone/prednisolone daily dose <10 mg

(continued)

Treatment Modifications (continued)

Adverse Event	Grade/Severity	Treatment Modification
	G4 rash or confirmed SJS or TEN	Avoid skin irritants, avoid sun exposure, topical emollients recommended. Administer oral or topical antihistamines for itching. Administer 1–2 mg/kg intravenously (methyl)prednisolone and convert to oral steroids 0.5–2 mg/kg prednisone/prednisolone each day or its equivalent only after a response. Taper over at least 4 weeks when the rash improves to G1. Permanently discontinue nivolumab and ipilimumab
Encephalitis	Confusion or altered behavior, headaches, alteration in Glasgow Coma Scale, motor or sensory deficits, speech abnormality, may or may not be febrile	Initially withhold nivolumab and ipilimumab, but permanently discontinue nivolumab and ipilimumab if there is no doubt as to diagnosis. Exclude bacterial and ideally viral infections prior to high-dose steroids. Administer oral prednisone/prednisolone at a dose of 0.5–2 mg/kg/day or its equivalent. When symptoms improve, begin a slow corticosteroid taper over at least 4–8 weeks. If symptoms are severe, administer 1–2 mg/kg intravenously (methyl)prednisolone and convert to 0.5–2 mg/kg prednisone/prednisolone orally each day or its equivalent only after a response. Consider concurrent empiric antiviral (intravenous acyclovir) and antibacterial therapy
Aseptic meningitis	Headache, photophobia, neck stiffness with fever or may be afebrile, vomiting; normal cognition/cerebral function (distinguishes from encephalitis)	
Other syndromes include neurosarcoidosis, posterior reversible leukoencephalopathy syndrome (PRES), Vogt-Koyanagi-Harada syndrome, demyelination, vasculitic encephalopathy, and generalized seizures		
Transverse myelitis	Acute or subacute neurologic signs/symptoms of motor/sensory/autonomic origin; most have sensory level; often bilateral symptoms	Initially withhold nivolumab and ipilimumab, but permanently discontinue nivolumab and ipilimumab if there is no doubt as to diagnosis. Administer 2 mg/kg intravenously (methyl)prednisolone or consider 1 g/day and convert to 0.5–2 mg/kg prednisone/prednisolone orally each day or its equivalent only after a response. When symptoms improve, begin a slow corticosteroid taper over at least 4–8 weeks. Plasmapheresis may be required if steroids do not bring about improvement
Myocarditis	G3	Permanently discontinue nivolumab and ipilimumab. Administer 2 mg/kg intravenously (methyl)prednisolone or consider 1 g/day and convert to 0.5–2 mg/kg prednisone/prednisolone orally each day or its equivalent only after a response. When symptoms improve, begin a slow corticosteroid taper over at least 4–8 weeks. If no response, add MMF 500–1000 mg twice daily. If worse on MMF, consider adding tacrolimus
Peripheral neurologic toxicity	Moderate: some interference with ADL, symptoms concerning to patient	Withhold nivolumab and ipilimumab. Initial observation reasonable or initiate prednisone/prednisolone 0.5–1 mg/kg (if progressing, eg, from mild) and/or pregabalin or duloxetine for pain. When symptoms improve, begin a slow corticosteroid taper over at least 4 weeks. Resume nivolumab and ipilimumab upon symptom control, or when prednisone/prednisolone daily dose <10 mg
	Severe: limits self-care and aids warranted, life-threatening, eg, respiratory problems	Permanently discontinue nivolumab and ipilimumab. Administer 1–2 mg/kg intravenously (methyl)prednisolone and convert to 0.5–2 mg/kg prednisone/prednisolone orally each day or its equivalent only after a response. Taper over at least 4–8 weeks when symptoms improve to G1
Guillain-Barré syndrome	Progressive symmetrical muscle weakness with absent or reduced tendon reflexes—involves extremities, facial, respiratory, and bulbar and oculomotor muscles; dysregulation of autonomic nerves	Permanently discontinue nivolumab and ipilimumab. Use of steroids not recommended in idiopathic Guillain-Barré syndrome; however, a trial of (methyl)prednisolone 1–2 mg/kg is reasonable, converting to 0.5–2 mg/kg prednisone/prednisolone orally each day or its equivalent only after a response. If no improvement or worsening, plasmapheresis or IVIG indicated

(continued)

Treatment Modifications (*continued*)

Adverse Event	Grade/Severity	Treatment Modification
Myasthenia gravis	Fluctuating muscle weakness (proximal limb, trunk, ocular, eg, ptosis/diplopia or bulbar) with fatigability, respiratory muscles may also be involved	Permanently discontinue nivolumab and ipilimumab. Administer pyridostigmine at an initial dose of 30 mg three times daily. Administer oral prednisone/prednisolone at a dose of 0.5–2 mg/kg/day or its equivalent or 1–2 mg/kg intravenously (methyl)prednisolone depending on the severity of symptoms. If begin with intravenous, convert to 0.5–2 mg/kg prednisone/prednisolone orally each day or its equivalent only after a response. If no improvement or worsening, plasmapheresis or IVIG may be considered. Additional immunosuppressants used in myasthenia gravis include azathioprine, cyclosporine, and mycophenolate. Avoid certain medications, eg, ciprofloxacin, beta-blockers, that may precipitate cholinergic crisis
Other syndromes including motor and sensory peripheral neuropathy, multifocal radicular neuropathy/plexopathy, autonomic neuropathy, phrenic nerve palsy, cranial nerve palsies (eg, facial nerve, optic nerve, hypoglossal nerve)		Permanently discontinue nivolumab and ipilimumab. Administer oral prednisone/prednisolone at a dose of 0.5–2 mg/kg/day or its equivalent or 1–2 mg/kg intravenously (methyl)prednisolone depending on the severity of symptoms. If begin with intravenous, convert to 0.5–2 mg/kg prednisone/prednisolone orally each day or its equivalent only after a response
Arthralgia	G1 (mild pain with inflammation, erythema or joint swelling)	Continue nivolumab and ipilimumab. Administer acetaminophen (paracetamol) and ibuprofen
	G2 (moderate pain with inflammation, erythema or joint swelling that limits ADLs)	Withhold nivolumab and ipilimumab. Administer higher doses of acetaminophen (paracetamol) and ibuprofen and use diclofenac or naproxen or etoricoxib. If inadequately controlled, consider intra-articular steroid injections for large joints or administer oral prednisone/prednisolone at a dose of 0.5–2 mg/kg/day or its equivalent. When improves to G1, begin a slow corticosteroid taper over at least 4 weeks. If does not respond adequately, then administer 0.5–1 mg/kg intravenously (methyl)prednisolone and convert to 0.5–2 mg/kg prednisone/prednisolone orally each day or its equivalent only after a response, followed by a taper over at least 4 weeks when improves to G1. Resume nivolumab and ipilimumab upon symptom control, or when prednisone/prednisolone daily dose <10 mg
	G3 (severe pain; irreversible joint damage; disabling; limits self-care ADL)	Withhold nivolumab and ipilimumab. Administer 0.5–1 mg/kg intravenously (methyl)prednisolone and convert to 0.5–2 mg/kg prednisone/prednisolone orally each day or its equivalent only after a response, followed by a taper over at least 4 weeks when improves to G1. In severe cases, infliximab or another anti–TNF alpha drug may be required for improvement of arthritis. Resume nivolumab and ipilimumab upon symptom control, or when prednisone/prednisolone daily dose <10 mg
Other	First occurrence of other G3	Withhold nivolumab and ipilimumab. Administer oral prednisone/prednisolone at a dose of 0.5–2 mg/kg/day or its equivalent. When improves to G1, begin a slow corticosteroid taper over at least 4 weeks. Resume nivolumab and ipilimumab upon symptom control, or when prednisone/prednisolone daily dose <10 mg
	Recurrence of same G3	Permanently discontinue nivolumab and ipilimumab. Administer 1–2 mg/kg intravenously (methyl)prednisolone and convert to 0.5–2 mg/kg prednisone/prednisolone orally each day or its equivalent only after a response. Taper over at least 4–8 weeks when symptoms improve to G1
	Life-threatening or G4	
	Requirement for ≥10 mg/day prednisone or equivalent for >12 weeks	Permanently discontinue nivolumab and ipilimumab
	Persistent G2/3 adverse reactions lasting ≥12 weeks	

ADL, activities of daily living; ALT, alanine aminotransferase; AST, aspartate aminotransferase; ATG, anti–thymocyte globulin; SJS, Stevens-Johnson syndrome; TEN, toxic epidermal necrolysis; ULN, upper limit of normal

Notes on general supportive care:
- Steroid taper in most cases will proceed over a minimum of 1 month but if symptoms improve rapidly, a 2-week taper can be considered. If steroids are administered for more than 4 weeks, consider PCP prophylaxis (cotrimoxazole 480 mg twice daily M/W/F or inhaled pentamidine if has cotrimoxazole allergy), regular random blood glucose, Vitamin D level, and starting calcium/Vitamin D supplementation per guidelines

Patient Population Studied

This randomized, stratified, open-label, phase 3 trial included 1096 adult patients with previously untreated RCC and compared treatment with nivolumab plus ipilimumab to sunitinib. Patients were eligible if they had RCC with a clear cell component, measurable disease (according to RECIST v1.1), adequate organ function, and a Karnofsky performance score of ≥70%. Patients were excluded if they had previously received systemic therapy for RCC (with the exception of one previous adjuvant or neoadjuvant therapy, not including VEGF-targeting drugs, for completely resectable renal cell carcinoma if the reoccurrence occurred ≥6 months after the last dose), if they had CNS metastases or an autoimmune disease, or if they were taking glucocorticoids or immunosuppressants. This study enrolled patients from all IMDC risk categories; however, the primary efficacy analysis was designed to investigate overall survival, progression free survival, and objective response only in those patients with IMDC intermediate and poor risk disease.

Efficacy (N = 1096)

Efficacy Variable	Nivolumab + Ipilimumab (N = 550)	Sunitinib (N = 546)	Between-group Comparison
Survival in ITT population (N = 550 in nivolumab + ipilimumab arm, N = 546 in sunitinib arm)			
Median OS—months (95% CI)	NR (NE–NE)	37.9 (32.2–NE)	HR 0.71 (95% CI 0.59–0.86); P = 0.0003
OS rate at 30 months—% (95% CI)	64 (60–68)	56 (52–60)	—
Median PFS—months (95% CI)	9.7 (8.1–11.1)	9.7 (8.3–11.1)	HR 0.85 (95% CI 0.73–0.98); P = 0.027
PFS rate at 30 months—% (95% CI)	28 (24–32)	18 (14–22)	—
Survival in intermediate- or poor-risk patients (N = 425 in nivolumab + ipilimumab arm, N = 422 in sunitinib arm)			
Median OS—months (95% CI)	NR (35.6–NE)	26.6 (22.1–33.4)	HR 0.66 (95% CI 0.54–0.80); P <0.0001
OS rate at 30 months—% (95% CI)	60 (55–64)	47 (43–52)	—
Median PFS—months (95% CI)	8.2 (6.9–10.0)	8.3 (7.0–8.8)	HR 0.77 (95% CI 0.65–0.90); P = 0.0014
PFS rate at 30 months—% (95% CI)	28 (23–33)	12 (8–16)	—
Survival in intermediate- or poor-risk patients with <1% PD-L1 expression (N = 284 in nivolumab + ipilimumab arm, N = 100 in sunitinib arm)			
Median OS*—months (95% CI)	NR (28.2–NE)	NR (24.0–NE)	HR 0.73 (95% CI 0.56–0.96)
OS rate at 12 months*—% (95% CI)	80 (75–84)	75 (70–80)	—
OS rate at 18 months*—% (95% CI)	74 (69–79)	64 (58–70)	—
Median PFS*—months	11.0	10.4	HR 1.00 (95% CI 0.80–1.26)
Survival in intermediate- or poor-risk patients with ≥1% PD-L1 expression (N = 100 in nivolumab + ipilimumab arm, N = 114 in sunitinib arm)			
Median OS*—months (95% CI)	NR (NE–NE)	19.6 (14.8–NE)	HR 0.45 (95% CI 0.29–0.71)
OS rate at 12 months*—% (95% CI)	86 (77–91)	66 (56–74)	—
OS rate at 18 months*—% (95% CI)	81 (71–87)	53 (43–62)	—
Median PFS*—months	22.8	5.9	HR 0.46 (95% CI 0.31–0.67)
Survival in favorable-risk patients (N = 125 in nivolumab + ipilimumab arm, N = 124 in sunitinib arm)			
Median OS*—months (95% CI)	NR (NE–NE)	NR (NE–NE)	HR 1.22 (95% CI 0.73–2.04); P = 0.44
Median PFS*—months (95% CI)	13.9 (9.9–17.9)	19.9 (15.1–23.5)	HR 1.23 (95% CI 0.90–1.69); P = 0.19
OS rate at 30 months*—% (95% CI)	80 (72–86)	85 (77–90)	—
PFS rate at 30 months*—% (95% CI)	29 (21–38)	35 (26–34)	—

(continued)

Efficacy (N = 1096) (continued)

Response

CR, ITT population—n/N (%)	58/550 (11)	10/546 (2)	—
ORR, ITT population†—n/N (%) [95% CI]	227/550 (41) [37–46]	186/546 (34) [30–38]	P = 0.015
Median DOR*—months (95% CI)	NR (24.7–NE)	18.0 (13.8–22.2)	HR 0.51 (95% CI 0.38–0.68)
CR, intermediate or poor risk—n/N (%)	48/425 (11)	5/422 (1)	—
ORR, intermediate or poor risk†—n/N (%) [95% CI]	178/425 (42) [37–47]	126/422 (29) [25–34]	P = 0.0001
ORR, intermediate or poor risk with <1% PD-L1 expression*†—% (95% CI)	37 (32–43)	28 (23–34)	P = 0.0252
ORR, intermediate or poor risk with ≥1% PD-L1 expression*† —% (95% CI)	58 (48–68)	22 (15–31)	P <0.001
CR, favorable risk*—n/N (%)	10/125 (8)	5/124 (4)	—
ORR, favorable risk*†—n/N (%) [95% CI]	49/125 (39) [31–48]	62/124 (50) [41–59]	P = 0.14

*Exploratory analyses
†Response rate exact two-sided CIs and P values were determined using the Clopper-Pearson method
ITT, intention to treat; OS, overall survival; CI, confidence interval; NR, not reached; NE, not estimable; HR, hazard ratio; PFS, progression-free survival; CR, complete response; ORR, overall response rate
Note: patients in this study were randomized to treatment groups using block stratification according to International Metastatic Renal Cell Carcinoma Database Consortium (IMDC) prognostic risk score (favorable = 0, intermediate = 1–2, poor = 3–6), and geographical region (USA vs Canada and Europe vs rest of the world). All stratified analyses were adjusted according to these strata, where applicable. Of the 550 patients randomized to ipilimumab + nivolumab and 546 patients randomized to sunitinib, 547 and 535 patients received their assigned study drug, respectively. Among these groups, 425 and 422 patients had intermediate or poor risk and 125 and 124 had favorable risk, respectively. Treatment groups had similar baseline characteristics, but baseline PD-L1 expression was lower and the incidence of previous nephrectomy was higher in both treatment groups in favorable-risk patients than in intermediate- or poor-risk patients or in the full intention-to-treat population, which included all patients randomized. Overall survival, progression-free survival, and duration of response were estimated with the Kaplan-Meier method; CIs and HRs were calculated for these outcomes using a stratified Cox proportional hazards model, and P values were calculated using two-sided stratified log-rank tests. All data in this table except for subgroup analyses according to PD-L1 expression were reported in an updated publication, Motzer RJ et al. Lancet Oncol 2019;20:1370–85. The median follow-up was 32.4 months (IQR, 13.4–36.3; minimum, 30 months) for overall survival. PD-L1 expression subgroup analyses were reported in the original publication, Motzer RJ et al. N Engl J Med 2018;378:1277–1290, or its supplementary appendix. In this paper, the median follow-up was 25.2 months (minimum 17.5) for overall survival. Response rates, progression-free survival, and duration of response were determined by the investigator according to RECIST v1.1 criteria except for analyses of PD-L1 expression subgroups, which were evaluated by an independent radiology review committee (IRRC). All outcomes related to response were also reported in the original paper, but were evaluated by an IRRC; these data were not included in the table except for PD-L1 subgroups

Adverse Events (N = 1082)

Event	Nivolumab + Ipilimumab (N = 547)		Sunitinib (N = 535)	
Treatment-related adverse events leading to discontinuation	22%		12%	
Treatment-related death*	8 deaths		4 deaths	

	Grade 1–2 (%)	Grade 3–4 (%)	Grade 1–2 (%)	Grade 3–4 (%)
All events	47	46	35	63
Fatigue	33	4	40	9
Pruritis	28	<1	9	0
Diarrhea	23	4	47	5
Rash	20	1	13	0
Nausea	18	1	37	1
Increased lipase level	6	10	4	7
Hypothyroidism	15	<1	25	<1

(continued)

Adverse Events (N = 1082) (continued)

	Grade 1–2 (%)	Grade 3–4 (%)	Grade 1–2 (%)	Grade 3–4 (%)
Decreased appetite	12	1	24	<1
Asthenia	12	1	15	2
Vomiting	10	<1	19	2
Anemia	6	<1	11	4
Dysgeusia	6	0	33	<1
Stomatitis	4	0	25	3
Dyspepsia	3	0	18	0
Mucosal inflammation	2	0	26	3
Hypertension	1	<1	24	16
Palmar-plantar erythrodysesthesia	<1	0	34	9
Thrombocytopenia	<1	0	13	5

Adverse events were included in the table if they were reported in ≥15% of patients in either group and were considered by the investigators to be related to treatment. Adverse effects were graded according to the National Cancer Institute Common Terminology Criteria for Adverse Events (NCI-CTCAE) v4.0 in patients who received at least one dose of their assigned treatment

*Causes of death in the nivolumab + ipilimumab group were pneumonitis, pneumonia and aplastic anemia, immune-mediated bronchitis, lower gastrointestinal hemorrhage, the hemophagocytic syndrome, sudden death, liver toxic effects, and lung infection (1 each); in the sunitinib group deaths were due to cardiac arrest (2), heart failure (1), and multiple organ failure (1)

Immune-mediated adverse events occurred in 436 patients in the nivolumab + ipilimumab group and 35% of those patients received high-dose glucocorticoids (≥40 mg of prednisone equivalents per day) in response. All adverse event data included in the table were reported in Motzer RJ et al. N Engl J Med 2018;378:1277–1290

Therapy Monitoring

1. Monitor patients for signs and symptoms of infusion-related reactions including pyrexia, chills, flushing, hypotension, dyspnea, wheezing, back pain, abdominal pain, and urticaria
2. Initially at the time of each dose, and eventually every 6–12 weeks, perform a total body skin examination with attention to *all* mucous membranes as well as a complete review of systems
3. Monitor patients for signs and symptoms of pneumonitis. Evaluate patients with suspected pneumonitis with chest x-ray, CT, and pulse oximetry. For ≥2 toxicity, may include nasal swab, sputum culture and sensitivity, blood culture and sensitivity, and urine culture and sensitivity
4. Monitor patients for signs and symptoms of colitis. Encourage patients to report diarrhea immediately to any member of the health care team
5. Draw AST, ALT, and bilirubin prior to each infusion and/or weekly if there are Grade 1 liver function test elevations. Note, no treatment is recommended for G1 LFT abnormalities. For ≥2 toxicity, work up for other causes of elevated LFTs including viral hepatitis
6. Use basic metabolic panel (Na, K, CO_2, glucose) and patient history as screening tools for hypophysitis including hypopituitarism and adrenal insufficiency. If in doubt, evaluate AM adrenocorticotropic hormone (ACTH) and cortisol levels. Consider ACTH stimulation test for indeterminate results
7. Assess thyroid function at the start of treatment, periodically during treatment, and as indicated based on clinical evaluation, and for clinical signs and symptoms of thyroid disorders. Test for TSH and free thyroxine (FT4) every 4–6 weeks as part of routine clinical monitoring of therapy or for case detection in symptomatic patients
8. Measure glucose at baseline and with each treatment during the first 12 weeks and every 6 weeks thereafter
9. Obtain a serum creatinine prior to every dose. If creatinine is found to be newly elevated, consider holding therapy while other potential causes are evaluated. Note, routine urinalysis is not necessary other than to rule out urinary tract infections, etc
10. Obtain a complete rheumatologic history and perform an examination of all peripheral joints for tenderness, swelling, and range of motion. Examine the spine. Consider plain x-ray/imaging to exclude metastases and evaluate joint damage (erosions), if appropriate
11. In patients at high risk for infections and in appropriately selected patients based on an infectious disease evaluation, draw screening laboratories (HIV, hepatitis A and B, and blood QuantiFERON for TB) to prepare patients to start infliximab

METASTATIC • CLEAR-CELL • FIRST-LINE
RENAL CELL CARCINOMA REGIMEN: AVELUMAB + AXITINIB

Motzer RJ et al. N Engl J Med 2019;380:1103–1115
Protocol for: Motzer RJ et al. N Engl J Med 2019;380:1103–1115
Supplementary appendix to: Motzer RJ et al. N Engl J Med 2019;380:1103–1115
BAVENCIO (avelumab) prescribing information. Rockland, MA: EMD Serono, Inc; revised May 2019
INLYTA (axitinib) prescribing information. New York, NY: Pfizer Labs; revised January 2020

Premedications for avelumab:
Acetaminophen 500–650 mg; administer orally 30–60 minutes prior to starting avelumab administration
Diphenhydramine 25–50 mg (or an equivalent H_1 antihistamine); administer orally 30–60 minutes *or* intravenously 30 minutes prior to starting avelumab administration
• Primary prophylaxis against infusion-related reactions is given during the first 4 avelumab doses
• Premedication after the fourth avelumab dose may be administered based upon clinical judgment and the presence and severity of infusion-related reactions encountered during previously administered avelumab doses
Avelumab 800 mg; administer intravenously over 60 minutes in 250 mL 0.9% sodium chloride injection or 0.45% sodium chloride injection, every 2 weeks (total dosage/cycle = 800 mg)

Notes:
• Administer avelumab with an administration set that contains a sterile, nonpyrogenic, low-protein-binding in-line filter with pore size of 0.2 μm
• Avelumab can cause severe or life-threatening infusion-related reactions
  ▪ Monitor patients for signs and symptoms of infusion-related reactions, including pyrexia, chills, flushing, hypotension, dyspnea, wheezing, back pain, abdominal pain, and urticaria
    ○ Infusion-related reactions have included severe (G3) and life-threatening (G4) reactions after premedication with an antihistamine and acetaminophen
    ○ Infusion-related reactions may occur after avelumab administration is completed
  ▪ Interrupt or slow the administration rate for mild or moderate infusion-related reactions
  ▪ *Stop* administration and permanently discontinue avelumab for G ≥3 severity infusion-related reactions

Axitinib 5 mg; administer orally twice daily (approximately every 12 hours), continually, until disease progression (total dose/week = 70 mg)

Notes:
• Axitinib should be swallowed whole (no breaking, crushing, or chewing) with water
• Axitinib may be administered without respect to food ingestion
• Advise patients to avoid grapefruit products while taking axitinib
• Instruct patients who vomit or miss a dose of axitinib to avoid taking an additional dose. Take the next prescribed dose at the usual time
• Patients who tolerate axitinib for at least 6 consecutive weeks with no adverse reactions G >2, who remain normotensive (blood pressure ≤150/90 mm Hg), and are not receiving anti-hypertension medications may have their dose increased to 7 mg twice daily, and further to 10 mg twice daily using the same criteria
• Avoid use of concomitant strong CYP3A4/5 inhibitors. If a strong CYP3A4/5 inhibitor must be co-administered, a dose decrease of axitinib by approximately half is recommended. Subsequent doses can be increased or decreased based on individual safety and tolerability. If co-administration of a strong inhibitor is discontinued, the axitinib dose should be returned (after 3–5 elimination half-lives of the inhibitor) to that used prior to initiation of the strong CYP3A4/5 inhibitor
• The axitinib starting dose should be reduced by approximately half in patients with baseline moderate hepatic impairment (Child-Pugh class B)
• If axitinib is interrupted, patients receiving antihypertensive medications should be monitored for hypotension. The plasma half-life of axitinib is 2–4 hours and blood pressure usually decreases within 1–2 days following dose interruption

Antiemetic prophylaxis
Emetogenic potential of axitinib is **MINIMAL TO LOW**
Emetogenic potential of avelumab is **MINIMAL**
See Chapter 42 for antiemetic recommendations

Hematopoietic growth factor (CSF) prophylaxis
Primary prophylaxis is **NOT** indicated
See Chapter 43 for more information

Antimicrobial prophylaxis
Risk of fever and neutropenia is **LOW**
  Antimicrobial primary prophylaxis to be considered:
  • Antibacterial—not indicated
  • Antifungal—not indicated
  • Antiviral—not indicated unless patient previously had an episode of HSV

(continued)

(continued)

Diarrhea management
Latent or delayed-onset diarrhea*:
    Loperamide 4 mg orally initially after the first loose or liquid stool, *then* 2–4 mg orally every 2–4 hours or **diphenoxylate hydrochloride** 2.5 mg with **atropine sulfate** 0.025 mg (eg, Lomotil)

*Abigerges D et al. J Natl Cancer Inst 1994;86:446–449
Rothenberg ML et al. J Clin Oncol 2001;19:3801–3807
Wadler S et al. J Clin Oncol 1998;16:3169–3178

Treatment Modifications

RECOMMENDED DOSE MODIFICATIONS FOR AXITINIB

Dose level +2	10 mg orally twice per day
Dose level +1	7 mg orally twice per day
Starting dose (level 1)	5 mg orally twice per day
Dose level −1	3 mg orally twice per day
Dose level −2	2 mg orally twice per day
Dose level −3	Discontinue axitinib*

Grade/Severity	Treatment Modification
The patient has tolerated axitinib at a dose of 5 mg twice per day for ≥2 weeks without G >2 treatment-related adverse reactions, is normotensive (blood pressure ≤150/90 mm Hg), and is not receiving anti-hypertension medication	Increase the dose of axitinib to dose level +1 (7 mg orally twice per day)
The patient has tolerated axitinib at a dose of 7 mg twice per day for ≥2 weeks without G >2 treatment-related adverse reactions, is normotensive (blood pressure ≤150/90 mm Hg), and is not receiving anti-hypertension medication	Increase the dose of axitinib to dose level +2 (10 mg orally twice per day)
Any hypertension	Treat as needed with standard anti-hypertensive therapy
Persistent hypertension despite use of maximal anti-hypertensive medications	Reduce the dosage of axitinib by 1 dosage level
Evidence of hypertensive crisis	Discontinue axitinib*
Urine dipstick >1+ for protein	Continue axitinib at the same dose pending results of a 24-hour urine protein
Urine protein ≥3 g/24 hours	Withhold axitinib until urine protein is <3 g/24 hours, then resume axitinib at 1 lower dose level*
Grade 3 diarrhea (not immune-related)	Optimize antidiarrheal regimen and reduce the dose of axitinib by 1 dose level
Grade 4 diarrhea (not immune-related)	Withhold axitinib until recovery to G ≤1, then resume axitinib with the dose reduced by 1 dose level and with optimization of the antidiarrheal regimen
Grade 2 AST, ALT, or bilirubin elevation (not immune-related)	Increase the frequency of LFT monitoring. Withhold axitinib until improvement to G ≤1 or baseline, then resume axitinib at the same dosage
Grade ≥3 AST, ALT, or bilirubin elevation (not immune-related)	Increase the frequency of LFT monitoring. Withhold axitinib until improvement to G ≤1 or baseline, then resume axitinib with the dosage reduced by 1 dose level
Bleeding occurs which requires medical intervention	Withhold axitinib until resolution of bleeding*
Patient requires elective surgery	Withhold axitinib for ≥2 days prior to elective surgery. Do not resume axitinib for at least 2 weeks following major surgery and until adequate wound healing has occurred*

(continued)

Treatment Modifications (*continued*)

Grade/Severity	Treatment Modification
RPLS is suspected (symptoms of headache, seizure, lethargy, confusion, blindness, and/or other visual and neurologic disturbances along with hypertension of any severity)	Withhold axitinib until clarification of the patient's neurologic status (ie, with an emergent brain MRI) has occurred*
RPLS is confirmed	Discontinue axitinib.* The safety of reinitiating axitinib in a patient who has experienced RPLS is unknown.
Patient has moderate hepatic impairment (Child-Pugh class B)	Decrease the starting dose of axitinib by approximately 50% and then increase or decrease the dose based on individual safety and tolerability
Patient requires concomitant use of a strong CYP3A4/5 inhibitor (eg, ketoconazole, itraconazole, posaconazole, clarithromycin, atazanavir, indinavir, nefazodone, nelfinavir, ritonavir, saquinavir, telithromycin, and voriconazole)	If concomitant use of the CYP3A4/5 inhibitor is unavoidable, then decrease the dose of axitinib by approximately 50% and then increase or decrease the dose based on individual safety and tolerability. If the strong CYP3A4/5 inhibitor is subsequently discontinued, then resume the axitinib dose that was used prior to initiation of the CYP3A4/5 inhibitor after 3–5 CYP3A4/5 inhibitor half-lives have transpired
Patient requires concomitant use of a moderate or strong CYP3A4/5 inducer (eg, rifampin, dexamethasone, phenytoin, carbamazepine, rifabutin, rifapentine, phenobarbital, St. John's Wort, bosentan, efavirenz, etravirine, modafinil, nafcillin)	Avoid concomitant use of a moderate or strong CYP3A4/5 inducer with axitinib

*If the patient is receiving antihypertensive medications, monitor closely for development of hypotension if axitinib is withheld or discontinued
AST, aspartate aminotransferase; ALT, alanine aminotransferase; LFT, liver function test; RPLS, reversible posterior leukoencephalopathy syndrome; MRI, magnetic resonance imaging

RECOMMENDED DOSE MODIFICATIONS FOR AVELUMAB

Adverse Event	Grade/Severity	Treatment Modification
Infusion reaction	Clinically significant but not severe infusion reaction	Interrupt the infusion in patients with clinically significant infusion reactions and consider resuming at a slower rate following resolution. If decision is made to restart, begin at ≤50% of the rate prior to the reaction and increase in 50% increments every 30 minutes if well tolerated. Infusions may be restarted at the full rate during the next cycle
	G3/4 (severe infusion reaction—pyrexia, chills, flushing, hypotension, dyspnea, wheezing, back pain, abdominal pain, and urticaria). Not rapidly responsive to brief interruption of infusion	Stop infusion and administer appropriate medical therapy (eg, epinephrine, corticosteroids, intravenous antihistamines, bronchodilators, and/or oxygen). Discontinue avelumab
Colitis	G1	Loperamide 4 mg as starting dose, then 2 mg before each meal and after each loose stool until without diarrhea for 12 hours, with maximum of 16 mg loperamide per day. If G1 diarrhea or colitis persists >14 days, add prednisolone 0.5–1 mg/kg (non–enteric coated) or consider oral budesonide 9 mg daily if no bloody diarrhea
	G2/3 diarrhea or colitis	Withhold avelumab. Loperamide 4 mg as starting dose, then 2 mg before each meal and after each loose stool until without diarrhea for 12 hours, with maximum of 16 mg loperamide per day. Administer oral prednisone/prednisolone at a dosage of 0.5–2 mg/kg/day or its equivalent. When symptoms improve to G1, begin a slow corticosteroid taper over at least 4 weeks. Resume avelumab upon symptom control, or when prednisone/prednisolone daily dose <10 mg
	G4 diarrhea or colitis	Permanently discontinue avelumab. Loperamide 4 mg as starting dose, then 2 mg before each meal and after each loose stool until without diarrhea for 12 hours, with maximum of 16 mg loperamide per day. Administer 1–2 mg/kg intravenous (methyl)prednisolone and convert to 0.5–2 mg/kg prednisone/prednisolone orally each day or its equivalent only after a response. Taper over at least 4 weeks when symptoms improve. If symptoms do not improve over 72 hours or worsen, perform flexible sigmoidoscopy/colonoscopy to document colitis, then begin infliximab 5 mg/kg (if no perforation, sepsis, TB, hepatitis, NYHA III/IV CHF). If no response, add MMF 500–1000 mg twice daily. If worse on MMF, consider addition of tacrolimus or ATG

(*continued*)

Treatment Modifications (*continued*)

Adverse Event	Grade/Severity	Treatment Modification
Pneumonitis	G2	Withhold avelumab. Start *Pneumocystis* prophylaxis (while patient is receiving a glucocorticoid dose equivalent to ≥20 mg of prednisone daily for 4 weeks or longer) and coverage with empiric antibiotics. Administer oral prednisone/prednisolone at a dosage of 1–2 mg/kg/day or its equivalent. When symptoms improve to G1, begin a slow corticosteroid taper over at least 4 weeks. If response is not adequate after 48 hours, administer 2–4 mg/kg intravenous (methyl)prednisolone and convert to 0.5–2 mg/kg prednisone/prednisolone orally each day or its equivalent only after a response, followed by a taper over at least 6 weeks when symptoms improve to G1, titrating to symptoms. Resume avelumab upon symptom control, or when prednisone/prednisolone daily dose <10 mg
	G3/4	Permanently discontinue avelumab. Start *Pneumocystis* prophylaxis (while patient is receiving a glucocorticoid dose equivalent to ≥20 mg of prednisone daily for 4 weeks or longer); cover with empiric antibiotics. Administer 2–4 mg/kg intravenous (methyl)prednisolone and convert to 1–2 mg/kg prednisone/prednisolone orally each day or its equivalent only after a response, followed by a taper over at least 8 weeks when symptoms improve to G1, titrating to symptoms. If, when initially treated, improvement does not occur within 48–72 hours, begin infliximab 5 mg/kg (if no perforation, sepsis, TB, hepatitis, NYHA III/IV CHF). If no response to infliximab, add MMF 500–1000 mg twice daily. Consider MMF, especially if concurrent hepatic toxicity
Hepatitis	G2 (AST or ALT >3–5× ULN or total bilirubin >1.5–3× ULN)	Withhold avelumab. Administer oral prednisone/prednisolone at a dosage of 1–2 mg/kg/day or its equivalent. When symptoms improve to G1, begin a slow corticosteroid taper over at least 4 weeks. Resume avelumab upon symptom control, or when prednisone/prednisolone daily dose <10 mg
	G3/4 (AST or ALT >5× ULN or total bilirubin >3× ULN)	Permanently discontinue avelumab. Administer 1–2 mg/kg intravenous (methyl)prednisolone and convert to 0.5–2 mg/kg prednisone/prednisolone orally each day or its equivalent only after a response. Taper over at least 6 weeks when symptoms improve. If no response, add MMF 500–1000 mg twice daily. If worse on MMF, consider adding tacrolimus or ATG
Hypophysitis	G2/3 (moderate symptoms, ie, headache but no visual disturbance or fatigue/mood alteration but hemodynamically stable, no electrolyte disturbance)	Administer analgesia as needed for headache. Withhold avelumab. Administer oral prednisone/prednisolone at a dosage of 0.5–2 mg/kg/day or its equivalent. When symptoms improve to G1, begin a slow corticosteroid taper over at least 4 weeks. If no improvement in 48 hours, administer 1–2 mg/kg intravenous (methyl)prednisolone and convert to 0.5–2 mg/kg prednisone/prednisolone orally each day or its equivalent only after a response. Taper over at least 4 weeks when symptoms improve to 5 mg prednisone/prednisolone or equivalent; do not stop steroids. Resume avelumab upon symptom control, or when prednisone/prednisolone daily dose <10 mg
	G4 (severe mass effect symptoms, ie, severe headache, any visual disturbance, or severe hypoadrenalism, ie, hypotension, severe electrolyte disturbance)	Permanently discontinue avelumab. Administer analgesia as needed for headache. Administer 1–2 mg/kg intravenous (methyl)prednisolone and convert to 0.5–2 mg/kg prednisone/prednisolone orally each day or its equivalent only after a response. Taper over at least 4 weeks when symptoms improve to 5 mg prednisone/prednisolone or equivalent; do not stop steroids
Adrenal insufficiency	G2	Withhold avelumab. Administer oral prednisone/prednisolone at a dosage of 0.5–2 mg/kg/day or its equivalent. When symptoms improve to G1, begin a slow corticosteroid taper over at least 4 weeks. Serially assess adrenal function and continue steroids at replacement doses (20–40 mg hydrocortisone daily ~2/3 dose in morning upon awakening and ~1/3 at 4 PM) until recovery of adrenal function is documented. Resume avelumab upon symptom control, or when prednisone/prednisolone daily dose <10 mg
	G3/4	Permanently discontinue avelumab. Administer oral prednisone/prednisolone at a dosage of 0.5–2 mg/kg/day or its equivalent. When improves to G1, begin a slow corticosteroid taper over at least 4 weeks. Serially assess adrenal function and continue steroids at replacement doses (20–40 mg hydrocortisone daily ~2/3 dose in morning upon awakening and ~1/3 at 4 PM) until recovery of adrenal function is documented

(*continued*)

Treatment Modifications (*continued*)

Adverse Event	Grade/Severity	Treatment Modification
Type 1 diabetes mellitus	G3 hyperglycemia	Withhold avelumab. Admit to hospital to manage hyperglycemia. Role of corticosteroids in preventing complete loss of insulin-producing cells is unknown and not recommended. Resume avelumab upon symptom control, or when prednisone/prednisolone daily dose <10 mg
	G4 hyperglycemia	Permanently discontinue avelumab. Admit to hospital to manage hyperglycemia. Role of corticosteroids in preventing complete loss of insulin-producing cells is unknown and use is not recommended
Nephritis and renal dysfunction	G2/3 (serum creatinine 1.5–6× ULN)	Withhold avelumab. Administer oral prednisone/prednisolone at a dosage of 0.5–2 mg/kg/day or its equivalent. When symptoms improve to G1, begin a slow corticosteroid taper over at least 4 weeks. If response is not adequate, administer 0.5–1 mg/kg intravenous (methyl)prednisolone and convert to 0.5–2 mg/kg prednisone/prednisolone orally each day or its equivalent only after a response, followed by a taper over at least 4 weeks when symptoms improve to G1. Resume avelumab upon symptom control, or when prednisone/prednisolone daily dose <10 mg
	G4 (serum creatinine >6× ULN)	Permanently discontinue avelumab. Administer 0.5–1 mg/kg intravenous (methyl)prednisolone and convert to 0.5–2 mg/kg prednisone/prednisolone orally each day or its equivalent only after a response, followed by a taper over at least 4 weeks when symptoms improve to G1
Skin	G1/2	Continue avelumab. Avoid skin irritants, avoid sun exposure; topical emollients recommended. Topical steroid (mild strength for G1, moderate/potent strength for G2) cream once or twice daily ± oral or topical antihistamines for itching
	G3 rash or suspected SJS or TEN	Withhold avelumab. Avoid skin irritants, avoid sun exposure; topical emollients recommended. Administer oral or topical antihistamines for itching. Administer oral prednisone/prednisolone at a dosage of 0.5–2 mg/kg or its equivalent daily for 3 days followed by a slow corticosteroid taper over at least 4 weeks when the rash improves to G1. If rash does not respond adequately, administer 0.5–1 mg/kg intravenous (methyl)prednisolone and convert to 0.5–2 mg/kg prednisone/prednisolone orally each day or its equivalent only after a response, followed by a taper over at least 4 weeks when the rash improves to G1. Resume avelumab upon symptom control, or when prednisone/prednisolone daily dose <10 mg
	G4 rash or confirmed SJS or TEN	Avoid skin irritants, avoid sun exposure; topical emollients recommended. Administer oral or topical antihistamines for itching. Administer 1–2 mg/kg intravenous (methyl)prednisolone and convert to oral steroids 0.5–2 mg/kg prednisone/prednisolone each day or its equivalent only after a response. Taper over at least 4 weeks when the rash improves to G1. Permanently discontinue avelumab
Encephalitis	Confusion or altered behavior, headaches, alteration in Glasgow Coma Scale, motor or sensory deficits, speech abnormality; may or may not be febrile	Initially withhold avelumab, but permanently discontinue avelumab if there is no doubt as to diagnosis. Exclude bacterial and ideally viral infections prior to high-dose steroids. Administer 1–2 mg/kg intravenous (methyl)prednisolone for 5 days or oral prednisone/prednisolone at a dosage of 0.5–2 mg/kg/day or its equivalent. When symptoms improve, begin a slow corticosteroid taper over at least 4–8 weeks. If symptoms are severe, administer 1–2 mg/kg intravenous (methyl)prednisolone and convert to 0.5–2 mg/kg prednisone/prednisolone orally each day or its equivalent only after a response. Consider concurrent empiric antiviral (intravenous acyclovir) and antibacterial therapy
Aseptic meningitis	Headache, photophobia, neck stiffness with fever, or may be afebrile, vomiting; normal cognition/cerebral function (distinguishes from encephalitis)	

Other syndromes include neurosarcoidosis, posterior reversible leukoencephalopathy syndrome (PRES), Vogt-Koyanagi-Harada syndrome, demyelination, vasculitic encephalopathy, and generalized seizures

Transverse myelitis	Acute or subacute neurologic signs/symptoms of motor, sensory, autonomic origin; most have sensory level; often bilateral symptoms	Initially withhold avelumab, but permanently discontinue avelumab if there is no doubt as to diagnosis. Administer 2 mg/kg intravenous (methyl)prednisolone or consider 1 g/day and convert to 0.5–2 mg/kg prednisone/prednisolone orally each day or its equivalent only after a response. When symptoms improve, begin a slow corticosteroid taper over at least 4–8 weeks. Plasmapheresis may be required if steroids do not bring about improvement

(*continued*)

Treatment Modifications (continued)

Adverse Event	Grade/Severity	Treatment Modification
Myocarditis	G3	Permanently discontinue avelumab. Administer 2 mg/kg intravenous (methyl)prednisolone or consider 1 g/day and convert to 0.5–2 mg/kg prednisone/prednisolone orally each day or its equivalent only after a response. When symptoms improve, begin a slow corticosteroid taper over at least 4–8 weeks. If no response, add MMF 500–1000 mg twice daily. If worse on MMF, consider adding tacrolimus
Peripheral neurologic toxicity	Moderate: some interference with ADL, symptoms concerning to patient	Withhold avelumab. Initial observation reasonable or initiate prednisone/prednisolone 0.5–1 mg/kg (if progressing, eg, from mild) and/or pregabalin or duloxetine for pain. When symptoms improve, begin a slow corticosteroid taper over at least 4 weeks. Resume avelumab upon symptom control, or when prednisone/prednisolone daily dose <10 mg
	Severe: limits self-care and aids warranted, life-threatening, eg, respiratory problems	Permanently discontinue avelumab. Administer 1–2 mg/kg intravenous (methyl)prednisolone and convert to 0.5–2 mg/kg prednisone/prednisolone orally each day or its equivalent only after a response. Taper over at least 4–8 weeks when symptoms improve to G1
Guillain-Barré syndrome	Progressive symmetrical muscle weakness with absent or reduced tendon reflexes—involves extremities; facial, respiratory, and bulbar and oculomotor muscles; dysregulation of autonomic nerves	Permanently discontinue avelumab. Use of steroids not recommended in idiopathic Guillain-Barré syndrome; however, a trial of (methyl)prednisolone 1–2 mg/kg is reasonable, converting to 0.5–2 mg/kg prednisone/prednisolone orally each day or its equivalent only after a response. If no improvement or worsening, plasmapheresis or IVIG indicated
Myasthenia gravis	Fluctuating muscle weakness (proximal limb, trunk, ocular, eg, ptosis/diplopia or bulbar) with fatigability; respiratory muscles may also be involved	Permanently discontinue avelumab. Administer pyridostigmine at an initial dose of 30 mg 3 times daily. Administer oral prednisone/prednisolone at a dosage of 0.5–2 mg/kg/day or its equivalent or 1–2 mg/kg intravenous (methyl)prednisolone, depending on the severity of symptoms. If treatment begins with intravenous drug, convert to 0.5–2 mg/kg prednisone/prednisolone orally each day or its equivalent only after a response. If no improvement or worsening, plasmapheresis or IVIG may be considered. Additional immunosuppressants used in myasthenia gravis include azathioprine, cyclosporine, and mycophenolate. Avoid certain medications, eg, ciprofloxacin, beta-blockers, that may precipitate cholinergic crisis

Other syndromes, including motor and sensory peripheral neuropathy, multifocal radicular neuropathy/plexopathy, autonomic neuropathy, phrenic nerve palsy, cranial nerve palsies (eg, facial nerve, optic nerve, hypoglossal nerve)

Arthralgia	G1 (mild pain with inflammation, erythema, or joint swelling)	Continue avelumab. Administer acetaminophen (paracetamol) and ibuprofen
	G2 (moderate pain with inflammation, erythema, or joint swelling that limits ADLs)	Withhold avelumab. Administer higher doses of acetaminophen (paracetamol) and ibuprofen and use diclofenac or naproxen or etoricoxib. If inadequately controlled, consider intra-articular steroid injections for large joints or administer oral prednisone/prednisolone at a dosage of 0.5–2 mg/kg/day or its equivalent. When symptoms improve to G1, begin a slow corticosteroid taper over at least 4 weeks. If response is not adequate, administer 0.5–1 mg/kg intravenous (methyl)prednisolone and convert to 0.5–2 mg/kg prednisone/prednisolone orally each day or its equivalent only after a response, followed by a taper over at least 4 weeks when symptoms improve to G1. Resume avelumab upon symptom control, or when prednisone/prednisolone daily dose <10 mg
	G3 (severe pain; irreversible joint damage; disabling; limits self-care ADLs)	Withhold avelumab. Administer 0.5–1 mg/kg intravenous (methyl)prednisolone and convert to 0.5–2 mg/kg prednisone/prednisolone orally each day or its equivalent only after a response, followed by a taper over at least 4 weeks when symptoms improve to G1. In severe cases, infliximab or another anti–TNF alpha drug may be required for improvement of arthritis. Resume avelumab upon symptom control, or when prednisone/prednisolone daily dose <10 mg

(continued)

Treatment Modifications (*continued*)

Adverse Event	Grade/Severity	Treatment Modification
Other	First occurrence of other G3	Withhold avelumab. Administer oral prednisone/prednisolone at a dosage of 0.5–2 mg/kg/day or its equivalent. When symptoms improve to G1, begin a slow corticosteroid taper over at least 4 weeks. Resume avelumab upon symptom control, or when prednisone/prednisolone daily dose <10 mg
	Recurrence of same G3	Permanently discontinue avelumab. Administer 1–2 mg/kg intravenous (methyl)prednisolone and convert to 0.5–2 mg/kg prednisone/prednisolone orally each day or its equivalent only after a response. Taper over at least 4–8 weeks when symptoms improve to G1
	Life-threatening or G4	
	Requirement for ≥10 mg/day prednisone or equivalent for >12 weeks	Permanently discontinue avelumab
	Persistent G2/3 adverse reactions lasting ≥12 weeks	

ADL, activities of daily living; ALT, alanine aminotransferase; AST, aspartate aminotransferase; ATG, anti–thymocyte globulin; IVIG, intravenous immunoglobulin; MMF, mycophenolate mofetil; NYHA, New York Heart Association; SJS, Stevens-Johnson syndrome; TEN, toxic epidermal necrolysis; ULN, upper limit of normal

Notes on general supportive care: Steroid taper in most cases will proceed over a minimum of 1 month, but if symptoms improve rapidly, a 2-week taper can be considered. If steroids are administered for more than 4 weeks, administer PCP prophylaxis (cotrimoxazole 480 mg twice daily M/W/F or inhaled pentamidine if cotrimoxazole allergy), regular random blood glucose, Vitamin D level, and starting calcium/Vitamin D supplementation per guidelines

Patient Population Studied

This randomized, stratified, open-label phase 3 trial included 886 adult patients with previously untreated, advanced RCC and compared treatment with avelumab plus axitinib to sunitinib. Patients were eligible if they had advanced RCC with a clear cell component, ≥1 measurable lesion, an ECOG PS of 0 or 1, and adequate organ function. Patients were excluded if they had active CNS metastases, an autoimmune disease, or current or previous use of glucocorticoids or other immunosuppressants within 7 days before randomization

Efficacy (N = 886)

	Avelumab + Axitinib (N = 442)	Sunitinib (N = 444)	—
Median progression-free survival, patients with PD-L1–positive tumors (N = 560)*†	13.8 months (95% CI 11.1–NE)	7.2 months (95% CI 5.7–9.7)	HR 0.61 (95% CI 0.47–0.79); P <0.001; repeated CI 0.43–0.92
Overall survival rate at data cutoff, patients with PD-L1–positive tumors (N = 560)*†	86.3%	84.8%	HR 0.82 (95% CI 0.53–1.28); P = 0.38; repeated CI 0.46–2.40
Median progression-free survival, all patients	13.8 months (95% CI 11.1–NE)	8.4 months (95% CI 6.9–11.1)	HR 0.69 (95% CI 0.56–0.84); P <0.001
Overall survival rate at data cutoff, all patients	85.7%	83.1%	HR 0.78 (95% CI 0.55–1.08); P = 0.14
Objective response rate, patients with PD-L1–positive tumors (N = 560)*	55.2% (95% CI 49.0–61.2)	25.5% (95% CI 20.6–30.9)	OR 3.73 (95% CI 2.53–5.37)
Complete response rate, patients with PD-L1–positive tumors (N = 560)*	4.4%	2.1%	—
Objective response rate, all patients	51.4% (95% CI 46.6–56.1)	25.7% (95% CI 21.7–30.0)	OR 3.10 (95% CI 2.30–4.15)
Complete response rate, all patients	3.4%	1.8%	—

(*continued*)

Efficacy (N = 886) (continued)

	Avelumab + Axitinib (N = 442)	Sunitinib (N = 444)	—
Objective response rate, favorable-risk patients[‡]	68.1%	37.5%	OR 3.56 (95% CI 1.87–6.77)
Objective response rate, intermediate-risk patients[‡]	51.3%	25.4%	OR 3.10 (95% CI 2.13–4.52)
Objective response rate, poor-risk patients[‡]	30.6%	11.3%	OR 3.47 (95% CI 1.33–9.72)

*PD-L1 status was considered positive when ≥1% of immune cells stained positive for PD-L1 within the tumor area of the tested sample for a given patient. The staining was performed and assessed at a central laboratory using the Ventana PD-L1 (SP263) assay. Of 886 patients randomized, 560 patients (63.2%) had PD-L1–positive tumors (270 patients in the avelumab + axitinib group and 290 patients in the sunitinib group). This constituted 69.0% of 812 patients for whom tumor samples were available for PD-L1 assessment

[†]Because the investigators used a group-sequential design for the trial, they applied the repeated confidence interval method to the primary outcome measures and these repeated confidence intervals were reported in the column on the right after the unadjusted, but stratified, 95% confidence interval.

[‡]Patients with favorable risk had an International Metastatic Renal Cell Carcinoma Database Consortium (IMDC) score of 0, those with intermediate risk had a score of 1 or 2, and those with poor risk had a score of 3 to 6

HR, hazard ratio; CI, confidence interval; NE, not estimable; OR, odds ratio

Note: progression-free survival and overall survival were estimated using the Kaplan-Meier method and a stratified log-rank test was used to generate two-sided P Values. Progression-free survival and response analyses were assessed by a blinded independent central review according to RECIST v1.1 criteria. Objective response rates and exact two-sided 95% CIs were calculated using the Clopper-Pearson method. All data included in this table were reported in Motzer RJ et al. N Engl J Med 2019; 380(12):1103–15 or its supplementary appendix, with median follow-up times for various outcomes and treatment groups of between 8.4 and 12.0 months

Adverse Events (N = 873)

Event	Avelumab + Axitinib (N = 434)		Sunitinib (N = 439)	
Dose reduction due to adverse event	42.2%		42.6%	
Dose discontinuation due to adverse event	7.6%		13.4%	
Death due to drug toxicity	3 (0.7%)		1 (0.2%)	
	G1/2 (%)	G ≥3 (%)	G1/2 (%)	G ≥3 (%)
Any adverse event	28	71	28	72
Diarrhea	56	7	45	3
Hypertension	24	26	19	17
Fatigue	38	3	36	4
Nausea	33	1	38	2
Palmar-plantar erythrodysesthesia syndrome	28	6	29	4
Dysphonia	30	<1	3	0
Decreased appetite	24	2	28	<1
Hypothyroidism	25	<1	14	<1
Stomatitis	22	2	23	<1
Cough	23	<1	19	0
Headache	20	<1	16	<1
Dyspnea	17	3	11	2
Arthralgia	19	<1	11	<1
Decreased weight	17	3	6	<1

(*continued*)

Adverse Events (N = 873) (continued)

	G1/2 (%)	G ≥3 (%)	G1/2 (%)	G ≥3 (%)
Vomiting	18	<1	18	2
Back pain	17	<1	13	2
Constipation	18	0	15	0
Increased ALT level	11	6	9	3
Chills	16	<1	8	0
Asthenia	12	3	13	3
Increased AST level	11	4	10	2
Rash	14	<1	11	<1
Mucosal inflammation	13	1	13	1
Pruritis	14	0	5	0
Abdominal pain	12	1	8	2
Dysgeusia	13	0	32	0
Pyrexia	13	0	14	<1
Infusion-related reaction	11	2	0	0
Pain in extremity	12	<1	10	<1
Dizziness	11	<1	10	<1
Oropharyngeal pain	10	0	6	0
Dry skin	10	0	10	0
Peripheral edema	9	<1	10	<1
Epistaxis	9	0	11	0
Dyspepsia	8	0	19	0
Anemia	4	2	15	8
Thrombocytopenia	3	<1	13	6
Decreased platelet count	2	0	9	5
Neutropenia	1	<1	11	8
Decreased neutrophil count	<1	0	5	6

Immune-related adverse events		
Immune-related adverse events	38.2%	—
Immune-related adverse events ≥3	9%	—
Immune-related thyroid disorders	24.7%	—
Administration of high dose corticosteroids for immune-related adverse event (≥40 mg of prednisone equivalents)	11.1%	—

ALT, alanine aminotransferase; AST, aspartate aminotransferase
G1/2 adverse events included in the table if they were reported in ≥10% of patients in either group. Adverse events G≥3 included if reported in ≥5% of patients. Adverse events included occurred during treatment, but were not necessarily treatment-related or causally related to drug treatment. Death due to toxicity of trial drug occurred in 3 (0.7%) patients in the avelumab + axitinib group (sudden death, myocarditis, and necrotizing pancreatitis) and 1 (0.2%) patient in the sunitinib group (intestinal perforation). The most frequent immune-related events were immune-related thyroid disorders, reported in 24.7% of patients who received avelumab + axitinib

Therapy Monitoring

Monitoring for Avelumab:

1. Premedicate with antihistamine and acetaminophen prior to the first 4 infusions. Monitor patients for signs and symptoms of infusion-related reactions, including pyrexia, chills, flushing, hypotension, dyspnea, wheezing, back pain, abdominal pain, and urticaria

2. Initially at the time of each dose, and eventually every 6–12 weeks, perform a total body skin examination with attention to *all* mucous membranes, as well as a complete review of systems

3. Monitor patients for signs and symptoms of pneumonitis. Evaluate patients with suspected pneumonitis with chest x-ray, CT scan, and pulse oximetry. For toxicity ≥2, may include nasal swab, sputum culture and sensitivity, blood culture and sensitivity, and urine culture and sensitivity

4. Monitor patients for signs and symptoms of colitis. Encourage patients to report diarrhea immediately to any member of the health care team

5. Draw AST, ALT, and bilirubin prior to each infusion and/or weekly if there are G1 LFT elevations. *Note:* no treatment is recommended for G1 LFT abnormalities. For toxicity ≥2, work up for other causes of elevated LFTs, including viral hepatitis

6. Use basic metabolic panel (Na, K, CO_2, glucose) and patient history as screening tools for hypophysitis, including hypopituitarism and adrenal insufficiency. If in doubt, evaluate morning adrenocorticotropic hormone (ACTH) and cortisol levels. Consider ACTH stimulation test for indeterminate results

7. Assess thyroid function at the start of treatment, periodically during treatment, and as indicated based on clinical evaluation, and for clinical signs and symptoms of thyroid disorders. Test for TSH and free thyroxine (FT4) every 4–6 weeks as part of routine clinical monitoring of therapy or for case detection in symptomatic patients

8. Measure glucose at baseline and with each treatment during the first 12 weeks and every 6 weeks thereafter

9. Obtain a serum creatinine level prior to every dose. If creatinine is found to be newly elevated, consider holding therapy while other potential causes are evaluated. *Note:* routine urinalysis is not necessary other than to rule out urinary tract infections, etc

10. Obtain a complete rheumatologic history and perform an examination of all peripheral joints for tenderness, swelling, and range of motion. Examine the spine. Consider plain x-ray/imaging to exclude metastases and evaluate joint damage (erosions), if appropriate

11. In patients at high risk for infections and in appropriately selected patients based on an infectious disease evaluation, draw screening laboratories (HIV, hepatitis A and B, and blood QuantiFERON for TB) to prepare patients to start infliximab

Monitoring for Axitinib:

1. *At baseline, week 2, week 4, and every 4 weeks thereafter:* clinical assessments including medical history and physical examination, vital signs, ALT, AST, total bilirubin, and CBC with differential. Control blood pressure prior to initiation of axitinib

2. *At screening, after 6 and 12 weeks of therapy, and every 8 weeks thereafter:* tumor assessments. Thyroid function tests. Spot urine for protein measurement (if spot urine dipstick >1+ for protein, perform a 24-hour urine protein)

METASTATIC • CLEAR-CELL • FIRST-LINE
RENAL CELL CARCINOMA REGIMEN: PAZOPANIB HYDROCHLORIDE

Sternberg CN et al. J Clin Oncol 2010;28:1061–1068
VOTRIENT (pazopanib) prescribing information. East Hanover, NJ: Novartis Pharmaceuticals Corporation; May 2017

Pazopanib 800 mg; administer orally once daily at least 1 hour before or 2 hours after a meal, continually, until disease progression (total dose/week = 5600 mg)

Notes:
- Tablets are swallowed whole (without breaking, chewing, or crushing)
- Patients who delay taking pazopanib at a regularly scheduled time may take a missed dose if the interval remaining before the next regularly scheduled dose is ≥12 hours
- Advise patients not to use drugs that increase gastric pH concurrently with pazopanib. Short-acting antacid products are preferable to histamine (H2) receptor antagonists and proton pump inhibitor medications. If used concomitantly, antacid administration should be separated from pazopanib ingestion by several hours
- Use caution in patients with hepatic dysfunction
  - In patients with baseline moderate hepatic impairment, administer pazopanib 200 mg orally once daily
  - The safety of pazopanib in patients with pre-existing severe hepatic impairment, defined as total bilirubin >3 × ULN with any level of ALT, is unknown. Treatment with pazopanib is not recommended in patients with severe hepatic impairment
  - Check LFTs monthly for the first 4 months on treatment (per FDA prescribing label), then monitoring can be reduced to every 3 months if tolerability is achieved
- Monitor patients electrocardiographically at baseline and periodically thereafter

Antiemetic prophylaxis
Emetogenic potential of axitinib is **MINIMAL TO LOW**
See Chapter 42 for antiemetic recommendations

Hematopoietic growth factor (CSF) prophylaxis
Primary prophylaxis is **NOT** *indicated*
See Chapter 43 for more information

Antimicrobial prophylaxis
Risk of fever and neutropenia is **LOW**
  Antimicrobial primary prophylaxis to be considered:
  - Antibacterial—not indicated
  - Antifungal—not indicated
  - Antiviral—not indicated unless patient previously had an episode of HSV

Diarrhea management
Latent or delayed-onset diarrhea*:
  Loperamide 4 mg orally initially after the first loose or liquid stool, *then* 2–4 mg orally every 2–4 hours or **diphenoxylate hydrochloride** 2.5 mg with **atropine sulfate** 0.025 mg (eg, Lomotil)

*Abigerges D et al. J Natl Cancer Inst 1994;86:446–449
Rothenberg ML et al. J Clin Oncol 2001;19:3801–3807
Wadler S et al. J Clin Oncol 1998;16:3169–3178

Treatment Modifications

PAZOPANIB DOSE MODIFICATIONS

Pazopanib dose levels	
Starting dose	800 mg each day
Dose level −1	600 mg each day
Dose level −2	400 mg each day
Dose level −3	200 mg each day
Dose level −4	Discontinue

(continued)

Treatment Modifications (*continued*)

Adverse Event	Treatment Modification
Hepatotoxicity	
Isolated AST or ALT elevations between 3–8× ULN (see note below)	Continue pazopanib with great care. Obtain weekly LFTs until ALT returns to G1 or baseline
AST or ALT elevations >3× ULN concurrently with bilirubin elevations >2× ULN (see note below)	Discontinue pazopanib permanently and monitor patients closely until resolution of LFT abnormalities
Isolated AST or ALT elevations of >8× ULN	Interrupt pazopanib until ALT elevation returns to G1 or baseline. If potential benefits for reinitiating pazopanib outweigh risks of hepatotoxicity, then reintroduce pazopanib at no more than 400 mg daily and measure LFTs weekly for 8 weeks
Recurrent AST or ALT elevations >3× ULN following its reintroduction for transient ALT elevation	Discontinue pazopanib permanently and monitor patients closely until resolution of LFT abnormalities
Total bilirubin >3× ULN with any level of ALT before the start of treatment with pazopanib	The safety of pazopanib in this setting is unknown; use with caution. Administer 200 mg daily
Proteinuria	
24-hour urine protein ≥3 grams	Withhold pazopanib until urine protein is <3 g/24 hours, then resume pazopanib at 1 lower dose level. For recurrent episodes despite dose reduction, discontinue pazopanib
Nephrotic syndrome	Discontinue pazopanib
Diarrhea	
G1/2 diarrhea	Focus on treatment for symptoms designed to resolve the diarrhea. No dose modifications for G1/2 diarrhea unless G2 diarrhea persists for >2 weeks
G2 diarrhea that persists ≥2 weeks	Follow guidelines for G3/4 diarrhea (below)
If diarrhea cannot be controlled with preventive measures outlined, and is G3/4 or worsens by one grade level (G3 to G4) while on pazopanib, and is not alleviated by symptomatic treatment within 48 hours	Hold pazopanib. Also, withhold pazopanib if persistent G2 diarrhea while on pazopanib is not alleviated by treatment for symptoms (persistent defined as lasting for >2 weeks)
If pazopanib is held for >3 weeks and diarrhea does not resolve to G ≤1	Discontinue therapy
If within 3 weeks of withholding pazopanib, diarrhea resolves to G≤1	Restart pazopanib at 1 dose level less than the dose level administered at the time toxicity developed
If G3/4 diarrhea or persistent G2 diarrhea recurs at reduced pazopanib doses (persistent defined as lasting for >2 weeks)	Again, withhold pazopanib until the toxicity resolves to CTCAE G ≤1, at which time pazopanib should be restarted at 1 dose level less than the dose level administered at the time toxicity developed. Treatment for symptoms may continue indefinitely as a preventive measure
If G3/4 diarrhea or persistent G2 diarrhea recurs at a dose of 200 mg once daily (persistent defined as lasting for >2 weeks)	Discontinue therapy
If diarrhea does not recur at reduced pazopanib doses with or without continued treatment for symptoms	The dose of pazopanib may be increased 1 dose level to the dose level that was being administered at the time diarrhea developed. If toxicity recurs following the increase, then follow the guidelines above, with the exception that when drug is restarted the pazopanib dose should be reduced 1 dose level
Hypertension	
Severe hypertension not controlled with medical management	Hold pazopanib pending further evaluation and treatment of hypertension
Severe hypertension despite optimal medical management	Consider reducing the dose of pazopanib or discontinuing it altogether. Discontinue if hypertension remains severe despite dosage reduction
Hypertensive crisis or hypertensive encephalopathy or reversible posterior leukoencephalopathy syndrome (RPLS)	Discontinue pazopanib

(*continued*)

Treatment Modifications (*continued*)

QTc Abnormalities

Patients with a history of QT-interval prolongation, patients taking antiarrhythmics or other medications that may prolong QT interval, and those with relevant preexisting cardiac disease	Use with caution
QTc prolongation defined as: • A single measurement of ≥550 ms • An increase of ≥100 ms from baseline • Two consecutive measurements (within 48 hours of each other) that were ≥500 ms but ≤550 ms • An increase of ≥60 ms, but <100 ms from baseline to a value ≥480 ms	Hold pazopanib until QTc <480 ms, then resume pazopanib at 1 dose level lower

Other Adverse Reactions

G3/4 fatigue	Reduce pazopanib 1 dose level
Clinically significant active infection	Institute appropriate anti-infective therapy and consider interrupting or discontinuing pazopanib for serious infections
Interstitial lung disease/pneumonitis	Discontinue pazopanib
Thrombotic microangiopathy, thrombotic thrombocytopenic purpura, or hemolytic uremic syndrome	Discontinue pazopanib
History of hemoptysis, cerebral, or clinically significant gastrointestinal hemorrhage while receiving pazopanib or in the past 6 months	Discontinue or avoid pazopanib
Patients with increased risk of arterial thrombotic events	Discontinue or avoid pazopanib
Onset of hypothyroidism	Treat hypothyroidism and monitor carefully
Planned elective surgery	Stop pazopanib at least 7 days prior to scheduled surgery. The decision to resume pazopanib after surgery should be based on clinical judgment of adequate wound healing
Wound dehiscence	Discontinue pazopanib

Drug Interactions

Concomitant use of a strong CYP3A4 inhibitor (eg, ketoconazole, ritonavir, clarithromycin) is required	Reduce pazopanib dose to 400 mg; further reduce to 200 mg if adverse effects are observed. The goal is to adjust the pazopanib AUC to the range observed without inhibitors. However, there are no clinical data with this dose adjustment in patients receiving strong CYP3A4 inhibitors
Concomitant use of strong CYP3A4 34 inducers (eg, rifampin)	Do not administer pazopanib
Concomitant use of a drug metabolized by CYP3A4, CYP2D6, or CYP2C8 that has a narrow therapeutic index	Pazopanib is a weak inhibitor of CYP3A4, CYP2D6, and CYP2C8 and may inhibit the metabolism of concomitantly administered drugs that are substrates of these enzymes. Use caution and consider increased monitoring and/or dose reduction of the sensitive substrate per the clinical judgment of the medically responsible health care provider
Patient requires treatment with simvastatin	Concomitant use of simvastatin with pazopanib is associated with a higher rate of ALT elevation
Patient requires treatment with a medication that raises the gastric pH	Short-acting antacid products are preferable to histamine (H2) receptor antagonists and proton pump inhibitor medications. If used concomitantly, antacid administration should be separated from pazopanib ingestion by several hours

Note: pazopanib is a UGT1A1 inhibitor. Mild, indirect (unconjugated) hyperbilirubinemia may occur in patients with Gilbert syndrome. Patients with only a mild indirect hyperbilirubinemia, known Gilbert syndrome, and elevation in ALT >3× ULN should be managed per the recommendations outlined for isolated ALT elevations

Efficacy (N = 290)*

Pazopanib Response Rate, Overall Study Population		95% CI
Complete response	<1%	—
Partial response	30%[†]	25.1–35.6
Median duration of response, weeks	58.7	52.1–68.1
Median time to response, weeks	11.9	9.4–12.3
Pazopanib Response Rate, Subsets		
Treatment-naïve population	32%	24.3–38.9
Cytokine pre-treated subpopulation	29%	21.2–36.5

Progression-Free Survival[‡]		HR vs Placebo
Pazopanib, overall study population	9.2 months	0.46 (0.34–0.62)
Pazopanib, treatment-naïve population	11.1 months	0.40 (0.27–0.60)
Pazopanib, cytokine pre-treated subpopulation	7.4 months	0.54 (0.35–0.84)
Placebo	2.8–4.2 months	—

*RECIST (Therasse P et al. J Natl Cancer Inst 2000;92:205–216)
[†]Median duration = 58.7 weeks
[‡]Prespecified subgroup analyses showed that PFS was improved for patients treated with pazopanib compared with placebo regardless of MSKCC risk category, sex, age, or ECOG PS (HR range: 0.40–0.52; P <0.001 by log-rank test for all)

Mixed-Model Repeated-Measures Analyses for QoL Change from Baseline

Model	Number of Patients		Difference[†]	95% CI	P Value
	Pazopanib	Placebo*			
EORTC Quality of Life Questionnaire-C30: Global Health Status/QoL by Week					
6	243	110	−1.90	−5.84–2.04	0.34
12	219	81	−2.82	−7.17–1.53	0.20
18	191	61	−2.05	−6.95–2.86	0.41
24	164	49	0.39	−4.47–5.25	0.88
48	96	24	−0.67	−6.48–5.14	0.82

Model	Pazopanib	Placebo*	Difference[†]	95% CI	P Value
EuroQuol Questionnaire–5D Index by Week					
6	253	125	0.01	−0.04–0.05	0.84
12	219	86	−0.04	−0.09–0.01	0.08
18	196	62	−0.02	−0.08–0.04	0.50
24	166	51	−0.03	−0.09–0.04	0.44
48	98	24	0.03	−0.03–0.10	0.33

(continued)

Efficacy (N = 290)* (continued)

Model	Number of Patients		Difference†	95% CI	P Value
	Pazopanib	Placebo*			
EQ–5D Visual Analog Scale by Week					
6	239	111	1.85	−2.41–6.12	0.39
12	212	80	0.06	−4.79–4.91	0.98
18	189	60	−0.08	−5.04–4.89	0.98
24	161	49	−0.15	−4.83–4.53	0.95
48	95	23	−1.97	−9.02–5.09	0.58

*More patients in the placebo arm discontinued study treatment because of disease progression compared with patients in the pazopanib arm
†The minimal important differences for the questionnaires have been previously established as 5–10 for the EORTC-QLQ-C30, 0.08 for the EQ–5D Index, and 7 for the EQ–5D VAS. Values greater than 0 indicate a trend in favor of pazopanib, and values less than 0 indicate a trend in favor of placebo

Toxicity (N = 290 Pazopanib; 145 Placebo)*

Adverse Event†	Placebo	Pazopanib		
	% Any Grade	% Any Grade	% G3	% G4
Diarrhea	13	52	3	<1
Hypertension	15	40	4	—
Hair color changes	4	38	<1	—
Nausea	13	26	<1	—
Anorexia	14	22	2	—
Vomiting	11	21	2	<1
Fatigue	11	19	2	—
Asthenia	12	14	3	—
Abdominal pain	2	11	2	—
Headache	7	10	—	—
Clinical Chemistry‡				
ALT increase	32	53	10	2
AST increase	27	53	7	<1
Hyperglycemia	47	41	<1	—
Total bilirubin increase	15	36	3	<1
Hypophosphatemia	16	34	4	—
Hypocalcemia	35	33	1	1
Hyponatremia	35	31	4	1
Hypomagnesemia	13	11	3	—
Hypoglycemia	4	17	—	<1

(continued)

Toxicity (N = 290 Pazopanib; 145 Placebo)* *(continued)*

Hematologic[‡]				
Leukopenia	9	37	—	—
Neutropenia	9	34	1	<1
Thrombocytopenia	7	32	<1	<1
Lymphocytopenia	34	31	4	<1

*NCI Common Terminology Criteria for Adverse Events v3.0
[†]Adverse events with an incidence of ≥10% in the pazopanib arm are displayed
[‡]Clinical laboratory abnormalities with an incidence of ≥30% in the pazopanib arm or with a 5% increase in incidence in the pazopanib arm compared with the placebo arm are displayed

Therapy Monitoring

1. *At baseline, day 8, every 3 weeks until week 24, and every 4 weeks thereafter:* physical examinations, vital signs, with blood pressure monitoring and clinical laboratory evaluations. Serum chemistries, particularly: calcium, magnesium, and potassium

2. *Electrocardiograms:* baseline and periodic (as clinically indicated) monitoring of electrocardiograms and maintenance of electrolytes (eg, calcium, magnesium, potassium) within the normal range should be performed

3. *Thyroid function tests:* monitor every 12 weeks. If thyroid-stimulating hormone levels are abnormal, evaluations of free triiodothyronine and thyroxine should be obtained

4. *Urine protein:* assess proteinuria by urine dipstick and/or urinary protein creatinine ratio. Patients with a urine dipstick reading ≥2+ should undergo further assessment with a 24-hour urine collection

5. *LFTs:* monitor at baseline and at weeks 3, 5, 7, and 9. Thereafter, monitor at month 3 and month 4 (or more often if clinically indicated), and then periodically

6. Thereafter, monitor at month 3 and at month 4, and as clinically indicated. Periodic monitoring should then continue after month 4.

7. *Gastrointestinal perforation:* although gastrointestinal perforation with pazopanib is rare, monitor for symptoms of gastrointestinal perforation or fistula

8. *Response assessment:* every 2–3 cycles

METASTATIC • CLEAR-CELL • FIRST-LINE
RENAL CELL CARCINOMA REGIMEN: SUNITINIB (STANDARD 4 WEEKS ON/2 WEEKS OFF SCHEDULE)

Motzer RJ et al. N Engl J Med 2013;369:722–31.

Sunitinib malate 50 mg; administer orally once daily, continually, without regard for meals, in 6-week cycles consisting of 4 consecutive weeks of daily treatment followed by 2 weeks without treatment, until disease progression (total dose/6-week cycle = 1400 mg)

Notes:
- Patients who delay taking sunitinib malate at a regularly scheduled time may take a missed dose if the interval remaining before the next regularly scheduled dose is ≥12 hours
- If possible, avoid concomitant use of strong CYP3A4 inhibitors and inducers. If a concomitant strong CYP3A4 inhibitor must be used, decrease sunitinib malate to 37.5 mg/dose. If a concomitant strong CYP3A4 inducer must be used, consider increasing sunitinib malate to 87.5 mg/dose while monitoring closely for side effects
- Patients using sunitinib malate should be advised to avoid consuming grapefruit juice for as long as they continue to use sunitinib malate

Supportive Care: Hand-Foot Reaction
For patients who develop a hand-foot reaction, use topical emollients (eg, Aquaphor), topical and/or oral steroids, antihistamine agents (H_1-receptor antagonists), or pyridoxine 50–150 mg/day orally

Antiemetic prophylaxis
Emetogenic potential is **LOW**
See Chapter 42 for antiemetic recommendations

Hematopoietic growth factor (CSF) prophylaxis
Primary prophylaxis is **NOT** indicated
See Chapter 43 for more information

Antimicrobial prophylaxis
Risk of fever and neutropenia is **LOW**
   Antimicrobial primary prophylaxis to be considered:
- Antibacterial—not indicated
- Antifungal—not indicated
- Antiviral—not indicated unless patient previously had an episode of HSV

Diarrhea management
Latent or delayed-onset diarrhea*:
   Loperamide 4 mg orally initially after the first loose or liquid stool, *then* 2–4 mg orally every 2–4 hours or **diphenoxylate hydrochloride** 2.5 mg with **atropine sulfate** 0.025 mg (eg, Lomotil)

*Abigerges D et al. J Natl Cancer Inst 1994;86:446–449
Rothenberg ML et al. J Clin Oncol 2001;19:3801–3807
Wadler S et al. J Clin Oncol 1998;16:3169–3178

Treatment Modification

SUNITINIB DOSE MODIFICATIONS

Sunitinib Dose Levels	
Starting dose (Level 1)	50 mg once daily, 4 weeks on/2 weeks off
Dose Level −1	37.5 mg once daily, 4 weeks on/2 weeks off
Dose Level −2	25 mg once daily, 4 weeks on/2 weeks off
Dose Level −3	Discontinue sunitinib

(continued)

Treatment Modification (*continued*)

Adverse Event	Treatment Modification
Cutaneous Toxicities	
Rash G ≥2	Withhold sunitinib and provide immediate symptomatic treatment. When toxicity resolves to G ≤1, restart sunitinib at 1 dose level lower than the dose level administered at the time toxicity developed. Treatment for symptoms may continue indefinitely as a preventive measure *Note: discontinue therapy if sunitinib is withheld >3 weeks*
Recurrence of G3/4 cutaneous toxicity at reduced doses of sunitinib	Withhold sunitinib and provide immediate symptomatic treatment. When toxicity resolves to G ≤1, restart sunitinib at 1 dose level lower than the dose level administered at the time toxicity developed. Treatment for symptoms may continue indefinitely as a preventive measure
Recurrence of G3/4 cutaneous toxicity at dose level −2 of sunitinib	Discontinue therapy
Cutaneous toxicity does not recur at reduced sunitinib doses with or without continued treatment for symptoms	Sunitinib dose may be increased 1 dose level to that administered at the time cutaneous toxicity developed. If toxicity recurs following the increase, then again withhold sunitinib and provide immediate symptomatic treatment. When toxicity resolves to G ≤1, restart sunitinib at 1 dose level lower than the dose level administered at the time toxicity developed. Treatment for symptoms may continue indefinitely as a preventive measure
Diarrhea	
G1/2 diarrhea (increase of 4–6 stools/day over baseline; limiting instrumental ADLs)	Focus on treatment for symptoms designed to resolve the diarrhea. No dose modifications are made for G1/2 diarrhea unless G2 diarrhea persists >2 weeks
G2 diarrhea persisting >2 weeks	Follow the guidelines below for G3/4 diarrhea
G2 diarrhea lasting >2 weeks *or* G3/4 diarrhea *or* diarrhea that worsens by 1 grade while on sunitinib	Withhold sunitinib until diarrhea resolves to G ≤1. If resolution occurs within 3 weeks of holding treatment, restart sunitinib at 1 dose level lower than the dose level administered at the time diarrhea developed *Note: discontinue therapy if sunitinib is withheld >3 weeks*
Recurrence of G2 diarrhea lasting >2 weeks *or* G3/4 diarrhea at reduced sunitinib doses and dose level is −1	Withhold sunitinib until toxicity resolves to G ≤1, then restart sunitinib at dose level −2. Treatment for symptoms may continue indefinitely as a preventive measure
Recurrence of G2 diarrhea lasting >2 weeks or G3/4 diarrhea at dose level −2	Discontinue therapy
Diarrhea does not recur at reduced sunitinib doses with or without continued treatment for symptoms	Sunitinib dose may be increased 1 dose level to the dose level administered at the time the diarrhea developed. If toxicity recurs following the increase, then again withhold sunitinib and provide immediate symptomatic treatment. When toxicity resolves to G ≤1, restart sunitinib at 1 dose level lower than the dose level administered at the time toxicity developed. Treatment for symptoms may continue indefinitely as a preventive measure
Hypertension	
Note: patients should have their blood pressure checked once weekly during their first 24 weeks of therapy and for an 8-week period after an adjustment in their sunitinib dose	
G1 hypertension (SBP 120–139 or DBP 80–89 mm Hg)	Continue sunitinib at same dose and schedule
G2 asymptomatic hypertension (SBP 140–159 or DBP 90–99 mm Hg if previously WNL; change in baseline medical intervention indicated; recurrent or persistent (≥24 hours); symptomatic increase DBP >20 mm Hg or to >140/90 mm Hg; monotherapy indicated initiated)	Treat with antihypertensive medications and continue sunitinib at same dose and schedule

(*continued*)

Treatment Modification (*continued*)

Adverse Event	Treatment Modification
G2 symptomatic, or persistent G2 despite antihypertensive medications, or DBP ≥110 mm Hg, or G3 hypertension (SBP ≥160 or DBP ≥100 mm Hg; medical intervention indicated; >1 drug or more intensive therapy than previously used indicated)	Withhold sunitinib and treat with antihypertensive medications until symptoms resolve and diastolic BP <100 mm Hg. Then continue sunitinib at 1 dose level lower *Note: discontinue therapy if sunitinib is withheld >3 weeks*
G4 hypertension (life-threatening consequences; urgent intervention indicated)	Discontinue therapy

Miscellaneous

G3/4 hepatotoxicity (ALT/AST >5× ULN if baseline was normal; >5× baseline if baseline was abnormal; bilirubin >3× ULN if baseline was normal; >3× baseline if baseline was abnormal)	Withhold sunitinib until LFTs resolve to baseline or G ≤1. If resolution occurs within 3 weeks of holding treatment, restart sunitinib at 1 dose level lower than the dose level administered at the time hepatotoxicity was noted *Note: discontinue therapy if sunitinib is withheld >3 weeks or if worsening occurs during the period of observation off therapy*
Any other G3/4 nonhematologic toxicity (eg, persistent nausea, vomiting, despite maximum supportive treatment)	Withhold treatment until toxicity improves to G ≤1, then resume with dose reduced by 1 level
Wound dehiscence or poor wound healing	Interrupt sunitinib until wound has adequately healed
LVEF decrease by ≥10% to <LLN, clinical heart failure syndrome, necrotizing fasciitis, EM, SJS, TEN, or TMA	Permanently discontinue sunitinib
Proteinuria	If urine dipstick ≥2+, obtain 24-hour urine protein. If 24-hour urine protein ≥3 g, interrupt treatment. Resume treatment when 24-hour urine protein ≤1 g. Resume sunitinib at 1 dose level lower
Repeat episodes of 24-hour urine protein ≥3 g despite dose reductions or nephrotic syndrome	Discontinue sunitinib
Co-administration of potent CYP3A4 inhibitors (eg, ketoconazole, itraconazole, voriconazole, clarithromycin, atazanavir, ritonavir, telithromycin)	Reduce sunitinib dose
Co-administration of potent CYP3A inducers (eg, rifampin, phenytoin, phenobarbital, carbamazepine)	Increase sunitinib dose (to a maximum of 87.5 mg daily)

EM, erythema multiforme; LLN, lower limit of normal; LVEF, left ventricular ejection fraction; SJS, Stevens-Johnson syndrome; TEN, toxic epidermal necrolysis; TMA, thrombotic microangiopathy
Dose adjustment for renal impairment:
- Creatinine clearance ≥30 mL/min: no initial adjustment necessary
- End-stage renal disease (ESRD) on hemodialysis: no initial adjustment necessary. Sunitinib exposure is 47% lower in patients with ESRD on hemodialysis, and doses may need to be increased gradually up to 2-fold based on tolerability

Patient Population Studied

The COMPARZ study was an international, randomized, open-label, phase 3 trial that involved 1110 adult patients with advanced or metastatic RCC with a clear cell histologic component and compared treatment with pazopanib to sunitinib. Participants were eligible if they had not received systemic treatment previously and had measurable disease according to RECIST. Additionally, participants had to have a Karnofsky performance status score of ≥70 and adequate organ function. Patients were excluded if they had brain metastases, poorly controlled hypertension, or a history of cardiac or vascular conditions within 6 months before screening. Participants were randomized 1:1 to receive pazopanib or sunitinib. Randomization was done in permuted blocks of four, stratified according to Karnofsky performance-status score, level of lactate dehydrogenase, and history of nephrectomy

Efficacy (N = 1110)

Endpoint	Pazopanib Group (N = 557)	Sunitinib Group (N = 553)	Between-group Comparison
Median progression-free survival*	8.4 months (95% CI 8.3–10.9)	9.5 months (95% CI 8.3–11.1)	HR 1.05 (95% CI 0.9–1.22)
Patients with partial response	170 patients (31%)	134 patients (24%)	—
Patients with complete response	1 (0.2%)	3 (0.5%)	—
Objective response rate	31%	25%	P = 0.03
Median overall survival	28.4 months (95% CI 26.2–35.6)	29.3 months (95% CI 25.3–32.5)	HR 0.91 (95% CI 0.76–1.08); P = 0.28[†]

*Imaging to determine disease assessment was reevaluated by an independent review committee whose members were unaware of treatment assignments to assess progression-free survival and tumor response according to RECIST version 1.0.
[†]Stratified log-rank test
HR, hazard ratio, CI, confidence interval

Adverse Events (N = 1102)

Event	Pazopanib Group (N = 554) Grade 1/2 (%)	Pazopanib Group (N = 554) Grade 3/4 (%)	Sunitinib Group (N = 548) Grade 1/2 (%)	Sunitinib Group (N = 548) Grade 3/4 (%)
Increased risk with sunitinib[†]				
Fatigue[‡]	44	11	45	18
Hand-foot syndrome[‡]	23	6	38	12
Dysgeusia	25	<1	36	0
Rash	17	1	22	1
Constipation	16	1	23	1
Dyspepsia	14	0	23	1
Stomatitis	13	1	26	1
Hypothyroidism	12	0	23	<1
Pain in a limb	11	<1	16	1
Mucosal inflammation[‡]	10	1	23	3
Peripheral edema	10	<1	16	<1
Epistaxis	8	<1	17	1
Pyrexia	9	<1	15	1
Increased blood LDH	6	<1	10	1
Increased blood thyrotropin	6	0	12	0
GERD	2	<1	9	<1

Event	Pazopanib Group (N = 554) Grade 1/2 (%)	Pazopanib Group (N = 554) Grade 3/4 (%)	Sunitinib Group (N = 548) Grade 1/2 (%)	Sunitinib Group (N = 548) Grade 3/4 (%)
Yellow skin	1	0	15	0
Leukopenia[‡€]	42	1	72	6
Thrombocytopenia[‡€]	37	4	56	22
Lymphocytopenia[‡€]	33	5	40	15
Neutropenia[‡€]	32	5	48	20
Anemia[‡€]	29	2	53	7
Hypophosphatemia[‡€]	32	4	43	9
Hypoalbuminemia[€]	32	1	40	2
Increased creatinine[€]	31	1	44	2
Hypomagnesemia[‡]	22	<1	22	2
Hypermagnesemia[‡€]	10	2	13	5
Increased risk with pazopanib[§]				
Changes in hair color	30	0	9	<1
Weight loss	14	1	5	<1
Alopecia	14	0	8	0
Increased AST[‖]	49	12	57	3
Increased ALT[§‖]	43	17	38	5
Increased total bilirubin[§]	32	4	24	3

(continued)

Adverse Events (N = 1102) *(continued)*

Event	Pazopanib Group (N = 554)		Sunitinib Group (N = 548)	
	Grade 1/2 (%)	Grade 3/4 (%)	Grade 1/2 (%)	Grade 3/4 (%)
Increased alkaline phosphatase‖	25	3	23	1
Hypoglycemia§	14	<1	10	1
Changes in hair color	30	0	9	<1

GERD, gastroesophageal reflux disease; AST, aspartate aminotransferase; ALT, alanine aminotransferase

*Adverse events listed included those that occurred in more than 10% of patients. The events were displayed to indicate a difference in relative risk between the groups, deemed a significant difference in relative risk if the 95% confidence interval for relative risk did not include unity. The confidence intervals were not corrected for multiple comparisons

†The relative risk of an event of any grade was significantly higher with sunitinib than with pazopanib

‡The relative risk of a Grade 3 or 4 event was significantly higher with sunitinib than with pazopanib

§The relative risk of an event of any grade was significantly higher with pazopanib than with sunitinib

¶The relative risk of an event of any grade was significantly higher with sunitinib than with pazopanib

‖The relative risk of a Grade 3 or 4 event was significantly higher with pazopanib than with sunitinib

Note: increased levels of lactate dehydrogenase and blood thyrotropin are not graded according to the Common Terminology Criteria for Adverse Events and were reported as adverse events when the investigator considered them clinically significant. The median duration of treatment was similar in both groups (8.0 months in the pazopanib group and 7.6 months in the sunitinib group). The proportion of patients who discontinued the intervention due to adverse events was 24% in the pazopanib group and 20% in the sunitinib group

Therapy Monitoring

1. *Prior to the first cycle of sunitinib:* electrocardiogram (for assessment of QTc interval), echocardiogram, CBC with differential, platelet count, LFTs, serum chemistries, blood glucose, blood pressure, thyroid-stimulating hormone, urine dipstick and/or urinary protein–creatinine ratio, physical examination (including dermatologic examination)
2. *Prior to each cycle of sunitinib:* CBC with differential, platelet count, LFTs, serum chemistries, blood glucose, blood pressure, thyroid-stimulating hormone, urine dipstick and/or urinary protein–creatinine ratio, physical examination (including dermatologic examination)
3. Hepatotoxicity, including liver failure, has been observed. Monitor LFTs before initiation of treatment, during each cycle of treatment, and as clinically indicated
4. Cardiac toxicity including declines in LVEF to below LLN and cardiac failure including death have occurred. Monitor patients for signs and symptoms of congestive heart failure
5. Prolonged QT intervals and torsades de pointes have been observed. Use with caution in patients at higher risk for developing QT interval prolongation. When using sunitinib, monitoring with on-treatment electrocardiograms and electrolytes should be considered monthly at first or when the dose is increased and less frequently thereafter
6. Hypertension may occur. Monitor blood pressure and treat as indicated under Treatment Modifications
7. Thyroid dysfunction may occur. Monitor thyroid function tests every 3 months. Treat hypothyroidism accordingly
8. Temporary interruption of therapy with sunitinib is recommended in patients undergoing major surgical procedures. *Note:* there is limited clinical experience regarding the timing of re-initiation of therapy following major surgical intervention. Therefore, the decision to resume sunitinib therapy following a major surgical intervention should be based on clinical judgment of recovery from surgery
9. Monitor adrenal function in case of stress such as surgery, trauma, or severe infection

METASTATIC • CLEAR-CELL • FIRST-LINE
RENAL CELL CARCINOMA REGIMEN: SUNITINIB (ALTERNATIVE 2 WEEKS ON/1 WEEK OFF SCHEDULE)

Jonasch E et al. J Clin Oncol 2018;36:1588–1593

Sunitinib malate 50 mg; administer orally once daily, continually, without regard for meals, in 3-week cycles consisting of 2 consecutive weeks of daily treatment followed by 1 week without treatment, until disease progression (total dose/3-week cycle = 700 mg)

Notes:

- Patients who delay taking sunitinib malate at a regularly scheduled time may take a missed dose if the interval remaining before the next regularly scheduled dose is ≥12 hours

- If possible, avoid concomitant use of strong CYP3A4 inhibitors and inducers. If a concomitant strong CYP3A4 inhibitor must be used, decrease sunitinib malate to 37.5 mg/dose. If a concomitant strong CYP3A4 inducer must be used, consider increasing sunitinib malate to 87.5 mg/dose while monitoring closely for side effects

- Patients using sunitinib malate should be advised to avoid consuming grapefruit juice for as long as they continue to use sunitinib malate

Supportive Care: Hand-Foot Reaction
For patients who develop a hand-foot reaction, use topical emollients (eg, Aquaphor), topical and/or oral steroids, antihistamine agents (H_1-receptor antagonists), or pyridoxine 50–150 mg/day orally

Antiemetic prophylaxis
Emetogenic potential is **LOW**
See Chapter 42 for antiemetic recommendations

Hematopoietic growth factor (CSF) prophylaxis
Primary prophylaxis is **NOT** indicated
See Chapter 43 for more information

Antimicrobial prophylaxis
Risk of fever and neutropenia is **LOW**
  Antimicrobial primary prophylaxis to be considered:
- Antibacterial—not indicated
- Antifungal—not indicated
- Antiviral—not indicated unless patient previously had an episode of HSV

Diarrhea management
Latent or delayed-onset diarrhea*:
  Loperamide 4 mg orally initially after the first loose or liquid stool, *then* 2–4 mg orally every 2–4 hours or **diphenoxylate hydrochloride** 2.5 mg with **atropine sulfate** 0.025 mg (eg, Lomotil)

*Abigerges D et al. J Natl Cancer Inst 1994;86:446–449
Rothenberg ML et al. J Clin Oncol 2001;19:3801–3807
Wadler S et al. J Clin Oncol 1998;16:3169–3178

Treatment Modification

SUNITINIB DOSE MODIFICATIONS

Sunitinib Dose Levels	
Starting dose (Level 1)	50 mg once daily, 2 weeks on/1 week off
Dose Level −1	50 mg once daily, 1 week on/3 days off alternating with 50 mg 1 week on/4 days off
Dose Level −2	37.5 mg once daily, 2 weeks on/1 week off
Dose Level −3	37.5 mg once daily, 1 week on/3 days off alternating with 37.5 mg 1 week on/4 days off
Dose Level −4	25 mg once daily, 2 weeks on/1 week off
Dose Level −5	25 mg once daily, 1 week on/3 days off alternating with 25 mg 1 week on/4 days off
Dose Level −6	Discontinue sunitinib

(continued)

Treatment Modification (*continued*)

Adverse Event	Treatment Modification
Cutaneous Toxicities	
Rash G ≥2	Withhold sunitinib and provide immediate symptomatic treatment. When toxicity resolves to G ≤1, restart sunitinib at 1 dose level lower than the dose level administered at the time toxicity developed. Treatment for symptoms may continue indefinitely as a preventive measure *Note: discontinue therapy if sunitinib is withheld >3 weeks*
Recurrence of G3/4 cutaneous toxicity at reduced doses of sunitinib	Withhold sunitinib and provide immediate symptomatic treatment. When toxicity resolves to G ≤1, restart sunitinib at 1 dose level lower than the dose level administered at the time toxicity developed. Treatment for symptoms may continue indefinitely as a preventive measure
Recurrence of G3/4 cutaneous toxicity at dose level −5 of sunitinib	Discontinue therapy
Cutaneous toxicity does not recur at reduced sunitinib doses with or without continued treatment for symptoms	Sunitinib dose may be increased 1 dose level to that administered at the time cutaneous toxicity developed. If toxicity recurs following the increase, then again withhold sunitinib and provide immediate symptomatic treatment. When toxicity resolves to G ≤1, restart sunitinib at 1 dose level lower than the dose level administered at the time toxicity developed. Treatment for symptoms may continue indefinitely as a preventive measure
Diarrhea	
G1/2 diarrhea (increase of 4–6 stools/day over baseline; limiting instrumental ADLs)	Focus on treatment for symptoms designed to resolve the diarrhea. No dose modifications are made for G1/2 diarrhea unless G2 diarrhea persists >2 weeks
G2 diarrhea persisting >2 weeks	Follow the guidelines below for G3/4 diarrhea
G2 diarrhea lasting >2 weeks *or* G3/4 diarrhea *or* diarrhea that worsens by 1 grade while on sunitinib	Withhold sunitinib until diarrhea resolves to G ≤1. If resolution occurs within 3 weeks of holding treatment, restart sunitinib at 1 dose level lower than the dose level administered at the time diarrhea developed *Note: discontinue therapy if sunitinib is withheld >3 weeks*
Recurrence of G2 diarrhea lasting >2 weeks *or* G3/4 diarrhea at reduced sunitinib doses	Withhold sunitinib until toxicity resolves to G ≤1, then restart sunitinib at 1 lower dose level. Treatment for symptoms may continue indefinitely as a preventive measure
Recurrence of G2 diarrhea lasting >2 weeks or G3/4 diarrhea at dose level −5	Discontinue therapy
Diarrhea does not recur at reduced sunitinib doses with or without continued treatment for symptoms	Sunitinib dose may be increased 1 dose level to the dose level administered at the time the diarrhea developed. If toxicity recurs following the increase, then again withhold sunitinib and provide immediate symptomatic treatment. When toxicity resolves to G ≤1, restart sunitinib at 1 dose level lower than the dose level administered at the time toxicity developed. Treatment for symptoms may continue indefinitely as a preventive measure
Hypertension	
Note: patients should have their blood pressure checked once weekly during their first 24 weeks of therapy and for an 8-week period after an adjustment in their sunitinib dose	
G1 hypertension (SBP 120–139 or DBP 80–89 mm Hg)	Continue sunitinib at same dose and schedule
G2 asymptomatic hypertension (SBP 140–159 or DBP 90–99 mm Hg if previously WNL; change in baseline medical intervention indicated; recurrent or persistent [≥24 hours]; symptomatic increase DBP >20 mm Hg or to >140/90 mm Hg; monotherapy indicated initiated)	Treat with antihypertensive medications and continue sunitinib at same dose and schedule
G2 symptomatic, or persistent G2 despite antihypertensive medications, or DBP ≥110 mm Hg, or G3 hypertension (SBP ≥160 or DBP ≥100 mm Hg; medical intervention indicated; >1 drug or more intensive therapy than previously used indicated)	Withhold sunitinib and treat with antihypertensive medications until symptoms resolve and diastolic BP <100 mm Hg. Then continue sunitinib at 1 dose level lower *Note: discontinue therapy if sunitinib is withheld >3 weeks*
G4 hypertension (life-threatening consequences; urgent intervention indicated)	Discontinue therapy

(*continued*)

Treatment Modification (*continued*)

Miscellaneous

G3/4 hepatotoxicity (ALT/AST >5× ULN if baseline was normal; >5× baseline if baseline was abnormal; bilirubin >3× ULN if baseline was normal; >3× baseline if baseline was abnormal)	Withhold sunitinib until LFTs resolve to baseline or G ≤1. If resolution occurs within 3 weeks of holding treatment, restart sunitinib at 1 dose level lower than the dose level administered at the time hepatotoxicity was noted *Note: discontinue therapy if sunitinib is withheld >3 weeks or if worsening occurs during the period of observation off therapy*
Any other G3/4 nonhematologic toxicity (eg, persistent nausea, vomiting, despite maximum supportive treatment)	Withhold treatment until toxicity improves to G ≤1, then resume with dose reduced by 1 level
Wound dehiscence or poor wound healing	Interrupt sunitinib until wound has adequately healed
LVEF decrease by ≥10% to <LLN, clinical heart failure syndrome, necrotizing fasciitis, EM, SJS, TEN, or TMA	Permanently discontinue sunitinib
Proteinuria	If urine dipstick ≥2+, obtain 24-hour urine protein. If 24-hour urine protein ≥3 g, interrupt treatment. Resume treatment when 24-hour urine protein ≤1 g. Resume sunitinib at 1 dose level lower
Repeat episodes of 24-hour urine protein ≥3 g despite dose reductions or nephrotic syndrome	Discontinue sunitinib
Co-administration of potent CYP3A4 inhibitors (eg, ketoconazole, itraconazole, voriconazole, clarithromycin, atazanavir, ritonavir, telithromycin)	Reduce sunitinib dose
Co-administration of potent CYP3A inducers (eg, rifampin, phenytoin, phenobarbital, carbamazepine)	Increase sunitinib dose (to a maximum of 87.5 mg daily)

EM, erythema multiforme; LLN, lower limit of normal; LVEF, left ventricular ejection fraction; SJS, Stevens-Johnson syndrome; TEN, toxic epidermal necrolysis; TMA, thrombotic microangiopathy

Dose adjustment for renal impairment:
- Creatinine clearance ≥30 mL/min: no initial adjustment necessary
- End-stage renal disease (ESRD) on hemodialysis: no initial adjustment necessary. Sunitinib exposure is 47% lower in patients with ESRD on hemodialysis, and doses may need to be increased gradually up to 2-fold based on tolerability

Patient Population Studied (N = 60)

This single-arm, open-label, phase 2 trial included 60 adult patients with treatment-naïve renal cell carcinoma and evaluated treatment with an alternate 2 weeks on, 1 week off schedule of sunitinib. Patients were eligible for the study if they had histologically or cytologically confirmed, metastatic clear cell RCC, measurable or evaluable disease (according to RECIST v1.0), an ECOG performance status of 0 or 1, and relatively normal organ and bone marrow function. Patients were excluded if they had received previous treatment with sunitinib or any other systemic treatment for metastatic disease (except for prior neoadjuvant therapy if completed > 6 months before registration and not discontinued due to toxicity), if they had received previous major surgery or radiation therapy within 4 weeks of starting treatment, if they had CNS metastases, NYHA class II or greater congestive heart failure, serious cardiovascular condition or procedure within 6 months of registration, or HIV/AIDS

Efficacy (N = 59)

Efficacy Variable	Sunitinib (N = 59)
Response	
ORR—n/N (%) [95% CI]	33/59 (56) [42.4–68.8]
CR rate—n/N (%)	1/59 (2)
PR rate—n/N (%)	32/59 (54)
PD rate—n/N (%)	7/59 (12)
PFS	
Median PFS—months (95% CI)	13.7 (10.9–16.3)
OS	
Median OS—months (95% CI)	NR (24.5–NR)

CI, confidence interval; NR, not reached; PFS, progression-free survival; OS, overall survival; ORR, objective response rate; CR, complete response; PR, partial response; PD, progressive disease

Note: although 60 patients were enrolled, only 59 patients received study drug treatment and were included in efficacy assessments. Median PFS and OS and their corresponding 95% CIs were estimated using the Kaplan-Meier method. Determinations of response and PFS were made by the investigator according to RECIST v1.0 criteria. Data in the table were reported in Jonasch et al, 2018, which had a median follow-up time of 17 months

Adverse Events (N = 59)

Event	Sunitinib (N = 59)	
	Any grade—%	Grade ≥3—n/N (%) [95% CI]
G ≥3 fatigue, diarrhea, or hand-foot syndrome	Not applicable	15/59 (25) [15.0–38.4]
Fatigue	78	8/59 (14) [6.0–25.0]
Diarrhea	76	5/59 (8) [2.8–18.7]
Hand-foot syndrome	54	3/59 (5) [1.1–14.1]
Miscellaneous safety outcomes—n/N (%) [95% CI]		
Schedule/dose reduction due to Grade ≥3 adverse event	29/59 (49) [37.5–64.1]	
Discontinuation due to toxicity	6/59 (10) [not reported]	

Note: adverse events were included in the table if they were described in the text of the results section of the paper or in a toxicity table. For additional toxicities, refer to Figure 2 in Jonasch E et al. J Clin Oncol 2018;36:1588–1593. Adverse events were graded according to the National Cancer Institute Common Terminology Criteria for Adverse Events (NCI-CTCAE) v4.03 in all patients who received study treatment and those reported were considered treatment-related. There was only 1 (1%) adverse event of ≥ 4 reported, a Grade 4 neutropenia. Reasons for discontinuation of study drug treatment were osteonecrosis, proteinuria, neutropenia, congestive heart failure, gout, and general intolerance

Therapy Monitoring

1. *Prior to the first cycle of sunitinib:* electrocardiogram (for assessment of QTc interval), echocardiogram, CBC with differential, platelet count, LFTs, serum chemistries, blood glucose, blood pressure, thyroid-stimulating hormone, urine dipstick and/or urinary protein–creatinine ratio, physical examination (including dermatologic examination)
2. *Prior to each cycle of sunitinib:* CBC with differential, platelet count, LFTs, serum chemistries, blood glucose, blood pressure, thyroid-stimulating hormone, urine dipstick and/or urinary protein–creatinine ratio, physical examination (including dermatologic examination)
3. Hepatotoxicity, including liver failure, has been observed. Monitor LFTs before initiation of treatment, during each cycle of treatment, and as clinically indicated
4. Cardiac toxicity including declines in LVEF to below LLN and cardiac failure including death have occurred. Monitor patients for signs and symptoms of congestive heart failure
5. Prolonged QT intervals and torsades de pointes have been observed. Use with caution in patients at higher risk for developing QT interval prolongation. When using sunitinib, monitoring with on-treatment electrocardiograms and electrolytes should be considered monthly at first or when the dose is increased and less frequently thereafter
6. Hypertension may occur. Monitor blood pressure and treat as indicated under Treatment Modifications
7. Thyroid dysfunction may occur. Monitor thyroid function tests every 3 months. Treat hypothyroidism accordingly
8. Temporary interruption of therapy with sunitinib is recommended in patients undergoing major surgical procedures. *Note:* there is limited clinical experience regarding the timing of re-initiation of therapy following major surgical intervention. Therefore, the decision to resume sunitinib therapy following a major surgical intervention should be based on clinical judgment of recovery from surgery
9. Monitor adrenal function in case of stress such as surgery, trauma, or severe infection

METASTATIC • CLEAR-CELL • FIRST-LINE
RENAL CELL CARCINOMA REGIMEN: CABOZANTINIB

Choueiri TK et al. N Engl J Med 2015;373:1814–1823
Protocol for: Choueiri TK et al. N Engl J Med 2015;373:1814–1823
Supplementary appendix to: Choueiri TK et al. N Engl J Med 2015;373:1814–1823
Choueiri TK et al. Lancet Oncol 2016;17:917–927
Motzer RJ et al. Br J Cancer 2018;118:1176–1178
CABOMETYX (cabozantinib) prescribing information. Alameda, CA: Exelixis, Inc; revised January 2020

Cabozantinib tablets (Cabometyx®) 60 mg orally at least 2 hours after or at least 1 hour before eating food, once daily, continually, until disease progression (total dose/week = 420 mg)
Notes:
• Tablets are swallowed whole. Do not crush cabozantinib tablets
• Do not substitute cabozantinib tablets (CABOMETYX) with cabozantinib capsules (COMETRIQ)
• Do not take a missed dose within 12 hours of the next scheduled dose
• In light of the fact that 60% of patients starting at the 60-mg dose had a subsequent dose reduction and 10% discontinued the medication because of adverse effects, clinicians are advised to consider the following:
  ▪ Avoid the use of concomitant strong CYP3A4 inhibitors. For patients who require treatment with a strong CYP3A4 inhibitor, reduce the daily cabozantinib dose by 20 mg. Resume the dose that was used prior to initiating the CYP3A4 inhibitor 2 to 3 days after discontinuing a strong inhibitor
  ▪ Avoid use of strong CYP3A4 inducers. For patients who require treatment with a strong CYP3A4 inducer, increase the daily cabozantinib dose by 20 mg *only if tolerability on the dose without the inducer has been convincingly demonstrated*. Resume the dose that was used prior to initiating a CYP3A4 inducer 2 to 3 days after discontinuing a strong inducer. The daily cabozantinib dose should not exceed 80 mg
  ▪ *Patients with hepatic impairment:* With moderate hepatic impairment (Child-Pugh class B), reduce the starting dose of cabozantinib to 40 mg once daily. Avoid use of cabozantinib in patients with severe hepatic impairment (Child-Pugh class C)

Supportive Care
Antiemetic prophylaxis
Emetogenic potential is **MINIMAL–LOW**
See Chapter 42 for antiemetic recommendations

Hematopoietic growth factor (CSF) prophylaxis
Primary prophylaxis is **NOT** *indicated*
See Chapter 43 for more information

Antimicrobial prophylaxis
Risk of fever and neutropenia is **LOW**
  Antimicrobial primary prophylaxis to be considered:
  • Antibacterial—not indicated
  • Antifungal—not indicated
  • Antiviral—not indicated unless patient previously had an episode of HSV

Diarrhea management
Latent or delayed-onset diarrhea*:
  Loperamide 4 mg orally initially after the first loose or liquid stool, *then* 2–4 mg orally every 2–4 hours or **diphenoxylate hydrochloride** 2.5 mg with **atropine sulfate** 0.025 mg (eg, Lomotil)

*Abigerges D et al. J Natl Cancer Inst 1994;86:446–449
Rothenberg ML et al. J Clin Oncol 2001;19:3801–3807
Wadler S et al. J Clin Oncol 1998;16:3169–3178

Hand-foot reaction (palmar-plantar erythrodysesthesia, PPE)
Use topical emollients (eg, Aquaphor), topical or orally administered steroids, antihistamines, or pyridoxine 50 to 200 mg/day

Treatment Modifications

RECOMMENDED DOSE MODIFICATIONS FOR CABOZANTINIB

Starting dose (level 1)	60 mg orally once daily
Dose level −1	40 mg orally once daily
Dose level −2	20 mg orally once daily
Dose level −3	Consider discontinuing cabozantinib or consider resuming at 20 mg orally once daily, if tolerable, at the discretion of the medically responsible health care provider

Grade/Severity	Treatment Modification
G ≥3 hemorrhage	Permanently discontinue cabozantinib
Development of a gastrointestinal perforation or Grade 4 fistula	
Acute MI	
Serious arterial or VTE event requiring medical intervention	
Any hypertension	Treat as needed with standard anti-hypertensive therapy
Persistent hypertension despite use of maximal anti-hypertensive medications	Withhold cabozantinib until blood pressure is adequately controlled, then resume cabozantinib with the dosage reduced by 1 dosage level
Evidence of hypertensive crisis or severe hypertension that cannot be controlled with anti-hypertensive therapy	Discontinue cabozantinib
Intolerable Grade 2 diarrhea	Optimize antidiarrheal regimen. Withhold cabozantinib until improvement to G ≤1, then resume cabozantinib with the dosage reduced by 1 dose level
Grade ≥3 diarrhea not manageable with standard antidiarrheal treatments	
Intolerable Grade 2 palmar-plantar erythrodysesthesia syndrome (skin changes [eg, peeling, blisters, bleeding, edema, or hyperkeratosis] with pain; limiting instrumental ADL)	Withhold cabozantinib until improvement to G ≤1, then resume cabozantinib with the dosage reduced by 1 dose level
Grade 3 palmar-plantar erythrodysesthesia syndrome (severe skin changes [eg, peeling, blisters, bleeding, edema, or hyperkeratosis] with pain; limiting self-care ADL)	
Patient requires dental surgery or an invasive dental procedure	If possible, withhold cabozantinib for ≥3 weeks prior to the procedure to reduce risk of osteonecrosis of the jaw and poor wound healing
Osteonecrosis of the jaw	Withhold cabozantinib until complete resolution, then reduce the cabozantinib dosage by 1 dose level
Patient requires elective surgery	If possible, withhold cabozantinib for ≥3 weeks prior to elective surgery and for ≥2 weeks after major surgery and until adequate wound healing, whichever is longer
RPLS is suspected (symptoms of headache, seizure, lethargy, confusion, blindness, and/or other visual and neurologic disturbances along with hypertension of any severity)	Withhold cabozantinib until clarification of the patient's neurologic status (ie, with an emergent brain MRI) has occurred
RPLS is confirmed	Discontinue cabozantinib. The safety of reinitiating cabozantinib in a patient who has experienced RPLS is unknown
Urine dipstick >1+ for protein	Continue cabozantinib at the same dose pending results of a 24-hour urine protein
Urine protein ≥3 g/24 hours	Withhold cabozantinib until urine protein is <3 g/24 hours, then resume cabozantinib at 1 lower dose level. Consider increasing the frequency of urine protein monitoring upon resumption of cabozantinib
Nephrotic syndrome	Discontinue cabozantinib treatment

(continued)

Treatment Modifications (*continued*)

Other Adverse Reactions

Other intolerable G2 adverse reactions	Withhold cabozantinib until improvement to G ≤1 or baseline, then reduce the cabozantinib dosage by 1 dose level
Other G ≥3 adverse reactions	

Hepatic Impairment

Moderate hepatic impairment (Child-Pugh class B)	Decrease the starting dose of cabozantinib to 40 mg once daily

Drug Interactions

Patient requires concomitant use of a strong CYP3A4 inhibitor (eg, atazanavir, clarithromycin, indinavir, itraconazole, ketoconazole, nefazodone, nelfinavir, ritonavir, saquinavir, telithromycin, voriconazole)	Reduce the daily cabozantinib dose by 20 mg. Resume the dose that was used prior to initiating the CYP3A4 inhibitor 2 to 3 days after discontinuing a strong inhibitor
Patient requires concomitant use of a strong CYP3A4 inducer (eg, carbamazepine, phenobarbital, phenytoin, rifabutin, rifampin, rifapentine, St. John's Wort)	Increase the daily cabozantinib dose by 20 mg only if tolerability on the dose without the inducer has been convincingly demonstrated. Resume the dose that was used prior to initiating a CYP3A4 inducer 2 to 3 days after discontinuing a strong inducer. The daily cabozantinib dose should not exceed 80 mg

MI, myocardial infarction; VTE, venous thromboembolic event; RPLS, reversible posterior leukoencephalopathy syndrome; UPCR, urine protein to creatinine ratio; MRI, magnetic resonance imaging; ADL, activities of daily living

Patient Population Studied (N = 658)

This randomized, stratified, open-label, phase 3 trial included 658 adult patients with previously treated RCC and compared treatment with cabozantinib to everolimus. Patients were eligible if they had advanced or metastatic RCC with a clear cell component and measurable disease (by RECIST v1.1) who were previously treated with at least one VEGFR-targeting tyrosine kinase inhibitor and whose disease progressed radiographically during treatment or within 6 months after the most recent dose of the VEGFR inhibitor; patients also had to have a Karnofsky performance score of ≥ 70% and adequate organ and marrow function. Patients were excluded if they had received treatment with an mTOR inhibitor or cabozantinib, treatment with any type of small molecule tyrosine kinase inhibitor within 2 weeks of randomization, treatment with any anticancer antibody within 4 weeks of randomization, radiation therapy for bone metastasis within 2 weeks or any other radiation within 4 weeks, if they had known brain metastases not adequately treated with radiotherapy and/or surgery and were not stable for at least 3 months before randomization, a history of uncontrolled, clinically significant illness, if they were being treated with oral anticoagulants or platelet inhibitors, or if they were chronically taking corticosteroids or other immunosuppressive agents

Efficacy (N = 658)

Efficacy Variable	Cabozantinib (N = 330)	Everolimus (N = 328)	Between-group Comparison
PFS (N = 187 cabozantinib arm, N = 188 everolimus arm), first interim analysis*			
Median PFS—months (95% CI)	7.4 (5.6–9.1)	3.8 (3.7–5.4)	HR 0.58 (95% CI 0.45–0.75); P <0.001
OS (N = 330 cabozantinib arm, N = 328 everolimus arm), first interim analysis			
Median OS—months (95% CI)	NR	NR	HR 0.67 (95% CI 0.51–0.89); P = 0.005, NS†
OS (N = 330 cabozantinib arm, N = 328 everolimus arm), unplanned second interim analysis‡			
Median OS—months (95% CI)	21.4 (18.7–NE)	16.5 (14.7–18.8)	HR 0.66 (95% CI 0.53–0.83); P = 0.00026)
OS (N = 330 cabozantinib arm, N = 328 everolimus arm), long-term follow-up§			
Median OS—months	21.4	17.1	HR 0.70 (95% CI 0.58–0.85); P = 0.0002
Response (N = 330 cabozantinib arm, N = 328 everolimus arm)			
ORR—n/N (%) [95% CI]	57/330 (17) [13–22]	11/328 (3) [2–6]	P <0.0001
CR rate—n/N	0/330	0/328	—

*The primary end point was PFS (Choueiri TK et al. N Engl J Med 2015;373:1814–23)
†From the prespecified interim analysis of OS. In this analysis, the significance boundary for OS required a P value of <0.0019. Choueiri TK et al. N Engl J Med 2015;373:1814–1823
‡A P value ≤0.0163 was considered significant for this overall survival analysis. Choueiri TK et al. Lancet Oncol 2016;17:917–927
§Median duration of follow-up was 28 months (IQR, 25–30)
CI, confidence interval; HR, hazard ratio; NS, not significant, PFS, progression-free survival; OS, overall survival; NR, not reported; ORR, objective response rate; CR, complete response; PR, partial response
Note: patients were randomized with stratification for the number of previous VEGFR-targeting tyrosine kinase inhibitors (1 or ≥2) received by subjects and prognostic risk category (favorable, intermediate, or poor), according to the Memorial Sloan Kettering Cancer Center (MSKCC) criteria. Efficacy performed in the intention-to-treat population

Adverse Events (N = 653)

Event	Cabozantinib (N = 331)			Everolimus (N = 322)		
	G1/2 (%)	G3 (%)	G4 (%)	G1/2 (%)	G3 (%)	G4 (%)
Any adverse event	21	63	8	32	52	0
Diarrhea	62	13	0	26	2	0
Fatigue	48	11	0	40	7	0
Nausea	48	5	0	29	<1	0
Decreased appetite	44	3	0	35	1	0
PPES	35	8	0	5	1	0
Vomiting	32	2	0	14	1	0
Weight decreased	32	3	0	13	0	0
Constipation	27	<1	0	20	<1	0
Dysgeusia	24	0	0	9	0	0
Hypothyroidism	23	0	0	<1	<1	0
Hypertension	22	15	0	4	4	0
Dysphonia	21	1	0	5	0	0
Cough	20	<1	0	33	1	0
Stomatitis	20	2	0	22	2	0
Mucosal inflammation	18	2	0	20	3	<1
Dyspnea	17	3	0	26	3	1
AST increased	17	2	0	6	<1	0
Back pain	16	2	0	13	2	0
Rash	16	1	0	29	1	0
Asthenia	15	5	0	14	2	0
Abdominal pain	15	4	0	8	2	0
ALT increased	14	2	<1	6	<1	0

Event	Cabozantinib (N = 331)			Everolimus (N = 322)		
	G1/2 (%)	G3 (%)	G4 (%)	G1/2 (%)	G3 (%)	G4 (%)
Pain in extremity	14	2	0	10	<1	0
Muscle spasms	14	0	0	5	0	0
Arthralgia	13	<1	0	14	1	0
Headache	13	<1	0	13	<1	0
Anemia	13	6	0	23	17	0
Dizziness	12	<1	0	7	0	0
Dyspepsia	12	<1	0	5	0	0
Peripheral edema	12	0	0	22	2	0
Hypomagnesemia	12	2	3	2	0	0
Dry skin	11	0	0	11	0	0
Proteinuria	11	2	0	9	1	0
Flatulence	10	0	0	2	0	0
Insomnia	10	0	0	10	<1	0
Pyrexia	9	1	0	18	1	0
Pruritus	8	0	0	15	<1	0
Blood creatinine increased	5	<1	0	12	0	0
Hypertriglyceridemia	5	1	0	10	2	1
Hyperglycemia	5	1	<1	14	5	0
Epistaxis	4	0	0	14	0	0

Adverse events included if they were G1–2 and reported in ≥ 10% of patients in either group, regardless of whether the adverse events were considered by the investigator to be related to study treatment. Adverse events were graded according to the National Cancer Institute Common Terminology Criteria for Adverse Events (NCI-CTCAE) v4.0.
Choueiri TK et al. Lancet Oncol 2016;17:917–927

Therapy Monitoring

1. *Prior to initiation of cabozantinib:* CBC with differential and platelet count, vital signs, liver function tests, serum electrolytes, oral examination. Control hypertension prior to initiation of cabozantinib
2. Monitor regularly for:
   • Hypertension
   • Signs and symptoms of bleeding
   • Signs and symptoms of fistulas and perforations, including abscess and sepsis
   • Diarrhea
   • Spot urine for protein measurement every 4–8 weeks (if spot urine dipstick >2+ for protein, perform a 24-hour urine protein)
   • Signs and symptoms of osteonecrosis of the jaw
     – Perform an oral examination prior to initiation of cabozantinib and periodically during treatment.
     – Advise patients regarding good oral hygiene practices
     – Withhold cabozantinib for ≥3 weeks prior to scheduled dental surgery or invasive dental procedures, if possible.
     – Withhold cabozantinib for development of osteonecrosis of the jaw until complete resolution
3. Withhold cabozantinib for ≥3 weeks prior to elective surgery (including dental surgery) and for ≥2 weeks after major surgery and until adequate wound healing, whichever is longer

METASTATIC • CLEAR-CELL • SUBSEQUENT THERAPY
RENAL CELL CARCINOMA REGIMEN: LENVATINIB + EVEROLIMUS

Motzer RJ et al. Lancet Oncol 2015;16:1473–1482
Supplementary appendix to: Motzer RJ et al. Lancet Oncol 2015;16:1473–1482
LENVIMA (lenvatinib) prescribing information. Woodcliff Lake, NJ: Eisai Inc; Revised February 2020
AFINITOR (everolimus) prescribing information. East Hanover, NJ: Novartis Pharmaceuticals Corporation; Revised January 2020

Lenvatinib 18 mg per dose; administer orally once daily, without regard to food, continuously until disease progression (total dosage/week = 126 mg)

- Lenvatinib capsules should ideally be swallowed whole. Patients who have difficulty swallowing whole lenvatinib capsules may instead place the appropriate combination of whole capsules necessary to administer the required dose in 15 mL of water or apple juice in a glass container for at least 10 minutes. After 10 minutes, the contents of the glass container should be stirred for at least 3 minutes and then the resulting mixture should be swallowed orally. After drinking, rinse the glass container with an additional 15 mL of water or apple juice and swallow the liquid to ensure complete administration of the lenvatinib dose
- A missed dose of lenvatinib may be taken up to 12 hours before a subsequently scheduled dose
- Reduce the lenvatinib starting dose to 10 mg per dose, administered orally once daily for severe (Child-Pugh class C) hepatic impairment
- Reduce the lenvatinib starting dose to 10 mg per dose, administered orally once daily for severe (creatinine clearance <30 mL/minute) renal impairment
- Patients with pre-existing hypertension should have blood pressure adequately controlled (blood pressure ≤150/90 mmHg) prior to initiation of treatment with lenvatinib

Everolimus 5 mg/dose; administer orally, once daily either consistently with food or without food, continually until disease progression (total dosage/week = 35 mg)

Notes:
- Patients who delay taking everolimus at a regularly scheduled time should be instructed to administer the missed dose if the delay is ≤6 hours following the normal time of administration. If the delay is >6 hours, take the next dose at the next regularly scheduled time
- Dexamethasone alcohol-free mouthwash used concomitantly with everolimus decreases the incidence of stomatitis (Rugo HS et al. Lancet Oncol 2017;18:654–662):
  - **Dexamethasone 0.5 mg/5 mL alcohol-free oral solution** 10 mL/dose; swish for 2 minutes and then expectorate four times per day during treatment with everolimus
- Everolimus is a substrate for cytochrome P450 (CYP) CYP3A subfamily enzymes and P-glycoprotein (P-gp). Avoid everolimus use with a concomitant P-gp inhibitor and strong CYP3A4 inhibitor. If everolimus must be used with a concomitant P-gp inhibitor and moderate CYP3A4 inhibitor, reduce the dose of everolimus. Avoid concomitant use of St. John's Wort. If concurrent use with a P-gp and strong CYP3A4 inducer is required, consider doubling the everolimus dose
- Advise patients to not consume grapefruit and grapefruit juice as they may inhibit CYP3A in the gut wall and increase the bioavailability of everolimus
- Everolimus undergoes extensive hepatic metabolism. Reduce the everolimus dose in patients with mild (Child-Pugh class A) hepatic dysfunction by 25%, moderate (Child-Pugh class B) hepatic dysfunction by 50%, and severe (Child-Pugh class C) hepatic dysfunction by 75% (if benefits outweigh risks)

Supportive Care
Antiemetic prophylaxis
Emetogenic potential of lenvatinib is **MODERATE TO HIGH**
Emetogenic potential of everolimus is **MINIMAL TO LOW**
See Chapter 42 for antiemetic recommendations
Hematopoietic growth factor (CSF) prophylaxis
Primary prophylaxis is **NOT** indicated
See Chapter 43 for more information

Antimicrobial prophylaxis
Risk of fever and neutropenia is **LOW**
  Antimicrobial primary prophylaxis to be considered:
- Antibacterial—not indicated
- Antifungal—not indicated
- Antiviral—not indicated unless patient previously had an episode of HSV

Prophylaxis and treatment for mucositis/stomatitis
General advice:
- Dexamethasone alcohol-free mouthwash used concomitantly with everolimus decreases the incidence of stomatitis (Rugo HS, et al. Lancet Oncol 2017;18:654–662):

(continued)

(*continued*)

- **Dexamethasone 0.5 mg/5 mL alcohol-free oral solution** 10 mL/dose; swish for 2 minutes and then expectorate four times per day during treatment with everolimus
- Otherwise, standard prophylaxis and treatment for mucositis/stomatitis

Diarrhea management
Latent or delayed-onset diarrhea*:
  Loperamide 4 mg orally initially after the first loose or liquid stool, *then* 2–4 mg orally every 2–4 hours or **diphenoxylate hydrochloride** 2.5 mg with **atropine sulfate** 0.025 mg (eg, Lomotil)

*Abigerges D et al. J Natl Cancer Inst 1994;86:446–449
Rothenberg ML et al. J Clin Oncol 2001;19:3801–3807
Wadler S et al. J Clin Oncol 1998;16:3169–3178

Treatment Modifications

RECOMMENDED DOSE MODIFICATIONS FOR LENVATINIB

Starting dose	18 mg by mouth once daily
Dose Level –1	14 mg by mouth once daily
Dose Level –2	10 mg by mouth once daily
Dose Level –3	8 mg by mouth once daily
Dose Level –4	Discontinue lenvatinib

For adverse reactions common to both lenvatinib and everolimus, prioritize reducing the lenvatinib dose first

Lenvatinib Dose Modification—Cardiovascular Toxicity

Adverse Event	Treatment Modification
Either of the following: • G2 hypertension (SBP 140–159 mm Hg or DBP 90–99 mm Hg) • G3 hypertension (SBP ≥160 mm Hg or DBP ≥100 mm Hg) on suboptimal antihypertensive therapy	Continue lenvatinib at the same dose and optimize antihypertensive therapy. Monitor blood pressure frequently
G3 hypertension (SBP ≥160 mm Hg or DBP ≥100 mm Hg) persistent despite optimal antihypertensive therapy	Withhold lenvatinib until hypertension controlled to G ≤2, then resume lenvatinib at one lower dose level. Monitor blood pressure frequently
G4 hypertension (life-threatening consequences [eg, malignant hypertension, transient or permanent neurologic deficit, hypertensive crisis]; urgent intervention indicated)	Permanently discontinue lenvatinib
G3 cardiac dysfunction	Withhold lenvatinib until cardiac dysfunction improves to G ≤1 or baseline, then resume lenvatinib at one lower dose level or discontinue lenvatinib depending upon the severity and persistence of cardiac dysfunction
G4 cardiac dysfunction	Permanently discontinue lenvatinib
QTc prolongation (>500 ms, or >60 ms increase from baseline)	Withhold lenvatinib until QTc improves to ≤480 ms or baseline, then resume at one lower dose level. Correct hypomagnesemia and/or hypokalemia if applicable
Arterial thromboembolic event	Permanently discontinue lenvatinib

Lenvatinib Dose Modification—Gastrointestinal Toxicity

Gastrointestinal perforation	Permanently discontinue lenvatinib
G3/4 fistula formation	Permanently discontinue lenvatinib

(*continued*)

Treatment Modifications (continued)

Adverse Event	Treatment Modification
Either of the following: • G1 diarrhea • G2 diarrhea lasting ≤2 weeks	Continue current lenvatinib dose and optimize antidiarrheal medications
Any of the following: • G2 diarrhea lasting >2 weeks • G3 diarrhea • G4 diarrhea developing in a patient not receiving an optimal antidiarrheal regimen	Withhold lenvatinib until diarrhea resolves to G ≤1 or baseline, then resume lenvatinib at 1 lower dose level. Antidiarrheal treatment for symptoms may continue indefinitely as a preventive measure
Recurrent or persistent G4 diarrhea in a patient receiving an optimal antidiarrheal regimen	Permanently discontinue lenvatinib

Lenvatinib Dose Modification—Hepatic Toxicity and Hepatic Impairment

G3/4 hepatotoxicity (ALT/AST >5× ULN, bilirubin >3× ULN)	Withhold lenvatinib until hepatotoxicity improves to G ≤1, then resume lenvatinib at one lower dose level or discontinue lenvatinib depending upon the severity and persistence of hepatotoxicity
Hepatic failure	Permanently discontinue lenvatinib
Severe hepatic impairment (Child-Pugh class C)	Reduce initial lenvatinib dose to 10 mg orally once daily

Lenvatinib Dose Modification—Renal Toxicity and Renal Impairment

G3/4 AKI (SCr >3× baseline or >4 mg/dL; hospitalization indicated; life-threatening consequences; dialysis indicated)	Initiate prompt evaluation and correction of dehydration if applicable. Withhold lenvatinib until toxicity improves to G ≤1 or baseline, then resume at one lower dose level or discontinue lenvatinib depending upon the severity and persistence of renal impairment
Severe renal impairment (CrCl <30 mL/min*)	Reduce initial lenvatinib dose to 10 mg orally once daily
Urine dipstick proteinuria ≥2+	Continue lenvatinib at current dose and obtain a 24-hour urine protein
Proteinuria ≥2 grams in 24 hours	Withhold lenvatinib until <2 grams of proteinuria per 24 hours, then resume lenvatinib at one lower dose level
Nephrotic syndrome	Permanently discontinue lenvatinib

Lenvatinib Dose Modification—Other Toxicities

RPLS	Withhold lenvatinib until fully resolved, then resume at a reduced dose or discontinue depending on severity and persistence of neurologic symptoms
Planned elective surgery	Withhold lenvatinib for at least 6 days prior to scheduled surgery. Resume lenvatinib after surgery based on clinical assessment of adequate wound healing
Patient with wound-healing complications	Permanently discontinue lenvatinib
Other toxicities (eg, hand-foot skin reaction, rash, nausea/vomiting, stomatitis, hemorrhage, etc) • Other persistent/intolerable G2 toxicities • Other G3 toxicities	Withhold lenvatinib until toxicity improves to G ≤1 or baseline, then resume lenvatinib at one lower dose level
G4 laboratory abnormality	Withhold lenvatinib until toxicity improves to G ≤1 or baseline, then resume lenvatinib at one lower dose level
Other G4 toxicity	Permanently discontinue lenvatinib

*CrCl calculated using the Cockcroft-Gault equation using actual body weight

SBP, systolic blood pressure; DBP, diastolic blood pressure; ALT, alanine aminotransferase; AST, aspartate aminotransferase; AKI, acute kidney injury; SCr, serum creatinine; CrCl, creatinine clearance; RPLS, reversible posterior leukoencephalopathy syndrome

LENVIMA (lenvatinib) prescribing information. Woodcliff Lake, NJ: Eisai Inc; Revised February 2020

(continued)

Treatment Modifications (*continued*)

RECOMMENDED DOSE MODIFICATIONS FOR EVEROLIMUS

Starting dose level	5 mg orally once daily
Dose level −1	5 mg orally once every other day
Dose level −2	Discontinue everolimus

For adverse reactions common to both lenvatinib and everolimus, prioritize reducing the lenvatinib dose first

Adverse Event	Dose Modification
Radiologic changes suggestive of noninfectious pneumonitis with few or no symptoms	Can continue everolimus therapy without dose alteration but with careful monitoring
Radiologic changes suggestive of noninfectious pneumonitis with moderate symptoms	Withhold everolimus until symptoms improve. Consider using corticosteroids. If symptoms improve, consider reintroducing everolimus one dose lower with careful continued monitoring
Radiologic changes suggestive of noninfectious pneumonitis with severe symptoms	Discontinue everolimus. Consider using corticosteroids
Diagnosis of a medically significant infection	Withhold everolimus and institute appropriate treatment promptly. Consider discontinuing everolimus
Diagnosis of invasive systemic fungal infection	Discontinue everolimus and treat with appropriate antifungal therapy
G1/2 stomatitis	Withhold everolimus and administer topical treatments (avoid alcohol- or peroxide-containing mouthwashes as they may exacerbate the condition). Do not use antifungal agents unless fungal infection has been diagnosed. If symptoms improve to G <1, everolimus treatment may begin with either the same dose or one dose level lower
G3 stomatitis	Withhold everolimus and administer topical treatments (avoid alcohol- or peroxide-containing mouthwashes as they may exacerbate the condition). Do not use antifungal agents unless fungal infection has been diagnosed. If symptoms improve to G <1, everolimus treatment may begin with one dose level lower
Recurrent G3 or G4 stomatitis	Discontinue everolimus
Elevated blood glucose	Withhold everolimus and correct before restarting everolimus

AFINITOR (everolimus) prescribing information. East Hanover, NJ: Novartis Pharmaceuticals Corporation; revised 2020 January

Patient Population Studied

This international, multicenter, randomized, phase 2, open-label trial included 153 adult patients with histologically verified clear cell RCC who had radiographic evidence of progressive advanced or metastatic renal cell carcinoma within 9 months of stopping prior therapy. Eligible participants had one previous disease progression with VEGF-targeted therapy, an Eastern Cooperative Oncology Group (ECOG) performance status of 0 or 1, and adequately controlled blood pressure (BP ≤150/90 mmHg). Patients were excluded if they had brain metastases. Participants were randomized 1:1:1 to receive either lenvatinib + everolimus, single-agent lenvatinib, or single-agent everolimus

Efficacy (N = 153)

Efficacy Variable	L + E (N = 51)	L (N = 52)	E (N = 50)	Between-group Comparison
Progression-free survival				
Median PFS, months (95% CI)	14.6 (5.9–20.1)	7.4 (5.6–10.2)	5.5 (3.5–7.1)	**L+E vs E** HR 0.40 (95% CI 0.24–0.68); P = 0.005, adjusted P = 0.0011
PFS at 6 months (95% CI)	64% (48–76)	63% (48–75)	39% (24–53)	
PFS at 12 months (95% CI)	51% (35–65)	34% (21–48)	21% (10–36)	**L+E vs L** HR 0.66 (95% CI 0.39–1.10); P = 0.12, adjusted P = 0.096 **L vs E** HR 0.61 (95% CI 0.38–0.98); P = 0.048
Objective response				
Compete response	2%	0	0	**L+E vs E; ORR** RR 7.2 (95% CI 2.3–22.5); P <0.0001
Partial response	41%	27%	6%	**L+E vs L; ORR** RR 1.6 (95% CI 0.9–2.8); P = 0.10 **L vs E; ORR** RR 4.5 (95% CI 1.4–14.7); P = 0.0067
Stable disease	41%	52%	62%	—
Progressive disease	4%	6%	24%	—
Not assessed	12%	15%	8%	—
Overall survival (at June 13, 2014)				
Median OS, months (95% CI)	25.5 (5.9–20.1)	18.4 (13.3–NE)	17.5 (11.8–NE)	**L+E vs E** HR 0.55 (95% CI 0.30–1.01); P = 0.062
OS at 12 months (95% CI)	74% (60–84)	71% (57–82)	62% (47–74)	**L+E vs L** HR 0.74 (95% CI 0.40–1.36); P = 0.30
OS at 18 months (95% CI)	67% (51–78)	54% (39–67)	47% (31–62)	**L vs E** HR 0.74 (95% CI 0.42–1.31); P = 0.29
Overall survival (post-hoc updated analysis at December 10, 2014)				
Median OS, months (95% CI)	25.5 (16.4–NE)	19.1 (13.6–26.2)	15.4 (11.8–19.6)	**L+E vs E** HR 0.51 (95% CI 0.30–0.88); P = 0.024
OS at 12 months (95% CI)	75% (60–84)	71% (57–82)	62% (47–74)	**L+E vs L** HR 0.75 (95% CI 0.43–1.30); P = 0.32
OS at 18 months (95% CI)	65% (50–76)	56% (41–68)	41% (27–54)	**L vs E** HR 0.68 (95% CI 0.41–1.14); P = 0.12

PFS, progression-free survival; CI, confidence interval; L, lenvatinib; E, everolimus; HR, hazard ratio; ORR, objective response rate; RR, rate ratio; NE, not evaluable
Note: the median duration of follow-up for overall survival at the post-hoc updated analysis with data cutoff date of December 10, 2014 was 24.2 months (IQR, 20.1–27.4) in the lenvatinib + everolimus arm, 22.3 months (IQR, 18.7–27.0) in the lenvatinib arm, and 25.0 months (IQR, 21.5–26.1) in the everolimus arm

Adverse Events (N = 153)

Event	Lenvatinib + Everolimus (N = 51)		Single-agent Lenvatinib (N = 52)		Single-agent Everolimus (N = 50)	
	G1/2 (%)	G3/4 (%)	G1/2 (%)	G3/4 (%)	G1/2 (%)	G3/4 (%)
Any TEAE	28	72	15	79	46	50
Diarrhea	65	20	60	12	32	2
Decreased appetite	45	6	54	4	18	0
Fatigue or asthenia	45	14	42	8	36	2
Vomiting	37	8	35	4	10	0
Nausea	35	6	54	8	16	0
Cough	37	0	15	2	30	0
Hypercholesterolemia	31	2	10	2	16	0
Decreased weight	29	2	42	6	8	0
Stomatitis	29	0	23	2	40	2
Hypertriglyceridemia	27	8	10	4	16	8
Hypertension	27	14	31	17	8	2
Peripheral edema	27	0	15	0	18	0
Upper abdominal pain	26	4	27	4	10	0
Hypothyroidism	24	0	35	2	2	0
Arthralgia	24	0	25	0	14	0
Dyspnea	22	2	19	2	14	8
Dysphonia	20	0	37	0	4	0
Pyrexia	20	2	10	0	8	2
Epistaxis	18	0	8	0	22	0
Proteinuria	18	4	12	19	12	2
Rash	18	0	17	0	22	0
Hyperglycemia	16	0	6	0	12	10
Back pain	16	4	21	0	14	0
Headache	16	2	21	4	8	2
Insomnia	16	2	14	0	2	0
Increased TSH	14	0	4	0	2	0
Musculoskeletal chest pain	14	2	10	2	4	0
Constipation	12	0	37	0	18	0
Dyspepsia	12	0	10	2	10	0
Nasopharyngitis	12	0	6	0	12	0

(continued)

Adverse Events (N = 153) (continued)

Event	Lenvatinib + Everolimus (N = 51)		Single-agent Lenvatinib (N = 52)		Single-agent Everolimus (N = 50)	
	G1/2 (%)	G3/4 (%)	G1/2 (%)	G3/4 (%)	G1/2 (%)	G3/4 (%)
Oral pain	12	0	10	0	2	0
Pruritis	12	0	6	0	14	0
Dry skin	10	0	6	0	6	0
Mouth ulceration	10	0	0	0	8	2
Musculoskeletal pain	10	0	12	2	2	0
Pain in extremity	10	0	10	2	6	0
Toothache	10	0	6	0	2	0
Anemia	8	8	6	2	14	12
Palmar-plantar erythrodysesthesia syndrome	8	0	15	0	4	0
Lethargy	6	0	14	0	4	0
Myalgia	6	0	12	2	2	0
Upper respiratory tract infection	6	0	14	0	10	0
Dry mouth	4	0	12	0	6	0
Exertional dyspnea	4	0	2	0	10	0
Lower respiratory tract infection	2	0	0	8	10	2

TSH, thyroid-stimulating hormone; TEAE, treatment-emergent adverse event
Note: includes TEAEs (Grade 1–2) with a frequency of ≥10% in any treatment group

Therapy Monitoring

1. Lenvatinib:
   - Check ALT, AST, bilirubin, and alkaline phosphatase at baseline, every 2 weeks for 2 months, and then at least monthly thereafter
   - Check BUN and serum creatinine at baseline and then periodically
   - Check serum calcium at baseline and at least monthly
   - Check TSH and free thyroxine (FT4) every 4–6 weeks
   - Monitor urine dipstick for protein at baseline and then periodically during treatment. If 2+, then perform a 24-hour urine collection for protein
   - Monitor blood pressure at baseline, after 1 week, every 2 weeks for 2 months, and then at least monthly thereafter
   - Check an electrocardiogram (ECG) at baseline and periodically in patients at increased risk for QT prolongation (eg, congenital long QT syndrome, heart failure, bradyarrhythmias, or in patients taking concomitant medications known to prolong the QT interval)
   - Monitor periodically for signs and symptoms of cardiac dysfunction, arterial thrombosis, reversible posterior leukoencephalopathy syndrome (RPLS), fistula formation, gastrointestinal perforation, and wound-healing complications

2. Everolimus:
   - *Baseline and periodically:* CBC with differential and platelet count, ALT, AST, bilirubin, alkaline phosphatase, BUN, and serum creatinine. Fasting serum glucose and lipid panel
   - Monitor for symptoms of pulmonary toxicity, infection, and stomatitis
   - Everolimus may impair wound healing; use caution and strongly consider withholding therapy in the peri-surgical period
   - Advise patients to avoid live vaccines and close contact with those who have received live vaccines

METASTATIC • CLEAR-CELL • SUBSEQUENT THERAPY

RENAL CELL CARCINOMA REGIMEN: NIVOLUMAB

Motzer RJ et al. N Engl J Med 2015;373:1803–1813
Protocol for: Motzer RJ et al. N Engl J Med 2015;373:1803–1813
Supplementary appendix to: Motzer RJ et al. N Engl J Med 2015;373:1803–1813
OPDIVO (nivolumab) prescribing information. Princeton, NJ: Bristol-Myers Squibb Company; revised September 2019

Nivolumab 240 mg; administer intravenously over 30 minutes in a volume of 0.9% NS or D5W, not to exceed 160 mL and sufficient to produce a nivolumab concentration within the range 1–10 mg/mL, every 2 weeks until disease progression (total dosage/2-week cycle = 240 mg)
- Administer nivolumab through an administration set that contains a sterile, non-pyrogenic, low-protein-binding in-line filter with pore size within the range of 0.2–1.2 μm
- Nivolumab can cause severe infusion-related reactions

or

Nivolumab 480 mg; administer intravenously over 30 minutes in a volume of 0.9% NS or D5W not to exceed 160 mL and sufficient to produce a nivolumab concentration within the range 1–10 mg/mL, every 4 weeks until disease progression (total dosage/4-week cycle = 480 mg)
- Administer nivolumab through an administration set that contains a sterile, non-pyrogenic, low-protein-binding in-line filter with pore size within the range of 0.2–1.2 μm
- Nivolumab can cause severe infusion-related reactions

Supportive Care
Antiemetic prophylaxis
Emetogenic potential with nivolumab is **MINIMAL**
See Chapter 42 for antiemetic recommendations

Hematopoietic growth factor (CSF) prophylaxis
Primary prophylaxis is **NOT** indicated
See Chapter 43 for more information

Antimicrobial prophylaxis
Risk of fever and neutropenia is **LOW**
Antimicrobial primary prophylaxis to be considered:
- Antibacterial—not indicated
- Antifungal—not indicated
- Antiviral—not indicated unless patient previously had an episode of HSV

Treatment Modifications

RECOMMENDED DOSE MODIFICATIONS FOR NIVOLUMAB

Adverse Event	Grade/Severity	Treatment Modification
Infusion reaction	Clinically significant but not severe infusion reaction	Interrupt the infusion in patients with clinically significant infusion reactions and consider resuming at a slower rate following resolution. If decision is made to restart, begin at ≤50% of the rate prior to the reaction and increase in 50% increments every 30 minutes if well tolerated. Infusions may be restarted at the full rate during the next cycle
	G3/4 (severe infusion reaction—pyrexia, chills, flushing, hypotension, dyspnea, wheezing, back pain, abdominal pain, and urticaria). Not rapidly responsive to brief interruption of infusion	Stop infusion and administer appropriate medical therapy (eg, epinephrine, corticosteroids, intravenous antihistamines, bronchodilators, and/or oxygen). Discontinue nivolumab
Colitis	G1	Loperamide 4 mg as starting dose then 2 mg before each meal and after each loose stool until without diarrhea for 12 hours, with maximum of 16 mg loperamide per day. If G1 diarrhea or colitis persists >14 days, then add prednisolone 0.5–1 mg/kg (non-enteric-coated) or consider oral budesonide 9 mg daily if no bloody diarrhea

(continued)

Treatment Modifications (*continued*)

Adverse Event	Grade/Severity	Treatment Modification
	G2/3 diarrhea or colitis	Withhold nivolumab. Loperamide 4 mg as starting dose then 2 mg before each meal and after each loose stool until without diarrhea for 12 hours, with maximum of 16 mg loperamide per day. Administer oral prednisone/prednisolone at a dose of 0.5 to 2 mg/kg/day or its equivalent. When improves to G1, begin a slow corticosteroid taper over at least 4 weeks. Resume nivolumab upon symptom control, or when prednisone/prednisolone daily dose <10 mg
	G4 diarrhea or colitis	Permanently discontinue nivolumab. Loperamide 4 mg as starting dose then 2 mg before each meal and after each loose stool until without diarrhea for 12 hours, with maximum of 16 mg loperamide per day. Administer 1–2 mg/kg IV (methyl)prednisolone and convert to 0.5–2 mg/kg prednisone/prednisolone orally each day or its equivalent only after a response. Taper over at least 4 weeks when symptoms improve. If does not improve over 72 hours or worsens, perform flexible sigmoidoscopy/colonoscopy to document colitis then begin infliximab 5 mg/kg (if no perforation/sepsis/TB/hepatitis/NYHA III/IV CHF). If no response, add MMF 500–1000 mg twice daily. If worse on MMF, consider addition of tacrolimus or ATG
Pneumonitis	G2	Withhold nivolumab. Consider *Pneumocystis* prophylaxis depending on the clinical context and coverage with empiric antibiotics. Administer oral prednisone/prednisolone at a dose of 1–2 mg/kg/day or its equivalent. When improves to G1, begin a slow corticosteroid taper over at least 4 weeks. If does not respond adequately after 48 hours, then administer 2–4 mg/kg IV (methyl)prednisolone and convert to 0.5–2 mg/kg prednisone/prednisolone orally each day or its equivalent only after a response, followed by a taper over at least 6 weeks when symptoms improve to G1, titrating to symptoms. Resume nivolumab upon symptom control, or when prednisone/prednisolone daily dose <10 mg
	G3/4	Permanently discontinue nivolumab. Consider *Pneumocystis* prophylaxis depending on the clinical context; cover with empiric antibiotics. Administer 2–4 mg/kg IV (methyl)prednisolone and convert to 1–2 mg/kg prednisone/prednisolone orally each day or its equivalent only after a response, followed by a taper over at least 8 weeks when symptoms improve to G1, titrating to symptoms. If when initially treated improvement does not occur within 48–72 hours, begin infliximab 5 mg/kg (if no perforation/sepsis/TB/hepatitis/NYHA III/IV CHF). If no response to infliximab, add MMF 500–1000 mg twice daily. Consider MMF especially if has concurrent hepatic toxicity
Hepatitis	G2 (AST or ALT >3–5× ULN or total bilirubin >1.5–3× ULN)	Withhold nivolumab. Administer oral prednisone/prednisolone at a dose of 1 to 2 mg/kg/day or its equivalent. When improves to G1, begin a slow corticosteroid taper over at least 4 weeks. Resume nivolumab upon symptom control, or when prednisone/prednisolone daily dose <10 mg
	G3/4 (AST or ALT >5× ULN or total bilirubin >3× ULN)	Permanently discontinue nivolumab. Administer 1–2 mg/kg IV (methyl)prednisolone and convert to 0.5–2 mg/kg prednisone/prednisolone orally each day or its equivalent only after a response. Taper over at least 6 weeks when symptoms improve. If no response, add MMF 500–1000 mg twice daily. If worse on MMF, consider adding tacrolimus or ATG
Hypophysitis	G2/3 (moderate symptoms, ie, headache but no visual disturbance or fatigue/mood alteration but hemodynamically stable, no electrolyte disturbance)	Administer analgesia as needed for headache. Withhold nivolumab. Administer oral prednisone/prednisolone at a dose of 0.5 to 2 mg/kg/day or its equivalent. When improves to G1, begin a slow corticosteroid taper over at least 4 weeks. If no improvement in 48 hours, administer 1–2 mg/kg IV (methyl)prednisolone and convert to 0.5–2 mg/kg prednisone/prednisolone orally each day or its equivalent only after a response. Taper over at least 4 weeks when symptoms improve to 5 mg prednisone/prednisolone or equivalent; do not stop steroids. Resume nivolumab upon symptom control, or when prednisone/prednisolone daily dose <10 mg
	G4 (severe mass effect symptoms, ie, severe headache, any visual disturbance or severe hypoadrenalism, ie, hypotension, severe electrolyte disturbance)	Permanently discontinue nivolumab. Administer analgesia as needed for headache. Administer 1–2 mg/kg IV (methyl)prednisolone and convert to 0.5–2 mg/kg prednisone/prednisolone orally each day or its equivalent only after a response. Taper over at least 4 weeks when symptoms improve to 5 mg prednisone/prednisolone or equivalent; do not stop steroids

(*continued*)

Treatment Modifications (*continued*)

Adverse Event	Grade/Severity	Treatment Modification
Adrenal insufficiency	G2	Withhold nivolumab. Administer oral prednisone/prednisolone at a dose of 0.5 to 2 mg/kg/day or its equivalent. When improves to G1, begin a slow corticosteroid taper over at least 4 weeks. Serially assess adrenal function and continue steroids at replacement doses (20–40 mg hydrocortisone daily ~2/3 dose in AM upon awakening and ~1/3 at 4 PM) until recovery of adrenal function is documented. Resume nivolumab upon symptom control, or when prednisone/prednisolone daily dose <10 mg
	G3/4	Permanently discontinue nivolumab. Administer oral prednisone/prednisolone at a dose of 0.5 to 2 mg/kg/day or its equivalent. When improves to G1, begin a slow corticosteroid taper over at least 4 weeks. Serially assess adrenal function and continue steroids at replacement doses (20–40 mg hydrocortisone daily ~2/3 dose in AM upon awakening and ~1/3 at 4 PM) until recovery of adrenal function is documented
Type 1 diabetes mellitus	G3 hyperglycemia	Withhold nivolumab. Admit to hospital to manage hyperglycemia. Role of corticosteroids in preventing complete loss of insulin-producing cells is unknown and not recommended. Resume nivolumab upon symptom control, or when prednisone/prednisolone daily dose <10 mg
	G4 hyperglycemia	Permanently discontinue nivolumab. Admit to hospital to manage hyperglycemia. Role of corticosteroids in preventing complete loss of insulin-producing cells is unknown and not recommended
Nephritis and renal dysfunction	G2/3 (serum creatinine 1.5–6× ULN)	Withhold nivolumab. Administer oral prednisone/prednisolone at a dose of 0.5 to 2 mg/kg/day or its equivalent. When improves to G1, begin a slow corticosteroid taper over at least 4 weeks. If does not respond adequately, then administer 0.5–1 mg/kg IV (methyl)prednisolone and convert to 0.5–2 mg/kg prednisone/prednisolone orally each day or its equivalent only after a response, followed by a taper over at least 4 weeks when improves to G1. Resume nivolumab upon symptom control, or when prednisone/prednisolone daily dose <10 mg
	G4 (serum creatinine >6× ULN)	Permanently discontinue nivolumab. Administer 0.5–1 mg/kg IV (methyl)prednisolone and convert to 0.5–2 mg/kg prednisone/prednisolone orally each day or its equivalent only after a response, followed by a taper over at least 4 weeks when improves to G1
Skin	G1/2	Continue nivolumab. Avoid skin irritants, avoid sun exposure, topical emollients recommended. Topical steroid (mild strength for G1, moderate/potent strength for G2) cream once or twice daily ± oral or topical antihistamines for itching
	G3 rash or suspected SJS or TEN	Withhold nivolumab. Avoid skin irritants, avoid sun exposure, topical emollients recommended. Administer oral or topical antihistamines for itching. Administer oral prednisone/prednisolone at a dose of 0.5–2 mg/kg or its equivalent daily for 3 days followed by a slow corticosteroid taper over at least 4 weeks when the rash improves to G1. If does not respond adequately, then administer 0.5–1 mg/kg IV (methyl)prednisolone and convert to 0.5–2 mg/kg prednisone/prednisolone orally each day or its equivalent only after a response, followed by a taper over at least 4 weeks when the rash improves to G1. Resume nivolumab upon symptom control, or when prednisone/prednisolone daily dose <10 mg
	G4 rash or confirmed SJS or TEN	Avoid skin irritants, avoid sun exposure, topical emollients recommended. Administer oral or topical antihistamines for itching. Administer 1–2 mg/kg IV (methyl)prednisolone and convert to oral steroids 0.5–2 mg/kg prednisone/prednisolone each day or its equivalent only after a response. Taper over at least 4 weeks when the rash improves to G1. Permanently discontinue nivolumab

(*continued*)

Treatment Modifications (continued)

Adverse Event	Grade/Severity	Treatment Modification
Encephalitis	Confusion or altered behavior, headaches, alteration in Glasgow Coma Scale, motor or sensory deficits, speech abnormality, may or may not be febrile	Initially withhold nivolumab, but permanently discontinue nivolumab if there is no doubt as to diagnosis. Exclude bacterial and ideally viral infections prior to high-dose steroids. Administer oral prednisone/prednisolone at a dose of 0.5–2 mg/kg/day or its equivalent. When symptoms improve, begin a slow corticosteroid taper over at least 4–8 weeks. If symptoms are severe, administer 1–2 mg/kg IV (methyl)prednisolone and convert to 0.5–2 mg/kg prednisone/prednisolone orally each day or its equivalent only after a response. Consider concurrent empiric antiviral (IV acyclovir) and antibacterial therapy
Aseptic meningitis	Headache, photophobia, neck stiffness with fever or may be afebrile, vomiting; normal cognition/cerebral function (distinguishes from encephalitis)	
Other syndromes include neurosarcoidosis, posterior reversible leukoencephalopathy syndrome (PRES), Vogt-Koyanagi-Harada syndrome, demyelination, vasculitic encephalopathy, and generalized seizures		
Transverse myelitis	Acute or subacute neurologic signs/symptoms of motor/sensory/autonomic origin; most have sensory level; often bilateral symptoms	Initially withhold nivolumab, but permanently discontinue nivolumab if there is no doubt as to diagnosis. Administer 2 mg/kg IV (methyl)prednisolone or consider 1 g/day and convert to 0.5–2 mg/kg prednisone/prednisolone orally each day or its equivalent only after a response. When symptoms improve, begin a slow corticosteroid taper over at least 4–8 weeks. Plasmapheresis may be required if steroids do not bring about improvement
Myocarditis	G3	Permanently discontinue nivolumab. Administer 2 mg/kg IV (methyl)prednisolone or consider 1 g/day and convert to 0.5–2 mg/kg prednisone/prednisolone orally each day or its equivalent only after a response. When symptoms improve, begin a slow corticosteroid taper over at least 4–8 weeks. If no response, add MMF 500–1000 mg twice daily. If worse on MMF, consider adding tacrolimus
Peripheral neurologic toxicity	Moderate: some interference with ADL, symptoms concerning to patient	Withhold nivolumab. Initial observation reasonable or initiate prednisone/prednisolone 0.5–1 mg/kg (if progressing, eg, from mild) and/or pregabalin or duloxetine for pain. When symptoms improve, begin a slow corticosteroid taper over at least 4 weeks. Resume nivolumab upon symptom control, or when prednisone/prednisolone daily dose <10 mg
	Severe: limits self-care and aids warranted, life-threatening, eg, respiratory problems	Permanently discontinue nivolumab. Administer 1–2 mg/kg IV (methyl)prednisolone and convert to 0.5–2 mg/kg prednisone/prednisolone orally each day or its equivalent only after a response. Taper over at least 4–8 weeks when symptoms improve to G1
Guillain-Barré syndrome	Progressive symmetrical muscle weakness with absent or reduced tendon reflexes—involves extremities, facial, respiratory, and bulbar and oculomotor muscles; dysregulation of autonomic nerves	Permanently discontinue nivolumab. Use of steroids not recommended in idiopathic Guillain-Barré syndrome; however, a trial of (methyl)prednisolone 1–2 mg/kg is reasonable, converting to 0.5–2 mg/kg prednisone/prednisolone orally each day or its equivalent only after a response. If no improvement or worsening, plasmapheresis or IVIG indicated
Myasthenia gravis	Fluctuating muscle weakness (proximal limb, trunk, ocular, eg, ptosis/diplopia or bulbar) with fatigability, respiratory muscles may also be involved	Permanently discontinue nivolumab. Administer pyridostigmine at an initial dose of 30 mg three times daily. Administer oral prednisone/prednisolone at a dose of 0.5 to 2 mg/kg/day or its equivalent or 1–2 mg/kg IV (methyl)prednisolone depending on the severity of symptoms. If begin with IV, convert to 0.5–2 mg/kg prednisone/prednisolone orally each day or its equivalent only after a response. If no improvement or worsening, plasmapheresis or IVIG may be considered. Additional immunosuppressants used in myasthenia gravis include azathioprine, cyclosporine, and mycophenolate. Avoid certain medications, eg, ciprofloxacin, beta-blockers, that may precipitate cholinergic crisis
Other syndromes including motor and sensory peripheral neuropathy, multifocal radicular neuropathy/plexopathy, autonomic neuropathy, phrenic nerve palsy, cranial nerve palsies (eg, facial nerve, optic nerve, hypoglossal nerve)		Permanently discontinue nivolumab. Administer oral prednisone/prednisolone at a dose of 0.5 to 2 mg/kg/day or its equivalent or 1–2 mg/kg IV (methyl)prednisolone depending on the severity of symptoms. If begin with IV, convert to 0.5–2 mg/kg prednisone/prednisolone orally each day or its equivalent only after a response

(continued)

Treatment Modifications (*continued*)

Adverse Event	Grade/Severity	Treatment Modification
Arthralgia	G1 (mild pain with inflammation, erythema, or joint swelling)	Continue nivolumab. Administer acetaminophen (paracetamol) and ibuprofen
	G2 (moderate pain with inflammation, erythema, or joint swelling that limits ADLs)	Withhold nivolumab. Administer higher doses of acetaminophen (paracetamol) and ibuprofen and use diclofenac or naproxen or etoricoxib. If inadequately controlled, consider intra-articular steroid injections for large joints or administer oral prednisone/prednisolone at a dose of 0.5 to 2 mg/kg/day or its equivalent. When improves to G1, begin a slow corticosteroid taper over at least 4 weeks. If does not respond adequately, then administer 0.5–1 mg/kg IV (methyl)prednisolone and convert to 0.5–2 mg/kg prednisone/prednisolone orally each day or its equivalent only after a response, followed by a taper over at least 4 weeks when improves to G1. Resume nivolumab upon symptom control, or when prednisone/prednisolone daily dose <10 mg
	G3 (severe pain; irreversible joint damage; disabling; limits self-care ADL)	Withhold nivolumab. Administer 0.5–1 mg/kg IV (methyl)prednisolone and convert to 0.5–2 mg/kg prednisone/prednisolone orally each day or its equivalent only after a response, followed by a taper over at least 4 weeks when improves to G1. In severe cases, infliximab or another anti–TNF alpha drug may be required for improvement of arthritis. Resume nivolumab upon symptom control, or when prednisone/prednisolone daily dose <10 mg
Other	First occurrence of other G3	Withhold nivolumab. Administer oral prednisone/prednisolone at a dose of 0.5 to 2 mg/kg/day or its equivalent. When improves to G1, begin a slow corticosteroid taper over at least 4 weeks. Resume nivolumab upon symptom control, or when prednisone/prednisolone daily dose <10 mg
	Recurrence of same G3	Permanently discontinue nivolumab. Administer 1–2 mg/kg IV (methyl)prednisolone and convert to 0.5–2 mg/kg prednisone/prednisolone orally each day or its equivalent only after a response. Taper over at least 4–8 weeks when symptoms improve to G1
	Life-threatening or G4	
	Requirement for ≥10 mg/day prednisone or equivalent for >12 weeks	Permanently discontinue nivolumab
	Persistent G2/3 adverse reactions lasting ≥12 weeks	

ADL, activities of daily living; ALT, alanine aminotransferase; AST, aspartate aminotransferase; ATG, anti–thymocyte globulin; SJS, Stevens-Johnson syndrome; TEN, toxic epidermal necrolysis; ULN, upper limit of normal

Notes on general supportive care:
- Steroid taper in most cases will proceed over a minimum of 1 month but if symptoms improve rapidly, a 2-week taper can be considered. If steroids are administered for more than 4 weeks, consider PCP prophylaxis (cotrimoxazole 480 mg twice daily M/W/F or inhaled pentamidine if has cotrimoxazole allergy), regular random blood glucose, Vitamin D level, and starting calcium/Vitamin D supplementation per guidelines

Patient Population Studied

Checkmate-025 was a randomized, open-label, phase 3 trial that included 821 adult patients with advanced renal cell carcinoma and compared treatment with nivolumab to everolimus as second-line treatment. Patients were eligible for the study if they had histologically confirmed advanced or metastatic RCC with a clear cell component, measurable disease (according to RECIST v1.1 criteria), if they had received one or two previous regimens of antiangiogenic therapy, if they had disease progression during or after the last treatment regimen and within 6 months of study enrollment, and if they had had a Karnofsky performance status of ≥70% at enrollment. Patients were excluded if they had received >3 previous regimens of systemic anticancer agents, if they had CNS metastases, if they had received treatment with an mTOR inhibitor, or if they had a condition requiring treatment with glucocorticoids (at a dose of >10 mg prednisone equivalents)

Efficacy (N = 821)

Efficacy Variable	Nivolumab (N = 410)	Everolimus (N = 411)	Between-group Comparison
OS			
Median OS—months (95% CI)	25.0 (21.8–NE)	19.6 (17.6–23.1)	HR 0.73 (98.5%CI, 0.57–0.93); P = 0.002*
PFS			
Median PFS—months (95% CI)	4.6 (3.7–5.4)	4.4 (3.7–5.5)	HR 0.88 (95% CI 0.75–1.03); P = 0.11
Response[†]			
ORR—n/N (%)	103/410 (25)	22/411 (5)	OR 5.98 (95% CI 3.68–9.72)[†]
CR rate—n/N (%)	4/410 (<1)	2/411 (<1)	—
PR rate—n/N (%)	99/410 (24)	20/411 (5)	—
Median duration of response—months (range)	12.0 (0–27.6)	12.0 (0–22.2)	—
OS in patients with ≥1% PD-L1 expression (N = 94 in nivolumab group, N = 97 in everolimus group)[‡]			
Median OS—months (95% CI)	21.8 (16.5–28.1)	18.8 (11.9–19.9)	HR 0.79 (95% CI 0.53–1.17)
OS in patients with <1% PD-L1 expression (N = 276 in nivolumab group, N = 299 in everolimus group)[‡]			
Median OS—months (95% CI)	27.4 (21.4–NE)	21.2 (17.7–26.2)	HR 0.77 (95% CI 0.60–0.97)

*This result met the prespecified criterion for superiority and led to the study being stopped early and considered the final analysis
[†]Response was assessed by the investigator according to RECIST v1.1 criteria. Between-group differences and CIs of response rates were estimated with the Cochran-Mantel-Haenszel method of weighting, with adjustment for stratification factors. ORR and its corresponding 95% CI were estimated using the Clopper-Pearson method
[‡]Tumor PD-L1 membrane expression (<1% vs ≥1 % and < 5% vs ≥5%) was assessed at a central laboratory using a Dako PD-L1 immunohistochemical staining method. PD-L1 expression was quantifiable in tumor samples from 92% of patients (90% in the nivolumab group and 94% in the everolimus group). Overall, 24% of patients with quantifiable PD-L1 expression had ≥1% PD-L1 expression and 76% had <1% PD-L1 expression
CI, confidence interval; HR, hazard ratio; NE, not estimable; PFS, progression-free survival; OS, overall survival; OR, odds ratio; ORR, objective response rate; CR, complete response; PR, partial response; PD-L1, programmed death-ligand 1
Note: randomization was stratified by region, MSKCC prognostic risk group (0: favorable risk vs 1: intermediate risk vs 2–3: poor risk), and the number of previous antiangiogenic therapy regimens (1 vs 2) for advanced RCC. Efficacy analyses were performed on all patients randomized. OS, PFS, and duration of response were estimated using Kaplan-Meier methods. HRs and CIs for OS and PFS were estimated by fitting a stratified Cox proportional hazards model and between-group differences for OS and PFS were compared using a stratified log-rank test. Data in the table were reported in Motzer et al, 2015 and its supplementary appendix. Data in this paper were collected with a minimum follow-up time of 14 months

Adverse Events (N = 803)

Event	Nivolumab (N = 406)	Everolimus (N = 397)
Dose reductions	Not allowed	26%
Treatment-related adverse events leading to discontinuation	8%	13%
Deaths related to therapy	None	2 (septic shock and acute bowel ischemia)

	Nivolumab (N = 406)		Everolimus (N = 397)	
	Any Grade (%)	Grade 3/4 (%)	Any Grade (%)	Grade 3/4 (%)
Any adverse event	79	19	88	37
Fatigue	33	2	34	3

	Nivolumab (N = 406)		Everolimus (N = 397)	
Nausea	14	<1	17	1
Pruritis	14	0	10	0
Diarrhea	12	1	21	1
Decreased appetite	12	<1	21	1
Rash	10	<1	20	1
Cough	9	0	19	0
Anemia	8	2	24	8
Dyspnea	7	1	13	1
Peripheral edema	4	0	14	1
Pneumonitis	4	1	15	3

(continued)

Adverse Events (N = 803) (continued)

	Nivolumab (N = 406)		Everolimus (N = 397)	
Mucosal inflammation	3	0	19	3
Dysgeusia	3	0	13	0
Hyperglycemia	2	1	12	4
Stomatitis	2	0	29	4
Hypertriglyceridemia	1	0	16	5

	Nivolumab (N = 406)		Everolimus (N = 397)	
Epistaxis	1	0	10	0

Note:
- Adverse events were considered treatment-related and were included in the table if they were reported in ≥10% of patients in either group
- Adverse events were graded according to the National Cancer Institute Common Terminology Criteria for Adverse Events (NCI-CTCAE) v4.0
- Treatment continued after RECIST v1.1-assessed progression in 44% of patients in nivolumab group and 46% of patients in everolimus group because the investigator determined there was continued clinical benefit of treatment

Therapy Monitoring

1. Initially at the time of each dose, and eventually every 6–12 weeks, perform a total body skin examination with attention to *all* mucous membranes as well as a complete review of systems
2. Monitor patients for signs and symptoms of pneumonitis. Evaluate patients with suspected pneumonitis with chest x-ray, CT, and pulse oximetry. For ≥2 toxicity, may include nasal swab, sputum culture and sensitivity, blood culture and sensitivity, and urine culture and sensitivity
3. Monitor patients for signs and symptoms of colitis. Encourage patients to report diarrhea immediately to any member of the health care team
4. Draw AST, ALT, and bilirubin prior to each infusion and/or weekly if there are Grade 1 liver function test elevations. Note, no treatment is recommended for G1 LFT abnormalities. For ≥2 toxicity, work up for other causes of elevated LFTs including viral hepatitis
5. Use basic metabolic panel (Na, K, CO_2, glucose) and patient history as screening tools for hypophysitis including hypopituitarism and adrenal insufficiency. If in doubt, evaluate am adrenocorticotropic hormone (ACTH) and cortisol levels. Consider ACTH stimulation test for indeterminate results
6. Thyroid function at the start of treatment, periodically during treatment, and as indicated based on clinical evaluation, and for clinical signs and symptoms of thyroid disorders. Test for TSH and free thyroxine (FT4) every 4–6 weeks as part of routine clinical monitoring of therapy or for case detection in symptomatic patients
7. Measure glucose at baseline and with each treatment during the first 12 weeks and every 6 weeks thereafter
8. Obtain a serum creatinine prior to every dose. If creatinine is found to be newly elevated, consider holding therapy while other potential causes are evaluated. Note, routine urinalysis is not necessary other than to rule out urinary tract infections, etc
9. Obtain a complete rheumatologic history and perform an examination of all peripheral joints for tenderness, swelling, and range of motion. Examine the spine. Consider plain x-ray/imaging to exclude metastases and evaluate joint damage (erosions), if appropriate
10. In patients at high risk for infections and in appropriately selected patients based on an infectious disease evaluation, draw screening laboratories (HIV, hepatitis A and B, and blood QuantiFERON for TB) to prepare patients to start infliximab

METASTATIC • CLEAR-CELL • SUBSEQUENT THERAPY
RENAL CELL CARCINOMA REGIMEN: TEMSIROLIMUS

Hudes G et al. N Engl J Med 2007;356:2271–2281
TORISEL (temsirolimus) prescribing information. Philadelphia, PA: Wyeth Pharmaceuticals Inc; revised March 2018

Premedication:

Diphenhydramine 25–50 mg; administer intravenously approximately 30 minutes before each dose of temsirolimus as prophylaxis against hypersensitivity reactions (other histamine H$_1$-receptor antagonists may be substituted)

Temsirolimus 25 mg; administer diluted in 250 mL 0.9% sodium chloride injection intravenously over 30–60 minutes once weekly until disease progression (total dose/week = 25 mg)

Notes:

- Prepare the final temsirolimus dilution in either bottles (glass or polypropylene) or plastic bags (polypropylene, polyolefin) protected from light
- Infuse temsirolimus through a non-diethylhexylpthalate (non-DEHP), non-polyvinylchloride (non-PVC), polyethylene-lined administration set containing an in-line polyethersulfone filter with a pore size of ≤5 μm. Alternatively, a polyethersulfone end-filter with a pore size ranging from 0.2 μm to 5 μm may be used in place of an in-line filter
- The concomitant use of strong cytochrome P450 (CYP) CYP3A4 inhibitors should be avoided. If a strong CYP3A4 inhibitor must be administered, a temsirolimus dose reduction to 12.5 mg/week should be considered. However, there are no clinical data with this dose adjustment in patients receiving strong CYP3A4 inhibitors
- If a concomitantly administered strong CYP3A4 inhibitor is discontinued, a washout period of approximately 1 week should be allowed before the temsirolimus dose is adjusted back to the dose used prior to initiation of the strong CYP3A4 inhibitor
- The use of concomitant strong CYP3A4 inducers should be avoided. If a strong CYP3A4 inducer must be administered, a temsirolimus dose increase from 25 mg/week up to 50 mg/week should be considered. However, there are no clinical data with this dose adjustment in patients receiving strong CYP3A4 inducers
- If a concomitantly administered strong CYP3A4 inducer is discontinued, the temsirolimus dose should be returned to the dose used prior to initiation of the strong CYP3A4 inducer
- Patients with mild hepatic impairment (bilirubin >1 to 1.5× ULN or AST >ULN but bilirubin ≤ULN) should be administered temsirolimus at a reduced dose of 15 mg per week
- Temsirolimus has immunosuppressive properties and may predispose patients to infections
- Elevations in serum glucose can occur with temsirolimus. When possible, optimal glucose and lipid control should be achieved before starting a patient on temsirolimus

Supportive Care

Antiemetic prophylaxis
Emetogenic potential is **MINIMAL**
See Chapter 42 for antiemetic recommendations

Hematopoietic growth factor (CSF) prophylaxis
Primary prophylaxis is **NOT** *indicated*
See Chapter 43 for more information

Antimicrobial prophylaxis
Risk of fever and neutropenia is **LOW**
Antimicrobial primary prophylaxis to be considered:
- Antibacterial—not indicated
- Antifungal—not indicated. Consider prophylaxis for *P. jirovecii* (eg, cotrimoxazole) in patients receiving concomitant treatment with corticosteroids or other immunosuppressive agents
- Antiviral—not indicated unless patient previously had an episode of HSV

Oral care
Standard prophylaxis and treatment for mucositis/stomatitis

(continued)

Treatment Modifications

TEMSIROLIMUS

Starting dose level	25 mg IV once per week
Dose level −1	20 mg IV once per week
Dose level −2	15 mg IV once per week
Dose level −3	Discontinue temsirolimus

Adverse Event	Dose Modification
Severe hypersensitivity/infusion reaction	Interrupt the temsirolimus infusion for at least 30–60 minutes depending on the severity of the reaction. At the discretion of the medically responsible health care provider, treatment may be resumed at a slower rate (up to 60-minute infusion duration) following administration of an H_1-receptor antagonist (eg, diphenhydramine 25–50 mg IV, if not previously administered) and/or an H_2-receptor antagonist (eg, famotidine 20 mg IV or ranitidine 50 mg IV)
Diagnosis of an invasive fungal infection	Discontinue temsirolimus and treat with appropriate antifungal therapy
Radiologic changes suggestive of noninfectious pneumonitis with no symptoms	Can continue temsirolimus therapy without dose alteration but with careful monitoring
Radiologic changes suggestive of noninfectious pneumonitis with mild–moderate symptoms	Withhold temsirolimus until symptoms improve. Consider administering corticosteroids. If symptoms improve, consider reintroducing temsirolimus one dose lower depending on the individual clinical circumstances with careful continued monitoring. Consider administering prophylaxis for opportunistic infections (eg, *P. jirovecii*) in patients requiring prolonged corticosteroids
Radiologic changes suggestive of noninfectious pneumonitis with severe symptoms (including a decrease in DL_{CO} on pulmonary function tests)	Discontinue temsirolimus and consider administering high doses of corticosteroids. Consider administering prophylaxis for opportunistic infections (eg, *P. jirovecii*) in patients requiring prolonged corticosteroids
ANC <1000/mm^3 or platelet count <75,000/mm^3	Withhold therapy. Resume temsirolimus when symptoms improve to G ≤2 with temsirolimus dose reduced by 5 mg/week to a dose not less than 15 mg/week
Nephrotic syndrome	Permanently discontinue temsirolimus
Any nonhematologic G3/4 toxicity	Withhold therapy. Resume temsirolimus when symptoms improve to G ≤2 with temsirolimus dose reduced by 5 mg/week to a dose not less than 15 mg/week
G1/2 stomatitis	Administer topical treatments (avoid alcohol- or peroxide-containing mouthwashes as they may exacerbate the condition). Do not use antifungal agents unless fungal infection has been diagnosed. Focus on pain control, oral hygiene, and ensuring adequate nutrition and hydration
Mild hepatic impairment (bilirubin >1 to 1.5× ULN or AST >ULN but bilirubin ≤ULN)	Administer temsirolimus at a reduced dose of 15 mg per week

Adapted in part from TORISEL (temsirolimus) prescribing information. Philadelphia, PA: Wyeth Pharmaceuticals Inc; revised March 2018

Patient Population Studied

A group of 626 patients were randomly assigned to receive interferon (207), temsirolimus (209), or a combination of interferon and temsirolimus (210). Eligibility criteria included patients with histologically confirmed advanced RCC (stage IV or recurrent disease) and a Karnofsky performance score of ≥60 (on a scale of 0–100, with higher scores indicating better performance) who had not previously received systemic therapy for renal cancer. A fasting level of total cholesterol of no more than 350 mg/dL (≤9.1 mmol/L) and a triglyceride level of no more than 400 mg/dL (≤4.5 mmol/L) were required. At least 3 of the following 6 predictors of short survival were required: (a) a serum lactate dehydrogenase level ≥1.5 times the upper limit of normal range; (b) a hemoglobin level less than the lower limit of normal range; (c) a corrected serum calcium level >10 mg/dL (>2.5 mmol/L); (d) <1 year from initial diagnosis of renal cell carcinoma to randomization; (e) a Karnofsky performance score of 60 or 70; or (f) metastases in multiple organs

Efficacy (N = 209)*

Percent objective response rate	8.6 (range: 4.8–12.4)
Median overall survival (95% CI), months	10.9 (range: 8.6–12.7)
Median progression-free survival (95% CI), months	5.5 (range: 3.9–7.0)
Median time to treatment failure (95% CI), months	3.8 (range: 3.5–3.9)

*RECIST (Therasse P et al. J Natl Cancer Inst 2000;92:205–216)

Toxicity (N = 208)*

Adverse Event	% All Grades	% G3/4
Asthenia	51	11
Rash	47	4
Nausea	37	2
Anorexia	32	3
Pain	28	5
Dyspnea	28	9
Infection	27	5
Diarrhea	27	1
Peripheral edema	27	2
Fever	24	1
Abdominal pain	21	4
Stomatitis	20	1
Constipation	20	0
Back pain	20	3
Vomiting	19	2
Weight loss	19	1
Headache	15	1
Chills	8	1
Laboratory Abnormalities		
Anemia	45	20
Hyperlipidemia	27	3
Hyperglycemia	26	11
Hypercholesterolemia	24	1
Increased creatinine level	14	3
Thrombocytopenia	14	1
Increased aspartate aminotransferase level (AST)	8	1
Neutropenia	7	3
Leukopenia	6	1

*NCI Common Terminology Criteria for Adverse Events v3.0

Therapy Monitoring

1. *Baseline and periodically:*
   - ALT, AST, bilirubin, alkaline phosphatase, BUN, and serum creatinine
   - Urine dipstick for protein. If >1+, consider obtaining a 24-hour urine for protein
   - Fasting serum glucose and lipid panel. When possible, achieve optimal glucose and lipid control prior to initiation of temsirolimus
   - Chest x-ray or chest computed tomography (CT) scan to assess for pneumonitis
   - Monitor for symptoms of pulmonary toxicity, infection, hyperglycemia, bowel perforation, nephrotic syndrome, and stomatitis
2. *Baseline and weekly:*
   - CBC with differential and platelet count
   - Monitor for infusion reactions
3. Temsirolimus may impair wound healing; use caution and strongly consider withholding therapy in the peri-surgical period
4. Advise patients to avoid live vaccines and close contact with those who have received live vaccines
5. Complete treatment of any pre-existing invasive fungal infections prior to initiating temsirolimus

METASTATIC • CLEAR-CELL • SUBSEQUENT THERAPY
RENAL CELL CARCINOMA REGIMEN: AXITINIB

Motzer RJ et al. Lancet Oncol 2013;14:552–562
Rini BI et al. Lancet 2011;378:1931–1939
Rini BI et al. Clin Genitourin Cancer 2015;13:540–547
INLYTA (axitinib) prescribing information. New York, NY: Pfizer Labs; revised January 2020

Axitinib 5 mg; administer orally twice daily (approximately every 12 hours), continually, until disease progression (total dose/week = 70 mg)
Notes:
- Axitinib should be swallowed whole (no breaking, crushing, or chewing) with water
- Axitinib may be administered without respect to food ingestion
- Advise patients to avoid grapefruit products while taking axitinib
- Instruct patients who vomit or miss a dose of axitinib to avoid taking an additional dose. The next prescribed dose should be taken at the usual time
- Patients who tolerate axitinib for at least two consecutive weeks with no adverse reactions G >2, who remain normotensive (blood pressure ≤150/90 mm Hg), and are not receiving anti-hypertension medications may have their dose increased to 7 mg twice daily, and further to 10 mg twice daily using the same criteria
- The concomitant use of strong CYP3A4/5 inhibitors should be avoided. Selection of an alternate concomitant medication with no or minimal CYP3A4/5 inhibition potential is recommended. If a strong CYP3A4/5 inhibitor must be co-administered, a dose decrease of axitinib by approximately half is recommended. Subsequent doses can be increased or decreased based on individual safety and tolerability. If co-administration of a strong inhibitor is discontinued, the axitinib dose should be returned (after 3–5 elimination half-lives of the inhibitor) to that used prior to initiation of the strong CYP3A4/5 inhibitor
- The axitinib starting dose should be reduced by approximately half in patients with baseline moderate hepatic impairment (Child-Pugh class B)
- If axitinib is interrupted, patients receiving antihypertensive medications should be monitored for hypotension. The plasma half-life of axitinib is 2–4 hours and blood pressure usually decreases within 1–2 days following dose interruption

Antiemetic prophylaxis
Emetogenic potential of axitinib is **MINIMAL TO LOW**
See Chapter 42 for antiemetic recommendations

Hematopoietic growth factor (CSF) prophylaxis
Primary prophylaxis is **NOT** indicated
See Chapter 43 for more information

Antimicrobial prophylaxis
Risk of fever and neutropenia is **LOW**
   Antimicrobial primary prophylaxis to be considered:
- Antibacterial—not indicated
- Antifungal—not indicated
- Antiviral—not indicated unless patient previously had an episode of HSV

Diarrhea management
Latent or delayed-onset diarrhea*:
   Loperamide 4 mg orally initially after the first loose or liquid stool, *then* 2–4 mg orally every 2–4 hours or **diphenoxylate hydrochloride** 2.5 mg with **atropine sulfate** 0.025 mg (eg, Lomotil)

*Abigerges D et al. J Natl Cancer Inst 1994;86:446–449
Rothenberg ML et al. J Clin Oncol 2001;19:3801–3807
Wadler S et al. J Clin Oncol 1998;16:3169–3178

Treatment Modifications

RECOMMENDED DOSE MODIFICATIONS FOR AXITINIB

Dose level +2	10 mg orally twice per day
Dose level + 1	7 mg orally twice per day
Starting dose (level 1)	5 mg orally twice per day
Dose level −1	3 mg orally twice per day
Dose level −2	2 mg orally twice per day
Dose level −3	Discontinue axitinib*

Grade/Severity	Treatment Modification
The patient has tolerated axitinib at a dose of 5 mg twice per day for ≥2 weeks without G >2 treatment-related adverse reactions, is normotensive (blood pressure ≤150/90 mm Hg), and is not receiving anti-hypertension medication	Increase the dose of axitinib to dose level +1 (7 mg orally twice per day)
The patient has tolerated axitinib at a dose of 7 mg twice per day for ≥2 weeks without G >2 treatment-related adverse reactions, is normotensive (blood pressure ≤150/90 mm Hg), and is not receiving anti-hypertension medication	Increase the dose of axitinib to dose level +2 (10 mg orally twice per day)
Any hypertension	Treat as needed with standard anti-hypertensive therapy
Persistent hypertension despite use of maximal anti-hypertensive medications	Reduce the dosage of axitinib by 1 dosage level
Evidence of hypertensive crisis	Discontinue axitinib*
Urine dipstick >1+ for protein	Continue axitinib at the same dose pending results of a 24-hour urine protein
Urine protein ≥3 g/24 hours	Withhold axitinib until urine protein is <3 g/24 hours, then resume axitinib at 1 lower dose level*
Grade 3 diarrhea	Optimize antidiarrheal regimen and reduce the dose of axitinib by 1 dose level
Grade 4 diarrhea	Withhold axitinib until recovery to G ≤1, then resume axitinib with the dose reduced by 1 dose level and with optimization of the antidiarrheal regimen
Grade 2 AST, ALT, or bilirubin elevation	Increase the frequency of LFT monitoring. Withhold axitinib until improvement to G ≤1 or baseline, then resume axitinib at the same dosage
Grade ≥3 AST, ALT, or bilirubin elevation	Increase the frequency of LFT monitoring. Withhold axitinib until improvement to G ≤1 or baseline, then resume axitinib with the dosage reduced by 1 dose level
Bleeding occurs which requires medical intervention	Withhold axitinib until resolution of bleeding*
Patient requires elective surgery	Withhold axitinib for ≥2 days prior to elective surgery. Do not resume axitinib for at least 2 weeks following major surgery and until adequate wound healing has occurred*
RPLS is suspected (symptoms of headache, seizure, lethargy, confusion, blindness, and/or other visual and neurologic disturbances along with hypertension of any severity)	Withhold axitinib until clarification of the patient's neurologic status (ie, with an emergent brain MRI) has occurred*
RPLS is confirmed	Discontinue axitinib.* The safety of reinitiating axitinib in a patient who has experienced RPLS is unknown
Patient has moderate hepatic impairment (Child-Pugh class B)	Decrease the starting dose of axitinib by approximately 50% and then increase or decrease the dose based on individual safety and tolerability

(continued)

Treatment Modifications (*continued*)

Grade/Severity	Treatment Modification
Patient requires concomitant use of a strong CYP3A4/5 inhibitor (eg, ketoconazole, itraconazole, posaconazole, clarithromycin, atazanavir, indinavir, nefazodone, nelfinavir, ritonavir, saquinavir, telithromycin, and voriconazole)	If concomitant use of the CYP3A4/5 inhibitor is unavoidable, then decrease the dose of axitinib by approximately 50% and then increase or decrease the dose based on individual safety and tolerability. If the strong CYP3A4/5 inhibitor is subsequently discontinued, then resume the axitinib dose that was used prior to initiation of the CYP3A4/5 inhibitor after 3–5 CYP3A4/5 inhibitor half-lives have transpired
Patient requires concomitant use of a moderate or strong CYP3A4/5 inducer (eg, rifampin, dexamethasone, phenytoin, carbamazepine, rifabutin, rifapentine, phenobarbital, St. John's Wort, bosentan, efavirenz, etravirine, modafinil, nafcillin)	Avoid concomitant use of a moderate or strong CYP3A4/5 inducer with axitinib

*If the patient is receiving antihypertensive medications, monitor closely for development of hypotension if axitinib is withheld or discontinued
AST, aspartate aminotransferase; ALT, alanine aminotransferase; LFT, liver function test; RPLS, reversible posterior leukoencephalopathy syndrome; MRI, magnetic resonance imaging

Patient Population Studied

The Axitinib Second-line (AXIS) trial was a multicenter, phase 3, open-label, randomized trial that compared axitinib versus sorafenib in 723 patients with advanced RCC. Eligible patients had RCC with clear cell histology and had progression of disease after one previous systemic therapy (sunitinib, bevacizumab plus interferon alfa, temsirolimus, or cytokines). Participants were required to have measurable disease, an Eastern Cooperative Oncology Group (ECOG) performance status score of ≤1, and blood pressure of ≤140/90 mmHg (antihypertensive medications were allowed). Randomization was stratified by ECOG performance status and previous treatment and patients were randomized 1:1 to receive axitinib or sorafenib

Efficacy (N = 723)

All Patients

Efficacy Variable	Axitinib (N = 361)	Sorafenib (N = 362)	Between-group Comparison
Median OS, months—(95% CI)	20.1 (16.7–23.4)	19.2 (17.5–22.3)	HR 0.969 (95% CI 0.80–1.174) P = 0.3744*
Median PFS, months—(95% CI)	8.3 (6.7–9.2)	5.7 (4.7–6.5)	HR 0.656 (95% CI 0.552–0.779) P <0.0001
Objective response rate, n/N (%)	82/361 (23)	45/362 (12)	P = 0.0001

Patients previously treated with sunitinib

	Axitinib (N = 194)	Sorafenib (N = 195)	Between-group Comparison
Median OS, months—(95% CI)	15.2 (12.8–18.3)	16.5 (13.7–19.2)	HR 0.997 (95% CI 0.782–1.27) P = 0.4902*
Median PFS, months—(95% CI)	6.5 (5.7–7.9)	4.4 (2.9–4.7)	HR 0.719 (95% CI 0.572–0.903) P = 0.0022

Patients previously treated with cytokines

	Axitinib (N = 126)	Sorafenib (N = 125)	Between-group Comparison
Median OS, months—(95% CI)	29.4 (24.5–NE)	27.8 (23.1–34.5)	HR 0.813 (95% CI 0.555–1.191) P = 0.1435*
Median PFS, months—(95% CI)	12.2 (10.2–15.5)	8.2 (6.6–9.5)	HR 0.505 (95% CI 0.373–0.684) P <0.0001

OS, overall survival; CI, confidence interval; HR, hazard ratio; PFS, progression-free survival; NE, not estimable
*One-sided stratified log-rank test

Adverse Events (N = 714)

Event	Axitinib (N = 359)		Sorafenib (N = 355)	
	G1–2 (%)	G3–5 (%)	G1–2 (%)	G3–5 (%)
Diarrhea	43	11	44	8
Hypertension	25	17	18	12
Fatigue	27	10	24	4
Decreased appetite	27	4	24	2
Nausea	28	2	18	1
Dysphonia	28	0	12	0
Hand-foot syndrome	22	6	34	17
Hypothyroidism	20	<0.5	8	0
Weight decreased	16	3	15	3
Asthenia	14	4	11	2
Vomiting	17	1	13	0
Mucosal inflammation	15	1	11	1
Stomatitis	14	1	12	<0.5
Rash	13	<0.5	27	4
Constipation	13	<0.5	13	<0.5
Proteinuria	10	3	7	1
Dysgeusia	11	0	8	0
Headache	10	1	7	0
Arthralgia	9	1	5	<0.5
Dry skin	10	0	10	0
Alopecia	4	0	33	0
Pruritus	6	0	13	0
Pain in extremity	9	<0.5	9	1
Erythema	3	0	10	<0.5

Adverse events included in the table are those that were considered to be treatment-related and that were reported in ≥10% of patients in either group

Therapy Monitoring

1. *At baseline, week 2, week 4, and every 4 weeks thereafter:* clinical assessments including medical history and physical examination, vital signs, ALT, AST, total bilirubin, and CBC with differential. Control blood pressure prior to initiation of axitinib

2. *At screening, after 6 and 12 weeks of therapy, and every 8 weeks thereafter:* tumor assessments. Thyroid function tests. Spot urine for protein measurement (if spot urine dipstick >1+ for protein, perform a 24-hour urine protein)

METASTATIC • NON-CLEAR CELL • FIRST-LINE

RENAL CELL CARCINOMA REGIMEN: SUNITINIB

Tannir NM et al. Eur Urol 2012;62:1013–1019

Sunitinib malate 50 mg; administer orally once daily, continually, without regard for meals, in 6-week cycles consisting of 4 consecutive weeks of daily treatment followed by 2 weeks without treatment, until disease progression (total dose/6-week cycle = 1400 mg)

Notes:

- Patients who delay taking sunitinib malate at a regularly scheduled time may take a missed dose if the interval remaining before the next regularly scheduled dose is ≥12 hours

- If possible, avoid concomitant use of strong CYP3A4 inhibitors and strong CYP3A4 inducers. If a concomitant strong CYP3A4 inhibitor must be used, decrease sunitinib malate to 37.5 mg/dose. If a concomitant strong CYP3A4 inducer must be used, consider increasing sunitinib malate to 87.5 mg/dose while monitoring closely for side effects

- Patients using sunitinib malate should be advised to avoid consuming grapefruit juice for as long as they continue to use sunitinib malate

Supportive Care: Hand-Foot Reaction

For patients who develop a hand-foot reaction, use topical emollients (eg, Aquaphor), topical and/or oral steroids, antihistamine agents (H_1-receptor antagonists), or pyridoxine 50–150 mg/day orally

Antiemetic prophylaxis
Emetogenic potential is **LOW**
See Chapter 42 for antiemetic recommendations

Hematopoietic growth factor (CSF) prophylaxis
Primary prophylaxis is **NOT** *indicated*
See Chapter 43 for more information

Antimicrobial prophylaxis
Risk of fever and neutropenia is **LOW**
   Antimicrobial primary prophylaxis to be considered:
   - Antibacterial—not indicated
   - Antifungal—not indicated
   - Antiviral—not indicated unless patient previously had an episode of HSV

Diarrhea management
Latent or delayed-onset diarrhea*:
   Loperamide 4 mg orally initially after the first loose or liquid stool, *then* 2–4 mg orally every 2–4 hours or **diphenoxylate hydrochloride** 2.5 mg with **atropine sulfate** 0.025 mg (eg, Lomotil)

(continued)

Patient Population Studied

This single-arm, phase 2 trial evaluated the use of sunitinib in 57 adult patients with non–clear cell RCC. Eligible participants had histologically confirmed non–clear cell RCC of any subtype. Patients with clear cell RCC with ≥20% sarcomatoid features also were permitted to enroll. In addition, participants were required to have measurable disease, an Eastern Cooperative Oncology Group performance status of ≤2, adequate hematologic, hepatic, cardiac, and renal function, ≤2 prior therapies, and no previous treatment with vascular endothelial growth factor (VEGF)-directed tyrosine kinase inhibitors (TKIs). Prior therapy with angiogenesis inhibitors that were not anti-VEGF TKIs was permitted. All patients received sunitinib

Efficacy (N = 55)

Histology	Median PFS, Months (95% CI)	Best Response by RECIST		
		PR (%)	Disease Control Rate PR + SD (%)	PD (%)
Entire group (N = 55)	2.7 (1.4–5.4)	3 (5)	3 + 29 (58)	23 (42)
Papillary (N = 25)	1.6 (1.4–5.4)	0 (0)	0 + 12 (48)	13 (52)
Unclassified (N = 8)	3.2 (1.4–NA)	1 (13)	1 + 4 (63)	3 (37)
Sarcomatoid (N = 7)	1.4 (1.3–NA)	0 (0)	0 + 3 (43)	4 (57)
Collecting duct/renal medullary (N = 6)	3.1 (1.4–NA)	0 (0)	0 + 4 (67)	2 (33)
Chromophobe (N = 5)	12.7 (8.5–NA)	2 (40)	2 + 3 (100)	0 (0)
Thyroid-like follicular (N = 1)*	33+	0 (0)	0 + 1 (100)	0 (0)
Translocation (N = 1)†	1.0	0 (0)	0 + 0 (0)	1 (100)
Tubulocystic (N = 1)†	9.8	0 (0)	0 + 1 (100)	0 (0)
Mucinous tubular and spindle (N = 1)†	6.5	0 (0)	0 + 1 (100)	0 (0)

PFS, progression-free survival; CI, confidence interval; RECIST, Response Evaluations Criteria in Solid Tumors; PR, partial response; SD, stable disease; PD, progressive disease
*During the study period, the patient experienced stable disease. There was no progressive disease observed
†Time to progressive disease

Adverse Events (N = 57)

Event	All Patients (N = 57)	
	Grade 3 (%)	Grade 4 (%)
Fatigue*	28.1%	0
Hypertension	28.1%	0
Neutropenia	17.5%	1.8%
Pain	12.3%	0
Mucositis/stomatitis	8.8%	1.8%
Thrombocytopenia	5.3%	3.5%

(continued)

(*continued*)

*Abigerges D et al. J Natl Cancer Inst 1994;86:446–449
Rothenberg ML et al. J Clin Oncol
2001;19:3801–3807
Wadler S et al. J Clin Oncol 1998;16:3169–3178

Therapy Monitoring

1. *Prior to the first cycle of sunitinib:* electrocardiogram (for assessment of QTc interval), echocardiogram, CBC with differential, platelet count, LFTs, serum chemistries, blood glucose, blood pressure, thyroid-stimulating hormone, urine dipstick and/or urinary protein–creatinine ratio, physical examination (including dermatologic examination)

2. *Prior to each cycle of sunitinib:* CBC with differential, platelet count, LFTs, serum chemistries, blood glucose, blood pressure, thyroid-stimulating hormone, urine dipstick and/or urinary protein–creatinine ratio, physical examination (including dermatologic examination)

3. Hepatotoxicity, including liver failure, has been observed. Monitor LFTs before initiation of treatment, during each cycle of treatment, and as clinically indicated

4. Cardiac toxicity including declines in LVEF to below LLN and cardiac failure including death have occurred. Monitor patients for signs and symptoms of congestive heart failure

5. Prolonged QT intervals and torsades de pointes have been observed. Use with caution in patients at higher risk for developing QT interval prolongation. When using sunitinib, monitoring with on-treatment electrocardiograms and electrolytes should be considered monthly at first or when the dose is increased and less frequently thereafter

6. Hypertension may occur. Monitor blood pressure and treat as indicated under Treatment Modifications

7. Thyroid dysfunction may occur. Monitor thyroid function tests every 3 months. Treat hypothyroidism accordingly

8. Temporary interruption of therapy with sunitinib is recommended in patients undergoing major surgical procedures. *Note:* there is limited clinical experience regarding the timing of re-initiation of therapy following major surgical intervention. Therefore, the decision to resume sunitinib therapy following a major surgical intervention should be based on clinical judgment of recovery from surgery

9. Monitor adrenal function in case of stress such as surgery, trauma, or severe infection

Adverse Events (N = 57) (*continued*)

Event	All Patients (N = 57)	
	Grade 3 (%)	Grade 4 (%)
Anemia	8.8%	0
Leukopenia	5.3%	0
Hyperuricemia	0	5.3%
Hyponatremia	5.3%	0
Diarrhea	5.3%	0
Sensory neuropathy	5.3%	0
Nausea	5.3%	0
Anorexia	3.5%	0
Hypophosphatemia	3.5%	0
Vomiting	3.5%	0
Dysphagia	0	1.8%
Motor neuropathy	1.8%	0
Hemorrhage/bleeding	0	1.8%
Non-neutropenic fever	1.8%	0
Left ventricular diastolic dysfunction	1.8%	0
Hyperbilirubinemia	1.8%	0
Hemolysis	1.8%	0
Transaminitis	1.8%	0
Elevated lipase	1.8%	0
Myocardial infarction	0	1.8%
Hypoalbuminemia	1.8%	0
Hypomagnesemia	1.8%	0
Thrombosis/embolism	0	1.8%
Dyspnea	1.8%	0
Rash/desquamation	1.8%	0
Hand-foot skin reaction	1.8%	0
Febrile neutropenia	1.8%	0
Hypokalemia	1.8%	0
Syncope/near syncope	1.8%	0
Dehydration	1.8%	0
Hypocalcemia	1.8%	0

*Fatigue also included asthenia, lethargy, and malaise
Note: reported are treatment-emergent adverse events of Grade 3 or higher that occurred in at least 1 of 57 patients. There was also 1 death (1.8%) within 30 days of discontinuation of the study drug

METASTATIC • NON-CLEAR CELL • FIRST-LINE
RENAL CELL CARCINOMA REGIMEN: CABOZANTINIB

Martínez Chanzá N et al. Lancet Oncol 2019;20:581–590
Supplementary appendix to: Martínez Chanzá N et al. Lancet Oncol 2019;20:581–590
CABOMETYX (cabozantinib) prescribing information. Alameda, CA: Exelixis, Inc; revised January 2020

Cabozantinib tablets (Cabometyx®) 60 mg orally at least 2 hours after or at least 1 hour before eating food, once daily, continually, until disease progression (total dose/week = 420 mg)

Notes:

- Tablets are swallowed whole. Do not crush cabozantinib tablets
- Do not substitute cabozantinib tablets (CABOMETYX) with cabozantinib capsules (COMETRIQ)
- Do not take a missed dose within 12 hours of the next scheduled dose
- In light of the fact that 60% of patients starting at the 60-mg dose had a subsequent dose reduction and 10% discontinued the medication because of adverse effects, clinicians are advised to consider the following:

  - *Patients Taking CYP3A4 Inhibitors*
    - Avoid the use of concomitant strong CYP3A4 inhibitors (eg, atazanavir, clarithromycin, indinavir, itraconazole, ketoconazole, nefazodone, nelfinavir, ritonavir, saquinavir, telithromycin, voriconazole)
    - For patients who require treatment with a strong CYP3A4 inhibitor, reduce the daily cabozantinib dose by 20 mg. Resume the dose that was used prior to initiating the CYP3A4 inhibitor 2 to 3 days after discontinuing a strong inhibitor

  - *Patients Taking Strong CYP3A4 Inducers*
    - Avoid use of strong CYP3A4 inducers (eg, carbamazepine, phenobarbital, phenytoin, rifabutin, rifampin, rifapentine) concomitantly with cabozantinib if alternative therapy is available
    - Inform patients not to ingest foods or nutritional supplements (eg, St. John's Wort [*Hypericum perforatum*]) known to induce cytochrome P450 activity
    - For patients who require treatment with a strong CYP3A4 inducer, increase the daily cabozantinib dose by 20 mg *only if tolerability on the dose without the inducer has been convincingly demonstrated*. Resume the dose that was used prior to initiating a CYP3A4 inducer 2 to 3 days after discontinuing a strong inducer. The daily cabozantinib dose should not exceed 80 mg

  - *Patients with hepatic impairment*
    - In patients with moderate hepatic impairment (Child-Pugh class B), reduce the starting dose of cabozantinib to 40 mg once daily
    - Avoid use of cabozantinib in patients with severe hepatic impairment (Child-Pugh class C)

Supportive Care
Antiemetic prophylaxis
Emetogenic potential is **MINIMAL–LOW**
See Chapter 42 for antiemetic recommendations

Hematopoietic growth factor (CSF) prophylaxis
Primary prophylaxis is **NOT** indicated
See Chapter 43 for more information

Antimicrobial prophylaxis
Risk of fever and neutropenia is **LOW**
  Antimicrobial primary prophylaxis to be considered:
  - Antibacterial—not indicated
  - Antifungal—not indicated
  - Antiviral—not indicated unless patient previously had an episode of HSV

Diarrhea management
Latent or delayed-onset diarrhea*:
Loperamide 4 mg orally initially after the first loose or liquid stool, *then* 2–4 mg orally every 2–4 hours or **diphenoxylate hydrochloride** 2.5 mg with **atropine sulfate** 0.025 mg (eg, Lomotil)

*Abigerges D et al. J Natl Cancer Inst 1994;86:446–449
Rothenberg ML et al. J Clin Oncol 2001;19:3801–3807
Wadler S et al. J Clin Oncol 1998;16:3169–3178

Hand-foot reaction (palmar-plantar erythrodysesthesia, PPE)
- For patients who develop a hand-foot reaction, use topical emollients (eg, Aquaphor), topical or orally administered steroids, antihistamine agents (H_1-receptor antagonists), or pyridoxine
- Pyridoxine may provide relief for discomfort/pain associated with PPE although the mechanism through which this occurs remains unclear
- The suggested pyridoxine starting dose is 50 mg/day, which may be increased to a maximum of 200 mg/day

Treatment Modifications

RECOMMENDED DOSE MODIFICATIONS FOR CABOZANTINIB

Starting dose (level 1)	60 mg orally once daily
Dose level −1	40 mg orally once daily
Dose level −2	20 mg orally once daily
Dose level −3	Consider discontinuing cabozantinib or consider resuming at 20 mg orally once daily, if tolerable, at the discretion of the medically responsible health care provider

Grade/Severity	Treatment Modification
G ≥3 hemorrhage	Permanently discontinue cabozantinib
Development of a gastrointestinal perforation or G4 fistula	
Acute MI	
Serious arterial or VTE event requiring medical intervention	
Any hypertension	Treat as needed with standard anti-hypertensive therapy
Persistent hypertension despite use of maximal anti-hypertensive medications	Withhold cabozantinib until blood pressure is adequately controlled, then resume cabozantinib with the dosage reduced by 1 dosage level
Evidence of hypertensive crisis or severe hypertension that cannot be controlled with anti-hypertensive therapy	Discontinue cabozantinib
Intolerable G2 diarrhea	Optimize antidiarrheal regimen. Withhold cabozantinib until improvement to G ≤1, then resume cabozantinib with the dosage reduced by 1 dose level
Grade ≥3 diarrhea not manageable with standard antidiarrheal treatments	
Intolerable G2 palmar-plantar erythrodysesthesia syndrome (skin changes [eg, peeling, blisters, bleeding, edema, or hyperkeratosis] with pain; limiting instrumental ADL)	Withhold cabozantinib until improvement to G ≤1, then resume cabozantinib with the dosage reduced by 1 dose level
Grade 3 palmar-plantar erythrodysesthesia syndrome (severe skin changes [eg, peeling, blisters, bleeding, edema, or hyperkeratosis] with pain; limiting self-care ADL)	
Patient requires dental surgery or an invasive dental procedure	If possible, withhold cabozantinib for ≥3 weeks prior to the procedure to reduce risk of osteonecrosis of the jaw and poor wound healing
Osteonecrosis of the jaw	Withhold cabozantinib until complete resolution, then reduce the cabozantinib dosage by 1 dose level
Patient requires elective surgery	If possible, withhold cabozantinib for ≥3 weeks prior to elective surgery and for ≥2 weeks after major surgery and until adequate wound healing, whichever is longer
RPLS is suspected (symptoms of headache, seizure, lethargy, confusion, blindness, and/or other visual and neurologic disturbances along with hypertension of any severity)	Withhold cabozantinib until clarification of the patient's neurologic status (ie, with an emergent brain MRI) has occurred
RPLS is confirmed	Discontinue cabozantinib. The safety of reinitiating cabozantinib in a patient who has experienced RPLS is unknown
Urine dipstick >1+ for protein	Continue cabozantinib at the same dose pending results of a 24-hour urine protein
Urine protein ≥3 g/24 hours	Withhold cabozantinib until urine protein is <3 g/24 hours, then resume cabozantinib at 1 lower dose level. Consider increasing the frequency of urine protein monitoring upon resumption of cabozantinib
Nephrotic syndrome	Discontinue cabozantinib treatment

(continued)

Treatment Modifications (*continued*)

Other Adverse Reactions

Other intolerable G2 adverse reactions	Withhold cabozantinib until improvement to G ≤1 or baseline, then reduce the cabozantinib dosage by 1 dose level
Other G ≥3 adverse reactions	

Hepatic Impairment

Moderate hepatic impairment (Child-Pugh class B)	Decrease the starting dose of cabozantinib to 40 mg once daily

Drug Interactions

Patient requires concomitant use of a strong CYP3A4 inhibitor (eg, atazanavir, clarithromycin, indinavir, itraconazole, ketoconazole, nefazodone, nelfinavir, ritonavir, saquinavir, telithromycin, voriconazole)	Reduce the daily cabozantinib dose by 20 mg. Resume the dose that was used prior to initiating the CYP3A4 inhibitor 2 to 3 days after discontinuing a strong inhibitor
Patient requires concomitant use of a strong CYP3A4 inducer (eg, carbamazepine, phenobarbital, phenytoin, rifabutin, rifampin, rifapentine, St. John's Wort)	Increase the daily cabozantinib dose by 20 mg only if tolerability on the dose without the inducer has been convincingly demonstrated. Resume the dose that was used prior to initiating a CYP3A4 inducer 2 to 3 days after discontinuing a strong inducer. The daily cabozantinib dose should not exceed 80 mg

MI, myocardial infarction; VTE, venous thromboembolic event; RPLS, reversible posterior leukoencephalopathy syndrome; UPCR, urine protein to creatinine ratio; MRI, magnetic resonance imaging; ADL, activities of daily living

Patient Population Studied

This retrospective cohort study included 112 patients with RCC and evaluated the effect of treatment with cabozantinib. Patients were eligible for the study if they had histologically confirmed non–clear cell RCC and if they received cabozantinib for metastatic disease during any treatment line. Patients were excluded if they had mixed tumors with clear cell components. Patients in the cohort had histopathologic disease considered as papillary (59%), Xp11.2 translocation (15%), unclassified (13%), chromophobe (9%), and collecting duct (4%). Within the cohort, sarcomatoid features were evident in 27% of patients. International Metastatic Renal Cell Carcinoma Database Consortium (IMDC) risk group cohort breakdown was favorable (8%), intermediate (63%), poor (26%), and unknown (3%)

Efficacy (N = 112)

Efficacy Variable	Cabozantinib (N = 112)
Survival and treatment failure analyses (N = 112)	
Median PFS—months (95% CI)	7.0 (5.7–9.0)
Median OS—months (95% CI)	12.0 (9.2–17.0)
OS at 6 months—% (95% CI)	79 (70–86)
OS at 12 months—% (95% CI)	51 (39–62)
Median TTF—months (95% CI)	6.7 (5.5–8.6)
Proportion of patients treatment failure-free at 6 months—% (95% CI)	55 (44–64)
Proportion of patients treatment failure-free at 12 months—% (95% CI)	27 (18–38)
Response (N = 112 patients total, 108 of which were evaluable)*	
ORR—n/N (%) [95% CI]	30/112 (27) [19–36]
CR rate—n/N (%)	1/112 (<1)
PR rate—n/N (%)	29/112 (26)

(*continued*)

Efficacy (N = 112) (continued)

Efficacy Variable	Cabozantinib (N = 112)
SD rate—n/N (%)	53/112 (47)
Proportion of patients with overall clinical benefit—n/N (%) [95% CI][†]	83/112 (74) [65–82]

*Clopper-Pearson exact 95% CIs for ORR and overall clinical benefit analysis refer to the percentage of patients, not the number of patients
[†]Overall benefit defined as any of CR, PR, or SD occurring while on treatment and is calculated as CR + PR + SD
CI, confidence interval; PFS, progression-free survival; OS, overall survival; TTF, time to treatment failure; ORR, objective response rate; CR, complete response; PR, partial response; SD, stable disease; IQR, interquartile range
Note: all data was obtained from a retrospective analysis of the included cohort from electronic medical records. OS, PFS, and TTF were estimated using Kaplan-Meier methods. PFS and response (according to RECIST [version not specified]) by either the site investigator or, preferably, official radiology evaluation. Four patients were not evaluable for tumor response (thus affecting PFS, TTF, proportion of patients treatment failure-free, and response analyses) because they were on cabozantinib for less than the cutoff duration of 8 weeks of treatment required for analysis. To be conservative, they were considered non-responders. Data in the table were reported in Chanza et al, 2019. Data were collected from patients treated from roughly 2015 to 2018 and the median follow-up time was 11 months (IQR, 6–18)

Subgroup Analysis				
Group/Subgroup	ORR n/N (%) [95% CI]	Clinical Benefit n/N (%) [95% CI]*	Median TTF Months (95% CI)	OS at 12 Months % (95% CI)
Histologic groups (N = 112 total; individual subgroup n values reported below)				
Papillary (N = 66)	18/66 (27) [17–40]	48/66 (73) [60–83]	6.9 (4.6–10.1)	46 (31–60)
Xp11.2 (n = 17)	5/17 (29) [10–56]	14/17 (82) [57–96]	8.3 (4.6–NR)	69 (36–87)
Unclassified (n = 15)	2/15 (13) [2–40]	10/15 (67) [38–88]	6.0 (1.4–9.9)	36 (8–67)
Chromophobe (n = 10)	3/10 (30) [7–65]	7/10 (70) [35–93]	5.7 (1.1–7.8)	60 (16–87)
Collecting duct (n = 4)	2/4 (50) [7–93]	4/4 (100) [40–99]	NC	NC
Presence of sarcomatoid features (N = 81 total; individual subgroup n values reported below)				
Present (n = 30)	6/30 (20) [8–39]	23/30 (77) [58–90]	5.1 (2.8–6.2)	25 (8–47)
Absent (n = 51)	13/51 (25) [14–40]	34/51 (67) [52–79]	7.4 (4.6–11.0)	48 (31–64)
IMDC risk group (N = 109 total; individual subgroup n values reported below)				
Favorable (n = 9)	5/9 (56) [21–86]	8/9 (89) [52–99]	11.0 (6.2–NR)	67 (19–90)
Intermediate (n = 71)	15/71 (21) [12–32]	52/71 (73) [61–83]	6.0 (4.6–7.8)	51 (36–64)
Poor (n = 29)	9/29 (31) [15–51]	21/29 (72) [53–87]	8.0 (3.7–15.9)	46 (23–66)

*Overall benefit defined as any of CR, PR, or SD occurring while on treatment and is calculated as ORR + stable disease rate
CI, confidence interval; TTF, time to treatment failure; NR, not reached; NC, not calculated; IMDC, International Metastatic Renal Cell Carcinoma Database Consortium; ORR, objective response rate
Note: Clopper-Pearson exact 95% CIs for ORR and overall clinical benefit analysis refer to the percentage of patients, not the number of patients. Four patients were not evaluable for tumor response (thus affecting TTF and response analyses) because they were on cabozantinib for less than the cutoff duration of 8 weeks of treatment required for analysis. To be conservative, they were considered non-responders

Adverse Events (N = 112)

Event	Cabozantinib (N = 112)		
	G1/2 (%)	G3 (%)	Unknown Grade (%)
Fatigue	38	2	13
Diarrhea	23	3	8
Skin toxicity*	16	4	11
Nausea	21	0	8
Hypertension	20	4	4
Transaminitis	17	1	4
Mucositis	13	1	6
Hypothyroidism	11	0	4
Vomiting	5	0	4
Thrombocytopenia	5	1	0
Dyspnea	3	0	2
Proteinuria	0	1	2
Neutropenia	3	0	0
Other	4	3	9
Treatment discontinued	66% (disease progression [85%], toxicity [7%], patient preference [3%], physician preference [1%], and other [4%])		
Treatment interrupted or discontinued	39%		
Dose adjustments	46% (due to treatment-related adverse events)		
Deaths on treatment	None ascribed to cabozantinib		

*Skin toxicity included rash and palmar-plantar erythrodysesthesia
Adverse events included in the table were considered drug-related and were recorded after the date of first cabozantinib dose and within 30 days of the last dose. Adverse events were graded according to the National Cancer Institute Common Terminology Criteria for Adverse Events (NCI-CTCAE) v4.0 in all patients included in the study

Therapy Monitoring

1. *Prior to initiation of cabozantinib:* CBC with differential and platelet count, vital signs, liver function tests, serum electrolytes, oral examination
   - Control hypertension prior to initiation of cabozantinib
2. *Monitor regularly for:*
   - Hypertension
   - Signs and symptoms of bleeding. Avoid initiation of cabozantinib in patients with a recent history of hemorrhage (eg, hemoptysis, hematemesis, or melena)
   - Signs and symptoms of fistulas and perforations, including abscess and sepsis
   - Diarrhea
   - Spot urine for protein measurement every 4–8 weeks (if spot urine dipstick >1+ for protein, perform a 24-hour urine protein)
   - Signs and symptoms of osteonecrosis of the jaw. Perform an oral examination prior to initiation of cabozantinib and periodically during treatment. Withhold cabozantinib for ≥3 weeks prior to scheduled dental surgery or invasive dental procedures, if possible
3. Withhold cabozantinib for ≥3 weeks prior to elective surgery (including dental surgery) and for ≥2 weeks after major surgery and until adequate wound healing, whichever is longer

METASTATIC • NON-CLEAR CELL • SUBSEQUENT THERAPY

RENAL CELL CARCINOMA REGIMEN: LENVATINIB + EVEROLIMUS

Schwartz C et al. Clin Genitourin Cancer 2017;15:e903–e906
Motzer RJ et al. Lancet Oncol 2015;16:1473–1482
Supplementary appendix to: Motzer RJ et al. Lancet Oncol 2015;16:1473–1482
LENVIMA (lenvatinib) prescribing information. Woodcliff Lake, NJ: Eisai Inc; revised February 2020
AFINITOR (everolimus) prescribing information. East Hanover, NJ: Novartis Pharmaceuticals Corporation; revised January 2020

Lenvatinib 18 mg per dose; administer orally once daily, without regard to food, continuously until disease progression (total dosage/week = 126 mg)
- Lenvatinib capsules should ideally be swallowed whole. Patients who have difficulty swallowing whole lenvatinib capsules may instead place the appropriate combination of whole capsules necessary to administer the required dose in 15 mL of water or apple juice in a glass container for at least 10 minutes. After 10 minutes, the contents of the glass container should be stirred for at least 3 minutes and then the resulting mixture should be swallowed orally. After drinking, rinse the glass container with an additional 15 mL of water or apple juice and swallow the liquid to ensure complete administration of the lenvatinib dose
- A missed dose of lenvatinib may be taken up to 12 hours before a subsequently scheduled dose
- Reduce the lenvatinib starting dose to 10 mg per dose, administered orally once daily for severe (Child-Pugh class C) hepatic impairment
- Reduce the lenvatinib starting dose to 10 mg per dose, administered orally once daily for severe (creatinine clearance <30 mL/minute) renal impairment
- Patients with pre-existing hypertension should have blood pressure adequately controlled (blood pressure ≤150/90 mmHg) prior to initiation of treatment with lenvatinib

Everolimus 5 mg/dose; administer orally, once daily either consistently with food or without food, continually until disease progression (total dosage/week = 35 mg)
Notes:
- Patients who delay taking everolimus at a regularly scheduled time should be instructed to administer the missed dose if the delay is ≤6 hours following the normal time of administration. If the delay is >6 hours, take the next dose at the next regularly scheduled time
- Dexamethasone alcohol-free mouthwash used concomitantly with everolimus decreases the incidence of stomatitis (Rugo HS et al. Lancet Oncol 2017;18:654–662):
- **Dexamethasone 0.5 mg/5 mL alcohol-free oral solution** 10 mL/dose; swish for 2 minutes and then expectorate four times per day during treatment with everolimus
- Everolimus is a substrate for cytochrome P450 (CYP) CYP3A subfamily enzymes and P-glycoprotein (P-gp). If everolimus must be used with a concomitant P-gp inhibitor and moderate CYP3A4 inhibitor, reduce the dose. If concurrent use with a P-gp and strong CYP3A4 inducer is required, consider doubling the everolimus dose
- Advise patients to not consume grapefruit and grapefruit juice as they may inhibit CYP3A in the gut wall and increase the bioavailability of everolimus
- Everolimus undergoes extensive hepatic metabolism. Reduce the everolimus dose in patients with mild (Child-Pugh class A) hepatic dysfunction by 25%, moderate (Child-Pugh class B) hepatic dysfunction by 50%, and severe (Child-Pugh class C) hepatic dysfunction by 75% (if benefits outweigh risks)

Supportive Care
Antiemetic prophylaxis
Emetogenic potential of lenvatinib is **MODERATE TO HIGH**
Emetogenic potential of everolimus is **MINIMAL TO LOW**
See Chapter 42 for antiemetic recommendations

Hematopoietic growth factor (CSF) prophylaxis
Primary prophylaxis is **NOT** *indicated*
See Chapter 43 for more information

Antimicrobial prophylaxis
Risk of fever and neutropenia is **LOW**
  Antimicrobial primary prophylaxis to be considered:
  - Antibacterial—not indicated
  - Antifungal—not indicated
  - Antiviral—not indicated unless patient previously had an episode of HSV

Oral care
Standard prophylaxis and treatment for mucositis/stomatitis

(continued)

(*continued*)

Diarrhea management
Latent or delayed-onset diarrhea*:
    Loperamide 4 mg orally initially after the first loose or liquid stool, *then* 2–4 mg orally every 2–4 hours or **diphenoxylate hydrochloride** 2.5 mg with **atropine sulfate** 0.025 mg (eg, Lomotil)

*Abigerges D et al. J Natl Cancer Inst 1994;86:446–449
Rothenberg ML et al. J Clin Oncol 2001;19:3801–3807
Wadler S et al. J Clin Oncol 1998;16:3169–3178

Treatment Modifications

RECOMMENDED DOSE MODIFICATIONS FOR LENVATINIB

Starting dose	18 mg by mouth once daily
Dose Level –1	14 mg by mouth once daily
Dose Level –2	10 mg by mouth once daily
Dose Level –3	8 mg by mouth once daily
Dose Level –4	Discontinue lenvatinib

For adverse reactions common to both lenvatinib and everolimus, prioritize reducing the lenvatinib dose first

Lenvatinib Dose Modification—Cardiovascular Toxicity

Adverse Event	Treatment Modification
Either of the following: • G2 hypertension (SBP 140–159 mm Hg or DBP 90–99 mm Hg) • G3 hypertension (SBP ≥160 mm Hg or DBP ≥100 mm Hg) on suboptimal antihypertensive therapy	Continue lenvatinib at the same dose and optimize antihypertensive therapy. Monitor blood pressure frequently
G3 hypertension (SBP ≥160 mm Hg or DBP ≥100 mm Hg) persistent despite optimal antihypertensive therapy	Withhold lenvatinib until hypertension controlled to G ≤2, then resume lenvatinib at one lower dose level. Monitor blood pressure frequently
G4 hypertension (life-threatening consequences [eg, malignant hypertension, transient or permanent neurologic deficit, hypertensive crisis]; urgent intervention indicated)	Permanently discontinue lenvatinib
G3 cardiac dysfunction	Withhold lenvatinib until cardiac dysfunction improves to G ≤1 or baseline, then resume lenvatinib at one lower dose level or discontinue lenvatinib depending upon the severity and persistence of cardiac dysfunction
G4 cardiac dysfunction	Permanently discontinue lenvatinib
QTc prolongation (>500 ms, or >60-ms increase from baseline)	Withhold lenvatinib until QTc improves to ≤480 ms or baseline, then resume at one lower dose level. Correct hypomagnesemia and/or hypokalemia if applicable
Arterial thromboembolic event	Permanently discontinue lenvatinib

Lenvatinib Dose Modification—Gastrointestinal Toxicity

Gastrointestinal perforation	Permanently discontinue lenvatinib
G3/4 fistula formation	Permanently discontinue lenvatinib
Either of the following: • G1 diarrhea • G2 diarrhea lasting ≤2 weeks	Continue current lenvatinib dose and optimize antidiarrheal medications

(*continued*)

Treatment Modifications (continued)

Adverse Event	Treatment Modification
Any of the following: • G2 diarrhea lasting >2 weeks • G3 diarrhea • G4 diarrhea developing in a patient not receiving an optimal antidiarrheal regimen	Withhold lenvatinib until diarrhea resolves to G ≤1 or baseline, then resume lenvatinib at 1 lower dose level. Antidiarrheal treatment for symptoms may continue indefinitely as a preventive measure
Recurrent or persistent G4 diarrhea in a patient receiving an optimal antidiarrheal regimen	Permanently discontinue lenvatinib
Lenvatinib Dose Modification—Hepatic Toxicity and Hepatic Impairment	
G3/4 hepatotoxicity (ALT/AST >5× ULN, bilirubin >3× ULN)	Withhold lenvatinib until hepatotoxicity improves to G ≤1, then resume lenvatinib at one lower dose level or discontinue lenvatinib depending upon the severity and persistence of hepatotoxicity
Hepatic failure	Permanently discontinue lenvatinib
Severe hepatic impairment (Child-Pugh class C)	Reduce initial lenvatinib dose to 10 mg orally once daily
Lenvatinib Dose Modification—Renal Toxicity and Renal Impairment	
G3/4 AKI (SCr >3× baseline or >4 mg/dL; hospitalization indicated; life-threatening consequences; dialysis indicated)	Initiate prompt evaluation and correction of dehydration if applicable. Withhold lenvatinib until toxicity improves to G ≤1 or baseline, then resume at one lower dose level or discontinue lenvatinib depending upon the severity and persistence of renal impairment
Severe renal impairment (CrCl <30 mL/min*)	Reduce initial lenvatinib dose to 10 mg orally once daily
Urine dipstick proteinuria ≥2+	Continue lenvatinib at current dose and obtain a 24-hour urine protein
Proteinuria ≥2 grams in 24 hours	Withhold lenvatinib until <2 grams of proteinuria per 24 hours, then resume lenvatinib at one lower dose level
Nephrotic syndrome	Permanently discontinue lenvatinib
Lenvatinib Dose Modification—Other Toxicities	
RPLS	Withhold lenvatinib until fully resolved, then resume at a reduced dose or discontinue depending on severity and persistence of neurologic symptoms
Planned elective surgery	Withhold lenvatinib for at least 6 days prior to scheduled surgery. Resume lenvatinib after surgery based on clinical assessment of adequate wound healing
Patient with wound-healing complications	Permanently discontinue lenvatinib
Other toxicities (eg, hand-foot skin reaction, rash, nausea/vomiting, stomatitis, hemorrhage, etc) Other persistent/intolerable G2 toxicities Other G3 toxicities	Withhold lenvatinib until toxicity improves to G ≤1 or baseline, then resume lenvatinib at one lower dose level
G4 laboratory abnormality	Withhold lenvatinib until toxicity improves to G ≤1 or baseline, then resume lenvatinib at one lower dose level
Other G4 toxicity	Permanently discontinue lenvatinib

*CrCl calculated using the Cockcroft-Gault equation using actual body weight
SBP, systolic blood pressure; DBP, diastolic blood pressure; ALT, alanine aminotransferase; AST, aspartate aminotransferase; AKI, acute kidney injury; SCr, serum creatinine; CrCl, creatinine clearance; RPLS, reversible posterior leukoencephalopathy syndrome
LENVIMA (lenvatinib) prescribing information. Woodcliff Lake, NJ: Eisai Inc; revised February 2020

(continued)

Treatment Modifications (*continued*)

RECOMMENDED DOSE MODIFICATIONS FOR EVEROLIMUS

Starting dose level	5 mg orally once daily
Dose level −1	5 mg orally once every other day
Dose level −2	Discontinue everolimus

For adverse reactions common to both lenvatinib and everolimus, prioritize reducing the lenvatinib dose first

Adverse Event	Dose Modification
Radiologic changes suggestive of noninfectious pneumonitis with few or no symptoms	Can continue everolimus therapy without dose alteration but with careful monitoring
Radiologic changes suggestive of noninfectious pneumonitis with moderate symptoms	Withhold everolimus until symptoms improve. Consider using corticosteroids. If symptoms improve, consider reintroducing everolimus one dose lower with careful continued monitoring
Radiologic changes suggestive of noninfectious pneumonitis with severe symptoms	Discontinue everolimus. Consider using corticosteroids
Diagnosis of a medically significant infection	Withhold everolimus and institute appropriate treatment promptly. Consider discontinuing everolimus
Diagnosis of invasive systemic fungal infection	Discontinue everolimus and treat with appropriate antifungal therapy
G1/2 stomatitis	Withhold everolimus and administer topical treatments (avoid alcohol- or peroxide-containing mouthwashes as they may exacerbate the condition). Topical steroids are highly effective, eg, dexamethasone/normal saline 3.3 mg/5 mL, swish and spit three times daily for diffuse stomatitis or triamcinolone oral paste 0.1% for isolated ulcers. Do not use antifungal agents unless fungal infection has been diagnosed. If symptoms improve to G <1, everolimus treatment may begin with either the same dose or one dose level lower
G3 stomatitis	Withhold everolimus and administer topical treatments (avoid alcohol- or peroxide-containing mouthwashes as they may exacerbate the condition). Topical steroids are highly effective, eg, dexamethasone/normal saline 3.3 mg/5 mL, swish and spit three times daily. Do not use antifungal agents unless fungal infection has been diagnosed. If symptoms improve to G <1, everolimus treatment may begin with one dose level lower
Recurrent G3 or G4 stomatitis	Discontinue everolimus
Elevated blood glucose	Withhold everolimus and correct before restarting everolimus

AFINITOR (everolimus) prescribing information. East Hanover, NJ: Novartis Pharmaceuticals Corporation; revised January 2020

Patient Population Studied

This case report describes a 52-year-old male with recurrent (bone metastases) biopsy-proven chromophobe type renal cell carcinoma (chRCC) following a left radical nephrectomy performed 17 months previously. First-line therapy with temsirolimus was initiated. The patient experienced progressive disease and underwent palliative radiation for a right hip metastasis and was then transitioned to second-line nivolumab. He completed 18 doses of nivolumab until disease progression occurred, including new lung metastases. Due to the patient's young age and good performance status, third-line treatment with lenvatinib (14 mg by mouth daily) and everolimus (5 mg by mouth daily) was initiated

Efficacy (N = 1)

After 26 weeks of therapy with lenvatinib and everolimus, the patient's bone disease was stable, his disease burden progressively decreased, and no new foci of metastatic disease were observed

Adverse Events (N = 1)

The patient in the case report tolerated the regimen well without significant toxicity or dose reduction. For additional safety data, refer to the description of this regimen within this chapter for metastatic clear cell RCC

Therapy Monitoring

Lenvatinib:

1. Check ALT, AST, bilirubin, and alkaline phosphatase at baseline, every 2 weeks for 2 months, and then at least monthly thereafter

2. Check BUN and serum creatinine at baseline and then periodically

3. Check serum calcium at baseline and at least monthly

4. Check TSH and free thyroxine (FT4) every 4–6 weeks

5. Monitor urine dipstick for protein at baseline and then periodically during treatment. If 2+, then perform a 24-hour urine collection for protein

6. Monitor blood pressure at baseline, after 1 week, every 2 weeks for 2 months, and then at least monthly thereafter

7. Check an electrocardiogram (ECG) at baseline and periodically in patients at increased risk for QT prolongation (eg, congenital long QT syndrome, heart failure, bradyarrhythmias, or in patients taking concomitant medications known to prolong the QT interval)

8. Monitor periodically for signs and symptoms of cardiac dysfunction, arterial thrombosis, reversible posterior leukoencephalopathy syndrome (RPLS), fistula formation, gastrointestinal perforation, and wound-healing complications

Everolimus:

1. *Baseline and periodically:*
   - CBC with differential and platelet count, ALT, AST, bilirubin, alkaline phosphatase, BUN, and serum creatinine
   - Fasting serum glucose and lipid panel
   - Monitor for symptoms of pulmonary toxicity, infection, and stomatitis

2. Everolimus may impair wound healing; use caution and strongly consider withholding therapy in the peri-surgical period

3. Advise patients to avoid live vaccines and close contact with those who have received live vaccines

METASTATIC • NON-CLEAR CELL • SUBSEQUENT THERAPY
RENAL CELL CARCINOMA REGIMEN: NIVOLUMAB

Koshkin VS et al. J Immunother Cancer 2018;6:9
OPDIVO (nivolumab) prescribing information. Princeton, NJ: Bristol-Myers Squibb Company; revised September 2019

Nivolumab 240 mg; administer intravenously over 30 minutes in a volume of 0.9% NS or D5W, not to exceed 160 mL and sufficient to produce a nivolumab concentration within the range 1–10 mg/mL, every 2 weeks until disease progression (total dosage/2-week cycle = 240 mg)
- Administer nivolumab through an administration set that contains a sterile, non-pyrogenic, low-protein-binding in-line filter with pore size within the range of 0.2–1.2 μm
- Nivolumab can cause severe infusion-related reactions

or

Nivolumab 480 mg; administer intravenously over 30 minutes in a volume of 0.9% NS or D5W not to exceed 160 mL and sufficient to produce a nivolumab concentration within the range 1–10 mg/mL, every 4 weeks until disease progression (total dosage/4-week cycle = 480 mg)
- Administer nivolumab through an administration set that contains a sterile, non-pyrogenic, low-protein-binding in-line filter with pore size within the range of 0.2–1.2 μm
- Nivolumab can cause severe infusion-related reactions

Supportive Care
Antiemetic prophylaxis
Emetogenic potential with nivolumab is **MINIMAL**
See Chapter 42 for antiemetic recommendations

Hematopoietic growth factor (CSF) prophylaxis
Primary prophylaxis is **NOT** indicated
See Chapter 43 for more information

Antimicrobial prophylaxis
Risk of fever and neutropenia is **LOW**
 Antimicrobial primary prophylaxis to be considered:
- Antibacterial—not indicated
- Antifungal—not indicated
- Antiviral—not indicated unless patient previously had an episode of HSV

Treatment Modifications

RECOMMENDED DOSE MODIFICATIONS FOR NIVOLUMAB

Adverse Event	Grade/Severity	Treatment Modification
Infusion reaction	Clinically significant but not severe infusion reaction	Interrupt the infusion in patients with clinically significant infusion reactions and consider resuming at a slower rate following resolution. If decision is made to restart, begin at ≤50% of the rate prior to the reaction and increase in 50% increments every 30 minutes if well tolerated. Infusions may be restarted at the full rate during the next cycle
	G3/4 (severe infusion reaction—pyrexia, chills, flushing, hypotension, dyspnea, wheezing, back pain, abdominal pain, and urticaria). Not rapidly responsive to brief interruption of infusion	Stop infusion and administer appropriate medical therapy (eg, epinephrine, corticosteroids, intravenous antihistamines, bronchodilators, and/or oxygen). Discontinue nivolumab
Colitis	G1	Loperamide 4 mg as starting dose then 2 mg before each meal and after each loose stool until without diarrhea for 12 hours, with maximum of 16 mg loperamide per day. If G1 diarrhea or colitis persists >14 days, then add prednisolone 0.5–1 mg/kg (non-enteric-coated) or consider oral budesonide 9 mg daily if no bloody diarrhea

(continued)

Treatment Modifications (continued)

Adverse Event	Grade/Severity	Treatment Modification
	G2/3 diarrhea or colitis	Withhold nivolumab. Loperamide 4 mg as starting dose then 2 mg before each meal and after each loose stool until without diarrhea for 12 hours, with maximum of 16 mg loperamide per day. Administer oral prednisone/prednisolone at a dose of 0.5 to 2 mg/kg/day or its equivalent. When improves to G1, begin a slow corticosteroid taper over at least 4 weeks. Resume nivolumab upon symptom control, or when prednisone/prednisolone daily dose <10 mg
	G4 diarrhea or colitis	Permanently discontinue nivolumab. Loperamide 4 mg as starting dose then 2 mg before each meal and after each loose stool until without diarrhea for 12 hours, with maximum of 16 mg loperamide per day. Administer 1–2 mg/kg IV (methyl)prednisolone and convert to 0.5–2 mg/kg prednisone/prednisolone orally each day or its equivalent only after a response. Taper over at least 4 weeks when symptoms improve. If does not improve over 72 hours or worsens, perform flexible sigmoidoscopy/colonoscopy to document colitis then begin infliximab 5 mg/kg (if no perforation/sepsis/TB/hepatitis/NYHA III/IV CHF). If no response, add MMF 500–1000 mg twice daily. If worse on MMF, consider addition of tacrolimus or ATG
Pneumonitis	G2	Withhold nivolumab. Consider *Pneumocystis* prophylaxis depending on the clinical context and coverage with empiric antibiotics. Administer oral prednisone/prednisolone at a dose of 1–2 mg/kg/day or its equivalent. When improves to G1, begin a slow corticosteroid taper over at least 4 weeks. If does not respond adequately after 48 hours, then administer 2–4 mg/kg IV (methyl)prednisolone and convert to 0.5–2 mg/kg prednisone/prednisolone orally each day or its equivalent only after a response, followed by a taper over at least 6 weeks when symptoms improve to G1, titrating to symptoms. Resume nivolumab upon symptom control, or when prednisone/prednisolone daily dose <10 mg
	G3/4	Permanently discontinue nivolumab. Consider *Pneumocystis* prophylaxis depending on the clinical context; cover with empiric antibiotics. Administer 2–4 mg/kg IV (methyl)prednisolone and convert to 1–2 mg/kg prednisone/prednisolone orally each day or its equivalent only after a response, followed by a taper over at least 8 weeks when symptoms improve to G1, titrating to symptoms. If when initially treated improvement does not occur within 48–72 hours, begin infliximab 5 mg/kg (if no perforation/sepsis/TB/hepatitis/NYHA III/IV CHF). If no response to infliximab, add MMF 500–1000 mg twice daily. Consider MMF especially if has concurrent hepatic toxicity
Hepatitis	G2 (AST or ALT >3–5× ULN or total bilirubin >1.5–3× ULN)	Withhold nivolumab. Administer oral prednisone/prednisolone at a dose of 1 to 2 mg/kg/day or its equivalent. When improves to G1, begin a slow corticosteroid taper over at least 4 weeks. Resume nivolumab upon symptom control, or when prednisone/prednisolone daily dose <10 mg
	G3/4 (AST or ALT >5× ULN or total bilirubin >3× ULN)	Permanently discontinue nivolumab. Administer 1–2 mg/kg IV (methyl)prednisolone and convert to 0.5–2 mg/kg prednisone/prednisolone orally each day or its equivalent only after a response. Taper over at least 6 weeks when symptoms improve. If no response, add MMF 500–1000 mg twice daily. If worse on MMF, consider adding tacrolimus or ATG
Hypophysitis	G2/3 (moderate symptoms, ie, headache but no visual disturbance or fatigue/ mood alteration but hemodynamically stable, no electrolyte disturbance)	Administer analgesia as needed for headache. Withhold nivolumab. Administer oral prednisone/ prednisolone at a dose of 0.5 to 2 mg/kg/day or its equivalent. When improves to G1, begin a slow corticosteroid taper over at least 4 weeks. If no improvement in 48 hours, administer 1–2 mg/kg IV (methyl)prednisolone and convert to 0.5–2 mg/kg prednisone/prednisolone orally each day or its equivalent only after a response. Taper over at least 4 weeks when symptoms improve to 5 mg prednisone/prednisolone or equivalent; do not stop steroids. Resume nivolumab upon symptom control, or when prednisone/prednisolone daily dose <10 mg
	G4 (severe mass effect symptoms, ie, severe headache, any visual disturbance or severe hypoadrenalism, ie, hypotension, severe electrolyte disturbance)	Permanently discontinue nivolumab. Administer analgesia as needed for headache. Administer 1–2 mg/kg IV (methyl)prednisolone and convert to 0.5–2 mg/kg prednisone/prednisolone orally each day or its equivalent only after a response. Taper over at least 4 weeks when symptoms improve to 5 mg prednisone/prednisolone or equivalent; do not stop steroids
Adrenal insufficiency	G2	Withhold nivolumab. Administer oral prednisone/prednisolone at a dose of 0.5 to 2 mg/kg/day or its equivalent. When improves to G1, begin a slow corticosteroid taper over at least 4 weeks. Serially assess adrenal function and continue steroids at replacement doses (20–40 mg hydrocortisone daily ~2/3 dose in AM upon awakening and ~1/3 at 4 PM) until recovery of adrenal function is documented. Resume nivolumab upon symptom control, or when prednisone/prednisolone daily dose <10 mg

(continued)

Treatment Modifications (continued)

Adverse Event	Grade/Severity	Treatment Modification
	G3/4	Permanently discontinue nivolumab. Administer oral prednisone/prednisolone at a dose of 0.5 to 2 mg/kg/day or its equivalent. When improves to G1, begin a slow corticosteroid taper over at least 4 weeks. Serially assess adrenal function and continue steroids at replacement doses (20–40 mg hydrocortisone daily ~2/3 dose in AM upon awakening and ~1/3 at 4 PM) until recovery of adrenal function is documented
Type 1 diabetes mellitus	G3 hyperglycemia	Withhold nivolumab. Admit to hospital to manage hyperglycemia. Role of corticosteroids in preventing complete loss of insulin-producing cells is unknown and not recommended. Resume nivolumab upon symptom control, or when prednisone/prednisolone daily dose <10 mg
	G4 hyperglycemia	Permanently discontinue nivolumab. Admit to hospital to manage hyperglycemia. Role of corticosteroids in preventing complete loss of insulin-producing cells is unknown and not recommended
Nephritis and renal dysfunction	G2/3 (serum creatinine 1.5–6× ULN)	Withhold nivolumab. Administer oral prednisone/prednisolone at a dose of 0.5 to 2 mg/kg/day or its equivalent. When improves to G1, begin a slow corticosteroid taper over at least 4 weeks. If does not respond adequately then administer 0.5–1 mg/kg IV (methyl)prednisolone and convert to 0.5–2 mg/kg prednisone/prednisolone orally each day or its equivalent only after a response, followed by a taper over at least 4 weeks when improves to G1. Resume nivolumab upon symptom control, or when prednisone/prednisolone daily dose <10 mg
	G4 (serum creatinine >6× ULN)	Permanently discontinue nivolumab. Administer 0.5–1 mg/kg IV (methyl)prednisolone and convert to 0.5–2 mg/kg prednisone/prednisolone orally each day or its equivalent only after a response, followed by a taper over at least 4 weeks when improves to G1
Skin	G1/2	Continue nivolumab. Avoid skin irritants, avoid sun exposure, topical emollients recommended. Topical steroid (mild strength for G1, moderate/potent strength for G2) cream once or twice daily ± oral or topical antihistamines for itching
	G3 rash or suspected SJS or TEN	Withhold nivolumab. Avoid skin irritants, avoid sun exposure, topical emollients recommended. Administer oral or topical antihistamines for itching. Administer oral prednisone/prednisolone at a dose of 0.5–2 mg/kg or its equivalent daily for 3 days followed by a slow corticosteroid taper over at least 4 weeks when the rash improves to G1. If does not respond adequately, then administer 0.5 –1 mg/kg IV (methyl)prednisolone and convert to 0.5–2 mg/kg prednisone/prednisolone orally each day or its equivalent only after a response, followed by a taper over at least 4 weeks when the rash improves to G1. Resume nivolumab upon symptom control, or when prednisone/prednisolone daily dose <10 mg
	G4 rash or confirmed SJS or TEN	Avoid skin irritants, avoid sun exposure, topical emollients recommended. Administer oral or topical antihistamines for itching. Administer 1–2 mg/kg IV (methyl)prednisolone and convert to oral steroids 0.5–2 mg/kg prednisone/prednisolone each day or its equivalent only after a response. Taper over at least 4 weeks when the rash improves to G1. Permanently discontinue nivolumab
Encephalitis	Confusion or altered behavior, headaches, alteration in Glasgow Coma Scale, motor or sensory deficits, speech abnormality, may or may not be febrile	Initially withhold nivolumab, but permanently discontinue nivolumab if there is no doubt as to diagnosis. Exclude bacterial and ideally viral infections prior to high-dose steroids. Administer oral prednisone/prednisolone at a dose of 0.5–2 mg/kg/day or its equivalent. When symptoms improve, begin a slow corticosteroid taper over at least 4–8 weeks. If symptoms are severe, administer 1–2 mg/kg IV (methyl)prednisolone and convert to 0.5–2 mg/kg prednisone/prednisolone orally each day or its equivalent only after a response. Consider concurrent empiric antiviral (IV acyclovir) and antibacterial therapy
Aseptic meningitis	Headache, photophobia, neck stiffness with fever or may be afebrile, vomiting; normal cognition/cerebral function (distinguishes from encephalitis)	
Other syndromes include neurosarcoidosis, posterior reversible leukoencephalopathy syndrome (PRES), Vogt-Koyanagi-Harada syndrome, demyelination, vasculitic encephalopathy, and generalized seizures		

(continued)

Treatment Modifications (*continued*)

Adverse Event	Grade/Severity	Treatment Modification
Transverse myelitis	Acute or subacute neurologic signs/symptoms of motor/sensory/autonomic origin; most have sensory level; often bilateral symptoms	Initially withhold nivolumab, but permanently discontinue nivolumab if there is no doubt as to diagnosis. Administer 2 mg/kg IV (methyl)prednisolone or consider 1 g/day and convert to 0.5–2 mg/kg prednisone/prednisolone orally each day or its equivalent only after a response. When symptoms improve, begin a slow corticosteroid taper over at least 4–8 weeks. Plasmapheresis may be required if steroids do not bring about improvement
Myocarditis	G3	Permanently discontinue nivolumab. Administer 2 mg/kg IV (methyl)prednisolone or consider 1 g/day and convert to 0.5–2 mg/kg prednisone/prednisolone orally each day or its equivalent only after a response. When symptoms improve, begin a slow corticosteroid taper over at least 4–8 weeks. If no response, add MMF 500–1000 mg twice daily. If worse on MMF, consider adding tacrolimus
Peripheral neurologic toxicity	Moderate: some interference with ADL, symptoms concerning to patient	Withhold nivolumab. Initial observation reasonable or initiate prednisone/prednisolone 0.5–1 mg/kg (if progressing, eg, from mild) and/or pregabalin or duloxetine for pain. When symptoms improve, begin a slow corticosteroid taper over at least 4 weeks. Resume nivolumab upon symptom control, or when prednisone/prednisolone daily dose <10 mg
	Severe: limits self-care and aids warranted, life-threatening, eg, respiratory problems	Permanently discontinue nivolumab. Administer 1–2 mg/kg IV (methyl)prednisolone and convert to 0.5–2 mg/kg prednisone/prednisolone orally each day or its equivalent only after a response. Taper over at least 4–8 weeks when symptoms improve to G1
Guillain-Barré syndrome	Progressive symmetrical muscle weakness with absent or reduced tendon reflexes—involves extremities, facial, respiratory, and bulbar and oculomotor muscles; dysregulation of autonomic nerves	Permanently discontinue nivolumab. Use of steroids not recommended in idiopathic Guillain-Barré syndrome; however, a trial of (methyl)prednisolone 1–2 mg/kg is reasonable, converting to 0.5–2 mg/kg prednisone/prednisolone orally each day or its equivalent only after a response. If no improvement or worsening, plasmapheresis or IVIG indicated
Myasthenia gravis	Fluctuating muscle weakness (proximal limb, trunk, ocular, eg, ptosis/diplopia or bulbar) with fatigability, respiratory muscles may also be involved	Permanently discontinue nivolumab. Administer pyridostigmine at an initial dose of 30 mg three times daily. Administer oral prednisone/prednisolone at a dose of 0.5 to 2 mg/kg/day or its equivalent or 1–2 mg/kg IV (methyl)prednisolone depending on the severity of symptoms. If begin with IV, convert to 0.5–2 mg/kg prednisone/prednisolone orally each day or its equivalent only after a response. If no improvement or worsening, plasmapheresis or IVIG may be considered. Additional immunosuppressants used in myasthenia gravis include azathioprine, cyclosporine, and mycophenolate. Avoid certain medications, eg, ciprofloxacin, beta-blockers, that may precipitate cholinergic crisis
Other syndromes including motor and sensory peripheral neuropathy, multifocal radicular neuropathy/plexopathy, autonomic neuropathy, phrenic nerve palsy, cranial nerve palsies (eg, facial nerve, optic nerve, hypoglossal nerve)		Permanently discontinue nivolumab. Administer oral prednisone/prednisolone at a dose of 0.5 to 2 mg/kg/day or its equivalent or 1–2 mg/kg IV (methyl)prednisolone depending on the severity of symptoms. If begin with IV, convert to 0.5–2 mg/kg prednisone/prednisolone orally each day or its equivalent only after a response
Arthralgia	G1 (mild pain with inflammation, erythema, or joint swelling)	Continue nivolumab. Administer acetaminophen (paracetamol) and ibuprofen
	G2 (moderate pain with inflammation, erythema, or joint swelling that limits ADLs)	Withhold nivolumab. Administer higher doses of acetaminophen (paracetamol) and ibuprofen and use diclofenac or naproxen or etoricoxib. If inadequately controlled, consider intra-articular steroid injections for large joints or administer oral prednisone/prednisolone at a dose of 0.5 to 2 mg/kg/day or its equivalent. When improves to G1, begin a slow corticosteroid taper over at least 4 weeks. If does not respond adequately, then administer 0.5–1 mg/kg IV (methyl)prednisolone and convert to 0.5–2 mg/kg prednisone/prednisolone orally each day or its equivalent only after a response, followed by a taper over at least 4 weeks when improves to G1. Resume nivolumab upon symptom control, or when prednisone/prednisolone daily dose <10 mg
	G3 (severe pain; irreversible joint damage; disabling; limits self-care ADL)	Withhold nivolumab. Administer 0.5–1 mg/kg IV (methyl)prednisolone and convert to 0.5–2 mg/kg prednisone/prednisolone orally each day or its equivalent only after a response, followed by a taper over at least 4 weeks when improves to G1. In severe cases, infliximab or another anti–TNF alpha drug may be required for improvement of arthritis. Resume nivolumab upon symptom control, or when prednisone/prednisolone daily dose <10 mg

(*continued*)

Treatment Modifications (*continued*)

Adverse Event	Grade/Severity	Treatment Modification
Other	First occurrence of other G3	Withhold nivolumab. Administer oral prednisone/prednisolone at a dose of 0.5 to 2 mg/kg/day or its equivalent. When improves to G1, begin a slow corticosteroid taper over at least 4 weeks. Resume nivolumab upon symptom control, or when prednisone/prednisolone daily dose <10 mg
	Recurrence of same G3	Permanently discontinue nivolumab. Administer 1–2 mg/kg IV (methyl)prednisolone and convert to 0.5–2 mg/kg prednisone/prednisolone orally each day or its equivalent only after a response. Taper over at least 4–8 weeks when symptoms improve to G1
	Life-threatening or G4	
	Requirement for ≥10 mg/day prednisone or equivalent for >12 weeks	Permanently discontinue nivolumab
	Persistent G2/3 adverse reactions lasting ≥12 weeks	

ADL, activities of daily living; ALT, alanine aminotransferase; AST, aspartate aminotransferase; ATG, anti–thymocyte globulin; SJS, Stevens-Johnson syndrome; TEN, toxic epidermal necrolysis; ULN, upper limit of normal

Notes on general supportive care:
Steroid taper in most cases will proceed over a minimum of 1 month but if symptoms improve rapidly, a 2-week taper can be considered. If steroids are administered for more than 4 weeks, consider PCP prophylaxis (cotrimoxazole 480 mg twice daily M/W/F or inhaled pentamidine if has cotrimoxazole allergy), regular random blood glucose, Vitamin D level, and starting calcium/Vitamin D supplementation per guidelines

Patient Population Studied

This multicenter retrospective analysis included 41 adult patients with non–clear cell renal cell carcinoma (nccRCC) who received at least one dose of nivolumab. Patient eligibility criteria included histologically confirmed nccRCC, presence of metastatic disease, at least one dose of nivolumab monotherapy administered, and available clinical and imaging data prior to initiation of treatment

Efficacy (N = 41)

Best Treatment Response According to RECIST v 1.1 by RCC Histology

Histology	PR, n/N (%)	SD, n/N (%)	PD, n/N (%)	Non-evaluable, n
Papillary (N = 16)	2/14 (2)	3/14 (21)	9/14 (64)	2
Unclassified (N = 14)	4/11 (36)	3/11 (27)	4/11 (36)	3
Chromophobe (N = 5)	0/4 (0)	3/4 (75)	1/4 (25)	1
Collecting duct (N = 4)	1/4 (25)	0/4 (0)	3/4 (75)	0
MTSCC (N = 1)	0/1 (0)	1/1 (100)	0/1 (0)	0
Translocation (N = 1)	0/1 (0)	0/1 (0)	1/1 (100)	0
All histologies (N = 41)	7/35 (20)	10/35 (29)	18/35 (51)	6

Survival, all histologies, N = 41

Median PFS, months (95% CI)	3.5 (1.9–5.0)
Median OS, months	Not reached

RECIST, Response Criteria in Solid Tumors version 1.1; RCC, Renal Cell Carcinoma; PR, partial response; SD, stable disease; PD, progressive disease; MTSCC, Mucinous Tubular and Spindle Cell Carcinoma; PFS, progression-free survival; CI, confidence interval; OS, overall survival
Note: no complete responses were observed. The median duration of therapy was 3.0 months (range 0–13.1) and the median number of doses of nivolumab was 7 (range 1–28). Median follow-up was 8.5 months (range, 1–28)

Adverse Events (N = 41)

Event	Nivolumab (N = 41)	
	G1/2 (%)	G3/4 (%)
Fatigue/malaise	10	2
Fever	3	7
Rash/Skin toxicity	5	5
Hypothyroidism	7	0
Diarrhea	3	2
Arthralgia	5	0
Myalgia/myositis	5	0
Adrenal insufficiency	5	0
Peripheral edema	5	0
Third-degree heart block	0	2
Respiratory failure	0	2
Headache	0	2
Aphasia	2	0
Infusion reaction	2	0
Diabetes	2	0
Uveitis	2	0
Hypertension	2	0
Hypophysitis	2	0
Cough	2	0
Lymphadenopathy	2	0
Back pain	2	0

Note: treatment-related adverse events and grading were determined via retrospective chart review

Therapy Monitoring

1. Initially at the time of each dose, and eventually every 6–12 weeks, perform a total body skin examination with attention to *all* mucous membranes as well as a complete review of systems

2. Monitor patients for signs and symptoms of pneumonitis. Evaluate patients with suspected pneumonitis with chest x-ray, CT, and pulse oximetry. For ≥2 toxicity, may include nasal swab, sputum culture and sensitivity, blood culture and sensitivity, and urine culture and sensitivity

3. Monitor patients for signs and symptoms of colitis. Encourage patients to report diarrhea immediately to any member of the health care team

4. Draw AST, ALT, and bilirubin prior to each infusion and/or weekly if there are Grade 1 liver function test elevations. Note, no treatment is recommended for G1 LFT abnormalities. For ≥2 toxicity, work up for other causes of elevated LFTs including viral hepatitis

5. Use basic metabolic panel (Na, K, CO_2, glucose) and patient history as screening tools for hypophysitis including hypopituitarism and adrenal insufficiency. If in doubt, evaluate AM adrenocorticotropic hormone (ACTH) and cortisol levels. Consider ACTH stimulation test for indeterminate results

6. Assess thyroid function at the start of treatment, periodically during treatment, and as indicated based on clinical evaluation, and for clinical signs and symptoms of thyroid disorders. Test for TSH and free thyroxine (FT4) every 4–6 weeks as part of routine clinical monitoring of therapy or for case detection in symptomatic patients

7. Measure glucose at baseline and with each treatment during the first 12 weeks and every 6 weeks thereafter

8. Obtain a serum creatinine prior to every dose. If creatinine is found to be newly elevated, consider holding therapy while other potential causes are evaluated. Note, routine urinalysis is not necessary other than to rule out urinary tract infections, etc

9. Obtain a complete rheumatologic history and perform an examination of all peripheral joints for tenderness, swelling, and range of motion. Examine the spine. Consider plain x-ray/imaging to exclude metastases and evaluate joint damage (erosions), if appropriate

10. In patients at high risk for infections and in appropriately selected patients based on an infectious disease evaluation, draw screening laboratories (HIV, hepatitis A and B, and blood QuantiFERON for TB) to prepare patients to start infliximab

METASTATIC • NON-CLEAR CELL • SUBSEQUENT THERAPY
RENAL CELL CARCINOMA: PAZOPANIB

Buti S et al. Clin Genitourin Cancer 2017;15:e609–e614
VOTRIENT (pazopanib) prescribing information. East Hanover, NJ: Novartis Pharmaceuticals Corporation; revised May 2017

Pazopanib 800 mg; administer orally once daily at least 1 hour before or 2 hours after a meal, continually, until disease progression (total dose/week = 5600 mg)

Notes:

- Tablets are swallowed whole (without breaking, chewing, or crushing). Oral bioavailability was increased after crushing tablets and when ingested concurrently with a high-fat or low-fat meal, resulting in increased systemic exposure (AUC [0–72 hour]) and maximum concentration achieved

- Patients who delay taking pazopanib at a regularly scheduled time may take a missed dose if the interval remaining before the next regularly scheduled dose is ≥12 hours

- Advise patients not to use drugs that increase gastric pH concurrently with pazopanib. Short-acting antacid products are preferable to histamine (H2) receptor antagonists and proton pump inhibitor medications. If used concomitantly, antacid administration should be separated from pazopanib ingestion by several hours

- Use caution in patients with hepatic dysfunction

  - In patients with baseline moderate hepatic impairment, administer pazopanib 200 mg orally once daily

  - The safety of pazopanib in patients with pre-existing severe hepatic impairment, defined as total bilirubin >3× ULN with any level of ALT, is unknown. Treatment with pazopanib is not recommended in patients with severe hepatic impairment

Antiemetic prophylaxis
Emetogenic potential of axitinib is **MINIMAL TO LOW**
See Chapter 42 for antiemetic recommendations

Hematopoietic growth factor (CSF) prophylaxis
Primary prophylaxis is **NOT** *indicated*
See Chapter 43 for more information

Antimicrobial prophylaxis
Risk of fever and neutropenia is **LOW**
  Antimicrobial primary prophylaxis to be considered:
  - Antibacterial—not indicated
  - Antifungal—not indicated
  - Antiviral—not indicated unless patient previously had an episode of HSV

Diarrhea management
Latent or delayed-onset diarrhea*:
  Loperamide 4 mg orally initially after the first loose or liquid stool, *then* 2–4 mg orally every 2–4 hours or **diphenoxylate hydrochloride** 2.5 mg with **atropine sulfate** 0.025 mg (eg, Lomotil)

*Abigerges D et al. J Natl Cancer Inst 1994;86:446–449
Rothenberg ML et al. J Clin Oncol 2001;19:3801–3807
Wadler S et al. J Clin Oncol 1998;16:3169–3178

Treatment Modifications

PAZOPANIB DOSE MODIFICATIONS

Pazopanib Dose Levels	
Starting dose	800 mg each day
Dose level −1	600 mg each day
Dose level −2	400 mg each day
Dose level −3	200 mg each day
Dose level −4	Discontinue

(continued)

Treatment Modifications (continued)

Adverse Event	Treatment Modification
Hepatotoxicity	
Isolated ALT elevations between 3–8× ULN (see note below)	Continue pazopanib with great care. Obtain weekly LFTs until ALT returns to G1 or baseline
ALT elevations >3× ULN concurrently with bilirubin elevations >2× ULN (see note below)	Discontinue pazopanib permanently and monitor patients closely until resolution of LFT abnormalities
Isolated ALT elevations of >8× ULN	Interrupt pazopanib until ALT elevation returns to G1 or baseline. If potential benefits for reinitiating pazopanib outweigh risks of hepatotoxicity, then reintroduce pazopanib at no more than 400 mg daily and measure LFTs weekly for 8 weeks
Recurrent ALT elevations >3× ULN following its reintroduction for transient ALT elevation	Discontinue pazopanib permanently and monitor patients closely until resolution of LFT abnormalities
Total bilirubin >3× ULN with any level of ALT before the start of treatment with pazopanib	The safety of pazopanib in this setting is unknown; use with caution. Administer 200 mg daily
Proteinuria	
24-hour urine protein ≥3 grams	Withhold pazopanib until urine protein is <3 g/24 hours, then resume pazopanib at 1 lower dose level. For recurrent episodes despite dose reduction, discontinue pazopanib
Nephrotic syndrome	Discontinue pazopanib
Diarrhea	
G1/2 diarrhea	Focus on treatment for symptoms designed to resolve the diarrhea. No dose modifications for G1/2 diarrhea unless G2 diarrhea persists for >2 weeks
G2 diarrhea that persists ≥2 weeks	Follow guidelines for G3/4 diarrhea (below)
If diarrhea cannot be controlled with preventive measures outlined, and is G3/4 or worsens by one grade level (G3 to G4) while on pazopanib, and is not alleviated by symptomatic treatment within 48 hours	Hold pazopanib. Also, withhold pazopanib if persistent G2 diarrhea while on pazopanib is not alleviated by treatment for symptoms (persistent defined as lasting for >2 weeks)
If pazopanib is held for >3 weeks and diarrhea does not resolve to G ≤1	Discontinue therapy
If within 3 weeks of withholding pazopanib, diarrhea resolves to G ≤1	Restart pazopanib at 1 dose level less than the dose level administered at the time toxicity developed
If G3/4 diarrhea or persistent G2 diarrhea recurs at reduced pazopanib doses (persistent defined as lasting for >2 weeks)	Again, withhold pazopanib until the toxicity resolves to CTCAE G ≤1, at which time pazopanib should be restarted at 1 dose level less than the dose level administered at the time toxicity developed. Treatment for symptoms may continue indefinitely as a preventive measure
If G3/4 diarrhea or persistent G2 diarrhea recurs at a dose of 200 mg once daily (persistent defined as lasting for >2 weeks)	Discontinue therapy
If diarrhea does not recur at reduced pazopanib doses with or without continued treatment for symptoms	The dose of pazopanib may be increased 1 dose level to the dose level that was being administered at the time diarrhea developed. If toxicity recurs following the increase, then follow the guidelines above, with the exception that when drug is restarted the pazopanib dose should be reduced 1 dose level
Hypertension	
Severe hypertension not controlled with medical management	Hold pazopanib pending further evaluation and treatment of hypertension
Severe hypertension despite optimal medical management	Consider reducing the dose of pazopanib or discontinuing it altogether. Discontinue if hypertension remains severe despite dosage reduction
Hypertensive crisis or hypertensive encephalopathy or reversible posterior leukoencephalopathy syndrome (RPLS)	Discontinue pazopanib

(continued)

Treatment Modifications (*continued*)

QTc Abnormalities

Patients with a history of QT-interval prolongation, patients taking antiarrhythmics or other medications that may prolong QT interval, and those with relevant preexisting cardiac disease	Use with caution
QTc prolongation defined as: • A single measurement of ≥550 ms • An increase of ≥100 ms from baseline • Two consecutive measurements (within 48 hours of each other) that were ≥500 ms but ≤550 ms • An increase of ≥60 ms, but <100 ms from baseline to a value ≥480 ms	Hold pazopanib until QTc <480 ms, then resume pazopanib at 1 dose level lower

Other Adverse Reactions

G3/4 fatigue	Reduce pazopanib 1 dose level
Clinically significant active infection	Institute appropriate anti-infective therapy and consider interrupting or discontinuing pazopanib for serious infections
Interstitial lung disease/pneumonitis	Discontinue pazopanib
Thrombotic microangiopathy, thrombotic thrombocytopenic purpura, or hemolytic uremic syndrome	Discontinue pazopanib
History of hemoptysis, cerebral, or clinically significant gastrointestinal hemorrhage while receiving pazopanib or in the past 6 months	Discontinue or avoid pazopanib
Patients with increased risk of arterial thrombotic events	Discontinue or avoid pazopanib
Onset of hypothyroidism	Treat hypothyroidism and monitor carefully
Planned elective surgery	Stop pazopanib at least 7 days prior to scheduled surgery. The decision to resume pazopanib after surgery should be based on clinical judgment of adequate wound healing
Wound dehiscence	Discontinue pazopanib

Drug Interactions

Concomitant use of a strong CYP3A4 inhibitor (eg, ketoconazole, ritonavir, clarithromycin) is required	Reduce pazopanib dose to 400 mg; further reduce to 200 mg if adverse effects are observed. The goal is to adjust the pazopanib AUC to the range observed without inhibitors. However, there are no clinical data with this dose adjustment in patients receiving strong CYP3A4 inhibitors
Concomitant use of strong CYP3A4 34 inducers (eg, rifampin)	Do not administer pazopanib
Concomitant use of a drug metabolized by CYP3A4, CYP2D6, or CYP2C8 that has a narrow therapeutic index	Pazopanib is a weak inhibitor of CYP3A4, CYP2D6, and CYP2C8 and may inhibit the metabolism of concomitantly administered drugs that are substrates of these enzymes. Use caution and consider increased monitoring and/or dose reduction of the sensitive substrate per the clinical judgment of the medically responsible health care provider
Patient requires treatment with simvastatin	Concomitant use of simvastatin with pazopanib is associated with a higher rate of ALT elevation
Patient requires treatment with a medication that raises the gastric pH	Short-acting antacid products are preferable to histamine (H2) receptor antagonists and proton pump inhibitor medications. If used concomitantly, antacid administration should be separated from pazopanib ingestion by several hours

Note: patients with only a mild indirect hyperbilirubinemia, known Gilbert syndrome, and elevation in ALT >3× ULN should be managed per the recommendations outlined for isolated ALT elevations

Patient Population Studied (N = 37)

The PANORAMA study was a multicenter retrospective analysis involving 37 adult patients with advanced non–clear cell RCC who were treated with first-line pazopanib. Patients were required to have received at least 2 weeks of therapy for stage IV disease

Baseline Characteristics of Patients (N = 37)

Characteristic	n (%)
Median age, years (range)	65 (44–80)
Female gender	11 (30)
Histology	
Papillary type 1	8
Papillary type 2	7
Papillary NOS	4
Chromophobe	9 (24)
Xp11 translocation	1 (3)
Unclassified	8 (22)
Grading (Fuhrman) (%)	
Grade 1–2	6 (16)
Grade 3	12 (32)
Grade 4	6 (16)
NA	13 (35)
Stage at Diagnosis (%)	
I–III	20 (54)
IV	17 (46)
Nephrectomy (%)	
Yes	28 (76)
No	9 (24)
ECOG Performance Status	
0	21 (57)
1	10 (27)
2–3	6 (16)
MSKCC Score Risk Group	
Good	8 (22)
Intermediate	25 (67)
Poor	4 (11)

Efficacy (N = 37)

Efficacy Variable	Pazopanib (N = 37)
Response rate (RECIST 1.1), n (%)	
Partial response	10 (27)
Complete response	0 (0)
Stable disease	20 (54)
Progressive disease	6 (16)
Not evaluable	1 (3)
Progression-free survival	
Median (95% CI), mo	15.9 (5.9–25.8)
PFS rate at 6 months	71%
PFS rate 12 months	55%
Overall survival	
Median (95% CI), mo	17.3 (11.5–23.0)
OS rate at 12 months	64%
OS rate 24 months	35%

RECIST, Response Evaluation Criteria in Solid Tumors; CI, confidence interval; PFS, progression-free survival; OS, overall survival
Note: median follow-up was 24.4 months (95% CI 16.6–31.1)

Adverse Events (N = 37)

Event	Pazopanib (N = 37) G1/2 (%)	Pazopanib (N = 37) G ≥3 (%)
Asthenia	35	8
Diarrhea	30	3
Hypertension	19	NR
Dyspepsia/epigastralgia	8	NR
Mucositis	5	NR
Loss of appetite/hyporexia	3	NR
Hyperbilirubinemia	4	NR
Hypertransaminasemia	4	5
Thrombocytopenia	3	NR
Anemia	4	8
Neutropenia	5	NR
Hypophosphoremia	3	NR
Hypertriglyceridemia	3	NR
Hypothyroidism	8	NR
Dysgeusia	8	NR
Cutaneous toxicity*	4	NR
Nausea/vomiting	4	NR
Heart failure	3	NR
Sleepiness	3	NR
Bleeding†	3	NR

Note: grading of adverse events was according to the National Cancer Institute Common Terminology Criteria for Adverse Events, version 4.0
NR, none reported
*Includes discoloration of hairs and cutis, hand-foot syndrome, dermatitis
†Includes melena, hemoptysis, and epistaxis

(*continued*)

Patient Population Studied
(N = 37) *(continued)*

IMDC Score Risk Group

Good	9 (24)
Intermediate	18 (49)
Poor	8 (22)
NA	2 (5)

Neutrophil/Lymphocyte Ratio (%)

≥3	8 (22)
<3	24 (65)
NA	5 (13)

Number of Metastatic Sites (%)

1	11 (30)
2	17 (46)
3–5	9 (24)

Type of Metastatic Site (%)

Lung	19 (51)
Nodes	19 (51)
Bone	11 (30)
Liver	8 (22)
Peritoneum	6 (16)
Other	11 (30)

NOS, not otherwise specified; NA, not assessed/available; ECOG, Eastern Cooperative Oncology Group; MSKCC, Memorial Sloan Kettering Cancer Center; IMDC, International Metastatic Renal Cell Carcinoma Database Consortium

Therapy Monitoring

1. *At baseline, day 8, every 3 weeks until week 24, and every 4 weeks thereafter:* physical examinations, vital signs, with blood pressure monitoring and clinical laboratory evaluations. Serum chemistries, particularly: calcium, magnesium, and potassium

2. *Electrocardiograms:* baseline and periodic (as clinically indicated) monitoring of electrocardiograms and maintenance of electrolytes (eg, calcium, magnesium, potassium) within the normal range should be performed

3. *Thyroid function tests:* monitor every 12 weeks. If thyroid-stimulating hormone levels are abnormal, evaluations of free triiodothyronine and thyroxine should be obtained

4. *Urine protein:* assess proteinuria by urine dipstick and/or urinary protein creatinine ratio. Patients with a urine dipstick reading ≥2+ should undergo further assessment with a 24-hour urine collection

5. *LFTs:* monitor at baseline and at weeks 3, 5, 7, and 9. Thereafter, monitor at month 3 and month 4 (or more often if clinically indicated), and then periodically

6. Thereafter, monitor at month 3 and at month 4, and as clinically indicated. Periodic monitoring should then continue after month 4

7. *Gastrointestinal perforation:* although gastrointestinal perforation with pazopanib is rare, monitor for symptoms of gastrointestinal perforation or fistula

8. *Response assessment:* every 2–3 cycles

METASTATIC • NON-CLEAR CELL • SUBSEQUENT THERAPY
RENAL CELL CARCINOMA REGIMEN: AXITINIB

Park I et al. Clin Genitourin Cancer 2018;16:e997–e1002
INLYTA (axitinib) prescribing information. New York, NY: Pfizer Labs; revised January 2020

Axitinib 5 mg; administer orally twice daily (approximately every 12 hours), continually, until disease progression (total dose/week = 70 mg)
Notes:
- Axitinib should be swallowed whole (no breaking, crushing, or chewing) with water
- Axitinib may be administered without respect to food ingestion
- Advise patients to avoid grapefruit products while taking axitinib
- Instruct patients who vomit or miss a dose of axitinib to avoid taking an additional dose. Take the next prescribed dose at the usual time
- Patients who tolerate axitinib for at least 6 consecutive weeks with no adverse reactions G >2, who remain normotensive (blood pressure ≤150/90 mm Hg), and are not receiving anti-hypertension medications may have their dose increased to 7 mg twice daily, and further to 10 mg twice daily using the same criteria
- Avoid use of concomitant strong CYP3A4/5 inhibitors. If a strong CYP3A4/5 inhibitor must be co-administered, a dose decrease of axitinib by approximately half is recommended. Subsequent doses can be increased or decreased based on individual safety and tolerability. If co-administration of a strong inhibitor is discontinued, the axitinib dose should be returned (after 3–5 elimination half-lives of the inhibitor) to that used prior to initiation of the strong CYP3A4/5 inhibitor
- The axitinib starting dose should be reduced by approximately half in patients with baseline moderate hepatic impairment (Child-Pugh class B)
- If axitinib is interrupted, patients receiving antihypertensive medications should be monitored for hypotension. The plasma half-life of axitinib is 2–4 hours and blood pressure usually decreases within 1–2 days following dose interruption

Antiemetic prophylaxis
Emetogenic potential of axitinib is **MINIMAL TO LOW**
See Chapter 42 for antiemetic recommendations

Hematopoietic growth factor (CSF) prophylaxis
Primary prophylaxis is **NOT** *indicated*
See Chapter 43 for more information

Antimicrobial prophylaxis
Risk of fever and neutropenia is **LOW**
   Antimicrobial primary prophylaxis to be considered:
- Antibacterial—not indicated
- Antifungal—not indicated
- Antiviral—not indicated unless patient previously had an episode of HSV

Diarrhea management
Latent or delayed-onset diarrhea*:

   Loperamide 4 mg orally initially after the first loose or liquid stool, *then* 2–4 mg orally every 2–4 hours or **diphenoxylate hydrochloride** 2.5 mg **with atropine sulfate** 0.025 mg (eg, Lomotil)

*Abigerges D et al. J Natl Cancer Inst 1994;86:446–449
Rothenberg ML et al. J Clin Oncol 2001;19:3801–3807
Wadler S et al. J Clin Oncol 1998;16:3169–3178

Treatment Modifications

RECOMMENDED DOSE MODIFICATIONS FOR AXITINIB

Dose level +2	10 mg orally twice per day
Dose level + 1	7 mg orally twice per day
Starting dose (level 1)	5 mg orally twice per day
Dose level −1	3 mg orally twice per day
Dose level −2	2 mg orally twice per day
Dose level −3	Discontinue axitinib*

(continued)

Treatment Modifications (*continued*)

Grade/Severity	Treatment Modification
The patient has tolerated axitinib at a dose of 5 mg twice per day for ≥2 weeks without G >2 treatment-related adverse reactions, is normotensive (blood pressure ≤150/90 mm Hg), and is not receiving anti-hypertension medication	Increase the dose of axitinib to dose level +1 (7 mg orally twice per day)
The patient has tolerated axitinib at a dose of 7 mg twice per day for ≥2 weeks without G >2 treatment-related adverse reactions, is normotensive (blood pressure ≤150/90 mm Hg), and is not receiving anti-hypertension medication	Increase the dose of axitinib to dose level +2 (10 mg orally twice per day)
Any hypertension	Treat as needed with standard anti-hypertensive therapy
Persistent hypertension despite use of maximal anti-hypertensive medications	Reduce the dosage of axitinib by 1 dosage level
Evidence of hypertensive crisis	Discontinue axitinib*
Urine dipstick >1+ for protein	Continue axitinib at the same dose pending results of a 24-hour urine protein
Urine protein ≥3 g/24 hours	Withhold axitinib until urine protein is <3 g/24 hours, then resume axitinib at 1 lower dose level*
Grade 3 diarrhea	Optimize antidiarrheal regimen and reduce the dose of axitinib by 1 dose level
Grade 4 diarrhea	Withhold axitinib until recovery to G ≤1, then resume axitinib with the dose reduced by 1 dose level and with optimization of the antidiarrheal regimen
Grade 2 AST, ALT, or bilirubin elevation	Increase the frequency of LFT monitoring. Withhold axitinib until improvement to G ≤1 or baseline, then resume axitinib at the same dosage
Grade ≥3 AST, ALT, or bilirubin elevation	Increase the frequency of LFT monitoring. Withhold axitinib until improvement to G ≤1 or baseline, then resume axitinib with the dosage reduced by 1 dose level
Bleeding occurs that requires medical intervention	Withhold axitinib until resolution of bleeding*
Patient requires elective surgery	Withhold axitinib for ≥2 days prior to elective surgery. Do not resume axitinib for at least 2 weeks following major surgery and until adequate wound healing has occurred*
RPLS is suspected (symptoms of headache, seizure, lethargy, confusion, blindness, and/or other visual and neurologic disturbances along with hypertension of any severity)	Withhold axitinib until clarification of the patient's neurologic status (ie, with an emergent brain MRI) has occurred*
RPLS is confirmed	Discontinue axitinib.* The safety of reinitiating axitinib in a patient who has experienced RPLS is unknown
Patient has moderate hepatic impairment (Child-Pugh class B)	Decrease the starting dose of axitinib by approximately 50% and then increase or decrease the dose based on individual safety and tolerability
Patient requires concomitant use of a strong CYP3A4/5 inhibitor (eg, ketoconazole, itraconazole, posaconazole, clarithromycin, atazanavir, indinavir, nefazodone, nelfinavir, ritonavir, saquinavir, telithromycin, and voriconazole)	If concomitant use of the CYP3A4/5 inhibitor is unavoidable, then decrease the dose of axitinib by approximately 50% and then increase or decrease the dose based on individual safety and tolerability. If the strong CYP3A4/5 inhibitor is subsequently discontinued, then resume the axitinib dose that was used prior to initiation of the CYP3A4/5 inhibitor after 3–5 CYP3A4/5 inhibitor half-lives have transpired
Patient requires concomitant use of a moderate or strong CYP3A4/5 inducer (eg, rifampin, dexamethasone, phenytoin, carbamazepine, rifabutin, rifapentine, phenobarbital, St. John's Wort, bosentan, efavirenz, etravirine, modafinil, nafcillin)	Avoid concomitant use of a moderate or strong CYP3A4/5 inducer with axitinib

*If the patient is receiving antihypertensive medications, monitor closely for development of hypotension if axitinib is withheld or discontinued
AST, aspartate aminotransferase; ALT, alanine aminotransferase; LFT, liver function test; RPLS, reversible posterior leukoencephalopathy syndrome; MRI, magnetic resonance imaging

Patient Population Studied (N = 40)

This was a prospective, multicenter, open-label, single-arm, phase 2 trial involving 40 adult patients with histologically confirmed RCC without a clear cell component that was not amenable to curative treatment with local therapies and that had progressed during or after prior treatment with temsirolimus. Eligible histologies included papillary, chromophobe, MiT family translocation, medullary, and unclassified RCC. Patients were required to have an Eastern Cooperative Oncology Group performance status of ≤1. Patients were excluded if they had an extensive sarcomatoid component, collecting duct carcinoma, poorly controlled hypertension (blood pressure ≥150/90 mm Hg despite optimal antihypertensive therapy), prior treatment with VEGF-targeting agents, or a requirement for concurrent treatment with a potent CYP3A4 inducer or inhibitor. All patients were treated with axitinib initially at 5 mg orally twice per day with the option to escalate doses to 7 mg twice per day and then to a maximum dose of 10 mg twice per day

Baseline Characteristics of Patients

Characteristic	n (%)
Median age, years (range)	59 (22–84)
Female gender	14 (35.0)
Histology	
Papillary type 1	1 (2.5)
Papillary type 2	24 (60.0)
Papillary NOS	1 (2.5)
Chromophobe	4 (10.0)
MiT family translocation	7 (17.5)
Others	3 (7.5)
ECOG performance status	
0	3 (7.5)
1	37 (92.5)
IMDC risk group	
Favorable	5 (12.5)
Intermediate	29 (72.5)
Poor	6 (15.0)
Previous treatment	
Nephrectomy	33 (82.5)
Temsirolimus	40 (100)
Cytokine	3 (7.5)
Cytotoxic chemotherapy	1 (2.5)
Line of axitinib treatment	
Second	36 (90.0)
Third	4 (10.0)

NOS, not otherwise specified; ECOG, Eastern Cooperative Oncology Group; IMDC, International Metastatic Renal Cell Carcinoma Database Consortium

Efficacy (N = 40)

Best Overall Response of Patients and Response According to Histology

Histology	Best Response, n (%)				PFS	OS	Total N
	PR	SD	PD	NA	Median (95% CI), mo	Median (95% CI), mo	
Full cohort	15 (37.5)	12 (30.0)	11 (27.5)	2 (5.0)	7.4 (5.2–9.5)	12.1 (6.4–17.7)	40 (100)
Papillary type 1	0	0	1 (100)	0	3.5 (0–10.9)*	8.3 (4.1–12.5)*	1 (100)
Papillary type 2	9 (37.5)	6 (25.0)	8 (33.3)	1 (4.1)			24 (100)
Papillary NOS	1 (100.0)	0	0	0			1 (100)
Chromophobe	1 (25.0)	3 (75.0)	0	0	11.0	22.2	4 (100)
MiT family translocation	4 (57.1)	2 (28.5)	1 (14.3)	0	11.1 (7.6–14.6)	16.9	7 (100)

PFS, progression-free survival; OS, overall survival; PR, partial response; SD, stable disease; NA, not assessable; CI, confidence interval; NOS, not otherwise specified
Includes patients with papillary type 1, papillary type 2, and papillary NOS histology
Note: median follow-up duration was 14.7 months (95% CI 10.8–18.6)

Adverse Events (N = 40)

Event	Axitinib (N = 40)		Event	Axitinib (N = 40)	
	All Grades (%)	G ≥3 (%)		All Grades (%)	G ≥3 (%)
Hypertension	55.0	20.0	Bleeding	15.0	2.5
Palmar-plantar erythrodysesthesia syndrome	37.5	0	Insomnia	15.0	0
Anorexia	32.5	0	Nausea	12.5	0
Cough	30.0	0	Skin rash	12.5	0
Constipation	27.5	0	Mucosal inflammation	12.5	0
Oral mucositis	27.5	0	Abdominal pain	12.5	0
Diarrhea	27.5	0	Flank pain	12.5	0
Hoarseness	25.0	0	Pelvic pain	12.5	0
Back pain	25.0	0	Depression	10.0	0
Infection	22.5	2.5	Dyspnea	10.0	0
Headache	20.0	0	Vomiting	10.0	0
Dyspepsia	17.5	0	Hypothyroidism	10.0	0
Fatigue	17.5	10.0	Myalgia	10.0	0
Proteinuria	15.0	7.5	Toothache	10.0	0

Adverse events included if they occurred in 10% of patients during axitinib therapy

Therapy Monitoring

1. *At baseline, week 2, week 4, and every 4 weeks thereafter:* clinical assessments including medical history and physical examination, vital signs, ALT, AST, total bilirubin, and CBC with differential. Control blood pressure prior to initiation of axitinib
2. *At screening, after 6 and 12 weeks of therapy, and every 8 weeks thereafter:* tumor assessments. Thyroid function tests. Spot urine for protein measurement (if spot urine dipstick >1+ for protein, perform a 24-hour urine protein)

METASTATIC • NON-CLEAR CELL • SUBSEQUENT THERAPY
RENAL CELL CARCINOMA REGIMEN: TEMSIROLIMUS

Venugopal B et al. BMC Urol 2013;13:26
TORISEL (temsirolimus) prescribing information. Philadelphia, PA: Wyeth Pharmaceuticals Inc; Revised March 2018

Premedication:
Diphenhydramine 25–50 mg; administer intravenously ~30 minutes before each dose of temsirolimus as prophylaxis against hypersensitivity reactions (other histamine H_1-receptor antagonists may be substituted)

Temsirolimus 25 mg; administer diluted in 250 mL 0.9% sodium chloride injection intravenously over 30–60 minutes once weekly until disease progression (total dose/week = 25 mg)
Notes:
- Prepare the final temsirolimus dilution in either bottles (glass or polypropylene) or plastic bags (polypropylene, polyolefin) protected from light
- Infuse temsirolimus through a non-diethylhexylpthalate (non-DEHP), non-polyvinylchloride (non-PVC), polyethylene-lined administration set containing an in-line polyethersulfone filter with a pore size of ≤5 μm. Alternatively, a polyethersulfone end-filter with a pore size ranging from 0.2 μm to 5 μm may be used in place of an in-line filter
- The concomitant use of strong cytochrome P450 (CYP) CYP3A4 inhibitors should be avoided. Ingestion of grapefruit products (fruit, juice) may also increase plasma concentrations of sirolimus (a major metabolite of temsirolimus) and should be avoided. If a strong CYP3A4 inhibitor must be administered, a temsirolimus dose reduction to 12.5 mg/week should be considered
- If a concomitantly administered strong CYP3A4 inhibitor is discontinued, a washout period of approximately 1 week should be allowed before the temsirolimus dose is adjusted back to the dose used prior to initiation of the strong CYP3A4 inhibitor
- The use of concomitant strong CYP3A4 inducers should be avoided. If a strong CYP3A4 inducer must be administered, a temsirolimus dose increase from 25 mg/week up to 50 mg/week should be considered
- If a concomitantly administered strong CYP3A4 inducer is discontinued, the temsirolimus dose should be returned to the dose used prior to initiation of the strong CYP3A4 inducer
- Patients with mild hepatic impairment (bilirubin >1 to 1.5× ULN or AST >ULN but bilirubin ≤ULN) should be administered temsirolimus at a reduced dose of 15 mg per week
- Elevations in serum glucose can occur with temsirolimus. When possible, optimal glucose and lipid control should be achieved before starting a patient on temsirolimus

Supportive Care
Antiemetic prophylaxis
Emetogenic potential is **MINIMAL**
See Chapter 42 for antiemetic recommendations

Hematopoietic growth factor (CSF) prophylaxis
Primary prophylaxis is **NOT** indicated
See Chapter 43 for more information

Antimicrobial prophylaxis
Risk of fever and neutropenia is **LOW**
  Antimicrobial primary prophylaxis to be considered:
  - Antibacterial—not indicated
  - Antifungal—not indicated. Consider prophylaxis for *P. jirovecii* (eg, cotrimoxazole) in patients receiving concomitant treatment with corticosteroids or other immunosuppressive agents.
  - Antiviral—not indicated unless patient previously had an episode of HSV

Oral care
Standard prophylaxis and treatment for mucositis/stomatitis

Treatment Modifications

TEMSIROLIMUS

Starting dose level	25 mg IV once per week
Dose level −1	20 mg IV once per week
Dose level −2	15 mg IV once per week
Dose level −3	Discontinue temsirolimus

Adverse Event	Dose Modification
Severe hypersensitivity/infusion reaction	Interrupt the temsirolimus infusion for at least 30–60 minutes depending on the severity of the reaction. At the discretion of the medically responsible health care provider, treatment may be resumed at a slower rate (up to 60 minute infusion duration) following administration of an H_1-receptor antagonist (eg, diphenhydramine 25–50 mg IV, if not previously administered) and/or an H_2-receptor antagonist (eg, famotidine 20 mg IV or ranitidine 50 mg IV)
Diagnosis of an invasive fungal infection	Discontinue temsirolimus and treat with appropriate antifungal therapy
Radiologic changes suggestive of noninfectious pneumonitis with no symptoms	Can continue temsirolimus therapy without dose alteration but with careful monitoring
Radiologic changes suggestive of noninfectious pneumonitis with mild–moderate symptoms	Withhold temsirolimus until symptoms improve. Consider administering corticosteroids. If symptoms improve, consider reintroducing temsirolimus one dose lower depending on the individual clinical circumstances with careful continued monitoring. Consider administering prophylaxis for opportunistic infections (eg, *P. jirovecii*) in patients requiring prolonged corticosteroids
Radiologic changes suggestive of noninfectious pneumonitis with severe symptoms (including a decrease in DL_{CO} on pulmonary function tests)	Discontinue temsirolimus and consider administering high doses of corticosteroids. Consider administering prophylaxis for opportunistic infections (eg, *P. jirovecii*) in patients requiring prolonged corticosteroids
ANC <1000/mm³ or platelet count <75,000/mm³	Withhold therapy. Resume temsirolimus when symptoms improve to G ≤2 with temsirolimus dose reduced by 5 mg/week to a dose not less than 15 mg/week
Nephrotic syndrome	Permanently discontinue temsirolimus
Any nonhematologic G3/4 toxicity	Withhold therapy. Resume temsirolimus when symptoms improve to G ≤2 with temsirolimus dose reduced by 5 mg/week to a dose not less than 15 mg/week
G1/2 stomatitis	Administer topical treatments (avoid alcohol- or peroxide-containing mouthwashes as they may exacerbate the condition). Do not use antifungal agents unless fungal infection has been diagnosed. Focus on pain control, oral hygiene, and ensuring adequate nutrition and hydration
Mild hepatic impairment (bilirubin >1 to 1.5× ULN or AST >ULN but bilirubin ≤ULN)	Administer temsirolimus at a reduced dose of 15 mg per week

Adapted in part from TORISEL (temsirolimus) prescribing information. Philadelphia, PA: Wyeth Pharmaceuticals Inc; revised March 2018

Patient Population Studied

This was a case report involving a 36-year-old female patient with metastatic chromophobe RCC with skeletal metastases. The patient underwent a cytoreductive nephrectomy and radiation to vertebral metastases. After disease progression was noted upon completion of 2 cycles of sunitinib, the patient was treated with temsirolimus 25 mg IV once per week along with zoledronic acid

Efficacy (N = 1)

The patient's pain and mobility improved after 8 weeks of treatment. A bone scan demonstrated reduced isotope uptake and a CT scan demonstrated disease stabilization. The response duration was 20 months

Adverse Events (N = 1)

The patient developed temsirolimus-induced pneumonitis after 13 months of treatment. The pneumonitis was steroid-responsive but recurred upon re-challenge with full-dose temsirolimus. The recurrent pneumonitis again improved with corticosteroid treatment and the patient was re-commenced on temsirolimus at a reduced dose of 20 mg per week. The patient also experienced Grade 1 nail changes and Grade 1 lethargy. For additional information, refer to the regimen description within this chapter for treatment of clear cell RCC

Therapy Monitoring

1. *Baseline and periodically:*
   - ALT, AST, bilirubin, alkaline phosphatase, BUN, and serum creatinine
   - Urine dipstick for protein. If >1+, consider obtaining a 24-hour urine for protein
   - Fasting serum glucose and lipid panel. When possible, achieve optimal glucose and lipid control prior to initiation of temsirolimus
   - Chest x-ray or chest computed tomography (CT) scan to assess for pneumonitis
   - Monitor for symptoms of pulmonary toxicity, infection, hyperglycemia, bowel perforation, nephrotic syndrome, and stomatitis
2. *Baseline and weekly:*
   - CBC with differential and platelet count
   - Monitor for infusion reactions
3. Temsirolimus may impair wound healing; use caution and strongly consider withholding therapy in the peri-surgical period
4. Advise patients to avoid live vaccines and close contact with those who have received live vaccines

36. Sarcomas

Brigitte Widemann, MD, Srivandana Akshintala, MBBS, MPH, and Jean-Yves Blay, MD

PRIMARY MALIGNANT BONE TUMORS

Epidemiology

Incidence:	3600 (male: 2120; female: 1480. Estimated new cases for 2020 in the United States) 1.1 per 100,000 males, 0.8 per 100,000 females
Deaths:	Estimated 1720 in 2020 (male: 1000; female: 720)
Median age:	42 years
Male to female ratio:	1.5:1

American Cancer Society. *Cancer Facts & Figures 2020*. Atlanta: American Cancer Society; 2020

2020 WHO Classification of Malignant Bone Tumors

1. **Chondrogenic tumors**
   Chondrosarcoma, grades 1
   Chondrosarcoma, grades 2
   Chondrosarcoma, grades 3
   Periosteal chondrosarcoma
   Clear cell chondrosarcoma
   Mesenchymal chondrosarcoma
   Dedifferentiated chondrosarcoma
2. **Osteogenic tumors**
   Low-grade central osteosarcoma
   Osteosarcoma NOS
      Conventional osteosarcoma
      Telangiectatic osteosarcoma
      Small cell osteosarcoma
   Parosteal osteosarcoma
   Periosteal osteosarcoma
   High-grade surface osteosarcoma
   Secondary osteosarcoma
3. **Fibrogenic tumors**
   Fibrosarcoma NOS
4. **Vascular tumors of bone**
   Epithelioid hemangioendothelioma NOS
   Angiosarcoma
5. **Osteoclastic giant cell-rich tumors**
   Giant cell tumor of bone, malignant
6. **Notochordal tumors**
   Chordoma NOS
      Chondroid chordoma

Poorly differentiated chordoma
Dedifferentiated chordoma
7. **Other mesenchymal tumors of bone**
   Adamantinoma of long bones
      Dedifferentiated adamantinoma
   Leiomyosarcoma NOS
   Pleomorphic sarcoma, undifferentiated
   Bone metastases
8. **Hematopoietic neoplasms of bone**
   Plasmacytoma of bone
   Malignant lymphoma, non-Hodgkin, NOS
   Hodgkin disease, NOS
   Diffuse large B-cell lymphoma NOS
   Follicular lymphoma NOS
   Marginal zone B-cell lymphoma NOS
   T-cell lymphoma NOS
   Anaplastic large cell lymphoma NOS
   Malignant lymphoma, lymphoblastic, NOS
   Burkitt lymphoma NOS
   Langerhans cell histiocytosis NOS
   Langerhans cell histiocytosis, disseminated
   Erdheim-Chester disease
   Rosai-Dorfman disease

Adapted from: Choi JH, Ro JY. Adv Anat Pathol 2021;28:119–138. (note: non-malignant tumors have been omitted from this list)

Work-up

1. History and physical examination
2. *Laboratory tests:* CBC with differential; electrolytes including calcium, phosphorus, and magnesium; renal function tests including blood urea nitrogen (BUN) and creatinine; liver function tests including liver enzymes and total bilirubin; alkaline phosphatase; lactate dehydrogenase
3. Plain films of affected bone
4. CT scan of chest, abdomen, and pelvis (particularly chest because 80% of metastatic lesions occur here). CT scan may be performed in conjunction with FDG-PET. High resolution chest CT scan should be performed
5. MRI with gadolinium contrast to ascertain extent of the tumor, involvement of surrounding neurovascular structures, invasion of the adjacent joint, and the presence of skip metastases
6. Technetium-99 bone scan to identify skip lesions within affected bones or distant metastatic disease
7. Whole body 18-fluoro-deoxyglucose positron emission tomography (FDG-PET)/CT is more routinely being performed particularly for Ewing sarcoma
8. Bilateral bone marrow aspirate and biopsy for light microscopy examination in the case of Ewing sarcoma
9. No radiologic studies are pathognomonic, so bone biopsy remains essential to diagnosis
10. Echocardiogram or MUGA scan to determine cardiac ejection fraction as clinically indicated
11. Audiogram before cisplatin chemotherapy
12. Fertility preservation to be offered when feasible

Surgical Staging

The surgical system as described by Enneking et al. is based on the GTM classification. Stage is determined by 3 different subcategories: grade (G), location or site (T), and lymph node involvement and metastases (M)

Grade (G)	
G1	Low grade, uniform cell type without atypia, few mitoses
G2	High grade, atypical nuclei, mitoses pronounced

Site (T)	
T1	Intracompartmental = Confined within limits of periosteum
T2	Extracompartmental = Breach in an adjacent joint cartilage, bone cortex (or periosteum) fascia lata, quadriceps, and joint capsule

Lymph Node Involvement and Metastases (M)	
M0	No identifiable skip lesions or distant metastases
M1	Any skip lesions, regional lymph nodes, or distant metastases

Enneking Staging System of Malignant Bone Tumors

Stage		G	T	M
IA	Low grade, intracompartmental	G1	T1	M0
IB	Low grade, extracompartmental	G1	T2	M0
IIA	High grade, intracompartmental	G2	T1	M0
IIB	High grade, extracompartmental	G2	T2	M0
IIIA	Low or high grade, intracompartmental with metastases	G1/2	T1	M1
IIIB	Low or high grade, extracompartmental with metastases	G1/2	T2	M1

Enneking WF et al. Clin Orthop 1980;153:106–120

Clinical Staging

AJCC 8th Edition Staging

Primary Tumor (T)

Appendicular Skeleton, Trunk, Skull, and Facial Bones

TX Primary tumor cannot be assessed
T0 No evidence of primary tumor
T1 Tumor ≤ 8 cm in greatest dimension
T2 Tumor >8 cm in greatest dimension
T3 Discontinuous tumors in the primary bone site

Spine

TX Primary tumor cannot be assessed
T0 No evidence of primary tumor
T1 Tumor confined to 1 vertebral segment or 2 adjacent segments
T2 Tumor confined to three adjacent vertebral segments
T3 Tumor confined to ≥4 adjacent vertebral segments, or any nonadjacent vertebral segments
T4 Extension into the spinal canal or great vessels
  T4a Extension into the spinal canal
  T4b Evidence of gross vascular invasion or tumor thrombus in the great vessels

Pelvis

TX Primary tumor cannot be assessed
T0 No evidence of primary tumor
T1 Tumor confined to one pelvic segment with no extraosseous extension
  T1a Tumor ≤ 8 cm in greatest dimension
  T1b Tumor > 8 cm in greatest dimension

Histologic Grading Systems for Assessing Response to Induction Chemotherapy in Osteosarcoma

Salzer-Kuntschik

I:	No viable cells
II:	Single viable tumor cells or cluster <0.5 cm
III:	Viable tumor <10%
IV:	Viable tumor 10–50%
V:	Viable tumor >50%
VI:	No effect on chemotherapy

Picci

Total response:	No viable tumor
Good response:	90–99% necrosis
Fair response:	60–89% necrosis
Poor response:	<60% necrosis

Huvos (Wunder et al)

IV:	No histologic evidence of viable tumor
III:	Only scattered foci of viable tumor cells (<10% vital tumor tissue)
II:	Areas of necrosis with areas of viable tumor (10–50% vital tumor tissue)
I:	Little or no chemotherapy effect

Picci P et al. Cancer 1985;56:1515–1521
Salzer-Kuntschik M et al. Pathologe 1983;4:135–141
Wunder JS et al. J Bone Joint Surg Am 1998;80: 1020–1033

(continued)

Clinical Staging (continued)

T2 Tumor confined to 1 pelvic segment with extraosseous extension or 2 segments without extraosseous extension

    T2a Tumor ≤ 8 cm in greatest dimension

    T2b Tumor > 8 cm in greatest dimension

T3 Tumor spanning 2 pelvic segments with extraosseous extension

    T3a Tumor ≤ 8 cm in greatest dimension

    T3b Tumor > 8 cm in greatest dimension

T4 Tumor spanning 3 pelvic segments or crossing the sacroiliac joint

    T4a Tumor involves sacroiliac joint and extends medial to the sacral neuroforamen

    T4b Tumor encasement of external iliac vessels or presence of gross tumor thrombus in major pelvic vessels

Regional Lymph Node (N)

NX Regional lymph nodes cannot be assessed*

N0 No regional lymph node metastasis

N1 Regional lymph node metastasis

*Because of the rarity of lymph node involvement in bone sarcomas, the designation NX may not be appropriate, and cases should be considered N0 unless clinical node involvement clearly is evident

Distant Metastasis (M)

M0 No distant metastasis

M1 Distant metastasis

    M1a Lung

    M1b Bone or other distant sites

Grade

GX Grade cannot be assessed

G1 Well differentiated, low grade

G2 Moderately differentiated, high gradre

G3 Poorly differentiated, high grade

Stage Grouping (applies to Appendicular Skeleton, Trunk, Skull, and Facial Bones)

IA	G1,X	T1	N0	M0
IB	G1,X	T2	N0	M0
	G1,X	T3	N0	M0
IIA	G2,3	T1	N0	M0
IIB	G2,3	T2	N0	M0
III	G2,3	T3	N0	M0
IVA	Any G	Any T	N0	M1a
IVB	Any G	Any T	N1	Any M
IVB	Any G	Any T	Any N	M1b

Amin MB et al, editors. AJCC Cancer Staging Manual. 8th ed. New York: Springer; 2017

5-Year Survival

Nonmetastatic (80% of Patients at Diagnosis)	
Good histologic response (>90% necrosis)	75%
Poor histologic response (<90% necrosis)	55%
Metastatic (20% of patients at diagnosis)	20%

Expert Opinion

Primary Bone Tumors

General

1. Rare, account for <0.2% of malignant tumors

2. *Relatively high incidence in children and adolescents,* although even in the young, benign bone tumors are more common

3. Considerably outnumbered by metastases to the bone in older patients

4. Presentations:

    • Nonmechanical pain or night pain around the knee are cause for concern

    • Swelling only if tumor extends through the cortex distending periosteum

Expert Opinion (*continued*)

5. Referral to reference center is strongly encouraged

6. Frequently difficult to recognize as malignant by clinicians, radiologists, as well as pathologists → major diagnostic difficulties in nonspecialized centers

7. Ideally, all cases of suspected bone tumor should be discussed at a multidisciplinary team meeting

Diagnosis and Local Staging

1. Conventional radiographs in two planes should be the first investigation

2. CT in the case of a diagnostic problem or doubt, to visualize calcification, periosteal bone formation, cortical destruction, or soft-tissue involvement

3. When malignancy is suspected on radiographs, the next step is MRI, in particular for limbs

4. General staging to assess the extent of distant disease includes (also see individual histologies)

   • Technetium-99 bone scan

   • High resolution chest CT

   • FDG-PET is being used more commonly especially in Ewings sarcoma, and may be more sensitive in detecting metastasis. However its role in staging, response assessment, and overall patient management needs further evaluation. Bone scan may be omitted if FDG-PET scan is being performed.

5. Whole-body MRI and FDG-PET/MRI under evaluation for staging and treatment assessment

Biopsy

1. Experienced physician(s) should biopsy suspicious sites, as exact staging of disease has impact on treatment and outcome

2. Principles of biopsy:

   • Determine stage before the biopsy → may guide location of biopsy

   • Minimal contamination of normal tissues

   • A core needle biopsy guided by ultrasound, x-ray, or CT is often adequate for obtaining a pathologic diagnosis

   • Samples for microbiologic culture as well as histology

   • Samples should be snap-frozen for future studies

   • An experienced pathologist should evaluate samples. The opinion of an expert bone pathologist may be required.

   • Excisional biopsy is contraindicated because it may contaminate tissue compartments, unless this approach has previously been discussed by a team of multidisciplinary sarcoma experts

   • Open biopsy requires a longitudinal incision

   • In aggressive and malignant tumors of bone, consider biopsy tract contaminated with tumor and removed together with the resection specimen to avoid local recurrences

3. Spinal column involvement: avoid laminectomy or decompression resulting in incomplete resection unless necessary to relieve spinal cord compression

Prevention and Management of Pathologic Fracture

1. Pathologic fractures may disseminate tumor cells into surrounding tissues and increase the risk of local recurrence

2. Patients with weakened bone → immobilize following biopsy with an external splint. In cases of fracture, internal fixation is contraindicated as it disseminates tumor further into both bone and soft tissues, increasing the risk of local recurrence. Neoadjuvant chemotherapy used with expectation of a good response will allow fracture hematoma to contract and allow subsequent resection

3. If response to chemotherapy is poor or in tumors unlikely to respond → consider early surgery obtaining wide margins including amputation

4. Consider postoperative radiotherapy to decrease the risk of local recurrence

Systemic Therapy
(Also see individual histologies)

1. Strongly consider treatment in reference centers or networks

2. High-grade osteosarcoma, Ewing sarcoma, malignant fibrous histocytoma/undifferentiated pleomorphic sarcoma (MFH/UPS) of the bone, and other spindle cell sarcomas should receive primary chemotherapy

Surgery
(Also see individual histologies)

1. Surgery should be performed only after adequate preoperative staging, and, depending on the tumor, primary chemotherapy

2. Striving to obtain adequate surgical margins → narrower margins are associated with an increased risk of local recurrence

3. If possible perform a wide en-bloc resection

   • General *intracompartmental* resection

   • Occasionally *extracompartmental* resection if entire bone/muscle compartment can be removed easily

4. If postoperative radiotherapy is likely, risk areas and close margins should be identified with clips

5. Surgical reconstruction varies; discuss with patient

(*continued*)

Expert Opinion (continued)

Follow-up

1. The goal is to detect local recurrence or metastatic disease when early treatment is still possible and might be effective
2. Follow-up includes physical exam of tumor site and assessment of function. Imaging evaluation to consider includes local imaging and chest X-Ray/CT scan with or without bone scan or FDG-PET scan
3. Recommended intervals for follow-up after completion of chemotherapy:
   - Every 6 weeks to 3 months for the first 2 years
   - Every 2–4 months for years 3–4
   - Every 6 months for years 5–10
   - Every 6–12 months thereafter

Note: these suggested intervals of follow-up need to be balanced against evidence that excessive exposure to radiation may increase the risk of developing leukemia, especially in children

3. Recommended intervals for follow-up for low-grade bone sarcoma
   - Every 6 months for 2 years, and then annually
4. Late metastases as well as local recurrences and functional deficits may occur >10 years after diagnosis, and there is no universally accepted stopping point for tumor surveillance
5. It is important to evaluate long-term toxicity of therapy for >10 years. Secondary cancers and leukemia, particularly acute myeloid leukemia, may occur

Hogendoorn PCW et al. ESMO/EUROBONET Working Group Bone sarcomas: ESMO Clinical Practice Guidelines for diagnosis, treatment and follow-up. Ann Oncol 2010;21 Suppl 5:v204–v213

Osteosarcoma

Background:

1. Most frequent primary cancer of bone (incidence: 0.2–0.3/100,000/year)
2. Higher incidence in adolescents (0.8–1.1/100,000/year at ages 15–19 years); accounts for >10% of all solid cancers
3. Male to female ratio: 1.4:1
4. Usually arises in the metaphysis of a long bone, most commonly around the knee. Involvement of the axial skeleton and craniofacial bones occurs primarily in adults
5. Risk factors:
   - Previous radiation therapy
   - Paget disease of bone
   - Germ-line abnormalities (Rb mutations, p53 mutations)

Staging and risk assessment:

1. 75% arise around the knee
2. Typically, there is pain that begins insidiously, gradually becomes constant, may be present at night, and is often nonmechanical in nature. Localized swelling and limitation of joint movement are later findings.
3. 10 to 20% of patients are diagnosed with metastatic disease (lung most common site)
4. Work-up and staging
   - Scans to detect lung and bone metastasis
5. Adverse prognostic or predictive factors:
   - Detectable metastases
   - Poor histologic response to preoperative chemotherapy
   - Axial or proximal extremity site
   - Large tumor volume
   - Elevated serum alkaline phosphatase or lactate dehydrogenase (LDH)
   - Older age, >40 years
   - Paget disease

Treatment: General

1. Changes in the size and ossification of tumor are not reliable indicators of response to neoadjuvant chemotherapy
2. Sequential dynamic MRI that evaluate changes in vascularity are reliable
3. Assessment of response usually is apparent only after several cycles of chemotherapy → do not discontinue and change chemotherapy regimen early

Expert Opinion (*continued*)

Treatment: Local therapy considerations
1. Surgery is the main form of local therapy.
2. Radiation has limited role but may be appropriate in highly selected cases or for palliation. Consider boost techniques to increase local dose, including intensity-modulated radiotherapy (IMRT), proton therapy, or samarium

Treatment: Multimodality
Localized disease
1. High-grade tumors should receive primary chemotherapy
2. Curative treatment for high-grade osteosarcoma = surgery + chemotherapy Compared with surgery alone, multimodal treatment of high-grade osteosarcoma increases DFS probabilities from 10–20% to >60%
3. Goal of surgery is to safely remove the tumor and preserve as much function as possible → consider limb salvage
4. Whenever possible, patients should receive chemotherapy in the context of prospective trials
5. Agents with activity
   - Doxorubicin
   - Cisplatin
   - High-dose methotrexate
   - Ifosfamide
6. Combinations:
   - Doxorubicin and cisplatin frequently are the basis of treatment
   - Evidence exists that combinations with methotrexate and/or ifosfamide might provide additional benefit over 2-drug schedules
   - Ideal combination and optimal treatment durations (commonly given over periods of 6–12 months) are yet to be defined
7. Most current protocols include a period of preoperative chemotherapy → although not proven to add survival benefit over postoperative chemotherapy alone
8. Extent of histologic response to preoperative chemotherapy offers important prognostic information
9. The multimodal treatment principles were generated in children, adolescents, and young adults with high-grade central osteosarcoma, but also relate to adults at least up to the age of 60 years
10. Chemotherapy also is recommended for older patients with osteosarcoma using protocols extrapolated from those designed for pediatric/adolescent patients. Methotrexate is often omitted in regimens for adults aged >25 years. A combination of doxorubicin, ifosfamide and cisplatin is often used in this case (Piperno-Neumann S et al. Int J Cancer 2020;146:413–423)
11. Extraosseous osteosarcoma: Use high-grade soft-tissue sarcoma or osteosarcoma regimens. No consensus among experts as to best approach

Metastatic disease
1. Some patients with a limited number of metastasis in a single organ have very similar or even identical prognosis to the prognosis of patients with localized disease, with surgical removal of all known metastatic lesions
2. ~30% of all patients with primary metastatic osteosarcoma and >40% of those who achieve a complete surgical remission become long-term survivors

Recurrent disease
1. Treatment is primarily surgical. Complete removal of all metastases must be attempted
2. Prognosis is poor, with long-term post-relapse survival <20%. However, >1/3 with second surgical remission survive for >5 years
3. Multiple recurrences may be curable as long as they are resectable, and repeated thoracotomies are often warranted
4. Role of second-line chemotherapy is less well-defined than that of surgery and there is no accepted standard regimen
5. Choice may take into account the prior disease-free interval, and often includes ifosfamide, with or without etoposide, with or without carboplatin. Regorafenib was demonstrated to improve progression-free survival in recurrent disease

Ewing Sarcoma and Primitive Neuroectodermal Tumor (PNET)
Background:
1. Second most common primary malignant bone cancer
2. Occurs most frequently in children and adolescents (median age: 15 years)
3. Male to female ratio: 1.5:1
4. ~25% pelvic bones/~50% extremity tumors, ≈16% chest wall, ≈6% spine
5. Occasionally arises in soft tissue

Staging and risk assessment:
1. All are high-grade tumors
2. Almost all share common gene rearrangement involving the EWS gene on chromosome 22. Most involve reciprocal translocation
3. 20–25% of patients are diagnosed with metastatic disease (10% lung, 10% bones/bone marrow, 5% combinations or others)

(continued)

Expert Opinion (continued)

4. Work-up and staging
   - Scan to detect lung and bone metastases
   - Perform bilateral bone marrow biopsy and aspirate (unilateral in the unaffected side for pelvic primary). Note: Although bone marrow biopsies are still routinely performed and considered standard of care, some recent data suggests that in the era of FDG-PET, bone marrow aspirate/biopsy may be less important.
   - Most are recognized with classical hematoxylin and eosin (H&E) stain and immunohistochemistry. Translocation detection by FISH or RT-PCR is highly recommended and is mandatory when diagnosis by light microscopy techniques is in doubt
5. Adverse prognostic or predictive factors:
   - Metastatic disease at diagnosis. The presence of bone metastases is associated with a poorer outcome than lung/pleura metastases (<20% compared with 20–40% 5-year survival)
   - Tumor size or volume
   - Serum LDH levels
   - Axial localization
   - Older age (>15 years)
   - Poor histologic response to preoperative chemotherapy
   - Incomplete or no surgery is possible (II, B)

Treatment: General
1. Change in the size of soft-tissue mass on on MRI is a rather reliable indicator of response
2. Dynamic MRI is not as reliable in evaluating response to treatment as in osteosarcoma
3. Sequential FDG-PET might be of value

Treatment: Local therapy considerations
1. Radiation-responsive tumor, radiotherapy in combination with chemotherapy achieves local control
2. For local therapy give radiotherapy alone only if complete surgery is not possible
3. Incomplete surgery, even when combined with postoperative radiotherapy, is not superior to radiotherapy alone and should be avoided
4. Postoperative radiotherapy should be given in case of inadequate surgical margins
5. Consider postoperative radiotherapy for patients who do not achieve a good response to chemotherapy (ie, >10% viable tumor cells)

Treatment: Multimodality
Localized disease
1. Successful therapy requires systemic therapy with local control
2. Should receive primary chemotherapy
3. Complete surgery, where feasible, best modality for local control
4. With surgery or radiotherapy alone, the 5-year survival is <10%
5. Current multimodality approaches include chemotherapy. Survival is ~60–70% in localized and ~20–40% in metastatic disease
6. Agents considered most active
   - Doxorubicin
   - Cyclophosphamide
   - Ifosfamide
   - Vincristine
   - Dactinomycin
   - Etoposide
7. Most protocols are based on 4- to 6-drug combinations. Current trials initially employ 3–6 cycles of chemotherapy after biopsy, followed by local therapy, then 6–10 cycles of chemotherapy (treatment duration ~10–12 months)
8. Chemotherapy intensity with time-compressed treatment cycles is positively associated with outcome. However, high-dose chemotherapy with stem cell transplantation is still investigational in high-risk localized Ewing sarcoma
9. Treatment of adult patients follows the same principles as for younger patients, but be aware of tolerability of treatment
10. Extra-skeletal Ewing sarcoma: same approach as for bone Ewing sarcoma

Metastatic disease
1. Patients with metastases at diagnosis have a worse prognosis; bone or bone marrow metastases are associated with a 5-year survival <20%
2. Patients treated with regimens similar to those for localized disease or on clinical trials
3. Experience with intensive or time-compressed chemotherapy has not shown improvement in outcomes thus far. High-dose chemotherapy followed by autologous stem cell transplantation is sometimes incorporated, but evidence of benefit is pending

(continued)

Expert Opinion (*continued*)

4. With lung metastases, whole-lung irradiation may confer a survival advantage
5. Surgical resection of residual metastases is less well defined

Recurrent disease
1. With recurrent disease, 5-year survival is <20%, although relapse >2 years from initial diagnosis is associated with a better outcome
2. Doxorubicin often cannot be used because of the cumulative lifetime dosages already administered
3. The choice of chemotherapy in relapse is not standardized:
   - Alkylating agents (cyclophosphamide, high-dose ifosfamide) in combination with topoisomerase inhibitors (etoposide, topotecan), *or*
   - Irinotecan with temozolomide

Chondrosarcoma
Background:
1. Most frequent bone sarcoma of adults (~0.1/100,000 per year), most common age 30–60 years
2. Male to female ratio: ~1:1
3. The majority are staged as low grade (grade I) rather than high grade (grades II–III)
4. Most arise centrally in the diametaphyseal region of long bones, but can also occur in flat bones
5. Per sarcoma evidence-based diagnosis and management, pain is present frequently, insidious and progressive → pain at the site of a cartilaginous lesion suggest malignancy

Staging and risk assessment:
1. Differentiation is difficult between benign enchondroma or osteochondroma and malignant grade I chondrosarcoma
2. Although they are extremely rare in hands and feet, lesions found in long bones and central cartilaginous lesions should be considered potential low-grade chondrosarcoma until proved otherwise
3. Inoperable, locally advanced, and metastatic lesions have poor prognosis because of resistance to radiotherapy and chemotherapy
4. Prognosis depends on histologic grade; however, assessing grade is difficult

Treatment: Multimodality
1. Low-grade chondrosarcoma are unlikely to metastasize, but may recur locally
   - Central chondrosarcoma in long bones can be managed with curettage with/without adjuvant (e.g. phenol, cement, cryotherapy)
   - Peripheral chondrosarcoma should be surgically excised with covering of normal tissue
2. Higher-grade chondrosarcomas and all chondrosarcomas of the pelvis or axial skeleton should be surgically excised with wide margins
3. Recent evidence suggests mesenchymal chondrosarcoma may be chemotherapy sensitive → consider for adjuvant or neoadjuvant therapy
4. Dedifferentiated chondrosarcoma
   - Uncertainty about chemotherapy sensitivity; often treated like osteosarcoma, but with a poorer outcome
   - There is a high risk of local recurrence following excision, particularly in the presence of a pathologic fracture
5. Role of of radiotherapy is limited but may be appropriate in highly selected cases or for palliation

Spindle Cell Sarcomas of Bone (Malignant Fibrous Histiocytoma/Fibrosarcoma of Bone [MFH/FS])
Background:
1. Heterogeneous group of tumors including:
   - Fibrosarcoma (FS)
   - Malignant fibrous histiocytoma (MFH)/ Undifferentiated pleomorphic sarcoma (UPS)
   - Leiomyosarcoma
   - Undifferentiated sarcoma
2. 2–5% of primary bone malignancies
3. Similar age group as chondrosarcoma
4. Similar skeletal distribution as osteosarcoma
5. Typically present with pain and have a high incidence of fracture at presentation

Staging and risk assessment:
1. Typically present in an older patient with a lytic lesion in bone
2. Differential diagnosis includes a metastasis
3. Pathologic fractures are common

Treatment:
1. Treatment strategies are similar to those used for osteosarcoma, with chemotherapy and complete en-bloc resection including any soft-tissue component

OSTEOSARCOMA • FIRST-LINE

OSTEOSARCOMA REGIMEN: HIGH-DOSE METHOTREXATE + DOXORUBICIN + CISPLATIN (MAP, EURAMOS-1)

Bielack SS et al. J Clin Oncol 2015;33:2279–2287
Marina NM et al. Lancet Oncol 2016;17:1396–1408
Meyers PA et al. J Clin Oncol 2005;23:2004–2011
Smeland S et al. Eur J Cancer 2019;109:36–50
Whelan JS et al. Ann Oncol 2015;26:407–414

Treatment Schedule for Methotrexate + Doxorubicin + Cisplatin (MAP) According to EURAMOS-1

Drugs	Week														
	1	2	3	4	5	6	7	8	9	10	11	12	13	14	15
Doxorubicin (A)	A					A					Surgery	A			
Cisplatin (P)	P					P						P			
Methotrexate (M)				M	M				M	M					M

Drugs	Week													
	16	17	18	19	20	21	22	23	24	25	26	27	28	29
Doxorubicin (A)		A					A				A			
Cisplatin (P)		P												
Methotrexate (M)	M				M	M			M	M			M	M

Hydration before and after each dose of cisplatin: ≥1000 mL 0.45% sodium chloride injection (0.45% NS); administer intravenously over a minimum of 2–4 hours

Cisplatin 60 mg/m^2/dose; administer intravenously in 150–1000 mL 0.9% sodium chloride injection (0.9% NS) over 4 hours on days 1 and 2 of each week in which cisplatin is administered (total dosage/cycle = 120 mg/m^2)

Note: Encourage patients to increase oral intake of nonalcoholic fluids, and monitor serum electrolytes and replace as needed (potassium, magnesium, sodium). Other hydration regimens may be employed as clinically appropriate (e.g., for pediatric patients)

Doxorubicin 37.5 mg/m^2 per day; administer intravenously in 50–1000 mL 0.9% NS or 5% dextrose injection (D5W) over 24 hours for 2 consecutive days, on days 1 and 2 of each week in which doxorubicin is administered (total dosage/cycle = 75 mg/m^2)

Hydration for methotrexate: 1500–3000 mL/m^2 per day; administer intravenously. Use a solution containing a total amount of sodium not >0.9% NS (ie, ≤154 mEq sodium/1000 mL) by intravenous infusion during methotrexate administration and for at least 24 hours afterward
• Fluid administration may commence 2–12 hours before starting methotrexate, depending on a patient's fluid status
• Urine output should be at least 100 mL/hour before starting methotrexate infusion
• Maintain hydration at a rate that maintains urine output ≥100 mL/hour until the serum methotrexate concentration is <0.1 μmol/L
• Urine pH should be increased within the range ≥7.0 to ≤8.0 to enhance methotrexate solubility and ensure elimination
  ▪ Adverse effects attributable to methotrexate are related to systemic methotrexate concentrations *and* the duration for which concentrations are maintained

Sodium bicarbonate 50–150 mEq/1000 mL is added to the parenteral solution to maintain urine pH ≥7.0 to ≤8.0

Base Solution Sodium Content	Sodium Bicarbonate Additive	Total Sodium Content
0.45% Sodium Chloride Injection (0.45% NS)		
77 mEq/L	50–75 mEq	127–152 mEq/L
0.2% Sodium Chloride Injection (0.2% NS)		
34 mEq/L	100–125 mEq	134–159 mEq/L
5% Dextrose Injection (D5W)		
0 mEq/L	125–150 mEq	125–150 mEq/L

(continued)

(*continued*)

D5W/0.45% NS		
77 mEq/L	50–75 mEq	127–152 mEq/L

D5W/0.2% NS		
34 mEq/L	100–125 mEq	134–159 mEq/L

Methotrexate 12,000 mg/m^2 (maximum dose = 20,000 mg); administer intravenously in 500–2000 mL 0.9% NS or D5W (or saline and dextrose combinations) over 4 hours on day 1 of each week in which methotrexate is administered (total dosage/cycle = 12,000 mg/m^2; maximum dose/cycle = 20,000 mg)

Note: For logistical practicality and efficiency, parenteral admixtures containing methotrexate may include a portion, or all of the fluid and sodium bicarbonate needed to meet hydration and urinary alkalinization requirements during methotrexate administration

Leucovorin 15 mg (fixed dose); administer intravenously in 25–250 mL 0.9% NS or D5W over 15 minutes every 6 hours, starting 24 hours after methotrexate administration *began* and continuing until the serum methotrexate concentration is <0.1 μmol/L (ie, <1 × 10^{-7} mol/L, or <100 nmol/L)

Note: Leucovorin may be administered orally after completing 1 day of parenteral administration if patients are compliant, are not vomiting, and have no other potentially mitigating complications

Leucovorin 10 mg (fixed dose); administer orally every 6 hours until the serum methotrexate concentration is <0.1 μmol/L (ie, <1 × 10^{-7} mol/L, or <100 nmol/L)

Leucovorin rescue for delayed methotrexate excretion:
- Hydration, urinary alkalinization, and a more intensive leucovorin regimen are required if methotrexate excretion is delayed (eg, worsening renal function, effusions present)
- If 24 hours after the completion of methotrexate administration a patient's serum creatinine is increased by ≥50% above the baseline value, or if serum methotrexate concentration is ≥5 μmol/L (≥5 × 10^{-6} mol/L), increase the leucovorin dosage and schedule to 100 mg/m^2 per dose intravenously (*not* orally) every 3 hours until serum methotrexate level is <0.1 μmol/L (<1 × 10^{-7} mol/L, <100 nmol/L); then resume leucovorin 10 mg/dose orally or intravenously every 6 hours until serum methotrexate concentration is <0.05μmol/L (<5 × 10^{-8} mol/L, or <50 nmol/L), or until undetectable (if the lower limit of assay sensitivity is ≥0.05 μmol/L [≥5 × 10^{-8} mol/L, or ≥50 nmol/L])

Supportive Care
Antiemetic prophylaxis
Emetogenic potential during cycles with cisplatin + doxorubicin is **HIGH**. *Potential for delayed symptoms*
Emetogenic potential with doxorubicin alone is **MODERATE**
Emetogenic potential with methotrexate is **MODERATE**
See Chapter 42 for antiemetic recommendations

Hematopoietic growth factor (CSF) prophylaxis
Primary prophylaxis is indicated with 1 of the following:
    Filgrastim (G-CSF) 5 mcg/kg per day by subcutaneous injection, *or*
    Pegfilgrastim (pegylated filgrastim) 6 mg/0.6 mL by subcutaneous injection for 1 dose
- Begin use at least 24 hours after doxorubicin is completed
- Continue daily filgrastim use after the neutrophil nadir until ANC ≥5000/mm^3
- Discontinue daily filgrastim use at least 24 hours before administering myelosuppressive treatment. Do not administer pegfilgrastim within 14 days before administering myelosuppressive treatment
See Chapter 43 for more information

Antimicrobial prophylaxis
Risk of fever and neutropenia is HIGH
Antimicrobial primary prophylaxis is recommended:
- Antibacterial—consider fluoroquinolone prophylaxis; *Pneumocystis jirovecii* prophylaxis is recommended (eg, cotrimoxazole; do not administer with or close to the administration of high dose methotrexate)
- Antifungal—recommended
- Antiviral—antiherpes antivirals (eg, acyclovir, famciclovir, valacyclovir)

Oral care
Standard prophylaxis and treatment for mucositis/stomatitis

Treatment Modifications

Dose Modifications for Doxorubicin/Cisplatin

Adverse Event	Dose Modification
On Day 1 of cycle ANC <0.75 x 10^9/L; Platelets < 75 x 10^9/L	Delay and repeat within 3-4 days until criteria are met. Retreat at full dose unless previous dose reduction. For a delay >7 days use filgrastim starting at least 24 hours after chemotherapy and continuing until WBC after nadir is >5,000/uL If delayed >7 days despite filgrastim then reduce cisplatin by 25%.
Febrile neutropenia accompanied by either sepsis or a microbiologically documented infection	Administer filgrastim starting at least 24 hours after chemotherapy and continuing until WBC after nadir is >5,000/μL Consider reducing cisplatin dosage by 25% if there are persistent delays >7 days in therapy administration despite filgrastim
Recurrence of febrile neutropenia accompanied by either sepsis or a microbiologically documented infection requiring prolonged hospitalization	Reduce cisplatin dosage by 25%.
G4 mucositis or typhlitis or repeated G3 mucositis	Delay until resolved & decrease subsequent doxorubicin to 60 mg/m²/cycle
Audiology: >30 dB at ≤2kHz	Discontinue cisplatin
LVEF <50% or SF <28%	Repeat echo or MUGA in one week. If echo or MUGA within normal range proceed with chemotherapy. If LVEF does not normalize, discontinue doxorubicin
Serum creatinine >2 x baseline or GFR <70 mL/min/1.73 m²	Delay one week. If renal function does not improve, omit cisplatin and give doxorubicin alone. Resume cisplatin if GFR ≥70 mL/min/1.73 m²
Elevated total bilirubin	<table><tr><td>**Bilirubin level**</td><td>**% of doxorubicin dose**</td></tr><tr><td>0–21 μmol/L (0 -1.24 mg/dL)</td><td>100%</td></tr><tr><td>22–35 μmol/L (1.25-2.09 mg/dL)</td><td>75%</td></tr><tr><td>36–52 μmol/L (2.1-3.05 mg/dL)</td><td>50%</td></tr><tr><td>53–86 μmol/L (3.06-5.0 mg/dL)</td><td>25%</td></tr><tr><td>>87 μmol/L (>5.0 mg/dL)</td><td>0%</td></tr></table>
G2 peripheral neurotoxicity	Reduce cisplatin by 25% in all future cycles
≥G3 peripheral neurotoxicity	Omit cisplatin in all future cycles

Dose Modifications for Methotrexate

Febrile neutropenia accompanied by sepsis or microbiologically documented infection	Delay until recovery according to standard practice
G3-4 mucositis or diarrhea after methotrexate	Consider leucovorin rescue adjustment. Reminder: exclude drugs interfering with excretion
G3-4 mucositis or diarrhea after methotrexate persisting for >1 week and present in week 4 of cycle	Omit Day 29 methotrexate (of this cycle only) and proceed to next cycle (or surgery)
GFR <70 mL/min/1.73m²	Delay until recovery. If renal function does not improve within 1 week, omit methotrexate and proceed to next possible cycle. If renal function subsequently improves, methotrexate can be resumed (Patients receiving doxorubicin alone may continue to receive the drug)
Elevated LFTs not induced by MTX	Delay one week. Give if ALT < 10X ULN
Elevated LFTs probably induced by MTX –i.e. up to 3 weeks after MTX	It is expected that patients receiving high dose methotrexate will develop hypertransaminasemia and occasionally hyperbilirubinemia. These elevations can last up to two weeks following the methotrexate infusion and will not be considered toxicity requiring discontinuation of methotrexate
Bilirubin >1.5 x ULN persisting > 3 weeks	Discontinue MTX

Patient Population Studied

EURAMOS-1 was an open-label, international, randomized, phase 3, controlled trial which aimed to optimize treatment based on histological response to neoadjuvant chemotherapy. The main eligibility criteria were: (1) high-grade localized or metastatic extremity or axial osteosarcoma deemed resectable; (2) age ≤40 years at diagnostic biopsy; (3) Karnofsky or Lansky status ≥60; (4) normal cardiac function (shortening fraction >28%); (5) normal hearing; (6) normal bone marrow with ANC ≥1.5 ×109/L (or WBC ≥3×109/L), and platelet count ≥100 000/μL; (7) serum bilirubin <1.5 × ULN; (8) normal serum creatinine; (9) no previous treatment for osteosarcoma, and if the osteosarcoma was a second malignancy, no previous chemotherapy; (10) life expectancy ≥3 months.

Baseline Characteristics of Registered Patients (n=2260)	
Male sex	1330 (59%)
Median age (quartiles)	14 years (11, 17)
Age 0-4 years	11 (0%)
Age 5-9 years	310 (14%)
Age 10-14 years	878 (39%)
Age 15-19 years	809 (36%)
Age 20-24 years	153 (7%)
Age 25-29 years	46 (2%)
Age 30-34 years	19 (1%)
Age 35-39 years	30 (1%)
Age 40 years	4 (0%)
Site and location of disease	
Proximal femur or humerus	293 (13%)
Other limb site	1837 (82%)
Axial or skeletal	108 (5%)
Missing primary site	22 (1%)
Pathological fracture at diagnosis	
No	1964 (88%)
Yes	273 (12%)
Unknown	23 (1%)
Localized disease	
Yes (no metastases)	1722 (77%)
No (yes metastases)	355 (16%)
Possible metastases	161 (7%)
Missing	23 (1%)
Lung metastases	
No	1782 (80%)
Possibly	156 (7%)
Yes	301 (13%)
Missing	21 (1%)
Other metastases	
No	2140 (96%)
Possibly	22 (1%)
Yes	76 (3%)
Missing	22 (1%)

Efficacy

Response to neoadjuvant MAP (n=2248)	
Patients with surgical resection specimen	2012/2248 (91%)
Good response to neoadjuvant MAP (≥90% necrosis)	979/2012 (49%)
Poor response to neoadjuvant MAP (<90% necrosis)	996/2012 (50%)
Unknown response to neoadjuvant MAP	37/2012 (2%)

Reference: Annals Oncol. 2015;26:407-414

Efficacy among good responders to neoadjuvant MAP randomized to receive standard adjuvant MAP/MA (n=359)	
EFS at 3 years	74% (95% CI, 69%-79%)
OS at 5 years	81% (95% CI, 74%-86%)

Median follow-up: 44 months
Reference: J Clin Oncol 2015;33:2279–2287

Efficacy in poor responders to neoadjuvant MAP randomized to receive standard adjuvant MAP/MA (n=308)	
EFS at 3 years	55% (95% CI, 49%-60%)
OS at 5 years	72% (95% CI, 67%-77%)

Median follow-up: 62.3 months
Reference: Lancet Oncol 2016;17:1396–1408

Efficacy in all patients registered to the EURAMOS-1 study who were without baseline metastases (M0) and who achieved complete surgical remission (CSR), regardless of randomization (n=1549)	
EFS at 3 years from surgery	70% (95% CI, 67%-72%)
EFS at 5 years from surgery	64% (95% CI, 61%-66%)
OS at 3 years from surgery	88% (95% CI, 86%-89%)
OS at 5 years from surgery	79% (95% CI, 77%-81%)

Median (IQR) follow-up: 57 months (39-74 months) from biopsy
Reference: Smeland S et al. Eur J Cancer 2019;109:36–50

Multivariable analysis for EFS among registered patients with M0-CSR status (n=1395)					
Characteristic	N	EFS events	Adjusted HR (95% CI)	p-value	Overall p-value
Site of tumor					0.039
Other limb site	1175	382	1.00	n/a	
Proximal femur/humerus	166	72	1.38 (1.06-1.80)	0.018	
Axial skeleton	54	27	1.29 (0.86-1.95)	0.214	
Age					0.003
Child	409	110	1.00	n/a	
Adolescent	689	250	1.43 (1.14-1.79)	0.002	
Adult	297	121	1.53 (1.17-1.99)	0.002	
Relative tumor volume					0.046
Small (<1/3 of uninvolved bone)	679	214	1.00	n/a	
Large (≥1/3 of uninvolved bone)	476	197	1.24 (1.00-1.52)	0.046	
Histological response					<0.001
Good (<10% viable tumor)	724	176	1.00	n/a	
Poor (≥10% viable tumor)	671	305	2.13 (1.76-2.58)	<0.001	

Reference: Smeland S et al. Eur J Cancer 2019;109:36–50
Note: table includes variables with overall p-value <0.05 only

(continued)

(*continued*)

Postoperative MAP [methotrexate, doxorubicin and cisplatin]

	Target cumulative standardized dose	Median cumulative standardized dose (IQR)	Target number of doses	Patients (%) who received target number of doses (n=302)	Received at least 80% of planned doseA (n=302)
Methotrexate (g/m²)	96	93·9 (80·0–97·1)	8–10	226 (75%)	235 (78%)
Doxorubicin (mg/m²)	300	296 (284–303)	4	250 (83%)	245 (81%)
Cisplatin (mg/m²)	240	239 (235–241)	2	277 (92%)	267 (88%)

APercentages calculated by dividing by number of patients who received at least one dose of study drug
Reference: Lancet Oncol 2016;17:1396–1408

Adverse Events

Postoperative Treatment-Related Adverse Events in Patients Assigned to MAP (Methotrexate, Doxorubicin, and Cisplatin), n=301

	Grade 1-2	Grade 3	Grade 4	Grade 5
Any toxicity	11 (4%)	26 (9%)	260 (86%)	1 (<1%)
Nonhematologic event	57 (19%)	197 (65%)	35 (12%)	1 (<1%)
Infection in patients with ANC ≥1 × 10⁹/mL	35/209 (17%)	48/209 (23%)	1/209 (<1%)	1/209 (<1%)
Left ventricular systolic dysfunction	42/290 (14%)	2/290 (1%)	0	
Neutropenia	16 (5%)	21 (7%)	247 (82%)	0
Thrombocytopenia	44/298 (15%)	50/298 (17%)	181/298 (61%)	0
Febrile neutropenia without documented infection	0/299	138/299 (46%)	11/299 (4%)	0
Anemia	*	19 (5%)	11 (4%)	0
Documented infection with ANC <1 x 10⁹/mL	19/300 (6%)	104/300 (35%)	4/300 (1%)	0
Leucopenia	*	2 (1%)	9 (3%)	0
Hypophosphatemia	70/286 (24%)	39/286 (14%)	4/286 (1%)	0
Mucositis or stomatitis	118/267 (44%)	84/267 (31%)	6/267 (2%)	0
Hypokalemia	*	1 (<1%)	0	0
Mood alteration	70/297 (24%)	2/297 (1%)	3/297 (1%)	0
Hypomagnesemia	*	1 (<1%)	3 (1%)	0
Abnormal creatinine concentration	41/300 (14%)	2/300 (1%)	1/300 (<1%)	0
Thrombosis, thrombus, or embolism	*	2 (1%)	1 (<1%)	0
Pain	*	10 (3%)	1 (<1%)	0
Abnormal bilirubin concentration	53/147 (36%)	7/147 (5%)	0	0
Encephalopathy	*	3 (1%)	0	0
Seizure	4/300 (1%)	0	1/300 (<1%)	0

(*continued*)

(*continued*)

Motor neuropathy	4/298 (1%)	12/298 (4%)	0	0
Hearing	60/270 (22%)	8/270 (3%)	0	0
Sensory neuropathy	39/299 (13%)	5/299 (2%)	0	0
Somnolence	2/300 (1%)	1/300 (<1%)	0	0
Confusion	5/298 (2%)	0	0	0
Typhlitis	6/298 (2%)	2/298 (1%)	0	0
Allergic reaction	*	2 (1%)	0	0
Urinary electrolyte wasting	20/275 (7%)	0	0	0
Glomerular filtration rate	22/255 (9%)	0	0	0
Hemorrhage, genitourinary bladder	13/297 (4%)	0	0	0

*Toxicities not routinely solicited; sites could report these only under "other" toxicities
Grade 1-2 adverse events are included if reported for at least 10% of patients
Reference: Lancet Oncol 2016;17:1396–1408

Worst grade toxicity during postoperative chemotherapy

	MAP (n=301)			
	Grade 3	Grade 4	Grade 5	Total Grade ≥3
Any Toxicity	26 (9%)	260 (86%)	1 (<1%)	287 (95%)
Nonhematologic events*	197 (65%)	35 (12%)	1 (<1%)	233 (77%)

*Any toxicity, excluding neutropenia, thrombocytopenia, anemia, and leucopenia
Reference: Lancet Oncol 2016;17:1396–1408

Therapy Monitoring

1. *Pretreatment evaluation:* Determination of LVEF by echocardiogram. Repeat LVEF determination prior to the fourth cycle of doxorubicin and at any time if clinical signs or symptoms of heart failure are present
2. *Before each cycle:* CBC with differential, serum electrolytes, BUN, and creatinine
3. *Prior to each dose of methotrexate:* CBC with differential, BUN, serum creatinine, estimated creatinine clearance (Cockroft-Gault method), AST, ALT, total bilirubin, electrolytes, serum bicarbonate, urine output, urine pH, review medication list for potential drug-drug interactions
4. *Following each dose of methotrexate, until methotrexate concentration is <0.1 μmol/L:*
   a. *Daily:* methotrexate concentration (draw first sample 24 hours after start of methotrexate infusion and repeat every 24 hours), CBC with differential, BUN, serum creatinine, AST, ALT, total bilirubin, weight, fluid balance
   b. *At least every 8 hours:* urine pH

FIRST-LINE

OSTEOSARCOMA REGIMEN: DOXORUBICIN + CISPLATIN + IFOSFAMIDE (API)

Piperno-Neumann S et al. Int J Cancer 2020;146:413-423
Supporting information for: Piperno-Neumann S et al. Int J Cancer 2020;146:413-423
Sarcome-09 Protocol available at: http://www.unicancer.fr/sites/default/files/S09-Protocole-version-amendee-6.1-VERSION-FINALE-11-avril-2013.pdf (accessed May 20, 2021)

Regimen overview: Neoadjuvant chemotherapy consisted of 3 cycles of doxorubicin + cisplatin + ifosfamide (API) alternating with 2 cycles of doxorubicin + ifosfamide (AI). Postoperative chemotherapy was determined based on risk group; localized patients with a good histological response (≥90% tumor necrosis at surgery) received 2 course of AI alternating with 2 courses of cisplatin + ifosfamide (PI). Patients with synchronous metastases, poor histological response (<90% necrosis), or unresectable primary site of disease received 5 cycles of etoposide + ifosfamide (EI).

Pre-Operative Chemotherapy Schedule According to the Sarcome-09 Study

	Week													
	1	2	3	4	5	6	7	8	9	10	11	12	13	14
Regimen	API			AI			API			AI			API	

API = doxorubicin + cisplatin + ifosfamide
AI = doxorubicin + ifosfamide

Post-Operative Chemotherapy Schedule for Patients with Localized Disease and Good Histological Response (≥90% Tumor Necrosis) According to the Sarcome-09 Study

	Week										
	1	2	3	4	5	6	7	8	9	10	11
Regimen	AI			PI		AI				PI	

AI = doxorubicin + ifosfamide
PI = cisplatin + ifosfamide

Post-Operative Chemotherapy Schedule for Patients with Synchronous Metastases, Poor Histological Response (<90% Tumor Necrosis), or Unresectable Primary According to the Sarcome-09 Study

	Week													
	1	2	3	4	5	6	7	8	9	10	11	12	13	14
Regimen	EI			EI			EI			EI			EI	

Doxorubicin + Cisplatin + Ifosfamide (API)

Doxorubicin 60 mg/m^2; administer by intravenous injection over 3–5 minutes on day 1, immediately prior to initiation of cisplatin hydration, during each cycle of API (total dosage/cycle = 60 mg/m^2)

Hydration before cisplatin: 3000 mL **5% Dextrose and 0.45% Sodium Chloride injection (D5W/0.45% NaCl)**; administer intravenously over 9 hours prior to starting the cisplatin infusion on day 1 during each cycle of API
   Note: The protocol specified that patients with <1500 mL urine output during the 9-hour pre-hydration period were to receive 250 mL of **10% mannitol** (25 grams) intravenously over 30 minutes

Cisplatin 100 mg/m^2; administer intravenously in 250 mL 0.9% Sodium Chloride injection (0.9% NS) over 3 hours on day 1, after completion of 9 hours of pre-hydration, during each cycle of API (total dosage/cycle = 100 mg/m^2)

Hydration after cisplatin: 2000 mL **D5W/0.45% NaCl**; administer intravenously over 8 hours after completion of the cisplatin infusion on day 1 of each cycle of API
   Note: Encourage patients to increase oral intake of nonalcoholic fluids, and monitor serum electrolytes and replace as needed (potassium, magnesium, sodium). Other hydration regimens may be employed as clinically appropriate (e.g., for pediatric patients)

Hydration prior to each dose of ifosfamide:
500 mL of **5% Dextrose injection (D5W)** containing 100 mEq (8.4 grams) of **Sodium Bicarbonate** additive; administer intravenously over 1 hour prior to the administration of ifosfamide for 2 consecutive days, days 2-3, of each cycle of API

(continued)

(continued)

Mesna 3600 mg/m^2 per dose; administer intravenously in 1000 mL D5W as a continuous infusion over 23 hours, starting at the same time as the ifosfamide infusion, for 2 consecutive days, days 2-3, of each cycle of API (total dosage/cycle = 7200 mg/m^2)

Ifosfamide 3000 mg/m^2 per dose; administer intravenously in 1000 mL 0.9% Sodium Chloride (0.9% NS) over 12 hours for 2 consecutive days, days 2-3, of each cycle of API (total dosage/cycle = 6000 mg/m^2)

Doxorubicin + Ifosfamide (AI)
Doxorubicin 60 mg/m^2; administer by intravenous injection over 3–5 minutes on day 1, immediately prior to initiation of ifosfamide pre-hydration, during each cycle of AI (total dosage/cycle = 60 mg/m^2)

Hydration prior to each dose of ifosfamide:
500 mL of **D5W** containing 100 mEq (8.4 grams) of **Sodium Bicarbonate** additive; administer intravenously over 1 hour prior to the administration of ifosfamide for 2 consecutive days, days 1-2, of each cycle of AI

Mesna 3600 mg/m^2 per dose; administer intravenously in 1000 mL D5W as a continuous infusion over 23 hours, starting at the same time as the ifosfamide infusion, for 2 consecutive days, days 1-2, of each cycle of AI (total dosage/cycle = 7200 mg/m^2)

Ifosfamide 3000 mg/m^2 per dose; administer intravenously in 1000 mL 0.9% NS over 12 hours for 2 consecutive days, days 1-2, of each cycle of AI (total dosage/cycle = 6000 mg/m^2)

Cisplatin + Ifosfamide (PI)
Hydration before cisplatin: 3000 mL **5% Dextrose and 0.45% Sodium Chloride injection (D5W/0.45% NaCl)**; administer intravenously over 9 hours prior to starting the cisplatin infusion on day 1 during each cycle of PI
   Note: The protocol specified that patients with <1500 mL urine output during the 9-hour pre-hydration period were to receive 250 mL of **10% mannitol** (25 grams) intravenously over 30 minutes

Cisplatin 100 mg/m^2; administer intravenously in 250 mL 0.9% NS over 3 hours on day 1, after completion of 9 hours of pre-hydration, during each cycle of PI (total dosage/cycle = 100 mg/m^2)

Hydration after cisplatin: 2000 mL **D5W/0.45% NaCl**; administer intravenously over 8 hours after completion of the cisplatin infusion on day 1 of each cycle of PI
   Note: Encourage patients to increase oral intake of nonalcoholic fluids, and monitor serum electrolytes and replace as needed (potassium, magnesium, sodium). Other hydration regimens may be employed as clinically appropriate (e.g., for pediatric patients)

Hydration prior to each dose of ifosfamide:
500 mL of **5% Dextrose injection (D5W)** containing 100 mEq (8.4 grams) of **Sodium Bicarbonate** additive; administer intravenously over 1 hour prior to the administration of ifosfamide for 2 consecutive days, days 2-3, of each cycle of API

Mesna 3600 mg/m^2 per dose; administer intravenously in 1000 mL D5W as a continuous infusion over 23 hours, starting at the same time as the ifosfamide infusion, for 2 consecutive days, days 2-3, of each cycle of API (total dosage/cycle = 7200 mg/m^2)
Ifosfamide 3000 mg/m^2 per dose; administer intravenously in 1000 mL 0.9% Sodium Chloride (0.9% NS) over 12 hours for 2 consecutive days, days 2-3, of each cycle of PI (total dosage/cycle = 6000 mg/m^2)

Etoposide + Ifosfamide (EI)
Etoposide 75 mg/m^2 per day; administer intravenously diluted with 0.9% NS to a concentration of 0.2–0.4 mg/mL over 60 minutes for 4 consecutive days, on days 1–4, every 21 days during each cycle of EI for 5 cycles (total dosage/cycle = 300 mg/m^2)

Hydration prior to each dose of ifosfamide:
500 mL of **D5W** containing 100 mEq (8.4 grams) of **Sodium Bicarbonate** additive; administer intravenously over 1 hour prior to the administration of ifosfamide for 4 consecutive days, days 1-4, every 21 days during each cycle of EI for 5 cycles

Mesna 3600 mg/m^2 per dose; administer intravenously in 1000 mL D5W as a continuous infusion over 23 hours, starting at the same time as the ifosfamide infusion, for 4 consecutive days, days 1-4, every 21 days during each cycle of EI for 5 cycles (total dosage/cycle = 14,400 mg/m^2)

Ifosfamide 3000 mg/m^2 per dose; administer intravenously in 1000 mL 0.9% NS over 12 hours for 4 consecutive days, days 1-4, every 21 days during each cycle of EI for 5 cycles (total dosage/cycle = 12,000 mg/m^2)

Supportive Care
Antiemetic prophylaxis
Emetogenic potential of API on days 1, 2, and 3 is **HIGH**. *Potential for delayed symptoms*
Emetogenic potential of AI on days 1 and 2 is **HIGH**. *Potential for delayed symptoms*
Emetogenic potential of PI on days 1 and 2 is **HIGH**. *Potential for delayed symptoms*
Emetogenic potential of EI on days 1, 2, 3, and 4 is **HIGH**. *Potential for delayed symptoms*
See Chapter 42 for antiemetic recommendations

(*continued*)

Hematopoietic growth factor (CSF) prophylaxis
Primary prophylaxis following each cycle of API, AI, PI, and EI is indicated with 1 of the following:
Filgrastim (G-CSF) 5 mcg/kg per day by subcutaneous injection, *or*
Pegfilgrastim (pegylated filgrastim) 6 mg/0.6 mL by subcutaneous injection for 1 dose
• Begin use at least 24 hours after completion of myelosuppressive chemotherapy
• Continue daily filgrastim use after the neutrophil nadir until ANC ≥5000/mm^3
• Discontinue daily filgrastim use at least 24 hours before administering myelosuppressive treatment. Do not administer pegfilgrastim within 14 days before administering myelosuppressive treatment
See Chapter 43 for more information

Antimicrobial prophylaxis
Risk of fever and neutropenia is HIGH
Antimicrobial primary prophylaxis is recommended:
• Antibacterial—consider administration of fluoroquinolone during periods of neutropenia, or no prophylaxis; *Pneumocystis jirovecii* prophylaxis is recommended (eg, cotrimoxazole)
• Antifungal—consider administration of fluconazole during periods of neutropenia, or no prophylaxis
• Antiviral—antiherpes antivirals (eg, acyclovir, famciclovir, valacyclovir)

Oral care
Standard prophylaxis and treatment for mucositis/stomatitis

Treatment Modifications

Adverse Event	Dose Modification		
On Day 1 of cycle ANC <0.75 x 10^9/L; Platelets < 75 x 10^9/L	Delay and repeat within 3-4 days until criteria are met. Retreat at full dose unless previous dose reduction. If delayed >7 days despite filgrastim then reduce cisplatin and/or doxorubicin and/or ifosfamide and/or etoposide doses by 25%.		
Febrile neutropenia accompanied by either sepsis or a microbiologically documented infection	Consider reducing cisplatin and/or doxorubicin and/or ifosfamide and/or etoposide doses by 25% in subsequent cycles		
G4 mucositis or typhlitis or repeated G3 mucositis	Delay until resolved & decrease subsequent cisplatin and/or doxorubicin and/or ifosfamide and/or etoposide doses by 25%		
Audiology: >30 dB at ≤2kHz	Consider discontinuation of cisplatin		
LVEF <50% or SF <28%	Repeat echo or MUGA in one week. If echo or MUGA within normal range proceed with chemotherapy. If LVEF does not normalize, discontinue doxorubicin		
Serum creatinine >2 x baseline or GFR <70 mL/min/1.73 m²	Delay one week. If renal function does not improve, omit cisplatin. Resume cisplatin if GFR ≥70 mL/min/1.73 m²		
Elevated total bilirubin		Bilirubin level	% of doxorubicin dose
		0–21 μmol/L (0 -1.24 mg/dL)	100%
		22–35 μmol/L (1.25-2.09 mg/dL)	75%
		36–52 μmol/L (2.1-3.05 mg/dL)	50%
		53–86 μmol/L (3.06-5.0 mg/dL)	25%
		>87 μmol/L (>5.0 mg/dL)	0%
G2 peripheral neurotoxicity	Reduce cisplatin by 25% in all future cycles		
≥G3 peripheral neurotoxicity	Omit cisplatin in all future cycles		
G2 renal toxicity- tubular (based on creatinine clearance, serum bicarbonate, need for electrolyte replacement, or TmP/GFR)	Reduce the ifosfamide and mesna doses by 25% in subsequent cycles		

(*continued*)

(*continued*)

≥G3 renal toxicity- tubular (based on creatinine clearance, serum bicarbonate, need for electrolyte replacement, or TmP/GFR)	Discontinue ifosfamide
Microscopic hematuria during ifosfamide therapy (>50 RBC/HPF) on >1 occasion	Discontinue ifosfamide for that cycle. If hematuria completely resolves, consider increasing the rate of intravenous fluids and/or the increasing the mesna dose in subsequent cycles
≥G2 non-infective hemorrhagic cystitis (related to ifosfamide)	Discontinue ifosfamide and provide appropriate supportive care
G2 encephalopathy during ifosfamide treatment	If persistent or distressing, then consider decreasing the ifosfamide and mesna dosages by 20%. If not contraindicated, treat with methylene blue 2 mg/kg (maximum dose of 50 mg) intravenously every 4-8 hours until resolution of symptoms, then consider prophylactic use at the same dose given every 6-8 hours in subsequent cycles.
≥G3 encephalopathy during ifosfamide treatment	Stop ifosfamide for this cycle. If not contraindicated, treat with methylene blue 2 mg/kg (maximum dose of 50 mg) intravenously every 4-8 hours until resolution of symptoms, then consider prophylactic use at the same dose given every 6-8 hours in subsequent cycles. Consider decreasing the ifosfamide and mesna dosages by 20% in subsequent cycles

Efficacy

Efficacy Variable	Result
Good histologic response at surgery	36/95 (38%; 95% CI, 28-48%)
3-year EFS	52% (95% CI, 42-61%)
5-year EFS	46% (95% CI, 36-56%)
3-year OS	66% (95% CI, 56-75%)
5-year OS	57% (95% CI, 47-67%)
5-year EFS among patients with metastatic disease (n=28)	21.4% (95% CI, 10.2-39.5%)
5-year OS among patients with metastatic disease (n=28)	14.5% (95% CI, 4.6-37.7%)

Abbreviations: CI, confidence interval; EFS, event-free survival; OS, overall survival

Adverse Events (n = 38)

Type of toxicity by Grade (%)	Patients Age > 25 years (N = 38)				
	None	G1	G2	G3	G4
AST/ALT elevation	47	34	13	5	0
Anemia	0	8	5	50	37
Auditory/ear toxicity	82	5	8	5	0
Bilirubin elevation	92	5	3	0	0
Cardiac toxicity	68	26	3	3	0
Central neurological toxicity	92	3	5	0	0
Constitutional symptoms	29	21	39	11	0
Dermatology/skin toxicity	76	18	5	0	0

Patient Population Studied

The French OS2006/Sarcome-09 study included patients ≤50 years of age with localized or metastatic high-grade osteosarcoma (n=106 total). Patients >25 years of age (n=66) received doxorubicin + cisplatin + ifosfamide (API-AI) and patients aged 18-25 years (n=40) could have received either API-AI or high-dose methotrexate-based treatment according to the center's preference. All patients were required to have normal baseline hematologic, renal, cardiac, and liver function. Among all enrolled patients, 74% had a primary tumor located in a limb whereas 26% had an axial primary tumor; 43% of patients had a primary tumor ≥10 cm; 92% had conventional histological subtype, 1% had telangiectasic subtye, 1% had surface high-grade subtypte, and 6% had "other" subtype; initial staging was localized in 74% and metastatic in 26% (metastatic sites included lung (19%), distant bone (2%), skip metastases (6%), and "other" (8%)].

(*continued*)

(continued)

Febrile neutropenia	32	0	0	61	8
Fever	63	24	13	0	0
Gastrointestinal toxicity	0	11	68	21	0
Headache	84	11	5	0	0
Hypocalcemia	24	41	30	3	3
Hypophosphatemia	62	0	27	5	5
Infection without neutropenia	68	11	18	3	0
Metabolic/laboratory toxicity	50	11	13	18	8
Miscellaneous	42	34	18	5	0
Mood alteration	82	3	16	0	0
Mucositis	55	24	16	5	0
Neutropenia	5	3	3	8	82
Peripheral neuropathy	79	11	8	3	0
Renal toxicity	68	26	3	0	3
Thrombocytopenia	3	5	11	13	68
Weight loss	24	32	34	11	0
Wound complication	100	0	0	0	0

Therapy Monitoring

1. *Pretreatment evaluation:* Determination of LVEF by echocardiogram. Repeat LVEF determination prior to the fourth cycle of doxorubicin and at any time if clinical signs or symptoms of heart failure are present
2. *Prior to each cycle:* Physical examination, ECOG PS, CBC with differential and platelet count, total bilirubin, ALT, AST, albumin, alkaline phosphatase, serum creatinine, BUN, calcium, carbon dioxide, chloride, glucose, potassium, sodium, and phosphate
3. *During cycles containing ifosfamide:*
    a. *Daily laboratory investigations:* serum creatinine, BUN, calcium, carbon dioxide, chloride, glucose, potassium, sodium, and phosphate
    b. *Every 8 hours (or with each void):* urine dipstick for blood (check microscopic urinalysis if >trace)
    c. *Other:* monitor fluid status (i.e., weight and intake/output) and for signs and symptoms of neurological toxicity
4. *At least twice per week between cycles:* CBC with differential and platelet count, serum creatinine, BUN, calcium, carbon dioxide, chloride, glucose, potassium, sodium, and phosphate

OSTEOSARCOMA • RECURRENT OR PROGRESSIVE

OSTEOSARCOMA REGIMEN: ETOPOSIDE + HIGH-DOSE IFOSFAMIDE + MESNA

Goorin AM et al. J Clin Oncol 2002;20:426–433

This regimen was initially developed for newly diagnosed osteosarcoma and included high-dose methotrexate, cisplatin, and doxorubicin as part of the continuation therapy. The protocol summarized here assumes that patients previously received high-dose methotrexate, cisplatin, and doxorubicin as part of their upfront therapy

Induction Chemotherapy

Start: Hour 0 End: Hour 1	**Etoposide** 100 mg/m^2 per day; administer intravenously in 250 mL/m^2 5% dextrose and 0.2% sodium chloride injection (D5W/0.2% NS) over 1 hour for 5 consecutive days, on days 1–5, every 21 days (total dosage/cycle = 500 mg/m^2)
Start: Hour 1 End: Hour 5	An admixture containing **ifosfamide** 3500 mg/m^2 + **mesna** 700 mg/m^2 per day; administer intravenously in 800 mL/m^2 D5W/0.2% NS over 4 hours, starting immediately after etoposide administration is completed, for 5 consecutive days, on days 1–5, every 21 days (total ifosfamide dosage/cycle = 17,500 mg/m^2)
Start: Hour 5 End: Hour 8	**Mesna** 700 mg/m^2 per day; administer by continuous intravenous infusion in 600 mL/m^2 D5W/0.2% NS over 3 hours, starting after ifosfamide administration is completed, for 5 consecutive days, on days 1–5, every 21 days
Start: Hour 8 End: Hour 14	**Hydration** with D5W/0.2% NS; administer intravenously at 150 mL/m^2 per hour for 6 hours for 5 consecutive days on days 1–5, every 21 days
Start: Hours 8, 11, and 14 End: 8:15, 11:15, and 14:15	**Mesna** 700 mg/m^2 per dose; administer intravenously diluted with 0.9% sodium chloride injection (0.9% NS) or 5% dextrose injection (D5W) to a concentration of 1–20 mg/mL, over 15 minutes, every 3 hours for 3 doses/day, starting 3 hours after ifosfamide administration is completed, for 5 consecutive days, on days 1–5, every 21 days (total mesna dosage/cycle = 17,500 mg/m^2; this total also includes hour 1 and hour 5 doses)
Start: Hour 14 End: Hour 24	**Hydration** with D5W/0.2% NS; administer intravenously at 100 mL/m^2 per hour for 10 hours for 5 consecutive days on days 1–5, every 21 days

Note: after 2 cycles of treatment, radiologic evaluation is completed and patients should have surgery for any metastatic sites of disease. Surgical removal of all metastatic sites is recommended when feasible

Continuation Chemotherapy

Start: Hour 0 End: Hour 1	**Etoposide** 100 mg/m^2 per day; administer intravenously in 250 mL/m^2 D5W/0.2% NS over 1 hour for 5 consecutive days, on days 1–5, every 21 days (total dosage/cycle = 500 mg/m^2)
Start: Hour 1 End: Hour 5	An admixture containing **ifosfamide** 2400 mg/m^2 + **mesna** 480 mg/m^2 per day; administer intravenously in 800 mL/m^2 D5W/0.2% NS over 4 hours, starting immediately after etoposide administration is completed, for 5 consecutive days, on days 1–5, every 21 days (total ifosfamide dosage/cycle = 12,000 mg/m^2)
Start: Hour 5 End: Hour 8	**Mesna** 480 mg/m^2 per day; administer intravenously in 600 mL/m^2 D5W/0.2% NS over 3 hours, starting after ifosfamide administration is completed, for 5 consecutive days, on days 1–5, every 21 days
Start: Hour 8 End: Hour 14	**Hydration** with D5W/0.2% NS; administer intravenously at 150 mL/m^2 per hour for 6 hours, for 5 consecutive days, on days 1–5, every 21 days
Start: Hours 8, 11, and 14 End: 8:15, 11:15, and 14:15	**Mesna** 480 mg/m^2 per dose; administer intravenously diluted with 0.9% NS or D5W to a concentration of 1–20 mg/mL, over 15 minutes, every 3 hours for 3 doses/day, starting 3 hours after ifosfamide administration is completed, for 5 consecutive days, on days 1–5, every 21 days (total mesna dosage/cycle = 12,000 mg/m^2; this total also includes hour 1 and hour 5 doses)
Start: Hour 14 End: Hour 24	**Hydration** with D5W/0.2% NS; administer intravenously at 100 mL/m^2 per hour for 10 hours for 5 consecutive days, on days 1–5, every 21 days

Supportive Care

Antiemetic prophylaxis

*Emetogenic potential is **MODERATE**. Potential for delayed symptoms*

See Chapter 42 for antiemetic recommendations

Hematopoietic growth factor (CSF) prophylaxis

Primary prophylaxis is indicated with 1 of the following:

Filgrastim (G-CSF) 5 μg/kg per day by subcutaneous injection, *or*

Pegfilgrastim (pegylated filgrastim) 6 mg/0.6 mL by subcutaneous injection for 1 dose

• Begin use on day 6, at least 24 hours after myelosuppressive chemotherapy is completed

(continued)

(continued)

- Continue daily filgrastim use after the neutrophil nadir until ANC ≥5000/mm³ on 2 measurements separated temporally by ≥12 hours
- Discontinue daily filgrastim use at least 24 hours before administering myelosuppressive treatment. Do not administer pegfilgrastim within 14 days before administering myelosuppressive treatment

See Chapter 43 for more information

Antimicrobial prophylaxis
Risk of fever and neutropenia is INTERMEDIATE
Antimicrobial primary prophylaxis to be considered:
- Antibacterial—consider a fluoroquinolone or no prophylaxis
- Antifungal—consider concomitant use of clotrimazole during periods of neutropenia
- Antiviral—antiherpes antivirals (eg, acyclovir, famciclovir, valacyclovir)

Oral care
Standard prophylaxis and treatment for mucositis/stomatitis

Treatment Modifications

Adverse Event	Dose Modification
Day 1 ANC <1000/mm³ or platelet count <120,000/mm³	Delay by 1 week. Re-treat at full dose unless delayed by >1 week despite use of G-CSF, in which case reduce the doses of both agents by 20%
Febrile neutropenia occurring in the prior cycle	Reduce the ifosfamide/mesna and etoposide doses by 20% in subsequent cycles and add G-CSF prophylaxis if not already receiving
SCr 1.5 × baseline	Delay by 1 week. If renal function does not improve, then discontinue ifosfamide
G2 renal toxicity—tubular (based on creatinine clearance, serum bicarbonate, need for electrolyte replacement, or TmP/GFR)	Reduce the ifosfamide and mesna doses by 20% in subsequent cycles
G ≥3 renal toxicity—tubular (based on creatinine clearance, serum bicarbonate, need for electrolyte replacement, or TmP/GFR)	Discontinue ifosfamide
Microscopic hematuria during ifosfamide therapy (>50 RBC/HPF) on >1 occasion	Discontinue ifosfamide for that cycle. If hematuria completely resolves, consider increasing the rate of intravenous fluids and/or the increasing the mesna dose in subsequent cycles
G ≥2 non-infective hemorrhagic cystitis (related to ifosfamide)	Discontinue ifosfamide and provide appropriate supportive care
G2 encephalopathy	If persistent or distressing, then consider decreasing the ifosfamide and mesna dosages by 20%. If not contraindicated, treat with methylene blue 2 mg/kg (maximum dose of 50 mg) intravenously every 4–8 hours until resolution of symptoms, then consider prophylactic use at the same dose given every 6–8 hours in subsequent cycles
G ≥3 encephalopathy	Stop ifosfamide for this cycle. If not contraindicated, treat with methylene blue 2 mg/kg (maximum dose of 50 mg) intravenously every 4–8 hours until resolution of symptoms, then consider prophylactic use at the same dose given every 6–8 hours in subsequent cycles. Consider decreasing the ifosfamide and mesna dosages by 20% in subsequent cycles

Patient Population Studied

A prospective phase 2/3 trial in 41 evaluable patients ≤30 years of age with measurable, newly diagnosed, biopsy-proven, high-grade, metastatic osteosarcoma with normal renal, hepatic, and bone marrow profile and ECOG performance status ≤2

Efficacy

Response Rate* (N = 23–41)

Combined pathologic + radiologic response (n = 39)	59% ± 8%
Pathologic response alone[†] (n = 23)	65% ± 10%
Radiologic response alone (n = 27)	52% ± 9%

*Assessed after 2 cycles of etoposide + ifosfamide with mesna
[†]As measured by necrosis of the primary tumor

Note:
1. Although few patients were treated, the response to ifosfamide and etoposide seemed to be dose dependent
2. This combination may be more active against bony metastases than other regimens

Adverse Events

Toxicities* (N = 41)

	% G3	% G4
Hematopoietic		
WBC count	2	83
ANC	2	29
Platelets	17	27
Hemoglobin	5	5
Nonhematopoietic		
Sepsis	10	—
Bacterial infection	7	—
Viral infection	2	—
Fanconi syndrome	7	—
Stomatitis	7	—
Sodium	2	—
Creatinine	2	—
Hematuria	2	—
Poor Karnofsky score	2	—
Vomiting	2	—
Potassium	2	—

*Toxicities listed are those pertaining only to the 2 cycles of induction chemotherapy using ifosfamide and etoposide

Therapy Monitoring

1. *Prior to each cycle:* Physical examination, ECOG PS, CBC with differential and platelet count, total bilirubin, ALT, AST, albumin, alkaline phosphatase, serum creatinine, BUN, calcium, carbon dioxide, chloride, glucose, potassium, sodium, and phosphate
2. *During chemotherapy administration:*
   a. *Daily laboratory investigations:* serum creatinine, BUN, calcium, carbon dioxide, chloride, glucose, potassium, sodium, and phosphate
   b. *Every 8 hours (or with each void):* urine dipstick for blood (check microscopic urinalysis if >trace)
   c. *Other:* monitor fluid status (ie, weight and intake/output) and for signs and symptoms of neurologic toxicity
3. *At least twice per week between cycles:* CBC with differential and platelet count, serum creatinine, BUN, calcium, carbon dioxide, chloride, glucose, potassium, sodium, and phosphate

OSTEOSARCOMA • RECURRENT OR PROGRESSIVE

OSTEOSARCOMA REGIMEN: GEMCITABINE + DOCETAXEL

Navid F et al. Cancer 2008;113:419–425

Gemcitabine 675 mg/m² per dose; administer intravenously, diluted in 0.9% sodium chloride injection (0.9% NS) to a concentration as low as 0.1 mg/mL, over 90 minutes for 2 doses, on days 1 and 8, every 21 days (total dosage/cycle = 1350 mg/m²)

Premedication for docetaxel:
Dexamethasone 8 mg/dose; administer orally twice daily for 3 days, starting 1 day before docetaxel administration (total dose/cycle = 48 mg)

Optional premedication for docetaxel:
- **Diphenhydramine HCl** 25 mg; administer orally 30–60 minutes *or* intravenously 5–30 minutes prior to docetaxel administration
- **Ranitidine** 150 mg; administer orally 30–60 minutes prior to docetaxel administration, *or*
- **Ranitidine** 50 mg; administer intravenously 5–30 minutes prior to docetaxel administration

Docetaxel 75–100 mg/m²; administer intravenously, in a volume of 0.9% NS or D5W sufficient to produce a docetaxel concentration within the range 0.3–0.74 mg/mL, over 60 minutes, on day 8 after completing gemcitabine administration, every 21 days (total dosage/cycle = 75–100 mg/m²)

Supportive Care
Antiemetic prophylaxis
Emetogenic potential is **LOW**
See Chapter 42 for antiemetic recommendations

Hematopoietic growth factor (CSF) prophylaxis
Primary prophylaxis is indicated with *1* of the following:
Filgrastim (G-CSF) 5 μg/kg per day by subcutaneous injection, *or*
Pegfilgrastim (pegylated filgrastim) 6 mg/0.6 mL by subcutaneous injection for one dose
- Begin use on cycle day 9—that is, 24 hours after myelosuppressive chemotherapy is completed
- Continue daily filgrastim use until ANC ≥10,000/mm³ on 2 measurements separated temporally by ≥12 hours
- Discontinue daily filgrastim use at least 24 hours before administering myelosuppressive treatment. Do not administer pegfilgrastim within 14 days before administering myelosuppressive treatment

See Chapter 43 for more information

Antimicrobial prophylaxis
Risk of fever and neutropenia is *LOW*
Antimicrobial primary prophylaxis to be considered:
- Antibacterial—not indicated
- Antifungal—not indicated
- Antiviral—not indicated unless patient previously had an episode of HSV

Patient Population Studied

A retrospective analysis of 22 patients with recurrent or progressive bone or soft-tissue sarcoma

Treatment Modifications

Adverse Event	Dose Modification
Febrile neutropenia or platelet count of <25,000/mm³ lasting >5 days	Reduce gemcitabine and docetaxel dosages by 25% in all subsequent cycles. Consider adding prophylactic G-CSF if not already using
ANC <1000/mm³ at start of next cycle	Withhold treatment until ANC ≥1000/mm³, then reduce gemcitabine and docetaxel dosages by 25%. Consider adding prophylactic G-CSF if not already using
Platelet count <100,000/mm³ at start of next cycle	Withhold treatment until platelet count ≥100,000/mm³, then reduce gemcitabine and docetaxel dosages by 25%
ANC <1000/mm³ or platelet count <100,000/mm³ despite 2-week delay	Discontinue therapy
Day 8 ANC 500–999/mm³ or day 8 platelet count 50,000–99,000/mm³	Reduce day 8 gemcitabine and docetaxel dosages by 25%
Day 8 ANC <500/mm³ or day 8 platelet count <50,000/mm³	Do not administer day 8 gemcitabine and docetaxel
Significant hypersensitivity reaction to docetaxel (hypotension, dyspnea, and angioedema requiring therapy)	Discontinue docetaxel
Unexplained new or worsening dyspnea or evidence of severe pulmonary toxicity	Withhold gemcitabine and assess for gemcitabine-related pulmonary toxicity. If confirmed, permanently discontinue gemcitabine
Hemolytic-uremic syndrome	Permanently discontinue gemcitabine for hemolytic uremic syndrome or severe renal impairment
Capillary leak syndrome	Permanently discontinue gemcitabine and docetaxel

(continued)

Efficacy

Tumor Response Categorization Using RECIST in 14 Patients by Disease Type*

Disease Type	Number of Patients	RECIST Category			
		CR	PR	SD	PD
Osteosarcoma[†]	10	0	3	1	6
Ewing sarcoma family of tumors[‡]	2	0	0	1	1
Malignant fibrous histiocytoma	1	1	0	0	0
Undifferentiated sarcoma	1	0	0	0	1
Total	14	1	3	2	8

Median number of cycles	4 (range: 1–13)
Median duration of PR/CR	3.8 months (range: 1.6–9.7+ months)
Median time to progressive disease	2.3 months (range: 0.8–14 months)
Number of patients dead and cause of death	19 (18 from PD and 1 from unknown cause)
Patients alive	3 with osteosarcoma (alive with disease at 7, 52, and 69 months after recurrence)

RECIST, Response Evaluation Criteria in Solid Tumors; CR, complete response; PR, partial response; SD, stable disease; PD, progressive disease (Therasse P et al. J Natl Cancer Inst 2000;92:205–216)

*Of the 22 patients, 8 were not evaluable for objective tumor response: 5 patients had tumors that did not qualify as target lesions as defined by RECIST, 3 patients had no evidence of disease by imaging studies at the initiation of gemcitabine and docetaxel treatment, and 1 patient died before undergoing imaging for response evaluation. Of the 5 patients with no target lesions, 4 had tumors measuring <1 cm and 1 had pleural-based lung disease. Lesions decreased in size in 2 of these patients, were stable in 2 patients, and progressed in 1 patient during therapy

[†]Duration of SD: 13 months

[‡]Duration of SD: 3.5 months

Treatment Modifications
(continued)

Posterior reversible encephalopathy syndrome	Permanently discontinue gemcitabine
G3/4 nonhematologic toxicity other than alopecia, fatigue, malaise, and nail changes	Hold chemotherapy up to 2 weeks until toxicity resolves to G ≤1. If toxicity does not resolve to G ≤1 within 2 weeks, discontinue therapy. Resume treatment if toxicity resolves to G ≤1 within 2 weeks, but reduce gemcitabine and docetaxel dosages by 25%
G3/4 nonhematologic toxicity other than alopecia, fatigue, malaise, and nail changes despite a 25% reduction in initial gemcitabine and docetaxel dosages	Hold chemotherapy up to 2 weeks until toxicity resolves to G ≤1. If toxicity does not resolve to G ≤1 within 2 weeks, discontinue therapy. Resume treatment if toxicity resolves to G ≤1 within 2 weeks, but reduce gemcitabine and docetaxel dosages by an additional 25%
G ≥3 liver function test abnormalities	Hold chemotherapy up to 2 weeks until toxicity resolves to G ≤1. If toxicity does not resolve to G ≤1 within 2 weeks, discontinue therapy. Resume treatment if toxicity resolves to G ≤1 within 2 weeks, but reduce gemcitabine and docetaxel dosages by 25%
G ≥3 liver function test abnormalities despite a 25% reduction in initial gemcitabine and docetaxel dosages	Hold chemotherapy up to 2 weeks until toxicity resolves to G ≤1. If toxicity does not resolve to G ≤1 within 2 weeks, discontinue therapy. Resume treatment if toxicity resolves to G ≤1 within 2 weeks, but reduce gemcitabine and docetaxel dosages by an additional 25%
G4 mucositis and diarrhea	Discontinue therapy
G2 neuropathy	Delay therapy 1 week. If symptoms do not resolve to G ≤1, reduce docetaxel dosage by 25%
G3 neuropathy	Discontinue docetaxel

Adverse Events

Grade 3/4 Toxicities in 22 Patients
(109 Courses of Gemcitabine + Docetaxel)*

Toxicity	Grade 3		Grade 4	
	Number of Events (%)	Number of Patients (%)	Number of Events (%)	Number of Patients (%)
Myelosuppression				
Anemia	14 (13)	7 (32)	2 (2)	2 (9)
Neutropenia	18 (17)	11 (50)	15 (14)	8 (36)
Thrombocytopenia	14 (13)	9 (41)	24 (22)	9 (41)
Gastrointestinal				
Diarrhea	2 (2)	2 (9)	—	—
Nausea	1 (1)	1 (5)	—	—
Vomiting	1 (1)	1 (5)	—	—
Colitis	1 (1)	1 (5)	—	—
Hepatic				
Elevated ALT/AST	5 (5)	3 (14)	—	—
Metabolic				
Hypokalemia	4 (4)	4 (18)	1 (1)	1 (5)
Hypophosphatemia	8 (7)	5 (23)	—	—
Hyperglycemia	1 (1)	1 (5)	—	—
Infection				
Without neutropenia	3 (3)	3 (14)	—	—
With neutropenia	1 (1)	1 (5)	—	—
Febrile neutropenia	3 (3)	2 (9)	—	—
Neurology				
Sensory neuropathy	1 (1)	1 (5)	—	—
Other				
Fluid retention	2 (2)	2 (9)	—	—

ALT, alanine aminotransferase; AST, aspartate aminotransferase
*Toxicities were graded according to National Cancer Institute Common Terminology Criteria for Adverse Events (v. 3.0)

Therapy Monitoring

1. *Prior to each treatment cycle:* physical examination, ECOG PS
2. *Day 1 and day 8 of each treatment cycle:* CBC with differential, serum electrolytes, magnesium and calcium, BUN, creatinine, and liver function tests
3. *Weekly CBC with leukocyte differential count:* at least the first 6 cycles of therapy
4. *After every 2 cycles of therapy:* tumor measurements

OSTEOSARCOMA • RECURRENT OR PROGRESSIVE
OSTEOSARCOMA REGIMEN: REGORAFENIB

Davis LE et al. J Clin Oncol 2019;37:1424–1431
Protocol for: Davis LE et al. J Clin Oncol 2019;37:1424–1431
Duffaud F et al. Lancet Oncol 2019;20:120–133
Supplementary appendix to: Duffaud F et al. Lancet Oncol 2019;20:120–133

Regorafenib 160 mg (or 82 mg/m^2 in patients aged 10–17 years with a body surface area 1.30–1.95 m^2); administer orally once daily for 21 consecutive days, days 1–21, followed by 7 days without treatment, every 28 days, until disease progression (total dose/28-day cycle = 3360 mg [or 1722 mg/m2 in patients aged 10–17 years with a body surface area 1.30–1.95 m^2])

Notes:
- Regorafenib tablets must be stored in the manufacturer's original container at room temperature between 20° and 25°C (68° and 77°F)
  - Regorafenib must not be repackaged in other vials or pill boxes
  - Regorafenib containers should be tightly closed after doses are removed
  - The bottle in which regorafenib is packaged contains a desiccant, which should remain in the container
  - Any unused regorafenib tablets are to be discarded 7 weeks after the container was initially opened
- Regorafenib should be taken about the same time each day
- If a dose is missed, it should be taken on the same day it was to have been taken—that is, patients should not take more than 1 dose on a single day to make up for 1 or more doses missed on previous days
- Tablets should be swallowed whole (no breaking, crushing, or chewing)
- Advise patients to avoid grapefruit products while taking regorafenib
- Regorafenib is taken with a low-fat meal that contains less than 600 calories and less than 30% fat
- Strong CYP3A4 inducers and strong CYP3A4 inhibitors: The concomitant use of strong CYP3A4 inducers (eg rifampin, phenytoin, carbamazepine, phenobarbital, and St. John's Wort) should be avoided. The concomitant use of strong CYP3A4 inhibitors (eg clarithromycin, grapefruit juice, itraconazole, ketoconazole, nefazodone, posaconazole, telithromycin, and voriconazole) should be avoided
- Breast cancer resistance protein (BCRP) substrates: The coadministration of regorafenib with a BCRP substrate (eg methotrexate, fluvastatin, atorvastatin) has the potential to increase plasma concentrations of the BCRP substrate. Monitor more closely for adverse effects related to the BCRP substrate and consult the BCRP substrate prescribing information for guidance if concurrent administration cannot be avoided

Supportive Care
Antiemetic prophylaxis
Emetogenic potential on is **MINIMAL–LOW**
See Chapter 42 for antiemetic recommendations

Hematopoietic growth factor (G-CSF) prophylaxis
Primary prophylaxis is NOT indicated
See Chapter 43 for more information

Antimicrobial prophylaxis
Risk of fever and neutropenia is *LOW*
  Antimicrobial primary prophylaxis to be considered:
  - Antibacterial—not indicated
  - Antifungal—not indicated
  - Antiviral—not indicated, unless patient previously had an episode of HSV

Hand-foot reaction (palmar-plantar erythrodysesthesia, PPE)
- For patients who develop a hand-foot reaction, use topical emollients (eg, Aquaphor), topical or orally administered steroids, antihistamine agents (H$_1$-receptor antagonists), or pyridoxine
- Pyridoxine may provide relief for discomfort/pain associated with PPE, although the mechanism through which this occurs remains unclear
- The suggested pyridoxine starting dose is 50 mg/day, which may be increased to a maximum of 200 mg/day

Diarrhea management*
Loperamide 4 mg orally initially after the first loose or liquid stool, *then* 2–4 mg orally every 2–4 hours or **diphenoxylate hydrochloride** 2.5 mg **with atropine sulfate** 0.025 mg (eg, Lomotil) 2 tablets orally four times daily until control has been achieved, after which the dose may be reduced to meet individual requirements

*Abigerges D et al. J Natl Cancer Inst 1994; 86:446–449
Rothenberg ML et al. J Clin Oncol 2001; 19:3801–3807
Wadler S et al. J Clin Oncol 1998; 16:3169–3178

Oral care
Standard prophylaxis and treatment for mucositis/stomatitis

Treatment Modifications

Recommended Dose Modifications for Regorafenib

Starting dose	160 mg once daily on days 1–21, every 28 days
Dose level −1	120 mg once daily on days 1–21, every 28 days
Dose level −2	80 mg once daily on days 1–21, every 28 days
Dose level −3	Discontinue regorafenib

Adverse Event	**Treatment Modification**
Dermatologic Toxicity	
First occurrence of G2 hand-foot skin reaction (HFSR) (palmar-plantar erythrodysesthesia [PPE]) of any duration at a regorafenib dose of 160 mg	Reduce regorafenib to a daily dose of 120 mg. If HFSR does not improve within 7 days despite dose reduction to 120 mg, then withhold therapy until toxicity resolves to G ≤1 at which time may resume regorafenib at a dose of 120 mg daily
G2 HFSR (palmar-plantar erythrodysesthesia [PPE]) that is recurrent or does not improve within 7 days despite dose reduction	Interrupt therapy for a minimum of 7 days for G3 HFSR until toxicity resolves to G ≤1 and resume regorafenib at one lower dose level
G3 HFSR (PPE) at a regorafenib dose of 160 mg	Withhold therapy for a minimum of 7 days and until toxicity resolves to G ≤1, then resume regorafenib at a daily dose of 120 mg
G3 HFSR (PPE) at a regorafenib dose of 120 mg	Withhold therapy for a minimum of 7 days and until toxicity resolves to G ≤1, then resume regorafenib at a daily dose of 80 mg
Other Toxicities	
G3 aspartate aminotransferase (AST)/alanine aminotransferase (ALT) elevation at a regorafenib dose of 160 mg	Resume regorafenib at a daily dose of 120 mg after toxicity resolves to G ≤1 only if the potential benefit outweighs the risk of hepatotoxicity
G3/4 adverse reaction at a regorafenib dose of 160 mg (except hepatotoxicity)	Withhold regorafenib until toxicity resolves to G ≤1 and resume regorafenib at a daily dose of 120 mg
G3/4 adverse reaction at the 120 mg dose (except hepatotoxicity or infection)	Withhold regorafenib until toxicity resolves to G ≤1 and resume regorafenib at a daily dose to 80 mg
Symptomatic G2 hypertension	Withhold therapy until symptoms resolve to G ≤1 and resume regorafenib at a daily dose of 80 mg
Worsening infection of any grade	Withhold therapy until resolution of infection, then resume regorafenib at same dose
Patient who undergoes elective surgery	Withhold regorafenib for ≥2 weeks prior to surgery and for ≥2 weeks after major surgery and until adequate wound healing, whichever is longer
Failure to tolerate 80 mg daily	Permanently discontinue regorafenib
Any G3/4 adverse reaction	
AST or ALT >20 × ULN	
AST or ALT >3 times ULN with concurrent bilirubin >2 times ULN	
Recurrence of AST or ALT >5 times ULN despite dose reduction to 120 mg	
Severe or life-threatening hemorrhage	
Gastrointestinal perforation or fistula	
Reversible posterior leukoencephalopathy syndrome (RPLS)	

Note: for any G4 adverse reaction, only resume if the potential benefit outweighs the risks

Treatment Administration

Duffaud et al. Lancet Oncol 2019;20:120–133

Starting dose	160 mg once daily on days 1–21, every 28 days
Dose level −1	120 mg once daily on days 1–21, every 28 days
Dose level −2	80 mg once daily on days 1–21, every 28 days
Dose level −3	Discontinue regorafenib

	Regorafenib				
Dose Reductions	Initially Assigned to Regorafenib (n = 26)	Received Regorafenib After Switch from Placebo (n = 10)	Subtotal (All Patients Who Received Regorafenib; n = 36)	Placebo (n = 12)	Patients Excluded from Efficacy Analysis (n = 5)
Duration of treatment, months	3.4 (2.1–7.6)	3.9 (1.6–6.3)	3.4 (1.6–7.0)	1.1 (0.9–1.3)	4.5 (1.0–5.3)
Dose reduction					
No	16 (62%)	6 (60%)	22 (61%)	11 (92%)	4 (80%)
Yes	10 (38%)	4 (40%)	14 (39%)	1 (8%)	1 (20%)
Reduction to dose level (−1)	7 (27%)	2 (20%)	9 (25%)	1 (8%)	0
Reduction to dose level (−2)	3 (11%)	2 (20%)	5 (14%)	0	1 (20%)

Data are median (IQR) or n (%)

Patient Population Studied

Duffaud et al. Lancet Oncol 2019;20:120–133

REGOBONE was a randomized, double-blind, phase 2 clinical trial designed by The French Sarcoma Group. The trial was designed as a basket study of four parallel independent cohorts of different histologic subtypes of metastatic bone cancers, to assess the activity and safety of regorafenib. Patients were enrolled in the following cohorts: osteosarcoma, Ewing sarcoma of bone, chondrosarcoma, and chordoma. In each parallel cohort, patients were randomly assigned (2:1) to receive either oral regorafenib or matching placebo

Patient Characteristics

	Regorafenib Group (n = 26)	Placebo Group (n = 12)	Excluded from Efficacy Analysis (n = 5)
Age, years	32 (21–50)	40 (29–43)	30 (23–43)
Sex			
Male	19 (73%)	5 (42%)	4 (80%)
Female	7 (27%)	7 (58%)	1 (20%)
ECOG performance status			
0	12 (46%)	2 (17%)	2 (40%)
1	14 (54%)	10 (83%)	2 (40%)
Unknown	0	0	1 (10%)
Presence of metastases			
No (locally advanced disease)	1 (4%)	0	2 (40%)
Yes	25 (96%)	12 (100%)	3 (60%)
Sites of metastases			
Lung	24 (92%)	10 (83%)	2 (40%)
Bone	6 (23%)	3 (25%)	0
Lymph node	3 (12%)	4 (33%)	0
Pleural	3 (12%)	1 (8%)	0

(continued)

Patient Population Studied (continued)

Previous lines of chemotherapy for metastatic disease			
1	21 (80%)	10 (83%)	3 (60%)
2	5 (20%)	2 (17%)	2 (40%)
0	0	0	0
Previous treatment at entry			
Doxorubicin	26 (100%)	12 (100%)	2 (40%)
Ifosfamide	24 (92%)	12 (100%)	3 (60%)
Cisplatin	25 (96%)	11 (92%)	1 (20%)
High-dose methotrexate	7 (27%)	3 (25%)	0
Etoposide	21 (81%)	5 (42%)	1 (20%)
Gemcitabine or docetaxel	3 (12%)	2 (16%)	0
Oral cyclophosphamide	3 (12%)	1 (8%)	2 (40%)

Data are median (IQR) or n (%)
ECOG, Eastern Cooperative Oncology Group

Davis et al. J Clin Oncol 2019;37:1424

SARC024 was a phase 2 clinical trial of the multikinase inhibitor regorafenib in specific sarcoma subtypes, including advanced osteosarcoma. After the release of the REGOBONE, the DSMC recommended closing the study after enrollment of 42 of 48 planned participants and 31 of the required 42 PFS events

Characteristic

	All Patients (N = 42)	Regorafenib (n = 22)	Placebo (n = 20)
Age, years—median [range]	37 [8–76]	33 [18–70]	47 [19–76]
Sex, No. male / female	20/22	6/16	14/6
Previous lines of therapy: 1 / >1	21/21	11/11	10/10
WHO performance status: 0–1 / 2	41/1 (98)	22/0 (100)	19/1 (95)
Primary tumor location			
Extremity	27 (64)	13 (59.1)	14 (70)
Head/neck	7 (17)	3 (13.6)	4 (20)
Pelvis/spine	4 (9.5)	3 (13.6)	1 (5)
Other	4 (9.5)	3 (14.6)	1 (5)
Histology			
Conventional osteosarcoma	33 (78.5)	17 (77.2)	16 (80)
Conventional chondroblastic	15 (36)	7 (31.8)	8 (40)
Conventional NOS	9 (21)	5 (22.7)	4 (20)
Conventional osteoblastic	5 (12)	3 (13.6)	2 (10)
Conventional osteoblastic and chondroblastic	3 (7)	1 (4.6)	2 (10)
Conventional fibroblastic	1 (2)	1 (4.6)	0 (0)
Other osteosarcoma*	4 (9.5)	1 (4.6)	3 (15)
Osteosarcoma NOS	5 (12)	4 (18.2)	1 (5)

Note: data are presented as No. (%) unless otherwise noted
*Other osteosarcoma includes juxtacortical, parosteal, and telangiectatic
NOS, not otherwise specified

Efficacy

Duffaud et al. Lancet Oncol 2019;20:120–133*

	Regorafenib Group (n = 26)	Placebo Group (n = 12)
No progression of disease at 8 weeks	17 (65%; 95% CI 47–)[†]	0
Response at 8 weeks		
Complete response	0	0
Partial response	2 (8%)	0
Stable disease	15 (58%)	0
Progressive disease	9 (35%)	12 (100%)
Median progression-free survival (weeks)	16.4 (95% CI 8.0–27.3)	4.1 (95% CI 3.0–5.7)
Progression-free survival at 12 weeks	62% (95% CI 40–77)	0
Progression-free survival at 24 weeks	35% (95% CI 17–52)	0

*Data are n (%) unless otherwise specified)
[†]One-sided 95% CI (due to the Fleming design)

Davis et al. J Clin Oncol 2019;37:1424

	Regorafenib	Placebo	Statistics
Partial response (RECIST*)	Three patients (13.6%)	0	
(PFS) (months; 95% CI)	3.6 mos (2.0–7.6)	1.7 mos (1.2–1.8)	HR 0.42; 95% CI, 0.21–0.85; P = 0.017
PFS at 8 weeks	79.0%	25.0%	P = 0.001
PFS at 16 weeks	44.4%	10.0%	P = 0.027
Median OS (months; 95% CI)[†‡]	11.1 mos (4.7–26.7)	13.4 mos (8.5–38.1)	HR 1.26; 95% CI, 0.51–3.13; P = 0.62

CI, confidence interval; PFS, progression-free survival; OS, overall survival
*These patients had received one, three, and five lines of prior therapy, respectively
[†]At the time of data cutoff, 20 (48%) of 42 patients were alive. Median follow-up among living patients was 7.4 months
[‡]Ten patients receiving placebo crossed over to active drug at time of progression

Adverse Events

Duffaud et al. Lancet Oncol 2019;20:120–133

	Regorafenib Group (n = 29)			Placebo Group (n = 14)		
	G1–2	G3	G4	G1–2	G3	G4
Blood and lymphatic system disorders						
Anemia	7 (24%)	0	0	1 (7%)	0	0
Lymphopenia	4 (14%)	1 (3%)	0	0	0	0
Thrombocytopenia	3 (10%)	0	0	0	0	0
Gastrointestinal disorders						
Diarrhea	11 (38%)	2 (7%)	0	1 (7%)	0	0
Nausea	7 (24%)	0	0	5 (36%)	0	0
Constipation	9 (31%)	2 (7%)	0	0	0	0
Abdominal pain	7 (24%)	0	0	0	0	0
Dry mouth	5 (17%)	0	0	1 (7%)	0	0
Vomiting	4 (14%)	0	0	1 (7%)	0	0
Stomatitis	4 (14%)	0	0	0	0	0

(continued)

Adverse Events (continued)

General disorders and administration site conditions						
Fatigue	23 (79%)	3 (10%)	0	6 (43%)	1 (7%)	0
Mucosal inflammation	9 (31%)	0	0	1 (7%)	0	0
Chest pain	3 (10%)	3 (10%)	0	1 (7%)	0	0
Fever	7 (24%)	0	0	0	0	0
Investigations						
Weight decreased	10 (35%)	0	0	0	1 (7%)	0
Blood alkaline phosphatase increase	5 (17%)	2 (7%)*	0	1 (7%)	0	0
Lymphocyte count decreased	5 (17%)	0	0	0	1 (7%)	0
Transaminases increased	5 (17%)	1 (3%)*	0	0	0	0
Blood bilirubin increased	5 (17%)	0	0	0	0	0
Gamma-glutamyl transferase phosphatase increase	5 (17%)	0	0	0	0	0
Hyperbilirubinemia	2 (7%)	1 (3%)	0	0	0	0
Lipase increase	0	1 (3%)*	0	0	0	0
Metabolism and nutrition disorders						
Decreased appetite	9 (31%)	1 (3%)	0	0	1 (7%)	0
Hypophosphatemia	2 (7%)	2 (7%)†	1 (3%)†	0	0	0
Hypokalemia	0	2 (7%)	0	0	1 (7%)	0
Musculoskeletal and connective tissue disorders						
Muscle spasms	5 (17%)	0	0	0	0	0
Back pain	4 (14%)	0	0	0	0	0
Myalgia	1 (3%)	0	0	0	1 (7%)	0
Muscle atrophy	0	0	0	0	1 (7%)	0
Nervous system disorders						
Headache	7 (24%)	0	0	1 (7%)	0	0
Dysgeusia	3 (10%)	0	0	0	0	0
Epilepsy	0	1 (3%)*	0	0	0	0
Anxiety	5 (17%)	0	0	0	0	0
Renal and urinary disorders						
Proteinuria	7 (24%)	0	0	1 (7%)	0	0
Respiratory, thoracic, and mediastinal disorders§						
Dysphonia	9 (31%)	0	0	1 (7%)	0	0
Dyspnea	7 (24%)	1 (3%)	0	2 (14%)	0	0
Cough	5 (17%)	0	0	2 (14%)	0	0
Pleural effusion	0	2 (7%)	0	0	0	0
Hemothorax	0	1 (3%)*	0	0	0	0
Respiratory distress	0	0	0	0	0	0
Skin and subcutaneous tissue disorders						
Hand-foot skin reaction	12 (41%)	3 (10%)†	0	1 (7%)	0	0
Other skin toxicity	12 (41%)	1 (3%)	1 (3%)	2 (14%)	0	0
Hypertension	5 (17%)	7 (24%)‡	0	2 (14%)	0	

Data are n (%).
*One patient had a related serious adverse event
†Two patients had a related serious adverse event
‡Three patients had a related serious adverse event. Several related serious adverse events could have occurred in one patient
§One Grade 5 with regorafenib = respiratory distress

Adverse Events (continued)

AEs Attributed to Treatment

Davis et al. J Clin Oncol 2019;37:1424

Adverse Event	Regorafenib (n = 22)		Placebo (n = 20)	
	All Grades	Grade ≥3	All Grades	Grade ≥3
Any	20 (91)	14 (64)	12 (60)	9 (45)
Hand-foot skin reaction	8 (36)	1 (5)	0	0
Hypertension	7 (32)	3 (14)	3 (15)	0
Nausea	5 (23)	0	4 (20)	1 (5)
Diarrhea	4 (18)	1 (5)	0	0
Oral mucositis	3 (14)	0	0	0
Maculopapular rash	3 (14)	2 (9)	0	0
Vomiting	3 (14)	0	1 (5)	1 (5)
Thrombocytopenia	2 (9)	2 (9)	0	0
Hypophosphatemia	2 (9)	2 (9)	1 (5)	1 (5)
Extremity pain	2 (9)	2 (9)	0	0

Therapy Monitoring

1. Prior to initiation of regorafenib: CBC with differential and platelet count, vital signs, liver function tests, serum electrolytes. Control hypertension prior to initiation of regorafenib

2. Monitor for:
   a. Liver function test abnormalities: obtain ALT, AST, and total bilirubin at least every 2 weeks during the first two months of treatment, and then at least monthly (or as clinically indicated) thereafter. In patients with elevated liver function tests, monitor ALT, AST, and total bilirubin weekly
   b. Hypertension: monitor blood pressure weekly for the first 6 weeks of treatment and then at least every cycle or as clinically indicated
   c. Cytopenias: obtain CBC with differential and platelet count periodically
   d. Hand-foot skin reaction (HFSR)/palmar-plantar erythrodysesthesia (PPE)
   e. Diarrhea
   f. Impaired wound healing
   g. Signs and symptoms of fistulas and perforations, including abscess and sepsis
   h. Signs and symptoms of bleeding
   i. Signs and symptoms of reversible posterior leukoencephalopathy syndrome (RPLS) (eg, seizures, severe headache, visual disturbances, confusion, altered mental status). Withhold regorafenib and perform an emergent brain MRI in patients with symptoms suspicious for RPLS
   j. In patients receiving concomitant warfarin monitor INR more frequently

3. Withhold regorafenib for ≥2 weeks prior to elective surgery and for ≥2 weeks after major surgery and until adequate wound healing, whichever is longer

OSTEOSARCOMA • RECURRENT OR PROGRESSIVE

OSTEOSARCOMA REGIMEN: CABOZANTINIB

Italiano A et al. Lancet Oncol 2020;21:446–455
Supplementary appendix to: Italiano A et al. Lancet 2020;21:446–455
CABOMETYX (cabozantinib) prescribing information. Alameda, CA: Exelixis, Inc; revised 2020 January

Cabozantinib tablets (CABOMETYX) 60 mg (or 40 mg/m^2 in patients <16 years old with body surface area <1.5 m^2); administer orally once daily at least 2 hours after or at least 1 hour before eating food, continually (total dose/week = 420 mg [or 280 mg/m^2 in patients <16 years old with body surface area <1.5 m^2]). Cycle length = 28 days
Notes:

- Tablets are swallowed whole. Do not crush cabozantinib tablets
- Do not substitute cabozantinib tablets (CABOMETYX) with cabozantinib capsules (COMETRIQ)
- Do not take a missed dose within 12 hours of the next scheduled dose
- Patients receive once-daily oral doses of cabozantinib until disease progression, or unacceptable toxicity
- *Patients with hepatic impairment or who are taking strong CYP3A4 inhibitors or inducers:* refer to TREATMENT MODIFICATIONS section for dose recommendations
- Inform patients not to ingest foods or nutritional supplements known to inhibit (eg, grapefruit products) or induce (eg, St. John's Wort) cytochrome P450 activity

Supportive Care
Antiemetic prophylaxis
Emetogenic potential is **MINIMAL–LOW**
See Chapter 42 for antiemetic recommendations

Hematopoietic growth factor (CSF) prophylaxis
Primary prophylaxis is NOT indicated
See Chapter 43 for more information

Antimicrobial prophylaxis
Risk of fever and neutropenia is *LOW*

Diarrhea management
Loperamide 4 mg; administer orally initially after the first loose or liquid stool, *then*
Loperamide 2 mg every 2 hours while awake; every 4 hours during sleep
Alternatively, a trial of **diphenoxylate hydrochloride** 2.5 mg **with atropine sulfate** 0.025 mg (eg, Lomotil) two tablets four times daily until control achieved

Treatment Modifications

RECOMMENDED DOSE MODIFICATIONS FOR CABOZANTINIB

Starting dose (level 1)	60 mg orally once daily
Dose level −1	40 mg orally once daily
Dose level −2	20 mg orally once daily
Dose level −3	Consider discontinuing cabozantinib or consider resuming at 20 mg orally once daily, if tolerable, at the discretion of the medically responsible health care provider

Grade/Severity	Treatment Modification
G ≥3 hemorrhage	Permanently discontinue cabozantinib
Development of a gastrointestinal perforation or Grade 4 fistula	
Acute MI	
Serious arterial or VTE event requiring medical intervention	
Any hypertension	Treat as needed with standard antihypertensive therapy
Persistent hypertension despite use of maximal antihypertensive medications	Withhold cabozantinib until blood pressure is adequately controlled, then resume cabozantinib with the dosage reduced by 1 dosage level
Evidence of hypertensive crisis or severe hypertension that cannot be controlled with antihypertensive therapy	Discontinue cabozantinib
Intolerable Grade 2 diarrhea	Optimize antidiarrheal regimen. Withhold cabozantinib until improvement to G ≤1, then resume cabozantinib with the dosage reduced by 1 dose level
Grade ≥3 diarrhea not manageable with standard antidiarrheal treatments	
Intolerable Grade 2 palmar-plantar erythrodysesthesia syndrome (skin changes [eg, peeling, blisters, bleeding, edema, or hyperkeratosis] with pain; limiting instrumental ADL)	Withhold cabozantinib until improvement to G ≤1, then resume cabozantinib with the dosage reduced by 1 dose level
Grade 3 palmar-plantar erythrodysesthesia syndrome (severe skin changes [eg, peeling, blisters, bleeding, edema, or hyperkeratosis] with pain; limiting self-care ADL)	
Patient requires dental surgery or an invasive dental procedure	If possible, withhold cabozantinib for ≥3 weeks prior to the procedure to reduce risk of osteonecrosis of the jaw and poor wound healing
Osteonecrosis of the jaw	Withhold cabozantinib until complete resolution, then reduce the cabozantinib dosage by 1 dose level
Patient requires elective surgery	If possible, withhold cabozantinib for ≥3 weeks prior to elective surgery and for ≥2 weeks after major surgery and until adequate wound healing, whichever is longer
RPLS is suspected (symptoms of headache, seizure, lethargy, confusion, blindness, and/or other visual and neurologic disturbances along with hypertension of any severity)	Withhold cabozantinib until clarification of the patient's neurologic status (ie, with an emergent brain MRI) has occurred
RPLS is confirmed	Discontinue cabozantinib. The safety of reinitiating cabozantinib in a patient who has experienced RPLS is unknown

(continued)

(continued)

Hand-foot reaction (palmar-plantar erythrodysesthesia, PPE)
Use topical emollients (eg, Aquaphor), topical or orally administered steroids, antihistamines, or pyridoxine 50 to 200 mg/day

Patient Population Studied

The CABONE trial was a multicenter, single-arm, phase 2 trial. Patients had to be at least 12 years of age, have histologically confirmed Ewing sarcoma or osteosarcoma, Eastern Cooperative Oncology Group performance status of 0–1. The number of previous lines of treatment was not limited. Histologic diagnosis of Ewing sarcoma had to be confirmed by fluorescence in-situ hybridization or RT-PCR for assessment of EWS gene rearrangement. All patients with osteosarcoma had centrally documented progressive disease

Patient Characteristics

	Ewing Sarcoma Group (n = 45)	Osteosarcoma Group (n = 45)
Sex		
Men	31 (69%)	27 (60%)
Women	14 (31%)	18 (40%)
Age, years		
Median (IQR)	33 (24–45)	34 (20–53)
<18	2 (4%)	6 (13%)
≥18	43 (96%)	39 (87%)
ECOG performance status		
0	15 (33%)	17 (38%)
1	29 (64%)	26 (58%)
2	1 (2%)	1 (2%)
3	0	1 (2%)
Metastatic sites		
Lung	32 (71%)	39 (87%)
Pleura	5 (11%)	4 (9%)
Bone	17 (38%)	10 (22%)
Liver	2 (4%)	1 (2%)
Other	8 (18%)	5 (11%)
Previous lines of treatment for advanced disease		
0*	3 (7%)	17 (38%)
1	12 (27%)	10 (22%)
2	13 (29%)	10 (22%)
>2	17 (38%)	8 (18%)

Data are n (%) unless otherwise indicated
ECOG, Eastern Cooperative Oncology Group

Treatment Modifications *(continued)*

Grade/Severity	Treatment Modification
Urine dipstick >1+ for protein	Continue cabozantinib at the same dose pending results of a 24-hour urine protein
Urine protein ≥3 g/24 hours	Withhold cabozantinib until urine protein is <3 g/24 hours, then resume cabozantinib at 1 lower dose level. Consider increasing the frequency of urine protein monitoring upon resumption of cabozantinib
Nephrotic syndrome	Discontinue cabozantinib treatment
Other Adverse Reactions	
Other intolerable Grade 2 adverse reactions	Withhold cabozantinib until improvement to G ≤1 or baseline, then reduce the cabozantinib dosage by 1 dose level
Other ≥Grade 3 adverse reactions	
Hepatic Impairment	
Mild to moderate hepatic impairment (Child-Pugh class A or B)	Decrease the starting dose of cabozantinib to 40 mg once daily
Severe hepatic impairment (Child-Pugh class C)	Avoid use of cabozantinib
Drug Interactions	
Patient requires concomitant use of a strong CYP3A4 inhibitor (eg, atazanavir, clarithromycin, indinavir, itraconazole, ketoconazole, nefazodone, nelfinavir, ritonavir, saquinavir, telithromycin, voriconazole)	Reduce the daily cabozantinib dose by 20 mg. Resume the dose that was used prior to initiating the CYP3A4 inhibitor 2 to 3 days after discontinuing a strong inhibitor
Patient requires concomitant use of a strong CYP3A4 inducer (eg, carbamazepine, phenobarbital, phenytoin, rifabutin, rifampin, rifapentine, St. John's Wort)	Increase the daily cabozantinib dose by 20 mg only if tolerability on the dose without the inducer has been convincingly demonstrated. Resume the dose that was used prior to initiating a CYP3A4 inducer 2 to 3 days after discontinuing a strong inducer. The daily cabozantinib dose should not exceed 80 mg

MI, myocardial infarction; VTE, venous thromboembolic event; RPLS, reversible posterior leukoencephalopathy syndrome; UPCR, urine protein to creatinine ratio; MRI, magnetic resonance imaging; ADL, activities of daily living

Efficacy

Note: six patients with Ewing sarcoma and three patients with osteosarcoma were not eligible for the efficacy assessment due to protocol deviations

	Ewing Sarcoma (n = 39)	Osteosarcoma (n = 42)
Median follow-up	31.3 months (95% CI 12.4–35.4)	31.1 months (95% CI 24.4–31.7)
Alive @ median follow-up	13 (33%)	10 (24%)
Receiving treatment @ median follow-up	3 (8%)	3 (7%)
CR	0	0
PR	10 (26%) (95% CI 13–42)	7 (17%)
SD	19 (49%)*	26 (62%)†
PD	8 (21%)	8 (19%)
Died during assessable period	26	32
PD during assessable period	32	40
Median progression-free survival	4.4 months (95% CI 3.7–5.6)	6.7 months (5.4–7.9)
Median overall survival	10.2 months (8.5–18.5)	10.6 months (7.4–12.5)
6-month non-progression	26% (13–42)	
Progression-free survival @ 6 mos	33% (19–48)	52% (36–66)
Progression-free survival @ 12 mos	18% (8–33)	9% (3–21)
Progression-free survival @ 24 mos	5% (<1–19)	9% (3–21)
Overall survival @ 6 mos	84% (68–93)	78% (62–88)
Overall survival @ 12 mos	48% (31–65)	38% (23–53)
Overall survival @ 24 mos	14% (4–31)	23% (11–38)
Metabolic response @ end cycle 1		
Partial metabolic response	13/31 (42%; 95% CI 25–61)	20 /31(65%)
Stable metabolic disease	9/31 (29%)	8 (26%)
Progressive metabolic disease	9 /31(29%)	3 (10%)

Progression-free survival according to metabolic response

	Ewing Sarcoma		Osteosarcoma	
Partial metabolic response	5.4 months (3.7–8.9)	Log-rank P = 0.002	7.2 months (4.7–10.9)	Log-rank P<0.0001
Stable metabolic disease	4.2 months (1.7–9.2)		4.5 months (1.8–9.5)	
Progressive metabolic disease	2.7 months (0.9–4.4)		1.8 months (0.8–1.9)	

*Including 15 (38%) with tumor shrinkage (range of tumor shrinkage −21.6% to −1.5%)
†Including 14 (33%) with tumor shrinkage (range −28.4% to −0.9%)

Therapy Monitoring

1. Prior to initiation of cabozantinib: CBC with differential and platelet count, vital signs, liver function tests, serum electrolytes, oral examination. Control hypertension prior to initiation of cabozantinib
2. Monitor regularly for:
   - Hypertension
   - Signs and symptoms of bleeding. Avoid initiation of cabozantinib in patients with a recent history of hemorrhage (eg, hemoptysis, hematemesis, or melena)
   - Signs and symptoms of fistulas and perforations, including abscess and sepsis
   - Signs and symptoms of palmar-plantar erythrodysesthesia
   - Diarrhea
   - Spot urine for protein measurement every 4–8 weeks (if spot urine dipstick >1+ for protein, perform a 24-hour urine protein)
   - Signs and symptoms of osteonecrosis of the jaw (jaw pain, osteomyelitis, osteitis, bone erosion, tooth or periodontal infection, toothache, gingival ulceration or erosion, persistent jaw pain or slow healing of the mouth or jaw after dental surgery)
3. Perform an oral examination prior to initiation of cabozantinib and periodically during treatment. Advise patients regarding good oral hygiene practices
4. Withhold cabozantinib for ≥3 weeks prior to scheduled dental surgery or invasive dental procedures, if possible
5. Withhold cabozantinib for ≥3 weeks prior to elective surgery (including dental surgery) and for ≥2 weeks after major surgery and until adequate wound healing, whichever is longer
6. Response assessment: every 2–3 cycles

Adverse Events

Event	Ewing Sarcoma (n = 45)			Osteosarcoma (n = 45)		
	Grade 1–2	Grade 3	Grade 4	Grade 1–2	Grade 3	Grade 4
Fatigue	26 (58%)	3 (7%)	0	29 (64%)	1 (2%)	0
Diarrhea	23 (51%)	2 (4%)	0	29 (64%)	1 (2%)	0
Oral mucositis	24 (53%)	1 (2%)	0	21 (47%)	3 (7%)	0
Hypothyroidism	22 (49%)	0	0	20 (44%)	0	0
AST increase	20 (44%)	2 (4%)	0	16 (36%)	3 (7%)	0
ALT increase	17 (38%)	2 (4%)	0	18 (40%)	2 (4%)	0
Nausea	19 (42%)	0	0	12 (27%)	0	0
Anorexia	21 (47%)	0	0	9 (20%)	0	0
Hair color changes	15 (33%)	0	0	15 (33%)	0	0
Palmar-plantar syndrome	11 (24%)	3 (7%)	0	16 (36%)	2 (4%)	0
Thrombocytopenia	13 (29%)	0	0	14 (31%)	2 (4%)	0
Dry skin	11 (24%)	0	0	16 (36%)	0	0
Dysgeusia	9 (20%)	0	0	13 (29%)	0	0
Weight loss	7 (16%)	3 (7%)	0	9 (20%)	0	0
Hypophosphatemia	5 (11%)	5 (11%)	0	10 (22%)	3 (7%)	0
Neutropenia	7 (16%)	2 (4%)	0	5 (11%)	3 (7%)	1 (2%)
Dysphonia	8 (18%)	0	0	4 (9%)	0	0
Alopecia	6 (13%)	0	0	6 (13%)	0	0
Abdominal pain	6 (13%)	0	0	5 (11%)	0	0
Hypomagnesaemia	8 (18%)	1 (2%)	1 (2%)	3 (7%)	2 (4%)	0
Anemia	4 (9%)	0	0	6 (13%)	1 (2%)	0
Vomiting	4 (9%)	0	0	6 (13%)	0	0
TSH increase	6 (13%)	0	0	4 (9%)	0	0
Hypokalemia	6 (13%)	0	0	4 (9%)	0	0
Headache	4 (9%)	0	0	6 (13%)	0	0
Proteinuria	6 (13%)	0	0	4 (9%)	0	0
Skin hypopigmentation	5 (11%)	0	0	5 (11%)	0	0
Constipation	5 (11%)	0	0	4 (9%)	0	0
Gastroesophageal reflux disease	3 (7%)	0	0	6 (13%)	0	0
Myalgia	6 (13%)	0	0	3 (7%)	0	0
ALP increase	2 (4%)	1 (2%)	0	6 (13%)	0	0
Erythema multiforme	4 (9%)	0	0	4 (9%)	0	0
Lipase increased	5 (11%)	3 (7%)	1 (2%)	2 (4%)	1 (2%)	1 (2%)
Pneumothorax	3 (7%)	1 (2%)	0	4 (9%)	4 (9%)	0
Dry mouth	1 (2%)	0	0	6 (13%)	0	0
Hypocalcemia	5 (11%)	0	0	2 (4%)	0	0
Epistaxis	3 (7%)	0	0	4 (9%)	0	0
Leucopenia	3 (7%)	0	0	3 (7%)	2 (4%)	0
Hypertension	3 (7%)	2 (4%)	0	2 (4%)	1 (2%)	0
Dysphagia	2 (4%)	0	0	3 (7%)	0	0
Hyperbilirubinemia	3 (7%)	0	0	2 (4%)	0	0
CPK increase	1 (2%)	0	0	4 (9%)	0	0
Cough	2 (4%)	0	0	3 (7%)	0	0
Maculopapular rash	4 (9%)	0	0	1 (2%)	0	0

Data are n (%)
G1/2 treatment-related adverse events and laboratory abnormalities reported in >5% of patients in one of the two cohorts
G3/4 events are shown
AST, aspartate aminotransferase; ALT, alanine aminotransferase; ALP, alkaline phosphatase; TSH, thyroid-stimulating hormone; CPK, creatine phosphokinase

PRIMARY MALIGNANT BONE TUMORS: EWING SARCOMA

Epidemiology

Incidence:	Estimated annual incidence from birth to age 20 years is 2.9/million population. Approximately 10% of patients are 20–30 years of age. Cases in patients >30 years of age are infrequent
Median age:	14 years; 90% of patients, <20 years of age
Mortality rate:	0.05/100,000 population
Male to female ratio:	Slightly more prevalent in males

American Cancer Society. *Cancer Facts & Figures 2020.* Atlanta: American Cancer Society; 2020
Gurney JG et al. Malignant bone tumors. In: Reis LAG et al (editors). Cancer incidence and survival among children and adolescents: United States SEER program, 1975–1995. NIH Pub. No. 99–4649. Bethesda, MD: National Cancer Institute SEER Program; 1999:99–110

Stage at Diagnosis

Nonmetastatic	80%
Metastatic	20%

5-Year Survival

Localized	60–70%
Metastatic	20%

Expert Opinion

Treatment of Ewing sarcoma is similar to that of osteosarcoma because it involves the use of neoadjuvant chemotherapy followed by local therapy (surgery or radiation), which is then followed by adjuvant chemotherapy

Chemotherapy
1. The most commonly used drugs are doxorubicin, vincristine, ifosfamide, etoposide, dactinomycin, and cyclophosphamide
2. The use of combination chemotherapy as part of a multidisciplinary approach has increased 5-year survival rates from <10% to approximately 60%

Local therapy
1. Local therapy in the treatment of Ewing sarcoma varies from surgery alone, to radiation alone, to a combination of both modalities, depending on where disease is located
2. Surgery remains the preferred route of local control. A wide surgical margin should be attempted
3. In contrast to osteosarcoma and the soft-tissue sarcomas, Ewing tumors are radiosensitive. Therefore, in patients in whom surgery is not possible or for those patients with marginal and intralesional surgery, radiation is an effective therapeutic option
4. The behavior of Ewing sarcoma and PNET (primitive neuroectodermal tumors) in adults is no different from their behavior in children

Adverse prognostic factors
1. Metastatic disease
2. Pelvic localization
3. Tumor diameter >8–10 cm
4. Age >15 years
5. Elevated LDH
6. Poor histologic response to preoperative chemotherapy
7. Radiation therapy as the only local treatment

Grier HE et al. N Engl J Med 2003;348:694–701
Verrill MW et al. J Clin Oncol 1997;15:2611–2621

Pathology

Ewing sarcoma family of tumors (includes primitive neuroectodermal tumors):
1. Rare tumors arising in the bone marrow from primitive neural crest elements
2. Constitute approximately 10% of bone sarcomas
3. Subtypes include:
   - Classic Ewing sarcoma (most commonly associated with bone)
   - Primitive neuroectodermal tumor (generally not associated with bones)
4. Distinguished immunohistochemically from other pediatric tumors by expression of the MIC2 gene
5. Most commonly detected translocation is t(11;22)(q24;q12), one of a series of related translocations that occur in >95% of the Ewing sarcoma family of tumors (including primitive neuroectodermal tumors)
6. The t(11;22) translocation joins the Ewing sarcoma gene *EWS* on chromosome 22 to friend leukemia insertion (*FLI 1*) on chromosome 11 (ie, t[11;22]).
Note: FLI1 is a member of the ETS (E-twenty six) family
7. The *EWS-FLI1* fusion transcript encodes a 68-kDa protein with 2 primary domains
   - *EWS* domain = a potent transcriptional activator
   - *FLI1* domain = a highly conserved *ETS* DNA-binding domain.
   The EWS-FLI1 fusion protein thus acts as an aberrant transcription factor
8. In an individual patient, t(11;22) fuses one of many observed combinations of exons from *EWS* and *FLI1* to form the fused message. Most common combination = *EWS* exon 7 fused to *FLI1* exon 6 ("7/6") in ~50–64% of tumors of the Ewing sarcoma family

NEWLY DIAGNOSED • EWING SARCOMA

EWING SARCOMA REGIMEN: INTERVAL COMPRESSED VINCRISTINE, DOXORUBICIN, AND CYCLOPHOSPHAMIDE ALTERNATING WITH IFOSFAMIDE AND ETOPOSIDE (AEWS0031 PROTOCOL)

Womer RB et al. J Clin Oncol 2012;30:4148–4154
Protocol for: Womer RB et al. J Clin Oncol 2012;30:4148–4154

Induction Chemotherapy Schedule for Interval Compressed Vincristine + Doxorubicin + Cyclophosphamide Alternating with Ifosfamide + Etoposide According to AEWS0031

Local Therapy	Treatment	Week											
		1	2	3	4	5	6	7	8	9	10	11	12
All	Vincristine (V)	V				V				V			
	Doxorubicin (D)	D				D				D			
	Cyclophosphamide (C)	C				C				C			
	Ifosfamide (I)			I				I				I	
	Etoposide (E)			E				E				E	

Consolidation Chemotherapy Schedule for Interval Compressed Vincristine + Doxorubicin + Cyclophosphamide Alternating with Ifosfamide + Etoposide According to AEWS0031

Local Therapy	Treatment	Week																
		13	14	15	16	17	18	19	20	21	22	23	24	25	26	27	28	29
Surgery Alone	Vincristine (V)			V				V				V				V		
	Doxorubicin (D)			D				D										
	Cyclophosphamide (C)			C				C				C				C		
	Ifosfamide (I)					I				I				I				I
	Etoposide (E)					E				E				E				E
	Surgery (S)	S																

Local Therapy	Treatment	Week																
		13	14	15	16	17	18	19	20	21	22	23	24	25	26	27	28	29
Radiation Therapy Alone	Vincristine (V)	V				V				V				V				
	Doxorubicin (D)	D												D				
	Cyclophosphamide (C)	C				C				C				C				
	Ifosfamide (I)			I				I				I				I		
	Etoposide (E)			E				E				E				E		
	Radiation (R)*	R																

(continued)

(*continued*)

Local Therapy	Treatment	Week																
		13	14	15	16	17	18	19	20	21	22	23	24	25	26	27	28	29
Surgery then Radiation Therapy	Vincristine (V)			V				V				V				V		
	Doxorubicin (D)			D												D		
	Cyclophosphamide (C)			C				C				C				C		
	Ifosfamide (I)					I				I				I				I
	Etoposide (E)					E				E				E				E
	Surgery (S)	S																
	Radiation (R) *			R														

*Refers to the *start* of radiation therapy

Notes:
- Doxorubicin should not be given during radiation therapy, except at the beginning of radiation therapy
- Primary tumor treatment commenced at week 13 and could have consisted of complete surgical excision with clear margins, surgery with radiation therapy for close or positive margins, or radiation therapy alone. Minimal adequate bony margins to avoid radiation therapy were defined as 1 cm (2 to 5 cm recommended), and minimal soft tissue margins were defined as 5 mm in muscle or fat or 2 mm with fascial planes. Radiation therapy doses were 45 Gy to the initial volume and 55.8 Gy to the final volume of unresected tumors, 50.4 Gy to extraosseous tumors with a complete response to chemotherapy, 45 Gy to vertebral bony primary tumors, and 45 Gy to pathologically involved lymph node areas. Preoperative radiotherapy was permitted with a dose of 45 Gy. Patients who were treated with planned radiation followed by consideration of later excision were treated with radiation during weeks 13–19 with surgery performed after week 29. Patients with chest wall primary tumors and ipsilateral pleural-based tumor nodules received 15 Gy to the hemithorax (12 Gy for patients <6 years old) and 36.6 Gy to any unresected gross pleural tumor. All radiation therapy was given in 1.8 Gy fractions

Cycles of vincristine, doxorubicin, and cyclophosphamide (VDC) + mesna or vincristine, and cyclophosphamide (VC) + mesna:

Vincristine 2 mg/m² per dose (maximum single dose = 2 mg); administer by intravenous infusion over 15 minutes in 25–50 mL 0.9% sodium chloride injection (0.9% NS) on day 1 (total dosage during the weeks in which vincristine is administered = 2 mg/m²; maximum dose/treatment = 2 mg)
- Dilute in 25 mL 0.9% NS for pediatric patients and in 50 mL 0.9% for adult patients

Doxorubicin 37.5 mg/m² per dose; administer by intravenous injection over 1–15 minutes on days 1 and 2 (total dosage during the weeks in which doxorubicin is administered = 75 mg/m²; total cumulative dosage permitted = 375 mg/m²)

Hydration for cyclophosphamide:
0.9% NS 750 mL/m²; administer intravenously over 1–2 hours prior to the start of cyclophosphamide on day 1. Then, encourage oral fluid ingestion or administer additional intravenous hydration (eg, 0.9% NS) at a rate of 100 mL/m²/hour continued until the last intravenous mesna dose has been administered

An admixture containing **cyclophosphamide** 1200 mg/m² + **mesna** 240 mg/m²; administer intravenously in 100–250 mL 0.9% sodium chloride injection (0.9% NS) or 5% dextrose injection (D5W) over 30–60 minutes on day 1 (total cyclophosphamide dosage during the weeks in which cyclophosphamide is administered = 1200 mg/m²)

Then, either:
Mesna 240 mg/m² per dose; administer intravenously diluted with 0.9% NS or D5W to a concentration of 1–20 mg/mL, over 15 minutes for 2 doses at 4 hours and 8 hours after cyclophosphamide administration is completed, on day 1 (total mesna dosage during the weeks in which cyclophosphamide is administered = 720 mg/m²; includes 240 mg/m² dose given with cyclophosphamide), *or*
Mesna 480 mg/m² per dose; administer orally for 2 doses at 2 hours and 6 hours after cyclophosphamide administration is completed on day 1 (total mesna dosage during the weeks in which cyclophosphamide is administered = 1200 mg/m²; includes 240 mg/m² dose given with cyclophosphamide)

Cycles of ifosfamide and etoposide (ie) + mesna:
Hydration during ifosfamide:
Administer 2000 mL/m² **0.9% NS** per day by intravenous infusion over 4–24 hours for 5 consecutive days, on days 1–5
If feasible, continue maintenance intravenous hydration during intervals between ifosfamide administration. Encourage oral fluid ingestion. Monitor daily weight, or if implemented in an inpatient setting, monitor fluid input and output. Replace electrolytes as medically appropriate

An admixture containing **ifosfamide** 1800 mg/m² + **mesna** 360 mg/m² per day; administer intravenously in a volume of 0.9% NS or D5W sufficient to produce ifosfamide concentrations between 0.6 and 20 mg/mL, over 60 minutes for 5 consecutive days, on days 1–5 (total ifosfamide dosage during the weeks in which ifosfamide is administered = 9000 mg/m²)
Then, either:
Mesna 360 mg/m² per dose; administer intravenously diluted with 0.9% NS or D5W to a concentration of 1–20 mg/mL, over 15 minutes for 2 doses per day at 4 hours and 8 hours after ifosfamide administration is completed, for 5 consecutive days, on days 1–5 (total mesna dosage during the weeks in which ifosfamide is administered = 5400 mg/m²; includes 360 mg/m² doses given daily with ifosfamide), *or*

(*continued*)

(*continued*)

Mesna 720 mg/m² per dose; administer orally for 2 doses per day at 2 hours and 6 hours after ifosfamide administration is completed, for 5 consecutive days, on days 1–5 (total mesna dosage during the weeks in which ifosfamide is administered = 9000 mg/m²; includes 360 mg/m² doses given daily with ifosfamide)

Etoposide 100 mg/m² per day; administer intravenously diluted with 0.9% NS to a concentration of 0.2–0.4 mg/mL over 60 minutes for 5 consecutive days, on days 1–5 (total etoposide dosage during weeks in which etoposide is administered = 500 mg/m²)
• The administration schedules for vincristine, doxorubicin, cyclophosphamide, ifosfamide, and etoposide appear in the table (above)

Supportive Care
Antiemetic prophylaxis
Emetogenic potential during cycles with vincristine, doxorubicin, and cyclophosphamide is **HIGH**. *Potential for delayed symptoms*
Emetogenic potential during cycles with vincristine and cyclophosphamide is **MODERATE**
Emetogenic potential during cycles with ifosfamide and etoposide is **MODERATE**
See Chapter 42 for antiemetic recommendations

Hematopoietic growth factor (CSF) prophylaxis
Primary prophylaxis is indicated with:
  Filgrastim (G-CSF) 5 μg/kg per day by subcutaneous injection
  • Begin use at least 24 hours after myelosuppressive chemotherapy is completed (that is, day 3 of VDC cycles, day 2 of VC cycles, and day 6 of IE cycles)
  • Continue daily filgrastim use for at least 7 days or until ANC ≥750/mm³, whichever comes last
  • Discontinue daily filgrastim use at least 24 hours before administering myelosuppressive treatment
See Chapter 43 for more information

Antimicrobial prophylaxis
Risk of fever and neutropenia is INTERMEDIATE
  Antimicrobial primary prophylaxis to be considered:
  • Antibacterial—consider a fluoroquinolone or no prophylaxis; *P. jirovecii* prophylaxis is recommended (eg, cotrimoxazole)
  • Antifungal—consider concomitant use of clotrimazole during periods of neutropenia
  • Antiviral—antiherpes antivirals (eg, acyclovir, famciclovir, valacyclovir)

Treatment Modifications

Hematologic Toxicity (Applies to VDC, VC, and IE Cycles)

Adverse Event	Dose Modification
Day 15 ANC <750/mm³ or platelet count <75,000/mm³	Delay initiation of the next cycle of chemotherapy until parameters are met
Day 22 (induction) or day 29 (consolidation) ANC <750/mm³, despite delay, first occurrence	Delay initiation of the next cycle of chemotherapy until parameters are met. Reduce doses of doxorubicin, cyclophosphamide, ifosfamide, (mesna), and etoposide by 25% in subsequent cycles. Increase doses by 25% in subsequent cycles if ANC criterion is met by day 18
Day 22 (induction phase) or day 29 (consolidation phase) ANC <750/mm³, despite delay, second occurrence	Delay initiation of the next cycle of chemotherapy until parameters are met. Reduce doses of doxorubicin, cyclophosphamide, ifosfamide, (mesna), and etoposide by a further 25% in subsequent cycles. Increase doses by 25% in subsequent cycles if ANC criterion is met by day 18

VINCRISTINE DOSE MODIFICATIONS

Neuropathy

G2 motor or sensory neuropathy	Administer full doses of vincristine
G ≥3 motor or sensory neuropathy	Administer vincristine with the dosage reduced by 50%. If the toxicity improves to G ≤1, then increase the dose to 75%, and then to 100% of the full dose as tolerated
Jaw pain	Continue vincristine at the current dose

Gastrointestinal Toxicity

G ≥3 constipation (obstipation with manual evacuation indicated; limiting self-care ADL)	Withhold vincristine and optimize laxative regimen. When toxicity improves to G ≤1, resume vincristine at full dose
G ≥3 ileus (severely altered GI function; TPN indicated)	

(*continued*)

Treatment Modifications (continued)

IFOSFAMIDE AND CYCLOPHOSPHAMIDE DOSE MODIFICATIONS FOR HEMATURIA

Transient microscopic hematuria (>50 RBC/HPF 1 or 2 times on two separate days)	No modification
Persistent microscopic hematuria (>50 RBC/HPF ≥3 times), or transient gross hematuria	Increase the rate of hydration to 3500–4000 mL/m²/day. Administer mesna as a continuous intravenous infusion (give mesna at a dose equal to 20 percent of the ifosfamide or cyclophosphamide dose [mixed with the cyclophosphamide or ifosfamide] and then administer mesna as a continuous intravenous infusion at an hourly rate equivalent to 10 percent of the ifosfamide or cyclophosphamide dose)
Persistent gross hematuria occurring during or following a cycle of therapy	Hold further ifosfamide/cyclophosphamide doses until the urine clears to less than gross hematuria or until the next cycle of therapy. Then, reinstitute ifosfamide or cyclophosphamide at full dose. Increase the rate of hydration and administer mesna as described above for persistent microscopic hematuria
Occurrence of a second episode of gross hematuria or persistence of microscopic hematuria on the continuous infusion mesna regimen	Continue the ifosfamide or cyclophosphamide when the urine clears to less than gross hematuria. Continue intravenous hydration at 3500–4000 mL/m²/day. Double the loading and infusion doses of mesna and continue to administer as a continuous infusion (ie, give mesna at a dose equal to 40 percent of the ifosfamide or cyclophosphamide dose [mixed with the cyclophosphamide or ifosfamide] and then administer mesna as a continuous intravenous infusion at an hourly rate equivalent to 20 percent of the ifosfamide or cyclophosphamide dose). Continue continuous infusion mesna for 48 hours after the last dose of ifosfamide/cyclophosphamide
Persistent gross hematuria despite "double dose, continuous infusion mesna regimen"	Discontinue the ifosfamide or cyclophosphamide

OTHER IFOSFAMIDE DOSE MODIFICATIONS

Development of significant Fanconi syndrome (ie, significant phosphorus wasting or significant bicarbonate wasting with any GFR, or GFR <50 mL/min/1.73m²)	In each subsequent course of ifosfamide + etoposide, replace ifosfamide with cyclophosphamide 2100 mg/m² intravenously over 1 hour on day 1 only (with a standard dose of mesna and with 5 days of etoposide)
G2 encephalopathy	If persistent or distressing, then decrease the ifosfamide and mesna dosages by 20%. If not contraindicated, treat with methylene blue 2 mg/kg (maximum dose of 50 mg) intravenously every 4–8 hours until resolution of symptoms, then consider prophylactic use at the same dose given every 6–8 hours in subsequent cycles
G3 encephalopathy	Stop ifosfamide for this cycle. If not contraindicated, treat with methylene blue 2 mg/kg (maximum dose of 50 mg) intravenously every 4–8 hours until resolution of symptoms, then consider prophylactic use at the same dose given every 6–8 hours in subsequent cycles. Decrease the ifosfamide and mesna dosages by 20% in subsequent cycles
G4 encephalopathy	Permanently discontinue ifosfamide. If not contraindicated, treat with methylene blue 2 mg/kg (maximum dose of 50 mg) intravenously every 4–8 hours until resolution of symptoms, then consider prophylactic use at the same dose given every 6–8 hours in subsequent cycles. Either decrease the ifosfamide and mesna dosages by 20% in subsequent cycles or replace ifosfamide with cyclophosphamide (as above for renal toxicity)
G ≥3 mucositis after IE cycle persisting beyond day 21 and unresponsive to maximum supportive care	Reduce the doses of ifosfamide/mesna and etoposide by 25% in subsequent cycles. If the mucositis was in part related to radiation therapy, then increase the chemotherapy doses back to full dose upon resolution of the toxicity

DOXORUBICIN DOSE MODIFICATIONS

LVEF is <45%	Discontinue doxorubicin. In subsequent VDC cycles, substitute doxorubicin with dactinomycin 1.25 mg/m² on day 1 only (maximum dose = 2.5 mg). For patients <1 year old, the dactinomycin dose is 0.025 mg/kg
G ≥3 mucositis after VDC cycle persisting beyond day 15 and unresponsive to maximum supportive care	Administer the total dose of doxorubicin as a continuous infusion over 24 hours rather than over 48 hours in the next course of VDC. If mucositis still recurs despite this, then reduce the dose of doxorubicin by 25% in subsequent VDC cycles

Patient Population Studied

Patients with a new diagnosis of Ewing sarcoma, peripheral neuroectodermal tumor, primitive neuroectodermal tumor, or Askin tumor. The primary site could be bone or soft tissue, but not intradural soft tissues. Patients could have no evidence of metastatic disease on a radionuclide bone scan, chest CT scan, and bilateral bone marrow aspirates and biopsies. One pulmonary or pleural nodule >1 cm in diameter or more than one nodule >0.5 cm in diameter on chest CT scan was considered evidence of metastasis. Patients with chest wall tumors and ipsilateral pleural effusions or pleural-based secondary nodules were considered to have localized disease, as were patients with clinically or pathologically involved regional lymph nodes. Chemotherapy had to begin within 30 days of initial biopsy

Demographic or Clinical Characteristic	Standard Timing: Regimen A		Intensive Timing: Regimen B		All Patients	
	No. of Patients	%	No. of Patients	%	No. of Patients	%
Age at diagnosis, years						
≤9	88	31	74	26	162	29
10–17	165	58	174	61	339	60
18+	31	11	36	13	67	12
Median	12		13		12	
Range	0–33		0–45		0–45	
Sex						
Male	154	54	154	54	308	54
Female	130	46	130	46	260	46
Race						
White	252	89	250	88	502	88
African American	8	3	6	2	14	2
Asian	8	3	8	3	16	3
Not reported/other	16	5	20	7	36	6
Ethnicity						
Not Hispanic	258	91	250	88	508	89
Hispanic	21	7	29	10	50	9
Not reported	5	2	5	2	10	3
Primary site (bone unless otherwise specified)						
Skull	18	6	13	5	31	5
Spine	14	5	30	11	44	8
Ribs	34	12	25	9	59	10
Sternum, scapula, or clavicle	15	5	15	5	30	5
Humerus	13	5	12	4	25	4
Radius, ulna, or bone of the hand	7	2	8	3	15	3
Pelvis	47	17	43	15	90	16
Femur	33	12	28	10	61	11
Tibia, fibula, patella, or bone of foot	51	18	43	15	94	17
Soft tissue	52	18	67	24	119	21

Efficacy

Patients were randomly assigned to the control regimen A or the experimental regimen B. Regimen A administered chemotherapy every 21 days, whereas regimen B administered chemotherapy every 14 days or as soon as blood count recovery permitted. Both regimens used 14 alternating cycles of VDC/IE with filgrastim, with identical per-cycle and total doses

	Regimen A	Regimen B	
5-year EFS rate	65%	73%	HR 0.74 (95% CI, 0.54–0.99); P = 0.48
5-year overall survival	77%	83%	HR 0.69 (95% CI, 0.47–1.0); P = 0.056
5-year cumulative local recurrence incidence	0.080 (95% CI, 0.052–0.12)	0.072 (95% CI, 0.045–0.11)	P = 0.74
5-year cumulative distant and combined local and distant relapse	0.23; 95% CI, 0.19–0.30	0.16; 95% CI, 0.13–0.23	P = 0.058

	All patients		
	≥18 years	<18 years	
EFS at 5 years	47%	72%,	P<0.001

Adverse Events

Toxicity	Regimen A: Standard Timing		Regimen B: Intensive Timing	
	No. of Cycles	%	No. of Cycles	%
Fever or infection				
Wound infection	35	1	27	0.7
Febrile neutropenia	221	6.2	266	7.3
Infection with neutropenia	166	4.6	172	4.7
Infection without neutropenia	80	2.2	72	2
Infection ANC unknown or other	18	0.5	13	0.3
Central line infection	51	1.4	38	1
Colitis or typhlitis	9	0.2	16	0.4
Total	580	16	604	16.4
Anorexia	46	1.3	48	1.3
Nausea	69	1.9	22	0.6
Vomiting	39	1	26	0.8
Stomatitis pharyngitis	80	2.2	104	2.9
Hypokalemia	54	1.5	42	1.2
Days in hospital per cycle				
Mean	5	5.1	—	—
Median	4	4	—	—

Note: patients were randomly assigned to the control regimen A or the experimental regimen B. Regimen A administered chemotherapy every 21 days, whereas regimen B administered chemotherapy every 14 days or as soon as blood count recovery permitted. Both regimens used 14 alternating cycles of VDC/IE with filgrastim, with identical per-cycle and total doses. Sixteen patients developed second malignancies, 9 on regimen A and 7 on regimen B (P = 0.62). There were 11 acute myeloid leukemias (5 on regimen A and 6 on regimen B), 3 osteosarcomas in radiation fields (2 on regimen A and 1 on regimen B), and 2 lymphomas (both on regimen A)
ANC, absolute neutrophil count

Therapy Monitoring

VDC and VC

1. *Prior to first dose of doxorubicin:* perform a thorough cardiac assessment, including history, physical examination, and determination of LVEF by echocardiogram or MUGA scan at baseline prior to initiation of doxorubicin. Reevaluate LVEF prior to the fourth cycle of VDC. Reevaluate LVEF if clinical symptoms of heart failure are present

2. *Before each cycle:* CBC with differential, total bilirubin, ALT, AST, albumin, alkaline phosphatase, serum creatinine, BUN, calcium, carbon dioxide, chloride, glucose, potassium, sodium, and phosphate, physical examination

3. *Twice per week:* CBC with differential until recovery from hematopoietic toxicity

IE

1. *Prior to each cycle:* CBC with differential, total bilirubin, ALT, AST, albumin, alkaline phosphatase, serum creatinine, BUN, calcium, carbon dioxide, chloride, glucose, potassium, sodium, and phosphate

2. *During chemotherapy administration:*
   a. *Daily laboratory investigations:* serum creatinine, BUN, calcium, carbon dioxide, chloride, glucose, potassium, sodium, and phosphate
   b. *Every 8 hours (or with each void):* urine dipstick for blood (check microscopic urinalysis if >trace)
   c. *Other:* monitor fluid status (ie, weight and intake/output) and for signs and symptoms of neurologic toxicity

3. *Twice per week:* CBC with differential until recovery from hematopoietic toxicity

NEWLY DIAGNOSED • EWING SARCOMA

EWING SARCOMA REGIMEN: VINCRISTINE, IFOSFAMIDE, DOXORUBICIN, AND ETOPOSIDE (VIDE) THEN VINCRISTINE, DACTINOMYCIN, AND IFOSFAMIDE (VAI) THEN VINCRISTINE, DACTINOMYCIN, AND CYCLOPHOSPHAMIDE (VAC) (EURO-EWING99-R1 PROTOCOL)

Le Deley M et al. J Clin Oncol 2014;32:2440–2448
Protocol for: Le Deley M et al. J Clin Oncol 2014;32:2440–2448
Supplementary appendix to: Le Deley M et al. J Clin Oncol 2014;32:2440–2448

<u>Induction Chemotherapy:</u> 6 cycles of VIDE
<u>Surgery:</u> following induction chemotherapy
<u>Adjuvant Therapy:</u> 1 cycle of VAI followed by 7 cycles of VAC
V, vincristine; I, ifosfamide; D, doxorubicin; E, etoposide; A, dactinomycin; C, cyclophosphamide

Induction chemotherapy cycles 1–6 (vincristine, ifosfamide, doxorubicin, etoposide [VIDE])
Vincristine 1.5 mg/m^2 (maximum single dose = 2 mg); administer by intravenous infusion over 15 minutes in 25–50 mL 0.9% sodium chloride injection (0.9% NS) on day 1, every 21 days, for 6 cycles (total dosage/3-week cycle = 1.5 mg/m^2; maximum dosage/3-week cycle = 2 mg)
• Dilute in 25 mL 0.9% NS for pediatric patients and in 50 mL 0.9% for adult patients

Ifosfamide
Mesna 1000 mg/m^2; administer intravenously diluted in a volume of 0.9% NS sufficient to produce a final mesna concentration ranging from 1–20 mg/mL, intravenously over 15 minutes one hour prior to the ifosfamide dose on day 1, every 21 days, for 6 cycles. *Then,*
Mesna 3000 mg/m^2; administer intravenously diluted in a volume of 0.9% NS sufficient to produce a final mesna concentration ranging from 1–20 mg/mL, by continuous infusion over 24 hours for 3 consecutive days, on days 1–3, beginning immediately after completion of the mesna bolus infusion on day 1, every 21 days, for 6 cycles (total dosage/3-week cycle = 10,000 mg/m^2 which includes the bolus infusion on day 1)
Hydration during ifosfamide:
Administer additional intravenous hydration (eg, 0.9% NS) to achieve a total rate of 2000 mL/m^2/day (taking into account volumes of diluent used for mesna, ifosfamide, doxorubicin, and etoposide administration) for the duration of ifosfamide treatment and continuing for 24 hours after the last dose
Ifosfamide 3000 mg/m^2 per day; administer intravenously in a volume of 0.9% NS or 5% dextrose injection (D5W) sufficient to produce ifosfamide concentrations between 0.6 and 20 mg/mL, over 1–3 hours for 3 consecutive days, on days 1–3, every 21 days, for 6 cycles (total dosage/3-week cycle = 9000 mg/m^2)

Doxorubicin 20 mg/m^2 per dose; administer intravenously in 25–1000 mL 0.9% NS or D5W over 4 hours, for 3 consecutive days on days 1–3, every 21 days, for 6 cycles (total dosage/3-week cycle = 60 mg/m^2)

Etoposide 150 mg/m^2 per day; administer intravenously diluted with 0.9% NS to a concentration of 0.2–0.4 mg/mL over 60 minutes for 3 consecutive days, on days 1–3, every 21 days, for 6 cycles (total dosage/3-week cycle = 450 mg/m^2)

Adjuvant chemotherapy cycle 7 (vincristine, dactinomycin, ifosfamide [VAI])
Vincristine 1.5 mg/m^2 (maximum single dose = 2 mg); administer by intravenous infusion over 15 minutes in 25–50 mL 0.9% NS on day 1 for 1 cycle (total dosage/3-week cycle = 1.5 mg/m^2; maximum dosage/3-week cycle = 2 mg)
• Dilute in 25 mL 0.9% NS for pediatric patients and in 50 mL 0.9% for adult patients

Dactinomycin 0.75 mg/m^2 per dose (maximum single dose = 1.5 mg); administer by intravenous injection over 3–5 minutes for 2 consecutive days, on days 1–2, for 1 cycle (total dosage/3-week cycle = 1.5 mg/m^2; maximum dosage/3-week cycle = 3 mg)

Ifosfamide
Mesna 1000 mg/m^2; administer intravenously diluted in a volume of 0.9% NS sufficient to produce a final mesna concentration ranging from 1–20 mg/mL, intravenously over 15 minutes one hour prior to the ifosfamide dose on day 1 for 1 cycle. *Then,*
Mesna 3000 mg/m^2; administer intravenously diluted in a volume of 0.9% NS sufficient to produce a final mesna concentration ranging from 1–20 mg/mL, by continuous infusion over 24 hours for 2 consecutive days, on days 1–2, beginning immediately after completion of the mesna bolus infusion on day 1, for 1 cycle (total dosage/3-week cycle = 7,000 mg/m^2 which includes the bolus infusion on day 1)
Hydration during ifosfamide:
Administer additional intravenous hydration (eg, 0.9% NS) to achieve a total rate of 2000 mL/m^2/day (taking into account volumes of diluent used for mesna and ifosfamide administration) for the duration of ifosfamide treatment and continuing for 24 hours after the last dose
Ifosfamide 3000 mg/m^2 per day; administer intravenously in a volume of 0.9% NS or D5W sufficient to produce ifosfamide concentrations between 0.6 and 20 mg/mL, over 1–3 hours for 2 consecutive days, on days 1–2, for 1 cycle (total dosage/3-week cycle = 6000 mg/m^2)

Adjuvant chemotherapy cycles 8–14 (vincristine, dactinomycin, cyclophosphamide [VAC])
Vincristine 1.5 mg/m^2 (maximum single dose = 2 mg); administer by intravenous infusion over 15 minutes in 25–50 mL 0.9% NS on day 1, every 21 days, for 6 cycles (total dosage/3-week cycle = 1.5 mg/m^2; maximum dosage/3-week cycle = 2 mg)
• Dilute in 25 mL 0.9% NS for pediatric patients and in 50 mL 0.9% for adult patients

Dactinomycin 0.75 mg/m^2 per dose (maximum single dose = 1.5 mg); administer by intravenous injection over 3–5 minutes for 2 consecutive days, on days 1–2, every 21 days, for 6 cycles (total dosage/3-week cycle = 1.5 mg/m^2; maximum dosage/3-week cycle = 3 mg)

(continued)

(continued)

Cyclophosphamide

Mesna 500 mg/m²; administer intravenously diluted in a volume of 0.9% NS sufficient to produce a final mesna concentration ranging from 1–20 mg/mL, intravenously over 15 minutes one hour prior to the cyclophosphamide dose on day 1, every 21 days, for 6 cycles. *Then,*
Mesna 1500 mg/m²; administer intravenously diluted in a volume of 0.9% NS sufficient to produce a final mesna concentration ranging from 1–20 mg/mL, by continuous infusion over 24 hours on day 1, beginning immediately after completion of the mesna bolus infusion, every 21 days, for 6 cycles (total dosage/3-week cycle = 2000 mg/m² which includes the bolus infusion on day 1)

Hydration during cyclophosphamide:
Administer additional intravenous hydration (eg, 0.9% NS) to achieve a total rate of 2000 mL/m²/day (taking into account volumes of diluent used for mesna and cyclophosphamide administration) continuing for 24 hours after the dose of cyclophosphamide

Cyclophosphamide 1500 mg/m²; administer intravenously, as either undiluted cyclophosphamide (20 mg/mL) or diluted in 100–1000 mL 0.9% NS or D5W, over 1–3 hours on day 1, every 21 days, for 6 cycles (total dosage/3-week cycle = 1500 mg/m²)

<u>Notes about local tumor control</u>:
• Surgery occurs after course 6 of VIDE
• RT (54.4 Gy) was administered if incomplete surgery or no surgery occurred
• A reduced RT dose (44.8 Gy) recommended for marginal excision of a protocol-defined, standard-risk tumor with good histologic response
• Postoperative RT was also recommended in tumors located in the vertebrae or chest wall (if associated with a pleural effusion)
• Postoperative RT applied during VAC consolidation therapy, ie, during courses 8–12

Supportive Care

Antiemetic prophylaxis
*Emetogenic potential during cycles with vincristine, ifosfamide, doxorubicin, and etoposide (VIDE) cycles on days 1–3 is **HIGH**. Potential for delayed symptoms*
*Emetogenic potential during the cycle with vincristine, dactinomycin, and ifosfamide (VAI) on days 1–2 is **HIGH**. Potential for delayed symptoms*
*Emetogenic potential during cycles with vincristine, dactinomycin, and cyclophosphamide (VAC) on days 1–2 is **MODERATE***
See Chapter 42 for antiemetic recommendations

Hematopoietic growth factor (CSF) prophylaxis
Primary prophylaxis is indicated with 1 of the following:
   Filgrastim (G-CSF) 5 μg/kg per day by subcutaneous injection, *or*
   Pegfilgrastim (pegylated filgrastim) 6 mg/0.6 mL by subcutaneous injection for 1 dose
   • Begin use at least 24 hours after myelosuppressive chemotherapy is completed (that is, day 4 of VIDE cycles and day 3 of VAI and VAC cycles)
   • Continue daily filgrastim use after the neutrophil nadir until ANC ≥5000/mm³ on 2 measurements separated temporally by ≥12 hours
   • Discontinue daily filgrastim use at least 24 hours before administering myelosuppressive treatment. Do not administer pegfilgrastim within 14 days before administering myelosuppressive treatment
See Chapter 43 for more information

Antimicrobial prophylaxis
Risk of fever and neutropenia is INTERMEDIATE
   Antimicrobial primary prophylaxis to be considered:
   • Antibacterial—consider a fluoroquinolone or no prophylaxis; *P. jirovecii* prophylaxis is recommended (eg, cotrimoxazole)
   • Antifungal—consider concomitant use of clotrimazole during periods of neutropenia
   • Antiviral—antiherpes antivirals (eg, acyclovir, famciclovir, valacyclovir)

Treatment Modifications

Induction VIDE (Cycles 1–6) and Adjuvant VAI (Cycle 7)

Adverse Event	Dose Modification
Day 22 ANC <1000/mm³ or platelet count <80,000/mm³	Delay initiation of the next cycle of chemotherapy until parameters are met. If delay is >6 days, reduce etoposide dose by 20% in subsequent cycles
Day 22 ANC <1000/mm³ or platelet count <80,000/mm³ despite reduction of etoposide dose by 20%	Reduce etoposide by another 20%. If necessary, omission of etoposide completely is preferred to dose reduction of other 3 drugs
G ≥3 neutropenic sepsis	Reduce etoposide dose by 20% in subsequent cycles
G ≥3 mucositis	

(continued)

Treatment Modifications (*continued*)

Adverse Event	Dose Modification
Recurrent G ≥3 neutropenic sepsis despite reduction of etoposide dose by 20%	Reduce etoposide by another 20%. If necessary, omission of etoposide completely is preferred to dose reduction of other 3 drugs
Recurrent G ≥3 mucositis despite reduction of etoposide dose by 20%	
G0/1 renal toxicity (GFR ≥60 mL/min/1.73 m², TmP/GFR ≥1.00 mmol/L, and serum bicarbonate ≥17.0 mmol/L)	Continue ifosfamide at the same dose
G2 renal toxicity (GFR 40–59 mL/min/1.73 m², or TmP/GFR 0.80–0.99 mmol/L, or serum bicarbonate 14.0–16.9 mmol/L)	Reduce the ifosfamide (and mesna) doses by 30%
G3 renal toxicity (GFR <40 mL/min/1.73 m², or TmP/GFR <0.80 mmol/L, or serum bicarbonate <14.0 mmol/L)	Substitute cyclophosphamide 1500 mg/m²/day on day 1 only (with mesna) for ifosfamide in subsequent VIDE and VAI cycles
GFR <60 mL/min/1.73m²	Reduce etoposide dose by 30%
FS <29% or LVEF <40%, or decrease by an absolute value of ≥10 percentile points from previous tests	Delay chemotherapy for 1 week and repeat echocardiography. If FS has recovered to ≥29%, then proceed to next course. If FS remains <29%, then omit doxorubicin and substitute with dactinomycin 0.75 mg/m² per dose (maximum single dose = 1.5 mg) administered by IV injection over 3–5 minutes on days 1–2
G ≥3 encephalopathy	Prolong ifosfamide infusion to 4–8 hours. If not contraindicated, treat with methylene blue 2 mg/kg (maximum dose of 50 mg) IV every 4–8 hours until resolution of symptoms, then consider prophylactic use at the same dose given every 6–8 hours in subsequent cycles. For recurrent G ≥3 toxicity, consider substituting cyclophosphamide 1500 mg/m²/day on day 1 only (with mesna) for ifosfamide in subsequent VIDE and VAI cycles

Adjuvant VAC (Cycles 8–14)

Adverse Event	Dose Modification
Day 22 ANC <1000/mm³ or platelet count <80,000/mm³	Delay initiation of the next cycle of chemotherapy until parameters are met. If delay is >6 days, then reduce cyclophosphamide and dactinomycin doses by 20% in subsequent cycles. For recurrence of toxicity, reduce cyclophosphamide and dactinomycin doses by another 20%
G ≥3 neutropenic sepsis	Reduce cyclophosphamide and dactinomycin doses by 20% in subsequent cycles. For recurrence of toxicity, reduce cyclophosphamide and dactinomycin doses by another 20%
G ≥3 mucositis	

Urologic Toxicity (Applies to VIDE, VAI, and VAC Cycles)

IFOSFAMIDE AND CYCLOPHOSPHAMIDE DOSE MODIFICATIONS FOR HEMATURIA

Transient microscopic hematuria (>50 RBC/HPF 1 or 2 times on two separate days)	No modification
Persistent microscopic hematuria (>50 RBC/HPF ≥3 times), or transient gross hematuria	Increase rate of hydration to 3500–4000 mL/m²/day
Persistent gross hematuria occurring during or following a cycle of therapy	Hold further ifosfamide or cyclophosphamide doses until urine clears to less than gross hematuria or until the next cycle of therapy. Then, reinstitute ifosfamide or cyclophosphamide at full dose. Increase the rate of hydration to 3500–4000 mL/m²/day
Occurrence of a second episode of gross hematuria or persistence of microscopic hematuria on the continuous infusion mesna regimen	Continue the ifosfamide or cyclophosphamide when the urine clears to less than gross hematuria. Continue intravenous hydration at 3500–4000 mL/m²/day. Double the loading and infusion doses of mesna. Continue continuous infusion mesna for 48 hours after last dose of ifosfamide/cyclophosphamide
Persistent gross hematuria despite "double dose mesna regimen"	Discontinue the ifosfamide or cyclophosphamide

VIDE, vincristine + ifosfamide + doxorubicin + etoposide; VAI, vincristine + dactinomycin + ifosfamide; ANC, absolute neutrophil count; GFR, glomerular filtration rate; TmP/GFR, ratio of tubular maximum reabsorption of phosphate to GFR; FS, fractional shortening; LVEF, left ventricular ejection fraction; IV, intravenously; VAC, vincristine + dactinomycin + cyclophosphamide; RBC, red blood cell; HPF, high-power field

Patient Population Studied

This trial was conducted in 202 European pediatric and adult oncology centers in 13 countries, via four national or cooperative groups. Eligible patients ≤50 years with a localized, biopsy-proven Ewing sarcoma classified as standard-risk disease, ie, either good histologic response to preoperative treatment (<10% cells), or small tumor (<200 mL) resected at diagnosis or with radiotherapy alone as local treatment. Patients who had preoperative radiotherapy were eligible provided both conditions were fulfilled

Baseline Characteristics, Overall and by Randomly Assigned Group

Patient or Tumor Characteristic	VAI Arm (n = 425) No. (%)	VAC Arm (n = 431) No. (%)	Total (n = 856) No. (%)
Sex			
Male	251 (59)	258 (60)	509 (59)
Female	174 (41)	173 (40)	347 (41)
Age, years			
<25	372 (88)	375 (87)	747 (87)
≥25	53 (12)	56 (13)	109 (13)
Estimated tumor volume, mL			
<200	299 (70)	314 (73)	613 (72)
≥200	124 (29)	113 (26)	237 (28)
Missing data	2 (0)	4 (1)	6 (1)
Tumor type			
Osseous lesion ± soft tissue component	364 (86)	363 (84)	727 (85)
Soft tissue only	61 (14)	68 (16)	129 (15)
Tumor site			
Pelvis	73 (17)	69 (16)	142 (17)
Abdomen	8 (2)	9 (2)	17 (2)
Spine	42 (10)	42 (10)	84 (10)
Chest	80 (19)	103 (24)	183 (21)
Head and neck	31 (7)	23 (5)	54 (6)
Upper extremity	41 (10)	34 (8)	75 (9)
Lower extremity	150 (35)	151 (35)	301 (35)
Metastatic disease at diagnosis			
No	425 (100)	430 (100)	855 (100)
Yes	0 (0)	1 (0)	1 (0)
Local treatment			
Surgery after VIDE courses ± RT	320 (75)	323 (75)	643 (75)
Initial surgery of primary ± RT	61 (14)	64 (15)	125 (15)
Local RT before surgery	8 (2)	9 (2)	17 (2)
Definitive RT	36 (8)	35 (8)	71 (8)
Histologic response			
Missing data or not applicable	106 (25)	108 (25)	214 (25)
No tumor (complete necrosis)	184 (43)	192 (45)	376 (44)
<1% tumor cells	16 (4)	20 (5)	36 (4)
1% to 4% tumor cells	43 (10)	36 (8)	79 (9)
5% to 9% tumor cells	68 (16)	60 (14)	128 (15)
Good response NOS	7 (2)	9 (2)	16 (2)
10% to 29% tumor cells	1 (0)	5 (1)	6 (1)
>50% tumor cells	0 (0)	1 (<1)	1 (<1)

NOS, not otherwise specified; RT, radiotherapy; VAC, vincristine, dactinomycin, and cyclophosphamide; VAI, vincristine, dactinomycin, and ifosfamide; VIDE, vincristine, ifosfamide, doxorubicin, and etoposide

Efficacy

Event-Free Survival and Overall Survival by Randomly Assigned Group (Intention-to-Treat Population, N = 856)

	VAI Arm (n = 425)	VAC Arm (n = 431)	Total (N = 856)
Event-free survival (EFS)			
Number of events	110	121	231
Progression/relapse	102	114	218
Local	30	34	64
Metastases	46	58	104
Combined	25	21	46
Site unknown	1	1	2
Secondary malignancy	7	5	12
Death as first event	1	2	3
Treatment-related death	0	1	1
Other cause	1	0	1
Cause unknown	0	1	1
3-year EFS from random assignment—% (95% CI)	78.2 (73.9–81.9)	75.4 (71.0–79.2)	76.8 (73.8–79.5)
3-year EFS difference—% (91.4%CI)	−2.8 (−7.8–2.2)		
Stratified HR$_{event}$ VAC/VAI—HR$_{event}$ (91.4%CI)	1.12 (0.89–1.41)		
Overall Survival (OS)			
No. of deaths	83	88	171
Resulting from progression/relapse	74	83	157
Treatment-related death related to EE99 protocol	0	1	1
Treatment-related death after second-line treatment	5	0	5
Secondary malignancy	3	1	4
Other cause	1	1	2
Unknown cause	0	2	2
3-year OS from random assignment—% (95% CI)	85.5 (81.7–88.6)	85.9 (82.2–89.0)	85.7 (83.1–87.9)
3-year OS difference—% (91.4%CI)	0.4 (3.8–4.6)		
Stratified HR$_{death}$ VAC/VAI—HR$_{death}$ (91.4%CI)	1.09 (0.84–1.42)		

Note: three cases of death reported as first event (VAC arm, one death of unknown cause in the VAC arm 1 month after the end of treatment and one anaphylactic shock after occurrence of pneumonia after the third course of VAC; VAI arm 5 years after the end of treatment)

HR$_{death}$, hazard ratio of death; HR$_{event}$, hazard ratio of events; VAC, vincristine + dactinomycin + cyclophosphamide; VAI, vincristine + dactinomycin + ifosfamide; VIDE, vincristine + ifosfamide + doxorubicin + etoposide

Therapy Monitoring

VIDE and VAI

1. *Prior to first dose of doxorubicin:* perform a thorough cardiac assessment, including history, physical examination, and determination of LVEF by echocardiogram or MUGA scan. Re-evaluate LVEF prior to the fifth cycle of VIDE. Re-evaluate LVEF if clinical symptoms of heart failure are present

2. *Before each cycle:* CBC with differential, total bilirubin, ALT, AST, albumin, alkaline phosphatase, serum creatinine, BUN, calcium, carbon dioxide, chloride, glucose, potassium, sodium, phosphate, and physical examination

3. *During chemotherapy administration:*
   a. *Daily laboratory investigations:* serum creatinine, BUN, calcium, carbon dioxide, chloride, glucose, potassium, sodium, and phosphate
   b. *Every 8 hours (or with each void):* urine dipstick for blood (check microscopic urinalysis if >trace)
   c. *Other:* monitor fluid status (ie, weight and intake/output) and for signs and symptoms of neurologic toxicity

4. *Twice per week:* CBC with differential until recovery from hematopoietic toxicity

VAC

1. *Prior to each cycle:* CBC with differential, total bilirubin, ALT, AST, albumin, alkaline phosphatase, serum creatinine, BUN, urinalysis, and physical examination

2. *During chemotherapy administration:*
   a. *Every 8 hours (or with each void):* urine dipstick for blood (microscopic urinalysis if >trace)
   b. *Other:* monitor fluid status (ie, weight and intake/output)

3. *Twice per week:* CBC with differential until recovery from hematopoietic toxicity

Adverse Events

Proportion of Patients Who Experienced Severe Toxicity by Randomly Assigned Group and Odds Ratio Estimated in Multivariable Models

Toxicity	VAI Arm Number* (Percent)	VAC Arm Number* (Percent)	Odds Ratio VAC/VAI (95% CI)	Nominal P Value
Severe hematologic toxicity, G ≥4	319/406 (79)	343/408 (84)	1.49 (1.03–2.2)	0.03
Anemia, G4	44/406 (11)	46/408 (11)	1.05 (0.68–1.62)	0.84
Leucopenia, G ≥4	256/406 (63)	283/408 (69)	1.36 (1.01–1.85)	0.04
Neutropenia, G ≥4	291/383 (76)	313/386 (81)	1.43 (0.99–2.1)	0.06
Thrombocytopenia, G ≥4	143/406 (35)	183/408 (45)	1.53 (1.15–2.0)	<0.001
Infection, G ≥4	168/404 (42)	176/409 (43)	1.08 (0.81–1.44)	0.62*
Other toxicity	215/408 (53)	207/410 (50)	0.92 (0.70–1.22)	0.56*
General condition, G ≥3	34/395 (9)	23/400 (5.8)	0.65 (0.37–1.12)	0.12*
Stomatitis, G ≥3	12/404 (3.0)	11/408 (2.7)	0.91 (0.40–2.1)	0.83*
Vomiting, G ≥3	26/405 (6.4)	19/407 (4.7)	0.72 (0.39–1.32)	0.29*
Diarrhea, G ≥3	8/404 (2.0)	5/408 (1.2)	0.61 (0.20–1.89)	0.40†
Skin toxicity, G ≥3	13/404 (3.2)	6/407 (1.5)	0.45 (0.17–1.20)	0.11†
Creatinine, G ≥2	8/403 (2.0)	8/408 (2.0)	0.99 (0.37–2.7)	0.98†
Proteinuria, G ≥2	7/345 (2.0)	5/354 (1.4)	0.69 (0.22–2.2)	0.53†
Hematuria, G ≥2	8/357 (2.2)	8/362 (2.2)	0.99 (0.37–2.7)	0.98†
Glomerular function, G ≥2	12/314 (3.8)	4/308 (1.3)	0.33 (0.11–1.04)	0.06†
Tubular function, G ≥2	71/229 (31)	34/208 (16)	0.41 (0.26–0.67)	<0.001‡
Hyperbilirubinemia, G ≥3	9/386 (2.3)	6\391 (1.5)	0.65 (0.23–1.85)	0.42‡
Transaminase elevation, G ≥3	14/402 (3.5)	16/40 (4.0)	1.15 (0.55–2.4)	0.71†
Cardiac toxicity, G ≥2	4/332 (1.2)	3/313 (1.0)	0.79 (0.18–3.6)	0.76†
LV-SF impairment, G ≥2	13/283 (4.6)	7/249 (2.8)	0.68 (0.26–1.77)	0.43‡
Central neurotoxicity, G ≥2	7/404 (1.7)	3/406 (0.7)	0.42 (0.11–1.64)	0.2†
Peripheral neurotoxicity, G ≥2	26/403 (6.5)	28/406 (6.9)	1.08 (0.62–1.89)	0.79‡

*Number indicates the number of patients who experienced at least one episode of severe toxicity among the patients evaluated for this type of toxicity. The number of patients varies across the table because of missing information for some specific toxicity items
†The odds ratios were estimated in univariable analysis because of the small number of patients with a severe toxicity. P values were not corrected for multiple tests
LV-SF, left ventricular shortening fraction; VAC, vincristine + dactinomycin + cyclophosphamide; VAI, vincristine + dactinomycin + ifosfamide
‡The odds ratios and P values were estimated in multivariable logistic regression, controlling for sex, age category, and data center

RECURRENT/REFRACTORY • EWING SARCOMA

EWING SARCOMA REGIMEN: CYCLOPHOSPHAMIDE + TOPOTECAN

Hunold A et al. Pediatr Blood Cancer 2006;47:795–800
Saylors RL III et al. J Clin Oncol 2001;19:3463–3469

Pretreatment hydration: 500 mL/m^2 0.9% sodium chloride injection (0.9% NS), *or* 0.45% sodium chloride injection, *or* 5% dextrose injection/0.45% sodium chloride injection; administer intravenously over 2–4 hours before starting chemotherapy

Cyclophosphamide 250 mg/m^2 per day; administer intravenously in 25–250 mL 0.9% NS or 5% dextrose injection (D5W) over 30 minutes for 5 consecutive days, on days 1–5, every 21 days (total dosage/cycle = 1250 mg/m^2)
Topotecan HCl 0.75 mg/m^2 per day; administer intravenously in 50–250 mL 0.9% NS or D5W over 30 minutes for 5 consecutive days, after cyclophosphamide on days 1–5, every 21 days (total dosage/cycle = 3.75 mg/m^2)

Posttreatment hydration: Hydration continues orally or intravenously at a rate of 3000 mL/m^2 per 24 hours until 24 hours after the last dose of chemotherapy is completed

Supportive Care
Antiemetic prophylaxis
Emetogenic potential is **MODERATE**
See Chapter 42 for antiemetic recommendations

Hematopoietic growth factor (CSF) prophylaxis
Primary prophylaxis is indicated with 1 of the following:
 Filgrastim (G-CSF) 5 µg/kg per day by subcutaneous injection, *or*
 Pegfilgrastim (pegylated filgrastim) 6 mg/0.6 mL by subcutaneous injection for 1 dose
 • Begin use at least 24 hours after myelosuppressive chemotherapy is completed (day 6)
 • Continue daily filgrastim use after the neutrophil nadir until ANC ≥5000/mm^3 on 2 measurements separated temporally by ≥12 hours
 • Discontinue daily filgrastim use at least 24 hours before administering myelosuppressive treatment. Do not administer pegfilgrastim within 14 days before administering myelosuppressive treatment
See Chapter 43 for more information

Antimicrobial prophylaxis
Risk of fever and neutropenia is INTERMEDIATE
 Antimicrobial primary prophylaxis to be considered:
 • Antibacterial—consider a fluoroquinolone or no prophylaxis; *P. jirovecii* prophylaxis is recommended (eg, cotrimoxazole)
 • Antifungal—consider concomitant use of clotrimazole during periods of neutropenia
 • Antiviral—antiherpes antivirals (eg, acyclovir, famciclovir, valacyclovir)

Patient Population Studied

A study of 91 pediatric patients with recurrent or refractory solid tumors, including Ewing sarcoma (n = 17), rhabdomyosarcoma (n = 15), and neuroblastoma (n = 13)

Efficacy

Ewing Sarcoma (n = 17)	
Complete response	12%
Partial response	24%
Rhabdomyosarcoma (n = 15)	
Complete response	0
Partial response	67%

Note: responses were observed in patients who had received >1 year of intensive alkylating agent therapy and/or ablative therapy with autologous stem cell rescue

Adverse Events (N = 307 Cycles)[*]

	% of Cycles with G3/4
Neutropenia	53
Thrombocytopenia	44
Anemia	27
Infection[†]	11
Nausea/vomiting	0.65
Hematuria[‡]	0.65
Perirectal mucositis	0.33
Transaminase elevation	0.33

[*]National Cancer Institute (USA) Common Toxicity Criteria, version 2.0
[†]Includes admissions for fever/neutropenia: 5 bacteremia or fungemia, 1 herpes zoster, 1 infectious cystitis
[‡]In 2 patients with history of hematuria on ifosfamide

Treatment Modifications

Topotecan

Topotecan starting dose	0.75 mg/m²/day × 5 days = 3.75 mg/m² every 3 weeks
Topotecan dose level −1	0.6 mg/m²/day × 5 days = 3 mg/m² every 3 weeks
Topotecan dose level −2	0.5 mg/m²/day × 5 days = 2.5 mg/m² every 3 weeks

Cyclophosphamide

Cyclophosphamide starting dose	250 mg/m²/day × 5 days = 1250 mg/m² every three weeks
Cyclophosphamide dose level −1	200 mg/m²/day × 5 days = 1000 mg/m² every three weeks
Cyclophosphamide dose level −2	160 mg/m²/day × 5 days = 800 mg/m² every three weeks

Adverse Event	Treatment Modifications
On day 1 of treatment ANC ≤1500/mm³ or platelets ≤100,000/mm³, or serum creatinine >1.5 mg/dL	Delay treatment by 1 week until ANC >1500/mm³ or platelets >100,000/mm³, or serum creatinine ≤1.5 mg/dL
On day 1 of treatment ANC ≤1000/mm³ or platelets ≤100,000/mm³, or serum creatinine >1.5 mg/dL	Delay treatment by 1 week until ANC >1000/mm³ or platelets >100,000/mm³, or serum creatinine ≤1.5 mg/dL
Febrile neutropenia (ANC <1000/mm³ with temperature >38°C or >100.4°F), or ANC <1000/mm³ for ≥7 days	Reduce topotecan and cyclophosphamide doses by 1 level and consider adding filgrastim in subsequent cycles, if applicable
Febrile neutropenia (ANC <1000/mm³ with temperature >38°C or >100.4°F), or ANC <1000/mm³ for ≥7 days despite 1 dose reduction; or ANC <500 at any time	Administer filgrastim in subsequent cycles. If already administering filgrastim, reduce topotecan and cyclophosphamide dosage by 1 level
Platelet nadir <50,000/mm³, or platelets <100,000/mm³ for ≥7 days; or platelet nadir <25,000/mm³ at any time	Reduce topotecan dosage by 1 level
G2/3 mucositis or diarrhea	
G4 mucositis or diarrhea	Reduce topotecan dosage by 1 level or consider discontinuing topotecan
Recurrent mucositis or diarrhea despite dosage reduction or persistence of mucositis/diarrhea >2 weeks beyond scheduled start of next cycle	Discontinue topotecan
Other G3/4 nonhematologic toxicity	Delay topotecan and cyclophosphamide until resolution to G ≤1, then reduce dosage of topotecan and cyclophosphamide by 1 level

Topotecan dose adjustments for renal impairment:
Creatinine clearance 46–60 mL/min: reduce topotecan dosage by 20%
Creatinine clearance 31–45 mL/min: reduce topotecan dosage by 25%
Creatinine clearance ≤30 mL/min: reduce topotecan dosage by 30%

Therapy Monitoring

1. *Daily during therapy:* urinalysis
2. *Twice weekly:* CBC with differential until recovery from hematopoietic toxicity
3. *Weekly:* physical examination
4. *Before each cycle:* serum creatinine, LFTs with bilirubin, serum electrolytes, including calcium, magnesium, and phosphorus
5. *Response evaluation:* after the first and second cycles, then after every 2 cycles

RECURRENT/REFRACTORY • EWING SARCOMA

EWING SARCOMA REGIMEN: TEMOZOLOMIDE + IRINOTECAN (5 DAYS × 2 DOSING)

Casey DA et al. Pediatr Blood Cancer 2009;53:1029–1034
Kurucu N et al. Pediatr Hematol Oncol 2015;32:50–59
Wagner LM et al. Pediatr Blood Cancer 2007;48:132–139

Temozolomide 100 mg/m^2 per day; administer orally for 5 consecutive days, on days 1–5, 1 hour before irinotecan, every 21–28 days (total dosage/cycle = 500 mg/m^2)
Notes:
- Temozolomide doses are rounded to the nearest 5 mg by using commercially available products
- Patients who vomit after taking temozolomide should be instructed to take their next dose at the next regularly scheduled time

Irinotecan 10–20 mg/m^2 per dose; administer intravenously, diluted with 5% dextrose injection to a concentration within the range of 0.12–2.8 mg/mL, over 90 minutes for 10 doses, on days 1–5 and days 8–12, every 21–28 days (total dosage/cycle = 100–200 mg/m^2)

Supportive Care
Antiemetic prophylaxis
Emetogenic potential is **MODERATE**
See Chapter 42 for antiemetic recommendations

Hematopoietic growth factor (CSF) prophylaxis
Primary prophylaxis is NOT indicated
See Chapter 43 for more information

Antimicrobial prophylaxis
Risk of fever and neutropenia is *LOW*
  Antimicrobial primary prophylaxis to be considered:
  - Antibacterial—not indicated
  - Antifungal—not indicated
  - Antiviral—not indicated unless patient previously had an episode of HSV

Acute cholinergic syndrome
Atropine sulfate 0.25–1 mg subcutaneously or intravenously if abdominal cramping or diarrhea develop during or within 1 hour after irinotecan administration
- If symptoms are severe, add as primary prophylaxis at least 30 minutes before irinotecan during subsequent cycles
- For irinotecan, acute cholinergic syndrome may be characterized by abdominal cramping, diarrhea, diaphoresis, hypotension, flushing, bradycardia, rhinitis, increased salivation, meiosis, and lacrimation

Diarrhea management
Latent or delayed-onset diarrhea*:
Loperamide 4 mg orally initially after the first loose or liquid stool, *then* 2–4 mg orally every 2–4 hours or **diphenoxylate hydrochloride** 2.5 mg **with atropine sulfate** 0.025 mg (eg, Lomotil)

*Abigerges D et al. J Natl Cancer Inst 1994;86:446–449
Rothenberg ML et al. J Clin Oncol 2001;19:3801–3807
Wadler S et al. J Clin Oncol 1998;16:3169–3178

Patient Population Studied

All patients had Ewing sarcoma and had experienced either progressive disease during initial therapy (n = 5) or relapsed within 2 years of diagnosis (n = 1). Twelve patients had metastatic disease at diagnosis, including 5 with bone and/or marrow metastases

Efficacy (N = 14)*

Complete response	1 (7%)
Partial response	3 (21%)
Minor response	3 (21%)
Median duration of response	30 (range: 12–64) weeks
Median time to progression	20 weeks
Marked symptomatic pain relief with reduction in medication usage†	7 (50%)

*WHO criteria; 2 patients started treatment with no measurable disease following other salvage therapies. Consequently, only 14 patients were fully evaluable for response
†In first course of therapy, irrespective of ultimate imaging response

Efficacy (N = 20)*

Casey DA et al. Pediatr Blood Cancer 2009;53:1029–1034

Best response achieved (n = 19)	
Complete response†	5 patients‡
Partial response	7 patients
Progressive disease	7 patients
Stable disease	0
Overall objective response	63%
Overall survival (n = 20)§	55%§
Median TTP	
All evaluable patients (n = 20)	8.3 months
Patients with recurrent ES (n = 14)	16.2 months
>2-year remission after primary diagnosis (n = 6)ᵉ	22.8 months
<2-year remission after primary diagnosis (n = 14)	3.7 months
Localized disease at initial diagnosis (n = 9)	16.4 months
Metastatic disease at initial diagnosis (n = 11)	2.4 months
Single-site disease recurrence	24.3 months
Multiple-site recurrence	2.4 months

*WHO criteria
†Each of the 5 completed 12 planned cycles of irinotecan/temozolomide; all were in remission with a median follow-up time of 28.3 months
‡Two patients disease free > additional radiation or chemotherapy. Five patients experienced PD > a median of 6 months and 9 cycles of therapy
§Eleven patients (55%) alive with median follow-up 25.7 months at conclusion of cohort analysis
ᵉFour of 6 achieved a CR and were in remission >12 cycles of therapy with a median follow-up time of 26.4 months

Treatment Modifications

Irinotecan Dose Levels*

Level 1 starting dosage	10–20 mg/m² per day
Level −1	7.5–15 mg/m² per day
Level −2	5–10 mg/m² per day

Temozolomide Dose Levels

Level 1 starting dosage	100 mg/m² per day orally on days 1–5
Level −1	75 mg/m² per day orally on days 1–5
Level −2	50 mg/m² per day orally on days 1–5

Adverse Event	Dose Modification
G1 ANC 1500–1999/mm³, or G1 thrombocytopenia during a cycle	Maintain dose and schedule
G2 ANC 1000–1499/mm³, or G2 thrombocytopenia during a cycle	Reduce dosage of both agents by 1 dosage level
G4 neutropenia >7 days duration	Reduce dosage of both agents for the following cycle by 1 dose level
G3/4 infection	
Day 21 ANC <1000/mm³, or platelet count <75,000/mm³	Delay start of next cycle by 1 week and reduce dosage of both agents 1 level
Day 28 ANC still <1000/mm³, or platelet count still <75,000/mm³	Delay start of next cycle by 1 additional week and reduce dosage of both agents 1 level
Day 35 ANC still <1000/mm³, or platelet count still <75,000/mm³	Discontinue therapy

Diarrhea in Children 2–15 Years of Age

Children 2–15 years, with first liquid stools	Begin oral loperamide liquid immediately with the first liquid stool at a dosage of 0.18 mg/kg per day (0.03 mg/kg administered orally every 4 hours). Maximum single dose for patients weighing <13 kg is 0.5 mg loperamide; for 13 to <20 kg, 1 mg; for 20 to <43 kg, initially 2 mg then subsequently 1 mg; and for ≥43 kg, initially 4 mg then subsequently 2 mg
G3/4 diarrhea within the first 24 hours	Hospitalize for optimal management. Begin loperamide 0.06 mg/kg every 4 hours. Maximum single dose for patients weighing <13 kg is 0.5 mg loperamide; for 13 to <20 kg, 1 mg; for 20 to <43 kg, initially 2 mg then subsequently 1 mg; and for ≥43 kg, initially 4 mg then subsequently 2 mg. Reduce irinotecan dosage for the following cycle by 1 dose level

Delayed Diarrhea in Patients >15 Years of Age

G1 (2–3 stools/day > baseline)	Maintain dose and schedule
G2 (4–6 stools/day > baseline)	Delay until diarrhea resolves to baseline, then reduce irinotecan dosage by 1 dosage level
G3 (7–9 stools/day > baseline)	Delay until diarrhea resolves to baseline, then reduce dosage of irinotecan by 1 dosage level
G4 (≥10 stools/day > baseline)	Delay until diarrhea resolves to baseline, then reduce dosage of irinotecan by 2 dosage levels

Other Nonhematologic Toxicities

Any G1 toxicity	Maintain dose and schedule
Any G2 toxicity	Hold treatment until toxicity resolves to G ≤1, then reduce dosage of both agents by 1 dosage level
Any G3 toxicity	Hold treatment until toxicity resolves to G ≤1, then reduce dosage of both agents by 1 dosage level
Any G4 toxicity	Hold treatment until toxicity resolves to G ≤1, then reduce dosage of both agents by 2 dosage levels

*Treatment should be stopped in case of recurrent toxicity at dose level −2, unless there is perceived clinical benefit from irinotecan that justifies continuation

André T et al. Eur J Cancer 1999;35:1343–1347
Camptosar irinotecan hydrochloride injection, product label. New York, NY: Pharmacia & Upjohn Company, Division of Pfizer, Inc.; August 2010
Douillard JY et al. Lancet 2000;355:1041–1047
Tournigand C et al. J Clin Oncol 2004;22:229–237

Adverse Events

154 Cycles of Irinotecan + Temozolomide*

Casey DA et al. Pediatr Blood Cancer 2009;53:1029–1034

Toxicity	No. G3	No. G4	Percent G3/4
Diarrhea	7	0	7 (4.5%)
Colitis	1	0	1 (0.6%)
Neutropenia	12	7	19 (12.3%)
Thrombocytopenia[†]	13	3	16 (10.4%)
Pneumonitis	1	0	1 (0.6%)
Hospitalizations			
Febrile neutropenia	—	2	1 (1.2%)
Diarrhea/dehydration	—	3	1 (1.9%)
Colitis	—	1	1 (0.6%)
Pneumonitis	—	1	1 (0.6%)

*National Cancer Institute (USA) Common Toxicity Criteria, version 2.0 (NCI-CTC v2.0)
[†]150 cycles/19 patients. One patient had thrombocytopenia prior to enrollment

Toxicity	21-Day Schedule	28-Day Schedule	Cumulative
Total number of patients	9	7	16
Total number of courses	67	28	95
Median courses per patient (range)	6 (2–17)	3 (1–7)	5 (1–17)
Courses with Grade 3–4 neutropenia	1 (2%) of 59[†]	1 (4%) of 28	2 (2%)[‡]
10 mg/m² per day	0 of 24	1 (5%) of 21	—
15 mg/m² per day	0 of 12	0 of 7	—
20 mg/m² per day	1 (4%) of 23	—	—
Courses with G3/4 thrombocytopenia	1 (2%) of 59[†]	2 (7%) of 28	3 (3%)[‡]
10 mg/m² per day	0 of 24	2 (10%) of 21	—
15 mg/m² per day	0 of 12	0 of 7	—
20 mg/m² per day	1 (4%) of 23	—	—
Courses with G3/4 vomiting	5 (7%) of 67	3 (11%) of 28	8 (8%)
10 mg/m² per day	0 of 32	0 of 21	—
15 mg/m² per day	4 (33%) of 12	3 (43%) of 7	—
20 mg/m² per day	1 (4%) of 23	—	—
Courses with G3/4 diarrhea	6 (9%)	4 (14%)	10 (11%)
10 mg/m² per day	0 of 32	0 of 21	—
15 mg/m² per day	4 (33%) of 12	4 (57%) of 7	—
20 mg/m² per day	2 (9%) of 23	—	—

*NCI-CTC, v.2.0
[†]Of 59 courses assessable for hematologic toxicity
[‡]Of 87 total courses assessable for hematologic toxicity

THERAPY MONITORING

1. *Prior to treatment:* complete medical history, clinical examination, performance status, hematologic and serum chemistries, cardiac evaluation in case of prior treatment with anthracyclines or mediastinal irradiation, and tumor target assessment
2. *Day 1 of each treatment cycle:* physical examination, ECOG PS, complete blood count with leukocyte differential count, liver function tests, and serum chemistries
3. *Weekly CBC with leukocyte differential count:* at least the first 6 cycles of therapy
4. *After every 2 cycles of therapy:* tumor measurements

RECURRENT/ REFRACTORY • EWING SARCOMA

EWING SARCOMA REGIMEN: TEMOZOLOMIDE + IRINOTECAN (5 DAYS) ± VINCRISTINE

Raciborska A et al. Pediatr Blood Cancer 2013;60:1621–1625
Palmerini E et al. Acta Oncol 2018;57:958–964

Temozolomide 125 mg/m^2 per day; administer orally for 5 consecutive days, on days 1–5, 1 hour before irinotecan, every 21 days (total dosage/cycle = 625 mg/m^2)
Notes:
- Temozolomide doses are rounded to the nearest 5 mg by using commercially available products
- Patients who vomit after taking temozolomide should be instructed to take their next dose at the next regularly scheduled time

Irinotecan 50 mg/m^2 per day; administer intravenously, diluted with 5% dextrose injection to a concentration within the range of 0.12–2.8 mg/mL, over 90 minutes for 5 doses, on days 1–5, every 21 days (total dosage/cycle = 250 mg/m^2)
±Vincristine 1.5 mg/m^2 (maximum dose = 2 mg); administer by intravenous infusion over 15 minutes in 25–50 mL 0.9% sodium chloride injection (0.9% NS) on day 1, every 21 days (total dosage/cycle = 1.5 mg/m^2; maximum dosage/cycle = 2 mg)
- Dilute in 25 mL 0.9% NS for pediatric patients and in 50 mL 0.9% for adult patients

Supportive Care
Antiemetic prophylaxis
Emetogenic potential is **MODERATE**
See Chapter 42 for antiemetic recommendations

Hematopoietic growth factor (CSF) prophylaxis
Primary prophylaxis is NOT indicated
See Chapter 43 for more information

Antimicrobial prophylaxis
Risk of fever and neutropenia is *LOW*
   Antimicrobial primary prophylaxis to be considered:
- Antibacterial—not indicated
- Antifungal—not indicated
- Antiviral—not indicated unless patient previously had an episode of HSV

(continued)

Treatment Modifications

Irinotecan Dose Levels*

Level 1 starting dosage	50 mg/m^2 per day IV on days 1–5
Level −1	37.5 mg/m^2 per day IV on days 1–5
Level −2	25 mg/m^2 per day IV on days 1–5

Temozolomide Dose Levels

Level 1 starting dosage	125 mg/m^2 per day orally on days 1–5
Level −1	100 mg/m^2 per day orally on days 1–5
Level −2	75 mg/m^2 per day orally on days 1–5

Vincristine Dose Levels

Level 1 starting dosage	1.5 mg/m^2 (maximum of 2 mg) IV on day 1
Level −1	1.2 mg/m^2 (maximum of 1.6 mg) IV on day 1
Level −2	1 mg/m^2 (maximum of 1.3 mg) IV on day 1

Adverse Event	Dose Modification
G1 ANC 1500–1999/mm^3, or G1 thrombocytopenia during a cycle	Maintain dose and schedule
G2 ANC 1000–1499/mm^3, or G2 thrombocytopenia during a cycle	Reduce dosage of irinotecan and temozolomide by 1 dosage level. Maintain the dosage of vincristine (if used)
G4 neutropenia >7 days duration G3/4 infection	Reduce dosage of irinotecan and temozolomide for the following cycle by one dose level. Maintain the dosage of vincristine (if used)
Day 21 ANC <1000/mm^3, or platelet count <75,000/mm^3	Delay start of next cycle by 1 week and then reduce the dosage of irinotecan and temozolomide by one level and maintain the same dosage of vincristine (if used).
Day 28 ANC remains <1000/mm^3, or platelet count remains <75,000/mm^3, despite delaying next cycle by 1 week	Delay start of next cycle by 1 additional week and reduce dosage of irinotecan and temozolomide by one level
Day 35 ANC remains <1000/mm^3, or platelet count remains <75,000/mm^3, despite delaying next cycle by 2 weeks	Discontinue therapy

Diarrhea in Children 2–15 Years of Age

Children 2–15 years, with first liquid stools	Begin oral loperamide liquid immediately with the first liquid stool at a dosage of 0.18 mg/kg per day (0.03 mg/kg administered orally every 4 hours). Maximum single dose for patients weighing <13 kg is 0.5 mg loperamide; for 13 to <20 kg, 1 mg; for 20 to <43 kg, initially 2 mg then subsequently 1 mg; and for ≥43 kg, initially 4 mg then subsequently 2 mg
G3/4 diarrhea within the first 24 hours	Hospitalize for optimal management. Begin loperamide 0.06 mg/kg every 4 hours. Maximum single dose for patients weighing <13 kg is 0.5 mg loperamide; for 13 to <20 kg, 1 mg; for 20 to <43 kg, initially 2 mg then subsequently 1 mg; and for ≥43 kg, initially 4 mg then subsequently 2 mg Reduce irinotecan dosage for the following cycle by 1 dose level

(continued)

(continued)

Acute cholinergic syndrome

Atropine sulfate 0.25–1 mg subcutaneously or intravenously if abdominal cramping or diarrhea develop during or within 1 hour after irinotecan administration

- If symptoms are severe, add as primary prophylaxis at least 30 minutes before irinotecan during subsequent cycles
- For irinotecan, acute cholinergic syndrome may be characterized by abdominal cramping, diarrhea, diaphoresis, hypotension, flushing, bradycardia, rhinitis, increased salivation, meiosis, and lacrimation

Diarrhea management

Latent or delayed-onset diarrhea*:
Loperamide 4 mg orally initially after the first loose or liquid stool, *then* 2–4 mg orally every 2–4 hours or **diphenoxylate hydrochloride** 2.5 mg **with atropine sulfate** 0.025 mg (eg, Lomotil)

*Abigerges D et al. J Natl Cancer Inst 1994;86:446–449
Rothenberg ML et al. J Clin Oncol 2001;19:3801–3807
Wadler S et al. J Clin Oncol 1998;16:3169–3178

Treatment Modifications (*continued*)

Delayed Diarrhea in Patients >15 Years of Age

G1 (2–3 stools/day > baseline)	Maintain dose and schedule
G2 (4–6 stools/day > baseline)	Delay until diarrhea resolves to baseline, then reduce irinotecan dosage by 1 dosage level
G3 (7–9 stools/day > baseline)	Delay until diarrhea resolves to baseline, then reduce dosage of irinotecan by 1 dosage level
G4 (≥10 stools/day > baseline)	Delay until diarrhea resolves to baseline, then reduce dosage of irinotecan by 2 dosage levels

Neurotoxicity

G1/2 peripheral neuropathy	Reduce vincristine one dose level (if used)
Recurrent or persistent G1/2 peripheral neuropathy despite reduction of vincristine one dose level	Reduce vincristine one additional dose level (if used)
G ≥3 peripheral neuropathy	Discontinue vincristine (if used)

Other Nonhematologic Toxicities

Any G1 toxicity	Maintain dose and schedule
Any G2 toxicity	Hold treatment until toxicity resolves to G ≤1, then reduce dosage of attributable agents by 1 dosage level
Any G3 toxicity	Hold treatment until toxicity resolves to G ≤1, then reduce dosage of attributable agents by 1 dosage level
Any G4 toxicity	Hold treatment until toxicity resolves to G ≤1, then reduce dosage of attributable agents by 2 dosage levels

*Treatment should be stopped in case of recurrent toxicity at dose level −2, unless there is perceived clinical benefit from irinotecan that justifies continuation
André T et al. Eur J Cancer 1999;35:1343–1347
Camptosar irinotecan hydrochloride injection, product label. New York, NY: Pharmacia & Upjohn Company, Division of Pfizer, Inc.; August 2010
Douillard JY et al. Lancet 2000;355:1041–1047
Tournigand C et al. J Clin Oncol 2004;22:229–237

Therapy Monitoring

1. *Prior to treatment:* complete medical history, clinical examination, performance status, hematologic and serum chemistries, cardiac evaluation in case of prior treatment with anthracyclines or mediastinal irradiation, and tumor target assessment
2. *Day 1 of each treatment cycle:* physical examination, ECOG PS, complete blood count with leukocyte differential count, serum chemistries, liver function tests
3. *Weekly CBC with leukocyte differential count:* at least the first 6 cycles of therapy
4. *After every 2 cycles of therapy:* tumor measurements

Patient Population Studied

Retrospective review of data of 22 patients with relapsed or refractory ES treated with the combination of vincristine + irinotecan + temozolomide during the period 2008–2012

Patient and Treatment Characteristics at Time of Original Diagnosis (n=22)

Gender: male/female	16/6
Median age in years	14.3
Primary tumor location	
Extremity	8
Pelvis	9
Others	5
Metastasis at initial diagnosis	14
Site of metastases at diagnosis	
Lungs	6
Bones	2
Lungs+bones	1
Lungs+CNS	1
Lungs+bone marrow	1
Bone marrow	1
Lungs+bones+lymph nodes	1
Lymph nodes	1
Local treatment at diagnosis	
Surgery only	8
RTX only	1
Both	9
Primary chemotherapy	
VIDE regimen	18
CWS regimen	4
Bone marrow transplant	7
Reason for VIT therapy	
First relapse	10
Progression on primary therapy	9
Poor response to first-line CHT	3
Median TTR in months	12.3

n, number; TTR, time to relapse

Efficacy and Adverse Events

	Sites of Disease	Courses	Best Response	Toxicity (G3–4)	Reason for Stopped Therapy	Treatment After VIT	Status (Last Follow-up in Months)
1	Primary (pelvis), bone marrow	9	PR	Diarrhea	Progression	DTIC, trofosfamide	AWD (12.9)
2	Lung	17	CR	None	Elective cessation	Surgery, HSCT second relapse—DTIC	AWD (46.5)
3	Primary (pelvis), lung	6	PR	None	Progression	VP	DOD (12.1)
4	Primary (chest wall)	3	SD	None	Progression	—	DOD (30.8)
5	Lung, bone marrow	1	PD	Diarrhea	Progression	VP	DOD (16.6)
6	Primary (pelvis), bone	2	PR	None	Poor pathological response	PACE	DOD (13.0)
7	Primary (humerus)	4	CR	None	Elective cessation	Surgery, RT	NED (2.1)
8	Bone	2	PD	↓Platelets ↓WBC	Progression	—	DOD (9.6)
9	Primary (pelvis)	8	CR	None	Elective cessation	HSCT	NED (8.5)
10	Primary (pelvis), bone	2	PD	None	Progression	—	DOD (2.2)
11	Lung	1	PD	None	Progression	—	DOD (2.5)
12	Lung	5	CR	None	Poor pathological response	PACE, HSCT	NED (2.9)
13	Primary (scapula), lung	2	PD	None	Progression	—	DOD (12.2)
14	Primary (pelvis), lung	4	PR	None	AML	HSCT, trofosfamide	AWD (27.2)
15	Lung	2	CR	Diarrhea	Elective cessation	HSCT	NED (2.2)
16	Primary (spine), lung	3	SD	None	Elective cessation	PACE, HSCT	NED (10.4)
17	Primary (sacrum), bone, lung	2	SD	None	Refusal of treatment	Chinese verbs	AWD (8.2)
18	Primary (pelvis), lung, marrow	4	PR	None	Elective cessation	HSCT	DOD (18.5)
19	Primary (pelvis), lung	4	PR	None	Elective cessation	HSCT	AWD (10.2)
20	Lung	2	PD	None	Progression	VP	DOD (2.2)
21	Primary (pelvis), marrow	5	PR	None	Elective cessation	Surgery	DOD (11.5)
22	Primary (pelvis), lung	3	PD	None	Progression	—	DOD (9.1)

CR, complete response; PR, partial response; SD, stable disease; PD, progression disease; DOD, death of disease; NED, no evidence of disease; AWD, alive with disease; PACE, cisplatin, Adriamycin, cyclophosphamide, teniposide; VP, etoposide; DTIC, dacarbazine; RT, radiotherapy; HSCT, hematopoietic stem cell transplant; AML, acute myelo-blastic leukemia

RECURRENT/REFRACTORY • EWING SARCOMA

EWING SARCOMA REGIMEN: HIGH-DOSE IFOSFAMIDE (HDIFO)

Ferrari S et al. Pediatr Blood Cancer 2009;52:581–584

Hydration:

0.9% Sodium chloride injection (0.9% NS) 1000 mL (or 500 mL/m^2 in pediatric patients); administer intravenously over 2 hours once, beginning 2 hours prior to the start of chemotherapy on day 1

Administer additional intravenous hydration to achieve a total rate of 2000 mL/m^2/day (taking into account volumes of diluent used for mesna and ifosfamide administration) for the duration of high-dose ifosfamide treatment and continuing for 12 hours after the last dose

Mesna 400 mg/m^2; administer intravenously, diluted in a convenient volume of 0.9% NS sufficient to produce a final mesna concentration ranging from 1–20 mg/mL, over 15 minutes to 1 hour, once just before the start of the ifosfamide + mesna admixture on day 1 only, *followed by:*
An admixture containing **ifosfamide** 3,000 mg/m^2 + **mesna** 3,000 mg/m^2; administer intravenously, diluted in a convenient volume of 0.9% NS sufficient to produce a final ifosfamide concentration within the range 0.6–20 mg/mL, by continuous infusion over 24 hours, for 5 consecutive days, on days 1–5 (total ifosfamide dosage/cycle = 15,000 mg/m^2), *followed on day 6 by:*

Mesna 1500 mg/m^2; administer intravenously diluted in a convenient volume of 0.9% NS sufficient to produce a final mesna concentration ranging from 1–20 mg/mL, by continuous infusion over 12 hours once beginning immediately after completion of the ifosfamide infusion on day 6 (total mesna dosage/cycle = 16,900 mg/m^2; includes mesna administered before, with, and following ifosfamide)

Notes:

- The second course of high-dose ifosfamide is started when the post-nadir ANC is >1,000/mL and post-nadir platelet count is >100,000/mL, and if there was no evidence of progressive disease (PD)
- Although mesna is used before ifosfamide administration, ifosfamide, like cyclophosphamide, has to be metabolized to active (and toxic) metabolites *before* there is a need to protect the uroepithelium. Consequently, pretreating with mesna may be of little value
- The investigators included potassium chloride and sodium bicarbonate additives with the mesna/ifosfamide admixture; however, this is not practiced routinely
- According to the authors, the treatment plan differed according to the response following 2 cycles of high-dose ifosfamide and according to the previous treatment.
  - Patients who experienced disease progression after the initial 2 cycles of high-dose ifosfamide discontinued the treatment program
  - Patients who had a response of stable disease (SD) or better and who had not previously undergone high-dose chemotherapy with autologous hematopoietic stem cell transplant (auto-HSCT) entered a chemotherapy protocol with leukapheresis for peripheral blood stem cell collection scheduled after cyclophosphamide (4 g/m^2 day 1), etoposide (200 mg/m^2/day, days 2–4), followed by G-CSF 10 μg/kg/day administered subcutaneously. The minimum number of CD34 cells to collect was 3×10^6/kg. A consolidation treatment was then administered with melphalan 140 mg/m^2 IV, busulfan 16 mg/kg orally (total dose) delivered over 4 days (four times a day) followed by reinfusion of autologous hemopoietic stem cells
  - In case of SD or better and previous treatment with high-dose chemotherapy auto-HSCT, patients received two more cycles of high-dose ifosfamide. Patients who showed PD were addressed to other treatment on a clinical basis

Supportive Care

Antiemetic prophylaxis

Emetogenic potential is **HIGH** *each day of ifosfamide administration*
See Chapter 42 for antiemetic recommendations

Hematopoietic growth factor (CSF) prophylaxis

Primary prophylaxis is indicated with:
   Filgrastim (G-CSF) 5 μg/kg per dose; administer by subcutaneous injection once per day, *or:*
   Pegfilgrastim (pegylated filgrastim) 6 mg/0.6 mL, by subcutaneous injection for one dose
- Begin use from 24–72 h after myelosuppressive chemotherapy is completed
- Continue daily filgrastim use until ANC ≥1500/mm^3 after the leukocyte nadir
- Discontinue daily filgrastim use at least 24 hours before administering myelosuppressive treatment
- Do not administer pegfilgrastim within 14 days before administering myelosuppressive treatment
See Chapter 43 for more information

Antimicrobial prophylaxis
Risk of fever and neutropenia is HIGH

   Antimicrobial primary prophylaxis to be considered:
- Antibacterial—not indicated
- Antifungal—not indicated
- Antiviral—not indicated unless patient previously had an episode of HSV

Treatment Modifications

Adverse Event	Dose Modification
Day 1 ANC <1000/mm³ or platelet count <75,000/mm³	Delay by 1 week. Re-treat at full dose unless delayed by >1 week despite use of filgrastim, in which case reduce the dose by 20%
Febrile neutropenia occurring in the prior cycle	Reduce the ifosfamide and mesna doses by 20% in subsequent cycles and add filgrastim prophylaxis if not already receiving
SCr 1.5 × baseline	Delay by 1 week. If renal function does not improve, then discontinue ifosfamide
G2 renal toxicity—tubular (based on creatinine clearance, serum bicarbonate, need for electrolyte replacement, or TmP/GFR)	Reduce the ifosfamide and mesna doses by 20% in subsequent cycles
G ≥3 renal toxicity—tubular (based on creatinine clearance, serum bicarbonate, need for electrolyte replacement, or TmP/GFR)	Discontinue ifosfamide
Microscopic hematuria during ifosfamide therapy (>50 RBC/HPF) on >1 occasion	Discontinue ifosfamide for that cycle. If hematuria completely resolves, consider increasing the rate of intravenous fluids and/or the increasing the mesna dose in subsequent cycles
G ≥2 non-infective hemorrhagic cystitis (related to ifosfamide)	Discontinue ifosfamide and provide appropriate supportive care
G2 encephalopathy	If persistent or distressing, then decrease the ifosfamide and mesna dosages by 20%. If not contraindicated, treat with methylene blue 2 mg/kg (maximum dose of 50 mg) intravenously every 4–8 hours until resolution of symptoms, then consider prophylactic use at the same dose given every 6–8 hours in subsequent cycles
G3 encephalopathy	Stop ifosfamide for this cycle. If not contraindicated, treat with methylene blue 2 mg/kg (maximum dose of 50 mg) intravenously every 4–8 hours until resolution of symptoms, then consider prophylactic use at the same dose given every 6–8 hours in subsequent cycles. Decrease the ifosfamide and mesna dosages by 20% in subsequent cycles
G4 encephalopathy	Permanently discontinue ifosfamide. If not contraindicated, treat with methylene blue 2 mg/kg (maximum dose of 50 mg) intravenously every 4–8 hours until resolution of symptoms

Patient Population Studied

A study by the Italian Sarcoma Group and the Associazione Italiana Ematologia Oncologia Pediatrica (AIEOP) evaluated the activity and toxicity associated with high-dose ifosfamide in patients with recurrent Ewing sarcoma family tumors (EFT). Eligible participants were aged 3 to 50 years with a diagnosis of bone EFT and a history of prior treatment with chemotherapy protocols including standard-dose ifosfamide. High-dose ifosfamide was administered for metastatic disease in 33 participants and for progression during neoadjuvant chemotherapy in 4 patients

Patient Population (n = 37)

Median age at study entry: 17 yr (range 6–45 yr)	
Male sex	62%
Median time to relapse/progression:	15.8 mo (range 9–152 mo)
Pattern of recurrence at study entry, n	
Monolateral lung metastases	1
Bilateral lung metastases	16
Multiple metastatic sites	20
Previous treatment with high-dose and peripheral blood stem cell rescue, n	12
Previous median (range) cumulative dose of chemotherapy	
Ifosfamide	72 g/m² (18–72)
Doxorubicin	400 mg/m² (80–400)
Cyclophosphamide	6.6 g/m² (1.2–10.4)
Etoposide	1.8 g/m² (0.9–2.1)
Vincristine	18 mg/m² (3–18)
Dactinomycin	6 mg/m² (0–6)

Efficacy (N = 35)

Two-year Survival Rate After High-Dose Ifosfamide

Overall 2-year survival rate, % (95% CI)	29 (11–46)
2-year survival rate for patients who had a response after HDIFO, % (95% CI)	51 (20–82)
2-year survival rate for patients who had stable disease after HDIFO, % (95% CI)	31 (0–66)
2-year survival rate for patients who had progressive disease after HDIFO, %	0

Median Survival Time After High-Dose Ifosfamide

Median (range) survival after HDIFO for responders in months	12.3 (9–39)
Median (range) survival after HDIFO for stable disease, in months	8.7 (2–40)
Median survival time after HDIFO for progressive disease, in months	2.5 (1–11)

Best Response, n (%)

Complete Response	2 (6)
Partial Response	10 (29)
Stable Disease	11 (32)
Progressive Disease	12 (34)

Treatment Response Based on Prior Therapy*

Previously treated with high-dose chemotherapy (n = 12), n (%)	3 (25)
Not previously treated with high-dose chemotherapy (n = 23), n (%)	10 (43)

Treatment Response Based on Age†

Patients <19 years of age (n = 15), n (%)	8 (53)
Patients ≥19 years of age (n = 20), n (%)	5 (25)

*P = 0.3
†P = 0.09
Note: 37 patients were enrolled in the study but two were not evaluable for response
HDIFO, high-dose ifosfamide; CI, confidence interval

Adverse Events (N = 36*)

	Grade (% Unless Specified)		
	G1–2	G3	G4
Neutropenia	—	—	97
Neutropenic fever	—	—	22
Thrombocytopenia	—	—	54
CNS toxicity	14	1 patient†	—

*Rates of adverse events were reported relative to the number of evaluable cycles. There were 72 cycles evaluable for toxicity throughout the study period
†One patient only completed the first cycle of high-dose ifosfamide due to Grade 3 CNS toxicity
Note: the use of filgrastim was mandatory in the study protocol. No cases of renal tubular acidosis, cardiac toxicity, or significant changes in serum creatinine were recorded. Methylene blue was added in 4 cases with reversal of encephalopathy
CNS, central nervous system

Therapy Monitoring

1. *Prior to each cycle:* physical examination, ECOG PS, CBC with differential and platelet count, total bilirubin, ALT, AST, albumin, alkaline phosphatase, serum creatinine, BUN, calcium, carbon dioxide, chloride, glucose, potassium, sodium, and phosphate
2. *During chemotherapy administration:*
   a. *Daily laboratory investigations:* serum creatinine, BUN, calcium, carbon dioxide, chloride, glucose, potassium, sodium, and phosphate
   b. *Every 8 hours (or with each void):* urine dipstick for blood (microscopic urinalysis if >trace)
   c. *Other:* monitor fluid status (ie, weight and intake/output) and for signs and symptoms of neurologic toxicity
3. *At least once per week between cycles:* CBC with differential and platelet count, serum creatinine, BUN, calcium, carbon dioxide, chloride, glucose, potassium, sodium, and phosphate
4. *After every 2 cycles of therapy:* tumor measurements

RECURRENT/REFRACTORY • EWING SARCOMA

EWING SARCOMA REGIMEN: TRABECTEDIN PLUS IRINOTECAN

Herzog J et al. Sarcoma. 2016;2016:7461783

Trabectedin premedication:

Dexamethasone 20 mg; administer intravenously 30 minutes prior to each trabectedin infusion on day 1, every 3 weeks (total dosage/cycle = 20 mg)

Trabectedin 1.5 mg/m^2; administer intravenously in 500 mL 0.9% sodium chloride or 5% dextrose injection through a central venous access device over 24 hours on day 1, every 3 weeks (total dosage/cycle = 1.5 mg/m^2), *plus:*

Irinotecan 90 mg/m^2 per dose; administered orally, at least 2 hours before or after food, once daily for six doses on days 3–5 and days 10–12, every 3 weeks (total dosage/cycle = 540 mg/m^2)

- There is no commercially available formulation of irinotecan labeled for oral administration. Irinotecan injection (preservative-free, 20 mg/mL solution) may be dispensed for oral use. Each daily dose should be dispensed in a plastic oral syringe and a full cycle (6 doses) dispensed with instructions to refrigerate (2°–8°C [36°–46°F]) and protect from light, under which conditions stability for up to 21 days has been demonstrated. Instruct the patient to dilute each dose in 50 mL CranGrape juice (Ocean Spray, Lakeville-Middleboro, MA, USA) immediately prior to administration
  Drengler RL et al. J Clin Oncol 1999;17:685–696
  Furman WL et al. J Clin Oncol 2006;24:563–570
- The authors note that irinotecan should be administered orally when possible. However, an option for intravenous administration at the same dose (90 mg/m^2/dose) is provided for patients who cannot tolerate oral irinotecan. However, the pharmacokinetics of orally administered irinotecan differ markedly from that of irinotecan administered intravenously (eg, median bioavailability 0.09 [range, 0.01–0.52]), so a direct 1:1 conversion may be ill-advised

Furman WL et al. J Clin Oncol 2006;24:563–570

Supportive Care

Antiemetic prophylaxis
Emetogenic potential of trabectedin is **MODERATE**
Emetogenic potential of irinotecan is **MODERATE**
See Chapter 42 for antiemetic recommendations

Hematopoietic growth factor (CSF) prophylaxis
Primary prophylaxis is NOT indicated
See Chapter 43 for more information

Antimicrobial prophylaxis
Risk of fever and neutropenia is *LOW*
  Antimicrobial primary prophylaxis to be considered:
  - Antibacterial—not indicated
  - Antifungal—not indicated
  - Antiviral—not indicated unless patient previously had an episode of HSV

Diarrhea management
- The potential for developing diarrhea and abdominal pain should be discussed with all patients and their caretakers, and instructions given to start loperamide immediately if these symptoms occur and to ensure adequate hydration is maintained. See Dose Modifications (below) for instructions

Latent or delayed-onset diarrhea:
Loperamide 4 mg orally initially after the first loose or liquid stool, *then*
Loperamide 2 mg orally every 2 hours during waking hours, *plus*
Loperamide 4 mg orally every 4 hours during hours of sleep
- Loperamide doses are for patients >15 years of age. Refer to Treatment Modifications section for dosing in younger patients
- Continue for at least 12 hours after diarrhea resolves
- Recurrent diarrhea after a 12-hour diarrhea-free interval is treated as a new episode
- Rehydrate orally with fluids and electrolytes during a diarrheal episode

Treatment Modifications

Trabectedin Dose Levels

Starting Dose Level	1.5 mg/m^2
Level −1	1.2 mg/m^2
Level −2	1 mg/m^2

Irinotecan Dose Levels*

Starting Dose Level	90 mg/m^2/dose orally
Level −1	75 mg/m^2/dose orally
Level −2	60 mg/m^2/dose orally

Adverse Event	Dose Modification
Day 21 ANC <1500/mm^3, or platelet count <100,000/mm^3	Delay start of next cycle by up to 3 weeks until ANC >1500/mm^3, and platelet count >100,000/mm^3 then reduce dose of irinotecan and trabectedin for the following cycle by one dose level
Day 42 ANC remains <1000/mm^3, or platelet count remains <75,000/mm^3, despite delaying next cycle by 3 weeks	Discontinue therapy
Platelet count <25,000/mm^3 during prior cycle	Reduce dose of trabectedin and irinotecan for the following cycle by one dose level
ANC <1000/mm^3 with fever/infection during prior cycle	
ANC <500/mm^3 lasting ≥5 days during prior cycle	
• LVEF less than lower limit of normal • G3/4 cardiac adverse event indicative of cardiomyopathy • Severe liver dysfunction in the prior treatment cycle • Capillary leak syndrome • Rhabdomyolysis	Discontinue trabectedin

(continued)

(continued)

- If a patient develops blood or mucus in stool, dehydration, or hemodynamic instability, or if diarrhea persists >48 hours despite loperamide, stop loperamide and hospitalize the patient for IV hydration
- Alternatively, a trial of **Diphenoxylate hydrochloride** 2.5 mg **with atropine sulfate** 0.025 mg (eg, Lomotil)
- Initial adult dose is 2 tablets 4 times daily until control has been achieved, after which the dose may be reduced to meet individual requirements. Control may often be maintained with as little as 2 tablets daily
- Clinical improvement of acute diarrhea is usually observed within 48 hours. If improvement of chronic diarrhea after treatment with a maximum daily dose of 8 tablets is not observed within 10 days, control is unlikely with further administration

Persistent diarrhea:
Octreotide 100–150 µg subcutaneously 3 times daily (adult dose). Maximum total daily adult dose is 1500 µg. Pediatric patients may initiate dosing at 1–10 µg/kg/dose every 8–12 hours (not to exceed 1500 µg per day)

Antibiotic primary prophylaxis and treatment during latent or delayed-onset diarrhea:
Consider the following to prevent or lessen irinotecan-associated diarrhea:
- Prophylactic oral **cefixime** 8 mg/kg (maximum dose of 400 mg) orally once daily, beginning 1–2 days prior to the start of irinotecan therapy and continuing until completion of the cycle, *alternatively:*
- **Cefpodoxime proxetil** 5 mg/kg/day per day orally twice daily with food (maximum dose of 200 mg twice daily)
  - Previous studies suggest prophylaxis with cephalosporin antibiotics can ameliorate irinotecan-associated diarrhea by reducing the enteric bacteria responsible for producing β-glucuronidase, which regenerates in the gut irinotecan's toxic metabolite, SN-38, by cleaving the glucuronide moiety from SN–38 (Wagner LM et al. Pediatr Blood Cancer 2008;50:201–207)
- Alternatively, **activated charcoal** at a dose equal to 5 times the irinotecan dose up to a maximum dose of 260 mg orally 3 times daily during irinotecan therapy (Michael M et al. J Clin Oncol 2004;22:4410–4417)

Antibiotic treatment during latent or delayed-onset diarrhea:
- A fluoroquinolone (eg, ciprofloxacin 500 mg orally every 12 hours) if absolute neutrophil count <500/mm^3 with or without accompanying fever in association with diarrhea Antibiotics should also be administered if a patient is hospitalized with prolonged diarrhea, and should be continued until diarrhea resolves

*Abigerges D et al. J Natl Cancer Inst 1994;86:446–449
Rothenberg ML et al. J Clin Oncol 2001;19:3801–3807
Wadler S et al. J Clin Oncol 1998;16:3169–3178

Patient Population Studied

This multinational case series included 12 patients with translocation-positive pediatric-type refractory and end-stage sarcomas who were deemed to have no conventional treatment options remaining. This case series reported the efficacy and toxicity of off-label, compassionate use chemotherapy with trabectedin and irinotecan. All patients had metastatic, progressive disease at the initiation of therapy and had been pretreated with standard chemotherapy protocols and at least one second-line therapy

Patient Population	
Median (range) age at diagnosis, years	18 (6–57)
Median (range) age at therapy initiation, years	26 (12–60)
Male sex	67%
Ewing sarcoma	67%
Prior therapy with irinotecan	50%
Median number of prior chemotherapy regimens	4
Prior radiation therapy	92%

Treatment Modifications
(continued)

• ALT or AST ≥2.5 × ULN • Creatine phosphokinase (CPK) ≥2.5 × ULN	Delay next dose of trabectedin for up to 3 weeks
• ALT or AST ≥5 × ULN • Creatine phosphokinase (CPK) ≥5 × ULN • ≥10% absolute decrease in LVEF from baseline	Reduce next dose of trabectedin by one dose level
• Total bilirubin ≥ULN	Delay next dose of trabectedin for up to 3 weeks until values recover to pre-treatment values then reduce next dose of trabectedin by one dose level

Diarrhea in Children 2–15 Years of Age

Children 2–15 years, with first liquid stools	Begin oral loperamide liquid immediately with the first liquid stool at a dosage of 0.18 mg/kg per day (0.03 mg/kg administered orally every 4 hours). Maximum single dose for patients weighing <13 kg is 0.5 mg loperamide; for 13 to <20 kg, 1 mg; for 20 to <43 kg, initially 2 mg then subsequently 1 mg; and for ≥43 kg, initially 4 mg then subsequently 2 mg
G3/4 diarrhea within the first 24 hours	Hospitalize for optimal management. Begin loperamide 0.06 mg/kg every 4 hours. Maximum single dose for patients weighing <13 kg is 0.5 mg loperamide; for 13 to <20 kg, 1 mg; for 20 to <43 kg, initially 2 mg then subsequently 1 mg; and for ≥43 kg, initially 4 mg then subsequently 2 mg. Reduce irinotecan dosage for the following cycle by 1 dose level

(continued)

Efficacy (N = 12)

Survival	
Median survival, months	6.4

Overall Survival by Response, Months (Range)

Patients with at least stable disease	**11.7 (3.0–25.8)**
Patients with no response	5.3 (2.2–9.2)

Best Response, n (%)

Partial remission	1 (8)
Stable disease	5 (42)
Progressive disease	6 (50)

Patients with Ewing Sarcoma (n = 7)*

Best response stable disease or better, n (%)	4 (57)
Median (range) survival with trabectedin-irinotecan†, months	6.6 (2.2–13.6)
Median (range) survival of matched-pairs†, months	5.8 (0.2–17.4)

*Of 8 patients with Ewing sarcoma, 7 were evaluable for response. One patient was censored
†A matched-pair analysis was conducted for patients with Ewing sarcoma using the blinded retrospective data from the EURO-E.W.I.N.G 99/EWING 2008 trial. Of 8 patients receiving trabectedin-irinotecan, 6 were matched successfully based on age, sex, metastasized primary disease, time to first relapse, number of relapses, and type of relapse. The matched pair analysis did not show a significant difference in survival between groups (P = 0.976). Median survival was observed to be longer with the trabectedin-irinotecan group (P = 0.808)

Adverse Events (N = 12)

Grade (%)	Grade 3	Grade 4
Hepatotoxicity	33	25
Pancytopenia*	—	33
Leukopenia	8	17
Febrile neutropenia	—	17
Mucositis	17	—
Infection	8	8
Diarrhea	8	8
Thrombocytopenia	—	8
Pancreatitis	8	—

*All patients experienced Grade 3 or Grade 4 hematologic toxicity though neutropenia was the most common

Therapy Monitoring

1. *Prior to each cycle:* physical examination, ECOG PS, CBC with differential and platelet count, liver function tests (total bilirubin, ALT, AST, albumin, alkaline phosphatase), serum creatinine, BUN, serum electrolytes, creatine phosphokinase, assessment of diarrhea (patients should have baseline bowel function without antidiarrheal therapy prior to commencement of each cycle)
2. *At least once per week:* CBC with differential and platelet count, serum creatinine, BUN, serum electrolytes, liver function tests
3. *Prior to each cycle and then every 2–3 months (or sooner if clinically indicated):* assessment of LVEF by echocardiogram or multigated acquisition scan
4. *After every 2 cycles of therapy:* tumor

Treatment Modifications
(continued)

Delayed Diarrhea in Patients >15 Years of Age

G1 (2–3 stools/day > baseline)	Maintain dose and schedule
G2 (4–6 stools/day > baseline)	Delay until diarrhea resolves to baseline, then reduce irinotecan dosage by 1 dosage level
G3 (7–9 stools/day > baseline)	Delay until diarrhea resolves to baseline, then reduce dosage of irinotecan by 1 dosage level
G4 (≥10 stools/day > baseline)	Delay until diarrhea resolves to baseline, then reduce dosage of irinotecan by 2 dosage levels

Other Nonhematologic Toxicities

Any G1 toxicity	Maintain dose and schedule
Any G2 toxicity	Hold treatment until toxicity resolves to G ≤1, then reduce dosage of both agents by 1 dosage level
Any G3 toxicity	Hold treatment until toxicity resolves to G ≤1, then reduce dosage of both agents by 1 dosage level
Any G4 toxicity	Hold treatment until toxicity resolves to G ≤1, then reduce dosage of both agents by 2 dosage levels

*Treatment should be stopped in case of recurrent toxicity at dose level −2, unless there is perceived clinical benefit from irinotecan that justifies continuation
André T et al. Eur J Cancer 1999;35:1343–1347
Camptosar irinotecan hydrochloride injection, product label. New York, NY: Pharmacia & Upjohn Company, Division of Pfizer, Inc.; August 2010
Douillard JY et al. Lancet 2000;355:1041–1047
Tournigand C et al. J Clin Oncol 2004;22:229–237

ADULT SOFT-TISSUE SARCOMAS (INCLUDING RHABDOMYOSARCOMA, BUT NOT INCLUDING GIST)

Epidemiology

Incidence:	13,130 (male: 7.470; female: 5,660. Estimated new cases for 2020 in the United States)
Deaths:	Estimated 5,350 in 2014 (male: 2,870; female: 2,480)
Male to female ratio:	1.2:1

American Cancer Society. *Cancer Facts & Figures 2020*. Atlanta: American Cancer Society; 2020

Cellular Classification of *Adult Soft-Tissue Sarcoma*

Soft-tissue sarcomas are classified histologically according to the soft-tissue cell of origin. The histologic grade reflects the metastatic potential of these tumors more accurately than the classic cellular classification listed below. Pathologists assign grade based on the number of mitoses per high-powered field, presence of necrosis, cellular and nuclear morphology, and the degree of cellularity. Discordance among expert pathologists can reach 40%

Alphabetical Listing of Major Diseases with Estimates of Percentage of *All Soft-Tissue Sarcomas*—Note, however, that the frequency of histologic type is site dependent

- Alveolar soft-part sarcoma (≤3%)
- Angiosarcoma (≤3%)
- Dermatofibrosarcoma protuberans (≤3%)
- Epithelioid sarcoma (≤3%)
- Extraskeletal chondrosarcoma (≤3%)
- Extraskeletal osteosarcoma (≤3%)
- Fibrosarcoma (≤3%)
- Gastrointestinal stromal tumor (GIST) (≤3%) (see separate section on GIST)
- **Leiomyosarcoma (~12%)**
- **Liposarcoma (~15–25%)**
- **Malignant fibrous histiocytoma (~28–40%)**
- Malignant hemangiopericytoma (≤3%)
- Malignant mesenchymoma (≤3%)
- Malignant schwannoma (≤3%)
- **Malignant peripheral nerve sheath tumor (MPNST) (~6%)**
- Peripheral neuroectodermal tumors (≤3%)
- *Rhabdomyosarcoma* **(~5%)** *(see separate section on rhabdomyosarcoma)*
- **Synovial sarcoma (~10%)**
- Sarcoma, NOS (not otherwise specified) (≤3%)

Abraham JA et al. Ann Surg Oncol 2007;14:1953–1967
Alvegård TA, Berg NO. J Clin Oncol 1989;7:1845–1851
Fayette J et al. Ann Oncol 2007;18:2030–2036
Fury MG et al. Cancer J 2005;11:241–247
Gaynor JJ et al. J Clin Oncol 1992;10:1317–1329
Marcus SG et al. Arch Surg 1993;128:1336–1343
Mendenhall WM et al. Cancer 2004;101:2503–2508
van Ruth S et al. Eur J Cancer 2002;38:1324–1328
de Pinieux G et al. PLoS One. 2021;16:e0246958

Disease Distribution

Extremity		45%
Lower		30%
Upper		15%
Intra-abdominal		38%
Visceral		21%
Retroperitoneal		17%
Trunk		10%
Head and Neck		5%

Samuel Singer, William D. Tap, David G. Kirsch, and Aimee M. Crago
Soft tissue sarcoma. In: *DeVita V, Lawrence T, Rosenberg S, eds. DeVita, Hellman, and Rosenberg's Cancer Principles & Practice of Oncology. 11th ed. (2019)*

Soft-Tissue Sarcomas, Other Than GIST

1. Fibrous tumors
   a. Fibrosarcoma:
      (1) Adult fibrosarcoma
      (2) Inflammatory fibrosarcoma
2. Fibrohistiocytic tumors
   a. Malignant fibrous histiocytoma
      (1) Storiform-pleomorphic
      (2) Myxoid (myxofibrosarcoma)
      (3) Giant cell (malignant giant cell tumor of the soft parts)
      (4) Inflammatory
3. Lipomatous
   a. Liposarcoma
      (1) Well-differentiated liposarcoma
         (a) Lipoma-like liposarcomas
         (b) Sclerosing liposarcoma
         (c) Inflammatory liposarcoma
      (2) Dedifferentiated liposarcoma
      (3) Myxoid or round cell liposarcoma
      (4) Pleomorphic liposarcoma
4. Smooth muscle tumors
   a. Leiomyosarcoma
   b. Epithelioid leiomyosarcoma
5. Skeletal muscle tumors
   a. Rhabdomyosarcoma
      (1) Embryonal rhabdomyosarcoma (includes botryoid rhabdomyosarcoma)
      (2) Spindle cell rhabdomyosarcoma
      (3) Alveolar rhabdomyosarcoma
      (4) Pleomorphic rhabdomyosarcoma
   b. Rhabdomyosarcoma with ganglionic differentiation (ectomesenchymoma)
6. Tumors of the blood and lymph nodes
   a. Epithelioid hemangioendothelioma
   b. Angiosarcoma and lymphangiosarcoma
   c. Kaposi sarcoma
7. Perivascular tumors
   a. Malignant glomus tumor (glomangiosarcoma)
   b. Malignant hemangiopericytoma
8. Synovial tumors

   a. Malignant giant cell tumor of tendon sheath
9. Neural tumors
   a. Malignant peripheral nerve sheath tumor (MPNST)
      (1) Malignant triton tumor (MPSNT with rhabdomyosarcoma)
      (2) Glandular MPNST
      (3) Epithelioid MPNST
   b. Malignant granular cell tumor
   c. Primitive neuroectodermal tumor
      (1) Neuroblastoma
      (2) Ganglioneuroblastoma
      (3) Neuroepithelioma (peripheral neuroectodermal tumor)
10. Paraganglionic tumors
    a. Malignant paraganglioma
11. Extraskeletal cartilaginous and osseous tumors
    a. Extraskeletal chondrosarcoma
       (1) Myxoid chondrosarcoma
       (2) Mesenchymal chondrosarcoma
    b. Extraskeletal osteosarcoma
12. Pluripotential mesenchymal tumors
    a. Malignant mesenchyma
13. Miscellaneous tumors
    a. Alveolar soft-part sarcoma
    b. Epithelioid sarcoma
    c. Malignant extrarenal rhabdoid tumor
    d. Desmoplastic small cell tumor
    e. Ewing sarcoma—extraskeletal
    f. Clear cell sarcoma
    g. Gastrointestinal stromal tumors
    h. Synovial sarcoma
    i. Dermatofibrosarcoma protuberans

DeVita V, Lawrence T, Rosenberg S, eds. DeVita, Hellman, and Rosenberg's Cancer Principles & Practice of Oncology. 11th ed. (2019)

Clinical Staging

TNM CLASSIFICATION FOR SOFT-TISSUE SARCOMA

The revised AJCC Cancer Staging Manual, Eighth edition classifies soft-tissue sarcoma based on TNM and tumor grade (G). The AJCC follows the grading system of the French Federation of Cancer Centers Sarcoma Group (FNCLCC). Tumor grade (G) is based on cellular differentiation, mitotic rate, and extent of necrosis, as outlined in the Table

HISTOLOGIC GRADE (G) FOR SOFT-TISSUE SARCOMA

Tumor Differentiation	Mitotic Count	Tumor Necrosis
Sarcoma closely resembling normal adult mesenchymal tissue (eg, low-grade leiomyosarcoma (1 point)	0–9 mitoses per 10 HPF (1 point)	No necrosis (0 points)
Sarcomas for which histologic typing is certain (eg, myxoid/round cell liposarcoma) (2 points)	10–19 mitoses per 10 HPF (2 points)	<50% tumor necrosis (1 point)
Embryonal and undifferentiated sarcomas, sarcomas of doubtful type, synovial sarcomas, soft tissue osteosarcoma, Ewing sarcoma/ primitive neuroectodermal tumor (PNET) of soft tissue (3 points)	≥20 mitoses per 10 HPF (3 points)	≥50% tumor necrosis (2 points)

Note: the scores for these variables are added to calculate the following G values:
- GX: Grade cannot be assessed
- G1: Total score of 2 or 3
- G2: Total score of 4 or 5
- G3: Total score of 6 or higher

Notes:
Histology and grade are critical components of staging
Lymph node involvement is not characteristic of most sarcomas except rhabdomyosarcoma and synovial, clear cell, vascular, and epithelioid sarcomas

Separate staging systems have been created based on anatomic location and type as follows:
- Soft-tissue sarcoma of the head and neck
- Soft-tissue sarcoma of the trunk and extremities
- Soft-tissue sarcoma of the abdomen and thoracic visceral organs
- Soft-tissue sarcoma of the retroperitoneum

Note: these guidelines do not pertain to the management of gastrointestinal stroma tumors (GISTs), rhabdomyosarcoma, Ewing sarcoma, desmoplastic round cell tumors, and primitive neuroectodermal tumors

Soft-Tissue Sarcoma of the Trunk and Extremities

TNM Classification for Soft-Tissue Sarcoma of the Trunk and Extremities

Primary tumor (T)

TX	Primary tumor cannot be assessed
T0	No evidence for primary tumor
T1	Tumor ≤5 cm in greatest dimension
T2	Tumor >5 cm to ≤10 cm in greatest dimension
T3	Tumor >10 cm to ≤15 cm in greatest dimension
T4	Tumor is >15 cm

Regional lymph nodes (N)

N0	No regional lymph node metastasis or nodes cannot be assessed
N1	Regional lymph node metastasis

Distant metastasis (M)

M0	No distant metastasis
M1	Distant metastasis

Histologic Grade (G)

GX	Grade cannot be assessed
G1	Grade 1
G2	Grade 2
G3	Grade 3

Grade is determined using the **French or FNCLCC system**, and is based on 3 factors:
- **Differentiation:** Cancer cells are given a score of 1 to 3, with 1 being assigned well-differentiated cells and 3 to poorly differentiated cells
- **Mitotic count:** Given a score from 1 to 3
- **Tumor necrosis:** Given a score from 0 to 2

GX: The grade cannot be assessed (because of incomplete information)
Grade 1 (G1): Total score of 2 or 3
Grade 2 (G2): Total score of 4 or 5
Grade 3 (G3): Total score of 6, 7 or 8

Anatomic Stage/Prognostic Groups

Stage	T	N	M	Histologic grade
Stage IA	T1	N0	M0	G1, GX
Stage IB	T2	N0	M0	G1, GX
	T3	N0	M0	G1, GX
	T4	N0	M0	G1, GX
Stage II	T1	N0	M0	G2, G3
Stage IIIA	T2	N0	M0	G2, G3
Stage IIIB	T3	N0	M0	G2, G3
	T4	N0	M0	G2, G3
Stage IV	Any T	N1	M0	Any G
	Any T	Any N	M1	Any G

Soft-Tissue Sarcoma of the Retroperitoneum

TNM Classification for Soft-Tissue Sarcoma of the Retroperitoneum

Primary tumor (T)

TX	Primary tumor cannot be assessed
T0	No evidence for primary tumor
T1	Tumor ≤5 cm in greatest dimension
T2	Tumor >5 cm to ≤10 cm in greatest dimension
T3	Tumor >10 cm to ≤15 cm in greatest dimension
T4	Tumor is >15 cm

Regional lymph nodes (N)

N0	No regional lymph node metastasis or nodes cannot be assessed
N1	Regional lymph node metastasis

Distant metastasis (M)

M0	No distant metastasis
M1	Distant metastasis

Histologic Grade (G)

GX	Grade cannot be assessed
G1	Grade 1
G2	Grade 2
G3	Grade 3

Grade is determined using the **French or FNCLCC system**, and is based on 3 factors:
- **Differentiation:** Cancer cells are given a score of 1 to 3, with 1 being assigned well-differentiated cells and 3 to poorly differentiated cells
- **Mitotic count:** Given a score from 1 to 3
- **Tumor necrosis:** Given a score from 0 to 2

GX: The grade cannot be assessed (because of incomplete information)
Grade 1 (G1): Total score of 2 or 3
Grade 2 (G2): Total score of 4 or 5
Grade 3 (G3): Total score of 6, 7 or 8

Anatomic Stage/Prognostic Groups

Stage	T	N	M	Histologic grade
Stage IA	T1	N0	M0	G1, GX
Stage IB	T2	N0	M0	G1, GX
	T3	N0	M0	G1, GX
	T4	N0	M0	G1, GX
Stage II	T1	N0	M0	G2, G3
Stage IIIA	T2	N0	M0	G2, G3
Stage IIIB	T3	N0	M0	G2, G3
	T4	N0	M0	G2, G3
	Any T	N1	M0	Any G
Stage IV	Any T	Any N	M1	Any G

Soft-Tissue Sarcoma of the Head and Neck

(Soft-tissue sarcoma of the head and neck is a new classification and anatomic staging and prognostic groups have not yet been defined due to a lack of data)

Tnm Classification for Soft-Tissue Sarcoma of the Head and Neck

Primary tumor (T)	
TX	Primary tumor cannot be assessed
T1	Tumor ≤2 cm in greatest dimension
T2	Tumor >2 cm to ≤4 cm in greatest dimension
T3	Tumor >4 cm
T4	Tumor with invasion of adjoining structures
T4a	Tumor with orbital invasion, skull base/dural invasion, invasion of central compartment viscera, involvement of facial skeleton or involvement of pterygoid muscles
T4b	Tumor with brain parenchymal invasion, carotid artery encasement, prevertebral muscle invasion or central nervous system involvement via perineural spread

Regional lymph nodes (N)	
N0	No regional lymph node metastasis or nodes cannot be assessed
N1	Regional lymph node metastasis

Distant metastasis (M)	
M0	No distant metastasis
M1	Distant metastasis

Note: regarding the newly described soft-tissue sarcoma of the "head and neck" in the eighth edition, each T factor has different criteria as shown. However, the prognostic stage groups of soft-tissue sarcomas in these sites are not defined

Soft-Tissue Sarcoma of the Abdomen and Thoracic Visceral Organs

(There is currently no recommended prognostic stage grouping)

TNM Classification for Soft-Tissue Sarcoma of the Abdomen and Thoracic Visceral Organs

Primary tumor (T)	
TX	Primary tumor cannot be assessed
T1	Organ confined
T2	Tumor extension into tissue beyond organ
T2a	Invades serosa or visceral peritoneum
T2b	Extension beyond serosa (mesentery)
T3	Invades another organ
T4	Multifocal involvement
T4a	Multifocal (2 sites)
T4b	Multifocal (3–5 sites)
T4b	Multifocal (>5 sites)

Regional lymph nodes (N)	
N0	No regional lymph node metastasis or nodes cannot be assessed
N1	Regional lymph node metastasis

Distant metastasis (M)	
M0	No distant metastasis
M1	Distant metastasis

Note: regarding the newly described soft-tissue sarcoma of the "abdomen and thoracic visceral organs" in the eighth edition, each T factor has different criteria as shown. However, the prognostic stage groups of soft-tissue sarcomas in these sites are not defined

Work-up

1. History and physical examination
2. *Laboratory tests:* CBC with differential; electrolytes including calcium, phosphorus, and magnesium; renal function tests including blood urea nitrogen (BUN) and creatinine; liver function tests including liver enzymes and total bilirubin; alkaline phosphatase; lactate dehydrogenase (LDH)
3. Radiologic imaging modality is variable and dictated by the site of disease. This involves a combination of plain x-rays, CT, MRI, and PET imaging. Although CT remains the imaging modality of choice in the staging of retroperitoneal soft-tissue sarcoma, MRI is used more frequently to stage soft-tissue sarcoma of the extremity
4. Bilateral bone marrow aspirate and biopsy for light microscopy examination in Ewing sarcoma (optional; Kopp LM et al. Pediatr Blood Cancer 2015;62:12–5.)
5. No radiologic studies are pathognomonic, so biopsy remains essential to diagnosis. Carefully plan biopsy to establish grade and histologic subtype and if needed molecular and cytogenetic studies
6. Echocardiogram or MUGA scan to determine cardiac ejection fraction as clinically indicated

SOFT-TISSUE SARCOMAS: ARISING FROM LIMBS AND SUPERFICIAL TRUNK

Expert Opinion

Note: levels of Evidence (I–V) and Grades of Recommendation (A–D) are as used by the American Society of Clinical Oncology

Casali PG, Blay JY. Soft tissue sarcomas: ESMO clinical practice guidelines for diagnosis, treatment and follow-up. ESMO/CONTICANET/EUROBONET Consensus Panel of experts. Ann Oncol 2010;21 Suppl 5:v198–v203.

Incidence

Adult soft-tissue sarcomas are rare tumors, with an estimated incidence averaging 5/100,000 population per year in Europe

Diagnosis and General Guidelines

- Multidisciplinary approach is mandatory in all cases; ideally in referral centers
- Enrollment in clinical trials is highly encouraged
- Biopsy options:
  - Standard approach: multiple core needle biopsies (using needles >16G)
  - Excisional biopsy may be the most practical option for superficial lesions <5 cm
  - Open biopsy is another option
- Frozen-section technique for immediate diagnosis is not encouraged
- Biopsy should be performed in such a way that the biopsy pathway and the scar can be safely removed on definitive surgery. The biopsy entrance point is preferably tattooed
- Tumor samples should be fixed in formalin (Bouin fixation should not be performed because it prevents molecular analysis)
- Recommend using a grading system that distinguishes 3 malignancy grades based on differentiation, necrosis, and mitotic rate (The Federation Nationale des Centres de Lutte Contre le Cancer [FNCLCC] grading system, also used by the WHO)
- If preoperative treatment was carried out, the pathology report should include a tumor response assessment. However, in contrast to osteosarcoma and Ewing sarcoma, no validated system is available at present, and no percentage of residual "viable cells" is considered to have a specific prognostic significance
- Collection of fresh-frozen tissue and tumor imprints (touch preps) with appropriate consent is encouraged, because new molecular pathology assessments could be made at a later stage

Stage Classification and Risk Assessment

- The American Joint Committee on Cancer (AJCC)/International Union against Cancer (UICC) stage classification system stresses the importance of the malignancy grade in sarcoma. However, its use in routine practice is limited
- Prognostic factors:
  1. Tumor grade
  2. Tumor size
  3. Tumor depth
  4. Tumor resectability

Staging Procedures

A chest spiral CT scan is mandatory for staging purposes
Depending on the histologic type and other clinical features, further staging assessments may be recommended (ie, regional lymph node clinical assessment for synovial sarcoma, epithelioid sarcoma, alveolar soft-part sarcoma, clear cell sarcoma; abdominal CT scan for myxoid liposarcoma, etc)

Treatment

Limited Disease

- Surgery is the standard treatment for all patients with adult type, localized soft-tissue sarcomas
- Standard surgical procedure is a wide excision with negative margins (R0). This implies removing the tumor with a rim of normal tissue around
- An excision with small margins may be acceptable in highly selected cases, in particular for extracompartmental atypical lipomatous tumors

Follow-up

- There are no published data to indicate the optimal routine follow-up policy of surgically treated patients with localized disease
- Malignancy grade affects the likelihood and speed at which relapses may take place. Risk assessment is based on:
  - Tumor grade
  - Tumor size
  - Tumor site
- High-risk patients generally relapse within 2–3 years
- Low-risk patients may relapse later, and relapse is less likely
- Relapses most often occur to the lungs
- Early detection of local or metastatic recurrence to the lungs may have prognostic implications. Lung metastases typically are asymptomatic at a stage in which they are suitable for surgery

Suggested follow-up for patients with high risk sarcoma is: every 3-4 months for 2 years and then every 6 months until year 5 and annually thereafter. Evaluation should typically focus on early detection of local or metastatic recurrence to lung. Suggested imaging include

- Non contrast chest CT for detection of pulmonary metastases (CXR may also be considered)
- Imaging of primary tumor with CT or MRI (ultrasound or clinial evaluation may be considered based on tumor site)
- FDG-PET, bone scan or MRI for detection of bony metastases if symptomatic

Suggested follow-up for low-grade sarcoma patients: followed for local relapse every 4–6 months, with chest X-rays or CT scan at more relaxed intervals in the first 3–5 years, then yearly

Roberts et al, J Am Coll Radiol 2016; 13:389–400.

5-Year Survival

Nonmetastatic (80% of Patients at Diagnosis)	
Stage II	70%
Stage III	25%
Metastatic (20% of Patients at Diagnosis)	20%

(continued)

Expert Opinion (*continued*)

Radiation Therapy (RT):

1. *High-grade, deep lesions, >5 cm:* Wide excision followed by RT
2. *High-grade, deep, <5 cm:* Surgery followed by RT
3. *Low-grade, superficial, >5 cm, and low-grade, deep, <5 cm STS:* RT occasionally used
4. *Low-grade, deep, >5 cm STS:* Discuss RT in a multidisciplinary fashion

Notes:

- RT is not given in the case of a truly compartmental resection of a tumor entirely contained within the compartment
- Overall, RT has been shown to improve local control, but not overall survival
- Timing and approach of RT depends on multiple factors and requires a multidisciplinary approach
- Postoperative RT: Follows marginal or R1 (microscopic residual disease) or R2 (gross residual disease) excisions, if these cannot be rescued through re-excision even outside of usual indications as described above; Dose 50–60 Gy, 1.8–2 Gy fractions, possibly with boosts up to 66 Gy
- Preoperative RT: 50 Gy. Preoperative RT allows for lower radiation dose to smaller target volume. Given risks and benefits of pre-operative RT, timing of RT should be individualized
- Intraoperative radiation therapy (IORT) and brachytherapy: In selected cases
- Local relapse: Approach parallels approach to primary local disease, except for a wider resort to preoperative or postoperative radiation therapy, if not previously performed
- For pediatric patients, the Children's Oncology Group (COG) recommends RT for high grade tumors that are either >5 cm (with chemotherapy) or ≤5 cm with R1 resection

Kaushal A, Citrin D. Surg Clin North Am. 2008; 88:629–46
Spunt et al. Lancet Oncol. 2020; 21:145–161

Surgery:

- Definitions:
  - R0 resection—No residual microscopic disease
  - R1 resection—Microscopic residual disease (presence of tumor cells on resection margins)
  - R2 resection—Gross residual disease
    - R1 resections: Consider reoperation if adequate margins can be achieved without major morbidity, taking into account tumor extent and tumor biology
- R2 surgery: Reoperation is mandatory, possibly with preoperative treatments if adequate margins cannot be achieved, or surgery is mutilating. In the latter case, the use of multimodal therapy with less-radical surgery requires shared decision making with the patient under conditions of uncertainty
- In nonresectable tumors, or those amenable only to mutilating surgery, options that can be considered include:
  - Chemotherapy and/or radiotherapy
  - Isolated hyperthermic limb perfusion with tumor necrosis factor α (TNF-α) + melphalan, if the tumor is confined to an extremity
  - Regional hyperthermia combined with chemotherapy

Note:

Adjuvant chemotherapy

- Might improve, or at least delay, distant and local recurrence in high-risk patients
- A meta-analysis found a statistically significant, limited benefit in terms of both survival and relapse-free survival. However, studies are conflicting, and a final demonstration of efficacy is lacking
- Therefore, while adjuvant chemotherapy is not standard treatment in adult-type soft-tissue sarcomas, it is being more frequently incorporated, especially for high-risk patients (having a G >1, deep, >5-cm tumor)
- Adjuvant chemotherapy is not used in histologies known to be insensitive to chemotherapy
- If the decision is made to use chemotherapy as upfront treatment, it may well be used preoperatively, at least in part. A local benefit may be gained, facilitating surgery.
- If used, adjuvant chemotherapy should consist of the combination chemotherapy regimens proven to be most active in advanced/extensive disease

(continued)

Expert Opinion (*continued*)

- In one large randomized phase 3 study (patients with G2–3, deep, >5-cm soft-tissue sarcomas), regional hyperthermia + systemic chemotherapy was associated with a local and disease-free survival advantage (no survival benefit demonstrated)

Extensive Disease
General guidelines:
- Metachronous resectable lung metastases without extrapulmonary disease are managed with complete excision of all lesions as standard treatment Chemotherapy may be added as an option in certain cases, although there is a lack of formal evidence that this improves results
- Chemotherapy is preferably given before surgery, in order to assess tumor response and thus modulate the length of treatment
- In the case of lung metastases being synchronous, in the absence of extrapulmonary disease, standard treatment is chemotherapy. Especially when patient benefit is achieved, surgery of lung metastases is an option
- Extrapulmonary disease is treated with chemotherapy as standard treatment
- In highly selected cases, surgery of responding metastases may be offered as an option following a multidisciplinary evaluation

Chemotherapy and targeted therapies:
- Standard chemotherapy is based on **anthracyclines** as first-line treatment
- No formal demonstration that multiagent chemotherapy is superior to single-agent chemotherapy with doxorubicin alone in terms of overall survival. However, a higher response rate may be expected in a number of sensitive histologic types according to several, although not all, randomized clinical trials
- Multiagent chemotherapy with **anthracyclines plus ifosfamide** may be the treatment of choice, especially when a tumor response is felt to give an advantage and patient performance status is good
- In angiosarcoma, **taxanes** are an alternative option
- **Imatinib** is standard medical therapy for rare patients with dermatofibrosarcoma protuberans whose disease is not amenable to nonmutilating surgery or with metastases requiring medical therapy
- **Sorafenib** can induce responses and prolong PFS patients with progressive, refractory, or symptomatic desmoid tumors
- **Crizotinib** has shown activity in metastatic or inoperable ALK positive inflammatory myofibroblastic tumors
- After failure of **anthracycline-based chemotherapy** or if an anthracycline cannot be used, the following criteria may apply (although it lacks high-level evidence):
  - Patients who have already received chemotherapy may be treated with **ifosfamide**, if they did not receive it previously
  - **High-dose ifosfamide** ($\sim$14 g/m^2) may be an option for patients who have already received standard-dose ifosfamide
  - **Trabectedin** is a second-line option. It has proved effective in leiomyosarcoma and liposarcoma and is FDA approved for these indications in the USA after treatment with an anthracycline. Responses have also been observed in synovial sarcoma and other histotypes; however, it is not currently approved for use in the United States outside the context of a clinical trial
  - Single agent **gemcitabine** was also shown to have antitumor activity in leiomyosarcoma as a single agent
    - Eribulin is also approved in the USA for unresectable or metastatic liposarcoma
  - **Dacarbazine** has some activity as second-line therapy (mostly in leiomyosarcoma). It could also be combined **with gemcitabine**. One randomized trial has demonstrated a survival advantage with the combination of gemcitabine and dacarbazine (DTIC) over DTIC alone
    - Targeted therapies such as **pazopanib** have been identified as having some activity in advanced disease
  - **Best supportive care** is an option for pretreated patients with advanced soft-tissue sarcoma, particularly when secondary and later treatment options have already been used
- *Pretreated patients with advanced disease are candidates for clinical studies*

SOFT-TISSUE SARCOMAS: RHABDOMYOSARCOMA

Epidemiology

Incidence: 4.5 cases per million with 350 estimated new cases in the United States per year; rhabdomyosarcoma represents 50% of all diagnosed soft-tissue sarcomas in 0-14 years age group. Male to female ratio is 1.37:1

Staging

Risk stratification is based on clinical group (determined post-operative), pre-treatment clinical staging, as well as histological subtype:
1. Determine the group (I, II, III, or IV)
2. Determine the stage (1, 2, 3, or 4)
3. Use the group and stage assignment together with histological subtype and age to assign a risk category. Recent protocols have incorporated FOXO1 status instead of histology for risk stratification.

Group classification system: A surgicopathologic grouping system with groups defined by the extent of disease and by the extent of initial surgical resection after pathologic review of the tumor specimens
Staging classification system: Classifies tumors based on primary site and size
Risk classification system: Used to assess the risk of recurrence as low, intermediate, and high risk; combines the clinical group and stage information

Group Classification System

Group	Extent of Disease and Initial Surgical Resection After Pathologic Review of Specimen	%*
I	Localized disease that is completely resected with no regional nodal involvement	14
IIA	Localized, grossly resected tumor with microscopic residual disease but no regional node involvement	20
IIB	Locoregional disease with tumor-involved lymph nodes with complete resection and no residual disease	
IIC	Locoregional disease with tumor-involved lymph nodes, grossly resected, but with evidence of microscopic residual tumor at the primary site and/or histologic involvement of the most distal regional node (from the primary site) in the dissection	
III	Localized, gross residual disease including incomplete resection or biopsy of the primary site	48
IV	Distant metastatic disease present at the time of diagnosis	18

*Percentage of all rhabdomyosarcomas

Staging Classification System

Stage	Description
1	Localized disease involving the orbit or head and neck (excluding parameningeal sites) or genitourinary region (excluding bladder/prostate sites) or biliary tract (**favorable sites**)
2	Localized disease of any other primary site not included in stage 1 (**unfavorable sites**). Primary tumor must be ≤5 cm in diameter with no clinical regional lymph node involvement by tumor
3	Localized disease of any other primary site not included in stage 1 (**unfavorable sites**). These patients differ from stage 2 patients by having primary tumors >5 cm in diameter and/or regional node involvement
4	Metastatic disease at diagnosis

Lawrence W Jr, Anderson JR, Gehan EA, Maurer H. Cancer. 1997; 80:1165–70.

Pathology

Embryonal Embryonal Botryoid* Spindle*	60–70%	Higher incidence in the 0–4 years age group
Alveolar	20%	Similar incidence throughout childhood
Pleomorphic	10–20%	Occurs predominantly in adults beyond 6th decade

*These subtypes are associated with more favorable outcomes

Disease Sites at Diagnosis

Site	%
Parameningeal*	23
Nonparameningeal head and neck	8
Bladder and prostate	11
Non-bladder and prostate genitourinary†	16
Limbs	16
Orbit	9
Other	17

*Sites in anatomic proximity to the base of the skull and adjacent meninges; eg, nasopharynx and middle ear
†Genitourinary other than bladder and prostate that include paratesticular, vagina, and uterus
Stevens MCG. Lancet Oncol 2005;6:77–84

5-Year Survival

Low risk	>90%
Intermediate risk	55–70%
High risk	20–25%

Children's Oncology Group (COG) Risk Classification System

Risk Group	Histology	Stage	Group
Low risk	ERMS	1	I/II,
		1	III for orbit only
		2	I/II
Intermediate risk	ERMS	1	III (non-orbit)
		2/3	III
		3	I/II
		4	IV, <10 years old
	ARMS	1-3	I-III
High risk	ERMS	4	IV ≥10 years
	ARMS	4	4

Expert Opinion

1. Disease prognosis is related to the age of the patient, site of origin, tumor size, histological subtype, FOXO1 fusion status, resectability, presence of metastases, number of metastatic sites, presence of lymph node involvement, and the unique biologic characteristics of the rhabdomyosarcoma tumor cells
2. Majority of alveolar rhabdomyosarcoma (ARMS) have translocation of FOXO1 gene with PAX 3 (t(2;13)(q35;q14)) or less commonly PAX7 (t(1;13)(p36;q14))
3. Fusion negative RMS is associated with embryonal histology and also with several tumor predisposition syndromes such as Li Fraumeni, Beckwith-Wiedemann (LOI at 11p15.5), NF1
4. RMS may occur at any location in the body and the variability with which rhabdomyosarcoma presents at different anatomic sites has a strong effect on treatment strategies
5. Work-up and staging
   • MRI or CT of primary site and regional lymph nodes
   • CT chest. May be performed with FDG-PET scan, however CT chest should be of diagnostic quality. May be omitted in certain patients with ERMS with clinically uninvolved nodes
   • FDG-PET/CT is being used more commonly and may be more sensitive for detection of lymph nodes and bone metastases. It is also being evaluated for assessing response to therapy
   • Bone scan. May be omitted if FDG-PET/CT is performed. May be omitted for certain patients (such as with ERMS and clinically uninvolved nodes and no lung metastases)
   • Bilateral bone marrow aspiration and biopsy. May be omitted in certain patients (such as with ERMS and clinically uninvolved nodes, and no lung or bone metastases)
   • Cerebrospinal fluid cytology for parameningeal/paraspinal tumors
   • Lymph node assessment depending on clinical/imaging findings or tumor location (paratesticular/extremity)

Treatment: General
1. Tumor response by conventional anatomic imaging has not shown to correlate with outcome in two COG studies but correlation has been observed in studies by Italian and German groups
2. Sequential FDG-PET might be of value

Treatment: Local therapy considerations
1. Radiation-responsive tumor and radiotherapy alone may accomplish local control
2. Upfront excision of primary tumor performed, if possible without causing major functional or cosmetic deficits. If not feasible, initial biopsy performed.

Expert Opinion (continued)

3. Delayed primary resection after initial systemic therapy can be considered in certain cases if complete surgical resection may significantly reduce radiation dose

Treatment: Multimodality
1. Successful therapy typically requires systemic therapy with local control
2. Agents considered most active
   - Vincristine
   - Actinomycin
   - Cyclophosphamide
   - Ifosfamide
   - Irinotecan
   - Vinorelbine

Metastatic disease
1. Prognosis is poor with 3 year FFS 25%

2. Patients treated with regimens similar to those for localized disease, or with addition of other active agents (such as doxorubicin, etoposide), or on clinical trials

3. Age at diagnosis <1 or ≥10 years, unfavorable primary site, bone and/or bone marrow involvement, ≥3 metastatic sites are adverse prognostic factors (Oberlin risk factors)

Recurrent disease
1. Disease relapse can be local, distant (lung, bone, bone marrow) or both

2. Survival is poor with 5 yr OS ~17% after 1st relapse. A small group of patients with favorable factors have 5-year survival of 50% (patients with botryoid histology, or ERMS stage 1 or group 1 at initial diagnosis with locoregional relapse)

3. Treatment options include chemotherapy and surgical resection (when complete resection feasible for local/regional relapse or resection of metastatic sites for palliation)

Barr FG. J Pediatr Hematol Oncol 1997;19:483–491
Arndt CAS et al. Cancer Treatment Revs 2018; 68: 94–101
Weiss et al J Clin Oncol 2013; 31:3226–32 (PMID: 23940218)
Oberlin et al J Clin Oncol 2008; 26(14):2384–9 (PMID 18467730)
Pappo et al J Clin Oncol 1999; 17(11):3487–93 (PMID: 10550146)

PREVIOUSLY UNTREATED • NONMETASTATIC • RHABDOMYOSARCOMA

RHABDOMYOSARCOMA (LOW RISK, SUBSET A) REGIMEN: VINCRISTINE + DACTINOMYCIN (D9602)

Raney RB et al. J Clin Oncol 2011;29:1312–1318

Treatment Schedule for Vincristine + Dactinomycin According to D9602

Drugs	0	1	2	3	4	5	6	7	8	9	10	11	12	13	14	15	16
							Week										
Vincristine (V)	V	V	V	V	V	V	V	V	V				V	V	V	V	V
Dactinomycin (A)	A			A			A*			A			A			A	
Radiation therapy (RT)				RT†													

	17	18	19	20	21	22	23	24	25	26	27	28	29	30	31	32	33
							Week										
Vincristine (V)	V	V	V	V				V	V	V	V	V	V	V	V	V	
Dactinomycin (A)		A			A			A			A			A			A

	34	35	36	37	38	39	40	41	42	43	44	45	46	47	48
						Week									
Vincristine (V)		V	V	V	V	V	V	V	V	V					
Dactinomycin (A)			A			A			A			A			

*Omit dactinomycin (A) at week 6 in patients who initiate RT at week 3

†Radiation therapy is delivered in conventional fashion using megavoltage equipment in 1.8 Gy fractions once daily for 5 days per week. The total dose was 36 Gy for stage 1 group IIA patients and 45 Gy for stage 1 group III N0 orbit patients. Patients with group II or III tumors initiate RT at week 3

Vincristine 1.5 mg/m² per dose (maximum single dose = 2 mg); administer by intravenous infusion over 15 minutes in 25–50 mL 0.9% sodium chloride injection (0.9% NS) on day 1 (total dosage during the weeks in which vincristine is administered = 1.5 mg/m²; maximum dose/treatment = 2 mg)

Age	Vincristine dose
≥3 years	1.5 mg/m²/dose (maximum single dose = 2 mg)
1 to <3 years	0.05 mg/kg/dose
<1 year	0.025 mg/kg/dose

Pediatric patients: Dilute in 25 mL 0.9% NS
Adult patients: Dilute in 50 mL 0.9% NS

Dactinomycin 0.045 mg/kg (maximum single dose = 2.5 mg); administer by intravenous injection over 1–2 minutes on day 1 (total dosage during the weeks in which dactinomycin is administered = 0.045 mg/kg; maximum dose/cycle = 2.5 mg)

Age	Dactinomycin dose
≥1 year	0.045 mg/kg/dose (maximum single dose = 2.5 mg)
<1 year	0.025 mg/kg/dose

Supportive Care:
Antiemetic prophylaxis
Emetogenic potential during weeks with vincristine, dactinomycin, and cyclophosphamide is **HIGH**. *Potential for delayed symptoms*
Emetogenic potential on days with vincristine and cyclophosphamide is **HIGH**
Emetogenic potential on days with vincristine alone is **MINIMAL**
See Chapter 42 for antiemetic recommendations

Hematopoietic growth factor (CSF) prophylaxis
Primary prophylaxis is NOT indicated
See Chapter 43 for more information

Antimicrobial prophylaxis
Risk of fever and neutropenia is *LOW*
    Antimicrobial primary prophylaxis to be CONSIDERED:
- Antibacterial—not indicated
- Antifungal—not indicated
- Antiviral—not indicated unless patient previously had an episode of HSV

Treatment Modifications

Vincristine and Dactinomycin

Note: administer vincristine regardless of peripheral blood counts

Hepatic Impairment

Direct bilirubin <3.1 mg/dL	Administer full dose vincristine and dactinomycin
Direct bilirubin 3.1–5.0 mg/dL	Reduce the dosages of vincristine and dactinomycin by 50%
Direct bilirubin 5.1–6.0 mg/dL	Reduce the dosages of vincristine and dactinomycin by 75%
Direct bilirubin >6.0 mg/dL	Withhold vincristine and dactinomycin and administer the next scheduled doses if direct bilirubin has improved

Neuropathy (See Grading Below)

G2 motor or sensory neuropathy	Administer vincristine with the dosage reduced by 50%. If the toxicity improves to G ≤1, then increase the dose for 75% of the full dose.
G ≥3 moto or sensory neuropathy	Withhold vincristine until toxicity improves to G ≤2, then resume vincristine with the dosage reduced by 50%
Jaw pain	Continue vincristine at the current dose

Gastrointestinal Toxicity

G ≥3 constipation (obstipation with manual evacuation indicated; limiting self-care ADL)	Withhold vincristine and optimize laxative regimen. When toxicity improves to G ≤1, resume vincristine with the dosage reduced by 50%. If the toxicity does not recur, then re-escalate the vincristine dose back to full dose.
G ≥3 ileus (severely altered GI function; TPN indicated)	
G ≥3 mucositis	Withhold dactinomycin until toxicity resolves to G <1, then reduce subsequent doses by 25%. Do not delay or reduce the dose of vincristine

Motor Neuropathy Grading

Grade 1	Subjective weakness, but no deficits detected under neurologic exam
Grade 2	Weakness that alters fine motor skills (buttoning shirt, writing or drawing, using eating utensils) or gait without abrogating ability to perform these tasks
Grade 3	Unable to perform fine motor tasks (buttoning shirt, writing or drawing, using eating utensils) or unable to ambulate without assistance
Grade 4	Paralysis

Sensory Neuropathy Grading

Grade 1	Paresthesias, pain, or numbness that do not require treatment or interfere with extremity function
Grade 2	Paresthesias, pain, or numbness that is controlled by non-narcotic medications or alter (without causing loss of function) fine motor skills (buttoning shirt, writing or drawing, using eating utensils) or gait without abrogating ability to perform these tasks
Grade 3	Paresthesias or pain that is controlled by narcotics, or interfere with extremity function (gait, fine motor skills as outlined above) or quality of life (loss of sleep, ability to perform normal activities severely impaired)
Grade 4	Complete loss of sensation or pain that is not controlled by narcotics

Patient Population Studied

Patients eligible for registration on D9602 were younger than 50 years, previously untreated, with a low risk of recurrence. Patients with ERMS or embryonal ectomesenchymoma in stage 1 groups I/IIA, group III orbit, and stage 2 group I were assigned to subgroup A. Patients with ERMS with stage 1 group III nonorbital tumors, groups IIB/C, stage 2 group II, and stage 3 group I/II were assigned to subgroup B

Characteristics of Patients with Low-risk ERMS Treated on the D9602 Study with Chemotherapy, with or Without Conventional Radiotherapy (n = 342)*

Characteristic	Condition and Regimen		Total (N = 342)
	ERMS/ VA (n = 264)	ERMS/ VAC (n = 78)	
	Number (%)	Number (%)	Number (%)
Age, years			
<5	94 (36)	36 (46)	130 (38)
5–9	93 (35)	14 (18)	107 (31)
10–14	44 (17)	19 (24)	63 (18)
15+	33 (13)	9 (12)	42 (12)
Sex			
Male	184 (70)	35 (45)	219 (64)
Female	80 (30)	43 (55)	123 (36)
Race/ethnicity			
White	201 (77)	45 (58)	246 (73)
Black	33 (13)	16 (21)	49 (14)
Hispanic	20 (8)	12 (15)	32 (9)
Other	7 (3)	5 (6)	12 (4)
Stage			
1	252 (97)	55 (72)	307 (91)
2	8 (3)	9 (12)	17 (5)
3	0	12 (16)	12 (4)
Group			
I	122 (47)	5 (6)	127 (38)
IIA	62 (24)	16 (21)	78 (23)
IIB	0	12 (16)	12 (4)
IIC	0	5 (6)	5 (1)
III	77 (30)	39 (51)	116 (34)
Primary site			
GU, not B/P			
Paratestis	108 (41)	17 (22)	125 (37)
Other GU	19 (7)	18 (24)	37 (11)
Orbit	96 (37)	2 (3)	98 (29)
Head and neck	29 (11)	13 (17)	42 (12)
Parameningeal	0	3 (4)	3 (1)
Extremity	2 (1)	4 (5)	6 (2)
Other sites	7 (3)	19 (25)	26 (8)
Tumor size, cm			
≤5	215 (83)	38 (51)	253 (76)
>5	44 (17)	37 (49)	81 (24)
Invasiveness			
T1 (noninvasive)	246 (95)	44 (59)	290 (87)
T2 (invasive)	13 (5)	30 (41)	43 (13)
Nodal status			
N0	259 (99)	58 (76)	317 (94)
N1	0	17 (22)	17 (5)
NX	1 (<1)	1 (1)	2 (1)

*Some data on race/ethnicity, stage, group, primary site, tumor size and invasiveness, and nodal status were missing in both treatment groups
ERMS, embryonal rhabdomyosarcoma; VA, vincristine and dactinomycin; VAC, vincristine, dactinomycin, cyclophosphamide; GU, not B/P, genitourinary tract, not bladder or prostate; NX, regional lymph node status unknown

Efficacy

Outcomes Among Three Subcategories of D9602 Patients, Compared with Similar Patients from IRSG Protocols III and IV

Parameter	IRS-III No.	IRS-III %	IRS-IV No.	IRS-IV %	D9602 No.	D9602 %
Stage I, group IIA, No. of patients	52		43		62	
Site of primary tumor						
Orbit	23	44	20	47	18	29
Nonparameningeal head/neck	21	40	7	16	14	23
Paratestis	4	8	11	26	18	29
Other GU, not bladder/prostate	4	8	5	12	11	18
Biliary tract	0		0		1	2
Protocol chemotherapy	VA		VAC/VAI/VIE		VA	
Protocol radiotherapy, Gy	41.4		41.4		36	
5-year failure-free survival		85		98		81
5-year overall survival		94		100		94
5-year cumulative incidence of local-only failure		11		2		15
5-year cumulative incidence of other failure		4		0		4
Group III orbit tumors, No. of patients	71		50		77	
Protocol chemotherapy	VA		VAC/VAI/VIE		VA	
Protocol radiotherapy, Gy	45.0 or 50.4		50.4 or 59.4		45.0	
5-year failure-free survival		79		94		86
5-year overall survival		95		100		96
5-year cumulative incidence of local-only failure		16		4		14
5-year cumulative incidence of other failure		3		0		0
Stages 2 + 3, group IIA, No. of patients	38		28		16	
Site of primary tumor						
Extremity	12	32	4	14	2	13
Retroperitoneum/trunk	9	24	4	14	6	38
Bladder/prostate	6	16	9	32	3	19
Parameningeal	5	13	8	29	3	19
Other	6	16	3	11	2	13
Protocol chemotherapy	VA		VAC/VAI/VIE		VAC	
Protocol radiotherapy, Gy	41.4		41.4		36	
5-year failure-free survival		76		88		94
5-year overall survival		78		92		100
5-year cumulative incidence of local-only failure		14		7		0
5-year cumulative incidence of other failure		11		4		6

IRSG, Intergroup Rhabdomyosarcoma Study Group; GU, genitourinary tract; VA, vincristine + dactinomycin; VAC, vincristine + dactinomycin + cyclophosphamide; I, ifosfamide; E, etoposide (randomized in IRS-IV)

Adverse Events

Hepatopathy with abdominal distension and right upper quadrant abdominal pain with/without other signs of sinusoidal obstruction syndrome*	5 patients—one died of sepsis and the others recovered*
Severe mucositis	2 patients
Hematuria	1 patient treated with VAC
Decreased absolute neutrophil count lower than 500/μL in patients receiving VA	14% to 34%
Decreased absolute neutrophil count lower than 500/μL in patients receiving VAC	60% to 95%

*After drug dose reductions no further cases of hepatopathy were reported

Therapy Monitoring

1. *Before each dose of vincristine and/or dactinomycin:* serum creatinine, LFTs with bilirubin, serum electrolytes, including calcium, magnesium, and phosphorus, CBC with differential, physical examination
2. *Response evaluation:* at week 12, 24, 36, and 48

PREVIOUSLY UNTREATED • NONMETASTATIC • RHABDOMYOSARCOMA

RHABDOMYOSARCOMA (LOW RISK, SUBSET A) REGIMEN: VINCRISTINE + DACTINOMYCIN + CYCLOPHOSPHAMIDE (VAC) FOLLOWED BY VA (ARST0331)

Walterhouse DO et al. J Clin Oncol 2014;32:3547–3552

Treatment Schedule According to ARST0331

Treatment	Week																							
	1	2	3	4	5	6	7	8	9	10	11	12	13	14	15	16	17	18	19	20	21	22	23	24
Vincristine (V)	V	V	V	V	V	V	V	V	V				V	V	V	V	V	V	V	V	V			
Dactinomycin (D)	A			A			A			A			A			A*			A			A		
Cyclophosphamide (C)	C			C			C			C														
Radiotherapy (RT)													RT†											

*Omit dactinomycin (A) at week 16 in patients receiving radiation therapy

†Begin RT in week 13 (applies to group II or III patients only). RT could be delivered as three-dimensional conformal RT, intensity-modulated RT, proton-beam RT, or brachytherapy. Radiotherapy was administered in 1.8 Gy fractions once daily for 5 days per week. Total doses were based on the extent of residual disease; no RT for group I tumors, 36 Gy for group IIA tumors, 41.4 Gy for group IIB/C tumors, and 45 Gy for group III orbit tumors

Note: the administration schedules for vincristine, dactinomycin, and cyclophosphamide appears in the table above

Vincristine 1.5 mg/m^2 per dose (maximum single dose = 2 mg); administer by intravenous infusion over 15 minutes in 25–50 mL 0.9% sodium chloride injection (0.9% NS) on day 1 (total dosage during the weeks in which vincristine is administered = 1.5 mg/m^2; maximum dose/treatment = 2 mg)

Age	Vincristine Dose
≥3 years	1.5 mg/m^2/dose (maximum single dose = 2 mg)
1 to <3 years	0.05 mg/kg/dose
<1 year	0.025 mg/kg/dose

Pediatric patients: Dilute in 25 mL 0.9% NS
Adult patients: Dilute in 50 mL 0.9% NS

Dactinomycin 0.045 mg/kg (maximum single dose = 2.5 mg); administer by intravenous injection over 1–2 minutes on day 1 (total dosage during the weeks in which dactinomycin is administered = 0.045 mg/kg; maximum dose/cycle = 2.5 mg)

Age	Dactinomycin Dose
≥1 year	0.045 mg/kg/dose (maximum single dose = 2.5 mg)
<1 year	0.025 mg/kg/dose

Hydration for cyclophosphamide:
0.9% NS 750 mL/m^2; administer intravenously over 1–2 hours prior to the start of cyclophosphamide, followed by additional intravenous hydration (eg, 0.9% NS) at a rate of 100 mL/m^2/hour continued until the last mesna dose has been administered

Mesna 240 mg/m^2 per dose; administer intravenously, diluted in a convenient volume of 0.9% NS sufficient to produce a final mesna concentration ranging from 1–20 mg/mL, over 15 minutes administered just before, 4 hours after, and 8 hours after the start of the cyclophosphamide infusion on day 1 (total dosage during the weeks in which cyclophosphamide is administered = 720 mg/m^2)

Age	Mesna Dose
≥3 years	240 mg/m^2/dose
<3 years	8 mg/kg/dose

Cyclophosphamide 1200 mg/m^2; administer intravenously in 100–1000 mL 0.9% NS or 5% dextrose injection (D5W) over 60 minutes, on day 1 (total dosage during the weeks in which cyclophosphamide is administered = 1200 mg/m^2)

Age	Cyclophosphamide Dose
≥3 years	1200 mg/m^2/dose
<3 years	40 mg/kg/dose

(continued)

(continued)

Supportive Care:
Antiemetic prophylaxis
Emetogenic potential during weeks with cyclophosphamide and/or dactinomycin is **MODERATE**.
Emetogenic potential on days with vincristine alone is **MINIMAL**
See Chapter 42 for antiemetic recommendations

Hematopoietic growth factor (CSF) prophylaxis
Primary prophylaxis MAY be indicated with:
Filgrastim (G-CSF) 5 μg/kg per day by subcutaneous injection
- Begin use from 24 hours after myelosuppressive chemotherapy is completed—that is, day 2 during cycles containing cyclophosphamide
- Filgrastim may be given on days when vincristine is administered alone
- Continue daily filgrastim use until ANC ≥15,000/mm³
- Discontinue daily filgrastim use at least 24 hours before administering resuming myelosuppressive treatment (containing dactinomycin or cyclophosphamide)
See Chapter 43 for more information

Antimicrobial prophylaxis
Risk of fever and neutropenia is *INTERMEDIATE*
Antimicrobial primary prophylaxis to be considered:
- Antibacterial—consider a fluoroquinolone or no prophylaxis; *P. jirovecii* prophylaxis is recommended (eg, cotrimoxazole)
- Antifungal—consider concomitant use of clotrimazole during periods of neutropenia
- Antiviral—antiherpes antivirals (eg, acyclovir, famciclovir, valacyclovir)

Treatment Modifications

Vincristine, Dactinomycin, and Cyclophosphamide Dose Modifications

Note: administer vincristine regardless of peripheral blood counts

Hepatic Impairment

Direct bilirubin <3.1 mg/dL	Administer full doses of chemotherapy
Direct bilirubin 3.1–5.0 mg/dL	Reduce the dosages of vincristine and dactinomycin by 50%
Direct bilirubin 5.1–6.0 mg/dL	Reduce the dosages of vincristine and dactinomycin by 75%
Direct bilirubin >6.0 mg/dL	Withhold vincristine and dactinomycin and administer the next scheduled doses if direct bilirubin has improved

Neuropathy (See Grading Below)

G2 motor or sensory neuropathy	Administer vincristine with the dosage reduced by 50%. If the toxicity improves to G ≤1, then increase the dose for 75% of the full dose
G ≥3 motor or sensory neuropathy	Withhold vincristine until toxicity improves to G ≤2, then resume vincristine with the dosage reduced by 50%
Jaw pain	Continue vincristine at the current dose

Gastrointestinal Toxicity

G ≥3 constipation (obstipation with manual evacuation indicated; limiting self-care ADL)	Withhold vincristine and optimize laxative regimen. When toxicity improves to G ≤1, resume vincristine with the dosage reduced by 50%. If the toxicity does not recur, then re-escalate the vincristine dose back to full dose
G ≥3 ileus (severely altered GI function; TPN indicated)	
G ≥3 mucositis	Withhold cyclophosphamide, mesna, and dactinomycin until toxicity resolves to G <1, then reduce subsequent doses of these medications by 25%. Do not delay or reduce the dose of vincristine.

(continued)

Patient Population Studied

Eligible for subset one of ARST0331 if:
- Age <50 years at the time of diagnosis
- Previously untreated
- Embryonal rhabdomyosarcoma, botryoid or spindle-cell variants
- Primitive ectomesenchymoma with embryonal rhabdomyosarcoma histology
- Stage I/II group I/II tumor or stage I group III orbit tumor
- Started protocol therapy within 42 days of diagnosis
- Staging ipsilateral retroperitoneal lymph node dissection required for boys age >10 years with paratestis tumors
- Regional lymph node sampling required for histologic evaluation in patients with extremity tumors

Demographic and Clinical Characteristics of Eligible Patients Enrolled on Subset One of ARST0331

Characteristic	Subset One (n = 271)	
	No.	%
Age, years		
< 5	101	37
5–9	76	28
10–14	48	18
15–21	41	15
> 21	5	2

(continued)

Treatment Modifications (continued)

Urologic Toxicity

Transient microscopic hematuria (>50 RBC/HPF 1 or 2 times)	Double the rate of post-hydration and continue mesna
Persistent microscopic hematuria (>50 RBC/HPF ≥3 times), or transient gross hematuria	Double the rate of post-hydration, continue hydration for at least 24 hours, and increase the total daily mesna dose to be equivalent to 100% of the cyclophosphamide dose
Persistent gross hematuria	Discontinue cyclophosphamide until urine clears to microscopic hematuria, then resume with the cyclophosphamide dose reduced to 50% of the full dose with post-hydration and mesna administered as per above for persistent microscopic hematuria. Escalate the cyclophosphamide dose to 75% and 100% of the full dose as tolerated. Consider urology consultation

Hematologic Toxicity

ANC <750/mm^3 or platelet count <75,000/mm^3 on a day that dactinomycin or cyclophosphamide is due	Delay the cyclophosphamide, mesna, and dactinomycin doses by 1 week. Consider use of G-CSF in subsequent cycles for delays related to neutropenia. If counts recover, then administer the full doses. If counts do not recover, then reduce the cyclophosphamide, mesna, and dactinomycin doses by 25%

Grading of Adverse Events

Motor Neuropathy Grading

Grade 1	Subjective weakness, but no deficits detected under neurologic exam
Grade 2	Weakness that alters fine motor skills (buttoning shirt, writing or drawing, using eating utensils) or gait without abrogating ability to perform these tasks
Grade 3	Unable to perform fine motor tasks (buttoning shirt, writing or drawing, using eating utensils) or unable to ambulate without assistance
Grade 4	Paralysis

Sensory Neuropathy Grading

Grade 1	Paresthesias, pain, or numbness that do not require treatment or interfere with extremity function
Grade 2	Paresthesias, pain, or numbness that is controlled by non-narcotic medications or alter (without causing loss of function) fine motor skills (buttoning shirt, writing or drawing, using eating utensils) or gait without abrogating ability to perform these tasks
Grade 3	Paresthesias or pain that is controlled by narcotics, or interfere with extremity function (gait, fine motor skills as outlined above) or quality of life (loss of sleep, ability to perform normal activities severely impaired)
Grade 4	Complete loss of sensation or pain that is not controlled by narcotics

Patient Population Studied
(continued)

Sex		
Male	202	75
Female	69	25
Histology		
Botryoid	28	10
Embryonal	186	69
Spindle cell	57	21
Stage		
I	251	93
II	20	7
Group		
I	137	51
IIA	52	19
IIB	11	4
IIC	9	3
III	62	23
Primary site		
Extremity	5	2
GU, non-BP		
Other	18	7
Paratestis	118	44
Head and neck	30	11
Orbit	82	30
Other	14	5
PM/PM extension	4	1
Tumor size, cm		
≤5	223	82
>5	48	18
Tumor invasion		
T1	250	92
T2	21	8
Nodal status		
N0	247	91
N1	18	7
Nx	6	2

BP, bladder/prostate; GU, genitourinary; PM, parameningeal

Efficacy

Outcome

Entire cohort

Long-term FFS rate	With a median follow-up of 4.3 years, observed 35 failures versus 48.4 expected failures (P = 0.05) based on the outcome for patients in subgroup A of D9602. "Reasonably confident not worse than 83%"
Estimated 3-year FFS rate	89% (95% CI, 85–92)
Estimated 3-year OS rate	98% (95% CI, 95–99)

Patients with stage I group IIB/C (node positive) or stage II group II ERMS (n = 30)

Estimated 3-year FFS	90% (95% CI, 72–97)
Estimated 3-year OS	96% (95% CI, 78–99)

Patients with paratestis tumors (n = 118)

Estimated 3-year FFS	93% (95% CI, 87–96)
Estimated 3-year OS	99% (95% CI, 94–99)

Patients with orbit tumors (n = 82)

Estimated 3-year FFS	86% (95% CI, 77–92)
Estimated 3-year OS	97% (95% CI, 90–99)

Patients with tumors in all other sites combined (n = 71)

Estimated 3-year FFS	86% (95% CI, 75–92)
Estimated 3-year OS	97% (95% CI, 88–99)

Patients with stage I/II group IIA tumors who received 36 Gy (n = 52)

Estimated 3-year FFS	90% (95% CI, 77–96)
Estimated 3-year OS	96% (95% CI, 84–99)

Recurrences

Entire cohort

3-year cumulative incidence rate of local failure alone	6.7%
3-year cumulative incidence rate for any local failure with/without regional or distant failure	7.6%
3-year cumulative incidence rate for any regional failure with/without distant failure	1.5%
3-year cumulative incidence rate for any distant failure with/without local or regional failure	3.4%

Patients with stage I/II group IIA tumors (n = 52)

3-year cumulative incidence rate of local failure	8.1%

Patients with group III orbit tumors (n = 62)

3-year cumulative incidence rate of local failure	11.5%

Adverse Events

- No unexpected Grade 4 toxicities and no deaths
- Five cases of hepatopathy (<2%). Two cases classified as mild by protocol guidelines and three as moderate. All patients with hepatopathy recovered fully

Therapy Monitoring

1. *Before each dose of chemotherapy:* serum creatinine, LFTs with bilirubin, serum electrolytes, including calcium, magnesium, and phosphorus, CBC with differential, physical examination
2. *Before each dose of cyclophosphamide and as clinically indicated:* urinalysis
3. *Response evaluation:* at weeks 13 and 24

PREVIOUSLY UNTREATED • NONMETASTATIC RHABDOMYOSARCOMA

RHABDOMYOSARCOMA (LOW RISK, SUBSET B) REGIMEN: VINCRISTINE + DACTINOMYCIN + CYCLOPHOSPHAMIDE (D9602)

Raney RB et al. J Clin Oncol 2011;29:1312–1318

Treatment Schedule for Vincristine + Dactinomycin + Cyclophosphamide According to D9602

Drugs	0	1	2	3	4	5	6	7	8	9	10	11	12	13	14	15	16
Vincristine (V)	V	V	V	V	V	V	V	V	V				V	V	V	V	V
Dactinomycin (A)	A			A			A*			A			A			A*	
Cyclophosphamide (C)	C			C			C			C			C			C	
Radiation (RT)				RT†									RT†				

	17	18	19	20	21	22	23	24	25	26	27	28	29	30	31	32	33
Vincristine (V)	V	V	V	V				V	V	V	V	V	V	V	V	V	
Dactinomycin (A)		A*			A			A			A			A*			A*
Cyclophosphamide (C)		C						C			C			C			
Radiation (RT)												RT†					

	34	35	36	37	38	39	40	41	42	43	44	45	46	47	48
Vincristine (V)			V	V	V	V	V	V	V	V	V				
Dactinomycin (A)			A			A			A			A			
Cyclophosphamide (C)			C			C			C						

*Omit dactinomycin (A) at week 6 in patients who initiate RT at week 3. Omit dactinomycin (A) at weeks 15 and 18 in patients who initiate RT at week 12. Omit dactinomycin (A) at weeks 30 and 33 in patients who initiate RT at week 28

†Patients with group II or III tumors, initiated RT in week 3. Patients with vaginal primaries and tumor-involved regional lymph nodes, initiated RT in week 12. Patients with vaginal primaries and negative nodes whose repeat biopsies show persistent viable tumor cells, initiated RT in week 28. RT is delivered in conventional fashion using megavoltage equipment in 1.8 Gy fractions once daily for 5 days per week. The total dose was 36 Gy for stages 2/3 group IIA patients (subgroup B)

Vincristine 1.5 mg/m² per dose (maximum single dose = 2 mg); administer by intravenous infusion over 15 minutes in 25–50 mL 0.9% sodium chloride injection (0.9% NS) on day 1 (total dosage during the weeks in which vincristine is administered = 1.5 mg/m²; maximum dose/treatment = 2 mg)

Age	Vincristine Dose
≥3 years	1.5 mg/m²/dose (maximum single dose = 2 mg)
1 to <3 years	0.05 mg/kg/dose
<1 year	0.025 mg/kg/dose

Pediatric patients: Dilute in 25 mL 0.9% NS
Adult patients: Dilute in 50 mL 0.9% NS

Dactinomycin 0.045 mg/kg (maximum single dose = 2.5 mg); administer by intravenous injection over 1–2 minutes on day 1 (total dosage during the weeks in which dactinomycin is administered = 0.045 mg/kg; maximum dose/cycle = 2.5 mg)

Age	Dactinomycin Dose
≥1 year	0.045 mg/kg/dose (maximum single dose = 2.5 mg)
<1 year	0.025 mg/kg/dose

(continued)

(*continued*)

Hydration during cyclophosphamide:
Administer additional intravenous hydration (eg, 0.9% NS) to achieve a total rate of 2000 mL/m^2/day (taking into account volumes of diluent used for mesna and cyclophosphamide) continuing for 24 hours after the cyclophosphamide dose

An admixture containing **cyclophosphamide** 2200 mg/m^2 + **mesna** 120 mg/m^2; administer intravenously in 100–1000 mL 0.9% NS or 5% dextrose injection (D5W) over 10–30 minutes, on day 1 (total dosage during the weeks in which cyclophosphamide is administered = 2200 mg/m^2)

Age	Cyclophosphamide Dose	Mesna Dose
≥3 years	2200 mg/**m**^{2}	120 mg/**kg**/dose
1 to <3 years	73 mg/**kg**/dose	4 mg/**kg**/dose
<1 year	36 mg/**kg**/dose	2 mg/**kg**/dose

followed by

Mesna 1200 mg/m^2; administer intravenously in 250–1000 mL of 0.9% NS or D5W over 24 hours (rate of 50 mg/m^2 per hour), starting immediately after each dose of cyclophosphamide (total dosage during the weeks in which cyclophosphamide is administered = 1320 mg/m^2; includes 120 mg/m^2; administered with cyclophosphamide)

Age	Mesna Dose
≥3 years	1200 mg/**m**^{2} per dose
1 to <3 years	40 mg/**kg**/dose
<1 year	20 mg/**kg**/dose

The administration schedules for vincristine, dactinomycin, and cyclophosphamide appears in the table (above)

Supportive Care: Antiemetic prophylaxis
Emetogenic potential during weeks with dactinomycin, cyclophosphamide, and ± vincristine is **HIGH**. *Potential for delayed symptoms*
Emetogenic potential during weeks with cyclophosphamide and vincristine is **HIGH**. *Potential for delayed symptoms*
Emetogenic potential on days with dactinomycin alone is **MODERATE**
Emetogenic potential on days with vincristine alone is **MINIMAL**
See Chapter 42 for antiemetic recommendations

Hematopoietic growth factor (CSF) prophylaxis
Primary prophylaxis is indicated with:
  Filgrastim (G-CSF) 5 μg/kg per day by subcutaneous injection
  • Begin use from 24 hours after myelosuppressive chemotherapy is completed—that is, day 2 during cycles containing cyclophosphamide
  • Filgrastim may be given on days when vincristine is administered alone
  • Continue daily filgrastim use until ANC ≥15,000/mm^3
  • Discontinue daily filgrastim use at least 24 hours before administering resuming myelosuppressive treatment (containing dactinomycin or cyclophosphamide)
See Chapter 43 for more information

Antimicrobial prophylaxis
Risk of fever and neutropenia is HIGH
  Antimicrobial primary prophylaxis is recommended:
  • Antibacterial—consider fluoroquinolone prophylaxis; *P. jirovecii* prophylaxis is recommended (eg, cotrimoxazole)
  • Antifungal—recommended
  • Antiviral—antiherpes antivirals (eg, acyclovir, famciclovir, valacyclovir)

Treatment Modifications

Vincristine, Dactinomycin, and Cyclophosphamide Dose Modifications

Note: administer vincristine regardless of peripheral blood counts

Hepatic Impairment	
Direct bilirubin <3.1 mg/dL	Administer full doses of chemotherapy
Direct bilirubin 3.1–5.0 mg/dL	Reduce the dosages of vincristine and dactinomycin by 50%
Direct bilirubin 5.1–6.0 mg/dL	Reduce the dosages of vincristine and dactinomycin by 75%
Direct bilirubin >6.0 mg/dL	Withhold vincristine and dactinomycin and administer the next scheduled doses if direct bilirubin has improved

Neuropathy (See Grading Below)	
G2 motor or sensory neuropathy	Administer vincristine with the dosage reduced by 50%. If the toxicity improves to G ≤1, then increase the dose for 75% of the full dose
G ≥3 motor or sensory neuropathy	Withhold vincristine until toxicity improves to G ≤2, then resume vincristine with the dosage reduced by 50%
Jaw pain	Continue vincristine at the current dose

Gastrointestinal Toxicity	
G ≥3 constipation (obstipation with manual evacuation indicated; limiting self-care ADL) G ≥3 ileus (severely altered GI function; TPN indicated)	Withhold vincristine and optimize laxative regimen. When toxicity improves to G ≤1, resume vincristine with the dosage reduced by 50%. If the toxicity does not recur, then re-escalate the vincristine dose back to full dose
G ≥3 mucositis	Withhold cyclophosphamide, mesna, and dactinomycin until toxicity resolves to G <1, then reduce subsequent doses of these medications by 25%. Do not delay or reduce the dose of vincristine

Urologic Toxicity	
Transient microscopic hematuria (>50 RBC/HPF 1 or 2 times)	Double the rate of post-hydration and continue mesna
Persistent microscopic hematuria (>50 RBC/HPF ≥3 times), or transient gross hematuria	Double the rate of post-hydration, continue hydration for at least 24 hours, and increase the total daily mesna dose to be equivalent to 100% of the cyclophosphamide dose
Persistent gross hematuria	Discontinue cyclophosphamide until urine clears to microscopic hematuria, then resume with the cyclophosphamide dose reduced to 50% of the full dose with post-hydration and mesna administered as per above for persistent microscopic hematuria. Escalate the cyclophosphamide dose to 75% and 100% of the full dose as tolerated. Consider urology consultation

Hematologic Toxicity	
ANC <750/mm³ or platelet count <75,000/mm³ on a day that dactinomycin or cyclophosphamide is due	Delay the cyclophosphamide, mesna, and dactinomycin doses by 1 week. Consider use of G-CSF in subsequent cycles for delays related to neutropenia. If counts recover, then administer the full doses. If counts do not recover, then reduce the cyclophosphamide, mesna, and dactinomycin doses by 25%

Grading of Adverse Events

Motor Neuropathy Grading

Grade 1	Subjective weakness, but no deficits detected under neurologic exam
Grade 2	Weakness that alters fine motor skills (buttoning shirt, writing or drawing, using eating utensils) or gait without abrogating ability to perform these tasks
Grade 3	Unable to perform fine motor tasks (buttoning shirt, writing or drawing, using eating utensils) or unable to ambulate without assistance
Grade 4	Paralysis

Sensory Neuropathy Grading

Grade 1	Paresthesias, pain, or numbness that do not require treatment or interfere with extremity function
Grade 2	Paresthesias, pain, or numbness that is controlled by non-narcotic medications or alter (without causing loss of function) fine motor skills (buttoning shirt, writing or drawing, using eating utensils) or gait without abrogating ability to perform these tasks
Grade 3	Paresthesias or pain that is controlled by narcotics, or interfere with extremity function (gait, fine motor skills as outlined above) or quality of life (loss of sleep, ability to perform normal activities severely impaired)
Grade 4	Complete loss of sensation or pain that is not controlled by narcotics

Patient Population Studied

Eligible for registration if:
• Age <50 years at the time of diagnosis
• Previously untreated
• Low risk of recurrence
• Subgroup A = Patients with embryonal rhabdomyosarcoma or embryonal ectomesenchymoma in stage 1 groups I/IIA, group III orbit, and stage 2 group I
• Subgroup B = Embryonal rhabdomyosarcoma with stage 1 group III nonorbital tumors, groups IIB/C, stage 2 group II, and stage 3 group I/II

Characteristics of Patients with Low-risk ERMS Treated on the D9602 Study with Chemotherapy, with or Without Conventional Radiotherapy (n = 342)

Characteristic ERMS/VA (n = 264)	Condition and Regimen				Total (N = 342)	
	ERMS/ VAC (n = 78)					
	No.	%	No.	%	No.	%
Age, years						
<5	94	36	36	46	130	38
5–9	93	35	14	18	107	31
10–14	44	17	19	24	63	18
15+	33	13	9	12	42	12
Sex						
Male	184	70	35	45	219	64
Female	80	30	43	55	123	36
Race/ethnicity						
White	201	77	45	58	246	73
Black	33	13	16	21	49	14
Hispanic	20	8	12	15	32	9
Other	7	3	5	6	12	4
Stage						
1	252	97	55	72	307	91
2	8	3	9	12	17	5
3	0		12	16	12	4
Group						
I	122	47	5	6	127	38
IIA	62	24	16	21	78	23
IIB	0		12	16	12	4
IIC	0		5	6	5	1
III	77	30	39	51	116	34
Primary site						
GU, not B/P						
Paratestis	108	41	17	22	125	37
Other GU	19	7	18	24	37	11
Orbit	96	37	2	3	98	29
Head and neck	29	11	13	17	42	12
Parameningeal	0		3	4	3	1

(continued)

Patient Population Studied (continued)

Characteristic ERMS/ VA (n = 264)	Condition and Regimen				Total (N = 342)	
	ERMS/ VAC (n = 78)					
	No.	%	No.	%	No.	%
Extremity	2	1	4	5	6	2
Other sites	7	3	19	25	26	8
Tumor size, cm						
≤5	215	83	38	51	253	76
>5	44	17	37	49	81	24
Invasiveness						
T1 (noninvasive)	246	95	44	59	290	87
T2 (invasive)	13	5	30	41	43	13
Nodal status						
N0	259	99	58	76	317	94
N1	0		17	22	17	5
NX	1	<1	1	1	2	1

Note: some data on race/ethnicity, stage, group, primary site, tumor size and invasiveness, and nodal status were missing in both treatment groups
ERMS, embryonal rhabdomyosarcoma; VA, vincristine and dactinomycin; VAC, vincristine, dactinomycin, cyclophosphamide; GU, not B/P, genitourinary tract, not bladder or prostate; NX, regional lymph node status unknown

Efficacy

All 342 Patients	
Estimated 5-year FFS rate	88% (95% CI, 84–91)
Estimated OS rate	97% (95% CI, 94–98)
5-year cumulative incidence rate of isolated distant metastases	0.9% (n = 3 patients)
5-year cumulative incidence rate of isolated local recurrence	8.5% (n = 28)
5-year cumulative incidence rate of isolated regional lymph-node recurrence	0.7% (n = 2)
5-year cumulative incidence rate of combined recurrences	1.5% (n = 6)
Primary sites of 39 recurrences	Orbit = 10; Head/neck nonorbital = 8; Vagina = 7; Paratestis = 6; Biliary = 2; Cervix uteri = 1; Vulva = 1; Extremity = 1; Other sites = 2; Unknown = 1
13 deaths	12 due to progressive tumor; one from *Staphylococcus* sepsis
Five-year FFS rate in subgroup A patients	89% (95% CI, 84–92)
Five-year FFS rate in subgroup B patients	85% (95% CI, 74–91)
Five-year FFS rate in subgroup A patients for 108 paratesticular patients	96% (95% CI, 90–99)
Five-year OS rate in subgroup A patients for 108 paratesticular patients	100%
Five-year FFS rate in 16 subgroup A girls with GU tumors	52% (95% CI, 23–74)
Five-year OS rate in 16 subgroup A girls with GU tumors	92% (95% CI, 57–99)

Adverse Events

- Five patients developed hepatopathy, with abdominal distension and right upper quadrant abdominal pain with/without other signs of sinusoidal obstruction syndrome; one died of sepsis and the others recovered. After drug dose reductions, no further cases of hepatopathy were reported
- Two patients had severe mucositis
- A patient treated with VAC developed hematuria attributed to cyclophosphamide
- Rates of decreased absolute neutrophil count lower than 500/μL were 14% to 34% in patients receiving VA and 60% to 95% in patients receiving VAC

Efficacy (continued)

Outcomes Among Three Subcategories of D9602 Patients Comparison With Similar Patients from IRSG Protocols III and IV

Parameter	IRS-III No.	IRS-III %	IRS-IV No.	IRS-IV %	D9602 No.	D9602 %
Stage I, group IIA, number of patients	52	100	43	100	62	100
Site of primary tumor						
Orbit	23	44	20	47	18	29
Nonparameningeal head/neck	21	40	7	16	14	23
Paratestis	4	8	11	26	18	29
Other GU, not bladder/prostate	4	8	5	12	12	19
Protocol chemotherapy	VA		VAC/ VAI/ VIE		VA	
Protocol radiotherapy, Gy	41.4		41.4		36	
5-year failure-free survival		85		98		81
5-year overall survival		94		100		94
5-year cumulative incidence of local-only failure		11		2		15
5-year cumulative incidence of other failure		4		0		4
Group III orbit tumors, number of patients	71	100	50	100	77	100
Protocol chemotherapy	VA		VAC/ VAI/ VIE		VA	
Protocol radiotherapy, Gy	45.0 or 50.4		50.4 or 59.4		45.0	
5-year failure-free survival		79		94		86
5-year overall survival		95		100		96
5-year cumulative incidence of local-only failure		16		4		14
5-year cumulative incidence of other failure		3		0		0
Stages 2 + 3, group IIA, number of patients	38	100	28	100	16	100
Site of primary tumor						
Extremity	12	32	4	14	2	13
Retroperitoneum/trunk	9	24	4	14	6	38
Bladder/prostate	6	16	9	32	3	19
Parameningeal	5	13	8	29	3	19
Other	6	16	3	11	2	13
Protocol chemotherapy	VA		VAC/ VAI/ VIE		VAC	
Protocol radiotherapy, Gy	41.4		41.4		36	
5-year failure-free survival		76		88		94
5-year overall survival		78		92		100
5-year cumulative incidence of local-only failure		14		7		0
5-year cumulative incidence of other failure		11		4		6

IRSG, Intergroup Rhabdomyosarcoma Study Group; GU, genitourinary tract; VA, vincristine and dactinomycin; VAC, vincristine, dactinomycin, cyclophosphamide; I, ifosfamide; E, etoposide (randomized in IRS-IV)

Therapy Monitoring

1. *Daily during therapy with cyclophosphamide, and as clinically indicated:* urinalysis
2. *Before each cycle:* serum creatinine, LFTs with bilirubin, serum electrolytes, including calcium, magnesium, and phosphorus
3. *Weekly:* physical examination
4. *Twice per week:* CBC with differential until recovery from hematopoietic toxicity
5. *Response evaluation:* at weeks 12, 24, and end of therapy

PREVIOUSLY UNTREATED • NONMETASTATIC • RHABDOMYOSARCOMA

RHABDOMYOSARCOMA (NOT LOW RISK) REGIMEN: VINCRISTINE + DACTINOMYCIN + CYCLOPHOSPHAMIDE (VAC, PER D9803) ± MAINTENANCE THERAPY (PER RMS 2005)

Arndt CAS et al. J Clin Oncol 2009;27:5182–5188
Bisogno G et al. Lancet Oncol 2019;20:1566–1575

Note: regarding "not low risk" designation—In the US categorized as intermediate risk; in Europe corresponds most closely to high risk. Currently either VAC ± maintenance or VAC/VI ± maintenance is used for those designated "not low risk" based on recent results comparing outcomes of ARST0531 (VAC/VI regimen) to D9803
VAC/VI regimen from Hawkins et al (see VAC/VI ± maintenance, Hawkins et al)
VAC regimen ± maintenance from Crist et al or Arndt et al (see VAC ± maintenance, Crist et al)
See also IVA regimen + maintenance VC, Bisogno et al

Treatment Schedule for Vincristine + Dactinomycin + Cyclophosphamide According to D9803

Drugs	Week 0	1	2	3	4	5	6	7	8	9	10	11	12	13	14	15	16
Vincristine (V)	V	V	V	V	V	V	V	V	V	V	V	V	V			V	
Dactinomycin (A)	A			A*			A*			A			A			*	
Cyclophosphamide (C)	C			C			C			C			C			C	
Radiation (RT)													RT†				

	Week 17	18	19	20	21	22	23	24	25	26	27	28	29	30	31	32	33
Vincristine (V)		V	V	V	V	V	V	V			V			V			V
Dactinomycin (A)		*			A			A			A			A			A
Cyclophosphamide (C)		C			C			C			C			C			C

	Week 34	35	36	37	38	39	40	41	42
Vincristine (V)	V	V	V			V			
Dactinomycin (A)			A			A			
Cyclophosphamide (C)			C			C			

*Withhold dactinomycin during weeks 3 and 6 in patients with parameningeal rhabdomyosarcoma with intracranial extension who initiate RT after week 0 VAC. For these patients, give dactinomycin as added therapy during weeks 15 and 18.
†See details regarding RT in Radiation Therapy table, below
Note: at week 12 excision of the tumor in group III patients was encouraged if it could be achieved with negative margins and with organ preservation and without loss of form or function. In these cases the radiation dose was adjusted according to the amount of residual tumor. Selected patients who responded poorly to induction chemotherapy were recommended to proceed to preoperative RT followed by second-look surgery at week 24

Vincristine 1.5 mg/m^2 per dose (maximum single dose = 2 mg); administer by intravenous infusion over 15 minutes in 25–50 mL 0.9% sodium chloride injection (0.9% NS) on day 1 (total dosage during the weeks in which vincristine is administered = 1.5 mg/m^2; maximum dose/treatment = 2 mg)

Age	Vincristine Dose
≥3 years	1.5 mg/m^2 per dose (maximum single dose = 2 mg)
1 to <3 years	0.05 mg/kg/dose
<1 year	0.025 mg/kg/dose

Pediatric patients: Dilute in 25 mL 0.9% NS
Adult patients: Dilute in 50 mL 0.9% NS

(continued)

(*continued*)

Dactinomycin 0.045 mg/kg (maximum single dose = 2.5 mg); administer by intravenous injection over 1–2 minutes on day 1 (total dosage during the weeks in which dactinomycin is administered = 0.045 mg/kg; maximum dose/cycle = 2.5 mg)

Age	Dactinomycin Dose
≥1 year	0.045 mg/kg (maximum single dose = 2.5 mg)
<1 year	0.025 mg/kg/dose

Hydration during cyclophosphamide:
Administer additional intravenous hydration (eg, 0.9% NS) to achieve a total rate of 2000 mL/m^2/day (taking into account volumes of diluent used for mesna and cyclophosphamide) continuing for 24 hours after the cyclophosphamide dose

An admixture containing **cyclophosphamide** 2200 mg/m^2 + **mesna** 120 mg/m^2; administer intravenously in 100–1000 mL 0.9% NS or 5% dextrose injection (D5W) over 10–30 minutes, on day 1 (total dosage during the weeks in which cyclophosphamide is administered = 2200 mg/m^2)

Age	Cyclophosphamide Dose	Mesna Dose
≥3 years	2200 mg/**m^2**/dose	120 mg/**m^2**/dose
1 to <3 years	73 mg/**kg**/dose	4 mg/**kg**/dose
<1 year	36 mg/**kg**/dose	2 mg/**kg**/dose

followed by

Mesna 1200 mg/m^2; administer intravenously in 250–1000 mL of 0.9% NS or D5W over 24 hours (rate of 50 mg/m^2 per hour), starting immediately after each dose of cyclophosphamide (total dosage during the weeks in which cyclophosphamide is administered = 1320 mg/m^2; includes 120 mg administered with cyclophosphamide)

Age	Mesna Dose
≥3 years	1200 mg/**m^2**/dose
<3 years	40 mg/**kg**/dose
<1 year	20 mg/**kg**/dose

The administration schedules for vincristine, dactinomycin, and cyclophosphamide appears in the table (above)

Radiation Therapy (RT)

Group	Time to Initiate RT	Total Dose of RT
Group I N0* (alveolar or undifferentiated tumors)	2–3 days after week 12 chemotherapy	36 Gy
Group II* (alveolar or undifferentiated tumors) at diagnosis	2–3 days after week 12 chemotherapy	36 Gy (node negative) 41.4 Gy (node positive)
Group III,* completely resected with negative margins at week 12	2–3 weeks after surgery	36 Gy
Group III,* with microscopic residual tumor after resection at week 12	2–3 weeks after surgery	41.4 Gy
Group III,* in complete remission by imaging and biopsy at week 12	2–3 days after week 12 chemotherapy (or longer delay if biopsy results not yet available)	41.4 Gy
Other group III* patients at diagnosis	2–3 days after week 12 chemotherapy	45 Gy (orbit) 50.4 Gy (all other sites)
Patients with parameningeal rhabdomyosarcoma with intracranial extension*	Begin at week 1 as soon as possible after completion of first VAC chemotherapy	50.4 Gy

*At diagnosis
Notes:
- Withhold dactinomycin during radiation therapy
- Megavoltage photon and/or electron beams were used, and brachytherapy was permitted in select cases. Proton therapy was not used.
- RT is delivered in 1.8 Gy fractions once daily for 5 days per week

Arndt CAS et al. J Clin Oncol 2009; 27:5182–5188
Supplement to: Casey DL et al. Cancer 2019; 125:3242–3248

(*continued*)

(continued)

Note: following completion of VAC according to D9803, consider administration of maintenance therapy with vinorelbine + cyclophosphamide as per the RMS 2005 protocol (Bisogno G et al. Lancet Oncol 2019;20:1566–1575). Refer to regimen entitled IFOSFAMIDE+ VINCRISTINE + DACTINOMYCIN (IVA) PLUS MAINTENANCE THERAPY (VINORELBINE + CYCLOPHOSPHAMIDE) for details

Supportive Care: Antiemetic prophylaxis
Emetogenic potential during weeks with dactinomycin, cyclophosphamide, and vincristine is **HIGH**. *Potential for delayed symptoms*
Emetogenic potential during weeks with cyclophosphamide and vincristine is **HIGH**. *Potential for delayed symptoms*
Emetogenic potential on days with vincristine alone is **MINIMAL**
See Chapter 42 for antiemetic recommendations

Hematopoietic growth factor (CSF) prophylaxis
Primary prophylaxis is indicated with:
Filgrastim (G-CSF) 5 μg/kg per day by subcutaneous injection
- Begin use from 24 hours after myelosuppressive chemotherapy is completed—that is, day 2 during cycles containing cyclophosphamide
- Filgrastim may be given on days when vincristine is administered alone
- Continue daily filgrastim use until ANC ≥15,000/mm^3
- Discontinue daily filgrastim use at least 24 hours before administering resuming myelosuppressive treatment (containing dactinomycin or cyclophosphamide)

See Chapter 43 for more information

Antimicrobial prophylaxis
Risk of fever and neutropenia is HIGH
Antimicrobial primary prophylaxis is recommended:
- Antibacterial—consider fluoroquinolone prophylaxis; *P. jirovecii* prophylaxis is recommended (eg, cotrimoxazole)
- Antifungal—recommended
- Antiviral—antiherpes antivirals (eg, acyclovir, famciclovir, valacyclovir)

Treatment Modifications

Vincristine, Dactinomycin, and Cyclophosphamide Dose Modifications

Note: administer vincristine regardless of peripheral blood counts

Hepatic Impairment	
Direct bilirubin <3.1 mg/dL	Administer full doses of chemotherapy
Direct bilirubin 3.1–5.0 mg/dL	Reduce the dosages of vincristine and dactinomycin by 50%
Direct bilirubin 5.1–6.0 mg/dL	Reduce the dosages of vincristine and dactinomycin by 75%
Direct bilirubin >6.0 mg/dL	Withhold vincristine and dactinomycin and administer the next scheduled doses if direct bilirubin has improved
Neuropathy (See Grading Below)	
G2 motor or sensory neuropathy	Administer vincristine with the dosage reduced by 50%. If the toxicity improves to G ≤1, then increase the dose for 75% of the full dose
G ≥3 motor or sensory neuropathy	Withhold vincristine until toxicity improves to G ≤2, then resume vincristine with the dosage reduced by 50%
Jaw pain	Continue vincristine at the current dose
Gastrointestinal Toxicity	
G ≥3 constipation (obstipation with manual evacuation indicated; limiting self-care ADL)	Withhold vincristine and optimize laxative regimen. When toxicity improves to G ≤1, resume vincristine with the dosage reduced by 50%. If the toxicity does not recur, then re-escalate the vincristine dose back to full dose
G ≥3 ileus (severely altered GI function; TPN indicated)	
G ≥3 mucositis	Withhold cyclophosphamide, mesna, and dactinomycin until toxicity resolves to G <1, then reduce subsequent doses of these medications by 25%. Do not delay or reduce the dose of vincristine

(continued)

Treatment Modifications (*continued*)

Urologic Toxicity

Transient microscopic hematuria (>50 RBC/HPF 1 or 2 times)	Double the rate of post-hydration and continue mesna
Persistent microscopic hematuria (>50 RBC/HPF ≥3 times), or transient gross hematuria	Double the rate of post-hydration, continue hydration for at least 24 hours, and increase the total daily mesna dose to be equivalent to 100% of the cyclophosphamide dose
Persistent gross hematuria	Discontinue cyclophosphamide until urine clears to microscopic hematuria, then resume with the cyclophosphamide dose reduced to 50% of the full dose with post-hydration and mesna administered as per above for persistent microscopic hematuria. Escalate the cyclophosphamide dose to 75% and 100% of the full dose as tolerated. Consider urology consultation

Hematologic Toxicity

ANC <750/mm³ or platelet count <75,000/mm³ on a day that dactinomycin or cyclophosphamide is due	Delay the cyclophosphamide, mesna, and dactinomycin doses by 1 week. Consider use of G-CSF in subsequent cycles for delays related to neutropenia. If counts recover, then administer the full doses. If counts do not recover, then reduce the cyclophosphamide, mesna, and dactinomycin doses by 25%

Grading of Adverse Events

Motor Neuropathy Grading

Grade 1	Subjective weakness, but no deficits detected under neurologic exam
Grade 2	Weakness that alters fine motor skills (buttoning shirt, writing or drawing, using eating utensils) or gait without abrogating ability to perform these tasks
Grade 3	Unable to perform fine motor tasks (buttoning shirt, writing or drawing, using eating utensils) or unable to ambulate without assistance
Grade 4	Paralysis

Sensory Neuropathy Grading

Grade 1	Paresthesias, pain, or numbness that do not require treatment or interfere with extremity function
Grade 2	Paresthesias, pain, or numbness that is controlled by non-narcotic medications or alter (without causing loss of function) fine motor skills (buttoning shirt, writing or drawing, using eating utensils) or gait without abrogating ability to perform these tasks
Grade 3	Paresthesias or pain that is controlled by narcotics, or interfere with extremity function (gait, fine motor skills as outlined above) or quality of life (loss of sleep, ability to perform normal activities severely impaired)
Grade 4	Complete loss of sensation or pain that is not controlled by narcotics

Patient Population Studied

Intermediate-risk rhabdomyosarcoma defined as stages 2 and 3, clinical group III embryonal (including botryoid and spindle cell) rhabdomyosarcoma, all nonmetastatic alveolar (defined as any part of the tumor having an alveolar component) rhabdomyosarcoma, undifferentiated sarcoma (UDS), or ectomesenchymoma. Previous analysis suggested that patients with stage 4, clinical group IV embryonal RMS who were younger than age 10 had an outcome similar to the intermediate-risk group; therefore, this subgroup of patients was also included

Previously untreated patients younger than age 50 who began therapy within 42 days after initial biopsy. If primary re-excision of tumor was the definitive operation, patients were classified according to clinical group after this operation, provided it was performed within 42 days of the initial procedure and before beginning protocol-specified chemotherapy

(*continued*)

Patient Population Studied (continued)

Baseline Characteristics of 617 Eligible Patients Enrolled on COG D9803

Baseline Characteristic	Randomized VAC (n = 264)		Randomized VAC/VTC (n = 252)		Nonrandomized VAC (n = 101)	
	Count	%	Count	%	Count	%
Sex						
Male	167	63	167	66	54	53
Female	97	37	85	34	47	47
Age, years						
<1	12	5	5	2	1	1
1–9	184	70	173	69	68	67
10+	68	26	74	29	32	32
Race/ethnicity						
White	177	67	170	67	70	69
Black	35	13	31	12	15	15
Hispanic	30	11	30	12	14	14
Other	22	8	21	8	2	2
Histology (composite)						
Embryonal	119	46	106	43	62	62
Alveolar	122	47	126	51	30	30
UDS	11	4	5	2	1	1
RMS, NOS	9	3	12	5	7	7
Tumor size (composite)						
≤5 cm	99	39	108	44	41	41
>5 cm	158	61	139	56	59	59
Primary site (composite)						
Extremity	45	18	46	19	0	
GU/BP	47	18	48	19	0	
Parameningeal	57	22	58	23	99	99
Retroperitoneal/perineal	50	19	35	14	0	
Other	58	23	62	25	1	1
Tumor stage (composite)						
1	38	15	46	18	0	
2	60	23	63	25	34	34
3	140	54	121	48	59	59
4	19	7	20	8	7	7
Group (composite)						
I	20	8	12	5	0	
II	34	13	42	17	1	1
III	184	72	175	70	92	92
IV	19	7	21	8	7	7
Regional lymph nodes (composite)						
N0	217	82	196	78	79	78
N1	40	15	53	21	21	21
NX	7	3	3	1	1	1
Tumor invasion (composite)						
T1	136	53	127	51	17	17
T2	120	47	121	49	83	83

Note: the percentage values are calculated within each column among patients with nonmissing data. Composite variables reflect central review data if available; otherwise, the value reported by the institution was used

COG, Children's Oncology Group; VAC, vincristine, dactinomycin, and cyclophosphamide; VAC/VTC, VAC alternating with vincristine, topotecan, and cyclophosphamide; UDS, undifferentiated sarcoma; RMS, rhabdomyosarcoma; NOS, not otherwise specified; GU, genitourinary; BP, bladder and prostate

Efficacy

Outcome by Treatment Stratum and Regimen

Treatment Stratum	4-Year FFS				
	VAC		VAC/VTC		
	No.	%	No.	%	p*
Estimated 4-year FFS rates		73%		68%	0.3
Estimated OS at 4 years		79%		79%	0.9
ERMS, stage 2/3, group III	106	76	99	73	0.7
ERMS, group IV, age <10 years	19	64	18	56	0.6
ARMS/UDS, stage 1 or group I	51	77	55	88	0.3
ARMS/UDS, stage 2/3, group II/III	88	68	80	52	0.05
PM with ICE	101	68			

Details of Treatment Failure

4-year local failure rate		16.5%		18.5%	0.5
4-year regional failure rates involving regional lymph nodes with or without local or distant recurrence		4.5%		4.8%	0.9
4-year distant failure rate, involving any metastatic disease		10.5%		13%	0.4

*Log-rank test
FFS, failure-free survival; VAC, vincristine, dactinomycin, and cyclophosphamide; VAC/VTC, VAC alternating with vincristine, topotecan, and cyclophosphamide; ERMS, embryonal rhabdomyosarcoma; ARMS, alveolar rhabdomyosarcoma; UDS, undifferentiated sarcoma; PM with ICE, parameningeal rhabdomyosarcoma with intracranial extension

Comparative Analysis—This Study and IRS-IV

	This Study	IRS-IV	P
Estimated OS at 4 years for VAC and VAC/VTC	79%	77%	

Treatment Outcome: PME

Four-year FFS for patients with PME assigned to VAC	68% (n = 101)	61% (n = 87)	0.4
Four-year OS for patients with PME assigned to VAC	71%, (n = 101)	65% (n = 87)	0.4

Outcome by Risk Group Stratum—Four-year FFS Rates

For alveolar/UDS stage 1 or group I patients	83%	74%
For embryonal, stage 2/3, group III patients	74%	77%
For PME patients	68%	62%
For alveolar/UDS stage 2/3 and group II/III patients	60%	57%
For patients <10 years with embryonal group IV disease	59%	36%

Adverse Events

Grade 3/4 Toxicities	VAC	VAC/VTC	
Febrile neutropenia	85%	78%	P = 0.04
Anemia	55%	58%	
Clinically documented infection	54%	55%	
Leukopenia	60%	62%	
Lymphopenia	22%	26%	
Neutropenia	63%	65%	
Thrombocytopenia	51%	53%	

Other toxicities

Severe hepatopathy	2.8% (n = 17)	3.1% incidence for VAC on IRS-IV	
Second malignancies	n = 11	n = 6	P = 0.6

Therapy Monitoring

1. *Daily during therapy with cyclophosphamide, and as clinically indicated:* urinalysis
2. *Before each cycle:* serum creatinine, LFTs with bilirubin, serum electrolytes, including calcium, magnesium, and phosphorus
3. *Weekly:* physical examination
4. *Twice per week:* CBC with differential until recovery from hematopoietic toxicity
5. *Response evaluation:* at weeks 12, 24, and end of therapy

PREVIOUSLY UNTREATED • NONMETASTATIC • RHABDOMYOSARCOMA

RHABDOMYOSARCOMA (NOT LOW RISK) REGIMEN: VINCRISTINE + DACTINOMYCIN + CYCLOPHOSPHAMIDE (VAC)/VINCRISTINE + IRINOTECAN (VI) (PER ARST0531) ± MAINTENANCE THERAPY (PER RMS 2005)

Hawkins DS et al. J Clin Oncol 2018;36:2770–2777
Casey DL et al. Cancer 2019;125:3242–3248
Bisogno G et al. Lancet Oncol 2019;20:1566–1575

Note: regarding "not low risk" designation—In the United States categorized as intermediate risk; in Europe corresponds most closely to high risk. Currently either VAC ± maintenance or VAC/VI ± maintenance is used for those designated "not low risk" based on recent results comparing outcomes of ARST0531 (VAC/VI regimen) to D9803
VAC/VI regimen from Hawkins et al
VAC regimen ± maintenance from Crist et al or Arndt et al (see VAC ± maintenance, Crist et al, or Arndt et al)
See also IVA regimen + maintenance VC, Bisogno et al

Treatment Schedule for VAC/VI According to ARST0531

Drugs	Week														
	1	2	3	4	5	6	7	8	9	10	11	12	13	14	15
Vincristine (V)	V	V	V	V	V	V	V	V	V	V	V	V	V		
Dactinomycin (A)	A												A		
Cyclophosphamide (C)	C									C			C		
Irinotecan (I)				I			I								
Radiation (RT)				RT											

	Week														
	16	17	18	19	20	21	22	23	24	25	26	27	28	29	30
Vincristine (V)	V	V		V	V		V	V	V	V	V		V		
Dactinomycin (A)							A						A		
Cyclophosphamide (C)							C						C		
Irinotecan (I)	I			I						I					

	Week														
	31	32	33	34	35	36	37	38	39	40	41	42	43		
Vincristine (V)	V	V	V	V			V	V		V					
Dactinomycin (A)				A						A					
Cyclophosphamide (C)				C						C					
Irinotecan (I)	I						I								

Note: response evaluations occurred at weeks 15 and 30 and at the completion of therapy. For patients >24 months of age, definitive RT was the planned local control modality. Delayed primary resection was allowed, but not encouraged. For patients age ≤24 months, individualized local control approaches, including delayed primary excision and response-adapted RT, were permitted. RT began at week 4 and was delivered in once-daily 1.8 Gy fractions administered 5 days per week. Target cumulative RT dose depended on clinical group, tumor site, node status, and histology at study entry

Vincristine 1.5 mg/m^2 per dose (maximum single dose = 2 mg); administer by intravenous infusion over 15 minutes in 25–50 mL 0.9% sodium chloride injection (0.9% NS) on day 1 (total dosage during the weeks in which vincristine is administered = 1.5 mg/m^2; maximum dose/treatment = 2 mg)

Age	Vincristine Dose
≥3 years	1.5 mg/m^2/dose (maximum single dose = 2 mg)
1 to <3 years	0.05 mg/kg/dose
<1 year	0.025 mg/kg/dose

Pediatric patients: Dilute in 25 mL 0.9% NS
Adult patients: Dilute in 50 mL 0.9% NS

(continued)

(continued)

Dactinomycin 0.045 mg/kg (maximum single dose = 2.5 mg); administer by intravenous injection over 1–2 minutes on day 1 (total dosage during the weeks in which dactinomycin is administered = 0.045 mg/kg; maximum dose/cycle = 2.5 mg)

Age	Dactinomycin Dose
≥1 year	0.045 mg/**kg**/dose (maximum single dose = 2.5 mg)
<1 year	0.025 mg/**kg**/dose

Hydration for cyclophosphamide:
0.9% NS 750 mL/m²; administer intravenously over 1–2 hours prior to the start of cyclophosphamide on day 1. Then, encourage oral fluid ingestion or administer additional intravenous hydration (eg, 0.9% NS) at a rate of 100 mL/m²/hour continued until the last intravenous mesna dose has been administered

Mesna 240 mg/m² per dose; administer intravenously, diluted in a convenient volume of 0.9% NS sufficient to produce a final mesna concentration ranging from 1–20 mg/mL, over 15 minutes administered just before, 4 hours after, and 8 hours after the start of the cyclophosphamide infusion on day 1 (total dosage during the weeks in which cyclophosphamide is administered = 720 mg/m²)

Cyclophosphamide 1200 mg/m²; administer intravenously in 100–1000 mL 0.9% NS or 5% dextrose injection (D5W) over 60 minutes, on day 1 (total dosage during the weeks in which cyclophosphamide is administered = 1200 mg/m²)

Age	Cyclophosphamide Dose	Mesna Dose
≥1 year	1200 mg/**m²**	240 mg/**m²** per dose
<1 year	40 mg/**kg**/dose	8 mg/**kg**/dose

Irinotecan 50 mg/m² per dose (maximum dose 100 mg); administer intravenously, diluted with 5% dextrose injection to a concentration within the range of 0.12–2.8 mg/mL, over 60 minutes once daily for 5 consecutive days on days 1–5 (total dosage during the weeks in which irinotecan is administered = 250 mg/m²)

Note: following completion of VAC/VI according to ARST0531, consider administration of maintenance therapy with vinorelbine + cyclophosphamide as per the RMS 2005 protocol (Bisogno G et al. Lancet Oncol 2019;20:1566–1575). Refer to regimen entitled IFOSFAMIDE + VINCRISTINE + DACTINOMYCIN (IVA) PLUS MAINTENANCE THERAPY (VINORELBINE + CYCLOPHOSPHAMIDE) for details

Supportive Care: Antiemetic prophylaxis
Emetogenic potential during weeks with dactinomycin, cyclophosphamide, and vincristine is **HIGH**. *Potential for delayed symptoms*
Emetogenic potential on days when irinotecan + vincristine is administered is **MODERATE**
Emetogenic potential on days with vincristine alone is **MINIMAL**
See Chapter 42 for antiemetic recommendations

Hematopoietic growth factor (CSF) prophylaxis
Primary prophylaxis is indicated with:
    Filgrastim (G-CSF) 5 µg/kg per day by subcutaneous injection
- Begin use from 24 hours after myelosuppressive chemotherapy is completed—that is, day 2 during VAC cycles and day 2 during vincristine and cyclophosphamide (VC) cycles
- Filgrastim may be given on days when vincristine is administered alone
- Continue daily filgrastim use until ANC ≥15,000/mm³
- Discontinue daily filgrastim use at least 24 hours before administering resuming myelosuppressive treatment (containing dactinomycin, cyclophosphamide, or irinotecan)
- Primary prophylaxis is not required following vincristine and irinotecan (VI) cycles
See Chapter 43 for more information

Antimicrobial prophylaxis
Risk of fever and neutropenia is HIGH
    Antimicrobial primary prophylaxis is recommended:
- Antibacterial—consider fluoroquinolone prophylaxis; *P. jirovecii* prophylaxis is recommended (eg, cotrimoxazole)
- Antifungal—recommended
- Antiviral—antiherpes antivirals (eg, acyclovir, famciclovir, valacyclovir)

Acute cholinergic syndrome
Atropine sulfate 0.25–1 mg subcutaneously or intravenously if abdominal cramping or diarrhea develop during or within 1 hour after irinotecan administration
- If symptoms are severe, add as primary prophylaxis at least 30 minutes before irinotecan during subsequent cycles

(continued)

(*continued*)

- For irinotecan, acute cholinergic syndrome may be characterized by abdominal cramping, diarrhea, diaphoresis, hypotension, flushing, bradycardia, rhinitis, increased salivation, meiosis, and lacrimation

Diarrhea management

- The potential for developing diarrhea and abdominal pain should be discussed with all patients and their caretakers, and instructions given to start loperamide immediately if these symptoms occur and to ensure adequate hydration is maintained. See Dose Modifications (below) for instructions

Latent or delayed-onset diarrhea*:

Loperamide 4 mg orally initially after the first loose or liquid stool, *then*

Loperamide 2 mg orally every 2 hours during waking hours, *plus*

Loperamide 4 mg orally every 4 hours during hours of sleep

- Loperamide doses are for patients >15 years of age. Refer to Treatment Modifications section for dosing in younger patients
- Continue for at least 12 hours after diarrhea resolves
- Recurrent diarrhea after a 12-hour diarrhea-free interval is treated as a new episode
- Rehydrate orally with fluids and electrolytes during a diarrheal episode
- If a patient develops blood or mucus in stool, dehydration, or hemodynamic instability, or if diarrhea persists >48 hours despite loperamide, stop loperamide and hospitalize the patient for IV hydration
- Alternatively, a trial of **diphenoxylate hydrochloride** 2.5 mg **with atropine sulfate** 0.025 mg (eg, Lomotil)
- Initial adult dose is 2 tablets 4 times daily until control has been achieved, after which the dose may be reduced to meet individual requirements. Control may often be maintained with as little as 2 tablets daily
- Clinical improvement of acute diarrhea is usually observed within 48 hours. If improvement of chronic diarrhea after treatment with a maximum daily dose of 8 tablets is not observed within 10 days, control is unlikely with further administration

Persistent diarrhea:

Octreotide 100–150 μg subcutaneously 3 times daily (adult dose). Maximum total daily adult dose is 1500 μg. Pediatric patients may initiate dosing at 1–10 μg/kg/dose every 8–12 hours (not to exceed 1500 μg per day)

Antibiotic primary prophylaxis and treatment during latent or delayed-onset diarrhea:

Consider the following to prevent or lessen irinotecan-associated diarrhea:

- Prophylactic oral **cefixime** 8 mg/kg (maximum dose of 400 mg) orally once daily, beginning 1–5 days prior to the start of irinotecan therapy and continuing until day 21 of the VI course, *alternatively:*
- **Cefpodoxime proxetil** 5 mg/kg/day per day orally twice daily with food (maximum dose of 200 mg twice daily)
  - Previous studies suggest prophylaxis with cephalosporin antibiotics can ameliorate irinotecan-associated diarrhea by reducing the enteric bacteria responsible for producing β-glucuronidase, which regenerates in the gut irinotecan's toxic metabolite, SN–38, by cleaving the glucuronide moiety from SN–38 (Wagner LM et al. Pediatr Blood Cancer 2008;50:201–207)
- Alternatively, **activated charcoal** at a dose equal to 5 times the irinotecan dose up to a maximum dose of 260 mg orally 3 times daily during irinotecan therapy (Michael M et al. J Clin Oncol 2004;22:4410–4417)

Antibiotic treatment during latent or delayed-onset diarrhea:

- A fluoroquinolone (eg, ciprofloxacin 500 mg orally every 12 hours) if absolute neutrophil count <500/mm³ with or without accompanying fever in association with diarrhea. Antibiotics should also be administered if a patient is hospitalized with prolonged diarrhea, and should be continued until diarrhea resolves

*Abigerges D et al. J Natl Cancer Inst 1994;86:446–449
Rothenberg ML et al. J Clin Oncol 2001;19:3801–3807
Wadler S et al. J Clin Oncol 1998;16:3169–3178

Treatment Modifications

Vincristine, Dactinomycin, Cyclophosphamide, and Irinotecan

Note: administer vincristine regardless of peripheral blood counts

Hepatic Impairment	
Direct bilirubin <3.1 mg/dL	Administer full doses of all chemotherapy
Direct bilirubin 3.1–5.0 mg/dL	Reduce the dosages of vincristine, dactinomycin, and irinotecan by 50%
Direct bilirubin 5.1–6.0 mg/dL	Reduce the dosages of vincristine, dactinomycin, and irinotecan by 75%
Direct bilirubin >6.0 mg/dL	Withhold vincristine, dactinomycin, and irinotecan and administer the next scheduled doses if direct bilirubin has improved

(*continued*)

Treatment Modifications (continued)

Neuropathy (See Grading Below)

G2 motor or sensory neuropathy	Administer vincristine with the dosage reduced by 50%. If the toxicity improves to G ≤1, then increase the dose for 75% of the full dose
G ≥3 motor or sensory neuropathy	Withhold vincristine until toxicity improves to G ≤2, then resume vincristine with the dosage reduced by 50%
Jaw pain	Continue vincristine at the current dose

Gastrointestinal Toxicity (Except Diarrhea)

G ≥3 constipation (obstipation with manual evacuation indicated; limiting self-care ADL)	Withhold vincristine and optimize laxative regimen. When toxicity improves to G ≤1, resume vincristine with the dosage reduced by 50%. If the toxicity does not recur, then re-escalate the vincristine dose back to full dose
G ≥3 ileus (severely altered GI function; TPN indicated)	
G ≥3 mucositis	Withhold cyclophosphamide, mesna, and dactinomycin until toxicity resolves to G <1, then reduce subsequent doses of these medications by 25%. Do not delay or reduce the dose of vincristine or irinotecan

Diarrhea in Children 2–15 Years of Age Related to Irinotecan

Children 2–15 years, with first liquid stools	Begin oral loperamide liquid immediately with the first liquid stool at a dosage of 0.18 mg/kg per day (0.03 mg/kg administered orally every 4 hours). Maximum single dose for patients weighing <13 kg is 0.5 mg loperamide; for 13 to <20 kg, 1 mg; for 20 to <43 kg, initially 2 mg then subsequently 1 mg; and for ≥43 kg, initially 4 mg then subsequently 2 mg
G3/4 diarrhea within the first 24 hours	Hospitalize for optimal management. Begin loperamide 0.06 mg/kg every 4 hours. Maximum single dose for patients weighing <13 kg is 0.5 mg loperamide; for 13 to <20 kg, 1 mg; for 20 to <43 kg, initially 2 mg then subsequently 1 mg; and for ≥43 kg, initially 4 mg then subsequently 2 mg. Reduce irinotecan dosage for the following cycle by 30% and initiate prophylaxis with cefixime or cefpodoxime proxetil if not already being used

Delayed Diarrhea in Patients >15 Years of Age Related to Irinotecan

G1 (2–3 stools/day > baseline)	Maintain irinotecan dose and schedule
G2 (4–6 stools/day > baseline)	Delay irinotecan until diarrhea resolves to baseline
G3 (7–9 stools/day > baseline)	Delay until diarrhea resolves to baseline, then reduce dosage of irinotecan by 30%
G4 (≥10 stools/day > baseline)	Delay until diarrhea resolves to baseline, then reduce dosage of irinotecan by at least 30%

Urologic Toxicity

Transient microscopic hematuria (>50 RBC/HPF 1 or 2 times)	Double the rate of post-hydration and continue mesna
Persistent microscopic hematuria (>50 RBC/HPF ≥3 times), or transient gross hematuria	Double the rate of post-hydration, continue hydration for at least 24 hours, and increase the total daily mesna dose to be equivalent to 100% of the cyclophosphamide dose
Persistent gross hematuria	Discontinue cyclophosphamide until urine clears to microscopic hematuria, then resume with the cyclophosphamide dose reduced to 50% of the full dose with post-hydration and mesna administered as per above for persistent microscopic hematuria. Escalate the cyclophosphamide dose to 75% and 100% of the full dose as tolerated. Consider urology consultation

Hematologic Toxicity

ANC <750/mm³ or platelet count <75,000/mm³ on day 1 of a VAC or VI cycle	Delay chemotherapy by 1 week. Consider use of G-CSF in subsequent cycles for delays related to neutropenia, if not already being used. If counts recover, then administer full chemotherapy doses. If counts do not recover, then reduce the dose of cyclophosphamide, mesna, and dactinomycin doses by 25% or the dose of irinotecan by 30% for the next cycle for which the same drug is due

(continued)

Treatment Modifications (continued)

Grading of Adverse Events

Motor neuropathy grading

Grade 1	Subjective weakness, but no deficits detected under neurologic exam
Grade 2	Weakness that alters fine motor skills (buttoning shirt, writing or drawing, using eating utensils) or gait without abrogating ability to perform these tasks
Grade 3	Unable to perform fine motor tasks (buttoning shirt, writing or drawing, using eating utensils) or unable to ambulate without assistance
Grade 4	Paralysis

Sensory Neuropathy Grading

Grade 1	Paresthesias, pain, or numbness that do not require treatment or interfere with extremity function
Grade 2	Paresthesias, pain, or numbness that is controlled by non-narcotic medications or alter (without causing loss of function) fine motor skills (buttoning shirt, writing or drawing, using eating utensils) or gait without abrogating ability to perform these tasks
Grade 3	Paresthesias or pain that is controlled by narcotics, or interfere with extremity function (gait, fine motor skills as outlined above) or quality of life (loss of sleep, ability to perform normal activities severely impaired)
Grade 4	Complete loss of sensation or pain that is not controlled by narcotics

Patient Population Studied

Intermediate-risk rhabdomyosarcoma (RMS) RMS was defined as ERMS (including botryoid and spindle cell variants) or ectomesenchymoma, stages II and III, clinical group 3, and any ARMS without distant metastases. For the purpose of analysis, botryoid and spindle cell RMS and ectomesenchymoma were classified with ERMS. Tumors with mixed histologic elements were classified by the majority component. Other major eligibility criteria were no prior chemotherapy or radiation therapy (RT); age <50 years; initiation of therapy within 42 days of diagnostic biopsy; and adequate renal, hepatic, and bone marrow function

Clinical Characteristics (n = 221)

Clinical Characteristic	Number	Percentage
Gender—male/female	120/106	53/47
Age, years		
0–0.99 13 6	20	9
1–9.99	129	57
≥10	77	34
Race		
White	167	74
Black	28	12
Asian	7	3
Other/unknown	24	11

(continued)

Efficacy

EFS and OS Rates VAC/VI
(VAC, Vincristine + Dactinomycin + Cyclophosphamide; VI, Vincristine + Irinotecan)

Patient Category	4-Year EFS, % (95% CI)	4-Year OS, % (95% CI)
All patients	59 (51–66)	72 (65–79)
ARMS only	51 (39–62)	66 (55–77)
ERMS/NOS/other	64 (54–73)	76 (68–84)

ARMS, alveolar rhabdomyosarcoma; EFS, event-free survival; ERMS, embryonal rhabdomyosarcoma; NOS, not otherwise specified; OS, overall survival

Patient Population Studied
(continued)

Ethnicity		
Hispanic or Latino	21	9
Non-Hispanic/ Latino	195	86
Unknown	10	4
RMS histology		
Embryonal	123	54
Alveolar	94	42
NOS/unknown	9	4
Clinical group—1/2/3	6/24/196	3/11/87
Stage—I/II/III	18/64/144	8/28/64
Maximum tumor size, cm*		
<5	101	45
5–9.99	101	45
≥10	23	10
T stage—T1/ T2	99/127	44/56
Regional lymph node status— N0/N1/ Nx	171/54/1	76/24/0.4
Primary site		
Orbit	4	2
Head or neck	15	7
Parameningeal	104	46
GU, bladder/ prostate	29	13
GU, nonbladder/ prostate	2	1
Extremity	29	13
Retroperitoneal/ perineal	26	12
Trunk	12	5
Other	5	2

*Data missing for three patients
GU, genito-urinary; N0, no clinical or radiographic evidence of regional lymph node involvement; N1, clinical and/or radiographic evidence of regional lymph node involvement; NOS, not otherwise specified; Nx, regional lymph nodes not evaluated; RMS, rhabdomyosarcoma; T1, confined to the organ of origin; T2, extends beyond organ of origin; VAC, vincristine, dactinomycin, and cyclophosphamide; VI, vincristine and irinotecan

Adverse Events

Percent With Toxicity With ≥10% Frequency in Any Reporting Period*

Grade 3 or 4 Toxicity	Week 1–15	Week 16–30	Week 31–43
Anemia	19.5	8.9	8.9
Anorexia	13.7	3.0	2.1
Diarrhea	15.9	10.8	2.6
Febrile neutropenia	10.6	18.1	6.8
Infections and infestations	10.6	5.9	6.3
Lymphopenia	15.9	22.2	22.1
Oral mucositis	18.6	2.5	1.1
Neutropenia	58.4	64.5	57.4
Peripheral motor neuropathy	3.5	10.8	7.4
Thrombocytopenia	5.3	11.8	6.8
Leukopenia	27.9	34.5	31.1

*Includes those who had a Grade 3/4 toxicity provided the toxicity had been reported in ≥10% of patients
VAC, vincristine, dactinomycin, and cyclophosphamide; VI, vincristine and irinotecan

Therapy Monitoring

1. *Daily during therapy with cyclophosphamide, and as clinically indicated:* urinalysis
2. *Before each cycle:* serum creatinine, LFTs with bilirubin, serum electrolytes, including calcium, magnesium, and phosphorus
3. *Weekly:* physical examination
4. *Twice per week:* CBC with differential until recovery from hematopoietic toxicity
5. *Response evaluation:* at weeks 12, 24, and end of therapy

PREVIOUSLY UNTREATED • NONMETASTATIC • RHABDOMYOSARCOMA

RHABDOMYOSARCOMA (NOT LOW RISK) REGIMEN: IFOSFAMIDE + VINCRISTINE + DACTINOMYCIN (IVA) PLUS VINORELBINE + CYCLOPHOSPHAMIDE MAINTENANCE THERAPY (RMS 2005)

Bisogno G et al. Lancet Oncol 2019;20:1566–1575
RMS 2005 Protocol, v1.3, May 2012. Available from https://www.skion.nl/workspace/uploads/Protocol-EpSSG-RMS–2005–1–3-May–2012_1.pdf [accessed 23 August 2020]

Induction therapy:

Treatment Schedule for IVA Induction According to RMS 2005

Drugs

Week	1	2	3	4	5	6	7	8	9	10	11	12	13	14	15
Vincristine (V)	V	V	V	V	V	V	V			V			V		
Dactinomycin (A)	A			A			A			A			A		
Ifosfamide (I)	I			I			I			I			I		
Radiation (RT)													RT		

Week	16	17	18	19	20	21	22	23	24	25	26	27
Vincristine (V)	V			V			V			V		
Dactinomycin (A)	A*			A			A			A		
Ifosfamide (I)	I			I			I			I		

*Week 16 dactinomycin is omitted during radiation therapy
Note: response evaluation occurred at week 9 to plan local treatment (surgery, RT, or both) which was then implemented at week 13. When a residual mass was identified, surgical resection was recommended when feasible, always followed by RT in cases of incomplete resection. RT doses ranged from 41.4 Gy to 50.4 Gy depending on tumor histology, response to chemotherapy, and surgical outcome. RT was delivered in once-daily 1.8 Gy fractions administered 5 days per week
For large tumors that responded poorly to chemotherapy, a boost of 5.4 Gy (1.8 Gy/fraction × 3 fractions) was recommended

Vincristine 1.5 mg/m^2 per dose (maximum single dose = 2 mg); administer by intravenous infusion over 15 minutes in 25–50 mL 0.9% sodium chloride injection (0.9% NS) on day 1 (total dosage during the weeks in which vincristine is administered = 1.5 mg/m^2; maximum dose/week = 2 mg)

Age	Vincristine Dose
Age ≥12 months and weight ≥10 kg	1.5 mg/**m**^{2}/dose (maximum single dose = 2 mg)
Age <12 months or with weight <10 kg	0.05 mg/**kg**/dose

Pediatric patients: Dilute in 25 mL 0.9% NS
Adult patients: Dilute in 50 mL 0.9% NS

Dactinomycin 1.5 mg/m^2 (maximum single dose = 2 mg); administer by intravenous injection over 1–2 minutes on day 1 (total dosage during the weeks in which dactinomycin is administered = 1.5 mg/m^2; maximum dose/week = 2 mg)

Age	Dactinomycin Dose
Age ≥12 months and weight ≥10 kg	0.045 mg/**kg**/dose (maximum single dose = 2.5 mg)
Age <12 months or with weight <10 kg	0.05 mg/**kg**/dose

Hydration during ifosfamide:
Administer additional intravenous hydration (eg, 0.9% NS) to achieve a total rate of 2000 mL/m^2/day (taking into account volumes of diluent used for mesna and ifosfamide administration) for the duration of ifosfamide treatment and continuing for 12 hours after the last dose

Ifosfamide 3000 mg/m^2 per day; administer intravenously, diluted in 0.9% NS or 5% dextrose injection (D5W) to a concentration within the range of 0.6–20 mg/mL, over 3 hours for 2 consecutive days, on days 1–2 (total dosage during the weeks in which ifosfamide is administered = 6000 mg/m^2)

(continued)

(continued)

Age	Ifosfamide Dose
Age ≥12 months and weight ≥10 kg	3000 mg/m^2/dose
Age 3 months to <12 months or with weight <10 kg	100 mg/kg/dose
Age 1 months to <3 months	50 mg/kg/dose

Mesna utilization strategies, include:

Mesna 3000 mg/m^2 per day; administer by continuous intravenous infusion, diluted in a convenient volume of 0.9% NS or D5W sufficient to produce a final mesna concentration ranging from 1–20 mg/mL, over 12 hours starting simultaneously with ifosfamide, on days 1–2; *or:*

Age	Mesna Dose
Age ≥12 months and weight ≥10 kg	3000 mg/m^2/dose
Age 3 months to <12 months or with weight <10 kg	100 mg/kg/dose
Age 1 months to <3 months	50 mg/kg/dose

Mesna 750 mg/m^2 per dose; administer intravenously, in convenient volume of 0.9% NS or D5W sufficient to produce a final mesna concentration ranging from 1–20 mg/mL, over 15–30 minutes every 3 hours for 4 doses per day on days 1–2. The first dose is given when ifosfamide commences (ie, hours 0, 3, 6, and 9)

Age	Mesna Dose
Age ≥12 months and weight ≥10 kg	750 mg/m^2/dose
Age 3 months to <12 months or with weight <10 kg	25 mg/kg/dose
Age 1 months to <3 months	12.5 mg/kg/dose

Notes:
- If tolerated, drug dose should be increased by 25–30% at each cycle to full dose by body weight
- Ifosfamide should not be given in children less than 3 months in the initial cycle(s); however, it should be administered in the subsequent courses as the child grows up and providing the chemotherapy is well tolerated
- In patients with body surface area >2 m^2 the chemotherapy dose should not exceed the dose calculated for a BSA of 2 m^2 (observe maximum single dose 2 mg for VCR and ACT-D). The dose given to obese patients should be calculated based on regular body weight

Supportive Care: Antiemetic prophylaxis
*Emetogenic potential during weeks with ifosfamide, vincristine, ± dactinomycin is **HIGH**. Potential for delayed symptoms*
*Emetogenic potential on days with vincristine alone is **MINIMAL***
See Chapter 42 for antiemetic recommendations

Hematopoietic growth factor (CSF) prophylaxis
Primary prophylaxis is indicated with:
Filgrastim (G-CSF) 5 μg/kg per day by subcutaneous injection
- Begin use from 24 hours after myelosuppressive chemotherapy is completed—that is, day 3 during IVA cycles and day 3 during ifosfamide and vincristine (IV) cycles
- Filgrastim may be given on days when vincristine is administered alone
- Continue daily filgrastim use until ANC ≥15,000/mm^3
- Discontinue daily filgrastim use at least 24 hours before administering resuming myelosuppressive treatment (containing dactinomycin, cyclophosphamide, or irinotecan)
- Primary prophylaxis is not required following vincristine and irinotecan (VI) cycles
See Chapter 43 for more information

Antimicrobial prophylaxis
Risk of fever and neutropenia is HIGH
Antimicrobial primary prophylaxis is recommended:
- Antibacterial—consider fluoroquinolone prophylaxis; *P. jirovecii* prophylaxis is recommended (eg, cotrimoxazole)
- Antifungal—recommended
- Antiviral—antiherpes antivirals (eg, acyclovir, famciclovir, valacyclovir)

(continued)

(continued)

Maintenance Therapy:
Cyclophosphamide 25 mg/m² per dose; administer orally, once daily in the morning, continuously, on days 1–28, every 28 days, for 6 cycles (total dosage/28-day cycle = 700 mg/m²)
Note: cyclophosphamide is only available in 25 mg and 50 mg capsules. Thus, it may be necessary to modify the schedule of administration (ie, by using different doses on different days) in order to attain a weekly cumulative dose as close to 175 mg/m² as possible

Vinorelbine 25 mg/m² per dose; administer by intravenous infusion in a volume of 0.9% NS or D5W sufficient to produce a vinorelbine concentration within the range 0.5–2 mg/mL, over 10 minutes, for 3 doses on days 1, 8, and 15, every 28 days, for 6 cycles (total dosage/28-day cycle = 75 mg/m²)

Supportive Care: Antiemetic prophylaxis
Emetogenic potential of oral cyclophosphamide is **MINIMAL TO LOW**
Emetogenic potential of vinorelbine is **MINIMAL**
See Chapter 42 for antiemetic recommendations

Hematopoietic growth factor (CSF) prophylaxis
Primary prophylaxis is NOT indicated during maintenance therapy

Antimicrobial prophylaxis
Risk of fever and neutropenia during maintenance is HIGH
   Antimicrobial primary prophylaxis is recommended:
   • Antibacterial—consider fluoroquinolone prophylaxis; *P. jirovecii* prophylaxis is recommended (eg, cotrimoxazole)
   • Antifungal—recommended
   • Antiviral—antiherpes antivirals (eg, acyclovir, famciclovir, valacyclovir)

Treatment Modifications

Vincristine, Dactinomycin, Ifosfamide (Induction)

Note: **administer vincristine regardless of peripheral blood counts**

Hepatic Impairment	
Direct bilirubin <3.1 mg/dL	Administer full doses of all chemotherapy
Direct bilirubin 3.1–5.0 mg/dL	Reduce the dosages of vincristine and dactinomycin by 50%. Reduce the ifosfamide/mesna doses by 75%
Direct bilirubin 5.1–6.0 mg/dL	Reduce the dosages of vincristine, dactinomycin, and ifosfamide/mesna by 75%
Direct bilirubin >6.0 mg/dL	Withhold vincristine, dactinomycin, and ifosfamide/mesna and administer the next scheduled doses if direct bilirubin has improved
Veno-occlusive disease (VOD) vod appears related to the administration of different drugs, dactinomycin in particular. Predisposing factors have not been found to identify patients at risk	Withhold dactinomycin until the main abnormalities have returned to normal. Then re-institute therapy with half the dose. If tolerated, the dactinomycin dose may be increased progressively in the following cycles. If the symptoms reappear during dactinomycin treatment, this drug should be withdrawn permanently

Renal Impairment or Renal Toxicity	
SCr 1.5 × baseline	Delay ifosfamide by 1–7 days; administer hydration. If renal function does not improve, then discontinue ifosfamide
G2 renal toxicity—tubular (based on creatinine clearance, serum bicarbonate, need for electrolyte replacement, or TmP/GFR)	Reduce the ifosfamide/mesna doses by 25% in subsequent cycles
G ≥3 renal toxicity—tubular (based on creatinine clearance, serum bicarbonate, need for electrolyte replacement, or TmP/GFR)	Discontinue ifosfamide

Neuropathy (See Grading Below)	
G2 motor or sensory neuropathy	Administer vincristine with the dosage reduced by 50%. If the toxicity improves to G ≤1, then increase the dose for 75% of the full dose
G ≥3 motor or sensory neuropathy	Withhold vincristine until toxicity improves to G ≤2, then resume vincristine with the dosage reduced by 50%
Jaw pain	Continue vincristine at the current dose

(continued)

Treatment Modifications (*continued*)

Gastrointestinal Toxicity

G ≥3 constipation (obstipation with manual evacuation indicated; limiting self-care ADL) G ≥3 ileus (severely altered GI function; TPN indicated)	Withhold vincristine and optimize laxative regimen. When toxicity improves to G ≤1, resume vincristine with the dosage reduced by 50%. If the toxicity does not recur, then re-escalate the vincristine dose back to full dose
G ≥3 mucositis	Withhold ifosfamide/mesna and dactinomycin until toxicity resolves to G <1, then reduce subsequent doses of these medications by 25%. Do not delay or reduce the dose of vincristine

Urologic Toxicity

Transient microscopic hematuria (>50 RBC/HPF 1 or 2 times)	Double the rate of post-hydration and continue mesna
Persistent microscopic hematuria (>50 RBC/HPF ≥3 times), or transient gross hematuria	Double the rate of post-hydration and continue mesna. Consider prolonging the duration of intravenous hydration
Persistent gross hematuria	Discontinue ifosfamide until urine clears to microscopic hematuria, then resume with the ifosfamide dose reduced to 50% of the full dose with post-hydration and mesna administered as per above for persistent microscopic hematuria. Escalate the ifosfamide dose to 75% and 100% of the full dose as tolerated. Consider urology consultation. Only recurrent macroscopic hematuria is an indication for discontinuing ifosfamide, in which case cyclophosphamide at a dose of 1500 mg/m^2 per course may be substituted

Encephalopathy

G2 encephalopathy	If persistent or distressing, then decrease the ifosfamide and mesna dosages by 25%. If not contraindicated, treat with methylene blue 2 mg/kg (maximum dose of 50 mg) intravenously every 4–8 hours until resolution of symptoms, then consider prophylactic use at the same dose given every 6–8 hours in subsequent cycles
G3 encephalopathy	Stop ifosfamide for this cycle. If not contraindicated, treat with methylene blue 2 mg/kg (maximum dose of 50 mg) intravenously every 4–8 hours until resolution of symptoms, then consider prophylactic use at the same dose given every 6–8 hours in subsequent cycles. Decrease the ifosfamide and mesna dosages by 25% in subsequent cycles
G4 encephalopathy	Permanently discontinue ifosfamide. If not contraindicated, treat with methylene blue 2 mg/kg (maximum dose of 50 mg) intravenously every 4–8 hours until resolution of symptoms

Hematologic Toxicity

ANC <1000/mm^3 or platelet count <80,000/mm^3 on day 1 of an IVA cycle	Delay chemotherapy by 1 week. Consider use of G-CSF in subsequent cycles for delays related to neutropenia, if not already being used. If counts recover, then administer full chemotherapy doses. If counts do not recover, then reduce the dose of ifosfamide, mesna, and dactinomycin by 25%
Neutropenic fever in the prior cycle	Add G-CSF in subsequent cycles if not already being used. Reduce the dose of ifosfamide, mesna, and dactinomycin by 25%

Cyclophosphamide and Vinorelbine (Maintenance) Dose Modifications

Hematologic Toxicity

ANC <1000/mm^3 or platelet count <80,000/mm^3 at any time during maintenance therapy, first occurrence	Withhold cyclophosphamide and vinorelbine until improvement of ANC to ≥1,000/mm^3 and platelet count to ≥80,000/mm^3. In subsequent cycles, continue cyclophosphamide at the same dose and omit the day 15 vinorelbine dose
ANC <1000/mm^3 or platelet count <80,000/mm^3 at any time during maintenance therapy, second occurrence	Withhold cyclophosphamide and vinorelbine until improvement of ANC to ≥1,000/mm^3 and platelet count to ≥80,000/mm^3. In subsequent cycles, continue cyclophosphamide at the same dose and administer vinorelbine on days 1 and 8 with the dosage reduced by 33%. Continue to omit the day 15 vinorelbine dose

Grading of Adverse Events

Motor Neuropathy Grading

Grade 1	Subjective weakness, but no deficits detected under neurologic exam
Grade 2	Weakness that alters fine motor skills (buttoning shirt, writing or drawing, using eating utensils) or gait without abrogating ability to perform these tasks

(*continued*)

Treatment Modifications (continued)

Grade 3	Unable to perform fine motor tasks (buttoning shirt, writing or drawing, using eating utensils) or unable to ambulate without assistance
Grade 4	Paralysis

Sensory Neuropathy Grading

Grade 1	Paresthesias, pain, or numbness that do not require treatment or interfere with extremity function
Grade 2	Paresthesias, pain, or numbness that is controlled by non-narcotic medications or alter (without causing loss of function) fine motor skills (buttoning shirt, writing or drawing, using eating utensils) or gait without abrogating ability to perform these tasks
Grade 3	Paresthesias or pain that is controlled by narcotics, or interfere with extremity function (gait, fine motor skills as outlined above) or quality of life (loss of sleep, ability to perform normal activities severely impaired)
Grade 4	Complete loss of sensation or pain that is not controlled by narcotics

Patient Population Studied

The high-risk group comprised patients with nonmetastatic, incompletely resected, embryonal rhabdomyosarcoma occurring at unfavorable sites, age ≥10 years or tumor size >5 cm, or both; those with any nonmetastatic embryonal rhabdomyosarcoma with nodal involvement; or those with any nonmetastatic alveolar rhabdomyosarcoma without nodal involvement. Patients in the low-risk, standard-risk, and very-high-risk groups were not eligible for this study and were treated according to specific recommendations included in the RMS 2005 study

Clinical Characteristics of Randomized Patients by Treatment Group

	Stop Treatment (n = 186) [n (%)]	Maintenance Chemotherapy (n = 185) [n (%)]
Age at diagnosis, years		
≤1 year	2 (1%)	11 (6%)
>1–9 years	143 (77%)	136 (74%)
10–17 years	36 (19%)	34 (18%)
≥18 years	5 (3%)	4 (2%)
Sex—female / male	82 (44%) / 104 (56%)	80 (43%) / 105 (57%)
Histology of rhabdomyosarcoma		
Alveolar	62 (33%)	61 (33%)
Botryoid	5 (3%)	11 (6%)
Embryonal	113 (61%)	109 (59%)
Not otherwise specified	4 (2%)	2 (1%)
Spindle cells or leiomyomatous	2 (1%)	2 (1%)
Pathology—favorable / unfavorable	120 (65%) / 66 (35%)	122 (66%) / 63 (34%)
Presence of *FOXO*, *PAX3* or *PAX*7 translocation— no / yes / not done	85 (46%) / 41 (22%) / 60 (32%)	102 (55%) / 43 (23%) / 40 (22%)
Post-surgical tumor staging (IRS)		
Group I	5 (3%)	5 (3%)
Group II	20 (11%)	21 (11%)
Group III	161 (86%)	159 (86%)
Primary tumor invasiveness		
T1: localized to the organ or tissue of origin	88 (47%)	72 (39%)
T2: extending beyond tissue or organ of origin	97 (52%)	108 (58%)
Tx: insufficient information about primary tumor	1 (1%)	5 (3%)
Tumor size—≤5 cm / >5 cm / not evaluable	61 (33%) / 125 (67%)	52 (28%) / 130 (70%) / 3 (2%)

(continued)

Patient Population Studied (*continued*)

Regional lymph node involvement		
N0: no evidence of lymph node involvement	154 (83%)	148 (80%)
N1: evidence of regional lymph node involvement	29 (16%)	31 (17%)
Nx: no information about lymph node involvement	3 (2%)	6 (3%)
Site of origin of primary tumor		
Orbit	7 (4%)	5 (3%)
Head and neck non-parameningeal	11 (6%)	14 (8%)
Parameningeal	56 (30%)	64 (35%)
Bladder prostate	25 (13%)	27 (15%)
Genitourinary non-bladder prostate	5 (3%)	7 (4%)
Extremities	36 (19%)	27 (15%)
Other sites	46 (25 %)	41 (22%)
Subgroup risk—E / F / G	91 (49%) / 29 (16%) / 66 (35%)	91 (49%) / 31 (17%) / 63 (34%)

Efficacy

	Stop Treatment (n = 186)	Maintenance Chemotherapy (n = 185)	P Value
All events	54	40	
Local relapse or regional lymph node relapse	37 (69%)	26 (65%)	
Local or regional lymph node relapse and metastasis	6 (11%)	3 (8%)	
Median time to relapse calculated from the randomization date to the event was	6.9 months (IQR 3.0–16.1)	10.1 months (IQR 6.9–15.4)	
Metastases	10 (19%)	10 (25%)	
Death	1* (2%)	1† (3%)	
5-year disease-free survival—ITT	69.8% (95% CI 62.2–76.2)	77.6% (95% CI 70.6–83.2)	HR 0.68 (95% CI 0.45–1.02); P = 0.061
5-year overall survival—ITT	73.7% (95% CI 5.8–80.1)	86.5% (95% CI 80.2–90.9)	HR 0.52 (95% CI 0.32–0.86); P = 0.0097
5-year disease-free survival—Per protocol analysis	69.6% (95% CI 62.0–76.0)	77.8% (95% CI 70.8–83.4	HR 0.67 (95% CI 0.44–1.01); P = 0.053
5-year overall survival—Per protocol analysis	73.5% (95% CI 65.6–79.9)	86.3% (95% CI 79.9–90.8)	HR 0.53 (95% CI 0.32–0.87); P = 0.011

Note: a post-hoc exploratory subgroup analysis, taking into account clinical variables known to be of prognostic value, showed no differences in any subgroup of patients between the two groups

Adverse Events

Adverse Events Reported in 181 Patients During Maintenance Chemotherapy*

Toxicity	G1/2	G3	G4
Hematologic toxicity			
Anemia	128 (71%)	16 (9%)	3 (2%)
Leucopenia	26 (14%)	86 (48%)	50 (28%)
Neutropenia	16 (9%)	66 (37%)	82 (45%)
Thrombocytopenia	28 (16%)	1 (1%)	1 (1%)
Nonhematologic toxicity			
Cardiac	1 (1%)	—	—
Infection	33 (18%)	56 (31%)	—
Fever and neutropenia	4 (2%)	44 (24%)	—
Fever without neutropenia	26 (14%)	9 (5%)	—
Other infection	3 (2%)	3 (2%)	—
Nephrotoxicity	14 (8%)	1 (1%)	—
Neurology	21 (12%)	2 (1%)	1 (1%)
Nausea or vomiting	34 (19%)	1 (1%)	—
Gastrointestinal	41 (23%)	9 (5%)	—
Allergy	4 (2%)	—	—
Dermatological	7 (4%)	1 (1%)	—
Other	37 (20%)	1 (1%)	—

*Data are n (%)

Therapy Monitoring

Induction therapy:

1. *At least daily during therapy with ifosfamide, and as clinically indicated:* urinalysis
2. *Before each cycle:* serum creatinine, LFTs with bilirubin, serum electrolytes, including calcium, magnesium, and phosphorus
3. *Weekly:* physical examination
4. *Twice per week:* CBC with differential until recovery from hematopoietic toxicity
5. *Response evaluation:* at week 9 and end of therapy

Maintenance therapy:

1. *Before each 4-week maintenance cycle:* serum creatinine, LFTs with bilirubin, serum electrolytes including calcium, magnesium, and phosphorus, CBC with differential
2. *Weekly:* physical examination, CBC with differential

PREVIOUSLY UNTREATED • METASTATIC • RHABDOMYOSARCOMA

RHABDOMYOSARCOMA REGIMEN: VINCRISTINE + DACTINOMYCIN + CYCLOPHOSPHAMIDE (VAC, PER IRS-IV)

Crist WM et al. J Clin Oncol 2001;19:3091–3102
Lager JJ et al. J Clin Oncol 2006;24:3415–3422

Treatment Schedule for Vincristine + Dactinomycin + Cyclophosphamide According to IRS-IV

Drugs	Week																
	0	1	2	3	4	5	6	7	8	9	10	11	12	13	14	15	16
Vincristine (V)	V	V	V	V	V	V	V	V	V	V	V	V	V				V
Dactinomycin (A)	A*			A*			A			✻			✻				A
Cyclophosphamide (C)	C			C			C			C			C				C
Radiation (RT)										RT							

	Week																
	17	18	19	20	21	22	23	24	25	26	27	28	29	30	31	32	33
Vincristine (V)				V	V	V	V	V	V				V	V	V	V	V
Dactinomycin (A)				A			A						A			A	
Cyclophosphamide (C)				C			C						C			C	

	Week												
	34	35	36	37	38	39	40	41	42	43	44	45	46
Vincristine (V)	V				V	V	V	V	V	V			
Dactinomycin (A)					A			A					
Cyclophosphamide (C)					C			C					

*Withhold dactinomycin during weeks 3 and 6 in patients with parameningeal rhabdomyosarcoma with intracranial extension who initiate RT after week 0 VAC. For these patients, give dactinomycin as added therapy during weeks 9 and 12

Vincristine 1.5 mg/m² per dose (maximum single dose = 2 mg); administer by intravenous infusion over 15 minutes in 25–50 mL 0.9% sodium chloride injection (0.9% NS) on day 1 (total dosage during the weeks in which vincristine is administered = 1.5 mg/m²; maximum dose/treatment = 2 mg). Dilute in 25 mL 0.9% NS for pediatric patients and in 50 mL 0.9% for adult patients

Dactinomycin 0.015 mg/kg/dose (maximum single dose = 0.5 mg); administer by intravenous injection over 1–2 minutes once per day for 5 consecutive days on days 1–5 (total dosage during the weeks in which dactinomycin is administered = 0.075 mg/kg; maximum dose/cycle = 2.5 mg)

Hydration during cyclophosphamide:
Administer additional intravenous hydration (eg, 0.9% NS) to achieve a total rate of 2000 mL/m²/day (taking into account volumes of diluent used for mesna and cyclophosphamide) continuing for 24 hours after the cyclophosphamide dose

An admixture containing **cyclophosphamide** 2200 mg/m² + **mesna** 120 mg/m²; administer intravenously in 100–1000 mL 0.9% NS or 5% dextrose injection (D5W) over 10–30 minutes, on day 1 (total dosage during the weeks in which cyclophosphamide is administered = 2200 mg/m²), *followed by*

Mesna 1200 mg/m²; administer intravenously in 250–1000 mL of 0.9% NS or D5W over 24 hours (rate of 50 mg/m² per hour), starting immediately after each dose of cyclophosphamide (total dosage during the weeks in which cyclophosphamide is administered = 1320 mg/m²; includes 120 mg administered with cyclophosphamide)

Notes:
• The administration schedules for vincristine, dactinomycin, and cyclophosphamide appears in the table (above)
• Drug doses were reduced by 50% for infants less than 1 year of age to avoid excessive toxicity. Subsequent doses were increased to 75% and then to 100%, if tolerated

(continued)

(*continued*)

Supportive Care: Antiemetic prophylaxis
Emetogenic potential during weeks with dactinomycin, cyclophosphamide, and vincristine is **HIGH**. *Potential for delayed symptoms*
Emetogenic potential during weeks with cyclophosphamide and vincristine is **HIGH**. *Potential for delayed symptoms*
Emetogenic potential on days with vincristine alone is **MINIMAL**
See Chapter 42 for antiemetic recommendations

Hematopoietic growth factor (CSF) prophylaxis
Primary prophylaxis is indicated with:
Filgrastim (G-CSF) 5 µg/kg per day by subcutaneous injection
- Begin use from 24 hours after myelosuppressive chemotherapy is completed—that is, day 6 during VAC cycles and day 2 during vincristine and cyclophosphamide (VC) cycles
- Filgrastim may be given on days when vincristine is administered alone
- Continue daily filgrastim use until ANC ≥15,000/mm³
- Discontinue daily filgrastim use at least 24 hours before administering resuming myelosuppressive treatment (containing dactinomycin or cyclophosphamide)

See Chapter 43 for more information

Antimicrobial prophylaxis
Risk of fever and neutropenia is HIGH
Antimicrobial primary prophylaxis is recommended:
- Antibacterial—consider fluoroquinolone prophylaxis; *P. jirovecii* prophylaxis is recommended (eg, cotrimoxazole)
- Antifungal—recommended
- Antiviral—antiherpes antivirals (eg, acyclovir, famciclovir, valacyclovir)

Treatment Modifications

Vincristine, Dactinomycin, and Cyclophosphamide Dose Modifications

Note: administer vincristine regardless of peripheral blood counts

Hepatic Impairment	
Direct bilirubin <3.1 mg/dL	Administer full doses of chemotherapy
Direct bilirubin 3.1–5.0 mg/dL	Reduce the dosages of vincristine and dactinomycin by 50%
Direct bilirubin 5.1–6.0 mg/dL	Reduce the dosages of vincristine and dactinomycin by 75%
Direct bilirubin >6.0 mg/dL	Withhold vincristine and dactinomycin and administer the next scheduled doses if direct bilirubin has improved

Neuropathy (See Grading Below)	
G2 motor or sensory neuropathy	Administer vincristine with the dosage reduced by 50%. If the toxicity improves to G ≤1, then increase the dose for 75% of the full dose
G ≥3 motor or sensory neuropathy	Withhold vincristine until toxicity improves to G ≤2, then resume vincristine with the dosage reduced by 50%
Jaw pain	Continue vincristine at the current dose

Gastrointestinal Toxicity	
G ≥3 constipation (obstipation with manual evacuation indicated; limiting self-care ADL)	Withhold vincristine and optimize laxative regimen. When toxicity improves to G ≤1, resume vincristine with the dosage reduced by 50%. If the toxicity does not recur, then re-escalate the vincristine dose back to full dose
G ≥3 ileus (severely altered GI function; TPN indicated)	
G ≥3 mucositis	Withhold cyclophosphamide, mesna, and dactinomycin until toxicity resolves to G <1, then reduce subsequent doses of these medications by 25%. Do not delay or reduce the dose of vincristine

(*continued*)

Treatment Modifications (*continued*)

Urologic Toxicity

Transient microscopic hematuria (>50 RBC/HPF 1 or 2 times)	Double the rate of post-hydration and continue mesna
Persistent microscopic hematuria (>50 RBC/HPF ≥3 times), or transient gross hematuria	Double the rate of post-hydration, continue hydration for at least 24 hours, and increase the total daily mesna dose to be equivalent to 100% of the cyclophosphamide dose
Persistent gross hematuria	Discontinue cyclophosphamide until urine clears to microscopic hematuria, then resume with the cyclophosphamide dose reduced to 50% of the full dose with post-hydration and mesna administered as per above for persistent microscopic hematuria. Escalate the cyclophosphamide dose to 75% and 100% of the full dose as tolerated. Consider urology consultation

Hematologic Toxicity

ANC <750/mm^3 or platelet count <75,000/mm^3 on a day that dactinomycin or cyclophosphamide is due	Delay the cyclophosphamide, mesna, and dactinomycin doses by 1 week. Consider use of G-CSF in subsequent cycles for delays related to neutropenia. If counts recover, then administer the full doses. If counts do not recover, then reduce the cyclophosphamide, mesna, and dactinomycin doses by 25%

Grading of Adverse Events

Motor Neuropathy Grading

Grade 1	Subjective weakness, but no deficits detected under neurologic exam
Grade 2	Weakness that alters fine motor skills (buttoning shirt, writing or drawing, using eating utensils) or gait without abrogating ability to perform these tasks
Grade 3	Unable to perform fine motor tasks (buttoning shirt, writing or drawing, using eating utensils) or unable to ambulate without assistance
Grade 4	Paralysis

Sensory Neuropathy Grading

Grade 1	Paresthesias, pain, or numbness that do not require treatment or interfere with extremity function
Grade 2	Paresthesias, pain, or numbness that is controlled by non-narcotic medications or alter (without causing loss of function) fine motor skills (buttoning shirt, writing or drawing, using eating utensils) or gait without abrogating ability to perform these tasks
Grade 3	Paresthesias or pain that is controlled by narcotics, or interfere with extremity function (gait, fine motor skills as outlined above) or quality of life (loss of sleep, ability to perform normal activities severely impaired)
Grade 4	Complete loss of sensation or pain that is not controlled by narcotics

Patient Popluation Studied

Analysis of pooled individual patient data from five phase 2 window studies of high-risk rhabdomyosarcoma performed between 1988 and 2000. These data were compared with data of individual patients treated on IRS-III. Eligible patients were younger than 21 years old and had newly diagnosed stage IV/group IV pathologically proven rhabdomyosarcoma or undifferentiated sarcoma and no exposure to chemotherapy or radiotherapy

Patient Characteristics

Characteristic	IRS-III		ID		VM		IE		Topo		TC		Irino	
	No.	%	No.	%	No.	%	No.	%	No.	%	No.	%	No.	%
Age, years														
<5	15	13	14	15	10	20	7	17	6	15	8	14	5	25
5–9	21	18	14	15	15	29	11	26	8	21	10	18	2	10
10–14	50	43	35	36	14	27	14	33	9	23	26	46	5	25
15+	29	25	33	34	12	24	10	24	16	41	13	23	8	40
Sex														
Male	62	54	50	52	26	51	19	45	21	54	31	54	10	50
Female	53	46	46	48	25	49	23	55	18	46	26	46	10	50
Race														
White	89	77	67	72	31	61	28	67	29	74	34	60	13	65
Black	13	11	13	14	10	20	7	17	5	13	15	26	3	15
Other	13	11	13	14	10	20	7	17	5	13	8	14	4	20
Histology														
Alveolar	58	50	56	58	30	59	29	69	24	62	35	61	16	80
Embryonal	26	23	18	19	9	18	5	12	5	13	10	18	2	10
Undifferentiated	13	11	8	8	1	2	3	7	1	3	5	9	1	5
Other	18	16	14	15	11	22	5	12	9	23	7	12	1	5
Primary site														
Extremity	45	39	39	41	17	33	17	40	10	26	21	38	9	45
Head and neck	4	3	4	4	2	4	1	2	0	0	0	0	1	5
Intrathoracic	1	1	4	4	1	2	3	7	0	0	0	0	0	0
Genitourinary	4	3	3	3	4	8	1	2	6	15	7	13	2	10
Parameningeal	11	10	3	3	6	12	6	14	2	5	0	0	0	0
Paratestis	5	4	3	3	5	10	2	5	1	3	6	11	2	10
Perineum	2	2	5	5	1	2	1	2	4	10	1	2	1	5
Retroperitoneum	20	17	15	16	8	16	6	14	10	26	8	15	3	15
Trunk	12	10	12	13	2	4	3	7	4	10	7	13	0	0
Other	11	10	8	8	5	10	2	5	2	5	5	9	2	10
Tumor size, cm														
<5	24	27	17	21	7	14	8	20	7	18	12	23	5	25
≥5	64	73	65	79	43	86	33	80	31	82	40	77	15	75
Tumor invasion														
T1	13	20	11	16	6	12	2	5	5	13	5	10	2	10
T2	52	80	56	84	44	88	39	95	33	87	47	90	18	90
Nodal involvement														
N0	46	54	27	36	16	33	16	42	12	32	24	48	5	25
N1	39	46	49	64	32	67	22	58	25	68	26	52	15	75

IRS, Intergroup Rhabdomyosarcoma Study; ID, ifosfamide/doxorubicin; VM, vincristine/melphalan; IE, ifosfamide/etoposide; Topo, topotecan; TC, topotecan/cyclophosphamide; Irino, irinotecan

Efficacy

Response to VAC in Patients Experiencing Treatment Failure with Window Therapy

Therapy	Response to VAC		
	≥PR		<PR
	No.	%	
Alkylator window			
Ifosfamide/Etoposide failure	3		7
Vincristine/Melphalan failure	3		12
Topotecan/Cyclophosphamide failure	4		13
Subtotal	10*	24	32
Topoisomerase I poison window			
Topotecan failure	9		8
Irinotecan failure	2		2
Subtotal	11*	53	10
Total	21	33	42

*P = 0.05 (Fisher's exact test)
VAC, vincristine, dactinomycin, and cyclophosphamide; PR, partial response

Adverse Events

Not provided

Treatment Monitoring

1. *Daily during therapy with cyclophosphamide, and as clinically indicated:* urinalysis
2. *Before each cycle:* serum creatinine, LFTs with bilirubin, serum electrolytes, including calcium, magnesium, and phosphorus
3. *Weekly:* physical examination
4. *Twice per week:* CBC with differential until recovery from hematopoietic toxicity
5. *Response evaluation:* at weeks 9, 20, 29, and end of therapy

PREVIOUSLY UNTREATED • METASTATIC • RHABDOMYOSARCOMA

RHABDOMYOSARCOMA REGIMEN: INTENSIVE MULTIAGENT THERAPY (ARST0431)

Weigel BJ et al. J Clin Oncol 2016;34:117–122
Protocol for: Weigel BJ et al. J Clin Oncol 2016;34:117–122
https://clinicaltrials.gov/ct2/show/NCT00354744 [accessed 29 August 2020]

ARST0431 Treatment Schedule

Drugs	Week																	
	1*	2	3	4	5	6	7	8	9	10	11	12	13	14	15	16	17	18
Vincristine (V)	V	V	V	V	V		V	V			V	V			V	V		
Irinotecan (Irin)	Irin			Irin														
Doxorubicin (D)							D				D				D			
Cyclophosphamide (C)							C				C				C			
Ifosfamide (Ifos)									Ifos				Ifos				Ifos	
Etoposide (E)									E				E				E	

	Week																	
	19	20	21	22	23	24	25	26	27	28	29	30	31	32	33	34	35	36
Vincristine (V)		V	V	V	V	V				V	V			V	V		V	
Irinotecan (Irin)		Irin			Irin													
Doxorubicin (D)										D				D				
Dactinomycin (A)																	A	
Cyclophosphamide (C)										C				C			C	
Ifosfamide (Ifos)								Ifos				Ifos						
Etoposide (E)								E				E						
Radiation therapy (RT)			RT															

	Week																	
	37	38	39	40	41	42	43	44	45	46	47†	48	49	50	51	52	53	54
Vincristine (V)		V			V	V	V	V			V	V		V	V			
Dactinomycin (A)		A			A			A										
Cyclophosphamide (C)		C			C			C										
Irinotecan (Irin)											Irin			Irin				

*Patients with intracranial extension or spinal cord compression begin radiation therapy (RT) during week 1 and omit doxorubicin during week 7
†Previously unradiated metastatic sites may be irradiated during weeks 47–51
Note: radiation therapy to the primary tumor and to metastatic sites begins at week 20 for most patients

Vincristine 1.5 mg/m² per dose (maximum single dose = 2 mg); administer by intravenous infusion over 15 minutes in 25–50 mL 0.9% sodium chloride injection (0.9% NS) on day 1 (total dosage during the weeks in which vincristine is administered = 1.5 mg/m²; maximum dose/treatment = 2 mg)
• Administer vincristine before irinotecan when treatments coincide on the same day
• Dilute in 25 mL 0.9% NS for pediatric patients and in 50 mL 0.9% for adult patients

Irinotecan 50 mg/m² per dose (maximum single dose = 100 mg); administer intravenously, diluted with 5% dextrose injection (D5W) to a concentration within the range of 0.12–2.8 mg/mL, over 60 minutes once daily for 5 consecutive days on days 1–5 (total dosage during the weeks in which irinotecan is administered = 250 mg/m²; maximum dosage during the weeks in which irinotecan is administered = 500 mg)
• Administer irinotecan after vincristine when treatments coincide on the same day

Ifosfamide + mesna:

Hydration during ifosfamide:
Administer additional intravenous hydration (eg, 0.9% NS) to achieve a total rate of 2000 mL/m²/day (taking into account volumes of diluent used for mesna, ifosfamide, and etoposide administration) for the duration of ifosfamide treatment and continuing for 24 hours after the last dose. If feasible, continue maintenance intravenous hydration during intervals between ifosfamide administration. Encourage oral fluid ingestion. Monitor daily weight, or if implemented in an inpatient setting, monitor fluid input and output. Replace electrolytes as medically appropriate

(continued)

(continued)

An admixture containing **ifosfamide** 1800 mg/m^2 + **mesna** 360 mg/m^2 per day; administer intravenously in a volume of 0.9% NS or D5W sufficient to produce ifosfamide concentrations between 0.6 and 20 mg/mL, over 60 minutes for 5 consecutive days, on days 1–5 (total ifosfamide dosage during the weeks in which ifosfamide is administered = 9000 mg/m^2); *then, either:*

Mesna 360 mg/m^2 per dose; administer intravenously diluted with 0.9% NS or D5W to a concentration of 1–20 mg/mL, over 15 minutes for 2 doses per day at 4 hours and 8 hours after ifosfamide administration is completed, for 5 consecutive days, on days 1–5 (total mesna dosage during the weeks in which ifosfamide is administered = 5400 mg/m^2; includes 360 mg/m^2 doses given daily with ifosfamide), *or*
Mesna 720 mg/m^2 per dose; administer orally for 2 doses per day at 2 hours and 6 hours after ifosfamide administration is completed, for 5 consecutive days, on days 1–5 (total mesna dosage during the weeks in which ifosfamide is administered = 9000 mg/m^2; includes 360 mg/m^2 doses given daily with ifosfamide)

Etoposide 100 mg/m^2 per day; administer intravenously diluted with 0.9% NS to a concentration of 0.2–0.4 mg/mL over 30–60 minutes for 5 consecutive days, on days 1–5 (total dosage during the weeks in which etoposide is administered = 500 mg/m^2)

Doxorubicin 37.5 mg/m^2 per day; administer intravenously in 50–1000 mL 0.9% NS or D5W over 24 hours for 2 consecutive days, on days 1–2 (total dosage during the weeks in which doxorubicin is administered = 75 mg/m^2)

Cyclophosphamide + mesna:
Hydration for cyclophosphamide:
0.9% NS 750 mL/m^2; administer intravenously over 1–2 hours prior to the start of cyclophosphamide on day 1. Then, encourage oral fluid ingestion or administer additional intravenous hydration (eg, 0.9% NS) at a rate of 100 mL/m^2/hour continued until the last intravenous mesna dose has been administered

An admixture containing **cyclophosphamide** 1200 mg/m^2 + **mesna** 240 mg/m^2; administer intravenously in 100–250 mL 0.9% NS or D5W over 30–60 minutes on day 1 (total dosage during the weeks in which cyclophosphamide is administered = 1200 mg/m^2); *then, either:*

Mesna 240 mg/m^2 per dose; administer intravenously diluted with 0.9% NS or D5W to a concentration of 1–20 mg/mL, over 15 minutes for 2 doses at 4 hours and 8 hours after cyclophosphamide administration is completed, on day 1 (total mesna dosage during the weeks in which cyclophosphamide is administered = 720 mg/m^2; includes 240 mg/m^2 dose given with cyclophosphamide), *or*
Mesna 480 mg/m^2 per dose; administer orally for 2 doses at 2 hours and 6 hours after cyclophosphamide administration is completed on day 1 (total mesna dosage during the weeks in which cyclophosphamide is administered = 1200 mg/m^2; includes 240 mg/m^2 dose given with cyclophosphamide)

Dactinomycin 0.045 mg/kg (maximum dose = 2.5 mg); administer by intravenous injection over 1–5 minutes on day 1 (total dosage during the weeks in which dactinomycin is administered = 0.045 mg/kg; maximum dose = 2.5 mg)
- The administration schedules for vincristine, irinotecan, ifosfamide, etoposide, doxorubicin, dactinomycin, cyclophosphamide, and radiation therapy appear in the table (above)

Pediatric Age-Based Dose Adjustments

Medication	Age	Dose
Vincristine	≥3 years	1.5 mg/m^2 IV × 1 dose (maximum dose, 2 mg)
	≥1 and <3 years	0.05 mg/kg IV × 1 dose (maximum dose, 2 mg)
	<1 year	0.025 mg/kg IV × 1 dose
Ifosfamide	≥1 year	1800 mg/m^2 per dose IV × 5 doses
	<1 year	Reduce initial dose to 50% of the full dose calculated on a square-meter basis*†
Etoposide	≥1 year	100 mg/m^2 per dose IV × 5 doses
	<1 year	Reduce initial dose to 50% of the full dose calculated on a square-meter basis*
Doxorubicin	≥1 year	37.5 mg/m^2 per day IV × 2 days
	<1 year	Reduce initial dose to 50% of the full dose calculated on a square-meter basis*
Cyclophosphamide	≥3 years	1200 mg/m^2 IV × 1 dose
	<3 years	40 mg/kg IV × 1 dose†
Dactinomycin	≥1 year	0.045 mg/kg IV × 1 dose (maximum dose, 2.5 mg)
	<1 year	0.025 mg/kg IV × 1 dose

*If tolerated (ie, no delay in administration of the next cycle because of delayed count recovery or delayed resolution of other toxicities and no serious toxicities), consider increasing to 75% and then to 100% of the calculated full doses
†Intravenous mesna doses should be reduced so that the intravenous mesna dose is equivalent to 20% of the daily cyclophosphamide or ifosfamide dose. Oral mesna doses should be equivalent to 40% of the daily cyclophosphamide or ifosfamide dose

(continued)

(continued)

Supportive Care: Antiemetic prophylaxis
Emetogenic potential during days with irinotecan ± vincristine is **MODERATE**
Emetogenic potential on days with vincristine alone is **MINIMAL**
Emetogenic potential on days with vincristine + doxorubicin + cyclophosphamide (VDC) is **HIGH**. *Potential for delayed symptoms*
Emetogenic potential on days with doxorubicin alone is **MODERATE**
Emetogenic potential on days with ifosfamide + etoposide (IE) is **MODERATE**
Emetogenic potential during weeks with vincristine + dactinomycin + cyclophosphamide (VAC) is **MODERATE**
See Chapter 42 for antiemetic recommendations

Hematopoietic growth factor (CSF) prophylaxis
Primary prophylaxis is indicated with:
Filgrastim (G-CSF) 5 μg/kg per day by subcutaneous injection
- Begin use from 24 hours after myelosuppressive chemotherapy is completed—that is, day 6 during ifosfamide + etoposide (IE) cycles, day 4 during vincristine + doxorubicin + cyclophosphamide (VDC) cycles, and day 2 during vincristine + dactinomycin + cyclophosphamide (VAC) cycles
- Filgrastim may be given on days when vincristine is administered alone
- Continue daily filgrastim use for at least 7 days or until ANC ≥750/mm³, whichever comes last
- Discontinue daily filgrastim use at least 24 hours before administering resuming myelosuppressive treatment (containing dactinomycin, doxorubicin, cyclophosphamide, ifosfamide, etoposide, or irinotecan)
See Chapter 43 for more information

Antimicrobial prophylaxis
Risk of fever and neutropenia is HIGH
Antimicrobial primary prophylaxis is recommended:
- Antibacterial—consider fluoroquinolone prophylaxis; *P. jirovecii* prophylaxis is recommended (eg, cotrimoxazole)
- Antifungal—recommended
- Antiviral—antiherpes antivirals (eg, acyclovir, famciclovir, valacyclovir)

Acute cholinergic syndrome
Atropine sulfate 0.25–1 mg subcutaneously or intravenously if abdominal cramping or diarrhea develop during or within 1 hour after irinotecan administration
- If symptoms are severe, add as primary prophylaxis at least 30 minutes before irinotecan during subsequent cycles
- For irinotecan, acute cholinergic syndrome may be characterized by abdominal cramping, diarrhea, diaphoresis, hypotension, flushing, bradycardia, rhinitis, increased salivation, meiosis, and lacrimation

Diarrhea management
- The potential for developing diarrhea and abdominal pain should be discussed with all patients and their caretakers, and instructions given to start loperamide immediately if these symptoms occur and to ensure adequate hydration is maintained. See Dose Modifications (below) for instructions

Latent or delayed-onset diarrhea*:
Loperamide 4 mg orally initially after the first loose or liquid stool, *then*
Loperamide 2 mg orally every 2 hours during waking hours, *plus*
Loperamide 4 mg orally every 4 hours during hours of sleep
- Loperamide doses are for patients >15 years of age. Refer to Treatment Modifications section for dosing in younger patients
- Continue for at least 12 hours after diarrhea resolves
- Recurrent diarrhea after a 12-hour diarrhea-free interval is treated as a new episode
- Rehydrate orally with fluids and electrolytes during a diarrheal episode
- If a patient develops blood or mucus in stool, dehydration, or hemodynamic instability, or if diarrhea persists >48 hours despite loperamide, stop loperamide and hospitalize the patient for IV hydration
- Alternatively, a trial of **diphenoxylate hydrochloride** 2.5 mg **with atropine sulfate** 0.025 mg (eg, Lomotil)
- Initial adult dose is 2 tablets 4 times daily until control has been achieved, after which the dose may be reduced to meet individual requirements. Control may often be maintained with as little as 2 tablets daily
- Clinical improvement of acute diarrhea is usually observed within 48 hours. If improvement of chronic diarrhea after treatment with a maximum daily dose of 8 tablets is not observed within 10 days, control is unlikely with further administration

Persistent diarrhea:
Octreotide 100–150 μg subcutaneously 3 times daily (adult dose). Maximum total daily adult dose is 1500 μg. Pediatric patients may initiate dosing at 1–10 μg/kg/dose every 8–12 hours (not to exceed 1500 μg per day)
Antibiotic primary prophylaxis and treatment during latent or delayed-onset diarrhea:
Consider the following to prevent or lessen irinotecan-associated diarrhea:
- Prophylactic oral **cefixime** 8 mg/kg (maximum dose of 400 mg) orally once daily, beginning 1–5 days prior to the start of irinotecan therapy and continuing until day 21 of the VI course, *alternatively:*

(continued)

(continued)

- **Cefpodoxime proxetil** 5 mg/kg/day per day orally twice daily with food (maximum dose of 200 mg twice daily)
  - Previous studies suggest prophylaxis with cephalosporin antibiotics can ameliorate irinotecan-associated diarrhea by reducing the enteric bacteria responsible for producing β-glucuronidase, which regenerates in the gut irinotecan's toxic metabolite, SN-38, by cleaving the glucuronide moiety from SN-38 (Wagner LM et al. Pediatr Blood Cancer 2008;50:201–207)
- Alternatively, **activated charcoal** at a dose equal to 5 times the irinotecan dose up to a maximum dose of 260 mg orally 3 times daily during irinotecan therapy (Michael M et al. J Clin Oncol 2004;22:4410–4417)

Antibiotic treatment during latent or delayed-onset diarrhea:
- A fluoroquinolone (eg, ciprofloxacin 500 mg orally every 12 hours) if absolute neutrophil count <500/mm³ with or without accompanying fever in association with diarrhea. Antibiotics should also be administered if a patient is hospitalized with prolonged diarrhea, and should be continued until diarrhea resolves

*Abigerges D et al. J Natl Cancer Inst 1994;86:446–449
Rothenberg ML et al. J Clin Oncol 2001;19:3801–3807
Wadler S et al. J Clin Oncol 1998;16:3169–3178

Treatment Modifications

Hematologic Toxicity (applies to VI, VDC, VAC, and IE cycles)

Adverse Event	Dose Modification
ANC <750/mm³, platelet count <75,000/mm³, GFR <70 mL/min/1.73 m², total bilirubin >1.5 × ULN, or ALT >2.5 × ULN	Delay initiation of the next cycle of VI, VDC, VAC, or IE until parameters are met
Initiation of chemotherapy (VDC and IE) cycles is delayed by >1 week for slow neutrophil recover (ANC <750/mm³) during weeks 9, 11, 13, 15, 17, 28, 30, and 32	Decrease doxorubicin, cyclophosphamide, ifosfamide, and etoposide doses by 25% in subsequent cycles (decrease mesna doses accordingly). If ANC still does not recover by day 22 of subsequent cycles, reduce doses by a further 25 percent. Increase doses by 25 percent in subsequent cycles if ANC criterion is met by day 18
Initiation of VAC is delayed by >1 week for slow neutrophil recover (ANC <750/mm³ or platelet count <75,000/mm³) during weeks 35, 38, 41, and 44; or ANC <750/mm³ for >1 week	Decrease dactinomycin and cyclophosphamide doses by 25% in the next cycle (decrease mesna doses accordingly). May increase chemotherapy doses in subsequent cycles as tolerated

Hepatic Impairment (Applies to VI, VDC, VAC, and IE Cycles)

Total bilirubin < 2.1 mg/dL	Full doses of vincristine, dactinomycin, and irinotecan
Total bilirubin 2.1—4.0 mg/dL	Administer 50% of the full doses of vincristine and dactinomycin and administer 60% of the full dose of irinotecan
Total bilirubin 4.1—6.0 mg/dL	Administer 25% of the full dose of vincristine, administer 50% of the full dose of dactinomycin, and administer 30% of the full dose of irinotecan
Total bilirubin > 6.0 mg/dL	Do not give vincristine; administer 50% of the full dose of dactinomycin and administer 30% of the full dose of irinotecan

VINCRISTINE DOSE MODIFICATIONS
Note: **administer vincristine regardless of peripheral blood counts**

Neuropathy (See Grading Below)

G2 motor or sensory neuropathy	Administer vincristine with the dosage reduced by 50%. If the toxicity improves to G ≤1, then increase the dose for 75% of the full dose
G ≥3 motor or sensory neuropathy	Withhold vincristine until toxicity improves to G ≤2, then resume vincristine with the dosage reduced by 50%
Jaw pain	Continue vincristine at the current dose

Gastrointestinal Toxicity

G ≥3 constipation (obstipation with manual evacuation indicated; limiting self-care ADL)	Withhold vincristine and optimize laxative regimen. When toxicity improves to G ≤1, resume vincristine with the dosage reduced by 50%. If the toxicity does not recur, then re-escalate the vincristine dose back to full dose
G ≥3 ileus (severely altered GI function; TPN indicated)	

(continued)

Treatment Modifications (*continued*)

IRINOTECAN DOSE MODIFICATIONS

Myelosuppression

ANC <750/mm³ or platelet count <75,000/mm³ at the time of scheduled irinotecan	Delay until parameters are met. If recovery requires >1 week delay, then reduce the dose of irinotecan in the next course by 30% to 35 mg/m²/day (maximum single dose = 70 mg)

Diarrhea in Children 2–15 Years of Age Related to Irinotecan

Children 2–15 years, with first liquid stools	Begin oral loperamide liquid immediately with the first liquid stool at a dosage of 0.18 mg/kg per day (0.03 mg/kg administered orally every 4 hours). Maximum single dose for patients weighing <13 kg is 0.5 mg loperamide; for 13 to <20 kg, 1 mg; for 20 to <43 kg, initially 2 mg then subsequently 1 mg; and for ≥43 kg, initially 4 mg then subsequently 2 mg
G3/4 diarrhea	Hospitalize for optimal management. Begin loperamide 0.06 mg/kg every 4 hours. Maximum single dose for patients weighing <13 kg is 0.5 mg loperamide; for 13 to <20 kg, 1 mg; for 20 to <43 kg, initially 2 mg then subsequently 1 mg; and for ≥43 kg, initially 4 mg then subsequently 2 mg Reduce irinotecan dosage for the following cycle by 70% and initiate prophylaxis with cefixime or cefpodoxime proxetil if not already being used

Delayed Diarrhea in Patients >15 Years of Age Related to Irinotecan

G1 (2–3 stools/day > baseline)	Maintain irinotecan dose and schedule
G2 (4–6 stools/day > baseline)	Delay irinotecan until diarrhea resolves to baseline
G3 (7–9 stools/day > baseline)	Delay until diarrhea resolves to baseline, then reduce dosage of irinotecan by 70%
G4 (≥10 stools/day > baseline)	Delay until diarrhea resolves to baseline, then reduce dosage of irinotecan by 70%

IFOSFAMIDE DOSE MODIFICATIONS

Transient microscopic hematuria (>50 RBC/HPF 1 or 2 times)	Double the rate of post-hydration. Consider increasing the dose of mesna so that the total daily mesna dose is equivalent to 100% of the daily ifosfamide dose; consider administering mesna by a continuous infusion strategy
Persistent microscopic hematuria (>50 RBC/HPF ≥3 times), or transient gross hematuria	Withhold ifosfamide until hematuria has been clear for >1 week, then resume ifosfamide with the dosage reduced by 50%. Administer mesna by a continuous infusion strategy, with the total daily mesna dosage increased to be equivalent to 100% of the daily ifosfamide dose. Increase the ifosfamide dose to 100% as tolerated in subsequent cycles
Estimated creatinine clearance decreases by ≥33% from baseline or estimated creatinine clearance is <50 mL/min/1.73 m² in the absence of dehydration	Delay by 1 week. If parameters are still not met, then in each subsequent course of ifosfamide + etoposide, replace ifosfamide with cyclophosphamide 700 mg/m²/day intravenously over 1 hour on days 1, 2, and 3; administer mesna with cyclophosphamide
Development of significant Fanconi syndrome (symptoms include renal phosphorus wasting, renal bicarbonate wasting, renal potassium wasting, glycosuria, proteinuria, and reduced GFR)	In each subsequent course of ifosfamide + etoposide, replace ifosfamide with cyclophosphamide 700 mg/m²/day intravenously over 1 hour on days 1, 2, and 3; administer mesna with cyclophosphamide
G2 encephalopathy	If persistent or distressing, then decrease the ifosfamide and mesna dosages by 20%. If not contraindicated, treat with methylene blue 2 mg/kg (maximum dose of 50 mg) intravenously every 4–8 hours until resolution of symptoms, then consider prophylactic use at the same dose given every 6–8 hours in subsequent cycles
G3 encephalopathy	Stop ifosfamide for this cycle. If not contraindicated, treat with methylene blue 2 mg/kg (maximum dose of 50 mg) intravenously every 4–8 hours until resolution of symptoms, then consider prophylactic use at the same dose given every 6–8 hours in subsequent cycles. Decrease the ifosfamide and mesna dosages by 20% in subsequent cycles
G4 encephalopathy	Permanently discontinue ifosfamide. If not contraindicated, treat with methylene blue 2 mg/kg (maximum dose of 50 mg) intravenously every 4–8 hours until resolution of symptoms, then consider prophylactic use at the same dose given every 6–8 hours in subsequent cycles. Either decrease the ifosfamide and mesna dosages by 20% in subsequent cycles or replace ifosfamide with cyclophosphamide (as above for renal toxicity)
G ≥3 mucositis after IE cycle persisting beyond day 21 and unresponsive to maximum supportive care	Reduce the doses of ifosfamide/mesna and etoposide by 25% in subsequent cycles. If the mucositis was in part related to radiation therapy, then increase the chemotherapy doses back to full dose upon resolution of the toxicity

(*continued*)

Treatment Modifications (continued)

DOXORUBICIN DOSE MODIFICATIONS

LVEF is <45%	Discontinue doxorubicin. In subsequent VDC cycles, substitute doxorubicin with dactinomycin 1.25 mg/m² on day 1 only (maximum dose = 2.5 mg). For patients <1 year old, the dactinomycin dose is 0.025 mg/kg
G ≥3 mucositis after VDC cycle persisting beyond day 15 and unresponsive to maximum supportive care	Administer the total dose of doxorubicin as a continuous infusion over 24 hours rather than over 48 hours in the next course of VDC. If mucositis still recurs despite this, then reduce the dose of doxorubicin by 25% in subsequent VDC cycles

DACTINOMYCIN DOSE MODIFICATIONS

Hepatopathy (See Diagnosis and Grading Below)

Mild hepatopathy	In subsequent VAC cycles, administer dactinomycin and cyclophosphamide with the dosages reduced by 50%. Refer to instructions above for "hepatic impairment" for vincristine dosage. If tolerated, then administer the full dose in subsequent courses
Moderate or severe hepatopathy	Discontinue all therapy

CYCLOPHOSPHAMIDE DOSE MODIFICATIONS

Urologic Toxicity

Transient microscopic hematuria (>50 RBC/HPF 1 or 2 times)	Double the rate of post-hydration and continue mesna
Persistent microscopic hematuria (>50 RBC/HPF ≥3 times), or transient gross hematuria	Double the rate of post-hydration, continue hydration for at least 24 hours, and increase the total daily mesna dose to be equivalent to 100% of the cyclophosphamide dose
Persistent gross hematuria	Discontinue cyclophosphamide until urine clears to microscopic hematuria, then resume (in subsequent cycles) with the cyclophosphamide dose reduced to 50% of the full dose with post-hydration and mesna administered as per above for persistent microscopic hematuria. Escalate the cyclophosphamide dose to 100% of the full dose as tolerated. Consider urology consultation

Grading of Adverse Events

Criteria for Diagnosis of Hepatopathy

Pathologic confirmation by liver biopsy, *or:*
reversal of portal venous flow by ultrasound, *or:*
Two or more of the following:
• Bilirubin >1.4 mg/dL
• Unexplained weight gain >10% of baseline weight or ascites
• Hepatomegaly or right upper quadrant pain without other explanation

Hepatopathy Grading

Mild hepatopathy	Total bilirubin ≤6 mg/dL, weight gain of ≤5% of baseline of non-cardiac origin, reversible hepatic dysfunction
Moderate hepatopathy	Total bilirubin >6 mg/dL and <20 mg/dL, weight gain >5% of baseline of non-cardiac origin, clinically or radiologically detected ascites, reversible hepatic dysfunction
Severe hepatopathy	Total bilirubin >20 mg/dL and/or ascites compromising respiratory function and/or renal deterioration and/or hepatic encephalopathy which may or may not be reversible

Motor Neuropathy Grading

Grade 1	Subjective weakness, but no deficits detected under neurologic exam
Grade 2	Weakness that alters fine motor skills (buttoning shirt, writing or drawing, using eating utensils) or gait without abrogating ability to perform these tasks
Grade 3	Unable to perform fine motor tasks (buttoning shirt, writing or drawing, using eating utensils) or unable to ambulate without assistance
Grade 4	Paralysis

Sensory Neuropathy Grading

Grade 1	Paresthesias, pain, or numbness that do not require treatment or interfere with extremity function
Grade 2	Paresthesias, pain, or numbness that is controlled by non-narcotic medications or alter (without causing loss of function) fine motor skills (buttoning shirt, writing or drawing, using eating utensils) or gait without abrogating ability to perform these tasks
Grade 3	Paresthesias or pain that is controlled by narcotics, or interfere with extremity function (gait, fine motor skills as outlined above) or quality of life (loss of sleep, ability to perform normal activities severely impaired)
Grade 4	Complete loss of sensation or pain that is not controlled by narcotics

Patient Population

Patient and Tumor Characteristics

Characteristic	
Age	
Age <1 year	3 (3)
Age 1–9 years	38 (35)
Age 10–20 years	61 (56)
Age ≥21 years	7 (6)
Sex: male/female	60 (55)/49 (45)
Histology	
Alveolar	64 (59)
Embryonal	36 (33)
Other 9 (8)	
Primary site	
Extremity 19 (17)	
GI 7 (6)	
GU	21 (19)
Head and neck	4 (4)
Intrathoracic	3 (3)
PM	11 (10)
Perineum	11 (10)
Retroperitoneum	14 (13)
Trunk	11 (10)
Other	8 (7)
Tumor size	
≤5 cm / >5 cm	22 (20) / 87 (80)
Regional lymph node involvement	
No / yes / not evaluated	35 (32) / 65 (60) / 9 (8)

GU, genitourinary; PM, parameningeal

Efficacy

Outcome by Oberlin Risk Group

		% (95% CI) by Risk Group		
Outcome	All Patients	≤1 Risk Factor (n = 43)	≥2 Risk Factors (n = 66)	ERMS at Age <10 Years (n = 20)
3-year EFS	38 (29 to 48)	69 (52 to 82)	20 (11 to 30)	60 (36 to 78)
3-year OS	56 (46 to 66)	79 (62 to 89)	14 (11 to 18)	79 (54 to 92)

	Patients on ARST0431	Patients with ERMS	Alveolar RMS (ARMS) on ARST0431	Alveolar RMS (ARMS) on IRS-IV/IRS-IV pilot
5-year EFS	45 (34 to 54)	60 (42 to 74)	16 (8 to 28)	15 (9 to 24)

EFS, event-free survival; ERMS, embryonal rhabdomyosarcoma; OS, overall survival

Adverse Events

Grades 3 to 5 Toxicities Seen in 5% of Patients by Reporting Period

	No. (%) of Toxicities by Reporting Period*			
Toxicity	Weeks 1–6 n = 107	Weeks 7–19 n = 98	Weeks 20–34 n = 87	Weeks 35–54 n = 70
Febrile neutropenia with documented infection	3 (2.8)	22 (22)	27 (32)	8 (11.4)
Febrile neutropenia, no documented infection	2 (1.9)	30 (30.6)	27 (31.0)	9 (12.9)
Diarrhea	19 (17.8)	2 (2.0)	17 (19.5)	9 (12.9)
Infection with G1–2 neutrophils, all sites	14 (13)	11 (11.2)	13 (15)	10 (14.2)
Anorexia	14 (13.1)	9 (9.2)	10 (11.5)	1 (1.4)
Dehydration	11 (10.3)	3 (3.1)	5 (5.7)	3 (4.3)
Hypokalemia	9 (8.4)	8 (8.2)	10 (11.5)	3 (4.3)
Mucositis oral examination	3 (2.8)	7 (7.1)	5 (5.7)	—
Nausea	9 (8.4)	6 (6.1)	6 (6.9)	4 (5.7)
Mucositis oral functional	1 (0.9)	6 (6.1)	5 (6.9)	1 (5.7)
Weight loss	3 (2.8)	2 (2.0)	6 (6.9)	4 (5.7)
Radiation dermatitis	—	—	66.9	—
Abdominal pain	7 (6.5)	2 (2)	6 (6.9)	2 (2.9)
Vomiting	6 (5.6)	4 (4.1)	5 (5.7)	5 (7.1)
Sensory neuropathy	—	2 (2)	5 (5.7)	1 (1.4)
ALT elevation	5 (4.7)	3 (3.1)	5 (5.7)	2 (2.9)
Colitis	6 (5.6)	—	1 (1.1)	1 (1.4)
Eligible patients with G3–5 toxicity in course	57 (52)	67 (68)	69 (79)	39 (55)

*Numbers of patients in each RP are the total number of patients with data for that RP

Treatment Monitoring

VI

1. *Prior to cycle start and weekly:* CBC with differential; serum creatinine; LFTs with bilirubin; serum electrolytes, including calcium, magnesium, and phosphorus; physical examination. Monitor for diarrhea

VDC and VAC

1. *Prior to first dose of doxorubicin:* perform a thorough cardiac assessment, with determination of LVEF by echocardiogram or MUGA scan at baseline prior to initiation of doxorubicin. Reevaluate LVEF prior to the fourth cycle of VDC. Reevaluate LVEF if clinical symptoms of heart failure are present

2. *Before each cycle:* serum creatinine; LFTs with bilirubin; serum electrolytes, including calcium, magnesium, and phosphorus; physical examination

3. *Before each vincristine dose:* physical examination

4. *Twice per week:* CBC with differential until recovery from hematopoietic toxicity

IE

1. *Prior to cycle:* CBC with differential, total bilirubin, ALT, AST, albumin, alkaline phosphatase, serum creatinine, BUN, calcium, carbon dioxide, chloride, glucose, potassium, sodium, and phosphate

2. *During chemotherapy administration:*

   a. *Daily laboratory investigations:* serum creatinine, BUN, calcium, carbon dioxide, chloride, glucose, potassium, sodium, and phosphate

   b. *Every 8 hours (or with each void):* urine dipstick for blood (check microscopic urinalysis if >trace)

   c. *Other:* monitor fluid status (ie, weight and intake/output) and for signs and symptoms of neurologic toxicity

3. *Twice per week:* CBC with differential, serum creatinine, BUN, calcium, carbon dioxide, chloride, glucose, potassium, sodium, and phosphate

Response evaluation: At weeks 6, 19, 34, and 54

RELAPSED/REFRACTORY • RHABDOMYOSARCOMA
RHABDOMYOSARCOMA REGIMEN: VINORELBINE + CYCLOPHOSPHAMIDE + TEMSIROLIMUS

Mascarenhas L et al. J Clin Oncol 2019;37:2866–2874

Hydration for cyclophosphamide:
0.9% NS 750 mL/m²; administer intravenously over 1–2 hours prior to the start of cyclophosphamide on day 1, every 21 days, for up to 12 cycles. Then, encourage oral fluid ingestion or administer additional intravenous hydration (eg, 0.9% NS) at a rate of 100 mL/m²/hour continued until the last intravenous mesna dose has been administered

An admixture containing **cyclophosphamide** 1200 mg/m² + **mesna** 240 mg/m²; administer intravenously in 100–250 mL 0.9% NS or D5W over 30–60 minutes on day 1, every 21 days, for up to 12 cycles (total cyclophosphamide dosage per 21-day cycle = 1200 mg/m²); *then, either:*

Mesna 240 mg/m² per dose; administer intravenously diluted with 0.9% NS or D5W to a concentration of 1–20 mg/mL, over 15 minutes for 2 doses at 4 hours and 8 hours after cyclophosphamide administration is completed, on day 1 (total mesna dosage per 21-day cycle = 720 mg/m²; includes 240 mg/m² dose given with cyclophosphamide), *or*
Mesna 480 mg/m² per dose; administer orally for 2 doses at 2 hours and 6 hours after cyclophosphamide administration is completed on day 1 (total mesna dosage per 21-day cycle = 1200 mg/m²; includes 240 mg/m² dose given with cyclophosphamide)

Premedication for temsirolimus:
Diphenhydramine 25–50 mg (*adult dose*) *or* 0.5 mg/kg (*pediatric dose*; maximum dose 50 mg); administer intravenously approximately 30 minutes before each dose of temsirolimus as prophylaxis against hypersensitivity reactions (other histamine H₁-receptor antagonists may be substituted) on days 1, 8, and 15, every 21 days, for up to 12 cycles
Temsirolimus 15 mg/m² per dose (maximum single dose, 30 mg); administer diluted in 250 mL 0.9% sodium chloride injection (0.9% NS) intravenously over 30–60 minutes once weekly for 3 doses on days 1, 8, and 15, every 21 days, for up to 12 cycles (total dosage/21-day cycle = 45 mg/m²; maximum dosage/21-day cycle = 90 mg)
Notes:
- Withhold temsirolimus during radiation therapy, if applicable
- The standard volume of 0.9% NS for dilution of temsirolimus is 250 mL. For pediatric patients, consider a reduced volume of 0.9% NS sufficient to produce a final concentration between 0.04–1 mg/mL (ARST1431 Protocol. http://rpc.mdanderson.org/rpc/credentialing/files/ARST1431_ProtocolDoc_032216.pdf [accessed 29 August 2020])
- Prepare the final temsirolimus dilution in either bottles (glass or polypropylene) or plastic bags (polypropylene, polyolefin) protected from light
- Infuse temsirolimus through a non-diethylhexylphthalate (non-DEHP), non-polyvinylchloride (non-PVC), polyethylene-lined administration set containing an in-line polyethersulfone filter with a pore size of ≤5 μm. Alternatively, a polyethersulfone end-filter with a pore size ranging from 0.2 μm to 5 μm may be used in place of an in-line filter

Vinorelbine 25 mg/m² per dose; administer by intravenous infusion in a volume of 0.9% NS or D5W sufficient to produce a vinorelbine concentration within the range 0.5–2 mg/mL, over 10 minutes, for 2 doses on days 1 and 8, every 21 days, for up to 12 cycles (total dosage/21-day cycle = 50 mg/m²)

Supportive Care: Antiemetic prophylaxis
Emetogenic potential on day 1 is **MODERATE**
Emetogenic potential on days 8 and 15 is **MINIMAL**
See Chapter 42 for antiemetic recommendations

Hematopoietic growth factor (CSF) prophylaxis
Primary prophylaxis is indicated with:
  Filgrastim (G-CSF) 5 μg/kg per day by subcutaneous injection
  - Begin use from 24 hours after myelosuppressive chemotherapy is completed—that is, day 9
  - Filgrastim may be given on day 15 when temsirolimus is administered alone
  - Continue daily filgrastim use for at least 7 days or until post-nadir ANC ≥2000/mm³, whichever comes last
  - Discontinue daily filgrastim use at least 24 hours before administering resuming myelosuppressive treatment (vinorelbine and cyclophosphamide)
See Chapter 43 for more information

Antimicrobial prophylaxis
Risk of fever and neutropenia is INTERMEDIATE
Antimicrobial primary prophylaxis to be considered:
- Antibacterial—consider a fluoroquinolone or no prophylaxis; *P. jirovecii* prophylaxis is recommended (eg, cotrimoxazole)
- Antifungal—consider concomitant use of clotrimazole during periods of neutropenia
- Antiviral—antiherpes antivirals (eg, acyclovir, famciclovir, valacyclovir)

(continued)

(continued)

Prophylaxis and treatment for mucositis/stomatitis
General advice:
- Encourage patients to maintain intake of nonalcoholic fluids
- Evaluate patients for oral pain and provide analgesic medications
- Consider histamine (H$_2$-subtype) receptor antagonists (eg, ranitidine, famotidine), or a proton pump inhibitor for epigastric pain

Patients with intact oral mucosa:
- Clean the mouth, tongue, and gums by brushing after every meal and at bedtime with an ultra-soft toothbrush with fluoride toothpaste
- Floss teeth gently every day unless contraindicated. If gums bleed and hurt, avoid bleeding or sore areas, but floss other teeth
- Patients may use saline or commercial bland, nonalcoholic rinses: Do not use mouthwashes that contain alcohols

If mucositis or stomatitis is present:
- Keep the mouth moist utilizing water, ice chips, sugarless gum, sugar-free hard candies, or a saliva substitute
- Rinse mouth several times a day to remove debris
  - Use a solution of ¼ teaspoon (1.25 g) each of baking soda and table salt (sodium chloride) in 1 quart (~950 mL) of warm water. Follow with a plain water rinse
  - Do not use mouthwashes that contain alcohols
- Advise patients who develop mucositis to:
  - Choose foods that are easy to chew and swallow
  - Take small bites of food, chew slowly, and sip liquids with meals
  - Encourage soft, moist foods such as cooked cereals, mashed potatoes, and scrambled eggs
  - For trouble swallowing, soften food with gravies, sauces, broths, yogurt, or other bland liquids
  - Avoid sharp, crunchy foods; hot, spicy, or highly acidic foods (eg, citrus fruits and juices); sugary foods; toothpicks; tobacco products; alcoholic drinks

Treatment Modifications

TEMSIROLIMUS

Starting dose level	15 mg/m^2 (maximum dose = 30 mg) IV once per week
Dose level −1	12 mg/m^2 (maximum dose = 24 mg) IV once per week
Dose level −2	9 mg/m^2 (maximum dose = 18 mg) IV once per week
Dose level −3	Discontinue temsirolimus
Adverse Event	**Dose Modification**
Severe hypersensitivity/infusion reaction	Interrupt the temsirolimus infusion for at least 30–60 minutes depending on the severity of the reaction. At the discretion of the medically responsible health care provider, treatment may be resumed at a slower rate (up to 60 minute infusion duration) following administration of an H$_1$-receptor antagonist (if not previously administered) and/or an H$_2$-receptor antagonist
Diagnosis of an invasive fungal infection	Discontinue temsirolimus and treat with appropriate antifungal therapy
Radiologic changes suggestive of noninfectious pneumonitis with no symptoms	Can continue temsirolimus therapy without dose alteration but with careful monitoring
Radiologic changes suggestive of noninfectious pneumonitis with mild-moderate symptoms	Withhold temsirolimus until symptoms improve. Consider administering corticosteroids. If symptoms improve, consider reintroducing temsirolimus one dose lower depending on the individual clinical circumstances with careful continued monitoring. Consider administering prophylaxis for opportunistic infections (eg, *P. jirovecii*) in patients requiring prolonged corticosteroids
Radiologic changes suggestive of noninfectious pneumonitis with severe symptoms (including a decrease in DL$_{CO}$ on pulmonary function tests)	Discontinue temsirolimus and consider administering high doses of corticosteroids. Consider administering prophylaxis for opportunistic infections (eg, *P. jirovecii*) in patients requiring prolonged corticosteroids
ANC <1000/mm^3 or platelet count <75,000/mm^3	Withhold therapy. Resume temsirolimus when symptoms improve to G ≤2 with temsirolimus dose reduced by 1 dose level
Nephrotic syndrome	Permanently discontinue temsirolimus

(continued)

Treatment Modifications (continued)

Adverse Event	Dose Modification
Any nonhematologic G3/4 toxicity related to temsirolimus	Withhold therapy. Resume temsirolimus when symptoms improve to G ≤2 with temsirolimus dose reduced by 1 dose level
G1/2 stomatitis	Administer topical treatments (avoid alcohol- or peroxide-containing mouthwashes as they may exacerbate the condition). Do not use antifungal agents unless fungal infection has been diagnosed. Focus on pain control, oral hygiene, and ensuring adequate nutrition and hydration
Mild hepatic impairment (bilirubin >1 to 1.5 × ULN or AST >ULN but bilirubin ≤ULN)	Administer temsirolimus at a reduced dose

Adapted in part from: TORISEL (temsirolimus) prescribing information. Philadelphia, PA: Wyeth Pharmaceuticals Inc; revised 2018 March

CYCLOPHOSPHAMIDE AND VINORELBINE DOSE MODIFICATIONS

Hematologic Toxicity

ANC <1000/mm^3 or platelet count <75,000/mm^3 on day 1	Withhold all therapy. Delay initiation of the cycle by at least 1 week and when parameters are met. If delayed by >1 week, then reduce the dose of cyclophosphamide/mesna by 25%
Neutropenic fever, or ANC <500/mm^3 for > 7 days, or G4 thrombocytopenia occurring during a cycle	Withhold all therapy until resolution of toxicity. Reduce the dose of cyclophosphamide/mesna and vinorelbine by 25% in subsequent cycles. Add prophylactic G-CSF if not already using

Pulmonary Toxicity

Pulmonary toxicity (acute bronchospasm, interstitial pneumonitis, acute respiratory distress syndrome) attributable to vinorelbine	Discontinue vinorelbine

Urologic Toxicity

Transient microscopic hematuria (>50 RBC/HPF 1 or 2 times)	Double the rate of post-hydration and continue mesna
Persistent microscopic hematuria (>50 RBC/HPF ≥3 times), or transient gross hematuria	Double the rate of post-hydration, continue hydration for at least 24 hours, and increase the total daily mesna dose to be equivalent to 100% of the cyclophosphamide dose
Persistent gross hematuria	Discontinue cyclophosphamide until urine clears to microscopic hematuria, then resume (in subsequent cycles) with the cyclophosphamide dose reduced to 50% of the full dose with post-hydration and mesna administered as per above for persistent microscopic hematuria. Escalate the cyclophosphamide dose to 100% of the full dose as tolerated. Consider urology consultation

Hepatic Impairment

Total bilirubin 2.1–3.0 mg/dL	Reduce the vinorelbine dose by 50%
Total bilirubin >3 mg/dL	Reduce the vinorelbine dose by 75%

Neuropathy

G2 motor or sensory neuropathy	Administer vinorelbine with the dosage reduced by 50%. If the toxicity improves to G ≤1, then increase the dose to 75% of the full dose
G ≥3 motor or sensory neuropathy	Withhold vinorelbine until toxicity improves to G ≤2, then resume vinorelbine with the dosage reduced by 50%
G ≥3 constipation (obstipation with manual evacuation indicated; limiting self-care ADL)	Withhold vinorelbine and optimize laxative regimen. When toxicity improves to G ≤1, resume vinorelbine with the dosage reduced by 50%. If the toxicity does not recur, then re-escalate the vinorelbine dose back to full dose
G ≥3 ileus (severely altered GI function; TPN indicated)	

Patient Population Studied

Phase 2 trial from the Children's Oncology Group (ARST0921) designed to prioritize bevacizumab or temsirolimus for additional investigation in rhabdomyosarcoma (RMS) when combined with cytotoxic chemotherapy. Eligible participants were <30 years of age with biopsy-proven RMS at first relapse or disease progression. Patients with primary refractory disease (first progression after ≥1 cycle of cyclophosphamide or ifosfamide-containing chemotherapy without a prior response) also were eligible. Additionally, patients were required to have an ECOG PS of ≤2. Patients were randomized 1:1 to receive cytotoxic chemotherapy with bevacizumab or temsirolimus

Patient Population

Characteristic, no (%)	Vinorelbine + Cyclophosphamide + Bevacizumab (n = 44)	Vinorelbine + Cyclophosphamide + Temsirolimus (n = 42)
Age, years		
< 10	19 (43)	13 (31)
10–19	20 (46)	24 (57)
> 19	5 (11)	5 (12)
Male sex	22 (50)	23 (55)
Histology		
Embryonal	15 (34)	17 (40)
Alveolar	27 (61)	25 (60)
Other	2 (5)	0
Primary site at original diagnosis		
Head/neck/orbit	3 (7)	3 (7)
Parameningeal	13 (29)	9 (21)
GU non-bladder/prostate	1 (2)	2 (5)
Bladder/prostate	2 (5)	5 (12)
Extremity	12 (27)	12 (29)
Retroperitoneum/perineum	8 (18)	6 (14)
Intrathoracic/trunk	3 (7)	3 (7)
Other	2 (5)	2 (5)
Primary tumor size at diagnosis, cm		
≤5	17 (39)	12 (29)
>5	27 (61)	30 (71)
Distant metastases at diagnosis	26 (59)	24 (57)
Site of recurrence		
Local only	8 (18)	14 (33)
Regional only	5 (12)	2 (5)
Metastatic only	23 (52)	20 (48)
Local and regional	2 (5)	3 (7)
Local and metastatic	1 (2)	3 (7)
Regional and metastatic	4 (9)	0
Local, regional, and metastatic	1 (2)	0

GU, genitourinary

Therapy Monitoring

1. *Day 1 of each cycle*: ALT, AST, bilirubin, alkaline phosphatase, BUN, serum creatinine, urinalysis
2. *At least once per week*:
   a. CBC with differential and platelet count, physical examination
3. *Baseline and periodic monitoring for temsirolimus*:
   a. Urine dipstick for protein. If >1+, consider obtaining a 24-hour urine for protein
   b. Fasting serum glucose and lipid panel. When possible, achieve optimal glucose and lipid control prior to initiation of temsirolimus
   c. Chest x-ray or chest computed tomography (CT) scan to assess for pneumonitis
   d. Monitor for symptoms of pulmonary toxicity, infection, hyperglycemia, bowel perforation, nephrotic syndrome, and stomatitis
   e. Monitor for infusion reactions during administration of each dose of temsirolimus

Temsirolimus notes:
- Temsirolimus may impair wound healing; use caution and strongly consider withholding therapy in the peri-surgical period
- Advise patients to avoid live vaccines and close contact with those who have received live vaccines
- Complete treatment of any pre-existing invasive fungal infections prior to initiating temsirolimus

Efficacy

Efficacy Variable	Vinorelbine + Cyclophosphamide + Bevacizumab (n = 44)	Vinorelbine + Cyclophosphamide + Temsirolimus (n = 42)	Between-group Comparison
Event-Free Survival, % (95% CI)			
At 6 months	54.6 (39.8–69.3)	69.1 (55.1–83)	P = 0.0182*
At 12 months	18.2 (6.8–29.6)	40.5 (25.6–55.3)	Estimated HR for treatment failure 1.71 (95% CI 1.08–2.69)
At 24 months	6.8 (0–14.3)	19.1 (7.2–30.9)	
Overall Survival, % (95% CI)			
At 6 months	84.1 (73.3–94.9)	90.5 (81.6–99.4)	**P = 0.2311†**
At 12 months	59.1 (44.6–73.6)	78.4 (65.8–91.1)	
At 24 months	29.6 (16.1–43)	39.2 (24.2–54.2)	
Response After 6 Weeks of Treatment (Bevacizumab n = 40; Temsirolimus n = 36)			
ORR‡, % (95% CI)	28 (13.7–41.3)	47 (31.5–63.2)	P = 0.12
Complete response, no (%)	4 (10)	5 (14)	—
Partial response, no (%)	7 (18)	13 (36)	—
Progressive disease, no (%)	11 (28)	4 (11)	—

*Event-free survival probability, two-sided P value
†Overall survival probability, two-sided P value
‡Objective response rate refers to complete response plus partial response
CI, confidence interval; HR, hazard ratio; ORR, objective response rate

Adverse Events

Toxicity (%) (N = 84)	Cycle 1–2		Cycle 3–5		Cycle 6–8		Cycle 9–12	
	BEV (n = 42)	TEM (n = 42)	BEV (n = 27)	TEM (n = 34)	BEV (n = 22)	TEM (n = 22)	BEV (n = 14)	TEM (n = 13)
Febrile neutropenia	11.9	26.2	18.5	17.6	13.6	18.2	14.3	23.1
Oral mucositis	2.4	11.9	0	0	4.5	0	0	7.7
Hypokalemia	2.4	11.9	3.7	5.9	4.5	0	0	0

*Two patients were randomly assigned to BEV but did not receive bevacizumab and were excluded.
Note: reported are Grade 3 or greater toxicities occurring in at least 10% of participants in either arm during the reporting periods. There were three dose-limiting toxicities in the BEV arm (one Grade 3 hypertension, one Grade 3 bleeding, and one Grade 3 oral mucositis). There were eight dose-limiting toxicities in the TEM arm (four Grade 3 oral mucositis, two Grade 3 hypertriglyceridemia, one Grade 3 pneumonitis, and one Grade 3 elevation of ALT that did not resolve to less than Grade 1 in 14 days)
BEV, bevacizumab; TEM, temsirolimus

RELAPSED/REFRACTORY • RHABDOMYOSARCOMA
RHABDOMYOSARCOMA REGIMEN: VINORELBINE

Kuttesch JF et al. Pediatr Blood Cancer 2009;53:590–593

Vinorelbine 30 mg/m² per dose; administer by intravenous infusion in a volume of 0.9% NS or D5W sufficient to produce a vinorelbine concentration within the range 0.5–2 mg/mL, over 10 minutes, once per week for 6 doses on days 1, 8, 15, 22, 29, and 36, every 56 days (8 weeks), for up to 10 cycles (total dosage/56-day cycle = 180 mg/m²)

Supportive Care: Antiemetic prophylaxis
Emetogenic potential is MINIMAL
See Chapter 42 for antiemetic recommendations

Hematopoietic growth factor (CSF) prophylaxis
Primary prophylaxis is NOT indicated
See Chapter 43 for more information

Antimicrobial prophylaxis
Risk of fever and neutropenia is INTERMEDIATE
Antimicrobial primary prophylaxis to be considered:
- Antibacterial—consider a fluoroquinolone or no prophylaxis; *P. jirovecii* prophylaxis is recommended (eg, cotrimoxazole)
- Antifungal—consider concomitant use of clotrimazole during periods of neutropenia
- Antiviral—antiherpes antivirals (eg, acyclovir, famciclovir, valacyclovir)

Treatment Modifications

Vinorelbine Dose Modifications

Hematologic Toxicity	
ANC <1500/mm³ or platelet count <75,000/mm³ on day 1	Delay initiation of the cycle by at least 1 week and until parameters are met
ANC is ≥1500/mm³ on day 8, 15, 22, 29, or 36 in a patient who has not had a dose delay for neutropenia of >1 week duration and who has not experienced a prior neutropenic fever	Proceed with full dose of vinorelbine
ANC is 1000–1499/mm³ on day 8, 15, 22, 29, or 36 in a patient who has not had a dose delay for neutropenia of >1 week duration and who has not experienced a prior neutropenic fever	Proceed with vinorelbine with the dose reduced by 50% from the full dose
ANC is <1000/mm³ on day 8, 15, 22, 29, or 36 in a patient who has not had a dose delay for neutropenia of >1 week duration and who has not experienced a prior neutropenic fever	Withhold vinorelbine. Repeat neutrophil count in 1 week. If ANC is ≥1000/mm³, then proceed with vinorelbine administration based on ANC count as described above
ANC is ≥1500/mm³ on day 8, 15, 22, 29, or 36 in a patient who has had a prior dose delay for neutropenia of >1 week duration or who has not experienced a prior neutropenic fever	Proceed with vinorelbine reduced by 25% from the full dose
ANC is 1000–1499/mm³ on day 8, 15, 22, 29, or 36 in a patient who has had a prior dose delay for neutropenia of >1 week duration or who has not experienced a prior neutropenic fever	Proceed with vinorelbine with the dose reduced by 62.5% from the full dose
ANC is <1000/mm³ on day 8, 15, 22, 29, or 36 in a patient who has had a prior dose delay for neutropenia of >1 week duration or who has not experienced a prior neutropenic fever	Withhold vinorelbine. Repeat neutrophil count in 1 week. If ANC is ≥1000/mm³, then proceed with vinorelbine administration based on ANC count as described above
Pulmonary Toxicity	
Pulmonary toxicity (acute bronchospasm, interstitial pneumonitis, acute respiratory distress syndrome) attributable to vinorelbine	Discontinue vinorelbine
Hepatic Impairment	
Total bilirubin 2.1–3.0 mg/dL	Reduce the vinorelbine dose by 50%
Total bilirubin >3 mg/dL	Reduce the vinorelbine dose by 75%

(continued)

Treatment Modifications (*continued*)

Neuropathy	
G2 motor or sensory neuropathy	Administer vinorelbine with the dosage reduced by 50%. If the toxicity improves to G ≤1, then increase the dose to 75% of the full dose
G ≥3 motor or sensory neuropathy	Withhold vinorelbine until toxicity improves to G ≤2, then resume vinorelbine with the dosage reduced by 50%
G ≥3 constipation (obstipation with manual evacuation indicated; limiting self-care ADL)	Withhold vinorelbine and optimize laxative regimen. When toxicity improves to G ≤1, resume vinorelbine with the dosage reduced by 50%. If the toxicity does not recur, then re-escalate the vinorelbine dose back to full dose
G ≥3 ileus (severely altered GI function; TPN indicated)	

Patient Population Studied

Patients were required to be ≤21 years of age when originally diagnosed with STS, CNS tumors, or NB. Patients were required to have received no more than two prior chemotherapy regimens

Demographic and Pretreatment Characteristics of Participants (N=50)

Age at diagnosis (years)—median (range)	8.5 (0–20)
Age at study entry (years)—median (range)	10 (1–25)
Sex—male/female	24 (48%)/26 (52%)
Race	
White	32 (64%)
Hispanic	10 (20%)
African American	6 (12%)
Native American	1 (2%)
Native Hawaiian	1 (2%)
Prior hematopoietic stem cell transplant	
Yes (neuroblastoma [8], glioblastoma [3], sarcoma [2])	13 (26%)
No	35 (70%)
Not reported	2 (4%)
Prior radiation: yes / no	45 (90%) / 5 (10%)
Bone marrow involvement: yes (neuroblastoma [5]) / no	5 (10%) / 45 (90%)
Performance status at study entry	
Asymptomatic and fully active	17 (34%)
Symptomatic, fully ambulatory, restricted in physically strenuous activity	20 (40%)
Symptomatic, ambulatory, capable self-care, >50% of walking hours out of bed	12 (24%)
Not reported	1 (2%)

Efficacy

Response to Vinorelbine by Tumor Type

	Soft-Tissue Sarcoma		CNS tumor	Neuroblastoma	Total
	RMS	Non-RMS			
Complete response	1	0	0	0	1 (2%)
Partial response	3	0	2	0	5 (10%)
Stable disease	6	3	3	3	15 (30%)
Progressive disease	1	6	17	5	29 (58%)
Total	20		22	8	50

RMS, rhabdomyosarcoma; Non-RMS, non-rhabdomyosarcoma

Adverse Events

	$33.75\,mg/m^2$ Vinorelbine* (n = 35)	$30\,mg/m^2$ Vinorelbine* (n = 15)	All Patients (n = 50)
G3/4 neutropenia during the initial two courses of therapy	25/35 (71%)	10/15 (67%)	35/50 (70%)
Delay in therapy and/or dose modification	9/35 (26%) (including 5 with initial bone marrow involvement of disease)	0/15	9/50 (18%)
Anemia	—	—	10 /50 20%
Grade 3 sensory neuropathy	—	—	4/50 (8%)

*Starting vinorelbine dose

Therapy Monitoring

1. *Weekly:* CBC with differential, ALT, AST, bilirubin, alkaline phosphatase, physical examination

RELAPSED/REFRACTORY • RHABDOMYOSARCOMA

RHABDOMYOSARCOMA REGIMEN: VINCRISTINE + IRINOTECAN + TEMOZOLOMIDE

Defachelles AS et al. J Clin Oncol 2019;37(suppl_15):10000
Setty BA et al. Pediatr Blood Cancer 2018;65:e26728

Vincristine 1.5 mg/m^2 per dose (maximum single dose = 2 mg); administer by intravenous infusion over 15 minutes in 25–50 mL 0.9% sodium chloride injection for 2 doses on days 1 and 8, every 21 days (total dosage/21-day cycle = 3 mg/m^2; maximum dosage/21-day cycle = 4 mg)
• Patients who weigh <10 kg should receive a vincristine dose of 0.05 mg/kg
• Dilute in 25 mL 0.9% NS for pediatric patients and in 50 mL 0.9% for adult patients

Irinotecan 50 mg/m^2 per dose; administer intravenously, diluted with 5% dextrose injection to a concentration within the range of 0.12–2.8 mg/mL, over 60 minutes once daily for 5 consecutive days on days 1–5, every 21 days (total dosage/21-day cycle = 250 mg/m^2)

Temozolomide 125 mg/m^2 per day; administer orally for 5 consecutive days, on days 1–5, every 21 days (total dosage/21-day cycle = 625 mg/m^2)
Notes:
• In the absence of G ≥2 toxicity during cycle 1, consider increasing the temozolomide dose in subsequent cycles as follows: **Temozolomide** 150 mg/m^2 per day; administer orally for 5 consecutive days, on days 1–5, every 21 days (total dosage/21-day cycle = 750 mg/m^2)
• Temozolomide doses are rounded to the nearest 5 mg by using commercially available products
• Patients who vomit after taking temozolomide should be instructed to take their next dose at the next regularly scheduled time

Supportive Care
Antiemetic prophylaxis
Emetogenic potential of irinotecan is **MODERATE**
Emetogenic potential of oral temozolomide is **MODERATE TO HIGH**
Emetogenic potential of vincristine is **MINIMAL**
See Chapter 42 for antiemetic recommendations

Hematopoietic growth factor (CSF) prophylaxis
Primary prophylaxis is NOT indicated
See Chapter 43 for more information

Antimicrobial prophylaxis
Risk of fever and neutropenia is INTERMEDIATE
  Antimicrobial primary prophylaxis to be considered:
  • Antibacterial—consider a fluoroquinolone or no prophylaxis; *P. jirovecii* prophylaxis is recommended (eg, cotrimoxazole)
  • Antifungal—consider concomitant use of clotrimazole during periods of neutropenia
  • Antiviral—antiherpes antivirals (eg, acyclovir, famciclovir, valacyclovir)

Acute cholinergic syndrome
Atropine sulfate 0.25–1 mg subcutaneously or intravenously if abdominal cramping or diarrhea develop during or within 1 hour after irinotecan administration
• If symptoms are severe, add as primary prophylaxis at least 30 minutes before irinotecan during subsequent cycles
• For irinotecan, acute cholinergic syndrome may be characterized by abdominal cramping, diarrhea, diaphoresis, hypotension, flushing, bradycardia, rhinitis, increased salivation, meiosis, and lacrimation

Diarrhea management
• The potential for developing diarrhea and abdominal pain should be discussed with all patients and their caretakers, and instructions given to start loperamide immediately if these symptoms occur and to ensure adequate hydration is maintained. See Dose Modifications (below) for instructions
Latent or delayed-onset diarrhea*:
Loperamide 4 mg orally initially after the first loose or liquid stool, *then*
Loperamide 2 mg orally every 2 hours during waking hours, *plus*
Loperamide 4 mg orally every 4 hours during hours of sleep
• Loperamide doses are for patients >15 years of age. Refer to Treatment Modifications section for dosing in younger patients
• Continue for at least 12 hours after diarrhea resolves
• Recurrent diarrhea after a 12-hour diarrhea-free interval is treated as a new episode
• Rehydrate orally with fluids and electrolytes during a diarrheal episode
• If a patient develops blood or mucus in stool, dehydration, or hemodynamic instability, or if diarrhea persists >48 hours despite loperamide, stop loperamide and hospitalize the patient for IV hydration
• Alternatively, a trial of **diphenoxylate hydrochloride** 2.5 mg **with atropine sulfate** 0.025 mg (eg, Lomotil)
• Initial adult dose is 2 tablets 4 times daily until control has been achieved, after which the dose may be reduced to meet individual requirements. Control may often be maintained with as little as 2 tablets daily

(continued)

(continued)

- Clinical improvement of acute diarrhea is usually observed within 48 hours. If improvement of chronic diarrhea after treatment with a maximum daily dose of 8 tablets is not observed within 10 days, control is unlikely with further administration

Persistent diarrhea:

> **Octreotide** 100–150 μg subcutaneously 3 times daily (adult dose). Maximum total daily adult dose is 1500 μg. Pediatric patients may initiate dosing at 1–10 μg/kg/dose every 8–12 hours (not to exceed 1500 μg per day)

Antibiotic primary prophylaxis and treatment during latent or delayed-onset diarrhea:

Consider the following to prevent or lessen irinotecan-associated diarrhea:

- Prophylactic oral **cefixime** 8 mg/kg (maximum dose of 400 mg) orally once daily, beginning 1–2 days prior to the start of irinotecan therapy and continuing until completion of the cycle, *alternatively:*

- **Cefpodoxime proxetil** 5 mg/kg/day per day orally twice daily with food (maximum dose of 200 mg twice daily)

  - Previous studies suggest prophylaxis with cephalosporin antibiotics can ameliorate irinotecan-associated diarrhea by reducing the enteric bacteria responsible for producing β-glucuronidase, which regenerates in the gut irinotecan's toxic metabolite, SN-38, by cleaving the glucuronide moiety from SN-38 (Wagner LM et al. Pediatr Blood Cancer 2008;50:201–207)

- Alternatively, **activated charcoal** at a dose equal to 5 times the irinotecan dose up to a maximum dose of 260 mg orally 3 times daily during irinotecan therapy (Michael M et al. J Clin Oncol 2004;22:4410–4417)

Antibiotic treatment during latent or delayed-onset diarrhea:

- A fluoroquinolone (eg, ciprofloxacin 500 mg orally every 12 hours) if absolute neutrophil count <500/mm^3 with or without accompanying fever in association with diarrhea. Antibiotics should also be administered if a patient is hospitalized with prolonged diarrhea, and should be continued until diarrhea resolves

*Abigerges D et al. J Natl Cancer Inst 1994;86:446–449
Rothenberg ML et al. J Clin Oncol 2001;19:3801–3807
Wadler S et al. J Clin Oncol 1998;16:3169–3178

Treatment Modifications

Irinotecan Dose Levels	
Starting dosage	50 mg/m^2 per day intravenously on days 1–5
Level −1	37.5 mg/m^2 per day intravenously on days 1–5
Level −2	25 mg/m^2 per day intravenously on days 1–5
Temozolomide Dose Levels	
Level +1	150 mg/m^2 per day orally on days 1–5
Starting dosage	125 mg/m^2 per day orally on days 1–5
Level −1	100 mg/m^2 per day orally on days 1–5
Level −2	75 mg/m^2 per day orally on days 1–5
Vincristine Dose Levels	
Starting dosage	1.5 mg/m^2 per dose (maximum dose = 2 mg) intravenously on days 1 and 8
Level −1	1 mg/m^2 per dose (maximum dose = 1.5 mg) intravenously on days 1 and 8
Level −2	0.75 mg/m^2 per dose (maximum dose = 1 mg) intravenously on days 1 and 8
Adverse Event	**Dose Modification**
Hematologic Toxicity	
Day 1 ANC <1000/mm^3 or platelet count <75,000/mm^3	Delay start of next cycle by 1 week and until parameters are met, and reduce doses of irinotecan and temozolomide by 1 level
G4 neutropenia >7 days duration	Reduce doses of irinotecan and temozolomide by 1 level in subsequent cycles
G4 thrombocytopenia (any duration)	
G3/4 infection	

(continued)

Treatment Modifications (*continued*)

Diarrhea in Children 2–15 Years of Age

Children 2–15 years, with first liquid stools	Begin oral loperamide liquid immediately with the first liquid stool at a dosage of 0.18 mg/kg per day (0.03 mg/kg administered orally every 4 hours). Maximum single dose • <13 kg is 0.5 mg loperamide • 13 to <20 kg, 1 m • 20 to <43 kg, initially 2 mg then 1 mg • ≥43 kg, initially 4 mg then 2 mg
G3/4 diarrhea	Hospitalize for optimal management. Begin loperamide 0.06 mg/kg every 4 hours. <u>Maximum single dose:</u> • <13 kg is 0.5 mg loperamide • 13 to <20 kg, 1 mg • 20 to <43 kg, initially 2 mg then 1 mg • ≥43 kg, initially 4 mg then 2 mg Reduce irinotecan dosage for the following cycle by 1 dose level

Delayed Diarrhea in Patients >15 Years of Age

G1 (2–3 stools/day > baseline)	Maintain irinotecan dose and schedule
G2 (4–6 stools/day > baseline)	Delay irinotecan until diarrhea resolves to baseline, then reduce irinotecan dosage by 1 dosage level
G3 (7–9 stools/day > baseline)	Delay irinotecan until diarrhea resolves to baseline, then reduce dosage of irinotecan by 1 or 2 dosage level
G4 (≥10 stools/day > baseline)	Delay irinotecan until diarrhea resolves to baseline, then reduce dosage of irinotecan by 2 dosage levels

Neuropathy

G2 motor or sensory neuropathy	Administer vincristine with dosage reduced by 50%. If the toxicity improves to G ≤1, then increase the dose for 75% of the full dose
G ≥3 motor or sensory neuropathy	Withhold vincristine until toxicity improves to G ≤2, then resume vincristine with dosage reduced by 50%
Jaw pain	Continue vincristine at the current dose
G ≥3 constipation (obstipation with manual evacuation indicated; limiting self-care ADL)	Withhold vincristine and optimize laxative regimen. When toxicity improves to G ≤1, resume vincristine with the dosage reduced by 50%. If the toxicity does not recur, then re-escalate the vincristine dose back to full dose
G ≥3 ileus (severely altered GI function; TPN indicated)	

Other Nonhematologic Toxicities

Any G1 toxicity	Maintain dose and schedule
Any intolerable G2 toxicity	Hold treatment until toxicity resolves to G ≤1, then reduce dosage of the attributable agent(s) by 1 dose level
Any G3 toxicity	Hold treatment until toxicity resolves to G ≤1, then reduce dosage of the attributable agent(s) by 1 dosage level
Any G4 toxicity	Hold treatment until toxicity resolves to G ≤1, then reduce dosage of the attributable agent(s) by 2 dosage levels

Patient Population Studied

The VIT–0910 trial, an EpSSG-ITCC randomized phase 2 trial, evaluated efficacy and safety of VI and VIT in patients aged 0.5–50 years with relapsed/refractory RMS. Median age was 11 years (0.75–46), 120 pts (60 VIT, 60 VI) recruited in 37 European centers. 89% relapsed RMS

Efficacy

	VIT	VI	Statistics
ORR	24/55 (44%)	18/58 (31%)	Adjusted OR, 0.50; 95% CI, 0.22–1.12; P = 0.09
PFS	—	—	Adjusted HR, 0.65; 95% CI, 0.43–0.97; P = 0.036
OS	—	—	HR, 0.53; 95% CI, 0.33–0.83; P = 0.005

Note: PFS and OS results were similar when only relapsed patients were included
CI, confidence interval; ORR, objective response rate (PR + CR); CR, complete response; PR, partial response; HR, hazard ratio; OR, odds ratio; PFS, progression-free survival; OS, overall survival

Adverse Events

Adverse events G ≥3 were more frequent in VIT compared to VI, but only hematologic toxicity was significantly increased (81% for VIT; 59% for VI; odds ratio, 1.36; 95% CI, 1.06–1.76; P = 0.02)

Therapy Monitoring

1. *Prior to chemotherapy on days 1 and 8:* serum creatinine; LFTs with bilirubin; serum electrolytes, including calcium, magnesium, and phosphorus; physical examination
2. *Weekly:* CBC with differential

UNRESECTABLE • SOFT-TISSUE SARCOMA

SOFT-TISSUE SARCOMA REGIMEN: DOXORUBICIN

Bramwell VHC et al. Cochrane Database Syst Rev 2003;2003(3):CD003293
O'Bryan RM et al. Cancer 1973;32:1–8
O'Bryan RM et al. Cancer 1977;39:1940–1948

Doxorubicin 60 mg/m²; administer by intravenous injection over 3–5 minutes on day 1, every 21 days (total dosage/cycle = 60 mg/m²)

Note:
1. Single-agent doxorubicin remains the standard therapy for palliation of metastatic disease
2. Although some advocate higher dosages up to 70–75 mg/m² per dose, the accumulated evidence does not convincingly support the use of these higher doses

Supportive Care

Antiemetic prophylaxis
Emetogenic potential is **MODERATE**
See Chapter 42 for antiemetic recommendations

Hematopoietic growth factor (CSF) prophylaxis
Primary prophylaxis may be indicated
See Chapter 43 for more information

Antimicrobial prophylaxis
Risk of fever and neutropenia is *LOW*
Antimicrobial primary prophylaxis to be considered:
- Antibacterial—not indicated
- Antifungal—not indicated
- Antiviral—not indicated unless patient previously had an episode of HSV

Oral care
Standard prophylaxis and treatment for mucositis/stomatitis

Treatment Modifications

Adverse Event	Dose Modification
WBC <3000/mm³ or platelets <100,000/mm³	Delay treatment 1 week until WBC ≥3000/mm³ and platelets ≥100,000/mm³
>2-week delay in start of cycle	Reduce doxorubicin dose by 15 mg/m²
WBC nadir <1000/mm³ or platelet nadir <29,500/mm³	Reduce doxorubicin dosage by 30 mg/m²
WBC nadir 1000–1499/mm³ or platelet nadir 30,000–49,500/mm³	Reduce doxorubicin dosage by 15 mg/m²
G ≥3 mucositis	Reduce doxorubicin dosage by 10–15 mg/m²
Doxorubicin total cumulative lifetime dosage ≥400–450 mg/m²	Obtain frequent MUGA scans to monitor cardiac function
A fall in ejection fraction (possible guidelines: resting cardiac ejection fraction decreased ≥10–15 percentage points below baseline or to <35–40%)	Discontinue therapy

Patient Population Studied

Patients with metastatic or unresectable locoregional recurrent soft-tissue sarcoma

Efficacy

O'Bryan RM et al. Cancer 1973;32:1–8 (N = 64)

	Partial Response*
All histologies (N = 64)	21 (32.8%)
Fibrosarcomas (n = 14)	2 (14.3%)
Leiomyosarcoma (n = 8)	3 (37.5%)
Hemangiosarcoma (n = 3)	2 (66.7%)
Other (n = 12)	4 (33.3%)
Rhabdomyosarcomas (n = 11)	3 (27.3%)
Osteogenic sarcoma (n = 9)	5 (55.5%)
Ewing sarcoma (n = 7)	2 (28.6%)

*Includes only patients who received 2 courses of doxorubicin

O'Bryan RM et al. Cancer 1977;39:1940–1948 (N = 98)

Risk Category and Dose (N = 98)	Partial Response
Good risk; 75 mg/m² (n = 41)	15 (37%)
Good risk; 60 mg/m² (n = 10)	2 (20%)
Good risk; 45 mg/m² (n = 28)	5 (18%)
Poor risk; 50 mg/m² (n = 9)	1 (11%)
Poor risk; 25 mg/m² (n = 10)	0

*Patients were classified as "good risk" if in the opinion of the investigator they were able to tolerate 75 mg/m² for 3 doses. Poor-risk patients were expected to tolerate 50 mg/m² for 3 doses. The latter included those older than 65 years of age, those with prior radiation therapy or chemotherapy, and those with poor tolerance of myelosuppressive therapy

Bramwell VHC et al. Cochrane Database Syst Rev 2003;2003(3):CD003293
- Median survival ranged from 7.7 to 12.0 months with single agent doxorubicin and from 7.3 to 12.7 months with combination chemotherapy
- Overall survival data for pooling were extracted directly from survival curves for six trials with a total of 2097 patients. None of the studies detected any significant differences in survival between single agent doxorubicin and combination chemotherapy

(continued)

Adverse Event (N = 472; N = 818)

O'Bryan RM et al. Cancer 1973;32:1–8 (N = 472)

Toxicity			No. of Patients (%)
Hematologic			
WBC/mm^3	or	Platelets/mm^3	
3000–4000	or	75,000–100,000	91 (19.3)
2000–2999	or	50,000–74,500	113 (23.9)
1000–1999	or	25,000–49,500	91 (19.3)
<1000	or	<25,000	52 (11)
Nonhematologic			
Mild gastrointestinal toxicity			40 (8.5)
Moderate gastrointestinal toxicity			152 (32.2)
Severe gastrointestinal toxicity			10 (2.1)

O'Bryan RM et al. Cancer 1977;39:1940–1948 (N = 818)

Hematologic Toxicity			% of Patients		
Dosage (mg/m^2)			75	60	45
WBC/mm^3	or	Platelets/mm^3			
3000–4000	or	75,000–100,000	3	13	19
2000–2999	or	50,000–74,500	28	31	6
1000–1999	or	25,000–49,500	27	23	31
<1000	or	<25,000	14	15	13

O'Bryan RM et al. Cancer 1977;39:1940–1948 (N = 818)

Congestive Heart Failure: According to Cumulative Dosage	
Cumulative Dosage	**No. of Patients (%)**
<200 mg/m^2 (n = 491)	1 (0.2)
201–300 mg/m^2 (n = 145)	2 (1.4)
301–400 mg/m^2 (n = 84)	5 (5.9)
401–550 mg/m^2 (n = 98)	5 (5.1)
Total (N = 818)	13 (1.6)

General Summary of Toxicities	
Myelosuppression	Dose-limiting toxicity. Leukopenia more common than thrombocytopenia or anemia; nadir usually on days 10–14 with recovery by day 21 after treatment
Nausea and vomiting	Moderate severity on the day of treatment; delayed symptoms (>24 hours after treatment) uncommon
Mucositis and diarrhea	Common, but not dose limiting
Cardiotoxicity (acute)	Incidence not related to dosage. Presents within 3 days after treatment as arrhythmias, conduction abnormalities, ECG changes, pericarditis, and/or myocarditis. Usually transient and asymptomatic
Cardiotoxicity (chronic)	Dosage-dependent dilated cardiomyopathy associated with congestive heart failure. Risk increases with increasing cumulative doses
Strong vesicant	Avoid extravasation
Skin	Hand-foot syndrome, with skin rash, swelling, erythema, pain, and desquamation. Onset at 5–6 weeks after starting treatment. Hyperpigmentation of nails, rarely skin rash, urticaria. Potential for radiation recall
Alopecia	Common, but generally reversible within 3 months after discontinuing doxorubicin
Infusion reactions	Signs and symptoms include flushing, dyspnea, facial swelling, headache, back pain, chest and/or throat tightness, and hypotension. May occur with a first treatment. Symptoms resolve within several hours to a day after discontinuing doxorubicin
Urine discoloration	Red-orange discoloration usually within 1–2 days after drug administration

Efficacy (continued)

- Pooled analysis of mortality data across six studies did not detect a statistically significant difference between single-agent and combination doxorubicin-based chemotherapy at 1 year (OR = 0.87; 95% CI, 0.73 to 1.05; P = 0.14 with the random effects model) or at 2 years (OR = 0.84; 95% CI, 0.67 to 1.05; P = 0.13 with the random effects model)
- The conclusions of the meta-analysis did not significantly change when the data were restricted to the four trials using combinations of known active agents (mortality OR = 0.89; 95% CI, 0.72–1.09; P = 0.3 at 1 year; OR, 0.90; 95% CI, 0.69–1.16; P = 0.4 at 2 years; with both models)

Therapy Monitoring

1. *During treatment cycles:* CBC with differential weekly, liver function tests prior to each dose
2. *At baseline, after reaching a cumulative doxorubicin dose of 250–300 mg/m^2, and then before each cycle after a cumulative doxorubicin dosage of 400–450 mg/m^2:* cardiac ejection fraction

UNRESECTABLE • SOFT-TISSUE SARCOMA

SOFT-TISSUE SARCOMA REGIMEN: DOXORUBICIN + IFOSFAMIDE

Le Cesne A et al. J Clin Oncol 2000;18:2676–2684

Hydration and mannitol diuresis:
1000 mL 5% dextrose and 0.9% sodium chloride injection (D5W/0.9% NS); administer intravenously over 2 hours, starting 2 hours before the start of chemotherapy
Mannitol may be given to patients who have received adequate hydration
Mannitol 20% 200 mL; administer intravenously over 30 minutes, starting 1 hour before the start of chemotherapy. It is *essential* to continue hydration after mannitol administration

Doxorubicin 50 mg/m^2; administer by intravenous injection over 3–5 minutes, on day 1, every 21 days (total dosage/cycle = 50 mg/m^2), *followed by:*
Mesna 600 mg/m^2; administer intravenously, diluted with 0.9% sodium chloride injection (0.9% NS) or 5% dextrose injection (D5W) to a concentration within the range of 1–20 mg/mL, over 15 minutes just before the start of the ifosfamide + mesna admixture (see Note below), *followed by:*
An admixture containing **ifosfamide** 5000 mg/m^2 + **mesna** 2500 mg/m^2; administer intravenously, diluted in a volume of D5W/0.9% NS sufficient to produce an ifosfamide concentration within the range of 0.6–20 mg/mL, over 24 hours, on day 1, every 21 days (total ifosfamide dosage/cycle = 5000 mg/m^2), *followed by:*
Mesna 1250 mg/m^2; administer intravenously in 2000 mL D5W/0.9% NS over 12 hours, on day 2 after completing administration of the ifosfamide + mesna admixture, every 21 days (total mesna dosage/cycle = 4350 mg/m^2; includes mesna administered before and with ifosfamide)
Note: although the use of mesna before ifosfamide administration was reported by the investigators, ifosfamide must be metabolized to active (and toxic) metabolites *before* there is a need to protect the uroepithelium. Consequently, pretreating with mesna may be of little value

Supportive Care
Antiemetic prophylaxis
Emetogenic potential is **HIGH**
See Chapter 42 for antiemetic recommendations

Hematopoietic growth factor (CSF) prophylaxis
Primary prophylaxis is indicated with 1 of the following:
  Filgrastim (G-CSF) 5 μg/kg per day by subcutaneous injection, *or*
  Pegfilgrastim (pegylated filgrastim) 6 mg/0.6 mL by subcutaneous injection for 1 dose
  • Begin use from 24–72 hours after myelosuppressive chemotherapy is completed
  • Continue daily filgrastim use until ANC ≥10,000/mm^3 on 2 measurements separated temporally by ≥12 hours
  • Discontinue daily filgrastim use at least 24 hours before administering myelosuppressive treatment. Do not administer pegfilgrastim within 14 days before administering myelosuppressive treatment
See Chapter 43 for more information

Antimicrobial prophylaxis
Risk of fever and neutropenia is INTERMEDIATE
  Antimicrobial primary prophylaxis to be considered:
  • Antibacterial—consider a fluoroquinolone or no prophylaxis
  • Antifungal—consider concomitant use of clotrimazole during periods of neutropenia
  • Antiviral—antiherpes antivirals (eg, acyclovir, famciclovir, valacyclovir)

Oral care
Prophylaxis and treatment for mucositis/stomatitis
  General advice:
  • Encourage patients to maintain intake of nonalcoholic fluids
  • Evaluate patients for oral pain and provide analgesic medications
  • Consider histamine (H$_2$-subtype)–receptor antagonists (eg, ranitidine, famotidine), or a proton pump inhibitor for epigastric pain
  • *Lactobacillus* sp.–containing probiotics may be beneficial in preventing diarrhea
  Patients with intact oral mucosa:
  • Clean the mouth, tongue, and gums by brushing after every meal and at bedtime with an ultra-soft toothbrush with fluoride toothpaste
  • Floss teeth gently every day unless contraindicated. If gums bleed and hurt, avoid bleeding or sore areas, but floss other teeth
  • Patients may use saline or commercial bland, nonalcoholic rinses
    ▪ Do not use mouthwashes that contain alcohols
  If mucositis or stomatitis is present:
  • Keep the mouth moist utilizing water, ice chips, sugarless gum, sugar-free hard candies, or a saliva substitute

(continued)

(continued)

- Rinse mouth several times a day to remove debris
  - Use a solution of ¼ teaspoon (1.25 g) each of baking soda and table salt (sodium chloride) in 1 quart (~950 mL) of warm water. Follow with a plain water rinse
  - Do not use mouthwashes that contain alcohols
- Foam-tipped swabs (eg, Toothettes) are useful in moisturizing oral mucosa, but ineffective for cleansing teeth and removing plaque
- Advise patients who develop mucositis to:
  - Choose foods that are easy to chew and swallow
  - Take small bites of food, chew slowly, and sip liquids with meals
  - Encourage soft, moist foods such as cooked cereals, mashed potatoes, and scrambled eggs
  - For trouble swallowing, soften food with gravies, sauces, broths, yogurt, or other bland liquids
  - Avoid sharp, crunchy foods; hot, spicy, or highly acidic foods (eg, citrus fruits and juices); sugary foods; toothpicks; tobacco products; alcoholic drinks

Treatment Modifications

Adverse Event	Dose Modification
Day 1 ANC <1500/mm³ or platelet count <100,000/mm³	Delay by 1 week. Re-treat at full dose unless delayed by >1 week despite use of G-CSF, in which case reduce the doses of doxorubicin and ifosfamide by 20%
Febrile neutropenia occurring in the prior cycle	Reduce the doses of doxorubicin and ifosfamide by 20% in subsequent cycles and add G-CSF prophylaxis if not already receiving
SCr 1.5× baseline	Delay by 1 week. If renal function does not improve, then discontinue ifosfamide
G2 renal toxicity—tubular (based on creatinine clearance, serum bicarbonate, need for electrolyte replacement, or TmP/GFR)	Reduce the ifosfamide and mesna doses by 20% in subsequent cycles
G ≥3 renal toxicity—tubular (based on creatinine clearance, serum bicarbonate, need for electrolyte replacement, or TmP/GFR)	Discontinue ifosfamide
Microscopic hematuria during ifosfamide therapy (>50 RBC/HPF) on >1 occasion	Discontinue ifosfamide for that cycle. If hematuria completely resolves, consider increasing the rate of intravenous fluids and/or the increasing the mesna dose in subsequent cycles
G ≥2 non-infective hemorrhagic cystitis (related to ifosfamide)	Discontinue ifosfamide and provide appropriate supportive care
G2 encephalopathy	If persistent or distressing, then decrease the ifosfamide and mesna dosages by 20%. If not contraindicated, treat with methylene blue 2 mg/kg (maximum dose of 50 mg) intravenously every 4–8 hours until resolution of symptoms, then consider prophylactic use at the same dose given every 6–8 hours in subsequent cycles.
G ≥3 encephalopathy	Stop ifosfamide for this cycle. If not contraindicated, treat with methylene blue 2 mg/kg (maximum dose of 50 mg) intravenously every 4–8 hours until resolution of symptoms, then consider prophylactic use at the same dose given every 6–8 hours in subsequent cycles. Consider decreasing the ifosfamide and mesna dosages by 20% in subsequent cycles
Nonhematologic life-threatening toxicity	Discontinue therapy
G ≥3 mucositis	Reduce doxorubicin dosage by 10–15 mg/m²
Doxorubicin total cumulative lifetime dosage ≥400–450 mg/m²	Obtain frequent MUGA scans to monitor cardiac function
A fall in ejection fraction (possible guidelines: resting cardiac ejection fraction decreased ≥10–15 percentage points below baseline or to <35–40%)	Discontinue doxorubicin

Patient Population Studied

A study of 294 adult patients with metastatic or unresectable locoregional recurrent soft-tissue sarcoma randomly assigned to receive ifosfamide with either standard-dose doxorubicin (50 mg/m²; n = 147) or intensified doxorubicin (75 mg/m²; n = 133) with sargramostim support

Efficacy

Efficacy (N = 147)

Complete response	3.4%
Partial response	17.7%
Early death from toxicity	1 patient
Median duration of response	47 weeks

Note: combination chemotherapy may produce a higher response rate than single-agent therapy, but toxicity is greater and survival advantages for the more aggressive regimens have not been reproducibly reported

Adverse Events

Toxicity* (N = 147)

Toxicity	% of Patients or Levels
Hematologic	
G3/4 WBC	86
G3/4 ANC	92
Median ANC nadir (all cycles)	200/mm³
Range of ANC nadir (all cycles)	0–5500/mm³
Infection	4.6
G3/4 platelets	8
Median platelet nadir (all cycles)	141,000/mm³
Range of platelet nadir (all cycles)	5–323,000/mm³
Nonhematologic	
G3/4 asthenia	4.5
G3/4 stomatitis	3.9
G3/4 vomiting	10
G2/3 myocardial insufficiency	1.3
G ≥2 diarrhea	6.5
G3/4 fever	2.6
G ≥2 flu-like syndrome	1
G ≥2 bone pain/myalgia	6

*National Cancer Institute (USA) Common Toxicity Criteria, version 2.0

Therapy Monitoring

1. *Prior to each cycle:* physical examination, ECOG PS, CBC with differential and platelet count, total bilirubin, ALT, AST, albumin, alkaline phosphatase, serum creatinine, BUN, calcium, carbon dioxide, chloride, glucose, potassium, sodium, and phosphate

2. *During ifosfamide and mesna administration:*
   a. *Daily laboratory investigations:* serum creatinine, BUN, calcium, carbon dioxide, chloride, glucose, potassium, sodium, and phosphate
   b. *Every 8 hours (or with each void):* urine dipstick for blood (check microscopic urinalysis if >trace)
   c. *Other:* monitor fluid status (ie, weight and intake/output) and for signs and symptoms of neurologic toxicity

3. *At least once per week between cycles:* CBC with differential and platelet count, serum creatinine, BUN, calcium, carbon dioxide, chloride, glucose, potassium, sodium, and phosphate

4. *At baseline, after reaching a cumulative doxorubicin dose of 250–300 mg/m², and then before each cycle after a cumulative doxorubicin dosage of 400–450 mg/m²:* cardiac ejection fraction

5. *After every 2 cycles of therapy:* tumor measurements

UNRESECTABLE • SOFT-TISSUE SARCOMA

SOFT-TISSUE SARCOMA REGIMEN: EPIRUBICIN + IFOSFAMIDE

Gronchi A et al. Lancet Oncol 2017;18:812–22
Supplementary appendix to: Gronchi A et al. Lancet Oncol 2017;18:812–22

Hydration during ifosfamide:
Administer additional intravenous hydration (eg, **0.9% sodium chloride injection [0.9% NS]**) over 4–24 hours to achieve a total rate of 2000 mL/m^2/day (taking into account volumes of diluent used for administration of mesna and ifosfamide) for the duration of ifosfamide treatment on days 1–3. If feasible, continue maintenance intravenous hydration during intervals between ifosfamide administration. Encourage oral fluid ingestion. Monitor daily weight, or if implemented in an inpatient setting, monitor fluid input and output. Replace electrolytes as medically appropriate

Mesna 1000 mg/m^2 per dose; administer intravenously diluted with 0.9% NS or 5% dextrose injection (D5W) to a concentration of 1–20 mg/mL, over 15 minutes for 3 doses administered 15 minutes prior to each ifosfamide dose and repeated 4 hours and 8 hours after ifosfamide administration, for 3 consecutive days on days 1–3, every 21 days, for 3 cycles (total mesna dosage/cycle = 9000 mg/m^2)

Ifosfamide 3000 mg/m^2 per dose; administer intravenously in a volume of 0.9% NS or D5W sufficient to produce ifosfamide concentrations between 0.6 and 20 mg/mL, over 1–3 hours for 3 consecutive days, on days 1–3, every 21 days, for 3 cycles (total dosage/3-week cycle = 9000 mg/m^2)

Epirubicin 60 mg/m^2 per dose; administer by intravenous injection over 3–5 minutes for 2 consecutive days on days 1–2, every 21 days, for 3 cycles (total dosage/cycle = 120 mg/m^2)

Supportive Care
Antiemetic prophylaxis
*Emetogenic potential is **HIGH***
See Chapter 42 for antiemetic recommendations

Hematopoietic growth factor (CSF) prophylaxis

(continued)

Treatment Modifications

Adverse Event	Dose Modification
Day 1 ANC <1000/mm^3 or platelet count <100,000/mm^3	Delay cycle until parameters are met
ANC <500/mm^3 for ≥5 days	Administer 75% of the full doses of epirubicin, ifosfamide, and mesna in subsequent cycles. For recurrent toxicity, reduce to 66% of full doses
Platelet count <25,000/mm^3	
G ≥3 other nonhematologic toxicity	
Febrile neutropenia occurring in the prior cycle	
G ≥3 mucositis	
SCr 1.5 × baseline	Delay by 1 week. If renal function does not improve, then discontinue ifosfamide
G2 renal toxicity—tubular (based on creatinine clearance, serum bicarbonate, need for electrolyte replacement, or TmP/GFR)	Reduce the ifosfamide and mesna doses by 25% in subsequent cycles
G ≥3 renal toxicity—tubular (based on creatinine clearance, serum bicarbonate, need for electrolyte replacement, or TmP/GFR)	Discontinue ifosfamide
G ≥2 non-infective hemorrhagic cystitis (related to ifosfamide)	Discontinue ifosfamide and provide appropriate supportive care
G2 encephalopathy	If persistent or distressing, then decrease the ifosfamide and mesna dosages by 25%. If not contraindicated, treat with methylene blue 2 mg/kg (maximum dose of 50 mg) intravenously every 4–8 hours until resolution of symptoms, then consider prophylactic use at the same dose given every 6–8 hours in subsequent cycles.
G ≥3 encephalopathy	Stop ifosfamide for this cycle. If not contraindicated, treat with methylene blue 2 mg/kg (maximum dose of 50 mg) intravenously every 4–8 hours until resolution of symptoms, then consider prophylactic use at the same dose given every 6–8 hours in subsequent cycles. Consider decreasing the ifosfamide and mesna dosages by 25% in subsequent cycles
Epirubicin total cumulative lifetime dosage ≥900 mg/m^2	Frequently evaluate left ventricular ejection fraction
A fall in ejection fraction (possible guidelines: resting cardiac ejection fraction decreased ≥10–15 percentage points below baseline or to <35–40%)	Discontinue epirubicin

Patient Population Studied

This international, open-label, randomized, controlled, phase 3 trial was designed to compare a short full-dose standard regimen (epirubicin plus ifosfamide) with a histotype-tailored regimen when used as neoadjuvant chemotherapy for high-risk soft-tissue sarcoma. Eligible patients were ≥18 years of age with histologically proven localized soft-tissue sarcoma, originating in an extremity or trunk wall, with a high malignancy grade (grade 3 according to the Federation Nationale des Centres de Lutte Contre le Cancer grading system or grade 2 with > 50% necrosis at baseline), deeply located, and 5 cm or longer in diameter during baseline radiologic assessment. Additionally, participants were required to have an ECOG PS of < 1 and adequate bone marrow, renal, hepatic, and cardiac function. Key exclusion criteria included presence of distant metastases, previous chemotherapy or radiotherapy

(continued)

Primary prophylaxis is indicated with 1 of the following:

Filgrastim (G-CSF) 5 μg/kg per day by subcutaneous injection, *or*

Pegfilgrastim (pegylated filgrastim) 6 mg/0.6 mL by subcutaneous injection for 1 dose

- Begin use from 24–72 hours after myelosuppressive chemotherapy is completed
- Continue daily filgrastim use until ANC ≥10,000/mm^3 on 2 measurements separated temporally by ≥12 hours
- Discontinue daily filgrastim use at least 24 hours before administering myelosuppressive treatment. Do not administer pegfilgrastim within 14 days before administering myelosuppressive treatment

See Chapter 43 for more information

Antimicrobial prophylaxis
Risk of fever and neutropenia is INTERMEDIATE

Antimicrobial primary prophylaxis to be considered:

- Antibacterial—consider a fluoroquinolone or no prophylaxis
- Antifungal—consider concomitant use of clotrimazole during periods of neutropenia
- Antiviral—antiherpes antivirals (eg, acyclovir, famciclovir, valacyclovir)

Oral care
Standard prophylaxis and treatment for mucositis/stomatitis

Patient Population

Characteristic	Standard Chemotherapy (n = 144)	Histology-tailored Chemotherapy (n = 142)
Mean age (SD), years	48.33 (12.70)	49.47 (13.45)
Size (mm)		
Mean (SD)	112.99 (52.68)	111.30 (71.36)
Histology, no (%)		
High-grade myxoid liposarcoma	36 (25)	28 (20)
Synovial sarcoma	36 (25)	34 (24)
Malignant peripheral nerve sheath tumor	15 (10)	12 (8)
Leiomyosarcoma	12 (8)	16 (11)
Undifferentiated pleomorphic sarcoma	45 (31)	52 (37)
Site, n/N (%)		
Thoracic wall	4/124 (3)	3/119 (3)
Abdominal wall	2/124 (2)	2/119 (2)
Paravertebral	4/124 (3)	0
Shoulder girdle	13/124 (10)	7/119 (6)
Upper limb	8/124 (6)	8/119 (7)
Pelvic girdle	10/124 (8)	18/119 (15)
Lower limb	83/124 (67	81/119 (68)

SD, standard deviation

Efficacy

Efficacy Variable	Standard Chemotherapy (n = 144)	Histotype-tailored Chemotherapy (n = 142)	Between-group Comparison
Disease-free survival rate at 46 months, % (95% CI)	62 (48–77)	38 (22–55)	Stratified log-rank P = 0.004; HR 2.00 (95% CI 1.22–3.26); P = 0.006
Overall survival rate at 46 months, % (95% CI)	89 (78–99)	64 (27–100)	Log-rank P = 0.033; HR 2.867 (95% CI 1.104–6940); P = 0.034
Local failure-free survival rate at 46 months, % (95% CI)	86 (74–97)	85 (77–92)	HR 1.990; (95% CI 0.833–4.757); P = 0.11
Distant metastases-free survival rate at 46 months, % (95% CI)	74 (59–88)	45 (26–65)	HR 2.147; (95% CI 1.172–3.930); P = 0.011

Therapy Monitoring

1. *Prior to each cycle:* physical examination, ECOG PS, CBC with differential and platelet count, total bilirubin, ALT, AST, albumin, alkaline phosphatase, serum creatinine, BUN, calcium, carbon dioxide, chloride, glucose, potassium, sodium, and phosphate

2. *During ifosfamide and mesna administration:*
   a. *Daily laboratory investigations:* serum creatinine, BUN, calcium, carbon dioxide, chloride, glucose, potassium, sodium, and phosphate
   b. *Every 8 hours (or with each void):* urine dipstick for blood (check microscopic urinalysis if >trace)
   c. *Other:* monitor fluid status (ie, weight and intake/output) and for signs and symptoms of neurologic toxicity

3. *At least once per week between cycles:* CBC with differential and platelet count, serum creatinine, BUN, calcium, carbon dioxide, chloride, glucose, potassium, sodium, and phosphate

4. *At baseline, after reaching a cumulative epirubicin dose of 600 mg/m², and then before each cycle after a cumulative epirubicin dosage of 900 mg/m²:* cardiac ejection fraction

5. *After every 2 cycles of therapy:* tumor measurements

Efficacy (continued)

Best Response, %* (n = 189; Standard Chemotherapy n = 100; Histotype-tailored Chemotherapy n = 89)

Complete Response	0	0	—
Partial Response	16	11	—
Stable Disease	76	80	—
Progressive Disease	8	9	—

*Of the 239 patients assessable for objective treatment response, only 189 patients had a local radiologic review
Note: at the time of the third futility analysis, the study was closed in advance to further recruitment for futility
CI, confidence interval; HR, hazard ratio

Adverse Events

Grade (%)	Standard Chemotherapy (Epirubicin + Ifosfamide) (n = 125)			Histotype-tailored Chemotherapy (n = 114)		
	G1–2	G3	G4	G1–2	G3	G4
Anemia	81	17	2	99	1	0
Leukopenia	48	10	42	86	6	8
Neutropenia	40	9	51	78	7	15
Thrombocytopenia	83	10	7	97	2	1
Febrile neutropenia	74	14	11	96	4	1
ALT increased	99	1	0	98	2	0
AST increased	99	1	0	97	3	0
GGT increased	98	2	0	98	1	1
Creatinine increased	100	0	0	99	1	0
Diarrhea	99	1	0	98	2	0
Mucositis oral	98	2	0	99	1	0
Nausea	98	2	0	96	4	0
Vomiting	98	1	1	98	2	0
Limb edema	100	0	0	99	1	0
Fatigue	94	6	0	96	4	0
Fever	97	2	1	100	0	0
Allergic reaction	100	0	0	99	1	0
Infection	97	2	2	96	4	1
Hypokalemia	98	1	1	99	1	0
Encephalopathy	99	1	0	100	0	0
Respiratory disorders	99	1	0	100	0	0
Cardiac disorders	100	0	0	99	1	0

ALT, alanine aminotransferase; AST, aspartate aminotransferase; GGT, γ-glutamyltransferase

RECURRENT OR PROGRESSIVE • SOFT-TISSUE SARCOMA

SOFT-TISSUE SARCOMA REGIMEN: GEMCITABINE + DOCETAXEL OR GEMCITABINE ALONE

Maki RG et al. J Clin Oncol 2007;25:2755–2763

Gemcitabine 900 mg/m² per dose; administer intravenously, diluted in 0.9% sodium chloride injection (0.9% NS) to a concentration as low as 0.1 mg/mL, over 90 minutes for 2 doses, on days 1 and 8, every 21 days (total dosage/cycle = 1800 mg/m²)

Premedication for docetaxel:
Dexamethasone 8 mg/dose; administer orally twice daily for 3 days, starting 1 day before docetaxel administration (total dose/cycle = 48 mg)

Docetaxel 100 mg/m²; administer intravenously, in a volume of 0.9% NS or 5% dextrose injection sufficient to produce a docetaxel concentration within the range 0.3–0.74 mg/mL, over 60 minutes, on day 8 after completing gemcitabine administration, every 21 days (total dosage/cycle = 100 mg/m²)

Or single agent gemcitabine as follows:
Gemcitabine 1200 mg/m² per dose; administer intravenously, diluted in 0.9% NS to a concentration as low as 0.1 mg/mL, over 2 hours for 2 doses, on days 1 and 8, every 21 days (total dosage/cycle = 2400 mg/m²)

Notes:
- Patients with prior pelvic irradiation should begin therapy with gemcitabine or gemcitabine and docetaxel dosages decreased by 25%
- The investigators concluded that gemcitabine + docetaxel yielded superior progression-free and overall survival in comparison with gemcitabine alone, but with increased toxicity for the combination

Supportive Care
Antiemetic prophylaxis
Emetogenic potential is LOW
See Chapter 42 for antiemetic recommendations

Hematopoietic growth factor (CSF) prophylaxis
Primary prophylaxis is indicated (following gemcitabine + docetaxel) or may be indicated (following single agent gemcitabine) with 1 of the following:
Filgrastim (G-CSF) 5 µg/kg per day by subcutaneous injection, *or*
Pegfilgrastim (pegylated filgrastim) 6 mg/0.6 mL by subcutaneous injection for 1 dose
- Begin use on cycle day 9—that is, 24 hours after myelosuppressive chemotherapy is completed
- Continue daily filgrastim use until ANC ≥10,000/mm³ on 2 measurements separated temporally by ≥12 hours
- Discontinue daily filgrastim use at least 24 hours before administering myelosuppressive treatment. Do not administer pegfilgrastim within 14 days before administering myelosuppressive treatment
See Chapter 43 for more information

Antimicrobial prophylaxis
Risk of fever and neutropenia is LOW
Antimicrobial primary prophylaxis to be considered:
- Antibacterial—not indicated
- Antifungal—not indicated
- Antiviral—not indicated unless patient previously had an episode of HSV

Treatment Modifications

Adverse Event	Dose Modification
Febrile neutropenia or platelet count of <25,000/mm³ lasting >5 days	Reduce gemcitabine and docetaxel dosages by 25% in all subsequent cycles. Consider adding prophylactic G-CSF if not already using
ANC <1000/mm³ at start of next cycle	Withhold treatment until ANC ≥1000/mm³, then reduce gemcitabine and docetaxel dosages by 25%. Consider adding prophylactic G-CSF if not already using
Platelet count <100,000/mm³ at start of next cycle	Withhold treatment until platelet count ≥100,000/mm³, then reduce gemcitabine and docetaxel dosages by 25%
ANC <1000/mm³ or platelet count <100,000/mm³ despite 2-week delay	Discontinue therapy
Day 8 ANC 500–999/mm³ or day 8 platelet count 50,000–99,000/mm³	Reduce day 8 gemcitabine and docetaxel dosages by 25%
Day 8 ANC <500/mm³ or day 8 platelet count <50,000/mm³	Do not administer day 8 gemcitabine and docetaxel
Significant hypersensitivity reaction to docetaxel (hypotension, dyspnea, and angioedema requiring therapy)	Discontinue docetaxel
Unexplained new or worsening dyspnea or evidence of severe pulmonary toxicity	Withhold gemcitabine and assess for gemcitabine-related pulmonary toxicity. If confirmed, permanently discontinue gemcitabine
Hemolytic-uremic syndrome	Permanently discontinue gemcitabine for hemolytic uremic syndrome or severe renal impairment

(continued)

Efficacy

Efficacy (N = 73)

Outcome	Percent of Patients (Number of Patients)	
	Gemcitabine + Docetaxel	Gemcitabine Alone
Complete response	3% (2)	0
Partial response	14% (10)	8% (4)
SD ≥24 weeks	15% (11)	18% (9)
SD <24 weeks	38% (28)	35% (17)
Disease progression	25% (18)	37% (18)
Not assessable	4% (3)	2% (1)
Median progression-free survival	6.2 months	3 months
Median overall survival	17.9 months	11.5 months

Best Response by Histology*

Histology (# of Patients with Histology)	Number of Patients in Each Category					
	CR	PR	SD ≥24 wks	SD <24 wks	PD	NA
Gemcitabine + Docetaxel (n = 73)						
Leiomyosarcoma (29)	—	5	3	13	8	—
MFH/HGUPS (11)	1	3	3	2	1	1
Liposarcoma (8)						
Well differentiated/dedifferentiated	—	—	—	4	—	1
Myxoid-round cell	—	—	—	—	—	—
Pleomorphic	—	2	—	1	—	—
Synovial sarcoma (5)	—	—	1	1	2	1
Malignant peripheral nerve sheath tumor (4)	—	—	1	—	3	—
Unclassified sarcoma (1)	—	—	—	1	—	—
Fibrosarcoma (3)	—	—	1	2	—	—
Rhabdomyosarcoma (2)	1	—	—	—	1	—
Other sarcoma histology (10)	—	—	2	4	4	—
Gemcitabine Alone (n = 49)						
Leiomyosarcoma (9)	—	1	2	5	1	—
MFH/HGUPS (8)	—	2	2	1	3	—
Liposarcoma (11)						
Well differentiated/dedifferentiated	—	—	2	3	3	—
Myxoid-round cell	—	—	—	2	1	—
Pleomorphic	—	—	—	—	—	—
Synovial sarcoma (4)	—	—	1	1	2	—

(continued)

Treatment Modifications
(continued)

Adverse Event	Dose Modification
Capillary leak syndrome	Permanently discontinue gemcitabine and docetaxel
Posterior reversible encephalopathy syndrome	Permanently discontinue gemcitabine
G3/4 nonhematologic toxicity other than alopecia, fatigue, malaise, and nail changes	Hold chemotherapy up to 2 weeks until toxicity resolves to G ≤1. If toxicity does not resolve to G ≤1 within 2 weeks, discontinue therapy. Resume treatment if toxicity resolves to G ≤1 within 2 weeks, but reduce gemcitabine and docetaxel dosages by 25%
G3/4 nonhematologic toxicity other than alopecia, fatigue, malaise, and nail changes despite a 25% reduction in initial gemcitabine and docetaxel dosages	Hold chemotherapy up to 2 weeks until toxicity resolves to G ≤1. If toxicity does not resolve to G ≤1 within 2 weeks, discontinue therapy. Resume treatment if toxicity resolves to G ≤1 within 2 weeks, but reduce gemcitabine and docetaxel dosages by an additional 25%
G ≥3 liver function test abnormalities	Hold chemotherapy up to 2 weeks until toxicity resolves to G ≤1. If toxicity does not resolve to G ≤1 within 2 weeks, discontinue therapy. Resume treatment if toxicity resolves to G ≤1 within 2 weeks, but reduce gemcitabine and docetaxel dosages by 25%

(continued)

Efficacy (continued)

Malignant peripheral nerve sheath tumor (2)	—	—	—	1	1	—
Unclassified sarcoma (4)	—	—	1	2	1	—
Fibrosarcoma (3)	—	—	1	—	2	—
Rhabdomyosarcoma (0)	—	—	—	—	—	—
Other sarcoma histology (7)	1	—	—	2	4	—

*Includes one Response Evaluation Criteria in Solid Tumors Group (RECIST) unconfirmed PR on each arm: gemcitabine (MFH/HGUPS); gemcitabine-docetaxel (uterine leiomyosarcoma)

CR, complete response; PR, partial response; PD, progressive disease; SD, stable disease; NA, not assessable; MFH/HGUPS, malignant fibrous histiocytoma/high-grade undifferentiated pleomorphic sarcoma

Adverse Events

Toxicity	Percent of Patients	
	Gemcitabine + Docetaxel (N = 49)	Gemcitabine Alone (N = 73)
G3/4 neutrophils*	16%	28%
G3 hemoglobin	7%	13%
Blood transfusion	16%	20%
G3/4 platelets	40%	35%
Platelet transfusion	15%	11%
Febrile neutropenia	5%	7%
G3/4 pulmonary	7%	6%
G3/4 fatigue	16%	8%
G3 myalgias or muscle weakness	8%	2%
All other G3†	23%	2%

*National Cancer Institute Common Terminology Criteria for Adverse Events, version 3.0

†Includes (1 each except as noted): deep venous thrombosis/pulmonary embolus (n = 5), nausea/vomiting or anorexia (n = 4), lymphopenia (n = 4), edema (n = 3), GI bleeding (n = 2), high serum glucose, abdominal pain, diarrhea, mucositis, cough, pleural effusion, hiccups, bone pain, back spasm/pain, rash, nail changes, hypokalemia

Therapy Monitoring

1. *Prior to each treatment cycle:* physical examination, ECOG PS
2. *Day 1 and day 8 of each treatment cycle:* CBC with differential, serum electrolytes, magnesium and calcium, BUN, creatinine, and liver function tests
3. *Weekly CBC with leukocyte differential count:* at least the first 6 cycles of therapy
4. *After every 2 cycles of therapy:* tumor measurements

Treatment Modifications
(continued)

Adverse Event	Dose Modification
G ≥3 liver function test abnormalities despite a 25% reduction in initial gemcitabine and docetaxel dosages	Hold chemotherapy up to 2 weeks until toxicity resolves to G ≤1. If toxicity does not resolve to G ≤1 within 2 weeks, discontinue therapy. Resume treatment if toxicity resolves to G ≤1 within 2 weeks, but reduce gemcitabine and docetaxel dosages by an additional 25%
G4 mucositis and diarrhea	Discontinue therapy
G2 neuropathy	Delay therapy 1 week. If symptoms do not resolve to G ≤1, reduce docetaxel dosage by 25%
G3 neuropathy	Discontinue docetaxel

Patient Population Studied

Patients with a diagnosis of recurrent or progressive soft-tissue sarcoma (excluding GI stromal tumor and Kaposi sarcoma); age >10 years; zero to 3 prior chemotherapy regimens; ECOG PS ≤2; peripheral neuropathy Grade ≤1 by National Cancer Institute (USA) Common Terminology Criteria for Adverse Events, version 3.0

ADVANCED/ PROGRESSIVE • SOFT-TISSUE SARCOMA • LIPOSARCOMA • LEIOMYOSARCOMA

SOFT-TISSUE SARCOMA; MYXOID LIPOSARCOMA METASTATIC LIPOSARCOMA/ LEIOMYOSARCOMA REGIMEN: TRABECTEDIN

Demetri GD et al. J Clin Oncol 2016;34:786–793
Demetri GD et al. J Clin Oncol 2009;27:4188–4196
Garcia-Carbonero R et al. J Clin Oncol 2004;22:1480–1490
Grosso F et al. Lancet Oncol 2007;8:595–602

Trabectedin premedication:
Dexamethasone 20 mg; administer intravenously 30 minutes prior to each trabectedin infusion on day 1, every 3 weeks (total dosage/cycle = 20 mg)

Trabectedin 1.5 mg/m²; administer intravenously in 500 mL 0.9% sodium chloride or 5% dextrose injection through a central venous access device over 24 hours on day 1, every 3 weeks (total dosage/cycle = 1.5 mg/m²)

Supportive Care
Antiemetic prophylaxis
Emetogenic potential is **MODERATE**
See Chapter 42 for antiemetic recommendations

Hematopoietic growth factor (CSF) prophylaxis
Primary prophylaxis may be indicated with 1 of the following:

Filgrastim (G-CSF) 5 µg/kg per day by subcutaneous injection, *or*
Pegfilgrastim (pegylated filgrastim) 6 mg/0.6 mL by subcutaneous injection for 1 dose
- Begin use from 24–72 hours after myelosuppressive chemotherapy is completed
- Continue daily filgrastim use until ANC ≥10,000/mm³ on 2 measurements separated temporally by ≥12 hours
- Discontinue daily filgrastim use at least 24 hours before administering myelosuppressive treatment. Do not administer pegfilgrastim within 14 days before administering myelosuppressive treatment

See Chapter 43 for more information

(continued)

Treatment Modifications

Trabectedin Dose Levels

	Normal hepatic function or mild hepatic impairment at baseline (bilirubin >1–1.5 × ULN and any AST or ALT)	Moderate hepatic impairment at baseline (bilirubin >1.5 to 3 × ULN and AST and ALT <8 × ULN)
Starting dose level	1.5 mg/m²	0.9 mg/m²
Level −1	1.2 mg/m²	0.6 mg/m²
Level −2	1 mg/m²	0.3 mg/m²

Adverse Event	Dose Modification
Day 21 ANC <1500/mm³, or platelet count <100,000/mm³	Delay start of next cycle by up to 3 weeks until ANC >1500/mm³ and platelet count >100,000/mm³
Day 42 ANC remains <1000/mm³, or platelet count remains <75,000/mm³, despite delaying next cycle by 3 weeks	Discontinue therapy
Platelet count <25,000/mm³ during prior cycle	Reduce dose of trabectedin for the following cycle by one dose level
ANC <1000/mm³ with fever/infection during prior cycle	
ANC <500/mm³ lasting ≥5 days during prior cycle	
• LVEF less than lower limit of normal • G3/4 cardiac adverse event indicative of cardiomyopathy • Severe liver dysfunction in the prior treatment cycle • Capillary leak syndrome • Rhabdomyolysis	Discontinue trabectedin
Any of the following day 21 laboratory values: • ALT, AST, or alkaline phosphatase >2.5 × ULN • Creatine phosphokinase (CPK) >2.5 × ULN • Total bilirubin >ULN	Delay next dose of trabectedin for up to 3 weeks
Any occurrence of the following in the previous cycle: • ALT or AST >5 × ULN • Alkaline phosphatase >2.5 × ULN • Creatine phosphokinase (CPK) >5 × ULN • Total bilirubin >ULN • Asymptomatic ≥10% absolute decrease in LVEF from baseline but still ≥LLN	Reduce next dose of trabectedin by one dose level
Other G ≥3 nonhematologic toxicity	Delay next dose of trabectedin for up to 3 weeks until toxicity recovers to G ≤1 or baseline, then reduce next dose of trabectedin by one dose level

Patient Populations Studied

Demetri GD et al. J Clin Oncol 2016; 34:786–793
Patients were eligible if they were ≥15 years; had unresectable, locally advanced or metastatic liposarcoma or leiomyosarcomas; and were previously treated with at least either a combination of an anthracycline and ifosfamide or an anthracycline plus one or more additional cytotoxic chemotherapy regimen(s). Patients required an Eastern Cooperative Oncology Group performance status score of 1 or lower

(continued)

Antimicrobial prophylaxis
Risk of fever and neutropenia is *LOW*
 Antimicrobial primary prophylaxis to be considered:
 • Antibacterial—not indicated
 • Antifungal—not indicated
 • Antiviral—not indicated unless patient previously had an episode of HSV

Therapy Monitoring

1. *Prior to each cycle:* physical examination, ECOG PS, CBC with differential and platelet count, liver function tests (total bilirubin, ALT, AST, albumin, alkaline phosphatase), serum creatinine, BUN, serum electrolytes, creatine phosphokinase
2. *At least once per week:* CBC with differential and platelet count, serum creatinine, BUN, serum electrolytes, liver function tests
3. *Prior to each cycle and then every 2–3 months (or sooner if clinically indicated):* assessment of LVEF by echocardiogram or multigated acquisition scan
4. *After every 2 cycles of therapy:* tumor measurements

Patient Populations Studied *(continued)*

Baseline Demographic and Disease Characteristics

Variable	No. (%) of Patients	
	Trabectedin (n = 345)	Dacarbazine n = 173)
Age, years—median (range)	57 (18.0–81.0)	56 (17.0–79.0)
Sex—male/female	107 (31) / 238 (69)	47 (27) / 126 (73)
Baseline BMI, kg/m²—median (range)	28.21 (14.5–78.1)	27.05 (13.3–66.7)
Histology		
Leiomyosarcoma	252 (73)	126 (73)
Uterine	134 (39)	78 (45)
Nonuterine	118 (34)	48 (28)
Liposarcoma	93 (27)	47 (27)
Myxoid 6 round cell	38 (11)	19 (11)
Pleomorphic	10 (3)	3 (2)
Dedifferentiated	45 (13)	25 (15)
Baseline ECOG performance status score—0/1	171 (50) / 174 (50)	86 (50) / 87 (50)
Lines of prior chemotherapy		
1	38 (11)	23 (13)
2	160 (46)	75 (43)
3	87 (25)	43 (25)
4	37 (11)	21 (12)
>4	23 (7)	11 (6)
Best response to last line of previous chemotherapy		
Complete response	4 (1)	3 (2)
Partial response	28 (8)	14 (8)
No change (stable disease)	114 (33)	51 (30)
Progression of disease	198 (57)	103 (60)
Unknown/missing	1 (0)	2 (1)
Previous surgery for malignancy—yes / no	327 (95) / 18 (5)	158 (91) / 15 (9)
Previous radiotherapy for malignancy—yes / no	176 (51) /169 (49)	80 (46) / 93 (54)
Time from initial diagnosis to random assignment, months—median (range)	33.94 (2.5–318.5)	27.10 (1.6–267.1)
Time from last disease progression to random assignment, months—median (range)	0.85 (0.0–13.7)	0.82 (0.1–9.8)

Note: percentages were calculated with the number of patients randomly assigned to each treatment group as the denominator
BMI, body mass index; ECOG, Eastern Cooperative Oncology Group

Efficacy

Demetri GD et al. J Clin Oncol 2016;34:786–793

Summary of Key Progression-Free Survival/Radiographic Progression-Free Survival Results

Variable			Survival Measure			
	PFS-INV (n = 518)	rPFS-INV (n = 518)	rPFS-INV (Audited Subset; n = 304)	rPFS-INV (Unaudited Subset; n = 214)	rPFS-IR (Audited Subset; n = 304)	rPFS-IR (Overall Estimate)
HR*	0.55	0.57	0.58	0.54	0.55	0.54
95% CI	0.44–0.70	0.45–0.72	0.43–0.79	0.37–0.80	0.40–0.75	0.41–0.71

*HR was calculated as the hazard in the trabectedin treatment group divided by the hazard in the dacarbazine treatment group
HR, hazard ratio; INV, investigator assessed; IR, independent radiologist; PFS, progression-free survival; rPFS, radiographic progression-free survival

Endpoints That Reflect Disease Control

Endpoint	Trabectedin n = 345)	Dacarbazine (n = 173)	HR/OR (95% CI)*	P
PFS, months	4.2	1.5	0.55 (0.44–0.70)	<0.001
TTP, months	4.2	1.5	0.52 (0.41–0.66)	<0.001
No. (%) of ORR	34 (9.9)	12 (6.9)	1.47 (0.72–3.2)	0.33
DOR, months	6.5	4.2	0.47 (0.17–1.32)	0.14
No. (%) with SD as best response	177 (51)	60 (35)	—	—
Duration of SD, months	6.01	4.17	0.45 (0.30–0.67)	<0.001
% of CBR	34	19	2.3 (1.45–3.7)	<0.001

*HR was calculated as the hazard in the trabectedin treatment group, divided by the hazard in the dacarbazine treatment group
CBR, clinical benefit rate; DOR, duration of response; HR, hazard ratio; OR, odds ratio; ORR, objective response rate; PFS, progression-free survival; SD, stable disease; TTP, time to progression

Adverse Events

Demetri GD et al. J Clin Oncol 2016;34:786–793

Most Common Adverse Events

Adverse Event	No. (%) Adverse Events by Treatment and Grade					
	Trabectedin (n = 340)			Dacarbazine (n = 155)		
	All G	G3	G4	All G	G3	G4
Nausea	247 (73)	18 (5)	0	76 (49)	3 (2)	0
Fatigue	228 (67)	20 (6)	0	79 (51)	2 (1)	1 (1)
Neutropenia	165 (49)	70 (21)	56 (16)	45 (29)	17 (11)	15 (10)
Alanine aminotransferase increased	154 (45)	85 (25)	4 (1)	9 (6)	1 (1)	0
Vomiting	149 (44)	16 (5)	0	33 (21)	2 (1)	0
Anemia	134 (39)	49 (14)	0	45 (29)	17 (11)	1 (1)
Constipation	121 (36)	3 (1)	0	44 (28)	0	0
Aspartate aminotransferase increased	120 (35)	40 (12)	4 (1)	8 (5)	0	0
Decreased appetite	116 (34)	7 (2)	0	31 (20)	0	1 (1)
Diarrhea	115 (34)	6 (2)	0	35 (23)	0	0
Thrombocytopenia	101 (30)	27 (8)	31 (9)	56 (36)	15 (10)	13 (8)
Dyspnea	84 (25)	12 (4)	1 (<1)	30 (19)	1 (1)	0
Peripheral edema	83 (24)	3 (1)	0	21 (14)	1 (1)	0
Headache	78 (23)	1 (<1)	0	29 (19)	0	0
Blood alkaline phosphatase increased	69 (20)	5 (1)	0	11 (7)	0	0
Cough	61 (18)	1 (<1)	0	32 (21)	0	0

Note: most common adverse events occurred with ≥20% frequency

UNRESECTABLE • LEIOMYOSARCOMA
LEIOMYOSARCOMA REGIMEN: GEMCITABINE + DOCETAXEL

Hensley ML et al. J Clin Oncol 2002;20:2824–2831

Gemcitabine 900 mg/m^2 per dose; administer intravenously, diluted in 0.9% sodium chloride injection (0.9% NS) to a concentration as low as 0.1 mg/mL, over 90 minutes for 2 doses, on days 1 and 8, every 21 days (total dosage/cycle = 1800 mg/m^2)

Premedication for docetaxel:
Dexamethasone 8 mg/dose; administer orally twice daily for 3 days, starting 1 day before docetaxel administration (total dose/cycle = 48 mg)

Docetaxel 100 mg/m^2; administer intravenously, in a volume of 0.9% NS or 5% dextrose injection (D5W) sufficient to produce a docetaxel concentration within the range 0.3–0.74 mg/mL, over 60 minutes on day 8 after gemcitabine, every 21 days (total dosage/cycle = 100 mg/m^2)

Notes:
• Patients previously treated with radiation therapy should receive *reduced* dosages as follows:

Gemcitabine 675 mg/m^2 per dose; administer intravenously, diluted in 0.9% NS to a concentration as low as 0.1 mg/mL, over 90 minutes for 2 doses, on days 1 and 8, every 21 days (total dosage/cycle = 1350 mg/m^2)

Premedication for docetaxel:
Dexamethasone 8 mg/dose; administer orally twice daily for 3 days, starting 1 day before docetaxel administration (total dose/cycle = 48 mg)

Docetaxel 75 mg/m^2; administer intravenously in a volume of 0.9% NS or D5W sufficient to produce a docetaxel concentration within the range 0.3–0.74 mg/mL over 60 minutes on day 8 after gemcitabine, every 21 days (total dosage/cycle = 75 mg/m^2)

• Patients who continue to respond after receiving 6 cycles may receive 2 additional cycles of therapy

Supportive Care
Antiemetic prophylaxis
Emetogenic potential is **LOW**
See Chapter 42 for antiemetic recommendations

Hematopoietic growth factor (CSF) prophylaxis
Primary prophylaxis is indicated with **1** *of the following:*
  Filgrastim (G-CSF) 5 μg/kg per day by subcutaneous injection, *or*
  Pegfilgrastim (pegylated filgrastim) 6 mg/0.6 mL by subcutaneous injection for 1 dose
  • Begin use on cycle day 9—that is, 24 hours after myelosuppressive chemotherapy is completed
  • Continue daily filgrastim use until ANC ≥10,000/mm^3 on 2 measurements separated temporally by ≥12 hours
  • Discontinue daily filgrastim use at least 24 hours before administering myelosuppressive treatment. Do not administer pegfilgrastim within 14 days before administering myelosuppressive treatment
See Chapter 43 for more information

Antimicrobial prophylaxis
Risk of fever and neutropenia is *LOW*
  Antimicrobial primary prophylaxis to be considered:
  • Antibacterial—not indicated
  • Antifungal—not indicated
  • Antiviral—not indicated unless patient previously had an episode of HSV

Treatment Modifications

Treatment Modifications	
Adverse Event	**Dose Modification**
Febrile neutropenia or platelet count of <25,000/mm^3 lasting >5 days	Reduce gemcitabine and docetaxel dosages by 25% in all subsequent cycles. Consider adding prophylactic G-CSF if not already using
ANC <1000/mm^3 at start of next cycle	Withhold treatment until ANC ≥1000/mm^3, then reduce gemcitabine and docetaxel dosages by 25%. Consider adding prophylactic G-CSF if not already using
Platelet count <100,000/mm^3 at start of next cycle	Withhold treatment until platelet count ≥100,000/mm^3, then reduce gemcitabine and docetaxel dosages by 25%
ANC <1000/mm^3 or platelet count <100,000/mm^3 despite 2-week delay	Discontinue therapy

(continued)

Treatment Modifications (continued)

Adverse Event	Dose Modification
Day 8 ANC 500–999/mm^3 or day 8 platelet count 50,000–99,000/mm^3	Reduce day 8 gemcitabine and docetaxel dosages by 25%
Day 8 ANC <500/mm^3 or day 8 platelet count <50,000/mm^3	Do not administer day 8 gemcitabine and docetaxel
Significant hypersensitivity reaction to docetaxel (hypotension, dyspnea, and angioedema requiring therapy)	Discontinue docetaxel
Unexplained new or worsening dyspnea or evidence of severe pulmonary toxicity	Withhold gemcitabine and assess for gemcitabine-related pulmonary toxicity. If confirmed, permanently discontinue gemcitabine
Hemolytic-uremic syndrome	Permanently discontinue gemcitabine for hemolytic uremic syndrome or severe renal impairment
Capillary leak syndrome	Permanently discontinue gemcitabine and docetaxel
Posterior reversible encephalopathy syndrome	Permanently discontinue gemcitabine
G3/4 nonhematologic toxicity other than alopecia, fatigue, malaise, and nail changes	Hold chemotherapy up to 2 weeks until toxicity resolves to G ≤1. If toxicity does not resolve to G ≤1 within 2 weeks, discontinue therapy. Resume treatment if toxicity resolves to G ≤1 within 2 weeks, but reduce gemcitabine and docetaxel dosages by 25%
G3/4 nonhematologic toxicity other than alopecia, fatigue, malaise, and nail changes despite a 25% reduction in initial gemcitabine and docetaxel dosages	Hold chemotherapy up to 2 weeks until toxicity resolves to G ≤1. If toxicity does not resolve to G ≤1 within 2 weeks, discontinue therapy. Resume treatment if toxicity resolves to G ≤1 within 2 weeks, but reduce gemcitabine and docetaxel dosages by an additional 25%
G ≥3 liver function test abnormalities	Hold chemotherapy up to 2 weeks until toxicity resolves to G ≤1. If toxicity does not resolve to G ≤1 within 2 weeks, discontinue therapy. Resume treatment if toxicity resolves to G ≤1 within 2 weeks, but reduce gemcitabine and docetaxel dosages by 25%
G ≥3 liver function test abnormalities despite a 25% reduction in initial gemcitabine and docetaxel dosages	Hold chemotherapy up to 2 weeks until toxicity resolves to G ≤1. If toxicity does not resolve to G ≤1 within 2 weeks, discontinue therapy. Resume treatment if toxicity resolves to G ≤1 within 2 weeks, but reduce gemcitabine and docetaxel dosages by an additional 25%
G4 mucositis and diarrhea	Discontinue therapy
G2 neuropathy	Delay therapy 1 week. If symptoms do not resolve to G ≤1, reduce docetaxel dosage by 25%
G3 neuropathy	Discontinue docetaxel

Efficacy

Leiomyosarcoma (LMS) (N = 34)*		
Best Response	Percent (Number of Patients)	95% CI
Complete response	8.8 % (3)	
Partial response	44% (15)	
Minor response/stable disease	23.5% (8)	
Progression of disease	26.5% (9)	
Overall objective response†	53% (18)	35–70%
Median duration of response	4 months	3 months–NR‡
Median progression-free survival	5.6 months	4.3–9.9 months
Progression-free at 6 months	47%	32–68%
Median overall survival	17.9 months	11.6 months—NR
Alive at 6 months	66%	49–88%
Patients Previously Treated with Doxorubicin ± Ifosfamide (N = 16)		
Overall objective response	50% (8)	

NR, Not reached
*RECIST criteria
†Among 5 patients with non-uterine primary LMS, 2 (40%) had PRs
‡Among 18 patients who achieved a complete or partial response

Patient Population Studied

Patients with histologically confirmed leiomyosarcoma (LMS) of the uterus or of other primary site that was considered unresectable for cure and who had received zero to 2 previous chemotherapy regimens for treatment of LMS

Adverse Events

Toxicity*
(N = 34 Patients/160 Cycles)

	Grade 3		Grade 4	
	Number of Patients	%	Number of Patients	%
Neutropenia	5	15	2	6
Thrombocytopenia	9	26	1	3
Neutropenia and fever	—	—	2	6
Anemia	4	12	1	3
Dyspnea	5	15	2	6
Diarrhea	3	9	1	3
Fatigue	7	21	—	—
Sensory neuropathy	2	6	—	—
Allergic reaction	1	3	—	—
Venous thrombosis	—	—	1	3

*National Cancer Institute (USA), Common Toxicity Criteria, version 2.0

Therapy Monitoring

1. *Prior to each treatment cycle:* physical examination, ECOG PS
2. *Day 1 and day 8 of each treatment cycle:* CBC with differential, serum electrolytes, magnesium and calcium, BUN, creatinine, and liver function tests
3. *Weekly CBC with leukocyte differential count:* at least the first 6 cycles of therapy
4. *After every 2 cycles of therapy:* tumor measurements

METASTATIC/INOPERABLE • LIPOSARCOMA • PREVIOUS ANTHRACYCLINE BASED THERAPY

METASTATIC OR INOPERABLE LIPOSARCOMA PREVIOUSLY TREATED WITH ANTHRACYCLINE BASED THERAPY REGIMEN: ERIBULIN

Demetri GD et al. J Clin Oncol 2017;35:3433–3439

Eribulin mesylate 1.4 mg/m^2 per dose*; administer (undiluted) by slow intravenous injection over 2–5 minutes for 2 doses on days 1 and 8, every 21 days (total dosage/cycle = 2.8 mg/m^2)
• Do not dilute in or administer through an intravenous line containing solutions with dextrose. Do not administer in the same intravenous line concurrent with the other medicinal products

*Dosage Recommendations for Impaired Liver and Renal Function

Condition	Dosage (Days 1 and 8; 21-day Cycle)
Mild hepatic impairment (Child-Pugh A)	1.1 mg/m^2 per dose (total dosage/cycle = 2.2 mg/m^2)
Moderate hepatic impairment (Child-Pugh B)	0.7 mg/m^2 per dose (total dosage/cycle = 1.4 mg/m^2)
Moderate or severe renal impairment (creatinine clearance: 15–49 mL/min [0.25–0.82 mL/s])	1.1 mg/m^2 per dose (total dosage/cycle = 2.2 mg/m^2)

Supportive Care
Antiemetic prophylaxis
Emetogenic potential is LOW
See Chapter 42 for antiemetic recommendations

Hematopoietic growth factor (CSF) prophylaxis
Primary prophylaxis is NOT indicated
See Chapter 43 for more information

Antimicrobial prophylaxis
Risk of fever and neutropenia is *LOW*
Antimicrobial primary prophylaxis to be considered:
• Antibacterial—not indicated
• Antifungal—not indicated
• Antiviral—not indicated, unless patient previously had an episode of HSV

Treatment Modifications

Eribulin Mesylate Dosage Levels

Dosage Level 1	1.4 mg/m^2
Dosage Level –1	1.1 mg/m^2
Dosage Level –2	0.7 mg/m^2

Adverse Events	Treatment Modifications
ANC <1000/mm^3 on cycle days 1 or 8	Hold eribulin mesylate. Administer when ANC >1000/mm^3
Platelet count <75,000/mm^3 on cycle days 1 or 8	Hold eribulin mesylate. Administer when platelet count >75,000/mm^3
Nonhematologic toxicities G ≥3 on cycle days 1 or 8	Hold eribulin mesylate. Administer when toxicities < G2
ANC <1000/mm^3 on cycle day 8 resolved by day 15	Give eribulin mesylate at a dosage decreased by 1 dose level but do not administer less than 0.7 mg/m^2. Initiate a subsequent cycle no sooner than 2 weeks later
Platelet count <75,000/mm^3 on cycle day 8 resolved by day 15	
Nonhematologic toxicities G ≥3 on cycle day 8 resolved to G ≤2 by day 15	

(continued)

Treatment Modifications (continued)

Adverse Events	Treatment Modifications
ANC <1000/mm³ on cycle day 8 and still <1000/mm³ on day 15	Omit day 8 eribulin mesylate dose
Platelet count <75,000/mm³ on cycle day 8 and still <75,000/mm³ on day 15	
Nonhematologic toxicities G ≥3 on cycle day 8 and still G ≥3 on day 15	
ANC <500/mm³ for >7 days	Permanently decrease eribulin mesylate dosage by one dosage level but do not administer less than 0.7 mg/m²
ANC <1000/mm³ with fever or infection	
Platelet count <25,000/mm³	
Platelet count <50,000/mm³ requiring transfusion	
Nonhematologic toxicities G ≥3	
Omission or delay of a day 8 dose during the previous cycle for toxicity	

Note: after any dosage decrease, do not re-escalate eribulin mesylate dosages during subsequent treatments

Patient Population Studied

This randomized, open-label, phase 3 trial (NCT01327885) included patients with advanced (locally recurrent, locally advanced, or metastatic) liposarcoma or leiomyosarcoma incurable by surgery or radiotherapy. Eligible patients had received ≥2 prior chemotherapy regimens, including an anthracycline. Patients with well-differentiated liposarcoma were excluded. Patients were randomized 1:1 to receive eribulin or dacarbazine, with stratification based on disease type, geographic region, and number of prior regimens

Patient Population (Liposarcoma Subgroup)		
Characteristic	Eribulin (n = 71)	Dacarbazine (n = 72)
Median age, years (range)	55 (32–83)	57 (34–83)
Age <65 (%) / age ≥65 (%)	77.5 / 22.5	75 / 25
Male sex (%)	53.5	70.8
Race, %		
White	73.2	70.8
Black or African American	0	2.8
Asian	5.6	5.6
Other or NA	21.1	21.1
ECOG PS (%) 0 / 1 /2	49.3 / 47.9 / 2.8	33.3 / 58.3 / 8.3
Histology subcategory (%)		
Dedifferentiated	43.7	47.2
Myxoid/round cell	40.8	36.1
Pleomorphic	15.5	16.7
Tumor grade (%)—high / intermediate / not done	53.5 / 45.1 / 1.4	54.2 / 44.4 / 1.4
Geographic region, %		

(continued)

Patient Population Studied (continued)

Patient Population (Liposarcoma Subgroup)		
Characteristic	Eribulin (n = 71)	Dacarbazine (n = 72)
United States and Canada	35.2	34.7
Western Europe, Australia, Israel	50.7	51.4
Eastern Europe, Latin America, Asia	14.1	13.9
Median age at diagnosis, years (range)	48 (22–82)	51 (30–82)
Previous anticancer regimens (%)—1/2/3/4/>4	0/52.1/25.4/12.7/9.9	2.8/45.8/30.6/5.6/15.3
Type of previous anticancer therapy (%)		
Neoadjuvant	8.5	11.1
Adjuvant	19.7	12.5
Therapeutic	100	98.6
Maintenance	2.8	6.9
Unknown	1.4	1.4
1 Previous neoadjuvant regimen (%)	7	11.1
1 Previous adjuvant regimen (%)	18.3	12.5

ECOG, Eastern Cooperative Group; NA, not applicable; PS, performance status

Efficacy

Efficacy Variable	Eribulin (n = 71)	Dacarbazine (n = 72)	Between-group Comparison
Median OS, months (95% CI)	15.6 (10.2–18.6)	8.4 (5.2–10.1)	HR 0.511 (95% CI 0.35–0.75) $P<0.001$
Median PFS, months	2.9	1.7	HR 0.521 (95% CI 0.35–0.78) $P = 0.0015$
PFS @ 12 weeks (%) (95% CI)	40.8 (29.3–53.2)	19.4 (11.1–30.5)	OR 2.8 (95% CI 1.3–6.0)
Patients with SD (%)	64.8	44.4	—

Note: data reported represent the subgroup analysis of patients with advanced liposarcoma
CI, confidence interval; HR, hazard ratio; OR, odds ratio; OS, overall survival; PFS, progression-free survival

Adverse Events

	Eribulin (n = 70)	Dacarbazine (n = 72)
Treatment-emergent Adverse Events with Frequency of ≥10% in Either Arm, no (%)		
Abdominal pain	17 (24.3)	12 (16.7)
Alopecia	28 (40.0)	1 (1.4)
Anemia	18 (25.7)	25 (34.7)
Arthralgia	7 (10.0)	0

(continued)

Treatment Monitoring

1. *Prior to each cycle:* CBC with differential, liver function tests, BUN, serum creatinine, physical examination (with attention to peripheral neuropathy)

2. *Prior to day 8 dose:* CBC with differential, physical examination (with attention to peripheral neuropathy)

3. *If G3/4 hematologic toxicity occurs or if fever or infection occurs:* frequent monitoring of CBC with differential

4. Consider periodic monitoring with electrocardiograms (ECGs) and electrolytes in patients with congestive heart failure, bradyarrhythmias, electrolyte abnormalities, or who are taking medications that are known to prolong the QT interval. Avoid use in patients with congenital long QT syndrome

Adverse Events (continued)

	Eribulin (n = 70)	Dacarbazine (n = 72)
Asthenia	12 (17.1)	17 (23.6)
Back pain	9 (12.9)	8 (11.1)
Constipation	20 (28.6)	17 (23.6)
Decreased appetite	16 (22.9)	22 (30.6)
Diarrhea	13 (18.6)	14 (19.4)
Dizziness	8 (11.4)	7 (9.7)
Dysgeusia	9 (12.9)	4 (5.6)
Dyspepsia	7 (10.0)	3 (4.2)
Dyspnea	9 (12.9)	11 (15.3)
Fatigue	28 (40.0)	23 (31.9)
Headache	9 (12.9)	4 (5.6)
Insomnia	9 (12.9)	1 (1.4)
Leukopenia	11 (15.7)	3 (4.2)
Myalgia	7 (10.0)	1 (1.4)
Nausea	27 (38.6)	32 (44.4)
Neutropenia	27 (38.6)	13 (18.1)
Neutrophil count decreased	8 (11.4)	3 (4.2)
Peripheral sensory neuropathy	16 (22.9)	2 (2.8)
Pyrexia	17 (24.3)	11 (15.3)
Stomatitis	9 (12.9)	7 (9.7)
Thrombocytopenia	3 (4.3)	15 (20.8)
Upper respiratory tract infection	8 (11.4)	2 (2.8)
Urinary tract infection	9 (12.9)	2 (2.8)
Vomiting	13 (18.6)	16 (22.2)
Treatment-emergent Adverse Events of Grade ≥3 with Frequency of ≥5% in Either Arm, no (%)		
Anemia	4 (5.7)	8 (11.1)
Leukopenia	7 (10.0)	2 (2.8)
Neutropenia	19 (27.1)	11 (15.3)
Neutrophil count decreased	7 (10.0)	1 (1.4)
Thrombocytopenia	0	8 (11.1)
White blood cell count decreased	4 (5.7)	4 (5.6)

DERMATOFIBROSARCOMA PROTUBERANS (DFSP) WITH PDGFB REARRANGEMENT

DERMATOFIBROSARCOMA PROTUBERANS (DFSP) WITH PDGFB REARRANGEMENT REGIMEN: IMATINIB MESYLATE

Rutkowski P et al. J Clin Oncol 2010;28:1772–1779

Note: dermatofibrosarcoma protuberans (DFSP) is a dermal sarcoma typically carrying a translocation between chromosomes 17 and 22 that generates functional platelet-derived growth factor B (PDGFB)

Starting dose: **Imatinib mesylate** 400 mg/day; administer orally with food and a large glass of water (total dose/week = 2800 mg)

Dose escalation: **Imatinib mesylate** 600–800 mg/day; administer orally with food and a large glass of water (total dose/week = 4200–5600 mg)

Notes:
- 400- and 600-mg doses may be given once daily, or, alternatively, may be split into 2 equal doses, one given during morning hours and a second dose during the evening
- 800-mg daily doses should be given as two 400-mg doses, one during morning hours and a second dose during the evening
- For patients unable to swallow the film-coated tablets, imatinib mesylate may be dispersed in a glass of water or apple juice. The required number of tablets should be placed in an appropriate volume of beverage (approximately 50 mL for a 100-mg tablet, and 200 mL for a 400-mg tablet) and stirred with a spoon. The suspension should be administered immediately after the tablets have completely disintegrated

Note: response rates and TTP did not differ between patients taking 400 mg daily versus 400 mg twice a day

Supportive Care
Antiemetic prophylaxis
Emetogenic potential is **MINIMAL TO LOW**
See Chapter 42 for antiemetic recommendations

Hematopoietic growth factor (CSF) prophylaxis
Primary prophylaxis is NOT indicated
See Chapter 43 for more information

Antimicrobial prophylaxis
Risk of fever and neutropenia is *LOW*
Antimicrobial primary prophylaxis to be considered:
- Antibacterial—not indicated
- Antifungal—not indicated
- Antiviral—not indicated unless patient previously had an episode of HSV

Diarrhea management*
Loperamide 4 mg orally initially after the first loose or liquid stool, *then* 2–4 mg orally every 2–4 hours or **diphenoxylate hydrochloride** 2.5 mg **with atropine sulfate** 0.025 mg (eg, Lomotil)

*Abigerges D et al. J Natl Cancer Inst 1994;86:446–449
Rothenberg ML et al. J Clin Oncol 2001;19:3801–3807
Wadler S et al. J Clin Oncol 1998;16:3169–3178

Treatment Modifications

Dosage Levels*
800 mg
600 mg
400 mg
300 mg
200 mg

Adverse Event	Treatment Modification
Hematologic[f]	
G1/2	No modifications
Recurrence of a G2 toxicity	Hold imatinib until toxicity resolves to G ≤1; then restart at 1 lower dose level
First episode of a G3/4 toxicity	Hold imatinib until toxicity resolves to G ≤1; then restart at the same dose
Second episode of a G3/4 toxicity	Hold imatinib until toxicity resolves to G ≤1; then restart at 1 lower dose level
Recurrent G2/3/4 at a reduced dose	Hold imatinib until toxicity resolves to G ≤1; then restart at 1 dose level lower, or for recurrent G4, consider discontinuing imatinib
Nonhematologic	
G1	No dose modifications
First episode of a G2 toxicity	Hold imatinib until toxicity resolves to G ≤1; then restart at the same dose
Recurrence of a G2 toxicity (second G2)	Hold imatinib until toxicity resolves to G ≤1; then restart at 1 lower dose level
G3/4	Hold imatinib until toxicity resolves to G ≤1; then restart at 1 lower dose level
Recurrent G2/3/4 at a reduced dose	Hold imatinib until toxicity resolves to G ≤1; then restart at 1 dose level lower, or for recurrent G4, consider discontinuing imatinib

*No dose modifications for anemia. Growth factors were allowed but not recommended

Patient Population Studied

Patients from 2 distinct phase 2 trials of imatinib (400–800 mg daily) in patients with locally advanced or metastatic dermatofibrosarcoma protuberans (DFSP) were conducted and closed prematurely, one in Europe (European Organization for Research and Treatment of Cancer [EORTC]) with 14-week progression-free rate as the primary endpoint and the other in North America (Southwest Oncology Group [SWOG]) with confirmed objective response rate as the primary endpoint. In the EORTC trial, confirmation of *PDGFB* rearrangement was required, and surgery was undertaken after 14 weeks if feasible. The SWOG study confirmed t(17;22) after enrollment

Efficacy

Dermatofibrosarcoma Protuberans (DFSP) Best Response by Subtype (N = 24)

	Number of Patients					
	Partial Response*		Stable Disease		Progressive Disease	
	Imatinib (mg/day)					
	400	800	400	800	400	800
DFSP classic	2	4	3	2	—	—
DFSP fibrosarcomatous	2	3	1	—	—	2
DFSP pigmented	—	—	—	—	—	1
Not DFSP	—	—	—	—	1	—

All patients (N = 24)	45.9% (11/24)
Primary tumors	71% (5/7)
Locally recurrent tumors N = 12)	33% (4/12)

Response, Progression, and Survival Status of Patients with Dermatofibrosarcoma Protuberans After Imatinib Therapy in the EORTC and SWOG Trials

Response, Progression, and Survival Status	EORTC (N = 16)		SWOG (N = 8)		Total (N = 24)	
	No.	%	No.	%	No.	%
Response at 14–16 Weeks						
Partial response	5	31.3	4	50	9	37.5
Stable disease	6	37.5	2	25	8	33.3
Progressive disease	3	18.8	1	12.5	4	16.7
Not evaluable	2	12.4	1	12.5	3	12.5
Best Overall Response						
Partial response (confirmed)	3	18.8	4	50	7	29.2
Partial response (resected)	4	25	0	0	4	16.7
Stable disease	4	25	2	25	6	25
Progressive disease	3	18.8	1	12.5	4	16.6
Not evaluable	2	12.5	1	12.5	3	12.5
Progression Status						
Progression-free	8	50	4	50	12	50
Progression	8	50	4	50	12	50
Survival Status						
Alive	10	62.5	8	100	18	75
Dead	6	37.5	0	0	6	25
Cause of Death						
Progression	5	31.3	0	0	5	20.8

*Four PRs not confirmed—resection of residual disease after >14 weeks of therapy
EORTC, European Organization for Research and Treatment of Cancer; SWOG, Southwest Oncology Group

Adverse Events

Adverse Events from Imatinib Reported in Patients with DFSP*

Adverse Event	EORTC (N = 16)						SWOG (N = 8)						Total (N = 24)					
	No.	%	No.	%	No.	%	No.	%	No.	%	No.	%	No.	%	No.	%	No.	%
Leukopenia	4	25	2	12.5	1	6.3	2	25	0	0	0	0	6	25	2	8.3	1	4.2
Neutropenia	2	12.5	1	6.3	2	12.5	0	0	0	0	2	25	2	8.3	1	4.2	4	16.7
Thrombocytopenia	1	6.3	0	0	1	6.3	0	0	0	0	0	0	1	4.2	0	0	1‡	4.2
Anemia	11	68.8	4	25	0	0	1	12.5	0	0	1	12.5	12	50	4	16.7	1	4.2
Bilirubin	4	25	1	6.3	1	6.3	0	0	0	0	0	0	4	16.7	1	4.2	1	4.2
AST increase	4	25	1	6.3	1	6.3	2	25	0	0	0	0	6	25	1	4.2	1‡	4.2
Hypertension†	1	6.3	1	6.3	0	0	0	0	0	0	0	0	1	4.2	1	4.2	0	0
Fatigue	3	18.8	2	12.5	2	12.5	5	62.5	0	0	2	25	8	33.3	2	8.3	4	16.7
Rash	4	25	1	6.3	1	6.3	3	37.5	0	0	0	0	7	29.2	1	4.2	1	4.2
Anorexia	2	12.5	0	0	0	0	2	25	0	0	0	0	4	16.7	0	0	0	0
Diarrhea	3	18.8	3	18.8	0	0	1	12.5	0	0	1	12.5	4	16.7	3	12.5	1	4.2
Nausea	3	18.8	2	12.5	1	6.3	4	50	0	0	0	0	7	29.2	2	8.3	1	4.2
Vomiting	1	6.3	0	0	2	12.5	1	12.5	0	0	0	0	2	8.3	0	0	2	8.3
H&N edema†	6	37.5	0	0	0	0	5	62.5	0	0	0	0	11	45.8	0	0	0	0
L/T/V edema†	6	37.5	1	6.3	1	6.3	5	62.5	0	0	0	0	11	45.8	1	4.2	1	4.2
Pain	3	18.8	0	0	0	0	0	0	0	0	1	12.5	3	12.5	0	0	1	4.2

*National Cancer Institute (USA), Common Terminology Criteria for Adverse Events, version 3.0
†Hypertension, arterial hypertension; H&N edema, head and neck edema; L/T/V edema: limbs/truncal/visceral edema
‡Grade 4; two toxic Grade 4 events were noted in one patient with preexisting liver disturbances and alcohol abuse history: thrombocytopenia and increased serum AST
DFSP, Dermatofibrosarcoma protuberans; EORTC, European Organization for Research and Treatment of Cancer; SWOG, Southwest Oncology Group

Therapy Monitoring

1. *Day 7 and at least monthly for 6 months, then every 3 months:* history and physical examination
2. *Weekly:* complete blood count with leukocyte differential count
3. *Twice monthly first 2 months, then monthly for 6, then every 3 months:* liver function tests
4. *At end of month 2 and every 3 months thereafter:* radiographic assessments were using the same modality as had been performed at baseline

ADULTS/PEDIATRIC (16 YEARS AND OLDER) • METASTATIC/ LOCALLY ADVANCED • EPITHELIOID SARCOMA AND *INI1 LOSS* NOT ELIGIBLE FOR COMPLETE RESECTION

ADULTS/PEDIATRIC PATIENTS AGED 16 YEARS AND OLDER WITH METASTATIC OR LOCALLY ADVANCED EPITHELIOID SARCOMA AND *INI1 LOSS* NOT ELIGIBLE FOR COMPLETE RESECTION REGIMEN: TAZEMETOSTAT

Chi S et al. Pediatric Blood and Cancer. 2018 ASPHO abstracts, 31 March 2018
Stacchiotti S et al. J Clin Oncol 2019;37(15s: 11003) [abstract 11003 from 2019 ASCO Annual Meeting]
TAZVERIK (tazemetostat) prescribing information. Cambridge, MA: Epizyme, Inc.; revised 2020 June

Tazemetostat 800 mg per dose; administer orally, twice per day, with our without food, continuously, until disease progression (total dosage/ week = 11,200 mg)

Notes:

• The accelerated approval of tazemetostat is contingent on the results of a confirmatory trial

• Swallow tablets whole. Do not take an additional dose if a dose is missed or vomiting occurs after tazemetostat, but continue with the next scheduled dose

• Advise patients to avoid consuming grapefruit products while taking tazemetostat

Recommended Dose Reductions of Tazemetostat for Unavoidable Concomitant Use of a Moderate CYP3A Inhibitor

Current Dosage	Adjusted Dosage
800 mg orally twice daily	400 mg orally twice daily
600 mg orally twice daily	400 mg for first dose and 200 mg for second dose
400 mg orally twice daily	200 mg orally twice daily

Notes:

• Avoid concomitant use of tazemetostat with strong CYP3A4 inhibitors and moderate-strong CYP3A4 inducers

• Coadministration of tazemetostat with CYP3A substrates, including hormonal contraceptives, can result in decreased concentrations and reduced efficacy of CYP3A substrates

Supportive Care

Antiemetic prophylaxis
Emetogenic potential is **MINIMAL TO LOW**
See Chapter 42 for antiemetic recommendations

Hematopoietic growth factor (CSF) prophylaxis
Primary prophylaxis is NOT indicated
See Chapter 43 for more information

Antimicrobial prophylaxis
Risk of fever and neutropenia is *LOW*
 Antimicrobial primary prophylaxis to be considered:
 • Antibacterial—not indicated
 • Antifungal—not indicated
 • Antiviral—not indicated unless patient previously had an episode of HSV

Treatment Modifications

TAZEMETOSTAT DOSE MODIFICATIONS

Tazemetostat Dose Levels	
Starting dose	800 mg orally twice daily
Dose level (−1)	600 mg orally twice daily
Dose level (−2)	400 mg orally twice daily
Dose level (−3)	Discontinue tazemetostat

(continued)

Treatment Modifications (*continued*)

Adverse Reaction	Severity	Dosage Modification
Neutropenia	ANC <1000/mm³	• Withhold until neutrophil count is greater than or equal to 1×10^9/L or baseline —For first occurrence, resume at same dose —For second and third occurrence, resume at reduced dose —Permanently discontinue after fourth occurrence
Thrombocytopenia	Platelet count <50,000/mm³	• Withhold until platelet count is greater than or equal to 75×10^9/L or baseline —For first and second occurrence, resume at reduced dose —Permanently discontinue after third occurrence
Anemia	Hemoglobin <8 g/dL	• Withhold until improvement to G ≤1 or baseline, then resume at same or reduced dose
Other adverse reactions	Grade 3	• Withhold until improvement to G ≤1 or baseline —For first and second occurrence, resume at reduced dose —Permanently discontinue after third occurrence
	Grade 4	• Withhold until improvement to G ≤1 or baseline —For first occurrence, resume at reduced dose —Permanently discontinue after second occurrence

Efficacy

Cohort 5 (62 Patients)—Median Follow-up of 13.8 Months

ORR	15% (9) 95% CI, 7%–26%
CR	1 1.6% (1)
PR	13% (8)
Median duration of response	4 to 24+ months
Median overall survival (OS)	82.4 weeks (95% CI, 47.4–not estimable)
Median progression-free survival (PFS)	23.7 weeks (95% CI, 14.7–25.7)

Cohort 6 (44 Patients)—Median Follow-up of 11.8 Months

ORR	11% (5)
CR	2.3% (1)
PR	9.1% (4)
Median duration of response	3.5 to 18.2+ months

Pooled Analysis—Cohort 5 + 6 (106 Patients)—Median Follow-up of 12.8 Months

ORR	13.2% (14)
CR	1.9% (2)
PR	11.3% (12)
Median duration of response	3.5 to 24+ months

*FDA noted that a significant limitation of the analysis is that not all of each patient's burden of disease was measured at baseline or followed for response

Note: sixty-eight percent of patients had a reduction in tumor burden, and 27% of patients with radiologic progression via RECIST criteria maintained stable disease after disease progression with continued use of tazemetostat

Patient Population Studied

Efficacy was investigated in a single-arm cohort (cohort 5) of a multicenter trial (study EZH–202) in patients with histologically confirmed, metastatic, or locally advanced epithelioid sarcoma. Patients were required to have INI1 loss (detected using local tests) and an Eastern Cooperative Oncology Group performance status of 0–2. Patients received 800 mg of tazemetostat orally twice daily until disease progression or unacceptable toxicity

Patient Population

Ethnicity	
White	76%
Asian	11%
Proximal disease	44%
ECOG performance status of 0 or 1	92%
ECOG performance status 2	8%
Prior surgery	77%
Prior chemotherapy	61%

Adverse Events

Tazemetostat (N = 62)
Adverse Reactions (≥10%) in Patients Receiving Tazemetostat in Cohort 5 of Study EZH–202

Adverse Reaction	All Grades (%)	G3/4 (%)
General		
Pain*	52	7
Fatigue†	47	1.6
Gastrointestinal		
Nausea	36	0
Vomiting	24	0
Constipation	21	0
Diarrhea	16	0
Abdominal pain‡	13	1.6
Metabolism and nutrition		
Decreased appetite	26	4.8
Respiratory, thoracic and mediastinal		
Cough	18	0
Dyspnea§	16	4.8
Vascular		
Hemorrhage¶	18	4.8
Nervous system		
Headache	18	0
Blood and lymphatic system		
Anemia	16	13
Investigations		
Weight decreased	16	7

*Includes tumor pain, pain in extremity, non-cardiac chest pain, flank pain, back pain, arthralgia, bone pain, cancer pain, musculoskeletal pain, myalgia, neck pain
†Includes fatigue and asthenia
‡Includes abdominal pain, gastrointestinal pain, abdominal pain lower
§Includes dyspnea and dyspnea exertional
¶Includes wound hemorrhage, rectal hemorrhage, pulmonary hemorrhage, hemorrhage intracranial, cerebral hemorrhage, hemoptysis

Note: regarding safety, the most common all-grade adverse events (AEs) of patients enrolled in cohort 5 included pain, fatigue, nausea, decreased appetite, vomiting, and constipation. Grade ≥3 AEs occurred in 48% of patients, which most commonly included anemia (13%), pain and decreased weight (7%), and hemorrhage, decreased appetite, dyspnea, and pleural effusion (4.8% each). Serious AEs included hemorrhage (6.5%), pleural effusion (6.5%), dyspnea (5%), cellulitis (3.2%), and pain (3.2%)

Note:
- Serious adverse reactions occurred in 37% of patients receiving tazemetostat. Serious adverse reactions in ≥3% of patients who received tazemetostat were hemorrhage, pleural effusion, skin infection, dyspnea, pain, and respiratory distress
- One patient (2%) permanently discontinued tazemetostat due to an adverse reaction of altered mood
- Dosage interruptions due to an adverse reaction occurred in 34% of patients who received tazemetostat. The most frequent adverse reactions requiring dosage interruptions in ≥3% were hemorrhage, increased alanine aminotransferase (ALT), and increased aspartate aminotransferase (AST). There were no deaths related to tazemetostat
- Dose reduction due to an adverse reaction occurred in one (2%) patient who received tazemetostat; the dose was reduced in this patient for decreased appetite
- The safety and effectiveness of tazemetostat in pediatric patients aged <16 years have not been established

(*continued*)

Adverse Events (*continued*)

Select Laboratory Abnormalities (≥10%) Worsening from Baseline in Patients Receiving Tazemetostat in Cohort 5 of Study EZH–202

Laboratory Abnormality	All Grades (%)	Grade ≥3 (%)
Hematology		
Decreased hemoglobin	49	15
Decreased lymphocytes	36	13
Decreased white blood cell count	19	0
Chemistry		
Increased triglycerides	36	3.3
Increased glucose	33	1.6
Decreased sodium	30	1.7
Decreased phosphate	28	1.7
Decreased albumin	23	0
Increased alkaline phosphatase	23	1.7
Decreased potassium	20	1.7
Increased aspartate aminotransferase	18	3.5
Decreased calcium	16	0
Decreased glucose	16	0
Increased partial thromboplastin time	15	5
Increased alanine aminotransferase	14	3.4
Increased creatinine	12	0
Increased potassium	12	0

Therapy Monitoring

1. Tazemetostat may increase the risk of developing a secondary malignancy including T-cell lymphoblastic lymphoma, myelodysplastic syndrome (MDS), and acute myeloid leukemia (AML). Monitor with frequent CBC and perform bone marrow examination if indicated. Across clinical trials of 668 adults who received tazemetostat 800 mg twice daily, MDS or AML occurred in 0.6% of patients

2. Advise females of reproductive potential to use effective nonhormonal contraception during treatment with tazemetostat and for 6 months after the final dose. Tazemetostat can render some hormonal contraceptives ineffective

ADVANCED SOFT-TISSUE SARCOMA • PRIOR CHEMOTHERAPY • PROGRESSIVE DESMOID TUMORS

ADVANCED SOFT-TISSUE SARCOMA (PRIOR CHEMOTHERAPY) PROGRESSIVE DESMOID TUMORS REGIMEN: PAZOPANIB

Glade Bender JL et al. J Clin Oncol 2013;31(24):3034–3043
Toulmonde M et al. Lancet Oncol 2019;20:1263–1272
van der Graaf et al. Lancet 2012;379:1879–1886

Adult Dose	Pediatric Dose (Using Intact 200-mg Tablets)	Pediatric Dose (Using Extemporaneously Compounded Suspension)
Pazopanib 800 mg; administer orally once daily at least 1 hour before or 2 hours after a meal, continually, until disease progression (total dose/week = 5600 mg)	Pazopanib 450 mg/m^2 (maximum dose = 800 mg); administer orally once daily at least 1 hour before or 2 hours after a meal, continually, until disease progression (total dose/week = 3150 mg/m^2; maximum dose/week = 5600 mg)	Pazopanib 160 mg/m^2; administer as a 50 mg/mL suspension prepared with Ora-Sweet (Paddock Laboratories, Minneapolis, MN) orally once daily at least 1 hour before or 2 hours after a meal, continually, until disease progression (total dose/week = 1120 mg/m^2)

Notes:
- Pazopanib is commercially available as a 200 mg film-coated tablet. Tablets are swallowed whole (without breaking, chewing, or crushing)
- Administration of pazopanib as a suspension is associated with increased bioavailability. Specifically, an increase in AUC (0–72) of 33% and increase in C(max) of 29% has been observed. Heath EI et al. Invest New Drugs 2012;30:1566–1574
- Patients who delay taking pazopanib at a regularly scheduled time may take a missed dose if the interval remaining before the next regularly scheduled dose is ≥12 hours
- Advise patients not to use drugs that increase gastric pH concurrently with pazopanib. Short-acting antacid products are preferable to histamine (H2) receptor antagonists and proton pump inhibitor medications. If used concomitantly, antacids administration should be separated from pazopanib ingestion by several hours
- Use caution in patients with hepatic dysfunction
  - In patients with baseline moderate hepatic impairment administer pazopanib 200 mg orally once daily (recommendation applies to adult dose using intact tablets)
  - The safety of pazopanib in patients with pre-existing severe hepatic impairment, defined as total bilirubin >3 × ULN with any level of ALT, is unknown. Treatment with pazopanib is not recommended in patients with severe hepatic impairment
- Monitor patients electrocardiographically at baseline and periodically thereafter

Antiemetic prophylaxis
Emetogenic potential of axitinib is **MINIMAL TO LOW**
See Chapter 42 for antiemetic recommendations

Hematopoietic growth factor (CSF) prophylaxis
Primary prophylaxis is NOT indicated
See Chapter 43 for more information

Antimicrobial prophylaxis
Risk of fever and neutropenia is *LOW*
  Antimicrobial primary prophylaxis to be considered:
  - Antibacterial—not indicated
  - Antifungal—not indicated
  - Antiviral—not indicated unless patient previously had an episode of HSV

Diarrhea management (adults)*
Loperamide 4 mg orally initially after the first loose or liquid stool, *then* 2–4 mg orally every 2–4 hours or **diphenoxylate hydrochloride** 2.5 mg **with atropine sulfate** 0.025 mg (eg, Lomotil)

*Abigerges D et al. J Natl Cancer Inst 1994;86:446–449
Rothenberg ML et al. J Clin Oncol 2001;19:3801–3807
Wadler S et al. J Clin Oncol 1998;16:3169–3178

Treatment Modifications

Pazopanib Dose Modifications

	Adult Daily Dose	Pediatric Daily Dose (Intact Tablets)	Pediatric Daily Dose (Extemporaneously Compounded Suspension)
Starting dose	800 mg	450 mg/m^2 (NTE 800 mg)	160 mg/m^2
Dose level (−1)	600 mg	337.5 mg/m^2 (NTE 600 mg)	120 mg/m^2
Dose level (−2)	400 mg	225 mg/m^2 (NTE 400 mg)	80 mg/m^2
Dose level (−3)	200 mg	112.5 mg/m^2 (NTE 200 mg)	40 mg/m^2
Dose level (−4)	Discontinue	Discontinue	Discontinue

NTE, not to exceed

Adverse Event	Treatment Modification
Hepatotoxicity	
Isolated ALT elevations between 3–8 × ULN (see note below)	Continue pazopanib with great care. Obtain weekly LFTs until ALT returns to G1 or baseline
ALT elevations >3 × ULN concurrently with bilirubin elevations >2 × ULN (see note below)	Discontinue pazopanib permanently and monitor patients closely until resolution of LFT abnormalities
Isolated ALT elevations of >8 × ULN	Interrupt pazopanib until ALT elevation returns to G1 or baseline. If potential benefit for reinitiating pazopanib outweigh risks of hepatotoxicity, then reintroduce pazopanib at no more than dose level −2 dose (eg, 400 mg daily for adults) and measure LFTs weekly for 8 weeks
Recurrent ALT elevations >3× ULN following its reintroduction for transient ALT elevation	Discontinue pazopanib permanently and monitor patients closely until resolution of LFT abnormalities
Total bilirubin >3 × ULN with any level of ALT before the start of treatment with pazopanib	The safety of pazopanib in this setting is unknown; use with caution. Administer 200 mg daily (refers to adult dose)
Proteinuria	
24-hour urine protein ≥3 g	Withhold pazopanib until urine protein is <3 g/24 hours, then resume pazopanib at 1 lower dose level. For recurrent episodes despite dose reduction, discontinue pazopanib
Nephrotic syndrome	Discontinue pazopanib
Diarrhea	
G1/2 diarrhea	Focus on treatment for symptoms designed to resolve the diarrhea. No dose modifications for G1/2 diarrhea unless G2 diarrhea persists for >2 weeks
G2 diarrhea that persists ≥2 weeks	Follow guidelines for G3/4 diarrhea (below)
If diarrhea cannot be controlled with preventive measures outlined, and is G3/4 or worsens by one grade level (G3 to G4) while on pazopanib, and is not alleviated by symptomatic treatment within 48 hours	Hold pazopanib. Also, withhold pazopanib if persistent G2 diarrhea while on pazopanib is not alleviated by treatment for symptoms (persistent defined as lasting for >2 weeks)
If pazopanib is held for >3 weeks and diarrhea does not resolve to G ≤1	Discontinue therapy
If within 3 weeks of withholding pazopanib diarrhea resolves to G ≤1	Restart pazopanib at 1 dose level less than the dose level administered at the time toxicity developed
If G3/4 diarrhea or persistent G2 diarrhea recurs at reduced pazopanib doses (persistent defined as lasting for >2 weeks)	Again, withhold pazopanib until the toxicity resolves to CTCAE G ≤1, at which time pazopanib should be restarted at 1 dose level less than the dose level administered at the time toxicity developed. Treatment for symptoms may continue indefinitely as a preventive measure

(continued)

Treatment Modifications (*continued*)

Adverse Event	Treatment Modification
If G3/4 diarrhea or persistent G2 diarrhea recurs at a dose of 200 mg once daily (persistent defined as lasting for >2 weeks)	Discontinue therapy
If diarrhea does not recur at reduced pazopanib doses with or without continued treatment for symptoms	The dose of pazopanib may be increased 1 dose level to the dose level that was being administered at the time diarrhea developed. If toxicity recurs following the increase, then follow the guidelines above, with the exception that when drug is restarted the pazopanib dose should be reduced 1 dose level
Hypertension	
Severe hypertension not controlled with medical management	Hold pazopanib pending further evaluation and treatment of hypertension
Severe hypertension despite optimal medical management	Consider reducing the dose of pazopanib or discontinuing it altogether. Discontinue if hypertension remains severe despite dosage reduction
Hypertensive crisis or hypertensive encephalopathy or reversible posterior leukoencephalopathy syndrome (RPLS)	Discontinue pazopanib
QTc Abnormalities	
Patients with a history of QT-interval prolongation, patients taking antiarrhythmics or other medications that may prolong QT interval, and those with relevant preexisting cardiac disease	Use with caution
QTc prolongation defined as: A single measurement of ≥550 ms An increase of ≥100 ms from baseline Two consecutive measurements (within 48 hours of each other) that were ≥500 ms but ≤550 ms An increase of ≥60 ms, but <100 ms from baseline to a value ≥480 ms	Hold pazopanib until QTc <480 ms, then resume pazopanib at 1 dose level lower
Other Adverse Reactions	
G3/4 fatigue	Reduce pazopanib 1 dose level
Clinically significant active infection	Institute appropriate anti-infective therapy and consider interrupting or discontinuing pazopanib for serious infections
Interstitial lung disease/pneumonitis	Discontinue pazopanib
Thrombotic microangiopathy, thrombotic thrombocytopenic purpura, or hemolytic uremic syndrome	Discontinue pazopanib
History of hemoptysis, cerebral, or clinically significant gastrointestinal hemorrhage while receiving pazopanib or in the past 6 months	Discontinue or avoid pazopanib
Patients with increased risk of arterial thrombotic events	Discontinue or avoid pazopanib
Onset of hypothyroidism	Treat hypothyroidism and monitor carefully
Planned elective surgery	Stop pazopanib at least 7 days prior to scheduled surgery. The decision to resume pazopanib after surgery should be based on clinical judgment of adequate wound healing
Wound dehiscence	Discontinue pazopanib
Drug Interactions	
Concomitant use of a strong CYP3A4 inhibitor (eg, ketoconazole, ritonavir, clarithromycin) is required	Reduce pazopanib dose to 400 mg; further reduce to 200 mg if adverse effects are observed (refers to adult dose). The goal is to adjust the pazopanib AUC to the range observed without inhibitors. However, there are no clinical data with this dose adjustment in patients receiving strong CYP3A4 inhibitors

(*continued*)

Treatment Modifications (*continued*)

Adverse Event	Treatment Modification
Concomitant use of strong CYP3A4 34 inducers (eg, rifampin)	Do not administer pazopanib
Concomitant use of a drug metabolized by CYP3A4, CYP2D6, or CYP2C8 that has a narrow therapeutic index	Pazopanib is a weak inhibitor of CYP3A4, CYP2D6, and CYP2C8 and may inhibit the metabolism of concomitantly administered drugs that are substrates of these enzymes. Use caution and consider increased monitoring and/or dose reduction of the sensitive substrate as per the clinical judgment of the medically responsible health care provider
Patient requires treatment with simvastatin	Concomitant use of simvastatin with pazopanib is associated with a higher rate of ALT elevation
Patient requires treatment with a medication that raises the gastric pH	Short-acting antacid products are preferable to histamine (H2) receptor antagonists and proton pump inhibitor medications. If used concomitantly, antacids administration should be separated from pazopanib ingestion by several hours

Note: pazopanib is a UGT1A1 inhibitor. Mild, indirect (unconjugated) hyperbilirubinemia may occur in patients with Gilbert syndrome. Patients with only a mild indirect hyperbilirubinemia, known Gilbert syndrome, and elevation in ALT $>3 \times$ ULN should be managed as per the recommendations outlined for isolated ALT elevations

Patient Population Studied

Van der Graaf et al. Lancet 2012;379:1879–1886

Patients with angiogenesis inhibitor-naive, metastatic soft-tissue sarcoma, progressing despite previous standard chemotherapy, were randomly 2:1 to receive either pazopanib 800 mg once daily or placebo, with no subsequent crossover. The primary endpoint was progression-free survival

Baseline Characteristics of Patients		
	Placebo Group (n = 123)	Pazopanib Group (n = 246)
Sex—male / female	54 (44%) / 69 (56%)	99 (40%) / 147 (60%)
WHO performance status 0 / 1	56 (46%) / 67 (54%)	113 (46%) / 133 (54%)
Age (years)—median (range)	51.9 (18.8–78.6)	56.7 (20.1–83.7)
Histologic grade—low / intermediate / high	3 (2%) / 30 (24%) / 90 (73%)	24 (10%) / 63 (26%) / 159 (65%)
Primary site involved—no / yes / unknown / missing	69 (56%) / 25 (20%) / 29 (24%)	131 (53%) / 62 (25%) / 53) 21%)
Liver involved—no /yes / missing	77 (63%) / 37 (30%) / 9 (7%)	163 (66%) / 67 (27%) / 16 (7%)

Data are n (%), unless otherwise stated

Toulmonde M et al. Lancet Oncol 2019;20:1263–1272

Open-label, phase 2 trial that enrolled adults (≥18 years) with progressive desmoid tumors, with documented progressive disease according to Response Evaluation Criteria in Solid Tumors version 1.1 based on two imaging assessments obtained within less than a 6-month interval. Participants were randomly assigned (2:1) to oral pazopanib 800 mg per day for up to 1 year or to an intravenous regimen combining vinblastine (5 mg/m^2 per dose) and methotrexate (30 mg/m^2 per dose), administered weekly for 6 months and then every other week for 6 months. The primary endpoint was proportion of patients who had not progressed at 6 months in the first 43 patients who had received one complete or two incomplete cycles of pazopanib

Baseline Characteristics		
	Pazopanib (n = 48)	Methotrexate and Vinblastine (n = 24)
Median age (range)	35 (18–78)	42 (21–79)
Sex—female / male	31 (65%) / 17 (35%)	15 (63%) / 9 (38%)
ECOG PS 0 / 1	34 (71%) / 14 (29%)	18 (75%) / 6 (25%)

(*continued*)

Patient Population Studied (continued)

Baseline Characteristics

Location		
Limbs and girdles	27 (56%)	9 (38%)
Internal trunk or mesenteric	13 (27%)	13 (54%)
Trunk wall	7 (15%)	2 (8%)
Head and neck	1 (2%)	0
Mutational status		
CTNNB1 T41A	15 (31%)	10 (42%)
CTNNB1 S45P	9 (19%)	4 (17%)
CTNNB1 S45F	8 (17%)	2 (8%)
APC gene	6 (13%)	2 (8%)
No mutation identified/Unknown	10 (21%)	3 (26%)
Gardner's syndrome yes / no	7 (15%) / 41 (85%)	4 (17%) / 20 (83%)
Previous treatment		
Hormonal therapy	11 (23%)	2 (8%)
Tyrosine kinase inhibitor	3 (6%)	2 (8%)
Chemotherapy	4 (8%)	0
COX2 inhibitor	27 (56%)	13 (54%)
Surgery	22 (46%)	8 (33%)
Radiotherapy	7 (15%)	1 (4%)
Number of previous systemic lines 0/1/2/3	11 (23%)/17 (35%)/13 (27%)/7 (15%)	6 (25%)/13 (54%)/1 (4%)/4 (17%)

Glade Bender JL et al J Clin Oncol 2013;31(24):3034–3043

Patients ≥2 and <22 years of age with recurrent or refractory solid or primary CNS tumors were eligible. Patients with CNS involvement could not have new or ≥ three foci of punctate hemorrhage on baseline MRI. Patients in part 2b (DCE-MRI cohort) had a diagnosis of STS, did not require anesthesia for imaging, and were younger than age 25 years. Other eligibility criteria included performance status ≥50; QTc <450 ms; and stable thyroxine supplementation if hypothyroid. Exclusion criteria included the following: active bleeding, intratumoral hemorrhage, or bleeding diathesis; history of thromboembolic events; treatment with antiplatelet or antithrombotic agents; recent or planned major surgery; impaired wound healing; abdominal fistula, perforation, or abscess; uncontrolled infection

Demographics and Clinical Characteristics of Eligible Patients

Characteristic	Number of Patients			
	Dose Escalation Part 1 (n = 25)	Suspension Part 2a (n = 16)	Imaging Part 2b (n = 10)	Total (n = 51)
Age, years—median (range)	13.4 (5.0–21.7)	10.5 (3.8–19.2)	17.2 (8.3–23.9)	12.9 (3.8–23.9)
Sex—male/female	13 / 12	8 / 8	5 / 5	26 / 25
Prior chemotherapy regimens—median (range)	1 (0–7)	2 (1–15)	3 (1–6)	2 (0–15)
Prior radiation therapy	18	14	7	39
Prior VEGF-blocking therapy	7	5	3	15

(continued)

Patient Population Studied (*continued*)

Demographics and Clinical Characteristics of Eligible Patients

Characteristic	Dose Escalation Part 1 (n = 25)	Suspension Part 2a (n = 16)	Imaging Part 2b (n = 10)	Total (n = 51)
Diagnosis				
Sarcoma				28
Rhabdomyosarcoma		1	4	5
Osteosarcoma	1	3		4
Synovial sarcoma	3	1		4
Ewing sarcoma	2	1		3
Alveolar soft part sarcoma	2		1	3
Clear cell sarcoma			2	2
Desmoplastic small round cell		1	1	2
Other soft-tissue sarcoma		3	2	5
Brain tumor				17
High-grade glioma	3	3		6
Ependymoma	3	1		4
Low-grade glioma	2			2
Germ cell	2			2
Medulloblastoma/PNET	2			2
Atypical teratoid/rhabdoid		1		1
Embryonal				3
Hepatoblastoma	1	1		2
Wilms tumor	1			1
Other				3
Melanoma	2			2
Renal cell	1			1

PNET, primitive neuroectodermal tumor; VEGF, vascular endothelial growth factor

Efficacy

van der Graaf et al. Lancet 2012;379:1879–1886

	Placebo (n = 123)	Pazopanib (n = 239–246)
Median treatment duration—weeks, (IQR)	8.1 (4–13.6)	16.4 (6.3–30)
Relative dose intensity	100%	96%
Treatment interruption	11 (9%)	118 (49%)

(*continued*)

Efficacy (continued)

van der Graaf et al. Lancet 2012;379:1879–1886

	Placebo (n = 123)	Pazopanib (n = 239–246)
Dose reductions	5 (4%)	92 (39%)
Treatment discontinuation for PD	118 (96%)	167 (70%)
Treatment discontinuation for toxicity	1 (1%)	34 (14%)
Median follow-up—months (IQR)	14.6 (11.3–19)	14.9 (11.0–18.2)
Response to therapy		
PR	0/123 (0%)	14/246 (6%)
SD	47 (38%)	164 (67%)
PD	70 (57%)	57 (23%)
Death	6 (5%)	3 (1%)*
Disease progression	106	168
Death due to disease	78	137
Median PFS—months (95% CI)	4.6 (3.7–4.8)	1.6 (0.9–1.8)
	HR 0.31; 95% CI 0.24–0.4; P = 0.0001	
Median OS—months (95% CI)	10.7 (8.7–12.8)	12.5 (10.6–14.8)
	HR 0.86; 95% CI 0.67–1.11; P = 0.2514[†]	

*In the pazopanib group, 3% of patients could not be assessed
[†]Favorable prognostic factors in patients treated with pazopanib according to the multivariable model were a good performance status (HR for 0 vs 1 was 0.73; 95% CI 0.54–0.99; P = 0.045) and low or intermediate tumor grade (HR for I and II vs III was 0.63; 95% CI 0.45–0.87; P = 0.006). Predictive analysis for histology subtype was done with Cox models with interaction terms; the interaction was not significant
CI, confidence interval; IQR, inter-quartile range; OS, overall survival; PD, progressive disease; PFS, progression-free survival; PR, partial response; SD, stable disease

Toulmonde M et al. Lancet Oncol 2019;20:1263–1272

Note: four patients were not eligible for activity assessment; 66 were included: 46 in the pazopanib group of whom the first 43 patients were included in the primary endpoint analyses, and 20 patients in the methotrexate–vinblastine group, 19 included

6-month progression-free	83.7% (95% CI 69.3–93.2)	45.0% (95% CI 23.1–68.5)
1-year PFS	85.6% (95% CI 70.7–93.2)	79.0% (95% CI 53.2–91.5)
2-year PFS	67.2% (95% CI 49.0–81.9)	79.0% (95% CI 53.2–91.5)
2-, 3-, and 4-year OS	97.3% (95% CI 82.3–99.6)	100% (95% CI not applicable)
Partial response	17/46 (37.0%) (95% CI 23.2–52.5)	5/20 (25%) (95% CI 8.7–49.1)
Stable disease	27/46 (58.7%) (95% CI 43.2–73.0)	10/20 (50%) (95% CI 27.2–72.8)
Progressive disease	2/46 (4.4%) (95% CI 0.1–14.8)	4/20 (20%) (95% CI 5.7–43.7)

CI, confidence interval; OS, overall survival PFS, progression-free survival

Glade Bender JL et al. J Clin Oncol 2013;31(24):3034–3043

- One patient with desmoplastic small round cell tumor achieved a sustained partial response (PR) after 14 cycles and completed 24 cycles of protocol therapy
- One patient with hepatoblastoma had a PR by cycle 4, maintained for 12 cycles, but was removed from study for recurrent neutropenia
- Eight patients had stable disease for ≥6 months (alveolar soft part sarcoma, n = 2; synovial sarcoma, osteosarcoma, alveolar rhabdomyosarcoma, mesenchymal chondrosarcoma, gastrointestinal stromal sarcoma, and myxopapillary ependymoma, n = 1 each)
- All but one patient with clinical benefit had Css >20 μg/mL, and all five patients who received therapy for a year or more had Css ≥30 μg/mL

Adverse Events

Common Adverse Events
van der Graaf et al. Lancet 2012;379:1879–1886

	Placebo Group (n = 123)			Pazopanib Group (n = 239)		
	All Grades	**G3**	**G4**	**All Grades**	**G3**	**G4**
Fatigue	60 (49%)	6 (5%)	1 (1%)	155 (65%)	30 (13%)	1 (<1%)
Diarrhea	20 (16%)	1 (1%)	0	138 (58%)	11 (5%)	0
Nausea	34 (28%)	2 (2%)	0	129 (54%)	8 (3%)	0
Weight loss	25 (20%)	0	0	115 (48%)	0	0
Hypertension	8 (7%)	4 (3%)	0	99 (41%)	16 (7%)	0
Anorexia	24 (20%)	0	0	95 (40%)	14 (6%)	0
Hair hypopigmentation	3 (2%)	0	0	92 (38%)	0	0
Vomiting	14 (11%)	1 (1%)	0	80 (33%)	8 (3%)	0
Dysgeusia	5 (4%)	0	0	64 (27%)	0	0
Rash or desquamation	13 (11%)	0	0	43 (18%)	1 (<1%)	0
Mucositis	4 (3%)	0	0	29 (12%)	3 (1%)	0

Data are n (%)

Treatment-related Adverse Events During the Treatment Period
Toulmonde M et al. Lancet Oncol 2019;20:1263–1272

	Pazopanib Group (n = 48)			Methotrexate and Vinblastine Group (n = 22)		
	Grade 1–2	**G3**	**G4**	**G1–2**	**G3**	**G4**
Fatigue	36 (75%)	3 (6%)	0	14 (64%)	1 (5%)	0
Diarrhea	31 (65%)	7 (15%)	0	7 (32%)	0	0
Nausea and vomiting	(54%)	0	0	16 (73%)	0	0
Headache	19 (40%)	1 (2%)	0	3 (14%)	0	0
Palmar-plantar syndrome	16 (33%)	1 (2%)	0	0	0	0
Anorexia	16 (33%)	0	0	4 (18%)	0	0
Mucositis oral	13 (27%)	0	0	7 (32%)	0	0
Dysgeusia	13 (27%)	0	0	2 (9%)	0	0
Hypertension	12 (25%)	9 (19%)	1 (2%)	0	0	0
ASAT or ALAT increase	10 (21%)	2 (4%)	0	2 (9%)	3 (14%)	1 (5%)
Hypothyroidism	10 (21%)	0	0	0	0	0
Arthralgia	9 (19%)	0	0	0	0	0
Myalgia	8 (17%)	0	0	4 (18%)	1 (5%)	0
Abdominal pain	8 (17%)	0	0	1 (5%)	0	0
Skin hypopigmentation	8 (17%)	0	0	0	0	0
Alopecia	6 (13%)	0	0	4 (18%)	0	0
Dry skin	6 (13%)	0	0	0	0	0
Other gastrointestinal	5 (10%)	1 (2%)	0	0	0	0
Gastrointestinal pain	4 (8%)	1 (2%)	0	3 (14%)	0	0
Other investigations	4 (8%)	1 (2%)	0	1 (5%)	2 (9%)	0
Neutropenia	3 (6%)	3 (6%)	1 (2%)	2 (9%)	9 (41%)	1 (5%)

(continued)

Adverse Events (continued)

	Pazopanib Group (n = 48)			Methotrexate and Vinblastine Group (n = 22)		
	Grade 1–2	G3	G4	G1–2	G3	G4
Bilirubin increase	3 (6%)	0	0	2 (9%)	0	0
Other hepatobiliary	2 (4%)	1 (2%)	0	2 (9%)	3 (14%)	0
Paresthesia	2 (4%)	0	0	5 (23%)	1 (5%)	0
Constipation	2 (4%)	0	0	8 (36%)	0	0
Anemia	0	1 (2%)	0	5 (23%)	0	0
Thromboembolic event	0	1 (2%)	0	0	0	0

Note: data are n (%); treatment-related adverse events that were reported in either study group in >5% of patients for Grade 1–2 and any for Grades 3 and 4 are shown; no deaths due to adverse events were reported; patients could have >1 adverse event
ALAT, alanine aminotransferase. ASAT, aspartate aminotransferase

Toxicity Related to Pazopanib Therapy
Glade Bender JL et al. J Clin Oncol 2013;31(24):3034–3043

	No. of Patients							
	Maximum Grade per Patient During Cycle 1				Maximum Grade per Patient Across All Subsequent Cycles			
Toxicity Type	G1	G2	G3	G4	G1	G2	G3	G4
TABLET FORMULATION (PARTS 1 AND 2B)*								
GI/metabolic[†]								
Diarrhea	12	4	—	—	7	2 (1‡)	—	—
Nausea	9	2	—	—	6	1	—	—
Vomiting	9	3	—	—	5	2	—	—
Abdominal pain	2	2	—	—	1	2	—	—
Anorexia	2	2	—	—	1	—	1‡	—
ALT increased	8	1	—	—	4	1‡	1‡	—
AST increased	8	—	—	—	7	1	—	—
Serum amylase increased	3	1	1‡	—	1	3	—	—
Lipase increased	1	2	—	1‡	1	1	1‡	—
Hyperglycemia	4	—	—	—	7	1	—	—
Hypophosphatemia	2	1	1	—	2	4	—	—
Constitutional[†]								
Fatigue	9	4	—	—	3	2	—	—
Headache	6	5	—	—	1	3	—	—
Dizziness	6	—	—	—	—	—	—	—
Back/tumor pain	2	1	1‡	—	—	—	1‡	—
Rash maculopapular/hand-foot	1	3	—	—	1	1	1‡	—
Hematologic[§]								
Thrombocytopenia	8	1	—	—	11	—	—	—
Absolute lymphocyte count	5	—	1	—	5	7	—	—
Absolute neutrophil count	3	5	1	—	3	6	4	1‡
Anemia	1	1	—	—	6	1	2 (1‡)	—

(continued)

Adverse Events (*continued*)

Toxicity Type	G1	G2	G3	G4	G1	G2	G3	G4
MTKI class targeted[†]								
Proteinuria	5	2	1[‡]	—	8	1	—	—
Hypertension	3	6	2[‡]	—	3	5	—	—
Left ventricular systolic dysfunction	3	1	—	—	4	2	—	—
Sinus bradycardia	4	—	—	—	3	—	—	—
Hypothyroidism	4	1	—	—	5	3	—	—
SUSPENSION FORMULATION (PART 2A)[ϵ]								
GI/metabolic[†]								
Diarrhea	4	—	—	—	2	—	—	—
Nausea	3	—	—	—	2	—	—	—
Vomiting	3	1	—	—	—	—	—	—
Abdominal pain	2	—	—	—	—	—	—	—
ALT increased	3	—	2[‡]	—	2	1	—	—
AST increased	2	1	—	—	2	—	—	—
Constitutional[†]								
Fatigue	2	1	—	—	1	—	—	—
Headache	2	—	—	—	1	1	—	—
Hematologic[§]								
Thrombocytopenia	3	—	—	—	—	—	—	—
Absolute lymphocyte count	2	—	2	—	1	—	—	—
Absolute neutrophil count	2	1	1	—	1	—	—	—
Anemia	1	—	—	—	1	1	—	—
MTKI class targeted[†]								
Proteinuria	4	—	—	—	2	—	—	—

*Cycle 1, n = 33 cycles; cycles 2 to 23, n = 148 cycles

[†]Nonhematologic toxicities related to protocol therapy that occurred in more than 10% of patients as determined in the first cycle of protocol therapy

[‡]Dose-limiting toxicity

[§]Hematologic toxicities independent of frequency and attribution

[ϵ]Cycle 1, n = 15 cycles; cycles 2 to 8, n = 22 cycles

MTKI, multitargeted tyrosine kinase receptor inhibitor

Therapy Monitoring

1. *At baseline, day 8, every 3 weeks until week 24, and every 4 weeks thereafter:* physical examinations, vital signs, with blood pressure monitoring and clinical laboratory evaluations. Serum chemistries, particularly: calcium, magnesium, and potassium

2. *Electrocardiograms:* baseline and periodic (as clinically indicated) monitoring of electrocardiograms and maintenance of electrolytes (eg, calcium, magnesium, potassium) within the normal range should be performed

3. *Thyroid function tests:* monitor every 12 weeks. If thyroid-stimulating hormone levels are abnormal, evaluations of free triiodothyronine and thyroxine should be obtained

4. *Urine protein:* assess proteinuria by urine dipstick and/or urinary protein creatinine ratio. Patients with a urine dipstick reading ≥2+ should undergo further assessment with a 24-hour urine collection

5. *LFTs:* monitor at baseline and at weeks 3, 5, 7, and 9. Thereafter, monitor at month 3 and month 4 (or more often if clinically indicated), and then periodically

6. Thereafter, monitor at month 3 and at month 4, and as clinically indicated. Periodic monitoring should then continue after month 4.

7. *Gastrointestinal perforation:* although gastrointestinal perforation with pazopanib is rare, monitor for symptoms of gastrointestinal perforation or fistula

8. *Response assessment:* every 2–3 cycles

ADVANCED • REFRACTORY • DESMOID TUMORS
ADVANCED AND REFRACTORY DESMOID TUMORS REGIMEN: SORAFENIB

Gounder MM et al. N Engl J Med 2018;379:2417–2428
Widemann BC et al. Clin Cancer Res 2012;18: 6011–22

Adult Dose	Pediatric Dose (Using Intact 200-mg Tablets)
Sorafenib 400 mg; administer orally once daily at least 1 hour before or 2 hours after a meal, continually, until disease progression (total dose/week = 2800 mg)	**Sorafenib** 200 mg/m^2 per dose (maximum single dose = 400 mg); administer orally twice per day at least 1 hour before or 2 hours after meals, continually, until disease progression (total dose/week = 2800 mg/m^2; maximum dose/week = 5600 mg)

Notes:
- Sorafenib is commercially available as a 200-mg film-coated tablet
- Patients who delay taking a sorafenib dose at a regularly scheduled time should take the next dose at the next regularly scheduled time
- Avoid concomitant use of strong CYP3A4 inducers with sorafenib

Supportive Care
Antiemetic prophylaxis
Emetogenic potential: **MINIMAL TO LOW**
See Chapter 42 for antiemetic recommendations

Hematopoietic growth factor (CSF) prophylaxis
Primary prophylaxis is NOT indicated
See Chapter 43 for more information

Antimicrobial prophylaxis
Risk of fever and neutropenia is LOW
  Antimicrobial primary prophylaxis to be considered:
  - Antibacterial—not indicated
  - Antifungal—not indicated
  - Antiviral—not indicated, unless patient previously had an episode of HSV

Diarrhea management (adults)
Latent or delayed-onset diarrhea*:
Loperamide 4 mg orally initially after the first loose or liquid stool, *then* 2–4 mg orally every 2–4 hours or **diphenoxylate hydrochloride** 2.5 mg **with atropine sulfate** 0.025 mg (eg, Lomotil)

*Abigerges D et al. J Natl Cancer Inst 1994;86:446–449
Rothenberg ML et al. J Clin Oncol 2001;19:3801–3807
Wadler S et al. J Clin Oncol 1998;16:3169–3178

Treatment Modifications

Sorafenib Dose Levels

	Adult Dose	Pediatric Dose (Intact 200-mg Tablets)
Starting dose level	400 mg daily	200 mg/m^2/dose (maximum dose = 400 mg) twice per day
Dose level (−1)	200 mg daily	100 mg/m^2/dose (maximum dose = 200 mg) twice per day, or 200 mg/m^2 (maximum dose = 400 mg) daily
Dose level (−2)	Discontinue	100 mg/m^2 (maximum dose = 200 mg) daily, or 200 mg/m^2 (maximum dose = 400 mg) every other day
Dose level (−3)	—	Discontinue

(continued)

Treatment Modifications (*continued*)

Adverse Event	Dose Modification
Cardiovascular Toxicity	
G ≥2 cardiac ischemia and/or infarction	Permanently discontinue sorafenib
G3 congestive heart failure	Interrupt until G ≤1; resume treatment with dose decrease one dose level. If no recovery after 30 day interruption, discontinue treatment unless the patient is deriving clinical benefit. If two dose reductions are insufficient, discontinue treatment
G4 congestive heart failure	Permanently discontinue sorafenib
G ≥2 hemorrhage requiring medical intervention	Permanently discontinue sorafenib
G2 hypertension (asymptomatic and diastolic pressure 90–99 mm Hg)	Treat with antihypertensive therapy. Continue dosing as scheduled and closely monitor blood pressure
G2 hypertension (symptomatic/persistent) *OR* G2 symptomatic increase by >20 mm Hg (diastolic) or >140/90 mm Hg if previously within normal limits *OR* Grade 3	Interrupt treatment and treat with antihypertensives until symptoms resolve and diastolic blood pressure <90 mm Hg. When resume treatment, reduce dose one dose level. If needed, reduce another dose level. If two dose reductions are insufficient, discontinue treatment
G4 hypertension	Permanently discontinue sorafenib
Any grade gastrointestinal perforation	Permanently discontinue sorafenib
QT prolongation: QTc >500 ms or an increase from baseline of ≥60 ms	Interrupt. Correct electrolyte abnormalities (magnesium, potassium, calcium). Monitor electrolytes and electrocardiograms. Use medical judgment before restarting
Hepatic Toxicity	
Severe drug-induced liver injury: G >3 ALT in the absence of another cause; AST/ALT >3 × ULN with bilirubin >2 × ULN in the absence of another cause	Permanently discontinue sorafenib
Any grade alkaline phosphatase increase in the absence of known bone pathology and G ≤2 or worse bilirubin increase	
INR ≥1.5, ascites, and/or encephalopathy in the absence of underlying cirrhosis or other organ failure considered to be due to severe drug-induced liver	
Nonhematologic Toxicity	
G2 nonhematologic toxicity	Treat on time. Decrease dose one dose level. If two dose reductions are insufficient, discontinue treatment
First occurrence G3 nonhematologic toxicity	Interrupt until G ≤2, then resume with dose decreased one dose level. If two dose reductions are insufficient, discontinue treatment
G3 nonhematologic toxicity without improvement within 7 days	Interrupt until G ≤2, then resume with dose decreased two dose levels. If two dose reductions are insufficient, discontinue treatment
Second or third occurrence of G3 nonhematologic toxicity	Interrupt until G ≤2, then resume with dose decreased two dose levels. If two dose reductions are insufficient, discontinue treatment
Fourth occurrence of G3 nonhematologic toxicity or G4 nonhematologic toxicity	Permanently discontinue sorafenib
Dermatologic Toxicity	
First occurrence of G2 dermatologic toxicity (painful erythema and swelling of the hands or feet and/or discomfort affecting the patient's normal activities)	Continue treatment with sorafenib and consider topical therapy for symptomatic relief. If no improvement within 7 days, interrupt sorafenib treatment until toxicity resolves to G0/1

(*continued*)

Treatment Modifications (*continued*)

Adverse Event	Dose Modification
First occurrence of G2 dermatologic toxicity (painful erythema and swelling of the hands or feet and/or discomfort affecting the patient's normal activities) without improvement within 7 days at the reduced dose	Interrupt sorafenib treatment until toxicity resolves to G0/1. Then resume treatment with the sorafenib dose decreased by one dose level
Second and third occurrence of G2 dermatologic toxicity (painful erythema and swelling of the hands or feet and/or discomfort affecting the patient's normal activities)	
Fourth occurrence of G2 dermatologic toxicity	Discontinue sorafenib treatment
First occurrence of G3 dermatologic toxicity (moist desquamation, ulceration, blistering, or severe pain of the hands or feet, resulting in inability to work or perform activities of daily living)	Interrupt sorafenib treatment until toxicity resolves to G0/1. Then resume treatment with the sorafenib dose decreased by one dose level
Second occurrence of G3 dermatologic toxicity (moist desquamation, ulceration, blistering, or severe pain of the hands or feet, resulting in inability to work or perform activities of daily living)	Interrupt sorafenib treatment until toxicity resolves to G0/1. Then resume treatment with the sorafenib dose decreased by one dose level
Third occurrence of G3 dermatologic toxicity	Discontinue sorafenib treatment

Note on dermatologic toxicity: Following improvement of G2/3 dermatologic toxicity to G0/1 after at least 28 days of treatment on a reduced dose of sorafenib, the dose of sorafenib may be increased one dose level from the reduced dose. Approximately 50% of patients requiring a dose reduction for dermatologic toxicity are expected to meet these criteria for resumption of the higher dose and roughly 50% of patients resuming the previous dose are expected to tolerate the higher dose (that is, maintain the higher dose level without recurrent G2 or higher dermatologic toxicity)

Patient Population Studied

Gounder MM et al. N Engl J Med 2018;379:2417–2428

Patients ≥18 years of age with histologically documented desmoid tumor (aggressive fibromatosis) with measurable disease and radiographic progression of ≥10% in maximum unidimensional measurement within the previous 6 months, recurrent or primary disease that was deemed inoperable or as requiring extensive surgery, or symptomatic disease. No minimum or maximum number of previous systemic treatments was stipulated

Demographic and Clinical Characteristics of the Patients at Randomization

Characteristic	Placebo (n = 37)	Sorafenib (n = 50)
Median age—years (range)	37 (21–67)	37 (18–72)
Female sex—no. (%)	26 (70)	34 (68)
ECOG performance-status score—0 / 1 no. (%)	22 (59) / 15 (41)	35 (70) / 15 (30)
Sum of target lesions at randomization—median cm (range)	7.6 (2.6–26.5)	8.4 (1.2–19.3)
BPI worst pain score at randomization—no. (%)		
0–2	14 (38)	17 (34)
3–6	14 (38)	21 (42)
7–10	9 (24)	12 (24)
Intra-abdominal disease—no. (%)	16 (43)	16 (32)

(*continued*)

Patient Population Studied (*continued*)

Demographic and Clinical Characteristics of the Patients at Randomization

Characteristic	Placebo (n = 37)	Sorafenib (n = 50)
Primary tumor site—no. (%)		
Abdominal	16 (43)	14 (28)
Extra-abdominal	18 (49)	32 (64)
Both abdominal and extra-abdominal	3 (8)	4 (8)
Previous radiation therapy—no. (%)	3 (8)	6 (12)
Previous systemic therapy—no. (%)	15 (41)	18 (36)
Previous surgical resection—no. (%)	18 (49)	23 (46)
Disease status—no./total no. (%)		
Newly diagnosed	19/37 (51)	26/48 (54)
Recurrent	18/37 (49)	22/48 (46)
Trial inclusion criteria—no. (%)		
Disease determined to be unresectable or to require surgery with unacceptably high associated morbidity	28 (76)	44 (88)
Progression detected by radiographic imaging within 6 months before randomization	16 (43)	19 (38)
Symptomatic disease with BPI worst pain score ≥3 and consideration of pain narcotic introduction or escalation	11 (30)	16 (32)

Efficacy

Gounder MM et al. N Engl J Med 2018;379:2417–2428

- Of 87 patients who underwent randomization, 84 (97%) were included in the analysis of primary and secondary endpoints
- Median follow-up of 27.2 months (interquartile range, 22.0–31.7)
- Surviving patients: 83

	Sorafenib	Placebo	Statistics
1-year PFS rate	89% (95% CI, 80–99)	46% (95% CI, 32–67)	HR 0.13; 95% CI, 0.05–0.31; P<0.001
2-year PFS rate	81% (95% CI, 69–96)	36% (95% CI, 22–57),	
Disease progression	12% of the patients (6/49)*	63% of the patients (22 of 35)*	—
ORR	33% (95% CI, 20–48)	20% (95% CI, 8–37)	—
CR	2% (1/49)	0% (0/35)	—
PR	31% (15/49)	20% (7/35)	—
Mean best percentage change in sum of target lesions	−26% (range, −100 to 7)	−12% (range, −85 to 32)	—
Median time to RECIST defined response	9.6 months (IQR, 6.6–16.7)	13.3 (IQR, 11.2–31.1)	—
Earliest RECIST-defined partial response	2.2 months	8.8 months	—

*Clinical deterioration in the absence of radiographic evidence was sole indicator of progression in 2 patients in the sorafenib group and 9 patients in the placebo

CI, confidence interval; HR, hazard ratio; IQR, interquartile range; ORR, objective response rate = CR + PR; PFS, progression-free survival

Adverse Events

Gounder MM et al. N Engl J Med 2018;379:2417–2428

Incidence of Adverse Events of Any Cause According to Initially Assigned Trial Regimen*

	Event Sorafenib (n = 49)		Placebo (n = 36)	
	G1/2	G3/4	G1/2	G3/4
Event	Number of Patients (%)			
Any adverse event	26 (53)	23 (47)	25 (69)	9 (25)
Events during receipt of trial with incidence ≥10%†				
Palmar-plantar erythrodysesthesia syndrome	34 (69)	1 (2)	8 (22)	0
Rash				
Any rash or skin disorder	36 (73)	7 (14)	15 (42)	0
Papulopustular	24 (49)	6 (12)	6 (17)	0
Acneiform	6 (12)	0	0	0
Maculopapular	7 (14)	0	1 (3)	0
Skin or subcutaneous tissue disorders—other	7 (14)	1 (2)	5 (14)	0
Pruritus	7 (14)	0	0	0
Fatigue	33 (67)	3 (6)	22 (61)	1 (3)
Hypertension	27 (55)	4 (8)	14 (39)	0
Diarrhea	25 (51)	0	12 (33)	0
Nausea	24 (49)	0	14 (39)	1 (3)
Myalgia	18 (37)	1 (2)	12 (33)	0
Alopecia	18 (37)	0	3 (8)	0
Arthralgia	17 (35)	1 (2)	9 (25)	0
Abdominal pain	15 (31)	1 (2)	9 (25)	4 (11)
Anorexia	15 (31)	0	9 (25)	0
Constipation	11 (22)	0	4 (11)	0
Oral mucositis	11 (22)	0	6 (17)	0
Vomiting	10 (20)	1 (2)	6 (17)	2 (6)
Anemia	8 (16)	1 (2)	2 (6)	1 (3)
Increase in alanine aminotransferase level	7 (14)	0	4 (11)	0
Decrease in platelet count	6 (12)	2 (4)	1 (3)	0
Hyperglycemia	6 (12)	1 (2)	3 (8)	0
Peripheral sensory neuropathy	6 (12)	0	1 (3)	0
Increase in aspartate aminotransferase level	5 (10)	1 (2)	3 (8)	0
Increase in blood bilirubin level	5 (10)	0	3 (8)	1 (3)
Decrease in neutrophil count	5 (10)	0	2 (6)	0
Dry skin	5 (10)	0	1 (3)	0
Headache	4 (8)	0	6 (17)	0
Decrease in white-cell count	3 (6)	0	6 (17)	0
Musculoskeletal connective-tissue disorders—other	3 (6)	0	4 (11)	0

*Events that occurred while the patient was taking the initially assigned trial regimen (before crossover) are shown. Adverse events were graded according to the Common Terminology Criteria for Adverse Events (CTCAE), version 4.03. The events reported reflect the maximum severity in each category for a given patient during the treatment period; multiple occurrences of the same event in a single patient were counted once, at the highest grade at which it occurred. All 85 patients were included in the assessment of safety
†Events that had an incidence of 10% or higher in either trial group are shown. One patient in the sorafenib group died from disease-related bowel perforation (not shown in this table) that was judged by the investigators not to have been related to the drug; no other Grade 5 events occurred

Therapy Monitoring

1. *At baseline, weekly for the first 6 weeks, then periodically:* blood pressure measurement
2. *Electrocardiograms:* baseline and periodic (as clinically indicated) monitoring of electrocardiograms and maintenance of electrolytes (eg, calcium, magnesium, potassium) within the normal range should be performed
3. *At baseline, around day 8, then every 4–8 weeks:* physical examination, vital signs, with blood pressure monitoring and clinical laboratory evaluations. Serum chemistries, particularly: calcium, magnesium, potassium, and liver function tests
4. *Gastrointestinal perforation, hemorrhage, cardiovascular events:* monitor for symptoms of gastrointestinal perforation or fistula, hemorrhage, and cardiovascular events
5. *Wound healing:* hold sorafenib for ≥10 days before elective surgery. Hold sorafenib for ≥14 days after major surgery and until adequate wound healing has occurred

MALIGNANT • PERIPHERAL NERVE SHEATH TUMORS
MALIGNANT PERIPHERAL NERVE SHEATH TUMORS REGIMEN: IFOSFAMIDE + DOXORUBICIN AND IFOSFAMIDE + ETOPOSIDE

Higham CS et al. Sarcoma 2017;2017:8685638
Supplementary appendix to: Higham CS et al. Sarcoma 2017;2017:8685638

Regimen overview: the regimen consists of a total of 8 cycles of chemotherapy. Two 21-day cycles of AI (doxorubicin + ifosfamide) are given, followed by two 21-day cycles of IE (ifosfamide + etoposide). Evaluation of response occurs after cycle 4 followed by local control (surgery, radiation therapy [RT], or both) if feasible. Patients who undergo RT receive 2 cycles of IE during RT followed by two additional cycles of AI (AI-AI-IE-IE-IE/RT-IE/RT-AI-AI). Patients who undergo surgery alone receive 2 cycles of adjuvant AI followed by 2 cycles of adjuvant IE (AI-AI-IE-IE-surgery-AI-AI-IE-IE)

Cycles of doxorubicin + ifosfamide (AI):
Hydration during ifosfamide:

Administer additional intravenous hydration (eg, **0.9% sodium chloride injection [0.9% NS]**) over 4–24 hours to achieve a total rate of 2000 mL/m^2/day (taking into account volumes of diluent used for mesna and ifosfamide administration) for the duration of ifosfamide treatment on days 1–5. If feasible, continue maintenance intravenous hydration during intervals between ifosfamide administration. Encourage oral fluid ingestion. Monitor daily weight, or if implemented in an inpatient setting, monitor fluid input and output. Replace electrolytes as medically appropriate

An admixture containing **ifosfamide** 1800 mg/m^2 + **mesna** 360 mg/m^2 per day; administer intravenously in a volume of 0.9% NS or 5% dextrose injection (D5W) sufficient to produce ifosfamide concentrations between 0.6 and 20 mg/mL, over 60 minutes for 5 consecutive days, on days 1–5, every 21 days (total ifosfamide dosage/cycle = 9000 mg/m^2)
Then, either:
Mesna 360 mg/m^2 per dose; administer intravenously diluted with 0.9% NS or D5W to a concentration of 1–20 mg/mL, over 15 minutes for 2 doses per day at 4 hours and 8 hours after ifosfamide administration is completed, for 5 consecutive days, on days 1–5, every 21 days (total mesna dosage/cycle = 5400 mg/m^2; includes 360 mg/m^2 doses given daily with ifosfamide), *or*

Mesna 720 mg/m^2 per dose; administer orally for 2 doses per day at 2 hours and 6 hours after ifosfamide administration is completed, for 5 consecutive days, on days 1–5, every 21 days (total mesna dosage/cycle = 9000 mg/m^2; includes 360 mg/m^2 doses given daily with ifosfamide)
Note: in the study, mesna was administered for a protracted duration. The above dosing schemes are instead derived from American Society of Clinical Oncology Clinical Practice Guidelines (Hensley ML et al. J Clin Oncol 2008;27:127–145)

Doxorubicin 37.5 mg/m^2; administer by intravenous injection over 3–5 minutes, for 2 doses on days 1 and 2, every 21 days (total dosage/cycle = 75 mg/m^2)
- *Note:* use of dexrazoxane for cardioprotection was allowed per institutional guidelines, but was not mandatory. Although not described in the article, in lieu of dexrazoxane, may also consider administering the total doxorubicin dose as a continuous intravenous infusion (eg, over 48 hours) for cardioprotection

Cycles of ifosfamide + etoposide (IE):
Hydration during ifosfamide:

Administer additional intravenous hydration (eg, **0.9% NS**) over 4–24 hours to achieve a total rate of 2000 mL/m^2/day (taking into account volumes of diluent used for mesna, ifosfamide, and etoposide administration) for the duration of ifosfamide treatment on days 1–5. If feasible, continue maintenance intravenous hydration during intervals between ifosfamide administration. Encourage oral fluid ingestion. Monitor daily weight, or if implemented in an inpatient setting, monitor fluid input and output. Replace electrolytes as medically appropriate

An admixture containing **ifosfamide** 1800 mg/m^2 + **mesna** 360 mg/m^2 per day; administer intravenously in a volume of 0.9% NS or 5% dextrose injection (D5W) sufficient to produce ifosfamide concentrations between 0.6 and 20 mg/mL, over 60 minutes for 5 consecutive days, on days 1–5, every 21 days (total ifosfamide dosage/cycle = 9000 mg/m^2)
Then, either:
Mesna 360 mg/m^2 per dose; administer intravenously diluted with 0.9% NS or D5W to a concentration of 1–20 mg/mL, over 15 minutes for 2 doses per day at 4 hours and 8 hours after ifosfamide administration, for 5 consecutive days, on days 1–5, every 21 days (total mesna dosage/cycle = 5400 mg/m^2; includes 360 mg/m^2 doses given daily with ifosfamide), *or*

Mesna 720 mg/m^2 per dose; administer orally for 2 doses per day at 2 hours and 6 hours after ifosfamide administration, for 5 consecutive days, on days 1–5, every 21 days (total mesna dosage/cycle = 9000 mg/m^2; includes 360 mg/m^2 doses given daily with ifosfamide)
Note: in the study, mesna was administered for a protracted duration. The above dosing schemes are instead derived from American Society of Clinical Oncology Clinical Practice Guidelines (Hensley ML et al. J Clin Oncol 2008; 27:127–145)

Etoposide 100 mg/m^2 per day; administer intravenously diluted with 0.9% NS to a concentration of 0.2–0.4 mg/mL over 60 minutes for 5 consecutive days, on days 1–5, every 21 days (total dosage/cycle = 500 mg/m^2)

(continued)

(continued)

Supportive Care (applies to AI and IE cycles)
Antiemetic prophylaxis
Emetogenic potential is **MODERATE**
See Chapter 42 for antiemetic recommendations

Hematopoietic growth factor (CSF) prophylaxis
Primary prophylaxis is indicated with 1 of the following:
Filgrastim (G-CSF) 5 µg/kg per day by subcutaneous injection, *or*
Pegfilgrastim (pegylated filgrastim) 6 mg/0.6 mL by subcutaneous injection for 1 dose
- Begin use from 24–72 hours after myelosuppressive chemotherapy is completed
- Continue daily filgrastim use until post-nadir ANC ≥1500/mm³ on 2 measurements separated temporally by ≥12 hours
- Discontinue daily filgrastim use at least 24 hours before administering myelosuppressive treatment. Do not administer pegfilgrastim within 14 days before administering myelosuppressive treatment

See Chapter 43 for more information

Antimicrobial prophylaxis
Risk of fever and neutropenia is INTERMEDIATE
Antimicrobial primary prophylaxis to be considered:
- Antibacterial—consider a fluoroquinolone or no prophylaxis
- Antifungal—consider concomitant use of clotrimazole during periods of neutropenia
- Antiviral—antiherpes antivirals (eg, acyclovir, famciclovir, valacyclovir)

Treatment Modifications

Doxorubicin, Ifosfamide, and Etoposide Treatment Modifications

Adverse Event	Dose Modification
Day 1 ANC <1500/mm³ or platelet count <100,000/mm³	Delay by 1 week. Re-treat at full dose unless delayed by >1 week despite use of G-CSF, in which case reduce the doses of both agents by 20% in the subsequent treatment cycle
Febrile neutropenia occurring in the prior cycle	Reduce the doses of both agents by 20% in subsequent cycles and add G-CSF prophylaxis if not already receiving
SCr 1.5 × baseline	Delay by 1 week. If renal function does not improve, then discontinue ifosfamide
G2 renal toxicity—tubular (based on creatinine clearance, serum bicarbonate, need for electrolyte replacement, or TmP/GFR)	Reduce the ifosfamide and mesna doses by 20% in subsequent cycles
G ≥3 renal toxicity—tubular (based on creatinine clearance, serum bicarbonate, need for electrolyte replacement, or TmP/GFR)	Discontinue ifosfamide
Microscopic hematuria during ifosfamide therapy (>50 RBC/HPF) on >1 occasion	Discontinue ifosfamide for that cycle. If hematuria completely resolves, consider increasing the rate of intravenous fluids and/or the increasing the mesna dose in subsequent cycles
G ≥2 non-infective hemorrhagic cystitis (related to ifosfamide)	Discontinue ifosfamide and provide appropriate supportive care
G2 encephalopathy	If persistent or distressing, then decrease the ifosfamide and mesna dosages by 20%. If not contraindicated, treat with methylene blue 2 mg/kg (maximum dose of 50 mg) intravenously every 4–8 hours until resolution of symptoms, then consider prophylactic use at the same dose given every 6–8 hours in subsequent cycles
G ≥3 encephalopathy	Stop ifosfamide for this cycle. If not contraindicated, treat with methylene blue 2 mg/kg (maximum dose of 50 mg) intravenously every 4–8 hours until resolution of symptoms, then consider prophylactic use at the same dose given every 6–8 hours in subsequent cycles. Consider decreasing the ifosfamide and mesna dosages by 20% in subsequent cycles
Nonhematologic life-threatening toxicity	Discontinue therapy

(continued)

Treatment Modifications (*continued*)

Adverse Event	Dose Modification
G ≥3 mucositis	Reduce doxorubicin or etoposide dosage by 20% in subsequent cycles
Doxorubicin total cumulative lifetime dosage ≥400–450 mg/m²	Obtain frequent MUGA scans to monitor cardiac function
A fall in ejection fraction (possible guidelines: resting cardiac ejection fraction decreased ≥10–15 percentage points below baseline or to <35–40%)	Discontinue doxorubicin

Patient Population Studied

Children and adults (no upper or lower age limit) with measurable, high-grade (stage III per AJCC TNM staging system) or metastatic (stage IV) sporadic or NF1-associated malignant peripheral nerve sheath tumors (MPNST) not previously treated with chemotherapy for MPNST were eligible for the study

Patient Characteristics at Enrollment and Response Evaluation

Stratum	NF1 MPNST	Sporadic MPNST
Eligible patients enrolled	34	14
Male/female	22/12	9/5
Median age: years (range)	33 (8–66)	40 (13–72)
Race (%)		
White, non-Hispanic	14 (41%)	11 (79%)
Black	13 (38%)	2 (14%)
Hispanic	4 (12%)	0 (0%)
Other/unknown	3 (9%)	1 (7%)
ECOG score: 0/1/2	4/24/6	6/5/3
Disease: localized/metastatic	18/16	5/9
Location		
Head	2	0
Neck	3	1
Chest	10	4
Abdomen/pelvis	9	5
Spine	5	1
Upper extremity	3	1
Lower extremity	2	2

Efficacy

Response Evaluation > Cycle 4	28	9	37
	NF1 MPNST	Sporadic MPNST	Total
Complete response	—	—	
Partial response	5 (17.9%; 95% CI 6.1–36.9%)	4 (44.4%; 95% CI 13.7–78.8%)	9
Stable disease	20	4	24
Progressive disease	3	1	4
Objective response rate	17.9%	44.4%	

Notes:
- Of the 48 patients, 37 were evaluable for response (28 NF1, 9 sporadic MPNST)
- Patients were deemed nonevaluable for the following reasons; PI decision (n = 2), early local control (n = 3), patient withdrawal (n = 4), death during cycle 1 (n = 1) due to internal hemorrhage unrelated to therapy, and noncompliance (n = 1)

Adverse Events

- Eight patients had dose reductions of chemotherapy
- Of the eight, three for neurotoxicity associated with ifosfamide
- Serious adverse events with possible, probable, or definite relationship were reported for nine patients with NF1 and four patients with sporadic MPNST including febrile neutropenia (n = 6), anemia (n = 4), altered mental status, aphasia, and somnolence (n = 4) attributed to ifosfamide and secondary acute myeloid leukemia 1 year after completion of treatment in one patient with NF1 MPNST

Therapy Monitoring

1. *Prior to each cycle:* physical examination, ECOG PS, CBC with differential and platelet count, total bilirubin, ALT, AST, albumin, alkaline phosphatase, serum creatinine, BUN, calcium, carbon dioxide, chloride, glucose, potassium, sodium, and phosphate
2. *During ifosfamide and mesna administration:*
   a. *Daily laboratory investigations:* serum creatinine, BUN, calcium, carbon dioxide, chloride, glucose, potassium, sodium, and phosphate
   b. *Every 8 hours (or with each void):* urine dipstick for blood (check microscopic urinalysis if >trace)
   c. *Other:* monitor fluid status (ie, weight and intake/output) and for signs and symptoms of neurologic toxicity
3. *At least once per week between cycles:* CBC with differential and platelet count, serum creatinine, BUN, calcium, carbon dioxide, chloride, glucose, potassium, sodium, and phosphate
4. *At baseline, after reaching a cumulative doxorubicin dose of 250–300 mg/m², and then before each cycle after a cumulative doxorubicin dosage of 400–450 mg/m²:* cardiac ejection fraction
5. *After every 2 cycles of therapy:* tumor measurements

METASTATIC/INOPERABLE • ALK POSITIVE • INFLAMMATORY MYOFIBROBLASTIC TUMORS

METASTATIC OR INOPERABLE ALK POSITIVE INFLAMMATORY MYOFIBROBLASTIC TUMORS REGIMEN: CRIZOTINIB

Mossé YP et al. J Clin Oncol 2017;35:3215–3221
Schöffski P et al. Lancet Respir Med 2018;6:431–441

Adult Dose	Pediatric Dose
Crizotinib 250 mg per dose; administer orally twice daily, continually with or without food (total dose/week = 3500 mg)	**Crizotinib** 280 mg/m^2 per dose; administer orally twice daily, continually with or without food (total dose/week = 3920 mg/m^2)

Notes:
- Crizotinib is commercially available as a 200-mg and 250-mg capsule
- Swallow crizotinib capsules whole
- If a patient misses a dose, advise the patient to take it as soon as remembered unless it is less than 6 hours until the next dose, in which case, advise the patient not to take the missed dose. If a patient vomits after taking a dose of crizotinib, advise the patient not to take an extra dose, but to take the next dose at the regular time
- In patients with moderate hepatic impairment (any AST and total bilirubin >1.5 × ULN and ≤3 × ULN), reduce the starting dose to 200 mg orally twice daily (refers to adult dose)
- In patients with severe hepatic impairment (any AST and total bilirubin >3 × ULN), reduce the starting dose to 250 mg orally once daily (refers to adult dose)
- In patients with severe renal impairment (ClCr <30 mL/min, calculated using the modified Cockcroft-Gault equation) not requiring dialysis, reduce the starting dose to 250 mg orally once daily (refers to adult dose)
- Drug/food interactions
  - Advise patients to avoid consuming grapefruit products while taking crizotinib
  - Avoid concomitant use of strong CYP3A4 inducers with crizotinib
  - If concomitant use of a strong CYP3A4 inhibitor is unavoidable, then reduce the starting crizotinib dose to 250 mg once daily (refers to adult dose)
  - Avoid concomitant use with sensitive CYP3A substrates
  - Avoid concomitant use with drugs that prolong the QT interval
  - Avoid concomitant use with drugs that cause bradycardia (eg, beta-blockers, non-dihydropyridine calcium channel blockers, clonidine, and digoxin)

Supportive Care

Antiemetic prophylaxis
Emetogenic potential: **MODERATE TO HIGH**
See Chapter 42 for antiemetic recommendations

Hematopoietic growth factor (CSF) prophylaxis
Primary prophylaxis is NOT indicated
See Chapter 43 for more information

Antimicrobial prophylaxis
Risk of fever and neutropenia is *LOW*
  Antimicrobial primary prophylaxis to be considered:
  - Antibacterial—not indicated
  - Antifungal—not indicated
  - Antiviral—not indicated, unless patient previously had an episode of HSV

Diarrhea management

Latent or delayed-onset diarrhea*:
Loperamide 4 mg orally initially after the first loose or liquid stool, *then* 2–4 mg orally every 2–4 hours or **diphenoxylate hydrochloride** 2.5 mg **with atropine sulfate** 0.025 mg (eg, Lomotil)

*Abigerges D et al. J Natl Cancer Inst 1994;86:446–449
Rothenberg ML et al. J Clin Oncol 2001;19:3801–3807
Wadler S et al. J Clin Oncol 1998;16:3169–3178

Treatment modifications

CRIZOTINIB DOSE ADJUSTMENTS

	Adult Dose	Pediatric Dose
Starting dose	250 mg orally twice per day	280 mg/m² per dose orally twice/day
Dose level (−1)	200 mg orally twice per day	215 mg/m² per dose orally twice/day
Dose level (−2)	250 mg orally daily	165 mg/m² per dose orally twice/day
Dose level (−3)	Discontinue	Discontinue

Adverse Event	Dose Modification
Hematologic Toxicity*	
G3 hematologic toxicity	Withhold until recovery to G ≤2, then resume at the same dose schedule
G4 hematologic toxicity	Withhold until recovery to G ≤2, then resume at 1 lower dose level
Nonhematologic Toxicity	
G3/4 alanine aminotransferase (ALT) or aspartate aminotransferase (AST) elevation with G ≤1 total bilirubin	Withhold until recovery to G ≤1 or baseline, then resume at 1 lower dose level
G2/3/4 ALT or AST elevation with concurrent G2/3/4 total bilirubin elevation (in the absence of cholestasis or hemolysis)	Permanently discontinue crizotinib
Any grade pneumonitis[†]	Permanently discontinue crizotinib
G3 QTc prolongation	Withhold until recovery to G ≤1, then resume at 1 lower dose level
Grade 4 QTc prolongation	Permanently discontinue crizotinib
Bradycardia[‡] (symptomatic, may be severe and medically significant, medical intervention indicated)	Withhold until recovery to asymptomatic bradycardia or to a heart rate of ≥60 bpm. Evaluate concomitant medications known to cause bradycardia. If contributing concomitant medication is identified and discontinued, or its dose is adjusted, resume at previous dose upon recovery. If no contributing concomitant medication is identified, or if contributing concomitant medications are not discontinued or dose modified, resume at reduced dose upon recovery
Bradycardia[‡,§] (life-threatening consequences, urgent intervention indicated)	Permanently discontinue if no contributing concomitant medication is identified. If contributing concomitant medication is identified and discontinued, or its dose is adjusted, resume at dose level −2 (refers to adult dose of 250 mg daily) upon recovery to asymptomatic bradycardia or to a heart rate of ≥60 bpm, with frequent monitoring
Visual loss (G4 ocular disorder)	Discontinue during evaluation of severe vision loss

*Except lymphopenia (unless associated with clinical events, eg, opportunistic infections)
[†]Not attributable to other pulmonary disease, infection, or radiation effect
[‡]Heart rate <60 beats per minute (bpm)
[§]Permanently discontinue for recurrence
Note: toxicities graded based on National Cancer Institute (NCI) Common Terminology Criteria for Adverse Events (CTCAE), version 4.0

Patient Population Studied

Mossé YP et al. J Clin Oncol 2017;35:3215–3221

A study from the Children's Oncology Group (COG) involved 26 patients with relapsed or refractory *ALK*-positive anaplastic large cell lymphoma (ALCL) and 14 patients with metastatic or inoperable *ALK*-positive inflammatory myofibroblastic tumors (IMTs). Patients aged ≤22 years with recurrent ALCL or unresectable IMT for >12 months and underlying *ALK*-fusion were eligible. Patients with IMT were eligible without prior exposure to therapeutic agents. Additionally, patients were required to meet COG eligibility criteria for performance status and organ function (bone marrow, renal, and liver function)

(continued)

Patient Population Studied (*continued*)

Patient Population

Characteristic	IMT (n = 14)
Median age, years (range)	7.0 (2.0–13.5)
Male sex (%)	36
Race: White/Black/Asian/Unknown (%)	71/7/0/21
Number of prior therapies: 0 / 1–2 / 3–4 (%)	14/64/21
Prior therapy	
Chemotherapy (%)	29
Surgery (%)	57
Anti-inflammatory (%)	29

IMT, inflammatory myofibroblastic tumor

Schöffski P et al. Lancet Respir Med 2018;6:431–441

Baseline Characteristics of Patients with Inflammatory Myofibroblastic Tumors Treated with Crizotinib

	ALK-positive Patients (n = 12)	*ALK*-negative Patients (n = 8)	Total (n = 20)
Age (years)			
Median (IQR)	35.5 (27.0–55.5)	59.5 (43.0–67.0)	45.5 (29.0–62.0)
Range	21.0–69.0	15.0–78.0	15.0–78.0
Eastern Cooperative Oncology Group performance status			
0	7 (58%)	4 (50%)	11 (55%)
1	5 (42%)	3 (38%)	8 (40%)
2	0	1 (13%)	1 (5%)
Sex			
Male	6 (50%)	5 (63%)	11 (55%)
Female	6 (50%)	3 (38%)	9 (45%)
Previous major surgery	7 (58%)	3 (38%)	10 (50%)
Previous systemic cancer therapy	6 (50%)	2 (25%)	8 (40%)
Chemotherapy	5 (42%)	2 (25%)	7 (35%)
Other cancer therapy	2 (17%)	1 (13%)	3 (15%)
Previous systemic treatments			
Neoadjuvant	0	0	0
Adjuvant	1 (8%)	0	1 (5%)
Palliative treatment			
1st line	5 (42%)	2 (25%)	7 (35%)
2nd line	2 (17%)	2 (25%)	4 (20%)
3rd line	1 (8%)	0	1 (5%)
4th line	1 (8%)	0	1 (5%)
5th line	1 (8%)	0	1 (5%)

Data are n (%) unless stated otherwise
ALK, anaplastic lymphoma kinase

Efficacy

Mossé YP et al. J Clin Oncol 2017;35:3215–3221

Outcome	IMT (n = 14)
ORR, %	86 (95% CI 57–98)
CR, no (%)	5 (36)
PR, no (%)	7 (50)
SD, no (%)	2 (14)
PD, no (%)	0
Median therapy duration, yr	1.63 (95% CI 0.55–2.3)
Time to first PR/CR, days	28.5 (95% CI 27–134)

IMT, inflammatory myofibroblastic tumor; ORR, objective response rate; CI, confidence interval; CR, complete response; PR, partial response; SD, stable disease; PD, progressive disease

Schöffski P et al. Lancet Respir Med 2018;6:431–441

Response Assessment and Activity Summary According to Investigator Assessment

	ALK-positive Patients (n = 12)	ALK-negative Patients (n = 7)	Total (n = 19)
Best RECIST 1.1 response			
Confirmed CR	2 (17%)	0	2 (11%)
Confirmed PR	4 (33%)	1 (14%)	5 (26%)
Non-confirmed PR	1 (8%)	0	1 (5%)
SD	5 (42%)	5 (71%)	10 (53%)
PD	0	1 (14%)	1 (5%)
Confirmed OR	6 (50%; 21.1–78.9)	1 (14%; 0.0–57.9)	7 (37%; 16.3–61.6)
Disease control	12 (100%; 73.5–100.0)	6 (86%; 42.1–99.6)	18 (95%; 74.0–99.9)
Progression-free survival			
Alive without PD	8 (67%)	3 (43%)	11 (58%)
PD or death	4 (33%)	4 (57%)	8 (42%)
12-month PFS	9 (73%; 37.9–90.6)	4 (54%; 13.2–82.5)	13 (67%; 39.9–83.5)
Survival status			
Alive	10 (83%)	4 (57%)	14 (74%)
Dead	2 (17%)	3 (43%)	5 (26%)
Reason for death			
Progression of IMFT	1 (8%)	3 (43%)	4 (21%)
Cardiovascular disease	1 (8%)	0	1 (5%)
12-month survival	10 (82%; 44.7–95.1)	6 (83%; 27.3–97.5)	16 (82%; 54.7–93.9)

Data are n (%) or n (%, 95% CI)
ALK, anaplastic lymphoma kinase; CR, complete response; IMFT, inflammatory myofibroblastic tumors; OR, objective response; PD, progressive disease; PFS, progression-free survival; PR, partial response; RECIST, Response Evaluation Criteria in Solid Tumors; SD, stable disease

Adverse Events

Mossé YP et al. J Clin Oncol 2017;35:3215–3221

Adverse Events G3/4 (n = 40)	ALCL 165 mg/m^2		ALCL 280 mg/m^2		IMT	
	No. of Patients	No. of Events	No. of Patients	No. of Events	No. of Patients	No. of Events
Total	2	5	27	47	9	31
ALT increased	0	0	1	1	0	0
Anemia	0	0	1	1	0	0
Diarrhea	0	0	1	1	1	1
Limb edema	0	0	0	0	1	1
Febrile neutropenia	0	0	1	1	0	0
Infective myositis	0	0	1	1	0	0
Lymphocyte count decreased	0	0	1	1	0	0
Neutrophil count decreased	2	5	14	33	6	28
Platelet count decreased	0	0	1	1	-	-
Sinus bradycardia	0	0	0	0	1	1
Skin and subcutaneous tissue disorder	0	0	1	1	0	0
Skin infection	0	0	1	1	0	0
Vomiting	0	0	1	1	0	0
WBC count decreased	0	0	3	4	0	0

ALT, alanine aminotransferase; WBC, white blood cell

Treatment-related Nonhematologic Adverse Events Occurring in ≥10% of Patients
Schöffski P et al. Lancet Respir Med 2018;6:431–441

	Grade 1	Grade 2	Grade 3	Grade 4
All adverse events	9 (45%)	6 (30%)	2 (10%)	1 (5%)
Eye disorders				
Blurred vision	8 (40%)	1 (5%)	—	—
Conjunctivitis	1 (5%)	—	—	—
Dry eye	2 (10%)	2 (10%)	—	—
Flashing lights	3 (15%)	—	—	—
Optic nerve disorder	2 (10%)	—	—	—
Other eye disorders	5 (25%)	—	—	—
Gastrointestinal disorders				
Abdominal pain	1 (5%)	—	—	—
Bloating	1 (5%)	—	—	—
Constipation	3 (15%)	2 (10%)	—	—
Diarrhea	6 (30%)	1 (5%)	—	—

(continued)

Adverse Events (continued)

	Grade 1	Grade 2	Grade 3	Grade 4
Dyspepsia	2 (10%)	1 (5%)	—	—
Esophagitis	2 (10%)	—	—	—
Flatulence	2 (10%)	—	—	—
Mucositis oral	2 (10%)	—	—	—
Nausea	6 (30%)	5 (25%)	—	—
Vomiting	5 (25%)	2 (10%)	—	—
General disorders and administration site conditions				
Edema limbs	5 (25%)	—	—	—
Fatigue	5 (25%)	3 (15%)	1 (5%)	—
Fever	1 (5%)	—	—	—
Pain	2 (10%)	—	—	—
Other general disorders	—	—	—	—
Hepatobiliary disorders	—	—	—	—
Investigations				
Gamma glutamyl transpeptidase increased	1 (5%)	—	—	—
Weight loss	1 (5%)	1 (5%)	—	—
Anorexia	1 (5%)	1 (5%)	—	—
Musculoskeletal and connective tissue disorders	1 (5%)	1 (5%)	—	—
Nervous system disorders				
Dizziness	2 (10%)	—	—	—
Dysgeusia	5 (25%)	—	—	—
Headache	1 (5%)	1 (5%)	—	—
Peripheral motor neuropathy	3 (15%)	—	—	—
Respiratory, thoracic, and mediastinal disorders				
Cough	—	1 (5%)	—	—
Dyspnea	—	1 (5%)	—	—
Skin and subcutaneous tissue disorders				
Alopecia	3 (15%)	—	—	—
Dry skin	2 (10%)	—	—	—
Pruritus	2 (10%)	—	—	—
Rash maculopapular	3 (15%)	—	—	—
Hypertension	1 (5%)	1 (5%)	—	—

Data are n (%) in 20 patients

Treatment Monitoring

1. *Monthly and as clinically indicated:* complete blood counts (CBC) including differential white blood cell counts
2. *Every 2 weeks during the first 2 months, then monthly, then as clinically indicated:* liver function tests, including ALT, AST, and total bilirubin. In patients with elevated liver function tests, increase the frequency of monitoring
3. *If G3/4 clinical or laboratory abnormalities are observed or if fever or infection occurs:* frequent monitoring of complete blood counts (CBC) including differential white blood cell counts and liver function tests
4. Consider periodic monitoring with electrocardiograms (ECGs) and electrolytes in patients with congestive heart failure, bradyarrhythmias, electrolyte abnormalities, or who are taking medications that are known to prolong the QT interval
5. Monitor heart rate and blood pressure regularly. Crizotinib may cause bradycardia
6. Crizotinib may cause severe visual loss. Advise patients to promptly report vision changes. Perform an ophthalmologic examination promptly for any reports of visual loss
7. Crizotinib may cause interstitial lung disease. Advise patients to promptly report pulmonary symptoms and evaluate any new symptoms promptly

METASTATIC/INOPERABLE • UNDIFFERENTIATED PLEOMORPHIC • DEDIFFERENTIATED • LIPOSARCOMA

METASTATIC OR INOPERABLE UNDIFFERENTIATED PLEOMORPHIC OR DEDIFFERENTIATED LIPOSARCOMA REGIMEN: PEMBROLIZUMAB

Tawbi HA et al. Lancet Oncol 2017;18:1493–1501
Supplementary appendix to: Tawbi HA et al. Lancet Oncol 2017;18:1493–1501
KEYTRUDA (pembrolizumab) prescribing information. Whitehouse Station, NJ: Merck & Co., Inc; revised 2020 June

Pembrolizumab 200 mg; administer intravenously over 30 minutes in a volume of 0.9% sodium chloride injection (0.9% NS) or 5% dextrose injection (D5W) sufficient to produce a pembrolizumab concentration within the range 1–10 mg/mL every 3 weeks, until disease progression (total dose/3-week cycle = 200 mg)

May consider an alternative pembrolizumab dose and schedule per the U.S. FDA regimens approved (for other indications) on April 28, 2020:
Pembrolizumab 400 mg; administer intravenously over 30 minutes in a volume of 0.9% NS or D5W sufficient to produce a pembrolizumab concentration within the range 1–10 mg/mL every 6 weeks, until disease progression (total dose/6-week cycle = 400 mg)

Notes:
- Administer pembrolizumab with an administration set that contains a sterile, non-pyrogenic, low protein-binding in-line or add-on filter with pore size within the range of 0.2–5 micrometers
- Pembrolizumab can cause severe or life-threatening infusion-related reactions, including hypersensitivity and anaphylaxis

Antiemetic prophylaxis
Emetogenic potential of pembrolizumab is **MINIMAL**
See Chapter 42 for antiemetic recommendations

Hematopoietic growth factor (CSF) prophylaxis
Primary prophylaxis is NOT indicated
See Chapter 43 for more information

Antimicrobial prophylaxis
Risk of fever and neutropenia is *LOW*
Antimicrobial primary prophylaxis to be considered:
- Antibacterial—not indicated
- Antifungal—not indicated
- Antiviral—not indicated unless patient previously had an episode of HSV

Dose Adjustments

RECOMMENDED DOSE MODIFICATIONS FOR PEMBROLIZUMAB

Adverse Event	Grade/Severity	Treatment Modification
Infusion reaction	Clinically significant but not severe infusion reaction	Interrupt the infusion in patients with clinically significant infusion reactions and consider resuming at a slower rate following resolution. If decision is made to restart, begin at ≤50% of the rate prior to the reaction and increase in 50% increments every 30 minutes if well tolerated. Infusions may be restarted at the full rate during the next cycle
	G3/4 (severe infusion reaction—pyrexia, chills, flushing, hypotension, dyspnea, wheezing, back pain, abdominal pain, and urticaria). Not rapidly responsive to brief interruption of infusion	Stop infusion and administer appropriate medical therapy (eg, epinephrine, corticosteroids, intravenous antihistamines, bronchodilators, and/or oxygen). Discontinue pembrolizumab
Colitis	G1	Loperamide 4 mg as starting dose then 2mg before each meal and after each loose stool until without diarrhea for 12 hours, with maximum of 16 mg loperamide per day. If G1 diarrhea or colitis persists >14 days, then add prednisolone 0.5–1 mg/kg (non-enteric coated) or consider oral budesonide 9 mg daily if no bloody diarrhea

(continued)

Dose Adjustments (*continued*)

Adverse Event	Grade/Severity	Treatment Modification
	G2/3 diarrhea or colitis	Withhold pembrolizumab. Loperamide 4 mg as starting dose then 2mg before each meal and after each loose stool until without diarrhea for 12 hours, with maximum of 16 mg loperamide per day. Administer oral prednisone/prednisolone at a dose of 0.5 to 2 mg/kg/day or its equivalent. When improves to G1, begin a slow corticosteroid taper over at least 4 weeks. Resume pembrolizumab upon symptom control, or when prednisone/prednisolone daily dose <10 mg
	G4 diarrhea or colitis	Permanently discontinue pembrolizumab. Loperamide 4 mg as starting dose then 2 mg before each meal and after each loose stool until without diarrhea for 12 hours, with maximum of 16 mg loperamide per day. Administer 1–2 mg/kg IV (methyl) prednisolone and convert to 0.5–2 mg/kg prednisone/prednisolone orally each day or its equivalent only after a response. Taper over at least 4 weeks when symptoms improve. If does not improve over 72 hours or worsens, perform flexible sigmoidoscopy/colonoscopy to document colitis then begin infliximab 5 mg/kg (if no perforation/sepsis/TB/hepatitis/NYHA III/IV CHF). If no response, add MMF 500–1000 mg twice daily. If worse on MMF, consider addition of tacrolimus or ATG
Pneumonitis	G2	Withhold pembrolizumab. Consider *Pneumocystis* prophylaxis depending on the clinical context and coverage with empiric antibiotics. Administer oral prednisone/prednisolone at a dose of 1–2 mg/kg/day or its equivalent. When improves to G1, begin a slow corticosteroid taper over at least 4 weeks. If does not respond adequately after 48 hours, then administer 2–4 mg/kg IV (methyl)prednisolone and convert to 0.5–2 mg/kg prednisone/prednisolone orally each day or its equivalent only after a response, followed by a taper over at least 6 weeks when symptoms improve to G1, titrating to symptoms. Resume pembrolizumab upon symptom control, or when prednisone/prednisolone daily dose <10 mg
	G3/4	Permanently discontinue pembrolizumab. Consider *Pneumocystis* prophylaxis depending on the clinical context; cover with empiric antibiotics. Administer 2–4 mg/kg IV (methyl) prednisolone and convert to 1–2 mg/kg prednisone/prednisolone orally each day or its equivalent only after a response, followed by a taper over at least 8 weeks when symptoms improve to G1, titrating to symptoms. If, when initially treated, improvement does not occur within 48–72 hours, begin infliximab 5 mg/kg (if no perforation/sepsis/TB/hepatitis/NYHA III/IV CHF). If no response to infliximab, add MMF 500–1000 mg twice daily. Consider MMF especially if has concurrent hepatic toxicity
Hepatitis	G2 (AST or ALT >3–5 × ULN or total bilirubin >1.5–3 × ULN)	Withhold pembrolizumab. Administer oral prednisone/prednisolone at a dose of 1 to 2 mg/kg/day or its equivalent. When improves to G1, begin a slow corticosteroid taper over at least 4 weeks. Resume pembrolizumab upon symptom control, or when prednisone/prednisolone daily dose <10 mg
	G3/4 (AST or ALT >5 × ULN or total bilirubin >3 × ULN)	Permanently discontinue pembrolizumab. Administer 1–2 mg/kg IV (methyl) prednisolone and convert to 0.5–2 mg/kg prednisone/prednisolone orally each day or its equivalent only after a response. Taper over at least 6 weeks when symptoms improve. If no response, add MMF 500–1000 mg twice daily. If worse on MMF, consider adding tacrolimus or ATG
Hypophysitis	G2/3 (moderate symptoms, ie, headache but no visual disturbance or fatigue/mood alteration but hemodynamically stable, no electrolyte disturbance)	Administer analgesia as needed for headache. Withhold pembrolizumab. Administer oral prednisone/prednisolone at a dose of 0.5 to 2 mg/kg/day or its equivalent. When improves to G1, begin a slow corticosteroid taper over at least 4 weeks. If no improvement in 48 hours, administer 1–2 mg/kg IV (methyl)prednisolone and convert to 0.5–2 mg/kg prednisone/prednisolone orally each day or its equivalent only after a response. Taper over at least 4 weeks when symptoms improve to 5 mg prednisone/prednisolone or equivalent; do not stop steroids. Resume pembrolizumab upon symptom control, or when prednisone/prednisolone daily dose <10 mg
	G4 (severe mass effect symptoms, ie, severe headache, any visual disturbance or severe hypoadrenalism, ie, hypotension, severe electrolyte disturbance)	Permanently discontinue pembrolizumab. Administer analgesia as needed for headache. Administer 1–2 mg/kg IV (methyl)prednisolone and convert to 0.5–2 mg/kg prednisone/prednisolone orally each day or its equivalent only after a response. Taper over at least 4 weeks when symptoms improve to 5 mg prednisone/prednisolone or equivalent; do not stop steroids

(*continued*)

Dose Adjustments (*continued*)

Adverse Event	Grade/Severity	Treatment Modification
Adrenal insufficiency	G2	Withhold pembrolizumab. Administer oral prednisone/prednisolone at a dose of 0.5 to 2 mg/kg/day or its equivalent. When improves to G1, begin a slow corticosteroid taper over at least 4 weeks. Serially assess adrenal function and continue steroids at replacement doses (20–40 mg hydrocortisone daily ~2/3 dose in AM upon awakening and ~1/3 at 4 PM) until recovery of adrenal function is documented. Resume pembrolizumab upon symptom control, or when prednisone/prednisolone daily dose <10 mg
	G3/4	Permanently discontinue pembrolizumab. Administer oral prednisone/prednisolone at a dose of 0.5 to 2 mg/kg/day or its equivalent. When improves to G1 begin a slow corticosteroid taper over at least 4 weeks. Serially assess adrenal function and continue steroids at replacement doses (20–40 mg hydrocortisone daily ~2/3 dose in AM upon awakening and ~1/3 at 4 PM) until recovery of adrenal function is documented
Type 1 diabetes mellitus	G3 hyperglycemia	Withhold pembrolizumab. Admit to hospital to manage hyperglycemia. Role of corticosteroids in preventing complete loss of insulin-producing cells is unknown and not recommended. Resume pembrolizumab upon symptom control, or when prednisone/prednisolone daily dose <10 mg
	G4 hyperglycemia	Permanently discontinue pembrolizumab. Admit to hospital to manage hyperglycemia. Role of corticosteroids in preventing complete loss of insulin-producing cells is unknown and not recommended
Nephritis and renal dysfunction	G2/3 (serum creatinine 1.5–6 × ULN)	Withhold pembrolizumab. Administer oral prednisone/prednisolone at a dose of 0.5 to 2 mg/kg/day or its equivalent. When improves to G1, begin a slow corticosteroid taper over at least 4 weeks. If does not respond adequately, then administer 0.5–1 mg/kg IV (methyl)prednisolone and convert to 0.5–2 mg/kg prednisone/prednisolone orally each day or its equivalent only after a response, followed by a taper over at least 4 weeks when improves to G1. Resume pembrolizumab upon symptom control, or when prednisone/prednisolone daily dose <10 mg
	G4 (serum creatinine >6 × ULN)	Permanently discontinue pembrolizumab. Administer 0.5–1 mg/kg IV (methyl)prednisolone and convert to 0.5–2 mg/kg prednisone/prednisolone orally each day or its equivalent only after a response, followed by a taper over at least 4 weeks when improves to G1
Skin	G1/2	Continue pembrolizumab. Avoid skin irritants, avoid sun exposure, topical emollients recommended. Topical steroid (mild strength for G1, moderate/potent strength for G2) cream once or twice daily ± oral or topical antihistamines for itching
	G3 rash or suspected SJS or TEN	Withhold pembrolizumab. Avoid skin irritants, avoid sun exposure, topical emollients recommended. Administer oral or topical antihistamines for itching. Administer oral prednisone/prednisolone at a dose of 0.5–2 mg/kg or its equivalent daily for 3 days followed by a slow corticosteroid taper over at least 4 weeks when the rash improves to G1. If does not respond adequately, then administer 0.5–1 mg/kg IV (methyl)prednisolone and convert to 0.5–2 mg/kg prednisone/prednisolone orally each day or its equivalent only after a response, followed by a taper over at least 4 weeks when the rash improves to G1. Resume pembrolizumab upon symptom control, or when prednisone/prednisolone daily dose <10 mg
	G4 rash or confirmed SJS or TEN	Avoid skin irritants, avoid sun exposure, topical emollients recommended. Administer oral or topical antihistamines for itching. Administer 1–2 mg/kg IV (methyl)prednisolone and convert to oral steroids 0.5–2 mg/kg prednisone/prednisolone each day or its equivalent only after a response. Taper over at least 4 weeks when the rash improves to G1. Permanently discontinue pembrolizumab

(*continued*)

Dose Adjustments (*continued*)

Adverse Event	Grade/Severity	Treatment Modification
Encephalitis	Confusion or altered behavior, headaches, alteration in Glasgow Coma Scale, motor or sensory deficits, speech abnormality, may or may not be febrile	Initially withhold pembrolizumab, but permanently discontinue pembrolizumab if there is no doubt as to diagnosis. Exclude bacterial and ideally viral infections prior to high-dose steroids. Administer oral prednisone/prednisolone at a dose of 0.5–2 mg/kg/day or its equivalent. When symptoms improve, begin a slow corticosteroid taper over at least 4–8 weeks. If symptoms are severe, administer 1–2 mg/kg IV (methyl)prednisolone and convert to 0.5–2 mg/kg prednisone/prednisolone orally each day or its equivalent only after a response. Consider concurrent empiric antiviral (IV acyclovir) and antibacterial therapy
Aseptic meningitis	Headache, photophobia, neck stiffness with fever or may be afebrile, vomiting; normal cognition/cerebral function (distinguishes from encephalitis)	
Other syndromes include neurosarcoidosis, posterior reversible leukoencephalopathy syndrome (PRES), Vogt-Koyanagi-Harada syndrome, demyelination, vasculitic encephalopathy, and generalized seizures		
Transverse myelitis	Acute or subacute neurologic signs/symptoms of motor/sensory/autonomic origin; most have sensory level; often bilateral symptoms	Initially withhold pembrolizumab, but permanently discontinue pembrolizumab if there is no doubt as to diagnosis. Administer 2 mg/kg IV (methyl)prednisolone or consider 1 g/day and convert to 0.5–2 mg/kg prednisone/prednisolone orally each day or its equivalent only after a response. When symptoms improve, begin a slow corticosteroid taper over at least 4–8 weeks. Plasmapheresis may be required if steroids do not bring about improvement
Myocarditis	G3	Permanently discontinue pembrolizumab. Administer 2 mg/kg IV (methyl)prednisolone or consider 1 g/day and convert to 0.5–2 mg/kg prednisone/prednisolone orally each day or its equivalent only after a response. When symptoms improve, begin a slow corticosteroid taper over at least 4–8 weeks. If no response, add MMF 500–1000 mg twice daily. If worse on MMF, consider adding tacrolimus
Peripheral neurologic toxicity	Moderate: some interference with ADL, symptoms concerning to patient	Withhold pembrolizumab. Initial observation reasonable or initiate prednisone / prednisolone 0.5–1 mg/kg (if progressing, eg, from mild) and/or pregabalin or duloxetine for pain. When symptoms improve, begin a slow corticosteroid taper over at least 4 weeks. Resume pembrolizumab upon symptom control, or when prednisone/prednisolone daily dose <10 mg
	Severe: limits self-care and aids warranted, life-threatening, eg, respiratory problems	Permanently discontinue pembrolizumab. Administer 1–2 mg/kg IV (methyl) prednisolone and convert to 0.5–2 mg/kg prednisone/prednisolone orally each day or its equivalent only after a response. Taper over at least 4–8 weeks when symptoms improve to G1
Guillain-Barré syndrome	Progressive symmetrical muscle weakness with absent or reduced tendon reflexes—involves extremities, facial, respiratory, and bulbar and oculomotor muscles; dysregulation of autonomic nerves	Permanently discontinue pembrolizumab. Use of steroids not recommended in idiopathic Guillain-Barré syndrome; however, a trial of (methyl)prednisolone 1–2 mg/kg is reasonable, converting to 0.5–2 mg/kg prednisone/prednisolone orally each day or its equivalent only after a response. If no improvement or worsening, plasmapheresis or IVIG indicated
Myasthenia gravis	Fluctuating muscle weakness (proximal limb, trunk, ocular, eg, ptosis/diplopia or bulbar) with fatigability, respiratory muscles may also be involved	Permanently discontinue pembrolizumab. Administer pyridostigmine at an initial dose of 30 mg three times daily. Administer oral prednisone/prednisolone at a dose of 0.5 to 2 mg/kg/day or its equivalent or 1–2 mg/kg IV (methyl)prednisolone depending on the severity of symptoms. If begin with IV, convert to 0.5–2 mg/kg prednisone/prednisolone orally each day or its equivalent only after a response. If no improvement or worsening, plasmapheresis or IVIG may be considered. Additional immunosuppressants used in myasthenia gravis include azathioprine, cyclosporine, and mycophenolate. Avoid certain medications, eg, ciprofloxacin, beta-blockers, that may precipitate cholinergic crisis

(*continued*)

Dose Adjustments (*continued*)

Adverse Event	Grade/Severity	Treatment Modification
Other syndromes including motor and sensory peripheral neuropathy, multifocal radicular neuropathy/plexopathy, autonomic neuropathy, phrenic nerve palsy, cranial nerve palsies (eg, facial nerve, optic nerve, hypoglossal nerve)		Permanently discontinue pembrolizumab. Administer oral prednisone/prednisolone at a dose of 0.5 to 2 mg/kg/day or its equivalent or 1–2 mg/kg IV (methyl)prednisolone depending on the severity of symptoms. If begin with IV, convert to 0.5–2 mg/kg prednisone/prednisolone orally each day or its equivalent only after a response
Arthralgia	G1 (mild pain with inflammation, erythema, or joint swelling)	Continue pembrolizumab. Administer acetaminophen (paracetamol) and ibuprofen
	G2 (moderate pain with inflammation, erythema, or joint swelling that limits ADLs)	Withhold pembrolizumab. Administer higher doses of acetaminophen (paracetamol) and ibuprofen and use diclofenac or naproxen or etoricoxib. If inadequately controlled, consider intra-articular steroid injections for large joints or administer oral prednisone/prednisolone at a dose of 0.5 to 2 mg/kg/day or its equivalent. When improves to G1, begin a slow corticosteroid taper over at least 4 weeks. If does not respond adequately, then administer 0.5–1 mg/kg IV (methyl)prednisolone and convert to 0.5–2 mg/kg prednisone/prednisolone orally each day or its equivalent only after a response, followed by a taper over at least 4 weeks when improves to G1. Resume pembrolizumab upon symptom control, or when prednisone/prednisolone daily dose <10 mg
	G3 (severe pain; irreversible joint damage; disabling; limits self-care ADL)	Withhold pembrolizumab. Administer 0.5–1 mg/kg IV (methyl)prednisolone and convert to 0.5–2 mg/kg prednisone/prednisolone orally each day or its equivalent only after a response, followed by a taper over at least 4 weeks when improves to G1. In severe cases, infliximab or another anti-TNF alpha drug may be required for improvement of arthritis. Resume pembrolizumab upon symptom control, or when prednisone/prednisolone daily dose <10 mg
Other	First occurrence of other G3	Withhold pembrolizumab. Administer oral prednisone/prednisolone at a dose of 0.5 to 2 mg/kg/day or its equivalent. When improves to G1, begin a slow corticosteroid taper over at least 4 weeks. Resume pembrolizumab upon symptom control, or when prednisone/prednisolone daily dose <10 mg
	Recurrence of same G3	Permanently discontinue pembrolizumab. Administer 1–2 mg/kg IV (methyl)prednisolone and convert to 0.5–2 mg/kg prednisone/prednisolone orally each day or its equivalent only after a response. Taper over at least 4–8 weeks when symptoms improve to G1
	Life-threatening or G4	
	Requirement for ≥10 mg/day prednisone or equivalent for >12 weeks	Permanently discontinue pembrolizumab
	Persistent G2/3 adverse reactions lasting ≥12 weeks	

ADL, activities of daily living; ALT, alanine aminotransferase; AST, aspartate aminotransferase; ATG, anti-thymocyte globulin; SJS, Stevens-Johnson Syndrome; TEN, toxic epidermal necrolysis; ULN, upper limit of normal

Notes on general supportive care:
• Steroid taper in most cases will proceed over a minimum of 1 month, but if symptoms improve rapidly, a 2-week taper can be considered. If steroids are administered for more than 4 weeks, consider PCP prophylaxis (cotrimoxazole 480 mg twice daily M/W/F or inhaled pentamidine if has cotrimoxazole allergy), regular random blood glucose, VitD level and starting calcium/VitD supplementation as per guidelines

Patient Population Studied

A two-cohort, single-arm, open-label, phase 2 trial conducted by members of the Sarcoma Alliance for Research through Collaboration (SARC028) assessed the safety and activity of pembrolizumab in patients with advanced soft-tissue sarcoma or bone sarcoma. Eligible patients had histologic evidence of metastatic or surgically unresectable locally advanced sarcoma and were aged ≥18 years in the soft-tissue sarcoma group and ≥12 years in the bone sarcoma group. Participants were required to have an ECOG PS ≤1. Patients were permitted to have received up to 3 prior lines of systemic therapy. Key exclusion criteria included active brain metastases, active autoimmune disease or syndrome (except vitiligo, resolved childhood asthma, or atopy), chronic use of steroids or immunosuppressants, or prior therapy with anti-PD-1 or PD-L1 antibodies

Patient Population		
Characteristic	**Bone Sarcoma (n = 42)**	**Soft-tissue Sarcoma (n = 42)**
Median age, years (range; IQR)	33 (16–70; 22–48)	3 (18–81; 45–63)
Male sex (%)	62	64
Number of previous therapies (%)		
One	19	19
Two	38	41
Three	43	41
Previous treatment in a metastatic setting (%)		
No	38	48
Yes	62	52

IQR, interquartile range

Efficacy

Best Response by Sarcoma Histology (n = 80)				
Sarcoma Histology	**CR**	**PR**	**SD**	**PD**
Soft-tissue sarcomas (n = 40)	1 (3)	6 (15)	15 (38)	18 (45)
Leiomyosarcoma (n = 10)	0	0	6 (60)	4 (40)
Undifferentiated pleomorphic sarcoma (n = 10)	1 (10)	3 (30)	3 (30)	3 (30)
Liposarcoma (n = 10)	0	2 (20)	4 (40)	4 (40)
Synovial sarcoma (n = 10)	0	1 (10)	2 (20)	7 (70)
Bone sarcomas (n = 40)	0	2 (5)	9 (23)	29 (73)
Chondrosarcoma (n = 5)	0	1 (20)	1 (20)	3 (60)
Ewing sarcoma (n = 13)	0	0	2 (15)	11 (85)
Osteosarcoma (n = 22)	0	1 (5)	6 (27)	15 (68)

Other Efficacy Outcomes	**Soft-tissue Sarcoma (n = 40)**	**Bone Sarcoma (n = 40)**
Median duration of response, weeks (IQR)	33 (23–49)	43 (25–61)
Median progression-free survival, weeks	18 (95% CI 8–21)	8 (95% CI 7–9)

CR, complete response; PR, partial response; SD, stable disease; PD, progressive disease; IQR, interquartile range; CI, confidence interval

Adverse Events

	Bone Sarcoma (n = 42)			Soft-tissue Sarcoma (n = 42)		
	G1–2 (%)	G3 (%)	G4 (%)	G1–2 (%)	G3 (%)	G4 (%)
Overall	2	7	2	2	7	0
Pulmonary embolism	—	—	—	—	2	—
Adrenal insufficiency	—	—	—	2	2	—
Interstitial nephritis	—	2	—	—	—	—
Infectious pneumonia	—	2	—	—	—	—
Bone pain	—	2	—	—	—	—
Hypoxia	—	—	2	—	—	—
Pleural effusion	—	2	—	—	—	—
Pneumonitis	2	—	—	—	2	—

Notes: No Grade 5 adverse events related to treatment were reported during the trial

Therapy Monitoring

1. Initially at the time of each dose, and eventually every 6–12 weeks, perform a total body skin examination with attention to *ALL* mucous membranes as well as a complete review of systems
2. Monitor patients for signs and symptoms of pneumonitis. Evaluate patients with suspected pneumonitis with chest x-ray, CT, and pulse oximetry. For ≥2 toxicity, may include nasal swab, sputum culture and sensitivity, blood culture and sensitivity, and urine culture and sensitivity
3. Monitor patients for signs and symptoms of colitis. Encourage patients to report diarrhea immediately to any member of the health care team
4. Draw AST, ALT, and bilirubin prior to each infusion and/or weekly if there are G1 liver function test elevations. Note, no treatment is recommended for G1 LFT abnormalities. For ≥2 toxicity, work up for other causes of elevated LFTs including viral hepatitis
5. Use basic metabolic panel (Na, K, CO_2, glucose) and patient history as screening tools for hypophysitis including hypopituitarism and adrenal insufficiency. If in doubt, evaluate AM adrenocorticotropic hormone (ACTH) and cortisol levels. Consider ACTH stimulation test for indeterminate results
6. Assess thyroid function at the start of treatment, periodically during treatment, and as indicated based on clinical evaluation, and for clinical signs and symptoms of thyroid disorders. Test for TSH and free thyroxine (FT4) every 4 to 6 weeks as part of routine clinical monitoring on therapy or for case detection in symptomatic patients
7. Measure glucose at baseline and with each treatment during the first 12 weeks and every 6 weeks thereafter
8. Obtain a complete rheumatologic history and perform an examination of all peripheral joints for tenderness, swelling, and range of motion. Examine the spine. Consider plain x-ray/imaging to exclude metastases and evaluate joint damage (erosions), if appropriate
9. Response evaluation: every 2 to 4 months

SOFT-TISSUE SARCOMAS: GI STROMAL TUMORS (GIST)

Epidemiology

Incidence: 4000–6000 estimated cases in the United States annually
Male to female ratio: 1:1
Gastrointestinal stromal tumors (GIST) account for <1% of all primary tumors of the gastrointestinal tract

Site of Disease	% of Patients
Stomach	60–70
Small bowel	20–30
Other*	10

*Large bowel, esophagus, rectum, mesentery, and omentum

Work-up

1. History and physical examination
2. *Laboratory tests:* complete blood count with differential, electrolytes, BUN, creatinine, LFTs
3. Contrast-enhanced CT scan of chest, abdomen, and pelvis
4. FDG-PET scan can complement conventional CT helping to differentiate benign from malignant tissue (Van den Abbeele A, Badawi R. Eur J Cancer 2002;38[Suppl 5]:S60–S65)
5. Upper endoscopy or endoscopic ultrasound-guided (EUS) fine-needle biopsy to obtain a tissue diagnosis. EUS can usually accurately differentiate leiomyoma and leiomyosarcoma

Expert Opinion

1. GIST consist of mesenchymal tumors that arise from the interstitial cells of Cajal (ICC) in the myenteric plexus
2. Incidence reported as 12,394 cases/1,000,000/year (de Pinieux G et al. PLoS One 2021;16:e0246958)
3. Because nearly all GIST express the cell surface tyrosine kinase receptor, KIT, immunohistochemical staining facilitates the diagnosis. The DOG1 marker is also very specific and sensitive in KIT-negative GIST
4. More than 85% of patients with GIST have activating *KIT* or *PDGFR-α* mutations (platelet-derived growth factor receptor-α) [Blay JY et al. Nat Rev Dis Primers 2021;7:22.]
5. Oncogenic mutations result in activation of *KIT* and its downstream pathways leading to uncontrolled cell division and resistance to apoptosis
6. Treatment of GIST should be done in reference centers
7. Complete surgical resection remains the gold standard in the treatment of localized GIST ≥2 cm. There is no consensus for therapy of small GIST (<2 cm). The goal of surgery is to remove all disease with negative resection margins. This is accomplished in up to 60% of GIST. Because nodal metastases are rare, lymphadenectomy is unnecessary. However, peritoneal surfaces and liver should be closely examined at laparotomy for evidence of metastatic spread
8. About 40-50% of GIST patients develop recurrence after surgery despite macroscopically complete resection. The median time to recurrence is 1.5–2 years, All GIST > 2 cm are at risk for recurrence. Rectal GIST < 2cm are also at risk. Primary tumor size, mitotic rate and tumor location are the most important prognostic factors. Molecular features also predict for clinical behavior. For example, KIT exon 11 deletions in codon 557 exhibit particularly aggressive behavior.
9. GIST is considered resistant to standard chemotherapy regimens for sarcomas such as doxorubicin and ifosfamide
10. Imatinib (STI571/Glivec/Gleevec) is an orally administered small-molecule selective tyrosine kinase inhibitor that is active in GIST (Demetri et al). Imatinib inhibits the activity of tyrosine kinases such as Bcr-Abl, PDGFR-α, and the stem cell factor receptor c-*KIT*. As a competitive antagonist of ATP binding, imatinib blocks the ability of the kinases to transfer phosphate groups from ATP to tyrosine residues on substrate proteins, interrupting signal transduction
11. Clinical response to imatinib and survival rates seem to correlate with the presence or absence of certain *KIT* mutations: Mutations in exon 11 that encodes the intracellular juxtamembrane domain account for ~70% of cases and are associated with an 85% response rate to imatinib

Histologic Classification

Cell Type	% of Tumors
Spindle	70
Epithelioid	20
Mixed	10

KIT Mutations

Mutation	Site	% Incidence
Exon 11	Juxtamembrane domain	67
Exon 9	External domain	17
Exon 13	TK1	2
Exon 17	TK2	2
None*		13

*KIT/PDGFRT wild-type GIST encompasses 10-15% of GIST. Succinate-dehydrogenase deficiency accounts for a subset of wild-type GIST

Expert Opinion (*continued*)

12. Imatinib is less effective in GIST bearing mutations of KIT other than those of exon 11. Imatinib is ineffective in GIST bearing the D842V PDGFRA mutation. Imatinib is also ineffective in GIST without mutations in KIT or PDGFRA

13. The mutational status of *KIT* also seems to influence the progression-free survival, with longer survival in patients who harbor exon 11 mutations compared with those lacking an exon 11 mutation (Singer et al)

14. Because PDGFR-α is also an imatinib substrate, some tumors without *KIT* mutations respond to imatinib. However, unlike *KIT* mutations, most *PDGFR-α* mutations occur in the kinase domain and are unresponsive to imatinib

15. Over time, acquired resistance to imatinib is seen in over 80% of patients with advanced GIST. In view of the high likelihood of resistance in these patients, imatinib is now recommended in the adjuvant setting. It is possible that it will have its maximal effect in the setting of minimal disease

16. The ACOSOG Z9001 trial demonstrated that the risk of recurrence in patients with resected GIST could be reduced by 1 year of adjuvant imatinib. Subsequently, the SSGXVIII/AIO trial demonstrated that 3 years of adjuvant imatinib was superior to 1 year of therapy in patients at high risk of recurrence after surgery by prolonging both recurrence-free survival and overall survival

17. For imatinib resistant GIST, several other therapies have been approved in many countries:

    a. Sunitinib for metastatic GIST resistant to imatinib

    b. Regorafenib for GIST refractory to imatinib and sunitinib

    c. Ripretinib for GIST after treatment with three or more kinases

    d. A fifth TKI, avapritinib is active and approved in GIST bearing mutations on PDGFRA, in particular the imatinib-resistant D842V mutation.

Demetri GD et al. N Engl J Med 2002;347:472–480
Singer S et al. J Clin Oncol 2002;20:3898–3905

GIST SARCOMA • ADJUVANT

GIST SARCOMA ADJUVANT REGIMEN: IMATINIB MESYLATE FOR 1 YEAR (ACOSOG Z9001)

DeMatteo RP et al. Lancet 2009;373:1097–1104

Imatinib mesylate 400 mg/day; administer orally with food and a large glass of water (total dose/week = 2800 mg)
Notes:
• For patients unable to swallow the film-coated tablets, imatinib mesylate may be dispersed in a glass of water or apple juice. The required number of tablets should be placed in an appropriate volume of beverage (approximately 50 mL for a 100-mg tablet, and 200 mL for a 400-mg tablet) and stirred with a spoon. The suspension should be administered immediately after the tablets have completely disintegrated

Supportive Care
Antiemetic prophylaxis
Emetogenic potential is **MINIMAL TO LOW**
See Chapter 42 for antiemetic recommendations

Hematopoietic growth factor (CSF) prophylaxis
Primary prophylaxis is NOT indicated
See Chapter 43 for more information

Antimicrobial prophylaxis
Risk of fever and neutropenia is *LOW*
   Antimicrobial primary prophylaxis to be considered:
   • Antibacterial—not indicated
   • Antifungal—not indicated
   • Antiviral—not indicated unless patient previously had an episode of HSV

Diarrhea management*
Loperamide 4 mg orally initially after the first loose or liquid stool, *then* 2–4 mg orally every 2–4 hours or **diphenoxylate hydrochloride** 2.5 mg **with atropine sulfate** 0.025 mg (eg, Lomotil)

*Abigerges D et al. J Natl Cancer Inst 1994; 86:446–449
Rothenberg ML et al. J Clin Oncol 2001; 19:3801–3807
Wadler S et al. J Clin Oncol 1998; 16:3169–3178

Dose Modifications

Imatinib Dosage Levels*

Initial dose	400 mg/day
First dose reduction	300 mg/day
Second dose reduction	200 mg/day

Hematologic*

G1/2	No modifications
Recurrence of a G2 toxicity	Hold imatinib until toxicity resolves to G ≤1, then restart at 1 lower dose level
First episode of a G3/4 toxicity	Hold imatinib until toxicity resolves to G ≤1, then restart at the same dose
Second episode of a G3/4 toxicity	Hold imatinib until toxicity resolves to G ≤1, then restart at 1 lower dose level
Recurrent G2/3/4 at a reduced dose	Hold imatinib until toxicity resolves to G ≤1, then restart at 1 lower dose level, or for recurrent G4, consider discontinuing imatinib

(continued)

Dose Modifications (*continued*)

Nonhematologic	
G1	No dose modifications
First episode of a G2 toxicity	Hold imatinib until toxicity resolves to G ≤1, then restart at the same dose
Recurrence of a G2 toxicity (second G2)	Hold imatinib until toxicity resolves to G ≤1, then restart at 1 lower dose level
G3/4	Hold imatinib until toxicity resolves to G ≤1, then restart at 1 lower dose level
Recurrent G2/3/4 at a reduced dose	Hold imatinib until toxicity resolves to G ≤1, then restart at 1 dose level lower, or for recurrent G4, consider discontinuing imatinib

*No dose modifications for anemia. Growth factors were allowed but not recommended

Patient Population Studied

Randomized phase 3, double-blind, placebo-controlled, multicenter trial. Eligible patients had complete gross resection of a primary GIST ≥3 cm in size and positive for the KIT protein by immunohistochemistry. Patients were randomly assigned to imatinib 400 mg (n = 359) or to placebo (n = 354) daily for 1 year after surgical resection. Patients and investigators were blinded to the treatment assignments. Patients assigned to placebo were eligible to crossover to imatinib treatment in the event of tumor recurrence. The primary endpoint was recurrence-free survival, and analysis was by intention-to-treat. Accrual was stopped early because the trial results crossed the interim analysis efficacy boundary for recurrence-free survival in favor of imatinib

Efficacy

(N = 359)

Median Follow-up for Surviving Patients = 19.7 Months

	Imatinib	Placebo	Hazard Ratio Imatinib vs Placebo
Estimated 1-year recurrence-free survival	98% (95% CI, 96–100)	83% (95% CI, 78–88)	0.35 (95% CI, 0.22–0.53) (P<0.0001)
Recurrence free survival tumor size >3 and <6 cm			0.23 (95% CI, 0.07–0.79) (P<0.011)
Recurrence free survival tumor size >6 and <10 cm			0.50 (95% CI, 0.25–0.98) (P<0.041)
Recurrence free survival tumor size >10 cm			0.29 (95% CI, 0.16–0.55) (P<0.0001)
Overall survival			0.66 (95% CI, 0.22–2.03) (P = 0.47)
Tumor recurrence or death at median follow-up of 19.7 months			30 (8%)

Adverse Events

(N = 359)				
Dose reduction or interruption, or both			59 (16%)	
Dose reduction or interruption, because of adverse events			52 (15%)	

	Grade, Number (%)*			
	Grade 1	Grade 2	Grade 3	Grade 4
Toxicity, all patients, all toxicities	81 (24%)	148 (44%)	86 (26%)	15 (4%)
Neutropenia	23 (6%)	26 (7%)	7 (2%)	5 (1%)
Fatigue	117 (33%)	20 (5%)	5 (1%)	2 (<1%)
Dermatitis	54 (15%)	15 (4%)	11 (3%)	0
Abdominal pain	61 (17%)	25 (7%)	12 (3%)	0
Nausea	78 (22%)	14 (4%)	8 (2%)	0
Vomiting	37 (10%)	9 (2%)	8 (2%)	0
Diarrhea	79 (22%)	17 (4%)	10 (2%)	0
ALT	38 (11%)	9 (2%)	7 (2%)	2 (<1%)
AST	31 (9%)	4 (1%)	4 (1%)	3 (<1%)
Edema	220 (65%)	32 (9%)	7 (2%)	0
Hyperglycemia	27 (8%)	9 (2%)	2 (<1%)	0
Hypokalemia	28 (8%)	0	4 (1%)	0
Syncope	1 (<1%)	0	4 (1%)	0
Dyspnea	13 (3%)	1 (1%)	4 (1%)	0

*Grade 5:3 (1%)
ALT, alanine aminotransferase; AST, aspartate aminotransferase

Therapy Monitoring

1. *Day 7 and at least monthly for 6 months, then every 3 months:* history and physical examination
2. *Weekly:* complete blood count with leukocyte differential count
3. *Twice monthly first 2 months, then monthly × 6, then every 3 months:* liver function tests
4. *Every 3 months for the first 2 years, and every 6 months for the next 3 years:* CT scans with intravenous and oral contrast (or MRI with intravenous contrast) of the abdomen and pelvis

GIST SARCOMA • ADJUVANT

GIST SARCOMA ADJUVANT REGIMEN: IMATINIB MESYLATE FOR 3 YEARS (SSGXVIII/AIO)

Joensuu H et al. JAMA 2012;307:1265–1272
Joensuu H et al. J Clin Oncol 2016;34:244–250

Imatinib mesylate 400 mg/day; administer orally with food and a large glass of water (total dose/week = 2800 mg)
Notes:
- For patients unable to swallow the film-coated tablets, imatinib mesylate may be dispersed in a glass of water or apple juice. The required number of tablets should be placed in an appropriate volume of beverage (approximately 50 mL for a 100-mg tablet, and 200 mL for a 400-mg tablet) and stirred with a spoon. The suspension should be administered immediately after the tablets have completely disintegrated

Supportive Care
Antiemetic prophylaxis
Emetogenic potential is **MINIMAL TO LOW**
See Chapter 42 for antiemetic recommendations

Hematopoietic growth factor (CSF) prophylaxis
Primary prophylaxis is NOT indicated
See Chapter 43 for more information

Antimicrobial prophylaxis
Risk of fever and neutropenia is *LOW*
Antimicrobial primary prophylaxis to be considered:
- Antibacterial—not indicated
- Antifungal—not indicated
- Antiviral—not indicated unless patient previously had an episode of HSV

Diarrhea management*
Loperamide 4 mg orally initially after the first loose or liquid stool, *then* 2–4 mg orally every 2–4 hours or **diphenoxylate hydrochloride** 2.5 mg **with atropine sulfate** 0.025 mg (eg, Lomotil)

*Abigerges D et al. J Natl Cancer Inst 1994;86:446–449
Rothenberg ML et al. J Clin Oncol 2001;19:3801–3807
Wadler S et al. J Clin Oncol 1998;16:3169–3178

Patient Population Studied

Joensuu H et al. J Clin Oncol 2016;34:244–250
A randomized phase 3 multicenter trial of adjuvant imatinib as treatment of operable GIST with a high risk of recurrence (SSGXVIII/AIO) according to the modified consensus criteria (Fletcher CDM et al. Hum Pathol 2002;33:459–465). Eligible patients had complete gross resection and of a primary GIST positive that was for the KIT protein by immunohistochemistry
Patients must also have a high risk of recurrence
- Tumor diameter >10 cm
- Tumor mitosis count >10/50 high-power fields, *or*
- Tumor rupture spontaneously or at surgery
Patients were randomly assigned to imatinib 400 mg daily for 1 or 3 years after surgical resection. Stratification: (a) R0 resection, no tumor rupture; (b) R1 resection *or* tumor rupture

(continued)

Treatment Modifications

Imatinib Dosage Levels*	
Initial dose	400 mg/day
First dose reduction	300 mg/day
Second dose reduction	200 mg/day

Hematologic*	
G1/2	No modifications
First episode of a G3/4 toxicity	Hold imatinib until toxicity resolves to G ≤1, then restart at the same dose
Second episode of a G3/4 toxicity	Hold imatinib until toxicity resolves to G ≤1, then restart at 1 lower dose level
Recurrent G3/4 at a reduced dose	Hold imatinib until toxicity resolves to G ≤1, then restart at 1 dose level lower, or for recurrent G4, consider discontinuing imatinib

Nonhematologic	
G1	No dose modifications
First episode of a G2 toxicity	Hold imatinib until toxicity resolves to G ≤1, then restart at the same dose
Recurrence of a G2 toxicity (second G2)	Hold imatinib until toxicity resolves to G ≤1, then restart at 1 lower dose level
G3/4	Hold imatinib until toxicity resolves to G ≤1, then restart at 1 lower dose level
Recurrent G2/3/4 at a reduced dose	Hold imatinib until toxicity resolves to G ≤1, then restart at 1 dose level lower, or for recurrent G4, consider discontinuing imatinib

*No dose modifications for anemia. Growth factors were allowed but not recommended

Patient Population Studied (*continued*)

Demographic and Clinical Characteristics in the Intention-To-Treat Population

	Adjuvant Imatinib Therapy			
	12 Months (n = 199)		36 Months (n = 198)	
Characteristic	No.	%	No.	%
Median (range) age, years	62 (23–84)		60 (22–81)	
Sex—male / female	104/95	52/48	97/101	49/51
Median (range) body mass index, kg/m²	24.5 (16.6–42.1)		24.9 (15.2–42.8)	
ECOG performance status—0 / 1 / 2	169/26/2	85/13/1	170/27/0	86/14/0
Resected intra-abdominal metastases—yes / no	13/186	7/93	11/187	6/94
Tumor location				
Stomach	97	49	105	53
Small intestine	74	37	62	31
Colon or rectum	16	8	19	10
Esophagus	1	1	1	1
Retroperitoneal space	3	2	5	3
Other / not available	7/1	4/1	5/1	3/1
Median (range) tumor diameter, cm	9 (2–35)		10 (2–40)	
Tumor mitotic count (per 50 microscope high-power fields, by central assessment)				
<6	86	43	98	49
6–10	29	15	25	13
>10	74	37	59	30
Tumor rupture before or at surgery—no / yes	164/35	82/18	154/44	78/22
Mutation location				
KIT exon 9	12	6	14	7
KIT exon 11	130	65	129	65
KIT exon 13	3	2	2	1
PDGFRA exon 12 or 18	25	13	21	11
PDGFRA exon 18 at codon D842	18	9	15	8
None, wild-type KIT and PDGFRA	18	9	14	7
Not available	11	6	18	9

Note: percentages may not equal 100% because of rounding or missing data

ECOG, Eastern Cooperative Oncology Group; GIST, GI stromal tumor

Efficacy

Joensuu H et al. J Clin Oncol 2016;34:244–250

(Median Follow-up: 90 Months)

	Duration of Adjuvant Imatinib	
Efficacy Endpoints	12 Months N = 199*	36 Months N = 198*
Recurrence-free survival ITT population†	102 (51.3%)	124 (62.6%)
Recurrence-free survival ITT population 5 years†	52.3%	71.1%
	HR, 0.6; 95% CI, 0.44–0.81; P<0.001	
Hazard of tumor recurrence between the groups during the first year > assignment	HR, 0.65; 95% CI, 0.27–1.59	
Hazard of tumor recurrence between the groups during study months 12 and 36	HR, 0.22; 95% CI, 0.13 to 0.38; P<0.001 (smaller in 3-year than in 1-year group)	
Hazard of tumor recurrence between the groups after study month 36	HR, 1.40; 95% CI, 0.87–2.26	
Overall survival at 5 years in ITT population‡	85.3%	91.9%
	HR, 0.60; 95% CI, 0.37–0.97; P = 0.036	

Cause of Death

GIST	25 (13%)	12 (6%)
Another cause with recurrence of GIST	6 (3%)	2 (1%)
Another cause, no GIST recurrence	5 (3%)	2 (1%)

*ITT cohort

Adverse Events

Joensuu H et al. JAMA 2012;307:1265–1272

(See Also Data from Imatinib for 1 Year and Imatinib in Metastatic Disease)

	Duration of Adjuvant Imatinib		
	12 Months (N = 194*)	36 Months N = 198*	P Value
Any adverse event	192 (99%)	198 (100%)	0.24
G3/4 event	39 (20%)	65 (33%)	0.006
Cardiac event	8 (4%)	4 (2%)	0.26
Second cancer	14 (7%)	13 (7%)	0.84
Death, possibly imatinib-related	1 (1%)	0	0.49
Discontinued imatinib, no GIST recurrence	25 (13%)	51 (26%)	0.001

Most Frequent Adverse Events

	Any Grade			G3/4		
	% Any Grade		P Value	% G3/4		P Value
Duration of Imatinib	12 Months	36 Months		12 Months	36 Months	
Anorexia	72	80	0.08	1	1	1
Periorbital edema	59	74	0.002	1	1	1
Elevated LDH	43	60	0.001	0	0	—
Fatigue	48	48	1	1	1	0.62
Nausea	45	51	0.23	2	1	0.37
Diarrhea	44	54	0.044	1	2	0.37
Leukopenia	35	47	0.014	2	3	0.75
Muscle cramps	31	49	<0.001	1	1	1

*Safety cohort

Therapy Monitoring

First year:
1. *Every 1–3 months:* history and physical examination
2. *Every 2–12 weeks:* complete blood counts with leukocyte differential and serum chemistry
3. *Every 6 months:* CT/MRI of abdomen and pelvis

Years 2 and 3:
1. *Every 6 months:* history and physical examination
2. *Every 6 months:* complete blood counts with leukocyte differential and serum chemistry
3. *Every 6 months:* CT/MRI of abdomen and pelvis

GIST SARCOMA • ADJUVANT

GIST SARCOMA ADJUVANT (5 YEARS) REGIMEN: IMATINIB MESYLATE

Raut CP et al. JAMA Oncol 2018;4:e184060
Supplements to: Raut CP et al. JAMA Oncol 2018;4:e184060

Imatinib mesylate 400 mg/day; administer orally with food and a large glass of water (total dose/week = 2800 mg)
Notes:
• For patients unable to swallow the film-coated tablets, imatinib mesylate may be dispersed in a glass of water or apple juice. The required number of tablets should be placed in an appropriate volume of beverage (approximately 50 mL for a 100-mg tablet, and 200 mL for a 400-mg tablet) and stirred with a spoon. The suspension should be administered immediately after the tablets have completely disintegrated

Supportive Care
Antiemetic prophylaxis
Emetogenic potential is MINIMAL TO LOW
See Chapter 42 for antiemetic recommendations

Hematopoietic growth factor (CSF) prophylaxis
Primary prophylaxis is NOT indicated
See Chapter 43 for more information

Antimicrobial prophylaxis
Risk of fever and neutropenia is *LOW*
Antimicrobial primary prophylaxis to be considered:
• Antibacterial—not indicated
• Antifungal—not indicated
• Antiviral—not indicated unless patient previously had an episode of HSV

Diarrhea management*
Loperamide 4 mg orally initially after the first loose or liquid stool, *then* 2–4 mg orally every 2–4 hours or **diphenoxylate hydrochloride** 2.5 mg **with atropine sulfate** 0.025 mg (eg, Lomotil)

*Abigerges D et al. J Natl Cancer Inst 1994;86:446–449
Rothenberg ML et al. J Clin Oncol 2001;19:3801–3807
Wadler S et al. J Clin Oncol 1998;16:3169–3178

Treatment Modifications

Imatinib Dosage Levels*

Initial dose	400 mg/day
First dose reduction	300 mg/day
Second dose reduction	200 mg/day

Hematologic*

G1/2	No modifications
First episode of a G3/4 toxicity	Hold imatinib until toxicity resolves to G ≤1, then restart at the same dose
Second episode of a G3/4 toxicity	Hold imatinib until toxicity resolves to G ≤1, then restart at 1 lower dose level
Recurrent G3/4 at a reduced dose	Hold imatinib until toxicity resolves to G ≤1, then restart at 1 dose level lower, or for recurrent G4, consider discontinuing imatinib

Nonhematologic

G1	No dose modifications
First episode of a G2 toxicity	Hold imatinib until toxicity resolves to G ≤1, then restart at the same dose
Recurrence of a G2 toxicity (second G2)	Hold imatinib until toxicity resolves to G ≤1, then restart at 1 lower dose level
G3/4	Hold imatinib until toxicity resolves to G ≤1, then restart at 1 lower dose level
Recurrent G2/3/4 at a reduced dose	Hold imatinib until toxicity resolves to G ≤1, then restart at 1 dose level lower, or for recurrent G4, consider discontinuing imatinib

*No dose modifications for anemia

Patient Population Studied

The PERSIST–5 trial was a prospective, single-arm, non-randomized, open-label, phase 2 trial that assessed 5 years of adjuvant imatinib therapy for primary gastrointestinal stromal tumor (GIST). Eligible patients were aged ≥18 years with primary GIST expressing KIT confirmed by immunohistochemistry who had received macroscopically complete resection within 12 weeks prior to initiation of imatinib therapy. All participants had an ECOG PS ≤1, intermediate- to high-risk of recurrence (primary GIST at any site, ≥2 cm or larger with ≥5 mitoses per 50 high-power field or non-gastric primary GIST measuring ≥5 cm)

Patient Population (n = 91)

Median (range) age, years	60 (30–90)
Male sex	53%
Race	
Caucasian	80%
Black	11%
Asian	4%
Native American / Pacific Islander /Other	4%
ECOG Performance Status—0 / 1	65% / 35%
Primary lesion location	
Stomach	55%
Small bowel	36%
Other	9%
Median (range) tumor size, cm	6.5 (2.3–30.0)
Median (range) mitoses, count per 50 HPF	7 (0–87)
Risk stratification—intermediate / high	26% / 74%
Resection margins—R0 / R1 / unknown	99% / 0 / 1
Median (range) time from diagnosis to imatinib, weeks	10.3 (3.1–23.9)
Median (range) time from surgery to imatinib, weeks	9.6 (3.1–12.3)
Prior adjuvant imatinib prior to enrollment	7%
Median (range) duration of prior adjuvant imatinib, days	21.5 (9–29)

ECOG, Eastern Cooperative Oncology Group; HPR, high-power field

Efficacy

Efficacy Outcome (n = 91)	
Median (range) treatment duration, mo	55.1 (0.5–60.6)
5-year recurrence-free survival, % (95% CI)	90 (80–95)
Recurrent disease, no (%)*	7 (8)
5-year overall survival rate, % (95% CI)	95 (86–99)

*Seven patients experienced recurrent disease, including one during therapy with imatinib (*PDGFRA*-D842V mutation) and six after discontinuing imatinib therapy
CI, confidence interval

Adverse Events

Grade (%) (N = 91)	All Grade	Grade 3–4
Nausea	61.5	1.1
Diarrhea	49.5	2.2
Fatigue	37.4	1.1
Periorbital edema	33.0	0
Muscle spasms	31.9	1.1
Vomiting	26.4	0
Rash	23.1	0
Peripheral edema	16.5	0
Abdominal pain	12.1	2.2
Anemia	11.0	1.1
Flatulence	11.0	0

Note: all patients experienced at least one adverse event

Therapy Monitoring

First year:
1. *Every 1–3 months:* history and physical examination
2. *Every 2–12 weeks:* complete blood counts with leukocyte differential and serum chemistry
3. *Every 6 months:* CT/MRI of abdomen and pelvis

Years 2 to 5:
1. *Every 6 months:* history and physical examination
2. *Every 6 months:* complete blood counts with leukocyte differential and serum chemistry
3. *Every 6 months initially (years 2–3), then every 6–12 months (years 4–5):* CT/MRI of abdomen and pelvis

METASTATIC/SURGICALLY UNRESECTABLE • GIST SARCOMA

METASTATIC/SURGICALLY UNRESECTABLE GIST SARCOMA REGIMEN: IMATINIB MESYLATE

Blanke CD et al. J Clin Oncol 2008;26:626–632
Verweij J et al. Lancet 2004;364:1127–1134

Starting dose: **Imatinib mesylate** 400 mg/day; administer orally with food and a large glass of water (total dose/week = 2800 mg)
Dose escalation: **Imatinib** 600–800 mg/day; administer orally with food and a large glass of water (total dose/week = 4200–5600 mg)

Notes:
- 400- and 600-mg doses may be given once daily, or, alternatively, may be split into 2 equal doses, one given during morning hours and a second dose during the evening
- 800-mg daily doses should be given as two 400-mg doses, one during morning hours and a second dose during the evening
- For patients unable to swallow the film-coated tablets, imatinib mesylate may be dispersed in a glass of water or apple juice. The required number of tablets should be placed in an appropriate volume of beverage (approximately 50 mL for a 100-mg tablet, and 200 mL for a 400-mg tablet) and stirred with a spoon. The suspension should be administered immediately after the tablets have completely disintegrated

Supportive Care
Antiemetic prophylaxis
Emetogenic potential is **MINIMAL TO LOW**
See Chapter 42 for antiemetic recommendations

Hematopoietic growth factor (CSF) prophylaxis
Primary prophylaxis is NOT indicated
See Chapter 43 for more information

Antimicrobial prophylaxis
Risk of fever and neutropenia is LOW
Antimicrobial primary prophylaxis to be considered:
- Antibacterial—not indicated
- Antifungal—not indicated
- Antiviral—not indicated unless patient previously had an episode of HSV

Diarrhea management*
Loperamide 4 mg orally initially after the first loose or liquid stool, *then* 2–4 mg orally every 2–4 hours or **diphenoxylate hydrochloride** 2.5 mg **with atropine sulfate** 0.025 mg (eg, Lomotil)

*Abigerges D et al. J Natl Cancer Inst 1994;86:446–449
Rothenberg ML et al. J Clin Oncol 2001;19:3801–3807
Wadler S et al. J Clin Oncol 1998;16:3169–3178

Patient Population Studied

A total of 746 patients metastatic or surgically unresectable GIST were eligible for this phase 3 open-label clinical trial. At registration, patients were randomly assigned to either standard- or high-dose imatinib with close interval follow-up. If objective progression occurred by RECIST, patients on the standard-dose arm could reregister to the trial and receive the high-dose imatinib regimen. Patients were required to have measurable or nonmeasurable, visceral or intra-abdominal, biopsy-proven GIST, which were not surgically curable. Tumors had to express CD117 by immunohistochemical staining. Any number of prior chemotherapy regimens was allowed

Treatment Modifications

Imatinib Dose Levels*

800 mg
600 mg
400 mg
300 mg
200 mg

Hematologic*

G1/2	No modifications
Recurrence of a G2 toxicity	Hold imatinib until toxicity resolves to G ≤1, then restart with dose decreased by 1 dose level
First episode of a G3/4 toxicity	Hold imatinib until toxicity resolves to G ≤1, then restart at the same dose
Second episode of a G3/4 toxicity	Hold imatinib until toxicity resolves to G ≤1, then restart with dose decreased by 1 dose level
Recurrent G2/3/4 at a reduced dose	Hold imatinib until toxicity resolves to G ≤1, then restart with dose decreased by 1 dose level, or, for recurrent G4 adverse effects, consider discontinuing imatinib

Nonhematologic

G1	No dose modifications
First episode of a G2 toxicity	Hold imatinib until toxicity resolves to G ≤1, then restart at the same dose
Recurrence of a G2 toxicity (second G2)	Hold imatinib until toxicity resolves to G ≤1, then restart with dose decreased by 1 dose level
G3/4	Hold imatinib until toxicity resolves to G ≤1, then restart with dose decreased by 1 dose level
Recurrent G2/3/4 at a reduced dose	Hold imatinib until toxicity resolves to G ≤1, then restart with dose decreased by 1 dose level, or for recurrent G4 adverse effects, consider discontinuing imatinib

*No dose modifications for anemia. Hematopoietic growth factors are allowed but not recommended

Efficacy

Blanke CD et al. J Clin Oncol 2008;26:626–632

Response	400 mg/day* Number	%	800 mg/day Number	%
Complete response	17	5	12	3
Partial response	137	40	148	42
Stable/no response	85	25	76	22
Progressive disease/early death	42	12	37	10
Assessment inadequate	34	10	52	15
Total	345	100	349	100

*After progression on 400 mg/day, 33% of patients who crossed over to 800 mg/day achieved either an objective response or stable disease

Best Overall Response to Treatment (Intention-to-treat Analysis)
Verweij J et al. Lancet 2004;364:1127–1134; RECIST

	400 mg Once Daily (n = 473)	400 mg Twice Daily (n = 473)
Complete response	5%	6%
Partial response	45%	48%
No change	32%	32%
Progression	13%	9%
Not assessable	5%	5%

Notes: These studies confirmed the effectiveness of imatinib as primary systemic therapy for patients with incurable GIST but showed limited advantage to higher dose (800 mg) treatment. The authors concluded:
- It appears reasonable to initiate therapy with 400 mg daily and to consider dose escalation on progression of disease (Blanke CD et al. J Clin Oncol 2008; 26:626–632)
- If response induction is the only aim of treatment, a daily dose of 400 mg of imatinib is sufficient; however, a dose of 400 mg twice daily achieves significantly longer progression-free survival

Adverse Event

Blanke CD et al. J Clin Oncol 2008;26:626–632; **National Cancer Institute (USA), Common Toxicity Criteria, version 2.0 (NCI CTC v2.0)**

Adverse Events	400 mg/day (n = 344) %G3	%G4	%G5	800 mg/day (n = 347) %G3	%G4	%G5
Death, cause undetermined	0	0	0	0	0	1
Allergy/ immunology	0	0	0	<0.5	0	0
Auditory/hearing	0	0	0	<0.5	0	0
Blood/bone marrow	15	4	<0.5	19	8	0
Cardiovascular, arrhythmia	2	0	0	1	0	<0.5
Cardiovascular, general	4	1	0	10	2	0
Constitutional symptoms	4	1	0	8	1	<0.5
Dermatology/ skin	4	<0.5	0	7	<0.5	0
Gastrointestinal	8	1	0	15	1	0

Adverse Events	400 mg/day (n = 344) %G3	%G4	%G5	800 mg/day (n = 347) %G3	%G4	%G5
Hemorrhage	4	1	1	8	2	1
Hepatic	4	0	0	2	1	<0.5
Infection/febrile neutropenia	4	1	0	5	1	1
Metabolic/ laboratory	2	0	0	2	1	0
Musculoskeletal	1	0	0	1	0	0
Neurology	3	1	0	2	0	1
Ocular/visual	0	0	0	1	0	0
Pain	10	1	0	11	1	0
Pulmonary	2	1	0	4	0	0
Renal/ genitourinary	1	0	0	1	1	0
Syndrome	0	0	0	<0.5	0	0

(continued)

Adverse Events (*continued*)

Verweij J et al. Lancet 2004; 364:1127–1134*†

	400 mg Once Daily (n = 470)				400 mg Twice Daily (n = 472)			
	%G1	%G2	%G3	%G4	%G1	%G2	%G3	%G4
Any side effect	21	46	26	6.2	8.7	40	43	7.6
Anemia	55	27	5.5	1.5	41	40	12	5.1
Leucopenia	27	13	2.7	—	29	16	2.1	0.4
Granulocytopenia	20	13	4.3	2.7	19	17	4.7	2.3
Thrombocytopenia	3.8	0.6	1	0.4	4	1.3	0.4	0.8
Edema	50	18	2.7	0.2	42	36	8.7	0.4
Fatigue	45	19	6	—	38	31	11	0.2
Fever	8.3	2.7	0.8	—	13	3.2	1.3	—
Pruritus	12	3.6	0.8	—	15	7.6	1.5	—
Rash	17	7.2	2.3	—	26	16	5.1	0.2
Anorexia	16	7.8	1.7	0.2	25	13	1.7	—
Constipation	11	3.8	0.8	0.2	13	4	1.5	—
Diarrhea	34	12	1.5	0.2	36	15	5.3	—
Nausea	36	10	2.5	—	36	21	3.2	—
Vomiting	18	5.3	2.5	0.2	23	13	2.8	—
Bleeding	7.2	<1	2.5	0.2	14	0.6	6.4	1.7
Infection	7.2	7.2	2.5	0.2	8.7	7.6	4.4	0.2
Dizziness	9.4	1.4	0.2	—	11	1.9	0.4	—
Arthralgia	11	2.3	—	—	12	3.2	0.8	—
Headache	13	3.2	0.2	—	11	1.7	0.8	—
Myalgia	19	5.7	0.2	—	19	7.4	1	—
Pleuritic pain	34	13	4	0.4	30	18	7	0.2
Cough	11	1.7	0.2	—	11	2.8	0.2	—
Dyspnea	—	8.3	3	0.2	—	13	3.4	1
Renal or genitourinary	9.1	3.4	0.4	0.2	10	4.7	2.1	0.6

*NCI CTC v2.0
†Data are the percentage of patients who started treatment per protocol

Therapy Monitoring

1. *Day 7 and at least monthly for 6 months, then every 3 months:* history and physical examination
2. *Weekly:* complete blood count with leukocyte differential
3. *Twice monthly for the first 2 months, then monthly for 6 months, then every 3 months:* liver function tests
4. *At the end of month 2, and every 3 months thereafter:* radiographic assessments using the same modality as had been performed at baseline

MALIGNANT • METASTATIC/SURGICALLY UNRESECTABLE • GIST SARCOMA

METASTATIC/SURGICALLY UNRESECTABLE GIST SARCOMA REGIMEN: SUNITINIB

George S et al: Eur J Cancer 2009;45:1959–1968
Demetri GD et al. Lancet 2006;368:1329–1338

Sunitinib malate 50 mg per dose; administer orally once daily, continually, without regard for meals, in 6-week cycles consisting of 4 consecutive weeks of daily treatment followed by 2 weeks without treatment, until disease progression (total dose/6-week cycle = 1400 mg)

Alternate continuous schedule:
Sunitinib malate 37.5 mg per dose; administer orally once daily, continually, without regard for meals, until disease progression (total dose/week = 262.5 mg)

Notes:
- Patients who delay taking sunitinib malate at a regularly scheduled time may take a missed dose if the interval remaining before the next regularly scheduled dose is ≥12 hours
- Dose interruption and dose modifications in 12.5-mg increments or decrements are recommended based on individual safety and tolerability
- Strong CYP3A4 inhibitors may increase sunitinib plasma concentrations
  - When medically appropriate, replace concomitant strong CYP3A4 inhibitors with medications that do not or minimally inhibit CYP3A4
  - A dose reduction should be considered if sunitinib must be co-administered with a strong CYP3A4 inhibitor
- CYP3A4 inducers such as rifampin may decrease sunitinib plasma concentrations
  - When medically appropriate, replace concomitant CYP3A4 inducers with medications that do not or minimally induce CYP3A4
  - A dose increase for sunitinib should be considered if sunitinib must be co-administered with a CYP3A4 inducer
  - *Dose adjustment for renal impairment:*
    - Creatinine clearance ≥30 mL/min: No initial adjustment necessary
    - End-stage renal disease (ESRD) on hemodialysis: No initial adjustment necessary. Sunitinib exposure is 47% lower in patients with ESRD on hemodialysis, and doses may need to be increased gradually up to 2-fold based on tolerability

Supportive Care
Antiemetic prophylaxis
Emetogenic potential is **MINIMAL TO LOW**
See Chapter 42 for antiemetic recommendations

Hematopoietic growth factor (CSF) prophylaxis
Primary prophylaxis is NOT indicated
See Chapter 43 for more information

Antimicrobial prophylaxis
Risk of fever and neutropenia is *LOW*
  Antimicrobial primary prophylaxis to be considered:
  - Antibacterial—not indicated
  - Antifungal—not indicated
  - Antiviral—not indicated unless patient previously had an episode of HSV

Diarrhea management*
Loperamide 4 mg orally initially after the first loose or liquid stool, *then* 2–4 mg orally every 2–4 hours or **diphenoxylate hydrochloride** 2.5 mg **with atropine sulfate** 0.025 mg (eg, Lomotil)

*Abigerges D et al. J Natl Cancer Inst 1994;86:446–449
Rothenberg ML et al. J Clin Oncol 2001;19:3801–3807
Wadler S et al. J Clin Oncol 1998;16:3169–3178

Hand-foot reaction (palmar-plantar erythrodysesthesia, PPE)
- For patients who develop a hand-foot reaction, use topical emollients (eg, Aquaphor), topical or orally administered steroids, antihistamine agents (H_1-receptor antagonists), or pyridoxine
- Pyridoxine may provide relief for discomfort/pain associated with PPE, although the mechanism through which this occurs remains unclear
- The suggested pyridoxine starting dose is 50 mg/day, which may be increased to a maximum of 200 mg/day

Treatment Modifications

Sunitinib Dose Levels

	4 Weeks on/2 Weeks off Schedule	Continuous Schedule
Dose level +1*	—	50 mg once daily, continuously
Starting dose	50 mg once daily, 4 weeks on/2 weeks off	37.5 mg once daily, continuously
Dose Level (−1)	37.5 mg once daily, 4 weeks on/2 weeks off	25 mg once daily, continuously
Dose Level (−2)	25 mg once daily, 4 weeks on/2 weeks off	Discontinue sunitinib
Dose Level −3	Discontinue sunitinib	—

*Consider escalating to 50 mg/day for patients experiencing treatment-related nonhematologic adverse effects (AEs) of G ≤1 or hematologic AEs of G ≤2 during the first 8 weeks of therapy

Adverse Event	Treatment Modification
Cutaneous Toxicities	
Rash G ≥2	Withhold sunitinib and provide immediate symptomatic treatment. When toxicity resolves to G ≤1, restart sunitinib at 1 dose level lower than the dose level administered at the time toxicity developed. Treatment for symptoms may continue indefinitely as a preventive measure *Note: discontinue therapy if sunitinib withheld >3 weeks*
Recurrence of G3/4 cutaneous toxicity at reduced doses of sunitinib	Withhold sunitinib and provide immediate symptomatic treatment. When toxicity resolves to G ≤1, restart sunitinib at 1 dose level lower than the dose level administered at the time toxicity developed. Treatment for symptoms may continue indefinitely as a preventive measure
Recurrence of G3/4 cutaneous toxicity at dose level −2 of sunitinib	Discontinue therapy
Cutaneous toxicity does not recur at reduced sunitinib treatment doses with or without continued for symptoms	Sunitinib dose may be increased 1 dose level to that administered at the time cutaneous toxicity developed. If toxicity recurs following the increase, then again withhold sunitinib and provide immediate symptomatic treatment. When toxicity resolves to G ≤1, restart sunitinib at 1 dose level lower than the dose level administered at the time toxicity developed. Treatment for symptoms may continue indefinitely as a preventive measure
Diarrhea	
G1/2 diarrhea (increase of 4–6 stools/day over baseline; limiting instrumental ADLs)	Focus on treatment for symptoms designed to resolve the diarrhea. No dose modifications are made for G1/2 diarrhea unless G2 diarrhea persists >2 weeks
G2 diarrhea persisting >2 weeks	Follow the guidelines below for G3/4 diarrhea
G2 diarrhea lasting >2 weeks *or* G3/4 diarrhea *or* diarrhea that worsens by 1 grade while on sunitinib	Withhold sunitinib until diarrhea resolves to G ≤1. If resolution occurs within 3 weeks of holding treatment, restart sunitinib at 1 dose level lower than the dose level administered at the time diarrhea developed *Note: discontinue therapy if sunitinib withheld >3 weeks*
Recurrence of G2 diarrhea lasting >2 weeks *or* G3/4 diarrhea at reduced sunitinib doses and dose level is (−1)	Withhold sunitinib until toxicity resolves to G ≤1, then restart sunitinib at dose level −2. Treatment for symptoms may continue indefinitely as a preventive measure
Recurrence of G2 diarrhea lasting >2 weeks or G3/4 diarrhea at dose level (−2)	Discontinue therapy
Diarrhea does not recur at reduced sunitinib doses with or without continued treatment for symptoms	Sunitinib dose may be increased 1 dose level to the dose level administered at the time the diarrhea developed. If toxicity recurs following the increase, then again withhold sunitinib and provide immediate symptomatic treatment. When toxicity resolves to G ≤1, restart sunitinib at 1 dose level lower than the dose level administered at the time toxicity developed. Treatment for symptoms may continue indefinitely as a preventive measure

(continued)

Treatment Modifications (continued)

Hypertension

Note: patients should have their blood pressure checked once weekly during their first 24 weeks of therapy and for an 8-week period after an adjustment in their sunitinib dose

G1 hypertension (SBP 120–139 or DBP 80–89 mm Hg)	Continue sunitinib at same dose and schedule
G2 asymptomatic hypertension (SBP140–159 or DBP 90–99 mm Hg if previously WNL; change in baseline medical intervention indicated; recurrent or persistent [≥24 hours]; symptomatic increase DBP >20 mm Hg or to >140/90 mm Hg; monotherapy indicated initiated)	Treat with antihypertensive medications and continue sunitinib at same dose and schedule
G2 symptomatic, or persistent G2 despite antihypertensive medications, or DBP ≥110 mm Hg, or G3 hypertension (SBP ≥160 or DBP ≥100 mm Hg; medical intervention indicated; >1 drug or more intensive therapy than previously used indicated)	Withhold sunitinib and treat with antihypertensive medications until symptoms resolve and diastolic BP <100 mm Hg. Then continue sunitinib at 1 dose level lower *Note: discontinue therapy if sunitinib withheld >3 weeks*
G4 hypertension (life-threatening consequences; urgent intervention indicated)	Discontinue therapy

Miscellaneous

G3/4 hepatotoxicity (ALT/AST >5 × ULN if baseline was normal; >5 × baseline if baseline was abnormal; bilirubin >3 × ULN if baseline was normal; >3 × baseline if baseline was abnormal)	Withhold sunitinib until LFTs resolve to baseline or G ≤1. If resolution occurs within 3 weeks of holding treatment, restart sunitinib at 1 dose level lower than the dose level administered at the time hepatotoxicity was noted *Note: discontinue therapy if sunitinib withheld >3 weeks or if worsening occurs off therapy*
Any other G3/4 nonhematologic toxicity (eg, persistent nausea, vomiting, despite maximum supportive treatment)	Withhold treatment until toxicity improves to G ≤1, then resume with dose reduced by 1 level
Wound dehiscence or poor wound healing	Interrupt sunitinib until wound has adequately healed
LVEF decrease by ≥10% to <LLN, clinical heart failure syndrome, necrotizing fasciitis, EM, SJS, TEN, or TMA	Permanently discontinue sunitinib
Proteinuria	If urine dipstick ≥2+, obtain 24-hour urine protein. If 24-hour urine protein ≥3 g, interrupt treatment. Resume treatment when 24-hour urine protein ≤1 g. Resume sunitinib at 1 dose level lower
Repeat episodes of 24-hour urine protein ≥3 g despite dose reductions or nephrotic syndrome	Discontinue sunitinib
Coadministration of potent CYP3A4 inhibitors (eg, ketoconazole, itraconazole, voriconazole, clarithromycin, atazanavir, ritonavir, telithromycin)	Reduce sunitinib dose
Coadministration of potent CYP3A inducers (eg, rifampin, phenytoin, phenobarbital, carbamazepine)	Increase sunitinib dose (to a maximum of 87.5 mg daily)

EM, erythema multiforme; LLN, lower limit of normal; LVEF, left ventricular ejection fraction; SJS, Stevens-Johnson syndrome; TEN, toxic epidermal necrolysis; TMA, thrombotic microangiopathy

Patient Population Studied

Demetri GD et al. Lancet 2006;368:1329–1338

Patients with histologically proven malignant gastrointestinal stromal tumor that was not amenable to surgery, radiation, or a combination of different approaches with curative intent. Patients also must have had confirmed objective failure of previous imatinib therapy based either on progression of disease or unacceptably severe toxic effects during imatinib therapy that precluded further treatment. The last imatinib should have been administered at least 2 weeks before randomization

(continued)

Patient Population Studied (continued)

Baseline Characteristics and Disease and Treatment History (ITT Population)

	Sunitinib (n = 207)	Placebo (n = 105)
Age (years)—median (range)	58.0 (23–84)	55.0 (23–81)
Sex		
Sex—male / female	132 (63.8%) / 75 (36.2%)	64 (61.0%) / 41 (39.0%)
Female		
ECOG status 0/1	92 (44.4%) / 113 (54.6%)	48 (45.7%) / 55 (52.4%)
GIST histology		
Spindle cell	125 (60.4%)	74 (70.5%)
Mixed spindle + epithelioid	33 (15.9%)	13 (12.4%)
Epithelioid	17 (8.2%)	7 (6.7%)
Other	31 (15.0%)	10 (9.5%)
Missing	1 (0.5%)	1 (1.0%)
Tumor burden at baseline (mm)—median (range)	233 (26–722)	239 (29–749)
Maximum dose of imatinib therapy (mg)—median (range)	800 (300–1600)	800 (400–1600)
Duration imatinib therapy (weeks)—median (range)	105.3 (0.3–205.1)	106.9 (11.4–187.7)
Imatinib therapy outcome		
Progression within 6 mos	36 (17.4%)	17 (16.2%)
Progression after >6 mos	162 (78.3%)	84 (80.0%)
Intolerance	9 (4.3%)	4 (3.8%)
Best response to imatinib		
Complete response	6 (2.9%)	1 (1.0%)
Partial response	51 (24.6%)	36 (34.3%)
Stable disease	87 (42.0%)	36 (34.3%)
Progressive disease	58 (28.0%)	30 (28.6%)

George S et al: Eur J Cancer 2009;45:1959–1968

Open-label, multicenter, phase 2 study with patients randomized (1:1) to receive continuous daily oral sunitinib either in the morning or in the evening. The starting sunitinib dose was 37.5 mg/day. Patients still experiencing clinical benefit after 1 year were offered continued sunitinib treatment on a separate treatment-continuation protocol, follow-up on which is ongoing

Baseline Characteristics, Therapy Details, and Disposition of Patients Treated with Sunitinib on a Continuous Daily Dosing Schedule

	All Patients (N = 60)	
	n	%
Baseline characteristics		
Sex—male / female	28 / 32	47 / 53
Median age (range), years	59 (24–84)	
ECOG performance status—0 / 1 / 2	34 / 25 / 1	57 / 42 / 1

(continued)

Patient Population Studied

Baseline Characteristics, Therapy Details, and Disposition of Patients Treated with Sunitinib on a Continuous Daily Dosing Schedule

	All Patients (N = 60)	
	n	%
Prior imatinib therapy		
Reason for discontinuation		
Tumor progression / intolerance	57 / 3	95 / 5
Median maximum dose (range), mg/day	800 (200–1200)	
Median duration of treatment (range), weeks	109 (2–269)	
Best response: CR / PRT / SD / PD	3 / 17 / 29 / 11	5 / 28 / 48 / 18
Continuous daily dosing of sunitinib		
Median number of cycles started (range)	11 (1–24)	
Median number of weeks on treatment (range)	46 (2–93)	
Median number of weeks administered (range)	40 (0.4–91)	
Dose interruptions	46	77
Median percentage of days with interruptions (range)	4 (0–46)	
Most common AEs leading to interruption		
Neutropenia	8	17*
Diarrhea	7	15*
Asthenia	6	13*
Vomiting	6	13*
Dose escalations to 50 mg	2	3
Reductions back to 37.5 mg	1	50†
Dose reductions	14	23
From 37.5 mg to 25 mg	14	23
From 25 mg to 12.5 mg	3	5
Escalations back to 25 mg and 37.5 mg	8	57†
Most common AEs leading to reduction		
Asthenia	2	14‡
Fatigue	2	14‡
Stomatitis	2	14‡
Patient disposition		
Completed	26	43
Discontinuations	34	57

(continued)

Patient Population Studied (*continued*)

Baseline Characteristics, Therapy Details, and Disposition of Patients Treated with Sunitinib on a Continuous Daily Dosing Schedule

	All Patients (N = 60)	
	n	**%**
Primary reason for discontinuation		
Disease progression	21	62[§]
Death	7[¶]	21[§]
Adverse event	4	12[§]
Other cancer treatment	2	6[§]

*Percentage based on all patients with dose interruptions
[†]Percentage of patients who returned to original dose after dose escalation or reduction
[‡]Percentage based on all patients with dose reductions
[§]Percentage based on all patients who discontinued
[¶]Due to disease progression (n = 3), adverse event (n = 3; one peritonitis and one bilateral stroke, both disease-related; one treatment-related septic shock) and unknown (n = 1)

Efficacy

Demetri GD et al. Lancet 2006;368:1329–1338

Endpoint	Sunitinib Duration (95% CI)	Placebo Duration (95% CI)	Hazard Ratio HR (95% CI)
Median time to tumor progression for the ITT population*	27.3 weeks (16–32.1)	6.4 weeks (4.4–10)	HR 0.33 (0.23–0.47) P<0.0001
Median duration of progression-free survival	24.1 weeks (11.1–28.3)	6 weeks (4.4–9.9)	HR 0.33 (0.24–0.47) P<0.0001
Percent progression-free ≥26 weeks[†]	16% (33)	1% (1)	—
Overall survival[‡]			HR 0.49 (0.29–0.83) P = 0.007
Median time to tumor response	10.4 weeks (9.7–16.1)		

Response Rates

	Partial Response	Stable Disease	Progressive Disease
Best tumor response (ITT population)	7% (14)[§,¶]	58% (120)	19% (39)
Patients who entered study > disease progression on imatinib (N = 198)	5.1% (10)		
Patients who crossed over to sunitinib from placebo group (N = 59)	10.2% (3.8–20.8)	7% (4)**	
Patients classified as intolerant to imatinib and randomized to sunitinib (N = 9)	44% (4)[††]		11% (1)

*Central radiology assessment
[†]26 weeks (~6 months) predefined as point most clinicians agree clinically meaningful
[‡]Despite option to cross over. Also note that since > half the patients in sunitinib group were still alive at interim analysis, a median overall survival value could not be calculated
[§]Although low, higher than with placebo (7% [14] vs. none; 95% CI 3.7–11.1%; P = 0.006)
[¶]Only 3 of 14 had progression at interim analysis, so duration of response could not be reliably estimated; observed duration of response for the 3 patients: 15.9–29.9 weeks
**Stable disease for at least 26 weeks after crossover
[††]Although numbers small, seemed better in patients intolerant of imatinib than in those resistant to imatinib

Efficacy (continued)

Clinical response to continuous daily dosing of sunitinib

George S et al: Eur J Cancer 2009;45:1959–1968

Objective Response	All Patients (N = 60)		Morning Dosing (n = 30)		Evening Dosing (n = 30)	
	n	%	n	%	n	%
PR	8	13	3	10	5	17
SD	40	67	20	67	20	67
≥12 weeks	33	55	19	63	14	47
≥24 weeks	24	40	12	40	12	40
PD	6	10	2	7	4	13
Not evaluable	6	10	5	17	1	3
Clinical benefit* rate (95% CI)	32	53 (40–66)	15	50 (31–69)	17	57 (37–75)

*CR + PR + SD ≥24 weeks

Adverse Events

Demetri GD et al. Lancet 2006;368:1329–1338 (N = 202)

Adverse Events That Occurred with a Frequency of at Least 5% Greater with Sunitinib Than Placebo in Per-protocol Population*

Nonhematologic	Number (%)		
	Grade 1/2	Grade 3	Grade 4
Fatigue	58 (29%)	10 (5%)	0
Diarrhea	52 (26%)	7 (3%)	0
Skin discoloration	50 (25%)	0	0
Nausea	47 (23%)	1 (1%)	0
Anorexia	38 (19%)	0	0
Dysgeusia	36 (18%)	0	0
Stomatitis	30 (15%)	1 (1%)	0
Vomiting	30 (15%)	1 (1%)	0
Hand-foot syndrome	19 (9%)	9 (4%)	0
Rash	24 (12%)	2 (1%)	0
Asthenia	18 (9%)	6 (3%)	0
Mucosal inflammation	24 (12%)	0	0
Dyspepsia	22 (11%)	1 (1%)	0

Nonhematologic	Number (%)		
Hypertension	15 (8%)	6 (3%)	0
Epistaxis	14 (7%)	0	0
Hair-color changes	14 (7%)	0	0
Dry mouth	13 (6%)	0	0
Glossodynia	11 (6%)	0	0
Hematologic			
Anemia	117 (58%)	7 (4%)	0
Leucopenia	104 (52%)	7 (4%)	0
Neutropenia	86 (43%)	17 (8%)	3 (2%)
Lymphopenia	80 (40%)	18 (9%)	1 (1%)
Thrombo-cytopenia	72 (36%)	8 (4%)	1 (1%)

*National Cancer Institute (USA), Common Terminology Criteria for Adverse Events, version 3.0

(continued)

Adverse Events (continued)

George S et al: Eur J Cancer 2009;45:1959–1968

Adverse Event or Laboratory Abnormality	Grades 1 and 2				Grade 3				Grade 4				Any Grade	
	Morning (n = 30)		Morning (n = 30)		Morning (n = 30)		Evening (n = 30)		Morning (n = 30)		Evening (n = 30)		All Patients (n = 60)	
	n	%	n	%	n	%	n	%	n	%	n	%	n	%
Treatment-related Nonhematologic Adverse Events (Occurring in ≥15% of Patients)														
Diarrhea	10	33	9	30	4	13	1	3	0	0	0	0	24	40
Asthenia	10	33	6	20	2	7	4	13	0	0	0	0	22	37
Fatigue	10	33	6	20	1	3	3	10	0	0	0	0	20	33
Hypertension	6	20	6	20	3	10	2	7	0	0	0	0	17	28
Nausea	8	27	7	23	0	0	1	3	0	0	0	0	16	27
Hand-foot syndrome	8	27	5	17	0	0	2	7	0	0	0	0	15	25
Vomiting	9	30	5	17	0	0	0	0	0	0	0	0	14	23
Hair color changes	7	23	6	20	0	0	0	0	0	0	0	0	13	22
Stomatitis	6	20	5	17	1	3	1	3	0	0	0	0	13	22
Anorexia	5	17	6	20	1	3	0	0	0	0	0	0	12	20
Mucosal inflammation	3	10	8	27	0	0	0	0	0	0	0	0	11	18
Upper abdominal pain	5	17	6	20	0	0	0	0	0	0	0	0	11	18
Increased blood TSH	5	17	4	13	0	0	0	0	0	0	0	0	9	15
Hematologic Laboratory Abnormalities														
Hemoglobin	23	77	21	70	2	7	2	7	1	3	1	3	50	83
Leukocytes	19	63	21	70	5	17	2	7	0	0	0	0	47	78
Neutrophils	11	37	15	50	5	17	3	10	0	0	0	0	34	57
Lymphocytes	7	23	6	20	8	27	7	23	1	3	0	0	29	48
Platelets	12	40	10	33	1	3	1	3	0	0	0	0	24	40

TSH, thyroid stimulating hormone

Therapy Monitoring

1. *Prior to the first cycle of sunitinib:* electrocardiogram (for assessment of QTc interval), echocardiogram, CBC with differential, platelet count, LFTs, serum chemistries, blood glucose, blood pressure, thyroid-stimulating hormone, urine dipstick and/or urinary protein:creatinine ratio, physical examination (including dermatologic examination)

2. *Prior to each cycle of sunitinib:* CBC with differential, platelet count, LFTs, serum chemistries, blood glucose, blood pressure, thyroid-stimulating hormone, urine dipstick and/or urinary protein:creatinine ratio, physical examination (including dermatologic examination)

3. Hepatotoxicity, including liver failure, has been observed. Monitor LFTs before initiation of treatment, during each cycle of treatment, and as clinically indicated

4. Cardiac toxicity including declines in LVEF to below LLN and cardiac failure including death have occurred. Monitor patients for signs and symptoms of congestive heart failure

5. Prolonged QT intervals and torsades de pointes have been observed. Use with caution in patients at higher risk for developing QT interval prolongation. When using sunitinib, monitoring with on-treatment electrocardiograms and electrolytes should be considered monthly at first or when the dose is increased and less frequently thereafter

6. Hypertension may occur. Monitor blood pressure and treat as indicated under TREATMENT MODIFICATIONS

7. Thyroid dysfunction may occur. Monitor thyroid function tests every 3 months. Treat hypothyroidism accordingly

8. Temporary interruption of therapy with sunitinib is recommended in patients undergoing major surgical procedures. *Note:* there is limited clinical experience regarding the timing of re-initiation of therapy following major surgical intervention. Therefore, the decision to resume sunitinib therapy following a major surgical intervention should be based on clinical judgment of recovery from surgery

9. Monitor adrenal function in case of stress such as surgery, trauma, or severe infection

METASTATIC/SURGICALLY UNRESECTABLE GIST SARCOMA

METASTATIC/SURGICALLY UNRESECTABLE GIST SARCOMA REGIMEN: REGORAFENIB

Demetri GD et al. Lancet 2013;381:295–302

Regorafenib 160 mg per dose; administer orally once daily for 21 consecutive days, days 1–21, followed by 7 days without treatment, every 28 days, until disease progression (total dose/28-day cycle = 3360 mg)

Notes:
- Regorafenib tablets must be stored in the manufacturer's original container at room temperature between 20° and 25°C (68° and 77°F)
- Regorafenib should be taken about the same time each day
- If a dose is missed, it should be taken on the same day it was to have been taken—that is, patients should not take more than 1 dose on a single day to make up for 1 or more doses missed on previous days
- Tablets should be swallowed whole (no breaking, crushing, or chewing)
- Advise patients to avoid grapefruit products while taking regorafenib
- Regorafenib is taken with a low-fat meal that contains less 600 calories and less than 30% fat
- The concomitant use of strong CYP3A4 inducer (eg rifampin, phenytoin, carbamazepine, phenobarbital, and St. John's Wort) should be avoided
- The concomitant use of strong CYP3A4 inhibitor (eg clarithromycin, grapefruit juice, itraconazole, ketoconazole, nefazodone, posaconazole, telithromycin, and voriconazole) should be avoided

Supportive Care
Antiemetic prophylaxis
Emetogenic potential on is **MINIMAL–LOW**
See Chapter 42 for antiemetic recommendations

Hematopoietic growth factor (G-CSF) prophylaxis
Primary prophylaxis is NOT indicated
See Chapter 43 for more information

Antimicrobial prophylaxis
Risk of fever and neutropenia is *LOW*
  Antimicrobial primary prophylaxis to be considered:
  - Antibacterial—not indicated
  - Antifungal—not indicated
  - Antiviral—not indicated, unless patient previously had an episode of HSV

Hand-foot reaction (palmar-plantar erythrodysesthesia, PPE)
- For patients who develop a hand-foot reaction, use topical emollients (eg, Aquaphor), topical or orally administered steroids, antihistamine agents (H_1-receptor antagonists), or pyridoxine
- Pyridoxine may provide relief for discomfort/pain associated with PPE, although the mechanism through which this occurs remains unclear
- The suggested pyridoxine starting dose is 50 mg/day, which may be increased to a maximum of 200 mg/day

Diarrhea management
Latent or delayed-onset diarrhea[*]:
Loperamide 4 mg orally initially after the first loose or liquid stool, *then* 2–4 mg orally every 2–4 hours or **diphenoxylate hydrochloride** 2.5 mg **with atropine sulfate** 0.025 mg (eg, Lomotil)

*Abigerges D et al. J Natl Cancer Inst 1994;86:446–449
Rothenberg ML et al. J Clin Oncol 2001;19:3801–3807
Wadler S et al. J Clin Oncol 1998;16:3169–3178

Oral care
Standard prophylaxis and treatment for mucositis/stomatitis

Treatment Modifications

RECOMMENDED DOSE MODIFICATIONS FOR REGORAFENIB

Starting dose	160 mg once daily on days 1–21, every 28 days
Dose level (−1)	120 mg once daily on days 1–21, every 28 days
Dose level (−2)	80 mg once daily on days 1–21, every 28 days
Dose level (−3)	Discontinue regorafenib

Adverse Event	Treatment Modification
Dermatologic Toxicity	
First occurrence of G2 hand-foot skin reaction (HFSR) (palmar-plantar erythrodysesthesia [PPE]) of any duration at a regorafenib dose of 160 mg	Reduce regorafenib to a daily dose of 120 mg. If HFSR does not improve within 7 days despite dose reduction to 120 mg, then withhold therapy until toxicity resolves to G ≤1 at which time may resume regorafenib at a dose of 120 mg daily.
G2 HFSR, (palmar-plantar erythrodysesthesia [PPE]) that is recurrent or does not improve within 7 days despite dose reduction	Interrupt therapy for a minimum of 7 days for G3 HFSR until toxicity resolves to G ≤1 and resume regorafenib at one lower dose level
G3 HFSR (PPE) at a regorafenib dose of 160 mg	Withhold therapy for a minimum of 7 days and until toxicity resolves to G ≤1, then resume regorafenib at a daily dose of 120 mg
G3 HFSR (PPE) at a regorafenib dose of 120 mg	Withhold therapy for a minimum of 7 days and until toxicity resolves to G ≤1, then resume regorafenib at a daily dose of 80 mg
Other Toxicities	
G3 aspartate aminotransferase (AST)/ alanine aminotransferase (ALT) elevation at a regorafenib dose of 160 mg	Resume regorafenib at a daily dose of 120 mg after toxicity resolves to G ≤1 only if the potential benefit outweighs the risk of hepatotoxicity
G3/4* adverse reaction at a regorafenib dose of 160 mg (except hepatotoxicity)	Withhold regorafenib until toxicity resolves to G ≤1 and resume regorafenib at a daily dose of 120 mg
G3/4* adverse reaction at the 120 mg dose (except hepatotoxicity or infection)	Withhold regorafenib until toxicity resolves to G ≤1 and resume regorafenib at a daily dose to 80 mg
Symptomatic G2 hypertension	Withhold therapy until symptoms resolve to G ≤1 and resume regorafenib at a daily dose of 80 mg
Worsening infection of any grade	Withhold therapy until resolution of infection, then resume regorafenib at the same dose
Patient will undergo elective surgery	Withhold regorafenib for ≥2 weeks prior to surgery and for ≥2 weeks after major surgery and until adequate wound healing, whichever is longer
Failure to tolerate 80 mg daily	Permanently discontinue regorafenib
Any NCI CTCAE v3.0 G3 or G4 adverse reaction	
Any occurrence of AST or ALT >20 times the upper limit of normal (ULN)	
Any occurrence of AST or ALT >3 times ULN with concurrent bilirubin >2 times ULN	
Recurrence of AST or ALT >5 times ULN despite dose reduction to 120 mg	
Severe or life-threatening hemorrhage	
Gastrointestinal perforation or fistula	
Reversible posterior leukoencephalopathy syndrome (RPLS)	

*For any G4 adverse reaction, only resume if the potential benefit outweighs the risks

Patient Population Studied

The GRID trial was an international, multicenter, randomized, placebo-controlled, phase 3 trial designed to assess the efficacy and safety of regorafenib in patients with metastatic or unresectable gastrointestinal stromal tumor (GIST) after progression or failure of imatinib and sunitinib. Eligible patients had histologically confirmed metastatic or unresectable GIST with at least failure of imatinib (disease progression or drug intolerance) and sunitinib (disease progression). Patients were permitted to have received other systemic agents with the exception of any VEGFR inhibitors (other than sunitinib). Participants were also required to have ECOG PS of ≤1

Patient Population

Characteristic	Regorafenib (n = 133)	Placebo (n = 66)
Median age, yr (IQR)	60 (51–67)	61 (48–66)
Male sex, %	64	64
Ethnic group, %		
White	68	68
Black or African American	0	2
Asian	26	24
Not reported/ missing	7	6
ECOG performance status, %		
0	55	56
1	45	44
Previous systemic anticancer therapy, %		
2 lines	56	59
> 2 lines	44	41
Duration of previous imatinib therapy, %		
≤6 months	14	6
6–18 months	20	11
>18 months	67	83

IQR, interquartile range; ECOG, Eastern Cooperative Oncology Group

Efficacy

Efficacy Variable	Regorafenib (n = 133)	Placebo (n = 66)	Between-group Comparison
Survival Outcomes			
Overall survival events, %	22	26	HR 0.77 (95% CI 0.42–1.41) P = 0.199
Median PFS*, mo (IQR)	4.8 (1.4–9.2)	0.9 (0.9–1.8)	HR 0.27 (95% CI 0.19–0.39) P<0.0001
PFS at 3 months, % (95% CI)	60 (51–68)	11 (3–18)	—
PFS at 6 months, % (95% CI)	38 (29–48)	0	—
Median PFS—months (IQR)	7.4 (2.7–NC)	1.7 (0.9–2.7)	HR 0.22 (95% CI 0.14–0.35) P<0.0001
Response			
Complete response, no (%)	0	0	—
Partial response, no (%)	6 (4.5)	1 (1.5)	—
Overall response rate, %	4.5	1.5	—
Stable disease†, no (%)	95 (71.4)	22 (33.3)	—
Disease control rate, no, (%)	70 (52.6)	6 (9.1)	95% CI –52.72 to –32.49; P<0.0001

*Median progression-free survival determined by blinded central review
†Defined as stable disease occurring at any time and for any duration
HR, hazard ratio; CI, confidence interval; PFS, progression-free survival; IQR, interquartile range; NC, not calculable

Adverse Events

	Regorafenib (n = 132*)			Placebo (n = 66)		
	Any Grade (%)	Grade 3 (%)	Grade 4 (%)	Any Grade (%)	Grade 3 (%)	Grade 4 (%)
Any event	98	58	2	68	8	2
Hand-foot skin reaction	56	20	0	14	0	0
Hypertension	49	23	1	17	3	0
Diarrhea	40	5	0	5	0	0
Fatigue	39	2	0	27	0	0
Oral mucositis	38	2	0	8	2	0
Alopecia	24	2	0	2	0	0
Hoarseness	22	0	0	5	0	0
Anorexia	21	0	0	8	0	0
Rash, maculopapular	18	2	0	3	0	0
Nausea	16	2	0	9	2	0
Constipation	15	1	0	6	0	0
Myalgia	14	1	0	9	0	0
Voice alteration	11	0	0	3	0	0

*Excluding one patient who did not receive the study treatment

Therapy Monitoring

1. *Prior to each cycle:* liver function tests, blood pressure, physical examination (including dermatologic examination)
2. *Weekly during the first 6 weeks:* blood pressure
3. *At least every 2 weeks during cycles 1–2:* liver function tests (increase frequency to at least once per week in patients with elevated liver function tests until improved to <3 × ULN or baseline)
4. *In patients receiving concomitant warfarin therapy:* monitor INR frequently
5. *Periodically:* advise patients to report signs/symptoms of infection, hemorrhage, gastrointestinal perforation or fistula, hand-foot skin reaction, cardiac ischemia, or reversible posterior leukoencephalopathy syndrome (seizure, severe headache, visual disturbances, confusion or altered mental status)
6. Withhold regorafenib for ≥2 weeks prior to elective surgery. Do not administer for at least 2 weeks following major surgery and until adequate wound healing. The safety of resumption of regorafenib after resolution of wound healing complications has not been established

METASTATIC/SURGICALLY UNRESECTABLE GIST SARCOMA

METASTATIC/SURGICALLY UNRESECTABLE GIST SARCOMA REGIMEN: RIPRETINIB

Blay JY et al. Lancet Oncol 2020:21:923–934
QINLOCK (ripretinib) prescribing information. Waltham, MA: Deciphera Pharmaceuticals, LLC; revised 2020 May

Ripretinib 150 mg per dose; administer orally, once daily, with or without food, until disease progression (total dosage/week = 1050 mg)
Notes:
- Advise patients to swallow tablets whole and to take ripretinib at the same time each day
- Advise patients to take a missed dose if <8 hours have passed since the missed scheduled dose. Advise patients not to take an additional dose if vomiting occurs after taking ripretinib and to continue with their next scheduled dose
- Advise patients to store ripretinib in the original container at room temperature (20°C to 25°C [68°F to 77°F])
- Avoid strong CYP3A4 inducer (eg rifampin, phenytoin, carbamazepine, phenobarbital, and St. John's Wort)
- Avoid strong CYP3A4 inhibitor (eg clarithromycin, grapefruit juice, itraconazole, ketoconazole, nefazodone, posaconazole, telithromycin, and voriconazole)

Supportive Care
Antiemetic prophylaxis
Emetogenic potential on is **MINIMAL–LOW**
See Chapter 42 for antiemetic recommendations

Hematopoietic growth factor (G-CSF) prophylaxis
Primary prophylaxis is NOT indicated
See Chapter 43 for more information

Antimicrobial prophylaxis
Risk of fever and neutropenia is *LOW*
  Antimicrobial primary prophylaxis to be considered:
  - Antibacterial—not indicated
  - Antifungal—not indicated
  - Antiviral—not indicated, unless patient previously had an episode of HSV

Hand-foot reaction (palmar-plantar erythrodysesthesia, PPE)
- For patients who develop a hand-foot reaction, use topical emollients (eg, Aquaphor), topical or orally administered steroids, antihistamine agents (H_1-receptor antagonists), or pyridoxine
- Pyridoxine may provide relief for discomfort/pain associated with PPE, although the mechanism through which this occurs remains unclear
- The suggested pyridoxine starting dose is 50 mg/day, which may be increased to a maximum of 200 mg/day

Diarrhea management*
Loperamide 4 mg orally initially after the first loose or liquid stool, *then* 2–4 mg orally every 2–4 hours or **diphenoxylate hydrochloride** 2.5 mg **with atropine sulfate** 0.025 mg (eg, Lomotil)

*Abigerges D et al. J Natl Cancer Inst 1994;86:446–449
Rothenberg ML et al. J Clin Oncol 2001;19:3801–3807
Wadler S et al. J Clin Oncol 1998;16:3169–3178

Oral care
Standard prophylaxis and treatment for mucositis/stomatitis

Treatment Modifications

RECOMMENDED DOSE MODIFICATIONS FOR RIPRETINIB

Ripretinib Dose Levels	
Starting dose	150 mg daily
Dose level −1	100 mg daily
Dose level −2	Discontinue ripretinib

(continued)

Treatment Modifications (continued)

Adverse Event*	Treatment Modification
Dermatologic Toxicity	
G2 palmar-plantar erythrodysesthesia syndrome	• Withhold ripretinib until G ≤1 or baseline. If recovered within 7 days, resume ripretinib at same dose; otherwise resume at reduced dose • Consider re-escalating ripretinib if maintained at G ≤1 or baseline for at least 28 days • If PPES recurs, withhold ripretinib until G ≤1 or baseline and then resume ripretinib at a reduced dose regardless of time to improvement
G3 palmar-plantar erythrodysesthesia syndrome	• Withhold ripretinib for ≥7 days or until G ≤1 or baseline (maximum 28 days). Resume ripretinib at a reduced dose • Consider re-escalating ripretinib if maintained at G ≤1 or baseline for ≥28 days
Skin lesion suspicious for cutaneous squamous cell carcinoma is present	Excise lesion and submit for dermatopathologic evaluation. Continue ripretinib at the same dose
Cardiac Toxicity	
G3 hypertension	• If symptomatic, withhold ripretinib until symptoms have resolved and blood pressure is controlled • If blood pressure is controlled to G ≤1 or baseline, resume ripretinib at the same dose; otherwise, resume ripretinib at reduced dose • If G3 hypertension recurs, withhold ripretinib until symptoms have resolved and blood pressure is controlled. Resume ripretinib at a reduced dose
G4 hypertension	Permanently discontinue ripretinib
G ≥3 left ventricular systolic dysfunction	Permanently discontinue ripretinib
Musculoskeletal Toxicity	
G2 arthralgia or myalgia	• Withhold ripretinib until G ≤1 or baseline. If recovered within 7 days, resume ripretinib at same dose; otherwise resume ripretinib at reduced dose • Consider re-escalating ripretinib if maintained at G ≤1 or baseline for at least 28 days • If arthralgia or myalgia recurs, withhold ripretinib until G ≤1 or baseline and then resume ripretinib at a reduced dose regardless of time to improvement
G3 arthralgia or myalgia	• Withhold ripretinib for ≥7 days or until G ≤1 or baseline (maximum 28 days). Resume ripretinib at reduced dose • Consider re-escalating ripretinib if maintained at G ≤1 or baseline for ≥28 days
Other Adverse Reactions	
Other G ≥3 adverse reactions	• Withhold ripretinib until G ≤1 or baseline (maximum 28 days), and then resume ripretinib at a reduced dose; otherwise permanently discontinue • Consider re-escalating ripretinib if no recurrence of the adverse reaction for ≥28 days • If G ≥3 adverse reaction recurs, permanently discontinue ripretinib

*Toxicities are graded per National Cancer Institute Common Terminology Criteria for Adverse Events version 4.03 (NCI CTCAE v4.03)

Patient Population Studied

Double-blind, randomized, placebo-controlled, phase 3 study in patients with a diagnosis of gastrointestinal stromal tumor, an Eastern Cooperative Oncology Group (ECOG) performance status of 0–2, and had progressed on at least imatinib, sunitinib, and regorafenib, or had documented intolerance to any of these treatments despite dose modifications

Baseline Patient Characteristics		
	Ripretinib Group (n = 85)	**Placebo Group (n = 44)**
Median age, years	59 (29–82)	65 (33–83)
Sex—male / female	47 (55%) / 38 (45%)	26 (59%) / 18 (41%)
Race—White / Non-white / Not reported	64 (75%) / 13 (15%) / 8 (9%)	33 (75%) / 7 (16%) / 4 (9%)

(continued)

Patient Population Studied (continued)

Baseline Patient Characteristics

	Ripretinib Group (n = 85)	Placebo Group (n = 44)
Region—USA / Non-USA	40 (47%) / 45 (53%)	20 (46%) / 24 (55%)
Number of previous therapies—3 / 4–7	54 (64%) / 31 (36%)	27 (61%) / 17 (39%)
ECOG performance status—0/1or2	37 (44%) / 48 (56%)	17 (39% /) 27 (61%)
Primary tumor site		
Gastric	40 (47%)	18 (41%)
Jejunum or ileum	20 (24%)	8 (18%)
Mesenteric or omental	6 (7%)	6 (14%)
Other	7 (8%)	4 (9%)
Duodenum	2 (2%)	8 (18%)
Colon or rectum	9 (11%)	0
Unknown	1 (1%)	0
Sum of longest diameters of target lesions (mm), median (range)	123 (28–495)	142 (17–412)
Primary mutation (central testing of tumor tissue)		
KIT exon 9	14 (17%)	6 (14%)
KIT exon 11	47 (55%)	28 (64%)
Other *KIT*	2 (2%)	2 (5%)
PDGFRA	3 (4%)	0
KIT and *PDGFRA* wild-type	7 (8%)	3 (7%)
Not available or not done	12 (14%)	5 (11%)

Note: data are median (IQR), n (%), or median (range), and percentages might not add up to 100 due to rounding
ECOG, Eastern Cooperative Oncology Group; *KIT*, KIT proto-oncogene, receptor tyrosine kinase; *PDGFRA*, platelet-derived growth factor receptor α

Efficacy

	Ripretinib Group (n = 85)	Placebo Group (n = 44)	P Value
Confirmed objective response	8 (9%; 4–18)	0 (0%; 0–8)	0.0504
Complete response	0 (0%; 0–4)	0 (0%; 0–8)	—
Partial response	8 (9%; 4–18)	0 (0%; 0–8)	—
Stable disease (6 weeks)	56 (66%; 55–76)	9 (20%; 10–35)	—
Stable disease (12 weeks)	40 (47%; 36–58)	2 (5%; 1–16)	—
Progressive disease	16 (19%; 11–29)	28 (64%; 48–78)	—
Not evaluable	4 (5%)	3 (7%)	—
No response assessment	1 (1%)	4 (9%)	—
Median time to best response	1.9 mos (IQR 1.0–2.7).		
Median time to progression	6.4 mos (95% CI 4.6–8.4)	1.0 mos (0.9–1.)	

(continued)

Efficacy (continued)

	Ripretinib Group (n = 85)	Placebo Group (n = 44)	P Value
Median OS	15.1 mos (95% CI 12.3–15.1)	6.6 mos (4.1–11.6)	HR 0.36, 95% CI 0.21–0.62
Estimated OS at 6 months	84.3% (95% CI 74.5–90.6)	55.9% (39.9–69.2)	
Estimated OS at 12 months	65.4% (51.6–76.1)	25.9% (7.2–49.9)	

Data are n (%; 95% CI) or n (%)
CI, confidence interval; HR, hazard ration; OS, overall survival

Adverse Events

	Ripretinib Group (n = 85)			Placebo Group (n = 43)		
	G1–2	G3	G4	G1–2	G3	G4
Alopecia	42 (49%)	—	—	1 (2%)	—	—
Myalgia	23 (27%)	1 (1%)	—	4 (9%)	0	—
Nausea	21 (25%)	1 (1%)	—	1 (2%)	0	—
Fatigue	20 (24%)	2 (2%)	—	6 (14%)	1 (2%)	—
PPES	18 (21%)	0	—	0	0	—
Diarrhea	17 (20%)	1 (1%)	0	2 (5%)	1 (2%)	0
Constipation	13 (15%)	0	0	3 (7%)	0	0
Decreased appetite	12 (14%)	1 (1%)	0	2 (5%)	1 (2%)	0
Weight loss	13 (15%)	0	—	3 (7%)	0	—
Blood bilirubin increased	12 (14%)	0	0	0	0	0
Arthralgia	10 (12%)	0	—	0	0	—
Muscle spasms	10 (12%)	0	—	2 (5%)	0	—
Hypertension	4 (5%)	3 (4%)	0	1 (2%)	0	0
Lipase increase	4 (5%)	4 (5%)	0	0	0	0
Pain in extremity	5 (6%)	1 (1%)	—	1 (2%)	0	—
Hypophosphatemia	3 (4%)	2 (2%)	0	0	0	0
Anemia	2 (2%)	0	1 (1%)	1 (2%)	2 (5%)	1 (2%)
Blood triglycerides increase	1 (1%)	1 (1%)	0	0	0	0
Dermatosis	1 (1%)	1 (1%)	0	0	0	0
Dehydration	1 (1%)	0	0	0	1 (2%)	0
GERD	1 (1%)	1 (1%)	—	0	0	—
Upper GI hemorrhage	0	1 (1%)	0	0	0	0

Data are n (%). Treatment-related treatment-emergent adverse events are listed that occurred in ≥10% of patients in either treatment group or were reported as Grade 3 or 4 in either treatment group are shown. Adverse event grade ratings specified by Common Terminology Criteria for Adverse Events version 4.03
GERD, gastroesophageal reflux disease; PPES, palmar-plantar erythrodysesthesia syndrome

Therapy Monitoring

1. *Prior to therapy and periodically during treatment:* CBC with differential, liver function tests, serum chemistries, physical exam (including dermatologic evaluation for palmar plantar erythrodysesthesia syndrome and cutaneous squamous cell carcinoma)
2. Monitor blood pressure at baseline. Adequately control blood pressure prior to initiating ripretinib. Monitor blood pressure as clinically indicated during treatment, and initiate or adjust antihypertensive therapy as appropriate
3. Assess left ventricular ejection fraction by echocardiogram or MUGA scan prior to initiating ripretinib and during treatment, as clinically indicated
4. Withhold ripretinib for ≥1 week prior to elective surgery. Do not administer for at least 2 weeks following major surgery and until adequate wound healing. The safety of resumption of ripretinib after resolution of wound healing complications has not been established

METASTATIC • SURGICALLY UNRESECTABLE • GIST

SARCOMA REGIMEN: AVAPRITINIB

Heinrich M et al. Lancet Oncol 2020;21:935–46
AYVAKIT (avapritinib) prescribing information. Cambridge, MA: Blueprint Medicines Corporation; revised 2020 January

Avapritinib 300 mg; administer orally, once daily on an empty stomach, at least 1 hour before and 2 hours after a meal, until disease progression (total dose/week = 2100 mg)

Notes:
• If a dose is missed, it should be taken as long as at least 8 hours remain until the next regularly scheduled dose
• In case of vomiting, do not administer an additional dose
• The concomitant use of moderate or strong CYP3A4 inducer should be avoided
• The concomitant use of strong CYP3A4 inhibitors should be avoided
• If concomitant use of a moderate CYP3A4 inhibitor is unavoidable, then reduce the starting dosage of avapritinib to 100 mg once daily

Supportive Care
Antiemetic prophylaxis
Emetogenic potential is **MODERATE-HIGH**
See Chapter 42 for antiemetic recommendations

Hematopoietic growth factor (CSF) prophylaxis
Primary prophylaxis is NOT indicated
See Chapter 43 for more information

Antimicrobial prophylaxis
Risk of fever and neutropenia is LOW
Antimicrobial primary prophylaxis is recommended:
• Antibacterial—not indicated
• Antifungal—not indicated
• Antiviral—not indicated, unless patient previously had an episode of HSV

Treatment Modifications

Avapritinib	
Starting Dosage	300 mg orally once daily
Dose level -1	200 mg orally once daily
Dose level -2	100 mg orally once daily
Dose level -3	Discontinue avapritinib

Adverse Event	Dose Modification
G1/2 intracranial hemorrhage, first occurrence	Withhold avapritinib until resolution, then resume at a reduced dose.
G1/2 intracranial hemorrhage, subsequent occurrence	Permanently discontinue avapritinib
G3/4 intracranial hemorrhage	Permanently discontinue avapritinib
G1 CNS effects*	Continue avapritinib at the same dose or withhold until improvement to baseline or resolution. Resume at the same or reduced dose.
G2/3 CNS effects*	Withhold avapritinib until improvement to baseline, G1, or resolution. Then resume at the same dose or reduced dose.
G4 CNS effects*	Permanently discontinue avapritinib
Other G3/4 adverse reactions	Withhold avapritinib until improvement to ≤G2. Resume at same dose or reduced dose, as clinically appropriate.

(continued)

Treatment Modifications (continued)

Concomitant use of a moderate CYP3A4 inhibitor cannot be avoided	Reduce the starting dosage of avapritinib to 100 mg once daily
Concomitant use of a moderate or strong CYP3A4 inducer is unavoidable	Do not administer avapritinib
Concomitant use of a strong CYP3A4 inhibitor cannot be avoided	Do not administer avapritinib

*CNS effects include but are not limited to cognitive impairment, dizziness, sleep disorders, mood disorders, speech disorders, hallucinations
Note: severity is defined according to the National Cancer Institute Common Terminology Criteria for Adverse Events version 5.0
Reference: AYVAKIT (avapritinib) prescribing information. Cambridge, MA: Blueprint Medicines Corporation; revised 2020 January

Patient Population Studied

NAVIGATOR was a two-part, open-label, dose-escalation (n=46) and dose-expansion (n=36), phase 1, international study involving adult patients with unresectable GIST. The dose-expansion phase required patients to have a PDGFRA D842V-mutant GIST (regardless of prior therapy) or GIST with other mutations that progressed on imatinib ± other TKIs. Patients with a PDGFRA D842V-mutation were analyzed separately (n=56 across both parts of the trial).

Efficacy

Best-Confirmed Response by Central Assessment per mRECIST v1.1 Among Patients with PDGFRA D842V-mutant GIST

	All doses (n=56)	300 mg (n=28)
Complete response	5 (9%)	1 (4%)
Partial response	44 (79%)	25 (89%)
Overall response*	49 (88%; 95% CI 76-95%)	26 (93%; 95% CI 77-99%)
Stable disease	7 (13%)	2 (7%)
Clinical benefit†	55 (98%; 95% CI 90-100%)	28 (100%; 95% CI 88-100%)
Progressive disease	0	0

*complete response + partial response
†complete response or partial response or stable disease lasting ≥16 weeks
Reference: Heinrich M et al. Lancet Oncol 2020;21:935-46

Survival Data

Progression-Free Survival (PFS)

PFS at 3 months	100%
PFS at 6 months	94%
PFS at 12 months	81%

Overall Survival (OS)

OS at 6 months	100%
OS at 12 months	91%
OS at 24 months	81%

Median follow-up at data cutoff of November 16, 2018 was 15.9 months (IQR 9.2-24.9)

Adverse Events

	Avapritinib 300 mg (n=32)			
	Grade 1-2 (%)	Grade 3 (%)	Grade 4 (%)	Grade 5 (%)
Any related adverse event	34	59	6	0
Nausea	69	0	0	0
Fatigue	38	3	0	0
Diarrhea	41	6	0	0
Periorbital edema	34	3	0	0
Anemia	34	22	0	0
Decreased appetite	38	0	0	0
Vomiting	16	0	0	0
Memory impairment	31	0	0	0
Hair color changes	25	0	0	0
Increased lacrimation	22	0	0	0
Peripheral edema	31	0	0	0
Blood bilirubin increased	22	3	0	0
Face edema	34	0	0	0
Dysgeusia	22	0	0	0
Hypophosphatemia	9	3	0	0
Neutropenia	19	9	0	0
Dizziness	19	0	0	0
Dyspepsia	13	0	0	0
Alopecia	13	0	0	0
Eyelid edema	16	0	0	0
Leukopenia	9	0	0	0
Headache	13	0	0	0
Hyperbilirubinemia	6	3	0	0
Dry mouth	6	0	0	0
Pleural effusion	9	3	0	0
Cognitive disorder	13	0	0	0
Dry skin	9	0	0	0
Hypomagnesemia	13	0	0	0
Rash	3	0	0	0
Decreased weight	9	0	0	0
Decreased neutrophil count	6	6	3	0
Vertigo	6	0	0	0
Lymphopenia	0	3	0	0
Hypocalcemia	0	3	0	0
Mental impairment	3	3	0	0
Peripheral neuropathy	3	3	0	0
Delirium	0	3	0	0

Therapy Monitoring

1. *Pretreatment evaluation:*
   a. Testing to determine the presence of a PDGFRAA exon 18 mutation to select patients appropriate for avapritinib therapy .
   b. Pregnancy test in female patients of reproductive potential
   c. Complete metabolic panel and CBC with differential at baseline and then periodically
2. Monitor for signs and symptoms of intracranial hemorrhage
3. Monitor for signs and symptoms of CNS toxicity (eg, cognitive impairment, dizziness, sleep disorders, mood disorders, speech disorders, and hallucinations). Advise patients not to drive or operate hazardous machinery if they are experiencing CNS adverse reactions

37. Testicular Cancer

Darren R. Feldman, MD

Epidemiology

Incidence: 9610 estimated new cases for 2020 in the United States
5.9 per 100,000 males per year
Most common malignancy in males ages 15–39

Deaths: Estimated 440 in 2020

Median age: 33 years

American Cancer Society Facts and Figures 2020: Special Section: Cancer in Adolescents and Young Adults
Siegel RL et al. CA Cancer J Clin 2020;70:7–30
Surveillance, Epidemiology and End Results (SEER) Program, available from http://seer.cancer.gov [accessed in 2020]

Frequency of Stage at Presentation

	Seminoma	Nonseminoma
Stage I	85%	60%
Stage II	10%	20%
Stage III	5%	20%

Frequency of IGCCCG Risk Groups at Diagnosis for Patients Requiring Chemotherapy

IGCCCG Risk Group	Seminoma	Nonseminoma	All
Good	90%	56%	60%
Intermediate	10%	28%	26%
Poor	N/A	16%	14%

IGCCCG, International Germ Cell Cancer Collaborative Group; GCT germ cell tumor
Biggs M, Schwartz S. Cancer of the testis. In Ries LAG et al (editors). SEER Survival Monograph: Cancer Survival Among Adults: U.S. SEER Program, 1988–2001. Bethesda, MD: National Cancer Institute; 2007.
Bosl G et al. In Devita V et al (editors). Cancer: Principles and Practice of Oncology. Philadelphia: Lippincott Williams and Wilkins; 2008:1463–1485
International Germ Cell Cancer Collaborative Group (IGCCCG). J Clin Oncol 1997;15:594–603
Siegel R et al. CA Cancer J Clin 2014;64:9–29

Pathology

Germ Cell Tumors (95%)

1. Derived from germ cell neoplasia in situ (GCNIS)
   a. Seminoma
   b. Nonseminoma
      i) Embryonal carcinoma
      ii) Trophoblastic tumor
         – Choriocarcinoma
         – Other trophoblastic tumors
      iii) Yolk-sac tumor, postpubertal type
      iv) Teratoma, postpubertal type
         – Teratoma with somatic malignancy
2. Not derived from GCNIS
   a. Spermatocytic tumor
   b. Yolk-sac tumor, prepubertal type
   c. Teratoma, prepubertal type

Note: Most common nonseminoma histology is a mixture of ≥2 histologies. Pure teratoma represents a fully malignant GCT

Non–Germ Cell Tumors (5%)

1. Sex cord-stromal (gonadal stromal) tumors
   a. Leydig cell
   b. Sertoli cell tumor
   c. Granulosa cell tumor
   d. Tumors in the fibroma-thecoma group
   e. Mixed and unclassified sex-cord stromal tumors
2. Both germ cell and gonadal stromal elements
   a. Gonadoblastoma
3. Adnexal and paratesticular tumors
   a. Mesothelioma
   b. Carcinoma of rete testis
4. Miscellaneous neoplasms
   a. Carcinoid
   b. Lymphoma
   c. Sarcoma
   d. Other

Moch H et al. World Health Organization Classification of Tumours of the Urinary System and Male Genital Organs. 4th ed. Lyon: IARC Press; 2016

Work-up

Suspicious Testicular Mass (by History or Exam)	Confirmed Testicular Mass (by Ultrasound)	Seminoma or Nonseminoma (S/P Orchiectomy)
History and physical	STM if not yet done	STM
AFP, hCG, and LDH (serum tumor markers [STM])	CBC, complete metabolic profile	CBC, complete metabolic profile
CBC, complete metabolic profile	CT A/P + either CXR or CT chest	**Nonseminoma:** CT A/P if >4 weeks since prior; CT chest if not previously performed **Seminoma:** CT A/P and CXR if >4 weeks since prior
Scrotal ultrasound	Bone scan or brain MRI, *only* if clinically indicated; sperm banking should be discussed/ considered in the setting of an atrophic or absent contralateral testis	Bone scan or brain MRI, *only* if clinically indicated Discussion of sperm banking if further treatment (surgery, chemotherapy, or XRT) is required

Caveats Regarding Work-up

1. CT chest should be part of the work-up staging for nonseminoma, whereas CXR can suffice for seminoma
2. There is a higher risk of brain metastasis among patients with diffuse lung metastases, choriocarcinoma histology, and hCG >1000 mIU/L and especially when hCG is >100,000 mIU/L (Feldman DR et al. J Clin Oncol 2016;34:345–351)

Staging

T: Primary Tumor Staging

pTx	Primary tumor cannot be assessed
pT0	No evidence of primary tumor
pTis	Germ cell neoplasia in situ
pT1	Tumor limited to testis (including rete testis invasion) without lymphovascular invasion
pT1a*	Tumor smaller than 3 cm in size
pT1b*	Tumor 3 cm or larger in size
pT2	Tumor limited to the testis (including rete testis invasion) with lymphovascular invasion OR tumor invading hilar soft tissue or epididymis or penetrating visceral mesothelial layer covering the external surface of tunica albuginea with or without lymphovascular invasion
pT3	Tumor directly invades spermatic cord soft tissue with or without lymphovascular invasion
pT4	Tumor invades scrotum with or without lymphovascular invasion

*Subclassification of pT1 applies only to pure seminoma

N: Regional Lymph Nodes Clinical Staging

cNX	Regional lymph nodes (LN) cannot be assessed
cN0	No regional LN metastasis
cN1	LN mass ≤2 cm in greatest dimension; or multiple LN, none >2 cm
cN2	LN mass >2 cm but not >5 cm in greatest dimension; or multiple LN, any 1 mass >2 cm but not >5 cm
cN3	Lymph node mass >5 cm in greatest dimension

N: Regional Lymph Nodes Pathologic Staging

pNX	Regional LN cannot be assessed
pN0	No regional LN metastasis
pN1	Metastasis with a lymph node mass ≤2 cm in greatest dimension and ≤5 lymph nodes positive, none >2 cm
pN2	Positive LN >2 cm but <5 cm in greatest dimension; or >5 positive LN, none >5 cm; or evidence of extranodal extension
pN3	Positive lymph node >5 cm in greatest dimension

M: Metastatic Disease Staging

M0	No distant metastasis
M1	Distant metastasis
M1a	Non-retroperitoneal nodal or pulmonary metastases
M1b	Non-pulmonary visceral metastases

S: Serum Tumor Markers Staging

Sx	Markers not available or not performed
S0	Marker levels within normal limits
S1	LDH <1.5× upper limit of normal (ULN) and human chorionic gonadotropin, beta subunit (hCG) <5000 mIU/L and alpha-fetoprotein (AFP) <1000 ng/mL
S2	LDH 1.5–10× ULN or hCG 5000–50,000 mIU/L or AFP 1000–10,000 ng/mL
S3	LDH >10× ULN or hCG >50,000 mIU/L or AFP >10,000 ng/mL

Caveats Regarding Staging

1. Although AJCC version 8 is provided as the most recent version, the authors prefer use of AJCC version 7 for the purposes of clinical management. In particular: (a) the use of pT1b for seminomas >3 cm in size may confuse some practitioners because it applies only to seminoma and can be mistaken for stage I-B which refers to pT2 cN0 M0 S0 tumors; (b) hilar tissue involvement by tumor is considered pT2 (and therefore stage I-B when combined with cN0, M0, and S0) in AJCC version 8 but in the author's opinion should be managed like pT1 (stage I-A) nonseminoma; and (c) discontinuous involvement of the spermatic cord is considered M1a disease in AJCC version 8 but in the setting of disease localized to the testis should be managed like stage I rather than advanced testicular cancer

2. Except for pTis and pT4, extent of tumor is classified by radical orchiectomy. Use pTx in absence of orchiectomy

3. Histology (seminoma vs nonseminoma) is incorporated into the risk classification system but not AJCC stage

4. Serum tumor markers (STM) for staging and IGCCCG risk prognostication should be drawn after orchiectomy or other tissue diagnosis but before chemotherapy. Elevated preoperative STM must be repeated postorchiectomy after marker half-life has been evaluated

TNM Stage Grouping		IGCCCG Risk Group Classification		
Stage	**TNM**	**Risk Group (5-Year DFS)**	**Seminoma (Criteria)**	**Nonseminoma (Criteria)**
0	pTis, N0, M0, S0	Good	Any primary site. Absence of nonpulmonary visceral metastasis. Normal AFP, any level hCG or LDH	*Must fulfill all of the following criteria:* Primary site not mediastinum (testis/retroperitoneal primary); absence of nonpulmonary visceral metastasis; markers S0 or S1
I	pT1–4, N0, M0, Sx	Nonseminoma (56% of cases) 5-y PFS 89% 5-y survival 92% Seminoma (90% of cases) 5-y PFS 82% 5-y survival 86%		
IA	pT1, N0, M0, S0			
IB	pT2–T4, N0, M0, S0			
IS	Any pT/Tx, N0, M0, S1–3			
II	Any pT/Tx, N1–3, M0, Sx	Intermediate	Any primary site. Presence of nonpulmonary visceral metastasis Normal AFP, any level hCG or LDH	*Must fulfill all of the following criteria:* Primary site not mediastinum (testis/retroperitoneal primary); absence of nonpulmonary visceral metastasis; and markers S2
IIA	Any pT/Tx, N1, M0, S0–1	Nonseminoma (28% of cases) 5-y PFS 75% 5-y survival 80% Seminoma (10% of cases) 5-y PFS 67% 5-y survival 72%		
IIB	Any pT/Tx, N2, S0–1			
IIC	Any pT/Tx, N3, S0–1			
III	Any pT/Tx, Any N, M1a, Sx			
IIIA	Any pT/Tx, Any N, M1a, S0–1	Poor	N/A—Seminomas are never poor risk	*Must fulfill at least 1 of the following criteria:* Primary site mediastinum; or presence of nonpulmonary visceral metastases; or markers S3
IIIB	Any pT/Tx, Any N, M1a, S2 Any pT/Tx, N1–3, M0, S2	Nonseminoma (16% of cases) 5-y PFS 41% 5-y survival 48% Seminoma (seminomas are not classified as poor prognosis)		
IIIC	Any pT/Tx, N1–N3, M0, S3 Any pT/Tx, Any N, M1a, S3 Any pT/Tx, Any N, M1b, Any S			

Amin MB et al (editors). AJCC Cancer Staging Manual. 8th ed. New York: Springer; 2017
International Germ Cell Cancer Collaborative Group (IGCCCG). J Clin Oncol 1997;15:594–603

Expert Opinion

I. Caveats

1. A testicular mass is malignant until proven otherwise. Radical inguinal orchiectomy is the indicated surgical procedure for all testicular masses; transscrotal orchiectomy and testicular biopsy are not recommended

2. Patients with seminoma and an elevated AFP level or any nonseminomatous histology, including teratoma, should be treated as a nonseminoma. Be careful of *stable* minimal elevations since they usually do not represent NSGCT (Wymer KM et al. Ann Oncol 2017;28:899–902)

3. Pure testicular teratoma should be treated as a fully malignant nonseminoma

4. Primary mediastinal site and level of serum tumor markers (STMs) do not affect prognosis for seminoma patients

5. Sperm banking should be discussed with patients after orchiectomy before initiation of any further therapy

6. There is a ~2% lifetime risk of developing a contralateral testicular tumor; self-exam and MD exam are recommended at regular intervals. Such tumors are treated as new primary GCTs

II. Treatment Recommendations by AJCC Stage and Histology

A. Nonseminomas
Stage I
- Stage IA: surveillance is the preferred option for compliant patients. The risk of recurrence is ~20% and if the disease recurs, >95% patients can be cured with chemotherapy (CT) using EP or BEP. For noncompliant patients, nerve-sparing retroperitoneal lymph node dissection (RPLND) may be preferred
- Stage IB: risk of relapse is ~50%. RPLND, surveillance, or 1 cycle of BEP are all options. RPLND results in the least likelihood of patients receiving chemotherapy
- Stage IS: CT should be administered (EP × 4 or BEP × 3 for S1; BEP × 4 for S2–S3)

Stage II (S0 and S1 STM only; S2 and S3 STM qualify as stage IIIB and IIIC, respectively)
- If adenopathy >2 cm or bilateral *or* STM are persistently elevated after orchiectomy, EP × 4 or BEP × 3 should be given
- If adenopathy <2 cm and unilateral/unifocal *and* STM are normal, RPLND or CT (EP × 4 or BEP × 3) can be considered depending on clinical circumstances. Following postchemotherapy RPLND, patients with complete resection should receive 2 cycles of EP if findings reveal pathologic stage IIB (pN2) (McHugh DJ et al. J Clin Oncol 2020;38:1332–1337)

Stage III
- Treatment is based on IGCCCG risk classification
- Patients in the good-risk category should be given either EP × 4 or BEP × 3
- Patients in the intermediate- or poor-risk categories should be given BEP × 4
- VIP × 4 (etoposide, ifosfamide, cisplatin) is as effective as BEP × 4 in patients with poor-risk GCT, but VIP is associated with greater toxicity (primarily hematologic). VIP can be considered for patients in whom bleomycin is contraindicated (ie, pulmonary disease)

Residual masses
- In general, all sites of residual masses after completion of CT should be resected, if possible. PET is not routinely indicated for evaluation of post-CT residual masses

B. Seminomas
Stage I
- The risk of recurrence is 15–20%. The 3 treatment options are active surveillance, adjuvant radiation therapy (RT), and adjuvant carboplatin
- Surveillance is the preferred option for compliant patients since RT and carboplatin overtreat ≥80% of patients. RT increases the risk of secondary cancers, and data on the long-term risks with carboplatin are lacking
- RT, 2000–2500 cGy is an option for noncompliant patients but recognition of the increased incidence of secondary intra-abdominal malignancies has rapidly led to less frequent use. Carboplatin may be an alternative option for noncompliant patients but long-term follow-up is lacking such that the frequency of late relapses and late toxicity have not been established. For these reasons, the author does not use carboplatin in his practice (van de Wetering RAW et al. J Clin Oncol 2018;36:837–840)

Stage II
- Stage IIA: RT (3000–3500 cGy) to retroperitoneal and ipsilateral pelvic lymph nodes or CT (EP × 4 or BEP × 3) (Garcia-del-Muro X et al. J Clin Oncol 2008;26:5416–5421; Tandstad T et al. J Clin Oncol 2011;29:719–725)
- Small stage IIB (single node <3 cm): either RT (≥3600 cGy) or CT with EP × 4 or BEP × 3 but CT is preferred by most experts
- Large (>3 cm) or multinodal stage IIB, all stage IIC and stage III: Treatment is with chemotherapy based on IGCCCG risk stratification. EP × 4 or BEP × 3 are used for good-risk seminoma, BEP × 4 is used for intermediate-risk disease. Seminoma patients are never poor-risk

Residual masses
- Surgery is more difficult with seminoma and carries a higher complication rate
- PET scan is recommended to evaluate residual masses >3 cm. Additional treatment (surgical or medical) or diagnostic procedure may be indicated for PET-positive residual masses >3 cm. PET-negative lesions >3 cm require no further treatment, just active surveillance. Since teratoma is rarely an issue with seminoma, false-negative results are uncommon

(continued)

Expert Opinion (*continued*)

III. Salvage Therapy

- The International Prognostic Factor Study Group (IPFSG) model estimates the prognosis of patients at the time of initial salvage chemotherapy. It is based on nearly 1600 patients from 11 countries who were treated with a standard-of-care initial salvage chemotherapy regimen. The authors identified seven factors associated with adverse prognosis including primary mediastinal tumor site, poor response to initial chemotherapy, short disease-free interval after first-line chemotherapy, presence of liver, bone, or brain metastasis, degree of hCG elevation, and degree of elevation of AFP. Using these factors, patients are assigned an individual score that allocates them into 1 of 5 groups, ranging from very low risk to very high risk with vastly different PFS and OS rates

IPFSG Model

Prognostic Group	Score	No. of Patients	Percent of Patients	2-Yr PFS	3-Yr OS
Very low	−1	76	13.0	75.1	77.0
Low	0	132	22.6	51.0	65.6
Intermediate	1	219	37.4	40.1	58.3
High	2	122	20.9	25.9	27.1
Very high	3	36	6.1	5.6	6.1

- Two general approaches are used for initial salvage management including either conventional-dose chemotherapy (CDCT) or high-dose chemotherapy (HDT) with autologous stem cell transplant (ASCT)
- CDCT generally consists of ifosfamide plus cisplatin plus a third agent not used as part of the patient's first-line regimen. The most common third agents are either paclitaxel in the TIP regimen or vinblastine in the VeIP regimen
- HDCT typically consists of sequential cycles of high-dose carboplatin plus etoposide, each followed by autologous stem cell reinfusion. Two or three high-dose cycles are used in most HDCT regimens
- The optimal approach (CDCT vs HDCT) to initial salvage treatment remains controversial. Only one randomized study (IT-94) investigated this question and found no improvement in outcome for the HDCT arm. However, IT-94 used only one high-dose cycle in the HDCT arm, limiting conclusions about sequential HDCT. In addition, >25% of the patients randomized to the HDCT arm never received the high-dose cycle. The consideration of other flaws, as well as retrospective data demonstrating improved outcomes with initial salvage HDCT over CDCT (such as in the IPFSG database), leads to the current conclusion that the optimal approach is an open-ended question. A randomized trial of standard vs high-dose therapy for all salvage patients is ongoing in the United States and Europe (Trial of Initial salvage chemotherapy for patients with **GER**m cell tumors; **TIGER**, NCT02375204) and participation is encouraged. (Lorch A et al. J Clin Oncol 2010;28:4906–4911; Feldman DR et al. J Cancer 2011; 2:374–377)
- There are no randomized data comparing two salvage CDCT regimens to one another. In the absence of such data, the author prefers TIP (paclitaxel, ifosfamide, and cisplatin) as his initial salvage CDCT regimen of choice. VeIP and similar regimens achieved an approximately 50% complete response rate and 25% durable remission rate when used as initial salvage treatment of GCT patients relapsing at least 4 weeks after first-line chemotherapy. In contrast, TIP was studied as initial salvage treatment of patients who achieved a CR or PR-negative markers lasting at least 6 months to first-line chemotherapy and led to a complete response rate of 70% with 63% durable remission rate. While patient selection likely played a role in the superior efficacy observed with TIP, similar results have never been achieved with any other salvage CDCT regimen

IV. Chemotherapy for Special Populations

- *Viable GCT upon resection after completing first-line chemotherapy:* administer 2 additional cycles of adjuvant chemotherapy with EP
- *Late relapses:* defined as relapse after ≥2 years of being in remission after chemotherapy. These tumors tend to be more chemoresistant and difficult to cure than relapses occurring ≤2 years after completing treatment. Surgery is the treatment of choice when possible. When surgery is not possible, TIP (50% durable CR rate in 14 patients) and cisplatin plus epirubicin (30% durable CR rate in 21 patients) are 2 regimens that have shown promise. High-dose chemotherapy may be indicated in selected patients. Referral to a specialist center is recommended. Investigational treatments should be considered
- *Intermediate- or poor-risk patients with severe lung disease:* VIP can be substituted for BEP with equivalent efficacy but increased hematologic toxicity
- *Pulmonary toxicity developing during BEP × 3 for good-risk disease or BEP × 4 for intermediate/poor risk disease:* if DLCO or TVC decrease by ≥25% or there is physical exam or CXR evidence of bleomycin toxicity, then discontinuation of bleomycin is indicated with continuation of treatment with EP. Patients who require discontinuation of bleomycin prior to completing 3 full cycles of BEP for good-risk disease should be given additional cycles of EP until a total of 4 cycles of chemotherapy have been administered. Suggest adding ifosfamide if bleomycin toxicity develops before the third cycle of BEP in patients with intermediate- and poor-risk disease

(*continued*)

Expert Opinion (*continued*)

V. **Mesna Dosing Schedules**
- Ifosfamide 1200 mg/m² per day for 5 days
  a. Mesna 120 mg/m² by short intravenous infusion when ifosfamide administration commences, followed immediately afterward by mesna 1200 mg/m² per day given by continuous intravenous infusion for 5 consecutive days (total dosage/5 days = 6120 mg/m²)
  b. Mesna 1200 mg/m² per day given intravenously for 5 consecutive days prepared as an admixture (in the same container) with ifosfamide (total dosage/5 days = 6000 mg/m²)
  c. Mesna 400 mg/m² per dose given intravenously when ifosfamide administration commences, and at 4 and 8 hours after ifosfamide for 3 doses per day such that equal total doses of mesna and ifosfamide are given daily; ie, 1200 mg/m² per day (total dosage/5 days = 6000 mg/m²)
- Ifosfamide 1500 mg/m² per day for 4 days
  a. Mesna 1500 mg/m² per day prepared as an admixture (in the same container) with ifosfamide (total dosage/4 days = 6000 mg/m²)
  b. Mesna 500 mg/m² per dose given intravenously with ifosfamide, and then at 4 hours and 8 hours after ifosfamide to equal the total amount of ifosfamide given daily; ie, 1500 mg/m² (total dosage/4 days = 6000 mg/m²)
  c. Mesna 500 mg/m² per dose given intravenously when ifosfamide administration commences followed by mesna 1000 mg/m² per dose given orally at 4 and 8 hours after ifosfamide (for total of 2500 mg/m² mesna per day; total dosage/4 days from IV + oral routes = 10,000 mg/m²)

VI. **Follow-up Schedules**
- Follow-up guidelines based on disease stage, histology (seminoma vs nonseminoma), and treatment type (radiation, chemotherapy, surgery, surveillance) have been published by various groups, primarily based on expert opinion rather than direct evidence from clinical trials. One commonly used set of guidelines is published by the National Comprehensive Cancer Network (NCCN) (www.nccn.org). Other guidelines also are available

For follow-up schedules, the author considers the starting point to be the first day of definitive treatment (surgery, radiation, or chemotherapy) resulting in expected cure. For patients with metastatic disease who receive chemotherapy followed by surgery, the first day of the first cycle is considered to be the start of year 1 unless adjuvant therapy is required for persistent viable disease. When adjuvant chemotherapy is required, the start date of adjuvant therapy is used to mark the start of year 1

De Santis M et al. J Clin Oncol 2004;22:1034–1039
Einhorn LH et al. N Engl J Med 2007;357:340–348
Motzer RJ et al. Cancer 1991;67:1305–1310
Rabbani F et al. Urology 2003;62:1092–1096

FIRST-LINE

TESTICULAR CANCER REGIMEN: ETOPOSIDE + CISPLATIN (EP)

Bosl GJ et al. J Clin Oncol 1988;6:1231–1238
Bajorin et al. J Clin Oncol 1993;11:598
Kondagunta et al. J Clin Oncol 2005;23:9290

Hydration for cisplatin: Administer intravenously 0.9% sodium chloride injection, USP (0.9% NS) to ensure a urinary output of at least 100 mL/hour prior to each dose of cisplatin. Hydration should be continued until the patient has completed chemotherapy and is able to take adequate oral liquids to prevent dehydration. Monitor and replace electrolytes/magnesium as needed

Etoposide 100 mg/m^2 per day; administer intravenously diluted in 0.9% NS to a concentration within the range of 0.2–0.4 mg/mL over 60 minutes, for 5 consecutive days, days 1–5, every 21 days for 4 cycles (total dosage/cycle = 500 mg/m^2)

Cisplatin 20 mg/m^2 per day; administer intravenously in 25–250 mL 0.9% NS over 30–60 minutes for 5 consecutive days, on days 1–5, every 21 days for 3–4 cycles (total dosage/cycle = 100 mg/m^2)

EP × 4 indicates 4 cycles

Supportive Care

Antiemetic prophylaxis
Emetogenic potential on days 1–5: **HIGH**. *Potential for delayed emetic symptoms*
See Chapter 42 for antiemetic recommendations

Hematopoietic growth factor (CSF) prophylaxis
Secondary prophylaxis is indicated in patients <50 years of age who have experienced neutropenic fever, and primary prophylaxis in patients >50 years of age or those who have received previous radiation therapy or chemotherapy for another cancer:
  Filgrastim (G-CSF) 5 mcg/kg per day by subcutaneous injection, *or*
  Pegfilgrastim (pegylated filgrastim) 6 mg/0.6 mL by subcutaneous injection for 1 dose
  • Begin use from 24–72 hours after myelosuppressive chemotherapy is completed
See Chapter 43 for more information

Antimicrobial prophylaxis
Risk of fever and neutropenia is **LOW**
  Antimicrobial primary prophylaxis to be considered:
  • Antibacterial—not indicated
  • Antifungal—not indicated
  • Antiviral—not indicated, unless patient previously had an episode of HSV

Treatment Modifications

Toxicity	MSKCC*	Indiana
Neutropenia day 1	Delay by 1 week unless WBC ≥2500/mm^3 *and* ANC ≥500/mm^{3*}; consider granulocyte colony-stimulating factor (G-CSF) with next cycle	No delay. Hold etoposide on day 5 if ANC still ≤2500/mm^{3†,‡}; consider G-CSF with next cycle
Febrile neutropenia (FN) or prior irradiation or age ≥50	Add G-CSF	Add G-CSF or reduce etoposide dosage by 25%†
FN despite G-CSF	Consider prophylactic antibiotic next cycle	Reduce etoposide dosage by 25%‡
Serum creatinine (Cr) ≥3.0 mg/dL (≥265.2 µmol/L)	Delay until Cr <3.0 mg/dL & CrCl creatinine clearance ≥50 mL/min (≥0.83 mL/s), then give full dose or substitute carboplatin if Cr does not return to <3.0 mg/dL or CrCl ≥50 mL/min	Delay until Cr <3.0 mg/dL‡

*Motzer R et al. Cancer 1990;66:857–861
†Einhorn L et al. J Clin Oncol 1989;7:387–391
‡Nichols CR et al. J Clin Oncol 1998;16:1287–1293

Patient Population Studied

Patients with good-risk GCT not previously treated with chemotherapy

Bajorin D et al. J Clin Oncol 1993;11:598–606
Bosl GJ et al. J Clin Oncol 1988;6:1231–1238
Culine S et al. Ann Oncol 2007;18:917–924
Kondagunta GV et al. J Clin Oncol 2005;9290–9294

Efficacy (EP × 4 for Good-Risk Patients)*

Author	Year	N	CR/FR	DurFR	OS†	Median Follow-up (Months)†
Bosl	1988	82	93%	82%	NR	26
Bajorin	1993	134	90%	87%	NR	22
Kondagunta*	2005	289	98%	92%	94%	92
Culine	2007	126	97%	86%	93%	53

CR/FR, complete or favorable response; DurFR, durable favorable response; OS, overall survival; NR, not reported
Favorable response: CR of any duration or PR with negative markers lasting ≥2 years
*Not a randomized controlled trial
†OS and median follow-up are 4-year actuarial rates

Toxicity

Bajorin D et al. J Clin Oncol 1993;11:598–606

Hematologic Toxicity	Percentage
Fever and neutropenia	23
Required RBC transfusion	13
Required platelets transfusion	3

Nonhematologic Toxicity

	% G1	% G2	% G3	% G4
Ototoxicity	23			
Neuropathy	31			
Mucositis	14			
Transaminitis		10		
Raynaud phenomenon*	None			

*Raynaud phenomenon reported in separate trial of EP × 4 for good-risk patients (de Wit R et al. J Clin Oncol 1997;15:1837–1843)

Therapy-Related Deaths N (%)	2 (1.5%)

Therapy Monitoring

1. *Every cycle:* CBC with differential, comprehensive metabolic profile, and serum tumor markers
2. *Response evaluation:* CT scan chest, abdomen, and pelvis and tumor markers after completion of cycle 4

FIRST-LINE

TESTICULAR CANCER REGIMEN: BLEOMYCIN, ETOPOSIDE, AND CISPLATIN (BEP)

Nichols CR et al. J Clin Oncol 1998;16:1287–1293

Hydration for cisplatin: 0.9% NS; administer intravenously to insure a urine output of ≥100 mL/hour prior to each dose of cisplatin and continue until the patient has completed chemotherapy and is able to take adequate oral liquids to prevent dehydration. We give 500 mL of 0.9% NS over 1 hour before cisplatin while premedications and etoposide are infused, and an additional 500 mL of 0.9% NS over 1 hour after cisplatin. Electrolytes/magnesium replaced as needed. Other hydration schedules are feasible

Bleomycin 30 units/week; administer by intravenous injection, weekly for 3–4 cycles (ie, 9–12 weeks; total dose/9-week course = 270 units; total dose/12-week course = 360 units)

Etoposide 100 mg/m² per day; administer intravenously diluted in 0.9% NS to a concentration within the range of 0.2–0.4 mg/mL over 30–60 minutes for 5 consecutive days on days 1–5, every 21 days for 3–4 cycles (total dosage/cycle = 500 mg/m²)

Cisplatin 20 mg/m² per day; administer intravenously in 25–250 mL 0.9% NS over 30–60 minutes for 5 consecutive days on days 1–5, every 21 days for 3–4 cycles (total dosage/cycle = 100 mg/m²)

BEP × 3 indicates 3 consecutive cycles; BEP × 4 indicates 4 consecutive cycles

Supportive Care

Antiemetic prophylaxis
Emetogenic potential on days 1–5: **HIGH**. *Potential for delayed symptoms*
Emetogenic potential on days with bleomycin alone: **MINIMAL**
See Chapter 42 for antiemetic recommendations

Hematopoietic growth factor (CSF) prophylaxis
Primary prophylaxis is indicated with one of the following:
Filgrastim (G-CSF) 5 mcg/kg per day by subcutaneous injection, *or*
Pegfilgrastim (pegylated filgrastim) 6 mg/0.6 mL by subcutaneous injection for 1 dose
• Begin use from 24–72 hours after myelosuppressive chemotherapy is completed
See Chapter 43 for more information

Antimicrobial prophylaxis
Risk of fever and neutropenia is **LOW**
Antimicrobial primary prophylaxis to be considered:
• Antibacterial—not indicated
• Antifungal—not indicated
• Antiviral—not indicated, unless patient previously had an episode of HSV

Patient Population Studied

Bleomycin, Etoposide, and Cisplatin × 3 (BEP × 3)
Indication/population studied: Good-risk GCT patients not previously treated with chemotherapy

Culine S et al. Ann Oncol 2007;18:917–924
de Wit R et al. J Clin Oncol 2001;19:1629–1640
Einhorn L et al. J Clin Oncol 1989;7:387–391
Loehrer P et al. J Clin Oncol 1995;13:470–476
Toner G et al. Lancet 2001;357:739–745

Bleomycin, Etoposide, and Cisplatin × 4 (BEP × 4)
Indication/population studied: Patients with intermediate- or poor-risk GCT not previously treated with chemotherapy

de Wit R et al. Br J Cancer 1995;71:1311–1314
Hinton S et al. Cancer 2003;97:1869–1875
Motzer R et al. J Clin Oncol 2007;25:247–256
Nichols C et al. J Clin Oncol 1991;9:1163–1172
Nichols CR et al. J Clin Oncol 1998;16:1287–1293

Toxicity (BEP × 4)

Hematologic Toxicity	% G3	% G4
Any hematologic toxicity	39	34

Nonhematologic Toxicity	% G3/G4
Nausea/vomiting	7
Neurologic	7
Infection	5
Pulmonary	5

Therapy-Related Deaths	N (%)
Pulmonary or pulmonary hemorrhage	3 (2)
Sepsis	3 (2)
Cerebral hemorrhage	1 (1)

Nichols CR et al. J Clin Oncol 1998;16:1287–1293

Toxicity (BEP × 3)

Hematologic Toxicity	Percentage
Leukocytes <1000/mm³	9
Fever and leukopenia (<2000/mm³ and T ≤38°C)	15
Platelet count is <25,000/mm³	3

Nonhematologic Toxicity	% G1	% G2	% G3	% G4
Pulmonary	13		1	
Ototoxicity	10	13	—	—
Sensory Neuropathy	20	4		—
Fatigue	39	21		—
Raynaud phenomenon*	8%			

*Raynaud phenomenon reported in regimen of BEP × 4 (not BEP × 3) for good-risk patients (de Wit R et al. J Clin Oncol 1997;15:1837–1843)
de Wit R et al. J Clin Oncol 2001;19:1629–1640

Efficacy (BEP × 3; Good Risk): Randomized Phase 3 Trials

Author	Year	N	CR/FR	DurFR	OS	Median Follow-up (Months)
Einhorn	1989	88	98%	92%	94%	NR*
Loehrer	1995	86	94%	86%	95%	49
de Wit	2001	397	97%	90%	97%	NR†
Toner	2001	83	88%	90%	96%	33
Culine	2007	132	95%	91%	96%	53‡

CR/FR, complete or favorable response; DurFR, durable favorable response; OS, overall survival; NR, not reported
Favorable response: CR of any duration or PR with negative markers lasting 2 years
*All patients had ≥1 year follow-up
†DurFR and OS assessed at 2 years
#DurFR and OS assessed at 4 years

Efficacy (BEP × 4: Intermediate- and Poor-Risk): Randomized Phase 3 Trials

Author	Year	N	CR/FR	DurFR	OS	Median Follow-up (Months)
Nichols	1991	77	73%	61%	74%	NR
de Wit	1995	105	72%	80%	80%	NR*
Hinton	2003	115	NR	55%	63%	88
Motzer	2007	111	55%	48%	72%	NR†

CR/FR, complete or favorable response; DurFR, durable favorable response; OS, overall survival; NR, not reported
Favorable response: CR of any duration or PR with negative markers lasting ≥2 years
*DurFR and OS assessed at 5 years
†DurFR assessed at 1 year and OS at 2 years

Treatment Modifications

Adverse Events	Treatment Modifications
Myelosuppression not improving during the first 4 days of therapy	Omit day 5 etoposide. Administer full-dose cisplatin
Febrile neutropenia	Add filgrastim during ongoing cycle and subsequent cycles so as to administer full-dose chemotherapy
Febrile neutropenia while receiving filgrastim	Reduce etoposide dosage by 25%
Clinical (rales or inspiratory lag) or radiographic evidence of pulmonary toxicity or fibrosis	Discontinue bleomycin

Repeated treatment cycles should begin on schedule without regard for the degree of myelosuppression noted on the day of scheduled treatment. Daily CBC is obtained to document marrow recovery

Therapy Monitoring

1. *Every cycle:* CBC with differential, comprehensive metabolic profile, serum tumor markers, and evaluation for bleomycin pulmonary toxicity (Indiana—lung exam[1,2], MSKCC—PFTs[3])
2. After completion of BEP × 3 or BEP × 4, repeat CT scan of chest, abdomen, and pelvis, and tumor markers

[1]Loehrer P et al. J Clin Oncol 1995;13:470–476
[2]Nichols CR et al. J Clin Oncol 1998;16:1287–1293
[3]Bosl GJ et al. J Clin Oncol 1988;6:1231–1238

FIRST-LINE

TESTICULAR CANCER REGIMEN: ETOPOSIDE + IFOSFAMIDE + CISPLATIN (VIP × 4)

Nichols CR et al. J Clin Oncol 1998;16:1287–1293

Indication:
Alternative initial therapy for intermediate- or poor-risk GCT patients who are not candidates for BEP (usually because of pulmonary compromise)

Order of administration: etoposide → cisplatin → ifosfamide/mesna
Hydration: 1000 mL 0.9% NS; administer intravenously over 2 hours. Consider additional intravenous fluid if medically appropriate until the patient has completed chemotherapy and is able to take adequate oral liquids to prevent dehydration. Monitor and replace electrolytes/magnesium as needed
Etoposide 75 mg/m^2 per day; administer intravenously diluted in 0.9% NS to a concentration within the range of 0.2–0.4 mg/mL over 60 minutes for 5 consecutive days on days 1 to 5, every 21 days for 4 cycles (total dosage/cycle = 375 mg/m^2)
Cisplatin 20 mg/m^2 per day; administer intravenously in 25–250 mL 0.9% NS over 30–60 minutes for 5 consecutive days on days 1–5, every 21 days for 4 cycles (total dosage/cycle = 100 mg/m^2)
Ifosfamide 1200 mg/m^2 per day; administer intravenously in 0.9% NS or D5W sufficient to produce a concentration within the range of 0.6 and 20 mg/mL, over 30–120 minutes for 5 consecutive days on days 1–5, every 21 days for 4 cycles (total dosage/cycle = 6000 mg/m^2)
Mesna 120 mg/m^2; administer by intravenous injection on day 1 just before or coincident with the start of ifosfamide administration, followed by mesna 1200 mg/m^2 per day; administer by continuous intravenous infusion over 24 hours for 5 consecutive days on days 1–5, every 21 days for 4 cycles (total dosage/cycle = 6120 mg/m^2). (See Expert Opinion for alternative administration schemes)

Supportive Care
Antiemetic prophylaxis
Emetogenic potential on days 1–5: **HIGH**. *Potential for delayed symptoms*
See Chapter 42 for antiemetic recommendations

Hematopoietic growth factor (CSF) prophylaxis
Primary prophylaxis is indicated with one of the following:
 Filgrastim (G-CSF) 5 mcg/kg per day by subcutaneous injection, *or*
 Pegfilgrastim (pegylated filgrastim) 6 mg/0.6 mL by subcutaneous injection for 1 dose
 • Begin use from 24–72 hours after myelosuppressive chemotherapy is completed
 • Discontinue daily filgrastim use if WBC >10,000/mm^3 on 2 consecutive daily measurements
See Chapter 43 for more information

Antimicrobial prophylaxis
Risk of fever and neutropenia is **INTERMEDIATE**
 Antimicrobial primary prophylaxis to be considered:
 • Antibacterial—consider a fluoroquinolone or no prophylaxis; *P. jirovecii* prophylaxis is recommended (eg, cotrimoxazole)
 • Antifungal—consider use during neutropenia and for anticipated mucositis
 • Antiviral—antiherpes antivirals (eg, acyclovir)

Therapy Monitoring

1. *Every cycle:* CBC with differential, comprehensive metabolic profile, and serum tumor markers
2. *Response evaluation:* CT scan of chest, abdomen, and pelvis, and tumor markers after completion of cycle 4

Patient Population Studied (N = 135)

Primarily intermediate- or poor-risk GCT patients not previously treated with chemotherapy

Nichols C et al. J Clin Oncol 1998;16:1287–1293

Toxicity

Hematologic Toxicity	% G3	% G4	% G5
Any hematologic toxicity	28	60	1

Nonhematologic Toxicity	% G3/G4
Nausea/vomiting	9
Neurologic	8
Infection	6
Genitourinary	5

Therapy-Related Deaths	Percentage
Sepsis	3
Cerebral hemorrhage	1

Nichols CR et al. J Clin Oncol 1998;16:1287–1293

Dose Modification

Toxicity	MSKCC	Indiana
Neutropenia day 1	Delay cycle by 1 week	No delay. Hold etoposide on day 5 if ANC still ≤2500/mm^3*
Thrombocytopenia and bleeding (TB), febrile neutropenia (FN), or prior irradiation	TB—delay until platelet count is ≥100,000/mm^3 FN—add G-CSF	Reduce etoposide dosage by 25%*
Serum creatinine >3 mg/dL (>265.2 μmol/L)	Delay cisplatin until Cr <3 mg/dL and creatinine clearance ≥50 mL/min (≥0.83 mL/s). Contact GCT high-dose experts for advice on subsequent use of cisplatin, ifosfamide, and etoposide, regardless of whether the creatinine returns to normal or not	

*Nichols CR et al. J Clin Oncol 1998;16:1287–1293

Efficacy

	Percentage
CR to chemotherapy alone	48
CR to chemotherapy + surgery	6
Partial response	22
Favorable response*	63
Failure-free survival at 2 years[†]	64
Overall survival at 2 years	74

*Includes patients with partial response and negative markers without relapse for ≥2 years
[†]Includes patients with partial responses (marker-negative or marker-positive) who did not have progression within 2 years

Nichols CR et al. J Clin Oncol 1998;16:1287–1293

	IGCCCG Classification		
	Good Risk (N = 13)	Intermediate Risk (N = 39)	Poor Risk (N = 92)
OS	92%	77%	62%
PFS	92%	72%	56%

Hinton S et al. Cancer 2003;97:1869–1875 (Long-term follow-up of patients in Nichols study [cited above] but with patients reclassified by IGCCCG risk status. Median follow-up for both OS and PFS was 7.3 years)

SUBSEQUENT THERAPY

TESTICULAR CANCER REGIMEN: PACLITAXEL + IFOSFAMIDE + CISPLATIN (TIP × 4)

Kondagunta GV et al. J Clin Oncol 2005;23:6549–6555

Indications:

1. First-line salvage chemotherapy for patients who relapsed after a complete response or partial response with negative markers lasting >6 months
2. Other patients who are not candidates for high-dose chemotherapy or have progressed after high-dose therapy and have not received paclitaxel

Premedication for paclitaxel: **Dexamethasone** 20 mg/dose; administer orally or intravenously for 2 doses at 14 and 7 hours prior to paclitaxel, plus **diphenhydramine** 50 mg and **cimetidine** 300 mg; administer both intravenously 1 hour prior to paclitaxel
Paclitaxel 250 mg/m^2; administer intravenously in 0.9% sodium chloride injection (0.9% NS) or 5% dextrose injection (D5W) to yield a final concentration within the range of 0.3 and 1.2 mg/mL over 24 hours on day 1, every 21 days for 4 cycles (total dosage/cycle = 250 mg/m^2)
Hydration: 1000 mL 0.9% NS; administer intravenously over 2 hours on days 2–5 before or during ifosfamide administration. Consider additional intravenous fluid if medically appropriate until the patient has completed chemotherapy and is able to take adequate oral liquids to prevent dehydration. Monitor and replace electrolytes/magnesium as needed
Ifosfamide 1500 mg/m^2 per day; administer intravenously in 0.9% NS or D5W to produce a concentration within the range of 0.6 and 20 mg/mL, over 2–3 hours for 4 consecutive days on days 2–5, every 21 days for 4 cycles (total dosage/cycle = 6000 mg/m^2)
Mesna 500 mg/m^2 per dose; administer intravenously in D5W to yield a concentration of 20 mg/mL, for 3 doses/day starting just before or coincident with the start of ifosfamide, with repeated doses at 4 and 8 hours after ifosfamide for 4 consecutive days on days 2–5, every 21 days for 4 cycles (total daily dosage = 1500 mg/m^2; total dosage/cycle = 6000 mg/m^2) (See Expert Opinion for alternative administration schemes)
Cisplatin 25 mg/m^2 per day; administer intravenously in 25–250 mL 0.9% NS, over 30–60 minutes for 4 consecutive days on days 2–5, every 21 days for 4 cycles (total dosage/cycle = 100 mg/m^2)

Supportive Care
Antiemetic prophylaxis
Emetogenic potential on day 1: LOW
Emetogenic potential on days 2–5: HIGH. Potential for delayed symptoms
See Chapter 42 for antiemetic recommendations

Hematopoietic growth factor (CSF) prophylaxis
Primary prophylaxis is indicated with one of the following:
Filgrastim (G-CSF) 5 mcg/kg per day by subcutaneous injection, *or*
Pegfilgrastim (pegylated filgrastim) 6 mg/0.6 mL by subcutaneous injection for 1 dose
• Begin use from 24–72 hours after myelosuppressive chemotherapy is completed
• Discontinue daily filgrastim use if WBC ≤10,000/mm3 on 2 consecutive daily measurements
See Chapter 43 for more information

Antimicrobial prophylaxis
Risk of fever and neutropenia is INTERMEDIATE
Antimicrobial primary prophylaxis to be considered:
• Antibacterial—consider a fluoroquinolone or no prophylaxis
• Antifungal—consider use during neutropenia
• Antiviral—antiherpes antivirals (eg, acyclovir) if history of multiple or severe HSV outbreaks

Dose Modifications

Toxicity	Modification
ANC <450/mm^3 on day 1	Delay until ANC >450/mm^3
Platelet count <75,000/mm^3 on day 1	Delay until platelet count is >75,000/mm^3
Platelets <10,000/mm^3 *or* platelets <50,000/mm^3 with bleeding	Transfuse platelets to >10,000/mm^3 if no bleeding, and to >50,000/mm^3 if bleeding
Hgb <8 g/dL	Transfuse RBC to keep Hgb >8 g/dL

Kondagunta GV et al. J Clin Oncol 2005;23:6549–6555

Therapy Monitoring

1. CBC with differential weekly
2. Comprehensive metabolic profile and serum tumor markers once to twice per cycle
3. *Response assessment:* CT scan of chest, abdomen, and pelvis, and tumor markers after completion of 4 cycles

Patient Population Studied (N = 46)

GCT patients fulfilling *all* of the following 3 criteria:
1. Gonadal primary tumor
2. Prior therapy with cisplatin-based treatment totaling 6 or fewer cycles
3. Prior CR or PR with negative markers lasting >6 months from completion of first-line chemotherapy

Kondagunta GV et al. J Clin Oncol 2005;23:6549–6555

Toxicity

Hematologic Toxicity	Percentage
Febrile neutropenia	48

Nonhematologic Toxicity	Percentage
Grade 3 neuropathy	7
Grade 4 or 5 nephrotoxicity	7
Grade 3 elevation of transaminases	2
Therapy-related deaths	2

Kondagunta GV et al. J Clin Oncol 2005;23:6549–6555

Efficacy (N = 46)

	Percentage
CR	70
Chemotherapy alone	63
Chemotherapy + surgery	7
IR	30
PR, marker negative	4
Other	26
Relapse From CR	7
Continuously NED*	63
Two-year overall survival	78

CR (complete response): disappearance of all clinical, radiographic, and biochemical evidence of disease for at least 4 weeks
IR (incomplete response): failure to achieve CR to chemotherapy with or without surgery, including patients who were observed to have failure of serum tumor marker normalization
NED (no evidence of disease)
*Median follow-up of 68 months

SUBSEQUENT THERAPY

TESTICULAR CANCER REGIMEN: VINBLASTINE + IFOSFAMIDE + CISPLATIN (VeIP × 4)

Loehrer PJ Sr et al. J Clin Oncol 1998;16:2500–2504

Indications:

1. First-line salvage chemotherapy for patients who relapsed after achieving a complete response or partial response with negative markers lasting >6 months

2. Other patients who progressed on or after first-line therapy who are not candidates for high-dose chemotherapy or progressed after high-dose therapy

Vinblastine 0.11 mg/kg per day; administer by intravenous injection over 1–2 minutes on 2 consecutive days, on days 1 and 2, every 3 weeks for 4 cycles (total dosage/cycle = 0.22 mg/kg)

Hydration: Administer 0.9% NS intravenously to insure a urine output of ≥100 mL/hour prior to each dose of cisplatin. Continue intravenous hydration until a patient has completed chemotherapy and is able to take adequate oral liquids to prevent dehydration
Suggested: 0.9% NS 500 mL over 1 hour before cisplatin and an additional 500 mL of 0.9% NS over 1 hour after cisplatin. Electrolytes/magnesium replaced as needed. Other hydration schedules are feasible

Cisplatin 20 mg/m² per day; administer intravenously in 25–250 mL of 0.9% NS over 30–60 minutes for 5 consecutive days on days 1–5, every 3 weeks for 4 cycles (total dosage/cycle = 100 mg/m²)

Ifosfamide 1200 mg/m² per day; administer intravenously in 0.9% NS or D5W sufficient to produce a concentration within the range of 0.6 and 20 mg/mL, over 30–60 minutes for 5 consecutive days on days 1–5, every 3 weeks for 4 cycles (total dosage/cycle = 6000 mg/m²)

Mesna 500 mg/m² per dose; administer intravenously in 25–50 mL 0.9% NS or D5W, over 15–30 minutes starting simultaneously with ifosfamide, followed by mesna 1200 mg/m² per day by continuous intravenous infusion in a volume of 0.9% NS, D5W (or dextrose and saline combinations) sufficient to produce a concentration of 20 mg/mL over 24 hours for 5 consecutive days on days 1–5, every 3 weeks for 4 cycles (total dosage/cycle = 6500 mg/m²). (See Expert Opinion for alternative administration schemes)

Supportive Care
Antiemetic prophylaxis
Emetogenic potential on days 1–5: **HIGH**. *Potential for delayed symptoms*
See Chapter 42 for antiemetic recommendations

Hematopoietic growth factor (CSF) prophylaxis
Primary prophylaxis is indicated with one of the following:
Filgrastim (G-CSF) 5 mcg/kg per day by subcutaneous injection, *or*
Pegfilgrastim (pegylated filgrastim) 6 mg/0.6 mL by subcutaneous injection for one dose
- Begin use from 24–72 hours after myelosuppressive chemotherapy is completed
- Discontinue daily filgrastim use if WBC >10,000/mm³ on 2 consecutive daily measurements
See Chapter 43 for more information

Antimicrobial prophylaxis
Risk of fever and neutropenia is **INTERMEDIATE**
  Antimicrobial primary prophylaxis to be considered:
  - Antibacterial—consider a fluoroquinolone or no prophylaxis
  - Antifungal—consider use during neutropenia and for anticipated mucositis
  - Antiviral—antiherpes antivirals (eg, acyclovir) if history of multiple or severe HSV outbreaks

Dose Modification

Toxicity	Modification
Neutropenia on day 1	No delay. Omit ifosfamide on day 5 if ANC still ≤2500/mm³
Thrombocytopenia and bleeding, febrile neutropenia (FN), or prior irradiation	Reduce etoposide and vinblastine dosages by 25%*
Platelet count <100,000/mm³ on day 5	Omit day 5 of ifosfamide*
Serum creatinine >2 mg/dL (>176.8 μmol/L)	Decrease ifosfamide dosage by 25%*
>10 RBCs/HPF	Hold ifosfamide and continue mesna and hydration until <10 RBCs/HPF

*Loehrer PJ Sr et al. J Clin Oncol 1998;16:2500–2504

Therapy Monitoring

1. Weekly CBC with differential
2. Comprehensive metabolic profile and serum tumor markers once to twice per cycle
3. *Response assessment:* CT scan of chest, abdomen, and pelvis, and tumor markers after completion of 4 cycles

Patient Population Studied (N = 145)

Second-line therapy for GCT patients who progressed during or after first-line chemotherapy

Loehrer PJ Sr et al. J Clin Oncol 1998;16:2500–2504

Toxicity

Hematologic Toxicity	Percentage
Febrile neutropenia	71
Required RBC transfusions	49
Required platelet transfusions	27

Nonhematologic Toxicity	Percentage
Renal insufficiency (Cr >4 mg/dL, 353.6 μmol/L)	6
Irreversible renal insufficiency	1
Secondary hematologic malignancies	1
Treatment-related deaths	2

Efficacy

Response	Percentage
CR	50
Chemotherapy alone	42
Chemotherapy + surgery	7
IR	50
Relapse From CR	24
Continuously NED	24

Progression-Free (PFS) and Overall Survival (OS)	
Median PFS	4.7 years
Median OS	1.3 years
OS at 2 years	38%
OS at 7 years	32%

CR (complete response): complete disappearance of all objective evidence of disease (clinical and radiographic) with normalization of hCG and AFP for at least 1 month
IR (incomplete response): any response that did not meet criteria of CR
NED (no evidence of disease) after VeIP + surgery

38. Thymic Malignancies

Chul Kim, MD, MPH, and Giuseppe Giaccone, MD, PhD

Epidemiology

Incidence: 0.13 cases per 100,000 (0.2–1.5% of all malignancies)
Median age: 40–60 years
Male to female ratio: 1:1

Engels EA, Pfeiffer RM. Int J Cancer 2003;105:546–551
Schmidt-Wolf IGH et al. Ann Hematol 2003;82:69–76
Tomiak EM, Evans WK. Crit Rev Oncol Hematol 1993;15:113–124

Stage at presentation:
(Masaoka Staging System)

Stage I:	32%
Stage II:	23%
Stage III:	34%
Stage IV:	11%

Pathology

Several histologic classifications of thymomas have been proposed. There is general agreement that the epithelial cells represent the malignant cells in this tumor type and the lymphocytic cells are considered benign

Classification of Thymic Epithelial Tumors

Muller-Hermelink	WHO Type	Levine and Rosai
Thymoma	Thymoma	Thymoma
Medullary type	Type A	Encapsulated
Mixed type	Type AB	—
Predominantly cortical	Type B1	Malignant type I (invasive)
Cortical type	Type B2	—
Well-differentiated carcinoma	Type B3	—
Thymic carcinoma	Type C	Malignant type II

Levine GD, Rosai J. Hum Pathol 1978;9:495–515
Müller-Hermelink HK, Marx A. Curr Opin Oncol 2000;12:426–433
Okumura M et al. Cancer 2002;94:624–632

Work-up

1. CT scan of the thorax
2. Extrathoracic disease such as metastases to the kidney, bone, liver, and brain are rare. Consequently, an extensive work-up for disease outside the thorax is not indicated in the absence of symptoms
3. Pleural or pericardial dissemination represents the most common form of metastatic involvement
4. Proper intrathoracic staging is surgical

Ströbel P et al. Blood 2002;100:159–166
Thomas CR Jr et al. J Clin Oncol 1999;17:2280–2289

Five-Year Survival

Stage I	96–100%
Stage II	86–96%
Stage III	56–69%
Stage IV	11–50%

Schneider PM et al. Ann Surg Oncol 1997;4:46–56

Expert Opinion

- Despite their rarity as a group of cancers, thymic epithelial tumors (TETs) are among the most common cancers of the anterior mediastinum in adults
- The clinical course can vary from relatively indolent in the case of some thymomas to highly aggressive in the case of thymic carcinomas
- Thymomas are often associated with a variety of autoimmune conditions; myasthenia gravis is the most common
- Complete surgical resection should be attempted whenever feasible
- Multimodality treatment is frequently required for locally advanced TETs
- Chemotherapy is offered to patients with advanced stages III to IV TETs. The evidence for these recommendations is derived from small phase 2 studies in either the neoadjuvant or refractory/recurrent disease setting
- Platinum-based combination chemotherapy is the standard of care for unresectable, advanced disease. A combination of cisplatin, doxorubicin, and cyclophosphamide (PAC) or cisplatin and etoposide (EP) are usually used as first-line regimens. More recently, the combination of carboplatin and paclitaxel has been introduced and appears to have reasonable activity in thymic carcinomas in particular[1–3]
- The molecular pathogenesis of TETs is gradually being unraveled. Sunitinib demonstrated anti-tumor activity in thymic carcinomas
- The role of immune checkpoint inhibitors in the treatment of TETs is being actively investigated and results indicate activity but also a higher incidence of autoimmune disorders[4]

References:
[1] Hirai F et al. Ann Oncol 2015;26:363–368
[2] Igawa S et al. Lung Cancer 2010;67:194–197
[3] Lemma GL et al. J Clin Oncol 2011;29:2060–2065
[4] Giaccone GJ et al. Lancet Oncol 2018;19:347–355

Prospective Chemotherapy Trials in Advanced-Stage Inoperable TETs

Reference	Regimen	Stage	Patients	CR + PR	mOS*
Anthracycline-containing Regimen					
Loehrer et al.	CDDP + **DOX** + CTX	IV	30	50	3.2
Fornasiero et al.	CDDP + **DOX** + CTX + VCR	III/IV	32	90	1.25
Non-anthracycline-containing Regimen					
Giaccone et al.	CDDP + VP–16	IV	16	56	4.3
Highley et al.	Ifosfamide	III/IV	13	46	N/R
Loehrer et al.	VP-16 + Ifosfamide + CDDP	IV	28	32	2.5
Grassin et al.	VP-16 + Ifosfamide + CDDP	IV	16	25	N/R
Lemma et al.	CDDP + Paclitaxel	IV	44	35	N/R
Gbolahan et al.	Pemetrexed	IV	27	19	2.4

Abbreviations: CDDP, cisplatin; CR, complete response; CTX, cyclophosphamide; DOX, doxorubicin; mOS, median overall survival; Not reported; PR, partial response; VCR, vincristine; VP–16, etoposide
*Median overall survival in years

Adapted from Kelly RJ et al. J Clin Oncol 2011;29:4820–4827

Fornasiero A et al. Cancer 1991;68:30–33
Gbolahan OB et al. J Thorac Oncol 2018;13:1940–1948
Giaccone G et al. J Clin Oncol 1996;14:814–820
Grassin F et al. J Thorac Oncol 2010;5:893–897
Highley MS et al. J Clin Oncol 1999;17:2737–2744
Lemma GL et al. J Clin Oncol 2008;26(Suppl):428s
Loehrer PJ et al. Cancer 2001;91:2010–2015
Loehrer PJ et al. J Clin Oncol 1994;12:1164–1168

Staging

Primary Tumor (T)*†

TX	Primary tumor not assessed
T0	No evidence of primary tumor
T1	Tumor encapsulated or extending into the mediastinal fat; may involve the mediastinal pleura
T1a	Tumor with no mediastinal pleura involvement
T1b	Tumor with direct invasion of mediastinal pleura
T2	Tumor with direct invasion of the pericardium (either partial or full thickness)
T3	Tumor with direct invasion into any of the following: lung, brachiocephalic vein, superior vena cava, phrenic nerve, chest wall, or extrapericardial pulmonary artery or veins
T4	Tumor with invasion into any of the following: aorta (ascending, arch, or descending), arch vessels, intrapericardial pulmonary artery, myocardium, trachea, esophagus

*Involvement must be microscopically confirmed in pathologic staging, if possible
†T categories are defined by "levels" of invasion; they reflect the highest degree of invasion regardless of how many other (lower-level) structures are invaded. T1, level 1 structures: thymus, anterior mediastinal fat, mediastinal pleura; T2, level 2 structures: pericardium; T3, level 3 structures: lung, brachiocephalic vein, superior vena cava, phrenic nerve, chest wall, hilar pulmonary vessels; T4, level 4 structures: aorta (ascending, arch, or descending), arch vessels, intrapericardial pulmonary artery, myocardium, trachea, esophagus

Regional Lymph Nodes (N)*

NX	Regional lymph nodes cannot be assessed
N0	No regional lymph node metastasis
N1	Metastasis in anterior (perithymic) lymph nodes
N2	Metastasis in deep intrathoracic or cervical lymph nodes

*Involvement must be microscopically confirmed in pathologic staging, if possible

Distant Metastasis (M)

M0	No pleural, pericardial, or distant metastasis
M1	Pleural, pericardial, or distant metastasis
M1a	Separate pleural or pericardial nodule(s)
M1b	Pulmonary intraparenchymal nodule or distant organ metastasis

Group	T	N	M
I	T1a,b	N0	M0
II	T2	N0	M0
IIIA	T3	N0	M0
IIIB	T4	N0	M0
IVA	Any T	N1	M0
IVA	Any T	N0,1	M1a
IVB	Any T	N2	M0, M1a
IVB	Any T	Any N	M1b

Amin MB et al (editors). AJCC Cancer Staging Manual. 8th ed. New York: Springer; 2017
Detterbeck FC et al. J Thorac Oncol 2014;9(9 Suppl 2):S65–S72.

ADVANCED DISEASE • FIRST-LINE

THYMIC MALIGNANCIES REGIMEN: DOXORUBICIN + CISPLATIN + VINCRISTINE + CYCLOPHOSPHAMIDE (ADOC)

Berruti A et al. Br J Cancer 1999;81:841–845

Hydration before cisplatin: ≥1000 mL 0.9% sodium chloride injection (0.9% NS); administer intravenously over 2–4 hours before chemotherapy commences. Monitor and replace electrolytes/magnesium as needed

Doxorubicin 40 mg/m^2; administer by intravenous injection over 3–5 minutes, on day 1, every 3 weeks (total dosage/cycle = 40 mg/m^2)

Cisplatin 50 mg/m^2; administer intravenously in 50–250 mL 0.9% NS over 1 hour on day 1, every 3 weeks (total dosage/cycle = 50 mg/m^2)

Hydration after cisplatin: Administer intravenously 1000 mL 0.9% NS over a minimum of 2 hours. Monitor and replace magnesium and other electrolytes as needed

Vincristine 0.6 mg/m^2; administer by intravenous injection over 1–2 minutes, on day 2, every 3 weeks (total dosage/cycle = 0.6 mg/m^2)

Cyclophosphamide 700 mg/m^2; administer intravenously in 50–150 mL 0.9% NS or 5% dextrose injection over 15 minutes, on day 4, every 3 weeks (total dosage/cycle = 700 mg/m^2)

Supportive Care

Antiemetic prophylaxis

Emetogenic potential on day 1 is **HIGH.** *Potential for delayed symptoms*

Emetogenic potential on day 2 is **MINIMAL**

Emetogenic potential on day 4 is **MODERATE**

See Chapter 42 for antiemetic recommendations

Hematopoietic growth factor (CSF) prophylaxis

Primary prophylaxis is **NOT** *indicated*

See Chapter 43 for more information

Antimicrobial prophylaxis

Risk of fever and neutropenia is **LOW**

  Antimicrobial primary prophylaxis to be considered:

- Antibacterial—not indicated
- Antifungal—not indicated
- Antiviral—not indicated unless patient previously had an episode of HSV

Note: Encourage patients to increase oral fluids intake on the days on which cisplatin and cyclophosphamide are administered

Use of steroids is discouraged, except for patients with myasthenia gravis who were previously receiving a stable dose of steroids

Treatment Modifications

Adverse Event	Dose Modification
ANC <1500/mm^3 or platelet count <100,000/mm^3	Delay therapy a maximum of 2 weeks until ANC >1500/mm^3 or platelet count >100,000/mm^3
2-week delay	Decrease dosage of all 4 drugs
Serum creatinine 1.6–2 mg/dL (141–177 μmol/L)	Hold therapy until serum creatinine <1.6 mg/dL (<141 μmol/L), then reduce cisplatin dosage by 25%
Serum creatinine ≥2 mg/dL (≥177 μmol/L)	Hold therapy until serum creatinine <1.6 mg/dL (<141 μmol/L), then reduce cisplatin dosage by 50%

Therapy Monitoring

1. *Pretreatment evaluation:* H&P, CBC with differential, serum electrolytes, creatinine, LFTs, ECG, CT chest and abdomen, and anterior mediastinotomy with mediastinal biopsy, determination of LVEF by echocardiogram
2. *Before each treatment cycle:* CBC with differential and serum creatinine
3. *Response evaluation:* Complete restaging including CT of chest and abdomen every 2–4 cycles

Patient Population Studied

A study of 16 patients with unresectable locally advanced nonmetastatic thymomas and locally advanced disease after radical surgery. Ten patients with stage III disease, and 6 patients with Stage IVa disease. Three patients had recurrent disease after previous surgery

Efficacy (N = 16)*

Complete response	6.25%
Partial response	75%
Stable disease	12.5%
Progressive disease	6.25%

*WHO criteria

Toxicity* (N = 16 patients/68 Cycles)

	% G3/4
Neutropenia	12.5
Anemia	—
Nausea/vomiting	6.25
Nephrotoxicity	—

*WHO criteria

Notes

1. Patients who achieve a CR or PR are referred for surgery after 4 cycles of ADOC chemotherapy
2. Additional ADOC is administered to patients with residual disease that is not surgically resectable for a maximum of 6 cycles
3. Patients with histologic evidence of malignancy at surgery receive fractionated RT (total dose = 45 Gy) followed by 2 additional cycles of ADOC

ADVANCED DISEASE • FIRST-LINE

THYMIC MALIGNANCIES REGIMEN: CISPLATIN + ETOPOSIDE

Giaccone G et al. J Clin Oncol 1996;14:814–820

Hydration before cisplatin: 1000 mL 0.9% sodium chloride injection (0.9% NS); administer intravenously over a minimum of 1 hour. Complete infusion before commencing cisplatin administration

Cisplatin 60 mg/m^2; administer intravenously in 50–500 mL of 0.9% NS over 60 minutes on day 1, every 3 weeks (total dosage/cycle = 60 mg/m^2)

Hydration after cisplatin: 1000 mL 0.9% NS; administer intravenously over a minimum of 2 hours. Monitor and replace magnesium and other electrolytes as needed

Etoposide 120 mg/m^2 per day; administer intravenously over 60 minutes, diluted in 0.9% NS or 5% dextrose injection to a concentration within the range of 0.2–0.4 mg/mL, for 3 consecutive days, days 1–3, every 3 weeks (total dosage/cycle = 360 mg/m^2)

Notes: Patients who tolerate treatment well and do not progress can receive up to 8 consecutive cycles of therapy. Use of steroids is discouraged, except for patients with myasthenia gravis previously receiving a stable dose of steroids

Supportive Care

Antiemetic prophylaxis
Emetogenic potential on day 1 is **HIGH.** *Potential for delayed symptoms*
Emetogenic potential on days 2 and 3 is **LOW**
See Chapter 42 for antiemetic recommendations

Hematopoietic growth factor (CSF) prophylaxis
Primary prophylaxis is **NOT** *indicated*
See Chapter 43 for more information

Antimicrobial prophylaxis
Risk of fever and neutropenia is **LOW**
   Antimicrobial primary prophylaxis to be considered:
   • Antibacterial—not indicated
   • Antifungal—not indicated
   • Antiviral—not indicated unless patient previously had an episode of HSV

Treatment Modifications

Adverse Event	Dose Modification
ANC <1500/mm^3 or platelet count <100,000/mm^3	Delay therapy a maximum of 2 weeks until ANC >1500/mm^3 and platelet count >100,000/mm^3
>2-week delay	Decrease dosage of both drugs by 25%

Dose reductions are also made based on nadir counts. If the leukocyte nadir and/or platelet nadir was 1000–1999/mm^3 or 50,000–74,999/mm^3 respectively, the doses of both drugs were reduced by 25% for subsequent cycles; if the nadirs were <1000/mm^3 and/or <50,000/mm^3 respectively, the doses of both drugs were reduced by 50% for subsequent cycles

| Serum creatinine 1.6–2 mg/dL (141–177 µmol/L) | Hold therapy until serum creatinine <1.6 mg/dL (<141 µmol/L), then reduce cisplatin dosage by 25% |
| Serum creatinine ≥1.5 mg/dL (≥133 µmol/L and remained elevated for more than 2 weeks after the scheduled time of the next cycle) | Hold therapy until serum creatinine <1.5 mg/dL (<133 µmol/L), then reduce cisplatin dosage by 50% |

Patient Population Studied

A study of 16 patients with recurrent or metastatic malignant thymoma that was considered incurable by excision and/or radiation therapy. Patients who previously received chemotherapy were eligible if they had not received cisplatin or etoposide. Patients receiving corticosteroids were not eligible for the study if previous radiation therapy

Efficacy (N = 15)

Complete response	5 (33%)
Partial response	4 (27%)
Stable disease	6 (40%)
Progressive disease	0 (0%)
Median survival	51.6 months

Toxicity* (N = 28)

	% G3–4
Hematologic	
Leukopenia	51
Thrombocytopenia	—
Anemia	—
Hemorrhage	—
Nonhematologic	
Infection	6
Nausea and vomiting	81
Diarrhea	6
Alopecia	69
Mucositis	6
Peripheral neuropathy	—
Phlebitis	—

*CTC

Therapy Monitoring

1. *Pretreatment evaluation:* H&P, CBC with differential, serum creatinine, LFTs, electrolytes, chest x-ray; CT scan of the chest and other tumor sites as indicated; creatinine clearance if adequacy of renal function is in doubt

2. *Before each treatment cycle:* H&P, CBC with differential, serum creatinine, LFTs, and electrolytes

3. *Response evaluation every 2 cycles:* CT scans of chest/abdomen

ADVANCED DISEASE • FIRST-LINE

THYMIC MALIGNANCIES REGIMEN: CISPLATIN + DOXORUBICIN + CYCLOPHOSPHAMIDE (PAC)

Loehrer PJ Sr et al. J Clin Oncol 1997;15:3093–3099
Loehrer PJ et al. J Clin Oncol 1994;12:1164–1168

Prechemotherapy hydration: ≥1000 mL 0.9% sodium chloride injection (0.9% NS); administer intravenously over a minimum of 2 hours. Monitor and replace magnesium and other electrolytes as needed
Cisplatin 50 mg/m²; administer intravenously in 50–150 mL of 0.9% NS over 15–30 minutes, on day 1, every 3 weeks (total dosage/cycle = 50 mg/m²)
Doxorubicin 50 mg/m²; administer by intravenous injection over 3–5 minutes, on day 1, every 3 weeks (total dosage/cycle = 50 mg/m²)
Cyclophosphamide 500 mg/m²; administer intravenously in 50–150 mL of 0.9% NS or 5% dextrose injection over 15–60 minutes, on day 1, every 3 weeks (total dosage/cycle = 500 mg/m²)
Postchemotherapy hydration: ≥1000 mL 0.9% NS; administer intravenously over a minimum of 2 hours on day 1, after chemotherapy is completed

Supportive Care
Antiemetic prophylaxis
Emetogenic potential on day 1 is **HIGH.** *Potential for delayed symptoms*
See Chapter 42 for antiemetic recommendations

Hematopoietic growth factor (CSF) prophylaxis
Primary prophylaxis is **NOT** *indicated*
See Chapter 43 for more information

Antimicrobial prophylaxis
Risk of fever and neutropenia is **LOW**
   Antimicrobial primary prophylaxis to be considered:
   • Antibacterial—not indicated
   • Antifungal—not indicated
   • Antiviral—not indicated unless patient previously had an episode of HSV

Note: Use of steroids is discouraged, except for patients with myasthenia gravis previously receiving a stable dose of steroids

Patient Population Studied

A study of 23 patients with limited-stage, unresectable thymoma or thymic carcinoma. Patients with limited-stage disease were defined as those patients with disease that could be encompassed by a single radiation therapy portal

Efficacy (N = 23)

Complete response	21.7%
Partial response	47.8%
Progressive disease	4.3%
Median survival	93 months

Toxicity* (N = 26)

	% G1	% G2	% G3	% G4
Hematologic				
Worst hematologic	19	23	12	42
Nonhematologic				
Emesis	15	23	15	—
Diarrhea	8	8	—	—
Infection	12	12	—	—
Cardiac	—	—	4	—
Mucositis	19	—	—	—
Neurologic/clinical	19	—	4	—
Genitourinary	23	4	—	—
Hepatic	19	—	—	—
Worst nonhematologic	23	42	23	8

*Eastern Cooperative Oncology Group scale

Treatment Modifications

Adverse Event	Dose Modification
ANC <1500/mm³ or platelet count <100,000/mm³	Delay therapy a maximum of 2 weeks until ANC >1500/mm³ or platelet count >100,000/mm³
2-week delay	Decrease dosage of all 3 drugs
Serum creatinine 1.6–2 mg/dL (141–177 µmol/L)	Hold therapy until serum creatinine <1.6 mg/dL (<141 µmol/L) then reduce cisplatin dosage by 25%
Serum creatinine ≥2 mg/dL (≥ 177 µmol/L)	Hold therapy until serum creatinine <1.6 mg/dL (<141 µmol/L), then reduce cisplatin dosage by 50%

Therapy Monitoring

1. *Pretreatment evaluation:* H&P, CBC with differential, serum creatinine, LFTs, electrolytes, chest x-ray; creatinine clearance if adequacy of renal function is in doubt
2. *Before each treatment cycle:* H&P, CBC with differential, serum creatinine, LFTs, and electrolytes
3. *Disease evaluation every 2 cycles:* Response evaluated before starting RT

Notes

1. Patients who achieve a CR or PR after 2 or 4 cycles of chemotherapy are referred for RT (total dose = 5400 cGy) to primary tumor and mediastinal and bilateral hilar lymph nodes
2. A maximum of 6 additional cycles of PAC chemotherapy may be administered after completing RT

ADVANCED DISEASE • FIRST-LINE

THYMIC MALIGNANCIES REGIMEN: PACLITAXEL + CARBOPLATIN

Lemma GL et al. J Clin Oncol 2011;29:2060–2065

Premedication (primary prophylaxis against hypersensitivity reactions from paclitaxel):
Dexamethasone 20 mg intravenously 30–60 minutes before paclitaxel
Diphenhydramine 25 mg by intravenous injection 15–30 minutes before paclitaxel
Cimetidine 300 mg (or **ranitidine** 50 mg, or **famotidine** 20 mg, or an equivalent histamine receptor [H_2]-subtype antagonist); intravenously over 15–30 minutes, 30–60 minutes before starting paclitaxel administration

Paclitaxel 225 mg/m^2 intravenously in a volume of 0.9% sodium chloride injection or 5% dextrose injection (D5W) sufficient to produce a solution with concentration within the range 0.3–1.2 mg/mL over 3 hours, on day 1, every 3 weeks (total dosage/cycle = 225 mg/m^2)
Carboplatin [calculated dose] AUC = 6 mg/mL × min; intravenously in 50–150 mL D5W over 30 minutes, on day 1, every 3 weeks (total dosage/cycle calculated to produce an AUC = 6 mg/mL × min) (see equation below)
Dexamethasone 8 mg/dose orally every 12 hours for 6 doses after chemotherapy if G ≥2 arthralgias/myalgias occur
• In patients who develop arthralgia or myalgia, include dexamethasone as prophylaxis against recurrent symptoms during subsequent treatment cycles

Carboplatin dose calculation is based on formulae developed to achieve consistent drug exposure within and among patients. Area under the plasma concentration versus time curve (AUC) is the targeted pharmacokinetic end point used to obtain consistent exposure

The method of Calvert et al:
Current product labeling for carboplatin approved by the U.S. Food and Drug Administration describes dose calculation based on a formula described by Calvert et al:

$$\text{Total carboplatin dose (mg)} = (\text{target AUC}) \times (\text{GFR} + 25)$$

In practice, creatinine clearance (CrCl) is used in place of glomerular filtration rate (GFR). CrCl can be measured from a 24-hour urine collection or estimated from any among several equations, such as the method of Cockcroft and Gault:

$$\text{For males, CrCl} = \frac{(140 - \text{age [year]}) \times (\text{body weight [kg]})}{72 \times (\text{serum creatinine [mg/dL]})}$$

$$\text{For females, CrCl} = \frac{(140 - \text{age [year]}) \times (\text{body weight [kg]})}{72 \times (\text{serum creatinine [mg/dL]})} \times 0.85$$

Note: On October 8, 2010, the U.S. Food and Drug Administration (FDA) identified a potential safety issue with carboplatin dosing based on recent changes in the measurement of serum creatinine. By the end of 2010, all clinical laboratories in the United States will use the standardized Isotope Dilution Mass Spectrometry (IDMS) method to measure serum creatinine, which could result in an overestimation of the GFR in some patients with normal renal function. A carboplatin dose calculated with an IDMS-measured serum creatinine result using the Calvert formula could exceed an expected exposure (AUC) and result in increased drug-related toxicity
Provided actual GFR measurements are made to assess renal function, carboplatin can be safely dosed according to the Calvert formula described in product labeling
If GFR (or creatinine clearance) is estimated based on serum creatinine measurements by the IDMS method, the FDA recommended for patients with normal renal function capping an estimated GFR at 125 mL/min for any targeted AUC value. No greater estimated GFR values should be used

U.S. FDA. Carboplatin dosing. [online] May 23, 2013. Available from: http://www.fda.gov/AboutFDA/CentersOffices/OfficeofMedicalProductsandTobacco/CDER/ucm228974.htm

Calvert AH et al. J Clin Oncol 1989;7:1748–1756
Cockcroft DW , Gault MH. Nephron 1976;16:31–41
Jodrell DI et al. J Clin Oncol 1992;10:520–528
Sørensen BT et al. Cancer Chemother Pharmacol 1991;28:397–401

(continued)

Patient Population Studied

A phase 2 study of carboplatin and paclitaxel in 46 patients with unresectable thymoma or thymic carcinoma. Patients previously treated with preoperative or adjuvant chemotherapy for thymic malignancy were allowed to enroll, if disease-free survival before recurrence was longer than 1 year

Toxicity (N = 46)

Adverse Event	G3	G4
Neutropenia	NR	24.4
Febrile neutropenia	2.2	2.2
Sensory neuropathy	13.3	0

National Cancer Institute Common Toxicity Criteria, version 2.0

(continued)

Supportive Care
Antiemetic prophylaxis
Emetogenic potential is at least **MODERATE**
See Chapter 42 for antiemetic recommendations

Hematopoietic growth factor (CSF) prophylaxis
Primary prophylaxis is **NOT** *indicated*
See Chapter 43 for more information

Antimicrobial prophylaxis
Risk of fever and neutropenia is **LOW**
   Antimicrobial primary prophylaxis to be considered:
   • Antibacterial—not indicated
   • Antifungal—not indicated
   • Antiviral—not indicated unless patient previously had an episode of HSV

Therapy Monitoring

1. *Pretreatment evaluation:* H&P, performance status (PS) evaluation, CBC with differential, metabolic profile including LFTs, CT scan of the chest and abdomen, pregnancy test (in females with childbearing potential)
2. *Before each cycle:* H&P, PS evaluation, CBC with differential, metabolic profile including LFTs, assessment of toxicity
3. *Response evaluation:* Every 2 cycles

Efficacy (N = 44)

Thymoma (N = 21)		
ORR (N = 21)*	42.9% (9)	90% CI, 24.5–62.8
CR (N = 21)*	14.3% (3)	
PR (N = 21)*	28.6% (6)	
Median PFS	16.7 months	95% CI, 7.2–19.8
Median OS	Not reached	Median follow up = 59.4 months
Median duration of response	16.9 months	95% CI, 3.1–22.0
Thymic Carcinoma (N = 23)		
ORR (N = 22)	21.7% (5)	90% CI, 9.0–40.4
CR (N = 22)	(0)	
PR (N = 22)	21.7 (5)	
Median PFS	5 months	95% CI, 3.0–8.3
Median OS	20 months	95% CI, 5.0–43.6
Median duration of response	4.5 months	95% CI, 3.4–9.9

*For patients with thymoma, no significant differences among various histologies were noted with respect to objective responses (A/AB v B1/B2 vs thymoma-NOS; P = 0.49), but the numbers were not large enough to make meaningful conclusions

Note: patients with thymoma have marginally improved PFS (logrank P = 0.06) and OS (logrank P = 0.01) compared with patients with thymic carcinoma. Cox regression analysis shows that the hazard ratio of thymic carcinoma over thymoma is 3.0 (95% CI, 1.2–7.8; P = 0.02) and 2.1 (95% CI, 1.0–4.5; P = 0.06) for OS and PFS, respectively

Treatment Modifications

Adverse Event	Treatment Modification
On day 1 of a cycle ANC <1500/mm³ or platelet count <100,000/mm³	Withhold paclitaxel and carboplatin until ANC ≥1500/mm³ and platelet count ≥100,000/mm³ for a maximum delay of 2 weeks
Delay of >2 weeks in reaching ANC >1500/mm³ and platelet count >100,000/mm³	Discontinue paclitaxel and carboplatin
After paclitaxel 225 mg/m² and carboplatin target AUC = 6 mg/mL × min: 1. Fever and neutropenia (ANC <500/mm³ with fever >38°C) *or* 2. A delay of next cycle by >7 days for ANC <1500/mm³, *or* 3. ANC <500/mm³ >7 days	Reduce paclitaxel dosage to 175 mg/m² and carboplatin dose to target AUC = 5 mg/mL × min every 3 weeks
After paclitaxel 175 mg/m² and carboplatin target AUC = 5 mg/mL × min: 1. Fever and neutropenia (ANC <500/mm³ with fever >38°C) *or* 2. A delay of next cycle by >7 days for ANC <1500/mm³, *or* 3. ANC <500/mm³ >7 days	Reduce paclitaxel dosage to 140 mg/m² and carboplatin dose to target AUC = 4 mg/mL × min every 3 weeks
After paclitaxel 140 mg/m² and carboplatin target AUC = 4 mg/mL × min: 1. Fever and neutropenia (ANC <500/mm³ with fever >38°C) *or* 2. A delay of next cycle by >7 days for ANC <1500/mm³, *or* 3. ANC <500/mm³ >7 days	Discontinue paclitaxel and carboplatin
Platelet count <50,000/mm³ at a paclitaxel dose of 225 mg/m² and carboplatin dose of AUC = 6 mg/mL × min every 3 weeks	Reduce paclitaxel dosage to 175 mg/m² and carboplatin dose to target AUC = 5 mg/mL × min every 3 weeks
Platelet count <50,000/mm³ at a paclitaxel dose of 175 mg/m² and carboplatin dose of AUC = 5 mg/mL × min every 3 weeks	Discontinue paclitaxel and carboplatin
G3/4 sensory neuropathy at a paclitaxel dose of 225 mg/m² and carboplatin dose of AUC = 6 mg/mL × min every 3 weeks	Withhold paclitaxel and carboplatin until toxicity G ≤1, then reduce paclitaxel dosage to 175 mg/m² and carboplatin dose to target AUC = 5 mg/mL × min every 3 weeks
G2 neurotoxicity	Reduce paclitaxel dosage to 200 mg/m²
G3 neurotoxicity	Reduce paclitaxel dosage to 175 mg/m²
G3/4 sensory neuropathy after paclitaxel 175 mg/m² and carboplatin dose of AUC = 5 mg/mL × min every 3 weeks	Withhold paclitaxel and carboplatin until toxicity G ≤1, then reduce paclitaxel dosage to 140 mg/m² and carboplatin dose to target AUC = 4 mg/mL × min every 3 weeks
G3/4 sensory neuropathy after paclitaxel 140 mg/m² and carboplatin dose of AUC = 4 mg/mL × min every 3 weeks	Discontinue paclitaxel and carboplatin
G2 arthralgia/myalgia despite dexamethasone	Reduce paclitaxel dosage to 200 mg/m²
G3 arthralgia/myalgia despite dexamethasone	Reduce paclitaxel dosage to 175 mg/m²
G ≥2 AST or G ≥3 bilirubin	Hold paclitaxel
Moderate hypersensitivity	Patient may be retreated
Severe hypersensitivity	Discontinue therapy
Chest pain or arrhythmia during chemotherapy	Immediately stop chemotherapy and evaluate the patient
Symptomatic arrhythmias, or ≥ second-degree AV block, or an ischemic event	Discontinue therapy

ADVANCED DISEASE • SECOND-LINE

THYMIC MALIGNANCIES REGIMEN: CAPECITABINE + GEMCITABINE

Palmieri G et al. Ann Oncol 2010;21:1168–1172
Palmieri G et al. Future Oncol 2014;10:2141–2147

Capecitabine 650 mg/m^2 per dose orally twice daily with approximately 200 mL of water within 30 minutes after a meal for 28 doses on days 1–14 every 3 weeks (total dosage/cycle = 18,200 mg/m^2)

Gemcitabine 1000 mg/m^2 per dose; intravenously in 50–250 mL 0.9% sodium chloride injection over 30 minutes for 2 doses, on days 1 and 8, every 3 weeks (total dosage/cycle = 2000 mg/m^2)

Notes:

- Capecitabine is given for 2 consecutive weeks followed by 1 week without treatment
- Doses are given as combinations of 500-mg and 150-mg tablets
- If a dose is missed, do not double the next dose; continue with the original schedule
- Advise patients to stop taking capecitabine and to contact their medical care provider if they develop:
  1. Diarrhea: an additional 4 bowel movements per day in excess of what is normal, or any diarrhea at night
  2. Vomiting: more than once in a 24-hour period
  3. Nausea or anorexia
  4. Stomatitis
  5. Hand-foot syndrome
  6. Fever or infection

Supportive Care

Antiemetic prophylaxis
Emetogenic potential on days *1–14* is **LOW**
See Chapter 42 for antiemetic recommendations

Hematopoietic growth factor (CSF) prophylaxis
Primary prophylaxis is **NOT** indicated
See Chapter 43 for more information

Antimicrobial prophylaxis
Risk of fever and neutropenia is **LOW**
  Antimicrobial primary prophylaxis to be considered:
  - Antibacterial—not indicated
  - Antifungal—not indicated
  - Antiviral—not indicated unless patient previously had an episode of HSV

Diarrhea management

Latent or delayed-onset diarrhea*:
Loperamide 4 mg orally initially after the first loose or liquid stool, *then* 2–4 mg orally every 2–4 hours or **diphenoxylate hydrochloride** 2.5 mg **with atropine sulfate** 0.025 mg (e.g., Lomotil®)

*Abigerges D et al. J Natl Cancer Inst 1994;86:446–449
Rothenberg ML et al. J Clin Oncol 2001;19:3801–3807
Wadler S et al. J Clin Oncol 1998;16:3169–3178

Hand-foot reaction (palmar-plantar erythrodysesthesia, PPE)

For patients who develop a hand-foot reaction, use topical emollients (eg, Aquaphor), topically or orally administered steroids, antihistamine agents (H$_1$-receptor antagonists), or pyridoxine. Pyridoxine may provide relief for discomfort/pain associated with PPE although the mechanism through which this occurs remains unclear

- The suggested pyridoxine starting dose is 50 mg/day, which may be increased to a maximum of 200 mg/day
- Patients who develop G1/2 PPE while receiving doxorubicin HCl liposome injection may receive a fixed daily dose of pyridoxine 200 mg. This may allow for treatment to be completed without dosage reduction, treatment delay, or recurrence of PPE

Patient Population Studied

A phase 2 study of capecitabine and gemcitabine in 30 patients with metastatic thymic epithelial tumors. All had previously received chemotherapy, including a platinum agent in first-line treatment

Patient Characteristics (N = 30)

	Number of Patients (%)
Gender	
Male	18 (60)
Female	12 (40)
Median age (range), 54 years (48–61 years)	
Histology	
Thymoma	22 (73.3)
B1	3 (10)
B1/B2	1 (3)
B2	9 (30)
B2/B3	3 (10)
B3	6 (20)
Thymic carcinoma	8 (26.7)
Stage IVA	8 (26.7)
Stage IVB	22 (73.3)
ECOG performance status	
0	16 (53.3)
1	11 (36.7)
2	3 (10)
Prior therapy	
Thymectomy	13 (43.3)
Mediastinal radiotherapy	13 (43.3)
Neoadjuvant chemotherapy	6 (20)
Chemotherapy for metastatic disease	30 (100)
Median number of previous lines of systemic therapy, 3 (range, 2–3)	

(continued)

Efficacy (N = 30)

Outcome	Result
Overall response rate	12 (40%)
ORR, thymic carcinoma (N = 8)	3 (37.5%)
Complete response	3 (10%)
Partial response	9 (30%)
Stable disease	15 (5%)
Progressive disease	3 (10%)
Median number of cycles	8 (range: 5–17)
Overall survival at 1 year	27 (90%)
Overall survival at 2 years	20 (66.7%)
Median progression-free survival	11 months (range: 6.5–16.5 months)
Median progression-free survival, thymoma (N = 22)	11 months (range: 8.5–16.5 months)
Median progression-free survival, thymic carcinoma (N = 8)	6 months (range: 3–10 months)

Toxicity (N = 30)

Adverse Event	% G1/2	% G3	% G4
Neutropenia	76.7	26.7	6.7
Anemia	43.3	16.7	0
Thrombocytopenia	43.3	16.7	0
Nausea/vomiting	23.3	6.7	0
Diarrhea	30	6.7	0
Alopecia	13.3	0	0
Hand-foot syndrome	30	13.3	0

National Cancer Institute Common Terminology Criteria for Adverse Events, version 3.0

Patient Population Studied
(continued)

	Number of Patients (%)
Previous first-line chemotherapy	
Cisplatin-doxorubicin-prednisone-cyclophosphamide	20 (66.7)
Carboplatin-doxorubicin-prednisone-cyclophosphamide	3 (10)
Carboplatin-etoposide	5 (16.7)
Cisplatin-doxorubicin-cyclophosphamide	2 (6.7)
Previous second-line chemotherapy	
Carboplatin-etoposide	11 (36.7)
Cetuximab	1 (3.3)
Imatinib	8 (26.7)
Octreotide + prednisone	10 (33.3)
Time from end of previous chemotherapy to relapse	
≤2 months	19 (63.3)
>2 months	11 (36.7)
Sites of metastases	
Pleura	30 (100)
Lung	20 (66.7)
Lymph nodes	18 (60)
Soft tissues	6 (20)
Liver	6 (20)
Bone	5 (16.7)
Myocardial tissue	3 (10)
Brain	1 (3.3)
Paraneoplastic syndrome	
B lymphopenia	19 (63.3)
Hypogammaglobulinemia	20 (66.7)
Myasthenia gravis	14 (46.7)
Autoimmune diabetes	2 (6.7)
Psoriasis	1 (3.3)
Pure red cell aplasia	1 (3.3)

Treatment Modifications

Adverse Event	Dose Modification
First G2 nonhematologic toxicity	Hold capecitabine and gemcitabine and resume after adverse events resolve to G ≤1. No change in dosage required
Second G2 nonhematologic toxicity	Hold capecitabine and gemcitabine and resume after adverse events resolve to G ≤1. Reduce dosage of both drugs by 25%
Third G2 nonhematologic toxicity	Hold capecitabine and gemcitabine and resume after adverse events resolve to G ≤1. Reduce dosage of both drugs by 50%
Fourth G2 nonhematologic toxicity	Discontinue capecitabine and gemcitabine
First G3 or G4 hematologic or nonhematologic toxicity	Hold capecitabine and gemcitabine and resume after adverse events resolve to G ≤1. Reduce dosages of both drugs by 50%
Second G3 or G4 hematologic or nonhematologic toxicity	Discontinue capecitabine and gemcitabine
G3 or G4 toxicity persisting for >3 weeks	Discontinue capecitabine and gemcitabine
Diarrhea, nausea, and vomiting	Treat symptomatically. Resume previous dosage if toxicity is adequately controlled within 2 days after initiating treatment. If control takes longer, reduce the capecitabine dosage or if symptoms occur despite prophylaxis, reduce the capecitabine dosage by 25–50%
ANC 1000–1499/mm^3, WBC 1000–1999/mm^3, or platelets 50,000–99,999/mm^3 on day of treatment	Proceed with treatment, but decrease both drug dosages by 25%
ANC and WBC <1000/mm^3 or platelets <50,000/mm^3 on day of treatment	Hold treatment until ANC and WBC are >1000/mm^3 and platelets >50,000/mm^3. Resume treatment with gemcitabine dosage reduced by 50%
WHO G4 nonhematologic adverse events	Hold treatment until resolution to G ≤1, then resume with both drug dosages decreased by 50%

Adapted in part from NCI of Canada CTC

Therapy Monitoring

1. *Before each cycle:* H&P, PS evaluation, CBC with differential, metabolic profile including LFTs, assessment of toxicity
2. *Every week:* CBC with differential, metabolic profile including LFTs
3. *Response evaluation:* Every 2 cycles

ADVANCED DISEASE • SECOND-LINE
THYMIC MALIGNANCIES REGIMEN: SUNITINIB

Remon J et al. Lung Cancer 2016;97:99–104
Thomas A et al. Lancet Oncol 2015;16:177–186
Supplement to: Thomas A et al. Lancet Oncol 2015;16:177–186

Sunitinib malate 50 mg/dose; administer orally once daily, continually, without regard for meals, in 6-week cycles consisting of 4 consecutive weeks of daily treatment followed by 2 weeks without treatment (total dose/6-week cycle = 1400 mg)

Treatment note:
• Patients who delay taking sunitinib at a regularly scheduled time may take a missed dose if the interval remaining before the next regularly scheduled dose is ≥12 hours

Supportive Care

Antiemetic prophylaxis
Emetogenic potential is **LOW**
See Chapter 42 for antiemetic recommendations

Hematopoietic growth factor (CSF) prophylaxis
Primary prophylaxis is **NOT** *indicated*
See Chapter 43 for more information

Antimicrobial prophylaxis
Risk of fever and neutropenia is **LOW**
  Antimicrobial primary prophylaxis to be considered:
  • Antibacterial—not indicated
  • Antifungal—not indicated
  • Antiviral—not indicated unless patient previously had an episode of HSV

Hand-foot skin reaction
For patients who develop a hand-foot skin reaction, use topical emollients (eg, Aquaphor), topical and/or oral steroids, antihistamine agents (H_1-receptor antagonists), or pyridoxine 50–150 mg/day orally

Diarrhea management
Latent or delayed-onset diarrhea*:
  Loperamide 4 mg orally initially after the first loose or liquid stool, *then* 2–4 mg orally every 2–4 hours or **diphenoxylate hydrochloride** 2.5 mg **with atropine sulfate** 0.025 mg (e.g., Lomotil®)

*Abigerges D et al. J Natl Cancer Inst 1994; 86:446–449
Rothenberg ML et al. J Clin Oncol 2001; 19:3801–3807
Wadler S et al. J Clin Oncol 1998; 16:3169–3178

Patient Population Studied

The open-label, single-arm, phase 2 study of 40 patients with chemotherapy-refractory histologically confirmed advanced thymoma (N = 16) or thymic carcinoma (N = 24). Eligible patients were aged ≥18 years, had Eastern Cooperative Oncology Group (ECOG) performance status ≤2, disease progression after failure of ≥1 previous line of platinum-based chemotherapy, and life expectancy >3 months. Patients who had hypertension were not eligible. All patients received sunitinib

---

Efficacy (N = 40)

	Patients with Thymoma	Patients with Thymic Carcinoma
Complete or partial response*	6%	26%
Median progression-free survival	8.5 months	7.2 months
Median overall survival	15.5 months	Not reached
Median duration of response	—	16.4 months

*Primary end point. Responses were confirmed ≥4 weeks after initial documentation
Note: Mean duration of treatment was 6.9 months for patients with thymoma and 6.1 months for patients with thymic carcinoma. Median follow-up was 17 months

Therapy Monitoring

1. *Prior to the first cycle of sunitinib:* physical examination, electrocardiogram, CBC with differential, platelet count, liver function tests, serum chemistries, blood glucose, blood pressure, and thyroid function tests

2. CBC, hepatic panel and mineral panel at the start of each cycle

3. Hepatotoxicity, including liver failure, has been observed. Monitor liver function tests before initiation of treatment, during each cycle of treatment, and as clinically indicated

4. Cardiac toxicity including declines in LVEF to below LLN and cardiac failure including death have occurred. Monitor patients for signs and symptoms of congestive heart failure

5. Prolonged QT intervals and torsades de pointes have been observed. Use with caution in patients at higher risk for developing QT interval prolongation. When using sunitinib, monitoring with on-treatment electrocardiograms and electrolytes should be considered monthly at first or when the dose is increased and less frequently thereafter

6. Hypertension may occur. Monitor blood pressure and treat as indicated under Treatment Modifications

7. Thyroid dysfunction may occur. Monitor thyroid function tests every 3 months. Treat hypothyroidism accordingly

8. Temporary interruption of therapy with sunitinib is recommended in patients undergoing major surgical procedures. *Note:* There is limited clinical experience regarding the timing of re-initiation of therapy following major surgical intervention. Therefore, the decision to resume sunitinib therapy following a major surgical intervention should be based upon clinical judgment of recovery from surgery

9. Monitor adrenal function in case of stress such as surgery, trauma or severe, infection

10. *Response assessment:* imaging every 2–3 months

Treatment Modifications

SUNITINIB	
Sunitinib Dose Levels	
Starting dose (Level 1)	50 mg once daily, 4 weeks on/2 weeks off
Dose Level −1	37.5 mg once daily, 4 weeks on/2 weeks off
Dose Level −2	25 mg once daily, 4 weeks on/2 weeks off
Dose Level −3	Discontinue sunitinib

Adverse Event	Treatment Modification
Cutaneous Toxicities	
Rash ≥G2	Withhold sunitinib and provide immediate symptomatic treatment. When toxicity resolves to G ≤1, restart sunitinib at 1 dose level lower than the dose level administered at the time toxicity developed. Treatment for symptoms may continue indefinitely as a preventive measure. *Note: Discontinue therapy if sunitinib is withheld >3 weeks*
Recurrence of G3/4 cutaneous toxicity at reduced doses of sunitinib	Withhold sunitinib and provide immediate symptomatic treatment. When toxicity resolves to G ≤1, restart sunitinib at 1 dose level lower than the dose level administered at the time toxicity developed. Treatment for symptoms may continue indefinitely as a preventive measure
Recurrence of G3/4 cutaneous toxicity at dose level −2 of sunitinib	Discontinue therapy
Cutaneous toxicity does not recur at reduced sunitinib doses with or without continued treatment for symptoms	Sunitinib dose may be increased 1 dose level to that administered at the time cutaneous toxicity developed. If toxicity recurs following the increase, then again withhold sunitinib and provide immediate symptomatic treatment. When toxicity resolves to G ≤1, restart sunitinib at 1 dose level lower than the dose level administered at the time toxicity developed. Treatment for symptoms may continue indefinitely as a preventive measure

(continued)

Treatment Modifications (*continued*)

Diarrhea

G1/2 diarrhea (increase of 4–6 stools/day over baseline; limiting instrumental ADL)	Focus on treatment for symptoms designed to resolve the diarrhea. No dose modifications are made for G1/2 diarrhea unless G2 diarrhea persists >2 weeks
G2 diarrhea lasting >2 weeks *or* G3/4 diarrhea *or* diarrhea that worsens by 1 grade while on sunitinib	Withhold sunitinib until diarrhea resolves to G ≤1. If resolution occurs within 3 weeks of holding treatment, restart sunitinib at 1 dose level lower than the dose level administered at the time diarrhea developed *Note: Discontinue therapy if sunitinib is withheld >3 weeks*
Recurrence of G2 diarrhea lasting >2 weeks *or* G3/4 diarrhea at reduced sunitinib doses and dose level is −1	Withhold sunitinib until the toxicity resolves to G ≤1, at which time sunitinib should be restarted at dose level −2. Treatment for symptoms may continue indefinitely as a preventive measure
Recurrence of G2 diarrhea lasting >2 weeks or G3/4 diarrhea at dose level −2	Discontinue therapy
Diarrhea does not recur at reduced sunitinib doses with or without continued treatment for symptoms	Sunitinib dose may be increased 1 dose level to the dose level administered at the time the diarrhea developed. If toxicity recurs following the increase, then again withhold sunitinib and provide immediate symptomatic treatment. When toxicity resolves to G ≤1, restart sunitinib at 1 dose level lower than the dose level administered at the time toxicity developed. Treatment for symptoms may continue indefinitely as a preventive measure

Hypertension

Note: Patients should have their blood pressure checked once weekly during their first 24 weeks of therapy and for an 8-week period after an adjustment in their sunitinib dose

G1 hypertension (SBP 120–139 or DBP 80–89 mm Hg)	Continue sunitinib at same dose and schedule
G2 asymptomatic hypertension (SBP 140–159 or DBP 90–99 mm Hg if previously WNL; change in baseline medical intervention indicated; recurrent or persistent [≥24 hrs]; symptomatic increase DBP >20 mm Hg or to >140/90 mm Hg; monotherapy indicated initiated)	Treat with antihypertensive medications and continue sunitinib at same dose and schedule
G2 symptomatic, or persistent G2 despite antihypertensive medications, or DBP ≥110 mm Hg, or G3 hypertension (SBP ≥160 or DBP ≥100 mm Hg; medical intervention indicated; >1 drug or more intensive therapy than previously used indicated)	Withhold sunitinib and treat with antihypertensive medications until symptoms resolve and diastolic BP <100 mm Hg. Then continue sunitinib at 1 dose level lower *Note: Discontinue therapy if sunitinib is withheld >3 weeks*
G4 hypertension (life-threatening consequences; urgent intervention indicated)	Discontinue therapy

Miscellaneous

G3/4 hepatotoxicity (ALT/AST >5× ULN if baseline was normal; >5× baseline if baseline was abnormal; bilirubin >3× ULN if baseline was normal; >3× baseline if baseline was abnormal)	Withhold sunitinib until LFTs resolve to baseline or G ≤1. If resolution occurs within 3 weeks of holding treatment, restart sunitinib at 1 dose level lower than the dose level administered at the time hepatotoxicity was noted *Note: Discontinue therapy if sunitinib is withheld >3 weeks or if worsening occurs during the period of observation off therapy*
Proteinuria	If urine dipstick ≥2+, obtain 24-hour urine protein. If 24-hour urine protein ≥3 grams, interrupt treatment. Resume treatment when 24-hour urine protein ≤1 gram. Resume sunitinib at one lower dose level
Repeat episodes of 24-hour urine protein ≥3 grams despite dose reductions or nephrotic syndrome	Discontinue sunitinib
Co-administration of potent CYP3A4 inhibitors (eg, ketoconazole, itraconazole, voriconazole, clarithromycin, atazanavir, ritonavir, telithromycin)	Reduce sunitinib dose (to a minimum of 37.5 mg once daily, 4 weeks on/2 weeks off)
Co-administration of potent CYP3A inducers (eg, rifampin, phenytoin, phenobarbital, dexamethasone, carbamazepine, St. John's wort)	Increase sunitinib dose (to a maximum of 87.5 mg once daily, 4 weeks on/2 weeks off)

Women of childbearing potential should be advised of the potential hazard to the fetus and to avoid becoming pregnant

Adverse Events (N = 40)

Grade (%)*	Grade 1–2	Grade 3	Grade 4	Grade 5
Nonhematologic				
Fatigue	78	20	0	0
Increased aspartate aminotransferase level	65	3	0	0
Oral mucositis	45	20	0	0
Hypoalbuminemia	63	3	0	0
Diarrhea	50	5	0	0
Anorexia	48	0	0	0
Hypertension	33	13	0	0
Increased alanine aminotransferase level	43	3	0	0
Nausea	43	0	0	0
Palmar-plantar erythrodysesthesia	33	3	0	0
Dyspepsia	35	0	0	0
Dysgeusia	33	0	0	0
Vomiting	33	0	0	0
Hypophosphatemia	23	8	0	0
Increased bilirubin level	23	3	0	0
Increased alkaline phosphatase level	23	0	0	0
Hypocalcemia	23	0	0	0
Oral pain	23	0	0	0
Edema of the limbs	23	0	0	0
Edema of the face	20	0	0	0
Abdominal pain	20	0	0	0
Hyponatremia	10	8	0	0
Alopecia	18	0	0	0
Hypothyroidism	18	0	0	0
Maculopapular rash	18	0	0	0
Dyspnea	13	3	0	0
Headache	13	3	0	0
Gastro-esophageal reflux disease	13	0	0	0
Hypomagnesemia	13	0	0	0
Noncardiac chest pain	13	0	0	0
Peripheral sensory neuropathy	13	0	0	0
Cough	10	0	0	0
Dry mouth	10	0	0	0

(continued)

Adverse Events (N = 40) (continued)

Grade (%)*	Grade 1–2	Grade 3	Grade 4	Grade 5
Nonhematologic				
Dry skin	10	0	0	0
Weight loss	10	0	0	0
Decreased ejection fraction	0	8	0	0
Tumor pain	0	5	0	0
Cardiac arrest	0	0	0	3
Hypoxia	0	3	0	0
Lung infection	0	3	0	0
Pancreatitis	0	3	0	0
Cholecystitis	0	3	0	0
Hypokalemia	0	3	0	0
Hyperkalemia	0	3	0	0
Hematologic				
Decreased lymphocyte count	58	8	13	0
Decreased white blood cells	65	10	0	0
Decreased neutrophil count	63	10	0	0
Decreased platelet count	60	5	5	0
Anemia	68	0	3	0
Febrile neutropenia	0	3	0	0

*According to the National Cancer Institute Common Toxicity Criteria for Adverse Events, version 4.0
Note: Grade 1/2 toxicities are included in the table if events occurred in ≥10% of patients. Only treatment-related adverse events are included. The highest grade per event per patient is included

39. Thyroid Cancer

Livia Lamartina, MD, PhD

Epidemiology

Incidence: Estimated U.S. incidence in 2020: 52,890 (male: 12,720; female: 40,170)
Estimated new cases: 15.8 per 100,000 persons (based on 2012–2016 cases)

Deaths: Estimated U.S. deaths in 2020: 2,180

- One of the few cancers that had increased in incidence over the past several years primarily due to the increased detection of occult papillary thyroid carcinomas on incidental screening techniques. The incidence plateaued from 2014 to 2015 and slowly declines starting from 2016
- Mainly affects young people. Nearly 2 of 3 cases are found in people between the ages of 20 and 55 years

Surveillance, Epidemiology and End Results (SEER) Program, available from http://seer.cancer.gov [accessed in 2020]

Pathology

Epithelial (Differentiated) Carcinomas	Incidence	Other Cell Types	Incidence
Papillary carcinomas	85%	**Medullary carcinoma**	<5%
Classic papillary	(75)	**Anaplastic carcinomas**	2%
Follicular variant	(15)	**Lymphoma**	Very rare
Tall cell variant	(4)	**Angiomatoid neoplasms**	Very rare
Columnar cell variant	(<1)	**Mucoepidermoid carcinomas**	Very rare
Diffuse sclerosing variant	(3)	**Malignant adult thyroid teratomas**	Very rare
Oxyphilic (Hürthle cell) variant	(2)	**Carcinomas with thymic features**	Very rare
Follicular carcinomas	2–5%	**Paragangliomas**	Very rare
Classic follicular	(76)		
Oxyphilic (Hürthle cell) variant	(20)		
Insular carcinoma	(4)		

Fagin JA et al. N Engl J Med 2016;375:1054–1067
Fagin JA et al. N Engl J Med 2016;375:2307
LiVolsi VA. Surgical Pathology of the Thyroid. Philadelphia, PA: WB Saunders, 1990

Papillary thyroid cancer (PTC)
1. Develops from thyroid follicular cells
2. Usually found in 1 lobe; only 10–20% appear in both lobes
3. Lymph node metastases are more frequent than distant metastases
4. Mutations in BRAF V600E (T1799A) occurs in 6–80% of patients
5. Recently, encapsulated noninvasive (ie, no signs of vascular or tumor capsule invasiveness) follicular variants of PTC have been reclassified as a benign entity and renamed "noninvasive follicular thyroid neoplasms with papillary-like nuclear features," thereby significantly reducing the number of patients who are considered to have thyroid cancer

Nikiforov YE et al. JAMA Oncol 2016;2:1023–1029

Follicular thyroid cancer (FTC)
1. Develops from the follicular cells in the normal thyroid
2. Mutations of codon 61 of N-*RAS* (N2) have been reported in as many as 19% of FTCs. Distant metastases are more frequent than lymph node metastases, namely in FTC with extensive vascular invasion (up to 46%)

Grani G et al. Lancet Diabetes Endocrinol 2018;6:500–514

Hürthle cell carcinoma
1. Usually assumed to be a variant of FTC, has been recognized as a separate entity in the last WHO classification
2. Both lymph node and distant metastases are frequent in Hürthle cell carcinoma

(continued)

(continued)

Medullary thyroid cancer (MTC)

1. Accounts for <5% of thyroid cancers
2. Develops in the C cells of the thyroid
3. Occurs in a familial form as multiple endocrine neoplasia type 2 (MEN 2A and MEN 2B2) and as a sporadic form (~80% of cases)
4. Germline mutations in the *RET* (**RE**arranged during **T**ransfection) protooncogene cause hereditary MTC (MEN 2A and MEN 2B). Up to 50% of patients with sporadic MTC have somatic *RET* mutations
5. MEN 2B: *RET* mutations most often in codons 918 and 883
6. MEN 2A: *RET* mutations most common in codons 609, 611, 618, 620, 630, 634, 768, 790, 791, 804, or 891
7. The constitutively active RET oncoproteins associated with MTC are sensitive to agents that inhibit RET kinase providing a rationale for targeting *RET* in patients with MTC

Anaplastic thyroid cancer (ATC)

1. Rare and fast-growing tumors. The majority present with extensive local invasion. All ATCs are classified as stage 4 disease
2. A poorly differentiated thyroid cancer originates from differentiated thyroid cancer. Approximately 50% of ATCs occur with either a prior or a coexistent differentiated carcinoma
3. The most common mutations are in *P53* and *CTNNB1*. *BRAFV600E*, while not common, has emerged as a mutation with therapeutic options
4. Work-up and treatment of ATC should be performed as rapidly as possible

Work-up

Initial Work-up of Thyroid Nodule

Thyroid nodule in clinically euthyroid patient

1. TSH level
2. Ultrasound of thyroid and neck lymph nodes with standardized sonographic scoring classification (TIRADS)
3. Fine-needle aspiration (FNA) is recommended for patients with nodules ≥1 cm with highly suspicious features on ultrasound, ≥1.5 cm for nodules with intermediate or moderately suspicious nodules, and ≥2–2.5 cm for low suspicious nodules
4. Nodules with benign features (purely cystic or entirely spongiform nodules) *should not* be submitted to FNA

Note: No role for thyroid scanning unless thyrotoxic (TSH suppressed):
• If thyrotoxic and palpated nodule is "hot" on scan, it is likely benign and biopsy is unnecessary. Refer to an endocrinologist
• If nodule is "cold," proceed to FNA

Durante C et al. JAMA 2018;319:914–924

Neck lymph node

1. FNA biopsy with thyroglobulin or calcitonin in washout fluid is appropriate for suspicious or indeterminate lymph nodes if the result would impact management (eg, positive result would result in treatment)

Leenhardt L et al. Eur Thyroid J 2013;2:147–159

Mass at site distant from neck

1. Biopsy (resection) and immunohistochemistry for thyroglobulin; calcitonin

Initial Work-up (Histologic Diagnosis Established)

Papillary or follicular carcinomas and their subtypes (usually iodine avid)

1. *Do not use iodinated contrast for radiography of any type of papillary or follicular carcinomas* within 2 months of a radioiodine treatment or a radioiodine scan
2. *Preop:*
   • Neck ultrasound or neck MRI
   • Cervical and chest CT (*use contrast if no radioiodine treatment or scan is scheduled within 2 months*) or MRI for patients with clinical suspicion of advanced disease (fixed, bulky substernal lesions, extensive lymph node involvement)
   • Evaluate vocal cord mobility
3. *Postop:*
   • ¹³¹I scanning (see below)
   • Thyroglobulin (TG) level

(continued)

Work-up (continued)

Dedifferentiated papillary/follicular cancers (iodine nonavid, often not apparent initially)

1. *CT scans* (*use contrast if no radioiodine treatment or scan is scheduled within 2 months*): Often "fused" with PET scans

2. *Preop:*
   - Neck ultrasound or neck MRI
   - Cervical and chest CT (*use contrast if no radioiodine treatment or scan is scheduled within 2 months*) or MRI for patients with clinical suspicion of advanced disease (fixed, bulky substernal lesions, extensive lymph node involvement)
   - Evaluate vocal cord mobility

3. *Postop:*
   - ^{131}I scanning (see below)
   - Thyroglobulin (TG) level

4. *PET scans* (*^{18}F-deoxyglucose*): Sensitivity enhanced with recombinant human TSH pretreatment

5. Radiographic bone surveys (may not be needed if PET scan is negative and all other scans do not demonstrate any obvious evidence of disease in bone)

Medullary thyroid carcinoma

1. Neck ultrasound

2. Evaluate vocal cord mobility

3. Serum calcitonin level

4. Serum CEA level

5. Complete metabolic panel; including calcium

6. Screen for the presence of a pheochromocytoma in patients with MEN2A and MEN2B

7. In all cases of MTC, collect blood for genetic testing for the presence of a *RET* germline mutation

8. Provide genetic counseling for patients found to have a *RET* germline mutation

Anaplastic carcinoma

1. Cross-sectional CT scan (with contrast) or MRI, and PET/CT of the neck and chest, and ultrasound of the neck

2. Consider bone scan

3. May need restaging at 2- to 4-week intervals because of rapid rate of tumor progression

4. **Work-up and treatment of ATC should be performed as rapidly as possible**

Staging

Separate T definitions are used for (1) papillary, follicular, poorly differentiated, Hürthle cell, and anaplastic thyroid carcinoma and (2) medullary thyroid cancer. Separate stage groupings are used for (1) papillary or follicular (differentiated), (2) anaplastic (undifferentiated), and (3) medullary thyroid carcinoma

AJCC TNM DEFINITIONS

Regional Lymph Nodes (N)

Regional lymph nodes are the central compartment, lateral cervical, and upper mediastinal lymph nodes

NX	Regional lymph nodes cannot be assessed
N0	No regional lymph node metastasis
N0a	One or more cytologically or histologically confirmed benign lymph nodes
N0b	No radiologic or clinical evidence of locoregional lymph node metastasis
N1	Regional lymph node metastasis
N1a	Metastasis to level VI or VII (pretracheal, paratracheal, or prelaryngeal/Delphian, or upper mediastinal) lymph nodes. This can be unilateral or bilateral disease
N1b	Metastasis to unilateral, bilateral, or contralateral lateral neck lymph nodes (levels I, II, III, IV, or V) or retropharyngeal lymph nodes

Primary Tumor (T) for papillary, follicular, poorly differentiated, Hürthle cell, and anaplastic thyroid carcinoma

All categories may be subdivided: (s) solitary tumor and (m) multifocal tumor (the largest determines the classification)

TX	Primary tumor cannot be assessed
T0	No evidence of primary tumor
T1	Tumor 2 cm or less in greatest dimension, limited to the thyroid
T1a	Tumor 1 cm or less, limited to the thyroid
T1b	Tumor more than 1 cm but not more than 2 cm in greatest dimension, limited to the thyroid
T2	Tumor more than 2 cm but not more than 4 cm in greatest dimension, limited to the thyroid
T3	Tumor more than 4 cm in greatest dimension limited to the thyroid, or gross extrathyroidal extension invading only strap muscles
T3a	Tumor more than 4 cm in greatest dimension limited to the thyroid
T3b	Gross extrathyroidal extension invading only strap muscles (sternohyoid, sternothyroid, thyrohyoid, or omohyoid muscles) from a tumor of any size
T4	Includes gross extrathyroidal extension beyond the strap muscles
T4a	Gross extrathyroidal extension invading subcutaneous soft tissues, larynx, trachea, esophagus, or recurrent laryngeal nerve from a tumor of any size
T4b	Gross extrathyroidal extension invading prevertebral fascia or encasing the carotid artery or mediastinal vessels from a tumor of any size

Primary Tumor (T) for Medullary Thyroid Cancer

TX	Primary tumor cannot be assessed
T0	No evidence of primary tumor
T1	Tumor 2 cm or less in greatest dimension, limited to the thyroid
T1a	Tumor 1 cm or less, limited to the thyroid
T1b	Tumor more than 1 cm but not more than 2 cm in greatest dimension, limited to the thyroid
T2	Tumor more than 2 cm but not more than 4 cm in greatest dimension, limited to the thyroid
T3	Tumor more than 4 cm in greatest dimension limited to the thyroid, or with extrathyroidal extension
T3a	Tumor more than 4 cm in greatest dimension limited to the thyroid
T3b	Gross extrathyroidal extension invading only strap muscles (sternohyoid, sternothyroid, thyrohyoid, or omohyoid muscles) from a tumor of any size
T4	Advanced disease
T4a	Moderately advanced disease; tumor of any size with gross extrathyroidal extension into the nearby tissues of the neck, including subcutaneous soft tissue, larynx, trachea, esophagus, or recurrent laryngeal nerve
T4b	Very advanced disease; tumor of any size with extension toward the spine or into nearby large blood vessels, gross extrathyroidal extension invading the prevertebral fascia, or encasing the carotid artery or mediastinal vessels

Distant Metastasis (M)

M0	No distant metastasis (no pathologic M0; use clinical M to complete stage group)
M1	Distant metastasis

(continued)

Staging (continued)

AJCC STAGE GROUPINGS

Papillary or Follicular (Differentiated) Thyroid Cancer

Younger than 55 Years

Stage	T	N	M
I	Any T	Any N	M0
II	Any T	Any N	M1

55 Years and Older

Stage	T	N	M
I	T1	N0/NX	M0
	T2	N0/NX	M0
II	T1	N1	M0
	T2	N1	M0
	T3a/T3b	Any N	M0
III	T4a	Any N	M0
IVA	T4b	Any N	M0
IVB	Any T	Any N	M1

Anaplastic Thyroid Carcinoma

All anaplastic carcinomas are considered stage IV

Group	T	N	M
IVA	T1–T3a	N0/NX	M0
IVB	T1–T3a	N1	M0
	T3b	Any N	M0
	T4	Any N	M0
IVC	Any T	Any N	M1

Medullary Thyroid Carcinoma

Stage	T	N	M
I	T1	N0	M0
II	T2	N0	M0
	T3	N0	M0
III	T1–3	N1a	M0
IVA	T4a	Any N	M0
	T1–3	N1b	M0
IVB	T4b	Any N	M0
IVC	Any T	Any N	M1

Amin MB et al (editors). AJCC Cancer Staging Manual. 8th ed. New York: Springer; 2017

Expert Opinion

Surgical Treatment

1. *Cytologically (or clinically) suspicious or indeterminate thyroid nodule:* Ipsilateral complete lobectomy and isthmusectomy followed by completion (during initial or subsequent procedure) of total thyroidectomy if malignancy confirmed, *unless there is a solitary intrathyroidal papillary carcinoma of ≤4 cm of maximum diameter with no lymphadenopathy, no vascular invasion, and no aggressive histologic type*
2. *Thyroid biopsy or extrathyroidal site biopsy positive for cancer:* Total thyroidectomy ± ipsilateral and central modified node dissection unless it is *a solitary intrathyroidal papillary carcinoma of ≤4 cm of maximum diameter with no lymphadenopathy, no vascular invasion, and no aggressive histologic type* and no local or distant metastases—in which case perform a lobectomy only
3. *Grossly invasive tumor or bilateral disease:* Total thyroidectomy with bilateral and central modified node dissection
4. Medullary thyroid carcinoma requires total thyroidectomy with bilateral central neck dissections. It is important to exclude the presence of a pheochromocytoma prior to thyroidectomy. Adrenalectomy should be performed for pheochromocytoma prior to performing thyroidectomy
5. Anaplastic carcinoma requires as complete a local resection as possible, often despite grossly invasive disease. Initially unresectable tumor might be resected after a partial course of external beam radiation therapy. In all cases of thyroidectomy, the parathyroid glands must be preserved, either by avoiding their resection or autografting those that are resected

Radioactive Iodine (^{131}I) for Papillary and Follicular Carcinomas Including Hürthle Cell Carcinoma

Indications:
1. Always indicated in high risk:
   - Macroscopic invasion of tumor into the perithyroidal soft tissues
   - R2 incomplete tumor resection
   - Presence of distant metastases
   - Postoperative serum thyroglobulin suggestive of distant metastases
   - Pathologic lymph node metastases of 3 cm or more
   - FTC with extensive vascular invasion (more than 4 foci of vascular invasion)

(continued)

Expert Opinion (continued)

2. Consider in intermediate risk:
   - Microscopic extrathyroidal extension of the tumor into the perithyroidal soft tissues
   - Aggressive histotype (eg, tall cell, hobnail variant, columnar cell carcinoma)
   - PTC with vascular invasion
   - Clinically evident lymph-node metastasis
   - More than 5 lymph node metastases of less than 3 cm
   - Multifocal papillary microcarcinoma with microscopic extrathyroidal extension
   - Tumors harboring BRAFV600E mutations
3. Usually not indicated in low risk:
   - Intrathyroidal tumor with no local or distant metastases
   - R0 or R1 resection
   - No aggressive histotype
   - No vascular invasion
   - No clinical evidence of lymph node metastases or less than 5 microscopic (ie, <2 mm) central compartment metastases

Diagnostic 131I WBS and TG may assist radioiodine treatment decision

If the ^{131}I WBS is positive	Treat with [131]I. Obtain ^{131}I WBS (posttreatment WBS) 48–72 hours after ^{131}I therapy. Value of subsequent treatments is based on verifying uptake on posttreatment WBS and/or significant decrease of stimulated TG
If the ^{131}I WBS is negative *and* if TG level is undetectable	No treatment. Resume levothyroxine therapy. Confirm absence of dedifferentiated disease (see 4–7 above)

Initial ablation for papillary and follicular carcinomas
1. *High risk:* 100–200 mCi empiric dosing or treat to maximal red marrow tolerance (200 REM, ascertain with whole body/blood dosimetry analysis) with thyroid hormone withdrawal preparation
2. *Intermediate risk:* 30 mCi empiric dosing with rhTSH preparation or 100 mCi empiric dosing with either *recombinant human TSH* or thyroid hormone withdrawal preparation (see below)
3. *Low-risk disease with no metastases:* 30 mCi empiric dosing with *recombinant human TSH* preparation (see below)

[131]*I treatment or diagnostic WBS preparation:*
a) *Thyroid hormone withdrawal protocol:*
   - *~6 weeks before scan:* Stop levothyroxine therapy. Continue without levothyroxine >6 weeks if needed until TSH >30 mIU/L (first 4 weeks on **liothyronine sodium** 25 mcg orally twice per day)
   - *2 weeks before and during scan:* Institute low-iodine diet
b) *Recombinant human TSH (thyrotropin alfa, Thyrogen) protocol:*
   - *2 weeks before and during scan:* Institute low-iodine diet
   - *Days 1 and 2:* Administer **recombinant human TSH** 0.9 mg/day intramuscularly for 2 consecutive days
   - *Day 3:* Administer ^{131}I orally
   - *Day 5:* Perform ^{131}I WBS (≥30 min/view; ≥140,000 counts)
   - *Day 5:* Obtain serum TG, antithyroglobulin autoantibody, and TSH levels

Management Following Thyroidectomy: Papillary or Follicular Carcinomas (and Their Subtypes) and Medullary Thyroid Carcinoma
Papillary or Follicular Carcinomas (and their subtypes)
Assess response to treatment at 6–12 months
1. TG levels (monitor for presence of interfering anti-TG antibodies) *Note:* The "normal range" for TG in this situation is "undetectable"
2. Antithyroglobulin autoantibodies occur in 20% of patients and interfere with the TG assay making it insensitive, but can sometimes be a surrogate marker for persistent disease
3. Physical exams, patient neck self-exams
4. Neck ultrasound
Further imaging is indicated in case of clinical suspicion of persistent disease
1. CT of chest
2. PET scans if ^{131}I WBS is negative but TG is positive. Sensitivity correlates with tumor dedifferentiation and hexokinase I expression
3. Radiographic bone survey

(continued)

Expert Opinion *(continued)*

Medullary Thyroid Carcinoma

1. Calcitonin and CEA levels

2. Neck ultrasound

3. Complete CT survey (with contrast)

4. Consider hepatic MRI and radiographic bone survey

Subsequent Radioiodine Treatments for:

• Pathologic ^{131}I WBS

• Stimulated TG >10 ng/mL and negative scans (including PET)

Treatment: 100-mCi empiric dosing with posttreatment ^{131}I imaging

Follow-up Treatments for M1 Disease

1. Empiric dose of 100 mCi or single dose to maximal red marrow tolerance (200 REM; ascertain with whole-body/blood dosimetry analysis)

2. Repeat treatment every 6 months then every 12 months until clinical benefit is evident (imaging and TG improvement)

Repeat Surgery

Indications:

1. Resection of macroscopic residual disease before [131]I

2. Localized non—iodine-avid tumor

3. Distant critical sites (eg, spinal cord, brain)

4. Bone metastases

5. Isolated distant metastases and palliation of recurrent disease

Suppression of TSH with Levothyroxine—Papillary and Follicular Carcinomas Including Hürthle Cell Carcinoma

Indication: for high-risk patients before first disease assessment and in patients with persistent morphologic disease

Goal: TSH ≤0.1 mIU/L or 0.1–0.5 mIU/L in case of atrial fibrillation or severe osteoporosis

Note: May use a β-adrenergic blocker to mitigate tachycardia and risk of late left ventricular hypertrophy

• In high-risk patients with no evidence of disease at the 6–12 months assessment, TSH can be allowed to rise between 0.1 and 0.5 mIU/L for 5 years then to 0.5–2 mIU/L thereafter

• In intermediate- and low-risk patients with no evidence of disease, TSH goal is in the normal low range, ie, 0.5–2 mIU/L

• In case of detectable TG in the biochemical incomplete response range (above 1 ng/mL on levothyroxine treatment or above 10 ng/mL under stimulation), in the absence of morphologic evidence of disease, mild suppression (TSH goal 0.1–0.5 mIU/L) should be considered, provided the absence of atrial fibrillation or severe osteoporosis

Bisphosphonate Therapy

Consider bisphosphonate therapy in patients with papillary, follicular, or medullary thyroid carcinoma who have symptomatic bone metastases or who have extensive disease that is not symptomatic, but who may need intervention if they progress

External Beam Radiation Therapy

Indications:

1. Patients with unresectable ATC should be managed by chemotherapy followed by external beam radiotherapy

2. Palliation of distant sites of disease

Selected Multimodal Approaches

Anaplastic carcinoma: Complete primary resection followed by local external beam radiation. Restage to detect early recurrence or distant disease, then treat with chemotherapy using these sites to assess response

Systemic Chemotherapy

1. Clearly effective in thyroid lymphoma

2. Necessary (although usually futile) in anaplastic thyroid cancer

3. Should be considered in patients with symptomatic/metastatic MTC. See vandetanib regimen below

[18]F FDG-PET Scans

As with most cancers, recommendations regarding the use of PET scans in thyroid cancer are not evidence based at this time. In very few instances will a PET scan result alter management. General recommendations can be summarized as follows:

1. *Initial work-up of a thyroid nodule:* Although increased FDG accumulation may heighten suspicion and help identify a thyroid nodule as malignant, the poor sensitivity and high cost do not support the use of PET imaging as a tool for diagnosis

2. *DTC:* In patients considered intermediate- and high-risk, PET may have some utility in:

   • Assessing the extent of disease in patients with metastases, and

   • Assessing patients with high thyroglobulin (TG) levels and negative ^{131}I scans. In these patients, a positive PET may indicate dedifferentiation associated with tumor aggressiveness

3. *MTC:* The role of PET is limited

4. *ATC:* PET can help assess the extent of disease

Three-Year Survival

Papillary Thyroid Cancer	
Stage I	100%
Stage II	100%
Stage III*	96%
Stage IV*	45%

Follicular Thyroid Cancer	
Stage I	100%
Stage II	100%
Stage III*	79%
Stage IV*	47%

Medullary Thyroid Cancer	
Stage I	100%
Stage II	97%
Stage III	78%
Stage IV	24%

Anaplastic Thyroid Cancer	
Stage IV†	9%

*All stages III and IV patients with follicular or papillary thyroid cancer are, by definition, more than 55 years old
†All anaplastic carcinomas are considered stage IV

Definition of Refractory Thyroid Cancer

1. For thyroid cancer originating from follicular cells, papillary and follicular carcinomas including Hürthle cell carcinoma, and poorly differentiated thyroid cancer, any of the following:

   - *Absence of radioiodine uptake on ^{131}I Scan*
   - *Absence of radioiodine uptake in at least one lesion despite the presence of radioiodine-avid lesions*
   - *Morphologic progression within 12 months from radioiodine treatment, despite significative radioiodine uptake*

Fugazzola L et al. Eur Thyroid J 2019;8:227–245

Note: After a cumulative radioiodine activity above 600 mCi, complete remission is anecdotal and further radioiodine treatments are usually not recommended

2. Medullary thyroid cancer with unresectable locally advanced or distant metastatic disease
3. Anaplastic thyroid cancer should always be considered as refractory and should be proactively treated

Smallridge RC et al. Thyroid 2012; 22:1104–1139

ADVANCED • RADIOACTIVE IODINE-REFRACTORY • DIFFERENTIATED

THYROID CANCER REGIMEN: SORAFENIB TOSYLATE

Brose MS et al. Lancet 2014;384:319–328

Sorafenib tosylate 400 mg administer orally every 12 hours (eg, morning and evening) continually in 28-day cycles (total dose/day = 800 mg; total dose/cycle = 22,400 mg)

Notes:

- Patients should swallow tablets whole with approximately 250 mL (8 oz) of water. Tablets may be taken with or without food
- Special precautions: Sorafenib is metabolized by cytochrome P450 (CYP) CYP3A subfamily enzymes and has been shown in preclinical studies to inhibit multiple CYP isoforms. Therefore, all patients who are taking concomitant medications metabolized by CYP enzymes should be closely observed for side effects associated with concomitantly administered medications. Special caution should be used with any of the following medications: ketoconazole, itraconazole, voriconazole, ritonavir, clarithromycin, cyclosporine, carbamazepine, phenytoin, and phenobarbital. Furthermore, patients taking medications with a low therapeutic index (eg, warfarin, quinidine, digoxin) should be monitored proactively. *Patients using sorafenib should be advised to avoid consuming grapefruit products for as long as they continue to use sorafenib*

Note: Patients receive once-daily oral doses of sorafenib until disease progression or unacceptable toxicity

Supportive Care: Hand-foot Reaction

For patients who develop a hand-foot reaction, use topical emollients (eg, Aquaphor), topical and/or oral steroids, antihistamine agents (H_1-receptor antagonists), or pyridoxine 50–150 mg/day orally

Antiemetic prophylaxis
Emetogenic potential is **MINIMAL**
See Chapter 42 for antiemetic recommendations

Hematopoietic growth factor (CSF) prophylaxis
Primary prophylaxis is **NOT** indicated
See Chapter 43 for more information

Antimicrobial prophylaxis
Risk of fever and neutropenia is **LOW**
   Antimicrobial primary prophylaxis to be considered:
- Antibacterial—not indicated
- Antifungal—not indicated
- Antiviral—not indicated unless patient previously had an episode of HSV

Diarrhea management

Latent or delayed-onset diarrhea:
- **Loperamide** 4 mg orally initially after the first loose or liquid stool, *then*
- **Loperamide** 2 mg orally every 2 hours during waking hours, *plus* **loperamide** 4 mg orally every 4 hours during hours of sleep

Persistent diarrhea:
- **Octreotide** 100–150 mcg subcutaneously 3 times daily. Maximum total daily dose is 1500 mcg

Antibiotic therapy during latent or delayed-onset diarrhea:
A fluoroquinolone (eg, **ciprofloxacin** 500 mg orally every 12 hours) if absolute neutrophil count $<500/mm^3$ with or without accompanying fever in association with diarrhea
- Antibiotics should also be administered if patient is hospitalized with prolonged diarrhea and should be continued until diarrhea resolves

Abigerges D et al. J Natl Cancer Inst 1994;86:446–449
Rothenberg ML et al. J Clin Oncol 2001;19:3801–3807
Wadler S et al. J Clin Oncol 1998;16:3169–3178

Treatment Modifications

Sorafenib Dose Levels

Starting dose: Level 1	400 mg every morning; 400 mg every evening
Level −1	200 mg every morning; 400 mg every evening
Level −2	200 mg every morning; 200 mg every evening
Level −3	200 mg once daily

Adverse Event	Dose Modification
Cutaneous Toxicities	
Rash G ≥2	Hold sorafenib and provide immediate symptomatic treatment
If treatment is withheld for more than 3 weeks because of cutaneous toxicity	Discontinue therapy
When toxicity resolves to G ≥1	Restart sorafenib at one dose level less than the dose level administered at the time toxicity developed. Treatment for symptoms may continue indefinitely as a preventive measure
If cutaneous toxicity G3/4 recurs at reduced sorafenib doses	Again, hold sorafenib until the toxicity resolves to G ≤1, at which time sorafenib should be restarted at one dose level lower than the dose level administered at the time toxicity developed. Treatment for symptoms may continue indefinitely as a preventive measure
If cutaneous toxicity G3/4 recurs at dose levels −2 or lower	Discontinue therapy
If cutaneous toxicity does not recur at reduced sorafenib doses with or without continued treatment for symptoms	The dose of sorafenib may be increased one dose level to the dose level administered at the time cutaneous toxicity developed. If toxicity recurs following the increase, then follow the guidelines above, with the exception that when drug is restarted, the sorafenib dose should be reduced one dose level
Diarrhea	
G1/2 diarrhea	Focus on treatment for symptoms designed to resolve the diarrhea. No dose modifications will be made for G1/2 diarrhea unless G2 diarrhea persists for more than 2 weeks
If G2 diarrhea persists for more than 2 weeks	Follow the guidelines below for G3/4 diarrhea
If diarrhea cannot be controlled with the preventive measures outlined, and is G3/4, or worsens by one grade level (G3 to G4) while on sorafenib and is not alleviated within 48 hours by antidiarrheal treatment	Hold sorafenib. Also, withhold sorafenib if persistent G2 diarrhea is not alleviated by antidiarrheal treatment while sorafenib use continues (persistent is defined as lasting for >2 weeks)
If sorafenib is held for more than 3 weeks and diarrhea does not resolve to G ≤1	Discontinue therapy
If within 3 weeks of withholding sorafenib, diarrhea resolves to G ≤1	Restart sorafenib at one dose level less than the dose level administered at the time toxicity developed
If G3/4 diarrhea or persistent G2 diarrhea recurs at reduced doses of sorafenib (persistent is defined as lasting >2 weeks)	Again, withhold sorafenib until the toxicity resolves to CTCAE G ≤1, at which time sorafenib should be restarted at one dose level lower than the dose level administered at the time toxicity developed. Treatment for symptoms may continue indefinitely as a preventive measure
If G3/4 diarrhea or persistent G2 diarrhea recurs at dose level −2 (persistent defined as lasting for >2 weeks)	Discontinue therapy
If diarrhea does not recur at reduced sorafenib doses with or without continued treatment for symptoms	The dose of sorafenib may be increased one dose level to the dose level administered at the time the diarrhea developed. If toxicity recurs following the increase, then follow the guidelines above, with the exception that when drug is restarted, the sorafenib dose should be reduced one dose level

(continued)

Treatment Modifications (*continued*)

Adverse Event	Dose Modification
Hypertension	
Note: Patients should have their blood pressure checked once weekly during their first 24 weeks of therapy and for an 8-week period after an adjustment in their sorafenib dose	
G1 hypertension	Continue sorafenib at same dose and schedule
G2 asymptomatic	Treat with antihypertensive medications and continue sorafenib at same dose and schedule
G2 symptomatic, or persistent G2 despite antihypertensive medications, or diastolic BP >110 mm Hg, or G3 hypertension	Treat with antihypertensive medications. Hold sorafenib (maximum 3 weeks until symptoms resolve and diastolic BP <100 mm Hg); then continue sorafenib at one dose level lower. *Note:* Discontinue therapy if sorafenib is withheld >3 weeks
G4 hypertension	Discontinue therapy

Patient Population Studied

Multicenter, double-blind, placebo-controlled trial conducted in 417 patients with locally advanced or metastatic radioactive iodine-refractory differentiated thyroid cancer (papillary, follicular [including Hürthle cell], and poorly differentiated) that had progressed within the past 14 months according to Response Evaluation Criteria in Solid Tumors (RECIST). Radioactive iodine-refractory differentiated thyroid cancer was defined as the presence of at least one target lesion without iodine uptake; or patients whose tumors had iodine uptake and either progressed after one radioactive iodine treatment within the past 16 months, or progressed after two radioactive iodine treatments within 16 months of each other (with the last such treatment administered more than 16 months ago), or received cumulative radioactive iodine activity of at least 22.3 GBq (≥600 mCi). Prior low-dose chemotherapy for radiosensitization was allowed. Patients had papillary (57%), follicular (25%), and poorly differentiated (10%) carcinomas. 96.4% (402/417) of patients had distant metastases, most frequently in the lungs (359/417 [86.1%]), lymph nodes (214/417 [51.3%]), and bone (113/417 [27.1%]). Approximately half of the patients were male, the median age was 63 years, 68% had no uptake of radioactive iodine (RAI), and 34% had received a cumulative dose of at least 600 mCi of RAI. The median cumulative RAI activity administered prior to study entry was 400 mCi

Efficacy (N = 417)

Variable	Sorafenib (N = 207)	Placebo (N = 210)
Progression-free survival (PFS)	10.8 months (95% CI 9.1–12.9)	5.8 months (95% CI 5.3–7.8)
	HR = 0.587 (95% CI, 0.46–0.76, P <0.001)	
Median treatment duration	10.6 months	6.5 months
Overall survival*	HR 0.88 (95% CI, 0.54–1.19, P = 0.14)	
Percentage of Patients		
Partial response[†]	12.2%	0.5%
Reduction in size of target lesions	73%	27%
PR + stable disease ≥6 months	41.8%	33.2%

CI, confidence interval

*Overall survival was not statistically significantly different in patients who received sorafenib tosylate compared with patients who received placebo. Note that following investigator-determined disease progression, 157 (75%) patients randomly assigned to receive the placebo crossed over to open-label sorafenib tosylate, and it remains uncertain if this may have impacted or will impact the OS analysis

[†]Duration of response = 10.2 months

Therapy Monitoring

1. *Every 6 weeks to 3 months:* Physical examination and routine laboratory tests
2. *Response assessment:* Every 2–3 cycles. A cycle defined as 28 days of oral therapy

Toxicity (N = 416)

	Sorafenib (n = 207)			Placebo (n = 209)		
	Any Grade	Grade 3	Grade 4	Any Grade	Grade 3	Grade 4
Hand–foot skin reaction	158 (76.3%)	42 (20.3%)	—	20 (9.6%)	0	—
Diarrhea	142 (68.6%)	11 (5.3%)	1 (0.5%)	32 (15.3%)	2 (1.0%)	0
Alopecia	139 (67.1%)	—	—	16 (7.7%)	—	—
Rash or desquamation	104 (50.2%)	10 (4.8%)	0	24 (11.5%)	0	0
Fatigue	103 (49.8%)	11 (5.3%)	1 (0.5%)	53 (25.4%)	3 (1.4%)	0
Weight loss	97 (46.9%)	12 (5.8%)	—	29 (13.9%)	2 (1.0%)	—
Hypertension	84 (40.6%)	20 (9.7%)	0	26 (12.4%)	5 (2.4%)	0
Anorexia	66 (31.9%)	5 (2.4%)	0	10 (4.8%)	0	0
Oral mucositis (functional/symptomatic)	48 (23.2%)	1 (0.5%)	1 (0.5%)	7 (3.3%)	0	0
Pruritus	44 (21.3%)	2 (1.0%)	—	22 (10.5%)	0	—
Nausea	43 (20.8%)	0	0	24 (11.5%)	0	0
Headache	37 (17.9%)	0	0	15 (7.2%)	0	0
Cough	32 (15.5%)	0	—	32 (15.3%)	0	—
Constipation	31 (15.0%)	0	0	17 (8.1%)	1 (0.5%)	0
Dyspnea	30 (14.5%)	10 (4.8%)	0	28 (13.4%)	4 (1.9%)	2 (1.0%)
Neuropathy: sensory	30 (14.5%)	2 (1.0%)	0	13 (6.2%)	0	0
Abdominal pain not otherwise specified	29 (14.0%)	3 (1.4%)	0	8 (3.8%)	1 (0.5%)	0
Pain, extremity (limb)	28 (13.5%)	1 (0.5%)	0	18 (8.6%)	1 (0.5%)	0
Dermatology, other	27 (13.0%)	2 (1.0%)	0	5 (2.4%)	0	0
Voice changes	25 (12.1%)	1 (0.5%)	0	6 (2.9%)	0	0
Fever	23 (11.1%)	2 (1.0%)	1 (0.5%)	10 (4.8%)	0	0
Vomiting	23 (11.1%)	1 (0.5%)	0	12 (5.7%)	0	0
Back pain	22 (10.6%)	2 (1.0%)	0	22 (10.5%)	2 (1.0%)	1 (0.5%)
Pain, other	22 (10.6%)	1 (0.5%)	0	16 (7.7%)	1 (0.5%)	0
Pain, throat, pharynx, or larynx	21 (10.1%)	0	0	8 (3.8%)	0	0
Laboratory						
Metabolic or laboratory— other*	74 (35.7%)	0	0	35 (16.7%)	0	0
Serum TSH increase(MedDRA)*	69 (33.3%)	0	0	28 (13.4%)	0	0
Hypocalcemia	39 (18.8%)	12 (5.8%)	7 (3.4%)	10 (4.8%)	1 (0.5%)	2 (1.0%)
Increased alanine transaminase	26 (12.6%)	5 (2.4%)	1 (0.5%)	9 (4.3%)	0	0
Increased aspartate aminotransferase	23 (11.1%)	2 (1.0%)	0	5 (2.4%)	9	0

ADVANCED • RADIOACTIVE IODINE-REFRACTORY • DIFFERENTIATED

THYROID CANCER REGIMEN: LENVATINIB

Schlumberger M et al. N Engl J Med 2015;372:621–630
Supplementary appendix to: Schlumberger M et al. N Engl J Med 2015;372:621–630
Protocol for: Schlumberger M et al. N Engl J Med 2015;372:621–630
Lenvima (lenvatinib) prescribing information. Woodcliff Lake, NJ: Eisai Inc; revised August 2018
http://www.lenvima.com/pdfs/dosing-guide.pdf

Lenvatinib 24 mg per dose; administer orally once daily, without regard to food, continuously until disease progression (total dosage/week = 168 mg)

- Lenvatinib capsules should ideally be swallowed whole. Patients who have difficulty swallowing whole lenvatinib capsules may instead place the appropriate combination of whole capsules necessary to administer the required dose in 15 mL of water or apple juice in a glass container for at least 10 minutes. After 10 minutes, the contents of the glass container should be stirred for at least 3 minutes and then the resulting mixture should be swallowed. After drinking, rinse the glass container with an additional 15 mL of water or apple juice and swallow the liquid to ensure complete administration of the lenvatinib dose

- A missed dose of lenvatinib may be taken up to 12 hours before a subsequently scheduled dose

- Reduce the lenvatinib starting dose to 14 mg per dose, administered orally once daily for severe (Child-Pugh class C) hepatic impairment

- Reduce the lenvatinib starting dose to 14 mg per dose, administered orally once daily for severe (creatinine clearance <30 mL/minute) renal impairment

- Patients with pre-existing hypertension should have blood pressure adequately controlled (blood pressure ≤150/90 mm Hg) prior to initiation of treatment with lenvatinib

Note: Patients receive once-daily oral doses of Lenvatinib until disease progression, or unacceptable toxicity

Supportive Care
Antiemetic prophylaxis
Emetogenic potential is **MODERATE**
See Chapter 42 for antiemetic recommendations

Hematopoietic growth factor (CSF) prophylaxis
Primary prophylaxis is **NOT** *indicated*
See Chapter 43 for more information

Antimicrobial prophylaxis
Risk of fever and neutropenia is **LOW**
  Antimicrobial primary prophylaxis to be considered:
- Antibacterial—not indicated
- Antifungal—not indicated
- Antiviral—not indicated unless patient previously had an episode of HSV

Diarrhea management
Latent or delayed-onset diarrhea:
- **Loperamide** 4 mg orally initially after the first loose or liquid stool, *then*
- **Loperamide** 2 mg orally every 2 hours during waking hours, *plus* **loperamide** 4 mg orally every 4 hours during hours of sleep

Persistent diarrhea:
- **Octreotide** 100–150 mcg subcutaneously 3 times daily. Maximum total daily dose is 1500 mcg

Antibiotic therapy during latent or delayed-onset diarrhea:
A fluoroquinolone (eg, **ciprofloxacin** 500 mg orally every 12 hours) if absolute neutrophil count <500/mm³ with or without accompanying fever in association with diarrhea
- Antibiotics should also be administered if patient is hospitalized with prolonged diarrhea and should be continued until diarrhea resolves

Abigerges D et al. J Natl Cancer Inst 1994;86:446–449
Rothenberg ML et al. J Clin Oncol 2001;19:3801–3807
Wadler S et al. J Clin Oncol 1998;16:3169–3178

Treatment Modifications

Lenvatinib

Starting dose	24 mg by mouth once daily
Dose Level −1	20 mg by mouth once daily
Dose Level −2	14 mg by mouth once daily
Dose Level −3	10 mg by mouth once daily
Dose Level −4	Discontinue lenvatinib

Cardiovascular Toxicity

Adverse Event	Treatment Modification
Either of the following: • G2 hypertension (SBP 140–159 mm Hg or DBP 90–99 mm Hg) • G3 hypertension (SBP ≥160 mm Hg or DBP ≥100 mm Hg) on suboptimal antihypertensive therapy	Continue lenvatinib at the same dose and optimize antihypertensive therapy. Standard options include calcium channel blockers, angiotensin-converting enzyme inhibitors (ACEi), angiotensin II receptor blockers (ARB), diuretics/thiazides, and b-adrenoceptor blockers. Monitor blood pressure frequently
G3 hypertension (SBP ≥160 mm Hg or DBP ≥100 mm Hg) persistent despite optimal antihypertensive therapy	Withhold lenvatinib until hypertension controlled to ≤G2, then resume lenvatinib at one lower dose level. Optimize antihypertensive therapy if existing therapy felt suboptimal. Standard options include calcium channel blockers, ACEi, ARB, diuretics/thiazides, and b-adrenoceptor blockers Monitor blood pressure frequently
G4 hypertension (life-threatening consequences [eg, malignant hypertension, transient or permanent neurologic deficit, hypertensive crisis]; urgent intervention indicated)	Permanently discontinue lenvatinib
G3 cardiac dysfunction	Withhold lenvatinib until cardiac dysfunction improves to G ≤1, then resume lenvatinib at one lower dose level or discontinue lenvatinib depending upon the severity and persistence of cardiac dysfunction
G4 cardiac dysfunction	Permanently discontinue lenvatinib
QTc prolongation (>500 ms, or >60 ms increase from baseline)	Withhold lenvatinib until QTc improves to ≤480 ms or baseline, then resume at one lower dose level. Correct hypomagnesemia and/or hypokalemia if applicable
Arterial thromboembolic event	Permanently discontinue lenvatinib

Gastrointestinal Toxicity

Gastrointestinal perforation	Permanently discontinue lenvatinib
G3/4 fistula formation	Permanently discontinue lenvatinib
Either of the following: • G1 diarrhea • G2 diarrhea lasting ≤2 weeks	Continue current lenvatinib dose and optimize antidiarrheal medications. First-line therapeutic interventions include loperamide or diphenoxylate/atropine; budesonide or tincture of opium also may be used
Any of the following: • G2 diarrhea lasting >2 weeks • G3 diarrhea • G4 diarrhea developing in a patient not receiving an optimal antidiarrheal regimen	Withhold lenvatinib until diarrhea resolves to £G1 or baseline, then resume lenvatinib at 1 lower dose level. Antidiarrheal treatment for symptoms may continue indefinitely as a preventive measure. First-line therapeutic interventions include loperamide or diphenoxylate/atropine; budesonide or tincture of opium also may be used
Recurrent or persistent G4 diarrhea in a patient receiving an optimal antidiarrheal regimen	Permanently discontinue lenvatinib
G1 stomatitis	Good oral hygiene is the first prophylactic measure. Encourage brushing teeth after each meal and rinsing with salt-water and baking soda mouthwash solutions (1/2 teaspoon baking soda in 8 ounces of water). Additional oral care recommendations include use of a soft toothbrush and fluoride toothpaste without tartar or whitening control during treatment. Topical lidocaine or steroid ointment may also be helpful for painful ulcerations
G ≥2 stomatitis	Interrupt lenvatinib. Conduct oral hygiene as described for G1 stomatitis. Resume lenvatinib only after stomatitis is resolved. Consider dose reduction if severity G ≥3 or if stomatitis recurs despite optimal prophylaxis

(continued)

Treatment Modifications (*continued*)

Hepatic Toxicity and Hepatic Impairment

G3/4 hepatotoxicity (ALT/AST >5× ULN, bilirubin >3× ULN)	Withhold lenvatinib until hepatotoxicity improves to G ≤1, then resume lenvatinib at one lower dose level or discontinue lenvatinib depending upon the severity and persistence of hepatotoxicity
Hepatic failure	Permanently discontinue lenvatinib
Severe hepatic impairment (Child-Pugh class C)	Reduce initial lenvatinib dose to 14 mg orally once daily

Renal Toxicity and Renal Impairment

G3/4 AKI (SCr >3× baseline or >4 mg/dL; hospitalization indicated; life-threatening consequences; dialysis indicated)	Initiate prompt evaluation and correction of dehydration if applicable. Withhold lenvatinib until toxicity improves to G ≤1 or baseline, then resume at one lower dose level or discontinue lenvatinib depending upon the severity and persistence of renal impairment
Severe renal impairment (CrCl <30 mL/min)	Reduce initial lenvatinib dose to 14 mg orally once daily
Urine dipstick proteinuria ≥2+	Continue lenvatinib at current dose and obtain a 24-hour urine protein
Proteinuria ≥2 g in 24 hours	Withhold lenvatinib until <2 g of proteinuria per 24 hours, then resume lenvatinib at one lower dose level
Nephrotic syndrome	Permanently discontinue lenvatinib

Palmar-plantar erythrodysesthesia syndrome

Palmar-plantar erythrodysesthesia syndrome	Withhold lenvatinib. Encourage patient to reduce exposure of the hands and feet to hot water, avoid tight footwear, and limit damage caused by vigorous exercise. When the AE has resolved to G ≤1, resume treatment at same dose or at one lower dose level

Hemorrhage

G3 hemorrhage	Discontinue lenvatinib or withhold until resolved to G ≤1. Once resolved, resume lenvatinib at a reduced dose or discontinue its use. Make decisions depending on the severity of the hemorrhagic event
G4 hemorrhage	Discontinue lenvatinib

Other Toxicities

Fatigue/asthenia	Managing fatigue/asthenia can be difficult. The initial step is to identify any treatable cause, if one exists (eg, anemia, thyroid dysfunction, poor sleep, or depression). If no underlying etiology can be identified, treatment for fatigue includes supportive care with adequate nutrition, exercise, and implementation of stress-reducing techniques. Consider lenvatinib dose interruption if a patient complains of moderate to severe fatigue
Reversible posterior leukoencephalopathy syndrome (RPLS)	Withhold lenvatinib until fully resolved. Depending on the severity and persistence of neurological symptoms as well as the benefit from lenvatinib, resume at a reduced dose or discontinue
Planned elective surgery	Discontinue lenvatinib about one week before any surgical procedure and resume only after wound healing is adequate
Patient with wound-healing complications	Permanently discontinue lenvatinib
• Other persistent/intolerable G2 toxicities • Other G3 toxicities	Withhold lenvatinib until toxicity improves to G ≤1 or baseline, then resume lenvatinib at one lower dose level
Other G4 toxicity	Permanently discontinue lenvatinib
G4 laboratory abnormality	Withhold lenvatinib until toxicity improves to G ≤1 or baseline, then resume lenvatinib at one lower dose level

Note: Lenvatinib can cause fetal harm. Advise females of reproductive potential of the potential risk to a fetus and to use effective contraception during treatment with lenvatinib and for at least 30 days after the last dose

SBP, systolic blood pressure; DBP, diastolic blood pressure; ALT, alanine aminotransferase; AST, aspartate aminotransferase; AKI, acute kidney injury; SCr, serum creatinine; CrCl, creatinine clearance

Patient Population Studied

The international, multicenter, randomized, double-blind, placebo-controlled, phase 3 study involved 392 patients with pathologically confirmed, differentiated thyroid cancer. Eligible patients were aged >18 years, had evidence of [131]iodine-refractory disease, and had radiologic evidence of progression within the previous 13 months. Patients who had received more than one prior treatment with a tyrosine kinase inhibitor were not eligible. Participants were randomly assigned in a 2:1 ratio to receive lenvatinib (24 mg once daily) or placebo

Therapy Monitoring

1. Monitor blood pressure. For optimal outcome, provide patients individualized BP thresholds at which health care providers should be contacted for advice

2. Prior to starting therapy, perform a urinalysis and measure the protein:creatinine ratio. Perform routine testing for proteinuria throughout treatment

3. Monitor cardiac function clinically. Obtain a baseline echocardiogram before the start of lenvatinib

4. Lenvatinib can interfere with and delay wound healing. Discontinue lenvatinib about 1 week before any surgical procedure and resume only after wound healing is adequate

5. Monitor for palmar-plantar erythrodysesthesia syndrome. Encourage frequent examination of the soles of the feet and palms and removal of any existing hyperkeratotic areas and calluses present, which can then be protected by cushioning and treated with moisturizing creams and keratolytic agents

6. Assess thyroid function prior to initiation of lenvatinib treatment and then monitor monthly. Adjust thyroid-replacement medication as necessary

7. Schedule a dental visit prior to treatment with lenvatinib and assess for stomatitis regularly

8. Patients taking blood thinners, who have undergone previous bowel surgery, or have a history of inflammatory bowel disease or diverticulitis, are at increased risk for bowel perforation and gastrointestinal bleeding. Monitor carefully

9. *Every 2–3 months:* Imaging to assess response. Serum markers can be considered/obtained at each visit if they have been shown to be of value in following the patient's disease status

Efficacy (N = 392)

	Lenvatinib (n = 261)	Placebo (n = 131)	
Median progression-free survival	18.3 months	3.6 months	HR 0.21, 95% CI 0.14–0.31; P <0.001
Objective response rate*	64.8%	1.5%	OR 28.87, 95% CI 12.46–66.86; P <0.001
Median overall survival	41.6 (31.2 to NE)	34.5 (21.7 to NE)	HR 0.73, 95% CI 0.50–1.07; P = 0.10

*Objective response rate includes patients with either a complete or partial response to treatment; NE, not estimable
Note: Median duration of follow-up was 17.1 months

Adverse Events (N = 392)

	Lenvatinib (N = 261)		Placebo (N = 131)	
Grade (%)*	Grade 1–2	Grade ≥3	Grade 1–2	Grade ≥3
Any event	21	76	50	10
Hypertension	26	42	7	2
Diarrhea	51	8	8	0
Fatigue or asthenia	50	9	25	2
Decreased appetite	45	5	12	0
Decreased weight	37	10	9	0
Nausea	39	2	13	<1
Stomatitis	31	4	4	0
Palmar-plantar erythrodysesthesia syndrome	28	3	<1	0
Proteinuria	21	10	2	0
Vomiting	27	2	6	0
Headache	25	3	6	0
Dysphonia	23	1	3	0
Arthralgia	18	0	<1	0
Dysgeusia	17	0	2	0
Rash	16	<1	2	0
Constipation	14	<1	8	0
Myalgia	13	2	2	0
Dry mouth	13	<1	4	0
Upper abdominal pain	13	0	4	0
Abdominal pain	11	<1	0	<1
Peripheral edema	11	<1	0	0
Alopecia	11	0	4	0
Dyspepsia	10	0	0	0
Oropharyngeal pain	10	<1	<1	0
Hypocalcemia	4	3	0	0
Pulmonary embolism	0	3	0	2

*According to the National Cancer Institute Common Terminology Criteria for Adverse Events, version 4.0
Note: Any-grade treatment-related adverse events that occurred in ≥10% and/or Grade ≥3 treatment-related adverse events that occurred in ≥2% of patients are included in the table. Treatment-related deaths occurred in six (2.3%) of the lenvatinib group (owing to pulmonary embolism, hemorrhagic stroke, general deterioration of health, and three cases reported as deaths or sudden deaths but not otherwise specified). Adverse events resulting in discontinuation of treatment were reported in 14.2% and 2.3% of the lenvatinib and placebo groups, respectively

ADVANCED • MEDULLARY
THYROID CANCER REGIMEN: VANDETANIB

Wells SA Jr et al. J Clin Oncol 2010;28:767–772
Wells SA Jr et al. J Clin Oncol 2012;30:134–141

Vandetanib 100–300 mg per day; administer orally, continually (total dose/week = 700–2100 mg)
Note:
- Patients should take vandetanib once daily at the same time each day. Vandetanib may be administered with or without food. Tablets should be swallowed whole (without chewing)
- If a patient misses a scheduled dose of vandetanib, they may take the missed dose if the next scheduled dose is not due to be taken within the next 12 hours
- If <12 hours remain before the next scheduled dose is due, the patient should not take the missed dose but should wait and take the next regularly scheduled dose
- If the patient vomits ≤15 minutes after taking vandetanib, another dose may be administered. The dose may only be repeated once
- If a patient vomits >15 minutes after an oral dose was administered, no attempt to supplement or replace the dose should be made
- If vandetanib tablets cannot be swallowed whole, they may be dispersed in a glass containing 2 ounces of non-carbonated water and stirred for approximately 10 minutes until the tablet is dispersed (tablets will not completely dissolve)

Note: Patients receive once-daily oral doses of vandetanib 300 mg until disease progression, or unacceptable toxicity

Note: **Although the starting dose is 300 mg per day, a majority of patients will experience an adverse event, making a dose reduction necessary.** In the study cited:
1. Vandetanib dose was reduced or interrupted in 24 patients because of adverse events, most commonly diarrhea (n = 7)
2. Among the 24 patients who required dose reduction or interruption, 21 patients had a combination of dose reduction and dose interruption and 3 patients had a dose interruption without dose reduction
3. Some patients required more than a single dose reduction
4. For patients who required dose reductions, vandetanib was decreased to:
   200 mg/day (60%, 18/30)
   150 mg/day (3%, 1/30)
   100 mg/day (23%, 7/30)
   50 mg/day (6.6%, 2/30)
5. The median time to first dose reduction was 4.9 months (95% CI, 2.7–8.4 months)

Supportive Care
Antiemetic prophylaxis
Emetogenic potential is **MINIMAL–LOW**
See Chapter 42 for antiemetic recommendations

Hematopoietic growth factor (CSF) prophylaxis
Primary prophylaxis is **NOT** *indicated*
See Chapter 43 for more information

Antimicrobial prophylaxis
Risk of fever and neutropenia is **LOW**
   Antimicrobial primary prophylaxis to be considered:
   - Antibacterial—not indicated
   - Antifungal—not indicated
   - Antiviral—not indicated unless patient previously had an episode of HSV

Treatment Modifications

Vandetanib Dose Levels

Starting dose: Level 1	300 mg
Level −1	200 mg
Level −2	100 mg
Level −3	50 mg (100 mg every other day)

Adverse Event	Dose Modification

Cutaneous Toxicities

Adverse Event	Dose Modification
Rash G ≥2	Hold vandetanib and provide *immediate* symptomatic treatment
If treatment held for more than 3 weeks because of cutaneous toxicity	Discontinue therapy
When toxicity resolves to G ≤1	Restart vandetanib at 1 dose level lower than that administered at the time the toxicity developed. Symptomatic treatment may continue indefinitely as a preventive measure
If cutaneous toxicity G3/4 recurs at reduced doses of vandetanib	Again, hold vandetanib until the toxicity resolves to G ≤1, at which time vandetanib should be restarted at 1 dose level lower than that administered at the time the toxicity developed. Symptomatic treatment may continue indefinitely as a preventive measure
If cutaneous toxicity G3/4 recurs at dose level −2 or lower	Discontinue therapy
If with or without continued symptomatic treatment the cutaneous toxicity does not recur at the reduced doses of vandetanib	The dose of vandetanib may be increased 1 dose level to that which was being administered at the time the cutaneous toxicity developed. If toxicity recurs following this increase, then follow the guidelines above, with the exception that when drug is restarted the vandetanib dose should be reduced 1 dose level

Diarrhea

Adverse Event	Dose Modification
G1/2 diarrhea	Focus on symptomatic treatment designed to resolve the diarrhea. No dose modifications will be made for G1/2 diarrhea unless G2 diarrhea persists for more than 2 weeks
If G2 diarrhea persists for more than 2 weeks	Then the guidelines below for G3/4 diarrhea should be followed
If the diarrhea cannot be controlled with the preventive measures outlined and is G3/4, or worsens by 1 grade level (G3 to G4) while on vandetanib and is not alleviated by symptomatic treatment within 48 hours	Hold vandetanib. Also, if persistent G2 diarrhea (persistent defined as lasting for more than 2 weeks) while on vandetanib is not alleviated by symptomatic treatment, hold vandetanib
If vandetanib is held for more than 3 weeks and the diarrhea does not resolve to G ≤1	Discontinue therapy
If within 3 weeks of holding therapy the diarrhea resolves to G ≤1	Restart vandetanib at 1 dose level lower than that administered at the time the toxicity developed
If diarrhea that is G3/4 or persistent G2 (persistent defined as lasting for more than 2 weeks) recurs at the reduced doses of vandetanib and this is greater than dose level −1	Again, hold vandetanib until the toxicity resolves to CTCAE G ≤1, at which time vandetanib should be restarted at 1 dose level lower than that administered at the time the toxicity developed. Symptomatic treatment may continue indefinitely as a preventive measure
If diarrhea that is G3/4 or persistent G2 (persistent defined as lasting for more than 2 weeks) recurs at dose level −2	Discontinue therapy
If with or without continued symptomatic treatment the diarrhea does not recur at the reduced doses of vandetanib	The dose of vandetanib may be increased 1 dose level to that which was being administered at the time the diarrhea developed. If toxicity recurs following this increase, then follow the guidelines above, with the exception that when drug is restarted the vandetanib dose should be reduced 1 dose level

Hypertension

Note: Patients should have their blood pressure checked once per week during their first 24 weeks of therapy or for any 8-week period after any adjustment is made in their vandetanib dose

(continued)

Treatment Modifications (*continued*)

Adverse Event	Dose Modification
G1 hypertension	Continue vandetanib at same dose and schedule
G2 asymptomatic	Treat with antihypertensive medications and continue vandetanib at same dose and schedule
G2 symptomatic or persistent G2 despite antihypertensive medications or diastolic BP >110 mm Hg or G3 hypertension	Treat with antihypertensive medications. Hold vandetanib (maximum 3 weeks until symptoms resolve and diastolic BP <100 mm Hg); then continue vandetanib at 1 dose level lower *Note:* If vandetanib is held more than 3 weeks, then discontinue therapy
G4	Discontinue therapy

QTc Abnormalities

ECGs and electrolytes should be checked 3 times per week if there are any QTc abnormalities noted

QTc prolongation defined as: • A single measurement of ≥550 ms • An increase of ≥100 ms from baseline • Two consecutive measurements (within 48 hours) ≥500 ms but <550 ms • An increase of ≥60 ms but <100 ms from baseline to a value ≥480 ms	Hold vandetanib until QTc <480 ms, then resume vandetanib at 1 dose level lower

Patient Population Studied

Baseline Demographics and Patient Characteristics

Characteristic	Vandetanib (300 mg) (n = 231) No.	%	Placebo (n = 100) No.	%
Sex				
Male	134	58	56	56
Female	97	42	44	44
Mean age, years	50.7		53.4	
WHO performance status				
0	154	67	58	58
1	67	29	38	38
2	10	4	4	4
Disease type				
Hereditary	28	12	5	5
Sporadic or unknown	203	88	95	95
Locally advanced	14	6	3	3
Metastatic	217	94	97	97
Hepatic	154	67	64	64
Lymph nodes	135	58	68	68
Respiratory	126	54	60	60

(*continued*)

Toxicity

Common Adverse Events (Safety Population)

Adverse Event	Vandetanib (300 mg) (n = 231) Number	%	Placebo (n = 99) Number	%
Any grade occurring with an incidence ≥10% overall				
Diarrhea	130	56	26	26
Rash	104	45	11	11
Nausea	77	33	16	16
Hypertension	73	32	5	5
Fatigue	55	24	23	23
Headache	59	26	9	9
Decreased appetite	49	21	12	12
Acne	46	20	5	5
Asthenia	34	14	11	11
Vomiting	34	14	7	7
Back pain	21	9	20	20
Dry skin	35	15	5	5
Insomnia	30	13	10	10
Abdominal pain	33	14	5	5
Dermatitis acneiform	35	15	2	2

(*continued*)

Patient Population Studied (continued)

Characteristic	Vandetanib (300 mg) (n = 231)		Placebo (n = 100)	
	No.	%	No.	%
Neck	33	14	17	17
No. of organs involved (excluding thyroid)				
0 or 1	29	13	8	8
≥2	202	87	92	92
Prior systemic therapy for MTC				
0	141	61	58	58
≥1	90	39	42	42
RET mutation				
Positive	137	59	50	50
Negative	2	1	6	6
Unknown	92	40	44	44

MTC, medullary thyroid cancer; *RET*, rearranged during transfection

Toxicity (continued)

Adverse Event	Vandetanib (300 mg) (n = 231)		Placebo (n = 99)	
	Number	%	Number	%
Nasopharyngitis	26	11	9	9
ECG QT prolonged*	33	14	1	1
Weight decreased	24	10	9	9
Grade ≥3 occurring with an incidence of ≥2% on either arm				
Diarrhea	25	11	2	2
Hypertension	20	9	0	
ECG QT prolonged*	18	8	1	1
Fatigue	13	6	1	1
Decreased appetite	9	4	0	
Rash	8	4	1	1
Asthenia	6	3	1	1
Dyspnea	3	1	3	3
Back pain	1	0.4	3	3
Syncope	0		2	2

*As defined according to the National Cancer Institute's Common Terminology Criteria for Adverse Events, v3 (and protocol-defined QTc prolongation)

Efficacy

Progression-Free Survival	Vandetanib		Placebo		HR	OR	95% CI	P Value
	# Events/# Pts	%	# Events/# Pts	%				
Primary analysis	73/231		51/100		0.46		0.31–0.69	<0.001
Predefined sensitivity analyses								
Cox proportional hazards model	73/231		51/100		0.46		0.32–0.68	<0.001
Per protocol analysis	71/215		48/91		0.45		0.30–0.68	<0.001
Whitehead's method	73/231		51/100		0.51		0.35–0.72	<0.001
Excluding data from open-label phase	64/231		59/100		0.27		0.18–0.41	<0.001
Investigator RECIST assessments	101/231		62/100		0.40		0.27–0.58	<0.001

(continued)

Efficacy (continued)

Progression-Free Survival	Vandetanib		Placebo					
	# Events/# Pts	%	# Events/# Pts	%	HR	OR	95% CI	P Value
Secondary efficacy end points								
Objective response rate		45		13	5.48		2.99–10.79	<0.001
Disease control rate		87		71	2.64		1.48–4.69	0.001
Calcitonin biochemical response rate		69		3	72.9		26.2–303.2	<0.001
CEA biochemical response rate		52		2	52.0		16.0–320.3	<0.001

HR, hazard ratio; OR, odds ratio; RECIST, Response Evaluation Criteria in Solid Tumors

Objective Response Rate: Summary of Subgroup Analyses (Randomized Phase)

Patient Subgroup and Randomized Treatment	No. of Patients	Responses	
		No.	%
Hereditary MTC			
Vandetanib, 300 mg	28	13	46.4
Placebo	5	0	
Sporadic *RET* mutation positive			
Vandetanib, 300 mg	110	57	51.8
Placebo	45	0	
Sporadic *RET* mutation negative			
Vandetanib, 300 mg	2	0	
Placebo	6	0	
Sporadic *RET* mutation unknown			
Vandetanib, 300 mg	91	31	34.1
Placebo	44	1	2.3
Sporadic *M918T* mutation positive			
Vandetanib, 300 mg	101	55	54.5
Placebo	41	0	
Sporadic *M918T* mutation negative			
Vandetanib, 300 mg	55	17	30.9
Placebo	39	1	2.6
Sporadic *M918T* mutation unknown			
Vandetanib, 300 mg	48	16	33.3
Placebo	17	0	

MTC, medullary thyroid cancer; *RET*, rearranged during transfection

Therapy Monitoring

1. *Prior to initiation of vandetanib:* CBC with differential and platelet count, vital signs, liver function tests, serum electrolytes, ECG
2. Control hypertension prior to initiation of vandetanib
3. *Monitor regularly for:*
   - Hypertension
   - Signs and symptoms of bleeding. Avoid initiation of cabozantinib in patients with a recent history of hemorrhage (eg, hemoptysis, hematemesis, or melena)
   - Signs and symptoms of fistulas and perforations, including abscess and sepsis
   - Signs and symptoms of palmar-plantar erythrodysesthesia
   - Diarrhea
   - Spot urine for protein measurement every 4–8 weeks (if spot urine dipstick >1+ for protein, perform a 24 hour urine protein).
   - Signs and symptoms of osteonecrosis of the jaw (jaw pain, osteomyelitis, osteitis, bone erosion, tooth or periodontal infection, toothache, gingival ulceration or erosion, persistent jaw pain or slow healing of the mouth or jaw after dental surgery)
4. *Response assessment:* Every 2–3 cycles

ADVANCED • MEDULLARY
THYROID CANCER REGIMEN: CABOZANTINIB

Elisei R et al. J Clin Oncol 2013;31:3639–3646
COMETRIQ (cabozantinib) prescribing information. Alameda, CA: Exelixis, Inc; revised January 2020

Cabozantinib capsules (Cometriq®) 140 mg orally at least 2 hours after or at least 1 hour before after eating food, continually (total dose/week = 980 mg)

Notes:

• Capsules are swallowed whole (without opening or breaking)

• Do not substitute cabozantinib tablets (CABOMETYX) for cabozantinib capsules (COMETRIQ)

• Do not take a missed dose within 12 hours of the next scheduled dose

• In light of the fact that 79% of patients starting at the 140-mg dose had a subsequent dose reduction and 27% discontinued the medication because of adverse effects, clinicians are advised to consider the following:

  ▪ *Patients Taking CYP3A4 Inhibitors*

    – Avoid the use of concomitant strong CYP3A4 inhibitors

    – For patients who require treatment with a strong CYP3A4 inhibitor, reduce the daily cabozantinib dose by 40 mg. Resume the dose that was used prior to initiating the CYP3A4 inhibitor 2–3 days after discontinuing a strong inhibitor

    – Inform patients not to ingest grapefruit products or nutritional supplements known to inhibit cytochrome P450 activity

  ▪ *Patients Taking Strong CYP3A4 Inducers*

    – Avoid use of strong CYP3A4 inducers

    – Inform patients not to ingest foods or nutritional supplements (eg, St. John's wort [*Hypericum perforatum*] known to induce cytochrome P450 activity

    – For patients who require treatment with a strong CYP3A4 inducer, increase the daily cabozantinib dose by 40 mg *only if tolerability on the dose without the inducer has been convincingly demonstrated*. Resume dose used prior to initiating a CYP3A4 inducer 2 to 3 days after discontinuing a strong inducer. The daily cabozantinib dose should not exceed 180 mg

  ▪ *Patients with hepatic impairment*

    – In patients with mild (Child-Pugh class A) or moderate (Child-Pugh class B) hepatic impairment, reduce the starting dose of cabozantinib to 80 mg once daily

    – Avoid use of cabozantinib in patients with severe hepatic impairment (Child-Pugh class C)

    – *Note:* Patients receive once-daily oral doses of cabozantinib until disease progression, or unacceptable toxicity

Supportive Care
Antiemetic prophylaxis
Emetogenic potential is **MINIMAL–LOW**
See Chapter 42 for antiemetic recommendations

Hematopoietic growth factor (CSF) prophylaxis
Primary prophylaxis is **NOT** *indicated*
See Chapter 43 for more information

Antimicrobial prophylaxis
Risk of fever and neutropenia is **LOW**
  Antimicrobial primary prophylaxis to be considered:

  • Antibacterial—not indicated

  • Antifungal—not indicated

  • Antiviral—not indicated unless patient previously had an episode of HSV

Diarrhea management
Latent or delayed onset diarrhea:
Loperamide 4 mg; administer orally initially after the first loose or liquid stool, *then*
Loperamide 2 mg every 2 hours while awake; every 4 hours during sleep
Alternatively, a trial of **diphenoxylate hydrochloride** 2.5 mg **with atropine sulfate** 0.025 mg (eg, Lomotil) two tablets four times daily until control achieved.

Hand-foot reaction (palmar-plantar erythrodysesthesia, PPE)
Use topical emollients (eg, Aquaphor), topical or orally administered steroids, antihistamines, or pyridoxine 50 to 200 mg/day

Dose Modifications

RECOMMENDED DOSE MODIFICATIONS FOR CABOZANTINIB

Starting dose (level 1)	140 mg orally once daily
Dose level −1	100 mg orally once daily
Dose level −2	60 mg orally once daily
Dose level −3	Consider discontinuing cabozantinib or consider resuming at 60 mg orally once daily, if tolerable, at the discretion of the medically responsible health care provider

Grade/Severity	Treatment Modification
G ≥3 hemorrhage	Permanently discontinue cabozantinib
Development of a gastrointestinal perforation or Grade 4 fistula	
Acute MI	
Serious arterial or VTE event requiring medical intervention	
Any hypertension	Treat as needed with standard antihypertensive therapy
Persistent hypertension despite use of maximal antihypertensive medications	Withhold cabozantinib until blood pressure is adequately controlled, then resume cabozantinib with the dosage reduced by 1 dosage level
Evidence of hypertensive crisis or severe hypertension that cannot be controlled with antihypertensive therapy	Discontinue cabozantinib
Intolerable Grade 2 diarrhea	Optimize antidiarrheal regimen. Withhold cabozantinib until improvement to G ≤1, then resume cabozantinib with the dosage reduced by 1 dose level
Grade ≥3 diarrhea not manageable with standard antidiarrheal treatments	
Intolerable Grade 2 palmar-plantar erythrodysesthesia syndrome (skin changes [eg, peeling, blisters, bleeding, edema, or hyperkeratosis] with pain; limiting instrumental ADL)	Withhold cabozantinib until improvement to G ≤1, then resume cabozantinib with the dosage reduced by 1 dose level
Grade 3 palmar-plantar erythrodysesthesia syndrome (severe skin changes [eg, peeling, blisters, bleeding, edema, or hyperkeratosis] with pain; limiting self-care ADL)	
Patient requires dental surgery or an invasive dental procedure	If possible, withhold cabozantinib for ≥3 weeks prior to the procedure to reduce risk of osteonecrosis of the jaw and poor wound healing
Osteonecrosis of the jaw	Withhold cabozantinib until complete resolution, then reduce the cabozantinib dosage by 1 dose level
Patient requires elective surgery	If possible, withhold cabozantinib for ≥3 weeks prior to elective surgery and for ≥2 weeks after major surgery and until adequate wound healing, whichever is longer
RPLS is suspected (symptoms of headache, seizure, lethargy, confusion, blindness, and/or other visual and neurologic disturbances along with hypertension of any severity)	Withhold cabozantinib until clarification of the patient's neurological status (ie, with an emergent brain MRI) has occurred
RPLS is confirmed	Discontinue cabozantinib. The safety of reinitiating cabozantinib in a patient who has experienced RPLS is unknown
Urine dipstick >1+ for protein	Continue cabozantinib at the same dose pending results of a 24-hour urine protein
Urine protein ≥3 g/24 hours	Withhold cabozantinib until urine protein is <3 g/24 hours, then resume cabozantinib at 1 lower dose level. Consider increasing the frequency of urine protein monitoring upon resumption of cabozantinib
Nephrotic syndrome	Discontinue cabozantinib treatment

(continued)

Dose Modifications (*continued*)

Other Adverse Reactions

Other intolerable Grade 2 adverse reactions	Withhold cabozantinib until improvement to G ≤1 or baseline, then reduce the cabozantinib dosage by 1 dose level
Other ≥Grade 3 adverse reactions	

Hepatic Impairment

Mild to moderate hepatic impairment (Child-Pugh class A or B)	Decrease the starting dose of cabozantinib to 80 mg once daily

Drug Interactions

Patient requires concomitant use of a strong CYP3A4 inhibitor (eg, atazanavir, clarithromycin, indinavir, itraconazole, ketoconazole, nefazodone, nelfinavir, ritonavir, saquinavir, telithromycin, voriconazole)	Reduce the daily cabozantinib dose by 40 mg. Resume the dose that was used prior to initiating the CYP3A4 inhibitor 2 to 3 days after discontinuing a strong inhibitor
Patient requires concomitant use of a strong CYP3A4 inducer (eg, carbamazepine, phenobarbital, phenytoin, rifabutin, rifampin, rifapentine, St. John's wort)	Increase the daily cabozantinib dose by 40 mg only if tolerability on the dose without the inducer has been convincingly demonstrated. Resume the dose that was used prior to initiating a CYP3A4 inducer 2–3 days after discontinuing a strong inducer. The daily cabozantinib dose should not exceed 180 mg

MI, myocardial infarction; VTE, venous thromboembolic event; RPLS, reversible posterior leukoencephalopathy syndrome; UPCR, urine protein to creatinine ratio; MRI, magnetic resonance imaging; ADL, activity of daily living
Adapted in part from: COMETRIQ (cabozantinib) prescribing information. Alameda, CA: Exelixis, Inc; revised January 2020

Patient Population Studied

Locally advanced or metastatic medullary thyroid cancer. All had RECIST-documented progressive disease within 14 months before screening, although the interval between scans was not fixed. There were no limits on the number of prior therapies; 95% had ECOG 0/1 PS. RET mutation status was "positive" in 46%, "negative" in 14%, and unknown in 40%. Of the studied population, 51% had bone metastases at baseline

Efficacy

	Cabozantinib	Placebo	Statistics
Median PFS, independent review (months)	11.2	4.0	HR 0.28 (95% CI: 0.19–0.40); P <0.0001
Median PFS, investigator (months)	13.8	3.1	HR 0.29 (95% CI: 0.21–0.42); P <0.0001
1-year PFS	47.3%	7.2%	—
ORR, independent review	28%	0	P <0.0001
Median duration of response (months)	14.6	—	—
Mean calcitonin levels during first 3 months	↓ 45%	↑ 57%	—

Toxicity

Adverse Event (>25% incidence)	Cabozantinib (N = 214) 6.7 months		Placebo (N = 109) 3.4 months	
Median Duration of Exposure	All Grades	G3/4	All Grades	G3/4
Diarrhea	135 (63%)	34 (16%)	36 (33%)	2 (2%)
Hand-foot skin reaction	107 (50%)	27 (13%)	2 (2%)	—
Decreased weight	102 (48%)	10 (5%)	11 (10%)	—
Decreased appetite	98 (46%)	10 (5%)	17 (16%)	1 (1%)
Nausea	92 (43%)	3 (1%)	23 (21%)	—
Fatigue	87 (41%)	20 (9%)	31 (28%)	3 (3%)
Dysgeusia	73 (34%)	1 (0.5%)	6 (6%)	—
Hair color changes	72 (34%)	1 (0.5%)	1 (1%)	—
Stomatitis	62 (29%)	4 (2%)	3 (3%)	—
Constipation	57 (27%)	—	6 (6%)	—
Hypertension	70 (33%)	18 (8%)	5 (5%)	1 (1%)
Hemorrhage	54 (25%)	7 (3%)	17 (16%)	1 (1%)
Venous thrombosis	12 (6%)	8 (4%)	3 (3%)	2 (2%)
GI perforation	7 (3%)	7 (3%)	0	0
Non–GI fistula	8 (4%)	4 (2%)	0	0
Death within 30 days of treatment	5.6%		2.8%	
Required dose reduction	79%		—	
Discontinued use	27%		—	

Therapy Monitoring

1. *Prior to initiation of cabozantinib:* CBC with differential and platelet count, vital signs, liver function tests, serum electrolytes, oral examination. Control hypertension prior to initiation of cabozantinib

2. *Monitor regularly for:*
   - Hypertension
   - Signs and symptoms of bleeding. Avoid initiation of cabozantinib in patients with a recent history of hemorrhage (eg, hemoptysis, hematemesis, or melena)
   - Signs and symptoms of fistulas and perforations, including abscess and sepsis
   - Signs and symptoms of palmar-plantar erythrodysesthesia
   - Diarrhea
   - Spot urine for protein measurement every 4–8 weeks (if spot urine dipstick >1+ for protein, perform a 24-hour urine protein).
   - Signs and symptoms of osteonecrosis of the jaw (jaw pain, osteomyelitis, osteitis, bone erosion, tooth or periodontal infection, toothache, gingival ulceration or erosion, persistent jaw pain, or slow healing of the mouth or jaw after dental surgery)

3. Perform an oral examination prior to initiation of cabozantinib and periodically during treatment. Advise patients regarding good oral hygiene practices

4. Withhold cabozantinib for ≥3 weeks prior to scheduled dental surgery or invasive dental procedures, if possible

5. Withhold cabozantinib for ≥3 weeks prior to elective surgery (including dental surgery) and for ≥2 weeks after major surgery and until adequate wound healing, whichever is longer

6. *Response assessment:* Every 2–3 cycles

ANAPLASTIC

THYROID CANCER REGIMEN: DOXORUBICIN AND RADIATION WITH DEBULKING SURGERY

Nilsson O et al. World J Surg 1998;22:25–30
Tennvall J et al. Cancer 1994;74:1348–1354

TREATMENT A

Preoperative treatment:
Doxorubicin 20 mg/dose; administer by intravenous injection over 3–5 minutes starting 1–2 hours before radiation therapy, weekly, for 3 weeks (total dose/3-week course = 60 mg)
Radiation 100 cGy per fraction twice daily for 30 fractions with a minimum of 6 hours between fractions 5 days/week to a target dose of 3000 cGy in 3 weeks

Debulking surgery:
Around week 5 approximately 10–14 days after completing preoperative radiation therapy

Postoperative treatment:
Doxorubicin 20 mg/dose; administer by intravenous injection over 3–5 minutes, weekly, starting 1–2 hours before radiation therapy (total dose/week = 20 mg)
Radiation 100 cGy per fraction twice daily for 16 fractions with a minimum of 6 hours between fractions 5 days/week to a target dose of 1600 cGy (total cumulative radiation including preoperative dose = 4600 cGy over approximately 70 days)

Additional doxorubicin:
Doxorubicin 20 mg/dose; administer by intravenous injection over 3–5 minutes, weekly, in patients considered to be in "reasonably good condition" (maximum dosage/complete treatment = 750 mg/m^2)
Note: Doxorubicin is administered as a fixed dose (20 mg), but cumulative dosage is calculated as mg/m^2

Supportive Care

Antiemetic prophylaxis
Emetogenic potential on days doxorubicin is administered is **MODERATE**
See Chapter 42 for antiemetic recommendations

Hematopoietic growth factor (CSF) prophylaxis
Primary prophylaxis is **NOT** *indicated*
See Chapter 43 for more information

Antimicrobial prophylaxis
Risk of fever and neutropenia is **LOW**
Antimicrobial primary prophylaxis to be considered:
- Antibacterial—not indicated
- Antifungal—not indicated
- Antiviral—not indicated unless patient previously had an episode of HSV

TREATMENT B

Preoperative treatment:
Doxorubicin 20 mg/dose; administer by intravenous injection over 3–5 minutes, weekly, starting 1–2 hours before radiation therapy for 3 weeks (total dose/3-week course = 60 mg)
Radiation 130 cGy/per fraction twice daily for 23 fractions with a minimum of 6 hours between fractions, 5 days/week to a target dosage of 3000 cGy

Debulking surgery:
Around week 4 (approximately 2 weeks after completing preoperative radiation therapy)

Postoperative treatment:
Doxorubicin 20 mg/week; administer by intravenous injection over 3–5 minutes, weekly, starting 1 hour before radiation therapy (total dose/week = 20 mg)
Radiation 130 cGY/per fraction twice daily for 12 fractions with a minimum of 6 hours between fractions 5 days/week to a target dosage of 1600 cGY (total cumulative radiation dose including preoperative dose = 4600 cGy over approximately 50 days)

Additional doxorubicin:
Doxorubicin 20 mg/week; administer by intravenous injection over 3–5 minutes, weekly, in patients considered to be in "reasonably good condition" (maximum dosage/complete treatment = 400–440 mg)

Treatment Modifications

Postoperative doxorubicin was administered to patients with good performance status and in the absence of disease progression

Patient Population Studied

A study of 33 patients with anaplastic thyroid carcinoma treated with combined radiation, chemotherapy, and surgery. In later review, 160 patients were studied

Efficacy (N = 33)

	Treatment	
	A (n = 16)	B (n = 17)
Median survival	3.5 months	4.5 months
Local control	5 patients	11 patients
Local failure*	6 patients	2 patients
Persistent local disease*	5 patients	3 patients

*Cause of death
1. 24% of patient deaths attributed to local failure
2. 48% of patients had no signs of local recurrence
3. Preoperative doxorubicin and concomitant hyperfractionated radiation therapy converted unresectable tumors into a resectable state in 23 patients

Toxicity (N = 33)

1. WHO Grades I and II mucosal and skin toxicity
2. Hematologic toxicity not observed
3. Treatment-related toxicities did not prevent any patient from completing planned treatment

Therapy Monitoring

1. *Weekly:* CBC with differential
2. *Before each treatment:* CBC with differential and left ventricular ejection fraction evaluation
3. *Every 2–3 cycles:* Imaging studies to evaluate response and left ventricular ejection fraction evaluation

Notes

Doxorubicin has been used historically; however, as a single agent, it is not considered an effective chemotherapeutic drug for anaplastic carcinoma

ANAPLASTIC

THYROID CANCER REGIMEN: 96-HOUR CONTINUOUS-INFUSION PACLITAXEL AND WEEKLY PACLITAXEL

Ain KB et al. Thyroid 2000;10:587–594

Continuous 96-Hour IV Infusion

Optional premedication* (Primary prophylaxis against hypersensitivity reactions from paclitaxel):
Dexamethasone 20 mg/dose; administer orally for 2 doses on the evening before and the morning of chemotherapy before paclitaxel *plus*
Diphenhydramine 50 mg for 1 dose; administer by intravenous injection 30 minutes before paclitaxel *and*
Ranitidine 50 mg or **cimetidine** 300 mg for 1 dose; administer by intravenous infusion in 25–100 mL 0.9% sodium chloride injection (0.9% NS) or 5% dextrose injection (D5W) over 5–30 minutes given 30 minutes before paclitaxel

*The incidence of hypersensitivity reactions with 96-hour continuous infusion of paclitaxel is much lower than with other paclitaxel regimens, and in most patients, premedication is not required. If a premedication regimen is not used, observe the patient carefully for at least 1 hour in the first cycle to ensure that no reaction occurs. If a reaction occurs, immediately stop paclitaxel infusion and administer the suggested premedication regimen, substituting intravenous dexamethasone

Paclitaxel 30–35 mg/m^2 per day; administer by continuous intravenous infusion in a volume of 0.9% NS or D5W sufficient to produce a solution with concentration within the range 0.3–1.2 mg/mL over 24 hours for 4 consecutive days, on days 1–4, every 3 weeks, for up to 6 cycles (total dosage/cycle for 30 mg/m^2 per day = 120 mg/m^2 for 35 mg/m^2 per day = 140 mg/m^2)

Intermittent Weekly Administration (Bible KC et al. Thyroid 2021;31:337–386)
Note: Subsequent clinical experience suggests that optimal use of paclitaxel uses a 1-hour infusion of 60–90 mg/m^2 given weekly continuing until there is progressive disease or limiting toxicity.

Primary prophylaxis against hypersensitivity reactions from paclitaxel:
Dexamethasone 10 mg/dose; administer orally for 2 doses at 12 hours and 6 hours before paclitaxel (total dose/week = 20 mg), *or*
Dexamethasone 20 mg; administer intravenously over 10–15 minutes, 30–60 minutes before starting paclitaxel (total dose/week = 20 mg)
Diphenhydramine 50 mg; administer by intravenous injection 30 minutes before paclitaxel, *and:*
Ranitidine 50 mg or **cimetidine** 300 mg; administer intravenously in 25–100 mL of 0.9% NS or D5W over 5–30 minutes, 30 minutes before paclitaxel

Paclitaxel 60–90 mg/m^2; administer by intravenous infusion in a volume of 0.9% NS or D5W sufficient to produce a solution with concentration of 0.3–1.2 mg/mL over 1 hour once per week (total dosage/week = 60–90 mg/m^2)

Supportive Care
Antiemetic prophylaxis
Emetogenic potential is **LOW**
See Chapter 42 for antiemetic recommendations

Hematopoietic growth factor (CSF) prophylaxis
Primary prophylaxis may be indicated
See Chapter 43 for more information

Antimicrobial prophylaxis
Risk of fever and neutropenia is **LOW**
  Antimicrobial primary prophylaxis to be considered:
  • Antibacterial—not indicated

  • Antifungal—not indicated

  • Antiviral—not indicated unless patient previously had an episode of HSV

Treatment Modifications

Adverse Event	Dose Modification
96-Hour Continuous Infusion Paclitaxel	
G2 hematologic adverse events	Hold paclitaxel until adverse events resolve to G1 or disappear, then resume paclitaxel with dosage reduced by 25%
G2/3 gastrointestinal, neurologic, cardiac, musculoskeletal toxicities, or mucositis	
G4 or unremitting G3 adverse events	Discontinue paclitaxel
ANC nadir <500/mm^3, platelet nadir <50,000/mm^3, or febrile neutropenia	Reduce paclitaxel dosage by 25%
Day 1 ANC <1500/mm^3 or platelets <100,000/mm^3	Delay chemotherapy until ANC > 1500/mm^3 and platelets >100,000/mm^3 for maximum delay of 2 weeks
Weekly Paclitaxel	
Day 1 ANC <1500/mm^3 or platelets <100,000/mm^3	Delay chemotherapy until ANC <1500/mm^3 and platelets >100,000/mm^3 for maximum delay of 2 weeks
Delay of <2 weeks in reaching ANC <1500/mm^3 and platelets >100,000/mm^3	Discontinue therapy
G2 neurotoxicity	Reduce paclitaxel dosage to 135 mg/m^2
G3 neurotoxicity	Discontinue paclitaxel
G2 arthralgia/myalgia despite dexamethasone prophylaxis	Reduce paclitaxel dosage to 135 mg/m^2
G3 arthralgia/myalgia despite dexamethasone prophylaxis	Discontinue paclitaxel
Moderate hypersensitivity	Patient may be retreated
Severe hypersensitivity	Discontinue therapy

Patient Population Studied

A study of 20 patients with metastatic anaplastic thyroid cancer

Efficacy* (N = 19)

Partial responses	47%
Complete responses	5%
Disease stabilization	5%
Progressive disease	42%
Therapeutic response	Median survival: 32 weeks
No therapeutic response	Median survival: 10 weeks

*From WHO criteria

Toxicity* (N = 11/8)

(Paclitaxel 140 mg/m², n = 11[†])

	G1	G2
Nausea	6	1
Alopecia	3	—
Vomiting	2	—
Diarrhea	3	—
Fever	1	2

(Paclitaxel 120 mg/m², n = 8[‡])

	G1	G2
Nausea	1	—
Alopecia	1	—
Stomatitis	1	—
Fatigue	1	—
Neutropenia	—	1

*NCI Common Terminology Criteria for Adverse Events
[†]Patients who received paclitaxel 35 mg/m² per day for 4 days (total dosage/cycle = 140 mg/m²)
[‡]Patients who received paclitaxel 30 mg/m² per day for 4 days (total dosage/cycle = 120 mg/m²)

Therapy Monitoring

1. *Before every cycle:* CBC with differential, platelet count, and LFTs
2. *Radiologic studies:* Every 2 cycles

ANAPLASTIC

THYROID CANCER REGIMEN: DABRAFENIB + TRAMETINIB

Keam B et al. Ann Oncol 2018;29(suppl_8):viii645–viii648
Data supplement to: Subbiah V et al. J Clin Oncol 2018;36:7–13

Note: The U.S. Food and Drug Administration approval for dabrafenib + trametinib in patients with anaplastic thyroid cancer is limited to patients with BRAF V600E mutation and no satisfactory locoregional treatment options

Dabrafenib 150 mg per dose; administer orally twice daily, at least 1 hour before or 2 hours after meals, continuously until disease progression or unacceptable toxicity (total dose/week = 2100 mg), *plus:*
Treatment notes:
• Advise patients NOT to open, crush, or break dabrafenib capsules

• Missed doses may be taken up to 6 hours before a subsequently scheduled dose

• Dabrafenib is a substrate for metabolism catalyzed by CYP2C8 and CYP3A4. Avoid concomitant use of dabrafenib with strong CYP3A4 or strong CYP2C8 inhibitors when possible. If concomitant use of a strong CYP3A4 or CYP2C8 inhibitor is unavoidable, monitor closely for toxicities. If concomitant use of a strong CYP3A4 or strong CYP2C8 inducer is unavoidable, monitor closely for loss of efficacy

• Dabrafenib has been shown in experimental studies in vitro to induce CYP3A4 and CYP2C9. As a result, dabrafenib decreases systemic exposure to *S*-warfarin and *R*-warfarin. Monitor international normalized ratio (INR) levels closely in patients receiving warfarin during the initiation or discontinuation of dabrafenib

Trametinib 2 mg per dose; administer orally once daily, at least 1 hour before or 2 hours after a meal at approximately the same time each day, continuously until disease progression or unacceptable toxicity (total dose/week = 14 mg)
Treatment note:
• Missed doses may be taken up to 12 hours before a subsequently scheduled dose

Supportive Care
Antiemetic prophylaxis
Emetogenic potential is **LOW**
See Chapter 42 for antiemetic recommendations

Hematopoietic growth factor (CSF) prophylaxis
Primary prophylaxis is **NOT** *indicated*
See Chapter 43 for more information

Antimicrobial prophylaxis
Risk of fever and neutropenia is **LOW**
    Antimicrobial primary prophylaxis to be considered:
    • Antibacterial—not indicated

    • Antifungal—not indicated

    • Antiviral—not indicated unless patient previously had an episode of HSV

Diarrhea management
Latent or delayed onset diarrhea*:
    Loperamide 4 mg orally initially after the first loose or liquid stool, *then*
    Loperamide 2 mg orally every 2 hours during waking hours, *plus*
    Loperamide 4 mg orally every 4 hours during hours of sleep

Treatment Modifications

Dabrafenib

Starting dose	150 mg by mouth twice a day
Dose Level −1	100 mg by mouth twice a day
Dose Level −2	75 mg by mouth twice a day
Dose Level −3	50 mg by mouth twice a day
Dose Level −4	Permanently discontinue dabrafenib

Trametinib

Starting dose	2 mg by mouth once daily
Dose Level −1	1.5 mg by mouth once daily
Dose Level −2	1 mg by mouth once daily
Dose Level −3	Permanently discontinue trametinib

Adverse Event	Dose Modification
New Primary Malignancy Adverse Events	
New primary non-cutaneous RAS mutation-positive malignancy	Permanently discontinue dabrafenib; continue trametinib without modification, if appropriate
New primary non-melanoma cutaneous malignancy	Continue dabrafenib and trametinib at the same dose. Refer patient to dermatologist for management of non-melanoma cutaneous malignancy
Cardiac Adverse Events	
Asymptomatic, absolute decrease in LVEF of ≥10% but <20% from baseline that is below LLN	Interrupt trametinib for up to 4 weeks. If LVEF improves to ≥LLN, then resume trametinib at one lower dose level. If LVEF does not improve to ≥LLN, then permanently discontinue trametinib. Continue dabrafenib without modification
Symptomatic CHF—absolute decrease in LVEF by ≥20% from baseline that is below LLN	Permanently discontinue trametinib. Interrupt dabrafenib. If LVEF improves to ≥LLN and an absolute decrease ≤10% compared to baseline, then resume dabrafenib at the same dose
Ocular Adverse Events	
Patient reports loss of vision or other visual disturbances	Interrupt dabrafenib and trametinib until ophthalmologic status is clarified. Urgently (within 24 hours) perform ophthalmologic evaluation
Uveitis, including iritis and iridocyclitis	If mild or moderate uveitis does not respond to ocular therapy, or for severe uveitis, interrupt dabrafenib for up to 6 weeks. If improved to G0/1, then resume at the same dose or at a lower dose level. If G ≥2 uveitis persists for >6 weeks, then permanently discontinue dabrafenib. Continue trametinib without modification
Retinal pigment epithelial detachments	Interrupt trametinib for up to 3 weeks. If improved, resume trametinib at the same or lower dose level. If not improved, then resume trametinib at one lower dose level, or permanently discontinue trametinib. Continue dabrafenib without modification
Retinal vein occlusion	Permanently discontinue trametinib. Continue dabrafenib without modification
Pulmonary Adverse Events	
Dyspnea, cough, fever, and radiologic abnormalities—pneumonitis is suspected	Interrupt trametinib until pulmonary status is clarified. Continue dabrafenib without modification
Interstitial lung disease/pneumonitis is confirmed	Permanently discontinue trametinib. Continue dabrafenib without modification

(continued)

Treatment Modifications (*continued*)

Febrile Adverse Events

Fever of 38.5°C to 40°C	Interrupt dabrafenib until fever resolves. Increase fluid intake and administer antipyretics (eg, acetaminophen) as needed. Consider monitoring renal function as clinically indicated. Upon resolution of fever, resume dabrafenib at the same or a lower dose level
Fever of >40°C	Interrupt dabrafenib until fever resolves. Increase fluid intake, administer antipyretics (eg, acetaminophen) as needed, and monitor renal function closely. Upon resolution of fever, resume dabrafenib at a lower dose level along with prophylactic antipyretics, or permanently discontinue dabrafenib
Fever ≥38.5°C complicated by rigors, hypotension, dehydration, or renal failure	Interrupt dabrafenib and trametinib until fever resolves. Increase fluid intake, administer antipyretics (eg, acetaminophen) as needed, and monitor renal function closely. Administer corticosteroids (eg, prednisone 10 mg daily) for ≥5 days if there is no evidence of active infection. Upon resolution of fever, resume dabrafenib at a lower dose level along with prophylactic antipyretics, or permanently discontinue dabrafenib. Upon resolution of fever, resume trametinib at the same or a lower dose level
Recurrent fever ≥38.5°C	Interrupt dabrafenib and trametinib until fever resolves. Increase fluid intake and administer antipyretics (eg, acetaminophen) as needed. In the absence of evidence of active infection, administer corticosteroids (eg, prednisone 10 mg daily) for ≥5 days if fever persists for >3 days or if fever is associated with complications such as dehydration, hypotension, renal failure, or severe chills/rigors. Upon resolution of fever, resume dabrafenib at a lower dose level along with prophylactic antipyretics, or permanently discontinue dabrafenib. Upon resolution of fever, resume trametinib at the same dose level, or optionally at a lower dose level if temperature was ≥40°C or associated with complications

Dermatologic Adverse Events

Intolerable G2 dermatologic toxicity G3/4 dermatologic toxicity	Interrupt dabrafenib and trametinib for up to 3 weeks. If improved, resume dabrafenib at one lower dose level and resume trametinib at one lower dose level. If not improved, permanently discontinue both dabrafenib and trametinib

Hemorrhagic Adverse Events

G3 hemorrhage	Interrupt dabrafenib and trametinib. If bleeding is improved to G0/1, resume dabrafenib at the next lower dose level and resume trametinib at the next lower dose level
G4 hemorrhage	Permanently discontinue dabrafenib and trametinib

Venous Thromboembolism Events

Uncomplicated DVT or PE	Interrupt trametinib for up to 3 weeks. If improved to G0/1 within 3 weeks, resume trametinib at one lower dose level Continue dabrafenib without modification
Life-threatening PE	Permanently discontinue trametinib Interrupt dabrafenib until toxicity resolves to G0/1, then resume at a lower dose level, or permanently discontinue dabrafenib

Other Adverse Events

Other intolerable G2 toxicities*† Other G3 toxicities*†	Interrupt dabrafenib and trametinib. If improved to G0/1, resume dabrafenib at one lower dose level and resume trametinib at one lower dose level. If not improved, permanently discontinue dabrafenib and trametinib
First occurrence of any other G4 toxicity*†	Interrupt dabrafenib and trametinib until toxicity improves to G0/1. If toxicity improves to G0/1, then resume at dabrafenib at one lower dose level or permanently discontinue dabrafenib. If toxicity improves to G0/1, then resume trametinib at one lower dose level or permanently discontinue trametinib
Recurrent other G4 toxicity*†	Permanently discontinue dabrafenib and trametinib
Known G6PD deficiency	Monitor closely for hemolytic anemia with dabrafenib

*Dose modifications are not recommended for dabrafenib when administered with trametinib for the following adverse reactions attributable to trametinib: retinal vein occlusion, retinal pigment epithelial detachment, interstitial lung disease/pneumonitis, and uncomplicated venous thromboembolism. Dose modification of dabrafenib is not required for new primary cutaneous malignancies
†Dose modifications are not recommended for trametinib when administered with dabrafenib for the following adverse reactions attributable to dabrafenib: non-cutaneous malignancies and uveitis. Dose modification of trametinib is not required for new primary cutaneous malignancies
LVEF, left ventricular ejection fraction; LLN, lower limit of normal; CHF, congestive heart failure; G6PD, glucose–6-phosphate dehydrogenase; DVT, deep vein thrombosis; PE, pulmonary embolism

Patient Population Studied

This was a multicenter, non-randomized, open-label, phase 2 basket study (NCT02034110) evaluating the combination of dabrafenib and trametinib in adult patients with a variety of pre-specified tumor types, including anaplastic thyroid cancer, harboring BRAF V600E mutations. Patients with anaplastic thyroid cancer were eligible if they were not potentially curable by surgical resection alone and if they had already previously received standard of care treatment and had an Eastern Cooperative Oncology Group performance status of ≤2. Patients were excluded if they had received prior treatment with BRAF or MEK inhibitors. Twenty-eight patients with anaplastic thyroid cancer enrolled—median age 70 years, 82% had prior radiation therapy, and 46% had received ≥1 prior line of systemic chemotherapy

Efficacy (N = 27)

	Dabrafenib + Trametinib (N = 27)
	Investigator Assessment
Overall response rate	18/27 (67%; 95% CI, 46–84)
Duration of response ≥6 months*	12/18 (67%)
Median progression-free survival	1.2 years (95% CI, 0.4–NR)
Median overall survival	1.7 years (95% CI, 0.7–NR)

At the time of data cut-off, 8 out of the 18 responses were ongoing
NR; not reached
Note: Data shown are from the intent-to-treat population; 25 of the 28 patients had central confirmation of BRAF^V600E mutation
Keam B et al. Ann Oncol 2018;29(suppl_8):viii645–viii648

Adverse Events

	Dabrafenib + Trametinib (n = 163 patients enrolled in 8/9 histologies)
Grade (%)*	All grades
Any adverse event	96
Pyrexia	50
Fatigue	36

	Dabrafenib + Trametinib (n = 28 patients enrolled in the anaplastic thyroid cancer cohort)
Grade (%)*	Grades 3–4
Anemia	25
Hyponatremia	21
Pneumonia	21

Keam B et al. Ann Oncol 2018;29 (suppl_8):viii645–viii648

Therapy Monitoring

1. *Prior to the start of therapy in women of child-bearing potential:* pregnancy test
2. *Prior to the start of therapy and repeated every 2 months during therapy and for 6 months after cessation of therapy:* dermatologic evaluation
3. *Prior to the start of therapy, 1 month after the start of therapy, and then every 2–3 months while on therapy:* assess left ventricular ejection fraction
4. *Periodically monitor for:*
   - Signs and symptoms of uveitis (eg, changes in vision, photophobia, ocular pain); perform an ophthalmologic examination in patients with new visual symptoms
   - Febrile reactions
   - Blood glucose levels
   - Signs and symptoms of colitis and/or gastrointestinal perforation
   - Signs and symptoms of venous thromboembolism
   - Signs and symptoms of hemorrhage
   - Signs of hemolytic anemia in patients with known glucose–6-phosphate dehydrogenase deficiency
   - Signs and symptoms of interstitial lung disease

RET-MUTANT MEDULLARY • RET FUSION-POSITIVE THYROID CANCER

THYROID CANCER REGIMEN: SELPERCATINB

Retevmo (selpercatinib) prescribing information. Indianapolis, IN: Lilly USA; 2020

Note: The U.S. Food and Drug Administration approval for selpercatinib in patients with refractory thyroid cancer is limited to patients older than 12 years old and with RET mutation or RET fusion. The approval is based on overall response rate and response duration but is contingent upon verification on confirmatory trials that are ongoing

Selpercatinib (40- and 80-mg capsules)
Starting dose:
— Body weight <50 kg 120 mg orally every 12 hours
— Body weight ≥50 kg 160 mg orally every 12 hours
— Severe hepatic impairment: 80 mg every 12 hours
• The capsules should be swallowed whole and not chewed or crushed
• Selpercatinib can be taken with or without food
• If a dose is missed, it should be taken within 6 hours, otherwise it should be not taken
• Avoid acid-reducing agents. If antacid use is needed:
  — For proton pump inhibitors, selpercatinib should be taken with a low-fat meal (approximately 390 calories and 10 g of fat)
  — For H_2 receptor antagonist take selpercatinib 2 hours before or 10 hours after
  — For locally acting antacids, take selpercatinib 2 hours before or 2 hours after
• Avoid strong and moderate CYP3A inhibitors. If strong and moderate CYP3A inhibitors are needed, reduce selpercatinib dose

Current dose	Recommended dose with concomitant use of	
	A moderate CYP3A inhibitor	A strong CYP3A inhibitor
120 mg bid	80 mg orally twice daily	40 mg orally twice daily
160 mg bid	120 mg orally twice daily	80 mg orally twice daily

• Avoid strong and moderate CYP3A inducers
• Avoid CYP2C8 and CYP3A substrates. If CYP2C8 and CYP3A substrates are needed, modify the substrate dosage

Selpercatinib should be stopped 7 days before surgery and resumed after 2 weeks and adequate wound healing
Pregnancy and lactation are contraindicated

Supportive Care
Antiemetic prophylaxis
Emetogenic potential is **LOW**
See Chapter 42 for antiemetic recommendations

Hematopoietic growth factor (CSF) prophylaxis
Primary prophylaxis is **NOT** *indicated*
See Chapter 43 for more information

Antimicrobial prophylaxis
Risk of fever and neutropenia is **LOW**
  Antimicrobial primary prophylaxis to be considered:
  • Antibacterial—not indicated
  • Antifungal—not indicated
  • Antiviral—not indicated unless patient previously had an episode of HSV

Diarrhea management
Latent or delayed onset diarrhea*:
  Loperamide 4 mg orally initially after the first loose or liquid stool, *then*
  Loperamide 2 mg orally every 2 hours during waking hours, *plus*
  Loperamide 4 mg orally every 4 hours during hours of sleep
  • Continue for at least 12 hours after diarrhea resolves
  • Recurrent diarrhea after a 12-hour diarrhea-free interval is treated as a new episode
  • Rehydrate orally with fluids and electrolytes during a diarrheal episode
  • If diarrhea persists >48 hours despite loperamide, stop loperamide and hospitalize the patient for IV hydration

Treatment Modifications

Patient weight	≥50 kg	<50 kg
Starting dose	160 mg bid	120 mg bid
First dose reduction	120 mg bid	80 mg bid
Second dose reduction	80 mg bid	40 mg bid
Third dose reduction	40 mg bid	40 mg once

Adverse Event	Dose Modification
Hepatotoxicity	
G3/4 AST and or ALT (increased >5.0× ULN)	Stop selpercatinib. Monitor AST and ALT weekly until G1 or baseline values. Resume at reduced dose by two dose levels; monitor AST and ALT weekly. Dose can be progressively increased by one level every 2 weeks to the dose taken at the moment of G3/4 hepatotoxicity if there is no recurrence of hepatotoxicity
Hypertension	
Grade 3 (systolic BP ≥160 mm Hg or diastolic BP ≥100 mm Hg) despite optimal antihypertensive treatment	Stop selpercatinib. Monitor until G1 or baseline level. Resume at reduced dose
Grade 4 (hypertension with life-threatening consequences, eg, malignant hypertension, transient or permanent neurologic deficit, hypertensive crisis)	Discontinue selpercatinib
QT interval prolongation	
QTc ≥501 ms on ≥2 separate ECGs	Stop selpercatinib. Monitor until G1 or baseline level. Resume at reduced dose
Torsade de pointes or polymorphic ventricular tachycardia or signs/symptoms of serious arrhythmia	Discontinue selpercatinib
Bleeding	
G3 (moderate symptoms, medical intervention or minor cauterization indicated) or G4 (transfusion, radiologic, endoscopic, or elective operative intervention indicated)	Stop selpercatinib. Monitor until G1 or baseline level. Discontinue for life threatening bleeding
Hypersensitivity	
Any grade	Stop selpercatinib. Initiate corticosteroids. Monitor until resolution. Resume at reduced dose by 3 dose levels. Increase progressively by one dose level per week until the dose taken at the moment of hypersensitivity onset and then taper corticosteroids
Other adverse events	
Grade 3 or 4	Stop selpercatinib. Monitor until Grade 1 or baseline level. Resume at reduced dose

Patient Population Studied

The efficacy of selpercatinib was evaluated in patients with RET-mutant MTC enrolled in a multicenter, open-label, multi-cohort clinical trial (LIBRETTO–001, NCT03157128) that evaluated the efficacy of selpercatinib in patients with refractory RET-mutant MTC and RET fusion-positive thyroid cancer. The patients enrolled could have been previously treated with other tyrosine kinase inhibitors (TKI) or be treatment-naïve

Efficacy

Efficacy in RET-mutant MTC Previously Treated with Other TKIs (N = 55)

(Fifty-five patients with RET-mutant MTC who had been previously treated with cabozantinib or vandetanib had a median age of 57 years [range: 17 to 84]; 66% were male. ECOG performance status was ≤1 [95%] or 2 [5%], and 98% of patients had distant metastases. Median number of previous treatment lines was 2 [range: 1–8])

	Selpercatinib
Overall response rate assessed by blinded independent central review	37/55 (69%; 95% CI, 55–81)
Partial response	5/55 (9%)
Duration of response ≥6 months	42/55 (76%)
Median progression-free survival	NE (95% CI, 19.1–NE)

NE; not estimable

Efficacy in RET-Mutant MTC not Previously Treated with Vandetanib or Cabozantinib (N = 88)

(Eighty-eight patients with RET-mutant MTC were cabozantinib and vandetanib treatment-naïve, had a median age of 58 years [range: 15 to 82]; 66% were male. ECOG performance status was ≤1 [97%] or 2 [3.4%]. All patients [100%] had distant metastases, 72% were treatment-naïve while 8% had received 1 or 2 prior systemic therapies [including 8% kinase inhibitors, 4.5% chemotherapy, 2.3% anti-PD1/PD-L1 therapy, and 1.1% radioactive iodine])

(continued)

Toxicity

Adverse Event (>15% Incidence)	% G1–2	% G3–4
Gastrointestinal		
Increased AST	51	8
Increased ALT	45	9
Dry mouth	39	0
Diarrhea	37	3.4
Constipation	25	0.6
Nausea	23	0.6
Abdominal pain	23	1.9
Vomiting	15	0.3
Vascular		
Hypertension	35	18
Prolonged QT interval	17	4
General		
Fatigue	35	2
Edema (generalized or localized)	33	0.3
Skin		
Rash	27	0.7
Nervous system		
Headache	23	1.4
Respiratory		
Cough	18	0
Dyspnea	16	2.3
Blood and lymphatic system		
Hemorrhage	15	1.9
Decreased leukocytes	43	1.6
Decreased platelets	33	2.7
Laboratory abnormalities		
Increased glucose	44	2.2
Decreased albumin	42	0.7
Decreased calcium	41	3.8
Increased creatinine	37	1
Increased alkaline phosphatase	36	2.3
Increased total cholesterol	31	0.1
Decreased sodium	27	7
Decreased magnesium	24	0.6
Increased potassium	24	1.2
Increased bilirubin	23	2
Decreased glucose	22	0.7

Treatment Monitoring

1. Before treatment initiation: CBC with differential and platelet count, vital signs, liver function tests, serum electrolytes, electrocardiogram QTc
2. Pregnancy test and recommend an effective contraception method
3. Monitor blood pressure and treat hypertension if needed, do not start treatment in patients with uncontrolled hypertension

Efficacy (continued)

	Selpercatinib
Overall response rate assessed by blinded independent central review	64/88 (73%; 95% CI, 62–82)
Complete response	10/88 (11%)
Partial response	54/88 (61%)
Duration of response ≥6 months	54/88 (61%)
Median progression-free survival	22 (95% CI, NE–NE)

NE, not estimable

Efficacy in RET Fusion-Positive Thyroid Cancer (N = 27)

(Twenty-seven patients with RET fusion-positive thyroid cancer had a median age of 54 years [range: 20 to 88]; 52% were male. ECOG performance status was ≤1 [89%] or 2 [11%]. All patients had distant metastases. Histotype was papillary [78%], poorly differentiated [11%], anaplastic [7%], and Hürthle cell thyroid cancer [4%]. Nineteen patients received previous systemic treatments [median number of previous treatment lines: 3; range: 1 – 7]. Eight patients were systemic treatment-naïve)

	Selpercatinib	
	Previously Treated (N = 19)	Systemic Treatment Naïve (N = 8)
Overall response rate by blinded independent central review	15/19 (79%; 95% CI, 54–94)	8/8 (100%; 95% CI, 63–100)
Complete response	1/19 (5.3%)	1/8 (12.5%)
Partial response	14/19 (74%)	7/8 (88%)
Duration of response ≥6 months	16/19 (87%)	6/8 (75%)
Median progression-free survival	18.4 (7.6—NE)	NE (95% CI, NE-NE)

NE; not estimable

40. Tissue-Agnostic Therapies

Tito Fojo, MD, PhD, and Susan E. Bates, MD

Tissue-agnostic cancer therapeutics treat cancers based on the mutations they harbor, and it is this genetic change and not the tissue of origin that has led to their regulatory approvals. To date, tissue-agnostic therapeutics have been developed for tumors harboring NTRK mutations, those with mismatch repair deficiencies, and those with high tumor mutational burden. Tissue-agnostic cancer therapeutics are the ultimate goal of precision oncology, and it is hoped additional targets will be added and the number of such drugs will grow

Expert Opinion

NTRK Fusions

- NTRK gene fusions, also called neurotrophic tyrosine receptor kinase gene fusions, lead to abnormal proteins called TRK fusion proteins. *NTRK* gene fusions involve either *NTRK1*, *NTRK2*, or *NTRK3*—the genes that encode the neurotrophin receptors TRKA, TRKB, and TRKC, respectively
- Usually intra- and inter-chromosomal rearrangements result in hybrid genes with the 3′ sequences of *NTRK1*, *NTRK2*, or *NTRK3* containing the kinase domain juxtaposed to the 5′ sequences of a different gene. The fusion results in a chimeric oncoprotein characterized by ligand-independent constitutive activation of the TRK kinase
- The fusions result in oncogenic drivers in both adult and pediatric tumors
- *NTRK* fusions were originally identified in colorectal and papillary thyroid carcinomas but have since been found in multiple tumors from both adult and pediatric patients. These cancers can be grouped into two general categories according to the frequency at which these fusions are detected. For example, in select series of patients the prevalence of the *ETV6–NTRK3* fusion exceeds 90% in mammary analogue secretory carcinoma (MASC), secretory breast carcinoma, congenital mesoblastic nephroma (cellular or mixed subtypes), and infantile fibrosarcomas. *NTRK* fusions are also found at lower and much lower frequencies in other cancers

Frequency of NTRK Fusions in Cancer

Tumor Type	NTRK Gene Fusions Involved	Frequency
Breast secretory carcinoma	NTRK3	96%
Infantile fibrosarcoma	NTRK3	95.5%
Mammary analogue secretory carcinoma (MASC)′	NTRK3	89.1%
(Cellular and mixed) Congenital mesoblastic nephroma	NTRK3	72%
Spitz tumors and spitzoid melanoma	NTRK1	16.4%
Papillary thyroid carcinoma	NTRK1,3	8.8%
Intrahepatic cholangiocarcinoma	NTRK1	3.6%
Astrocytoma	NTRK2	3.1%
High-grade glioma	NTRK1,2,3	2.1%
Uterine sarcoma	NTRK1,3	2.1%
GIST (pan-negative)	NTRK3	1.9%
Lung cancer	NTRK1,2	1.7%
Thyroid carcinoma	NTRK1,3	1.2%
Glioblastoma	NTRK1,2	1.2%
Sarcoma	NTRK1	1.0%

(continued)

Expert Opinion (continued)

Ph-like ALL	NTRK3	0.7%
Colorectal cancer	NTRK1,3	0.61%
Melanoma	NTRK3	0.3%
Head and neck cancer	NTRK2,3	0.24%
Invasive breast cancer	NTRK3	<0.1%
Other: Renal cell carcinoma, pancreatic cancer, breast cancer, histiocytosis, multiple myeloma, and dendritic cell neoplasms	Various	<1%

Adapted from: https://oncologypro.esmo.org/oncology-in-practice/anti-cancer-agents-and-biological-therapy/targeting-ntrk-gene-fusions/overview-of-cancers-with-ntrk-gene-fusion/ntrk-gene-fusions-as-oncogenic-drivers/epidemiology-of-cancers-with-ntrk-gene-fusion

- These fusions can be detected using a variety of methods, including tumor DNA and RNA sequencing and plasma cell–free DNA profiling
- The clinical detection of *NTRK* fusions has predominantly been based on NGS

Techniques to Detect NTRK Gene Fusions

Technique	Use
NGS	Detects known and novel fusions with breakpoints in DNA or RNA
RT-PCR	Detects known fusion transcripts in RNA
FISH	Detects gene rearrangements in DNA that may generate a fusion transcript
IHC	Useful in detecting TRK protein*

*IHC can detect the TRK protein expression only
FISH, fluorescence in situ hybridization; IHC, immunohistochemistry
Adapted from: https://oncologypro.esmo.org/oncology-in-practice/anti-cancer-agents-and-biological-therapy/targeting-ntrk-gene-fusions/importance-of-testing-of-cancers-with-ntrk-gene-fusions

Algorithm for *NTRK* gene fusion testing*

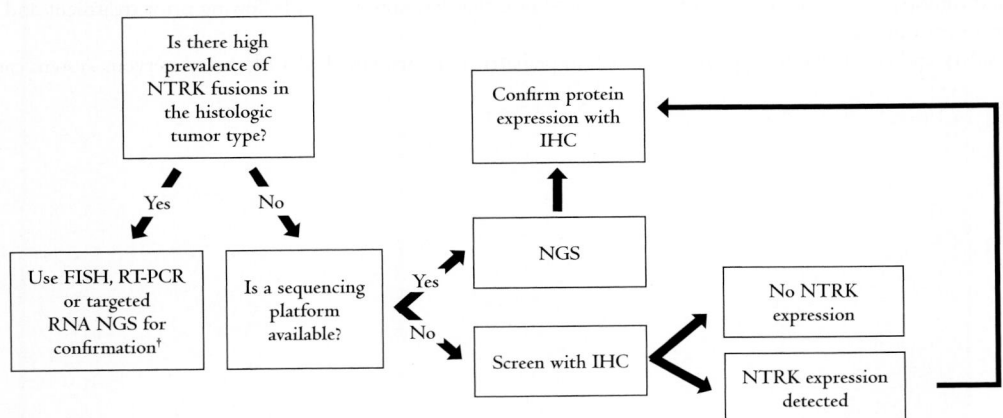

*Based on ESMO 2019 guidelines for *NTRK* fusion detection and guidelines for TRK fusion cancer in children by Albert et al. 2019; †Limited data using RT-PCR for *NTRK* fusion detection. Abbreviations: FISH, fluorescence *in situ* hybridization; IHC, immunohistochemistry; NGS, next-generation sequencing; RT-PCR, reverse transcriptase-polymerase chain reaction.

- Treatment of cancers bearing *NTRK* fusions with TRK inhibitors—initially with larotrectinib and then also with entrectinib—is associated with high response rates regardless of tumor histology
- While durable disease control is achieved in many patients, cancers harboring *NTRK* fusions eventually develop resistance that in some cases is mediated by acquired mutations in the *NTRK* kinase domain. Second-generation TRK inhibitors, including LOXO-195 and TPX-0005, are in clinical trials. Drugs approved by regulatory agencies include larotrectinib and entrectinib

LAROTRECTINIB

The FDA label states:

Larotrectinib (VITRAKVI) is a kinase inhibitor indicated for the treatment of adult and pediatric patients with solid tumors that:

– Have a neurotrophic receptor tyrosine kinase (*NTRK*) gene fusion without a known acquired resistance mutation

– Are metastatic or where surgical resection is likely to result in severe morbidity

– Have no satisfactory alternative treatments or that have progressed following treatment

ENTRECTINIB

The FDA label states:

Adult and pediatric patients 12 years of age and older with solid tumors that:

– Have a neurotrophic tyrosine receptor kinase (*NTRK)* gene fusion without a known acquired resistance mutation

– Are metastatic or where surgical resection is likely to result in severe morbidity

– Have progressed following treatment or have no satisfactory alternative therapy

Note: This indication was approved under accelerated approval based on tumor response rate and durability of response. Continued approval for this indication may be contingent upon verification and description of clinical benefit in the confirmatory trials

- The FDA indication for pediatric patients 12 years of age and older with tumors harboring *NTRK* fusions relied on efficacy data obtained primarily in adults, but safety was demonstrated in 30 pediatric patients

- Entrectinib was also approved for the treatment of adults with metastatic, *ROS1*-positive non-small cell lung cancer (NSCLC). Clinical trials of entrectinib in 51 adults with *ROS1*-positive lung cancer achieved an overall response rate of 78% (40/51), with a complete response rate in 5.9% (3/51). In 55% of those with a response (22/40), the duration lasted 12 months or longer

MSI-High/Mismatch Repair Deficiencies

PEMBROLIZUMAB

The FDA label states:

Microsatellite-instability-high cancer

For the treatment of adult and pediatric patients with unresectable or metastatic, microsatellite instability-high (MSI-H) or mismatch repair deficient

- Solid tumors that have progressed following prior treatment and who have no satisfactory alternative treatment options or

- Colorectal cancer that has progressed following treatment with a fluoropyrimidine, oxaliplatin, and irinotecan

Limitations of Use: The safety and effectiveness of pembrolizumab in pediatric patients with MSI-H central nervous system cancers have not been established

Tumor Mutational Burden-High (TMB-H) Cancer

PEMBROLIZUMAB

The FDA label states:

Tumor mutational burden-high cancer

For the treatment of adult and pediatric patients with unresectable or metastatic tumor mutational burden-high (TMB-H) (≥10 mutations/ megabase [mut/Mb]) solid tumors, as determined by an FDA-approved test, that have progressed following prior treatment and who have no satisfactory alternative treatment options

Limitations of Use: The safety and effectiveness of pembrolizumab in pediatric patients with TMB-H central nervous system cancers have not been established

METASTATIC NTRK GENE FUSION-POSITIVE TUMORS
TISSUE-AGNSOTIC REGIMEN: LAROTRECTINIB

Drilon A et al. N Engl J Med 2018;378:731–739
Vitrakvi (larotrectinib) prescribing information. Whippany, NJ: Bayer HealthCare Pharmaceuticals Inc.; 2019 July

Dosage in adult and pediatric patients with body surface area (BSA) ≥1 m²:
Larotrectinib 100 mg/dose; administer orally, twice daily, with or without food, continually until disease progression (total dose/week = 1400 mg)

Dosage in pediatric patients with BSA <1 m²:
Larotrectinib 100 mg/m²/dose; administer orally, twice daily, with or without food, continually until disease progression (total dose/week = 1400 mg/m²)

Notes on larotrectinib administration:
• Larotrectinib is indicated for metastatic tumors harboring neurotrophic receptor tyrosine kinase (NTRK) gene fusions without satisfactory alternative treatments where surgical resection is likely to result in severe morbidity and have progressed following treatment
• Dosage forms and strengths: capsules: 25 mg and 100 mg; oral solution: 20 mg/mL
• Larotrectinib is metabolized predominantly by CYP3A4. Refer to treatment modification section for initial dose adjustment recommendations for patients requiring concurrent treatment with strong CYP3A4 inhibitors or strong CYP3A4 inducers
• Larotrectinib is a weak inhibitor of CYP3A4 activity; coadministration of larotrectinib with midazolam, a probe substrate for CYP3A4, increased the AUC_{0-inf} and C_{max} of midazolam by 1.7-fold. If coadministration of larotrectinib with a sensitive CYP3A4 substrate is unavoidable, then anticipate and monitor closely for adverse effects associated with the sensitive CYP3A4 substrate

Advise patients to:
• Swallow larotrectinib capsules whole. Do not chew or crush the capsules
• In case of vomiting after taking a dose of larotrectinib, wait and take the next dose at your next scheduled time
• If a dose of larotrectinib is missed, take it as soon as you remember unless your next scheduled dose is due within 6 hours. Take the next dose at your regular time
• Avoid grapefruit and grapefruit juice while taking larotrectinib
• Store larotrectinib capsules at room temperature: 20°C to 25°C (68°F to 77°F)
• Store larotrectinib oral solution under refrigeration: 2°C to 8°C (36°F to 46°F). Discard any unused oral solution remaining after 90 days of first opening the bottle
• Avoid driving or operating machinery if experiencing adverse neurologic effects

Supportive Care
Antiemetic prophylaxis
Emetogenic potential is **MINIMAL TO LOW**
See Chapter 42 for antiemetic recommendations

Hematopoietic growth factor (CSF) prophylaxis
Primary prophylaxis is **NOT** indicated
See Chapter 43 for more information

Antimicrobial prophylaxis
Risk of fever and neutropenia is **LOW**
Antimicrobial primary prophylaxis to be considered:
• Antibacterial—not indicated
• Antifungal—not indicated
• Antiviral— not indicated unless patient previously had an episode of HSV

Treatment Modification

Recommended Dosage Modifications for Larotrectinib for Adverse Reactions

	Adult and Pediatric Patients with Body Surface Area ≥1.0 m²	Pediatric Patients with Body Surface Area <1.0 m²
Dosage Modification		
First	75 mg orally twice daily	75 mg/m² orally twice daily
Second	50 mg orally twice daily	50 mg/m² orally twice daily
Third	100 mg orally once daily	25 mg/m² orally twice daily

Permanently discontinue larotrectinib in patients who are unable to tolerate larotrectinib after three dose modifications

(continued)

Treatment Modification (*continued*)

Larotrectinib

Adverse Event	Treatment Modification
Any G3/4 adverse event	Withhold larotrectinib until adverse event resolves or improves to baseline or G1. If symptoms resolve within 4 weeks resume larotrectinib at one lower dosage
Any G3/4 adverse event lasting more than 4 weeks despite drug discontinuation	Discontinue larotrectinib
Co-administration of a strong CYP3A4 inhibitor cannot be avoided	Reduce the dose of larotrectinib by 50%. After the inhibitor has been discontinued for 3 to 5 elimination half-lives, resume the larotrectinib dose taken prior to initiating the CYP3A4 inhibitor
Co-administration of a strong CYP3A4 inducer cannot be avoided	Double the larotrectinib dose. After the inducer has been discontinued for 3 to 5 elimination half-lives, resume the larotrectinib dose taken prior to initiating the CYP3A4 inducer
Moderate (Child-Pugh B) or severe (Child-Pugh C) hepatic impairment	Start with 50% dose of larotrectinib

Efficacy

Overall Response Rate, According to Investigator and Central Assessment*

Response	Investigator Assessment (N = 55)	Central Assessment (N = 55)
	Percentage	
Overall response rate (95% CI)[†]	80 (67–90)	75 (61–85)
Best response		
Partial response	64[‡]	62
Complete response	16	13
Stable disease	9	13
Progressive disease	11	9
Could not be evaluated	0	4

Median time to response, median in months (range)	1.8 months (0.9 to 6.4)
Duration of response, median in months (range)	Not reached; median follow-up of 8.3 months (0.03+ to 24.9+)
Progression-free survival	Not reached; median follow-up duration of 9.9 months (range, 0.7 to 25.9+)
Percent with response at 1 year	71% ongoing
Percent progression-free at 1 year	55% progression-free

- As of the data-cutoff date, 86% (38/44) of patients with a response were continuing to receive treatment or had undergone surgery that was intended to be curative
- Two children with locally advanced infantile fibrosarcoma had sufficient tumor shrinkage during treatment to allow for limb-sparing surgery with curative intent. Pathologic assessment confirmed negative margins (R0 surgery). These two patients remained progression-free without larotrectinib after 4.8 months and 6.0 months of follow-up

*Percentages may not total 100 because of rounding
[†]The best overall response was derived from the responses as assessed at specified time points according to the Response Evaluation Criteria in Solid Tumors, version 1.1
[‡]Data include one patient who had a partial response that was pending confirmation at the time of the database lock. The response was subsequently confirmed, and the patient's treatment and response were ongoing at time of publication

Patient Population Studied

The trial enrolled patients with consecutively and prospectively identified cancers harboring TRK fusions, detected by molecular profiling as routinely performed at each site, into one of three protocols: (1) a phase 1 study involving adults; (2) a phase 1–2 study involving children; or (3) a phase 2 study involving adolescents and adults. The primary end point for the combined analysis was the overall response rate according to independent review. Secondary end points included duration of response, progression-free survival, and safety

Demographic and Clinical Characteristics of the 55 Patients

Characteristic	Value
Age	
Median (range)—years	45.0 (0.3–76.0)
Distribution—no. (%)	
<2 years	6 (11)
2–5 years	5 (9)
6–14 years	1 (2)
15–39 years	12 (22)
≥40 years	31 (56)
Sex—no. (%)	
Male	29 (53)
Female	26 (47)

(*continued*)

Toxicity

Adverse Events

Adverse Event*	Adverse Events, Regardless of Attribution					Treatment-Related Adverse Events		
	G1	**G2**	**G3**	**G4**	**Any Grade**	**G3**	**G4**	**Any Grade**
	Percentage of Patients with Event							
Increased ALT or AST level	31	4	7	0	42	5	0	38
Fatigue	20	15	2	0	36	0	0	16
Vomiting	24	9	0	0	33	0	0	11
Dizziness	25	4	2	0	31	2	0	25
Nausea	22	7	2	0	31	2	0	16
Anemia	9	9	11	0	29	2	0	9
Diarrhea	15	13	2	0	29	0	0	5
Constipation	24	4	0	0	27	0	0	16
Cough	22	4	0	0	25	0	0	2
Increased body weight	11	5	7	0	24	0	0	11
Dyspnea	9	9	0	0	18	0	0	2
Headache	13	4	0	0	16	0	0	2
Pyrexia	11	2	2	2	16	0	0	0
Arthralgia	15	0	0	0	15	0	0	2
Back pain	5	9	0	0	15	0	0	0
Decreased neutrophil count	0	7	7	0	15	2	0	9

*The adverse events listed are those that occurred in at least 15% of patients, regardless of attribution. The relatedness of the treatment to adverse events was determined by the investigators
ALT, alanine aminotransferase; AST, aspartate aminotransferase

Therapy Monitoring

1. Monthly CBC with differential and compete metabolic panel including LFTs every 2 weeks during the first month of treatment, then monthly thereafter, and as clinically indicated
2. Tumor assessments every 8 weeks for 1 year, then every 12 weeks thereafter until disease progression

Patient Population Studied
(*continued*)

ECOG performance status score—no. (%)*	
0	24 (44)
1	27 (49)
2	4 (7)
No. of previous systemic chemotherapies—no. (%)	
0 or 1	27 (49)
2	9 (16)
≥3	19 (35)
Tumor type—no. (%)	
Salivary-gland tumor	12 (22)
Other soft-tissue sarcoma†	11 (20)
Infantile fibrosarcoma	7 (13)
Thyroid tumor	5 (9)
Colon tumor	4 (7)
Lung tumor	4 (7)
Melanoma	4 (7)
GIST	3 (5)
Cholangiocarcinoma	2 (4)
Appendix tumor	1 (2)
Breast tumor	1 (2)
Pancreatic tumor	1 (2)
CNS metastases—no. (%)	
No	54 (98)
Yes	1 (2)
TRK gene—no. (%)	
NTRK1	25 (45)
NTRK2	1 (2)
NTRK3	29 (53)

CNS, central nervous system; GIST gastrointestinal stromal tumor; TRK, tropomyosin receptor kinase
*Eastern Cooperative Oncology Group (ECOG) performance status scores range from 0 to 5, with higher scores indicating greater disability
†Subtypes of other soft-tissue sarcomas included myopericytoma (in two patients), sarcoma that was not otherwise specified (in two), peripheral-nerve sheath tumor (in two), spindle-cell tumor (in three), infantile myofibromatosis (in one), and inflammatory myofibroblastic tumor of the kidney (in one)

METASTATIC NTRK GENE FUSION-POSITIVE TUMORS

TISSUE-AGNOSTIC REGIMEN: ENTRECTINIB

Doebele RC et al. Lancet Oncol 2020;21:271–282
Rozlytrek (entrectinib) prescribing information. South San Francisco, CA: Genentech USA, Inc.; 2019 August

Entrectinib (see dosage in table below); administer orally, once daily, with or without food, continually until disease progression

Entrectinib Dosage	
Adult Patients	**Recommended Dosage (Orally Once Daily)**
Irrespective of Body Surface Area (BSA)	600 mg
Pediatric Patients (Adolescents) ≥12 Years of Age	
BSA greater than 1.50 m^2	600 mg
BSA 1.11 to 1.50 m^2	500 mg
BSA 0.91 to 1.10 m^2	400 mg

Notes on entrectinib administration:
• Entrectinib is indicated for treatment of patients with metastatic solid tumors harboring neurotrophic receptor tyrosine kinase (NTRK) gene fusions in the absence of a known acquired resistance mutation. Appropriate patients should have no satisfactory alternative treatments, be unsuitable for surgical resection, and have progressed following prior treatment(s)
• Dosage form and strengths: capsules—100 mg and 200 mg
• Entrectinib is metabolized predominantly by CYP3A4. Refer to treatment modification section for initial dose adjustment recommendations for patients requiring concurrent treatment with moderate or strong CYP3A4 inhibitors. Avoid coadministration of entrectinib with moderate or strong CYP3A4 inducers

Advise patients to:
• Swallow entrectinib capsules whole. Do not open, crush, chew, or dissolve the contents of the capsules
• In case of vomiting immediately after taking a dose of entrectinib, repeat the dose of entrectinib
• If a dose of entrectinib is missed, take it as soon as you remember unless your next scheduled dose is due within 12 hours. Take the next dose at your regular time
• Avoid grapefruit and grapefruit juice while taking entrectinib
• Avoid driving or operating machinery if experiencing adverse neurologic effects

Supportive Care
Antiemetic prophylaxis
Emetogenic potential is **MINIMAL TO LOW**
See Chapter 42 for antiemetic recommendations

Hematopoietic growth factor (CSF) prophylaxis
Primary prophylaxis is **NOT** *indicated*
See Chapter 43 for more information

Antimicrobial prophylaxis
Risk of fever and neutropenia is **LOW**
Antimicrobial primary prophylaxis to be considered:
• Antibacterial—not indicated
• Antifungal—not indicated
• Antiviral— not indicated unless patient previously had an episode of HSV

Treatment Modification

Dosing in Pediatric Patients 12 Years and Older (Adolescents)

	Adults and Pediatric Patients 12 Years and Older with BSA >1.50 m² (Orally Once Daily)	Pediatric Patients 12 Years and Older with BSA of 1.11 to 1.50 m² (Orally Once Daily)	Pediatric Patients 12 Years and Older with BSA of 0.91 to 1.10 m² (Orally Once Daily)
Action			
First dose reduction	400 mg	400 mg	300 mg
Second dose reduction*	200 mg	200 mg	200 mg

*For a subsequent modification, permanently discontinue entrectinib in patients who are unable to tolerate entrectinib after two dose reductions

Recommended Dosage Modifications for Entrectinib for Adverse Reactions

Adverse Reaction*	Dosage Modification
Co-administration of moderate/strong CYP3A inhibitors cannot be avoided	• Adult and pediatric patients 12 years and older with BSA >1.50 m², reduce the dose of entrectinib • Pediatric patients 12 years and older with a BSA ≤1.50 m², avoid co-administration with entrectinib
Co-administration of moderate/strong CYP3A inducers cannot be avoided	• If co-administration cannot be avoided do not give entrectinib
G2/3 congestive heart failure	• Withhold entrectinib until recovered to ≤G1. For patients with myocarditis, with or without a decreased ejection fraction, MRI or cardiac biopsy may be required to make the diagnosis. For new-onset or worsening CHF, withhold entrectinib, reassess LVEF, and institute appropriate medical management • Resume at reduced dose or permanently discontinue entrectinib based on severity of CHF or worsening LVEF
G4 congestive heart failure	• Permanently discontinue entrectinib
Intolerable G2	• Withhold entrectinib until recovery to ≤G1 or to baseline • Resume at same dose or reduced dose, as clinically appropriate
G3 central nervous system effects	• Withhold entrectinib until recovery to ≤G1 or to baseline • Resume at reduced dose
G4 central nervous system effects	• Permanently discontinue entrectinib
G3 hepatotoxicity	• Withhold entrectinib until recovery to ≤G1 or to baseline • Resume at same dose if resolution occurs within 4 weeks • Permanently discontinue if adverse reaction does not resolve within 4 weeks • Resume at a reduced dose for recurrent G3 events that resolve within 4 weeks
G4 hepatotoxicity	• Withhold entrectinib until recovery to ≤G1 or to baseline • Resume at reduced dose if resolution occurs within 4 weeks • Permanently discontinue if adverse reaction does not resolve within 4 weeks • Permanently discontinue for recurrent Grade 4 events
ALT or AST >3× ULN with concurrent total bilirubin >1.5 × ULN (in the absence of cholestasis or hemolysis)	• Permanently discontinue entrectinib
Symptomatic or G4 hyperuricemia	• Initiate urate-lowering medication • Withhold entrectinib until improvement of signs or symptoms • Resume entrectinib at same or reduced dose
QTc greater than 500 ms	• Withhold entrectinib until QTc interval recovers to baseline • Resume at same dose if factors that cause QT prolongation are identified and corrected • Resume at reduced dose if other factors that cause QT prolongation are not identified

(continued)

Treatment Modification (continued)

Torsade de pointes; polymorphic ventricular tachycardia; signs/symptoms of serious arrhythmia	• Permanently discontinue entrectinib
G ≥2 vision disorders	• Dose or reduced dose, as clinically appropriate
G3/4 anemia or neutropenia	• Withhold entrectinib until recovery to G ≤2. Resume at the same dose or reduced dose, as clinically appropriate
G3/4 other clinically relevant adverse reactions	• Withhold entrectinib until adverse reaction resolves or improves to recovery or improvement to G1 or baseline. Resume at the same or reduced dose, if resolution occurs within 4 weeks. Permanently discontinue if adverse reaction does not resolve within 4 weeks. Permanently discontinue for recurrent G4 events

*Severity as defined by National Cancer Institute Common Terminology Criteria for Adverse Events (NCI CTCAE) version 4.0

Efficacy

Efficacy Outcomes

	Efficacy-Evaluable Population (N = 54)	Patients with Baseline CNS Disease (N = 12)*†	Patients with No Baseline CNS Disease (N =42)
Best overall response			
Proportion of patients achieving a response	31 (57%)	6 (50%)	25 (60%)
Complete response	4 (7%)	0	4 (10%)
Partial response	27 (50%)	6 (50%)	21 (50%)
Stable disease	9 (17%)	4 (33%)	5 (12%)
Progressive disease	4 (7%)	0	4 (10%)
Non-complete response or progressive disease	3 (6%)	0	3 (7%)
Missing or unevaluable‡	7 (13%)	2 (17%)	5 (12%)
Median duration of response	10.4 (7.1–NE)	NE	12.9 (7.1–NE)
Median progression-free survival, months	11.2 (8.0–14.9)	7.7 (4.7–NE)	12.0 (8.7–15.7)

Response According to NTRK Fusion

	NTRK1 Fusions	NTRK3 Fusions	NTRK3 Fusions
Proportion achieving a response	13/22 (59%; 95% CI 36.4–79.3)	0/1 (0%)	18/31 (58%; 95% CI 39.1–75.5)

Response According to Histology

Histology	Response Rate
Mammary analogue secretory carcinoma	6/7 (86%; 95% CI, 42–100)

(continued)

Patient Population Studied

An integrated database comprising three pivotal datasets collected from ongoing phase 1 or 2 clinical trials (ALKA-372-001, STARTRK-1, and STARTRK-2), which enrolled patients ≤18 years with metastatic or locally advanced NTRK fusion-positive solid tumors. All patients had received entrectinib orally at a dose of at least 600 mg once per day. All patients had an Eastern Cooperative Oncology Group performance status of 0–2 and could have received previous anti-cancer therapy (except previous TRK inhibitors). The primary end points were the proportion of patients with an objective response and median duration of response, evaluated by blinded independent central review in the efficacy-evaluable population (ie, patients with solid tumors harboring NTRK fusions who were TRK inhibitor–naive and had received at least one dose of entrectinib). Overall safety-evaluable population included patients from STARTRK-1, STARTRK-2, ALKA-372-001, and STARTRK-NG (NCT02650401; treating young adult and pediatric patients [aged ≤21 years]), who received at least one dose of entrectinib, regardless of tumor type or gene rearrangement

Most patients had a NTRK1 or NTRK3 fusion; the most frequently represented gene fusion was ETV6–NTRK3, which was identified in 25 patients (46%). Two other frequent gene fusions, TPM3–NTRK1 (in four patients [7%]) and TPR–NTRK1 (four [7%]), were reported. Ten tumor types were treated, with at least 19 distinct histologies represented; the predominant tumor types were sarcoma (in 13 patients [24%]), NSCLC (ten [19%]), and mammary analogue secretory carcinoma of the salivary gland (seven [13%])

(continued)

Patient Population Studied
(continued)

Baseline Characteristics

Age, years	58 (48–67)
Sex	
Female	32 (59%)
Male	22 (41%)
Race	
White	43 (80%)
Asian	7 (13%)
Other	4 (7%)
Eastern Cooperative Oncology Group performance status	
0	23 (43%)
1	25 (46%)
2	6 (11%)
Previous lines of systemic therapy	
0	20 (37%)
1	11 (20%)
2	14 (26%)
3	4 (7%)
≥4	5 (9%)
Previous treatment*	
Chemotherapy	46 (85%)
Targeted therapy	13 (24%)
Hormonal therapy	9 (17%)
Immunotherapy	7 (13%)
CNS metastases at baseline	
Yes	12 (22%)
No	42 (78%)
Previous radiotherapy to the brain	
Yes	7 (13%)
No	47 (87%)
Time from end of previous radiotherapy of the brain to first dose of entrectinib†	

(continued)

Efficacy *(continued)*

Breast cancer	5/6 (83%; 95% CI, 36–100)
NSCLC	7/10 (70%; 95% CI, 35–93)
Pancreatic cancer	2/3 (67%; 95% CI, 9–99)
Sarcoma	6/13 (46%; 95% CI, 19–75)
Colorectal cancer	1/4 (25%; 95% CI, 1–81)
Thyroid cancer	1/5 (20%; 95% CI, 1–72)

Data are n (%) or median (95% CI)
*CNS disease status determined by the investigator
†According to blinded independent central review assessment, 11 (20%) of 54 patients had brain metastases at baseline and, in this population, six patients (55%; 95% CI, 23.4–83.3) had an intracranial response according to blinded independent review. Seven (64%) of these 11 patients had previously received radiotherapy to the brain
‡Missing or unevaluable included patients with no post-baseline scans available, missing subsets of scans at all time points, or patients who discontinued before obtaining adequate scans to evaluate or confirm response
Median intracranial duration of response according to blinded independent central review was not estimable (95% CI 5.0 to not estimable). At data cutoff, five patients with intracranial disease at baseline had an intracranial progression-free survival event, and median intracranial progression-free survival according to blinded independent central review assessment was 14 months (95% CI 5.1 to not estimable)
NE, not estimable

Toxicity

Treatment-related Adverse Events

Adverse Event	NTRK Fusion-positive Safety-evaluable Population* (n = 68)			Overall Safety-evaluable Population† (n = 355)		
	G1/2	G3	G4	G1/2	G3	G4
Clinical events						
Dysgeusia	32 (47%)	0	0	146 (41%)	1 (<1%)	0
Constipation	19 (28%)	0	0	83 (23%)	1 (<1%)	0
Fatigue	19 (285)	5 (7%)	0	89 (25%)	10 (3%)	0
Diarrhea	18 (27%)	1 (2%)	0	76 (21%)	5 (1%)	0
Edema peripheral	16 (24%)	1 (2%)	0	49 (14%)	1 (<1%)	0
Dizziness	16 (24%)	1 (2%)	0	88 (25%)	2 (1%)	0
Paresthesia	11 (16%)	0	0	67 (19%)	0	0
Nausea	10 (15%)	0	0	74 (21%)	0	0
Vomiting	9 (13%)	0	0	48 (14%)	0	0
Arthralgia	8 (12%)	0	0	42 (12%)	2 (1%)	0
Myalgia	8 (12%)	0	0	52 (15%)	2 (1%)	0
Weight increased	8 (12%)	7 (10%)	0	51 (14%)	18 (5%)	0
Muscular weakness	6 (9%)	1 (2%)	0	22 (6%)	3 (1%)	0
Asthenia	5 (7%)	0	0	28 (8%)	2 (1%)	0

(continued)

Toxicity (continued)

Peripheral sensory neuropathy	4 (6%)	1 (2%)	0	20 (6%)	4 (1%)	0
Rash	4 (6%)	0	0	18 (5%)	2 (1%)	0
Disturbance in attention	3 (4%)	0	0	13 (4%)	1 (<1%)	0
Pain of skin	3 (4%)	0	0	9 (3%)	1 (<1%)	0
Localized edema	2 (3%)	1 (2%)	0	3 (1%)	1 (<1%)	0
Hyperesthesia	2 (3%)	0	0	22 (6%)	1 (<1%)	0
Ataxia	2 (3%)	0	0	9 (3%)	3 (1%)	0
Dehydration	2 (3%)	0	0	5 (1%)	2 (1%)	0
Diplopia	1 (2%)	1 (2%)	0	4 (1%)	1 (<1%)	0
Hypotension	1 (2%)	1 (2%)	0	14 (4%)	2 (1%)	0
Pyrexia	1 (2%)	0	0	7 (2%)	1 (<1%)	0
Pruritus	1 (2%)	0	0	15 (4%)	1 (<1%)	0
Hypoxia	1 (2%)	0	0	! (<1%)	1 (<1%)	0
Fall	1 (2%)	0	0	6 (2%)	1 (<1%)	0
Osteoarthritis	0	1 (2%)	0	2 (1%)	1 (<1%)	0
Laboratory abnormalities						
Blood creatinine increased	12 (18%)	1(2%)	0	52 (15%)	2 (1%)	0
AST increased	7 (10%)	0	1 (2%)	35 (10%)	3 (1%)	1 (<1%)
ALT increased	6 (9%)	0	1 (2%)	30 (9%)	3 (15)	1 (<1%)
Neutrophil count decreased	4 (6%)	0	0	13 (4%)	8 (2%)	0
Neutropenia	3 (4%)	2 (3%)	0	9 (3%)	9 (3%)	0
Anemia	5 (7%)	8 (12%)	0	27 (10%)	16 (5%)	0
Platelet count decreased	2 (3%)	0	0	4 (1%)	0	1 (<1%)
Hyperuricemia	2 (3%)	0	2 (3%)	14 (4%)	0	5 (1%)
Hypophosphatemia	2 (3%)	2 (3%)	0	6 (2%)	4 (1%)	0
Lymphocyte count decreased	1 (2%)	0	0	4 (1%)	1 (<1%)	0
Blood uric acid increased	0	0	1 (2%)	3 (<1%)	0	1 (<1%)
Dysarthria	0	0	0	5 (1%)	2 (1%)	0
Anorectal disorder	0	0	0	0	0	1 (<1%)
Generalized edema	0	0	0	5 (15)	2 (1%)	0

Patient Population Studied
(continued)

	<2 months	2 (29%)
	2 to <6 months	4 (57%)
	≥6 months	1 (14%)
Tumor type		
	Sarcoma‡	13 (24%)
	NSCLC	10 (19%)
	Mammary analogue secretory carcinoma (salivary)	7 (13%)
	Breast	6 (11%)
	Thyroid	5 (9%)
	Colorectal	4 (7%)
	Neuroendocrine	3 (6%)
	Pancreatic	3 (6%)
	Gynecologic	2 (4%)
	Ovarian	1 (2%)
	Endometrial	1 (2%)
	Cholangiocarcinoma	1 (2%)

Data are median (IQR) and n (%)
*Patient might have received multiple or combination therapies, resulting in the sum of previous treatments being >100%
†Patients with baseline CNS metastases
‡Subtypes of soft tissue sarcoma included cervical adenosarcoma (n = 1), dedifferentiated chondrosarcoma (n = 1), endometrial stromal sarcoma (n = 1), follicular dendritic cell sarcoma (n = 1), gastrointestinal stromal tumor (n = 1; wild-type gastrointestinal stromal tumor, succinate dehydrogenase complex subunit B immunohistochemistry—tumor cells retain normal expression), malignant peripheral nerve sheath tumor (n = 1), and sarcoma not otherwise specified (n = 7)
NSCLC, non-small cell lung cancer

(continued)

Therapy Monitoring

1. CBC with differential and platelet count at least monthly
2. Assess left ventricular ejection fraction prior to initiation of entrectinib in patients with symptoms or known risk factors for CHF. Monitor patients for clinical signs and symptoms of congestive heart failure (CHF). For patients with myocarditis, with or without a decreased ejection fraction, MRI or cardiac biopsy may be required to make the diagnosis
3. Monitor liver tests, including ALT and AST, every 2 weeks during the first month of treatment, then monthly thereafter, and as clinically indicated
4. Assess serum uric acid levels prior to initiation and periodically during treatment with entrectinib. Monitor patients for signs and symptoms of hyperuricemia. Initiate treatment with urate-lowering medications as clinically indicated and withhold entrectinib for signs and symptoms of hyperuricemia
5. Monitor patients who have or who are at risk for QTc interval prolongation. Assess QT interval and electrolytes at baseline and periodically during treatment
6. Conduct ophthalmological evaluations as appropriate
7. Entrectinib increases the risk of fractures. Promptly evaluate patients with signs or symptoms (eg, pain, changes in mobility, deformity) of fractures

Toxicity (continued)

Electrocardiogram QT prolonged	0	0	0	5 (1%)	1 (<1%)	0
Lipase increased	0	0	0	2 (1%	2 (1%)	
Amylase increased	0	0	0	1 (<1%)	3 (1%)	0
Increased blood creatine phosphokinase	0	0	0	2 (<1%)	1 (<1%)	1 (<1%)
Hyponatremia	0	0	0	3 (1%)	2 (1%)	0
Hypermagnesemia	0	1 (2%)	0	0	1 (<1%)	0
Hypoalbuminemia	0	0	0	0	1 (<1%)	0
Pulmonary edema	0	0	0	0	2 (1%)	0
Mental status changes	0	0	0	0	2 (1%)	0
Agitation	0	0	0	0	1 (<1%)	0
Mood altered	0	0	0	0	1 (<1%)	0
Orthostatic hypotension	0	0	0	2 (1%)	1 (<1%)	0
Hypertension	0	0	0	0	1 (<1%)	0
Cardiac failure	0	1 (2%)	0	0	2 (1%)	0
Cardiac failure congestive	0	1 (2%)	0	0	1 (<1%)	0
Myocarditis	0	0	0	0	0	1 (<1%)

Data are n (%). Adverse events were encoded using MedDRA (version 21.0)

*All patients with *NTRK* gene fusions who received ≥1 dose of entrectinib, regardless of dose or duration of follow-up

†All patients from STARTRK–1, STARTRK–2, ALKA–372–001, and STARTRK-NG (regardless of tumor type or gene rearrangement) who received ≥1 dose of entrectinib. No deaths due to adverse events were reported

ALT, alanine aminotransferase; AST=aspartate aminotransferase

MICROSATELLITE INSTABILITY-HIGH OR MISMATCH REPAIR DEFICIENT SOLID TUMORS

TISSUE AGNOSTIC REGIMEN: PEMBROLIZUMAB

KEYNOTE–016 [NCT01876511] Le DT et al. N Engl J Med 2015;372:2509–2520
KEYNOTE–164 [NCT02460198] Le DT et al. J Clin Oncol 2020;38:11–19
KEYNOTE–158 [NCT02628067] Marabelle A et al. J Clin Oncol 2020;38:1–10
KEYNOTE–012 [NCT01848834]
KEYNOTE–028 [NCT02054806]
Keytruda (pembrolizumab) prescribing information. Whitehouse Station, NJ: Merck & Co., Inc.; 2020 November

Pembrolizumab 200 mg for adults or 2 mg/kg (up to 200 mg) for pediatric patients; administer intravenously over 30 minutes in a volume of 0.9% sodium chloride injection (0.9% NS) or 5% dextrose injection (D5W) sufficient to produce a pembrolizumab concentration within the range 1–10 mg/mL every 3 weeks for up to 24 months (total dose/3-week cycle = 200 mg in adult patients or 2 mg/kg up to 200 mg in pediatric patients)

Alternative pembrolizumab dose and schedule for adult patients per the U.S. FDA regimens approved on April 28, 2020:

Pembrolizumab 400 mg; administer intravenously over 30 minutes in a volume of 0.9% NS or D5W sufficient to produce a pembrolizumab concentration within the range 1–10 mg/mL every 6 weeks for up to 24 months (total dose/6-week cycle = 400 mg)

Note:
- Administer pembrolizumab with an administration set that contains a sterile, non-pyrogenic, low-protein-binding in-line or add-on filter with pore size within the range of 0.2–5 μm
- Pembrolizumab can cause severe or life-threatening infusion-related reactions, including hypersensitivity and anaphylaxis

Supportive Care
Antiemetic prophylaxis
Emetogenic potential is **MINIMAL**
See Chapter 42 for antiemetic recommendations

Hematopoietic growth factor (CSF) prophylaxis
Primary prophylaxis is **NOT** indicated
See Chapter 43 for more information

Antimicrobial prophylaxis
Risk of fever and neutropenia is **LOW**
Antimicrobial primary prophylaxis to be considered:
- Antibacterial—not indicated
- Antifungal—not indicated
- Antiviral—not indicated unless patient previously had an episode of HSV

Treatment Modification

Recommended Dose Modifications for Pembrolizumab

Adverse Reaction	Grade/Severity	Dose Modification
Colitis	G1	Prednisolone 0.5–1 mg/kg (non-enteric coated) or consider oral budesonide 9 mg daily if no bloody diarrhea
	G2/3 diarrhea or colitis	Withhold pembrolizumab. Loperamide 4 mg as starting dose then 2 mg before each meal and after each loose stool until without diarrhea for 12 hours, with maximum of 16 mg loperamide per day. Administer oral prednisone/prednisolone at a dose of 0.5 to 2 mg/kg/day or its equivalent. When improves to G1 begin a slow corticosteroid taper over at least 4 weeks. Resume pembrolizumab upon symptom control, or when prednisone/prednisolone daily dose <10 mg
	G4 diarrhea or colitis	Permanently discontinue pembrolizumab. Loperamide 4 mg as starting dose then 2 mg before each meal and after each loose stool until without diarrhea for 12 hours, with maximum of 16 mg loperamide per day. Administer 1–2 mg/kg IV (methyl)prednisolone and convert to 0.5–2 mg/kg prednisone/prednisolone orally each day or its equivalent only after a response. Taper over at least 4 weeks when symptoms improve. If does not improve over 72 hours or worsens, perform flexible sigmoidoscopy/colonoscopy to document colitis then begin infliximab 5 mg/kg (if no perforation/sepsis/TB/hepatitis/NYHA III/IV CHF). If no response add MMF 500–1000 mg twice daily. If worse on MMF, consider addition of tacrolimus or ATG

(continued)

Treatment Modification (*continued*)

Pneumonitis	G2	Withhold pembrolizumab. Consider pneumocystis prophylaxis depending on the clinical context and coverage with empiric antibiotics. Administer oral prednisone/prednisolone at a dose of 1–2 mg/kg/day or its equivalent. When improves to G1 begin a slow corticosteroid taper over at least 4 weeks. If does not respond adequately after 48 hours then administer 2–4 mg/kg IV (methyl)prednisolone and convert to 0.5–2 mg/kg prednisone/prednisolone orally each day or its equivalent only after a response, followed by a taper over at least 6 weeks when symptoms improve to G1, titrating to symptoms. Resume pembrolizumab upon symptom control, or when prednisone/prednisolone daily dose <10 mg
	G3/4	Permanently discontinue pembrolizumab. Consider *Pneumocystis* prophylaxis depending on the clinical context; cover with empiric antibiotics. Administer 2–4 mg/kg IV (methyl)prednisolone and convert to 1–2 mg/kg prednisone/prednisolone orally each day or its equivalent only after a response, followed by a taper over at least 8 weeks when symptoms improve to G1, titrating to symptoms. If when initially treated improvement does not occur within 48–72 hours begin infliximab 5 mg/kg (if no perforation/sepsis/TB/hepatitis/NYHA III/IV CHF). If no response to infliximab add MMF 500–1000 mg twice daily. Consider MMF especially if has concurrent hepatic toxicity
Hepatitis	G2 (AST or ALT >3–5× ULN or total bilirubin >1.5–3× ULN)	Withhold pembrolizumab. Administer oral prednisone/prednisolone at a dose of 1 to 2 mg/kg/day or its equivalent. When improves to G1 begin a slow corticosteroid taper over at least 4 weeks. Resume pembrolizumab upon symptom control, or when prednisone/prednisolone daily dose <10 mg
	G3/4 (AST or ALT >5× ULN or total bilirubin >3× ULN)	Permanently discontinue pembrolizumab. Administer 1–2 mg/kg IV (methyl)prednisolone and convert to 0.5–2 mg/kg prednisone/prednisolone orally each day or its equivalent only after a response. Taper over at least 6 weeks when symptoms improve. If no response add MMF 500–1000 mg twice daily. If worse on MMF, consider adding tacrolimus or ATG
Hypophysitis	G2/3 (moderate symptoms, ie, headache but no visual disturbance or fatigue/mood alteration but hemodynamically stable, no electrolyte disturbance)	Administer analgesia as needed for headache. Withhold pembrolizumab. Administer oral prednisone/prednisolone at a dose of 0.5 to 2 mg/kg/day or its equivalent. When improves to G1 begin a slow corticosteroid taper over at least 4 weeks. If no improvement in 48 hours administer 1–2 mg/kg IV (methyl)prednisolone and convert to 0.5–2 mg/kg prednisone/prednisolone orally each day or its equivalent only after a response. Taper over at least 4 weeks when symptoms improve to 5 mg prednisone/prednisolone or equivalent; do not stop steroids. Resume pembrolizumab upon symptom control, or when prednisone/prednisolone daily dose <10 mg
	G4 (severe mass effect symptoms, ie, severe headache, any visual disturbance or severe hypoadrenalism, ie, hypotension, severe electrolyte disturbance)	Permanently discontinue pembrolizumab. Administer analgesia as needed for headache. Administer 1–2 mg/kg IV (methyl)prednisolone and convert to 0.5–2 mg/kg prednisone/prednisolone orally each day or its equivalent only after a response. Taper over at least 4 weeks when symptoms improve to 5 mg prednisone/prednisolone or equivalent; do not stop steroids
Adrenal insufficiency	G2	Withhold pembrolizumab. Administer oral prednisone/prednisolone at a dose of 0.5 to 2 mg/kg/day or its equivalent. When improves to G1 begin a slow corticosteroid taper over at least 4 weeks. Serially assess adrenal function and continue steroids at replacement doses (20–40 mg hydrocortisone daily ~2/3 dose in AM upon awakening and ~1/3 at 4 PM) until recovery of adrenal function is documented. Resume pembrolizumab upon symptom control, or when prednisone/prednisolone daily dose <10 mg
	G3/4	Permanently discontinue pembrolizumab. Administer oral prednisone/prednisolone at a dose of 0.5 to 2 mg/kg/day or its equivalent. When improves to G1 begin a slow corticosteroid taper over at least 4 weeks. Serially assess adrenal function and continue steroids at replacement doses (20–40 mg hydrocortisone daily ~2/3 dose in AM upon awakening and ~1/3 at 4 PM) until recovery of adrenal function is documented
Type 1 diabetes mellitus	G3 hyperglycemia	Withhold pembrolizumab. Admit to hospital to manage hyperglycemia. Role of corticosteroids in preventing complete loss of insulin producing cells is unknown and not recommended. Resume pembrolizumab upon symptom control, or when prednisone/prednisolone daily dose <10 mg
	G4 hyperglycemia	Permanently discontinue pembrolizumab. Admit to hospital to manage hyperglycemia. Role of corticosteroids in preventing complete loss of insulin producing cells is unknown and not recommended

(*continued*)

Treatment Modification (*continued*)

Nephritis and renal dysfunction	G2/3 (serum creatinine 1.5–6× ULN)	Withhold pembrolizumab. Administer oral prednisone/prednisolone at a dose of 0.5 to 2 mg/kg/day or its equivalent. When improves to G1 begin a slow corticosteroid taper over at least 4 weeks. If does not respond adequately then administer 0.5–1 mg/kg IV (methyl) prednisolone and convert to 0.5–2 mg/kg prednisone/prednisolone orally each day or its equivalent only after a response, followed by a taper over at least 4 weeks when improves to G1. Resume pembrolizumab upon symptom control, or when prednisone/prednisolone daily dose <10 mg
	G4 (serum creatinine >6× ULN)	Permanently discontinue pembrolizumab. Administer 0.5–1 mg/kg IV (methyl)prednisolone and convert to 0.5–2 mg/kg prednisone/prednisolone orally each day or its equivalent only after a response, followed by a taper over at least 4 weeks when improves to G1
Skin	G1/2	Continue pembrolizumab. Avoid skin irritants, avoid sun exposure, topical emollients recommended. Topical steroid (mild strength for G1, moderate/potent strength for G2) cream once or twice daily ± oral or topical antihistamines for itching
	G3 rash or suspected SJS or TEN	Withhold pembrolizumab. Avoid skin irritants, avoid sun exposure, topical emollients recommended. Administer oral or topical antihistamines for itching. Administer oral prednisone/prednisolone at a dose of 0.5–2 mg/kg or its equivalent daily for 3 days followed by a slow corticosteroid taper over at least 4 weeks when the rash improves to G1. If does not respond adequately then administer 0.5–1 mg/kg IV (methyl)prednisolone and convert to 0.5–2 mg/kg prednisone/prednisolone orally each day or its equivalent only after a response, followed by a taper over at least 4 weeks when the rash improves to G1. Resume pembrolizumab upon symptom control, or when prednisone/prednisolone daily dose <10 mg
	G4 rash or confirmed SJS or TEN	Avoid skin irritants, avoid sun exposure, topical emollients recommended. Administer oral or topical antihistamines for itching. Administer 1–2 mg/kg IV (methyl)prednisolone and convert to oral steroids 0.5–2 mg/kg prednisone/prednisolone each day or its equivalent only after a response. Taper over at least 4 weeks when the rash improves to G1. Permanently discontinue pembrolizumab
Encephalitis	Confusion or altered behavior, headaches, alteration in Glasgow Coma Scale, motor or sensory deficits, speech abnormality, may or may not be febrile	Initially withhold pembrolizumab, but permanently discontinue pembrolizumab if there is no doubt as to diagnosis. Exclude bacterial and ideally viral infections prior to high-dose steroids. Administer oral prednisone/prednisolone at a dose of 0.5–2 mg/kg/day or its equivalent. When symptoms improve begin a slow corticosteroid taper over at least 4–8 weeks. If symptoms are severe administer 1–2 mg/kg IV (methyl)prednisolone and convert to 0.5–2 mg/kg prednisone/prednisolone orally each day or its equivalent only after a response. Consider concurrent empiric antiviral (IV acyclovir) and antibacterial therapy
Aseptic meningitis	Headache, photophobia, neck stiffness with fever or may be afebrile, vomiting; normal cognition/cerebral function (distinguishes from encephalitis)	
Other syndromes include neurosarcoidosis, posterior reversible leukoencephalopathy syndrome (PRES), Vogt-Koyanagi-Harada syndrome, demyelination, vasculitic encephalopathy, and generalized seizures		
Transverse myelitis	Acute or subacute neurologic signs/symptoms of motor/sensory/autonomic origin; most have sensory level; often bilateral symptoms	Initially withhold pembrolizumab, but permanently discontinue pembrolizumab if there is no doubt as to diagnosis. Administer 2 mg/kg IV (methyl)prednisolone or consider 1 g/day and convert to 0.5–2 mg/kg prednisone/prednisolone orally each day or its equivalent only after a response. When symptoms improve begin a slow corticosteroid taper over at least 4–8 weeks. Plasmapheresis may be required if steroids do not bring about improvement
Myocarditis	G3	Permanently discontinue pembrolizumab. Administer 2 mg/kg IV (methyl)prednisolone or consider 1 g/day and convert to 0.5–2 mg/kg prednisone/prednisolone orally each day or its equivalent only after a response. When symptoms improve begin a slow corticosteroid taper over at least 4–8 weeks. If no response add MMF 500–1000 mg twice daily. If worse on MMF, consider adding tacrolimus

(*continued*)

Treatment Modification (continued)

Peripheral neurologic toxicity	Moderate: some interference with ADL, symptoms concerning to patient	Withhold pembrolizumab. Initial observation reasonable or initiate prednisone/prednisolone 0.5–1 mg/kg (if progressing, eg, from mild) and/or pregabalin or duloxetine for pain. When symptoms improve begin a slow corticosteroid taper over at least 4 weeks. Resume pembrolizumab upon symptom control, or when prednisone/prednisolone daily dose <10 mg
	Severe: limits self-care and aids warranted, life threatening, eg, respiratory problems	Permanently discontinue pembrolizumab. Administer 1–2 mg/kg IV (methyl)prednisolone and convert to 0.5–2 mg/kg prednisone/prednisolone orally each day or its equivalent only after a response. Taper over at least 4–8 weeks when symptoms improve to G1
Guillain-Barré syndrome	Progressive symmetrical muscle weakness with absent or reduced tendon reflexes—involves extremities, facial, respiratory and bulbar and oculomotor muscles; dysregulation of autonomic nerves	Permanently discontinue pembrolizumab. Use of steroids not recommended in idiopathic Guillain-Barré syndrome; however, a trial of (methyl)prednisolone 1–2 mg/kg is reasonable, converting to 0.5–2 mg/kg prednisone/prednisolone orally each day or its equivalent only after a response. If no improvement or worsening, plasmapheresis or IVIG indicated
Myasthenia gravis	Fluctuating muscle weakness (proximal limb, trunk, ocular, eg, ptosis/diplopia or bulbar) with fatigability, respiratory muscles also may be involved	Permanently discontinue pembrolizumab. Administer pyridostigmine at an initial dose of 30 mg three times daily. Administer oral prednisone/prednisolone at a dose of 0.5–2 mg/kg/day or its equivalent or 1–2 mg/kg IV (methyl)prednisolone depending on the severity of symptoms. If begin with IV convert to 0.5–2 mg/kg prednisone/prednisolone orally each day or its equivalent only after a response. If no improvement or worsening, plasmapheresis or IVIG may be considered. Additional immunosuppressants used in myasthenia gravis include azathioprine, cyclosporine, and mycophenolate. Avoid certain medications, eg, ciprofloxacin, beta-blockers, that may precipitate cholinergic crisis
Other syndromes including motor and sensory peripheral neuropathy, multifocal radicular neuropathy/plexopathy, autonomic neuropathy, phrenic nerve palsy, cranial nerve palsies (eg, facial nerve, optic nerve, hypoglossal nerve)		Permanently discontinue pembrolizumab. Administer oral prednisone/prednisolone at a dose of 0.5 to 2 mg/kg/day or its equivalent or 1–2 mg/kg IV (methyl)prednisolone depending on the severity of symptoms. If begin with IV convert to 0.5–2 mg/kg prednisone/prednisolone orally each day or its equivalent only after a response
Arthralgia	G1 (mild pain with inflammation, erythema, or joint swelling)	Continue pembrolizumab. Administer acetaminophen (paracetamol) and ibuprofen
	G2 (moderate pain with inflammation, erythema or joint swelling that limits ADLs)	Withhold pembrolizumab. Administer higher doses of acetaminophen (paracetamol) and ibuprofen and use diclofenac or naproxen or etoricoxib. If inadequately controlled, consider intra-articular steroid injections for large joints or administer oral prednisone/prednisolone at a dose of 0.5–2 mg/kg/day or its equivalent. When improves to G1 begin a slow corticosteroid taper over at least 4 weeks. If does not respond adequately then administer 0.5–1 mg/kg IV (methyl)prednisolone and convert to 0.5–2 mg/kg prednisone/prednisolone orally each day or its equivalent only after a response, followed by a taper over at least 4 weeks when improves to G1. Resume pembrolizumab upon symptom control, or when prednisone/prednisolone daily dose <10 mg
	G3 (severe pain; irreversible joint damage; disabling; limits self-care ADL)	Withhold pembrolizumab. Administer 0.5–1 mg/kg IV (methyl)prednisolone and convert to 0.5–2 mg/kg prednisone/prednisolone orally each day or its equivalent only after a response, followed by a taper over at least 4 weeks when improves to G1. In severe cases, infliximab or another anti-TNF alpha drug may be required for improvement of arthritis. Resume pembrolizumab upon symptom control, or when prednisone/prednisolone daily dose <10 mg
Other	First occurrence of other G3	Withhold pembrolizumab. Administer oral prednisone/prednisolone at a dose of 0.5 to 2 mg/kg/day or its equivalent. When improves to G1 begin a slow corticosteroid taper over at least 4 weeks. Resume pembrolizumab upon symptom control, or when prednisone/prednisolone daily dose <10 mg
	Recurrence of same G3	Permanently discontinue pembrolizumab. Administer 1–2 mg/kg IV (methyl)prednisolone and convert to 0.5–2 mg/kg prednisone/prednisolone orally each day or its equivalent only after a response. Taper over at least 4–8 weeks when symptoms improve to G1
	Life-threatening or G4	
	Requirement for ≥10 mg/day prednisone or equivalent for >12 weeks	Permanently discontinue pembrolizumab
	Persistent G2/3 adverse reactions lasting ≥12 weeks	

ADL, activities of daily living; ALT, alanine aminotransferase; AST, aspartate aminotransferase; ATG, anti-thymocyte globulin; SJS, Stevens-Johnson Syndrome; TEN, toxic epidermal necrolysis; ULN, upper limit of normal

(continued)

Treatment Modification (continued)

<u>Notes on general supportive care</u>:
• Steroid taper in most cases will proceed over a minimum of 1 month but if symptoms improve rapidly a 2-week taper can be considered. If steroids are administered for more than 4 weeks, consider PCP prophylaxis (cotrimoxazole 480 mg twice daily M/W/F or inhaled pentamidine if patient has cotrimoxazole allergy), regular random blood glucose, VitD level, and starting calcium/VitD supplementation as per guidelines

<u>Notes on pregnancy and breast feeding</u>:
• Pembrolizumab can cause fetal harm. If used during pregnancy, or if the patient becomes pregnant during treatment, apprise the patient of the potential hazard to a fetus. Females of reproductive potential should use highly effective contraception during treatment and for 4 months after the last dose of pembrolizumab
• It is not known whether pembrolizumab is excreted in human milk. Therefore, it is recommended that women discontinue nursing during treatment with and for 4 months after the final dose of pembrolizumab

Efficacy

Efficacy Results for Patients with MSI-H/dMMR Cancer

Endpoint	Pembrolizumab (n = 149)
Objective response rate	
ORR (95% CI)	39.6% (31.7, 47.9)
Complete response rate	7.4%
Partial response rate	32.2%
Response duration	
Median in months (range)	NR (1.6+, 22.7+)
% with duration ≥6 months	78%

NR, not reached

Response by Tumor Type

	N	Objective Response Rate n (%) 95% CI	DOR range (Months)
CRC	90	32 (36%) (26%, 46%)	(1.6+, 22.7+)
Non-CRC	59	27 (46%) (33%, 59%)	(1.9+, 22.1+)
Endometrial cancer	14	5 (36%) (13%, 65%)	(4.2+, 17.3+)
Biliary cancer	11	3 (27%) (6%, 61%)	(11.6+, 19.6+)
Gastric or GE junction cancer	9	5 (56%) (21%, 86%)	(5.8+, 22.1+)
Pancreatic cancer	6	5 (83%) (36%, 100%)	(2.6+, 9.2+)
Small intestinal cancer	8	3 (38%) (9%, 76%)	(1.9+, 9.1+)
Breast cancer	2	PR, PR	(7.6, 15.9)
Prostate cancer	2	PR, SD	9.8+
Bladder cancer	1	NE	
Esophageal cancer	1	PR	18.2+
Sarcoma	1	PD	
Thyroid cancer	1	NE	
Retroperitoneal adenocarcinoma	1	PR	7.5+
Small cell lung cancer	1	CR	8.9+
Renal cell cancer	1	PD	

CR, complete response; NE, not evaluable; PD, progressive disease; PR, partial response; SD, stable disease

PATIENT POPULATION STUDIED

KEYNOTE–016 [NCT01876511] Le et al. N Engl J Med 2015;372:2509–2520
KEYNOTE–164 [NCT02460198] Le et al. J Clin Oncol 2020;38:11–19
KEYNOTE–158 [NCT02628067] Marabelle et al. J Clin Oncol 2020;38:1–10
KEYNOTE–012 [NCT01848834]
KEYNOTE–028 NCT02054806]

The efficacy of pembrolizumab was investigated in patients with MSI-H or mismatch repair–deficient (dMMR), solid tumors enrolled in one of five uncontrolled, open-label, multi-cohort, multi-center, single-arm trials. Patients received either pembrolizumab 200 mg every 3 weeks or pembrolizumab 10 mg/kg every 2 weeks. The major efficacy outcome measures were ORR as assessed by blinded independent central radiologist (BICR) review according to RECIST v1.1 and duration of response

N = 149 with MSI-H or dMMR Cancers Across 5 Trials

Median age	55 years (36% age 65 or older);
Gender M/F	56%/44%
Race	77% White, 19% Asian, 2% Black
ECOG PS 0/1	36%/64%
Stage of disease	98% metastatic/2% locally advanced
Median number of prior therapies for metastatic or unresectable disease	2 (84% with metastatic CRC and 53% with other solid tumors ≥2 prior lines of therapy

CRC, colorectal cancer

Therapy Monitoring

1. Before therapy: History and physical exam, CBC with differential, renal and liver function tests, serum electrolytes

2. Prior to each cycle: CBC with differential, serum electrolytes, BUN, serum creatinine, serum bilirubin, AST and ALT. For ≥2 LFT elevations work up for other causes of elevated LFTs including viral hepatitis

3. CBC with differential initially also at day 10–14

4. Observe closely for hypersensitivity reactions, especially during the first and second infusions

5. Initially at the time of each dose, and eventually every 6–12 weeks, perform a total-body skin examination with attention to *all* mucous membranes as well as a complete review of systems

6. Monitor patients for signs and symptoms of pneumonitis. Evaluate patients with suspected pneumonitis with chest x-ray, CT, and pulse oximetry. For ≥2 toxicity may include nasal swab, sputum culture and sensitivity, blood culture and sensitivity, and urine culture and sensitivity

7. Monitor patients for signs and symptoms of colitis. Encourage patients to report diarrhea immediately to any member of the health care team

8. Use basic metabolic panel (Na, K, CO_2, glucose) and patient history as screening tools for hypophysitis including hypopituitarism and adrenal insufficiency. If in doubt evaluate am adrenocorticotropic hormone (ACTH) and cortisol levels. Consider ACTH stimulation test for indeterminate results

9. Thyroid function at the start of treatment, periodically during treatment, and as indicated based on clinical evaluation) and for clinical signs and symptoms of thyroid disorders. Test for TSH and free thyroxine (FT4) every 4–6 weeks as part of routine clinical monitoring on therapy or for case detection in symptomatic patients

10. Measure glucose at baseline and with each treatment during the first 12 weeks and every 6 weeks thereafter

11. Obtain a complete rheumatologic history and perform an examination of all peripheral joints for tenderness, swelling, and range of motion. Examine the spine. Consider plain x-ray/imaging to exclude metastases and evaluate joint damage (erosions), if appropriate

12. Every 2–3 months: CT scans to assess response

Toxicity

KEYNOTE–016 [NCT01876511] Le et al. N Engl J Med 2015;372:2509–2520

Adverse Events Occurring in >5% of Patients (N = 41)

Adverse Event (%)	All Grades	Grade 3 or 4
Any	98	41
Anemia	20	17
Lymphopenia	20	20
Sinus tachycardia	10	0
Dry skin	12	0
Rash or pruritus	24	0
Thyroiditis, hypothyroidism, or hypophysitis	10	0
Abdominal pain	24	0
Anorexia	10	0
Constipation	20	0
Diarrhea	24	5
Dry mouth	12	0
Nausea	12	0
Bowel obstruction	7	7
Elevated alanine aminotransferase	7	5
Pancreatitis*	15	0
Hypoalbuminemia	10	10
Hyponatremia	7	7
Arthralgia	17	0
Myalgia	15	0
Dizziness	10	0
Headache	17	0
Insomnia	7	0
Allergic rhinitis	29	0
Cough	10	0
Dyspnea	15	0
Upper respiratory infection	7	0
Cold intolerance	15	0
Edema	10	0
Fatigue	32	0
Fever	12	0
Pain	34	0

*All pancreatitis cases were asymptomatic
Of note, there was 1 case of pneumonitis reported (2% incidence)

TUMOR MUTATIONAL BURDEN-HIGH SOLID TUMORS
TISSUE AGNOSTIC REGIMEN: PEMBROLIZUMAB

Marabelle A et al. Lancet Oncol 2020;21:1353–1365
Keytruda (pembrolizumab) prescribing information. Whitehouse Station, NJ: Merck & Co., Inc.; 2020 November

Pembrolizumab 200 mg for adults or 2 mg/kg (up to 200 mg) for pediatric patients; administer intravenously over 30 minutes in a volume of 0.9% sodium chloride injection (0.9% NS) or 5% dextrose injection (D5W) sufficient to produce a pembrolizumab concentration within the range 1–10 mg/mL every 3 weeks for up to 24 months (total dose/3-week cycle = 200 mg in adult patients or 2 mg/kg up to 200 mg in pediatric patients)

Alternative pembrolizumab dose and schedule for adult patients per the U.S. FDA regimens approved on April 28, 2020:

Pembrolizumab 400 mg; administer intravenously over 30 minutes in a volume of 0.9% NS or D5W sufficient to produce a pembrolizumab concentration within the range 1–10 mg/mL every 6 weeks for up to 24 months (total dose/6-week cycle = 400 mg)

Note:
- Administer pembrolizumab with an administration set that contains a sterile, non-pyrogenic, low-protein-binding in-line or add-on filter with pore size within the range of 0.2–5 μm
- Pembrolizumab can cause severe or life-threatening infusion-related reactions, including hypersensitivity and anaphylaxis

Supportive Care
Antiemetic prophylaxis
Emetogenic potential is **MINIMAL**
See Chapter 42 for antiemetic recommendations

Hematopoietic growth factor (CSF) prophylaxis
Primary prophylaxis is **NOT** indicated
See Chapter 43 for more information

Antimicrobial prophylaxis
Risk of fever and neutropenia is **LOW**
Antimicrobial primary prophylaxis to be considered:
- Antibacterial—not indicated
- Antifungal—not indicated
- Antiviral—not indicated unless patient previously had an episode of HSV

Treatment Modification

Recommended Dose Modifications for Pembrolizumab

Adverse Reaction	Grade/Severity	Dose Modification
Colitis	G1	Prednisolone 0.5–1 mg/kg (non-enteric-coated) or consider oral budesonide 9 mg daily if no bloody diarrhea
	G2/3 diarrhea or colitis	Withhold pembrolizumab. Loperamide 4 mg as starting dose then 2 mg before each meal and after each loose stool until without diarrhea for 12 hours, with maximum of 16 mg loperamide per day. Administer oral prednisone/prednisolone at a dose of 0.5 to 2 mg/kg/day or its equivalent. When improves to G1 begin a slow corticosteroid taper over at least 4 weeks. Resume pembrolizumab upon symptom control, or when prednisone/prednisolone daily dose <10 mg
	G4 diarrhea or colitis	Permanently discontinue pembrolizumab. Loperamide 4 mg as starting dose then 2 mg before each meal and after each loose stool until without diarrhea for 12 hours, with maximum of 16 mg loperamide per day. Administer 1–2 mg/kg IV (methyl)prednisolone and convert to 0.5–2 mg/kg prednisone/prednisolone orally each day or its equivalent only after a response. Taper over at least 4 weeks when symptoms improve. If does not improve over 72 hours or worsens, perform flexible sigmoidoscopy/colonoscopy to document colitis then begin infliximab 5 mg/kg (if no perforation/sepsis/TB/hepatitis/NYHA III/IV CHF). If no response add MMF 500–1000 mg twice daily. If worse on MMF, consider addition of tacrolimus or ATG

(continued)

Treatment Modification (*continued*)

Pneumonitis	G2	Withhold pembrolizumab. Consider *Pneumocystis* prophylaxis depending on the clinical context and coverage with empiric antibiotics. Administer oral prednisone/prednisolone at a dose of 1–2 mg/kg/day or its equivalent. When improves to G1 begin a slow corticosteroid taper over at least 4 weeks. If does not respond adequately after 48 hours then administer 2–4 mg/kg IV (methyl)prednisolone and convert to 0.5–2 mg/kg prednisone/prednisolone orally each day or its equivalent only after a response, followed by a taper over at least 6 weeks when symptoms improve to G1, titrating to symptoms. Resume pembrolizumab upon symptom control, or when prednisone/prednisolone daily dose <10 mg
	G3/4	Permanently discontinue pembrolizumab. Consider *Pneumocystis* prophylaxis depending on the clinical context; cover with empiric antibiotics. Administer 2–4 mg/kg IV (methyl)prednisolone and convert to 1–2 mg/kg prednisone/prednisolone orally each day or its equivalent only after a response, followed by a taper over at least 8 weeks when symptoms improve to G1, titrating to symptoms. If when initially treated improvement does not occur within 48–72 hours begin infliximab 5 mg/kg (if no perforation/sepsis/TB/hepatitis/NYHA III/IV CHF). If no response to infliximab add MMF 500–1000 mg twice daily. Consider MMF especially if has concurrent hepatic toxicity
Hepatitis	G2 (AST or ALT >3–5× ULN or total bilirubin >1.5–3× ULN)	Withhold pembrolizumab. Administer oral prednisone/prednisolone at a dose of 1 to 2 mg/kg/day or its equivalent. When improves to G1 begin a slow corticosteroid taper over at least 4 weeks. Resume pembrolizumab upon symptom control, or when prednisone/prednisolone daily dose <10 mg
	G3/4 (AST or ALT >5× ULN or total bilirubin >3× ULN)	Permanently discontinue pembrolizumab. Administer 1–2 mg/kg IV (methyl)prednisolone and convert to 0.5–2 mg/kg prednisone/prednisolone orally each day or its equivalent only after a response. Taper over at least 6 weeks when symptoms improve. If no response add MMF 500–1000 mg twice daily. If worse on MMF, consider adding tacrolimus or ATG
Hypophysitis	G2/3 (moderate symptoms, ie, headache but no visual disturbance or fatigue/mood alteration but hemodynamically stable, no electrolyte disturbance)	Administer analgesia as needed for headache. Withhold pembrolizumab. Administer oral prednisone/prednisolone at a dose of 0.5 to 2 mg/kg/day or its equivalent. When improves to G1 begin a slow corticosteroid taper over at least 4 weeks. If no improvement in 48 hours administer 1–2 mg/kg IV (methyl)prednisolone and convert to 0.5–2 mg/kg prednisone/prednisolone orally each day or its equivalent only after a response. Taper over at least 4 weeks when symptoms improve to 5 mg prednisone/prednisolone or equivalent; do not stop steroids. Resume pembrolizumab upon symptom control, or when prednisone/prednisolone daily dose <10 mg
	G4 (severe mass effect symptoms, ie, severe headache, any visual disturbance or severe hypoadrenalism, ie, hypotension, severe electrolyte disturbance)	Permanently discontinue pembrolizumab. Administer analgesia as needed for headache. Administer 1–2 mg/kg IV (methyl)prednisolone and convert to 0.5–2 mg/kg prednisone/prednisolone orally each day or its equivalent only after a response. Taper over at least 4 weeks when symptoms improve to 5 mg prednisone/prednisolone or equivalent; do not stop steroids
Adrenal insufficiency	G2	Withhold pembrolizumab. Administer oral prednisone/prednisolone at a dose of 0.5 to 2 mg/kg/day or its equivalent. When improves to G1 begin a slow corticosteroid taper over at least 4 weeks. Serially assess adrenal function and continue steroids at replacement doses (20–40 mg hydrocortisone daily ~2/3 dose in AM upon awakening and ~1/3 at 4 PM) until recovery of adrenal function is documented. Resume pembrolizumab upon symptom control, or when prednisone/prednisolone daily dose <10 mg
	G3/4	Permanently discontinue pembrolizumab. Administer oral prednisone/prednisolone at a dose of 0.5 to 2 mg/kg/day or its equivalent. When improves to G1 begin a slow corticosteroid taper over at least 4 weeks. Serially assess adrenal function and continue steroids at replacement doses (20–40 mg hydrocortisone daily ~2/3 dose in AM upon awakening and ~1/3 at 4 PM) until recovery of adrenal function is documented

(continued)

Treatment Modification (*continued*)

Type 1 diabetes mellitus	G3 hyperglycemia	Withhold pembrolizumab. Admit to hospital to manage hyperglycemia. Role of corticosteroids in preventing complete loss of insulin producing cells is unknown and not recommended. Resume pembrolizumab upon symptom control, or when prednisone/prednisolone daily dose <10 mg
	G4 hyperglycemia	Permanently discontinue pembrolizumab. Admit to hospital to manage hyperglycemia. Role of corticosteroids in preventing complete loss of insulin producing cells is unknown and not recommended
Nephritis and renal dysfunction	G2/3 (serum creatinine 1.5–6× ULN)	Withhold pembrolizumab. Administer oral prednisone/prednisolone at a dose of 0.5 to 2 mg/kg/day or its equivalent. When improves to G1 begin a slow corticosteroid taper over at least 4 weeks. If does not respond adequately then administer 0.5–1 mg/kg IV (methyl)prednisolone and convert to 0.5–2 mg/kg prednisone/prednisolone orally each day or its equivalent only after a response, followed by a taper over at least 4 weeks when improves to G1. Resume pembrolizumab upon symptom control, or when prednisone/prednisolone daily dose <10 mg
	G4 (serum creatinine >6× ULN)	Permanently discontinue pembrolizumab. Administer 0.5–1 mg/kg IV (methyl)prednisolone and convert to 0.5–2 mg/kg prednisone/prednisolone orally each day or its equivalent only after a response, followed by a taper over at least 4 weeks when improves to G1
Skin	G1/2	Continue pembrolizumab. Avoid skin irritants, avoid sun exposure, topical emollients recommended. Topical steroid (mild strength for G1, moderate/potent strength for G2) cream once or twice daily ± oral or topical antihistamines for itching
	G3 rash or suspected SJS or TEN	Withhold pembrolizumab. Avoid skin irritants, avoid sun exposure, topical emollients recommended. Administer oral or topical antihistamines for itching. Administer oral prednisone/prednisolone at a dose of 0.5–2 mg/kg or its equivalent daily for 3 days followed by a slow corticosteroid taper over at least 4 weeks when the rash improves to G1. If does not respond adequately then administer 0.5–1 mg/kg IV (methyl)prednisolone and convert to 0.5–2 mg/kg prednisone/prednisolone orally each day or its equivalent only after a response, followed by a taper over at least 4 weeks when the rash improves to G1. Resume pembrolizumab upon symptom control, or when prednisone/prednisolone daily dose <10 mg
	G4 rash or confirmed SJS or TEN	Avoid skin irritants, avoid sun exposure, topical emollients recommended. Administer oral or topical antihistamines for itching. Administer 1–2 mg/kg IV (methyl)prednisolone and convert to oral steroids 0.5–2 mg/kg prednisone/prednisolone each day or its equivalent only after a response. Taper over at least 4 weeks when the rash improves to G1. Permanently discontinue pembrolizumab
Encephalitis	Confusion or altered behavior, headaches, alteration in Glasgow Coma Scale, motor or sensory deficits, speech abnormality, may or may not be febrile	Initially withhold pembrolizumab, but permanently discontinue pembrolizumab if there is no doubt as to diagnosis. Exclude bacterial and ideally viral infections prior to high-dose steroids. Administer oral prednisone/prednisolone at a dose of 0.5–2 mg/kg/day or its equivalent. When symptoms improve begin a slow corticosteroid taper over at least 4–8 weeks. If symptoms are severe administer 1–2 mg/kg IV (methyl)prednisolone and convert to 0.5–2 mg/kg prednisone/prednisolone orally each day or its equivalent only after a response. Consider concurrent empiric antiviral (IV acyclovir) and antibacterial therapy
Aseptic meningitis	Headache, photophobia, neck stiffness with fever or may be afebrile, vomiting; normal cognition/cerebral function (distinguishes from encephalitis)	
Other syndromes include neurosarcoidosis, posterior reversible leukoencephalopathy syndrome (PRES), Vogt-Koyanagi-Harada syndrome, demyelination, vasculitic encephalopathy, and generalized seizures		
Transverse myelitis	Acute or subacute neurologic signs/symptoms of motor/sensory/autonomic origin; most have sensory level; often bilateral symptoms	Initially withhold pembrolizumab, but permanently discontinue pembrolizumab if there is no doubt as to diagnosis. Administer 2 mg/kg IV (methyl)prednisolone or consider 1 g/day and convert to 0.5–2 mg/kg prednisone/prednisolone orally each day or its equivalent only after a response. When symptoms improve begin a slow corticosteroid taper over at least 4–8 weeks. Plasmapheresis may be required if steroids do not bring about improvement

(continued)

Treatment Modification (continued)

Myocarditis	G3	Permanently discontinue pembrolizumab. Administer 2 mg/kg IV (methyl)prednisolone or consider 1 g/day and convert to 0.5–2 mg/kg prednisone/prednisolone orally each day or its equivalent only after a response. When symptoms improve begin a slow corticosteroid taper over at least 4–8 weeks. If no response add MMF 500–1000 mg twice daily. If worse on MMF, consider adding tacrolimus
Peripheral neurologic toxicity	Moderate: some interference with ADL, symptoms concerning to patient	Withhold pembrolizumab. Initial observation reasonable or initiate prednisone/prednisolone 0.5–1 mg/kg (if progressing, eg, from mild) and/or pregabalin or duloxetine for pain. When symptoms improve begin a slow corticosteroid taper over at least 4 weeks. Resume pembrolizumab upon symptom control, or when prednisone/prednisolone daily dose <10 mg
	Severe: limits self-care and aids warranted, life threatening, eg, respiratory problems	Permanently discontinue pembrolizumab. Administer 1–2 mg/kg IV (methyl)prednisolone and convert to 0.5–2 mg/kg prednisone/prednisolone orally each day or its equivalent only after a response. Taper over at least 4–8 weeks when symptoms improve to G1
Guillain-Barré syndrome	Progressive symmetrical muscle weakness with absent or reduced tendon reflexes—involves extremities, facial, respiratory and bulbar and oculomotor muscles; dysregulation of autonomic nerves	Permanently discontinue pembrolizumab. Use of steroids not recommended in idiopathic Guillain-Barré syndrome; however, a trial of (methyl)prednisolone 1–2 mg/kg is reasonable, converting to 0.5–2 mg/kg prednisone/prednisolone orally each day or its equivalent only after a response. If no improvement or worsening, plasmapheresis or IVIG indicated
Myasthenia gravis	Fluctuating muscle weakness (proximal limb, trunk, ocular, eg, ptosis/diplopia or bulbar) with fatigability, respiratory muscles also may be involved	Permanently discontinue pembrolizumab. Administer pyridostigmine at an initial dose of 30 mg three times daily. Administer oral prednisone/prednisolone at a dose of 0.5 to 2 mg/kg/day or its equivalent or 1–2 mg/kg IV (methyl)prednisolone depending on the severity of symptoms. If begin with IV convert to 0.5–2 mg/kg prednisone/prednisolone orally each day or its equivalent only after a response. If no improvement or worsening, plasmapheresis or IVIG may be considered. Additional immunosuppressants used in myasthenia gravis include azathioprine, cyclosporine, and mycophenolate. Avoid certain medications, eg, ciprofloxacin, beta-blockers, that may precipitate cholinergic crisis
Other syndromes including motor and sensory peripheral neuropathy, multifocal radicular neuropathy/plexopathy, autonomic neuropathy, phrenic nerve palsy, cranial nerve palsies (eg, facial nerve, optic nerve, hypoglossal nerve)		Permanently discontinue pembrolizumab. Administer oral prednisone/prednisolone at a dose of 0.5 to 2 mg/kg/day or its equivalent or 1–2 mg/kg IV (methyl)prednisolone depending on the severity of symptoms. If begin with IV convert to 0.5–2 mg/kg prednisone/prednisolone orally each day or its equivalent only after a response
Arthralgia	G1 (mild pain with inflammation, erythema or joint swelling)	Continue pembrolizumab. Administer acetaminophen (paracetamol) and ibuprofen
	G2 (moderate pain with inflammation, erythema or joint swelling that limits ADLs)	Withhold pembrolizumab. Administer higher doses of acetaminophen (paracetamol) and ibuprofen and use diclofenac or naproxen or etoricoxib. If inadequately controlled, consider intra-articular steroid injections for large joints or administer oral prednisone/prednisolone at a dose of 0.5 to 2 mg/kg/day or its equivalent. When improves to G1 begin a slow corticosteroid taper over at least 4 weeks. If does not respond adequately then administer 0.5–1 mg/kg IV (methyl)prednisolone and convert to 0.5–2 mg/kg prednisone/prednisolone orally each day or its equivalent only after a response, followed by a taper over at least 4 weeks when improves to G1. Resume pembrolizumab upon symptom control, or when prednisone/prednisolone daily dose <10 mg
	G3 (severe pain; irreversible joint damage; disabling; limits self-care ADL)	Withhold pembrolizumab. Administer 0.5–1 mg/kg IV (methyl)prednisolone and convert to 0.5–2 mg/kg prednisone/prednisolone orally each day or its equivalent only after a response, followed by a taper over at least 4 weeks when improves to G1. In severe cases, infliximab or another anti-TNF alpha drug may be required for improvement of arthritis. Resume pembrolizumab upon symptom control, or when prednisone/prednisolone daily dose <10 mg

(continued)

Treatment Modification (*continued*)

Other	First occurrence of other G3	Withhold pembrolizumab. Administer oral prednisone/prednisolone at a dose of 0.5 to 2 mg/kg/day or its equivalent. When improves to G1 begin a slow corticosteroid taper over at least 4 weeks. Resume pembrolizumab upon symptom control, or when prednisone/prednisolone daily dose <10 mg
	Recurrence of same G3	Permanently discontinue pembrolizumab. Administer 1–2 mg/kg IV (methyl)prednisolone and convert to 0.5–2 mg/kg prednisone/prednisolone orally each day or its equivalent only after a response. Taper over at least 4–8 weeks when symptoms improve to G1
	Life-threatening or G4	
	Requirement for ≥10 mg/day prednisone or equivalent for >12 weeks	Permanently discontinue pembrolizumab
	Persistent G2/3 adverse reactions lasting ≥12 weeks	

ADL, activities of daily living; ALT, alanine aminotransferase; AST, aspartate aminotransferase; ATG, anti-thymocyte globulin; SJS, Stevens-Johnson Syndrome; TEN, toxic epidermal necrolysis; ULN, upper limit of normal

Notes on general supportive care:
- Steroid taper in most cases will proceed over a minimum of 1 month but if symptoms improve rapidly a 2-week taper can be considered. If steroids are administered for more than 4 weeks, consider PCP prophylaxis (cotrimoxazole 480 mg twice daily M/W/F or inhaled pentamidine if has cotrimoxazole allergy), regular random blood glucose, VitD level, and starting calcium/VitD supplementation as per guidelines

Notes on pregnancy and breast feeding:
- Pembrolizumab can cause fetal harm. If used during pregnancy, or if the patient becomes pregnant during treatment, apprise the patient of the potential hazard to a fetus. Females of reproductive potential should use highly effective contraception during treatment and for 4 months after the last dose of pembrolizumab
- It is not known whether pembrolizumab is excreted in human milk. Therefore, it is recommended that women discontinue nursing during treatment with and for 4 months after the final dose of pembrolizumab

Efficacy

Efficacy Results for Patients with TMB-H Cancer Treated with Pembrolizumab

Endpoint	TMB ≥10 mut/Mb (n = 102)*	TMB ≥13 mut/Mb (n = 70)
Objective response rate		
ORR (95% CI)	29% (21 to 39)	37% (26 to 50)
Complete response rate	4%	3%
Partial response rate	25%	34%
Response duration	n = 30	n = 26
Median in months (range)†	NR (2.2+ to 34.8+)	NR (2.2+ to 34.8+)
% with duration ≥12 months	57%	58%
% with duration ≥24 months	50%	50%

*Median follow-up of 11.1 months
†From product-limit (Kaplan-Meier) method for censored data
+Denotes ongoing response
ORR, overall response rate; CI, confidence interval; NR, not reached

Keytruda (pembrolizumab) prescribing information. Whitehouse Station, NJ: Merck & Co., Inc.; 2020 November
Marabelle A et al. Lancet Oncol 2020;21:1353–1365

Patient Population Studied

Marabelle A et al. Lancet Oncol 2020;21:1353–1365
Keytruda (pembrolizumab) prescribing information. Whitehouse Station, NJ: Merck & Co., Inc.; 2020 November

The efficacy of pembrolizumab was investigated in patients with TMB-H solid tumors enrolled in 1 of 10 cohorts (A through J) of KEYNOTE-158 (NCT02628067) in a prospectively planned, retrospective analysis. KEYNOTE-158 was a multicenter, non-randomized, open-label trial that evaluated pembrolizumab in patients with a variety of previously treated unresectable or metastatic solid tumors. The major efficacy outcome measures were ORR as assessed by blinded independent central radiologist (BICR) review according to RECIST v1.1 and duration of response. Prespecified cutoffs for defining TMB-H were ≥10 and ≥13 mutations per megabase

Baseline Characteristics

N = 102 with TMB-H (≥10 mut/Mb)	
Median age	61 years (34% age 65 or older)
Male gender	34%
White race	81%
ECOG PS 0/1	41%/58%
At least 2 prior lines of therapy	56%

Marabelle A et al. Lancet Oncol 2020;21:1353–1365

Efficacy (*continued*)

Response by Tumor Type (TMB ≥10 mut/Mb)

	N	Objective Response Rate		Duration of Response Range (Months)
		n (%)	95% CI	
Overall*	102	30 (29%)	21–39	2.2+ to 34.8+
Small cell lung cancer	34	10 (29%)	15–47	4.1 to 32.5+
Cervical cancer	16	5 (31%)	11–59	3.7+ to 34.8+
Endometrial cancer	15	7 (47%)	21–73	8.4+ to 33.9+
Anal cancer	14	1 (7%)	0.2–34	18.8+
Vulvar cancer	12	2 (17%)	2–48	8.8 to 11.0
Neuroendocrine cancer	5	2 (40%)	5–85	2.2+ to 32.6+
Salivary cancer	3	PR, SD, PD	—	31.3+
Thyroid cancer	2	CR, CR	—	8.2 to 33.2+
Mesothelioma cancer	1	PD	—	N/A

Note: No TMB-H patients were identified in the cholangiocarcinoma cohort

+ Denotes ongoing response

TMB, tumor mutational burden; CI, confidence interval; PR, partial response; SD, stable disease; PD, progressive disease; CR, complete response; N/A, not applicable

Keytruda (pembrolizumab) prescribing information. Whitehouse Station, NJ: Merck & Co., Inc.; 2020 November

Therapy Monitoring

1. Before therapy: History and physical exam, CBC with differential, renal and liver function tests, serum electrolytes
2. Prior to each cycle: CBC with differential, serum electrolytes, BUN, serum creatinine, serum bilirubin, AST and ALT. For ≥2 LFT elevations, work up for other causes of elevated LFTs including viral hepatitis
3. CBC with differential initially also at day 10–14
4. Observe closely for hypersensitivity reactions, especially during the first and second infusions
5. Initially at the time of each dose, and eventually every 6–12 weeks, perform a total-body skin examination with attention to *all* mucous membranes as well as a complete review of systems
6. Monitor patients for signs and symptoms of pneumonitis. Evaluate patients with suspected pneumonitis with chest x-ray, CT, and pulse oximetry. For ≥2 toxicity may include nasal swab, sputum culture and sensitivity, blood culture and sensitivity, and urine culture and sensitivity

(*continued*)

Toxicity

Treatment-Related Adverse Events (n = 105)

Adverse Event (%)	Grade 1–2	Grade 3	Grade 4	Grade 5
Treatment-related adverse events*				
Any	49	13	1	1
Fatigue	16	0	0	0
Asthenia	11	1	0	0
Hypothyroidism	12	0	0	0
Decreased appetite	10	0	0	0
Pruritus	10	0	0	0
Colitis	1	2	0	0
Pneumonitis	2	1	0	0
Anemia	1	1	0	0
Chest pain	1	1	0	0
Gamma-glutamyltransferase increased	1	1	0	0
Hyponatremia	1	1	0	0
Pneumonia	0	0	0	1
Sepsis	0	0	1	0

(*continued*)

Toxicity (*continued*)

Lower abdominal pain	0	1	0	0
Acute respiratory distress syndrome	0	1	0	0
Drug-induced liver injury	0	1	0	0
Fulminant type 1 diabetes	0	1	0	0
Hepatocellular injury	0	1	0	0
Hypotension	0	1	0	0
Primary adrenal insufficiency	0	1	0	0
Secondary adrenal insufficiency	0	1	0	0
Thrombocytopenia	0	1	0	0
Immune-mediated adverse events and infusion reactions				
Any	16	9	0	0
Hypothyroidism	13	0	0	0
Hyperthyroidism	8	0	0	0
Colitis	2	2	0	0
Pneumonitis	3	1	0	0
Infusion reactions	3	0	0	0
Adrenal insufficiency	0	2	0	0
Severe skin reactions	1	1	0	0
Hepatitis	0	1	0	0
Nephritis	1	0	0	0
Pancreatitis	0	1	0	0
Type 1 diabetes	0	1	0	0

*Treatment-related adverse events occurring with a frequency of ≥10% and all grade 3–5 adverse events irrespective of frequency are included in this section
Marabelle A et al. Lancet Oncol 2020;21:1353–1365

Therapy Monitoring (*continued*)

7. Monitor patients for signs and symptoms of colitis. Encourage patients to report diarrhea immediately to any member of the health care team

8. Use basic metabolic panel (Na, K, CO_2, glucose) and patient history as screening tools for hypophysitis including hypopituitarism and adrenal insufficiency. If in doubt evaluate AM adrenocorticotropic hormone (ACTH) and cortisol levels. Consider ACTH stimulation test for indeterminate results

9. Thyroid function at the start of treatment, periodically during treatment, and as indicated based on clinical evaluation) and for clinical signs and symptoms of thyroid disorders. Test for TSH and free thyroxine (FT4) every 4–6 weeks as part of routine clinical monitoring on therapy or for case detection in symptomatic patients

10. Measure glucose at baseline and with each treatment during the first 12 weeks and every 6 weeks thereafter

11. Obtain a complete rheumatologic history and perform an examination of all peripheral joints for tenderness, swelling, and range of motion. Examine the spine. Consider plain x-ray/imaging to exclude metastases and evaluate joint damage (erosions), if appropriate

12. Every 2–3 months: CT scans to assess response

41. Vaginal Cancer

Leslie Boyd, MD, and Franco Muggia, MD

Epidemiology

Incidence:	6230 (Estimated new cases for 2020 in the United States)
	Incidence of clear cell adenocarcinoma as a result of in utero diethylstilbestrol (DES) exposure estimated at 1/1000
Deaths:	Estimated 1450 in 2020
Median age:	Squamous cell cancer (60–65 years); DES-related adenocarcinoma/clear cell (19 years)

Stage at presentation	
Localized	33.1%
Regional	35.5%
Distant	17.1%
Unstaged	14.3%

Daling JR et al. Gynecol Oncol 2002;84:263–270
Siegel R et al. CA Cancer J Clin 2020;70:7–30
Surveillance, Epidemiology and End Results (SEER) Program, available from http://seer.cancer.gov [accessed in 2020]
Tedeschi C et al. J Low Genit Tract Dis 2005;9:11–18

Pathology

Histologic Classification of Vaginal Neoplasia

VAIN (VAginal Intraepithelial Neoplasms)

These are pre-malignant lesions of the vaginal squamous epithelium that can develop primarily in the vagina or as an extension from the cervix. Histologically, VAIN is defined in the same way as cervical intraepithelial neoplasia (CIN). Classification includes three grades: Grade 1 (VAIN I = mild dysplasia); Grade 2 (VAIN II = moderate dysplasia); and Grade 3 (VAIN III = severe dysplasia or carcinoma in situ)

Invasive carcinoma:

1. Squamous cell carcinoma	88%
2. Adenocarcinoma	5%
3. Other epithelial cell types (adenosquamous, adenoid cystic, undifferentiated)	1–2%
4. Mesenchymal tumors (leiomyosarcoma, sarcoma botryoides, endometrioid sarcoma)	2%
5. Mixed epithelial and mesenchymal tumors	<1%
6. Other histologies (melanoma, sarcoma, yolk sac tumors, lymphoma, carcinoid, small cell)	3–4%

Higinia R et al. Vagina. In: Hoskins WJ et al (editors). Principles and Practice of Gynecologic Oncology. 4th ed. Philadelphia: Lippincott-Raven; 2005:707–742
Zaino RJ et al. Diseases of the vagina. In: Blaustein's Pathology of the Female Genital Tract. 5th ed. New York: Springer-Verlag; 2002:178–195

Work-up

VAIN (vaginal intraepithelial neoplasia):

1. H&P, including bimanual examination, palpation, and colposcopic examination of the vagina, vulva, and cervix
2. Multiple site-directed biopsies, including cervical and vulvar biopsies, to rule out invasive disease and metastatic lesions

Invasive carcinoma:

1. H&P including bimanual examination and palpation of vagina
2. Multiple site-directed biopsies, including cervical biopsies to rule out invasive disease and primary cervical cancer
3. Studies allowable for staging as per FIGO* guidelines: chest x-ray, cystoscopy, proctosigmoidoscopy, and intravenous pyelogram. Although not part of staging, pelvic MRI or CT scan may aid in planning of patient care
4. If clinically warranted, barium enema and CAT scan or MRI

Staging is best performed by gynecologic and radiation oncologists with the patient under general anesthesia. Additional biopsies of the vagina should be done to determine the limits of abnormal vaginal mucosa

*International Federation of Gynecology and Obstetrics (FIGO)
Hoskins WJ et al (editors). Principles and Practice of Gynecologic Oncology. 2nd ed. Philadelphia: Lippincott-Raven; 1997

Staging

TNM Category	FIGO Stage	Primary Tumor (T)
TX		Primary tumor cannot be assessed
T0		No evidence of primary tumor
T1	I	Tumor confined to vagina
T1a	I	Tumor confined to the vagina, measuring ≤2.0 cm
T1b	I	Tumor confined to the vagina, measuring >2.0 cm
T2	II	Tumor invades paravaginal tissues but not to pelvic sidewall
T2a	II	Tumor invades paravaginal tissues but not to pelvic wall, measuring ≤2.0 cm
T2b	II	Tumor invades paravaginal tissues but not to pelvic wall, measuring >2.0 cm
T3	III	Tumor extends to the pelvic sidewall*, and/or causing hydronephrosis or nonfunctioning kidney
T4	IVA	Tumor invades mucosa of the bladder or rectum and/or extends beyond the true pelvis (bullous edema is not sufficient evidence to classify a tumor as T4)

*Pelvic sidewall is defined as the muscle, fascia, neurovascular structures, or skeletal portions of the bony pelvis. On rectal examination, there is no cancer-free space between the tumor and pelvic sidewall

TNM Category	FIGO Stage	Regional Lymph Nodes (N)
NX		Regional lymph nodes cannot be assessed
N0		No regional lymph node metastasis
N0(i+)		Isolated tumor cells in regional lymph node(s) no greater than 0.2 mm
N1	III	Pelvic or inguinal lymph node metastasis

TNM Category	FIGO Stage	Distant Metastasis (M)
M0		No distant metastasis (no pathologic M0; use clinical M to complete stage group)
M1	IVB	Distant metastasis

Staging*

	T	N	M
IA	T1a	N0	M0
IB	T1b	N0	M0
IIA	T2a	N0	M0
IIB	T2b	N0	M0
III	T1	N1	M0
	T2	N1	M0
	T3	N1	M0
	T3	N0	M0
IVA	T4	Any N	M0
IVB	Any T	Any N	M1

Amin MB et al (editors). AJCC Cancer Staging Manual. 8th ed. New York: Springer; 2017

Expert Opinion

General:

1. Vaginal neoplasms are quite rare and are considered primary only if neither the vulva nor the cervix is involved at the time of diagnosis
2. A carcinoma involving the upper vagina and cervix should be considered a cervical primary and managed accordingly
3. Histologically most vaginal carcinomas are squamous, and chemotherapeutic management is usually based on extrapolation from experience with cervical carcinoma, given similarities in location, pattern of spread, histologic appearance, relation to HPV, and response to radiation therapy

Therapeutic Principles:

1. *Vaginal intraepithelial neoplasia (VAIN):* Treated with local modalities such as CO_2 laser ablation, topical fluorouracil, local radiation, imiquimod, or surgical excision. Regression rates are excellent. Close cytologic surveillance is warranted

(continued)

Expert Opinion (*continued*)

2. *Stages I and II:* Standard treatment by gynecologic or radiation oncologists is highly effective

3. *Stages III and IVA:* Radiation therapy alone has yielded suboptimal results. Reports of combined chemoradiation have been more encouraging, and because of similarities with cervical cancer, cisplatin-based chemoradiation has been advocated as standard therapy

4. *Stage IVB and recurrences are not amenable to locoregional therapy:* Anthracyclines and platinum compounds as single agents or in combinations have some activity, but experience is limited to small case series. Taxane-based therapy also is reasonable, particularly for adenocarcinoma. Considering the rarity of cases, care providers should consider clinical trials

Curtin JP et al. J Clin Oncol 2001;19:1275–1278
Dancuart F et al. Int J Radiat Oncol Biol Phys 1988;14:745–749
Davis KP et al. Gynecol Oncol 1991;42:131–136
Evans LS et al. Int J Radiat Oncol Biol Phys 1988;15:901–906
Grisbgy PW. Curr Treat Options Oncol 2002;3:125–130
Higinia R et al. Vagina. In: Hoskins WJ et al (editors). Principles and Practice of Gynecologic Oncology. 4th ed. Philadelphia: Lippincott-Raven; 2005:707–742
Kucera H, Vavra N. Gynecol Oncol 1991;40:12–16
Piver MS et al. Am J Obstet Gynecol 1978;131:311–313

LOCALLY ADVANCED

VAGINAL CANCER REGIMEN: CISPLATIN + FLUOROURACIL + RADIATION THERAPY

Roberts WS et al. Gynecol Oncol 1991;43:233–236

Hydration before cisplatin: 1000 mL 0.9% sodium chloride injection (0.9% NS); administer intravenously over a minimum of 2 hours
Cisplatin 50 mg/m²; administer intravenously in 100–1000 mL 0.9% sodium chloride injection (0.9% NS), over 6 hours on day 1, every 4 weeks for 2 cycles (total dosage/4-week cycle = 50 mg/m²)

Followed by:
Fluorouracil 1000 mg/m² per day; administer as a continuous intravenous infusion in 250–2000 mL 0.9% NS or 5% dextrose injection over 24 hours for 4 consecutive days, on days 1–4, every 4 weeks for 2 cycles (total dosage/4-week cycle = 4000 mg/m²)

Hydration after cisplatin: 1000 mL 0.9% sodium chloride injection (0.9% NS); administer intravenously over a minimum of 2 hours. Encourage patients to increase oral intake of non-alcoholic fluids, and provide electrolyte replacement as needed (potassium, magnesium, sodium)
Concurrent with chemotherapy administer radiation therapy as follows:
External beam radiation with 20-MeV linear accelerator, 180 cGy/day fractions to a total dose of 4000–5000 cGy to the whole pelvis, ± periaortic radiation to a dose of 3600–4500 cGy
±
Additional external pelvic irradiation to limited fields to a total dose of 6480 cGy
±
Additional brachytherapy starting 2–3 weeks after external beam radiation

Supportive Care
Antiemetic prophylaxis
Emetogenic potential on day 1: **HIGH**. *Potential for delayed symptoms*
Emetogenic potential on days 2–4: **LOW**
See Chapter 42 for antiemetic recommendations

Hematopoietic growth factor (CSF) prophylaxis
Primary prophylaxis is **NOT** *indicated*
See Chapter 43 for more information

Antimicrobial prophylaxis
Risk of fever and neutropenia is **LOW**
  Antimicrobial primary prophylaxis to be considered:
  • Antibacterial—not indicated
  • Antifungal—not indicated
  • Antiviral—not indicated unless patient previously had an episode of HSV

Patient Population Studied

Study of 67 patients with advanced carcinomas of the lower female genital tract that were not amenable to resection, among whom 7 had vaginal cancers. Of the 7 patients with vaginal cancer, 5 had stage III disease and 2 had recurrent disease

Efficacy*

Complete clinical response (all histologies)	85%
Partial response (all histologies)	9%
Stable disease (all histologies)	3%

*Not stated for the subset of patients with vaginal cancer. However, 3 of 7 patients with vaginal cancer were without recurrence or failure of the treatment for a median follow-up of 13 months

Treatment Modifications

Roberts WS et al. Gynecol Oncol 1991;43:233–236
Whitney CW et al. J Clin Oncol 1999;17:1339–1348

Adverse Events	Treatment Modifications
Serum creatinine ≥1.7 mg/dL (≥29.1 μmol/L)	Hold cisplatin until serum creatinine returns to pre-treatment level, then reduce dosage by 50% in subsequent cycles
WBC ≤3000/mm³ or platelet ≤100,000/mm³	Delay cisplatin and fluorouracil until WBC ≥3000/mm³ and platelet count ≥100,000/mm³
>2-week delay in start of cycle	Reduce cisplatin and fluorouracil dosages by 50% each
G3/4 hematologic toxicity	Hold radiation therapy until hematologic toxicity is G ≤2

Whitney et al. utilized a similar regimen for patients with cervical cancer; 91% completed both chemotherapy courses and had similar completion rates for radiation therapy

Toxicity

Acute Toxicities

Neutropenia and thrombocytopenia	1 patient*
Radiation enteritis	5 patients†
Nausea, vomiting, and diarrhea	Very common
Renal, hepatic, or neurologic	Not significant

Delayed Toxicities

Rectovaginal fistula	3 patients‡
Radiation proctitis	1 patient‡
Small bowel fistula	2 patients‡
Soft tissue necrosis	2 patients‡
Hemorrhagic cystitis	1 patient

*Resulted in 8- to 14-day treatment delay
†Resulted in 8- to >14-day treatment delay
‡Required surgery

Therapy Monitoring

Weekly: CBC with differential, LFTs, electrolytes, and creatinine

LOCALLY ADVANCED

VAGINAL CANCER REGIMEN: NEOADJUVANT CISPLATIN + EPIRUBICIN

Zanetta G et al. Gynecol Oncol 1997;64:431–435

Hydration before cisplatin with ≥1000 mL 0.9% sodium chloride injection intravenously over a minimum of 2 hours

Cisplatin 50 mg/m² per dose intravenously in 50–250 mL 0.9% NS over 30–60 minutes once weekly for 9 doses (total dosage/9-week course = 450 mg/m²)

Hydration after cisplatin with ≥1000 mL 0.9% NS intravenously over a minimum of 2 hours
Notes: Encourage increased oral intake of nonalcoholic fluids. Goal is to achieve a urine output ≥100 mL/hour. Monitor and replace electrolytes as needed (potassium, magnesium, sodium)
Epirubicin HCl 70 mg/m² per dose intravenously by injection over 3–5 minutes *or* in 25–250 mL 0.9% NS or 5% dextrose injection over 15–20 minutes every 3 weeks, weeks 1, 4, and 7, for 3 doses (total dosage/9-week course = 210 mg/m²)

Supportive Care
Antiemetic prophylaxis
Emetogenic potential is **HIGH**. *Potential for delayed symptoms*
See Chapter 42 for antiemetic recommendations

Hematopoietic growth factor (CSF) prophylaxis
Primary prophylaxis is indicated with:
  Filgrastim (G-CSF) 5 mcg/kg per day by subcutaneous injection daily for 5 days
  • Begin use on the day after cisplatin (± epirubicin) is administered
  • Discontinue daily filgrastim use at least 24 hours before administering myelosuppressive treatment
See Chapter 43 for more information

Antimicrobial prophylaxis
Risk of fever and neutropenia is **LOW**
  Antimicrobial primary prophylaxis to be considered:
  • Antibacterial—not indicated
  • Antifungal—not indicated
  • Antiviral—not indicated unless patient previously had an episode of HSV

Oral care
Prophylaxis and treatment for mucositis/stomatitis
  General advice:
  • Encourage patients to maintain intake of nonalcoholic fluids
  • Evaluate patients for oral pain and provide analgesic medications
  • Consider histamine (H₂-subtype) receptor antagonists (eg, ranitidine, famotidine) or a proton pump inhibitor for epigastric pain
  • *Lactobacillus* sp.-containing probiotics may be beneficial in preventing diarrhea
  Patients with intact oral mucosa:
  • Clean the mouth, tongue, and gums by brushing after every meal and at bedtime with an ultrasoft toothbrush with fluoride toothpaste
  • Floss teeth gently every day unless contraindicated. If gums bleed and hurt, avoid bleeding or sore areas, but floss other teeth
  • Patients may use saline or commercial bland, nonalcoholic rinses
    ▪ Do not use mouthwashes that contain alcohols
  If mucositis or stomatitis is present:
  • Keep the mouth moist utilizing water, ice chips, sugarless gum, sugar-free hard candies, or a saliva substitute
  • Rinse mouth several times a day to remove debris
    ▪ Use a solution of ¼ teaspoon (1.25 g) each of baking soda and table salt (sodium chloride) in 1 quart (~950 mL) of warm water. Follow with a plain water rinse
    ▪ Do not use mouthwashes that contain alcohol

(continued)

Treatment Modifications

Adverse Event	Treatment Modification
ANC <2000/mm³ or platelets <75,000/mm³ on day of treatment	Delay treatment for 1 week

Patient Population Studied

The study population included 20 patients with locally advanced cervical adenocarcinoma (bulky IB–IIA, IIB) and 2 subjects with vaginal adenocarcinoma; mean age was 51 years (range: 15–67 years). Disease histology was adenocarcinoma in 18 subjects and adenosquamous in 4 subjects. Those with stages IB–IIA cervical carcinomas and those with vaginal adenocarcinoma were required to have tumors >4 cm in diameter, as assessed by alginate mold. All patients had a performance status <2 according to the World Health Organization criteria. Staging was done according to the International Federation of Gynecology and Obstetrics

(*continued*)

- Foam-tipped swabs (eg, Toothettes) are useful in moisturizing oral mucosa, but ineffective for cleansing teeth and removing plaque
- Advise patients who develop mucositis to:
  - Choose foods that are easy to chew and swallow
  - Take small bites of food, chew slowly, and sip liquids with meals
  - Encourage soft, moist foods such as cooked cereals, mashed potatoes, and scrambled eggs
  - For trouble swallowing, soften food with gravies, sauces, broths, yogurt, or other bland liquids
  - Avoid sharp, crunchy foods; hot, spicy, or highly acidic foods (eg, citrus fruits and juices); sugary foods; toothpicks; tobacco products; alcoholic drinks

Additional therapies given:
- In operable patients, Piver 3 radical hysterectomy with pelvic lymphadenectomy and aortic node sampling was performed within 30 days after the completion of chemotherapy
- Histologic analysis of all surgical specimens assessed the extent of cervical, vaginal, and parametrial disease and the status of all surgical margins and lymph nodes
- Patients with surgical detection of positive lymph nodes, parametrial infiltration, or peritoneal spread received adjuvant treatments
- Postoperative radiotherapy consisted of 4500 cGy with 18 MeV photons, given by means of a field up to L4–L5 in the case of negative nodes, and up to T11–T12 in the case of positive common iliac nodes for subjects with stable disease or minimal response
- Subjects achieving a good clinical response to neoadjuvant treatment received additional chemotherapy "in order to confirm this response"

Efficacy

Number enrolled	22
Received more than 1 dose of therapy	21
Completed all planned therapy	19
Underwent surgery	18
Complete clinical response	2
Complete response at surgery	0
Microscopic residual tumor	4*
Macroscopic residual tumor	14

With median follow-up of 22 months for surviving patients

Experienced recurrence	8[†]
Died of recurrent or persistent disease	5
Alive with tumor	3
Alive without evidence of recurrence	14

*At time of the report 2 were alive with no evidence of disease at 32 and 47 months; 1 was alive with tumor; and 1 died of disease at 33 months after first diagnosis
[†]In 4/8 patients with positive nodes at time of surgery, 2/10 without nodal metastases, and 2/4 not undergoing surgery

Treatment Monitoring

1. Weekly CBC with differential
2. Weekly serum electrolytes, BUN, and creatinine
3. Echocardiogram for determination of left ventricular ejection fraction at baseline and then if needed for signs or symptoms suggestive of congestive heart failure

Toxicity (N = 21*)

Grade	G0–1	G2	G3	G4
Leucopenia	5	6	8	2[†]
Thrombocytopenia	13	4	3	1
Anemia	11	6	4	—
Mucositis	18	2	1	—
Nephrotoxicity	4	—	1*	—
Neurotoxicity	18	3	—	—
Fever	17	2	2	—
Nausea/vomiting	—	12	9	—
Cardiac	—	—	—	—
Alopecia	—	9	12	—
Completed 9 courses of treatment	19/22 (86%)			
No delays in administration	3/19			
Delays in administration	16/19			
Duration of delays in administration	1–5 weeks			

*One patient refused further treatment after first course (*Note:* a course of therapy was inconsistently defined as "… the administration of cisplatin and epirubicin [weeks 1, 4, and 7] or the administration of cisplatin alone [weeks 2, 3, 5, 6, 8, and 9].")
[†]Two subjects requiring discontinuation of the treatment; 19 received the planned dose of drug without reduction

METASTATIC • RECURRENT

VAGINAL CANCER REGIMEN: DOXORUBICIN (SINGLE AGENT)

Piver MS et al. Am J Obstet Gynecol 1978;131:311–313

Doxorubicin 60–90 mg/m^2; administer by slow intravenous injection over 3–5 minutes on day 1, every 4 weeks (total dosage/cycle = 60 to 90 mg/m^2)

Supportive Care
Antiemetic prophylaxis
Emetogenic potential: **MODERATE**
See Chapter 42 for antiemetic recommendations

Hematopoietic growth factor (CSF) prophylaxis
Primary prophylaxis is **NOT** indicated
See Chapter 43 for more information

Antimicrobial prophylaxis
Risk of fever and neutropenia is **LOW**
Antimicrobial primary prophylaxis to be considered:
- Antibacterial—not indicated
- Antifungal—not indicated
- Antiviral—not indicated unless patient previously had an episode of HSV

Patient Population Studied

Cervical or vaginal malignancies; 7 of 100 patients with advanced vaginal squamous cell carcinoma

Efficacy

(N = 7 Patients with Vaginal Cancer)

Complete response	1 patient
Partial response	1 patient*

*Treated with combination doxorubicin, cyclophosphamide, and fluorouracil

Toxicity

Myelosuppression	Dose-limiting toxicity. Leukopenia more common than thrombocytopenia or anemia. Nadir usually on days 10–14, with recovery by day 21 after treatment
Nausea and vomiting	Moderate severity on the day of treatment; delayed symptoms (>24 hours after treatment) uncommon
Mucositis and diarrhea	Common, but not dose limiting
Cardiotoxicity (acute)	Incidence not related to dosage. Presents within 3 days after treatment as arrhythmias, conduction abnormalities, ECG changes, pericarditis, and/or myocarditis. Usually transient and asymptomatic
Cardiotoxicity (chronic)	Dosage-dependent dilated cardiomyopathy associated with congestive failure. Risk increases with cumulative doses >550 mg/m^2
Strong vesicant	Avoid extravasation
Skin	Hand-foot syndrome, with skin rash swelling, erythema, pain, and desquamation. Onset at 5–6 weeks after starting treatment. Hyperpigmentation of nails, rarely skin rash, urticaria. Potential for radiation recall
Alopecia	Common, but generally reversible within 3 months after discontinuing doxorubicin
Infusion reactions	Signs and symptoms include flushing, dyspnea, facial swelling, headache, back pain, chest and/or throat tightness, and hypotension. May occur with a first treatment. Symptoms resolve within several hours to a day after discontinuing doxorubicin
Urine discoloration	Red-orange discoloration usually within 1–2 days after drug administration

Chu E, DeVita VT Jr (editors). Physicians' Cancer Chemotherapy Drug Manual 2001. Sudbury, MA: Jones and Bartlett; 2001

Treatment Modifications

Adverse Events	Treatment Modifications
WBC <3000/mm^3 and platelet counts <100,000/mm^3	Delay start of next cycle until WBC >3000/mm^3 and platelet counts >100,000/mm^3
>2-week delay in start of cycle	Reduce doxorubicin dose by 15 mg/m^2
Doxorubicin total cumulative lifetime dosage ≥550 mg/m^2	Obtain frequent MUGA scans to monitor cardiac function

Therapy Monitoring

1. *Before each treatment with doxorubicin (every 4 weeks):* H&P, CBC with differential, serum electrolytes, LFTs, BUN, and serum creatinine
2. Echocardiogram for determination of left ventricular ejection fraction at baseline and then as needed for signs or symptoms suggestive of congestive heart failure. For patients who reach a total cumulative doxorubicin dose of 550 mg/m^2, repeat an echocardiogram every 1–2 cycles if continued administration of doxorubicin is planned

Piver MS et al. Am J Obstet Gynecol 1978;131:311–313

METASTATIC • RECURRENT

VAGINAL CANCER REGIMEN: CISPLATIN (SINGLE AGENT)

Thigpen JT et al. Gynecol Oncol 1986;23:101–104

Hydration before cisplatin: ≥1000 mL 0.9% sodium chloride injection (0.9% NS) administered intravenously over a minimum of 3–4 hours

Cisplatin 50 mg/m²; administer intravenously in 50–250 mL 0.9% NS at a rate of 1 mg/min on day 1, every 3 weeks, (total dosage/cycle = 50 mg/m²)

Hydration after cisplatin: ≥1000 mL 0.9% sodium chloride injection (0.9% NS) administered intravenously over a minimum of 3–4 hours. Encourage patients to increase oral intake of nonalcoholic fluids, and provide electrolyte replacement as needed (potassium, magnesium, sodium)

Supportive Care
Antiemetic prophylaxis
Emetogenic potential: **HIGH**. *Potential for delayed symptoms*
See Chapter 42 for antiemetic recommendations

Hematopoietic growth factor (CSF) prophylaxis
Primary prophylaxis is **NOT** *indicated*
See Chapter 43 for more information

Antimicrobial prophylaxis
Risk of fever and neutropenia is **LOW**
  Antimicrobial primary prophylaxis to be considered:
  • Antibacterial—not indicated
  • Antifungal—not indicated
  • Antiviral—not indicated unless patient previously had an episode of HSV

Patient Population Studied

Study of 22 patients with advanced or recurrent vaginal cancers

Efficacy (N = 22)

One complete response out of 22 evaluable patients with vaginal cancer (most were heavily pretreated)

Toxicity (N = 22)

Hematologic Toxicities			
	% G1	% G2	
Leukopenia*	9	13.6	
Thrombocytopenia†	9	—	

Nonhematologic Toxicities			
	Mild	Moderate	Severe
Nephrotoxicity‡	27	—	—
Nausea/vomiting§	9	45	4.5
Fatigue	9	4.5	4.5

*Lowest WBC nadir = 2000 leukocytes/mm³
†Lowest platelet nadir = 126,000 platelets/mm³
‡Dose-limiting toxicity in 35–40%
§Most common adverse effect

Treatment Modifications

Adverse Events	Treatment Modifications
Serum creatinine ≥1.7 mg/dL (≥29.1 µmol/L)	Hold treatment until creatinine returns to pretreatment level, then reduce cisplatin dosage in subsequent cycles by 50%
G3/4 ototoxicity	Hold treatment until G ≤2 then reduce cisplatin dosage in subsequent cycles by 50%
G3/4 neurotoxicity	Hold treatment until G ≤2 then reduce cisplatin dosage in subsequent cycles by 50%

Toxicities Reported in other Studies

Neurotoxicity	Usually peripheral sensory neuropathy with bilateral paresthesia and anesthesia in a "stocking-and-glove" distribution. Risk increases with high individual doses and cumulatively. Motor and autonomic neuropathies may also occur. Neurotoxic effects may be irreversible
Ototoxicity	High-frequency hearing loss and tinnitus
Hypersensitivity	Facial edema, wheezing, bronchospasm, and hypotension within minutes of drug exposure
Hepatic	Transient increases in LFTs
Gustatory	Dysgeusia (metallic taste) and loss of appetite

Chu E, DeVita VT Jr (editors). Physicians' Cancer Chemotherapy Drug Manual 2001. Sudbury, MA: Jones and Bartlett; 2001:100–105
Thigpen JT et al. Gynecol Oncol 1986;23:101–104

Therapy Monitoring

Before each treatment with cisplatin (every 4 weeks): H&P, paying attention to history and objective findings of neurotoxicity, CBC with differential, LFTs, serum electrolytes, and creatinine

METASTATIC • RECURRENT

VAGINAL CANCER REGIMEN: PACLITAXEL (SINGLE AGENT)

Curtin JP et al. J Clin Oncol 2001;19:1275–1278

Premedications:
Dexamethasone 20 mg per dose; administer orally or intravenously for 2 doses, 14 hours and 7 hours before starting paclitaxel
Diphenhydramine 50 mg; administer by intravenous injection 30 minutes before starting paclitaxel
Ranitidine 50 mg; administer intravenously in 25–100 mL of 0.9% sodium chloride injection (0.9% NS) or 5% dextrose injection (D5W), over 30–60 minutes, 30 minutes before starting paclitaxel
Paclitaxel 170 mg/m^{2*}; administer by continuous intravenous infusion diluted in 0.9% NS or D5W to a concentration within the range 0.3 and 1.2 mg/mL, over 24 hours on day 1, every 3 weeks (total dosage/cycle = 170 mg/m^{2*})

*Patients who previously received radiation treatment to the pelvis should be treated initially with a paclitaxel dosage of 135 mg/m². This may be increased according to the guidelines under dose modification

Supportive Care
Antiemetic prophylaxis
Emetogenic potential: LOW
See Chapter 42 for antiemetic recommendations

Hematopoietic growth factor (CSF) prophylaxis
Primary prophylaxis may be indicated
See Chapter 43 for more information

Antimicrobial prophylaxis
Risk of fever and neutropenia is LOW
Antimicrobial primary prophylaxis to be considered:
- Antibacterial—not indicated
- Antifungal—not indicated
- Antiviral—not indicated unless patient previously had an episode of HSV

Treatment Modifications

Paclitaxel dosage levels:
110 mg/m² (minimum dosage to be administered)
135 mg/m²
170 mg/m²
200 mg/m² (maximum dosage to be administered)

Adverse Events	Treatment Modifications*
ANC <1500/mm³	Hold treatment until ANC ≥1500/mm³
Platelet count <100,000/mm³	Hold treatment until platelets ≥100,000/mm³
G1 hematologic toxicity	Increase paclitaxel dosage by 1 level
G2/3 hematologic toxicity	Administer same paclitaxel dosage
G4 hematologic toxicity	Decrease paclitaxel dosage by 1 level
G2 nonobstructive renal toxicity	Decrease paclitaxel dosage by 1 level
G3 hepatic toxicity	
G3 mucositis	
G4 GOG nonhematologic toxicity	

*Based on adverse events during previous cycles

Patient Population Studied

Study of 42 patients with advanced nonsquamous cell cervical cancer who had either no benefit from or progressive disease on standard chemotherapy

Toxicity (N = 42)

Toxicity Grades*					
Toxicity†	0	1	2	3	4
Hematologic Toxicities					
Leukopenia	5	3	11	16	7
Neutropenia	7	1	3	5	26
Thrombocytopenia	35	5	1	1	0
Anemia	21	7	10	4	0
Nonhematologic Toxicities					
Nausea/vomiting	28	7	7	0	0
Gastrointestinal	31	5	5	0	1
Alopecia	16	7	19	0	0
Neurotoxicity	28	4	9	1	0
Edema	41	0	0	1	0

*Number of patients with toxicity
†The table identifies only toxicities where at least 1 patient experienced a G3 or G4 toxicity

(continued)

Efficacy

Complete response	9.5%
Partial response	21.5%
Median duration of response	4.8 months

Therapy Monitoring

Before each treatment: H&P, paying attention to history and objective findings of neurotoxicity, CBC with differential, LFTs, electrolytes, and creatinine

Toxicity (N = 42) *(continued)*

Other Toxicities

Febrile neutropenia	8 patients
Alopecia	26 patients
Mucositis	2 patients
Myalgia and arthralgia	Infrequent
Bradycardia Grade 2	Incidence not specified

SECTION II. Antiemetics, Growth Factors, and Drug Preparation

42. Prophylaxis and Treatment of Chemotherapy- and Radiation-Induced Nausea and Vomiting

Thomas E. Hughes, PharmD, BCOP

Chemotherapy-Induced Nausea and Vomiting (CINV)

Neurotransmitters and their receptor targets implicated in CINV
- Serotonin and the serotonin subtype 3 (5-HT_3) receptor
- Dopamine and the dopamine subtype 2 (D_2) receptor
- Substance P and the neurokinin subtype 1 (NK_1) receptor
- Histamine, acetylcholine, opioids, and their respective receptors

Two Phases of CINV

Acute phase
- Occurs during the first 24 hours after exposure to emetogenic chemotherapy and is mediated by release of serotonin from enterochromaffin cells within GI tract
- Actual time of onset varies depending on the chemotherapeutic agent

Delayed phase
- Substance P and the NK_1 receptor may be more important than serotonin in delayed CINV
- Delayed CINV was initially described with cisplatin
- Delayed CINV has also been described with other chemotherapeutic agents, including carboplatin, cyclophosphamide, and the anthracyclines
- Although the onset of delayed emesis was initially defined as that which occurs 24 hours postchemotherapy, more recent evidence suggests that referable symptoms may occur as early as 16 hours after cisplatin
- The incidence of delayed vomiting after cisplatin is greatest during the 24-hour period from 48 to 72 hours after treatment, and, thereafter, declines progressively

Anticipatory Nausea and Vomiting

- Development is associated with poor emetic control during prior administration of chemotherapy
- Prevention is the best approach
- Pharmacologic interventions are usually not successful, but behavioral methods with systemic desensitization are effective and have been used with some success

Radiation-induced Nausea and Vomiting (RINV)

- The emetic risk associated with radiation therapy is primarily based on the site of radiation. Patients receiving total-body, upper-abdomen, and craniospinal irradiation incur the greatest risk for nausea and vomiting. Risk categories based on site are provided in Table 42–9

Antiemetic Principles[1–5]

- 5-HT_3 receptor antagonists demonstrate comparable efficacy at equivalent doses. In general, they can be used interchangeably based on convenience, availability, and cost. Clinical trials and subsequent meta-analysis studies have demonstrated that palonosetron is more effective than other 5-HT_3 receptor antagonists in preventing CINV, particularly in the delayed phase. However, these trials did not include NK_1 receptor antagonists within the trial design and many did not consistently include corticosteroids such as dexamethasone. Clinical practice guidelines from the Multinational Association of Supportive Care in Cancer (2016) suggest that palonosetron is preferred in moderately emetogenic chemotherapy when dexamethasone is not included and in AC (anthracycline plus cyclophosphamide) chemotherapy when an NK1 receptor antagonist is not included.[3,4] The National Comprehensive Cancer Network (NCCN) antiemesis guideline (version 2.2020) recommends palonosetron as the preferred 5-HT_3 receptor antagonist in prophylaxis for high and moderate emetic risk categories when an NK_1 receptor antagonist is not included in the regimen.[2] The NCCN antiemesis guidelines also recommend subcutaneous granisetron extended-release injection as a preferred 5-HT_3 receptor antagonist when used with dexamethasone without an NK_1 receptor antagonist. This recommendation is based on a phase 3 comparative trial that demonstrated that subcutaneous extended-release granisetron was non-inferior to IV palonosetron in patients receiving highly or moderately emetogenic chemotherapy.[2,17,18] The 2017 and 2020 updates of the American Society of Clinical Oncology (ASCO) clinical practice guidelines on antiemetics supports the use of any of the available 5-HT_3 receptor antagonists in CINV prophylaxis.[1,5] For RINV prophylaxis and rescue therapy, granisetron and ondansetron are the preferred 5-HT_3 receptor antagonists due to a larger body of evidence for these agents[1,2,5]
- The lowest established proven dose of each 5-HT_3 receptor antagonist should be used
- Single-dose prophylactic regimens of 5-HT_3 receptor antagonists and corticosteroids for acute-phase CINV prophylaxis are effective and preferred

(continued)

Antiemetic Principles[1-5] (continued)

- At biologically equivalent doses, oral antiemetic regimens are equivalent to intravenous antiemetic regimens
- All patients receiving chemotherapy should have antiemetics available on a PRN basis for breakthrough nausea and vomiting. Rescue agents should be selected to complement, not duplicate, the prophylactic regimen (ie, select drugs from a different pharmacologic class)
- For CINV prophylaxis where there is a high emetic potential (emetic incidence of >90%), a four-drug antiemetic regimen that includes a 5-HT$_3$ receptor antagonist, a corticosteroid, an NK$_1$ receptor antagonist, and olanzapine is recommended as the preferred regimen for adult patients (Table 42–5). The NCCN antiemesis guidelines and the 2020 update of the ASCO antiemetic guidelines both recommend the four-drug regimen that includes olanzapine for adults based on a phase 3 randomized clinical trial that demonstrated a higher complete response and less nausea throughout the study period with the addition of olanzapine.[1,2,5,19] The NCCN antiemesis guidelines[2] also recommend two three-drug regimens as alternatives, and these regimens also are included in Table 42–5
- For CINV prophylaxis where there is a moderate emetic potential (emetic incidence of 30–90%), a two- or three-drug antiemetic regimen that includes a 5-HT$_3$ receptor antagonist and a corticosteroid with or without an NK-1 receptor antagonist or olanzapine is recommended for adult patients (Table 42–5)
- A 5-HT$_3$ receptor antagonist or a corticosteroid alone is the recommended prophylactic regimen for chemotherapy with low emetic potential (emetic incidence of 10–30%). Alternative single-agent regimens also may be considered, such as metoclopramide or prochlorperazine
- For RINV prophylaxis where there is a high emetic potential, a two-drug antiemetic regimen that includes a 5-HT$_3$ receptor antagonist and dexamethasone is recommended
- For RINV prophylaxis where there is a moderate emetic potential, prophylaxis with a 5-HT$_3$ receptor antagonist with or without dexamethasone is recommended
- Rescue therapy with a 5-HT$_3$ receptor antagonist, dexamethasone, or a dopamine receptor antagonist is recommended for patients receiving radiation therapy with a low or minimal emetic risk. For brain irradiation, dexamethasone is the preferred agent
- For concurrent chemotherapy and radiation therapy, the antiemetic regimen chosen should be based on the emetic risk level of the chemotherapy agent, unless the risk level of the radiation therapy is higher. If prophylaxis for CINV has completed and radiation therapy is administered alone during a combination regimen, the antiemetic regimen should then be based on the emetic risk level of the radiation rather than using rescue therapy for the chemotherapy agents as needed

Table 42–1. Antiemetic Pharmacologic Classes and Class Side Effects

Pharmacologic Class	Agents/Generic Name (Trade Name) (U.S. FDA Approved)	Side-Effect Profile[6-16]
5-HT$_3$ receptor antagonists	Dolasetron (Anzemet) Granisetron (Kytril, Sancuso) Ondansetron (Zofran) Palonosetron (Aloxi)	Headache [C] Constipation [I] Light-headedness or dizziness [I] Transient elevations in liver enzymes [I] *ECG interval changes:* Prolongation of PR, QTc, and JT, and widening of QRS (especially dolasetron) [R]
Corticosteroids	Dexamethasone (Decadron, generic products) Methylprednisolone (Solu-Medrol, generic products)	Hyperglycemia Mood changes Increased appetite Diarrhea Perineal irritation with rapid IV administration of dexamethasone Fluid retention
NK$_1$ receptor antagonists	Aprepitant (Emend) Fosaprepitant (Emend) Netupitant-palonosetron (Akynzeo) Fosnetupitant-palonosetron (Akynzeo) Rolapitant (Varubi)	In randomized trials, treatment side effects were similar with or without an NK$_1$ receptor antagonist
Dopaminergic antagonists: phenothiazines	Chlorpromazine (Thorazine, generic products) Perphenazine (Trilafon, generic products) Prochlorperazine (Compazine, generic products) Promethazine (Phenergan, generic products)	Extrapyramidal side effects* Sedation Anticholinergic effects Hypotension with rapid IV administration, hypersensitivity Hepatotoxicity Cholestatic jaundice Leukopenia and agranulocytosis Hormonal dysfunction Neuroleptic malignant syndrome† Cardiovascular effects‡

(continued)

Table 42–1. (*continued*)

Pharmacologic Class	Agents/Generic Name (Trade Name) (U.S. FDA Approved)	Side-Effect Profile[6–16]
Dopaminergic antagonists: butyrophenones	Droperidol (Inapsine) Haloperidol (Haldol, generic products)	Extrapyramidal side effects* Sedation Agitation Dizziness Chills Hallucinations Hypotension or hypertension Prolongation of ECG intervals (QT prolongation) Arrhythmias (eg, torsades de pointes)
Substituted benzamides	Metoclopramide (Reglan) Trimethobenzamide (Tigan)	Sedation Diarrhea Extrapyramidal side effects* Neuroleptic malignant syndrome† Hypotension Arrhythmias
Benzodiazepines	Lorazepam (Ativan) Alprazolam (Xanax)	Sedation Lethargy Weakness Impaired coordination
Cannabinoids	Dronabinol (Marinol) Nabilone (Cesamet)	Mood changes Memory loss Euphoria Dysphoria Hallucinations Sedation Paranoid ideation Ataxia Motor incoordination Blurred vision Hunger Cardiovascular effects§ Syncope
Atypical antipsychotics	Olanzapine (Zyprexa) Mirtazapine (Remeron)	Sedation Extrapyramidal side effects* Neuroleptic malignant syndrome† Weight gain, hyperglycemia, and other features of metabolic syndrome may be seen with high doses and prolonged use
Antihistamines	Diphenhydramine (Benadryl, generic products) Hydroxyzine (Atarax, generic products) Meclizine (Antivert, generic products)	Sedation Dry mouth Constipation Blurred vision
Anticholinergics	Scopolamine (Transderm Scōp)	Dry mouth Somnolence Sedation Constipation

*Extrapyramidal side effects: akathisia, dyskinesias, parkinsonism, acute dystonias (oculogyric crisis, torticollis)

†Neuroleptic malignant syndrome: hyperthermia, severe extrapyramidal dysfunction (eg, severe hypertonicity of skeletal muscles, altered mental status and/or level of consciousness, and autonomic instability)

‡Phenothiazine cardiovascular effects include hypotension, syncope, hypertension, bradycardia, and various ECG changes (nonspecific, reversible Q- and T-wave abnormalities). Cases of sudden death also have been reported, presumably secondary to ventricular arrhythmias

§The cardiovascular adverse effects of cannabinoid therapy: hypotension, hypertension, syncope, tachycardia, palpitations, vasodilation, and facial flushing

C, common; I, infrequent; R, rare. For other agents, order of frequency is less clear

Table 42–2. Pharmacokinetic Parameters of 5-HT₃ Receptor Antagonists[6–11]

Parameter	Ondansetron (0.15 mg/kg IV)	Granisetron (40 µg/kg IV)	Dolasetron* (Oral)	Palonosetron (10 µg/kg IV)
Half-life (hours)	3.5–5.5[‡]	8.95[†]	7.9[†]	40[‡]
Protein binding	70–76%	65%	77%	62%
Oral bioavailability	56%	60%	75%	NR
Metabolism CYP enzymes	Hepatic CYP3A4 (major) CYP2D6, CYP1A2	Hepatic CYP3A4	Hepatic CYP2D6 (major) CYP3A4 (minor)	Hepatic CYP2D6 (major) CYP3A4, 1A2
Urinary excretion (parent compound)	5%	12%	61%	40%
Decreased clearance in elderly Dosage adjustment in elderly	Yes No	Yes No	No No	No No
Decreased clearance in hepatic dysfunction Dosage adjustment in hepatic dysfunction	Yes Yes (in severe dysfunction)	Yes No	Yes No	No No
Decreased clearance in renal dysfunction Dosage adjustment in renal dysfunction	Yes No	No No	Yes No	Yes No

*Dolasetron is rapidly converted to the active metabolite hydrodolasetron. All reported parameters refer to hydrodolasetron
[†]Data from adult cancer patients
[‡]Data from studies in healthy volunteers

Table 42–3. Classification of Emetic Risk of Parenteral Antineoplastic Agents[1–3]

Emetic Potential	Chemotherapy Drug	
High Frequency of emesis >90%	Anthracycline/cyclophosphamide combination[1,2,3] Carboplatin (AUC ≥4 mg/mL per minute)[2] Carmustine (>250 mg/m²)[2] Cisplatin[1,2,3] Cyclophosphamide (>1500 mg/m²)[1,2,3] Dacarbazine[1,2,3] Doxorubicin (≥60 mg/m²)[2] Epirubicin (>90 mg/m²)[2] Ifosfamide (≥2 g/m² per dose)[2] Mechlorethamine[1,2,3] Streptozocin[1,2,3]	
Moderate Frequency of emesis 30–90%	Aldesleukin (IL-2) (>12–15 million IU/m²)[2] Arsenic Trioxide[1] Azacitidine[1,2,3] Bendamustine[1,2,3] Busulfan[1,2] Carboplatin (AUC <4 mg/mL/min)[2] Carmustine (≤250 mg/m²)[2] Clofarabine[1,2,3] Cyclophosphamide (<1500 mg/m²)[1,2,3] Cytarabine (>1000 mg/m²)[1,3] Dactinomycin[2] Daunorubicin[1,2,3] Daunorubicin and cytarabine, liposome[1,2] Dinutuximab[2] Doxorubicin (<60 mg/m²)[2] Epirubicin (≤90 mg/m²)[2]	Fam-trastuzumab deruxtecan-nxki[1,2] Idarubicin[1,2,3] Ifosfamide (<2 g/m² per dose)[2] Interferon alfa (≥10 million IU/m²)[2] Irinotecan[1,2,3] Irinotecan liposome injection[1,2] Melphalan[2] Methotrexate (≥250 mg/m²)[2] Oxaliplatin[1,2,3] Pentostatin* Romidepsin[1,3] Temozolomide[1,2,3] Thiotepa[1,3] Trabectedin[1,2,3]

(continued)

Table 42–3. (*continued*)

Emetic Potential	Chemotherapy Drug	
Low Frequency of emesis 10–30%	Ado-trastuzumab emtansine[1,2,3] Aldesleukin (IL-2) (<12 million IU/m^2)[2] Axicabtagene ciloleucel[1,2] Belinostat[1,2,3] Blinatumomab[1,3] Bortezomib[1,3] Brentuximab vedotin[1,2,3] Cabazitaxel[1,2,3] Carfilzomib[1,2,3] Cetuximab[1,3] Copanlisib[1,2] Cytarabine (<1000 mg/m^2)[1,3] Decitabine[1] Docetaxel[1,2,3] Doxorubicin, liposomal[1,2,3] Elotuzumab[1] Eribulin[1,2,3] Etoposide[1,2,3] Floxuridine[2] Fluorouracil[1,2,3] Gemcitabine[1,2,3] Gemtuzumab ozogamicin[1,2] Inotuzumab ozogamicin[1,2]	Ipilimumab[3] Ixabepilone[1,2,3] Methotrexate (>50 to <250 mg/m^2)[2] Mitomycin[1,2,3] Mitoxantrone[1,2,3] Mogamulizumab[2] Moxetumomab pasudotox[1,2] Necitumumab[1,2] Nelarabine[1] Olaratumab[2] Omacetaxine mepesuccinate[2] Paclitaxel[1,2,3] Paclitaxel, albumin-bound suspension[1,2,3] Panitumumab[1,3] Pemetrexed[1,2,3] Pertuzumab[1,3] Polatuzumab vedotin[2] Pralatrexate[2] Tagraxofusp[1,2] Talimogene laherparepvec[2] Temsirolimus[1,3] Teniposide* Tisagenlecleucel[1,2] Topotecan[1,2,3] Ziv-aflibercept[1,2,3]
Minimal Frequency of emesis <10%	Alemtuzumab[2] Atezolizumab[1,2] Asparaginase[2] Avelumab[1,2] Bevacizumab[1,2,3] Bleomycin[1,2,3] Cemiplimab[1,2] Cladribine[1,2,3] Daratumumab[1,2] Durvalumab[1,2] Fludarabine[1,2,3] Methotrexate (<50 mg/m^2)[2] Nivolumab[1,2,3] Obinutuzumab[1,2] Ofatumumab[1,2,3]	Pegaspargase[2] Peginterferon[2] Pembrolizumab[1,2] Ramucirumab[1,2] Rituximab[1,2,3] Rituximab/hyaluronidase human injection[2] Siltuximab[2] Trastuzumab[1,2,3] Trastuzumab and hyaluronidase-oysk[2] Valrubicin[2] Vinblastine[1,2,3] Vincristine[1,2,3] Vincristine, liposome injection[2] Vinorelbine[1,2,3]

Classifications are adapted from references 1–3. Each agent is referenced to a specific guideline. When discrepancies existed among guidelines, the author classified the agent on personal opinion and referenced the guideline that supported the classification chosen. If the agent was not classified by a clinical guideline or the clinical guideline classification was in doubt, the classification was based on the incidence of emesis documented in product labeling
*Classified based on the incidence of emesis documented in product labeling

Table 42–4. Classification of Emetic Risk of Oral Antineoplastic Agents[1–3]

Emetic Potential	Chemotherapy Drug	
Moderate to High Frequency of emesis ≥30%	Altretamine (hexamethylmelamine)[1,2,3] Avapritinib[1,2] Binimetinib[2] Bosutinib[1,3] Busulfan (≥4 mg/day)[2] Ceritinib[1,2,3] Crizotinib[1,2,3] Cyclophosphamide (≥100 mg/m^2/day)[2] Dabrafenib[2] Enasidenib[1,2]	Etoposide[2] Fedratinib[1] Lenvatinib[1,2] Lomustine (single day)[2] Midostaurin[1,2] Mitotane[2] Niraparib[1,2] Olaparib[2] Procarbazine[1,2,3] Rucaparib[1,2] Selinexor[1,2] Temozolomide[1,2,3]

(*continued*)

Table 42–4. (*continued*)

Emetic Potential	Chemotherapy Drug	
Minimal to Low Frequency of emesis <30%	Abemaciclib[2]	Lenalidomide[1,2,3]
	Acalabrutinib[1,2]	Lorlatinib[1,2]
	Afatinib[1,2,3]	Melphalan[1,2,3]
	Alectinib[1,2]	Mercaptopurine[2]
	Alpelisib[1,2]	Methotrexate[1,2,3]
	Axatinib[1,2,3]	Neratinib[1,2]
	Bexarotene[1,2]	Nilotinib[1,2,3]
	Brigatinib[1,2]	Osimertinib[1,2]
	Busulfan (<4 mg/day)[2]	Palbociclib[1,2]
	Cabozantinib[2]	Panobinostat[1,2]
	Capecitabine[1,2,3]	Pazopanib[1,2,3]
	Chlorambucil[1,2,3]	Pexidartinib[1]
	Cobimetinib[1,2]	Pomalidomide[1,2,3]
	Cyclophosphamide (<100 mg/m²/day)[2]	Ponatinib[1,2,3]
	Dacomitinib[1,2]	Regorafinib[1,2,3]
	Dasatinib[1,2,3]	Ribociclib[2]
	Duvelisib[1,2]	Ruxolitinib[1,2,3]
	Entrectinib[1,2]	Sonidegib[1,2]
	Erdafitinib[1,2]	Sorafenib[1,2,3]
	Erlotinib[1,2,3]	Sunitinib[1,2,3]
	Estrumustine[1]	Talazoparib tosylate[1,2]
	Everolimus[1,2,3]	Thalidomide[1,2,3]
	Gefitinib[1,2,3]	Thioguanine[1,2,3]
	Gilteritinib[1,2]	Topotecan[1,2]
	Glasdegib[1,2]	Trametinib[1,2]
	Hydroxyurea[1,2,3]	Tretinoin[2]
	Ibrutinib[1,3]	Trifluridine/tipiracil[2]
	Idelalisib[1,2,3]	Vandetanib[1,2,3]
	Imatinib[2]	Vemurafenib[1,2,3]
	Ivosidenib[1,2]	Venetoclax[1,2]
	Ixazomib[1,2]	Vismodegib[1,2,3]
	Lapatinib[1,2,3]	Vorinostat[1,2,3]
	Larotrectinib[1,2]	Zanubrutinib[1,2]

Classifications are adapted from references 1–3. The moderate to high (emetic risk >30%) and the minimal to low classification (emetic risk <30%) are grouped together consistent with ASCO and NCCN antiemetic guidelines (references 1 and 2). The MASCC Antiemetic Guidelines differentiate all four emetic risk categories (reference 3). Each agent is referenced to a specific guideline. When discrepancies existed among guidelines, the author classified the agent on personal opinion and referenced the guideline that supported the classification chosen

Table 42–5. Antiemetic Regimens for Prophylaxis of CINV for Parenteral Chemotherapy (Adults)[1–5]

Emetic Potential	Acute Nausea and Vomiting Antiemetic Regimen (First 24 Hours, Day 1)	Delayed Nausea and Vomiting Antiemetic Regimen (>24 Hours, Days 2–4)	Notes and Comments
High Frequency of emesis >90%	5-HT$_3$ antagonist + dexamethasone + NK$_1$ antagonist + olanzapine (**preferred regimen**; all given as single doses 30–60 minutes prior to chemotherapy) *Alternative regimens* 5-HT$_3$ antagonist + dexamethasone + NK$_1$ antagonist *or* Palonosetron* + dexamethasone + olanzapine	Dexamethasone + olanzapine on days 2–4 + aprepitant (if aprepitant PO used on day 1) on days 2,3 Dexamethasone on days 2–4 + aprepitant (if aprepitant PO used on day 1) on days 2,3 Olanzapine on days 2–4	See Table 42–3 for emetic risk classification of parenteral chemotherapy agents and regimens Agents associated with delayed CINV include cisplatin, carboplatin, cyclophosphamide, anthracyclines (eg, doxorubicin, epirubicin) and drug combinations that include these agents See Table 42–6 for dosing recommendations for antiemetic agents Dexamethasone should *not* be used with certain immunotherapy or cellular therapy regimens (eg, aldesleukin or CAR T-cell therapies). Dexamethasone may be included in the prophylactic antiemetic regimen when checkpoint inhibitors are utilized in combination with emetogenic chemotherapy.[1]

(*continued*)

Table 42–5. (*continued*)

Emetic Potential	Acute Nausea and Vomiting Antiemetic Regimen (First 24 Hours, Day 1)	Delayed Nausea and Vomiting Antiemetic Regimen (>24 Hours, Days 2–4)	Notes and Comments
Moderate Frequency of emesis 30–60%	5-HT$_3$ antagonist + dexamethasone ± NK$_1$ antagonist or olanzapine (all given as single doses 30–60 minutes prior to chemotherapy)	Dexamethasone on days 2, 3 *or* Aprepitant on days 2, 3 (if PO aprepitant used on day 1) + dexamethasone on days 2, 3 *or* Olanzapine on days 2, 3 (if olanzapine used on day 1) *or* 5-HT$_3$ antagonist on days 2, 3	See above Prophylaxis on days 2 and 3 can be individualized and prioritized for regimens that carry a higher risk for delayed nausea and vomiting. A three-drug regimen that contains either an NK$_1$ antagonist or olanzapine should be considered for moderate emetogenic regimens for patients with higher patient-related risk factors and in patients with prior treatment failures with a two-drug regimen
Low Frequency of emesis 10–30%	Dexamethasone (a single dose 30–60 minutes prior to chemotherapy *or* 5-HT$_3$ antagonist (a single dose 30–60 minutes prior to chemotherapy) *or* Dopaminergic antagonist (a single dose 30–60 minutes prior to chemotherapy)	Not necessary	Dopaminergic antagonists include prochlorperazine, chlorpromazine, haloperidol, metoclopramide, perphenazine, and promethazine
Minimal Frequency of emesis <10%	Antiemetic prophylaxis is usually not necessary	Not necessary	See above

*The NCCN antiemesis guideline[2] recommends palonosetron as the preferred 5-HT$_3$ receptor antagonist in combination antiemetic regimens that do not include an NK$_1$ receptor antagonist

Table 42–6. **Dosing Recommendations for CINV Prophylaxis (Adults) for Moderate to Highly Emetic Parenteral Chemotherapy[1–5]**

Agent	Acute CINV Prophylaxis (Day 1)*			Delayed CINV Prophylaxis (Days 2–5)	Dosage Forms
	Oral (PO)	Intravenous (IV)	Other		
5-HT$_3$ receptor antagonists					
Dolasetron mesylate (Anzemet)	100 mg PO	Not recommended		100 mg PO daily for 2–4 days	Injection Tablets: 50 mg, 100 mg
Granisetron HCl (Kytril)	2 mg PO	1 mg or 0.01 mg/kg IV		1 mg PO twice daily for 2–4 days	Injection Tablets: 1 mg
Granisetron extended-release injection (Sustol)			10 mg by subcutaneous injection administered as a single dose at least 30 minutes prior to emetogenic treatment		Injection
Granisetron transdermal system (Sancuso)	NA	NA	Apply 1 patch to the upper outer arm 24–48 hours before chemotherapy Patches are removed a minimum of 24 hours after emetogenic treatment is completed, and may be worn for up to 7 days		Transdermal system: 52-cm² patch delivers 3.1 mg/24 hours

(*continued*)

Table 42–6. (*continued*)

Agent	Acute CINV Prophylaxis (Day 1)*			Delayed CINV Prophylaxis (Days 2–5)	Dosage Forms
	Oral (PO)	Intravenous (IV)	Other		
Ondansetron HCl (Zofran)	16–24 mg PO	8 mg or 0.15 mg/kg IV		8 mg PO twice daily for 2–4 days	Injection Tablets: 4 mg, 8 mg, 24 mg Oral solution: 4 mg/5 mL Orally disintegrating tablets: 4 mg, 8 mg
Ondansetron oral soluble film (Zuplenz)	High emetic risk: 24 mg PO, 30 minutes before emetogenic treatment Moderate emetic risk: 8 mg PO, 30 minutes before emetogenic treatment, then 8 mg PO 8 hours after emetogenic treatment	NA		8 mg PO every 12 hours for 1–2 days	Oral soluble film: 4 mg, 8 mg
Palonosetron HCl (Aloxi)	NA	0.25 mg IV		NA	Injection
Palonosetron/ netupitant (PO) or fosnetupitant (IV) (Akynzeo)	0.5 mg PO (with 300 mg netupitant), 60 minutes prior to emetogenic treatment	0.25 mg IV (with 235 mg fosnetupitant), 30 minutes prior to emetogenic treatment		NA	Injection Capsule: 300 mg netupitant and 0.5 mg of palonosetron

Notes:
- Because of its long half-life, palonosetron is usually given as a single dose prior to moderately and highly emetogenic chemotherapy with demonstrable efficacy against developing delayed CINV symptoms on subsequent days
- When utilized as prophylaxis in a multiple-day chemotherapy regimen, alternative palonosetron administration strategies have been employed (eg, days 1, 3, and 5, during a chemotherapy regimen in which cisplatin 20 mg/m² is given daily for 5 consecutive days)

Corticosteroids

Agent	Oral (PO)	Intravenous (IV)	Other	Delayed	Dosage Forms
Dexamethasone phosphate (Decadron)	8–20 mg PO	8–20 mg IV		4 mg twice daily *or* 8 mg PO daily *or* 8 mg twice daily for 2–4 days	Injection Tablets: numerous tablet strengths
Methylprednisolone sodium succinate (Solu-Medrol)	NA	40–125 mg IV		NA	Injection

Notes:
- For highly emetogenic chemotherapy, dexamethasone doses of 20 mg have been shown to be more efficacious than lower doses. In moderately emetogenic chemotherapy, doses greater than 8 mg have not been shown superior to an 8-mg dose
- Dexamethasone doses should be reduced when combined with aprepitant, fosaprepitant, or netupitant due to inhibition of CYP3A4 by these NK$_1$ receptor antagonists. When combined with aprepitant, IV doses of dexamethasone should be reduced by 25%, and PO doses of dexamethasone should be reduced by 50%. A 12-mg dose of dexamethasone on day 1 of chemotherapy for acute prophylaxis in combination with aprepitant or netupitant is the only dexamethasone dose evaluated in large randomized trials. Dose reduction of dexamethasone is not required when combined with rolapitant

(*continued*)

Table 42–6. (*continued*)

| Agent | Acute CINV Prophylaxis (Day 1)* | | | Delayed CINV Prophylaxis (Days 2–5) | Dosage Forms |
	Oral (PO)	Intravenous (IV)	Other		
NK₁ Receptor Antagonists					
Aprepitant (Emend)	125 mg PO	NA		80 mg PO daily for 2 days	Capsules: 80 mg, 125 mg Oral Suspension: 125 mg
Fosaprepitant (Emend)	NA	150 mg IV		Not evaluated	Injection
Netupitant/ palonosetron	300 mg PO (with 0.5 mg palonosetron)	NA		NA	Capsule: 300 mg netupitant and 0.5 mg of palonosetron
Rolapitant	180 mg PO	166.5 mg IV		NA	Injection Tablet: 90 mg

Notes:
- Aprepitant has been evaluated only in single-day chemotherapy regimens and therefore is recommended to be given for 3 days, with an initial dose of aprepitant 125 mg on the day of chemotherapy plus 80 mg/day on days 2 and 3 after emetogenic treatment. If utilized in a multiple-day chemotherapy regimen, longer durations may be indicated (80 mg/day); however, the safety data with longer use of aprepitant are not well established
- Fosaprepitant has been evaluated in 2 dosing formats. It has been used in a 3-day regimen with fosaprepitant 115 mg IV on day 1, followed by 80 mg/day orally on days 2 and 3 after chemotherapy. It has also been studied in a single-dose regimen with fosaprepitant 150 mg on day 1 prior to chemotherapy with no additional aprepitant doses administered subsequently during the same course of emetogenic treatment. The single-dose 150 mg fosaprepitant regimen was shown to be non-inferior to the alternative 3-dose aprepitant regimen in a randomized study of patients receiving a highly emetogenic, cisplatin-based chemotherapy regimen and is the only current FDA-approved dosing regimen in adults[14]
- Drug interaction considerations with NK₁ receptor antagonists[13–16]
  - Aprepitant/fosaprepitant is a substrate, moderate inhibitor, and inducer of CYP3A4 when used at doses utilized in CINV prophylaxis. In addition, aprepitant/fosaprepitant can induce CYP2C9. Drug interactions of note include dexamethasone, pimozide, benzodiazepines, oral contraceptives, and warfarin
  - Netupitant is a substrate and moderate inhibitor of CYP3A4. Drug interactions of note with netupitant include dexamethasone and benzodiazepines
  - Rolapitant is a substrate of CYP3A4 but is neither an inducer nor an inhibitor of CYP3A4. Rolapitant is a moderate inhibitor of CYP2D6 and an inhibitor of breast cancer resistance protein (BCRP) and P-glycoprotein. Drug interactions of note include CYP2D6 substrates with a narrow therapeutic index (eg, thioridazine, pimozide) and BCRP substrates with a narrow therapeutic index (eg, methotrexate, topotecan, irinotecan)

*For chemotherapy/biologic regimens where emetogenic agents are given either multiple times within the same day or by continuous IV infusions, alternative multiple-dose antiemetic regimens may be indicated
†Delayed CINV has been associated with cisplatin, carboplatin, cyclophosphamide, and anthracyclines (eg, doxorubicin, epirubicin)
NA, not applicable

Table 42–7. Antiemetic Regimens for Prophylaxis of CINV for Oral Chemotherapy (Adults)[2]

Emetic Potential	Antiemetic Regimen	Drug and Dosing Recommendations (Order Does Not Imply Preference)
Moderate to High Frequency of emesis ≥30%	5-HT₃ receptor antagonist (scheduled prior to chemotherapy and continued daily)	Dolasetron 100 mg PO once daily
		Granisetron 1 mg to 2 mg PO once daily or 1 mg PO twice daily or 3.1 mg/24 hour transdermal patch every 7 days
		Ondansetron 8 mg to 16 mg PO once daily or 8 mg PO twice daily
Minimal to Low Frequency of emesis < 30%	PRN antiemetics Consider escalation to scheduled antiemetics prior to chemotherapy and continued daily based on symptoms	See Table 42–8 for treating CINV
		If escalated to scheduled daily antiemetics, consider the following regimens based on NCCN Antiemesis guidelines[2]
		Metoclopramide 10–20 mg PO daily and then every 6 hours PRN (maximum 40 mg/day)
		or
		Prochlorperazine 10 mg PO daily and then every 6 hours PRN (maximum 40 mg/day)
		or
		5-HT₃ receptor antagonist (as noted above for moderate to high emetic risk)

Table 42–8. Antiemetics for Treatment of Chemotherapy-Induced Nausea and Vomiting (Adults)

Pharmacologic Classes/Agents	Dosage Form	Adult Dosages, Routes, and Schedules
Atypical antipsychotic		
Olanzapine (Zyprexa, others)	Tablets Oral disintegrating tablets	5–10 mg PO once daily
Dopaminergic antagonists: phenothiazines		
Chlorpromazine (Thorazine, others)	Oral solution	10–25 mg PO every 4–6 hours
	Tablets	10–25 mg PO every 4–6 hours
	Injection	25–50 mg IVPB/IM every 4–6 hours*
Perphenazine (Trilafon)	Tablets	2–4 mg PO every 8 hours
Prochlorperazine (Compazine, others)	Tablets	5–10 mg PO every 6 hours
	Suppositories	25 mg PR every 12 hours
	Injection	5–10 mg IV/IM every 6 hours*
Promethazine (Phenergan)	Tablets	12.5–25 mg PO every 4–6 hours
	Suppositories	12.5–25 mg PR every 4–6 hours
	Injection	12.5–25 mg IV every 4–6 hours†
Dopaminergic antagonists: butyrophenones		
Haloperidol (Haldol, others)	Tablets	0.5–2 mg PO every 6 hours
	Injection	0.5–2 mg IV/IM every 6 hours*
Substituted benzamide		
Metoclopramide (Reglan, others)	Tablets	10–40 mg (or 0.5 mg/kg) PO every 6 hours
	Injection	10–40 mg (or 0.5 mg/kg) IV every 6 hours‡
Corticosteroids		
Dexamethasone	Tablets/oral solution	4–10 mg PO every 6–12 hours
	Injection	4–10 mg IV every 6–12 hours
Methylprednisolone	Injection	20–125 mg IV/IM every 6 hours
Benzodiazepines§		
Alprazolam (Xanax)	Tablets	0.125–0.5 mg PO every 8 hours
Lorazepam (Ativan)	Tablets	0.5–1 mg PO every 6–12 hours
	Injection	0.5–1 mg IV every 6–12 hours
Cannabinoids		
Dronabinol (Marinol)	Capsules	2.5–10 mg PO every 6 hours
Nabilone (Cesamet)	Capsules	1–2 mg PO every 8–12 hours

*Rapid IV administration may induce hypotension. See product labeling for rate recommendation. Administer by slow IV push or by IV infusion (eg, over 30 minutes)
†Promethazine injection is a potential vesicant. Use caution with intravenous administration, particularly during administration into a peripheral vein. Drug dilution and administration by IV infusion are techniques that may reduce vascular irritation
‡Greater metoclopramide doses have been utilized for the prophylaxis of CINV for highly emetic chemotherapy
§Benzodiazepines lack intrinsic antiemetic effects and should not be used as single agents against emetogenic chemotherapy
IM, intramuscular; IV, intravenous; IVPB, IV piggyback (IV infusion of short duration); PO, orally; PR, per rectum (suppository)

Table 42–9. Antiemetic Regimens for Prophylaxis of RINV (Adults)[1–5]

Emetic Potential	Antiemetic Regimen	Drug and Dosing Recommendations (Order Does Not Imply Preference)
High Frequency of emesis ≥90% Radiation site: Total body irradiation	5-HT$_3$ receptor antagonist + dexamethasone	Administer once or twice daily prior to radiation therapy and the day after each fraction) 5-HT$_3$ receptor antagonist[†]: Granisetron 2 mg PO once daily or 1 mg PO twice daily or 1 mg (or 0.01 mg/kg IV once daily Ondansetron 8 mg PO or 8 mg (or 0.15 mg/kg) IV once to twice daily Corticosteroid: Dexamethasone 4 mg PO or IV once daily
Moderate Frequency of emesis 30–90% Radiation site: Upper abdomen* Craniospinal	5-HT$_3$ receptor antagonist ± (optional) dexamethasone (administer prior to each fraction)	Administer once or twice daily prior to radiation therapy and the day after each fraction) 5-HT$_3$ receptor antagonist[†]: Granisetron 2 mg PO once daily or 1 mg PO twice daily or 1 mg (or 0.01 mg/kg IV once daily Ondansetron 8 mg PO or 8 mg (or 0.15 mg/kg) IV once to twice daily Corticosteroid: Dexamethasone 4 mg PO or IV once daily
Low Frequency of emesis 10–30% Radiation site: Brain Head and neck Thorax Pelvis	PRN rescue therapy with: 5-HT$_3$ receptor antagonist *or* Dexamethasone (preferred agent for brain irradiation) *or* Dopamine receptor antagonist	5-HT$_3$ receptor antagonist[†]: Granisetron 2 mg PO once daily or 1 mg PO twice daily or 1 mg (or 0.01 mg/kg IV once daily PRN Ondansetron 8 mg PO or 8 mg (or 0.15 mg/kg) IV three times daily PRN Corticosteroid: Dexamethasone 4 mg PO/IV PRN titrated up to a maximum of 16 mg/day Dopamine receptor antagonist: Prochlorperazine 5–10 mg PO/IV every 6 hours PRN Metoclopramide 5–20 mg PO/IV every 6 hours PRN
Minimal Frequency of emesis <10% Radiation site: Extremities Breast	PRN rescue therapy with: 5-HT$_3$ receptor antagonist *or* Dexamethasone *or* Dopamine receptor antagonist	See above recommendations for low emetic risk

*Upper-abdomen radiation defined by ASCO Antiemetic Guidelines as the anatomic region that extends from the superior border of the 11th thoracic vertebra to the inferior border of the third lumbar vertebra[5]
[†]Granisetron and ondansetron are the preferred 5-HT$_3$ receptor antagonists per ASCO and NCCN guidelines due to a larger body of evidence for these agents[1,2,5]

References

1. Hesketh PJ et al. Antiemetics: ASCO Guideline Update. J Clin Oncol 2020; 38(24):2782–2797
2. NCCN Clinical Practice Guidelines in Oncology. Antiemesis version 2.2020, April 23, 2020. Available from: http://www.nccn.org
3. Roila F et al. 2016 MASCC and ESMO guideline update for the prevention of chemotherapy- and radiotherapy-induced nausea and vomiting and of nausea and vomiting in advanced cancer patients. Ann Oncol 2016;27(suppl 5):v119–v133
4. MASCC/ESMO. Antiemetic Guidelines. 2016. Available from: http://www.mascc.org/antiemetic-guidelines
5. Hesketh PJ et al. Antiemetics: American Society of Clinical Oncology clinical practice guideline update. J Clin Oncol 2017; 35(28):3240–3261
6. Zofran (ondansetron hydrochloride) injection for intravenous or intramuscular use [package insert]. Research Triangle Park, NC: GlaxoSmithKline; March 2017
7. Zofran (ondansetron hydrochloride) Tablets, Zofran ODT (ondansetron) Orally Disintegrating Tablets, Zofran (ondansetron hydrochloride) Oral Solution [package insert]. East Hanover, NJ: Novartis Pharmaceuticals Corporation; August 2017
8. Kytril (granisetron hydrochloride) tablets, oral solution [package insert]. Nutley, NJ: Roche Laboratories, Inc.; March 2010
9. Kytril (granisetron hydrochloride) injection for intravenous use [package insert]. South San Francisco, CA: Genentech USA, Inc.; April 2011
10. Anzemet (dolasetron mesylate) tablets [package insert]. Parsippany, NJ: Validus Pharmaceuticals; June 2016
11. Aloxi (palonosetron HCl) injection for intravenous use [package insert]. Woodcliff Lake, NJ: Eisai, Inc.; December 2015
12. Davidson TG. Causes and prevention of chemotherapy-induced emesis. Philadelphia: Medical Education Systems, Inc.; 1996;34–.5
13. Emend (aprepitant) capsules and oral suspension [package insert]. Whitehouse Station, NJ: Merck & Co., Inc.; November 2019
14. Emend (fosaprepitant) for injection, for intravenous use [package insert]. Whitehouse Station, NJ: Merck & Co., Inc.; April 2020
15. Varubi (rolapitant) tablets and injectable emulsion [package insert]. Lake Forest, IL: TerSara Therapeutics LLC; September 2018
16. Akynzeo (netupitant and palonosetron) capsules and (fosnetupitan and palonosetron) injection [package insert]. Lugano, Switzerland: Helsinn Healthcare SA.; May 2020
17. Sustol (granisetron) extended-release injection [package insert], San Diego, CA: Heron Therapeutics; May 2017
18. Raftopoulos H et al. Comparison of an extended-release formulation of granisetron (APF530) versus palonosetron for the prevention of chemotherapy-induced nausea and vomiting associated with moderately or highly emetogenic chemotherapy: Results of a prospective, randomized, double-blind, noninferiority phase 3 trial. Support Care Cancer 2015;23:3281–3288
19. Navari RM et al. Olanzapine for the prevention of chemotherapy-induced nausea and vomiting. N Engl J Med 2016;375:134–142

43. Indications for Growth Factors in Hematology-Oncology

Gerard P. Mascara, PharmD, BCOP and Tito Fojo, MD, PhD

Febrile Neutropenia

Epidemiology

Febrile neutropenia is a major dose-limiting toxicity of chemotherapy. Studies have demonstrated that selective use of colony-stimulating factors (CSFs) in patients at high risk for complications of neutropenia can enhance cost-effectiveness by reducing the risk, severity, and duration of febrile neutropenia

NCI Common Terminology Criteria for Adverse Events (CTCAE) Version 5.0 Neutrophil Count Decreased[1]

Grade	ANC
0	Normal
1	≥1500/mm³ to LLN
2	≥1000 to <1500/mm³
3	≥500 to <1000/mm³
4	<500/mm³

ANC, absolute neutrophil count; LLN, lower limit of normal range

WHO Toxicity Criteria[2]

Grade	AGC
0	≥2000/mm³
1	1500–1900/mm³
2	1000–1400/mm³
3	500–900/mm³
4	<500/mm³

AGC, absolute granulocyte count; WHO, World Health Organization

Examples of Regimens with >20% Risk of Febrile Neutropenia[3]

Cancer Type	Regimen
Acute lymphoblastic leukemia	Use of growth factor varies according to protocol
Bladder cancer	Dose-dense MVAC (methotrexate, vinblastine, doxorubicin, cisplatin)
Bone cancer	VAI (vincristine, doxorubicin or dactinomycin, ifosfamide)
	VDC-IE (vincristine, doxorubicin or dactinomycin, and cyclophosphamide alternating with ifosfamide and etoposide)
	Cisplatin, doxorubicin
	VDC (vincristine, doxorubicin or dactinomycin, cyclophosphamide)
	VIDE (vincristine, ifosfamide, doxorubicin or dactinomycin, etoposide)
Breast cancer	Dose-dense AC→T (doxorubicin, cyclophosphamide, paclitaxel)
	Docetaxel, cyclophosphamide ± trastuzumab
	TAC (docetaxel, doxorubicin, cyclophosphamide)
	TC(H) (docetaxel, carboplatin, ± trastuzumab)
Colorectal cancer	FOLFOXIRI (fluorouracil, leucovorin, oxaliplatin, irinotecan)
Head and neck squamous cell carcinoma	TPF (docetaxel, cisplatin, fluorouracil)
Hodgkin lymphoma	A+AVD (brentuximab vedotin, doxorubicin, vinblastine, dacarbazine)
	Escalated BEACOPP (bleomycin, etoposide, doxorubicin, cyclophosphamide, vincristine, procarbazine, prednisone)
Kidney cancer	Doxorubicin, gemcitabine
Non-Hodgkin lymphoma	Dose-adjusted EPOCH (etoposide, prednisone, vincristine, cyclophosphamide, doxorubicin ± rituximab)
	ICE (ifosfamide, carboplatin, etoposide ± rituximab)
	Dose-dense CHOP-14 (cyclophosphamide, doxorubicin, vincristine, prednisone ± rituximab)
	MINE (mesna, ifosfamide, mitoxantrone, etoposide ± rituximab)
	ESHAP (etoposide, methylprednisolone, cisplatin, cytarabine ± rituximab)
	Hyper-CVAD (cyclophosphamide, vincristine, doxorubicin, dexamethasone, ± rituximab)
	DHAP (dexamethasone, cisplatin, cytarabine ± rituximab)
Melanoma	Dacarbazine-based combinations (with: cisplatin, vinblastine, aldesleukin [IL-2], interferon alfa)

(continued)

Treatment Overview

Indications for CSFs per ASCO 2015 Guidelines[4]

Prophylaxis in patients undergoing myelosuppressive chemotherapy

- As primary prophylaxis in patients at high risk (>20%) of developing FN based on patient-, disease-, and treatment-related factors*

- As primary prophylaxis in patients with diffuse aggressive lymphomas aged ≥65 years treated with curative chemotherapy (CHOP or more aggressive regimens), particularly in patients with comorbidities[†]

- As primary prophylaxis in patients receiving dose-dense or dose-intense regimens supported by convincing efficacy data, eg:
  - Dose-dense chemotherapy regimens used in the adjuvant treatment of high-risk breast cancer*
  - Dose-dense MVAC (methotrexate, vinblastine, doxorubicin, cisplatin) for the treatment of urothelial cancer[†]
  - Interval-compressed (every 14 days) VDC (vincristine, doxorubicin, cyclophosphamide) alternating with IE (ifosfamide/etoposide) for treatment of pediatric Ewing sarcoma*

- As secondary prophylaxis in patients who experienced a neutropenic complication during a prior cycle of chemotherapy given without CSF use when a reduced chemotherapy dose or treatment delay might compromise disease-free or overall survival or treatment outcome*

Adjunctive Therapy for FN

- Patients with FN who are at high risk for infection-associated complications or poor clinical outcomes, as an adjunct to antibiotic therapy*
  - Risk factors for poor outcome include:
    - Sepsis syndrome
    - Age >65 years
    - ANC <100/mm^3
    - Expected duration of neutropenia >10 days
    - Pneumonia
    - Invasive fungal infection
    - Other clinically documented infections
    - Hospitalization at fever onset
    - Prior episode(s) of neutropenic fever

(continued)

Examples of Regimens with >20% Risk of Febrile Neutropenia[3] *(continued)*

Multiple myeloma	DT-PACE (dexamethasone, thalidomide, cisplatin, doxorubicin, cyclophosphamide, etoposide ± bortezomib)
Ovarian cancer	Topotecan ± bevacizumab
	Docetaxel
Pancreatic adenocarcinoma	FOLFIRINOX (fluorouracil, leucovorin, irinotecan, oxaliplatin)
Soft tissue sarcoma	MAID (mesna, doxorubicin, ifosfamide, dacarbazine)
	Doxorubicin
	Doxorubicin/ifosfamide
Small cell lung cancer	Topotecan
Testicular cancer	VeIP (vinblastine, ifosfamide, cisplatin)
	VIP (etoposide, ifosfamide, cisplatin)
	TIP (paclitaxel, ifosfamide, cisplatin)

Preparations[5–13]

Products	Approved Route(s) of Administration	Commercially Available Strengths
Filgrastim and biosimilars	Subcutaneous, intravenous	Vials containing 300 μg/1 mL or 480 μg/1.6 mL Prefilled syringes (with needle guard) containing 300 μg/0.5 mL or 480 μg/0.8 mL
tbo-Filgrastim	Subcutaneous	Prefilled syringes (with needle guard)* containing 300 μg/0.5 mL or 480 μg/0.8 mL Prefilled syringes (without needle guard)[†] containing 300 μg/0.5 mL or 480 μg/0.8 mL Vials containing 300 μg/1 mL or 480 μg/1.6 mL
Pegfilgrastim and biosimilars	Subcutaneous	Prefilled syringe containing 6 mg/0.6 mL
Pegfilgrastim kit with on-body injector	Subcutaneous	Prefilled syringe containing pegfilgrastim 6.4 mg/0.64 mL that delivers 6 mg/0.6 mL when used with the copackaged on-body injector

*For administration by a health care professional only
[†]For administration by a patient or caregiver

ASCO 2015 guidelines state that pegfilgrastim, filgrastim, tbo-filgrastim, filgrastim-sndz (and other biosimilars, as they become available) can be used for the prevention of treatment-related neutropenia. Factors to consider when choosing an agent include convenience, cost, and clinical situation[4]

Only Neupogen and Neulasta products have a U.S. Food and Drug Administration (FDA)-approved indication for increasing survival in patients acutely exposed to myelosuppressive doses of radiation.[5,9] Biosimilar products do not carry this indication

tbo-Filgrastim was approved in the United States through an original biologics license application prior to the adoption of a standard biosimilar regulatory pathway. Therefore, it is not considered a biosimilar to Neupogen. The FDA-approved prescribing information includes only one approved indication for tbo-filgrastim compared with six approved indications for Neupogen.[5,8] The approved indication is for adult and pediatric patients 1 month and older for reduction in the duration of severe neutropenia in patients with nonmyeloid malignancies receiving myelosuppressive anticancer drugs associated with a clinically significant incidence of febrile neutropenia

Treatment Overview
(continued)

HSCT

- Patients requiring mobilization of peripheral-blood progenitor cells, either alone, after chemotherapy, or in combination with plerixafor as clinically appropriate*

- Patients who have undergone autologous HSCT* or allogeneic HSCT‡ to reduce the duration of severe neutropenia

Hematopoietic Subsyndrome of Acute Radiation Syndrome

- Patients exposed to lethal doses of TBI, but not doses high enough to lead to certain death as a result of injury to other organs†

*High-quality evidence, strong recommendation
†Intermediate-quality evidence, moderate strength recommendation
‡Low-quality evidence, weak recommendation
CSF, colony stimulating factor; FN, febrile neutropenia; ANC, absolute neutrophil count; HSCT, hematopoietic stem cell transplant; TBI, total body irradiation

The chemotherapy regimens given as examples increase a patient's risk of developing febrile neutropenia. Additional risk factors to be considered when evaluating a patient's overall risk of febrile neutropenia according to the ASCO guidelines include:[4]

- Age ≥65 years
- Advanced disease
- Previous chemotherapy or radiation therapy
- Bone marrow involvement with tumor
- Preexisting conditions including:
  - Neutropenia
  - Infection/open wounds
  - Recent surgery
- Poor performance status
- Poor nutritional status
- Poor renal function
- Cardiovascular disease
- Multiple comorbid conditions
- HIV infection
- Liver dysfunction, especially elevated bilirubin

NCI Common Terminology Criteria for Adverse Events (CTCAE) Version 5.0 Febrile Neutropenia[1]

Grade	
3	ANC <1000/mm^3 with a single temperature >38.3°C (>101°F) or a sustained temperature ≥38°C (≥100.4°F) for more than 1 hour
4	Life-threatening consequences; urgent intervention indicated
5	Death

1. NCI, CTCAE, National Cancer Institute (USA) Common Terminology Criteria for Adverse Events, version 5.0. At: https://ctep.cancer.gov/protocoldevelopment/electronic_applications/docs/ctcae_v5_quick_reference_5x7.pdf [accessed November 19, 2020]
2. WHO Handbook for Reporting Results of Cancer Treatment. World Health Organization Offset Publication No. 48. Geneva, 1979. At: https://apps.who.int/iris/bitstream/handle/10665/37200/WHO_OFFSET_48.pdf [accessed December 6, 2020]
3. Hematopoietic growth factors. Version 2.2020. NCCN Clinical Practice Guidelines in Oncology (NCCN Guidelines). National Comprehensive Cancer Network, Inc., 2013. At: http://www.nccn.org [accessed November 19, 2020]
4. Smith TJ et al. J Clin Oncol 2015;33:3199–3212
5. Neupogen (filgrastim) prescribing information. Thousand Oaks, CA: Amgen Inc.; June 2018
6. ZARXIO (filgrastim-sndz) prescribing information. Princeton, NJ: Sandoz Inc.; February 2017
7. NIVESTYM (filgrastim-aafi) prescribing information. Lake Forest, IL: Hospira, Inc.; July 2018
8. GRANIX (tbo-filgrastim) prescribing information. North Wales, PA: Teva Pharmaceuticals USA, Inc.; April 2020
9. NEULASTA (pegfilgrastim) injection for subcutaneous use; prescribing information. Thousand Oaks, CA: Amgen, Inc.; January 2020
10. UDENYCA (pegfilgrastim-cbqv) injection for subcutaneous use; prescribing information. Redwood City, CA: Coherus BioSciences, Inc.; September 2019
11. FULPHILA (pegfilgrastim-jmdb) injection for subcutaneous use; prescribing information. Rockford, IL: Mylan Institutional LLC; June 2020
12. ZIEXTENZO (pegfilgrastim-bmez) injection for subcutaneous use; prescribing information. Princeton, NJ: Sandoz Inc.; September 2020
13. NYVEPRIA (pegfilgrastim-apgf) injection for subcutaneous use; prescribing information. New York, NY: Pfizer Inc.; June 2020

REGIMEN

FILGRASTIM (G-CSF, NEUPOGEN, AND BIOSIMILARS)

Patients with cancer receiving myelosuppressive chemotherapy:[1–3]
Filgrastim (or biosimilar) 5 μg/kg per day; administer by subcutaneous injection, short intravenous infusion (over 15–30 minutes), or continuous subcutaneous or intravenous infusion beginning 1–3 days after completion of chemotherapy and continuing until ANC reaches 10,000/mm³ or clinically sufficient neutrophil count is achieved after nadir

Notes:
- Calculated doses may be rounded to use the most economical combination of available products (commercial vials and syringes contain either 300 μg or 480 μg)
- FDA-approved labeling indicates subcutaneous or intravenous administration for up to 2 weeks after expected chemotherapy-induced ANC nadir
- It is recommended not to use filgrastim within 24 hours before or 24 hours after chemotherapy administration

Dose Adjustment:
- Dosages may be increased in increments of 5 μg/kg per dose for each chemotherapy cycle, according to the duration and severity of the ANC nadir

Patients with cancer receiving bone marrow/peripheral blood stem cell transplants (BMT/PBPCT):
Filgrastim (or biosimilar) 10 μg/kg per day; administer by intravenous infusion over 4 or 24 hours or as a continuous 24-hour subcutaneous infusion
Note: Administer at least 24 hours after cytotoxic chemotherapy, and at least 24 hours after bone marrow infusion

Dosage adjustment:
- When ANC >1000/mm³ for 3 consecutive days, reduce dose to 5 μg/kg per day
- If ANC remains >1000/mm³ for 3 more consecutive days, discontinue G-CSF
- If ANC decreases to <1000/mm³, resume at 5 μg/kg per day
- If ANC decreases to <1000/mm³ at any time during administration of 5 μg/kg per day, increase G-CSF dosage to 10 μg/kg per day and follow dose adjustment guidelines

Peripheral blood progenitor cells (PBPCs) collection:
Filgrastim 10 μg/kg/day; administer by subcutaneous injection

Notes:
- The optimal timing and duration of growth factor stimulation have not been determined
- Administration is recommended to begin 4 days before the first leukapheresis and continued until the last leukapheresis

Severe chronic neutropenia (SCN):
Congenital neutropenia
Filgrastim 6 μg/kg per dose; administer by subcutaneous injection twice daily, continually
Idiopathic or cyclic neutropenia
Filgrastim 5 μg/kg per day; administer by subcutaneous injection, continually

Notes:
- Chronic daily administration is needed to maintain clinical benefit
- ANC should not be used as the sole indication of efficacy
  - Dosages should be individually adjusted based on a patient's clinical course as well as ANC
- In a postmarketing surveillance study, median daily doses were 6 μg/kg (congenital neutropenia), 2.1 μg/kg (cyclic neutropenia), and 1.2 μg/kg (idiopathic neutropenia). In rare instances patients with congenital neutropenia have required dosages ≥100 μg/kg per day

Notes on dosing:
- The recommendations listed apply only to adult patients
- Doses for obese patients should be calculated on actual body weight, including morbidly obese patients
- Do not empirically reduce doses in elderly patients because of patient age

(continued)

Efficacy[1–3]

- In a phase 3 placebo-controlled trial of patients with small cell lung cancer, filgrastim use reduced the incidence of febrile neutropenia after chemotherapy by 36% (76% vs 40%; P<0.001)
- An increase in ANC is seen approximately 24 hours after beginning filgrastim administration
- A 50% decrease in circulating neutrophils occurs within 1–2 days after discontinuing filgrastim use, which returns to pretreatment levels within 4–7 days
- In patients with AML receiving induction chemotherapy, filgrastim use reduced the median time to ANC recovery by 5 days (P<0.0001), the median duration of fever by 1.5 days (P = 0.009), and resulted in a statistically significant reduction in duration of intravenous antibiotic use and hospitalization
- In patients with AML receiving consolidation therapy, filgrastim significantly reduced the incidence of severe neutropenia, time to neutrophil recovery, the incidence and duration of fever, and the duration of intravenous antibiotic use and hospitalization
- After BMT, patients who received filgrastim support had a statistically significant reduction in the median number of days of severe neutropenia (21.5 vs 10 days) and in the number of days of febrile neutropenia (13.5 vs 5 days)
- In mobilized PBPCs, both CFU-GM and CD34+ cells were increased by more than 10-fold from baseline on day 5, and remained increased with leukapheresis. During engraftment, filgrastim-treated patients had significantly fewer days of platelet transfusion (median 6 vs 10 days), fewer days of RBC transfusion (median 2 vs 3 days), and significantly shorter time to recover a sustained ANC ≥500/mm³
- In 120 patients with severe chronic neutropenia, filgrastim treatment resulted in significant benefits in the incidence and duration of infection, fever, antibiotic use, and oropharyngeal ulcers

(continued)

Preparation for intravenous administration:
- Filgrastim may be diluted in 5% dextrose injection (D5W) to a concentration within the range of 5–15 μg/mL
  - Dilution to concentrations <5 μg/mL is not recommended
- The diluted product must be protected from adsorption to container and administration set surfaces by adding albumin (human) to the vehicle solution (D5W) to a final concentration of 2 mg/mL *BEFORE* adding filgrastim
- *Do not* dilute filgrastim with sodium chloride–containing solutions
  - Admixture in saline solutions may cause precipitation
- The needle cover of prefilled syringes contains dry natural rubber (a latex derivative), which may cause allergic reactions in sensitive individuals. This does not apply to all available products (including biosimilars); therefore consult individual product labeling for detailed information

Adverse Events

Adverse Events Reported Among Patients with Cancer Receiving Myelosuppressive Chemotherapy and GCSF Support in Clinical Trials[1–3]

Allergic reactions (<1 in 4000)	Dyspnea (9%)	Fever and neutropenia (13%)
Alopecia (18%)	Fatigue (11%)	Pain, unspecified (2%)
Anorexia (9%)	Fever (12%)	Skeletal pain (22%)
Chest pain (5%)	Generalized weakness (4%)	Skin rash (6%)
Constipation (5%)	Headache (7%)	Sore throat (4%)
Cough (6%)	Mucositis (12%)	Stomatitis (5%)
Diarrhea (14%)	Nausea/Vomiting (57%)	

- Bone pain was reported more frequently in patients treated at high dosages, 20–100 μg/kg per day administered intravenously compared with low dosages of 3–10 μg/kg per day administered subcutaneously. Bone pain is generally controlled with nonopioid analgesics but may infrequently require opioids
- Spontaneously reversible, mild-to-moderate increases in serum uric acid, lactate dehydrogenase, and alkaline phosphatase, occurred in 27–58% of 98 patients receiving cytotoxic chemotherapy

Adverse Events Reported Postmarketing[1–3]
1. Splenomegaly and splenic rupture, including fatalities
2. Acute respiratory distress syndrome (ARDS)
3. Anaphylaxis
4. Alveolar hemorrhage and hemoptysis
5. Sickle cell crisis, including fatalities
6. Glomerulonephritis
7. Capillary leak syndrome
8. Myelodysplastic syndrome and acute myelogenous leukemia in patients with congenital neutropenia
9. Thrombocytopenia
10. Cutaneous vasculitis
11. Aortitis
12. Sweet's syndrome (acute febrile neutrophilic dermatosis)
13. Decreased bone density and osteoporosis in pediatric patients with severe chronic neutropenia (SCN) receiving chronic CSF treatment

Indications[1–3]

Patients with neoplastic diseases
- Use after myelosuppressive chemotherapy to reduce the incidence of febrile neutropenia
- Patients with acute myeloid leukemia receiving induction or consolidation chemotherapy
- Use after BMT in patients undergoing myeloablative chemotherapy
- Peripheral blood progenitor cell (PBPC) collection

Patients *with non-neoplastic* diseases
- Increase survival in patients acutely exposed to myelosuppressive doses of radiation (note: this indication is limited to Neupogen and not biosimilar products)
- Severe chronic neutropenia

Therapy Monitoring

1. *During G-CSF therapy after cytotoxic chemotherapy:* CBC with differential, before chemotherapy and twice weekly
2. *After BMT:* CBC with differential at least 3 times per week
3. *During initiation of therapy for severe chronic neutropenia:* CBC with differential twice weekly for the first 4 weeks and for 2 weeks following dose adjustment, then monthly if ANC is stable during the first year of treatment. Thereafter, regular CBC evaluation is recommended as clinically indicated and at least quarterly
4. *PBPC collection:* CBC with differential after 4 days of G-CSF, and consider dose modifications if WBC is >100,000/mm^3

Notes

1. The manufacturer recommends against CSF use 24 hours before or after cytotoxic chemotherapy, as well as simultaneous CSF use with chemotherapy and radiation
2. Patients must be instructed to report abdominal or shoulder tip pain, prompting evaluation for splenomegaly or splenic rupture, especially healthy donors receiving filgrastim for mobilization of PBPC
3. Patients must be instructed to report symptoms associated with respiratory distress, prompting evaluation for acute respiratory distress syndrome (ARDS)
4. Use with caution in patients with sickle cell disease; sickle cell crises have been reported following therapy. Only physicians qualified by specialized training or experience in the treatment of patients with sickle cell disorders should prescribe filgrastim for such patients, and only after careful consideration of the potential risks and benefits
5. Safety has not been established in patients with chronic myeloid leukemia (CML) or myelodysplastic syndromes (MDS)
6. In all clinical studies of the use of G-CSF for PBPC collection, G-CSF was administered after reinfusion of the collected cells
7. G-CSF is contraindicated in patients with a hypersensitivity to *Escherichia coli*–derived proteins, filgrastim, or any component of the formulation (sorbitol, polysorbate 80)
8. Patients should be referred to the Patient Information portion of product labeling, which provides information about neutrophils, neutropenia, safety, and efficacy. If home administration is desired, a puncture-resistant container for the disposal of used syringes and needles should be provided[1–3]

1. Neupogen (filgrastim) prescribing information. Thousand Oaks, CA: Amgen Inc.; June 2018
2. ZARXIO (filgrastim-sndz) prescribing information. Princeton, NJ: Sandoz Inc.; February 2017
3. NIVESTYM (filgrastim-aafi) prescribing information. Lake Forest, IL: Hospira, Inc.; July 2018

REGIMEN

TBO-FILGRASTIM (GRANIX)

Patients with non-myeloid malignancies receiving myelosuppressive chemotherapy:[1]
tbo-Filgrastim 5 μg/kg per day; administer by subcutaneous injection beginning 1–3 days after completion of chemotherapy and continuing until ANC has recovered to the normal range after nadir

Notes:
- Calculated doses may be rounded to use the most economical combination of available products (commercial vials and syringes contain either 300 μg or 480 μg
- It is recommended not to use tbo-filgrastim within 24 hours before or 24 hours after chemotherapy administration
- Doses for obese patients should be calculated on actual body weight, including morbidly obese patients
- tbo-Filgrastim and all of its components are not made with natural rubber latex

Efficacy

- tbo-Filgrastim was evaluated in a multinational, multicenter, randomized, controlled, phase 3 study involving 348 chemotherapy-naïve breast cancer patients receiving doxorubicin (60 mg/m²) and docetaxel (75 mg/m²). Patients were randomly assigned to receive daily injections of placebo, 5 μg/kg/day tbo-filgrastim, or 5 μg/kg/day of a non-US-approved Neupogen product starting 1 day after chemotherapy and continuing until post-nadir ANC of ≥10,000/mm³ was reached and for a minimum of 5 and maximum of 14 days

Treatment Group	tbo-Filgrastim	Neupogen	Placebo/tbo-Filgrastim*
Full analysis set (n = 348)	(n = 140)	(n = 136)	(n = 72)
Mean duration of severe neutropenia			
Cycle 1	1.1 days	1.1 days	3.8 days
ANCOVA (CI)[†]	0.028 (−0.261, 0.316)		
Cycle 4	0.7 days	0.7 days	0.6 days
Mean ANC nadir			
Cycle 1	700/mm³	700/mm³	200/mm³
ANCOVA (CI)[†]	−0.001 (−0.190, 0.189)		
Cycle 4	1000/mm³	1000/mm³	1100/mm³
Mean time to ANC recovery			
Cycle 1	8.0 days	7.8 days	14.0 days
ANCOVA (CI)[†]	0.207 (−0.425, 0.838)		
Cycle 4	7.6 days	7.1 days	7.2 days
Incidence of febrile neutropenia[‡]			
Cycle 1	12.1%	12.5%	36.1%
Across all cycles	20.7%	22.1%	41.7%

*Patients in this group received placebo in cycle 1 and tbo-filgrastim afterwards (including in cycle 4)
[†]ANCOVA estimate and 2-sided 95% CI for difference tbo-filgrastim minus filgrastim in cycle 1
[‡]Observed or protocol-defined febrile neutropenia
ANC, absolute neutrophil count; ANCOVA, analysis of covariance; CI, confidence interval
del Giglio A et al. BMC Cancer 2008;8:332

Adverse Events

Adverse Events Reported Among Patients with Cancer Receiving Myelosuppressive Chemotherapy and GCSF Support in Clinical Trials[1]

Bone pain (3.4%)
Severe leukocytosis, WBC >100,000/mm³ (<1%)
Myalgia
Headache
Vomiting

Warnings and/or Adverse Events Reported Postmarketing[1]

1. Splenomegaly and splenic rupture, including fatalities
2. Acute respiratory distress syndrome (ARDS)
3. Anaphylaxis
4. Alveolar hemorrhage and hemoptysis
5. Sickle cell crisis, including fatalities
6. Glomerulonephritis
7. Capillary leak syndrome
8. Thrombocytopenia
9. Cutaneous vasculitis
10. Aortitis
11. Sweet's syndrome (acute febrile neutrophilic dermatosis)
12. Asthenia
13. Diarrhea
14. Fatigue

Indication[1]

Patients with neoplastic diseases
- Use after myelosuppressive chemotherapy in adult and pediatric patients 1 month and older with non-myeloid malignancies

Therapy Monitoring

1. CBC with differential, before chemotherapy and twice weekly

Notes

1. The manufacturer recommends against CSF use 24 hours before or after cytotoxic chemotherapy, as well as simultaneous CSF use with chemotherapy and radiation

2. Patients must be instructed to report abdominal or shoulder tip pain, prompting evaluation for splenomegaly or splenic rupture

3. Patients must be instructed to report symptoms associated with respiratory distress, prompting evaluation for acute respiratory distress syndrome (ARDS)

4. Use with caution in patients with sickle cell disease; sickle cell crises have been reported following therapy. Only physicians qualified by specialized training or experience in the treatment of patients with sickle cell disorders should prescribe filgrastim for such patients, and only after careful consideration of the potential risks and benefits

5. tbo-Filgrastim is contraindicated in patients with a history of serious allergic reactions to filgrastim products, pegfilgrastim products, or any component of the formulation (sorbitol, polysorbate 80)

6. Patients should be referred to the Patient Information and Instructions for Use portions of product labeling, which provides information about neutrophils, neutropenia, safety, efficacy, and administration instructions. If home administration is desired, a puncture-resistant container for the disposal of used syringes and needles should be provided[1]

1. GRANIX (tbo-filgrastim) prescribing information. North Wales, PA: Teva Pharmaceuticals USA, Inc.; April 2020

REGIMEN

PEGFILGRASTIM (PEGYLATED G-CSF, NEULASTA, AND BIOSIMILARS)

Patients with cancers receiving myelosuppressive chemotherapy:[1–5]
Pegfilgrastim (or biosimilar) 6 mg; administer subcutaneously once per chemotherapy cycle

Notes:
- A 6-mg fixed dose is recommended for adult patients whose body weight is ≥45 kg
- Administer doses at least 24 hours after cytotoxic chemotherapy is completed and at least 14 days before the next administration of cytotoxic chemotherapy
- The brand-name pegfilgrastim product, Neulasta, and currently available biosimilar products are available as prefilled syringes containing pegfilgrastim 6 mg/0.6 mL intended for manual subcutaneous injection. In addition, the brand-name Neulasta product is also available in a kit (Neulasta Onpro) containing a prefilled syringe containing pegfilgrastim 6.4 mg/0.64 mL that delivers 6 mg/0.6 mL when used with the copackaged on-body injector
- Recommended injection sites for the manual injection are outer upper arm, abdomen >2 inches from the umbilicus, the front of the middle thighs, and upper outer area of the buttocks
- Dosing of pegfilgrastim for patients weighing <45 kg is provided in the table below:

Dosing of Pegfilgrastim for Pediatric Patients Weighing <45 kg

Body Weight	Pegfilgrastim Dose	Volume to Administer
<10 kg*	See below*	See below*
10–20 kg	1.5 mg	0.15 mL
21–30 kg	2.5 mg	0.25 mL
31–44 kg	4 mg	0.4 mL

*For pediatric patients weighing <10 kg, administer 0.1 mg/kg (0.01 mL/kg) of pegfilgrastim
Notes:
- Pegfilgrastim prefilled syringes do not bear graduation marks and are therefore unsuitable for direct administration to patients who require a dose of <6 mg/0.6 mL
- Pegfilgrastim administered by on-body injector has not been evaluated in pediatric patients

Information and instructions specific to Neulasta Onpro (administration by on-body injector):[1]
- Neulasta Onpro contains an acrylic adhesive. Do not use the product in patients who have had prior reactions to acrylic adhesive
- Neulasta Onpro is not indicated for pediatric patients or for treatment of hematopoietic subsyndrome of acute radiation syndrome
- Refer to the current Neulasta Onpro FDA-approved prescribing information for complete administration details
- Instructions for health care provider:
  1. Remove the Neulasta Onpro kit from the refrigerator and allow to equilibrate to room temperature for 30 minutes
  2. Choose an injection site, either the triceps area or abdomen (except 2-inch area surrounding navel). Choose the flattest site possible. Do not use the triceps area if there is not a caregiver available to monitor the status of the on-body injector. Avoid scar tissue, areas with moles, areas with excessive hair (unless trimmed close to the skin), surgical sites, areas where skin folds are present, or areas where belts, waistbands, or tight clothing may interfere with the on-body injector
  3. Clean the injection site with alcohol and allow to completely dry
  4. Grasp the Neulasta prefilled syringe by the syringe barrel, inspect the syringe and its contents, remove the gray needle cap, and expel air bubbles from the syringe
  5. Insert the Neulasta prefilled syringe needle at a 90-degree angle completely into the medicine port on the blue needle cover on the on-body injector. Push the plunger rod to empty the entire syringe contents. During filling, the device will beep and the status light will flash amber, which indicates there are 3 minutes remaining to apply the on-body injector to the patient

(continued)

Adverse Events

Adverse Events Reported in Clinical Trials[1–5]

≥10% of patients

Bone pain*	31%

<10% of patients

Pain in extremity	9%
Leukocytosis (WBC >100,000/mm³)	<1%

*Bone pain is generally controlled with nonopioid analgesics but may infrequently require opioid use

Adverse Events Reported Postmarketing[1–5]

1. Splenic rupture
2. Sickle cell crisis
3. Allergic reactions, including urticaria, rash, generalized erythema, flushing, or anaphylaxis
4. ARDS
5. Sweet's syndrome
6. Cutaneous vasculitis
7. Injection-site reactions
8. Capillary leak syndrome
9. Aortitis
10. Glomerulonephritis

A randomized trial comparing naproxen to placebo for prevention of pegfilgrastim-related bone pain was shown to reduce the mean AUC for pain (6.04 vs 7.71; P = 0.037), overall incidence of bone pain (61.1% vs 71.3%; P = 0.020), maximum pain score (2.59 vs 3.40; P = 0.005), duration of bone pain (1.92 vs 2.40 days; P = 0.009), and incidence of severe (>5 on a scale of 1–10) bone pain (19.2% vs 27.0%; P = 0.048). The median onset to peak pain score was 3 days for both groups. In the experimental group, naproxen 500 mg orally twice per day was administered starting on the day of pegfilgrastim administration and continued for 5–8 days[7]

(*continued*)

6. Verify that the on-body injector is full by checking the fill indicator and verify that the amber light is flashing

7. Firmly lift and remove the blue needle cover away from the on-body injector

8. Carefully peel away both pull tabs to reveal the adhesive, taking care to avoid touching the adhesive and automatic needle area with hands or gloves

9. Before the cannula deploys, and while the status light is still flashing amber, securely and firmly apply the on-body injector to the chosen injection site, ensuring that the adhesive does not become folded or wrinkled

10. After 3 minutes, the status light will change from an amber color to green, indicating that the cannula has automatically been inserted

11. Verify the quality of adhesion before sending the patient home. If folding or wrinkling is present in front of the cannula window or in any place that might prevent the on-body injector from remaining securely adhered to the skin, start again with a new kit

12. Record the dose delivery information in the patient instructions including when the on-body injector was applied, when the dose will begin (27 hours after application), and health care provider contact information

13. Review the patient instructions for use with the patient. Ensure that the patient understands that the on-body injector will flash a slow green light to indicate proper functioning. After 27 hours, a series of beeps will indicate that the dose delivery will begin in two minutes. The dose delivery takes approximately 45 minutes to complete, during which time the on-body injector will rapidly flash a green light. The patient should monitor the on-body injector closely during the administration period. When dose delivery is complete, the device will emit a long beep and the indicator light will change to solid green, at which time the patient may remove the device and dispose of it in a sharps disposal container

14. Advise the patient to notify their health care provider if the red error light is on, if the adhesive is noticeable wet (saturated), if there is leaking from the on-body injector, or if the on-body injector is dislodged as this may indicate the need for a replacement dose

Therapy Monitoring

Recommended only with regard to patient's hematologic status and ability to tolerate myelosuppressive chemotherapy[1–5]

Efficacy

• In a phase 3 trial in patients with breast cancer (stages II–IV) who received combination chemotherapy with doxorubicin 60 mg/m^2 and docetaxel 75 mg/m^2, the efficacy of pegfilgrastim was similar to that of filgrastim based on the duration of severe neutropenia (1.8 days vs 1.6 days) and the incidence of febrile neutropenia (13% vs 20%)[1–6]

• Pegfilgrastim is primarily eliminated by neutrophil receptor binding. Consequently, pegfilgrastim concentrations decline rapidly at the onset of neutrophil recovery[1–5]

• In two randomized controlled trials, pegfilgrastim was similar to filgrastim in the number of days of severe neutropenia during cycles 2–4 of chemotherapy[1–5]

• In a placebo-controlled trial, pegfilgrastim was found to lower the incidence of febrile neutropenia compared to placebo (1% vs 17% P<0.001), decrease hospitalizations (1% vs 14%), and decrease anti-infective use (2% vs 10%)[1–5]

Notes

1. Safety and efficacy have not been established for PBPC mobilization

2. Allergic reactions including anaphylaxis, skin rash, generalized erythema, flushing, and urticaria have been reported. In rare cases, allergic reactions including anaphylaxis recurred within days after initial anti-allergic treatment was discontinued. Patients should report flushing, dizziness, rash, and any signs or symptoms of infection

3. Patients must be instructed to report upper left abdominal or shoulder tip pain, prompting evaluation for splenomegaly or splenic rupture

4. Patients must be instructed to report symptoms of respiratory distress including shortness of breath, prompting evaluation for acute respiratory distress syndrome

5. Use with caution in patients with sickle cell disease; sickle cell crises have been reported following therapy with filgrastim, the active component of pegfilgrastim. Only physicians qualified by specialized training or experience in the treatment of patients with sickle cell disorders should administer pegfilgrastim

6. The needle cover of some available products contains dry natural rubber (a latex derivative), which may cause allergic reactions in sensitive individuals. Consult individual product package labeling to confirm the presence or absence of rubber or latex in patients with a known allergy to latex

7. The G-CSF receptor through which pegfilgrastim and filgrastim act has been found on tumor cell lines. The possibility that pegfilgrastim acts as a growth factor for any tumor type, including myeloid malignancies and myelodysplasia, diseases for which pegfilgrastim is not approved, cannot be excluded[1–5]

1. NEULASTA (pegfilgrastim) injection for subcutaneous use; prescribing information. Thousand Oaks, CA: Amgen, Inc.; January 2020

2. UDENYCA (pegfilgrastim-cbqv) injection for subcutaneous use; prescribing information. Redwood City, CA: Coherus BioSciences, Inc.; September 2019

3. FULPHILA (pegfilgrastim-jmdb) injection for subcutaneous use; prescribing information. Rockford, IL: Mylan Institutional LLC; June 2020

4. ZIEXTENZO (pegfilgrastim-bmez) injection for subcutaneous use; prescribing information. Princeton, NJ: Sandoz Inc.; September 2020

5. NYVEPRIA (pegfilgrastim-apgf) injection for subcutaneous use; prescribing information. New York, NY: Pfizer Inc.; June 2020

6. Green MD et al. Ann Oncol 2003;14;29–35

7. Kirshner JJ et al. J Clin Oncol 2012;30:1974–1979

REGIMEN
SARGRAMOSTIM (GM-CSF, LEUKINE)

Following induction chemotherapy in AML (adults):

Sargramostim 250 μg/m^2 per day; administer by intravenous infusion over 4 hours until ANC >1500/mm^3 for 3 consecutive days or a maximum of 42 days is reached

Notes:

- Start therapy on day 11 of cycle or 4 days after completion of induction chemotherapy if the bone marrow on day 10 is hypoblastic with <5% blasts
- This regimen may be repeated if a second cycle of induction chemotherapy is needed
- Interrupt or reduce the dose by half if ANC is >20,000 cells/mm^3
- Discontinue immediately if leukemia regrows

Mobilization of peripheral blood progenitor cells (PBPCs):

Sargramostim 250 μg/m^2 per day; administer by intravenous infusion over 24 hours or by subcutaneous injection once daily throughout the entire course of PBPC collection

Note:

Reduce dose by 50% if WBC >50,000 cells/mm^3

Following transplantation of autologous PBPCs:

Sargramostim 250 μg/m^2 per day; administer by intravenous infusion over 24 hours or by subcutaneous injection once daily beginning immediately after the infusion of PBPCs and continuing until ANC >1500 cells/mm^3 for 3 consecutive days

Myeloid reconstitution after autologous or allogeneic BMT:

Sargramostim 250 μg/m^2 per day; administer by intravenous infusion over 2 hours beginning 2–4 hours after bone marrow infusion and ≥24 hours after the last dose of chemotherapy or radiation therapy. Patients should not receive sargramostim until the post–marrow infusion ANC is <500 cells/mm^3. Continue therapy until ANC >1500 cells/mm^3 for 3 consecutive days

Notes:

1. If blast cells appear or progression of the underlying disease occurs, discontinue use immediately
2. Interrupt or reduce the dosage by half if ANC is >20,000 cells/mm^3

BMT failure or engraftment delay:

Sargramostim 250 μg/m^2 per day; administer by intravenous infusion over 2 hours for 14 consecutive days

Notes:

- If engraftment has not occurred within 7 days after completing sargramostim therapy, repeat the course of **sargramostim** 250 μg/m^2 per day by intravenous infusion over 2 hours for 14 consecutive days
- If engraftment has not occurred within 7 days after completing a second course of sargramostim, administer **sargramostim** 500 μg/m^2 per day by intravenous infusion over 2 hours for 14 consecutive days. If there is still no improvement, it is unlikely that further dose escalation will be beneficial
- If blast cells appear or progression of the underlying disease occurs, discontinue use immediately

Notes on dosing:

- If a severe adverse reaction occurs, temporarily reduce the sargramostim dosage by 50% or temporarily interrupt administration until the reaction abates
- Doses recommended are for adult patients
- Doses for obese patients should be calculated on actual body weight, including use in morbidly obese patients
- Do not empirically reduce doses in elderly patients because of patient age

Preparation of solution:

Sargramostim for intravenous infusion must be diluted with 0.9% sodium chloride injection (0.9% NS). If the final concentration of sargramostim is <10 μg/mL, albumin (human) must be added to the vehicle solution (0.9% NS) to produce a final albumin concentration of 0.1% *BEFORE* adding sargramostim to prevent sargramostim adsorption to the product container and administration set tubing

- To produce a vehicle solution with an albumin concentration of 0.1% suitable for diluting sargramostim

Add 1 mL 5% albumin (human) to 49 mL 0.9% NS, *or*

Add 0.2 mL 25% albumin (human) to 49.8 mL 0.9% NS

When administered by subcutaneous injection, sargramostim should be used without further dilution

Efficacy

- After AML 7+3 induction therapy, sargramostim significantly shortened the duration of neutropenia compared with placebo[1] (ANC <500/mm^3 by 4 days, ANC <1000/mm^3 by 7 days), decreased the incidence of Grade 3–5 infection (10% and 36%, respectively) and death from infection (6% and 15%, respectively), and significantly shortened the time to neutrophil recovery
- A retrospective review of PBPC collections from patients with cancer treated with sargramostim 250 µg/m^2 per day showed significantly higher numbers of granulocyte-macrophage colony-forming units (CFU-GM) than those collected without mobilization (11.41 × 10^4 CFU-GM/kg and 0.96 × 10^4 CFU-GM/kg, respectively)[1]
- In a historical controlled study of patients with lymphoma or myeloid leukemia who experienced BMT failure or engraftment delay, patients who received sargramostim with autologous transplantation achieved a median survival of 474 days versus 161 days for historical controls who had not received GM-CSF[1]
- Similarly, after failure of allogeneic hematopoietic progenitor cell transplantation, the median survival was 97 days in a group of patients who received sargramostim versus 35 days for the historical control patients who had not received GM-CSF[1]

Indications

1. Following induction chemotherapy in AML
2. Mobilization of PBPCs for collection and myeloid reconstitution after autologous PBPC transplantation
3. Myeloid reconstitution after autologous or allogeneic BMT
4. BMT failure or engraftment delays[1]

Therapy Monitoring

CBC with differential twice weekly during therapy. Monitoring of renal and hepatic function is recommended at least biweekly in patients displaying renal or hepatic dysfunction prior to initiation of treatment. Body weight and hydration status should be carefully monitored during administration. Interrupt therapy or reduce dose by half for excessive leukocytosis as defined by manufacturer: ANC >20,000 cells/mm^3 or WBC >50,000 cells/mm^3

Notes

1. Use with caution in patients with:
   a. Pre-existing cardiac disease
   b. Hypoxia, lung disease, or pulmonary symptoms
   c. Fluid retention
   d. Renal or hepatic impairment
   e. Rapid increase in peripheral blood counts
2. Use with caution in children
3. Discontinue GM-CSF immediately if blast cells appear after bone marrow infusion. It is possible that GM-CSF may act as a growth factor for tumor cells; use caution with patients with any malignancy with myeloid characteristics
4. Contraindications
   a. Patients with known hypersensitivity to GM-CSF, yeast-derived products, or any component of the sargramostim formulations, including:
      i. Mannitol, sucrose, tromethamine in both liquid and lyophilized formulations
      ii. Benzyl alcohol in the liquid formulation (do not administer to neonates, infants, pregnant women, and nursing mothers, as benzyl alcohol may cause "gasping syndrome")
   b. Concomitant sargramostim use with cytotoxic chemotherapy and radiation therapy
      i. Commence administering sargramostim at least 24 hours after completing myelosuppressive chemotherapy or radiation therapy, and discontinue use at least 24 hours before resuming myelosuppressive chemotherapy or radiation therapy administration
   c. Patients with >10% leukemic myeloid blasts in the bone marrow or peripheral blood
5. Efficacy of GM-CSF has not been assessed in AML patients <55 years of age[1]

Adverse Events

Adverse Events Reported in >30% of Patients Receiving GM-CSF Support in Clinical Trials[1]

Fever*	Stomatitis
Nausea	Alopecia
Diarrhea	Edema
Vomiting	Anorexia
Weight loss	Hypertension
Headache	Rash
Malaise	GI disorders
Asthenia*	Neurotoxicity
Hyperglycemia	Abdominal pain
Hypoalbuminemia	Liver toxicity
Infections	Genitourinary disorders
Pulmonary toxicity	

*These systemic events were generally mild to moderate, and were usually prevented or reversed by the administration of analgesics and antipyretics such as acetaminophen

Adverse Events Associated with the First Administration of Sargramostim[1]

1. Respiratory distress
2. Hypoxia
3. Flushing
4. Hypotension
5. Syncope
6. Tachycardia

These signs have been reported to occur following the first administration of sargramostim in a particular cycle, and have resolved with symptomatic treatment. They usually do not recur with subsequent doses in the same cycle of treatment

Adverse Events Reported Postmarketing[1]

1. Infusion-related reactions (eg, dyspnea, hypoxia, flushing, hypotension, syncope, and/or tachycardia)
2. Serious allergic reactions/hypersensitivity (eg, anaphylaxis, skin rash, urticaria, generalized erythema, and flushing)
3. Effusions and capillary leak syndrome
4. Supraventricular arrhythmias
5. Leukocytosis including eosinophilia
6. Thromboembolic events
7. Pain (eg, chest, abdominal, back, joint pain)
8. Injection-site reactions

1. LEUKINE (sargramostim) prescribing information. Lexington, MA: Partner Therapeutics, Inc.; May 2018

Chemotherapy-Induced Anemia

Epidemiology

Incidence rates of 50–60% for chemotherapy-induced anemia have been reported in retrospective reviews of patients with non-myeloid malignancies who were receiving myelosuppressive chemotherapy and who have required red blood cell (RBC) transfusion during therapy[1]

Agent/Regimen	Malignancy	Anemia Cases	
		% G1/2	% G3/4[2]
Paclitaxel	Breast cancer	93	7
Docetaxel	NSCLC	73–85	2–10
Docetaxel	Ovarian cancer	58–60	27–42
CHOP	Non-Hodgkin lymphoma	49	17
Topotecan	Ovarian cancer	67	32
Cisplatin/etoposide	SCLC	59	16–55
Fluorouracil	Colorectal cancer	50–54	5–8
Vinorelbine	Breast cancer	67–71	5–14
Cisplatin/cyclophosphamide	Ovarian cancer	43	9
Fluorouracil/carboplatin	Head and neck	42	14
Paclitaxel-doxorubicin	Breast cancer	78–84	8–11
Paclitaxel-carboplatin	NSCLC	10–59	5–34

NCI, CTCAE, Version 5.0 Criteria, Anemia[3]

Grade	Severity	Hemoglobin
0	None	WNL
1	Mild	10.0 g/dL to < lower limit of normal
2	Moderate	8.0 to <10 g/dL
3	Severe	<8 g/dL; transfusion indicated
4	Life-threatening	Urgent intervention indicated
5	Death	—

Preparations

1. Epoetin alfa (Procrit, Epogen) and biosimilars (eg, Retacrit, epoetin alfa-epbx)
2. Darbepoetin alfa (Aranesp)

Treatment Overview[4–9]

Oncology Indications for ESA therapy
- Cancer patients with myelosuppressive chemotherapy-related anemia (Hgb <10 g/dL)
  - Note that RBC transfusion is the standard option for treatment of anemia
  - ESAs are not indicated for patients receiving myelosuppressive therapy when the anticipated outcome is cure
  - When using ESAs target the minimum Hgb concentration necessary to avoid RBC transfusion
  - Do not initiate ESAs in patients who are anticipated to receive <2 additional months of chemotherapy
- Patients with incurable, nonmyeloid, hematologic malignancies (myeloma, non-Hodgkin lymphoma, and chronic lymphocytic leukemia) who are undergoing myelosuppressive chemotherapy should not be considered for ESA therapy until after the initial assessment of hematologic response from chemotherapy has been completed. Use caution in patients with multiple myeloma receiving concomitant immunomodulatory drugs due to higher risk of venous thromboembolism
- Anemic patients with lower risk myelodysplastic syndrome and a serum erythropoietin level of ≤500 IU/L. Patients who have lower baseline RBC transfusion dependence (<2 units/month) or those with an even lower serum erythropoietin level of <200 IU/L are most likely to respond to ESAs[10,11]

(continued)

Treatment Overview[4–9] (*continued*)

- Prior to initiation of an ESA for any of the above indications, rule out other treatable causes of anemia by considering the following baseline investigations, as clinically appropriate:[4]
  - History and physical examination, including drug exposure
  - Peripheral blood smear ± bone marrow biopsy
  - Iron studies (iron, total iron-binding capacity [TIBC], transferrin saturation [TSAT, goal ≥20%], ferritin (goal ≥100 ng/mL])*
  - Folate*
  - Vitamin B12*
  - Hemoglobinopathy screening
  - Reticulocyte count
  - Assessment for occult blood loss
  - BUN and serum creatinine
  - Erythropoietin level
  - Thyroid stimulating hormone
  - Direct antiglobulin test (patients with CLL, NHL, or autoimmune disease)

*Monitor at baseline and periodically during therapy; correct deficiencies if necessary

Discontinuation of ESA therapy
- Discontinue ESAs following the completion of a chemotherapy course (no plan to resume treatment)
- Discontinue ESA therapy in patients who do not respond within 6–8 weeks (<1–2 g/dL increase in Hgb or no reduction in transfusion requirements)

Major toxicity concerns
- ESAs increase the risk of thromboembolism and vascular arterial events by 50–75%. Use caution in patients who are at higher risk for venous thromboembolism
- The possibility that ESAs can act as a growth factor for any tumor type, particularly myeloid malignancies, cannot be excluded. ESAs shortened overall survival and/or increased the risk of tumor progression or recurrence in some clinical studies in patients with breast, non-small cell lung, head and neck, lymphoid, and cervical cancers.[5–9] To decrease these risks, as well as the risk of serious cardio- and thrombovascular events, use the lowest dose needed to avoid red blood cell transfusion[4–8]
- Blood pressure should be carefully monitored and controlled prior to initiation and during treatment with ESAs
- Pure red blood cell aplasia (PRCA) has been reported in a limited number of patients. If a patient shows evidence of PRCA (severe anemia and low reticulocyte count), withhold treatment and evaluate patient for neutralizing antibodies to erythropoietin; contact the product manufacturer to perform assays for binding and neutralizing antibodies. If PRCA is detected, do not restart or switch to any other ESA[5–8]
- There have been rare reports of potentially serious allergic reactions to ESAs
- Contraindications to ESA therapy are uncontrolled hypertension, PRCA that begins after ESA treatment, and serious allergic reactions to ESAs

Additional considerations for use
- Epoetin alfa increases the reticulocyte count within 10 days of initiation, followed by increases in the RBC count, Hgb, and Hct, usually within 2–6 weeks
- ASCO guidelines state that iron replacement with either oral or IV iron may be used as an adjunct to ESA therapy in patients with or without iron deficiency[4]
  - A 2016 Cochrane Review evaluated 8 randomized controlled trials (12 comparisons) involving 2087 patients that compared ESA plus iron supplementation to ESA alone[12]
    - Iron supplementation was associated with improved hematopoietic response (RR, 1.17; 95% CI, 1.09–1.26; P<0.0001; 1712 patients)
    - Use of IV iron was associated with improved hematopoietic response (RR 1.20; 95% CI, 1.10–1.31; P<0.00001; 1321 patients) whereas use of oral iron did not impact hematopoietic response (RR 1.04; 95% CI, 0.87–1.24; P = 0.68; 391 patients)
- The Epogen, Procrit, Retacrit, and Aranesp package inserts include two additional documents: a "Medication Guide" and "A Patient Instructions for Use." The Medication Guide provides patients with important information necessary for safe and effective use of Epogen, Procrit, Retacrit, and Aranesp. Under FDA regulations, a Medication Guide must be distributed to all patients to whom the products are dispensed
- Prescribers should discuss with their patients the benefits of treatment with ESAs and the potential and demonstrated risks of ESAs for thrombovascular events (myocardial infarction, stroke, venous thromboembolism, thrombosis of vascular access), increased risk of tumor progression or recurrence, and shortened survival time of cancer patients before starting or continuing therapy with ESAs
- In the United States, the Centers for Medicare and Medicaid Services (CMS) has ruled that Medicare will not underwrite the cost of ESAs for patients whose Hgb concentration is >10 g/dL, as stated in the July 2007 National Coverage Determination on ESAs. Currently, CMS does not make a distinction in ESA coverage between curative and palliative goals[13]
- In June 2008, the European Medicines Agency recommended that the ESAs prescribing information state that "blood transfusion should be the preferred method of correcting anemia in patients suffering cancer"[14]

(*continued*)

Treatment Overview[4–9] (*continued*)

- If home use is prescribed for a patient, the patient should be thoroughly instructed in the importance of proper disposal and cautioned against reusing needles, syringes, or drug product. A puncture-resistant container should be available for the disposal of used syringes and needles, and guidance provided on disposal of full containers

Randomized, Controlled Trials with Decreased Survival and/or Decreased Locoregional Control[5–8]

Tumor Type	Hgb Target (g/dL)	Achieved Hgb (g/dL) [Median (Q1, Q3)]	Primary Endpoint	Adverse Outcome in ESA Arm
Chemotherapy Trials				
Metastatic breast cancer (n = 2098)[15]	Minimum concentration to avoid transfusion, not to exceed 12 g/dL	11.6 (10.7, 12.1)	Progression-free survival	Decreased progression-free and overall survival
Metastatic breast cancer (BEST Study) (n = 939)[16]	12–14	12.9 (12.2, 13.3)	12-month overall survival	Decreased 12-month survival
Lymphoid (20000161) (n = 344)[17]	13–15 (M) 13–14 (F)	11 (9.8, 12.1)	Proportion of patients achieving a Hgb response	Decreased overall survival
Early breast cancer (PREPARE Study) (n = 733)[18]	12.5–13	13.1 (12.5, 13.7)	Relapse-free and overall survival	Decreased 3-year relapse-free and overall survival
Cervical cancer (GOG 191) (n = 114)[19]	12–14 g/dL	12.7 (12.1, 13.3)	Progression-free and overall survival and locoregional control	Decreased 3-year progression-free and overall survival and locoregional control

Q1, 25th percentile; Q3, 75th percentile

1. Groopman JE, Itri LM. J Natl Cancer Inst 1999;91:1616–1634
2. Cancer- and chemotherapy-induced anemia. Version 2.2014. NCCN Clinical Practice Guidelines in Oncology (NCCN Guidelines). National Comprehensive Cancer Network, Inc., 2014. At: http://www.nccn.org [accessed December 30, 2013]
3. NCI, CTCAE, National Cancer Institute (USA) Common Terminology Criteria for Adverse Events, version 5.0. At: http://ctep.cancer.gov/protocolDevelopment/electronic_applications/ctc.htm [accessed December 5, 2020]
4. Bohlius J et al. J Clin Oncol 2019;37:1336–1351
5. Aranesp (darbepoetin alfa) injection, for intravenous or subcutaneous use; prescribing information. Thousand Oaks, CA: Amgen Inc.; January 2019
6. PROCRIT (epoetin alfa) injection, for intravenous or subcutaneous use; prescribing information. Horsham, PA: Janssen Products, LP; July 2018
7. Epogen (epoetin alfa) injection, for intravenous or subcutaneous use; prescribing information. Thousand Oaks, CA: Amgen Inc.; July 2018
8. Retacrit (epoetin alfa-epbx) injection, for intravenous or subcutaneous use; prescribing information. New York, NY: Pfizer Inc.; August 2020
9. Bennett CL et al. JAMA 2008;299:914–924
10. Fenaux P et al. Leukemia 2018;32:2648–2658
11. Hellström-Lindberg E et al. Blood 1998;92:68–75
12. Mhaskar R et al. Cochrane Database Syst Rev 2016;2:CD009624
13. Centers for Medicaid & Medicare Services. National coverage determination (NCD) for erythropoiesis stimulating agents (ESAs) in cancer and related neoplastic conditions. Publication number 100–3, version 1, effective date 7/30/2007 [accessed December 5, 2020, at cms.gov]
14. European Medicine Agency Press Release: Doc. Ref. EMEA/CHMP/333963/2008–corr. London, 26 June. At: www.ema.europa.eu/docs/en_GB/document_library/Press_release/2009/11/WC500015069.pdf [accessed December 5, 2020]
15. Leyland-Jones B et al. J Clin Oncol 2016;34:1197–1207
16. Leyland-Jones B et al. J Clin Oncol 2005;23:5960–5972
17. Hedenus M et al. Br J Haematol 2003;122:394–403
18. Untch M et al. Ann Oncol 2011;22:1999–2006
19. Thomas G et al. Gynecol Oncol 2008;108:317–325

REGIMEN

EPOETIN ALFA, INCLUDING BIOSIMILARS (EPOGEN, PROCRIT, RETACRIT)

In patients with non-myeloid malignancies where anemia is due to the effect of myelosuppressive chemotherapy, and, after initiating epoetin therapy, there are planned at least two additional months of chemotherapy:

- Therapy *should not* be initiated if Hgb ≥10 g/dL
- ESA treatment should target the lowest Hgb level that will avoid RBC transfusion
- ESA therapy is not indicated for patients receiving chemotherapy with curative intent

Adult cancer patients receiving myelosuppressive chemotherapy:[1-4]

Epoetin alfa (or biosimilar) 40,000 units; administer by subcutaneous injection once weekly*, or

Epoetin alfa (or biosimilar) 150 units/kg; administer by subcutaneous injection 3 times per week

Note: off-label alternative regimens with extended dosing intervals have also been described:

Epoetin alfa (or biosimilar) 80,000 units; administer by subcutaneous injection every 2 weeks[5] or

Epoetin alfa (or biosimilar) 120,000 units; administer by subcutaneous injection every 3 weeks[6]

*This schedule is more convenient and more practical than a 3-times-weekly regimen

Pediatric patients (ages 5–18 years) with cancer who are receiving myelosuppressive chemotherapy:

Epoetin alfa (or biosimilar) 600 units/kg; administer by intravenous injection once weekly (maximum weekly dose = 40,000 units)

Treatment Modifications[1-4,7]

Epoetin-alfa (and Biosimilars) Treatment Modifications		
Type of Modification	Parameter	Dose Modification
Dose reduction for overcorrection of Hgb	• Hgb reaches a level needed to avoid transfusion *or* • Hgb increases >1 g/dL during any 2-week period	Reduce dose by 25%
Dose withholding for overcorrection of hemoglobin	• Hgb exceeds a level needed to avoid transfusion*	Withhold dose until Hgb approaches a level at which transfusions may be required, then resume epoetin alfa (or biosimilar) use at 25% less than the dose previously administered
Treatment modifications for hypertension	• Uncontrolled hypertension	Withhold or reduce the dose if blood pressure becomes difficult to control. Advise patient to comply with antihypertensive therapy and dietary restrictions
Dose increase for insufficient response	• Hgb increase is ≤1 g/dL and remains <10 g/dL after 4 weeks of therapy	• *Adult weekly dosing:* increase dose to 60,000 units by subcutaneous injection once weekly • *Adult TIW dosing:* increase dose to 300 units/kg three times weekly • *Pediatric weekly dosing:* increase dose to 900 units/kg by intravenous injection once weekly (maximum weekly dose = 60,000 units)
Discontinuation criteria	• Hgb response after 8 weeks of use is <1 g/dL or transfusion is still required • Following completion of a chemotherapy course[†] • If a serious allergic reaction or severe cutaneous reaction occurs • If the patient develops pure red cell aplasia (notify manufacturer to coordinate testing for binding and neutralizing antibodies to erythropoietin). Do not switch to another ESA	

*The CMS NCD defines the threshold for withholding therapy as ≥10 g/dL or a hematocrit of ≥30%
[†]The CMS NCD states that the duration for each course of chemotherapy includes the 8-week period following the final dose of myelosuppressive chemotherapy in a regimen
Hgb, hemoglobin; TIW, three times per week; CMS NCD, Centers for Medicare & Medicaid Services National Coverage Determination; ESA, erythropoiesis stimulating agent

Therapy Monitoring

Until a maintenance dose is established and after any dose adjustment: monitor Hgb weekly until the hemoglobin level is stable and sufficient to minimize the need for RBC transfusion
After Hgb stabilizes: monitor Hgb at regular intervals
Monitor iron, folate, and vitamin B_{12} status before and during treatment. Supplementation is recommended if serum ferritin <100 μg/L or serum transferrin saturation <20%, or folate or vitamin B_{12} are less than the range of normal concentrations

Efficacy

- Among 344 anemic patients with cancer receiving epoetin alfa (n = 174) or placebo (n = 170) concomitantly with chemotherapy, 14% vs 28% (P<0.001), respectively, required transfusion support during weeks 5–16 after starting ESA treatment[1-3]
- Incidence of RBC transfusion (entire study period) for the epoetin-alfa and placebo arms was 25.3% and 39.6% (P = 0.005), respectively[8]
- Over the course of the study, 73% of patients who receive epoetin-alfa achieved a ≥2-g/dL increase in Hgb compared with 32% of patients receiving placebo (P<0.0001), despite the fact that the transfusion rate was greater in the placebo group[8]
- Epoetin alfa therapy was not associated with improvement in Functional Assessment of Cancer Therapy (FACT) anemia fatigue subscale (+3 in the epoetin-alfa arm vs +0.6 in the placebo arm; P = 0.18). However, hemoglobin responders (irrespective of treatment arm) did demonstrate improvements in this score of +5.1 compared with −2.1 for the nonresponders (P = 0.006)[8]

Cycle Number	Mean Hemoglobin (g/dL)	
	Placebo Arm	Epoetin-alfa Arm
0 (baseline)	9.4	9.5
1	9.6	10.7
2	10.1	11.7
3	10.3	12.4
4	10.5	12.6

P<0.001 at each study time point after baseline[8]

Indications[1-4]

Patients with neoplastic diseases
- Anemia from concomitantly administered chemotherapy for incurable nonmyeloid malignancies receiving chemotherapy for a minimum of 2 months
- In addition to the FDA-approved indications, ASCO/ASH 2019 guidelines recognize ESA use in low-risk myelodysplasia

Patients with non-neoplastic diseases
- Anemia from chronic kidney disease (CKD)
- Zidovudine-related anemia in HIV patients
- Reduction of allogeneic blood transfusion in patients who receive elective, noncardiac, nonvascular surgery

Adverse Events

Adverse Events Reported Among Patients with Cancer Receiving Chemotherapy and Epoetin Alfa Support in Clinical Trials[1-3]

≥10% of Patients

Nausea (35%)	Arthralgia (10%)
Vomiting (20%)	Stomatitis (10%)
Myalgia (10%)	

1–9% of Patients

Cough (9%)	Weight decrease (9%)
Leukopenia (8%)	Bone pain (7%)
Rash (7%)	Hyperglycemia (6%)
Insomnia (6%)	Headache (5%)
Depression (5%)	Dysphagia (5%)
Hypokalemia (5%)	Thrombosis (5%)

Adverse Events Reported Postmarketing

Seizures	Serious allergic reactions
Pure red cell aplasia	Porphyria
Injection site reactions, including irritation and pain	Severe cutaneous reactions

Notes[1-3]

1. Epoetin alfa increases the risk of seizures in patients with CKD. Patients should be monitored closely and contact their prescriber for new-onset seizures, premonitory symptoms, or change in seizure frequency
2. Epoetin alfa (and biosimilars) are contraindicated in patients with hypersensitivity to any component of the formulation (see table below for excipient content)
3. Patients with uncontrolled hypertension should not receive epoetin alfa (or biosimilars)
4. ESA therapy increased the risks for myocardial infarction, stroke, congestive heart failure, and fatal thrombotic events (1.1% in patients with cancer participating in clinical trials). An increase in Hgb >1 g/dL over 2 weeks may contribute to these risks
5. Multiple-dose vials contain benzyl alcohol, which is contraindicated in neonates, infants, pregnant women, and nursing mothers, as it may cause "gasping syndrome"

Available Epoetin Alfa (and Biosimilar) Formulations[1-3]

Brand (Generic) Name	Strengths	Each mL Also Contains the Following Excipients:
Procrit (epoetin alfa) and Epogen (epoetin alfa)	2000 units/1 mL SDV 3000 units/1 mL SDV 4000 units/1 mL SDV 10,000 units/1 mL SDV	**Albumin** (human) (2.5 mg), citric acid (0.06 mg), sodium chloride (5.9 mg), and sodium citrate (5.8 mg) in SWFI
	20,000 units/2 mL MDV* 20,000 units/1 mL MDV	**Albumin** (human) (2.5 mg), **benzyl alcohol** (1%), sodium chloride (8.2 mg), citric acid (0.11 mg), and sodium citrate (1.3 mg) in SWFI
Procrit (epoetin alfa)	40,000 units/1 mL SDV	**Albumin** (human) (2.5 mg), citric acid (0.0068 mg), sodium chloride (5.8 mg), sodium citrate (0.7 mg), sodium phosphate dibasic anhydrate (1.8 mg), and sodium phosphate monobasic monohydrate (1.2 mg) in SWFI
Retacrit (epoetin alfa-epbx)	2000 units/1 mL SDV 3000 units/1 mL SDV 4000 units/1 mL SDV 10,000 units/1 mL SDV	Calcium chloride dihydrate (0.01 mg), glycine (7.5 mg), isoleucine (1 mg), leucine (1 mg), L-glutamic acid (0.25 mg), phenylalanine (0.5 mg), polysorbate 20 (0.1 mg), sodium chloride (2.4 mg), sodium phosphate dibasic anhydrous (4.9 mg), sodium phosphate monobasic monohydrate (1.3 mg), and threonine (0.25 mg), in SWFI
	20,000 units/2 mL MDV* 20,000 units/1 mL MDV	**Benzyl alcohol** (8.5 mg), L-methionine (0.45 mg), polysorbate 20 (0.04 mg), sodium phosphate dibasic anhydrous (0.09 mg), sodium phosphate monobasic monohydrate (2.67 mg), and sucrose (60 mg) in SWFI

Clinically relevant considerations with regard to excipient content include presence of benzyl alcohol (risks in neonates, infants, pregnant women, and lactating women), human albumin (some patients may have a religious objection to receipt of fractions from blood plasma, including human albumin), and any excipient to which the patient has a history of allergic reaction

*Product concentration is 10,000 units/mL

SDV, single-dose vial; SWFI, sterile water for injection; MDV, multiple-dose vial

1. PROCRIT (epoetin alfa) injection, for intravenous or subcutaneous use; prescribing information. Horsham, PA: Janssen Products, LP; July 2018
2. Epogen (epoetin alfa) injection, for intravenous or subcutaneous use; prescribing information. Thousand Oaks, CA: Amgen Inc.; July 2018
3. RETACRIT (epoetin alfa-epbx) injection, for intravenous or subcutaneous use; prescribing information. New York, NY: Pfizer Inc.; August 2020
4. Bohlius J et al. J Clin Oncol 2019;37:1336–1351
5. Henry DH et al. Curr Med Res Opin 2006;22:1403–1413
6. Steensma DP et al. J Clin Oncol 2006;24:1079–1089
7. Centers for Medicaid & Medicare Services. National coverage determination (NCD) for erythropoiesis stimulating agents (ESAs) in cancer and related neoplastic conditions. Publication number 100–3, version 1, effective date 7/30/2007 [accessed December 5, 2020, at cms.gov]
8. Witzig TE et al. J Clin Oncol 2005;23:2606–2617

REGIMEN

DARBEPOETIN ALFA (ARANESP)

In adult patients with metastatic, nonmyeloid malignancies receiving myelosuppressive chemotherapy:
- Therapy *should not* be initiated if Hgb is ≥10 g/dL
- ESA treatment should target the lowest Hgb level that will avoid RBC transfusion
- ESA therapy is not indicated for patients receiving chemotherapy with curative intent

Patients with cancer who are receiving myelosuppressive chemotherapy[1]:
Darbepoetin alfa 2.25 µg/kg; administer by subcutaneous injection, once weekly, *or*
Darbepoetin alfa 500 µg; administer by subcutaneous injection, once every 3 weeks

Alternative, fixed-dose, off-label, initial dosing regimens recommended in NCCN guidelines[2]:
Darbepoetin alfa 100 µg; administer by subcutaneous injection, once weekly, *or*
Darbepoetin alfa 200 µg; administer by subcutaneous injection, once every 2 weeks[3], *or*
Darbepoetin alfa 300 µg; administer by subcutaneous injection, once every 3 weeks[4]

Note: NCCN Guidelines recommend the above alternative fixed dosages schedules over the FDA-approved dosages to support the administration of the lowest possible dosage while maintaining maximum efficacy[2]

Therapy Monitoring[1]

Until a maintenance dose established and after any dose adjustment: Monitor Hgb weekly until hemoglobin is stable and sufficient to minimize the need for RBC transfusion
After Hgb stabilized: Monitor Hgb at regular intervals

Monitor iron, folate, and vitamin B$_{12}$ status before and during treatment. Supplementation is recommended if serum ferritin <100 µg/L or serum transferrin saturation <20%, or folate or vitamin B$_{12}$ are less than the range of normal concentrations

Treatment Modifications

Darbepoetin Alfa Treatment Modifications[1,5]

Titration for Inadequate Response
(Inadequate Response Defined as Hgb Increase of ≤1 g/dL and Remains <10 g/dL After 6 Weeks of Therapy)

Initial Dosing Schedule	Dose Modification
2.25 µg/kg weekly	Increase dose to up to 4.5 µg/kg by subcutaneous injection every week
500 µg every 3 weeks	Not applicable
100 µg (fixed dose) weekly	Increase dose to up to 150–200 µg (fixed dose) by subcutaneous injection every week
200 µg (fixed dose) every 2 weeks	Increase dose to up to 300 µg (fixed dose) by subcutaneous injection every 2 weeks
300 µg (fixed dose) every 3 weeks	Increase dose to up to 500 µg (fixed dose) by subcutaneous injection every 3 weeks

Other Treatment Modifications

Type of Modification	Parameter(s)	Dose Modification
Dose reduction for overcorrection of Hgb	• Hgb reaches a level needed to avoid transfusion *or* • Hgb increases >1 g/dL during any 2-week period	Reduce dose by 40%
Dose withholding for overcorrection of hemoglobin	• Hgb exceeds a level needed to avoid transfusion*	Withhold dose until Hgb approaches a level at which transfusions may be required, then resume darbepoetin alfa use at 40% less than the dose previously administered
Treatment modifications for hypertension	• Uncontrolled hypertension	Withhold or reduce the dose if blood pressure becomes difficult to control. Advise patient to comply with antihypertensive therapy and dietary restrictions
Discontinuation criteria	• Hgb response after 8 weeks of use is <1 g/dL or transfusion is still required • Following completion of a chemotherapy course† • If a serious allergic reaction or severe cutaneous reaction occurs • If the patient develops pure red cell aplasia (notify manufacturer to coordinate testing for binding and neutralizing antibodies to erythropoietin). Do not switch to another ESA	

*The CMS NCD defines the thresholds for withholding therapy as ≥10 g/dL or a hematocrit of ≥30%
†The CMS NCD states that the duration for each course of chemotherapy includes the 8-week period following the final dose of myelosuppressive chemotherapy in a regimen
Hgb, hemoglobin; CMS NCD, Centers for Medicare & Medicaid Services National Coverage Determination; ESA, erythropoiesis-stimulating agent

Indications[1,5]

Patients with neoplastic diseases
- Anemia from concomitantly administered chemotherapy that is expected to continue for a minimum of 2 months (non-curative intent) in patients with metastatic, nonmyeloid malignancies
- In addition to the FDA-approved indications, ASCO/ASH 2019 guidelines recognize ESA use in low-risk myelodysplasia

Patients with non-neoplastic diseases
Anemia associated with chronic renal failure, including patients on dialysis and patients not on dialysis

Efficacy

Darbepoetin once-weekly 2.25-µg/kg dosing was studied in advanced lung cancer patients (both SCLC and NSCLC) with Hgb values <11g/dL who were receiving platinum-containing chemotherapy regimens. At 12 weeks, a significantly lower proportion of patients who received darbepoetin vs placebo required a RBC transfusion (26% and 50%, respectively; P<0.001)[6]

Efficacy of darbepoetin 500 µg administered once every 3 weeks versus 2.25 µg/kg weekly was studied in patients with Hgb <11g/dL undergoing cytotoxic chemotherapy. Seventy-two percent of patients required dose reductions in the every-3-weeks group, whereas 77% required dose reductions in the once-weekly group. Twenty-three percent of patients in the once-every-3-weeks group required RBC transfusion, and 28% of the weekly group required RBC transfusion[1,7]

Efficacy of darbepoetin 300 µg administered once every 3 weeks (off-label dosing) was evaluated in a phase 2 study comparing darbepoetin alfa 300 µg (n = 118) or 500 µg (n = 120) administered subcutaneously every 3 weeks. The study was a factorial design that also evaluated the effect of intravenous iron supplementation. Similar proportions of patients in the 300-µg arm versus the 500-µg arm reached the target hemoglobin concentration of ≥11 g/dL (75% and 78%, respectively)[4]

Adverse Events

Adverse Events Reported in Clinical Trials[1]

≥10% of Patients	
Edema (12.8%)	Abdominal pain (13.2%)

<10% of Patients	
Thromboembolic adverse reactions (5.1%)	Arterial adverse reactions (1.1%)
Myocardial infarction (0.6%)	Venous adverse reactions (4.1%)
Pulmonary embolism (1.5%)	Cerebrovascular disorders* (1.3%)

*Cerebrovascular disorders encompass CNS hemorrhages and cerebrovascular accidents (ischemic and hemorrhagic)

Adverse Events Reported Postmarketing[1]

1. Seizures
2. Pure red cell aplasia
3. Serious allergic reactions
4. Severe cutaneous reactions

Notes

1. Darbepoetin alfa increases the risk of seizure in patients with CKD; monitor patients for changes in seizure frequency or premonitory symptoms
2. Patients with uncontrolled hypertension, PRCA, or allergy to any component of Aranesp should not receive darbepoetin alfa
   - Aranesp, packaged in vials and prefilled syringes contains darbepoetin alfa and polysorbate 80, sodium chloride, sodium phosphate dibasic anhydrous, and sodium phosphate monobasic monohydrate, in water for injection, USP
3. Darbepoetin alfa should be discontinued after completion of a chemotherapy course
4. The needle cover of the prefilled syringe contains dry natural rubber (a derivative of latex), which may cause allergic reactions in individuals sensitive to latex
5. Rare cases of allergic reactions, including skin rash, anaphylactic reactions, angioedema, bronchospasm, and urticaria have been reported
6. *Do not use* darbepoetin alfa that has been shaken or frozen
7. Aranesp is supplied in single-dose vials containing darbepoetin alfa in the following concentrations 25 µg/1 mL, 40 µg/1 mL, 60 µg/1 mL, 100 µg/1 mL, 200 µg/1 mL, and 300 µg/1 mL
8. Aranesp is supplied in single-dose prefilled syringes containing 10 µg/0.4 mL, 25 µg/0.42 mL, 40 µg/0.4 mL, 60 µg/0.3 mL, 100 µg/0.5 mL, 150 µg/0.3 mL, 200 µg/0.4 mL, 300 µg/0.6 mL, and 500 µg/1 mL

Conversion of Epoetin Alfa to Darbepoetin Alfa in Adult Patients with CKD on Dialysis[1]

Epoetin Alfa (Units/wk)	Darbepoetin Alfa (µg/wk)
<2499	6.25
2500–4999	12.5
5000–10,999	25
11,000–17,999	40
18,000–33,999	60
34,000–89,999	100
≥90,000	200

1. Aranesp (darbepoetin alfa) injection, for intravenous or subcutaneous use; prescribing information. Thousand Oaks, CA: Amgen Inc.; January 2019
2. Hematopoietic growth factors. Version 2.2020. NCCN Clinical Practice Guidelines in Oncology (NCCN Guidelines). National Comprehensive Cancer Network, Inc., 2020. At: http://www.nccn.org [accessed December 6, 2020]
3. Thames WA et al. Pharmacotherapy 2004;24:313–323
4. Auerbach M et al. Am J Hematol 2010;85:655–663
5. Bohlius J et al. J Clin Oncol 2019;37:1336–1351
6. Vansteenkiste J et al. J Natl Cancer Inst 2002;94:1211–1220
7. Canon JL et al. J Natl Cancer Inst 2006;98:273–284

44. Guidelines for Chemotherapy Dosage Adjustment

Timothy J. George, PharmD, BCOP, Pamela W. McDevitt, PharmD, BCOP, Carla A. Hively, RPh, BCOP,
Gerard P. Mascara, PharmD, BCOP, and Tito Fojo, MD, PhD

Child-Pugh Liver Function Classification

Assessment	Degree of Abnormality	Score
Encephalopathy grade	None	1
	1 or 2	2
	3 or 4	3
Ascites	Absent	1
	Slight	2
	Moderate	3
Total bilirubin (mg/dL)	<2	1
	2–3	2
	>3	3
Serum albumin (g/dL)	>3.5	1
	2.8–3.5	2
	<2.8	3
Prothrombin time (seconds prolonged)	<4	1
	4–6	2
	>6	3

Mild hepatic impairment	=	Child-Pugh class A	=	Score 5–6
Moderate hepatic impairment	=	Child-Pugh class B	=	Score 7–9
Severe hepatic impairment	=	Child-Pugh class C	=	Score 10–15

Calculation of Creatinine Clearance (CrCl)
Timed Urine Collection
(Often Used to Approximate Glomerular Filtration Rate [GFR])
Requirements: Timed Urine Collection (Time, Urine Volume, and Creatinine Concentration) and Serum Creatinine Concentration

Creatinine clearance (mL/min)	=	$\dfrac{U_{Cr} \times U_{vol}}{Cr \times T_{min}}$
Corrected CrCl (mL/min × 1.73 m²)	=	$\dfrac{CrCl \times 1.73\,m^2}{BSA\,(m^2)}$

Calculation of Creatinine Clearance (CrCl)
Cockcroft and Gault Formula
Requirements: Weight, Age, and Serum Creatinine Concentration

Males CrCl	=	$\dfrac{[BW \times (140 - Age)]}{(72 \times SCr)}$
Females CrCl	=	$\dfrac{0.85 \times [BW \times (140 - Age)]}{(72 \times SCr)}$

Cockcroft and Gault Formula:
- CrCl in mL/min
- BW = body weight in kg
- Age in years
- SCr in mg/dL

Note: estimating ideal body weight in (kg)
Males: IBW = 50 kg + 2.3 kg for each inch over 5 feet
Females: IBW = 45.5 kg + 2.3 kg for each inch over 5 feet
Note: if the ABW (actual body weight) is less than the IBW, use the ABW for calculating the CrCl

Calculation of Estimated Glomerular Filtration Rate (eGFR)
Modification of Diet in Renal Disease (MDRD) Formula
Requirements: Age, Race, Sex, Serum Creatinine Concentration

$$eGFR = 175 \times (SCr)^{-1.154} \times (Age)^{-0.203} \times (0.742 \text{ if female}) \times (1.212 \text{ if Black})$$

MDRD formula:
- eGFR in mL/min/1.73 m²
- Age in years
- Standardized SCr in mg/dL

Guidelines for Chemotherapy Dosage Adjustments

Generic Drug Name	Hepatic Dysfunction			Renal Dysfunction	
	Bilirubin	AST/SGOT and/or ALT/SGPT	Percent Dosage/Dose Administered	Creatinine Clearance (CrCl), Estimated Glomerular Filtration Rate (eGFR), or Serum Creatinine (SCr)	Percent Dosage/Dose Administered
Abemaciclib[1]	Child-Pugh class C (severe hepatic impairment)		Reduce frequency from twice daily to once daily	CrCl ≥30–89 mL/min	No dose adjustment necessary
				CrCl <30 mL/min or requiring hemodialysis	No data available; however, no requirement for dose reduction is anticipated because only 3% of a dose is excreted into the urine
Abiraterone acetate[2]	Child-Pugh class B (moderate hepatic impairment prior to starting treatment)		Reduce dose to 250 mg once daily	No dose adjustment necessary	
	Child-Pugh class C (severe hepatic impairment prior to starting treatment)		Has not been studied in this population: avoid		
	Bilirubin >3 × ULN during treatment	ALT and/or AST >5 × ULN during treatment	Interrupt treatment. Restart 750 mg once daily after LFTs return to baseline or AST and ALT ≤2.5 × ULN and bilirubin <1.5 × ULN		
	Bilirubin >3 × ULN while receiving 750 mg once daily	ALT and/or AST >5 × ULN during treatment with 750 mg once daily	Interrupt treatment. Restart 500 mg once daily after LFTs return to baseline or AST and ALT ≤2.5 × ULN and l bilirubin <1.5 × ULN		
	Bilirubin >3 × ULN while receiving 500 mg once daily	ALT and/or AST >5 × ULN during treatment with 500 mg once daily	Discontinue treatment		
Acalabrutinib[3]	Child-Pugh class C (severe hepatic impairment)		Do not administer	eGFR ≥30 mL/min/1.73m²	No dose adjustment necessary
				eGFR <30 mL/min/1.73m² or requiring hemodialysis	No data available; however, no requirement for dose reduction is anticipated because only 12% of a dose is excreted into the urine (<2% as unchanged drug)
ado-Trastuzumab emtansine[4]	Child-Pugh class A (mild hepatic impairment) or Child-Pugh class B (moderate hepatic impairment)		No effect on DM1 and DM1-containing metabolite concentrations. Parent drug AUC 38% lower (class A) or 67% lower (class B) in cycle 1 but then similar in cycle 3	Mild to moderate renal impairment (CrCl 30–89 mL/min)	No dosage adjustments necessary
	Child-Pugh class C (severe hepatic impairment)		No clinical trials have been conducted	Severe renal impairment (CrCl <30 mL/min)	No clinical trials have been conducted

(continued)

Generic Drug Name	Hepatic Dysfunction			Renal Dysfunction	
	Bilirubin	AST/SGOT and/or ALT/SGPT	Percent Dosage/Dose Administered	Creatinine Clearance (CrCl), Estimated Glomerular Filtration Rate (eGFR), or Serum Creatinine (SCr)	Percent Dosage/Dose Administered
Afatinib[5]	Child-Pugh class A (mild hepatic impairment) or Child-Pugh class B (moderate hepatic impairment)		No dosage adjustment necessary	eGFR 15–29 mL/min/1.73 m²	Reduce starting dose to 30 mg daily
	Child-Pugh class C (severe hepatic impairment)		Limited data available. Monitor closely for toxicity	eGFR ≥30 mL/min/1.73 m²	No starting dose adjustment necessary
Aldesleukin[6]	No dosage adjustments necessary			SCr >4.5 mg/dL	Hold or discontinue treatment. Resume when SCr <4 mg/dL
				SCr ≥4.0 mg/dL in presence of severe volume overload, acidosis, or hyperkalemia	Hold or discontinue treatment. Resume when SCr <4 mg/dL and fluid and electrolyte status are stable
				Renal failure requiring dialysis >72 hours while receiving an earlier course of therapy	Treatment contraindicated
				Persistent oliguria or urine output <10 mL/hour for 16–24 hours with rising serum creatinine	Withhold dose; may resume when urine output >10 mL/hour with serum creatinine decrease of >1.5 mg/dL or normalization
Alectinib[7]	Child-Pugh class C (severe hepatic impairment)		Administer 450 mg twice daily	CrCl ≥30 mL/min	No dose adjustment necessary
				CrCl <30 mL/min or hemodialysis	No safety data available
				Note: renal toxicity occurs with alectinib and may require dose interruption, reduction, and/or discontinuation	
Alemtuzumab[8]	No dosage adjustments necessary			No dosage adjustments necessary	
Alitretinoin[9]	No dosage adjustments necessary			No dosage adjustments necessary	
Alpelisib[10]	No dosage adjustments necessary			CrCl 30–90 mL/min	No dose adjustment necessary
				CrCl <30 mL/min	No data available; however, no requirement for dose reduction is anticipated because only 14% of a dose is excreted into the urine (2% as unchanged drug)
Amifostine[11]	No dosage adjustments necessary			No dosage adjustments necessary	
Apalutamide[12]	Child-Pugh class A or B (mild to moderate hepatic impairment)		No dose adjustment necessary	eGFR 30–89 mL/min/1.73 m²	No dose adjustment necessary
	Child-Pugh class C (severe hepatic impairment)		No data available	eGFR <30 mL/min/1.73 m²	No data available

(continued)

Drug	Hepatic impairment		Renal impairment	
Anagrelide[13]	Moderate hepatic impairment	Starting dose of 0.5 mg/day must be maintained for 1 week with cardiovascular monitoring. Do not increase dose more than 0.5 mg/day during any week. Measure liver function tests before and during treatment	No dosage adjustments necessary, but monitor renal function closely	
	Severe hepatic impairment	Do not administer		
Anastrozole[14]	Mild to moderate hepatic impairment	No dosage adjustments necessary	No dosage adjustments necessary	
	Severe hepatic impairment	No data available		
Arsenic trioxide[15]	Child-Pugh class C (severe hepatic impairment)	Limited data available. Monitor closely for toxicity	CrCl <30 mL/min	Monitor closely; may require dosage reduction
			Dialysis patients	Has not been studied
Asparaginase (E. coli or E. chrysanthemi sources)[16,17]	Specific guidelines for dosage adjustments in hepatic impairment are not available; however, these patients may be at increased risk for toxicity. Evaluate hepatic enzymes and bilirubin pretreatment and periodically during treatment. Use caution in patients with a history of coagulopathy		Specific guidelines for dosage adjustments in renal impairment not available; it appears that no dosage adjustments are needed	
Atezolizumab[18]	No formal recommendation, but dosage adjustment seems unnecessary. Refer to FDA prescribing information for recommendations on management of autoimmune hepatitis		No formal recommendation, but dosage adjustment seems unnecessary. Refer to FDA prescribing information for recommendations on management of autoimmune nephritis	
Avapritinib[19]	Bilirubin ≤ ULN / AST > ULN	No dose adjustment necessary	CrCl 30–89 mL/min	No dose adjustment necessary
	Bilirubin >1 to 1.5 × ULN / Any AST		CrCl ≤29 mL/min	No data available. Note that 18% of a dose is excreted in the urine (0.23% as unchanged drug)
	Bilirubin >3 × ULN / Any AST	No data available		
Avelumab[20]	No formal recommendation, but dosage adjustment seems unnecessary. Refer to FDA prescribing information for recommendations on management of autoimmune hepatitis		No formal recommendation, but dosage adjustment seems unnecessary. Refer to FDA prescribing information for recommendations on management of autoimmune nephritis	
Axitinib[21]	Child-Pugh class A (mild hepatic impairment)	No dosage adjustment necessary	Mild to severe renal impairment (CrCl 15 to <89 mL/min)	No dosage adjustment necessary
	Child-Pugh class B (moderate hepatic impairment)	Reduce starting dosage by approximately 50%	End-stage renal disease (CrCl <15 mL/min)	Use is not recommended as it has not been studied. Use only with caution
	Child-Pugh class C (severe hepatic impairment)	Not recommended as it has not been studied		

(continued)

Generic Drug Name	Hepatic Dysfunction			Renal Dysfunction	
	Bilirubin	AST/SGOT and/or ALT/SGPT	Percent Dosage/Dose Administered	Creatinine Clearance (CrCl), Estimated Glomerular Filtration Rate (eGFR), or Serum Creatinine (SCr)	Percent Dosage/Dose Administered
Azacitidine for injection[22]	Pre-existing severe hepatic impairment		No data available. Use caution and monitor closely for toxicity	CrCl <30 mL/min	No dosage adjustment necessary. Exposure after multiple dosing is increased by 41%; use with caution
				Unexplained elevations of BUN or SCr	Delay next cycle until values return to normal or baseline and reduce dosage by 50%
				Unexplained reduction in serum bicarbonate to <20 mEq/L	Reduce dosage by 50%
Azacitidine for oral use[23]	Bilirubin ≤ ULN	AST > ULN	No dose adjustment necessary	CrCl 15–29 mL/min	No dosage adjustment necessary
	Bilirubin 1 to 1.5 × ULN	Any AST			
	Bilirubin > 1.5× ULN	Any AST	No data available		
Belantamab mafodotin-blmf[24]	Bilirubin ≤ ULN	AST > ULN	No dose adjustment necessary	eGFR 30–89 mL/min/1.73 m²	No dose adjustment necessary
	Bilirubin 1 to ≤1.5 × ULN	Any AST		eGFR <30 mL/min/1.73 m² or hemodialysis	No data available
	Bilirubin >1.5 × ULN	Any AST	No data available		
Belinostat[25]	Bilirubin ≤ ULN	AST > ULN	No dose adjustment necessary	CrCl >39 mL/min	No dose adjustment necessary
	Bilirubin 1 to ≤1.5 × ULN	Any AST		CrCl ≤39 mL/min	No data available
	Bilirubin >1.5 × ULN	Any AST	No data available		
Bendamustine[26]	1.5–3 × ULN	AST or ALT 2.5–10 × ULN	Do not administer	CrCl <30 mL/min	Do not administer
	>3 × ULN		Do not administer		
Bevacizumab[27]	No dosage adjustments necessary			No dosage adjustments necessary	
Bexarotene for oral use[28]	No specific studies have been conducted in patients with hepatic insufficiency. Less than 1% of a dose is excreted in the urine unchanged and there is in vitro evidence of extensive hepatic contribution to bexarotene elimination, thus hepatic impairment would be expected to lead to greatly decreased clearance. Use with great caution in this population			No formal studies have been conducted in patients with renal insufficiency. However, renal insufficiency may result in significant protein binding changes and may alter pharmacokinetics of bexarotene, so use caution	

(continued)

Drug	Hepatic impairment criteria	Hepatic impairment recommendation	Renal impairment criteria	Renal impairment recommendation
Bicalutamide[29]	No adjustment required for mild, moderate, or severe hepatic impairment. Use caution with moderate to severe impairment. Consider periodic LFTs during long-term therapy. Discontinue if ALT >2 × ULN or jaundice develops		No dosage adjustment is necessary	
Binimetinib[30]	Bilirubin >1.5 × ULN, Any AST	Administer 30 mg twice daily	No dosage adjustment is necessary	
Bleomycin sulfate[31,32]	Not studied in patients with hepatic impairment; adjustment for hepatic impairment may be needed		Dosage recommendations using Cockcroft and Gault formula	
			CrCl ≥50 mL/min	Administer 100% of dosage
			CrCl 40–49 mL/min	Administer 70% of dosage
			CrCl 30–39 mL/min	Administer 60% of dosage
			CrCl 20–29 mL/min	Administer 55% of dosage
			CrCl 10–19 mL/min	Administer 45% of dosage
			CrCl 5–9 mL/min	Administer 40% of dosage
			Continuous renal replacement therapy (CRRT)	Administer 75% of dose
			Note: terminal elimination half-life increases exponentially as the creatinine clearance decreases. Administration of nephrotoxic drugs with bleomycin may affect its renal clearance	
Blinatumomab[33]	No dose adjustment necessary		CrCl ≥30 mL/min	No dose adjustment necessary
			CrCl <30 mL/min or hemodialysis	No data available
Bosutinib[34]	Mild, moderate, and severe hepatic impairment	200 mg/day	CrCl 30–50 mL/min	300 mg/day (first-line, chronic-phase CML) or 400 mg/day (advanced-phase CML or ≥2nd line)
			CrCl <30 mL/min	200 mg/day (first-line, chronic-phase CML) or 300 mg/day (advanced-phase CML or ≥2nd line)
Bortezomib[35]	Bilirubin ≤ULN, AST >ULN	No dose adjustment necessary	No dosage adjustments necessary	
	Bilirubin >1–1.5 × ULN, Any AST	No dose adjustment necessary	*Note:* dialysis may reduce concentrations, so the drug should be administered postdialysis	
	Bilirubin >1.5 × ULN, Any AST	Reduce dosage to 0.7 mg/m² in the first cycle. Consider escalation to 1 mg/m² or further reduction to 0.5 mg/m² in subsequent cycles based on tolerability		

(continued)

Generic Drug Name	Hepatic Dysfunction			Renal Dysfunction	
	Bilirubin	AST/SGOT and/or ALT/SGPT	Percent Dosage/Dose Administered	Creatinine Clearance (CrCl), Estimated Glomerular Filtration Rate (eGFR), or Serum Creatinine (SCr)	Percent Dosage/Dose Administered
Brentuximab vedotin[36]	Child-Pugh class A (mild hepatic impairment), usual dosage of 1.2 mg/kg (maximum 120 mg) every 2 weeks		Reduce dosage to 0.9 mg/kg (maximum 90 mg) every 2 weeks	CrCl <30 mL/min	Do not administer
	Child-Pugh class A (mild hepatic impairment), usual dosage of 1.8 mg/kg (maximum 180 mg) every 3 weeks		Reduce dosage to 1.2 mg/kg (maximum 120 mg) every 3 weeks		
	Child-Pugh class B or C (moderate or severe hepatic impairment)		Do not administer		
Brigatinib[37]	Child-Pugh class C (severe hepatic impairment)		Reduce the dose by approximately 40% (i.e. from 180 mg to 120 mg, 120 mg to 90 mg, or from 90 mg to 60 mg)	CrCl 15–29 mL/min	Reduce the dose by approximately 50% (i.e. from 180 mg to 90 mg or from 90 mg to 60 mg)
Busulfan[38,39,40]	Has not been administered in clinical studies to patients with hepatic impairment. Undergoes extensive hepatic metabolism. Dosage adjustment may be necessary, although specific guidelines are not available. When used in patients with hepatic impairment, therapeutic drug monitoring is highly recommended			Renal excretion is insignificant	
Cabazitaxel[41]	Bilirubin >1 to ≤1.5 × ULN	Any	Reduce dose to 20 mg/m²	Renal impairment not requiring hemodialysis	No dosage adjustment necessary
	Bilirubin ≤1.5 × ULN	AST >1.5 × ULN	Reduce dose to 20 mg/m²		
	Bilirubin >1.5 to ≤3 × ULN	Any	Reduce dose to 15 mg/m²	End-stage renal disease (CrCl <15 mL/min/1.73 m²)	Monitor carefully during treatment
	Bilirubin >3 × ULN	Any	Do not administer		
Cabozantinib capsules (Cometriq)[42]	Child-Pugh class A or B (mild or moderate hepatic impairment)		Reduce starting dose to 80 mg	Mild to moderate renal impairment (eGFR ≥30 mL/min/1.73 m²)	No dosage adjustment necessary
	Child-Pugh class C (severe hepatic impairment)		Do not administer	Severe renal impairment (eGFR <30 mL/min/1.73 m² or requiring hemodialysis)	Has not been studied
Cabozantinib tablets (Cabometyx)[43]	Child-Pugh class B (moderate hepatic impairment)		Reduce starting dose to 40 mg	Mild to moderate renal impairment (eGFR ≥30 mL/min/1.73 m²)	No dosage adjustment necessary
	Child-Pugh class C (severe hepatic impairment)		Do not administer	Severe renal impairment (eGFR <30 mL/min/1.73 m² or requiring hemodialysis)	Has not been studied

(continued)

Drug	Hepatic condition		Recommendation	Renal condition	Recommendation
Capecitabine[44,45,46]	Mild to moderate hepatic dysfunction caused by liver metastases		No dosage adjustment necessary. Monitor carefully	CrCl 51–80 mL/min	No dosage adjustment necessary
	Severe hepatic dysfunction		No data available	CrCl 30–50 mL/min	Reduce dosage to 75%
				CrCl <30 mL/min	Do not administer
Caplacizumab-yhdp[47]	Severe hepatic impairment		No data available. Monitor closely due to the potential for increased bleeding risk	No dose adjustment necessary	
Capmatinib[48]	Mild, moderate, or severe hepatic impairment		No dose adjustment necessary	CrCl ≥30 mL/min	No dose adjustment necessary
				CrCl <30 mL/min	No data available
Carboplatin[32,46,49]	No dosage adjustments necessary for initial therapy			Patients with CrCl values <60 mL/min are at ↑ risk of severe bone marrow suppression. Incidence of severe leukopenia, neutropenia, or thrombocytopenia has been about 25% with the tiered dosage modifications shown below (*Note:* dose modification for impaired renal function is not necessary for carboplatin doses based on systemic exposure [AUC] calculations, such as the methods described by Calvert et al, Chatelut et al, and Bénézét et al)	
				CrCl 41–59 mL/min	250 mg/m² (Day 1)
				CrCl 16–40 mL/min	200 mg/m² (Day 1)
				CrCl ≤15 mL/min	No guidelines available
				Hemodialysis	Administer 50% of dosage
				Continuous ambulatory peritoneal dialysis (CAPD)	Administer 25% of dosage
				Continuous renal replacement therapy (CRRT)	200 mg/m²
Carfilzomib[50]	Bilirubin 1–3× ULN	Any AST	Reduce dose by 25%	Mild, moderate, and severe renal impairment	No dosage adjustment necessary
	Bilirubin ≤ ULN	AST > ULN	Reduce dose by 25%	Hemodialysis	Administer after dialysis
	Bilirubin >3× ULN	Any AST	Not recommended as it has not been studied		
Carmustine[51]	Dosage adjustment may be necessary, but no specific guidelines are available			CrCl 46–60 mL/min	Administer 80% of dosage
				CrCl 31–45 mL/min	Administer 75% of dosage
				CrCl <30 mL/min	Consider alternative therapy
Cemiplimab-rwlc[52]	No formal recommendation, but dosage adjustment seems unnecessary. Refer to FDA prescribing information for recommendations on management of autoimmune hepatitis			No formal recommendation, but dosage adjustment seems unnecessary. Refer to FDA prescribing information for recommendations on management of autoimmune nephritis	
	Child-Pugh class A or B (mild or moderate hepatic impairment)		No dose adjustment necessary	CrCl ≥30 mL/min	No dose adjustment necessary

(continued)

Generic Drug Name	Hepatic Dysfunction			Renal Dysfunction	
	Bilirubin	AST/SGOT and/or ALT/SGPT	Percent Dosage/Dose Administered	Creatinine Clearance (CrCl), Estimated Glomerular Filtration Rate (eGFR), or Serum Creatinine (SCr)	Percent Dosage/Dose Administered
Ceritinib[53]	Child-Pugh class C (severe hepatic impairment)		Reduce the dose by approximately 33% (round to nearest multiple of 150 mg strength)	CrCl <30 mL/min	No data available. Only 1.3% of an administered dose is excreted in the urine
Cetuximab[54]	No dosage adjustments necessary			No dosage adjustments necessary	
Chlorambucil[32,55]	Hepatic metabolism into active and inactive metabolites. Dosage adjustment may be needed in patients with hepatic impairment			*Note:* renal excretion of chlorambucil and phenylacetic acid mustard accounts for <1% of elimination	
				CrCl 10–50	Administer 75% of dosage
				CrCl <10 mL/min	Administer 50% of dosage
				Hemodialysis	Administer 50%; no supplemental dosing
				Peritoneal dialysis	Administer 50%; no supplemental dosing
Cisplatin[56]	No dosage adjustments necessary			Curative intent, GFR 50–59 mL/min	Administer 75%
				Curative intent, GFR 40–49 mL/min	Administer 50%
				Curative intent, GFR <40 mL/min	Do not administer
				Curative intent, hemodialysis	Consider administering 50%
				Palliative intent, GFR 50–59 mL/min	Administer 75%
				Palliative intent, GFR <50 mL/min	Do not administer
				Palliative intent, hemodialysis	Do not administer. Consider carboplatin as an alternative
Cladribine[32,57]	No specific dosage adjustment guidelines are available due to lack of data. Caution should be used in patients with hepatic impairment			CrCl 10–50 mL/min	Adult: 75% of dosage
				CrCl <10 mL/min	Adult: 50% of dosage
Clofarabine[56,58]	Safety not established. Use with caution			*Note:* up to 60% of an administered dose is excreted unchanged in the urine	
				CrCl 30–60 mL/min	Reduce dose by 50%
				CrCl <30 mL/min or hemodialysis	No data available; not recommended
Cobimetinib[59]	Mild, moderate, or severe hepatic impairment		No dose adjustment necessary	CrCl ≥30 mL/min	No dose adjustment necessary
				CrCl <30 mL/min	No data available
Copanlisib[60]	Bilirubin ≤ ULN	ALT > ULN	No dose adjustment necessary	CrCl ≥15 mL/min	No dose adjustment necessary
	Bilirubin >1 to 1.5 × ULN	Any AST	No dose adjustment necessary		
	Child-Pugh class B (moderate hepatic impairment)		Reduce the dose to 45 mg	CrCl <15 mL/min or hemodialysis	No data available
	Child-Pugh class C (severe hepatic impairment)		No data available		

(*continued*)

Drug	Hepatic function	Hepatic adjustment	Renal function	Renal adjustment
Crizanlizumab-tmca[61]	No data available. Likely metabolized into small peptides and amino acids		No data available. Likely metabolized into small peptides and amino acids	
Crizotinib[62]	Bilirubin >1.5 to ≤3 × ULN / Any AST	Reduce dosage to 200 mg twice daily	CrCl 30–90 mL/min	No dosage adjustments necessary
	Bilirubin >3 × ULN / Any AST	Reduce dosage to 250 mg once daily	CrCl <30 mL/min	Reduce dosage to 250 mg once daily
Cyclophosphamide[32,51,56]	Mild-moderate impairment	No dose adjustment necessary	CrCl 10–29 mL/min	Administer 75-100% of the normal dose
	Severe impairment	Use is not recommended due to risk of reduced efficacy	CrCl <10 mL/min	Administer 50%, 75%, or 100% of the normal dose
Cytarabine[56,63]	Cytarabine 100–200 mg/m² per dose: No dose adjustment necessary		Cytarabine 100–200 mg/m² per dose: No dose adjustment necessary	
	High-dose cytarabine ≥1000 mg/m² per dose: Bilirubin >3 × ULN / Any AST	Administer 25–50% of dose; may increase subsequent doses in the absence of toxicities	High-dose cytarabine ≥1000 mg/m² per dose: GFR = 31–59 mL/min/1.73 m²	Administer 50% of dosage
			GFR ≤30 mL/min/1.73 m²	Do not administer
			Hemodialysis	Administer 50% of dosage, start hemodialysis 4–5 hours after administration
			High-dose cytarabine ≥2000 mg/m² per dose: SCr 1.5–1.9 mg/dL or an ↑ from baseline of 0.5–1.2 mg/dL	Reduce dosage to 1000 mg/m² per dose
			SCr ≥2 mg/dL or ↑ from baseline of >1.2 mg/dL	Reduce dosage to 100 mg/m² per day as a continuous infusion
Dabrafenib[64]	Bilirubin ≤ ULN / AST > ULN	No dose adjustment necessary	GFR 30–89 mL/min/1.73 m²	No dose adjustment necessary
	Bilirubin >1 to ≤1.5 × ULN / Any AST	No dose adjustment necessary	GFR <30 mL/min/1.73 m²	No data available. *Note:* urinary excretion accounts for 23% of elimination (recovered from urine as metabolites only)
	Bilirubin >1.5 × ULN / Any AST	Exposure may be increased; limited data available. Use with caution and monitor closely for toxicity		
Dacarbazine[56]	Bilirubin >1 to 3 × ULN / Any AST	No dose adjustment necessary in the absence of concomitant renal impairment	GFR ≥30 mL/min without hepatic impairment	No dose adjustment necessary
	Bilirubin ≤ ULN / AST > ULN	Do not administer	GFR <30 mL/min or hemodialysis	Administer 70% of the dose
	Bilirubin >3 × ULN / Any AST	Do not administer		

(continued)

Generic Drug Name	Hepatic Dysfunction			Renal Dysfunction	
	Bilirubin	AST/SGOT and/or ALT/SGPT	Percent Dosage/Dose Administered	Creatinine Clearance (CrCl), Estimated Glomerular Filtration Rate (eGFR), or Serum Creatinine (SCr)	Percent Dosage/Dose Administered
Dacomitinib[65]	Mild, moderate, or severe hepatic impairment		No dose adjustment necessary	CrCl ≥30 mL/min	No dose adjustment necessary
				CrCl <30 mL/min	No data available. Note that only 3% of an administered dose is eliminated renally (<1% as parent drug)
Dactinomycin[56]	Bilirubin >1 to 3 × ULN	Any AST	No dose adjustment necessary. Note that hepatotoxicity (eg, sinusoidal obstruction syndrome) related to therapy may require dose modification or discontinuation	No dosage adjustment necessary	
	Bilirubin ≤ ULN	AST >ULN			
	Bilirubin >3 × ULN	Any AST	Do not administer		
	Bilirubin ≤3 × ULN	Any AST	No dose adjustment necessary		
Daratumumab[66]	Bilirubin >3 × ULN	Any AST	No data available; therefore, no formal recommendation, though dosage adjustment seems unnecessary	CrCl ≥15 mL/min	No dosage adjustment necessary
Darbepoetin alfa[67]	No dosage adjustment necessary			No dosage adjustment necessary	
Darolutamide[68]	Child-Pugh class A (mild hepatic impairment)		No dosage adjustment necessary	eGFR ≥30 mL/min/1.73 m²	No dosage adjustment necessary
	Child-Pugh class B (moderate hepatic impairment)		Reduce dosage to 300 mg twice daily	eGFR 15–29 mL/min/1.73 m², not receiving hemodialysis	Reduce dosage to 300 mg twice daily
	Child-Pugh class C (severe hepatic impairment)		No data available	eGFR ≤15 mL/min/1.73 m² or hemodialysis	No data available
Dasatinib[69]	No dosage adjustments necessary. Note: after administering a 70-mg dose, compared to subjects with normal liver function, patients with moderate hepatic impairment (Child-Pugh class B) had decreases in dose normalized C_{max} and AUC of 47% and 8%, respectively; patients with severe hepatic impairment (Child-Pugh class C) had dose normalized C_{max} decreased by 43% and AUC decreased by 28% compared to normal controls. These differences in C_{max} and AUC are not clinically relevant			Currently no clinical studies on renal insufficiency. Less than 4% of dasatinib and its metabolites are excreted via the kidney	
Daunorubicin HCl[70]	Bilirubin 1.2–3.0 mg/dL		Administer 75% of dosage	SCr >3 mg/dL	Administer 50% of dosage
	Bilirubin >3 mg/dL		Administer 50% of dosage		

(continued)

Drug	Hepatic Function		Renal Function	
Daunorubicin and cytarabine, liposome for injection[71]	Bilirubin ≤3 mg/dL	No dose adjustment necessary	CrCl ≥30 mL/min	No dose adjustment necessary
	Bilirubin >3 mg/dL	No data available. Do not administer	CrCl <30 mL/min or end-stage renal disease	No data available
Decitabine for injection[72]	No data exist on the use of decitabine in patients with hepatic dysfunction; therefore, it should be used with caution. If bilirubin and/or ALT is >2 × ULN temporarily hold until resolution		No data exist on the use of decitabine in patients with renal dysfunction; therefore, it should be used with caution. If SCr >2 mg/dL, temporarily withhold decitabine until resolution	
Decitabine and cedazuridine, for oral use[73]	Bilirubin >1 to 1.5 × ULN / Any AST	No dose adjustment necessary	CrCl ≥60 mL/min	No dose adjustment necessary
	Bilirubin ≤ ULN / AST >ULN	No dose adjustment necessary	CrCl 30–59 mL/min	No dose adjustment necessary; monitor frequently for adverse reactions
	Bilirubin >1.5 × ULN / Any AST	No data available	CrCl <30 mL/min or end-stage renal disease	No data available
Defibrotide[74]	No dose adjustment necessary. Metabolism is by nucleases, nucleotidases, nucleosidases, deaminases, and phosphorylases. Incubation of defibrotide with cultured human hepatocytes suggests insignificant levels of hepatic metabolism		End-stage renal disease	No dose adjustment necessary. Not removed by hemodialysis. Exposure (AUC) is ↑ by 50–60% and peak concentrations are ↑ by 35–37%
Denosumab[75]	No clinical trials have been conducted		CrCl <30 mL/min or hemodialysis	Use with caution; may be at greater risk for hypocalcemia. Ensure adequate vitamin D and calcium supplementation if not contraindicated
Dexrazoxane[76]	No dosage reductions necessary		CrCl <40 mL/min	Administer 50% of dosage
Docetaxel[77,78,79,80]	Bilirubin > ULN / Any AST or ALT	Do not administer	No dosage reductions necessary. *Note: not removed by hemodialysis; may be administered before or after hemodialysis*	
	Any bilirubin / AST or ALT >1.5 × ULN and alkaline phosphatase >2.5 × ULN	Do not administer		
	Any bilirubin / AST or ALT >5 × ULN and/or alkaline phosphatase >5 × ULN	Do not administer		
	Bilirubin <ULN / ALT or AST >1 to ≤1.5 × ULN	No dose reduction necessary		
	Bilirubin <ULN / ALT or AST >1.5 to ≤5 × ULN and alkaline phosphatase >2.5 to ≤5 × ULN	Administer 80% of dosage		
	Bilirubin <ULN / ALT or AST >2.5 to ≤5 × ULN and alkaline phosphatase ≤2.5 × ULN	Administer 80% of dosage		

(continued)

Generic Drug Name	Hepatic Dysfunction			Renal Dysfunction	
	Bilirubin	AST/SGOT and/or ALT/SGPT	Percent Dosage/Dose Administered	Creatinine Clearance (CrCl), Estimated Glomerular Filtration Rate (eGFR), or Serum Creatinine (SCr)	Percent Dosage/Dose Administered
Doxorubicin HCl[81,82,83]	Bilirubin 1.2–3 mg/dL		Administer 50% of dosage	No dosage reductions necessary	
	Bilirubin 3.1–5 mg/dL		Administer 25% of dosage		
	Bilirubin >5 mg/dL		Contraindicated		
Doxorubicin HCl liposomal[82,84,85]	Bilirubin 1.2–3 mg/dL		Administer 75% of dosage initially, then escalate to full dose if tolerated	No dosage reductions necessary	
	Bilirubin >3 mg/dL		Administer 50% of dosage initially, then escalate to 75% dosage, and then to full dosage, as tolerated		
Durvalumab[86]	No formal recommendation, but dosage adjustment seems unnecessary. Refer to FDA prescribing information for recommendations on management of autoimmune hepatitis			No formal recommendation, but dosage adjustment seems unnecessary. Refer to FDA prescribing information for recommendations on management of autoimmune nephritis	
Duvelisib[87]	No dose adjustment necessary			No dose adjustment necessary	
Elotuzumab[88]	Bilirubin >1 to 1.5 × ULN	Any AST	No dose adjustment necessary	No dose adjustment necessary	
	Bilirubin ≤ ULN	AST >ULN	No dose adjustment necessary		
	Bilirubin >1.5 × ULN	Any AST	No data available		
Eltrombopag[89]	Child-Pugh class A, B, or C hepatic impairment (aplastic anemia indication)		Reduce initial dose by 50%. If baseline ALT or AST are > 6 × ULN, then do not initiate therapy until ALT and AST are 5 × ULN	CrCl >80 mL/min	No dose adjustment necessary
	Child-Pugh class A, B, or C hepatic impairment (ITP indication)		Reduce initial dose by 50%	CrCl 30–80 mL/min	No dose adjustment necessary; AUC is ↓ by 32–36%; effect on unbound eltrombopag exposure is unknown
	Child-Pugh class A, B, or C hepatic impairment (HCV-associated thrombocytopenia indication)		No dose adjustment necessary	CrCl <30 mL/min	No dose adjustment necessary; AUC is ↓ by 60%; effect on unbound eltrombopag exposure is unknown
Enasidenib[90]	Bilirubin ≤ ULN	AST >ULN	No dose adjustment necessary	CrCl ≥30 mL/min	No dose adjustment necessary
	Bilirubin 1 to 1.5 × ULN	Any AST	No dose adjustment necessary		
	Bilirubin >1.5 × ULN	Any AST	No data available	CrCl <30 mL/min	No data available. Note that only 11% of an administered dose is excreted in the urine (0.4% as parent drug)

Note: enasidenib inhibits UGT1A1, resulting in an elevation of bilirubin to ≥2 × ULN in 37% of patients. If bilirubin increases to >3 × ULN for ≥2 weeks, then reduce the dose to 50 mg daily. If bilirubin improves to <2 × ULN subsequently, then resume the usual 100 mg daily dose

(continued)

Drug	Hepatic impairment condition		Hepatic adjustment	Renal impairment condition	Renal adjustment
Encorafenib[91]	Child-Pugh class A (mild hepatic impairment)		No dose adjustment necessary	CrCl ≥30 mL/min	No dose adjustment necessary
	Child-Pugh class B or C (moderate or severe hepatic impairment)		No data available	CrCl <30 mL/min	No data available
Enfortumab vedotin-ejfv[92]	Bilirubin ≤ ULN	AST >1 to 2.5 × ULN	No dose adjustment necessary; a 48% ↑ in unconjugated MMAE AUC was observed	No dose adjustment necessary	
	Bilirubin 1 to 1.5 × ULN	AST ≤2.5 × ULN			
	Bilirubin >1.5 × ULN	—	No data available. Do not administer		
	—	AST or ALT >2.5 × ULN			
Entrectinib[93]	Bilirubin ≤1.5 × ULN		No dose adjustment necessary	CrCl ≥30 mL/min	No dose adjustment necessary
	Bilirubin >1.5x ULN		No data available	CrCl <30 mL/min	No data available. Note that only 3% of an administered dose is excreted in the urine
Enzalutamide[94]	Mild, moderate, or severe hepatic impairment		No dosage adjustments necessary	Creatinine clearance 30 to ≤89 mL/min	No dosage adjustment necessary
				CrCl <30 mL/min	No clinical trials have been conducted
Epirubicin HCl[46,95,96]	Bilirubin 1.2–3 mg/dL	AST ≤4 × ULN	Administer 50% of dosage	CrCl <50 mL/min	No dosage adjustments necessary
		AST 2–4 × ULN	Administer 50% of dosage		
	Bilirubin >3 mg/dL to ≤5 mg/dL	Any AST	Administer 25% of dosage	SCr >5 mg/dL	Dosage adjustment required; no specific guidelines
	Bilirubin ≤5 mg/dL	AST >4 × ULN	Administer 25% of dosage		
	Severe hepatic impairment (Child-Pugh class C, or bilirubin >5 mg/dL)		Use is contraindicated		
Epoetin Alfa[97]	No dosage adjustments necessary			No dosage adjustments necessary	
Erdafitinib[98]	Bilirubin ≤ ULN	AST > ULN	No dose adjustment necessary	eGFR ≥30 mL/min/1.73 m²	No dose adjustment necessary
	Bilirubin 1 to 1.5 × ULN	Any AST	No dose adjustment necessary	eGFR <30 mL/min/1.73 m² or hemodialysis	No data available
	Bilirubin >1.5× ULN	Any AST	No data available		
Eribulin mesylate[99]	Child-Pugh class A (mild hepatic impairment)		Reduce dose to 1.1 mg/m²	CrCl ≥50 mL/min	No dose adjustment necessary
	Child-Pugh class B (moderate hepatic impairment)		Reduce dose to 0.7 mg/m²	CrCl 15–49 mL/min	Reduce dose to 1.1 mg/m²
	Child-Pugh class C (severe hepatic impairment)		Use has not been studied	CrCl <15 mL/min	No clinical trials have been conducted

(continued)

Generic Drug Name	Hepatic Dysfunction			Renal Dysfunction	
	Bilirubin	AST/SGOT and/or ALT/SGPT	Percent Dosage/Dose Administered	Creatinine Clearance (CrCl), Estimated Glomerular Filtration Rate (eGFR), or Serum Creatinine (SCr)	Percent Dosage/Dose Administered
Erlotinib HCl[100,101]	In vitro and in vivo data suggest erlotinib is cleared primarily by the liver. However, erlotinib exposure was similar in patients with moderately impaired hepatic function (Child-Pugh B) and patients with adequate hepatic function, including patients with primary liver cancer or hepatic metastases			No dosage adjustments necessary. Less than 9% of a single dose is excreted in the urine	
	Direct bilirubin 1–7 mg/dL, or AST >3 × ULN		Administer 50% dosage initially. Escalate dosage if tolerated		
	Note: erlotinib dosing should be interrupted or discontinued in patients with pre-existing hepatic impairment if changes in liver function are severe such as doubling of total bilirubin and/or tripling of transaminases in the setting				
Estramustine phosphate sodium[102]	No dosage adjustments necessary			No dosage adjustments necessary	
Etoposide[56,103,104]	Bilirubin <2.9 mg/dL and normal albumin and renal function		No dose adjustment necessary	CrCl 10–50 mL/min	Administer 75% dosage; increase if tolerated
	Bilirubin ≥2.9 mg/dL or reduced albumin levels		Administer 50% dosage initially; consider increasing if tolerated	CrCl <10 mL/min	Not studied, consider further dose reduction (eg, to 50% dosage)
	Note: decreased albumin increases unbound drug concentration and increases hematologic toxic effects			Hemodialysis	Not dialyzable. Administer 75% dosage. No supplemental dosing needed
Everolimus[105]	Hepatic Dosing for Oncologic Indications			Renal Dosing for Oncologic Indications	
	Child-Pugh class A		Reduce initial dosage to 7.5 mg daily; decrease to 5 mg daily if not tolerated		
	Child-Pugh class B		Reduce initial dosage to 5 mg daily; decrease to 2.5 mg daily if not tolerated	No dosage adjustments necessary	
	Child-Pugh class C		Reduce initial dosage to 2.5 mg daily if benefit outweighs risk		
Exemestane[106]	No dosage adjustments necessary			No dosage adjustments necessary	
Fam-trastuzumab deruxtecan-nxki[107]	Bilirubin ≤ ULN	AST > ULN	No dose adjustment necessary	eGFR ≥30 mL/min/1.73 m²	No dose adjustment necessary
	Bilirubin >1 to 1.5 × ULN	Any AST	No dose adjustment necessary		
	Bilirubin >1.5 × to 3x ULN	Any AST	No dose adjustment necessary. Monitor more closely for toxicity	eGFR <30 mL/min/1.73 m² or hemodialysis	No data available
	Bilirubin >3 × ULN	Any AST	No data available		

(continued)

Drug	Hepatic Function		Hepatic Dosage Adjustment	Renal Function	Renal Dosage Adjustment
Fedratinib[108]	Bilirubin ≤ ULN	AST > ULN	No dose adjustment necessary	CrCl ≥60 mL/min	No dose adjustment necessary
	Bilirubin >1 to 3 × ULN	Any AST	No dose adjustment necessary	CrCl 30–59 mL/min	No dose adjustment necessary. Monitor more closely for adverse effects
	Bilirubin >3 × ULN	Any AST	No data available; do not administer	CrCl 15–29 mL/min	Reduce dosage to 200 mg once daily
Filgrastim[109]	No dosage adjustments necessary			No dosage adjustments necessary	
Floxuridine[110,111]	1.2 × ULN	Alkaline phosphatase 1.2 × ULN	Administer 80% of dosage	Dosage adjustment may be necessary. No specific guidelines are available	
	1.5 × ULN	AST or ALT 3 × baseline or alkaline phosphatase 1.5 × ULN	Administer 50% of dosage		
	2 × ULN	AST or ALT >3 × baseline or alkaline phosphatase 2 × ULN	No recommendations available		
Fludarabine[32,112]	Dosage adjustments may be necessary. No specific guidelines are available			CrCl 50–79 mL/min in adults	Administer 80% of IV dosage
				CrCl 30–49 mL/min in adults	Administer 60–75% of IV dosage
				CrCl <30 mL/min in adults	Administer 0–50% of IV dosage
				Hemodialysis	Administer 50% of the IV dose after dialysis
				Continuous ambulatory peritoneal dialysis (CAPD)	Administer 50% of IV dosage
				Continuous renal replacement therapy (CRRT)	Administer 75% of IV dosage
Fluorouracil[46,56,111,113]	>5 mg/dL		Do not administer	No dose adjustment necessary	
	Increased bilirubin: no relation to fluorouracil clearance; no adjustment needed				
Fluoxymesterone[114]	Severe hepatic impairment		Contraindicated	Severe renal impairment	Contraindicated
Flutamide[115]	Severe hepatic impairment		Contraindicated	No dosage adjustments necessary	
Fostamatinib disodium hexahydrate[116]	No dose adjustment necessary for baseline hepatic impairment. Note: can cause elevated ALT and AST. If ALT or AST ↑ by >3 × ULN, manage toxicity with dose interruption, dose reduction, or discontinuation as described in the FDA-approved prescribing information			No dose adjustment necessary	
Fulvestrant[117]	Child-Pugh class A (mild hepatic impairment)		No dosage adjustments necessary	No dosage adjustments necessary	
	Child-Pugh class B (moderate hepatic impairment)		Reduce maintenance and initial doses to 250 mg		
	Child-Pugh class C (severe hepatic impairment)		Use has not been evaluated		

(continued)

Generic Drug Name	Hepatic Dysfunction			Renal Dysfunction	
	Bilirubin	AST/SGOT and/or ALT/SGPT	Percent Dosage/Dose Administered	Creatinine Clearance (CrCl), Estimated Glomerular Filtration Rate (eGFR), or Serum Creatinine (SCr)	Percent Dosage/Dose Administered
Gefitinib[118]	Moderate to severe impairment as a result of metastases		No dosage adjustments necessary		No dosage adjustments necessary
Gemcitabine HCl[56,119,120]	Bilirubin ≤1.6 mg/dL	AST > ULN	No dose adjustment necessary	No dosage adjustments necessary. In hemodialysis patients, initiate hemodialysis 6–12 hours after gemcitabine administration	
	Bilirubin >1.6 mg/dL	Any AST	Reduce initial dosage by 20%; increase as tolerated		
Gemtuzumab ozogamicin[121]	Use extra caution when administering in patients with hepatic impairment due to a higher risk of sinusoidal obstruction syndrome			No dosage adjustments necessary	
Gilteritinib[122]	Child-Pugh class A or B (mild or moderate hepatic impairment)		No dose adjustment necessary	CrCl ≥30 mL/min	No dose adjustment necessary
	Child-Pugh class C (severe hepatic impairment)		No data available	CrCl <30 mL/min	No data available
Glasdegib[123]	No dose adjustment necessary			eGFR ≥30 mL/min	No dose adjustment necessary
				eGFR <30 mL/min	No dose adjustment necessary; monitor closely for adverse effects (eg, QTc prolongation)
Goserelin acetate[124]	No dosage adjustments necessary			No dosage adjustments necessary	
Hydroxyurea[125,126]	Moderate to severe hepatic impairment		Dosage adjustments may be necessary, but specific guidelines not available. Monitor CBC frequently	CrCl ≥60 mL/min	No dose adjustment necessary
				CrCl <60 mL/min	Administer 50% dosage
				Hemodialysis	Administer 50% dosage; on dialysis days, administer following dialysis
Ibritumomab tiuxetan[127]	No dosage adjustments necessary			No dosage adjustments necessary	
Ibrutinib[128,129,130]	Child-Pugh class A (mild hepatic impairment)		Reduce dosage to 140 mg daily (FDA) or 280 mg daily (EMA)	CrCl >25 mL/min	No dosage adjustment necessary
	Child-Pugh class B (moderate hepatic impairment)		Reduce dosage to 70 mg daily (FDA) or 140 mg daily (EMA)	CrCl <25 mL/min or hemodialysis	No data are available; however, dose adjustment is not expected to be necessary since <10% of a dose is excreted in the urine (all as metabolites)
	Child-Pugh class C (severe hepatic impairment)		Do not administer		

(continued)

Drug	Hepatic criteria	Hepatic adjustment	Renal criteria	Renal adjustment
Idarubicin HCl[32,56]	Bilirubin 2.6–5 mg/dL	Administer 50% dosage	GFR >50 mL/min	No dose adjustment necessary
	Bilirubin >5 mg/dL	Do not administer	GFR 30–50 mL/min	Administer 75–100% of dosage
			GFR <30 mL/min or hemodialysis	Administer 50–67% of dosage
Idelalisib[131]	Bilirubin >ULN to ≤1.5 × ULN	No dose adjustment necessary	No dose adjustment necessary	
	ALT or AST >ULN to ≤2.5 × ULN	No dose adjustment necessary		
	Bilirubin >1.5 × ULN	No dose adjustment necessary; limited safety and efficacy data; monitor closely		
	ALT or AST >2.5 × ULN			
	Note: fatal and/or serious hepatotoxicity occurs in 16–18% of patients			
Ifosfamide[51,111,132]	Bilirubin >3 mg/dL	Administer 25% of dosage	CrCl 46–60 mL/min	Administer 80% of dosage
	Other dosage adjustments may be necessary, but no specific guidelines are available		CrCl 31–45 mL/min	Administer 75% of dosage
			CrCl <30 mL/min	Administer 70% of dosage
			Hemodialysis	No supplemental dose needed
Imatinib mesylate[133,134]	Bilirubin >3–10 × ULN / Any AST	Administer 75% of dose	CrCl 40–59 mL/min	600 mg = maximum recommended dose
			CrCl 20–39 mL/min	Decrease starting dose by 50% and increase as tolerated to a maximum dosage of 400 mg
			CrCl <20 mL/min	Dose adjustment may be necessary, specific guidelines not available. Two patients with severe renal impairment tolerated 100 mg/day
Inotuzumab ozogamicin[135]	Bilirubin ≤ 1.5 × ULN / AST and ALT ≤ 2.5 × ULN	No dose adjustment necessary	No dose adjustment necessary	
	Bilirubin > 1.5 × ULN / AST or ALT > 2.5 × ULN	Limited safety data. Do not administer (unless hyperbilirubinemia due to Gilbert's syndrome or hemolysis)		
Interferon alfa[136]	No dosage adjustments necessary		No dosage adjustments necessary	
Ipilimumab[137]	No formal recommendation, but dosage adjustment seems unnecessary. Refer to FDA prescribing information for recommendations on management of autoimmune hepatitis		No formal recommendation, but dosage adjustment seems unnecessary. Refer to FDA prescribing information for recommendations on management of autoimmune nephritis	

(continued)

Generic Drug Name	Hepatic Dysfunction			Renal Dysfunction	
	Bilirubin	AST/SGOT and/or ALT/SGPT	Percent Dosage/Dose Administered	Creatinine Clearance (CrCl), Estimated Glomerular Filtration Rate (eGFR), or Serum Creatinine (SCr)	Percent Dosage/Dose Administered
Irinotecan HCl[138,139,140,141]	3-weekly irinotecan dosing (usual dose 350 mg/m² every 3 weeks)			Use caution; not recommended for use in patients on dialysis	
	≤1.5 × ULN		350 mg/m²		
	1.51–3 × ULN		200 mg/m²		
	>3 × ULN		Not recommended		
	Once weekly irinotecan dosing (usual dose 125 mg/m² for 4 of 6 weeks)				
	1.5–3 × ULN	AST/ALT ≤5 × ULN	60 mg/m²		
	1.5–3 × ULN	AST/ALT 5.1–20 × ULN	40 mg/m²		
	3.1–5 × ULN	AST/ALT ≤5 × ULN	50 mg/m²		
	≤1.5 × ULN	AST/ALT 5.1–20 × ULN	60 mg/m²		
	Special note: when administered in combination with other agents, or as a single-agent, a reduction in the starting dose by at least 1 level of irinotecan should be considered for patients known to be homozygous for the UGT1A1*28 allele				
Irinotecan liposome[142]	Bilirubin > ULN		No recommended dose available. Among patients with a bilirubin 1–2 mg/dL in a population PK study, SN38 steady state concentrations were ↑ by 37%	CrCl ≥30 mL/min	No dose adjustment necessary
				CrCl <30 mL/min	No data available
Isatuximab-irfc[143]	No dosage adjustments necessary			No dosage adjustments necessary	
Isotretinoin[144]	Empiric dose reductions are recommended in patients with hepatitis or abnormal liver enzymes			No dosage adjustments necessary	
Ivosidenib[145]	Child-Pugh class A or B (mild or moderate hepatic impairment)		No dose adjustment necessary	eGFR ≥ 30 mL/min/1.73m²	No dose adjustment necessary
	Child-Pugh class C (severe hepatic impairment)		No data available. Consider risks and potential benefits.	eGFR < 30 mL/min/1.73m², or hemodialysis	No data available. Consider risks and potential benefits

(continued)

Drug	Condition	Recommendation
Ixabepilone[146]	≤1 × ULN (AST and ALT ≤2.5 × ULN)	No dosage adjustments necessary. If administering with capecitabine, do not need a dosage adjustment
	≤1.5 × ULN (AST and ALT 2.5–10 × ULN)	Reduce dosage to 32 mg/m²
	1.5–3 × ULN (AST and ALT ≤10 × ULN)	Reduce dosage to 20 mg/m² dosage in subsequent cycles may be escalated up to, but not exceed, 30 mg/m² if tolerated
	>3 × ULN (AST or ALT >10 × ULN)	Do not administer
	>1 × ULN (AST and ALT >2.5 × ULN)	If administering with capecitabine, ixabepilone use is contraindicated
	CrCl >30 mL/min	No dosage adjustment necessary
	CrCl <50 mL/min	Combination therapy with capecitabine has not been studied
Ixazomib[147]	Moderate (total bilirubin >1.5–3 × ULN) or severe (total bilirubin >3 × ULN) hepatic impairment	3 mg orally once a week on days 1, 8, and 15 of a 28-day treatment cycle
	CrCl <30 mL/min or dialysis	3 mg orally once a week on days 1, 8, and 15 of a 28-day treatment cycle. May be given without regard to dialysis timing
Lapatinib[148]	Child-Pugh class C (severe hepatic impairment)	Dose reduction to 750 mg/day (HER2-positive metastatic breast cancer indication) or 1000 mg/day (hormone receptor–positive, HER2-positive breast cancer indication)
	Minimal renal elimination (<2%)	Dosage adjustments may not be necessary
Lanreotide[149]	No dose adjustments provided for carcinoid/gastroenteropancreatic neuroendocrine tumors	
	No dose adjustments provided for carcinoid/gastroenteropancreatic neuroendocrine tumors	
Larotrectinib[150]	Child-Pugh class A (mild hepatic impairment)	No dosage adjustment
	Child-Pugh classes B and C (moderate to severe hepatic impairment)	Reduce initial dosage by 50%
		No dosage adjustments necessary
Lenalidomide[151]		No dosage adjustments necessary

Dosage recommendations using Cockroft and Gault formula

	Combination therapy for MM and MCL	Combination therapy for FL and MZL	MDS and maintenance therapy following auto-HSCT for MM
CrCl 30–60 mL/min	10 mg daily	10 mg daily	5 mg daily
CrCl <30 mL/min (not requiring dialysis)	15 mg every 48 hours	5 mg daily	2.5 mg daily
CrCl <30 mL/min (requiring dialysis)	5 mg once daily. On dialysis days, administer the dose following dialysis	5 mg once daily. On dialysis days, administer the dose following dialysis	2.5 mg once daily. On dialysis days, administer the dose following dialysis

(continued)

Generic Drug Name	Hepatic Dysfunction			Renal Dysfunction	
	Bilirubin	AST/SGOT and/or ALT/SGPT	Percent Dosage/Dose Administered	Creatinine Clearance (CrCl), Estimated Glomerular Filtration Rate (eGFR), or Serum Creatinine (SCr)	Percent Dosage/Dose Administered
Lenvatinib[152]	Child-Pugh class C (severe hepatic impairment)		Endometrial or renal cell cancer—reduce to 10 mg daily; Thyroid cancer—reduce to 14 mg daily; Hepatocellular carcinoma—no dose adjustment provided	CrCl <30 mL/min	Endometrial or renal cell cancer: 10 mg daily; Hepatocellular carcinoma: No dose adjustment provided; Thyroid cancer: 14 mg daily
Letrozole[153]	Child-Pugh classes A and B (mild to moderate hepatic impairment)		No dose adjustments necessary	CrCl >10 mL/min	No dose adjustments necessary
	Child-Pugh class C (severe hepatic impairment) and cirrhosis		Reduce dose to 2.5 mg every other day		
Leucovorin calcium[154]	No dosage adjustments necessary			No dosage adjustments necessary	
Leuprolide acetate[114]	No dosage adjustments necessary			No dosage adjustments necessary	
Lomustine[46,111,56,155]	Dosage adjustments may be necessary, but no specific guidelines are available. Use caution in patients with hepatic dysfunction			CrCl 30–50 mL/min	Administer 75% dosage
				CrCl <30 mL/min	Avoid use
Lorlatinib[156]	Mild hepatic impairment (Total bilirubin ≤ ULN with AST > ULN or total bilirubin >1 to 1.5 times ULN with any AST)		No dosage adjustments necessary	CrCl 30–89 mL/min	No dosage adjustments necessary
	Moderate to severe hepatic impairment		Recommended dose has not been established	CrCl <30 mL/min	Recommended dose has not been established
Lurbinectedin[157]	Mild hepatic impairment (total bilirubin ≤ ULN with AST > ULN or total bilirubin >1 to 1.5 times ULN with any AST)		No dosage adjustment necessary	CrCl 30–89 mL/min	No clinically significant differences in pharmacokinetics seen; need for adjustment unlikely
	Moderate to severe hepatic impairment		No dose provided/not studied	CrCl <30 mL/min	No dose provided/not studied
Luspatercept-aamt[158]	Mild to severe hepatic impairment (total bilirubin ≤ ULN and AST or ALT > ULN, or total bilirubin > ULN and any AST or ALT)		No dosage adjustments necessary; pharmacokinetics not altered	eGFR ≥30 mL/min/1.73m²	No dosage adjustments necessary; pharmacokinetics not altered
	AST or ALT >3 × ULN		No dose provided/not studied	eGFR < 30 mL/min/1.73m²	No dose provided/not studied

(continued)

Drug	Hepatic impairment criteria	Hepatic recommendation	Renal impairment criteria	Renal recommendation
Lutetium Lu 177 dotatate[159]	Mild or moderate hepatic impairment	No dosage adjustments necessary	CrCl ≥30 mL/min	No dose adjustment necessary. Monitor renal function closely in mild to moderate impairment due to risk of toxicity
	Severe hepatic impairment (total bilirubin > 3 × ULN and any AST)	No dose provided/not studied	CrCl <30 mL/min	No dose provided/not studied
Megestrol acetate[160]	No dosage adjustments necessary		No dosage adjustments necessary	
Melphalan or melphalan HCl[39,161,162,163]	No dosage adjustments necessary		CrCl 30–59 mL/min	Oral regimens in MM: Reduce by 25%; High dose for autologous transplant in MM: Reduce to 140 mg/m²
			CrCl 15–29 mL/min	Oral regimens in MM: Reduce by 25%; High dose for autologous transplant in MM: Reduce to 140 mg/m²
			CrCl <15 mL/min	Oral regimens in MM: Reduce by 50%; High dose for autologous transplant in MM: Reduce to 140 mg/m²
			Hemodialysis	Oral regimens in MM: Reduce by 50%; High dose for autologous transplant in MM: Reduce to 100–140 mg/m²
Mercaptopurine[32,46,164]	Dosage adjustment may be necessary, but no specific guidelines are available. Use lowest recommended dose and monitor for toxicity		CrCl <50 mL/min	Use lowest recommended dose and monitor for toxicity. May increase interval to every 36–48 hours
Mesna[165]	Dosage adjustment may be necessary, but no specific guidelines are available		Dosage adjustment may be necessary, but no specific guidelines are available	
Methotrexate[46,111,166,167]	3.1–5.0 mg/dL — ALT and AST >3 × ULN	Administer 75% dosage	High-dose methotrexate: CrCl ≥100 mL/min	No dose adjustment necessary
	>5 mg/dL	Do not administer	CrCl 50–99 mL/min	Calculate dose as percent reduction of CrCl measurement below 100 mL/min
			CrCl < 50 mL/min	Avoid use
				For low or intermediate methotrexate—consult specific regimen for guidance in pediatric and adult patients. Renal adjustments required for CrCl <50 mL/min and in the setting of continuous renal replacement therapy. Avoid use in hemodialysis whenever possible
Midostaurin[168]	Mild (total bilirubin >1 to 1.5 times ULN or AST > ULN) or moderate (total bilirubin 1.5 to 3 times ULN and any AST) impairment	No dosage adjustments necessary; pharmacokinetics not altered	CrCl >30 mL/min	No dosage adjustments necessary; pharmacokinetics not altered
	Severe impairment (total bilirubin >3 times ULN and any AST)	No dose adjustment provided/not studied	CrCl 15–29 mL/min	No dose adjustment provided/not studied
Mitomycin[46,56,169]	Dosage adjustment may be necessary, but no specific guidelines are available. Clearance is affected primarily by metabolism in the liver, but metabolism occurs in other tissues as well		CrCl <30 mL/min or SCr >1.7 mg/dL	Do not administer
			Continuous ambulatory peritoneal dialysis (CAPD)	Administer 75% of dosage

(continued)

Generic Drug Name	Hepatic Dysfunction			Renal Dysfunction	
	Bilirubin	AST/SGOT and/or ALT/SGPT	Percent Dosage/Dose Administered	Creatinine Clearance (CrCl), Estimated Glomerular Filtration Rate (eGFR), or Serum Creatinine (SCr)	Percent Dosage/Dose Administered
Mitotane[170]	Dosage adjustment may be necessary, but no specific guidelines are available. Monitoring serum levels is recommended				No dosage adjustments necessary
Mitoxantrone HCl[171]	Clearance reduced in hepatic impairment. For total bilirubin >3.4 mg/dL, AUC increased threefold. Consider dose adjustment, but specific guideline unavailable				No dosage adjustments provided/not studied
Mogamulizumab-kpkc[172]	Mild (total bilirubin >1 to 1.5 times ULN or AST > ULN) or moderate (total bilirubin 1.5 to 3 times ULN and any AST) impairment		No dosage adjustments expected to be necessary; pharmacokinetics not altered	CrCl <90 mL/min	No dosage adjustments expected to be necessary; pharmacokinetics not altered
	Severe impairment (total bilirubin >3 times ULN and any AST)		No dose adjustment provided/not studied		
Moxetumomab pasudotox-tdfk[173]	Mild impairment (total bilirubin ≤ ULN and AST > ULN or total bilirubin >1 to 1.5 times ULN and any AST)		No dosage adjustments expected to be necessary; pharmacokinetics not altered	CrCl 30–89 mL/min	No dosage adjustments expected to be necessary; pharmacokinetics not altered
	Moderate to severe impairment (total bilirubin >1.5 times ULN)		No dose adjustment provided/not studied	CrCl ≤29 mL/min	Avoid use
Necitumumab[174]	Mild to moderate hepatic impairment		No dosage adjustments expected to be necessary; pharmacokinetics not altered	No dosage adjustments expected to be necessary; pharmacokinetics not altered	
	Severe hepatic impairment		No dosage adjustments provided/not studied		
Nelarabine[175]	Total bilirubin >3 × ULN		Monitor closely for toxicities	CrCl <50 mL/min	Clearance reduced with renal impairment. Monitor closely for toxicities
Neratinib[176]	Child-Pugh classes A and B (mild to moderate hepatic impairment)		No dosage adjustments required	No dosage adjustments expected to be necessary; PK not altered	
	Child-Pugh class C (severe hepatic impairment)		Decrease initial dose to 80 mg daily		
Nilotinib[177]	Newly diagnosed Ph+ CML			Effects in patients with renal impairment are unknown. Metabolites with minimal renal excretion; dosage adjustments for renal dysfunction may not be needed	
	Child-Pugh class A, B, or C (mild, moderate, or severe hepatic impairment)		200 mg twice daily. Increase to 300 mg twice daily if tolerated		
	Resistant or intolerant Ph+ CML				
	Child-Pugh class A or B (mild or moderate hepatic impairment)		300 mg twice daily. Increase to 400 mg twice daily if tolerated		
	Child-Pugh class C (severe hepatic impairment)		200 mg twice daily; increase to 300 mg twice daily and then further to 400 mg twice daily based on patient tolerability		

(continued)

Drug	Hepatic Impairment		Renal Impairment	
Nilotinib[177]	During treatment		No dosage adjustments necessary	
	3 × ULN	Withhold treatment, monitor bilirubin; resume treatment at 400 mg once daily when bilirubin returns to ≤1.5 × ULN		
	ALT or AST >5 × ULN	Withhold treatment, monitor transaminases; resume treatment at 400 mg once daily when ALT or AST return to <2.5 × ULN		
Nilutamide[178]	Dosage adjustment may be necessary, but no specific guidelines are available			
	Severe hepatic impairment	Contraindicated		
	Jaundice during treatment / ALT >2 × ULN during treatment	Discontinue		
Niraparib[179]	Mild hepatic impairment	No dosage adjustment necessary	CrCl 30–89 mL/min	No dosage adjustment necessary
	Moderate to severe hepatic impairment	No dose adjustment provided/not studied	CrCl < 30 mL/min	No dose adjustment provided/not studied
Nivolumab[180]	Mild (total bilirubin >1 to 1.5 times ULN or AST > ULN) or moderate (total bilirubin 1.5 to 3 times ULN and any AST) impairment	No dosage adjustments expected to be necessary; pharmacokinetics not altered. Refer to FDA prescribing information for management of autoimmune hepatitis	eGFR ≥15 mL/min/1.73m²	No dosage adjustments expected to be necessary; pharmacokinetics not altered. Refer to FDA prescribing information for management of autoimmune nephritis
	Severe impairment (total bilirubin >3 times ULN and any AST)	No dose adjustment provided/not studied. Refer to FDA prescribing information for management of autoimmune hepatitis		
Obinutuzumab[181]	No formal studies in patients with hepatic impairment have been conducted		CrCl ≤30 mL/min	No data
			CrCl >30 mL/min	No effect on PK
Octreotide acetate[182]	Established liver cirrhosis	Initial dose: 10 mg IM every 4 weeks. Titrate based upon response	Non-dialysis-dependent renal impairment	No dosage adjustments necessary
			Dialysis-dependent renal impairment	Initial dose: 10 mg IM every 4 weeks. Titrate based upon response
Ofatumumab[183]	No formal studies in patients with hepatic impairment have been conducted		CrCl ≥30 mL/min	No dosage adjustments expected to be necessary; pharmacokinetics not altered

(continued)

Generic Drug Name	Hepatic Dysfunction — Bilirubin	AST/SGOT and/or ALT/SGPT	Percent Dosage/Dose Administered	Renal Dysfunction — Creatinine Clearance (CrCl), Estimated Glomerular Filtration Rate (eGFR), or Serum Creatinine (SCr)	Percent Dosage/Dose Administered
Olaparib[184]	Child-Pugh class A or B (mild or moderate hepatic impairment)		No dose adjustment necessary	CrCl >50 mL/min	No dose adjustment necessary
				CrCl 31–50 mL/min	Reduce dose to 200 mg twice daily
	Child-Pugh class C (severe hepatic impairment)		No dose adjustment provided/not studied	CrCl ≤30 mL/min	No dose adjustment provided/not studied
Omacetaxine mepesuccinate[185]	No clinical trials have been conducted			No clinical trials have been conducted	
Osimertinib[186]	Child-Pugh A and B or Total bilirubin ≤ ULN and AST > ULN or Total bilirubin 1 to 3 × ULN and any AST		No dose adjustment necessary	CrCl ≥15 mL/min	No dose adjustment necessary
	Total bilirubin > 3 × ULN and any AST		No dose adjustment provided/not studied	CrCl <15 mL/min	No dose adjustment provided/not studied
Oxaliplatin[187,188]	No dosage adjustments necessary			CrCl <30 mL/min	Reduce initial dose from 85 mg/m² to 65 mg/m²
Paclitaxel[189,190]	24-hour infusion			No dosage adjustments necessary	
	≤1.5 mg/dL	*and* <2 × ULN	135 mg/m²		
	≤1.5 mg/dL	*and* 2–10 × ULN	100 mg/m²		
	1.6–7.5 mg/dL	*and* <10 × ULN	50 mg/m²		
	>7.5 mg/dL	*or* ≥10 × ULN	Do not administer		
	3-hour infusion				
	≤1.25 × ULN	*and* <10 × ULN	175 mg/m²		
	1.26–2.0 × ULN	*and* <10 × ULN	135 mg/m²		
	2.01–5.0 × ULN	*and* <10 × ULN	90 mg/m²		
	>5.0 × ULN	*or* ≥10 × ULN	Do not administer		

(continued)

Drug	Parameter	Metastatic breast cancer	Non-small cell lung cancer	Pancreatic adenocarcinoma	Renal function
Paclitaxel protein-bound particles[191]	Total bilirubin > 1.5 to ≤ 3 × ULN AND AST ≤ 10 × ULN	Reduce to 200 mg/m²	Reduce to 80 mg/m²	Not recommended	CrCl ≥30 mL/min — No dosage adjustments necessary
	Total bilirubin > 3 to ≤5 × ULN and AST ≤10 × ULN	Reduce to 200 mg/m²	Reduce to 80 mg/m²	Not recommended	CrCl <30 mL/min — No dose adjustment provided/not studied
	Total bilirubin > 5 × ULN or AST > 10 × ULN	Not recommended	Not recommended	Not recommended	
Palbociclib[192]	Child-Pugh class A or B (mild or moderate hepatic impairment)	No dosage adjustments necessary	CrCl ≥15 mL/min — No dosage adjustments necessary		
	Child-Pugh class C (severe hepatic impairment)	Reduce dose to 75 mg once daily for 21 days (28 day cycle)	CrCl <15 mL/min or hemodialysis — No dose adjustment provided/not studied		
Pamidronate disodium[193]	Mild to moderate hepatic impairment	No dosage adjustments necessary	CrCl <30 mL/min or SCr >3 mg/dL — Do not administer, or administer with caution. Limited data exist—consider dose reductions and longer administration times		
	Severe hepatic impairment	Not studied	Multiple myeloma: 90 mg over 4–6 hours unless renal impairment is preexisting then consider reduced initial dose		
Panitumumab[194]		No formal recommendation but dosage adjustment seems unnecessary	No formal recommendation but dosage adjustment seems unnecessary		
Panobinostat[195]	Mild impairment (bilirubin ≤1× ULN and AST >1× ULN, or bilirubin >1.0 to 1.5× ULN and any AST)	Reduce initial dose to 15 mg			
	Moderate impairment (bilirubin >1.5× to 3.0× ULN, any AST)	Reduce initial dose to 10 mg	CrCl <80 mL/min — No dosage adjustment required. No data in ESRD and dialysis		
	Severe impairment	Avoid use			
Pazopanib HCl[196]	Preexisting moderate dysfunction (total bilirubin 1.5 to 3 × ULN) and Any ALT value	Reduce to 200 mg once daily	No dosage adjustments necessary		
	Preexisting total bilirubin >3 × ULN and Any ALT level	Do not administer			
Pegaspargase[197]	No dosage adjustments provided. Effects on pharmacokinetics unknown. Contraindicated in severe hepatic impairment	No dosage adjustments provided. Effects on pharmacokinetics unknown			

(continued)

Generic Drug Name	Hepatic Dysfunction			Renal Dysfunction	
	Bilirubin	AST/SGOT and/or ALT/SGPT	Percent Dosage/Dose Administered	Creatinine Clearance (CrCl), Estimated Glomerular Filtration Rate (eGFR), or Serum Creatinine (SCr)	Percent Dosage/Dose Administered
Pegfilgrastim[198]	No dosage adjustments seem to be necessary, but PK profiles in patients with hepatic insufficiency have not been assessed				No dosage adjustments necessary
Pemetrexed disodium[199]	No dosage adjustments necessary			CrCl <80 mL/min	Use caution with concomitant NSAIDs
				CrCl <45 mL/min	Insufficient data. Do not administer
Pembrolizumab[200]	Mild (total bilirubin between 1 to 1.5 × ULN or AST > ULN)		No dosage adjustments expected to be necessary; PK not altered. Refer to FDA prescribing information for management of autoimmune hepatitis	eGFR >15 mL/min/1.73m²	No dosage adjustments necessary; PK not altered. Refer to FDA prescribing information for management of autoimmune nephritis
	Moderate (total bilirubin 1.5 to 3 × ULN and any AST) or severe (total bilirubin >3 × ULN and any AST) impairment		No dose adjustment provided/not studied. Refer to FDA prescribing information for management of autoimmune hepatitis		
Pemigatinib[201]	Mild (total bilirubin > ULN to 1.5 × ULN or AST > ULN) or moderate hepatic impairment (total bilirubin >1.5–3 × ULN with any AST)		No dosage adjustments necessary	Glomerular filtration rate (GFR) ≥30 to <90 mL/min (per MDRD equation)	No dosage adjustments necessary
	Severe hepatic impairment (total bilirubin >3 × ULN with any AST)		No dose adjustment provided/not studied	Glomerular filtration rate (GFR) <30 mL/min (per MDRD equation)	No dose adjustment provided/not studied
Pentostatin[56,202]	No dosage adjustments necessary			CrCl ≥60 mL/min	No dosage adjustment necessary
				CrCl 40–59 mL/min	Reduce to 3 mg/m²
				CrCl 35–39 mL/min	Reduce to 2 mg/m²
				CrCl <35 mL/min	Avoid use
Pertuzumab[203]	Mild, moderate, and severe hepatic impairment		No clinical trials have been conducted	CrCl 30 to ≤90 mL/min	No dosage adjustment necessary
				CrCl <30 mL/min	No clinical trials have been conducted
Pexidartinib[204]	Mild hepatic impairment (total bilirubin >1 to 1.5 × ULN with any AST)		No dosage adjustments necessary	CrCl 15–89 mL/min	Reduce dose to 200 mg in the morning and 400 mg in the evening
	Moderate (total bilirubin >1.5 to 3 × ULN and any AST) to severe (total bilirubin >3 to 10 × ULN and any AST)		No dose adjustment provided; pharmacokinetics not fully characterized		

(continued)

Drug	Hepatic impairment	Hepatic dosage adjustment	Renal impairment	Renal dosage adjustment
Plerixafor[205]	No dosage adjustments necessary		CrCl >50 mL/min	No dosage adjustments necessary. 0.24 mg/kg; maximum dose: 40 mg/day
			CrCl ≤50 mL/min	0.16 mg/kg; maximum dose: 27 mg/day
Pomalidomide[206]	Mild or moderate hepatic impairment (Child-Pugh A or B) — Kaposi sarcoma	Reduce to 3 mg daily	CrCl ≥15 mL/min to 60 mL/min — Kaposi sarcoma	No dosage adjustments provided; pharmacokinetics not altered
	Mild or moderate hepatic impairment (Child-Pugh A or B) — Multiple myeloma	Reduce to 3 mg daily	CrCl ≥15 mL/min to 60 mL/min — Multiple myeloma	No dosage adjustments provided; pharmacokinetics not altered
	Severe hepatic impairment (Child-Pugh C) — Kaposi sarcoma	Reduce to 3 mg daily	Hemodialysis dependent — Kaposi sarcoma	Reduce to 4 mg daily (give after dialysis)
	Severe hepatic impairment (Child-Pugh C) — Multiple myeloma	Reduce to 2 mg daily	Hemodialysis dependent — Multiple myeloma	Reduce to 3 mg daily (give after dialysis)
Ponatinib HCl[207]	Mild, moderate, or severe hepatic impairment (Child-Pugh A, B, or C)	Reduce to 30 mg daily		No dose adjustment provided/not studied
Polatuzumab vedotin-piiq[208]	Mild hepatic impairment (bilirubin >ULN to 1.5 × ULN or AST greater than ULN)	No dosage adjustment necessary	CrCl 30 to 89 mL/min	No dosage adjustments provided; pharmacokinetics not altered
	Moderate to severe hepatic impairment (AST or ALT >2.5 × ULN or total bilirubin >1.5 × ULN)	Avoid administration	CrCl < 30 mL/min	No dose adjustment provided/not studied
Pralatrexate[209]	>1.5 mg/dL; ALT or AST >2.5 × ULN; or AST or ALT >5 × ULN if known hepatic lymphoma	No clinical trials have been conducted	eGFR > 30 mL/min/1.73 m²	No dosage adjustment necessary
			eGFR 15 to <30 mL/min/1.73 m²	Reduce dose to 15 mg/m²
Pralsetinib[210]	Mild hepatic impairment (total bilirubin >1 to 1.5 × ULN with any AST)	No dosage adjustment necessary	CrCl 30 to 89 mL/min	No dosage adjustment necessary
	Moderate (total bilirubin >1.5 to 3 × ULN and any AST) to severe (total bilirubin >3 to 10 × ULN and any AST)	No dose adjustment provided/not studied	CrCl < 30 mL/min	No dose adjustment provided/not studied
Procarbazine HCl[111]	AST or ALT 1.6 to 6 × ULN	Administer 75% of dose		No dose adjustment provided/not studied
	Bilirubin >5 mg/dL and AST or ALT >3 × ULN	Avoid use		
Radium Ra 223 Dichloride[211]	Mild hepatic impairment	No dosage adjustment necessary	CrCl 30 to 89 mL/min	No dosage adjustment necessary
	Moderate to severe hepatic impairment	No dosage adjustments provided; pharmacokinetics unlikely to be altered	CrCl <30 mL/min	No dose adjustment provided/not studied

(continued)

Generic Drug Name	Hepatic Dysfunction			Renal Dysfunction	
	Bilirubin	AST/SGOT and/or ALT/SGPT	Percent Dosage/Dose Administered	Creatinine Clearance (CrCl), Estimated Glomerular Filtration Rate (eGFR), or Serum Creatinine (SCr)	Percent Dosage/Dose Administered
Raloxifene HCl[212]	Safety and efficacy have not been established in patients with hepatic impairment. Use with caution			Safety and efficacy have not been established in patients with moderate or severe renal impairment. Use with caution	
Ramucirumab[213]	Mild (total bilirubin < ULN and AST > ULN or total bilirubin >1 to 1.5 × ULN and any AST) or moderate (total bilirubin >1.5 to 3 × ULN and any AST) hepatic impairment		No dosage adjustments necessary. Use with caution with Child-Pugh B or C cirrhosis	CrCl ≥15 mL/min	No dose adjustment necessary. Pharmacokinetics not altered
	Severe hepatic impairment (total bilirubin >3 times ULN and any AST)		No dose adjustment provided/not studied. Use with caution with Child-Pugh B or C cirrhosis		
Ravulizumab-cwvz[214]	No dosage adjustments necessary			No dosage adjustments necessary	
Regorafenib[215]	Mild (total bilirubin ≤ULN and AST >ULN, or total bilirubin >ULN to ≤1.5 times ULN) or moderate (total bilirubin >1.5 to ≤3 times ULN and any AST) hepatic impairment		No dosage adjustments necessary	CrCl ≥15 mL/min	No dosage adjustment necessary
	Severe hepatic impairment (total bilirubin >3x ULN)		Not recommended as it has not been studied		
Ribociclib[216]	Mild hepatic impairment (Child-Pugh A)		No dosage adjustments necessary	End-stage renal disease or hemodialysis	No dose adjustment provided/not studied
	Moderate or severe hepatic impairment (Child-Pugh B or C)		Reduce to 400 mg daily	eGFR ≥30 mL/min/1.73 m²	No dosage adjustment necessary
				eGFR 15 to <30 mL/min/1.73 m²	Reduce to 200 mg daily
Ripretinib[217]	Mild (total bilirubin ≤ ULN and AST > ULN, or total bilirubin > ULN to ≤1.5 × ULN)		No dosage adjustments necessary	CrCl ≥30 mL/min	No dosage adjustment necessary
	Moderate to severe (total bilirubin >1.5 × ULN and any AST) hepatic impairment		No dose adjustment provided/not studied	CrCl <30 mL/min	No dose adjustment provided/not studied
Rituximab[218]	No dose adjustment necessary			No dose adjustment necessary	

(continued)

Drug	Hepatic Impairment	Hepatic Dosage	Renal Impairment	Renal Dosage
Romidepsin[219]	Mild	No dosage adjustment necessary	CrCl ≥15 mL/min	No dose adjustments necessary; pharmacokinetics not altered
	Moderate (bilirubin >1.5 × ULN to ≤3 × ULN and any AST)	Reduce to 7 mg/m²	CrCl <15 mL/min	No dose adjustment provided/not studied
	Severe (bilirubin >3 × ULN and any AST)	Reduce to 5 mg/m²		
Romiplostim[220]	No clinical studies have been conducted in patients with hepatic impairment. Use caution in this population		No clinical studies have been conducted in patients with renal impairment. Use caution in this population	
Rucaparib[221]	Mild hepatic impairment (total bilirubin ≤ ULN and AST > ULN, or total bilirubin between 1.0 to 1.5 × ULN and any AST)	No dosage adjustments necessary	CrCl ≥30 mL/min	No dosage adjustments necessary
	Moderate to severe hepatic impairment (total bilirubin > 1.5 × ULN)	No dose adjustment provided/not studied	CrCl <30 mL/min or hemodialysis	No dose adjustment provided/not studied

Ruxolitinib[222]

Myelofibrosis patients

	Hepatic Impairment			Renal Impairment		
Child-Pugh class A, B, or C	Platelets >150 × 10⁹/L	No dose reduction necessary	CrCl 15–59 mL/min	Platelets >150 × 10⁹/L	No dose reduction necessary	
	Platelets 100 to 150 × 10⁹/L	10 mg twice daily		Platelets 100–150 × 10⁹/L	10 mg twice daily	
	Platelets 50–100 × 10⁹/L	5 mg daily		Platelets 50–100 × 10⁹/L	5 mg daily	
	Platelets < 50 × 10⁹/L	Do not administer		Platelets <50 × 10⁹/L	Do not administer	
			Hemodialysis	Platelets >200 × 10⁹/L	20 mg once after dialysis session	
				Platelets 100–200 × 10⁹/L	15 mg once after dialysis session	

Polycythemia vera patients

	Hepatic Impairment		Renal Impairment	
	Child-Pugh class A, B, or C	5 mg twice daily	CrCl 15–59 mL/min	5 mg twice daily
			Hemodialysis	10 mg once after dialysis session

Acute graft versus host disease patients

	Hepatic Impairment		Renal Impairment	
	Stage 3 or 4 liver GVHD	No dose adjustment necessary. Monitor CBC more frequently; consider 5 mg once daily	CrCl 15–59 mL/min	5 mg once daily
			Hemodialysis	5 mg once after dialysis session

(continued)

Generic Drug Name	Hepatic Dysfunction: Bilirubin	Hepatic Dysfunction: AST/SGOT and/or ALT/SGPT	Hepatic Dysfunction: Percent Dosage/Dose Administered	Renal Dysfunction: Creatinine Clearance (CrCl), Estimated Glomerular Filtration Rate (eGFR), or Serum Creatinine (SCr)	Renal Dysfunction: Percent Dosage/Dose Administered
Sacituzumab govitecan-hziy[223]	Mild hepatic impairment (bilirubin less than or equal to 1.5 × ULN and AST/ALT < 3 ULN)		No dosage adjustments necessary	CrCl ≥30 mL/min	No dosage adjustments necessary
	Moderate or severe hepatic impairment		No dose adjustment provided/not studied. Exposure of active metabolite (SN-38) may be increased	CrCl <30 mL/min	No dose adjustment provided/not studied. Active metabolite (SN-38) excretion minimally excreted through kidneys
Sargramostim[224]	No dosage adjustments necessary			No dosage adjustments necessary	
Selinexor[225]	Mild hepatic impairment		No dosage adjustments necessary	CrCl ≥15 mL/min	No dosage adjustments necessary. Pharmacokinetics not altered
	Moderate or severe hepatic impairment		No dose adjustment provided/not studied	CrCl <15 mL/min	No dose adjustment provided/not studied
Selpercatinib[226]	Mild (total bilirubin > 1 to 1.5 × ULN with any AST) or moderate (total bilirubin > 1.5 to 3 × ULN and any AST) hepatic impairment		No dosage adjustments necessary	CrCl ≥30 mL/min	No dosage adjustments necessary
	Severe (total bilirubin > 3 to 10 × ULN and any AST) hepatic impairment		Reduce to 80 mg BID	CrCl <30 mL/min	No dose adjustment provided/not studied
Selumetinib[227]	Mild hepatic impairment (Child-Pugh A)		No dosage adjustments necessary	No dosage adjustments necessary	
	Moderate hepatic impairment (Child-Pugh B)		Reduce to 20 mg/m² BID		
	Severe hepatic impairment (Child-Pugh C)		No dosage adjustment established. Unbound $AUC_{0\text{-}INF}$ increased 3.2-fold		
Siltuximab[228]	Mild or moderate hepatic impairment (Child-Pugh A or B)		No dose adjustments necessary; pharmacokinetics not altered	CrCl ≥15 mL/min	No dose adjustments necessary; pharmacokinetics not altered
	Severe hepatic impairment (Child-Pugh C)		No dose adjustment provided/not studied	CrCl <15 mL/min	No dose adjustment provided/not studied
Sipuleucel-T[229]	No dosage adjustments seem to be necessary, but no pharmacokinetic profiles in patients with hepatic insufficiency have been assessed			No dosage adjustments seem to be necessary, but no pharmacokinetic profiles in patients with renal insufficiency have been assessed	

(continued)

Drug	Hepatic impairment	Recommendation	Renal impairment	Recommendation
Sonidegib[230]	Mild, moderate, or severe hepatic impairment (Child-Pugh A, B, or C)	No dosage adjustments provided; pharmacokinetics not altered	CrCl 30–89 mL/min	No dosage adjustments provided; pharmacokinetics not altered
			CrCl <30 mL/min	No dose adjustment provided/not studied
Sorafenib tosylate[231,232]	≤1.5 × ULN	400 mg BID	No dosage adjustments necessary for renal impairment. Pharmacokinetics unknown in hemodialysis population	
	1.5–3 × ULN	200 mg BID		
	3–10 × ULN	Do not administer		
Streptozocin[46,233,234]	No dosage adjustments seem to be necessary, but follow liver function tests carefully		CrCl 10–50 mL/min	Administer 75% of dosage
			CrCl <10 mL/min	Administer 50% of dosage
			Note: renal toxicity is dose related and cumulative; may be severe or fatal. Minimize adverse effects by basing dosage on clinical, renal, hematologic, and hepatic responses and tolerance of the patient	
Sunitinib malate[235]	Child-Pugh class A or B (mild to moderate hepatic impairment)	No dosage adjustments necessary	No dosage adjustments necessary. However, compared to subjects with normal renal function, the sunitinib exposure is 47% lower in subjects with ESRD on hemodialysis. Therefore, the subsequent dosages may be increased gradually up to twofold based on safety and tolerability	
	Child-Pugh class C (severe hepatic impairment)	No information available		
Tafasitamab-cxix[236]	Mild hepatic impairment (total bilirubin < ULN and AST > ULN, or total bilirubin between 1.0 to 1.5 × ULN and any AST)	No dosage adjustments necessary; pharmacokinetics not altered	CrCl ≥30 mL/min	No dosage adjustments necessary; pharmacokinetics not altered
	Moderate to severe hepatic impairment (total bilirubin > 1.5 × ULN)	No dose adjustment provided/not studied	CrCl <30 mL/min	No dose adjustment provided/not studied
Tagraxofusp-erzs[237]	Mild (total bilirubin ≤ ULN and AST > ULN, or total bilirubin > ULN to ≤1.5 × ULN) or moderate (total bilirubin >1.5 to ≤3 × ULN and any AST) hepatic impairment	No dosage adjustments necessary; pharmacokinetics not altered	eGFR ≥ 30 mL/min/1.73 m²	No dosage adjustments necessary; pharmacokinetics not altered. Renal toxicity during treatment requires interruption
	Severe hepatic impairment (total bilirubin >3x ULN)	No dose adjustment provided/not studied	eGFR 15 to <30 mL/min/1.73 m²	No dose adjustment provided/not studied. Renal toxicity during treatment requires interruption
Talazoparib[238]	Mild hepatic impairment (total bilirubin < ULN and AST > ULN, or total bilirubin between 1.0 to 1.5 × ULN and any AST)	No dosage adjustments necessary	CrCl ≥60 mL/min	No dosage adjustments necessary
			CrCl 30–59 mL/min	Reduce to 0.75 mg daily
	Moderate to severe hepatic impairment (total bilirubin > 1.5 × ULN)	No dose adjustment provided/not studied	CrCl 15–29 mL/min	Reduce to 0.5 mg daily
			CrCl <15 mL/min	No dose adjustment provided/not studied

(continued)

Generic Drug Name	Hepatic Dysfunction			Renal Dysfunction	
	Bilirubin	AST/SGOT and/or ALT/SGPT	Percent Dosage/Dose Administered	Creatinine Clearance (CrCl), Estimated Glomerular Filtration Rate (eGFR), or Serum Creatinine (SCr)	Percent Dosage/Dose Administered
Tamoxifen citrate[239]	No dosage adjustments necessary			No dosage adjustments necessary	
Tazemetostat[240]	Mild hepatic impairment (total bilirubin >1 to 1.5 × ULN or AST > ULN)		No dosage adjustments necessary	No dosage adjustments necessary	
	Moderate (total bilirubin >1.5 to 3 times ULN) or severe (total bilirubin >3 times ULN)		No dose adjustment provided/not studied		
Temozolomide[241]	Child-Pugh class A or B (mild to moderate hepatic impairment)		No dosage adjustments necessary	CrCl ≥36 mL/min	No dosage adjustments necessary
	Child-Pugh class C (severe hepatic impairment)		No dose adjustment provided/not studied Use caution in patients with severe hepatic impairment	CrCl <36 mL/min	No dosage adjustment provided. Use caution in patients with severe renal impairment
Temsirolimus[242]	Mild hepatic impairment (bilirubin >1 to 1.5× ULN or AST > ULN but bilirubin ≤ ULN)		Reduce dose to 15 mg/week	No dosage adjustments necessary	
	Moderate to severe hepatic impairment (bilirubin > 1.5 × ULN)		Contraindicated		
Teniposide[56,243]	Dosage adjustments may be necessary in patient with significant hepatic impairment. Avoid in severe hepatic impairment			Dosage adjustment may be necessary, but no specific guidelines are available	
Thalidomide[244]	No dosage adjustments necessary			No dosage adjustments necessary	
Thioguanine[245]	No formal recommendation but dosage adjustments are recommended in patients with hepatic impairment			No dosage adjustments necessary	
Thiotepa[246]	Mild (bilirubin >1 to 1.5× ULN or AST > ULN but bilirubin ≤ ULN) hepatic impairment		No dosage adjustment necessary	CrCl ≥60 mL/min	No dosage adjustment necessary
	Moderate (bilirubin >1.5 to 3 × ULN and any AST) or severe (bilirubin >3 × ULN and any AST) hepatic impairment		No formal recommendation, but dose reduction may be necessary. Monitor for toxicity due to possible increased plasma levels of thiotepa	CrCl <60 mL/min	No formal recommendation, but dose reduction may be necessary. Monitor for toxicity due to possible increased plasma levels of thiotepa

(continued)

Drug	Condition	Recommendation
Topotecan HCl[247,248]	**Intravenous formulation**	
	CrCl >40 mL/min	No dosage adjustment necessary
	CrCl 20–39 mL/min	Reduce dosage to 0.75 mg/m²
	CrCl <20 mL/min	Insufficient data
	Oral formulation	
	CrCl 30–49 mL/min	Reduce dosage to 1.5 mg/m²/day
	CrCl <30 mL/min	Reduce dosage to 0.6 mg/m²/day
Toremifene citrate[56,249]		No dose adjustments provided by manufacturer. Half-life may be prolonged in hepatic impairment. Consider 50% reduction in severe hepatic impairment
		No dosage adjustments necessary; pharmacokinetics not altered
Trabectedin[250]	Moderate hepatic impairment (bilirubin levels >1.5 to 3 × ULN, and AST and ALT < 8 × ULN)	Reduce to 0.9 mg/m²
	Severe hepatic impairment (bilirubin levels > 3 × ULN, and any AST and ALT)	Do not administer
	CrCl ≥30 mL/min	No dosage adjustments necessary
	CrCl <30 mL/min	No dosage adjustment provided/not studied
Trametinib dimethyl sulfoxide[251]	Mild hepatic impairment (total bilirubin >1 to 1.5 × ULN or AST > ULN)	No dosage adjustment necessary
	Moderate (total bilirubin >1.5 to 3 times ULN) or severe (total bilirubin > 3 times ULN)	No dosage adjustment provided/not studied
	eGFR ≥30 mL/min/1.73 m²	No dosage adjustment necessary
	eGFR <30 mL/min/1.73 m²	No dosage adjustment provided/not studied
Trastuzumab[252]		No dosage adjustments necessary
		No dosage adjustments necessary
Tretinoin[253]		No dose adjustment provided/not studied. Consider temporary interruption for bilirubin or transaminases >5 × ULN
		No dose adjustment provided/not studied. Consider interruption of therapy for renal impairment related to differentiation syndrome
Trifluridine/ tipiracil[254]	Mild hepatic impairment (total bilirubin < ULN and AST > ULN, or total bilirubin between 1.0 to 1.5 × ULN and any AST)	No dosage adjustment necessary
	Moderate (total bilirubin > 1.5 to 3 times ULN) or severe (total bilirubin > 3 times ULN)	Do not administer
	CrCl ≥30 mL/min	No dosage adjustments necessary
	CrCl 15–29 mL/min	Reduce dose to 20 mg/m²
	CrCl <15 mL/min	No dose adjustment provided/not studied
Tucatinib[255]	Child-Pugh class A or B (mild to moderate hepatic impairment)	No dose adjustment necessary
	Child-Pugh class C (severe hepatic impairment)	Reduce to 200 mg BID
	CrCl ≥30 mL/min	No dose adjustment necessary
	CrCl <30 mL/min	Recommend against use due to combination with capecitabine

(continued)

Generic Drug Name	Hepatic Dysfunction			Renal Dysfunction	
	Bilirubin	AST/SGOT and/or ALT/SGPT	Percent Dosage/Dose Administered	Creatinine Clearance (CrCl), Estimated Glomerular Filtration Rate (eGFR), or Serum Creatinine (SCr)	Percent Dosage/Dose Administered
Valrubicin[256]	Dosage adjustments do not appear to be necessary due to route of administration and low absorption, but no specific guidelines are available			Dosage adjustments do not appear to be necessary due to route of administration and low absorption, but no specific guidelines are available	
Vandetanib[56,257]	Child-Pugh classes A, B, and C (mild to severe hepatic impairment)		No formal recommendations provided, but dose adjustment unlikely to be necessary	CrCl <50 mL/min	Reduce starting dose to 200 mg
Vemurafenib[258]	1–3 × ULN		No dosage adjustments necessary	CrCl 30–89 mL/min	No dosage adjustments necessary
	>3 × ULN		Need for dosage adjustments has not been determined. Use with caution	CrCl <29 mL/min	Need for dosage adjustments has not been determined. Use with caution
Venetoclax[259]	Child-Pugh class A or B (mild to moderate hepatic impairment)		No dosage adjustments necessary	CrCl ≥15 mL/min	No dose adjustments necessary. Monitor closely for tumor lysis syndrome
	Child-Pugh class C (severe hepatic impairment)		Reduce daily dose by 50%	CrCl <15 mL/min	No dose adjustments provided/not studied
Vinblastine sulfate[56,111,260]	1.5–3 mg/dL		Administer 50% dosage	No dosage adjustments necessary	
	>3 mg/dL		Do not administer		
Vincristine sulfate[56,111,261]	1.5–3 mg/dL		Administer 50% dosage	No dosage adjustments necessary	
	>3 mg/dL		Do not administer		
Vincristine sulfate liposome[56,262]	Child-Pugh class A or B (mild to moderate hepatic impairment)		No dosage adjustments necessary	No clinical trials have been conducted, but no dosage adjustments expected to be necessary	
	Child-Pugh class C (severe hepatic impairment)		Avoid unless benefits outweigh risks. Consider 50% dose reduction		
Vinorelbine tartrate[263,264]	2.1–3 mg/dL		Administer 50% dosage	No dosage adjustments necessary	
	3.1–5 mg/dL		Administer 25% dosage		
	>5 mg/dL		Do not administer		
	Diffuse liver metastases		Administer 50% dosage		
Vismodegib[265]	No dosage adjustments necessary			No dosage adjustments necessary	

(continued)

Drug	Hepatic Impairment	Hepatic Dosage Adjustment	Renal Impairment	Renal Dosage Adjustment
Vorinostat[266,267]	Mild to moderate hepatic impairment (bilirubin 1 to 3 × ULN or AST > ULN)	Reduce to 300 mg daily		No dosage adjustments necessary; minimal renal excretion.
	Severe hepatic impairment (bilirubin > 3 × ULN)	Reduce daily dose by at least 50%		
Voxelotor[268]	Child-Pugh class A or B (mild to moderate hepatic impairment)	No dose adjustment necessary	CrCl ≥15 mL/min	No dosage adjustments necessary
	Child-Pugh class C (severe hepatic impairment)	Reduce to 1000 mg daily		
Zanubrutinib[269]	Child-Pugh class A or B (mild to moderate hepatic impairment)	No dose adjustment necessary	CrCl ≥30 mL/min	No dosage adjustments necessary
	Child-Pugh class C (severe hepatic impairment)	Reduce to 80 mg BID	CrCl <30 mL/min	No dosage adjustments provided; monitor closely
ziv-Aflibercept[270]	Mild (total bilirubin ≤ ULN and AST > ULN, or total bilirubin > ULN to ≤1.5 × ULN) or moderate (total bilirubin >1.5 to ≤3 × ULN and any AST) hepatic impairment	No dosage adjustments necessary		No dosage adjustments necessary
	Severe hepatic impairment (total bilirubin >3× ULN)	No dose adjustment provided/not studied		
Zoledronic acid[271]		Data is not adequate to provide guidelines on dosage selection and adjustment or how to safely use zoledronic acid in patients with hepatic impairment	*Dose recommendations using Cockcroft and Gault formula*	
			CrCl ≥60 mL/min	4 mg
			CrCl 50–59 mL/min	3.5 mg
			CrCl 40–49 mL/min	3.3 mg
			CrCl 30–39 mL/min	3 mg
			CrCl ≤30 mL/min	Use not recommended
			Hypercalcemia of malignancy with SCr >4.5 mg/dL	Consider treatment only after considering risks vs benefits. Use not recommended
			Bone metastases with SCr >3.0 mg/dL	Use not recommended

1. Verzenio (abemaciclib) product label. Indianapolis, IN: Lilly USA, LLC; March 2020
2. Zytiga (abiraterone) prescribing information. Horsham, PA: Janssen Biotech, Inc.; October 2020
3. Calquence (acalabrutinib) product label. Wilmington, DE: AstraZeneca Pharmaceuticals LP; November 2019
4. Kadcyla (ado-trastuzumab emtansine) prescribing information. South San Francisco, CA: Genentech, Inc.; September 2020
5. Gilotrif (afatinib) prescribing information. Ridgefield, CT: Boehringer Ingelheim Pharmaceuticals, Inc.; October 2019
6. Proleukin (aldesleukin) prescribing information. Yardley, PA: Clinigen, Inc.; September 2019
7. Alecensa (alectinib) product label. South San Francisco, CA: Genentech USA, Inc; June 2018
8. Campath (Alemtuzumab) product label. Cambridge, MA: Genzyme Corporation; October 2020
9. Panretin (alitretinoin) prescribing information. Woodcliff Lake, NJ: Eisai, Inc.; June 2018
10. Piqray (alpelisib) product label. East Hanover, NJ: Novartis Pharmaceuticals Corporation; September 2020
11. Ethyol (amifostine) product label. Yardley, PA: Clinigen, Inc.; December 2019
12. Erleada (apalutamide) product label. Horsham, PA: Janssen Products, LP; November 2020
13. Agrylin (anagrelide) prescribing information. Lexington, MA: Takeda Pharmaceuticals America, Inc.; August 2020
14. Arimidex (anastrozole) product label. Baudette, MN: ANI Pharmaceuticals, Inc.; August 2019
15. Trisenox (arsenic trioxide) product label. Parsippany, NJ: Teva Pharmaceuticals USA, Inc.; October 2020
16. Elspar (asparaginase) package insert. Deerfield, IL: Lundbeck; April 2010
17. Erwinaze (asparaginase *Erwinia chrysanthemi*) product label. Palo Alto, CA: Jazz Pharmaceuticals, Inc.; December 2019
18. Tecentriq (atezolizumab) product label. South San Francisco, CA: Genentech, Inc.; December 2020
19. Ayvakit (avapritinib) product label. Cambridge, MA: Blueprint Medicines Corporation; January 2020
20. Bavencio (avelumab) product label. Rockland, MA: EMD Serono, Inc.; November 2020
21. Inlyta (axitinib) product label. New York, NY: Pfizer Labs; June 2020
22. Vidaza (azacitidine) product label. Summit, NJ: Celgene Corporation; March 2020
23. Onureg (azacitidine) product label. Summit, NJ: Celgene Corporation; September 2020
24. Blenrep (belantamab mafodotin-blmf) product label. Research Triangle Park, NC: GlaxoSmithKline LLC; August 2020
25. Beleodaq (belinostat) product label. East Windsor, NJ: Acrotech Biopharma LLC; January 2020
26. Treanda (bendamustine) product label. North Wales, PA: Teva Pharmaceuticals USA, Inc.; November 2019
27. Avastin (bevacizumab) product label. South San Francisco, CA: Genentech Inc.; December 2020
28. Targretin (bexarotene) product label. Bridgewater, NJ: Bausch Health US, LLC.; April 2020
29. Casodex (bicalutamide) product label. Baudette, MN: ANI Pharmaceuticals, Inc.; August 2019
30. Mektovi (binimetinib) product label. Boulder, CO: Array BioPharma Inc.; October 2020
31. Bleomycin (product label). Lake Forest, IL: Hospira, Inc.; May 2018
32. Aronoff GR, Bennett WM, Berns JS et al. Drug Prescribing in Renal Failure: Dosing Guidelines for Adults and Children, 5th ed. Philadelphia, PA: American College of Physicians; 2007
33. Blincyto (blinatumomab) product label. Thousand Oaks, California: Amgen Inc.; March 2020
34. Bosulif (bosutinib) product label. New York, NY: Pfizer Labs; June 2020
35. Velcade (bortezomib) product label. Cambridge, MA: Millennium Pharmaceuticals Inc.; April 2019
36. Adcetris (brentuximab vedotin) prescribing information. Bothell, WA: Seagen Inc.; October 2019
37. Alunbrig (brigatinib) product label. Cambridge, MA: Takeda Pharmaceutical Company Limited; May 2020
38. Busulfex (busulfan) product label. Rockville, MD: Otsuka America Pharmaceutical, Inc.; March 2020
39. Bodge MN et al. Biol Blood Marrow Transplant 2014;20:908–919
40. Bodge MN et al. Biol Blood Marrow Transplant 2014;20:622–629
41. Jevtana (cabazitaxel) product label. Bridgewater, NJ: Sanofi-Aventis; December 2020
42. Cometriq (cabozantinib) product label. Alameda, CA: Exelixis, Inc.; October 2020
43. Cabometyx (cabozantinib) product label. Alameda, CA: Exelixis, Inc.; July 2020
44. Xeloda (capecitabine) product label. South San Francisco, CA: Genentech USA, Inc.; February 2019
45. Twelves C et al. Clin Cancer Res 1999;5:1696–1702
46. Eklund JW et al. Oncology (Williston Park) 2005;19:1057–1063
47. Cablivi (caplacizumab-yhdp) product label. Cambridge, MA: Genzyme Corporation; September 2020
48. Tabrecta (capmatinib) product label. East Hanover, New Jersey: Novartis Pharmaceuticals Corporation; May 2020
49. Paraplatin (carboplatin) product label. Princeton, NJ: Bristol-Myers Squibb; November 2010
50. Kyprolis (carfilzomib) product label. Thousand Oaks, CA: Onyx Pharmaceuticals, Inc.; August 2020
51. Kintzel PE, Dorr RT. Cancer Treat Rev 1995;21:33–64
52. Libtayo (cemiplimab-rwlc) product label. Tarrytown, NY: Regeneron Pharmaceuticals, Inc.; November 2020
53. Zykadia (ceritinib) product label. East Hanover, NJ: Novartis Pharmaceuticals Corporation; March 2019
54. Erbitux (cetuximab) product label. Indianapolis, IN: ImClone LLC; November 2020
55. Leukeran (chlorambucil) product label. Grand Bay, Mauritius: Aspen Global Inc.; March 2017
56. Supplement to: Krens SD et al. Lancet Oncol 2019;20:e201–e208
57. Cladribine product label. Rockford, IL: Mylan Institutional LLC; March 2018
58. Clolar (clofarabine) product label. Cambridge, MA: Genzyme Corporation; December 2019
59. Cotellic (cobimetinib) product label. South San Francisco, CA: Genentech, Inc.; January 2018
60. Aliqopa (copanlisib) product label. Whippany, NJ: Bayer HealthCare Pharmaceuticals, Inc.; December 2020
61. Adakveo (crizanlizumab-tmca) product label. East Hanover, New Jersey: Novartis Pharmaceuticals Corporation; November 2019
62. Xalkori (crizotinib) product label. New York, NY: Pfizer Labs; June 2019
63. Smith G et al. J Clin Oncol 1997;15:833–839
64. Tafinlar (dabrafenib) product label. East Hanover, New Jersey: Novartis Pharmaceuticals Corporation; April 2020
65. Vizimpro (dacomitinib) product label. New York, NY: Pfizer Labs; December 2020
66. Darzalex (daratumumab). Horsham, PA: Janssen Biotech, Inc.; August 2020
67. Aranesp (darbepoetin alfa) prescribing information. Thousand Oaks, CA: Amgen Inc.; January 2019
68. Nubeqa (darolutamide) product label. Whippany, NJ: Bayer HealthCare Pharmaceuticals Inc.; July 2019
69. Sprycel (dasatinib) package insert. Princeton, NJ: Bristol-Myers Squibb Company; December 2018
70. Daunorubicin HCl product label. Irvine, CA: Teva Parenteral Medicines, Inc.; September 2012
71. Vyxeos (daunorubicin and cytarabine liposome) product label. Palo Alto, CA: Jazz Pharmaceuticals, Inc.; July 2019
72. Dacogen (decitabine) product label. Rockville, MD: Otsuka America Pharmaceutical, Inc.; June 2020
73. Inqovi (cedazuridine and decitabine) product label. Princeton, NJ: Taiho Oncology, Inc.; July 2020
74. Defitelio (defibrotide sodium) product label. Palo Alto, CA: Jazz Pharmaceuticals, Inc.; March 2016
75. Xgeva (denosumab) product label. Thousand Oaks, CA: Amgen Inc.; June 2020
76. Dexrazoxane product label. Rockford, IL: Mylan Institutional LLC; April 2018
77. Taxotere (docetaxel) product label. Bridgewater, NJ: Sanofi Aventis Pharmaceuticals; December 2019
78. Janus N et al. Ann Oncol 2010;21:1395–403
79. Clarke SJ, Rivory LP. Clin Pharmacokinet 1999;36:99–114
80. Hooker AC et al. Clin Pharmacol Ther 2008;84:111–118
81. Adriamycin (doxorubicin) package insert. Eatontown, NJ: Hikma Pharmaceuticals USA Inc.; October 2019
82. Donelli MG et al. Pharmacokinetics of anticancer agents in patients with impaired liver function. Eur J Cancer 1998;34:33–46
83. Benjamin RS et al. Cancer 1974;33:19–27
84. Doxil (doxorubicin liposomal) product label. Deerfield, IL: Baxter Healthcare Corporation; August 2019
85. Caelyx pegylated liposomal product label (EMA). Beerse, Belgium: Janssen Pharmaceutica NV; March 2020
86. Imfinzi (durvalumab) product label. Wilmington, DE: AstraZeneca Pharmaceuticals LP; November 2020
87. Copiktra (duvelisib) product label. Needham, MA: Verastem, Inc.; July 2019
88. Empliciti (elotuzumab) product label. Princeton, NJ: Bristol-Myers Squibb Company; October 2019
89. Promacta (eltrombopag) product label. East Hanover, NJ: Novartis Pharmaceuticals Corporation; April 2020
90. Idhifa (enasidenib mesylate) product label. Summit, NJ: Celgene Corporation; November 2020
91. Braftovi (encorafenib) product label. Boulder, CO: Array BioPharma Inc.; April 2020
92. Padcev (enfortumab vedotin-ejfv). Bothell, WA: Seattle Genetics, Inc.; December 2019
93. Rozlytrek (entrectinib) product label. South San Francisco, CA: Genentech USA, Inc.; August 2019
94. Xtandi (enzalutamide) product label. Northbrook, IL: Astellas Pharma US, Inc.; October 2020
95. Ellence (epirubicin HCl) product label. New York, NY: Pharmacia & Upjohn Co; July 2019
96. Dobbs NA et al. Eur J Cancer 2003;39:580–586
97. Procrit (epoetin alfa) product label. Thousand Oaks, CA: Amgen, Inc.; July 2018
98. Balversa (erdafitinib) product label. Horsham, PA: Janssen Products LP; July 2020
99. Halaven (eribulin mesylate) product label. Woodcliff Lake, NJ: Eisai Inc.; December 2017
100. Tarceva (erlotinib) product label. South San Francisco, CA: Genentech USA, Inc.; October 2016
101. Miller AA et al. J Clin Oncol 2007;25:3055–3060
102. Emcyt (estramustine phosphate sodium) product label. New York, NY: Pharmacia & Upjohn Company; June 2007

103. Etoposide capsules product label. Morgantown, WV: Mylan Pharmaceuticals, Inc.; April 2016

104. Joel SP et al. J Clin Oncol 1996;14:257–267

105. Afinitor (everolimus) product label. East Hanover, NJ: Novartis Pharmaceutical Co; March 2020

106. Aromasin (exemestane) product label. New York, NY: Pharmacia and Upjohn; May 2018

107. Enhertu (fam-trastuzumab deruxtecan-nxki) product label. Basking Ridge, NJ: Daiichi Sankyo Inc.; December 2019

108. Inrebic (fedratinib) product label. Summit, NJ: Celgene Corporation; August 2019

109. Neupogen (filgrastim) product label. Thousand Oaks, CA: Amgen Inc.; June 2018

110. Floxuridine product label. Lake Zurich, IL: Fresenius Kabi USA, LLC; August 2016

111. Floyd J et al. Semin Oncol 2006;33:50–67

112. Fludarabine product label. Parsippany, NJ: Actavis Pharma, Inc; June 2014

113. Fleming GF et al. Ann Oncol 2003;14:1142–1147

114. Halotestin (fluoxymesterone) product label. Maple Grove, MN: Pharmacia and Upjohn Company; May 2002

115. Flutamide product label. Chestnut Ridge, NY: Par Pharmaceutical, Inc.; October 2017

116. Tavalisse (fostamatinib disodium hexahydrate) product label. South San Francisco, CA: Rigel Pharmaceuticals, Inc.; April 2018

117. Faslodex (fulvestrant) product label. Wilmington, DE: AstraZeneca Pharmaceuticals LP; October 2020

118. Iressa (gefitinib) product label. Wilmington, DE: AstraZeneca Pharmaceuticals LP; May 2019

119. Gemzar (gemcitabine) package insert. Indianapolis, IN: Eli Lilly; February 2011

120. Venook AP et al. J Clin Oncol 2000;18:2780–2787

121. Mylotarg (gemtuzumab ozogamicin) product label. Philadelphia, PA: Wyeth Laboratories LLC; June 2020

122. Xospata (gilteritinib) product label. Northbrook, IL: Astellas Pharma US, Inc.; May 2019

123. Daurismo (glasdegib) product label. New York, NY: Pfizer Labs; March 2020

124. Zoladex (goserelin) product label. Lake Forest, IL: TerSera Therapeutics LLC; February 2019

125. Hydrea (hydroxyurea) product label. Princeton, New Jersey: Bristol-Myers Squibb Company; December 2020

126. Siklos (hydroxyurea) product label. Bryn Mawr, PA: Medunik USA; May 2019

127. Zevalin (ibritumomab tiuxetan) prescribing information. East Windsor, NJ: Acrotech Biopharma LLC; September 2019

128. Imbruvica (ibrutinib) product label. Sunnyvale, CA: Pharmacyclics LLC; December 2020

129. Imbruvica (ibrutinib) summary of product characteristics (EMA). Beerse, Belgium: Janssen-Cilag International NV; September 2020

130. de Jong J et al. Leuk Lymphoma 2017;58:185–194

131. Zydelig (idelalisib) product label. Foster City, CA: Gilead Sciences, Inc; October 2020

132. Ifex (ifosfamide) product label. Deerfield, IL: Baxter Healthcare Corporation; July 2018.

133. Gleevec (imatinib) package insert. East Hanover, NJ: Novartis Pharmaceuticals Corporation; August 2020

134. Eckel F et al. Oncology 2005;69:363–371

135. Besponsa (inotuzumab ozogamicin) product label. Philadelphia, PA: Wyeth Pharmaceuticals LLC; March 2018

136. Intron A (interferon alfa–2b) product label. Whitehouse Station, NJ: Merck Sharp & Dohme Corp.; August 2019

137. Yervoy (ipilimumab) prescribing information. Princeton, NJ: Bristol-Myers Squibb Company; November 2020

138. Camptosar (irinotecan) package insert. New York, NY: Pharmacia & Upjohn Company; January 2020

139. Venook AP et al. Ann Oncol 2003;14:1783–1790

140. Raymond E et al. Clin Cancer Res 2006;20:4303–4312

141. Schaaf LJ et al. Clin Cancer Res 2006;12:3782–3791

142. Onivyde (irinotecan liposome injection) product label. Cambridge, MA: Ipsen Biopharmaceuticals, Inc.; December 2020

143. Sarclisa (isatuximab) product label. Bridgewater, NJ: Sanofi-Aventis U.S. LLC; March 2020

144. Claravis (isotretinoin) product label. North Wales, PA: Teva Pharmaceuticals USA, Inc.; April 2018

145. Tibsovo (ivosidenib) product label. Cambridge, MA: Agios Pharmaceuticals, Inc.; May 2019

146. Ixempra (ixabepilone) prescribing information. Princeton, NJ: R-Pharm US LLC; January 2016

147. Ninlaro (ixazomib) prescribing information. Cambridge, MA: Takeda Pharmaceutical Company Limited; March 2020

148. Tykerb (lapatinib) prescribing information. Baltimore, MD: Lupin Pharmaceuticals, Inc.; September 2020

149. Somatuline depot (lanreotide acetate) prescribing information. Cambridge, MA: Ipsen Biopharmaceuticals, Inc.; September 2019

150. Vitrakvi (larotrectinib) prescribing information. Stamford, CT: Loxo Oncology, Inc.; December 2018

151. Revlimid (lenalidomide) prescribing information. Summit, NJ: Celgene Corporation; October 2019

152. Lenvima (lenvatinib) prescribing information. Woodcliff Lake, NJ: Eisai Inc.; November 2020

153. Femara (letrozole) prescribing information. East Hanover, NJ: Novartis Pharmaceuticals Corporation; May 2020

154. Lexi-Drugs Online. Leucovorin. Lexi-Comp, Inc. 2020 [Accessed December 11, 2020]

155. Gleostine (lomustine) prescribing information. Miami, FL: NextSource Biotechnology, LLC.; September 2018

156. Lorbrena (lorlatinib) prescribing information. New York, NY: Pfizer Laboratories Div Pfizer Inc.; June 2020

157. Zepzelca (lurbinectedin) prescribing information. Palo Alto, CA: Jazz Pharmaceuticals Inc.; June 2020

158. Reblozyl (luspatercept-aamt) prescribing information. Summit, NJ: Celgene Corporation; April 2020

159. Lutathera (lutetium Lu 177 dotatate) prescribing information. Millburn, NJ: Advanced Accelerator Applications USA, Inc.; May 2020

160. Megace (megestrol acetate) prescribing information. Chestnut Ridge, NY: Par Pharmaceutical, Inc.; October 2018

161. Dimopoulos MA et al. J Clin Oncol 2016;34:1544–1557

162. Alkeran (melphalan) prescribing information. Weston, FL: ApoPharma USA, Inc.; May 2017

163. King PD, Perry MC. Oncologist 2001;6:162–176

164. Purinethol (mercaptopurine) prescribing information. Coral Springs, FL: Florida Pharmaceutical Product, LLC.; May 2020

165. Mesnex (mesna) prescribing information. Deerfield, IL: Baxter Healthcare Corporation; December 2018

166. Batchelor T et al. J Clin Oncol 2003;21:1044–1049

167. Superfin D et al. Oncologist 2007;12:1070–1083

168. Rydapt (midostaurin) prescribing information. East Hanover, NJ: Novartis Pharmaceuticals Corporation; November 2020

169. Mutamycin (mitomycin for injection) prescribing information. Durham, NC: Accord BioPharma Inc.; September 2016

170. Lysodren (mitotane) prescribing information. Princeton, NJ: Bristol-Myers Squibb; November 2019

171. Novantrone (mitoxantrone) prescribing information. Lake Forest, IL: Hospira, Inc.; May 2018

172. Poteligeo (mogamulizumab-kpkc) prescribing information. Bedminster, NJ: Kyowa Kirin, Inc.; August 2018

173. Lumoxiti (moxetumomab pasudotox-tdfk injection) prescribing information. Wilmington, DE: AstraZeneca Pharmaceuticals LP; January 2019

174. Portrazza (necitumumab injection) prescribing information. Indianapolis, IN: Eli Lilly and Company; May 2017

175. Arranon (nelarabine injection) prescribing information. East Hanover, NJ: Novartis Pharmaceuticals Corporation; July 2019

176. Nerlynx (neratinib) prescribing information. Los Angeles, CA: Puma Biotechnology, Inc.; December 2020

177. Tasigna (nilotinib) prescribing information. East Hanover, NJ: Novartis Corporation; September 2019

178. Nilandron (nilutamide) prescribing information. Dublin, Ireland: Concordia Pharmaceuticals, Inc.; January 2020

179. Zejula (niraparib) prescribing information. Research Triangle Park, NC: Glaxo SmithKline LLC.; April 2020

180. Opdivo (nivolumab) prescribing information. Princeton, NJ: Bristol-Meyers Squibb Company; November 2020

181. Gazyva (obinutuzumab) prescribing information. South San Francisco, CA: Genentech, Inc.; March 2020

182. Sandostatin LAR (octreotide) prescribing information. East Hanover, NJ: Novartis Pharmaceuticals Corporation; April 2019

183. Arzerra (ofatumumab) prescribing information. East Hanover, NJ: Novartis Pharmaceuticals Corporation; August 2016

184. Lynparza (olaparib) prescribing information. Wilmington, DE: AstraZeneca Pharmaceuticals LP; December 2020

185. Synribo (omacetaxine mepesuccinate) prescribing information. North Wales, PA: Teva Pharmaceuticals USA, Inc.; November 2019

186. Targrisso (osimertinib) prescribing information. Wilmington, DE: AstraZeneca Pharmaceuticals LP; December 2020

187. Eloxatin (oxaliplatin) prescribing information. Deerfield, IL: Baxter Healthcare Corporation; April 2020

188. Doroshow JH et al. Semin Oncol 2003;30:14–19

189. Taxol (paclitaxel) prescribing information. Lake Forest, IL: Hospira, Inc; May 2018

190. Venook AP et al. J Clin Oncol 1998;16:1811–1819

191. Abraxane (paclitaxel protein-bound particles) prescribing information. Bridgewater, NJ: Abraxis Bioscience, LLC; August 2020

192. Ibrance (palbociclib) prescribing information. New York, NY: Pfizer Laboratories Div Pfizer Inc.; November 2019

193. Aredia (pamidronate disodium) prescribing information. Lake Forest, IL: Akorn-Strides, LLC; November 2008

194. Vectibix (panitumumab) prescribing information. Thousand Oaks, CA: Amgen, Inc.; June 2017

195. Farydak (panobinostat) prescribing information. East Hanover, NJ: Novartis Pharmaceuticals Corporation; June 2016

196. Votrient (pazopanib) prescribing information. East Hanover, NJ: Novartis Pharmaceuticals Corporation; August 2020

197. Oncaspar (pegaspargase) Injection, prescribing information. Boston, MA: Servier Pharmaceuticals LLC; June 2020

198. Neulasta (pegfilgrastim) prescribing information. Thousand Oaks, CA: Amgen, Inc.; January 2020

199. Alimta (pemetrexed) prescribing information. Indianapolis, IN: Eli Lilly and Co; January 2019

200. Keytruda (pembrolizumab) prescribing information. Whitehouse Station, NJ: Merck & Co., Inc.; November 2020

201. Pemazyre (pemigatinib) prescribing information. Wilmington, DE: Incyte Corporation; April 2020

202. Nipent (pentostatin for injection) prescribing information. Lake Forest, IL: Hospira, Inc.; October 2019

203. Perjeta (pertuzumab) prescribing information. South San Francisco, CA: Genentech, Inc.; January 2020

204. Turalio (pexidartinib) prescribing information. Basking Ridge, NJ: Daiichi Sankyo, Inc.; April 2020

205. Mozobil (plerixafor) prescribing information. Cambridge, MA: Genzyme Corporation; August 2020

206. Pomalyst (pomalidomide) prescribing information. Summit, NJ: Celgene Corporation; May 2020

207. Iclusig (ponatinib) prescribing information. Cambridge, MA: Takeda Pharmaceutical Company Limited; July 2020

208. Polivy (polatuzumab vedotin-piiq) prescribing information. South San Francisco, CA: Genentech, Inc.; September 2020

209. Folotyn (pralatrexate) prescribing information. Westminster, CO: Allos Therapeutics Inc.; November 2016

210. Gavreto (pralsetinib) prescribing information. Cambridge, MA: Blueprint Medicines Corporation; September 2020

211. Xofigo (radium ra 223 dichloride injection) prescribing information. Whippany, NJ: Bayer HealthCare Pharmaceuticals Inc.; December 2019

212. Evista (raloxifene) prescribing information. North Wales, PA: Teva Pharmaceuticals USA, Inc.; July 2018.

213. Cyramza (ramucirumab) prescribing information. Indianapolis, IN: Eli Lilly and Co; June 2020

214. Ultomiris (ravulizumab-cwvz) prescribing information. Boston, MA: Alexion Pharmaceuticals Inc.; October 2020

215. Stivarga (regorafenib) prescribing information. Whippany, NJ: Bayer HealthCare Pharmaceuticals Inc.; December 2020

216. Kisqali (ribociclib) prescribing information. East Hanover, NJ: Novartis Pharmaceuticals Corporation; July 2020

217. Qinlock (ripretinib) prescribing information. Waltham, MA: Deciphera Pharmaceuticals, LLC; October 2020

218. Rituxan (rituximab) prescribing information. South San Francisco, CA: Genentech, Inc.; August 2020

219. Istodax (romidepsin) prescribing information. Summit, NJ: Celgene Corporation; October 2020

220. Nplate (romiplostim) prescribing information. Thousand Oaks, CA: Amgen, Inc.; November 2020

221. Rubraca (rucaparib) prescribing information. Boulder, CO: Clovis Oncology, Inc.; October 2020

222. Jakafi (ruxolitinib) prescribing information. Wilmington, DE: Incyte Corporation; February 2020.

223. Trodelvy (sacituzumab govitecan-hziy) prescribing information. Morris Plains, NJ: Immunomedics, Inc.; April 2020

224. Leukine (sargramostim) prescribing information. Bridgewater, NJ: Sanofi-Aventis U.S. LLC; March 2018

225. Xpovio (Selinexor) prescribing information. Newton, MA: Karyopharm Therapeutics, Inc.; December 2020

226. Retevmo (selpercatinib) prescribing information. Indianapolis, IN: Eli Lilly and Company; May 2020

227. Koselugo (selumetinib) prescribing information. Wilmington, DE: AstraZeneca Pharmaceuticals LP; May 2020

228. Sylvant (siltuximab) prescribing information. Horsham, PA: Janssen Biotech, Inc; May 2018

229. Provenge (sipuleucel-T) prescribing information. Seattle, WA: Dendreon Pharmaceuticals LLC; July 2017

230. Odomzo (sonidegib) prescribing information. Cranbury, NJ: Sun Pharmaceutical Industries Inc.; May 2019

231. Nexavar (sorafenib) prescribing information. Wayne, NJ: Bayer HealthCare Pharmaceuticals, Inc.; July 2020

232. Miller AA et al. J Clin Oncol 2009;11:1800–1805

233. Zanosar (streptozocin sterile powder) prescribing information. Irvine, CA: Teva Parenteral Medicines, Inc.; May 2020

234. Lexi-Drugs Online. Streptozocin. Lexi-Comp, Inc. 2021 [Accessed January 2, 2021]

235. Sutent (sunitinib) prescribing information. New York, NY: Pfizer Inc.; August 2020

236. Monjuvi (tafasitamab-cxix) prescribing information. Boston, MA: Morphosys US Inc.; July 2020

237. Elzonris (tagraxofusp-erzs) prescribing information. New York, NY: Stemline Therapeutics, Inc.; December 2018

238. Talzenna (talazoparib) prescribing information. New York, NY: Pfizer, Inc.; October 2020

239. Soltamox (tamoxifen) prescribing information. Morgantown, WV: Mylan Pharmaceuticals, Inc.; April 2013

240. Tazverik (tazemetostat) prescribing information. Cambridge, MA: Epizyme, Inc.; July 2020

241. Temodar (temozolomide) prescribing information. Whitehouse Station, NJ: Merck & Co., Inc.; November 2019

242. Torisel (temsirolimus) prescribing information. Lake Zurich, IL: Fresenius Kabi USA, LLC; March 2020

243. Vumon (teniposide) prescribing information. Paramus, NJ: WG Critical Care, LLC; April 2015

244. Thalomid (thalidomide) prescribing information. Summit, NJ: Celgene Corporation; June 2019

245. Tabloid (thioguanine) prescribing information. Mason, OH: Aspen Global Inc.; May 2018

246. Tepadina (thiotepa injection) prescribing information. Bridgewater, NJ: Amneal Pharmaceuticals LLC; March 2020

247. Hycamtin (topotecan capsule) prescribing information. East Hanover, NJ: Novartis Pharmaceuticals Corporation; September 2018

248. Hycamtin (topotecan hydrochloride injection) prescribing information. Bedford, OH: Bedford Laboratories; April 2016

249. Fareston (toremifene) prescribing information. Piscataway, NJ: Novadoz Pharmaceuticals LLC.; February 2020

250. Yondelis (trabectedin) prescribing information. Horsham, PA: Janssen Inc.; June 2020

251. Mekinist (trametinib) prescribing information. East Hanover, NJ: Novartis Pharmaceuticals Corporation, Inc.; June 2020

252. Herceptin (trastuzumab) prescribing information. South San Francisco, CA: Genentech, Inc.; November 2018

253. Vesanoid (tretinoin) prescribing information. Livonia, MI: Major Pharmaceuticals; January 2017

254. Lonsurf (trifluridine/tipiracil) prescribing information. Princeton, NJ: Taiho Oncology, Inc.; February 2019

255. Tuksya (tucatinib) prescribing information. Bothell, WA: Seattle Genetics, Inc.; April 2020

256. Valstar (valrubicin) prescribing information. Malvern, PA: Endo Pharmaceuticals Solutions Inc.; October 2019

257. Caprelsa (vandetanib) prescribing information. Cambridge, MA: Genzyme Corporation; June 2020

258. Zelboraf (vemurafenib) prescribing information. South San Francisco, CA: Genentech USA, Inc.; November 2017

259. Venclexta (venetoclax) prescribing information. North Chicago, IL: AbbVie Inc.; November 2020

260. Velban (vinblastine sulfate) prescribing information. Lake Zurich, IL: Fresenius Kabi USA, LLC; November 2016

261. Vincasar (vincristine sulfate) prescribing information. Lake Forest, IL: Hospira, Inc.; September 2020

262. Marqibo (vincristine sulfate, liposomal injection) prescribing information. East Windsor, NJ: Acrotech Biopharma LLC; June 2020

263. Navelbine (vinorelbine tartrate) prescribing information. Parsippany, NJ: Actavis Pharma, Inc.; January 2020

264. Robieux I et al. Clin Pharmacol Ther 1996;59:32–40

265. Erivedge (vismodegib) prescribing information. South San Francisco, CA: Genentech, Inc.; July 2020.

266. Zolinza (vorinostat) prescribing information. Whitehouse Station, NJ: Merck & Co., Inc.; January 2020

267. Ramalingam SS et al. J Clin Oncol 2010;28:4507–4512

268. Oxbryta (voxelotor) prescribing information. South San Francisco, CA: Global Blood Therapeutics Inc.; November 2019.

269. Brukinsa (zanubrutinib) prescribing information. San Mateo, CA: BeiGene USA, Inc.; November 2019.

270. Zaltrap (ziv-aflibercept) prescribing information. Bridgewater, NJ: Sanofi-Aventis U.S. LLC; December 2020

271. Zometa (zoledronic acid) prescribing information. Lake Zurich, IL: Fresenius Kabi USA, LLC; March 2018

45. Drug Preparation and Administration

Gerard P. Mascara, PharmD, BCOP

The following tables describe appropriate handling and storage, as well as drug product preparation and administration procedures, for antineoplastics and other selected medications often used concomitantly. The tables describe drug use under a variety of commonly encountered conditions, but they do not identify all applications or conditions of product stability and compatibility. Likewise, the tables are not an exhaustive list of marketed products and should not be construed as an endorsement for any manufacturer's products or discriminating against products that were not specifically identified. Clinicians are advised to refer to product labeling for more complete information about individual products and up-to-date reference sources for information about drug compatibility and stability

The information contained in this chapter is derived from contemporary product labeling approved by the U.S. Food and Drug Administration (FDA), pharmaceutical manufacturers' websites, and, in some cases, published studies and personal communications with pharmaceutical manufacturers

Occasionally, the package insert component of product labeling for drugs that have received FDA approval for commercial use is prefaced by prominent precautionary and warning summaries circumscribed by a rectangular border, commonly referred to as *black box warnings*, or, simply, *boxed warnings*. The boxed warnings reproduced in this chapter faithfully recapitulate the most current versions of manufacturers' product labeling available lacking only referent citations to information located elsewhere within product labeling. Referents are replaced here by an ellipsis (...). Health care providers are urged to consult the most current versions of product labeling and primary medical publications for more information.

In 2001, the FDA Office of Generic Drugs requested manufacturers of 16 similarly named drug pairs to voluntarily revise the appearance of those established drug names by enhancing distinguishing elements of otherwise very similar (look-alike) names. The Name Differentiation Project of 2001 encouraged manufacturers to supplement their applications with revised labeling that incorporated "Tall Man" letters within drug names to aid visual differentiation between those drug names with a goal toward minimizing medication errors by inappropriate drug selection, ie, capitalizing letters that aid in distinguishing between similar generic and proprietary drug names. With the exception of section titles, labeled identities, compendial names, and boxed warnings, drug names appear in this chapter with the Tall Man names and conventions established and recommended by the FDA and the Institute for Safe Medication Practices, Horsham, PA (www.ismp.org/sites/default/files/attachments/2017-11/tallmanletters.pdf [accessed November 17, 2020])

Key to Abbreviations

0.45% NaCl	0.45% Sodium chloride injection, USP	D5W/0.9% NS	5% Dextrose and 0.9% sodium chloride injection, USP
0.9% NS	0.9% Sodium chloride injection, USP	D5W/LR	5% Dextrose injection in lactated Ringer's injection, USP
1/6-M SLI	Sodium lactate injection, USP (1/6 molar [1.9%] sodium lactate)	D5W/RI	5% Dextrose injection in Ringer's injection, USP
3% NaCl	3% Sodium chloride injection (hypertonic)	DEHP	di-2-ethylhexyl phthalate (a plasticizing ingredient commonly used in flexible PVC containers)
AKA	Also known as		
ALT	Alanine aminotransferase	LRI	Lactated Ringer's injection, USP
ANC	Absolute neutrophil count	NDC	National Drug Code
AST	Aspartate aminotransferase	NF	"National Formulary," a portion of the official American pharmaceutical compendia, *United States Pharmacopeia-National Formulary*
AUC	Area under the concentration versus time curve		
B0.9% NS	Bacteriostatic (antimicrobially preserved) 0.9% sodium chloride injection		
BSA	Body surface area	PE	Polyethylene
BWFI	Bacteriostatic water for injection, USP	PICC	Peripherally inserted central catheter
CrCl	Creatinine clearance	PK	Pharmacokinetic
CYP	A prefix denoting cytochrome P450 enzymes	PVC	Polyvinyl chloride
CSF	Cerebrospinal fluid	Q.S.	*Quantum sufficit* or *quantum satis* [Latin]: "As much as is sufficient"
D10W	10% Dextrose injection, USP		
D2.5W	2.5% Dextrose injection, USP	RI	Ringer's injection, USP
D2.5W/0.45% NaCl	2.5% Dextrose and 0.45% sodium chloride injection, USP	SICC	Subclavian-inserted central catheter
D5W	5% Dextrose injection, USP	SWFI	(Sterile) Water for injection, USP
D5W/0.2% NaCl	5% Dextrose and 0.20% sodium chloride injection, USP	ULN	Upper limit of normal
D5W/0.33% NaCl	5% Dextrose and 0.33% sodium chloride injection, USP	USP	United States Pharmacopeia/U.S. Pharmacopeial Convention
D5W/0.45% NaCl	5% Dextrose and 0.45% sodium chloride injection, USP	VAD	Vascular access device (eg, catheter, port, other cannula)

ado-TRASTUZUMAB

KADCYLA (ado-trastuzumab emtansine) prescribing information. South San Francisco, CA: Genentech, Inc. May 2019

Do Not Substitute KADCYLA for or with Trastuzumab

WARNING: HEPATOTOXICITY, CARDIAC TOXICITY, EMBRYO-FETAL TOXICITY

- Hepatotoxicity: Serious hepatotoxicity has been reported, including liver failure and death in patients treated with KADCYLA. Monitor serum transaminases and bilirubin prior to initiation of KADCYLA treatment and prior to each KADCYLA dose. Reduce dose or discontinue KADCYLA as appropriate in cases of increased serum transaminases or total bilirubin …
- Cardiac Toxicity: KADCYLA administration may lead to reductions in left ventricular ejection fraction (LVEF). Evaluate left ventricular function in all patients prior to and during treatment with KADCYLA. Withhold treatment for clinically significant decrease in left ventricular function …
- Embryo-Fetal Toxicity: Exposure to KADCYLA can result in embryo-fetal death or birth defects. Advise patients of these risks and the need for effective contraception …

Boxed Warning for KADYCLA (ado-trastuzumab emtansine) prescribing information

Product Identification, Preparation, Storage, and Stability

- Ado-trastuzumab emtansine contains the humanized anti-HER2 IgG1, trastuzumab, covalently linked to the microtubule inhibitory drug DM1 (a maytansine derivative) via the stable thioether linker MCC (4-[*N*-maleimidomethyl] cyclohexane-1-carboxylate). Emtansine refers to the MCC-DM1 complex
- The commercial product, KADCYLA, is a sterile, white to off-white, preservative-free, lyophilized powder in individually packaged, single-use vials that contain ado-trastuzumab emtansine 100 mg (NDC 50242-088-01) or 160 mg (NDC 50242-087-01)
- Store intact vials under refrigeration at 2–8°C (35.6–46.4°F) until time of reconstitution
- *Do not freeze or shake* intact vials

Reconstitution:
- In order to prevent medication errors, it is important to check the vial labels to ensure that the drug being prepared and administered is KADCYLA (ado-trastuzumab emtansine), *NOT* trastuzumab
- Using a sterile syringe, slowly inject SWFI diluent into vials containing ado-trastuzumab emtansine as follows:

Vial Contents (ado-Trastuzumab Emtansine)	SWFI Volume for Reconstitution	ado-Trastuzumab Emtansine Concentration after Reconstitution
100 mg	5 mL	20 mg/mL
160 mg	8 mL	

- Swirl vials gently until the drug substance is completely dissolved
  - *Do not shake* vials to aid dissolution, to avoid foaming
- After reconstitution, each vial contains ado-trastuzumab emtansine 20 mg/mL, polysorbate 20 0.02% (w/v), sodium succinate 10 mmol/L, and sucrose 6% (w/v), with a pH = 5.0
- Inspect the reconstituted drug product (20 mg/mL) for particulates and discoloration
  - The solution should be clear to slightly opalescent, free of visible particulates, and colorless to pale brown
  - *Do not use* the reconstituted solution if it contains visible particulates or is cloudy or discolored
- The reconstituted lyophilized drug product should be used immediately following reconstitution, or, if not used immediately, reconstituted product may be stored for up to 24 hours under refrigeration at 2–8°C (35.6–46.4°F). *Do not freeze*
- Discard all unused ado-trastuzumab emtansine stored under refrigeration after 24 hours

Note: The reconstituted product contains no preservative and is intended for single use only

Dilution:
- Calculate the volume of concentrated reconstituted ado-trastuzumab emtansine solution (20-mg/mL) needed to prepare a patient's dose
- With a syringe, aseptically transfer from one or more vials the volume needed to a parenteral product container prefilled with 250 mL 0.9% NS
  - *Do not use* 5% dextrose injection as a diluent/vehicle solution
- Mix the diluted drug product by repeated gentle inversion of the container to avoid foaming
- After dilution, ado-trastuzumab emtansine admixture should be used immediately, but if not used immediately, it may be stored under refrigeration (2–8°C) for up to 24 hours prior to use
  - The time under refrigeration for storing diluted ado-trastuzumab emtansine (24 h) is in addition to the time allowed for storing the reconstituted concentrated solution (20 mg/mL) in vials (24 h)
- Do not freeze or shake the diluted drug product

Selected incompatibility:
- Do not mix ado-trastuzumab emtansine with other medicinal products in the same container

Recommendations for Drug Administration and Ancillary Care

General:

- In order to prevent medication errors it is important to check the vial labels to ensure that the drug being prepared and administered is KADCYLA (ado-trastuzumab emtansine), *NOT* trastuzumab
  - In order to improve traceability of biological pharmaceutical products and prevent medication errors, the complete generic name or a distinguishing proprietary (brand) name of the administered product should be clearly recorded in a patient's medical records

Administration:

- *Do not mix* ado-trastuzumab emtansine with other medicinal products in the same container or during administration
- *Do not substitute* ado-trastuzumab emtansine for trastuzumab *or* trastuzumab for ado-trastuzumab emtansine
- The recommended dose of ado-trastuzumab emtansine is 3.6 mg/kg, given as an intraVENous infusion every 3 weeks (21-day cycles)
  - *Do not administer* KADCYLA at dosages greater than 3.6 mg/kg
  - *Do not administer* ado-trastuzumab emtansine by intraVENous injection or bolus
  - *Do not re-escalate* ado-trastuzumab emtansine dosages after a dosage reduction is made

Event	Administration	Monitoring	
First infusion	• Administer intraVENously over 90 minutes	• Observe patients closely during the infusion and for at least 90 minutes following the initial dose for fever, chills, and other infusion-related reactions	• Patients should be observed closely for infusion-related reactions, especially during the first infusion • Administration should be slowed or interrupted if a patient develops an infusion-related reaction
Second and subsequent infusions	• Administer intraVENously over 30 minutes if prior administrations were well tolerated • Subsequent doses may be administered at the dosage and rate previously tolerated during the most recently administered treatment	• Observe patients during the infusion and for ≥30 minutes after administration	• Permanently discontinue KADCYLA for life-threatening infusion-related reactions

- Administer ado-trastuzumab emtansine intraVENously only with a 0.22-μm, inline, polyethersulfone filter
- If a planned dose is delayed or missed, it should be administered as soon as possible
  - *Do not wait* until the next planned cycle
  - The schedule of administration should be adjusted to maintain a 3-week interval between doses

Notes:

- FDA-approved product labeling for ado-trastuzumab emtansine includes recommendations for treatment modifications for concomitant use with potentially interacting medications, co-morbid conditions, and adverse effects associated with treatment, including: increased serum liver transaminases (AST and ALT), hyperbilirubinemia, or both conditions, and hepatic toxicity including nodular regenerative liver hyperplasia; left ventricular dysfunction, thrombocytopenia, pulmonary toxicity, and peripheral neuropathy (refer to current product labeling for detailed recommendations)
  - Management may require temporary delays, interruption, dose reduction, or treatment discontinuation
- Infusion-related reactions associated with ado-trastuzumab emtansine reported in clinical trials were characterized by one or more of the following: flushing, chills, pyrexia, dyspnea, hypotension, wheezing, bronchospasm, and tachycardia, and one episode of a serious allergic/anaphylactic reaction
  - The overall frequency of infusion-related reactions reported in one randomized trial was 1.4%
  - In most patients, reactions resolved over the course of several hours to a day after ado-trastuzumab emtansine administration was discontinued
  - Interrupt ado-trastuzumab emtansine treatment in patients who develop severe infusion-related reactions
  - ado-trastuzumab emtansine should be permanently discontinued in the event of life-threatening infusion-related reactions

ALDESLEUKIN

PROLEUKIN (aldesleukin) prescribing information. Yardley, PA: Clinigen, Inc.; September 2019

WARNINGS

Therapy with Proleukin (aldesleukin) should be restricted to patients with normal cardiac and pulmonary functions as defined by thallium stress testing and formal pulmonary function testing. Extreme caution should be used in patients with a normal thallium stress test and a normal pulmonary function test who have a history of cardiac or pulmonary disease

Proleukin should be administered in a hospital setting under the supervision of a qualified physician experienced in the use of anticancer agents. An intensive care facility and specialists skilled in cardiopulmonary or intensive care medicine must be available

Proleukin administration has been associated with capillary leak syndrome (CLS), which is characterized by a loss of vascular tone and extravasation of plasma proteins and fluid into the extravascular space. CLS results in hypotension and reduced organ perfusion, which may be severe and can result in death. CLS may be associated with cardiac arrhythmias (supraventricular and ventricular), angina, myocardial infarction, respiratory insufficiency requiring intubation, gastrointestinal bleeding or infarction, renal insufficiency, edema, and mental status changes

Proleukin treatment is associated with impaired neutrophil function (reduced chemotaxis) and with an increased risk of disseminated infection, including sepsis and bacterial endocarditis. Consequently, preexisting bacterial infections should be adequately treated prior to initiation of Proleukin therapy. Patients with indwelling central lines are particularly at risk for infection with gram-positive microorganisms. Antibiotic prophylaxis with oxacillin, nafcillin, ciprofloxacin, or vancomycin has been associated with a reduced incidence of staphylococcal infections

Proleukin administration should be withheld in patients developing moderate to severe lethargy or somnolence; continued administration may result in coma

Boxed Warning for PROLEUKIN (aldesleukin) prescribing information

Product Identification, Preparation, Storage, and Stability

- Proleukin is supplied in individually boxed single-use vials containing aldesleukin 22 million International Units (IU) as a sterile, white to off-white, preservative-free, lyophilized powder (equivalent to a protein mass of 1.3 mg). NDC 76310-022-01
  - Aldesleukin biologic potency is determined by a lymphocyte proliferation bioassay and is expressed in IU as established by the World Health Organization 1st International Standard for Interleukin 2 (human)
- Store intact vials (in original carton) and reconstituted and diluted aldesleukin under refrigeration at 2°C–8°C (36°F–46°F). Protect from light. *Do not* freeze aldesleukin
- Reconstitute the contents of a vial with 1.2 mL of SWFI to produce a clear, colorless to slightly yellow solution with a biologic potency of 18 million IU aldesleukin/mL (equivalent to 1.1 mg of aldesleukin protein per milliliter)
  - Each milliliter of the reconstituted product also contains 50 mg mannitol and 0.19 mg sodium dodecyl sulfate, buffered with disodium hydrogen

phosphate dihydrate (1.12 mg) and sodium dihydrogen phosphate dihydrate (0.19 mg) to a pH of 7.5 (range 7.2–7.8)
  - During reconstitution, direct the stream of SWFI at the side wall of a vial rather than directly into the drug powder and gently swirl vials to avoid excessive foaming
- *Do not shake* vials to dissolve aldesleukin
- For intraVENous administration, dilute aldesleukin *only* with D5W to a final concentration between 0.5 and 1.1 million IU/mL (30–70 μg/mL; see chart below). Drug delivery may be adversely affected by aldesleukin concentrations <30 μg/mL or >70 μg/mL

Aldesleukin (million IU)	Diluent Volume (D5W)
5–11	10 mL
7.5–16.5	15 mL
12.5–27.5	25 mL
25–55	50 mL
50–110	100 mL

- Either glass bottles or PVC bags are acceptable containers for aldesleukin, but plastic containers provide more consistent drug delivery than glass containers
- Reconstituted and diluted aldesleukin solutions are stable for up to 48 hours at 2–25°C (36–77°F), but the Proleukin product does not contain a preservative
- Store reconstituted and diluted solutions under refrigeration, but allow diluted aldesleukin to warm to room temperature before administering it to a patient

Selected incompatibility:
- *Do not combine* aldesleukin with other drugs in the same container
- *Do not reconstitute or dilute* aldesleukin with 0.9% NS or antimicrobially preserved diluents, which may increase protein aggregation

Recommendations for Drug Administration and Ancillary Care

General:

- Dose modification for toxicity should be accomplished by withholding or interrupting a dose rather than reducing the dose to be administered
- See Chapter 43 for recommended use in renal dysfunction
- Bring aldesleukin solution to room temperature before administration
- Administer aldesleukin by intraVENous infusion over 15 minutes
- *Do not filter* aldesleukin either during preparation or administration
- Complete administration within 48 hours after reconstitution

Pharmacodynamic interactions:

- Aldesleukin may affect CNS function, which may be exacerbated by concomitant administration of drugs with psychotropic activity—for example, opioids, analgesics, antiemetics, sedatives, hypnotics
- Aldesleukin may increase the nephrotoxic, myelotoxic, cardiotoxic, or hepatotoxic effects of other drugs if given concurrently
- Impaired kidney and liver function associated with aldesleukin use may delay elimination and increase the risk of adverse events from concomitantly administered medications
- Hypersensitivity reactions that consisted of erythema, pruritus, and hypotension have been reported in patients who received combination regimens containing sequential high-dose aldesleukin and antineoplastic agents, specifically: dacarbazine, CISplatin, tamoxifen, and interferon alfa. Adverse reactions occurred within hours after administration of chemotherapy and required medical intervention in some patients[1]
- In patients who received aldesleukin and interferon alfa concurrently:
  - The incidence of myocardial injury, including myocardial infarction, myocarditis, ventricular hypokinesia, and severe rhabdomyolysis, appears to be increased[2]
  - Exacerbation or initial presentation of autoimmune and inflammatory disorders has been observed, including: crescentic IgA glomerulonephritis, oculobulbar myasthenia gravis, inflammatory arthritis, thyroiditis, bullous pemphigoid, and Stevens-Johnson syndrome
- Glucocorticoids have been shown to reduce aldesleukin-induced side effects, including fever, renal insufficiency, hyperbilirubinemia, confusion, and dyspnea, but concomitant use should be avoided to preclude compromising aldesleukin's antitumor effectiveness[3]
- Beta-blockers and other antihypertensives may potentiate aldesleukin's hypotensive effects
- Aldesleukin use followed by administration of iodinated radiographic contrast media is associated with acute, atypical adverse reactions, including fever, chills, nausea, vomiting, pruritus, rash, diarrhea, hypotension, edema, and oliguria, with onset commonly within 1–4 hours after the administration of contrast media. In some cases, the reactions resemble the immediate side effects caused by aldesleukin administration; however, other than a temporal relationship between aldesleukin and iodinated contrast media administration, the cause of aldesleukin-associated contrast reactions is not known. Although most events were reported to occur when contrast media was given within 4 weeks after the last dose of aldesleukin, events were also reported to occur when contrast media was given several months after aldesleukin[4,5,6,7,8,9]

ALEMTUZUMAB

CAMPATH (alemtuzumab) prescribing information. Cambridge, MA: Genzyme Corporation; June, 2020

WARNINGS
CYTOPENIAS, INFUSION REACTIONS, and INFECTIONS

<u>Cytopenias</u>: Serious, including fatal, pancytopenia/marrow hypoplasia, autoimmune idiopathic thrombocytopenia, and autoimmune hemolytic anemia can occur in patients receiving CAMPATH. Single doses of CAMPATH greater than 30 mg or cumulative doses greater than 90 mg per week increase the incidence of pancytopenia …

<u>Infusion-Related Reactions</u>: CAMPATH administration can result in serious, including fatal, infusion-related reactions. Carefully monitor patients during infusions and withhold CAMPATH for Grade 3 or 4 infusion-related reactions. Gradually escalate CAMPATH to the recommended dose at the initiation of therapy and after interruption of therapy for 7 or more days …

<u>Immunosuppression/Infections</u>: Serious, including fatal, bacterial, viral, fungal, and protozoan infections can occur in patients receiving CAMPATH. Administer prophylaxis against *Pneumocystis jirovecii* pneumonia (PCP) and herpes virus infections …

Boxed Warning for "CAMPATH (alemtuzumab), Injection for intravenous use"; June 2020 product label; Genzyme Corporation, Cambridge, MA

Change in Product Availability

- As of September 4, 2012, Campath (alemtuzumab) injection for treatment of B-cell chronic lymphocytic leukemia was withdrawn from commercial availability in the United States
- Genzyme Corporation, the American distributor, announced activation of the "US Campath Distribution Program," which " …was developed to ensure continued access to Campath (alemtuzumab) for appropriate patients"
- An announcement advised visitors, "Campath will no longer be available commercially, but will be provided through the Campath Distribution Program free of charge. In order to receive Campath, the health care provider is required to document and comply with certain requirements"
- The website provides contact telephone numbers for more information:
  - Clinigen Group: 1-877-768-4303
  - Genzyme Medical Information: 1-800-745-4447, Option #2
  - URL: www.clinigengroup.com/direct/en-gb/products/detail/alemtuzumab/ (last accessed 13 October 2020).

Product Identification, Preparation, Storage, and Stability

- Campath is packaged in clear, glass, single-use vials containing 30 mg alemtuzumab/mL NDC: 58468-0357-3 (3 vials per carton) and NDC 58468-0357-1 (single vial per carton)
  - Campath is a sterile, clear, colorless, preservative-free, isotonic solution for injection containing alemtuzumab 30 mg/mL at pH 6.8–7.4
  - Each milliliter of the commercial product also contains 8 mg sodium chloride, 1.44 mg dibasic sodium phosphate, 0.2 mg potassium chloride, 0.2 mg monobasic potassium phosphate, 0.1 mg polysorbate 80, and 0.0187 mg disodium edetate dihydrate
- Store intact vials under refrigeration at 2–8°C (36–46°F); protect vials from direct sunlight
- *Do not freeze* alemtuzumab. If the product is accidentally frozen, thaw at 2–8°C before use
- *Do not shake* vials before use
  1. Withdraw from a vial into a syringe an amount of alemtuzumab needed to prepare a patient's dose
     a. 0.1 mL Campath solution for a 3-mg dose
     b. 0.33 mL Campath solution for a 10-mg dose
     c. 1 mL Campath solution for a 30-mg dose
  2. Inject the amount of drug needed to prepare a patient's dose into 100 mL of 0.9% NS or D5W in a plastic parenteral product container
  3. Gently invert the bag to mix the solution
- Diluted alemtuzumab solutions may be stored at room temperature (15°C–30°C; 59°F–86°F) or under refrigeration 2–8°C (36–46°F). Protect from light
- The commercial drug product contains no antimicrobial preservatives. Use the product within 8 hours after dilution

Selected incompatibility:
- Alemtuzumab is compatible with PVC bags and PVC- or polyethylene-lined PVC administration sets
- No data are available concerning the compatibility of alemtuzumab with other drugs. Do not add or simultaneously infuse other drugs through the same intraVENous line with alemtuzumab

Recommendations for Drug Administration and Ancillary Care

General:

- Administer alemtuzumab only by intraVENous infusion over ≥2 hours
- Do not administer alemtuzumab by direct intraVENous injection or bolus injection

Infusion reactions and dose escalation:

- Alemtuzumab administration can result in serious infusion reactions commonly including: pyrexia, chills, hypotension, urticaria, and dyspnea
  - G3 and G4 pyrexia and/or chills occurred in approximately 10% of previously untreated patients and in approximately 35% of previously treated patients
  - The occurrence of infusion reactions was greatest during the initial week of treatment and decreased with subsequent doses
  - All patients were pretreated with antipyretics and antihistamines; additionally, 43% of previously untreated patients received glucocorticoid prior to alemtuzumab
- Gradual escalation to the recommended maintenance dose/schedule is required when initiating therapy and after treatment interruptions ≥7 days. Generally, escalation to a 30-mg dose can be accomplished in 3–7 days as follows:
  1. Initiate treatment with alemtuzumab 3 mg intraVENously over 2 hours
  2. After a 3-mg DAILY dose is tolerated (ie, infusion-related toxicities are Grade ≤2), escalate DAILY dose to 10 mg/day and continue until tolerated
  3. After a 10-mg DAILY dose is tolerated (infusion-related toxicities Grade ≤2), escalate to a maintenance dose and schedule of alemtuzumab 30 mg/dose on 3 nonconsecutive days for 3 doses per week (eg, Monday, Wednesday, and Friday) for a total treatment duration of 12 weeks, including the period of dose escalation

Concomitant medications:

- Give premedication 30 minutes before the first alemtuzumab dose, before dose escalations, and as clinically indicated, with:
  - **DiphenhydrAMINE** 50 mg orally or intraVENously
  - **Acetaminophen** 500–1000 mg orally
- Treat severe infusion-related events with:
  - **Hydrocortisone** intraVENously (anaphylactoid reactions)
  - **Meperidine** intraVENously (chills, rigors)
  - **EPINEPHrine 1:1000** (1 mg/mL) intraMUSCularly (preferred) or SUBCUTaneously (anaphylactoid reactions)
  - **EPINEPHrine 1:10,000** (0.1 mg/mL) intraVENously with cardiac monitoring (airway edema, severe bronchospasm, hypotension)
- Give antibacterial and antiviral primary prophylaxis during treatment and continue for at least 2 months after the last dose of alemtuzumab is administered or until CD4+ lymphocyte counts are ≥200/mm^3, whichever event occurs later, with:
  - **Cotrimoxazole** (trimethoprim 160 mg + sulfamethoxazole 800 mg) orally, twice daily for 3 days/week (or equivalent anti-PCP prophylaxis)
  - **Famciclovir** 250 mg orally twice daily (or equivalent anti-herpesvirus prophylaxis)

AMIFOSTINE

ETHYOL (amifostine) prescribing information. Yardley, PA: Clinigen, Inc.; December 2019

Product Identification, Preparation, Storage, and Stability

- ETHYOL is a sterile, lyophilized, white powder supplied in single-dose vials (NDC 76310-017-01). Each vial contains 500 mg of amifostine on the anhydrous base. A carton contains 3 vials (NDC 76310-017-50)
- Store intact vials at controlled room temperature, 20–25°C (68–77°F)
- Reconstitute amifostine with 9.7 mL of 0.9% NS to produce a solution with concentration of 500 mg amifostine/10 mL
- Amifostine should be further diluted in PVC containers with 0.9% NS to concentrations ranging from 5 to 40 mg/mL
- The reconstituted drug product (50 mg/mL) and diluted amifostine solutions are chemically stable for up to 5 hours at approximately 25°C and for up to 24 hours under refrigeration (2–8°C; 35.6–46.4°F)

Selected incompatibility:

- Product labeling advises admixture with solutions other than 0.9% NS with or without other (unspecified) additives is not recommended

Recommendations for Drug Administration and Ancillary Care

General:

- Administer intraVENously (see indication-specific recommendations below)
- Provide adequate hydration before amifostine infusion
- Administer antiemetic primary prophylaxis before amifostine
  - Emetic risk is related to amifostine dosage: low risk, ≤300 mg/m^2; moderate risk, >300 mg/m^2 (NCCN Clinical Practice Guidelines in Oncology [NCCN Guidelines]: Antiemesis, V.2.2020. National Comprehensive Cancer Network, Inc., 2020. [Accessed July 23, 2020, at www.nccn.org])
- At the 910 mg/m^2 dose, monitor a patient's blood pressure before, at least every 5 minutes during amifostine administration, at the end of the infusion, and thereafter as clinically indicated
- At the 200 mg/m^2 dose, monitor a patient's blood pressure before and at the end of the infusion and thereafter as clinically indicated
- Keep patients in a supine position during the amifostine infusion. Interrupt amifostine administration if systolic blood pressure (SBP) decreases significantly from baseline as follows:

Baseline SBP (mm Hg)	Decrease in SBP That Warrants Interrupting Amifostine Infusion
<100	20 mm Hg
100–119	25 mm Hg
120–139	30 mm Hg
140–179	40 mm Hg
≥180	50 mm Hg

- If BP returns to normal within 5 minutes and the patient is asymptomatic, resume administration to complete the planned dose
- If the planned dose cannot be administered, decrease the amifostine dosage during subsequent chemotherapy cycles from 910 mg/m^2 to 740 mg/m^2

To reduce cumulative renal toxicity with chemotherapy:

- Administer antiemetic primary prophylaxis before amifostine, including dexamethasone 20 mg intraVENously, a serotonin receptor (5-HT$_3$ subtype) antagonist, *plus* additional antiemetics as appropriate for the chemotherapy utilized
- Administer amifostine 910 mg/m^2 once daily by intraVENous infusion over 15 minutes, starting 30 minutes before chemotherapy
  - A 15-minute infusion is better tolerated than longer infusions

To decrease moderate to severe xerostomia from head and neck radiation:

- Administer antiemetic primary prophylaxis before amifostine, for example, a 5-HT$_3$ antagonist ± additional antiemetics if clinically appropriate
- Administer amifostine 200 mg/m^2 once daily by intraVENous infusion over 3 minutes, 15–30 minutes before standard-fraction radiation therapy (ie, 1.8–2 Gy/fraction)
- Monitor blood pressure at least before and immediately after the infusion, and thereafter as clinically indicated

ARSENIC TRIOXIDE

TRISENOX (arsenic trioxide) prescribing information. North Wales, PA: Teva Pharmaceuticals USA, Inc.; June 2019
ARSENIC TRIOXIDE prescribing information. Vernon Hills, IL: Nexus Pharmaceuticals, Inc.; May 2017

WARNING: DIFFERENTIATION SYNDROME, CARDIAC CONDUCTION ABNORMALITIES AND ENCEPHALOPATHY INCLUDING WERNICKE'S

Differentiation Syndrome: Patients with acute promyelocytic leukemia (APL) treated with TRISENOX have experienced symptoms of differentiation syndrome, which can be fatal if not treated. Symptoms may include fever, dyspnea, acute respiratory distress, pulmonary infiltrates, pleural or pericardial effusions, weight gain or peripheral edema, hypotension, and renal, hepatic, or multiorgan dysfunction, in the presence or absence of leukocytosis. If differentiation syndrome is suspected, immediately initiate high-dose corticosteroid therapy and hemodynamic monitoring until resolution of signs and symptoms. Temporary discontinuation of TRISENOX may be required …

Cardiac Conduction Abnormalities: Arsenic trioxide can cause QTc interval prolongation, complete atrioventricular block, and a torsade de pointes-type ventricular arrhythmia, which can be fatal. Before initiating therapy, assess the QTc interval, correct pre-existing electrolyte abnormalities, and consider discontinuing drugs known to prolong QTc interval. Do not administer TRISENOX to patients with ventricular arrhythmia or prolonged QTcF …

Encephalopathy: Serious encephalopathy, including Wernicke's, has occurred in patients treated with TRISENOX. Wernicke's is a neurologic emergency. Consider testing thiamine levels in patients at risk for thiamine deficiency. Administer parenteral thiamine in patients with or at risk for thiamine deficiency. Monitor patients for neurological symptoms and nutritional status while receiving TRISENOX. If encephalopathy is suspected, immediately interrupt TRISENOX and initiate parenteral thiamine. Monitor until symptoms resolve or improve and thiamine levels normalize …

Boxed Warning for TRISENOX (arsenic trioxide) prescribing information

---

Product Identification, Preparation, Storage, and Stability

- **Warning:** arsenic trioxide is available in two different concentrations: 12-mg vials (2 mg/mL) and 10-mg vials (1 mg/mL). Carefully check the vial label at the time of dose preparation to ensure that the appropriate concentration is used for preparation calculations

- Trisenox is packaged in a carton containing 10 single-dose glass vials containing 12 mg arsenic trioxide (2 mg/mL) formulated as a sterile, nonpyrogenic, preservative-free, clear solution of arsenic trioxide in SWFI using sodium hydroxide and dilute hydrochloric acid to adjust to pH 8 (range 7.5–8.5). NDC 63459-601-06 (package of 10 vials)

- Various generic formulations of arsenic trioxide may be packaged in single-dose glass vials containing 10 mg arsenic trioxide (1 mg/mL) formulated as a sterile, nonpyrogenic, preservative-free, clear solution of arsenic trioxide in SWFI using sodium hydroxide and dilute hydrochloric acid to adjust to pH 8 (range 7.5–8.5)

- Store intact vials at 20–25°C (68–77°F). Temperature excursions are permitted to 15–30°C (59–86°F). Do not freeze

- Dilute arsenic trioxide in 100–250 mL of 0.9% NS or D5W immediately after withdrawing the drug product from an ampule. Unused drug should be discarded in a manner appropriate for hazardous drugs

- Diluted arsenic trioxide solutions are chemically and physically stable for 24 hours when stored at room temperature and for up to 48 hours under refrigeration

Selected incompatibility:

Arsenic trioxide should not be mixed with other drugs

Recommendations for Drug Administration and Ancillary Care

General:

- See Chapter 43 for recommended use in renal and hepatic dysfunction
- Administer arsenic trioxide by intraVENous infusion over 2 hours. The duration of administration may be extended to 4 hours for patients who experience acute vasomotor reactions
- A central VAD is not required for administering arsenic trioxide

ECG changes:

- QT/QTc prolongation should be expected during treatment with arsenic trioxide, and torsade de pointes and complete heart block have been reported
- In clinical trials of newly diagnosed patients with low-risk APL, 11% experienced QTc prolongation >450 ms for men and >460 ms for women throughout treatment cycles. In the clinical trial of patients with relapsed or refractory APL, >460 ECG tracings from 40 patients evaluated for QTc prolongation, 16 patients (40%) demonstrated at least 1 QTc interval >500 ms
- The risk of QTc prolongation may be higher in patients who have baseline QTc prolongation, who are treated with concomitant medications known to prolong the QT interval, who have congestive heart failure, who are receiving medications known to cause potassium wasting (eg, diuretics, amphotericin), or who have other conditions that cause hypokalemia or hypomagnesemia
- Prior to initiating therapy, discontinue (when feasible) other medications that prolong the QT interval, assess the QTc interval by electrocardiogram (ECG), and correct pre-existing electrolyte abnormalities (goal serum potassium >4 mEq/L, goal serum magnesium >1.8 mg/dL)
- Guidelines recommend assessing the QTc interval at least twice per week by ECG. QT interval should be corrected for heart rate using an alternative formula other than the classical Bazett correction (eg, Fridericia, Hodges, or Sagie/Framingham should be used). Very high-risk patients may warrant telemetered ECG monitoring. If the QT (or QTc for patients with heart rate >60 beats per minute) interval is prolonged longer than 500 ms, arsenic trioxide should be withheld, electrolytes (potassium and magnesium) should be repleted, and other medications with potential to prolong the QT interval should be discontinued if possible. Arsenic may be resumed (initially at a 50% reduced dose, then later increased to full dose) upon repletion of electrolytes and improvement of the QT/QTc interval to ~460 ms[10]

ASPARAGINASE, *ERWINIA CHRYSANTHEMI*

ERWINAZE (asparaginase *Erwinia chrysanthemi*) prescribing information. Palo Alto, CA: Jazz Pharmaceuticals, Inc.; December 2019

Product Identification, Preparation, Storage, and Stability

Erwinaze is a sterile, white lyophilized powder supplied in clear, 3-mL, glass vials. Each carton of the commercial product contains 5 vials (NDC 57902-249-05). Each vial (NDC 57902-249-01) contains 10,000 IU of asparaginase *Erwinia chrysanthemi*

- Store intact vials and cartons under refrigeration at 2–8°C (36–46°F)
- Protect intact vials and the reconstituted drug product from light

Reconstitution:

- Slowly inject 1 or 2 mL of preservative-free 0.9% NS against the inner vial wall
- *DO NOT* forcefully inject the diluent solution directly into the drug powder

Diluent Volume	Product Concentration
1 mL	10,000 IU/mL
2 mL	5000 IU/mL

- Dissolve the drug powder by gentle mixing or swirling after adding preservative-free 0.9% NS diluent. *DO NOT* shake or invert vials to solubilize the drug product
- After reconstitution, asparaginase *Erwinia chrysanthemi* should be a clear, colorless solution. Discard the reconstituted product if visible particles or protein aggregates are present
- *DO NOT* freeze or refrigerate asparaginase *Erwinia chrysanthemi* solutions
- Within 15 minutes of reconstitution, withdraw the calculated dose from the vial into a polypropylene syringe
- If preparing a dose for intraVENous administration, then slowly inject the reconstituted solution into an IV infusion bag containing 100 mL of 0.9% NS acclimatized to room temperature. Do not shake or squeeze the IV bag
- Reconstituted and diluted product solutions should be administered within 4 hours from the time of reconstitution. Do not refrigerate or freeze reconstituted or diluted solutions

Recommendations for Drug Administration and Ancillary Care

General:
- See Chapter 43 for recommended use in hepatic dysfunction
- Administer asparaginase *Erwinia chrysanthemi* in a setting with resuscitation equipment and other agents necessary to treat anaphylaxis

IntraMUSCular administration:
- Volumes for injection >2 mL should be distributed among 2 or more injection sites

IntraVENous administration:
- Administer over 1 to 2 hours and within 4 hours after reconstitution

To substitute asparaginase *Erwinia chrysanthemi* for a dose of pegaspargase:
- For each planned dose of pegaspargase, the recommended dose of asparaginase *Erwinia chrysanthemi* is 25,000 International Units/m^2 administered intraMUSCularly or intraVENously 3 times per week (eg, Monday, Wednesday, and Friday) for 6 doses
- When administered intraVENously, consider monitoring nadir (pre-dose) serum asparaginase activity (NSAA) levels and switching to intraMUSCular administration if desired NSAA levels are not achieved

ATEZOLIZUMAB

TECENTRIQ (atezolizumab) prescribing information. South San Francisco, CA: Genentech, Inc.; May 2020

Product Identification, Preparation, Storage, and Stability

- TECENTRIQ is a sterile, colorless to slightly yellow, preservative-free solution in individually boxed single-dose vials that contain either: atezolizumab 840 mg/14 mL (NDC 50242-918-01) formulated in glacial acetic acid (11.5 mg), L-histidine (43.4 mg), polysorbate 20 (5.6 mg), and sucrose (575.1 mg) with a pH of 5.8, or atezolizumab 1200 mg/20 mL (NDC 50242-917-01) formulated in glacial acetic acid (16.5 mg), L-histidine (62 mg), polysorbate 20 (8 mg), and sucrose (821.6 mg) with a pH of 5.8

- Store intact vials under refrigeration at 2–8°C (36–46°F) in original carton to protect from light
- Do not freeze or shake intact vials

Dilution:

- Inspect vials for particulate matter and discoloration prior to use. Discard if solution is cloudy, discolored, or visible particles are observed
- Dilute to a final concentration between 3.2 mg/mL and 16.8 mg/mL in a PVC, polyethylene, or polyolefin (PO) infusion bag containing 0.9% NS

- Mix diluted solution by gentle inversion. Do not shake
- Administer immediately once prepared. Diluted solution may be stored at room temperature for no more than 6 hours (including administration time) from the time of preparation or under refrigeration 2–8°C (35–46°F) for no more than 24 hours (including administration time) from the time of preparation

Selected incompatibility:

- Do not co-administer other drugs through the same intravenous line

Recommendations for Drug Administration and Ancillary Care

General:

- The effect of severe renal impairment or severe hepatic impairment on the PK of atezolizumab is unknown
- Do not administer as an intraVENous push or bolus

Administration:

- The recommended dose of atezolizumab is indication and regimen specific. Atezolizumab may be dosed at 840 mg every 2 weeks, 1200 mg every 3 weeks, or 1680 mg every 4 weeks. See current FDA-approved label for indications, dosages, and schedules
- Administer the first infusion over 60 minutes. If well-tolerated, subsequent infusions may be given over 30 minutes
- May be administered with or without a sterile, non-pyrogenic, low-protein-binding inline filter (pore size of 0.2–0.22 μm)

Adverse events and treatment modifications:

- Immune-mediated adverse events can occur with atezolizumab. Some of these adverse events can be severe or life-threatening
- Refer to the current FDA-approved product label for detailed warnings and recommendations regarding treatment modifications for pneumonitis, hepatitis, colitis or diarrhea, endocrinopathies, other immune-mediated adverse reactions, infections, persistent G2 or G3 adverse reactions (excluding endocrinopathies) or recurrent G3 or G4 adverse reactions according to the NCI CTCAE version 4.0
  - Permanently discontinue atezolizumab if unable to reduce steroid dose for adverse reactions to ≤10 mg prednisone per day (or equivalent) within 12 weeks after last dose
- Severe or life-threatening infusion-related reactions have occurred in patients treated with atezolizumab. Infusion reactions occurred in 1.3% of 2616 patients across trials of various cancers using atezolizumab as a single agent (G3 0.2%)
  - Interrupt or slow the administration rate in patients with mild or moderate infusion-related reactions. Consider premedications with subsequent doses
  - Permanently discontinue atezolizumab in patients who experience infusion reactions G ≥3

AVELUMAB

BAVENCIO (avelumab) prescribing information. Rockland, MA: EMD Serono, Inc.; June 2020

Product Identification, Preparation, Storage, and Stability

- BAVENCIO is a sterile, preservative-free, nonpyrogenic, clear, colorless to slightly yellow solution in individually boxed single-dose vials (NDC 44087-3535-1) that contain avelumab (200 mg/10 mL). Each mL contains avelumab (20 mg), D-mannitol (51 mg), glacial acetic acid (0.6 mg), polysorbate 20 (0.5 mg), sodium hydroxide (0.3 mg), and SWFI. The pH range of the solution is 5.0–5.6
- Store intact vials under refrigeration at 2–8°C (36–46°F) in original package to protect from light
- Do not freeze or shake intact vials

Dilution:
- Inspect vials for particulate matter and discoloration prior to use. Discard if solution is cloudy or discolored, or if visible particles are observed
- Withdraw the required volume of avelumab from the vial(s) and inject into a 250-mL infusion bag containing either 0.9% NS or 0.45% NaCl
- Gently invert the bag to mix the diluted solution. Avoid foaming or excessive shearing
- Protect diluted solution from light. Do not freeze or shake

- Store at room temperature up to 25°C (77°F) for no more than 4 hours from the time of dilution or under refrigeration 2–8°C (36–46°F) for no more than 24 hours from the time of dilution. If refrigerated, allow the diluted solution to come to room temperature prior to administration

Selected incompatibility:
- Do not co-administer with other drugs through the same intraVENous line

Recommendations for Drug Administration and Ancillary Care

General:
- The effect of severe hepatic impairment on the PK of avelumab is unknown

Administration:
- The recommended dose of avelumab is 800 mg every 2 weeks. See current FDA-approved label for indications
- Prior to the first four infusions, premedicate patients with an antihistamine and acetaminophen
- Premedication after the fourth avelumab dose may be administered based upon clinical judgment and the presence and severity of infusion-related reactions encountered during previously administered avelumab doses
- Administer diluted solution over 60 minutes with an administration set that contains a sterile, non-pyrogenic, low-protein-binding inline filter with pore size of 0.2 μm

Adverse events and treatment modifications:
- Refer to the current FDA-approved product label for detailed recommendations regarding treatment modifications for pneumonitis, hepatitis, colitis, endocrinopathies, nephritis and renal dysfunction, and other immune-mediated adverse reactions
- Infusion-related reactions occurred in 25% of patients treated with avelumab in clinical trials, including nine (0.5%) G3 and three (0.2%) G4 reactions. Reactions may be severe or life-threatening
  - Monitor for signs and symptoms of infusion-related reactions including pyrexia, chills, flushing, hypotension, dyspnea, wheezing, back pain, abdominal pain, and urticaria
  - Interrupt or slow the rate of infusion for mild or moderate infusion-related reactions. Stop and permanently discontinue for severe G ≥3 infusion-related reactions

Selected precautions:
- Immune-mediated adverse events can occur with avelumab. Some of these adverse events can be severe or life-threatening. Refer to the current FDA-approved label for detailed warnings
- Severe and fatal cardiovascular events have occurred in combination with axitinib. Optimize management of cardiovascular risk factors such as hypertension, diabetes, or dyslipidemia

AZACITIDINE

VIDAZA (azacitidine for injection) prescribing information. Summit, NJ: Celgene Corporation; March, 2020
AZACITIDINE prescribing information. Parsippany, NJ: Actavis Pharma, Inc.; July 2020

Product Identification, Preparation, Storage, and Stability

- AzaCITIDine for injection is packaged in single-dose vials containing 100 mg azaCITIDine as a sterile, lyophilized, white to almost white powder. Excipient content varies among available products
  - Store intact vials at 25°C (77°F); temperature excursions are permitted to 15–30°C (59–86°F)
  - Note: maximum storage times for reconstituted and diluted azaCITIDine may vary between available products; refer to current product label for details

Preparation for SUBCUTaneous administration:

1. Reconstitute lyophilized azaCITIDine powder by slowly injecting 4 mL of SWFI into a vial
2. Vigorously shake or roll the vial until a uniform cloudy suspension is formed. The resulting suspension contains 25 mg azaCITIDine per milliliter

Preparation for *immediate* SUBCUTaneous administration:

1. Divide doses >4 mL (>100 mg) equally into two syringes
2. Store reconstituted azaCITIDine suspension for up to 1 hour at room temperature, but the product must be administered within 1 hour after reconstitution

Preparation for *delayed* SUBCUTaneous administration:

1. Reconstituted azaCITIDine may be kept in the vial or drawn into a syringe
2. Divide doses >4 mL (>100 mg) equally into 2 syringes
3. Immediately place the product under refrigeration (2–8°C; 36–46°F)

a. If refrigerated SWFI was used in reconstituting azaCITIDine, the reconstituted product may be stored under refrigeration (2–8°C) for up to 22 hours
b. If *non*-refrigerated SWFI was used in reconstituting azaCITIDine, the reconstituted product may be stored under refrigeration (2–8°C) for up to 8 hours, or for one hour if stored at room temperature (25°C [77°F])

4. After removal from refrigeration, the suspension may be allowed to equilibrate to room temperature for up to 30 minutes before administration

Preparation for *delayed* intraVENous administration:

1. Reconstitute an appropriate number of vials to achieve the desired dose. Inject 10 mL SWFI into each vial and vigorously shake or roll the vial until all solids are dissolved. The resulting solution should be clear and will contain azaCITIDine 10 mg/mL
2. Withdraw a volume of azaCITIDine solution appropriate to deliver the desired dose and inject it into 50–100 mL of 0.9% NS or LRI
3. After reconstitution for intraVENous administration, azaCITIDine may be stored at 25°C, but administration must be completed within 1 hour after reconstitution

Selected incompatibilities:

- D5W , Hespan (6% hetastarch [hydroxyethyl starch] in 0.9% NS), and solutions that contain bicarbonate have the potential to increase the rate of azaCITIDine degradation and should be avoided

Recommendations for Drug Administration and Ancillary Care

General:

- See Chapter 43 for recommended use in renal and hepatic dysfunction
- If patients experience an unexplained decrease in serum bicarbonate concentration to <20 mEq/L during or after treatment with azaCITIDine, the dosage should be decreased by 50% during the next treatment cycle
- If patients experience an unexplained increase in BUN or serum creatinine during treatment, the next cycle should be delayed until laboratory values return to normal or baseline and azaCITIDine dosage should be decreased by 50% on the next treatment course
- AzaCITIDine and its metabolites are substantially renally excreted. Elderly individuals and other patients with impaired renal function may be at increased risk of toxicity from azaCITIDine

For SUBCUTaneous administration only:

- Doses >4 mL (>100 mg) should be divided equally into 2 syringes and injected into 2 separate sites. Rotate sites for each injection (thigh, abdomen, or upper arm)
- New injections should be given at least 1 inch from an old site and never into areas where the site is tender, bruised, red, or hard
- For azaCITIDine suspension that is not administered immediately after preparation:
  - After removal from refrigeration, allow the suspension to equilibrate to room temperature for up to 30 minutes before administration
  - Resuspend the product before administration to provide a homogeneous suspension by vigorously shaking a vial or rolling syringes between the palms until a uniform cloudy suspension is formed

For IntraVENous administration:

- After reconstitution and further dilution, administer the total azaCITIDine dose over a period of 10–40 minutes
- Administration must be completed within 1 hour after initial reconstitution

BELINOSTAT

BELEODAQ (belinostat for injection) prescribing information. East Windsor, NJ: Acrotech Biopharma LLC; January 2020

Product Identification, Preparation, Storage, and Stability

- BELEODAQ (belinostat for injection) is a sterile, yellow, lyophilized powder supplied in a single-dose vial that contains belinostat 500 mg (NDC 72893-002-01) and 1000 mg of the inactive ingredient L-Arginine, USP
- Store intact vials at room temperature 20–25°C (68–77°F); temperature excursions to 15–30°C (59–86°F) are permitted

Reconstitution:
- Using a sterile syringe, slowly inject 9 mL of SWFI diluent into the vial containing belinostat

- Swirl vials gently until the drug substance is completely dissolved and no visible particles remain
- After reconstitution, each vial contains belinostat 50 mg/mL
- The reconstituted lyophilized drug product may be stored for up to 12 hours at ambient temperature (15–25°C; 59–77°F)

Dilution:
- Calculate the volume of concentrated reconstituted belinostat 50 mg/mL solution needed to prepare a patient's dose

- With a syringe, aseptically transfer from one or more vials the volume needed to a parenteral product container prefilled with 250 mL 0.9% NS
  - *Do not use* if cloudiness or particulates are observed in the diluted solution
- After dilution, the belinostat admixture may be stored at ambient temperature (15–25°C; 59–77°F) for up to 36 hours, inclusive of the infusion time

Recommendations for Drug Administration and Ancillary Care

General:
- See Chapter 43 for recommended use in patients with hepatic dysfunction
  - There are insufficient data to recommend a belinostat dose in patients with creatinine clearance ≤39 mL/minute or in patients with moderate and severe hepatic dysfunction (total bilirubin >1.5 × upper limit of normal)

Administration:
- The recommended dose of belinostat is 1000 mg/m^2, given as an intraVENous infusion through a 0.22-μm inline filter over 30 minutes once daily on days 1–5 of a 21-day cycle
- The duration of administration may be extended to 45 minutes in patients who experience infusion site pain or other infusion-related symptoms
- Reduce the starting dose of belinostat to 750 mg/m^2 in patients known to be homozygous for the UGT1A1*28 allele
- A central VAD is not required for administering belinostat

Adverse events and treatment modifications:
- Refer to the current FDA-approved product label for detailed recommendations regarding treatment modifications for management of hematologic toxicities (eg, G4 thrombocytopenia, G4 neutropenia) and G ≥3 nonhematologic toxicities
  - Initiation of a cycle should be delayed in patients with a day 1 absolute neutrophil count <1000/mm^3, day 1 platelet count <50,000/mm^3, day 1 nonhematologic toxicity G ≥3, or evidence of an active infection

Potential drug interaction:
- UGT1A1 is primarily responsible for the metabolism of belinostat. UGT1A1 inhibitors (eg, gemfibrozil, ketoconazole, atazanavir, indinavir) have a potential to increase belinostat concentration and their use should be avoided

Selected precautions:
- In patients at high risk for the tumor lysis syndrome (eg, high tumor burden, renal dysfunction, rapidly progressing disease, markedly elevated LDH, baseline abnormalities in laboratory indices of tumor lysis syndrome [potassium, phosphate, uric acid, calcium, serum creatinine]), consider frequent monitoring of laboratory indices of tumor lysis syndrome, intraVENous hydration, and prophylaxis with a xanthine oxidase inhibitor (eg, allopurinol) during the first cycle
- Belinostat may cause nausea, vomiting, and/or diarrhea. Proactively advise patients on warning signs and appropriate self-care measures, including proper use of antiemetic and antidiarrheal medications

BENDAMUSTINE HYDROCHLORIDE

TREANDA (bendamustine hydrochloride) prescribing information. North Wales, PA: Teva Pharmaceuticals USA, Inc.; November 2019
Note: Although TREANDA (bendamustine hydrochloride) (product formulated in solution) received FDA approval in September 2013, it is currently (as of August 2020) not commercially available within the USA
BENDEKA (bendamustine hydrochloride injection) prescribing information. North Wales, PA: Teva Pharmaceuticals USA, Inc.; October 2019

Product Identification, Preparation, Storage, and Stability

Product Comparison

	BENDEKA Solution	TREANDA Lyophilized Powder	TREANDA Solution
How supplied	100 mg/4 mL in multiple-dose vials	25 mg or 100 mg in single-dose vials	45 mg/0.5 mL or 180 mg/2 mL in single-dose vials
Excipients	Propylene glycol, monothioglycerol in polyethylene glycol 400, and possibly sodium hydroxide	Mannitol	Propylene glycol and DMA
Concentration	25 mg/mL	5 mg/mL after reconstitution with 5 mL (25 mg vial) or 20 mL (100 mg vial) SWFI	90 mg/mL
Dilution	0.9% NS, D2.5W/0.45% NaCl, or D5W to final concentration 1.85–5.6 mg/mL. Typical volume is 50 mL	0.9% NS or D2.5W/0.45% NaCl to final concentration 0.2–0.6 mg/mL. Typical volume is 500 mL	0.9% NS or D2.5W/0.45% NaCl to final concentration 0.2–0.7 mg/mL. Typical volume is 500 mL
Infusion time	10 minutes for both CLL and NHL	30 minutes for CLL 60 minutes for NHL	30 minutes for CLL 60 minutes for NHL
Device compatibility	No DMA-related device compatibility issues	No DMA-related device compatibility issues	Incompatible with devices that contain polycarbonate or ABS, including most CSTDs
Product storage	Refrigerated in original carton. After first use, store vial refrigerated in original carton for up to 28 days. Not recommended for >6 dose withdrawals	Up to 25°C (77°F) with excursions up to 30°C (86°F) in original package to protect from light	Refrigerated in original carton to protect from light
Admixture stability	• 6 hours at RT and room light when diluted with 0.9% NS or D2.5W/0.45% NaCl • 3 hours at RT and room light when diluted with D5W • 24 hours when refrigerated	• 3 hours at RT and room light • 24 hours when refrigerated	• 2 hours at RT and room light • 24 hours when refrigerated

DMA, N N-dimethylacetamide; CLL, chronic lymphocytic leukemia; NHL, Non-Hodgkin Lymphoma; ABS, acrylonitrile-butadiene-styrene; CSTDs, Closed System Transfer Devices; RT, room temperature
Note: RT = 15–30°C (59–86°F); refrigerated = 2–8°C (36–46°F)
TREANDA (bendamustine hydrochloride) prescribing information. North Wales, PA: Teva Pharmaceuticals USA; November 2019
BENDEKA (bendamustine hydrochloride injection) prescribing information. North Wales, PA: Teva Pharmaceuticals USA, Inc.; October 2019

BENDEKA (Bendamustine HCl Injection); (100 mg/4 mL solution in a multiple-dose vial)
• BENDEKA is supplied as a sterile, clear, colorless to yellow, preservative-free, ready-to-dilute solution. Each mL contains 25 mg of bendamustine hydrochloride, 0.1 mL of propylene glycol, USP, 5 mg of monothioglycerol, NF, in polyethylene glycol 400, NF. Sodium hydroxide may have been used to adjust the acidity of polyethylene glycol 400. BENDEKA is packaged in individual cartons of 5 mL clear multiple-dose vials containing 100 mg of bendamustine hydrochloride as a clear, and colorless to yellow ready-to-dilute solution (NDC 63459-348-04 100 mg/4 mL)
• Store intact vials under refrigeration at 2–8°C (35–46°F) in the original carton to protect from light
• BENDEKA is in a multiple-dose vial. If additional dose withdrawal from the same vial is intended, retain the partially used vial in the original package to protect from light and store refrigerated for up to 28 days from first use. Each vial is not recommended for more than a total of 6 dose withdrawals. Although BENDEKA does not contain any antimicrobial preservatives, the product is bacteriostatic

(continued)

Product Identification, Preparation, Storage, and Stability *(continued)*

- At room temperature, BENDEKA is a clear, colorless to yellow ready-to-dilute solution. When refrigerated, the contents may partially freeze. Allow the vial to reach room temperature (15–30°C or 59–86°F) prior to use. Do not use the product if particulate matter is observed after achieving room temperature
- BENDEKA is a cytotoxic drug. Follow applicable special handling and disposal procedures
- Using proper aseptic technique, withdraw the volume needed for the required dose from the 25 mg/mL solution as per the table in the FDA-approved product label and immediately transfer the solution to a 50 mL infusion bag with one of the following diluents: 0.9% NS, D2.5W/0.45% NaCl, or D5W
- The resulting final concentration should be within 1.85 mg/mL–5.6 mg/mL. Thoroughly mix the contents of the infusion bag. The admixture should be a clear, colorless to yellow solution
- If diluted with 0.9% NS, D2.5W/0.45% NaCl, the final admixture is stable for 6 hours at room temperature (15–30°C or 59–86°F) and room light or 24 hours refrigerated (2–8°C or 36–46°F)
- If diluted with D5W, the final admixture is stable for 3 hours at room temperature (15–30°C or 59–86°F) and room light or 24 hours refrigerated (2–8°C or 36–46°F)
- Infuse over 10 minutes intraVENously

TREANDA (Bendamustine HCl for injection); (25 mg or 100 mg lyophilized powder in single-dose vials)
- TREANDA is available in single-dose, individually packaged, amber glass vials containing a sterile, non-pyrogenic, white to off-white, lyophilized powder available in two presentations:
  - 25 mg bendamustine HCl with 42.5 mg mannitol, USP; NDC 63459-390-08; *and*
  - 100 mg bendamustine HCl with 170 mg mannitol, USP; NDC 63459-391-20
- Store intact vials at temperatures up to 25°C (77°F); temperature excursions are permitted up to 30°C (86°F)
- Vials should be stored in the original packaging carton to protect bendamustine HCl from light
- Reconstitute the commercial products only with SWFI as follows:

Bendamustine HCl Content	SWFI (Diluent) Volume	Resulting Bendamustine HCl Concentration
25 mg	5 mL	5 mg/mL
100 mg	20 mL	

  - Shake well to yield a clear and colorless to pale yellow solution with pH of 2.5–3.5
  - The lyophilized powder should completely dissolve within 5 minutes. If particulate matter is observed, the reconstituted product should not be used
- Within 30 minutes after reconstitution, transfer an amount of bendamustine HCl sufficient to prepare a patient's dose to a parenteral product container with a volume of 0.9% NS or D2.5W/0.45% NaCl sufficient to produce a clear and colorless to slightly yellow solution with a concentration within the range of 0.2–0.6 mg/mL
- Thoroughly mix the diluted product
- After reconstitution and dilution as described, the drug product is stable for 24 hours if stored under refrigeration (2–8°C [36–46°F]), or for 3 hours if stored at room temperature (15–30°C [59–86°F]) and exposed to room light
- Administration must be completed within the duration of known product stability
  - TREANDA contains no antimicrobial preservatives. The admixture should be prepared as close as possible to the time of use

TREANDA (Bendamustine HCl injection); (45 mg/0.5 mL or 180 mg/2 mL solution in single-dose vials)
- TREANDA is packaged in single-dose, individually cartoned, amber glass vials containing a clear, colorless-to-yellow solution of bendamustine HCl with a concentration of 90 mg/mL. The commercial product is available in two presentations:
  - Bendamustine HCl 45 mg/0.5 mL with propylene glycol, USP (162 mg) and *N,N*-dimethylacetamide, EP (293 mg); NDC 63459-395-02, *or*
  - Bendamustine HCl 180 mg/2 mL with propylene glycol, USP, (648 mg) and *N,N*-dimethylacetamide, EP (1172 mg); NDC 63459-396-02
  - Each vial contains 0.2 mL of excess drug (overfill)
- Store intact vials under refrigeration at 2–8°C (35.6–46.4°F) in the original packaging carton to protect bendamustine HCl from light
- **Warning: Do not use TREANDA injection (product in solution) with devices that contain polycarbonate or acrylonitrile-butadiene-styrene (ABS), including most closed system transfer devices (CSTDs). If using a syringe to withdraw and transfer TREANDA Injection from the vial into the infusion bag, only use a polypropylene syringe with a metal needle and a polypropylene hub to withdraw and transfer TREANDA Injection into the infusion bag. After dilution of TREANDA Injection into the infusion bag, devices that contain polycarbonate or ABS, including infusion sets, may be used**

(continued)

Product Identification, Preparation, Storage, and Stability (*continued*)

- Using a polypropylene syringe with a metal needle and polypropylene hub, aseptically transfer a volume of concentrated bendamustine HCl solution sufficient to prepare a patient's dose to a parenteral product container already containing a volume of 0.9% NS or D2.5W/0.45% NaCl sufficient to produce a clear, colorless-to-yellow solution with a concentration within the range 0.2–0.7 mg/mL
- Thoroughly mix the diluted product
- After dilution, the admixture is stable for 24 hours if stored under refrigeration (2–8°C), or for 2 hours if stored at room temperature (15–30°C [59–86°F]) and exposed to room light
- Administration must be completed within the duration of known product stability
  - TREANDA contains no antimicrobial preservatives. The admixture should be prepared as close as possible to the time of use

Recommendations for Drug Administration and Ancillary Care

General:

- See Chapter 43 for recommended use in renal and hepatic dysfunction
- Do not use bendamustine in patients with CrCl <30 mL/min
- Do not use in patients with moderate to severe hepatic impairment (total bilirubin 1.5–3 × ULN and AST or ALT 2.5–10 × ULN or total bilirubin >3 × ULN) since the PK of bendamustine is unknown in these populations
- Dosages and administration rates vary between FDA-approved indications and between available products. Refer to above table and current FDA-approved product labels for the product being used for details

Potential drug interactions:

- CYP1A2 catalyzes bendamustine metabolism to its active metabolites, γ-hydroxy-bendamustine (M3) and *N*-desmethyl-bendamustine (M4)
  - CYP1A2 inhibitors (eg, fluvoxamine, ciprofloxacin) have a potential to increase bendamustine concentration and decrease concentrations of its active metabolites in plasma
  - Conversely, CYP1A2 inducers (eg, omeprazole, tobacco use) potentially may decrease plasma concentrations of bendamustine and its active metabolites
- In vitro studies suggest that P-glycoprotein (MDR1, ABCB1), breast cancer resistance protein (BCRP, ABCG2, MXR1), and other efflux transporters may have a role in bendamustine transport
- Based on in vitro data, bendamustine is not likely to inhibit metabolism via human CYP1A2, CYP2C9/10, CYP2D6, CYP2E1, or CYP3A4/5, or to induce the metabolism of cytochrome P450 substrates

BEVACIZUMAB

AVASTIN (bevacizumab) prescribing information. South San Francisco, CA: Genentech, Inc.; May 2020

Product Identification, Preparation, Storage, and Stability

- Avastin is packaged in individually boxed, single-use, glass vials in 2 presentations containing either 100 mg or 400 mg bevacizumab preservative-free solution in a uniform concentration of 25 mg/mL
- Carton of one vial (100 mg/4 mL) NDC 50242-060-01 or carton of 10 vials NDC 50242-060-10
- Carton of one vial (400 mg/16 mL) NDC 50242-061-01 or carton of 10 vials NDC 50242-061-10
- Store intact vials under refrigeration at 2–8°C (35.6–46.4°F) in the original carton to protect them from light
- *Do not freeze or shake* Avastin
- The commercial product contains a clear to slightly opalescent, colorless to pale brown, sterile solution of bevacizumab with pH = 6.2
  - The 100-mg product is formulated in 240 mg α,α-trehalose dihydrate, 23.2 mg sodium phosphate (monobasic, monohydrate), 4.8 mg sodium phosphate (dibasic, anhydrous), 1.6 mg polysorbate 20, and SWFI
  - The 400-mg product is formulated in 960 mg α,α-trehalose dihydrate, 92.8 mg sodium phosphate (monobasic, monohydrate), 19.2 mg sodium phosphate (dibasic, anhydrous), 6.4 mg polysorbate 20, and SWFI
- Withdraw from a vial an amount of bevacizumab sufficient to prepare a patient's dose and add it to a volume of 0.9% NS sufficient to produce a total volume of (Q.S.) 100 mL in a PVC or polyolefin container. Gently invert the container to mix diluted bevacizumab solution. Discard any unused bevacizumab that remains in a vial
- *Do not mix* bevacizumab with dextrose solutions
- After dilution, bevacizumab solutions may be stored at 2–8°C for up to 8 hours
- After dilution in 0.9% NS, bevacizumab was stable for up to 24 hours under the following conditions:

Bevacizumab Concentrations (mg/mL)	Storage Temperatures	Results
0.9 2.25 6.6 12.5 16.5	30°C	No significant changes in protein concentration, pH, turbidity, or potency
1 12.5	2–8°C 30°C	No change in protein concentration, turbidity, or potency

Genentech Medical Communications, Genentech, Inc., data on file, April 13, 2004
Bing CM et al: Extended stability for Parenteral Drugs, 4th ed., Bethesda, MD: American Society of Health-System Pharmacists; 2009

Selected incompatibility:

- Do not mix bevacizumab with dextrose solutions

Recommendations for Drug Administration and Ancillary Care

General:

- *Do not administer* bevacizumab by direct intraVENous injection or bolus injection
- Administer bevacizumab by intraVENous infusion after chemotherapy. The *INITIAL DOSE* is given over 90 minutes. If a dose given over 90 minutes was well tolerated, the administration duration may be decreased to 60 minutes during a subsequent infusion. If a 60-minute infusion was well tolerated, subsequent treatments may be administered over 30 minutes
- *Do not administer, mix, or flush* bevacizumab with dextrose solutions

Selected Precautions

- **See current FDA-approved product label for detailed warnings and precautions**
- Serious, and sometimes fatal, gastrointestinal perforation occurred at a higher incidence in patients receiving Avastin compared to patients receiving chemotherapy. Perforation can be complicated by intra-abdominal abscess, fistula formation, and the need for diverting ostomies. The majority of perforations occurred within 50 days of the first dose
- Discontinue Avastin in patients with wound healing complications requiring medical intervention. Withhold for at least 28 days prior to elective surgery. Do not administer for at least 28 days following surgery and until the wound is fully healed
- Avastin can result in two distinct patterns of bleeding: minor hemorrhage, which is most commonly Grade 1 epistaxis, and serious hemorrhage, which in some cases has been fatal. Severe or fatal hemorrhage, including hemoptysis, gastrointestinal bleeding, hematemesis, CNS hemorrhage, epistaxis, and vaginal bleeding, occurred up to 5-fold more frequently in patients receiving Avastin compared to patients receiving chemotherapy alone

BLEOMYCIN SULFATE

BLEOMYCIN (bleomycin) prescribing information. Lake Forest, IL: Hospira, Inc.; June 2018
BLEOMYCIN (bleomycin) prescribing information. North Wales, PA: Teva Pharmaceuticals USA, Inc.; February 2016

WARNINGS

It is recommended that Bleomycin for Injection be administered under the supervision of a qualified physician experienced in the use of cancer chemotherapeutic agents. Appropriate management of therapy and complications is possible only when adequate diagnostic and treatment facilities are readily available

Pulmonary fibrosis is the most severe toxicity associated with Bleomycin for Injection

The most frequent presentation is pneumonitis occasionally progressing to pulmonary fibrosis. Its occurrence is higher in elderly patients and in those receiving greater than 400 units total [cumulative] dose, but pulmonary toxicity has been observed in young patients and those treated with low doses

A severe idiosyncratic reaction consisting of hypotension, mental confusion, fever, chills, and wheezing has been reported in approximately 1% of lymphoma patients treated with Bleomycin for Injection

Boxed Warning for BLEOMYCIN (bleomycin) prescribing information. Lake Forest, IL: Hospira, Inc.; June 2018

Product Identification, Preparation, Storage, and Stability

- Bleomycin is generically available as a lyophilized powder for reconstitution for injection in individually packaged vials
- Each vial contains sterile bleomycin sulfate equivalent to 15 units or 30 units of bleomycin
  - Sulfuric acid or sodium hydroxide are used, if necessary, to adjust product pH
- Store intact vials under refrigeration at 2–8°C (36–46°F)
- One unit of bleomycin activity corresponds to the formerly used 1 mg of bleomycin activity. The term milligram activity is a misnomer and was changed to units to be more precise
  - Commercial products are a mixture of bleomycin glycopeptides. Measurement in activity units is a more precise indication of drug potency
- Reconstitute with 0.9% NS, SWFI, or BWFI as follows:

Bleomycin Content/Vial	0.9% NS for IntraVENous or Intrapleural Administration		0.9% NS, SWFI, or BWFI for SUBCUTaneous or IntraMUSCular Administration	
		Diluent Volumes		
15 units	5 mL	Bleomycin concentration = 3 units/mL	1 mL	Bleomycin concentration = 15 units/mL
30 units	10 mL		2 mL	

- For *intrapleural administration* as a sclerosing agent, further dilute bleomycin 60 units in 50–100 mL of 0.9% NS
- *Do not reconstitute or dilute* bleomycin with dextrose-containing solutions
  - Bleomycins A$_2$ and B$_2$ potencies decrease after reconstitution or dilution in dextrose-containing solutions, which does not occur in 0.9% NS[11]
- After reconstitution in 0.9% NS, bleomycin is stable for 24 hours at room temperature
- Bleomycin is compatible with glass, PVC, and high-density polyethylene containers[10], and with polyethylene, PVC, and polybutadiene administration sets[12]

Recommendations for Drug Administration and Ancillary Care

General:

- See Chapter 43 for recommended use in patients with renal dysfunction
- Bleomycin is given by slow intraVENous injection over 10 minutes; by intraVENous infusion; and by the intraMUSCular, intrapleural, and SUBCUTaneous routes
- Bleomycin may be filtered during administration with filter membranes composed of cellulose ester,[11,13] cellulose nitrate/cellulose acetate ester,[14] or tetrafluoroethylene polymer (Teflon [DuPont]), without a significant loss of drug potency

Idiosyncratic reactions:

- In approximately 1% of patients with lymphoma treated with bleomycin, a severe idiosyncratic reaction, similar to anaphylaxis, has been reported, consisting of: hypotension, mental confusion, fever, chills, and wheezing. Treatment is symptomatic including volume expansion, vasopressors, antihistamines, and glucocorticoids. The reaction may be immediate or delayed for several hours, and usually occurs after a first or second dose
  - Consequently, current FDA approved product labeling recommends because of the possibility of an anaphylactoid reaction, patients with lymphoma should receive not more than 2 units of bleomycin for the first 2 doses. If no acute reaction occurs, then the regular dosage schedule may be followed
    - The absence of hypersensitivity to test doses (≤2 units bleomycin) does not preclude hypersensitivity phenomena during subsequent administration at full treatment dosages
- Renal insufficiency markedly alters bleomycin elimination. Bleomycin terminal elimination half-life increases exponentially as creatinine clearance decreases
  - Patients with impaired renal function should be treated with caution and their renal function should be carefully monitored during the administration of bleomycin. Bleomycin dosage reduction may be required in renally impaired patients
  - See Chapter 43 for modifying bleomycin dosage in renal impairment

For intrapleural administration:

- Administer bleomycin through a thoracostomy tube after excess pleural fluid drainage and confirming complete lung expansion. The thoracostomy tube is clamped after bleomycin instillation. The patient is moved from the supine to the left and right lateral positions several times during the next 4 hours. The clamp is then removed and thoracostomy tube suction is reestablished. The amount of time a thoracostomy tube remains in place following sclerosis is dictated by the clinical situation. The intrapleural injection of topical anesthetics or systemic narcotic analgesia is generally not required

BLINATUMOMAB

BLINCYTO (blinatumomab) prescribing information. Thousand Oaks, CA: Amgen Inc.; March 2020

WARNING: CYTOKINE RELEASE SYNDROME and NEUROLOGICAL TOXICITIES

- Cytokine Release Syndrome (CRS), which may be life-threatening or fatal, occurred in patients receiving BLINCYTO. Interrupt or discontinue BLINCYTO and treat with corticosteroids as recommended …
- Neurological toxicities, which may be severe, life-threatening, or fatal, occurred in patients receiving BLINCYTO. Interrupt or discontinue BLINCYTO as recommended …

Boxed Warning for BLINCYTO (blinatumomab) prescribing information. Thousand Oaks, CA: Amgen Inc.; March 2020

Product Identification, Preparation, Storage, and Stability

- Each package (NDC 55513-160-01) contains 1 vial of BLINCYTO (blinatumomab) and 1 vial of IV solution stabilizer:
  - BLINCYTO is available as a preservative-free, sterile, white to off-white, lyophilized powder composed of blinatumomab (35 μg), citric acid monohydrate (3.35 mg), lysine hydrochloride (23.23 mg), polysorbate 80 (0.64 mg), trehalose dihydrate (95.5 mg), and sodium hydroxide to adjust pH to 7.0. After reconstitution with 3 mL of preservative-free SWFI, the resulting concentration is 12.5 μg/mL blinatumomab
  - IV solution stabilizer is available as a single-dose glass vial containing a sterile, preservative-free, colorless to slightly yellow, clear solution composed of citric acid monohydrate (52.5 mg), lysine hydrochloride (2283.8 mg), polysorbate 80 (10 mg), sodium hydroxide to adjust pH to 7.0, and SWFI. The IV solution stabilizer is intended to coat the IV bag PRIOR TO addition of reconstituted BLINCYTO to prevent adhesion of blinatumomab to IV bags and tubing
- Store intact BLINCYTO and IV solution stabilizer vials in the original package refrigerated at 2–8°C (36–46°F). Protect from light until time of use. Do not freeze. BLINCYTO and IV solution stabilizer vials may be stored for a maximum of 8 hours at room temperature 23°C to 27°C (73°F to 81°F) in the original carton to protect from light
- Because the product vials are preservative-free, it is important to strictly observe aseptic technique when preparing the infusion solution. The solution must be prepared in a USP 797–compliant facility in an ISO Class 5 laminar flow hood or better. The admixing area must have appropriate environmental specifications as confirmed by periodic monitoring. Personnel involved in product preparation must be trained in aseptic manipulations and admixing of oncology drugs, must wear appropriate protective clothing and gloves, and must ensure that gloves and surfaces have been disinfected
- **It is very important that the instructions for preparation (including admixing) and administration provided in the current FDA-approved product label are strictly followed to minimize medication errors (including underdose and overdose). It is strongly recommended to refer to the current label for the most up-to-date information. Call 1-800-772-6436 if you have questions about the reconstitution and preparation**
- Reconstitute BLINCYTO with preservative-free SWFI. *DO NOT* use IV solution stabilizer for reconstitution of BLINCYTO
- **BLINCYTO may be prepared as a 24-hour (preservative-free), 48-hour (preservative-free), or 168-hour (with preservative) infusion. The 168-hour infusion option is not recommended for patients who weigh <22 kg due to concern for adverse effects related to excessive benzyl alcohol exposure. The choice between these options should be made by the treating health care provider**

Reconstitution:

- Determine the number of BLINCYTO vials needed for a dose and infusion duration
- Reconstitute each BLINCYTO vial with 3 mL of preservative-free SWFI by directing the water along the walls of the BLINCYTO vial and not directly on the lyophilized powder to yield a solution containing 12.5 μg/mL blinatumomab
- Gently swirl the contents of the vial to avoid excessive foaming to yield. Do not shake. The resulting solution should appear clear to slightly opalescent and colorless to slightly yellow. Discard the vial if the solution is cloudy or has precipitated

Dilution (24-hour and 48-hour infusions):

- Verify the prescribed dose and infusion duration for each BLINCYTO infusion bag. To minimize errors, use the specific volumes described in the following tables to prepare the BLINCYTO infusion bag
- Aseptically add 270 mL of 0.9% NS to the empty IV bag
- Aseptically transfer 5.5 mL of IV solution stabilizer to the IV bag containing 0.9% NS. Gently mix the contents of the bag to avoid foaming. Discard the vial containing unused IV solution stabilizer
- Aseptically transfer the required volume of reconstituted BLINCYTO solution into the IV bag containing 0.9% NS and IV solution stabilizer. Gently mix the contents of the bag to avoid foaming. Discard the vial containing unused BLINCYTO

(continued)

Product Identification, Preparation, Storage, and Stability *(continued)*

- Under aseptic conditions, attach the IV tubing to the IV bag with the sterile 0.2-μm inline filter. Ensure that the IV tubing is compatible with the infusion pump
- Remove air from the IV bag. This is particularly important for use with an ambulatory infusion pump
- Prime the IV tubing only with the solution in the bag containing the FINAL prepared BLINCYTO solution for infusion
- Store refrigerated at 2–8°C (36–46°F) if not used immediately

Dilution (24-hour and 48-hour infusions):
- Verify the prescribed dose and infusion duration for each BLINCYTO infusion bag. To minimize errors, use the specific volumes described in the following tables to prepare the BLINCYTO infusion bag
- Aseptically add 90 mL of B0.9% NS (containing 0.9% benzyl alcohol) to the empty IV bag
- Aseptically transfer 2.2 mL of IV solution stabilizer to the IV bag containing B0.9% NS. Gently mix the contents of the bag to avoid foaming. Discard the vial containing unused IV solution stabilizer
- Aseptically transfer the required volume of reconstituted BLINCYTO solution into the IV bag containing B0.9% NS and IV solution stabilizer. Gently mix the contents of the bag to avoid foaming. Discard the vial containing unused BLINCYTO
- Aseptically transfer the required volume of 0.9% NS to the IV bag to obtain a final volume of 110 mL. Gently mix the contents of the bag to avoid foaming
- Under aseptic conditions, attach the IV tubing to the IV bag. Ensure that the IV tubing is compatible with the infusion pump. **Do** *not* **use an inline filter for a 168-hour bag**
- Remove air from the IV bag. This is particularly important for use with an ambulatory infusion pump
- Prime the IV tubing only with the solution in the bag containing the *FINAL* prepared BLINCYTO solution for infusion
- Store refrigerated at 2–8°C (36–46°F) if not used immediately

Blinatumomab Infusion Options (for Patients Who Weigh ≥45 kg)

Intended Infusion Duration	Blinatumomab Dose	Volume 0.9% NS	Volume B0.9% NS (Contains 0.9% Benzyl Alcohol)	IV Solution Stabilizer* Volume	Reconstituted Blinatumomab Solution Volume (Blinatumomab Content)	Final Bag Volume†	Infusion Rate, Duration, and Delivered Dose of Blinatumomab
24-hour bag	9 μg per day	270 mL	Not applicable	5.5 mL	0.83 mL (10.375 μg)	276.33 mL	10 mL/hour intraVENously, for 24 hours only, to deliver a dose of 9 μg over 24 hours
48-hour bag	9 μg per day	270 mL	Not applicable	5.5 mL	1.7 mL (21.25 μg)	277.2 mL	5 mL/hour intraVENously, for 48 hours only, to deliver an approximate dose of 18 μg over 48 hours
24-hour bag	28 μg per day	270 mL	Not applicable	5.5 mL	2.6 mL (32.5 μg)	278.1 mL	10 mL/hour intraVENously, for 24 hours only, to deliver a dose of 28 μg over 24 hours
48-hour bag	28 μg per day	270 mL	Not applicable	5.5 mL	5.2 mL (65 μg)	280.7 mL	5 mL/hour intraVENously, for 48 hours only, to deliver an approximate dose of 56 μg over 48 hours
168-hour bag	28 μg per day	1 mL	90 mL	2.2 mL	16.8 mL (210 μg)	110 mL	0.6 mL/hour intraVENously, for 168 hours only, to deliver an approximate dose of 196 μg over 168 hours

*The specified volume of IV solution stabilizer is transferred to the IV bag containing either 0.9% NS [for 24-hour and 48-hour bags] or B0.9% NS (containing 0.9% benzyl alcohol) [for 168-hour bags] before the transfer of the specified volume of reconstituted blinatumomab. The IV solution stabilizer is *NOT* to be used for reconstitution of blinatumomab

(continued)

Product Identification, Preparation, Storage, and Stability *(continued)*

				Blinatumomab Infusion Options (for Patients Who Weigh <45 kg)				
Intended Infusion Duration	Blinatumomab Dose	IV Solution Stabilizer° Volume	Volume B0.9% NS (Contains 0.9% Benzyl Alcohol)	BSA (m²) Range	Volume 0.9% NS	Reconstituted Blinatumomab Solution Volume (Blinatumomab Content)	Final Bag Volume	Infusion Rate, Duration, and Delivered Dose of Blinatumomab
24-hour bag	5 μg/m² per day	5.5 mL	Not applicable	1.5–1.59	270 mL	0.7 mL (8.75 μg)	276.2 mL	10 mL/hour intraVENously, for 24 hours only, to deliver an approximate dose of 5 μg/m² over 24 hours
				1.4–1.49	270 mL	0.66 mL (8.25 μg)	276.16 mL	
				1.3–1.39	270 mL	0.61 mL (7.625 μg)	276.11 mL	
				1.2–1.29	270 mL	0.56 mL (7 μg)	276.06 mL	
				1.1–1.19	270 mL	0.52 mL (6.5 μg)	276.02 mL	
				1–1.09	270 mL	0.47 mL (5.875 μg)	275.97 mL	
				0.9–0.99	270 mL	0.43 mL (5.375 μg)	275.93 mL	
				0.8–0.89	270 mL	0.38 mL (4.75 μg)	275.88 mL	
				0.7–0.79	270 mL	0.33 mL (4.125 μg)	275.83 mL	
				0.6–0.69	270 mL	0.29 mL (3.625 μg)	275.79 mL	
				0.5–0.59	270 mL	0.24 mL (3 μg)	275.74 mL	
				0.4–0.49	270 mL	0.2 mL (2.5 μg)	275.7 mL	
48-hour bag	5 μg/m² per day	5.5 mL	Not applicable	1.5–1.59	270 mL	1.4 mL (17.5 μg)	276.9 mL	5 mL/hour intraVENously, for 48 hours only, to deliver an approximate dose of 10 μg/m² over 48 hours
				1.4–1.49	270 mL	1.3 mL (16.25 μg)	276.8 mL	
				1.3–1.39	270 mL	1.2 mL (15 μg)	276.7 mL	
				1.2–1.29	270 mL	1.1 mL (13.75 μg)	276.6 mL	
				1.1–1.19	270 mL	1 mL (12.5 μg)	276.5 mL	
				1–1.09	270 mL	0.94 mL (11.75 μg)	276.44 mL	
				0.9–0.99	270 mL	0.85 mL (10.625 μg)	276.35 mL	
				0.8–0.89	270 mL	0.76 mL (9.5 μg)	276.26 mL	
				0.7–0.79	270 mL	0.67 mL (8.375 μg)	276.17 mL	
				0.6–0.69	270 mL	0.57 mL (7.125 μg)	276.07 mL	
				0.5–0.59	270 mL	0.48 mL (6 μg)	275.98 mL	
				0.4–0.49	270 mL	0.39 mL (4.875 μg)	275.89 mL	
24-hour bag	15 μg/m² per day	5.5 mL	Not applicable	1.5–1.59	270 mL	2.1 mL (26.25 μg μg)	277.6 mL	10 mL/hour intraVENously, for 24 hours only, to deliver an approximate dose of 15 μg/m² over 24 hours
				1.4–1.49	270 mL	2 mL (25 μg)	277.5 mL	
				1.3–1.39	270 mL	1.8 mL (22.5 μg)	277.3 mL	
				1.2–1.29	270 mL	1.7 mL (21.25 μg)	277.2 mL	
				1.1–1.19	270 mL	1.6 mL (20 μg)	277.1 mL	
				1–1.09	270 mL	1.4 mL (17.5 μg)	276.9 mL	
				0.9–0.99	270 mL	1.3 mL (16.25 μg)	276.8 mL	
				0.8–0.89	270 mL	1.1 mL (13.75 μg)	276.6 mL	
				0.7–0.79	270 mL	1 mL (12.5 μg)	276.5 mL	
				0.6–0.69	270 mL	0.86 mL (10.75 μg)	276.36 mL	
				0.5–0.59	270 mL	0.72 mL (9 μg)	276.22 mL	
				0.4–0.49	270 mL	0.59 mL (7.375 μg)	276.09 mL	

(continued)

Product Identification, Preparation, Storage, and Stability *(continued)*

Blinatumomab Infusion Options (for Patients Who Weigh <45 kg)

Intended Infusion Duration	Blinatumomab Dose	IV Solution Stabilizer* Volume	Volume B0.9% NS (Contains 0.9% Benzyl Alcohol)	BSA (m²) Range	Volume 0.9% NS	Reconstituted Blinatumomab Solution Volume (Blinatumomab Content)	Final Bag Volume	Infusion Rate, Duration, and Delivered Dose of Blinatumomab
48-hour bag	15 μg/m² per day	5.5 mL	Not applicable	1.5–1.59	270 mL	4.2 mL (52.5 μg)	279.7 mL	5 mL/hour intraVENously, for 48 hours only, to deliver an approximate dose of 30 μg/m² over 48 hours
				1.4–1.49	270 mL	3.9 mL (48.75 μg)	279.4 mL	
				1.3–1.39	270 mL	3.7 mL (46.25 μg)	279.2 mL	
				1.2–1.29	270 mL	3.4 mL (42.5 μg)	278.9 mL	
				1.1–1.19	270 mL	3.1 mL (38.75 μg)	278.6 mL	
				1–1.09	270 mL	2.8 mL (35 μg)	278.3 mL	
				0.9–0.99	270 mL	2.6 mL (32.5 μg)	278.1 mL	
				0.8–0.89	270 mL	2.3 mL (28.75 μg)	277.8 mL	
				0.7–0.79	270 mL	2 mL (25 μg)	277.5 mL	
				0.6–0.69	270 mL	1.7 mL (21.25 μg)	277.2 mL	
				0.5–0.59	270 mL	1.4 mL (17.5 μg)	276.9 mL	
				0.4–0.49	270 mL	1.2 mL (15 μg)	276.7 mL	
168-hour bag	15 μg/m² per day	2.2 mL	90 mL	1.5–1.59	3.8 mL	14 mL (175 μg)	110 mL	0.6 mL/hour intraVENously, for 168 hours only, to deliver an approximate dose of 105 μg/m² over 168 hours
				1.4–1.49	4.7 mL	13.1 mL (163.75 μg)	110 mL	
				1.3–1.39	5.6 mL	12.2 mL (152.5 μg)	110 mL	
				1.2–1.29	6.5 mL	11.3 mL (141.25 μg)	110 mL	
				1.1–1.19	7.4 mL	10.4 mL (130 μg)	110 mL	
				1–1.09	8.3 mL	9.5 mL (118.75 μg)	110 mL	
				0.9–0.99	9.2 mL	8.6 mL (107.5 μg)	110 mL	

*The specified volume of IV solution stabilizer is transferred to the IV bag containing either 0.9% NS [for 24-hour and 48-hour bags] or B0.9% NS (containing 0.9% benzyl alcohol) [for 168-hour bags] before the transfer of the specified volume of reconstituted blinatumomab. The IV solution stabilizer is *NOT* to be used for reconstitution of blinatumomab

†168-hour bag is not recommended for patients who weigh <22 kg

Storage Time for Reconstituted BLINCYTO Vial and Prepared BLINCYTO Infusion Bags

	Maximum Storage Time	
	Room Temperature 23°C–27°C (73°F–81°F)	Refrigerated 2–8°C (36–46°F)
Reconstituted BLINCYTO Vial	4 hours	24 hours
Prepared BLINCYTO Infusion Bag *(Preservative-free)*	48 hours*	8 days
Prepared BLINCYTO Infusion Bag *(with Preservative)*	7 days*	14 days

*Storage time includes infusion time. If the prepared BLINCYTO infusion bag is not administered within the time frames and temperatures indicated, it must be discarded; it should not be refrigerated again

Selected incompatibility:
- BLINCYTO is incompatible with DEHP. Use polyolefin, PVC DEHP-free, or ethyl vinyl acetate (EVA) infusion bags/pump cassettes. Use polyolefin, PVC DEHP-free, or EVA intraVENous tubing sets.

(continued)

Recommendations for Drug Administration and Ancillary Care

General:

- See Chapter 43 for recommended use in patients with renal and hepatic dysfunction
- No formal PK studies have been completed in patients with hepatic or renal impairment

Administration:

Administration of BLINCYTO as a 24-hour or 48-hour infusion

- Administer BLINCYTO as a continuous intraVENous infusion at a constant flow rate using an infusion pump. The pump should be programmable, lockable, and non-elastomeric, and it should have an alarm
- The starting volume (270 mL) is more than the volume administered to the patient (240 mL) to account for the priming of the intraVENous tubing and to ensure that the patient will receive the full dose of BLINCYTO
- Infuse prepared BLINCYTO final infusion solution according to the instructions on the pharmacy label on the prepared bag at one of the following constant infusion rates:
  - Infusion rate of 10 mL/hour for a duration of 24 hours, *OR*
  - Infusion rate of 5 mL/hour for a duration of 48 hours
- Administer prepared BLINCYTO final infusion solution using intraVENous tubing that contains a sterile, non-pyrogenic, low-protein-binding, 0.2-μm inline filter
- **Important Note: Do not flush the BLINCYTO infusion line or intraVENous catheter, especially when changing infusion bags. Flushing when changing bags or at completion of infusion can result in excess dosage and complications thereof. When administering via a multi-lumen venous catheter, infuse BLINCYTO through a dedicated lumen**
- At the end of the infusion, discard any unused BLINCYTO solution in the intraVENous bag and intraVENous tubing in accordance with local requirements

Administration of BLINCYTO as a 168-hour infusion

- Administer BLINCYTO as a continuous intraVENous infusion at a constant flow rate using an infusion pump. The pump should be programmable, lockable, and non-elastomeric, and it should have an alarm
- The final volume of infusion solution (110 mL) is more than the volume administered to the patient (100 mL) to account for the priming of the intraVENous tubing and to ensure that the patient will receive the full dose of BLINCYTO
- **Do *NOT* use an inline filter for a 168-hour bag**
- Infuse prepared BLINCYTO final infusion solution according to the instructions on the pharmacy label on the prepared bag at an infusion rate of 0.6 mL/hour for a duration of 7 days (168 hours)
- **Important Note: Do not flush the BLINCYTO infusion line or intraVENous catheter, especially when changing infusion bags. Flushing when changing bags or at completion of infusion can result in excess dosage and complications thereof. When administering via a multi-lumen venous catheter, infuse BLINCYTO through a dedicated lumen**
- At the end of the infusion, discard any unused BLINCYTO solution in the intraVENous bag and intraVENous tubing in accordance with local requirements

Blinatumomab Dosing and Premedications for Treatment of MRD-positive B-cell ALL		
Cycle	Patient Weight ≥45 kg (Fixed Dose)	Patient Weight <45 kg (BSA-based Dose)
Induction Cycle 1		
Premedications	*Adult patients:* predniSONE 100 mg IV or equivalent (eg, dexamethasone 16 mg) 1 hour prior to initiation of blinatumomab on day 1 *Pediatric patients:* dexamethasone 5 mg/m² (NTE 20 mg) 1 hour prior to initiation of blinatumomab on day 1 and when restarting an infusion after an interruption of ≥4 hours	
Daily blinatumomab dose on days 1–28	28 μg/day	15 μg/m²/day (NTE 28 μg/day)
Days 29–42	14-day treatment-free interval	

(*continued*)

Recommendations for Drug Administration and Ancillary Care *(continued)*

Blinatumomab Dosing and Premedications for Treatment of MRD-positive B-cell ALL

Cycle	Patient Weight ≥45 kg (Fixed Dose)	Patient Weight <45 kg (BSA-based Dose)
Consolidation Cycles 2–4		
Premedications	*Adult patients:* predniSONE 100 mg IV or equivalent (eg, dexamethasone 16 mg) 1 hour prior to initiation of blinatumomab on day 1 *Pediatric patients:* none	
Daily blinatumomab dose on days 1–28	28 μg/day	15 μg/m²/day (NTE 28 μg/day)
Days 29–42	14-day treatment-free interval	

MRD, minimal residual disease; ALL, acute lymphoblastic leukemia; BSA, body surface area; NTE, not to exceed
A treatment course consists of 1 cycle of induction and up to 3 cycles of consolidation. Cycle length is 42 days
Hospitalization is recommended for the first 3 days of the first cycle and the first 2 days of the second cycle. For all subsequent cycle starts and re-initiations (eg, if treatment is interrupted for 4 or more hours), supervision by a health care professional or hospitalization is recommended

Blinatumomab Dosing for Treatment of Relapsed or Refractory B-cell ALL

Cycle	Patient Weight ≥45 kg (Fixed Dose)	Patient Weight <45 kg (BSA-based Dose)
Induction Cycle 1		
Premedications	*Adult patients:* dexamethasone 20 mg 1 hour prior to initiation of blinatumomab on day 1 and prior to a step dose (eg, cycle 1 day 8), and when restarting an infusion after an interruption of ≥4 hours *Pediatric patients:* dexamethasone 5 mg/m² (NTE 20 mg) 1 hour prior to initiation of blinatumomab on day 1 and prior to a step dose (eg, cycle 1 day 8), and when restarting an infusion after an interruption of ≥4 hours	
Daily dose on days 1–7	9 μg/day	5 μg/m²/day (NTE 9 μg/day)
Daily dose on days 8–28	28 μg/day	15 μg/m²/day (NTE 28 μg/day)
Days 29–42	14-day treatment-free interval	14-day treatment-free interval
Induction Cycle 2		
Premedications	*Adult patients:* dexamethasone 20 mg 1 hour prior to initiation of blinatumomab on day 1 and when restarting an infusion after an interruption of ≥4 hours *Pediatric patients:* none	
Daily dose on days 1–28	28 μg/day	15 μg/m²/day (NTE 28 μg/day)
Days 29–42	14-day treatment-free interval	
Consolidation Cycles 3–5		
Premedications	*Adult patients:* dexamethasone 20 mg 1 hour prior to initiation of blinatumomab on day 1 and when restarting an infusion after an interruption of ≥4 hours *Pediatric patients:* none	
Daily dose on days 1–28	28 μg/day	15 μg/m²/day (NTE 28 μg/day)
Days 29–42	14-day treatment-free interval	

(continued)

Recommendations for Drug Administration and Ancillary Care (*continued*)

Blinatumomab Dosing for Treatment of Relapsed or Refractory B-cell ALL

Cycle	Patient Weight ≥45 kg (Fixed Dose)	Patient Weight <45 kg (BSA-based Dose)
Continued Therapy Cycles 6–9		
Premedications	*Adult patients:* dexamethasone 20 mg 1 hour prior to initiation of blinatumomab on day 1 and when restarting an infusion after an interruption of ≥4 hours *Pediatric patients:* none	
Daily dose on days 1–28	28 μg/day	15 μg/m²/day (NTE 28 μg/day)
Days 29–84	56-day treatment-free interval	

ALL, acute lymphoblastic leukemia; BSA, body surface area; NTE, not to exceed

A treatment course consists of up to 2 cycles of induction, up to 3 cycles of consolidation, and up to 4 cycles of continued therapy. Cycle length during induction and consolidation is 42 days. Cycle length during continued therapy is 84 days

Hospitalization is recommended for the first 9 days of the first cycle and the first 2 days of the second cycle. For all subsequent cycle starts and re-initiation (eg, if treatment is interrupted for 4 or more hours), supervision by a health care professional or hospitalization is recommended

Concomitant medications:

- Refer to the preceding tables for details regarding corticosteroid premedication based on indication, cycle, and age
- Consider administration of prophylaxis for the tumor lysis syndrome in the appropriate clinical context
- Consider administration of prophylactic antimicrobials as clinically indicated

Adverse events and treatment modifications:

- Refer to the current FDA-approved product label for detailed warnings and treatment modifications for missed doses (dose interruptions), cytokine release syndrome, neurological toxicity, pancreatitis, tumor lysis syndrome, prolonged neutropenia, hepatotoxicity, and other clinically relevant G ≥3 adverse reactions
- Advise patients to refrain from driving and engaging in hazardous occupations or activities such as operating heavy or potentially dangerous machinery while BLINCYTO is being administered

Potential drug interactions:

- Do not administer live virus vaccines for at least the 2 weeks prior to the start of BLINCYTO treatment, during treatment, and until immune recovery following the last cycle
- Transient release of cytokines induced by BLINCYTO may occur, most commonly during the initial 9 days of cycle 1 and in the initial 2 days of cycle 2. Cytokines may cause transient suppression of CYP450 enzyme activity; monitor patients closely who are taking sensitive substrates of CYP450 enzymes during these periods

BORTEZOMIB

VELCADE (bortezomib) prescribing information. Cambridge, MA: Millennium Pharmaceuticals, Inc.; April 2019
BORTEZOMIB (bortexomib) prescribing information. Visakhapatnam, India: Dr. Reddy's Laboratories Ltd; October 2019
BORTEZOMIB (bortezomib) prescribing information. Lake Zurich, IL: Fresenius Kabi USA, LLC.; September 2018

Product Identification, Preparation, Storage, and Stability	VELCADE (Bortezomib) for Injection	BORTEZOMIB (Bortexomib) Injection, Powder, Lyophilized, for Solution	BORTEZOMIB (Bortezomib) Injection, Powder, Lyophilized, for Solution
Distributor	Millennium Pharmaceuticals, Inc.	Dr. Reddy's Laboratories, Inc	Fresenius Kabi USA, LLC
NDC number	63020-049-01	43598-865-60	63323-721-10
Product description	Supplied in individually packaged 10-mL vials as a sterile, white to off-white, preservative-free, lyophilized powder containing bortezomib (3.5 mg) and mannitol, USP (35 mg). The product is provided as a mannitol boronic ester which, in reconstituted form, consists of the mannitol ester in equilibrium with its hydrolysis product, the monomeric boronic acid. The drug substance exists in its cyclic anhydride form as a trimeric boroxine	Supplied in individually packaged 10-mL vials as a sterile, white to off-white lyophilized cake or powder containing bortezomib (3.5 mg), citric acid, USP (10 mg), and tromethamine, USP (8.4 mg). The product is provided as a citric acid boronic ester which, in reconstituted form, consists of the citric acid ester in equilibrium with its hydrolysis product, the monomeric boronic acid. The drug substance exists in its cyclic anhydride form as a trimeric boroxine	Supplied in individually packaged 10-mL vials as a sterile, white to off-white lyophilized cake or powder containing bortezomib (3.5 mg), boric acid (10.5 mg), glycine (25 mg). Solubility of bortezomib (as the monomeric boronic acid) in water is 3.3–3.8 mg/mL in a pH range of 2–6.5
Storage of intact vials	25°C (77°F) with excursions permitted from 15–30°C (59–86°F) in original package to protect from light	20–25°C (68–77°F) in original package to protect from light	20–25°C (68–77°F) with excursions permitted from 15–30°C (59–86°F) in original package to protect from light
Preparation for intraVENous injection (1 mg/mL solution)	• Reconstitute bortezomib powder with 3.5 mL of 0.9% NS to produce a clear, colorless solution with concentration = 1 mg bortezomib/mL • Apply the appropriate included sticker to the prepared syringe to alert practitioners of the correct route of administration		
Preparation for SUBCUTaneous injection (2.5 mg/mL solution)	• Reconstitute bortezomib powder with 1.4 mL of 0.9% NS to produce a clear, colorless solution with concentration = 2.5 mg bortezomib/mL • Apply the appropriate included sticker to the prepared syringe to alert practitioners of the correct route of administration	Product is not approved for SUBCUTaneous use	Product is not approved for SUBCUTaneous use
Stability and storage of reconstituted products	The reconstituted products may be stored in the original vials or in syringes at 25°C (77°F), and should be administered within 8 hours after reconstitution if exposed to normal indoor lighting		

Recommendations for Drug Administration and Ancillary Care

General:

- See Chapter 43 for recommended use in patients with renal and hepatic dysfunction

Caution:

- Exercise caution in calculating the volume of bortezomib to be administered
  - For the brand name VELCADE product, which is approved for both SUBCUTaneous and intraVENous administration, note that different volumes of 0.9% NS diluent are used to reconstitute the product for the different routes of administration
  - The concentration of reconstituted VELCADE for SUBCUTaneous administration (2.5 mg/mL) is greater than the concentration of reconstituted VELCADE for intraVENous administration (1 mg/mL)
- Stickers that identify the intended route of administration are provided with all bortezomib products and should be placed on syringes containing prepared doses as a safeguard against administration via an unintended route
- The reconstituted products are suitable for direct injection

IntraVENous Administration:

- For administration by intraVENous injection over 3–5 seconds

SUBCUTaneous Administration:

- When administered SUBCUTaneously (note, this applies to only the brand name VELCADE product), rotate injection sites (thigh or abdomen). Administer repeated injections at least 1 inch from a previously injected site, and never where a site is tender, bruised, erythematous, or indurated
- If local injection site reactions occur after SUBCUTaneous administration of VELCADE prepared in a concentration of 2.5 mg/mL, a less-concentrated solution (1 mg/mL) may be administered SUBCUTaneously. Alternatively, consider intraVENous administration

Potential for drug interactions:

- Bortezomib is a substrate for metabolism by CYP3A4, CYP2C19, and CYP1A2
  - Concomitant administration with potent inhibitors or inducers of CYP3A subfamily enzymes has been shown to alter bortezomib's pharmacokinetic behavior
  - Avoid use of bortezomib with potent inhibitors or inducers of CYP3A subfamily enzymes

BRENTUXIMAB VEDOTIN

ADCETRIS (brentuximab vedotin) prescribing information. Bothell, WA: Seattle Genetics, Inc.; October 2019

WARNING: PROGRESSIVE MULTIFOCAL LEUKOENCEPHALOPATHY (PML)

JC virus infection resulting in PML and death can occur in patients receiving ADCETRIS …

Boxed Warning for ADCETRIS (brentuximab vedotin) prescribing information. Bothell, WA: Seattle Genetics, Inc.; October 2019

Product Identification, Preparation, Storage, and Stability

- ADCETRIS (brentuximab vedotin) for injection is supplied as a sterile, white to off-white, preservative-free, lyophilized cake or powder in individually boxed single-use vials containing 50 mg brentuximab vedotin. NDC 51144-050-01
  - The reconstituted product contains a solution of brentuximab vedotin 5 mg/mL with 70 mg/mL trehalose dihydrate, 5.6 mg/mL sodium citrate dihydrate, 0.21 mg/mL citric acid monohydrate, and 0.20 mg/mL polysorbate 80 and water for injection. The pH is approximately 6.6
- Store intact vials at 2–8°C (36–46°F) in the original carton to protect brentuximab vedotin from light
- *Caution:* calculate a patient's dose and the number of ADCETRIS vials required to prepare a dose. A dose for patients weighing >100 kg should be calculated based on a weight of 100 kg

- *Reconstitution*
  1. Reconstitute brentuximab vedotin with 10.5 mL of SWFI, to produce a solution containing 5 mg brentuximab vedotin/mL
  2. Direct the stream of SWFI toward the vial wall, not directly into the drug product
  3. Gently swirl vial to aid drug dissolution. *Do not shake* a vial to aid dissolution
  4. The reconstituted solution should be clear to slightly opalescent, colorless, and free of visible particulates. Following reconstitution, dilute brentuximab vedotin immediately, or store the solution at 2–8°C and use it within 24 hours after reconstitution. *Do not freeze* brentuximab vedotin
  5. Discard any unused portion of brentuximab vedotin left in a vial

- *Dilution*
  1. Immediately add reconstituted brentuximab vedotin (5 mg/mL) to a parenteral product container containing a minimum volume of 100 mL 0.9% NS, D5W, or LRI to achieve a final diluted concentration within the range 0.4–1.8 mg/mL brentuximab vedotin
  2. Gently invert the product container to mix the solution
  3. Following dilution, administer brentuximab vedotin solution immediately, or store the solution at 2–8°C and use the product within 24 hours after reconstitution. *Do not freeze* brentuximab vedotin

Recommendations for Drug Administration and Ancillary Care

General:

- The recommended initial dosage and schedule of brentuximab vedotin varies according to indication
  - Doses for patients whose body weight is >100 kg should be calculated based on a weight of 100 kg; that is, the maximum single brentuximab vedotin dose is 180 mg
  - *Do not administer* brentuximab vedotin by direct intraVENous injection or over a period <30 minutes

Cautions:

- In vitro, the binding of monomethyl auristatin E (MMAE, the microtubule disrupting portion of brentuximab vedotin) to human plasma proteins ranged from 68–82%. MMAE is not likely to displace or to be displaced by highly protein-bound drugs
- *In vitro*, MMAE was a substrate but was not a potent inhibitor of the P-glycoprotein transport protein (P-gp, ABCB1, MDR1)
- *In vitro* data indicate that MMAE is largely eliminated in urine and feces as unchanged drug; however, a small portion of MMAE is a substrate for metabolism by CYP3A4/5. In vitro studies using human liver microsomes indicate MMAE inhibits CYP3A4/5 but not other CYP isoforms
  - Avoid concomitant use of brentuximab vedotin with potent inhibitors and inducers of CYP3A subfamily enzymes
- Concomitant use of brentuximab vedotin and bleomycin is contraindicated because of a greater incidence rate of noninfectious pulmonary toxicity with concurrent use than a historic comparison of the incidence of pulmonary toxicity reported with the ABVD (DOXOrubicin, bleomycin, vinBLAStine, dacarbazine) regimen

(continued)

Recommendations for Drug Administration and Ancillary Care (*continued*)

Adverse events:

- Infusion-related reactions, including anaphylaxis, have occurred with brentuximab vedotin. Continually monitor patients during drug administration
  - If anaphylaxis occurs, immediately and permanently discontinue brentuximab vedotin administration and administer appropriate medical therapy
  - In the event of less-severe manageable infusion-related reactions, interrupt brentuximab vedotin administration and institute appropriate medical management
    - Patients who experience an infusion-related hypersensitivity reaction should receive prophylaxis against hypersensitivity reactions before retreatment with brentuximab vedotin
    - Medications for hypersensitivity prophylaxis may include acetaminophen, an antihistamine, and a glucocorticoid
- Peripheral neuropathy should be managed using a combination of dose delay and dosage reduction (see FDA-approved prescribing information for details)
- JC virus infection resulting in PML and death has been reported in patients treated with brentuximab vedotin
  - Other possible contributory factors include prior therapies and underlying disease that may cause immunosuppression
  - Consider a diagnosis of PML in any patient presenting with new-onset signs and symptoms of CNS abnormalities
  - Evaluation for PML includes, but is not limited to, consultation with a neurologist, brain MRI, and lumbar puncture or brain biopsy
  - Withhold brentuximab vedotin for any suspected case of PML and discontinue use if a diagnosis of PML is confirmed
  - Recommendations for management of neutropenia vary by indication (refer to the FDA-approved prescribing information for details). Patients receiving brentuximab vedotin in combination with chemotherapy should receive primary prophylaxis with G-CSF

BUSULFAN

BUSULFEX (busulfan) prescribing information. Rockville, MD: Otsuka America Pharmaceutical, Inc.; March 2020
BUSULFAN (busulfan injection) prescribing information. Rockford, IL: Mylan Institutional LLC; May 2019

WARNING: MYELOSUPPRESSION

BUSULFEX (busulfan) Injection causes severe and prolonged myelosuppression at the recommended dosage. Hematopoietic progenitor cell transplantation is required to prevent potentially fatal complications of the prolonged myelosuppression …

Boxed Warning for BUSULFEX (busulfan) prescribing information. Rockville, MD: Otsuka America Pharmaceutical, Inc.; March 2020

Product Identification, Preparation, Storage, and Stability

- BUSULFEX (busulfan) injection is supplied as a clear, colorless, sterile solution in 10-mL, single-use, clear glass vials each containing busulfan 60 mg/10 mL (6 mg/mL) dissolved in *N,N*-dimethylacetamide (DMA) 33% (v/v) and polyethylene glycol 400, 67% (v/v). NDC 59148-070-90
- BUSULFEX is distributed as a unit carton containing 8 vials. NDC 59148-070-91
- Store intact vials under refrigeration at 2–8°C (36–46°F)

Dilution for clinical use:
- The solubility of busulfan in water is 100 mg/L and the pH of BUSULFEX diluted to approximately 0.5 mg busulfan/mL in 0.9% NS or D5W as recommended reflects the pH of the diluent used, and ranges from 3.4 to 3.9
- BUSULFEX must be diluted for clinical use with either 0.9% NS or D5W
  - The volume of diluent should be 10 times the volume of BUSULFEX solution, such that the final concentration of busulfan for clinical use is approximately 0.5 mg/mL
- Mix busulfan thoroughly by inverting the product container several times
- After dilution in 0.9% NS or D5W, BUSULFEX is stable at room temperature, 25°C (77°F), for up to 8 hours, but administration must be completed within that time[15]
- After dilution in 0.9% NS, BUSULFEX is stable under refrigeration at 2–8°C for up to 12 hours, but administration must be completed within that time

Preparation and administration precautions:
- *Do not use* polycarbonate syringes or polycarbonate filter needles in transferring or administering busulfan solutions
- *Do not inject* BUSULFEX solution (6 mg/mL) into a parenteral product container that does not contain 0.9% NS or D5W
  - Always add BUSULFEX to a diluent (vehicle) solution, not the reverse

Selected incompatibility:
- *Do not mix* BUSULFEX with another solution unless compatibility is known

---

Recommendations for Drug Administration and Ancillary Care

General:
- See Chapter 43 for recommended use in patients with hepatic dysfunction
- Select an administration set with minimal intraluminal priming volume (≤5 mL) to administer busulfan
- Prime the administration set tubing with diluted busulfan solution to allow accurate determination of the start of busulfan administration
  - It is important to accurately identify administration starting and completion times in order to modify busulfan dosage based on its pharmacokinetic behavior in individual patients
- A rate-controlling device (infusion pump) should be used to administer diluted busulfan by intraVENous infusion via a central VAD over 2 hours
  - More rapid administration has not been tested and is not recommended

- Before starting and after completing busulfan administration, flush the patient's VAD with approximately 5 mL of 0.9% NS or D5W. *Do not mix* BUSULFEX with another solution unless compatibility is known
  - Flushing is particularly important if blood samples for pharmacokinetically guided busulfan dose adjustment must be acquired from the same VAD used to administer the drug

Concomitant drug use:
- Busulfan crosses the blood–brain barrier and induces seizures. All patients should receive anticonvulsant prophylaxis with phenytoin prior to starting busulfan
  - Although phenytoin decreases busulfan AUC_{plasma} by 15%, other anticonvulsants may increase busulfan AUC_{plasma}, and

increase the risk of venoocclusive disease or seizures
  - Busulfan pharmacokinetics were studied in patients treated with phenytoin, and its clearance at the recommended dose may be less and exposure (AUC) greater in patients not treated with phenytoin
  - Plasma busulfan exposure should be monitored in cases where other anticonvulsants must be used
- Acetaminophen use should be avoided within 72 hours before and concurrently with busulfan use
  - Busulfan is eliminated via conjugation with glutathione. Acetaminophen is known to decrease glutathione concentrations in blood and tissues. Concurrent use with busulfan may result in reduced busulfan clearance, potentially prolonged systemic exposure to busulfan, and enhanced adverse effects

(*continued*)

Recommendations for Drug Administration and Ancillary Care *(continued)*

- Itraconazole decreases busulfan clearance by up to 25%
- MetroNIDAZOLE decreases busulfan clearance to an extent even greater than that observed with metroNIDAZOLE
- Decreased clearance of busulfan was observed with concomitant use of deferasirox. Therefore, discontinue iron chelating agents prior to administration of busulfan

Busulfan dosage as a component of the "BuCy" conditioning regimen before hematopoietic stem cell transplantation:

- The usual adult dosage is based on the lesser of either ideal or actual body weight, and is 0.8 mg/kg per dose, every 6 hours, for a total of 16 doses (total daily dosage = 3.2 mg/kg per day for 4 consecutive days, or a total dosage/4-day course = 12.8 mg/kg)
- Busulfan clearance is best predicted when doses are based on adjusted ideal body weight (AIBW)
  - Dose calculations based on actual body weight, ideal body weight, or other factors can produce significant differences in busulfan clearance among lean, normal, and obese patients
- Busulfan dosage in obese patients is based on adjusted ideal body weight as follows:

*Ideal body weight and adjusted ideal body weight calculations (**IBW** and **AIBW**, respectively):*

- IBW for men (kg) = $50 + 0.91 \times$ ([height in cm] $- 152$)
- IBW for women (kg) = $45 + 0.91 \times$ ([height in cm] $- 152$)
- AIBW men and women (kg) = IBW $+ 0.25 \times$ ([actual body weight] $-$ IBW)
- Where available, pharmacokinetic monitoring may be considered to optimize therapeutic targeting
  - Therapeutic target $AUC_{plasma} = 1125$ $\mu M \cdot min$

CABAZITAXEL

JEVTANA (cabazitaxel) prescribing information. Bridgewater, NJ: Sanofi-Aventis U.S. LLC; March 2020

WARNING: NEUTROPENIA AND HYPERSENSITIVITY

<u>Neutropenia</u>: Neutropenic deaths have been reported. Monitor for neutropenia with frequent blood cell counts. JEVTANA is contraindicated in patients with neutrophil counts of ≤1500 cells/mm^3. Primary prophylaxis with G-CSF is recommended in patients with high-risk clinical features …

<u>Severe hypersensitivity</u>: Severe hypersensitivity reactions can occur and may include generalized rash/erythema, hypotension, and bronchospasm. Severe hypersensitivity reactions require immediate discontinuation of the JEVTANA infusion and administration of appropriate therapy. Patients should receive premedication. JEVTANA is contraindicated in patients who have a history of severe hypersensitivity reactions to cabazitaxel or to other drugs formulated with polysorbate 80 …

Boxed Warning for JEVTANA (cabazitaxel) prescribing information. Bridgewater, NJ: Sanofi-Aventis U.S. LLC; March 2020

Product Identification, Preparation, Storage, and Stability

- JEVTANA (cabazitaxel) injection 60 mg/1.5 mL (NDC 0024-5824-11) is supplied as a kit consisting of 2 vials in a blister pack in 1 carton, including:
  - One single-use vial contains 60 mg of cabazitaxel (anhydrous and solvent-free) in 1.5 mL of polysorbate 80 (1.56 g) as a sterile, nonpyrogenic, clear yellow to brownish-yellow, viscous solution. Each milliliter of the concentrated drug product contains cabazitaxel (anhydrous) 40 mg and 1.04 g of polysorbate 80
  - One vial contains Diluent for JEVTANA, a clear, colorless, sterile, nonpyrogenic solution containing 13% (w/w) ethanol in water for injection, approximately 5.7 mL
- Both the JEVTANA injection and Diluent for JEVTANA vials contain excess drug and diluent solutions (overfill), respectively, to compensate for volume lost during preparation
- Store JEVTANA injection and Diluent for JEVTANA at 25°C (77°F); temperature excursions are permitted between 15–30°C (59–86°F)
- *Do not refrigerate* JEVTANA Injection and Diluent for JEVTANA
- JEVTANA requires 2 dilutions before it may be administered to patients:
  - The concentrated drug product should be diluted only with the supplied Diluent for JEVTANA, followed by dilution in either 0.9% NS or D5W
  - Do not use PVC infusion containers or polyurethane administration sets during preparation or administration of JEVTANA

Initial dilution:
1. With a syringe, aseptically withdraw the entire contents of a Diluent for JEVTANA vial and inject it into a vial containing the JEVTANA drug product
   a. When transferring the diluent, direct the needle onto the inside wall of the drug product vial and inject slowly to limit foaming
2. Remove the syringe and needle and gently mix the initially diluted solution by repeated inversions for at least 45 seconds to assure a homogeneous mixture of the drug and diluent. *Do not shake* initially diluted JEVTANA to avoid foaming
3. Let the solution stand for a few minutes to allow any foam to dissipate, and check that the solution is homogeneous and contains no visible particulate matter
   a. It is not required that all foam dissipate prior to continuing preparation
   b. The resulting initially diluted JEVTANA solution (10 mg cabazitaxel/mL) requires further dilution before it may be given to patients

Caution: Secondary dilution must be completed within 30 minutes after completing initial dilution to obtain a product appropriate for administration to patients

Secondary dilution:
1. With a syringe, aseptically withdraw an amount of the initially diluted JEVTANA solution (10 mg cabazitaxel/mL) appropriate for a patient's dose and transfer it to a volume of 0.9% NS or D5W to produce a cabazitaxel concentration within the range 0.1–0.26 mg/mL
   a. Product concentrations must not exceed 0.26 mg cabazitaxel/mL. Discard any unused portion of the initially diluted JEVTANA solution
2. Thoroughly mix the secondarily diluted product by manual rotation and by gently inverting the container
3. After the second dilution in either 0.9% NS or D5W , JEVTANA should be used within 8 hours if maintained at ambient temperatures (including the 1-hour administration time), or may be used within 24 hours after preparation (including the 1-hour administration time) if stored under refrigeration at 2–8°C (36–46°F)

Cautions: JEVTANA should not be mixed with any other drugs

Chemical and physical stability of cabazitaxel solution has been demonstrated for 24 hours under refrigerated conditions; however, both the initially diluted and secondarily diluted solutions are supersaturated. Consequently, if crystals or particulates appear in either solution, the solutions must not be used and should be discarded

Recommendations for Drug Administration and Ancillary Care

General:

- See Chapter 43 for recommended use in patients with renal and hepatic dysfunction
- Cabazitaxel is administered intraVENously over 60 minutes in combination with predniSONE 10 mg/day administered orally, continually throughout treatment with cabazitaxel

Primary prophylaxis against hypersensitivity reactions:

- At least 30 minutes before each dose of cabazitaxel give the following medications intraVENously to decrease the risk or severity of hypersensitivity:
  - A histamine H1-subtype receptor antagonist, for example, dexchlorpheniramine 5 mg, diphenhydrAMINE 25 mg, or equivalent antihistamine, *plus*
  - A glucocorticoid, for example, dexamethasone 8 mg, or another steroid at a glucocorticoid-equivalent dose, *plus*
  - A histamine H_2-subtype receptor antagonist, for example, raNITIdine 50 mg or equivalent
- After secondary dilution, JEVTANA solution (concentration 0.1–0.26 mg cabazitaxel/mL) should be administered intraVENously over 60 minutes at room temperature through an inline filter with nominal pore size of 0.22 μm
- Although it is recommended the secondarily diluted solution should be used immediately, storage time can be longer under specific conditions:
  - Up to 8 hours after preparation if maintained at ambient temperatures (including the 1-hour administration time), *or*
  - Up to 24 hours after preparation (including the 1-hour administration time) if stored under refrigeration at 2–8°C

Caution with medications given concomitantly:

- Cabazitaxel is a substrate for metabolism catalyzed by CYP3A subfamily enzymes
  - *Avoid concomitant use* of strong CYP3A subfamily enzyme inhibitors, which may increase systemic exposure to cabazitaxel (eg, atazanavir, clarithromycin, indinavir, itraconazole, ketoconazole, nefazodone, nelfinavir, ritonavir, saquinavir, telithromycin, voriconazole). If coadministration of a strong CYP3A4 inhibitor is unavoidable, then consider reducing the cabazitaxel dose by 25%

CARBOPLATIN

Carboplatin prescribing information. Lake Forest, IL: Hospira, Inc.; April 2018
CARBOPLATIN–carboplatin injection, solution (50-, 150-, and 450-mg multidose vials) prescribing information. Irvine, CA: Teva Parenteral Medicines, Inc.; January 2016
CARBOPLATIN INJECTION prescribing information. Lake Zurich, IL: Fresenius Kabi USA, LLC.; March 2017

WARNING

Carboplatin injection should be administered under the supervision of a qualified physician experienced in the use of cancer chemotherapeutic agents. Appropriate management of therapy and complications is possible only when adequate treatment facilities are readily available

Bone marrow suppression is dose related and may be severe, resulting in infection and/or bleeding. Anemia may be cumulative and may require transfusion support. Vomiting is another frequent drug-related side effect

Anaphylactic-like reactions to carboplatin have been reported and may occur within minutes of carboplatin injection administration. EPINEPHrine, corticosteroids, and antihistamines have been employed to alleviate symptoms

---

Boxed Warnings for Carboplatin prescribing information. Lake Forest, IL: Hospira, Inc.; April 2018

Product Identification, Preparation, Storage, and Stability

- CARBOplatin is marketed as branded and generic products from several manufacturers in multidose (*or multiuse*) vials containing 50 mg, 150 mg, 450 mg, or 600 mg CARBOplatin per vial
- CARBOplatin injection is a sterile aqueous solution of CARBOplatin at a concentration of 10 mg/mL (1%); the pH of a 1% solution of CARBOplatin is 5–7
- Store unopened vials under temperature conditions indicated for individual products, generally within a range between 20°C and 25°C (68°F and 77°F). Available products often indicate temperature excursions to 15–30°C (59–86°F) are permitted. Protect unopened vials from light
- CARBOplatin injection in multidose vials maintain microbial, chemical, and physical stability for up to 14 days (Teva Pharmaceuticals USA product) or 15 days

(Hospira, Inc. product) at 25°C following multiple needle entries
- CARBOplatin injection is supplied as a ready-to-use solution or it may be further diluted to concentrations as low as 0.5 mg/mL with either D5W or 0.9% NS. After dilution, CARBOplatin may be stored at room temperature (25°C [77°F]) for up to 8 hours before use

Selected incompatibility:

- Avoid admixture with solutions with pH >6.5 (eg, solutions containing fluorouracil or sodium bicarbonate)
- Avoid admixture with mesna
- Aluminum reacts with CARBOplatin, causing precipitation and loss of drug potency. *Do not prepare or administer* CARBOplatin with needles or administration sets that contain aluminum parts that may come into contact with the drug

Recommendations for Drug Administration and Ancillary Care

General:

- See Chapter 43 for recommended use in patients with renal dysfunction
- Administer CARBOplatin intraVENously over at least 15 minutes. Pre- or post-treatment hydration and forced diuresis are not required
- Prescriptions and medication orders should identify the drug by its complete generic name, "CARBOplatin," to prevent confusion with other platinum compounds

CARFILZOMIB

KYPROLIS (carfilzomib) prescribing information. Thousand Oaks, CA: Onyx Pharmaceuticals, Inc.; August 2020

Product Identification, Preparation, Storage, and Stability

- KYPROLIS (carfilzomib) for injection is supplied in individually cartoned single-use vials as a sterile, white to off-white, lyophilized cake or powder
  - Each 10 mg vial contains carfilzomib (10 mg), sulfobutylether beta-cyclodextrin (500 mg), anhydrous citric acid (9.6 mg), and sodium hydroxide to adjust the product pH to 3.5. NDC 76075-103-01
  - Each 30 mg vial contains carfilzomib (30 mg), sulfobutylether beta-cyclodextrin (1500 mg), anhydrous citric acid (28.8 mg), and sodium hydroxide to adjust the product pH to 3.5. NDC 76075-102-01
  - Each 60 mg vial contains carfilzomib (60 mg), sulfobutylether beta-cyclodextrin (3000 mg), anhydrous citric acid (57.7 mg), and sodium hydroxide to adjust the product pH to 3.5. NDC 76075-101-01
- Store unopened vials under refrigeration between 2°C and 8°C (36°F and 46°F) in the original packaging to protect carfilzomib from light
- Preparation:
  1. Remove a vial from refrigeration just prior to use
  2. Slowly inject the appropriate volume of SWFI (see table) by directing the solution onto the inside vial wall, not into the drug product to minimize foaming

Reconstitution Volumes for Carfilzomib	
Strength	**Volume of SWFI Required for Reconstitution**
10 mg vial	5 mL
30 mg vial	15 mL
60 mg vial	29 mL

  3. Gently swirl or slowly and repeatedly invert the vial for approximately 1 minute, or until the drug cake or powder has completely dissolved. DO NOT SHAKE carfilzomib to avoid generating foam
  4. If foaming occurs, set the vial aside for approximately 5 minutes, to allow the foam to dissipate
  5. After reconstitution, the resulting solution should be clear and colorless and contains carfilzomib at a concentration of 2 mg/mL
- Carfilzomib stability

Storage Conditions After Reconstitution (Carfilzomib 2 mg/mL)	Stability as a Function of Product Container*		
	Vial	Syringe	Diluted with D5W and Stored in a Plastic Container (Bag)
Refrigeration (2–8°C)	24 hours		
Room temperature (15–30°C [59–86°F])	4 hours		

*Total time from reconstitution to administration should not exceed 24 hours

  6. Reconstituted carfilzomib may be administered directly by intraVENous infusion or in a 50-mL to 100-mL parenteral product container containing D5W. Do not administer as an intraVENous push or bolus. When administering in an intraVENous bag, use a 21-gauge or larger needle to withdraw the calculated dose from the vial
  7. Discard vials containing unused drug solution

Recommendations for Drug Administration and Ancillary Care

Supportive Care:

Hydration
- Prior to administering carfilzomib, evaluate a patient's fluid status to ensure they are well hydrated
- Patients should receive hydration with carfilzomib to reduce the risk of developing renal toxicity and tumor lysis syndrome (TLS)
  - Overall, TLS occurred in <1% of patients, but patients with multiple myeloma and a high tumor burden should be considered at greater risk for TLS
  - Monitor for evidence of TLS during treatment, and manage promptly
  - Interrupt carfilzomib treatments until TLS is resolved
- Maintain patients' fluid volume status and monitor blood chemistries closely throughout treatment with carfilzomib
  - During cycle 1:
    - Give 250–500 mL 0.9% NS or another fluid intraVENously as clinically appropriate before each carfilzomib dose
    - Give an additional 250–500 mL of fluids intraVENously as needed after completing each carfilzomib dose
  - During repeated treatment cycles, continue intraVENous hydration as needed
- Monitor patients for fluid overload

Prophylaxis against hypersensitivity/infusion-related reactions
- Hypersensitivity reactions may occur immediately after or during the first 24 hours after carfilzomib administration
- Infusion-related reactions may be characterized by any of the following: fever, chills, arthralgia, myalgia, facial flushing, facial edema, vomiting, weakness, shortness of breath, hypotension, syncope, chest tightness, angina
- To mitigate the incidence and severity of infusion reactions, premedicate with the recommended dose of dexamethasone for monotherapy or dexamethasone administered as part of the combination therapy (see FDA-approved prescribing information for details). Dexamethasone should be given orally or intraVENously prior to each carfilzomib dose during cycle 1. Continue or resume prophylaxis with dexamethasone orally or intraVENously if symptoms develop or reappear during subsequent cycles

General:

- Carfilzomib is administered only by intraVENous infusion. The treatment schedule and infusion duration vary depending on the regimen being utilized
- Flush with 0.9% NS or D5W the administration set tubing and VAD through which carfilzomib is given immediately before beginning and after completing carfilzomib administration
- Provide thromboprophylaxis for patients being treated with carfilzomib in combination with other therapies. Consider avoiding use of oral contraceptives or hormonal contraception associated with a risk of thrombosis
- Consider antiviral prophylaxis to decrease the risk of herpes zoster infection
- Do not mix carfilzomib with other medicinal products or administer it through the same intraVENous VAD with other medicinal products

Carfilzomib dose calculation:

- Carfilzomib dose is calculated using a patient's actual BSA calculated at baseline. Patients with a BSA >2.2 m² should receive a dose based upon a BSA of exactly 2.2 m²
- There is no need to make dose adjustments for changes in body weight ≤20%

Carfilzomib dosage escalation:

- Dosages may be escalated based on tolerance; refer to the FDA-approved prescribing information for details

CARMUSTINE

CARMUSTINE prescribing information. East Brunswick, NJ: Heritage Pharmaceuticals Inc.; September 2019

WARNING: MYELOSUPPRESSION and PULMONARY TOXICITY

Myelosuppression
Carmustine for Injection causes suppression of marrow function (including thrombocytopenia and leukopenia), which may contribute to bleeding and overwhelming infections … Monitor blood counts weekly for at least 6 weeks after each dose. Adjust dosage based on nadir blood counts from the prior dose … Do not administer a repeat course of Carmustine for Injection until blood counts recover

Pulmonary Toxicity
Carmustine for Injection causes dose-related pulmonary toxicity. Patients receiving greater than 1400 mg/m² cumulative dose are at significantly higher risk than those receiving less. Delayed pulmonary toxicity can occur years after treatment, and can result in death, particularly in patients treated in childhood …

Boxed Warning for CARMUSTINE prescribing information. East Brunswick, NJ: Heritage Pharmaceuticals Inc.; September 2019

Product Identification, Preparation, Storage, and Stability[16]

- Carmustine for Injection, NDC 23155-649-41, packaging includes 2 containers, including:
  - One vial containing 100 mg of carmustine as sterile, lyophilized, pale-yellow flakes or a congealed mass
  - A vial containing 3 mL of sterile dehydrated alcohol injection, USP, which is used to initially dissolve carmustine before attempting further dilution with aqueous media
- Store the unopened vial of the dry drug and the diluent vial under refrigeration at 2–8°C (36–46°F). Intact vials containing the drug product, carmustine, are stable for at least 3 years if stored under refrigeration at 2–8°C, but for only 7 days if stored at room temperature (up to 25°C [≤77°F]). The lyophilized formulation does not contain a preservative and is intended for a single use
  - *Caution:* Carmustine for Injection has a low melting point (30.5–32°C [86.9–89.6°F])
    - Exposure of the drug to this or greater temperatures will cause the drug to liquefy, becoming an oily film on the interior surface of a vial—a sign of decomposition indicating affected vials should be discarded
    - If upon receipt appropriate storage during transportation is in question, immediately examine the vial containing carmustine in each individual carton by holding it to a bright light for inspection
    - If carmustine appears as a very small amount of dry flakes or a dry congealed mass, the product is suitable for use and should be refrigerated immediately

Preparation
1. Dissolve carmustine with 3 mL of the supplied diluent (dehydrated alcohol injection, USP)
2. *Only after* the drug product has been completely dissolved, aseptically add 27 mL of SWFI
   a. The resulting solution is clear, colorless to yellowish, and contains 3.3 mg carmustine/mL in 10% ethanol
      - After reconstitution as recommended, carmustine is stable for 8 hours at room temperature (25°C) if it is protected from light exposure, and for at least 24 hours if stored under refrigeration and protected from light
        - Reconstituted vials should be examined for crystal formation prior to use
        - If crystals are observed, they may be re-dissolved by warming the vial to room temperature with agitation

Administration
- For administration to patients, carmustine should be further diluted to a concentration of 0.2 mg/mL with D5W and *stored only* in glass or polyolefin parenteral product containers[17]
- Carmustine adsorption to PVC, ethylene vinyl acetate (EVA), and polyurethane containers results in substantial drug loss as a result of drug adsorption to the container material. Administer Carmustine for Injection solution from the glass bottles or polypropylene container only. Ensure that polypropylene containers used are PVC free and DEHP free

Stability as a Function of Carmustine Concentration and Storage Temperature[18,19]

Diluent Solution	Carmustine Concentration	Storage Temperature	Duration of Stability
D5W	0.5–1 mg/mL	25°C (77°F)	4 hours
	0.1–1 mg/mL	4°C (39.2°F)	24 hours

- Initial solubilization with ethanol produces a carmustine solution that can be very irritating to vascular endothelium during intraVENous administration. Consequently, several investigators have evaluated alternative preparation schemes to decrease or eliminate ethanol from carmustine for intraVENous administration. Although these methods are not advocated by the product manufacturer, and may present some logistical challenges with respect to material resources, two methods for producing an ethanol-free solution for intraVENous administration are described below

Alternative Preparation Schemes

Method 1:[20]
- To a vial containing 100 mg carmustine, add 30 mL of preservative-free D5W
- Heat the vial to 60°C (140°F) in a water bath for 5 minutes, and, during heating, vigorously shake the vial 3 times
- The preparation scheme produces a solution with a carmustine concentration of 3.3 mg/mL and a stability half-life of 46 hours
  - The investigators demonstrated an 8% loss in concentration after product filtration
  - Although carmustine must be diluted before it is administered to patients, the investigators did not describe secondary dilution

Method 2:[21]
- To a vial containing 100 mg carmustine, add 25 mL of preservative-free D5W warmed to 37°C (98.6°F)
- Shake the vial by hand or in a water bath warmed to 37°C for approximately 5 minutes
- The preparation scheme produces a solution with a carmustine concentration of ~4 mg/mL and a mean stability half-life of 6.8 hours
  - When prepared with ethanol according to the manufacturer's instruction, carmustine must be diluted before it is administered to patients. Tepe et al. did not describe secondary dilution

Selected incompatibility:
- Avoid admixture with solutions of pH >6 (eg, solutions containing sodium bicarbonate)[22]
- Photodegradation occurs after exposure to strong light sources (>500 lux; >46 foot-candles)

Recommendations for Drug Administration and Ancillary Care[23]

General:
- See Chapter 43 for recommended use in patients with renal and hepatic dysfunction
- Administer by intraVENous infusion over at least 2 hours. Do not exceed an administration rate of 1.66 mg/m^2/minute
  - Carmustine is irritating to vascular endothelium largely because of the ethanol used to initially dissolve the drug. Administration over <2 hours may produce sensations of intense pain and burning at the site of administration
- *Use only* polyethylene or polyethylene-lined administration sets
  - A substantial amount of carmustine may be lost from solution as a result of adsorption to the surfaces of ethylene vinyl acetate, PVC, and polyurethane product containers and administration sets
- *Do not* mix carmustine with solutions containing sodium bicarbonate
- Carmustine should not be given more frequently than every 6 weeks

CETUXIMAB

ERBITUX (cetuximab) prescribing information. Branchburg, NJ: ImClone LLC; December 2019

WARNING: INFUSION REACTIONS and CARDIOPULMONARY ARREST

Infusion Reactions: ERBITUX can cause serious and fatal infusion reactions. . . Immediately interrupt and permanently discontinue ERBITUX for serious infusion reactions . . .

Cardiopulmonary Arrest: Cardiopulmonary arrest or sudden death occurred in patients with squamous cell carcinoma of the head and neck receiving ERBITUX with radiation therapy or a cetuximab product with platinum-based therapy and fluorouracil. Monitor serum electrolytes, including serum magnesium, potassium, and calcium, during and after ERBITUX administration . . .

Boxed Warning for ERBITUX (cetuximab) prescribing information. Branchburg, NJ: ImClone LLC; December 2019

Product Identification, Preparation, Storage, and Stability

- ERBITUX is supplied in individually packaged, single-use vials containing cetuximab 100 mg/50 mL (NDC 66733-948-23) or 200 mg/100 mL (NDC 66733-958-23) as a sterile, preservative-free, clear and colorless, injectable liquid with pH = 7.0–7.4
  - The commercial product contains cetuximab 2 mg/mL with 8.48 mg/mL sodium chloride, 1.88 mg/mL sodium phosphate dibasic heptahydrate, 0.41 mg/mL sodium phosphate monobasic monohydrate, and SWFI

- Store vials under refrigeration at 2–8°C (36–46°F). *Do not freeze* the product
- The product may contain a small amount of visible, white, amorphous cetuximab particulates
  - Increased particulate formation may occur at temperatures ≤0°C (≤32°F)
- Cetuximab stored in parenteral product containers is chemically and physically stable for up to 12 hours at 2–8°C and for up to 8 hours at controlled room temperature (20–25°C; 68–77°F)

- Discard any unused cetuximab within 8 hours or within 12 hours after preparation for products maintained at controlled room temperature or under refrigeration (2–8°C), respectively
- Discard any unused portions of cetuximab remaining in a vial
- *Do not shake or dilute* cetuximab solution

Recommendations for Drug Administration and Ancillary Care

General:
- Administer cetuximab by intraVENous infusion with an infusion pump or syringe pump
- *Do not administer* cetuximab by direct intraVENous injection or bolus injection
- Do not shake or dilute cetuximab solution

Premedication:
- Give primary prophylaxis against infusion-related reactions with an antihistamine (H$_1$-receptor) antagonist (eg, diphenhydrAMINE 50 mg IV, *or* equivalent H$_1$ antagonist) 30–60 minutes before a first dose of cetuximab
  - Infusion reactions have occurred in 15–21% of patients across studies, and included: pyrexia, chills, rigors, dyspnea, bronchospasm, angioedema, urticaria, hypertension, and hypotension
    - Grades 3 and 4 infusion reactions occurred in 2–5% of patients, and were fatal in 1 patient

- Premedication for subsequent cetuximab doses should be based upon clinical judgment and the presence and severity of infusion reactions during prior doses

Administration:
- Administer cetuximab through a low protein binding, 0.22-μm, inline filter (placed as proximal to the patient as practical)
- Administer cetuximab 400 mg/m^2 doses over 2 hours (120 min); administer 250 mg/m^2 doses over 1 hour (60 min)
  - The *MAXIMUM INFUSION RATE* should be ≤5 mL/min (≤10 mg/min), which is ≤300 mL/hour (≤600 mg/hour)
  - Use 0.9% NS to flush the line at the end of infusion

Patient monitoring:
- A 1-hour observation period is recommended after completing cetuximab administration in a setting with resuscitation equipment and other agents necessary to treat anaphylaxis (eg, EPINEPHrine, bronchodilators, oxygen, and parenteral steroids and antihistamines)
  - Continue monitoring to confirm resolution of an acute event in patients who required treatment for infusion reactions
  - Longer observation periods may be required in patients who experience infusion reactions
- Patients should be periodically monitored for hypomagnesemia, hypocalcemia, and hypokalemia, during and following cetuximab administration. The same electrolyte analyses should be continually monitored for approximately 8 weeks after the last dose administered, that is, a period of time commensurate with the half-life and persistence of cetuximab

(continued)

Recommendations for Drug Administration and Ancillary Care (continued)

- The onset of electrolyte abnormalities has been reported to occur from days to months after cetuximab administration. Electrolyte supplementation may be necessary in some patients and, in severe cases, intraVENous replacement may be required. The time to resolution of electrolyte abnormalities is not known

Patient counseling:

Advise patients:
- To report signs and symptoms of infusion reactions such as fever, chills, or breathing problems

- Of the risk of cardiopulmonary arrest or sudden death and to report any history of coronary artery disease, congestive heart failure, or arrhythmias
- To contact their health care provider immediately for new or worsening cough, chest pain, or shortness of breath
- Who are females of reproductive potential of the potential risk to a fetus and to use effective contraception during cetuximab treatment and for 2 months following the last dose

- That breastfeeding is not recommended during and for 2 months following the last dose of cetuximab therapy
- To limit sun exposure (use sunscreen, wear hats) while receiving cetuximab and for 2 months following the last dose of cetuximab and to notify their health care provider of any sign of acne-like rash, conjunctivitis, blepharitis, or decreased vision

CISPLATIN

CISPLATIN prescribing information. Lake Zurich, IL: Kabi USA, LLC.; March 2017
CISPLATIN prescribing information. Paramus, NJ: WG Critical Care, LLC; April 2015
CISPLATIN prescribing information. Paramus, NJ: WG Critical Care, LLC: April 2019

WARNING: NEPHROTOXICITY, PERIPHERAL NEUROPATHY, NAUSEA AND VOMITING, and MYELOSUPPRESSION.

- Nephrotoxicity: cisplatin for injection can cause severe renal toxicity, including acute renal failure. Severe renal toxicities are dose-related and cumulative. Ensure adequate hydration and monitor renal function and electrolyte. Consider dose reductions or alternative treatments in patients with renal impairment …
- Peripheral Neuropathy: cisplatin for injection can cause dose-related peripheral neuropathy that becomes more severe with repeated courses of the drug …
- Nausea and Vomiting: cisplatin for injection can cause severe nausea and vomiting. Use highly effective antiemetic premedication …
- Myelosuppression: cisplatin for injection can cause severe myelosuppression with fatalities due to infections. Monitor blood counts accordingly. Interruption of therapy may be required …

Boxed Warning for CISPLATIN prescribing information. Paramus, NJ: WG Critical Care, LLC: April 2019
- Prescriptions and medication orders should identify the drug by its complete generic name, CISPLATIN, to prevent confusion with other platinum compounds
- Product labeling advises pharmacists to contact health care providers who prescribe CISplatin dosages >100 mg/m^2 per cycle for dose confirmation as doses above this threshold are rarely used

---

Product Identification, Preparation, Storage, and Stability

- CISplatin is generically available from several manufacturers in vials in at least 2 presentations, including:
  - A sterile, clear, light yellow, aqueous solution for injection (CISplatin injection, solution)
    - Commercially available products contain 50 mg, 100 mg, or 200 mg CISplatin in individually packaged, multiple-dose, amber vials
      - Each milliliter contains CISplatin 1 mg and sodium chloride 9 mg
      - Additional excipients may be present in some product formulations
    - CISplatin Injection (1 mg/mL) must be diluted before it is administered to patients
  - A white to light yellow lyophilized powder for reconstitution (CISplatin injection, powder, lyophilized, for solution)
    - The commercially available product contains CISplatin (50 mg) along with sodium chloride, USP (450 mg) and mannitol, USP (500 mg) in individually packaged, single-dose, amber vials (NDC 44567-530-01)

  - Reconstitute lyophilized CISplatin with 50 mL of SWFI to obtain a solution containing 1 mg CISplatin and sodium chloride 9 mg/mL
  - Reconstituted CISplatin (1 mg/mL) must be diluted before it is administered to patients
- Consult product labeling for manufacturer recommendations about acceptable storage temperatures for intact vials
  - Acceptable storage temperatures for products in solution (CISplatin injection) vary within a range from 15°C (59°F) or 20°C (68°) for a lower temperature limit to an upper limit of 25°C (77°F)
  - The commercial product formulated as a lyophilized powder for reconstitution (NDC 44567-530-01) specifies storage at 20–25°C (68–77°F) with excursions permitted to 15–30°C (59–86°F)
- *Do not store* CISplatin in solution (1 mg/mL) under refrigeration, under which condition it is more likely to precipitate
- Protect unopened containers from light
- Dilute CISplatin in a convenient volume of fluid. The diluting fluid *MUST CONTAIN* a chloride concentration ≥0.225% sodium chloride (≥38.5 mEq/L), for example,

0.45% NaCl, 0.9% NS, 3% NaCl, and saline and dextrose solutions with chloride concentrations >0.225%[24]
- Mannitol is compatible and may be added to diluted CISplatin solutions
- Protect CISplatin solutions that are not used within 6 hours after preparation from exposure to light
- CISplatin that remains in an amber vial after initial entry is stable for 28 days if protected from light or for 7 days under fluorescent room lighting

Selected incompatibility:

- *Aluminum* reacts with CISplatin causing precipitation and loss of drug potency
  - *Do not prepare or administer* CISplatin with needles or administration sets that contain aluminum parts that may come into contact with the drug
- *Do not dilute* CISplatin in solutions with chloride content less than the concentration found in 0.225% NaCl, that is, *not less than* 38.5 mEq/L
- CISplatin is incompatible in admixtures with mesna

Recommendations for Drug Administration and Ancillary Care

General:

- See Chapter 43 for recommended use in patients with renal dysfunction
- Hydration with 1000–2000 mL of fluid administered intraVENously is recommended starting at least 2 hours before CISplatin administration commences

- Consider continuing hydration during and after CISplatin administration is completed, particularly in patients who receive a diuretic before, during, or after CISplatin to augment urine formation
- Maintain increased hydration via oral, parenteral, or both routes, and urine

output for at least 24 hours after CISplatin administration
- Administer CISplatin intraVENously. Infusion duration generally is within a range of 15–120 minutes, but may be prolonged in some regimens (8–24 hours)

CLADRIBINE

CLADRIBINE prescribing information. Lake Zurich, IL: Fresenius Kabi USA, LLC.; August 2016
CLADRIBINE prescribing information. Rockford, IL: Mylan Institutional LLC.; March 2018

WARNING

Cladribine injection should be administered under the supervision of a qualified physician experienced in the use of antineoplastic therapy. Suppression of bone marrow function should be anticipated. This is usually reversible and appears to be dose dependent. Serious neurological toxicity (including irreversible paraparesis and quadriparesis) has been reported in patients who received cladribine injection by continuous infusion at high doses (4 to 9 times the recommended dose for Hairy Cell Leukemia). Neurologic toxicity appears to demonstrate a dose relationship; however, severe neurological toxicity has been reported rarely following treatment with standard cladribine dosing regimens

Acute nephrotoxicity has been observed with high doses of cladribine (4 to 9 times the recommended dose for Hairy Cell Leukemia), especially when given concomitantly with other nephrotoxic agents/therapies

Boxed Warning for CLADRIBINE prescribing information. Rockford, IL: Mylan Institutional LLC.; March 2018

Product Identification, Preparation, Storage, and Stability

- Cladribine injection is generically available packaged in single-use, individually packaged, clear glass vials containing cladribine 10 mg/10 mL (1 mg/mL) as a sterile, clear, colorless, preservative-free, isotonic solution
  - Each milliliter of commercially available products also contains 1 mg cladribine and 9 mg (0.15 mEq) of sodium chloride
  - The solution has a pH in the range of 5.5–8.0. Phosphoric acid and/or dibasic sodium phosphate may have been added to adjust the pH to 6.3 ± 0.3
- Store intact vials under refrigeration 2–8°C (36–46°F) and protected from light during storage
- Cladribine *must be diluted* before administration

24-Hour drug supply (daily bag exchanges):
- Transfer the required amount of cladribine necessary to provide treatment for a single day through a sterile, disposable, hydrophilic syringe filter with pore size 0.22 μm into a parenteral product container containing 500 mL of 0.9% NS
  - Compared with dilution in 0.9% NS, dilution in D5W increases the rate of cladribine degradation and is not recommended
  - Cladribine admixtures in 0.9% NS in PVC containers (eg, Viaflex Container, Baxter Healthcare Corporation, Deerfield, IL) are chemically and physically stable for at least 24 hours at room temperature under normal fluorescent lighting

(continued)

Recommendations for Drug Administration and Ancillary Care

General:
- See Chapter 43 for recommended use in patients with renal and hepatic dysfunction
- Administer only by intraVENous infusion over 2–24 hours
- Cladribine should be administered promptly, or, after dilution, stored under refrigeration (2–8°C [36–46°F]) for not more than 8 hours before starting administration
- Cladribine should not be mixed with other drugs or additives or administered simultaneously with other drugs via a common intraVENous line

Product Identification, Preparation, Storage, and Stability (*continued*)

7-Day drug supply:

- A 7-day infusion solution should only be prepared with B0.9% NS (preserved with 0.9% benzyl alcohol) as follows:

  1. Add to a plastic container an amount of cladribine needed for a 7-day supply of medication

  2. Add to the same plastic container a calculated amount of B0.9% NS sufficient to produce a total volume of (Q.S.) 100 mL

     a. Both cladribine and the diluent solution should be transferred into a parenteral product container through a sterile, disposable, hydrophilic syringe filter with pore size 0.22 μm to minimize the risk of microbial contamination

     b. Inject cladribine through the filter first followed by the B0.9% NS vehicle solution to flush into the product container any cladribine remaining in the filter

        - Solutions prepared with B0.9% NS for individuals weighing >85 kg may have reduced preservative effectiveness because of displacement of the benzyl alcohol-containing diluent by the volume of drug, that is, >53.6 mg in a total volume to deliver of 100 mL

        - Admixtures prepared with antimicrobially preserved diluent have demonstrated acceptable chemical and physical stability for at least 7 days in a SIMS Deltec, Inc., MEDICATION CASSETTE Reservoir

  3. Aseptically connect to the drug product container (reservoir) any tubing that will be used to connect the reservoir to a patient's VAD during drug administration

  4. Aseptically remove air from the product container and any connected tubing

  5. Aseptically cap with a sterile Luer locking cap, closure, or seal any tubing attached to the drug reservoir for storage if the product is not immediately connected to a patient's VAD after preparation is completed

- Cladribine may precipitate when exposed to low temperatures, but can be resolubilized by warming at ambient room temperature and vigorous shaking

- *Do not* attempt to resolubilize cladribine by heating or microwaving

- Freezing does not adversely affect the solution. If freezing occurs, thaw at room temperature, but *do not* thaw cladribine by radiant thermal or microwave heating

- After thawing, vials are stable until the expiration date on the product label if stored under refrigeration

- *Do not* refreeze cladribine

- Any unused portion of cladribine remaining in a single-use vial should be discarded

CLOFARABINE

CLOLAR (clofarabine) prescribing information. Cambridge, MA: Genzyme Corporation; December 2019
CLOFARABINE prescribing information. Lake Zurich, IL: Fresenius Kabi USA, LLC.; March 2020
CLOFARABINE prescribing information. Weston, FL: Apotex Corp.; January 2020

Product Identification, Preparation, Storage, and Stability

- Clofarabine is packaged in 20-mL-capacity, glass, single-use vials containing 20 mL of a clear, practically colorless, preservative-free, sterile solution of clofarabine 1 mg/mL (20 mg/20 mL)
  - The commercial products are formulated in 20 mL of unbuffered 0.9% NS. The pH range of the solutions is 4.5–7.5

- Store intact vials at 25°C (77°F). Temperature excursions are permitted to 15–30°C (59–86°F)
- Clofarabine solution must be filtered before dilution. Use a sterile filter with a pore size equal to 0.2 μm either when aspirating the drug into a syringe *or* when expelling drug from the syringe into a diluent solution

- Dilute clofarabine with a volume of 0.9% NS or D5W sufficient to produce a concentration between 0.15 and 0.4 mg/mL before administering it to patients
- Diluted solutions may be stored at 15–30°C, but must be used within 24 hours after preparation

Recommendations for Drug Administration and Ancillary Care

General:
- See Chapter 43 for comments about use in patients with renal and hepatic dysfunction
- Administer diluted clofarabine solutions by intraVENous infusion over 2 hours
- Provide supportive care, such as intraVENous fluids, allopurinol, and alkalinize urine throughout a 5-day treatment course to reduce the effects of tumor lysis and other adverse events
- Monitor patients taking medications known to affect blood pressure. Monitor cardiac function during clofarabine administration
  - Avoid medications that produce or exacerbate hypotension during the days on which clofarabine is administered
- Evaluate and monitor patients receiving clofarabine treatment for signs and symptoms of cytokine release (eg, tachypnea, tachycardia, hypotension, pulmonary edema) that could develop into systemic inflammatory response syndrome (SIRS), capillary leak syndrome, and organ dysfunction

- Immediately discontinue clofarabine in the event of clinically significant signs or symptoms of SIRS or capillary leak syndrome and provide appropriate supportive measures, which may include steroids, diuretics, and albumin
  - Glucocorticoid prophylaxis (eg, hydrocortisone 100 mg/m² per day for 3 days [days 1–3]) may prevent signs or symptoms of SIRS or capillary leak syndrome
- Monitor renal and hepatic function closely during a 5-day treatment course with clofarabine
  - In patients with creatinine clearance of 30–60 mL/minute, reduce the initial clofarabine dose by 50%. No recommendation on dose is available for patients with creatinine clearance <30 mL/minute or for those requiring hemodialysis. In pediatric patients, 49–60% of a dose was renally eliminated as unchanged drug within 24 hours after administration

- Avoid medications that adversely affect kidney and liver function during the days on which clofarabine is administered
- Clofarabine should be immediately discontinued if Grade ≥3 increases in serum creatinine or bilirubin are observed during treatment
  - Clofarabine treatment may resume after a patient's condition has stabilized and organ function has returned to baseline, generally with a 25% reduction in clofarabine dose
- Discontinue clofarabine administration if a Grade 4 noninfectious nonhematologic adverse event occurs

Selected incompatibility:
- Do not administer other medications through the same intraVENous line as clofarabine
  - Clofarabine compatibility with other drugs is not yet known

COPANLISIB

ALIQOPA (copanlisib) prescribing information. Whippany, NJ: Bayer HealthCare Pharmaceuticals Inc; February 2020

Product Identification, Preparation, Storage, and Stability

- ALIQOPA (copanlisib) is a sterile, white to slightly yellowish, lyophilized powder supplied as a carton including one single-use vial that contains 60 mg copanlisib free base equivalent to 69.1 mg copanlisib dihydrochloride (NDC 50419-385-01) and the following inactive ingredients: citric acid anhydrous, mannitol, and sodium hydroxide
- Store intact vials under refrigeration at 2–8°C (35.6–46.4°F) until time of reconstitution

Reconstitution:
- Using a 5-mL sterile syringe with needle, slowly inject 4.4 mL of 0.9% NS diluent through the disinfected stopper surface into the vial containing copanlisib
- Gently shake the injection vial for 30 seconds to dissolve the lyophilized solid and then allow to stand for one minute to allow the bubbles to rise to the surface
- Repeat the gentle shaking and settling procedure if any undissolved substance is observed
- The reconstitution procedure should yield a solution that is colorless to slightly yellowish, free of visible particles, and that contains copanlisib 15 mg/mL
- The reconstituted copanlisib solution may be stored for up to 24 hours under refrigeration at 2–8°C (36–46°F)
- Discard any unused reconstituted solution appropriately

Dilution:
- With a sterile syringe, withdraw the required volume of concentrated reconstituted copanlisib 15 mg/mL solution needed to prepare a patient's dose according to the table below and inject the contents of the syringe into a parenteral product container prefilled with 100 mL 0.9% NS. Mix the dose well by inverting

Desired Copanlisib Dose	Volume of Reconstituted Copanlisib 15 mg/mL Solution Required
60 mg	4 mL
45 mg	3 mL
30 mg	2 mL

- After dilution, the copanlisib admixture may be stored for up to 24 hours under refrigeration at 2–8°C (35.6–46.4°F)
- Avoid exposure of the copanlisib admixture to direct sunlight
- Discard any unused diluted solution appropriately

Selected incompatibility:

- Mix only with 0.9% NS solution. Do not mix or inject copanlisib with other drugs or diluents

Recommendations for Drug Administration and Ancillary Care

General:
- See Chapter 43 for recommended use in patients with hepatic dysfunction
- Reduce the copanlisib dose to 45 mg in patients with moderate hepatic impairment (Child-Pugh B)
- There is insufficient data available to recommend a dose of copanlisib in patients with end stage renal disease (CrCl <15 mL/min by Cockcroft Gault equation)

Administration:
- The recommended dose of copanlisib is 60 mg, given as an intraVENous infusion over 60 minutes once daily on days 1, 8, and 15 of a 28-day cycle
- Allow the diluted copanlisib solution to adapt to ambient temperature before use following refrigeration, when applicable
- Ensure a minimum of 7 days between any two consecutive infusions

Concomitant medications:
- Considering that the incidence of severe *Pneumocystis jiroveci* pneumonia (PJP) was 0.6% in clinical trials, consider prescribing a medication for primary prophylaxis of PJP in susceptible individuals. Patients who have recovered from PJP should receive secondary prophylaxis throughout copanlisib therapy

Adverse events and treatment modifications:
- Refer to the current FDA-approved product label for detailed recommendations regarding treatment modifications for management of infections (including PJP), hyperglycemia, hypertension, noninfectious pneumonitis, neutropenia, severe cutaneous reactions, thrombocytopenia, and other G ≥3 toxicities (toxicities graded according to NCI CTCAE v4.03)
  - Administration of a dose requires that the following parameters be met: absence of infection, fasting blood glucose <160 mg/dL or random/non-fasting blood glucose <200 mg/dL, systolic blood pressure <150 mm Hg and diastolic blood pressure <90 mm Hg, absence of G ≥2 noninfectious pneumonitis, ANC ≥500/mm³, absence of severe cutaneous reaction G ≥3, platelet count ≥25,000/mm³, and absence of other toxicities G ≥3

Potential drug interactions:
- CYP3A4 is responsible for >90% of copanlisib metabolism. Avoid use of strong CYP3A4 inducers with copanlisib. If concomitant use of a strong CYP3A4 inhibitor is unavoidable, then reduce the copanlisib dose to 45 mg

CYCLOPHOSPHAMIDE

Cyclophosphamide prescribing information. Deerfield, IL: Baxter Healthcare Corporation; March 2017

Product Identification, Preparation, Storage, and Stability

- Cyclophosphamide is available as a sterile white powder for reconstitution for injection in individually packaged single-use vials containing 500 mg (NDC 10019-955-01), 1000 mg (NDC 10019-956-01), or 2000 mg (NDC 10019-957-01) of cyclophosphamide monohydrate
- Store cyclophosphamide at temperatures ≤25°C (≤77°F)
- Cyclophosphamide may melt if exposed to high temperatures during transportation or storage
  - Melted cyclophosphamide appears as a clear or yellowish viscous liquid usually found in connection with portions of the drug that have remained in powdered form, or as droplets that have become separated from a portion of the drug that remains in powdered form
  - *Do not use* cyclophosphamide that exhibits signs of melting
- Commercially marketed cyclophosphamide products do not contain antimicrobial preservatives
- Reconstitute cyclophosphamide with 0.9% NS* or SWFI†, as follows:

Cyclophosphamide Content per Vial	Diluent Volume	Cyclophosphamide Concentration After Reconstitution
500 mg	25 mL	20 mg/mL
1000 mg	50 mL	
2000 mg	100 mL	

*After reconstitution with 0.9% NS, cyclophosphamide is suitable for direct intraVENous, intraMUSCular, intraperitoneal, or intrapleural injection

†Reconstitution with SWFI yields a hypotonic product, which should not be administered by intraVENous injection, but may be administered by intraVENous infusion after further dilution with 1 of the following solutions: D5W , 0.45% NaCl, 0.9% NS, D5W/RI, D5W/0.9% NS, LRI, sodium lactate injection, USP (1/6 molar sodium lactate)

- After reconstituting cyclophosphamide with SWFI, the resulting solution is hypotonic. Reconstitution with SWFI and 0.9% NS to a concentration of 20 mg/mL yields solutions with the following osmolarity:

Cyclophosphamide and Diluent	Osmolarity
100 mg cyclophosphamide in 5 mL of SWFI	74 mOsm/L
100 mg cyclophosphamide in 5 mL of 0.9% NS	374 mOsm/L

- After adding a diluent solution, shake cyclophosphamide vials vigorously to dissolve the drug powder
  - If cyclophosphamide does not readily and completely dissolve, allow the vials to stand for a few minutes and, if necessary, resuming shaking
- Reconstitution to a concentration of 20 mg cyclophosphamide/mL with 0.9% NS yields a product that is chemically and physically stable for 24 hours at room temperature or for 6 days under refrigeration (2–8°C [35.6–46.4°F]). Cyclophosphamide that is reconstituted with SWFI should not be stored but rather should be further diluted immediately
- After reconstitution with 0.9% NS or SWFI to a concentration of 20 mg cyclophosphamide per milliliter, the reconstituted solution may be further diluted
  - Product labeling identifies cyclophosphamide stability diluted to a minimum concentration of 2 mg/mL with three vehicle solutions as follows:

Solution	Storage Temperature	
	Room Temperature	Refrigeration
0.45% NaCl	Up to 24 hours	Up to 6 days
D5W	Up to 24 hours	Up to 36 hours
D5W/0.9% NS	Up to 24 hours	Up to 36 hours

Recommendations for Drug Administration and Ancillary Care

General:

- After reconstitution with 0.9% NS to a concentration of 20 mg cyclophosphamide/mL the drug product is suitable for administration by direct intraVENous injection, intraVENous infusion, intraMUSCular intraperitoneal, or intrapleural injection
- Solutions prepared by reconstituting cyclophosphamide with SWFI are hypotonic, and *are not recommended* for intraVENous injection, but may be administered by intraVENous infusion if further diluted with any of the following solutions: D5W , 0.45% NaCl, 0.9% NS, D5W/RI, D5W/0.9% NS, LRI, sodium lactate injection, USP

CYTARABINE

Cytarabine injection PHARMACY BULK PACKAGE—NOT FOR DIRECT INFUSION prescribing information. Lake Forest, IL: Hospira, Inc.; June 2020
Cytarabine injection NOT FOR INTRATHECAL USE—CONTAINS BENZYL ALCOHOL FOR INTRAVENOUS OR SUBCUTANEOUS USE ONLY prescribing information. Lake Forest, IL: Hospira, Inc.; June 2020
Cytarabine injection for intravenous, intrathecal, and subcutaneous use only; prescribing information. Lake Forest, IL: Hospira, Inc.; June 2020

WARNING

Only physicians experienced in cancer chemotherapy should use Cytarabine Injection

For induction therapy, patients should be treated in a facility with laboratory and supportive resources sufficient to monitor drug tolerance and protect and maintain a patient compromised by drug toxicity. The main toxic effect of Cytarabine Injection is bone marrow suppression with leukopenia, thrombocytopenia, and anemia. Less serious toxicity includes nausea, vomiting, diarrhea and abdominal pain, oral ulceration, and hepatic dysfunction

The physician must judge possible benefit to the patient against known toxic effects of this drug in considering the advisability of therapy with Cytarabine Injection. Before making this judgment or beginning treatment, the physician should be familiar with … [all other elements of product labeling]

Boxed Warning for Cytarabine injection for intravenous, intrathecal, and subcutaneous use only; prescribing information. Lake Forest, IL: Hospira, Inc.; June 2020

Product Identification, Preparation, Storage, and Stability

- Cytarabine is generically available from several manufacturers. Products are currently available in solution formulations only, though historically were also available in a lyophilized (powder) formulation. Presentations include products packaged for a single use or multiple doses, and for pharmaceutical admixture and compounding (eg, *Pharmacy Bulk Package*)

Cautions: Among products in solution (ie, "cytarabine injection …"):
  - Cytarabine concentrations are not consistently the same among available products. Presentations include a 20-mg/mL concentration and a 100-mg/mL concentration
  - Products may or may not contain an antimicrobial preservative
- In general, cytarabine products are stored at controlled room temperatures around 20–25°C (68–77°F), with temperature excursions permitted to 15–30°C (59–86°F)
  - Acceptable storage temperatures vary among products from different manufacturers
  - Refer to product packaging and labeling for storage conditions appropriate for different products
- *Do not use* bacteriostatically preserved drug and diluent products for intraTHECAL use and for preparing cytarabine for high-dose treatments (dosages ≥1000 mg/m²)

For intraVENous or SUBCUTaneous use:
  - *Do not use* preservative-containing products when preparing cytarabine doses ≥1000 mg/m²
- Products may be further diluted to a convenient volume in 0.9% NS or D5W

For intraTHECAL use:
- *Do not use* preservative-containing products when preparing cytarabine doses for intraTHECAL use
- Cytarabine for intraTHECAL use may *only* be further diluted with *PRESERVATIVE-FREE* 0.9% NS to produce a solution with concentration ≤20 mg/mL. Typical administration volumes range from 5 to 10 mL, and should closely approximate the volume of cerebrospinal fluid removed
- Admixtures with hydrocortisone sodium succinate for intraTHECAL administration (with or without methotrexate) should be prepared just before use and administered as soon as possible (within minutes) after preparation because of the instability of the hydrocortisone component

Caution: **Do not use an antimicrobially preserved diluent to prepare cytarabine for intraTHECAL use**

Recommendations for Drug Administration and Ancillary Care

General:
- See Chapter 43 for recommended use in patients with renal and hepatic dysfunction
- Administer by intraVENous, intraTHECAL, or SUBCUTaneous routes
  - Use products prepared for intraTHECAL administration immediately after they are prepared
- If cytarabine is given intraMUSCularly, administration sites should be rotated
- Although the amount of drug administered is a modulating factor, patients generally can tolerate higher total doses given by rapid intraVENous injection than by slow infusion because of cytarabine's rapid inactivation and the relatively brief cellular exposure to cytotoxic concentrations that occur after rapid administration

DACARBAZINE

Dacarbazine prescribing information. Eatontown, NJ: Hikma Pharmaceuticals USA Inc.; March 2020
DACARBAZINE prescribing information. Parsippany, NJ: Teva Pharmaceuticals USA, Inc.; February 2020
DACARBAZINE prescribing information. Schaumburg, IL: APP Pharmaceuticals LLC; January 2008

WARNING

It is recommended that dacarbazine be administered under the supervision of a qualified physician experienced in the use of cancer chemotherapeutic agents.

1. Hemopoietic depression is the most common toxicity with dacarbazine …
2. Hepatic necrosis has been reported …
3. Studies have demonstrated this agent to have a carcinogenic and teratogenic effect when used in animals
4. In treatment of each patient, the physician must weigh carefully the possibility of achieving therapeutic benefit against the risk of toxicity

Boxed Warning (excerpt) from:
Dacarbazine prescribing information. Eatontown, NJ: Hikma Pharmaceuticals USA Inc.; March 2020
DACARBAZINE prescribing information. Parsippany, NJ: Teva Pharmaceuticals USA, Inc.; February 2020
DACARBAZINE prescribing information. Schaumburg, IL: APP Pharmaceuticals LLC; January 2008

Product Identification, Preparation, Storage, and Stability

- Dacarbazine is generically available from several manufacturers. In general, the drug is packaged in single-use, amber glass vials, containing either 100 mg or 200 mg dacarbazine per vial
  - Commercial formulations also include mannitol and citric acid
  - Packaging varies among manufacturers' products, including: individually packaged vials and boxes containing 10 vials
- Dacarbazine is a white to pale yellow solid that is sensitive to light
- Store intact vials under refrigeration at 2–8°C (36–46°F) and protect from light exposure
- Reconstitute dacarbazine with SWFI as follows:

Dacarbazine Content per Vial	Diluent (SWFI) Volume	Dacarbazine Concentration After Reconstitution
100 mg	9.9 mL	10 mg/mL
200 mg	19.7 mL	

- The resulting clear, yellowish solution has a pH from 3.0 to 4.0 and is highly sensitive to degradation as a result of exposure to light[25]
- The reconstituted solution is suitable for intraVENous injection, or it may be further diluted in up to 250 mL of D5W or 0.9% NS and given by intraVENous infusion
- Product labeling includes the following stability information:
  - After reconstitution, dacarbazine solution (10 mg/mL) may be stored in the product vial at 4°C (39.2°F) for up to 72 hours or at normal room temperature and (fluorescent) lighting conditions for up to 8 hours[28]
  - After dilution in D5W or 0.9% NS, the resulting product may be stored at 4°C (39.2°F) for up to 24 hours or under normal room conditions (ambient temperature and artificial lighting) for up to 8 hours[26]
  - See comments under "Dacarbazine Degradation," below
- Change in solution color from pale yellow or ivory to pink or red is a sign of decomposition
  - Dacarbazine solutions that exhibit changes in color toward pink or red should not be used

Recommendations for Drug Administration and Ancillary Care

General:

- See Chapter 43 for recommended use in patients with renal and hepatic dysfunction
- Administer dacarbazine only by intraVENous routes:
  - By intraVENous injection over 1 minute *or* by intraVENous infusion over 15–30 minutes
- Cover parenteral product containers containing dacarbazine solutions with light-opaque materials (bags, aluminum foil)
- Use opaque or light-resistant (light-shielded) VAD to administer dacarbazine, or cover VAD used to administer dacarbazine to protect the drug from light; eg, with opaque sleeves or by wrapping tubing with aluminum foil

Dacarbazine degradation:

- Dacarbazine degrades to active and potentially toxic products, including 2-azahypoxanthine by photolysis[25,27] and hydrolysis
- Photodegradation products are associated with adverse effects encountered during dacarbazine administration, including local venous pain, nausea, and vomiting
  - In small case series, venous pain ± other symptoms and signs of toxicity were eliminated or reduced during administration in a room illuminated by a red photographic lamp[28] and when the drug in vials and VAD tubing was protected from light exposure[29]

- Dacarbazine degradation is accelerated by light exposure and storage temperature
  - Sunlight causes more rapid photolysis than fluorescent lighting[30]
  - For dacarbazine exposed to sunlight during preparation or administration:
    - Cover parenteral containers with opaque material or foil during administration[30,31]
    - Use light-resistant or opaque administration sets, or wrap tubing with opaque material or foil during administration[30,31]
  - Prepare dacarbazine just before it is used, or store reconstituted and diluted products under refrigeration and protected from light until used[26,30]

DACTINOMYCIN

DACTINOMYCIN prescribing information. Rockford, IL: Mylan Institutional LLC; April 2019
COSMEGEN (dactinomycin for injection) prescribing information. Lebanon, NJ: Recordati Rare Diseases Inc.; August 2018

Product Identification, Preparation, Storage, and Stability

- DACTINomycin is marketed in individually packaged, single-use vials containing DACTINomycin 500 μg (0.5 mg) and 20 mg mannitol as a sterile, yellow to orange, lyophilized powder
- Store intact vials at 20–25°C (68–77°F). Temperature excursions to 15–30°C (59–86°F) are permitted. Protect vials from light and humidity
- Reconstitute the drug product by injecting 1.1 mL of SWFI (without preservative) into a vial to produce a clear, gold-colored solution that contains approximately 500 μg (0.5 mg) DACTINomycin per milliliter
  - Reconstituted DACTINomycin is chemically stable, but the product does not contain an antimicrobial preservative
  - Diluents preserved with benzyl alcohol or parabens may cause drug precipitation and *should not* be used to reconstitute DACTINomycin
- *Do not filter* DACTINomycin during preparation. Filtration through cellulose ester filters may remove DACTINomycin from the solution being filtered
- DACTINomycin may be added to the tubing or side arm of a rapidly flowing intraVENous infusion of D5W or 0.9% NS. Alternatively, it may be prepared as an admixture in the same solutions for administration by intraVENous infusion or isolation perfusion techniques
  - DACTINomycin may be prepared as an admixture in 0.9% NS or D5W to concentrations >10 μg/mL (>0.01 mg/mL) in glass or PVC containers for intraVENous infusion
  - DACTINomycin is reported to be most stable at pH 5–7[32]
- Use a "2-needle technique" if DACTINomycin is to be injected percutaneously directly into a vein without the use of an infusion
  - DACTINomycin is corrosive to skin, irritating to the eyes and respiratory tract mucosa, highly toxic by the oral route, and a vesicant if extravasated
- The "2-needle technique" prevents soft-tissue exposure to DACTINomycin that remains on the external surfaces of needles used to reconstitute the drug product

Two-needle technique for preparing DACTINomycin:

1. Use 1 sterile needle to reconstitute and withdraw from a vial a measured amount of DACTINomycin needed to deliver a patient's dose
2. Aspirate all drug solution from the needle and needle hub into the syringe, and replace the first needle with a second sterile needle
3. With a second sterile needle on the syringe, carefully express air without expelling drug from the tip of the needle and inject DACTINomycin through an injection port into the tubing of a rapidly running intraVENously administered solution

Recommendations for Drug Administration and Ancillary Care

General:

- See Chapter 43 for recommended use in patients with hepatic dysfunction
- For intraVENous administration *only*, by direct intraVENous injection over approximately 1 minute or intraVENous infusion over 15–30 minutes
- Final prepared products must be used within 4 hours of initial reconstitution when stored at ambient room temperature
  - DACTINomycin should be diluted *only* with 0.9% NS or D5W for intraVENous infusion
  - *Caution:* After initial reconstitution with SWFI, further dilution with SWFI decreases DACTINomycin osmolality, which may result in an extremely hypotonic solution. Depending on administration rate and blood flow, administration of hypotonic solutions may result in some degree of intravascular hemolysis
- The dosage for DACTINomycin is calculated in micrograms (μg)
  - Dosage calculations for obese or edematous patients should be performed on the basis of ideal body weight
- Please review the 2-needle technique for direct intraVENous injection (see above). The procedure prevents soft-tissue exposure to DACTINomycin that remains on the external surfaces of needles used during drug preparation
- *Do not filter* DACTINomycin during administration
- Filtration through 0.22-μm pore size filter membranes composed of cellulose ester (cellulose nitrate/cellulose acetate) or polytetrafluoroethylene (PTFE, Teflon) was shown to remove a substantial portion of DACTINomycin from the solution being filtered[14,33]
- Filtration through a 0.22-μm pore size cellulose ester filter membranes resulted in approximately 13% of the total amount of filtered DACTINomycin bound by the filter[34]

Caution: DACTINomycin is a vesicant and may cause severe local soft-tissue necrosis if administered by injection into soft tissues or extravasated

DARATUMUMAB

DARZALEX (daratumumab) prescribing information. Horsham, PA: Janssen Biotech, Inc.; June 2020

Product Identification, Preparation, Storage, and Stability

- DARZALEX (daratumumab) is a colorless to pale yellow, preservative-free solution available in individually boxed single-dose vials containing either 100 mg/5 mL or 400 mg/20 mL daratumumab. The pH of the solutions is 5.5
- The 5 mL vial (NDC 57894-502-05) contains daratumumab (100 mg), glacial acetic acid (0.9 mg), mannitol (127.5 mg), polysorbate 20 (2 mg), sodium acetate trihydrate (14.8 mg), sodium chloride (17.5 mg), and SWFI
- The 20 mL vial (NDC 57894-502-20) contains daratumumab (400 mg), glacial acetic acid (3.7 mg), mannitol (510 mg), polysorbate 20 (8 mg), sodium acetate trihydrate (59.3 mg), sodium chloride (70.1 mg), and SWFI
- Store intact vials under refrigeration at 2–8°C (36–46°F) in the original carton to protect from light
- *Do not freeze or shake* intact vials

Dilution:
- Use aseptic technique during product preparation
- Inspect the product visually for the presence of opaque particulate matter, discoloration, or other foreign particles
- Remove a volume of diluent from parenteral product container that is equivalent to the required volume of DARZALEX (daratumumab). The infusion bag must be composed of PVC, polypropylene (PP), polyethylene (PE), or polyolefin blend (PP + PE)
- Using a sterile syringe, withdraw the required volume of DARZALEX (daratumumab) and dilute by adding it to the infusion bag containing 0.9% NS. Refer to the table in the "Recommendations for Drug Administration and Ancillary Care" section for the appropriate volume of diluent
- Gently invert the parenteral product container to mix. Do not shake

- Do not use the dilute solution if visibly opaque particles, discoloration, or foreign particles are observed. Note that the presence of very small, translucent to white proteinaceous particles is considered normal
- The diluted solution should be infused immediately at room temperature 15°C–25°C (59°F–77°F) in room light. The diluted solution may be kept at room temperature for up to 15 hours, which includes the infusion time. If not used immediately, the diluted solution may be stored for up to 24 hours under refrigerated conditions 2°C–8°C (36°F–46°F) protected from light. Do not freeze

Selected incompatibility:
- Do not infuse DARZALEX (daratumumab) with any other agents concomitantly in the same intraVENous line. Only dilute DARZALEX (daratumumab) with 0.9% NS

Recommendations for Drug Administration and Ancillary Care

General:
- No dose adjustment is necessary for patients with renal impairment (CrCl 15–89 mL/min), mild hepatic impairment (total bilirubin 1 to 1.5 × ULN, or AST > ULN), or moderate hepatic impairment (total bilirubin >1.5 to 3 × ULN and any AST)
- There are no PK data in patients with severe hepatic impairment (total bilirubin >3 × ULN and any AST)

Administration:
- The usual dose of daratumumab is 16 mg/kg (based on actual body weight) administered intraVENously. Refer to the current FDA-approved product label for details regarding various schedules of administration. Note that the initial dose may optionally be split over two consecutive days (ie, 8 mg/kg on day 1 and day 2)
- Daratumumab must be administered by a health care professional in a setting with immediate access to emergency equipment and appropriate medical support to manage infusion-related reactions
- If the diluted solution was stored in the refrigerator, allow the solution to come to room temperature prior to administration
- Administer by intraVENous infusion with a flow regulator and using an intraVENous tubing infusion set (composed of PP, PE, PVC, polyurethane, or polybutadiene) with a 0.2- or 0.22-μm inline, sterile, non-pyrogenic, low-protein-binding polyethersulfone filter

Dilution Volumes and Infusion Rates of Daratumumab Administration

	Dilution Volume	Initial Rate (First Hour)	Rate Increment*	Maximum Rate
Week 1 infusion				
Option 1 (Single dose infusion)				
Week 1 Day 1 (16 mg/kg)	1000 mL	50 mL/hour	50 mL/hour every hour	200 mL/hour

(continued)

Recommendations for Drug Administration and Ancillary Care (continued)

Dilution Volumes and Infusion Rates of Daratumumab Administration

	Dilution Volume	Initial Rate (First Hour)	Rate Increment*	Maximum Rate
Option 2 (Split dose infusion)				
Week 1 Day 1 (8 mg/kg)	500 mL	50 mL/hour	50 mL/hour every hour	200 mL/hour
Week 1 Day 2 (8 mg/kg)	500 mL	50 mL/hour	50 mL/hour every hour	200 mL/hour
Week 2 (16 mg/kg) infusion†	500 mL	50 mL/hour	50 mL/hour every hour	200 mL/hour
Subsequent (Week 3 and onwards, 16 mg/kg) infusions‡	500 mL	100 mL/hour	50 mL/hour every hour	200 mL/hour

*Consider incremental escalation of the infusion rate only in the absence of infusion-related reactions
†Use a dilution volume of 500 mL for the 16 mg/kg dose only if there were no infusion-related reactions the previous week. Otherwise, use a dilution volume of 1000 mL
‡Use a modified initial rate (100 mL/hour) for subsequent infusions (ie, week 3 onwards) only if there were no infusion-related reactions during the previous infusion. Otherwise, continue to use instructions indicated in the table for the week 2 infusion rate

Concomitant medications:

Pre-infusion Medications (administered 1–3 hours before each infusion)
- Corticosteroid (long- or intermediate-acting):
  - Monotherapy daratumumab: administer 100 mg methylPREDNISolone (or equivalent) intraVENously. Consider reducing the dose to 60 mg (or equivalent) beginning with the third infusion either orally or intraVENously
  - Combination therapy daratumumab: administer dexamethasone 20 mg (or equivalent) orally or intraVENously. When dexamethasone is the background regimen-specific corticosteroid, the dexamethasone dose that is part of the background regimen will serve as premedication on daratumumab infusion days. Do not administer background regimen-specific corticosteroids (eg, predniSONE) on daratumumab infusion days when patients have received dexamethasone (or equivalent) as a premedication
- Acetaminophen 650–1000 mg orally
- DiphenhydrAMINE 25–50 mg (or equivalent) orally or intraVENously

Post-infusion Medications:
- Corticosteroid (long- or intermediate-acting):
  - Monotherapy daratumumab: administer 20 mg methylPREDNISolone (or equivalent) orally for 2 days starting the day after daratumumab administration
  - Combination therapy daratumumab: consider administering oral methylPREDNISolone at a dose of ≤20 mg (or equivalent) beginning the day after daratumumab administration. If a background regimen-specific corticosteroid (eg, dexamethasone, predniSONE) is administered the day after daratumumab administration, additional corticosteroids may not be needed
- Consider prescribing short- and long-acting bronchodilators and inhaled corticosteroids to patients with chronic obstructive pulmonary disease following the first 4 daratumumab infusions. In the absence of prior major infusion-related reactions, consider discontinuing these additional post-infusion medications after the fourth infusion
- Initiate antiviral prophylaxis to prevent herpes zoster reactivation (eg, acyclovir, valACYclovir, or famciclovir) within 1 week after starting daratumumab and for 3 months after the last infusion

Adverse events and treatment modifications:
- Refer to the current FDA-approved product label for detailed warnings and treatment modifications for missed doses, infusion-related reactions, and hematologic toxicities. No dose reductions are recommended
- Among patients treated with daratumumab in clinical trials (n=2066), infusion-related reactions were reported in 37% with the week 1 infusion (16 mg/kg), 2% with the week 2 infusion, and cumulatively 6% with subsequent infusions. Less than 1% of patients had a G3/4 reaction at week 2 or later. The median (range) onset of infusion-related reactions was 1.5 hours (0–72.8), and 36% of patients required a modification of the infusion due to reactions. Nearly all reactions occurred during the infusion or within 4 hours of completion with the use of post-infusion medication. Prior to routine use of post-infusion medications, infusion-related reactions occurred up to 48 hours after infusion
- In a clinical trial (CASSIOPEIA) where patients interrupted daratumumab therapy for a median (range) of 3.75 months (2.4–6.9) to undergo autologous stem cell transplant, the incidence of infusion reaction with the first dose of post-transplant daratumumab was 11% (patients resumed using the most recent rate/dilution volume prior to interruption). In the EQUULEUS trial, patients underwent the first daratumumab infusion split over two days (ie, 8 mg/kg on day 1 and day 2). The incidence of all-grade reaction was 42% (36% with week 1 day 1, 4% with week 1 day 2, and 8% with subsequent infusions)

(continued)

Recommendations for Drug Administration and Ancillary Care (*continued*)

- Administer required pre- and post-infusion medications and monitor vital signs frequently during the infusion. Interrupt the infusion for any grade infusion-related reaction and provide appropriate medical management
  - For G1–2 reactions, upon resolution of symptoms, resume the infusion at ≤50% of the rate at which the reaction occurred. In the absence of further reaction symptoms, escalate the infusion rate at increments and intervals as clinically appropriate up to a maximum rate of 200 mL/hour
  - For G3 reactions, follow the same guidance as for G1–2 reactions; the procedure may be repeated once in case of recurrent G3 symptoms. Permanently discontinue daratumumab upon the third occurrence of G3 infusion-related reaction
  - Permanently discontinue daratumumab for G4 infusion-related reactions or for anaphylactic reactions

Potential drug interactions:

- Daratumumab binds to CD38 expressed on red blood cells (RBCs) and therefore may result in a false positive indirect antiglobulin test, which may persist for up to 6 months following the last infusion. Check blood type and screen tests prior to the first infusion. Inform the blood bank that a patient has received daratumumab
- Daratumumab, an IgG kappa monoclonal antibody, may be detected on serum protein electrophoresis and immunofixation assays

DARATUMUMAB AND HYALURONIDASE-fihj

DARZALEX FASPRO (daratumumab and hyaluronidase-fihj) prescribing information. Horsham, PA: Janssen Biotech, Inc.; May 2020

Product Identification, Preparation, Storage, and Stability

- To prevent medication errors, check the vial labels to ensure that the drug being prepared and administered is DARZALEX FASPRO (daratumumab and hyaluronidase-fihj) for SUBCUTaneous use. Do not administer DARZALEX FASPRO (daratumumab and hyaluronidase-fihj) intraVENously
- DARZALEX FASPRO (daratumumab and hyaluronidase-fihj) is a combination of daratumumab and hyaluronidase. Daratumumab is a human IgG1 kappa

monoclonal antibody directed against CD38. Recombinant human hyaluronidase is an endoglycosidase used to increase the dispersion and absorption of co-administered drugs when administered SUBCUTaneously
- DARZALEX FASPRO (daratumumab and hyaluronidase-fihj) is a sterile, colorless to yellow, preservative-free, clear to opalescent solution available in individually boxed single-dose vials (NDC 57894-503-01) containing 15 mL of ready-to-use solution

comprising daratumumab (1800 mg), hyaluronidase (30,000 units), L-histidine (4.9 mg), L-histidine hydrochloride monohydrate (18.4 mg), L-methionine (13.5 mg), polysorbate 20 (6 mg), sorbitol (735.1 mg), and SWFI
- Store intact vials under refrigeration at 2–8°C (36–46°F) in the original carton to protect from light
- *Do not freeze or shake* intact vials

Recommendations for Drug Administration and Ancillary Care

General:
- The usual dose of DARZALEX FASPRO (daratumumab and hyaluronidase-fihj) is 1800 mg/30,000 units (1800 mg daratumumab and 30,000 units hyaluronidase) administered SUBCUTaneously over approximately 3–5 minutes. Refer to the current FDA-approved product label for details regarding various schedules of administration
- DARZALEX FASPRO (daratumumab and hyaluronidase-fihj) should be administered by a health care professional
- No dose adjustment is necessary for patients with renal impairment (CrCl 15–89 mL/min) or mild hepatic impairment (total bilirubin 1 to 1.5 × ULN and AST > ULN). There are no PK data in patients with moderate or severe hepatic impairment

Preparation:
- DARZALEX FASPRO (daratumumab and hyaluronidase-fihj) is supplied as a ready-to-use product that requires no reconstitution or further dilution
- Remove the vial from the refrigerator and allow it to equilibrate to ambient temperature 15–30°C (59–86°F). Store the intact vial at ambient temperature and lighting for up to 24 hours. Avoid direct sunlight. Do not shake intact vials
- Using a sterile syringe (composed of polypropylene [PP] or polyethylene [PE]) and a stainless steel transfer needle, withdraw 15 mL of solution from the vial

- Replace the transfer needle with a syringe closing cap. Label the syringe according to institutional standards and with a peel-off label
- Attach the hypodermic stainless steel injection needle or SUBCUTaneous infusion set (composed of PP, PE, or PVC) immediately prior to SUBCUTaneous administration to prevent needle clogging
- Visually inspect the contents of the syringe for opaque particulate matter, discoloration, and foreign particles prior to administration
- Once DARZALEX FASPRO (daratumumab and hyaluronidase-fihj) has been withdrawn from its original vial, it should be used immediately. If not used immediately, it may be stored for up to 4 hours at ambient temperature and lighting

Administration:
- Inject DARZALEX FASPRO (daratumumab and hyaluronidase-fihj) into the SUBCUTaneous tissue of the abdomen approximately 7.5 cm (3 inches) to the right or left of the navel over approximately 3–5 minutes. Never inject into areas where the skin is red, bruised, tender, or hard, or areas where there are scars. No data are available on performing the injection at other sites of the body. Rotate injection sites for successive injections
- If the patient experiences pain during the administration of DARZALEX FASPRO (daratumumab and hyaluronidase-fihj), the injection should be paused and/or slowed.

A second injection site may be chosen on the opposite side of the abdomen to deliver the remainder of the dose
- Do not administer other medications for SUBCUTaneous use at the same sites as DARZALEX FASPRO (daratumumab and hyaluronidase-fihj)

Concomitant medications:
Pre-Administration Medications (administered 1–3 hours before each dose)
- Corticosteroid (long- or intermediate-acting):
  - <u>Monotherapy</u>: administer 100 mg methylPREDNISolone (or equivalent) orally or intraVENously. Consider reducing the dose to 60 mg (or equivalent) beginning with the third injection
  - <u>Combination therapy</u>: administer dexamethasone 20 mg (or equivalent) orally or intraVENously. When dexamethasone is the background regimen-specific corticosteroid, the dexamethasone dose that is part of the background regimen will serve as premedication on DARZALEX FASPRO (daratumumab and hyaluronidase-fihj) injection days. Do not administer background regimen-specific corticosteroids (eg, predniSONE) on DARZALEX FASPRO (daratumumab and hyaluronidase-fihj) injection days when patients have received dexamethasone (or equivalent) as a premedication

(continued)

Recommendations for Drug Administration and Ancillary Care (continued)

- Acetaminophen 650–1000 mg orally
- DiphenhydrAMINE 25–50 mg (or equivalent) orally or intraVENously

Post-Administration Medications:
- Corticosteroid (long- or intermediate-acting):
  - Monotherapy: administer 20 mg methylPREDNISolone (or equivalent) orally for 2 days starting the day after injection
  - Combination therapy: consider administering oral methylPREDNISolone at a dose of ≤20 mg (or equivalent) beginning the day after DARZALEX FASPRO (daratumumab and hyaluronidase-fihj) injection. If a background regimen-specific corticosteroid (eg, dexamethasone, predniSONE) is administered the day after injection, additional corticosteroids may not be needed
  - In the absence of a major systemic administration-related reaction after the first 3 injections of DARZALEX FASPRO (daratumumab and hyaluronidase-fihj), consider discontinuing the administration of post-administration corticosteroids (excluding any background regimen-specific corticosteroid)
- Consider prescribing short- and long-acting bronchodilators and inhaled corticosteroids to patients with chronic obstructive pulmonary disease following the first 4 daratumumab and hyaluronidase-fihj injections. In the absence of prior major systemic administration-related reactions, consider discontinuing these additional post-administration medications after the fourth injection
- Initiate antiviral prophylaxis to prevent herpes zoster reactivation (eg, acyclovir, valACYclovir, or famciclovir) within 1 week after starting daratumumab and for 3 months after the last injection

Adverse events and treatment modifications:

- Refer to the current FDA-approved product label for detailed warnings and treatment modifications for missed doses and hematologic toxicities. No dose reductions are recommended
- Advise patients that systemic administration-related reactions and local cutaneous reactions may occur, sometimes with a delayed onset >24 hours after administration. In clinical studies (n=490), the incidence of systemic reactions was 11% (G2, 3.9%; G3, 1.4%). Median (range) onset was 3.7 hours (9 minutes to 3.5 days); 87% of reactions occurred on the day of administration. The incidence of systemic reactions declined with subsequent doses (first injection, 10%; second injection, 0.2%; subsequent injections [cumulative], 0.8%). The incidence of local cutaneous reactions was 8% (G2, 0.6%). Median (range) onset was 7 minutes (0 minutes–4.7 days)

Potential drug interactions:

- Daratumumab binds to CD38 expressed on red blood cells (RBCs) and therefore may result in a false positive indirect antiglobulin test which may persist for up to 6 months following the last injection. Check blood type and screen tests prior to the first injection. Inform the blood bank that a patient has received a daratumumab-containing product
- Daratumumab, an IgG kappa monoclonal antibody, may be detected on serum protein electrophoresis and immunofixation assays

DAUNORUBICIN AND CYTARABINE LIPOSOME FOR INJECTION

VYXEOS (daunorubicin and cytarabine) prescribing information. Palo Alto, CA: Jazz Pharmaceuticals, Inc; July 2019

WARNING: DO NOT INTERCHANGE WITH OTHER DAUNORUBICIN AND/OR CYTARABINE-CONTAINING PRODUCTS

- VYXEOS has different dosage recommendations than daunorubicin hydrochloride injection, cytarabine injection, daunorubicin citrate liposome injection, and cytarabine liposome injection. Verify drug name and dose prior to preparation and administration to avoid dosing errors …

Boxed Warning for VYXEOS (daunorubicin and cytarabine) prescribing information. Palo Alto, CA: Jazz Pharmaceuticals, Inc; July 2019

Product Identification, Preparation, Storage, and Stability

- DAUNOrubicin and cytarabine liposome for injection contains a combination of DAUNOrubicin and cytarabine (1:5 molar ratio) encapsuled in liposomes. The liposome membrane is composed of distearoylphosphatidylcholine (DSPC), distearoylphosphatidylglycerol (DSPG), and cholesterol in a 7:2:1 molar ratio
- DAUNOrubicin and cytarabine liposome for injection is a sterile, preservative-free, purple, lyophilized cake supplied in a single-dose vial. Each vial (NDC 68727-745-01) contains DAUNOrubicin (44 mg), cytarabine (100 mg), and the following inactive ingredients: DSPC (454 mg), DSPG (132 mg), cholesterol HP (32 mg), copper gluconate (100 mg), triethanolamine (4 mg), and sucrose (2054 mg). Cartons containing 2 vials (NDC 68727-745-02) or 5 vials (NDC 6 8727-745-05) are available
- Store intact unreconstituted vials under refrigeration at 2–8°C (36–46°F), in an upright position, and in their original carton (to protect from light) until time of reconstitution
- DAUNOrubicin and cytarabine liposome for injection is a cytotoxic drug. Follow applicable special handling and disposal procedures

Reconstitution:
- Calculate the VYXEOS dose based on the DAUNOrubicin component and the individual patient's BSA, then calculate the number of vials needed based on the DAUNOrubicin dose
- Remove the required number of vials from the refrigerator and allow to equilibrate to room temperature for 30 minutes
- Using a sterile syringe, inject 19 mL of SWFI into the vial and immediately start a 5-minute timer
- Carefully swirl the contents of the vial for 5 minutes while gently inverting the vial every 30 seconds. Do not heat, vortex, or shake vigorously
- After reconstitution, let the vial rest for 15 minutes to yield an opaque, purple, homogenous dispersion, essentially free of visible particulates, that contains 2.2 mg/mL DAUNOrubicin and 5 mg/mL of cytarabine. If the reconstituted product is not diluted into a parenteral product container immediately, it may be stored in the refrigerator at 2–8°C (36–46°F) for up to 4 hours

Dilution:
- Gently invert each vial 5 times prior to withdrawing the reconstituted product for further dilution.

- Calculate the volume of reconstituted product required using the following formula:

$$[\text{volume required (mL)} = \text{dose of DAUNOrubicin (mg/m}^2) \times \text{patient's BSA (m}^2) \div 2.2 \text{ (mg/mL)}]$$

- Using a sterile syringe, aseptically withdraw the calculated volume of the reconstituted product from the vial(s) and transfer it to a parenteral product container containing 500 mL of 0.9% NS or D5W. There may be residual unused product remaining in the vial, which should be discarded
- Gently invert the parenteral product container to mix the solution, yielding a deep purple, translucent, homogenous dispersion, free from visible particulates
- If the diluted infusion solution is not used immediately, store in the refrigerator at 2–8°C (36–46°F) for up to 4 hours

Selected incompatibility:
- Do not mix DAUNOrubicin and cytarabine liposome for injection with other drugs or administer as an infusion with other drugs

Recommendations for Drug Administration and Ancillary Care

General:

- Assess cardiac function, complete blood counts, liver and renal function tests before induction and before each consolidation cycle
- Dose adjustment is not required for patients with mild or moderate renal impairment (CrCl 30–89 mL/min) or in patients with bilirubin ≤3 mg/dL. Data are lacking in patients with a bilirubin >3 mg/dL or with severe renal impairment (CrCl 15–29 mL/min) or end-stage renal disease
- Prior to each dose, calculate the patient's prior cumulative anthracycline exposure. Use of the product is not recommended in patients whose lifetime anthracycline exposure has reached the commonly accepted maximum cumulative limits of 550 mg/m^2 (or 400 mg/m^2 in those with prior mediastinal radiation exposure)
- See Chapter 43 for recommended use in patients with hepatic dysfunction

Administration:

- The typical course of VYXEOS for the treatment of adult patients with newly diagnosed therapy-related AML or AML with myelodysplasia-related changes consists of 1–2 cycles of induction and up to 2 cycles of consolidation at the doses and schedules listed in the following table:

Cycle	VYXEOS Dose and Schedule
First induction	(DAUNOrubicin 44 mg/m^2 and cytarabine 100 mg/m^2) liposome days 1, 3, and 5
Second induction*	(DAUNOrubicin 44 mg/m^2 and cytarabine 100 mg/m^2) liposome days 1 and 3
Consolidation	(DAUNOrubicin 29 mg/m^2 and cytarabine 65 mg/m^2) liposome days 1 and 3

*Only for patients failing to achieve a response with the first induction cycle

Note: The second induction cycle (when indicated) is administered 2–5 weeks after the start of the first cycle. The first consolidation cycle is administered between 5–8 weeks after the start of the last induction cycle. The second consolidation cycle is administered 5–8 weeks after the start of the first consolidation cycle in patients who do not show disease progression

- DAUNOrubicin and cytarabine liposome for injection is to be administered as a constant intraVENous infusion over 90 minutes via an infusion pump through a central VAD or PICC. An inline membrane filter with pore diameter ≥15 μm may be used for the intraVENous infusion. Flush the line after administration with 0.9% NS or D5W
- Prior to administration, inspect the diluted infusion solution for discoloration and particulate matter. Do not use the product if it contains visible particles

Concomitant medications:

- Administer prophylactic antiemetics before treatment with DAUNOrubicin and cytarabine liposome for injection.
- Medications to prevent hypersensitivity reactions are not required for primary prophylaxis. However, antihistamines and/or corticosteroids should be considered as secondary prophylaxis prior to reexposure in patients with prior mild hypersensitivity reaction symptoms and should be administered upon rechallenge in patients with prior moderate symptoms

Adverse events and treatment modifications:

- Refer to the current FDA-approved product label for detailed recommendations regarding treatment modifications for missed doses, hypersensitivity reactions, and cardiotoxicity
- Do not start a consolidation cycle if the ANC is <500/mm^3 or if the platelet count is <50,000/mm^3
- Serious or fatal hypersensitivity reactions, including anaphylactic reactions, have occurred with DAUNOrubicin and cytarabine liposome for injection. Monitor closely for signs and symptoms of hypersensitivity reactions. If a mild reaction occurs, interrupt the infusion and manage symptoms. Upon resolution of symptoms, reinitiate the infusion at 50% of the prior rate. Consider premedication with antihistamines and/or corticosteroids for subsequent doses. If a moderate reaction occurs, discontinue the infusion for that day and manage symptoms. For subsequent doses, administer premedication with antihistamines and/or corticosteroids prior to initiating the infusion at the same rate. If a severe or life-threatening reaction occurs, discontinue DAUNOrubicin and cytarabine liposome for injection permanently, treat symptoms as clinically indicated, and monitor the patient until resolution of symptoms
- DAUNOrubicin and cytarabine liposome for injection is contraindicated in patients with a history of serious hypersensitivity reaction to cytarabine, DAUNOrubicin, or any component of the formulation

Potential drug interactions:

- Monitor cardiac function more frequently when coadministered with other cardiotoxic agents
- Monitor hepatic function more frequently when coadministered with hepatotoxic agents

Selected precautions:

- **Hemorrhage:** serious or fatal hemorrhagic events associated with prolonged thrombocytopenia have occurred. Monitor blood counts regularly until recovery and transfuse platelets as required
- **Cardiotoxicity:** DAUNOrubicin and cytarabine liposome for injection contains DAUNOrubicin, an anthracycline medication with a known risk of cardiotoxicity. Prior exposure to anthracyclines or mediastinal radiotherapy, pre-existing cardiac disease, or concomitant use of other cardiotoxic medications may increase the risk of DAUNOrubicin-induced cardiac toxicity. Calculate the lifetime cumulative anthracycline dose prior to administration of each dose of DAUNOrubicin and cytarabine liposome for injection and ensure that the patient will not exceed threshold values of 550 mg/m^2 (or 400 mg/m^2 if prior mediastinal radiation). Prior to the first induction cycle, obtain an electrocardiogram and assess the left ventricular ejection fraction (LVEF) by multi-gated radionuclide angiography (MUGA) or echocardiography (ECHO). Repeat a MUGA or ECHO for LVEF determination prior to consolidation and then as clinically indicated. DAUNOrubicin and cytarabine liposome injection is not recommended in patients with LVEF that is less than the lower limit of normal. Discontinue therapy in patients with impaired cardiac function unless the benefit of treatment outweighs its risks
- **Tissue necrosis:** DAUNOrubicin has been associated with severe local tissue necrosis at sites of drug extravasation. DAUNOrubicin and cytarabine liposome for injection is to be administered by intraVENous infusion only through a central VAD or PICC. Monitor the infusion site closely for signs and symptoms of extravasation. Do not administer it by the intramuscular or subcutaneous route
- **Copper overload:** reconstituted DAUNOrubicin and cytarabine liposome for injection contains 5 mg/mL copper gluconate (equivalent to 0.7 mg/mL elemental copper). Use caution and exercise appropriate monitoring in patients with copper-related metabolic disorders such as Wilson's disease; refer to the current FDA-approved product label for detailed recommendations

DAUNORUBICIN HYDROCHLORIDE

DAUNORUBICIN HYDROCHLORIDE prescribing information. Eatontown, NJ: West-Ward Pharmaceuticals; May 2015
DAUNORUBICIN HYDROCHLORIDE prescribing information. Irvine, CA: Teva Parenteral Medicines, Inc.; September 2012

WARNINGS

1. Daunorubicin hydrochloride injection must be given into a rapidly flowing intravenous infusion. It must never be given by the intramuscular or subcutaneous route. Severe local tissue necrosis will occur if there is extravasation during administration

2. Myocardial toxicity manifested in its most severe form by potentially fatal congestive heart failure may occur either during therapy or months to years after termination of therapy. The incidence of myocardial toxicity increases after a total cumulative dose exceeding 400 to 550 mg/m^2 in adults, 300 mg/m^2 in children more than 2 years of age, or 10 mg/kg in children less than 2 years of age

3. Severe myelosuppression occurs when used in therapeutic doses; this may lead to infection or hemorrhage

4. It is recommended that daunorubicin hydrochloride be administered only by physicians who are experienced in leukemia chemotherapy and in facilities with laboratory and supportive resources adequate to monitor drug tolerance and protect and maintain a patient compromised by drug toxicity. The physician and institution must be capable of responding rapidly and completely to severe hemorrhagic conditions and/or overwhelming infection

5. Dosage should be reduced in patients with impaired hepatic or renal function

Boxed Warning for DAUNORUBICIN HYDROCHLORIDE prescribing information. Eatontown, NJ: West-Ward Pharmaceuticals; May 2015 and DAUNORUBICIN HYDROCHLORIDE prescribing information. Irvine, CA: Teva Parenteral Medicines, Inc.; September 2012

Product Identification, Preparation, Storage, and Stability

- DAUNOrubicin HCl injection (solution) is generically available from several manufacturers. It was historically also available as a lyophilized (powder) formulation. DAUNOrubicin is a sterile, deep red product packaged in glass single-use vials

  ▪ DAUNOrubicin HCl injection (solution) is available in vials containing 20 mg/4 mL (packaged in cartons containing 10 vials) or 50 mg/10 mL (individually packaged) DAUNOrubicin base

- Storage:

  ▪ Store intact DAUNOrubicin HCl injection (solution) vials under refrigeration at 2–8°C (36–46°F)

- Protect DAUNOrubicin from exposure to light by storing unused vials in their packaging carton

Stability (solution formulations):

- DAUNOrubicin HCl injection (formulations already in solution) are stable for 24 hours at 15–30°C (59–86°F)

- DAUNOrubicin HCl diluted with D5W (pH = 4.36) or 0.9% NS (pH = 5.20 or 6.47) to a concentration of 98 μg/mL (estimated) in PVC containers stored at 25°C, 4°C, or −20°C was stable for 43 days under all conditions evaluated[35]

  ▪ DAUNOrubicin HCl for injection reconstituted with SWFI and diluted with 0.9% NS or D5W to an estimated concentration of 98 μg/mL stored in PVC containers for 43 days did not degrade during or after 11 repeated cycles of freezing (−20°C) and thawing at ambient temperature (25°C)[35]

- DAUNOrubicin HCl for injection reconstituted with SWFI to a concentration of 2 mg/mL was stable for at least 43 days when stored in polypropylene syringes at 4°C[35]

- DAUNOrubicin solutions undergo photodegradation

  ▪ The rate and extent of photodegradation are inversely related to DAUNOrubicin concentrations in solution[36]

    ○ At DAUNOrubicin concentrations ≥100 μg/mL (≥0.1 mg/mL) stored at 25°C for 168 h under artificial room lighting (four 65/80-watt fluorescent tubes mounted approximately 1 m above the samples), little or no photodegradation occurred in clear or amber glass or opaque polyethylene containers[36]

    ○ At DAUNOrubicin concentrations ≥500 μg/mL (≥0.5 mg/mL), no special precautions are necessary to protect freshly prepared solutions from exposure to artificial light or sunlight[36]

Selected incompatibility:

- Product labeling recommends *not mixing* DAUNOrubicin with heparin or other drugs

Recommendations for Drug Administration and Ancillary Care

General:

- See Chapter 43 for recommended use in patients with renal and hepatic dysfunction

- A calculated dose is withdrawn into a syringe with 10–15 mL of 0.9% NS for intraVENous injection

- Inject DAUNOrubicin into the tubing or side-arm of a rapidly flowing intraVENous infusion of D5W or 0.9% NS

- Severe hepatic or renal impairment may enhance adverse effects associated with DAUNOrubicin

  ▪ Clinical laboratory evaluation of hepatic and renal function should be completed before administering DAUNOrubicin. Consult recommendations for modifying DAUNOrubicin dosage and schedule in hepatic or renal impairment

Caution: DAUNOrubicin is a vesicant and can produce severe local soft-tissue necrosis if extravasation occurs. *NEVER inject DAUNOrubicin by the intraMUSCular, SUBCUTaneous, or intraTHECAL routes*

- The current standard of care for managing anthracycline extravasation, including extravasation of DAUNOrubicin, is a 3-day course of intraVENously administered dexrazoxane (Totect, Savene)

- Advise patients DAUNOrubicin HCl may transiently impart a red discoloration to urine after administration

DECITABINE

DECITABINE prescribing information. Princeton, NJ: Dr. Reddy's Laboratories Inc.; July 2020
DECITABINE prescribing information. Cranbury, NJ: Sun Pharmaceutical Industries, Inc.; July 2020
DACOGEN (decitabine) prescribing information. Rockville, MD: Otsuka America Pharmaceutical, Inc.; June 2020

Product Identification, Preparation, Storage, and Stability

- Decitabine is a sterile, lyophilized, white to almost-white powder. It is commercially available in two different formulations:
  - The brand product and the majority of generic products are presented in individually packaged clear, colorless, single-use, 20-mL, glass vials containing 50 mg decitabine, 68 mg monobasic potassium phosphate (potassium dihydrogen phosphate), and 11.6 mg sodium hydroxide
  - One generic product (Sun Pharmaceutical Industries, Inc.) is presented as a "kit" containing two separate vials (NDC 47335-361-41). The drug product consists of a clear, colorless, tubular, single-use, 20-mL, glass vial containing 50 mg decitabine (NDC 47335-361-40). The diluent is provided as a clear, colorless solution consisting of 68 mg monobasic potassium phosphate, 11.6 mg sodium hydroxide, and 10 mL SWFI (NDC 47335-362-40)
- Store intact cartons at 20–25°C (68–77°F); the labeling for some products allows temperature excursions to 15–30°C (59–86°F)
- Caution: *BEFORE BEGINNING* reconstitution, evaluate whether decitabine administration will begin within 15 minutes after the lyophilized product is reconstituted
  - Decitabine hydrolyzes spontaneously after reconstitution
  - If drug administration commences within 15 minutes after reconstitution began, there is no need to used prechilled diluents to further dilute reconstituted decitabine, but preparation should not commence until just before the drug is needed
  - If drug administration is to begin >15 minutes after reconstitution, use prechilled solutions (2–8°C

[35.6–46.4°F]) of 0.9% NS or D5W to further dilute reconstituted decitabine
- For the brand product and generic products that are supplied without an included diluent, reconstitute the drug product vial with 10 mL of room temperature (20–25°C) SWFI to produce a solution with concentration of 5 mg decitabine/mL. For the generic product supplied as a "kit" (NDC 47335-36141), instead reconstitute the vial with 10 mL of the supplied "diluent for Decitabine for Injection" at room temperature (20–25°C) to produce a solution with concentration of 5 mg decitabine/mL
- After powdered decitabine is completely dissolved, immediately withdraw with a syringe the calculated volume of drug needed for a patient's dose from a vial and transfer it into a sterile plastic or glass parenteral product container containing a volume of 0.9% NS or D5W sufficient to produce a decitabine concentration between 0.1–1.0 mg/mL
  - If decitabine cannot be used within 15 minutes after diluent was introduced into a vial, the product should be promptly refrigerated. Storage times vary according to various product labels; the brand name product and most generic products allow for storage for up to 4 hours after reconstitution if prechilled solution was used for dilution. Labeling for the generic product supplied as a "kit" (NDC 47335-36141) allows for storage for up to 4 hours after reconstitution if prechilled solution was used for dilution
  - Reconstituted and diluted products that have not been used within the time limits identified above and all materials potentially contaminated with decitabine during product preparation should be discarded as hazardous waste

Recommendations for Drug Administration and Ancillary Care

General:
- See Chapter 43 for recommended use in patients with renal and hepatic dysfunction
- If decitabine is not prepared with chilled solutions and promptly refrigerated after preparation, administration *MUST BEGIN* within 15 minutes after reconstitution
- If decitabine was prepared with chilled solutions and stored under refrigeration promptly after preparation, administration *MAY BEGIN* up to 4 hours after reconstitution [or up to 7 hours after reconstitution if the generic product supplied as a "kit" (NDC 47335-36141) is used]
  - Drug administration should begin promptly after stored products are transferred from refrigeration to room temperature conditions

DEXRAZOXANE

Utilized as a Cardioprotectant

DEXRAZOXANE prescribing information. Eatontown, NJ: West-Ward Pharmaceuticals; December 2018
DEXRAZOXANE prescribing information. Hyderabad-500043, India: Gland Pharma Limited; December 2016
DEXRAZOXANE prescribing information. Morristown, NJ: Almaject, Inc.; May 2019
DEXRAZOXANE prescribing information. Pine Brook, NJ: Alvogen, Inc; July 2017
DEXRAZOXANE prescribing information. Princeton, NJ: Fosun Pharma USA Inc.; March 2019
DEXRAZOXANE prescribing information. Boca Raton, FL: Breckenridge Pharmaceutical, Inc.; April 2017
DEXRAZOXANE HYDROCHLORIDE prescribing information. Rockford, IL: Mylan Institutional LLC; April 2019

Product Identification, Preparation, Storage, and Stability

	Dexrazoxane for Injection (Generic)	
Product and manufacturer	**Mylan Institutional LLC** -*250 mg vial:* NDC 67457-207-25 -*500 mg vial:* NDC 67457-208-50	**West-Ward Pharmaceuticals (Hikma Pharmaceuticals USA Inc.)** -*250 mg vial:* NDC 0143-9247-01 -*500 mg vial:* NDC 0143-9248-01 **Gland Pharma Limited** -*500 mg vial:* NDC 68083-195-01 **Almaject, Inc** -*500 mg vial:* NDC 72611-716-01 **Alvogen, Inc** -*500 mg vial:* NDC 47781-578-07 **Breckenridge Pharmaceutical, Inc** -*500 mg vial:* NDC 51991-942-98
Product presentation	Packaged in cartons containing two single-use vials: 1. A vial containing sterile, pyrogen-free, lyophilized dexrazoxane HCl equivalent to dexrazoxane 250 mg *or* dexrazoxane 500 mg 2. A vial containing 0.167 mol/L (0.167 M, 1/6 Molar, M/6) sodium lactate injection, USP, for reconstitution	Packaged in cartons containing sterile, pyrogen-free, lyophilized dexrazoxane HCl equivalent to dexrazoxane 250 mg or dexrazoxane 500 mg
Formulation excipients	Hydrochloric acid, NF, is added to adjust product pH	
Diluent	• 25 mL sodium lactate injection, USP, 0.167 mol/L is packaged with dexrazoxane for injection 250 mg • 50 mL sodium lactate injection, USP, 0.167 mol/L is packaged with dexrazoxane for injection 500 mg	• Reconstituted *only* with SWFI • Diluent is not included in products
Reconstitution	Dexrazoxane for Injection *must be* reconstituted with 0.167 M sodium lactate injection, USP, to produce a solution with a concentration of 10 mg/mL, thus: | Dexrazoxane Content per Vial	Diluent Volume (0.167 M Sodium Lactate, USP)
---	---
250 mg	25 mL
500 mg	50 mL | • pH for the reconstituted solution is within the range of 3.5–5.5	Must be reconstituted with SWFI to produce a solution with a concentration of 10 mg/mL, thus: | Dexrazoxane Content per Vial	Diluent Volume (SWFI)
---	---
250 mg	25 mL
500 mg	50 mL	 • pH for the reconstituted solution is within the range of 1.0–3.0
Dilution for clinical use	• The reconstituted solution may be transferred to a parenteral product container and diluted with either 0.9% NS or D5W to a concentration within the range of 1.3–5 mg/mL • All unused dexrazoxane solutions should be discarded	• The reconstituted solution must be transferred to a parenteral product container and diluted *only* with LRI to a concentration within the range of 1.3–3 mg/mL • The resulting solution pH is within the range of 3.5–5.5 • All unused dexrazoxane solutions should be discarded
Storage	Store intact vials at 20–25°C (68–77°F)	

(continued)

Product Identification, Preparation, Storage, and Stability (*continued*)

Stability	• Dexrazoxane (10 mg/mL) is stable for 6 hours after the time of reconstitution with 0.167 M sodium lactate injection when stored at controlled room temperature, 20–25°C, or under refrigeration, 2–8°C (35.6–46.4°F) • Diluted dexrazoxane is stable for 6 hours when stored at controlled room temperature or under refrigeration	• Dexrazoxane (10 mg/mL) is stable for 30 minutes after reconstitution with SWFI when stored at room temperature, or for up to 3 hours if stored under refrigeration, 2–8°C (36–46°F) • After dilution in LRI, dexrazoxane is stable for 1 hour at controlled room temperature, or for up to 4 hours if stored under refrigeration
Selected incompatibility	• Product labeling recommends *not* mixing dexrazoxane with other drugs	

Recommendations for Dexrazoxane Utilization as a Cardioprotectant

General:

• See Chapter 43 for recommended use in patients with hepatic dysfunction

Administration:

Product Source	Route and Rate of Administration
Mylan Institutional LLC	• Administer dexrazoxane by slow intraVENous injection *or* a rapid intraVENous infusion over a period of <30 minutes due to the temporal relationship between dexrazoxane and DOXOrubicin administration • After completing the infusion of dexrazoxane for injection, and prior to a total elapsed time of 30 minutes (from the beginning of the dexrazoxane for injection infusion), the intraVENous injection of DOXOrubicin should be given
West-Ward Pharmaceuticals (Hikma Pharmaceuticals USA Inc.) Gland Pharma Limited Almaject, Inc Alvogen, Inc Breckenridge Pharmaceutical, Inc	• Administer dexrazoxane *only* by intraVENous infusion over a period of 15 minutes • Administer DOXOrubicin within 30 minutes after the completion of dexrazoxane for injection infusion

• Recommended dosage ratios of dexrazoxane to DOXOrubicin:
  ▪ Patients with creatinine clearance ≥40 mL/min (≥0.66 mL/s), dexrazoxane to DOXOrubicin ratio is 10:1; eg, 500 mg dexrazoxane/m²: 50 mg DOXOrubicin/m²
  ▪ Patients with creatinine clearance <40 mL/min (<0.66 mL/s), dexrazoxane to DOXOrubicin ratio is 5:1; eg, 250 mg dexrazoxane/m²: 50 mg DOXOrubicin/m²

DEXRAZOXANE

Utilized in Treating Anthracycline Extravasation

TOTECT (dexrazoxane hydrochloride) prescribing information. Nashville, TN: Cumberland Pharmaceuticals Inc.; December 2019

Product Identification, Preparation, Storage, and Stability

- TOTECT is packaged as individually boxed, single-dose, 50-mL, type I glass vials containing dexrazoxane 500 mg (free base) and hydrochloric acid added for pH adjustment kit (NDC 66220-110-01)
- Store the unreconstituted product in its carton to protect it from light at 25°C (77°F). Temperature excursions are permitted to 15–30°C (59–86°F)

	Option 1 for Preparation (Prepare with SWFI and LRI)	Option 2 for Preparation (Prepare with 0.167M Sodium Lactate Injection and 0.9% NS)
Reconstitution	Reconstitute each 500 mg dexrazoxane vial with 50 mL of SWFI to produce a solution containing dexrazoxane 10 mg/mL	1. To prepare 50 mL of a 0.167M sodium lactate injection solution, add 1.67 mL of 5 mEq/mL sodium lactate injection to 50 mL SWFI 2. Reconstitute each 500 mg dexrazoxane vial with 50 mL of the 0.167M sodium lactate injection solution prepared in step 1 to produce a solution containing dexrazoxane 10 mg/mL
Dilution for clinical use	Withdraw the calculated volume of the reconstituted solution and dilute into an infusion bag containing 1000 mL LRI	Withdraw the calculated volume of the reconstituted solution and dilute into an infusion bag containing 1000 mL 0.9% NS
Stability	Reconstituted vials are stable for 30 minutes after reconstitution at ambient temperature The final product diluted in LRI is stable for 4 hours at room temperature or for 12 hours refrigerated between 2–8°C (36–46°F)	Reconstituted vials are stable for 30 minutes after reconstitution at ambient temperature The final product diluted in 0.9% NS is stable for 4 hours at room temperature or for 12 hours refrigerated between 2–8°C (36–46°F)
Selected incompatibility	Do not mix or administer with any other drug during the infusion	

Recommendations for Drug Administration and Ancillary Care for Dexrazoxane

Utilized as an Antidote for Anthracycline[*] Extravasations

General:

- Dexrazoxane dosage should be decreased by 50% in persons whose creatinine clearance is <40 mL/min (<0.66 mL/s)
- Dimethylsulfoxide (DMSO) should not be applied topically to treat anthracycline extravasations in patients who are receiving dexrazoxane
  - Anecdotal clinical reports and experimental evidence in mice indicate concomitant use of topical DMSO at the site of anthracycline extravasation decreases the efficacy of systemically administered dexrazoxane
- Dexrazoxane is a cytotoxic drug and may produce myelosuppression additive to what is expected from antineoplastic treatments
- Reversible increases in liver enzymes (serum AST, ALT, bilirubin) may follow dexrazoxane use

Dosage and administration:

- Cooling packs (if used) should be removed from an extravasation site at least 15 minutes before dexrazoxane administration to improve blood flow to the affected site
  - Vasoconstriction caused by local hypothermia may compromise dexrazoxane distribution to the affected area
- **Dexrazoxane administration must begin within 6 hours** after an extravasation event to be optimally effective
- Administer dexrazoxane via a large-caliber vein:

Day 1   Dexrazoxane 1000 mg/m² (maximum recommended single dose = 2000 mg) intraVENously over 1–2 hours, via an administration site not affected by the extravasation

Day 2[†]   Dexrazoxane 1000 mg/m² (maximum recommended single dose = 2000 mg) intraVENously over 1–2 hours via an administration site not affected by the extravasation

Day 3[†]   Dexrazoxane 500 mg/m² (maximum recommended single dose = 1000 mg) intraVENously over 1–2 hours via an administration site not affected by the extravasation (total dosage/3-day course = 2500 mg/m²; maximum recommended dose/3-day course = 5000 mg)

[*]Anthracyclines, including DAUNOrubicin, DOXOrubicin, epirubicin, and IDArubicin
[†]Product labeling recommends administering successive 24 hours (±3 hours) after a previously administered dose

DOCETAXEL

[*One-vial formulation*] TAXOTERE (docetaxel) prescribing information. Bridgewater, NJ: Sanofi-Aventis U.S. LLC; December 2019
Docetaxel prescribing information. Lake Forest, IL: Hospira, Inc.; July 2020
Docetaxel prescribing information. Bridgewater, NJ: Winthrop U.S.; May 2020
Docetaxel prescribing information. Princeton, NJ: Sandoz Inc.; May 2020
Docetaxel prescribing information. Durham, NC: Accord Healthcare, Inc.; July 2020

WARNING: TOXIC DEATHS, HEPATOTOXICITY, NEUTROPENIA, HYPERSENSITIVITY REACTIONS, and FLUID RETENTION

Treatment-related mortality associated with docetaxel is increased in patients with abnormal liver function, in patients receiving higher doses, and in patients with non-small cell lung carcinoma and a history of prior treatment with platinum-based chemotherapy who receive docetaxel as a single agent at a dose of 100 mg/m^2 ...

Avoid the use of Docetaxel Injection in patients with bilirubin > upper limit of normal (ULN), or to patients with AST and/or ALT >1.5 × ULN concomitant with alkaline phosphatase >2.5 × ULN. Patients with elevations of bilirubin or abnormalities of transaminase concurrent with alkaline phosphatase are at increased risk for the development of severe neutropenia, febrile neutropenia, infections, severe thrombocytopenia, severe stomatitis, severe skin toxicity, and toxic death. Patients with isolated elevations of transaminase >1.5 × ULN also had a higher rate of febrile neutropenia. Measure bilirubin, AST or ALT, and alkaline phosphatase prior to each cycle of Docetaxel Injection ...

Do not administer Docetaxel Injection to patients with neutrophil counts of <1500 cells/mm^3. Monitor blood counts frequently as neutropenia may be severe and result in infection ...

Do not administer Docetaxel Injection to patients who have a history of severe hypersensitivity reactions to docetaxel or to other drugs formulated with polysorbate 80 ... Severe hypersensitivity reactions have been reported in patients despite dexamethasone premedication. Hypersensitivity reactions require immediate discontinuation of the Docetaxel Injection infusion and administration of appropriate therapy ...

Severe fluid retention occurred in 6.5% (6/92) of patients despite use of dexamethasone premedication. It was characterized by one or more of the following events: poorly tolerated peripheral edema, generalized edema, pleural effusion requiring urgent drainage, dyspnea at rest, cardiac tamponade, or pronounced abdominal distention (due to ascites) ...

Boxed Warning for Docetaxel prescribing information. Lake Forest, IL: Hospira, Inc.; July 2020

Product-Specific Identification, Storage, and Stability

Product Name (Manufacturer or Distributor)	Product Identification	Vial Storage
[*One-vial formulation*] TAXOTERE (Sanofi-Aventis U.S. LLC)	[*One-vial formulation*] TAXOTERE (DOCEtaxel) Injection Concentrate, Intravenous infusion (IV) is a sterile, non-pyrogenic, pale yellow to brownish-yellow, nonaqueous solution in *single-use* vials containing 20 mg DOCEtaxel (anhydrous), 0.54 g polysorbate 80, and 0.395 g dehydrated alcohol solution per milliliter in two presentations: • TAXOTERE (DOCEtaxel) Injection Concentrate 20 mg DOCEtaxel in 1 mL in 50/50 (v/v) ratio polysorbate 80/dehydrated alcohol in a blister pack in 1 carton (NDC 0075-8003-01) TAXOTERE (DOCEtaxel) injection concentrate 80 mg DOCEtaxel in 4 mL in 50/50 (v/v) ratio polysorbate 80/dehydrated alcohol in a blister pack in 1 carton (NDC 0075-8004-04)	Store TAXOTERE vials between 2–25°C (36–77°F) in the original packaging to protect the product from bright light Freezing does not adversely affect the product
[*One-vial formulation*] DOCEtaxel injection, concentrate (Winthrop U.S.)	[*One-vial formulation*] DOCEtaxel injection concentrate, for intravenous use is a sterile, non-pyrogenic, pale yellow to brownish-yellow, nonaqueous solution in *single-use* vials containing 20 mg DOCEtaxel (anhydrous), 0.54 g polysorbate 80, and 0.395 g dehydrated alcohol solution per milliliter in three presentations: • DOCEtaxel 20 mg in 1 mL of 50/50 (v/v) ratio polysorbate 80/dehydrated alcohol in a blister pack in 1 carton (NDC 0955-1020-01) • DOCEtaxel 80 mg in 4 mL of 50/50 (v/v) ratio polysorbate 80/dehydrated alcohol in a blister pack in 1 carton (NDC 0955-1021-04) • DOCEtaxel 160 mg in 8 mL of 50/50 (v/v) ratio polysorbate 80/dehydrated alcohol in a blister pack in 1 carton (NDC 0955-1022-08)	Store at 2–25°C (35.6° –77°F) in the original packaging to protect the product from bright light Freezing does not adversely affect the product

(continued)

Product-Specific Identification, Storage, and Stability (*continued*)

Product Name (Manufacturer or Distributor)	Product Identification	Vial Storage
DOCEtaxel Injection (Hospira, Inc.)	DOCEtaxel Injection is a sterile, non-pyrogenic, clear, colorless to pale yellow, nonaqueous solution, available in individually packaged vials in a *single-use* formulation: • DOCEtaxel 20 mg/2 mL (NDC 0409-0201-02); and in individually packaged *multiple-dose* vials in 2 presentations: • DOCEtaxel 80 mg/8 mL (NDC 0409-0201-10) *and* • DOCEtaxel 160 mg/16 mL (NDC 0409-0201-20) Each milliliter of solution contains 10 mg DOCEtaxel (anhydrous) in 260 mg polysorbate 80, NF; 4 mg citric acid, USP; 23% (v/v) dehydrated alcohol, USP; and PEG 300, NF	Store at 20–25°C (68–77°F) in the original packaging carton to protect the product from bright light Freezing does not adversely affect the product. After first use and following multiple needle entries and product withdrawals, DOCEtaxel injection multiuse vials are stable for up to 28 days when stored between 2° and 8°C (36° and 46°F) and protected from light
DOCEtaxel Injection (Sandoz)	DOCEtaxel Injection is a sterile, non-pyrogenic, clear, colorless to pale yellow solution in *multiple-dose* vials available in 3 presentations: • DOCEtaxel 20 mg/2 mL (NDC 66758-050-01), • DOCEtaxel 80 mg/8 mL (NDC 66758-050-02), • DOCEtaxel 160 mg/16 mL (NDC 66758-050-03) Each milliliter of solution contains 10 mg DOCEtaxel, 275.9 mg alcohol 96% (v/v), 4 mg citric acid, 648 mg PEG 300, and 80 mg polysorbate 80	Store intact vials at 2–25°C (36–77°F) in the original packaging to protect from bright light. Freezing does not adversely affect the product After initial entry, the multiple dose vials are stable for 28 days when stored between 2° and 8°C (36° and 46°F) and at room temperature, with or without protection from light
DOCEtaxel injection, concentrate (Accord Healthcare, Inc)	DOCEtaxel Injection is a sterile, non-pyrogenic, pale-yellow to brownish-yellow solution in *multiple-dose* vials containing 20 mg DOCEtaxel (anhydrous), 520 mg polysorbate 80, and 395 mg dehydrated alcohol solution in three presentations: • DOCEtaxel 20 mg/mL (NDC 16729-267-63), • DOCEtaxel 80 mg/4 mL (NDC 16729-267-64), • DOCEtaxel 160 mg/8 mL (NDC 16729-267-65)	Store intact vials between 15° –25°C (59° –77°F) in the original packaging to protect from bright light. Freezing does not adversely affect the product After initial entry, the multiple dose vials are stable for 28 days when stored at room temperature, with protection from light

General Guidance

• Do not use plasticized PVC equipment or devices that will come into contact with DOCEtaxel solutions during drug preparation or administration
  ▪ Phthalate plasticizers (including DEHP; di-2-ethylhexyl phthalate) may be leached from PVC containers and administration sets
• Glass, polypropylene, and polyolefin devices and equipment, and containers and tubing with surfaces in contact with drug products composed of those materials are appropriate for use in manipulating, containing, and administering DOCEtaxel solutions and minimize patient exposure to phthalate plasticizers[17]

Product-Specific Preparation and Stability

• If vials are removed from refrigeration, allow the vials to stand at room temperature for approximately 5 minutes before proceeding (when applicable)

Dilute the concentrated drug product:

1. Use only a 21-gauge needle to withdraw the drug product from a vial
   • Larger bore needles (eg, 18- and 19-gauge) may result in stopper coring and introduce particulate matter into the drug product
2. With a calibrated syringe, aseptically withdraw the amount of DOCEtaxel solution required for a patient's dose and transfer it into an appropriate parenteral product bag or bottle containing a volume of either 0.9% NS or D5W sufficient to produce a final DOCEtaxel concentration within the range 0.3–0.74 mg/mL
   • *CAUTION: Product concentrations vary among commercial DOCEtaxel injection products; some products are supplied at a DOCEtaxel concentration of 10 mg/mL while others are supplied at a concentration that is 2 times greater, that is, 20 mg/mL*
   • Product concentrations *must not exceed* 0.74 mg DOCEtaxel per milliliter

(*continued*)

Product-Specific Preparation and Stability (*continued*)

3. Thoroughly mix the admixture by manual rotation and by gently inverting the product container

Product (Manufacturer)	NDC Number	Stability of Prepared Infusion
TAXOTERE (Sanofi-Aventis U.S. LLC)	NDC 0075-8003-01 NDC 0075-8004-04	Stable for 6 hours (inclusive of infusion time) if stored between 2–25°C (36–77°F) Additionally, physical and chemical stability has been demonstrated in non-PVC bags up to 48 hours when stored between 2–8°C (36–46°F)
DOCEtaxel injection, concentrate (Winthrop U.S.)	NDC 0955-1020-01 NDC 0955-1021-04 NDC 0955-1022-08	Stable for 6 hours (inclusive of infusion time) if stored between 2–25°C (36–77°F) Additionally, physical and chemical stability has been demonstrated in non-PVC bags up to 48 hours when stored between 2–8°C (36–46°F)
DOCEtaxel Injection (Hospira, Inc.)	NDC 0409-0201-02 NDC 0409-0201-10 NDC 0409-0201-20	Stable for 4 hours (inclusive of infusion time) if stored between 2–25°C (36–77°F)
DOCEtaxel Injection (Sandoz)	NDC 66758-050-01 NDC 66758-050-02 NDC 66758-050-03	Stable for 4 hours (inclusive of infusion time) if stored between 2–25°C (36–77°F). Do not freeze infusion solution
DOCEtaxel injection, concentrate (Accord Healthcare, Inc)	NDC 16729-267-63 NDC 16729-267-64 NDC 16729-267-65	Stable for 6 hours (inclusive of infusion time) if stored between 2–25°C (36–77°F) Additionally, physical and chemical stability has been demonstrated in non-PVC bags up to 48 hours when stored between 2–8°C (36–46°F)

- *Caution:* Product labeling for all of the above product formulations except those distributed by Accord Healthcare, Inc. include a warning about product stability after dilution:
  - DOCEtaxel infusion solution is supersaturated; therefore, over time, crystals may appear in solution
  - Solutions in which crystals or particulate matter appear should not be used but should be discarded

Recommendations for Drug Administration and Ancillary Care

Premedication:
- See Chapter 43 for recommended use in patients with renal and hepatic dysfunction
- FDA-approved product labeling recommends that all patients who are treated with DOCEtaxel should receive a steroid before, during, and after DOCEtaxel administration to reduce the incidence and severity of fluid retention and the severity of hypersensitivity reactions
  - For patients with hormone-refractory metastatic prostate cancer already receiving predniSONE concurrently:
    - **Dexamethasone** 8 mg/dose for 3 doses, at 12 hours, 3 hours, and 1 hour before DOCEtaxel administration
  - Other patients:
    - **Dexamethasone** 8 mg orally twice daily for 3 days (6 doses), starting 1 day before DOCEtaxel administration

General:
- Visually inspect the infusion product for particulate matter or discoloration prior to administration. All DOCEtaxel-containing solutions that are not clear or appear to contain a precipitate should be discarded

- Administer DOCEtaxel by intraVENous infusion over one hour at ambient room temperature (<25°C; <77°F) and lighting conditions
- To minimize patient exposure to phthalate plasticizers (eg, DEHP), which may be leached from PVC containers and administration sets, administer DOCEtaxel *only* through polyethylene-lined administration sets

Potential drug interactions:
- DOCEtaxel is a substrate for metabolism by CYP3A4 and for extracellular transport by P-glycoprotein (MDR1, ABCB1)
  - Avoid concomitant use of DOCEtaxel with potent inhibitors and inducers of CYP3A subfamily enzymes and P-glycoprotein

Hypersensitivity reactions:
- Patients should be observed closely for hypersensitivity reactions, especially during the first and second infusions
  - Hypersensitivity reactions may occur within a few minutes after initiating DOCEtaxel administration

- Severe hypersensitivity reactions characterized by generalized rash/erythema, hypotension and/or bronchospasm, or very rarely fatal anaphylaxis, have been reported in patients who received steroid premedication
  - Severe hypersensitivity reactions require immediate discontinuation of the DOCEtaxel administration and aggressive supportive therapy
  - Patients with a history of severe hypersensitivity reactions should not be rechallenged with DOCEtaxel
- Minor events, including flushing, rash with or without pruritus, chest tightness, back pain, dyspnea, drug fever, or chills, have been reported and resolved after discontinuing DOCEtaxel administration and instituting appropriate therapy
- Treatment interruption is not required for minor reactions such as flushing or localized skin reactions

DOXORUBICIN HYDROCHLORIDE

ADRIAMYCIN (doxorubicin hydrochloride) prescribing information. Eatontown, NJ: West-Ward Pharmaceuticals; December 2018
ADRIAMYCIN (doxorubicin hydrochloride) prescribing information. Eatontown, NJ: West-Ward Pharmaceuticals; March 2018

WARNING: CARDIOMYOPATHY, SECONDARY MALIGNANCIES, EXTRAVASATION AND TISSUE NECROSIS, and SEVERE MYELOSUPPRESSION

- Cardiomyopathy: Myocardial damage, including acute left ventricular failure can occur with doxorubicin. The risk of cardiomyopathy is proportional to the cumulative exposure with incidences from 1% to 20% for cumulative doses from 300 mg/m^2 to 500 mg/m^2 when doxorubicin is administered every 3 weeks. The risk of cardiomyopathy is further increased with concomitant cardiotoxic therapy. Assess LVEF before and regularly during and after treatment with doxorubicin …
- Secondary Malignancies: Secondary acute myelogenous leukemia (AML) and myelodysplastic syndrome (MDS) occur at a higher incidence in patients treated with anthracyclines, including doxorubicin …
- Extravasation and Tissue Necrosis: Extravasation of doxorubicin can result in severe local tissue injury and necrosis requiring wide excision of the affected area and skin grafting. Immediately terminate the drug, and apply ice to the affected area …
- Severe myelosuppression resulting in serious infection, septic shock, requirement for transfusions, hospitalization, and death may occur …

Boxed Warning (excerpt) for ADRIAMYCIN (doxorubicin hydrochloride) prescribing information. Eatontown, NJ: West-Ward Pharmaceuticals; December 2018

Product Identification, Preparation, Storage, and Stability

- **DOXOrubicin Hydrochloride for Injection, USP** (ADRIAMYCIN for injection, USP; West-Ward Pharmaceuticals), is a sterile, red-orange, lyophilized powder packaged in single-dose vials as follows:

Content DOXOrubicin HCl	No. Vials/Package Unit	NDC No.
10 mg/vial	Individually boxed	0143-9275-01
50 mg/vial	Individually boxed	0143-9277-01

- Store intact vials (unreconstituted drug product) at room temperature, 20–25°C (68–77°F) in the packaging carton to protect them from light
- Reconstitute the lyophilized powder with 0.9% NS as follows to produce a final concentration of 2 mg DOXOrubicin HCl/mL:

DOXOrubicin HCl Content per Vial	Diluent (0.9% NS) Volume
10 mg	5 mL
50 mg	25 mL

- After adding the diluent, vials should be shaken and the contents allowed to dissolve
- After initially entering a sealed vial, DOXOrubicin solution is stable for 7 days at room temperature and under normal room light (100 foot-candles) and for 15 days at 2–8°C (35.6–46.4°F). Protect DOXOrubicin from exposure to sunlight. Promptly discard partially used vials
- Storage of reconstituted vials under refrigeration can result in the formation of a gelled product which can be returned to a slightly viscous, mobile solution after placement at controlled room temperature for 2–4 hours
- One hundred twenty-four days after reconstitution to a concentration of 2 mg/mL and storage in the manufacturer's original glass vials at 4°C (39.2°F) and 23°C (73.4°F), DOXOrubicin retained >90% of its initial concentration, remained clear, and had exhibited no changes in pH or absorbance by ultraviolet-visible spectrophotometry[37]
  - Mass balance analysis indicated approximately 3.5% of DOXOrubicin stored at 23°C and about 1% stored at 4°C had degraded at 124 days after reconstitution[37]
- Protect DOXOrubicin from exposure to sunlight. Promptly discard partially used vials

(continued)

Product Identification, Preparation, Storage, and Stability (*continued*)

- **DOXOrubicin hydrochloride injection, USP**, is available from several manufacturers. The products contain a red-orange, sterile, isotonic solution with a concentration of 2 mg DOXOrubicin HCl/mL. Products may be packaged individually or are sold in cartons containing multiple vials:

DOXOrubicin HCl Content
10 mg in 5 mL, single-dose vials
20 mg in 10 mL, single-dose vials
50 mg in 25 mL, single-dose vials
150 mg in 75 mL, multiple-dose vials
200 mg in 100 mL, multiple-dose vials

  - Store vials under refrigeration at 2–8°C (36–46°F) in their packaging carton to protect them from light
    - Storage of DOXOrubicin HCl solution for injection under refrigeration can result in the formation of a gelled product. The gelled product will return to a slightly viscous to mobile solution after 2 hours to a maximum of 4 hours equilibration at controlled room temperature 15–30°C (59–86°F)
    - After preparing a single dose, discard any unused portion of products formulated for a single use
    - Unused solution remaining in multidose containers should be discarded after the recommended storage times
- DOXOrubicin HCl Injection (2 mg/mL) and DOXOrubicin HCl for Injection after reconstitution (2 mg/mL) are suitable for intraVENous injection but may also be diluted for administration to patients
  - Dilution in 0.9% NS, D5W, or LRI to concentrations as low as 0.01 mg/mL results in products stable for at least 24 hours when stored at room temperature under fluorescent lighting or in the dark
    - DOXOrubicin stability is inversely related to solution concentration
  - DOXOrubicin has been shown to adsorb to PVC containers
    - The proportion of a dose lost to sorption may be expected to vary inversely with the surface area of a container with which the drug is in contact
    - The concentration of DOXOrubicin diluted with 0.9% NS (estimated concentration, 95.2 µg/mL) stored in 100-mL-capacity PVC containers at 4°C was shown to decrease over a period of 8 days, possibly representing initial adsorption to container surfaces followed by a protracted absorption and migration into the container matrix before equilibration was achieved, or adsorption of DOXOrubicin degradation products to container surfaces similar to the parent compound[35]
      - Loss of DOXOrubicin due to adsorption was (1) greater from solutions in which the vehicle solution was 0.9% NS in comparison with D5W, and (2) greatest at higher storage temperatures (25°C > 4°C > –20°C), and (3) greater at solution pH of 5.20 and 6.47 (0.9% NS) than at pH of 4.36 (D5W) at all temperature conditions evaluated
  - DOXOrubicin HCl solutions (estimated concentration, 95.2 µg/mL) stored in PVC containers at 25°C, 4°C, or –20°C was more stable at more acidic solution pH under the conditions of pH evaluated (4.36, 5.20, and 6.47)[35]
  - DOXOrubicin HCl for injection reconstituted with SWFI and diluted with 0.9% NS or D5W to an estimated concentration of 95.2 µg/mL stored in PVC containers for 43 days did not degrade during or after 11 repeated cycles of freezing (–20°C) and thawing at ambient temperature (25°C)[35]
  - DOXOrubicin HCl for injection reconstituted with SWFI to a concentration of 2 mg/mL was stable for at least 43 days when stored in polypropylene syringes at 4°C[35]

(continued)

Recommendations for Drug Administration and Ancillary Care

General:
- See Chapter 43 for recommended use in patients with hepatic dysfunction
- Administer DOXOrubicin by slow intraVENous injection into the tubing of a freely running intraVENous infusion of 0.9% NS or D5W. The tubing should be attached to a needle or cannula inserted preferably into a large vein. If possible, avoid veins over joints and in extremities with compromised venous or lymphatic drainage
- The rate of administration is dependent on vein size and DOXOrubicin dosage, but a dose should be administered over not less than 3–5 minutes
- *Caution:* DOXOrubicin is a powerful vesicant and can produce severe local soft tissue necrosis if extravasation occurs. DOXOrubicin *must not be given* by the intraMUSCular, SUBCUTaneous, or intraTHECAL routes
  - The current standard of care for managing anthracycline extravasation, including extravasation of DOXOrubicin, is a 3-day course of intraVENously administered dexrazoxane (Totect)
- Erythematous streaking along a vein as well as facial flushing may indicate an administration rate that is too rapid. Burning or stinging sensations may be indicative of perivenous infiltration and the infusion should be immediately terminated, and, if resumed, restarted in another vein. Extravasation may also occur painlessly

Inadvertent exposure:
- DOXOrubicin HCl spills and leaks on environmental surfaces should be treated with dilute sodium hypochlorite (1% available chlorine) solution, preferably by soaking, and then rinsing with water
- In case of skin contact, thoroughly wash the affected area with soap and water or sodium bicarbonate solution. *Do not abrade* the skin by using a scrub brush
- Treat accidental contact with the eyes immediately by copious lavage with water

Product Identification, Preparation, Storage, and Stability (*continued*)

- DOXOrubicin solutions undergo photodegradation
  - The rate and extent of photodegradation are inversely related to DOXOrubicin concentrations in solution[36] and directly related to solution pH (rate of degradation increases at pH >5.0)[35]
  - At DOXOrubicin concentrations ≥100 µg/mL (≥0.1 mg/mL) stored at 25°C for 168 h under artificial room lighting (four 65/80-watt fluorescent tubes mounted approximately 1 m above the samples), little or no photodegradation occurred in clear or amber glass or opaque polyethylene containers[36]
    - A 10-fold difference in lability to photodegradation was demonstrated for DOXOrubicin at a concentration of 0.01 mg/mL than a concentration of 0.1 mg/mL
  - At DOXOrubicin concentrations ≥500 µg/mL (0.5 mg/mL), no special precautions are necessary to protect freshly prepared solutions from exposure to artificial light or sunlight[36]

Selected incompatibility:

- Antimicrobially preserved diluents are not recommended for use in reconstituting DOXOrubicin for injection (lyophilized powder formulations)
- *Do not mix* DOXOrubicin with heparin or fluorouracil. The admixtures are incompatible and will precipitate
- *Do not mix* DOXOrubicin with alkaline solutions (eg, solutions containing sodium bicarbonate), which may cause hydrolytic degradation of DOXOrubicin

DOXORUBICIN HYDROCHLORIDE LIPOSOME INJECTION

DOXIL (doxorubicin hydrochloride liposome injection) prescribing information. Deerfield, IL: Baxter Healthcare Corporation; August 2019
Doxorubicin Hydrochloride Liposome Injection prescribing information. Cranbury, NJ: Sun Pharmaceutical Industries, Inc.; May 2020

WARNING: CARDIOMYOPATHY and INFUSION-RELATED REACTIONS

- Doxorubicin hydrochloride liposome injection can cause myocardial damage, including acute left ventricular failure. The risk of cardiomyopathy was 11% when the cumulative anthracycline dose was between 450 mg/m2 to 550 mg/m2. Assess left ventricular cardiac function prior to initiation of doxorubicin hydrochloride liposome injection and during and after treatment …
- Serious, life-threatening, and fatal infusion-related reactions can occur with doxorubicin hydrochloride liposome injection. Acute infusion-related reactions occurred in 11% of patients with solid tumors. Withhold doxorubicin hydrochloride liposome injection for infusion-related reactions and resume at a reduced rate. Discontinue doxorubicin hydrochloride liposome injection infusion for serious or life-threatening infusion-related reactions …

Boxed Warning for Doxorubicin Hydrochloride Liposome Injection prescribing information. Cranbury, NJ: Sun Pharmaceutical Industries, Inc.; May 2020

Product Identification, Preparation, Storage, and Stability

Characteristics common to both products:
- Both products contain DOXOrubicin HCl, >90% of which is encapsulated in a proprietary liposome carrier
  - Both products are sometimes referred to as liposomal DOXOrubicin and "PEGylated DOXOrubicin," because the microscopic liposomes in which DOXOrubicin is encapsulated are formulated with surface-bound methoxypolyethylene glycol, which protects the liposomes from detection by the mononuclear phagocyte system and increases the circulation time in blood
- DOXOrubicin HCl liposome injection is a translucent, red, liposomal dispersion; it is neither clear nor a solution
- Store unopened vials at 2–8°C (36–46°F)
  - DOXOrubicin HCl liposome injection does not contain any antimicrobial preservatives or bacteriostatic agents
- Avoid freezing DOXOrubicin HCl liposome injection. Prolonged freezing may adversely affect liposomal drug products
  - Freezing for periods <1 month does not appear to adversely affect DOXOrubicin HCl liposome injection

- Dilute DOXOrubicin HCl liposome injection with D5W before administration as follows:

Note: Do not dilute DOXOrubicin HCl liposome injection with any solution other than D5W

Dose to Administer	Volume of D5W for Dilution
≤90 mg	250 mL
>90 mg	500 mL

- After dilution, the products will not clarify, but remain a translucent, red, liposomal dispersion
- After dilution, liposomal DOXOrubicin should be refrigerated (2–8°C) and used within 24 hours
- *Do not filter* liposomal DOXOrubicin either before or after dilution
- Available products (brand name and several generics) include individually packaged vials containing DOXOrubicin HCl at a concentration of 2 mg/mL. Two presentations are available:
  - 20 mg DOXOrubicin HCl/10 mL in glass, single-use vials, and
  - 50 mg DOXOrubicin HCl/25 mL in glass, single-use vials

Characteristics common to all products:
- Each milliliter of both products also contains ammonium sulfate (approximately) 0.6 mg, histidine as a buffer, sucrose to maintain isotonicity, and hydrochloric acid and/or sodium hydroxide to maintain a pH of 6.5
- The pegylated liposome carriers are composed of cholesterol 3.19 mg/mL, fully hydrogenated soy phosphatidylcholine (HSPC) 9.58 mg/mL, and *N*-(carbonyl-methoxypolyethylene glycol 2000)-1,2-distearoyl-sn-glycero-3-phosphoethanolamine sodium salt (MPEG-DSPE) 3.19 mg/mL

Selected incompatibilities (both products):
- *Do not mix* liposomal DOXOrubicin with other drugs
- *Do not mix* liposomal DOXOrubicin with solutions that contain a bacteriostatic agent, such as benzyl alcohol

Recommendations for Drug Administration and Ancillary Care

General:

- See Chapter 43 for recommended use in patients with hepatic dysfunction
- Liposomal DOXOrubicin must be diluted before administration
- Administer liposomal DOXOrubicin by intraVENous infusion:
  - Give doses ≤60 mg over 60 minutes
  - Doses >60 mg should initially be administered no more rapidly than 1 mg/minute (60 mg/hour) to minimize the risk of adverse reactions during infusion
  - If no reactions are observed, the delivery rate may be increased to complete administration over one hour
  - Infusion reactions may respond to slowing the rate of administration or temporarily interrupting treatment, and resuming administration at a slower rate after signs and symptoms abate
    - Infusion-related adverse events have included life-threatening and fatal allergic or anaphylactoid reactions

- Infusion-related adverse events have included one or more of the following:
  - Flushing, shortness of breath, facial swelling, headache, chills, chest pain, back pain, chest and throat tightness, fever, tachycardia, pruritus, rash, cyanosis, syncope, bronchospasm, asthma, apnea, hypotension
- *Do not filter* liposomal DOXOrubicin during administration
- *Do not rapidly flush* an administration set used to administer liposomal DOXOrubicin to complete drug delivery
  - Utilize a technique to empty an administration set containing liposomal DOXOrubicin that will not substantially increase the rate at which the dose was being administered
- *Caution:* liposomal DOXOrubicin has been associated with vesicant reactions after extravasation and may produce severe local necrosis if infiltration into soft tissues occurs[38]

- Extravasation may occur during intraVENous administration with or without an accompanying stinging or burning sensation, and in spite of easy blood aspiration (good blood return) from the vascular access device through which liposomal DOXOrubicin is administered
- If signs or symptoms of extravasation occur during liposomal DOXOrubicin administration, the infusion should be immediately discontinued at the affected access site, but may be restarted in another vein
  - Liposomal DOXOrubicin *must never be given* by the intraMUSCular or SUBCUTaneous routes

Note:
- Advise patients that liposomal DOXOrubicin after treatment may impart a reddish-orange color to urine and other body fluids, a nontoxic reaction due to the color of the product that will dissipate as the drug is eliminated from the body

DURVALUMAB

IMFINZI (durvalumab) prescribing information. Wilmington, DE: AstraZeneca Pharmaceuticals LP; June 2020

Product Identification, Preparation, Storage, and Stability

- IMFINZI is a sterile, clear to opalescent, colorless to slightly yellow preservative-free solution in individually boxed single-dose vials that contain either 120 mg of durvalumab in 2.4 mL (NDC 0310-4500-12) or 500 mg of durvalumab in 10 mL (NDC 0310-4611-50). Each mL of the above solutions contains durvalumab (50 mg), L-histidine (2 mg), L-histidine hydrochloride monohydrate (2.7 mg), α, α-trehalose dihydrate (104 mg), Polysorbate 80 (0.2 mg) and SWFI
- Store intact vials under refrigeration at 2–8°C (36–46°F) in original carton to protect from light

- Do not freeze or shake intact vials

Dilution:

- Visibly inspect drug product for particulate matter and discoloration prior to administration. Discard the vial if the solution is cloudy or discolored, or if visible particles are observed
- Withdraw the required volume from the vial(s) of durvalumab and transfer to an intraVENous bag containing 0.9% NS or D5W to a final concentration of 1 to 15 mg/mL

- Mix by gentle inversion. Do not shake. Do not freeze
- Diluted solution should be used immediately. If not administered immediately, the total time from vial puncture to the start of administration should not exceed 24 hours in a refrigerator at 2–8°C (36–46°F) or 8 hours at room temperature 25°C (77°F)

Selected incompatibility:

- Do not co-administer other drugs through the same infusion line

Recommendations for Drug Administration and Ancillary Care

General:

- The effect of severe renal impairment (CrCl 15–29 mL/min), moderate hepatic impairment (bilirubin > 1.5 to 3 × ULN and any AST), or severe hepatic impairment (bilirubin > 3 × ULN and any AST) on the PK of durvalumab is unknown

Administration:

- The recommended dose of durvalumab is 10 mg/kg every 2 weeks for urothelial carcinoma or unresectable stage III non-small cell lung cancer
- The recommended dose of durvalumab is 1500 mg (fixed dose) in combination with chemotherapy every 3 weeks for 4 cycles, followed by 1500 mg (fixed dose) every 4 weeks as a single agent for extensive stage small cell lung cancer
  - Note if patients have a body weight of <30 kg, they must receive weight-based dosing of durvalumab 20 mg/kg

- Administer durvalumab prior to chemotherapy when given on the same day
- Administer intraVENously over 60 minutes through an intraVENous line containing a sterile, low-protein-binding 0.2- or 0.22-μm inline filter

Adverse events and treatment modifications:

- Immune-mediated adverse events can occur with durvalumab. Some of these adverse events can be severe or life-threatening
- Refer to the current FDA-approved label for detailed warnings and recommendations regarding treatment modifications for pneumonitis, hepatitis, colitis or diarrhea, hyperthyroidism or thyroiditis, adrenal insufficiency, hypophysitis/hypopituitarism, type 1 diabetes mellitus, nephritis, rash or dermatitis, infection, other G ≥3 immune-mediated adverse reactions and persistent G2 or G3 adverse reaction (excluding endocrinopathies)

- Permanently discontinue atezolizumab if unable to reduce steroid dose for adverse reactions to ≤10 mg prednisone per day (or equivalent) within 12 weeks after last dose
- Durvalumab can cause severe or life-threatening infusion-related reactions. In clinical trials enrolling 1889 patients with various cancers, infusion-related reactions occurred in 2.2% including Grade 3 (0.3%)
  - Monitor patients for signs and symptoms of infusion-related reactions. Interrupt, slow the rate of, or permanently discontinue durvalumab based on the severity. For Grade 1 or 2 infusion-related reactions, consider using premedications with subsequent doses

ELOTUZUMAB

EMPLICITI (elotuzumab) prescribing information. Princeton, NJ: Bristol-Myers Squibb Company; October 2019

Product Identification, Preparation, Storage, and Stability

- EMPLICITI (elotuzumab) is supplied as a sterile, nonpyrogenic, preservative-free, white to off-white, lyophilized powder cake in individually boxed single-use vials:
  - NDC 0003-2291-11 contains elotuzumab (300 mg) along with the following inactive ingredients: citric acid monohydrate (2.44 mg), polysorbate 80 (3.4 mg), sodium citrate (16.6 mg), and sucrose (510 mg)
  - NDC 0003-4522-11 contains elotuzumab (400 mg) along with the following inactive ingredients: citric acid monohydrate (3.17 mg), polysorbate 80 (4.4 mg), sodium citrate (21.5 mg), and sucrose (660 mg)
- Store intact vials at 2–8°C (36–46°F) in the original carton to protect from light until the time of use. Do not freeze or shake

Reconstitution:
- Using a sterile syringe of an appropriate volume and ≤18-gauge needle, reconstitute each 300-mg vial with 13 mL SWFI and each 400-mg vial with 17 mL SWFI yielding solutions with a post-reconstitution concentration of 25 mg/mL elotuzumab

- Note that each vial contains overfill to allow for withdrawal of 12 mL (300 mg) and 16 mL (400 mg), respectively
- Note that it is normal to experience a slight back pressure during injection of SWFI
- Gently swirl the solution by rotating the vial in an upright position to dissolve the lyophilized cake. Invert the vial a few times to dissolve any powder that may be deposited on top of the vial or stopper. Avoid vigorous agitation. *DO NOT* shake. Dissolution of the lyophilized powder should occur in <10 minutes
- After the remaining solids are completely dissolved, allow the reconstituted solution to stand for 5–10 minutes, resulting in a colorless to slightly yellow, clear to slightly opalescent solution. Discard the solution if any particulate matter or discoloration is observed

Dilution:
- Withdraw the required volume for the individual patient's dose from each vial, up to a maximum of 16 mL from each 400 mg vial and 12 mL from each 300 mg vial

- Further dilute with a sufficient volume of either 0.9% NS or D5W into an infusion bag made of polyvinyl chloride or polyolefin such that the final infusion concentration falls within the range of 1 mg/mL and 6 mg/mL and that the volume of diluent (0.9% NS or D5W) does not exceed 5 mL/kg of patient weight
- The elotuzumab infusion should be completed within 24 hours from the reconstitution of the elotuzumab lyophilized powder. If the final diluted product is not used immediately, it may be stored at 2–8°C (36–46°F) and protected from light for up to 24 hours (a maximum of 8 hours of the total 24 hours can be at room temperature, 20–25°C [68–77°F] and room light)

Selected incompatibility:
- Do not mix elotuzumab with, or administer as an infusion with, other medicinal products

Recommendations for Drug Administration and Ancillary Care

Administration and Concomitant Medications:
- Refer to the following tables for details regarding elotuzumab dosing, schedule, premedications, and concomitant therapy for current FDA-approved indications

Recommended Dosing Schedule of Elotuzumab in Combination with Lenalidomide and Dexamethasone								
Cycle	28-Day Cycles 1 and 2				28-Day Cycles 3+			
Day of Cycle	1	8	15	22	1	8	15	22
Premedication*	✓	✓	✓	✓	✓		✓	
Elotuzumab (mg/kg) IV	10	10	10	10	10		10	
Lenalidomide (25 mg) orally	Days 1–21				Days 1–21			
Dexamethasone† (mg) orally	28	28	28	28	28	40	28	40
Dexamethasone‡ (mg) IV	8	8	8	8	8		8	

*Premedicate with the following 45 to 90 minutes prior to elotuzumab infusion: 8 mg IV dexamethasone, H1 blocker: diphenhydrAMINE (25 to 50 mg orally or intraVENously) or equivalent; H2 blocker: raNITIdine (50 mg IV) or equivalent; acetaminophen (650 to 1000 mg orally)
†Oral dexamethasone (28 mg) taken between 3 and 24 hours before elotuzumab infusion
‡IV dexamethasone 45–90 minutes before elotuzumab infusion
IV, intraVENous

(continued)

Recommendations for Drug Administration and Ancillary Care (*continued*)

Recommended Dosing Schedule of Elotuzumab in Combination with Pomalidomide and Dexamethasone

Day of cycle	28-Day Cycles 1 and 2				28-Day Cycles 3+			
	1	**8**	**15**	**22**	**1**	**8**	**15**	**22**
Premedication*	✓	✓	✓	✓	✓			
Elotuzumab (mg/kg) IV	10	10	10	10	20			
Pomalidomide (4 mg) orally	Days 1–21				Days 1–21			
Dexamethasone† (mg) orally ≤75 years old	28	28	28	28	28	40	40	40
Dexamethasone† (mg) orally >75 years old	8	8	8	8	8	20	20	20
Dexamethasone‡ (mg) IV	8	8	8	8	8			

*Premedicate with the following 45 to 90 minutes prior to elotuzumab infusion: 8 mg IV dexamethasone, H1 blocker: diphenhydrAMINE (25 to 50 mg orally or IV) or equivalent; H2 blocker: raNITIdine (50 mg IV) or equivalent; acetaminophen (650 to 1000 mg orally)
†Oral dexamethasone taken between 3 and 24 hours before elotuzumab infusion
‡IV dexamethasone 45–90 minutes before elotuzumab infusion
IV, intraVENous

Elotuzumab Infusion Instructions

Elotuzumab 10 mg/kg	First infusion	Infuse initially at 0.5 mL/min (30 mL/hour) for the first 30 minutes. If tolerated, increase to 1 mL/min (60 mL/hour) for 30 minutes. If tolerated, increase to 2 mL/min (120 mL/hour) for the remainder of the infusion
	Second infusion	Infuse initially at 3 mL/min (180 mL/hour) for the first 30 minutes. If tolerated, increase to 4 mL/min (240 mL/hour) for the remainder of the infusion
	Third and subsequent infusions	Infuse at 5 mL/min (300 mL/hour) for the entire infusion
Elotuzumab 20 mg/kg	First infusion (of 20 mg/kg dose)	Infuse at 3 mL/min (180 mL/hour) for the first 30 minutes. If tolerated, increase to 4 mL/min (240 mL/hour) for the remainder of the infusion
	Second and subsequent infusions (of 20 mg/kg dose)	Infuse at 5 mL/min (300 mL/hour) for the entire infusion

Note:
- Administer elotuzumab intraVENously using an automated infusion pump through an administration set that contains a sterile, nonpyrogenic, low-protein-binding inline filter with pore size within the range of 0.2–1.2 μm
- Elotuzumab can cause severe infusion-related reactions. Symptoms may include fever, chills, hypertension or hypotension, and bradycardia. The incidence of infusion-related reactions in the ELOQUENT-2 study was 10% and in the ELOQUENT-3 study was 3.3%

Adverse events and treatment modifications:

- If the dose of one drug in the regimen is delayed, interrupted, or discontinued, the treatment with the other drugs may continue as scheduled. However, if dexamethasone is delayed or discontinued, then base the decision on whether to administer elotuzumab on clinical judgment with regard to the risk of hypersensitivity reaction

Adverse Event	Treatment Modification
G1 infusion-related reaction	Continue elotuzumab infusion and provide supportive care. Monitor vital signs every 30 minutes during the infusion and for 2 hours after infusion completion
G2–4 infusion-related reactions	Interrupt elotuzumab infusion and provide supportive care. Consider permanent discontinuation of elotuzumab and emergency care for severe reactions. Monitor vital signs every 30 minutes during the infusion and for 2 hours after infusion completion. Upon resolution to G≤1, resume elotuzumab infusion at 0.5 mL/min (30 mL/hour) and gradually increase the infusion rate every 30 minutes, as tolerated, in increments of 0.5 mL/min (30 mL/hour) until the rate at which the infusion-related reaction occurred is reached. In the absence of a recurrent infusion-related reaction, continue the standard dose escalation regimen as described in the FDA-approved product label. If the infusion-related reaction recurs, discontinue the remainder of the elotuzumab infusion for that day
G ≥3 elevation of liver enzymes	Withhold elotuzumab. After resolution to baseline values, continuation of treatment may be considered

Potential drug-laboratory test interaction:

Elotuzumab is a humanized IgG kappa monoclonal antibody that can be detected on both the serum protein electrophoresis and immunofixation assays used in the monitoring of multiple myeloma patients

ENFORTUMAB VEDOTIN-ejfv

PADCEV (enfortumab vedotin-ejfv) prescribing information. Bothell, WA: Seattle Genetics, Inc; December 2019

Product Identification, Preparation, Storage, and Stability

- Enfortumab vedotin-ejfv is an antibody drug conjugate composed of a fully human anti-Nectin-4 IgG1 kappa monoclonal antibody conjugated to the small molecule microtubule disrupting agent monomethyl auristatin E (MMAE) by a cleavable linker
- PADCEV (enfortumab vedotin-ejfv) for injection is supplied as a sterile, white to off-white, preservative-free, lyophilized powder in individually boxed single-use vials containing either 20 mg (NDC 51144-020-01) or 30 mg (NDC 51144-030-01) of enfortumab vedotin-ejfv
  - The reconstituted products contain a solution of enfortumab vedotin-ejfv (10 mg/mL) plus histidine (1.4 mg/mL), histidine hydrochloride monohydrate (2.31 mg/mL), polysorbate 20 (0.2mg/mL), and trehalose dihydrate (55 mg/mL). The pH is approximately 6.0
- Store intact vials at 2–8°C (36–46°F) in the original carton. Do not freeze or shake
- Enfortumab vedotin-ejfv is a cytotoxic drug. Follow applicable special handling and disposal procedures. During all reconstitution and preparation steps, use appropriate aseptic technique

Reconstitution
- Calculate a dose based on the patient's weight to determine the number and strength of PADCEV vials required. *Caution:* a dose for patients weighing >100 kg should be calculated based on a weight of 100 kg
- Reconstitute each 20 mg vial with 2.3 mL of SWFI and reconstitute each 30 mg vial with 3.3 mL of SWFI to produce solution(s) containing 10 mg/mL enfortumab vedotin-ejfv. Direct the stream of SWFI toward the vial wall, when possible, and not directly into the drug product
- Slowly swirl each vial until the contents are completely dissolved, then allow the reconstituted vial(s) to settle for at least 1 minute until bubbles have disappeared. *Do not shake* a vial to aid dissolution. Do not expose to direct sunlight
- The reconstituted solution should be clear to slightly opalescent, colorless to light yellow, and free of visible particulates. Discard any vial with visible particulates or discoloration
- Following reconstitution, dilute enfortumab vedotin-ejfv immediately, or store the solution at 2–8°C and use it within 4 hours after reconstitution. *Do not freeze* enfortumab vedotin-ejfv. Discard any unused vials with reconstituted solution beyond the recommended storage time

Dilution
- Withdraw the calculated dose amount of reconstituted enfortumab vedotin-ejfv solution (10 mg/mL) from the vial(s) and transfer into an infusion bag
- Dilute enfortumab vedotin-ejfv with a sufficient volume of 0.9% NS, D5W, or LRI to achieve a final diluted concentration within the range 0.3–4 mg/mL enfortumab vedotin-ejfv
- Mix the diluted solution by gentle inversion yielding a clear to slightly opalescent, colorless to light yellow solution. *Do not shake the bag.* Do not expose to direct sunlight
- Prior to administration, inspect the diluted infusion solution for discoloration and particulate matter. Do not use the product if it contains visible particles or if discoloration is observed
- Following dilution, administer enfortumab vedotin-ejfv immediately, or store the diluted solution at 2–8°C and use the product within 8 hours. *Do not freeze* enfortumab vedotin-ejfv

Selected incompatibility:
- *DO NOT* mix enfortumab vedotin-ejfv with, or administer as an infusion with, other medicinal products

Recommendations for Drug Administration and Ancillary Care

General:
- Dose adjustment is not required for patients with mild, moderate, or severe renal impairment, or in patients with mild (Child-Pugh A) hepatic impairment. Although enfortumab vedotin-ejfv has not been evaluated in patients with moderate (Child-Pugh B) or severe (Child-Pugh C) hepatic impairment, another antibody drug conjugate containing MMAE, brentuximab vedotin, was associated with a higher rate of adverse events in this population. Therefore, the use of enfortumab vedotin is not recommended in patients with moderate or severe hepatic impairment based on extrapolated data
- See Chapter 43 for recommended use in patients with hepatic dysfunction

Administration:
- The typical dose of enfortumab vedotin-ejfv for adult patients with locally advanced or metastatic urothelial cancer is 1.25 mg/kg (up to a maximum of 125 mg for patients weighing ≥100 kg) administered as an intraVENous infusion over 30 minutes on days 1, 8, and 15 of a 28-day cycle until disease progression or unacceptable toxicity
- Ensure adequate venous access is present prior to administering enfortumab vedotin-ejfv

Concomitant medications:
- *Dry eye prophylaxis (primary prophylaxis is optional):* prescribe a **lubricating ophthalmic** solution (active and inert ingredients vary by brand); administer 2 drops by intraocular instillation into each eye 4 times per day starting with the first enfortumab vedotin-ejfv dose (if used as primary prophylaxis) or at the onset of symptoms. Advise patients to report any new onset or worsening ocular symptoms and consider ophthalmological evaluation as clinically indicated. Treatment-related dry eye events occurred in 36% of patients in clinical studies

Adverse events and treatment modifications:
- Refer to the current FDA-approved product label for detailed recommendations

(continued)

Recommendations for Drug Administration and Ancillary Care (*continued*)

regarding treatment modifications for hyperglycemia (blood glucose >250 mg/dL), peripheral neuropathy G ≥2, skin reactions G ≥3, other nonhematologic toxicities G ≥3, thrombocytopenia G ≥2, and other hematologic toxicities G ≥3.

Potential drug interactions:
- Strong CYP3A4 inhibitors may increase exposure to free MMAE which may lead to increased incidence and/or severity of toxicities. If concomitant use of a strong CYP3A4 inhibitor is unavoidable, then monitor closely for signs and symptoms of toxicity

Selected precautions:
- **Hyperglycemia:** in EV-201, 8% of patients developed G3/4 hyperglycemia and patients with baseline hemoglobin A1C ≥8% were excluded. Monitor blood glucose in patients with, or at risk for (eg, elevated body mass index or baseline A1C) diabetes mellitus or hyperglycemia. Withhold enfortumab vedotin-ejfv for blood glucose >250 mg/dL

- **Peripheral neuropathy:** peripheral neuropathy occurred in 49% of patients in clinical trials; Grade 3 reactions occurred in 2%. Monitor closely for new or worsening symptoms and consider dose interruption, dose reduction, or permanent discontinuation
- **Ocular disorders:** ocular disorders occurred in 46% of 310 patients treated with enfortumab vedotin-ejfv. The majority involved the cornea and included keratitis, blurred vision, limbal stem cell deficiency, and other events associated with dry eyes. Dry eye symptoms occurred in 36% of patients and blurry vision in 14%. Consider primary prophylaxis with artificial tears. Advise patients to report new onset or persistent ocular symptoms and refer the patient for an ophthalmic exam. Ophthalmic topical steroids may be considered following an exam. Consider dose interruption or reduction for symptomatic ocular disorders
- **Skin reactions:** skin reactions occurred in 54% of 310 patients treated with enfortumab vedotin-ejfv in clinical

trials. Twenty-six percent of patients had a maculopapular rash and 30% had pruritus. G3/4 reactions occurred in 10% of patients and included symmetrical drug-related intertriginous and flexural exanthema (SDRIFE), bullous dermatitis, exfoliative dermatitis, and palmar-plantar erythrodysesthesia. Monitor for skin reactions and consider topical steroids and antihistamines as clinically indicated. Withhold enfortumab vedotin-ejfv for G3 reactions and permanently discontinue for G4 or recurrent G3 reactions
- **Infusion site extravasation:** of 310 patients treated with enfortumab vedotin-ejfv in clinical trial, 1.3% experienced skin and soft tissue reactions characterized by erythema, swelling, increased temperature, and pain. One percent of patients developed extravasation reactions with secondary cellulitis, bullae, or exfoliation. Ensure adequate venous access is present prior to administering enfortumab vedotin-ejfv and monitor for signs and symptoms of extravasation during and following administration

EPIRUBICIN HYDROCHLORIDE

ELLENCE (epirubicin hydrochloride injection) prescribing information. New York, NY: Pharmacia & Upjohn Co., Division of Pfizer Inc.; July 2019
EPIRUBICIN HYDROCHLORIDE prescribing information. Eatontown, NJ: West-Ward Pharmaceuticals; December 2018

WARNING: CARDIAC TOXICITY, SECONDARY MALIGNANCIES, EXTRAVASATION AND TISSUE NECROSIS, and SEVERE MYELOSUPPRESSION

- **Cardiac Toxicity:** Myocardial damage, including acute left ventricular failure, can occur with [Epirubicin HCl]. The risk of cardiomyopathy is proportional to the cumulative exposure with incidence rates from 0.9% at a cumulative dose of 550 mg/m^2, 1.6% at 700 mg/m^2, and 3.3% at 900 mg/m^2. The risk of cardiomyopathy is further increased with concomitant cardiotoxic therapy. Assess left ventricular ejection fraction (LVEF) before and regularly during and after treatment with [Epirubicin HCl] …

- **Secondary Malignancies:** Secondary acute myelogenous leukemia (AML) and myelodysplastic syndrome (MDS) occur at a higher incidence in patients treated with anthracyclines, including [Epirubicin HCl] …

- **Extravasation and Tissue Necrosis:** Extravasation of [Epirubicin HCl] can result in severe local tissue injury and necrosis requiring wide excision of the affected area and skin grafting. Immediately terminate the drug and apply ice to the affected area …

- **Severe myelosuppression** resulting in serious infection, septic shock, requirement for transfusions, hospitalization, and death may occur …

Boxed Warning from ELLENCE (epirubicin hydrochloride injection) prescribing information. New York, NY: Pharmacia & Upjohn Co., Division of Pfizer Inc.; July 2019

Product Identification, Preparation, Storage, and Stability

- **EpiRUBicin HCl injection** is available in individually packaged single-use vials containing a sterile, preservative-free, ready-to-use, clear, red solution containing 2 mg epiRUBicin hydrochloride/mL
- EpiRUBicin HCl was previously commercially available as a lyophilized powder which has been discontinued
  - Product presentations include vials containing 50 mg and 200 mg epiRUBicin HCl
    - Inactive ingredients include sodium chloride, USP, and SWFI. Product pH is adjusted to 3.0 with hydrochloric acid, NF
  - Store unopened vials under refrigeration between 2° and 8°C (36° and 46°F), but *do not freeze* epiRUBicin
    - Storage at refrigerated temperatures can result in the formation of a gelled product, which will return to a slightly viscous to mobile solution after 2 hours to a maximum of 4 hours equilibration at controlled room temperature (15–25°C [59–77°F])
    - EpiRUBicin HCl for injection reconstituted with SWFI and diluted with D5W or 0.9% NS (to pH = 4.36 or 5.20, respectively) was stable for up to 43 days when stored in PVC containers at 25°C, 4°C, or –20°C (–4°F)[35]
      - EpiRUBicin HCl solutions (estimated concentration, 95.2 µg/mL) stored in PVC containers was more stable at more acidic solution pH under the conditions of pH evaluated (4.36, 5.20, and 6.47)
      - A significant loss in potency (≥10%) occurred at 20 days for epiRUBicin HCl admixtures in 0.9% NS (pH = 6.47) stored in PVC at 25°C, but not for epiRUBicin admixtures in 0.9% NS (pH = 5.20) stored in PVC at 25°C
      - EpiRUBicin HCl for injection reconstituted with SWFI and diluted with 0.9% NS or D5W to an estimated concentration of 95.2 µg/mL stored in PVC containers for 43 days did not degrade during or after 11 repeated cycles of freezing (–20°C) and thawing at ambient temperature (25°C)
      - Adsorption of epiRUBicin (diluted in D5W or 0.9% NS to a concentration of ~95.2 mg/mL) to PVC container surfaces during the 8 days after admixture preparation correlated inversely with solution pH (4.36 < 5.20 < 6.47) and directly with storage temperatures (25°C > 4°C > –20°C)[35]
        - Drug loss from PVC mini-bags appeared to be due to a combination of epiRUBicin degradation and adsorption to container surfaces
  - EpiRUBicin solutions undergo photodegradation
    - The rate and extent of photodegradation are inversely related to epiRUBicin concentrations in solution[36] and directly related to solution pH (rate of degradation increases at pH >5.0)[35]
      - At epiRUBicin concentrations ≥100 µg/mL (≥0.1 mg/mL) stored at 25°C for 168 h under artificial room lighting (four 65/80-watt fluorescent tubes mounted approximately 1 m above the samples), little or no photodegradation occurred in clear or amber glass or opaque polyethylene containers[36]
      - At epiRUBicin concentrations ≥500 µg/mL (0.5 mg/mL), no special precautions are necessary to protect freshly prepared solutions from exposure to artificial light or sunlight[36]
- EpiRUBicin HCl solution is suitable for direct intraVENous administration
- Use epiRUBicin HCl solution within 24 hours after first penetrating vial stoppers
- Discard partially used vials after dose preparation

Selected incompatibility:

- *Do not mix* epiRUBicin with other drugs in the same container
- EpiRUBicin is most stable at pH 4–5, and hydrolyzes spontaneously at alkaline pH
- EpiRUBicin is chemically incompatible with heparin and fluorouracil

Recommendations for Drug Administration and Ancillary Care

General:

- See Chapter 43 for recommended use in patients with renal and hepatic dysfunction
- Administer epiRUBicin by slow intraVENous injection into the tubing of a freely running intraVENous infusion of 0.9% NS or D5W over 3–20 minutes, depending on the dosage to be given and vein size
- Initial therapy within a dosage range of 100–120 mg/m² should generally be administered over 15–20 minutes
  - The administration time may be proportionally decreased, for lesser dosages, but SHOULD NOT BE <3 minutes
- Do *not* inject epiRUBicin directly into a vein because of the risk of extravasation, which may occur even in the presence of adequate blood return during aspiration. Venous sclerosis may result from injection into small vessels or repeated injections into the same vein
- Avoid administration into veins over joints or in extremities with compromised venous or lymphatic drainage
- *Caution:* EpiRUBicin is a vesicant and can produce severe local soft tissue necrosis if extravasation occurs. EpiRUBicin *must not be given* by the intraMUSCular. SUBCUTaneous, or intraTHECAL routes
  - The current standard of care for managing anthracycline extravasation, including extravasation of epiRUBicin, is a 3-day course of intraVENously administered dexrazoxane (Totect)
- Erythematous streaking along the vein through which epiRUBicin is administered and facial flushing may indicate too rapid an administration rate, and may precede local phlebitis or thrombophlebitis. Burning or stinging sensations may be indicative of perivenous infiltration and the infusion should be immediately terminated and resumed in another vein. Perivenous infiltration may occur painlessly

Caution:

- Do not administer epiRUBicin in combination with other cardiotoxic agents unless the patient's cardiac function is closely monitored
  - Administering epiRUBicin after stopping treatment with other cardiotoxic agents may also increase the risk of developing cardiotoxicity
  - Avoid when possible epiRUBicin therapy for up to 24 weeks after a last dose of trastuzumab
    - Monitor cardiac function carefully if epiRUBicin is used within 24 weeks after stopping trastuzumab
  - Concomitant use of epiRUBicin with cardioactive compounds that could cause heart failure (eg, calcium channel blockers) requires close monitoring of cardiac function throughout treatment
- Coadministration of cimetidine increased epiRUBicin's mean AUC by 50% and decreased its plasma clearance by 30%
- EpiRUBicin administered immediately before or after DOCEtaxel did not affect the systemic exposure of epiRUBicin, but increased the systemic exposure (mean AUC) of epirubicinol (~10% the cytotoxic activity of epiRUBicin) and 7-deoxydoxorubicin aglycone (inactive) when DOCEtaxel was administered immediately after epiRUBicin compared to epiRUBicin alone
- EpiRUBicin had no effect on the exposure of DOCEtaxel whether it was administered before or after DOCEtaxel
- EpiRUBicin administered immediately before or after PACLitaxel increased the systemic exposure of epiRUBicin, epirubicinol, and 7-deoxydoxorubicin aglycone
  - EpiRUBicin had no effect on the exposure of PACLitaxel whether it was administered before or after PACLitaxel
- It is likely that epiRUBicin use concurrently with radiotherapy may sensitize tissues to the cytotoxic actions of irradiation
- EpiRUBicin administration after ionizing radiation therapy may induce an inflammatory recall reaction involving previously irradiated tissues

Inadvertent exposure:

- EpiRUBicin HCl spills and leaks on environmental surfaces should be treated with dilute sodium hypochlorite (1% available chlorine) solution, preferably by soaking, and then rinsing with water
- In case of skin contact, thoroughly wash the affected area with soap and water or sodium bicarbonate solution. *Do not abrade* the skin by using a scrub brush
- Treat accidental contact with the eyes immediately by copious lavage with water

ERIBULIN MESYLATE

HALAVEN (eribulin mesylate) prescribing information. Woodcliff Lake, NJ: Eisai Inc.; December 2017

Product Identification, Preparation, Storage, and Stability

- HALAVEN is a clear, colorless, sterile solution for intraVENous administration. Each vial contains 1 mg of eriBULin mesylate per 2 mL of solution (0.5 mg/mL) in ethanol:water (5:95)
- The commercial product is packaged in individually packaged single-use vials (NDC 62856-389-01)
- Store intact vials in their original cartons at 25°C (77°F). Temperature excursions are permitted to 15–30°C (59–86°F). *Do not* freeze eriBULin mesylate. Store intact vials in their original cartons
- With a syringe, withdraw a volume of eriBULin mesylate appropriate for a patient's dose
- Undiluted eriBULin mesylate is suitable for direct intraVENous administration, or the drug product may be diluted in 100 mL of 0.9% NS
- Undiluted eriBULin mesylate may be stored in a syringe for up to 4 hours at room temperature or for up to 24 hours under refrigeration 4°C (~40°F)
- Diluted solutions of eriBULin mesylate may be stored for up to 4 hours at room temperature or for up to 24 hours under refrigeration 4°C (~40°F)
- Discard partially used and empty vials

Selected incompatibility:
- *Do not dilute or administer* eriBULin mesylate through an administration set containing dextrose solutions
- *Do not administer* eriBULin mesylate through an administration set with other medications

Recommendations for Drug Administration and Ancillary Care

General:
- See Chapter 43 for recommended use in patients with renal and hepatic dysfunction
- Administer eriBULin mesylate by intraVENous injection over 2–5 minutes

Caution:
- ECG monitoring is recommended if therapy is initiated in patients with congestive heart failure, bradyarrhythmias, and drugs known to prolong the QT interval, including Class Ia and III anti-arrhythmics, and electrolyte abnormalities
- The effect of eriBULin mesylate on the QTc interval was assessed in an open-label, uncontrolled, multicenter, single-arm, dedicated QT trial. A total of 26 patients with solid tumors received eriBULin mesylate 1.4 mg/m^2 on days 1 and 8 of a 21-day cycle
  - A delayed QTc prolongation was observed on day 8, without prolongation observed on day 1
  - The maximum mean QTcF change from baseline (95% upper confidence interval) was 11.4 ms (19.5 ms; 95% upper confidence interval)
- Correct hypokalemia or hypomagnesemia prior to administering eriBULin mesylate and monitor serum potassium and magnesium periodically during therapy
- Avoid administering eriBULin mesylate to patients with congenital long QT syndrome

ETOPOSIDE

ETOPOSIDE INJECTION prescribing information. Eatontown, NJ: West-Ward Pharmaceuticals; October 2012
TOPOSAR (etoposide injection, USP) prescribing information. North Wales, PA: Teva Pharmaceuticals USA, Inc.; October 2015
Bristol-Myers Oncology Division. VePesid stability above 0.4 mg/mL. April 26, 1993

WARNINGS

[Etoposide injection] should be administered under the supervision of a qualified physician experienced in the use of cancer chemotherapeutic agents. Severe myelosuppression with resulting infection or bleeding may occur

---

Boxed Warning (excerpt) for TOPOSAR (etoposide injection, USP) prescribing information. North Wales, PA: Teva Pharmaceuticals USA, Inc.; October 2015

Product Identification, Preparation, Storage, and Stability

- Etoposide is generically available from several manufacturers. In general, etoposide injection, USP, is a viscous, clear, colorless to light yellow solution containing etoposide 20 mg/mL at pH 3–4
- Etoposide is sparingly soluble in water. Consequently, etoposide is made more miscible with water by means of organic solvent excipients, including: either polysorbate 80 or modified polysorbate 80, with polyethylene glycol 300, and dehydrated alcohol
  - Additional excipient components vary among manufacturers' products
- Available presentations include multidose vials containing 100, 500, or 1000 mg etoposide
- Store intact vials and diluted solutions at controlled room temperature of 20–25°C (68–77°F)
  - Unopened vials of etoposide injection are stable for 24 months at room temperature (25°C [77°F])
- Commercially marketed etoposide (20 mg/mL) *MUST BE DILUTED* before administration with either D5W or 0.9% NS to a concentration between 0.2 and 0.4 mg/mL in either glass or plastic containers
  - After dilution, product stability is affected by the concentration of etoposide and storage temperatures

- Solutions with concentrations >0.1 mg/mL are supersaturated and potentially may precipitate
- The time to precipitation at concentrations ≤0.4 mg/mL is unpredictable and may occur earlier than the times indicated in the following table, particularly if etoposide is stored at cool temperatures or is agitated, as may occur during administration with a peristaltic pump

Etoposide Concentration	Duration of Stability
0.1 mg/mL	96 hours
0.2 mg/mL	96 hours*
0.4 mg/mL	24–48* hours
0.6 mg/mL	8 hours
1 mg/mL	2 hours

*At 25°C (77°F), normal room fluorescent lighting, in both glass and plastic containers

Selected incompatibility:
- Devices made of acrylic or ABS plastic (acrylonitrile, butadiene, and styrene polymer) may crack and leak when used with undiluted etoposide injection

Recommendations for Drug Administration and Ancillary Care

General:
- See Chapter 43 for recommended use in patients with renal and hepatic dysfunction
- *Do not administer* etoposide by rapid intraVENous injection. Administer etoposide by intraVENous infusion over at least 30–60 minutes to prevent hypotension. Longer infusion durations may be used when clinically appropriate for the volume of fluid that must be administered

FAM-TRASTUZUMAB DERUXTECAN-nxki

ENHERTU (fam-trastuzumab deruxtecan-nxki) prescribing information. Basking Ridge, NJ: Daiichi Sankyo, Inc.; December 2019

Do Not Substitute ENHERTU for or with trastuzumab or ado-trastuzumab emtansine

WARNING: INTERSTITIAL LUNG DISEASE and EMBRYO-FETAL TOXICITY

- Interstitial Lung Disease (ILD) and pneumonitis, including fatal cases, have been reported with ENHERTU. Monitor for and promptly investigate signs and symptoms including cough, dyspnea, fever, and other new or worsening respiratory symptoms. Permanently discontinue ENHERTU in all patients with Grade 2 or higher ILD/pneumonitis. Advise patients of the risk and the need to immediately report symptoms …
- Embryo-Fetal Toxicity: Exposure to ENHERTU during pregnancy can cause embryo-fetal harm. Advise patients of these risks and the need for effective contraception …

Boxed Warning for ENHERTU (fam-trastuzumab deruxtecan-nxki) prescribing information. Basking Ridge, NJ: Daiichi Sankyo, Inc.; December 2019

Product Identification, Preparation, Storage, and Stability

- Fam-trastuzumab deruxtecan-nxki is an antibody-drug conjugate that contains a humanized anti-HER2 IgG1 monoclonal antibody, covalently linked to a topoisomerase inhibitor via a tetrapeptide-based cleavable linker
- ENHERTU (fam-trastuzumab deruxtecan-nxki) is supplied as a sterile, white to yellowish white, preservative-free, lyophilized powder in individually boxed single-use vials containing fam-trastuzumab deruxtecan-nxki (100 mg) (NDC 65597-406-01) along with the following inactive ingredients: L-histidine (4.45 mg), L-histidine hydrochloride monohydrate (20.2 mg), polysorbate 80 (1.5 mg), and sucrose (450 mg)
  - Following reconstitution with 5 mL SWFI, the reconstituted product contains a solution of fam-trastuzumab deruxtecan 20 mg/mL. The pH is 5.5
- Store intact vials at 2–8°C (36–46°F) in the original carton to protect from light until the time of reconstitution. Do not freeze. Do not shake the reconstituted or diluted solution
- Fam-trastuzumab deruxtecan is a cytotoxic drug. Follow applicable special handling and disposal procedures. During all reconstitution and preparation steps, use appropriate aseptic technique

Reconstitution:
- In order to prevent errors, check the vial labels to ensure that the drug being prepared and administered is ENHERTU (fam-trastuzumab deruxtecan) and *NOT* trastuzumab or ado-trastuzumab emtansine
- Calculate a dose based on the patient's weight to determine the number of ENHERTU (fam-trastuzumab deruxtecan) vials required and the total volume of reconstituted product solution required
- Reconstitute each 100-mg vial by using a sterile syringe to slowly inject 5 mL of SWFI into each vial to yield a final concentration of 20 mg/mL
- Slowly swirl each vial until the contents are completely dissolved. *Do not shake* a vial to aid dissolution
- The reconstituted solution should be clear and colorless to light yellow, and free of visible particulates. Discard any vial that is cloudy, discolored, or that contains visible particulates
- Following reconstitution, dilute fam-trastuzumab deruxtecan immediately, or store the solution at 2–8°C and use it within 24 hours after reconstitution. *Do not freeze* fam-trastuzumab deruxtecan. The product does not contain a preservative; discard any unused vials with reconstituted solution beyond the recommended storage time

Dilution
- Withdraw the calculated dose amount of reconstituted fam-trastuzumab deruxtecan solution (20 mg/mL) from the vial(s) and transfer into an infusion bag containing 100 mL of D5W. ENHERTU (fam-trastuzumab deruxtecan) is compatible with infusion bags made of PVC or polyolefin (copolymer of ethylene and polypropylene)
- Mix the diluted solution by gentle inversion. *Do not shake the bag.*
- Cover the infusion bag to protect from light
- Following dilution, administer fam-trastuzumab deruxtecan immediately, or store the diluted solution at either room temperature for up to 4 hours (including preparation and infusion) or in a refrigerator at 2–8°C for up to 24 hours, protected from light. *Do not freeze* fam-trastuzumab deruxtecan
- Prior to administration, inspect the diluted infusion solution for discoloration and particulate matter. Do not use the product if it contains visible particles or if discoloration or cloudiness is observed

Selected incompatibility:
- *DO NOT* mix fam-trastuzumab deruxtecan with sodium chloride injection, USP
- *DO NOT* mix fam-trastuzumab deruxtecan with other drugs or administer other drugs through the same intraVENous line

Recommendations for Drug Administration and Ancillary Care

General:

- To prevent medication errors, check the product label prior to administration to ensure that it contains ENHERTU (fam-trastuzumab deruxtecan) and *NOT* trastuzumab or ado-trastuzumab emtansine

- Dose adjustment is not required for patients with mild (CrCl ≥60 and <90 mL/min) or moderate (CrCl ≥30 and <60 mL/min) renal impairment, or in patients with mild (total bilirubin ≤ULN and any AST >ULN or total bilirubin >1 to 1.5 × ULN and any AST) or moderate (total bilirubin >1.5 to 3 × ULN and any AST) hepatic impairment. In patients with moderate hepatic impairment, monitor closely for potential increased toxicities related to the topoisomerase inhibitor, DXd. Data are insufficient to recommend a dose of fam-trastuzumab deruxtecan in patients with severe renal impairment and severe hepatic impairment (total bilirubin >3 to 10 × ULN and any AST)

- See Chapter 43 for recommended use in patients with hepatic dysfunction

Administration:

- The typical dose of fam-trastuzumab deruxtecan for adult patients with unresectable or metastatic HER2-positive breast cancer is 5.4 mg/kg administered as an intraVENous infusion on day 1 only of a 21-day cycle until disease progression or unacceptable toxicity. The first infusion is administered over 90 minutes. If prior infusion(s) were well tolerated, subsequent infusions may be administered over 30 minutes

- Administer fam-trastuzumab deruxtecan-nxki through an administration set composed of either polyolefin or polybutadiene that contains an inline polyethersulfone or polysulfone filter with pore size of either 0.20 or 0.22 μm

- *DO NOT* administer as an intraVENous push or bolus

- Slow or interrupt the infusion rate if the patient develops infusion-related symptoms

- Permanently discontinue fam-trastuzumab deruxtecan in case of severe infusion reactions

- If a planned dose is delayed or missed, administer as soon as possible; do not wait until the next planned cycle. Adjust the schedule of administration to maintain a 3-week interval between doses. Administer the infusion at the dose and rate the patient tolerated in the most recent infusion

Adverse events and treatment modifications:

- Refer to the current FDA-approved product label for detailed recommendations regarding treatment modifications (eg, temporary interruption, dose reduction, or permanent discontinuation) for infusion-related reactions, interstitial lung disease/pneumonitis (any grade), neutropenia (ANC <1000/mm³), febrile neutropenia (ANC <1000/mm³ and temperature >38.3°C or a temperature of 38°C sustained for >1 hour), symptomatic congestive heart failure, and left ventricular dysfunction

- Do not re-escalate the fam-trastuzumab deruxtecan dose after a dose reduction is made

Selected precautions:

- **Interstitial Lung Disease (ILD)/ Pneumonitis:** refer to the aforementioned black box warning. Additionally, if ILD/pneumonitis is suspected, withhold fam-trastuzumab deruxtecan while pulmonary status is clarified. Evaluate promptly with radiographic imaging and other tests as clinically indicated and consider consultation with a pulmonologist. When G1 ILD/pneumonitis is confirmed, consider corticosteroid treatment (eg, ≥0.5 mg/kg/day prednisolone or equivalent

and then gradually tapered) and withhold fam-trastuzumab deruxtecan until complete resolution then either maintain the current dose (if resolution occurs in ≤28 days from the date of onset) or reduce the dosage by 1 dose level (if resolution occurs in >28 days). If G ≥2 or higher ILD/pneumonitis is confirmed, then promptly administer corticosteroid treatment (eg, ≥1 mg/kg/day prednisolone or equivalent initially and continued until improvement, and then tapered gradually [eg, over 4 weeks]) and permanently discontinue fam-trastuzumab deruxtecan

- **Neutropenia:** severe neutropenia, including neutropenic fever, may occur with fam-trastuzumab deruxtecan. Among 234 patients in clinical trials, 16% of patients experienced Grade 3 or 4 events. Monitor complete blood counts prior to each dose

- **Left Ventricular Dysfunction:** left ventricular dysfunction has been observed in patients treated with fam-trastuzumab deruxtecan and other HER2-directed therapies. Among 234 patients in clinical trials, two cases (0.9%) of asymptomatic reductions in left ventricular ejection fraction (LVEF) were reported. Fam-trastuzumab deruxtecan has not been evaluated in patients with a history of clinically significant cardiac disease or in patients with baseline LVEF <50%. Assess LVEF prior to initiation of fam-trastuzumab deruxtecan and at regular intervals during treatment as clinically indicated

- **Embryo-Fetal Toxicity:** fam-trastuzumab deruxtecan may cause fetal harm. For female patients of reproductive potential, verify pregnancy status and advise the patient to use effective contraception during treatment and for 7 months following the last dose. Advise male patients with female partners of reproductive potential to use effective contraception during treatment and for 4 months following the last dose

FLOXURIDINE (FUDR)

FLOXURIDINE prescribing information. Eatontown, NJ: West-Ward Pharmaceuticals Corp.; January 2017
FLOXURIDINE prescribing information. Lake Zurich, IL: Fresenius Kabi USA, LLC.; August 2016

WARNING

It is recommended that floxuridine be given only by or under the supervision of a qualified physician who is experienced in cancer chemotherapy and intra-arterial drug therapy and is well versed in the use of potent antimetabolites

Because of the possibility of severe toxic reactions, all patients should be hospitalized for initiation of the first course of therapy

---

Boxed Warning for FLOXURIDINE prescribing information. Eatontown, NJ: West-Ward Pharmaceuticals Corp.; January 2017

Product Identification, Preparation, Storage, and Stability

- Floxuridine for injection USP is available generically as a sterile, nonpyrogenic, white to off-white, odorless, lyophilized powder for reconstitution packaged in individually packaged 5-mL vials containing 500 mg of floxuridine
- Intact vials should be stored at 20–25°C (68–77°F)
- Reconstitute floxuridine with SWFI 5 mL to yield a solution containing approximately 100 mg floxuridine/mL
- The reconstituted drug product (100 mg/mL) should be stored under refrigeration 2–8°C (36–46°F) for no longer than 2 weeks
- An appropriate amount of the reconstituted solution (100 mg/mL) is then diluted with a volume of 0.9% NS or D5W appropriate for delivery device used to administer the drug product intra-arterially
  - Floxuridine administration is best achieved by utilizing a rate-controlling device able to overcome pressure in large arteries and ensure a uniform drug delivery rate

Selected incompatibility:
- Floxuridine is optimally stable at pH = 4–7. Avoid admixture with highly acidic or alkaline solutions

Recommendations for Drug Administration and Ancillary Care

General:
- See Chapter 43 for recommended use in patients with hepatic dysfunction
- Floxuridine has received FDA approval only for administration by continuous regional intra-arterial infusion

FLUDARABINE PHOSPHATE

FLUDARABINE PHOSPHATE prescribing information. Lake Forest, IL: Hospira, Inc.; May 2018
FLUDARABINE prescribing information. Lake Zurich, IL: Fresenius Kabi USA, LLC.; September 2016

WARNING: [Fludarabine] … should be administered under the supervision of a qualified physician experienced in the use of antineoplastic therapy. [Fludarabine] … can severely suppress bone marrow function. When used at high doses in dose-ranging studies in patients with acute leukemia, [Fludarabine] … was associated with severe neurologic effects, including blindness, coma, and death. This severe central nervous system toxicity occurred in 36% of patients treated with doses approximately four times greater (96 mg/m^2/day for 5 to 7 days) than the recommended dose. Similar severe central nervous system toxicity, including coma, seizures, agitation and confusion, has been reported in patients treated at doses in the range of the dose recommended for chronic lymphocytic leukemia.

Instances of life-threatening and sometimes fatal autoimmune phenomena such as hemolytic anemia, autoimmune thrombocytopenia/thrombocytopenic purpura (ITP), Evans syndrome, and acquired hemophilia have been reported to occur after one or more cycles of treatment with [Fludarabine] … Patients undergoing treatment with [Fludarabine] … should be evaluated and closely monitored for hemolysis.

In a clinical investigation using [Fludarabine] … in combination with pentostatin (deoxycoformycin) for the treatment of refractory chronic lymphocytic leukemia (CLL), there was an unacceptably high incidence of fatal pulmonary toxicity. Therefore, the use of [Fludarabine] … in combination with pentostatin is not recommended

FLUDARABINE PHOSPHATE prescribing information. Lake Forest, IL: Hospira, Inc.; May 2018

Product Identification, Preparation, Storage, and Stability

Fludarabine Phosphate for Injection, USP (lyophilized product for reconstitution)

- Fludarabine phosphate for injection, USP, is available generically in individually packaged, clear, glass, single-use vials containing a sterile, white, lyophilized, solid cake of fludarabine phosphate 50 mg with mannitol 50 mg and sodium hydroxide to adjust pH to 7.7
- Storage temperatures vary among the manufacturers' products, that is, storage at room temperature or under refrigeration
  - Consult product labeling for product-specific recommendations for storage
- Reconstitute fludarabine with 2 mL of SWFI to produce a solution containing 25 mg fludarabine phosphate/mL at a pH within the range 7.2–8.2
- The solid cake should fully dissolve in ≤15 seconds

Fludarabine Phosphate Injection, USP (product in solution)

- Fludarabine phosphate injection is available generically in individually packaged, glass, single-use vials containing a clear, sterile solution of fludarabine phosphate 50 mg/2 mL (25 mg/mL), with mannitol, USP, 50 mg, SWFI (Q.S.), and sodium hydroxide to adjust pH to 6.8. The pH range for the final product is 6.0–7.1
- Store fludarabine phosphate injection under refrigeration at 2–8°C (35.6–46.4°F)
- Neither the lyophilized drug products nor products in solution contain an antimicrobial preservative and should be used within 8 hours after first entering a vial
- Fludarabine phosphate may be further diluted in 100–125 mL of D5W or 0.9% NS in glass or plastic containers
- *Do not mix* fludarabine phosphate with other drugs

Recommendations for Drug Administration and Ancillary Care

General:

- See Chapter 43 for recommended use in patients with renal dysfunction
- Administer fludarabine intraVENously over approximately 30 minutes
- *Caution:* The use of fludarabine phosphate, USP, in combination with pentostatin (*AKA* deoxycoformycin) for the treatment of refractory chronic lymphocytic leukemia in adults, is associated with an unacceptably high incidence of fatal pulmonary toxicity. Therefore, concomitant use of fludarabine phosphate with pentostatin is not recommended

Inadvertent exposure:

- In case of contact with skin or mucous membranes, thoroughly wash the affected area with soap and water. *Do not abrade* the skin by using a scrub brush
- Treat accidental contact with the eyes immediately by copious lavage with water

FLUOROURACIL

Fluorouracil Injection, solution, for intravenous use, Pharmacy Bulk Package—Not for Direct Infusion; prescribing information. Lake Zurich, IL: Fresenius Kabi USA, LLC.; April 2017

Product Identification, Preparation, Storage, and Stability

- Fluorouracil Injection, USP, is available generically from several manufacturers. Presentations include products packaged for single use and for pharmaceutical admixture and compounding (*pharmacy bulk package*)
- Fluorouracil injection, USP, is available in cartons of 10 single-use vials containing a sterile, nonpyrogenic, colorless to faint yellow solution of fluorouracil, 500 mg/10 mL or 1000 mg/20 mL
  - Each milliliter of the drug product contains fluorouracil 50 mg and water for injection. Sodium hydroxide may be added during manufacturing to adjust pH to approximately 9.2
- Pharmacy bulk packages are *only* for use in a pharmacy admixture service
  - Pharmacy bulk package vials contain either 2500 mg (in 50 mL) or 5000 mg (in 100 mL)
  - Packaging varies among manufacturers, and includes individually packaged vials and cartons containing multiple vials
  - *Directions for proper use of a pharmacy bulk package (not for direct infusion) (excerpted and paraphrased)*
    - The 50- and 100-mL pharmacy bulk packages are for use in a pharmacy admixture service only in a suitable work area, such as a laminar flow hood

- Container closures may be penetrated only 1 time, utilizing a suitable sterile transfer device or dispensing set that allows measured distribution of the contents
  - The use of a syringe with a needle is not recommended because multiple vial entries increase the potential of microbial and particulate contamination
  - Complete fluid transfers from a pharmacy bulk package within a maximum time of 4 hours after initial closure entry
- Fluorouracil should be stored at room temperature, but specific recommendations for storage temperature vary among manufacturers' products
  - Consult product labeling for product-specific storage instructions
  - Do not refrigerate or freeze fluorouracil
- Fluorouracil is subject to photodegradation and should be protected from light. Store the product in its original packaging carton until vials are used
  - Fluorouracil is characteristically colorless to faint yellow; the color results from the presence of free fluorine. Dark yellow indicates degradation and may result from prolonged storage in excessive heat or

exposure to light. Discolored solutions should be discarded
  - Although fluorouracil solution may discolor slightly during storage, its potency and safety are not adversely affected
- Fluorouracil may be given undiluted or diluted in a volume of dextrose or sodium chloride solutions, or solutions in which dextrose and sodium chloride are combined, appropriate for a particular application
- Discard any unused portion of fluorouracil remaining in single-use vials and in pharmacy bulk packages at 4 hours after initial vial entry

Selected incompatibility:

- Prepare, store, and administer fluorouracil with plastic containers and administration sets[39,40]
  - Fluorouracil adsorbs to glass surfaces more extensively than plastic surfaces (polyvinyl chloride, polyethylene, polypropylene)
- Fluorouracil and leucovorin calcium should not be combined in the same product container
- Fluorouracil should not be combined in the same product container with DOXOrubicin or simultaneously administered through the same administration set or VAD lumen

Recommendations for Drug Administration and Ancillary Care

General:

- See Chapter 43 for recommended use in patients with renal and hepatic dysfunction
- Fluorouracil injection, USP, may be given by direct intraVENous injection over

≤2 minutes or as an intraVENous infusion for durations of minutes to days
- Fluorouracil also has been given by prolonged infusion intra-arterially and by regional venous perfusion (eg, via the portal vein)

- Fluorouracil solutions may be given via peripheral or central vascular access; however, the undiluted solution has an osmolality of 650 mOsm/kg, has a pH of approximately 9.2 (range: 8.6–9.4), and can be irritating to small veins

GEMCITABINE HYDROCHLORIDE

GEMZAR (gemcitabine for injection) prescribing information. Indianapolis, IN: Lilly USA, LLC; May 2019
GEMCITABINE prescribing information. Lake Zurich, IL: Fresenius Kabi USA, LLC.; September 2019
GEMCITABINE prescribing information. Lake Forest, IL: Hospira, Inc. June 2019
INFUGEM (gemcitabine in sodium chloride injection) prescribing information. Cranbury, NJ: Sun Pharmaceuticals, Inc.; December 2019

Product Identification, Preparation, Storage, and Stability

- Gemcitabine HCl is available generically from several manufacturers. Presentations vary among manufacturers' products

Gemcitabine for Injection, USP (lyophilized product for reconstitution)

- Gemcitabine for Injection is individually packaged in single-use vials containing 200 mg, 1000 mg, or 2000 mg of gemcitabine (expressed as free base) formulated as a sterile, white to off-white lyophilized powder with mannitol (200 mg, 1000 mg, or 2000 mg, respectively), and sodium acetate. Hydrochloric acid and/or sodium hydroxide may have been added to adjust product pH
- Store intact vials at controlled room temperature 20–25°C (68–77°F); temperature excursions between 15° and 30°C (59° and 86°F) are permitted
- Reconstitute gemcitabine with 0.9% NS (without preservatives) to produce a clear, colorless to light straw-colored solution with concentration equal to 38 mg/mL
  - Reconstitute gemcitabine as follows:

Gemcitabine Content per Vial	Volume of 0.9% NS Diluent per Vial	Gemcitabine Concentration After Reconstitution
200 mg	5 mL	38 mg/mL
1000 mg	25 mL	
2000 mg	50 mL	

Gemcitabine has limited solubility in aqueous media. Reconstitution to concentrations >40 mg/mL may prevent complete solubilization
- Shake vials to which 0.9% NS was added to aid gemcitabine dissolution

Gemcitabine Injection, USP (product in solution)

- Gemcitabine injection is individually packaged in single-use vials containing 200 mg, 1000 mg, or 2000 mg of gemcitabine (expressed as free base) at a concentration of 38 mg gemcitabine per milliliter formulated as a sterile, clear, colorless to light straw-colored solution in SWFI. Hydrochloric acid and/or sodium hydroxide may have been added to adjust product pH
- Store intact vials under refrigeration at 2–8°C (36–46°F)

INFUGEM (gemcitabine in 0.9% NS, ready to infuse bags)

- INFUGEM (gemcitabine in 0.9% NS) is individually packaged in single-dose, premixed, ready-to-infuse, aluminum-overwrapped, intraVENous infusion bags containing 1200 mg, 1300 mg, 1400 mg, 1500 mg, 1600 mg, 1700 mg, 1800 mg, 1900 mg, 2000 mg, and 2200 mg of gemcitabine (expressed as free base) at a concentration of 10 mg gemcitabine per milliliter formulated as a sterile, clear, colorless solution in 0.9% NS. Hydrochloric acid and/or sodium hydroxide may have been added to adjust product pH
- Store intact infusion bags at 20–25°C (68–77°F); temperature excursions to 15–30°C (59–86°F) are permitted. Do not freeze (crystallization may occur)
- Select the INFUGEM premixed bag(s) that allow for a variance of up to 5% of the BSA-calculated dose as described in the FDA-approved prescribing information. Use another formulation of gemcitabine for patients who require a dose <1150 mg
- Infuse all doses of INFUGEM over 30 minutes. If two premixed infusion bags are required to achieve the prescribed dose, infuse the total volume of both bags over 30 minutes

Instructions common to formulations that require further preparation (Gemcitabine for Injection, USP [lyophilized product for reconstitution] and Gemcitabine Injection, USP [product in SWFI])

- *Do not refrigerate* reconstituted gemcitabine solutions to prevent crystallization
- Prior to administration, the appropriate amount of drug must be further diluted with 0.9% NS to concentrations as low as 0.1 mg/mL
- When prepared as directed, diluted gemcitabine solutions are stable for 24 hours at 20–25°C (68–77°F)
- Discard any unused portion of gemcitabine solutions
- Gemcitabine is compatible with either glass or PVC containers and PVC administration sets

Recommendations for Drug Administration and Ancillary Care

General:

- See Chapter 43 for recommended use in patients with renal and hepatic dysfunction
- Administer gemcitabine by intraVENous infusion over 30 minutes

Treatment strategies and other factors affecting gemcitabine pharmacokinetics:

- Gemcitabine has been administered intraVENously at a fixed dose rate (FDR) of 10 mg/m² per min

Notes: Experimental data have demonstrated that small increases in intracellular concentrations of gemcitabine's active triphosphate metabolite profoundly affect its intracellular AUC; the kinetics of interaction with deoxycytidine kinase, and a fixed gemcitabine administration rate of 10 mg/m² per minute, maximizes the rate at which the metabolite accumulates in peripheral blood mononuclear cells

This observation is the basis for clinical trials with FDR gemcitabine administration, which attempt to correlate increases in intracellular gemcitabine triphosphate concentrations with improved objective treatment outcomes[41]

- Population pharmacokinetic analyses of combined single- and multiple-dose studies showed gemcitabine's volume of distribution (V_d) was significantly influenced by duration of administration and patients' sex
- Gemcitabine's V_d increases directly with its duration of administration (70–285-minute durations)
- Administration durations >60 minutes and administration at intervals more frequent than once weekly have been shown to increase the incidence of clinically significant adverse events
- Gemcitabine clearance is decreased in females[42] (vs males) and the elderly,[43] resulting in higher concentrations of gemcitabine for any given dose

Caution:

- Enhanced tissue injury typically associated with radiation toxicity is associated with concurrent use of gemcitabine and radiation therapies given together or ≤7 days apart:
  - Gemcitabine has radiosensitizing activity. Toxicity associated with concurrent use of gemcitabine and radiation therapies is dependent on multiple factors, including gemcitabine dosage, the frequency of gemcitabine administration, radiation dose, radiotherapy planning technique, and type and target volume of irradiated tissues
- Gemcitabine clearance has been shown to be decreased by concurrent use of CISplatin
- If Gemcitabine Injection or diluted solutions contact the skin or mucosa, immediately wash the skin thoroughly with soap and water or rinse the mucosa with copious amounts of water
  - Acute dermal irritation has not been observed in animal studies, but 2 of 3 rabbits exhibited drug-related systemic toxicities (death, hypoactivity, nasal discharge, shallow breathing) due to dermal absorption

GEMTUZUMAB OZOGAMICIN

MYLOTARG (gemtuzumab ozogamicin) prescribing information. Philadelphia, PA: Wyeth Pharmaceuticals LLC a subsidiary of Pfizer, Inc; June 2020

WARNING: HEPATOTOXICITY

- Hepatotoxicity, including severe or fatal hepatic veno-occlusive disease (VOD), also known as sinusoidal obstruction syndrome (SOS), has been reported in association with the use of MYLOTARG as a single agent, and as part of a combination chemotherapy regimen. Monitor frequently for signs and symptoms of VOD after treatment with MYLOTARG …

MYLOTARG (gemtuzumab ozogamicin) prescribing information. Philadelphia, PA: Wyeth Pharmaceuticals LLC a subsidiary of Pfizer, Inc; June 2020

Product Identification, Preparation, Storage, and Stability

- Gemtuzumab ozogamicin is composed of a CD33-directed monoclonal humanized IgG4 kappa monoclonal antibody covalently linked to the cytotoxic agent N-acetyl gamma calicheamicin
- MYLOTARG is a sterile, white to off-white, preservative-free, lyophilized cake or powder supplied in a carton (NDC 0008-4510-01) containing one 4.5 mg single-dose vial. Each single-dose vial delivers 4.5 mg gemtuzumab ozogamicin along with the following inactive ingredients: dextran 40 (41.0 mg), sodium chloride (26.1 mg), sodium phosphate dibasic anhydrous (2.7 mg), sodium phosphate monobasic monohydrate (0.45 mg), and sucrose (69.8 mg)
- Store intact vials under refrigeration at 2–8°C (35–46°F) in the original carton to protect from light. *DO NOT FREEZE*

Reconstitution:
- MYLOTARG is a cytotoxic drug. Follow applicable special handling and disposal procedures
- Use appropriate aseptic technique and protect the reconstituted and diluted solution from light

- Allow drug product, vials to reach ambient temperature for approximately 5 minutes prior to reconstitution
- Reconstitute each vial with 5 mL of SWFI to obtain a concentration of 1 mg/mL of MYLOTARG that delivers 4.5 mL (4.5 mg)
- Gently swirl the vial to aid dissolution. *DO NOT SHAKE*
- Inspect the reconstituted solution for particulates and discoloration. The reconstituted solution may contain small white to off-white, opaque to translucent, and amorphous to fiber-like particles
- Use reconstituted solution immediately or after being refrigerated at 2–8°C (36–46°F) for up to 1 hour. *PROTECT FROM LIGHT. DO NOT FREEZE*

Dilution:
- Calculate the required volume of the reconstituted solution needed to obtain the appropriate dose according to patient BSA. Withdraw this amount from the vial(s) using a syringe. *PROTECT FROM LIGHT.* Discard any unused reconstituted solution left in the vial

- **Doses must be mixed to a concentration between 0.075 mg/mL and 0.234 mg/mL**
- Doses <3.9 mg must be prepared for administration by syringe. Add the reconstituted MYLOTARG solution to a syringe with an appropriate volume of 0.9% NS
- Doses ≥3.9 mg are to be diluted in a syringe or an IV bag in an appropriate volume of 0.9% NS
- Gently invert the infusion container to mix the diluted solution. *DO NOT SHAKE*
- If not used immediately, store at room temperature 15–25°C (59–77°F) for up to 6 hours, which includes the 2-hour infusion time and 1 hour, if needed, to allow the refrigerated diluted solution to equilibrate to room temperature. The diluted solution can be refrigerated at 2–8°C (36–46°F) for up to 12 hours which includes up to 1 hour in the vial post-reconstitution. *PROTECT FROM LIGHT* and *DO NOT FREEZE*

Selected incompatibility:
- Do not mix MYLOTARG with, or administer as an infusion with, other medicinal products

Recommendations for Drug Administration and Ancillary Care

General:
- See Chapter 43 for recommended use in patients with hepatic dysfunction
- The PK of gemtuzumab ozogamicin in patients with severe renal impairment (CrCl 15–29 mL/min), moderate hepatic impairment (total bilirubin > 1.5 to 3 × ULN), and severe hepatic impairment (total bilirubin >3 × ULN) are unknown
- Consider cytoreduction (eg, with hydroxyurea) in patients with WBC ≥30,000/mm³ prior to gemtuzumab ozogamicin administration

Administration:
- The recommended dose of gemtuzumab ozogamicin in combination with DAUNOrubicin and cytarabine for induction is 3 mg/m² (up to one 4.5-mg vial) on days 1, 4, and 7 for adults with newly diagnosed de novo CD33-positive acute myeloid leukemia (AML). For the consolidation cycles, the recommended dose is 3 mg/m² (up to one 4.5-mg vial) on day 1 in combination with DAUNOrubicin and cytarabine
  - Note for patients requiring a second induction cycle: do *NOT* administer MYLOTARG during the second induction. Up to 2 consolidation cycles may be given
- The recommended dose of gemtuzumab ozogamicin for induction as a single-agent for newly diagnosed CD33-positive AML in adults is 6 mg/m² (*NOT* limited to one 4.5-mg vial) on day 1, and 3 mg/m² (*NOT* limited to one 4.5-mg vial) on day 8. For continuation (up to 8 cycles), the recommended dose of gemtuzumab ozogamicin is 2 mg/m² (*NOT* limited to

one 4.5-mg vial) as a single agent on day 1 every 4 weeks
- The recommended dose of gemtuzumab ozogamicin for relapsed or refractory CD33-positive AML as a single agent for adults is 3 mg/m² (up to one 4.5-mg vial) on days 1, 4, and 7. Treatment in the relapsed or refractory setting consists of a single course
- **Use an inline 0.2-μm polyethersulfone filter for infusion of MYLOTARG**
- Protect the intraVENous bag from light using a light-blocking cover during infusion. The infusion line does not need to be protected from light
- Infuse the diluted solution over 2 hours

Concomitant medications:
- Premedicate adults with acetaminophen 650 mg orally and diphenhydrAMINE 50 mg orally or intraVENously 1 hour prior to MYLOTARG dosing and 1 mg/kg methylPREDNISolone or an equivalent dose of an alternative corticosteroid within 30 minutes prior to infusion of MYLOTARG
- In patients at high risk for tumor lysis syndrome, consider frequent monitoring of laboratory indices of tumor lysis syndrome, intraVENous hydration, and prophylaxis with a xanthine oxidase inhibitor (eg, allopurinol)

Adverse events and treatment modifications:
- Refer to the current FDA-approved product label for detailed recommendations regarding treatment modifications for thrombocytopenia, neutropenia, hepatotoxicity, and other severe or life-threatening nonhematologic toxicities

- Life-threatening or fatal infusion-related reactions can occur during or within 24 hours following infusion of MYLOTARG. Signs and symptoms of an infusion-related reaction may include fever, chills, hypotension, tachycardia, hypoxia, and respiratory failure. Premedication is recommended. Monitor vital signs frequently during infusion and for at least 1 hour post-infusion
- Interrupt infusion immediately for patients who develop evidence of infusion reaction, especially dyspnea, bronchospasm, or hypotension. Initiate appropriate medical management
- For mild, moderate, or severe infusion-related reactions, once symptoms resolve, consider resuming the infusion at no more than half the rate at which the reaction occurred. Discontinue MYLOTARG in patients who develop signs or symptoms of anaphylaxis, including severe respiratory symptoms or clinically significant hypotension

Selected precautions:
- MYLOTARG is myelosuppressive and can cause fatal or life-threatening hemorrhage due to prolonged thrombocytopenia. Assess blood counts prior to each dose and monitor frequently after treatment until resolution of cytopenias. Monitor patients for signs and symptoms of bleeding
- When administering MYLOTARG to patients who have a history of or predisposition for QTc prolongation, who are taking medicinal products that are known to prolong QT interval, and in patients with electrolyte disturbances, obtain electrocardiograms and electrolytes prior to the start of treatment and as needed during administration

GLUCARPIDASE

VORAXAZE (glucarpidase) prescribing information. West Conshohocken, PA: BTG International Inc.; August 2019

Product Identification, Preparation, Storage, and Stability

- VORAXAZE is marketed in individually packaged, single-use, glass vials as a sterile, preservative-free, white, lyophilized powder containing 1000 units of glucarpidase per vial, with lactose monohydrate 10 mg, Tris-HCl 0.6 mg, and zinc acetate dihydrate 2 μg (NDC 50633-210-11)
  - Glucarpidase potency units correspond with the enzymatic cleavage of 1 μmol/L of methotrexate per minute at 37°C (98.6°F)
- Store glucarpidase under refrigeration at 2–8°C (36–46°F). *Do not freeze* glucarpidase. Do not use glucarpidase after the expiration date on the vial
- Reconstitute the contents of a vial with 1 mL of 0.9% NS
- Gently roll and tilt vials to dissolve the lyophilized powder. *Do not shake* vials to aid dissolution
- Inspect the product to ensure product dissolution and discard vials in which the solution is not clear, colorless, and free of particulate matter
- Use reconstituted glucarpidase immediately, or store it under refrigeration at 2–8°C (36–46°F) for up to 4 hours if it is not used immediately
- Discard any unused reconstituted product

Recommendations for Drug Administration and Ancillary Care

General:

- Administer glucarpidase 50 units/kg of body weight as a single intraVENous injection over 5 minutes. Flush intraVENous lines through which glucarpidase is given before and after administering glucarpidase

Caution:

- Leucovorin is a substrate for glucarpidase. Do not administer leucovorin within 2 hours before or after glucarpidase
  - No dose adjustment is recommended for a continuing leucovorin regimen because leucovorin doses/dosages and schedules are based on a patient's methotrexate concentrations before glucarpidase is administered
- Glucarpidase is a carboxypeptidase produced by recombinant DNA technology in genetically modified *Escherichia coli*
  - Serious allergic reactions, including anaphylactic reactions, may occur. The most common adverse reactions (incidence >1%) associated with glucarpidase are paresthesia, flushing, nausea and/or vomiting, hypotension, and headache

Monitoring methotrexate concentration/interference with assay:

- Methotrexate concentrations within 48 hours following administration of glucarpidase can only be reliably measured by a chromatographic method
- DAMPA (4-deoxy-4-amino-N^{10}-methylpteroic acid), an inactive metabolite of methotrexate resulting from treatment with glucarpidase, interferes with methotrexate concentration measurements using immunoassays, resulting in erroneous measurements that overestimate methotrexate concentrations
- Because of DAMPA's long half-life (approximately 9 hours), measurement of methotrexate using immunoassays is unreliable for samples collected within 48 hours after glucarpidase administration

Continuation and timing of leucovorin rescue:

- Continue to administer leucovorin after glucarpidase is administered. *Do not administer* leucovorin within 2 hours before or after a glucarpidase dose because leucovorin is a substrate for glucarpidase
- For the first 48 hours after administering glucarpidase, give the same leucovorin doses/dosages and schedules as had been given prior to glucarpidase
- Leucovorin doses/dosages and schedule at times >48 hours after glucarpidase are based on the measured methotrexate concentration
- Do not discontinue leucovorin therapy based on the determination of a single methotrexate concentration less than the threshold for starting or continuing leucovorin treatment
- Leucovorin rescue should be continued until methotrexate concentrations have been maintained below the leucovorin treatment threshold for a minimum of 3 days

IDARUBICIN HYDROCHLORIDE

Idamycin PFS (idarubicin hydrochloride injection) prescribing information. New York, NY: Pharmacia & Upjohn Company, Division of Pfizer, Inc.; August 2019

WARNINGS

1. [IDArubicin hydrochloride] … should be given slowly into a freely flowing intravenous infusion. It must never be given intramuscularly or subcutaneously. Severe local tissue necrosis can occur if there is extravasation during administration

2. As is the case with other anthracyclines, the use of [IDArubicin hydrochloride] … can cause myocardial toxicity leading to congestive heart failure. Cardiac toxicity is more common in patients who have received prior anthracyclines or who have pre-existing cardiac disease

3. As is usual with antileukemic agents, severe myelosuppression occurs when [IDArubicin hydrochloride] … is used at effective therapeutic doses

4. It is recommended that [IDArubicin hydrochloride] … be administered only under the supervision of a physician who is experienced in leukemia chemotherapy and in facilities with laboratory and supportive resources adequate to monitor drug tolerance and protect and maintain a patient compromised by drug toxicity. The physician and institution must be capable of responding rapidly and completely to severe hemorrhagic conditions and/or overwhelming infection

5. Dosage should be reduced in patients with impaired hepatic or renal function …

Boxed Warnings for Idamycin PFS (idarubicin hydrochloride injection) prescribing information. New York, NY: Pharmacia & Upjohn Company, Division of Pfizer, Inc.; August 2019

Product Identification, Preparation, Storage, and Stability

IDArubicin HCl is available generically from several manufacturers

- IDArubicin HCl Injection is packaged in single-use vials containing a sterile, red-orange, isotonic parenteral preservative-free solution of IDArubicin at a uniform concentration of 1 mg/mL
- Product presentations include vials containing IDArubicin 5, 10, or 20 mg
- Store IDArubicin HCl injection (solution) under refrigeration 2–8°C (35.6–46.4°F) in their packaging carton to protect them from light
- IDArubicin HCl 1 mg/mL is suitable for direct administration to patients. It also

may be diluted to a concentration as low as 0.01mg/mL in 0.9% NS or D5W, or to a concentration of 0.1 mg/mL in LRI
- IDArubicin is compatible with PVC, glass, and polypropylene containers
- *Note:* IDArubicin HCl solutions in 0.9% NS exhibit a low level of haziness that is visible under high-intensity light and measurable with a turbidimeter. The haziness increases to maximum with increasing drug dilution from a concentration of 1 mg/mL to 0.05 mg/mL. The haze is not indicative of drug instability or incompatibility[44]

Selected incompatibility:

- IDArubicin is subject to photodegradation, and its susceptibility is inversely related to the concentration of IDArubicin in solution. Protection from light is not necessary if IDArubicin is used promptly after preparation, but product containers should be protected from light exposure when IDArubicin is not administered within a few hours after preparation
- IDArubicin is physically incompatible with heparin (precipitation occurs)
- IDArubicin is degraded by contact with alkaline solutions

Recommendations for Drug Administration and Ancillary Care

General:
- See Chapter 43 for recommended use in patients with renal and hepatic dysfunction
- Administer IDArubicin by slow intraVENous injection over 10–15 minutes into the tubing of a freely running intraVENous infusion of 0.9% NS or D5W, or by intraVENous infusion after dilution

- *Caution:* IDArubicin is a vesicant and may produce severe local soft-tissue necrosis if extravasation occurs. IDArubicin *must not be given* by the intraMUSCular, SUBCUTaneous, or intraTHECAL routes
  - The current standard of care for managing anthracycline extravasation, including extravasation of IDArubicin, is a 3-day course of intraVENously administered dexrazoxane (Totect)

IFOSFAMIDE

IFOSFAMIDE prescribing information. Parsippany, NJ: Teva Pharmaceuticals USA, Inc.; February 2020
IFEX (ifosfamide injection, powder, for solution, intravenous use) prescribing information. Deerfield, IL: Baxter Healthcare Corporation; July 2017

WARNING: MYELOSUPPRESSION, NEUROTOXICITY, and UROTOXICITY

Myelosuppression can be severe and lead to fatal infections. Monitor blood counts prior to and at intervals after each treatment cycle. CNS toxicities can be severe and result in encephalopathy and death. Monitor for CNS toxicity and discontinue treatment for encephalopathy. Nephrotoxicity can be severe and result in renal failure. Hemorrhagic cystitis can be severe and can be reduced by the prophylactic use of mesna …

Boxed Warnings for IFOSFAMIDE prescribing information. Parsippany, NJ: Teva Pharmaceuticals USA, Inc.; February 2020

Product Identification, Preparation, Storage, and Stability

Ifosfamide injection (product supplied in solution)
- Ifosfamide injection is available in individually boxed single-use vials containing a sterile solution of either 1000 mg/20 mL or 3000 mg/60 mL, in a concentration of 50 mg ifosfamide/mL
- Commercial formulations also contain monobasic sodium phosphate, dibasic sodium phosphate, and SWFI, but products vary in the amount of excipients present
- Store ifosfamide injection under refrigeration at 2–8°C (36–46°F)

Ifosfamide for injection (product supplied as powder)
- Ifosfamide for injection, USP, is available in individually boxed single-use vials containing 1000 mg or 3000 mg ifosfamide without excipient ingredients

- Store intact vials at controlled room temperature 20–25°C (68–77°F). Protect ifosfamide from temperatures >30°C (>86°F)
- Reconstitute lyophilized ifosfamide with SWFI or BWFI (preserved with benzyl alcohol or parabens) as follows: Benzyl alcohol-containing solutions can reduce the stability of ifosfamide

Ifosfamide Content per Vial	Diluent Volume	Ifosfamide Concentration After Reconstitution
1000 mg	20 mL	50 mg/mL
3000 mg	60 mL	

Instructions common to both products
- After adding a diluent solution, shake vials to dissolve ifosfamide powder

- Ifosfamide must be completely dissolved before the product may be used
- After reconstitution, ifosfamide may be diluted to obtain concentrations within the range of 0.6–20 mg/mL in any of the following fluids: D5W, 0.9% NS, LRI, D2.5W, 0.45% NaCl, or D5W/0.9% NS
  - Mesna may be prepared as an admixture with ifosfamide (both present in the same container) without compromising the stability of either product
- Ifosfamide is physically and chemically stable in a variety of parenteral product containers, including those made of glass, ethylene and propylene copolymers, PVC plasticized with phthalates, and other polyolefin materials
- Ifosfamide solutions should be refrigerated and used within 24 hours after preparation

---

Recommendations for Drug Administration and Ancillary Care

General:
- See Chapter 43 for recommended use in patients with renal and hepatic dysfunction
- On days when ifosfamide is administered, give intraVENous or oral fluid hydration consisting of *at least* 2000 mL/day greater than a patient's routine daily fluid consumption. Aggressive hydration has been shown to decrease the urothelial toxicity associated with ifosfamide
- Mesna should be used to reduce the incidence of urothelial hemorrhage
  - When given concomitantly with ifosfamide, mesna protects the urinary tract from exposure to reactive ifosfamide metabolites that are highly concentrated in urine

  - Mesna may be added to the same container as ifosfamide without compromising the stability of either product
- Administer ifosfamide by intraVENous infusion over a minimum of 30 minutes
- Ifosfamide is nephrotoxic and urotoxic
  - Evaluate glomerular and tubular kidney function before, during, and after ifosfamide treatment

Monitor:
- Urinary sediment for the presence of erythrocytes and other signs of urotoxicity/nephrotoxicity
- Serum and urine chemistries, including phosphorus and potassium
- Urinalysis prior to each ifosfamide dose

  - If microscopic hematuria (>10 RBCs/HPF) is present, subsequent administration should be withheld until hematuria completely resolves. Further ifosfamide administration should be given with vigorous oral or parenteral hydration
  - Use ifosfamide with caution, if at all, in patients with active urinary tract infections

Inadvertent exposure:
- In case of skin contact, thoroughly wash the affected area with soap and water. *Do not abrade* the skin by using a scrub brush
- Treat accidental contact with mucous membranes and the eyes immediately by copious lavage with water

INOTUZUMAB OZOGAMICIN

BESPONSA (inotuzumab ozogamicin) prescribing information. Philadelphia, PA: Wyeth Pharmaceuticals LLC a subsidiary of Pfizer Inc; March 2018

WARNING: HEPATOTOXICITY, INCLUDING HEPATIC VENO-OCCULUSIVE DISEASE (VOD) (ALSO KNOWN AS SINUSOIDAL OBSTRUCTION SYNDROME) and INCREASED RISK OF POST-HEMATOPOIETIC STEM CELL TRANSPLANT (HSCT) NON-RELAPSE MORTALITY

- Hepatotoxicity, including fatal and life-threatening VOD, occurred in patients with relapsed or refractory acute lymphoblastic leukemia (ALL) who received BESPONSA. The risk of VOD was greater in patients who underwent HSCT after BESPONSA treatment; use of HSCT conditioning regimens containing 2 alkylating agents and last total bilirubin level ≥ upper limit of normal (ULN) before HSCT were significantly associated with an increased risk of VOD. Other risk factors for VOD in patients treated with BESPONSA included ongoing or prior liver disease, prior HSCT, increased age, later salvage lines, and a greater number of BESPONSA treatment cycles. Elevation of liver tests may require dosing interruption, dose reduction, or permanent discontinuation of BESPONSA. Permanently discontinue treatment if VOD occurs. If severe VOD occurs, treat according to standard medical practice …
- There was higher post-HSCT non-relapse mortality rate in patients receiving BESPONSA, resulting in a higher day 100 post-HSCT mortality rate …

Boxed Warning for BESPONSA (inotuzumab ozogamicin) prescribing information. Philadelphia, PA: Wyeth Pharmaceuticals LLC a subsidiary of Pfizer Inc; March 2018

Product Identification, Preparation, Storage, and Stability

- Inotuzumab ozogamicin is composed of a CD22-directed monoclonal humanized IgG4 kappa monoclonal antibody covalently linked to the cytotoxic agent N-acetyl gamma calicheamicin
- BESPONSA is a sterile, white to off-white, preservative-free, lyophilized powder in individually boxed single-dose vials that contain 0.9 mg inotuzumab ozogamicin (NDC 0008-0100-01). Inactive ingredients are polysorbate 80 (0.36 mg), sodium chloride (2.16 mg), sucrose (180 mg), and tromethamine (8.64 mg)
- Store intact vials under refrigeration at 2–8°C (36–46°F) in the original carton to protect from light. Do not freeze
- BESPONSA is a cytotoxic drug. Follow applicable special handling and disposal procedures
- Protect the reconstituted and diluted BESPONSA solutions from light. Do not freeze the reconstituted or diluted solution
- The maximum time from reconstitution through the end of administration should be ≤8 hours, with ≤4 hours between reconstitution and dilution

Reconstitution:
- Reconstitute each vial with 4 mL SWFI to obtain the reconstituted concentration of 0.25 mg/mL of inotuzumab ozogamicin with a deliverable volume of 3.6 mL (0.9 mg)
- Gently swirl the vial to aid dissolution. ***DO NOT SHAKE***
- Inspect the reconstituted solution for particulates and discoloration. The reconstituted solution should be clear to opalescent, colorless to slightly yellow, and essentially free of visible foreign matter

Dilution:
- Calculate the required volume of the reconstituted solution needed to obtain the appropriate dose according to the patient's BSA. Withdraw this amount from the vial(s) using a syringe. Discard any unused reconstituted BESPONSA solution left in the vial
- Add reconstituted solution to an infusion container with 0.9% NS to make a total volume of 50 mL. An infusion container made of PVC (DEHP- or non-DEHP-containing), polyolefin (polypropylene and/or polyethylene), or ethylene vinyl acetate (EVA) is recommended
- Gently invert the infusion container to mix the diluted solution. ***DO NOT SHAKE***

Product Identification, Preparation, Storage, and Stability (continued)

Storage Times and Conditions for Reconstituted and Diluted BESPONSA Solution*

Reconstituted Solution	Diluted Solution		
	After Start of Dilution	Administration	
Use immediately or after being refrigerated (2–8°C; 36–46°F) for up to 4 hours. *PROTECT FROM LIGHT. DO NOT FREEZE*	Use immediately or after storage at room temperature (20–25°C; 68–77°F) for up to 4 hours or being refrigerated (2–8°C; 36–46°F) for up to 3 hours. *PROTECT FROM LIGHT. DO NOT FREEZE*	If the diluted solution is refrigerated (2–8°C; 36–46°F), allow it to equilibrate at room temperature (20–25°C; 68–77°F) for approximately 1 hour prior to administration. Administer diluted solution within 8 hours of reconstitution as a 1-hour infusion at a rate of 50 mL/h at room temperature (20–25°C; 68–77°F). *PROTECT FROM LIGHT*	

*Maximum time from reconstitution through end of administration ≤8 hours

Selected incompatibility:

• Do not mix inotuzumab ozogamicin or administer as an infusion with other medicinal products

Recommendations for Drug Administration and Ancillary Care

General:

• See Chapter 43 for recommended use in patients with hepatic dysfunction
• The safety and efficacy of inotuzumab ozogamicin in patients with end-stage renal disease with or without hemodialysis is unknown
• There is insufficient data in patients with moderate and severe hepatic impairment (total bilirubin >1.5 ULN)

Administration:

The recommended dose of inotuzumab ozogamicin is outlined in the following table:

Inotuzumab Ozogamicin Dosing and Schedule Based on Cycle and Response to Treatment

	Day 1	Day 8*	Day 15*	Total Dosage per Cycle
Dosing regimen for cycle 1				
Dose	0.8 mg/m²	0.5 mg/m²	0.5 mg/m²	Total dosage during cycle 1 for *all* patients = 1.8 mg/m²
Cycle length	21 days†			
Dosing regimen for subsequent cycles depending on response to treatment				
Patients who *have* achieved a CR or CRi:				
Dose	0.5 mg/m²	0.5 mg/m²	0.5 mg/m²	Total dosage during subsequent cycles for patients *with* CR or CRi = 1.5 mg/m²
Cycle length‡	28 days			
Patients who *have not* achieved a CR or CRi:				
Dose	0.8 mg/m²	0.5 mg/m²	0.5 mg/m²	Total dosage during subsequent cycles for patients *without* CR or CRi = 1.8 mg/m²
Cycle length‡	28 days			

*± 2 days (maintain a minimum of 6 days between doses)
†Cycle length may be extended up to 28 days to allow for recovery from toxicity and for patients who achieve a complete remission (CR) or CR with incomplete count recovery (CRi)
‡If the patient is planned to undergo a future hematopoietic stem cell transplant (HSCT), then administer up to 2 cycles. If CR or CRi with measurable residual disease (MRD) negativity has not been achieved after 2 cycles, then consider administering a third cycle. If no HSCT is planned, then administer up to a maximum of 6 cycles

• Infuse the diluted solution for 1 hour at a rate of 50 mL/h at room temperature 20–25°C (68–77°F). Infusion lines made of PVC (DEHP- or non-DEHP-containing), polyolefin (polypropylene and/or polyethylene), or polybutadiene are recommended. *PROTECT FROM LIGHT*

(continued)

Recommendations for Drug Administration and Ancillary Care (*continued*)

- If the diluted solution is refrigerated 2–8°C (36–46°F), allow it to equilibrate at room temperature 20–25°C (68–77°F) for approximately 1 hour prior to administration
- Filtration of the diluted solution is not required. However, if the diluted solution is filtered, polyethersulfone (PES)-, polyvinylidene fluoride (PVDF)-, or hydrophilic polysulfone (HPS)-based filters are recommended. Do not use filters made of nylon or mixed cellulose ester (MCE)

Concomitant medications:

- For patients with circulating lymphoblasts, cytoreduction with a combination of hydroxyurea, steroids, and/or vinCRIStine to a peripheral blast count of ≤10,000/mm^3 is recommended prior to the first dose
- Premedication with a corticosteroid, antipyretic, and antihistamine is recommended prior to dosing. Patients should be observed during and for at least 1 hour after the end of infusion for symptoms of infusion-related reactions

Adverse events and treatment modifications:

- Refer to the current FDA-approved product label for detailed recommendations regarding treatment modifications for neutropenia, thrombocytopenia, hepatotoxicity, and nonhematologic toxicities G ≥2
- BESPONSA doses within a treatment cycle (ie, days 8 and/or 15) do not need to be interrupted due to neutropenia or thrombocytopenia, but dosing interruptions within a cycle are recommended for nonhematologic toxicities. If the dose is reduced due to BESPONSA-related toxicity, the dose must not be re-escalated
- Infusion-related reactions were reported in 4/164 patients (2%) in the INO-VATEALL trial. These were all G2 and generally occurred in cycle 1 shortly after the end of infusion
- Premedication is recommended, and patients should be monitored closely during and for at least 1 hour after the end of infusion. Signs and symptoms of infusion-related reactions include fever, chills, rash, or breathing problems
- Interrupt infusion and institute appropriate medical management if an infusion-related reaction occurs. Depending on the severity of the infusion-related reaction, consider discontinuation of the infusion or administration of steroids and antihistamines. For severe or life-threatening infusion reactions, permanently discontinue

Potential drug interactions:

- Concomitant use of BESPONSA with drugs known to prolong the QT interval or induce Torsades de Pointes may increase the risk of a clinically significant QTc interval prolongation

Selected precautions:

- Monitor complete blood counts prior to each dose of BESPONSA and monitor for signs and symptoms of infection, bleeding/hemorrhage, or other effects of myelosuppression during treatment with BESPONSA. As appropriate, administer prophylactic anti-infectives and employ surveillance testing during and after treatment with BESPONSA
- Administer BESPONSA with caution in patients who have a history of or predisposition for QTc prolongation, who are taking medicinal products that are known to prolong QT interval, and in patients with electrolyte disturbances. Obtain electrocardiograms (ECGs) and electrolytes prior to the start of treatment, after initiation of any drug known to prolong QTc, and periodically monitor as clinically indicated during treatment

INTERFERON ALFA-2b

INTRON A prescribing information. Whitehouse Station, NJ: Merck & Co., Inc.; August 2019

WARNING

Alpha interferons, including INTRON A, cause or aggravate fatal or life-threatening neuropsychiatric, autoimmune, ischemic, and infectious disorders. Patients should be monitored closely with periodic clinical and laboratory evaluations. Patients with persistently severe or worsening signs or symptoms of these conditions should be withdrawn from therapy. In many but not all cases these disorders resolve after stopping INTRON A therapy …

Boxed Warnings for INTRON A prescribing information. Whitehouse Station, NJ: Merck & Co., Inc.; August 2019

Product Identification, Preparation, Storage, and Stability

- INTRON A is available in several formulations and package formats. The products in solution packaged in vials are *not recommended* for intraVENous administration
- INTRON A powder for injection is packaged as a kit containing two vials:
  - One single-use vial contains interferon alfa-2b as a white- to cream-colored powder, *plus*
  - One single-use vial contains Diluent for INTRON A (sterile water for injection, USP) 5 mL/vial
- The following presentations are available:

Amount of Recombinant Interferon Alfa-2b per Vial	Volume of Diluent (SWFI)	Interferon Alfa-2b Concentration After Reconstitution	NDC Number
10 million IU (0.038 mg/vial*)	1 mL	10 million IU/mL	0085-4350-01
18 million IU (0.069 mg/vial*)		18 million IU/mL	0085-4351-01
50 million IU (0.192 mg/vial*)		50 million IU/mL	0085-4352-01

Each milliliter of the reconstituted solution also contains 20 mg glycine, 2.3 mg dibasic sodium phosphate, 0.55 mg monobasic sodium phosphate, and 1 mg albumin (human)†
*Based on the specific activity of approximately 2.6×10^8 IU/mg protein, as measured by HPLC assay
†The addition of albumin prevents drug adsorption to containers and administration set surfaces during drug preparation and administration

- Store recombinant interferon alfa-2b powder for injection between 2° and 8°C (36° and 46°F) both before and after reconstitution
- Prepare a solution for intraVENous infusion immediately before use by adding 1 mL of SWFI (diluent included in product packaging) to a vial containing Intron A powder for injection. Discard the unused portion of SWFI diluent
  - Interferon alfa-2b products formulated as solutions are *not recommended* for intraVENous administration
- Vials may be gently swirled to hasten dissolving the powdered drug product
- Dilute an amount of interferon appropriate for a patient's dose in a bag (typically 100 mL) containing 0.9% NS to produce a solution with an interferon alfa concentration ≥10 million IU/100 mL

Recommendations for Drug Administration and Ancillary Care

General:
- Premedication with acetaminophen may mitigate fever that often follows interferon alfa-2b administration
- Allow refrigerated solutions to come to room temperature before commencing administration
- Administration before sleep may mitigate a patient's experience of "flu-like" symptoms (fever, headache, chills, myalgias, fatigue) that are frequently associated with interferon alfa-2b administration
- Administer interferon alfa-2b by intraVENous infusion over 20 minutes

IPILIMUMAB

YERVOY (ipilimumab) prescribing information. Princeton, NJ: Bristol-Myers Squibb Company; October 2020

Product Identification, Preparation, Storage, and Stability

- YERVOY is a sterile, preservative-free, clear to slightly opalescent, colorless to pale yellow solution for intraVENous infusion, which may contain a small amount of visible, translucent-to-white, amorphous ipilimumab particulates
- The commercial product is supplied in single-use vials containing either 50 mg/10 mL (NDC 0003-2327-11) or 200 mg/40 mL (NDC 0003-2328-22)
  - Each milliliter of solution contains 5 mg ipilimumab at a pH = 7, with the following inactive ingredients: diethylene triamine pentaacetic acid 0.04 mg, mannitol 10 mg, polysorbate 80 (vegetable origin) 0.1 mg, sodium chloride 5.85 mg, tris hydrochloride 3.15 mg (buffer), and SWFI
- Store unused vials under refrigeration at 2–8°C (36–46°F) protected from light. *Do not freeze* the product
- Ipilimumab *must be diluted* before administration

Preparation
- *Do not shake* ipilimumab
- Discard vials containing a cloudy solution, if there is pronounced discoloration (solution may have pale yellow color), or with the appearance of foreign particulate matter other than translucent-to-white, amorphous particles
- Allow vials to stand at room temperature for approximately 5 minutes before diluting the product for clinical use
- With a syringe, withdraw a volume of ipilimumab appropriate for a patient's dose and transfer it to a sterile parenteral product container
- Dilute the drug with 0.9% NS or D5W to a concentration within the range of 1–2 mg/mL. Mix the diluted solution by gently inverting the parenteral product container
  - Store the diluted solution for no more than 24 hours under refrigeration at 2–8°C (36–46°F) or at room temperature (20–25°C [68–77°F])
- Discard partially used and empty vials

Recommendations for Drug Administration and Ancillary Care

General:
- *Do not mix* ipilimumab during preparation or administration with fluids and medications other than 0.9% NS or D5W
- Administer diluted ipilimumab intraVENously through a sterile, nonpyrogenic, low-protein-binding, 1.2-μm pore size inline filter. The duration of the infusion and the recommended sequence of administration (when used as part of combination therapy) depend on the indication; refer to the current FDA-approved prescribing information for details
- Flush administration sets used to administer ipilimumab with 0.9% NS or D5W after completing drug administration

IRINOTECAN HYDROCHLORIDE

Camptosar (irinotecan hydrochloride) prescribing information. New York, NY: Pharmacia & Upjohn Co., Division of Pfizer Inc; January 2020
IRINOTECAN HYDROCHLORIDE prescribing information. Lake Forest, IL: Hospira, Inc.; May 2020

WARNING: DIARRHEA and MYELOSUPPRESSION

- Early and late forms of diarrhea can occur. Early diarrhea may be accompanied by cholinergic symptoms which may be prevented or ameliorated by atropine. Late diarrhea can be life-threatening and should be treated promptly with loperamide. Monitor patients with diarrhea and give fluid and electrolytes as needed. Institute antibiotic therapy if patients develop ileus, fever, or severe neutropenia. Interrupt CAMPTOSAR and reduce subsequent doses if severe diarrhea occurs …
- Severe myelosuppression may occur …

Boxed Warning for Camptosar (irinotecan hydrochloride) prescribing information. New York, NY: Pharmacia & Upjohn Co., Division of Pfizer Inc; January 2020

Product Identification, Preparation, Storage, and Stability

- Irinotecan Hydrochloride Injection is generically available
- Commercially available presentations include:
  - Individually packaged, single-use amber glass vials containing a sterile, pale yellow, clear, aqueous solution
  - Each milliliter of solution contains 20 mg of irinotecan hydrochloride (on the basis of the trihydrate salt), 45 mg of sorbitol, NF, and 0.9 mg of lactic acid, USP
  - Solution pH has been adjusted to 3.5 (range, 3.0–3.8) with sodium hydroxide or hydrochloric acid
  - Single-dose amber glass vials contain 40 mg (2 mL), 100 mg (5 mL), 300 mg (15 mL), or 500 mg (25 mL) of irinotecan (on the basis of the trihydrate salt)

Irinotecan Content	
In Amber Glass Vials	**In Amber-colored Polypropylene (CYTOSAFE) Vials**
40 mg (2 mL)	40 mg (2 mL)
100 mg (5 mL)	100 mg (5 mL)
500 mg (25 mL)	300 mg (15 mL)

- Store intact vials at controlled room temperature (20–25°C [68–77°F]) in the original packaging carton to protect the drug product from light until it is used. Excursions are permitted to 15–30°C (59–86°F)
- Irinotecan *must be diluted* before administration with D5W (preferred) or 0.9% NS to a concentration within the range of 0.12–2.8 mg/mL
- After dilution, irinotecan is physically and chemically stable for up to 24 hours at room temperature (approximately 25°C [77°F]) under ambient fluorescent lighting
- After dilution in D5W, solutions stored at approximately 2–8°C (36–46°F) and protected from light are physically and chemically stable for 48 hours
- *Do not refrigerate* admixtures prepared with 0.9% NS to prevent the formation of visible particulates
- *Avoid* freezing irinotecan and admixtures containing irinotecan, which may result in drug precipitation
- Commercially available products contain no antimicrobial preservatives; therefore, product labeling recommends using irinotecan admixtures as follows:

Vehicle Solution	Storage Temperature (After Preparation)	Shelf-life/Expiry Time (After Preparation)
D5W	2–8°C (36–46°F)	24 hours
D5W *or* 0.9% NS	15–30°C (59–86°F)	4 hours
D5W *or* 0.9% NS*	15–30°C (59–86°F)	12 hours
	2–8°C (36–46°F)	24 hours

*Under strictly maintained aseptic conditions; infusion should be completed before the aforementioned expiry times [Camptosar (irinotecan hydrochloride) prescribing information]

(*continued*)

Product Identification, Preparation, Storage, and Stability (continued)

Selected incompatibilities:

- Irinotecan in its active lactone form is maximally stable at pH ≤6. *Avoid admixture* with neutral or alkaline solutions[45]
- Irinotecan is susceptible to photodegradation
  - Photodegradation occurs at any solution pH, but is accelerated at neutral and alkaline pH in comparison with acidic pH[46,47]
  - The extent of photodegradation appears to be inversely related to irinotecan concentration in solution[48]
  - Although there is experimental evidence that indicates light protection may not be necessary during clinical use,[49] given the compound's propensity for photodegradation, protection from light exposure is a simple and prudent measure to employ toward maintaining product quality[48]

Recommendations for Drug Administration and Ancillary Care

General:

- See Chapter 43 for recommended use in patients with renal and hepatic dysfunction
- Administer irinotecan intraVENously over 90 minutes
- Irinotecan has anticholinesterase activity
  - Patients may experience cholinergic symptoms during or shortly after receiving irinotecan, including rhinitis, increased salivation, miosis, lacrimation, diaphoresis, hypotension, flushing, bradycardia, and intestinal hyperperistalsis that may cause abdominal cramping and diarrhea
- Atropine 0.25–1 mg intraVENously or SUBCUTaneously may be administered prophylactically or therapeutically to patients who experience cholinergic symptoms in association with irinotecan
- Irinotecan is metabolically activated to SN-38 by carboxyl esterase enzymes primarily in the liver

- SN-38 is a substrate for phase 2 metabolism by polymorphically expressed uridine diphosphate glucuronosyltransferase enzymes, particularly UGT1A1
  - Approximately 10% of the North American population expresses homozygously *UGT1A1*28* alleles (also known as a UGT1A1 7/7 genotype) and, consequently, experiences greater exposure to SN-38 and is at greater risk for neutropenia from irinotecan than are persons who express wild-type *UGT1A1* alleles (*AKA* UGT1A1 6/6 genotype)
- Initial irinotecan dose should be decreased by at least one level for persons who homozygously express *UGT1A1*28* alleles
  - The degree to which irinotecan doses should be decreased cannot be predicted
  - Second and subsequent doses should be based on an individual's tolerance of prior treatment

- Irinotecan and SN-38 metabolism and elimination are susceptible to perturbation by potent CYP3A4 inducers (carBAMazepine, PHENobarbital, phenytoin, rifabutin, rifAMPin, St. John's Wort) and inhibitors of CYP3A4 (ketoconazole), UGT1A1 (SORAfenib), or both CYP3A4 and UGT1A1 enzymes (atazanavir)

Inadvertent exposure:

- In case of skin contact, immediately and thoroughly wash the affected area with soap and water. *Do not abrade* the skin by using a scrub brush
- Treat accidental contact with mucous membranes immediately by thoroughly flushing the affected area with water

IRINOTECAN LIPOSOME INJECTION

ONIVYDE (irinotecan liposome injection) prescribing information. Basking Ridge, NJ: Ipsen Biopharmaceuticals, Inc; June 2017

WARNINGS: SEVERE NEUTROPENIA AND SEVERE DIARRHEA

- Fatal neutropenic sepsis occurred in 0.8% of patients receiving ONIVYDE. Severe or life-threatening neutropenic fever or sepsis occurred in 3% and severe or life-threatening neutropenia occurred in 20% of patients receiving ONIVYDE in combination with fluorouracil and leucovorin. Withhold ONIVYDE for absolute neutrophil count below 1500/mm^3 or neutropenic fever. Monitor blood cell counts periodically during treatment …
- Severe diarrhea occurred in 13% of patients receiving ONIVYDE in combination with fluorouracil and leucovorin. Do not administer ONIVYDE to patients with bowel obstruction. Withhold ONIVYDE for diarrhea of Grade 2–4 severity. Administer loperamide for late diarrhea of any severity. Administer atropine, if not contraindicated, for early diarrhea of any severity …

Boxed Warning for ONIVYDE (irinotecan liposome injection) prescribing information. Basking Ridge, NJ: Ipsen Biopharmaceuticals, Inc; June 2017

Product Identification, Preparation, Storage, and Stability

- ONIVYDE is a sterile, white to slightly yellow opaque isotonic liposomal dispersion. Each 10-mL single-dose vial contains 43 mg irinotecan free base at a concentration of 4.3 mg/mL (NDC 15054-0043-1). The liposome is a unilamellar lipid bilayer vesicle, approximately 110 nm in diameter, which encapsulates an aqueous space containing irinotecan in a gelated or precipitated state as the sucrose octasulfate salt

- ONIVYDE is a cytotoxic drug. Follow applicable special handling and disposal procedures
- Store ONIVYDE at 2°C to 8°C (36°F to 46°F). Do *NOT* freeze. Protect from light

Dilution
- Withdraw the calculated volume of ONIVYDE from the vial. Dilute ONIVYDE in 500 mL D5W or 0.9% NS and mix diluted solution by gentle inversion
- Protect diluted solution from light
- Administer diluted solution within 4 hours of preparation when stored at room temperature or within 24 hours of preparation when stored under refrigerated conditions (2°C to 8°C [36°F to 46°F]). Allow diluted solution to come to room temperature prior to administration

Recommendations for Drug Administration and Ancillary Care

General:
- See Chapter 43 for recommended use in patients with hepatic dysfunction
- No data are available for use in patients with bilirubin >2 mg/dL

Administration:
- Recommended dose of ONIVYDE is 70 mg/m^2 intraVENous infusion every 2 weeks in combination with fluorouracil and leucovorin for the treatment of metastatic adenocarcinoma of the pancreas
- Administer a corticosteroid and an antiemetic 30 minutes prior to ONIVYDE infusion
- Administer ONIVYDE prior to leucovorin and fluorouracil
- Infuse diluted solution intraVENously over 90 minutes. Do not use inline filters. Discard unused portion

Adverse events and treatment modifications:
- Refer to the current FDA-approved product label for detailed recommendations regarding treatment modifications for management of interstitial lung disease, anaphylactic reaction and other G ≥3 adverse events graded according to the NCI CTCAE v 4.0

Potential drug interactions
- Irinotecan and SN-38 metabolism and elimination are susceptible to perturbation by potent CYP3A4 inducers (carBAMazepine, PHENobarbital, phenytoin, rifabutin, rifAMPin, St. John's Wort) and inhibitors of CYP3A4 (clarithromycin, indinavir, itraconazole, lopinavir, nefazodone, nelfinavir, ritonavir, saquinavir, telaprevir, voriconazole), UGT1A1 (gemfibrozil), or both CYP3A4 and UGT1A1 enzymes (ketoconazole)

Patient Monitoring:
- Irinotecan has anticholinesterase activity. Patients may experience cholinergic symptoms during or shortly after receiving irinotecan, including rhinitis, increased salivation, miosis, lacrimation, diaphoresis, hypotension, flushing, bradycardia, and intestinal hyperperistalsis that may cause abdominal cramping and diarrhea

- Atropine 0.25–1 mg intraVENously or SUBCUTaneously may be administered prophylactically or therapeutically to patients who experience cholinergic symptoms in association with irinotecan
- Irinotecan is metabolically activated to SN-38 by carboxyl esterase enzymes primarily in the liver
- SN-38 is a substrate for phase 2 metabolism by polymorphically expressed uridine diphosphate glucuronosyltransferase enzymes, particularly UGT1A1
- Approximately 10% of the North American population expresses homozygously *UGT1A1*28* alleles (also known as a UGT1A1 7/7 genotype) and, consequently, experiences greater exposure to SN-38 and is at greater risk for neutropenia from irinotecan than are persons who express wild-type *UGT1A1* alleles (*AKA* UGT1A1 6/6 genotype)
- Initial irinotecan dosage should be decreased for persons who homozygously express *UGT1A1*28* alleles

ISATUXIMAB-irfc

SARCLISA (isatuximab-irfc) prescribing information. Bridgewater, NJ: Sanofi-Aventis U.S. LLC; March 2020

Product Identification, Preparation, Storage, and Stability

- SARCLISA (isatuximab-irfc) is a sterile, clear to slightly opalescent, colorless to slightly yellow, preservative-free solution, essentially free of visible particles available in individually boxed single-dose vials containing either 100 mg/5 mL (NDC 0024-0654-01) or 500 mg/25 mL (NDC 0024-0656-01). Each milliliter contains isatuximab-irfc (20 mg), histidine (1.46 mg), histidine hydrochloride monohydrate (2.22 mg), polysorbate 80 (0.2 mg), sucrose (100 mg), and SWFI. The pH is 6.0
- Store intact vials under refrigeration at 2–8°C (36–46°F) in the original carton to protect from light
- *Do not freeze or shake* intact vials

Dilution:
- Use aseptic technique during product preparation
- Inspect the product visually for the presence of particulate matter and discoloration
- Calculate the individual patient's dose based on actual patient weight measured prior to each cycle. More than one vial of SARCLISA (isatuximab-irfc) may be required
- Remove a volume of diluent from the 250-mL 0.9% NS or D5W diluent bag that is equivalent to the required volume of SARCLISA (isatuximab-irfc) injection. The infusion bag must be composed of polyolefins, polyethylene, polypropylene, PVC with DEHP or ethyl vinyl acetate

- Using a sterile syringe, withdraw the required volume of SARCLISA (isatuximab-irfc) injection and dilute by adding it to the infusion bag containing 0.9% NS or D5W to achieve the appropriate concentration for infusion
- Gently invert the bag to mix. Do not shake
- If the diluted solution is not used immediately, it must be used within 48 hours when stored refrigerated at 2–8°C, followed by 8 hours (including the infusion time) at room temperature

Selected incompatibility:
- Do not co-administer other drugs through the same intravenous line

Recommendations for Drug Administration and Ancillary Care

General:

- No dose adjustment is necessary for patients with renal impairment (estimated glomerular filtration rate <90 mL/min/1.73 m^2) or mild hepatic impairment (total bilirubin 1 to 1.5 × ULN, or AST > ULN). There are no PK data in patients with moderate (total bilirubin >1.5 × to 3 × ULN and any AST) or severe (total bilirubin >3 × ULN and any AST) hepatic impairment

Administration:

- The usual dose of isatuximab-irfc in combination with pomalidomide and dexamethasone for the treatment of multiple myeloma is 10 mg/kg intravenously every week for 4 weeks (cycle 1), followed by every 2 weeks (cycles 2 and beyond). Treatment cycle length is 28 days
- Isatuximab-irfc must be administered by a health care professional in a setting with immediate access to emergency equipment and appropriate medical support to manage infusion-related reactions
- Administer by intravenous infusion using an intravenous tubing infusion set (composed of polyethylene, PVC with or without DEHP, polybutadiene, or polyurethane) with a 0.22-μm inline filter (composed of polyethersulfone, polysulfone, or nylon)

Infusion Rates of SARCLISA (Isatuximab-irfc) Administration (Diluted to 250 mL)

Infusion	Initial Rate	Absence of Infusion-Related Reaction	Rate Increment	Maximum Rate
First	25 mL/hour	For 60 minutes	25 mL/hour every 30 minutes	150 mL/hour
Second	50 mL/hour	For 30 minutes	50 mL/hour for 30 minutes then increase by 100 mL/hour every 30 minutes	200 mL/hour
Subsequent	200 mL/hour	—	—	200 mL/hour

Note: increase of the infusion rate should only occur in the absence of an infusion-related reaction

Concomitant medications:

Pre-infusion Medications (administered 15–60 minutes before each infusion):
- Dexamethasone 40 mg orally or intravenously (or 20 mg in patients ≥75 years of age). Note that this dose corresponds to the total dose to be administered only once before infusion as part of both the premedication regimen and the backbone treatment for multiple myeloma
- Acetaminophen 650–1000 mg orally (or equivalent)

(continued)

Recommendations for Drug Administration and Ancillary Care *(continued)*

- ○ DiphenhydrAMINE 25–50 mg orally or intravenously (or equivalent). Note that the intravenous form is recommended for at least the first 4 doses
- ○ An H2 antagonist
- Consider the use of prophylactic antimicrobials during treatment, when indicated
- Consider the use of granulocyte colony-stimulating factor during treatment, when indicated
- Refer to current FDA-approved product labels for details regarding the use of other antineoplastic agents (eg, pomalidomide, dexamethasone) in combination with isatuximab

Adverse events and treatment modifications:

- Refer to the current FDA-approved product label for detailed warnings and treatment modifications for missed doses, infusion-related reactions, hematologic toxicities, and G4 neutropenia (ANC <500/mm^3). No dose reductions are recommended
- Infusion-related reactions were reported in 39% of patients. All reactions started during the first infusion and resolved on the same day in 98% of cases. Common symptoms included dyspnea, cough, chills, and nausea. Severe signs and symptoms included hypertension and dyspnea. Monitor vital signs frequently during the infusion. G1/2 reactions should be managed by infusion interruption and appropriate medical care. Upon improvement, resume the infusion at 50% of the initial infusion rate. If symptoms do not recur, increase to the initial rate after 30 minutes. If tolerated, then increase according to the usual instructions. Permanently discontinue isatuximab-irfc if symptoms do not improve after interruption, if symptoms recur after interruption, or in cases of G3/4 infusion-related reactions

Potential drug interactions:

- Isatuximab-irfc binds to CD38 expressed on red blood cells (RBCs) and therefore may result in a false positive indirect antiglobulin test. Check blood type and screen tests prior to the first infusion. Consider phenotyping prior to initiation of treatment. Inform the blood bank that a patient is receiving isatuximab-irfc and that blood compatibility testing can be resolved using dithiothreitol-treated RBCs
- Isatuximab-irfc, an IgG kappa monoclonal antibody, may be detected on serum protein electrophoresis and immunofixation assays

IXABEPILONE

IXEMPRA Kit (ixabepilone) prescribing information. Halle/Westfalen, Germany: Baxter Oncology GmbH; January 2016. Diluent for IXEMPRA manufactured by Baxter Oncology GmbH. Distributed by R-Pharm US LLC, Princeton, NJ

WARNING: TOXICITY IN HEPATIC IMPAIRMENT

IXEMPRA (ixabepilone) in combination with capecitabine is contraindicated in patients with AST or ALT >2.5 × ULN or bilirubin >1 × ULN due to increased risk of toxicity and neutropenia-related death …

Boxed Warning for IXEMPRA Kit (ixabepilone) prescribing information. Halle/Westfalen, Germany: Baxter Oncology GmbH; January 2016

Product Identification, Preparation, Storage, and Stability

- IXEMPRA is supplied as a kit containing one sterile, nonpyrogenic, single-use vial of ixabepilone as a lyophilized white powder, labeled: "IXEMPRA for Injection"

- The lyophilized drug product is packaged with a vial of a sterile, nonpyrogenic diluent solution of 52.8% (w/v) purified polyoxyethylated castor oil and 39.8% (w/v) dehydrated alcohol, USP, labeled: "Diluent for IXEMPRA"

- The commercial product is marketed in 2 presentations:

1 Vial IXEMPRA for Injection (Ixabepilone Content)	1 Vial of Diluent for IXEMPRA (Diluent Volume)	NDC Number
15 mg	8 mL	70020-1910-1
45 mg	23.5 mL	70020-1911-1

Note: To compensate for withdrawal losses, vials labeled 15 mg Ixempra for injection contain 16 mg of ixabepilone and vials labeled 45 mg Ixempra for injection contain 47 mg of ixabepilone

- Commercial IXEMPRA Kit must be stored under refrigeration at 2–8°C (36–46°F) and retained in the original packaging until time of use to protect it from light

- Prior to constituting Ixempra for injection, both drug and diluent vials should be removed from the refrigerator and allowed to stand at room temperature for approximately 30 minutes

- When diluent vials are first removed from the refrigerator, a white precipitate may be observed within the vials. The precipitate will dissolve to form a clear solution after the diluent warms to room temperature

- Only the diluent supplied in a kit should be used to reconstitute Ixempra (ixabepilone) for injection

Reconstitution:

- With a syringe, aseptically withdraw the diluent and slowly inject it into the copackaged vial containing lyophilized ixabepilone:

  - To a vial containing 15 mg of ixabepilone, add 8 mL of diluent

  - To a vial containing 45 mg of ixabepilone, add 23.5 mL of diluent

- Gently swirl and invert the vial until the lyophilized powder is completely dissolved

- After reconstitution, concentrated ixabepilone solution (2 mg/mL) should be further diluted with an appropriate fluid as soon as possible, but may be stored in the vial (*not the syringe*) for a maximum of 1 hour at room temperature and room lighting

Dilution:

- Before administration, concentrated ixabepilone solution (2 mg/mL) must be further diluted in a DEHP-free parenteral product container (generally, non-PVC containers)

- Aseptically withdraw and measure with a calibrated syringe an amount of concentrated ixabepilone solution required for a patient's dose, and transfer it to a DEHP-free parenteral product bag or bottle containing a volume of solution sufficient to produce a final ixabepilone concentration within the range 0.2–0.6 mg/mL (typically 250 mL)

- Fluids appropriate for diluting ixabepilone have in common a pH within the range of 6.0–9.0, which is required to maintain ixabepilone stability. Other infusion fluids should not be used

- The following parenteral fluids are appropriate for diluting ixabepilone:

  - Lactated Ringer injection, USP

  - Plasma-Lyte A injection pH 7.4 (multiple electrolytes injection, type 1, USP) (Baxter Healthcare Corporation)

  - 0.9% Sodium chloride injection, USP, with pH adjusted with sodium bicarbonate injection, USP

    ○ When using 0.9% NS as a vehicle for clinical use, the solution pH must be adjusted to 6.0–9.0 *before* concentrated ixabepilone solution (2 mg/mL) is added to the vehicle solution

    ○ To 250 mL or 500 mL of 0.9% NS, add:

    ○ 2 mL of Sodium bicarbonate injection, USP 8.4% (w/v) solution, *or*

    ○ 4 mL of Sodium bicarbonate injection, USP 4.2% (w/v) solution

- Thoroughly mix diluted ixabepilone by manually rotating the product container

- The diluted product is stable at room temperature and room light for a maximum of 6 hours; the infusion must be completed within this period

Recommendations for Drug Administration and Ancillary Care

Premedication:

- All patients must receive primary prophylaxis against hypersensitivity reactions approximately 1 hour before ixabepilone administration commences, including:
  - A histamine H_1-subtype receptor antagonist, for example, diphenhydrAMINE 50 mg or equivalent H_1 antihistamine administered orally, *plus*
  - A histamine H_2-subtype receptor antagonist, for example, raNITIdine 150–300 mg or equivalent H_2 antihistamine administer orally

- In addition to pretreatment with H_1 and H_2 antihistamines, patients who previously experienced a hypersensitivity reaction associated with ixabepilone administration require steroid premedication, for example, dexamethasone 20 mg administered intraVENously 30 minutes before infusion, *or* dexamethasone 20 mg administered orally 60 minutes before starting ixabepilone administration

General:

- See Chapter 43 for recommended use in patients with renal and hepatic dysfunction

- DEHP-free administration sets must be used to administer ixabepilone
- Ixabepilone must be administered through an inline filter with a pore size within the range of 0.2–1.2 μm
- The durations of administration recommended for 40 mg ixabepilone/m^2 is 3 hours, and 4 hours for 60 mg ixabepilone/m^2
  - Other dosages, administration schedules, and durations of administration have been evaluated in clinical trials

LEUCOVORIN CALCIUM

LEUCOVORIN CALCIUM prescribing information. Schaumburg, IL: SAGENT Pharmaceuticals; October 2017
LEUCOVORIN CALCIUM prescribing information. Schaumburg, IL: SAGENT Pharmaceuticals; April 2016
LEUCOVORIN CALCIUM prescribing information. Lake Zurich, IL: Fresenius Kabi USA, LLC; April 2018
LEUCOVORIN CALCIUM prescribing information. Lake Zurich, IL; Fresenius Kabi USA, LLC; May 2018

Product Identification, Preparation, Storage, and Stability

Leucovorin calcium for injection (lyophilized powder formulation):
• Leucovorin calcium for injection is generically available in a variety of presentations, including:
  ▪ 50 mg/vial packaged in cartons of 10 single-use vials
  ▪ 100 mg/vial individually packaged in single-use vials *or* in cartons of 10 single-use vials
  ▪ 200 mg/vial individually packaged in single-use vials
  ▪ 350 mg/vial individually packaged in single-use vials
  ▪ 500 mg/vial individually packaged in single-use vials
• Leucovorin calcium for injection is a sterile, lyophilized powder indicated for intraMUSCular or intraVENous administration. In general, the lyophilized powdered products do not contain an antimicrobial preservative
• Store leucovorin calcium for injection at room temperature
  ▪ *Note:* Storage temperature requirements for leucovorin calcium for injection vary among different manufacturers' products
  ▪ Consult product labeling for product-specific storage temperature recommendations
• Retain vials in their packaging carton to protect the drug product from light until they are used
• Reconstitute leucovorin calcium for injection with BWFI (preserved with benzyl alcohol)* or SWFI as follows:

Amount of Leucovorin Calcium per Vial	Volume of Diluent per Vial	Concentration After Reconstitution
50 mg	5 mL	10 mg/mL
100 mg	10 mL	
200 mg	20 mL	
350 mg	17.5 mL	20 mg/mL
500 mg	50 mL	10 mg/mL

*FDA-approved product labeling recommends reconstituting leucovorin with SWFI for dosages >10 mg/m² (for adult patients) because of the amount of benzyl alcohol present in BWFI. *Avoid* administering benzyl alcohol-containing products to adolescents and younger patients

• After reconstitution with BWFI, the resulting solution must be used within 7 days. If reconstituted with SWFI, use the product immediately and discard any unused portion

Leucovorin calcium injection (product in solution):
• Leucovorin calcium injection, USP, is available in individually boxed, single-use vials containing leucovorin calcium 500 mg (per 50 mL) or 100 mg (per 10 mL) in a sterile, preservative-free solution indicated for intraMUSCular or intraVENous administration
• Each milliliter of solution contains leucovorin calcium equivalent to 10 mg leucovorin, USP, with sodium chloride and sodium hydroxide and/or hydrochloric acid to adjust solution to an alkaline pH, which varies among different manufacturers' products (range: pH 6.5–8.5)
• Store leucovorin calcium injection under refrigeration at 2–8°C (36–46°F). Retain vials in their packaging carton to protect the drug product from light until they are used
• Discard any unused portion

Instructions common to both leucovorin calcium for injection and leucovorin calcium injection:
• Leucovorin calcium may be further diluted with D5W, 0.9% NS, D5W/0.9% NS, D10W, RI, or LRI for clinical use

Selected incompatibility:
• *Do not mix* leucovorin with fluorouracil. Admixture results in particulate formation

Recommendations for Drug Administration and Ancillary Care

General:

- For intraVENous or intraMUSCular administration
- Administer leucovorin intraVENously over *at least* 3 minutes
- *Do not administer* leucovorin intraVENously more rapidly than 160 mg/min because of the rate at which calcium will be injected
  - For solutions reconstituted from (lyophilized) leucovorin calcium for injection:

Leucovorin Concentration in Solution	Volume of Solution Containing 160 mg Leucovorin
10 mg/mL	16 mL
20 mg/mL	8 mL

- One milligram of leucovorin calcium contains:

Calcium	0.004 mEq
Calcium	0.002 mmol
Leucovorin	0.002 mmol

Caution:

- In treating an accidental overdose of intraTHECALly administered folic acid antagonists, *do not administer* leucovorin intraTHECALly; leucovorin may be harmful or fatal if given intraTHECALly
- Concomitant use of leucovorin with trimethoprim-sulfamethoxazole (cotrimoxazole) for the acute treatment of *Pneumocystis jirovecii* (formerly *Pneumocystis carinii*) pneumonia in patients with HIV infection was associated with increased rates of treatment failure and morbidity in a placebo-controlled study
- High doses of leucovorin by intraVENous, intraMUSCular, or oral routes may reduce the efficacy of intraTHECALly administered methotrexate

LEVOLEUCOVORIN CALCIUM

Fusilev (levoleucovorin) prescribing information. East Windsor, NJ: Acrotech Biopharma LLC.; January 2020
KHAPZORY (levoleucovorin) prescribing information. East Windsor, NJ: Acrotech Biopharma LLC.; March 2020

Product Identification, Preparation, Storage, and Stability

- LEVOleucovorin is the levorotatory isomeric form of racemic *d,l*-leucovorin, the pharmacologically active isomer of leucovorin [(6-*S*)-leucovorin], present as the calcium salt

Fusilev Injection, for intravenous use (product in solution):

- Fusilev injection is provided in 50-mg single-use vials containing a sterile solution of either 175 mg LEVOleucovorin in 17.5 mL (NDC 72893-013-01) or 250 mg LEVOleucovorin in 25 mL (NDC 72893-014-01)
- Each milliliter of solution contains LEVOleucovorin calcium pentahydrate equivalent to 10 mg LEVOleucovorin and 8.3 mg sodium chloride. Sodium hydroxide is used to adjust solution pH to 8.0 (6.5–8.5). Fusilev injection does not contain an antimicrobial preservative
- Store LEVOleucovorin in solution under refrigeration at 2–8°C (36–46°F) in its packaging carton to protect the drug product from light until vial contents are used
- Fusilev injection (LEVOleucovorin in solution, 10 mg/mL) may be further diluted to a concentration = 0.5 mg/mL in 0.9% NS or D5W
- Fusilev injection (LEVOleucovorin in solution) diluted in 0.9% NS or D5W stored at room temperature *must be used* within 4 hours after preparation

Fusilev for injection (lyophilized product):

- Fusilev for injection is provided in 50-mg single-use vials containing a sterile lyophilized powder consisting of 64 mg LEVOleucovorin calcium pentahydrate (equivalent to 50 mg LEVOleucovorin) and 50 mg mannitol per 50-mg vial. Sodium hydroxide and hydrochloric acid are used to adjust product pH during manufacture (NDC 72893-009-01).

Fusilev for injection does not contain an antimicrobial preservative

- Store Fusilev for injection (lyophilized product) at 20° to 25°C (68–77°F) in its packaging carton to protect the drug product from light until vial contents are used. Temperature excursions are permitted from 15° to 30°C (59–86°F)
- Reconstitute the lyophilized product (Fusilev for injection 50-mg vial) with 5.3 mL of sterile 0.9% NS to produce a solution with LEVOleucovorin concentration of 10 mg/mL

  - *Do not use* preserved diluent solutions
- The reconstituted solution (10 mg/mL) may be immediately diluted to concentrations within a range of 0.5–5 mg/mL in 0.9% NS or D5W
- After reconstitution (10 mg/mL), dilution in D5W, and storage at room temperature, LEVOleucovorin *must be used* within 4 hours after preparation
- After reconstitution (10 mg/mL) and dilution in 0.9% NS, LEVOleucovorin solutions stored at room temperature *must be used* within 12 hours after preparation
- *Do not use* LEVOleucovorin if cloudiness or a precipitate is observed in solution

Selected incompatibility:

- *Do not mix* LEVOleucovorin with fluorouracil. Admixture results in particulate formation
- *Do not administer* LEVOleucovorin in an admixture with other drug products or in diluent or vehicle solutions other than 0.9 NS or D5W

KHAPZORY for injection (lyophilized product):

- KHAPZORY for injection is provided in single-use vials containing LEVOleucovorin

175-mg (NDC 72893-004-01) or 300-mg (NDC 72893-006-01) as a sterile, white to yellowish lyophilized powder. Vials also contain sodium hydroxide (29.6 mg and 50.7 mg, respectively) and mannitol (105 mg and 180 mg, respectively) and may also contain additional sodium hydroxide and/or hydrochloric acid to adjust the pH during manufacture

- Store KHAPZORY for injection at 20° to 25°C (68–77°F) in its packaging carton to protect the drug product from light until vial contents are used. Temperature excursions are permitted from 15° to 30°C (59–86°F)
- Reconstitute KHAPZORY for injection with sterile 0.9% NS as follows:

KHAPZORY for Injection Reconstitution

Amount of LEVOleucovorin per Vial	Volume of Diluent (0.9% NS) per Vial	Concentration After Reconstitution
175 mg	3.6 mL	50 mg/mL
300 mg	6.2 mL	

- *Do not use* preserved diluent solutions
- The reconstituted KHAPZORY solution (50 mg/mL) may be stored at room temperature for up to 12 hours protected from light
- The reconstituted KHAPZORY solution (50 mg/mL) may be immediately diluted to concentrations within a range of 0.5–5 mg/mL in 0.9% NS or D5W
- After reconstitution of KHAPZORY, further dilution in either 0.9% NS or D5W, and storage at room temperature protected from light, KHAPZORY *must be used* within 12 hours after preparation
- *Do not use* KHAPZORY if cloudiness or a precipitate is observed in solution

Recommendations for Drug Administration and Ancillary Care

General:

- LEVOleucovorin dose or dosage is one-half (50%) the dose or dosage recommended for racemic *d,l*-leucovorin
- Fusilev and KHAPZORY are indicated only for intraVENous administration. *Do not administer* LEVOleucovorin intraTHECALly
- *Do not inject* Fusilev products (which contain calcium) more rapidly than 160 mg/min because of the rate at which calcium will be injected
  - One milligram of LEVOleucovorin calcium (Fusilev formulations) contains:

Calcium	0.004 mEq
Calcium	0.002 mmol
LEVOleucovorin	0.002 mmol

- Concomitant use of racemic leucovorin with trimethoprim-sulfamethoxazole (cotrimoxazole) for the acute treatment of *Pneumocystis jirovecii* (formerly *Pneumocystis carinii*) pneumonia in patients with HIV infection was associated with increased rates of treatment failure and morbidity in a placebo-controlled study

LURBINECTEDIN

ZEPZELCA (lurbinectedin for injection) prescribing information. Palo Alto, CA: Jazz Pharmaceuticals, Inc; January 2020

Product Identification, Preparation, Storage, and Stability

- Lurbinectedin for injection is supplied as a sterile, preservative-free, white to off-white lyophilized powder in a single-dose clear glass vial
- Each carton (NDC 68727-712-01) includes one single-dose vial containing lurbinectedin (4 mg), sucrose (800 mg), lactic acid (22.1 mg), and sodium hydroxide (5.1 mg)
- Store unopened vials refrigerated at 2° to 8°C (36° to 46°F)
- Lurbinectedin is a hazardous drug. Follow applicable special handling and disposal procedures

Reconstitution:
- Inject 8 mL of SWFI into the vial, yielding a solution containing 0.5 mg/mL lurbinectedin. Shake the vial until complete dissolution
- Visually inspect the solution for particulate matter and discoloration. The reconstituted solution is a clear, colorless or slightly yellowish solution, essentially free of visible particles
- Calculate the required volume of reconstituted solution as follows:
    - $$\text{Volume (mL)} = \frac{\text{Body Surface Area (m}^2) \times \text{Individual Dose (mg/m}^2)}{0.5 \text{ mg/mL}}$$

Dilution:
- For administration through a central VAD, withdraw the appropriate amount of reconstituted solution from the vial and add to an infusion container containing at least 100 mL of diluent (0.9% NS or D5W)
- For administration through a peripheral venous line, withdraw the appropriate amount of reconstituted solution from the vial and add to an infusion container containing at least 250 mL of diluent (0.9% NS or D5W)
- If not used immediately after reconstitution or dilution, the lurbinectedin solution can be stored prior to administration for up to 24 hours following reconstitution, including infusion time, at either room temperature/ambient light or under refrigeration at 2°C–8°C (36°F–46°F) conditions

Recommendations for Drug Administration and Ancillary Care

General:
- See Chapter 43 for recommended use in patients with hepatic dysfunction
- The effects of severe renal impairment (ClCr < 30 mL/min) and moderate or severe hepatic impairment (total bilirubin > 1.5 × ULN and any AST) on the pharmacokinetics of lurbinectedin have not been studied

Administration:
- Recommended dose is 3.2 mg/m² by intraVENous infusion over 60 minutes every 21 days for patients with small cell lung cancer with disease progression on or after platinum-based chemotherapy

Adverse events and treatment modifications:
- Refer to the current FDA-approved product label for detailed recommendations regarding treatment modifications for management of neutropenia, thrombocytopenia, and hepatotoxicity graded according to the NCI CTCAE v 4.0

Potential drug interactions:
- Avoid coadministration with strong or moderate CYP3A inhibitors. If coadministration cannot be avoided, consider dose reduction of lurbinectedin if clinically indicated
- Avoid coadministration with strong or moderate CYP3A inducers

Selected precautions:
- Initiate treatment only if absolute neutrophil count is ≥1500 cells/mm³ and platelet count is ≥100,000/mm³

MELPHALAN HYDROCHLORIDE

ALKERAN (melphalan hydrochloride) prescribing information. Weston, FL: ApoPharma USA Inc.; November 2018
EVOMELA (melphalan for injection, for intravenous use) prescribing information. East Windsor, NJ: Acrotech Biopharma LLC; March 2020

WARNING: SEVERE BONE MARROW SUPPRESSION, HYPERSENSITIVITY, and LEUKEMOGENICITY

- Severe bone marrow suppression with resulting infection or bleeding may occur. Controlled trials comparing intravenous (IV) melphalan to oral melphalan have shown more myelosuppression with the IV formulation. Monitor hematologic laboratory parameters …
- Hypersensitivity reactions, including anaphylaxis, have occurred in approximately 2% of patients who received the IV formulation of melphalan. Discontinue treatment with Evomela for serious hypersensitivity reactions …
- Melphalan produces chromosomal aberrations in vitro and in vivo. Evomela should be considered potentially leukemogenic in humans …

Boxed Warning for EVOMELA (melphalan for injection, for intravenous use) prescribing information. East Windsor, NJ: Acrotech Biopharma LLC; March 2020

WARNING

Melphalan should be administered under the supervision of a qualified physician experienced in the use of cancer chemotherapeutic agents. Severe bone marrow suppression with resulting infection or bleeding may occur. Controlled trials comparing intravenous (IV) to oral melphalan have shown more myelosuppression with the IV formulation. Hypersensitivity reactions, including anaphylaxis, have occurred in approximately 2% of patients who received the IV formulation. Melphalan is leukemogenic in humans. Melphalan produces chromosomal aberrations in vitro and in vivo and, therefore, should be considered potentially mutagenic in humans

Boxed Warning for ALKERAN (melphalan hydrochloride) prescribing information. Weston, FL: ApoPharma USA Inc.; November 2018

Product Identification, Preparation, Storage, and Stability

Alkeran (melphalan hydrochloride for injection):

- Alkeran (melphalan hydrochloride for injection) is supplied in a carton containing (1) one single-use, clear, glass vial containing freeze-dried melphalan hydrochloride equivalent to 50 mg melphalan and the inactive ingredient povidone 20 mg as a sterile, nonpyrogenic, freeze-dried powder, and (2) one 10-mL, clear, glass vial of sterile, nonpyrogenic sterile diluent for melphalan hydrochloride for injection containing 200 mg sodium citrate, 6 mL of propylene glycol, 0.52 mL of ethanol (96%), and SWFI to a total of (Q.S.) 10 mL
- Store Alkeran (melphalan hydrochloride for injection) at room temperature and protect from light
  - *Note:* Storage temperature requirements for melphalan hydrochloride for injection vary among different manufacturers' products
  - Consult product labeling for product-specific storage temperature recommendations

Preparation of Alkeran (melphalan hydrochloride for injection) for administration:

1. Reconstitute Alkeran (melphalan hydrochloride for injection) by *rapidly injecting* 10 mL of the supplied diluent directly into the vial of lyophilized powder using a sterile needle (20-gauge or larger) and syringe
   a. Melphalan is practically insoluble in water and has a pKa_1 of ~2.5
2. Immediately *shake the vial vigorously* until a clear solution is obtained. This provides a 5-mg/mL solution of melphalan. Rapid addition of the diluent followed by immediate vigorous shaking is important for proper dissolution.
3. Immediately withdraw into a syringe an amount of reconstituted melphalan solution appropriate for a patient's dose and dilute it in 0.9% NS, to a concentration ≤0.45 mg/mL
   a. The time between melphalan reconstitution, dilution, and administration should be kept to a minimum because the diluted solution is unstable

b. Within 30 minutes after melphalan reconstitution with sterile diluent for melphalan hydrochloride for injection, a citrate derivative of melphalan has been detected
c. After further dilution with 0.9% NS, nearly 1% of the labeled strength of melphalan hydrolyzes every 10 minutes
d. A precipitate forms if the reconstituted solution is stored at 5°C (41°F). *Do not refrigerate* the reconstituted product

EVOMELA (melphalan for injection):

- EVOMELA (melphalan for injection) is supplied in a carton containing a single-use 20-mL vial containing melphalan hydrochloride (56 mg) (equivalent to 50 mg of melphalan free base) and Betadex sulfobutyl ether sodium, NF (2700 mg) as a white to off-white lyophilized powder
- Store EVOMELA (melphalan for injection) at room temperature (25°C [77°F]) in the original carton to protect from light. Excursions to 15° to 30°C (59–86°F) are permissible

(continued)

Product Identification, Preparation, Storage, and Stability (*continued*)

Preparation of EVOMELA (melphalan for injection) for administration:

1. Reconstitute EVOMELA (melphalan for injection) with 8.6 mL 0.9% NS to provide a solution with a nominal melphalan concentration of 50 mg/10 mL (5 mg/mL)

a. Reconstituted EVOMELA (melphalan for injection) is stable for 24 hours at refrigerated temperature (5°C) and for 1 hour at room temperature

2. Withdraw into a syringe an amount of reconstituted EVOMELA (melphalan for injection) solution appropriate for a

patient's dose and dilute it an appropriate volume of 0.9% NS to obtain a final concentration = 0.45 mg/mL

a. The diluted EVOMELA (melphalan for injection) solution is stable for 4 hours at room temperature in addition to the 1 hour following reconstitution

Recommendations for Drug Administration and Ancillary Care

General:

• See Chapter 43 for recommended use in patients with renal dysfunction
• Recommended infusion duration differs by product:
  ▪ Administer Alkeran (melphalan hydrochloride for injection) by intraVENous infusion over 15–20 minutes (at least 15 minutes). Complete Alkeran (melphalan hydrochloride for injection) administration within 60 minutes after reconstitution, as reconstituted and diluted solutions are unstable
  ▪ Administer EVOMELA (melphalan for injection) by intraVENous infusion over 30 minutes via an injection port

or central VAD. Do not administer by direct injection into a peripheral vein. Administer by injecting slowly into a fast-running IV infusion via a central VAD. Complete EVOMELA (melphalan for injection) administration within 4 hours after dilution, as diluted solutions are unstable

Caution:

• Severe renal failure has been reported in patients treated with a single dose of intraVENously administered melphalan followed by standard oral doses of cycloSPORINE
• CISplatin may affect melphalan pharmacokinetics by inducing renal

dysfunction and secondarily decreasing melphalan clearance
• IntraVENously administered melphalan may decrease the threshold for lung toxicity associated with carmustine
• The incidence of severe hemorrhagic necrotic enterocolitis has been reported to increase in pediatric patients when nalidixic acid and intraVENously administered melphalan are given simultaneously

Inadvertent exposure:

• If melphalan HCl contacts skin or mucosa, immediately wash the affected area with soap and water

MESNA

MESNEX (mesna) prescribing information. Deerfield, IL: Baxter Healthcare Corporation; December 2018

Product Identification, Preparation, Storage, and Stability

- Mesna injection is a sterile, nonpyrogenic, clear, colorless, aqueous solution for intraVENous administration in clear, glass, multidose vials packaged individually or in greater quantities
- Each milliliter of mesna injection contains mesna 100 mg; edetate disodium 0.25 mg; benzyl alcohol 10.4 mg as a preservative, (Q.S.) SWFI, and sodium hydroxide to adjust solution to an alkaline pH that varies among different manufacturers' products (range: pH 6.5–8.5)
- Store mesna at room temperature, 20–25°C (68–77°F). Product-specific recommendations for storage temperatures

may identify permissible temperature excursions
- Multidose vials may be stored and used for up to 8 days after initial vial entry
- For intraVENous administration mesna injection (100 mg/mL) may be diluted by admixture (1 mL of mesna injection added to 4 mL of a compatible solution) with any of the following fluids to produce a concentration of 20 mg mesna/mL: D5W, D5W/0.2% NaCl, D5W/0.33% NaCl, D5W/0.45% NaCl, 0.9% NS, LRI
- Diluted mesna solutions (20 mg/mL) are chemically and physically stable for 24 hours at 25°C (77°F)

- Additional compatibility and stability data indicate mesna is stable at room temperature for at least 24 hours when diluted to concentration of 1 mg/mL in 0.9% NS, D5W, D5W/0.45% NaCl, and LRI[50]
- Mesna is compatible in admixture (prepared in the same container) with both ifosfamide and cyclophosphamide

Selected incompatibility:
- Mesna is *not compatible* and should not be mixed in a container or in administration set tubing with CISplatin or CARBOplatin

Recommendations for Drug Administration and Ancillary Care

General:
- See Chapter 43 for comments about use in patients with renal and hepatic dysfunction
- Mesna may be administered by intraVENous injection, intermittent intraVENous infusion over 15–30 minutes, or continuous intraVENous infusion during ifosfamide or cyclophosphamide administration and for periods afterward
- If mesna tablets are not available for use, the parenteral product also may be given orally, diluted just before use in a small volume (60–120 mL; 2–4 oz) of a chilled carbonated beverage to mask the drug's unpleasant flavor
- Avoid exposing mesna injection to the air. Mesna spontaneously oxidizes to dimesna on exposure to oxygen
- FDA-approved product labeling describes intermittent administration of mesna with ifosfamide as follows:

IntraVENous administration:
- Mesna in a dosage equal to 20% (w/w) of the ifosfamide dosage is given at the same

time as ifosfamide, and then at 4 hours and 8 hours after ifosfamide administration began; that is, the total daily mesna dose is approximately 60% of the daily ifosfamide dose

IntraVENous and oral administration:
- Mesna in a dosage equal to 20% (w/w) of the ifosfamide dosage is given intraVENously at the same time as ifosfamide, and then mesna tablets are given orally at 2 hours and 6 hours after each ifosfamide dose with each oral doses equal to 40% of the ifosfamide dose; that is, the total daily mesna dose is approximately equal to the daily ifosfamide dose

Caution:
- Allergic reactions to mesna, ranging from mild hypersensitivity to systemic anaphylactic reactions, have been reported
- Mesna injection does not prevent urothelial toxicity in all patients
  - Advise patients who receive mesna with ifosfamide or cyclophosphamide who are not receiving parenterally

administered fluids to drink at least 1 quart (≥1000 mL) per day on days of treatment and for several days afterward
  - A morning specimen of urine should be examined microscopically for the presence of hematuria each day prior to ifosfamide therapy
  - To reduce the risk of hematuria, mesna must be administered with each dose of ifosfamide
  - Mesna is not effective in reducing the risk of hematuria caused by other pathologic conditions, for example, thrombocytopenia
- Multidose vials containing benzyl alcohol should not be used in neonates or infants and should be used with caution in older pediatric patients

Interaction with laboratory test:
- A false-positive test for urinary ketones may arise in patients treated with mesna injection. In this test, a red-violet color develops, which, with the addition of glacial acetic acid, will return to violet

METHOTREXATE

METHOTREXATE prescribing information. Lake Zurich, IL: Fresenius Kabi USA, LLC.; April 2016
METHOTREXATE prescribing information. Lake Forest, IL: Hospira, Inc.; May 2018
METHOTREXATE prescribing information. Eatontown, NJ: West-Ward Pharmaceuticals; August 2018

WARNINGS

FOR INTRATHECAL AND HIGH-DOSE THERAPY, USE THE PRESERVATIVE-FREE FORMULATION OF METHOTREXATE. DO NOT USE THE PRESERVED FORMULATION FOR INTRATHECAL OR HIGH-DOSE THERAPY BECAUSE IT CONTAINS BENZYL ALCOHOL

METHOTREXATE SHOULD BE USED ONLY IN LIFE-THREATENING NEOPLASTIC DISEASES, OR IN PATIENTS WITH PSORIASIS OR RHEUMATOID ARTHRITIS WITH SEVERE, RECALCITRANT, DISABLING DISEASE WHICH IS NOT ADEQUATELY RESPONSIVE TO OTHER FORMS OF THERAPY

DEATHS HAVE BEEN REPORTED WITH THE USE OF METHOTREXATE IN THE TREATMENT OF MALIGNANCY, PSORIASIS, AND RHEUMATOID ARTHRITIS

PATIENTS SHOULD BE CLOSELY MONITORED FOR BONE MARROW, LIVER, LUNG, AND KIDNEY TOXICITIES …

PATIENTS SHOULD BE INFORMED BY THEIR PHYSICIAN OF THE RISKS INVOLVED AND BE UNDER A PHYSICIAN'S CARE THROUGHOUT THERAPY

THE USE OF METHOTREXATE HIGH-DOSE REGIMENS RECOMMENDED FOR OSTEOSARCOMA REQUIRES METICULOUS CARE … HIGH-DOSE REGIMENS FOR OTHER NEOPLASTIC DISEASES ARE INVESTIGATIONAL AND A THERAPEUTIC ADVANTAGE HAS NOT BEEN ESTABLISHED

- Methotrexate has been reported to cause fetal death and/or congenital anomalies. Therefore, it is not recommended for women of childbearing potential unless there is clear medical evidence that the benefits can be expected to outweigh the considered risks. Pregnant women with psoriasis or rheumatoid arthritis should not receive methotrexate …

- Methotrexate elimination is reduced in patients with impaired renal functions, ascites, or pleural effusions. Such patients require especially careful monitoring for toxicity, and require dose reduction or, in some cases, discontinuation of methotrexate administration

- Unexpectedly severe (sometimes fatal) bone marrow suppression, aplastic anemia, and gastrointestinal toxicity have been reported with concomitant administration of methotrexate (usually in high dosage) along with some nonsteroidal anti-inflammatory drugs (NSAIDs) …

- Methotrexate causes hepatotoxicity, fibrosis, and cirrhosis, but generally only after prolonged use. Acutely, liver enzyme elevations are frequently seen. These are usually transient and asymptomatic, and also do not appear predictive of subsequent hepatic disease. Liver biopsy after sustained use often shows histologic changes, and fibrosis and cirrhosis have been reported; these latter lesions may not be preceded by symptoms or abnormal liver function tests in the psoriasis population. For this reason, periodic liver biopsies are usually recommended for psoriatic patients who are under long-term treatment. Persistent abnormalities in liver function tests may precede appearance of fibrosis or cirrhosis in the rheumatoid arthritis population …

- Methotrexate-induced lung disease, including acute or chronic interstitial pneumonitis, is a potentially dangerous lesion, which may occur acutely at any time during therapy and has been reported at low doses. It is not always fully reversible and fatalities have been reported. Pulmonary symptoms (especially a dry, nonproductive cough) may require interruption of treatment and careful investigation

- Diarrhea and ulcerative stomatitis require interruption of therapy: otherwise, hemorrhagic enteritis and death from intestinal perforation may occur

- Malignant lymphomas, which may regress following withdrawal of methotrexate, may occur in patients receiving low-dose methotrexate and, thus, may not require cytotoxic treatment. Discontinue methotrexate first and, if the lymphoma does not regress, appropriate treatment should be instituted

- Like other cytotoxic drugs, methotrexate may induce "tumor lysis syndrome" in patients with rapidly growing tumors. Appropriate supportive and pharmacologic measures may prevent or alleviate this complication

- Severe, occasionally fatal, skin reactions have been reported following single or multiple doses of methotrexate. Reactions have occurred within days of oral, intramuscular, intravenous, or intrathecal methotrexate administration. Recovery has been reported with discontinuation of therapy …

- Potentially fatal opportunistic infections, especially *Pneumocystis carinii* pneumonia, may occur with methotrexate therapy

- Methotrexate given concomitantly with radiotherapy may increase the risk of soft tissue necrosis and osteonecrosis

Boxed Warning for METHOTREXATE prescribing information. Eatontown, NJ: West-Ward Pharmaceuticals; August 2018

Product Identification, Preparation, Storage, and Stability

- Methotrexate is generically available in a variety of product strengths in liquid and lyophilized formulations
- Store methotrexate at room temperature and protected from light
  - *Note:* Storage temperature requirements for methotrexate vary among different manufacturers' products
  - Consult product labeling for product-specific storage temperature recommendations
- The lyophilized products (1-g vials) are reconstituted with 19.4 mL of an appropriate sterile, preservative-free diluent such as D5W or 0.9% NS to a concentration = 50 mg methotrexate/mL. When high doses of methotrexate are administered by intraVENous infusion, the total dose of reconstituted product is further diluted

- Protect methotrexate products from light. Methotrexate is susceptible to photodegradation, the extent of which correlates inversely with methotrexate concentration and is exacerbated by admixture with sodium bicarbonate
- After reconstitution, lyophilized formulations and methotrexate injection (25 mg/mL product supplied as an isotonic liquid) are suitable for direct intraVENous injection
- Methotrexate may also be further diluted for clinical use. A therapeutic indication often determines the volume in which a dose is prepared and administered—that is, whether dilution is necessary, or clinically or logistically appropriate. Compatible diluents include 0.9% NS, D5W, and combinations of saline and dextrose

For intraTHECAL injection and high-dose regimens:
- Use only preservative-free methotrexate and diluent solutions

For intraTHECAL injection:
- Use preservative-free 0.9% NS to dilute methotrexate for intraTHECAL injection to a concentration within the range of 1–2.5 mg/mL
- Admixtures with hydrocortisone sodium succinate for intraTHECAL administration (with or without cytarabine) should be prepared just before use and administered as soon as possible (within minutes) after preparation because of the instability of the hydrocortisone component

Recommendations for Drug Administration and Ancillary Care

General:
- See Chapter 43 for recommended use in patients with renal and hepatic dysfunction
- Methotrexate may be given parenterally by direct intraVENous injection, short intraVENous infusions over <1 hour, or continuous intraVENous infusions for periods up to 24–36 hours, and by the intraMUSCular, intra-arterial, and intraTHECAL routes

For intraVENous use:
- The duration of methotrexate administration varies among treatment protocols and published reports, and in the case of moderate- and high-dose regimens ($\geq$100 mg/m^2), often correlates with schemes for concomitant hydration, urinary alkalinization, serum level monitoring and expectations for the rate at which methotrexate will be eliminated, and leucovorin rescue

For intraTHECAL injection:
- Use *only products that do not contain antimicrobial preservatives* (eg, alcohols, parabens)
- Cerebrospinal fluid volume is dependent on age, *not* body surface area (BSA); therefore, methotrexate doses for intraTHECAL use should be based on patient age, *not* BSA

- Administration should be completed as soon as possible after product preparation
- When possible, inject methotrexate in a volume equivalent to the volume of cerebrospinal fluid removed

Selected drug interactions:
- Avoid concomitant use of nonsteroidal anti-inflammatory drugs (NSAIDs) or salicylates with methotrexate, particularly at dosages and treatment schedules used in oncology
  - NSAIDs and salicylates may compete for renal tubular secretion of methotrexate, thus decreasing the rate of methotrexate elimination and enhancing its toxicity
  - Use caution during concomitant use of NSAIDs or salicylates with methotrexate, such as doses and schedules used in immunologic and rheumatologic indications
- Penicillins and probenecid also diminish renal tubular transport and elimination of methotrexate. Serum or plasma methotrexate concentrations should be carefully monitored if methotrexate is given concurrently with these drugs
- Trimethoprim/sulfamethoxazole (cotrimoxazole) has been reported rarely to increase bone marrow suppression in patients receiving methotrexate, probably

by competition for renal tubular secretion, additive antifolate effect, or a combination of factors
- Methotrexate increases concentrations of mercaptopurine in plasma during concomitant use
- Folate deficiency states may increase methotrexate toxicity; however, vitamin preparations containing folic acid or its derivatives may decrease responses to systemically administered methotrexate
- Methotrexate volume of distribution approximates the distribution of body water; that is, methotrexate distributes and slowly exits from third-space fluid compartments (eg, pleural or pericardial effusions or ascites), which may result in a prolonged elimination and unexpected toxicity. It is advisable to evacuate significant third-space fluid accumulations before treatment and to monitor serum or plasma methotrexate levels until they are no longer detectable (optimally, $\leq$0.01 μmol/L [$\leq$10^{-8} mol/L])
- Lesions of psoriasis may be aggravated by concomitant exposure to ultraviolet radiation. Radiation dermatitis and dermal inflammation and injuries associated with thermal and solar burns may be exacerbated and "recalled" by subsequent use of methotrexate

MITOMYCIN

MUTAMYCIN prescribing information. Durham, NC: Accord Healthcare, Inc.; September 2016

WARNING

Mitomycin should be administered under the supervision of a qualified physician experienced in the use of cancer chemotherapeutic agents. Appropriate management of therapy and complications is possible only when adequate diagnostic and treatment facilities are readily available

Bone marrow suppression, notably thrombocytopenia and leukopenia, which may contribute to overwhelming infections in an already compromised patient, is the most common and severe of the toxic effects of mitomycin …

Hemolytic Uremic Syndrome (HUS), a serious complication of chemotherapy consisting primarily of microangiopathic hemolytic anemia, thrombocytopenia, and irreversible renal failure, has been reported in patients receiving systemic mitomycin. The syndrome may occur at any time during systemic therapy with mitomycin as a single agent or in combination with other cytotoxic drugs; however, most cases occur at doses ≥60 mg of mitomycin. Blood product transfusion may exacerbate the symptoms associated with this syndrome

The incidence of the syndrome has not been defined

Boxed Warning (excerpt) for MUTAMYCIN prescribing information. Durham, NC: Accord Healthcare, Inc.; September 2016

Product Identification, Preparation, Storage, and Stability

MitoMYcin for Injection

- MitoMYcin is available generically in individually packaged multiuse vials containing a dry mixture of mitoMYcin with mannitol

  - Available presentations include:
    - MitoMYcin 5 mg with 10 mg of mannitol
    - MitoMYcin 20 mg with 40 mg of mannitol
    - MitoMYcin 40 mg with 80 mg of mannitol

- Store intact vials at 25°C (77°F), with temperature excursions permitted between 15° and 30°C (59° and 86°F)

  - MitoMYcin is heat stable and has a high melting point, but avoid exposure to temperatures >40°C (>104°F)

- Protect mitoMYcin from exposure to light by storing vials in their packaging cartons

- Reconstitute mitoMYcin as follows:

Amount of MitoMYcin per Vial	Volume of SWFI Diluent	MitoMYcin Concentration After Reconstitution
5 mg	10 mL	0.5 mg/mL
20 mg	40 mL	
40 mg	80 mL	

- After adding the diluent, shake the vials to dissolve mitoMYcin. If the product does not dissolve immediately, allow it to stand at room temperature until a solution is obtained

- After reconstitution with SWFI, the product is stable for 14 days under refrigeration or 7 days at room temperature protected from light

- Store reconstituted mitoMYcin solutions (0.5 mg/mL) under refrigeration 2–8°C (36–46°F) protected from light

- Discard reconstituted solutions after 14 days if the product was stored under refrigeration. If unrefrigerated, discard after 7 days

- Reconstituted mitoMYcin (0.5 mg/mL) is suitable for intraVENous administration, but the product may be further diluted to a concentration of 20–40 μg/mL (0.02–0.04 mg/mL) in the following fluids at room temperature:[51]

Vehicle/Diluent Solution	Duration of Stability
D5W	3 hours
0.9% NS	12 hours
1/6-M SLI (sodium lactate injection, USP)	24 hours

- MitoMYcin stability is highly dependent on solution pH: it is most stable at pH ~7[52,53]

Recommendations for Drug Administration and Ancillary Care

MitoMYcin for Injection

General:

- See Chapter 43 for recommended use in patients with renal and hepatic dysfunction

- MitoMYcin may be injected directly into any suitable vein, but preferably is injected into the side arm of a freely flowing intraVENous infusion

- MitoMYcin diluted in 20–50 mL of SWFI or 0.9% NS has also been given intravesically into the urinary bladder as a treatment for transitional cell carcinoma

Caution:

- MitoMYcin is a powerful vesicant and may produce severe local soft-tissue necrosis if extravasation occurs

MITOXANTRONE HYDROCHLORIDE

MITOXANTRONE prescribing information. Lake Forest, IL: Hospira, Inc.; May 2018

WARNING

Mitoxantrone Injection, USP (concentrate), should be administered under the supervision of a physician experienced in the use of cytotoxic chemotherapy agents

Mitoxantrone Injection, USP (concentrate), should be given slowly into a freely flowing intravenous infusion. It must *never* be given subcutaneously, intramuscularly, or intra-arterially. Severe local tissue damage may occur if there is extravasation during administration …

NOT FOR INTRATHECAL USE. Severe injury with permanent sequelae can result from intrathecal administration …

Except for the treatment of acute nonlymphocytic leukemia, mitoxantrone therapy generally should not be given to patients with baseline neutrophil counts of less than 1500 cells/mm^3. In order to monitor the occurrence of bone marrow suppression, primarily neutropenia, which may be severe and result in infection, it is recommended that frequent peripheral blood cell counts be performed on all patients receiving mitoxantrone

Cardiotoxicity

Congestive heart failure (CHF), potentially fatal, may occur either during therapy with mitoxantrone or months to years after termination of therapy. Cardiotoxicity risk increases with cumulative mitoxantrone dose and may occur whether or not cardiac risk factors are present. Presence or history of cardiovascular disease, radiotherapy to the mediastinal/pericardial area, previous therapy with other anthracyclines or anthracenediones, or use of other cardiotoxic drugs may increase this risk. In cancer patients, the risk of symptomatic CHF was estimated to be 2.6% for patients receiving up to a cumulative dose of 140 mg/m^2. To mitigate the cardiotoxicity risk with mitoxantrone, prescribers should consider the following:

All Patients

- All patients should be assessed for cardiac signs and symptoms by history, physical examination, and ECG prior to start of mitoxantrone therapy
- All patients should have baseline quantitative evaluation of left ventricular ejection fraction (LVEF) using appropriate methodology (echocardiogram, multi-gated radionuclide angiography [MUGA], MRI, etc.)

Multiple Sclerosis Patients

- MS patients with a baseline LVEF below the lower limit of normal should not be treated with mitoxantrone
- MS patients should be assessed for cardiac signs and symptoms by history, physical examination and ECG prior to each dose
- MS patients should undergo quantitative reevaluation of LVEF prior to each dose using the same methodology that was used to assess baseline LVEF. Additional doses of mitoxantrone should not be administered to multiple sclerosis patients who have experienced either a drop in LVEF to below the lower limit of normal or a clinically significant reduction in LVEF during mitoxantrone therapy
- MS patients should not receive a cumulative mitoxantrone dose greater than 140 mg/m^2
- MS patients should undergo yearly quantitative LVEF evaluation after stopping mitoxantrone to monitor for late occurring cardiotoxicity …

Secondary Leukemia

Mitoxantrone therapy in patients with MS and in patients with cancer increases the risk of developing secondary acute myeloid leukemia

Boxed Warning (excerpt) for MITOXANTRONE prescribing information. Lake Forest, IL: Hospira, Inc.; May 2018

Product Identification, Preparation, Storage, and Stability

- MitoXANTRONE injection, USP (concentrate), is available generically in individually packaged multidose vials containing a sterile, nonpyrogenic, dark blue, aqueous solution of mitoXANTRONE HCl
  - Available presentations include:
    MitoXANTRONE 20 mg/10 mL
    MitoXANTRONE 25 mg/12.5 mL
    MitoXANTRONE 30 mg/15 mL
- Each milliliter of the concentrated solution contains 2 mg mitoXANTRONE (free base equivalent), with sodium chloride 0.80% (w/v), sodium acetate anhydrous 0.005% (w/v), acetic acid 0.046% (w/v)

and SWFI. The solution has a pH of 3–4.5 and contains sodium 0.14 mEq/mL, but does not contain antimicrobial preservatives. At least one generic product additionally includes sodium metabisulfite (0.01% w/v)

- Store MitoXANTRONE injection, USP at room temperature 20–25°C (68–77°F). *Do not* freeze mitoXANTRONE. The prescribing information for one product indicates that cartons and vials must be stored upright
- If vials are used to prepare >1 dose, the portion of undiluted mitoXANTRONE concentrate remaining in a vial should

be stored no longer than 7 days at temperatures within the range of 15–25°C (59–77°F), or for up to 14 days under refrigeration (2–8°C [36–46°F])

- MitoXANTRONE concentrate *must be diluted* prior to use to at least 50 mL with either 0.9% NS, D5W, or 0.9% NS/D5W, and used immediately

Selected incompatibility:
- MitoXANTRONE admixture with heparin may result in precipitation
- MitoXANTRONE should not be mixed in the same parenteral product container with other drugs

Recommendations for Drug Administration and Ancillary Care

General:
- See Chapter 43 for comments about use in patients with hepatic dysfunction
- MitoXANTRONE is usually given as a short, intraVENous infusion over 5–30 minutes into the side arm of a freely flowing intraVENous solution, or it may be given by continuous intraVENous infusion over 24 hours
- *Do not administer* a dose of MitoXANTRONE over <3 minutes
- *Caution:* MitoXANTRONE is a vesicant drug and may produce severe local soft-tissue necrosis if extravasation occurs

- MitoXANTRONE *must not be administered* intraTHECALly or intra-arterially, or SUBCUTaneously, intraMUSCularly, or by other infiltrative routes into soft tissues
- Signs and symptoms of extravasation may include burning, pain, pruritus, erythema, swelling, blue discoloration, or ulceration at the injection site, but extravasation may occur with or without accompanying discomfort and even if blood returns well on aspiration of a patient's VAD
- Advise patients mitoXANTRONE may impart a blue-green color to their urine for 24 hours after administration, and

discoloration of the sclera (blue) may also occur

Inadvertent exposure:
- Skin accidentally exposed to mitoXANTRONE should be rinsed copiously with warm water
- If the eyes are involved, standard irrigation techniques should be used immediately

MOXETUMOMAB PASUDOTOX-tdfk

LUMOXITI (moxetumomab pasudotox-tdfk) prescribing information. Rockville, MD: Innate Pharma, Inc; April 2020

WARNING: CAPILLARY LEAK SYNDROME and HEMOLYTIC UREMIC SYNDROME

- Capillary Leak Syndrome (CLS), including life-threatening cases, occurred in patients receiving LUMOXITI. Monitor weight and blood pressure; check labs, including albumin, if CLS is suspected. Delay dosing or discontinue LUMOXITI as recommended …
- Hemolytic Uremic Syndrome (HUS), including life-threatening cases, occurred in patients receiving LUMOXITI. Monitor hemoglobin, platelet count, serum creatinine, and ensure adequate hydration. Discontinue LUMOXITI in patients with HUS …

Boxed Warning for LUMOXITI (moxetumomab pasudotox-tdfk) prescribing information. Rockville, MD: Innate Pharma, Inc; April 2020

Product Identification, Preparation, Storage, and Stability

- Moxetumomab pasudotox-tdfk is a CD22-directed cytotoxin. Moxetumomab pasudotox-tdfk is composed of a recombinant, murine immunoglobulin variable domain genetically fused to a truncated form of *Pseudomonas* exotoxin, PE38, that inhibits protein synthesis
- LUMOXITI, is a sterile, preservative-free, white to off-white lyophilized cake or powder. Each carton contains one single-dose vial that contains 1 mg moxetumomab pasudotox-tdfk, glycine (80 mg), polysorbate 80 (0.2 mg), sodium phosphate monobasic monohydrate (3.4 mg), sucrose (40 mg), and sodium hydroxide to adjust pH to 7.4 (NDC 73380-4700-1)
- The IV Solution Stabilizer is packaged separately from LUMOXITI. Each carton (NDC 73380-4715-9) contains one single-dose vial of Solution Stabilizer. Do not use the IV Solution Stabilizer to reconstitute LUMOXITI
- IV Solution Stabilizer is supplied as a sterile, preservative-free, colorless to slightly yellow, clear solution free from visible particles in a 1-mL single-dose vial. Each vial contains citric acid monohydrate (0.7 mg), polysorbate 80 (6.5 mg), sodium citrate dihydrate (6.4 mg), and SWFI. The pH is 6
- Only one vial of IV Solution Stabilizer should be used per administration of LUMOXITI
- Store intact vials of LUMOXITI and IV solution stabilizer under refrigeration at 2–8°C (35–46°F) until time of reconstitution in the original cartons to protect from light
- Do not freeze or shake intact vials

Reconstitution:
- Use proper aseptic technique to reconstitute and dilute moxetumomab pasudotox-tdfk
- Calculate the dose (mg) and the number of LUMOXITI vials (1 mg/vial) to be reconstituted. *DO NOT* round down for partial vials
- Reconstitute each LUMOXITI (1 mg/vial) with 1.1 mL SWFI. The resulting 1-mg/mL solution allows a withdrawal volume of 1 mL
- Direct the SWFI along the walls of the vial and not directly at the lyophilized cake or powder
- *DO NOT* reconstitute LUMOXITI vials with the IV Solution Stabilizer
- Gently swirl the vial until completely dissolved. Invert the vial to ensure all cake or powder in the vial is dissolved. Do not shake. Use reconstituted solution immediately. *DO NOT STORE* reconstituted vials
- Visually inspect that the reconstituted solution is clear to slightly opalescent, colorless to slightly yellow, and free from visible particles. Do not use if solution is cloudy, discolored, or contains any particles

Dilution:
- **Add the IV Solution Stabilizer to the infusion bag prior to adding LUMOXITI solution to the infusion bag. Vial of IV Solution Stabilizer is packaged separately**
- Obtain a 50-mL 0.9% NS infusion bag
- Add 1 mL IV Solution Stabilizer to the infusion bag containing 50 mL 0.9% NS. Only 1 vial of IV Solution Stabilizer should be used per administration of LUMOXITI
- Gently invert the bag to mix the solution. Do not shake
- Withdraw the required volume of LUMOXITI for the patient's individualized dose from the reconstituted vial(s)
- Inject LUMOXITI into the infusion bag containing 50 mL 0.9% NS and 1 mL IV Solution Stabilizer
- Gently invert the bag to mix the solution. Do not shake. Discard any partially used or empty vials
- Use diluted solution immediately or after storage at room temperature 20C° to 25°C (68F° to 77°F) for up to 4 hours or store refrigerated at 2°C to 8°C (36°F to 46°F) for up to 24 hours. *PROTECT FROM LIGHT. DO NOT FREEZE. DO NOT SHAKE*

Selected incompatibility:
- **Reconstitute LUMOXITI vials with SWFI only**
- Do not mix or administer LUMOXITI as an infusion with other medicinal products

Recommendations for Drug Administration and Ancillary Care

General:
- The PK of moxetumomab pasudotox-tdfk in patients with moderate to severe hepatic impairment (total bilirubin >1.5 ULN) or severe renal impairment (CrCl ≤ 29 mL/min) are unknown

Administration:
- The recommended dose of moxetumomab pasudotox-tdfk is 0.04 mg/kg per dose
- Individualize dosing based on the patient's actual body weight prior to the first dose of the first treatment cycle
- Changes in dose due to fluctuations in weight should only be made between cycles when a change in weight of >10% is observed from the baseline weight used to calculate the first dose of cycle 1. Do not change the dose within a cycle
- Administer over 30 minutes as an intraVENous infusion on days 1, 3, and 5 of each 28-day cycle. Continue for a maximum of 6 cycles, disease progression, or unacceptable toxicity
- After the infusion, flush the intraVENous administration line with of 0.9% NS at the same rate as the infusion. This ensures that the full LUMOXITI dose is delivered
- If the diluted solution is refrigerated 2°C to 8°C (36°F to 46°F), allow it to equilibrate at room temperature 20°C to 25°C (68°F to 77°F) for no more than 4 hours prior to administration. Administer diluted solution within 24 hours of reconstitution. *PROTECT FROM LIGHT*

Concomitant medications:
- Pre- and post-infusion hydration:
  - 0.9% NS 1000 mL (or 500 mL if weight <50 kg); administer intraVENously over 2–4 hours prior to and following each moxetumomab pasudotox-tdfk infusion on days 1, 3, and 5

- Thromboprophylaxis
  - Consider low-dose aspirin on days 1 through 8 of each 28-day cycle
- Moxetumomab pasudotox-tdfk premedications (given 30–90 minutes prior to each LUMOXITI infusion:
  - A histamine-1 receptor antagonist (eg, hydrOXYzine or diphenhydrAMINE)
  - Acetaminophen
  - A histamine-2 receptor antagonist (eg, raNITIdine, famotidine, or cimetidine)
- If history of prior severe infusion-related reaction, then add a corticosteroid before each infusion thereafter
- Moxetumomab pasudotox-tdfk post-infusion medications:
  - Consider oral antihistamines and antipyretics for up to 24 hours following LUMOXITI infusions
  - An oral corticosteroid (eg, 4 mg dexamethasone) is recommended to decrease nausea and vomiting
  - Maintain adequate oral fluid intake. Advise all patients to adequately hydrate with up to 3 L (twelve 8-oz glasses) of oral fluids (eg, water, milk, or juice) per 24 hours on days 1 through 8 of each 28-day cycle. In patients under 50 kg, up to 2 L (eight 8-oz glasses) per 24 hours is recommended

Adverse events and treatment modifications:
- Refer to the current FDA-approved product label for detailed recommendations regarding treatment modifications (withholding or discontinuation) for CLS, HUS, and increased creatinine
- In study 1053, infusion-related reactions occurred in 50% (40/80) of patients. Grade 3 infusion-related events, as defined, occurred in 11% (9/80) of LUMOXITI-treated patients. Premedications are recommended with antihistamines and antipyretics

- Infusion-related reactions can occur with any cycle. Monitor for signs and symptoms of infusion-related reactions including: chills, cough, dizziness, dyspnea, feeling hot, flushing, headache, hypertension, hypotension, myalgia, nausea, pyrexia, sinus tachycardia, tachycardia, vomiting, or wheezing
- If a severe infusion-related reaction occurs, interrupt the LUMOXITI infusion and institute appropriate medical management. Administer an oral or intraVENous corticosteroid approximately 30 minutes before resuming, or before the next LUMOXITI infusion

Selected precautions:
- Before every infusion, check weight and blood pressure. If weight has increased by 5.5 pounds (2.5 kg) or 5% or greater from day 1 of the cycle and the patient is hypotensive, promptly check for peripheral edema, hypoalbuminemia, and respiratory symptoms, including shortness of breath and cough. If CLS is suspected, check for a decrease in oxygen saturation and evidence of pulmonary edema and/or serosal effusions
- Before every infusion check hemoglobin, platelet count, and serum creatinine
- If HUS is suspected, promptly check blood LDH, indirect bilirubin, and blood smear schistocytes for evidence of hemolysis
- Renal toxicity can occur. Monitor renal function prior to each infusion of LUMOXITI, and as clinically indicated throughout treatment. Delay LUMOXITI dosing in patients with Grade ≥ 3 elevations in creatinine, or upon worsening from baseline by ≥2 grades
- Electrolyte abnormalities can occur. Monitor serum electrolytes prior to each dose and on day 8 of each treatment cycle. Monitoring mid-cycle is also recommended

NELARABINE

ARRANON (nelarabine) prescribing information. East Hanover, NJ: Novartis Pharmaceuticals Corporation; July 2019

WARNING: NEUROLOGIC ADVERSE REACTIONS

Severe neurologic adverse reactions have been reported with the use of ARRANON. These adverse reactions have included altered mental states including severe somnolence, central nervous system effects including convulsions, and peripheral neuropathy ranging from numbness and paresthesias to motor weakness and paralysis. There have also been reports of adverse reactions associated with demyelination, and ascending peripheral neuropathies similar in appearance to Guillain-Barré syndrome ...

Full recovery from these adverse reactions has not always occurred with cessation of therapy with ARRANON. Monitor frequently for signs and symptoms of neurologic toxicity during treatment with ARRANON. Discontinue ARRANON for neurologic adverse reactions of NCI Common Toxicity Criteria for Adverse Events (CTCAE) Grade 2 or greater ...

Boxed Warning for ARRANON (nelarabine) prescribing information. East Hanover, NJ: Novartis Pharmaceuticals Corporation; July 2019

Product Identification, Preparation, Storage, and Stability

- ARRANON is packaged in type I, clear, glass vials containing a clear, colorless sterile solution of nelarabine 250 mg in 50 mL
- Each milliliter of solution contains 5 mg nelarabine with sodium chloride 4.5 mg and SWFI in a total volume of (Q.S.) 50 mL; solution pH is within the range 5.0–7.0. The product is packaged individually (NDC 0078-0683-61) or in cartons containing 6 vials (NDC 0007-0683-06)
- Store ARRANON at 20–25°C (68–77°C). Temperature excursions to 15–30°C (59–86°F) are permitted
- Preparation for administration:
  - *Do not dilute* ARRANON prior to administration. Transfer a volume of nelarabine appropriate for a patient's dose into a PVC or glass container
- Undiluted nelarabine is stable in PVC and glass containers for up to 8 hours at temperatures up to 30°C (86°F)

Recommendations for Drug Administration and Ancillary Care

General:

- See Chapter 43 for recommended use in patients with renal and hepatic dysfunction
- Administer nelarabine intraVENously over 2 hours for adult patients and over 1 hour for pediatric patients

NIVOLUMAB

OPDIVO (nivolumab) prescribing information. Princeton, NJ: Bristol-Myers Squibb Company; June 2020

Product Identification, Preparation, Storage, and Stability

- OPDIVO is a sterile, preservative-free, non-pyrogenic, clear to opalescent, colorless to pale-yellow liquid that may contain light (few) particles available in individually boxed single-dose vials containing nivolumab 40 mg/4 mL (NDC 0003-3772-11), nivolumab 100 mg/10 mL (NDC 0003-3774-12), or nivolumab 240 mg/24 mL (NDC 0003-3734-13). Each mL of the above nivolumab solutions contains nivolumab (10 mg), mannitol (30 mg), pentetic acid (0.008 mg), polysorbate 80 (0.2 mg), sodium chloride (2.92 mg), sodium citrate dihydrate (5.88 mg), and SWFI. May contain hydrochloric acid and/or sodium hydroxide to adjust pH to 6
- Store intact vials under refrigeration at 2–8°C (35–46°F) protect from light by storing in the original package until the time of use
- Do not freeze or shake intact vials

Dilution:
- Nivolumab is a clear to opalescent, colorless to pale-yellow solution. Visually inspect for particulate matter and discoloration. Discard if cloudy, discolored, or contains extraneous particulate matter other than a few translucent-to-white, proteinaceous particles
- Dilute nivolumab with either 0.9% NS or D5W to a final concentration ranging from 1 to 10 mg/mL. The total volume of infusion must not exceed 160 mL for patients with body weight ≥ 40 kg. For patients <40 kg do not exceed a total volume of infusion of 4 mL/kg of body weight
- Mix diluted solution by gentle inversion. Do not shake
- Store diluted solution either at room temperature for no more than 8 hours from the time of preparation to end of infusion or under refrigeration at 2–8°C (36–46°F) for no more than 24 hours from the time of preparation to end of infusion. Discard if not used within these times. Do not freeze

Selected incompatibility:
- Do not co-administer other drugs through the same intraVENous line

Recommendations for Drug Administration and Ancillary Care

General:
- Nivolumab has not been studied in patients with severe hepatic impairment (bilirubin > 3 × ULN and any AST).

Administration:
- The recommended dose of nivolumab is 240 mg every 2 weeks or 480 mg every 4 weeks as a single agent
  - Note weight-based dosing at 3 mg/kg is recommended for MSI-H or dMMR metastatic colorectal cancer for pediatric patients age 12 years and older weighing <40 kg
- Refer to the current FDA-approved product label for dosing of nivolumab in combination with other therapeutic agents
- Administer the infusion over 30 minutes through an intraVENous line containing a sterile, non-pyrogenic, low-protein-binding, inline filter (pore size of 0.2 to 1.2 μm)
- Administer OPDIVO in combination with other therapeutic agents as follows:
  - With ipilimumab: administer OPDIVO first followed by ipilimumab on the same day
  - With platinum-doublet chemotherapy: administer OPDIVO first followed by platinum-doublet chemotherapy on the same day

- With ipilimumab and platinum doublet chemotherapy: administer OPDIVO first followed by ipilimumab and then platinum-doublet chemotherapy on the same day
- Use separate infusion bags and filters for each infusion
- Flush the intraVENous line at the end of infusion

Adverse events and treatment modifications:
- Immune-mediated adverse events can occur with nivolumab. Some of these adverse events can be severe or life-threatening
- Refer to the current FDA-approved product label for warnings and detailed recommendations regarding treatment modifications for colitis, pneumonitis, hepatitis, hypophysitis, adrenal insufficiency, type 1 diabetes mellitus, nephritis and renal dysfunction, skin rash, encephalitis or other G3 adverse reactions according to NCI CTCAE v4
  - Permanently discontinue nivolumab if unable to reduce steroid dose for adverse reactions to ≤10 mg prednisone per day (or equivalent) >12 weeks after last dose
  - Permanently discontinue nivolumab for G2 or G3 adverse reaction (excluding endocrinopathy) lasting ≥12 weeks after the last dose
- Permanently discontinue for Grade 3 myocarditis or other life-threatening G4 adverse reactions
- OPDIVO can cause severe infusion-related reactions which have been reported in <1% of patients in clinical trials. Interrupt or slow the rate of infusion in patients with mild or moderate infusion-related reactions. Discontinue OPDIVO in patients with severe or life-threatening infusion-related reactions
- Note when OPDIVO is administered in combination with ipilimumab, if OPDIVO is withheld, ipilimumab should also be withheld

Selected precaution:
- Fatal and other serious complications can occur in patients who receive allogeneic hematopoietic stem cell transplantation (HSCT) before or after being treated with a PD-1 receptor–blocking antibody such as nivolumab. Follow patients closely for transplant-related complications and intervene promptly. Consider the benefit versus risk of treatment with a PD-1 receptor–blocking antibody prior to or after an allogeneic HSCT

OBINUTUZUMAB

GAZYVA (obinutuzumab) prescribing information. South San Francisco, CA: Genentech, Inc.; March 2020

WARNING: HEPATITIS B VIRUS REACTIVATION and PROGRESSIVE MULTIFOCAL LEUKOENCEPHALOPATHY

- Hepatitis B Virus (HBV) reactivation, in some cases resulting in fulminant hepatitis, hepatic failure, and death, can occur in patients receiving CD20-directed cytolytic antibodies, including GAZYVA. Screen all patients for HBV infection before treatment initiation. Monitor HBV-positive patients during and after treatment with GAZYVA. Discontinue GAZYVA and concomitant medications in the event of HBV reactivation …

- Progressive Multifocal Leukoencephalopathy (PML) including fatal PML, can occur in patients receiving GAZYVA …

Boxed Warning for GAZYVA (obinutuzumab) prescribing information. South San Francisco, CA: Genentech, Inc.; March 2020

Product Identification, Preparation, Storage, and Stability

- GAZYVA is supplied individually packaged, single-use vials that contain obinutuzumab as a sterile, clear, colorless to slightly brown, preservative-free, concentrated solution
- Each vial of concentrated drug product contains 1000 mg obinutuzumab per 40 mL (25 mg/mL) formulated in L-histidine/L-histidine hydrochloride 20 mmol/L, trehalose 240 mmol/L, and poloxamer 188 0.02% at a pH = 6.0 (NDC 50242-070-01)
- Store intact vials at 2–8°C (36–46°F) protected from light
- *Do not freeze* and *do not shake* the drug product
- Preparation:

Chronic Lymphocytic Leukemia

Cycles and Days of Treatment	Amount of Obinutuzumab per Dose	Instructions
Cycle 1: Dilution to a concentration within the range of 0.4–4 mg/mL		
Day 1	100 mg	1. With a sterile syringe, withdraw 40 mL of solution from a vial of GAZYVA (obinutuzumab)
Day 2	900 mg	2. Transfer 4 mL (100 mg) of the concentrated drug product into a parenteral product container already containing 100 mL of 0.9% NS for immediate use
		3. Transfer the remaining 36 mL (900 mg) of the concentrated drug product into a second parenteral product container already containing 250 mL of 0.9% NS for use on day 2
		4. Mix the diluted drug products by repeated gentle inversion of the product container. *Do not shake* the drug product
		5. Store the second container under refrigeration (2–8°C) for up to 24 hours; *do not freeze* the drug product
		6. After storage under refrigeration, allow diluted obinutuzumab to come to room temperature before use
Days 8 and 15	1000 mg	1. With a sterile syringe, withdraw 40 mL (1000 mg) of concentrated obinutuzumab from a vial
		2. Transfer 40 mL into a parenteral product container already containing 250 mL of 0.9% NS
		3. Mix the diluted drug product by repeated gentle inversion of the product container. *Do not shake* the drug product
		4. For microbiological stability, the solution may be stored under refrigeration (2–8°C) for up to 24 hours; *do not freeze* the drug product
Cycles 2–6: Dilution to a concentration within the range of 0.4–4 mg/mL		
Day 1	1000 mg	1. With a sterile syringe, withdraw 40 mL (1000 mg) of concentrated obinutuzumab from a vial
		2. Transfer 40 mL into a parenteral product container already containing 250 mL of 0.9% NS
		3. Mix the diluted drug product by repeated gentle inversion of the product container. *Do not shake* the drug product
		4. For microbiological stability, the solution may be stored under refrigeration (2–8°C) for up to 24 hours; *do not freeze* the drug product

(continued)

Product Identification, Preparation, Storage, and Stability (continued)

Follicular Lymphoma

Cycles and Days of Treatment	Amount of Obinutuzumab per Dose	Instructions
Cycle 1: Dilution to a concentration within the range of 0.4–4 mg/mL		
Days 1, 8, and 15	1000 mg	1. With a sterile syringe, withdraw 40 mL (1000 mg) of concentrated obinutuzumab from a vial 2. Transfer 40 mL into a parenteral product container already containing 250 mL of 0.9% NS 3. Mix the diluted drug product by repeated gentle inversion of the product container. *Do not shake the* drug product 4. For microbiological stability, the solution may be stored under refrigeration (2–8°C) for up to 24 hours; *do not freeze* the drug product
Cycles 2–6 or 2–8: Dilution to a concentration within the range of 0.4–4 mg/mL		
Day 1	1000 mg	1. With a sterile syringe, withdraw 40 mL (1000 mg) of concentrated obinutuzumab from a vial 2. Transfer 40 mL into a parenteral product container already containing 250 mL of 0.9% NS 3. Mix the diluted drug product by repeated gentle inversion of the product container. *Do not shake the* drug product 4. For microbiological stability, the solution may be stored under refrigeration (2–8°C) for up to 24 hours; *do not freeze* the drug product
Monotherapy: Dilution to a concentration within the range of 0.4–4 mg/mL		
Every 2 months for up to 2 years	1000 mg	1. With a sterile syringe, withdraw 40 mL (1000 mg) of concentrated obinutuzumab from a vial 2. Transfer 40 mL into a parenteral product container already containing 250 mL of 0.9% NS 3. Mix the diluted drug product by repeated gentle inversion of the product container. *Do not shake the* drug product 4. For microbiological stability, the solution may be stored under refrigeration (2–8°C) for up to 24 hours; *do not freeze* the drug product

• Product labeling recommends administering obinutuzumab solutions immediately after dilution; however, diluted products may be stored under refrigeration for up to 24 hours

- -

Recommendations for Drug Administration and Ancillary Care

Administration as Recommended in Product Labeling (version dated March 2020)

Premedication:

• Premedication before each use to decrease the risk of infusion-related reactions (IRR) in patients with chronic lymphocytic leukemia (CLL) and follicular lymphoma (FL)*

Day of Treatment Cycle	Patients Who Require Premedication	Premedication	Timing Relative to Obinutuzumab Administration
Cycle 1: CLL Day 1, Day 2 FL Day 1	All patients	High-potency glucocorticoid†‡, intraVENously; ie: **Dexamethasone** 20 mg, *or* **MethylPREDNISolone** 80 mg	Complete administration ≥1 hour before starting obinutuzumab
		Acetaminophen 650–1000 mg orally	≥30 minutes before starting obinutuzumab
		Antihistamine§; eg: **DiphenhydrAMINE** 50 mg	

(continued)

Recommendations for Drug Administration and Ancillary Care (continued)

Day of Treatment Cycle	Patients Who Require Premedication	Premedication	Timing Relative to Obinutuzumab Administration
All subsequent infusions, CLL or FL	All patients	Acetaminophen 650–1000 mg orally	≥30 minutes before starting obinutuzumab
	Patients with an IRR (G 1–2) during the previous infusion	Acetaminophen 650–1000 mg orally	≥30 minutes before starting obinutuzumab
		Antihistamine[§]; eg: DiphenhydrAMINE 50 mg	
	Patients with a G3 IRR during the previous infusion OR Patients with a lymphocyte count >25,000/mm^3 before the next treatment	High-potency glucocorticoid[†], intraVENously; ie: Dexamethasone 20 mg, or MethylPREDNISolone 80 mg	Complete administration ≥1 hour before starting obinutuzumab
		Acetaminophen 650–1000 mg orally	≥30 minutes before starting obinutuzumab
		Antihistamine[§]; eg: DiphenhydrAMINE 50 mg	

[*]Among 45 patients who received recommended premedication and obinutuzumab divided into two doses given on two consecutive days (100 mg followed by 900 mg on days 1 and 2, respectively), 21 patients (47%) experienced a reaction with the first 1000 mg and <2% thereafter
[†]Hydrocortisone is not recommended because it has not been effective in reducing the rate of infusion reactions
[‡]If a glucocorticoid-containing chemotherapy regimen is administered on the same day as GAZYVA, the glucocorticoid can be administered as an oral medication if given at least 1 hour prior to GAZYVA, in which case additional intraVENous glucocorticoid as premedication is not required
[§]Antihistamine (H$_1$-receptor subtype antagonists)

Administration:

• *Administer* obinutuzumab only as an intraVENous infusion through a dedicated line
• *Do not administer* as an intraVENous push or bolus
  ▪ After storage under refrigeration, allow diluted obinutuzumab to come to room temperature before use
  ▪ No incompatibilities have been observed between GAZYVA and PVC or polyolefin containers and administration sets
• GAZYVA (obinutuzumab) should be administered only by health care professionals with appropriate medical support to manage severe infusion reactions that can be fatal if they occur
• Administration rates: initial rate and rate escalation

Dose of GAZVYA in Chronic Lymphocytic Leukemia (CLL) Patients

Cycle	Day	Obinutuzumab Dose	Administration Rate
1	1	100 mg	Administer at 25 mg/hour over 4 hours *DO NOT* increase the infusion rate
	2	900 mg	If no IRR occurred during the prior infusion, then initiate administration at 50 mg/hour If tolerated, the administration rate may be increased in increments of 50 mg/hour every 30 minutes to a maximum rate of 400 mg/hour If an IRR occurred during the prior infusion, then initiate administration at 25 mg/hour If tolerated, the administration rate may be increased in increments of 50 mg/hour every 30 minutes to a maximum rate of 400 mg/hour
	8	1000 mg	If no IRR occurred during the prior infusion and the final infusion rate was at least 100 mg/hour, then administration may begin at a rate of 100 mg/hour, and, if tolerated, may be increased by100-mg/hour increments every 30 minutes to a maximum rate of 400 mg/hour If an IRR occurred during the prior infusion, then administration may begin at a rate of 50 mg/hour, and, if tolerated, may be increased by 50-mg/hour increments every 30 minutes to a maximum rate of 400 mg/hour
	15		
2–6	1		

▪ Obinutuzumab is administered for 6 cycles; each cycle is 28 days in duration
▪ If a planned dose is missed, administer the missed dose as soon as possible and adjust the dosing schedule accordingly
▪ If appropriate, patients who do not complete the day 1, cycle 1 dose may proceed to the day 2, cycle 1 dose

(continued)

Recommendations for Drug Administration and Ancillary Care *(continued)*

Dose of GAZVYA in Follicular Lymphoma (FL) Patients

Cycle	Day	Obinutuzumab Dose	Administration Rate
Cycle 1 (loading doses)	1	1000 mg	Initiate administration at 50 mg/hour. If tolerated, the administration rate may be increased in increments of 50 mg/hour every 30 minutes to a maximum rate of 400 mg/hour
	8	1000 mg	If no IRR or an IRR of Grade 1 occurred during the prior infusion and the final infusion rate was at least 100 mg/hour, then administration may begin at a rate of 100 mg/hour and, if tolerated, may be increased by 100-mg/hour increments every 30 minutes to a maximum rate of 400 mg/hour
	15	1000 mg	
Cycles 2–6 or 2–8	1	1000 mg	
Monotherapy	Every 2 months for up to 2 years	1000 mg	If an IRR of Grade 2 or higher occurred during the prior infusion, then administration may begin at a rate of 50 mg/hour and, if tolerated, may be increased by 50-mg/hour increments every 30 minutes to a maximum rate of 400 mg/hour

- Obinutuzumab is administered for 6–8 cycles, followed (2 months after the last induction obinutuzumab dose) by obinutuzumab monotherapy given every 2 months for up to 2 years. The number of cycles and cycle length depends upon which chemoimmunotherapy regimen is chosen
- If a planned dose is missed, administer the missed dose as soon as possible and adjust the dosing schedule accordingly
- Infusion-related reactions (IRR)
- If a patient experiences an infusion reaction of any grade during obinutuzumab administration, adjust drug delivery as follows:

Reaction Grade (G)	Intervention
G4 (life threatening)	Immediately *STOP* administration and permanently discontinue treatment with obinutuzumab
G3 (severe)	1. Interrupt infusion and manage symptoms 2. After symptoms resolve, consider restarting obinutuzumab administration at no more than half the rate used at the time that an infusion reaction occurred 3. If the patient does not experience any further infusion-reaction symptoms, rate escalation may again be attempted at increments and intervals appropriate for the treatment cycle and dose *Caution:* Permanently discontinue treatment with obinutuzumab if a patient experiences G3 infusion-related symptoms when re-challenged *Note:* For CLL patients only, the cycle 1 day 1 infusion rate may be increased back up to 25 mg/hour after 1 hour but not increased further
G1–2 (mild–moderate)	1. Promptly decrease the rate, or interrupt administration and treat symptoms 2. After symptoms resolve, continue or resume administration 3. If the patient does not experience any further infusion-reaction symptoms, rate escalation may again be attempted at increments and intervals appropriate for the treatment cycle and dose *Note:* For CLL patients only, the cycle 1 day 1 infusion rate may be increased back up to 25 mg/hour after 1 hour but not increased further

- Additional recommendations for pharmacological support:
- For patients with a high tumor burden or high circulating absolute lymphocyte counts (>25,000/mm^3), premedicate with **anti-hyperuricemics** (eg, allopurinol), and implement or ensure **hydration** appropriate for potential tumor lysis syndrome (TLS) starting 12–24 hours before obinutuzumab treatment begins
- Hypotension may occur during obinutuzumab administration
  - Consider withholding antihypertensive medications for 12 hours before obinutuzumab administration, during treatment with obinutuzumab, and for the first hour after obinutuzumab administration until blood pressure is stable
  - For patients at increased risk of hypertensive crisis as a consequence of withholding antihypertensive medications, consider the benefits versus the risks of withholding hypertensive medications

(continued)

Recommendations for Drug Administration and Ancillary Care (*continued*)

- **Antimicrobial prophylaxis** is strongly recommended for neutropenic patients throughout obinutuzumab treatment
  - Consider antiviral and antifungal prophylaxis
  - *Do not administer* obinutuzumab to patients with an active infection
  - Patients with a history of recurring or chronic infections may be at increased risk of infection
- Immunization with live virus vaccines is not recommended during treatment and until B-cell recovery

Monitoring:

- Obinutuzumab can cause severe and life-threatening infusion reactions during and within 24 hours after administration
  - Of CLL patients who received recommended premedication and the initial 1000 mg of obinutuzumab divided into two doses given on two consecutive days (100 mg and 900 mg on days 1 and 2, respectively), 47% experienced an infusion reaction
    - A decrease from 89% of patients who did not receive premedication or "split dose" treatment experienced infusion reactions
  - Infusion reactions can also occur with subsequent infusions
  - Symptoms may include hypotension, tachycardia, dyspnea, and respiratory symptoms (eg, bronchospasm, larynx and throat irritation, wheezing, laryngeal edema)
  - Other common symptoms include nausea, vomiting, diarrhea, hypertension, flushing, headache, pyrexia, and chills
  - Institute medical management for infusion reactions as needed (eg, glucocorticoids, EPINEPHrine, bronchodilators, oxygen)
  - Closely monitor patients throughout obinutuzumab administration
  - Patients with pre-existing cardiac or pulmonary conditions may be at greater risk of experiencing more severe reactions
    - Monitor more frequently during and after obinutuzumab administration
- Acute renal failure, hyperkalemia, hypocalcemia, hyperuricemia, and/or hyperphosphatemia associated with TLS also can occur within 12–24 hours after the first treatment
  - Correct electrolyte abnormalities, monitor renal function, fluid balance, and administer supportive care, including dialysis as indicated
- During the FDA registration trial for CLL, obinutuzumab in combination with chlorambucil caused:
  - G3/4 neutropenia in 34% of patients
    - Patients with G3/4 neutropenia should be monitored frequently until neutropenia resolves
    - Anticipate, evaluate, and treat any symptoms or signs of developing infection
    - Neutropenia onset can be >28 days after treatment completion and may persist >28 days
  - G3/4 thrombocytopenia in 12% of patients
    - In 5% of patients, an acute thrombocytopenia occurred within 24 hours after obinutuzumab administration
- Approximately 13% (9/70) of patients tested positive for anti-obinutuzumab antibodies at one or more time points during a 12-month follow-up period after obinutuzumab treatment
  - Neutralizing activity of anti-obinutuzumab antibodies has not been assessed

OFATUMUMAB

ARZERRA (ofatumumab) prescribing information. East Hanover, NJ: Novartis Pharmaceuticals Corporation; August 2016

WARNING: HEPATITIS B VIRUS REACTIVATION and PROGRESSIVE MULTIFOCAL LEUKOENCEPHALOPATHY

- Hepatitis B Virus (HBV) reactivation can occur in patients receiving CD20-directed cytolytic antibodies, including ARZERRA, in some cases resulting in fulminant hepatitis, hepatic failure, and death …
- Progressive Multifocal Leukoencephalopathy (PML) resulting in death can occur in patients receiving CD20-directed cytolytic antibodies, including ARZERRA …

Boxed Warning for ARZERRA (ofatumumab) prescribing information. East Hanover, NJ: Novartis Pharmaceuticals Corporation; August 2016

Product Identification, Preparation, Storage, and Stability

- ARZERRA is a sterile, clear to opalescent, colorless, preservative-free liquid concentrate (20 mg/mL) for dilution and intraVENous administration provided in single-use glass vials with a latex-free rubber stopper and an aluminum overseal
- Each vial contains either: 100 mg ofatumumab in 5 mL of solution, *or* 1000 mg ofatumumab in 50 mL of solution
  - The commercial product is available in the following presentations:
  - A carton containing 3 single-use, 100-mg/5-mL vials: NDC 0078-06900-61
    - Single vials labeled NDC 0078-0669-61
  - A carton containing 1 single-use, 1000-mg/50-mL vial: NDC 0078-0690-61
- Store intact vials under refrigeration between 2° and 8°C (36° and 46°F), but do not freeze. Protect vials from light
- *Do not shake* vials containing ofatumumab
- The solution should not be used if discolored or cloudy, or if foreign particulate matter is present
- Dilute *all* ofatumumab doses in 0.9% NS to deliver a volume of (Q.S.) 1000 mL, as follows:

Ofatumumab Dose	Volume of Ofatumumab Concentrate (20 mg/mL) Needed	Volume of 0.9% NS Needed
300 mg	15 mL	985 mL
1000 mg	50 mL	950 mL
2000 mg	100 mL	900 mL

- Mix the diluted product by gently inverting the container
- *Do not mix* ofatumumab with other drugs or fluids
- Store diluted ofatumumab solutions under refrigeration at 2–8°C (36–46°F)

Recommendations for Drug Administration and Ancillary Care

Premedication:

- FDA-approved product labeling recommends patients receive the following premedications from 2 hours to 30 minutes before each ofatumumab dose:

Infusion Number	Previously Untreated CLL, Relapsed CLL or Extended Treatment in CLL		Refractory CLL		
	1 and 2	3 and beyond*	1, 2, and 9	3 to 8	10 to 12
IntraVENous corticosteroid (prednisoLONE or equivalent)	50 mg	0–50 mg†	100 mg	0–100 mg†	50–100 mg‡
Oral acetaminophen	1000 mg				
Oral or intraVENous antihistamine (H1-receptor subtype antagonist)	DiphenhydrAMINE 50 mg or cetirizine 10 mg (or equivalent)				

*Up to 13 infusions in previously untreated CLL; up to 7 infusions in relapsed CLL, up to 14 infusions in extended treatment in CLL
†Corticosteroid may be reduced or omitted for subsequent infusions if a Grade 3 or greater infusion-related adverse event did not occur with the preceding infusion(s)
‡PrednisoLONE may be given at reduced dose of 50 mg to 100 mg (or equivalent) if a Grade 3 or greater infusion-related adverse event did not occur with infusion 9

(continued)

Recommendations for Drug Administration and Ancillary Care (*continued*)

Doses and schedules:

- Recommended doses and administration schedules of ofatumumab vary by indication:
  - Previously untreated CLL (in combination with chlorambucil): 300 mg on day 1, followed 1 week later by 1000 mg on day 8 (cycle 1), followed by 1000 mg on day 1 of subsequent 28-day cycles for a minimum of 3 cycles until best response or a maximum of 12 cycles
  - Relapsed CLL (in combination with fludarabine and cyclophosphamide): 300 mg on day 1, followed 1 week later by 1000 mg on day 8 (cycle 1), followed by 1000 mg on day 1 of subsequent 28-day cycles for a maximum of 6 cycles
  - Extended treatment in CLL (single-agent extended treatment): 300 mg on day 1, followed 1 week later by 1000 mg on day 8, followed by 1000 mg 7 weeks later and every 8 weeks thereafter for up to a maximum of 2 years
  - Refractory CLL (single-agent, up to 12 doses): 300 mg on day 1, followed 1 week later by 2000 mg weekly for 7 doses (infusions 2–8), followed 4 weeks later by 2000 mg every 4 weeks for 4 doses (infusions 9–12)

Escalating administration rates:

- If ofatumumab is well tolerated, administration rates may be escalated every 30 minutes as follows:

Infusion Rates in Previously Untreated Chronic Lymphocytic Leukemia (CLL) (with Chlorambucil), Relapsed CLL (with Fludarabine and Cyclophosphamide), and Extended Monotherapy Treatment in CLL

Interval After Starting Ofatumumab Administration (Minutes)	Administration Rates for the First and Subsequent Ofatumumab Doses	
	Dose 1[*] (mL/hour)	Subsequent Infusions[†] (mL/hour)
0–30	12	25
31–60	25	50
61–90	50	100
91–120	100	200
121–150	200	400
151–180	300	400
>180	400	400

[*]Dose 1: Ofatumumab 300 mg in 1000 mL 0.9% NS (0.3 mg/mL)
[†]Subsequent Doses: Ofatumumab 1000 mg in 1000 mL 0.9% NS (1 mg/mL)

Infusion Rates in Refractory Chronic Lymphocytic Leukemia

Interval After Starting Ofatumumab Administration (Minutes)	Administration Rates for the First, Second, Third, and Subsequent Ofatumumab Doses		
	Dose 1[*] (mL/hour)	Dose 2[†] (mL/hour)	Doses 3–12[†] (mL/hour)
0–30	12	12	25
31–60	25	25	50
61–90	50	50	100
91–120	100	100	200
>120	200	200	400

[*]Dose 1: Ofatumumab 300 mg in 1000 mL 0.9% NS (0.3 mg/mL)
[†]Doses 2–12: Ofatumumab 2000 mg in 1000 mL 0.9% NS (2 mg/mL)

(*continued*)

Recommendations for Drug Administration and Ancillary Care (*continued*)

General:
- Administer ofatumumab with an infusion pump and administration set
- Flush the tubing through which ofatumumab is administered with 0.9% NS before and after each dose
- Start ofatumumab administration within 12 hours after product preparation
- Ofatumumab concentrate contains no antimicrobial preservatives
  - Discard diluted ofatumumab solutions within 24 hours after product preparation

Infusion-related hypersensitivity reactions:
- Ofatumumab can cause serious infusion reactions manifesting as bronchospasm, dyspnea, laryngeal edema, pulmonary edema, flushing, hypertension, hypotension, syncope, cardiac ischemia/infarction, back pain, abdominal pain, pyrexia, rash, urticaria, and angioedema
- Infusion reactions occur more frequently with the first 2 infusions:
  - Among 154 patients, infusion reactions occurred in 44% on the day of the first infusion (300 mg), 29% on the day of the second infusion (2000 mg), and less frequently during subsequent administration
- Intervene medically for severe infusion reactions, including angina and other signs and symptoms of myocardial ischemia

Modifying ofatumumab treatment for infusion reactions:
- Interrupt ofatumumab administration for infusion reactions of any severity
  - For G1–4 infusion reactions, if the infusion reaction resolves or remains G ≤2, resume infusion (at the discretion of the medically responsible health care provider) with the following modifications according to the initial grade of the reaction:
    - Grade 1 or 2: Resume administration at 50% the previous administration rate
    - Grade 3 or 4: Resume administration at a rate of 12 mL/hour
- After resuming ofatumumab administration, the infusion rate may be increased according to the tables above ("Escalating Administration Rates"), based on patient tolerance
- Consider permanently discontinuing treatment in patients who experience an anaphylactic reaction to ofatumumab or in those in whom the infusion reaction does not resolve to G ≤2 despite medical intervention

OMACETAXINE MEPESUCCINATE

SYNRIBO (omacetaxine mepesuccinate) prescribing information. North Wales, PA: Teva Pharmaceuticals USA, Inc.; November 2019

Product Identification, Preparation, Storage, and Stability

- SYNRIBO for injection is a sterile, preservative-free, white to off-white, lyophilized powder in individually packaged, clear, glass, 8-mL-capacity, single-use vials. Each vial contains 3.5 mg omacetaxine mepesuccinate and mannitol; NDC 63459-177-14
- Store unused vials at 20–25°C (68–77°F); temperature excursions are permitted from 15–30°C (59–86°F). Maintain omacetaxine mepesuccinate in its packaging carton until used to protect the drug from light

- Reconstitute omacetaxine mepesuccinate with 1 mL 0.9% NS
- After addition of the diluent, gently swirl the vial until a clear solution is obtained
- The lyophilized powder should be completely dissolved in <1 minute
- The resulting solution will contain 3.5 mg omacetaxine mepesuccinate per milliliter with pH between 5.5 and 7.0
- Withdraw from the vial into a syringe the patient-specific dose of omacetaxine mepesuccinate. Attach a capped needle appropriate for SUBCUTaneous injection

- Promptly discard any unused solution after completing dose preparation
- Avoid contact with the skin. If omacetaxine mepesuccinate comes into contact with skin, immediately and thoroughly wash exposed areas with soap and water
- Use omacetaxine mepesuccinate within 12 hours after reconstitution when stored at room temperature (20–25°C [68–77°F]) and within 6 days (144 hours) after reconstitution if the product is stored under refrigeration (2–8°C [35.6–46.4°F])

Recommendations for Drug Administration and Ancillary Care

General:

- Omacetaxine mepesuccinate is administered by SUBCUTaneous injection
- Omacetaxine mepesuccinate must be reconstituted by a health care professional in a health care facility
- In patients deemed to be appropriate candidates for self-administration or for administration by a non-health care professional caregiver, provide training on proper handling, storage conditions, administration, disposal, and clean-up of accidentally spilled product. Ensure that necessary supplies are available, including but not limited to:
  - Reconstituted omacetaxine mepesuccinate supplied in a syringe with capped needle for SUBCUTaneous injection. Syringe(s) should be filled with reconstituted omacetaxine mepesuccinate to the patient-specific dose by a health care professional in a health care facility prior to dispensing to the patient for home administration
  - Protective eyewear
  - Gloves

- An appropriate biohazard container
- Absorbent pads for placement of administration materials and for accidental spillage
- Alcohol swabs
- Gauze pads
- Ice packs or cooler for transportation of reconstituted omacetaxine mepesuccinate syringes

Caution:

- FDA-approved recommendations for omacetaxine mepesuccinate use include different dose schedules for induction and maintenance dosing
- In addition to hematologic adverse effects (decreased leukocyte, platelet, and erythrocyte counts), omacetaxine mepesuccinate can induce glucose intolerance and hyperglycemia, and 1 patient during clinical development experienced hyperosmolar nonketotic hyperglycemia
  - Monitor blood glucose concentrations frequently, especially in patients with diabetes or risk factors for diabetes

- Avoid omacetaxine mepesuccinate in patients with poorly controlled diabetes mellitus until good glycemic control has been established
- Omacetaxine mepesuccinate is not a substrate of CYP450 enzymes in vitro
  - Omacetaxine mepesuccinate and its primary metabolite, 4'-desmethylhomoharringtonine (4'-DMHHT), do not inhibit major CYP450 enzymes in vitro at concentrations that can be expected clinically
  - The potential for omacetaxine mepesuccinate or 4'-DMHHT to induce CYP450 enzymes has not been determined
- Omacetaxine mepesuccinate is a substrate for transport by P-glycoprotein (P-gp, ABCB1, MDR1) in vitro
  - Omacetaxine mepesuccinate and 4'-DMHHT do not inhibit P-gp-mediated efflux of the P-gp substrate, loperamide, in vitro at concentrations that can be expected clinically

OXALIPLATIN

Oxaliplatin prescribing information. Haikou, China: Qilu Pharmaceutical (Hainan) Co., Ltd.; June 2020
Oxaliplatin prescribing information. Haikou, China: Qilu Pharmaceutical (Hainan) Co., Ltd.; June 2016

WARNING: HYPERSENSITIVITY REACTIONS, INCLUDING ANAPHYLAXIS

Serious and fatal hypersensitivity adverse reactions, including anaphylaxis, can occur with oxaliplatin for injection within minutes of administration and during any cycle. [Oxaliplatin] is contraindicated in patients with hypersensitivity reactions to oxaliplatin and other platinum-based drugs. . . Immediately and permanently discontinue [oxaliplatin] for hypersensitivity reactions and administer appropriate treatment for management of the hypersensitivity reaction . . .

Boxed Warning for Oxaliplatin prescribing information. Haikou, China: Qilu Pharmaceutical (Hainan) Co., Ltd.; June 2020

Product Identification, Preparation, Storage, and Stability

Oxaliplatin for Injection (lyophilized powder):

- Oxaliplatin is supplied in individually packaged, clear, glass, single-use vials containing 50 mg oxaliplatin with lactose monohydrate 450 mg, *or* 100 mg of oxaliplatin with lactose monohydrate 900 mg as a sterile, preservative-free, lyophilized powder for reconstitution
- Store the lyophilized powder under normal lighting conditions at 20–25°C (68–77°F); temperature excursions to 15–30°C (59–86°F) are permitted

Reconstitution of lyophilized oxaliplatin:
- *Important:* Reconstitution or final dilution must *never* be performed with a sodium chloride solution or other chloride-containing solutions
- Reconstitute oxaliplatin lyophilized powder for solution as follows:

Oxaliplatin Content per Vial	Volume of Diluent (SWFI *or* D5W)	Resulting Oxaliplatin Concentration
50 mg	10 mL	5 mg/mL
100 mg	20 mL	

- After reconstitution in the original vial, oxaliplatin solution (5 mg/mL) may be stored for up to 24 hours under refrigeration, 2–8°C (36–46°F)
- Reconstituted oxaliplatin (5 mg/mL) must be diluted in 250–500 mL of D5W before administration to patients
- After dilution in 250–500 mL of D5W, oxaliplatin solutions are stable for up to 6 hours if stored at room temperature, 20–25°C, or up to 24 hours under refrigeration, 2–8°C
- Oxaliplatin for injection is not light sensitive

Oxaliplatin concentrate (solution):

- Oxaliplatin concentrate is supplied in individually packaged, clear, glass, single-use vials
- Product formulations and presentations vary among manufacturers, but include vials containing 50 mg, 100 mg, or 200 mg of oxaliplatin as a sterile, preservative-free, aqueous solution at a concentration of 5 mg oxaliplatin/mL in SWFI ± additional excipients
- Store oxaliplatin solution at 25°C (77°F); temperature excursions to 15–30°C are permitted. Do not freeze and protect from light (keep in original outer packaging carton)
- Oxaliplatin concentrate (5 mg/mL) must be diluted in 250–500 mL of D5W before administration to patients
- After dilution in 250–500 mL of D5W, oxaliplatin solutions are stable for up to 6 hours if stored at room temperature (20–25°C), or up to 24 hours under refrigeration (2–8°C)
- *Important:* Oxaliplatin concentrate dilution must never be performed with a sodium chloride solution or other chloride-containing solutions
- Protection from light exposure is not required after dilution

Selected incompatibility:

- Oxaliplatin in solution is incompatible and must not be mixed or administered simultaneously through the same infusion line with alkaline medications or media (eg, fluorouracil)
- Do not use aluminum needles or administration sets containing aluminum parts that may come into contact with oxaliplatin-containing solutions. Aluminum has been reported to cause degradation of platinum compounds

Recommendations for Drug Administration and Ancillary Care

General:
- See Chapter 43 for recommended use in patients with renal dysfunction
- Oxaliplatin administration does not require prehydration
- Oxaliplatin is usually given by intraVENous infusion over 2 hours
  - Increasing the infusion time from 2 hours to 6 hours decreases maximum oxaliplatin concentrations by an estimated 32% and may mitigate acute toxicities
- Administration sets and VAD used to administer oxaliplatin should be flushed with D5W after completing oxaliplatin infusion before using them to administer any other medications
- Do not use aluminum needles or administration sets containing aluminum parts that may come into contact with oxaliplatin solutions. Aluminum has been reported to cause degradation of platinum compounds
- Prescriptions and medication orders should identify the drug by its complete generic name, oxaliplatin

Altered platinum exposure in renal impairment:
- The AUC of platinum in plasma ultrafiltrate increases as renal function decreases. The mean AUC of unbound platinum in patients with mild (creatinine clearance 50–80 mL/min [Clcr 0.83–1.33 mL/s]), moderate (Clcr 30 to <50 mL/min[0.5 to <0.83 mL/s]), and severe renal (Clcr <30 mL/min [<0.5 mL/s]) impairment is increased by approximately 40%, 95%, and 342%, respectively, compared to patients with Clcr >80 mL/min (>1.33 mL/s)
- Consult recommendations for oxaliplatin use in renal impairment

Neuropathy associated with exposure to cold temperatures:
- Oxaliplatin is associated with 2 types of neuropathy, including an acute, reversible, primarily peripheral, sensory neuropathy
  - Onset is within hours or 1–2 days after administration; it characteristically resolves within 14 days but frequently recurs with subsequent oxaliplatin treatment
- Symptoms may be precipitated or exacerbated by exposure to cold temperature or cold objects and usually present as transient paresthesia, dysesthesia, and hypoesthesia in the hands, feet, perioral area, or throat. Jaw spasm, abnormal tongue sensation, dysarthria, eye pain, and a feeling of chest pressure also have been observed
- Patients should be instructed to avoid cold drinks and use of ice (eg, prophylaxis against mucositis and palliation for pain with mucositis), and should cover skin exposed to cold temperatures

Inadvertent exposure:
- In case of skin contact, immediately and thoroughly wash the affected area with soap and water
- In case of contact with mucous membranes, thoroughly flush the affected area with water

PACLITAXEL

PACLITAXEL prescribing information. North Wales, PA: Teva Pharmaceuticals USA; July 2015

WARNING

Paclitaxel injection should be administered under the supervision of a physician experienced in the use of cancer chemotherapeutic agents. Appropriate management of complications is possible only when adequate diagnostic and treatment facilities are readily available

Anaphylaxis and severe hypersensitivity reactions characterized by dyspnea and hypotension requiring treatment, angioedema, and generalized urticaria have occurred in 2 to 4% of patients receiving paclitaxel in clinical trials. Fatal reactions have occurred in patients despite premedication. All patients should be pretreated with corticosteroids, diphenhydrAMINE, and H_2 antagonists … Patients who experience severe hypersensitivity reactions to paclitaxel injection should not be rechallenged with the drug

Paclitaxel injection therapy should not be given to patients with solid tumors who have baseline neutrophil counts of less than 1500 cells/mm^3 and should not be given to patients with AIDS-related Kaposi's sarcoma if the baseline neutrophil count is less than 1000 cells/mm^3. In order to monitor the occurrence of bone marrow suppression, primarily neutropenia, which may be severe and result in infection, it is recommended that frequent peripheral blood cell counts be performed on all patients receiving paclitaxel injection

---

Boxed Warning for PACLITAXEL prescribing information. North Wales, PA: Teva Pharmaceuticals USA; July 2015

Product Identification, Preparation, Storage, and Stability

- PACLitaxel is generically available from several manufacturers. Available presentations vary among manufacturers' products, but include individually packaged, multidose, glass vials, containing: 30 mg (in 5 mL), 100 mg (in 16.7 mL), 150 mg (in 25 mL), or 300 mg (in 50 mL)

- PACLitaxel injection is a clear, colorless to slightly yellow, viscous, concentrated solution. Each milliliter contains PACLitaxel, USP, 6 mg formulated in a solvent system consisting of polyoxyl 35 castor oil, NF (*AKA* polyoxyethylated castor oil; Cremophor EL), 527 mg; and dehydrated alcohol 49.7% (v/v). Some products may contain additional excipients

- Store unopened vials at 20–25°C (68–77°F) in the original package

  - Neither freezing nor refrigeration adversely affects PACLitaxel stability

  - Components in PACLitaxel injection may precipitate under refrigeration, but will redissolve upon reaching room temperature with little or no agitation

    ○ Precipitation and redissolution under these circumstances do not affect product quality

  ○ Discard vials in which PACLitaxel solution remains cloudy after warming to room temperature and gentle agitation, or if an insoluble precipitate is observed

- For clinical use, *concentrated PACLitaxel must be diluted* to a concentration within the range 0.3–1.2 mg/mL with 0.9% NS, D5W, D5W/0.9% NS, or D5W/RI in a polyolefin container

- *Avoid bringing PACLitaxel into contact* with containers, syringes, tubing, and other materials made of PVC during drug preparation and administration

- PACLitaxel-containing solutions characteristically leach DEHP and other phthalate plasticizers from flexible PVC containers and infusion sets[54,55,56,57]

  - PACLitaxel solutions should be stored in glass, polypropylene, or polyolefin[17] containers and administered through polyethylene- or polyolefin-lined administration sets

    ○ *Caution:* Use of vented administration sets with rigid (glass) parenteral product containers has been associated with PACLitaxel solution dripping from the air vent, presumably as a result of

surfactant wetting the hydrophobic air vent (inlet) filter[58]

  ○ *Caution: Do not use* chemotherapy dispensing pins and similar solution transfer devices with spikes with PACLitaxel, as they can cause a vial's stopper to collapse and compromise the sterility of its contents

- After dilution in 0.9% NS or D5W, PACLitaxel solutions are physically and chemically stable for up to 48 hours at ambient temperature (20–23°C [68–73.4°F]) and fluorescent lighting[59,60,61]

  - Product labeling stipulates PACLitaxel solutions are stable at ambient temperature (approximately 25°C [77°F]) and lighting conditions for up to 27 hours after dilution to a concentration within the range 0.3–1.2 mg/mL in D5W/0.9% NS or D5W/RI

- PACLitaxel should be inspected visually for particulate matter and discoloration before administration whenever solution and container permit. After preparation, PACLitaxel solutions may show haziness, which is attributed to the presence of surfactant in the commercial product[62]

Recommendations for Drug Administration and Ancillary Care

General:

- See Chapter 43 for recommended use in patients with hepatic dysfunction
- Use non-PVC containers, administration sets, and filters to administer PACLitaxel. *Avoid vented* administration sets
  - Glass, polyethylene, and polyolefin containers and polyethylene- or polyolefin-lined administration sets are compatible
- After dilution within the recommended concentration range (0.3–1.2 mg/mL), PACLitaxel may unpredictably precipitate in a product container or administration set tubing. The mechanisms underlying spontaneous precipitation and predisposing conditions are not well defined. Consequently, care providers should remain vigilant for drug precipitation throughout the duration of PACLitaxel administration
- *Administer PACLitaxel through an inline filter* with a filter membrane pore size ≤0.22 μm. Filtration does not cause significant losses in potency
  - Use of filter devices that incorporate short inlet and outlet PVC-coated tubing has not resulted in significant leaching of DEHP
- Administer PACLitaxel by intraVENous infusion over periods from 1 to ≥24 hours (commonly, 3 hours)

Primary prophylaxis against hypersensitivity reactions:

- PACLitaxel treatment is contraindicated in patients who have a history of hypersensitivity reactions to PACLitaxel or other drugs formulated in polyoxyl 35 castor oil, NF (eg, cycloSPORINE, teniposide)
- All patients should receive primary prophylaxis against hypersensitivity reactions, particularly with PACLitaxel infusion duration ≤3 hours. Prophylaxis may consist of:
  - I. **Dexamethasone** 20 mg; administer orally or intraVENously for 2 doses, at approximately 12 hours and 6 hours before PACLitaxel (in treatment of Kaposi's sarcoma, each dexamethasone dose is decreased to 10 mg per dose on the same administration schedule), *plus*
  - 2. **DiphenhydrAMINE** (or an equivalent H_1 antihistamine) 50 mg; administer intraVENously 30–60 minutes before PACLitaxel, *and*
  - 3. **RaNITIdine** 50 mg *or* **cimetidine** 300 mg (or an equivalent H_2 antihistamine); administer intraVENously 30–60 minutes before PACLitaxel administration

Hypersensitivity reactions:

- Refer to the boxed "WARNING" (above) excerpted from current product labeling
- The most frequent hypersensitivity symptoms observed during severe reactions were dyspnea, flushing, chest pain, and tachycardia. Abdominal pain, pain in the extremities, diaphoresis, and hypertension also were noted
- Minor symptoms such as flushing, skin reactions, hypotension, dyspnea, or tachycardia do not require interruption of therapy
- Immediately discontinue PACLitaxel for severe reactions and utilize aggressive symptom-appropriate therapy

Selected drug interactions:

- In a phase 1 clinical trial in which PACLitaxel and CISplatin were given in sequence, myelosuppression was more profound when PACLitaxel was given after CISplatin than with the alternate sequence (ie, PACLitaxel before CISplatin). Pharmacokinetic data demonstrated a decrease in PACLitaxel clearance of approximately 33% when PACLitaxel was administered after CISplatin
- PACLitaxel metabolism is catalyzed by CYP2C8 and CYP3A4. Exercise caution when PACLitaxel is administered concomitantly with substrates, inhibitors, and inducers of either CYP2C8 or CYP3A4
- PACLitaxel has been shown to decrease the rate of DOXOrubicin metabolism when PACLitaxel is given concomitantly in sequence before the other drug. A pharmacokinetic study in which the sequence of administration of PACLitaxel and DOXOrubicin alternated during 2 consecutive treatment cycles revealed DOXOrubicin plasma concentrations at the end of infusion were increased by an average of 70% and DOXOrubicin clearance was decreased approximately 30% when PACLitaxel is given first compared with the alternative sequence. Similarly, the incidence of G2/3 mucositis was 70% with the PACLitaxel-followed-by-DOXOrubicin sequence versus only 10% with the reverse sequence
- Patients exhibited an 80% mean increase in DOXOrubicin AUC and a mean decrease in clearance of 71% when liposomal DOXOrubicin hydrochloride DOXIL was given concomitantly with weekly PACLitaxel
- PACLitaxel significantly increased the bioavailability of epiRUBicin and slowed recovery from neutropenia in patients with stages 2 or 3 breast cancer who received epiRUBicin either before or after a 3-hour infusion of PACLitaxel. EpiRUBicin AUC increased by 37% and maximum plasma concentration increased by 65%, while total clearance decreased by 25%. When epiRUBicin was given after PACLitaxel, ANC recovery occurred more slowly compared with the alternative administration sequence

Inadvertent exposure:

- If PACLitaxel injection solution contacts the skin, wash the skin immediately and thoroughly with soap and water
  - Following topical exposure, events have included tingling, burning, and redness
- If PACLitaxel injection contacts mucous membranes, thoroughly flush the affected area with water
- Upon inhalation, dyspnea, chest pain, burning eyes, sore throat, and nausea have been reported

PACLITAXEL PROTEIN-BOUND PARTICLES FOR INJECTABLE SUSPENSION

ABRAXANE prescribing information. Summit, NJ: Celgene Corporation; August 2020

WARNING: SEVERE MYELOSUPPRESSION

- Do not administer ABRAXANE therapy to patients with baseline neutrophil counts of less than 1500 cells/mm^3 ...
- Monitor for neutropenia, which may be severe and result in infection or sepsis ...
- Perform frequent complete blood cell counts on all patients receiving ABRAXANE

Boxed Warning for ABRAXANE prescribing information. Summit, NJ: Celgene Corporation; August 2020

Product Identification, Preparation, Storage, and Stability

- ABRAXANE is available in individually packaged single-use vials containing 100 mg of PACLitaxel bound to human albumin and approximately 900 mg albumin human containing sodium caprylate and sodium acetyltryptophanate as a sterile, white to yellow, lyophilized powder. NDC 68817-134-50
  - The product does not contain Cremophor or other solvents
- Store unopened vials at 20–25°C (68–77°F) in the original package to protect from bright light
- The following reconstitution procedure yields a suspension for intraVENous injection containing 5 mg PACLitaxel/mL:
  1. Slowly inject 20 mL of 0.9% NS against the inside wall of a product vial over a minimum of 1 minute. To prevent foaming, *do not inject* the diluent directly into the lyophilized drug
  2. After all diluent has been added to a vial, allow each vial to sit for a minimum of 5 minutes to ensure that the lyophilized drug is properly wetted, *then*
  3. Gently swirl and invert the vial slowly for at least 2 minutes until the drug is homogenously dispersed. Avoid aggressively agitating the vial contents to prevent foaming

  4. If foaming or clumping occurs, allow the solution to stand undisturbed for at least 15 minutes until foam subsides
- *Do not filter* ABRAXANE during preparation or administration
- Reconstituted ABRAXANE (5 mg PACLitaxel/mL) should be milky and homogenous without visible particulates. If particulates or drug settling are observed, gently invert affected product vials to completely resuspend the product before it is administered to a patient
- The reconstituted product may be stored under refrigeration at 2–8°C (36–46°F) for a maximum of 24 hours.
  - Although freezing and refrigeration do not adversely affect product stability, reconstituted ABRAXANE suspension should be stored in its original carton and protected from bright light
- Discard the reconstituted suspension if precipitates are observed
- Inject an amount of reconstituted ABRAXANE appropriate for a patient's dose into an empty, sterile PVC container
  - The use of medical devices containing silicone oil as a lubricant (ie, syringes and intraVENous bags) to reconstitute and administer ABRAXANE may result in the formation of proteinaceous strands.

- DEHP-free solution containers and administration sets are not necessary to prepare or administer ABRAXANE, but they may be used
- After transfer to a parenteral product container, the ABRAXANE suspension is stable at ambient temperature (approximately 25°C [77°F]) and lighting conditions for up to 4 hours and under refrigeration (2–8°C [36–46°F]) for up to 24 hours if protected from bright light. The total *combined* refrigerated storage time of reconstituted ABRAXANE in the vial and in the infusion bag is 24 hours. This may be followed by storage in the infusion bag at ambient temperature (approximately 25°C [77°F]) and lighting conditions for a maximum of 4 hours
- Suspended particles may settle if the product is not used soon after reconstitution. Ensure complete resuspension by mildly agitating ABRAXANE before it is used. Discard the diluted product if proteinaceous strands, particulate matter, or discoloration are observed
- Discard any unused reconstituted ABRAXANE after preparing a patient's dose

Recommendations for Drug Administration and Ancillary Care

General:

- See Chapter 43 for recommended use in patients with hepatic dysfunction
- Premedication to prevent hypersensitivity reactions is not required before administering ABRAXANE
- Administer ABRAXANE suspension intraVENously over 30 minutes when used for metastatic breast cancer and non-small cell lung cancer (NSCLC) indications and over 30–40 minutes when used for pancreatic ductal adenocarcinoma (PDAC)
  - When used for NSCLC, administer ABRAXANE immediately prior to CARBOplatin
  - When used for PDAC, administer ABRAXANE immediately prior to gemcitabine
  - Administration over 30 minutes may reduce the likelihood of infusion-related reactions in comparison with more protracted delivery durations
- It is not necessary to prepare or administer ABRAXANE with DEHP-free containers and administration sets, but they may be used
- *Do not filter* ABRAXANE during administration
- If ABRAXANE administration does not commence within 30 minutes after product preparation, the product container should be gently inverted (several repetitions) to resuspend the drug particles before commencing drug administration

PANITUMUMAB

Vectibix (panitumumab) prescribing information. Thousand Oaks, CA: Amgen Inc.; June 2017

WARNING: DERMATOLOGIC TOXICITY

<u>Dermatologic Toxicity:</u> Dermatologic toxicities occurred in 90% of patients and were severe (NCI-CTC Grade 3 and higher) in 15% of patients receiving Vectibix monotherapy …

Boxed Warning for Vectibix (panitumumab) prescribing information. Thousand Oaks, CA: Amgen Inc.; June 2017

Product Identification, Preparation, Storage, and Stability

- Vectibix is available in individually packaged single-use vials containing a sterile, colorless, preservative-free solution of panitumumab 20 mg/mL at a pH within the range 5.6–6.0 in the following presentations:

Panitumumab Content	Excipients Content	NDC Number
100 mg/5 mL	Sodium chloride 29 mg, sodium acetate 34 mg, and SWFI	55513-954-01
400 mg/20 mL	Sodium chloride 117 mg, sodium acetate 136 mg, and SWFI	55513-956-01

- Store vials in their packaging carton under refrigeration at 2–8°C (36–46°F) until time of use. Protect vials from direct exposure to sunlight and *do not freeze* the concentrated solution (20 mg/mL)
- The undiluted drug product may contain a small amount of visible translucent-to-white, amorphous, proteinaceous, panitumumab particulates
- *Do not shake* concentrated panitumumab solution (20 mg/mL)
- *Do not use* panitumumab if it appears to be discolored or cloudy, or if foreign matter is present
- Using a 21-gauge or larger gauge (smaller bore) hypodermic needle, withdraw from the vial the volume of concentrated panitumumab solution (20 mg/mL) necessary for a patient's dose and dilute as follows:

Panitumumab Dose	Vehicle Solution	Total Product Volume After Dilution (Q.S.)
≤1000 mg	0.9% NS	100 mL
>1000 mg		150 mL

Do not exceed a final concentration of 10 mg/mL

- Mix diluted solutions by repeatedly but gently inverting the product container. *Do not shake* diluted solutions
- Use diluted panitumumab solutions within 6 hours after dilution if stored at room temperature, or within 24 hours after dilution if stored under refrigeration at 2–8°C (36–46°F). *Do not freeze* diluted panitumumab solutions
- Discard any unused panitumumab remaining in a vial

Recommendations for Drug Administration and Ancillary Care

Determining appropriate utilization:

- Panitumumab is not indicated for patients with *RAS*-mutated metastatic colorectal cancer or for patients whom *RAS* mutation status is unknown. It is necessary to assess *RAS* mutation status to confirm the absence of a *RAS* mutation in exon 2 (codons 12 and 13), exon 3 (codons 59 and 61), and exon 4 (codons 117 and 146) of both *KRAS* and *NRAS* before administering panitumumab

General:

- See Chapter 43 for comments about use in patients with renal and hepatic dysfunction
- *Caution: Do not administer* panitumumab as an intraVENous injection (IV push *or* bolus)
- Flush administration set tubing and a patient's VAD with 0.9% NS before and after panitumumab administration
  - *Do not mix or administer* panitumumab with other medications, or add other medications to solutions containing panitumumab
  - Administer panitumumab intraVENously via a peripheral or central VAD with a rate controlling device; that is, an infusion pump
- Administer doses ≤1000 mg over 60 minutes. If the first infusion is tolerated, administer subsequent infusions over 30–60 minutes
- Administer doses >1000 mg over 90 minutes
- During administration, the fluid pathway must include a low-protein-binding inline filter with pore size 0.2 or 0.22 μm

Infusion reactions:

- Severe infusion reactions including anaphylactoid and fatal reactions

have occurred during panitumumab administration and on the day of administration
  - The utility of medications as prophylaxis against infusional toxicities is unknown
  - Appropriate medical resources for the treatment of severe infusion reactions should be available during panitumumab administration
- Dose modifications for infusion reactions
  - Decrease the administration rate by 50% in patients who experience a mild or moderate (Grades 1 or 2) infusion reaction for the duration of that infusion
  - Terminate panitumumab administration in patients who experience more severe infusion reactions
  - Depending on the severity and/or persistence of a reaction, permanently discontinue panitumumab

Dermatologic Toxicities:

- First occurrence of G3 dermatologic reaction: withhold 1–2 doses of panitumumab. If the reaction improves to <G3, reinitiate panitumumab at the original dose
- Second occurrence of G3 dermatologic reaction: withhold 1–2 doses of panitumumab. If the reaction improves to <G3, reinitiate panitumumab at 80% of the original dose
- Third occurrence of G3 dermatologic toxicity: withhold 1–2 doses of panitumumab. If the reaction improves to <G3, reinitiate panitumumab at 60% of the original dose
- Fourth occurrence of G3 dermatologic toxicity: permanently discontinue panitumumab

- Any occurrence of a G4 dermatologic toxicity, or for a G3 dermatologic reaction that does not recover after withholding 1 or 2 doses: permanently discontinue panitumumab

Additional selected potentially severe adverse effects:

- Interstitial lung disease (ILD), including fatalities, has been reported in patients treated with panitumumab
  - Interrupt panitumumab therapy for the acute onset or worsening of pulmonary symptoms
  - Discontinue panitumumab therapy if ILD is confirmed
- Hypomagnesemia has been associated with panitumumab therapy. Hypocalcemia and hypokalemia also have been observed
  - Periodically monitor patients' electrolytes during and for 8 weeks after panitumumab therapy is discontinued
- Exposure to sunlight can exacerbate dermatological toxicities associated with panitumumab
  - Advise patients to wear sunscreen and hats and limit sun exposure while receiving panitumumab
- Keratitis and ulcerative keratitis, risk factors for corneal perforation, have been reported with panitumumab use
  - Monitor for evidence of keratitis or ulcerative keratitis, and interrupt or discontinue panitumumab for acute or worsening keratitis

PEGASPARGASE

Oncaspar (pegaspargase) prescribing information. Boston, MA: Servier Pharmaceuticals LLC; June 2020

Product Identification, Preparation, Storage, and Stability

- Oncaspar (pegaspargase) is asparaginase (L-asparagine amidohydrolase; identical 34.5-kDa subunits) produced by *Escherichia coli* that is covalently conjugated to monomethoxypolyethylene glycol (mPEG; MW ~5 kDa). Approximately 69–82 molecules of mPEG are linked to L-asparaginase
  - Pegaspargase activity is expressed in International Units
  - One International Unit of L-asparaginase is defined as the amount of enzyme required to generate 1 micromole of ammonia per minute at pH 7.3 and 37°C
- The commercial product, Oncaspar, is supplied in type I, single-use vials containing a clear, colorless, preservative-free, isotonic, sterile solution in phosphate-buffered saline at pH 7.3
  - Each milliliter of solution contains pegaspargase 750 International Units, dibasic sodium phosphate, USP 5.58 mg, monobasic sodium phosphate, USP 1.20 mg, and sodium chloride, USP 8.50 mg in water for injection, USP
- Oncaspar vials contain pegaspargase 3750 International Units (L-asparaginase) per 5 mL solution (NDC 72694-954-01)
- Store Oncaspar under refrigeration at 2–8°C (36–46°F). Unopened vials may be stored at room temperature (2–8°C [36–46°F]) for no more than 48 hours
- *Do not shake or freeze* Oncaspar. Protect vials from exposure to light

Recommendations for Drug Administration and Ancillary Care

Administration:

- The recommended dosage of pegaspargase for patients ages ≤21 years is 2500 International Units/m² BSA for administration by intraMUSCular or intraVENous routes not more frequently than every 14 days
- The recommended dosage of pegaspargase for patients ages >21 years is 2000 International Units/m² BSA for administration by intraMUSCular or intraVENous routes not more frequently than every 14 days
- *IntraMUSCular administration:* Oncaspar is suitable for intraMUSCular injection without further modification
  - The volume at a single injection site should be ≤2 mL. Dose volumes >2 mL should be administered in two or more injection sites
- *IntraVENous administration:* Transfer a volume of pegaspargase appropriate for a patient's dose to a parenteral product container with 100 mL of 0.9% NS or D5W. Administer pegaspargase intraVENously over 1–2 hours ("piggybacked" or as a secondary infusion) into a running intraVENous infusion of the same fluid used for dilution (either 0.9% NS or D5W)

- Diluted pegaspargase should be used immediately. If immediate use is not possible, store diluted pegaspargase solutions under refrigeration at 2–8°C
- Storage after dilution should not exceed 48 hours from the time of preparation to completion of administration
- Protect diluted pegaspargase from direct exposure to sunlight
- *Do not administer* Oncaspar if the drug product has been frozen, stored at room temperatures 15–25°C (59–77°F) for >48 hours, or shaken or vigorously agitated

Potentially serious adverse events:

- Oncaspar is contraindicated in patients with a history of serious hypersensitivity reactions, including anaphylaxis, to Oncaspar or to any of its excipients, in patients with a history of severe thrombosis with prior L-asparaginase therapy, in patients with a history of pancreatitis related to prior L-asparaginase therapy, in patients with a history of serious hemorrhagic events with prior L-asparaginase therapy, and in patients with severe hepatic impairment
- Allergic reactions may occur in association with pegaspargase administration

- Persons with known hypersensitivity to other forms of asparaginase are at increased risk of developing a serious allergic reaction
- Observe patients for one hour after pegaspargase administration in a setting with resuscitation equipment and medications necessary for treating anaphylaxis (eg, oxygen and injectable EPINEPHrine, steroids, antihistamines)
- Discontinue pegaspargase in patients who experience serious allergic reactions
- Patients should be informed of the possibility of serious allergic reactions, including anaphylaxis, and to immediately report any swelling or difficulty breathing
- Thrombotic events, including sagittal sinus thrombosis, can occur in persons who receive pegaspargase
  - Discontinue pegaspargase in patients who develop serious thrombotic events
  - Patients should be advised to immediately report a severe headache, swelling of extremities, acute shortness of breath, chest pain, severe abdominal pain, excessive thirst, increase in the volume or frequency of urination, unusual bleeding or bruising, or jaundice after receiving pegaspargase

PEGINTERFERON ALFA-2b

SYLATRON (peginterferon alfa-2b) prescribing information. Whitehouse Station, NJ: Merck Sharp & Dohme Corp.; August 2019

WARNING: DEPRESSION AND OTHER NEUROPSYCHIATRIC DISORDERS

The risk of serious depression, with suicidal ideation and completed suicides, and other serious neuropsychiatric disorders is increased with alpha interferons, including SYLATRON. Permanently discontinue SYLATRON in patients with persistently severe or worsening signs or symptoms of depression, psychosis, or encephalopathy. These disorders may not resolve after stopping SYLATRON …

Boxed Warning for SYLATRON (peginterferon alfa-2b) prescribing information. Whitehouse Station, NJ: Merck Sharp & Dohme Corp.; August 2019

Product Identification, Preparation, Storage, and Stability

- SYLATRON, peginterferon alfa-2b, is a covalent conjugate of recombinant alfa-2b interferon with monomethoxy polyethylene glycol (PEG)
  - The specific activity of pegylated interferon alfa-2b is approximately 0.7×10^8 international units/mg protein
- Each vial contains peginterferon alfa-2b as a sterile, white to off-white lyophilized powder, and dibasic sodium phosphate anhydrous 1.11 mg, monobasic sodium phosphate dihydrate 1.11 mg, polysorbate 80 0.074 mg, and sucrose 59.2 mg, in the following presentations:

Each SYLATRON Package Contains:

Labeled Peginterferon alfa-2b Content	Actual Product Contents	NDC No.
200 μg	One vial of peginterferon alfa-2b powder (296 μg), one 5 mL vial of SWFI*, 2 B-D Safety Lok syringes with 1/2 inch 27-gauge needles and safety sleeve, and 2 alcohol swabs	0085-4347-01
300 μg	One vial of peginterferon alfa-2b powder (444 μg), one 5 mL vial of SWFI*, 2 B-D Safety Lok syringes with 1/2 inch 27-gauge needles and safety sleeve, and 2 alcohol swabs	0085-4348-02
600 μg	One vial of peginterferon alfa-2b powder (888 μg), one 5 mL vial of SWFI*, 2 B-D Safety Lok syringes with 1/2 inch 27-gauge needles and safety sleeve, and 2 alcohol swabs	0085-4349-01

*Advise patients that the SWFI vials supplied contain an excess amount of diluent and only 0.7 mL should be withdrawn to reconstitute SYLATRON. Discard the unused portion of SWFI; do not save or reuse

- SYLATRON should be stored at 25°C (77°F); temperature excursions are permitted to 15–30°C (59–86°F). *Do not freeze* SYLATRON
- Reconstitute SYLATRON products with SWFI as follows:

(continued)

Recommendations for Drug Administration and Ancillary Care

General:
- Give primary prophylaxis against febrile reactions with acetaminophen 500–1000 mg orally 30 minutes before a first dose of peginterferon alfa-2b, and as needed for subsequent doses
- *Do not withdraw* more than 0.5 mL of reconstituted solution from each vial
- Administer SYLATRON by SUBCUTaneous injection. Rotate injection sites

Contraindications:
- SYLATRON is contraindicated in patients with:
  - A history of anaphylaxis to peginterferon alfa-2b or interferon alfa-2b
  - Autoimmune hepatitis
  - Hepatic decompensation (Child-Pugh scores >6 [classes B and C])

Potential for drug interactions:
- In healthy subjects who received metabolic probe drugs before and after 2 doses of peginterferon alfa-2b 3 μg/kg, the geometric mean AUC_{last} for caffeine (CYP1A2 probe substrate) was increased by 36% and for desipramine (CYP2D6 probe substrate) was increased by 30%. No meaningful changes in exposure of probe substrates for CYP2C9 and CYP3A4 activity were observed

(continued)

Product Identification, Preparation, Storage, and Stability (continued)

Labeled Peginterferon alfa-2b Content (Actual Content) per Vial	Volume of SWFI for Reconstitution	Deliverable Peginterferon alfa-2b	Reconstituted Product Concentration
200 μg (296 μg)	0.7 mL	200 μg in 0.5 mL	40 μg/0.1 mL
300 μg (444 μg)		300 μg in 0.5 mL	60 μg/0.1 mL
600 μg (888 μg)		600 μg in 0.5 mL	120 μg/0.1 mL

- Gently swirl vials to dissolve lyophilized peginterferon alfa-2b powder. *Do not shake* vials
- Visually inspect the solution for particulate matter and discoloration prior to administration. Discard vials containing a discolored or cloudy solution, or if particulates are present
- If the reconstituted solution is not used immediately, store it under refrigeration at 2–8°C (36–46°F) for no more than 24 hours. *Do not freeze* Sylatron
  - Discard any unused reconstituted solution after 24 hours
- *Do not withdraw* more than 0.5 mL of reconstituted solution from each vial

Recommendations for Drug Administration and Ancillary Care (continued)

Advice and instructions for patients and their personal caregivers:

- Peginterferon alfa-2b may be administered with antipyretics at bedtime to minimize common "flu-like" symptoms (chills, fever, muscle aches, joint pain, headaches, tiredness)
- Maintain hydration with nonalcoholic fluids if patients are experiencing "flu-like" symptoms
- Immediately report any symptoms of depression or suicidal ideation to their health care provider during treatment and for up to 6 months after the last dose
- A female patient using peginterferon alfa-2b who becomes pregnant should promptly consult her health care provider for guidance about continuing use
- Do not re-use or share syringes and needles
- Instruct patients how to properly disposal of peginterferon alfa-2b vials, syringes, and hypodermic needles
- Advise patients that the SWFI vials supplied contain an excess amount of diluent and only 0.7 mL should be withdrawn to reconstitute SYLATRON. Discard the unused portion of SWFI. Do not save or reuse

PEMBROLIZUMAB

KEYTRUDA (pembrolizumab) prescribing information. Whitehouse Station, NJ: Merck Sharp & Dohme Corp.; June 2020

Product Identification, Preparation, Storage, and Stability

- KEYTRUDA is a sterile, clear to slightly opalescent, colorless to slightly yellow, preservative-free solution in single-dose vials that contain 100 mg of pembrolizumab in 4 mL of solution. Each 1 mL of solution contains 25 mg of pembrolizumab and is formulated in L-histidine (1.55 mg), polysorbate 80 (0.2 mg), sucrose (70 mg), and SWFI (NDC 0006-3026-02). A carton containing two 100-mg pembrolizumab vials also is available (NDC 0006-3026-04)
- Store intact vials under refrigeration at 2–8°C (36–46°F) in the original carton to protect from light
- Do not freeze or shake intact vials

Dilution:
- The solution is clear to slightly opalescent, colorless to slightly yellow. Visibly inspect the solution for particulate matter and discoloration. Discard the vial if visible particles are observed
- Withdraw the required volume from the vial(s) of pembrolizumab and transfer into an intraVENous bag containing 0.9% NS or D5W to a final concentration between 1 to 10 mg/mL
- **Mix diluted solution by gentle inversion.** Do not shake
- Store the diluted solution at either room temperature for no more than 6 hours from

the time of dilution (including duration of the infusion) or under refrigeration at 2–8°C (36–46°F) for no more than 96 hours from the time of dilution
- If refrigerated, allow the diluted solution to come to room temperature prior to administration. Do not shake. Do not freeze
- Discard after 6 hours at room temperature or after 96 hours under refrigeration

Selected incompatibility:
- Do not co-administer with other drugs through the same infusion line

Recommendations for Drug Administration and Ancillary Care

General:
- The impact of moderate or severe hepatic impairment on the PK of pembrolizumab is unknown

Administration:
- The recommended dose of pembrolizumab is 200 mg every 3 weeks or 400 mg every 6 weeks for adults
- Refer to the current FDA-approved product label for specific indications as well as for details on agents administered in combination with pembrolizumab for certain cancers
- Administer intraVENously over 30 minutes through an intraVENous line containing a sterile, non-pyrogenic, low-protein-binding 0.2- to 5-µm inline or add-on filter

Adverse events and treatment modifications:
- Immune-mediated adverse events can occur with pembrolizumab. Some of these adverse events can be severe or life-threatening

- Refer to the current FDA-approved product label for detailed warnings and recommendations regarding treatment modifications for immune-mediated adverse reactions including pneumonitis, colitis, hepatitis, endocrinopathies, nephritis, skin adverse reactions or other G ≥3 immune-mediated adverse reactions, hematologic toxicity in patients with classical Hodgkin lymphoma or primary mediastinal large B-cell lymphoma and persistent G2 or G3 adverse reactions (excluding endocrinopathy)
  - Permanently discontinue pembrolizumab if unable to reduce steroid dose for adverse reactions to ≤10 mg prednisone per day (or equivalent) >12 weeks after last dose
  - Permanently discontinue pembrolizumab for G2 or G3 adverse reaction (excluding endocrinopathy) lasting ≥12 weeks after the last dose
- Pembrolizumab can cause severe or life-threatening infusion-related reactions, including hypersensitivity and anaphylaxis,

which have been reported in 6 (0.2%) of 2799 patients receiving pembrolizumab. Monitor for signs and symptoms of infusion-related reactions including rigors, chills, wheezing, pruritus, flushing, rash, hypotension, hypoxemia, and fever
  - For G1 or G2 infusion-related reactions interrupt or slow the rate of infusion
  - For severe (G3) and life-threatening (G4) infusion-related reactions, stop the infusion and permanently discontinue

Selected precautions:
- Immune-mediated complications, including fatal events, occurred in patients who underwent allogeneic hematopoietic stem cell transplantation (HSCT) after being treated with pembrolizumab. Follow patients closely for early evidence of complications and intervene promptly
- Consider the benefit of treatment with pembrolizumab versus the risk of possible GVHD in patients with a history of allogeneic HSCT

PEMETREXED DISODIUM

ALIMTA (pemetrexed for injection) prescribing information. Indianapolis, IN: Eli Lilly US LLC; January 2019

Product Identification, Preparation, Storage, and Stability

- ALIMTA is available in individually packaged, sterile, single-use vials containing PEMEtrexed disodium as a white to either light-yellow or green-yellow lyophilized powder in the following presentations:

PEMEtrexed Disodium Equivalent to PEMEtrexed (Labeled PEMEtrexed Content)	Excipients	NDC Number
100 mg	106 mg mannitol	0002-7640-01
500 mg	500 mg mannitol	0002-7623-01

Note: Hydrochloric acid and/or sodium hydroxide may have been added to adjust pH

- PEMEtrexed for injection, should be stored at 25°C (77°F); temperature excursions are permitted to 15–30°C (59–86°F)

- Reconstitute PEMEtrexed disodium with preservative-free 0.9% NS as follows:

Labeled PEMEtrexed Content[*]	Diluent Volume	Resulting Concentration
100 mg	4.2 mL	25 mg/mL
500 mg	20 mL	

[*]Alimta vials contain an excess of PEMEtrexed to facilitate delivery of the labeled amount

- Gently swirl each vial until lyophilized PEMEtrexed powder is completely dissolved
- The resulting reconstituted solution (25 mg/mL) is clear, ranges in color from colorless to yellow or green-yellow without adversely affecting product quality
- Reconstituted PEMEtrexed solution (25 mg/mL) must be further diluted with preservative-free 0.9% NS to a total volume of (Q.S.) 100 mL

- ALIMTA is compatible with standard PVC parenteral product containers and administration sets
- PEMEtrexed disodium is chemically and physically stable after reconstitution (25 mg/mL) and dilution in preservative-free 0.9% NS (to a volume of Q.S. 100 mL) for up to 24 hours after initial reconstitution, when stored under refrigeration at 2–8°C (36–46°F),[63] or ambient room temperatures and lighting
- ALIMTA does not contain antimicrobial preservatives. Discard any unused portion

Selected incompatibility:
- ALIMTA is physically incompatible with solutions containing calcium, including Ringer injection, USP, and lactated Ringer injection, USP
- Coadministration of PEMEtrexed with other drugs and diluents has not been studied, and, therefore, is not recommended

Recommendations for Drug Administration and Ancillary Care

General:
- See Chapter 43 for recommended use in patients with renal dysfunction
- Administer PEMEtrexed intraVENously over 10 minutes

Supportive ancillary care:
- To reduce treatment-related hematologic and gastrointestinal toxicities, patients treated with PEMEtrexed should take folic acid 400–1000 μg orally daily beginning 7 days prior to the first dose of PEMEtrexed and continuing throughout treatment and for 21 days after the last dose of PEMEtrexed
- Give 1 intraMUSCular injection of vitamin B$_{12}$ (cyanocobalamin) 1000 μg 1 week before the first dose of PEMEtrexed and every 3 cycles thereafter (ie, approximately every 9 weeks). Repeated vitamin B$_{12}$

injections may be given the same day as PEMEtrexed
- Do not substitute orally administered vitamin B$_{12}$ for a vitamin B$_{12}$ product administered intraMUSCularly
- Primary prophylaxis with dexamethasone (or an equivalent glucocorticoid) reduces the incidence and severity of cutaneous reactions in patients treated with PEMEtrexed. In clinical trials, dexamethasone 4 mg orally was given twice daily for 3 consecutive days: the day before, the day of, and the day after PEMEtrexed administration

Selected potential drug interactions:
Nonsteroidal anti-inflammatory drugs (NSAIDs)
- Ibuprofen 400 mg administered 4 times daily decreases PEMEtrexed clearance by approximately 20% (and increases

AUC by 20%) in patients with normal renal function. The effect of greater doses of ibuprofen on PEMEtrexed pharmacokinetics is unknown
- In patients with creatinine clearances between 45 mL/min and 79 mL/min who are also taking ibuprofen, avoid administration of ibuprofen for 2 days before, the day of, and for 2 days after PEMEtrexed administration. If ibuprofen administration cannot be avoided, then monitor more closely for PEMEtrexed adverse effects including myelosuppression, renal toxicity, and gastrointestinal toxicity.

Competition for organic anion transporter 3
- In vitro studies indicate that PEMEtrexed is a substrate of organic anion transporter 3 (OAT3), which may play a role in active secretion of PEMEtrexed

PENTOSTATIN

NIPENT (pentostatin for injection) prescribing information. Lake Forest, IL: Hospira, Inc.; October 2019

WARNING

NIPENT should be administered under the supervision of a physician qualified and experienced in the use of cancer chemotherapeutic agents. The use of higher doses than those specified ... is not recommended. Dose-limiting severe renal, liver, pulmonary, and CNS toxicities occurred in Phase 1 studies that used NIPENT at higher doses (20–50 mg/m² in divided doses over 5 days) than recommended

In a clinical investigation in patients with refractory chronic lymphocytic leukemia using NIPENT at the recommended dose in combination with fludarabine phosphate, 4 of 6 patients entered in the study had severe or fatal pulmonary toxicity. The use of NIPENT in combination with fludarabine phosphate is not recommended

Boxed Warning for NIPENT (pentostatin for injection) prescribing information. Lake Forest, IL: Hospira, Inc.; October 2019

Product Identification, Preparation, Storage, and Stability

- Pentostatin for injection is available in individually packaged single-dose vials containing 10 mg of pentostatin (NDC 0409-0801-01) as a sterile, apyrogenic, lyophilized, white to off-white powder with mannitol, USP, 50 mg. The pH of the final product is maintained within the range 7.0–8.5 by addition of sodium hydroxide or hydrochloric acid
- Store intact vials under refrigeration at 2–8°C (36–46°F)
- Reconstitute pentostatin with 5 mL of SWFI to obtain a solution

with concentration equal to 2 mg pentostatin/mL
- After reconstitution, pentostatin solution is suitable for direct intraVENous injection, or it may be diluted in 25–50 mL of D5W or 0.9% NS to concentrations within the range 0.18–0.33 mg/mL. Pentostatin does not interact with PVC parenteral product containers or administration sets
- Pentostatin in intact vials is stable when stored under refrigeration at 2–8°C (36–46°F) until the expiration date on package labeling

- After reconstitution (2 mg/mL) with or without further dilution (0.18–0.33 mg/mL) and storage at room temperature under ambient light, pentostatin manufacturers recommend using the product within 8 hours, as it does not contain antimicrobial preservatives
- Spills and wastes should be treated with a 5% sodium hypochlorite solution prior to disposal

---

Recommendations for Drug Administration and Ancillary Care

General:

- See Chapter 43 for recommended use in patients with renal dysfunction
- Administer pentostatin intraVENously by rapid injection over 5 minutes, or by infusion over 20–30 minutes
- Give intraVENous hydration with D5W/0.45% NS, 500–1000 mL before pentostatin administration plus 500 mL of D5W after pentostatin is given

Selected potential drug interactions:

- Pentostatin has been shown to enhance the effects of vidarabine, a purine nucleoside with antiviral activity. The combined use of vidarabine and pentostatin may result in an increase in adverse reactions associated with each drug
- The combined use of pentostatin and fludarabine phosphate is not recommended because it may be associated with an increased risk of fatal pulmonary toxicity

- Acute pulmonary edema and hypotension, leading to death, have been reported in patients treated with pentostatin in combination with carmustine, etoposide, and high-dose cyclophosphamide as part of a conditioning regimen prior to hematopoietic stem cell transplantation

Inadvertent release:

- Spills and wastes should be treated with a 5% sodium hypochlorite solution prior to disposal

PERTUZUMAB

PERJETA (pertuzumab) prescribing information. South San Francisco, CA: Genentech, Inc.; August 2020

WARNING: LEFT VENTRICULAR DYSFUNCTION and EMBRYO-FETAL TOXICITY

- **Left Ventricular Dysfunction:** PERJETA can result in subclinical and clinical cardiac failure manifesting as decreased LVEF and CHF. Evaluate cardiac function prior to and during treatment. Discontinue PERJETA treatment for a confirmed clinically significant decrease in left ventricular function …

- **Embryo-fetal Toxicity:** Exposure to PERJETA can result in embryo-fetal death and birth defects. Advise patients of these risks and the need for effective contraception …

PERJETA (pertuzumab) prescribing information. South San Francisco, CA: Genentech, Inc.; August 2020

Product Identification, Preparation, Storage, and Stability

- PERJETA is supplied in single-use vials containing a sterile, clear to slightly opalescent, colorless to pale brown, preservative-free solution of pertuzumab 420 mg/14 mL (30 mg/mL) with 20 mmol/L L-histidine acetate (pH 6.0), 120 mmol/L sucrose, and 0.02% polysorbate 20 (NDC 50242-145-01)

- Store vials under refrigeration at 2–8°C (36–46°F) until time of use in their outer packaging carton to protect pertuzumab from light. *Do not freeze* pertuzumab. *Do not shake* vials containing pertuzumab

- Preparation for clinical use:

  - Transfer to a PVC or non-PVC polyolefin parenteral product container containing 250 mL of 0.9% NS a volume of pertuzumab appropriate for a patient's dose

  - *Do not use* dextrose solutions to dilute pertuzumab

  - Mix the diluted solution by gentle inversion. *Do not shake* the admixture

- If pertuzumab solution is not used immediately after dilution, it can be stored under refrigeration (2–8°C) for up to 24 hours

- Do not mix pertuzumab with other drugs

Recommendations for Drug Administration and Supportive Care

HER2 testing is prerequisite to using pertuzumab:

- Detection of HER2 protein overexpression or HER2 gene amplification in tumor specimens is necessary in selecting patients for whom pertuzumab therapy is appropriate, because these are the only patients studied and for whom benefit has been shown

- HER2 status should be assessed by laboratories with demonstrated proficiency in the specific technology being utilized to avoid unreliable results

- Improper assay performance, including use of suboptimally fixed tissue, failure to utilize specified reagents, deviation from specific assay instructions, and failure to include appropriate controls for assay validation can lead to unreliable results

General:

- Pertuzumab is administered intraVENously every 3 weeks

- Dose for initial treatment, and if the interval between 2 consecutive pertuzumab doses is ≥6 weeks:

  - Pertuzumab 840 mg administered intraVENously over 60 minutes

- Dose for repeated treatments, and if the interval between consecutive pertuzumab doses is <6 weeks:

  - Pertuzumab 420 mg administered intraVENously over 30–60 minutes every 3 weeks

- Refer to the current FDA-approved prescribing information for detailed recommendations regarding sequence of medication administration, monitoring and management of infusion-related reactions and hypersensitivity reactions, monitoring of left ventricular ejection fraction, and treatment modifications for left ventricular dysfunction

PERTUZUMAB, TRASTUZUMAB, AND HYALURONIDASE-zzxf

PHESGO (pertuzumab, trastuzumab, and hyaluronidase-zzxf) prescribing information. South San Francisco, CA: Genentech, Inc.; June 2020

WARNING: CARDIOMYOPATHY, EMBRYO-FETAL TOXICITY, and PULMONARY TOXICITY

Cardiomyopathy
PHESGO administration can result in subclinical and clinical cardiac failure. The incidence and severity was highest in patients receiving PHESGO with anthracycline-containing chemotherapy regimens. Evaluate cardiac function prior to and during treatment with PHESGO. Discontinue PHESGO treatment in patients receiving adjuvant therapy and withhold PHESGO in patients with metastatic disease for clinically significant decrease in left ventricular function …

Embryo-Fetal Toxicity
Exposure to PHESGO can result in embryo-fetal death and birth defects, including oligohydramnios and oligohydramnios sequence manifesting as pulmonary hypoplasia, skeletal abnormalities, and neonatal death. Advise patients of these risks and the need for effective contraception …

Pulmonary Toxicity
PHESGO administration can result in serious and fatal pulmonary toxicity. Discontinue PHESGO for anaphylaxis, angioedema, interstitial pneumonitis, or acute respiratory distress syndrome. Monitor patients until symptoms completely resolve …

Boxed Warning for PHESGO (pertuzumab, trastuzumab, and hyaluronidase-zzxf) prescribing information. South San Francisco, CA: Genentech, Inc.; June 2020

Product Identification, Preparation, Storage, and Stability

- PHESGO is for SUBCUTaneous use only in the thigh; do not administer intraVENously. PHESGO has different dosage and administration instructions than intraVENous pertuzumab, intraVENous trastuzumab, and SUBCUTaneous trastuzumab when administered alone. Do not substitute PHESGO for or with pertuzumab, trastuzumab, ado-trastuzumab emtansine, or fam-trastuzumab deruxtecan

- PHESGO (pertuzumab, trastuzumab, and hyaluronidase-zzxf) is a combination of pertuzumab, trastuzumab, and hyaluronidase. Pertuzumab is a humanized monoclonal antibody directed against the extracellular dimerization domain of HER2. Trastuzumab is a humanized IgG1 kappa monoclonal antibody directed against the extracellular domain of HER2. Recombinant human hyaluronidase is an endoglycosidase used to increase the dispersion and absorption of co-administered drugs when administered SUBCUTaneously

- PHESGO (pertuzumab, trastuzumab, and hyaluronidase-zzxf) is available in individually packaged single-dose vials containing a sterile, colorless to slightly brownish, clear to opalescent, preservative-free, ready-to-use solution in the following presentations:

  - PHESGO (pertuzumab, trastuzumab, and hyaluronidase-zzxf): pertuzumab (1200 mg), trastuzumab (600 mg), hyaluronidase (30,000 units), α,α-trehalose (397 mg), L-histidine (6.75 mg), L-histidine hydrochloric monohydrate (53.7 mg), L-methionine (22.4 mg), polysorbate 20 (6 mg), and sucrose (685 mg) in 15 mL with a pH of 5.5 (NDC 50242-245-01). Each milliliter contains 80 mg pertuzumab, 40 mg trastuzumab, and 2000 units hyaluronidase

  - PHESGO (pertuzumab, trastuzumab, and hyaluronidase-zzxf): pertuzumab (600 mg), trastuzumab (600 mg), hyaluronidase (20,000 units), α,α-trehalose (397 mg), L-histidine (4.4 mg), L-histidine hydrochloric monohydrate (36.1 mg), L-methionine (14.9 mg), polysorbate 20 (4 mg), and sucrose (342 mg) in 10 mL with a pH of 5.5 (NDC 50242-260-01). Each milliliter contains 60 mg pertuzumab, 60 mg trastuzumab, and 2000 units hyaluronidase

- Store intact vials under refrigeration at 2–8°C (36–46°F) in the original carton to protect from light. Do not freeze or shake

Recommendations for Drug Administration and Ancillary Care

General:

- The usual initial "loading" dose of PHESGO (pertuzumab, trastuzumab, and hyaluronidase-zzxf) is 1200 mg/600 mg/30,000 units (1200 mg pertuzumab, 600 mg trastuzumab, and 30,000 units hyaluronidase) in 15 mL administered SUBCUTaneously into the thigh over approximately 8 minutes
- The usual initial "maintenance" dose of PHESGO (pertuzumab, trastuzumab, and hyaluronidase-zzxf) is 600 mg/600 mg/20,000 units (600 mg pertuzumab, 600 mg trastuzumab, and 20,000 units hyaluronidase) in 10 mL administered SUBCUTaneously into the thigh over approximately 5 minutes every 3 weeks
- No adjustment in the doses are required for patient body weight or concomitant chemotherapy regimen. Refer to the current FDA-approved product label for details regarding duration of use based on the indication
- When transitioning from intraVENous pertuzumab and trastuzumab, if <6 weeks have elapsed since the last intraVENous dose, administer the PHESGO (pertuzumab, trastuzumab, and hyaluronidase-zzxf) maintenance dose. If ≥6 weeks have elapsed, then begin with the loading dose
- When used in combination with an anthracycline-based regimen for early breast cancer, pertuzumab, trastuzumab, and hyaluronidase-zzxf should be initiated only after completion of anthracycline
- When used in combination with docetaxel or paclitaxel, administer the pertuzumab, trastuzumab, and hyaluronidase-zzxf first, followed by the taxane

Preparation:

- To prevent medication errors, it is important to check the vial labels to ensure that the drug being prepared and administered is PHESGO (pertuzumab, trastuzumab, and hyaluronidase-zzxf) and not intraVENous pertuzumab,

or intraVENous trastuzumab, or SUBCUTaneous trastuzumab

- PHESGO (pertuzumab, trastuzumab, and hyaluronidase-zzxf) is supplied as a ready-to-use product that requires no reconstitution or further dilution
- Visually inspect the contents of the vial for particulate matter or discoloration
- Using a sterile syringe [composed of polypropylene (PP), polycarbonate, polyethylene, polyurethane, PVC, or fluorinated ethylene PP] and a stainless-steel transfer needle, withdraw the required volume of solution from the appropriate vial (depending upon whether preparing a loading dose or maintenance dose)
- Replace the transfer needle with a syringe closing cap. Label the syringe according to institutional standards and with a peel-off label
- Once PHESGO (pertuzumab, trastuzumab, and hyaluronidase-zzxf) has been withdrawn from its original vial, it should be used immediately. If not used immediately, it may be stored for up to 24 hours under refrigeration at 2–8°C (36°F–46°F) or for up to 4 hours at room temperature 20–25°C (68°F–77°F)

Administration:

- PHESGO (pertuzumab, trastuzumab, and hyaluronidase-zzxf) must be administered by a health care professional. Ensure that medications and emergency equipment to manage systemic hypersensitivity reactions are immediately available
- Attach the hypodermic stainless-steel injection needle (3/8–5/8' 25G–27G) immediately prior to SUBCUTaneous administration to prevent needle clogging followed by volume adjustment, if necessary
- Inject PHESGO (pertuzumab, trastuzumab, and hyaluronidase-zzxf) SUBCUTaneously into the thigh. The dose is administered over 8 minutes (loading dose) or 5 minutes (maintenance doses). Alternate between the left and right thigh only and choose a site at least 1 inch (2.5 cm) from the prior injection site. Do not

split the dose between two syringes or two sites of administration. Never inject into areas where the skin is red, bruised, tender, or hard. Do not administer other medications for SUBCUTaneous use at the same sites

Concomitant medications:

Pre-Administration Medications:

- Use of premedications is not necessary for primary prophylaxis of administration-related systemic reactions. Consider implementation of secondary prophylaxis in patients who have experienced a prior reversible G1/2 reaction with an analgesic, antipyretic, or antihistamine

Adverse events and treatment modifications:

- Refer to the current FDA-approved product label for detailed warnings and treatment modifications for delayed/missed doses, cardiomyopathy, pulmonary toxicity, and hypersensitivity/administration-related reactions. No dose reductions are recommended
- Advise patients that severe administration-related reactions may occur. In the FeDeriCa study, the incidence of hypersensitivity and administration-related reactions was 1.2% and 21%, respectively. The most common administration-related reactions were injection-site reaction and injection-site pain
- Observe patients for signs and symptoms of hypersensitivity or administration-related reactions for at least 30 minutes after the initial dose and for at least 15 minutes after each maintenance dose

Potential drug interactions:

When feasible, avoid anthracycline-based therapy for up to 7 months after stopping PHESGO (pertuzumab, trastuzumab, and hyaluronidase-zzxf) due to a higher risk of cardiotoxicity. If anthracyclines are used, carefully monitor the patient's cardiac function

POLATUZUMAB VEDOTIN-piiq

POLIVY (polatuzumab vedotin-piiq) prescribing information. South San Francisco, CA: Genentech, Inc.; June 2019

Product Identification, Preparation, Storage, and Stability

- Polatuzumab vedotin-piiq contains the humanized immunoglobulin G1 (IgG1) monoclonal antibody specific for human CD79b covalently linked to the small molecule anti-mitotic agent monomethyl auristatin E (MMAE) via a protease-cleavable linker maleimidocaproyl-valine-citrulline-p-aminobenzyloxycarbonyl (mc-vc-PAB)
- POLIVY (polatuzumab vedotin-piiq for injection) is a sterile, white to grayish-white, preservative-free, lyophilized powder that has a cake-like appearance in individually boxed single-dose vials (NDC 50242-105-01) that contain polatuzumab vedotin-piiq (140 mg), polysorbate-20 (8.4 mg), sodium hydroxide (3.80 mg), succinic acid (8.27 mg), and sucrose (288 mg). The pH of the reconstituted solution is 5.3
- Store intact vials under refrigeration at 2–8°C (36–46°F) until time of reconstitution
- Do not freeze or shake intact vials

Reconstitution:
- Calculate the dose, total volume of reconstituted solution needed, and number of vials of polatuzumab vedotin-piiq. Reconstitute immediately prior to dilution
- Using a sterile syringe, slowly inject 7.2 mL of SWFI diluent into the vial containing polatuzumab vedotin-piiq directed toward the wall of the vial. Swirl until completely dissolved. Do not shake. Inspect for particulate and discoloration prior to dilution
- The reconstituted vial contains 20 mg/mL polatuzumab vedotin-piiq
- Store at 2–8°C (36–46°F) for up to 48 hours or at 9–25°C (47–77°F) up to a maximum of 8 hours prior to dilution. Discard when cumulative storage time prior to dilution exceeds 48 hours
- Do not freeze or expose to direct sunlight

Dilution:
- Dilute polatuzumab vedotin-piiq to a final concentration of 0.72–2.7 mg/mL in an intraVENous infusion bag containing 50 mL of 0.9% NS, 0.45% NaCl or D5W
- Gently mix by slowly inverting the bag. Do not shake. Inspect for particulates and discard if present. Do not freeze or expose to direct sunlight
- Store diluted polatuzumab vedotin-piiq as below in the table:

Diluent Used	Diluted Polatuzumab Vedotin-piiq Solution Storage Conditions
0.9% NS	Up to 24 hours at 2–8°C (35–46°F) or up to 4 hours at 9–25°C (47–77°F)
0.45% NaCl	Up to 18 hours at 2–8°C (35–46°F) or up to 4 hours at 9–25°C (47–77°F)
D5W	Up to 36 hours at 2–8°C (35–46°F) or up to 6 hours at 9–25°C (47–77°F)

- Limit transportation to 30 minutes at 9°C to 25°C or 12 hours at 2°C to 8°C. The total storage plus transportation times of the diluted product should not exceed the storage duration specified above in the table
- Agitation stress can result in aggregation of the product. Limit agitation of diluted product during preparation and transportation to the site of administration. Do not use automated systems for transportation such as pneumatic tube systems or automated carts. If the prepared solution must be transported to a separate facility, then remove air from the infusion bag to prevent aggregation. If air is removed, an infusion set with a vented spike is required to ensure accurate dosing during the infusion

Recommendations for Drug Administration and Ancillary Care

General:

- See Chapter 43 for recommended use in patients with hepatic dysfunction
- There are insufficient data to recommend a dose of polatuzumab vedotin-piiq in patients with CrCl <30 mL/min or with end-stage renal disease with or without dialysis
- There are insufficient data to recommend a dose of polatuzumab vedotin-piiq in patients with AST or ALT >2.5 × ULN or total bilirubin >1.5 × ULN or liver transplantation

Administration:

- The recommended dose of polatuzumab vedotin-piiq is 1.8 mg/kg administered intraVENously over 90 minutes every 21 days for 6 cycles in combination with bendamustine and a riTUXimab product
- If a planned dose is missed, administer as soon as possible and then adjust the schedule of administration to maintain a 21-day interval between doses
- Administer using a dedicated infusion line equipped with a sterile, non-pyrogenic, low-protein-binding, inline or add-on filter (0.2- or 0.22-μm pore size) and a catheter
- Administer the first infusion over 90 minutes. Observe for infusion reactions for a minimum of 90 minutes after completion of the infusion. If well tolerated, subsequent infusions may be administered over 30 minutes. Observe for infusion reactions for a minimum of 30 minutes after completion of the infusion

Concomitant medications:

- If not already administered, administer an antihistamine (eg, diphenhydrAMINE) and antipyretic (eg, acetaminophen) at least 30 minutes prior to polatuzumab vedotin-piiq
- Administer prophylaxis for *Pneumocystis jiroveci pneumonia (PJP)* and herpes-virus throughout treatment with polatuzumab vedotin-piiq
- Consider prophylactic granulocyte colony stimulating factor administration for neutropenia

Adverse events and treatment modifications:

- Refer to the current FDA-approved product label for detailed recommendations regarding treatment modifications for infusion-related reactions, G ≥2 peripheral neuropathy, G ≥3 neutropenia, or G ≥3 thrombocytopenia
- Polatuzumab vedotin-piiq can cause infusion-related reactions. These can be delayed as late as 24 hours afterwards. With premedication, 7% of patients (12/173) in Study GO29365 reported infusion-related reactions. The reactions were Grade 1 in 67%, Grade 2 in 25%, and Grade 3 in 8%. Symptoms included fever, chills, flushing, dyspnea, hypotension, and urticaria
- Monitor for infusion-related reactions during the infusion and for at least 90 minutes after completion of the first dose. If the previous infusion was well tolerated, monitoring following completion of the subsequent dose may be reduced to 30 minutes
- If an infusion-related reaction occurs, interrupt the infusion and institute the appropriate medical management. Refer to the current FDA-approved product label for guidance on resuming or discontinuing polatuzumab vedotin-piiq infusion after an infusion-related reaction

Potential drug interactions:

- Concomitant use with CYP3A inhibitors may increase unconjugated MMAE AUC and concomitant use with CYP3A inducers may decrease unconjugated MMAE

Selected precautions:

- Monitor for peripheral neuropathy. Neuropathy is primarily sensory but can be motor and sensorimotor. Monitor for symptoms of peripheral neuropathy such as hypoesthesia, hyperesthesia, paresthesia, dysesthesia, neuropathic pain, burning sensation, weakness, or gait disturbance. New or worsening peripheral neuropathy may require a delay, dose reduction, or discontinuation of polatuzumab vedotin-piiq
- In patients at high risk for tumor lysis syndrome (eg, high tumor burden, renal dysfunction, rapidly progressing disease, markedly elevated LDH, baseline abnormalities in laboratory indices of tumor lysis syndrome [potassium, phosphate, uric acid, calcium, serum creatinine]), consider frequent monitoring of laboratory indices of tumor lysis syndrome, intraVENous hydration, and prophylaxis with a xanthine oxidase inhibitor (eg, allopurinol) during the first cycle
- Serious and fatal infections can occur in patients treated with polatuzumab vedotin-piiq. Closely monitor for signs and symptoms of infections
- Myelosuppression and hepatotoxicity can occur with polatuzumab vedotin-piiq. Closely monitor complete blood counts, liver enzymes and bilirubin

PRALATREXATE

FOLOTYN (pralatrexate injection) prescribing information. East Windsor, NJ: Acrotech Biopharma LLC; September 2020

Product Identification, Preparation, Storage, and Stability

- FOLOTYN is available in individually packaged, single-use, clear, glass, vials (type I) containing a preservative-free, sterile, isotonic, nonpyrogenic, clear, yellow, aqueous solution of PRALAtrexate 20 mg in 1 mL (NDC 72893-003-01) *or* 40 mg in 2 mL (NDC 72893-005-01)
- Each milliliter of solution contains (racemic) PRALAtrexate 20 mg, sufficient

sodium chloride to produce an isotonic solution (280–300 mOsm), and sufficient sodium hydroxide and hydrochloric acid to adjust and maintain solution pH within the range of 7.5–8.5
- The commercially marketed product does not contain antimicrobial preservatives: used vials including any unused drug should be discarded after withdrawing a dose

- Store intact vials of FOLOTYN under refrigeration at 2–8°C (36–46°F) in the original packaging carton to protect the drug product from light
- Aseptically withdraw the calculated dose from the appropriate number of vial(s) into a syringe for immediate use. Do not dilute FOLOTYN

Recommendations for Drug Administration and Supportive Care

General:

- See Chapter 43 for recommendations for use in patients with renal and hepatic dysfunction
- Undiluted PRALAtrexate 30 mg/m^2 per dose is administered by intraVENous injection over 3–5 minutes into a freely flowing solution of 0.9% NS once weekly for 6 consecutive weeks in 7-week cycles
- Before administering any dose of PRALAtrexate:
  - Mucositis if present should be G ≤1
  - Platelet count should be ≥100,000/mm^3 for first dose and ≥50,000/mm^3 for all subsequent doses
  - ANC should be ≥1000/mm^3
- Omitted doses will not be made up at the end of a treatment cycle
- If PRALAtrexate dosage is decreased for toxicities, do not re-escalate dosage during subsequent treatments
- Refer to the current FDA-approved prescribing information for detailed recommendations regarding treatment modifications for mucositis, thrombocytopenia, neutropenia, and other adverse reactions

Supportive care:

- Patients should receive folic acid 1–1.25 mg/day orally starting 10 days

before first receiving PRALAtrexate, and continue use for 30 days after their last dose of PRALAtrexate
- Patients should receive cyanocobalamin (vitamin B$_{12}$) 1000 µg by intraMUSCular injection within 10 weeks before they first receive PRALAtrexate. Doses should be repeated every 8–10 weeks thereafter
  - Repeated cyanocobalamin injections may be given on the same day when PRALAtrexate is given
  - Folic acid and cyanocobalamin supplementation potentially mitigate against treatment-related hematologic toxicity and mucositis

Potential drug interactions:

- Coadministration of increasing doses of probenecid resulted in delayed PRALAtrexate clearance and a commensurate increase in exposure
- In vitro studies using human hepatocytes, liver microsomes, S9 fractions, and recombinant human CYP enzymes showed PRALAtrexate is not significantly metabolized by CYP enzymes or phase II hepatic glucuronidases
- In vitro studies indicated that PRALAtrexate does not induce or inhibit the activity of CYP enzymes at clinically achievable concentrations

- In vitro, PRALAtrexate is a substrate for the breast cancer resistance protein (BCRP, ABCG2), MRP2 (ABCC2), multidrug resistance associated protein 3 (MRP3, ABCC3), and organic anion transport protein (OATP) OATP1B3 transporter systems at concentrations of PRALAtrexate that can be reasonably expected clinically
- PRALAtrexate is not a substrate for the P-glycoprotein (P-gp, ABCB1), OATP1B1, organic cation transporter 2 (OCT2), organic anion transporter (OAT) OAT1, and OAT3 transporter systems
- In vitro, PRALAtrexate inhibits MRP2 and MRP3 transporter systems at PRALAtrexate concentrations that can be reasonably expected clinically
  - MRP3 is a transport protein that may affect the transport of etoposide and teniposide
- In vitro, PRALAtrexate did not significantly inhibit the P-gp, BCRP, OCT2, OAT1, OAT3, OATP1B1, and OATP1B3 transporter systems at PRALAtrexate concentrations that can be reasonably expected clinically

RAMUCIRUMAB

CYRAMZA (ramucirumab) prescribing information. Indianapolis, IN: Eli Lilly and Company; July 2020

Product Identification, Preparation, Storage, and Stability

- CYRAMZA is a sterile, clear to slightly opalescent and colorless to slightly yellow, preservative-free solution in individually boxed single-dose vials that contain either ramucirumab 100 mg/10 mL (NDC 0002-7669-01) or ramucirumab 500 mg/50 mL(NDC 0002-7678-01). CYRAMZA is formulated in glycine (9.98 mg/mL), histidine (0.65 mg/mL), histidine monohydrochloride (1.22 mg/mL), polysorbate 80 (0.1 mg/mL), sodium chloride (4.383 mg/mL), and SWFI. The pH of the solution is 6.0

- Store intact vials under refrigeration at 2–8°C (35–46°F) in the original carton to protect from light until time of use
- Do not freeze or shake intact vials

Dilution:
- Visually inspect for particulate matter and discoloration prior to dilution
- Calculate the dose and required volume of ramucirumab
- Withdraw the required volume of ramucirumab and further dilute only with 0.9% NS in an intraVENous infusion container to a final volume of 250 mL

- Do not shake. Gently invert the container to ensure adequate mixing
- Do not freeze. Store diluted solution for no more than 24 hours refrigerated at 2–8°C (36–46°F) or 4 hours at ambient temperature below 25°C (77°F)

Selected incompatibility:
- Do not mix ramucirumab with dextrose-containing solutions
- Do not co-infuse with other electrolytes or medications

Recommendations for Drug Administration and Ancillary Care

General:
- No dose adjustment is recommended for patients with mild hepatic impairment (total bilirubin within ULN and AST > ULN or total bilirubin 1 to 1.5 times ULN and any AST)
- No dose adjustment is recommended for patients with moderate hepatic impairment (total bilirubin >1.5 to 3 × ULN and any AST)
- Note that clinical deterioration was reported in patients with Child-Pugh B or C cirrhosis who received single-agent ramucirumab. The effect of severe hepatic impairment (total bilirubin >3 × ULN and any AST) is unknown
- Renal impairment (CrCl 15–89 mL/min as calculated by Cockcroft-Gault) had no meaningful effect on the PK of ramucirumab

Administration:
- The recommended dose of ramucirumab is 8 mg/kg every 2 weeks or 10 mg/kg every 2 to 3 weeks. Refer to the current FDA-approved label for specific indications and regimens. Ramucirumab may be used as a single agent or in combination regimens
- Administer diluted ramucirumab solution via infusion pump through a separate infusion line. Use of a protein-sparing 0.22-μm filter is recommended
- Administer the first infusion intraVENously over 60 minutes. If

first infusion is tolerated, all subsequent infusions may be given over 30 minutes
- Flush the line with sterile 0.9% NS at the end of the infusion

Concomitant medications:
- Prior to each ramucirumab infusion premedicate with an intraVENous histamine-1 antagonist (eg, diphenhydrAMINE)
- If patient experiences G1 or G2 infusion-related reaction, premedicate with a histamine-1 receptor antagonist, dexamethasone (or equivalent), and acetaminophen prior to each ramucirumab infusion

Adverse events and treatment modifications:
- Refer to the current FDA-approved product label for detailed recommendations regarding treatment modifications for hypertension, proteinuria, G ≥3 hemorrhage, or any grade gastrointestinal perforation, wound healing complications, or arterial thrombotic events graded according to the NCI CTCAE v 4.0
- Monitor proteinuria by urine dipstick and/or urine protein creatinine ratio. If the result of the urine dipstick is ≥2+, perform a 24-hour urine collection for protein measurement. Refer to the current FDA-approved package label for detailed guidance on proteinuria

- Infusion-related reactions (IRR) can be severe and life-threatening with ramucirumab. The majority of IRR occurred during or following a first or second ramucirumab infusion. Symptoms of IRR included rigors/tremors, back pain/spasms, chest pain and/or tightness, chills, flushing, dyspnea, wheezing, hypoxia, and paresthesia. In severe cases, symptoms included bronchospasm, supraventricular tachycardia, and hypotension. Incidence of all-grade IRR ranged from <1–9% in trials that recommended or required premedication. IRR G ≥3 incidence was <1%
  - Monitor patients during the infusion for signs and symptoms of an IRR in a setting with available resuscitation equipment
  - For G1 or G2 infusion-related reactions, reduce the infusion rate of ramucirumab by 50%. For G ≥3 infusion-related reactions, permanently discontinue ramucirumab

Selected precautions:
- Ramucirumab can cause serious adverse events including hemorrhage, gastrointestinal perforations, impaired wound healing, and arterial thrombotic events. Refer to the current FDA-approved label for detailed information
- Control hypertension prior to initiating treatment with ramucirumab and monitor at least every 2 weeks during treatment

RASBURICASE

ELITEK (rasburicase) prescribing information. Bridgewater, NJ: Sanofi-Aventis U.S. LLC; December 2019

WARNING: HYPERSENSITIVITY REACTIONS, HEMOLYSIS, METHEMOGLOBINEMIA, and INTERFERENCE WITH URIC ACID MEASUREMENTS

Hypersensitivity Reactions

Elitek can cause serious and fatal hypersensitivity reactions including anaphylaxis. Immediately and permanently discontinue Elitek in patients who experience a serious hypersensitivity reaction ...

Hemolysis

Do not administer Elitek to patients with glucose-6-phosphate dehydrogenase (G6PD) deficiency. Immediately and permanently discontinue Elitek in patients developing hemolysis. Screen patients at higher risk for G6PD deficiency (eg, patients of African or Mediterranean ancestry) prior to starting Elitek ...

Methemoglobinemia

Elitek can result in methemoglobinemia in some patients. Immediately and permanently discontinue Elitek in patients developing methemoglobinemia ...

Interference with Uric Acid Measurements

Elitek enzymatically degrades uric acid in blood samples left at room temperature. Collect blood samples in prechilled tubes containing heparin and immediately immerse and maintain sample in an ice water bath. Assay plasma samples within 4 hours of collection ...

Boxed Warning for ELITEK (rasburicase) prescribing information. Bridgewater, NJ: Sanofi-Aventis U.S. LLC; December 2019

Product Identification, Preparation, Storage, and Stability

- ELITEK is available in 2 presentations, including:
  - Cartons containing 3 single-use, 3-mL, colorless, glass vials, each containing rasburicase 1.5 mg *plus* 3 ampules each containing 1 mL diluent (NDC 0024-5150-10)
  - Individually packaged, single-use, 10-mL, colorless, glass vials containing rasburicase 7.5 mg *plus* 1 ampule containing 5 mL diluent (0024-5151-75)
- ELITEK is formulated as a sterile, white to off-white, lyophilized powder containing:

Rasburicase Content	Excipients	
	Rasburicase Vials	**Diluent Ampules**
1.5 mg	10.6 mg mannitol, 15.9 mg L-alanine, between 12.6 and 14.3 mg of dibasic sodium phosphate (lyophilized powder)	1 mL of SWFI and 1 mg poloxamer 188
7.5 mg	53 mg mannitol, 79.5 mg L-alanine, and between 63 and 71.5 mg dibasic sodium phosphate (lyophilized powder)	5 mL of SWFI and 5 mg poloxamer 188

- Store the copackaged drug product and diluent for reconstitution at 2–8°C (36–46°F) protected from light. *Do not freeze* rasburicase
- Reconstitute rasburicase as follows:

Rasburicase Content per Vial	Diluent Volume	Rasburicase Concentration After Reconstitution
1.5 mg	1 mL	1.5 mg/mL
7.5 mg	5 mL	

- Dissolve and mix rasburicase by gently swirling vials. *Do not shake* or vortex vials
- Inject a volume of reconstituted rasburicase (1.5 mg/mL) appropriate for a patient's dose into a volume of 0.9% NS sufficient to produce a total volume of (Q.S.) 50 mL
- Store reconstituted and diluted rasburicase solutions at 2–8°C
- Discard unused rasburicase solutions within 24 hours after reconstitution

Recommendations for Drug Administration and Ancillary Care

General:

- Rasburicase is administered intraVENously over 30 minutes, and may be given daily for up to 5 days
- Dosing for periods >5 days or administration of >1 course of treatment are not recommended
- Administer rasburicase through a separate line or flush line with at least 15 mL of 0.9% NS before starting and after completing rasburicase administration
- Do not filter rasburicase during administration
- Discard unused rasburicase solutions within 24 hours after reconstitution

Uric acid sample handling procedure:

- At room temperature, rasburicase causes enzymatic degradation of uric acid in blood, plasma, and serum samples potentially resulting in spuriously low plasma uric acid assay readings
  - The following special sample handling procedure must be followed to avoid ex vivo uric acid degradation:
1. Uric acid must be analyzed in plasma. Blood must be collected into prechilled tubes containing heparin anticoagulant
2. Immediately after collecting samples for uric acid measurement, immerse samples in an ice water bath
3. Plasma samples must be prepared by centrifugation in a precooled centrifuge (4°C [39.2°F])
4. Plasma must be maintained in an ice water bath and analyzed for uric acid within 4 hours after collection

Contraindication:

- Rasburicase is contraindicated in patients with G6PD deficiency because hydrogen peroxide is one of the major by-products of the conversion of uric acid to allantoin
- Immediately and permanently discontinue rasburicase administration in any patient who develops hemolysis
  - Institute appropriate patient monitoring and support measures (eg, transfusion support)
- Screen patients at high risk for G6PD deficiency (eg, patients of African or Mediterranean ancestry) before administering rasburicase
- Rasburicase is contraindicated in patients with a history of anaphylaxis or severe hypersensitivity to rasburicase or in patients with development of hemolytic reactions or methemoglobinemia with rasburicase

RITUXIMAB

Rituxan (rituximab) prescribing information. South San Francisco, CA: Genentech, Inc.; August 2020

WARNING: FATAL INFUSION-RELATED REACTIONS, SEVERE MUCOCUTANEOUS REACTIONS, HEPATITIS B VIRUS REACTIVATION and PROGRESSIVE MULTIFOCAL LEUKOENCEPHALOPATHY

Infusion-Related Reactions

RITUXAN administration can result in serious, including fatal, infusion-related reactions. Deaths within 24 hours of RITUXAN infusion have occurred. Approximately 80% of fatal infusion reactions occurred in association with the first infusion. Monitor patients closely. Discontinue RITUXAN infusion for severe reactions and provide medical treatment for Grade 3 or 4 infusion-related reactions …

Severe Mucocutaneous Reactions

Severe, including fatal, mucocutaneous reactions can occur in patients receiving Rituxan …

Hepatitis B Virus (HBV) Reactivation

HBV reactivation can occur in patients treated with Rituxan, in some cases resulting in fulminant hepatitis, hepatic failure, and death. Screen all patients for HBV infection before treatment initiation, and monitor patients during and after treatment with Rituxan. Discontinue Rituxan and concomitant medications in the event of HBV reactivation …

Progressive Multifocal Leukoencephalopathy (PML), including fatal PML, can occur in patients receiving Rituxan …

Boxed Warning for Rituxan (rituximab) prescribing information. South San Francisco, CA: Genentech, Inc.; August 2020

Product Identification, Preparation, Storage, and Stability

- Rituxan is available in single-use vials containing a sterile, preservative-free solution at a uniform concentration of 10 mg riTUXimab/mL in the following presentations:
  - RiTUXimab 100 mg in 10 mL (NDC 50242-051-21)
  - Carton containing ten riTUXimab 100 mg in 10 mL vials (NDC 50242-051-10), *and*
  - RiTUXimab 500 mg in 50 mL (NDC 50242-053-06)

- Store intact vials under refrigeration at 2–8°C (36–46°F). Protect riTUXimab vials from direct sunlight. *Do not freeze or shake* vials containing riTUXimab
- Withdraw from a vial an amount of riTUXimab appropriate for a patient's dose and dilute it in either D5W or 0.9% NS to a concentration within the range of 1–4 mg/mL
- Gently invert the parenteral product container to mix the solution

- After dilution to a concentration within the range of 1–4 mg/mL, riTUXimab solutions may be stored under refrigeration for up to 24 hours after preparation, and may then be removed from refrigeration to room temperature conditions and used within 48 hours after preparation
- Discard any partially used vials
- No incompatibilities between riTUXimab and PVC or polyethylene bags have been observed
- *Do not mix* riTUXimab with other drugs

Recommendations for Drug Administration and Ancillary Care

General:

- Rate of administration is constrained by individual patient tolerance, and generally always proceeds through a series of escalating rates to a maximum of 400 mg/hour
  - Do not administer riTUXimab by rapid intraVENous injection

Premedication:

- Primary prophylaxis against adverse infusion-related reactions is indicated prior to administering riTUXimab
  - **Acetaminophen** 650–1000 mg orally 30–60 minutes before riTUXimab administration, and an antihistamine (H_1 receptor antagonist), for example, **diphenhydrAMINE** 50–100 mg (or equivalent) orally or intraVENously 30–60 minutes before riTUXimab administration

Other concomitant medications:

- Labeled indications for rheumatoid arthritis, Wegener's granulomatosis, microscopic polyangiitis, and pemphigus vulgaris include recommendations for premedication with glucocorticoids

(continued)

Recommendations for Drug Administration and Ancillary Care (*continued*)

- Recommendations for antibiotic prophylaxis are specific to indications for riTUXimab treatment, including:
  - *Pneumocystis jirovecii* pneumonia (PJP) and antiherpetic viral prophylaxis for patients with chronic lymphocytic leukemia during and for up to 12 months after completing treatment
  - PCP prophylaxis for patients with Wegener's granulomatosis and microscopic polyangiitis during and for up to 6 months after completing treatment
  - Consider PCP prophylaxis for patients with pemphigus vulgaris during and following riTUXimab treatment

RiTUXimab dosage and administration:

- RiTUXimab dosages and administration schedules vary among its labeled indications
- Rate of administration is constrained by individual patient tolerance, and, at least during initial treatment, proceeds through a series of escalating rates to a standardized maximum rate:
  - If adverse reactions occur during riTUXimab administration, either decrease the administration rate or interrupt treatment depending on the type and severity of reaction
    - If riTUXimab administration was interrupted, and, after adverse symptoms resolve it is considered medically appropriate to resume treatment, restart riTUXimab at a rate decreased by at least 50% from the rate at which symptoms occurred
    - If riTUXimab is tolerated after resuming treatment, administration may continue without attempting to escalate the rate of administration, or rate escalation may be cautiously reattempted
- Initial treatment:
  - The recommended initial dose rate for first riTUXimab exposure and reexposure after a 3- to 6-month hiatus is 50 mg/hour. If no toxicity is seen, the dose rate may be escalated gradually in 50-mg/hour increments at 30-minute intervals to a maximum rate of 400 mg/hour
- Second and subsequent doses:
  - Standard administration scheme for second and subsequent infusions
    - Patients who tolerate initial riTUXimab treatment without experiencing infusion-related adverse effects, but for whom the 90-minute infusion scheme during subsequent treatments is considered inappropriate, may receive subsequent riTUXimab doses at the standard rate for repeated treatments, which is as follows:
      - Begin at an initial rate of 100 mg/hour for 30 minutes. If administration is well tolerated, the administration rate may be escalated gradually in 100-mg/hour increments at 30-minute intervals to a maximum rate of 400 mg/hour
  - 90-minute administration scheme for patients with " … *previously untreated follicular NHL and DLBCL* [who] … did not experience a Grade 3 or 4 infusion related adverse event during Cycle 1 … [and who are receiving riTUXimab] … with a glucocorticoid-containing chemotherapy regimen."*,†
    - If the first dose of riTUXimab was well tolerated, subsequent doses may be administered over 90 minutes with 20% of the total dose given during the first 30 minutes, and the remaining 80% of the total dose administered over the subsequent 60 minutes; eg:

Two-Step Rate Escalation	Volume to Administer (X mL)
First portion (0–30 minutes)	$\dfrac{\text{Total Dose (mg)}}{\text{RiTUXimab Concentration (mg/mL)}} \times 0.2 = \text{X mL (over 30 min)}$
Second portion (30–90 minutes)	$\dfrac{\text{Total Dose (mg)}}{\text{RiTUXimab Concentration (mg/mL)}} \times 0.8 = \text{X mL (over 60 min)}^{[4]}$

*Rituxan (rituximab) Injection for Intravenous Infusion; August 2020 product label
†*Special Note:* The 90-minute administration scheme is not recommended for patients with clinically significant cardiovascular disease or high circulating lymphocyte counts (≥5000/mm³) before cycle 2

Caution:
- Do not administer riTUXimab as a rapid intraVENous injection or bolus
- Vaccination with live virus vaccines is not recommended during and for an unspecified period after completing riTUXimab treatment
  - Persons with impaired immunity receiving treatment with riTUXimab may be at increased risk of acquiring an infection from household contacts who receive live virus vaccinations
    - Examples of live vaccines include intranasally administered influenza, measles, mumps, rubella, oral polio, BCG, yellow fever, varicella, and TY21a typhoid vaccines
- Individuals of childbearing potential should use effective contraception during and for at least 12 months after completing treatment

RITUXIMAB AND HYALURONIDASE HUMAN

RITUXAN HYCELA (rituximab and hyaluronidase human) prescribing information. South San Francisco, CA: Genentech, Inc.; May 2020

WARNING: SEVERE MUCOCUTANEOUS REACTIONS, HEPATITIS B VIRUS REACTIVATION, and PROGRESSIVE MULTIFOCAL LEUKOENCEPHALOPATHY

Severe Mucocutaneous Reactions: severe, including fatal, mucocutaneous reactions can occur in patients receiving rituximab-containing products, including RITUXAN HYCELA …

Hepatitis B Virus (HBV) Reactivation: HBV reactivation can occur in patients treated with rituximab-containing products, including RITUXAN HYCELA, in some cases resulting in fulminant hepatitis, hepatic failure, and death. Screen all patients for HBV infection before treatment initiation, and monitor patients during and after treatment with RITUXAN HYCELA. Discontinue RITUXAN HYCELA and concomitant medications in the event of HBV reactivation …

Progressive Multifocal Leukoencephalopathy (PML): PML, including fatal PML, can occur in patients receiving rituximab-containing products, including RITUXAN HYCELA …

Boxed Warning for RITUXAN HYCELA (rituximab and hyaluronidase human) prescribing information. South San Francisco, CA: Genentech, Inc.; May 2020

Product Identification, Preparation, Storage, and Stability

- To prevent medication errors, check the vial labels to ensure that the drug being prepared and administered is RITUXAN HYCELA (rituximab and hyaluronidase human) for SUBCUTaneous use. Do not administer RITUXAN HYCELA (rituximab and hyaluronidase human) intraVENously
- RITUXAN HYCELA (rituximab and hyaluronidase human) is a combination of rituximab and hyaluronidase human. Rituximab is a chimeric murine/human monoclonal IgG1 kappa antibody directed against CD20. Recombinant human hyaluronidase is an endoglycosidase used to increase the dispersion and absorption of co-administered drugs when administered SUBCUTaneously
- RITUXAN HYCELA (rituximab and hyaluronidase human) is available in individually packaged single-use vials containing a sterile, preservative-free, colorless to yellowish, clear to opalescent, ready-to-use solution in the following presentations:
  - RITUXAN HYCELA (rituximab and hyaluronidase human) 1400 mg rituximab and 23,400 units hyaluronidase human in 11.7 mL (NDC 50242-108-01), *and*
  - RITUXAN HYCELA (rituximab and hyaluronidase human) 1600 mg rituximab and 26,800 units hyaluronidase human in 13.4 mL (NDC 50242-109-01)
  - Each milliliter of the above solutions contains the following ingredients: rituximab (120 mg), hyaluronidase human (2000 Units), L-histidine (0.53 mg), L-histidine hydrochloride monohydrate (3.47 mg), L-methionine (1.49 mg), polysorbate 80 (0.6 mg), α,α-trehalose dihydrate (79.45 mg), and SWFI
- Store intact vials under refrigeration at 2–8°C (36–46°F) in the original carton to protect from light. Do not freeze

---

Recommendations for Drug Administration and Ancillary Care

General:

- RITUXAN HYCELA (rituximab and hyaluronidase human) is for SUBCUTaneous use only and should only be administered by a health care professional with appropriate medical support to manage severe reactions that can be fatal if they occur
- Initiate treatment with RITUXAN HYCELA (rituximab and hyaluronidase human) only after patients have received at least one full dose of a rituximab product by intraVENous infusion without experiencing severe adverse reactions. If patients are not able to receive one full dose by intraVENous infusion, they should continue subsequent cycles with a rituximab product by intraVENous infusion and not switch to RITUXAN HYCELA (rituximab and hyaluronidase human) until a full intraVENous dose is successfully administered
- RITUXAN HYCELA (rituximab and hyaluronidase human) is not indicated for the treatment of non-malignant conditions

Premedication:

- Primary prophylaxis against adverse infusion-related reactions is indicated prior to administering RITUXAN HYCELA (rituximab and hyaluronidase human)
  - **Acetaminophen** 650–1000 mg orally 30–60 minutes before RITUXAN HYCELA (rituximab and hyaluronidase human) administration, and an antihistamine (H_1 receptor antagonist), for example, **diphenhydrAMINE** 50–100 mg (or equivalent) orally or intraVENously 30–60 minutes before RITUXAN HYCELA (rituximab and hyaluronidase human) administration
  - Premedication with a glucocorticoid should also be considered

(continued)

Recommendations for Drug Administration and Ancillary Care *(continued)*

Other concomitant medications:

- Recommendations for antibiotic prophylaxis are specific to indications for RITUXAN HYCELA (rituximab and hyaluronidase human) treatment, including:

  - *Pneumocystis jirovecii* pneumonia (PJP) and antiherpetic viral prophylaxis for patients with chronic lymphocytic leukemia during and for up to 12 months after completing treatment

RITUXAN HYCELA (rituximab and hyaluronidase human) dosage and administration:

- RITUXAN HYCELA (rituximab and hyaluronidase human) dosages and administration schedules vary among its labeled indications. Refer to the current FDA-approved product label for approved indications, dosages, and schedules

Preparation:

- RITUXAN HYCELA (rituximab and hyaluronidase human) is supplied as a ready-to-use product that requires no reconstitution or further dilution
- Using a sterile 20-mL syringe and any length, narrow-gauge needle (eg, 25–30 gauge), withdraw the contents of the vial corresponding to the individual patient's dose based on the indication according to the FDA-approved product label.
- Label the syringe with the provided peel-off label
- Change the needle to a 1/2' to 5/8' long, narrow-gauge needle (eg, 25–30 gauge) immediately prior to SUBCUTaneous administration to prevent needle clogging
- Visually inspect the contents of the syringe for particulate matter and discoloration prior to administration. The product should be a clear to opalescent and colorless to yellowish liquid. Do not use if particulates or discoloration are present

- Once RITUXAN HYCELA (rituximab and hyaluronidase human) has been withdrawn from its original vial, it should be used immediately. If not used immediately, it may be stored at 2–8°C (36–46°F) for up to 48 hours and subsequently for 8 hours at room temperature up to 30°C (86°F) in diffuse light

Administration:

- Inject RITUXAN HYCELA (rituximab and hyaluronidase human) into the SUBCUTaneous tissue of the abdomen over approximately 5–7 minutes. Never inject into areas where the skin is red, bruised, tender, or hard, or areas where there are moles or scars. No data are available on performing the injection at other sites of the body

  - When the volume to be administered is 11.7 mL (corresponding to a dosage of 1400 mg rituximab and 23,400 Units hyaluronidase human), then inject SUBCUTaneously into the abdomen over approximately 5 minutes
  - When the volume to be administered is 13.4 mL (corresponding to a dosage of 1600 mg rituximab and 26,800 Units hyaluronidase human), then inject SUBCUTaneously into the abdomen over approximately 7 minutes

- If signs of a severe reaction are observed during the administration of RITUXAN HYCELA (rituximab and hyaluronidase human), the injection should be interrupted immediately and aggressive symptomatic treatment should be initiated as clinically indicated
- If administration of RITUXAN HYCELA (rituximab and hyaluronidase human) is interrupted, continue administering at the same site, or at a different site, but restricted to the abdomen
- Observe patients for at least 15 minutes following RITUXAN HYCELA

(rituximab and hyaluronidase human) administration

- Advise patients that local cutaneous reactions or injection-site reactions may occur, sometimes with a delayed onset >24 hours after administration. Symptoms may include pain, swelling, induration, hemorrhage, erythema, pruritus, and rash. In clinical studies, the incidence of local reactions was 16%, severity was mild or moderate, and the reactions were self-limiting with no specific treatment. Local reactions occurred most commonly following the first dose of RITUXAN HYCELA (rituximab and hyaluronidase human)
- Do not administer other medications for SUBCUTaneous use at the same sites as RITUXAN HYCELA (rituximab and hyaluronidase human)

Caution:

- Do not administer RITUXAN HYCELA (rituximab and hyaluronidase human) intraVENously
- Vaccination with live virus vaccines is not recommended during and for an unspecified period after completing RITUXAN HYCELA (rituximab and hyaluronidase human) treatment

  - Persons with impaired immunity receiving treatment with RITUXAN HYCELA (rituximab and hyaluronidase human) may be at increased risk of acquiring an infection from household contacts who receive live virus vaccinations

    - Examples of live vaccines include intranasally administered influenza, measles, mumps, rubella, oral polio, BCG, yellow fever, varicella, zoster vaccine live, and TY21a typhoid vaccines

- Individuals of childbearing potential should use effective contraception during and for at least 12 months after completing treatment

ROMIDEPSIN

ISTODAX (romidepsin) prescribing information. Summit, NJ: Celgene Corporation; June 2013
ROMIDEPSIN prescribing information. North Wales, PA: Teva Pharmaceuticals USA, Inc.; March 2020

Product Identification, Preparation, Storage, and Stability

ISTODAX (romiDEPsin) for injection, for intravenous use (kit containing lyophilized drug product and diluent):

- ISTODAX Kit (NDC 59572-984-01), includes in a single package 2 single-use vials

  - One vial contains romiDEPsin 11 mg and 22 mg of the bulking agent, povidone, USP, as a sterile, lyophilized, white powder

  - A second single-use vial contains 2.2 mL (deliverable volume) of a sterile clear solution of 80% (v/v) propylene glycol, USP, and 20% (v/v) dehydrated alcohol, USP, to be used as a diluent in reconstituting romiDEPsin

- Store ISTODAX Kit in its packaging carton at 20–25°C (68–77°F), temperature excursions are permitted between 15° and 30°C (59° and 86°F)

- Reconstitute romiDEPsin by slowly injecting 2.2 mL of the supplied diluent into the vial containing the lyophilized drug product

- Swirl the contents of the vial until there are no visible particles in the resulting solution. The reconstituted solution contains 5 mg romiDEPsin/mL, and is chemically stable for at least 8 hours at room temperature. The reconstituted vial will contain 2 mL of deliverable volume of drug product

- RomiDEPsin must be further diluted in 500 mL 0.9% NS before it may be given by intraVENous infusion (product label)

  - After dilution in 500 mL of 0.9% NS, romiDEPsin is chemically stable for at least 24 hours when stored at room temperature, but should be administered as soon as possible after dilution

RomiDEPsin injection, solution, concentrate (Teva Pharmaceuticals product in solution):

- RomiDEPsin injection (product in solution) is commercially available as a sterile, clear, colorless to pale yellow solution supplied in single-dose vials in two different strengths: 10 mg/2 mL (NDC 0703-3071-01) or 27.5 mg/5.5 mL (NDC 0703-4004-01)

  - Each milliliter of the commercial product contains romiDEPsin 5 mg, povidone 10 mg, DL-alpha-tocopherol 0.05 mg, dehydrated alcohol 157.8 mg (20.1% v/v), and propylene glycol 828.8 mg

- Store RomiDEPsin injection in its packaging carton to protect from light at 20–25°C (68–77°F); temperature excursions are permitted between 15° and 30°C (59° and 86°F)

- RomiDEPsin must be further diluted in 500 mL 0.9% NS before it may be given by intraVENous infusion (product label)

  - After dilution in 500 mL of 0.9% NS, romiDEPsin is chemically stable for at least 24 hours when stored at room temperature, but it should be administered as soon as possible after dilution

Recommendations for Drug Administration and Ancillary Care

General:

- See Chapter 43 for comments about use in patients with renal and hepatic dysfunction
- Administer romiDEPsin intraVENously over 4 hours

Electrolytes and cardiac monitoring:

- Serum potassium and magnesium should be monitored and, if results are found less than the lower limits of normal values, supplemented and remeasured to ensure replacement was adequate to obtain serum potassium and magnesium results within the range of normal values before romiDEPsin is administered
- Several treatment-emergent morphologic changes in ECGs were reported in clinical studies, including T-wave and ST-segment

changes; however, the clinical significance of ECG changes is unknown
- Consider ECG monitoring at baseline and periodically during treatment in patients:

  - With congenital long QT syndrome
  - With a history of significant cardiovascular disease
  - Who are taking anti-arrhythmic medicines or medicinal products that lead to significant QT interval prolongation

- RomiDEPsin was associated with a delayed concentration-dependent increase in heart rate in patients with advanced cancer with a maximum mean increase in heart rate of 20 beats/min occurring at 6 hours after start of romiDEPsin 14 mg/m^2 administered intraVENously over 4 hours

Potential drug interactions:

- Concomitant use of romiDEPsin and warfarin was reported to prolong the PT and increase INR. The mechanism for an interaction between romiDEPsin and warfarin has not been determined
- RomiDEPsin is highly protein bound in human plasma (92–94%) over the concentration range (50–1000 ng/mL). Specific binding to human serum albumin and α_1-acid-glycoprotein were 19.91% and 93.51%, respectively
- RomiDEPsin is a substrate for metabolism by CYP3A4

  - Monitor for toxicity related to increased romiDEPsin exposure in patients concomitantly using a strong CYP3A4 inhibitor

(continued)

Recommendations for Drug Administration and Ancillary Care (*continued*)

- Potent CYP3A4 inducers may decrease concentrations of romiDEPsin if used concomitantly and should also be avoided
  - Paradoxically, when given concomitantly with rifAMPin in a pharmacokinetic drug interaction trial, romiDEPsin exposure was increased by approximately 80% and 60% for $AUC_{0-\infty}$ and C_{max}, respectively; its clearance was decreased by 44% and volume of distribution was decreased by 52%

- The increase in exposure is likely due to rifAMPin's inhibition of an undetermined hepatic uptake process that is predominantly responsible for romiDEPsin disposition
- It is not known if other potent CYP3A4 inducers may also alter the romiDEPsin exposure
- RomiDEPsin is a substrate for the transport protein, ABCB1 (*AKA* P-glycoprotein, P-gp, MDR1)

- Concurrent use of romiDEPsin with drugs that inhibit ABCB1 may increase systemic exposure to romiDEPsin
- RomiDEPsin has also been found to inhibit BSEP (*AKA* bile salt export pump, ABCB11, sister of P-glycoprotein [sPgp]) and OATP1B1

SACITUZUMAB GOVITECAN-hziy

TRODELVY (sacituzumab govitecan-hziy) prescribing information. Morris Plains, NJ: Immunomedics, Inc; April 2020

WARNING: NEUTROPENIA and DIARRHEA

- Severe neutropenia may occur. Withhold TRODELVY for absolute neutrophil count below $1500/mm^3$ or neutropenic fever. Monitor blood cell counts periodically during treatment. Consider G-CSF for secondary prophylaxis. Initiate anti-infective treatment in patients with febrile neutropenia without delay . . .
- Severe diarrhea may occur. Monitor patients with diarrhea and give fluid and electrolytes as needed. Administer atropine, if not contraindicated, for early diarrhea of any severity. At the onset of late diarrhea, evaluate for infectious causes and, if negative, promptly initiate loperamide. If severe diarrhea occurs, withhold TRODELVY until resolved to < Grade 1 and reduce subsequent doses . . .

Boxed Warning for TRODELVY (sacituzumab govitecan-hziy) prescribing information. Morris Plains, NJ: Immunomedics, Inc; April 2020

Product Identification, Preparation, Storage, and Stability

- Do *NOT* substitute TRODELVY for or use with other drugs containing irinotecan or its active metabolite SN-38
- Sacituzumab govitecan-hziy contains three components: the humanized monoclonal antibody sacituzumab, the drug SN-38, and a hydrolysable linker called CL2A which links the humanized monoclonal antibody to SN-38
- TRODELVY is a sterile, off-white to yellowish, preservative-free, lyophilized powder in individually boxed single-dose glass vials (NDC 55135-132-01) that contain sacituzumab govitecan-hziy (180 mg), 2-(N-morpholino) ethane sulfonic acid (77.3 mg), polysorbate 80 (1.8 mg), and trehalose dihydrate (154 mg). The pH of the reconstituted solution is 6.5
- Store intact vials under refrigeration at 2–8°C (36–46°F) in the original carton to protect from light until time of reconstitution
- Do not freeze

Reconstitution:
- Sacituzumab govitecan-hziy is a cytotoxic drug. Follow applicable special handling and disposal procedures

- Allow the required number of vials to warm to room temperature
- Use a sterile syringe to slowly inject 20 mL of 0.9% NS into each 180 mg sacituzumab govitecan-hziy vial to yield a 10-mg/mL solution
- Gently swirl vials and allow to dissolve for up to 15 minutes. Do not shake. Inspect for particulate matter and discoloration prior to administration. Use immediately to prepare a diluted sacituzumab govitecan-hziy infusion solution

Dilution:
- Calculate the required volume of reconstituted sacituzumab govitecan-hziy needed to obtain the appropriate dose according to the patient's body weight. Withdraw this amount from the vial(s) used into a syringe. Discard any unused portion remaining in the vial(s)
- Slowly inject the required volume of reconstituted sacituzumab govitecan-hziy solution into a polypropylene infusion bag to minimize foaming. Do not shake the contents
- Dilute in a volume of 0.9% NS sufficient to produce a final concentration ranging

from 1.1–3.4 mg/mL and not to exceed 500 mL. For patients who weigh >170 kg, divide the total dose of sacituzumab govitecan-hziy equally between two polypropylene bags each containing 500 mL 0.9% NS and infuse sequentially such that the total volume of 1000 mL is infused over the proper duration of 1–3 hours, depending on dose number and prior infusion reaction history
- Use immediately after dilution. The sacituzumab govitecan-hziy solution can be stored refrigerated for up to 4 hours. After refrigeration at 2–8°C (36–46°F), administer diluted solution within 4 hours (including infusion time)

Selected incompatibility:
- Do not mix with any diluent besides 0.9% NS. The stability of the reconstituted product has not been determined with other diluents

Recommendations for Drug Administration and Ancillary Care

General:
- See Chapter 43 for recommended use in patients with hepatic dysfunction
- There are no data on the PK of sacituzumab govitecan-hziy in patients with renal impairment or end-stage renal disease (CrCL ≤30 mL/min)
- Sacituzumab govitecan-hziy exposure is unknown in patients with moderate or severe hepatic impairment
- Calculate the required dose of sacituzumab govitecan-hziy based on the patient's body weight at the beginning of each cycle (or more frequently if the patient's body weight changed by >10% since the previous administration)
- For intraVENous infusion only. Do not administer as an intraVENous push or bolus

Administration:
- The recommended dose of sacituzumab govitecan-hziy is 10 mg/kg as an intraVENous infusion once weekly on days 1 and 8 of a 21-day treatment cycle
- Administer first infusion over 3 hours. If well tolerated, administer subsequent infusions over 1 to 2 hours
- Flush the line with 20 mL of 0.9% NS after completion of the sacituzumab govitecan-hziy infusion

Concomitant medications:
- Premedicate with antipyretics (eg, acetaminophen) and H1 (eg, diphenhydrAMINE) and H2 (eg, raNITIdine or equivalent) blockers prior to infusion
- If the patient experienced a prior non-life-threatening hypersensitivity reaction and a corticosteroid was not already being administered for antiemetic purposes, then consider adding dexamethasone
- Patients who exhibit an excessive cholinergic response to treatment (eg, abdominal cramping, diarrhea, salvation) can receive premedication with atropine for subsequent treatments

Adverse events and treatment modifications:
- Refer to the current FDA-approved product label for detailed recommendations regarding treatment modifications for neutropenia including febrile neutropenia, G3–4 nausea, vomiting or diarrhea due to treatment not controlled with antiemetics and anti-diarrheal agents, or other severe (G3–4) non-neutropenic toxicities graded according to the NCI CTCAE v. 4.0
- Withhold treatment for ANC <1500/mm^3 on day 1 of any cycle or <1000/mm^3 on day 8 of any cycle
- Withhold treatment for G3–4 diarrhea at the time of scheduled treatment. Refer to current FDA-approved label for information regarding use of anti-diarrheals such as loperamide
- Hypersensitivity reactions within 24 hours of dosing occurred in 37% (151/408) of patients treated with sacituzumab govitecan-hziy. G3–4 hypersensitivity reactions occurred in 1% (6/408)
- Administer sacituzumab govitecan-hziy in a setting with immediate access to emergency equipment and medications for management of severe hypersensitivity reactions
- Observe patients during the infusion and for at least 30 minutes following the dose for signs and symptoms of infusion-related reactions

Potential drug interactions:
- UGT1A1 inhibitors (eg, gemfibrozil, ketoconazole, atazanavir, indinavir) may increase the incidence of adverse reactions due to potential increase in systemic exposure to SN-38. Avoid UGT1A1 inhibitors with sacituzumab govitecan-hziy
- UGT1A1 inducers (eg, carBAMazepine, phenytoin) may substantially reduce exposure to SN-38. Avoid UGT1A1 inducers with sacituzumab govitecan-hziy

Selected precautions:
- Patients who have reduced UGT1A1 activity (eg, patients who are homozygous or heterozygous for UGT1A1*28) may be at increased risk for toxicity related to sacituzumab govitecan-hziy and should be monitored closely and have doses adjusted as necessary based on treatment tolerance

STREPTOZOCIN

ZANOSAR prescribing information. Irvine, CA: Teva Parenteral Medicines, Inc.; September 2018

WARNING

ZANOSAR should be administered under the supervision of a physician experienced in the use of cancer chemotherapeutic agents

A patient need not be hospitalized but should have access to a facility with laboratory and supportive resources sufficient to monitor drug tolerance and to protect and maintain a patient compromised by drug toxicity. Renal toxicity is dose-related and cumulative and may be severe or fatal. Other major toxicities are nausea and vomiting which may be severe and at times treatment-limiting. In addition, liver dysfunction, diarrhea, and hematological changes have been observed in some patients. Streptozocin is mutagenic. When administered parenterally, it has been found to be tumorigenic or carcinogenic in some rodents

The physician must judge the possible benefit to the patient against the known toxic effects of this drug in considering the advisability of therapy with ZANOSAR. The physician should be familiar with the following text [contained within the U.S. FDA-approved prescribing information] before making a judgment and beginning treatment

Boxed Warning for ZANOSAR prescribing information. Irvine, CA: Teva Parenteral Medicines, Inc.; September 2018

Product Identification, Preparation, Storage, and Stability

- ZANOSAR is available as individually packaged, single-use vials containing streptozocin 1000 mg as a sterile, pale yellow, freeze-dried powder (NDC 0703-4636-01)
- Store intact vials under refrigeration at 2–8°C (36–46°F) and protected from light in the original packaging
- Reconstitute the product with 9.5 mL of either D5W or 0.9% NS. Each milliliter of the resulting pale-gold solution contains streptozocin 100 mg and citric acid 22 mg. Sodium hydroxide may have been added to adjust product pH. After reconstitution as directed, the solution pH will range from 3.5–4.5

- Reconstituted streptozocin (10 mg/mL) is stable at room temperature, 15–30°C (59–86°F), for 48 hours or for 96 hours under refrigeration
- The reconstituted product may be further diluted to a volume convenient for clinical use in either D5W or 0.9% NS
  - After dilution to 2 mg/mL in D5W or 0.9% NS, streptozocin is stable for 48 hours at room temperature and 96 hours under refrigeration

- The commercial product does not contain an antimicrobial preservative and the manufacturer recommends storage for not greater than 12 hours after reconstitution
- At concentrations from 10–200 μg/mL streptozocin exhibited no loss because of adsorption to filters made of mixed cellulose esters (nitrocellulose, Millex-GS; EMD Millipore Corporation, Billerica, MA) or PTFE (*AKA* Teflon, poly[tetrafluoroethylene]; Millex-FG [EMD Millipore Corporation])[14,33]

Recommendations for Drug Administration and Ancillary Care

General:

- See Chapter 43 for recommendations for use in patients with renal and hepatic dysfunction
- Administer streptozocin either by rapid intraVENous injection (push) or by intraVENous infusion over a period within the range of 15 minutes to 6 hours
- Streptozocin does not contain an antimicrobial preservative, the manufacturer recommends storage for not greater than 12 hours after reconstitution

Inadvertent exposure:

- In case of contact with skin or mucous membranes, thoroughly wash the affected area with soap and water

TEMOZOLOMIDE

TEMODAR (temozolomide) prescribing information. Whitehouse Station, NJ: Merck Sharp & Dohme Corp.; October 2017

Product Identification, Preparation, Storage, and Stability

- TEMODAR for Injection is supplied in single-use glass vials containing 100 mg temozolomide as a light tan to light pink, sterile, pyrogen-free, lyophilized powder with mannitol 600 mg, L-threonine 160 mg, polysorbate 80 120 mg, sodium citrate dihydrate 235 mg, and hydrochloric acid 160 mg (NDC 0085-1381-01)
- Store intact vials of TEMODAR for Injection under refrigeration at 2–8°C (36–46°F)

- Allow vials of TEMODAR for Injection to equilibrate to room temperature before reconstitution
- Reconstitute TEMODAR for Injection with 41 mL of SWFI to produce a solution containing 2.5 mg temozolomide per milliliter
- Gently swirl but *do not* shake vials to aid dissolution
- After reconstitution, store reconstituted temozolomide (2.5 mg/mL) at room temperature (25°C [77°F]) for up to 14 hours

- TEMODAR for Injection should not be diluted further after reconstituting the lyophilized drug product
- With a sterile syringe, aseptically transfer a volume of temozolomide appropriate for a patient's dose (up to 100 mg [40 mL] from each vial) into a 250 mL plastic parenteral product container
- The reconstituted product must be used within 14 hours, including the time for administration

Recommendations for Drug Administration and Ancillary Care

General:

- See Chapter 43 for recommendations for use in patients with renal and hepatic dysfunction
- Flush administration set tubing with 0.9% NS both before and after temozolomide administration
  - Temozolomide may be administered through an administration set only with 0.9% NS
  - The compatibility of temozolomide solutions with other fluids and medications is not known
- Administer temozolomide intraVENously over 90 minutes using an infusion control device (pump)

- Bioequivalence between oral and intraVENous administration has been established only when temozolomide was administered intraVENously over 90 minutes
- Administration over shorter or longer durations may result in suboptimal dosing, and potentially may alter the incidence of infusion-related adverse reactions
- Temozolomide must be used within 14 hours after reconstitution, which includes the administration time

Cautions:

- Administration of valproic acid decreases oral clearance of temozolomide by about

5%. The clinical implication of this effect is not known
- Temozolomide use is contraindicated in patients who have a history of hypersensitivity to dacarbazine because both drugs are metabolized to the active MTIC metabolite
- Adverse reactions probably related to treatment with intraVENously administered temozolomide that were not reported in studies using orally administered temozolomide, include pain, irritation, pruritus, warmth, swelling, and erythema at the infusion site, petechiae, and hematoma

TEMSIROLIMUS

TORISEL Kit (temsirolimus) prescribing information. Philadelphia, PA: Wyeth Pharmaceuticals, Inc.; March 2018
TEMSIROLIMUS prescribing information. Durham, NC: Accord Healthcare, Inc.; July 2018
TEMSIROLIMUS prescribing information. Visakhapatnam, India: Gland Pharma Limited; August 2019

Product Identification, Preparation, Storage, and Stability

- Temsirolimus injection is packaged as a kit consisting of two clear glass vials:
  - One single-use temsirolimus injection vial contains temsirolimus 25 mg/mL as a clear, colorless to light yellow, nonaqueous, ethanolic, sterile solution. Excipient content varies among commercially available products; consult individual product labeling for details. The temsirolimus injection vial contains 0.2 mL of excess drug (5 mg overfill) to ensure the ability to withdraw from a vial the recommended dose
  - One single-use diluent for temsirolimus injection vial contains a sterile solution of polysorbate 80 40.0% (w/v), polyethylene glycol 400 42.8% (w/v), and dehydrated alcohol 19.9% (w/v), in a deliverable volume of 1.8 mL. The diluent for temsirolimus injection vial also contains excess fluid to ensure the appropriate volume can be withdrawn from a vial
- Store temsirolimus injection kits at 2–8°C (36–46°F). Protect temsirolimus injection from light

Temsirolimus injection dilution

- Temsirolimus injection (25 mg/mL) requires two dilutions before administration to patients
- During handling and preparation of admixtures, temsirolimus injection should be protected from excessive room light and sunlight
- *Do not add* undiluted temsirolimus injection to aqueous solutions without initially combining it with the provided diluent for temsirolimus injection
- Temsirolimus should be diluted only with the supplied diluent for temsirolimus injection
- Direct addition of temsirolimus injection to aqueous solutions will result in drug precipitation

Initial dilution of temsirolimus injection (25 mg/mL) with supplied diluent for temsirolimus injection

- Transfer 1.8 mL of solution from the vial containing DILUENT for TORISEL to a vial containing the TORISEL drug product
  - The resulting solution contains 30 mg temsirolimus in 3 mL (10 mg/mL)
- Mix the vial contents by repeatedly inverting the vial
- Allow time for air bubbles to subside. The solution should be clear to slightly turbid, colorless to light-yellow, and essentially free from visible particulates
  - The temsirolimus concentrate-diluent mixture (10 mg/mL) is stable at <25°C for up to 24 hours
  - After the contents of the temsirolimus injection vial have been diluted with diluent for temsirolimus, the resulting solution contains approximately 35% alcohol
  - After admixture with the diluent for temsirolimus, the drug product contains polysorbate 80 (240 mg/mL), which is known to increase the rate of DEHP extraction from PVC
    - Avoid using phthalate-plasticized PVC transfer devices and containers when transferring diluent for temsirolimus

for initial drug dilution and during all subsequent phases of temsirolimus preparation and administration

Secondary dilution of the temsirolimus (10 mg/mL) concentrate-diluent mixture with 0.9% NS
- With a syringe, withdraw from a vial containing the required amount of temsirolimus concentrate-diluent mixture 10 mg/mL (the initially diluted product described above) and transfer it to an appropriate parenteral product container containing 250 mL of 0.9% NS
  - Parenteral product containers appropriate for preparing and administering temsirolimus should be composed of glass, polypropylene, or polyolefin
    - Non-PVC containers and administration sets are preferred, but if PVC materials must be used, they should not contain DEHP
- Mix the solutions by repeatedly inverting the product container, avoiding excessive shaking that may cause foaming
- Protect the temsirolimus admixture in 0.9% NS from excessive room light and sunlight

Selected incompatibilities:
- The stability of temsirolimus injection in solutions other than 0.9% NS has not been evaluated
- Temsirolimus is degraded by both acids and bases: avoid combinations of temsirolimus with agents capable of modifying solution pH
- Do not add other drugs or nutritional products to admixtures of temsirolimus injection after dilution in 0.9% NS

Recommendations for Drug Administration and Ancillary Care

General:
- See Chapter 43 for recommendations for use in patients with hepatic dysfunction
- After initial dilution with the diluent for temsirolimus injection, the product contains polysorbate 80, which is known to increase the rate of DEHP extraction from plasticized PVC devices in contact with the drug
- Administration sets in which the fluid pathway (the surface in contact with a fluid or drug) is lined with polyethylene are appropriate for administering temsirolimus
  - Polyethylene-lined administration sets prevent excessive loss of temsirolimus and DEHP leaching into the drug-containing solution
- Non-PVC administration sets are preferred, but if PVC materials must be used, they should not contain DEHP
- An inline polyethersulfone filter with a pore size ≤5 μm is recommended for administration to avoid the possibility of particles >5 μm from being administered

(continued)

Recommendations for Drug Administration and Ancillary Care (continued)

- Polyethersulfone filters with pore sizes from 0.2–5 μm are acceptable
  - Administration sets that do not have an integral inline filter may be used with an appropriate polyethersulfone filter added to the fluid pathway (at the end of an administration set closest to a patient)
  - The use of dual inline and add-on filters is not recommended

Premedication:
- Patients should receive an antihistamine (H_1 receptor antagonist), for example, **diphenhydrAMINE** 25–50 mg (or equivalent) administered intraVENously approximately 30 minutes before the start of each temsirolimus dose

Temsirolimus administration:
- Administer temsirolimus intraVENously over 30–60 minutes with a rate-controlling device (eg, a pump); administration should be completed within 6 hours after dilution in 0.9% NS

Infusion-related reactions:
- Hypersensitivity reactions during temsirolimus administration have included, but are not limited to: flushing, chest pain, dyspnea, hypotension, apnea, loss of consciousness, and anaphylaxis
  - Infusion reactions can occur very early during a first exposure to temsirolimus, but they may also occur with subsequent use
  - Monitor patients throughout temsirolimus administration; appropriate supportive care should be available
  - Interrupt temsirolimus administration in all patients who experience severe infusion reactions and administer medical interventions as appropriate
  - Give temsirolimus with caution to persons who have demonstrated hypersensitivity to temsirolimus, its metabolites (including sirolimus), polysorbate 80, any other component of the commercially available product, or antihistamines (H_1 receptor antagonists), which are recommended as premedication for all persons who receive treatment with temsirolimus
- In patients who develop a hypersensitivity reaction during temsirolimus administration:
  - Interrupt the infusion and observe the patient for at least 30–60 minutes (duration depending on the severity of the reaction)

- At the discretion of a treating physician, temsirolimus administration may resume after signs and symptoms of hypersensitivity abate and administering intraVENously an H_1 receptor antagonist, if one was not previously administered, and/or an H_2 receptor antagonist (eg, famotidine 20 mg or raNITIdine 50 mg) administered intraVENously approximately 30 minutes before restarting temsirolimus
  - Temsirolimus infusion may then be restarted at a slower rate (administration duration of up to 60 minutes)

Potential drug interactions:
- Temsirolimus has been shown to inhibit CYP2D6 and CYP3A4 in in vitro systems with human liver microsomes, but did not alter desipramine concentration in vivo when single 50-mg doses of desipramine (a CYP2D6 substrate) were administered to 26 healthy volunteers with and without temsirolimus 25 mg[64]
- Temsirolimus is a substrate of the efflux transporter P-glycoprotein (*AKA* P-gp, ABCB1, MDR1) in vitro. It is not yet clear whether temsirolimus can modify the pharmacokinetic behavior or may itself be affected by concomitant use with other ABCB1 substrates or drugs that perturb expression or function of ABCB1[65]
- Use with CYP3A subfamily inducers
  - Concomitant administration of temsirolimus with rifAMPin, a potent CYP3A4/5 inducer, had no significant effect on temsirolimus C_{max} (maximum concentration) and AUC (area under the concentration versus time curve) after intraVENous administration, but decreased sirolimus C_{max} by 65% and AUC by 56% compared to temsirolimus treatment without rifAMPin
  - St. John's Wort may decrease temsirolimus plasma concentrations unpredictably, and concomitant use with temsirolimus should be avoided
  - Strong CYP3A4/5 inducers such as dexamethasone, carBAMazepine, phenytoin, PHENobarbital, rifAMPin, and rifabutin may decrease sirolimus exposure
    - If a strong CYP3A4 inducer must be coadministered during treatment with temsirolimus, consider increasing temsirolimus dose from 25 to 50 mg/week
    - This temsirolimus dose is predicted to adjust the AUC to the range observed

without inducers; however, there are no clinical data with this dose adjustment in patients receiving strong CYP3A4 inducers
  - If a concomitantly administered strong inducer is discontinued, the temsirolimus dose should be returned to the dose used prior to initiation of a strong CYP3A4 inducer
- Use with CYP3A subfamily inhibitors:
  - Strong CYP3A4 inhibitors, such as atazanavir, clarithromycin, indinavir, itraconazole, ketoconazole, nefazodone, nelfinavir, ritonavir, saquinavir, and telithromycin, may increase sirolimus blood concentrations
  - Grapefruit juice may also increase sirolimus concentrations in plasma (a major metabolite of temsirolimus) and should be avoided
  - If a strong CYP3A4 inhibitor must be coadministered, consider temsirolimus dose reduction to 12.5 mg/week
    - This temsirolimus dose is predicted to adjust the AUC to the range observed without inhibitors; however, there are no clinical data with this dose adjustment in patients receiving strong CYP3A4 inhibitors
    - If a concomitantly administered strong inhibitor is discontinued, a washout period of approximately 1 week should be allowed before readjusting temsirolimus doses to what was used before strong CYP3A4 inhibitor was introduced or the recommended dose of temsirolimus with CYP3A subfamily inhibitors
- Combination treatment with temsirolimus and SUNItinib malate resulted in dose-limiting toxicities (G3/4 erythematous maculopapular rash, and gout/cellulitis requiring hospitalization) in 2 of 3 patients treated in a phase I study with temsirolimus 15 mg per week and SUNItinib 25 mg/day administered orally for 28 consecutive days, days 1–28, during a 6-week treatment cycle
- Persons receiving temsirolimus should not receive vaccination with live vaccines and should avoid close contact with persons who have received live vaccines during treatment
  - Examples of live vaccines include intranasally administered influenza, measles, mumps, rubella, and polio (oral), BCG, yellow fever, varicella, and TY21a typhoid vaccines

TENIPOSIDE

TENIPOSIDE prescribing information. Paramus, NJ: WG Critical Care, LLC; April 2015

WARNING

Teniposide injection is a cytotoxic drug which should be administered under the supervision of a qualified physician experienced in the use of cancer chemotherapeutic agents. Appropriate management of therapy and complications is possible only when adequate treatment facilities are readily available

Severe myelosuppression with resulting infection or bleeding may occur. Hypersensitivity reactions, including anaphylaxis-like symptoms, may occur with initial dosing or at repeated exposure to teniposide injection. EPINEPHrine, with or without corticosteroids and antihistamines, has been employed to alleviate hypersensitivity reaction symptoms

Boxed Warning for TENIPOSIDE prescribing information. Paramus, NJ: WG Critical Care, LLC; April 2015

Product Identification, Preparation, Storage, and Stability

- Teniposide injection is available in individually packaged, clear, colorless, glass ampules containing a clear, sterile, nonpyrogenic solution of teniposide in a nonaqueous medium intended for dilution with a suitable parenteral vehicle prior to intraVENous administration (NDC 44567-507-01)
  - Teniposide injection ampules contain teniposide 50 mg in 5 mL. Each milliliter of solution contains 10 mg teniposide with 30 mg benzyl alcohol, 60 mg *N,N*-dimethylacetamide, 500 mg purified polyoxyl 35 castor oil*, and 42.7% (v/v) dehydrated alcohol. Solution pH is adjusted to approximately 5 with maleic acid

*Polyoxyl 35 castor oil is further purified by Corden Pharma before use

- Store unopened ampules under refrigeration at 2–8°C (36–46°F). Freezing does not adversely affect the product
- Retain ampules in their original packaging to protect teniposide from light
- Dilute teniposide (10 mg/mL) with either D5W or 0.9% NS to obtain products with teniposide concentrations of 0.1 mg/mL, 0.2 mg/mL, 0.4 mg/mL, or 1 mg/mL
  - *Do not permit plastic* equipment or devices to remain in contact with undiluted teniposide. Prolonged exposure may cause syringes and other plastic solution transfer devices, tubing, and containers to soften or crack, which may increase the risk of drug leakage. The effect has not been reported with teniposide solutions after dilution
  - Teniposide solutions may leach phthalate plasticizers from PVC containers and administration set tubing. The extent of leaching correlates directly with the concentration of drug and the duration of exposure[55,66]
  - *Use only non-DEHP* containers and administration sets (glass or polyolefin[17] containers, polyolefin-lined administration sets) to prepare and administer teniposide. Stability and use times are identical in glass and plastic containers
- Teniposide stability at ambient room temperature and lighting conditions after dilution in D5W or 0.9% NS is as follows:

Teniposide Concentration	Duration of Stability
0.1 mg/mL	24 hours
0.2 mg/mL	
0.4 mg/mL	
1 mg/mL	4 hours

- Do not refrigerate teniposide solutions after dilution. Stability and use times are identical in glass and plastic parenteral product containers
- Although the undiluted product is clear, solutions may exhibit a slight opalescence after dilution due to its surfactant components
- Although solutions are chemically stable under the conditions indicated, precipitation still may occur unpredictably. Spontaneous precipitation has been reported during 24-hour infusions of teniposide diluted to the lowest recommended concentrations of 0.1–0.2 mg/mL, resulting in occlusion of central VADs
  - Precipitation depends upon the formation of crystallization nuclei. Once crystallization nuclei are formed, precipitation proceeds rapidly
  - Strategies to prevent precipitation include:
    1. After diluting teniposide, gently invert product containers, agitating the solution as little as possible to ensure a homogeneous admixture
    2. *Minimize the storage time* between teniposide dilution and administration
    3. *Do not permit* diluted teniposide to come into contact with other drugs and fluids

Selected incompatibility:

- Teniposide admixture with heparin can cause precipitation

Recommendations for Drug Administration and Ancillary Care

General:

- See Chapter 43 for comments about use in patients with renal and hepatic dysfunction
- Administer teniposide as soon as possible after preparation to avoid precipitation
- Administer teniposide intraVENously over at least 30–60 minutes to avoid hypotension associated with more rapid administration
- In general, administration sets designed for infusing intraVENous fat emulsion or PACLitaxel, and low-DEHP-containing nitroglycerin sets, are suitable for use with teniposide
- Thoroughly flush an administration apparatus used to administer teniposide and a patient's VAD with D5W or 0.9% NS before and after teniposide administration
- *Do not permit* diluted teniposide to come into contact with other drugs and fluids

Hypersensitivity reactions:

- Teniposide treatment has been associated with a hypersensitivity reaction variably manifested by chills, fever, urticaria, tachycardia, bronchospasm, dyspnea, hypertension or hypotension, rash, and facial flushing
- Hypersensitivity reactions may occur with a first dose of teniposide and may be life-threatening if not treated promptly
- Patients who experience hypersensitivity reactions to teniposide are at risk for recurrence of symptoms if rechallenged, and should only be retreated with teniposide if the antileukemic benefit already demonstrated clearly outweighs the risk of a probable hypersensitivity reaction
- Patients who are retreated with teniposide in spite of an earlier hypersensitivity reaction should receive prophylaxis against recurrent hypersensitivity reactions with glucocorticoids and antihistamines (H_1 receptor antagonists) and remain under careful clinical observation during and after teniposide administration
- All patients who receive teniposide should be under continuous observation for at least the first 60 minutes after administration commences and at frequent intervals thereafter. If symptoms or signs of anaphylaxis occur, teniposide administration should be stopped immediately, followed by the administration of EPINEPHrine, corticosteroids, antihistamines, vasopressor agents, or volume expanders as clinically appropriate at the discretion of a physician
  - An aqueous solution of EPINEPHrine 1:1000 (1 mg/mL) and a source of oxygen should be available at the bedside during teniposide administration
    - Promptly administer EPINEPHrine at the onset of anaphylaxis. IntraMUSCular administration is preferred to the SUBCUTaneous route because EPINEPHrine is better absorbed after intraMUSCular administration. There are no absolute contraindications to EPINEPHrine administration in anaphylaxis

Potential drug interactions:

- Patients with both Down syndrome (trisomy 21) and leukemia may be especially sensitive to myelosuppressive chemotherapy; that is, teniposide dosage initially should be reduced in these patients
  - Product labeling suggests teniposide should be given at half the usual dose
- Teniposide dosages during subsequent courses may then be modified in individual patients depending on the degree of myelosuppression and mucositis previously encountered in earlier courses
- In a study in which 34 different drugs were tested, therapeutically relevant concentrations of tolbutamide, sodium salicylate, and sulfamethizole displaced protein-bound teniposide in fresh human serum to a small but significant extent
  - Teniposide is very highly bound to plasma proteins (>99%); thus, small decreases in protein binding, whether because of hypoalbuminemia or displacement from plasma protein by other substances, may cause substantial increases in free drug levels that could result in potentiation of drug toxicity
  - Exercise caution when administering teniposide to hypoalbuminemic patients and those who are concomitantly receiving drugs implicated in protein displacement interactions
- Teniposide plasma kinetics were not altered when it was coadministered with methotrexate, but methotrexate clearance from plasma was slightly increased. An increase in intracellular levels of methotrexate was observed in vitro in the presence of teniposide

Inadvertent exposure:

- In case of skin contact, immediately and thoroughly wash the affected area with soap and water
- In case of contact with mucous membranes, thoroughly flush the affected area with water

THIOTEPA

TEPADINA (thiotepa) prescribing information. Bridgewater, NJ: Amneal Pharmaceuticals LLC; March 2020
THIOTEPA prescribing information. Eatontown, NJ: West-Ward Pharmaceuticals; January 2019

WARNING: SEVERE MYELOSUPPRESSION, CARCINOGENICITY

TEPADINA may cause severe marrow suppression, and high doses may cause marrow ablation with resulting infection or bleeding. Monitor hematologic laboratory parameters. Hematopoietic progenitor (stem) cell transplantation (HSCT) is required to prevent potentially fatal complications of the prolonged myelosuppression after high doses of TEPADINA . . .

TEPADINA should be considered potentially carcinogenic in humans . . .

Boxed Warning for TEPADINA (thiotepa) prescribing information. Bridgewater, NJ: Amneal Pharmaceuticals LLC; March 2020

Product Identification, Preparation, Storage, and Stability

TEPADINA (thiotepa for injection, product distributed by Amneal Pharmaceuticals LLC for ADIENNE SA)

- The commercial branded product TEPADINA is available in individually packaged single-use type I glass vials containing either 15 mg (NDC 70121-1630-1) or 100 mg (NDC 70121-1631-1) of thiotepa as a nonpyrogenic, sterile, lyophilized white powder for reconstitution and dilution for intravenous, intracavitary, or intravesical administration. The product does not contain an antimicrobial preservative
- Store intact TEPADINA vials under refrigeration at 2–8°C (36–46°F). Do not freeze
- Reconstitute thiotepa with SWFI to produce a solution with concentration of 10 mg/mL thiotepa

Reconstitution Volumes for TEPADINA

Strength	Volume of SWFI Required for Reconstitution	Thiotepa Concentration After Reconstitution*
15 mg/vial (NDC 70121-1630-1)	1.5 mL	10 mg/mL
100 mg/vial (NDC 70121-1631-1)	10 mL	

- The reconstituted TEPADINA solution, free of visible particular matter, may occasionally appear opalescent, which does not preclude further use after dilution

- Reconstituted TEPADINA solution (10 mg/mL) is stable for 8 hours under refrigeration at 2–8°C (36–46°F)
- The reconstituted TEPADINA solution hypotonic and must be diluted in 0.9% NS prior to administration as follows:

Calculated TEPADINA Dose	Dilution Volume (0.9% NS) to Produce a Product Appropriate for Administration
<250 mg	Appropriate volume to obtain a final thiotepa concentration of 0.5–1 mg/mL
250 mg to 500 mg	500 mL or appropriate volume to obtain a final concentration of 0.5–1 mg/mL
>500 mg	1000 mL or appropriate volume to obtain a final concentration of 0.5–1 mg/mL

- Following dilution, the TEPADINA solution is stable for up to 24 hours under refrigeration at 2–8°C (36–46°F) and for 4 hours when stored at 25°C (77°F). From a microbiological point of view, the product should be used immediately
- The recommended dose of TEPADINA for intravesical use in the treatment of superficial papillary carcinoma of the urinary bladder is 60 mg diluted in 60 mL of 0.9% NS. If the patient cannot retain 60 mL for 2 hours, then reduce the volume to 30 mL

- To eliminate haze in thiotepa solutions, filter the solutions through a 0.2-μm filter before or during administration
- Filtering does not alter thiotepa potency

Thiotepa for injection, USP (product distributed by West-Ward Pharmaceuticals)

- Thiotepa for injection, USP, is available in individually packaged single-use vials containing 15 mg of thiotepa as a nonpyrogenic, sterile, lyophilized powder for reconstitution for intraVENous, intracavitary, or intravesical administration (NDC 0143-9565-01) from West-Ward Pharmaceuticals. The product does not contain an antimicrobial preservative
- Store intact vials under refrigeration at 2–8°C (36–46°F). Protect thiotepa for injection, USP, from light at all times
- Reconstitute a vial labeled as containing 15 mg thiotepa for injection, USP with 1.5 mL SWFI to produce a solution with concentration of approximately 10.4 mg/mL, and pH within the range 5.5–7.5
  - The actual amount of thiotepa present in a vial and the amounts that can be retrieved from vials are as follows:

Labeled content per vial	15 mg
Actual content per vial	15.6 mg
Volume of diluent (SWFI) to be added	1.5 mL
Approximate retrievable volume per vial	1.4 mL
Approximate retrievable amount (mass) per vial	14.7 mg
Approximate reconstituted concentration	10.4 mg/mL

(continued)

Product Identification, Preparation, Storage, and Stability (*continued*)

- Store reconstituted thiotepa (10.4 mg/mL) under refrigeration at 2–8°C for up to 8 hours
- Reconstituted solutions should be clear. Solutions that are opaque or contain a precipitate should not be used
  - To eliminate haze in thiotepa solutions, filter the solutions through a 0.22-μm filter before or during administration (polysulfone membrane [Gelman's Sterile Aerodisc, Single Use] or triton-free mixed ester of cellulose/PVC [MILLEX-gs Filter Unit, Millipore Corp])
  - Filtering does not alter thiotepa potency

- Reconstitution with SWFI to 10.4 mg/mL and further dilution with 0.9% NS to concentrations ≥3 mg/mL produces a hypotonic solution. Greater dilution with 0.9% NS to concentrations of 0.5 mg/mL or 1 mg/mL produces nearly isotonic solutions (277 and 269 mOsm/kg, respectively)
- Dilution with 0.9% NS to concentrations <1.8 mg/mL are nearly isotonic; *but*
  - After dilution with 0.9% NS to a concentration <1 mg/mL, thiotepa solutions should be *used immediately* because of the formation of drug adducts with chloride[67,74]

- Both the amount and rate of chloro-adduct formation are inversely related to the concentration of thiotepa in solution[67]
- Storage under refrigeration slows the rate but does not eliminate chloro-adduct formation and loss of thiotepa potency[67]
- Dilute thiotepa (10.4 mg/mL) with 0.9% NS before clinical use
- Thiotepa diluted in D5W to 0.5 mg/mL and 5 mg/mL was stable in both PVC and polyolefin composition containers with no drug loss due to adsorption[68]

Recommendations for Drug Administration and Ancillary Care

General:
- See Chapter 43 for comments about use in patients with renal and hepatic dysfunction
- To eliminate haze in thiotepa solutions, a solution should be filtered through a 0.22-μm filter with hydrophilic polyethersulfone or cellulose ester filter membranes either before or during administration
  - Filtering does not alter thiotepa potency
- Thiotepa is usually given by rapid intraVENous administration, but has also been given by intravesical, intracavitary, intraTHECAL, intraMUSCular, and intratumoral routes

IntraVENous administration for adenocarcinoma of the breast or ovary:
- Thiotepa 0.3–0.4 mg/kg body weight may be given by rapid intraVENous injection over 5 minutes at 1- to 4-week intervals
- Thiotepa dosage must be carefully individualized. A slow response to thiotepa does not necessarily indicate a lack of effect. Increasing the frequency of repeated administration may only increase toxicity
- Initially, the higher dose in a given range is commonly administered. Maintenance dosages should be adjusted based on pretreatment blood counts (CBC with differential leukocyte and platelet counts)

High-dose intraVENous administration in pediatric patients with class 3 beta-thalassemia undergoing allogeneic hematopoietic stem cell transplantation (HSCT):
- The FDA-approved dosage of thiotepa which appears in the FDA-approved prescribing information is 5 mg/kg/dose

administered by intraVENous infusion over 3 hours, every 12 hours, for 2 doses on day −6 prior to HSCT, through a central VAD using an infusion set equipped with a 0.2-μm inline filter
  - Flush the central VAD with approximately 5 mL 0.9% NS prior to and following each thiotepa infusion
- Thiotepa and/or its active metabolites may be excreted in part through the skin in patients receiving high-dose therapy. Treatment may cause skin discoloration, pruritus, blistering, desquamation, and peeling that may be more severe in the groin, axillae, skin folds, in the neck area, and under dressings. During the period beginning with the first thiotepa infusion and ending 48 hours following the last thiotepa dose, take the following precautions:
  - Advise patients to shower or bathe with water at least twice per day
  - Change occlusive dressings and clean the covered skin at least twice per day
  - Change bed sheets daily

Intracavitary administration:
- Thiotepa 0.6–0.8 mg/kg body weight
- Tubing that is used to drain fluid from the body cavity often is used to instill thiotepa

Intravesical administration:
- Fluids are withheld for 8–12 hours before treatment. Thiotepa 60 mg in 30–60 mL of 0.9% NS is instilled into the bladder by a urethral catheter. For maximum effect, the solution should be retained for 2 hours. If it is not possible to retain 60 mL for 2 hours, the dose may be given in a volume

of 30 mL. A patient is repositioned every 15 minutes for maximum area contact
- The usual course of treatment is once weekly for 4 consecutive weeks
- A treatment course may be repeated if necessary, but second and third courses must be given with caution since bone-marrow depression may be increased
- Deaths have occurred after intravesical administration, caused by bone-marrow depression from systemically absorbed drug

IntraTHECAL administration:
- Thiotepa 2–10 mg/m^2 per dose, or a fixed dose of 10 mg/dose administered by either intralumbar or intraventricular routes, diluted with preservative-free 0.9% NS to a concentration of 1–5 mg/mL
- There is no PK advantage for intraTHECAL versus intraVENous administration[69]
  - Thiotepa clearance from the CSF is approximately 9 times greater than CSF bulk outflow, which results in disproportionate distribution throughout the neuraxis[69]
  - TEPA (*N,N',N'*-triethylenephosphoramide), thiotepa's active metabolite, is formed only after systemic administration, after which it readily crosses the blood–brain barrier[70]

Inadvertent exposure:
- In case of skin contact, immediately and thoroughly wash the affected area with soap and water
- In case of contact with mucous membranes, thoroughly flush the affected area with water

TOPOTECAN HYDROCHLORIDE

TOPOTECAN prescribing information. Durham, NC: Accord Healthcare, Inc.; April 2017
TOPOTECAN prescribing information. North Wales, PA: Teva Pharmaceuticals USA, Inc.; June 2019
TOPOTECAN prescribing information. Schaumburg, IL: SAGENT Pharmaceuticals; December 2017
TOPOTECAN prescribing information. Rockford, IL: Mylan Institutional LLC; March 2020
TOPOTECAN prescribing information. Lake Forest, IL: Hospira, Inc.; December 2019
TOPOTECAN HYDROCHLORIDE prescribing information. Sunrise, FL: Cipla USA, Inc.; November 2019
TOPOTECAN HYDROCHLORIDE prescribing information. Durham, NC: Accord Healthcare, Inc.; December 2019
HYCAMTIN (topotecan hydrochloride) prescribing information. East Hanover, NJ: Novartis Pharmaceuticals Corporation; October 2019

WARNING: MYELOSUPPRESSION

[Topotecan hydrochloride for injection] can cause severe myelosuppression. Administer first cycle only to patients with baseline neutrophil counts of greater than or equal to $1500/mm^3$ and platelet counts greater than or equal to $100,000/mm^3$. Monitor blood cell counts …

Boxed Warning for HYCAMTIN (topotecan hydrochloride) prescribing information. East Hanover, NJ: Novartis Pharmaceuticals Corporation; October 2019

Product Identification, Preparation, Storage, and Stability

Topotecan for Injection (lyophilized powder):
- Topotecan for injection is available generically as a sterile, lyophilized, buffered, light yellow to greenish powder in single-dose vials containing topotecan hydrochloride equivalent to 4 mg of topotecan as the free base, with mannitol 48 mg and tartaric acid 20 mg. Hydrochloric acid and sodium hydroxide may be used to adjust the product pH. Available products do not contain an antimicrobial preservative
  - Presentations vary by manufacturer, but include individually packaged vials and packages containing 5 vials
- Store intact vials protected from light in the original cartons at controlled room temperature between 20° and 25°C (68° and 77°F)
- Reconstitute lyophilized topotecan HCl with 4 mL of SWFI to produce a yellow to yellow-green solution with concentration equal to 1 mg/mL and a pH within the range 2.5–3.5
- After reconstitution with SWFI to a concentration of 1 mg topotecan HCl per milliliter, topotecan HCl 1 mg/mL, stored for 28 days at 4°C (39.2°F) or 25°C and protected from light, the drug product was found to be physically and chemically stable by HPLC analysis without color change or visible precipitation[71]
- After reconstitution with SWFI to a concentration of 1 mg topotecan/mL in the original product vials, storage either upright or inverted for 28 days at 5°C (41°F), 25°C, or 30°C (86°F), and protected from light, the drug product was found to be physically and chemically stable by stability-indicating HPLC analysis without change in color or clarity
  - The amount of topotecan remaining was >98% of the initial concentration in all solutions stored at 5°C (41°F), 25°C, or 30°C
  - There was no significant difference in the total amount of impurities and degradation products for samples stored at 5°C. In comparison, the total amount of impurities and degradation products increased for samples stored at 25°C or 30°C, more so for samples stored at 30°C
- After reconstitution with BWFI (preserved with benzyl alcohol) to a concentration of 1 mg/mL and further diluted in a PVC container, topotecan HCl stability was as follows:

Diluting/Vehicle Solution	Diluted Concentration	Storage Conditions	Loss of Topotecan
0.9% NS	10 µg/mL	Room temperature × 4 days	<3%
	500 µg/mL		
D5W	10 µg/mL		
	500 µg/mL		
BWFI	10 µg/mL	Room temperature × 21 days	<4%

- Dilute an amount of drug appropriate for a patient's dose in 50–250 mL of either 0.9% NS or D5W
- After dilution with 0.9% NS or D5W, solutions prepared with Topotecan for Injection are stable for at least 24 hours when stored at 20–25°C
- Topotecan 0.05 mg/mL diluted in 0.9% NS or D5W was stable for up to 24 hours at 23–24°C (73.4–75.2°F) and for up to 7 days at 5°C (41°F) in PVC, polyolefin, and glass parenteral product containers[72]
- Topotecan 0.025 mg/mL diluted in 0.9% NS or D5W was stable for up to 24 hours at 23–24°C and for up to 7 days at 5°C in PVC parenteral product containers.[72] At the topotecan concentrations and for the conditions studied:

(continued)

Product Identification, Preparation, Storage, and Stability (*continued*)

- ▪ There were no significant differences observed in stability between topotecan diluted in either 0.9% NS or D5W[72]
- ▪ Topotecan hydrochloride did not contribute to significant leaching of DEHP from PVC containers[72]
- Topotecan is susceptible to photodegradation during storage:
  - ▪ *Protect stored solutions* from light exposure[71]
  - ▪ Protection from light is not necessary during topotecan administration

Topotecan Injection (solution):

- Topotecan Injection is available generically in individually packaged vials containing a sterile, non-pyrogenic, clear, yellow solution of topotecan HCl
- Commercially available presentations include single-use vials containing 4 mg (4 mL) of topotecan and multiple-dose vials containing either 1 mg (1 mL) or 4 mg (4 mL) of topotecan
  - ▪ Each milliliter of solution contains topotecan hydrochloride equivalent to 1 mg of topotecan (free base), with 5 mg tartaric acid, NF, and SWFI. Hydrochloric acid and/or sodium hydroxide may be added to adjust product pH
- Storage of intact vials varies among manufacturers:
  - ○ Labeling for single-use vials indicates storage in the original carton to protect from light under refrigeration at 2–8°C (36–46°F) and protected from light in the original packaging carton
  - ○ Labeling for multiple dose vials (ie, the product distributed by Accord Healthcare Inc) indicates storage in the original carton to protect from light at room temperature (20–25°C [68–77°F]) with excursions permitted to 15–30°C (59–86°F)
    - ▫ Product supplied in a multiple dose vial is stable for 28 days after initial puncture when stored at room temperature
  - ○ Refer to individual package labeling to confirm appropriate storage conditions for intact vials
- Dilute an amount of Topotecan Injection (1 mg/mL) appropriate for a patient's dose in a minimum volume of 50 mL of 0.9% NS or D5W
- After dilution with 0.9% NS or D5W, solutions prepared with Topotecan Injection are stable to varying degrees based on information provided in the labeling of commercially available products:
  - ○ Topotecan injection distributed by Teva Pharmaceuticals USA, Inc and SAGENT Pharmaceuticals specify stability of diluted topotecan injection for up to 4 hours when stored at room temperature (20–25°C) and for up to 12 hours when stored under refrigeration (2–8°C)
  - ○ Topotecan injection distributed by Accord Healthcare Inc specifies stability of diluted topotecan injection for up to 4 hours when stored at room temperature (20–25°C) and for up to 24 hours when stored under refrigeration (2–8°C) in ambient lighting
  - ○ Topotecan injection distributed by Mylan Institutional LLC and Hospira, Inc. specify stability of diluted topotecan injection for up to 24 hours when stored at 20–25°C under ambient lighting
  - ○ Refer to individual package labeling to confirm appropriate storage conditions for diluted topotecan injection

Selected incompatibility:

- Topotecan is formulated with tartaric acid to maintain a pH between 2.5 and 3.5. Topotecan solubility and stability decrease with increasing pH; its lactone ring spontaneously hydrolyzes at pH >4

Recommendations for Drug Administration and Ancillary Care

General:

- See Chapter 43 for recommendations for use in patients with renal dysfunction
- Administer topotecan doses intraVENously over 30 minutes

Inadvertent exposure:

- In case of skin contact, immediately and thoroughly wash the affected area with soap and water
- In case of contact with mucous membranes, thoroughly flush the affected area with water

TRASTUZUMAB

HERCEPTIN (trastuzumab) prescribing information. South San Francisco, CA: Genentech, Inc.; November 2018

WARNING: CARDIOMYOPATHY, INFUSION REACTIONS, EMBRYO-FETAL TOXICITY, and PULMONARY TOXICITY

Cardiomyopathy
Herceptin administration can result in sub-clinical and clinical cardiac failure. The incidence and severity was highest in patients receiving Herceptin with anthracycline-containing chemotherapy regimens.
Evaluate left ventricular function in all patients prior to and during treatment with Herceptin. Discontinue Herceptin treatment in patients receiving adjuvant therapy and withhold Herceptin in patients with metastatic disease for clinically significant decrease in left ventricular function . . .

Infusion Reactions; Pulmonary Toxicity
Herceptin administration can result in serious and fatal infusion reactions and pulmonary toxicity. Symptoms usually occur during or within 24 hours of Herceptin administration. Interrupt Herceptin infusion for dyspnea or clinically significant hypotension. Monitor patients until symptoms completely resolve. Discontinue Herceptin for anaphylaxis, angioedema, interstitial pneumonitis, or acute respiratory distress syndrome . . .

Embryo-Fetal Toxicity
Exposure to Herceptin during pregnancy can result in oligohydramnios and oligohydramnios sequence manifesting as pulmonary hypoplasia, skeletal abnormalities, and neonatal death. Advise patients of these risks and the need for effective contraception . . .

Boxed Warning for HERCEPTIN (trastuzumab) prescribing information. South San Francisco, CA: Genentech, Inc.; November 2018

Product Identification, Preparation, Storage, and Stability

- The commercial product HERCEPTIN is available in two presentations, a multiple-dose vial containing 420 mg HERCEPTIN copackaged with one vial (20 mL) of BWFI preserved with 1.1% benzyl alcohol, and a single-dose vial containing 150 mg HERCEPTIN

	HERCEPTIN 420 mg Multiple-Dose Vial	HERCEPTIN 150 mg Single-Dose Vial
NDC number	50242-333-01 (individual package)	50242-132-01 (individual package) 50242-132-10 (package of ten)
Description	Sterile, white to pale yellow, preservative-free, lyophilized powder under vacuum	
Included (copackaged) diluent	20 mL BWFI preserved with 1.1% benzyl alcohol	Not included
α,α-trehalose dihydrate	381.8 mg	136.2 mg
L-histidine HCl monohydrate	9.5 mg	3.4 mg
L-histidine	6.1 mg	2.2 mg
Polysorbate 20	1.7 mg	0.6 mg
Intact vial storage	2–8°C (36–46°F)	

Reconstitution:
- Slowly inject diluent (see table below) directly into the lyophilized powder cake

Reconstitution Volumes for HERCEPTIN

Strength	Diluent for Reconstitution	HERCEPTIN Concentration After Reconstitution	Storage of Reconstituted Solution
420 mg Multiple-Dose Vial (NDC 50242-333-01)	20 mL BWFI (included)	21 mg/mL	2°C to 8° C (36°F to 46°F) for up to 28 days *Do not freeze*
	20 mL SWFI[*]	21 mg/mL	Use immediately (consider as single-dose) Discard any unused portion
150 mg Single-Dose Vial (NDC 50242-132-01)	7.4 mL SWFI	21 mg/mL	Use immediately (single-dose) If not used immediately, store at 2°C to 8°C (36°F to 46°F) for up to 24 hours *Do not freeze*

[*]If SWFI is used instead of BWFI (for example, in a patient with known hypersensitivity to benzyl alcohol) to reconstitute a multiple-dose vial, then the reconstituted solution should be considered single-dose

Product Identification, Preparation, Storage, and Stability (continued)

- Gently swirl vials to aid reconstitution. *Do not shake* trastuzumab during reconstitution to avoid excessive foaming, which may make dissolution difficult and compromise the amount of solution that can be withdrawn from a vial
  - Trastuzumab may be sensitive to shear-induced stresses that can be produced during agitation or rapid expulsion from a syringe
  - Slight foaming is not unusual during reconstitution. After adding the diluent, allow vials to stand undisturbed for approximately 5 minutes

- Reconstituted trastuzumab (21 mg trastuzumab/mL) should be free of visible particulates, clear to slightly opalescent, and colorless to pale yellow

Dilution:
- After reconstitution, dilute an amount of trastuzumab appropriate for a patient's dose in 250 mL of 0.9% NS
- *Do not use* dextrose solutions to dilute trastuzumab
- Gently invert the container to mix the solution

- Trastuzumab is compatible with PVC and polyethylene containers
- Trastuzumab solutions diluted in 0.9% NS in PVC or polyethylene bags may be stored at 2–8°C (36–46°F) for up to 24 hours before use

Selected incompatibility:
- *Do not use* D5W to dilute trastuzumab
- *Do not mix or dilute* trastuzumab with other drugs

Recommendations for Drug Administration and Ancillary Care

General:
- Administer doses intraVENously over 90 minutes. If administration over 90 minutes is well tolerated, subsequent doses may be administered over 30–90 minutes
  - *Do not administer* trastuzumab by rapid injection techniques (push or bolus)
  - Observe patients for fever and chills and other infusion-associated symptoms
- *Do not mix or dilute* trastuzumab with other drugs

Infusion reactions:
- Infusion reactions consist of a symptom complex characterized by fever and chills, and on occasion included nausea, vomiting, pain (in some cases at tumor sites), headache, dizziness, dyspnea, hypotension, rash, and asthenia
- Decrease the rate of infusion for mild or moderate infusion reactions
- Severe reactions, including bronchospasm, anaphylaxis, angioedema, hypoxia, and severe hypotension, were usually reported during or immediately after an initial treatment. However, the onset and clinical course were variable, including:
  - Progressive worsening
  - Initial improvement followed by clinical deterioration, *or*
  - Delayed post-infusion events with rapid clinical deterioration
- For fatal events, death occurred within hours to days following a serious infusion reaction
- Interrupt trastuzumab administration in all patients who experience dyspnea, clinically significant hypotension, and provide medical therapy appropriate for signs and symptoms, which may include EPINEPHrine, corticosteroids, diphenhydrAMINE, bronchodilators, and oxygen
- Evaluate and carefully monitor patients who experience moderate and more severe infusion reactions until associated signs and symptoms completely resolve
- Discontinue trastuzumab in all patients who experience severe or life-threatening infusion reactions
- There are no data to guide the most appropriate method for identifying patients who may safely be retreated with trastuzumab after experiencing a severe infusion reaction
- Prophylaxis against severe hypersensitivity reactions with antihistamines and/or steroids may or may not prevent recurrent severe infusion reactions

Cardiomyopathy:
- Trastuzumab can cause left ventricular cardiac dysfunction, arrhythmias, hypertension, disabling cardiac failure, cardiomyopathy, and cardiac death, and an asymptomatic decline in left ventricular ejection fraction (LVEF)
- There is a 4- to 6-fold increase in the incidence of symptomatic myocardial dysfunction among patients who receive trastuzumab as a single agent or in combination therapy compared with those who do not receive trastuzumab; the highest absolute incidence occurs when trastuzumab is administered with an anthracycline
- Assess left ventricular ejection fraction (LVEF) before administering trastuzumab and at regular intervals during treatment

Cardiac monitoring:
- Conduct thorough cardiac assessment, including history, physical examination, and determine LVEF by echocardiogram or MUGA scan. The following schedule is recommended:
  - Baseline LVEF measurement immediately before initiating trastuzumab

  - LVEF measurements every 3 months during and after completing trastuzumab treatments
  - Repeat LVEF measurement at 4-week intervals if trastuzumab is withheld for significant left ventricular cardiac dysfunction
  - LVEF measurements every 6 months for at least 2 years after completing trastuzumab as a component of adjuvant therapy

Treatment modification for cardiac toxicity:
- Withhold trastuzumab for at least 4 weeks for either of the following:
  - ≥16% absolute decrease in LVEF from pretreatment values
  - LVEF below institutional limits of normal *and* ≥10% absolute decrease in LVEF from pretreatment values
- Trastuzumab may be resumed if, within 4–8 weeks, LVEF returns to normal limits and the absolute decrease from baseline is ≤15%
  - Whether it is safe to continue or resume trastuzumab treatment in patients with trastuzumab-induced left ventricular cardiac dysfunction has not been studied
  - Permanently discontinue trastuzumab for a persistent (>8 weeks) LVEF decline or for suspension of trastuzumab dosing on >3 occasions for cardiomyopathy

Pulmonary toxicity:
- Trastuzumab use is associated with serious and fatal pulmonary toxicity, including dyspnea, interstitial pneumonitis, pulmonary infiltrates, pleural effusions, non-cardiogenic pulmonary edema, pulmonary insufficiency and hypoxia, acute respiratory distress syndrome, and pulmonary fibrosis
  - Pulmonary toxicity may occur as sequelae of infusion-related reactions
  - Patients with symptomatic intrinsic lung disease or with extensive tumor involvement of the lungs, resulting in dyspnea at rest, appear to have more severe toxicity

TRASTUZUMAB AND HYALURONIDASE-oysk

HERCEPTIN HYLECTA (trastuzumab and hyaluronidase-oysk) prescribing information. South San Francisco, CA: Genentech, Inc.; February 2019

WARNING: CARDIOMYOPATHY, EMBRYO-FETAL TOXICITY, and PULMONARY TOXICITY

Cardiomyopathy

HERCEPTIN HYLECTA administration can result in sub-clinical and clinical cardiac failure. The incidence and severity was highest in patients receiving HERCEPTIN HYLECTA with anthracycline-containing chemotherapy regimens. Evaluate left ventricular function in all patients prior to and during treatment with HERCEPTIN HYLECTA. Discontinue HERCEPTIN HYLECTA treatment in patients receiving adjuvant therapy and withhold HERCEPTIN HYLECTA in patients with metastatic disease for clinically significant decrease in left ventricular function …

Pulmonary Toxicity

HERCEPTIN HYLECTA administration can result in serious and fatal pulmonary toxicity. Symptoms usually occur during or within 24 hours of HERCEPTIN HYLECTA administration. Discontinue HERCEPTIN HYLECTA for anaphylaxis, angioedema, interstitial pneumonitis, or acute respiratory distress syndrome … Monitor patients until symptoms completely resolve

Embryo-Fetal Toxicity

Exposure to HERCEPTIN HYLECTA during pregnancy can result in oligohydramnios and oligohydramnios sequence manifesting as pulmonary hypoplasia, skeletal abnormalities, and neonatal death. Advise patients of these risks and the need for effective contraception …

Boxed Warning for HERCEPTIN HYLECTA (trastuzumab and hyaluronidase-oysk) prescribing information. South San Francisco, CA: Genentech, Inc.; February 2019

Product Identification, Preparation, Storage, and Stability

- HERCEPTIN HYLECTA is for SUBCUTaneous use only. HERCEPTIN HYLECTA has different dosage and administration instructions than intraVENous trastuzumab products. Do not administer intraVENously
- Do not substitute HERCEPTIN HYLECTA for or with ado-trastuzumab emtansine
- HERCEPTIN HYLECTA (trastuzumab and hyaluronidase-oysk) is a combination of trastuzumab and hyaluronidase. Trastuzumab is a humanized IgG1 kappa monoclonal antibody directed against HER2. Recombinant human hyaluronidase is an endoglycosidase used to increase the dispersion and absorption of co-administered drugs when administered SUBCUTaneously
- HERCEPTIN HYLECTA (trastuzumab and hyaluronidase-oysk) is a sterile, colorless to yellowish, clear to opalescent, preservative-free, ready-to-use solution available in individually boxed single-dose 5 mL vials (NDC 50242-077-01) that contain trastuzumab (600 mg) and hyaluronidase (10,000 units). Each mL of solution contains trastuzumab (120 mg), hyaluronidase (2000 units), L-histidine (0.39 mg), L-histidine hydrochloride monohydrate (3.67 mg), L-methionine (1.49 mg), polysorbate 20 (0.4 mg), α,α-trehalose dihydrate (79.45 mg), and SWFI
- Store intact vials under refrigeration at 2–8°C (36–46°F) in the original carton to protect from light
- *Do not freeze or shake* intact vials

Recommendations for Drug Administration and Ancillary Care

General:

- The usual dose of HERCEPTIN HYLECTA (trastuzumab and hyaluronidase-oysk) is 600 mg/10,000 units (600 mg trastuzumab and 10,000 units hyaluronidase) administered SUBCUTaneously over approximately 2–5 minutes once every 3 weeks. No loading dose is required. No adjustment in the dose is required for patient body weight or concomitant chemotherapy regimen
- HERCEPTIN HYLECTA (trastuzumab and hyaluronidase-oysk) must be administered by a health care professional. Ensure that medications and emergency equipment to manage systemic hypersensitivity reactions are immediately available.
- To prevent medication errors, it is important to check the vial labels to ensure that the drug being prepared and administered is HERCEPTIN HYLECTA (trastuzumab and hyaluronidase-oysk) and not ado-trastuzumab emtansine or intraVENous trastuzumab

Preparation:

- HERCEPTIN HYLECTA (trastuzumab and hyaluronidase-oysk) is supplied as a ready-to-use product that requires no reconstitution or further dilution
- Visually inspect the contents of the vial for particulate matter or discoloration
- Using a sterile syringe (composed of polypropylene or polycarbonate) and a stainless steel transfer needle, withdraw 5 mL of solution from the vial under controlled and validated aseptic conditions
- Replace the transfer needle with a syringe closing cap. Label the syringe according to institutional standards and with a peel-off label
- Once HERCEPTIN HYLECTA (trastuzumab and hyaluronidase-oysk) has been withdrawn from its original vial, it should be used immediately. If not used immediately, it may be stored for up to 4 hours at room temperature not exceeding 30°C (86°F). Alternatively, it may be stored for up to 24 hours under refrigeration at 2–8°C, followed by up to 4 hours at room temperature (20–25°C). Protect from light. Do not shake or freeze

Administration:

- Attach the hypodermic stainless steel injection needle immediately prior to SUBCUTaneous administration to prevent needle clogging followed by volume adjustment to 5 mL, if necessary
- Inject HERCEPTIN HYLECTA (trastuzumab and hyaluronidase-oysk) SUBCUTaneously into the thigh over approximately 2–5 minutes. Alternate between the left and right thigh and choose a site at least 2.5 cm from the prior injection site. Never inject into areas where the skin is red, bruised, tender, or hard, or areas where there are moles or scars. Do not administer other medications for SUBCUTaneous use at the same sites

Concomitant medications:

Pre-Administration Medications:

- Use of premedications is not necessary for primary prophylaxis of administration-related systemic reactions. Consider implementation of secondary prophylaxis in patients who have experienced a prior reversible G1/2 reaction with an analgesic, antipyretic, or antihistamine

Adverse events and treatment modifications:

- Refer to the current FDA-approved product label for detailed warnings and treatment modifications for missed doses, cardiomyopathy, pulmonary toxicity, and hypersensitivity reactions. No dose reductions are recommended
- Advise patients that severe administration-related reactions may occur. In the SafeHER and HannaH trials, the incidence of all-grade (G3/4) anaphylaxis or hypersensitivity was 4.2% (<1%) and 9% (1%), respectively

Potential drug interactions:

When feasible, avoid anthracycline-based therapy for up to 7 months after stopping HERCEPTIN HYLECTA (trastuzumab and hyaluronidase-oysk) due to a higher risk of cardiotoxicity. If anthracyclines are used, carefully monitor the patient's cardiac function

VALRUBICIN

VALSTAR (valrubicin) prescribing information. Malvern, PA: Endo Pharmaceuticals Solutions Inc.; November 2012
VALRUBICIN prescribing information. Carlsbad, CA: Leucadia Pharmaceuticals; January 2019

Product Identification, Preparation, Storage, and Stability

- Valrubicin Intravesical Solution, USP, is available generically in single-use, clear, glass vials packaged in cartons containing 4 vials
- Each vial contains a sterile, nonpyrogenic, clear, red, nonaqueous solution of valrubicin at a concentration of 40 mg/mL in 50% polyoxyl castor oil and 50% dehydrated alcohol, USP, without preservatives or other additives
- Store vials under refrigeration at 2–8°C (36–46°F) in the packaging carton. *Do not freeze* valrubicin
- For each instillation, allow 4 vials (a total of 800 mg valrubicin) to warm slowly to room temperature, without heating
  - *Notes:*
    1. Valrubicin Intravesical Solution, USP, contains polyoxyl castor oil, which has been known to cause leaching of DEHP, a hepatotoxic plasticizer, from parenteral product containers and administration sets made from PVC
       a. Valrubicin solutions should be prepared and stored in glass, polypropylene, or polyolefin containers
       b. Only administration sets that do not contain DEHP in the fluid pathway (the surface in contact with a drug-containing solution) should be used to administer valrubicin, for example, polyethylene-lined administration sets
    2. At temperatures <4°C (<39°F), polyoxyl castor oil may begin to form a waxy precipitate
       a. If a vial is found to contain a precipitate, warm the vial in one's hands until the solution is clear
       b. A vial in which particulate matter is still seen after warming should not be used to prepare a dose
- Withdraw 20 mL of valrubicin (800 mg) from the 4 vials and dilute the concentrated product with 55 mL of 0.9% NS to produce 75 mL of a diluted solution (10.7 mg/mL)
- After dilution in 0.9% NS for administration is stable for 12 hours at temperatures up to 25°C (77°F)

Compatibility:
- Valrubicin should not be mixed with other drugs

Recommendations for Drug Administration and Ancillary Care

General:
- See Chapter 43 for comments about use in patients with renal and hepatic dysfunction
- For intraVESICAL administration in the urinary bladder only
  - *Do not administer* by the intraVENous or intraMUSCular routes
- *Caution:* Delay administration ≥2 weeks after transurethral resection or fulguration
- Valrubicin is recommended at a dose of 800 mg administered intravesically once weekly for 6 weeks
  - A urethral catheter should be inserted into a patient's bladder under aseptic conditions, the bladder drained, and 75 mL of diluted valrubicin solution (10.7 mg/mL) instilled slowly via gravity flow over a period of several minutes. The urethral catheter should then be withdrawn
  - The patient should retain the drug for 2 hours before voiding. At the end of a 2-hour retention period, patients should void
- Some patients will be unable to retain the drug for a full two hours and may void earlier than planned
- Patients should be instructed to maintain adequate hydration following treatment

Information for patients:
- Advise patients the major acute toxicities from valrubicin are symptoms related to bladder irritation that may occur during drug instillation and retention and for a limited period following voiding
  - Use valrubicin with caution in patients with severe irritable bladder symptoms: bladder spasm and spontaneous discharge of the intravesical instillate may occur
  - Clamping the urinary catheter is not advised but, if performed, should be executed with caution and under medical supervision
- Red-tinged urine is typical and should be expected during the first 24 hours after valrubicin administration
- Patients should immediately report to their physician prolonged irritable bladder symptoms or prolonged passage of red-colored urine

Contraindications:
- Valrubicin is contraindicated in patients with known hypersensitivity to anthracyclines or polyoxyl castor oil
- Patients with concurrent urinary tract infections should not receive valrubicin
- Valrubicin should not be administered to patients with a small bladder capacity, that is, unable to tolerate a 75-mL fluid instillation

VINBLASTINE SULFATE

VINBLASTINE SULFATE prescribing information. Lake Zurich, IL: Fresenius Kabi USA, LLC.; November 2016

WARNINGS

Caution: This preparation should be administered by individuals experienced in the administration of vinblastine sulfate. It is extremely important that the intravenous needle or catheter be properly positioned before any vinblastine sulfate is injected. Leakage into surrounding tissue during intravenous administration of vinblastine sulfate may cause considerable irritation. If extravasation occurs, the injection should be discontinued immediately, and any remaining portion of the dose should then be introduced into another vein. Local injection of hyaluronidase and the application of moderate heat to the area of leakage help disperse the drug and are thought to minimize discomfort and the possibility of cellulitis

FOR INTRAVENOUS USE ONLY—FATAL IF GIVEN BY OTHER ROUTES ...

[Treatment of patients given intrathecal vinBLAStine sulfate injection]

This product is for intravenous use only. It should be administered by individuals experienced in the administration of vinblastine sulfate. The intrathecal administration of vinblastine sulfate usually results in death. Syringes containing this product should be labeled, using the auxiliary sticker provided to state "FOR INTRAVENOUS USE ONLY—FATAL IF GIVEN BY OTHER ROUTES"

Extemporaneously prepared syringes containing this product must be packaged in an overwrap which is labeled "DO NOT REMOVE COVERING UNTIL MOMENT OF INJECTION. FOR INTRAVENOUS USE ONLY—FATAL IF GIVEN BY OTHER ROUTES"

After inadvertent intrathecal administration of vinca alkaloids, immediate neurosurgical intervention is required in order to prevent ascending paralysis leading to death. In a very small number of patients, life-threatening paralysis and subsequent death was averted but resulted in devastating neurological sequelae, with limited recovery afterward

There are no published cases of survival following intrathecal administration of vinblastine sulfate to base treatment on. However, based on the published management of survival cases involving the related vinca alkaloid vincristine sulfate[73,74,75], if vinblastine sulfate is mistakenly given by the intrathecal route, the following treatment should be initiated **immediately after the injection**:

1. Remove as much CSF as is safely possible through the lumbar access
2. Insertion of an epidural catheter into the subarachnoid space via the intervertebral space above initial lumbar access and CSF irrigation with lactated Ringer's [Injection, USP] solution. Fresh frozen plasma should be requested and, when available, 25 mL should be added to every 1 liter of lactated Ringer's [Injection, USP] solution
3. Insertion of an intraventricular drain or catheter by a neurosurgeon and continuation of CSF irrigation with fluid removal through the lumbar access connected to a closed drainage system. Lactated Ringer's [Injection, USP] solution should be given by continuous infusion at 150 mL/hour, or at a rate of 75 mL/hour when fresh frozen plasma has been added as above

The rate of infusion should be adjusted to maintain a spinal fluid protein level of 150 mg/dL

The following measures have also been used in addition but may not be essential:

Glutamic acid, 10 grams, has been given intravenously over 24 hours, followed by 500 mg three times daily by mouth for 1 month. Folinic acid has been administered intravenously as a 100 mg bolus and then infused at a rate of 25 mg/hour for 24 hours, then bolus doses of 25 mg every 6 hours for 1 week. Pyridoxine has been given at a dose of 50 mg every 8 hours by intravenous infusion over 30 minutes. Their roles in the reduction of neurotoxicity are unclear

Boxed Warnings for VINBLASTINE SULFATE prescribing information. Lake Zurich, IL: Fresenius Kabi USA, LLC.; November 2016

Product Identification, Preparation, Storage, and Stability

VinBLAStine Sulfate Injection:
- VinBLAStine sulfate injection (drug product in solution) is available generically in individually packaged multidose vials. Each milliliter contains vinBLAStine sulfate 1 mg, sodium chloride 9 mg, benzyl alcohol 0.9% (v/v) as a preservative, Q.S. SWFI, at a pH within the range 3.5–5.0

- Store under refrigeration 2–8°C (36–46°F) to assure extended stability
- Protect vinBLAStine sulfate from light by retaining vials in their packaging carton until time of use
- *Discard* partially used vials within 28 days after initial use

- VinBLAStine sulfate may be further diluted with a volume of 0.9% NS, D5W, or LRI that is convenient for administration
- Maximum stability for vinBLAStine sulfate in aqueous solutions is within the pH range 2–4.[76] VinBLAStine (base) may precipitate in solutions with pH >6

Recommendations for Drug Administration and Ancillary Care

Special Dispensing Information: When dispensing vinBLAStine sulfate injection in other than its original container (eg, a syringe), it is imperative that it be packaged in the provided overwrap that bears the following statement: "DO NOT REMOVE COVERING UNTIL MOMENT OF INJECTION. FOR INTRAVENOUS USE ONLY—FATAL IF GIVEN BY OTHER ROUTES"

A syringe containing a specific dose must be labeled, using the auxiliary sticker provided to state: "FOR INTRAVENOUS USE ONLY—FATAL IF GIVEN BY OTHER ROUTES"

General:

- See Chapter 43 for recommendations for use in patients with hepatic dysfunction
- VinBLAStine is for intraVENous use only
  - VinBLAStine sulfate (1 mg/mL) is suitable for direct intraVENous injection, or it may be injected into the tubing of a running intraVENous solution. In either case, injection may be completed in about 1 minute
- Drug loss due to adsorption was demonstrated for vinBLAStine sulfate administration through nylon or positively charged nylon filters[77]
  - VinBLAStine concentration was not affected by filtration through filter membranes made of cellulose acetate, cellulose nitrate/cellulose acetate ester, Teflon, or polysulfone[13,14,33]
- FDA-approved labeling recommends rinsing the syringe and needle by aspirating blood into the syringe after completing drug

injection before the needle is withdrawn. The procedure is intended to minimize the possibility of vinBLAStine extravasation after administration by venipuncture

- VinBLAStine doses should not be further diluted after reconstitution or given intraVENously for prolonged periods (≥15 minutes), unless administration technique is based on continuous infusion through central VADs, implanted "ports," or peripherally inserted central VADs (eg, PICC, SICC)
- Do not administer vinBLAStine by intraVENous injection into a lower extremity, or an extremity in which the circulation is impaired or potentially impaired by such conditions as compressing or invading neoplasm, phlebitis, or varicosity, because of the enhanced potential for treatment-related thrombosis
- *Caution:* VinBLAStine is a vesicant and may produce severe local soft-tissue necrosis if extravasation occurs
  - It is extremely important that the intraVENous needle or catheter be properly positioned before any vinBLAStine sulfate is injected
  - Leakage into surrounding tissue during intraVENous administration of vinBLAStine sulfate may cause considerable irritation
  - If extravasation occurs, the injection should be discontinued immediately, and any remaining portion of the dose should then be introduced into another vein
  - Local injection of hyaluronidase and the application of moderate heat to the area

of leakage help disperse the drug and minimize discomfort and the possibility of cellulitis

Potential drug interactions:

- Concomitant administration of phenytoin and vinBLAStine sulfate has been associated with decreased blood concentrations of the anticonvulsant and, consequently, increased seizure activity
  - Phenytoin dosage adjustment should be based on serial blood concentration monitoring
- VinBLAStine metabolism is mediated by CYP3A subfamily enzymes
  - Exercise caution in treating patients with vinBLAStine who are using drugs known to inhibit CYP3A subfamily enzymes and in patients with impaired hepatic function
    - Consult recommendations for vinBLAStine use in hepatic impairment
  - Enhanced toxicity has been reported in patients who received erythromycin, a CYP3A subfamily enzyme inhibitor, and vinBLAStine concomitantly

Inadvertent exposure:

- If accidental eye contamination occurs, severe irritation, or, if vinBLAStine was delivered under pressure, corneal ulceration may result
  - An exposed eye should be immediately and thoroughly irrigated with water
- 5% sodium hypochlorite bleach has been used to inactivate vinBLAStine sulfate spills on environmental surfaces[78]

VINCRISTINE SULFATE

VinCRIStine sulfate prescribing information. Lake Forest, IL: Hospira, Inc.; July 2020

WARNINGS

Caution—This preparation should be administered by individuals experienced in the administration of Vincristine Sulfate Injection, USP. It is extremely important that the intravenous needle or catheter be properly positioned before any vincristine is injected. Leakage into surrounding tissue during intravenous administration of Vincristine Sulfate Injection, USP, may cause considerable irritation. If extravasation occurs, the injection should be discontinued immediately, and any remaining portion of the dose should then be introduced into another vein. Local injection of hyaluronidase and the application of moderate heat to the area of leakage help disperse the drug and are thought to minimize discomfort and the possibility of cellulitis

FOR INTRAVENOUS USE ONLY—FATAL IF GIVEN BY OTHER ROUTES

See OVERDOSAGE section for the treatment of patients given intrathecal Vincristine Sulfate Injection, USP

WARNINGS

This preparation is for intravenous use only. It should be administered by individuals experienced in the administration of vincristine sulfate injection. The intrathecal administration of vincristine sulfate injection usually results in death

To reduce the potential for fatal medication errors due to incorrect route of administration, Vincristine Sulfate Injection should be diluted in a flexible plastic container and prominently labeled as indicated "FOR INTRAVENOUS USE ONLY—FATAL IF GIVEN BY OTHER ROUTES"

[Excerpted from "OVERDOSAGE" section:]

Treatment of patients following intrathecal administration of vincristine sulfate injection has included immediate removal of spinal fluid and flushing with Lactated Ringer's [Injection, USP], as well as other solutions and has not prevented ascending paralysis and death. In one case, progressive paralysis in an adult was arrested by the following treatment **initiated immediately after the intrathecal injection:**

1. As much spinal fluid was removed as could be safely done through lumbar access
2. The subarachnoid space was flushed with Lactated Ringer's [Injection, USP] ... infused continuously through a catheter in a cerebral lateral ventricle at the rate of 150 mL/h. The fluid was removed through a lumbar access
3. As soon as fresh frozen plasma became available, the fresh frozen plasma, 25 mL, diluted in 1 L of Lactated Ringer's [Injection, USP] ... was infused through the cerebral ventricular catheter at the rate of 75 mL/h with removal through the lumbar access. The rate of infusion was adjusted to maintain a protein level in the spinal fluid of 150 mg/dL
4. Glutamic acid, 10 [grams] ... was given intravenously over 24 hours followed by 500 mg 3 times daily by mouth for 1 month or until neurological dysfunction stabilized. The role of glutamic acid in this treatment is not certain and may not be essential

Boxed Warnings for VinCRIStine sulfate prescribing information. Lake Forest, IL: Hospira, Inc.; July 2020

Product Identification, Preparation, Storage, and Stability

- VinCRIStine sulfate injection, USP, is available generically (as of November 16, 2020 only from Hospira, Inc) in individually packaged single-use vials containing either 1 mg (NDC 61703-0309-06) or 2 mg (NDC 61703-0309-16) of vinCRIStine sulfate, both in a concentration of 1 mg/mL
- Each milliliter of VinCRIStine sulfate injection, USP, contains vinCRIStine sulfate 1 mg, mannitol 100 mg, and Q.S. SWFI. Sulfuric acid or sodium hydroxide may have been added to maintain product pH within the range 4–5
- VinCRIStine sulfate injection, USP, does not contain antimicrobial preservatives
- Store VinCRIStine sulfate injection, USP, vials upright under refrigeration at 2–8°C (36–46°F) in the carton in which vials are

packaged to protect the medication from light until it is used
- VinCRIStine should be diluted with a volume of 0.9% NS or D5W that is convenient for administration in a flexible plastic container and prominently labeled as indicated "FOR INTRAVENOUS USE ONLY—FATAL IF GIVEN BY OTHER ROUTES"
- *Avoid admixture* with other solutions
    - Maximum stability for vinCRIStine sulfate in aqueous solutions is within the pH range 4–6[79]
    - Product labeling recommends not preparing vinCRIStine in solutions that raise or lower the pH outside the range 3.5–5.5
    - After dilution with 0.9% NS to concentrations within the range,

0.0015–0.08 mg/mL, vinCRIStine sulfate solutions are stable for up to 24 hours when protected from light or up to 8 hours under normal light at 25°C (77°F)
    - After dilution with D5W to concentrations within the range, 0.0015–0.08 mg/mL, vinCRIStine sulfate solutions are stable for up to 4 hours under normal light at 25°C (77°F)

Selected incompatibility:
- When used in combination with asparaginase, vinCRIStine should be given 12–24 hours *before* asparaginase to minimize toxicity. Administering asparaginase before vinCRIStine may decrease vinCRIStine's hepatic clearance

Recommendations for Drug Administration and Ancillary Care

General:
- See Chapter 43 for recommendations for use in patients with hepatic dysfunction
- VinCRIStine is *for intraVENous use only*
- VinCRIStine sulfate injection *should not be given to patients* while they are receiving radiation therapy through fields that include the liver
- VinCRIStine sulfate diluted to a concentration of 25 µg/mL in 0.9% NS exhibited a 9% loss of potency due to adsorption during the first 60 min of delivery through PVC administration set tubing, but negligible loss during delivery through a polyethylene administration set under identical conditions[77]
    - The concentration of vinCRIStine sulfate delivered through the PVC tubing returned to full concentration at 1.5 h after drug delivery began (samples for analysis were collected every 30 min)[77]
- *Do not filter* vinCRIStine solutions:
    - Administration through cellulose acetate, cellulose nitrate, cellulose ester, nylon, or Teflon filters has demonstrated variable drug loss because of absorption. In general, the extent of drug loss as a result of filtration is inversely proportional to the concentration of vinCRIStine in solution

- *Caution:* VinCRIStine is a vesicant and may produce severe local soft-tissue necrosis if extravasation occurs
    - It is extremely important that the intraVENous needle or catheter be properly positioned before any vinCRIStine sulfate is injected
    - Leakage into surrounding tissue during intraVENous administration of vinCRIStine sulfate may cause considerable irritation
    - If extravasation occurs, the infusion should be discontinued immediately, and any remaining portion of the dose should then be introduced into another vein
    - Local injection of hyaluronidase and the application of moderate heat to the area of leakage help disperse the drug and minimize discomfort and the possibility of cellulitis

Potential drug interactions:
- Concomitant administration of phenytoin and vinCRIStine sulfate has been associated with decreased blood concentrations of the anticonvulsant, and, consequently, increased seizure activity
    - Phenytoin dosage adjustment should be based on serial blood concentration monitoring

- VinCRIStine metabolism is mediated by CYP3A subfamily enzymes
    - Concurrent administration of vinCRIStine sulfate with itraconazole (a known potent inhibitor of CYP3A subfamily enzymes) has been reported to cause an earlier onset and/or an increased severity of neuromuscular adverse effects presumably related to inhibition of vinCRIStine metabolism
    - Exercise caution in treating patients with vinCRIStine who are using drugs known to inhibit CYP3A subfamily enzymes and in patients with impaired hepatic function
        - Consult recommendations for vinCRIStine use in hepatic impairment

Inadvertent exposure:
- If accidental eye contamination occurs, severe irritation, or, if vinCRIStine was delivered under pressure, corneal ulceration may result
    - An eye exposed to vinCRIStine should be washed with water immediately and thoroughly
- 5% sodium hypochlorite bleach has been used to inactivate vinCRIStine sulfate spills on environmental surfaces[78]

VINCRISTINE SULFATE LIPOSOME INJECTION

Marqibo (vinCRIStine sulfate LIPOSOME injection) prescribing information. East Windsor, NJ: Acrotech Biopharma LLC; June 2020

WARNING: FOR INTRAVENOUS USE ONLY—FATAL IF GIVEN BY OTHER ROUTES

- Marqibo is for intravenous use only and fatal if given by other routes. Death has occurred with intrathecal administration ...
- Marqibo (vincristine sulfate LIPOSOME injection) has different dosage recommendations than vincristine sulfate injection. Verify drug name and dose prior to preparation and administration to avoid overdosage ...

Boxed Warning for Marqibo (vinCRIStine sulfate LIPOSOME injection) prescribing information. East Windsor, NJ: Acrotech Biopharma LLC; June 2020

Product Identification, Preparation, Storage, and Stability

- Marqibo (vinCRIStine sulfate liposome injection) is vinCRIStine encapsulated in liposomes
  - The active ingredient in Marqibo is vinCRIStine sulfate
  - The lipid components from which liposomes are formed are sphingomyelin and cholesterol at a molar ratio of approximately 60:40 (mol:mol)
- After preparation, each vial of Marqibo contains 5 mg vinCRIStine sulfate with mannitol 500 mg, sphingomyelin 73.5 mg, cholesterol 29.5 mg, sodium citrate 36 mg, citric acid 38 mg, sodium phosphate 355 mg, and sodium chloride 225 mg
- Marqibo appears as a white to off-white, translucent suspension, essentially free of visible foreign matter and aggregates
  - Approximate liposome mean diameter is 100 nm with >95% of vinCRIStine encapsulated in the liposomes
- A Marqibo Kit (NDC 72893-008-03) includes the following components:
  - VinCRIStine sulfate injection, USP
    - Each vial contains 5 mg/5 mL vinCRIStine sulfate (equivalent to 4.5 mg/5 mL vinCRIStine base) and 500 mg/5 mL mannitol; NDC 72893-012-05
  - Sphingomyelin/cholesterol liposome injection (103 mg/mL)
    - Each vial contains sphingomyelin 73.5 mg/mL, cholesterol 29.5 mg/mL, citric acid 33.6 mg/mL, sodium citrate 35.4 mg/mL, and ethanol ≤0.1%; NDC 72893-011-05
  - Sodium phosphate injection
    - Each vial contains dibasic sodium phosphate 355 mg/25 mL (14.2 mg/mL) and sodium chloride 225 mg/25 mL; NDC 72893-010-05
  - Flotation ring
  - Overlabel for sodium phosphate injection vial containing constituted Marqibo (vinCRIStine sulfate LIPOSOME injection), 5 mg/31 mL (0.16 mg/mL)
  - Infusion bag label
- Store Marqibo Kits under refrigeration at 2–8°C (36–46°F). *Do not freeze* the product

Product Preparation and Materials Required to Prepare Marqibo

1. Marqibo Kit
2. Water bath* or block heater[†]
3. Calibrated thermometer (scale graduations from 0–100°C [32–212°F])*
4. Calibrated electronic timer*
5. One sterile needle or another suitable venting device equipped with a sterile 0.2-μm filter
6. One 1-mL- or 3-mL-capacity sterile syringe with needle
7. One 5-mL-capacity sterile syringe with needle
8. Tongs[‡]

---

*The manufacturer will provide the water bath, calibrated thermometer, and calibrated electronic timer to the medical facility at the initial order of Marqibo and will replace them every 2 years. (Statement reprinted from Marqibo product label, June 2020; Acrotech Biopharma LLC)

[†]The manufacturer will provide the block heater to the medical facility at the initial order of Marqibo. The block heater will be replaced every 5 years. (Statement reprinted from Marqibo product label, June 2020; Acrotech Biopharma LLC)

[‡]The manufacturer will provide tongs to the medical facility at the initial order of Marqibo. (Statement reprinted from Marqibo product label, June 2020; Acrotech Biopharma LLC)

(continued)

Product Identification, Preparation, Storage, and Stability (continued)

General instructions:

- Call [1-888-292-9617] with questions about preparing Marqibo
- Aseptic technique must be strictly observed as no preservative or bacteriostatic agent is present in Marqibo
- Marqibo takes approximately 60–90 minutes to prepare
  - Persons who prepare Marqibo should have adequate time to prepare the drug without interruption or distraction because of the extensive monitoring of temperature and time required for preparation
- Deviations in temperature, time, and preparation procedures may fail to ensure proper encapsulation of vinCRIStine sulfate into liposomes
  - In the event preparation deviates from the instructions that follow, the components of a kit affected by the deviation should be discarded and a new Marqibo Kit used to prepare a dose

Engineering controls:

- The preparation steps that involve mixing sodium phosphate injection, sphingomyelin/cholesterol liposome injection, and VinCRIStine sulfate injection must be performed within a biologic safety cabinet or with engineering controls and by established safety procedures appropriate for the aseptic preparation of sterile injectable hazardous drugs
- The preparation steps that involve placing a vial in a water bath must be done outside of the aseptic preparation area
- *Do not use* with inline filters when preparing Marqibo. *Do not mix* Marqibo with other drugs

Preparation—nonaseptic environment:

Water Bath Process	Block Heater Process
1. Fill a water bath with water to a level ≥8 cm (≥3.2 inches) measured from the bottom and maintain this minimum water level throughout the procedure • The water bath will remain outside of an aseptic product preparation environment	1. Arrange the 3 heater blocks such that the block holding the constitution vial is centered between the two other blank heater blocks • The block heater will remain outside of an aseptic product preparation environment
2. Place a calibrated thermometer in the water bath to monitor water temperature and leave it in the water bath until the procedure has been completed	2. Place a calibrated thermometer in the block opening adjacent to the vial well to monitor temperature and leave it in the block opening until the procedure has been completed
3. Preheat the water bath to 63–67°C (145.4–152.6°F). Using the calibrated thermometer, maintain this water temperature until preparation is completed	3. Turn on the block heater and set the controller to 75°C. Using the calibrated thermometer, verify the block temperature has reached 73–77°C (163.4–170.6°F). Allow the heating block to equilibrate at this temperature range for 15 minutes and then maintain the temperature of the block within this range until preparation is completed

Preparation—aseptic environment:

1. Visually inspect each vial in the Marqibo Kit for particulate matter and discoloration prior to preparation, whenever solution and container permit. Do not use component products if a precipitate or foreign matter is present
2. Remove the caps from all vials and swab the vial septa (injection ports) with alcohol
3. Vent the vial containing sodium phosphate injection with a sterile venting needle equipped with a sterile 0.2-μm filter or another suitable venting device
   - Position the venting needle tip well above the liquid level before adding sphingomyelin/cholesterol liposome injection and VinCRIStine sulfate injection
4. With a syringe, transfer 1 mL of sphingomyelin/cholesterol liposome injection into the vial labeled sodium phosphate injection
5. With a different syringe, transfer 5 mL of VinCRIStine sulfate injection into the vial labeled sodium phosphate injection
6. Remove the venting needle from the vial containing the mixture of vinCRIStine sulfate, sphingomyelin/cholesterol liposome, and sodium phosphate, and gently invert the vial 5 times to mix. *Do not shake* the vial
7. If using the water bath method of preparation, then fit the flotation ring around the neck of the vial containing the mixture (*NOTE:* Skip this step if using the block heater method of preparation)

Preparation—nonaseptic environment:

Water Bath Process	Block Heater Process
1. Confirm the water bath temperature is 63–67°C (145.4–152.6°F) using the calibrated thermometer	1. Confirm the block heater temperature is 73–77°C (163.4–170.6°F) using the calibrated thermometer

(continued)

Product Identification, Preparation, Storage, and Stability (continued)

Water Bath Process	Block Heater Process
2. Remove from the aseptic preparation environment the vial containing the mixture of vinCRIStine sulfate, sphingomyelin/cholesterol liposome, and sodium phosphate, and place it into the water bath for 10 minutes using the calibrated electronic timer to measure the passage of time	2. Remove from the aseptic preparation environment the vial containing the mixture of vinCRIStine sulfate, sphingomyelin/cholesterol liposome, and sodium phosphate, and place it into the block heater for 18 minutes using the calibrated electronic timer to measure the passage of time
3. Monitor the water bath temperature to ensure the temperature is maintained at 63–67°C (145.4–152.6°F)	3. Monitor the block heater temperature to ensure the temperature is maintained at 73–77°C (163.4–170.6°F)
4. After placing the vial containing the vinCRIStine sulfate, sphingomyelin/cholesterol liposome, and sodium phosphate mixture into the water bath, record the "constitution start time" and water temperature on the Marqibo overlabel	4. After placing the vial containing the vinCRIStine sulfate, sphingomyelin/cholesterol liposome, and sodium phosphate mixture into the block heater, record the "constitution start time" and block heater temperature on the Marqibo overlabel
5. At the end of 10 minutes, confirm the water temperature is 63–67°C (145.4–152.6°F) using the calibrated thermometer, remove the vial from the water bath (use tongs to prevent burns), and remove the flotation ring from the vial	5. At the end of 18 minutes, confirm the block heater temperature is 73–77°C (163.4–170.6°F) using the calibrated thermometer and then remove the vial from the block heater (use tongs to prevent burns)
6. Record the final constitution time and the water temperature on the Marqibo overlabel	6. Record the final constitution time and the block heater temperature on the Marqibo overlabel
7. Dry the exterior of the vial containing the vinCRIStine sulfate, sphingomyelin/cholesterol liposome, and sodium phosphate mixture (subsequently referred to as "constituted Marqibo") with a clean paper towel, apply the Marqibo overlabel to the vial, and then, gently invert the vial 5 times to mix. *Do not shake* the vial	7. Apply the Marqibo overlabel to the vial containing the vinCRIStine sulfate, sphingomyelin/cholesterol liposome, and sodium phosphate mixture (subsequently referred to as "constituted Marqibo"), and then, gently invert the vial 5 times to mix. *Do not shake* the vial
8. Permit constituted Marqibo to equilibrate to controlled room temperature (15–30°C [59–86°F]) for at least 30 minutes	8. Permit constituted Marqibo to equilibrate to controlled room temperature (15–30°C [59–86°F]) for at least 30 minutes
9. After preparation is completed, store constituted Marqibo at controlled room temperature (15–30°C [59–86°F]) for no longer than 12 hours	9. After preparation is completed, store constituted Marqibo at controlled room temperature (15–30°C [59–86°F]) for no longer than 12 hours

Preparation—aseptic environment:

1. Return the vial containing constituted Marqibo to the aseptic preparation environment and swab the vial septum with alcohol
2. Calculate a patient's Marqibo dose based on their actual body surface area and the volume of Marqibo that corresponds to that volume
   • Constituted Marqibo contains 5 mg of vinCRIStine sulfate per 31 mL of solution (0.16 mg/mL)
3. From a prefilled parenteral product container containing a nominal volume of 100 mL of either 0.9% NS or D5W, withdraw a volume of solution corresponding to a patient's Marqibo dose
4. Transfer from a vial containing constituted Marqibo the volume of drug needed for a patient's dose and inject it into the container of solution prepared in the previous step to produce a diluted solution of constituted Marqibo with a total volume of 100 mL
5. Label the diluted drug product container according to applicable regulatory requirements

Preparation—nonaseptic environment:

1. Empty, clean, and dry the water bath after each use (does not apply if using the block heater method of preparation)

Recommendations for Drug Administration and Ancillary Care

General:

• Dosage recommendations for VinCRIStine sulfate liposome injection (2.25 mg/m² administer intraVENously over 1 hour once every 7 days) are different than those for nonliposomal vinCRIStine sulfate injection
• Verify drug name and dose prior to preparation and administration to avoid overdose

■ *Warnings: For intraVENous use only. Fatal if given by other routes*
• Administration should be completed within 12 hours after preparation was initiated

Potential drug interactions:

• VinCRIStine is a substrate for CYP3A subfamily enzymes; therefore, concomitant use of strong CYP3A inhibitors and inducers should be avoided

• VinCRIStine is also a substrate for the MDR1 transport protein (*AKA* ABCB1, P-glycoprotein [P-gp])
  ■ In the absence of information to guide concomitant use of Marqibo with potent MDR1 inhibitors or inducers, a conservative utilization strategy recommends avoiding concomitant use
• Marqibo is expected to interact with drugs known to interact with nonliposomal VinCRIStine sulfate

VINORELBINE TARTRATE

Vinorelbine Injection prescribing information. Schaumburg, IL: SAGENT Pharmaceuticals; April 2020

WARNING: MYELOSUPPRESSION

- Severe myelosuppression resulting in serious infection, septic shock, hospitalization, and death can occur ...
- Decrease the dose or withhold vinorelbine in accord with recommended dose modifications ...

Boxed Warning for Vinorelbine Injection prescribing information. Schaumburg, IL: SAGENT Pharmaceuticals; April 2020

Product Identification, Preparation, Storage, and Stability

- Vinorelbine injection, USP, is available in individually packaged single-use, glass vials containing vinorelbine tartrate equivalent to 10 mg vinorelbine/mL as a sterile, nonpyrogenic, preservative-free, clear, colorless to pale yellow solution in SWFI at a pH of approximately 3.5
  - Commercially available presentations include vials containing 10 mg vinorelbine in 1 mL or 50 mg vinorelbine in 5 mL

- Store intact vials of vinorelbine injection, USP, under refrigeration at 2–8°C (36–46°F), and in their packaging carton to protect the product from light. *Do not freeze* vinorelbine injection, USP
- Intact unused vials of vinorelbine injection, USP, are stable at temperatures up to 25°C (77°F) for up to 72 hours
- Vinorelbine injection, USP, must be diluted before administration with a compatible parenteral solution:

- In a parenteral product container (bag), dilute vinorelbine tartrate to a concentration within the range 0.5–2 mg/mL with 0.9% NS, D5W, 0.45% NaCl, D5W/0.45% NaCl, RI, or LRI
- Vinorelbine injection, USP, may be used for up to 24 hours under normal room light when stored at 5–30°C (41–86°F) in PVC containers

---

Recommendations for Drug Administration and Ancillary Care

General:

- See Chapter 43 for recommendations for use in patients with hepatic dysfunction
- Diluted vinorelbine should be administered intraVENously into the side port of a freely flowing intraVENous solution closest to the parenteral product container as follows:[80]
  - In a minibag, diluted to 0.5–2 mg/mL, administer by intraVENously over 6–10 minutes
- After vinorelbine administration is completed, flush the patient's VAD or administration set connected to a VAD

with ≥75 mL to 125 mL of a solution compatible with vinorelbine (eg, 0.9% NS, D5W, 0.45% NaCl, D5W/0.45% NaCl, RI, or LRI)

Caution:

- Vinorelbine is a substrate for metabolism catalyzed by CYP3A subfamily enzymes. Concurrent vinorelbine tartrate use with an inhibitor of this metabolic pathway or in patients with impaired hepatic function may cause an earlier onset and increased severity of adverse effects

- Administration of vinorelbine to patients who previously experienced soft-tissue damage from radiation therapy may result in radiation recall reactions within the areas that previously sustained injury

Inadvertent exposure:

- In case of contact with skin or mucous membranes, immediately wash the affected areas thoroughly with soap and water
- An eye exposed to vinorelbine tartrate should be washed with water immediately and thoroughly

ZIV-AFLIBERCEPT

ZALTRAP (ziv-aflibercept) prescribing information. Bridgewater, NJ: Sanofi-Aventis U.S. LLC; June 2020

Product Identification, Preparation, Storage, and Stability

- ZALTRAP is a sterile, clear, colorless to pale yellow, nonpyrogenic, preservative-free, solution supplied in single-use vials containing ziv-aflibercept 25 mg/mL in polysorbate 20 0.1%, sodium chloride 100 mmol/L, sodium citrate 5 mmol/L, sodium phosphate 5 mmol/L, and sucrose 20%, in SWFI, at a pH of 6.2
  - Commercial ZALTRAP (ziv-aflibercept 25 mg/mL) is available in 2 presentations, including:
    - ziv-Aflibercept 100 mg/4 mL, carton containing 1 single-use vial, NDC 0024-5840-01

- ziv-Aflibercept 200 mg/8 mL, carton containing 1 single-use vial, NDC 0024-5841-01
- Store unopened vials under refrigeration between 2° and 8°C (35.6° and 46.4°F) in the original packaging carton to protect ZALTRAP from light
- *Do not* use the product if the solution is discolored or cloudy or the solution contains particles
- *Do not* reenter a vial after initial entry
- Withdraw an amount of drug appropriate for a patient's dose and dilute it in a volume of 0.9% NS or D5W sufficient to produce

a final concentration of ziv-aflibercept within the range 0.6–8 mg/mL
  - Discard any unused portion of drug left in a vial
- Compatible product containers include those made of polyolefin or PVC plasticized with DEHP
- Store diluted ziv-aflibercept under refrigeration (2–8°C [35.6–46.4°F]) for up to 24 hours or at controlled room temperature 20°C to 25°C (68°F to 77°F) for up to 8 hours.
  - Discard any unused portion of a dose remaining at the end of treatment

Recommendations for Drug Administration and Ancillary Care

General:

- After dilution, ziv-aflibercept is administered intraVENously over 1 hour every 2 weeks before any component of the FOLFIRI combination chemotherapy regimen
- Administer ziv-aflibercept through an administration set made of 1 of the following materials:
  - PVC containing DEHP
  - DEHP-free PVC containing trioctyl-trimellitate (TOTM)
  - polypropylene
  - polyethylene-lined PVC
  - polyurethane
- Administer ziv-aflibercept through a polyethersulfone filter with pore size equal to 0.2 μm
  - Do not use filters made of polyvinylidene fluoride (PVDF) or nylon
- Do not mix ziv-aflibercept in the same container with other medicinal products or administer it through an intraVENous VAD at the same time as other medicinal products

- Discontinue ziv-aflibercept for:
  - Severe hemorrhage
  - Gastrointestinal perforation
  - Compromised wound healing
  - Fistula formation
  - Hypertensive crisis or hypertensive encephalopathy
  - Arterial thromboembolic events
  - Nephrotic syndrome or thrombotic microangiopathy
  - Reversible posterior leukoencephalopathy syndrome
- Temporarily suspend ziv-aflibercept:
- At least 4 weeks prior to elective surgery
  - For recurrent or severe hypertension, until controlled. Upon resuming treatment, permanently decrease the ziv-aflibercept dosage to 2 mg/kg
  - For proteinuria of 2 g/24 hours. Resume when proteinuria is <2 g/24 hours. For recurrent proteinuria, withhold ziv-aflibercept until proteinuria is <2 g/24 hours, and then, permanently decrease the ziv-aflibercept dosage to 2 mg/kg

- For toxicities related to irinotecan, fluorouracil, or leucovorin, refer to current prescribing information for those products

Selected Precautions

- **See current FDA-approved product label for detailed warnings and precautions**
- Patients treated with ZALTRAP have an increased risk of hemorrhage, including severe and sometimes fatal hemorrhagic events
- Gastrointestinal (GI) perforation including fatal GI perforation can occur in patients receiving ZALTRAP
- Withhold ZALTRAP for at least 4 weeks prior to elective surgery. Do not administer ZALTRAP for at least 4 weeks after major surgery and until wounds have adequately healed. For minor surgery such as central venous access port placement, biopsy, and tooth extraction, ZALTRAP may be initiated/resumed once the surgical wound is fully healed

General Reference

Trissell LA. Handbook on Injectable Drugs. 20th ed. Bethesda, MD: American Society of Health-System Pharmacists; 2018

Drug-Specific References

1 Heywood GR et al. Hypersensitivity reactions to chemotherapy agents in patients receiving chemoimmunotherapy with high-dose interleukin 2. J Natl Cancer Inst 1995;87:915–922

2 Kruit WH et al. Cardiotoxicity as a dose-limiting factor in a schedule of high dose bolus therapy with interleukin-2 and alpha-interferon. An unexpectedly frequent complication. Cancer 1994;74:2850–2856

3 Mier JW et al. Inhibition of interleukin-2-induced tumor necrosis factor release by dexamethasone: prevention of an acquired neutrophil chemotaxis defect and differential suppression of interleukin-2-associated side effects [see comment]. Blood 1990;76:1933–1940. Comment in: Blood 1991;78:1389–1390

4 Oldham RK et al. Contrast medium "recalls" interleukin-2 toxicity. J Clin Oncol 1990;8:942–943

5 Zukiwski AA et al. Increased incidence of hypersensitivity to iodine-containing radiographic contrast media after interleukin-2 administration. Cancer 1990;65:1521–1524

6 Abi-Aad AS et al. Metastatic renal cell cancer: interleukin-2 toxicity induced by contrast agent injection. J Immunother 1991;10:292–295

7 Fishman JE et al. Atypical contrast reactions associated with systemic interleukin-2 therapy. AJR Am J Roentgenol 1991;156:833–834

8 Choyke PL et al. Delayed reactions to contrast media after interleukin-2 immunotherapy. Radiology 1992;183:111–114

9 Shulman KL et al. Adverse reactions to intravenous contrast media in patients treated with interleukin-2. J Immunother Emphasis Tumor Immunol 1993;13:208–212

10 Sanz MA et al. Management of acute promyelocytic leukemia: updated recommendations from an expert panel of the European LeukemiaNet. Blood 2019;133:1630–1643

11 Koberda M et al. Stability of bleomycin sulfate reconstituted in 5% dextrose injection or 0.9% sodium chloride injection stored in glass vials or polyvinyl chloride containers. Am J Hosp Pharm 1990;47:2528–2529

12 De Vroe C et al. A study on the stability of three antineoplastic drugs and on their sorption by i.v. delivery systems and end-line filters. Int J Pharm 1990;65:49–56

13 Butler DL et al. Effect of inline filtration on the potency of low-dose drugs. Am J Hosp Pharm 1980;37:935–941

14 Pavlik EJ et al. Sensitivity to anticancer agents in vitro: standardizing the cytotoxic response and characterizing the sensitivities of a reference cell line. Gynecol Oncol 1982;14:243–261

15 Xu QA et al. Stability of busulfan injection admixtures in 5% dextrose injection and 0.9% sodium chloride injection. J Oncol Pharm Pract 1996;2:101–105

16 Arbus MH. Room temperature stability guidelines for carmustine. Am J Hosp Pharm 1988;45:531

17 Trissel LA et al. Drug compatibility with new polyolefin infusion solution containers. Am J Health Syst Pharm 2006;63:2379–2382

18 Hadji-Minaglou-Gonzalvez MF et al. Effects of temperature, solution composition, and type of container on the stability and absorption of carmustine. Clin Ther 1992;14:821–824

19 Favier M et al. Stability of carmustine in polyvinyl chloride bags and polyethylene-lined trilayer plastic containers. Am J Health Syst Pharm 2001;58:238–241

20 Levin VA, Levin EM. Dissolution and stability of carmustine in the absence of ethanol. Sel Cancer Ther 1989;5:33–35

21 Tepe P et al. BCNU stability as a function of ethanol concentration and temperature. J Neurooncol 1991;10:121–127

22 Colvin M et al. Stability of carmustine in the presence of sodium bicarbonate. Am J Hosp Pharm 1980;37:677–678

23 Fredriksson K et al. Stability of carmustine—kinetics and compatibility during administration. Acta Pharm Suec 1986;23:115–124

24 Cheung YW et al. Stability of cisplatin, iproplatin, carboplatin, and tetraplatin in commonly used intravenous solutions. Am J Hosp Pharm 1987;44:124–130

25 Horton JK, Stevens MFG. A new light on the photo-decomposition of the antitumour drug DTIC. J Pharm Pharmacol 1981;33:808–811

26 Shetty BV et al. Degradation of dacarbazine in aqueous solution. J Pharm Biomed Anal 1992;10:675–683

27 Dorr RT et al. Experimental dacarbazine antitumor activity and skin toxicity in relation to light exposure and pharmacologic antidotes. Cancer Treat Rep 1987;71:267–272

28 Baird GM, Willoughby MLN. Photodegradation of dacarbazine [letter]. Lancet 1978;2:681

29 Shukla VS. A device to prevent photodegradation of dacarbazine (DTIC). Clin Radiol 1980;31:239–240

30 El Aatmani M et al. Stability of dacarbazine in amber glass vials and polyvinyl chloride bags. Am J Health Syst Pharm 2002;59:1351–1356

31 Kirk B. The evaluation of a light-protective giving set. The photosensitivity of intravenous dacarbazine solutions. Intensive Ther Clin Monit 1987;78, 81, 82, 85, 86

32 Crevar GE, Slotnick IJ. A note on the stability of actinomycin D. J Pharm Pharmacol 1964;16:429–432

33 Pavlik EJ et al. Properties of anticancer agents relevant to in vitro determinations of human tumor cell sensitivity. Cancer Chemother Pharmacol 1983;11:8–15

34 Rusmin S et al. Effect of inline filtration on the potency of drugs administered intravenously. Am J Hosp Pharm 1977;34:1071–1074

35 Wood MJ et al. Stability of doxorubicin, daunorubicin and epirubicin in plastic syringes and minibags. J Clin Pharm Ther 1990;15:279–289

36 Wood MJ et al. Photodegradation of doxorubicin, daunorubicin and epirubicin measured by high-performance liquid chromatography. J Clin Pharm Ther 1990;15:291–300

37 Walker S et al. Doxorubicin stability in syringes and glass vials and evaluation of chemical contamination. Can J Hosp Pharm 1991;44:71–78, 88

38 Lokich J. Doxil extravasation injury: a case report. Ann Oncol 1999;10:735–736

39 Driessen O et al. Adsorption of fluorouracil on glass surfaces. J Pharm Sci 1978;67:1494–1495

40 Benvenuto JA et al. Stability and compatibility of antitumor agents in glass and plastic containers. Am J Hosp Pharm 1981;38:1914–1918

41 Tempero M et al. Randomized phase II comparison of dose-intense gemcitabine: thirty-minute infusion and fixed dose rate infusion in patients with pancreatic adenocarcinoma [see comment]. J Clin Oncol 2003;21:3402–8. Comment in: J Clin Oncol 2003;21:3383, 3384

42 Peters GJ et al. Clinical phase I and pharmacology study of gemcitabine (2, 2-difluorodeoxycytidine) administered in a two-weekly schedule. J Chemother 2007;19:212–221

43 Gusella M et al. Equilibrative nucleoside transporter 1 genotype, cytidine deaminase activity and age predict gemcitabine plasma clearance in patients with solid tumours. Br J Clin Pharmacol 2011;71:437–444

44 Trissel LA, Martinez JF. Idarubicin hydrochloride turbidity versus incompatibility. Am J Hosp Pharm 1993;50:1134–1137

45 Li WY, Koda RT. Stability of irinotecan hydrochloride in aqueous solutions. Am J Health Syst Pharm 2002;59:539–544

46 Dodds HM et al. Photodegradation of irinotecan (CPT-11) in aqueous solutions: identification of fluorescent products and influence of solution composition. J Pharm Sci 1997;86:1410–1416

47 Thiesen J, Krämer I. Physicochemical stability of irinotecan injection concentrate and diluted infusion solutions in PVC bags. J Oncol Pharm Pract 2000;6:115–121

48 Akimoto K et al. Photodegradation reactions of CPT-11, a derivative of camptothecin. II. Photodegradation behaviour of CPT-11 in aqueous solution. Drug Stability 1996;1:141–146

49 Dodds HM et al. The detection of photodegradation products of irinotecan (CPT-11, Campto, Camptosar), in clinical studies, using high-performance liquid chromatography/atmospheric pressure chemical ionisation/mass spectrometry. J Pharm Biomed Anal 1998;17:785–792

50 MESNA. In: Trissel LA et al, eds. NCI Investigational Drugs, Pharmaceutical Data 1987. NIH Publication 88-2141 ed. Bethesda (MD): U.S. Department of Health and Human Services, Public Health Service, National Institutes of Health, National Cancer Institute; 1987:57, 58

51 Dorr RT, Liddil JD. Stability of mitomycin C in different infusion fluids: compatibility with heparin and glucocorticosteroids. J Oncol Pharm Pract 1995;1:19–24

52 Beijnen JH et al. Qualitative aspects of the degradation of mitomycins in alkaline solution. J Pharm Biomed Anal 1985;3:71–79

53 Beijnen HN, Underberg WJM. Degradation of mitomycin C in acidic solution. Int J Pharm 1985;24:219–229

54 Waugh WN et al. Stability, compatibility, and plasticizer extraction of taxol (NSC-125973) injection diluted in infusion solutions and stored in various containers. Am J Hosp Pharm 1991;48:1520–1524

55 Pearson SD, Trissel LA. Leaching of diethylhexyl phthalate from polyvinyl chloride containers by selected drugs and formulation components. Am J Hosp Pharm 1993;50:1405–1409

56 Allwood MC, Martin H. The extraction of diethylhexylphthalate (DEHP) from polyvinyl chloride components of intravenous infusion containers and administration sets by paclitaxel injection. Int J Pharm 1996;127:65–71

57 Mazzo DJ et al. Compatibility of docetaxel and paclitaxel in intravenous solutions with polyvinyl chloride infusion materials. Am J Health Syst Pharm 1997;54:566–569

58 Trissel LA et al. Compatibility of paclitaxel injection vehicle with intravenous administration and extension sets. Am J Hosp Pharm 1994;51:2804–2810

(continued)

Drug-Specific References (*continued*)

59 Chin A et al. Paclitaxel stability and compatibility in polyolefin containers. Ann Pharmacother 1994;28:35–36

60 Xu Q et al. Stability of paclitaxel in 5% dextrose injection or 0.9% sodium chloride injection at 4, 22, or 32 °C. Am J Hosp Pharm 1994;51:3058–3060

61 Donyai P, Sewell GJ. Physical and chemical stability of paclitaxel infusions in different container types. J Oncol Pharm Pract 2006;12:211–222

62 Trissel LA, Bready BB. Turbidimetric assessment of the compatibility of taxol with selected other drugs during simulated Y-site injection. Am J Hosp Pharm 1992;49:1716–1719

63 Zhang Y, Trissel LA. Physical and chemical stability of pemetrexed in infusion solutions. Ann Pharmacother 2006;40:1082–1085

64 Boni J et al. Disposition of desipramine, a sensitive cytochrome P450 2D6 substrate, when coadministered with intravenous temsirolimus. Cancer Chemother Pharmacol 2009;64:263–270

65 Hofmeister CC et al. Phase I trial of lenalidomide and CCI-779 in patients with relapsed multiple myeloma: evidence for lenalidomide-CCI-779 interaction via P-glycoprotein [see comment]. J Clin Oncol 2011;29:3427–34. Comment in: J Clin Oncol 2012;30:340–342

66 Faouzi MA et al. Leaching of diethylhexyl phthalate from PVC bags into intravenous teniposide solution. Int J Pharm 1994;105:89–93

67 Murray KM et al. Stability of thiotepa (lyophilized) in 0.9% sodium chloride injection. Am J Health Syst Pharm 1997;54:2588–2591

68 Xu QA et al. Stability of thiotepa (lyophilized) in 5% dextrose injection at 4 and 23 °C. Am J Health Syst Pharm 1996;53:2728–2730

69 Blaney SM et al. Pharmacologic approaches to the treatment of meningeal malignancy. Oncology (Williston Park) 1991;5:107–116; discussion 123, 127

70 Strong JM et al. Pharmacokinetics of intraventricular and intravenous N,N',N'-triethylenethiophosphoramide (thiotepa) in rhesus monkeys and humans. Cancer Res 1986;46:6101–6104

71 Krämer I, Thiesen J. Stability of topotecan infusion solutions in polyvinylchloride bags and elastomeric portable infusion devices. J Oncol Pharm Pract 1999;5:75–82

72 Craig SB et al. Stability and compatibility of topotecan hydrochloride for injection with common infusion solutions and containers. J Pharm Biomed Anal 1997;16:199–205

73 Dyke RW. Treatment of inadvertent intrathecal injection of vincristine. N Engl J Med 1989;321:1270–1271

74 Michelagnoli MP et al. Potential salvage therapy for inadvertent intrathecal administration of vincristine. Br J Haematol 1997;99:364–367

75 Zaragoza MR et al. Neurologic consequences of accidental intrathecal vincristine: a case report. Med Pediatr Oncol 1995;24:61, 62

76 Vendrig DEMM et al. Degradation kinetics of vinblastine sulphate in aqueous solutions. Int J Pharm 1988;43:131–138

77 Francomb MM et al. Adsorption of vincristine, vinblastine, doxorubicin and mitozantrone to inline intravenous filters. Int J Pharm 1994;103:87–92

78 Johnson EG, Janosik JE. Manufacturers' recommendations for handling spilled antineoplastic agents. Am J Hosp Pharm 1989;46:318, 319

79 Beijnen JH et al. Stability of vinca alkaloid anticancer drugs in three commonly used infusion fluids. J Parenter Sci Technol 1989;43:84–87

80 deLemos ML. Vinorelbine and venous irritation: optimal parenteral administration [see comment]. J Oncol Pharm Pract 2005;11:79–81. Comment in: J Oncol Pharm Pract 2006;12:123

Index

For a listing of treatment regimens by cancer type, please see the Table of Contents.